# TRAUMA

# TRAUMA

## Sixth Edition

### EDITORS

**DAVID V. FELICIANO**, MD
*Professor of Surgery*
*Emory University School of Medicine*
*Chief of Surgery*
*Grady Memorial Hospital*
*Atlanta, Georgia*

**KENNETH L. MATTOX**, MD
*Professor and Vice Chairman*
*Department of Surgery*
*Baylor College of Medicine*
*Chief of Staff*
*Chief of Surgery*
*Ben Taub General Hospital*
*Houston, Texas*

**ERNEST E. MOORE**, MD
*Professor and Vice Chairman, Department of Surgery*
*University of Colorado at Denver and Health Sciences Center*
*Bruce M. Rockwell Distinguished Chair of Trauma Surgery*
*Rocky Mountain Regional Trauma Center*
*Chief of Surgery*
*Denver Health Medical Center*
*Denver, Colorado*

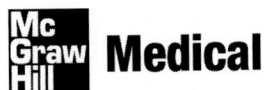

New York   Chicago   San Francisco   Lisbon   London   Madrid   Mexico City
Milan   New Delhi   San Juan   Seoul   Singapore   Sydney   Toronto

**Trauma, Sixth Edition**

Copyright © 2008 by The McGraw-Hill Companies, Inc. All rights reserved. Printed in the United States of America. Except as permitted under the United States Copyright Act of 1976, no part of this publication may be reproduced or distributed in any form or by any means, or stored in a data base or retrieval system, without the prior written permission of the publisher.

1 2 3 4 5 6 7 8 9 0 CCW/CCW 0 9 8 7

ISBN 978-0-07-146912-8
MHID 0-07-146912-5

This book was set in AGaramond Font by Aptara.
The editors were Marsha S. Loeb and Christie Naglieri.
The editorial assistant was Eric J. Klopfer.
The production supervisor was Sherri Souffrance.
Project management was provided by Aptara.
The designer was Janice Bielawa.
Courier printing was printer and binder.
This book is printed on acid-free paper.

**Library of Congress Cataloging-in-Publication Data**

Trauma / editors, David V. Feliciano, Kenneth L. Mattox, Ernest E. Moore. -- 6th ed.
p. ; cm.
Includes bibliographical references and index.
ISBN-13: 978-0-07-146912-8 (alk. paper)
ISBN-10: 0-07-146912-5 (alk. paper)
1. Wounds and injuries. 2. Traumatology. I. Feliciano, David V. II. Mattox, Kenneth L., 1938- III. Moore, Ernest Eugene.
[DNLM: 1. Wounds and Injuries. 2. Critical Care. 3. Surgical Procedures, Operative. WO 700 T7732 2008]
RD93.T67 2008
617.1-dc22
2007038022

*TRAUMA, Sixth Edition is dedicated*
*to our families, whose love, patience, and support*
*have allowed each of us to have a fulfilling career in surgery:*
*Grace S. Rozycki, MD, David J. Feliciano, Douglas D. Feliciano,*
*June Mattox, Kimber Mattox, Sarah V. Moore, MD, Hunter B. Moore,*
*Peter K. Moore. We hope that this edition will also be a fitting tribute*
*to the memories of our colleagues: C. James Carrico, MD*
*1935–2002, Peter Mucha, Jr, MD 1943–2006,*
*Charles J. Weigel, II, JD 1936–2006.*

# Contents

## Section I
## TRAUMA OVERVIEW

## Section II
## GENERALIZED APPROACHES TO THE
## TRAUMATIZED PATIENT

# Section III
# MANAGEMENT OF SPECIFIC INJURIES

# Contributors

**Maria M. Aaron, MD**
Associate Professor of Ophthalmology
Residency Program Director
Emory University School of Medicine
Emory Eye Center
Atlanta, Georgia
Chapter 21

**Charles A. Adams, Jr., MD**
Assistant Professor of Surgery
The Warren Alpert Medical School of Brown University
Providence, Rhode Island
Chapter 49

**David H. Ahrenholz, MD**
Associate Professor of Surgery
University of Minnesota Medical School
Associate Director
Regions Burn Center
St. Paul, Minnesota
Commentary on Chapter 51

**Jameel Ali, MD**
Professor of Surgery
University of Toronto
Chief, Region XII
American College of Surgeons, Committee on Trauma
Toronto, Ontario, Canada
Commentary on Chapter 11

**Reginald Alouidar, MD**
Fellow
Division of Trauma/Critical Care Surgery
University of Miami Miller School of Medicine
Miami, Florida
Chapter 47

**Juan A. Asensio, MD**
Professor of Surgery
The New Jersey Medical School
University of Medicine and Dentistry of New Jersey
UMDNJ - University Hospital
Newark, New Jersey
Chapter 28

**Dennis W. Ashley, MD**
Director of Trauma and Critical Care
Medical Center of Georgia
Professor of Surgery
Mercer University School of Medicine
Macon, Georgia
Commentary on Chapter 13

**Philip S. Barie, MD, MBA**
Professor of Surgery and Public Health
Chief
Division of Critical Care and Trauma
Director
Anne and Max A. Cohen Surgical Intensive Care Unit
Weill Cornell Medical College
New York, New York
Chapter 19

**Robert D. Barraco, MD, MPH**
Assistant Professor of Surgery
Penn State College of Medicine
Chief
Geriatric and Pediatric Trauma
Lehigh Valley Hospital
Allentown, Pennsylvania
Commentary on Chapter 62

**Michael B. Shapiro, MD**
Associate Professor of Surgery
Northwestern University Feinberg School of Medicine
Medical Director, Surgical Intensive Care Unit
Northwestern Memorial Hospital
Chicago
Commentary on Chapter 41

**Tiffany K. Bee, MD**
Assistant Professor of Surgery
University of Tennessee Health Science Center
Memphis, Tennessee
Chapter 32

**Walter L. Biffl, MD**
Associate Professor of Surgery
Denver Health Medical Center
University of Colorado School of Medicine Denver
Colorado
Chapter 49
Commentary on Chapter 63

**H. Scott Bjerke, MD**
Medical Director
Methodist Trauma Service and IPD Swat Medics
Associate Professor of Surgery
Indiana University School of Medicine
Indianapolis, Indiana
Chapter 48
Commentary on Chapter 8

**Ernest F.J. Block, MD, EMT-P**
Clinical Associate Professor of Surgery
University of Florida
Orlando Regional Medical Center
Orlando, Florida
Commentary on Chapter 61

**Elliot B. Bodfosky, MD**
Assistant Professor of Physical Medicine and Rehabilitation
UMDNJ Robert Wood Johnson Medical School
Chief
Department of Physical Medicine and Rehabilitation
UMDNJ Cooper University Hospital
Camden, New Jersey
Chapter 54

**Karen J. Brasel, MD, MPH**
Associate Professor of Surgery and Health Policy
Medical College of Wisconsin
Milwaukee, Wisconsin
Commentary on Chapter 2

**L. D. Britt, MD, MPH**
Brichouse Professor and Chairman
Eastern Virginia Medical School,
Norfolk, Virginia
Chapter 23

**Geoffrey Broocker, MD**
Walthour-DeLaPerriere Professor of Ophthalmology
Emory University School of Medicine
Chief of Service
Department of Ophthalmology
Grady Memorial Hospital
Atlanta, Georgia
Chapter 21

**Susan I. Brundage, MD, MPH**
Associate Professor of Trauma and Critical Care
Stanford University School of Medicine
Stanford, California
Commentary on Chapter 34

**Jon M. Burch, MD**
Professor of Surgery
University of Colorado at Denver and Health Sciences Center
Denver, Colorado
Chapter 35

**Tom Burdick, MD**
Assistant Professor of Radiology
University of Washington
Harborview Medical Center
Seattle, Washington
Chapter 16

**Lisa K. Cannada, MD**
Assistant Professor
University of Texas Southwestern Medical Center
Parkland Hospital
Dallas, Texas
Commentary on Chapter 24

**Eddy H. Carrillo, MD**
Director of Trauma Services
Memorial Regional Hospital
Hollywood, Florida
Commentary on Chapter 35

**David C. Chang, PhD, MPH, MBA**
Assistant Professor of Surgery
Johns Hopkins School of Medicine
Department of Health Policy and Management
Bloomberg School of Public Health
Baltimore, Maryland
Chapter 48

**Michael Chang, MD**
Professor of General Surgery
Wake Forest University School of Medicine
Director of Trauma/Burn Services
Wake Forest University Health Sciences
Winston-Salem, North Carolina
Commentary on Chapter 68

**David J. Ciesla, MD**
Associate Professor, Dept. of Surgery
University of South Florida
Director Division of Trauma and Surgical Critical Care
Tampa General Hospital
2 Columbia Drive G417
Tampa Florida
Chapter 68

**William G. Cioffi, MD**
Professor and Chairman
Brown Medical School
Surgeon-in-Chief
Rhode Island Hospital
Providence, Rhode Island
Chapter 49

**David L. Ciraulo, DO, MPH**
Clinical Associate Professor of Surgery
University of Vermont College of Medicine/University of New
    England College of Osteopathic Medicine
Director
Trauma Outreach and Surgical Emergency Preparedness
Maine Medical Center
Portland, Maine
Chapter 56

**Ian Civil, MD, ChB, MB**
Director of Trauma Services
Auckland City Hospital
Auckland, Grafton, New Zealand
Commentary on Chapter 44

**Michael Coburn, MD**
Associate Professor of Urology
Carlton-Smith Chair in Urologic Education
Vice Chairman for Academic Affairs
Baylor College of Medicine
Chief of Urology
Ben Taub General Hopsital
Houston, Texas
Chapter 39

**Raul Coimbra, MD, PhD**
Professor of Surgery
Chief
Division of Trauma, Surgical Critical Care, and Burns
University of California, San Diego Medical Center
Chapter 4
Commentary on Chapter 28

**Frederic J. Cole, Jr., MD**
Associate, Trauma Director
Legacy Emanuel Hospital and Health Center
Portland, OR
Chapter 23

**Edward E. Cornwell, III, MD**
Director
Adult Trauma Service
Johns Hopkins University School of Medicine
Baltimore Maryland
Chapter 48
Commentary on Chapter 3

**Robert L. Coscia, MD**
Assistant Professor of Surgery
Medical College of Wisconsin
Froedtert Memorial Lutheran Hospital
Milwaukee, Wisconsin
Commentary on Chapter 10

**C. Clay Cothren, MD**
Assistant Professor
University of Colorado Health Sciences Center
Attending Surgeon
Denver Health Medical Center
Denver, Colorado
Chapter 15
Commentary on Chapter 30

**H. Gill Cryer, MD, PhD**
Professor of Surgery
Chief of Trauma & Critical Care
University of California, Los Angeles
Los Angeles California
Chapter 65

**James G. Cushman, MD**
Associate Professor of Surgery
University of Maryland School of Medicine
R. Adams Cowley Shock Trauma Center
Baltimore, Maryland
Commentary on Chapter 9

**James W. Davis, MD**
Associate Professor of Clinical Surgery
University of California, San Francisco - Fresno
Chief of Trauma
University Medical Center
Fresno, California
Chapter 31

**Kimberly A. Davis, MD**
Associate Professor of Surgery
Chief of the Section of Trauma
Surgical Critical Care and Surgical Emergencies
Yale University School of Medicine
Trauma Director
Yale New Haven Hospital
New Haven, Connecticut
Commentary on Chapter 49

**Gerald B. Demarest, MD**
Associate Professor of Surgery
Director of Burns and Trauma
University of New Mexico
Albuquerque, New Mexico
Commentary on Chapter 48

**Demetrios Demetriades, MD, PhD**
Professor of Surgery
University of Southern California, Los Angeles
Director
Division of Trauma/SICU
Los Angeles County & University of Southern California
   Medical Center
Los Angeles, California
Chapter 30

**Christopher J. Dente, MD**
Assistant Professor Surgery
Emory University
Associate Director of Trauma
Grady Memorial Hospital
Atlanta, Georgia
Chapters 17, 37
Commentary on Chapter 65

**Rochelle A. Dicker, MD**
Assistant Professor of Surgery
University of California, San Francisco
San Francisco, California
Chapter 60
Commentary on Chapter 58

**Lawrence N. Diebel, MD**
Professor of Surgery
Wayne State University
Detroit, Michigan
Chapter 34

**James C. Duke, MD, MBA**
Associate Professor of Anesthesiology
University of Colorado Health Sciences Center
Associate Director of Anesthesiology
Denver Health Medical Center
Denver, Colorado
Chapter 18

**Chris Dunn, PhD**
Associate Professor of Psychiatry and Behavioral Sciences
University of Washington School of Medicine
Harborview Medical Center
Seattle, Washington
Chapter 45

**Soumitra R. Eachempati, MD**
Associate Professor of Surgery and Public Health
Weill Cornell Medical College
New York, New York
Chapter 19

**Alexander L. Eastman, MD**
Resident in General Surgery
University of Texas Southwestern Medical Center
Dallas, Texas
Commentary on Chapter 17

**Brent Eastman, MD**
N. Paul Whittier Chair of Trauma
Scripps Memorial Hospital
La Jolla, California
Chief Medical Officer
Scripps Health
San Diego, California
Commentary on Chapter 37

**Babak Eghbalieh, MD**
Chief Surgical Resident
University of California, San Francisco
University Medical Center - Fresno
Fresno, California
Chapter 31

**A. Peter Ekeh, MD**
Associate Professor of Surgery
Boonshoft School of Medicine
Wright State University
Miami Valley Hospital
Dayton, Ohio
Commentary on Chapter 40

**Timothy C. Fabian, MD**
Harwell Wilson Alumni Professor & Chairman
Department of Surgery
University of Tennessee Health Science Center
Memphis, Tennessee
Chapter 32

**Eugen Faist, MD**
Professor of Surgery
Ludwig-Maximilians-University
Munich, Germany
Chapter 67

**Samir M. Fakhry, MD**
Professor of Surgery
Virginia Commonwealth University - Inova Campus
Chief
Trauma and Surgical Critical Care Services
Associate Chair for Research and Education
Department of Surgery
Inova Fairfax Hospital
Falls Church, Virginia
Chapter 61

**Sam E. Farish, DMD**
Assistant Professor of Oral & Maxillofacial Surgery
Department of Surgery
Emory University School of Medicine
Chief of Oral & Maxillofacial Surgery
Atlanta VA Medical Center
Atlanta, Georgia
Commentary on Chapter 22

**David V. Feliciano, MD**
Professor of Surgery
Emory University School of Medicine
Chief of Surgery
Grady Memorial Hospital
Atlanta, Georgia
Chapters 37, 41
Commentary on Chapter 7

**Ricardo Ferrada, MD**
Professor of Surgery
Universidad del Valle
Cali, Colombia
Commentary on Chapter 25

**John Fildes, MD**
Professor and Vice Chair of Surgery
University of Nevada School of Medicine
Chief
Division of Trauma and Critical Care
University of Nevada School of Medicine
Las Vegas, Nevada
Commentary on Chapter 5

**Lewis Flint, MD**
Editor-in Chief
Selected Readings in General Surgery
Division of Education, American College of Surgeons
633 North St. Clair Street
Chicago, Illinois
Commentary on Chapter 38

**Raquel M. Forsythe, MD**
Assistant Professor of Surgery and Critical Care Medicine
University of Pittsburgh
Pittsburgh, Pennsylvania
Chapter 13

**Carolyn J. Fowler, MD**
Assistant Professor
Johns Hopkins Bloomberg School of Public Health
Johns Hopkins University School of Nursing
Baltimore, Maryland
Chapter 2

**Heidi L. Frankel, MD**
Professor of Surgery
University of Texas Southwestern
Dallas, Texas
Commentary on Chapters 17, 47

**Bradley D. Freeman, MD**
Associate Professor of Surgery
Washington University School of Medicine
St. Louis, Missouri
Commentary on Chapter 57

**Eric R. Frykberg, MD**
Professor of Surgery
University of Florida College of Medicine
Chief Division of General Surgery
Shanos Jacksonville Medical Center
Jacksonville, Florida
Chapter 44

**Richard L. Gamelli, MD**
The Robert J. Freeark Professor and Chairman
Department of Surgery
Chief
Burn Center
Loyola University Medical Center
Director
Burn & Shock Trauma Institute
Professor of Pediatrics
Loyola University Medical Center
Maywood, Illinois
Commentary on Chapter 50

**Luis M. García-Núñez, MD**
General and Trauma Surgeon
Department of Surgery
Central Military Hospital
National Defense Department
Professor
Military School of Health Professionals
University of Army and Air Force
National Defense Department
Distrito Federal, Mexico
Chapter 28

**Jennifer Garza, MD**
Resident in Pediatric Surgery
Oklahoma University Health Sciences Center
Oklahoma City, Oklahoma
Chapter 46

**Larry M. Gentilello, MD**
Professor of Surgery
Division of Burns, Trauma  and Critical Care
University of Texas Southwestern Medical School
Dallas, Texas
Chapters 45, 51

**David A. Gerber, MD**
Associate Professor of Surgery
University of North Carolina at Chapel Hill
Chapel Hill, North Carolina
Commentary on Chapter 52

**Ankush Gosain, MD**
Resident in General Surgery
Loyola University Medical Center
Chicago, Illinois
Chapter 62

**Ronald I. Gross, MD**
Assistant Professor of Traumatology
Emergency Medicine & Surgery
University of Connecticut School of Medicine
Associate Director of Trauma
Hartford Hospital
Commentary on Chapter 12

**Zbigniew Gugala, MD, PhD**
Assistant Professor
Department of Orthopedic Surgery and Rehabilitation
The University of Texas Medical Branch
Galveston, Texas
Chapter 24

**Mark Gunst, MD**
Assistant Instructor and Fellow
Division of Burn, Trauma, and Critical Care
Department of Surgery
University of Texas Southwestern Medical Center
Dallas, Texas
Commentary on Chapter 47

**James B. Haenel, RRT**
Denver Health Medical Center
The University of Colorado Health Sciences Center
Denver, Colorado
Chapter 63

**Brian G. Harbrecht, MD**
Professor of Surgery
Director of Trauma Services
University of Louisville
Louisville, Kentucky
Chapter 13

**Carl J. Hauser, MD**
Visiting Professor of Surgery
Harvard Medical School
Beth Israel Deaconess Medical Center
Boston, Massachusetts
Chapter 26

**Michael L. Hawkins, MD**
Professor of Surgery
Medical College of Georgia
Professor of Anesthesiology
Professor of Emergency Medicine
Medical College of Georgia
Augusta, Georgia
Commentary on Chapter 31

**David N. Herndon, MD**
Professor of Surgery
Jesse H. Jones Distinguished Chair in Burn Surgery
University of Texas Medical Branch
Chief of Staff and Director of Research
Shriners Hospitals for Children
Galveston, Texas
Chapter 50

**Asher Hirshberg, MD**
Associate Professor
The Michael E. DeBakey Department of Surgery
Baylor College of Medicine
Chief of Vascular Surgery
Ben Taub General Hospital
Houston, Texas
Chapter 9

**John B. Holcomb, MD, Col, MC, USA**
Commander
US Army Institute of Surgical Research
Fort Sam Houston, Texas
Chapter 55

**David B. Hoyt, MD**
John Connolly Professor of Surgery
Chairman
Department of Surgery
University of California, Irvine School of Medicine
Irvine, California
Chapter 4

**Joseph Huh, MD**
Assistant Professor of Surgery
Baylor College of Medicine
Chief of Cardiothoracic Surgery
Michael E DeBakey Veterans Affairs Medical Center
Houston, Texas
Chapter 25

**John P. Hunt, MD, MPH**
Associate Professor of Surgery
Louisiana State University Health Science Center - New Orleans
Section Chief
Trauma/Critical Care/General Surgery
Charity Hospital
New Orleans, Louisiana
Chapter 7

**Robert C. Jacoby, MD**
Assistant Professor of Surgery
University of California, Davis Medical Center
Sacramento, California
Chapter 33

**Donald Jenkins, MD**
Assistant Professor of Surgery
Uniformed Services University of the Health Sciences
Trauma Medical Director
Wilford Hall United States Air Force Medical Center
Lackland Air Force Base, San Antonio, Texas
Chapter 55

**Jeffrey L. Johnson, MD**
Assistant Professor of Surgery
University of Colorado Health Sciences Center
Director of SICU
Denver Health
Denver, Colorado
Chapter 63

**Ronald M. Jou, MD**
Littlefield Biodesign Innovation Fellow
Stanford University
Stanford, California
Commentary on Chapter 34

**Gregory J. Jurkovich, MD**
Professor of Surgery
University of Washington
Chief of Trauma
Harborview Medical Center
Seattle, Washington
Chapters 27, 59

**David A. Kappel, MD**
Clinical Professor of Surgery
West Virginia University
Morgantown, West Virginia
Commentary on Chapter 53

**Riyad Karmy-Jones, MD**
Medical Director
Thoracic and Vascular Surgery
Southwest Washington Medical Center
Vancouver, Washington
Chapter 27

**Jeffry L. Kashuk, MD**
Assistant Professor of Surgery
University of Colorado Health Sciences Center
Surgery and Trauma Services
Denver Health Medical Center
Denver, Colorado
Chapter 35
Commentary on Chapter 66

**Christopher R. Kaufman, MD, MPH**
Professor of Surgery
Uniformed Services University of the Health Sciences
Associate Medical Director
Trauma Services
Legacy Emanuel Hospital
Portland, Oregon
Chapter 11

**Aditya K. Kaza, MD**
Clinical Fellow
Department of Cardiovascular Surgery
Harvard Medical School
Children's Hospital Boston
Boston, Massachusetts
Chapter 52

**Robert M. Kellman, MD**
Professor and Chair
Department of Otolaryngology and Communication Sciences
SUNY Upstate Medical University
Syracuse, New York
Chapter 22

**Patrick D. Kilgo, MS**
Senior Associate Faculty
Department of Biostatistics
Emory University School of Public Health
Atlanta, Georgia
Chapter 5

**Joung Y. Kim, MD**
Assistant Professor
Emory University School of Medicine
Atlanta, Georgia
Chapter 21

**Fernando J. Kim, MD**
Assistant Professor
University of Colorado Health Sciences Center
Chief of Urology
Denver Health Medical Center
Director of Minimally Invasive Urological Oncology
Denver, Colorado
Commentary on Chapter 39

**Terry Kim, MD**
Associate Professor of Ophthalmology
Duke University School of Medicine
Director of Fellowship Programs
Associate Director
Cornea and Refractive Surgery
Duke University Eye Center
Durham, North Carolina
Commentary on Chapter 21

**M. Margaret Knudson, MD**
Professor of Surgery
University of California, San Francisco
Director
San Francisco Injury Center
San Francisco General Hospital
San Francisco, California
Chapter 40

**Rosemary A. Kozar, MD, PhD**
Associate Professor of Surgery
University of Texas - Houston Health Science Center
Houston, Texas
Chapter 64

**Kenneth A. Kudsk, MD**
Professor of Surgery
University of Wisconsin - Madison
Madison, Wisconsin
Chapter 66

**Anna M. Ledgerwood, MD**
Professor of Surgery
Wayne State University
Detroit Medical Center
Detroit, Michigan
Chapter 58

**Jong O. Lee, MD**
Assistant Professor of Surgery
University of Texas Medical Branch
Staff Surgeon
Shriners Hospital for Children
Galveston, Texas
Chapter 50

**Thomas P. Lehman, MD, PT**
Chief of Hand Surgery
Assistant Professor of Orthopedics
University of Oklahoma Health Sciences Center
Oklahoma City, Oklahoma
Chapter 42

**Scott Lemaire, MD**
Associate Professor and Director of Clinical and
    Translational Research
Division of Cardiothoracic Surgery
Michael E. DeBakey Department of Surgery
Baylor College of Medicine
Cardiovascular Surgery Staff
The Texas Heart Institute at St. Luke's Episcopal Hospital
Houston, Texas
Chapter 29

**Ari Leppaniemi, MD**
Chief of Emergency Surgery
Associate Professor
Meilahti Hospital
Department of Surgery
University of Helsinki
Helsinki, Finland
Adjunct Associate Professor
Uniformed Services University of the Health Sciences
Bethesda, Maryland
Commentary on Chapter 55

**Peter Letarte, MD**
Chief
Section of Neurosurgery
Heinz VA Medical Center
Maywood, Illinois
Chapter 20

**Ronald W. Lindsey, MD**
Professor and Chair
Department of Orthopedic Surgery & Rehabilitation
University of Texas
Medical Branch
Galveston, Texas
Chapter 24

**Ken F. Linnau, MD, MS**
NRSA Radiology Research Fellow
Department of Radilogy
University of Washington
Harborview Medical Center
Seattle, Washington
Chapter 16

**Kathleen R. Liscum, MD**
Associate Professor of Surgery
Baylor College of Medicine
Chief of General Surgery
Ben Taub General Hospital
Houston, Texas
Chapter 48

**David H. Livingston, MD**
Wesley J. Howe Professor of Surgery
UMDNJ - New Jersey Medical School
Director
New Jersey Trauma Center
UMDNJ - University Hospital
Newark, New Jersey
Chapter 26

**Albert Losken, MD**
Assistant Professor of Plastic Surgery
Emory University
Atlanta, Georgia
Chapter 53

**Lawrence Lottenberg, MD**
Associate Professor of Surgery & Anesthesiology
University of Florida College of Medicine
Gainesville, Florida
Commentary on Chapter 4

**Charles E. Lucas, MD**
Professor of Surgery
Wayne State University
Detroit Medical Center
Detroit, Michigan
Chapter 58

**Kathryn A. Lucas, JD**
Attorney at Law
Glendale, California
Chapter 58

**Fred Luchette, MD**
The Ambrose and Gladys Bowyer Professor of Surgery
Loyola University Stritch School of Medicine
Director Division of Trauma
Surgical Critical Care and Burns
Loyola University Medical Center
Maywood, Illinois
Chapter 62

**Ellen J. MacKenzie, PhD**
Professor and Chair
Johns Hopkins Bloomberg School of Public Health
Department of Health Policy & Management
Baltimore, Maryland
Chapter 2

**Robert C. Mackersie, MD**
Professor of Surgery
University of California, San Francisco
Director of Trauma
San Francisco General Hospital
San Francisco, California
Chapter 60

**Ronald V. Maier, MD**
Jane & Donald D. Trunkey Professor and Vice-Chair
Department of Surgery
University of Washington
Surgeon-in-Chief
Harborview Medical Center
Seattle, Washington
Chapter 3

**Mark A. Malangoni, MD**
Professor of Surgery
Case Western Reserve University
Chairperson
Department of Surgery
Surgeon-in-Chief
MetroHealth Medical Center
Cleveland, Ohio
Commentary on Chapter 19

**F. A. Mann, MD**
Seattle Radiologists, APC
Seattle, Washington
Chapter 16

**Alan B. Marr, MD**
Associate Professor of Clinical Surgery
Louisiana State Univeristy Health Sciences Center - New Orleans
Attending in Trauma and Critical Care
Medical Center of Louisiana in New Orleans
New Orleans, Louisiana
Chapter 7

**Kenneth L. Mattox, MD**
Professor and Vice Chairman
Department of Surgery
Baylor College of Medicine
Chief of Staff
Chief of Surgery
Ben Taub General Hospital
Houston, Texas
Chapters 25, 29
Commentary on Chapter 26

**Mary C. McCarthy, MD**
Professor of Surgery
Wright State University School of Medicine
Director of Trauma Services
Miami Valley Hospital
Dayton, Ohio
Commentary on Chapter 40

**Gary McGillivary, MD**
Assistant Professor of Orthopedic Surgery
Emory University School of Medicine
Atlanta, Georgia
Commentary on Chapter 42

**Mark G. McKenney, MD**
Chief
Division of Trauma & Surgical Critical Care
University of Miami
Miller School of Medicine,
Professor of Surgery
University of Miami/Jackson Memorial Medical Center
Miami, Florida
Chapter 47

**J. Wayne Meredith, MD**
Director
Division of Surgical Sciences
Professor and Chair
Department of General Surgery
Wake Forest University School of Medicine
Winston-Salem, North Carolina
Chapter 5
Commentary on Chapter 27

**Christopher P. Michetti, MD**
Assistant Profesor of Surgery
Virginia Commonwealth University
Trauma and Surgical Care Services
Fairfax Hospital
Falls Church, Virginia
Chapter 61

**Joseph P. Minei, MD**
Professor and Vice Chair
Department of Surgery
University of Texas Southwestern Medical Center
Surgeon-in-Chief
Parkland Memorial Hospital
Dallas, Texas
Commentary on Chapter 33

**Stuart E. Mirvis, MD**
Professor of Radiology
Section Head
Emergency Radiology
Department of Diagnostic Radiology
University of Maryland School of Medicine
Baltimore, Maryland
Commentary on Chapter 16

**Max B. Mitchell, MD**
Associate Professor of Surgery
University of Colorado
The Children's Hospital Heart Institute
Aurora, Colorado
Chapter 52

**Charles Mock, MD, PhD**
Professor
Department of Surgery and Epidemiology
University of Washington
Seattle, Washington
Chapter 3

**Ernest E. Moore, MD**
Professor and Vice Chairman
Department of Surgery
University of Colorado Health Sciences Center
Chief of Surgery and Trauma Services
Denver Health Medical Center
Denver, Colorado
Chapters 15, 68

**Frederick A. Moore, MD**
James H. "Red" Duke, Jr. Professor & Chairman
Chief
General Surgery and Trauma & Critical Care
University of Texas Health Science Center Houston
    Medical School
Houston, Texas
Chapters 64, 68

**John B. Moore, MD**
Assistant Director of SICU
University of Colorado Health Sciences Center
Denver Health Medical Center
Denver, Colorado
Commentary on Chapter 66

**Steven J. Morgan, MD**
Associate Professor
University of Colorado School of Medicine
Associate Director of Orthopedic Surgery
Denver Health Medical Center
Denver, Colorado
Chapter 43

**Richard J. Mullins, MD**
Professor of Surgery
Oregon Health & Sciences University
Portland, Oregon
Commentary on Chapter 6

**Lena M. Napolitano, MD**
Professor of Surgery
Division Chief
Acute Care Surgery, Trauma, Burn, Critical Care, and
    Emergency Surgery
Director
Surgical Critical Care
Associate Chair of Surgery for Critical Care
University of Michigan Health System
Commentary on Chapter 14

**Russell J. Nauta, MD**
Professor of Surgery
Harvard Medical School
Charman
Department of Surgery
Mt. Auburn Hospital
Cambridge, Massachusettes
Commentary Chapter 59

**Jeffrey M. Nicholas, MD**
Associate Professor of Surgery
Emory University School of Medicine
Deputy Chief of Surgery
Grady Memorial Hospital
Atlanta, Georgia
Commentary on Chapter 64

**M. Gage Ochsner, Jr., MD**
Professor of Surgery
Mercer University School of Medicine - Savannah Campus
Director of Trauma and Surgical Critical Care
Memorial Health University Medical Center
Savannah, Georgia
Commentary on Chapter 56

**Grant E. O'Keefe, MD, MPH**
Associate Professor of Surgery
School of Medicine
University of Washington
Seattle, Washington
Chapter 57

**Turner M. Osler, MD, MSc**
Research Professor
University of Vermont College of Medicine
Burlington, Vermont
Chapter 5

**Robert O'Toole, MD**
Assistant Professor of Orthopedics
University of Maryland
Attending Orthopedic Traumatologist
R.A. Cowley Shock Trauma Center
Baltimore, Maryland
Chapter 38

**H. Leon Pachter, MD**
The George David Stewart Professor and Chairman
Department of Surgery
New York University School of Medicine
New York, New York
Commentary on Chapter 32

**Michael Pasquale, MD**
Associate Professor of Surgery
Penn State College of Medicine
Chief
Division of Trauma/Surgical Critical Care
Vice Chairman
Department of Surgery
Lehigh Valley Hospital
Allentown, Pennsylvania
Chapter 6
Commentary on Chapter 62

**Andrew J. Patterson, MD, PhD**
Associate Professor of Anesthesia
Division of Critical Care Medicine
Director of Critical Care Research
Stanford University
Stanford, California
Commentary on Chapter 60

**Andrew B. Peitzman, MD**
Professor & Chief
Executive Vice Chairman
Division of General Surgery
Department of Surgery
University of Pittsburgh
Pittsburgh, Pennsylvania
Chapter 13

**Vincent J. Perciaccante, DDS**
Clinical Assistant Professor of Surgery
Division of Oral & Maxillofacial Surgery
Emory University School of Medicine
Chief, Oral & Maxillofacial Surgery
Grady Memorial Hospital
Atlanta, GA
Commentary on Chapter 22

**Scott R. Petersen, MD**
Clinical Professor of Surgery
University of Arizona
Medical Director of Trauma
St. Joseph's Hospital and Medical Center
Phoenix, Arizona
Chapter 14

**Steven L. Peterson, DVM, MD, MS**
Associate Professor of Surgery
The University of Colorado Health Sciences Center
Division of Reconstructive Surgery
Denver Health Medical Center
Denver, Colorado
Chapter 42

**Patrizio Petrone, MD**
Assistant Professor of Surgery
Chief, International Research Fellows
Division of Trauma Surgery & Critical Care
Department of Surgery
Keck School of Medicine, University of Southern California
Los Angeles, California
Chapter 28

**Frederic M. Pieracci, MD, MPH**
Fellow in Surgery and Public Health
Weill Cornell Medical College
New York, New York
Chapter 19

**Jean Francois Pittet, MD**
Associate Professor in Residence
Department of Anesthesia
University of California, San Francisco
San Francisco General Hopsital
San Francisco, California
Chapter 60

**Spiros G. Pneumaticos, MD**
Assistant Professor of Orthopedic Surgery
University of Athens Medical School
Athens, Greece
Adjunct Assistant Professor of Orthopedic Surgery
Baylor College of Medicine
Houston, Texas
Chapter 24

**Bruce M. Potenza, MD**
Associate Professor of Surgery
Division of Trauma Burns and Critical Care
University of California, San Diego School of Medicine
San Diego, California
Chapter 4

**Basil A. Pruitt, Jr., MD**
Clinical Professor of Surgery
University of Texas Health Science Center at San Antonio
Consultant
U.S. Army Institute of Surgical Research
San Antonio, Texas
Chapter 1

**Jeffrey H. Pruitt, MD**
Assistant Professor of Radiology
University of Texas Southwestern Medical Center
Associate Medical Director
Department of Radiology
Parkland Hospital
Dallas, Texas
Chapter 1

**Sally Raty, MD**
Interim Vice-Chair
Department of Anesthesiology
Baylor College of Medicine
Houston, Texas
Commentary on Chapter 18

**Sunil S. Rayan, MD**
Attending Surgeon
Division of Vascular and Endovascular Surgery
Scripps Memorial Hospital
La Jolla, California
Commentary on Chapter 37

**R. Lawrence Reed, II, MD**
Professor of Surgery
Loyola University Medical Center
Maywood, Illinois
Director
Surgical Intensive Care Unit
Edward Hines, Jr. Hospital
Chapter 51

**Peter Rhee, MD, MPH**
Professor of Surgery and Molecular Biology
Uniformed Services University of the Health Sciences
Associate Professor of Surgery
University of Southern California
Director of Navy Trauma Training Center
Attending Surgeon
Los Angeles County Medical Center
Los Angeles, California
Chapter 55

**Michael Rhodes, MD**
Professor of Surgery
Thomas Jefferson University
Chairman
Department of Surgery
Christiana Care Health System
Newark, Delaware
Chapter 6

**Charles F. Rinker II, MD**
General Surgeon
Past Director of Trauma
Bozeman Deaconess Hospital
Bozeman, Montana
Chapter 10

**Dave Roccaforte, MD**
Assistant Professor of Anesthesiology
New York University
Co-Director, SICU
Bellevue Hospital
New York, New York
Commentary on Chapter 9

**Aurelio Rodriguez, MD**
Professor of Surgery
Drexel University College of Medicine
Director of the Division of Trauma Surgery
Allegheny General Hospital
Shock Trauma Center
Pittsburgh, Pennsylvania
Commentary on Chapter 29

**Matthew L. Rontal, MD**
Attending Physician
Department of Otolaryngology
Craniofacial Institute
Providence Hospital
Southfield, Michigan
Chapter 22

**Steven E. Ross, MD**
Professor of Surgery
University of Medicine and Dentistry of New Jersey
Robert Wood Johnson - Camden
Head
Division of Trauma and Surgical Critical Care
Cooper University Hospital
Camden, New Jersey
Chapter 54

**Michael F. Rotondo, MD**
Professor and Chairman
Department of Surgery
The Brody School of Medicine
Chief of Trauma & Critical Care
Pitt County Memorial Hospital
Greenville, North Carolina
Chapter 12

**Grace S. Rozycki, MD, MBA, RDMS**
Professor of Surgery
Emory University School of Medicine
Director
Trauma and Surgical Critical Care
Grady Memorial Hospital
Atlanta, Georgia
Chapter 17

**Gordon S. Sacks, PharmD**
Clinical Associate Professor
University of Wisconsin - School of Pharmacy
Madison, Wisconsin
Chapter 66

**Scott G. Sagraves, MD**
Associate Professor of Surgery
The Brody School of Medicine
Attending Trauma Physician
Trauma Director
Pitt County Memorial Hospital
Greenville, North Carolina
Chapter 12

**Ali Salim, MD**
Assistant Professor of Surgery
University of Southern California
Keck School of Medicine
Los Angeles, California
Commentary on Chapter 23

**Joseph A. Salomone, III, MD**
Associate Professor of Emergency Medicine
Emergency Medical Services Director
University of Missouri at Kansas City School of Medicine
Truman Medical Center
Kansas City, Missouri
Chapter 8

**Jeffrey P. Salomone, MD, NREMT-P**
Associate Professor of Surgery
Emory University School of Medicine
Deputy Chief of Surgery (Administration)
Grady Memorial Hospital
Atlanta, Georgia
Chapter 8

**John Santaniello, MD**
Assistant Professor of Surgery
Loyola University Stritch School of Medicine
Attending Surgeon
Medical Director
Surgical Intensive Care Unit
Hines VA Hospital
Maywood, Illinois
Chapter 62

**Thomas M. Scalea, MD**
Francis X. Kelly Professor of Trauma Surgery
University of Maryland School of Medicine
Physician in Chief
R. Adams Cowley Shock Trauma Center
Baltimore, Maryland
Chapter 38

**Timothy G. Schaefer, MD**
Fellow in Plastic Surgery
Emory University
Atlanta, Georgia
Chapter 53

**Carol R. Schermer, MD, MPH**
Associate Professor of Surgery
Loyola University Chicago
Stritch School of Medicine
Division of Trauma and Critical Care
Loyola University Medical Center
Maywood IL
Commentary on Chapter 45

**Miren A. Schinco, MD**
Assistant Professor of Surgery
University of Florida College of Medicine
Chief
Division of Trauma and Critical Care
Shands Jacksonville Medical Center
Jacksonville, Florida
Chapter 44

**G. Douglas Schmitz, MD**
Clinical Adjunct Faculty
University of Wyoming Family Practice Program
Cheyenne, Wyoming
Chapter 10

**Carl I. Schulman, MD, MSPH**
Assistant Professor of Surgery
University of Miami Miller School of Medicine
Miami, Florida
Chapter 47

**Bradford G. Scott, MD**
Assistant Professor
Michael E. DeBakey Department of Surgery
Baylor College of Medicine
Houston, Texas
Commentary on Chapter 15

**Wade R. Smith, MD**
Associate Professor
University of Colorado Health Sciences Center
Director of Orthopedic Surgery
Co-Director of Orthopedic Trauma
Denver Health Medical Center
Denver, Colorado
Chapter 43

**R. Stephen Smith, MD, RDMS**
Professor of Surgery
University of Kansas School of Medicine – Wichita
Medical Director, Trauma and Surgical Critical Care
Via Christi Medical Center
Wichita, Kansas
Commentary on Chapter 54

**David A. Spain, MD**
Professor of Surgery
Chief of Trauma/Critical Care Surgery
Stanford University
Stanford, California
Commentary on Chapter 60

**Philip F. Stahel, MD**
Associate Professor of Orthopedic Surgery
University of Colorado School of Medicine
Denver Health Medical Center
Denver, Colorado
Chapter 43

**Luana Stanescu, MD**
Fellow
Department of Radiology and Body Imaging
University of Washington School of Medicine
Harborview Medical Center
Seattle, Washington
Chapter 16

**Michael Stein, MD**
Chairman
Israel Trauma Society
Director of Trauma & Attending Surgeon
Department of Surgery
The Rabin Medical Center
Beilinson Campus
Petach-Tikva, Israel
Sackler Faculty of Medicine
Tel-Aviv University
Tel-Aviv, Israel
Chapter 9

**Deborah M. Stein, MD**
Assistant Professor of Surgery
University of Maryland School of Medicine
Attending Surgeon
Medical Director
Acute Care
R. Adams Cowley Shock Trauma Center
Balitmore, Maryland
Chapter 38

**Steven Stylianos, MD**
Professor of Surgery
University of Miami Miller School of Medicine
Chief
Department of Pediatric Surgery
Miami Children's Hospital
Miami, Florida
Commentary on Chapter 46

**Kathryn M. Tchorz, MD**
Associate Professor of Surgery
Wright State University
Boonshoft School of Medicine
Miami Valley Hospital
Dayton, Ohio
Commentary on Chapter 36

**Eric A. Toschlog, MD**
Associate Professor of Surgery
The Brody School of Medicine
Attending Trauma Physician
Director of Surgical Critical Care
Pitt County Memorial Hospital
Greenville, North Carolina
Chapter 12

**Peter G. Trafton, MD**
Professor of Orthopedic Surgery
Brown University
Providence, Rhode Island
Chapter 43

**Heiko Trentzsch, MD**
Department of Surgery
Ludwig-Maximilians-University
Munich, Germany
Chapter 67

**Donald D. Trunkey, MD**
Professor of Surgery
Oregon Health & Science University
Portland, Oregon
Commentary on Chapter 1

**David W. Tuggle, MD**
Professor and Vice Chairman
Department of Surgery
Chief
Section of Pediatric Surgery
CMRI/Paula Milburn Miller Chair in Pediatric Surgery
The University of Oklahoma Health Sciences Center
Oklahoma City, Oklahoma
Chapter 46

**George C. Velmahos, MD, PhD, MSEd**
Professor of Surgery
Harvard Medical School
Chief Division of Trauma, Emergency Surgery, and Surgical
  Critical Care
Massachusetts General Hospital
Boston, Massachusetts
Chapters 30, 36

**Matthew J. Wall, Jr., MD**
Professor of Surgery
Michael E. DeBakey Department of Surgery
Baylor College of Medicine
Houston, Texas
Chapters 25, 29

**Jennifer J. Wan, MD**
Research Fellow
San Franciso Injury Center
University of California, San Francisco
Resident
University of California, San Francisco - East Bay
San Francisco, California
Chapter 40

**Jordan A. Weinberg, MD**
Assistant Professor of Surgery
University of Alabama at Birmingham
Memphis, Tennessee
Chapter 14

**Sharlon L. Weintraub, MD, MPH**
Assistant Professor of Surgery
Louisina State University School of Medicine
Staff Surgeon
Medical Center of Louisiana
New Orleans, Louisiana
Chapter 7

**Leonard J. Weireter, Jr., MD**
Professor of Surgery
Eastern Virginia Medical School
Norfolk, Virginia
Chapter 23

**Norman W. Weisbrodt, PhD**
Professor of Integrative Biology and Pharmacology
University of Texas Medical School at Houston
Houston, Texas
Chapter 64

**Michael A. West, MD, PhD**
Professor of Surgery
Division of Trauma/Critical Care
Northwestern University Feinberg School of Medicine
Chicago, Illinois
Commentary on Chapter 67

**Jack Wilberger, MD**
Professor and Chairman
Department of Neurosurgery
Senior Associate Dean
Drexel University College of Medicine
Allegheny General Hospital
Pittsburgh, Pennsylvania
Commentary on Chapter 20

**Mark Wilczynski, MD**
Resident
Department of Orthopedic Surgery
Emory University School of Medicine
Atlanta, Georgia
Commentary on Chapter 42

**David H. Wisner, MD**
Vice Chair and Professor of Surgery
University of California, Davis Health System
Sacramento, California
Chapter 33

**Douglas E. Wood, MD**
Professor and Chief
General Thoracic Surgery
University of Washington
Endowed Chair in Lung Cancer Research
Seattle, Washington
Chapter 27

**Amy D. Wyrzykowski, MD**
Assistant Professor of Surgery
Emory University School of Medicine
Associate Director of Surgical Critical Care
Grady Memorial Hospital
Atlanta, Georgia
Chapter 41

**Bruce H. Ziran, MD**
Associate Professor of Orthopedic Surgery
Northeast Ohio University College of Medicine
Director of Orthopedic Trauma
St. Elizabeth Health Center
Youngston, Ohio
Commentary on Chapter 43

# Foreword

The emerging new millennium has unveiled awe-inspiring breakthroughs in many domains. The Gordian knot of the genome has been severed, thus releasing a continuous stream of discoveries about our inner being. Technology has exploded as typified by ubiquitous, unwired communications, widespread use of industrial robots, cloning, and the marvelous exploration of interplanetary space. The field of medicine has shared in this modern industrial and technological revolution. Among the many examples of this expansion are the availability of highly accurate and more detailed magnetic resonance imaging, ultrasonography, and computed tomography, genetic engineering, and the application of robotic technology to the surgeons' armamentarium.

Many strategies for injury prevention have been developed in the new millennium, as well. The automotive industry has introduced assisted braking sensors, blind spot sensors, and improved restraint and airbag systems. Engineering creations, such as front distance sensors, will allow cars to be propelled along highways with greatly enhanced warning systems. The Occupational Safety and Health Administration has increased the protection of workers. The medical industry is expanding safety goals to prevent injury to patients and physicians with multiple innovations including retractable scalpels. Great advances are being made at reducing recidivism in our injured population. Screening and brief intervention programs are being applied more frequently for patients under the influence of alcohol or illicit substances, and these approaches should show much benefit in the near future.

With all of the progress made in the prevention of injury and reduced recidivism, why do we need this Sixth Edition? Sadly, the examples of man's inhumanity to man have kept pace with the recent gains in science, technology, medicine, prevention of injury, and patient reeducation. Drivers routinely push their vehicles beyond the limits of safety. This carelessness of course, is exaggerated when under the influence of alcohol or other substances. Motorcyclists persist in their efforts to have our legislative bodies repeal helmet laws. Our citizenry continues to resolve minor disputes with knives and guns in both our large cities and in our so-called peaceful suburbs. The world community has incorporated the scientific advances in weaponry into conflicts on the battlefields, which are often in the middle of large cities. A new technique for creating injury to innocent citizens, namely, the suicidal terroristic act, has created great havoc. More mass catastrophes, such as occurred at the World Trade Center, are waiting to occur. Injury will continue to be the number one cause of death and disability in young people throughout the world. And, the ravages of injury will continue to challenge our most experienced physicians in all specialties; hence, this Sixth Edition is truly needed.

This edition follows the format of the prior editions—namely, presenting the most current thinking by the brightest and the best. The text covers trauma from a global perspective with topics including penetrating wounds, blunt injury, gang violence, insect bites and stings, burns and radiation injury, geriatric and pediatric trauma, genetic influences, and the contributive effects of substance abuse. Each author incorporates appropriate historical vignettes and then progresses to the most current thinking regarding prevention, etiology, and definitive management in both the operating room and in the critical care suite. Excellent illustrations augment the written word. The authors pay appropriate respect to the different views of best therapy where there is controversy, but are sure to leave the reader with a compilation of his/her desired approaches to treatment. The complete bibliography that accompanies each chapter directs the reader to the differing opinions regarding the best therapy for each type of injury. The postoperative challenges of multiple organ failure after hemorrhagic shock and sepsis are thoroughly discussed.

The Sixth Edition has added four new topics that are vital to the trauma and acute care surgeon in the 21st century. Two of these new chapters, "Disaster Management" and "Weapons of Mass Destruction", are in response to the increased threat of terrorism and mass casualties. A third new chapter, "Acute Care Surgery," introduces the reader to the role that trauma surgeons will be fulfilling in the near future throughout the world. This chapter identifies the logic and efficiency of having on-call surgeons provide emergency care for both trauma and non-trauma emergencies. The fourth new chapter, "Gastrointestinal Failure," expands the reader's appreciation of the effects of shock and sepsis on the gut and outlines the optimal skills for providing nutritional support to the patient with multiple organ dysfunction.

This comprehensive text on trauma and its complications is an important treatise, which belongs in the library of all students, residents, and practitioners who care for or wish to be informed about care of the injured patient.

Charles E. Lucas, MD
Professor, Department of Surgery
Wayne State University School of Medicine
Detroit, Michigan

# Foreword to the First Edition

Death and taxes are the two most quoted inevitabilities of life; trauma qualifies as a legitimate third. Since trauma is a peculiarly surgical disease, surgeons have an overriding responsibility for the injured patient. From the beginning of what we choose to call civilization, the universal public image of the surgeon has been that of the citizen to whom the injured are brought.

If ever all other surgical disease is conquered, trauma will remain. Sooner or later every citizen is a patient. Whether terrorists endure, urban assassins thrive, conventional warfare flare, or atomic power be unleashed can only be conjectured. We can be certain, however, that the exploring child will tumble, the adventurous adolescent misjudge, the young sportsman overreach, the intoxicated adult crash, and the aged fall. Buildings will burn, vehicles will crash, and tornadoes will destroy.

Inconsistencies abound in our attitudes to trauma. As a nation, we talk about premature birth but little about premature death, even though trauma remains the greatest killer of our citizens between the ages of 1 and 44 years when most productive as breadwinners and parents. We properly stress the vital need for active measures to prevent birth accidents when we remain apathetic about other accidents. We view with horror the intoxicated obstetrician but tolerate the drunken driver. We insist on detailed privileges for individual physicians but not for all institutions that seek to manage injured patients. Our Congress, lobbied by interested scientists and lay persons, grants disproportionately vast sums of money to categorical diseases affecting much smaller numbers of citizens than does trauma. It may perhaps be reasonably argued that those interested in trauma have not stressed their case with sufficient vigor. We protect animals against the guns of hunters but accept with seeming equanimity the shame of the highest homicide rate in the Western World and possibly beyond. We devote public money to sports stadiums while neglecting our emergency medical services. We acquiesce in the repeal of helmet laws while we bemoan the cost of care for the thousands of vegetating humans produced each year by this legislative cowardice condoned in the name of personal freedom. The indictment is long and can be lengthened.

The litany is sad, well known, and widely ignored. Almost 100,000 die from accidents each year and 9 million more sustain disabling injuries. With an increase in the speed limit recently legislated, vehicular deaths will soon exceed 50,000 again and disabling injuries rise to approximately 2 million annually. The cost to the country is estimated at about $100 billion each year with vehicular accidents accounting for half of this. Approximately $25 billion more will be lost in wages, and medical expenses will be about $15 billion. Almost 10% of all hospital discharges will have originated in trauma and about 4 million citizens will be labeled with a capricious DRG that discriminates against the institutions that treat the most severely injured among them. Alcohol will continue to be a factor in more than half the motor vehicle accidents with few attempts made to curb its potential for carnage. Each U.S. citizen will have a 1 in 70 chance of being hospitalized for trauma this year and almost 50% of the male deaths due to trauma will occur in individuals under the age of 34. Two million citizens will be burned, approximately 100,000 hospitalized, and 10,000 will die.

As if inured to the presence of trauma, our society has chosen for the most part-or at least until very recent times-to accept trauma with a passivity reminiscent of that displayed by the ancients toward lightning and the bubonic plague. For the most part, public interest has flared only in times of military or civilian conflict. Over the years, a relatively small group of surgeons has viewed the care of the injured as their primary clinical responsibility while a still smaller cadre have concerned themselves with the scientific and sociologic aspects of the disease. Regrettably, the central governments of the world have conspicuously ignored the problem even when trauma takes the pride of their youth, hobbles their workers, and empties their coffers. Most citizens are sensitized to trauma only when a personal loss is suffered or when a national celebrity falls victim. Even then, the more for reform tends to be fleeting and surgeons and physicians as a group have been slow to fan the embers of heightened sensitivity. As yet, no sustained passion for prevention and cure, as typified by campaigns on cancer and cardiovascular disease, has been generated.

Happily, a perceptible change has occurred over the past 25 years. A sense of urgency is now discernible and a determination

"The First Edition was published in October, 1987."

to improve results is increasingly visible. Today, it is clearly recognized that trauma is a disease that can be identified, measured, and often prevented. The effects of trauma can be ameliorated and lives saved. While the needs of the injured patient have often been obscured by a veil shot through with institutional ambitions, personal gains, professional convenience, and public apathy, many holes have now been made in this fabric, which in some parts of the country has been virtually stripped away. The Committee on Trauma of the American College of Surgeons, aided increasingly by other medical and lay organizations, has been largely responsible for this change as it has sought to elevate the public recognition of trauma of that accorded to other major diseases. While doing this, these groups have stressed organization, efficiency, quality of care, and their individual responsibility of all health professionals involved with the injured patient. It is proper that surgeons should lead in the design of systems to prevent trauma. Surgeons should also lead in the rapid identification of the injured when such systems fail, the implementation of protocols for prehospital transport and care, the organization of hospital staffs and resources to permit optimal care, the collection of data for trauma registries which permit epidemiologic and clinical studies, the design of educational programs for physicians and others, and the pursuit or research whether managerial, fiscal, sociologic, basic, or clinical in nature. Finally, it is proper that surgeons should be deeply concerned with improving the much neglected phase of rehabilitation.

Education merits special comment. Since trauma knows no visceral boundaries and calls forth a profound physiologic response liable to affect every cell and system in the body simultaneously and to varying unpredictable degrees, an essential feature of the training of any surgeon is the ability to recognize priorities as if by instinct. The sequential application of resuscitative interventions should come naturally to any trained surgeon of whatever persuasion. Knowledge of advanced trauma life support skills should be as integral to a surgeon as a knowledge of the importance of sterility at the operating table.

Trauma does not lend itself well nor naturally to intellectual fragmentation. Organs cannot be viewed in isolation. The potential for organ failure-lung, kidney, intestine, cerebrum-originating from an anatomic distant site is omnipresent. The need for imaginative and logical mental projection into the patient's clinical future is therefore axiomatic. While important for all surgical lesions, nowhere is this skill more important than in the care of the acutely injured patient.

To this point, most textbooks, reflecting the rather narrow vision of trauma held by most physicians, have concentrated almost exclusively on the technical aspects of therapy. This volume is possibly the first to attempt to encompass their modern approach to trauma as an integrated, orderly, broad and thoughtful enterprise rather than a relatively crude prosaic venture. This comprehensive array of chapters ranges from the surgeon's inescapable responsibility for promoting the avoidance of trauma to the long neglected social, economic, and rehabilitative facets that we have found so difficult to engage. Samuel Johnson's observation that "man needs more often to be reminded than informed" is belied in the pages that follow as all who care for the injured patient will find much to instruct them. Trauma is the common thread that binds all surgeons together. It remains a stark reminder of our origins and our obligations.

Alexander J. Walt, MB, ChB, MS(Minn),
FRCS(Eng), FRCS(C),
Penberthy Professor and Chairman
Department of Surgery
Wayne State University
Chief of Surgery
Harper-Grace Hospitals
Detroit, Michigan

# Preface to the Sixth Edition

Over 22 years ago, the three editors of *TRAUMA* met with the original publishers of the textbook to plan the First Edition. Envisioned as a true, comprehensive reference for all involved with the care of injured patients, the book has continued to evolve over what are now six editions. The philosophy of the editors, however, has remained consistent. First, new chapters are added as the body of knowledge in trauma expands and areas of interest change in the trauma community. Second, the authors of 30-35% of the chapters are changed with each edition to bring new perspectives to a textbook that is published on a regular basis at relatively short intervals.

This Sixth Edition retains the format of previous editions with sections entitled Trauma Overview, Generalized Approaches to the Traumatized Patient, Management of Specific Injuries, Special Problems, and Management of Complications after Trauma. All aspects of trauma, including history, epidemiology, prevention, regionalization, scoring and outcomes, kinematics, prehospital care, response to mass casualties and disasters, rural trauma, evaluation and resuscitation in the emergency department, operative and nonoperative care for specific injuries, management of special problems, and critical care after trauma are discussed. Also, the Sixth Edition includes four new chapters entitled Disaster Management, Weapons of Mass Destruction, Acute Care Surgery, and Gastrointestinal Failure. These are all topics of great interest currently in the worldwide trauma community. In addition, 31% of the chapters now have new authors from new institutions. The authors of the commentaries have been changed from those in the Fifth Edition, as well. The Sixth Edition, therefore, is intended to be an up-to-date and one-stop comprehensive reference source that contains information on the entire continuum of trauma care.

Since the completion of the Fifth Edition, three special colleagues who made significant contributions to prior editions of *TRAUMA* have passed away. This Sixth Edition is dedicated to their memories and is a small token of appreciation for their teaching, friendship, and contributions to *TRAUMA*:

C. James Carrico, MD (l935-2002)-Friend, teacher, leader in the trauma community, renowned academic surgeon, and Role Model in American Surgery

Peter Mucha, Jr., MD (l943-2006)-Mentor, friend, charismatic inspiration to many, Mayo surgeon, and Innovative Leader in Trauma Care

Charles J. Weigel, II, JD (l936-2006)-Friend, teacher and advisor, founder of the South Texas Law Institute for Medical Studies, and Distinguished Professor of Law

## ACKNOWLEDGMENTS

An extraordinary number of individuals contribute to a comprehensive textbook of this size. The Editors are especially grateful for the efforts of the authors of the chapters and commentaries for their willingness to share their knowledge, expertise, and time and ensure that *TRAUMA* remains a standard in the field. Special thanks are extended to Dr. Charles E. Lucas, Professor of Surgery at Wayne State University School of Medicine and surgeon extraordinaire, for writing the Foreword to the Sixth Edition. In addition to mentoring the first editor, he has been a teacher and role model for an entire generation of surgeons who care for injured patients.

We are also indebted to the most tolerant and supportive staff from McGraw-Hill Medical Publishing Division-Marsha S. Loeb, Editor, and Christie Naglieri, Project Development Editor. They have endured delays, excuses, and revisions with remarkable professionalism and patience. We thank them for their commitment to excellence.

*TRAUMA* could not have been completed without the valiant efforts of our administrative assistants-Chuki King Valentine, Samantha Bucknor, Meg Lewis-Howe (DVF), Mary Allen and Lisa Villarreal(KLM), and Victoria Martin (EEM). They arranged schedules to permit writing and editing, typed manuscripts, communicated with authors and publishers, and coordinated many of the activities necessary to complete this Sixth Edition. We thank them for their many contributions to the textbook and for their friendship and loyalty.

Finally, we thank all of our families, mentors, teachers, friends in the field of trauma, and especially, faculty colleagues and surgical residents from Emory University, Baylor College of Medicine, and the University of Colorado.

David V. Feliciano, MD
Kenneth L. Mattox, MD
Ernest E. Moore, MD

# TRAUMA

# TRAUMA OVERVIEW

# History of Trauma Care

*Basil A. Pruitt, Jr.* ■ *Jeffrey H. Pruitt*

In the earliest times injury was frequent and varied from that due to falls to assaults by other humans and wild animals. Since most nonfatal injuries such as lacerations and fractures are visible, trauma care must have been a major component of early medical practice. Ancient physicians initially treated injuries by observation and only by tentative trial and error were surgical interventions developed. The surgeons of Egypt, surely some of the first trauma surgeons, are reported to have performed amputations, lithotomies, removal of cataracts, extraction of foreign bodies, and the dressing of wounds. Egyptian civilization, which began perhaps as early as 6000 BC and reached its peak around 3500 BC,[1] produced some of the earliest medical documents that serve as a baseline from which we can assess medical progress and improvements in trauma care. The Edwin Smith papyrus, dated 1600 BC, presents 48 cases of trauma described from head to foot, capita ad calcem, an approach that is still in use.[2] The Ebers papyrus, dated 1550 BC, recommended several topical applications for the treatment of injuries. Goat dung in fermenting yeast or a frog warmed in oil was recommended for burns, so was raw meat for crocodile bites. The effectiveness of such treatment was amplified by a specific incantation which in the case of a burn was delivered to the god Horus.[3]

Surgery developed to an unusually high level in ancient India (2500–500 BC) as recorded in three books that were considered to be sacred: the *Rig Veda*, the *Atharva Veda*, and the *Sushruta Samhita*. The *Rig Veda*, the *Atharva Veda*, and the other two original vedas, "Yajur" and "Sama", were written between 2000 and 1000 BC and the *Ayur Veda*, a "life science supplement" upon which Sushruta, the father of Hindu surgery, based his Samhita was added sometime in the 9th century BC. The Sushruta Samhita, which was probably written around 600 BC, classified operations into eight general types: incising, excising, scraping, puncturing, searching or probing, extracting, secreting fluids, and suturing. Sushruta described 125 surgical instruments and provided instructions for the use of each. The volume also detailed the character traits and temperament needed by surgeons, emphasized adequate

training, and described the use of models to prepare apprentices to perform surgery. Plastic surgery had its origin in this era since the repair of torn earlobes and those deformed by infection was described and reconstruction of the nose was rather commonplace. Cataract extraction was also described, as was the extraction of bladder stones and the manipulation and surgical extraction of a dead fetus from the uterus. In his description of operations, Sushruta emphasized the importance of adequate preparation of the surgeon, as well as cleanliness throughout the operative procedure.[3]

One of the earliest textbooks of medicine, the *Nei Ching* (Canon of Medicine), was written in ancient China by Huang Ti about 1100 BC, but apparently antedated to 2600 BC to increase its authority.[3] In that volume debridement is described in the management of dirty ulcers, for which the surgeon cut and scooped out the spoiled tissue.[4] The development of surgery in ancient China was impeded by the Confucian belief in the sanctity of the body which prohibited anatomical dissections. Consequently, Chinese surgeons had little anatomic knowledge and limited their practice to massage, acupuncture, and moxibustion. Hua T'o, considered to be the god of surgery by Chinese surgeons of the 2nd and 3rd centuries, was known for his moxibustion skills, his use of a mixture of opium and wine as an anesthetic, and his ability to foretell the sex of unborn children.[5]

## THE PRACTICE OF MEDICINE IN ANCIENT GREECE

In the 7th century BC, the Iliad was written to describe events and conflicts that occurred five or six centuries earlier. In that volume it is reported that Makaon, son of Asklepios, treated Menelaus for an arrow wound by removing the arrow, "sucking out the blood", and applying a healing salve originally given to Asklepios by the centaur Cheiron, who had raised Asklepios and taught him the healing arts.[6] That report is considered to be the first written description of the treatment of battle wounds.

The influence of the cult of Asklepios peaked in the 6th and 5th centuries BC as evidenced by the hundreds of temples of Asklepios present in the Greek empire. In those temples, considered by many to have been the first hospitals, treatment was a mix of religious supplication directed by priests and medical advice provided by the collection of physicians gathered near each temple. Pythagoras (circa 530 BC) was opposed to any surgical procedure lest it destroy the soul. Consequently, surgical procedures at the temples were limited to the incision of abscesses.[5]

The rise of Greek civilization marked a turning point in medicine. In the 6th century BC, the existing doctrine of disease as a mystic imbalance was challenged by two physicians of Miletos, Anaximander proposed water as the principle element and source of life, while Anaximenes made the same claims for air. In the 5th century BC several Greek schools laid the foundation of modern medicine. Two philosopher-scientist schools flourished at about the same time, one at Cnidos on the coast of Asia Minor and one at Cos, an island off the coast of Greece. Hippocrates, considered the father of modern medicine, lived and taught on the island of Cos.[5]

Surgery reached a high point in Greek civilization and many conditions are mentioned that were treated by either operative or manipulative means. In the 5th and 4th centuries BC, Hippocrates is believed to have authored some of the 72 medical books that were subsequently collectively titled "Corpus Hippocraticum." Fractures and dislocations, being of common occurrence, are given a great deal of attention in these writings. Wounds of all kinds were described and treatment was emphasized. The noun iatros, which means physician in modern Greek, originally meant "extractor of arrows" in ancient Greek.[7] Essentially, the Hippocratic school believed in keeping the wound at rest, adding little or nothing from the outside, and carefully coapting the edges of the wound to achieve healing.[8] Unfortunately, Hippocrates believed that wound inflammation was beneficially reduced by inducing pus formation as soon as possible.[5] It was a piece of Greek pottery from the 2nd century BC on which the word τραυμα meaning wound appears in the inscription, "the wound (trauma) that you have, we didn't do it…," that led to the use of the word *trauma* to describe a wound or injury (Figure 1-1).

After Hippocrates, Greek medicine reached a peak at Alexandria. Ptolemy, one of Alexander's generals, determined that the sum total of the world's knowledge should be housed in a library at Alexandria.[9] From that repository, the medical knowledge of the Greeks began to infiltrate Rome, taken there by Greek practitioners. Greek was the language of cultivated Romans, and the upper classes had their children taught by Greek tutors and derived their literature from Greek models. Medicine of the time was almost entirely that of the Greeks.[10]

## CONTRIBUTIONS OF THE ROMAN EMPIRE TO MEDICINE

The center of medical progress slowly shifted to the west. In 162, Galen (130–200 AD) moved from his birthplace, Pergamon, to Rome where his success in treating the wounds of gladiators resulted in his appointment as personal physician to the emperor Marcus Aurelius. In Galen's prolific writings (over 400) he described trepanning of the skull, intestinal or abdominal wall suture for penetrating abdominal wounds of the gladiators, removal of varicose veins, plastic surgery for cleft lip, and uvulectomy for coughing. Even so, his advocacy of suppuration as an essential and beneficial component of wound healing is credited with impeding surgical progress for a millennium.[11]

The Ayurvedic medical writings of Charaka provided detailed description of hospital systems in India in the 600 BC to 200 AD era which served as de facto blueprints for the Muslims who built the world's first great hospitals after their conquest of India.[5] The first system of hospitals in the Western world is said to have been developed by the Romans primarily for the military legions, not for the public at large.[3] Prior to that time wounded soldiers had been cared for in the homes of the rich; later tents were set up apart from military barracks as separate units. In 394, Fabiola, a Roman aristocrat, established the first Christian public hospital in Rome.[5] Early hospitals were also established in the Byzantine Empire which became the eastern part of the Roman Empire in the 1st century BC and the capital of the entire Roman Empire in 330 AD.

## MEDICAL ADVANCES DURING THE MIDDLE AGES

The Middle Ages or medieval period, which extended from 476 when Rome fell to the Goths to 1453 when Constantinople fell to the Turks, was a time in which little medical progress occurred and surgery was actually diminished. After the fall of Rome, the Persians preserved and promulgated Greek knowledge and in turn conveyed it to Arab conquerors.[12] After the Mohammedans rose to power and captured Alexandria (640 AD), the Arabs preserved and ultimately transmitted the science of the Greeks.[13] The Arab school began in 640 when Omar (Mahomat's successor) destroyed the Alexandrian school.[12] Arabian physicians, apparently heeding an aphorism of Hippocrates extolling the virtues of cautery, replaced most of operative surgery with cautery as their favored modality to control hemorrhage and create a dry wound surface.[14] However, Rhazes, a famous Arab surgeon of the 9th and 10th centuries (850–932), continued his surgical work and described the use of the strings from a harp (cat gut) to suture wounds.[15]

The rise of Christianity brought compassion for the sick and injured, who were previously isolated and shunned, and marked the beginning of compassionate care as we know it today.[10] During the early part of the medieval period (476–814, known as the Dark Ages)

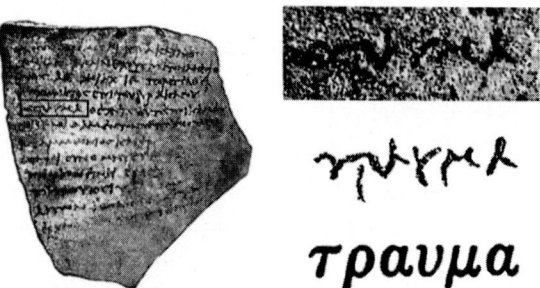

**FIGURE 1-1.** A statement on a piece of ancient Greek pottery, written by two brothers who deny beating up a third brother by stating, "the wound (trauma) that you have, we didn't do it….."

priests and monks developed what has been termed monastic medicine and monastic hospitals in which they provided care to the sick. That care, based on theological concepts which emphasized treatment by prayer and attributed results to God's will, had no place for operative intervention. Beginning in 1125 at Rheims a series of ecclesiastic edicts were issued to preserve traditional monastic lifestyle and limit involvement of the clergy in medical activities. The edict of the Council of Clermont in 1130 decreed that priests and monks should no longer practice medicine.[5] Consequently, the monastic hospitals either ceased to function or were subsequently taken over by lay physicians. In the absence of the clergy, hospital care deteriorated with little attention given to hygiene and cleanliness because of total ignorance of the cause of infection. For the next several centuries hospitals in civilian life were generally held in low regard and were commonly populated by the economically indigent.

The subsequent Ecclesia Abhorrent a Sanguine edicts of the Council of Tours in 1169 and of Pope Innocent III in 1215 which were issued to prohibit the clergy from any surgical activity, in essence defined surgeons as inferior to practitioners of general medicine and thereby separated medicine from surgery.[16,11] Collectively the edicts removed the stagnating effects of religious dogma on medical progress and opened medicine to the beneficial influence of scientific thinking and experimental observation on the part of secular practitioners.

Failure of the monasteries and cathedral schools of the Holy Roman Empire to provide an effective program of medical education resulted in a shift of medical education to the universities as they developed. The school of Salerno, at which the physicians had remained free of church control and female practitioners were accepted, was the site of the first re-emergence of western European medical education. Constantinus Africanus, a Carthaginian who became a prominent member of the early Salerno faculty, translated Greek and Arabic texts into Latin and made those teachings available to the Salerno students. King Roger II of Sicily issued a decree mandating passage of an examination proving the ability to cure patients and requiring a license to practice. Frederick II, the grandson of Roger and subsequent Emperor of the Holy Roman Empire, dictated in 1240 that all candidates for a medical license be publicly examined by masters of the Salerno school and established examination standards which classified medicine and surgery as equal disciplines. Two classes of surgeons were defined by Frederick, i.e., the first class questioned in Latin by three professors and the second class questioned by two teachers in Italian. A preceptor year was required before the candidate could take the examination and obtain a medical license.[5]

The "Bamberg Surgery", named after the principality in which it was found, describes the treatment of a variety of wounds and fractures including those of the skull and is considered to be the first (mid-12th century) surgical manuscript written by a faculty member of the Salernitan School. Two decades later, Ruggierio Frugardi, known as Roger of Salerno, authored the Practica Chirurgiae, the first independent systematic surgical text in the western world. That volume describes the treatment of fractures, both simple and compound, treatment of lacerated nerves, and in discussing the treatment of wounds recommends immediate extraction of foreign matter. The repair of an incomplete laceration of the intestine by suture of the intestinal wound over a wooden stent placed within the intestinal lumen is described.[5]

Even though the ecclesiastic edicts that abhorred bloodshed retarded surgical progress, the advance of surgery was maintained, to a degree, by faculty members of the University of Bologna. Hugo of Lucca and his son, Theodoric, were both keen observers, original thinkers, and innovative surgeons. Theodoric, who became Bishop of Cervia in 1256, conducted an extensive practice of surgery and in 1256 published Chirurgia in which he recorded his father's accomplishments and his own techniques and principles of surgical care.[5] Theodoric disputed the medical belief of the times that laudable pus and the healing of wounds by secondary intention were desirable. He taught the simple dry treatment of wounds as noted in the following quotation:

> For it is not necessary, as Roger and Roland have written, as many of their disciples teach, and as all modern surgeons profess, that pus should be generated in wounds. No error can be greater than this. Such a practice is indeed to hinder nature, to prolong the disease, and to prevent the conglutination and consolidation of the wound.[9]

Theodoric's name is also associated with medieval anesthesia on the basis of his description of a soporific sponge in the following passage:

> Some prescribed medicaments . . . send a patient to sleep, so that the incision may not be felt such as opium, the juice of the morel, hyoscyamus, mandrake, ivy, hemlock, and lettuce. A new sponge is soaked, by them, in these juices and left to dry in the sun; and when they have need of it, they put this sponge into warm water and then hold it under the nostrils of the patient until he goes to sleep. Then they perform the operation.[9]

One of the most important medical advances during the middle ages was the extension of the regulation of physician training and the licensing begun by King Roger II of Sicily. In the 15th century, the Guild of Barber Surgeons, which ultimately evolved into the Royal College of Surgeons, was chartered in England and the College de St. Côme regulated surgeons in the practice of surgery in France.[14] Some ideas of contagion developed and policies of public health were expanded and became a part of medical thought.

Surgeons who contributed much during this time were Henri de Mondeville who studied with Theodoric and Guy de Chauliac. De Mondeville made a major stand on the principle of avoiding suppuration by simple cleanliness, thus permitting the wound to heal by first intention. In his manuscript which he began in 1306 and entitled "Chirurgie" he enunciated the removal of foreign objects, control of bleeding, closure of the wound, and application of compresses soaked in hot wine as principles of wound care.[5] De Chauliac was unusual because, although he was a country boy, he had received an excellent education. He was an outstanding surgeon and attempted to have surgical operations put in the hands of qualified surgeons instead of the itinerant quacks who so often performed surgery in those days. He advanced the treatment of fractures by using a sling bandage for the arm and using weights with pully traction for the leg. In 1363, DeChauliac published a seven-part text entitled "La Grande Chirurgie" in which he recommended individualized wound care based on the characteristics of the wound and described the use of Theodoric's soporific sponge for analgesia. In the third volume of his magnum opus he enumerated the five components of wound care which included removal of foreign objects, rejoining of severed tissues, maintenance of tissue continuity, preservation of organ substance, and prevention of complications. Unfortunately, he was a committed proponent of laudable pus. The prominence of DeChauliac and the long term preeminence of La Grande Chirurgie obscured the earlier work of Theoderic and DeMondeville and earned DeChauliac the dubious reputation of having impeded progress in surgical wound care for over four centuries.[5,11,16]

## MEDICAL ADVANCES DURING THE RENAISSANCE

The period of the Renaissance, or the revival of learning, extended approximately from 1450 AD to 1600 AD. Although mysticism and superstition were still a major part of medical thought, science based on observation and experimentation was beginning to develop. Misconceptions about anatomy, some of which arose as a consequence of Galen's transposition of animal data to humans, were dispelled and corrected by the detailed studies of Vesalius. Those studies were published in 1543 as the copiously illustrated volume De Humani Corporis Fabrica Libri Septem.

In 1560, Leonardo Botallo recommended removing foreign material, trimming away dead tissue, and returning the affected tissue to as normal a condition as possible without mention of a need for suppuration.[17] That recommendation can be viewed as confirmation of a revolutionary change in wound care that occurred 24 years earlier. Ambroise Paré began his medical career as a "dissector" and surgeon's assistant at the Hotel Dieu in Paris before becoming an army surgeon in 1536. Paré is credited with reorienting wound care by noting the absence of inflammation and the benign condition of his patients when a lack of boiling oil (commonly used to sear wounds) forced him to omit that component of wound care during the siege of Turin. Paré wrote a compendium of Vesalius' Fabrica in the vernacular and thus made it accessible to all surgeons.[18] Because he wrote in his native tongue and was not a Latin scholar, he was ridiculed by his fellow physicians, but he possessed a clear mind, keen powers of observation, and a gift for original thought.

In the last decade of the 16th century William Clowes, considered to be the greatest surgeon of Elizabethan England, published a book for young surgeons based on his experience in the British Navy. In that volume, "A Prooved Practise for All Young Chirurgians, Concerning Burnings With Gunpowder, and Woundes Made With Gunshot, Sword, Halbard, Pyke…" published in 1588, he recommended debridement, extraction of foreign bodies, and avoidance of cautery in treating war wounds.[19] He also described suture closure of an abdominal gunshot wound after replacing eviscerated intestine which he had correctly deemed to be uninjured.

## MEDICAL ADVANCES DURING THE 17TH CENTURY

The 17th century was a period in which a number of great physicians made discoveries that brought about remarkable changes in medicine and for the first time provided a scientific basis for the advances in medicine which were to follow. In 1628 William Harvey[20] published his great work "De Motu Cordis" in which he described for the first time the circulation of the blood and the action of the heart as a muscular pump. In 1661, Malpighi discovered the capillaries and identified the connection between the arteries and veins previously described by Harvey. Those studies contributed directly to the understanding of the cardiovascular effects of trauma.

In 1656, Christopher Wren, otherwise known for his architectural accomplishments, demonstrated that medicines could be administered to animals by the intravenous route.[21] In 1666, Lower demonstrated that homologous blood could be directly transfused between animals.[22] The clinical application of Lower's work resulted in fatal transfusion reactions which led to legal proscriptions against blood transfusions until the problem of transfusion reactions was solved in the early 1900s. The 17th century closed with the new knowledge of the circulation of the blood; the beginnings of physiologic chemistry, microscopic anatomy, and histology; and some remarkable descriptions of clinical disease.

Unfortunately, the promise of scientific progress did not extend to wound care. In the latter half of the 17th century, Richard Wiseman, often cited as the "Father of English Surgery", accepted the theory of gunpowder as poison and reintroduced cautery for the treatment of war wounds and recommended bandaging such wounds with raw onions to counteract the effects of the gunpowder. He also recommended an onion–salt mixture for application to burns before blistering occurred. Wiseman could also be considered one of the fathers of vascular surgery. In 1672 he published "A Treatise of Wounds" in which he described a two-stage removal of an aneurysm from an artery in the upper limb of a cooper.[11]

## MEDICAL ADVANCES DURING THE 18TH CENTURY

The beginning of the 18th century saw the rise of the medical school at Vienna. It reached its peak about mid century with a very illustrious faculty. The science of physiology was expanded in the 18th century by the studies of the Englishman, Steven Hale, who, interestingly, was both a clergyman and an inventor. He originated artificial ventilation and was the first to measure blood pressure by inserting a long glass tube into the artery of a horse and measuring the height of the blood column.

During this century various gasses that occur in the atmosphere were discovered.[23] Carbon dioxide was identified by Black in 1757, hydrogen by Cavendish in 1766, nitrogen by Rutherford in 1772, and oxygen by Priestley and Scheele in 1771. It was, however, Antoine-Laurent Lavoisier who described the interchange of the gasses in the lungs and demonstrated that respiration was necessary to the process of oxidation in living tissue. These discoveries eventually led to an understanding of the role of blood pressure and respiration.

A professor at Padua for almost 50 years, Giovanni Battista Morgagni created the science of cellular pathology. Although we usually credit this to Virchow, he himself acknowledged that Morgagni was the first pathologist. Morgagni's classic work, not written and published until he was 79 years of age, consisted of five books including a total of 70 letters. Morgagni was the first to correlate postmortem findings with the clinical symptoms he saw in some 500 cases at autopsy. He provided a basis for medical study that is still used today, and discredited once and for all the humoral theories of disease promulgated by many famous physicians that had existed for centuries. From this time on, cellular structure would be evaluated in the study of trauma.

Two Scotsmen played an important and almost electrifying role in the 18th century. The first was William Hunter, who became the leading obstetrician in London and gave a course of private lectures on anatomic dissection, operative surgery, and bandaging. In 1768 he built the Anatomic Theater and Museum on Great Windmill Street, where he performed his teaching and trained some of the best English anatomists and surgeons of the period including his brother, John.[5] John Hunter was an interesting contrast to his brother William, having been a poor student and not very interested in much of anything until he joined his brother and was put to work helping in the dissecting room. John was fascinated by dissection, and not only was he a superb student but within a year he was teaching anatomy as well as continuing to learn surgery under such surgeons as Cheselden and Percival Pott.[5] It is fair to say that John Hunter converted surgery from a purely clinical activity into a science. He was an avid collector of animal specimens of all kinds, and developed a museum of over 13,000 such specimens. He trained many of the most gifted scientists and surgeons who were to come after him, including Jenner, Astley Cooper, and John Abernethy, as well as a number of budding American physicians.[5] John Hunter was the founder of experimental and surgical pathology and an expert in comparative physiology and experimental morphology. In 1763, on the basis of his experiences in military campaigns in France and Portugal, he began writing his book entitled *A Treatise on the Blood, Inflammation, and Gunshot Wounds*,[24] which was published in 1794 one year after his death. As noted below, this work stands as a monument to this outstanding scientist who had almost no education and taught himself and the world the experimental method.

Sir John Pringle contributed to trauma care in a slightly different way during this same period. He was the Surgeon General of the English Army from 1742 to 1758, and was considered by many to be the founder of military medicine and the originator of the Red Cross. Pringle was an excellent epidemiologist and as an early advocate of antisepsis is said to have coined the word antisepsis.[25] During the battle of Dettingen (1743), the English surgeons under Pringle's leadership made the suggestion, readily accepted by the French surgeons, that the hospitals on both sides be considered sanctuaries for the wounded and be mutually protected. This was readily agreed to by the leaders of both sides and the concept remained loosely in effect, not only through that war but until it was put on a permanent basis during the Geneva Convention of 1864.[26]

It would be unwise to leave the 18th century without mentioning American medicine which began to take shape in the 1700s as European physicians immigrated to the United States and U.S. physicians journeyed to Europe for training, such as that provided by John Hunter noted above. There had been only one medical publication in the American colonies in the 17th century and the first book in the 18th century was apparently nothing more than a reprint of an English text. As so often happens, the Revolutionary War brought American medicine into clear focus and was the basis for its development in the American colonies. In 1775, John Jones, who had studied with the Hunters in England and had founded the Kings College Medical School in New York, published a manual on the treatment of wounds and fractures for young military surgeons. The manual largely conformed to Hunter's recommendations with relatively minor modifications based on Jones' experience as a volunteer surgeon in the French and Indian Wars. Sutures were to be seldom employed, but when used were removed when the surgeon deemed wound union to have occurred often within 24 to 72 hours. The presence of pus and other signs of inflammation were considered to be signs of proper healing and their absence was considered ominous. Compound fractures were commonly amputated to avoid the risk of life-threatening infection. Bloodletting was a prominent feature of what was called exhaustive therapy, which also included enemata, emetics, and blistering agents as well.[27]

## MEDICAL ADVANCES DURING THE 19TH CENTURY

During the 19th century there were revolutionary changes in medical education and tremendous advances in trauma care brought about by social, political, and scientific changes. The political revolutions of France and the rest of Central Europe, which followed the revolution in the United States, changed the attitudes of people and brought about a new dimension to intellectual as well as political freedom. This intellectual freedom created a rebellion against dogmatism, charlatanism, and metaphysics which had earlier restricted human thought. The middle and lower classes began to participate in this intellectual freedom. The doors were open to the Universities, now free from political and religious control, and a new and bright horizon opened for everyone. Between 1842 and 1867 four events—the discovery of general anesthesia, the establishment of standards for hospital sanitation and hygiene, the publication of Virchow's Cellular Pathology, and the development of antiseptic surgery—set the stage for the future of medicine and advanced surgical care of the injured.

General anesthesia was a great American contribution to the medical world. The effectiveness of ether was demonstrated by Crawford Long in 1842 and by William Morton in 1846. Similarly, in 1847 James Simpson, Professor of Obstetrics at the University of Edinburgh, demonstrated the effectiveness of chloroform as yet another anesthetic agent.[5] Dr. Edward H. Barton first used ether to amputate a leg at the U.S. Army Hospital in Vera Cruz in 1847 during the Mexican-American War. That agent was used in at least a dozen more patients, but the senior army surgeon at that hospital deemed anesthetic agents to be "universally injurious" and terminated their use.[28] During the Civil War chloroform was the preferred agent in both armies as reported by H. H. McGuire, the Medical Director of the Stonewall Brigade of the Confederate States Army. McGuire reported that he and his staff had used chloroform in more than 28,000 cases without a death including its use when he amputated General Jackson's left arm and removed a round ball from his right hand.[29]

The control of operative pain increased the acceptance of surgery by both patients and surgeons. Anesthesia also permitted the surgeon to perform a more deliberate operation and to identify and ligate individual vessels and thereby reduce blood loss.[30] The use of anesthesia led to a new concept that hemostasis was a principle of operative surgery. Even so, one must remember that laudable pus was still the watchword of the day, and it was believed that pus was necessary to the healing of wounds. If secondary hemorrhage occurred because of infection or because of avulsion of sutures no replacement fluid was available and such bleeding could be fatal.

A second advance was brought about by the heroic efforts of Florence Nightingale and her staff of thirty-seven nurses who under the auspices of the British Sanitary Commission coordinated medical relief activities in hospitals and the hospital services during the Crimean War (1854–1856). Institution of sanitation and hygiene measures in the hospitals and in the living quarters of the troops established new standards for military hospitals and strikingly reduced death from disease which had reduced the original 25,000 member British force in the Crimea to 17,000 in the first year of the campaign.[31] Although hemorrhage remained a nemesis for the surgeon, infection began to come under control. The brilliant work of Louis Pasteur in France, and his discovery of bacteria as the source of infection, began to change the entire picture of trauma care.[32] Pasteur disposed of the theory of spontaneous generation by demonstrating that microorganisms were in the air and were the cause of putrefaction. Pasteur discovered the Streptococci and the Staphylococci, provided one of the earliest reports of sepsis when he described the toxic effects of bacteria, and developed vaccines for both animal and human infections.[11] A British surgeon, Joseph Lister, was despondent over the high mortality rate that accompanied compound fractures. When he learned of the work of Pasteur, Lister concluded that the high infection rate and subsequent death rate from compound fractures might be due to the same microorganisms. It was known at the time that carbolic acid was a powerful antiseptic, and Lister developed a machine to spray carbolic acid in the wounds and into the air surrounding operative sites.[33] As Lister reported in 1867, his technique reduced the death rate after amputation from 46% of 35 cases to 15% of 40 cases.[11] Antisepsis met with resistance from many surgeons who thought that it was nonsense to suggest that something that could not be seen was the cause of infection. The studies of Robert Koch, Professor of Hygiene and Bacteriology in Berlin, published in 1877 documented that bacteria caused wound infections and accelerated the acceptance of antisepsis.[5] Adoption of antisepsis throughout the world remarkably changed the outcome for trauma patients just as the studies of Holmes and those of Semmelweis identified the cause of childbed fever and changed the outcome for women giving birth.[34] The theory of asepsis with use of sterile operating garb, sterile drapes, and rubber gloves, and the sterilization of equipment and supplies was subsequently developed. The aseptic regimen, the standard in today's operating rooms, was completed in the early years of the 20th century when the use of surgical masks became common place.[35]

Virchow's publication of "Cellular Pathology" in 1860 revealed previously unappreciated cellular changes that expanded the knowledge of surgical pathology and the pathogenesis of surgical disease.[36] Subsequent clinical and laboratory studies at the cellular level based on Virchow's work were particularly important in unraveling the mechanisms underlying hemorrhagic shock in trauma patients.

The establishment of the Sheffield Scientific School at Yale University in 1869 is considered to have been the first attempt in the United States to provide training in the scientific method for potential clinical investigators.[37] In 1871, Dr. Henry P. Bowditch established the first university laboratory for experimental physiology

at Harvard Medical School.[37] The second laboratory of physiology was soon established at the Johns Hopkins University School of Medicine in 1876.[37] Simultaneously, in the last half of the 19th century, establishment of basic science laboratories at the German medical schools provided the environment in which what was called "physiological medicine" developed and was used to study clinical problems.[37] Studies at those and subsequently established laboratories led to the development of improved treatment of shock and wounds in injured patients.

Physiologically based clinical research involving trauma patients began even earlier in the 19th century in the U.S. Army when William Beaumont, on June 16, 1822, was called to see the penetrating abdominal wound of Alexis St. Martin. Beaumont's 238 experiments and observations on gastric physiology conducted on St. Martin over the next 11 years identified gastric acid production and the morphologic changes of the gastric mucosa associated with digestion, emotion, and injury.[38] In 1833 Beaumont published his findings in "Experiments and Observations on the Gastric Juice and the Physiology of Digestion."

## MEDICAL ADVANCES DURING THE 20TH CENTURY

During the 20th century the United States was involved in four major wars on foreign soil, each of which had a specific impact on the development of trauma surgery. Persistent problems with care of the severely injured were recognized at the beginning of the century and addressed by focused research during the major conflicts. The experience of the surgeons involved in each conflict and the results of combat casualty care research have subsequently been applied to improve the outcome of civilian trauma patients. Medical research activity in the military increased during each of the four major conflicts of the 20th century. In World War I (WWI), George Crile, who strongly advocated intravenous fluid therapy on the basis of his experimental use of sea water for the treatment of hemorrhagic shock, was placed in charge of the central laboratory of the American Expeditionary Forces where he extended his earlier studies.[39] Saline infusions as treatment for hypovolemia were not Crile's original idea, Thomas Latta had used saline infusions for the treatment of cholera patients way back in 1831.[40] In 1854 Buhl noted the similarity of volume losses in cholera patients and burn patients,[41] but it was not until 1901 that Parascondolo, in Naples, reported a good response of three burn patients to whom he had administered intravenous saline solutions.[42] Shortly thereafter, Haldor Snevé of St. Paul, Minnesota, reported eight patients with thermal injury to whom he administered normal saline orally, as chilled enemata, as transfusions, by hypodermoclysis, and as baths in which the patients were immersed.[43] Snevé's recommendations were largely ignored until Frank P. Underhill of Yale studied patients burned in the Rialto Theater fire of 1921.[44] He identified the severity of their postburn volume changes in his studies of blister fluid and focused attention on plasma loss. Subsequent experimental studies by Alfred Blalock and the clinical studies of Henry M. Harkins established a blood and plasma volume deficit as the cardinal feature of hemorrhagic and burn shock.[45,46] In 1930 Blalock further showed that hypovolemia due to mechanical trauma was characterized by a disproportionate plasma loss as compared to red cell loss.[47]

Subsequent studies by Cope and Moore in burn patients and Shires and colleagues in trauma patients have quantified the volume deficits subsequent to injury and identified the effects of such volume loss on organ and cell function.[48,49]

In 1932 Gerald Domagk patented Prontosil which was the first of a family of sulfonamides.[50] Domagk received a Nobel Prize in 1939 for this work. In 1941, sulfonamides became available for clinical use and were used both topically and systemically for the treatment of wounds. Studies by Frank Meleney ultimately demonstrated that the sulfonamides then in use did not influence the occurrence of wound infection and could actually physically impair wound healing by forming a thick crust.[51] In studies by German surgeons and the later studies by Mendelson and Lindsey, however, it was found that topical application of mafenide acetate, an $n^1$ unsubstituted sulfonamide, could prevent the development of gas gangrene in soft tissue wounds of patients for whom definitive treatment was delayed.[52] Penicillin, the first bactericidal antibiotic, was discovered in 1929 by Alexander Fleming but its clinical usefulness was not appreciated until the early years of World War II. Subsequent slow development of large-scale production delayed its clinical introduction until 1943 after which it quickly revolutionized the treatment of war wounds.[53]

In 1939 when World War II erupted and millions of Americans were sent to war, science was thrown into high gear. In the few short years between World War I, which first saw the airplane as a combat weapon, and World War II aviation had mushroomed, our methods of destruction had multiplied, and mechanization had taken over. World War II was a mechanized combat even though the foot soldiers still played a major role and unheard of warfare medical problems (such as extensive fragment wounds, wet lung, kidney failure, and problems peculiar to the new types of weapons used) were suddenly upon us. Massive amounts of money were thrown into scientific research during this period and many developments that were the result of this research had far-ranging effects on trauma care. The application of such new technology as sonar, radar, new electronic monitoring modalities, computers, and finally, atomic science led to significant improvement in the care of the trauma patient.

The Korean conflict brought about further advances in trauma care and use of the helicopter as a means for rapidly transporting the wounded. Helicopter transport permitted the severely wounded to receive surgical care close to the front in Mobile Army Surgical Hospital (MASH) units, from which (at times within 24 hours) they could then be transported in fixed wing aircraft to hospitals as far away as Japan and the Philippines. Rapid air evacuation provided a major improvement in the management of the wounded. Improved knowledge in the management of hemorrhagic shock and the provision of adequate supplies of blood and electrolyte solutions at the front also contributed to the reduction in mortality as did the surgery performed by Board-certified or Board-eligible surgeons. Antibiotic therapy had expanded since World War II and this provided the surgeon with new weapons against infection from battle wounds. Hemodialysis was performed in the theater of operations and the repair of vascular injuries became a reality and increased the salvage of severely injured limbs.

The Vietnam War followed soon after the Korean conflict and the lessons learned in World War II and Korea were promptly applied in Vietnam. The artificial kidney, which had been introduced as a support service in Korea, was again available in Vietnam.[54] However, the large volumes of crystalloid solution typically used to effect hemodynamic resuscitation of severely injured patients in the Vietnam conflict markedly reduced the occurrence of acute renal failure.[55] Such therapy appears to have given rise to other complications as indexed by the frequent occurrence of acute pulmonary failure and acute respiratory distress syndrome (ARDS), called Da Nang lung by some, in critically injured combat casualties.[56] Routine laboratory assays permitted scheduled monitoring of organ function and included arterial blood gas measurements that could be used to adjust mechanical ventilators which for the first time were widely used in the theater of operations. Monitoring of critically ill and injured casualties was enhanced by portable radiographic equipment and electronic monitoring devices such as the ultrasonic flow meter.

## FRACTURE FIXATION AND EARLY AMBULATION

The history of fracture treatment provides an excellent illustration of the effective synergy of increased physiologic understanding and new technology. In the 19th century the treatment of long-bone fractures underwent a revolutionary change when Samuel Gross used adhesive tape to apply traction.[57] Henry G. Davis later devised an elastic dressing to use in applying traction and that technique, modified by Gurdon Buck, became the standard treatment in the Union Army Medical Corps during the Civil War.[57] Although plaster fixation with antiseptic occlusion was the common treatment employed for bone and joint wounds during the Spanish American War,[39] Themistocles Gluck used nickel-coated steel plates and screws to immobilize fractures as early as 1885. Gluck also used intramedullary ivory pegs and nails for fracture immobilization.[57] Just Lucas-Championnière, in 1910, emphasized that movement not immobilization promoted the formation of callus,[58] and in 1916 Hey-Groves described both retrograde and direct intramedullary nailing.[57] In 1929, Böhler proposed treating long-bone fractures with closed reduction, plaster of paris dressings, and active ambulation.[59] The Rush brothers of Mississippi reported in 1937 on their experience with the use of intramedullary pin fixation of ulnar fractures.[59] It remained, however, for Gerhard Kuntscher to design a nail made of nonreactive, nontoxic $V^2A$ steel in the 1930s and use that nail in the treatment of German soldiers injured in World War II.[59] In 1942, Maatz described reaming the bone shaft to maximize nail width.[57] Subsequently, Robert Danis advocated axial compression and what he termed "primary suture" of the fractured bone to permit immediate movement of adjacent joints.[59] In the 1950s, M.E. Müller, M. Allgöwer, and H. Willenegger developed the Arbeitsgemeinschaft für Osteosynthesefragen (AO) system which entails atraumatic technique to achieve anatomic reduction and rigid internal fixation followed by early active mobilization.[59] Subsequent to the development of the AO system, Sarmiento designed a below-the-knee plaster of paris dressing for the treatment of tibial fractures with full weight bearing and unrestricted knee motion.[60] Both internal and external fixation which permit early ambulation and reduce the complications associated with prolonged immobilization improve the functional recovery of fracture patients.

## IMAGING AS RELATED TO TRAUMA PATIENTS

Imaging techniques discovered and developed in last years of the 19th century and throughout the 20th century have revolutionized both the diagnosis and treatment of trauma patients. Accuracy of diagnosis has been enhanced and that in turn has established a new equilibrium between nonoperative and operative care of trauma patients. Wilhelm Conrad Roentgen, Professor of Physics and Acting Rector of the University of Wurzburg, discovered X-rays, the first imaging modality in 1895. He received the first Nobel Prize in Physics in 1901 for that discovery. In 1923, Berberich and Hirsch first used strontium bromide as intravascular contrast media to opacify blood vessels of the extremities.. Brooks continued the development of angiography by using sodium iodide solutions in 1924 and Egas Moniz utilized sodium iodide solution for cerebral angiography in 1926.[61] Farinas is credited with being the first to describe insertion of an angiographic catheter into the abdominal aorta by way of the femoral artery in 1941.[62] Margolies et al first employed transcatheter embolization for pelvic trauma in 1972.[63]

In 1897, Tuffier reported making the urinary tract opaque to X-rays by placing a metal stylet within a ureteral catheter.[64] In 1904, Wulff opacified the urinary bladder with a mixture of bismuth subnitrate, starch, and water to demonstrate an anatomical anomaly.[65] In 1905, Voelcker and von Lichtenberg published an article on cystography using a colloidal silver preparation and they performed the first retrograde pyelographic examination using the same solution.[66] In 1923, Leonard G. Rowntree of the Mayo Clinic, first reported opacification of the kidneys, ureters, and bladder after administering both oral and intravenous preparations of sodium iodide. The concentration of that contrast material was too low to permit meaningful interpretation.[67] Between 1921 and 1927, Arthur Binz and his colleagues synthesized numerous pyridine compounds in search for an improved therapeutic agent for the treatment of syphilis.[68] After several trials and errors and modifications suggested by Moses Swick, Professor Binz produced the sodium salt of 5-iodo-2-pyridone-N-acetic acid which possessed high solubility, good tolerance, and urinary excretion which resulted in good visualization of the urinary tract as was described in a paper presented at the 9th Congress of the German Urologic Society in 1929.[69,70] Current urinary tract opacification agents represent modifications of that compound.

For imaging technology, 1971 and 1972 were the banner years. Kristensen and his associates published a case report in 1971 describing the use of ultrasound to identify splenic hematomas in blunt abdominal trauma victims.[71] Abdominal ultrasound examination has been used in Europe and Japan since that time for the evaluation of patients with blunt abdominal trauma. In the United States, surgeons have expanded the Focused Abdominal Sonogram for Trauma (FAST) examination to include assessment of the pericardial sac and the pleural cavities.[72,73] At many trauma centers in the United States the FAST exam, which is noninvasive, relatively inexpensive, and readily repeatable, has replaced diagnostic peritoneal lavage for the rapid identification of intraperitoneal hemorrhage due to organ injury. More recently, ultrasound has also been shown to be effective in the detection of posttraumatic pneumothoraces and fractures.[74,75]

In 1972, computed tomography (CT) was added to the diagnostic modalities available to the trauma surgeon. It was invented by Godfrey Hounsfield and Alan Cormack, who received a Nobel Prize for their invention in 1979.[76] Helical (also called spiral) CT, in the development of which Kalender et al played a major role in the late 1980s, is now widely used in the evaluation of trauma patients.[77] The most notable advance in CT technology has been the development of multidetector-row CT, which allows significantly shorter acquisition times and the ability to retrospectively reconstruct thinner sections and improve three-dimensional rendering, which can be important, for example, in better delineating spinal or pelvic fractures. A two-detector row CT was first introduced in 1992 with the development of the Elscint CT Twin, but it was not until 1998 that four-detector-row CT scanners were made widely available.[78] At present, clinically available machines have up to 64 physical rows of detectors, which are up to 64 times faster than a single detector row machine. Due to the significantly faster acquisition times and the ability to acquire very thin sections with multidetector scanners, CT angiography is becoming comparable to catheter angiography in its sensitivity in the detection of vascular injuries, adding the benefit of being able to evaluate the adjacent soft tissues.[79,80]

Magnetic resonance imaging (MRI) was also developed in 1972. In that year, Lauterbur produced the first two-dimensional proton MRI of a water sample and two years later produced an image of a live animal.[81] MRI is most often employed to identify otherwise inapparent spine injuries.

## WEAPONS, CAMPAIGNS, AND TRAUMA PIONEERS

The earliest weapon that man had at his disposal was his hand, particularly when doubled into a fist. It must not have taken too long to realize that the fists were no match for wild animals or even for other men who were bent on destruction. At some time, prehistoric man must have realized that to pick up a stick and use it as a club gave him more effective fire power, so to speak. Clubs and stones that could be thrown and thus work at some distance became the first weapons of warfare. As ancient man searched for better ways to hurl stones at greater distances the slingshot was developed. The precise time at which this discovery was made remains unknown. It certainly is mentioned in the Bible but probably occurred long before that.

Some time after the development of the slingshot, between 4000 and 3000 BC, the bow and arrow were developed, and for the first time an effective weapon that could be used at a distance was available. A soldier was able to strike at the enemy at some distance with the bow and arrow and thus gained the advantage over hand-to-hand combat with clubs and stones.

To provide protection from flying arrows as well as clubs and swords, armor was developed. The date of the first use of armor is unknown, but the Greeks had armor, as did the Romans and all civilizations since that time. This would place the development of armor around 400 AD. The first form of armor was the shield, either round or oblong in shape, which could ward off the blow of a club or deflect a flying arrow.

A more powerful bow and arrow was fashioned with the invention of the crossbow which came into common usage around 1300 AD. This provided greater fire power than had ever before been available because the crossbow was able to shoot an arrow a longer distance and provide greater penetration of the target. The race between firepower and armor protection has continued over the subsequent eight centuries and actually accelerated during each successive conflict.

## GUNPOWDER

It was not long after the development of the crossbow that gunpowder was invented and changed the entire picture of warfare. It is believed that gunpowder was invented in China and was originally used to make firecrackers rather than weapons.[4] The first reported use of gunpowder in warfare was in the Battle of Crecy in 1346 AD. By 1350, crude cannons had been invented and were firing solid metal balls of 700 or 2,000 pounds. The development of gunpowder clearly gave the soldier an enormous ability to hurl a heavy missile a long way and strike the enemy at a far greater distance than a bow and arrow could reach. The use of gunpowder also provided the ability to inflict greater destruction than the bow and arrow. The arrow had to strike the enemy in a vulnerable spot, and armor could protect against the penetration of an arrow in most parts of the body. Armor in its earliest form, however, was not effective against missiles fired from guns.

## EARLY GERMAN SURGEONS

### Heinrich von Pfolspeundt

In the late 15th and early 16th centuries, German surgeons made important contributions to the care of injured patients. In 1460, Heinrich von Pfolspeundt wrote, in manuscript form, the first book on trauma, *Bundth-Ertznei*, which means "bandage treatment." Von Pfolspeundt had extensive war experience,[9] on the basis of which he propounded the theory that gunshot wounds were poisoned by gunpowder.[5] That theory was used to justify cauterizing all war wounds and initiated a controversy that retarded progress in wound care for 300 years. Von Pfolspeundt also described the repair of injured bowel, but it was Hieronymus Brunschwig who in 1497 published "Dis Ist Das Buch Der Cirurgia Hantwirckung Der Wundartzny" which is considered the first report of the surgical treatment of abdominal war wounds.[82] Von Pfolspeundt wrote that wounds should be bound with clean white cloths, for unclean cloth could cause harm. He also stated that the physicians should wash their hands before beginning treatment.

### Hans von Gersdorff

Another German surgeon, Hans von Gersdorff, also acquired a rich experience in wound care through apprenticeship, travel, and military service.[9] After nearly 40 years in the army, he wrote a handbook of wound surgery entitled *Das Feldbuch der Wundarzney*, which was published in 1517. This book was written shortly after the development of movable type, and is one of the first books to contain a large number of illustrations, some in color. They illustrate operative techniques, instruments that were used at the time, and many other aspects of military life. Von Gersdorff appears to have been the first to use an ox bladder as a pressure dressing to control amputation wound bleeding. He developed, or at least reported on, the use of many mechanical devices, including the tripod screw-elevator for raising a depressed skull fragment, as well as a number of other devices for the reduction of fractures and dislocations and the correction of crooked limbs and stiff joints. Von Gersdorff supported the view that warm oil should be poured into wounds and that styptics should be used to control bleeding. He also recommended preoperative administration of opium.[5]

### Ambroise Paré

The beginning of modern wound surgery occurred in 1545 with the publication of a book by Ambroise Paré.[18] Paré, a military surgeon at the siege of Turin, was accustomed to treating wounds with boiling oil, which was poured into a wound in order to stop putrefaction and promote healing by suppuration. When Paré's supplies of boiling oil ran low, and he had no more, he simply dressed wounds with clean cloths and minimal medication. He was somewhat dumbfounded to find that on the following morning, the soldiers treated in this way were relatively free of pain, afebrile, and resting comfortably. The salutary results led Paré to resolve " . . . never so cruelly, to burne poor men wounded with gunshot."[83] His expression "I dressed him, and God healed him," became well known in medical history. Paré also used ligatures to control hemorrhage, although he was not the first to do this. Ligatures had been used off and on throughout the centuries, but in most instances the surgeon returned to styptics and cautery to control hemorrhage. Paré's rejection of cauterizing wounds and his reintroduction of ligatures revolutionized wound care. Like most steps forward, this was not readily accepted by the majority of surgeons, and the idea that suppuration was a sign of good wound healing continued until the 20th century. Paré served as surgeon to four successive kings of France, starting with Henry II, and eventually attained the position of chief surgeon.

## THE FRENCH AND INDIAN WAR

The French and Indian War (1754–1763) was the last of the four wars between France and England fought in North America during the period 1689–1763. In 1756, this war spread to Europe where it was called the Seven Years War. In 1761, William Hunter obtained a commission for his brother John as an army surgeon apparently as a form of rest therapy for the acute episode of tuberculosis that John developed during a four-year period of intensive specimen preparation. John served with the military during the last two years of the Seven Years War, first at Bell Isle in France and then in the peninsular campaign in Portugal.[11] In his book on gunshot wounds cited above, Hunter discussed wounds in general and was the first to differentiate between primary and secondary healing. He also distinguished between granulation tissue and epithelialization, and concisely described the contraction of the wound as a part of healing. His book finally resolved the gunpowder as poison controversy when Hunter declared that gunshot wounds should be treated like other wounds and that war surgery for shot injuries should be ordinary surgery.[24] Regrettably, Hunter did not believe in debriding wounds and allowed blood clots to remain in the wound. He also said that a gunshot wound should not be made larger and "should not be opened simply because it is a wound." Those recommendations ensured inadequate debridement and virtually guaranteed the appearance of "laudable pus" by the fourth post-injury day.

## AMERICAN REVOLUTIONARY WAR

Three leading American physicians of the time, John Morgan, William Shippen, Jr., and Benjamin Rush[84] each played a role in combat casualty care in the Revolutionary War. At the outbreak of the war the colonies were totally unprepared to provide care for the injured, and had even less medical organization. John Morgan had been educated at Edinburgh, graduating in 1762, and had worked with William Hunter and other famous British surgeons. In 1765, he helped establish the first American medical school at the College of Philadelphia. He became the second Surgeon General of the Continental Army.[85] The first Surgeon General, Benjamin Church, had been convicted of treason, dismissed from the Army, jailed in Connecticut, subsequently released from jail, and left the country bound for Martinique on the sloop Welcome which was lost at sea.[86]

After his October 16, 1775 election as Surgeon General by the Continental Congress, Morgan promptly set about to centralize medical care, direct the treatment of severe injuries to general hospitals, evaluate physician qualifications, and regulate the distribution of supplies (particularly that of rum and wine). His valiant efforts met with fierce resistance and managed to antagonize many of the regimental surgeons. After the British forces defeated the Americans in the Battle of Harlem Heights, he established a general hospital at Hackensack, New Jersey, where he himself provided surgical care for some of the 1000 sick and injured who promptly flooded the hospital. The surgical repertoire of the day was limited and included "setting" bones, removing "easily reached" bullets, amputations, and trepanning the skull. Shortages of medicines and supplies compromised even the limited care which could be given and Morgan was soon thereafter dismissed allegedly as a consequence of political maneuvering orchestrated by William Shippen.[85] Morgan demanded a court of inquiry, and after two years of deliberation was acquitted of all charges.

William Shippen also graduated from Edinburgh and fell under the influence of the Hunters and the Monros. Upon returning to the American continent in 1762 he began to give private and public instructions in anatomy and obstetrics and was the first public teacher of obstetrics in America. He, as was Morgan, was involved in organizing the medical school at the College of Philadelphia. In July 1776, Shippen was appointed by Congress as surgeon of a small "flying camp" (a mobile tent or hut with a few beds and a surgeon's table) in New Jersey and placed under Morgan's command. Shippen did not recognize Morgan's authority and in fact is said to have hoarded supplies to prevent their use by Morgan and to have exaggerated his successes and Morgan's difficulties in his campaign to have Morgan relieved.[85] Shippen's boasts of treating a large number of casualties with unprecedented salvage were impugned by Dr. James Tilton,[87] but Congress accepted Shippen's exaggerated reports and gave him command of all hospitals on the New Jersey

side of the Hudson and later designated him Surgeon General when Morgan was relieved. As soon as Congress acquitted Morgan he joined with Benjamin Rush to have Shippen court-martialed for "malpractice and misconduct in office." As in the case of Morgan, Shippen was acquitted in 1780. In a letter to Morgan, written sometime later, George Washington indicated that he considered the animosities between Morgan and Shippen to have been a major cause of the "calamities that befell the sick in 1776."[85] When the medical school of the College of Philadelphia was reconstituted at the University of Pennsylvania after the Revolutionary War, Shippen was appointed Professor of Anatomy and Surgery. Both Morgan and Rush promptly refused their professorships at that institution and petitioned, to no avail, to have Shippen removed.[85] In a few years Rush relented and accepted his professorship, but Morgan never accepted his appointment which was kept open until his death. Neither Shippen nor Morgan left much in the way of writings.

Benjamin Rush graduated from Edinburgh in 1768 and a year later became a Professor of Chemistry at the College of Philadelphia which eventually became the Medical College of the University of Pennsylvania. He was a physician to the Pennsylvania Hospital and founded the Philadelphia Dispensary, the first in the United States, and also served as Treasurer of the United States Mint. He was a signer of the Declaration of Independence and was a Surgeon General for the Middle Department of the Continental Army for two years during which time he was responsible for providing care for injured soldiers. His active participation in plots against George Washington imperiled his status during the war. After the war Rush became the nation's authority on exhaustive therapy which he recommended to such a degree and at such high doses of bleeding, diarrhea, salivation, sweating, vomiting, and skin blistering that his regimen was given the name of heroic therapy. This therapy was commonly applied to the injured no matter how severely their physiologic reserve had been compromised by the injury per se. Rush's prominence persisted long after his death and heroic therapy was a central theme of American medical treatment into the 1860s and the American Civil War as evidenced by the bleeding to which the wounded "Stonewall" Jackson was subjected.[31]

## DOMINIQUE JEAN LARREY

As a student in the latter half of the 18th century, Dominique Jean Larrey was taught the principles of debridement and excision by Pierre Joseph Desault. Desault used the term debridement to describe making a deep incision into the wound to explore and establish drainage. He also reintroduced the concept of excising injured tissue enunciated two centuries earlier by Botallo.[17] As a surgeon of one of the armies of the French Republic, Larrey used Desault's technique of wound care and added the concept of prompt surgical intervention before the shock of the injury per se, which rendered a wound relatively insensitive, could dissipate. To achieve that goal he designed a system of rapid casualty evacuation using a light horse-drawn "flying ambulance" which was so successful at the Battle of Metz in 1793 that the system was installed for all fourteen armies of the French Republic.[88] Larrey's surgical speed and skill which further reduced surgical stress were unparalleled as evidenced by his performance of 200 amputations at the Battle of Boradino in 1812 (one every 7.2 minutes).[89] The recovery of 75% of the patients upon whom he and his assistants operated was unprecedented.

Larrey expanded the role of the military surgeon to include more than care of the wound and encompass all aspects of patient care.[33] He worked to improve sanitation, procurement of food and supplies for the sick and the wounded, and training of medical personnel. He was also an epidemiologist and gave one of the best descriptions of frostbite that has ever been written. In his later years Larray demonstrated his versatility when he reported the successful treatment of twelve compound fracture patients using a benzoin-based antiseptic agent.[25] Napoleon thought so highly of his surgeon that he bequeathed 100,000 francs to Larrey and stated "He is the most virtuous man I have ever known."[90]

## THE ADVENT OF NURSING CARE

An inscription on limestone dated 1250 BC is the earliest written record of nurses who at that time principally cared for sick family members at home and also assisted priests in caring for the sick in the Egyptian temples. Nursing as a career was first developed in India at the monastic hospitals founded by Buddha in the 5th century BC. The oldest Christian nursing school was established in 370 AD at a time when care was apparently focused on counseling the terminally ill. In the late 4th century, Marcella, a wealthy Roman widow, converted her palatial home into a cloister for nursing nuns. For the next several centuries it was largely nuns and monks who provided what was essentially spiritual solace to the sick at the monastic hospitals.[11]

Nursing education began in 1836 at Kaiserswerth, Germany, under the leadership of Theodore Fliedner. In 1851, Florence Nightingale became a student at Fliedner's School, but apparently chaffed under Germanic discipline and left after three months. After a similar brief experience as a novice at a convent and several months with the sisters of Vincent de Paul in Paris, she was appointed matron at the London Harley Street Hospital for Gentlewomen during Illness and subsequently became superintendent of nurses at Kings College Hospital where she was considered somewhat of an authority on hospital sanitation and function.[11,26]

The previously noted staggering number of deaths of British troops in the first year of the Crimean War and the fact that more English soldiers were in hospitals because of infectious disease and malnutrition than were on active duty aroused the English Parliament and Queen Victoria who appointed a Sanitary Commission to oversee medical relief activities. Sidney Herbert, the British Secretary of War, gave Ms. Nightingale the mission of coordinating the relief effort and improving the deplorable conditions of the Hospital for English Forces at Scutarri.[31] She and the 37 nurses whom she had recruited quickly established sanitation, food services, nursing service, clean water, hospital laundry, bathrooms, and housecleaning, all of which reduced the death rate among the patients from 42% to 2%.[5] After Nightingale returned to England she established the first independent educational institution for training nurses in 1860, the Nightingale Training School for Nurses. As part of the required training she demanded that accurate hospital records be kept for each patient and she initiated the use of statistical assessment to determine the quality of a hospital's performance. Her two books, "Notes on Hospitals" published in 1859 and "Notes on Nursing" published in 1860, served as early basic textbooks for nursing schools around the world. As a result of Nightingale's efforts, there are nursing corps in all the major armies today.

## THE WAR BETWEEN THE STATES

The Crimean War had barely ended when the War Between the States broke out in America. This was perhaps the bloodiest war ever fought, including the world wars, and medical care was, at least initially, more disorganized and chaotic than in any other conflict. The lessons of previous wars had been ignored in the United States, so that at the outbreak of hostilities there was a poorly organized medical corps, literally no ambulance service, and no hospital system. All this reflected a disregard for the medical treatment of the wounded. Many generals thought that the medical supply wagons got in their way, and tried to avoid having them if possible. As a consequence of such neglect the Union army lost 110,070 men from battle wounds, and the Confederate army lost 94,000. The value of nursing care, which had been demonstrated by Florence Nightingale in the Crimean War, did not come into play until late in the Civil War. Oliver Wendell Holmes had delivered his paper on puerperal sepsis, demonstrating that childbed fever was a problem of contamination caused by dirty hands of physicians and others in attendance, but this was largely ignored.[33]

The magnitude of these deficiencies was evidenced by the typically delayed application of the generally inadequate care given to the casualties of both sides at the first Battle of Manassas. The hapless state of medical care caught the attention of the Sanitary Commission, founded in New York City by Henry W. Bellows, and patterned after the British Sanitary Commission. The Commission, which had been given official status by a June 13, 1861, executive order of Abraham Lincoln, dispatched Frederick Olmsted, its recently hired executive secretary, to survey the capabilities of the Medical Department and review the care provided or not provided during that first major battle of the Civil War. Olmsted's report documenting the number and magnitude of problems of the Union Army Medical Department stimulated the Commission to collaborate with Surgeon General William Hammond and play a major role in bringing about reform of the Union Army Medical Corps.[31]

After his appointment as Surgeon General in April 1862, William Hammond reorganized the Union Army Medical Department to increase centralization and improve the delivery of medical care. In August of 1862 the ambulance corps of the Army of the Potomac, developed by Dr. Jonathan Letterman, was authorized by Union Army General Orders Number 147 and was subsequently established in all Union armies.[91] Hospital construction received priority in both armies and by June 1863 there were 84,000 beds available for Union casualties alone. Both armies built and each Surgeon General, Hammond of the Union Army and Samuel Preston Moore of the Confederate Army, claimed to have originated pavilion-type hospitals. Each army also constructed specialty hospitals, small pox, eye and ear, and nervous system disease hospitals in the Union Army and orthopedic and hernia hospitals in the Confederate Army.[92]

Most wounds were left open, mainly because of expediency rather than the idea that healing was more likely with this method. When one realizes that the surgeons were largely untrained and often had to perform many procedures in a day, the wonder is not that so many died, but that so many survived. Three-quarters of the operations performed in the Civil War were amputations, and the mortality rate ranged from 15 or 20% for primary amputations of the forearm or foot to as high as 48% for primary amputation at the upper one-third of the thigh.[93] In contrast to the major advance provided by anesthesia, advances in wound care were modest because pus was still considered to be a laudable event and necessary for the healing of a wound. Secondary hemorrhage caused by infection following operative procedures was common and caused a great many deaths. Additionally, ligatures applied to blood vessels were left hanging out of the wound and were gently "tugged" on each day to hasten their removal. When the ligatures separated, if the vessel was not healed or thrombosed, secondary life threatening hemorrhage could occur even without overt infection. A major limitation of Civil War wound care was infection which was made virtually universal by the reuse of clothing, bedding, and even dressings, failure to cleanse hands or instruments, lack of general sanitation, and the misuse of antiseptic agents. The categories of infection ranged from erysipelas with a mortality rate of 8% to pyemia with a mortality rate of 97%. Tetanus had a mortality rate of 89%, but was fortunately relatively infrequent. The reduction of the 38% to 62% mortality rate associated with untreated hospital gangrene to only 2.6% when Middleton Goldsmith, a surgeon in the Union Army, applied topical bromine provided early evidence of the effectiveness of antiseptic agents.[94] By the end of the war bromine was being used as an antiseptic in most Union hospitals.

Other advances in combat casualty care included the preferential performance of primary as opposed to secondary amputation to reduce the risk of infection (Confederate surgeons observed a 24% survival advantage with primary amputation), and delay of primary amputation for a sufficient time to avoid the deleterious effects of "wound shock." For the first time whole blood infusion was carried out. Even though the blood was unmatched, no complications and an initial favorable systemic response were reported for each of the two patients given blood, one of whom expired twelve days later with diffuse uncontrollable bleeding from an amputation stump.[95] A surgeon in each army, N. R. Smith of the Confederate Medical Department and John D. Hodgen of the Union Army Medical Department, designed a splint for extension of a fractured limb that improved the management of casualties with skeletal trauma. One of the most important advances in trauma care during the Civil War is considered to be the institution of a competence-based physician and surgeon credentialing system by Jonathan Letterman in the Union Army.[31] C. J. Chisholm who was the first medical appointee for military service in the Confederate Army advocated that surgeons be examined by senior surgeons before being allowed to amputate limbs.[93]

At about the midpoint of the war, nurses were recruited and eventually given some stature, but nursing care was rudimentary. In general, nurses were not wanted by the surgeons or by the army, and their job was mainly to clean up slop pails, cook food, and perform similar duties. Clara Barton, initially a volunteer nurse, was virtually a one-person medical service and was of major help in recruiting nurses into the medical corps. In 1864 she was appointed superintendent of nurses for the Union Army of the James. She was the eventual founder of the American branch of the Red Cross in 1881.[96] She was in Cuba when the Battleship Maine blew up and nursed the resulting casualties. She later provided nursing support, equipment, and supplies for the casualties from the Battle of Santiago in the Spanish-American War in 1898.[92]

## FRANCO-PRUSSIAN WAR

Carl Reyher, a native of Latvia, served as a surgeon in the Prussian Army during the Franco-Prussian War of 1870–1871. From 1872–1877 he worked with von Bergmann at the medical school in Dorpat. Reyher was familiar with Lister's work and on the basis of the time he had spent studying in Edinburgh and his work with von Bergmann, who pioneered steam sterilization for surgical materials, he developed a strong interest in wound infections. When the Russo-Turkish War of 1877–1878 (the last of four such wars in the 19th century) began, Reyher enlisted as a surgeon in the Russian Army Medical Service. During the war, Reyher organized and completed a controlled study of the effectiveness of debridement of gunshot wounds.[5] He subsequently published a paper "Primary Debridement of Gunshot Wounds" in which he showed that the antiseptic treatment of wounds reduced the mortality from gunshot injuries and that the addition of early debridement, reduced the mortality even further.[25,33] Unfortunately, little attention was paid to his work and it was almost forgotten. Many surgeons who followed Reyher quoted his work, but always the portion on the antiseptic management of wounds and usually ignored the role of debridement.

## THE SPANISH-AMERICAN WAR

The Spanish-American War which lasted only five months, April to August 1898, was the first conflict in which antisepsis was widely employed to prevent infection in combat casualties. The antiseptic treatment of wounds began in the field with the application of the materials in the first-aid packet carried by each soldier. Following an initial debridement, treatment was continued by application of occlusive antiseptic dressings to wounds of the extremities, chest, and even abdomen. The effectiveness of such debridement and antiseptic occlusion reduced the amputation rate in casualties with open fractures and decreased mortality. It was noted that 35% of patients with penetrating abdominal wounds treated with antiseptic occlusive dressings survived, whereas both the American and Spanish surgeons reported that all patients with penetrating abdominal wounds who were operated upon expired.[92] Tetanus was a persistent risk and was associated with a 42% mortality.[97]

The significance of disease as compared to wounds in military conflicts was abundantly evident in this war in which the 3,681 deaths from disease exceeded by a factor of 12 the 293 deaths due to wounds.[92] Sanitation and hygiene measures were so primitive that the health of the army was considered good when as many as 20% of personnel were too sick to be effective.[98]

# WORLD WAR I

As World War I began, the controversy over whether laparotomy should be performed for penetrating abdominal wounds was unresolved and the policy of both the French and English armies was not to explore abdominal wounds. Although many surgeons recommended operative intervention for the treatment of penetrating abdominal wounds in civilian practice, they generally advised against laparotomy in the military setting on the stated basis of lack of hot water, absence of trained assistants, and concern that the time required would compromise the care of other less seriously wounded casualties. On the contrary, others beginning with von Pfolspeundt in the latter half of the 15th century had repaired wounded bowel and abdominal wounds, including Brunschwig in 1535, Larrey in 1798, and Bauden in the 1830s. James Marion Simms, who cared for combat casualties in the Franco-Prussian War, was a strong advocate for the surgical treatment of abdominal gunshot wounds, but the previously noted experience in the Spanish-American War and the discouraging experience reported by British surgeons in the Boer War supported nonoperative treatment and delayed general acceptance of prompt operative intervention (Table 1-1).[92]

The Russian princess, Viera Gedroitz, made an important contribution in resolving the laparotomy controversy. Dr. Gedroitz, who completed medical school and obtained surgical training and qualifications in Germany, outfitted a railway car as an operating room in which, during the Russio-Japanese War of 1904–1905, she performed 183 laparotomies on patients with penetrating abdominal wounds. The results she achieved, attributable in large part to her insistence that operation be limited to patients in whom the interval from time of injury to operation was three hours or less, were so good that the Russian Army adopted the procedure.[82] In analyzing the issue, the British surgeon Cuthbert Wallace attributed the failures of operative treatment to delay of surgical intervention

and he and Owen Richards became proponents of the operative management of casualties with penetrating abdominal wounds. Beginning in 1915, after a review of nonoperative management revealed that 118,000 soldiers with abdominal wounds had died, laparotomy became the standard of care on the Western Front. That policy was made possible by the use of motorized field ambulances for the prompt movement of patients to a facility where definitive treatment could be provided by highly qualified physicians. The frequent delay in transfer of the patients to such facilities compromised results and mortality remained in the 53% to 66% range in the operated patients.[92]

The high incidence of gas gangrene in patients injured in trench warfare was initially attributed to the microbial ecology of the area. The fields of France and Belgium were heavily cultivated with animal manure and the ground was laden with the spores of gas gangrene. Even so, the occurrence of clostridial infections was ultimately related to inadequate debridement and early wound closure.[17] At the Inter-Allied Surgical Conference held in Paris in 1917, the delegates established a policy for the management of war wounds, i.e., debridement and delayed closure. Primary closure was accepted only for wounds that were less than eight hours old. In addition to the general acceptance of prompt operative treatment for penetrating abdominal wounds, the care of soft tissue wounds was improved by the use of effective antiseptic irrigation as employed in the Carrel-Dehelly-Depage technique using Dakin's hypochlorite solution.[33] The availability and use of anti-tetanus serum essentially eliminated tetanus as a complication in the American casualties.[97]

After Roentgen's discovery of X-rays in 1895, radiographic equipment was rapidly developed and used by the U.S. military forces in the Spanish-American War. The weight and size of that equipment limited it to use in general hospitals and hospital ships where it was employed largely in the management of typhoid fever patients.[99] In World War I, improved radiographic equipment with

## TABLE 1-1

### Treatment of Penetrating Abdominal Wounds: 12th to 20th Centuries

| YEAR | CONFLICT | SURGEON | TREATMENT |
|------|----------|---------|-----------|
| 1170 | – | Roger of Salerno (Ruggierio Frugardi) | Suture of lacerated intestine over an intraluminal wooden stent |
| 1460 | Wars of the German Order | Heinrich von Pfolspeundt | Originated doctrine of poisoned gunshot wounds. Repaired bowel by transection and insertion of silver tube over which ends of bowel were tied |
| 1497 | German wars of late 15th century | Hieronymous Brunschwig | First published description of gunshot wound treatment by surgical repair; considered wounds poisoned |
| 1545 | Siege of Turin | Ambroise Paré | Reduced prolapsed bowel |
| 1800 | Napoleon's Egyptian campaign | Dominique-Jean Larrey | Successful exteriorization of transected ileum |
| 1830 | French-Algerian War | Lucien Baudens | Finger exploration to identify blood, feces, or gas. Two enterorrhaphies—one success |
| 1849 | The Caucasus War | Nicholai Pirogov | One successful enterorrhaphy |
| 1861–1865 | U.S. Civil War | Union and Confederate surgeons | Laparotomy "forgotten" |
| 1870–1871 | Franco-Prussian War | William MacCormac | Penetrating abdominal wounds all fatal—"no operation justified" |
| 1883 | French campaign in Tonkin | Henri Nimier | Nonoperative mortality 75% vs. operative mortality 62% |
| 1898 | Spanish-American War | U.S. and Spanish surgeons | Operation universally fatal for both sides |
| 1899–1902 | Boer War | William MacCormac | Operative mortality 69%—treatment abandoned |
| 1904–1905 | Russo-Japanese War | Princess Viera Gedroitz | 183 laparotomies with "great success" |
| 1914–1917 | World War I | Theodore Tuffier, Owen Richards | French and British policy changed from expectant to operative treatment in early 1915 |

fluoroscopic capability was used to facilitate localization of foreign bodies which improved wound debridement in casualties.[39] The availability of highly trained specialists, as exemplified by the neurosurgeon Harvey Cushing, whose work placed emphasis upon removal of all intracranial foreign bodies for which he developed a magnet to extract metallic fragments further increased salvage of the wounded and improved outcomes. Dr. Cushing's meticulous records of the thousands of cases that he operated upon formed an early neurosurgical trauma database.[100,101]

Recognition that at least a part of the problem of shock was due to blood or fluid loss led, as noted previously, to the early use of plasma transfusion and the infusion of salt containing fluid to replace lost blood volume. Even so, renal failure was a common complication in fatally injured patients. Discovery of three blood groups (A, B, and O) by Landsteiner in 1901 and the fourth, (AB) by Sturli and De Castello in 1902 made it possible for Dr. O.H. Robertson to establish the first military blood bank at which he prepared, stored, and administered compatible blood to the severely injured.[92,102,103]

The persistent high mortality and limitations in the care of casualties demonstrated the need to develop better treatments for the wounded, methods that would later be applicable to the civilian population. Dr. J.M.T. Finney, a member of Halsted's surgical faculty at Johns Hopkins and Chief Consultant in surgery for the American Expeditionary Forces, established a central laboratory to study the problem of shock in wounded soldiers. George Crile of Cleveland was placed in charge of that laboratory where he and Walter B. Canon conducted studies of shock in the wounded. Those studies, sponsored by the Medical Research Committee, documented the usefulness of salt-containing fluids given intravenously as treatment for hemorrhagic shock.[97] In the Canadian army, Fraser B. Gurd completed an extensive review and study of chronic osteomyelitis in wounded soldiers that led to refinements in fracture care.[104]

## WORLD WAR II

As World War II began, the American as well as the European forces were better equipped medically than they had been at the beginning of any other conflict. At the outset, as with any war, certain equipment was in short supply but the United States very quickly geared up its industrial might to provide all the supplies that would be needed as the military activity heightened. Whole blood and plasma fractions became available in massive quantities in the United States and it was rapidly prepared and shipped overseas under refrigeration, and was available at the battle front as needed.

The lessons of World War I were still relatively fresh in the minds of the surgeons of World War II, and after a brief relearning curve, all wounds were carefully debrided and left open for delayed closure. Two directives issued by the U.S. Army Surgeon General, Norman Kirk, in 1943 contributed to the improved outcomes of wounded soldiers in WWII and influenced surgical care for many years. A directive in April 1943 stated, "The guillotine or open-circular method of amputation is the procedure of choice in traumatic surgery under war conditions. Primary suture of all wounds of extremities under war conditions is never to be done."[105] In

October of that year, Circular Letter No. 178 was issued stating " . . . in large bowel injuries the damaged segment will be exteriorized by drawing it out through a separate incision, preferably in the flank."[106] In no case was the bowel to be resected and primary anastomosis performed.

At the urging of Colonel Edward D. Churchill, the surgical consultant for the U.S. Army in the Mediterranean theater of operations, a program of "early reparative surgery" was established in 1944.[107] Such treatment consisted of closure of the wound between the 4th and 10th postinjury day if the wound was clinically assessed to be "clean" no matter what bacteria were cultured from the wound surface. "Delayed primary closure" was performed on simple soft tissue wounds without penicillin therapy and complex wounds, i.e., those involving large volumes of muscle, bone, joint, nerves, or vessels, were closed and 40,000 units of penicillin were administered every three hours. The success of such treatment completely altered the military policy guiding the care of soft tissue wounds.

At the beginning of World War II, medical facilities which had been designed for the trench warfare of World War I were virtually immobile. Such medical units could not respond and provide the care needed by the wounded when the velocity of troop movement increased. Five special surgical teams known as auxiliary units or AUX units were formed under the command of Col. James C. Forsee. These teams which consisted of highly trained specialists designated by the surgical consultants and included anesthesiologists were deployed to augment the surgical capability of another treatment facility and overcome a relative shortage of highly qualified surgeons.[108] Several of these units became famous for their activities during various campaigns of World War II and served as the forerunners of the MASH units used in the Korean conflict. The Second Auxiliary Group had a particularly distinguished record as documented by marked improvement in mortality rates associated with injuries of the large bowel, small bowel, and liver. The thoracic surgery team of that group strikingly reduced the mortality of penetrating chest wounds from the 25% of WWI to 10% and reported "Wet Lung in War Casualties" which appears to have been a form of what is now called ARDS.[109]

The tradition of medical research in the U.S. Army was continued in World War II. Dr. Edward D. Churchill, the surgical consultant in the North African-Mediterranean theater of operations, identified the consequences of inadequate resuscitation in American casualties and in September 1944 was able to establish The Board for the Study of the Severely Wounded.[110] That unit conducted physiologic and biochemical studies focused on the whole body and organ-specific responses to injury and shock. In 1952 the results of those studies were published in "The Physiologic Effects of Wounds." That book was a landmark volume in the series "Surgery in World War II" edited by Dr. Michael DeBakey and published under the direction of the U.S. Army Surgeon General, Lieutenant General Leonard D. Heaton.[111] In the introduction to that volume, Dr. Churchill stated, "Cobwebs of theory and hypothesis were swept away by simple observations and precise definitions."[111] The Board for the Study of the Severely Wounded included surgeons, anesthesiologists, and pathologists who studied the pathophysiologic responses to injury during the nine months in which the Board was active. The cardiovascular response to injury was defined, postinjury hepatic dysfunction was described, and the effect of injury on renal function was studied to refine the diagnosis of renal failure and develop effective treatment of the consequence of prolonged shock. The use of alkali (sodium bicarbonate) in the treatment of shock was also evaluated, the crush syndrome studied, the general pathology of traumatic shock recorded, and a system to grade shock was developed.[111] Dr. Churchill took great pride in the fact that systemic and precise measurements were made that for the first time described the actual physiologic state of wounded man. He described three phases in the evolution of surgical knowledge during that war: identification of the problem, development of practical treatment, and documentation by scientific evidence.[111] Those three phases have characterized the process by which further improvements in combat casualty care and all trauma care have been achieved since then.

General Fred W. Rankin, who served in World War II as Director of the Surgery Division of the U.S. Army, noted that the percentage of combat casualties dying of wounds had decreased from the World War I level of 8.1% to 3.3%. He further noted that the mortality rates of patients with life threatening wounds of the head, chest, and abdomen had decreased by approximately two-thirds.[112] The mortality of penetrating abdominal wounds had decreased from 66% in World War I to 15% in World War II. The mortality associated with injury of specific viscera was also markedly decreased (Table 1-2). He attributed these improvements to the availability of excellently trained young surgeons at hospital facilities to minimize injury-operation interval, improved methods of resuscitation including the ready availability of blood and blood plasma, the availability of antibiotics, and improved means of transportation including aircraft to evacuate the wounded. Additionally, the development of formulae to predict the fluid needs of burn patients simplified resuscitation, ameliorated acute hypovolemia in burn patients, and prevented acute renal failure.[110]

The increased funding and multiplication of NIH Institutes after World War II were paralleled during and after World War II in the Army Medical Corps. A proliferation of categorical research units, the provision of secure funding, and ultimately the formation of an independent medical research and development command have ensured the continuity of clinical research activities focused on injury within the Army Medical Department. In 1947, the U.S. Army Surgical Research Unit, originally established in 1943 to define the role of antibiotics in the treatment of war wounds, was moved to San Antonio, Texas, and assigned a new mission. As a response to the massive number of burns produced by the detonation of atomic weapons, the unit was directed to care for burn and trauma patients, teach others about the care of the injured patient, and conduct both clinical and laboratory studies. That institute, renamed the U.S. Army Institute of Surgical

Research in 1969, has conducted multidisciplinary integrated clinical and laboratory research to generate information which has been used to improve the care and increase the survival of trauma and burn patients.[104]

## THE KOREAN CONFLICT

World War II was barely over and America was returning to a peacetime environment when the Korean conflict broke out in 1950. The medical corps was well equipped at this time, although seasoned surgeons were in short supply. The management of wounds was done much as it had been during World War II, with debridement and delayed primary closure. Whole blood, plasma, salt solutions, and antibiotics were available in ample quantities, as were adequate hospital facilities to care for the wounded. The MASH unit was developed as a mobile surgical hospital of 60 beds operating just behind the combat area but out of range of ordinary artillery.

The terrain of Korea was mountainous in many areas. Consequently, the movement of the wounded over hills and valleys was often difficult, and helicopters were pressed into service. These early helicopters had two pods on the outside, each carrying a wounded soldier from the front line to the MASH unit, the aeronautical reincarnation of Larrey's "flying ambulance."

Vascular surgery, which had begun to expand in the late 1940s, was performed in the Korean conflict and many limbs were saved using this technique. Contrary to the directive of April 1943, primary repair of combat incurred vascular injuries was undertaken for the first time as was the use of arterial homografts. In the course of their surgical practice in Korea, Dr. John H. Davis performed what is said to have been the first primary vascular repair in the U.S. Army and Dr. Frank Spencer introduced arterial repair including the use of arterial homografts into the U.S. Marine Corps at the Easy Medical Company U.S. Naval Hospital in July-August 1952.[114,115] The homografts represented a mixed blessing in light of the high subsequent failure rate of such implants in patients injured in the Vietnam conflict. Many of the surgeons in Korea were taught the methods of vascular repair on site and used those skills to salvage many limbs. A Registry of vascular injuries was started which has been continued in subsequent conflicts.

During the Korean conflict, Colonel William S. Stone, who had been involved in the formation of the Board for the Study of the Severely Wounded in World War II, played a key role in organizing the U.S. Army Surgical Research Team on which Dr. John Howard represented Walter Reed Army Medical Center and Dr. John H. Davis represented Brooke Army Medical Center. That team conducted physiologic and biochemical studies of combat casualties for whom they provided surgical care. They measured total body water and documented that the relatively high incidence of acute renal failure in casualties at the beginning of the conflict was a consequence of inadequate fluid resuscitation. Subsequent emphasis on the timely administration of sufficient volumes of electrolyte-containing solutions strikingly reduced the incidence of acute renal failure to a level of 0.5% of casualties in the latter years of that conflict.[97]

The research team established a hemodialysis center in the combat zone using the artificial kidney developed by Dr. Wilhelm Kolff

### TABLE 1-2

| Hospital Mortality of Wounded with Visceral Injury WWI and WWII[113] | | | | |
|---|---|---|---|---|
| | COLON | JEJUNUM AND ILEUM | DUODENUM | LIVER |
| WWI | 77% | 75% | 80% | 67% |
| WWII | | | | |
| British | 54% | 48% | | 41% |
| U.S. | 37% | 30% | 57% | 27% |

and initiated a program in which dialysis was performed as soon as serum potassium rose to 6 mEq per liter in order to minimize hyperkalemia-related mortality and developed a program of prophylactic dialysis to prevent the complications of uremia.[116] That team also identified the high output form of acute renal failure and conducted studies of vasoactive humoral factors in combat casualties.[117]

## THE VIETNAM WAR

The helicopter was increasingly important for the movement of the wounded in Vietnam, largely because of the jungle terrain and the inability to move by ambulance even when distances were short. The effectiveness of aeromedical transfer of injured patients by helicopter was documented by McCaughey et al. who reported that the average prehospital time for combat casualties treated at the U.S. Navy Hospital in Da Nang was only 80 minutes.[118] The short transit times resulted in the hospitals in Vietnam receiving patients so badly injured that in prior conflicts they would have died before admission. Even so the board-certified general surgeons and other surgical specialists who cared for the patients reduced the morbidity associated with ophthalmic injuries, chest wounds, head wounds, and penetrating abdominal wounds and achieved unprecedented survival rates. The progressive increase in casualty survival since Word War II has paralleled the progressive decrease in the time between injury and admission to a definitive treatment facility (Table 1-3).

In January 1968, topical mafenide acetate cream, an antimicrobial chemotherapeutic agent developed for burn wound care at the U.S. Army Institute of Surgical Research, was first used in the theater of operations. Such topical treatment of burn wounds reduced the occurrence of invasive burn wound infections and increased the salvage of patients with combat incurred burns.[119] In 1967 a burn patient holding center was established at a U.S. Army Hospital in Japan where patients burned in Vietnam were cared for until a burn flight team consisting of a surgeon and corpsmen from the Army Burn Center made their weekly trip to escort the burn patients and provide in-flight care on a direct flight from Japan to San Antonio, Texas. This system of staged intercontinental burn patient transfer was developed in collaboration with the U.S. Air Force and effected the transfer of 824 patients in 103 flights with only one in-flight death.

The Vietnam War further emphasized the need for new knowledge in many areas, as new postinjury complications such as Da Nang lung were seen for the first time. Clinical investigation within the theater of operations was also conducted in Vietnam. The Walter Reed Army Institute of Research Trauma Study Section, stationed originally at Dong Tam and later at Long Binh, utilized state-of-the-art assays and technology to study the physiologic changes that occurred in combat casualties.[110] That research team described the effect of chest injuries on both pulmonary and hemodynamic function and the hemodynamic consequences of respiratory insufficiency following trauma. Other studies included those of gastric acid secretion and stress ulcers in combat casualties, the bacteriology of war wounds (an extension of studies conducted by the research team in Korea), and a study of the effect of injury on serum levels of hepatic enzymes in combat casualties. A similar research unit was established at the U.S. Naval Hospital in Da Nang where studies on fluid resuscitation and postinjury respiratory failure were conducted.

## CONFLICTS SINCE VIETNAM

Inexplicably and unfortunately the U.S. Army Medical Corps has had no in-theater research units during the six conflicts since Vietnam. The absence of focused, militarily relevant research activity means that important research opportunities have gone and are going unrealized. During Operation Desert Shield/Desert Storm, the Institute of Surgical Research provided teams of burn specialists that were sited at selected evacuation hospitals to provide theater-wide burn coverage in Saudi Arabia for that conflict. The Institute also collaborated with the U.S. Air Force to reactivate the system of staged intercontinental aeromedical transfer that had worked so well for patients burned in Vietnam. For Operation Iraqi Freedom that system has again been reactivated and has successfully transported casualties burned in Iraq from a burn holding unit at a U.S. Army hospital in Germany to the U.S. Army Burn Center in San Antonio, Texas.

At the present time, Colonel John Holcomb and other personnel of the reorganized U.S. Army Institute of Surgical Research are directing and participating in individual research projects on resuscitation fluids, haemostatic agents, and field first-aid devices, but progress is less than would be generated by a dedicated surgical research unit in the theater of operation as was true in Vietnam and earlier conflicts. Perhaps, most importantly, both Army and Air Force personnel are working to establish for the first time an accurate and reliable trauma registry for use in the current and future conflicts.

Medicine is one of the few areas that benefit directly from warfare. Many of the technological advances in trauma care since World War I have resulted from knowledge and experience gained from research conducted in the conflicts that have occurred during the intervening eight decades. The benefits of modern combat casualty care are evident in the mere 2.5% death rate of casualties admitted to U.S. Army hospitals in Vietnam during a 21-month period.[17] The improvement in care is further

**TABLE 1-3**

### Mortality of Combat Casualties 1898–1973

| CONFLICT | MORTALITY[93] | | Injury to Admission Interval[119] (Hrs) |
|---|---|---|---|
| | All Wounds Admitted | Penetrating Abdominal Wounds | |
| Spanish-American War | 100%[a] 65%[b] | | |
| World War I | | | |
| British | | 60% | |
| American | 9.5% | 66% | 12–18 |
| World War II | | | |
| British | | 42% | |
| American | 3.3% | 24% | 10.4 |
| Korea | 2.5% | 12% | 4–6 |
| Vietnam | 2.3% | 9% | 1.2–5 |

[a]Operative treatment
[b]Nonoperative treatment

documented by the 0.7% death rate of all who served in Vietnam as compared to the 1.8% death rate in our Revolutionary War even though the fire power of modern weapons has increased exponentially since the days of musketry.[92]

## ORGANIZATIONS AND SOCIETIES

Several organizations and societies have contributed in a major way to the field of trauma care. Two of these stand out because of their role in bringing the care of the trauma patient into clear focus for the medical profession and the public. The first of these is the Committee on Trauma of the American College of Surgeons (ACS). The College, founded in 1913, appointed a committee on fractures in 1922, with Dr. Charles Scudder of Boston as Chairman. The ACS was engaged in trying to improve and standardize hospitals at this time. A report on the management of fractures was the first assignment of the committee, and its report was presented in 1923. From this early committee came the Committee on Trauma (COT), formalized in 1949. This committee has labored long and hard to improve all aspects of trauma care. Publication of "Early Care of the injured," which was written by the committee, has served the profession well. It has been replaced by sections on critical care and trauma in the American College of Surgeons publication "Care of the Surgical Patient." This publication is in loose-leaf form and is updated periodically so that it is always current.

The Committee on Trauma has also done much to educate surgeons in trauma care. Annual postgraduate courses in trauma and trauma care, the creation of posters for display in emergency departments, standards for ambulances, training and standard setting for rescue squads, and the categorization of hospitals are some of the Committee's activities. Multiple sub committees take on these various tasks. The Committee's educational activities have focused in recent years on the development and administration of the Advanced Trauma Life Support (ATLS) program in which the curriculum focuses on initial pre-trauma center care, triage, and transfer of severely injured patients. Literally thousands of surgeons have completed an ATLS provider or instructor course. Many hospitals now require that their Emergency Department physicians complete and pass the Advanced Burn Life Support (ABLS) course. In 1987, the Committee established a trauma center verification program under the auspices of which 85 Level I trauma centers are currently verified as are 89 Level II trauma centers, 28 Level III trauma centers, 12 Level I Pediatric Trauma Centers, and 3 Level II Pediatric Trauma Centers.

Perhaps the most important parts of the COT are its state committees on trauma. Each state has at least one such committee, and the larger states have several. This unique structure has provided the grassroots surgeon a role in developing better trauma care in the states. The states are grouped into regions, with a region chief, and all are active at the meetings of the central committee. This organization provides the opportunity for any surgeon to play an active role in improving trauma care, and many trauma surgeons have enhanced their stature by their activities in the ACS Committee on Trauma.

The second organization to have a major impact on the care of the trauma victim is the American Association for the Surgery of Trauma (AAST). President Kellogg Speed called the first annual meeting of what was then called the American Association for Traumatic Surgery to order on May 8, 1939.[110] The inauspicious nature of the name of the association was recognized almost immediately and changed to the American Association for the Surgery of Trauma at the second annual meeting. The founders of the association believed that the trauma patient was not receiving the best of care. The goals of the founders were to call attention to the problem, to promote scientific interchange regarding trauma care, and to bring various specialties to a common forum to improve trauma care. In 1959, the AAST voted to begin publication of a journal devoted to trauma. The first issue of the *Journal of Trauma* was published in 1961 and it has continued to grow in scope and stature since then.[120]

Today, all surgical specialties are represented in the AAST membership, and the scientific papers presented at its annual meeting cover all aspects of trauma care, both experimental and clinical. The cross-fertilization in this multidisciplinary society of experts has made the AAST unique in American surgery. With the direct input of the related surgical specialists, the Association has developed a scale for grading the severity of organ injury which has been widely accepted. The association now funds up to three research fellowships each year which are providing a stream of young investigators in the field of trauma care. It is expected that many of these young people will make a career as trauma surgeons.

In addition to the AAST, several new associations have been formed to further the cause of trauma care. The Eastern Association for the Surgery of Trauma (EAST) is made up of members of the eastern states who have a demonstrated interest in trauma care. EAST presents a broad-based scientific program at its annual meeting each January and has been developing and publishing, in the *Journal of Trauma*, practice management guidelines for the diagnosis and management of various injuries. The Western Trauma Association also has a very active scientific program and is made up of members interested in trauma from the western states. This organization has been active in organizing, conducting, and publishing, in the *Journal of Trauma*, the results of multi-institutional randomized controlled trials related to trauma. The Trauma Association of Canada (TAC) is very active in promulgating the cause of trauma care among surgeons in Canada. Scientific papers from the TAC are also published in the *Journal of Trauma*.

The American Trauma Society was founded in 1968 as an organization of physicians and laymen similar to the American Heart Association and the American Cancer Society. The goals of this organization are to provide public education and effect societal changes with respect to trauma epidemiology and develop effective prevention programs to reduce the incidence of trauma and increase the survival of trauma patients. The organization is young but vigorous and growing in stature each year as it assumes a leadership role in public education and trauma prevention.

The American Burn Association (ABA), founded in 1967, has also played a major role in improving the care of a subset of trauma patients, burn victims. Although its scientific programs relate primarily to experimental and clinical advances in burn care, these advances often relate to all types of trauma. The key papers from the ABA's meetings are published in the *Journal of Burn Care and*

*Rehabilitation* (recently renamed *Journal of Burn Care and Research*). A close association exists between the AAST and the ABA, since both work for improvement in the care of the trauma patient.

## THE FUTURE

Trauma is a multisystem disease, and as such, benefits from almost any advance in medical science. As we learn more about the physiology and biochemistry of various organ systems, we can provide better management for trauma victims. However, advancing scientific knowledge is only a part of the future. We also need to be able to compare groups of patients with various injuries in order to evaluate the best methods of treatment. As new and more sophisticated treatments are developed, we need to find out whether they are truly helpful, since they are often expensive and time consuming. Several methods of grading injury severity have been developed in an attempt to allow comparisons of various treatments. None of these methods has proved entirely satisfactory, yet there remains an intense need to be able to stratify patients on the basis of injury severity, in order to evaluate prevention and treatment methods.

Recognition of trauma as the unsolved epidemic of modern society must be accepted by the public, the government, and the medical profession. The landmark National Research Council Report "Accidental Death and Disability: the Neglected Disease of Modern Society" documented how little progress had been made by 1966 in developing effective injury control programs and identifying effective therapeutic interventions to prevent or correct the vital organ and cellular response to injury.[121] During the subsequent 17 years over two million Americans died from injuries and no coherent nationwide system of trauma care had been developed. Accordingly, Congress enacted a law authorizing the Secretary of the Department of Transportation to commission the National Academy of Sciences to conduct a study to determine the status of trauma care and delivery, the status of trauma research, and what could be done to improve the knowledge of injury. A multidisciplinary committee conducted public hearings and published their report "Injury in America" which documented that trauma remained "the neglected disease of modern society" and represented a continuing public health problem of enormous proportions in terms of loss of both money and productive years of life.[122] That report resulted in the development of a Center for Injury Control that is housed in the Centers for Disease Control and administered by that agency. The funding for the new center was provided by congressional appropriation and in the past decade the Center has provided support for a far-ranging program of research focused on all types of injury control.

Trauma is expensive, and it involves all of society, not just the injured person. Nevertheless, the society continues to resist helmet and seatbelt laws, gun control, fire safety, and other measures that can protect it against trauma. Institution of the prevention programs developed to address common causes of trauma would help prevent needless pain and suffering as well as death.

It is now generally recognized that not every physician or surgeon can provide the optimum care required by a trauma patient. Such management requires expertise on the part of the physician and proper backup facilities. For too long we have believed that anything done for the trauma patient is better than nothing. This is not true. Physicians do not undertake the care of a disease that they believe is outside their area of expertise. The specialization required for the treatment of the severely injured trauma patient can now be acquired in any of several trauma fellowships. Many trauma fellowships are configured to qualify the graduate to sit for the American Board of Surgery examination for added qualifications in surgical critical care. That certificate recognizes that the trauma surgeon must be able to provide care for the multisystem effects of trauma and the myriad complications encountered in caring for the trauma patient. The increasing ability to manage a variety of trauma patients nonoperatively has changed the complexion of trauma surgery and limited the scope of operative activity of trauma surgeons. At the present time, members of the AAST are working with representatives of other surgical specialties to address these changes and develop a curriculum for a proposed new specialty of Acute Care Surgery. Consideration is being given to enrichment of the residency experience of that "specialty-to-be" with extended rotations on the specialty services of neurosurgery, orthopaedics, vascular surgery including endoluminal procedures, noncardiac thoracic surgery, burn surgery, and perhaps even interventional radiology.

We must also provide increased training for personnel managing the prehospital phase of trauma patient care and develop an integrated transportation system with ground and air capability. Simultaneously, we must continue to categorize hospitals according to their ability to manage the patient. This includes categorization of both staffing and the support services required to manage the most severely injured patients which will permit the development of regional trauma systems. If we can accomplish these goals, the care of the trauma patient will be further improved and an increased number of productive survivors will be returned to society.

## REFERENCES

1. Davis NS: *History of Medicine.* Chicago: Cleveland Press, 1907.
2. Breasted JH: *The Edwin Smith Surgical Papyrus.* Chicago: University of Chicago Press, 1930.
3. Graham H: *Surgeons All.* New York: Philosophical Library, 1957, p. 35.
4. Lyons AS, Petrucelli RJ: *Medicine: An Illustrated History.* New York: Harry Abrams, 1978.
5. Rutkow IM: *Surgery: An Illustrated History.* St. Louis, MO: Mosby, 1993.
6. Homer: *The Iliad IV* (translated by Robert Fagles). New York, NY: Penguin Book, Book 4, 1990, p. 151.
7. Karger B, Sudhues H, Kneubuehl BP, Brinkmann B: Experimental arrow wounds-ballistics and traumatology. *J Trauma* 45:495–501, 1998.
8. Coar T: *The Aphorisms of Hippocrates* (translated by Thomas Coar). London: AJ Valpy, 1822.
9. Zimmerman LM, Veith I: *Great Ideas in the History of Surgery.* Baltimore: Williams & Wilkins, 1961.
10. Davis JH: Our Surgical Heritage. *Clinical Surgery.* St. Louis: Mosby, 1987.
11. Haeger K: *The Illustrated History of Surgery.* London: Harold Starke, 1989.
12. Watson LF: *Hernia.* St. Louis: Mosby, 1948, p. 24.
13. Olch PD, Harkins HN: Historical Survey of the Treatment of Inguinal Hernia. In: *Hernia* (eds Nyhus TM, Harkins HN). Philadelphia: JB Lippincott Co, 1964, p. 2.
14. Zimmerman LM, Anson BI: *Anatomy and Surgery of Hernia.* Baltimore: Williams & Wilkins, 1953, p. 2.
15. Haddad FS: Rhazes (842–932 AD). *J Lab Clin Med* 117:339–340, 1991.
16. Johnson PC: Guy de chauliac and the grand surgery. *Surg Gynecol Obstet* 169:172–174, 1989.
17. Whelan TJ, Burkhalter WE, Gomez A: *Management of War Wounds.* Advances in Surg, Vol. 3. Chicago: Year Book Medical Publishers, Inc., 1968, p. 257.
18. Keynes G: *The Apologie and Treatise of Ambroise Paré.* London: Falcon Educational Books, 1951.
19. Watt J: Some forgotten contributions of naval surgeons. *J R Soc Med* 78:753, 1983.

20. Harvey W: *Exercitatio Anatomica de Motu Cordis et Sanguinis in Animalibus* (The Keynes English translation of 1928). Classics of Medicine Library. Birmingham, AL: LB Adams, 1978.

21. Aldenberg H: An account of the rise and attempts of a way to convey liquors immediately into the mass of blood. *Philos Trans R Soc Lond B Biol Sci* 1:128, 1665.

22. Lower R: de Transfusione Sanguinis, 1665–1666 (translated by Hollingsworth MW). *Ann Med Hist* 10:213, 1928.

23. Castiglioni A: *A History of Medicine*. New York: Knopf, 1941.

24. Hunter J: *A Treatise on the Blood, Inflammation, and Gunshot Wounds*. Classics of Medicine Library. Birmingham, AL: LB Adams, 1982.

25. Wangensteen OH, Wangensteen SD: Successful pre-listerian antiseptic management of compact fracture: Crowther (1802) Larrey (1824) and Bennion (ca1840). *Surgery* 69:811, 1971.

26. Porter R: *The Greatest Benefit to Mankind*. New York: WW Norton & Co, 1997.

27. Rogers BO: Surgery in the revolutionary war. Contributions of John Jones (1729–1791). *Plast Reconstr Surg* 49:1, 1972.

28. Albin MS: The use of anesthetics during the civil war 1861–1864. *Pharm Hist* 42:99, 2000.

29. Albin MS: The wounding amputation, and death of Thomas Jonathan "Stonewall" Jackson—some medical and historical insights. *Bull Anesth Hist* 19:4, 2001.

30. Nuland SB: *The Origins of Anesthesia*. Classics of Medicine Library, Birmingham, AL: LB Adams, 1983.

31. Rutkow IM: *Bleeding in Blue and Gray: Civil War Surgery and the Evolution of American Medicine*. New York: Random House, 2005.

32. Mettler CC, Mettler FA: *History of Medicine*. Philadelphia: Blakiston, 1947.

33. Wangensteen OH, Wangensteen SD: *The Rise of Surgery: From Empiric Craft to Scientific Discipline*. Minneapolis: University of Minnesota Press, 1978.

34. Pruitt BA Jr: Cadaverus particles and infection in injured man. *Eur J Surg* 159:515, 1993.

35. Earle AS: The germ theory in America: Antisepsis and asepsis [1867–1990]. *Surgery* 65:508, 1969.

36. Virchow R: *Cellular Pathology* (translated by Frank Chance). London: Churchill, 1860.

37. Harvey AM: *Science at the Bedside: Clinical Research in American Medicine, 1905–1945*. Baltimore: Johns Hopkins University Press, 1981, p. 18.

38. Zollinger RM, Coleman DW: *The Influences of Pancreatic Tumors on the Stomach*. Springfield, IL: Charles C. Thomas, 1974, p. 158.

39. Ravitch MM: *A Century of Surgery 1880–1980 Vol. 1*. Philadelphia: JB Lippincott Company, 1981.

40. Latta T: Letter to the secretary of the central board of London. *Lancet* ii:274, 1832.

41. Buhl: Mitteilunger aus der pfeuferchen Klinik: Epidemische cholera. *Z Rationelle Med* 6:1, 1855.

42. Monafo WW: *The Treatment of Burns*. St. Louis, Green, 1970, p. 23.

43. Sneve H: The treatment of burns and skin grafting. *JAMA* XLV:1, 1905.

44. Underhill FP: The significance of anhydremia in extensive superficial burns. *JAMA* 95:852, 1930.

45. Blalock A: Experimental shock: VII. The importance of the local loss of fluid in the production of the low blood pressure after burns. *Arch Surg* 22:610, 1931.

46. Harkins HH: *The Treatment of Burns*. Springfield, IL: Thomas, 1942.

47. Blalock A: Experimental shock: The cause of the low blood pressure produced by muscle injury. *Arch Surg* 20:959, 1930.

48. Cope O, Moore FD: The redistribution of body water and the fluid therapy of the burned patient. *Ann Surg* 126:1010, 1947.

49. Shires GT, Brown FT, Canizaro PC: *Shock*. Philadelphia: Saunders, 1973 (chap 4).

50. Domagk G: A Contribution to the chemotherapy of bacterial infections. *Rev Infect Dis* 8:163, 1986.

51. Meleney FL: A statistical analysis of a study of the prevention of infection in soft part wounds, compound fractures and burns with special reference to the sulfonamides. *Surg Gynecol Obstet* 80:263, 1945.

52. Mendelson JA, Lindsey D: Sulfamylon (mafenide) and penicillin as expedient treatment of experimental massive open wounds with *C. perfringens* infection. *J Trauma* 2:239, 1962.

53. Keefer CS: *Penicillin: A Wartime Achievement*. Chapter L11 of Part Nine: Penicillin in Advances in Military Medicine (eds. Andrus EC, Bronk DW, Carden GA: Keefer CS, Lockwood JS, Wearn JT, Winternitz MC). An Atlantic Monthly Press Book. Boston, Little, Brown, and Company, 1948.

54. Butkus DE: Post-traumatic acute renal failure in combat casualties: A historic review. *Mil Med* 149:117, 1984.

55. Whelton A, Donadio JV Jr: Post-traumatic acute renal failure in Vietnam. *Johns Hopkins Med J* 124:95, 1969.

56. Eisman B: Introduction to conference. *J Trauma* 8:649, 1968.

57. Le Vay David: *The History of Orthopaedics*. Park Ridge, NJ: The Parthenon Published Group, 1990.

58. Rang M: *The Story of Orthopaedics*. Philadelphia: Saunders, 2000.

59. Peltier LF: *Fractures: A History and Iconography of Their Treatment*. San Francisco: Norman Publishing, 1990.

60. Sarmiento A: A functional below-the-knee cast for tibial fractures. *J Bone Joint Surg* 49A:855, 1967.

61. Parvez Z, ed: *Contrast Media: Biologic Effects and Clinical Application*, vol. I. Boca Raton, FL: CRC Press, 1987.

62. Fariñus PL: A new technique for the arteriographic examination of the abdominal aorta and its branches. *AJR Am J Roentgenol* 46:641, 1941.

63. Margolies NN, Ring EJ, Waltman AC, et al.: Arteriography in the management of hemorrhage from pelvic fractures. *N Engl J Med* 287:317, 1972.

64. Tuffier: *Sonde ureterale opaque*. In: "Traite de Chirurgie" 2nd ed. (eds. Duplay SE, Recluse P). Paris: Masson et Cie, 1897–1899, vol. 7, p. 412.

65. Wulff P: Verwendbarkeit der X-strahlen für die Diagnose der Blasendeformitäten. *Fortschr Geb Rontgenstr* 8:193, 1904.

66. Voelcker F, von Lichtenberg A. Die Gestalt der menschlichen Harnblase im Röntgenbilde. *Munch Med Wochenschr* 52:1576, 1905.

67. Osborne ED, Sutherland CG, Scholl AJ, Rowntree LG: Roentgenography of urinary tract during excretion of sodium iodide. *JAMA* 80:368, 1923.

68. Binz A: The chemistry of uroselectan. *J Urol* 25:297, 1931.

69. Swick M: Intravenous urography by means of the sodium salt of 5-iodo-2-pyridon-*n*-acetic acid. *JAMA* 95:1403, 1930.

70. Swick M: Intravenous urography by means of uroselectan. *Am J Surg* 8:405, 1930.

71. Kristensen JK, Buemann B, Kuehl E: Ultrasonic scanning in the diagnosis of splenic haematomas. *Acta Chir Scand* 137:653, 1971.

72. Rozycki GS, Ochsner MG, Jaffin JH, Champion HR: Prospective evaluation of surgeons' use of ultrasound in the evaluation of trauma patients. *J Trauma* 34:516, 1993.

73. Shackford SR: Focused ultrasound examinations by surgeons: The time is now (editorial). *J Trauma* 35:181, 1993.

74. Knudtson JL, Dort JM, Helmer SD, Smith RS: Surgeon-performed ultrasound for Pneumothorax in the trauma suite. *J Trauma* 56:527, 2004.

75. Marshburn TH, Legome E, Sargsyan A, et al.: Goal-directed ultrasound in the detection of long-bone fractures. *J Trauma* 57:329, 2004.

76. Spiral CT: *Principles, Technics, and Clinical Applications* (eds. Fishman E, Jeffrey RB). New York: Raven Press, 1995.

77. Kalender WA, Sissler W, Klotz E, Vock P: Spiral volumetric CT with single-breathhold technique, continuous transport, and continuous scanner rotation. *Radiology* 176:181, 1990.

78. Liang Y, Kruger RA: Dual-slice spiral versus single-slice spiral scanning: Comparison of the physical performance of two computed tomography scanners. *Med Phys* 213:205, 1996.

79. Busquets AR, Acosta JA, Colon E, et al.: Helical computed tomographic angiography for the diagnosis of traumatic arterial injuries of the extremities. *J Trauma* 56:625, 2004.

80. Berne JD, Norwood SH, McAuley CE, Villareal DH: Helical computed tomographic angiography: An excellent screening test for blunt cerebrovascular injury. *J Trauma* 57:11, 2004.

81. Luterbur PC: Image formation by induced local interactions: Examples employing nuclear magnetic resonance. *Nature* 243:190, 1973.

82. Adams DB: Abdominal gunshot wounds in warfare: A historical review. *Mil Med* 148:15, 1983.

83. Bagwell CE: Ambroise paré and the renaissance of surgery. *Surg Gynecol Obstet* 152:350, 1981.

84. Garrison FH: *An Introduction to the History of Medicine*. Philadelphia: Saunders, 1929.

85. Flexner JT: *Doctors on Horseback*. New York: Collier Books, 21, 1962.

86. Laughlin KR: Benjamin Church: Physician, patriot, and spy. *J Am Coll Surg* 192:215, 2001.

87. Saffon MH: The Tilton affair. *JAMA* 236:67, 1976.

88. DiGioia JM, Rocko JM, Swan KG: Baron Larrey. Modern military surgeon. *Am Surg* 49:226, 1983.

89. Wiese ER: Larrey, Napoleon's chief surgeon. *Ann Med Hist* 1:435, 1939.

90. Bechet PE: Jean Dominique Larrey. A great military surgeon. *Ann Med Hist* 9:428, 1937.

91. EMTs civil war style. *Civil War Times* 45:74, 2006.

92. Pruitt BA Jr: Combat casualty care and surgical progress. *Ann Surg* 243:715, 2006.

93. Cunningham HH: *Doctors in Gray: The Confederate Medical Service*. Baton Rouge, LA: Louisiana State University Press, 1993, p. 339.

94. Adams GW: *Doctors in Blue: The Medical History of the Union Army in the Civil War*. Baton Rouge, LA: Louisiana State University Press, 1996, p. 253.

95. Kuhns WJ: Blood transfusion in the civil war. *Transfusion* 5:92, 1965.

96. The World Book Encyclopedia, B Vol. 2. Chicago: World Book, Inc., 1995, p. 121.

97. Pruitt BA Jr: Centennial changes in surgical care and research. *Ann Surg* 232:287, 2000.

98. Sartin JS: Infectious diseases during the civil war: The triumph of the "Third army." *Clin Infect Dis* 16:580, 1993.

99. Schreiber W. The discovery of X-rays by Willhelm C. Roentgen 1895. *Med Bull US Army Eur* 43:3, 1986.

100. Tilney NL: The marrow of tragedy. *Surg Gynecol Obstet* 157:380, 1983.

101. Cushing H: *From a Surgeon's Journal 1915–1918*. Boston: Little Brown and Company, 1936, p. 50.

102. Landsteiner K: Zur Kenntnis der antifermentativen, lytischen und agglutinierenden Wirkungen des Blutserums und der Lymphe. *Zentralbl Bakteriol* [*Orig*] 27:357, 1900.

103. DeCastello A, Sturli A: Über die isoagglutine im serum gesunder und kranker Menschen. *Munch Med Wochenschr* 49:1090, 1902.

104. Pruitt BA Jr: The integration of clinical care and laboratory research. *Arch Surg* 130:461, 1995.

105. Wangensteen OH, Smith J, Wangensteen SD: Some highlights in the history of amputation reflecting lesions in wound healing. *Bull Hist Med* 41:97, 1967.

106. Poer DH: The Management of Colostomies. Chapter XXX. In: "*Surgery in World War II, Vol. II. General Surgery*" (ed. DeBakey, ME). Washington, D.C.: Office of the Surgeon General, Department of the Army, 1955, p. 340.

107. Churchill ED: The surgical management of the wounded in the Mediterranean theater at the time of the fall of Rome. *Ann Surg* 120:268, 1944.

108. DeBakey ME: History, the torch that illuminates: Lessons from military medicine. *Mil Med* 161:711, 1996.

109. Brewer LA III: The contributions of the second auxiliary surgical group to military surgery during World War II with special reference to Thoracic surgery. *Ann Surg* 197:318, 1983.

110. Pruitt BA Jr: Trauma care in war and peace: The Army/AAST synergism: 1992 fitts lecture. *J Trauma* 35:78, 1993.

111. *The Physiologic Effects of Wounds*. Washington, D.C.: The Board for the Study of the Severely Wounded, Medical Department, United States Army, Surgery in World War II, Office of the Surgeon General, 1952.

112. Rankin FW: Mission accomplished: The task ahead. *Ann Surg* 130:289, 1949.

113. Giddlings WP, Wolff LH: Factors of Mortality, Chapter XVI. In: "*Surgery in World War II, Vol. II, General Surgery*" (ed. DeBakey, ME). Washington, D.C.: Office of the Surgeon General, Department of the Army, 1955, p. 218.

114. Simeone FA: Studies of trauma and shock in man: William S. Stone's role in the military effort (1983 William S. Stone lecture). *J Trauma* 24:181, 1984.

115. Spencer FC: Historical vignette: The introduction of arterial repair into the U.S. marine corps, U.S. Naval hospital, in July–August 1952. *J Trauma* 60:906, 2006.

116. Smith LH Jr, Post RS, Teschan PE, et al.: Post-traumatic renal insufficiency in military casualties: II. Management, use of an artificial kidney, prognosis. *Am J Med* 18:187, 1955.

117. Teschan PE, Post RS, Smith LH Jr, et al.: Post-traumatic renal insufficiency in military casualties: I. Clinical characteristics. *Am J Med* 18:172, 1955.

118. McCaughey BG, Garrick J, Carey LC, Kelly JB: Naval support activity hospital, Danang, combat casualty study. *Mil Med* 153:109, 1988.

119. DiVincenti FC, Pruitt BA Jr, Moncrief JA, et al.: Clinical operation, burn center. In: *Annual Research Progress Report*. Houston, TX: U.S. Army Institute of Surgical Research, Fort Sam, Brooke Army Medical Center, Houston, Texas, 30 June 1969.

120. Peltier LF, Davis JH: A history of the American association for the surgery of trauma: The first 50 years. *J Trauma* 29:143, 1989.

121. *Accidental Death and Disability: The Neglected Disease of Modern Society*. Washington, D.C.: National Research Council, National Academy Press, 1966.

122. Committee on Trauma Research, National Research Council, and the Institute of Medicine: *Injury in America*. Washington, D.C.: National Academy Press, 1985.

# Commentary ■ DONALD D. TRUNKEY

This initial chapter in the 6th edition of *Trauma* by the Drs. Pruitt is elegant and comprehensive. They rightly point out the very close association of trauma care and war. In addition to trauma care, the history of trauma systems, shock, and resuscitation are also inextricably linked to armed conflicts. The origins of trauma systems can be traced to the early cultures of Greece, Rome, and India. King Ashoka was the third of the Maurya dynasty that waged war on Kalinga, a kingdom on his eastern border. His army had an ambulance service and well-equipped surgeons. Women accompanied the ambulances and prepared food, beverages, and assisted with wound dressings. In Arthashastra, a treatise on statecraft, economic policy and military strategy, Kautilya lays "the provision of comfort for men and animals."

A continent away, the Greeks also established a trauma system to treat and manage the warriors that had been wounded and described in the Iliad. This may be the first mention of a trauma system, as the wounded were carried off the battlefield and tended in special barracks called klisíai. The treatment was often primitive; fractures were splinted, and dislocations were reduced. Women would wash the wounds with warm water and dress them. Nothing was done to stop the bleeding, and in fact, the tourniquet was condemned in the Hippocratic collection. It was not until the mid-1500s that Ambroise Paré was credited for discovering the principle and application of the tourniquet.

A few centuries later, the Romans also established a very sophisticated trauma system. In the 1st and 2nd century AD, Roman generals provided special quarters, called valetudinaria, for the sick and wounded. At least 25 archeological remains of these valetudinaria have been found along the borders of the Roman Empire. Eleven of the trauma centers have been found in Roman Britannia, which is more than what currently exists. These hospitals for the wounded were very sophisticated. Open ventilation was stressed. Patient flow for patients, including triage, was based on the seriousness of their wounds. Surgical instruments as well as unmistakable medicinal herbs such as henbane (scopolamine) and dried poppies have been found in these remains.

Further development of trauma systems did not occur until the time of Larrey during the Napoleonic Wars. His contributions were clearly remarkable and included operating on the wounded as close to the battlefield as possible. He invented the flying ambulance, and he established teams of surgeons (17 teams during the march on Moscow) who could resuscitate and operate depending on where the heaviest casualties were. The 20th century saw the introduction of trauma systems into civilian practice in Austria in 1925, in Germany in 1975, and the United States beginning in 1966.

The concept of shock was not articulated until 290 years after Harvey described the circulation. The 17th and 18th century surgeons thought of shock in very prosaic terms. LeDran defined shock as "reflections drawn from experiences with gunshot wound." John Warren stated, "Shock is a momentary pause in the act of death," and Samuel Gross thought that shock was "the manifestation of the rude unhinging of the machinery of life." It was in 1918 that Walter B. Cannon, based on a three-month study of casualties during World War I, provided a definition of shock that is applicable even today. His description of shock is matched only by his intellectual and sound approach to resuscitation.

Pruitt and Pruitt point out that Thomas Lotta used saline infusion for the treatment of cholera patients in 1831. Simultaneously, W. B. O'Shaughnassy also treated patients with fluid and electrolytes for diarrhea. This work was then confirmed in 1850 by Karl Schmidt, but all these authors were essentially ignored. Between 1880 and 1882, Sydney Ringer showed that potassium was a normal constituent of physiologic fluids, and nine years later, Rudolph Matas reported successes with IV fluid administration, again for diarrhea and cholera. In 1915, three pediatricians described the chemical composition of diarrheal fluid as compared with normal stools in infants. Thirteen years later, Alexis F. Hartman, another pediatrician in St. Louis, described the chemical changes in the body as the result of certain diseases and developed fluid therapy based on the 1915 work. He gave this to seven medical students, and they had no undesirable effects. Six years later, it was used in children suffering cholera and

dysentery with a remarkable reduction in mortality from 60% down to 10%. The next major hurdle was to use blood. Work by Nuttal identified the blood types. Arthus and Pages showed that calcium was necessary for clotting, and Hustin described citrate anticoagulation. Robinson used citrated blood for combat casualties in WWI. The next major advance was the work by Shires in 1964 where he showed that in severe shock, there was depletion of the extracellular space above and beyond the predicted or measured loss of blood in patients. This physiologic concept had been predicted by Cannon, but Shires work conclusively showed the extent of the fluid loss with volume of distribution measurements.

History teaches us that few discoveries are really new, and our surgical forefathers were very innovative. As one sage noted, "Those who ignore history must be prepared to repeat it."

# Epidemiology

*Ellen J. MacKenzie* ■ *Carolyn J. Fowler*

The term *epidemiology* derives from the Greek word *epidemion*, which means "to visit." It is the study of the patterns of disease occurrence in human populations and the factors that influence these patterns.[1] The concepts of epidemiology, used in concert with those from other disciplines, including medicine, sociology, behavioral sciences, and biomechanics, are critical to the development of effective interventions for reducing injuries and their adverse consequences. *Descriptive epidemiology* refers to the distribution of disease or injury over time, place, and within or across specific subgroups of the population. It is important for understanding the impact of injury in a population and opportunities for intervention. *Analytic epidemiology*, in contrast, refers to the more detailed study of the determinants of observed distributions of disease in terms of causal factors. The epidemiologic framework traditionally identifies these factors as related to the *host* (i.e., characteristics intrinsic to the person), the *agent* (physical, chemical, nutritive, or infectious), and the *environment* (i.e., characteristics extrinsic to the individual that influence exposure or susceptibility to the agent). It is the understanding of how these multiple factors interact to increase the risk of injury and poor outcome that exemplifies the epidemiologic approach to the study of disease and injury; other disciplines typically focus on only one aspect of the epidemiologic triad. What further characterizes the unique role of epidemiology is its emphasis on the study of defined *populations*. Although it is true that injuries occur and are treated one at a time, it is only by studying patterns of occurrence across populations of individuals that we learn how best to prevent them. Indeed, as George W. Albee wrote, "No mass disorder afflicting mankind was ever brought under control or eliminated by attempts at treating the individual."[2]

Injuries result from acute exposure to physical agents such as mechanical energy, heat, electricity, chemicals, and ionizing radiation in amounts or at rates above or below the threshold of human tolerance.[3] The transfer of mechanical energy alone accounts for more than three-quarters of all injuries.[4] The extent and severity of injury is largely determined by the amount of energy concentrated outside the band of human tolerance. It is well known, however, that both the exposure to energy and the consequences of that exposure are greatly influenced by a variety of factors both within and beyond our control.[5] These concepts were first articulated in the late 1960s by William Haddon, who proposed a matrix approach for delineating the risk factors associated with the occurrence and severity of injury.[3] His phase-factor matrix retains the classic epidemiologic framework of host, agent, and environment but emphasizes the dynamic process of injury causation. The time sequence is divided into three phases: pre-event, event, and post-event. Factors in the pre-event phase determine whether the event (e.g., motor vehicle crash) will occur; factors in the event phase determine whether an injury will occur (as a result of the crash); and factors in the post-event phase influence the outcome from, or consequences of, the injury. These phases interact with the three sets of factors encountered in each phase, namely, host or human factors (including both biologic and behavioral factors), factors associated with the agent or vehicle of energy transfer such as a car or gun, and the environment. A variation of the original Haddon Matrix further separates the physical environment from the social, political, and economic environment. An example of the Haddon Matrix is displayed in Table 2-1 and is used here simply to illustrate the complexity of the multiple factors that contribute to the "cause" of any given injury. How this matrix is used to identify effective strategies for prevention is discussed in Chap. 3.

This chapter will begin with an overview of what is known in general about the epidemiology of injuries in the population and proceed to a more detailed discussion of the leading mechanisms of injury mortality and morbidity. The chapter ends with a discussion of the sources of injury information available on both a national and local level, as well as the challenges we face in monitoring trends in injury over time and place.

**TABLE 2-1**

**Haddon Phase-Factor Matrix**

| PHASES | FACTORS | | ENVIRONMENT | |
|---|---|---|---|---|
| | Host (Human) | Agent (Vehicle) | (Physical) | (Social) |
| Pre-event | Driver age, gender, driving experience, drug or alcohol use, vision, fatigue, frequency of travel, risk taking behavior | Vehicle speed, brakes, tires, road-holding ability, visibility (e.g., daytime running lights) | Road design and traffic flow, road conditions, whether, traffic density, traffic control (lights, signals), visibility | Speed restrictions, impared driving laws, licensing restrictions, road rage, seat belt and child restraint laws |
| Event | Age, pre-existing conditions (e.g., osteoporosis), restraint use | Vehicle speed, size, crash-worthiness, type of seat belts, airbag, interior surface hazards | Guardrails, median dividers, break-away poles, road side hazards | Entorcement of speed limits |
| Post-event | Age, comorbidities | Integrity of fuel system | Distance from emergency medical care, obstacles to extrication | EMS planning and delivery, bystander control, quality of trauma care, rehabilitation, compensation practices |

EMS, emergency medical services.

## OVERVIEW

### Overview of Injury and Its Relationship to Other Diseases

In the United States, injuries constitute the fourth leading cause of death over all ages (accounting for 6% of all deaths) and the leading cause of death among children, adolescents, and young adults aged 1 to 44 (Fig. 2-1).[6] In 2003 alone, 164,002 U.S. residents died as a result of an injury, translating into an overall rate of 55.9 injury deaths per 100,000 population.[7] Put in more immediate terms, over 400 people die of injuries in the United States each day; nearly 50 of these deaths are among our children and adolescents. Nearly 8 of every 10 deaths in young people aged 15 to 24 are injury related. Indeed, more young lives between the ages of 1 and 34 are lost to injury than to all other causes of death combined. The impact of injury as a cause of death among our young people is best summarized by comparing the total years of potential life lost before the age of 75 (YPLL-75) across the leading causes of death (Fig. 2-2). Injuries account for more premature deaths than either cancer, heart disease, or human immunodeficiency virus (HIV) infection.[7]

It is important to understand that 50% of all deaths occur within minutes of the injury either at the scene or en route to the hospital. These immediate deaths are typically the result of massive hemorrhage or severe neurologic injury. An additional 20–30% die primarily of neurologic dysfunction within several hours to 2 days postinjury. The remaining 10–20% die of infection or multiple organ failure many days or weeks after the injury.[8,9] Although the exact percent distributions of time to death vary by region of the country depending on both the mix of blunt versus penetrating trauma and the maturity of the emergency medical services (EMS) system,[10] it is evident that even the best EMS and trauma systems will be largely ineffective in preventing about one-half of all trauma deaths. Only efforts at preventing the occurrence of the injurious event or reducing the severity of the injury once it occurs will be effective in reducing the large numbers of immediate deaths.

Deaths are only the tip of the injury iceberg, however. Each year, 1.9 million people are hospitalized as the result of an acute injury and survive to discharge, and 27 million are treated in an emergency department.[7] Injuries account for an estimated 8% of all hospital discharges, 37% of all emergency department visits and 35% of all emergency medical services (EMS) transports. Many of these nonfatal injuries have far-reaching consequences in terms of reduced quality of life and high costs accrued to the health care system, employers, and society in general. It is estimated that the total lifetime costs associated with both fatal and nonfatal injuries occurring in the year 2000 amount to over $406 billion.[11] While costs associated with injury deaths account for a disproportionate share of the total (deaths account for less than 1% of all injuries but 35% of total injury costs), the majority (65%) of the costs are associated with nonfatal injuries. The costs for nonfatal injuries include direct expenditures for health care and other goods and services purchased as a result of the injury and the value of lost productivity due to temporary and permanent disabilities. Lost productivity costs associated with injury survivors represent 45% of the total lifetime costs of injury (Fig. 2-3). As a measure of the overall impact of injury on society, however, these costs are conservative as they do not take into account the pain, suffering, and reduced quality of life often associated with nonfatal injury. Estimates of the value individuals place on these consequences have been derived and are often used in studies of cost-benefit analyses of alternative strategies for preventing injury.[12]

## OVERALL INJURY PATTERNS BY AGE AND GENDER

As previously indicated, the majority of both fatal and nonfatal injuries occur among the young. Persons under the age of 45 account for approximately one-half of all injury fatalities and hospitalizations and over three-quarters (78%) of all emergency department visits.[7] Different patterns emerge, however, when one looks at the *risk* or *rate* of injury by age. Figure 2-4 displays

Age Groups

| Rank | <1 | 1-4 | 5-9 | 10-14 | 15-24 | 25-34 | 35-44 | 45-54 | 55-64 | 65+ | Total |
|---|---|---|---|---|---|---|---|---|---|---|---|
| 1 | Congenital Anomalies 5,621 | Unintentional Injury 1,717 | Unintentional Injury 1,096 | Unintentional Injury 1,522 | Unintentional Injury 15,272 | Unintentional Injury 12,541 | Unintentional Injury 16,766 | Malignant Neoplasms 49,843 | Malignant Neoplasms 95,692 | Heart Disease 563,390 | Heart Disease 685,089 |
| 2 | Short Gestation 4,849 | Congenital Anomalies 541 | Malignant Neoplasms 516 | Malignant Neoplasms 560 | Homicide 5,368 | Suicide 5,065 | Malignant Neoplasms 15,509 | Heart Disease 37,732 | Heart Disease 65,060 | Malignant Neoplasms 388,911 | Malignant Neoplasms 556,902 |
| 3 | SIDS 2,162 | Malignant Neoplasms 392 | Congenital Anomalies 180 | Suicide 244 | Suicide 3,988 | Homicide 4,516 | Heart Disease 13,600 | Unintentional Injury 15,837 | Chronic Low. Respiratory Disease 12,077 | Cerebro-vascular 138,134 | Cerebro-vascular 157,689 |
| 4 | Maternal Pregnancy Comp. 1,710 | Homicide 376 | Homicide 122 | Congenital Anomalies 206 | Malignant Neoplasms 1,651 | Malignant Neoplasms 3,741 | Suicide 6,602 | Liver Disease 7,466 | Diabetes Mellitus 10,731 | Chronic Low. Respiratory Disease 109,139 | Chronic Low. Respiratory Disease 126,382 |
| 5 | Placenta Cord Membranes 1,099 | Heart Disease 186 | Heart Disease 104 | Homicide 202 | Heart Disease 1,133 | Heart Disease 3,250 | HIV 5,340 | Suicide 6,481 | Cerebro-vascular 9,946 | Alzheimeris Disease 62,814 | Unintentional Injury 109,277 |
| 6 | Unintentional Injury 945 | Influenza & Pneumonia 163 | Influenza & Pneumonia 75 | Heart Disease 160 | Congenital Anomalies 451 | HIV 1,588 | Homicide 3,110 | Cerebro-vascular 6,127 | Unintentional Injury 9,170 | Influenza & Pneumonia 57,670 | Diabetes Mellitus 74,219 |
| 7 | Respiratory Distress 831 | Septicemia 85 | Septicemia 39 | Chronic Low. Respiratory Disease 81 | Influenza & Pneumonia 224 | Diabetes Mellitus 657 | Liver Disease 3,020 | Diabetes Mellitus 5,658 | Liver Disease 6,428 | Diabetes Mellitus 54,919 | Influenza & Pneumonia 65,163 |
| 8 | Bacterial Sepsis 772 | Perinatal Period 79 | Benign Neoplasms 38 | Influenza & Pneumonia 72 | Cerebro-vascular 221 | Cerebro-vascular 583 | Cerebro-vascular 2,460 | HIV 4,442 | Suicide 3,843 | Nephritis 35,254 | Alzheimeris Disease 63,457 |
| 9 | Neonatal Hemorrhage 649 | Chronic Low. Respiratory Disease 55 | Chronic Low. Respiratory Disease 37 | Benign Neoplasms 41 | Chronic Low. Respiratory Disease 191 | Congenital Anomalies 426 | Diabetes Mellitus 2,049 | Chronic Low. Respiratory Disease 3,537 | Nephritis 3,806 | Unintentional Injury 34,335 | Nephritis 42,453 |
| 10 | Circulatory System Disease 591 | Benign Neoplasms 51 | Cerebro-vascular 29 | Cerebro-vascular 40 | HIV 178 | Influenza & Pneumonia 373 | Influenza & Pneumonia 992 | Viral Hepatitis 2,259 | Septicemia 3,651 | Septicemia 26,445 | Septicemia 34,069 |

Source: National Vital Statistics System, National Center for Health Statistics, CDC.
Produced by: Office of Statistics and Programming, National Center for Injury Prevention and Control, CDC.

FIGURE 2-1. Ten leading causes of death by age group—2003. (Reproduced with permission from National Center for Injury Prevention and Control: Ten Leading Causes of Death, 2003. Atlanta: Centers for Disease Control, 2006.)

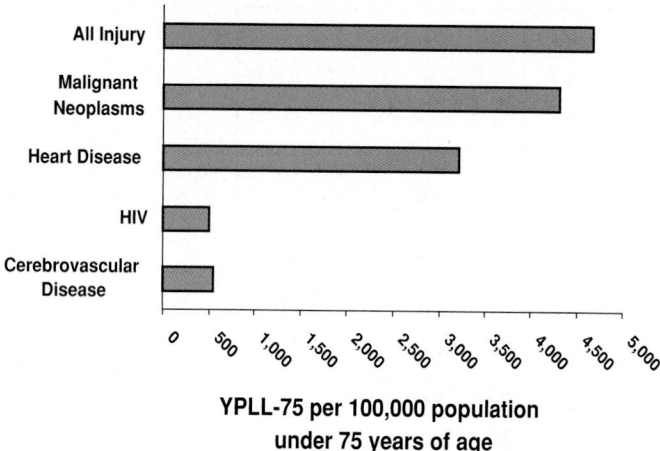

**FIGURE 2-2.** Years of potential life lost before age 75 (YPLL-75) by cause of death: United States, 2003.
*(Reproduced with permission from National Center for Injury Prevention and Control: Years of Potential Life Lost, 2003. Atlanta: Centers for Disease Control, 2006.)*

age-specific injury rates for males and females for deaths, hospitalizations, and emergency department visits separately. What is most striking about these figures is that the elderly aged 65 and older are actually at highest risk of both fatal injuries and injuries requiring hospitalization. The rate of injury death among persons aged 65 and older is 113 per 100,000 population; for persons aged 75 and older, it is 169 per 100,000—a rate that is three times higher than the rate for all ages combined. Although they comprised only 12% of the U.S. population in 2003, the elderly aged 65 and older accounted for approximately 25% of all injury deaths and 30% of injury-related hospitalizations. In light of the demographic changes occurring in the United States, these figures have profound implications for the health care system and society at large. The percentage of the population that is 65 and older is projected to

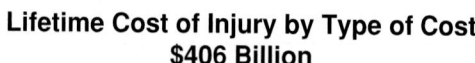

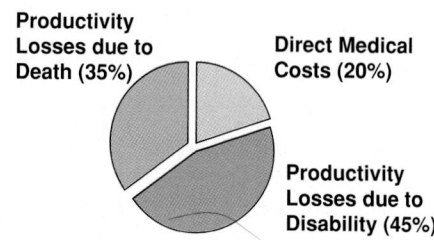

**FIGURE 2-3.** Total lifetime costs of injury by type of cost: These new estimates underscore the public health impact of injuries in terms of both health care costs and lost productivity. Injuries that occurred in 2000 will cost the U.S. health care system $80.2 billion in lifetime medical care costs. These high costs, however, are dwarfed by the costs associated with lost productivity resulting from premature death and disability. Injuries that occurred in 2000 will cost our society an estimated $326 billion in productivity losses: $142 billion for fatal injuries and $184 billion for nonfatal injuries.

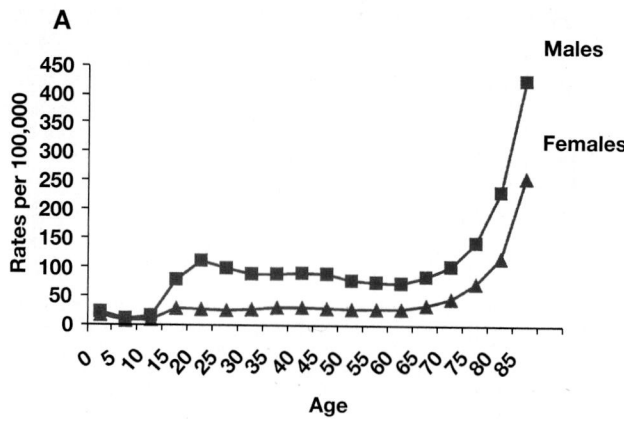

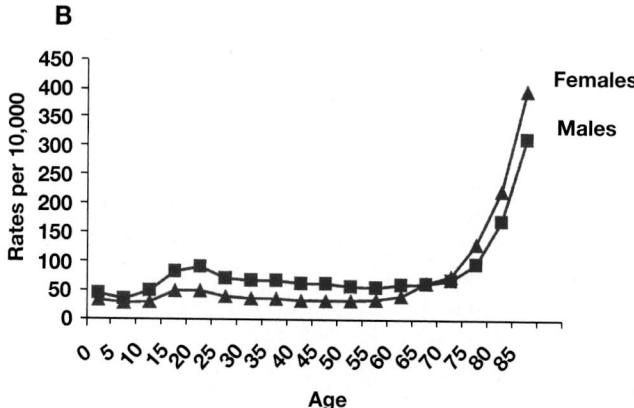

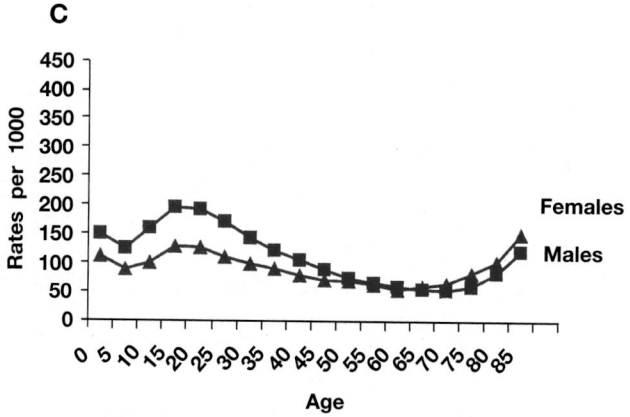

**FIGURE 2-4.** **(A)** Injury death rates by age and gender, United States, 1995. **(B)** Hospital discharge rates for injury by age and gender, United States, 1993–1994. **(C)** Average annual rate of emergency room visits for injury by age and gender, United States, 1992–1995.
*(Reproduced with permission from Fingerhut LA, Warner M. Injury Chartbook: Health, United States, 1996–97. Hyattsville, MD: National Center for Health Statistics, 1997.)*

increase from 12 to nearly 20% by the year 2030.[13] If we assume that age- and gender-specific rates of injury remain constant over the next couple of decades, we can expect that by the year 2030, elders 65 and older will account for approximately 40% of all injury deaths and hospitalizations. They will also account for an equal, if not higher, share of acute hospital costs for trauma.[14] Patterns of injury risk by age are considerably different for less severe injuries that are treated and discharged from the emergency department. The elderly aged 75 and older are at a comparatively low risk of minor injury. Rather, adolescents and young adults aged 15 to 24 are at highest risk of minor injury. Seventy percent of injury deaths and over one-half (56%) of nonfatal injuries occur among males.[7] However, the risk of injury by gender also varies by class of injury. In every age group except the very young (ages 0 to 9), the rate of injury death for males is more than twice as high as the rate for females. In contrast, males are only 1.3 times as likely as females to sustain a nonfatal injury. Furthermore, among older adults, the risk to females of nonfatal injury actually exceeds the risk to males. Among elders aged 65 and older, females are 1.3 times as likely as males to suffer a nonfatal injury.

## PATTERNS OF INJURY BY MECHANISM AND INTENT

Injuries are typically categorized by their mechanism, intent, and place of injury. Mechanism refers to the external agent or particular activities that cause the injury (e.g., motor vehicle, firearm, fall, or poisoning). Intent of the injury is classified as either unintentional (often referred to as accidental*), intentional (intentionally inflicted by someone, including the injured person him- or herself), or intent undetermined. Injuries resulting from legal interventions and operations of war are typically classified separately as in "other intent" category. Intentional injuries are further classified as assaults or homicides versus self-inflicted injuries or suicides. The classification system most often used in describing the specific mechanism and intent of injury is the International Classification of Diseases (ICD), promulgated by the World Health Organization[15] and modified for morbidity coding by the United States.[16] Standard ICD groupings of injuries by intent and mechanism have been developed and should be used as a minimum framework for tabulating injury counts and rates.[17] Detailed injury mortality data from 2000 are presented in Table 2-2 using this framework.[7]

The distribution of injuries by mechanism varies for deaths, hospitalizations, and emergency department visits (Table 2-3). The two leading mechanisms of injury death are related to motor vehicles and firearms, accounting for 29% and 18%, respectively, of all injury deaths in 2003. Taken together, they account for nearly one-half of all injury deaths. Falls and poisonings account for an additional 11% and 17% of all injury deaths. In contrast, the leading cause of nonfatal injury is falls, accounting for one-third of hospitalizations and one-quarter of emergency department visits. Transportation remains an important cause of injury requiring hospitalization and treatment in the emergency department (18% and 15% of hospitalizations and emergency department visits, respectively), whereas firearm injuries account for less than 1% of all nonfatal injuries. These differences in distribution by cause and class of injury underscore the lethality of injuries involving firearms and motor vehicles. Other common causes of nonfatal injuries include being hit by an object or person, poisonings, overexertion, and injuries resulting from a cutting or piercing instrument (including stabbings).

Nearly one-third (30%) of all injury deaths are intentional; in 2003, they accounted for 31,484 suicides (63% of all intentional deaths) and 18,155 homicides (37%). Firearms were involved in 67% of all homicides and 54% of all suicides.[7] The distribution of nonfatal injuries by intent is not as well understood. Intent is not uniformly recorded in the medical record, and when it is, this information is unreliable because it often represents only a conjecture on the part of the person completing the narrative. Rough estimates are that at least 5 to 15% of injury-related hospitalizations and emergency department visits are related to intentional injuries.[7,11,18]

Work occupies about 40% of waking hours for most adults (aged 22 to 65). More than 136 million civilian workers are employed in the United States, with some risk of injury present in most jobs. In 2004, 5764 fatal work injuries (4.0 per 100,000 workers) were reported by the Census of Fatal Occupational Injuries.[19] Overall, transportation-related incidents account for the majority (43%) of occupational injury deaths. Assaults and violent acts, contacts with objects and equipment, and falls accounted for an additional 14%, 18%, and 14%, respectively, of all fatal occupational injuries. It is important to note that approximately 1 in 10 occupational deaths in 2004 was a homicide. Firearm-related homicides comprise three-quarters of all occupational homicides.[19] Occupations at highest risk of fatal injury include fishers, timber cutters, and airplane pilots. The average number of fatal injuries, however, is highest for truck drivers (an average of 873 per year in 2004).[19]

In addition to the high death rate associated with work-related activities, it is estimated that over 13 million nonfatal occupational injuries occur each year.[20] Nearly one-half (46%) of these injuries are disabling.[21] Approximately one-third of nonfatal injuries are sustained by workers in nine industries (eating and drinking places, hospitals, nursing and personal care facilities, trucking and nonair courier services, grocery stores, department stores, motor vehicles and equipment, air transportation, and hotels and motels), with the highest incidence rate (13.7 per 100 full-time workers) reported in persons employed in nursing and personal care facilities.[20]

## DISTRIBUTION OF INJURIES BY THEIR NATURE AND SEVERITY

An understanding of the distribution of injuries by their nature and severity is important to efforts at establishing priorities for prevention as well as treatment and system development. Several systems for classifying the nature and severity of injury exist; some of these systems are described in Chap. 5. The most widely used classification is the Clinical Modification of the ICD.[16] The International Collaborative Effort on Injury Statistics published an injury diagnosis matrix that provides a uniform framework for using the ICD-9CM in categorizing injury diagnoses by the body region involved and the specific nature of the injury.[22] The use of this matrix is encouraged as it will ensure comparability of data across studies.

In the ensuing chapters, injuries to different body systems are described in detail. Here, we attempt to provide an overall population perspective on the incidence and principal mechanism of both fatal and nonfatal injuries to different body systems. The only comprehensive source of national data on the nature of injury death is death certificate data. However, these data have significant limitations due to variations in diagnosis, terminology, and reporting

---

*The term accident is generally avoided in the scientific literature as it incorrectly implies that injuries occur by chance and cannot be anticipated or prevented.

**TABLE 2-2**

## Deaths and Crude Death Rates for External Causes of Injury: United States, 2000

| MECHANISM | | MANNER OF DEATH | | | | |
| --- | --- | --- | --- | --- | --- | --- |
| | All | Unintentional | Suicide Deaths | Homicide | Other | Undetermined |
| All injury | 148,209 | 97,900 | 29,350 | 16,765 | 375 | 3,819 |
| Cut/pierce | 2,288 | 85 | 383 | 1,805 | – | 15 |
| Drowning | 4,073 | 3,482 | 321 | 39 | ... | 231 |
| Fall | 14,002 | 13,322 | 607 | 18 | ... | 55 |
| Fire and flame/hot substances | 3,907 | 3,487 | 162 | 181 | – | 77 |
| Firearm | 28,663 | 776 | 16,586 | 10,801 | 270 | 230 |
| Machinery | 676 | 676 | ... | ... | ... | ... |
| All transportation | 46,509 | 46,259 | 103 | 106 | – | 41 |
| MV traffic | 41,994 | 41,994 | ... | ... | ... | ... |
|   Occupant | 18,649 | 18,649 | ... | ... | ... | ... |
|   Motorcyclist | 2,704 | 2,704 | ... | ... | ... | ... |
|   Pedal cyclist | 572 | 572 | ... | ... | ... | ... |
|   Pedestrian | 4,598 | 4,598 | ... | ... | ... | ... |
|   Other | 12 | 12 | ... | ... | ... | ... |
|   Unspecified | 15,459 | 15,459 | ... | ... | ... | ... |
| Other pedal cycle | 168 | 168 | ... | ... | ... | ... |
| Other pedestrian | 1,272 | 1,272 | ... | ... | ... | ... |
| Other land transportation | 1,662 | 1,412 | 103 | 106 | ... | 41 |
| Other transportation | 1,413 | 1,413 | ... | ... | – | ... |
| Natural/environmental | 1,643 | 1,643 | ... | ... | ... | ... |
| Overexertion | 13 | 13 | ... | ... | ... | ... |
| Poisoning | 20,230 | 12,757 | 4,859 | 56 | 1 | 2,557 |
| Struck by/against | 1,292 | 938 | 2 | 349 | – | 3 |
| Suffocation | 12,098 | 5,648 | 5,688 | 658 | ... | 104 |
| Other specified | 1,970 | 1,238 | 278 | 325 | 81 | 48 |
| Not elsewhere classified | 2,261 | 903 | 216 | 964 | 22 | 156 |
| Not specified | 8,584 | 6,673 | 145 | 1,463 | 1 | 302 |

| | All | Unintentional | Suicide Deaths per 100,000 Population | Homicide | Other | Undetermined |
| --- | --- | --- | --- | --- | --- | --- |
| All injury | 53.8 | 35.6 | 10.7 | 6.1 | 0.1 | 1.4 |
| Cut/pierce | 0.8 | 0.0 | 0.1 | 0.7 | * | * |
| Drowning | 1.5 | 1.3 | 0.1 | 0.0 | ... | 0.1 |
| Fall | 5.1 | 4.8 | 0.2 | * | ... | 0.0 |
| Fire and flame/hot substances | 1.4 | 1.3 | 0.1 | 0.1 | * | 0.0 |
| Firearm | 10.4 | 0.3 | 6.0 | 3.9 | 0.1 | 0.1 |
| Machinery | 0.2 | 0.2 | ... | ... | ... | ... |
| All transportation | 16.9 | 16.8 | 0.0 | 0.0 | * | 0.0 |
| MV traffic | 15.3 | 15.3 | ... | ... | ... | ... |
|   Occupant | 6.8 | 6.8 | ... | ... | ... | ... |
|   Motorcyclist | 1.0 | 1.0 | ... | ... | ... | ... |
|   Pedal cyclist | 0.2 | 0.2 | ... | ... | ... | ... |
|   Pedestrian | 1.7 | 1.7 | ... | ... | ... | ... |
|   Other | * | * | ... | ... | ... | ... |
|   Unspecified | 5.6 | 5.6 | ... | ... | ... | ... |
| Other pedal cycle | 0.1 | 0.1 | ... | ... | ... | ... |
| Other pedestrian | 0.5 | 0.5 | ... | ... | ... | ... |
| Other land transportation | 0.6 | 0.5 | 0.0 | 0.0 | ... | 0.0 |
| Other transportation | 0.5 | 0.5 | ... | ... | * | ... |
| Natural/environmental | 0.6 | 0.6 | ... | ... | ... | ... |
| Overexertion | * | * | ... | ... | ... | ... |
| Poisoning | 7.3 | 4.6 | 1.8 | 0.0 | * | 0.9 |
| Struck by/against | 0.5 | 0.3 | * | 0.1 | * | * |

**TABLE 2-2** *(Continued)*

## Deaths and Crude Death Rates for External Causes of Injury: United States, 2000

| | All | Unintentional | Suicide<br>Deaths per 100,000 Population | Homicide | Other | Undetermined |
|---|---|---|---|---|---|---|
| Suffocation | 4.4 | 2.1 | 2.1 | 0.2 | ... | 0.0 |
| Other specified | 0.7 | 0.4 | 0.1 | 0.1 | 0.0 | 0.0 |
| Not elsewhere classified | 0.8 | 0.3 | 0.1 | 0.4 | 0.0 | 0.1 |
| Not specified | 3.1 | 2.4 | 0.1 | 0.5 | * | 0.1 |

Notes:

– cell has zero deaths

... not applicable; there is no code in matrix for this cell.

* no rate calculated when based on fewer than 20 deaths.

0.0 Quantity more than zero but less than 0.05.

US resident population (2000 estimate)= 275,264,999.

ICD 10 codes for these causes can be found at http://www.cdc.gov/nchs/data/ice/icd10_transcode.pdf. Injury deaths exclude deaths from adverse effects and complications of medical and surgical care (ICD-10 codes Y40-Y84, Y88);in 2000, there were 3,059 such deaths.Other includes legal intervention and war operations (95% due legal intervention). For additional information, contact Lois A. Fingerhut at Lfingerhut@cdc.gov

practices for injury by place and over time.[23,24] Rather, what is known about the overall nature of trauma deaths is largely based on a limited number of studies conducted in selected geographic regions using coroners' reports and autopsy records.[9,25,26] Although the results of these studies vary, they all point to some common themes. First, injuries to the central nervous system are the most common cause of injury death, accounting for 40 to 50% of the total; the second and third leading causes are hemorrhage, accounting for an additional 30 to 35% and multiple organ failure, accounting for 5–10%. In a study of trauma deaths in San Diego County, for instance, head injuries accounted for 40% of the deaths, and spinal cord injury another 8%. Hemorrhage was the cause of 30% of the injury deaths, most often associated with isolated cavity bleeding into the thorax or bleeding into both the abdomen and chest.[26]

The distribution of nonfatal injuries by nature and severity is quite different from that described above for fatal injuries. First, it is important to remember that the majority of injuries occurring each year are to isolated body systems and are associated with low threat to life. Even among injuries resulting in hospitalization, only about one-quarter have an Abbreviated Injury Scale (AIS)[27] score of 3 or above; only 10 to 15% typically require treatment at a Level I or Level II trauma center.[14,28] These more severe cases, however, use a disproportional share of hospital resources, accounting for approximately one-half of hospital charges associated with injury.[14]

Injuries to the lower and upper extremities constitute the leading cause of hospitalizations and emergency department visits related to nonfatal injury. They account for approximately one-half of all nonfatal occurrences (as classified by the principal diagnosis).[11,12] Slightly over one-third of hospitalizations for extremity injuries are for moderately severe to severe injuries as measured by an AIS score of 3 or above.[11] For many of these injuries, recovery can be long and expensive, and even optimal treatment can result in permanent impairment and disability.[29–33] Some of the most severe injuries can result in amputation, of which there are an estimated 3700 each year (excluding amputations to the fingers and toes).[34] The primary mechanism of extremity injuries resulting in hospitalization is falls, accounting for an estimated 30% of all upper extremity injuries and 50 to 60% of lower extremity injuries. Motor vehicle crashes are also an important contributor to hospitalizations for lower extremity injuries, especially among the young. Indeed, there is evidence accumulating to suggest that the relative number of significant injuries to the leg and foot are increasing due to the increasing number of vehicles with airbags.

**TABLE 2-3**

## Percent Distribution of Leading Mechanisms of Injury: United States, 2003

| MECHANISM | PERCENT DISTRIBUTION OF LEADING MECHANISM | | |
|---|---|---|---|
| | Deaths (%) | Hospital Discharges (%) | Treated and Released from the ED (%) |
| Transportation related | 29 | 18 | 15 |
| Falls | 11 | 36 | 27 |
| Firearms | 18 | 2 | <1 |
| Struck by/against | <1 | 6 | 21 |
| Cut/pierce | 2 | 4 | 9 |
| Fire/burn | 2 | 1 | 2 |
| Poisoning | 17 | 18 | 2 |
| Drowning/near drowning | 2 | <1 | <1 |
| Overexertion | <1 | 2 | 12 |
| Other mechanism | 18 | 12 | 11 |

(*Source:* http://www.cdc.gov/ncipc/wisqars/)

Airbags reduce the number of severe head injuries and deaths over-all, leaving a larger proportion of survivors hospitalized for their leg injuries, often resulting from intrusion of the toepan into the compartment of the vehicle. The use of machinery and tools is an important cause of upper extremity injuries, accounting for an estimated 20% of all hospitalized upper extremity injuries.

The second leading cause of injury hospitalization is head injury, accounting for 10 to 15% of the total, or approximately 230,000 hospitalizations per year.[35] Mild head injuries are also treated on an outpatient basis, comprising 2 to 5% of all injury-related emergency department visits or approximately one million per year.[36] Estimates of the total incidence of head injury vary widely and range between 152 and 367 per 100,000 population.[37,38] Although the majority of head injuries are classified as mild, conservative estimates suggest that between 70,000 and 90,000 people survive a significant head injury that often results in long-term disability.[39] Motor vehicle injuries (including motorcycle, bicycle, and pedestrian) constitute the leading cause of hospitalization for head injury in the United States, accounting for approximately one-third to one-half of all discharges with a principal diagnosis of head injury. Falls are the second leading cause of head injury hospitalizations, accounting for an additional 20 to 30% of the total.[40,41] The important role of sports-related head injury should not be overlooked, however. Approximately 300,000 such injuries occur each year. Although most are classified as concussions, there is increasing evidence to suggest that repeated mild brain injuries over an extended time or within a short period can have serious long-term consequences.[42,43]

Although spinal cord injuries account for a very small proportion of all nonfatal injuries (an estimated 15,000 to 20,000 hospitalizations per year),[11,44] they often result in significant physical and psychological deficits and have a substantial impact on the individual and society. It is estimated that nearly 200,000 people live in the United States with a disability related to a spinal cord injury.[45] Motor vehicles are the major cause of spinal cord injury, accounting for an estimated 30 to 60% of all injuries. Falls constitute the second-leading cause; they account for an additional 20 to 30% of all spinal cord injuries. Approximately 5 to 10% of all spinal cord injuries are due to diving.[44,45]

Musculoskeletal injury to the spinal column also accounts for a large proportion of hospitalizations and emergency department visits for injury and is a major source of impairment and disability, especially among workers. Overall estimates of the incidence of back injury are difficult to obtain, however, because of the difficulty in making a differential diagnosis among patients presenting with low back complaints. Work-related back injuries alone account for about one-fifth to one-quarter of all workers' compensation claims.[46] In 2001, the Bureau of Labor Statistics reported a total of 372,683 back injury cases that involved days away from work, a rate of 41.0 per 10,000 workers.[47] Rates of back injury vary considerably by industry, with the highest rates reported among machine operators, truck drivers, and nurses. Overexertion, including lifting, pulling, and throwing, is the most common cause of back injury.

## DISTRIBUTION OF INJURIES BY PLACE

The overall incidence and patterns of injury vary substantially across urban versus rural populations and across different regions of the country.[4] It is well known that unintentional injury death rates are highest in rural areas, whereas homicide rates are several times higher in central cities compared to rural and suburban communities. Interestingly, suicide exhibits the least variation by urban(rural differences. Injury death rates also vary by region of the country. Death rates for unintentional injury tend to be highest in the West and South, whereas suicide rates are highest in the West and homicide rates highest in the South. There is substantial state-by-state as well as county-by-county variation, however. Death rates by mechanism and intent by county for each state are now readily available and can be useful to local communities in identifying priorities for prevention initiatives.[48] To date, local data about nonfatal injuries are not uniformly available for examining trends by rurality or geographic region. The reasons for observed differences by rurality of the community and region of the country are complex and beyond the scope of this chapter. However, it is important to note that although differences in demographic composition of the population factor into the variation in rates, differences in the physical, social, and economic environment are equally, and in some cases, more important.

## TRENDS IN THE RATES OF INJURY OVER TIME

Over the past century, we have witnessed a substantial decline in the overall death rate due to injury.[4] Indeed, the Centers for Disease Control and Prevention in looking forward to the 21st century identified motor vehicle safety and safer workplaces as two of the top 10 greatest public health achievements of the last century.[49] Despite the number of miles traveled in motor vehicles today is 10 times higher than it was in the early 1900s, the annual motor vehicle death rate has declined from 18 per million vehicle miles traveled (VMT) in 1925 to 1.7 per million VMT in 1997, a 91% decrease (Fig. 2-5).[50] Similarly, data from the National Safety Council indicate that deaths from unintentional work-related

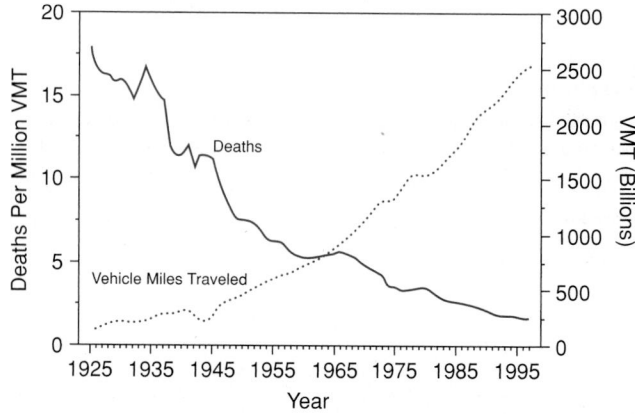

**FIGURE 2-5.** Motor-vehicle-related deaths per million vehicle miles traveled (VMT) and annual VMT, by year—United States, 1925–1997. *(Reproduced with permission from Mortal Morbid Weekly Rev 48(18). Atlanta, Georgia: Centers for Disease Control and Prevention, 1999.)*

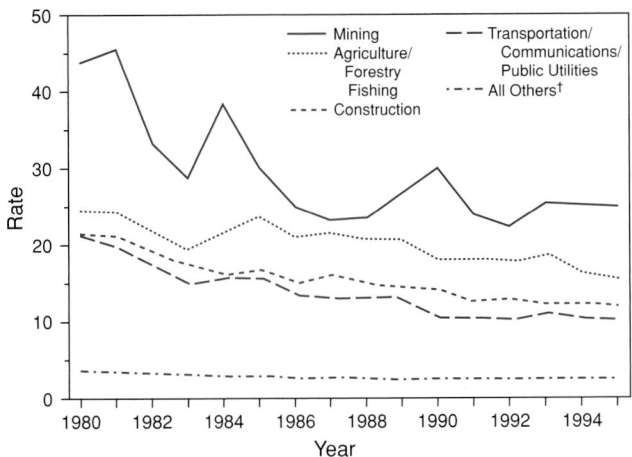

**FIGURE 2-6.** Occupational injury death rates by industry division and year—United States, 1980–1995.
*(Reproduced with permission from Mortal Morbid Weekly Rev 48(22). Atlanta, Georgia: Centers for Disease Control and Prevention, 1999.)*

injuries declined 89% from 37 per 100,000 workers in 1933 to 4 per 100,000 in 1997.[51] Data from the National Institute for Occupational Safety and Health indicate that the average rate of deaths from all occupational injuries decreased from 7.5 per 100,000 in 1980 to 4.3 per 100,000 workers in 1995 (Fig. 2-6). In contrast to the declining rates of motor-vehicle- and work-place-related injury death rates, the rate of homicides has fluctuated over the last decade with a low of about 6 per 100,000 in 1910 to a high of more than 11 per 100,000 in 1991. It has since been declining, reaching a low of 5.5 deaths per 100,000 in 2004. The suicide rate has remained relatively stable over the past century.[7]

Of particular note are the trends in deaths related to firearms. Beginning in the mid-1980s, the age-adjusted firearm death rate steadily increased, from 12.7 per 100,000 in 1985 to 15.6 per 100,000 in 1993.[6,7] This increase can be explained almost exclusively by an increase in firearm homicides among adolescents and young adults aged 15 to 34. In this age group alone, the firearm homicide rates increased 83% between 1985 and 1993, from 8.7 to 15.9 per 100,000. Since 1993, the rate of firearm deaths has steadily declined. The rate in 1999 was 10.6 per 100,000, the lowest in two decades. These declines are observed for both firearm homicides and suicides, although rates of decline were higher for firearm homicides. Declines in rates were consistent across age groups. Despite these encouraging statistics, there has been little change in this rate since 1993. In 2003, 30,136 people died from a firearm injury.[7]

## LEADING MECHANISMS OF MAJOR TRAUMA: MOTOR VEHICLES, FIREARMS, AND FALLS

In this section, the epidemiology of three leading mechanisms of major trauma—motor vehicles, firearms, and falls—will be described in more detail.

## MOTOR VEHICLE INJURIES

As previously stated, motor vehicles are the leading cause of injury death and the second leading cause of nonfatal injury in the United States. They account for approximately 45,000 deaths, 357,000 hospitalizations, and over 4 million emergency department visits each year, or an average of 123 deaths and over 10,000 nonfatal injuries each day.[7] Despite a small increase of 2% in motor vehicle death rates between 1993 and 1996, all age groups from 0 to 84 years have lower death rates today when compared with 1985 figures. Elders (over 85 years of age) are the only age group whose death rate in 1999 was greater than the 1985 rate, largely due to the increased mobility of the elderly. The elderly aged 75 and older are at relatively high risk of dying from motor vehicle injury (24.9 per 100,000 for ages 75 to 84 and 28.8 for ages 85 and older).[7,52]

Adolescents and young adults, however, are at highest risk of both fatal and nonfatal injuries due to motor vehicles. Their rates of death, hospitalization, and emergency department visits are approximately twice the rate for all ages combined.[7] Motor-vehicle-related injuries were the leading cause of all deaths among white males aged 15 to 24 and the second leading cause (behind firearms) for black males aged 15 to 24. In Fig. 2-7, motor vehicle injury death rates among males aged 15 to 24 (averaged across 1992 to 1995) are compared across several developed countries.[6] Only New Zealand had a higher death rate (63 per 100,000) than did the United States (41.0 per 100,000).

Males are more than twice as likely as females to die from a motor vehicle crash, with the largest male-to-female ratio (over three-fold) among adolescents and young adults aged 15 to 44. Males under the age of 45 are also more likely to be hospitalized as a result of a motor vehicle injury, although the gender differential is not as great as for fatalities. Males and females aged 45 and older, in contrast, are equally likely to be hospitalized.

Major factors contributing to the likelihood of a crash include speed, vehicle instability and braking deficiencies, inadequate road design, and alcohol intoxication. When a crash occurs, important determinants of the likelihood of an injury and its severity include the speed of impact, vehicle crashworthiness, and the use of safety devices and restraints, including seat belts, airbags, and helmets. When used, lap and shoulder belts reduce fatalities to front seat car occupants by 45% and the risk of moderate-to-critical injury by 50%. In 2006, mandatory seat belt laws were in place in all states except New Hampshire, although only 22 states and the District of Columbia have seat belt use laws that provide for primary enforcement.[52,53] The additional presence of an airbag in belted drivers provides increased protection, resulting in an estimated 51% reduction in fatality rate.[53,54] In 2004, more than 157 million cars and light trucks on U.S. roads had driver airbags; 139 million of these had dual airbags. There is little question that airbags are effective in reducing deaths as well as the incidence of severe head and chest injuries (by 75% and 66%, respectively). The National Highway Traffic Safety Administration (NHTSA) estimates that between 1987 and 2004, 16,904 lives were saved by airbags.[55]

Despite some success in reducing the role of alcohol in motor vehicle injuries, it remains a major factor in fatal crashes among adolescents and young adults. In 2005, approximately 39% of all traffic fatalities were alcohol related (i.e., either the driver, occupant, or pedestrian/pedal cyclist had a blood alcohol concentration of

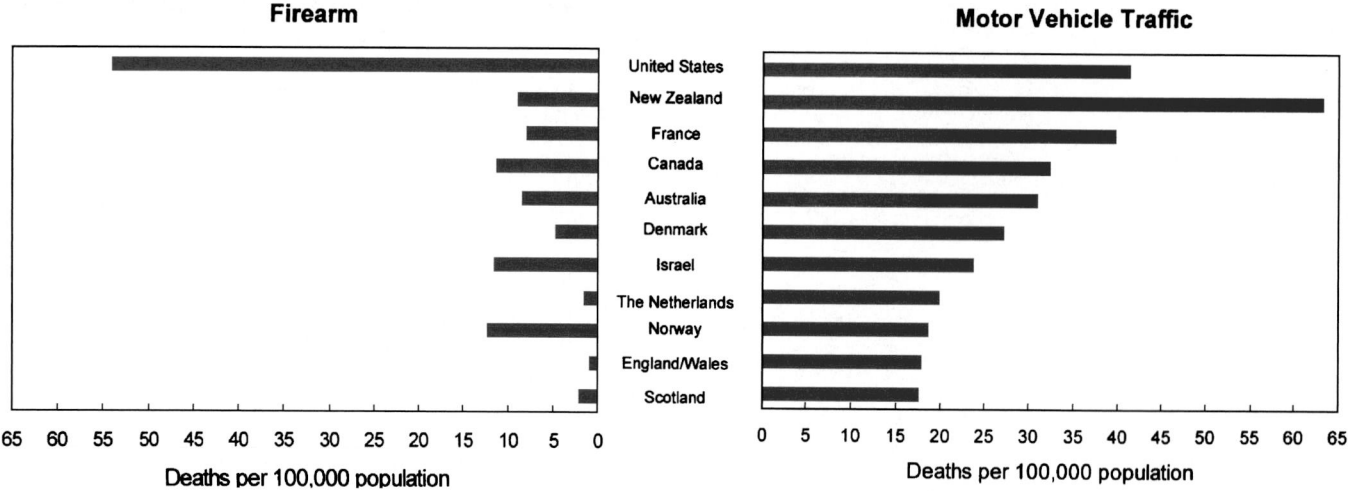

**FIGURE 2-7.** Firearm and motor vehicle traffic injury death rates, males 15 to 34, 1992–1995 for selected countries. *(Reproduced with permission from Annest JL, Conn JM, James SP. Inventory of Federal Data Systems in the United States. Atlanta: National Center for Injury Prevention and Control, 1996.)*

0.01 g/dL or greater).[56] Intoxication rates among drivers of all ages in fatal crashes are highest among motorcycle operators (27% had a blood alcohol concentration of 0.08 g/dL or greater) and lowest among drivers of large trucks (1%). They have decreased in all age groups since 1985, with the decline most dramatic among drivers aged 16 to 20, for whom the percentage intoxicated decreased from 47 to 13%. The NHTSA estimates that minimum-age drinking laws have reduced motor vehicle fatalities involving 18- to 20-year-old drivers by over 13%.[52] Nevertheless, in 2000, alcohol-involved crashes accounted for 21% of nonfatal crash costs, and 46% of fatal injury crash costs, or 22% of all motor vehicle crash costs—an economic expense to society of over $50 billion.[11,57]

## FIREARM-RELATED INJURIES

In 2003, there were 30,136 intentional and unintentional gun-related deaths in the United States—about 82 deaths every day.[7] Gun-related deaths are the second leading cause of injury death over all ages in the United States, responsible for 18% of all injury deaths. Furthermore, in three states and the District of Columbia, firearm-related deaths actually outnumbered motor-vehicle-related deaths in 1999. More than half (56%) of all gun deaths were suicides, and 39% were homicides. Unintentional fatalities claimed the lives of 730 people in 2003.[7]

Gun deaths disproportionately affect males and young people. For the age group of 10 to 34 years, firearms are the second leading cause of all deaths.[6,7] Between the ages of 15 and 34, the firearm death rates for males are about seven times the rates for females[6,7]; for young black males aged 15 to 34, guns have replaced motor vehicles as the leading mechanism of all injury deaths.[7] The rate of gun-related mortality is eight times higher in the United States than other high-income countries in the world.[58] (Fig. 2-7)

The majority of firearm deaths among males aged 15 to 34 in the United States (60%) are homicides, but an additional 35% are suicides. Youth suicide rates increased dramatically from 1980 to 1999,

largely due to gun-related suicides.[7] Although rates of gun suicides have declined in more recent years, in 2003 there were 809 suicides with guns among young people 10 to 19 years old. Although this rate of gun suicide among our young is alarming, it is important to note that the problem is most acute among the elderly. In 2003, there were 3295 firearm suicides among elders between the ages of 65 and 84; over 90% of these suicides were among males.[7]

Deaths related to guns, however, do not tell the whole story. It is estimated that for every firearm fatality, over two nonfatal firearm-related injuries occur.[7,59] In the year 2004, 64,389 persons were treated for nonfatal firearm-related injuries in the United States. Of these, 35,993 were injured severely enough to be hospitalized.[7] Males comprised 89% of all emergency department visits for firearm injury. For firearm injuries occurring in 2000, the estimated lifetime cost is more than $36 billion.[11] The cost of providing medical care alone is projected at $1.2 billion, with 80% of the hospital costs borne by the public.[11,60,61] More comprehensive estimates of the direct and social costs (including the impact of nonfatal injuries on quality of life) are estimated to exceed $80 billion per year.[62]

Of all firearm homicides in 2002 in which the type of gun was known, the majority (77%) involved handguns,[63] although increasing prevalence of gang warfare and use of assault weapons by drug traffickers may result in different patterns of firearm deaths. Although guns are present in about 35% of all U.S. households and carried by 17.4% of students on one or more days within a month,[64,65] they remain a virtually unregulated consumer product. The U.S. Consumer Product Safety Commission, the federal agency charged with protecting the public from unreasonable risks of injury and death associated with consumer products, is expressly prohibited from regulating firearms or ammunition. Yet, studies have shown that people who live in homes with guns are more likely to die from homicide and suicide in the home than are people who live in homes without guns.[66,67] The risk of a homicide of a household member is increased three times in homes with guns; the risk of a suicide is increased five times. In addition, family and intimate assaults involving firearms are 12 times more likely to result in death than are non-firearm-related assaults.[68] Although handguns are often marketed for self-protection, there is evidence to suggest that few firearm deaths in the home stem from acts of self-protection. Analysis of the U.S. Department of Justice's National Crime Survey reveals an average of about 108,000 defensive uses of guns in 1994 compared with about 1.3 million crimes committed with guns.[69] It is interesting to note that Americans generally support government regulation of guns as consumer products, especially regarding the safe design of guns.[64,70,71]

## FALLS

Although falls were responsible for fewer than 11% of injury deaths in 2003, they account for over one-third of all injury hospitalizations and over one-quarter of all injury-related visits to emergency departments.[7] Fall risk is greatest in the youngest and oldest members of our society, although the severity profile in these two groups is quite different. In children, falls are common but generally not severe. For children less than 5 years of age, falls are the leading cause of nonfatal injury and account for 45% of emergency department visits for injury; less than 3% of these visits, however, result in hospitalization.[7] This age group has the highest emergency department visit rate for falls (49.1 per 1000 persons). Approximately one-half of all pediatric falls occur at home and one-quarter at school.[72] Indeed, in children aged 0 to 4 years, the home is the site of most falls, which are usually from furniture or stairs.[73] Baby walkers are associated with more than 25,000 emergency department visits for injuries from falls annually.[74] In older children, falls are commonly on the level or associated with play and recreational activities such as playground equipment, bicycling, or sporting activities.[73] The estimated 54,000 fall-related hospitalizations and fewer than 125 deaths in children below the age of 15 are most often associated with falls from heights greater than 10 meters or two stories.[74] It has also been suggested that abuse may be involved in cases of fatal falls from lower heights.[75]

After childhood, death rates from falls increase steadily from 0.6 per 100,000 at 15 to 19 years to 4.7 per 100,000 for ages 55 to 64 and 38.5 per 100,000 for ages 65 and older. Fall deaths are mostly unintentional (96%), with suicide (4% of all falls) the main cause of intentional fall deaths. In adults of working age, most fatal falls are from buildings, ladders, and scaffolds, although falls on stairs increase in importance from age 45.[4] Gender ratios for injury deaths in adults differ by mechanism and appear driven by exposure (1.2:1 for all falls; 29:1 for falls from scaffolds).[4] Emergency department visit rates for falls are consistently higher for men up to the age of 44. From age 45, this trend reverses, and by age 65, emergency department visit rates and hospitalizations for falls in women are 2.7 times those of men.[18] This finding is consistent with the increased fracture risk in women after menopause and, specifically, those with osteoporosis.[76]

In the elderly, falls are an important cause of injury death (34% and 46% of injury deaths in people 65 and over and 85 and over, respectively).[4] The death rate from falls after age 85 (136.5 per 100,000) is over three times that for persons aged 75 to 84 years (41.1 per 100,000).[7] Falls are also the most common cause of nonfatal injury in the elderly, accounting for 58% of injury-related emergency department visits and nearly 80% of injury-related hospitalizations for persons aged 65 years and older. In the

United States, more than one-third of adults over the age of 65 will fall each year.[77] Of these, about one-quarter will be injured and another quarter will restrict their daily activities for fear of another fall.[78] Fractures occur in about 5% of falls.[76,79] Risk for hip fractures from falls increases dramatically with age. Elders over age 85 are 10 to 15 times as likely to sustain hip fractures as people aged 60 to 65.[80] Long hospitalizations and the fact that one-half of elderly persons cannot live independently after their hip fracture makes this an expensive and important public health problem.[11,81] In 2000, lifetime medical expenditures associated with falls totaled $26.9 billion and accounted for 34% of total direct medical costs for injuries.[11] Major risk factors for falls among the elderly include those related to the host (advanced age; history of previous falls; hypotension; psychoactive medications; dementia; difficulties with postural stability and gait; visual, cognitive, neurologic, or other physical impairment) and environmental hazards (loose rugs and loose objects on the floor, ice and slippery surfaces, uneven floors, poor lighting, unstable furniture, absent handrails on staircases).[4,82–86] Risk of falling increases linearly with number of risk factors present,[76,82] and it has been suggested that falls and some other geriatric syndromes may share a set of predisposing factors, all of which are potentially modifiable with combinations of environmental, rehabilitative, psychological, medical, or surgical interventions.[86–88]

## DATA SOURCES

The data used in this chapter to describe the epidemiology of injury were obtained from multiple sources, including ongoing surveillance systems as well as one-time surveys and targeted studies. Although comprehensive data on nonfatal injuries are still lacking in many areas, significant strides over the past decade in both the scope and quality of data collection have enhanced our understanding of the magnitude and impact of injury as a major public health problem. In this section, federal, state, and local sources of data on injury are discussed, as well as areas where improvement is necessary.

## NATIONAL DATA SOURCES

An inventory of national data systems identified over 30 sources of data on injury mortality, morbidity, and risk factors.[89,90] Eight of these systems provide data on work-related injuries; the remainder focus on injuries and injury deaths related to other unintentional and intentional injuries. Approximately one-half are ongoing surveillance systems. They vary in scope and the extent to which they provide information on mechanism and intent, nature and severity, risk factors, health services use and costs, and health outcomes. Comprehensive data on fatalities are available from vital statistics, although as previously noted, these data do not provide detailed information about the extent and nature of injury sustained.

Uniform data on nonfatal injuries treated in emergency departments (including those treated and released, transferred, or hospitalized) are now available from the National Electronic Injury Surveillance System-All Injury Program (NEISS-AIP).[91] The NEISS-AIP, a collaborative effort between the National Center for Injury Prevention and Control (NCIPC) and the U.S. Consumer Product Safety Commission (CPSC), collects information on approximately 600,000 injury-related emergency department visits to a nationally representative sample of 66 hospitals. The NEISS-AIP is the most comprehensive database on all nonfatal injuries currently available. These data, together with injury mortality data, can be easily accessed through WISQARS (Web-based Injury Statistics Query and Reporting System), an interactive database system supported by the NCIPC.[91]

Additional data on all injuries treated in an outpatient setting are also available from the National Health Interview Survey (NHIS), the National Ambulatory Medical Care Survey (NAMCS), and the National Hospital Ambulatory Medical Care Survey (NHAMCS). The NHIS relies on self-reports of injury events, whereas both the NAMCS and the NHAMCS consist of data abstracted from injury-related visits to hospital emergency departments, hospital outpatient departments, and/or physician offices. The NHAMCS has routinely included external cause codes since 1992, whereas the NAMCS did not add external cause codes until 1995 and the NHIS until 1997.

More detailed data on injuries resulting in hospitalization can be obtained from both the National Hospital Discharge Survey (NHDS) and the Healthcare Costs and Utilization Project (HCUP). Both of these data sources provide comprehensive estimates of the number of hospitalizations associated with injury although they are limited in scope and content (see discussion below regarding limitations of state hospital discharge data).

In addition to these sources of comprehensive data across all types and severities of injury, several sources of national data exist specific to a particular mechanism or intent. Examples include the Fatality Analysis Reporting System (FARS) and the National Automotive Sampling System (NASS) including the Crashworthiness Data System (CDS) for motor vehicle-related injuries; the National Traumatic Occupational Fatality Surveillance System and the Survey of Occupational Injuries and Illness for occupational injuries; and the National Crime Victimization Survey (NCVS) and the Uniform Crime Reporting System for intentional injuries (excluding suicides and self-inflicted injuries). These data systems are particularly useful for monitoring trends in injury rates specific to certain mechanisms and for identifying risk factors associated with their occurrence. Conspicuously absent has been an ongoing system of surveillance for violence-related injuries overall and firearm-related injuries, in particular. Development of a data collection system similar to that developed for motor vehicle crashes is an essential component to a nationwide effort at reducing the toll exacted by violence.[92,93] The development of a National Violent Death Reporting System (NVDRS) is currently underway and should provide much needed data in this regard.[94,95] The purpose of the reporting system is to collect objective, ongoing data for use in planning and evaluating policies aimed at reducing violent deaths. Similar to the FARS database for motor vehicle deaths, the NVDRS is designed to link records from multiple sources to help identify risk factors. As of 2004, 17 states were funded by the Centers for Disease Control to implement the NVDRS.

## STATE AND LOCAL SOURCES OF INJURY DATA

National data are critical for drawing attention to the magnitude of the injury problem, for monitoring the impact of federal legislation, and for examining variations in injury rates by region of

the country and by rural versus urban(suburban environments. They can also be useful in aggregating sufficient numbers of cases of a particular type of injury to analyze causal patterns. Often, however, national data are not sufficient for developing and sustaining injury prevention programs at the state and local level. State and local data are more likely to reflect injury problems specific to the local area and are therefore more useful in setting priorities and evaluating the impact of policies and programs. In addition, local data are typically more persuasive than are national data in advocating to establish a policy or funding of a program at the local level. Although some of the databases described earlier provide data at the state level, most are inadequate for these purposes.

Although availability of local injury data varies substantially by state and county, typical sources are described herein. Vital statistics and death certificate data are available for 100% of injury-related deaths. As previously discussed, however, these data are limited in the information they provide about the nature and circumstances of the injury and risk factors associated with the death. Medical examiner and coroner reports can be a useful adjunct to death certificate data, although the completeness and quality of these data vary substantially from state to state depending on the policies established for forensic investigations and full autopsies.[96,97] State and local data on trauma hospitalizations are generally available from two principal sources: uniform hospital discharge data and trauma registries. Currently, 90% of the states and the District of Columbia gather uniform hospital discharge data.[98] Although the scope of the data collected varies, most states obtain a minimum of information as defined by the Uniform Hospital Discharge Data Set. A significant limitation of these databases has been the lack of uniform ICD coding for identifying the mechanism, intent, and place of the injury.[99] This is changing, however. Now 26 states have mandates for the inclusion of external cause codes in their hospital discharge data systems, although fewer than 45% have more than 90% of their records E-coded.[98] Despite some limitations, these data systems are particularly well suited for examining the epidemiology of trauma-related hospitalizations as they maintain information on all hospitalizations regardless of where the patient is treated. Furthermore, the potential exists for using ICD-9CM coded discharges to assign severity scores.[100,101] They are limited, however, in that they typically do not include information on trauma deaths that occur at the scene, in transport, or in the emergency department. In addition, there is a potential for double-counting patients who are initially admitted to one hospital and transferred to another acute care facility. Although the percentage transferred is generally low (less than 3–5%), they may represent an important subgroup of patients.[99] Increasingly, databases are being constructed to facilitate the identification of these duplicate cases.

An additional source of information on hospitalized trauma is the trauma registry.[102] Compared to hospital discharge data, trauma registries typically include more detailed information about the cause, nature, and severity of the injury. Most registries will also include data on deaths occurring in both the emergency department and after admission to the hospital. Often, however, they collect information only on "major" trauma patients, generally excluding those patients who survive but stay in the hospital less than three days. Most statewide registries also collect data from trauma centers only. The American College of Surgeons Committee on Trauma

(ACSCOT) has developed a minimum data set recommended for use by all trauma centers in developing their registries. The National Trauma Data Bank (NTDB) has been established by the ACSCOT to collate uniform registry data from trauma centers and trauma systems across the country.[103] It now contains over 1.5 million cases from 565 U.S. trauma centers, representing 70% of Level I and 53% of Level II trauma centers. The NTDB publishes annual reports that contain the most up-to-date profile of hospital trauma care nationwide. Standard data reports are also accessible through *NTDB Online*. In general, trauma registries can provide useful information, especially for clinical research and continuous quality improvement initiatives. Great caution should be exercised, however, in using these databases for describing the epidemiology of trauma as they are not population-based; that is, they typically exclude data on "nonmajor" trauma patients and data on trauma patients treated at nontrauma center hospitals.

Uniform data on trauma patients treated and released from emergency departments, hospital clinics, and physicians' offices are generally less accessible on a county or state level. Significant efforts are being directed, however, in developing emergency department surveillance systems and uniform ambulatory care data systems that parallel those developed for hospital discharges.[104,105] In 2004, approximately 50% of the states and the District of Columbia had Statewide Hospital Emergency Department Data Systems (HEDDS) in place; this is double the number having these systems in 1997.[98] As these data systems are developed, it will be important to ensure that appropriate information is included about the cause and nature of the injury. Only 15 of the states with HEDDS currently mandate E-coding of their records.[98] Other data sources often available at the state and local levels that can be useful in studying the epidemiology of injury include routinely collected information from emergency medical services, police, fire departments, poison control centers, child protective services, and child death review teams.

The utility of existing data at the state and local level can be significantly enhanced by linking data across multiple data sources. As one can see from the previous discussion, single data sources are often limited in their content or scope of coverage, or both. In recent years, techniques have been developed to facilitate linkage of these databases to avoid the high costs of gathering new data.[106] Several states have now linked hospital discharge data, vital statistics, police accident reports, and prehospital run sheets to examine patterns and outcomes of motor-vehicle-related crashes.[107] Although careful attention must be given to issues of confidentiality when pursuing these data linkages, they provide tremendous opportunity for facilitating trauma research and evaluation.

## CONCLUSION

In this chapter, an overview of the epidemiology of trauma has been provided, with attention paid to its distribution across time, place, and specific demographic subgroups of the population. Although the focus has been on the epidemiology of trauma in the United States, it is important to recognize that many of the findings presented herein are not unique to the United States. Worldwide, injuries account for 1 in every 10 deaths. They are also estimated to account for 11% of the global burden of disease as measured by the number of disability-adjusted life years experienced by the world's population.[108–110] Rates of injury clearly vary by country, however, with the highest rates often found in developing areas undergoing rapid economic change and urbanization. In a report on the global burden of disease, it was estimated that road traffic injuries alone will rise from ninth place overall as a leading cause of disease burden to third place by the year 2020. Violence, which is currently in nineteenth place as a cause of disease burden, is expected to rise to twelfth place, and self-inflicted injuries from seventeenth place to fourteenth place.[108] These projections are staggering and underscore the importance of injury as a major source of death and disability now and in the future.

In summary, while significant strides have been made in reducing the rate at which people are injured, trauma remains a major public health problem. We must continue to find better and more efficient ways of treating injuries as they occur; it is also important that we continue to develop appropriate programs and policies that will prevent them from occurring in the first place. Only through primary prevention will we make major strides in reducing the toll that injuries exact on individuals and society at large. Studying the epidemiology of injuries provides us with the clues for understanding how, when, and with whom to intervene.

## REFERENCES

1. Lilienfeld AM, Lilienfeld DE: *Foundations of Epidemiology.* New York: Oxford University Press, 1980, p. 3.
2. Albee GW: Psychopathology, prevention and the just society. *J Prim Prev* 4:5, 1983.
3. Haddon W Jr: The changing approach to epidemiology, prevention, and amelioration of trauma: The transition to approaches etiologically rather than descriptively based. *Am J Pub Health* 58:1431, 1968.
4. Baker SP, O'Neill B, Ginsburg MJ, et al.: *The Injury Fact Book.* New York: Oxford University Press, 1992.
5. Robertson LS: *Injury Epidemiology.* New York: Oxford University Press, 1998.
6. Fingerhut LA, Warner M: *Injury Chartbook. Health, United States, 1996–97.* Hyattsville, MD: National Center for Health Statistics, 1997.
7. WISQARS fatal injuries: mortality reports. http://webappa.cdc.gov/sasweb/ncipc/mortrate.html. Accessed September 15, 2006.
8. Sauaia A, Moore FA, Moore EE, et al.: Epidemiology of trauma deaths: A reassessment. *J Trauma* 38:185, 1995.
9. Demetriades D, Kimbrell B, Salim A, et al.: Trauma deaths in the mature urban trauma system: is "trimodal" distribution a valid concept? *J Am Coll Surg* 201:343, 2005.
10. Meslin H, Criss EA, Judkins D, et al.: Fatal trauma: The modal distribution of time to death is a function of patient demographics and regional resources. *J Trauma* 43:433, 1997.
11. Finkelstein EA, Corso PS, Miller TR and Associates: *The Incidence and Economic Burden of Injuries in the Untied States.* New York, New York: Oxford University Press, 2006.
12. Miller TR, Pindus NM, Douglass JB, R et al.: *Databook on Nonfatal Injury: Incidence, Costs and Consequences.* Washington, D.C.: The Urban Institute Press, 1995.
13. U.S. interim projections by age, sex, race, and Hispanic origin. http://www.census.gov/ipc/www/usinterimproj/. Accessed September 15, 2006.
14. MacKenzie EJ, Morris JA, Smith GS, et al.: Acute hospital costs of trauma in the United States: Implications for regionalized systems of care. *J Trauma* 30:1096, 1990.
15. World Health Organization: *Manual for the International Statistical Classification of Diseases, Injuries, and Causes of Death, Based on the Recommendations of the Tenth Revision Conference, 1975.* Geneva: World Health Organization, 1977.
16. U.S. Department of Health and Human Services, Public Health Service, Health Care Financing Administration: *International Classification of Diseases, 9th rev; Clinical Modification,* 6th rev, October 1, 1996.
17. http://www.cdc.gov/nchs/about/otheract/ice/matrix10.htm. Accessed on 2006.
18. Burt CW, Fingerhut LA: *Injury Visits to Hospital Emergency Departments: United States, 1992–95.* Hyattsville, MD: National Center for Health Statistics, 1998.

19. Census of fatal occupational injuries (CFOI) - Current and revised data. http://www.bls.gov/iif/oshcfoi1.htm#2004. Accessed September 15, 2006.

20. U.S. Department of Labor, Bureau of Labor Statistics: *Workplace Injuries and Illnesses in 2000*. Washington, D.C.: USDL 1, 2001.

21. Leigh JP, Markowitz SB, Fahs M, et al.: Occupational injury and illness in the United States. *Arch Intern Med* 157:1557, 1997.

22. The Barell injury diagnosis matrix, classification by body region and nature of injury. http://www.cdc.gov/nchs/data/ice/final_matrix_post_ice.pdf. Accessed September 13, 2007.

23. Isreal RA, Rosenberg HA, Curtin LR: Analytic potential for multiple cause of death data. *Am J Epidemiol* 124:161, 1986.

24. Sosin DM, Sacks JJ, Smith SM: Head injury-associated deaths in the United States from 1979–1986. *JAMA* 362:2251, 1989.

25. Baker CC, Oppenheimer L, Stephens B, et al.: Epidemiology of trauma deaths. *Am J Surg* 140:144, 1980.

26. Shackford SR, Mackersie RC, Holbrook TL, et al.: The epidemiology of traumatic death: A population-based analysis. *Arch Surg* 128:571, 1993.

27. Committee on Injury Scaling: *The Abbreviated Injury Scale*. Des Plaines, IL: Association for the Advancement of Automotive Medicine, 1990.

28. Nathens AB, Jurkovich GJ, MacKenzie EJ, et al.: Resource-based assessment of trauma care in the United States. *J Trauma* 56:173, 2004.

29. Jurkovich GJ, Mock C, MacKenzie EJ, et al.: The sickness impact profile as a tool to evaluate functional outcome in trauma patients. *J Trauma* 39:625, 1995.

30. MacKenzie EJ, Morris JA, Jurkovich GJ, et al.: Return to work following injury: The role of economic, social and job-related factors. *Am J Pub Health* 88:1630, 1998.

31. MacKenzie EJ, Bosse MJ, Pollak AN et al.: Disability persists long-term following severe lower limb trauma: results of a seven year follow-up. *J Bone Joint Surg* 87:1801, 2005.

32. Wesson DE, Williams JI, Sapence LJ, et al.: Functional outcomes in pediatric trauma. *J Trauma* 29:589, 1989.

33. Holbrook T, Anderson J, Sieber W, et al.: Outcome after major trauma: 12-month and 18-month follow-up results from the Trauma Recovery Project. *J Trauma* 46:765, 1999.

34. Dillingham TR, Pezzin LE, Mackenzie EJ: Incidence, acute care length of stay and discharge to rehabilitation of traumatic amputee patients: An epidemiologic study. *Arch Phys Med Rehabil* 79:279, 1998.

35. Thurman DJ, Guerrero J: Trends in hospitalization associated with traumatic brain injury. *JAMA* 282:954, 1999.

36. Guerrero J, Thurman DJ, Sniezek JE: Emergency department visits associated with traumatic brain injury: United States, 1995–1996. *Brain Injury* 14:181, 2000.

37. Kraus JF: Epidemiologic features of injuries to the central nervous system. In Anderson DW, ed. *Neuroepidemiology: A Tribute to Bruce Schoenberg*. Boca Raton, FL: CRC Press, 1991, p. 333.

38. Langlois JA, Kegler SR, Butler JA, et al.: Traumatic brain injury-related hospital discharges results from a 14-state surveillance system, 1997. *MMWR Morb Mortal Wkly Rep* 52:1, 2003.

39. U.S. Department of Health and Human Services: *Interagency Head Injury Task Force Report*. Washington, D.C.: U.S. Department of Health and Human Services, 1989.

40. Frankowski RF, Annegers JF, Whitman S: The descriptive epidemiology of head trauma in the United States. In Becker DP, Povlishock JT, eds. *Central System Trauma Status Report: 1985*. Bethesda, MD: National Institute of Neurological and Communicative Disorders and Stroke, National Institutes of Health, 1985.

41. Sosin DM, Sniezek JE, Thurman DJ: Incidence of mild and moderate brain injury in the United States, 1991. *Brain Injury* 10:47, 1996.

42. Kelly J: Sports-related recurrent brain injuries—United States. *MMWR Morb Mortal Wkly Rep* 46:224, 1997.

43. Guskiewicz KM, McCrea M, Marshall SW, et al.: Cumulative effects associated with recurrent concussion in collegiate football players: The NCAA Concussion Study. *JAMA* 290:2549, 2003.

44. Kraus JF: Epidemiological aspects of acute spinal cord injury: A review of incidence, prevalence, causes and outcome. In Becker DP, Povlishock JT, eds. *Central System Trauma Status Report: 1985*. Bethesda, MD: National Institute of Neurological and Communicative Disorders and Stroke, National Institutes of Health, 1985.

45. Berkowitz M, O'Leary P, Kruse D, et al.: *Spinal Cord Injury: An Analysis of Medical And Social Costs*. New York: Demos Medical Publishing Inc., 1998.

46. Klein BP, Jensen RC, Sanderson LM: Assessment of workers compensation claims for back strains and sprains. *J Occup Med* 26:443, 1984.

47. U.S. Department of Health and Human Services, National Institute for Occupational Safety and Health (NIOSH): *Worker Health Chart book*, 2004. Washington, D.C.: DHHS(NIOSH) Pub No. 2004-146.

48. Injury maps. http://www.cdc.gov/ncipc/maps/default.htm. Accessed September 13, 2007.

49. Centers for Disease Control and Prevention: Ten great public health achievements—United States, 1900–1999. *MMWR Morb Mortal Wkly Rep* 48:241, 1999.

50. Centers for Disease Control and Prevention: Achievements in public health, 1900–1999. Motor vehicle safety: A 20th-century public health achievement. *MMWR Morb Mortal Wkly Rep* 48:369, 1999.

51. Centers for Disease Control and Prevention: Achievements in public health, 1900–1999: Improvements in workplace safety—United States, 1900–1999. *MMWR Morb Mortal Wkly Rep* 48:461, 1999.

52. National Highway Traffic Safety Administration: *Traffic Safety Facts, 2000*. Washington, D.C.: Department of Transportation, DOT. http://www-nrd.nhtsa.dot.gov/Pubs/TSF2000.PDF. Accessed September 13, 2007.

53. Traffic safety facts: Strengthening safety belt use. http://www.nhtsa.dot.gov/staticfiles/DOT/NHTSA/Rulemaking/Articles/Associated%20Files/13%20Strength%20Safety%20Belt%20Use.pdf. Accessed September 13, 2007.

54. National Highway Traffic Safety Administration: The third report to Congress on the effectiveness of occupant protection systems and their use. December 1996. http://www.nhtsa.dot.gov/cars/rules/rulings/208con2e.html. Accessed September 13, 2007.

55. Traffic safety facts: Occupant protection http://www-nrd.nhtsa.dot.gov/pdf/nrd-30/ncsa/TSF2004/809909.pdf. Accessed September 13, 2007.

56. Traffic safety facts: Driver alcohol involvement in fatal crashes by age group and vehicle type. http://www-nrd.nhtsa.dot.gov/pubs/810598.PDF. Accessed September 13, 2007.

57. Blincoe LJ, Seay A, Zaloshnja E, et al.: *The Economic Impact of Motor Vehicle Crashes, 2000*, Washington D.C.: National Highway Traffic Safety Administration, 2002. DOT HS 809 446.

58. Krug EG, Powell KE, Dahlberg LL: Firearm-related deaths in the United States and 35 other high- and upper-middle-income countries. *Intl J Epidemiol* 27:214, 1998.

59. Annest JL, Mercy JA, Gibson DR, et al.: National estimates of nonfatal firearm-related injuries: Beyond the tip of the iceberg. *JAMA* 283:1749, 1995.

60. Kizer KW, Vasser MJ, Harry RL, et al.: Hospitalization charges, costs and income for firearm-related injuries at a university trauma center. *JAMA* 273:1768, 1995.

61. Wintemute GJ, Wright MA: Initial and subsequent hospital costs of firearm injuries. *J Trauma* 33:556, 1992.

62. Cook PJ, Ludwig J: *Gun Violence: The Real Costs*. New York: Oxford University Press, 2000, p. 113.

63. Federal Bureau of Investigation: *Uniform Crime Reports for the United States: 2002*. Washington, D.C.: U.S. Department of Justice, 2003.

64. Johns Hopkins Center for Gun Policy and Research: *1998 National Gun Policy Survey: Questionnaire With Weighted Frequencies*. Baltimore, MD: The Johns Hopkins Center for Gun Policy and Research, 1999.

65. Grunbaum JA, Kann L, Kinchen ST, et al.: Youth Risk Behavior Surveillance, United States, 2001. *MMWR Morb Mortal Wkly Rep* 51:1, 2002.

66. Kellermann AL, Rivara FP, Rushforth NB, et al.: Gun ownership as a risk factor for homicide in the home. *N Engl J Med* 329:1084, 1993.

67. Kellermann AL, Rivara FP, Somes G, et al.: Suicide in the home in relation to gun ownership. *N Engl J Med* 327:467, 1992.

68. Saltzman LE, Mercy JA, O'Carroll PW, et al.: Weapon involvement and injury outcomes in family and intimate assaults. *JAMA* 267:3043, 1992.

69. Cook PJ, Ludwig J, Hemenway D: The gun debate's new mythical number: How many defensive uses per year? *J Policy Anal Management* 16:463, 1997.

70. Blendon RJ, Young JT, Hemenway D: The American public and the gun control debate. *JAMA* 275:1719, 1996.

71. Teret SP, Webster DW, Vernick JS, et al.: Support for new policies to regulate firearms: Results of two national surveys *NEJM* 339:813, 1998.

72. Scheidt P, Harel Y, Trumble AC, et al.: The epidemiology of nonfatal injuries among U.S. children and youth. *Am J Public Health* 85:932, 1995.

73. Committee on Injury and Poison Prevention, American Academy of Pediatrics: *Injury Prevention and Control for Children and Youth*, 3d ed. Elk Grove Village, IL: American Academy of Pediatrics, 1997.

74. Rivara FP, Alexander B, Johnston B, et al.: Population-based study of fall injuries in children and adolescents resulting in hospitalization or death. *Pediatrics* 92:61, 1993.

75. Chadwick D, Chin S, Salerno C, et al.: Deaths from falls in children: How far is fatal? *J Trauma* 31:1350, 1991.

76. Tinetti ME, Speechley M, Ginter SF: Risk factors for falls among elderly persons living in the community. *N Engl J Med* 319:1701, 1988.

77. Hausdorff JM, Rios DA, Edelber HK. Gait variability and fall risk in community-living older adults: a 1-year prospective study. *Arch Phys Med Rehabil* 82:1050, 2001.

78. Sterling DA, O'Connor JA, Bonadies J: Geriatric falls: injury severity is high and disproportionate to mechanism. *J Trauma* 50:116, 2001.

79. Wilkins K: Health care consequences of falls for seniors. *Health Reports* 10:47, 1999.

80. Melton LJ III, Riggs BL: Epidemiology of age-related fractures. In Avioli LV, ed. *The Osteoporotic Syndrome.* New York: Grune and Stratton, 1983.

81. Norris RJ: Medical costs of osteoporosis. *Bone* 13:S11, 1992.

82. Tinetti ME, Baker DI, McAvay G: A multifactorial intervention to reduce risk of falling among elderly people living in the community. *N Engl J Med* 331:821, 1994.

83. Tinetti ME, Speechley M: Prevention of falls among the elderly. *N Engl J Med* 320:1055, 1989.

84. Ray WA, Griffin MR, Schaffner W, et al.: Psychotropic drug use and the risk of hip fracture. *N Engl J Med* 316:363, 1987.

85. Sorock GS: Falls among the elderly: Epidemiology and prevention. *Am J Prev Med* 4:282, 1988.

86. Tinetti ME, Inouye SK, Gill TM, et al.: Shared risk factors for falls, incontinence, and functional dependence. *JAMA* 273:1348, 1995.

87. Gill TM, Williams CS, Robison JT, et al.: A population-based study of environmental hazards in the homes of older persons. *Am J Pub Health* 89:553, 1999.

88. Stevens JA, Olson S. Reducing falls and resulting hip fractures among older women. In CDC Recommendations Regarding Selected Conditions Affecting Women's Health. *MMWR Morb Mortal Wkly Rep* 49:3, 2000.

89. Annest JL, Conn JM, James SP: *Inventory of Federal Data Systems in the United States for Injury Surveillance, Research and Prevention Activities.* Atlanta: Centers for Disease Control and prevention, National Center for Injury Prevention and Control, May 1996.

90. Injury databases & published Statistics. http://www.injurycontrol.com /icrin/stats.htm. Accessed September 13, 2007.

91. WISQARS nonfatal injuries: Nonfatal injury Reports. http:// webappa.cdc.gov/sasweb/ncipc/nfirates.html. Accessed September 13, 2007.

92. Teret SP, Winemute GJ, Beilenson PL: The firearm fatality reporting system: A proposal. *JAMA* 267:3073, 1992.

93. Barber C, Hemenway D, Hargarten S, et al.: A "call to arms" for a national surveillance system on firearm injuries (editorial). *Am J Pub Health* 90:1191, 2000.

94. Azrael D, Barber C, Mercy J: Linking data to save lives: Recent progress in establishing a National Violent Death Reporting System. *Harvard Health Policy Rev* 2:38, 2001.

95. National Violent Death Reporting System. http://www.cdc.gov/ncipc/profiles/nvdrs/. Accessed September 13, 2007.

96. Dijkhuis H, Zwerling C, Parrish G, et al.: Medical examiner data in injury surveillance: A comparison with death certificates. *Am J Epidemiol* 139:637, 1994.

97. Combs DL, Parrish RG, Ing R: *Death Investigation in the United States and Canada.* Atlanta: Centers for Disease Control and Prevention, 1992.

98. How states are collecting and using cause of injury data: 2004 update to the 1997 report. http://www.cste.org/pdffiles/newpdffiles/ECodeFinal3705.pdf. Accessed September 13, 2007.

99. Smith GS, Langlois JA, Buechner JS: Methodological issues in using hospital discharge data to determine the incidence of hospitalized injuries. *Am J Epidemiol* 134:1146, 1991.

100. Sacco WJ, MacKenzie EJ, Champion HR. A comparison of alternative methods for assessing injury severity based on anatomic descriptors. *J Trauma* 47:441, 1999.

101. Meredith JW, Evans G, Kilgo PD, et al.: A comparison of the abilities of nine scoring algorithms in predicting mortality. *J Trauma* 53:621, 2002.

102. Rutledge R: The goals, development and use of trauma registries and trauma data sources in decision making in injury. *Surg Clin North Am* 75:305, 1995.

103. National Trauma Data Bank® (NTDB) http://www.facs.org/trauma/ntdb.html. Accessed September 13, 2007.

104. Garrison HG, Runyan CW, Tintinalli JE, et al.: Emergency department surveillance: An examination of issues and a proposal for a national strategy. *Ann Emerg Med* 42:81, 1994.

105. National Center for Injury Prevention and Control: *Data Elements for Emergency Department Systems.* Release 1.0. Atlanta, Centers for Disease Control and Prevention, 1997.

106. Johnson SW: So you want to link your data? DOT HS 808 426. Washington, D.C.: Department of Transportation, National Highway Traffic Safety Administration, 1996.

107. Crash Outcome Data Evaluation System (CODES). http://www-nrd.nhtsa. dot.gov/departments/nrd-30/ncsa/CODES.html. Accessed September 13, 2007.

108. Murray CJL, Lopez AD, eds: *The Global Burden of Disease.* Geneva, Switzerland: World Health Organization, 1996.

109. Peden M, McGee K, Sharma G: The injury chart book: A graphical overview of the global burden of injuries. Geneva, Switzerland: World Health Organization, 2002.

110. Peden M, Scurfield R, Sleet D, et al.: World report on road traffic injury prevention, Geneva, Switzerland: World Health Organization, 2004. http:// www.who.int/world-health-day/2004/infomaterials/world_report/en/. Accessed September 13, 2007.

# Commentary ■ KAREN J. BRASEL

Epidemiology is defined as the study of the patterns of disease occurrence in human populations and the factors that influence these patterns. Paraphrasing MacKenzie and Fowler, the purpose of injury epidemiology might be best stated as the foundation on which effective interventions to reduce injuries and their adverse consequences are based.

Haddon's Matrix is presented as the basic framework used for injury prevention, using the epidemiologic triad of the host, agent, and environment, and the time sequence of pre-event, event, and post-event occurrences. This matrix has been beneficial when applied to motor vehicle crashes, with injury prevention efforts focusing on the host (driver education, reducing driving under the influence), the agent (seatbelts, airbags, crumple zones), and the environment (merging lanes, guardrails, speed limits) at various points along the time sequence of injury. The myriad of successful prevention efforts that have reduced the burden of injury from motor vehicle crashes should suggest that very few motor vehicle crashes are truly accidents, but are predictable and preventable occurrences.

We have been less successful in applying Haddon's Matrix to other injuries, including firearm injuries. Prevention efforts targeting the host (firearm safety education, licensing requirements), agent (gun locks, fingerprint identification), and environment (laws restricting gun ownership and(or use) are possible, but have not been implemented to the same degree as have prevention efforts for unintentional injuries. As a result, the mortality rate for firearm injuries has changed little since 1993. It is likely that economic, political, social, and behavioral factors, mentioned very briefly, are responsible for some of the difference in the progress made in reducing the burden of injury from intentional injuries. A new data source, the National Violent Death Reporting System, should improve the epidemiologic data available on fatalities due to intentional injury, hopefully improving our ability to inform policy and prevention efforts.

One of the most important populations highlighted in the chapter is the elderly. Our population is aging, and geriatric trauma is increasing. The epidemiology of geriatric trauma is significantly different, and outcomes are worse. Worth repeating are the facts that those ( 65 years of age account for 25% of injury deaths and 30% of injury-related hospitalizations, despite accounting for only 12% of the overall population. We will all be caring for these patients, and need to learn how to best use the different epidemiology of the disease in the elderly to improve injury prevention efforts as well as clinical care.

Although it is true that "no mass disorder afflicting mankind was ever brought under control or eliminated by attempts at treating the individual," it is important to consider this chapter as a starting point for those practitioners who do focus on evaluating and treating individual patients with individual injuries. How do we know whether and which patients should be evaluated for thoracic aortic injury after a motor vehicle crash or fall, blunt cerebrovascular injury, thoracic spine injury in the presence of a cervical spine injury, intraabdominal injury with omental evisceration after a stab wound, intraabdominal injury in the presence of a seatbelt mark? Individual decision-making about evaluating for occult injuries is guided by the study of patterns of injury occurrence across populations, one of the principles of epidemiology. These patterns are then applied to the individual patient in the trauma bay. Although the chapter does not present the epidemiology of specific injuries, description by age, gender, mechanism, intent, nature and severity of injury, and place is a starting point for the answers to these questions. Given the vast number of physicians who treat injured patients on an occasional basis while also maintaining busy general practices, it is likely this principle that will be most helpful to them and their patients.

The chapter ends with a discussion about the data sources available for describing the epidemiology of trauma. In order to effectively combat the number one killer of young Americans, it is imperative that accurate data are collected that adequately describe this disease. We can't rest on the reduction of motor vehicle fatalities or the decline in workplace-related deaths highlighted in the section describing trends in rates of injury over time. It should be clear from the discussion about linkages between somewhat incomplete datasets that our data are currently imperfect, and that which we do have is not in a form usable by the majority of clinicians. Information most familiar to most trauma surgeons comes from the National Trauma Data Bank (NTDB), contributed to by the majority of Level I and Level II trauma centers. However, this information is not population-based and therefore does not describe the full impact of the disease. Although the American College of Surgeons Committee on Trauma has taken a step forward by requiring all verified trauma centers to contribute data to the NTDB, this will still be an incomplete picture of Injury in America. In order to have the complete picture, we must have data on those that die at the scene, those that die awaiting transfer, and those treated at nontrauma center hospitals. Accurate data will improve not only injury prevention efforts, but also our clinical care.

# Injury Prevention

*Ronald V. Maier* ■ *Charles Mock*

## INTRODUCTION

Trauma has been termed the "neglected disease of modern society." It is also now the costliest medical problem, with trauma costs nearly doubling since the mid-1990s.[1] Until recently, injuries were considered to be due to "accidents," or randomly occurring, unpredictable events. Injuries were thus regarded in a fundamentally different manner from other diseases, which are viewed as having defined and preventable causes. This viewpoint, on the part of the public, professionals, and policy makers, induced a nihilistic attitude and severely limited the development of injury prevention efforts.

Trauma, as with any other disease, should be approached from a scientific vantage point, with delineation of causative factors and with development of preventive strategies targeting such factors. This scientific approach has been successful in decreasing the toll of mortality and morbidity from most diseases. However, this same organized scientific approach has only recently been applied to the prevention of injury.[2–6]

The importance of injury prevention efforts is pointed out by trauma mortality patterns. One-third to one-half of trauma deaths still occur in the field,[7–9] before any possibility of treatment even by the most advanced trauma treatment system. Such deaths can only be decreased by prevention efforts. In terms of severely injured persons who survive long enough to be treated by prehospital personnel, very few "preventable deaths" occur in a modern trauma system with a well-run emergency medical system and designated trauma centers. Even among those who survive to reach the hospital, a significant portion of in-hospital deaths are directly related to head injuries and occur despite optimal use of currently available therapy.[10,11] Hence, injury prevention is critical to further significantly reduce the toll of death caused by trauma. Moreover, prevention efforts can also decrease the severity of injuries and thus the likelihood of disability that arises after trauma.

In the following chapter, the historical development of the scientific approach to prevention is discussed and practical considerations for implementation of prevention efforts and for assessment of their effectiveness are reviewed. The chapter will discuss how these basic principles have been successfully applied to the prevention of both unintentional and intentional injuries. Finally, the chapter will conclude with a discussion of surgeons' roles in injury prevention programs.

## SCIENTIFIC APPROACH TO PREVENTION OF INJURIES

### Historical Development of the Science of Injury Prevention

Early attempts at injury prevention were largely based on the premise that injured individuals had been careless or were "accident prone." Although this may be true in some circumstances, the resulting injury prevention strategies, limited to generic admonitions to be careful, were greatly limited in their scope and success.[6,12] The current foundation for the scientific approach to understanding the causation of injuries and to developing rational prevention programs was laid by several pioneers.

One of the earliest developments of the science of injury prevention was the work of Hugh DeHaven in the 1930s–40s. DeHaven demonstrated that during an injury producing event such as a crash or a fall, the body could withstand varying amounts of kinetic energy depending on how that energy was dissipated. He pointed out the possibility of disconnecting the linkage of "accident" and the resultant "injury."[13,14] He provided a biomechanical foundation for subsequent injury prevention work and introduced the concept of injury thresholds. His groundwork is credited with eventually leading to the introduction of automotive seatbelts.[6,12–15]

In the 1940s, John E. Gordon introduced the use of epidemiology to the evaluation of injury. He pointed out how, similar to any other disease, injuries occurred with recognizable patterns across time and populations. He also pointed out how, as with other diseases, injuries were the result of the interaction of the host, the agent of injury production, and the environment within which they interacted.[16]

The most notable of the early pioneers of injury prevention was William Haddon, the first director of the National Highway Traffic Safety Administration. Haddon advanced these early works and developed a systematic approach to the evaluation and prevention of injuries. He based his approach upon the recognition that virtually all injuries resulted from rapid and uncontrolled transfer of energy to the human body. Furthermore, such energy transfers were understandable and predictable and hence preventable. Haddon expanded Gordon's ideas on the interaction of the three factors of host, agent, and environment into what ultimately became known as Haddon's Matrix (Table 3-1). In this model, each of the three factors influences the likelihood of injury during each of the three phases: pre-event, event, and post-event. In the pre-event phase, each of the three factors influences the likelihood of an injury producing event, such as a crash, to occur. During the event phase, they influence the probability that such an event will result in an injury and determine the severity of that injury. During the post-event phase, these same components determine what ultimate consequences the injury will have. Table 3-1 gives examples of such interactions.[17]

Haddon provided a firm basis for the modern approach to injury control. The principles summarized in his Matrix have also served as guidelines for the development of prevention efforts. He went on to develop 10 strategies to dissociate potentially injury producing "energy" from the host. Most current strategies for prevention and control of injuries are conceptually derived from these 10 strategies. They are listed below with examples.

A. Pre-Event Phase

1. Prevent the creation of the hazard; prevent the development of the energy which would lead to a harmful transfer. For example, prevent manufacture of certain poisons, fireworks, or handguns.

2. Reduce the amount of the hazard. For example, reduce speeds of vehicles.

3. Prevent the release of the hazard that already exists. For example, placing a trigger lock on a handgun.

B. Event Phase

4. Modify the rate or spatial distribution of the release of the hazard from its source. For example, seatbelts, airbags.

5. Separate in time or space the hazard being released from the people to be protected. For example, separation of vehicular traffic and pedestrian walkways.

6. Separate the hazard from the people to be protected by a mechanical barrier. For example, protective helmets.

7. Modify the basic structure or quality of the hazard to reduce the energy load per unit area. For example, breakaway roadside poles, rounding sharp edges of a household table.

8. Make what is to be protected (both living and nonliving) more resistant to damage from the hazard. For example, fire and earthquake resistant buildings, prevention of osteoporosis.

C. Post-Event Phase

9. Detect and counter the damage already done by the environmental hazard. For example, emergency medical care.

10. Stabilize, repair, and rehabilitate the damaged object. For example, acute care, reconstructive surgery, physical therapy.[6,12,15,17]

## Practical Considerations in Injury Prevention Work

Almost all prevention efforts can be conceptually derived from Haddon's 10 strategies. However, implementing such strategies in the real world involves a variety of practical considerations. In general, interventions can be thought of as either being active or passive on the part of the person being protected. *Active* interventions involve a behavior change and require people to perform an act such as putting on a helmet, fastening a seatbelt, or using a trigger lock for a handgun. *Passive* interventions require no action on the part of those being protected and are built into the design of the agent or the environment, such as airbags or separation of vehicle routes and pedestrian walkways. In general, passive interventions are considered more reliable than active ones.[17,18] However, even passive interventions require an action on the part of some segment of society, such as passage of legislation to require certain safety features in automobiles.

**TABLE 3-1**

| **Examples of the Interactions of Phases and Factors within Haddon's Matrix of Injury Etiology** | | | |
|---|---|---|---|
| **PHASE** | **FACTOR** | | |
| | **Human/Host** | **Vector/Vehicle** | **Environment: Social and Physical** |
| PRE-EVENT | Driver intoxication<br>Experience | Condition of brakes, tires<br>Accessibility of moving parts in machinery in factories<br>Window bars at high elevations | Speed limits<br>Traffic regulations<br>Societal attitudes and laws on intoxicated driving<br>Highway design (road curvature, intersections, road conditions) |
| EVENT | Use of safety belts | Airbags<br>Collapsible steering column<br>Side impact protection | Highway design (guard rails, breakaway poles)<br>Societal attitudes and laws regarding seatbelt use |
| POST-EVENT | Age<br>Physical conditioning | Integrity of fuel system/fire proof gasoline tanks | Trauma care systems |

The accomplishment of injury prevention strategies in society can be undertaken through three primary modalities: (i) *legislation and enforcement*, (ii) *education and behavior change*, and (iii) *engineering and technology*. These are often referred to as the three "E's."

Enforcement and legislation can work at different governmental levels. For example, national or federal level legislation regulates safety features built into the design of motor vehicles. States define what constitutes drunk driving and establish the strictness with which such laws are enforced. Local governments establish safety-related building codes.

Education and behavior change were once the mainstay of injury prevention work. However, if used uncritically and without evaluation, they usually have limited effect.[19] Educational efforts need to be delivered in a well thought out manner, utilizing the techniques of social marketing, to succeed in actually effecting behavior change. Moreover, educational work is often most effective when coupled with other methods of injury prevention, such as informing the public of the risk of being apprehended and prosecuted under new and more stringent anti-drunk driving laws. Also, to be most effective, a committed and ongoing program is required.

Engineering and technology address a variety of issues, such as development of safer roadways, more effective safety features for automobiles, and automatic protection for manufacturing equipment.

These three main modalities are frequently complementary. For example, seatbelts are a technological development. Convincing people to adopt the behavior of using them requires education and is reinforced through legislation. Convincing legislators to pass seatbelt laws requires lobbying and education.[6] In the later sections of this chapter, specific examples of use of these modalities are discussed.

Certain common principles run through many successful injury prevention programs. These include a multidisciplinary approach, community involvement, and should involve ongoing evaluation of both the process and outcome of the program. Depending on the targeted injury type, a program might involve contributions from health care professionals, public health practitioners, epidemiologists, psychologists, manufacturers, traffic safety and law enforcement officials, experts in biomechanics, educators, and individuals associated with the media, advertising, and public relations. Health care professionals might include those in primary care, such as pediatricians, and those involved in acute trauma care. Finally, individual members of the public might be involved.[18,20]

There is frequently the need to organize several groups with diverse interests into a coalition focusing on one particular injury prevention goal. Such groups might include governmental agencies, such as the health department, schools, and transportation department. They might also include academic institutions, the media, community groups, private foundations, corporations, and medical associations.[20–22] Coordination of these diverse groups and interests is an important component of the overall prevention program and is often best performed by having one organization act as a "lead agency."[6]

Programs are more likely to be successful when they have specific objectives and focus on a few or even just one key intervention. In general, interventions which can be integrated into existing programs will be more sustainable than will be short-term, temporary programs. When a prevention program achieves ongoing support and commitment from the agency, organization, or community in which it is based, it can be considered to be "institutionalized"[6]. Such sustainability is especially necessary for interventions based on education and behavior change.

Funding for injury prevention is frequently a limiting factor, as these programs are almost always non-profit endeavors. However, much can be accomplished by utilizing available community resources. These can include volunteer labor, publicity from the media in the form of free advertising space or special interest stories, and gifts in kind, such as donations of safety devices from manufacturers. The greater the level of involvement of the community, the greater the availability of such resources. Hence, a key component of many injury prevention programs is to elicit and sustain the interest of the community.

A critical element of injury prevention programs, which is frequently given inadequate attention, is evaluation of effectiveness. This requires two main activities: evaluation of both the process and the outcome. Process evaluation can be regarded, in part, as quality assurance of the program. For example, are the various items in a public information campaign progressing at the scheduled rate? The main purpose of such evaluation is to provide feedback for modification of the intervention.

Most importantly, outcome assessment evaluates possible changes or impact in the incidence of injury. Ideally, outcomes would monitor the most severe consequences of injury, namely, fatalities and injuries producing disability. This may not always be possible, given the limitations of size of the target population and the influence of other factors influencing injury rates. In these circumstances, measurement of "proxy outcomes" can be suitable, if carefully chosen. These are outcomes which are more frequent and hence more easily measurable, but which are less important and which represent less tangible benefit than the more important outcomes. However, they should reflect or initiate a change ultimately in the more serious outcomes. For example, a program to promote bicycle helmet use would reasonably start by measuring changes in the percent of bicycle riders wearing a helmet rather than changes in head injuries or deaths. Such a program would be more likely to demonstrate changes in the proxy measure, helmet use, in a shorter period or in a smaller population, whereas serious head injuries and deaths are more likely to change only over longer periods. Using such measurable outcomes are critical to "document" the success of a program and hence to increase or sustain community "buy-in" and support.

Injury outcomes can be thought of as a hierarchy, with the highest level being fatalities. These are the most desirable to prevent, but the hardest in which to reliably evaluate changes, due to their relatively infrequent occurrence. The lower levels of the outcome hierarchy are the easiest in which to assess change, especially in small-scale projects. However, the lower levels have the disadvantage of being less directly and less definitely associated with ultimate decreases in the more serious outcomes. The list below indicates this hierarchy from most desirable, but more difficult to assess, to less important, but more easily measured:

1. Injury fatalities.
2. Injury admissions.
3. Injury cases treated as outpatients.
4. All injury cases.[1–3]
5. Direct observation of behavior or the physical environment.
6. Measures of self-reported behavior.
7. Measures of knowledge, attitudes, beliefs, or intentions.[6]

Factors which influence choice of outcome to measure include: size of project, size of population to be studied, specific intervention planned, and funding available. Larger programs should focus on more important and tangible outcomes such as injury fatalities and injury admissions. However, these are not usually possible for smaller programs. Moreover, if smaller programs are implementing an intervention which has had proven success in other areas or in similar circumstances, then changes in behavior or attitudes regarding this intervention may suffice to prove success.

Whichever outcome is chosen, it is important to build outcome assessment into the design of the prevention program. In this way baseline measurements can be obtained, which will subsequently enable comparisons before and after an intervention and comparisons of groups with and without an intervention.

Such outcomes assessment is useful for identifying strategies that have been successful and hence are worth promulgating on a wider scale. Outcome assessment is also useful for identifying those strategies that are not working and hence should be changed or discontinued.

## Ethical Issues

In circumstances where educational efforts seek to increase voluntary compliance with safety measures, ethical issues in injury prevention are minimal. Ethical issues usually arise with laws mandating compliance with safety practices. These issues typically involve the balancing of an individual's personal rights with the overall good of society. In circumstances where an individual's actions adversely affect others, the ethical questions are usually straightforward. For example, an individual's "right" to drink and then drive is easily deprived in favor of protecting other members of society from the potential harm of such an action. Similarly, laws mandating use of restraint seats for children in automobiles may be viewed as an infringement on the rights of their parents to choose how they wish to treat their children. However, the vulnerable state of children and the precedent of protecting them from potentially harmful acts of their parents is well established and such laws, once passed, have easily stood.

The difficult issues in injury prevention arise with laws to protect against injuries in which the potential victims are only harming themselves. One of the best examples of this is mandatory motorcycle helmet laws. Such laws have been opposed by motorcycle groups, who feel that they are only risking their own safety by riding without a helmet. Proponents of helmet laws have generally pointed to the societal costs of treatment of severely head injured motorcyclists as the rationale as to why the issue affects society as a whole.[23] Courts have consistently backed the latter view, as best summed up in the case of Simon vs. Sargent in Massachusetts:

"From the moment of the injury, society picks the person up off the highway; delivers him to a municipal hospital and municipal doctors; provides him with unemployment compensation, if after recovery, he cannot replace his lost job and, if the injury causes permanent disability, may assume the responsibility for his and his family's continued subsistence. We do not understand the state of mind that permits the plaintiff to think that only he himself is concerned."[24]

Ethical issues related to injury prevention will continue to evolve. Most activities in life require some degree of risk taking. Societal norms and legal standards as to what represents acceptable risk taking are continually shifting. As these values change and as injury prevention strategies evolve which might call upon legislation for mandatory compliance, new ethical issues will continue to arise.

## Political Issues

Even when scientifically proven and cost-effective, the acceptance by society and government of safety measures to prevent important causes of injury are often blocked by a variety of political issues.[3,25] In some cases, there is resistance to behavior change on the part of a specific segment of society. For example, motorcycle helmet laws are frequently challenged by motorcycle groups. Besides ethical issues, the actual alternating legislative enactment and repeal of state motorcycle helmet laws have been due to political pressures from motorcycle groups on one hand and safety advocates on the other.[3]

In other cases however, safety measures have been specifically blocked by the active efforts of special interests that would stand to loose financially. For example, one of the major advances in automotive safety in recent decades has been the enactment of the Federal Motor Vehicle Safety Standards (FMVSS). These have been estimated to have saved 10,000–20,000 lives per year since their initial enactment in the 1960s.[3,26–28] Despite their effectiveness, efforts to promote such safety advances are often hindered by lobbying from the automobile industry or opposition from anti-regulatory minded members of the government.[3,29]

Another example of political opposition involves efforts to legislate mandatory setting of hot water heater temperatures at 120–125°F. As will be described later, this is a tremendously effective strategy to prevent scald burns in young children. Initial work on such regulation was carried out at the state level. Despite the obvious low-cost and significant benefits of such laws, they were frequently opposed. As one particular example, the legislative fight to pass a 120°F water heater temperature bill in Wisconsin has been well documented.[25] This bill was opposed by legislators who considered it to be anti-business. Although a state level bill, it was lobbied against by national interests, such as the Gas Appliance Manufacturers Association, as representing too much government interference in their business. Such opposition was eventually overcome by lobbying from several groups, including the State Medical Association and the state chapter of the American Academy of Pediatrics, and by a public letter writing campaign.

Unfortunately, many other examples are also common. Among these is the opposition to efforts to promote responsible alcohol advertising on the part of alcohol manufacturers and retailers.[25] One of the more extreme examples is the vehement opposition to efforts to any limit on availability of firearms by the National Rifle Association and its allies in the gun manufacturing industry. Such groups have opposed even efforts such as closing the gun-show loophole, which has allowed convicted criminals to continue to purchase guns.

In addition to specific injury prevention issues, addressing deeper issues in our society is pertinent in protecting the health of the public from injury related death and disability. Virtually every form of injury is more common in the lower socio-economic strata of society. The inequities that produce this situation need to be confronted as well. This has been well stated by Christoffel and Gallagher in their recent book, *Injury Prevention and Public Health:* "Truly effective injury prevention interventions challenge the structural underpinnings of the status quo. Effective injury prevention means things like worker participation in production decisions, community involvement in land use policy, equitable distribution of risk...These are dangerous ideas; they challenge unbridled free-market competition. Yet they are necessary for long-term, meaningful advances in injury prevention."[3]

These deep-seated political challenges indicate the need for those who wish to promote injury prevention to develop skills in advocacy and lobbying. This includes becoming proficient at efforts such as testifying before legislatures, pushing behind the scenes as individuals or through organizations such as professional societies, publicly countering unproven or non-evidence based arguments used by safety opponents (such as motor cycle helmets increase the risk of crashes), and by working to mobilize public support for safety related measures. Simultaneously, this challenge places the burden on the injury prevention community to develop scientific, evidence-based proposals that can withstand the appropriate public scrutiny before imposing legislative constraints on selected components of society.

## STRATEGIES TO PREVENT UNINTENTIONAL INJURIES

The remaining portions of this chapter will demonstrate how Haddon's principles of injury causation and his strategies for prevention, as well as three main modalities for implementation (legislation, education, and technology), can be utilized in programs directed at specific types of both unintentional and intentional injury.

### Motor Vehicle and Transportation

Several well-established groups have been working in motor vehicle-related safety, including the National Highway Traffic Safety Administration (NHTSA), the Centers for Disease Control (CDC), state and local highway departments, as well as various injury prevention coalitions. Progress in road safety has been made along multiple avenues, as indicated by the examples given in Table 3-1. Some of those potentially warranting special discussion are detailed below.

### Safety Related Vehicle Design and Occupant Protection

Much has been accomplished to make motor vehicles safer. This includes engineering features that make it less likely for a vehicle to crash. This is referred to as crash avoidance and takes into account such features as brakes, headlights, triple brakelights, and signals. Automotive safety also includes engineering features that make occupant injury less likely in the event of a crash.[30] This is referred to as crashworthiness and takes into account such features as collapsible steering columns, shatter proof glass, and improved side impact protection. These improvements have resulted from both improved car design on the part of the automobile manufacturers and from regulations from NHTSA, in the form of Federal Motor Vehicle Safety Standards.

One of the greatest advances in automotive safety was the realization that a significant component of the injuries sustained in crashes were due to ejections and to secondary collision of the occupant with the vehicle interior after the vehicle had collided with another object. This understanding led to the development of seatbelts to allow occupants to "ride down" the crash, dissipating their kinetic energy more slowly and in a controlled fashion.

However, this accomplishment of engineering is an active intervention, requiring the occupant to decide to put on the belt each time they begin a new journey. Hence, convincing people to use seatbelts remains a major injury prevention challenge. Even though the addition of airbags has enhanced safety and is a completely passive intervention, concomitant use of seatbelts is required to optimize their benefit and avoid airbag-related injuries. Efforts to increase belt usage include both education and legislation. Legislation includes mandatory seatbelt laws. Although some form of such a law has been passed in most states, only 22 states have laws allowing primary enforcement. Belt usage in the United States remains incomplete, at 82% overall, including 86% in those states with primary enforcement and 78% in states with secondary enforcement of seatbelt laws.[31,32]

A particular subset of restraint use that warrants special attention is that of infant and child car seats and booster seats. These are necessitated by the fact that infants and children do not fit into adult size seatbelts and hence such seatbelts do not provide adequate protection for these age groups. The need for infant car seats was recognized many years ago. These are required by legislation in all states. These laws require infant/child harness seats which are appropriate for children aged 0–4 years. These have played a major part in decreasing occupant deaths for children aged 0–4 years from 682 deaths nationwide in 1994 to 513 deaths in 2001.[33,34]

The need for booster seats for children aged 4–9 years (under 4'9") has been more recently recognized. The need for these arises from the fact that adult seatbelts rarely fit children of this age group. The shoulder belt portion typically lies over the face, leading children to place it behind their backs. Likewise, the lap belt portion rides high, over the abdomen. These factors have been associated with intra-abdominal and spinal injuries, known as seatbelt syndrome.[35] Such factors have contributed to the minimal declines in occupant death rates for children of this age group.

Booster seats raise the child into a position where the shoulder belt fits more properly over the chest and shoulder and where the lap belt is properly positioned low, across the pelvis. Booster seats reduce severe injuries to child occupants.[36] The recognition of the importance of booster seats has led an increasing number of states (34 states as of 2006) to pass booster seat laws.[37]

### Helmets

Occupant protection is obviously difficult to engineer for motorcycles and bicycles due to the exposed position of the riders. However, head injuries are the primary cause of death and prolonged disability for crashes involving both types of vehicles.[4] Helmets have been shown to decrease the probability of a head injury during crashes, to decrease the severity of head injuries when they occur, and to decrease the probability of death in both bicycle and motorcycle crashes.[38-43] As with seatbelts, helmets are an active intervention and the challenge has been to get riders to wear them. Programs to accomplish this have involved both education and legislation. The two case studies at the end of this section of the chapter detail examples of each approach.

## Speed Limits

In the pre-crash, environmental segment of Haddon's Matrix, two factors which stand out are roadway design and traffic regulations, including speed limits. Safety aspects of roadway design have been greatly advanced by such features as greater use of limited access highways, which have eliminated the risk of head-on collisions and decreased intersection related conflicts. One of the most important safety related traffic regulations has been the speed limit. The nationwide 55 MPH speed limit contributed significantly to lowering the motor vehicle crash fatality rate. The move toward higher speed limits can be considered a societal sacrifice to directly appease personal freedom demands. As a consequence, the nation sustained a rise in motor vehicle related deaths in the early and mid 1990s.[31]

## Alcohol

Another of the major risk factors for motor vehicle crashes is alcohol impaired driving. Risk of a crash increases dramatically with increasing blood alcohol concentration (BAC). The risk of a crash increases five-fold at a BAC of 80 mg/dl; seven-fold at a BAC of 100 mg/dl; and 25-fold at 150 mg/dl.[6,44] On weekend nights, when a large percent of severe crashes occur, 3% of all drivers are legally intoxicated. Drunk driving is associated currently with 36% of all fatal crashes in the United States.[45]

In light of these dramatic facts, anti-drunk driving efforts have been a cornerstone of road safety efforts in the United States and most other developed nations. These have employed both educational and legislative approaches.[46] A great many anti-drunk driving educational campaigns have been undertaken by diverse groups such as NHTSA, state agencies, and citizen groups such as Mothers Against Drunk Driving. Many of these have targeted younger drivers, who are at especially high risk for drunk driving.[6]

In terms of legislation, all states have adopted per se laws, in which any driver with an alcohol level above a specified level is considered impaired, regardless of any witnessed driving infractions. This legal limit has now been decreased to 80 mg/dl in all states. Likewise, many states have moved toward zero tolerance laws for underage drivers.[31]

However, legislation must be linked to enforcement, because any law is only as good as its enforcement. Drunk-driving laws are enforced to extremely varying degrees in different jurisdictions. Random sobriety checkpoints and administrative license suspension are just two methods to increase enforcement effectiveness and should strongly be considered.[6]

Another avenue to pursue in the fight against drunk driving is identification of injured, alcohol impaired drivers following hospital admission. There is a documented high rate of recidivism among intoxicated trauma patients in general, and not only among drunk drivers. Hence, identification and appropriate treatment of injured persons with alcohol abuse problems is a means toward decreasing the level of alcohol related injury from all causes.[4,47,48] Blood alcohol screening on admission, accompanied by brief questioning, such as the Short Michigan Alcohol Screening Test (SMAST), Michigan Alcohol Screening Test (MAST), or CAGE, can detect patients at a high risk of alcohol related injury recidivism. The CAGE questionnaire consists of four basic questions: Have you every tried to Cut down on your drinking? Are you Annoyed when people complain about your drinking? Do you ever feel Guilty about your drinking? Do you ever drink Eye-Openers?[4,47,48]

Referring these patients for counseling or even engaging in very brief interventions by trained professionals in the hospital is a potentially effective way of getting these patients to decrease their alcohol intake. In a prospective, randomized, controlled trial of screening and brief intervention among admitted trauma patients, it was found that patients who had undergone this brief counseling demonstrated a long term (> one year) decrease in their alcohol intake. This group reduced their alcohol intake by more than 20 drinks per week compared to only 7 per week in patients not undergoing such brief counseling. In addition, there was a 43% reduction in new injuries in treated individual compared to controls.[49] Brief interventions generally entail one or more counseling sessions, adding up to less than one hour. These have been shown to be effective in the context of acute injury hospitalization for all except the most severely impaired patients. The reader is directed to the cited references for more details on brief intervention counseling methods.[47-49]

The effectiveness and importance of alcohol screening and brief intervention (SBI) has recently led the American College of Surgeons Committee on Trauma (ACSCOT) to add a requirement that SBI programs must be present to its list of requirements for trauma center verification for Level I and II trauma centers.

## Graduated Drivers Licensing Systems

A particularly high-risk group for crashes is new adolescent (16–17 year old) drivers. Rates of crashes and crash-related death are higher than for older drivers due to having less experience and skill coupled with more risk-taking behavior. Drivers aged 16–20 have an annual rate of involvement in fatal crashes of 62 / 100,000 licensed drivers, compared with 29 / 100,000 for the general public.[31]

One particularly effective method to decrease the crash rate in this age group has been graduated driver licensing (GDL). Details vary from state to state and between countries, however, several common features include: (1) new adolescent drivers first obtain a learner's permit which allows them to drive only while supervised by a licensed adult; (2) a provisional license is next obtained which allows new adolescent drivers to drive unsupervised only under restricted conditions, such as only during certain times of day (usually not late at night), and with restrictions on the numbers and ages of passengers (e.g., with only limited numbers of other adolescents). Progression from one stage to the next and to a full license can only occur after specified minimum time periods and is contingent upon the absence of traffic violations or at-fault crashes.[50]

GDL programs have been shown to be effective in decreasing rates of crashes and crash-related death among new adolescent drivers. For example, after institution of a GDL system for 16-year-old drivers in North Carolina, rates of fatal crashes involving 16-year-old drivers declined by 57%, from 5 to 2 per 10,000 population per year.[51]

As of 2006, a total of 47 states and several other countries have adopted GDL. However, only 21 such states have achieved a rating of "good" according to the scale developed by the Insurance Institute for Highway Safety, which takes into account the toughness of the restrictions and the length of the period after the 16th birthday for which these restrictions apply. Factors in this rating include the hour at which nighttime restrictions apply, the number of adolescent passengers that are allowed, and the age at which a full license may be obtained, among other criteria. The other states have been rated as fair, marginal, or poor, indicating that much work still needs to be done.[50]

## Residential Safety: Burns

Improved residential safety encompasses poisoning, suffocation, drowning, falls, and burns. In the United States, burns are the 4th leading cause of injury related mortality. There are three major causes of death and injury due to burns. House fires account for 75% of burn deaths, but only 4% of burn admissions, due to their high case fatality rate. Many of these deaths from fires are actually due to smoke inhalation.[5] Scalds from hot liquids and burns from clothing ignition each account for only about 3% of burn deaths, but these mechanisms account for a large percent of burn admissions (scalds –29%; clothing –10%).[10] Hence, burn prevention efforts have been oriented toward these three most common causes.

## House Fires

Most house fire deaths occur because of entrapment in burning buildings. In many cases, people do not know their building is on fire until it is too late to escape or to call the fire department. Many injuries and deaths could be prevented if people knew earlier that a fire had started and had time to escape. Therefore, a key component to injury prevention for house fires is the early warning system provided by smoke detectors.

Smoke detectors are an extremely effective injury prevention tool. They have been found to lower the potential for death in 86% of fires.[6] This is an example of the use of engineering in injury prevention. However, the tool is of no value if people do not use it. Use of smoke detectors has been promulgated by both education and legislation. Educational campaigns have been run on a regular basis by local fire departments and nonprofit groups, such as the Northwest Burn Foundation in Seattle. These activities educate people about the importance of having a smoke detector in their home and the need to change the batteries every 6–12 months. In addition, most states have laws that require placement of smoke detectors in all new buildings. These measures have been extremely effective. The percent of homes having smoke detectors rose from 5% in 1970 to 67% in 1982. Primarily based on increased use of smoke detectors, fire related deaths in the United States decreased by 20% between the 1970s and the 1980s.[6,10]

Other efforts to prevent deaths due to house fires have attempted to attack root causes.[52] Most house fires arise from: (1) faulty heating equipment, especially in lower income housing, and (2) ignition of mattresses or upholstered furniture from cigarettes. The first has been addressed primarily through legislation regarding housing codes. The second, cigarette-related fires, has been worked on by (a) educating people about the dangers of smoking in bed and by (b) laws which require mattresses to be made with less flammable materials.[6] Unfortunately, the most effective measure, manufacture of self-extinguishing cigarettes, has been effectively blocked, even though the technology exists. It is the impact of unbridled free enterprise.[25]

## Scalds

Young children, aged 0–4 years, account for half of scald injuries.[10] The leading cause is hot water, especially hot tap water used for bathing. A typical scenario is a child being bathed and the faucet being turned on too hot, either unintentionally by a child playing with the knobs or by an adult not realizing how hot the water is. Thus, a major prevention focus is lowering the temperature in hot water heaters. Hot water heaters can heat water as high as 160°F (71°C), which can produce a first degree burn in 1 second of exposure, and more severe burns with longer periods of exposure. However, temperatures of 125°F (52°C) require three or more minutes of exposure to produce burns. Hence, essentially all scald burns due to tap water can be prevented by keeping the temperature in hot water heaters to 125°F or less.[6,10]

Reduction in thermostat settings is the engineering aspect. To achieve this, injury prevention groups have been educating parents of the dangers of high temperatures for hot water heaters and the importance of lowering the thermostat on the heater. Liquid crystal thermometers have been made specifically for the purpose of checking the temperature at the faucet. As regards legislation, many states have introduced laws which require manufacturers to pre-set their hot water heaters at 120–125°F (49–52°C).[6] These scald prevention efforts have been very effective. Between the 1960s and the 1980s, scald-related deaths have decreased by over half for all age groups and by 75% for children.[10]

## Clothing Ignition

The second leading cause of burn-related admissions is ignition of clothing. This may happen from contact with stoves, electrical heating units (space heaters), cigarettes, matches, or other sources. The two major groups in whom these occur are young children, who do not realize the dangers, and the elderly, in whom reaction time is slowed.

One of the most notable examples of burn prevention efforts is in this field. Most of the clothing ignition burns to children occurred from sleepwear, which was formerly made of easily flammable fabrics. In the 1970s, the Children's Sleepwear Standard law required children's sleepwear to be made of less flammable materials and required that any new sleepwear products pass a flame test before being allowed in the market. These measures have resulted in a dramatic decrease in childhood clothing related burns to the point where burns related strictly to clothing ignition are very rare. However, a major problem remains in clothing ignition burns among the elderly, which currently account for over 75% of clothing ignition burns.[6,10]

## Two Contrasting Case Studies: Helmet Promotion

These two case studies address a similar issue, the use of protective helmets; in one case for bicycle riders and in the other for motorcycle riders. Both affect the crash phase and human factor of Haddon's Matrix (i.e., decreasing the likelihood of injury once an injury producing event has occurred). In addition, both involve the same concepts of Haddon's 10 principles of prevention, namely, separation of the hazard from the people to be protected by a mechanical barrier. This particular strategy has been shown to decrease the severity of head injuries in victims of both bicycle and motorcycle crashes.[38–43] From an implementation viewpoint, use of helmets for bicyclists and motorcyclists are both active interventions, requiring the rider to put on a helmet, voluntarily and repetitively, each time he/she performs the act of riding. The challenge in both circumstances has been to increase compliance with this behavior. However, due to selective social circumstances and pressures in the populations to be protected, very different modalities of implementation have been required.

## The Seattle Bicycle Helmet Campaign

The Seattle bicycle helmet campaign has been considered a model program in health promotion and injury prevention. It utilized a multidimensional approach, emphasizing a broad-based community coalition building and focusing on young elementary school-age children. The initial step consisted of a background survey of schoolchildren and their parents, undertaken to assess the current knowledge, attitudes, and practices regarding bicycle helmets. Over 1000 elementary school aged children and their parents were surveyed. Only 12% of children who had bicycles reported that they used helmets when they rode. Among the large majority of children who did not use helmets, three main barriers to helmet use were identified. (1) Parents were largely unaware of the danger of head injuries to bicycle riders and were also unaware of the effectiveness of helmets in preventing such injuries. (2) The price of helmets at the time was $40–60 and was considered too high. (3) Children were reluctant to wear helmets as most other children did not do so and hence wearing a helmet would result in them being viewed as "nerds."[53] These barriers subsequently became the main targets of the bicycle helmet campaign.

After this background survey, the Harborview Injury Prevention and Research Center (HIPRC) elicited the support and involvement of a number of organizations in forming a coalition to promote helmet use. This coalition relied on use of volunteer labor and gifts in kind. Members of this coalition included the Cascade Bicycle Club, local and state health departments, the Washington State Medical Association, the Parent Teachers Association (PTA), local television and radio stations, local sports figures, manufacturers of bicycle helmets, and Group Health Cooperative, the state's largest health maintenance organization. The HIPRC acted as the lead agency in the program and coordinated the activities of the other coalition members.[21,22,54]

The program focused on elementary school-aged children as these were felt to be most amenable to changes in behavior. Increasing parental awareness was primarily undertaken via the mass media. Air time was donated as a gift in kind from local radio and television stations for public service announcements about bicycle helmets. The media provided reports by the Level I Trauma Center at Harborview Medical Center to publicize, as human interest stories, head injuries to unhelmeted children bicyclists. Families of bicycle crash victims were asked if their child's case could be publicized on behalf of the helmet campaign. Compliance was usually high with these requests. The pediatricians and surgeons caring for these children played a key role in identifying their cases for publicity and also acted as spokespersons for helmets in the subsequent news stories. The trauma registry at Harborview Medical Center provided up to date statistics on bicycle trauma, which were popular with reporters and news broadcasters.

In addition to the direct mass media approach, articles on bicycle helmets appeared in the newsletters of the Washington State PTA and the Boy Scouts. Similar articles, directed at health care providers, also appeared in the newsletters of the Washington State Medical Association and the state chapter of the American Academy

of Pediatrics (AAP). Such items stressed the importance of injury prevention counseling in general and, in particular, about bicycle helmets, in primary care practices involving children. Through the state medical association, informational pamphlets were provided to physicians to distribute to their patients.

At the start of the campaign, helmets were primarily sold at specialty bicycle shops catering to adults and retailed for $40–60. Few stores that sold children's bicycles also sold helmets. A "partnership" was developed between the helmet coalition and Mountain Safety Research, a Seattle-based helmet manufacturer. This company mass produced and marketed helmets for children under a different label for $20–25. In exchange, retailers of bicycles who were involved with the coalition, agreed to attach "hang tags" on children's bicycles they sold to promote helmets. Large chain stores that sold children's bicycles were convinced to also provide helmets at reduced costs. The retail outlets likewise received public commendation and hence publicity from the state chapter of the AAP. In addition, helmets were made available through the PTA. Other cost lowering activities included distribution of discount coupons through physicians' offices, schools, and youth and community groups. Other helmet manufacturers eventually became involved in the campaign.

To promote helmet use among school-age children, bicycle safety programs were conducted in Seattle public elementary schools. These included posters, assemblies, and endorsements by local sports figures. Outside of school, bicycle rodeos and rallies were put on in city parks and other public sites, hosted by radio stations and the Cascade Bicycle Club. At these bicycling events, rewards were given to children wearing helmets, including coupons for free French fries and free tickets to Seattle Mariner baseball games.[21,22,54]

This campaign has been held annually since 1986 with most intensive activities from April through September each year.[21,22,54] The direct monetary costs of the program were primarily for printing and mailing. The only full-time personnel was a health educator for years two and three of the campaign. A public relations specialist was employed on a part-time basis for the most intensive periods of the campaign, during the riding season. Otherwise, the bulk of activities of the campaign were provided for by "in-kind" donations of services.[21]

A key element in the program was assessment, both of the process of the campaign and of its outcome. Process factors which were followed included: (i) number of discount coupons distributed and percent redeemed; and (ii) number of helmets sold. During the first two years of the campaign, 109,450 discount coupons were distributed, of which 4.7% were redeemed, a figure which is deemed very high by standards of product promotion. Discount coupons distributed at the bicycle rodeos and fairs were especially productive, with an 8.7% redemption rate. Seattle area bicycle helmet sales also rose dramatically during the early years of the campaign, from 1500 in 1986 to 20,000 in 1988.[21]

In terms of assessment of outcome, death or major neurologic disability related to bicycle crashes would be the most important to decrease. Given the proven efficacy of helmets at preventing severe head injuries and death in bicycle crashes,[42,43] it was felt that a change in helmet use behavior would be a reasonable surrogate measure of the program's effectiveness.[21,54] Observations on randomly chosen bicyclists were carried out throughout the Seattle area, utilizing a formal epidemiologic sampling strategy. To fully assess the effectiveness of the helmet campaign, such observations were carried out before the initiation of the public information campaign. Moreover, as a control for general societal trends in helmet use, similar observations were carried out simultaneously in Portland, Oregon, a city without a helmet promotion campaign at the time.[22,54] These observations were carried out on 8860 Seattle area bicycle riders from 1987 through 1993. During the first two years of the program, the percent of helmeted riders rose from 5% in 1987 to 16% in 1988, during which time the helmet use rates in Portland remained below 3%.[54] Helmet use rates in Seattle continued to rise to 62% in 1993.[55]

This helmet promotion campaign has continued for the past 15 years, becoming partially "institutionalized" in that pamphlets and other educational materials are available on a regular basis from the state medical association; helmets are now a routine item for sale at stores which sell children's bicycles; free helmets are available for all children on public assistance through the state welfare office; and many pediatricians and family practitioners routinely work injury prevention and bicycle helmet promotion into their counseling of families. In turn, over the years of the program, the program's success at decreasing the more serious sequelae of bicycle crashes has materialized. In a study of the population enrolled in the state's largest health maintenance organization, Group Health Cooperative, it was found that from 1987 to 1992, medically treated (admitted or emergency room) bicycle-related head injuries decreased by 72% among 5–9 year olds and by 78% among 10–14 year olds.[22] Likewise, at the state's only Level I trauma center, at Harborview Medical Center, among patients admitted for bicycle crashes, the proportion of patients with severe head injuries (Abbreviated Injury Scale (AIS) for head of 4 or 5) declined from 29% in 1986 to 11% in 1993. The mortality rate for admitted bicyclists also decreased from 7% in 1986–1990 to 3% in 1991–1993.[55]

## Washington State Motorcycle Helmet Law

In contrast to the bicycle helmet campaign, efforts to improve use of helmets by motorcyclists in Washington State have emphasized legislation. Mandatory motorcycle helmet laws have been the subject of nationwide debate. During the 1960s and 1970s many states enacted such legislation, primarily due to the threat of the withholding of federal highway funds. In 1976, Congress withdrew the U.S. Department of Transportation's authority to withhold highway funds based on individual states' helmet laws. Many states, including Washington, repealed their mandatory motorcycle helmet laws, primarily due to lobbying by motorcyclists groups. Increases in motorcycle related deaths and severe head injuries were noted nationwide.[6,23]

In Washington State, attempts were made to reinstitute a motorcycle helmet law during the 1980s. Such efforts were defeated twice in the legislature. A third and final lobbying effort by proponents of the helmet law utilized not only information on the terrible human consequences of preventable motorcycle related head trauma but also utilized data on the financial cost of these injuries. These data showed that not only does helmet use decrease the incidence of severe head injury by more than 50% but also that the average cost ($15,592) of an admission for motorcycle related trauma was increased dramatically by the presence of a severe head injury ($46,936), with even more costs accruing for subsequent rehabilitative and custodial care of those with these severe head injuries.[39] Of special interest to the state legislature was the fact that 63% of the costs of treatment for motorcycle related injuries

were borne by general public funds, primarily state Medicaid.[56] In part, because of these data showing the stake of taxpayers and the state budget in the motorcycle helmet debate, the Washington State Legislature passed a law the following year requiring helmets for all motorcycle drivers and passengers, effective June 7, 1990. Follow-up of the results of the reinstitution of the motorcycle helmet law has re-established the efficacy of this law. Among victims of motorcycle crashes admitted to the state's Level I trauma center, the proportion of those sustaining severe (AIS 4 or 5) head injuries declined from 20% before enactment of the helmet law to 9% afterward. The mortality rate declined from 10% to 6%.[55]

These case studies point out several important principles about injury prevention efforts. First, they show the need for multidisciplinary collaboration and point out the important role that surgeons and other clinicians caring for injured patients can play in both education and advocacy work. Second, they show the importance of considering the political and cultural environment in which the prevention effort is occurring. Parents were more than ready to listen to messages about the safety of their children, when those messages were properly delivered. Although many motorcyclists were utilizing helmets without a mandatory law, those who were not using helmets have been unlikely to appreciably respond to educational efforts, hence the need for legislation.[23] Advocacy for passage of this legislation was aided by publicizing information on the public costs of motorcycle trauma at a time when fiscal conservatism was a priority. Third, these efforts each focused on one key injury prevention strategy, rather than a wide array of activities, such as promotion of safe riding habits by riders of both types of vehicles. Although such efforts might be useful and should be promoted, intensive efforts, as in the helmet campaigns, are more likely to succeed when focused on a simple message.[21] Fourth, outcome assessment was a key component, especially of the bicycle campaign. Outcomes which were feasible to measure and which would reliably indicate the success of the campaign were chosen (e.g., change in behavior of wearing helmets). Assessment of this outcome was built into the design of the campaign, both in before-and-after comparisons and in comparisons with a control community. Lastly, both efforts were accomplished largely with a minimum of funding and in the case of the bicycle campaign with a generous input of volunteer labor.

## Nationwide Effectiveness of Prevention Efforts Aimed at Unintentional Injury

Other examples of successful prevention programs aimed at unintentional injuries abound, so do examples of the complementary use of the three primary injury prevention modalities. These have been applied particularly well to traffic related trauma. On a nationwide scale, this is especially well seen with promotion of restraints. The technological advancements, first of seatbelts and then the development of child safety seats and airbags have been complemented by promotion and education and by advocacy for legislation. Increased awareness of the importance of seatbelts has enabled passage of mandatory safety seats for children under four years old in all states and of mandatory seatbelt laws for all occupants in many states.[6,31,57]

The field of traffic related injury prevention has also been advanced by other means, including vehicle design, highway design, lower speed limits, increased minimum legal drinking age, and increased public awareness about and increased enforcement of laws against driving while intoxicated.[6,15,20] Similar advancements have been recorded in other types of unintentional injuries such as occupational injuries, residential injuries, and burn prevention.[10]

These advances in prevention, coupled with advances in trauma treatment, have reduced the death rate for unintentional injuries to some of the lowest rates recorded since statistics were first collected in the early part of the past century.[10] The accomplishments have been especially notable in the last two decades. During the 1980s and 1990s, the rate of death due to unintentional injury declined by 19%, from 42.8 deaths/100,000/year (1981) to 34.8/100,000/year (2000). Obviously, there is still much to do. In fact, there has been some erosion of gains in the past few years, with rates increasing from the nadir of 34.8 deaths/100,000/year in 2000 to 37.6/100,000/year in 2003.[58,59]

Priorities for future work in the prevention of unintentional injuries include: decreasing public acceptance of driving while intoxicated, especially among younger drivers; increasing use of seatbelts both through educational efforts and through advocacy for passage of mandatory seatbelt laws with provisions for primary enforcement in all states; further promotion of helmets for motorcyclists and bicyclists; and increased occupational safety especially in the highest risk professions of mining, construction, logging, and transportation.[18,20]

## STRATEGIES FOR PREVENTION OF INTENTIONAL INJURIES

Organized injury prevention efforts do not have as long a history for intentional injuries as it does for unintentional injuries. Prevention of intentional injuries has traditionally been the realm of the criminal justice system, with health care professionals and injury prevention personnel being relative newcomers. However, the same basic principles of injury etiology apply. Likewise, prevention work can be based on the development of strategies to identify and decrease risk factors. These strategies can use the same modalities of engineering, education, and enforcement to accomplish change in society.

Some of the prevention efforts that have been utilized against some of the more common forms of intentional injury will be reviewed briefly. Fatal intentional injury is commonly categorized as either homicide or suicide. However, it is important to remember that homicide is a final common pathway for several types of violent behavior, each of which produces many more non-fatal injuries. These include domestic violence, child abuse, elder abuse, and assaultive behavior in general. Prevention strategies for each of these are fairly different and examples will be considered separately.

### Assaultive Behavior

A minority of interpersonal violence occurs between strangers. The majority occurs between people who know each other and occurs in the course of interpersonal relationships which have evolved into conflicts. Hence, a focus for violence prevention has been to promote non-violent "conflict resolution." The teaching and promotion of conflict resolution skills has been undertaken within two broad categories of programs: school based and community based.[6,60–63]

### School Based Programs

These usually involve an educational curricula aimed at changing students' attitudes toward violence and teaching adaptive interpersonal skills for non-violent conflict resolution. Several standardized curricula are available, oriented for a variety of grades, from primary through high school. These curricula have been shown to change students' attitudes toward violence and to decrease interpersonal aggression in the short term. However, their long-term effectiveness at decreasing assaultive behavior is not known.[6]

An example of one such curriculum is *Second Step: A Violence Prevention Curriculum, Grades 1-3*. The curriculum consists of thirty, half-hour lessons. Each lesson involves the presentation of a social scenario, with an accompanying photograph. This scenario forms the basis for discussion and role playing by the students. Teachers who participate are usually given a two-day training session. The lessons are arranged in three groups: (1) empathy training; (2) impulse control; and (3) anger management.

In a study to evaluate the effectiveness of this curriculum, 12 elementary schools in King County, Washington State, were randomized to have the curriculum taught or to be a control. Observers rated specific children's interactions with other children and with teachers using a standardized social science behavior coding system. These observers were blinded as to whether or not a given school or specific children had received the curriculum. There was a decrease in physical aggression and an increase in neutral/prosocial behavior in the group receiving the curriculum compared with the control group. This was true at both 2 weeks and at 6 months after the course was taught. These changes were significant at both time periods, but less pronounced at 6 months. The ultimate effect on violent behavior in adolescence and adulthood remains unknown.[62]

### Community Based Programs

These programs focus on decreasing youth violence outside of the school environment. This has the advantage of reaching older adolescents and drop-outs. Some community based programs utilize conflict resolution education, similar to school based programs. Such education is delivered by public education campaigns and via neighborhood health centers. In some cases, high risk youths, such as those seen in emergency rooms for assaultive injuries, are identified and referred for violence prevention counseling.[64]

Some community based programs are parts of more general youth development programs, featuring mentoring, as well as recreational and cultural activities. These include some traditional approaches which have been active for years, such as the Boys Club. Such programs seek to decrease violent behavior as part of decreasing overall delinquency and drug dependency.

An example of a successful community based program is the Harlem Hospital Injury Prevention Program (HHIPP). This program, founded in 1988, sought to decrease childhood injuries from all causes, including violence. The program used a broad multidimensional approach, including educational programs on health and safety; increased environmental safety in parks and playgrounds; and increased availability of supervised recreational activities for children and adolescents. The program was community based, with the HHIPP acting as the lead agency in building a coalition which included neighborhood organizations and agencies of the local and state government.[60,61]

The results of these activities were evaluated using the Northern Manhattan Injury Surveillance System. The incidence of all injuries targeted by the HHIPP decreased by 44% after the institution of the program. Violent injuries decreased by 50%, in comparison to control communities, where such violent injuries increased by 93% during the study period.[60,61]

## Domestic Violence

Although a large proportion of all violent acts involve persons living in the same household, a specific subset of such violence warrants special attention. This is violence involving spouses or other intimate partners and hence is often know as intimate partner violence. The vast majority of such abuse involves a man injuring his female partner.

This is often regarded as a separate entity because of the interpersonal dynamics involved and the associated prevention implications. Domestic violence usually is a chronic, repetitive phenomenon. It is usually associated with psychological abuse and verbal intimidation. It is usually characterized by a man who seeks to dominate his partner both physically and emotionally and by a woman who is afraid to leave the relationship because of psychological and(or financial dependency. The more extreme forms of domestic violence, including homicide, are usually the endpoints of long abusive relationships.[6,65,66] It is the identification of domestic violence at its earlier stages upon which most preventive strategies are built.

For years, the mainstay of domestic violence prevention has been the criminal justice system. This has included both active interventions, such as restraining orders against abusive men, and deterrence by threat of punishment. None of the other newer interventions are likely to work unless such a system is functional. However, as traditionally used, the criminal justice system is underutilized primarily because many women are afraid to step forward and file complaints.

Hence, other modalities have been deemed necessary. These have included the use of hot lines, counseling services, and shelters for battered women. Another component of prevention has included early identification of battered women through the health care system. This has included identification in the setting of both emergency departments and primary care practices. Although many battered women may not volunteer information as to a history of battering, many are willing to divulge the information when asked. Hence, questioning about domestic violence is critical for screening and identification. Both the American Medical Association and the American College of Emergency Physicians strongly recommend routine screening for domestic violence.[65–68] Specific programs aimed at domestic violence have included programs to improve training of health care workers (including doctors, nurses, and receptionists) in such screening for domestic violence. This includes techniques for eliciting confidential information from victims, for establishing severity and risk, and for presenting options for safety and counseling. Such programs have been documented to improve screening and case identification of abused women.[6,65,66,69]

In addition, further work is needed to identify the most effective interventions, once a woman at risk for repeated domestic violence has been identified. The same rigor that has been applied to outcome assessments for unintentional injury needs to be applied for intentional injury. This implies a furthering of scientific inquiry into domestic violence and other forms of intentional injury. As one example of such evaluation, Holt et al. demonstrated that year-long restraining orders were more likely to lead to a decrease in subsequent acts of violence against women than short-term orders.[70]

## Suicide

High-risk groups for suicide include adolescents and young adults in all races, but especially Native Americans. Unlike other forms of intentional injury however, one of the highest risk groups is older white men.[10] A common problem with suicide prevention efforts is the relative lack of evaluation of their effectiveness. In part, this has been due to a difficulty in monitoring suicides due to underreporting. Also, the sporadic nature of actual suicides mandates very large sample sizes in order to assess effectiveness.[6] Thus, a variety of different prevention strategies have been utilized.

## Identification and Treatment of Individuals at High Risk of Suicide

Such identification has most often been done within the health care system, especially in emergency departments and primary care practices. Patients who present to an emergency department having just made an unsuccessful suicide attempt are obviously one high-risk group to identify. Identifying patients with depression or other "warning signs" of impending suicide within the context of a primary care practice, however, is much more difficult.[71]

In addition to a history of prior suicide attempt, studies have shown several risk factors for future attempts, including alcohol or substance abuse and mental illness, especially affective disorders.[72] However, none of these factors is sufficiently sensitive or specific to be a good screening test in and of itself. Special efforts to upgrade the training of primary care providers to improve recognition of these risk factors and to increase their familiarity with treatment for these disorders has shown some promise in improving the detection and treatment of high risk individuals.[73–76]

## Education Programs Aimed at General Public

These have most notably been utilized in school-based settings. The goals of such programs are to educate teachers, students, and parents about warning signs of impending suicide attempts and to provide them with information about available resources for help.[6,77]

## Crisis Intervention Services

Accessible self-referral resources for suicidal persons have included hot lines and personal counseling. In addition to the services they directly provide, these also function as an entry point into the mental health system. Such crisis intervention services have been the most frequently utilized suicide prevention strategies. However, their impact on lowering the suicide incidence rate has not been well demonstrated.[6,77]

## Reducing the Availability of the Means of Suicide

Reducing access to the means of suicide can be considered on both an individual and a societal level. It might seem that someone who wishes to commit suicide would find alternative means. However, most cases of suicide involve complex psychological processes in which both ambivalence and spontaneity play major roles. Elimination of a convenient and acceptable way to commit suicide may not lead to choosing another alternative, but rather to a decision not to complete the act.[6,77]

One of the best examples of the effects of decreasing the availability of the means of suicide was in England. Prior to the 1960s, half of the persons committing suicide in England used cooking gas to asphyxiate themselves. At the time, cooking gas was coal-based and consisted of 10–20% carbon monoxide. During the 1960s and 1970s, this was replaced by natural gas, both for safety and for economic reasons. The overall suicide rate in Britain decreased by 35% in the years after the gas supply had changed.[78,79] This example has obvious implications for the United States, where the majority of suicides are committed with firearms.

## The Roles of Alcohol and Firearms

As can be seen, there are a variety of interventions to decrease specific types of intentional injury, based on the human, psychological, and interpersonal factors at play. However, there are several common risk factors for all forms of intentional injury. These are the high frequency of involvement of alcohol and firearms. Between 30–60% of all homicides involve alcohol on the part of at least either the assailant or victim.[6] Alcohol involvement in suicides also appears frequent, although the exact percentages are more difficult to identify.[6,10] Similarly, firearms are used in 60% of suicides and 70% of homicides.[5,10]

Strategies to decrease the availability or impact of alcohol in society are also ways to decrease alcohol's involvement in intentional injuries. Such strategies include institution of a 21-year-old drinking age, higher alcohol excise taxes, and increased availability of alcohol rehabilitation services.[6] Hospital- and trauma center-based counseling interventions aimed at patients who present with any type of alcohol related injury are another strategy to consider, as discussed in the section on unintentional injury.[47–49]

Likewise, strategies to decrease the availability or impact of firearms are ways to decrease intentional injuries in general. However, probably no other aspect of injury prevention engenders a greater debate than this issue. Firearms are more common in American society than in almost any other developed country. The United States has higher rates of firearm related injury than any other developed country which is not at war. Attempts to decrease the availability of firearms have met with sustained, emotional resistance from Americans who consider unrestricted ownership of firearms a constitutionally guaranteed right.

However, it is important to recognize that communities with differing gun laws causing resultant differences in the prevalence of gun ownership also demonstrate decreases in homicide rates in those communities with more restrictive gun control laws.[80] Data on the effects of the institution of more restrictive gun ownership laws in a given area over time are less clear cut. However, the weight of the evidence does indicate a net reduction in firearm-related deaths from such laws.[5,81,82]

The CDC recommends a greater use of restrictive licensing for firearms, especially for handguns. Such gun control laws restrict possession of handguns to those with a clearly demonstrated need. The CDC also recommends greater enforcement of existing firearms laws, such as requiring waiting periods and background checks for those wishing to purchase guns.[6] In addition, another matter requiring attention is closing the current gun show sales loophole.

Other preventive measures directed at firearms include educational programs to teach safe gun handling, as a way primarily to decrease unintentional firearm injuries. However, similar to other generic nonfocused educational programs, the efficacy of such programs is not well demonstrated. Moreover, unintentional injuries account for only a small proportion of all firearm-related injuries.[6] Finally, there has been increased emphasis lately on safer storage of firearms. This includes keeping guns stored unloaded with ammunition stored separately. Other alternatives include the use of trigger locks and locked gun boxes. These devices allow a loaded gun to be kept more immediately available for those who feel the need to have such weapons rapidly available for self protection. All these techniques are felt to be ways to decrease not only unintentional firearms injuries, but also both assaultive and suicidal use of firearms.[83–85] In addition to social marketing efforts to promote use of these devices, mandated trigger locks on all guns sales is a currently proposed approach.

## RECENT GLOBAL INITIATIVES

This chapter primarily addresses the circumstances of North America and other high-income countries. However, the vast majority of injury-related deaths occur in low and middle-income countries (LMICs). This is because this is where the majority of people live; injury rates are higher; there have been limited application of organized injury prevention efforts; and trauma care systems are less than optimally developed. Moreover, injury rates are declining in most high-income countries, but rising, sometimes rapidly, in most LMICs.[86–89]

Many of the general injury prevention principles discussed in the current chapter are applicable under any circumstances. However, some of the specific applications need to vary to fit the circumstances of most of the world. This is due to varying injury mechanisms, resource restrictions, and cultural differences. There is a need to develop local injury prevention expertise and locally-applicable strategies.

After years of neglect by international agencies, injury control has been gradually receiving justifiable increases in attention worldwide. One of the groups spearheading these efforts has been the World Health Organization (WHO). Two recent landmark publications by the WHO have addressed two of the biggest injury problems, road traffic injury and violence. The *World Report on Road Traffic Injury Prevention* has helped raise awareness about the problem and to promote practical policy solutions for countries at varying economic levels worldwide.[90] The *World Report on Violence and Health* has emphasized the role that the health sector can have in violence prevention, in addition to sectors, such as criminal justice, that have traditionally been the foundation of violence prevention.[91] This report points out the complementary role that the health sector brings by its focus on changing the behavioral, social, and environmental factors that give rise to violence. Health also brings its focus on prevention, its scientific outlook, and its potential to coordinate multidisciplinary approaches.

Readers interested in learning more about the application of injury prevention programs in low and middle-income countries

## BOX 3-1    COMPONENTS OF A SUCCESSFUL INJURY PREVENTION PROGRAM

1. Identify a significant, eminently preventable, injury problem and a potential, eminently feasible, intervention.
   Problem should be a significant health problem, in terms of mortality or morbidity.
   Focus on injuries that are severe or common, or both.
   An effective intervention should exist, especially one which is being sub-optimally utilized in a given environment.
   Gather information on the extent of the problem and the effectiveness of possible interventions.
   Be able to communicate this information in terms understandable to the public, politicians, and other constituencies.

2. Identify and elicit the support of potential partners.
   Create a coalition of those with similar interests and goals.
   This coalition could include clinicians, public health practitioners, government, members of the lay public, insurance companies and other industry representatives, and others.
   Having one of these partners function as a "lead agency" is helpful to coordinate and stimulate the actions of the other partners.

3. Identify barriers to the use of the intervention. Such barriers could include:
   The knowledge and attitudes of the public.
   Available interventions may need to be modified or presented differently to certain high-risk groups.
   Lack of political will.
   Opposition by special interest groups.

4. Develop and implement a plan to address these barriers.
   Such a plan could involve a wide variety of actions and goals, such as, among other items:
   A public information campaign to change a dangerous behavior.
   A change in a law or the enforcement/application of a law.
   Change in the availability or characteristics of a product.
   Change in a hazardous environment.
   Surgeons and other clinicians can play key roles in all of the above, through actions, such as, among others:
   Bearing witness to the human toll of injury, so as to increase public and political will for changes.
   Advocacy for changes with local, state, and national government.
   Institute changes in injury prevention practice in their own institutions, such as with instituting alcohol interventions in hospitals.
   Injury prevention related counseling and advice for patients and their families.
   Successful programs usually involve:
   Multidisciplinary approach.
   Community involvement.
   Ongoing evaluation.
   Need to mobilize resources:
   Funding.
   Volunteer labor.
   Publicity/free advertising/human interest stories.
   Gifts-in-kind.
   More resources usually available with increased community interest and involvement.
   Other aspects of successful programs.
   Specific tasks assigned to specific partners.
   Set reasonable, meaningful, yet achievable goals.
   Regular meetings and updates by coalition members.

5. Evaluate the outcome of this program.
   Potential items to assess.
   Change in a law or its enforcement.
   Change in behavior, such as use of safety devices (e.g., smoke detectors, helmets).
   Decreases in rates of death or severe injury.
   Be prepared to change plans, if needed, based on feedback from outcome assessment.

6. Prevent the erosion of success.
   Most successful injury prevention campaigns are those that eventually become "institutionalized" and thus a regular part of the function of government or other groups.
   Guard against successful programs being rolled back by opposing interest groups or apathy by the public.

are encouraged to read these and other related[2,88,92] publications, as well as the WHO website (www.who.int/violence_injury_prevention/en/).

## CONCLUSION: THE SURGEON'S ROLE IN INJURY PREVENTION

Injury prevention efforts do work. Such efforts have had considerable success in lowering the toll of injury-related death and disability. These successes have been most notable in unintentional injury, especially due to road safety. Organized injury prevention work is also being increasingly applied to intentional injury. Obviously, much more remains to be done. This is especially true in light of recent setbacks in highway safety, motorcycle helmet use, and flame retardant clothing for children's sleepwear. In addition, the raising of speed limits in most states resulted in an increase in the motor vehicle crash death rate in the early 1990s with stagnation in the death rate thereafter.[31,57]

The accomplishments and successes of injury prevention programs rely on multidisciplinary input. Although many surgeons may not consider themselves as a usual part of injury prevention work, there is much they can contribute. In some injury prevention programs, they have played a pivotal role. Their contributions can be on both individual and societal levels. Surgeons, along with emergency physicians and prehospital providers, have more direct contact with acutely injured patients than do any other health care professionals. Hence, they are in a position to provide individual patient counseling regarding safety at a time when many injured persons are in a receptive state. Examples include emphasizing the importance of bicycle helmets to the parents of a child who has been injured bicycling without one and stressing the necessity of wearing a seatbelt to a motorist injured without one.

Perhaps one of the biggest roles for surgeons is to screen patients for alcohol abuse. Surgeons in hospitals that receive large numbers of injured persons should make sure that their hospitals institute mandatory screening, counseling, and referral programs, as now required by the American College of Surgeons for Level I and II trauma centers.

The voice of authority with which health care professionals speak allows them to be effective advocates for injury prevention educational campaigns and for legislation. Surgeons and other clinicians were instrumental in the public information campaigns that formed a component of the Seattle bicycle helmet campaign. Likewise, surgeons and other clinicians provided testimony in the motorcycle helmet debate which eventually led to the passage of numerous state motorcycle helmet laws.

Research is another avenue through which surgeons have and can contribute to injury prevention. This includes research that demonstrates the extent of a problem. For example, research on the costs of nonhelmeted motorcyclists in Washington State has provided useful data in the motorcycle helmet debate.[39,40,56] Such research also includes evaluation of the effectiveness of injury prevention programs.[55] In addition to such analytic research, surgeons have contributed to the development of systems to collect basic information on the extent of the toll from injury. For example, surgeons have been actively involved in the ongoing development of the National Violent Death Reporting System, created by the CDC. This system is seeking to provide information on the toll of violence in our society and to provide answers to questions about violence prevention strategies (www.cdc.gov/ncipc/profiles/nvdrs/facts.htm).

For surgeons and other clinicians wishing to get involved in injury prevention, many of the references cited in this chapter offer useful practical information. We especially recommend *Injury Prevention: Meeting the Challenge*, published by the CDC[6] and *Injury Prevention and Public Health* by Christoffel and Gallagher.[3] Finally, the American Association for the Surgery of Trauma and the American College of Surgeons both have prevention sections on their websites (http://www.aast.org and www.facs.org/trauma/inj-menu.html). These sites provide useful, practical information on injury prevention and on important injury-related legislation which is pending. They also have multiple links to other injury prevention resources, including a large number of local programs.

A summary of the components of a successful injury prevention program, with emphasis on a surgeon's involvement, is included in Box 3-1.

## REFERENCES

1. American Trauma Society. Trauma Watch, February 13, 2006.
2. Barss P, Smith G, Baker S et al.: *Injury Prevention: An International Perspective.* New York: Oxford University Press, 1998.
3. Christoffel T, Gallagher S: *Injury Prevention and Public Health.* Gaithersburg, MD: Aspen Publishers, Inc, 1999.
4. Rivara FP, Grossman DC, Cummings P: Injury prevention: First of two parts. *N Engl J Med* 337:543, 1997.
5. Rivara FP, Grossman DC, Cummings P: Injury prevention: Second of two parts. *N Engl J Med* 337:613, 1997.
6. The National Committee for Injury Prevention and Control: *Injury Prevention: Meeting the Challenge.* New York: Oxford University Press, 1989.
7. Baker CC, Oppenheimer L, Stephens B, et al.: Epidemiology of trauma deaths. *Am J Surg* 140:144, 1980.
8. Mock CN, Jurkovich GJ, nii-Amon-Kotei D, et al.: Trauma mortality patterns in three nations at different economic levels: Implications for global trauma system development. *J Trauma* 44:804, 1998.
9. Sauaia A, Moore FA, Moore EE, et al.: Epidemiology of trauma deaths: A reassessment. *J Trauma* 38:185, 1995.
10. Baker SP, O'Neill B, Ginsburg MJ, et al.: *The Injury Fact Book.* New York: Oxford University Press, 1992.
11. Valadka AB: Injury to the Cranium. In: Mattox, K., Feliciano, D. et al., eds. *Trauma,* 4th ed. New York, McGraw-Hill, 2000, p. 377.
12. Waller J: Injury: Conceptual shifts and preventive implications. *Annu Rev Public Health* 8:21, 1987.
13. DeHaven H: Mechanical analysis of survival in falls from heights of fifty to one hundred and fifty feet. *War Medicine* 2:586, 1942.
14. DeHaven H: Research on crash injuries (editorial). *JAMA* 131:524, 1946.
15. Moeller DW: *Environmental Health.* Cambridge, MA: Harvard University Press, 1992.
16. Gordon JE: The epidemiology of accidents. *Am J Pub Health* 39:504, 1949.
17. Haddon W: Advances in the epidemiology of injuries as a basis for public policy. *Public Health Reports* 95:411, 1980.
18. Hazinski MF, Francescutti LH, Lapidus GD, et al.: Pediatric injury prevention. *Ann Emerg Med* 22:456, 1993.
19. Insurance Institute for Highway Safety: Education alone won't make drivers safer. It won't reduce crashes. Insurance Institute for Highway Safety: Status Report 36:1, 2001.
20. Brown ST, Foege WH, Bender TR, et al.: Injury prevention and control: prospects for the 1990s. *Annu Rev Public Health* 11:251, 1990.
21. Bergman AB, Rivara FP, Richards DD, et al.: The Seattle children's bicycle helmet campaign. *AJDC* 144:727, 1990.
22. Rivara FP, Rogers LW, Thompson DC, et al.: The Seattle children's bicycle helmet campaign: Effects on helmet use and head injury admissions. *Pediatrics* 93:567, 1994.
23. McSwain NE, Belles A: Motorcycle helmets: Medical costs and the law. *J Trauma* 30:1189, 1990.
24. Simon v. Sargent FSM, (1972), affirmed in 409 U.S. 1020 (1972).
25. Bergman A: *Political Approaches to Injury Control at the State Level.* Seattle: University of Washington Press, 1992.

26. Robertson L: Automobile safety regulation in the United States. *Am J Pub Health* 71:818, 1981.

27. Robertson L: Automobile safety regulation. *Am J Pub Health* 74:1390, 1984.

28. Robertson LS: *Injury Epidemiology: Research and Control Strategies.* New York: Oxford University Press, 1998.

29. Nader R: *Unsafe At Any Speed: The Designed-In Dangers of the American Automobile.* New York: Grossman Publishers, 1965.

30. National Highway Traffic Safety Administration: NHTSA Crash Injury Research and Engineering Network (CIREN) Program Report (DOT HS 809 564). Washington, D.C.: NHTSA, 2002.

31. National Highway Traffic Safety Administration: *Traffic Safety Facts 2004.* Washington, DC: National Center for Statistics and Analysis, US DOT, 2005.

32. National Highway Traffic Safety Administration: www.nhtsa.dot.gov/people/NCSA, 2006.

33. Centers for Disease Control: WISQARS (Web-based Injury Statistics Query and Reporting System). Centers for Disease Control and Prevention [web page]. Available at: http://www.cdc.gov/ncipc/wisqars/. Accessed February 16, 2006.

34. Ebel B, Grossman D: Crash proof kids? An overview of current motor vehicle child occupant safety strategies. *Current Problems in Pediatric and Adolescent Health Care* 33:35, 2003.

35. Anderson P, Rivara F, Maier R, et al.: The epidemiology of seatbelt-associated injuries. *J Trauma* 31:60, 1991.

36. Durbin D, Elliott M, Winston F: Belt-positioning booster seats and reduction in risk of injury among children in vehicle crashes. *JAMA* 289:2835, 2003.

37. Insurance Institute for Highway Safety: www.iihs.org. Accessed February 16, 2006.

38. Evans L, Frick M: Helmet effectiveness in preventing motorcycle driver and passenger fatalities. *Accid Anal Prev* 6:447, 1988.

39. Offner PJ, Rivara FP, Maier R: The impact of motorcycle helmet use. *J Trauma* 32:636, 1992.

40. Rowland J, Rivara FP, Salzberg P, et al.: Motorcycle helmet use and injury outcome and hospitalization costs in Washington State. *Am J Publ Health* 86:41, 1996.

41. Sosin DM, Sacks JJ: Motorcycle helmet use laws and head injury prevention. *JAMA* 267:1649, 1992.

42. Thomas S, Acton C, Nixon J, et al.: Effectiveness of bicycle helmets in preventing head injury in children: case-control study. *BMJ* 308:173, 1994.

43. Thompson RS, Rivara FP, Thompson DC: Case-control study of the effectiveness of bicycle safety helmets. *N Engl J Med* 320:1361, 1989.

44. Borkenstein RF, Crowther RF, Shumate RP, et al.: The role of the drinking driver in traffic accidents. *Alcohol Drugs Behav* 2:8, 1974.

45. Voas RB, Wells J, Lestina D, et al.: Drinking and driving in the United States: The 1996 National Roadside Survey. *Accid Anal Prev* 30:267, 1998.

46. DeJong W, Hingson R: Strategies to reduce driving under the influence of alcohol. *Annu Rev Public Health* 19:359, 1998.

47. Dunn CW, Donovan DM, Gentilello LM: Practical guidelines for performing alcohol interventions in trauma centers. *J Trauma* 42:299, 1997.

48. Gentilello LM, Donovan DM, Dunn CW, et al.: Alcohol interventions in trauma centers. *JAMA* 274:1043, 1995.

49. Gentilello L, Rivara F, Donovan D, et al.: Alcohol interventions in a trauma center as a means of reducing the risk of injury recurrence. *Annals of Surgery* 230:473, 1999.

50. Insurance Institute for Highway Safety: Graduated Licensing: A Blueprint for North America. Available from: www.iihs.org/laws/state_laws/pdf/blueprint.pdf, 2006.

51. Foss R, Feaganes J, Rodgman E: Initial effects of graduated driver licensing on 16-year-old driver crashes in North Carolina. *JAMA* 286:1588, 2001.

52. Wanda L, Tenenbein M, Moffatt ME: House fire injury prevention update. *Injury Prevention* 5:217, 1999.

53. DiGuiseppi CG, Rivara FP, Koepsell TD: Attitudes toward bicycle helmet ownership and use by school-age children. *AJDC* 144:83, 1990.

54. DiGuiseppi CG, Rivara FP, Koepsell TD, et al.: Bicycle helmet use by children: Evaluation of a community-wide helmet campaign. *JAMA* 262:2256, 1989.

55. Mock CN, Maier RV, Boyle E, et al.: Injury prevention strategies to promote helmet use decrease severe head injury at a level I trauma center. *J Trauma* 39:29, 1995.

56. Rivara FP, Dicker BG, Bergman AB, et al.: The public cost of motorcycle trauma. *JAMA* 260:221, 1988.

57. National Center for Health Statistics: *Health, United States, 1996–97 and Injury Chartbook.* Hyattsville, Maryland: National Center for Health Statistics, 1997.

58. Centers for Disease Control: webapp.cdc.gov/sasweb/ncipc/mortrate.html. Accessed June 18, 2007.

59. National Safety Council: *Accident Facts.* Chicago: National Safety Council, 1990.

60. Davidson LL, Durkin MS, Kuhn L, et al.: The impact of the safe kids/healthy neighborhoods injury prevention program in Harlem, 1988 through 1991. *Am J Pub Health* 84:580, 1994.

61. Durkin MS, Kuhn L, Davidson LL, et al.: Epidemiology and prevention of severe assault and gun injuries to children in an urban community. *J Trauma* 41:667, 1996.

62. Grossman DC, Neckerman HJ, Koepsell TD, et al.: Effectiveness of a violence prevention curriculum among children in elementary school. *JAMA* 277:1605, 1997.

63. Wright J, Cheng T: Successful approaches to community violence intervention and prevention. *Pediatr Clin North Am* 45:459, 1998.

64. Prothrow-Stith D: The violence prevention project: a public health approach. *Sci Tech Human Values* 12:67, 1987.

65. El-Bayoumi G, Borum M, Haywood Y: Domestic violence in women. *Medl Clin North Am* 82:391, 1998.

66. Melvin S, Rhyne M: Domestic violence. *Adv Intern Med* 43:1, 1998.

67. American College of Emergency Physicians Policy Statement: *Emergency Medicine and Domestic Violence.* Dallas, Sept. 1994.

68. American Medical Association: *Diagnostic and Treatment Guidelines on Domestic Violence.* Chicago: American Medical Association, 1992.

69. Thompson RS, Rivara FP, Thompson DC, et al.: Identification and management of domestic violence: A randomized trial. *Am J Prev Med* 19:253, 2000.

70. Holt V, Kernic M, Lumley T, et al.: Civil protection orders and risk of subsequent police-reported violence. *JAMA* 288:589, 2002.

71. Mock CN, Grossman D, Mulder D, et al.: Detection of suicide risk during health care visits on a Native American reservation. *J Gen Internl Med* 11:519, 1996.

72. Fowler RC, Rich CL, Young D: San Diego suicide study, II: Substance abuse in young cases. *Arch Gen Psychiatry* 43:962, 1986.

73. Katon W, VonKorff M, Lin E, et al.. Collaborative management to achieve treatment guidelines: Impact on depression in primary care. *JAMA* 273:1026, 1995.

74. Rutz W, LVonKnorring, Walinder J: Frequency of suicide in Gotland after systematic postgraduate education of general practitioners. *Acta Psychiatr Scand* 80:151, 1989.

75. Rutz W, LVonKnorring, Walinder J: Long-term effects of an educational program for general practitioners given by the Swdish Committee for the Prevention and Treatment of Depression. *Acta Psychiatr Scand* 85:83, 1992.

76. Simon GE, VonKorff M: Recognition, managment, and outcomes of depression in primary care. *Arch Fam Med* 4:99, 1995.

77. O'Carroll P, Rosenberg M, Mercy J: Suicide. In: Rosenberg, M. & Fenley, M., eds. *Violence in America.* New York: Oxford University Press, 1991.

78. Brown JH: Suicide in Britain. *Arch Gen Psychiatry* 36:1119, 1979.

79. Kreitman N: The coal gas story: United Kingdom suicide rates, 1960–1971. *Br J Prev Soc Med* 30:89, 1976.

80. Sloan JH, Kellermann AL, Reay DT, et al.: Handgun regulations, crime, assaults, and homicide: A tale of two cities. *N Engl J Med* 319:1256, 1988.

81. Loftin C, McDowall D, Wiersema B, et al.: Effects of restrictive licensing of handguns on homicide and suicide in the District of Columbia. *N Engl J Med* 325:1615, 1991.

82. Rosengart M, Cummings P, Nathens A, et al.: An evaluation of state firearm regulations and homicide and suicide death rates. *Injury Prevention* 11:77, 2005.

83. Cummings P, Grossman DC, Rivara FP, et al.: State gun safe storage laws and child mortality due to firearms. *JAMA* 278:1084, 1997.

84. Denno DM, Grossman DC, Britt J, et al.: Safe storage of handguns: What do the police recommend. *Arch Pediatr Adolesc med* 150:927, 1996.

85. Grossman DC, Cummings P, Koepsell TD, et al.. Firearm safety counseling in primary care pediatrics: a randomized, controlled trial. *Pediatrics* 106:22, 2000.

86. Krug E: *Injury: A Leading Cause of the Global Burden of Disease* (WHO/HSC/PVI/99.11). Geneva: World Health Organization, 1999.

87. Krug EG, Sharma GK, Lozano R: The global burden of injuries. *Am J Pub Health* 90:523, 2000.

88. Mock C, Quansah R, Krishnan R, et al.: Strengthening the prevention and care of injuries worldwide. *Lancet* 363:2172, 2004.

89. Nantulya V, Reich M: The neglected epidemic: road traffic injuries in developing countries. *BMJ* 324:1139, 2002.

90. Peden M, Scurfield R, Sleet D, et al.: *World Report on Road Traffic Injury Prevention.* Geneva: World Health Organization, 2004.

91. Krug E, Dahlberg L, Mercy J, et al.: *World Report on Violence and Health.* Geneva: World Health Organization, 2002.

92. Berger LR, Mohan D: *Injury Control: A Global View.* Delhi: Oxford University Press, 1996.

# Commentary ■ EDWARD E. CORNWELL, III

Drs. Maier and Mock have masterfully set forth the history, strategies, components, and barriers involved in developing and maintaining an effective injury prevention program. This encyclopedic reference could not have emerged from a more appropriate University. The collaboration between the Division of Trauma and the Harborview Injury Prevention and Research Center at Harborview Medical Center has long served not only as a beacon of enlightenment resulting from productive injury research, but also as an example for the optimal curriculum for young trauma surgical academicians.

The Haddon's Matrix that depicts the interactions of factors that affect both the likelihood and the result of injuries has stood the test of time and continues to deserve a position of prominence in any chapter describing the framework of injury prevention. What will continue to change are societal norms and events that will have an impact on our culture in terms of the acceptability of certain behaviors. The result of these changes will be manifest through impact on the specific boxes found in Table 3-1 which demonstrates interaction between the phases (pre-event, event, post-event) and factors, (host, vehicle, environment) within Haddon's Matrix. Closer inspection of Table 3-1 with a view toward cultural changes in America's society over the last generation demonstrate why the authors are able to enumerate successes in reducing the impact of unintentional injuries, particularly those related to motor vehicle crashes. A generation of American children has grown up with the expectation that they will use seatbelts and frequently remind their parents to do the same. Concomitant improving frequency in the use of airbags, collapsible steering columns, and improvement of fuel systems lend promise for continued progress in decreasing traffic fatality rates.

Two other factors in post-event phase deserve special mention as recent developments that effect Haddon's Matrix. On the one hand is the human factor of the aging and progressively more obese American population. Time will tell if this generation of more mobile seniors being on the road translates into a post-event factor of worse physical conditioning that may affect the outcome of injury. Also deserving of mention is the environmental factor of a trauma care system. For many years, trauma surgeons and public health professionals have proclaimed the life-saving impact of trauma centers, yet true academic rigor was missing from such a proclamation because of the absence of information on the outcomes of injured patients who were taken to nontrauma centers. This gap in knowledge was recently filled by the National Study on Cost and Outcomes of Trauma (NSCOT) reported by McKenzie et al. which showed a survival benefit among critically injured patients taken to Level I trauma centers.

The American College of Surgeons Committee on Trauma has moved in accordance with the development of new knowledge. The Committee now offers consultation to states that wish to develop a trauma system, and has moved the requirement of Level I and Level II trauma centers to maintain an injury prevention program to a more specific mandate based on published successes: the mandate of maintaining a brief alcohol screening and intervention program.

## "Prevention of Intentional Injuries"

The ever-changing cultural environment in American society is responsible for the greater challenges seen in preventing death due to intentional injuries. The experience at an urban Level I trauma center at Johns Hopkins Hospital amplifies some of the challenges highlighted by the authors.

Improvement in overall mortality and timeliness of care was the result of the commitment of significant resources to the trauma service at Johns Hopkins Hospital. However, despite the overall improvement, there was no benefit for patients with gunshot wounds (GSW). Greater lethality of weaponry was suggested by the fact that 70% of patients with lethal GSW were in extremis or dead on arrival, and the majority of those leaving the ED "alive" who died later were victims of GSW to the head. There are certain injuries, such as GSW to the head and GSW to the thoracic aorta, that a carry a high mortality no matter how extensive the commitment of resources.

The particulars and demographics involved in the trauma service at the Johns Hopkins Hospital offer a less optimistic picture regarding the role of secondary prevention in the in-patient setting than is referenced in this chapter. A study of young (ages 15–24) alcohol and drug abusing trauma patients found a disproportionate number of high school dropouts, and patients with GSW, and a relative rarity in demonstrating introspection and readiness to change their abusive habits. Furthermore, these young patients ages (15–24) represent two-thirds of all GSW victims. Finally, we have identified that 80% of our trauma patients live within a 5 mile radius of the hospital. These data suggest that injury prevention efforts for this center should take the form of violence prevention for at-risk youths in the community setting. Currently, the program includes slide and video presentations to young males at a local Police Athletic League center, and hospital tours to visit disabled survivors of gun violence. A short-term improvement in attitudes toward conflict and aggression was demonstrated and published.

Sadly, the structured approach described herein competes poorly with trends in our culture at large. Recent visits of the executive offices of media production companies have emphasized the dominance of an American culture that glamorizes violence. Images that sensationalize violent acts reach millions of young people every day, while the previously described study of the outreach program analyzes only 90 kids over 1 year.

Accordingly, it was decided to incorporate an approach that seeks to reach influential adults (journalists, TV/radio personalities, politicians, athletes, and entertainers) with a graphic message that describes the tragic consequences of trivializing interpersonal injuries. This academic-community partnership may require new parameters in evaluating efficacy, as it attacks a generational problem. With this effort, we join the growing cadre of surgeons and other physicians and public health professionals who have resolved to extend the sphere of their influence beyond the hospital and university walls, and interact with a larger audience beyond our typical professional societies and scientific publications.

# Trauma Systems, Triage, and Transport

*David B. Hoyt* ■ *Raul Coimbra* ■ *Bruce M. Potenza*

## DEFINITION OF TRAUMA SYSTEM

A trauma system is an organized approach to acutely injured patients in a defined geographical area that provides full and optimal care and that is integrated with the local or regional Emergency Medical Service (EMS) system.

A system has to achieve cost-efficiency through the integration of resources with local health and EMS system to provide the full range of care (from prehospital to rehabilitation).[1-3]

Regionalization is an important aspect of trauma as a system because it facilitates the efficient use of health care facilities within a defined geographical area and the rational use of equipment and resources. Trauma care within a trauma system is multidisciplinary and is provided along a continuum that includes all phases of care.[2-8]

The major goal of a trauma system is to enhance the community health. This can be achieved by identifying risk factors in the community and creating solutions to decrease the incidence of injury, and by providing optimal care during the acute as well as the late phase of injury including rehabilitation, with the objective to decrease overall injury-related morbidity and mortality and years of life lost. Disaster preparedness is also an important function of trauma systems, and using an established trauma system network will facilitate the care of victims of natural disasters or terrorist attacks. The Model Trauma System Planning and Evaluation Standard has recently been completed by the U.S. Department of Health and Human Services.[9]

## THE NEED FOR TRAUMA SYSTEMS—HISTORY

The need for a trauma system seems obvious and intuitive. However, trauma is not yet recognized as a disease process. Many people still think of trauma as an accident. Trauma is an epidemic that affects all age groups with devastating personal, psychological, and economic consequences. Recent calculations have estimated the total cost of injury in the United States to be about $260 billion per year.[10]

Because of the association of injury and personal behavior, trauma is often predictable and preventable.

The modern approach to trauma care is based on lessons learned during war conflicts. Advances in rapid transport, volume resuscitation, wound care management of complex injuries, surgical critical care, early nutritional management, deep venous thrombosis prophylaxis were all derived from the military experience.

The American College of Surgeons Committee on Trauma (ACSCOT) was created in 1949 and evolved from the Committee on the Treatment of Fractures that was established in 1922. A specific trauma unit was opened in 1961 at the University of Maryland. In 1966, the National Academy of Sciences and the National Research Council published the important "white" paper entitled *Accidental Death and Disability: The Neglected Disease of Modern Society*.[11] The outgrowth of this document was the development and propagation of systems of trauma care. This publication increased public awareness and led to a federal agenda for trauma systems development. Two trauma centers were simultaneously formed in Chicago and San Francisco.

The Maryland Institute of Emergency Medicine became the first completely organized, statewide, regionalized system in 1973. Similar initiatives were taken in 1971 in Illinois,[6,12] where the designation of trauma centers was established by state law, and in Virginia in 1981, where a statewide trauma system based on volunteer participation and compliance with national standards as defined by the ACSCOT was established.

In 1973, the Emergency Medical Services Systems Act became law, providing guidelines and financial assistance for the development of regional EMS systems.[13] In addition, state and local efforts were initiated by using prehospital care systems to deliver patients to major hospitals where appropriate care could be provided.

Prehospital provider programs were formalized, and training programs were established for paramedics and emergency medical technicians.

At that time, major teaching hospitals in large cities were, by default, recognized as regional trauma centers. With strong academic leadership, these centers were able to develop regionalization of systems of trauma care by setting examples.

ACSCOT developed a task force to publish *Optimal Hospital Resources for the Care of the Seriously Injured* in 1976, establishing a standard for evaluation of care.[14] This document was the first to set out specific criteria for the categorization of hospitals as trauma centers. This document is periodically revised and is recognized nationally and internationally as the standard for hospitals aspiring to be trauma centers. The current version entitled *Resources for Optimal Care of the Injured Patient* was published in 2006.[4] It establishes criteria for prehospital and trauma care personnel and the importance of ongoing quality assessment. In addition, ACSCOT developed the Advanced Trauma Life Support (ATLS) course in 1980, which has contributed to the uniformity of initial care and the development of a common language for all care providers.[15]

In 1985, the National Research Council and the Institute of Medicine published *Injury in America: A Continuing Health Care Problem*. This document concluded that despite considerable funding used to develop trauma systems, little progress had been made toward reducing the burden of injury.[16] This document also reinforced the necessity of investments in epidemiological research and injury prevention. Following the publication of this document, the Centers for Disease Control (CDC) was chosen as the site for an injury research center, to coordinate efforts at the national level in injury control, injury prevention, and all other aspects of trauma care.

In 1987, the ACSCOT instituted the Verification/Consultation Program, which provided further resources and incentive for trauma system development and trauma centers' designation. More recently, the ACSCOT published a document entitled *Consultation for Trauma Systems* with the objective of providing guidelines for trauma system evaluation and enhancement.[17] In 1987, the American College of Emergency Physicians (ACEP) published *Guidelines for Trauma Care Systems*.[18] This document focused on the continuum of trauma care, and identified essential criteria for trauma care systems.

In 1988, the National Highway Safety Administration (NTHSA) established the Statewide EMS Technical Assessment Program and the Development of Trauma Systems Course, both important tools to assess the effectiveness of trauma systems components as well as for system development. NHTSA also developed standards for quality EMS, including trauma care.[19] The standard required that the trauma care system be fully integrated into the state's EMS system and have specific legislation (Table 4-1). The trauma care component must include designated trauma centers, transfer and triage guidelines, trauma registries, and initiatives in public education and injury prevention.

In 1990, the Trauma Systems Planning and Development Act created the Division of Trauma and EMS (DTEMS) within the Health Resources Tand Services Administration (HRSA) to improve emergency medical services and trauma care. Unfortunately, the program was not funded between 1995 and 2000 in many states that were in the process of developing trauma

systems.[20] Two initiatives from this legislation were noteworthy: (1) planning grants for statewide trauma system development were provided to states on a competitive basis, and (2) the Model Trauma Care System Plan was published as a consensus document.[21] The Model Trauma Care System Plan established an apolitical framework for measuring progress in trauma system development and set the standard for the promulgation of systems of trauma care. The program was again funded in fiscal year 2001 but lost funding in 2006. New legislation is being written to further this effort. The newest document for trauma system planning uses the public health care model of assessment, policy development, and evaluation of the outcome. With appropriate federal funding this approach will be very successful.[9]

## TABLE 4-1

### Criteria for Statewide Trauma Care System

Legal authority for designation
Formal process for designation
Use American College of Surgeon's standards
Use out-of-area survey teams
Number of trauma centers population- or volume-based
Triage criteria allow direct transport to trauma center
Monitoring systems in place
Full geographic coverage

*Source: West JG, Williams MJ, Trunkey DD, Wolferth CC. Trauma systems: Current Status-future challenges. JAMA 259:3597, 1988.*

## TRAUMA SYSTEMS DEVELOPMENT

The criteria for a statewide EMS and trauma systems have been determined and are identified in Table 4-2. The first step is to establish legal authority for the development of a system. This usually requires legislation at a state or local level that provides public agency authority. The next step in the development of a trauma system is to determine the need of such a system. In general, this has been done in communities by reviewing the outcome of trauma cases in the region. Traditionally, such reviews have focused on preventable deaths. The surgeon's role is critical in both leadership and commitment to establish a better standard of care.

## TABLE 4-2

### Emergency Medical Service System Components

Regulation and policy
Resource management
Human resources and training
Transportation
Facilities
Communications
Trauma systems
Public information and education
Medical direction
Evaluation

*Source: Development of Trauma Systems (DOT). Washington, DC, National Highway Traffic Safety Administration, 1988.*

The designated agency in combination with local trauma surgeons and other medical personnel develop criteria for the trauma system, determine which facilities will be designated trauma centers, and establish a trauma registry, a fundamental component of a quality assurance program.[4,22–27] (Fig. 4-1)

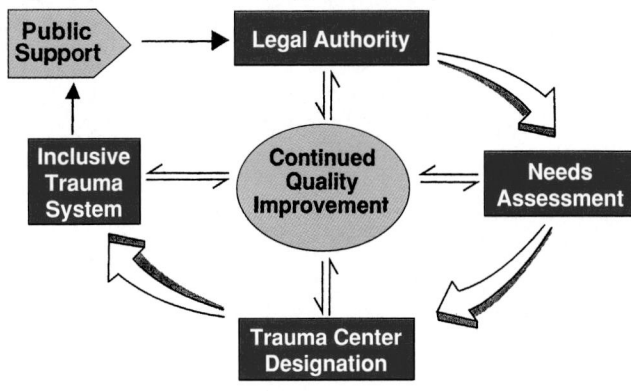

**FIGURE 4-1.** Regional trauma system development must progress in a sequential fashion; a comprehensive needs assessment is a pivotal early step.
*(Reproduced with permission from Moore EE. Trauma systems, trauma centers, and trauma surgeons: Opportunity in managed competition. J Trauma 39:1, 1995.)*

## TRAUMA SYSTEM COMPONENTS

The most significant improvement in the care of injured patients in the United States has occurred through the development of trauma systems. However, recent data show that only 50% of states in the United States have statewide trauma systems, about 20% have no trauma system at all.[28] The necessary elements of a trauma system are: access to care, prehospital care, hospital care, and rehabilitation, in addition to prevention, disaster medical planning, patient education, research, and rational financial planning. Prehospital communications, transport system, trained personnel, and qualified trauma care personnel for all phases of care are of utmost importance for a system's success (Fig. 4-1).

External peer review generally is used to verify specific hospital's capabilities and its ability to deliver the appropriate level of care. The verification process can be accomplished through the ACSCOT or by inviting experts in the field of trauma as outside reviewers. Finally, quality assessment and quality improvement is a vital component of the system, as it provides directions for improvement as well as constant evaluation of the system's performance and needs.

The Model Trauma Care System Plan introduced the concept of the "inclusive system"[21] (Fig. 4-2). Based on this model, trauma centers were identified by their ability to provide definitive care to the most critically injured. Approximately 15% of all trauma patients will benefit from the resources of a Level I or II trauma center. Therefore, it is appropriately expected in an inclusive system to encourage participation and to enhance capabilities of the smaller hospitals.

Surgical leadership is of fundamental importance in the development of trauma systems. Trauma systems cannot develop without the commitment of the surgeons of a hospital or community.

## PUBLIC INFORMATION, EDUCATION, AND INJURY PREVENTION

Death following trauma occurs in a tri-model distribution (Fig. 4-3). Effective trauma programs must also focus on injury prevention, since more than half of the deaths occur within minutes of injury, and will never be addressed by acute care.

Because trauma is not considered an important public health problem by the general population, efforts to increase awareness of the public as well as to instruct the public about how the system operates and how to access the system are important and mandatory. A recent Harris Poll conducted by the Anemia Trauma Society showed that most citizens value the importance of a trauma system with the same importance as fire and police services.[29] Trauma

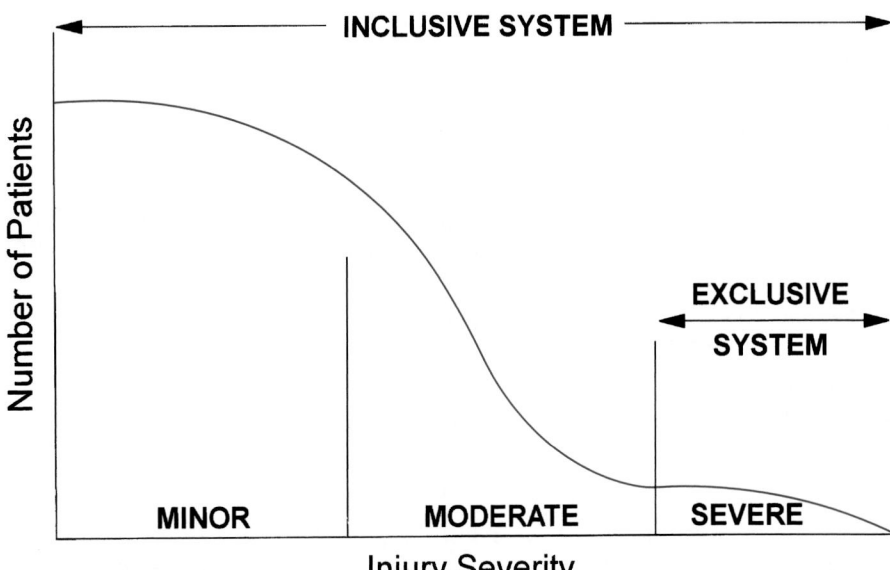

**FIGURE 4-2.** Diagram showing the growth of the trauma care system to become inclusive. Note that the number of injured patients is inversely proportional to the severity of their injuries.

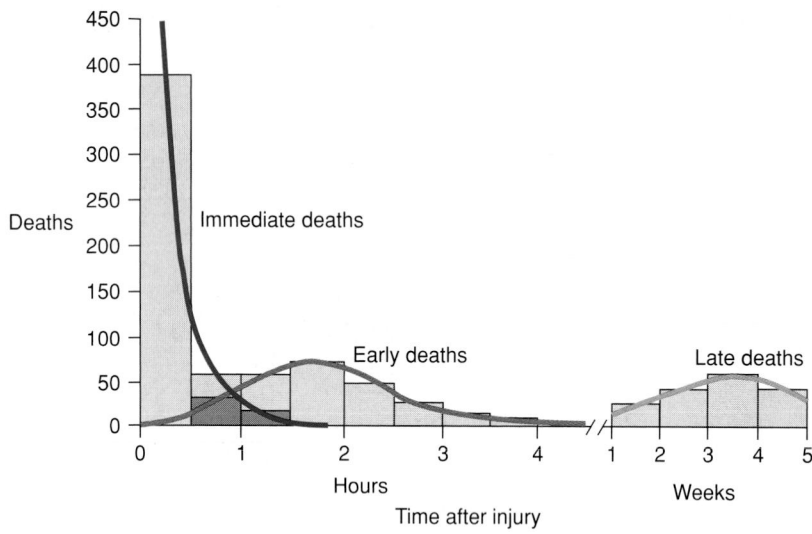

**FIGURE 4-3.** The trimodal distribution of trauma deaths. *(Reproduced with permission from Trunkey DD. Trauma. Sci Amer 249:28, 1983.)* *(Reproduced with permission from Lazar J. Greenfield, ed: Michael W. Mulholland, Keith Oldham, Gerald Zelenock, Keith Lillemoe, Assoc eds: Surgery, Scientific Principles And Practice, 3rd ed., 2001: p. 271: Lippincott Williams & Wilkins, Philadelphia, PA.)*

system must also focus on injury prevention based on data relevant to injuries and what interventions will likely reduce their occurrence. Identification of risk factors and high-risk groups, development of strategies to alter personal behavior through education or legislation, and other preventive measures have the greatest impact on trauma in the community, and over time, will have the greatest effect on nonfatalities.[30–35]

## HUMAN RESOURCES

Because the system cannot function optimally without qualified personnel, a quality system provides quality education to its providers. This includes all personnel along the trauma care continuum: physicians, nurses, emergency medical technicians (EMTs), and others who impact the patient and/or the patient's family.

## PREHOSPITAL

Trauma care prior to hospital arrival has a direct effect on survival. The system must ensure prompt access and dispatch of qualified personnel, appropriate care at the scene, and safe and rapid transport of the patient to the closest most appropriate facility.

The primary focus is on education of paramedical personnel to provide initial resuscitation, triage, and treatment of trauma patients. Effective prehospital care requires coordination between various public safety agencies and hospitals to maximize efficiency, minimize duplication of services, and provide care at a reasonable cost.

## COMMUNICATION SYSTEM

A reliable communications system is essential for providing optimal trauma care. Although many urban centers have used modern electronic technology to establish emergency systems, most rural communities have not. It must include universal access to emergency

telephone numbers (e.g., 911), trained dispatch personnel who can efficiently match EMS expertise with the patient's needs, and the capability of EMS personnel at the trauma incident to communicate with prehospital dispatch, with the trauma hospital, and with other units.

Access also requires that all users know how to enter the system. This can be achieved through public safety and information and school educational programs designed to educate health care providers and the public about emergency medical access.

## MEDICAL DIRECTION

Medical direction provides the operational matrix for care provided in the field. It grants freedom of action and limitations to EMTs who must rescue injured patients. The medical director is responsible for the design and implementation of field treatment guidelines, their timely revision, and their quality control. Medical direction can be "off line" in the form of protocols for training, triage, treatment, transport, and technical skill operations or "on line", given directly to the field provider.

## TRIAGE & TRANSPORT

The word triage derives from the French word meaning "to sort." When applied in a medical context, triage involves the initial evaluation of a casualty and the determination of the priority and level of medical care necessary for the victim.[36] The purpose of triage is to be selective, so that limited medical resources are allocated to patients who will receive the most benefit. Proper triage should ensure that the seriously injured patient be taken to a facility capable of treating these types of injuries—a trauma center. Patients with lesser severity of injuries may be transported to other appropriate medical facilities for care.

Each medical facility has its own unique set of medical resources. As such, triage principles may vary from one locale to another depending upon the resource availability. Likewise, established triage principles may be modified to handle multiple casualty incident or mass casualties. Then, a different set of triage criteria may be employed which will attempt to provide medical care to the greatest number of patients. In this scenario, some critically injured patients may not receive definitive care as this may consume an "unfair share" of resources. The goal of triage and acute medical care is to provide the greatest good to the greatest numbers.

From a historical perspective, war has been the catalyst for developing and refining the concept of medical triage. Dominique Jean Larrey, Napoleon's chief surgeon, was one of the first to prioritize the needs of the wounded on a mass scale. He believed ". . . it is necessary to always begin with the most dangerously injured, without regard to rank or distinction." He evacuated both friend and foe on the battlefield and rendered medical care to both. He refined his techniques for evacuation and determining medical priorities for injured patients over the 18 years and 60 battles while a member of the French army.[37]

During World War I, the English developed the "casualty clearing station," where the injured were separated based on the extent of their injuries. Those with relatively minor injuries received first aid, while those with more serious injuries underwent initial resuscitative measures prior to definitive care. As medical and surgical care of battlefield injuries expanded, a system of triage and tiered levels (echelons) of medical care was designed. Echelons of medical care and triage of single, multiple, and mass casualties remain the paradigm for military combat medical care.

There are five echelons (or levels) of care in the present military medicine. The first line of medical care is that which is provided by fellow soldiers. Principles of airway management, cessation of bleeding, and basic support are offered by fellow soldiers. Organized medical care begins with a medic or corpsman who participates in echelon 1 care. They are assigned to functional military units and serve as the initial medical evaluation and care of the injured patient. Echelon 2 is a battalion aid station or a surgical company. Resuscitation and basic life saving surgical procedures may be performed at these stations. Echelon 3 is a Mobile Army Surgical Hospital (MASH) or Fleet Surgical Hospital. Advanced surgical and medical diagnostic and therapeutic capabilities are available at these facilities. An Echelon 4 facility is larger and has enhanced medical capacity. Examples include a hospital ship (USNS Mercy or Comfort) or an out-of-country medical facility (Landstuhl Region Medical Center (Army), Germany). An Echelon 5 facility is a large tertiary and rehabilitative medical facility and is located within the home country (Naval Medical Center San Diego). Each increasing echelon has a more comprehensive medical and surgical capacity. As patients are identified on the battlefield, they are triaged and transferred to the next higher echelon for care. During the Vietnam War, air medical transport enabled the triage of a seriously injured soldier from the battlefield directly to a MASH unit.[38] The time to definitive surgical care was less than 2 hours compared to 6 hours during World War II.[39]

The lessons learned from the triage and treatment of combat casualties were slow to translate into civilian use. Injured patients, regardless of the severity of injury, were simply taken to the nearest hospital for treatment. Neither a triage system nor an organized approach to injury existed. The Advanced Trauma Life Support course was created in the late 1970s and with it the concept of requisite skills and facilities to treat injured patients emerged.[15]

## PURPOSE AND CHALLENGES OF TRIAGE

The purpose of triage is to match the patient with the optimal resources necessary to adequately and efficiently manage their injuries. It is a dynamic process of patient evaluation and reevaluation until the patient receives definitive care. The challenge of a triage system lies in correctly identifying which patient has injuries in need of a designated trauma center. Studies have demonstrated better outcomes in major trauma victims who have been treated at hospitals that have a commitment for this specialized care.[26] Of all trauma patients, only 7 to 15% have injuries that require the facilities of a dedicated trauma center.[15]

The ideal triage system would direct patients with serious injuries to the most appropriately staffed hospital while transporting those with less serious injuries to all other hospitals within the geographic area. Due to the complexities of patient evaluation and injury determination, "the perfect triage system" is yet to be developed.

The primary goal of an effective triage system is to identify which casualties are seriously injured and in need of immediate surgical or medical care. This requires a rapid evaluation of the patient and a decision about the level of emergency care that will be needed for the patient. Once this is determined they are matched and transported to the appropriate medical facility.[40] The triage physician often has limited resources, information, and time to make this important decision. While many triage methods can be used they often rely on physiologic, anatomic, and mechanism of injury information to assist in the triage decision. Once the patient has been routed to a treatment facility, information concerning the patient's injuries and physiologic state should be transmitted to the receiving facility if possible. This will give the receiving physician an opportunity to gather the appropriate personnel and equipment to treat the incoming casualty. A concise prehospital radio report will enable the receiving medical personnel to anticipate emergent equipment and personnel needs. In some instances, a direct operative resuscitation may be indicated to stabilize the patient.[41] In other cases, emergent airway control may be the primary concern. The few minutes of preparation, prior to the patient's arrival, may be the difference in patient survival.

The other goal is to define the "major trauma victim." While this term may be easy to conceptualize, it is very difficult to quantify. A precise definition is important so that triage, treatment, and outcomes can be compared. Prompt recognition of those patients who are in immediate risk of life (e.g., loss of airway or hemorrhagic shock), loss of a limb (ischemia) or will need immediate operative or life-saving interventions is paramount. These patients are in need of definitive care in an expedient fashion where delays in care may result in excess morbidity or mortality.

The Injury Severity Score (ISS) provides the means for a trauma system to retrospectively identify major trauma victims with an ISS of greater than 15 being a commonly accepted level.[42,43] Another definition of major trauma is provided by the Major Outcome Study (MTOS), which defines the trauma patient as all patients who died due to their injuries or were admitted to the hospital.[44] The threshold that defines the major trauma victim within a trauma system is based not only on the resources of a particular trauma center, but also on the inability of the nondesignated hospitals to consistently provide appropriate care for an injury exceeding the threshold. This may vary from system to system.

After a traumatic event, the effectiveness of a triage system should be analyzed based upon expected performance standards. Data monitoring and quality assessment tools should be applied after a disaster or after any one patient who has been treated so that system or operator errors can be identified and corrected. Each multiple casualty event presents unique problems to a triage system. Constant reevaluation and refinement are cornerstones for improved performance.

One of the accepted performance markers to an effective triage system is found in the determination of the undertriage and overtriage rates. *Undertriage* is defined as a triage decision that classifies a patient as not needing a higher level of care (e.g., trauma center), when in fact they do. This is false-negative triage classification.[45] *Undertriage* is a medical problem that may result in an adverse patient outcome. The receiving medical facility may not be adequate to diagnose and treat the trauma victim.

Defining an acceptable level of undertriage is dependent on how one defines the patient requiring trauma center care. One method is to identify all the potentially preventable causes. Using this method, a target undertriage rate would be 1% or less. Using a broader definition, undertriage would also result in patients being sent to institutions without the capability to render appropriate care. In this instance, an undertriage rate of 5–10% is accepted.[45]

Another method is to determine how many major trauma patients were incorrectly transported to a nontrauma center. If an ISS of greater than 16 or more is used to define the major trauma patient, undertriaged patients would be those patients (ISS >16), who were taken to a nontrauma center hospital. Using this method, an acceptable undertriage rate can be as high as 5%.[45]

*Overtriage* is a decision that incorrectly classifies a patient as needing a trauma center, although retrospective analysis suggests that such care was not justified. Overtriage has been said to result in over utilization of finite material, i.e., financial and human resources.[46,47]

## COMPONENTS OF TRIAGE TOOLS AND DECISION-MAKING

Trauma triage decisions are usually made within a limited time frame and are based on information that can be difficult to obtain. These decisions are based on evidence gathered in the field that estimates the potential for severe injury. Physiologic and anatomic criteria, mechanism of injury, and comorbid factors are used in the triage decision-making process. Unfortunately, all these criteria have limitations that affect their validity in certain situations. The judgment of experienced EMS personnel is also a key factor in triage.

## PHYSIOLOGIC CRITERIA

Physiologic data is felt to represent a snapshot into the well-being of an injured patient.[45] Physiologic criteria include measurements of basic life sustaining functions such as heart rate, blood pressure, respiratory rate and effort, level of consciousness, and temperature. The advantage of physiologic data is that it is readily assessable in

the field with a simple physical examination. This data can be ranked into a numerical format, which allows it to be quantified; and used in various trauma scoring systems such as the revised trauma score. The larger the deviation from normal, the more likely there is a severe injury. In this way, physiologic data may correlate to severity of injury and may predict serious injury or death. Patients who have sustained a mortal injury tend to have the greatest deviation in their vital signs.[48–50] The problem is that their ability to detect physiologic derangement is time-dependent. A single set of physiologic signs is only a snapshot to the patient's state. Patients who have sustained significant injury may not manifest physiologic changes immediately after the event and, as a result, are at risk for undertriage.[31] A significant injury may take some time to manifest life-threatening hemorrhage or tension pneumothorax. This is especially true of young, otherwise healthy adults who have significant physiologic compensation mechanisms that may mask the true extent of the injury.

## ANATOMIC CRITERIA

The anatomic location and external appearance of the injury aid in the immediate field triage decisions. This visual picture of the injured patient may be sufficient for an experienced triage officer to make a disposition decision without further evaluation. In a mass casualty event, rapid triage may be performed with a quick visual exam of the patient. Anatomic criteria that suggest triage to a trauma center may include, but are not limited to: penetrating injury to the head, neck, torso, or proximal extremity; two or more proximal long-bone fractures; pelvic fracture; flail chest; amputation proximal to the wrist or angle; limb paralysis; or greater than 10% total body surface area burn or inhalation injury.[51] Each regionalized trauma system must decide what constitutes significant anatomic injury as a triage criterion.[52]

Anatomic injury may be challenging to predict reliably based on physical examination in the field. Fracture of long bones, amputations, and skin and soft tissue injuries may appear devastating in the field but are rarely life threatening and may distract the field examiner as well as the patient from more subtle and serious injuries.

Significant blunt chest and abdominal injuries can have little external evidence of internal injury and initial physical examination lacks diagnostic accuracy.[53–57] Other significant injuries missed on initial examination include spine[58–60] and certain types of pelvic injuries. A[61] pelvic bony injury can be diagnosed on physical examination in the awake, cooperative patient[62,63]; however, a significant number of trauma victims have altered mental status due to head injury or ingestion of drugs or alcohol.[64–66]

The distinction between blunt and penetrating injury is an important triage distinction. Oftentimes there may be little external trauma to the patient. However, recognition of the penetrating wounds correlated with the likelihood of internal injury are needed to effectively triage these patients. Penetrating injuries to trunk and proximal extremities are of concern because of their proximity to vital structures; however, it is nearly impossible to know the direction or depth of penetration while in the field. Finally, the triage officer must expeditiously evaluate patients and not perform time-consuming physical examinations in the field which only slow down the triage process. Complex patients may be better served by urgent transport to a trauma center.

## MECHANISM OF INJURY

Evaluation is more than the simple determination of how a trauma injury occurred. To the trained eye, it can give information on the type, amount, and direction of force or energy applied to the body. Prehospital personnel, who view the effects of the forces that were applied during the injurious event, can estimate the amount of energy involved. This, in turn, helps predict the likelihood of injury.[67-69] Mechanisms of injury felt to have a high potential for major trauma include falls of more than 15 ft; motor vehicle accidents with a fatality at the scene, passenger ejection, prolonged extrication (>20 min), or major intrusion of the passenger compartment; pedestrians struck by a motor vehicle; motorcycle accidents of more than 20 mph; or any penetrating injuries to the head, neck, torso, or proximal extremities. When used as a triage criterion by itself, mechanism of injury results in the high over-triage rate. However, when combined with other triage components, such as physiologic indices and anatomic injury, mechanism of injury improves the sensitivity and specificity of the triage process.[69-71]

## AGE, COMORBID DISEASE, AND ENVIRONMENTAL CONCERNS

Age has been shown to impact the outcome of trauma victims and should be taken into consideration when triaging a patient. Elderly trauma victims, using a variety of definitions (i.e., >55 years old, >65 years old, etc.) have been shown to have increased morbidity and mortality compared to younger trauma victims.[72-77] When compared to young patients, the elderly are at risk for undertriage, because a similar amount of force may cause a greater magnitude of injury.[42,73]

The effect of age on morbidity and mortality is not as clear in the pediatric population.[78] There are significant differences in physiology and anatomy in the pediatric population that require specialized equipment, facilities, and personnel. Certainly, the optimal treatment involves identifying the unique resources needed to care for the injured child and having those available when needed. These differences are significant enough that specialized triage criteria have been developed for the pediatric population.[79,80]

Chronic diseases have also been shown to have a significant impact on morbidity and mortality in the trauma victim independent of age and injury severity.[81-83] Acute conditions such as ethanol or cocaine intoxication or systemic anticoagulation may also impact morbidity and mortality. Comorbidities such as cardiopulmonary, hepatic, renal disease, diabetes mellitus, malignancy, or neurologic disorders, have been found to have increased mortality rates compared to their disease-free counterparts.[84] The problem is that many times the associated medical condition of the patient cannot be ascertained in the prehospital arena unless the patient has identification such as a medical alert bracelet or a relative who can provide the necessary history to the field personnel.

### TABLE 4-3

**Commonly Used Trauma Triage Criteria**

**Physiologic and Anatomic Criteria**
Glasgow Coma Scale of 13 or less
Systolic blood pressure of 90 or less
Respiratory rate of 10 per minute or less, or greater than 29 per m
Sustained pulse rate of 120 per m or more
Head trauma with altered state of consciousness, hemiplegia, or uneven pupils
Penetrating injuries of the head, neck, torso, and extremities proximal to the elbow or knee
Chest trauma with respiratory distress or signs of shock

**Pelvic Fractures**
Amputations above the wrist or ankle

**Limb Paralysis**
Two or more proximal long bone fractures
Combination of trauma with burns
Mechanism of Injury and High Energy Impact
Fall of 20 feet or more
Patient struck by a vehicle moving 20 MPH or more
Patient ejected from a vehicle
Vehicle rollover with the patient unrestrained
High speed crash (initial speed of >40 MPH) with 20 inches of major front end deformity, 12 inches or more deformity into the passenger compartment
Patient was a survivor of a MVA where a death occurred in the same vehicle

**Other Criteria**
Age of less than 5 years old, or over 55 years old
History of cardiac disease, respiratory disease, insulin dependent diabetes, cirrhosis, or morbid obesity
Pregnancy
Immunosuppressed patients
Patients with bleeding disorders, or patients on anticoagulants
Burns of greater than 30% of body surface area in adults, or 15% body surface area in children
Burns of the head, hands, feet, or genital area
Inhalation injuries
Electrical burns
Burns associated with multiple trauma or severe medical problems

Environmental extremes can have serious consequences for the trauma patient. Hypothermia is known to have adverse physiologic effects, prolongs blood coagulation time, and contributes to mortality.[85-88] Prolonged heat exposure may lead to dehydration. Burn injuries require accurate assessment for resuscitation and wound care, as well as evaluation for potential inhalation injury. When combined with associated trauma, patient management can be complex.[89] (Table 4-3)

## PARAMEDIC JUDGMENT

A working familiarity of clear, concise, and reliable triage guidelines are essential for effective triage.[90] Experience and judgment of EMS personnel are crucial to this mission. EMS personnel are in a unique position to directly assess the trauma scene, ascertain the mechanism of injury, determine the extent of the patient's injuries, and estimate the patient's physiologic response. For example, a patient with a fractured femur due to a frontal, high-speed motor vehicle collision will be evaluated and triaged differently than will a patient with a femur fracture due to a low-speed collision. Paramedic triage is outlined in the prehospital trauma life support manual.[91]

Several studies have shown that prehospital field personnel judgment can be as good or better than the available triage scoring methods commonly in use[92,93] and, when combined with other triage criteria, improves on the identification of major trauma victims.[93–96] In a systematic review of Mulholland there was no conclusive evidence for/or against paramedic judgment in the field.[97] The one constant theme in triage at all levels of medical personnel was the level of clinical experience. Pointer and colleagues[98] studied the compliance of paramedics to established triage rules. Paramedics triage was best when evaluating triaging based upon a patient's injury patterns. Compliance was intermediate when based upon mechanism of injury and the lowest for patients evaluated for physiologic triage criteria. They demonstrated a paramedic undertriage rate of 9.6%, which is relatively close to the acceptable 5% or less undertriage rate.

## CURRENT FIELD METHODS FOR FIELD TRIAGE SCORING

In order for a triage scoring method to be acceptable for use in the field, it must meet certain criteria.[99,100] The components of the scoring scheme must be credible, meaning that they have some correlating relationship with the injuries being described. Because there is no "gold standard" to test the accuracy of the scoring scheme, the results of the scoring scheme must be in general agreement with other, currently accepted scoring methods.[101]

The triage scoring method must correlate with outcome. The scores that indicate more severe injury should identify the patients with worse outcomes. The better the correlation with outcome, the lower the undertriage and overtriage rates within a trauma care system. Outcomes for major trauma victims are usually classified as death, need for urgent/emergent surgical intervention, length of intensive care unit (ICU) and/or hospital stay, and major single-system or multisystem organ injuries.

The scoring scheme must also have inter and intra-observer reliability; that is, it should be able to be consistently applied between observers and by the same observer at another point in time with the same results. Finally, the scoring scheme must be practical and easily applied to trauma victims for a variety of mechanisms, by a variety of personnel without the need of specialized training or equipment.[102]

## SPECIFIC TRIAGE METHODS-DEFINITIONS

### Trauma Index

The Trauma Index was one of the earliest triage scoring methods, first reported in 1971 by Kirkpatrick and Youmans.[103] It included measures of five variables: blood pressure, respiratory status, central nervous system (CNS) status, anatomic region, and type of injury. One study showed some correlation with injury severity[104];

however, the Trauma Index never saw widespread use. A revision of the Trauma Index in 1990 reported undertriage and overtriage rates comparable to those of the Trauma Score, CRAMS, Prehospital Index, and Mechanism of Injury scales and correlated to the final ISS.[105]

### Glasgow Coma Scale

When Teasdale and Jennett first introduced the Glasgow Coma Scale (GCS),[106] it was intended as a description of the functional status of the CNS, regardless of the type of insult to the brain, and was never intended to be used as a prehospital assessment tool. The three components of the score reflect different levels of brain function with eye opening corresponding to the brainstem, motor response corresponding to CNS function, and verbal response corresponding to CNS integration.

Because the degree of injury to the CNS is considered to be a major determinant of outcome in trauma victims, many of the field triage tools measure CNS function, including the Trauma Score (TS),[107] the Revised Trauma Score (RTS),[108] the CRAMS scale,[109] and the Trauma Triage Rule.[107–110] Interpretation of GCS in the presence of an intubated patient diminishes the ability to use the GCS as a prehospital evaluation tool.[111] A more recent study found that the motor component of the GCS is almost as good as the Trauma Score and better than the ISS in predicting mortality. This suggests that the motor component score could be used to identify patients who are likely to require urgent trauma center care.[112]

### Triage Index, Trauma Score, Revised Trauma Score

The Triage Index (TI) was described in 1981, and analyzed physiologic parameters of an injured patient.[113] These variables were examined alone and in combination in an effort to make the TI more precise. One year later, Champion et al. modified the TI by adding systolic blood pressure and respiratory effort in an effort to be more discriminatory in patient severity identification. The resulting Trauma Score (TS) was designed to look at those physiologic parameters known to be associated with higher severity of injury if found to be abnormal.[107] Central to this idea was the fact that the known leading causes of traumatic death were related to dysfunction of the cardiovascular, respiratory, and central nervous system. The authors recommended trauma center care for trauma victims with a TS of 12 or less. The TS was revised in 1989 because of concerns about accurate assessment of capillary refill and respiratory effort at night as well as potential underestimation of CNS injury.[108] These components were deleted and the revised trauma score (r-TS) consists of three parameters: GCS, systolic blood pressure, and respiratory rate.

### CRAMS Scale

CRAMS stands for circulation, respiration, abdominal/thoracic, motor, and speech. It was first proposed as a simplified method of field triage.[109–114] These parameters are individually assessed and assigned a value corresponding to normal, mildly abnormal, or markedly abnormal. With a range of 0 to 10, a score of 8 or less signifies major trauma, indicating that the patient should be taken to a designated trauma center. Both retrospective and prospective studies have shown that the CRAMS method of triage is accurate in identifying major trauma victims with relatively high specificity and sensitivity and is easy to use.[114,115]

## Prehospital Index

The prehospital index (PHI) consists of field measurements of blood pressure, pulse, respiratory status, and level of consciousness, which were determined to have the best correlation with mortality or the need for surgery. A subsequent prospective multicenter validation study by the same authors showed that the PHI is accurate in predicting the need for life-saving surgery within 4 hours and death within 72 hours following injury.[116,117] Furthermore, the attachment of non time-dependent variables such as age, body region injured, and mechanism of injury to the PHI improved the predictive power to select those patients who were likely to need intensive care or a surgical procedure.

## Trauma Triage Rule

The Trauma Triage Rule (TTR) proposed by Baxt et al. consists of measurements of blood pressure, the GCS motor response, and the anatomic region and type of injury.[110] Rather than comparing the scoring method to traditional outcome measures to determine the factors that constitute a major trauma victim, major trauma was defined a priori as a systolic blood pressure of less than 85 mm Hg; a GCS motor component score of 5 or less; or penetrating trauma to the head, neck, or trunk. Retrospective review revealed major trauma victim identification with a sensitivity and specificity of 92%. The TTR was concluded to potentially reduce overtriage while maintaining an acceptable undertriage rate. However, it has not been adapted widely.

## Disaster Triage: START—Simple Triage and Rapid Treatment

In the event of a mass casualty or disaster, EMS personnel may utilize the START triage system initially developed to be used in earthquakes in California.[118] The object of this system is to triage large numbers of patients rapidly. It is relatively simple and can be used with limited training.[119] The focus of START is to evaluate four physiologic variables: the patient's ability to ambulate, respiratory function, systemic perfusion, and level of consciousness. It can be performed by lay and emergency personnel. Victims are usually divided into one of the four groups with color codes according to the timing of care delivery based on the clinical evaluation as follows: (a) green—minor injuries (walking wounded); (b) red—immediate; (c) yellow—delayed; and (d) black—unsalvageable or deceased.

If the patient is able to walk they are classified as a delayed transport, but if not, ventilation is assessed. If the respiratory rate is >30 the patient is an immediate transport. If the respiratory rate is <30, perfusion is assessed. A capillary refill of >2 seconds will mandate an immediate transport. If the capillary refill is <2 seconds the patient's level of consciousness is assessed. If the patient cannot follow commands, they are immediately transported; otherwise they are a delayed transport.[120] The Fire Department of New York used this system during the World Trade Center disaster. Unfortunately, due to the collapse of the buildings and

concern for the safety of the rescue workers, the START system came to a complete halt.[121] It resumed only when it was declared safe to approach ground zero.

In some systems the START system is coupled with severity scores: in the immediate category the trauma score varies from 3 to 10; in the urgent category the trauma score varies from 10 to 11, and in the delayed (nonurgent) group the trauma score is 12.

The triage principles are the same for children and adults. However, due to differences in physiology, response to insults, ability to talk and walk, and anatomic differences, disaster triage in the pediatric age group is not straightforward. Assessment tools have been proposed to increase the accuracy of the process but were found to have major limitations.

The START system is important in the triage of the severely injured trauma patient because those requiring surgical care are transported by air or ground ambulances to trauma centers distant enough from the incident where the number of victims is lower and the resources are still available to provide optimal care.

## Combination Methods

While most of the field triage criteria are based on physiologic criteria, there are other methods for assessing the severity of the potential injury to a trauma victim. As shown earlier in the chapter, mechanism of injury, anatomic region and type of injury, pre-existing illnesses, and paramedic judgment are important considerations in providing additional information in the field to help determine whether a patient requires transport to a designated trauma center. Combination field triage methods make use of this additional information by including it in the initial evaluation of the trauma victim.

## American College of Surgeons Field Triage System

The ACS Field Triage System is a more complete, advanced triage scoring scheme that is described in the Resources for Optimal Care of the Injured Patient. This decision scheme describes indications for transport of the trauma victim to a trauma center based on specific physiologic and anatomy of injury variables. In addition, mechanism of injury and comorbid factors are evaluated and, if specific criteria are met, may also indicate transport to a trauma center. Finally, if there is concern on the part of the prehospital medical personnel that the victim may have significant injuries, consideration is given to taking the patient to the designated trauma center. Figure 4-4 shows the triage decision scheme which is widely used throughout the country.

## APPLICATION OF TRIAGE PRINCIPLES FOR MULTIPLE PATIENT SCENARIOS

Triage principles may need to be modified to include triage of multiple patient and mass casualty situations.

### Single Patient

Triaging a single trauma victim is relatively straightforward. The prehospital care provider assesses the patient according to the

# FIELD TRIAGE DECISION SCHEME

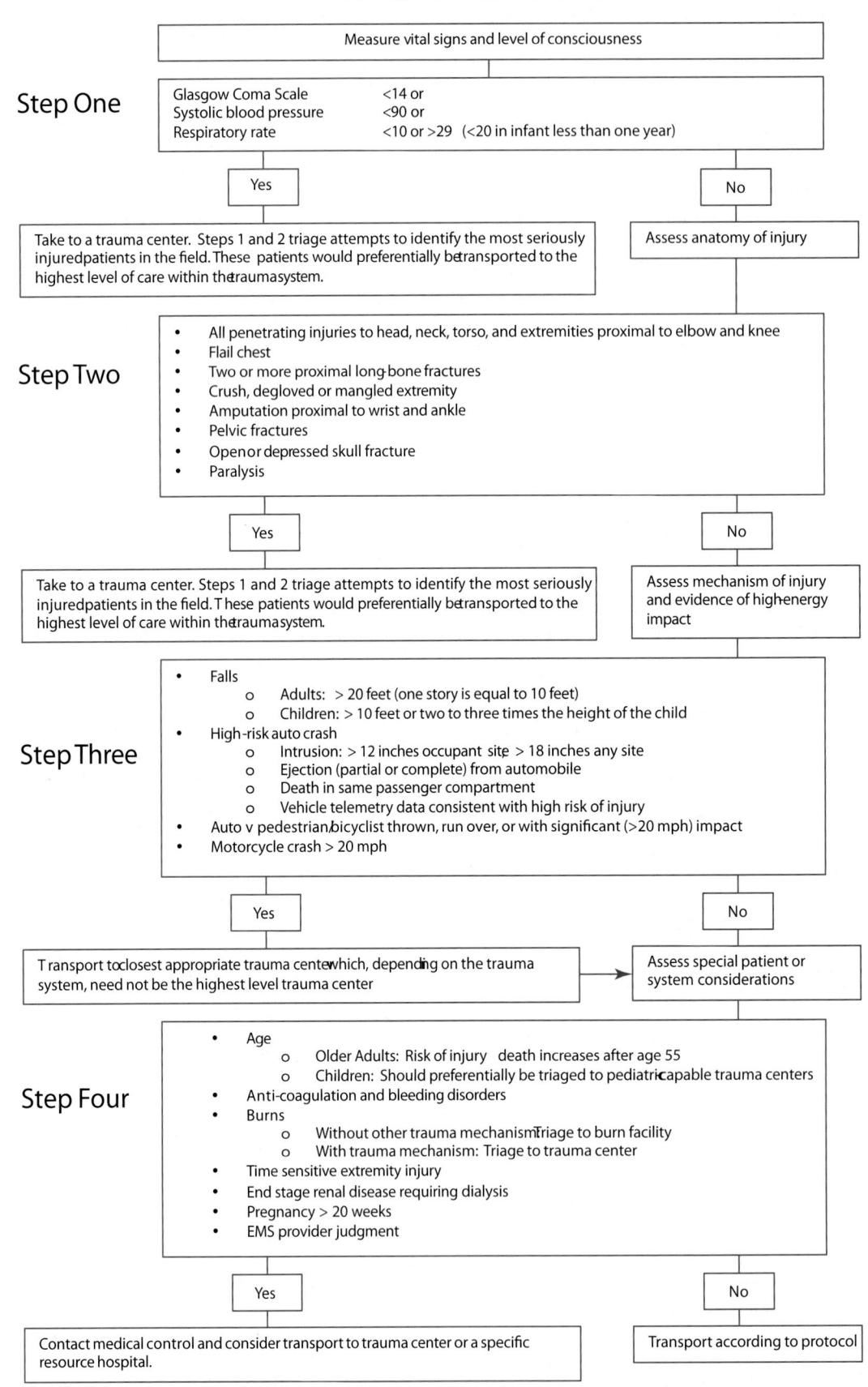

**FIGURE 4-4.** Prehospital triage decision scheme recommended by the American College of Surgeons *Committee on Trauma.*
*(Reproduced with permission from The American College of Surgeons Committee on Trauma. Resources for Optimal Care of the Injured Patient: 2006. Chicago, American College of Surgeons.)*

defined triage criteria for that particular regionalized trauma system. If the patient meets the criteria of a major trauma victim, he or she is transported to the nearest designated trauma center.

## Multiple Casualties

In the situation of multiple patients, such as seen with multiple cars involved in the same accident, the same essential principles apply; however, decisions must be made in the field as to which patients have priority. A state of multiple casualties occurs when the numbers of patients and injury severity do not exceed the hospital resources. Those patients who are identified as major trauma victims by field triage criteria have priority over those who appear less injured. All major trauma patients should be transported to a trauma center as long as the trauma center has adequate resources to manage all the patients effectively. This type of situation can stress local resources, and possible diversion of the less critically injured to another trauma center should be considered. Monitoring transports with online computer assistance allows for contemporaneous determination if one trauma center is overwhelmed.

## Mass Casualties

Triage in this situation is unique in that priorities are different from those in the single- or multiple-victim scenarios. In the instance of mass casualties, the resources of the designated trauma center, as well as the regional trauma system, are overwhelmed. When resources are inadequate to meet the needs of all the victims, priority shifts from providing care to those with the most urgent need to providing care to those with the highest probability of survival.

A severely injured patient, who would consume a large amount of medical resources, is now a lower triage priority. Despite the potential salvageability of this patient, the medical resources are focused on other patients who would benefit from advanced medical and surgical care. This method provides the greatest good for the greatest number of people. Field triage in this situation is probably the most difficult to perform as one has to make choices of quantity over quality with very limited amounts of information. These issues are further complicated when dealing with children.[122,123]

The most experienced and best-trained personnel available should make these field triage decisions. Physicians may be the best qualified to make these triage decisions; however, if they are the only receiving physicians available, direct patient care should take precedence and triage decisions would fall to other personnel. Patients are identified according to a triage code, based on the severity of injuries and likelihood of survival, and are treated accordingly.[124–126] Occasionally, there may be an indication for a specialized surgical triage team with the capability to render acute lifesaving care of an injured trapped patient.[127] In some disaster scenarios moving the intensive care into a disaster zone may be beneficial when evacuation of patients may be unrealistic due to logistical reasons.[128]

In order to optimize patient care in these situations, it is important for regionalized systems to periodically have mock disaster drills. These drills allow for the proper training of all individuals who might be involved as well as the identification and correction of potential problems.[126,129] With increasing terrorist

activity, specific triage algorithms have been developed for specific scenarios such as biologic, chemical, radiologic, or blast attacks.[130]

## Disaster Management

Events surrounding the recent terrorist attacks of the Oklahoma Federal Building, World Trade Center, the Pentagon, and natural disasters such as Katrina, should crystallize the resolve of all medical personnel to become educated and proficient in disaster management. The approach to disasters, whether natural or man-made, requires a coordinated relief effort of EMS, hospital, fire, police, and public works personnel. This multiorganizational operation can function in a crisis environment only if it well directed and controlled. The ability to assess a disaster scene, call in appropriate personnel to provide damage control, fire and rescue operations, and crowd control is dependent upon an organization structure which permits dynamic information processing and decision making of vital scene information.

The military uses the concept of command and control for its combat operations. Key personnel continually monitor and manage the battlefield situation. The Fire Service of the US Department of Forestry, in 1970, adapted command and control into an incident command structure.[118,121] Within this framework, a centralized group of disaster personnel work to command and control all of resources at the disaster site. Dynamic disaster scene information is processed at the incident command and decisions as to how best to engage the rescue resources are implemented.

The incident command center structure is composed of seven key groups. If the disaster is small in scope a single person may fill all seven areas. As the disaster increases in scope, more personnel are required to fulfill these functions. The incident commander is responsible for the entire rescue or recovery operation. Under the direction of the incident commander, are the seven group commanders: operations, logistics, planning, finance, safety, information, and liaison. Each of these section commanders has well-defined areas of authority and responsibility. Continuous on-scene information will be communicated to the command center. This will enable the incident command center to plan and direct the rescue or recovery operation. Thus, limited resources and key personnel will be directed to produce the greatest benefit.

The disaster scene is typically divided into zones of operation. Ground zero is the inner hazard zone where the fire and rescue operations occur. EMS and other nonessential personnel are kept out of this area. Rescued victims are brought out of this area to the EMS staging area. This is the second zone, a primary casualty receiving area, and it is here that EMS personnel perform triage and initial care for the patient. Disposition directly to the hospital may occur or the patient may be sent to a distant receiving area for care and ultimate triage and transport.

The distant casualty receiving areas provides for additional safety in the environment. This downstream movement of injured patients prevents the primary triage sites from being overrun. Transportation of the wounded from the primary receiving site is reserved for the most seriously injured patients. Thus, a tiered triage approach is developed. A temporary morgue is also set up at a distant site.

Typically, groups of patients, the walking wounded, will migrate toward the nearest medical treatment facility. This process is called convergence. Medical facilities will often set up a triage area in front of the emergency department to handle these patients. Present day medical teaching supports the treatment of any patient who arrives at an institution's doorstep. Perhaps thought should be given to transporting groups of these patients to secondary medical facilities so that the closer hospitals do not become overburdened with an influx of patients. The use of outpatient operating facilities is being considered for this purpose.

The final operational zone of the disaster site is the outer perimeter. Police permit only essential personnel access into the disaster site. Crowd and traffic control ensure the safety and security of the disaster scene as well as to provide emergency vehicles rapid transit to and from the site.

Disasters may be of a small scale such as an intra-facility fire or explosion and may remain only a local or regional problem. As was seen at the World Trade Center, the magnitude of a local disaster was of such proportions that a national response was needed to address the rescue and recovery efforts. The standard appeal for this today is to activate the National Disaster Medical System.

Interestingly, in some of the more recent natural disasters, there have been approximately 10–15% of the survivors who were seriously injured. The remaining people were either dead or had mild to moderate trauma. It becomes a pivotal task to rapidly sort through the survivors and identify the level of care needed by each patient. In the World Trade Center, the New York Fire Department and EMS utilized the START system. The initial scene casualties were from the planes striking the building. Fire and rescue personnel could not reach these patients. With the collapse of the first tower, rescue operations were aborted and attempts to evacuate rescue personnel became paramount.[121] Following the collapse, victims injured in the street or from the surrounding buildings required medical treatment. As rescue operations resumed, injured rescue workers began to arrive at medical treatment facilities. Unfortunately, there were only five survivors of the Twin Tower collapse with over 3000 fatalities, which included civilians and rescue personnel.

The experience in Israel with terrorist attacks has demonstrated that rapid and accurate triage is critical to decrease or minimize mortality. Therefore, it has been suggested that the best triage officer, at least in bombings and shooting massacres, which are the most common form of terrorist violence, is the trauma surgeon. This is important to guarantee that those in real need of immediate surgical attention are seen and treated in a timely fashion without inundating the hospitals with patients that can be treated at a later time.

Critical concepts have been learned from the Israeli experience. These include rapid and abbreviated care, unidirectional flow of casualties, minimization of the use of diagnostic tests, and relief of medical teams ever so often to maintain quality and effectiveness in care delivery. The concepts of damage control should be liberally applied in the operating room to free up resources for the next "wave" of injured individuals.[131–135]

In mass casualties, hospitals become overwhelmed very easily. Therefore, communication between hospitals is critical to distribute the casualties in an evenly fashion.

Surgeons should be familiar with the basic principles of mass casualty management. Trauma surgeons should be the leaders in this field, as trauma systems serve as a template for the triage, evacuation, and treatment of mass casualty victims. The American College of Surgeons has emphasized on this critical role for surgeons.[136]

## CURRENT EVIDENCE FOR TRIAGE GUIDELINES

There is little argument that a regionalized trauma system reduces the number of potentially preventable deaths due to trauma.[24,26,137] To do so, one must accurately select which trauma victim will benefit from the resources of a trauma center. The dilemma is two-fold: (1) which criteria should be used to define the "major trauma" victims, and (2) how are these patients identified in the field? Other relevant questions include: Does selective triage of patients in terms of hospital resources at the time of hospital admission benefit the major trauma patient, and, if so, what selection criteria are the most appropriate? Do transport times modify the definition of a major trauma victim, and does this influence outcome? Finally, do present field triage criteria provide adequate rates of undertriage and overtriage? Each of these questions will be addressed individually.

### Major Trauma Patient

The definition of a major trauma patient is a person who has sustained potentially life- or limb-threatening injuries and is based on retrospective analysis of the patient's injuries. The major trauma definition is used primarily to monitor field triage criteria as well as calculate undertriage and overtriage rates within a regional trauma system. Unfortunately, there is no absolute standard for the criteria that have been used when defining major trauma. The best that can be accomplished is to retrospectively compare quantified injury severity data to mortality and then use a predefined threshold as defining major trauma.

The Injury Severity Score (ISS) is a measure of physical injury, based on adding up the square of the three highest individual anatomic injury scores (Abbreviated Injury Scale [AIS], range 1 to 6) calculated from all of the patient's known injuries.[42] When used to define major trauma, an ISS of 15 or more has been the most frequently utilized threshold. Using this definition, a trauma victim must have a single anatomic injury score of 4, or two AIS 3 injuries in order to be categorized as sustaining "major trauma". Because ISS has been shown to have a good correlation with mortality over a wide range of ages[138] and different types of injuries,[138–141] it has been the most frequently utilized method for stratifying the injuries of patients for comparison with prehospital triage scores.[141–144] However, it has several shortcomings when used as a determinant of major trauma with regard to analysis of field triage criteria.

Several studies have shown that preventable deaths can occur with a single AIS 3 injury.[23,145] For example, a patient with a closed head injury and an AIS of 3 is at a higher risk of death than if the patient had a similar grade extremity injury. As a result, there is no consensus on the numeric value of ISS that defines major trauma. Stewart and colleagues used an ISS of greater than 12 to define their study population when they reported on the improvement in outcomes of motor vehicle accident victims after trauma center designation.[146] Similarly, Petrie and colleagues also used an ISS of greater than 12 when they reported on the improvement of outcomes of patients who had trauma team activation when compared to those who did not.[147] However, Morris and colleagues defined major trauma as a patient with an ISS of 20 or more when they reported on the ability of the Trauma Score to prospectively identify patients with life-threatening injuries.[148] Additionally, Norwood and coworkers stratified their patient sample into two groups based on injury severity scores—19 or less and 20 or more—when they reported on outcomes from a rural-based trauma center.[149] Thus, comparing studies that define major trauma becomes very difficult due to the differences in the ISS threshold.

A second problem with ISS is that it is based on injuries identified within specific anatomic regions and takes into account only one injury per body region.[150] Therefore, ISS may not be a sensitive indicator of certain types of injuries. Several studies have found that ISS is not as accurate in identifying the severity of the injury in penetrating or blunt[151] trauma, in which several organ systems may be injured within the same anatomic location. This has led to the development of specialized anatomic injury scoring systems such as the Penetrating Abdominal Trauma Index (PATI)[152] and, ultimately, the Organ Injury Scale (OIS)[153] that may more accurately reflect the severity of the injury. A modification to the calculation of ISS scoring has been introduced as the New Injury Severity Score (NISS), which is defined as the sum of the squares of the AIS scores of each of a patient's three most severe AIS injuries regardless of the body region in which they occur. This method has been found to be more predictive of survival, but may overestimate the severity of injury for lesser injury grades.[154,155] In addition, injury severity scoring may also be inaccurate. Rutledge found that the ISS fails to differentiate between severity of injury and mismanagement of injury and, as a result, assigns an increased injury severity to lesser injuries of inappropriately managed patients.[143]

Transport times may need to be included in the definition of the major trauma patient[143] when used for triage or interfacility transport purposes, particularly when they exceed 30 minutes. When time is added to lesser injuries before definitive care, then ongoing bleeding, the magnitude of the resuscitation, and the relative stability of the patient may increase the injury severity of otherwise equivalent injuries. A number of studies have shown that hemodynamic and respiratory dysfunction,[156] as well as mortality,[157] is increased with increasing transport times. As such, when long transport times are a problem and complications due to long transport and inadequate resuscitation can be anticipated, these patients should be considered for a higher level of care where critical care resources are more likely to be available. Patient transport modalities and point to trauma center time of transport are unique to each region. Goldstein et al. validated a transport decision process that utilized a modification of the prehospital index (the pretransport index) and documented the time and distance from a trauma center for these trauma transfer patients in British Columbia. The pretransport index adds onto the two PHI variables: intubation and pneumothorax. Accurate recognition of the more seriously injured patients and the knowledge of the quickest modality to transport the patient to a trauma center resulted in a quicker time to definitive time to care.[158] Utilization of the most appropriate mode for specific patient needs maximally utilize health care resources and dollars.

## Field Triage Scores

Triage scores that are based on physiologic data are accurate in doing so. Baxt and colleagues found that the TS, CRAMS scale, RTS, and the PHI have good correlation with the ISS and are able

to predict mortality with a sensitivity of at least 85%.[99] However, no single field triage scoring scheme has been universally accepted as the gold standard.[51] This is due, in part, to the fact that there is no agreed-upon standard that defines "major trauma" that allows for comparison of the individual triage scoring systems. An evidence-based analysis is limited by this problem. As a result, each of the individual scoring systems has its advocates as well as critics.

When Gormican[109] originally described the CRAMS scale, rather than using an ISS threshold to define major trauma, he defined it as the patient who died in the emergency department or went directly to the operating room (OR). Minor trauma was defined as a patient who was discharged home from the emergency department. Using a CRAMS score of 8 or less to signify major trauma, he found a sensitivity of 92% and a specificity of 98% in identifying major trauma victims. Others examined the ability of the CRAMS scale to accurately identify patients who required admission to the hospital or any operation for their injuries. Using this definition for major trauma, they found that a CRAMS score of 8 or less failed to identify two out of three patients.[93]

Champion, who constructed the Trauma Score by analyzing CNS, cardiovascular, and respiratory data, a priori defined major trauma as a TS of 12 or less because it correlated with a decreased probability of survival.[107] Ornato and colleagues' study showed that a TS of 12 or less also failed to identify two out of three patients who required admission or an operation.[93] Similar criticisms in the literature can be found for the prehospital index (PHI) for its failure to accurately identify patients requiring emergency surgery,[159] and the RTS for its low sensitivity in identifying patients requiring emergency treatment.[160] The addition of the variables of age, body region injured, mechanism of injury, comorbidity, and the PHI improved prediction of the PHI alone by 10% (sensitivity of 76 vs. 66%).[161] Unfortunately, the addition of mechanism of injury to the PHI was almost as accurate as all of the major descriptors.[162]

Baxt and coworkers reported that the physiologic based triage scores were unable to accurately identify survivors of major injuries, each score having a sensitivity and specificity of less than 70%.[49] Holcomb recently evaluated the utility of manual vital signs plus the GCS (motor and verbal scores) to predict the need for life-saving interventions in non closed head injured patients. In this group, patients with a weak radial arterial pulse had an 11-fold increase in the need for a life-saving intervention. A GCS verbal score of 2-3 in a non closed head injured patient had a six-fold while a GCS motor score of 2–3 had a 20-fold increase in the need for a life-saving intervention. An additional conclusion was that the addition of automated vital sign reporting, oxygen saturation monitors, or end tidal $CO_2$ monitors did not improve the predictive model of which patients might need a life-saving intervention.[163]

The incorporation of non-time-dependent data, such as mechanism of injury, anatomic injury, and comorbid factors, has been shown to make physiologic-based triage scores more sensitive in identifying the major trauma victim.[164,165] However, questions have also been raised as to whether this type of data identifies the major trauma patient. Its ability to do so appears to be dependent on the context in which it is used. For example, Cooper and colleagues found that mechanism of injury had a positive predictive value of only 6.9% when used to identify patients with an ISS of 16 or greater. They concluded that it did not justify bypass of local hospitals when used as a sole criterion for triage to a trauma center.[166]

There are conflicting reports when analyzing non-time-dependent criteria as a determinant of outcome in trauma patients. Smith and colleagues stratified patients into age over 65 and age under 65, and they found that pre-existing conditions did not significantly affect outcome. Age, however, was a significant determinant of mortality.[167] DeKeyser and colleagues compared the mortality and functional outcomes of patients who were stratified into three groups based on age: age 35 to 45, age 55 to 64, and age 65 and over. They found that there were no differences between the three groups in terms of ISS, mortality rates, or functional outcome.[168] Van der Sluis and colleagues also evaluated differences in mortality and long-term outcome between young and elderly patients. They analyzed two groups of patients with an ISS of 16 or greater: age 20 to 29 and age 60 and over. They reported that while there was a significant difference in terms of early mortality, survivors of both groups were discharged in equal percentages and their functional outcome two years after injury was essentially the same.[169]

A possible explanation for these contradictory findings may be that there are interactions between all the possible factors that have not been previously appreciated. Hill and colleagues analyzed multiple factors as possible determinants of outcome in major trauma patients (ISS >15). They found that preresuscitation GCS was the overall strongest predictor of mortality. However, when the patients were stratified into different GCS categories (GCS score 3, 4 to 12, and 13 to 15) and the same analysis was performed, they found that each group had a different factor that best predicted mortality. Systolic blood pressure was the strongest predictor of mortality in the GCS 3 group, ISS in the GCS 4 to 12 group, and age in the GCS 13 to 15 group.[170]

Finally, the use of non-time-dependent data requires that the prehospital personnel have enough training and experience to recognize, interpret, and report it to the physician. Burstein and coworkers reviewed the prehospital emergency medical services (EMS) reports for specific ACS mechanism of injury triage criteria and found that it was underreported in standard EMS reporting documentation. Reporting improved with the use of a structured data instrument that requested the presence or absence of the criteria.[171] A paramedic's ability to recognize and report this type of criteria may explain the discrepancy in studies reporting on the ability of paramedic judgment to correctly[172,173] or incorrectly[174] triage patients to a trauma center. The mechanism of injury does seem to have a correlation with the need for a higher intensity of medical care or operation. In a study by Santaneillo, nearly 50% of patients who met a mechanism of injury criteria needed an operative intervention.[175]

## In-Hospital Triage

Secondary, or in-hospital, triage complements field triage by stratifying the immediate needs of the trauma patient at the time of admission. The emphasis of this retriage is to direct the patient into the proper hospital area; urgent care, emergent care, trauma bay, or the operating room.[176] During a multiple casualty event, this in-hospital triage is essential to maximize hospital resource allocation and patient flow.

Tinkoff and colleagues reported on a two-tiered trauma response protocol.[177] They used field triage criteria to identify patients requiring either a surgery-supervised "trauma code" or an emergency medicine-supervised "trauma alert." Using this protocol, they found that accurate identification of the most seriously injured patients was achieved as demonstrated by the improved ability to predict those patients who would require direct disposition to the operating room or intensive care unit. Prehospital prediction models as well as admission systemic inflammatory response syndrome (SIRS) scores may be useful to predict the need for ICU services, and estimate length of stay and potential mortality of seriously injured patients.[178,179]

Hoyt and colleagues originally described predefined field criteria that indicated OR resuscitation.[41] Indications included cardiac arrest with one vital sign present, persistent hypotension despite field intravenous fluid, and uncontrolled external hemorrhage. They found that penetrating and blunt trauma patients who underwent operation in less than 20 minutes had a significantly greater probability of survival versus that predicted by MTOS data.

A more recent analysis of their 10-year experience with OR resuscitation shows the survival advantage predominates in the penetrating trauma victims.[180] Rhodes and coworkers used a variety of triage criteria to indicate need for OR resuscitation: systolic blood pressure of 80 mm Hg or less, penetrating torso trauma, multiple long-bone fractures, major limb amputation, extensive soft-tissue wounds, severe maxillofacial hemorrhage, and witnessed arrest.[181] The mean ISS and survival rate of all patients meeting these criteria was 29.3% and 70.4%, respectively, which was better than predicted by TRISS methodology. Finally, Barlow and colleagues have advocated triage of pediatric patients (age 16 and younger) directly to the OR based on mechanism of injury and have reported survival rates of 100% for patients admitted with stab wounds and 94% for patients admitted with gunshot wounds.[182,183]

Secondary triage has also been shown to benefit the hospital in terms of human and financial resources. DeKeyser and colleagues reported that the institution of a two-tiered, in-hospital trauma response system, based on patient status at the time of admission, reduced the cost of trauma care by more than $600,000 over a one-year period by reducing the utilization of personnel, operating room, laboratory work, and protective wear.[184] Secondary triage characteristics such as patient response to resuscitation measure, newly diagnosed major injuries, or the presence of markedly abnormal blood values such as elevated lactate levels portend the need for enhanced medical resources and ICU care.[185]

## Undertriage/Overtriage

The determination of the rates of undertriage and overtriage based on the use of each of the current field triage scoring methods would provide an answer to the main question of which method best identifies the major trauma patient in the field. The best method would have the lowest rates of both undertriage and overtriage. However, the variability over an equivalent definition of a major trauma patient make this type of analysis subject to criticism.

It is impossible to achieve perfect overtriage and undertriage rates using current field triage methods. West and colleagues found that the addition of non-time-dependent criteria to traditional physiologic triage criteria reduced the undertriage rate from 21 to 4.4%, when undertriage is defined as non-CNS-related motor vehicle accident deaths occurring in non-trauma-designated hospitals. However, depending on the definition of major trauma, overtriage ranged from 36 to 80%.[164]

Other factors also appear to confound analysis of undertriage and overtriage. Studies have found that major trauma patients (defined by ISS) were more likely to be undertriaged if they were elderly or had single-system injuries. Patients with minor injuries were more likely to be overtriaged if they were intoxicated, obese, or had an injury to the head or face. In reality, acceptable rates of undertriage and overtriage are dependent on how a trauma system defines major trauma and the type of field triage criteria employed.

The San Diego Trauma System has reported overtriage rates by comparing patients transported to those entered into the trauma registry using MTOS criteria.[185] Data regarding preventable deaths are also available because all non-trauma centers have trauma deaths reviewed. Using this approach the data suggest that combining physiologic and non-time-dependent criteria leads to an overtriage rate of approximately 35% and an undertriage rate of less than 1%. These rates have been found to be stable over time and would seem to be reasonable targets. Looked at another way, this translates to about 30% unnecessary transports, which calculates to 2,000 patients per year or about six patients per day. This amounts to no more than one to two extra patient evaluations per trauma center per day, hardly a significant overburden to a trauma system.

At present, a combination of methods may provide the most accurate field assessment of the seriously injured trauma victim and represents the current state of the art in identification of major trauma victims. A number of studies have shown that the sensitivity and specificity of physiologic based triage scoring methods are improved by the addition of anatomic and/or mechanistic injury data.[186] The addition of the mechanism of injury with the prehospital index did not improve the ability to identify seriously injured trauma patients.[162] The structure of triage decisions must be based on the individual trauma system's unique resources and capabilities in both the prehospital and hospital phases of care and then employed such that patient morbidity and mortality are minimized.

## Interhospital Transfer

Many trauma victims who live in rural communities do not have immediate access to a designated trauma center or regional trauma system. These patients are generally taken to the local community hospital for their initial care. While most are adequately cared for by these facilities, there are a significant number of patients who will require the services found only at a hospital dedicated to the overall care of the trauma patient. Previous studies have shown that these patients are at an increased risk of death.[187–189] Some of the factors that have been implicated in contributing to potentially avoidable mortality in this situation include failure to recognize the severity of the injury, lack of adequate resuscitative measures, and delay in or lack of necessary treatment procedures for stabilization.[190–193] It is imperative that the initial treating physician should be able to recognize that the trauma victim may have injuries that require diagnostic and/or therapeutic modalities beyond the scope of the initial receiving hospital. If this situation is identified, then transfer of the patient to a "higher level of care" is appropriate.

Interhospital transfers should occur from one facility to another that will provide the additional resources needed. This generally occurs from a Level III or IV hospital as part of a regionalized trauma system. Patients may also need care from specialized centers such as a burn center or a pediatric trauma center. However, one must recognize that the period of transport is one of potential instability for the patient, and the risks of transport must be balanced against the benefits of a higher level of care.[194–196]

Risk to the patient can be minimized with the use of proper equipment, personnel, and planning. The patient may need to undergo a period of resuscitation and stabilization prior to transfer.[197] Some patients may not stabilize and require more definitive intervention prior to transfer. Communication with the trauma center will assist in this determination as well as interventional planning. A patient with an unstable intra-abdominal hemorrhage may need a damage control surgery with abdominal packing in order to be stable enough for transfer. The trauma surgeon could be in constant communication with the outlying surgeon to assist in the decision making for the operative procedure. This concept is particularly important with distant interhospital transfers.[198–200] In addition to the medical aspects of interhospital transfer, physicians must also comply with certain federal and local legal regulations.[201,202] Failure to do so has serious ramifications for the transferring hospital as well as the individual physician.[203]

## Criteria for Interhospital Transfer

Identification of a trauma victim who may benefit from transfer to a designated trauma center is based on specific criteria. A number of factors must be examined when making this decision, including patient status and recognition of possible injuries and/or comorbid factors as well as the personnel and equipment resources necessary for optimal patient care.

Criteria for transfer are often not followed because of financial conflicts or failure to appreciate the long-term complexities of certain injuries.[204] This may be best addressed in a trauma system through a legislative process that defines which patients should be transferred to which level of care. The Colorado State Board of Health has published Rules and Regulations Pertaining to the Statewide Trauma System in which criteria for interhospital transfer have been defined.[205] Patient criteria are based primarily on physiologic and anatomic injury data (aortic tears, liver injuries requiring intraoperative packing, bilateral pulmonary contusions requiring nonconventional ventilation, etc.), and on the level of care (Level II, III, IV) that the patient's facility is able to provide. If the patient meets the criteria for that specific health care facility, then consultation with a Level I trauma surgeon and discussion of possibility for interhospital transfer is mandatory.

Interhospital transfer may be essential in multiple casualty events whereby a single hospital is overburdened by casualties. In this case the criteria for the transfer of patients changes in order to offload the primary hospital patient load. Good triage principles need to apply so that those patients who would benefit the most would be transferred.[206] These transfers may even occur between two equivalent level institutions in order to facilitate the distribution of trauma victims. As was demonstrated in the World Trade Center disaster, the walking wounded inundated the closest medical facilities to ground zero. This condition has the potential to make it more difficult to identify and treat the most seriously injured patients from the mass of patients who arrive at the hospital.[129]

## Methods of Transfer

Transfer of the trauma victim must be organized in a way that minimizes the risk to the patient during the transfer process. This includes establishing transfer protocols at the EMS and institutional levels prior to transport. It also includes the planning that is necessary after the decision for transfer is made in individual cases with respect to the type of equipment, mode of transport, and personnel necessary to maximize patient safety.

## Transfer Agreement

Minor delays can have adverse consequences for the major trauma victim; it is therefore necessary to expedite the transfer process once its need is recognized. Transfer agreements are established protocols between hospitals that ensure rapid and efficient passage of pertinent patient information prior to the actual transfer. This should include patient identification, history and physical examination findings, diagnostic and therapeutic procedures performed and their results, and the initial impression and a clear identification of the referring and receiving physicians.[207] This information then allows the trauma surgeon at the receiving hospital to suggest possible diagnostic or therapeutic maneuvers that may be required prior to transfer, such as intubation, insertion of a nasogastric tube, Foley catheter, or thoracostomy tube. It also allows for mobilization of resources, such as an ICU bed or operating room, at the receiving hospital in anticipation of possible injuries. The physicians involved should also discuss the mode of transportation, accompanying personnel, and equipment that may be needed for optimal transfer. Discussion should also include who will assume medical control of the patient during transport. Full documentation, including a summary of care from the referring hospital and copies of all studies, should accompany the patient to the receiving hospital.

## Transport Modality

The objective is to get the trauma victim to the receiving hospital as quickly and safely as possible. However, the mode of transportation is dependent on the availability of a particular mode, distance, geography, weather, patient status, and the skills of the transport personnel and equipment that will likely be needed during transport. This should be discussed between the referring and receiving physicians with each transfer. Knowledge of transporting agencies in the area and their availability should be ascertained as soon as the need for transport is recognized.

The patient should have appropriate monitoring of physiologic indices, including invasive monitoring, during the transport period. This may include monitoring of respiratory rate, cardiac rhythm and blood pressure, intracranial pressure, and central venous or pulmonary artery pressure. If the patient is intubated, end-tidal $CO_2$ should be monitored and the transport ventilator should have alarms to indicate disconnects and high airway pressures. The other additional equipment necessary for safe transport is that needed for effective ACLS/ATLS interventions and has been outlined in a number of publications.[208]

## Transport Team

The patient should be accompanied by at least two people in addition to the vehicle operator, one of whom should have requisite training in advanced airway management, intravenous therapy, cardiac dysrhythmia recognition and treatment, and advanced trauma life support.[209] If the transporting personnel do not have the necessary training or skills, a nurse or physician should accompany the patient during transport to ensure optimal care.

## IMPROVED OUTCOME FROM TRANSFER

Reduction in the morbidity and mortality of trauma patients who require the resources of a trauma center depends on early identification of the severely injured, proper initial stabilization, and safe interhospital transfer.[210] There is evidence that patients who sustain major trauma in a rural or small community setting are at an increased risk for adverse outcomes. Houtchens demonstrated a high incidence of departure from well-defined standards in the initial evaluation and management of major trauma victims in rural community hospitals.[192] Certo and colleagues reported on the care of fatally injured patients in a rural state.[189] They found that 22% of fatally injured patients with non-CNS injuries reaching the emergency department alive had potentially survivable injuries. Errors in initial volume replacement, airway control, and recognition of the need for surgical intervention were factors complicating the care of these patients.

Hicks and colleagues studied the adequacy of initial care of patients subsequently transferred to a trauma center with regard to neurologic, chest, abdominal, and orthopedic injuries.[191] They found major departures from accepted standards of care, promoted by the ASCOT and the American College of Emergency Physicians, in more than 70% of these cases. Martin and colleagues reviewed the care of patients initially treated at local community hospitals during initial management and subsequent transport to a referral trauma center.[190] Quality of care was assessed based on advanced trauma support (ATLS) guidelines. Their study reported life-threatening deficiencies in 5% and serious deficiencies in 80% of cases reviewed, including inadequate cervical spine immobilization, inadequate intravenous access, and inadequate oxygen delivery. Veenema and Rodewald demonstrated that, while initial triage and management of rural trauma victims at a Level III trauma center prior to Level I transfer provide outcomes similar to MTOS data, there were still unexpected deaths.[210]

Timely transfer of major trauma victims to trauma centers improves patient care and subsequent outcome. Trauma centers not only provide the resources for the early management of severely injured patients, they also can provide more extensive support for the patient beyond the initial 24 hours.[211–214]

There are few studies that have looked at specific criteria as markers for patients who would benefit from interhospital transfer. Lee and colleagues attempted to clarify specific anatomic criteria that would indicate the need for interhospital transfer from Level III centers.[215] They found that the presence of three or more rib fractures was a marker for potential serious injury, as evidenced by significant differences in outcome when compared to patients with one or two rib fractures. A subsequent population-based study confirmed that these patients have a significantly higher mortality rate, higher ISS, and longer ICU and overall hospital stay.[216] Clark and colleagues reviewed their experience with major hepatic trauma (Grade III or more) in patients transferred from rural facilities. However, they did not delineate specific transfer criteria.[217] Similar studies have looked at mechanistic and physiologic criteria as reasons for bypassing rural/local community hospitals[218] or determining the need for a specific transport modality.[219]

## MODE OF TRANSPORT-INTERFACILITY TRANSFER

The question of whether air or ground transport is more appropriate for the transfer of the trauma victim is dependent on a number of factors. This includes the distance to be traveled, geography, weather, and overall patient status. Because outcome is directly related to time to definitive care, the quickest mode of transport that ensures patient safety should be chosen. Several options are available at many major trauma centers, including traditional ground transport and helicopter and fixed-wing air transport. The data on transport modality may not directly correlate to interhospital transfer because much of it comes from analyzing transports from the scene of the accident rather than from one hospital to another.

Baxt and Moody found that patients transported from the scene of the accident by helicopter had a 52% reduction in mortality compared to those transported by ground.[220] Similar results were found by Moylan and colleagues when they looked at factors improving survival in multisystem trauma patients who were transported by air versus ground.[221] There were no differences in the prehospital times between these two sets of patients, and the air transported patients were more frequently intubated and transfused blood, and had larger volumes of fluid given than the ground-transported patients.

The main benefit of air transport appears to be its use for long-distance transport. Several studies have shown that there is an improved survival in patients who need higher level of care when transported by air,[222] and this benefit can be realized up to an 800-mile radius from the trauma center.[223] This mode of transport may not be appropriate for short-distance transfer due to prolonged response time for interhospital transport.[224] For local urban transport, helicopters offer no advantage over an organized ground transportation system,[225] and the increased cost for air transport, especially that of helicopters, is probably not justified.[226,227]

Trauma triage and the interhospital transfer process have many similarities. Both have the same goal: to minimize potentially avoidable deaths. In order to accomplish this, both attempt to accurately identify the trauma patient who will require the specialized skills and resources provided by a Level I or II trauma center. Both utilize the same type of limited information early in the course of events in order to make that decision.

While certain types of obvious injuries warrant expeditious transport of the trauma victim, it is best to look at all of the available information in terms of physiologic indices, mechanism of injury, comorbid factors, and known or suspected injuries. This approach allows one to assess potential problems that may be more appropriately handled at a major trauma center. If there is any doubt, it is in the patients' best interest to be taken to a facility providing the highest level of care available.

## TRAUMA CENTER FACILITIES AND LEADERSHIP

Hospital care of the injured patient requires commitments from specific facilities to provide administrative support, medical staff, nursing staff, and other support personnel.[228] The trauma center integrates the trauma care system by providing local or regional leadership. Trauma centers are categorized by level, as described below.[4]

### Level I Trauma Center

The Level I trauma center is a tertiary care hospital usually serving large inner city communities that demonstrates a leadership role in system development, optimal trauma care, quality improvement, education, and research. It serves as a regional resource for the provision of the most sophisticated trauma care, from resuscitation through rehabilitation managing large numbers of severely injured patients through immediate 24-hour availability of an attending trauma surgeon. Level I trauma centers address public education and prevention issues on a regional basis and provide continuing education for all levels of trauma care providers. They lead research efforts to advance care.

### Level II Trauma Center

The Level II trauma center also provides definitive care to the injured and may be the principal hospital in the community or may work together with a Level I trauma center, in an attempt to optimize resources and clinical expertise necessary to provide optimal care for the injured victim. Its approach to trauma is generally not as comprehensive as the Level I facility. The attending trauma surgeon's availability is equivalent and they must participate early in the care of the patient. Graduate education and research are not required.

### Level III Trauma Center

A Level III trauma center generally serves a community that lacks Level I or II facilities. Maximum commitment is required to assess, resuscitate, and, when necessary, provide definitive operative therapy. For the major trauma patient, the principal role of the Level III center is to stabilize the injured patient and effect safe transfer to a higher level of care when capabilities for definitive care are exceeded. Transfer agreements and protocols are essential in a Level III trauma center. Education program for health care personnel may be part of a Level III center's role, as the hospital may be the only designated trauma center in the community.

### Level IV Trauma Center

A Level IV trauma center is usually a hospital located in a rural area. Level IV trauma centers are expected to provide the initial evaluation and care to acutely injured patients. Transfer agreements and protocols must be in place, since most of these hospitals have no definitive surgical capabilities on a regular basis.

### Acute Care Facilities Within the System

Many general hospitals exist within a trauma care system but are not officially designated as trauma centers. Circumstances often exist in which less severely injured patients reach these hospitals and appropriate care is provided. The system should provide for interfacility transfer of patients if a major trauma patient is mistriaged and registry entry for injured patients managed at nondesignated facilities.

## Specialty Trauma Centers

Regional specialty facilities concentrate expertise in a specific discipline and serve as a valuable resource for patients with critical specialty oriented injuries. Examples include pediatric trauma, burns, spinal cord injuries, and hand (replantation) trauma. Where present, these facilities provide a valuable resource to the community and should be included in the design of the system.

## REHABILITATION

Rehabilitation is as important as prehospital and hospital care. It is often the longest and most difficult phase of the trauma care continuum for both patient and family. Only 1 of 10 trauma patients in the United States has access to adequate rehabilitation programs, although it is critically important to reintegrating the patient into society. Rehabilitation can be provided in a designated area within the trauma center or by agreement with a free-standing rehabilitation center.

## SYSTEM EVALUATION

A trauma system has to monitor its own performance over time and determine areas where improvement is needed. To achieve this goal, reliable data collection and analysis through a statewide or systemwide trauma registry is necessary. Information from each phase of care is important and must be linked with every other phase. Compatibility between data collection during different phases of care is important to accurately determine the effects of certain interventions on long-term outcome. The practical use of a system evaluation instrument is to identify where the system falls short operationally and allow for improvements in system design. This feedback mechanism must be part of the system plan for evaluation.

The implementation of trauma care systems coupled with trauma registry databases, injury severity indices, and measurable outcome indicators has led to improved validity for investigations across the entire spectrum of injury control research. The system also has to be evaluated, by the American College of Surgeons Committee on Trauma Verification Review Committee or by inviting experts as outside reviewers, in addition to internal review.

## TRAUMA SYSTEM QUALITY IMPROVEMENT (Q/I)

The systemwide QI program's most important role is to monitor the quality of trauma care from incident through rehabilitation and create solutions to correct identified problems. The purpose of

quality improvement is to provide care in a planned sequence, to measure compliance with defined standards of care, and to reduce variability and cost while maintaining quality. A comprehensive downloadable guide to this process is detailed on the American College of Surgeons website.[229]

It allows health care providers to monitor several aspects of medical care using explicit guidelines to identify problems that have a negative impact on patient outcome. This is accomplished by establishing standards of trauma care and a mechanism to monitor the trauma care provided (surveillance), usually with audit filters designed to identify outliers.

Errors occur due to the complexity of trauma care and because of the involvement of multiple providers. It is of fundamental importance to make a distinction between process complexity and human errors when developing a quality improvement program in trauma.[230–233]

A peer process must be established to review QA/QI problems.[26,234] The process must be accurately documented, corrective action instituted and applied uniformly across the system, and the results reassessed. These principles apply to systemwide QA/QI as well as to the process within the hospital. Corrective action is taken through changes in existing policies or protocols, through education targeted at the problem, or by restriction of privileges.

A successful trauma system monitors the performance of the Emergency Medical Services (EMS) agency and prehospital operations, individual trauma hospitals, and care in nondesignated hospitals.

The prehospital audit process should include timeliness of arrival, timeliness of transport, application of prehospital procedures and treatments, and outcomes. To develop this part of the quality improvement process extensive involvement by the regional authority, the regional medical director, the provider agencies, and the trauma hospitals is required.

Standards of care are defined in relation to the availability of resources and personnel, timeliness of physician response, diagnosis, and therapy. These standards have been defined by the ACS and published in the *Resources for Optimal Care of the Injured Patient*.[4,233] Guidelines or protocols are then developed and audit filters are established to monitor the guidelines. Audit filters are useful tools to provide continuous monitoring of established practices. Standard audit filters and complications that need to be monitored have been established by the ACSCOT and include timeliness of care, appropriateness of care, and death review. Tracking of complications and illnesses allows trends to be monitored over time. Death reviews should be conducted in an attempt to determine preventability. Guidelines reduce variability, and consequently, fewer errors are made.

The process of quality improvement requires accurate documentation and this is achieved by using the trauma registry. The trauma registry provides objective data to support continuous quality improvement. The registry should be designed to collect and calculate response times, admission diagnoses, diagnostic and therapeutic procedures, discharge diagnoses, complications, costs, and functional recovery.

The trauma coordinator is of utmost importance in making the quality-improvement process effective. This person assures timely recognition of problems, use of the registry to document problems, and that problems are resolved. Cases identified as noncompliant with established standards of care are reviewed at the hospital level and by a trauma medical audit committee overseeing the trauma system.[234]

Peer review identifies the problem, the results are documented and determination of problem recurrence is made, trends are identified, and a decision is made if more specific action for problem resolution is required.

Actions may include simple education of the staff or revision of the guidelines, or eventually development of new guidelines, hiring additional staff, or even removing a staff member. The monitoring process should continue after action was taken to determine its effectiveness. Quality-improvement processes in trauma are a multidisciplinary task.[235]

## STANDARDIZED DEFINITION OF ERRORS AND PREVENTABLE DEATH

The development of trauma systems led to a significant reduction in the number of preventable deaths after injury. A preventable death rate of less than 1–2% is now widely accepted as ideal in a trauma system. However, a small number of patients continue to die, or eventually, to develop complications that could otherwise be avoided or prevented. These errors occur in different phases of trauma care (resuscitative, operative, and critical care phases), and are named provider-related, as a group. These include events that lead to delays or errors in technique, judgment, treatment, or communication. A delay in diagnosis is defined as an injury-related diagnosis made greater than 24 hours after admission resulting in minimum morbidity. An error in diagnosis is an injury missed because of misinterpretation or inadequacy of physical examination or diagnostic procedures. An error in judgment is defined as a therapeutic decision or diagnostic modality employed contrary to available data. An error in technique occurs during the performance of a diagnostic or therapeutic procedure.[233]

According to the ACSCOT *Resources for Optimal Care of the Injured Patient: 2006* document, an event is defined as nonpreventable when it is a sequela of a procedure, disease, or injury for which reasonable and appropriate preventable steps had been observed and taken. Potentially preventable is an event or complication that is a sequela of a procedure, disease, or injury that has the potential to be prevented or substantially ameliorated. A preventable event or complication is an expected or unexpected sequela of a procedure, disease, or injury that could have been prevented or substantially ameliorated.[4]

With regard to mortality, the same definitions apply. Nonpreventable deaths are defined as fatal injuries despite optimal care, evaluated and managed appropriately accordingly to standard guidelines (ATLS), and with a probability of survival, estimated by using the TRISS methodology, of less than 25%. A potentially preventable death is defined as an injury or combination of injuries considered very severe but survivable under optimal conditions. Generally these are unstable patients at the scene who respond minimally to treatment. Evaluation and management are generally appropriate and suspected care, however, directly or indirectly is implicated in patient demise. The calculated probability of survival varies from 25% to 50%.

A preventable death usually includes an injury or combination of injuries considered survivable. Patients in this category are generally stable, or if unstable, respond adequately to treatment. The

evaluation or treatment is suspected in any way, and the calculated probability of survival is greater than 50%.

The causes of preventable deaths in trauma centers are different than those occurring at nontrauma hospitals. In nontrauma hospitals, preventable deaths occur because the severity or multiplicity of injuries is not fully appreciated, leading to delays in diagnosis, lack of adequate monitoring, and delays to definitive therapy. In trauma hospitals, the causes of preventable death include errors in judgment or errors in technique. In trauma centers the diagnostic modalities used are normally adequate, and delays in diagnosis or treatment are uncommon and have minimal impact on outcome.

These definitions are useful to monitor trauma system's performance and to compare different trauma systems. Once preventable death rate reaches a plateau after trauma system implementation, system performance should focus on tracking provider related complications. This approach has been proved adequate to identify problems and to implement solutions.[236,237]

## ANALYSIS OF TRAUMA SYSTEM PERFORMANCE

Different study designs have been used to evaluate trauma system effectiveness. The most common scientific approaches include panel review preventable death studies, trauma registry performance comparisons, and population-based studies. Panel review studies are conducted by a panel of experts in the field of trauma who review trauma-related deaths in an attempt to determine preventability. Well-defined criteria and standardized definitions regarding preventability have been used, but significant methodological problems (Table 4-4) can lead to inconsistencies in the results and interpretation of the data.[26,234,237–250]

Registry studies are frequently used to compare data from a trauma center or a trauma system with a national reference norm available, between trauma centers within the same system, or in the same trauma center at different periods.[251–266] The Major Trauma Outcome Study (MTOS)[255] has been used as the national reference, although several of its limitations have been recognized, compromising the reliability of the comparison with data from other systems or centers (Table 4-4). The advantages of registry-based studies include a detailed description of injury severity and physiologic data.

Population-based studies use information obtained from death certificates, hospital discharge claim data, or fatal accident reporting system (FARS) on all injured patients in a region. These methodologies of data collection and analysis are important to evaluate changes in outcome before and after, or at different time periods following the implementation of trauma systems in a defined region. Limited information on physiologic data, injury severity, and treatment is available.[267–284] The limitations of the most commonly used databases in population-based studies are described in Table 4-4.

The data on trauma system effectiveness published in the literature is difficult to interpret due to great variability in study design, type of analysis, and definition of outcome variables. In an attempt to review the existing evidence on the effectiveness of trauma systems, the Oregon Health Sciences University with support from the NTHSA and the National Center for Injury Prevention and Control of the CDC organized the Academic Symposium to

## TABLE 4-4

### Limitations of Current Trauma System Evaluation Studies

**Panel Studies**

Inconsistent definition of preventability
Case mix of the population
Size, composition, and expertise of the panel
Process and criteria to determine preventability
Inconsistent report of pre-hospital and autopsy data

**Registry-Based Studies**

Missing or incomplete data sets
Coding inconsistencies and errors
Inconsistent report of autopsy data
MTOS limitations
Outdated data set
Data is not population based
Mostly blunt trauma
Differences in trauma centers' level of care
Inconsistencies in trauma registry inclusion criteria
Lack of data on comorbid factors
Lack of data on long term follow-up

**Population-Based Studies**

Mechanism of injury, physiologic, and anatomic data usually not available
Autopsies not performed consistently in all trauma deaths
Limited number of secondary diagnoses in claims data
Autopsy findings not always included in claims data
Hospital discharge data is inaccurate in transfers and deaths in the Emergency Department
Inconsistencies in obtaining AIS scores
Outcome measure is in-hospital mortality. No long term or functional outcome data available

Evaluate Evidence Regarding the Efficacy of Trauma Systems, also known as the Skamania Symposium.[285]

Trauma care providers, policy makers, administrators, and researchers reviewed and discussed the available literature in an attempt to determine the impact of trauma systems on quality of patient care. The available literature on trauma system effectiveness does not contain class I (prospective randomized controlled trials) or class II (well designed, prospective or retrospective controlled cohort studies, or case-controlled studies). There are several class III (panel studies, case series, or registry-based) studies that were reviewed and discussed during the symposium. According to Mann et al. reviewing the published literature in preparation for the Skamania Symposium, it is appropriate to conclude that the implementation of trauma systems decreases hospital mortality of severely injured patients.[286] Independently of the used methodology (panel review, registry-based, or population-based), and despite the above-mentioned limitations of each study design, a decrease in mortality of 15% to 20% has been shown with the implementation of trauma systems.[287–293] The participants of the symposium also concluded that not only mortality, but functional outcomes, financial outcomes, patient satisfaction, and cost-effectiveness should be evaluated in future prospective, well-controlled studies.

Outcomes data is difficult to interpret due to differences in study design. One recent area of interest has been in comparing outcomes in inclusive and exclusive systems. As mentioned previously, in an inclusive system, care is provided to all injured patients and involves all acute care facilities, whereas in exclusive systems

specialized trauma care is provided only in high-level trauma centers that deliver definitive care. In inclusive systems, patients may be transferred to a higher level of care (trauma center) after initial stabilization based on the availability of resources and expertise in the initial treating facility. Two problems arise: (a) delay to transfer and (b) dilution of trauma centers' experience. Utter et al. have recently investigated whether mortality is lower in inclusive systems compared to exclusive systems. They concluded that severely injured patients are more likely to survive in states with the most inclusive trauma system, independent of the triage system in place. A possible explanation to these findings includes better initial care in referring hospitals.[294] A more recent study confirms a mortality reduction of 25% in patients under the age of 55.[137]

## SPECIAL PROBLEMS

Despite the experience acquired on trauma system development in the United States during the last three decades, trauma systems still face multiple problems and challenges. The financial aspect, linked to the problem of uncompensated care has led to the closure of several trauma centers and the collapse of some trauma systems. Alternative and stable sources for funding indigent care have to be part of an agenda for legislative action in support of trauma systems. Funds for prevention strategies should also be provided, targeting particularly the pediatric and the elderly population. Table 4-5 lists the actual problems faced by regionalized trauma

## TABLE 4-5

### Current Problems of Trauma Systems

Urban
Financial
Uncompensated care
Closure of trauma centers
Source of funding for indigent care
Over designations of trauma center
Rural
Sparse population
Long distances
Difficult patient access
Weather conditions
Delays in notification
Treatment delays due to interfacility transfer needs
Lack of medical oversight
Pediatric
Integral part of the system
Education
Elderly
Increased costs
Increased morbidity and mortality
Prevention
Lack of federal/state funding needs to be addressed in order to increase the number of states engaged in developing statewide or regional trauma systems in the US.
Funding required:
National Level: National Trauma system development
State/Local Level: To finance the EMS system
Research/Prevention/Avoidance of duplication

## TABLE 4-6

### Critical Targets for Future Trauma System Development

Regionalization of trauma care

Development of disaster preparedness

Identification of trauma as a disease process

Recognition of the continuum of care required

Recognition that trauma requires a multidisciplinary approach

Improving cost effectiveness

Coordination of resources, services, and special populations

Reimbursement, funding, and legislation

systems as documented through a SWOT analysis conducted by the Health Resources and Service Administration in 2003.[28]

One effort that has been developed recently is the Consultations for Trauma Systems document and accompanying process developed by the ACSCOT.[16] It follows previous efforts to develop trauma systems and the original Model Trauma System Care Plan.[21] Overall, it conveniently brings accepted expertise and standards in the field and attempts to evaluate and improve trauma systems. A more recent effort has led to the Model Trauma System Planning and Evaluation Program.[9] This is the most comprehensive tool available to help develop regional trauma systems.

Despite the realization that trauma systems reduce morbidity and mortality, there remain several barriers to full implementation. A trauma system agenda for the future has been recently written and endorsed as a template for going forward.[295] Critical elements are defined in Table 4-6. It is imagined that trauma systems when fully implemented will enhance community health through an organized system of injury prevention, acute care, and rehabilitation that is fully integrated into the public health system of a community. In addition to addressing the daily demands of trauma, it will form the basis for disaster preparedness and possess the distinct ability to identify risk factors and early interventions to prevent injuries in a community while integrating a delivery of optimal resources for patients who ultimately need acute trauma care.

The availability of federal dollars to assist in the development of trauma systems will be essential. At the same time, a developing consensus to build trauma systems that do not cover designated trauma centers yet meet the needs of all components of the trauma patient will be equally critical. The biggest challenge in the future will be the implementation of what we already know how to do. Developing the political and public will to do so remains the challenge before us.

## REFERENCES

1. West JG, Williams MJ, Trunkey DD, et al.: Trauma systems: Current status-future challenges. *JAMA* 259:3597, 1988.
2. Bazzoli GJ, MacKenzie EJ: Trauma centers in the United States: Identification and examination of key characteristics. *J Trauma* 38:103, 1995.
3. Bazzoli GJ, Madura KJ, Cooper GF, et al.: Progress in the development of trauma systems in the United States. Results of a national survey. *JAMA* 273:395, 1995.
4. American College of Surgeons Committee on Trauma: *Resources for Optimal Care of the Injured Patient: 2006.* Chicago, IL: American College of Surgeons, 2006.
5. Bazzoli GJ, Meersman PJ, Chan C: Factors that enhance continued trauma center participation in trauma systems. *J Trauma* 41:876, 1996.
6. Boyd DR: A symposium on The Illinois Trauma Program: A systems approach to the care of the critically injured. Introduction: A controlled systems approach to trauma patient care. *J Trauma* 13:275, 1973.
7. Eastman AB, Bishop GS, Walsh JC, et al.: The economic status of trauma centers on the eve of health care reform. *J Trauma* 36:835, 1994.
8. Eastman AB, Lewis FR Jr, Champion HR, et al.: Regional trauma system design: Critical concepts. *Am J Surg* 154:79, 1987.
9. U.S. Department of Health and Human Services, Health Resources and Services Administration, Trauma-EMS Systems Program: Model Trauma System Planning and Evaluation; Trauma Systems Collaborating with Public Health for Improved Injury Outcomes. 2006.
10. Bonnie RJ, Fulco CE, Liverman CT: *Magnitude and Costs. Reducing the burden of Injury. Advancing Prevention and Treatment.* Washington, D.C.: National Academy Press, 1999, p. 41.
11. *Accidental Death and Disability: The Neglected Disease of Modern Society.* Washington: National Academy of Sciences, 1966.
12. Boyd D, Dunea M, Flashner B: The Illinois plan for a statewide system of trauma centers. *Journal of Trauma* 13:24, 1973.
13. *Emergency Medical Services Systems Act of 1973, Public Law 93-154.* Washington, D.C., 1973.
14. Committee on Trauma, American College of Surgeons: Optimal hospital resources for care of the seriously injured. *Bull Am Coll Surg* 61:15, 1976.
15. American College of Surgeons Committee on Trauma: *Advanced Trauma Life Support Course: Instructor Manual.* Chicago, IL: American College of Surgeons, 2004.
16. National Research Council: *Injury in America: A Continuing Health Care Problem.* Washington, D.C.: National Academy Press, 1985.
17. Committee on Trauma, American College of Surgeons: *Consultation for Trauma Systems.* Chicago: American College of Surgeons, 1998.
18. American College of Emergency Physicians: Guidelines for Trauma Care Systems. *Ann Emerg Med* 16:459, 1987.
19. *Development of Trauma Systems* (DOT). Washington, D.C.: National Highway Traffic Safety Administration, 1988.
20. Bass RR, Gainer PS, Carlini A: Update on trauma system development in the US. *J Trauma* 47:S15, 1999.
21. *Model Trauma Care System Plan.* Rockville, MD: Department of Health and Human Services, Health Resources and Services Administration, 1992.
22. Detmer DE, Moylan JA, Rose J, et al.: Regional categorization and quality of care in major trauma. *J Trauma* 17:592, 1977.
23. West J, Trunkey D, Lim R: Systems of trauma care-A study of two counties. *Arch Surg* 114:455, 1979.
24. West JG, Cales RH, Gazzaniga AB: Impact of regionalization-The Orange County experience. *Arch Surg* 118:740, 1983.
25. Boyd DR, Cowley RA: Comprehensive regional trauma/ emergency medical services (EMS) delivery systems: The United States Experience. *World J Surg* 7:149, 1983.
26. Shackford SR, Hollingworth-Fridlund P, Cooper GF, et al.: The effect of regionalization upon the quality of trauma care as assessed by concurrent audit before and after institution of a trauma system: A preliminary report. *J Trauma* 26:812, 1986.
27. Mullins RJ, Veum-Stone J, Hedges JR, et al.: Influence of a statewide trauma system on location of hospitalization and outcome in injured patients. *J Trauma* 40:536, 1996.
28. U.S. Department of Health & Human Services. A 2002 National Assessment of State Trauma System Development, Emergency Medical Services Resources, and Disaster Readiness for Mass Casualty Events. 2003
29. American Trauma Society: Harris Poll. www.amtrauma.org. Accessed October 15, 2006.
30. Kraus JF, Peek C. McArthur DL, et al.: The effect of the 1992 California motorcycle helmet use law on motorcycle crash fatalities and injuries. *JAMA* 272:1506, 1994.
31. Lowe DK, Gately HL, Goss JR, et al.: Patterns of death, complication and error in management of motor vehicle accident victims: Implications for a regional system of trauma care. *J Trauma* 23:50, 1983.
32. Baker CC, Oppenheiner L, Stephens B, et al.: Epidemiology of trauma deaths. *Am J Surg* 140:144, 1980.
33. Shackford SR, Mackersie RC, Hollingsworth-Fridlund P, et al.: The epidemiology and pathology of traumatic death: A population-based analysis. *Arch Surg* 128:571, 1993.
34. Runyan CW, Gerken EA: Epidemiology and prevention of adolescent injury: A review and research agenda. *JAMA* 262:2273, 1989.
35. Potenza BM, Hoyt DB, Coimbra R, et al.: Trauma Research and Education Foundation: The epidemiology of serious and fatal injury in San Diego county over an 11-year period. *J Trauma* 56:68, 2004.
36. *Dorlands Illustrated Medical Dictionary*, 28th ed. Philadelphia: W.B. Saunders, 1994.
37. Burris DG, Welling DR, Rich NM: Dominique Jean Larrey and the principles of humanity in warfare. *J Am Coll Surg* 198:831, 2004.

38. *Emergency War Surgery. Second United States Revision of The Emergency War Surgery NATO Handbook.* Bowen TE, Bellamy R, eds. Department of Defense. Washington, D.C.: United States Government Printing Office, 1988.

39. Beebe GW, DeBakey ME, Thomas CC: *Battle Casualties: Incidence, Mortality, and Logistic Considerations.* Springfield, IL, 1952.

40. *National Association of Emergency Medical Technology, American College of Surgeons Committee on Trauma, Prehospital Trauma Life Support.* 6th ed. St. Louis: Mosby, 2004.

41. Hoyt DB, Shackford SR, McGill T, et al.: The impact of in-house surgeons and operating room resuscitation on outcome of traumatic injuries. *Arch Surg* 124:906, 1989.

42. Baker SP, O'Neill B: The injury severity score: An update. *J Trauma* 16:882, 1976.

43. Baker SP, O'Neill B, Hadden W, et al.: The injury severity score: A method for describing patients with multiple injuries and evaluating emergency care. *J Trauma* 14:187, 1974.

44. Champion HR, Copes WS, Sacco WJ, et al.: The major trauma outcome study: Establishing national norms for trauma care. *J Trauma* 30:1356, 1990.

45. Champion HR: *Triage.* In Cales RH, Heileg RW, eds. *Trauma Care Systems.* Rockville, MD: Aspen Publishers, 1986, p. 79.

46. Flancbaum L, Dougherty C, Brotman DN, et al.: DRGs and the "negative" trauma workup. *Ann Emerg Med* 19:741, 1990.

47. Hoff WS, Tinkoff GH, Lucke JF, Lehr S: Impact of minimal injuries on a level I trauma center. *J Trauma* 33:408, 1992.

48. Kirkpatrick JR, Youmans RL: Trauma index: An aid in evaluation of injury victims. *J Trauma* 11:711, 1971.

49. Baxt WB, Berry CC, Epperson MD: The failure of prehospital trauma prediction rules to classify trauma patients accurately. *Ann Emerg Med* 18:21, 1989.

50. Guzzo JL, Bochicchio GV, Napolitano LM, et al.: Predictions of outcomes in trauma: Anatomic or physiologic parameters? *J Am Coll Surg* 201:891, 2005.

51. Maslanka AM: Scoring systems and triage from the field. *Emerg Med Clin North Am* 11:15, 1993.

52. Kane G, Engelhardt R, Celentano J, et al.: Empirical development and evaluation of prehospital trauma triage instruments. *J Trauma* 25:482, 1985.

53. Mackersie RC, Tiwary AD, Shackford SR, et al.: Intra-abdominal injury following blunt trauma. Identifying the high-risk patient using objective risk factors. *Arch Surg* 124:809, 1989.

54. Miller FB, Cryer HM, Chiliduri S, et al.: Negative findings on laparotomy for trauma. *South Med J* 82:1231, 1989.

55. Landercasper J, Cogbill TH, Strutt PJ: Delayed diagnosis of flail chest. *Crit Care Med* 18:611, 1990.

56. Dunlop MG, Beattie TF, Preston PG, et al.: Clinical assessment and radiograph following blunt chest trauma. *Arch Emerg Med* 6:125, 1989.

57. Rizoli SB, Boulanger BR, McLellan BA, et al.: Injuries missed during initial assessment of blunt trauma patients. *Accid Anal Prev* 26:681, 1994.

58. Anderson S, Biros MH, Reardon RF: Delayed diagnosis of thoracolumbar fractures in multiple-trauma patients. *Acad Emerg Med* 3:832, 1996.

59. Frankel HL, Rozycki GS, Ochsner MG, et al.: Indications for obtaining surveillance thoracic and lumbar spine radiographs. *J Trauma* 37:673, 1994.

60. Lieberman IH, Webb JK: Cervical spine injuries in the elderly. *J Bone Joint Surg* 76B:877, 1994.

61. Lynch JM, Gardner MJ, Albanese CT: Blunt urogenital trauma in prepubescent female patients: More than meets the eye. *Pediatr Emerg Care* 11:372, 1995.

62. Koury HI, Peschiera JL, Welling RE: Selective use of pelvic roentgenograms in blunt trauma patients. *J Trauma* 34:236, 1993.

63. Salvino CK, Esposito TJ, Smith D, et al.: Routine pelvic x-rays in awake blunt trauma patients: A sensible policy? *J Trauma* 33:413, 1992.

64. Mackersie RC, Shackford SR, Garfin SR, et al.: Major skeletal injuries in the obtunded blunt trauma patient: A case for routine radiologic survey. *J Trauma* 28:1450, 1988.

65. Rivara FP, Jurkovich GJ, Gurney JG, et al.: The magnitude of acute and chronic alcohol abuse in trauma patients. *Arch Surg* 128:907, 1993.

66. Marx J: Alcohol and trauma. *Emerg Med Clin North Am* 8:929, 1990.

67. King AI, Yang KH: Research in biomechanics of occupant protection. *J Trauma* 38:570, 1995.

68. Grande CM: Mechanisms and patterns of injury: The key to anticipation in trauma management. *Crit Care Clin* 6:25, 1990.

69. Presswalla FB: The pathophysics and pathomechanics of trauma. *Med Sci Law* 18:239, 1978.

70. Lowe DK, Oh GR, Neely KW, et al.: Evaluation of injury mechanism as a criterion in trauma triage. *Am J Surg* 152:6, 1986.

71. Knopp R, Yanagi A, Kallsen G, et al.: Mechanism of injury and anatomic injury as criteria for prehospital trauma triage. *Ann Emerg Med* 17:895, 1988.

72. Knudson P, Frecceri CA, Delauteur SA: Improving the field triage of major trauma victims. *J Trauma* 28:602, 1988.

73. McCoy GF, Johnstone RA, Duthie RB: Injury to the elderly in road traffic accidents. *J Trauma* 29:494, 1989.

74. Shorr RM, Rodriguez A, Indeck MC, et al.: Blunt chest trauma in the elderly. *J Trauma* 29:234, 1989.

75. Morris JA, MacKensie EJ, Damiano AM, et al.: Mortality in trauma patients: The interaction between host factors and severity. *J Trauma* 30:1476, 1990.

76. Sauaia A, Moore FA, Moore EE, et al.: Early predictors of postinjury multiple organ failure. *Arch Surg* 129:39, 1994.

77. West JG: An autopsy method for evaluating care. *J Trauma* 21:32, 1981.

78. Nakayama DK, Copes WS, Sacco WJ: The effect of patient age upon survival in pediatric trauma. *J Trauma* 31:1521, 1991.

79. Eichelberger MR, Gotschall CS, Sacco WJ, et al.: A comparison of the trauma score, the revised trauma score and the pediatric trauma score. *Ann Emerg Med* 18:1053, 1989.

80. Phillips S, Rond PC III, Kelly SM, et al.: The need for pediatric-specific triage criteria: Results from the Florida Trauma Triage Study. *Pediatr Emerg Care* 12:394, 1996.

81. Milzman DP, Boulanger BR, Rodriguez A, et al.: Pre-existing disease in trauma patients: A predictor of fate independent of age and ISS. *J Trauma* 32:236, 1992.

82. Morris JA, MacKenzie EJ, Edelstein S: The effect of pre-existing conditions on mortality in trauma patients. *JAMA* 236:1942, 1990.

83. Sacco WJ, Copes WS, Bain LW Jr, et al.: Effect of preinjury illness on trauma patient survival outcome. *J Trauma* 35:538, 1993.

84. Milzman DP, Hinson D, Magnant CM: Overview and outcomes: Trauma and pre-existing disease. *Crit Care Clin* 9:633, 1993.

85. Fritsch DE: Hypothermia in the trauma patient. *AACN Clin Issues* 6:196, 1995.

86. Gentilello LM: Advances in the management of hypothermia. *Surg Clin North Am* 75:243, 1995.

87. Bernabei AF, Levison MA, Bender JS: The effects of hypothermia and injury severity on blood loss during trauma laparotomy. *J Trauma* 33:835, 1992.

88. Jurkovich GJ, Greiser WB, Luterman A, et al.: Hypothermia in trauma victims: An ominous predictor of survival. *J Trauma* 27:1019, 1987.

89. Dougherty W, Waxman K: The complexities of managing severe burns with associated trauma. *Surg Clin North Am* 76:923, 1996.

90. Janousek JT, Jackson DE, De Lorenzo RA, et al.: Mass casualty triage knowledge of military medical personnel. *Mil Med* 164:332, 1999.

91. Holcomb JB: The 2004 Fitts Lecture: Current Perspective on Combat Casualty Care. *J Trauma* 59:990, 2005.

92. Emerman CL, Shade B, Kubincanek J: A comparison of EMT judgement and prehospital trauma triage instruments. *J Trauma* 31:1369, 1991.

93. Ornato J, Milnek EJ, Craren EF, et al.: Ineffectiveness of the Trauma Score and the CRAMS Scale for accurately triaging patients to trauma centers. *Ann Emerg Med* 14:1061, 1985.

94. Esposito TJ, Offner PF, Jurkovich GJ, et al.: Do prehospital trauma center triage criteria identify major trauma victims? *Arch Surg* 130:171, 1995.

95. Richards JR, Ferrall SJ: Triage ability of emergency medical services providers and patient disposition: A prospective study. *Prehospital and Disaster Medicine* 14:174, 1999.

96. Leslie CL, Cushman M, McDonald GS, et al.: Management of multiple burn casualties in a high volume ED without a verified burn unit. *Am J Emerg Med* 19:469, 2001.

97. Mulholland SA, Gabbe BJ, Cameron P: Is Paramedic Judgment Useful in Prehospital Trauma Triage? *Injury* 36:1298, 2005.

98. Pointer JE, Levitt MA, Young JC, et al.: Can paramedics using guidelines accurately triage patients? *Ann Emerg Med* 38:268, 2001.

99. Detmer DE, Moylan JA, Rose J, et al.: Regional categorization and quality of care in major trauma. *J Trauma* 17:592, 1977.

100. Center for Health Systems Research and Analysis: *Report on the Trauma Severity Index Conference.* Madison, WI: University of Wisconsin, 1980.

101. Senkowski CK, McKenney MG: Trauma Scoring System: A Review. *J Am Coll Surg* 189:491, 1999.

102. Kuhls DA, Malone DL, McCarter RJ, et al.: Predictors of mortality in adult trauma patients: The physiologic trauma score is equivalent to the trauma and injury severity score. *J Am Coll Surg* 194:695, 2002.

103. Kirkpatrick JR, Youmans RL: Trauma index: An aide in evaluation of injury victims. *J Trauma* 14:934, 1971.

104. Hedges JR, Sacco WJ, Champion HR: An analysis of prehospital care of blunt trauma. *J Trauma* 22:989, 1982.

105. Smith JS Jr, Bartholomew MJ: Trauma index revisited: A better triage tool. *Crit Care Med* 18:174, 1990.

106. Teasdale G, Jennet B: Assessment of coma and impaired consciousness: A practical scale. *Lancet* 2:81, 1974.

107. Champion HR, Sacco WJ, Carnazzo AJ, et al.: Trauma score. *Crit Care Med* 9:672, 1981.

108. Champion HR, Sacco WJ, Copes WS, et al.: A revision of the trauma score. *J Trauma* 20:188, 1989.

109. Gormican SP: CRAM Scale: Field triage of trauma victims. *Ann Emerg Med* 11:132, 1982.

110. Baxt WG, Jones G, Fortlage D: The trauma triage rule: A new, resource-based approach to the prehospital identification of major trauma victims. *Ann Emerg Med* 19:1401, 1990.
111. Winkler JV, Rosen P, Alfry EJ: Prehospital use of the Glasgow Coma Scale in severe head injury. *J Emerg Med* 2:1, 1984.
112. Meredith W, Rutledge R, Hansen AR, et al.: Field triage of patients based upon the ability to follow commands: A study in 29,573 injured patients. *J Trauma* 38:129, 1995.
113. Champion HR, Sacco WJ, Hannan DS, et al.: Assessment of injury severity: The triage index. *Crit Care Med* 8:201, 1980.
114. Clemmer TP, Orme JF Jr, Thomas F, et al.: Prospective evaluation of the CRAMS scale for triaging major trauma. *J Trauma* 25:188, 1985.
115. Kilberg L, Clemmer TP, Clawson J, et al.: Effectiveness of implementing a trauma triage system on outcome: A prospective evaluation. *J Trauma* 28:1493, 1988.
116. Koehler JJ, Baer LJ, Malafa SA, et al.: Prehospital index: A scoring system for field triage of trauma victims. *Ann Emerg Med* 15:178, 1986.
117. Keohler JJ, Malafa SA, Hillesland J, et al.: A multicenter validation of the prehospital index. *Ann Emerg Med* 16:380, 1987.
118. Heide EA: *Disaster response: Principle of Preparation and Coordination.* St Louis, MO: Mosby Co., 1989.
119. Risavi BL, Salen PN, Heller MB, et al.: A two-hour intervention using START improves prehospital triage of mass casualty. *Prehosp Emerg Care* 5:197, 2001.
120. Hubble MW, Hubble JP: *Principles of Advanced Trauma Care.* Albany, New York: Delmar Publishing, 2002, p. 131.
121. Asaeda G: The day that the START triage system came to a STOP: Observations from the World Trade Center. *Acad Emerg Med* 9:255, 2002.
122. Eichelberger MR, Mangubat EA, Sacco WS, et al.: Comparative outcomes of children and adults suffering blunt trauma. *J Trauma* 28:430, 1988.
123. Maconochie I, Hodgetts T, Hall J. Planning for major incidents involving children by implementing a Delphi study. Letter to the Editor. *Arch Dis Child* 82:266, 2000.
124. Ryan JM, Sibson J, Howell G: Assessing injury severity during general war. Will the Military Triage system meet future needs? *J R Army Med Corps* 136:27, 1990.
125. Berkel FM, Sanner PH, Wolcott WB: *Disaster Medicine: Application for the Immediate Management and Triage of Civilian and Military Disaster Victims.* New York: Medical Examination Publishing Company, 1984.
126. Eisner ME, Waxman K, Mason GR: Evaluation of possible patient survival in a mock airplane disaster. *Am J Surg* 150:321, 1985.
127. Blank-Reid C, Santora TA: Developing and implementing a surgical response and physician triage team. *Disaster Manag Response* 1:41, 2003.
128. Grissom ET, Farmer JC: The provision of sophisticated critical care beyond the hospital: Lessons from physiology and military experiences that apply to civil disaster medical response. *Crit Care Med* 33:S13, 2005.
129. Kossman T, Wittling I, Buhren V, et al.: Transferred triage to a level I trauma center in a mass catastrophe of patients; many of them burns. *Acta Chir Plast* 33:145, 1991.
130. Subbarao I, Johnson C, Bond WF, et al.: Symptom-based, algorithmic approach for handling the initial encounter with victims of a potential terrorist attack. *Prehospital Disaster Med* 20:301, 2005.
131. Frykberg ER. Principles of mass casualty management following terrorist disasters. *Ann Surg* 239:319, 2004.
132. Einav S, Feigenberg Z, Weissman C, et al.: Evacuation priorities in mass-casualty terror-related events. Implications for contingency planning. *Ann Surg* 239:304, 2004.
133. Peleg K, Aharonson-Daniel L, Stein M, et al.. Gunshot and explosion injuries: Characteristics, outcomes, and implications for care of terror-related injuries in Israel. *Ann Surg* 239:311, 2004.
134. Almogy G, Belzberg H, Mintz Y, et al.: Suicide bombing attacks: Update and modifications of the protocol. *Ann Surg* 239:295, 2004.
135. Feliciano DV, Anderson GV, Rozycki GS, et al.: Management of casualties from the bombing at the centennial olympics. *Am J Surg* 176:538, 1995.
136. American College of Surgeons: Statement on disaster and mass casualty management by the American College of Surgeons. *Bull Am Coll Surg* 88:14, 2003.
137. MacKenzie EJ, Rivara FP, Jurkovich GJ, et al.: A national evaluation of the effect of trauma-center care on mortality. *N Engl J Med* 354:366, 2006.
138. Shedden PM, Moulton RJ, Sullivan I, et al.: Effect of population characteristics on head injury mortality. *Pediatr Neurosurg* 16:203, 1990–1991.
139. Chen RJ, Fang JF, Lin BC, et al.: Factors that influence the operative mortality after blunt hepatic injuries. *Eur J Surg* 161:811, 1995.
140. Kollmorgen DR, Murray KA, Sullivan JJ, et al.: Predictors of mortality in pulmonary contusion. *Am J Surg* 168:659, 1994.
141. Gaillard M, Herve C, Mandin L, et al.: Mortality prognostic factors in chest injury. *J Trauma* 14:93, 1990.
142. King RW, Plewa MC, Buderer NM, et al.: Injury severity determination: Requirements, approaches, and applications. *Ann Emerg Med* 3:1427, 1986.
143. Rutledge R: The Injury Severity Score is unable to differentiate between poor care and severe injury. *J Trauma* 40:944, 1996.
144. Rutledge R: Injury severity and probability of survival assessment in trauma patients using a predictive hierarchical network model derived from ICD-9 codes. *J Trauma* 38:590, 1995.
145. Trunkey DD, Lim RC: Analysis of 425 consecutive trauma fatalities: An autopsy study. *J Am Coll Emerg Phys* 3:368, 1974.
146. Stewart TC, Lane PL, Stefanits T: An evaluation of patient outcomes before and after trauma center designation using Trauma and Injury Severity Score analysis. *J Trauma* 39:1036, 1995.
147. Petrie D, Lane P, Stewart TC: An evaluation of patient outcomes comparing trauma team activated versus trauma team not activated using TRISS analysis. Trauma and Injury Severity Score. *J Trauma* 37:870, 1996.
148. Morris JA Jr, Auerbach PS, Marshall GA, et al.: The Trauma Score as a triage tool in the prehospital setting. *JAMA* 256:1319, 1986.
149. Norwood S, Myers MB: Outcomes following injury in a predominantly rural-population-based trauma center. *Arch Surg* 129:800, 1994.
150. Norwood S, Myers MB: Injury severity scoring: Perspectives in development and future directions. *Am J Surg* 129:43S, 1993.
151. Brenneman FD, Boulanger BR, McLellan BA, et al.: Measuring injury severity: Time for a change? *J Trauma* 44:580, 1998.
152. Moore EE, Dunn EL, Moore JB, et al.: Penetrating abdominal trauma index. *J Trauma* 21:439, 1981.
153. Moore EE, Shackford SR, Pachter HL, et al.: Organ injury scaling: Spleen, liver, and kidney. *J Trauma* 29:1664, 1989.
154. Osler T, Baker SP, Long W: A modification of the injury severity score that both improves accuracy and simplifies scoring. *J Trauma* 43:922, 1997.
155. Tay S, Sloan EP, Zun L, et al.: Comparison of the new injury severity score and the injury severity score. *J Trauma* 56:162, 2004.
156. Hedges JR, Feero S, Moore B, et al.: Factors contributing to paramedic onscene time during evaluation and management of blunt trauma. *Am J Emerg Med* 6:443, 1988.
157. Feero S, Hedges JR, Simmons E, et al.: Does out-of-hospital EMS time affect trauma survival? *Am J Emerg Med* 13:133, 1995.
158. Goldstein L, Doig CJ, Bates S, et al.: Adopting the pre-hospital index for interfacility helicopter transport: a proposal. *Int J Care of Injured* 34:3, 2005.
159. Plant JR, MacLeod DB, Korbeck J: Limitations of the prehospital index in identifying patients in need of a major trauma center. *Ann Emerg Med* 26:133, 1995.
160. Roorda J, Van Beeck EF, Stapert JW, et al.: Evaluation performance of the Revised Trauma Score as a triage instrument in the prehospital setting. *Injury* 27:163, 1996.
161. Kim Y, Jung KY, Kim C, et al.: Validation of the International Classification of Diseases 10th Edition-based Injury Severity Score (ICISS). *J Trauma* 48:280, 2000.
162. Bond RJ, Kortbeek JB, Preshaw RM: Field trauma triage: Combining mechanism of injury with the prehospital index for an improved trauma triage tool. *J Trauma* 43:283, 1997.
163. Holcomb JB, Salinas J, McManus JM, et al.: Manual vital signs reliably predict need for life-saving interventions in trauma patients. *J Trauma* 59:821, 2005.
164. West JG, Murdock MA, Baldwin LC, et al.: A method for evaluating field triage criteria. *J Trauma* 26:655, 1986.
165. Norcross ED, Ford DW, Cooper ME, et al.: Application of American College of Surgeons' field triage guidelines by pre-hospital personnel. *J Am Coll Surg* 181:539, 1995.
166. Cooper ME, Yarbrough DR, Zone-Smith L, et al.: Application of field triage guidelines by pre-hospital personnel: Is mechanism of injury a valid guideline for patient triage? *Am Surg* 61:363, 1995.
167. Smith DP, Enderson BL, Maull KI: Trauma in the elderly: Determinants of outcome. *South Med J* 83:171, 1990.
168. DeKeyser F, Carolan D, Trask A: Suburban geriatric trauma: The experiences of a level I trauma center. *Am J Crit Care* 4:379, 1995.
169. Van der Sluis CK, Klasen HJ, Eisma WH, et al.: Major trauma in young and old: What is the difference? *J Trauma* 40:78, 1996.
170. Hill DA, Delaney LM, Roncal S: A chi-square automatic interaction detection (CHAID) analysis of factors determining trauma outcomes. *J Trauma* 42:62, 1997.
171. Burstein JL, Henry MC, Alicandro JM, et al.: Evidence for and impact of selective reporting of trauma triage mechanism criteria. *Acad Emerg Med* 3:1011, 1996.
172. Fries GR, McCalla G, Levitt MA, et al.: A prospective comparison of paramedic judgement and the trauma triage rule in the prehospital setting. *Ann Emerg Med* 24:885, 1994.
173. Simmons E, Hedges JR, Irwin L, et al.: Paramedic injury severity perception can aid trauma triage. *Ann Emerg Med* 26:461, 1995.
174. Rouse A: Do ambulance crews triage trauma patients? *Arch Emerg Med* 8:185, 1991.

175. Santaniello JM, Esposito TJ, Luchette FA, et al.: Mechanism of injury does not predict acuity or level of service need: Field triage criteria revisited. *Surgery* 134:698, 2003.

176. Terregino CA, Reid JC, Marburger RK, et al.: Secondary emergency department triage (supertriage) and trauma team activation: Effects on resource utilization and patient care. *J Trauma* 43:61, 1997.

177. Tinkoff GH, O'Connor RE, Fulda GJ: Impact of a two-tiered trauma response in the emergency department: Promoting efficient resource utilization. *J Trauma* 41:735, 1996.

178. Gabbe BJ, Cameron PA, Wolkfe R, et al.: Prehospital prediction of intensive care unit stay and mortality in blunt trauma patients. *J Trauma* 49:647, 2000.

179. Napolitano LM, Ferrer T, McCarter RJ, et al.: Systemic inflammatory responses syndrome score at admission independently predicts mortality and length of stay in trauma patients. *J Trauma* 49:647, 2000.

180. Steele JT, Hoyt DB, Simons RK, et al.: Is operating room resuscitation a way to save time? *Am J Surg* 174:683, 1997.

181. Rhodes M, Brader A, Lucke J, et al.: Direct transport to the operating room for resuscitation of trauma patients. *J Trauma* 29:907, 1989.

182. Barlow B, Niemirska M, Gandhi RP: Stab wounds in children. *J Pediatr Surg* 18:926, 1983.

183. Barlow B, Neimirska M, Gandhi RP: Ten years' experience with pediatric gunshot wounds. *J Pediatr Surg* 17:927, 1982.

184. DeKeyser FG, Paratore A, Seneca RP et al.: Decreasing the cost of trauma care: A system of secondary inhospital triage. *Ann Emerg Med* 23:841, 1994.

185. *The San Diego County Trauma System Report*. San Diego County, CA: Department of Health Services, 1999.

186. Henry MC, Hollander JE, Alicandro JM: Incremental benefit of individual American College of Surgeons trauma triage criteria. *Acad Emerg Med* 3:992, 1996.

187. Baker SB, O'Neill B: Geographic variations in mortality from motor vehicle crashes. *N Engl J Med* 316:1384, 1987.

188. Cales RH, Trunkey DD: Preventable trauma deaths: A review of trauma care systems development. *JAMA* 254:1059, 1985.

189. Certo TF, Rogers FB, Pilcher DB: Review of care of fatally injured patients in a rural state: 5-year follow up. *J Trauma* 23:559, 1983.

190. Martin GD, Cogbill TH, Landercasper J, et al.: Prospective analysis of rural interhospital transfer of injured patients to a referral trauma center. *J Trauma* 30:1014, 1990.

191. Hicks TC, Danzl DF, Thomas DM, et al.: Resuscitation and transfer of trauma patients: A prospective study. *Ann Emerg Med* 11:296, 1982.

192. Houtchens BA: Major trauma in the rural mountain West. *J Am Coll Emerg Phys* 6:343, 1977.

193. Deane SA, Gaudry PL, Woods WP: Interhospital transfer in the management of acute trauma. *Aust N Z J Surg* 60:441, 1990.

194. Kanter R, Tompkins J: Adverse events during interhospital transport: Physiologic deterioration associated with pre-transport severity of illness. *Pediatrics* 84:43, 1989.

195. Andrews P, Piper I, Dearden N, et al.: Secondary insults during interhospital hospital transport of head-injured patients. *Lancet* 335:327, 1990.

196. Olson CM, Jastremski MS, Vilogi JP, et al.: Stabilization of patients prior to interhospital transport. *Am J Emerg Med* 5:33, 1987.

197. Rogers FB, Osler TM, Shackford SR, et al.: Study of the outcome of patients transferred to a level I hospital after stabilization at an outlying hospital in a rural setting. *J Trauma* 46:328, 1999.

198. McGinn GH, MacKenzie RE, Donnelly JA, et al.: Interhospital transfer of the critically ill trauma patient: The potential role of a specialist transport team in a trauma system. *J Accid Emerg Med* 13:90, 1996.

199. Harrahil M, Bartkus E: Preparing the trauma patient for transfer. *J Emerg Nurs* 16:25, 1990.

200. Hackel A: An organizational system for critical care transports. *Int Anesthesiol Clin* 25:1, 1987.

201. Dunn JD: Legal aspects of transfers. In Fromm RE, ed. *Problems in Critical Care: Critical Care Transport.* Philadelphia: JB Lippincott, 1990, p. 447.

202. Frew SA: *Patient Transfers: How to Comply With the Law.* Dallas: American College of Emergency Physicians, 1990.

203. Strobos J: Tightening the screw: Statutory and legal supervision of interhospital patient transfers. *Ann Emerg Med* 20:302, 1991.

204. Nathens AB, Maier RV, Copass MK, et al.: Payer status: The unspoken triage criterion. *J Trauma* 50:776, 2001.

205. State of Colorado, Board of Health: *Rules and Regulations Pertaining to the Statewide Trauma System-Chapter 2*: Area Trauma Advisory Councils, 1999.

206. Leibovici D, Gofrit ON, Heruti RJ, et al.: Interhospital patient transfer: A quality improvement indicator for prehospital triage in mass casualties. *Am J Emer Med* 14:91–93, 1997.

207. Committee on Trauma: Interhospital transfer of patients. *Bull Am Coll Surg* 69:29, 1984.

208. Guidelines Committee of the American College of Critical Care Medicine: Guidelines for the transfer of critically ill patients. *Crit Care Med* 21:931, 1993.

209. Moylan JA: Trauma injuries. Triage and stabilization for safe transfer. *Postgrad Med* 71:166, 1985.

210. Veenema KR, Rodewald LE: Stabilization of rural multiple trauma patients at Level III emergency departments before transfer to a Level I Regional Trauma Center. *Ann Emerg Med* 25:175, 1995.

211. Cone JB: Tertiary trauma care in a rural state. *Am J Surg* 160:652, 1990.

212. Gilmore KM, Clemmer TP, Orme JF: Commitment to trauma in a low population density area. *J Trauma* 21:883, 1981.

213. Mucha P, Farnell MB, Czech JM, et al.: A rural regional trauma center. *J Trauma* 23:337, 1983.

214. Wenneker WW, Murray DH, Ledwich T: Improved trauma care in a rural hospital after establishing a Level II trauma center. *Am J Surg* 160:655, 1990.

215. Lee RB, Morris JA Jr, Parker RS: Presence of three or more rib fractures as an indicator of need for interhospital transfer. *J Trauma* 29:795, 1989.

216. Lee RB, Bass SM, Morris JA Jr, et al.: Three or more rib fractures as an indicator for transfer to a Level I Trauma Center: A population-based study. *J Trauma* 30:689, 1990.

217. Clark DE, Cobean RA, Radke FR, et al.: Management of major hepatic trauma involving interhospital transfer. *Am Surg* 60:881, 1994.

218. Henry MC, Alicandro JM, Hollander JE, et al.: Evaluation of American College of Surgeons trauma triage criteria in a suburban and rural setting. *Am J Emerg Med* 14:124, 1996.

219. Rhodes M, Perline R, Aronson J, et al.: Field triage for on-scene helicopter transport. *J Trauma* 26:963, 1986.

220. Baxt WG, Moody P: The impact of a rotocraft aeromedical emergency care service on trauma mortality. *JAMA* 249:3047, 1983.

221. Moylan JA, Fitzpatrick KT, Beyer AF III, et al.: Factors improving survival in multisystem trauma patients. *Ann Surg* 27:679, 1988.

222. Boyd CR, Corse KM, Campbell RC: Emergency interhospital transport of the major trauma patient: Air versus ground. *J Trauma* 29:793, 1989.

223. Valenzuela TD, Criss EA, Copass MK, et al.: Critical care air transportation of the severely injured: Does long distance transport adversely affect survival? *Ann Emerg Med* 19:169, 1990.

224. Garrison HG, Benson NH, Whitley TW: Helicopter use by rural emergency departments to transfer trauma victims: A study of time-to-request intervals. *Am J Emerg Med* 7:384, 1989.

225. Schiller WR, Knox R, Zinnecker H, et al.: Effect of helicopter transport of trauma victims on survival in an urban trauma center. *J Trauma* 28:1127, 1988.

226. Thomas F, Wisham J, Clemmer TP, et al.: Outcome, transport times and costs of patients evacuated by helicopter versus fixed-wing aircraft. *West J Med* 153:40, 1990.

227. Morley AP: The costs and benefits of helicopter emergency ambulance services in England and Wales. *J Public Health Med* 18:67, 1996.

228. Lowe RJ, Baker RJ: Organization and function of trauma care units. *J Trauma* 13:285, 1973.

229. http://www.facs.org/dept/trauma/handbook.html. Accessed October 15, 2006.

230. Hoyt DB, Hollingsworth-Fridlund P, Winchell RJ, et al.: An analysis of recurrent process errors leading to provider-related complications on an organized trauma service: directions for care improvement. *J Trauma* 36:377, 1994.

231. Davis JW, Hoyt DB, McArdle MS, et al.: The significance of critical care errors in causing preventable death in trauma patients in a trauma system. *J Trauma* 31:813, 1991.

232. Davis JW, Hoyt DB, McArdle MS, et al.: An analysis of errors causing morbidity and mortality in a trauma system: a guide for quality improvement. *J Trauma* 32:660, 1992.

233. Hoyt DB, Hollingsworth-Fridlund P, Fortlage D, et al.: An evaluation of provider-related and disease-related morbidity in a Level 1 university trauma service: Directions for quality improvement. *J Trauma* 33:586, 1992.

234. Shackford SR, Hollingsworth-Fridlund P, McArdle MS, et al.: Assuring quality in a trauma system——The medical audit committee: Composition, cost, and results. *J Trauma* 27:866, 1987.

235. Hoyt DB, Hollingsworth-Fridlund P: Quality improvements in trauma systems. In Trunkey DD and Lewis FR. *Current Therapy of Trauma.* 4th ed. St. Louis, MO: Mosby, Inc, 1999, p. 23.

236. Lowe DK, Gately HL, Goss JR, et al.: Patterns of death, complications and errors in the management of motor vehicle accident victims: Implications for a regional system of trauma care. *J Trauma* 23:503, 1983.

237. Kreis DJ, Plasencia G, Augenstein D, et al.: Preventable trauma deaths: Dade County, Florida. *Trauma* 26:649, 1986.

238. Cales RH, Trunkey DD. Preventable trauma deaths. A review of trauma care systems development. *JAMA* 254:1059, 1985.

239. Dubois RW, Brook RH: Preventable deaths: Who, how often, and why? *Ann Intern Med* 109:582, 1988.

240. MacKenzie EJ, Steinwachs DM, Bone LR, et al.: Inter-rater reliability of preventable death judgments. The Preventable Death Study Group. *J Trauma* 33:292, 1992.

241. McDermott FT, Cordner SM, Tremayne AB, Consultative Committee on Road Traffic Fatalities in Victoria: Reproducibility of preventable death judgments and problem identification in 60 consecutive road trauma fatalities in Victoria, Australia. *J Trauma* 43:831, 1997.
242. Maio RF, Burney RE, Gregor MA, et al.: A study of preventable trauma mortality in rural Michigan. *J Trauma* 41:83, 1996.
243. Sampalis JS, Boukas S, Nikolis A, et al.: Preventable death classification: Interrater reliability and comparison with ISS-based survival probability estimates. *Accid Anal Prev* 27:199, 1995.
244. Wilson DS, McElligott J, Fielding LP: Identification of preventable trauma deaths: confounded inquiries? *J Trauma* 32:45, 1992.
245. Cales RH: Trauma mortality in Orange County: The effect of implementation of a regional trauma system. *Ann Emerg Med* 13:1, 1984.
246. Campbell S, Watkins G, Kreis D: Preventable deaths in a self-designated trauma system. *Am Surg* 55:478, 1989.
247. Guss DA, Meyer FT, Neuman TS, et al.: The impact of a regionalized trauma system on trauma care in San Diego County. *Ann Emerg Med* 18:1141, 1989.
248. Moylan JA, Detmer DE, Rose J, et al.: Evaluation of the quality of hospital care for major trauma. *J Trauma* 16:517, 1976.
249. Neuman TS, Bockman MA, Mood, et al.: An autopsy study of traumatic deaths; San Diego County, 1979. *Am J Surg* 144:722, 1982.
250. Thoburn E, Norris P, Flores R, et al.: System care improves trauma outcome: patient care errors dominate reduced preventable death rate. *J Emerg Med* 11:135, 1993.
251. Boyd CR, Tolson MA, Copes WS: Evaluating trauma care: The TRISS method. Trauma score and the injury severity score. *J Trauma* 27:370,1987.
252. Payne SR, Waller JA: Trauma registry and trauma center biases in injury research. *J Trauma* 29:424, 1989.
253. Jones JM, Redmond AD, Templeton J: Uses and abuses of statistical models for evaluating trauma care. *J Trauma* 38:89, 1995.
254. Waller JA, Skelly JM, Davis JH: Trauma center-related biases in injury research. *J Trauma* 38:325, 1995.
255. Champion HR, Copes WS, Sacco WJ, et al.: The major trauma outcome study: Establishing national norms for trauma care. *J Trauma* 30:1356, 1990.
256. Shackford SR, Mackersie RC, Hoyt DB, et al.: Impact of a trauma system on outcome of severely injured patients. *Arch Surg* 122:523, 1987.
257. Champion HR, Sacco WJ, Copes WS: Improvement in outcome from trauma center care. *Arch Surg* 127:333, 1992.
258. Sampalis JS, Lavoie A, Williams JI, et al.: Standardized mortality ratio analysis on a sample of severely injured patients from a large Canadian city without regionalized trauma care. *J Trauma* 33:205, 1992.
259. Cooper A, Barlow B, DiScala C, et al.: Efficacy of pediatric trauma care: Results of a population-based study. *J Pediatr Surg* 28:299, 1993.
260. Wald SL, Shackford SR, Fenwick J: The effect of secondary insults on mortality and long-term disability after severe head injury in a rural region without a trauma system. *J Trauma* 34:377, 1993.
261. Norwood S, Myers MB: Outcomes following injury in a predominantly rural-population-based trauma center. *Arch Surg* 129:800, 1994.
262. Karsteadt LL, Larsen CL, Farmer PD: Analysis of a rural trauma program using the TRISS methodology: A three-year retrospective study. *J Trauma* 36:395, 1994.
263. Norwood S, Fernandez L, England J: The early effects of implementing American College of Surgeons level II criteria on transfer and survival rates at a rurally based community hospital. *J Trauma* 39:240, 1995.
264. Stewart TC, Lane PL, Stefanits T: An evaluation of patient outcomes before and after trauma center designation using Trauma and Injury Severity Score analysis. *J Trauma* 39:1036, 1995.
265. Lane PL, Doig G, Stewart TC, et al.: Trauma outcome analysis and the development of regional norms. *Accid Anal Prev* 29:53, 1997.
266. Barquist E, Pizzutiello M, Tian L, et al.: Effect of trauma system maturation on mortality rates in patients with blunt injuries in the Finger Lakes region of New York State. *J Trauma* 49:63, 2000.
267. Clemmer TP, Orme JF Jr, Thomas FO, et al.: Outcome of critically injured patients treated at Level I trauma centers versus full-service community hospitals. *Crit Care Med* 13:861, 1985.
268. Ornato JP, Craren EJ, Nelson NM, et al.: Impact of improved emergency medical services and emergency trauma care on the reduction in mortality from trauma. *J Trauma* 25:575, 1985.
269. MacKenzie EJ, Steinwachs DM, Shankar B: Classifying trauma severity based on hospital discharge diagnoses. Validation of an ICD-9CM to AIS-85 conversion table. *Med Care* 27:412, 1989.
270. Stout N, Bell C: Effectiveness of source documents for identifying fatal occupational injuries: A synthesis of studies. *Am J Public Health* 81:725, 1991.
271. Romano PS, McLoughlin E: Unspecified injuries on death certificates: A source of bias in injury research. *Am J Epidemiol* 136:863, 1992.
272. Kane G, Wheeler NC, Cook S, et al.: Impact of the Los Angeles county trauma system on the survival of seriously injured patients. *J Trauma* 32:576, 1992.
273. Pollock DA, O'Neil JM, Parrish RG, et al.: Temporal and geographic trends in the autopsy frequency of blunt and penetrating trauma deaths in the United States. *JAMA* 269:1525, 1993.
274. Mullins RJ, Veum-Stone J, Helfand M, et al.: Outcome of hospitalized injured patients after institution of a trauma system in an urban area. *JAMA* 271:1919, 1994.
275. Kraus JF, Peek C, Silberman T, et al.: The accuracy of death certificates in identifying work-related fatal injuries. *Am J Epidemiol* 141:973, 1995.
276. Mullins RJ, Veum-Stone J, Hedges JR, et al.: Influence of a statewide trauma system on location of hospitalization and outcome of injured patients. *J Trauma* 40:536, 1996.
277. Hulka F, Mullins RJ, Mann NC, et al.: Influence of a statewide trauma system on pediatric hospitalization and outcome. *J Trauma* 42:514, 1997.
278. Mullins RJ, Mann NC, Hedges JR, et al.: Adequacy of hospital discharge status as a measure of outcome among injured patients. *JAMA* 279:1727, 1998.
279. Mullins RJ, Mann NC, Hedges JR, et al.: Preferential benefit of implementation of a statewide trauma system in one of two adjacent states. *J Trauma* 44:609, 1998.
280. Rogers FB, Shackford SR, Hoyt DB, et al.: Trauma deaths in a mature urban vs rural trauma system. A comparison. *Arch Surg* 132:376, 1997.
281. Rutledge R, Fakhry SM, Meyer A, et al.: An analysis of the association of trauma centers with per capita hospitalizations and death rates from injury. *Ann Surg* 218:512, 1993.
282. Rutledge R, Messick J, Baker CC, et al.: Multivariate population-based analysis of the association of county trauma centers with per capita county trauma death rates. *J Trauma* 33:29, 1992.
283. Smith JS Jr, Martin LF, Young WW, et al.: Do trauma centers improve outcome over non-trauma centers: The evaluation of regional trauma care using discharge abstract data and patient management categories. *J Trauma* 30:1533, 1990.
284. Nathens AB, Jurkovich GJ, Cummings P, et al.: The effect of organized systems of trauma on motor vehicle crash mortality. *JAMA* 283:1990, 2000.
285. Mullins RJ, Mann NC: Introduction to the academic symposium to evaluate evidence regarding the efficacy of trauma systems. *J Trauma* 47:S3, 1999.
286. Mann NC, Mullins RJ, Mackenzie EJ, et al.: Systematic review of published evidence regarding trauma system effectiveness. *J Trauma* 47:S25, 1999.
287. MacKenzie EJ: Review of evidence regarding trauma system effectiveness resulting from panel studies. *J Trauma* 47:S34, 1999.
288. Hoyt DB: Use of panel study methods. *J Trauma* 47:S42, 1999.
289. Trunkey DD: Invited commentary: Panel reviews of trauma mortality. *J Trauma* 47:S44, 1999.
290. Jurkovich GJ, Mock C: Systematic review of trauma system effectiveness based on registry comparisons. *J Trauma* 47:S46, 1999.
291. Pollock DA: Summary of the discussion: trauma registry data and TRISS evidence. *J Trauma* 47:S56, 1999.
292. Mullins RJ, Mann NC: Population-based research assessing the effectiveness of trauma systems. *J Trauma* 47:S59, 1999.
293. Hedges JR. Summary of the discussion: What have we learned about population-based investigations? *J Trauma* 47:S67, 1999.
294. Utter GH, Maier RV, Rivara FP, et al.: Inclusive trauma systems: Do they improve triage or outcomes of the severely injured? *J Trauma* 60:529, 2006.
295. Trauma System Agenda for the Future, NHTSA, 2002.

# Commentary ■ LAWRENCE LOTTENBERG

In this chapter, Hoyt, Coimbra, and Potenza have once again provided a comprehensive overview of trauma systems, triage and transport. This is a must-read for all governmental agencies dealing with trauma on a federal, state, and local level, and for all trauma medical directors and program managers. The authors have meticulously outlined the extensive history that has now evolved into the modern trauma system present in most of the United States today. However, the authors continue to remind us that although progress has been made, there are still several issues that must be dealt with in order to create the ideal comprehensive trauma system. These issues will be addressed below.

For this edition, the authors have included expanded comments and data on the anatomic and mechanism of injury criteria in field triage and hospital triage. The significance of age and body region injured to improve the predictive power to select patients likely to need intensive care or a surgical procedure are also included.

The authors have greatly expanded triage principles for multiple patient scenarios and a clear distinction between multiple and mass casualties help the reader begin to understand the challenges of disaster preparedness. The section on disaster management brings a new kind of disaster to the forefront, natural disasters, such as Hurricane Katrina. One overall theme in disaster management is how the trauma surgeon and the trauma community must be the leaders in organizing, preparing, and triaging in all mass casualty situations, even ones such as Katrina. Certainly the efforts of one of the editors (K.M.) in organizing the Atlantic and Gulf States Disaster Coalition in order that multiple states and regions affected by storms of such magnitude be able to talk to each other and share resources is a refreshing concept which was long overdue. This section concludes by reinforcing the Israeli experience with mass casualty and terrorist attacks and also emphasizes the key role trauma surgeons play, concluding the best triage officer is the trauma surgeon. Recently, the American College of Surgeons Committee on Trauma has initiated a superb course entitled Disaster Management and Emergency Preparedness that emphasizes on an "all hazards" approach and educates trauma physicians and other providers. It is hoped that this course will become the "gold standard" by which all disaster management is administered.

Hoyt and associates close this outstanding chapter with a call for more attention by our legislators to the problem of trauma funding. This will be a cog in the wheels of trauma system development. There are, however, many initiatives that can be taken to deal with this problem. The trauma community needs to continue to push the federal government for trauma funding and the recent HRSA document Model Trauma System Planning and Evaluation is certainly a starting point. Many, many stakeholders in federal government and state government as well as the trauma professionals have participated in this document and the fact that it uses a public health model to justify the need for federal support can only be a positive one.

My own personal experience in the state of Florida over the last 25 years has shown that being persistent and working side by side with our legislators can allow many initiatives to come to fruition. The State of Florida Department of Health Office of Trauma is now contracted with a state trauma medical director, who is a trauma surgeon and employs over one dozen trauma surgeons to sit on numerous committees that regulate trauma care. The state authorized and financed a recent trauma study entitled A Comprehensive Assessment of the Florida Trauma System that was administered by the trauma community and concluded that trauma is underfinanced throughout Florida but that outcomes are among the best in the nation. The study also addressed patient destinations and suggested only two or three more strategically located trauma centers to satisfy West's original criteria for a mature trauma system. That study resulted in the Florida legislature and the governor enacting the very first bill that will guarantee a recurring source of funds directly to the 21 (soon to be 22) trauma center hospitals in the state, via fines on traffic violations. These initiatives are not the end, but just the beginning. Certainly, using the data presented by Hoyt et al. should allow anyone to accomplish their goals.

# Injury Severity Scoring and Outcomes Research

*Patrick D. Kilgo* ■ *J. Wayne Meredith* ■ *Turner M. Osler*

## INTRODUCTION

Trauma severity scoring is defined simply as the quantification of the risk of an outcome following trauma. It is an amalgam that combines elements of clinical acumen and statistical theory to provide a single metric used to describe aspects of patient condition after some traumatic incident. The outcome of interest may be survival, hospital or ICU length of stay, performance of a procedure, or any other endpoint of interest.

Long before these "scores" are formally calculated, physicians use estimates of the severity of trauma based upon their clinical experience in managing their patients. Thus, severity scores are not typically used for clinical decision making in the acute setting but are used for field triage, referrals, outcomes prediction, epidemiological studies, and quality improvements. To the trauma outcomes researcher the scores are risk stratifiers, used to divide patients into subsets of risk so that other predictors of outcome may be evaluated. To administrators, score-based measures are a first step toward quality control "report cards" and improvements in health care delivery or injury prevention.

All these applications fall under the broad umbrella of risk adjustment or "case mix" adjustment, that is, the accounting of risk due to trauma severity so that other risk factors (time to treatment, mechanism, surgeon, injury prevention equipment, etc.) may be properly evaluated when examining outcomes. Risk adjustment might be as simple as defining classes of a variable to stratify risk groups or as complicated as using the risk adjustor in a multivariable regression model.[1]

In general, three types of risk adjustments (hereafter called scores) are calculated to account for trauma severity:

Anatomic Injury Scores

Physiologic Derangement Scores

Comorbidity Scores

Unlike other circumstantial factors (time to treatment, quality of care, etc) each of these factors are intrinsic to the patient and therefore important to understand and quantify.

## INJURY CODING

The accurate cataloging of injuries and clinical data precedes severity scoring. Most trauma-oriented care facilities have trained coding personnel on staff that transcribe clinician records of traumatic incidents into codes that capture individual injuries. The most advanced trauma-specific coding lexicon is the Abbreviated Injury Scale (AIS) which was first conceived as a system to define the type and severity of injuries arising from motor vehicle accidents and is currently in its 5th revision.[2] The AIS is a proprietary system that requires specialized training for medical records coding personnel. An AIS code consisted of a six-digit number followed by a consensus-derived severity designation after the decimal. The six digits classify the injury by region, type of anatomic structure, specific structure, and level. Of most interest is the "AIS severity", that is, the digit following the decimal which ranges from 1 to 6 and numerically describes the severity of the injury. An AIS severity of 1 is a superficial injury while a 6 is thought to be unsurvivable (see Table 5-1). The AIS 2004 revision contains over 2000 descriptors of injury and includes mappings to the Functional Capacity Index (FCI), a 10-dimensional quality of life measure.[3]

The International Classification of Diseases (ICD) coding system is over 100 years old and is currently in its 9th revision (ICD-9).[4] ICD-9 codes exist for over 10,000 medical conditions, about 2,000 of which are physical injuries. Smaller acute care centers code with ICD-9 while larger ACS-verified institutions will often code with both ICD-9 and AIS. ICD-9 codes are primarily used for administrative purposes, such as billing and event reporting. The trauma range in ICD-9 codes is 800.0 to 959.9. Unlike

**TABLE 5-1**

| AIS Components, Definition of 1–6 | |
|---|---|
| **AIS SEVERITY** | **ORDINAL DESCRIPTION** |
| 1 | Minor injury |
| 2 | Moderate injury |
| 3 | Serious injury |
| 4 | Severe injury |
| 5 | Critical injury |
| 6 | Virtually unsurvivable injury |

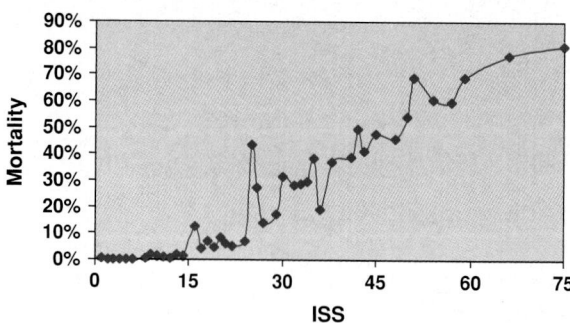

**FIGURE 5-1.** ISS versus actual mortality. This graph plots the mortality associated with each ISS value. Of note is the erratic choppiness of the curve, indicating that ISS is not a monotonically increasing function of mortality. It is characterized in places by steep decreases in mortality as ISS gets larger. Ideally, ISS would be considered nominal and not ordinal.

AIS which attaches an ordinal severity to each injury, ICD-9 codes are only nominal classifications and do not measure the severity of injury. AIS codes are generally preferred over ICD-9 because of its greater specificity of injury description but valid scores can be formulated from either system. Today, most countries use ICD-10; however, it is still not in use in the United States.[5]

## SEVERITY SCORES

### Anatomic Scores

Anatomic injury scores are the most developed types of risk adjustment following trauma. Many scores have been proposed in the literature but this review will be limited to scores that have gained practical acceptance. The majority of scoring algorithms are designed to predict mortality and are not specifically validated on other outcomes like length of stay (LOS) or functional status, though moderate correlations may exist. The AIS severity designation (ordinal 1 through 6) that accompanies each coded injury is the simplest form of a score. The maximum AIS (maxAIS), which is the largest AIS severity among a set of injuries within a patient, is highly associated with mortality but ignores information provided from other injuries.

In 1974, Baker et al. first posited a multiinjury score by introducing the Injury Severity Score (ISS).[6] ISS divides the body into six regions – head or neck, face, abdominal, chest, extremities, and external. Any patient that sustains an injury with AIS severity of 6 is automatically given an ISS score of 75. Otherwise, the largest AIS severity in each of the three most severely injured regions is subset and the sum of the squares of these AIS severities is computed to form ISS.

ISS correlates well with mortality and remains the most widely used anatomical scoring system. However, ISS has many limitations.[7] ISS is most often treated as a continuous, ordinal, monotonic function of mortality but it is in fact none of these (see Fig. 5-1).[8,9] There are 44 distinct values of ISS, some of which are possible in two different combinations of sums of squares. Optimally, each combination would be treated nominally (or as its own class) in terms of risk adjustment but in practice this seldom occurs. Further, ISS only considers one injury in each of the body regions and thus ignores important injury information. Because of these shortcomings we believe ISS should be retired and replaced by one of the more modern injury scores that are now available (see below).

Osler et al. formulated the New Injury Severity Score (NISS) to address some of the ISS shortcomings, specifically its omission of multiple occurrences of serious injuries within a body region.[10] NISS is the sum of the squares of the three most severe AIS severities, regardless of body region (and keeping the convention that an AIS of 6 automatically results in a NISS of 75). This permutation offers a slight prediction advantage but has several of the same shortcomings as ISS (see Fig. 5-2).

Copes et al. adjusted for body region differences and AIS severity with the Anatomic Profile Score (APS), in which three "modified components" are weighted to form a single scalar.[8] The mA component quantifies head/brain and spinal cord injuries, the mB component quantifies thorax and neck injuries, and the mC component quantifies all other injuries. The components themselves are defined as the square root of the sum of the squares of all serious injuries (AIS severity of 3, 4, 5, or 6) within their specified body region. Once the components are computed,

$$APS = .3199(mA) + .4381(mB) + .1406(mC) + .7961(\max AIS).$$

Although APS represents a logical approach to anatomic scoring it has failed to supplant ISS.

Mackenzie et al. made the first attempt to translate ICD-9 codes into the AIS lexicon, and thus allow AIS-based injury scoring

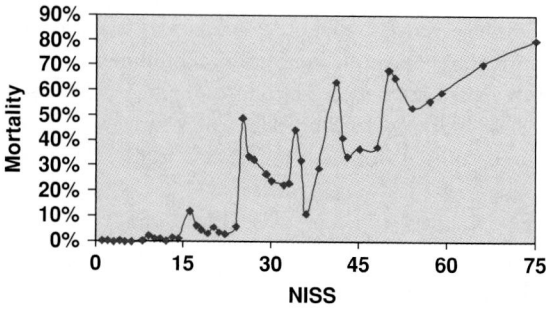

**FIGURE 5-2.** NISS versus actual mortality. This graph plots the mortality associated with each NISS value. The NISS curve is also very nonmonotonic, even more so than ISS.

approaches to be applied to data encoded using ICD-9 codes.[11] The resulting proprietary software is called ICDMAP-90 and is widely used to "map" ICD-9 codes to approximate AIS codes for each injury, from which ISS, NISS, APS, and other scores can be calculated. This approach has been utilized effectively to study trauma system outcomes.[12,13] However, the software has some limitations since AIS is so much more specific than ICD-9 that many ICD-9 codes do not have an exact AIS equivalent.

Osler et al. took an empirical estimation approach to injury severity estimation with the formulation of ICD-9 survival risk ratios (SRRs) and defined the International Classification of Diseases Injury Severity Score (ICISS) based upon these SRRs.[14] An SRR is an ICD-9 code-specific estimate of the survival probability associated with a particular injury. For a set of patients, the SRR for a particular injury code is the number of patients that survive an injury divided by the number of patients who display the injury. The ICISS score is the product of the SRRs corresponding to a patient's set of injuries and is bounded by 0 and 1. Though it resembles an overall probability, ICISS can only be considered a scalar since most SRRs are "contaminated" by patients with multiple injuries. Independent SRRs can be calculated from patients that only have an isolated injury but these are not available for all codes since many injuries rarely occur in isolation.[15]

ICISS offers several advantages over other anatomic scores and the ICDMAP-90 mapping software. First, because of its ICD-9 base coding lexicon, it can be used in any clinical setting, including smaller centers that typically do not perform AIS coding. Unlike the consensus-derived AIS scores, ICISS' empirical approach means that powerful statistical estimates of injury-specific survival can be computed if enough representative patients are available for study. Consequently, unlike ISS and NISS, ICISS is a smooth, if nonlinear, function of mortality (see Fig. 5-3). ICISS also has limitations including the fact that SRRs are database-specific and the degree to which they are applicable within disparate populations remains uncertain. SRRs are available from several sources including the National Trauma Data Bank (NTDB), which provides them to researchers free of charge.[16]

Like ICD-9 codes, AIS codes may also be treated nominally, ignoring the AIS severity and taking advantage of the code's specificity in injury classification. SRRs are available for AIS codes and

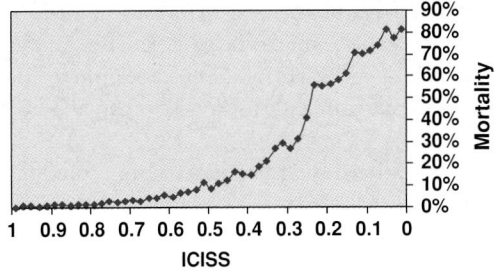

**FIGURE 5-3.** ICISS versus actual mortality. ICISS, unlike ISS and NISS, has a very smooth association with mortality, though it too is nonlinear. In the places where ICISS mortality decreases from one value to the next, the decrease is very slight, never more than about 7% and corrects itself quickly. Contrast these small decreases with the decreases seen in ISS and NISS, which can be as large as 20% from one value to the next and 30% in the span of two values.

the TRAIS score (the product of AIS SRRs) is the analog to ICISS. Kilgo et al. showed that ICISS and TRAIS behave very similarly in a large group of patients coded both ways (see Fig. 5-4) and that TRAIS outpredicts its AIS counterparts ISS, NISS, and APS.[17]

Researchers and administrators may ask: Which of these approaches is the best? Several large studies have compared these scores. Sacco et al. and Meredith et al. compared these anatomic scores in terms of their ability to predict mortality.[18,19] Both studies found that APS and ICISS better discriminate survivors from nonsurvivors than ISS, NISS, and the ICDMAP versions of ISS, NISS, and APS. A surprising finding was that MAXAIS performed better than its multi-injury counterparts ISS and NISS. Based on this result, Kilgo et al. showed that the patient's worst injury, regardless of the coding lexicon (ICD-9 or AIS) and the estimation approach (AIS consensus or empirical SRRs), was a better predictor of mortality than multi-injury scores, though there remains no consensus on this.[17]

Finally, in 1987, the American Association for the Surgery of Trauma (AAST) introduced the AAST Organ Injury Scale (OIS).[20] The goal of the scale was to standardize descriptive measures of intra-abdominal and intra-thoracic organ injuries into a common "grading" system. Like AIS, the OIS provides an ordinal scale to

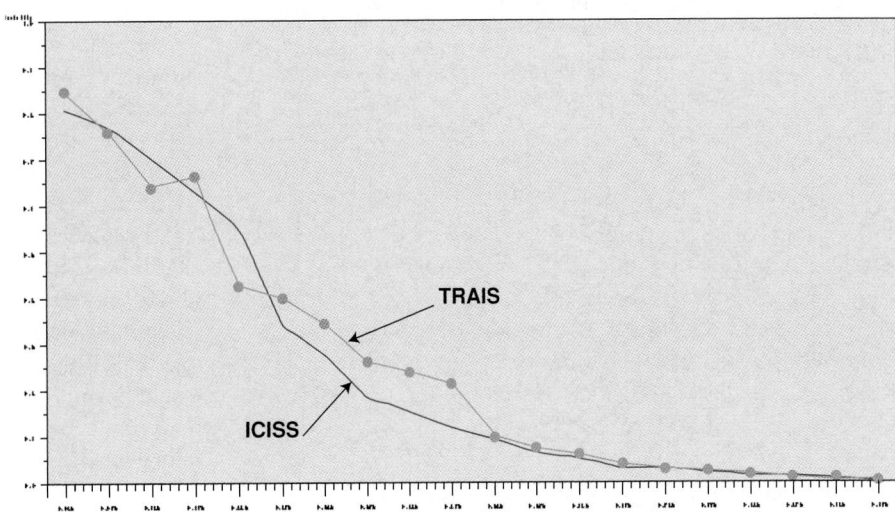

**FIGURE 5-4.** TRAIS and ICISS by mortality rate. ICISS and TRAIS behave very similarly in terms of their association with mortality (the vertical axis) despite being derived from two very different types of codes. This suggests that empirical approaches might obviate the inherent structure of the coding systems.

each level of organ disfigurement with Grade 1 injuries being relatively minor and Grade 5 injuries being destructive injuries that are thought to be fatal. These scales, originally developed by Moore et al. via a series of journal articles, exist for 32 organ and body region systems.[21–26]

Though descriptions using this lexicon are common, the scale has not been widely adopted into formal risk adjustment methods, though the potential exists for these scales to make an enduring impact on outcomes research. The validation of OIS should be carried out with a large representative database.

## Physiologic Status Scores

Physiologic status is a powerful predictor of mortality. Clinical markers including respiratory rate, systolic blood pressure, base deficit, and others are important prognosticators of outcome and are routinely used in triage and clinical management. However, these data are difficult to utilize in risk adjustment because they are ever-changing both spontaneously and in response to therapy, unlike anatomic injuries and pre-existing comorbidities which are fixed at the time of injury. The solution, albeit imperfect, is to use a "snapshot" of physiologic status at one point in time, usually immediately upon hospital arrival. Though there is no barrier to analyzing the change in these markers over time, it is most often impractical to collect multiple time point data in large studies.

Perhaps the most widely employed physiologic adjuster is the Glasgow Coma Scale (GCS), first proposed first by Teasdale and Jennett as a means to monitor postoperative craniotomy patients.[27,28] The GCS was subsequently adopted by trauma surgeons as a measure of overall physiologic derangement. The scale has three components – Eye, Verbal, and Motor – each of them with ordinal characterizations of severity (see Table 5-2). The scales can be summed to produce the Glasgow Coma Scale Score, often called just the GCS score. The GCS score is labeled a measure of brain injury but in actuality it measures brain *function*. It ranges from 3 (completely unresponsive) to 15 (completely responsive) and has been shown to be highly associated with survival. Osler et al. used the NTDB to show that the Glasgow Motor Component was almost as powerful as the full GCS score and had better statistical properties in general.[29] As such, the motor score alone could replace the full GCS score.

In 1983, Champion et al. first described an approach to combine clinical and observational physiologic data into one score, the Trauma Score, later updated to the Revised Trauma Score (RTS).[30,31] The RTS computes indexed values of GCS, systolic blood pressure, and respiratory rate by weighting them with logistic regression coefficients and summing them. The RTS score ranges from 0 to 7.84; lower scores translate into more physiologic derangement. RTS is highly associated with mortality and remains important in injury scoring through its contribution to the TRISS model (see below).

## Comorbidity Adjustments

Morris et al., among others, have identified several pre-existing conditions that worsen prognosis following trauma, most notably liver cirrhosis, COPD, congenital coagulopathy, diabetes, and congenital heart disease.[32] However, no trauma-specific score is available to adjust for these comorbidities, though adjustments such as the Deyo-Charlson scale are widely used in other disciplines.[33] The problem is difficult since so many pre-existing conditions exist, each of which may itself occur with variable severity. Further, many are relatively rare and confounded by age and may be inconsistently recorded. Hence, one accepted convention is to simply use patient age as a surrogate for comorbidities, since age is moderately associated with serious pre-existing disease. Another approach is to use the presence of individual comorbidities or classes of conditions (perhaps ICD-9 ranges) in risk adjustment methods. Either of these is acceptable but eventually a generalized score that incorporates all of this information might improve the accuracy of trauma scoring.

## Combined Scoring Systems

The three types of risk adjustments – anatomic, physiological, and comorbid – can be easily combined so that information from all three sources is used to predict outcomes. The first such attempt from Champion et al. resulted in the Trauma and Injury Severity Score (TRISS).[34] TRISS has become the standard tool to estimate survival probabilities. TRISS incorporates ISS (anatomic component), RTS (physiologic component), and an age indicator ($\leq$55, >55, comorbidity component) to estimate survival. Two separate equations, one each for blunt and penetrating patients, represent weighted sums of each of the three components and were calculated from data gathered in the Major Trauma Outcomes Study (MTOS).[35] From these equations, a probability of survival can be calculated for an individual patient. This probability (usually called the TRISS Score) can be used as a risk adjustor.

However, the TRISS approach has shortcomings.[36] It requires 8–10 variables (depending on the number of injuries used by ISS); failing to capture even a single predictor renders TRISS incalculable. This is the case in as many as 28% of all trauma cases. TRISS could be improved by replacing ISS with ISS squared or replacing it with a better anatomic predictor, accounting for comorbidities more accurately and updating the MTOS equations with more modern NTDB coefficients that reflect the advancements made since TRISS first appeared (see Table 5-3).[37]

**TABLE 5-2**

| Descriptors of GCS Components | | |
|---|---|---|
| **FUNCTION** | **DESCRIPTION** | **GCS SCALED VALUE** |
| Eye | Spontaneous | 4 |
| | To voice | 3 |
| | To pain | 2 |
| | None | 1 |
| Verbal Responses | Oriented | 5 |
| | Confused | 4 |
| | Inappropriate | 3 |
| | Incomprehensible | 2 |
| | None | 1 |
| Motor Response | Obeys commands | 6 |
| | Localizes pain | 5 |
| | Withdraw (pain) | 4 |
| | Flexion | 3 |
| | Extension (pain) | 2 |
| | None | 1 |

**TABLE 5-3**

**Equations for TRISS: Probability of Death = $1/(1+e^{-(LOGIT)})$ where Logit is Given by: $LOGIT = Intercept + \beta_{ISS}*(ISS) + \beta_{RTS}*(RTS) + \beta_{AGE}(AGE)$**

| | MTOS | | NTDB | |
|---|---|---|---|---|
| MECHANISM | Blunt | Penetrating | Blunt | Penetrating |
| Intercept | −0.4499 | −2.5355 | −2.17 | −0.36 |
| $\beta_{ISS}$ | .8085 | .9934 | 0.077 | 0.10 |
| $B_{RTS}$ | −0.0835 | −0.0651 | −0.49 | −0.68 |
| $B_{AGE}$ | −1.743 | −1.1360 | 1.85 | 1.12 |

Age is dichotomized as follows: 0–55 years=0, > 55 years=1.

Other TRISS-like models aim to account for all three risk adjustments. Champion et al. introduced the ASCOT score (A Severity Characterization of Trauma) to address some weaknesses in TRISS, in particular its poor prediction for certain types of trauma (e.g., penetrating torso trauma) and the reliance upon ISS.[38] Like TRISS, ASCOT relies upon anatomic descriptors, ED physiological status, age, and mechanism. However, instead of ISS, the Anatomic Profile (AP), which is the basis for the APS score, is used to adjust for anatomic severity.[8] Further, age is parsed into five ordinal categories rather than two. Similar to TRISS, all the values are statistically weighted in such a manner as to produce a probability of survival. Although ASCOT provides better predictions than TRISS, it has failed to replace TRISS as the standard survival predictor.

## STATISTICAL EVALUATION OF TRAUMA SEVERITY SCORES

Several statistical criteria are employed when evaluating the efficacy of the above scores. The choice of the model-based evaluation depends on the data type of the outcome. If the outcome is dichotomous (i.e., it takes on one of the two possible values), then logistic regression is warranted.[39,40] Logistic regression has two important functions. First, it establishes the relationships between the outcome and the predictors. Within logistic models, the strength of the association between predictors and outcomes is directly measured and inferences about statistical significance are made. Second, logistic regression returns an estimated probability of exposure of the outcome of interest. This estimated (expected) probability can be compared with the observed outcomes in the following ways:

Tests of Discrimination – a score that *discriminates* well is able to efficiently separate dichotomies (survivors from nonsurvivors, for example). Popular tests of discrimination include the area under the ROC curve and Harrell's c-index.[41,42]

Tests of Goodness-of-Fit – These tests measure the degree of agreement between observed and predicted probabilities. The Hosmer-Lemeshow statistic is probably used the most but it has severe limitations.[43] Many researchers prefer to graph predicted and observed classes and compare them visually.

Information Criterion Scores – Because models can be compared using different criteria (ROC, HL, etc.) that may disagree among themselves as to which model is preferred it is desirable to have a mathematically consistent approach to comparing models. Based upon the work of Kullbach and Leibler, it is possible to measure the distance between any two models in terms of the amount of information contained in each model.[44] In order to compare two models of a system (say, two models predicting death from trauma) it is enough to measure the Kullbach-Leibler distance from each putative model to the "true model." The "true model" is never known (of course, otherwise we would have no interest in modeling it), but by means of a mathematically rigorous sleight of hand it is possible to substitute another measure of information content, the Akaike Information Criterion (AIC), for the Kullbach-Leibler distance and avoid the need to explicitly specify the true model.[45] Fortuitously, the AIC is a simple function of the likelihood function (available from all standard statistical software) and the number of parameters estimated for the model of interest, and is thus straightforward to calculate. Once the AICs for each model are available it is a simple matter to order them and to further assign probabilities to each model as to the likelihood that it is, in fact, the true model.[46]

When the response is continuous, analysis of variance (ANOVA) methods including model R-square values, information criterion, and tests of significance of risk factors suffice to evaluate the accuracy of these scores.[47]

## RISK ADJUSTMENT RESEARCH APPROACHES

Risk adjustment using the above tools is increasingly simpler because of the advent of large relational databases and powerful, easily implemented statistical software. Researchers interested in risk adjustment should choose carefully which methods best accommodate their data constraints. Here are some factors to consider when planning a risk adjusted study:

### Database Type: Trauma Registry vs. Administrative

Trauma registries exist at most verified trauma centers for clinical documentation, research, and quality control purposes. These data include the pertinent medical records outcomes for each patient. In most cases, absent large amounts of missing data, full, TRISS-like risk models are fit and probabilities of survival are computed, if desired. This situation is optimal because the best available risk adjustments are derived from scoring approaches that use all three types of trauma severity adjustments.

Administrative databases, on the other hand, exist primarily for billing purposes and aren't meant specifically to be used for clinical research. In many cases administrative databases will have at least some injury ICD-9 codes but seldom do they have physiological data. Therefore, risk adjustments on administrative data are usually limited to anatomic severity adjustments.[48] If only a principal ICD-9 diagnosis code exists, then the worst injury approach is indicated and the SRR for this code is used for adjustments. If a complete set of injury codes is present, the evidence suggests that ICISS should be used.

## Empirical SRRs vs. AIS Severities: Which to Use?

AIS severities have the advantage of familiarity but studies show that SRR approaches account for more variance in the outcome, discriminate dichotomies better, and contain more information. The problem is that conglomerate scores such as TRISS and ASCOT use AIS severities and no established empirically-based alternative exists. Hence, it is advisable to take empirical approaches like TRAIS or ICISS when adjusting only with anatomic scores. Otherwise, TRISS-like combined scores that are AIS-based offer a substantial improvement over single anatomic adjustments.

## ICD-9 vs. AIS: Which to Use?

When the variables necessary for TRISS or ASCOT are available then AIS codes should be used. TRAIS may be calculated for any case where AIS codes are present, though it only represents the effect due to anatomic injury. Alternatively, when only ICD-9 codes are available (as with most administrative databases) then the literature suggests that the ICISS score be used rather than mapping software. When both types of codes are available the decision is more difficult and no consensus exists. AIS codes possess more specificity in describing the trauma landscape and have in the past been used for these types of adjustments. However, ICD-9 scores repeatedly have been shown to possess similar statistical properties. While most trauma surgeons will prefer AIS scoring, these decisions are usually guided by other facets of the study design.

## GENERAL STATISTICAL FRAMEWORK OF OUTCOMES RESEARCH

The goal of statistical hypothesis testing is to make inferences about populations based on samples from those populations. From these samples powerful inferences can be made if studies are properly designed and adequately powered. The mathematical "model" is usually the *modus operandi* for exploring relationships among variables. In general, three types of variables are used in the statistical modeling of data:

## Outcome Variables

Common outcomes in trauma research include mortality, ICU and hospital length of stay, the presence of some complication, functional status, and others. The data type of the outcome (continuous, dichotomous, ordinal, etc.) drives the type of model chosen.

## Predictor Variables

The variables whose effect on the outcome is of primary interest.

## Covariates

Variables that are known to influence the study outcome, but whose relationship to the outcome is not of primary interest, are included in a model. These variables are called covariates and their purpose is to account for as much of the variance in the outcome as possible. Sometimes called "confounders" or "nuisance variables," covariates are included in the model so that the association between predictors

and outcomes is properly ascribed. The significance of the covariates are of no interest; all that matters is the association of the predictors to the outcome *in the presence of* covariates. In observational and interventional studies, trauma severity scores are usually used as covariates, hence removing (or adjusting) the confounding effect coincident with some other predictor of interest.

## THE FUTURE OF TRAUMA SEVERITY SCORING

The very best scoring models available only account for about 55% of the variance in survival outcomes. This means there is vast room for methodology improvements in a field that is still relatively in its infancy. A better understanding of important clinical relationships between predictors and outcomes will carry the field forward. These include finding ways of adjusting for individual comorbidities and accounting for interactions of injuries. Further, better estimates of SRRs for all types of codes will result in improved prediction. Also, incorporating the OIS into common scoring algorithms is likely to vastly improve the prediction of outcomes.

Further, multiple imputation (MI) procedures that handle missing data now exist for patients with incomplete clinical records.[49] Missing data is a problem in severity approaches because some of the best scores require many variables. Far from "making up data," these MI procedures are akin to adding 0, or multiplying by 1; that is, they impute values that are representative of the nonmissing values and allow scores to be computed even when data are missing. These methods are computer-intensive but can easily be employed to make outcomes studies stronger by not excluding important observations.

Finally, and most importantly, outcomes other than survival need to be studied. The relationship between survival and trauma severity could be improved but in general is well understood. The FCI and other quality of life measures are a step in the right direction but more efforts need to be appropriated for studying the effect of trauma severity.

There are three basic sources of improvement in scoring methodology, regardless of outcome. First, the base coding lexicons can be refined so as to be as specific as possible. Second, point estimators of injury quantifiers need to be more accurate and uniform so that the precision of inferences are maximized. Third, better statistical tools need to be made available including cogent goodness-of-fit tests and more accurate modeling. Continuing to build on the achievements of the past 35 years will result in better adjustments and, consequently, better research studies in a field so vital to our public health system.

## REFERENCES

1. Iezzoni LI: *Risk Adjustment For Measuring Health Care Outcomes*, 3rd ed. Chicago: Health Administration Press, 2002.
2. Association for the Advancement of Automotive Medicine, Committee on Injury Scaling: *The Abbreviated Injury Scale 2005*. Des Plains, IL, 2005.
3. Mackenzie EJ, Damiano A, Miller T: The Development of the Functional Capacity Index. *J Trauma* 41:799, 1996.
4. American Medical Association, International Classification of Diseases, 9th revision, Clinical Modification, World Health Organization, Volumes 1 and 2, 1999.
5. American Medical Association, International Classification of Diseases, 10th revision, Clinical Modification, 2nd edition, World Health Organization, Volumes 1 and 2, 2004.

6. Baker SP, O'Neill B, Haddon W, Long WB: The severity score: A method for describing patients with multiple injuries an evaluating emergency care. *J Trauma* 14:187, 1974.

7. Linn S: The injury severity score—importance and uses. *Ann Epidemiol* 5:440, 1995.

8. Copes WS, Champion HR, Sacco WJ, et al.: Progress in characterizing anatomic injury. *J Trauma* 30:1200, 1990.

9. Kilgo PD, Meredith JW, Hensberry R: A note on the disjointed nature of the injury severity score. *J Trauma* 57:479; discussion 486, 2004.

10. Osler T, Baker SP, Long W: A modification to the Injury Severity Score that both improves accuracy and simplifies scoring. *J Trauma* 43:922, 1997.

11. MacKenzie EJ, Sacco WJ, et al.: *ICDMAP-90: A Users Guide.* Baltimore, MD: The Johns Hopkins University School of Public Health and Tri-Analytics, Inc., 1997.

12. MacKenzie EJ, Steinwachs DM, Ramzy AI: Evaluating performance of statewide regionalized systems of trauma care. *J Trauma* 30:681, 1990.

13. Mullins RJ, Veum-Stone J, Hefland M, et al.: Outcome of hospitalized injured patients after institution of a trauma system in an urban area. *JAMA* 271:1919, 1990.

14. Osler T, Rutledge R, Deis J, Bedrick, E: ICISS: An international classification of disease-based injury severity score. *J Trauma* 41:380, 1996.

15. Meredith JW, Kilgo PD, Osler TM: Independently derived survival risk ratios yield better estimates of survival than traditional survival risk ratios when using the ICISS. *J Trauma* 55:933, 2003.

16. Meredith JW, Kilgo PD, Osler TM: A fresh set of survival risk ratios derived from incidents in the National Trauma Data Bank from which the ICISS may be calculated. *J Trauma* 55:924, 2003.

17. Kilgo PD, Osler TM, Meredith JW: The worst injury predicts mortality outcome the best: Rethinking the role of multiple injuries in trauma outcome scoring. *J Trauma* 55:599, discussion 606, 2003.

18. Sacco WJ, MacKenzie EJ, Champion H: Comparison of alternative methods for assessing injury severity based on anatomic descriptors. *J Trauma* 47:441, 1999.

19. Meredith JW, Evans G, Patrick D: Kilgo A comparison of the abilities of nine scoring algorithms in predicting mortality. *J Trauma* 53:621, discussion 628, 2002.

20. http://www.aast.org/injury/injury.html - Organ Injury Scale

21. Moore EE, Shackford SR, Pachter HL: Organ injury scaling: Spleen, liver, and kidney. *J Trauma* 29:1664, 1989.

22. Moore EE, Cogbill TH, Malangoni MA: Organ injury scaling, II: Pancreas, duodenum, small bowel, colon, and rectum. *J Trauma* 30:1427, 1990.

23. Moore EE, Cogbill TH, Jurkovich GJ: Organ injury scaling, III: Chest wall, abdominal vascular, ureter, bladder, and urethra. *J Trauma* 33:337, 1992.

24. Moore EE, Malangoni MA, Cogbill TH: Organ injury scaling, IV: Thoracic vascular, lung, cardiac, and diaphragm. *J Trauma* 36:299, 1994.

25. Moore EE, Jurkovich GJ, Knudson MM: Organ injury scaling. VI: Extrahepatic biliary, esophagus, stomach, vulva, vagina, uterus (nonpregnant), uterus (pregnant), fallopian tube, and ovary. *J Trauma* 39:1069, 1995.

26. Moore EE, Malangoni MA, Cogbill: Organ injury scaling VII: Cervical vascular, peripheral vascular, adrenal, penis, testis, and scrotum. *J Trauma* 41:523, 1996.

27. Geasdale G, Murray G, Parker L et al.: Adding up the Glasgow Coma Score. *Acta Neurochir Suppl (Wien)* 28:13, 1979.

28. Segatore M, Way C: The Glasgow Coma Scale: Time for change. *Heart Lung* 21:548, 1992.

29. Healey C, Osler T, Rogers FB: Improving the Glasgow Coma Scale score: Motor score alone is a better predictor. *J Trauma* 54:671, discussion 678, 2003.

30. Champion HR, Sacco WJ, Carnazzo AJ et al.: Trauma score. *Crit Care Med* 9:672, 1981.

31. Champion HR, Sacco WJ, Copes WS et al.: A revision of the Trauma Score. *J Trauma* 29:623, 1989.

32. Morris J, MacKenzie E, Edelstein S: The effect of preexisting conditions on mortality in trauma patients. *JAMA* 263:1942,

33. Needham DM, Scales DC, Laupacis A: A systematic review of the Charlson comorbidity index using Canadian administrative databases: A perspective on risk adjustment in critical care research. *J Crit Care* 20:12, 2005.

34. Boyd C, Tolson M, Copes W: Evaluating trauma care: The TRISS method *J Trauma* 27:370, 1987.

35. Champion HR, Copes WS, Sacco WJ, et al.: The major trauma outcome study: Establishing national norms for trauma care. *J Trauma* 30:1356, 1990.

36. Gabbe B, Cameron P, Wolfe R: TRISS: Does it get better than this. *Acad Emer Med* 11:181, 2004.

37. Osler TM, Rogers FB, Badger GJ: A simple mathematical modification of TRISS markedly improves calibration. *J Trauma* 53:630, 2002.

38. Champion H, Copes W, Sacco W: A new characterization of injury severity. *J Trauma* 30:539, 1990.

39. Hosmer D, Lemeshow S: *Applied Logistic Regression,* 2nd ed. New York: John Wiley & Sons, Inc, 2000.

40. Harrell Frank: *Regression Modeling Strategies, Springer Series in Statistics.* New York: Springer.

41. Hanley J, McNeil B: The meaning and use of the area under a receiver operating characteristic (ROC) curve. *Radiology* 143:29, 1982.

42. Harrell Frank: *Regression Modeling Strategies, Springer Series in Statistics.* New York: Springer, p. 247.

43. Harrell Frank: *Regression Modeling Strategies, Springer Series in Statistics.* New York: Springer, p. 230.

44. Kullback S, Leibler RA: On information and sufficiency. *Annals of Mathematical Statistics* 22:79, 1951.

45. Harrell Frank: *Regression Modeling Strategies, Springer Series in Statistics.* New York: Springer, p. 202.

46. Burnham KP, Anderson DR: *Model Selection and Multi-Model Inference – A Practical Information-Theoretic Approach.* 2nd ed. New York: Springer-Verlag, 2002.

47. Neter J, Kutner M, Wasserman W et al.: *Applied Linear Statistical Models,* 4th ed. New York: McGraw-Hill/Irwin, 1996.

48. Clark D, Winchell J: Risk adjustment for injured patients uisng administrative databases. *J Trauma* 57:130, 2004.

49. Rubin, DB: Inference and missing data. *Biometrika* 63:581, 1976.

# Commentary ■ JOHN FILDES

Patrick Kilgo, Wayne Meredith, and Turner Osler have provided a detailed and comprehensive discussion of trauma severity scoring and its application in outcomes research. These scoring systems rely on data describing physiologic changes, anatomic injuries, and comorbid conditions. Physiologic status scores are powerful predictors of mortality. They use clinical data like Glasgow Coma Score, systolic blood pressure, respiratory rate, base deficit, and others. These measures change continuously based on the progression of disease and effects of therapy. This raises questions about when and how this data should be collected. Anatomic scoring systems have traditionally relied on coders and registrars with special training in the Abbreviated Injury Scale (AIS) to describe injuries and calculate the Injury Severity Score (ISS). The authors point out some of the shortcomings of this scoring system.

Issues like the relative weight of injuries to the brain and spine compared to chest or abdomen require additional qualification. In addition, the ISS considers only one injury in each of the body regions and thus ignores other important injuries. These issues combined with adequate training and data quality improvement have stimulated research for scoring systems that utilize ICD-9 codes. The authors have published data that ICD-9 based scoring systems may outpredict AIS-based systems. The release of AIS 2005 and eventual adoption of ICD-10 will fuel this discussion for the foreseeable future. Scoring systems that use comorbid conditions are extremely important. Sadly, they are the least well developed. Comorbidity scoring is essential for calculating risk adjusted outcomes in trauma similar to the risk adjustment outcomes that exist for cancer and heart disease. This hampers our ability to compare the outcomes of individual trauma surgeons and trauma centers. The current healthcare climate demands this and trauma is struggling to provide it. Clearly, this is a complicated issue that involves the quality of collecting comorbid conditions, complications, and deaths in an era where advanced directives play a role in the survival statistics.

The authors make several recommendations to improve injury severity scoring and outcomes measurement. They include the reduction of variance through improved data quality and elimination of missing data. They also recommend studying outcomes other than survival and improving the base coding lexicons like AIS and ICD-9 to be as specific as possible. These efforts will allow the development of better statistical models and the creation of new outcomes measures. To this end, The American College of Surgeons Committee on Trauma subcommittee for the National Trauma Data Bank (NTDB) collaborated with the Health Resources and Services Administration (HRSA) and other stakeholders to develop a national minimum standard trauma care dataset. This data dictionary is called the National Trauma Data Standard (NTDS). This minimum standard trauma care dataset is being embedded into all commercially supported trauma registry software. In addition, it is being adopted by state trauma systems. It is clear that high quality data is the result of high quality data collection. Errors and inconsistencies in data entry will lead to increased variability and degrade the reliability of these calculated measures. The NTDS uses standardized definitions, online education, and validity checking as software solutions to support high quality data collection. The vision is to aggregate the next generation of trauma data in the NTDB. This will provide the raw materials needed to advance the discipline of severity scoring and outcomes research.

## References

1. DE Clark, RJ Fantus (eds): American College of Surgeons National Trauma Data Bank® 2006, Version 6.0. © American College of Surgeons 2006.
2. NTDS can be found at www.ntdb.org.

# Trauma Outcomes

*Michael Pasquale* ■ *Michael Rhodes*

Since the Institute of Medicine (IOM) published *Crossing the Quality Chasm: A New Health System for the 21st Century*[1] and *Leadership by Example: Coordinating Government Roles in Improving Health Care Quality* (2002),[2] conversations among healthcare policymakers have shifted. Whereas the focus previously was on safety efforts, prevention of errors, and their application to public health programs, the emphasis now includes the implementation of quality improvement processes and outcomes measures across the health care system.

Outcomes are the results of care from the perspective of the patient, provider, payer, and society. The standard outcome parameters of mortality and morbidity have been extended to include length of stay, cost, quality of life, patient satisfaction, and compliance with guidelines. Outcome "tools" used to measure these parameters have included audits, surveys, severity scoring, registries, data banks, cost accounting, and research studies. Until very recently, trauma outcome research has been composed primarily of descriptive studies or retrospective analyses of data collected either retrospectively or prospectively.[3] Even with this limitation, many of these outcome studies have had an impact on the development of trauma centers and trauma systems and the legislation supporting them.[4,5] Trauma-related outcome studies have also influenced seat belt and air-bag legislation in the United States.[6] In addition, many trauma outcome studies have influenced the process of care throughout the world.[7]

Although cycling in severity over the past several decades, the medical-legal and malpractice crisis has been a constant challenge to medical practice, with a particular threat to the delivery of trauma care throughout the United States.[8,9] Annual malpractice premiums of more than $300,000 have been required for some neurosurgeons participating in trauma call. Trauma outcome studies are important in demonstrating the ranges of expected outcomes and supporting the observation that suboptimal outcome does not necessarily equate with bad or negligent care.[10] Adequate reimbursement for trauma care is also under siege.[11] Although the concept of outcome-based reimbursement for trauma care does not yet have traction in the United States, it has been suggested for other areas of medicine.[12] The availability of expected trauma outcomes will be essential in guiding appropriate documentation, coding, and compliance for reimbursement.[13]

Performance improvement in trauma care is the continuous evaluation of a trauma system and trauma providers through structured review of the process of care as well as the outcome.[14] Knowledge of expected outcomes is necessary to evaluate the processes of care and provide corrective action plans for identified opportunities for improvement. Two reports from the IOM have focused national attention on errors in medicine, and numerous patient safety initiatives have emerged.[15,16] Most of these initiatives are relevant to trauma care and are outcomes sensitive.

This chapter defines and reviews the importance of evidence-based medicine in trauma outcomes. The responsibilities of professional organizations, associations, and societies in trauma outcomes research are discussed, and critiques of current outcome parameters are provided. Representative cataloging of trauma outcome studies is developed, and initiatives for future direction are presented.

## EVIDENCE-BASED MEDICINE

Evidence-based medicine (EBM) has been defined as a method of patient care, decision making, and teaching that integrates high-quality research evidence with pathophysiologic reasoning, experience, and patient preference.[17] The discipline of EBM is derived from utilizing validated methodology to quantify the power of research for clinical decision making.[18] The idea is to base clinical decisions on the best available evidence and understand the power (or quality) of that evidence. EBM involves, at the core, a fundamental acknowledgement that our clinical convictions can be wrong. Additionally, we invariably underestimate the power of the placebo effect and assume that because most patients we treat in a certain way feel better, the treatment must be effective. It is only through double-blind, placebo-controlled, clinical trials that we

## TABLE 6-1

### Evidence-Based Classification of Outcome Studies

| EVIDENCE | DESCRIPTION |
| --- | --- |
| Class I | Prospective, randomized, controlled trials–the gold standard of clinical trials. However, some may be poorly designed, lack sufficient patient numbers, or suffer from other methodological inadequacies. |
| Class II | Clinical studies in which the data were collected prospectively; retrospective analyses based on clearly reliable data. Types of study so classified include observational studies, cohort studies, prevalence studies, and case control studies. |
| Class III | Most studies based on retrospectively collected data. Evidence used in this class indicates clinical series, databases, or registries, case reviews, case reports, and expert opinion. |
| Technology Assessment | The assessment of technology, such as devices for monitoring intracranial pressure, does not lend itself to classification in the format above. Thus, for technology assessment, devices were evaluated in terms of their accuracy, reliability, therapeutic potential, and cost-effectiveness. |

From Rhodes M, Fallon W Jr. How guidelines can serve as outcomes tools. J Surg Outcomes 2:9–18, 2003.

## TABLE 6-2

### Examples of Website Addresses for Evidence-Based Medicine

| | |
| --- | --- |
| www.ahrq.gov | Agency for Healthcare Research and Quality |
| www.aast.org | American Association for the Surgery of Trauma |
| www.facs.org | American College of Surgeons |
| www.cochrane.org | Cochrane Collaboration |
| www.east.org | Eastern Association for the Surgery of Trauma |
| www.clinicalevidence.com | Evidence-based Medicine |
| www.swsahs.nsw.gov .au/livtrauma | Liverpool Trauma |
| www.guidelines.gov | National Guidelines Clearinghouse |
| pedsccm.wustl.edu/EBJ/ EB_Resources.html | Resources for Practicing EBM |
| www.sccm.org | Society for Critical Care Medicine |
| www.swscongress.org | Southwestern Surgical Congress |
| www.ucl.ac.uk/primcare- popscit/research/uebpp.htm | Unit for Evidence-based Practice and Policy |

realize that patients treated with placebo also get better. It is not good enough for a treatment to work . . . it must be shown to work better than the placebo.

A review of EBM for trauma-related topics points out the somewhat uncomfortable fact that much of what trauma practitioners do is based on published evidence of limited certainty.[3] This, of course, indicated the direction for areas of future research. Much of the EBM in trauma care derived from trauma outcome studies. Several data classification schemes have been developed; the scheme most commonly used in trauma related topics is outlined in Table 6-1. The process of data classification is labor-intensive and usually requires the resources of professional societies and governmental organizations (Table 6-2). The growth of EBM outcome studies in the past decade has been profound; however, the impact on health care remains unclear.[19]

The relevant skills of EBM include precisely defining a patient problem, proficiently searching and critically appraising relevant information from the literature, and deciding whether, and how, to use this information in practice. These skills are now being incorporated into the training of primary care providers and continuing medical education. Efficient literature searching and proficient critical appraisal skills are necessary for the acquisition of valid and current information on the most important clinical and economic aspects of a disease. When evidence becomes the neutral arbiter of optimal practice, and all members of a multidisciplinary team are empowered to share relevant evidence, a more coordinated, holistic approach is likely to emerge. Evidence about the most effective methods of changing clinician behavior can be incorporated into disease management programs and thus, clinical and economic

outcomes can be improved by reducing variation around optimal practice. Randomized, controlled trials clearly are not possible for many clinical situations and, when available, may not have practical application. If adequate research is unavailable, no specific recommendations can be made, thus avoiding inappropriate decision making and allowing for clinical flexibility. By identifying the inadequacies in research, the concept of evidence-based medicine can help formulate a prioritized research agenda in a setting where random and systematic errors caused by different practice styles are minimized. Steps for developing an evidence-based disease management program include:

1. Formulate a clear definition of the disease, its scope, and its impact over time using a multidisciplinary team.

2. Develop comprehensive baseline information to understand current health care delivery and resource utilization.

3. Generate specific clinical and economic questions and search the literature.

4. Critically appraise and synthesize the evidence.

5. Evaluate the benefits, harms, and costs.

6. Develop evidence-based practice guidelines, clinical pathways, and protocols.

7. Create a system for process and outcome measurement and reporting.

8. Implement the evidence-based guidelines, pathways, and protocols.

9. Complete the quality improvement cycle.

## GUIDELINES, PATHWAYS, AND PROTOCOLS

The Agency for Healthcare Research and Quality (AHRQ) definition of **guidelines** as systematically developed statements designed to assist in clinical decision making has been expanded

**TABLE 6-3**

### Steps in Clinical Practice Guideline Development

1. Selection of topic
2. Selection of committee members
3. Clarification of scope and purpose
4. Listing of goals
5. Assessment of scientific evidence
6. Drafting and validation of document
7. Presentation of final guidelines
8. Implementation
9. Evaluations
10. Research/revise

*From: Agency for Healthcare Policy & Research (1991).*

**TABLE 6-4**

### Trauma-Surgical Critical Care Related Practice Management Guidelines

Primer on evidence-based medicine

Screening of blunt cardiac injury

Management of mild traumatic brain injury

Identifying cervical spine injuries following trauma

Penetrating intraperitoneal colon injuries

Management of venous thromboembolism in trauma patients

Nonoperative management of blunt injury to the liver and spleen

Prophylactic antibiotics in tube thoracostomy for traumatic hemopneumothorax

Diagnosis and management of blunt aortic injury

Prophylactic antibiotics in penetrating abdominal trauma

Prophylactic antibiotics in open fractures

Optimal timing of long bone fracture stabilization in polytrauma patients

Violence prevention programs

Management of penetrating trauma to the lower extremity revised 2002

Management of pelvic hemorrhage in pelvic fracture

Evaluation of blunt abdominal trauma

Geriatric trauma

Nutritional support

Emergency tracheal intubation following traumatic injury revised 2002

Endpoints of resuscitation

Evaluation of genitourinary trauma

Management of genitourinary trauma

Pain management in blunt chest trauma

Timing of tracheostomy

Diagnosis and management of injury in the pregnant patient

Surviving sepsis campaign guidelines for management of severe sepsis and septic shock

Guidelines for the acute medical management of severe traumatic brain injury in infants, children, and adolescents

Clinical practice guidelines for the sustained use of sedatives and analgesics in the critically ill adult

Clinical practice guidelines for sustained neuromuscular blockade in the critically ill adult patient

Guidelines for granting privileges for the performance of procedures in critically ill patients

Evidence-based guidelines for weaning and discontinuing ventilatory support

Guidelines for the management of intravascular catheter-related infections

to include evidence-based guidelines, which are outlines of generally accepted management approaches based on the best available evidence.[20] Thus, guidelines are developed utilizing the principles of EBM. These guidelines may be specific to a disease, problem, or process, but they are general in nature and include a series of recommendations rated by the power of the evidence. These documents are aimed at the appropriateness of care and are best developed through national organizations and societies.[21] The goals of such guidelines are to identify all treatment options and possible outcomes, weigh the benefits against the risks and costs, and, in the broadest context, factor in logistics, ethical, economic, societal, and legal considerations. Ideally, clinical practice guidelines are derived from the data sources available and used to guide health care professionals through a continuous quality improvement effort in which the process involved in health care delivery is analyzed, changes recommended, patient outcomes defined, variances from expected outcomes evaluated, and the process reassessed. Utilizing this approach, health care is delivered in an evidence-based outcome model. A step-by-step process for evidence-based outcome evaluation (EBOE), from which practice management guidelines are developed, has been established by the AHRQ (formerly the AHCPR).[22] The 10-step process ensures a combination of rigorous methodology and practical feasibility that can be adapted to clinical decision making at any institution (Table 6-3). In essence, the model consists of development, implementation, measurement, and revision stages.

The development, classification, and distribution of trauma and surgical critical care related evidence-based guidelines have progressed rapidly over the last decade (Table 6-4). However, the implementation of and outcome studies on the effect of the guidelines themselves are lagging behind.[23] It appears that the true value of evidence-based guideline implementation will require the electronic medical record with physician order entry and clinical decision support systems. These systems are currently evolving rapidly and are anticipated to facilitate guideline implementation and analysis of their impact.

**Pathways and protocols** are bedside and patient-side tools for the implementation of the nationally derived management guidelines. Pathways are designed to provide an overview of the entire care process and are primarily calendars of expected events designed to improve efficiency. They are usually specific to a diagnosis related group (DRG), disease, or procedure and are meant to provide a checklist for elements of care. Pathways have been used successfully for many entities, including coronary artery bypass procedures, knee replacement, hip replacement, and procedures relating to general surgery and trauma.[24,25] Because of the multi-DRG nature of trauma, pathways tend to be less useful in the critically injured. Clinical management protocols derived from evidence-based national guidelines[26] are institution specific algorithms that can be used as bedside instruments to effect care. Most experience to date has been with an annotated algorithm format following predetermined conventions of style, typically using "if, then" formats. Ventilator management protocols have been demonstrated to improve outcomes.[27] Pathways and protocols are frequently applied synergistically. For example, the pathway for blunt chest injury with rib fractures may incorporate a pain management protocol within its pathway. It must be emphasized that both protocols and pathways are developed from evidence-based guidelines.

## ORGANIZATIONS INVOLVED IN OUTCOME ANALYSIS

### Institute of Medicine (IOM)

The IOM is an independent think tank commissioned by the United States Congress to perform studies relating to the quality (among other aspects) of medicine in the United States. The results of these studies suggest that outcome studies should be sensitive to the high-profile initiatives of patient safety as outlined by the IOM. More importantly, the IOM reports have had a tremendous impact on how health care providers view outcomes.

In 1999, the IOM published the landmark report, *To Err Is Human: Building a Safer Health System*.[15] This report estimated that as many as 98,000 people die annually as a result of medical errors and calls for a national effort to make health care safe. Patient safety, a topic that had been little understood and even less discussed in care systems, became a frequent focus for health care leaders. Indeed, this concept was embraced by the trauma community and acknowledged by the American College of Surgeons – Committee on Trauma (ACSCOT) in 2004 when they officially changed the Performance Improvement Committee to the Performance Improvement and Patient Safety Committee. This name change brought about a redirection in the focus of the committee's efforts with a strong emphasis placed on patient safety.

A follow-up study published in 2005, *Five Years After To Err Is Human: What Have We Learned?*,[28] addressed the changes that had occurred in health care as a result of the original publication. The authors noted that small but consequential changes had been made with decreased medication errors leading to death, decreased complications related to anticoagulation, and decreased numbers of serious infections.[29–31] Despite this, the overall impact is hard to see in national statistics as no comprehensive nationwide monitoring system exists for patient safety, and a recent study by the AHRQ suggested little improvement.[32] Additionally, despite the message from the IOM that systems failures cause most injuries, most individuals still believe that the major cause of bad care is bad physicians.[33] Others claim however, that emphasis on systems, and particularly, not blaming individuals for errors, will weaken accountability for physician performance.[34] Leape and Berwick[28] conclude that although the fruits of the IOM report thus far are few, its impact on attitudes and organizations has been profound and a great deal about safety has been learned. The authors further acknowledge that the effects of the IOM report are evident in at least three important areas: viewing the task of error prevention, enlisting the support of stakeholders, and changing practice.

As far as viewing the task of error prevention, the IOM report changed the way health care providers think and talk abut medical errors and injury. Few individuals now doubt that preventable medical injuries are a serious problem and more are engaged in looking for what they can do about these injuries. The second major effect was to enlist a broad array of stakeholders, the first of which was the federal government through appropriations for patient safety research. This led to the development of a Center for Quality Improvement and Safety (established by the AHRQ) which has become a leader in education, training, and dissemination of patient safety practices. The AHRQ has also been an important

voice for safety through its support for evaluating best practices, demonstrations to enhance reporting of adverse events, errors, and near misses, its development of patient safety indicators now used by many hospitals, and its development of a roadmap of evidence-based best practices used by the National Quality Forum (NQF). The NQF has developed a consensus process that has generated standards for mandatory reporting[34] and created a list of high-impact evidence-based safe practices that the Joint Commission on Accreditation of Healthcare Organizations (JCAHO) and other organizations are now beginning to require hospitals to implement.[35,36] The Centers for Medicare and Medicaid Services and the Centers for Disease Control and Prevention have joined hands with more than 20 surgical organizations in a new program to reduce surgical complications.[37] The Accreditation Council on Graduate Medical Education (ACGME) and the American Board of Medical Specialties (ABMS) are engaged in a massive effort to define competencies and measures in each specialty, both for residency training and continuing evaluation of practicing physicians.[38] The Leapfrog Group[39] has strongly encouraged the adoption of a number of safer practices in hospitals, including computerized physician order entry systems, proper staffing of intensive care units, and the concentration of highly technical surgery services in high-volume centers. More recently, they have embraced the implementation of the NQF's Safe Practices.

The third effect of the IOM report was to accelerate the changes in practice needed to make health care safe. Following the 2002 publication by the NQF[34] of a list of 30 evidence-based safe practices ready for implementation, JCAHO required hospitals to implement 11 of these practices, including improving patient identification, communication, and surgical site verification.[35] Results of these changes are beginning to come in and time series data from hospitals and systems that have been working to improve safety are encouraging. The results achieved in implementing 12 practice changes are shown in Table 6-5.[31,40–47] The last major practice change that occurred in teaching hospitals was the work hour limitations promulgated by the ACGME and based on the relationships between fatigue and errors in the work place.[48–51]

Advances expected in the next five years include: implementation of the electronic medical record, wide diffusion of proven and safe practices (those suggested by NQF), expansion of training teamwork and safety practices, and full disclosure to patients following injury.

### Agency for Healthcare Research and Quality (AHRQ)

The AHRQ is a governmental agency that has created 12 centers throughout the United States commissioned to study evidence-based guidelines on a variety of topics, including trauma.[52] The agency has also identified clear opportunities for safety improvement relating to topics such as central catheters, enteral nutrition, antibiotic prophylaxis, prophylaxis for venous thromboembolism, and informed consent (Table 6-6).[53] They have prioritized issues such as hand-washing compliance, analgesia, computerized order entry with clinical decision support, nurse staffing for reduced morbidity, and prevention of urinary tract infections.

AHRQ has also established The National Guideline Clearinghouse™ (NGC),[54] a comprehensive database of evidence-based clinical practice guidelines and related documents. NGC was originally created by AHRQ in partnership with the AMA and the

**TABLE 6-5**

## Clinical Effectiveness of Safe Practices

| INTERVENTION | RESULTS |
|---|---|
| Perioperative antibiotic protocol | Surgical site infections decreased by 93%[a] |
| Physician computer order entry | 81% reduction of medical errors[38,39] |
| Pharmacist rounding with team | 66% reduction of preventable adverse drug events[40] |
| | 78% reduction of preventable adverse drug events[41] |
| Protocol enforcement | 95% reduction in central venous line infections[b] |
| | 92% reduction in central venous line infections[c] |
| Rapid response teams | Cardiac arrests decreased by 15%[42] |
| Reconciling medication practices | 90% reduction in medication errors[43] |
| Reconciling and standardizing medication practices | 60% reduction in adverse drug events over 12 months (from 7.6 per 1000 doses to 3.1 per 1000 doses)[43] |
| | 64% reduction in adverse drug events in 20 months (from 3.8 per 1000 doses to 1.39 per 1000 doses)[31] |
| Standardized insulin dosing | Hypoglycemic episodes decreased 63% (from 2.95% of patients to 1.1%)[44] |
| | 90% reduction in cardiac surgical wound infections (from 3.9%) of patients to 1.1%)[d] |
| Standardized warfarin dosing | Out-of-range INR decreased by 60% (from 25% of tests to 10%)[43] |
| Team training in labor and delivery | 50% reduction in adverse outcomes in preterm deliveries[e] |
| Trigger tool and automation | Adverse drug events reduced by 75% between 2001 and 2003[45] |
| Ventilator bundle protocol | Ventilator-associated pneumonias decreased by 62%[a] |

[a]J Whittington, written communication, March 2005.

[b]P. Pronovost, Johns Hopkins Hospital, written communication, January 2005.

[c]R. Shannon, written communication, January 2005.

[d]K. McKinley, Geisinger Clinic, written communication, April 2005.

[e]B. Sachs, Beth Israel Deaconess Medical Center, written communication, October 2004.

American Association of Health Plans (now America's Health Insurance Plans [AHIP]). The NGC mission is to provide physicians, nurses, other health professionals, health care providers, health plans, integrated delivery systems, purchasers, and others with an accessible mechanism for obtaining objective, detailed information on clinical practice guidelines and to further their dissemination, implementation, and use. The key components of NGC include:

1. Structured abstracts (summaries) about the guideline and its development.

2. Links to full-text guidelines, where available, and/or ordering information for print copies.

3. Palm-based PDA downloads of the Complete NGC Summary for all guidelines represented in the database.

**TABLE 6-6**

## Practices Rated Most Highly in Terms of Strength of the Evidence Supporting More Widespread Implementation

| ITEM | PATIENT SAFETY PROBLEM | PATIENT SAFETY PRACTICE | IMPLEMENTATION COST/COMPLEXITY |
|---|---|---|---|
| 1 | Venous thromboembolism (VTE) | Appropriate VTE prophylaxis | Low |
| 2 | Perioperative cardiac events in patients undergoing noncardiac surgery | Use of perioperative beta-blockers | Low |
| 3 | Central venous catheter-related bloodstream infections | Use of maximum sterile barriers during catheter insertion | Low |
| 4 | Surgical site infections | Appropriate use of antibiotic prophylaxis | Low |
| 5 | Missed, incomplete or not fully comprehended informed consent | Asking that patients recall and restate what they have been told during informed consent | Low |
| 6 | Ventilator-associated pneumonia | Continuous aspiration of subglottic secretions (CASS) | Medium |
| 7 | Pressure ulcers | Use of pressure relieving bedding materials | Medium |
| 8 | Morbidity due to central venous catheter insertion | Use of real-time ultrasound guidance during central line insertion | High |
| 9 | Adverse events related to chronic anticoagulation with warfarin | Patient self management using home monitoring devices | High |
| 10 | Morbidity and mortality in post-surgical and critically ill patients | Various nutritional strategies | Medium |
| 11 | Central venous catheter-related bloodstream infections | Antibiotic-impregnated catheters | Low |

From: Agency for Healthcare Research and Quality, 2001.

4. A guideline comparison utility that gives users the ability to generate side-by-side comparisons for any combination of two or more guidelines.

5. Unique guideline comparisons called guideline syntheses prepared by NGC staff, which compares guidelines covering similar topics, highlighting areas of similarity and difference. NGC Guideline Syntheses often provide a comparison of guidelines developed in different countries, providing insight into commonalities and differences in international health practices.

6. An electronic forum, NGC-L for exchanging information on clinical practice guidelines, their development, implementation, and use.

7. An annotated bibliography database where users can search for citations for publications and resources about guidelines, including guideline development and methodology, evaluation, implementation, and structure.[55]

## The Leapfrog Group

The Leapfrog Group is a business roundtable-sponsored initiative to mobilize employer purchasing power to initiate breakthrough improvements in safety and quality of health care for Americans. The consortium includes many of the Fortune 500 companies in the United States and other large private and public health care purchasers.[56] The Leapfrog Group recently identified three highly ranked and evidence-based characteristics for high-quality health care: (a) high volume in complex diseases and procedures, (b) the presence of an electronic medical record with physician order entry, and (c) the presence of intensivists in the intensive care unit. These evidence-based recommendations have been shown to substantially reduce medical error and mortality and should be considered in future outcome studies.

## Joint Commission on Accreditation of Healthcare Organizations

Most hospitals in the United States seek accreditation by the JCAHO, because lack of accreditation can jeopardize reimbursement and residency programs.[35] A JCAHO program known as Oryx requires accredited hospitals to capture and report on clinical performance indicators such as complication rates. Although not trauma-specific, this program may present opportunities for trauma outcome studies. Additionally, JCAHO has determined that effective leadership within an organization depends on:

1. Governance: sets the framework for supporting quality patient care, treatment, and services.

2. Management: an environment is created that enables a hospital to fulfill its mission and meet or exceed its goals. There are clear lines of responsibility and accountability.

3. Planning, designing, and providing services to accomplish the mission of the organization needs to be done by the leadership. In addition, they communicate objectives and coordinate efforts to integrate care, treatment, and services throughout the hospital.

4. Improving safety and quality of care must be a priority and the leadership must ensure that a process is in place to measure, assess, and improve the hospital's governance, management, clinical, and support functions.

5. Use of clinical practice guidelines (CPGS): The standards do not require the leaders to use clinical practice guidelines; however, they do provide a framework for developing and using them if the leaders choose to do so. A guideline provides an effective way to improve processes by reducing variance. A hospital's success in implementing and using clinical practice guidelines on an ongoing basis depends on the processes for reviewing, revising, and implementing the guidelines. Specifically in sections LD.5.10 it is noted that the hospital should consider CPGS when designing or improving processes as appropriate. LD.5.20 notes that when CPGS are used, the leaders must identify criteria for their selection and implementation. LD.5.30 states that appropriate leaders, practitioners, and health care professionals in the hospital review and approve CPGS selected for implementation. Lastly, LD.5.40 states that the leaders should evaluate the outcomes related to use of CPGS and determine steps to improve processes.

6. Teaching and coaching staff through mentoring and educational efforts are an essential leadership function.[57]

## American College of Surgeons

The American College of Surgeons – Committee on Trauma (ACSCOT) has long championed trauma outcome studies and evidence-based guidelines for trauma. The National Trauma Data Bank (NTDB) is designed to provide national and regional benchmarking through the collection of class III EBM where little or none exists today.[58] Although not totally population-based, the incidence and prevalence of trauma disease and trauma-related complications can be estimated more accurately from a large database. Data from the National Trauma Registry of the American College of Surgeons (TRACS) and a variety of other commercially available registries are downloaded from trauma centers or trauma systems to the NTDB. Although the accuracy of trauma registries has been challenged, they can provide local and regional trauma outcome data.[59,60] The ACS has recently opened the office of Continuous Quality Improvement (CQI), formerly the Office of Evidence-Based Surgery as part of its Division of Research and Optimal Patient Care.[61] The mission of the CQI is to promote the highest standards of surgical care through evaluation of surgical outcomes in clinical practice. The Division of Research and Optimal Patient Care encompasses three areas including trauma, cancer, and CQI. Each area has dedicated major resources toward the measurement of outcomes with the trauma department housing the NTDB, the cancer department housing the National Cancer Database, and CQI being responsible for the ACS-National Surgical Quality Improvement Program (NSQIP). It is anticipated that trauma outcome research will be a major emphasis of this office in collaboration with trauma-related academic societies.

During the mid-to-late 1980s, the Department of Veterans Affairs (VA) came under a great deal of public scrutiny over the quality of surgical care in their 133 VA hospitals. At issue were the operative mortality rates in the VA hospitals and the perception in Congress that these rates were significantly above the national (private sector) norm. To address the gap, Congress passed law 99–166 which mandated the VA to report its surgical outcomes annually on a risk-adjusted basis to factor in a patient's severity of illness and compare to the national averages. Realizing that these national averages did not exist, the VA embarked upon the National VA

Surgical Risk Study (NVASRS) in 44 VA medical centers.[62] The NVASRS was able to develop models for 30-day mortality and morbidity in nine surgical specialties. Additionally, they found that the risk-adjusted outcomes produced by the models matched quality of systems and processes in the 44 hospitals. Their work allowed, for the first time, a comparative measurement of the quality of surgical care in these specialties. The success of the NVASRS study encouraged the VA to establish an ongoing program for monitoring and improving the quality of surgical care across all medical centers, and the NSQIP was born. Results of the VA NSQIP study showed a 27% decline in operative mortality and a 45% drop in postoperative morbidity as well as a decrease in mean length of postoperative stay and improved patient satisfaction.[63] Such results have led to expansion of the program into the private sector under the auspices of the ACS.[64] The ACSCOT is reviewing the NSQIP data and seeking out ways to apply a similar outcomes methodology to the trauma population. Additionally, it has been noted that several of the surgical outcomes evaluated pertain to trauma patients.

An excellent example of such overlap comes from the Surgical Care Improvement Project (SCIP),[36] which is targeting a reduction in surgical complications. SCIP plans to focus on process, in an effort to decrease complications in four specific areas. The four targeted areas and examples of process changes associated with each are shown below:

1. Surgical site infections: administration of prophylactic antibiotics within 1 hour prior to surgery and control of perioperative serum glucose in major cardiac surgical patients.

2. Adverse cardiac events: administration of beta-blockers to eligible major noncardiac surgical patients during perioperative period and to those surgical patients with coronary artery disease during perioperative period.

3. Deep vein thrombosis: assess patient risk for VTE and administer appropriate perioperative prophylaxis.

4. Postoperative ventilator-related pneumonia: for major surgical patients on ventilation, without contraindications, postoperatively elevate head of bed greater than or equal to 30°.

It is readily apparent that trauma could benefit from following process improvements in all but the adverse cardiac events area.

In October 2005, the ACS launched its Evidence Based Reviews in Surgery (EBRS) educational program for ACS fellows, candidates, and resident members. EBRS is an Internet-based journal club designed to teach practicing general surgeons and residents critical appraisal skills.[65] The EBRS will consist of eight monthly packages per academic year, from October to May. Each package includes a clinical article that is relevant to the practice of general surgery, plus a methodological article that can be used to assist in the evaluation of the clinical article. In addition, methodological and clinical reviews are provided by experts in the field and surgeons may also participate in an expert-led listserv discussion of the article. It is hoped that participants will be able to evaluate the clinical article being reviewed, further their knowledge in the clinical topic, and learn critical appraisal skills that can be used to evaluate other articles that they read in the future. Selected articles cover a spectrum of important clinical and methodological topics including trauma, e.g., accuracy of FAST performed by trauma surgeons was one of the previous topics selected.

## National Institute of General Medical Sciences (NIGMS)[66]

Inflammation and the Host Response to Injury is funded as a "glue" grant by the NIGMS, a component of the National Institutes of Health (NIH). This collaborative research program sponsored by NIGMS is a new mechanism that encourages independently funded investigators to work together to solve a major biomedical research problem. The funds are intended to provide the "glue" to bring investigators together and allow them to work together interactively. Researchers in the program are leading the way to new knowledge about the role of inflammation in trauma injury. By profiling gene expression changes and other white blood cell molecular markers, scientists hope to identify an injured patient's fate: either recovery or multiple organ dysfunction syndrome (MODS). The patient-oriented research centers will identify patients with severe blunt trauma and burn injury, based upon strict entry criteria. Program researchers will focus on a cohort of subjects at high risk for MODS and death, documenting data describing injury severity, the development of organ failure, and ultimate clinical outcome. Clinical outcome data will be integrated with proteomic and genomic data gathered through the other core programs. To date, program researchers have established standard operating procedures for clinical care involving resuscitation of the trauma patient, management of acute respiratory failure, weaning from mechanical ventilation, and the diagnosis and treatment of ventilator-assisted pneumonia (VAP). The group is also developing strategic diagnostic criteria for complications to ensure consistent reporting and quality assessment of treatment and outcomes among the participating centers. Utilization of standard operating procedures (SOPs) along with standardized tracking of complications should pave the way for consistency in future multicenter trials assessing the impact of outcomes and interventional therapies in the severely injured patient population nationwide.

## OUTCOME PARAMETERS

The generally recognized outcome parameters in medicine are listed in Table 6-7. Survival and morbidity are traditional parameters that have been used in surgical research for decades. Although survival seems straightforward, the endpoint in time may vary considerably, including ICU, hospital, 30 days, 6 months, 1 year, and time to death. Many severity scoring and mortality prediction models have been developed. However, none is without defects, and precise definitions must be developed for measuring mortality in trauma outcome studies.

**TABLE 6-7**

### Outcome Parameters in Medicine

Survival (mortality)
Complications (morbidity)
Length of stay
Cost
Quality of life
Patient satisfaction
Compliance with guidelines

**TABLE 6-8**

### Top 25 Complications Associated With Survivors and Nonsurvivors

|  | NONSURVIVORS | SURVIVORS | TOTAL |
|---|---|---|---|
| Jaundice | 0 | 49 | 49 |
| Disseminated fungal infection | 11 | 209 | 220 |
| Esophageal intubation | 12 | 281 | 293 |
| Loss of operative reduction/fixation | 19 | 445 | 464 |
| Dehiscence/evisceration | 29 | 589 | 618 |
| Empyema | 41 | 658 | 699 |
| Bacteremia | 46 | 949 | 995 |
| Intra-abdominal abscess | 48 | 882 | 930 |
| Pancreatitis | 66 | 1138 | 1204 |
| Pulmonary embolus | 83 | 1652 | 1735 |
| Progression of original neurologic insult | 93 | 1590 | 1683 |
| Hypothermia | 128 | 2314 | 2442 |
| Pneumothorax | 147 | 2816 | 2963 |
| Compartment syndrome | 150 | 2846 | 2996 |
| Renal failure | 151 | 2945 | 3096 |
| DVT (lower extremity) | 161 | 2703 | 2864 |
| Cardiac arrest | 172 | 3198 | 3370 |
| Aspiration pneumonia | 179 | 3528 | 3707 |
| Wound infection | 182 | 3469 | 3651 |
| Skin breakdown | 197 | 3470 | 3667 |
| Coagulopathy | 230 | 4367 | 4597 |
| Acute respiratory distress syndrome (ARDS) | 293 | 5222 | 5515 |
| Myocardial infarction | 409 | 7173 | 7582 |
| Urinary tract infection | 570 | 9882 | 10452 |
| Pneumonia | 965 | 16445 | 17410 |
| None | 53,162 | 99,1861 | 104,5023 |

From: National Trauma Data Bank (NTDB), 2005.

The use of morbidity as an outcome parameter requires distinguishing between a complication and a pre-existing disease (i.e., a comorbidity) and providing a precise definition of the complication.[67] For example, a wound infection may require the recovery of an organism and documented treatment with antibiotics. Further differentiation between a superficial and a deep site infection may be necessary. Occasionally, more confounding is defining a denominator for determining comparative survival or morbidity rates. Should the denominator for a surgeon's wound infection rate be determined by the total number of patients undergoing surgery, or should it be determined by specific procedure, i.e., adjusted for the risk by contamination risk? Obviously, the latter is preferred, but sometimes the former is used in physician profiling. Information acquired from the National Trauma Data Bank shows the most common complications found in survivors and nonsurvivors (Table 6-8). Of course, further research is needed to determine if the patients died because of the complication or with the complication. In a study designed to quantify the costs associated with the development of complication in injury victims, 32 complications defined by the ACSCOT were analyzed using a linear regression model.[68] Six complications were found to be important predictors of cost, including acute respiratory distress syndrome (ARDS), acute renal failure, sepsis, pneumonia, decubitus ulceration, and wound infection. The 1201 individuals with these complications had an observed average cost of $47,457 compared with a predicted average cost of $23,266, with mean excess costs ranging from $7000 to $18,000 per complication.

In studying in-patient length of stay (LOS), different levels of intensity must be recognized, such as intensive care unit, step-down unit, floor, and so on, because these are not uniform among institutions. In addition, reduced hospital LOS must be measured by its effect on the patient's family, visiting nurses, physicians' offices, and unanticipated hospital readmission. Few systems have the sophistication to measure these effects accurately. Therefore, hospital LOS is, at best, a gross parameter of quality or outcome.[69]

In the past, trauma studies have used charges as a surrogate for cost. Such an arrangement has led to many flawed conclusions and is largely unsuitable in today's health care environment. The determination of true cost is challenging, because most hospital data systems were developed to track operational and capital expenditures rather than clinical care. To overcome this dilemma, techniques generally termed cost accounting have emerged.[70] These techniques require many assumptions that need to be clearly understood by clinicians. These assumptions factor in personnel time, resource utilization, supplies, overhead, and so on, by developing equations of proportionality based on expenditures, both direct and indirect as well as fixed and variable.

As with all outcome parameters, the cost of trauma care can be in the eye of the beholder. The payer is likely to know his or her cost with some precision, which usually reflects what he or she paid plus administrative costs. The patient usually perceives the cost as his or her out-of-pocket expenses plus lost wages. However, the cost to the providers has many confounding variables and is much less precise. The cost to society is even more abstract, and studies have revealed substantial variation in estimates.

Quality of life has been recognized by researchers for several decades as a desired outcome parameter. Table 6-9 provides a catalog of health-related quality-of-life measurement tools that have been reported in the trauma(critical care literature. Many of these tools are

**TABLE 6-9**

### Quality-Of-Life Measurement Tools

American Spinal Injury Association (ASIA) Score
Ashworth Scale
Barthel Index
Beck Depression Index
Craig Handicap Assessment and Reporting Technique (CHART)
Disability Rating Scale (DRS)
Frankel Score
Functional Capacity Index (FCI)
Functional Independence Measure (FIM)
Glasgow Outcome Scale (GOS)
Head Injury Symptom Checklist
Health Assessment Questionnaire (HAQ)
Impact on Family Scale
Index of Activities of Daily Living
Injury Impairment Scale (IIS)
Katz Adjustment Scale
Medical Rehabilitation Follow Along (MRFA)
Minnesota Multiphasic Personality Inventory (MMPI)
Musculoskeletal Functional Assessment (MFA)
Nottingham Health Profile
Patient Evaluation and Conference System (PECS)
Pediatric Evaluation of Disability Inventory (PEDI)
Quality of Well-Being (QWB) Scale
Rancho Scale of Cognitive Functioning
Rehabilitation Outcome Questionnaire
SF-36 Survey
Sickness Impact Profile (SIP)
Supervision Rating Scale (SRS)
Trauma Motor Index (TMI)
UCLA Activity Index

designed to measure the patient, family, and the provider perceptions of outcome. Some are labor-intensive and become impractical except for focused studies. The Functional Independence Measure (FIM), Glasgow Outcome Scale (GOS), Functional Capacity Index (FCI), Quality of Well-Being Scale, Sickness Impact Profile (SIP), and SF-36 Survey are among the most popular in trauma-related outcome studies. Many commercially available survey tools are religiously utilized by hospital and system administrators as measures of patient satisfaction (Table 6-10). Goals are frequently set to meet target scores, suggesting either improvement or decline in outcome.

Finally, measuring compliance with evidence-based guidelines can provide a measurement of outcomes.[71] Studies of compliance with the Advanced Trauma Life Support (ATLS) guidelines, as well

**TABLE 6-10**

### Patient Satisfaction Measurement Tools

Press Ganey
404 Columbia Place, South Bend, IN 46601
Picker Institute
1295 Boylston Street, Suite 100, Boston, MA 02215
Solution Point
1501 LBJ Freeway, Suite 440, Dallas, TX 75234
National Research Corporation (NRC)
1003 O Street, Lincoln, NB 68508
Partners in Quality (Parkside Associates)
205 West Touhy Avenue

as head injury guidelines, have provided several outcome studies.[72–74] Using guideline compliance as an outcome itself assumes that the desired outcome is compliance, inferring improvement in other standard patient outcomes based on the evidence on which the guidelines were developed. Therefore, caution is required in interpreting this outcome parameter.

## OUTCOME STUDIES

Many notable trauma-related outcome studies have emerged over the past decade. Table 6-11 lists a number of representative studies[75–104] that have been influential on guideline development as well as in providing direction for future research. These studies represent only a snapshot of the galaxy of studies that are emerging at an ever-increasing pace.[3] This encouraging trend must be tempered with the observation that critical care outcome studies appear to dwarf other trauma-related studies both in power and in volume. This reflects the fact that the environment of critical care, although replete with many confounding variables, lends itself to some element of measure and control, which can produce many more randomized, controlled trials. Because of the uncontrolled aspect of much of the prehospital, resuscitative, and operative phases of trauma care, studies from these areas, especially when measuring organ-specific injury, may have class II and class III studies as appropriate and useful goals. Numerous class III multi-institutional trials sponsored by academic societies provide valuable outcome data that would otherwise be unavailable.

The recently published, *A National Evaluation of the Effect of Trauma-Center Care on Mortality*, is the first major paper on the results of the National Study on Costs and Outcomes from Trauma (NSCOT).[105] The study analyzed the outcomes of 5190 adult trauma patients who received treatment at 18 Level 1 trauma centers and 51 nontrauma centers. The researchers also analyzed the characteristics of each hospital, such as the number of patients treated and types of specialty services available. After adjusting for factors such as severity of injury, patient age, and pre-existing medical conditions, the researchers found a 25% overall decrease in the risk of death following care in a trauma center compared to receiving care at a nontrauma center. The adjusted in-hospital death rate was 7.6% for patients treated at trauma centers compared to 9.5% for patients treated at nontrauma facilities. The mortality rate 1 year following the injury was 10.4% for patients at trauma centers compared to 13.8% for patients at nontrauma centers. Such outcomes data provide staff and community leaders with crucial information, so that they can make sound decisions regarding their trauma systems and the care that people receive after they are injured. The study group is currently in the process of writing the next major paper, which will describe the impact of trauma center care on functional outcomes at 12 months after injury. The group anticipates that there will be a number of other papers describing the impact of different aspects of care on outcome, as well as papers on the cost-effectiveness of care.

## FUTURE DIRECTION

Both interest in and funding of trauma outcome research appear to be increasing as measured by the activities of many academic societies and professional organizations. The completion of randomized,

**TABLE 6-11**

### Representative Trauma Outcome Studies

| AUTHORS/REFERENCE | YEAR | EVIDENCE CLASS | TOPIC |
|---|---|---|---|
| Trauma Systems/Centers | | | |
| Demetriades et al.[75] | 2005 | III | Outcomes with specific injuries in level I and II trauma centers |
| Ehrlich et al.[76] | 2005 | III | Patient care indicators after trauma designation |
| Glance LG et al.[77] | 2005 | III | Use of TRISS and ASCOT for benchmarking performance and quality improvement |
| van Olden et al.[78] | 2004 | III | Clinical impact of advanced trauma life support |
| Simons R et al.[79] | 2002 | | Outcomes after trauma center designation and accreditation |
| Nathens et al.[80] | 2001 | III | Multicenter study of the relationship between trauma center volume and outcomes |
| Age/Gender | | | |
| Larson et al.[81] | 2004 | III | Outcomes in pediatric trauma with air ambulance transportation from injury scene |
| Holbrook et al.[82] | 2001 | II | Gender differences on functional and psychological outcomes |
| Napolitano et al.[83] | 2001 | III | Gender differences in adverse outcomes |
| Osler et al.[84] | 2001 | III | Comparative survival in pediatric and adult trauma centers |
| Potaka et al.[85] | 2000 | III | Impact of pediatric trauma centers (registry study) |
| Ferrera et al.[86] | 2000 | III | Functional outcomes in admitted geriatric trauma victims |
| Prehospital | | | |
| Wang et al.[87] | 2004 | III | Outcome with out-of-hospital endotracheal intubation after traumatic brain injury |
| Eckstein et al.[88] | 2000 | III | Effect of prehospital advanced life support |
| Gausche et al.[89] | 2000 | II | Controlled trial of prehospital pediatric intubation |
| Jacobs et al.[90] | 1999 | III | Mortality outcome with air medical transport |
| Thoracic Trauma | | | |
| Maenza et al.[91] | 1996 | II | Large meta-analysis of blunt cardiac injury |
| Fabian et al.[92] | 1997 | III | Prospective multicenter study of blunt aortic injury |
| Abdominal Trauma | | | |
| Harbrecht et al.[93] | 2004 | II | Outcome of adult blunt splenic injuries at level I and II trauma centers |
| Demetriades et al.[94] | 2001 | III | Prospective multicenter study of penetrating colon injury |
| Peitzman et al.[95] | 2000 | III | Multi-institutional study of blunt splenic injury |
| Livingston et al.[96] | 1998 | III | Prospective multi-institutional study of discharge after negative abdominal computed tomography |
| Head and Spinal Cord Injuries | | | |
| Chan et al.[97] | 2005 | III | Outcome after traumatic spinal cord injury in tertiary center |
| Jones et al.[98] | 2005 | III | Incidence of VTE after spinal cord injury |
| Davis et al.[99] | 2003 | III | Outcome with severe traumatic brain injury after paramedic rapid sequence intubation |
| Vascular Injuries | | | |
| Dennis et al.[100] | 1998 | III | Long-term follow-up of occult vascular injuries |
| Intensive Care Unit | | | |
| Harrison et al.[101] | 2005 | III | Mortality and blood product use in traumatic hemorrhage |
| Gattinoni et al.[102] | 2001 | I | Randomized multicenter study of prone positioning for acute respiratory failure |
| ARDS Network[103] | 2000 | I | Randomized multicenter trial of low tidal volumes in ARDS |
| Hebert et al.[104] | 1999 | I | Randomized multicenter study of transfusion requirements in critical care |

controlled trials is accelerating and will provide valuable class I data. The product of this effort should foster the continued development of evidence-based guidelines to improve trauma care worldwide. The electronic patient record will enable a much more robust development of class II and class III data, especially when the record includes the prehospital and post-hospital outcomes. The components of the electronic record include (a) physician order entry, (b) clinical decision support systems, (c) documentation, and (d) picture archiving and communication systems (PACS) for cataloging images in a film-less fashion.

Registries as we now know them will be replaced by or incorporated into this technology. More sophisticated and validated severity adjusting tools will allow for more meaningful and consistent trauma outcome research. It is not clear that richer local, regional, and national trauma outcome research will promote further regionalization of trauma care, but the converging technologies in health care will likely create new models of trauma care delivery that will demand outcome-based direction.

Over the next several years, trauma organizations will be responsible for determining and defining which outcomes are important to follow and assure that data collection is complete and accurate. National benchmarks need to be established beyond "live, die" and our outcomes should direct our performance improvement initiatives. Such initiatives should be approached in an evidence-based fashion with attempts made to provide sound clinical practice guidelines.

# REFERENCES

1. Committee on Quality of Health Care in America, Institute of Medicine: *Crossing the Quality Chasm: A New Health System for the 21st Century.* Washington, D.C.: National Academy Press, 2001.

2. Committee on Enhancing Federal Healthcare Quality Programs, Institute of Medicine: Corrigan JM, Eden J, Smith BM, eds. *Leadership by Example: Coordinating Government Roles in Improving Health Care Quality.* Washington, D.C.: National Academy Press, 2002.

3. Fabian TC: Evidence-based medicine in trauma care: Whither goest thou? *J Trauma* 47:225, 1999.

4. West JG, Trunkey DD, Lim RC: Systems of trauma care. A study of two countries. *Arch Surg* 114:455, 1979.

5. Shackford SR, Mackersie RC, Hoyt DB, et al.: Impact of a trauma system on outcome of severely injured patients. *Arch Surg* 122:523, 1987.

6. National Highway Traffic Safety Administration: *The Third Report to Congress: Effectiveness of Occupant Protection Systems and Their Use.* Washington, D.C.: U.S. Department of Transportation, December 1996. http://www/nhtsa.dot.gov/. Accessed June 1, 2007.

7. Trunkey DD: Trauma. Accidental and intentional injuries account for more years of life lost in the U.S. than cancer and heart disease. Among the prescribed remedies are improved preventive efforts, speedier surgery and further research. *Sci Am* 249:28, 1983.

8. Crane M: Why premiums are soaring again. A new "malpractice crisis"? *Med Econ* 87:132, 2001.

9. Delaware Valley Healthcare Council: Trauma care is in critical condition. (Full-page advertisement from 12 trauma centers.) Philadelphia, PA: *The Philadelphia Inquirer,* Dec. 9, 2001.

10. Long WB: The use of trauma data bases to determine injury survivability (abstract). *J Trauma* 44:431, 1998.

11. Selzer D, Gomez G, Jacobson L, et al.: Public hospital-based level I trauma centers: Financial survival in the new millennium. *J Trauma* 51:301, 2001.

12. Finestone AJ: Reimbursement as incentive to improve physicians' quality of care. *JAMA* 286:1575, 2001.

13. Osler TM, Cohen M, Rogers FB, et al.: Trauma registry injury coding is superfluous: A comparison of outcome prediction based on trauma registry International Classification of Diseases—Ninth Revision (ICD-9) and hospital information system ICD-9 codes. *J Trauma* 43:253, 1997.

14. Maier RV, Rhodes M: Trauma performance improvement, In Rivara FP, Cummings P, Koepsell TD, et al. eds. *Injury Control. A Guide to Research and Program Evaluation.* Cambridge, United Kingdom: Cambridge University Press, 2001, p. 196.

15. Kohn LT, Corrigan JM, Donaldson MS, eds: *Institute of Medicine (US) Committee on Quality of Health Care in America. To Err Is Human: Building a Safer Health System.* Washington, D.C.: National Academy Press, 2000.

16. Institute of Medicine (US) Committee on Quality of Health Care in America: *Crossing the Quality Chasm: A New Health System for the 21st Century.* Washington, D.C.: National Academy Press, 2001.

17. Cook D: Evidence-based critical care medicine: A potential tool for change. *New Horiz* 6:20, 1998.

18. Guyatt GH, Sackett DL, Sinclair JC, et al.: Users' guides to the medical literature: IX. A method for grading health care recommendations. Evidence-Based Medicine Working Group. *JAMA* 274:1800, 1995.

19. Vincent J: Which therapeutic interventions in critical care medicine have been shown to reduce mortality in prospective, randomized, clinical trials? A survey of candidates for the Belgian Board Examination in Intensive Care Medicine. *Crit Care Med* 28:1616, 2000.

20. Institute of Medicine (US) Committee on Clinical Practice Guidelines, Field MJ, Lohr KN, eds: *Guidelines for Clinical Practice: From Development to Use.* Washington, D.C.: National Academy Press, 1992.

21. Pasquale M, Fabian TC: Practice management guidelines for trauma from the Eastern Association for the Surgery of Trauma. *J Trauma* 44:941, 1998.

22. Agency for Healthcare Policy & Research: *Interim Manual For Clinical Practice Guidelines Development.* Rockville, MD: Agency for Healthcare Policy and Research, 1991.

23. Cabana MD, Rand CS, Powe NR, et al.: Why don't physicians follow clinical practice guidelines? A framework for improvement. *JAMA* 282:1458, 1999.

24. Rhodes M: Guidelines, protocols and pathways for trauma care. In Trunkey DD, Lewis FR, eds. *Current Therapy of Trauma,* 4th ed. St Louis, MO: Mosby, 1999, p. 343.

25. Sesperez J, Wilson S, Jalaludin B, et al.: Trauma case management and clinical pathways: Prospective evaluation of their effect on selected patient outcomes in five key trauma conditions. *J Trauma* 50:643, 2001.

26. Bullock R, Chestnut RM, Cliffton G, et al.: *Guidelines for Management of Severe Head Injury.* New York, NY: The Brain Trauma Foundation, 1995.

27. Collin GR, Atkinson N, Furrow K, et al.: Decreasing the duration of mechanical ventilation through the use of a ventilator management protocol (abstract.) *Crit Care Med* 27:A110, 1999.

28. Leape LL, Berwick DM: Five years after *To Err Is Human*: What have we learned? *JAMA* 293:2384, 2005.

29. Joint Commission on Accreditation of Healthcare Organization: Sentinel event trends: Potassium chloride events by year. http://www.caho.org/NR/rdonlyres/E744A75A-32A7-4B73-A9EE-B5E64CDED821/0/se_trends_potassium_chlorid.gif. Accessed March 7, 2006.

30. Kelly JJ, Sweigard KW, Shields K, et al.: Eisenberg Patient Safety Awards: Safety, effectiveness, and efficiency: A Web-based virtual anticoagulation clinic. *Jt Comm J Qual Saf* 29:646, 2003.

31. Whittington J, Cohen H: OSF Healthcare's journey in patient safety. *Qual Manag Health Care* 13:53, 2004.

32. *2004 National Healthcare Quality Report.* Rockville, MD: Agency for Healthcare Research and Quality, 2004.

33. Blendon RJ, DesRoches CM, Brodie M, et al.: Views of practicing physicians and the public on medical errors. *N Engl J Med* 347:1933, 2002.

34. *Serious Reportable Events in Patient Safety: A National Quality Forum Consensus Report.* Washington, D.C.: National Quality Forum, 2002.

35. Joint Commission on Accreditation of Healthcare Organizations: *Improving hospital performance. 2002 Comprehensive Accreditation Manual of Hospital: The Official Handbook.* Oakbrook Terrace, IL: Joint Commission on Accreditation of Healthcare Organizations, 2002.

36. *Safe Practices for Better Health Care: A Consensus Report.* Washington, D.C.: National Quality Forum, 2003.

37. Surgical Care Improvement Project. A partnership for better care. http://www.medqic.org/scip/ Accessed March 8, 2006.

38. American Board of Medical Specialties: Status of MOC programs. http://www.abms.org/MOC.asp. Accessed March 8, 2006.

39. The Leapfrog Group: Patient safety: Leapfrog hospital safety standards. http://www.leapfroggroup.org/safety.htm. Accessed March 9, 2006.

40. Bates DW, Teich JM, Lee J, et al.: The impact of computerized physician order entry on medication error prevention. *J Am Med Inform Assoc* 6:313, 1999.

41. Bates DW, Gawande AA: Improving safety with information technology. *N Engl J Med* 348:2526, 2003.

42. Leape LL, Cullen DJ, Clapp MD, et al.: Pharmacist participation on physician rounds and adverse drug events in the intensive care unit. *JAMA* 282:267, 1999.

43. Kucukarslan SN, Peters M, Mlynarek M, et al.: Pharmacists on rounding teams reduce preventable adverse drug events in hospital general medicine units. *Arch Intern Med* 163:2014, 2003.

44. Landro L: The informed patient: Hospitals form "SWAT" teams to avert deaths. Wall Street Journal, December 1, 2004.

45. Rozich J, Resar R: Medication safety: One organization's approach to the challenge. *J Clin Outcomes Manage* 8:27, 2001.

46. Rozich J, Howard R, Justeson J, et al.: Standardization as a mechanism to improve safety in health care. *Jt Comm J Qual Saf* 30:5, 2004.

47. Institute for Healthcare Improvement: Reducing Adverse Drug Events: Missouri Baptist Medical Center. http://www.ihi.org/IHI/Topics/PatientSafety/Medication Systems/ImprovementStories/ReducingAdverseDrug EventsMissouriBaptistMedicalCenter.htm. Accessed March 7, 2006.

48. Samkoff JS, Jacques CH: A review of studies concerning effects of sleep deprivation and fatigue on residents' performance. *Acad Med* 66:687, 1991.

49. Pilcher JJ, Huffcutt AI: Effects of sleep deprivation on performance: A meta-analysis. *Sleep* 19:318, 1996.

50. Gaba DM, Howard SL: Fatigue among clinicians and the safety of patients. *N Engl J Med* 347:1249, 2002.

51. Harrison Y, Horne JA: The impact of sleep deprivation on decision making: A review. *J Exp Psychol Appl* 6:236, 2000.

52. *AHRQ: Evidence-based Practice Centers.* Rockville, MD: Agency for Healthcare Research and Quality, 1998.

53. Shojania KG, Duncan BW, McDonald KM, et al. (eds): *Making Health Care Safer. A Critical Analysis for Patient Safety Practices: Summary.* AHRQ Publication No. 01-E057. Rockville, MD: Agency for Healthcare Research and Quality, 2001. http://www.ahrq.gov/clinic/ptsafety/summary.htm. Accessed March 12, 2006.

54. National Guideline Clearinghouse™ (NGC) http://www.guideline.gov/ Accessed March 8, 2006.

55. National Guideline Clearinghouse™ (NGC) Annotated Bibliographies http://www.guideline.gov/ab/ab.aspx. Accessed March 8, 2006.

56. The Leapfrog Group. Who are members? http://www.leapfroggroup.org/about_us/who_are_members. Accessed March 9, 2006.

57. Joint Commission on Accreditation of Healthcare Organizations: *Improving Hospital Performance.* CAMH Refreshed Core, January 2005. Oakbrook Terrace, IL: Joint Commission on Accreditation of Healthcare Organizations, 2005.

58. Kincaid EH, Chang MC, Letton RW, et al.: Admission base deficit in pediatric trauma: A study using the National Trauma Data Bank. *J Trauma* 51:332, 2001.

59. Wynn A, Wise M, Wright MJ, et al.: Accuracy of administrative and trauma registry databases. *J Trauma* 51:64, 2001.

60. Owen JL, Bolenbaucher RM, Moore ML: Trauma registry databases: A comparison of data abstraction, interpretation and entry at two level I trauma centers. *J Trauma* 46:1100, 1999.

61. College establishes Office of Evidence-Based Surgery. *Bull AM Cool Surg* 86:30, 2001.

62. Daley J, Forbes MG, Young GJ, et al.: Validating risk-adjusted surgical outcomes: Site visit assessment of process and structure. National VA Surgical Risk Study. *J Am Coll Surg* 185:341, 1997.

63. Khuri SF, Daley J, Henderson W, et al.: The Department of Veterans Affairs' NSQIP: The first national, validated, outcome-based, risk-adjusted, and peer-controlled program for the measurement and enhancement of the quality of surgical care. National VA Surgical Quality Improvement Program. *Ann Surg* 228:491, 1998.

64. Dimick JB, Chen SL, Taheri PA, et al.: Hospital costs associated with surgical complications: A report from the private-sector National Surgical Quality Improvement Program. *J Am Coll Surg* 199:531, 2004.

65. McLeod RS: Evidence-based reviews in surgery: A new educational program for ACS Fellows, Candidates, and Resident Members. *Bull Am Coll Surg* 90:9, 2005.

66. National Institute of General Medical Sciences (NIGMS) www.nigms.nih.gov/About/Council/Minutes/January13-14_2005.htm. Accessed March 9, 2006.

67. American College of Surgeons Committee on Trauma: *Resources for Optimal Care of the Injured Patient: 1999.* Chicago: American College of Surgeons, 1998, p. 69.

68. O'Keefe GE, Maier RV, Diehr P, et al.: The complications of trauma and their associated costs in a level I trauma center. *Arch Surg* 132:920, 1997.

69. Taheri PA, Butz DA, Greenfield L: Length of stay has minimal impact on the cost of hospital admission. *J Am Coll Surg* 191:123, 2000.

70. Roberts RR, Frutos PW, Ciavarella GG, et al.: Distribution of variable vs fixed costs of hospital care. *JAMA* 281:644,1999.

71. Rhodes M, Fallon W JR: How guidelines can serve as outcomes tools. *J Surg Outcomes* 2:9, 1999.

72. Lewell M, McCauley W, Anderson SL: Review of the compliance with advanced trauma life support protocol among patients referred to a level I trauma centre (abstract). *Ann Emerg Med* 34:S31, 1999.

73. Palmer S, Bader MK, Qureshi A: The impact on outcomes in a community hospital setting of using the AANS traumatic brain injury guidelines. *J Trauma* 50:657, 2001.

74. Marion DW, Spiegel TP: Changes in the management of severe traumatic brain injury: 1991–1997. *Crit Care Med* 28:16, 2000.

75. Demetriades D, Martin M, Salim A, et al.: The effect of trauma center designation and trauma volume on outcome in specific severe injuries. *Ann Surg* 242:5127; discussion 517, 2005.

76. Ehrlich PF, McClellan WT, Wesson DE: Monitoring performance: Longterm impact of trauma verification and review. *J Am Coll Surg* 200:166, 2005.

77. Glance LG, Osler TM, Dick AW: Evaluating trauma center quality: Does the choice of the severity-adjustment model make a difference? *J Trauma* 58:1265, 2005.

78. van Olden, Meeuwis JD, Bolhuis HW, et al.: Clinical impact of advanced trauma life support. *Am J Emerg Med* 22:522, 2004.

79. Simons R, Kasic S, Kirkpatrick A, et al.: Relative importance of designation and accreditation of trauma centers during evolution of a regional trauma system. *J Trauma* 52:827; discussion 833, 2002.

80. Nathens AB, Jurkovich GJ, Maier RV, et al.: Relationship between trauma center volume and outcomes. *JAMA* 285:1164, 2001.

81. Larson JT, Dietrich AM, Abdessalam SF, et al.: Effective use of the air ambulance for pediatric trauma. *J Trauma* 56:89, 2004.

82. Holbrook TL, Hoyt DB, Anderson JP: The importance of gender on outcome after major trauma: Functional and psychologic outcomes in women versus men. *J Trauma* 50:270, 2001.

83. Napolitano LM, Greco ME, Rodriguez A, et al.: Gender differences in adverse outcomes after blunt trauma. *J Trauma* 50:274, 2001.

84. Osler TM, Vane DW, Tepas JJ, et al.: Do pediatric trauma centers have better survival rates than adult trauma centers? An examination of the National Pediatric Trauma Registry. *J Trauma* 50:96, 2001.

85. Ferrera PC, Bartfielf JM, D'Andrea CC: Outcomes of admitted geriatric trauma victims. *Am J Emerg Med* 18:575, 2000.

86. Potoka DA, Schall LC, Gardner MJ, et al.: Impact of pediatric trauma centers on mortality in a statewide system. *J Trauma* 49:237, 2000.

87. Wang HE, Peitzman AB, Cassidy LD, et al.: Out-of-hospital endotracheal intubation and outcome after traumatic brain injury. *Ann Emerg Med* 44:439, 2004.

88. Eckstein M, Chan L, Schneir A, et al.: Effect of prehospital advanced life support on outcomes of major trauma patients. *J Trauma* 48:643, 2000.

89. Gausche M, Lewis RJ, Stratton SJ, et al.: Effect of out-of hospital pediatric endotracheal intubation on survival and neurological outcome. *JAMA* 238:783, 2000.

90. Jacobs LM, Gabram SG, Sztajnkrycer MD, et al.: Helicopter air medical transport: Ten-year outcomes for trauma patients in a New England Program. *Conn Med* 63:677, 1999.

91. Maenza RL, Seaberg D, D'Amico F: A meta-analysis of blunt cardiac trauma: Ending myocardial confusion. *Am J Emerg Med* 14:237, 1996.

92. Fabian TC, Richardson JD, Croce MA, et al.: Prospective study of blunt aortic injury: Multicenter trial of the American Association for the Surgery of Trauma. *J Trauma* 42:374, 1997.

93. Harbrecht BG, Zenati MS, Ochoa JB, et al.: Management of adult blunt splenic injuries: Comparison between level I and level II trauma centers. *J Am Coll Surg* 198:232, 2004.

94. Demetriades D, Murray JA, Chan L, et al.: Penetrating colon injuries requiring resection: Diversion or primary anastomosis? An AAST prospective multicenter study. *J Trauma* 50:765, 2001.

95. Peitzman AB, Heil B, Rivera L, et al.: Blunt splenic injury in adults: Multi-institutional study of the Eastern Association for the Surgery of Trauma. *J Trauma* 49:177, 2000.

96. Livingston DH, Lavery RF, Passannante MR, et al.: Admission or observation is not necessary after a negative abdominal computed tomographic scan in patients with suspected blunt abdominal trauma: Results of a prospective, multi-institutional trial. *J Trauma* 44:273, 1998.

97. Chan SC, Chan AP: Rehabilitation outcomes following traumatic spinal cord injury in a tertiary spinal cord injury centre: A comparison with an international standard. *Spinal Cord* 43:489, 2005.

98. Jones T, Ugalde V, Franks P, Zhou H, et al.: Venous thromboembolism after spinal cord injury: Incidence, time course, and associated risk factors in 16,240 adults and children. *Arch Phys Med Rehab* 86:2240, 2005.

99. Davis DP, Hoyt DB, Ochs M, et al.: The effect of paramedic rapid sequence intubation on outcome in patients with severe traumatic brain injury. *J Trauma* 54:444, 2003.

100. Dennis JW, Frykberg ER, Veldenz HC, et al.: Validation of nonoperative management of occult vascular injuries and accuracy of physical examination alone in penetrating extremity trauma: 5- to 10-year follow-up. *J Trauma* 44:243, 1998.

101. Harrison TD, Laskosky J, Jazaeri O, et al.: "Low-dose" recombinant activated factor VII results in less blood and blood product use in traumatic hemorrhage. *J Trauma* 59:150, 2005.

102. Gattinoni L, Tognoni G, Presenti A, et al.: Effect of prone positioning on the survival of patients with acute respiratory failure. *N Engl J Med* 345:568, 2001.

103. The Acute Respiratory Distress Syndrome Network. Ventilation with lower tidal volumes as compared with traditional tidal volumes for acute lung injury and the acute respiratory distress syndrome. *N Engl J Med* 342:1301, 2000.

104. Hebert PC, Wells G, Blajchman MA, et al.: A Multicenter, randomized, controlled clinical trial of transfusion requirements in critical care. Transfusion Requirements in Critical Care Investigators, Canadian Critical Care Trials Group. *N Engl J Med* 340:409, 1999.

105. MacKenzie EJ, Rivara FP, Jurkovich GJ, et al.: A national evaluation of the effect of trauma-center care on morality. *N Engl J Med* 354:366, 2006.

# Commentary ■ RICHARD J. MULLINS

Dr Pasquale and Dr Rhodes emphasize that government agencies and multiple payer groups are demanding greater oversight of healthcare delivery. Major problems in contemporary medical care are errors, excessive costs for limited value, and unwarranted variations from evidence-based practice. Dr Pasquale and Dr Rhodes argue that trauma surgeons will need to modify their practice and develop valid, reliable, and accurately measured outcomes as the foundation for their response to critics who seek to impose reforms on the care of injured patients.

For decades trauma surgeons have been pathfinders in measuring outcomes. Since the 1970s trauma surgeons have championed trauma systems. In fully implemented regional trauma system, to designate a hospital as a trauma center the survival rate for patients' are expected to be within outcome standards. Trauma surgeons need to evaluate not just outcome, but also processes of care, which are treatments, diagnostic tests, and interventions that occur to injured patients as a consequence of surgeons' decisions. For example, what should the tracheostomy rate for a trauma center be? A lack of published evidence because of a scarcity of randomized control trials has limited the value of evidence-based processes of care as a measure of quality of care. Trauma surgeons should rely upon research as the best foundation for completing "the quality improvement cycle."

An idea incompletely discussed by Dr Pasquale and Dr Rhodes is the unique challenge of determining optimal outcome in elderly patients. Successful outcome is typically hospital survival. The most desirable outcome for some elders is being restored to independent living. A desirable outcome in the mind of health care provider may be in conflict with what the patients consider an acceptable outcome. The authors call for trauma surgeons to have greater reliance upon evidence-based practice of surgery. Guidelines, pathways, and protocols are mechanisms that reduce the unwarranted variation in practice. Enthusiasm for reducing treatment variations should be tempered by recognition that surgeons care for injured patients in a diverse environments. A single surgeon performing a lapartomy in a remote small hospital should readily remove a bleeding spleen that would be repaired by a professor of surgery leading a trauma team in Level 1 trauma center. In the rush to mandate compliance with guidelines, pathways, and protocols based upon evidence derived from ideal clinical circumstances trauma surgeons should permit flexibility related to nonideal circumstances.

The authors endorse greater use of electronic devices and information management technologies. Physical examination finding, radiographic findings, and laboratory data recorded in the electronic record can be linked to orders written by surgeons and provide concurrent oversight. The value of the electronic record remains hypothetical, and trauma surgeons may encounter substantial impediments to its real-time use. Inaccurate and missing data erode the practical value of the electronic record. Patient's multiple providers may have conflicting data in the record. Finally, there will always be the risk of simplification of a complex clinical course of events with the electronic record's preference to record one data point.

The authors appropriately credit the American College of Surgeons Committee on Trauma in its multiple efforts to improve the quality of care delivered to injured patients. Professional surgical organizations provide a context for surgeons to debate and reach consensus on standards. Working in the context of a credible national organization can enable, surgeons can lead the debate to define optimal, and not just low-cost, care.

In conclusion the authors have placed the issue of measuring trauma patient's outcome within the context of the nationwide call for reform in all of medical care. Trauma surgeons should heed the advice of Dr Pasquale and Dr Rhodes, and lead healthcare reforms through research that measures what is optimal treatment for injured patients. The authors conclude "outcomes are the results of care from the perspective of the patient, provider, payer, and society." A question that should always be debated is among these three stakeholders, who has priority? The editors of this text should consider revising the chapter's title to Quality of Trauma Care. As Avedis Donabedian, a leading healthcare policy scholar of the twentieth century emphasized, quality of medical care is measured with three major components; one is outcomes, but the other two, processes of care and structure, also need to be emphasized with equal intensity as trauma surgeons seek methods for improving the quality of care they delivered to trauma patients.

# Kinematics of Trauma

*John P. Hunt* ∎ *Sharon L. Weintraub* ∎ *Alan B. Marr*

**Kin·e·mat·ics** (*kn-mtks*) *n*: The branch of mechanics that studies the motion of a body or a system of bodies without consideration given to its mass or the forces acting on it. From Greek *knma, knmat-, motion.*[1]

As can be deduced from the derivation of the word *kinematics*, its essence revolves around motion. All injury, except thermal and radiation, are related to the interaction of the host and a moving object. Basic Newtonian mechanics, in conjunction with the anatomic and material properties of the host, explain many of the injuries and patterns of injury seen in penetrating as well as blunt trauma. Injury is related not only to the energy of the injuring element, but the interface of that element with the host. Specific configurations in trauma such as position in a motor vehicle compartment and collision pattern or trajectory of projectiles and position of victim typically yield specific injury patterns. Knowing the details of a traumatic event may aid the treating physician in detecting occult but predictable injuries.

This chapter has been organized in a stepwise fashion. First, the basic laws of physics and materials that dictate the interaction between the victim and the injuring implement are reviewed. This is followed by a more detailed examination of penetrating and blunt trauma and a synopsis of mechanisms specific to organs and body regions. It is hoped that this will offer the reader a better understanding of specific injury patterns, how they occur, and which injuries may result.

## BASIC PRINCIPLES

### Newton's Laws, Impulse, Momentum, Energy, and Work

Newton's first law states that every object will remain at rest or in uniform motion unless compelled to change its state by the action of an external force. This is taken as the definition of inertia. Newton's second law builds on the first and further defines a force ($F$) as equal to the product of the mass ($m$) and acceleration ($a$).

$$F = ma$$

The application of a force does not occur instantaneously, but over time. If both sides of the previous equation are multiplied by time, the following equation results:

$$F(t) = ma(t)$$

The product of force and time is known as impulse and multiplying acceleration by time yields velocity. The momentum ($p$) is defined to be the mass ($m$) of an object times its velocity ($v$).

$$p = mv$$

hence,

*Impulse = Change in momentum*

The important fact is that a force or impulse will cause a change in momentum, and, likewise, a change in momentum will generate a force.[2] This folds into Newton's third law, which states that for every action (force), there is an equal and opposite reaction.[3] An example of this is when two objects of equal velocity and mass strike each other their velocities are reduced to zero. As per Newton's second law each object applies a force to the other causing a change in momentum. This illustrates the law of conservation of momentum, which states the total momentum of a system will remain constant unless acted upon by an external force. The momentum of this two-object system is the same after a collision as it was prior to impact.[4]

The next important basic principles are of work and energy. Work ($W$) is defined as a force exerted over a distance and is frequently written as follows:

$$W = Fdx \text{ (See p. 142, 5th edition)}$$

with $F = ma$ and $a = vdv/dx$

which, after integration, yields the familiar formula for kinetic energy: $\frac{1}{2}mv^2$.

$$W = \frac{1}{2}\,mv_2^2 - \frac{1}{2}\,mv_1^2$$

Therefore, the work being done by a moving object, which interacts with a second object, equals the kinetic energy of the first object prior to doing work minus that after the interaction. More simply put, the work performed is equal to the change in kinetic energy of the first object.[5] When this interaction sets the other body in motion, the second body now has kinetic energy of its own, equal to the work done. James Joule described the first law of thermodynamics in 1840, which simply states that energy can be neither created nor destroyed.[6] This is an elastic collision because both kinetic energy and momentum are conserved and the colliding objects do not deform or conglomerate.

In trauma most collisions are inelastic. Inelastic collisions conserve momentum, but not kinetic energy. In these instances the kinetic energy "does work" in the deformation of materials even to the point where objects can conglomerate and form a single object. This is the hallmark of the inelastic collision.

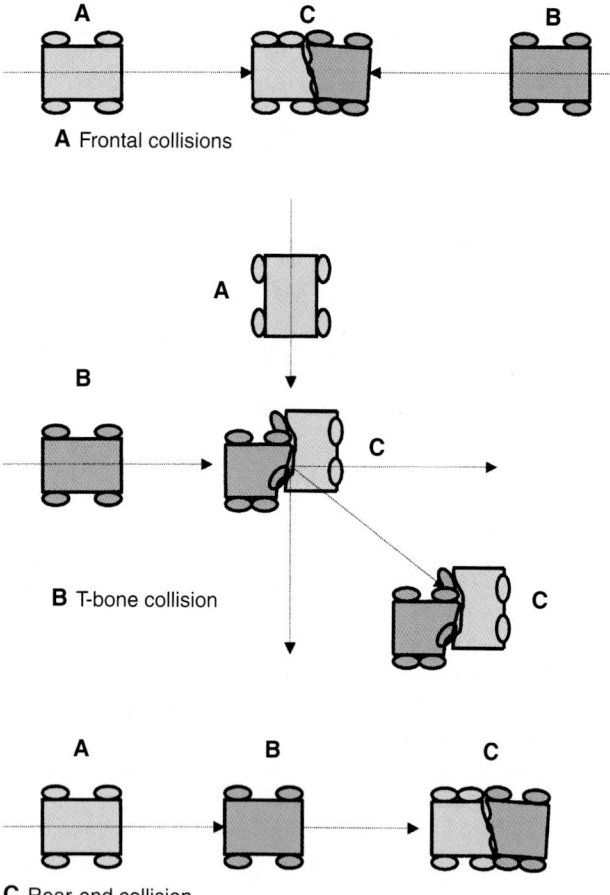

**A** Frontal collisions

**B** T-bone collision

**C** Rear-end collision

**FIGURE 7-1.** Energy and momentum available in various motor vehicle crash scenarios. **(A)** Frontal collisions have the greatest change in momentum over the shortest amount of time and hence the highest forces generated. **(B)** T-bone collision. When cars A and B collide their resultant momentum directs them toward their final position C, the individual momentums in the x and y axis are dissipated over a greater time resulting in smaller forces than head-on collision. **(C)** Rear-end collision. Since these vehicles move in the same direction, the change in momentum and forces generated are smaller.

Energy transfer and momentum conservation can be illustrated in the collision of two cars. Using Fig. 7-1 as an illustration, (A) represents a head-on collision of two cars with equal mass and velocity and thus equal kinetic energy and momentum. The momentums are equal, but in opposite directions. Thus, the total momentum for the system is 0 prior to the crash and, by the law of conservation of momentum, must be 0 after the crash. Upon impact, both cars will come to rest. It is as if one of the cars struck an immovable wall. Recalling Newton's second and third laws this sudden change in momentum represents a force, which is equally applied to both cars. Since the final velocity is 0, the final kinetic energy is 0, meaning that all the kinetic energy has been converted to work that stops the other car and causes deformation such as breaking glass, bending metal, and causing physical intrusion into the passenger compartment. If the momentum of car A was greater than that of car B, by having a greater mass or velocity, the resultant mass C will have momentum in the previous direction in which car A was traveling.

In T-bone type crashes the directions of the momentum of car A and B are perpendicular. Therefore, in the momentum axis of car A, car B has 0 momentum, and, in the momentum axis of car B, car A has no momentum. The conglomerate C conserves momentum in both the A and B axes with the resultant direction as shown in Fig. 7-1 (B). As a consequence, the changes in momentum and force generated are far less than that of a head-on collision. Also, C continues to have a velocity and, as such, kinetic energy. This means that some of the initial kinetic energy was not converted to work, and less damage to the automobiles will occur. In general, the closer to a head-on collision the greater the change in momentum and, thus, the greater the force generated.

In rear-end collisions, Fig. 7-1 (C), the momentum of both cars is typically in the same direction. Therefore, the change in momentum and resultant forces generated are typically small as is the conversion of kinetic energy to work. These principles apply to all collisions whether they are a bullet penetrating a victim, a car hitting a pedestrian, or a driver impacting the windshield.

## PROPERTIES OF BIOMATERIALS

### Stress, Strain, Elasticity, and Young's Modulus

When a force is applied to a particular material it is typically referred to as a stress, which is a load or force per unit area. This stress will cause deformation of a given material. Strain is the distance of the deformation caused by the stress, divided by the length of the material to which the stress was applied.[7]

Strain can be tensile, shear, compressive, or overpressure (a relative of compressive strain) (Fig. 7-2). Tensile strain of a particular structure or organ occurs as opposing forces are applied to the same region. The forces are opposite and concentrated upon a particular point. This essentially interrupts the integrity of the structure by pulling it apart.

Shear strain occurs as opposing forces are applied to a particular structure, but at different points within that structure. This can be caused by an application of opposing external forces or can arise from a relative differential in the change of momentum within a single structure or between structures that are attached to one another.[8]

Compressive strain is the direct deformation that occurs as a result of impact. The energy involved with a particular force

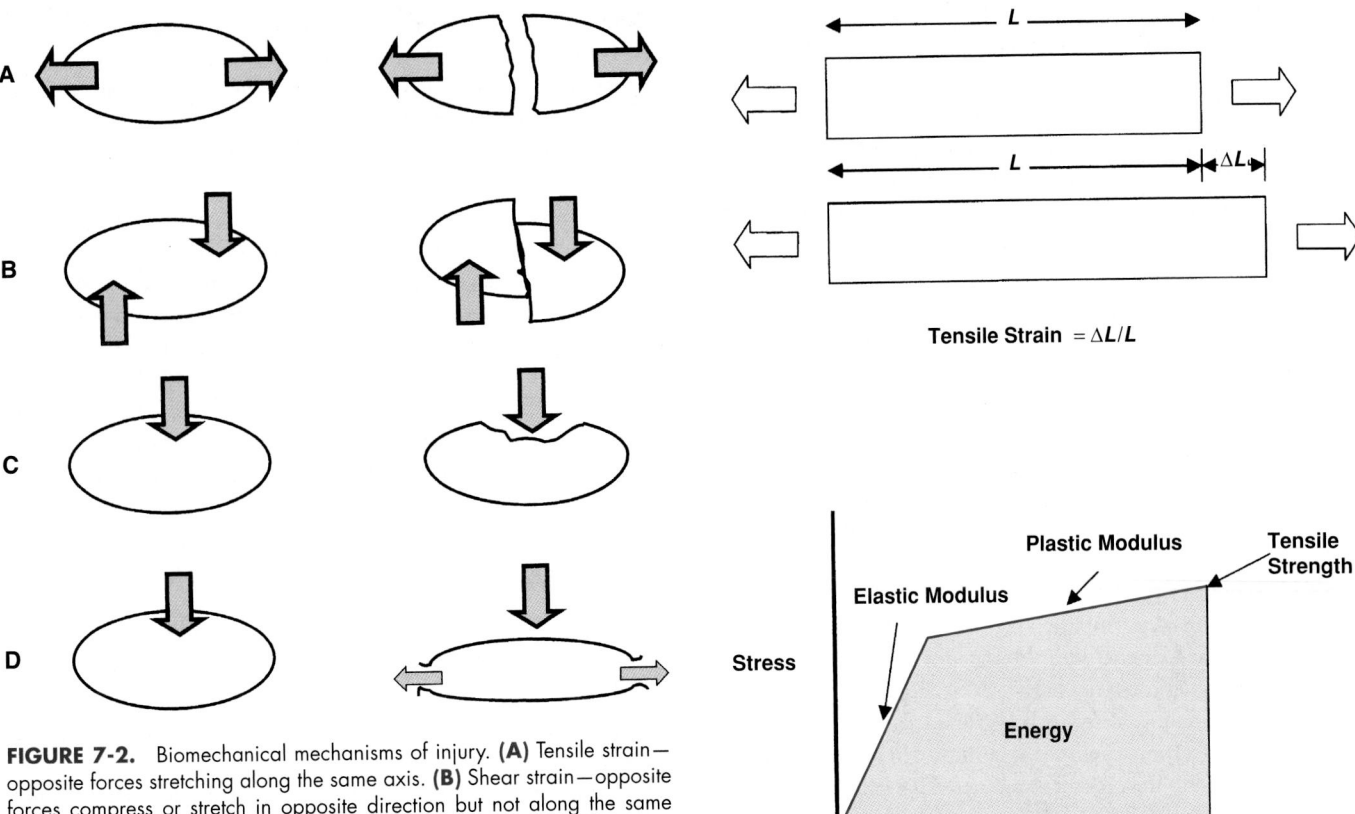

**FIGURE 7-2.** Biomechanical mechanisms of injury. **(A)** Tensile strain—opposite forces stretching along the same axis. **(B)** Shear strain—opposite forces compress or stretch in opposite direction but not along the same axis. **(C)** Compressive strain—stress applied to a structure usually causing simple deformation. **(D)** Overpressure—a compressive force increases the pressure within the viscus passing the "breaking point" of the wall.

**FIGURE 7-3.** The concept of stress, strain, elastic modulus, plastic modulus, tensile strength, and energy as demonstrated by a tensile stress applied to a given structure. The tensile strain is the change in length under a stress divided by the original length. This concept is applicable to compressive and shear strain. In the stress and strain relation the elastic modulus is the portion of the curve where permanent deformation does not occur as opposed to the plastic modulus where it does fracture or where tearing occurs at the tensile strength. The energy applied is the area under the curve.

does work on the structure causing a crushing-type injury resulting in deformation and interruption of the structural integrity of the injured organ. Overpressure is a type of compressive strain that is applied to a gas or fluid-filled cavity. The energy applied to a fluid- or gas-filled viscus can deform that structure and cause a decrease in the volume of the structure. Following Boyle's law

$$P_1 V_1 = P_2 V_2$$

The product of the pressure and the volume prior to an applied force must be equal to the product afterward.[4] Therefore, a decrease in its original volume will increase the pressure inside that viscus. If the rise in pressure, which is a force, overcomes the tensile strength of the viscus, it will rupture.[9]

When stress is plotted on the same graph as strain, there are several clear and distinct aspects to the curve. The elastic modulus is that part of the curve in which the force does not cause permanent deformation and a material is said to be more elastic if it restores itself more precisely to its original configuration.[10] The portion of the curve thereafter is called the plastic modulus and denotes when an applied stress will cause permanent deformation.[11] The tensile, compressive, or shear strength is the level of stress at which a fracture or tearing occurs.[12] This is also known as the "failure point." The area under the curve is the amount of energy that was applied to achieve the given stress and strain (Fig. 7-3).[13] In general, the higher the density of a particular tissue, the less elastic it is and the more energy is transferred to it in a collision. Lung tends not to absorb energy whereas the spleen, liver, or bone do.[14]

## PENETRATING TRAUMA AND BALLISTICS

One simple example of energy transfer is offered in the study of firearms and projectiles known as ballistics. Theodore Kocher first proposed that the kinetic energy possessed by the bullet was dissipated in four ways: namely, heat, energy used to move tissue radially outward, energy used to form a primary path by direct crush of the tissue, and energy expended in deforming the projectile.[15] Despite limited techniques for studying ballistics, Kocher was for the most part correct.

Our more extensive knowledge of the behavior of projectiles in a host comes from the observed performance of bullets in gelatin, which has properties similar to that of muscle and is thought to reflect the way in which energy is transferred through tissue. From such experiments several characteristics of a projectile piercing tissue have been described. These include: (a) penetration (the distance the projectile passes through tissue is reflected in the distance from the cut edge of the gelatin block to where the projectile comes to rest); (b) fragmentation (the pattern is assessed by biplaner x-rays and the degree reflected in the difference of the weight of the prefired projectile minus the weight of the collected fragments); (c) permanent cavity (the tissue disintegrated by direct contact with the missile and preserved in the gelatin); and (d) temporary cavity (the amount of "stretch" caused by the passing projectile). This is reflected by the distance from the edge of the permanent cavity to the outer perimeter of the cracks within the gelatin.[16]

The performance of the bullet and the injury sustained is reliant upon three factors: velocity, construction of the bullet, and composition of the target.[17] The prominent eighteenth-century surgeon John Hunter stated, "If the velocity of the ball is small, then the mischief is less in all, there is not so great a chance of being compounded with fractures of bones etc."[18] This astute observation reflects the exponential importance of velocity in determining the amount of kinetic energy that a particular projectile is capable of transmitting to a given target (kinetic energy $= \frac{1}{2} mv^2$). As such, high-velocity missiles will generally cause more tissue destruction than their lower velocity counterparts. The velocities and kinetic energies[19,20] of common handguns and rifles are listed in Table 7-1.

The amount of energy imparted (or work) to the tissue by a projectile is equal to the kinetic energy of the missile as it enters the tissue minus the kinetic energy as it leaves the tissue. Bullets are extremely aerodynamic, causing little disturbance while passing through the air. To some extent, this is similar in tissue (i.e., if the projectile moves with the point forward and passes in and out of the tissue, only a small portion of its kinetic energy will be transferred to the target). The characteristics of damage created along the track of a bullet are divided into two components, the temporary and the permanent cavities. The temporary cavity is the momentary stretch or movement of tissue away from the path of the bullet. This could be construed as an area of blunt trauma surrounding the tract of the projectile and the tissue involved corresponds to the elastic portion of Young's modulus. The temporary cavity increases in size with increasing velocity. The largest portion of the temporary cavity is on the surface where the velocity of the striking missile is the greatest.[20] The concept of the temporary cavity has been used to advocate excessive tissue debridement in high-velocity wounds. In truth,

postinjury observation of wound healing and animal experiments involving microscopic examination of tissue in the temporary cavity demonstrate that the momentary stretch produced does not usually cause cell death or tissue destruction.[21] As such, debridement of high-velocity injuries should be confined to obviously devitalized tissue.

The compressive stress of the projectile itself is what causes the permanent cavity, and the stress-strain relationship of the tissue involved is in the plastic portion or past the failure point of Young's modulus. Bullets can be constructed to alter their performance and increase the permanent cavity after they strike their target. This can be enhanced in four ways that all work by increasing the surface area of the projectile-tissue interface which facilitates the transfer of kinetic energy to the target. These include the following: (a) yaw, the deviation of the projectile in its longitudinal axis from the straight line of flight; (b) tumbling, the forward rotation around the center of mass; (c) deformation, a mushrooming of the projectile that increases the diameter of the projectile, usually by a factor of 2, increases the surface area, and, hence, the tissue contact area by four times; hollow point, soft nose, and dum-dum bullets all promote deformation; and (d) fragmentation, in which multiple projectiles can weaken the tissue in multiple places and enhance the damage rendered by cavitation. This usually occurs in high-velocity missiles. Nonfragmenting bullets will have a deeper penetration, whereas a fragmented projectile will not penetrate as deeply, but will affect a larger cross-sectional area.[22–24] If the bullet deforms, yaws, tumbles, or fragments, it will cause more tissue destruction. This occurs in deeper structures, not at the surface (Fig. 7-4).

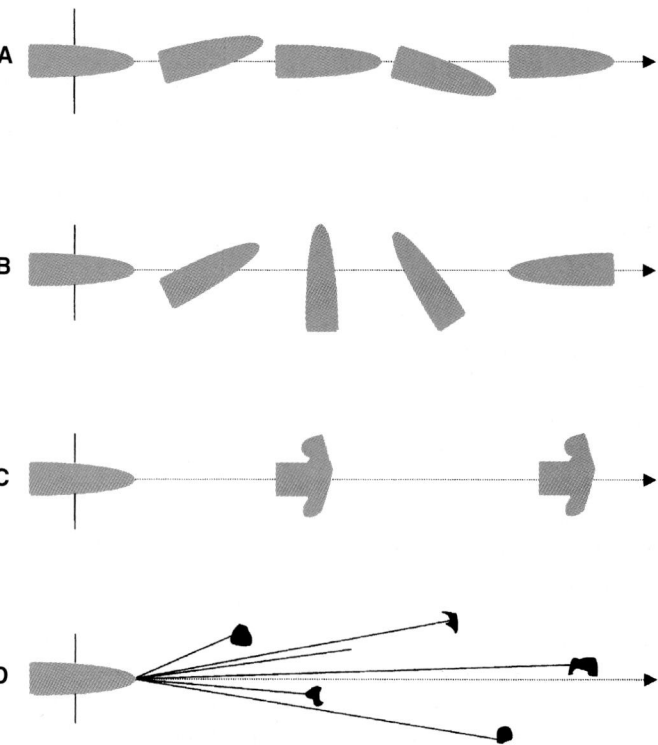

**FIGURE 7-4.** Yaw, tumble, deformation, and fragmentation. **(A)** Yaw describes deviation from flight path along the longitudinal axis. **(B)** Tumble is deviation in a "head over heels" manner. **(C)** Deformation occurs on impact and increases the actual surface area of the projectile. **(D)** Fragmentation involves the bullet scattering. All of these increase surface area of the projectile and tissue interface.

**TABLE 7-1**

| Velocity and Kinetic Energy Characteristics of Various Guns | | |
|---|---|---|
| **CALIBER** | **VELOCITY (ft/s)** | **MUZZLE ENERGY (ft-lb)** |
| Handguns | | |
| 0.25 in. | 810 | 73 |
| 0.32 in. | 745 | 140 |
| 0.357 in. | 1410 | 540 |
| 0.38 in. | 855 | 255 |
| 0.40 in. | 985 | 390 |
| 0.44 in. | 1470 | 1150 |
| 0.45 in. | 850 | 370 |
| 9 mm | 935 | 345 |
| 10 mm | 1340 | 425 |
| Long guns/military weapons | | |
| 0.243 Winchester | 3500 | 1725 |
| M-16 | 3650 | 1185 |
| 7.62 NATO | 2830 | 1535 |
| Uzi | 1500 | 440 |
| AK47 | 3770 | 1735 |

The characteristics of the tissue injured are also instrumental in determining the extent of the damage of the wound.[25] Tissue elasticity is a more significant determinant than is the energy transmitted to the tissue, when accounting for actual damage.[26] The actual destruction of the permanent cavity and stretch caused by the temporary cavity are better tolerated by more elastic tissues such as the lung as opposed to a more rigid tissue like bone. Wounds caused by knives are of very low energy and cause only a permanent cavity. With little energy transferred to the tissue, serious injury is caused by directly striking vital structures such as the heart, major vessels, lung, or abdominal organs.

## BLUNT TRAUMA MECHANISMS AND PATTERNS OF INJURY

The transfer of energy and application of forces in blunt trauma is frequently much more complex than that of penetrating trauma. The most frequent mechanisms of blunt trauma include motor vehicle crashes, motor vehicles striking pedestrians, and falls from a significant height. In these instances there are typically varying energies and forces in both the victim and the striking object. Other variables that complicate subsequent care include the larger surface area over which the energy is dispersed as compared to penetrating trauma and the multiple areas of contact that can disperse energy to different regions of the victim's body. The interactions and directions of these lines of force and energy dispersion are often instrumental in causing specific kinds of injury.

### Motor Vehicle Crashes

Although there are frequently confusing vectors for energy transfer and force in a victim of a motor vehicle crash, mortality is directly related to the total amount of energy and force available. This is demonstrated by the fact that mortality from motor vehicle crashes is accounted for in large part by head-on collisions with mortality rates up to 60%. Side impact collisions (20–35%) and rollovers (8–15%) have progressively lower mortality rates with rear-end collisions (3–5%) having the lowest.[27,28] Rollover crashes have a lower than expected mortality because the momentum is dissipated, and forces generated and projected to the passenger compartment are in a random pattern that frequently involves many different parts of the car. Although there are certain forces and patterns of energy exchange that occur in a motor vehicle crash, the vehicle itself does offer some degree of protection from the direct force generated by a collision. Patients who are ejected from their vehicle have the velocity of the vehicle as they are ejected and a significant momentum. They typically strike a relatively immobile object or the ground and undergo serious loads. Trauma victims who were ejected from the vehicle were four times more likely to require admission to an intensive care unit, had a five-fold increase in the average Injury Severity Score, were three times more likely to sustain a significant injury to the brain, and were five times more likely to expire secondary to their injuries.[29]

Understanding the changes in momentum, forces generated, and patterns of energy transfer between colliding vehicles is important. Yet, the behavior of the occupants of the passenger compartment in response to these is what helps identify specific patterns of injury. In frontal collisions the front of the vehicle decelerates as unrestrained front-seat passengers continue to move forward in keeping with Newton's first law. Lower extremity loads, particularly those to the feet and knees, occur early in the crash sequence, and are caused by the floorboard and dashboard that are still moving forward. Therefore, relative contact velocity and change in momentum are still low. Contact of the chest and head with the steering column and windshield occurs later in the crash sequence; therefore, contact velocities and deceleration, change in momentum, and contact force are higher.[27,30]

Types of injuries are dependent on the path the patient takes. The patient may slide down and under the steering wheel and dashboard. This may result in the knee first impacting the dashboard causing a posterior dislocation and subsequent injury to the popliteal artery. The next point of impact is the upper abdomen or chest. Compression and continued movement of solid organs results in lacerations to the liver or spleen. Compression of the chest can result in rib fractures, cardiac contusion, or pneumothorax from the lung being popped like a paper bag. Finally, the sudden stop can cause shear forces on the descending thoracic aorta resulting in a partial- or full-thickness tear. The other common path is for the occupant to launch up and over the steering wheel. The head then becomes the lead point and strikes the windshield with a starburst pattern resulting on the windshield. The brain can sustain direct contusion or can bounce within the skull causing brain shearing and contrecoup injury. Once the head stops, forces are transferred to the neck which may undergo hyperflexion, hyperextension, or compression injuries, depending on the angle of impact. Once the head and neck stop, the chest and abdomen strike the steering wheel with similar injuries to the down and under path.

Lateral collisions, specifically those that occur on the side of a seated passenger, can be devastating because of the small space between the striking car and the passenger. Therefore, resistance to slow momentum of the striking car prior to contact with the passenger is limited. If the side of the car provides minimal resistance the passenger can be exposed to the entire momentum change of the striking car. These loads are usually applied to the lateral chest, abdomen, and pelvis and, as such, injuries to the abdomen and thorax are more frequent in lateral collisions than in frontal collisions.[31] Injuries to the chest include rib fractures, flail chest, and pulmonary contusion. Lateral compression often causes injuries to the liver, spleen, and kidneys, as well. Finally, the femoral head can be driven through the acetabulum.

Rear-end collisions are classically associated with cervical whiplash-type injury and are a good example of Newton's first law at work. When the victim's car is struck from behind, the body, buttressed by the seat, undergoes a forward acceleration and change in momentum that the head does not. The inertia of the head tends to hold it in a resting position. The forward pull of the trunk causes a backward movement on the head causing hyperextension of the neck. Similarly, this injury pattern can also be seen in head-on collisions where a sudden deceleration of the trunk with a continued forward movement of the head is followed by a backward rotation resulting from recoil.[32,33]

### Pedestrian Injuries

Pedestrian injuries frequently follow a well-described pattern of injury depending on the size of the vehicle and the victim. Nearly 80% of adults struck by a car will have injuries to the lower extremities. This is intuitively obvious in that the level of a car's bumper is at the height of the patient's knee. This is the first contact point in this collision sequence, with the largest force being applied to the lower extremity. Those struck by a truck or other vehicle with a higher center of mass more frequently have serious injury to the chest and abdomen, since the initial force is applied to those regions. In the car-pedestrian interaction, the force, applied to the knee region, causes an acceleration of the lower portion of the body that is not shared by the trunk and head, which, by Newton's first law, tend to stay at rest. As the lower extremities are pushed forward they will act as a fulcrum bringing the trunk and head forcefully down on the hood of the car applying a secondary force to those regions, respectively. The typical injury pattern in this scenario is a tibia and fibula fracture, injury to the trunk such as rib fractures or rupture of the spleen, and injury to the brain.[34,35]

## Falls

Falls from height can result in a large amount of force transmitted to the victim. The energy absorbed by the victim at impact will be the kinetic energy at landing. This is related to the height from which the victim fell. The basic physics formula describing the conservation of energy in a falling body states that the product of mass, gravitational acceleration, and height, the potential energy prior to the fall, equals the kinetic energy as the object strikes the ground. With mass and gravitational acceleration being a constant for the falling body, velocity, and, therefore, momentum and kinetic energy are directly related to height.[4] The greater the change in momentum upon impact the larger the load or force applied to the victim. Injury patterns will vary depending upon which portion of the victim strikes the ground first and, hence, how the load is distributed.

The typical patient with injuries sustained in a free-fall has a mean fall height of just under 20 ft. One prospective study of injury patterns summarized the effects of falls from heights ranging between 5 and 70 ft. Fractures accounted for 76.2% of all injuries, with 19 to 22% sustaining spinal fractures and 3.7% showing a neurologic deficit.[36] Nearly 6% of patients had intra-abdominal injuries, with the majority requiring operative management for injury to a solid organ. Bowel and bladder perforation were observed in less than 1% of injuries.[37]

## ANATOMIC CONSIDERATIONS

### Injury to the Head (Brain and Maxillofacial Injury)

The majority of closed-head injuries are caused by motor vehicle collisions, with an incidence of approximately 1.14 million cases each year in the United States.[38,39] The severity of traumatic brain injury represents the single most important factor contributing to death and disability after trauma and may contribute independently to mortality when coexistent with extra-cranial injury.[33,40,41] Our knowledge of the biomechanics of injury to the brain comes from a combination of experiments conducted with porcine head models, bi-planer high-speed x-ray systems, and computer-driven finite element models.[42]

There are a multitude of mechanisms that occur under the broad heading of traumatic brain injury. They are all a consequence of loads applied to the head resulting in differing deceleration forces between components of the brain. Brain contusion can result from impact and the direct compressive strain associated with it. The indirect component of injury to the brain on the side opposite to that of impact is known as the *contrecoup* injury. This occurs because the brain is only loosely connected to the surrounding cranium. As a result, after a load is applied to the head causing a compressive strain at the point of impact and setting the skull in motion along the line of force, the motion of the brain lags behind the skull. As the skull comes to rest, or even recoils, the brain, still moving along the line of the initial load, will strike the calvarium on the opposite side and another compressive strain is generated. The existence of the coup-contrecoup injury mechanism is supported by clinical observation and has been confirmed by a three-dimensional finite element head model and pressure-testing data in cadavers.[43] It is even suspected that this forward acceleration of the brain relative to the skull may set up a tensile strain in the bridging veins causing their laceration and formation of a subdural hematoma.[44]

Injury to the superficial regions of the brain is explained by these linear principles; however, injury to the deep structures of the brain, such as diffuse axonal injury (DAI), is more complicated. Several authors have tried to explain DAI as a result of shear strain between different parts of the brain, but there is also another model known as the stereotactic phenomena. This model relies more on wave propagation and utilizes the concavity of the skull as a "collector," which focuses multiple wave fronts to a focal point deep within the brain, causing disruption of tissue even in the face of minimal injury at the surface of the brain.[45] This "wave propagation" through deeper structures within the brain, such as the reticular-activating system, with subsequent disruption of their structural integrity is thought to account for a loss of consciousness, the most frequent serious sign after blunt trauma to the brain.[46] An injury caused by shear strain is the laceration or contusion of the brainstem. This is explained by opposing forces applied to the brain and the spinal cord perpendicular to their line of orientation, with the spinal cord and brainstem being relatively fixed in relation to the mobile brain.

Maxillofacial injuries are associated with injuries to the head and brain in terms of mechanism and are a common presentation in motor vehicle trauma. The classic force vector that results in mid-face fractures is similar to that of traumatic brain injury and occurs when a motor vehicle occupant impacts the steering wheel, dashboard, or windshield. Nearly all of these subtypes of injury are secondary to compressive strain. This mechanism is associated with the greatest morbidity for the driver and front-seat passenger, while the forces are attenuated for the back-seat passenger impacting the more compliant front seat.

### Thoracic Injury

The primary mechanism of blunt trauma to the chest wall involves inward displacement of the body wall with impact. Musculoskeletal injury in the chest is dependent upon both the magnitude and rate of the deformation of the chest wall and is usually secondary to compressive strain from the applied load. Patterns of injury for the internal organs of the thorax frequently reflect the interactions between organs that are fixed and those that are relatively mobile and compressible. This arrangement allows for differentials in momentum between adjacent structures that lead to compressive, tensile, and shear stress.

The sternum is deformed and rib cage compressed with a blunt force to the chest. Depending on the force and rate of impact in a collision, ribs may fracture from compressive strain applied to their outer surface and consequent tensile strain on the inner aspects of the rib. Indirect fractures may occur due to stress concentration at the lateral and posterolateral angles of the rib. Furthermore, stress waves may propagate deeper into the chest resulting in small, rapid distortions or shear forces in an organ with significant pressure differential across its parenchymal surface (i.e., the air and tissue interface of the lung). This is thought to be the mechanism causing a pulmonary contusion.

Blunt intrusion into the hemithorax and pliable lung could also result in overpressure and cause a pneumothorax. A direct load applied to the chest compresses the lung and increases the pressure within this air-filled structure beyond the failure point of the alveoli and visceral pleura. This overpressure mechanism may also be seen with fluid (blood) instead of air in a blunt cardiac rupture. High-speed cine-radiography in an anterior blunt chest trauma model using a pig has demonstrated that the heart can be compressed to half of its precrash diameter with a doubling of the pressure within the cardiac chambers.[47] If the failure point is reached, rupture occurs with disastrous results.

There are several examples of indirect injury secondary to asynchronous motion of adjacent, connected structures and development of shear stress at sites of attachment.[48] Mediastinal vascular injury and bronchial injury are examples of this mechanism. Transaction of the thoracic aorta is a classic deceleration injury mediated by shear forces. This injury can occur in frontal or lateral impacts[49] and occurs because of the continued motion of the mobile and compressible heart in relation to an aorta that is tethered to more fixed structures. In frontal and lateral impacts the heart moves in a horizontal motion, relative to an aorta that is fixed to the spinal column by ligamentous attachments. This causes a shear force applied at the level of the ligamentum arteriosum. When the stress is applied in a vertical direction, such as a fall from a height in which the victim lands on the lower extremities, the relative discrepancy in momentum is in that plane and a tensile strain is generated at the root of the thoracic aorta (Fig. 7-5). Injury to a

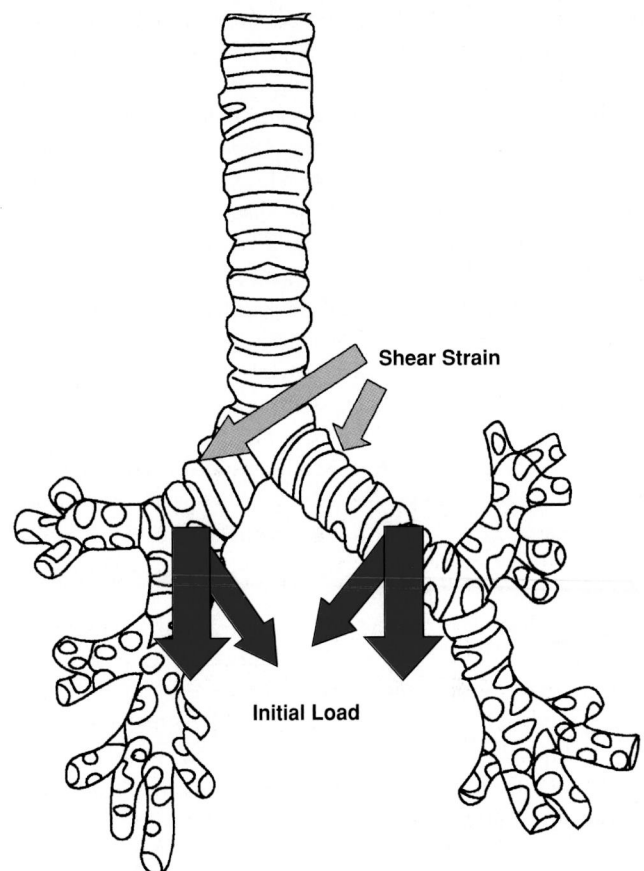

**FIGURE 7-6.** Mechanisms of injury for bronchial injury. The carina is tethered to the mediastinum and spinal complex while the lungs are extremely mobile, setting up shear strain in the mainstem bronchus upon horizontal or vertical deceleration.

major bronchus is another example of this mechanism. The relatively pliable and mobile lung generates a differential in momentum in a horizontal or vertical plane depending on the applied load as compared to the tethered trachea and carina. This creates a shear force at the level of the mainstem bronchus (Fig. 7-6) and explains why the majority of blunt bronchial injuries occur within 2 cm of the carina.

## Abdominal Injury

Abdominal organs are more vulnerable than those of the thorax because of the lack of protection by the sternum and ribs. A number of different mechanisms account for the spectrum of injury observed in blunt trauma to the abdomen. With regard to the solid abdominal organs, a direct compressive force, with parenchymal destruction, probably accounts for most observed injuries to the liver, spleen, and kidney. Yet, shear strain can also contribute to laceration of these organs. As with the previous description of strain forces, a point of attachment is required to exacerbate a differential in movement. This can occur at the splenic hilum resulting in vascular disruption at the pedicle or at the ligamentous attachments to the kidney and diaphragm. Shear forces in the liver revolve upon the attachments of the falciform ligament anteriorly and the hepatic veins posteriorly, explaining injuries to the parenchyma in these areas. Another significant injury related to this mechanism is that of injury to the renal artery. The renal artery is

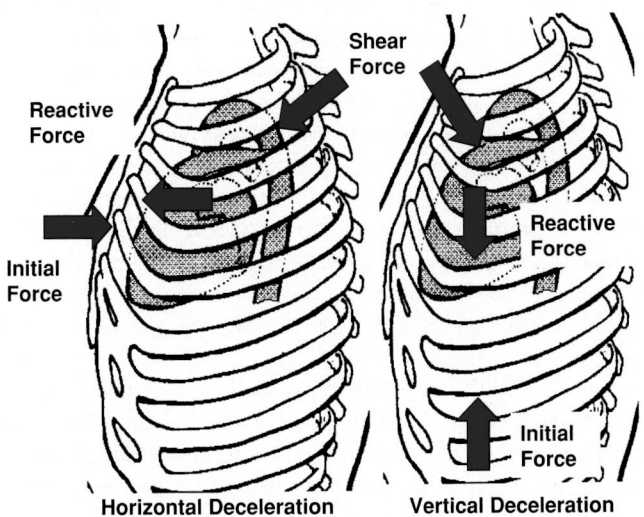

**FIGURE 7-5.** Various mechanisms for injury to the thoracic aorta. In a horizontal deceleration the heart and arch move horizontally away from the descending aorta causing shear strain and tearing at the ligamentum arteriosum. A vertical deceleration causes caudad movement of the heart, causing a strain at the root of the aorta.

attached proximally to the abdominal aorta, which is fairly immobile secondary to its attachments to the spinal column, and distally to the kidney, which has more mobility. A discrepancy in momentum between the two will exact a shear stain on the renal artery resulting in disruption.[50] This same relation to the spinal column occurs with the pancreas (Fig. 7-7). The relatively immobile spine and freely mobile pancreatic tail predispose to a differential in momentum between the two in a deceleration situation leading to fracture in the neck or body of the pancreas. The biomechanics of such injuries suggest that the body's tolerance to such forces decreases with a higher speed of impact, resulting in an injury of greater magnitude from a higher velocity collision.[13] Perforation of a hollow viscus in blunt trauma occurs in approximately 3% of victims.[51] The exact cause is a matter of debate. Some believe that it is related to compressive forces, which cause an effective "blowout" through generation of significant overpressure, while others believe that it is secondary to shear strains. Both explanations are plausible, and clinical observations have supported the respective conclusions. Most injuries to the small bowel occur within 30 cm of the ligament of Treitz or the ileocecal valve, which supports the shear force theory[52] (Fig. 7-7). Yet, injuries do occur away from these points of fixation. Also, experiments have documented that a "pseudo-obstruction" or temporarily closed loop under a load can develop bursting pressures as described by the overpressure theory.[53] Most likely, both proposed mechanisms are applicable in individual instances. The most common example of the pseudo-obstruction type is blunt rupture of the duodenum, where the pylorus and its retroperitoneal location can prevent adequate escape of gas and resultant high pressures that overcome wall strength.

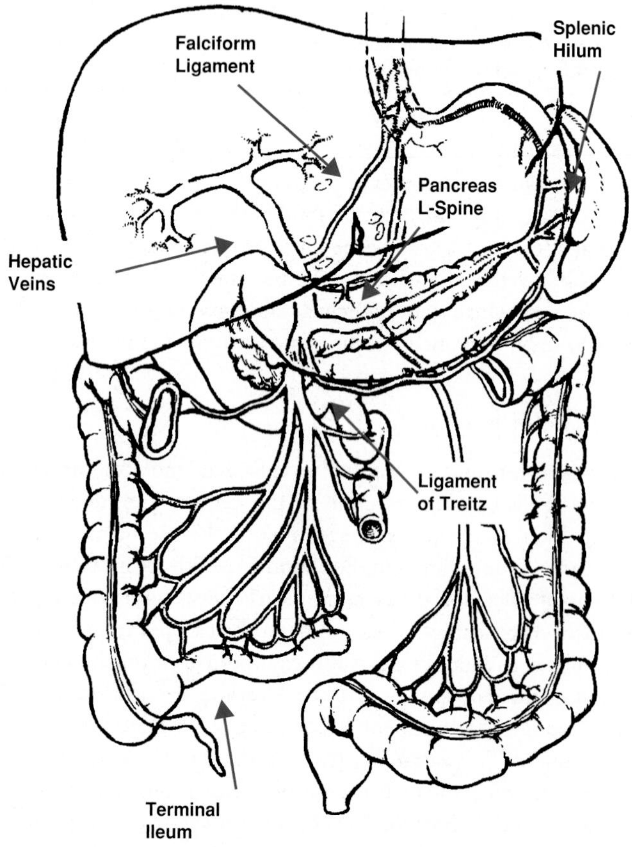

Another important example of overpressure is rupture of the diaphragm. The peritoneal cavity is also subject to Boyle's law. A large blunt force, such as that related to impact with the steering wheel applied to the anterior abdominal wall will cause a temporary deformation and decrease in the volume of the peritoneal cavity. This will subsequently raise intra-abdominal pressure. The weakest point of the cavity is the diaphragm with the left side being the preferred route of pressure release as the liver absorbs pressure and protects the right hemidiaphragm. The relative deformability of the lung on the other side of the diaphragm facilitates this.

## Musculoskeletal Injury

By far, the most common type of blunt injury in industrialized nations is to the musculoskeletal system. The ratio of orthopedic operations to general surgical, thoracic, and neurosurgical operations is nearly 5:1. As stated earlier, seatbelts and air bags have significantly decreased the incidence of major intracranial and abdominal injuries; however, they have not decreased the incidence of musculoskeletal trauma. While these are not usually fatal injuries, they often require operative repair and rehabilitation and can leave a significant proportion of patients with permanent disability.[54] With the advent of seatbelt laws, improved restraint systems, and air bags in motor vehicles, the incidence of lower extremity trauma, in particular, has increased. It is thought that these patients in the past may have suffered fatal injuries to the brain or torso and, therefore, their associated fractures of the femur, tibia, and fibula were not included in the overall list of injuries.

The type and extent of injury is determined by the momentum and kinetic energy associated with impact, underlying tissue characteristics, and angle of stress of the extremity. High-energy injuries can involve extensive loss of soft-tissue, associated neurovascular compromise, and highly comminuted fracture patterns. Low-energy injuries are often associated with crush or avulsion of soft tissue in association with simple fractures. Injuries to soft tissue are usually secondary to compressive strain with crush injury as an example. Tensile and shear strain mechanisms, however, are present with degloving and avulsion injuries, respectively.

Most of that written about musculoskeletal injury involves fractures of long bones. Although each fracture is probably a consequence of multiple stresses and strains, there are four basic biomechanisms (Fig. 7-8). In a lateral load applied to the mid shaft of a long bone, bowing will occur and compressive strain occurs in the cortex of the bone where the load is applied. The cortex on the opposite side of the bone will undergo tensile strain as the bone bows away from the load. Initially, small fractures will occur in the cortex undergoing tensile strain because bone is weaker under tension than it is under compression.[55] Once the failure point is reached on the far side from the load, the compressive strain increases markedly and the failure point for the side near the applied load is reached, also, resulting in a complete fracture. This mechanism can be seen in passengers in lateral collisions, pedestrians struck by a passenger car in the tibia and fibula region, or in the upper extremities from direct applied force such as assault with a blunt instrument.

**FIGURE 7-7.** Points of shear strain in blunt abdominal trauma. All of these points occur where a relatively fixed structure is adjacent to a mobile structure.

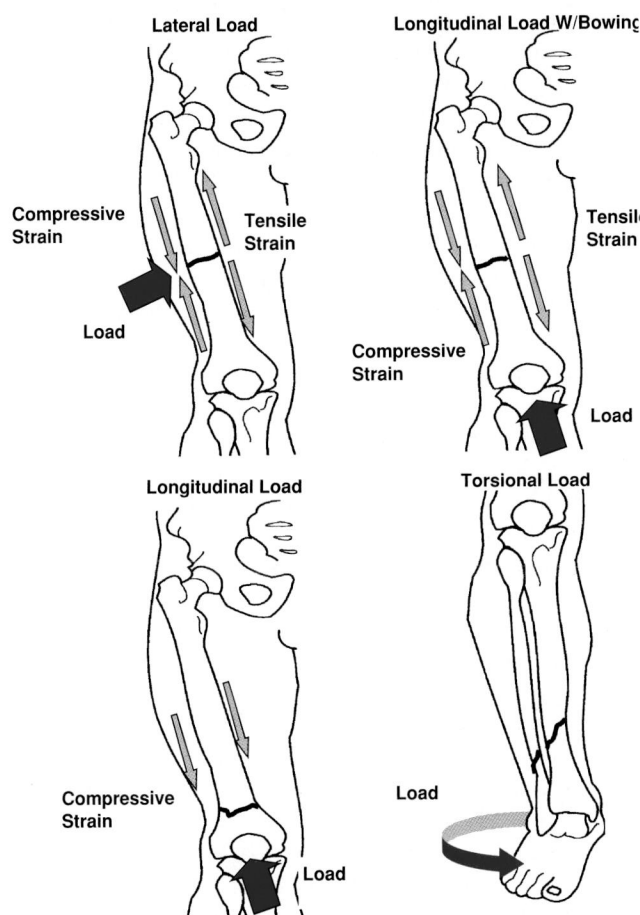

Lateral Load

Longitudinal Load W/Bowing

Compressive Strain

Tensile Strain

Load

Tensile Strain

Compressive Strain

Load

Longitudinal Load

Torsional Load

Compressive Strain

Load

Load

Load

**FIGURE 7-8.** Fracture mechanics. A lateral load causing "bowing" will create tensile strain in the cortex opposite the force and compressive strain in the adjacent cortex. If a longitudinal stress caused bowing, a similar strain pattern occurs. If no bowing occurs the strain is all compressive. A torsion load will cause a spiral fracture.

When a longitudinal load is placed on a long bone, bowing can also occur, and the compressive and tensile strain patterns will be similar to that previously described. If bowing does not occur, then only a compressive strain is seen and a compression fracture can occur. In the case of the femur this usually occurs distally with the shaft being driven into the condyles. These mechanisms can be seen in falls from a height but are more frequently seen in head-on collisions resulting in fractures of the femur or tibia. In these cases deceleration occurs and the driver's or passenger's feet receive a load from the floorboard or the knee receives a load from the dashboard upon deceleration. This causes a longitudinal force to be applied to the tibia or femur, respectively. A torsional load will cause the bone to fracture in a spiral pattern.

## Injury to the Spine and Whiplash

Injury to the vertebral column and spinal cord can be devastating and is frequently the result of a complex combination of specific anatomic features and transmitted forces. These can cause a wide variety of injury patterns distributed through the different portions of the spinal column. Deceleration forces in motor vehicle crashes, such as impact with the windshield, steering assembly, and instrument panel, inertial differences in the head and torso, or ejection

are responsible for both flexion and hyperextension injuries. While the biomechanics of transmission of force can be readily demonstrated for the spinal column's individual components (disks, vertebrae, etc.), a model demonstrating injury patterns in the intact spinal unit is lacking.[56]

The cervical spine is most frequently injured in motor vehicle crashes, due to its relatively unprotected position compared to the thoracic and lumbar regions. Injuries are related to flexion, extension, or lateral rotation, along with tension or compression forces generated during impact of the head. The direction and degree of loading with impact account for the different injury patterns in trauma to the cervical spine.[13] Approximately 65% of injury is related to flexion-compression, about 30% to extension-compression, and 10% to extension-tension injuries.[57] Fracture-dislocation of the vertebrae is related to flexion and extension mechanisms, while fracture of the facets is related to lateral-bending mechanisms. In contrast to trauma to the cervical spine, injury to the thoracic or lumbar spine is more likely related to compressive mechanisms. The rib cage and sternum likely provide stabilizing forces in motor vehicle crashes and lessen the risk of injury in these regions.

*Whiplash* refers to a pattern of injury seen often in motor vehicle collisions with a rear-end impact. The injury is usually a musculo-ligamentous sprain, but may be combined with injury to cervical nerve roots or the spinal cord. Patients typically experience neck pain and muscle spasm, although an additional spectrum of symptoms has been described.[58] The etiology of whiplash probably relates to acceleration and extension injury, with some rotational component in non-rear-impact crashes.

## Kinematics in Prevention

The ideas of William Haddon have become the cornerstone of injury prevention, and approximately a third of his strategies involve altering the interaction of the host and the environment.[59] Understanding forces and patterns of energy transfer have allowed the development of devices to reduce injury. Most of this understanding has been applied to the field of automotive safety.

The first set of design features revolve around the concept of decreasing the force transmitted to the passenger compartment. This includes the "crumple zone," which allows the front and rear ends of a car to collapse upon impact. The change in momentum the passenger compartment undergoes in a collision will, therefore, occur over a longer period. Going back to the impulse and momentum relation, this means less force will be transmitted to the passenger compartment. In terms of energy, work is done in the crumple zone and energy is expended before reaching the passenger compartment.[60] The second design feature directs the engine and transmission downward and not into the passenger compartment decreasing intrusion into the passenger compartment.

Passenger restraint systems, which include safety harnesses and child car seats, keep the passengers' velocity equal to that of the car and prevent the passengers from generating a differential in momentum and striking the interior of the car. They also more evenly distribute loads applied to the victim across a greater surface area thereby decreasing stress.

Even with restraint systems the occupants of a car can develop relative momentum and kinetic energy during a crash. This energy and momentum can be dissipated by air bags, which convert it into the work of compressing the gas within the device. The helmets used by cyclists and bicyclists work on a similar principle in that a compliant helmet absorbs some of the energy of impact, which is therefore not transmitted to the brain.

Many studies have demonstrated the benefits of using seatbelts and air bags with mortality reductions ranging from 41–72% for seatbelts, 63% for air bags, 80% for both, and 69% for child safety seats.[61] Seatbelts and air bags have also significantly reduced the incidence of injuries to the cervical spine, brain, and maxillofacial region by keeping the forward momentum of the passenger to a minimum and preventing the head from striking the windshield.[42] Also worth mentioning is the head-rest which has decreased whiplash-type injury by 70% by preventing a difference in momentum between the head and body and hyperextension of the neck in rear-end collisions.[62]

Despite their effectiveness, air bags can be responsible for injury in motor vehicle crashes. Approximately 100 air bag related deaths were confirmed by the National Highway Traffic Safety Administration (NHTSA) over a five-year period, many associated with improper restraint of small adults or children in front seat locations. Additionally, a spectrum of minor injuries such as corneal abrasion and facial lacerations can be seen in a low speed impact. Also of note are several injuries that can occur from the use of safety belts. Lap seatbelts can cause compressive injuries such as rupture of the bowel, pelvic fractures, and mesenteric tears and avulsions. They can also act as a fulcrum for the upper portion of the trunk and be associated with hyperflexion injuries such as compression fractures of the lumbar spine. As a consequence, newer automobiles are required to have the more extensive and protective lap and shoulder harness style belts. Even still, shoulder harnesses can cause intimal tears or thrombosis of the great vessels of the neck and thorax and fracture and dislocation of the cervical spine in instances of submarining, where the victim slides down under the restraint system.[63] Even when a shoulder harness system works as intended, clavicular and rib fractures or perforations of hollow viscera in the abdomen secondary to a compressive-type mechanism can occur.[64,65]

## Special Considerations

Pediatrics.    Differences have been noted between adults and children in both patterns of injury and physiologic response to injury. In one analysis of adults and children sustaining comparable degrees of injury from blunt trauma, significant differences were noted in the incidence of thoracic, spinal, and pelvic injuries in children. While the overall incidence of injury to the brain is higher in blunt pediatric trauma, thoracic and pelvic injuries occur less frequently.[66] Overall mortality is generally higher for adults than it is for children sustaining comparable degrees of injury. When assessed by mechanism, however, mortality is slightly higher for children in motor vehicle crashes.[67]

The most significant difference between adults and children is in the compliance of the bony structures. This difference is seen commonly in the resilience of the chest wall. The incidence of rib fractures, flail chest, hemo-pneumothorax, and injury to the thoracic aorta in children is significantly less than that in adults, though the incidence of pulmonary contusion is higher. Because of this resilience, the chest wall can absorb a greater impact in children while demonstrating less external sign of injury. In children the index of suspicion for a pulmonary contusion, in the absence of rib fractures, must be higher than in an adult.

Injury to the spinal cord is rare in children, representing only 1 to 2% of all pediatric trauma. The cervical spine is injured in the majority of cases (60 to 80%), compared to 30 to 40% in adult injury. The immature spinal column has incomplete ossification, a unique vertebral configuration, and ligamentous laxity, which accounts for this difference in pattern of injury. The proportionally larger head and less developed neck musculature of younger children (<10 years old) account for more torque and acceleration stress in the higher cervical spine during injury as well. Young children have high rates of dislocations and spinal cord injury without radiographic abnormality (SCIWORA), and these are more likely to be seen at the upper cervical levels. Since older children have a low fulcrum of cervical motion (C5–C6) and more ossification and maturity of the vertebral bodies and interspinous ligaments, they have a high incidence of fractures in the lower cervical spine.[68] SCIWORA is associated with 15 to 25% of all injuries to the cervical spine in pediatrics and represents a transient vertebral displacement and realignment during injury, resulting in damage to the spinal cord without injury to the vertebral column.

Nothing has reduced the incidence of injury to children and infants more than the mandatory use of safety belts and restraints. The problem still to be faced is the different contours and shapes with infant restraints. Also, there has been increased interest in the issue of pediatric restraint systems because of a number of injuries related to air bags. It is recommended that restrained infants and children not be placed in a front seat and that all children under age 12 ride in the rear seat. Injuries related to air bags have ranged from minor orthopedic trauma to fatal injury to the brain.[69]

Unfortunately, child abuse is a reality in the pediatric population and must be considered when evaluating a child who has been injured in less than clear circumstances or if a pediatric patient has multiple injuries of varying age. Although injury to soft tissue is the most common presentation, fractures follow as a close second. There is a high rate of spiral fractures of the humerus and femur secondary to a torsional force, applied by an adult grabbing the child's extremity in a twisting motion. Injury to the brain is the third most common injury, with skull fractures thought to be secondary to direct blows to the child's head or the dropping and throwing of the child. Intracranial hemorrhage has been noted in the "shaken impact syndrome" and is thought to result from significant acceleration and deceleration forces followed by direct force transfer with impact. Subdural and subarachnoid hemorrhages can often result, as blood vessels between the brain and skull are ruptured. Retinal hemorrhage may also be identified in this pattern of injury and occurs in approximately 3% of cases. Impact injury to the abdomen is common in such cases of child abuse and can result in injury to solid organs (liver, spleen, or kidney), duodenal hematoma (sometimes with delayed symptoms of intestinal obstruction), pancreatitis, injury to the colon or rectum, or mesenteric bleeding. In addition, falls from even very small heights may cause severe intracranial hemorrhage in the infant or child.[70]

## Pregnancy

Injury to pregnant women in motor vehicle crashes is estimated to account for 1500 to 5000 fetal deaths each year. There has been little investigation into specific forces and the kinematics of injury in pregnancy. Several studies have demonstrated that the most common cause of fetal demise in motor vehicle crashes with a viable mother is placental abruption. The biomechanics of this injury involves generation of tensile and shear forces, with the circumferential forces in the uterine wall inducing a shear strain across the placental surface, resulting in placental strain and subsequent abruption. Shorter women have a higher incidence of fetal demise with automotive crashes because of their close proximity to the steering wheel. As in other populations, restraints have been demonstrated to increase survival in both mother and fetus.[71]

## Geriatrics

Trauma remains a disease of the young, though there is a significant incidence of morbidity and mortality in the elderly population. Death from trauma represents the fifth leading cause of mortality in persons over 65 years of age. The most common mechanisms of injury in the elderly are falls, fires, and vehicular trauma.

When patients with similar injury levels are compared with respect to age and mortality, the incidence of fatality in older persons is five- to ten-fold higher than it is in the younger population. It is not the severity of injury that is crucial, but rather the incidence of comorbid factors in this population, especially cardiac and vascular disease. Most likely it is the patient's inability to demonstrate a cardiovascular reserve that is a contributing factor to their subsequent increased morbidity and mortality. The Injury Severity Score and other predictors of outcome do not hold up at the extremes of age, either geriatric or pediatric. Another significant finding in this population is that most (as many as 88%) of these patients never return to their previous level of independence.[72]

The incidence of falls in the geriatric population is high, with an annual incidence of approximately 30% in those over 65, and approximately 50% in those over 80 years of age. Falls account for approximately half the cases of geriatric trauma. Most falls in the elderly occur from standing with mortality secondary to the comorbid factors mentioned earlier.[73] The propensity for fracture is also increased secondary to a loss of bone density with aging, with hip fractures being one of the most common injuries.

## BLAST INJURY

Explosions are physical, chemical, or nuclear reactions involving a large, rapid release of energy. Primary blast injuries are those that result from the interaction of the initial blast wave with the body and represent a combination of stress and shear waves. The propagation of stress waves with high local forces along tissue planes with different physical properties leads to injury exemplified by blast lung. This consists of disruption of inter-alveolar septa, with hemorrhage and laceration of affected parenchyma. Tearing of the visceral pleura can result in pneumothorax or hemopneumothorax. Shear waves are also generated in primary blast injury, with similar propagation resulting in tearing of structures from their attachments and shearing of solid organs. Injuries to the mesentery and bowel reflect the propagation of these types of forces through the abdominal cavity.

Secondary blast injury refers to projectiles energized by the explosion and can result in penetrating or nonpenetrating impact-type wounds. Tertiary injury describes displacement of the body by externally applied blast forces. This results in traumatic amputations and crush injuries, as would occur with structural collapse. Quaternary blast injury refers to other mechanisms, such as flash burns, inhalation, and metabolic derangements from radiant, heat, and chemical forces generated during the explosion.[74,75]

## REFERENCES

1. *The American Heritage Dictionary of the English Language*, 4th ed. Houghton: Mifflin, 2000.
2. Dennis JT: The complete idiot's guide to physics. New York, NY: Alpha Books, 2006.
3. Newton I: *Philosophiae Naturalis Principia Mathematica*. Motte A, trans. 1729. Reprint. New York: Prometheus Books, 1995.
4. Cutnell J, Johnson K: *Physics*, 4th ed. New York, NY: Wiley, 1997.
5. Sears FW, Zemansky MW: *University Physics*. Reading, Mass: Addison-Wesley, 1949, p. 117.
6. Reif F: *Statistical Physics*. New York, NY: McGraw-Hill, 1967.
7. Weast RC: *CRC Handbook of Chemistry and Physics*. Boca Raton, FL: CRC Press, 1986.
8. Viano DC, King AI, Melvin JW, et al.: Injury biomechanics research: An essential element in the prevention of trauma. *Brit J Surg* 22:403, 1989.
9. McSwain N: *Kinematics of trauma*. In Mattox KL, Moore EE, Feliciano DV, eds. Trauma, 4th ed, New York: McGraw-Hill, 1996.
10. Halliday D, Resnick RE: *Fundamentals of Physics*, 3rd ed. New York: Wiley, 1988.
11. Hoadley BR: *Understanding Wood. A Craftsman's Guide To Wood Technology*. Newton, CT: The Taunton Press Inc., 1980, p. 107.
12. Pugh J, Dee R: *Properties Of Musculoskeletal Tissues And Biomaterials*. In Dee R, Mango E, Hurst LC, eds: Principles of Orthopaedic Practice. New York: McGraw-Hill, 1988, p. 134.
13. Frankel VH, Burstein AH: *Orthopaedic Biomechanics*. Philadelphia: Lea & Febinger, 1970.
14. Ryan JM, Rich NM, Dale RF, et al.: *Ballistic Trauma: Clinical Relevance in Peace And War*. New York, NY: Oxford University Press, 1997.
15. Fackler ML, Dougherty PJ: Theodor Kocher and the scientific foundation of wound ballistics. *Surg Gyn Obstet* 172:153, 1991.
16. Fackler ML, Malinowski JA: The wound profile: A visual method for qualifying gunshot wound components. *J Trauma* 25:522, 1985.
17. Williams M: *Practical Handgun Ballistics*. Springfield, IL: Charles C Thomas, 1980.
18. Hunter J: *A Treatise on the Blood, Inflammation and Gunshot Wounds*. John Richardson, London, 1794. Published posthumously by E. Home.
19. McSwain NE: *Ballistics*. In Ivatury RR, Cayten CG, eds. The Textbook of Penetrating Trauma. Media, Pennsylvania: Williams & Wilkins, 1996, p. 105.
20. Fackler ML, Bellamy RF, Malinkowski JA: Wounding mechanism of projectiles striking at more than 1.5 km/sec. *J Trauma* 26:250, 1986.
21. Fackler ML: Wound ballistics: A review of common misconceptions. *JAMA* 259:2730, 1988.
22. Fackler ML, Surinchak JS, Malinowski JA, et al.: Bullet fragmentation: A major cause of tissue disruption. *J Trauma* 24:35, 1984.
23. Swan KG, Swan RC: *Gunshot Wounds: Pathophysiology and Management*. Littleton, Massachusetts: PSG Publishing, 1980.
24. Fackler ML, Bellamy RF, Malinowski JA: A reconsideration of the wounding mechanism of very high velocity projectiles—Importance of projectile shape. *J Trauma* 28:S637, 1988.
25. Lindsey D: The idolatry of velocity, or lies, damn lies and ballistics. *J Trauma* 20:1068, 1980.
26. Fackler ML, Surinchak JS, Malinowski JA, et al.: Wounding potential of the Russian AK-47 assault rifle. *J Trauma* 24:263, 1984.
27. Mackay M: Mechanisms of injury and biomechanics: Vehicle design and crash performance. *World J Surg* 16:420, 1992.
28. Gikas PW: Mechanisms of injury in automobile crashes. *Clin Neurosurg* 19:175, 1972.
29. Gongora E, Acosta JA, Wang DSY, et al.: Analysis of motor vehicle ejection victims admitted to Level I trauma center. *J Trauma* 51:854, 2001.
30. Daffner RH, Ziad LD, Lupetin AR, et al.: Patterns of high-speed impact injuries in motor vehicle occupants. *J Trauma* 28:408, 1988.
31. Dischinger PC, Cushing BM, Kerns TJ: Injury patterns associated with direction of impact: Drivers admitted to trauma centers. *J Trauma* 35:454, 1993.
32. Punjabi MM, White AA: Basic biomechanics of the spine. *Neurosurgery* 7:76, 1980.
33. Swierzewski MJ, Feliciano DV, Lillis RP, et al.: Deaths from motor vehicle crashes: Patterns of injury in restrained and unrestrained victims. *J Trauma* 37:404, 1994.
34. Vestrup JA, Reid JDS: A profile of urban adult pedestrian trauma. *J Trauma* 29:741, 1989.

35. Lane PL, McClafferty KJ, Nowak ES: Pedestrians in real world collisions. *J Trauma* 36:231, 1994.
36. Helling TS, Watkins M, Evans LL, et al.: Low falls: An underappreciated mechanism of injury. *J Trauma* 46:453, 1999.
37. Velmahos GC, Demetriades D, Theodorou D, et al.: Patterns of injury in urban free falls. *World J Surg* 21:816, 1997.
38. Peek C, McArthur D, Hovda D, et al.: Early predictors of mortality in penetrating compared with closed brain injury. *Brain Injury* 15:804, 2001.
39. Guerrero JL, Thurman DJ, Sniezek JE: Emergency department visits associated with traumatic brain injury: United States 1995–1996. *Brain Injury* 14:181, 2000.
40. Gennarelli TA, Champion HR, Copes WS, et al.: Comparison of mortality, morbidity and severity of 59,713 head injured patients with 114,447 patients with extracranial injuries. *J Trauma* 37:962, 1994.
41. McMahon CG, Yates DW, Campbell FM: Unexpected contribution of moderate traumatic brain injury to death after major trauma. *J Trauma* 47:891, 1999.
42. Park HK, Fernandez II, Duchovny M, et al.: Experimental animal models of traumatic brain injury: Medical and biomechanical mechanisms. *Crit Rev Neurosurg* 26:44, 1999.
43. King AI, Ruan JS, Zhou C, et al.: Recent advances in biomechanics of brain injury research: A review. *J Neurotrauma* 12:651, 1995.
44. Gennarelli TA, Thibault LE: Biomechanics of acute subdural hematoma. *J Trauma* 22:680, 1982.
45. Holburn AS: Mechanics of head injury. *Lancet* 2:438, 1942.
46. Blumberg PC, Scott G, Manavais J, et al.: Staining of amyloid precursor to study axonal damage in mild head injury. *Lancet* 344:1055, 1994.
47. Cooper GJ, Maynard RL, Pearce BP, et al.: Cardiovascular distortion in experimental non-penetrating chest impacts. *J Trauma* 24:188, 1984.
48. Cooper GJ: Biophysics of impact injury to the chest and abdomen. *J R Army Med Corps* 135:58, 1989.
49. Shkrum MJ, McClafferty KJ, Green RN, et al.: Mechanisms of aortic injury in fatalities occurring in motor vehicle collisions. *J Forensic Sci* 44:44, 1999.
50. Rabinovici R, Ovadia P, Mathiak G, et al.: Abdominal injuries associated with lumbar spine fractures in blunt trauma. *Injury* 30:471, 1999.
51. Neugebauer H, Wallenboeck E, Hungerford M: Seventy cases of injuries of the small intestine by blunt abdominal trauma: A retrospective study from 1970 to 1994. *J Trauma* 46:116, 1999.
52. Dautrieve AH, Flacbaum L, Cox EF: Blunt intestinal trauma: A modern day review. *Ann Surg* 201:198, 1985.
53. Geoghegan T, Brush B: The mechanism of intestinal perforation from non-penetrating abdominal trauma. *Arch Surg* 73:455, 1956.
54. Morris S, Lenihan B, Duddy L, et al.: Outcome after musculoskeletal trauma treated in a regional hospital. *J Trauma* 49:461, 2000.
55. Harkess JW, Ramsey CW, Harkess JW: Biomechanics of fractures, in Rockwood CA, Green DP, Bucholz RW, eds: *Fractures in Adults*. New York: Lippincott, 1991, p. 1.
56. Panjabi MM, Whit AA: Basic biomechanics of the spine. *NeuroSurg* 7:76, 1980.
57. Viano DC: Causes and control of spinal cord injury in automotive crashes. *World J Surg* 16:410, 1992.
58. Pennie B, Agambar L: Patterns of injury and recovery in whiplash. *Injury* 22:57, 1991.
59. Haddon W: Energy damage and the ten countermeasure strategies. *J Trauma* 13:321, 1973.
60. Mashaw J: *The Struggle for Auto Safety*. Cambridge, MA: Harvard Press, 1990.
61. Cummings P, Weiss NS: Mortality reduction with air bag and seatbelt use in head-on passenger car collisions. *Am J Epidemiol* 154:387, 2001.
62. Viano DC, Olsen S: The effectiveness of active head restraint in preventing whiplash. *J Trauma* 51:959, 2001.
63. Miller PR, Fabian TC, Bee TK, et al.: Blunt cerebrovascular injuries—diagnosis and treatment. *J Trauma* 51:279, 2001.
64. Feliciano DV, Wall MJ: Patterns of injury. In Moore EE, Mattox KL, Feliciano DV, eds. *Trauma* 2nd ed. Norwalk, CT: Appleton & Lange, 1991, p. 81.
65. Hendey GW, Votey SR: Injuries in restrained motor vehicle accident victims. *Ann Emerg Med* 24:77, 1994.
66. Arbogast KB, Moll EK, Morris SD, et al.: Factors influencing pediatric injury in side impact collisions. *J Trauma* 51:469, 2001.
67. Snyder CL, Vivant NJ, Saltzman DA, et al.: Blunt trauma in adults and children: A comparative analysis. *J Trauma* 30:1239, 1990.
68. Kokoska ER, Keller MS, Rallo MC: Characteristics of pediatric cervical spine injuries. *J Ped Surg* 36:100, 2001.
69. Mehlman CT, Scott KA, Bernadette L: Orthopaedic injuries in children secondary to air bag deployment. *J Bone Joint Surg* 82:895, 2000.
70. Berkowitz CD: Pediatric abuse: New patterns of injury. *Emer Med Clin North Am* 13:321, 1995.
71. Pearlman MD, Klinich KD, Schneider LW: A comprehensive program to improve safety for pregnant women and fetuses in motor vehicle crashes: A preliminary report. *Am J Ob-Gyn* 182:5, 2000.
72. Tornetta P, Mostafavi H, Rinna J, et al.: Morbidity and mortality in elderly trauma patients. *J Trauma* 46:702, 1999.
73. Sterling DA, O'Conner JA, Bonadies J: Geriatric falls: Injury severity is high and disproportionate to mechanism. *J Trauma* 50:116, 2001.
74. Horrocks CL: Blast injuries: Biophysics, pathophysiology and management principles. *J R Army Med Corps* 147:28, 2001.
75. Hull JB: Traumatic amputation by explosive blast: Pattern of injury in survivors. *Brit J Surg* 79:1303, 1992.

# Commentary ■ DAVID V. FELICIANO

Each edition of *Trauma* has included this chapter describing the physical principles involved in the transfer of energy that results in injury to a patient. The principles described are quite old (Sir Isaac Newton, 1642–1727; James P. Joule, 1818–1889; etc.), but continue to apply and explain the injuries received by victims of motor vehicle or motorcycle crashes, assaults, falls, gunshot wounds and other common mechanisms of injury. When there is contact between a victim and an object (outside of a car, inside of a car, street, weapon, missile, etc.) over time, the kinetic energy transfer is related to the weight and velocity of the moving component(s) as explained in the well-known formula $\frac{1}{2}mv^2$. When the transfer of kinetic energy occurs as a force or stress, a variety of strains are caused that may exceed the "failure point" or "break point" of a given body part. Other than poisoning, drowning, burns, and bites and stings, all common mechanisms of blunt and penetrating trauma cause only three different types of injury – i.e.,

injury to the skin, buckle or fracture of bone, and rupture of part of or an entire organ such as a viscus or a vessel.

The authors have described the significantly higher mortality that results from head-on motor vehicle collisions (60%) as compared to those that are side impacts (20–35%), rollovers (8–15%), and rear end collisions (3–5%). They have emphasized the importance of wearing a restraint device in a motor vehicle as ejection after a crash results in a five times greater mortality for the victim.

They have once again commented on the reasons for multiple injuries in unrestrained drivers in motor vehicle crashes. Direct contact with the head (and brain) on the windshield, compressive injuries to the thoracic wall, lung, heart, liver, and spleen from contact with the steering wheel, and fractures and dislocations in the lower extremities from contact with the dashboard continue to constitute the "expressway syndrome" first described back in the 1960s. When lateral collisions occur in motor vehicles without reinforced doors or side airbags, injuries to the lateral thoracic wall, thoracoabdominal structures and the pelvic bones predominate.

The authors emphasize the classic triad of injuries sustained in auto-pedestrian crashes. With a first point of contact at the patient's knee or upper leg depending on braking of the vehicle, dislocations of the knee or fractures of the tibia-fibula are common injures. Fortunately, associated vascular injuries requiring operative repair occur in only 15–17% of patients with dislocations of the knee and in <2% of patients with routine tibial fractures (not Gustilo IIIB or IIIC open fractures). The trunk of the victim in an auto-pedestrian crash then makes contact with the hood of the automobile resulting in the standard set of blunt abdominal visceral injuries to the mesentery, spleen, and liver. The third part of the triad involves contact between the victim's head and windshield of the vehicle or with the ground after the victim falls off the hood. When one or two components of the triad are present upon initial evaluation of the victim in the emergency center, the others should be ruled out based on the physical examination and appropriate diagnostic testing.

Victims of falls from a height absorb kinetic energy at landing that is directly related to the height as mass and gravitational acceleration are constant for falling bodies. Therefore, the pattern of injury may be predicted when the height of the fall, position of the victim upon impact, and the density of the landing zone are known. The authors emphasize that fractures constitute 75% of all injuries in falls from a height and that intra-abdominal injuries occur in only 6% of victims.

The authors emphasize the important anatomic considerations that affect the magnitude of injuries to the skeletal systems and its contents. Direct injuries to the brain such as contusions and contrecoup injuries result from the size discrepancy between the cranial vault and the enclosed brain. This size difference is exaggerated in older patients and accounts for the significant increase in deaths from traumatic brain injuries in this group as compared to younger victims. Different theories to explain the unsettling and nonsurgical diagnosis of diffuse axonal injury are also described in the chapter.

In patients with thoracic trauma, the authors emphasize the horizontal movement of the victim's heart in frontal or lateral motor vehicle crashes while the descending thoracic aorta is fixed to the vertebral column. This is one postulated mechanism for the frequent rupture of the descending thoracic aorta at the ligamentum arteriosum in such crashes, though the actual structure of the aortic wall at the former site of the fetal ductus arteriosus may well be a contributing factor.

Intraabdominal injuries in motor vehicle crashes can result from direct compression from the lower rim of the steering wheel or from lap seatbelts that are positioned improperly over the abdomen instead of the pelvic bones. Injuries also result from shearing at ligamentous attachments of solid organs, at fixation points of the midgut, and at fixation points for retroperitoneal vascular structures such as the renal arteries.

In terms of prevention of injuries, the authors describe William Haddon's matrix and the many sites where interaction between a potential victim (host) and the environment may be altered. Changes in the design of motor vehicles including the addition of "crumple zones," downward direction of the transmission, and the addition of head rests, restraint devices, and air bags have changed the patterns of injury and lowered the mortality rates after motor vehicle crashes significantly over the last 50 years. This occurred as the number of vehicles on the road and the number of miles driven have continued to increase in the United States.

As a nice supplement to the chapter on "Pediatric Trauma" (Chap 46), the authors emphasize the different compliance of the skeletal system in children as compared to adults. The chest wall, in particular, may demonstrate no sign of injury such as a fractured rib in a child while there are significant intrathoracic injuries present. The interesting phenomenon of SCIWORA (spinal cord injury without radiographic abnormality) in 15–20% of children with injuries to the cervical spine is also discussed by the authors. There is also a comprehensive review of the injuries in children that result from child abuse.

This is a critical chapter in *Trauma*, 6th edition, as the understanding of kinematics of injury results in a greater likelihood that occult injuries will be detected and treated properly. The chapter is well written, well organized, enjoyable to read, comprehensive, and lays a foundation that every individual interested in trauma will be able to build on throughout his or her career.

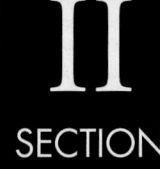

# GENERALIZED APPROACHES TO THE TRAUMATIZED PATIENT

# Prehospital Care

*Jeffrey P. Salomone* ■ *Joseph A. Salomone, III*

Critically injured patients must receive high-quality care from the earliest postinjury moment to have the best chance of survival. Most trauma victims first receive health care from the Emergency Medical Services (EMS) system, which is responsible for rendering aid and transporting the trauma patient to an appropriate facility.

The practice of medicine in the prehospital setting presents numerous challenges not encountered in the hospital. Hazardous materials along with environmental and climatic conditions may pose dangers to rescuers as well as to patients. If the patient is entrapped in a mangled vehicle or a collapsed building, there must be meticulous coordination of medical and rescue teams. Providers of prehospital care are expected to deliver high-quality medical care in situations that are austere and unforgiving and, often, for prolonged periods.

The role of the EMS system is far more complex than simply transporting the trauma victim to a medical facility. In most EMS systems in the United States, specially trained health care professionals are responsible for the initial assessment and management of the injured patient. Experience from the last several decades has shown that these paraprofessionals can safely perform many of the interventions that were previously performed only by physicians or nurses in the emergency department.

While many of these procedures have proven beneficial for victims of cardiac emergencies, critically injured patients may need two items not available on an ambulance—blood and a surgeon. As EMS systems mature and additional prehospital care research is conducted, the question is no longer, "What *can* the EMT do for the trauma patient in the prehospital setting?" but rather, "What *should* the EMT do?"

## HISTORICAL PERSPECTIVE

While the roots of prehospital trauma care can be traced back to military physicians, modern civilian prehospital trauma care began about four decades ago. J.D. "Deke" Farrington and Sam Banks instituted the first trauma course for ambulance personnel in 1962.[1] This course, initiated with the Chicago Committee on Trauma and the Chicago Fire Academy, marked the beginning of formal training in prehospital care of injured patients. Farrington is generally acknowledged as the father of modern EMS.[2]

In September 1966, the National Academy of Sciences and National Research Council published the landmark monograph, *Accidental Death and Disability: The Neglected Disease of Modern Society.*[3] This document argued that there were no standards for ambulances with respect to design, equipment, or training of personnel. As a direct result of this monograph, the Department of Transportation funded the development of the Emergency Medical Technician–Ambulance (EMT-A) curriculum, published in 1969. Continued public pressure resulted in the passage of the Emergency Medical Services (EMS) Systems Act of 1973 (PL 93-154). This act revolutionized EMS in this country and resulted in federal funding for the establishment of EMS systems.

In the late 1960s, J.F. Pantridge, an Irish physician practicing in Dublin, developed a mobile coronary care unit that was staffed by physicians.[4] He conceived of a system in which the victim of an acute myocardial infarction was stabilized at the scene by bringing advanced life support to the patient. The physicians worked to restore normal cardiac rhythm through medications and defibrillation at the location where the victim was stricken.

In the United States, the concept of advanced prehospital care involved training Emergency Medical Technicians (EMTs) to perform these life-saving skills. The original "paramedic" programs began in Los Angeles, California; Houston, Texas; Jacksonville, Florida; and Columbus, Ohio, and were often associated with fire departments. Paramedics were trained to serve as the "eyes and ears" of the physicians in their base hospitals and provide care under their direction.

While prehospital advanced life support proved beneficial for victims of cardiac emergencies, it was not until the 1980s that it became obvious that definitive care for trauma patients was fundamentally different than that for the cardiac patient. Efforts to restore circulating blood volume proved to be unsuccessful in the face of ongoing internal hemorrhage. The exsanguinating trauma patient requires operative intervention, and any action that delays the trauma patient's arrival in the operating room is ultimately detrimental to survival. During this period, significant controversy surrounded prehospital advanced life support for trauma patients as expert panels and editorialists debated its pros and cons.[5,6] Several studies documented the detrimental effect of prolonged attempts at field stabilization on seriously injured trauma patients,[7–9] while others showed that paramedics could employ advanced life support measures in an expeditious manner.[10–13]

## EMERGENCY MEDICAL SERVICES SYSTEM

The modern EMS system involves the integration of a number of complex components. Essential elements include the following: personnel, equipment, communications, transport modalities, medical control, and an ongoing quality improvement process. Different configurations of EMS systems result when these components are integrated in varying combinations. The EMS System represents a significant component of the trauma system, described elsewhere (see Chap. 4).

## PERSONNEL

While EMTs comprise the vast majority of prehospital care providers employed in the United States, a small number of nurses and physicians also deliver care in the out-of-hospital setting.

### Emergency Medical Technicians

The *National EMS Education and Practice Blueprint*, resulting from a consensus conference convened in 1993 by the National Highway Traffic Safety Administration (NHTSA), provides the basis for the levels of emergency medical technicians current utilized in the United States. The Blueprint divides the major areas of prehospital instruction and/or performance into 16 "core elements." For each core element, there are progressively increasing knowledge and skill objectives, representing a continuum of education and practice. The four levels of EMTs currently recognized are the First Responder, EMT-B, EMT-I, and EMT-P.[14]

### First Responder

This prehospital caregiver uses a limited amount of equipment to perform initial assessment and rudimentary intervention or aid other EMS providers. This term has also been applied to the first person who may arrive on scene with any training below the EMT-B level. This may include those individuals trained at the basic or advanced first-aid level of the American Red Cross.

### Emergency Medical Technician—Basic

The EMT-B has the knowledge and skills of the first responder but, in addition, is qualified to function as minimum staff for an ambulance. The current course work required to achieve this level is successful completion of the 110-hour course developed by the U.S. Department of Transportation. A new national standard curriculum for the EMT-B was developed and released by the NHTSA in 1994.[15] Upon completion of the course, the prospective EMT-B must pass written and practical examinations administered by either the National Registry of EMTs (NREMT) or the state, or both.

### Emergency Medical Technician—Intermediate

The EMT-I must have completed the EMT-B course, followed by an additional 150 to 200 hours of training.[16] The additional time is devoted to acquiring a more in-depth knowledge of pathophysiology and management of shock, advanced techniques of patient assessment, and advanced skills for airway management. The EMT-I is trained in intravenous access and can perform in-field fluid resuscitation with crystalloid solutions. The EMT-I level is probably the least well defined of all the levels, as training requirements vary dramatically from state to state.

### Emergency Medical Technician—Paramedic

In addition to the knowledge and skills of the previous levels, the EMT-P is trained in the use of a wider range of medications and the performance of a greater number of advanced skills. A new curriculum, approved by a national review team in 1997, requires approximately 1000 hours of didactic and practical training.[17] With the introduction of assessment-based management to field care, the paramedic educated under this model rises above the level of a mere technician and enters the realm of a true medical professional. The paramedic has had a major impact on the resuscitation of patients with cardiac or major medical problems and is very effective in urban areas in which response times are short.

The *EMS Education Agenda for the Future: A Systems Approach*, published by NHTSA in 1999, established the foundation for a more integrated system of training and credentialing prehospital care providers.[18] While many of the five components have been completed and integrated into the current EMS system, others remain in development or awaiting adoption by the individual states. The components are as follows:

The National EMS Core Content, describing the domain of prehospital care.

The National EMS Scope of Practice Model, categorizing the core content in to four new levels of EMTs: the Emergency Medical Responder, the EMT, the Advanced EMT, and the Paramedic.

The National EMS Education Standards, providing the requirements for educating each of these EMT levels.

National EMS Certification, board certification for each of the EMT levels, conducted by the National Registry of EMTs.

National EMS Educational Program Accreditation.

The Committee on Accreditation of Allied Health Education Programs (CAAHEP), established as a nonprofit organization in 1994, has developed an accreditation process for EMT training programs (Committee on Accreditation of EMS Programs). While some states require that all paramedic training programs be approved by CoAEMSP, many states have no such requirements. The status of EMT-Ps as health care professionals would be significantly elevated by requiring accreditation through this entity to standardize and maintain quality of education for paramedics. More recent data indicate that graduates of accredited EMT-P programs are more likely to successfully achieve certification by the National Registry of EMTs.[19]

## Nurses

Nurses occupy a unique position in the EMS system. They serve as prehospital providers (when dual trained), instructors, and proctors of quality improvement. Nursing education imparts an excellent understanding of patient care and the pathophysiology of disease processes and is a valuable source for the education of the EMT. Nurses may also be employed by EMS services as field observers and on-site instructors for continuing education. Nurses can provide insight to the EMTs on disease processes and the smooth integration of patient care from the field to the emergency department.

## Ground Nurses

When dual trained as a nurse and an EMT, the individual can function in the field as a prehospital provider under the auspices of EMT training. In the United States, nurses should not function in the prehospital setting until they are trained in field skills such as extrication, splinting, endotracheal intubation, and operation of an emergency vehicle as these skills are not part of the traditional nursing curriculum. Nurses are utilized by many critical care transport services to assist in the care of special patients (e.g., neonatal and cardiac). In this context, nurses can function to the extent of their nursing training, abilities, and license restrictions. Most states have not developed standards for the prehospital role of nurses. Because of the paucity of trained EMTs, nurses often serve as ambulance attendants in foreign countries.

## Flight Nurses

Almost all aeromedical services in the United States utilize nurses in the delivery of prehospital care and transport. The composition of the flight crews varies widely, and common configurations are two nurses, a nurse and a paramedic or EMT, or a physician with either a nurse or paramedic. In this context, nurses are limited in their roles just as in ground transport. They provide important knowledge and skills in critical care but, in most states, need to be paired with a partner who is licensed to perform in the prehospital arena. Nurses who are dual trained as both an EMT and a nurse can provide care in the prehospital phase under the auspices of their EMT training.

## Physicians

In the United States, it is unusual for physicians to directly participate in the provision of care to the injured patient in the field, although some aeromedical services utilize physicians as members of their flight crew. The physicians assigned to such crews are usually emergency medicine residents who rotate onto the aircraft as a formal part of their residency. Another use of physicians in the prehospital setting involves neonatologists or pediatric residents or fellows who staff units used for interfacility transport of critically ill infants.

In Europe and Central and South America it is common for physicians to function as primary members of the EMS team. Because of a surplus of physicians or a lack of attractive employment opportunities, physicians may work for an EMS service, either staffing an ambulance or responding in a separate vehicle. The standards of EMT training in the United States suggest that little is gained by employing physicians on EMS units, and this use of a valuable resource in the field is a challenging one to defend.

Physicians who happen upon the scene of a motor vehicle crash may be tempted to assume control of the patient despite the fact that they possess little experience caring for patients in the prehospital setting. In such situations, the physician should realize that the vast majority of EMTs are well-trained and capable of performing their job and that they work under the medical direction of a licensed physician. Additionally, should the physician begin to direct care for a patient, he or she must remain with the patient until care is formally transferred over to an accepting physician, either by radio communication or by face-to-face turnover in the emergency department. Failure to do so may constitute abandonment of the patient and leave the physician exposed to serious legal repercussions.

## SYSTEM DESIGN

Prior to the early 1970s, EMS in the United States were very rudimentary and focused primarily on transportation of patients. Actual medical care began only after the patient's arrival at the hospital. Today, numerous models of EMS systems exist, as the various elements of the system are combined in different ways. No definitive evidence exists that one model is superior in performance to any other, and community leaders design their system around the available resources in the community. An EMS service may be operated by a private company, a hospital, a fire department, a police department, or a governmentally funded agency solely responsible for emergency medical care (a public "third service"). Regardless of which agency provides EMS, prehospital care generally fits into one of two distinct categories, i.e., basic life support and advanced life support.[20]

## Basic Life Support

*Basic life support* (BLS) is a term used to describe a level of care that provides noninvasive emergency care. BLS involves providing basic airway management, supplemental oxygen, and rescue breathing; cardiopulmonary resuscitation (CPR); control of external hemorrhage; splinting; spinal immobilization; and uncomplicated childbirth. The goal of BLS care is to maintain breathing and circulation and transport the patient without causing further harm. The two most common types of BLS providers are the First Responder and Emergency Medical Technician–Basic (EMT-B). Many BLS services utilize automatic or semiautomatic external defibrillators

(AEDs) that identify ventricular fibrillation and deliver electrical countershocks. Because of the limited equipment and training, BLS systems are less costly to establish and maintain than are more advanced levels of care.

## Advanced Life Support

*Advanced life support* (ALS) describes care that involves the use of invasive procedures. EMS providers at the ALS level are capable of more sophisticated airway management, cardiac monitoring and defibrillation, insertion of intravenous lines, and administration of numerous medications. ALS systems utilize individuals trained at the EMT-I or EMT-P level.

In contrast to BLS systems, ALS systems provide advanced therapy to the patient at the scene, rather than waiting until arrival at a hospital to institute care. ALS systems have had impressive results in the care of cardiac patients, especially when CPR is started within 4 minutes of a cardiopulmonary arrest and advanced life support can be initiated within 8 minutes of the arrest. These types of systems, however, are very expensive to establish and maintain and place high demands on the personnel for education and maintenance of skills.

## Tiered Response Systems

An EMS system that is not purely BLS or ALS, but a combination of both, is called a *tiered response system*.[21] The goal of a tiered EMS system is to match the training level of the provider with the needs of the patient. The first level of care is usually BLS with the providers being either first responders or EMT-B personnel, typically from a public safety agency (e.g., fire or police) or EMS units staffed by EMT-Basics. In this model, BLS personnel would initiate transport if the patient did not require ALS procedures. If ALS interventions are needed, the BLS crews initiate basic care and attempt to stabilize the patient until the ALS unit arrives. A limited number of ALS units respond only when needed.

Proponents of this system argue that it functions in a more cost-effective manner, providing ALS-level care only to those patients who require it. This type of system offers the advantages of rapid BLS response times combined with the cost-effective utilization of ALS resources. In many communities, especially those in rural settings, a third tier of aeromedical transport may be present. This tier usually provides a slightly higher level of training and expertise, combined with the more rapid transport capabilities of the aircraft.

## EQUIPMENT

The American College of Surgeons Committee on Trauma (ACSCOT) joined with the American College of Emergency Physicians (ACEP) and the National Association of EMS Physicians to publish a document delineating the necessary equipment that should be stocked on an EMS unit.[22] This document includes separate recommendations for both BLS and ALS ambulances. It also provides that EMS units maintain equipment in sufficient sizes to adequately care for infants, children, and adults. In most jurisdictions, state law mandates the equipment carried by EMS

units, and administrative agencies periodically inspect ambulances to ensure that necessary equipment is present. Medical directors may also require that certain equipment or medications be added to units under their direction.

## COMMUNICATIONS

Communications comprise an essential component of the EMS system. The EMS dispatch center must be able to readily locate the unit closest to the incident and provide them with an exact location and description of the call. EMS units must also be able to communicate with other agencies that provide first responder care (i.e., the fire department) and those that serve an adjunctive role such as extrication and control of hazardous materials. EMS units must also have two-way communication with receiving facilities and with the physicians who provide medical oversight. EMS personnel may request specific orders from a physician when a patient's condition falls outside established treatment protocols.

## TRANSPORT MODALITIES

### Ground Units

EMS units operating on the ground may possess transport capabilities (i.e., an ambulance) or they may be a "quick response" unit that contains only equipment and personnel, and a separate ambulance is required for transport. Such quick response vehicles are common in rural areas or in tiered EMS systems. Ambulances should conform to size and performance specifications as outlined by governmental agencies and authoritative organizations and possess required equipment as described earlier.

Minimal staffing for a BLS unit is two EMT-Basics. In areas primarily covered by BLS units, a tiered response arrangement should be in place so that ALS back-up is available when needed.[20]

To qualify as an ALS unit, at least one member of the team must possess training beyond the EMT-Basic level. Most commonly, ALS units now are staffed by at least one EMT-P, although many ALS services utilize units staffed by two paramedics. Additional equipment and supplies must be available on the ALS unit to support the defined scope of practice.

## AIR MEDICAL EMS

### Rotor-Wing Aircraft

Helicopter evacuation of military casualties began during the Korean War, and matured during the Vietnam War.[23] The improvement noted in survival was largely attributed to the speed of evacuation to facilities capable of providing initial trauma care. Civilian air medical services were established in the United States as a result of the success during wartime and have proliferated throughout the industrialized world.

Significant controversy surrounds the utility of rotor-wing aircraft, especially in terms of improvements in patient outcome. Helicopter transport appears to be beneficial in rural locations and wilderness rescue.[24–26] While some studies have correlated an improvement in the outcome of victims of blunt trauma transported by helicopter,[27–30] others have found little or no benefit.[24,31,32] The benefits of on-scene helicopter response are also debatable in an urban or suburban setting when a well-trained ground EMS service is present.[33,34] A recent study by Diaz and coworkers demonstrated that ground transport is always faster than air medical transport when the distance from the scene to the trauma center is 10 miles or less, while helicopter transport was always faster when the scene was more than 45 miles from the trauma center.[35] The National Association of EMS Physicians (NAEMSP) has published guidelines for helicopter response to the trauma scene.[36]

There seems to be little debate that the transport of critically injured patients from a rural facility with limited resources to a major trauma center is beneficial for the patient.[37,38] The typical maximum transport radius for a helicopter service is 150 miles.

In the United States, air ambulances are most commonly operated by an EMS service or are hospital based; however, the Coast Guard, military, law enforcement agencies, or park services may also provide helicopter transport. Crew configurations vary from service to service. The two most common combinations are two flight nurses or a flight nurse and a paramedic. Helicopters are universally equipped as ALS units at a minimum and more commonly as compact intensive care units. There is an element of risk associated with air medical transport, and a study by Bledsoe and Smith documented a steady and marked increase in the number of crashes of medical helicopters over the decade of 1993 to 2002.[39]

## Fixed-Wing Aircraft

Fixed-wing aircraft are constrained by the need for a runway and, therefore, lack the versatility of rotor-wing units that can land at an accident scene or at a trauma center. With the additional time required to transport a patient to and from a local airport, fixed-wing aircraft only become more time-efficient when a patient requires transfer over a distance greater than about 150 miles. Aircraft equipped for aeromedical transport often serve to transfer patients to regional specialized facilities such as those for burns or spinal cord injuries, or to transplant centers. The equipment and supply requirements for fixed-wing aircraft are not as well defined as for ground or rotor-wing units.

## CONTINUOUS QUALITY IMPROVEMENT

Quality medical care is a vital issue in all areas of the health care system. Continuous quality improvement (CQI) is an ongoing cycle of evaluation, data collection, interpretation, and modifying the system to improve patient care. CQI is a never-ending cycle with the primary goal being improving the delivery of health care.[40]

Providing the best medical care possible requires a concerted effort to objectively evaluate care rendered, efficiency of the system, and equipment. Medical care and performance of the system are evaluated in a variety of ways to determine if care is rendered in a timely, efficient, and medically sound fashion. Finally, equipment must be reliable and durable in order to withstand the sometimes harsh conditions associated with the delivery of prehospital care.

## Care Rendered

The medical director and leadership of an EMS service must be able to objectively review the care rendered by the personnel they supervise. Evaluation of medical care can be separated into prospective, concurrent, and retrospective phases.

## Prospective Evaluation

This form of evaluation attempts to improve the level of care rendered prior to the actual delivery of the care. Evaluating continuing education programs and periodic assessment of skill performance are examples of prospective evaluation tools.

## Concurrent Evaluation

Concurrent evaluation involves direct observation of the EMT during the delivery of care. The medical director or a designated member of the staff of the EMS system (e.g., field training officer) accompanies the crew in order to observe the delivery of care in the field. Steps can be taken immediately to correct deficiencies and improve patient care.

## Retrospective Evaluation

Retrospective evaluation occurs after care has been delivered. This form of review is the easiest and least costly of the methods and comprises chart audits, case reviews, and debriefings to review the events of any particular EMS call. Trauma surgeons should participate in the retrospective evaluation of EMS services that transport patients to their facility. Such involvement helps EMS providers gain perspective into the entire spectrum of trauma care.

## System Efficiency

The evaluation process for any EMS system must determine the efficiency of all components involved in providing care to the patient. One method of evaluating efficiency of the system is to review notification time, response time, on-scene time, and transport time.

## Notification Time

The notification time for the EMS system can be viewed as the time interval between the injury and notification of the EMS dispatch center. In the United States, most requests for EMS arrive via the 911 phone system. Data from 1996 indicate that approximately 80% of the United States was covered by a dedicated 911 system and, at that time, only six states had 100% coverage by 911 service.[41] There is an additional time interval in many systems between the call being answered at the Public Safety Answering Point (PSAP) and the call being routed to the EMS dispatch center.

## Response Time

Response time is defined as the period that starts when an emergency call is received by the EMS dispatch center and ends with the arrival of the ambulance at the scene. This timeframe encompasses several actions as follows: (a) the call must be physically received; (b) the dispatcher must analyze the call and decide on the appropriate response; (c) the ambulance must be contacted and dispatched; and (d) the ambulance must leave its current location and travel to the scene. The final factor, ambulance travel time, is a function of location and availability of the ambulance, weather, and traffic conditions.

The desired response time for any system directly impacts the number of ambulances that the system requires. In order to meet the target response times, sufficient EMS units must be available to meet the expected number of emergency calls in the coverage area. While many urban systems have set a standard of 8 minutes that must be met 90% of the time, the ideal response time for trauma is unknown. A retrospective study failed to identify an association between shorter EMS response times and improved outcome in trauma patients.[42]

## On-Scene Time

The on-scene time is the interval from the arrival of EMS at the scene until their departure en route to the receiving facility. This time will vary according to environmental conditions, geography of the scene and location, accessibility of the patient, entrapment, injuries present, and requirements for packaging of the patient. When caring for a critically injured patient, the EMS personnel should strive to limit their on-scene time to 10 minutes or less.[43] A retrospective study of the outcome of seriously injured trauma patients (Injury Severity Score >15) in an urban setting demonstrated improved survival when the patient was transported by private vehicle compared to an ALS unit, primarily because the EMS crews were spending, on average, more than 20 minutes on scene.[44]

Approximately 85 to 90% of trauma patients encountered by EMS are not critically injured and, thus, do not require rapid packaging and immediate transport. Continuous monitoring of on-scene times should be performed to ensure that time is not being lost in the performance of futile procedures on patients with severe injuries.

## Transport Time

The length of time required to transport the patient from the scene to an appropriate facility is the final phase of the total prehospital period. The factors that affect this time are distance from the facility, weather, transport modality (air vs. ground) and traffic conditions, if transported by ground. The choice of a destination facility is a critical decision in the care of the critical patient. For the patient who requires emergent operative intervention to control hemorrhage, transport must be made to a hospital staffed and equipped to move the patient to the operating room immediately.

This generally means that closer hospitals that lack this capability are bypassed in favor of a trauma center farther away. EMS services must know the capabilities of the hospitals in their area, so that such decisions may be made in a logical fashion. Quality improvement reviews should address these issues in an ongoing manner.

## MEDICAL CONTROL

One of the most important relationships in EMS is that between the prehospital providers and the physician. In the United States, EMS personnel practicing at the ALS level can be thought of as physician extenders.[45] The Medical Practice Act spells out who may render care and under what circumstances.

State laws and regulations give EMS providers the authority to deliver care, but place the responsibility for EMT practice on the physician who agreed to supervise them. Many terms have been applied to this association, including *medical control, medical direction,* or *medical oversight.*

Medical direction of an EMS system is provided in a variety of fashions that differ from region to region. In some systems a single physician provides medical direction, and, in other circumstances, medical direction is carried out by a group of physicians acting collectively through a consensus process. In 1986, Holroyd and coauthors recommended that the EMS medical director be a physician with the following qualifications: (a) knowledge and demonstrated ability in planning and operation of prehospital EMS systems; (b) experience in the prehospital provision of emergency care for acutely ill or injured patients; (c) experience in the training and ongoing evaluation of all levels of participants in the prehospital care system; (d) knowledge and experience in the application of medical control to an EMS system; and (e) a knowledge of the administrative and legislative processes affecting regional and/or state prehospital EMS systems.[46]

The medical director must be interested in, and committed to, the day-to-day activities of the EMS service. The role of medical director for an EMS service is not limited to emergency physicians, and trauma/critical care surgeons are well suited to function in this role once they have gained the prerequisite knowledge of how EMS systems function. The National Association of EMS Physicians has developed a workshop for EMS medical directors.

Medical control is divided into two categories including indirect (off-line/protocols) and direct (on-line).[47]

### Indirect (Off-Line/Protocols)

This form of medical direction involves the development of written protocols and the review of EMT performance.[48] The amount of time required to accomplish these administrative duties varies with the size and complexity of the particular EMS system. The medical director's review of care is a CQI function and has been discussed previously.

Protocols are the overall steps in patient management that are to be followed by the prehospital provider at every patient contact. As an accurate diagnosis is often not possible in the field, protocols are usually developed based upon the patient's complaints or condition. For ease of memorization and integration with those of other conditions, many protocols are designed in an algorithmic fashion. Trauma surgeons should participate in the development of EMS protocols regarding care for injured patients in their region.

### Direct (On-Line)

Direct or on-line medical control by the medical director is clinical in nature.[49] This form of direction involves providing radio or telephone instructions to prehospital providers for conditions that are not covered in their protocols and direct observation of individual performance.

Early in the development of EMS systems, a great deal of emphasis was given to direct medical control. Many authorities believed that direct communication between the physician and the prehospital providers would be the mainstay of good prehospital care. Despite this, several studies have demonstrated that there is no difference in survival with and without on-line medical control and less time is spent in the field when there is no requirement to call the hospital.[48]

## TRAUMA EDUCATION FOR EMS PERSONNEL

Two continuing education courses have been developed to provide EMS personnel with the essential knowledge and skills to manage critically injured patients. Both courses have been promulgated nationally and internationally.

### Prehospital Trauma Life Support

The Prehospital Trauma Life Support (PHTLS) program was developed by the National Association of EMTs in cooperation with the ACSCOT.[43] The PHTLS course is based upon the tenets of the ATLS course developed by ACSCOT, but has been modified to meet the needs of the patient in the prehospital setting.[50] The central philosophy of the PHTLS course is that EMS providers, when given an appropriate fund of knowledge, can make appropriate decisions regarding patient care. Thus, the course emphasizes "principles" of management, rather than focusing on individual preferences or protocols.

A new edition of the course is produced every 4 years, one year after the revised ATLS course has been released. This strategy guarantees that PHTLS continues to disseminate any changes in treatment or philosophy that have been introduced in ATLS and ensures a seamless interface between the prehospital providers and personnel in the emergency department in the initial management of the trauma patient. PHTLS is currently taught throughout the United States and in almost 40 foreign countries.

### International Trauma Life Support

About the same time that PHTLS was developed by NAEMT, the Alabama Chapter of the American College of Emergency Physicians developed the BTLS course.[51] The course was subsequently transitioned to BTLS International, a not-for-profit organization, and, in 2005, changed the name to International Trauma Life Support. Like PHTLS, ITLS is also based upon the philosophies of ATLS and taught both in the United States and internationally.

## ASSESSMENT AND MANAGEMENT

Assessment and management of the injured patient in the prehospital setting should proceed in an orderly manner, despite the fact that the EMT must frequently make rapid decisions about patient care under adverse conditions. While the general approach is based upon that taught in the ATLS course, one important modification is that the EMT first performs a "scene assessment" prior to evaluating an individual patient. Next, a "primary survey" is conducted to identify life-threatening conditions and initiate immediate therapy.

At the end of the primary survey the EMT considers whether life-threatening or potentially life-threatening injuries have been identified. If so, the patient is expeditiously packaged and transported to the closest *appropriate* facility. Definitive care for severe, uncontrolled internal hemorrhage cannot be provided in the field, and surgery is usually required. Interventions such as direct pressure on a bleeding wound and infusion of intravenous fluids are not substitutes for rapid transportation to an appropriate facility with immediate surgical capabilities.

### Scene Assessment

In the prehospital setting, assessment of the patient actually begins before reaching the patient's side. As an EMS crew is dispatched to a scene, they begin to consider numerous factors that may play a role in caring for the patient, as well as ensuring their safety and that of the patient. These factors include such things as mechanism of injury, environmental conditions, and hazards present at the scene. The important aspects of this assessment can be divided into the following two key categories: safety and situation.

### Safety

Prehospital personnel must first evaluate the safety of the scene. EMS must not enter into a situation that puts their health and well-being at risk; to do otherwise puts them at risk of becoming patients as well. For example, EMS workers are dependent upon law enforcement personnel to ensure that the scene has been cleared of violent assailants and their weapons. In addition to their personal safety, the EMS providers need to consider concerns that threaten the safety of the patient. The scene of a traumatic incident may include dangers such as traffic, downed power lines, hazardous materials, and harsh environmental conditions. In light of incidents of terrorism there is heightened concern of chemical, biological, or nuclear contamination of a scene, or secondary devices planted with the intent of killing rescuers.

### Standard Precautions

One hazard ubiquitous to virtually all trauma scenes is blood. Blood and other body fluids may contain communicable diseases including hepatitis and human immunodeficiency viruses. In any patient encounter, healthcare workers are encouraged to employ measures to decrease the risk of contracting these pathogens. Standard precautions involve the use of impermeable gloves, gowns, masks, and goggles. In addition to wearing this protective gear, EMS providers must also exercise caution when handling sharp devices, such as needles that are contaminated with a patient's blood or body fluid.

### Situation

The second component of the scene assessment is evaluation of the situation. The EMS providers should consider the following issues: the number of patients and their ages; the need for specialized personnel or equipment (power company, heavy rescue); the need for additional EMS units, including summoning an air medical helicopter; the need for a physician at the scene to assist with triage; and the possibility that the traumatic event was triggered by a medical emergency (acute myocardial infarction or a cerebrovascular accident). Because the EMS personnel are essentially the "eyes and ears" of the emergency physician and trauma surgeon at the scene, they are in the position to observe key data about the mechanism of injury.

## Kinematics

A satisfactory understanding of the mechanism of injury assists in evaluating the patient for potential injuries (see Chap. 7). If the incident involves a motor vehicle crash, the EMS crew should evaluate the type of collision (frontal, rear, or lateral impact, etc.) and note the degree of damage to the vehicles. The location of the patient at the time of the crash and the use of restraints or protective gear is also valuable information. For penetrating trauma, the caliber of the weapon and distance from the assailant should be documented.

## Primary Survey (see Chap. 11)

After assessing the scene, EMS personnel perform a primary survey of the patient. As taught in ATLS, this survey serves to identify life-threatening or potentially life-threatening conditions. While it is taught in a stepwise A-B-C-D-E approach, one must remember that many aspects of this evaluation can be done simultaneously. EMS personnel employ a "treat as you go" philosophy, wherein care is initiated for life-threatening conditions as they are identified. Thus, the primary survey establishes a framework for setting priorities for management.

## Airway Management (see Chap. 12)

Management of the airway is given highest priority, but care must be taken not to aggravate a potential injury to the cervical spine. One EMS provider applies manual in-line stabilization to the head and neck while a coworker begins assessment and management of the airway. This stabilization of the cervical spine is continued until the patient is either completely immobilized on a long backboard or until it is determined that the patient does not require spinal immobilization.

All EMS providers, regardless of their level of training, must possess "essential skills" of airway management.[43] These skills include the following: manually clearing the patient's airway of foreign material; manually opening the airway using the trauma jaw thrust or trauma chin lift; suctioning the oropharynx; and inserting basic oral or nasal airways. An algorithm for prehospital management of the airway is provided (Fig. 8-1).[43]

## Endotracheal Intubation

Endotracheal intubation remains the "gold standard" to secure an airway in the prehospital setting. This skill is typically limited to advanced providers, though all levels of EMTs have now been taught to safely insert endotracheal tubes. The use of this technique is almost universally accepted at the EMT-P level throughout the United States. A limited number of communities have allowed EMT-Bs to be trained in endotracheal intubation. In most EMS systems, the success rate for endotracheal intubation exceeds 90%. The rate of eosphageal intubation has been demonstrated to be no greater than the in-hospital rate. With good, indirect medical control and field preceptors, training in endotracheal intubation can be successfully accomplished.[52]

Indications for endotracheal intubation in the field include the following:

Inability of patient to maintain an airway due to altered level of consciousness (Glasgow Coma Scale score <8)

Need for assisted ventilations

Threatened airway (e.g., respiratory burns, expanding hematoma of the neck)

Concern has arisen that endotracheal tubes placed in the prehospital setting may be misplaced or may become dislodged more commonly than previously believed.[53] Once endotracheal intubation has been performed, care should be taken to confirm proper placement using a combination of clinical assessments and adjunctive devices. The clinical assessments include presence of bilateral breath sounds and the absence of ventilatory sounds over the epigastrium, chest rise with ventilation, fogging of the endotracheal tube, and the provider watching the tube pass through the vocal cords. Adjuncts that help confirm a successful intubation include colorimetric $CO_2$ detectors, capnography, and the esophageal detector device.[54] Following intubation, the tube is carefully secured and its position checked each time the patient is moved. A recent publication suggests that continuous capnography in the prehospital setting may significantly reduce the incidence of misplaced or dislodged ET tubes.[55]

Because of the concern of potential fractures of the cervical spine, endotracheal intubation should be performed concurrently with in-line stabilization of the cervical spine.[56,57] While intubation is most commonly accomplished via the orotracheal route using a laryngoscope, other techniques can be utilized. These include blind nasotracheal intubation, digital intubation, and retrograde intubation.[58-60]

## Dual-Lumen Airways

Dual-lumen airways are devices that are inserted blindly through the mouth. Once in proper position, the EMT ventilates through each of the two lumens in order to determine whether the tube passed down the esophagus or into the trachea. Ventilations are then administered through the port that allows passage of air into the trachea. The two dual-lumen devices that are currently marketed are the pharyngotracheal lumen (PtL) airway (Gettig Pharmaceutical Instrument Company, Spring Hills, PA) and the Combitube (Nellcor, Typo Healthcare, Pleasanton, CA). Because of their design and the blind insertion, minimal training is necessary to achieve competency. This airway is a reasonable option when the EMS provider lacks the training to perform endotracheal intubation or when attempts at endotracheal intubation have proven unsuccessful.

## Laryngeal Mask Airway

The laryngeal mask airway (LMA) (LMA North America, San Diego, CA) consists of an inflatable silicone ring attached to a silicone tube. This device is blindly inserted into the hypopharynx so that the ring seals around the glottic opening. Ventilation is

# AIRWAY MANAGEMENT

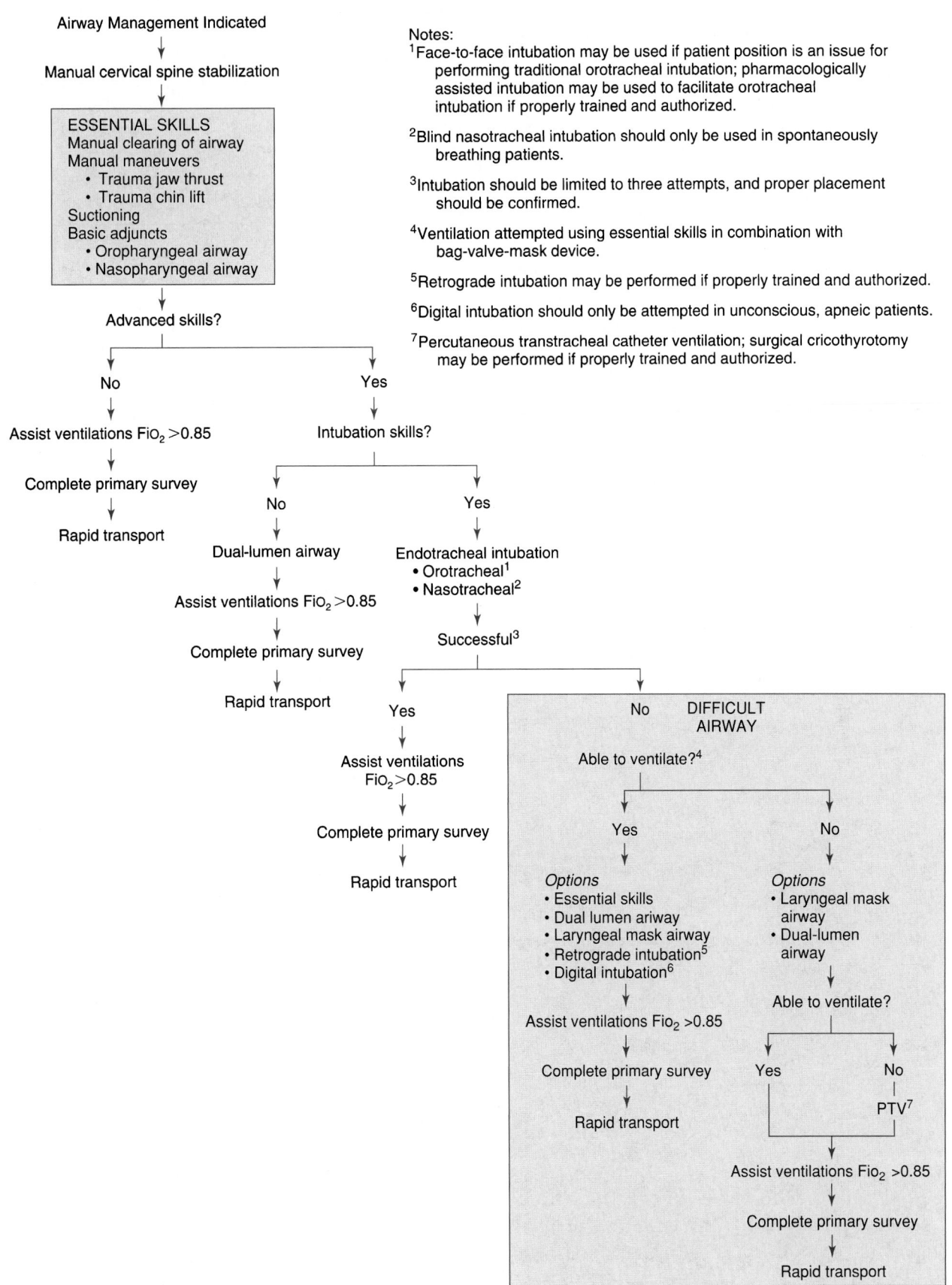

Notes:
[1] Face-to-face intubation may be used if patient position is an issue for performing traditional orotracheal intubation; pharmacologically assisted intubation may be used to facilitate orotracheal intubation if properly trained and authorized.

[2] Blind nasotracheal intubation should only be used in spontaneously breathing patients.

[3] Intubation should be limited to three attempts, and proper placement should be confirmed.

[4] Ventilation attempted using essential skills in combination with bag-valve-mask device.

[5] Retrograde intubation may be performed if properly trained and authorized.

[6] Digital intubation should only be attempted in unconscious, apneic patients.

[7] Percutaneous transtracheal catheter ventilation; surgical cricothyrotomy may be performed if properly trained and authorized.

**FIGURE 8-1.** Airway management.
*(Reproduced with permission from Salomone JP, Pons PT, McSwain NE, eds: PHTLS: Prehospital Trauma Life Support, 6th ed. St. Louis: Mosby, 2007, p. 125.)*

then provided through the tube. This device has replaced endotracheal intubation for general anesthesia in a significant percentage of shorter operations, especially in Great Britain. The risk of aspiration is higher than with endotracheal intubation; however, a newer model, the intubating LMA, allows passage of a tube into the trachea without the use of a laryngoscope. The LMA requires less training to achieve satisfactory competency. It is gradually gaining acceptance for EMS personnel who are not trained in intubation or as a backup airway when endotracheal intubation fails.[61]

## PERCUTANEOUS TRANSTRACHEAL VENTILATION

Percutaneous transtracheal ventilation (PTV) involves the insertion of a large-bore needle through the cricothyroid membrane and connecting it to high-pressure oxygen. The lungs are then insufflated periodically. This technique possesses the following advantages: it does not require paralysis; is less invasive than surgical cricothyroidotomy; affords easy access and insertion; and requires minimal education and very basic equipment. The technique has been demonstrated experimentally to be safe and effective even in the presence of complete obstruction of the airway.[62] While oxygenation is adequate, studies have shown that the patient may become hypercarbic. PTV is indicated when an injured patient is unable to be intubated and cannot be ventilated using a bag-mask-valve device, an LMA, or a dual-lumen airway.

### Surgical Cricothyroidotomy

Surgical cricothyroidotomy involves incising the skin and the cricothyroid membrane, followed by the insertion of a small endotracheal or tracheostomy tube. Because it is highly invasive, complications have included significant hemorrhage and injury to adjacent nerves, blood vessels, and the larynx. Aeromedical crews have utilized surgical cricothyroidotomy in the prehospital setting for several years.[63]

Groups from Indianapolis and Tucson have reported on the experience with this procedure when performed by ground ambulance crews.[64,65] Although these authors concluded that surgical cricothyroidotomy could be safely performed by paramedics assigned to ground units, many experts have argued that the procedure was excessively utilized. In the studies, between 10 and 20% of the total field airways were surgical, and, of these, 20 to 25% were performed as the *initial* technique of airway management. Well-trained aeromedical crews who have been allowed to perform this skill have demonstrated a much smaller need. In systems with tight medical control, EMS providers could consider this procedure when faced with the "can't intubate, can't ventilate" situation.

### Rapid Sequence Intubation

Many services now are allowing EMS providers to perform rapid sequence intubation (RSI). This involves the administration of a sedating agent and a neuromuscular block to facilitate endotracheal intubation. In skilled hands, this technique can aid effective airway control in patients when other methods fail or are otherwise unacceptable (e.g., the patient with trismus). The role of RSI in the prehospital setting is controversial, primarily because of the risks of losing a partially patent airway by administering a paralytic agent.

Several studies have documented that, with adequate medical control, EMS personnel can safely perform this procedure.[66–68] Data from a case-control study demonstrated an interesting paradox. While paramedics using RSI had a higher success rate at performing endotracheal intubation, the patients with suspected severe traumatic brain injury (TBI) intubated with RSI had a higher mortality than did those in the control group.[69] Davis et al. recently published the findings of an expert panel on the role of prehospital RSI.[70]

### Ventilatory Support

The patient's ventilatory status ("breathing") is next examined. If the patient's ventilatory rate is 10 or less, ventilations should be assisted with a bag-valve-mask (BVM) device connected to 100% oxygen. The tidal volume should be estimated if the patient is tachypneic. Rapid, shallow breaths indicate inadequate minute ventilation and require assistance with a BVM. Auscultation of breath sounds should be performed during the primary survey if the patient has an abnormal ventilatory rate. Most patients who have suffered an injury benefit from supplemental oxygen. Pulse oximetry should be monitored, and oxygen administered to maintain an $Spo_2 \geq 95\%$.

Prehospital care providers must exercise caution while providing ventilatory support, as deleterious effects may ensue. Hyperventilation by EMS personnel in one study was associated with increased mortality in patients with suspected TBI.[71] Additionally, data from animal models suggest that hyperventilation resulted in auto-PEEP (positive end-expiratory pressure) that further compromised the hemodynamic status of a hypovolemic swine.[72] For an adult patient, a reasonable tidal volume of 350–500 mL delivered at a rate of 10 breaths per minute is probably sufficient to maintain a satisfactory oxygen saturation while minimizing the risk of hyperventilation. Continuous pulse oximetry and capnography can help guide the ventilatory support.

### Circulation

Assessment of a patient's circulatory status involves examining for external hemorrhage and evaluating the adequacy of perfusion. Most life-threatening external hemorrhage can be controlled with direct pressure. If manpower is limited, a pressure dressing with gauze pads and an elastic bandage can be placed around an extremity. Should direct pressure alone not control bleeding in an extremity, a tourniquet should be applied just proximal to the site of hemorrhage and tightened until bleeding ceases. No published data documents any significant decrease in hemorrhage when a bleeding extremity is elevated, and such manipulation may result in the conversion of a closed fracture to an open one. The efficacy of applying pressure over "pressure points" in the axilla and groin has also not been studied in the prehospital setting and is labor-intensive. In the operating room, arterial tourniquets have been used safely for periods of 120–150 minutes. Options for a tourniquet include a blood pressure cuff, a cravat tied into a "Spanish windlass" or the use of a manufactured tourniquet.[73] A sample protocol for application of a tourniquet is shown (Fig. 8-2).

1. Attempt at direct pressure or pressure dressing must fail to control hemorrhage.

2. A commercially manufactured tourniquet, blood pressure cuff, or "Spanish windlass" is applied to the extremity just proximal to the bleeding wound.

3. The tourniquet is tightened until hemorrhage ceases, and then it is secured in place.

4. The time of tourniquet application is written on a piece of tape and secured to the tourniquet ("TK 21:45" indicates that the tourniquet was applied at 9:45 PM)

5. The tourniquet should be left uncovered so that the site can be monitored for recurrent hemorrhage.

6. Pain management should be considered unless the patient is in Class III or IV shock.

7. The patient should ideally be transported to a facility that has surgical capability.

**FIGURE 8-2.** Protocol for tourniquet application. *(Reproduced with permission from Salomone JP, Pons PT, McSwain NE, eds: PHTLS: Prehospital Trauma Life Support, 6th ed. St. Louis: Mosby, 2007, p. 182.)*

Several topical hemostatic agents have been approved by the FDA. Studies conducted by the military have shown that a chitosan dressing and Zeolite product (derived from volcanic rock) to be the most effective, although the latter agent has been associated with thermal injury as a result of an exothermic reaction that takes place when the material comes in contact with water.[74–76]

Perfusion is assessed primarily by evaluating pulse rate and quality, skin color, temperature, and moisture; however, prolonged capillary refill time may add further evidence that the patient is in shock. Time should not be taken in the primary survey to measure blood pressure. Even mild tachycardia (heart rate >100/minute) should always make one consider that the injured patient is hypovolemic. Significant tachycardia (>120/minute), weak peripheral pulses, and anxiety are associated with loss of 30 to 40% of the blood volume of an adult.[50]

## Traumatic Cardiopulmonary Arrest

Trauma patients who are found in cardiopulmonary arrest require special consideration. Unlike cardiopulmonary arrest associated with an acute myocardial infarction, most patients who suffer cessation of their vital signs prior to the arrival of EMS have exsanguinated. Cardiopulmonary resuscitation (CPR), defibrillation, antidysrhythmic medications, and crystalloid resuscitation will not reverse this. Attempts at resuscitation are typically futile and place the EMS personnel at unnecessary risk from automobile crashes during emergency transport and exposure to blood. The National Association of EMS Physicians and the ACSCOT have collaborated on a position paper that endorses the following guidelines[77]:

For victims of blunt trauma, resuscitation efforts may be withheld if the patient is pulseless and apneic upon the arrival of EMS.

For victims of penetrating trauma, resuscitation efforts may be withheld if there are no signs of life (papillary reflexes, spontaneous movement, or organized cardiac rhythm on the electrocardiogram greater than 40/minute).

Resuscitation efforts are not indicated when the patient has sustained an obviously fatal injury (such as decapitation) or when evidence exists of dependent lividity, rigor mortis, and decomposition.

Termination of resuscitation should be considered in trauma patients with an EMS-witnessed cardiopulmonary arrest and 15 minutes of unsuccessful resuscitation including CPR.

Termination of resuscitation should be considered for a patient with traumatic scardiopulmonary arrest who would require transport of greater than 15 minutes to reach an emergency department or trauma center.

Victims of drowning, lightning strike, or hypothermia, or those in whom the mechanism of injury does not correlate with the clinical situation (suggesting a nontraumatic cause) deserve special consideration before a decision is made to withhold or terminate resuscitation.

## Disability

During the primary survey, the EMS provider assesses neurologic function by evaluating the patient's Glasgow Coma Scale (GCS) score and pupillary response. The GCS score comprises three components including eyes, verbal, and motor.[78] If a painful stimulus is required to complete the assessment, the EMT can either apply pressure to the nail bed or squeeze the axillary tissue. If the patient has an altered level of consciousness (GCS <15), pupillary response to light is assessed. Any belligerent, combative, or uncooperative patient should be considered to be hypoxic or have a traumatic brain injury until proven otherwise. In a trauma patient, a GCS score of ≤13, seizure activity, or a motor or sensory deficit are all reasons for concern.

## Exposure and Environmental Control

The final part of the primary survey involves a quick scan of the patient's body to note any other potentially life-threatening injuries. In general, this requires removal of the patient's clothes, but environmental conditions and the presence of bystanders may make this impractical. Hypothermia from failure to preserve body heat can contribute to a serious coagulopathy in the trauma patient.

Heavy, dark colored woolen clothing may absorb significant amounts of blood. On occasion, patients may have more than one mechanism of injury; that is, blunt trauma from a motor vehicle crash that occurred while trying to flee the assailant who had shot them. Injuries cannot be treated unless they are identified.

## RESUSCITATION

Upon completion of the primary survey, the EMS provider determines whether or not the patient is critical (Fig. 8-3). Because the primary survey involves a "treat as you go" philosophy, airway management, ventilatory support, and control of external hemorrhage are initiated as the problems are identified. When a critically injured patient is identified (Table 8-1), scene time should ideally be less than 10 minutes.

If indicated, spinal immobilization should be performed expeditiously and the patient moved to the ambulance. Time is not taken to splint each individual fracture. For the critically injured patient, immobilization to the long backboard provides satisfactory immobilization of potential musculoskeletal injuries.

Because definitive care cannot be provided to the critically injured patient in the field, EMS personnel must realize that initiation of transport to the closest appropriate facility demonstrates good judgment. Trauma patients with abnormal physiology (altered vital signs) and those who meet specific anatomic injury criteria are best cared for in a recognized trauma center (see "Trauma Systems," Chap. 4). Protocols should be written so that EMS personnel may bypass a closer hospital in order to take a patient with life-threatening injuries to a trauma center.

## Fluid Therapy

Infusions of crystalloid solutions and blood transfusion are the mainstays of therapy for the in-hospital treatment of severe hypovolemic shock. Because it requires refrigeration and typing, blood is not available in the prehospital environment. Isotonic crystalloid solutions, such as lactated Ringer's or normal saline (0.9% sodium chloride), can be used for volume resuscitation. Although hypertonic saline (7.5% sodium chloride) initially showed promise, a meta-analysis of several studies failed to demonstrate an improvement in survival rates compared to those patients treated with isotonic solutions.[79]

En route to the receiving facility, the EMS providers should insert two large-bore (14- or 16-gauge) intravenous catheters in

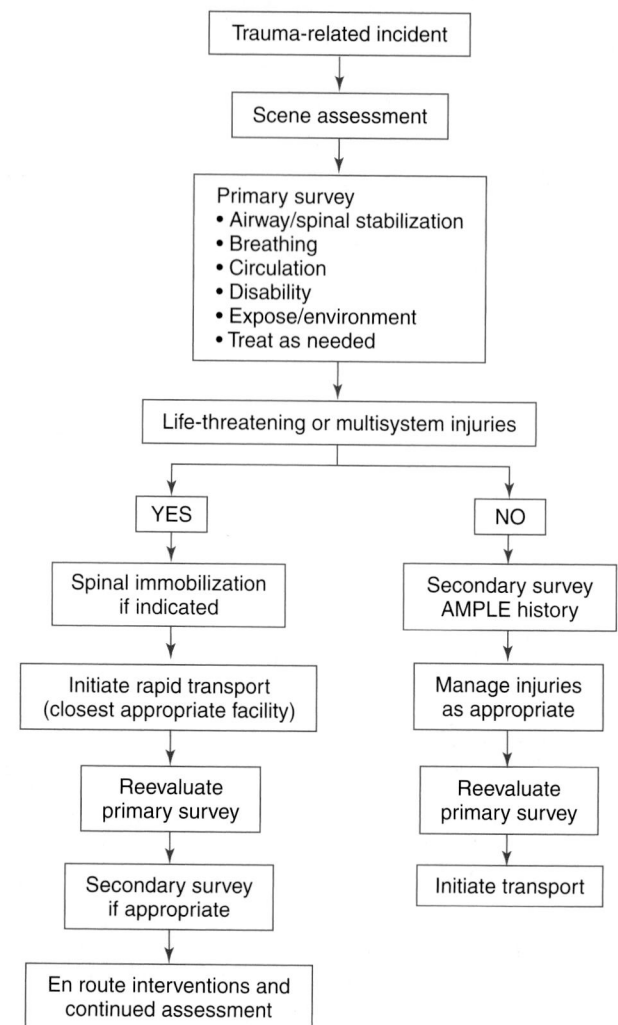

**FIGURE 8-3.**  Prehospital care overview.
*(Reproduced with permission from Salomone JP, Pons PT, McSwain NE, eds: PHTLS: Prehospital Trauma Life Support, 6th ed. St. Louis: Mosby, 2007, p. 488.)*

veins of the forearm or antecubital area. If possible, lactated Ringer's solution (or normal saline) should be warmed (102°F [38.8°C]) prior to administration. Fluid resuscitation in the prehospital setting must be based upon the clinical scenario.[43] If the patient has suspected uncontrolled hemorrhage in the thorax, abdomen, or retroperitoneum, fluid infusions should be titrated to maintain a systolic blood pressure (SBP) in the range of 80–90 mm Hg (mean arterial pressure of 60 to 65 mm Hg) in the hope of perfusing vital organs while limiting the risk of increased, uncontrollable internal hemorrhage. If the patient has a suspected injury to the central nervous system injury (TBI or injury to spinal cord), intravenous fluids should be administered at a rate sufficient to maintain the SBP at 90 mm Hg. If the patient has identifiable shock that resulted from external hemorrhage that has been controlled, a 1- to 2-L bolus of fluid should be infused as rapidly as possible and fluid titrated to maintain a normal pulse rate and blood pressure. If the patient again becomes hypotensive, further intravenous fluids should be titrated to maintain a systolic blood pressure in the range of 80 to 90 mm Hg.

Controversy exists regarding the role of therapy with intravenous fluids in the prehospital setting. No published study has

## TABLE 8-1

### Critical Trauma Patient

Limit scene time to 10 min or less when any of the following life-threatening conditions are present:

Inadequate or threatened airway

Impaired ventilation as demonstrated by the following:

Abnormally fast or slow ventilatory rate

Hypoxia (Spo$_2$ <95% even with supplemental oxygen)

Dyspnea

Open pnemothorax or flail chest

Suspected pneumothorax

Significant external hemorrhage or suspected internal hemorrhage

Abnormal neurologic status

GCS score ≤13

Seizure activity

Ssensory or motor deficit

Penetrating trauma to the head, neck, or torso. or proximal to the elbow and knee in the extremities

Amputation or near amputation proximal to the fingers or toes

Any trauma in the presence of the following:

History of serious medical conditions (e.g., coronary artery disease, chronic obstructive pulmonary disease, bleeding disorder)

Age >55

Hypothermia

Burns

Pregnancy

From: Salomone JP, Pons PT, Mcswain Ne (eds): Phtls: Prehospital Trauma Life Support, 6th ed. St. Louis: Mosby, 2007, p. 101.

ever demonstrated an improvement in survival resulting from the prehospital administration of fluids. One computer model of prehospital fluid therapy suggested that intravenous therapy is potentially beneficial when all of the following occur: (a) the bleeding rate is initially 25 to 100 mL/min; (b) the prehospital time exceeds 30 minute; and (c) the intravenous infusion rate is approximately equal to the bleeding rate.[80]

Opponents of prehospital fluid therapy cite data from animal models of uncontrolled internal hemorrhage. In these studies, attempts to improve blood pressure with crystalloid infusions have resulted in increased blood loss and mortality.[81–84] Data from a prospective, randomized prehospital trial of intravenous fluid therapy in patients with penetrating torso trauma found an improved outcome when intravenous fluids were withheld until operative control of hemorrhage was obtained.[85] Unfortunately, there were long delays until operation was performed in this study.

Although further studies will be needed to clarify this issue, EMS providers should never delay transport simply to initiate intravenous therapy. While one agent has progressed to a clinical trial in the civilian prehospital setting, no blood substitute has yet been approved for routine use by the FDA.

## SECONDARY SURVEY

Secondary survey refers to a more thorough history and physical examination. For the patient with life-threatening conditions identified in the primary survey, the EMS provider performs the secondary survey when those conditions have been addressed and are stable or improving and the patient is being transported. If the primary survey fails to indicate that the injured patient is critical, then the provider proceeds on to the secondary survey.

### AMPLE History

This brief history from the patient or family includes the following:

Allergies to medications

Prescription or over-the-counter Medications

Pertinent Past medical history

Last eaten

Recall of Events leading up to the injury

### Head-to-Toe Survey

This complete physical examination begins with obtaining a complete set of vital signs. Injuries to the head, neck, chest, abdomen, pelvis, and extremities are noted. The patient is then turned using the logroll maneuver, if spinal injury is suspected, and the patient's back is examined. Finally, a neurologic examination that involves reassessing the GCS score, pupillary reaction, and motor and sensory functions in the extremities is completed.

## SPECIFIC CONDITIONS

### Head Trauma

**Scalp Wounds.** Because of the high concentration of blood vessels in the skin and soft tissues of the face and neck, even a small wound can result in serious external hemorrhage. EMS providers and other healthcare workers often fail to appreciate that patients with a complex scalp wound may bleed sufficiently to develop shock. A compression dressing created with gauze pads and an elastic bandage often provides satisfactory control of hemorrhage.

### Traumatic Brain Injury

Traumatic brain injury (TBI) remains one of the leading causes of mortality in injured patients. Secondary brain injury refers to the extension of the original injury and may result from numerous causes. These include hypoxia, hypo- and hypercapnia, anemia, hypotension, hypo- and hyperglycemia, seizures, and intracranial hypertension as the result of edema or mass effect. Optimal prehospital care of the patient with TBI involves preventing secondary brain injury, maintaining cerebral perfusion pressure (mean arterial pressure minus intracranial pressure), and expeditious transfer to a facility capable of caring for the injury.

Patients with severe TBI may be unable to control their airway, and endotracheal intubation should be considered for patients with a GCS score of 8 or less. In one retrospective study, prehospital intubation was associated with a lower mortality in patients with TBI.[86] Ventilatory support should be administered and the patient maintained eucapneic as prophylactic hyperventilation is no longer indicated.[87,88] Blood loss should be minimized by controlling external sources and splinting fractures as appropriate. Because of the risk of

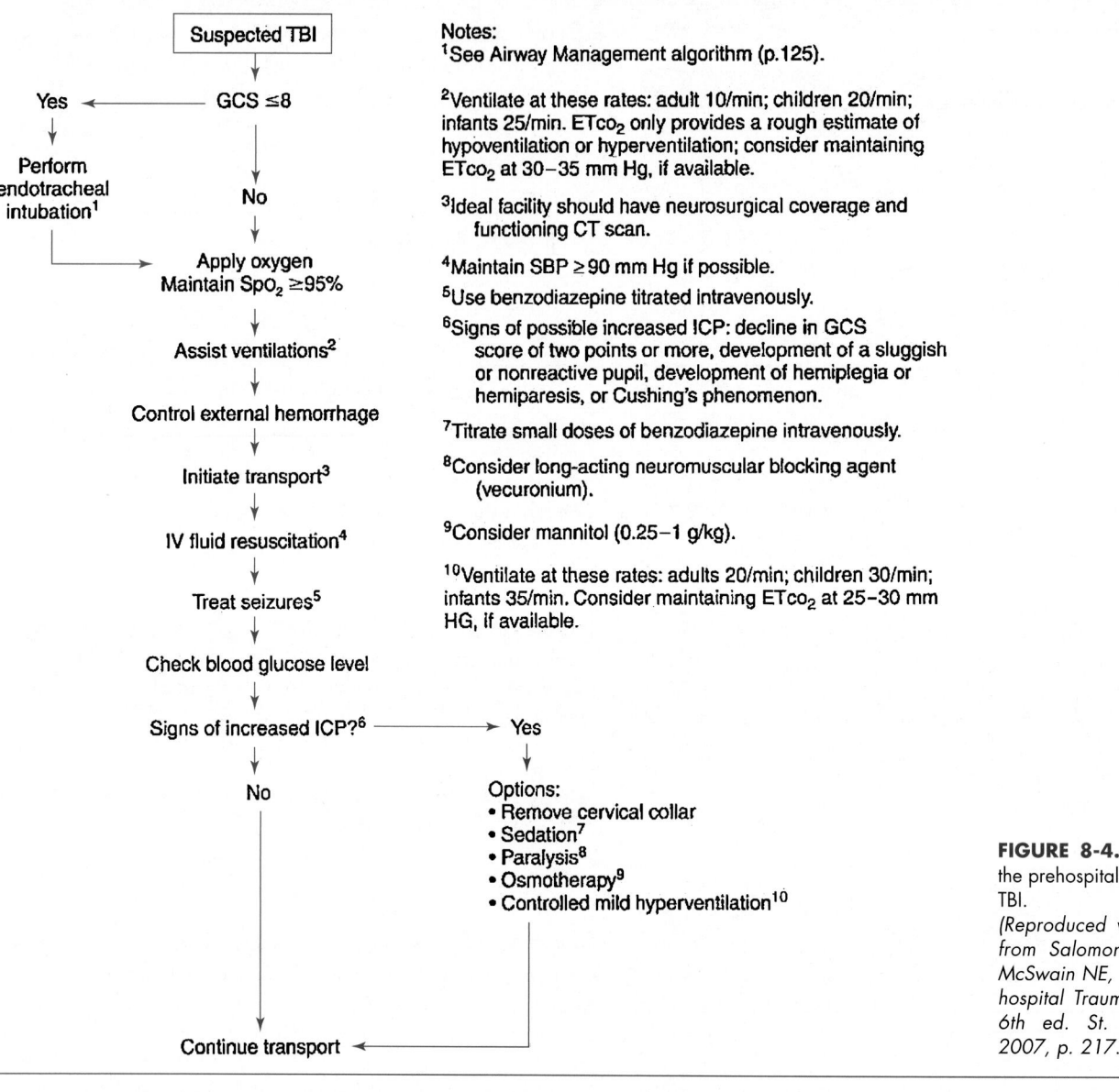

Notes:
[1]See Airway Management algorithm (p.125).

[2]Ventilate at these rates: adult 10/min; children 20/min; infants 25/min. ETco$_2$ only provides a rough estimate of hypoventilation or hyperventilation; consider maintaining ETco$_2$ at 30–35 mm Hg, if available.

[3]Ideal facility should have neurosurgical coverage and functioning CT scan.

[4]Maintain SBP ≥ 90 mm Hg if possible.

[5]Use benzodiazepine titrated intravenously.

[6]Signs of possible increased ICP: decline in GCS score of two points or more, development of a sluggish or nonreactive pupil, development of hemiplegia or hemiparesis, or Cushing's phenomenon.

[7]Titrate small doses of benzodiazepine intravenously.

[8]Consider long-acting neuromuscular blocking agent (vecuronium).

[9]Consider mannitol (0.25–1 g/kg).

[10]Ventilate at these rates: adults 20/min; children 30/min; infants 35/min. Consider maintaining ETco$_2$ at 25–30 mm HG, if available.

**FIGURE 8-4.** Algorithm for the prehospital management of TBI.
*(Reproduced with permission from Salomone JP, Pons PT, McSwain NE, eds: PHTLS: Prehospital Trauma Life Support, 6th ed. St. Louis: Mosby, 2007, p. 217.)*

an associated injury to the spine, patients with suspected TBI should undergo spinal immobilization. Intravenous fluids should be initiated en route to the receiving facility with a goal of maintaining the systolic blood pressure of at least 90 mm Hg. During prolonged transport, blood glucose can be monitored and dextrose administered if the patient is hypoglycemic. Benzodiazepines are appropriate for control of seizures, but they should be carefully titrated intravenously because of the risk of hypotension and respiratory depression.

Intracranial hypertension may cause cerebral herniation and brain death, but it cannot be measured in the prehospital setting. Signs of possible intracranial hypertension include the following: a decline in the GCS score of 2 points or more; development of a sluggish or nonreactive pupil; development of hemiplegia or hemiparesis; or Cushing's phenomena (bradycardia associated with arterial hypertension). An algorithm for the prehospital management of TBI has been developed (Fig. 8-4).[43]

## Thoracic Trauma (see Chaps. 26–29)

Flail Chest and Pulmonary Contusion.   In the prehospital setting, the administration of oxygen and ventilatory support are the primary therapies for a flail chest and suspected pulmonary contusion. Oxygen saturation should be kept at 95% or higher, ventilations should be assisted, and endotracheal intubation considered if the patient's tidal volume appears inadequate.

Tension Pneumothorax.   Tension pneumothorax should be suspected whenever the following three criteria are identified: increasing respiratory distress or difficulty ventilating with a BVM device; decreased or absent breath sounds; and hemodynamic compromise. Needle decompression of the pleural space can be life-saving.[43,89] The intravenous catheter inserted should be left in place; there is no need, however, to create a one-way ("flutter") valve as any air exchange through the catheter is clinically insignificant.

Open Pneumothorax.   An open pneumothorax should be sealed with an occlusive dressing. One of the four sides of the dressing can be left untaped so that air can decompress from the pleural space as needed. After an occlusive dressing has been applied to an open pneumothorax, any signs of a developing tension pneumothorax should prompt the EMS worker to remove the dressing.

**Pericardial Tamponade.** Pericardial tamponade is generally encountered following penetrating trauma to the heart; however, it may be a complication of a blunt cardiac rupture. In the prehospital setting, the classic symptoms of Beck's triad (elevated venous pressure, muffled heart tones, and hemodynamic compromise) may be difficult to identify. While some EMS systems permit ALS personnel to perform pericardiocentesis if pericardial tamponade is suspected, the emphasis should be placed on transporting that patient with a suspected tamponade to a facility that has immediate surgical capabilities.

## Abdominal Trauma (see Chaps. 30–40)

**Intra-Abdominal Hemorrhage.** In the absence of an obvious sign such as a bullet wound, intra-abdominal hemorrhage is difficult to identify in the prehospital setting, especially in the unconscious trauma patient. Unexplained hypovolemic shock should lead the EMS provider to suspect this condition. Management involves rapid transport to a facility that offers immediate operative intervention.

The pneumatic antishock garment (PASG) can be considered if the patient is hypotensive (systolic blood pressure <90 mm Hg), especially if the transport time is prolonged.[43,90,91] Research by Mattox et al. suggests that this device does not improve outcome in the urban setting where rapid transport to a trauma center is available. Their study was limited to patients with penetrating trauma, and those with a wound to the chest clearly had a worse outcome.[92] Other studies in New York and San Francisco, as well as the article by Mattox et al. from Houston, have demonstrated a beneficial effect in patients with severe hypotension (blood pressure less than 50 mm Hg).[93,94] No data exist regarding its use in prolonged transport as would be seen in suburban or rural settings.

**Pelvic Fractures (see Chap. 38).** The presence of a severe pelvic fracture may be suspected if the EMS provider finds instability on examination of the pelvis, especially if the patient has evidence of hypovolemic shock. The PASG may help tamponade bleeding in this setting.[43,90,95]

**Pregnancy (see Chap. 40).** Prehospital management of the injured pregnant patient focuses on adequately resuscitating the mother, especially if shock is present. In the third trimester, pregnant individuals may exhibit hypotension while lying supine due to compression of the inferior vena cava by the uterus. Supine hypotension is treated by gently rolling the mother into the left lateral decubitus position or, if immobilized on a long backboard, placing sufficient padding under the right side of the board to elevate it 30° or so. If hypotension does not correct with this measure, hemorrhagic shock should be suspected. Oxygen should be administered, and the patient transported to a facility that has both trauma and obstetrical capabilities.

## Spinal Trauma (see Chap. 24)

An algorithm has been developed that details the indications for spinal immobilization in the prehospital setting (Fig. 8-5).[43,96] Patients with penetrating trauma to the torso almost never have an unstable vertebral column.[97] Therefore, spinal immobilization is indicated in the setting of penetrating trauma only when the patient has a neurologic complaint or finding. In patients with blunt trauma, spinal immobilization should be performed if the patient has an altered level of consciousness (GCS score <15) or if spinal pain or tenderness, a neurologic deficit or complaint, or an anatomic deformity of the spine is present. In the absence of these findings, the mechanism of injury should be evaluated. If the mechanism is considered to be concerning, the patient should be evaluated for evidence of alcohol or drug intoxication, presence of a distracting injury, or the inability to communicate. If any of these are present, spinal immobilization should be performed. In their absence, spinal immobilization is not indicated.

## Musculoskeletal Trauma (see Chaps. 42–44)

**Hemorrhage.** Hemorrhage is the only immediately life-threatening condition associated with trauma to an extremity. External hemorrhage should be controlled with direct pressure or a pressure dressing, followed by a tourniquet if these measures fail. Internal hemorrhage is best managed in the field by immobilization of the extremity. In the critically injured patient, immobilization to a long backboard is sufficient stabilization. If the patient does not have life-threatening injuries, time can be taken to splint each suspected fracture individually. A traction splint provides reasonable pain control and will stabilize a suspected fracture of the femur.

**Amputation.** The ACSCOT has published guidelines for the management of amputated parts.[98] These include the following:

Cleansing the amputated part by gentle rinsing with lactated Ringer's solution

Wrapping the part in sterile gauze moistened with lactated Ringer's solution and placing it in a plastic bag

Labeling the bag or container and placing it in an outer container filled with crushed ice

The part should not be allowed to freeze, and it should be transported along with the patient to the closest appropriate facility.

**Pain Control.** Analgesics are indicated for an isolated injury to an extremity, but not in a patient with multisystem trauma.[43,99,100] After appropriately splinting the extremity, small doses of narcotics, titrated intravenously, may help relieve pain. The patient should be observed for side effects including hypotension and respiratory depression. Narcotics should not be administered in the trauma patient who exhibits signs of shock or when the patient appears to be under the influence of drugs and alcohol.

## TRIAGE

Disasters may be the result of natural phenomena, such as tornadoes, hurricanes, and earthquakes, or man-made in the case of a building collapse or terrorist event. When situations such as these occur, the EMS and healthcare systems must try to match their resources with the needs of the community. A *multiple-patient incident* refers to a situation where numerous individuals may be injured, but the EMS system possesses the ability to provide adequate care. In a *mass casualty incident*, the number of injured patients overwhelms the resources of the community, and additional aid from other locations is required. The number of patients involved in each of these circumstances may vary, depending upon the size of the EMS system and the resources of the community.

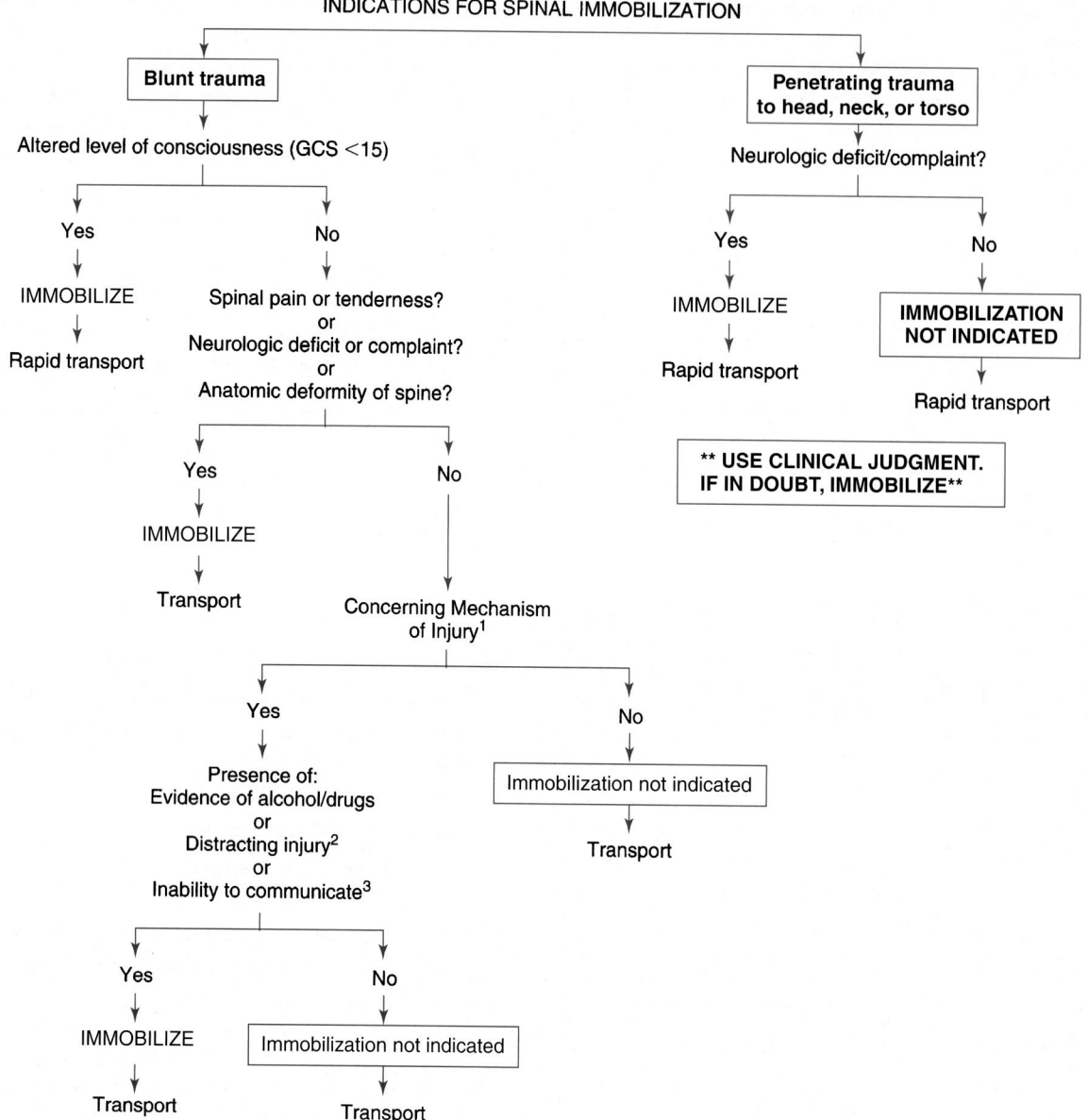

**FIGURE 8-5.** Indications for spinal immobilization.
*(Reproduced with permission from Salomone JP, Pons PT, McSwain NE, eds: PHTLS: Prehospital Trauma Life Support, 6th ed. St Louis: Mosby, 2007, p. 235.)*

Notes:
[1]Concerning Mechanisms of Injury
• Any mechanism that produced a violent impact to the head, neck, torso, or pelvis (e.g., assault, entrapment in structural collapse, etc.)
• Incidents producing sudden acceleration, deceleration, or lateral bending forces to the neck or torso (e.g., moderate- to high-speed (MVC), pedestrian struck, involvement in an explosion, etc.)
• Any fall, especially in the elderly persons
• Ejection or fall from any motorized or otherwise-powered transportation device (e.g., scooters, skateboards, bicycles, motor vehicles, motorcycles, or recreational vehicles)
• Victim of shallow-water diving incident

[2]Distracting Injury
  Any injury that may have the potential to impair the patient's ability to appreciate other injuries. Examples of distracting injuries include a) long-bone fracture; b) a visceral injury requiring surgical consultation; c) a large laceration, degloving injury, or crush injury; d) large burns, or e) any other injury producing acute functional impairment.
  (Adapted from Hoffman JR, Wolfson AB, Todd K., Mower WR: Selective cervical spine radiography in blunt trauma:methodology of the National Emergency X-Radiography Utilization Study [NEXUS], *Ann Emerg Med* 461, 1998.)

[3]Inability to communicate. Any patient who, for reasons not specified above, cannot clearly communicate so as to actively participate in their assessment. Examples: speech or hearing impaired, those who only speak a foreign language, and small children.

In either situation, EMS personnel and healthcare workers must employ the principles of triage in order that the most seriously injured patients receive care before those with minor injuries. A simple straightforward system that is easily taught has been developed to aid EMS providers in performing triage when faced with numerous injured patients.[43,101,102] A more comprehensive discussion of disaster care is presented in Chap. 9.

## PREHOSPITAL RESEARCH

Over the last decade the entire healthcare field has seen a growing trend toward evidence-based medicine. EMS, in general, and prehospital trauma care, specifically, are ripe for quality research to separate sound medical practice from conjecture. Management of the airway and fluid therapy are two areas that deserve intensive investigation in the prehospital setting. Far too few treatment protocols in EMS are based upon high-quality data. More commonly, protocols are written that include the biases of the authors and extrapolations from in-hospital care.

Several major obstacles to the development of quality EMS research exist.[103] Funding is woefully inadequate and integrated information systems are needed to link data on patient care with information on outcome. Few academic institutions possess a long-term commitment to EMS research. Governmental regulations regarding informed consent inhibit the conduct of research in the emergency situation, as well. Finally, EMS personnel lack an appreciation of the importance of research in their own field. As these challenges are overcome, new research will lead us to better care for our patients. NHTSA has published a document detailing numerous issues in prehospital care that are awaiting investigation.[104]

### TABLE 8-2

**Golden Principles of Prehospital Trauma Care**

1. Ensure the safety of the prehospital care providers and the patient
2. Assess the scene situation to determine the need for additional resources
3. Recognize the kinematics that produced the injuries
4. Use the primary survey approach to identify life-threatening conditions
5. Provide appropriate airway management while maintaining cervical spine stabilization
6. Support ventilation and deliver oxygen to maintain an $Spo_2 \geq 95\%$.
7. Control any significant external hemorrhage
8. Provide basic shock therapy, including restoring and maintaining normal body temperature and appropriately splinting musculoskeletal injuries
9. Consider the use of the pneumatic antishock garment for patients with decompensated shock (SBP <90 mm Hg).
10. Maintain manual spine stabilization until the patient is immobilized on a long backboard
11. For critically injured trauma patients, initiate transport to the closest appropriate facility within 10 min of arrival on scene
12. Initiate warmed, intravenous fluid replacement en route to the receiving facility
13. Ascertain the patient's medical history and perform a secondary survey when life-threatening conditions have been satisfactorily managed or have been rule out
14. Above all, do no further harm

*From: Salomone JP, Pons PT, Mcswain NE (eds): Phtls: Prehospital Trauma Life Support, 6th ed. St. Louis: Mosby, 2007, p. 489.*

## GOLDEN PRINCIPLES

In order for the injured patient to have the best chance of survival, there must be optimal prehospital care. A mere "scoop and run" by EMS personnel leaves the patient without support of vital functions during the transport to the hospital. Modern prehospital care involves the following:

Rapid assessment to identify life-threatening injuries

Key field interventions including management of the airway, ventilatory support with administration of oxygen, control of external hemorrhage, etc.

Rapid transport to the closest appropriate facility

The PHTLS program has summarized optimal prehospital trauma care into 14 golden principles (Table 8-2).[43] This approach to trauma care has been shown to improve the outcome of trauma victims. A study from Trinidad and Tobago compared the overall mortality of trauma patients following the introduction of PHTLS training with the period preceding PHTLS. The authors documented a decrease in mortality of about 33% following PHTLS training of EMS personnel.[105]

## REFERENCES

1. McSwain NE Jr: Pre-hospital care. In Feliciano DV, Moore EE, Mattox KL, eds. *Trauma*, 3rd ed. Stamford, CT: Appleton & Lange, 1996, p. 107.
2. Rockwood CA, Mann CM, Farrington JD, et al.: History of emergency medical services in the United States. *J Trauma* 16:299, 1976.
3. National Academy of Sciences(National Research Council: *Accidental Death and Disability: The Neglected Disease of Modern Society.* Rockville, MD: U.S. Department of Health, Education, and Welfare, 1966.
4. Pantridge JF, Adgey AA: Prehospital coronary care: The mobile coronary care unit. *Am J Cardiol* 24:666, 1969.
5. Border JR, Lewis FR, Aprahamian C, et al.: Panel: Prehospital trauma care—stabilize or scoop and run. *J Trauma* 23:708, 1983.
6. Trunkey DD: Is ALS necessary for pre-hospital trauma care? *J Trauma* 24:86, 1984.
7. Gervin AS, Fischer RP: The importance of prompt transport in salvage of patients with penetrating heart wounds. *J Trauma* 22:443, 1982.
8. Smith JP, Bodai BI, Hill AS, et al.: Prehospital stabilization of critically injured patients: A failed concept. *J Trauma* 25:65, 1985.
9. Ivatury RR, Nallathambi MN, Roberge RJ, et al.: Penetrating thoracic injuries: In-field stabilization vs. prompt transport. *J Trauma* 27:1066, 1987.
10. Jacobs LM, Sinclair A, Beiser A, et al.: Prehospital advanced life support: Benefits in trauma. *J Trauma* 24:8, 1984.
11. Pons PT, Honigman B, Moore EE, et al.: Prehospital advanced trauma life support for critical penetrating wounds to the thorax and abdomen. *J Trauma* 25:828, 1985.
12. Cwinn AA, Pons PT, Moore EE, et al.: Prehospital advanced trauma life support for critical blunt trauma victims. *Ann Emerg Med* 16:399, 1987.
13. Honigman B, Rohweder K, Moore EE, et al.: Prehospital advanced trauma life support for penetrating cardiac wounds. *Ann Emerg Med* 19:145, 1990.
14. *National Emergency Medical Services Education and Practice Blueprint.* Columbus, OH: National Registry of Emergency Medical Technicians, 1993.
15. U.S. Department of Transportation: *National Standard EMT—Basic Curriculum.* Washington, D.C.: U.S. Government Printing Office, 1994.
16. U.S. Department of Transportation: *National Standard EMT—Intermediate Curriculum.* Washington, D.C.: U.S. Government Printing Office, 1998.
17. U.S. Department of Transportation: *National Standard EMT—Paramedic Curriculum.* Washington, D.C.: U.S. Government Printing Office, 1998.
18. U.S. Department of Transportation, NHTSA: EMS education agenda for the future: A systems approach, available at www.nhtsa.dot.gov.
19. Dickison P, Hostler D, Platt TE, et al.: Program accreditation effect on paramedic credentialing examination success rate. *Prehosp Emerg Care* 10:224, 2006.
20. Mustalish AC, Post C: Appendix I: Scope and specificity of each component in EMS systems. In Kuehl AE, ed. *National Association of EMS Physicians: Prehospital Systems & Medical Oversight*, 2nd ed. St. Louis: Mosby Year Book, 1994, p. 24.
21. Giordana LM, Davidson SJ: Urban systems. In Kuehl AE, ed. *National Association of EMS Physicians: Prehospital Systems & Medical Oversight*, 2nd ed. St. Louis: Mosby Year Book, 1994, p. 35.

22. American College of Emergency Physicians, National Association of EMS Physicians and American College of Surgeons: Equipment for ambulances, 2006, available at www.facs.org/trauma/publications/ambulance.pdf

23. Neel S: Army aeromedical evacuation procedures in Vietnam: Implications for rural America. *JAMA* 204:99, 1968.

24. Fischer RP, Flynn TC, Miller PW, et al.: Urban helicopter response to the scene of injury. *J Trauma* 24:946, 1984.

25. Baxt WG, Moody P: The impact of a rotorcraft aeromedical emergency care service on trauma mortality. *JAMA* 249:3047, 1983.

26. Law DK, Law JK, Brennan R, et al.: Trauma operating room in conjunction with an air ambulance system: Indications, interventions, and outcomes. *J Trauma* 22:759, 1982.

27. Baxt WG, Moody P, Cleveland HC, et al.: Hospital-based rotorcraft aeromedical emergency care services and trauma mortality: A multicenter study. *Ann Emerg Med* 14:859, 1985.

28. Moront ML, Gotschall CS, Eichelberger MR: Helicopter transport of injured children: System effectiveness and triage criteria. *J Pediatr Surg* 31:1183, 1996.

29. Bartolacci RA, Munford BJ, Lee A, et al.: Air medical scene response to blunt trauma: Effect on early survival. *Med J Aust* 169:612, 1998.

30. Thomas SH, Harrison TH, Buras WR, et al.: Helicopter transport and blunt trauma mortality: A multicenter trial. *J Trauma* 52:136, 2002.

31. Cunningham P, Rutledge R, Baker CC, et al.: A comparison of the association of helicopter and ground transport with the outcome of injury in trauma patients transported from the scene. *J Trauma* 43:940, 1997.

32. Brathwaite CEM, Rosko M, McDowell R, et al.: A critical analysis of on-scene helicopter transport on survival in a statewide trauma system. *J Trauma* 45:140, 1998.

33. Schiller WR, Knox R, Zinnecker H, et al.: Effect of helicopter transport of trauma victims on survival in an urban trauma center. *J Trauma* 28:1127, 1988.

34. Schwartz RJ, Jacobs LM, Yaezel D: Impact of pre-trauma center care on length of stay and hospital charges. *J Trauma* 29:1611, 1989.

35. Diaz MA, Hendey GW, Bivins HG: When is the helicopter faster? A comparison of helicopter and ground ambulance transport times. *J Trauma* 58:148, 2005.

36. National Association of EMS Physicians: Air medical dispatch: Guidelines for trauma scene response. *Prehosp Disast Med* 7:75, 1992.

37. Urdaneta LF, Miller BK, Ringenberg BJ, et al.: Role of an emergency helicopter transport service in rural trauma. *Arch Surg* 122:992, 1987.

38. Boyd CR, Corse KM, Campbell RC: Emergency interhospital transport of the major trauma patient: Air versus ground. *J Trauma* 29:789, 1989.

39. Bledsoe BE, Smith MG: Medical helicopter accidents in the United States: A 10-year review. *J Trauma* 56:1325, 2004.

40. Swor RA, ed: *National Association of EMS Physicians: Quality Management in Prehospital Care.* St. Louis: Mosby Year Book, 1993.

41. National Highway Traffic Safety Administration: Public access, in *Emergency Medical Services: Agenda for the Future.* Washington, D.C.: U.S. Department of Transportation, 1996, p. 43.

42. Pons PT, Markovchick VJ: Eight minutes or less: Does the ambulance response time guideline impact trauma patient outcome? *J Emerg Med* 23:43, 2002.

43. Salomone JP, Pons PT, McSwain NE, eds: *PHTLS: Prehospital Trauma Life Support,* 6th ed. St. Louis: Mosby, 2007.

44. Demetriades D, Chan L, Cornwell E, et al.: Paramedic vs private transportation of trauma patients: Effect on outcome. *Arch Surg* 131:133, 1996.

45. McSwain NE Jr: EMS medical director. In McSwain NE Jr, Paturas JL, eds. *The Basic EMT: Comprehensive Prehospital Patient Care,* 2nd ed. St. Louis: Mosby Year Book, 2001, p. 42.

46. Holroyd BR, Knopp R, Kallsen G: Medical control: Quality assurance in prehospital care. *JAMA* 256:1027, 1986.

47. McSwain NE Jr: Medical control in prehospital care. *J Trauma* 24:172, 1984.

48. McSwain NE Jr: Indirect medical control. In Kuehl AE, ed. *National Association of EMS Physicians: Prehospital Systems & Medical Oversight,* 2nd ed. St. Louis: Mosby Year Book, 1994, p. 186.

49. Braun O: Direct medical control. In Kuehl AE, ed. *National Association of EMS Physicians: Prehospital Systems & Medical Oversight,* 2nd ed. St. Louis: Mosby Year Book, 1994, p. 196.

50. American College of Surgeons Committee on Trauma: *Advanced Trauma Life Support for Doctors,* 7th ed. Chicago: American College of Surgeons, 2004.

51. Campbell JE, ed: *Basic Trauma Life Support for Paramedics and Other Advanced Providers,* 5th ed. Upper Saddle River, NJ: Brady/Prentice Hall Health, 2004.

52. Stewart RP, Paris PM, Pelton GH, et al.: Effect of various training techniques on field endotracheal intubation success rates. *Ann Emerg Med* 13:1032, 1984.

53. Katz SH, Falk JL: Misplaced endotracheal tubes by paramedics in an urban emergency medical services system. *Ann Emerg Med* 31:32, 2001.

54. O'Connor RE, Swor RA: Verification of endotracheal tube placement following intubation. *Prehosp Emerg Care* 3:248, 1999.

55. Silvestri S, Ralls GA, Krauss B, et al.: The effectiveness of out-of-hospital use of continuous end-tidal carbon dioxide monitoring on the rate of unrecognized or misplaced intubations within a regional emergency medical services system. *Ann Emerg Med* 45:497, 2005.

56. Scannell G, Waxman K, Tominaga G, et al.: Orotracheal intubation in trauma patients with cervical fractures. *Arch Surg* 128:903, 1993.

57. Shatney CH, Brunner RD, Nguyen TQ: The safety of orotracheal intubation in patients with unstable cervical spine fracture or high spinal cord injury. *Am J Surg* 170:676, 1995.

58. Iserson KV: Blind nasotracheal intubation. *Ann Emerg Med* 10:468, 1981.

59. Hardwick WC, Bluhm D: Digital intubation. *J Emerg Med* 1:317, 1983.

60. McNamara RM: Retrograde intubation of the trachea. *Ann Emerg Med* 16:680, 1987.

61. Martin SE, Ochsner MG, Jarman RH, et al.: Use of the laryngeal mask airway in air transport when intubation fails. *J Trauma* 47:352, 1999.

62. Frame SB, Simon JM, Kerstein MD, et al.: Percutaneous transtracheal catheter ventilation (PTCV) in complete airway obstruction—A canine model. *J Trauma* 29:774, 1989.

63. Boyle MF, Hatton D, Sheets C: Surgical cricothyroidotomy performed by air ambulance flight nurses: A 5-year experience. *J Emerg Med* 11:41, 1993.

64. Jacobson LE, Gomez GA, Sobieray RJ, et al.: Surgical cricothyroidotomy in trauma patients: Analysis of its use by paramedics in the field. *J Trauma* 41:15, 1996.

65. Fortune JB, Judkins DG, Scanzaroli D, et al.: Efficacy of prehospital surgical cricothyroidotomy in trauma patients. *J Trauma* 42:832, 1997.

66. Hedges JR, Dronen SC, Feero S, et al.: Succinylcholine-assisted intubations in prehospital care. *Ann Emerg Med* 17:469, 1988.

67. Wayne MA, Friedland E: Prehospital use of succinylcholine: A 20-year review. *Prehosp Emerg Care* 3:107, 1999.

68. Ochs M, David D, Hoyt D, et al.: Paramedic-performed rapid sequence intubation of patients with severe head injuries. *Ann Emerg Med* 40:159, 2002.

69. Davis DP, Hoyt DB, Ochs M, et al.: The effect of paramedic rapid sequence intubation on outcome in patients with severe traumatic brain injury. *J Trauma* 54:444, 2003.

70. Davis DP, Fakhry SM, Wang HE, et al.: Paramedic rapid sequence intubation for severe traumatic brain injury: Perspectives from an expert panel. *Prehosp Emerg Care* 11:1, 2007.

71. Davis DP, Dunford JV, Poste JC, et al.: The impact of hypoxia and hyperventilation on outcome after paramedic rapid sequence intubation of severely head injured patients. *J Trauma* 57:1, 2004.

72. Pepe PE, Raedler C, Lurie KG: Emergency ventilatory management in hemorrhagic states: Elemental or detrimental? *J Trauma* 54:1048, 2003.

73. Walters TJ, Mabry RL: Use of tourniquets on the battlefield: A consensus panel report. *Mil Med* 170:770, 2005.

74. Pusateri AE, McCarthy S, Gregory KW, et al.: Effects of a chitosan-based hemostatic dressing on blood loss and survival in a model of severe venous hemorrhage and hepatic injury in swine. *J Trauma* 54:177, 2003.

75. Alam HB, Uy GB, Miller D, et al.: Comparative analysis of hemostatic agents in a swine model of lethal groin injury. *J Trauma* 54:1077, 2003.

76. McManus J, Hurtado T, Pusateri A, et al.: A case series describing thermal injury resulting from zeolite use for hemorrhage control in combat operations. *Prehosp Emerg Care* 11:67, 2007.

77. Hopson LR, Hirsch E, Delgado J, et al.: Guidelines for withholding or termination of resuscitation in prehospital traumatic cardiopulmonary arrest: Joint Position Statement of the National Association of EMS Physicians and the American College of Surgeons Committee on Trauma. *J Am Coll Surg* 196:106, 2003.

78. Teasdale G, Jennett B: Assessment of coma and impaired consciousness: A practical scale. *Lancet* 2:81, 1974.

79. Wade CE, Kramer GC, Grady JJ: Efficacy of hypertonic 7.5% saline and 6% dextran in treating trauma: A metaanalysis of controlled clinical trials. *Surgery* 122:609, 1997.

80. Lewis FR: Prehospital intravenous fluid therapy: Physiologic computer modeling. *J Trauma* 26:804, 1986.

81. Gross D, Landau EH, Assalia A, et al.: Is hypertonic saline resuscitation safe in "uncontrolled" hemorrhagic shock? *J Trauma* 28:751, 1988.

82. Gross D, Landau EH, Klin B, et al.: Quantitative measurement of bleeding following hypertonic saline therapy in "uncontrolled" hemorrhagic shock. *J Trauma* 29:79, 1989.

83. Krausz MM, Bar-Ziv M, Rabinovici R, et al.: "Scoop and run" or stabilize hemorrhagic shock with normal saline or small-volume hypertonic saline? *J Trauma* 33:6, 1992.

84. Craig RL, Poole GV: Resuscitation in uncontrolled hemorrhage. *Am Surg* 60:59, 1994.

85. Bickell WH, Wall MJ, Pepe PE, et al.: Immediate versus delayed fluid resuscitation for hypotensive patients with penetrating torso injuries. *N Engl J Med* 331:1105, 1994.

86. Winchell RJ, Hoyt DB: Endotracheal intubation in the field improves survival in patients with severe head injury. *Arch Surg* 132:592, 1997.

87. Muizelaar JP, Marmarou A, Ward JD, et al.: Adverse effects of prolonged hyperventilation in patients with severe brain injury: A randomized clinical trial. *J Neurosurg* 75:731, 1991.

88. Brain Trauma Foundation: *Guidelines for Prehospital Management of Traumatic Brain Injury.* New York: Brain Trauma Foundation, 2000, p. 39.

89. Eckstein M, Suyehara D: Needle thoracostomy in the prehospital setting. *Prehosp Emerg Care* 2:132, 1998.

90. McSwain NE Jr: Pneumatic anti-shock garment: State of the art 1988. *Ann Emerg Med* 17:506, 1988.

91. O'Connor RE, Domeier R: Use of the pneumatic antishock garment (PASG). *Prehosp Emerg Care* 1:36, 1997.

92. Mattox KL, Bickell W, Pepe PE, et al.: Prospective MAST study in 911 patients. *J Trauma* 29:1104, 1989.

93. Cayten CG, Berendt BM, Byren DW, et al.: A study of pneumatic antishock garments in severely hypotensive trauma patients. *J Trauma* 34:728, 1993.

94. Mackersie RC, Christensen JM, Lewis FR: The prehospital use of external counterpressure: Does MAST make a difference? *J Trauma* 24:882, 1984.

95. Richardson JD, Harty J, Amin M, et al.: Open pelvic fractures. *J Trauma* 22:533, 1982.

96. Domeier RM, National Association of EMS Physicians Standards and Clinical Practices Committee: Indications for prehospital spinal immobilization. *Prehosp Emerg Care* 3:251, 1997.

97. Cornwell EE, Chang DC, Bonar JP, et al.: Thoracolumbar immobilization for trauma patients with torso gunshot wounds: Is it necessary? *Arch Surg* 136:324, 2001.

98. Seyfer AE: *Guidelines for Management of Amputated Parts.* Chicago: American College of Surgeons, 1996.

99. White LJ, Cooper JD, Chambers RM, et al.: Prehospital use of analgesia for suspected extremity fractures. *Prehosp Emerg Care* 4:205, 2000.

100. Alonso-Serra HM, Wesley K: Prehospital pain management. *Prehosp Emerg Care* 7:482, 2003.

101. Arnold T, Cleary V, Groth S, et al.: *START.* Newport Beach, CA: Newport Beach Fire and Marine Department, 1994.

102. Risavi BL, Salen PN, Heller MB, et al.: A two-hour intervention using START improves prehospital triage of mass casualty incidents. *Prehosp Emerg Care* 5:197, 2001.

103. National Highway Traffic Safety Administration: EMS research, in *Emergency Medical Services: Agenda for the Future.* Washington, D.C.: U.S. Department of Transportation, 1996, p. 13.

104. U.S. Department of Transportation, NHTSA: National EMS research agenda, available at www.nhtsa.dot.gov.

105. Ali J, Adam RU, Gana TJ, et al.: Trauma patient outcome after the prehospital trauma life support program. *J Trauma* 42:1018, 1997.

# Commentary ■ H. SCOTT BJERKE

Surgeons, especially trauma surgeons, hold a special place in their hearts and minds for prehospital medical care. Historically, surgeons were the first paramedics and prehospital personnel, long before our profession was considered safe enough for admission into the "medical" fraternity as physicians. That pride of historical roots is most evident in the United Kingdom where, upon graduation, surgeons are no longer referred to as Doctor, but their title reverts back to Mister, as it was during our association with the Barber's and Surgeons Union. Upon the dissolution of the Union, the Barber's kept the red and white Barber's pole, but surgeons went on to develop ambulance transport systems in the Napoleonic Wars, write treatises on the cure for scurvy at sea and develop the art and science of surgical care in ever more technologically advanced hospitals and medical centers. Prehospital and emergency care is part of our genetic heritage as surgeons, and cannot be totally separated from our surgical souls.

As surgery has changed, so has prehospital medical care. Rapid assessment in the field, stabilization, triage, and safe transport without inflicting further damage was a surgeon's job in Napoleon's time but is now the province of the medic and paramedic. Prehospital care and management is a specific knowledge base that has taken on less importance in medical and surgical training as surgeons have become more facility-bound with our advancing technology. We have handed over the mantle of prehospital care to our medic and paramedic colleagues, who as the authors point out, at least in the United States, do a better job of maintaining those principles of rapid assessment, stabilization, and timely transport than we do as physicians under the same conditions. Physicians, no matter what their specialty, are no longer trained to function well in the prehospital setting as a primary part of their education. Prehospital care is a specific knowledge base and we as physicians will only be competent at it if we consciously add that specialized knowledge to our already extensive training. Like our patients and our colleagues in other specialties, we need to embrace our colleagues in the prehospital setting and not only participate in their education but also in their development

as professionals assisting with training, maintenance of training, oversight, and continuing education. We have passed on the actual mantle of prehospital care but we cannot relinquish the responsibility of participation and education in the development of those who now provide that service. If medicine had not recognized the "science" of surgery over 300 years ago we might still be teamed with the Barber's Union quibbling over ownership of the red and white pole.

The authors have succinctly and successfully taken the complex topic of prehospital care and explained, defined, and summarized the essential elements, as well as reminding us of our responsibilities to nurture and participate in the field. Well-trained professionals in the field, with continuing education and standardized certification with the guidance of physicians, will only improve our ability to provide the best of care to our patients and improve our profession. Though not yet well proven in a scientific sense, the communal sense of sharing of medical knowledge and expertise in the prehospital setting has captured the imagination of police departments, search and rescue providers, disaster planners, and even the Federal Government. Police SWAT teams now specially train medics (and occasionally physicians) to accompany them on warrants and raids to assure the quick availability of prehospital medical care for officers and civilian victims in urban combat like conditions. FEMA Urban Search and Rescue includes specialized medical training for medics, nurses, and physicians in disaster situations for both natural and man-made disasters while anti-terrorism teams include prehospital and medical personnel as advisors and consultants.

Prehospital care is evolving and advancing, and as surgeons we should be part of this development and evolution, not only because it enhances our patient outcomes but because it recognizes the continuity of medical care does not just start at the doors to the hospital but starts in homes, the workplace, and in specialized environments such as natural disasters and police interventions, and our medic and paramedic colleagues function as the first medical representatives the public sees before they arrive at the doors of our hospital institutions.

# Trauma Care in Mass Casualty Incidents

*Asher Hirshberg* ■ *Michael Stein*

## INTRODUCTION

Until recently, trauma care providers viewed a multiple or mass casualty incident (MCI) as a logistic and administrative problem that boils down to streamlining the flow of large numbers of patients through the emergency facilities of the hospital. The prevailing view was that care of the injured in these situations is essentially similar to normal daily practice, except for the need to perform triage and prioritize care.[1] It is therefore not surprising that the previous editions of this textbook did not dedicate a specific chapter to the trauma care aspects of MCIs.

This view has changed dramatically in the wake of 9/11 and the wave of urban terrorism that has been sweeping across the globe since the turn of the century. Today, trauma care providers know that regardless of the location, size, or trauma designation of their hospitals, a MCI is no longer a remote possibility but a palpable threat. At the same time, a series of large-scale natural disasters, particularly the tsunami in Southeast Asia in December 2004[2] and Hurricane Katrina which devastated New Orleans in August 2005,[3–5] focused public attention on the medical response to such catastrophes. Disaster planning and preparedness have become priorities, and trauma care providers are called upon to participate in these efforts in their institutions as well as at the regional and national levels.

A MCI presents a unique challenge to trauma systems because a large casualty load has a direct impact on the ability of the system to provide high-quality trauma care to the severely injured. Furthermore, urban terrorism confronts care providers with unusual injury patterns and unique clinical problems not seen in daily practice. Preparing for such incidents requires not only special planning and training but, more importantly, a different mindset.[6]

This chapter presents an overview of the medical response to MCIs *from the clinical perspective of a modern trauma system*. The aim is not to provide a comprehensive treatise on disaster medicine or hospital preparedness, but rather to focus on those aspects of the emergency response that directly affect patient care and are therefore particularly relevant for trauma care providers.

## GENERAL CONSIDERATIONS

### Goal of the Disaster Response

The common denominator of all MCIs and disasters is a discrepancy between a large number of casualties and the limited resources available to treat them. The underlying principle of disaster preparedness is "to do the greatest good for the greatest number" of casualties,[7,8] but it is important to understand the implications of this principle for trauma care.

A key characteristic of MCIs is that the overwhelming majority of casualties sustain only minor injuries. Regardless of the etiology or magnitude of the incident, only about 10–15% of survivors presenting to a trauma system are severely wounded. These patients obviously require the best possible trauma care immediately. However, most other casualties sustain minor or nonurgent injuries that do not require immediate life-saving care, or can tolerate significant delays.[9] For example, on March 11, 2004, ten bombs exploded almost simultaneously on four commuter trains and in four train stations in Madrid, Spain, resulting in 2062 casualties. The Gregorio Marañón University General Hospital received 312 casualties within approximately 3 hours, but only 29 were in critical condition and only seven underwent emergency surgery.[10]

Thus, from the trauma care perspective, a mass casualty incident is a "needle in a haystack" situation: a small group of severely injured patients who require immediate care is immersed within a much larger group of casualties who can tolerate delays and even some degree of suboptimal care. The ultimate goal of the disaster response is, therefore, to provide this small group of critically injured casualties with a level of care that approximates the care provided to similarly injured patients under normal circumstances. This goal has always been implicitly understood by trauma care providers and is certainly an expectation of the public, but it can only be achieved by diverting trauma assets and resources from the mildly injured to the critically wounded.[1]

The role of any modern trauma system is to establish and maintain a dedicated trauma service line for severely injured patients during normal daily operations. This service line is composed of trained trauma care providers and dedicated facilities and assets such as trauma resuscitation bays and trauma teams. The aim of an effective disaster response is to preserve this service line in the face of an unusually large casualty load. From the trauma care perspective, success in dealing with an urban bombing incident is not streamlining the flow of 40 or 60 casualties through the Emergency Department (ED), but rather preserving the capability to provide optimal trauma care to the four or five critically injured (but salvageable) casualties.[11]

## Classification of Disasters

MCIs can be classified according to their etiology (natural vs. manmade), duration, location, frequency, and other characteristics.[12,13] The magnitude of an incident can be defined by the level of emergency response required to cope with it rather than the absolute number of casualties. A Level I incident requires only local resources, whereas Level II and III incidents require regional or state/federal resources, respectively, representing ascending levels of magnitude.[13] This classification is retrospective, and therefore is more useful for analysis of past incidents than for real-time response to an evolving disaster.[12]

From the trauma care perspective, the most important distinction is between *multiple* and *mass casualty incidents*.[12,14] The casualty load of a multiple casualty incident is limited, so the hospital is able to cope using local resources without external help. Mass casualty incidents exceed the capabilities of a single hospital.

The quantitative definition of multiple and mass casualty incidents varies between institutions because it depends on local resources. While it is customary to point out that two severely injured patients arriving simultaneously can overwhelm a small community hospital,[1] it is often forgotten that even in busy trauma centers the routine trauma response envelope during normal working hours extends to no more than 4–5 severely injured patients arriving together. Larger casualty inflows will require mobilization of additional teams and resources outside the daily trauma response envelope. Cushman et al.[15] in reporting the medical response to 9/11 in New York City described hospital planning for two types of multiple casualty incidents: a limited or low-volume scenario that does not exceed the bed capacity of the Emergency Department (ED) and a high-volume scenario that requires the use of additional facilities and resources. However, in terms of the hospital trauma service line, the distinction between various degrees of multiple casualty incidents is less important than the fundamental difference between a multiple casualty incident (which implies an intact service line) and mass casualty (which implies a compromised or failing line).

How does the magnitude of the incident affect trauma care? Experienced providers know that an increase in casualty load beyond a certain limit will lead to degradation of trauma assets and resources, because critical casualties will compete for limited

resources.[1] The casualty load is defined quantitatively not only by the total number of patients that have arrived during an incident but also, and more importantly, by their arrival rate.[16] An intact trauma service line provides each arriving critical casualty with a trauma team, resuscitation bay, and available trauma-related resources such as CT scanner, operating room, and a bed in a surgical intensive care unit (SICU). The point beyond which this level of service cannot be maintained for new arrivals represents the surge capacity of the hospital trauma service line. Using a similar definition, surge capacity can also be defined for each trauma-related facility in the hospital.

In a *multiple casualty* incident, the casualty load is below surge capacity and therefore the trauma service line of the hospital remains intact. In a *mass casualty incident* the casualty load exceeds the surge capacity of a single institution. The term "mass casualty" thus implies a gradual failure of the trauma service line of the hospital, with a resulting degradation of the level of care for the severely wounded. In a *major medical disaster*, the casualty load exceeds the surge capacity of the trauma system(s) involved to such a degree that urgent trauma care for individual patients with life-threatening injuries is made impossible by the sheer number of casualties and lack of access to medical care. A recently published computer simulation[16] demonstrated the effect of an increasing casualty load on the availability of trauma assets and resources for the critically injured (Fig. 9-1). The upper flat portion of the curve represents a multiple casualty incident, where the level of care for critical casualties approximates the care given to a single patient on a normal working day. The steep portion represents a mass casualty situation with gradual failure of the trauma service line, and the lower flat portion represents a hospital overwhelmed by a major medical disaster. An effective disaster response increases the surge capacity of the trauma service line by shifting the sigmoid curve to

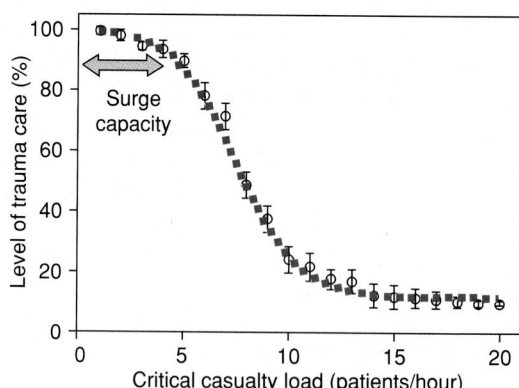

**FIGURE 9-1.** The graph depicts results of a computer simulation of the flow of urban bombing casualties through the trauma care facilities of a Level 1 trauma center (Data from Reference #16). The model demonstrates a sigmoid-shaped relationship between the casualty load (number of critical casualties arriving per hour) and the availability of trauma assets and resources (with the level of care for a single patient on a normal working day being 100%). The upper flat portion of the curve corresponds to a multiple casualty incident, the steep portion represents a mass casualty situation, and the lower flat portion represents a major medical disaster. The surge capacity of the hospital trauma assets is the maximal critical casualty load that can be managed without a precipitous drop in the level of care.

the right, resulting in a more graceful degradation instead of an abrupt drop in the level of care.[16]

## BLAST TRAUMA IN THE CIVILIAN SETTING

### Urban Bombing as a MCI

Not surprisingly, terror-related MCIs have become the most common reference scenarios for disaster planning, training, and response. However, it is important to keep in mind that the great majority of urban bombings result in limited multiple casualty incidents that do not overwhelm the trauma assets and resources of participating hospitals.[15,17,18] The coordinated simultaneous bombings in Madrid in March 2004 (2253 injured, 191 dead)[10] and London in July 2005 (approximately 700 injured, 56 dead)[19] represented deliberate attempts to produce large-scale and highly disruptive events with heavy casualty loads. However, the medical response to both incidents clearly showed that an emergency medical system of a large metropolitan area serves as an effective buffer by distributing casualties between hospitals. While the total number of live casualties may have been compatible with a mass casualty incident, each participating hospital faced only a multiple casualty scenario. A notable (though not well documented) exception was the US Embassy bombing in 1998 in Nairobi, Kenya, where several thousand casualties flooded the Kenyatta National Hospital, the only functioning trauma center in the city.[20]

From a review of published reports of past urban bombing incidents, it is impossible to infer how close the receiving hospitals came to their surge capacity. Clinical outcomes in large-scale events are typically reported as global statistics, such as critical mortality (the death rate of critically injured patients),[6] not in terms of preventable complications or deaths. In view of the high public profile of such incidents, it is unlikely that a systematic analysis of treatment delays or failures will ever be published from an urban bombing incident.

An urban bombing is an unusually severe form of trauma. In these incidents, up to one-third of hospital admissions have an Injury Severity Score of more than 15, as compared with only 10% in daily civilian practice.[21] On-scene mortality can also be very high.[17] The three factors that determine the overall number of casualties and the proportion of immediate deaths are the size of the explosive charge, structural failure of the building, and indoor detonation.[6,22–24]

When compared to an open space explosion, indoor detonation results in increased mortality and injury severity (particularly blast lung) among survivors. The blast wave, which rapidly dissipates in an open space, is reflected off the walls of the closed space, thereby greatly amplifying the damage. In comparing outdoor and indoor urban bombing incidents, Leibovici et al.[22] showed a six-fold increase in mortality and more than double the incidence of primary blast trauma among survivors of bus bombings.

Suicide bombers are a particularly devastating weapon of urban terrorism, since they specifically target crowded indoor locations or large gatherings in open spaces to maximize the blast effect.[25] The typical explosive vest that a suicide bomber carries around the torso consists of 5–12 kilograms of TNT-equivalent. Multiple small metal objects such as nails, screws, and bolts are added to the charge to increase secondary blast injuries. The explosion is lethal to the bomber and, depending on the specific circumstances of the detonation, results in some 50–150 casualties. Immediate mortality is around 10% in open-space explosions and up to 40–50% on a crowded bus.[18,22,23]

### Clinical and System Implications of Blast Trauma

Blast trauma is a *multidimensional injury* complex that often combines blast, penetrating, blunt, and burn mechanisms in the same patient.[21] This results in unusually challenging patterns of wounding. When compared with everyday civilian trauma, blast injuries result in higher injury severity and complexity, involve more anatomical regions, consume more hospital resources and are associated with higher in-hospital mortality.[21] The wounding of air-filled viscera as a direct result of the blast wave is defined as primary blast injury.[18,26] Penetrating trauma from shrapnel or flying fragments is secondary blast injury, and tertiary blast injury occurs when a casualty is propelled by the blast wind against a stationary object. The pathophysiology of blast trauma is discussed in detail in Chap. 55. The aim of this section is to provide an overview of the clinical presentation and management of blast injuries in the civilian setting and describe the implications of these unique injury patterns on the hospital disaster response.

### Ear Injury

The ear is the organ most susceptible to blast overpressure, and therefore rupture of the tympanic membrane is the most prevalent clinical sign of blast injury.[27] Less common injuries to the auditory system include ossicular discontinuity, or dislocation and bleeding in the middle ear, but vestibular damage is distinctly rare.[28–30] While the natural history of blast-induced eardrum perforation is usually benign with spontaneous healing in three of every four patients,[29] blast injury can result in various degrees of hearing loss.[29,30]

Tympanic membrane rupture is a useful marker of the proximity of a casualty to the detonation, but not a reliable predictor of blast lung injury.[31] Therefore, all casualties arriving from the scene of an urban bombing should be examined for tympanic membrane rupture in the ED and those in proximity to the blast should undergo at least an audiometric screening test to detect hearing impairment within 24 hours of injury regardless of the presence of symptoms.[18,30]

Casualties with eardrum perforation are often admitted for overnight observation, because of concerns for insidious respiratory deterioration due to blast lung injury. Although this concern is not evidence-based,[31] it nevertheless remains a common belief that governs discharge policies in many hospitals.

### Blast Lung Injury

Clinically important *blast lung injury* (BLI) occurs in 5–8% of live casualties in urban bombings. Almogy et al.[32] have shown that penetrating head and torso injuries, burns, and skull fractures are external signs associated with a high risk of developing BLI. Among early survivors from the explosion, the extent of BLI is the most important determinant of subsequent mortality.[26] The blast wave disrupts the alveolo-capillary interface, resulting in a clinical spectrum ranging from mild pulmonary contusion (with intra-alveolar hemorrhage) to full-blown ARDS with rapidly progressive oxygenation failure.[33] Other effects of the blast on the respiratory system include barotrauma (pneumothorax and broncho-alveolar fistula), air embolism, and mucosal damage to the upper airway.[18]

Pizov et al.[34] provided a detailed description of the clinical course and managment of BLI in a modern SICU environment in 15 survivors of bus explosions. Ten patients were extremely hypoxic on arrival in hospital and all but one required intubation and respiratory support within 2 hours of admission. A more recent series confirms this clinical course of rapid deterioration in severe cases.[33] However, the occasional casualty may gradually become symptomatic over many hours, sometimes as long as 48 hours after the explosion.[26] Mild BLI ($PaO_2/FIO_2$ ratio >200) presents with localized infiltrates on chest X-ray, is managed as a lung contusion and has a good prognosis. Severe BLI (P/F ratio <60) progresses to ARDS. It is associated with diffuse bilateral pulmonary infiltrates and with bronchopleural fistulae.[34] Air embolism is another recognized manifestation of BLI, and may well be a major cause of death at the scene in immediate fatalities with little or no external signs of injury.[25]

The mainstay of respiratory support in severe BLI are lung-protective ventilatory strategies similar to those employed in the management of patients with ARDS, typically using pressure-controlled ventilation modes that limit peak inspiratory pressure to 35 cm $H_2O$ and plateau pressures to around 25, and permissive hypercapnia if necessary.[35,36] The obvious tendency to limit IV fluid loading often conflicts with the need to optimize oxygen delivery by correcting hypovolemia due to the other effects of the blast (such as multiple penetrating injuries).[36]

Pneumothorax should be aggressively sought and immediately treated when identified. Although unsupported by evidence, some surgeons advocate empirical chest tube placement in every patient with severe BLI on positive-pressure ventilation.[18] Mortality is in excess of 60% in the most severe cases.[34]

Aschkenasy-Steuer et al.[36] provide a vivid description how an urban bombing incident taxes the critical care assets and resources of a large university hospital.[36] The presentation, within minutes, of several patients with rapidly deteriorating oxygenation and in need of emergency endotracheal intubation in the ED followed later by the need for advanced ventilatory support and invasive hemodynamic monitoring is a situation almost unique to an urban bombing scenario. The frequent presence of associated injuries further complicates matters and adds to the logistical effort involved. These patients require not only an SICU bed but, more importantly, the close, personal, and undivided attention of a team of experienced critical care providers. Under these circumstances, it is crucial to maintain operational flexibility in mobilizing and deploying the critical care assets of the hospital. In systems where the ICU is run by anesthesiologists or medical intensivists, early involvement of these providers by integrating them into the trauma teams in the ED receiving area facilitates the admission of critically injured patients to the ICU.[36]

## Intestinal Blast Trauma

Intestinal blast injury is rare in survivors of urban bombings, presenting in less than 2% of casualties. It is, however, the most common form of injury in immersion blast (underwater explosions). Intestinal blast injury spans a wide spectrum of severity from sub-serosal hemorrhage to full-thickness perforation.[37]

The major clinical problem with intestinal blast injury is delayed presentation.[37,38] Casualties may develop peritoneal signs as long as 48 hours or more after the explosion. Although blast injury has been reported throughout the entire length of the small bowel and colon, a report of three cases from a bus explosion described a propensity for the terminal ileum.[38] In each case, laparotomy revealed an isolated perforation of the terminal ileum with no evidence of peritonitis despite a 48-hour delay from the blast, suggesting that perforation occurred shortly before the onset of symptoms and supporting the concept of evolving trans-mural damage.

The operative dilemma is how much traumatized but nonperforated bowel to resect, since bruised or contused bowel may eventually progress to perforation.[37] The decision is an operative judgment call that must be tailored to the specific patient; however, an experimental study showed that larger contusions (>1.5 cm in the small bowel or >2 cm in the colon) are more likely to progress to perforation.[37]

## Secondary Blast Injury

Penetrating trauma from fragments of the bomb casing or other metal projectiles added to the explosive (such as nuts and bolts or steel pellets) is defined as secondary blast injury. Depending on their velocity, size, and shape, these projectiles cause a spectrum of injuries ranging from trivial skin lacerations to deep, life-threatening visceral wounds.[25]

An important implication of secondary blast injury for the hospital disaster plan is the extensive need for imaging to identify and locate penetrating fragments and to define their trajectories.[39] Physical examination is notoriously misleading in secondary blast injury: seemingly superficial lacerations may in fact hide a deep penetration of a metal fragment (Fig. 9-2). Plain radiographs can be useful to screen for radio-opaque foreign bodies in an anatomical region, but a single-shot radiograph will not distinguish between superficial and deep penetration, which often have totally different clinical significance. Adding a tangential view will help localize the foreign body.[40]

While there are no agreed guidelines for imaging casualties with suspected secondary blast injury, experienced providers use helical CT scanning to rapidly identify and locate multiple projectiles and to define their trajectories.[39,40] This very liberal approach to imaging, which is characteristic of an urban bombing incident, requires setting strict priorities and limiting access to scanners during the initial phase of the hospital response. In reality, the CT scanner is a classic bottleneck to casualty flow in an urban bombing incident.[25,41]

An often neglected aspect of secondary blast injury is significant external blood loss. Multiple projectiles may cause deep soft tissue lacerations that often bleed profusely. Since these injuries are often located in the posterior aspect of the torso and extremities, the associated blood loss is often underappreciated. Therefore, if the patient is taken emergently to the operating room, it is advisable to log-roll the patient and rapidly perform gauze packing of the wounds prior to celiotomy to prevent ongoing blood loss during the procedure.[42]

There is no consensus on the best surgical management of soft tissue wounds from multiple metal projectiles.[25] The principles of wound management call for debridement of each wound and

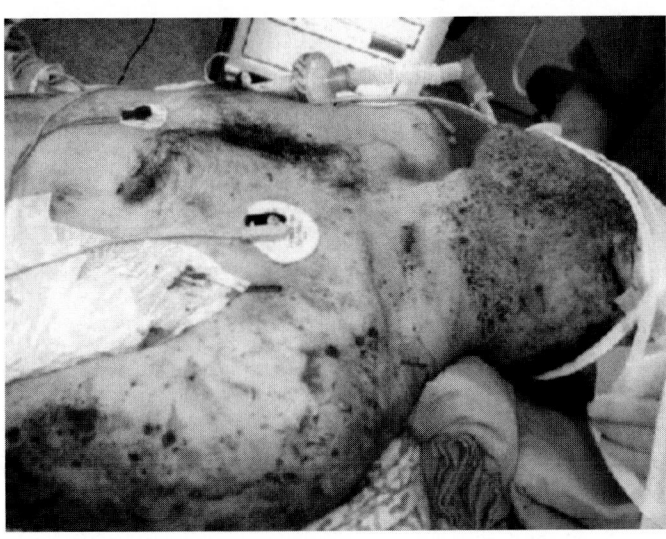

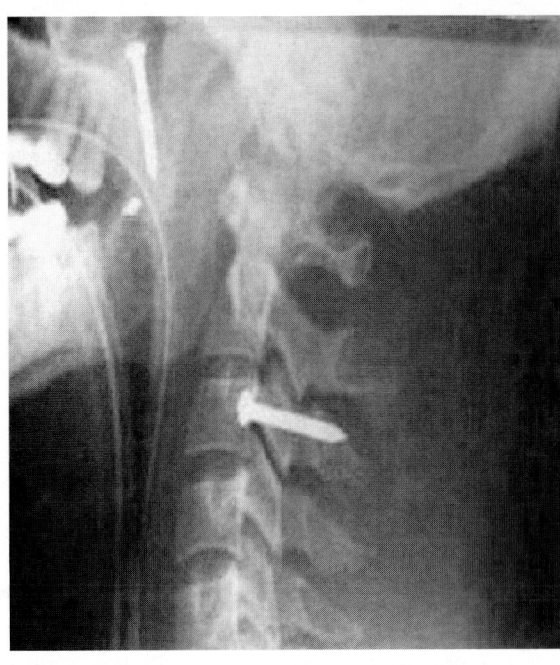

A

B

**FIGURE 9-2.** The unpredictability of secondary blast injury. Seemingly superficial lacerations on the head and neck of this casualty **(A)** hide deep penetration of two nails into the upper neck and oropharynx **(B)**.

removal of the embedded foreign body. However, this is often not a realistic option since debridement of multiple wounds in search of deeply embedded asymptomatic projectiles consumes valuable time and OR resources, and the dissection ends up causing more tissue destruction than the foreign body. A common-sense approach is to remove only troublesome projectiles (e.g., symptomatic, intra-articular, or infected). The great majority of wounds usually heal uneventfully.

The *human remains shrapnel* is a special kind of secondary blast injury. Penetration of biological material, typically consisting of small bone fragments originating from the suicide bomber, poses an unusual management problem to trauma care providers. In the first reported case in 2001,[43] a casualty from a suicide bombing presented with a small strange foreign body embedded in the neck. Exploration revealed a chip of bone which proved (on DNA testing) to originate from the suicide bomber, who was Hepatitis B positive. Similar cases have been reported since.[19,25,44]

## Tertiary and Quaternary Blast Injury

Tertiary blast injury occurs when casualties are propelled by the blast wind and collide with stationary objects.[18,26] The resulting injuries follow standard patterns of blunt trauma. However, when combined with other injuries sustained by the explosion in a MCI, tertiary blast injury may present unusual dilemmas in terms of prioritization and use of resources.

Quaternary blast injury refers to other injury mechanisms not included above, primarily burns and crush injuries.[18,26] Burns are a common finding in casualties of urban bombing incidents. Superficial "flash" burns (typically involving large body areas) are caused by the flame of the explosion itself, which is of very short duration. These burns are commonly found in fatalities at the scene and are

markers of proximity to the blast.[18,32] Another type of burn is caused by the ignition of clothes and other flammable materials, resulting in deep burns of variable extent, sometimes in conjunction with smoke and toxic inhalation injuries.

Urban bombing incidents that involve a large proportion of burn casualties pose an unusual burden on trauma systems. A prominent example was the Bali nightclub bombing in October 2002.[45,46] During the initial phase of hospital care of casualties from Bali, the major clinical challenge was dealing with other effects of the blast (such as complex penetrating trauma) in conjunction with the need for burn resuscitation and urgent wound management.[45] At later stages, the problems were septic complications from unusual multiresistant organisms and the sheer logistical effort of managing a large number of severely burned patients simultaneously. In an urban bombing, burn casualties are often brought to hospitals that do not have a dedicated burn service.[47] Secondary distribution to burn centers, if possible, is often in the patients' best interest.

## Other Injuries

*Traumatic amputation* from primary blast injury is uncommon and often considered a marker of a lethal injury because it denotes close proximity of the casualty to the explosive charge.[18,32] The precise mechanism of a traumatic amputation is not clear, but it is presumed to result from direct coupling of the blast wave with the tissue.[26]

Early *neurological impairment* after blast exposure has been attributed to air emboli in cerebral vessels or to diffuse axonal injury from direct effects of the blast overpressure on the brain.[48] Regardless of the precise mechanism, the clinical consequences of blast neurotrauma are EEG changes and a variety of mild neurological symptoms such as retrograde amnesia, mental blockage, apathy, psychomotor agitation, and anxiety.[49] Cernak et al.[50] identified long-term subtle neurological impairment in up to 30% of blast casualties one year after the incident.

Another clinical presentation that is attributed to the blast wave is *transient profound hemodynamic instability*, a syndrome consisting of bradycardia, hypotension (without peripheral vasoconstriction), and hypoxemia—all without any evidence of external injury.[51] In experimental studies, bradycardia occurs about 3 seconds after the primary blast, reaching maximal effect at 10–15 seconds. Hypotension, which may be severe, and short periods of apnea occur immediately after the blast. Experimental evidence suggests that this triad may be due to activation of a pulmonary vagally-mediated reflex.[51,52]

## Acute Stress Reaction and Posttraumatic Stress Disorder

Stress-related reactions and disorders are by far the most common health effect of an urban bombing incident, outweighing the incidence of physical injuries by an order of magnitude.[53] In the wake of the World Trade Center disaster on 9/11, symptoms of posttraumatic stress disorder (PTSD) were extremely prevalent among residents of lower Manhattan.[54] The psychological response to an urban bombing can be classified into anxiety-related and loss-related syndromes, with a significant amount of overlap between the two.[53]

*Acute stress reaction* is a normal response that occurs in some 20% of casualties admitted to hospital after a terror-related urban bombing.[25] It consists of an undifferentiated clinical picture of distress with shifting symptoms such as impaired response to external stimuli due to mental detachment, decreased situation awareness, and ability to listen, or overwhelming anxiety with physical signs such as tremor, hyperventilation, and sweating. The diagnosis of *acute stress disorder* is considered only when these symptoms persist for more than 48 hours. It is then also possible to discern more specific clusters of symptoms such as dissociation, re-experiencing, and avoidance. The diagnosis of PTSD is considered when the symptoms persist for more than 4 weeks.[53] PTSD is a chronic condition that is difficult to treat.

Casualties with acute stress reaction need an early intervention to help reduce the duration and intensity of their symptoms, with the aim of preventing progression along the sequence from stress reaction to stress disorder, and eventually PTSD. Acute stress reaction and disorder represent temporary psychological and physiological dysfunction that should correct itself within hours or days of the event. Early intervention (for an individual casualty or for a group), is crucial since the window of opportunity to prevent chronic debilitating PTSD is time-sensitive.

Trauma care providers must be aware of two important implications of acute stress reaction. First, these casualties must be separated from the physically injured so that their needs can best be addressed by a trained provider. Therefore, the hospital disaster plan must designate an appropriately located facility for acute stress intervention, away from the chaotic and stressful environment of the ED receiving area. The site should be staffed by a team of trained mental health care providers, and accept casualties after significant physical injury has been rapidly ruled out.[53] Second, trauma team leaders must be aware that their team members are susceptible to acute stress reaction while coping with an urban bombing incident, despite their trauma training and experience. These internal casualties must be identified rapidly and referred for early intervention.

## TRAUMA CARE ASPECTS OF THE PREHOSPITAL RESPONSE

### Time Line of a MCI

The time line of the scene response to a MCI follows a typical sequence, beginning with chaos immediately after the inciting event (e.g., bomb blast, stadium stampede, or plane crash) and ending with return to normal daily routine.[18] Understanding this sequence is germane to planning an effective medical response both at the scene and in the hospital.

The initial *chaos phase* begins with the inciting event and ends when a prehospital responder assumes command of the scene.[18] The hallmark of this phase is lack of organized medical effort. From the trauma care perspective, casualties with minor injuries, "walking wounded," and casualties with acute stress reaction escape from the scene and make their way to a nearby hospital, often assisted by family, strangers, and even public transportation. These casualties generate the first of the three waves of casualties arriving in hospital in an urban MCI. They do not receive any prehospital care and typically have low injury severity scores.[18]

The *organization phase* begins when a prehospital responder (usually a local EMS commander) assumes command at the scene and starts organizing the medical effort. From the trauma care perspective, the primary role of the scene commander is to initiate effective field triage that will identify casualties with life-threatening injuries and organize their priority-driven transport to hospitals.[55] By performing triage and assigning transfer priorities, the scene commander represents the first opportunity of the trauma system to reduce preventable mortality. The security and safety of the medical teams is a prime consideration and must be assured prior to initiating any kind of medical activity at the scene. One of the hallmarks of urban terrorism is the "second hit" phenomenon, whereby teams of responders rushing to provide care to casualties of the first blast are injured by a subsequent explosion in the same location.[6]

The duration of the *site-clearing* phase depends on the magnitude of the incident, the presence of structural collapse, and the need for prolonged extrication.[18] It ends when the last live casualty is transported from the scene.

The *late phase* is a poorly-defined period during which mild casualties who initially ran away from the scene decide to seek medical attention many hours later, often under pressure from family and friends. They typically present with superficial abrasions, minor phonal trauma, and many of them complain of symptoms related to acute stress reaction or disorder.[53]

The typical timeline of an urban MCI translates into three waves of casualties arriving in the ED (Fig. 9-3): a small group of early arrivals with minor injuries who escaped from the scene prior to the arrival of medical aid, the main casualty load presenting with a wide range of injury severities, and finally a slow ongoing trickle

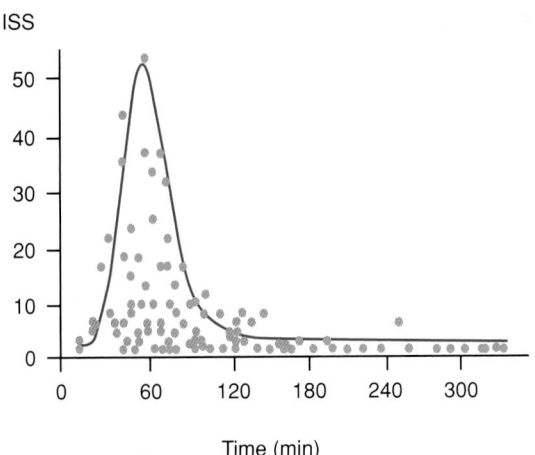

**FIGURE 9-3.** Injury Severity Score (ISS) vs. time of arrival in hospital of 128 casualties of an urban open-space suicide bombing. Jerusalem, September 4, 1997. The graph depicts the typical three waves of casualties: an initial small group of mild casualties, the main wave with a wide spectrum of injury severities and an ongoing tickle of late arrivals.

of late arrivals over many hours, typically presenting with minor physical injuries or acute stress reaction.[18]

## Trauma Care at the Scene

Reports of past incidents have shown that the time interval from injury to definitive care is a key determinant of mortality.[8] Rapid and priority-driven transport to a hospital is therefore of critical importance.[18]

In an urban MCI scenario, distances to nearby hospitals are short and transport is swift. In the recently reported cumulated Israeli experience from a large series of urban bombing incidents, the mean time to transport of the last critical casualty from the scene was 16 minutes from the blast.[55] Under these circumstances, the general philosophy of trauma care at the scene is "scoop and run." The emphasis is not on treating casualties but on determining correct priorities for their transport to hospital.[18,55] The only interventions performed at the scene (or en route to hospital) are airway management, ventilation, and control of external hemorrhage.

An important part of the first responders' role is to identify casualties that are obviously dead. CPR should not be initiated for pulseless casualties since it is futile and consumes precious resources. A major limb amputation from the blast denotes close proximity to the explosion and is usually lethal. Airway control (with cervical spine protection) is probably the single most important intervention in salvageable critical casualties.[18] However, since EMS teams adopt a "scoop and run" mentality, it is not surprisingly that a large proportion of casualties with a compromised airway undergo endotracheal intubation in the ED.[36]

In a rural or remote MCI, transport is often delayed because of limited means and long distances. This transport bottleneck may mandate some form of trauma care at the scene. It is in these rural or remote scenarios that deployment of a medical team to the scene, if feasible, makes sense from the trauma care perspective.[56] A special scenario is a mass casualty incident in a sports stadium, an airport, or any other location where access to the casualties and

egress from the scene are severely limited by physical constraints. The on-scene medical response in such incidents will usually combine elements of both urban and remote scenarios.

## Scene Triage

There are currently three major algorithms in use for triage at the scene of a MCI: Simple Triage And Rapid Treatment (START) triage (used mostly in the USA), Triage Sieve (used in the UK), and Careflight (used in Australia).[57] Regardless of the specific algorithm used, the aim is to provide a simple tool for rapidly sorting casualties into transport and treatment priorities.

START was developed in 1983 by the Hoag Hospital and the Newport Beach Fire Department and was modified in 1994.[58] Casualties are sorted into four categories: immediate, delayed, minor, and deceased. All walking casualties are designated as minor. Nonwalking casualties with a palpable radial pulse who are following commands are designated as delayed. Nonbreathing casualties are deceased, and the rest are designated as immediate. Color-coded tags are used to facilitate and expedite the triage process. JumpSTART is an adaptation of the START system for pediatric casualties using a more elaborate algorithm.[59]

The differences between the three field triage systems are minor since they use essentially similar clinical filters with slight variations.[60] For example, the Triage Sieve uses capillary refill or pulse rate instead of a palpable radial pulse as the hemodynamic filter. There is no convincing evidence that one system is superior to the others.[57,60]

## ORGANIZATION OF THE HOSPITAL RESPONSE

### The Hospital Disaster Response Envelope

The aim of the institutional emergency plan is to rapidly augment the surge capacity of the hospital disaster response envelope. This envelope consists of five key facilities: Emergency Department (ED) (including the trauma resuscitation area), operating rooms, intensive care units, blood bank, and emergency laboratory. An Emergency Operations Center (EOC) is established to coordinate the institutional effort.

Each key facility within the hospital response envelope activates a facility-specific disaster protocol. The movement of casualties through the ED and other trauma-related facilities in the hospital is essentially flow between decision points: a casualty does not enter nor leave a facility (such as a trauma resuscitation bay or a CT scanner) without someone making a decision. Therefore, the effective response of each facility to a large casualty load hinges on a small group of local managers and decision-makers whose decisions drive the entire effort.[1,11] In the ED these are the medical director, charge nurse, surgeon-in-charge, and triage officer.[1,61]

Full mobilization of the hospital disaster response envelope is time-consuming, disruptive to normal daily activities, costly—and often unnecessary. Multiple casualty incidents with limited casualty loads are much more common than catastrophic mass casualty scenarios. Therefore, some hospitals base their disaster plans on a tiered response.[15] There is a plan for a limited casualty load

(10–20 casualties, 2–4 critically injured) that relies on existing in-house staff and resources, while a plan for larger casualty loads uses staff reinforcements and, if necessary, additional facilities outside the ED receiving area.[25]

An effective scene response distributes a large casualty load among several hospitals, so that each hospital encounters only a multiple casualty incident. Thus, even multifocal or large-scale urban terrorist bombings were reported as "busy mornings" rather than overwhelming events in the participating hospitals.[10,15,17] In fact, there is not a single description in the trauma literature of a modern hospital ever being overwhelmed by a large casualty load to an extent that compromised the care of the severely wounded.

Occasionally, a small hospital with limited trauma capabilities may become overwhelmed by a large casualty load because it happens to be located in close proximity to the incident site. Under these unusual circumstances, one effective option is to offload casualties to other institutions by switching the emergency facilities of the hospital into a MASH-like operating mode, the so-called "triage hospital" (originally named "evacuation hospital").[62] The triage hospital functions as a forward triage and resuscitation facility, providing only resuscitative or immediately life-saving interventions. The great majority of casualties are transferred to other hospitals for definitive care.

This solution, while effective, cannot be improvised on the spot. Implementation requires not only pre-existing transfer agreements with other institutions but also careful planning to establish a pre-transfer intensive care facility where critically injured patients awaiting transfer can be safely monitored and treated.

## Trauma Aspects of Incident Command

Hospital disaster plans are traditionally based on a top-down organizational hierarchy. In the USA, the Hospital Emergency Incident Command System (HEICS) was introduced in 1991[8,63,64] and is currently in its third revision (Fig. 9-4). It is based on the concept of the Incident Command Structure (ICS), which was developed in the 1970s to streamline the field management of large-scale incidents.[8] The HEICS top-down structure puts an incident commander in overall charge of the institutional effort and clearly defines areas of responsibility and spans of control for managers in five domains: command, operations, planning, logistics, and finances. Medical care is within the responsibility of the Chief of Operations, through a Director of Medical Care. Similar organizational structures based on top-down hierarchies are used in other countries.

While these hierarchical command structures are useful as frameworks for disaster planning, implementing them during a real event is problematic. First, the great majority of incidents that a hospital is likely to encounter are limited urban incidents, where the dynamics are rapid and the duration is short. Thus, the incident is typically over long before the command and control structure has been deployed. The second disadvantage is structural rigidity, heavy reliance of up-and-down communication (which often is the first to fail in a real event), and delays between the time a problem is identified and the implementation of an effective solution. The severe shortcomings of the rigid top-down command structure were dramatically demonstrated during the rescue efforts and the disaster response to Hurricane Katrina in 2005.[5] An effective disaster response at any

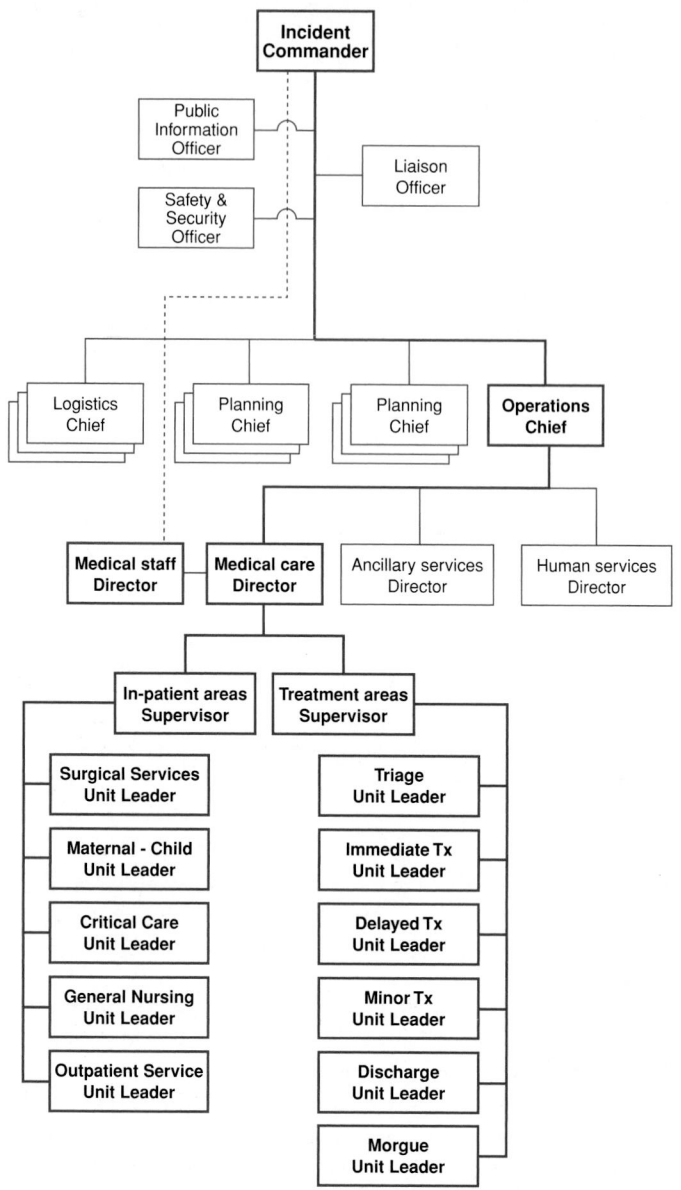

**FIGURE 9-4.** The general organizational structure of the Hospital Emergency Incident Command System (HEICS). (Data from Reference #63). The scheme emphasizes the medical chain of command in bold boxes, while nonmedical functions and elements are represented in lumped form.

level, including the hospital level, must be based on collaborative networks of local managers. These decision-makers understand the overarching goals of the hospital plan, are empowered to solve problems instead of merely reporting them up the chain of command, and are trained to improvise when necessary. Such collaborative network architectures provides flexibility, adaptability and speed, and are resilient in the face of unexpected failures of parts of the system.[5]

The HEICS and similar hierarchical command structures do not specifically address medical command issues, such as the ultimate responsibility for clinical decision making in trauma patients. During normal daily operations, a trauma team leader supervising a team working in a resuscitation bay has full autonomy in clinical decisions regarding treatment priorities and the use of resources. In a MCI, this autonomy is no longer possible because a large number of injured patients compete for the same resources and facilities. All key clinical decisions must therefore be reported to and coordinated by the surgeon-in-charge who supervises the trauma resuscitation area, has an overview of the institutional situation and is responsible for resource allocation.[42,61] The flow of casualties through the trauma resuscitation area of the ED and related facilities (such as the operating rooms and SICU) is driven by clinical decisions, and since resources are limited, these clinical decisions must be centralized. This is a fundamental difference between trauma care in MCIs as opposed to normal daily care of the injured. The surgeon-in-charge is not merely a coordinator or supervisor but actually makes key clinical decisions at the level of the individual patient.[42]

## Initiating the Hospital Response

The hospital disaster response is triggered when the hospital is alerted about a possible unusually large influx of casualties. Large parts of the disaster plan are generic regardless of the type or etiology of the incident.[12] The plan must make absolutely clear who is authorized to activate various levels of the institutional response, bearing in mind that this individual must be able to shoulder responsibility for an unnecessary or inappropriate activation based on erroneous information. The person authorized to initiate the response can be an upper-echelon hospital administrator or a local decision-maker in the ED (such as the charge nurse or the attending emergency physician). The former reflects the top-down command mentality and entails significant delays, especially outside normal working hours. The latter is more in line with the nimble approach of empowering local managers to make decisions, facilitating a rapid response.

There is typically a time lag between the notification that a MCI has occurred and the arrival of the first casualties. This time lag is a window of opportunity to initiate the critical first steps of the institutional response, and actions taken during these 10–15 minutes (in an urban scenario) may have a profound effect on the ensuing response. Upon notification, each facility participating in the hospital disaster response envelope initiates an emergency protocol tailored to the specific goals and needs of that facility. In generic terms, this entails suspension of normal daily activities and rapid mobilization of additional staff and resources in preparation for an unusually heavy workload.[36]

The HEICS recommends the use of call-up mechanisms to mobilize additional staff.[8] Each facility creates a list of contact information for their staff and a method for rapid notification of the staff upon activation of the plan. The HEICS also advocates the use of job-action sheets, a preprinted list of tasks for every role or function within the HEICS structure. The job action sheet contains a list of "things to do" for every staff member in a supervisory role, including tasks and responsibilities that come with the role. The sheet clearly defines their place in the command structure.

## Preparing the Emergency Department

Upon activation of the disaster plan, the ED puts in place a rapid evacuation plan to curtail normal activities and create physical space for a large number of incoming casualties.[12,36] Based on their medical conditions, ED patients can be rapidly discharged, admitted to the floors, or transferred to a predesignated location within the hospital so as not to be in the way of incoming casualties.

Another priority is to establish a triage function before the arrival of the first casualties.[12] To effectively control casualty flow, triage must be performed outside and not inside the ED.[1] Triage on the ambulance dock is only the first step in dynamic reiterative triage process that continues as each casualty is repeatedly re-examined, as described below.

The identity of the four key decision makers (medical director, charge nurse, surgeon-in-charge, and triage officer) and the command chain for both clinical and administrative decisions must be clear to the entire ED staff, including ad-hoc reinforcements mobilized through a call-up mechanism. The medical, nursing, and administrative staff of each treatment area must be briefed and assigned specific roles. For example, in the trauma resuscitation area, care providers are assigned to specific trauma teams, and each team is explicitly told that they will take the first, second, or third critically injured arrival.

Emergency equipment is deployed according to plan in pre-assigned treatment areas within the ED. The treatment area for mild casualties ("walking wounded" who can sit) is typically located outside the ED but in proximity to it. Casualties who need ED gurneys but are not critically injured are treated in the main ED receiving (or holding) area, while the severely wounded are treated in trauma resuscitation bays or shock rooms. An effective plan includes measures to augment the capacity of the trauma resuscitation area by adding improvised resuscitation bays, or by accommodating more than one casualty in each shock room.

## HOSPITAL CARE IN MASS CASUALTY INCIDENTS

There are two distinct phases in the trauma care of casualties arriving in hospital.[18,25] During the initial phase, the incident is still evolving, the hospital response envelope is still being mobilized, casualties are arriving, and their ultimate number is unknown. During this phase, the key concern is to preserve the trauma service line of the hospital by diverting trauma assets and resources to the severely wounded while offering a lesser level of care to all others. The definitive phase begins when casualties are no longer arriving, the total casualty load is known, and the disaster response envelope has been fully deployed. The key concern during this phase is to provide all casualties with optimal care in a graded, priority-driven fashion.

## Triage

Effective triage is a key component of the hospital disaster response. The traditional view of hospital triage is that a very experienced trauma care provider (typically a trauma surgeon or emergency physician)[1,7,15] stands at the ED entrance and rapidly sorts arriving casualties into treatment priorities, often using a color-coded tagging system.

Traditional teaching distinguishes between five triage categories: immediate, delayed, minimally injured, expectant, and dead[7] (Table 9-1). Experience from real incidents, however, has shown that it is it is often impossible to distinguish between "immediate" and "delayed" casualties based on a rapid cursory examination on

**TABLE 9-1**

**Hospital Triage Categories**

| TRADITIONAL | REALISTIC |
|---|---|
| Immediate | |
| *Unstable with life-threatening injuries* | |
| Expectant | |
| *Unsalvageable critical injuries* | To trauma resuscitation bay |
| Dead | |
| *No signs of life* | |
| Delayed | |
| *Stable patients that require treatment* | All others |
| Minimally injured | |
| *Walking wounded with minimal injuries* | |

the ambulance dock, especially with blast injuries.[1,7] It is also frequently impossible to pronounce a casualty dead without a cardiac monitor and a more thorough examination. Furthermore, the decision to declare a casualty "expectant" is fraught with problems when attempted on the ambulance dock.[65] The "expectant" designation often depends on the casualty load and on available resources: the same critical patient may be deemed potentially salvageable if the casualty load is light (or if the patient is an early arrival) or hopeless if the hospital is overwhelmed.[1]

For all these reasons, realistic triage at the ED door consists of sorting incoming casualties into two categories only: those referred to the trauma resuscitation area (and enter the dedicated trauma service line) and all others.[1,7,25] In a large-scale MCI, when the casualty load is expected to exceed the capacity of the ED, it makes sense to separate walking casualties (i.e., those who can sit in chairs and usually have minimal or no physical injuries) from nonwalking casualties who require an ED gurney and may harbor serious injuries.

Triage in MCIs is often grossly inaccurate. Overtriage is the assignment of noncritical casualties to the trauma resuscitation area.[6,7] The overtriage rate is defined as the percentage of noncritical casualties erroneously assigned to the trauma resuscitation area from among all casualties assigned to this area. Overtriage rates of 50% or more at the hospital door are routinely reported from MCIs[9] and are a source of concern since these "false positive" casualties compete with true critical casualties for the attention of trauma teams and for trauma resources.[16]

Undertriage is the erroneous assignment of a critical casualty to the noncritical area of the ED and may lead to delayed or suboptimal treatment of a critically injured patient. Reported undertriage rates are low because the denominator (total number of noncritical casualties) is large, but each case represents a medical error that may result in preventable morbidity or even mortality. While it is generally assumed that a high overtriage rate is the price the system pays for keeping undertriage rates very low,[6] in fact triage errors can lead to both high over- and high undertriage rates in the same incident.

Given the austere circumstances of triage at the ED door, there is no evidence that triage accuracy can be improved by assigning it to a more experienced trauma care provider.[1,7] Instead, a more practical approach is to accept that triage errors are inevitable, but their adverse consequences can be mitigated.[16] For example, increasing the capacity of the trauma service line (by adding teams

or improvising trauma bays) or improving the efficiency of the teams will mitigate the effects of overtriage.

Triage is not a single decision made at a specific service point. It is a dynamic, ongoing process where the initial evaluation on the ambulance dock is only the first step in an iterative process of repeated re-examination that continues at every subsequent service point.[7,14] As each casualty is reassessed again and again, errors made during initial triage at the ED door can be identified and corrected.

## The Initial Phase

While casualties are still arriving, the ultimate number is unknown and the disaster response envelope of the hospital is not fully deployed, the guiding principle is to conserve trauma assets and resources. The focus of concern is the ability to accommodate the next critical casualty.

Trauma care for severely injured patients who have entered the trauma service line of the hospital is essentially similar to everyday care, except that team leaders do not make independent decisions. All major decisions are referred to the surgeon-in-charge, who roams between shock rooms and acts as both coordinator and ultimate clinical decision-maker.[42] The emphasis is on expediency and rapid turnover of resuscitation bays. The most important tool used by the surgeon-in-charge is a list of casualties, with diagnoses and disposition for each critical casualty. Without such as list (whether preprinted, digital, or simply improvised on a piece of paper) the surgeon-in-charge will not be able to keep track of the severely injured.

During the initial phase of a MCI, trauma care for noncritical casualties is guided by the principle of minimal acceptable care.[18,25] This essentially means empirical care along the lines of first aid in the field, with the aim of buying time, delaying definitive care, and offloading the ED and other trauma assets and facilities (such as the CT scanners and the operating rooms). The concept of minimal acceptable care is based on the well-known observation that among casualties of war, some 65% will survive for a week after injury without any medical care,[66] and that non-operative management of these casualties can buy valuable time and improve survival. According to the principle of minimal acceptable care, a casualty with clinical suspicion of a long bone fracture will receive empirical splinting and analgesia and will be rapidly admitted to a floor bed without imaging. Penetrating abdominal trauma with peritoneal signs in a hemodynamically stable patient will be treated with intravenous fluids, antibiotics, nasogastric suction, analgesia, and admission to a floor bed.[18,25] One of the hallmarks of this temporizing philosophy is to limit access to the CT scanner only to patients in whom the scan is absolutely essential or potentially life-saving (such as a head injury with lateralizing signs or a deteriorating level of consciousness).

In many hospital disaster plans, noncritical casualties are managed in the ED by staff reinforcements from other facilities (such as inpatient wards or outpatient clinics) who often lack trauma experience and may not be familiar with ED routines and procedures. However, these staff reinforcements can examine a casualty and execute a management plan if guided and supervised by a trauma care provider familiar with the ED work environment.

The availability of operating rooms is rarely a major concern in a MCI during working hours, since only a small fraction of the casualty load requires emergency life-saving operative procedures. Based on the military concepts of far forward surgery, some authors advocate adopting damage control methods and techniques to shorten operative procedures and decrease turnover times in a MCI.[67] It certainly seems wasteful spending 2–3 hours on definitive repairs and closing the abdomen rather then doing a 45-minute damage-control procedure and leaving the abdomen open. However, experience from real MCIs[10,42] and predictions from computer simulations[16,41] have shown that in a large trauma center there is no logistical indication to perform damage control in urban bombing incidents, since operating room availability is virtually never a bottleneck. Furthermore, in choosing a damage control solution for logistical reasons, the cost of expediency is the need for an SICU bed and a ventilator for a patient with an open belly who could otherwise have been extubated following a definitive procedure and transferred to a floor bed.

The availability of SICU beds in a MCI is a perpetual source of concern since, in an urban bombing, roughly one in every four admitted casualties requires an SICU bed.[68] In many urban trauma centers there is a routine shortage of SICU beds on normal working days. Therefore, the hospital disaster plan must make provisions to generate an acceptable surge capacity in intensive care beds. This is typically accomplished by rapidly discharging convalescent nonventilated SICU patients to floor beds and by transferring appropriately selected patients to nonsurgical intensive care facilities within the hospital.[69,70] This process takes time—but so does the arrival of casualties in the SICU. Shamir et al.[69,70] showed that a critically injured patient undergoing resuscitation and evaluation in a trauma bay followed by a CT scan or angiography will need an SICU bed some 4 hours after arrival in hospital, and a patient undergoing surgery will arrive even later. This significant delay allows the SICU staff to prepare beds, transfer patients, and mobilize staff reinforcements. The postanesthesia care unit (PACU) is an excellent surge facility for ventilated critical patients.[70]

## The Definitive Care Phase

During the definitive phase, casualties are no longer arriving, their ultimate number is known, and the disaster response envelope of the hospital is fully deployed. It is now possible to take stock of all admitted casualties and to proceed with priority-driven definitive care.[18]

The trauma service of the hospital conducts detailed rounds on all admitted casualties and makes a treatment plan for each. The deliverables of these rounds are prioritized lists of patients in need of imaging, consults, operative procedures, or transfer to other institutions. In other words, the minimal acceptable care of the initial phase is transformed into optimal care in the definitive phase.

The definitive care of casualties consumes time and resources. Even a limited multiple casualty incident disrupts the normal daily activities of key hospital facilities for 24–48 hours. Return to normal daily activities is gradual and the time line differs between facilities. The ED can return to normal relatively quickly, but the operating rooms and surgical intensive care units may be overloaded and overworked, requiring special support for several days. Useful descriptions of a general ICU coping with a multiple casualty incident, the importance of relieving staff after

8–12 hours of work, and the use of staff reinforcements, nursing students, and volunteers were provided by Aschkenasy-Steuer et al.[36] and Shamir et al.[70]

During the definitive care phase, consideration should be given to the need for secondary distribution of casualties by transferring some of them to other institutions. Inter-hospital transfer of burn patients to a burn center is a self-evident example. Inter-hospital transfer during an MCI may also reflect triage errors at the scene, with severely injured patients sent to facilities that lack the trauma resources to provide definitive care for them.[71] Inter-hospital transfer is more problematic when the indication is not purely medical but mostly logistical, such as the wish to shorten waiting times for nonurgent operative procedures (e.g., internal fixation of a femur fracture). Financial and administrative barriers or considerations of institutional prestige often play a role in these decisions.

An urban bombing is an example of a short MCI, since the main body of casualties arrives within about 2 hours of the explosion. When structural collapse is involved, prolonged extrication and site clearing activities extend the initial phase, but there is still a clear distinction between the initial and definitive care phases. However, in other types of MCIs such as natural disasters or civilian trauma care in areas of conflict, an ongoing stream of casualties blurs the difference between the phases. The hospital disaster response must therefore include plans for such "ongoing MCIs," with strict rationing of staff working hours, maintenance of an ongoing emergency supply chain, and preparing for the possibility that hospital staff will have to reside in-house for many days.

The last formal step in the hospital response is a formal debriefing. This activity takes place as soon as possible after the event. Ideally, all staff (hospital and prehospital) who took part in the effort should participate. The debriefing should be carefully structured to cover all key areas of clinical and administrative activity, while allowing free input from any participant who wishes to make a significant point. The aim is to learn lessons and identify barriers to the hospital response that can later be incorporated into the hospital disaster plan.[72] Although not a primary goal of the debriefing, it also helps the hospital staff to cope with the psychological and emotional impacts of the incident.[73] The importance of a good and systematic debriefing session cannot be overemphasized.

## Role of the Trauma Surgeon

The role of trauma surgeons within the hospital disaster response is not well defined and varies between institutions and systems. The American College of Surgeons Committee on Trauma calls for a surgeon with trauma experience to perform triage at the ED door,[14] and indeed in many disaster plans, a very experienced trauma surgeon is assigned to this role.[15,42] However, as discussed above, this initial triage is grossly inaccurate even in the most experienced hands, and the function can be successfully fulfilled by another trauma care provider, not necessarily a surgeon or even a physician.[7] This is especially true if there is a limited number of surgeons with trauma experience in the institution. In performing triage at the ED door, leadership, crowd management skills, situation awareness, and the ability to remain calm under severe stress are probably more important qualities than expertise in trauma surgery.

Bearing in mind the core mission of preserving the dedicated trauma service line of the hospital, trauma surgeons with experience in multiple casualty incidents and particularly urban bombings focus their attention primarily on the severely wounded. Thus, the surgeon-in-charge in the ED maintains medical control of the entire trauma resuscitation area, roams between resuscitation bays, and makes clinical decisions on treatment priorities in conjunction with each trauma team leader.[42] If necessary, each trauma surgeon can supervise and direct several trauma teams.

The top-down hierarchical structure of the typical disaster plan (and the HIECIS) calls for a single medical director or command physician. However, the amount of administrative, logistic and clinical information flowing through the ED is too vast for a single individual—however experienced—to absorb, digest, and respond to effectively.[1,8] Under these circumstances, it makes sense to use a "dual command" structure where an administrative director (typically an emergency physician) assumes responsibility for running the facility, thus allowing the medical director (typically a trauma surgeon) to focus on clinical decisions.[8,56]

## TRAUMA CARE IN MAJOR NATURAL DISASTERS

There are fundamental differences between trauma care in an urban MCI and the medical response to a major natural disaster. In the former, a functioning trauma system is coping with an unusually large casualty load over a brief period of time (from hours to several days). In the latter, the catastrophic event compromises or destroys infrastructure and community support systems (including trauma and health care systems) in the disaster area. External assets and resources are therefore imported into the disaster area to reinforce, support or replace compromised local assets. The medical response spans over a much longer time line, measured in weeks, months, and years.[2]

Injuries encountered in casualties of major natural disasters follow predictable patterns.[74] In all major natural disasters, poverty is the single most important factor that determines the vulnerability of the affected population: poor countries or areas have weaker infrastructure, and poor people cannot afford to move to safer areas.

### Patterns of Injury

In a major earthquake, the most important wounding mechanisms are falling debris and entrapment underneath collapsed buildings. Most lives are saved by the immediate search and rescue actions of survivors in their immediate vicinity rather than by the organized (but delayed) efforts of external agencies. In the first hours after the event, casualties exhibit a wide range of extremity and visceral trauma,[75] but later the prevailing patterns are extremity injuries and a high incidence of crush injury.[75,76] Delayed extrication translates into a high incidence of crush syndrome and acute renal failure, as seen in 12% of hospitalized patients after the Marmara earthquake in Turkey in 1999.[77]

Following the tsunami in Southeast Asia in December 2004, the impact of the wall of water destroyed buildings, flooded infrastructures, and caused injuries from floating debris. The dead (primarily from drowning) outnumbered live casualties by a ratio of 2:1,[2] and the most prevalent injuries among survivors were extremity fractures and soft tissue wounds.[2,78]

The most common cause of death in a volcanic eruption is suffocation.[80] Injuries can be caused by falling rocks, exposure to ash (a strong respiratory and eye irritant), and inhalation of volcanic gases, as well as from associated mechanisms such as mudslides (causing crush injuries) and floods.[74]

### The Rapid Needs Assessment

A critical first step in the medical response to a major natural catastrophe is the rapid needs assessment.[80] This mission, carried out as soon as possible by a small team of experts, provides essential information for planning any subsequent relief effort.[81] A United Nations Disaster Assessment and Coordination (UNDAC) team (typically 2–6 experts) travels quickly to a disaster area to report on the immediate needs to the international community.[2,80]

The needs assessment defines the extent of the damage to local infrastructure and medical capabilities, the numbers of casualties and types of injuries, and the key priorities in terms of disaster aid and relief, in close collaboration with the local authorities and facilities. Not surprisingly, medical needs often assume a lower priority than essentials such as water, food, and shelter but are nevertheless an integral part of the assessment.

From the trauma care perspective, there are two distinct phases in the medical response to a major natural disaster. The major aim in the immediate phase in the days and weeks following the disaster is to provide acute trauma care for the injured, while during the late phase the goal is to support the reconstruction of local medical capabilities and services in the disaster area.

### Trauma Care in the Disaster Area

In the immediate aftermath of a major natural catastrophe, casualties exhibit a wide clinical spectrum of injuries.[75] However, by the time outside teams arrive to render surgical assistance and support, casualties with severe visceral injuries are either treated early or do not survive. The clinical focus shifts to the management of extremity injuries that may be neglected and infected, or to specific complications such as renal failure from crush syndrome.[76,77]

The management of extremity injuries in the disaster area during the initial phase is based on the principles of the field management of war wounds.[82–84]

The aim is to avoid complex or multistaged reconstructions in favor of straightforward procedures. Muscle compartments should be decompressed early. Nonviable and heavily contaminated (or infected) tissue should be excised, while carefully preserving intact skin.[84] The wound should be left open for delayed primary closure (or wound re-excision, if necessary). Mangled extremities should undergo early amputation with delayed primary closure of the stump.

During the late phase of the disaster response, the need arises for complex orthopedic and plastic reconstructions which sometimes require special expertise and resources (such as specific operative technology or rehabilitation facilities).[2] The surgical solution must be realistically tailored to the patient's needs and to the available resources.

The composition of a surgical/trauma team deployed to a disaster area is dictated by the clinical needs. A typical team should consist of torso and extremity surgeons with trauma experience, who are trained to work in an austere environment in a spirit of collaboration.

A decision must be made regarding the scope of surgical work that the team will undertake, and whether the mission should be extended to other medical domains beyond trauma.[2] In this era of surgical sub-specialization, extending the goals of the mission translates into a larger team which, while representing a wider scope of clinical expertise, may not be in the best interests of the mission.

Depending on the local circumstances in the disaster zone, the external team can function either as an independent facility akin to a field surgical unit, or in support of a local functioning hospital. Very close collaboration with local trauma care providers and resources is essential. An effective mission is typically based on a reliable needs assessment, is aimed at specific achievable goals, and is limited in scope and duration.[2]

## CONCLUSION

The central message of this chapter is that amid the chaos and emotional turmoil of a MCI, trauma care providers should not lose sight of their primary goal. This goal is to provide critically injured patients with a level of care comparable to the care given to similar patients under normal circumstances.[11] The mission of the trauma service in a MCI is to preserve the dedicated service line of the hospital for the severely wounded, a service line that is their field of daily activity and special expertise. From the trauma care perspective, preserving the capability to provide a high level of trauma care to a relatively small group of severely injured patients is the crux of the entire effort.[11]

Reports of past MCIs indicate that, with effective planning and preparation, modern urban trauma systems are remarkably resilient and able to maintain a high level of care for the critically injured. The response to the bombing at the Centennial Olympics in Atlanta in 1996[85] or the Rhode Island nightclub fire in February 2003[86] are just two examples of such resilience of well-prepared trauma systems in the face of a sudden and large casualty load. Ensuring an effective response to a MCI with outcomes that are comparable to normal daily trauma care is the responsibility of every trauma care provider.

## REFERENCES

1. Hirshberg A, Holcomb JB, Mattox KL: Hospital trauma care in multiple-casualty incidents: A critical view. *Ann Emerg Med* 37:647, 2001.
2. Ryan JM: Natural disasters: The surgeon's role. *Scand J Surg* 94:311, 2005.
3. Centers of Disease Control and Prevention (CDC): Assessment of health-related needs after Hurricanes Katrina and Rita–Orleans and Jefferson Parishes, New Orleans area, Louisiana, October 17–22, 2005. *MMWR Morb Mortal Wkly Rep* 55:38, 2006.
4. Centers of Disease Control and Prevention (CDC): Injury and illness surveillance in hospitals and acute-care facilities after Hurricanes Katrina And Rita–New Orleans area, Louisiana, September 25–October 15, 2005. *MMWR Morb Mortal Wkly Rep* 55:35, 2006.
5. Mattox KL: Hurricanes Katrina and Rita: Role of individuals and collaborative networks in mobilizing/coordinating societal and professional resources for major disasters. *Crit Care* 10:205, 2005.
6. Frykberg ER: Medical management of disasters and mass casualties from terrorist bombings: How can we cope? *J Trauma* 53:201, 2002.
7. Frykberg ER: Triage: Principles and practice. *Scand J Surg* 94:272, 2005.
8. O'Neill PA: The ABC's of disaster response. *Scand J Surg* 94:259, 2005.
9. Frykberg ER, Tepas JJ III: Terrorist bombings. Lessons learned from Belfast to Beirut. *Ann Surg* 208:569, 1988.
10. Gutierrez de Ceballos JP, Turegano FF, Perez DD, et al.: Casualties treated at the closest hospital in the Madrid, March 11, terrorist bombings. *Crit Care Med* 33:S107, 2005.
11. Hirshberg A: Multiple casualty incidents: Lessons from the front line. *Ann Surg* 239:322, 2004.
12. Hammond J: Mass casualty incidents: Planning implications for trauma care. *Scand J Surg* 94:267, 2005.
13. Waeckerle JF: Disaster planning and response. *N Engl J Med* 324:815, 1991.
14. ACS Committee on Trauma: Chapter 20—Mass casualties. In: *Resources for optimal care of the injured patient.* Chicago, American College of Surgeons, 1999, p. 87.
15. Cushman JG, Pachter HL, Beaton HL: Two New York City hospitals' surgical response to the September 11, 2001, terrorist attack in New York City. *J Trauma* 54:147, 2003.
16. Hirshberg A, Scott BG, Granchi T, et al.: How does casualty load affect trauma care in urban bombing incidents? A quantitative analysis. *J Trauma* 58:686, 2005.
17. Teague DC: Mass casualties in the Oklahoma City bombing. *Clin Orthop* 422:77, 2004.
18. Stein M, Hirshberg A: Medical consequences of terrorism. The conventional weapon threat. *Surg Clin North Am* 79:1537, 1999.
19. Ryan J, Montgomery H: The London attacks–preparedness: Terrorism and the medical response. *N Engl J Med* 353:543, 2005.
20. Macintyre AG, Weir S, Barbera JA: The international search and rescue response to the US Embassy bombing in Kenya: The medical team experience. *Prehospital Disaster Med* 14:215, 1999.
21. Kluger Y, Peleg K, Daniel-Aharonson L, et al.: The special injury pattern in terrorist bombings. *J Am Coll Surg* 199:875, 2004.
22. Leibovici D, Gofrit ON, Stein M, et al.: Blast injuries: Bus versus open-air bombings—a comparative study of injuries in survivors of open-air versus confined-space explosions. *J Trauma* 41:1030, 1996.
23. Katz E, Ofek B, Adler J, et al.: Primary blast injury after a bomb explosion in a civilian bus. *Ann Surg* 209:484, 1989.
24. Mayorga MA: The pathology of primary blast overpressure injury. *Toxicology* 121:17, 1997.
25. Stein M: Urban bombing: A trauma surgeon's perspective. *Scand J Surg* 94:286, 2005.
26. Born CT: Blast trauma: The fourth weapon of mass destruction. *Scand J Surg* 94:279, 2005.
27. Mellor SG: The relationship of blast loading to death and injury from explosion. *World J Surg* 16:893, 1992.
28. Walsh RM, Pracy JP, Huggon AM, et al.: Bomb blast injuries to the ear: The London Bridge incident series. *J Accid Emerg Med* 12:194, 1995.
29. Wolf M, Kronenberg J, Ben Shoshan J, et al.: Blast injury of the ear. *Mil Med* 156:651, 1991.
30. Mrena R, Paakkonen R, Back L, et al.: Otologic consequences of blast exposure: A Finnish case study of a shopping mall bomb explosion. *Acta Otolaryngol* 124:946, 2004.
31. Leibovici D, Gofrit ON, Shapira SC: Eardrum perforation in explosion survivors: Is it a marker of pulmonary blast injury? *Ann Emerg Med* 34:168, 1999.
32. Almogy G, Luria T, Richter E, et al.: Can external signs of trauma guide management? Lessons learned from suicide bombing attacks in Israel. *Arch Surg* 140:390, 2005.
33. Avidan V, Hersch M, Armon Y, et al.: Blast lung injury: Clinical manifestations, treatment, and outcome. *Am J Surg* 190:927, 2005.
34. Pizov R, Oppenheim-Eden A, Matot I, et al.: Blast lung injury from an explosion on a civilian bus. *Chest* 115:165, 1999.
35. Sorkine P, Szold O, Kluger Y, et al.: Permissive hypercapnia ventilation in patients with severe pulmonary blast injury. *J Trauma* 45:35, 1998.
36. Aschkenasy-Steuer G, Shamir M, Rivkind A, et al.: Clinical review: The Israeli experience: Conventional terrorism and critical care. *Crit Care* 9:490, 2005.
37. Cripps NP, Cooper GJ: Risk of late perforation in intestinal contusions caused by explosive blast. *Br J Surg* 84:1298, 1997.
38. Paran H, Neufeld D, Shwartz I, et al.: Perforation of the terminal ileum induced by blast injury: Delayed diagnosis or delayed perforation? *J Trauma* 40:472, 1996.
39. Sosna J, Sella T, Shaham D, et al.: Facing the new threats of terrorism: Radiologists' perspectives based on experience in Israel. *Radiology* 237:28, 2005.
40. Shaham D, Sella T, Goitein O, et al.: Terror attacks: The role of imaging. In Shemer J, Shoenfeld Y, eds. *Terror and Medicine: Medical aspects of biological, chemical and radiological terrorism.* Lengerich: Pabst Science Publishers, 2003, p. 394.
41. Hirshberg A, Stein M, Walden R: Surgical resource utilization in urban terrorist bombing: A computer simulation. *J Trauma* 47:545, 1999.
42. Almogy G, Belzberg H, Mintz Y, et al.: Suicide bombing attacks: Update and modifications to the protocol. *Ann Surg* 239:295, 2004.
43. Braverman I, Wexler D, Oren M: A novel mode of infection with hepatitis B: Penetrating bone fragments due to the explosion of a suicide bomber. *Isr Med Assoc J* 4:528, 2002.
44. Eshkol Z, Katz K: Injuries from biologic material of suicide bombers. *Injury* 36:271, 2005.

45. Kennedy PJ, Haertsch PA, Maitz PK: The Bali burn disaster: Implications and lessons learned. *J Burn Care Rehabil* 26:125, 2005.
46. Palmer DJ, Stephens D, Fisher DA, et al.: The Bali bombing: The Royal Darwin Hospital response. *Med J Aust* 179:358, 2003.
47. Leslie CL, Cushman M, McDonald GS, et al.: Management of multiple burn casualties in a high volume ED without a verified burn unit. *Am J Emerg Med* 19:469, 2001.
48. Cernak I, Wang Z, Jiang J, et al.: Ultrastructural and functional characteristics of blast injury-induced neurotrauma. *J Trauma* 50:695, 2001.
49. Cernak I, Savic J, Zunik G, et al.: Recognizing, scoring and predicting blast injuries. *World J Surg* 23:44, 1999.
50. Cernak I, Savic J, Ignjatovic D, et al.: Blast injury from explosive munitions. *J Trauma* 47:96, 1999.
51. Irwin RJ, Lerner MR, Bealer JF, et al.: Shock after blast wave injury is caused by a vagally mediated reflex. *J Trauma* 47:105, 1999.
52. Ohnishi M, Kirkman E, Guy RJ, et al.: Reflex nature of the cardiorespiratory response to primary thoracic blast injury in the anaesthetised rat. *Exp Physiol* 86:357, 2001.
53. Kutz I, Bleich A: Conventional, chemical and biological terror of mass destruction: Psychological aspects and psychiatric guidelines. In Shemer J, Shoenfeld Y, eds. *Terror and Medicine: Medical aspects of biological, chemical and radiological terrorism.* Lengerich: Pabst Science Publishers, 2003, p. 493.
54. Galea S, Ahern J, Resnick H, et al.: Psychological sequelae of the September 11 terrorist attacks in New York City. *N Engl J Med* 346:982, 2002.
55. Einav S, Feigenberg Z, Weissman C, et al.: Evacuation priorities in mass casualty terror-related events: Implications for contingency planning. *Ann Surg* 239:304, 2004.
56. Klein JS, Weigelt JA: Disaster management. Lessons learned. *Surg Clin North Am* 71:257, 1991.
57. Garner A, Lee A, Harrison K, et al.: Comparative analysis of multiple-casualty incident triage algorithms. *Ann Emerg Med* 38:541, 2001.
58. START Triage: Available at: http://www.start-triage.com. Accessed January 17, 2006.
59. Romig LE: Pediatric triage. A system to JumpSTART your triage of young patients at MCIs. *JEMS* 27:52, 2002.
60. Wallis L: START is not the best triage strategy. *Br J Sports Med* 36:473, 2002.
61. Avitzour M, Libergal M, Assaf J, et al.: A multicasualty event: Out-of-hospital and in-hospital organizational aspects. *Acad Emerg Med* 11:1102, 2004.
62. Klausner JM, Rozin RR: The evacuation hospital in civilian disasters. *Isr J Med Sci* 22:365, 1986.
63. HEICS III: Available at: http://www.emsa.ca.gov/Dms2/heics3.htm. Accessed January 17, 2006.
64. Zane RD, Prestipino AL: Implementing the Hospital Emergency Incident Command System: An integrated delivery system's experience. *Prehospital Disaster Med* 19:311, 2004.
65. Kennedy K, Aghababian RV, Gans L, et al.: Triage: Techniques and applications in decision making. *Ann Emerg Med* 28:136, 1996.
66. Coupland RM: Epidemiological approach to surgical management of the casualties of war. *BMJ* 308:1693, 1994.
67. Holcomb JB, Helling TS, Hirshberg A: Military, civilian, and rural application of the damage control philosophy. *Mil Med* 166:490, 2001.
68. Peleg K, Aharonson-Daniel L, Michael M, et al.: Patterns of injury in hospitalized terrorist victims. *Am J Emerg Med* 21:258, 2003.
69. Shamir MY, Weiss YG, Willner D, et al.: Multiple casualty terror events: The anesthesiologist's perspective. *Anesth Analg* 98:1746, 2004.
70. Shamir MY, Rivkind A, Weissman C, et al.: Conventional terrorist bomb incidents and the intensive care unit. *Curr Opin Crit Care* 11:580, 2005.
71. Leibovici D, Gofrit ON, Heruti RJ, et al.: Interhospital patient transfer: A quality improvement indicator for prehospital triage in mass casualties. *Am J Emerg Med* 15:341, 1997.
72. Kluger Y, Mayo A, Soffer D, et al.: Functions and principles in the management of bombing mass casualty incidents: Lessons learned at the Tel-Aviv Souraski Medical Center. *Eur J Emerg Med* 11:329, 2004.
73. Hammond J, Brooks J: The World Trade Center attack. Helping the helpers: The role of critical incident stress management. *Crit Care* 5:315, 2001.
74. Redmond AD: Natural disasters. *BMJ* 330:1259, 2005.
75. Kuwagata Y, Oda J, Tanaka H, et al.: Analysis of 2,702 traumatized patients in the 1995 Hanshin-Awaii earthquake. *J Trauma* 43:427, 1997.
76. Oda J, Tanaka H, Yoshioka T, et al.: Analysis of 372 patients with Crush syndrome caused by the Hanshin-Awaji earthquake. *J Trauma* 42:470, 1997.
77. Sever MS, Erek E, Vanholder R, et al.: Lessons learned from the Marmara disaster: Time period under the rubble. *Crit Care Med* 30:2443, 2002.
78. Dries D, Perry JF Jr: Tsunami disaster: a report from the front. *Crit Care Med* 33:1178, 2005.
79. Centers for Disease Control and Prevention (CDC): Key facts about volcanic eruptions. Available at: http://www.bt.cdc.gov/disasters/volcanoes/facts.asp. Accessed January 17, 2006.
80. Redmond AD: Needs assessment of humanitarian crises. *BMJ* 330:1320, 2005.
81. Centers for Disease Control and Prevention (CDC): Tropical Storm Allison rapid needs assessment–Houston, Texas, June 2001. *MMWR Morb Mortal Wkly Rep* 51:365, 2002.
82. Coupland RM: War wound excision. *Br J Surg* 77:833, 1990.
83. Coupland RM: Technical aspects of war wound excision. *Br J Surg* 76:663, 1989.
84. Mannion SJ, Chaloner E: Principles of war surgery. *BMJ* 330:1498, 2005.
85. Feliciano DV, Anderson GV Jr, Rozycki GS, et al.: Management of casualties from the bombing at the centennial Olympics. *Am J Surg* 176:538, 1998.
86. Mahoney EJ, Harrington DT, Biffl WL, et al.: Lessons learned from a nightclub fire: Institutional disaster preparedness. *J Trauma* 58:487, 2005.

## Commentary ■ JAMES G. CUSHMAN ■ DAVE ROCCAFORTE

It is difficult to overstate the degree to which the issue of disaster preparedness has been scrutinized in our society during this era of global terrorism and natural disasters. Necessity mandates study and analysis of our ability at *all* levels to respond to sudden surges in casualties. Correspondingly, the editors of the 6th edition of *Trauma* have added this chapter on trauma care in mass casualty incidents. Authors Hirshberg and Stein have emphasized, in this chapter and elsewhere, key concepts in the clinical preparation and response to such a surge. Their first point focuses not on the absolute number of casualties per se, but how the hospital's resources are suited to match both the number and rate of arrival of casualties. The authors define a multiple casualty incident (MCI) as (hospital) resources taxed but with optimal management preserved, whereas a mass casualty event (MCE) over-

whelms community and hospital resources and requires drastic changes in triage and treatment priorities. A second point made is one repeatedly emphasized by Frykberg and others: the majority of explosive urban MCIs result in few critically injured casualties relative to those killed or minimally wounded. The authors refer to several recent events including the train explosions in Spain and England as well as the plethora of bombing events in the Middle East to illustrate this association. The triage process, by which certain casualties are deemed critical and in need of definitive care, is emphasized as being continuous and dynamic. Definitive Care Area physicians, working routinely in the operating room and the Intensive Care Unit, must provide leadership on a multidisciplinary hospital disaster preparedness team. In the event of an actual MCI/MCE they will help implement the plan, being fully aware of the above concepts, as well as having helped define for the hospital its surge capacity (SC) in advance. The authors refer to SC as a point whereby resources are overwhelmed such that optimal care cannot be assured for newly arriving casualties. An alternate but related concept of SC would be an amount of increase in a system—whatever that system may be—that allows the system to expand while continuing to function adequately. (If you are out of wall oxygen sources, a portable tank might do; if you are out of wheelchairs, a rolling cardiac chair or even large office chair might do). These alternate resources and the process of obtaining them can and should be defined pre-event by whatever system is assessing its own capability. Early uses of the term SC by Smithson and Levy (2000), O'Toole (2001), and Kamarck (2002) support both forms of definition. Whether SC is conceptualized as a phase (of expanded services but with optimal care preserved) or a point (where such optimal care is no longer able to be provided) is less important than the understanding that any hospital may be called upon to expand their casualty flow capacity in the event of an MCI/MCE. Herein lies the early work required of any hospital disaster preparedness team, to be followed by exercises and practice. Like global warming, MCI/MCEs are upon us—thus the need for disaster planning. Unlike its climatic counterpart whose effects are daily measured and recorded globally, the impact of MCIs are experienced sporadically. The physician who takes an interest in disaster preparation should self-educate beginning with the chapter authors' provided literature review. Numerous online resources are also available. Falkenrath and his co-editors have written an outstanding primer on covert attack by use of biologic, chemical, and nuclear means.[1] Others have expanded on the Hirshberg-Stein concept of optimizing outcomes when casualty flow exceeds resources by focusing on definitive care areas.[2] Smithson, presently an expert at The Center for Strategic and International Studies (CSIS), offers a perspective on first responders and bioterrorism scenarios.[3] Clearly, more funding, study, and support is required for our first responders. According to one of their own, Ret. Lt. John McLoughlin, PAPD, "There is need in emergency preparedness for those in charge of response and action to ask and take advice from the Line Supervisor in their decision making. Emergency preparedness needs to come from the bottom up instead of the traditional top down to be the most effective." Today, when experts predict that "81 million may die" from pandemic H5N1 influenza, and that conceivably "there will be more opportunity for saving lives in the emergency medical response to a biological terrorist attack than in the response to a conventional (explosive) terrorist attack" (Simon, JAMA, 1997) it is clear that the scope of required reading, as well as preparation and practicing, must extend beyond the common conventional scenarios best known to surgeons with an interest in trauma. Of note, the problem solving, leadership, and triage skills requisite to manage explosive traumatic-type MCIs have much to offer in the all-hazards preparedness approach. Please: read, learn, prepare, collaborate, and participate.

## References

1. Falkenrath RA, Newman RD, Thayer BA. *America's Achilles' Heel: Nuclear, Biological, and Chemical Terrorism and Covert Attack.* Cambridge, MA: MIT Press, 2001.
2. Roccaforte JD, Cushman JG. Disaster preparedness, triage and surge capacity for hospital definitive care areas: optimizing outcomes when demands exceed resources. *Anesth Clin No Amer.* In Press, March, 2007.
3. Smithson A. The biological weapons threat and nonproliferation options: A Survey of senior U.S. decision makers and policy shapers. A CSIS report, available online at http://www.csis.org/media/csis/pubs/061129_biosurvey.pdf. Accessed December 27, 2006.

# Rural Trauma

*Charles F. Rinker, II* ■ *G. Douglas Schmitz*

## THE RURAL ENVIRONMENT

Seventy percent of the population of the United States lives in an urban environment, while 70% of the trauma deaths occur in a rural locale. "It is surprising that a disease that kills rural citizens at nearly twice the rate of urban citizens has not received more attention."[1,2] The chance of dying in a rural area from a severe injury sustained in a motor vehicle-pedestrian collision is three to four times greater than in urban areas.[3] The relative risk of a rural victim dying in a motor vehicle crash is 15:1 compared with a victim of an urban crash.[4] Death from motor vehicle crashes is inversely related to population density.[5] In fact, death rates from all unintentional injuries combined are generally 50% greater in rural, sparsely populated counties of the western United States than they are in the densely populated northeastern counties.[6,7] Pediatric deaths from injury in a rural setting are more frequent than they are in an urban setting, despite the recent increase in gunshot wounds in the urban population.[8] Autopsy studies have suggested preventable trauma death rates of 20 to 30% in rural populations.[9–12] What are the reasons for these differences?

In this chapter we will attempt to identify circumstances that make rural trauma care difficult and consider some solutions. An illustrative case will help to explain some of the unique features of trauma care outside an urban setting:

A 48-year-old real estate developer was mountain biking with friends in a national forest in the Rocky Mountains. While unhelmeted, he rode ahead of the group and down a steep slope. Several minutes later his companions found him unconscious at the bottom of a ravine, after he had apparently lost control of his mountain bike. One of the party rode out for help, which arrived in the form of a Basic Life Support (BLS) ambulance unit from the local ski area, approximately 45 minutes following the crash. The patient had to be extricated from a ravine and carried several hundred yards to the ambulance, which then had a one-hour trip to the nearest hospital, a Level III trauma center. Communication (hand-held radio) with the hospital was not possible until the ambulance exited a narrow mountain canyon about

15 minutes before arrival. His Glasgow Coma Scale (GCS) score on the scene and in the emergency department was 8. He was hemodynamically normal, but a computed tomography (CT) scan of the head showed a large epidural hematoma with >5-mm shift; no other injuries were identified. Following consultation with a neurosurgeon at the nearest Level II center (150 air miles away,) a general surgeon trained in emergency limited craniotomy (and following established local protocols) drilled a burr hole and enlarged it sufficiently to permit evacuation of the clot and to control the hemorrhage. The patient was transferred directly from the operating room to a helicopter, which flew him to the neurosurgeon for a formal craniotomy. He survived with a Glasgow Outcome Score of 4 and is now independent, although no longer able to function in his former capacity.

This true scenario could have any of the following plausible variables: unaccompanied victim hours or days to discovery; less accessible to rescuers; greater distance to hospital; lack of trauma team and trained surgeon; or adverse weather preventing air transport to Level II trauma center. He might have been a hunter injured by firearm or animal, a back-country skier caught in an avalanche, a rancher thrown from a horse, or the driver of a car on a remote rural road.

Remoteness, rugged beauty, and "nature" are powerful magnets for tourists, recreationists, and those seeking a quieter, less stressful lifestyle. Such visitors are often shocked to discover that medical services they take for granted at home are simply unavailable in a rural setting. In contrast, local residents tend to be independent, fatalistic and accepting of limitations, suspicious of outsiders, resistant to both change and regulations (helmet and seatbelt laws; gun control), and unaware of trauma as a public health problem because, in their limited experience, it is a rare event.[1,13]

## DEFINING RURAL

Rural spaces are sparsely populated and support only one-third as many physicians as do urban areas.[1] Specialists, and sometimes even primary care physicians, cannot make a living in communities under a certain population threshold. Lack of physicians skilled in rapid assessment and treatment of the critically injured has a significant effect on outcomes. Conversely, the number of physicians in a given county, and particularly emergency physicians who have taken Advanced Trauma Life Support (ATLS), is associated with lower trauma death rates.[14]

An urban area consists of a central city and its environs with a combined population of greater than 50,000 and a population density of 1000 or more per square mile. As far as the United States Bureau of the Census is concerned, everything else is rural. Not all rural environments, however, support farming, and many are surprisingly close to cities, but separated by geographic barriers such as mountains or large bodies of water. Residents of coastal Marin County, only a few miles north of San Francisco, may have difficulty accessing a trauma center because of intervening steep mountains, narrow roads, and local regulations prohibiting noisy and disruptive helicopters. San Diego County, home of a model trauma system, reports morbidity and mortality from delayed discovery of motor vehicle crash victims on remote county roads.[15] North Carolina is the tenth most populous state, but 29 counties in the eastern part of the state are served by a single trauma center, 12 counties have no general surgeon, 17 no orthopedic surgeon, and 23 no neurosurgeon. Only 14 can reach an emergency department staffed with emergency physicians in less than 30 minutes.[14] Virtually all regions of our country have many areas that are sparsely populated and relatively poor in resources. In the central and northern plains, one sees the combination of few people and great distance from urban centers as nowhere else in the lower 48 states. Alaska, of course, along with some portions of the northern Rocky Mountains, is more accurately described as a frontier area (six or fewer people per square mile.)

Rural, then, may be defined in accordance with census data based on metropolitan statistical areas, in terms of geography and distance, or by virtue of limited resources. In a recent analysis of the general surgery workforce, Thompson et al. identified significant differences between communities with a population between 10,000 and 50,000 (large rural) and those with 2500 to 10,000 residents (small, or isolated rural). Large rural towns are far more likely to have the necessary resources such as general surgery, medical and surgical subspecialties, Advanced Life Support (ALS) ambulance services and essential equipment to provide prompt and sophisticated trauma care.[16]

Environmental factors are also important as "rural trauma occurs in areas where geography, population density, weather, distance, or availability of professional and institutional resources combine to isolate the patient in an environment where access to definitive care is limited."[17] An alternate, somewhat more precise definition has been proposed as follows: ". . . A rural trauma region would be an area in which the population served is fewer than 2500, has a population density of fewer than 50 persons per square mile, has only basic life support prehospital care, has prehospital transport times that exceed 30 minutes on average, and is lacking in subspecialty coverage for specific injuries (such as a neurosurgeon to manage the patient with head injuries)."[1] In any event, though we may think we know it when we see it, it is apparent that "rural" is difficult to define.

## EPIDEMIOLOGY

There are reasons why few people live in rural locations. The climate may be harsh, the terrain rugged and remote from services, the roads badly engineered and maintained, communications rudimentary, and the economy marginal. Career opportunities for the young are limited, so the young leave. As a result, significant segments of the population are elderly, poor, poorly educated, and in ill health. Population density (low) and personal income (also low) are the strongest predictors of per-capita trauma death rates.[14] Nearly one-fourth of adults in this environment sustain some form of unintentional injury per year. The injuries are usually relatively minor, but, occasionally, they are major and/or fatal. Binge drinking and depression are strongly associated comorbid factors, and suicide accounts for 10% of all rural trauma deaths.[1,18] Elderly rural patients tend to start out with a lower Injury Severity Score (ISS) and are less likely to die at the scene, but have a higher complication rate and worse overall survival for comparable severity of injury. Based on data from the Major Trauma Outcome Study (MTOS), rural geriatric trauma patients fare less well than do an urban cohort.[19] In addition, older age and lower population density independently increase vehicle-related mortality.[20] A recent study by Wigglesworth compared two groups of five states each with the highest (Group 1) and lowest (Group 2) traffic death rates, respectively. Epidemiologic data from the Centers for Disease Control and Prevention (CDC) indicated that the fatality rates for falls, poisoning, drowning, fire, suffocation, homicide, and suicide conformed closely to the traffic death rates in the two groups of states. Group 1 states were rural, western, and below national averages for per capita income; Group 2 states were urban, eastern, and financially well-off.[21]

Unintentional blunt injury comprises about 90% of cases, largely because of the prevalence of motor-vehicle-related incidents and the paucity of assaults with firearms. The most common causes of fatal injury are auto crashes, suicide, homicide, and falls. For these and the next 10 most frequent causes, rural death rates exceed urban rates for all but poisonings. Some of the most hazardous occupations such as mining, logging, and farming are almost exclusively rural by their very nature.[22] Large animal injuries may occur on a farm or ranch in the course of daily work or in conjunction with such recreational pursuits as hunting, pleasure riding, or rodeo. Typical injuries are falls (horses), tramplings and gorings (bulls, wild game), and kicks (cows.)[23] Travel on rural highways entails the additional hazard of motor vehicle-wild animal collisions (elk, deer, bear, or moose.) A mature moose weighs half a ton or more. Drivers unfortunate enough to strike one risk significant injury to the brain or death.[24] Fatal accidents are significantly higher for loggers (140/100,000) than they are for workers in other industries (94/100,000), and are typically the result of being struck by falling trees, limbs, or snags. Crush injury between moving logs and encounters with heavy equipment are other common mechanisms, and access to care is often a problem.[25] Recreation also provides endless opportunities for serious injury and death. Small community hospitals bear the brunt of these misadventures, particularly when situated in proximity to ski hills, wilderness areas, national parks, and seashores or lakefronts. Risk-taking behavior by adventure seekers only magnifies the problem.

Most people feel safe in rural settings. The risk of violent assault and penetrating trauma is very low as noted above. Blunt trauma comprises 95% or more of the trauma case load at most rural community hospitals, 85% of which is minor or moderate (ISS<10) and can be treated without the need for transfer to a trauma center. Blunt trauma is less time-dependent, which is fortunate since it is far more difficult to mount a rapid response in a small community hospital. It can be subtle, however, requiring experience and a high index of suspicion to avoid missed injuries.[26] Motor vehicle crashes, although in aggregate the biggest killer in all areas of this country and the rest of the world, are sporadic events in small towns and the countryside.

In essence, the greatest problems confronting rural trauma care are access to the system and lack of resources. The challenge is to devise a system, ensure access, and make the most of limited resources.

## RURAL RESOURCES AND LIMITATIONS

### Discovery and Access to the System

In the minds of many students of the rural trauma problem, discovery and access are the most important explanations for high mortality rates. When people are scarce and distances between population centers great, the injured may be lost or misplaced, whether in the back country or on a remote highway.[1,13,27–29] Delays of hours are common, and, occasionally, days may pass before a victim can be found. In rural systems of care, time of crash until time of arrival at the hospital is more than an hour in 30% of cases, as opposed to 7% in urban systems.[30] Prolonged mean prehospital times have been reported in rural Vermont (105 minutes), upstate New York (96 minutes), northern California (55 minutes), rural Washington (48 minutes) and Georgia (40 minutes). Thus, the "golden hour" is often spent on the road, not in the hospital.[1] In extreme cases, crash victims in a snow-filled roadside ditch or ravine, or a hunter or back country nordic skier may not be found until spring break-up. Retrieval is equally challenging and often relies on the special skills of search-and-rescue volunteers equipped to go into swamps and tidal flats, high mountains, or dense forests and other wilderness areas. Even when a helicopter is at hand, victims must often be moved over rough terrain by litter, watercraft, snowmobile, all-terrain vehicle, horse, or other conveyance to a suitable and safe landing area. Fortunately, most guides and outfitters now carry global positioning satellite (GPS) units, cellular phones, and/or hand-held radios to facilitate rescues in emergency situations. If a hospital lacks a trauma program and leader, the response to a major trauma event tends to be disorganized. In the absence of field-to-hospital communication, the patient arrives unannounced. Obvious extremity injuries may overshadow more critical internal injuries and prompt a call for an orthopedic surgeon when a trauma team led by a general surgeon is more appropriate. Even when notification occurs, the physician in the emergency department may wait to see just how badly a patient is injured, instead of mobilizing the trauma team and alerting the helicopter for interhospital transfer. The opportunity to eliminate a critical rate-limiting step is then lost. The patient proceeds from scene to litter to ambulance to local hospital and then perhaps on to the next higher level sequentially, and precious time is wasted (see Table 10-1).

### TABLE 10-1

**Rural Resources and Limitations**

Discovery and access to system
Manpower
Communications
Transport
Facilities
Education and maintenance of skills

One of the most important steps a small hospital can take toward improving trauma care is the establishment of a trauma team. When possible, the team should be led by a general surgeon.[31–34] Criteria for team activation should be established, and team members should commit to come to the patient's bedside immediately when called. In very small hospitals lacking general surgery support, it is still possible to provide appropriate emergency care. The Rural Trauma Subcommittee of the American College of Surgeons Committee on Trauma conducted an informal survey of small rural hospitals and found that most could mobilize three health care providers most of the time including physician extenders, nurses, technicians (lab, X-ray, respiratory therapy), and clerks. Drawing on these resources (as well as primary care physicians, or surgeons, in slightly larger facilities) the committee's Rural Trauma Team Development Course trains these individuals in the team approach to the initial assessment, resuscitation, and transfer to definitive care for the injured patient. This one-day interactive course is patterned on ATLS, but is inexpensive to present and may be given in modular form. The program is coordinated through the state chair of the Committee on Trauma.[35] Obstacles to this logical solution include medical staff reluctance to get involved with trauma; fears that overtriage will place greater demands on surgeons; turf wars between ambulance services, hospitals, and communities; and financial incentives to treat patients locally rather than transport them. In addition, the Emergency Medical Transfer and Active Labor Act (EMTALA) may have the unintended consequence of discouraging efficient transfers within a trauma system.

## MANPOWER

Physicians are reluctant to practice in rural areas. Those who do likely grew up in a small town, were influenced by a mentor, or have an independent streak.[36] Those who will not have fears of being overworked, underpaid, and unable to obtain backup or guidance. Social and cultural deprivations may bear heavily on a spouse, and, if the spouse is unhappy, the sojourn will be brief. Patient volumes are insufficient to support specialty services, and generalists with little or no formal trauma training predominate. Such individuals are expected to treat a significant number of minor trauma cases, but also the occasional complex major trauma case for which they have not been trained. A study of five small hospitals in rural Washington and Idaho revealed that they averaged three patients per year with an ISS greater than 19, and each physician saw, on average, 0.6% of these patients.[37] Because trauma events are sporadic and infrequent, rural physicians may develop a fear of or aversion to care of the injured. Furthermore, despite evidence to the contrary,[38] general surgeons believe they are more likely to be sued by trauma patients.

In many communities, a nurse practitioner or autonomous physician's assistant is the town "doctor." Their educational background and experience, as well as that of their supervising physician, rarely includes exposure to sufficient cases of major injury. Ambulance workers are predominantly volunteers trained to advanced first aid, EMT (emergency medical technician)-Basic, or at most, EMT-I level, usually at their own expense. Their experience with trauma is also very limited, even though in some rural ambulance services trauma may be one-third to one-half of the case load.[39]

Outside the academic medical center it is uncommon for resident staff or independent practitioners to stay in-house after hours. In hospitals with less than 30 inpatient beds it is unusual to have emergency physicians. In many small communities, a nurse or physician's assistant is the only professional at the hospital on nights and weekends. The doctor may be at home or out of town and may or may not be willing to come in if called for a trauma emergency. If the doctor does come in, he or she will conduct the resuscitation with minimal assistance and limited equipment. Despite these shortcomings, there usually is no other choice since the next hospital may be many miles distant and may be no better equipped. It is for reasons such as these that it is so important for rural physicians, physician assistants, and nurses to take or audit the ATLS course and to become involved in a regional trauma system.

An effective emergency medical service (EMS) program is vital for proper trauma care. In most rural counties the fire department provides EMS, although private ambulance services are occasionally found. Rural EMS providers are a mixture of paid or unpaid volunteers, and most function at the basic EMT level. Their focus is on cardiopulmonary resuscitation (CPR), extrication, immobilization, and transport. Scene management is protocol driven. Training requires 100 hours, often paid out of pocket by the volunteer. Additional hours are required for more advanced levels, which permit intravenous insertion and defibrillation (198 hours), administration of some basic drugs (216 hours), and, at the paramedic level, intubation (548 hours). Unfortunately, the latter skill, which certainly could be lifesaving for many rural trauma victims, particularly those with severe injuries to the brain, requires constant practice. In low-volume systems, it is difficult to maintain proficiency. Consequently, because of time, expense, and infrequent need for advanced skills, it is unusual to find Advanced Life Support (ALS) providers in a rural service area. Despite suggestions that trauma death rates are lower in counties where ALS is available,[40] it is not likely that the current rural EMT manpower situation will change in the near future.

In some locations, unique solutions to local needs have been devised. When ALS is required, it is sometimes provided by an on-scene helicopter flight team or by rendezvous with an ALS ground unit during transport. Other communities have the ambulance stop at the local hospital or clinic to pick up a doctor or nurse on the way to the scene. Creative use of limited resources is one of the ongoing challenges of rural trauma care.

## COMMUNICATIONS

The original EMS legislation and subsequent funding bills recognized the need for effective and reliable communication between field and hospital. Rural regions have not always been successful in competing for these grant funds, and their communities either cannot afford to purchase necessary equipment or question the need. Distance and terrain make good equipment even more important, and dead zones where no communication is possible are common. Skilled dispatchers are hard to find in small towns. Physicians and nurses at the hospital may be unfamiliar with and wary of communications equipment, and, accordingly, reluctant to talk with field personnel to provide medical guidance. Consequently, ambulance personnel have little incentive to use the equipment even when it is serviceable. There are still locations where 911 is unavailable. In addition, enhanced 911, which pinpoints locations by street address, is not feasible in those outlying areas which lack street names and numerical addresses. Communication between the local hospital and regional trauma center may also be difficult and unrewarding. Local practitioners often complain of unpleasant encounters with flight crews, emergency room personnel at the receiving hospital, and surgical staff on the trauma service. Attending surgeons are infrequently available for telephone consultation, despite the fact that they are, in essence, being referred a patient by a colleague. Feedback and constructive criticism regarding transferred patients are frequently sought by referring physicians, but not often attainable. In addition, they may receive mixed messages including criticism for overtriage on the one hand to holding onto a patient too long on the other.

The net effect of problems in communication is that the rural practitioner ends up functioning in a relative vacuum, receiving little advance warning from the field, limited help at the hospital, and negative or no feedback from the regional center.

## TRANSPORT

Evacuation of rural trauma victims is generally accomplished by surface conveyances. If the victim is inaccessible to an ambulance, various methods, all of them slow, may be employed to convey the patient to a road. The ambulance may then need to negotiate a sequence of roads from unsurfaced or gravel to county or state highway. Even the latter may be narrow, winding, and poorly maintained. Most often the destination is the nearest hospital, which will vary in its capabilities, and may be many miles distant. Response times, which include travel from the dispatch site to scene, extrication or retrieval, packaging, and travel to the hospital, are sometimes measured in hours, not minutes, as previously noted.

Ambulance services may be freestanding or, more commonly, an integral part of the local fire department. Funding may be through a special ambulance district or as part of the county budget, jealously guarded by county commissioners.[26] Frequently, because of limited funding, the ambulance service may employ aging although lovingly maintained vehicles, which are limited in number. In Vermont, it is estimated that the average local ambulance is unavailable 15% of the time.[1] If an ambulance is in service on a call or out of service for maintenance, the next call might have to be answered by a crew in a neighboring district through mutual aid agreement. Multiple incidents or victims can easily overwhelm the transport system.

Helicopters can be used both for scene rescue and for interhospital transport. Ideally, evacuation from the scene of injury directly to the trauma center should afford the patient the best opportunity for recovery. In the urban environment, ground ALS has actually been shown to be preferable for relatively short distances, since it takes time to prepare the aircraft for flight. With flight times above 15 minutes, helicopters gain the advantage.[41] In Fresno County, California, a study of ground versus helicopter transport in a relatively flat, nonmountainous area served by one Level I trauma center concluded that, within 10 miles of the hospital, ground transport yielded the shortest 911–hospital interval. Beyond that distance, the simultaneous dispatch of ground and air transport was the most efficient: ground personnel could extricate and resuscitate in advance of the arrival of the helicopter. For surface transports of more than 45 miles, helicopter was faster even if dispatched after the ground unit.[42]

In the rural environment, provided the scene is within the range of aircraft without the need to refuel, direct transport may be worthwhile if the time to the local hospital by ground ambulance is greater than that of the helicopter flight.[43] If not, surface transport is preferable.[44] A helicopter may also be invaluable in wilderness rescue if a suitable landing site can be assured. The downside is that the aircraft are expensive ($900,000–$2,200,000 start-up; $500,000–$2,000,000 annual maintenance), hazardous (fatal accident rate 4.7/100,000 hour),[45] and have a limited range. They are also sensitive to weather and not always available. Although newer models are roomier, it is still difficult to examine, monitor, and resuscitate unstable patients while airborne. Finally, their effectiveness is open to question. In one study of scene (18.8%) and interhospital (79.5%) transports, the most severely injured patients (17%) died en route or shortly after arrival at the medical center, while 55% had relatively trivial injuries that did not require the use of the rotorcraft.[46] The group with intermediate severity of injury (27%) benefited from use of the helicopter, but was difficult to identify in advance. ISS was not used in this study, but, in another study of scene transports alone, the group that benefited appeared to be those with an ISS of 22 to 30.[45]

In the remote rural setting, helicopters are used primarily for interhospital transfers, following stabilization at the local facility. Even in this circumstance, the solution is not ideal. Once the initial outlay for equipment and personnel has been made, an incentive exists to use it, even when surface conveyance may be an acceptable alternative. Helicopters become an important part of the sponsoring hospital's marketing program. Overtriage reflected in an average ISS of 19 is a major problem that remains to be solved.[41,45] In some mature programs, as many as 55% of patients transported were determined retrospectively to have minor trauma. It would appear that continued refinement of triage criteria is necessary to ensure that helicopters are used judiciously and effectively.

Fixed-wing transfers are another option, but are restricted to interhospital transfer. These aircraft are fast and, when properly equipped, can function as an airborne intensive care unit.[47] Their use is common in the noncoastal western states in helping to bridge vast distances. Drawbacks include the 30 minutes or more needed to get the plane airborne, and the need to transport the victim by ground ambulance between airport and hospital on both ends of the transfer.

## FACILITIES

Urban trauma systems attempt to identify those hospitals with the resources and staff commitment to care for the critically injured patient and direct patients to those facilities, bypassing hospitals unable or unwilling to provide appropriate response and treatment. In less populated areas, where resources are not so abundant, bypass may not be an option. In the two decades following introduction of state EMS programs, most authors have asserted that rural community hospitals are the logical destination for critically injured.[9,12,19,33,44,48–51] Following stabilization, they can then be transferred to the nearest trauma center. Studies indicate that, while this time-honored principle still applies in remote areas, in some rural areas bypass may be possible. With improved triage criteria, astute prehospital personnel, and good communications, a system can allow for transport of some stable rural patients with severe injuries directly to the trauma center without stopping at the local hospital.[52–55] In rural Georgia, where one-third of all ambulance trips were trauma related, 50% of patients were taken to the local hospital, but the remainder could be taken directly to a regional trauma center or urban hospital. The more remote the county, the more likely the patient was taken first to the local hospital.[39] It is still true that in many rural systems, it is simply not feasible to transfer unstable patients, whether by ground or helicopter, directly and over long distance to a trauma center. Bypass of the local hospital is not appropriate in these circumstances. A corollary of this observation is that rural health care facilities should be prepared, within their capabilities, to manage properly the sporadic seriously injured patient. Unfortunately, as a result of trauma legislation, malpractice concerns, uncertainty regarding the appropriate role of the local hospital, and lack of surgeon commitment, many patients are now transferred to trauma centers when they could have been treated locally.[52]

In a few select locations, a Level I academic trauma center may be strategically situated close to a large rural referral base. (For purposes of this discussion, Levels I to IV are those defined by the American College of Surgeons Committee on Trauma.)[17] More commonly, particularly in the plains and mountainous western states, huge distances intervene between regional trauma centers, and there may be no Level I, or, in some cases, even a Level II. These trauma centers serve the population not only with equipment and technical expertise unavailable in smaller hospitals, but also through system development, performance improvement, professional and lay education, prevention programs, and rehabilitation services.

Some rural Level II centers are located close enough to a Level I that their job is primarily to share some of the burden of the trauma case load and education and outreach responsibilities.[31] Many serve a vast geographic area, however, and, accordingly, must assume a larger role. They will differ from a Level I in terms of lower volumes, mostly blunt trauma, surgeons who take calls from home, and lack of certain sophisticated services such as limb replantation or management of complex pelvic and acetabular fractures.[51] Most will provide helicopter and(or fixed-wing transport to their region. They may have resident house staff and medical students, but most do not. Leadership in education, outreach, performance improvement, and system development, normally the purview of Level I academic centers, become their mission.

A rural Level III trauma center, even though it may lack many of the capabilities of the regional Level II, is a critical resource that will receive patients from many smaller hospitals in its region.[2,33] It is expected to provide full-time emergency medicine, general surgical, orthopedic, and operating room availability. Size will vary from about 40 to 150 beds. Case volumes are low, approximately 50 to 125 trauma registry patients per annum, and most have an

ISS less than 15. In addition, the medical staff will usually have specialists in internal medicine, a variety of medical subspecialists, and family practitioners. Anesthesia is provided by anesthesiologists or nurse anesthetists. Services that are important to the care of trauma patients, but are usually unavailable, include neurosurgery, cardiovascular surgery, plastic and reconstructive surgery, interventional radiology, dialysis, comprehensive blood banking, in-house operating room team, and backup. Imaging services will include ultrasound and a CT scanner, while angiography, nuclear medicine, and magnetic resonance imaging may be available. The trauma team, taking calls from home, is committed to early evaluation and treatment of critically injured individuals, based on prehospital triage and timely notification from the field so that the team may be present when the patient arrives. Physicians in the emergency department and, sometimes, surgeons should provide both on-line and off-line medical direction for local ambulance services. The hospital has sufficient equipment and personnel to provide definitive care for the majority of patients, but must recognize those patients who exceed local capabilities and need rapid, efficient stabilization followed by transport to the next appropriate level of care. The trauma program, aided by a trauma registry, is expected to conduct ongoing performance improvement for itself and prehospital personnel and to provide outreach services to smaller hospitals within its catchment area. The rural Level III is more likely to encounter and provide definitive care for moderately injured patients (ISS 9 to 25) and to serve as a regional resource, than its urban or suburban conterpart.[53,54]

Level IV hospitals have surgical capability, but often only one surgeon, who accordingly cannot be available at all times.[29,31,33] With the aid of improved triage criteria and prompt assembly of the trauma team, a group of nondesignated, isolated rural hospitals (size 18 to 77 beds) in northern California demonstrated the ability to provide care to 266 patients (mean ISS 26) that exceeded Major Trauma Outcome Study norms. They lacked the financial resources to be designated by the state as Level III, but were able to provide operative and inpatient care under the proper circumstances. Above all, they demonstrated commitment to care of the injured, without which no hospital, regardless of other resources, will succeed as a trauma center.[56] In many small hospitals, however, those requiring surgical or inpatient care will usually need to be transferred early. Observation of patients with blunt injury to a solid organ is not advisable in this setting unless the surgeon and operating room staff commit to being available at a moment's notice if nonoperative management fails. The trauma team and trauma program will be led by a surgeon when possible, but will include family physicians, physician assistants, and nurse practitioners. Damage control surgery or operative stabilization before transport should be undertaken when indicated, provided the surgeon and operating room staff are available.

The Washington trauma system includes Level V trauma centers in its designation process. These are health care facilities lacking inpatient capability, but which commit to early availability for resuscitation, stabilization, and transport within the system. Some regions of California have developed Emergency Department Approved for Trauma (EDAT) in rural areas of the state to serve the same stabilization and transport function. Most hospitals in most states are undesignated, but also have an important role to play in an inclusive system.

## EDUCATION AND MAINTENANCE OF SKILLS

Severe trauma represents 5% or less of the workload of most rural general surgeons.[2,33,37] Rural health care workers at all levels have difficulty maintaining their skills because they will have few opportunities to exercise them. ATLS was designed specifically to teach physicians how to manage patients in the early minutes and hours after a critical injury. The target audience was the rural physician or surgeon who sees such patients infrequently and must cope with very limited resources to resuscitate and transfer such patients. It has now become the international standard for early care of the injured and has had a positive impact on rural trauma care. Pre-Hospital Trauma Life Support (PHTLS) has been developed in conjunction with ATLS to educate EMTs about trauma.

In the early 1980s and early 1990s, before the general dissemination of ATLS, most articles on rural trauma care were in agreement that a significant proportion of preventable trauma morbidity and mortality resulted from inappropriate care at the local hospital.[9,12,13,15,29] More recent studies indicate that, at least in some areas, patients are now being stabilized much more effectively before transport to the regional Level I or II trauma center, and delays in discovery, retrieval, and transport are the principal causes of death.[1,14,27,28,57-59] On the other hand, a recent report from Rhode Island, where ATLS is not mandated for emergency room staff, demonstrated frequent departure from ATLS guidelines, with resultant delays in transport to the centrally located Level I trauma center.[60]

New technology and techniques take time to arrive in rural areas. Expense and lack of need contribute to the delay. For instance, most rural surgeons and physicians in the emergency department will not encounter enough patients with serious abdominal injuries to become adept in the use of ultrasound to identify intra-abdominal hemorrhage. For them, time and expenditures for capital equipment may be better directed at more basic and utilitarian items. Ignorance of new methods, however, is not acceptable. Members of the trauma team should assume responsibility for remaining sufficiently current in the trauma literature and in ATLS. They should know how to evaluate and resuscitate severely injured patients, recognize the need for operative intervention before transfer, know when nonoperative management is appropriate and safe, and realize when a patient's needs exceed local resources.

Feedback on specific cases and trauma educational outreach programs are primary responsibilities of the leading trauma center in the area. Intramural offerings, particularly if based on local registry information, will help all members of the team to remain up to date. Prevention programs will help raise public awareness of the impact trauma has on individual lives and may assist in increasing support for the purchase of equipment and development of a regional trauma system.

## TREATMENT OPTIONS

### Stabilization and Transfer to Definitive Care

When a trauma patient is en route or has already arrived at a small hospital with limited resources, one of the most critical decisions to be made is whether the patient can be treated locally or whether transfer is necessary. Trauma outcome is directly related to time to definitive care. If it is clear from the field report that the victim's injuries will exceed local resources, that is the time to begin making transfer arrangements in order to eliminate the principal rate-limiting step (i.e., dispatch and arrival of the transport team and conveyance).[61] Hospitals that need to transfer patients frequently know in advance which trauma centers will receive them and have transfer agreements in effect.

Once the patient is in the emergency department, it is the responsibility of the surgeon or physician leading the team to recognize the need for transfer and initiate arrangements as soon as possible. From that point onward, all efforts should be directed at optimizing the patient's physiology. ATLS should be the guide to the resuscitation, and testing and interventions should be limited to essentials and should not delay the departure.[62] The team leader should speak directly with the receiving trauma surgeon and should avoid transferring care directly to a subspecialist (orthopedic surgeon, neurosurgeon, plastic surgeon.) If the receiving hospital is on diversion, their representatives should help the referring hospital find an alternate destination.

Federal law now governs transfer of patients from an emergency department to another hospital, to another area within the same hospital, or to home. Violation of the Emergency Medical Treatment and Active Labor Act (EMTALA) regulations can lead to draconian penalties for hospitals and individuals. Punishments include denial of the ability to care for Medicare and Medicaid patients, as well as civil liability. This set of rules, originally enacted in 1985 to prevent patient "dumping" (inappropriate transfer of unstable indigent patients from private to public emergency rooms), has been expanded to what is essentially a federal right to emergency care and a federal malpractice act. The receiving hospital is obligated to report whenever a patient was "unstable" or inappropriately transferred. A complaint by any concerned party must be investigated by the Office of the Inspector General (OIG).[63]

Most traumatic events will be viewed by the patient, although not necessarily by health care workers, as an emergency. Any patient has a right to request a medical screening exam (MSE) for a perceived emergency medical condition (EMC.) The hospital or clinic is required to determine by this exam whether or not an EMC in fact exists. If the patient has an EMC, "the hospital must stabilize the emergency condition, or, if it is unable to stabilize the patient, the hospital must transfer the patient to a hospital that is capable of stabilizing the emergency condition. Hospitals with specialized capabilities or facilities are required to accept transfers of patients who require such specialized services. . . ."[63] What constitutes an EMC, and the details of the MSE, are open to interpretation.

How are hospitals and physicians to respond (Table 8-2)? One strategy already being employed is for surgeons to refuse to take trauma calls and for hospitals to close their doors to injured patients. The ethical and legal ramifications of this approach are debatable and will undoubtedly be subjected to close scrutiny. The proactive response is for health care workers and facilities to familiarize themselves with the provisions of the law and to establish, in cooperation with each other, a trauma program that will be in compliance. Properly executed transfer agreements should, in most cases, streamline the process. It is likely that the strongest defense in any given instance will be the ability to demonstrate that actions were directed toward the patient's best interest. For the trauma patient, the following would be appropriate:

1. Prehospital triage protocols for identification of critically injured patients

2. A mechanism for ensuring early evaluation, at the bedside, by the appropriate surgeon or emergency medicine physician

3. Prompt initiation of resuscitation and stabilization measures

4. Early decision regarding the medical need for transfer

5. Consultation with the receiving hospital (ideally with the trauma surgeon)

6. Documentation of indications for, and acceptance of, transfer

7. Arrangement of the appropriate transfer team, conveyance, and equipment

8. Before transfer, stabilization of the patient's condition to the degree possible given the resource imitations of the transferring hospital

Managed care may also interfere with the orderly transfer of patients as established by a regional trauma system. Several types of problems have arisen. Payments for emergency and after-hours transfers have been denied for lack of prior authorization, even though such authorization was impossible to obtain at the time. Triage to a hospital within the managed care system may be mandated, even though that facility may not be an authorized trauma center. The American College of Surgeons has issued a statement condemning such practices and encouraging cooperation of managed care and trauma systems.[64]

## OPERATIVE STABILIZATION AND TRANSFER

Most patients respond to standard resuscitative measures and, once stabilized, can be admitted locally, discharged home, or transferred to a higher level of care. A small proportion, probably less than 10%, will be either transient or nonresponders and will remain hemodynamically abnormal despite continued skilled resuscitation. If the patient has multiple injuries, suffers from significant medical comorbidity, is at the extremes of age, or has injuries requiring subspecialty (i.e., neurosurgical) or complex intensive care, transfer will likely be necessary. The more remote the primary facility is, the greater the risk that the patient will deteriorate during transfer unless something is done to address the underlying problem, generally hemorrhage. In this circumstance, the local general or subspecialty surgeon should be prepared to operate and stabilize the patient before transfer. With a properly equipped transport vehicle, usually a fixed-wing aircraft or helicopter, the patient may often be transferred immediately into the hands of the flight team without any compromise of care.[47,65] Operative stabilization of this sort falls into two categories: definitive surgery and damage control surgery.

### Definitive Surgery

Under most circumstances a stabilizing procedure can be conducted and completed in conventional fashion, such that no further treatment will be required for that particular problem. Examples would include, but are not limited to the following:

1. Establishment of a surgical airway

2. Splenorrhaphy or splenectomy; hepatorrhaphy, resection and debridement, or insertion of perihepatic packs

3. Closure of evisceration

4. Closure of injuries to the gastrointestinal tract

5. Repair of truncal and extremity vascular injuries

6. Reduction of dislocations

7. Debridement and control of hemorrhage from open fractures in an extremity or mangled extremities

## Damage Control Surgery

Damage control operations followed by temporary closure of the abdomen have been described for a variety of truncal injuries[66–68] with an emphasis on limiting time in the operating room and avoiding the triad of acidosis, hypothermia, and coagulopathy. Candidates for these desperate measures typically have an overwhelming constellation of injuries. Most reports on damage control surgery and temporary closure techniques have come from urban trauma centers. Following a period of rewarming and correction of acidosis in the intensive care unit, the patient is then returned to surgery for definitive repair of the remaining injuries. Rural surgeons can apply the same principles. Occasional patients will have such complex injuries that definitive management exceeds the technical abilities or resources of the local surgeon and hospital, but may be amenable to temporizing maneuvers, followed by rapid transfer in an aircraft equipped as an airborne intensive care unit.[69] Examples include packing of the liver for complex hepatic injuries; peritoneal cleansing, hemorrhage control and stapling or rapid suture of multiple bowel perforations; temporary abdominal closure; and abbreviated thoracotomy, hemorrhage control, and temporary chest closure for patients with extensive pulmonary and thoracic vascular injuries.[70] If interventional radiology is not available locally, patients with unstable pelvic fractures may benefit from application of external fixators prior to transfer.

Injury to the brain remains the single greatest source of morbidity and mortality for trauma victims.[15] Many patients sustain their closed-head injuries far from the nearest neurosurgeon, and time becomes the enemy. Under most circumstances, the only option is to minimize secondary brain injury with appropriate ventilatory and pharmacologic maneuvers and expedite transfer.[71,72] A small proportion of these patients, however, will have lesions amenable to surgical drainage. While rural hospitals generally lack neurosurgical services, most hospitals in the United States now have CT scanners. General surgeons can be trained to perform yet another kind of damage control surgery: burr holes and/or limited craniotomy for decompression and hemorrhage control in patients with epidural or subdural hematomas noted on a CT scan.[73,74] When a patient with an injury to the brain shows signs of rapid deterioration and a delay of more than 90 minutes to definitive neurosurgical care is anticipated, consideration should be given to emergency decompression of the hematoma.[72,75] The necessary components are as follows:

1. A general surgeon trained in indications for and technique of burr holes with limited craniotomy

2. Closed-head injury with lateralizing signs and threatened herniation

3. Surgical lesion present on CT scan

4. Consultation with, and approval of, neurosurgeon at receiving trauma center

5. Limited craniotomy for decompression and hemorrhage control

6. Immediate transfer to definitive care.[71]

Prompt intervention may reduce morbidity and mortality.

## LOCAL DEFINITIVE CARE

Most trauma patients can be cared for at a local community hospital capable of offering continuous surgical care. "The mindset that a well-trained general surgeon is not able to care for many trauma patients must be corrected."[52] Although triage and transfer guidelines address anatomic, physiologic, and mechanism of injury parameters, there are few publications that describe specifically which patients might reasonably be cared for in small hospitals. Currently accepted examples are patients with isolated extremity fractures, minor burns, lacerations, hemo- and/or pneumothorax, multiple rib fractures, closed-head injury with GCS of 14 to 15, and a variety of organ and vessel injuries within the ability and comfort range of the attending surgeon. It is important for surgeons to remember that colleagues, nursing staff, and ancillary services must also be able to provide the necessary adjunctive care. Patients at the extremes of age, with multiple organ system involvement, with the need for prolonged ventilator support and/or intensive care, and with serious underlying illnesses will probably benefit from care in a trauma center under most circumstances. Patients should always be advised of the option to be transferred. It is important to be aware of pertinent state statutes or transfer guidelines used by the regional trauma system and to realize that in the event of misadventures, the burden of proof will rest with the doctor who chooses not to transfer a patient.

The management of patients with blunt injury to solid abdominal viscera (particularly spleen and liver) presents some difficult logistical problems for the rural surgeon. Most patients with injuries to the spleen or liver and normal hemodynamics can be managed without an operation. When an operation is necessary, the well-trained general surgeon is certainly fully capable of performing a splenectomy or splenorrhaphy. Major hepatic injuries have the potential for overwhelming the technical ability of the surgeon or the resources of a small blood bank, but may be amenable to simple suture repair, resectional debridement, or packing and immediate transfer. It is to the patient's advantage to be managed in the local hospital rather than be transferred to a distant Level I or II center, if it can be done safely. The problem lies with the patient who deteriorates unexpectedly, becomes hypotensive, and requires urgent surgery. In a hospital lacking house staff, immediate availability of the surgeon, and a plan for rapid preparation of the operating room, there is a small but real potential for death from exsanguinating hemorrhage. In these circumstances, a lower threshold for early operation or transfer is appropriate.[76]

When patients are selected properly for local treatment, a number of advantages accrue. It is generally more convenient for patient and family as friends, clergy, and support groups in the area provide moral support and can hasten recovery and reintegration into the community. Risks inherent in emergency transfers are eliminated. Use of local services keeps money in the community. Because most rural trauma is motor-vehicle-related, insurance coverage is better than average and supports the financial stability of the hospital. Finally, appropriate local care reduces the burden on busy regional trauma centers.[52,77]

A downside for many surgeons is that trauma of this sort, particularly in the era of observation of injuries to solid organs, is not very exciting and produces relatively few operations. Overseeing care for patients while subspecialists perform a variety of operative procedures does not appeal to many general surgeons. Hours are inconvenient, and trauma emergencies can wreak havoc with elective schedules. The high incidence of substance abuse in association with traumatic events is well-documented and may make evaluation and management of injured patients difficult or unpleasant. Surveys of surgeons' attitudes toward trauma reflect many of these concerns and yet, interestingly, demonstrate that rural surgeons are significantly more willing to accept these burdens than are their urban colleagues.[78,79] In fact, the opportunity to provide potentially life-saving treatment to friends, neighbors, or acquaintances and to see its long-term effects is one of the benefits of a general surgery practice in a small town.[52]

## Population Shifts

Population shifts in the coming years will have an impact on the problems of rural trauma. Although many parts of the Great Plains are becoming progressively depopulated, rural areas of the coastal regions, Rocky Mountains, Southwest, and Sunbelt states are experiencing an influx of young, active people who are tired of city life and eager for what small town America has to offer. Equipped with cell phones, modems, GPS-based equipment, and sport utility vehicles, these members of generation X (and their baby-boom parents) are very much into hiking, camping, climbing, skiing, and other activities that are best pursued in rural and frontier settings. They are affluent and well educated and accustomed to getting what they want. It is likely that, in order to support their desired lifestyles, they will expect or demand a trauma infrastructure that is sophisticated, efficient, effective, and comparable to what is available in a resource-rich environment. Whether they will be willing to pay for it through taxes or user fees is another matter. An important mission for rural systems will be convincing constituents of the importance of financial support for trauma activities.

## WIRELESS TECHNOLOGY

Many of the problems of rural communities could be mitigated with the use of technology for prevention and for discovery. In the decade of the 90s, rural EMS notification times (from time of motor vehicle crash) dropped from 9 to 7 minutes with the advent of wireless phones. In mountainous terrain, wireless communication is hampered by line-of-sight, but this problem is already being addressed through the installation of low power, short distance relay boxes. Vehicles produced by the leading automobile manufacturers can now include automatic crash notification (ACN) equipment. A combination of crash sensors, GPS devices, and a wireless phone allow for automatic phone activation on impact to notify EMS of the location and severity of a crash.[30]

Crash avoidance is possible with sensors installed in the roadway to measure road edge, lane tracking, intersections, and merging traffic. Vehicle sensors can assist with rear-end crash avoidance, vision enhancement, navigation and routing information, and driver condition. The development of smart highways will be expensive, however, and, predictably, rural areas will be the last to benefit. Improvements in crash protection will result from refinements of existing passive restraints (seatbelts, airbags) and structural characteristics of vehicles.

While the advances just described are specific for automobile occupants, wireless communication and location systems will also benefit hikers, hunters, workers, and others in the back country, provided they equip themselves with cell phones and GPS monitors. Another device under investigation is the personal status monitor (PSM), which is worn like a wristwatch and combines pulse, blood pressure, and arterial hemoglobin saturation with GPS.[80] The resulting improvement in notification and location will guide rescuers to victims more efficiently and eliminate much of the delay to definitive care that currently plagues rural EMS.

## TRANSPORT

Transport systems are another area where technology combined with a secure funding source could improve outcomes for trauma victims. Helicopters are very expensive, but may have the greatest potential for eliminating delay and downtime in the process of getting the right patient to the right hospital at the right time. Extended range, expanded capacity for onboard equipment and access to the patient, safer landing areas, and creative methods of funding are all possible areas for investigation. If national health policy moves toward regionalization of medical and surgical care, improved transport from scene or local hospital will be essential.

## TELEMEDICINE

If we are unable to improve on methods of transporting the patient to the trauma center, investigators are now actively studying strategies for bringing the trauma center to the patient. Telemedicine, particularly digital radiology, is already in use in many parts of the country. Outpatient follow-up of patients discharged from a trauma center to a remote rural area has been successfully accomplished using videoconferencing over T1 lines at 768 kbps. Cable-based broadband technology is increasingly available in rural areas and is an even faster mode of data transmission. Adjuncts include an analog electronic stethoscope, document cameras and close-up cameras with macro lenses, and a fax line for document transmission.[81] Satellite uplinks on emergency vehicles and appropriate audiovisual equipment can allow trauma experts at the medical center to observe a rescue in real time and offer suggestions regarding appropriate evaluations, interventions, and disposition at a distance.[82,83] Laptops and landlines have been used to transmit real-time images of trauma resuscitations at remote rural hospitals. In one case the trauma surgeon talked a local doctor through a life-saving cricothyroidotomy in a patient with an injury to the brain, and, in another, recommended a diagnostic peritoneal lavage that was positive and led to local laparotomy for control of abdominal hemorrhage prior to transfer.[84] The Internet has been used to transfer images to aid in assessing candidates for extremity replantation.[85] Limiting factors include money and infrastructure including T1 lines at 2 mbps, broadband fiberoptic lines at 155 mbps, and advanced communication satellite access at 622 mbps. Surgeons in Taiwan have recently reported on 35 patients with a total of 60 traumatic digital amputations who were evaluated at a distance with the aid of a camera phone to determine whether transfer for replantation was appropriate.[86]

The trauma service at the University of Vermont has developed a remote teleconsultation service to provide immediate access to the trauma surgeon for physicians and physician extenders in rural northern New York. Each of the on-call surgeons has a telemedicine workstation at home which can communicate by interactive video with a similar workstation at one of the nine participating community hospitals using three ISDN lines. (ISDN is a digital network capable of transmitting voice, video, and data over telephone lines at speeds up to 1.4 Mbps.) The surgeon can observe the physical exam, monitor vital signs, and view X-rays. In one case, the surgeon walked a physician's assistant through reduction of an elbow dislocation prior to transfer (3.5 hours by ground) to definitive care at the Level I trauma center. Adaptation of similar technology to moving ambulances is under development by the same group.[87] Medicolegal considerations, including licensure if the supervising doctor is in another state, and the essence of the doctor-patient relationship if she or he never physically encounter the patient, have yet to be resolved.

## TELEPRESENCE SURGERY

These strictures will also apply in another area under investigation, telepresence surgery, in which a surgeon uses a robotic system designed to make him feel as if he is actually at the remote site with the patient. Much of the research in this area has been sponsored by the Defense Advanced Research Projects Agency (DARPA) for the U.S. military to develop methods for safely operating on troops at or near a battlefield. If it can be done under those circumstances, it surely can be applied to less hostile rural environments. One limitation is the latent period required to transmit signals (currently 200 to 300 km by terrestrial cable, and 35 to 50 km by wireless transmission) at an acceptable delay of 200 minutes. Communications satellites, by comparison, have a latent period of 1.5 seconds.[88] Laparoscopic surgery lends itself ideally to this technology and has, in fact, been accomplished by specially trained surgeons performing cholecystectomies from a "remote" console within the same operating suite.[89,90] Efforts are underway to accomplish similar surgery at a much greater distance. The equipment utilized was originally designed for endoscopic coronary bypass surgery and has been used with success for that purpose, as well.[91] At the moment, the acquisition cost of one of these robotic systems is approximately 1 million dollars.

## TRAUMA SYSTEMS

Trauma systems are covered in depth elsewhere in this book. Most trauma experts are convinced that a systemic approach to trauma will be necessary in the future. Computer models are now available that can help policymakers decide where to place trauma hospitals and helicopters in order to best meet the trauma needs of a given region and population.[92] It is important to emphasize that a system will offer rural hospitals and health care workers the best opportunity to expand their limited resources. By pooling efforts with others in the region in common purpose, small hospitals benefit from educational and prevention services, improved patient transport, increased political influence, better financial support, and access to new technology. Failure to take advantage of these opportunities may consign a rural hospital and its patients to isolation and inadequate trauma care. "One of the most important functions of a trauma system is to ensure that patients do not die of simple injuries. Death caused by easily correctable and relatively minor injuries still occurs with an alarming frequency in the rural setting."[93]

## REFERENCES

1. Rogers FB, Shackford SR, Osler TM, et al.: Rural Trauma: The challenge for the next decade. J Trauma 47:802, 1999.
2. Wayne R: Rural trauma management. Am J Surg 157:463, 1989.
3. Muelleman RL, Walker RA, Edney JA: Motor vehicle deaths: A rural epidemic. J Trauma 35:717, 1993.
4. Maio RF, Green PE, Becker MP, et al.: Rural motor vehicle crash mortality: The role of crash severity and medical resources. Accid Anal Prev 24:631, 1992.
5. Baker SP, Whitfield RA, O'Neill B: Geographic variations in mortality from motor vehicle crashes. N Engl J Med 316:1384, 1987.
6. Baker SP, Whitfield RA, O'Neill B: County mapping of injury mortality. J Trauma 28:741, 1988.
7. Kearney PA, Stallones L, Swartz C, et al.: Unintentional injury death rates in rural Appalachia. J Trauma 30:1524, 1990.
8. Vane DW, Shackford SR: Epidemiology or rural traumatic death in children: A population-based study. J Trauma 38:867, 1995.
9. Certo TF, Rogers FB, Pilcher DB: Review of care of fatally injured patients in a rural state: 5-year follow up. J Trauma 23:559, 1983.
10. Esposito TJ, Sanddal ND, Hansen JD, et al.: Analysis of preventable trauma deaths and inappropriate care in a rural state. J Trauma 39:955, 1995.
11. West JG, Trunkey DD, Lim RC: Systems of trauma care: Study of two counties. Arch Surg 114:455, 1979.
12. Houtchens BA: Major trauma in the rural mountain West. J Amer Coll Emerg Med 6:343, 1977.
13. Waller JA: Urban-oriented methods: Failure to solve rural emergency care problems. JAMA 226:1441, 1973.
14. Rutledge R, Fakhry SM, Baker CC, et al.: A population-based study of the association of medical manpower with country trauma death rates in the United States. Ann Surg 218:547, 1994.
15. Shackford SR, Mackersie RC, Holbrook TL, et al.: The epidemiology of traumatic death: A population-based analysis. Arch Surg 128:571, 1993.
16. Thompson MJ, Lynge DC, Larson EH, et al.: Characterizing the General Surgery workforce in rural America. Arch Surg 140:74, 2005.
17. Heilman J: Rural trauma care. Resources for optimal care of the injured patient: 1999. Chicago: American College of Surgeons Committee on Trauma, 1998, p. 49.
18. Nordstrom DL, Zwerling C, Stromquist AM, et al.: Epidemiology of unintentional adult injury in a rural population. J Trauma 51:758, 2001.
19. Rogers FB, Osler TM, Shackford SR, et al.: A population-based study of geriatric trauma in a rural state. J Trauma 50:604, 2001.
20. Clark DE: Motor vehicle crash fatalities in the elderly: Rural versus urban. J Trauma 51:896, 2001.
21. Wigglesworth EC. Do some US states have higher(lower injury mortality rates than others? J Trauma 58:1144, 2005.
22. Pratt DS: Occupational health and the rural worker: Agriculture, mining and logging. J Rural Health 6:399, 1990.
23. Norwood S, McAuley C, Vallma VL, et al.: Mechanisms and patterns of injuries related to large animals. J Trauma 48:740, 2000.
24. Farrell TM, Sutton JE Jr, Clark DE, et al.: Moose-motor vehicle collisions: An increasing hazard in northern New England. Arch Surg 131:377, 1996.
25. Helmkamp JC, Derk SJ: Nonfatal logging-related injuries in West Virginia. J Occup Environ Med 41:967, 1999.
26. Robertson R, Mattox R, Collins T, et al.: Missed injuries in a rural area trauma center. Am J Surg 172:564, 1996.
27. Rogers FB, Osler TM, Shackford SR, et al.: Population-based study of hospital care in a rural state without a formal trauma system. J Trauma 50:409, 2001.
28. Rogers FB, Osler TM, Shackford Sr, et al.: Study of the outcome of patients transferred to a level I hospital after stabilization at an outlying hospital in a rural setting. J Trauma 46:328, 1999.
29. Martin GD, Cogbill TH, Landercasper JL, et al.: Prospective analysis of rural interhospital transfer of injured patients to a referral trauma center. J Trauma 30:1014, 1990.

30. Champion HR, Cushing B: Emerging technology for vehicular safety and emergency response to roadway crashes. *Surg Clin North Am* 79:1229, 1999.
31. Zulick LC, Dietz PA, Brooks K: Trauma experience of a rural hospital. *Arch Surg* 126:1427, 1991.
32. Bintz ML, Cogbill TH, Bacon J: Rural trauma care: Role of the general surgeon. *J Trauma* 41:462, 1996.
33. Rinker CF, Sabo RR: Operative management of rural trauma over a 10-year period. *Am J Surg* 158:548, 1989.
34. Sariego J: Impact of a formal trauma program on a small rural hospital in Mississippi. *South Med J* 93:182, 2000.
35. Foley T, Kessel J. Schmitz GD. RTTDC©: New course to improve rural trauma care. *Bull Am Coll Surg* 90:22, 2005.
36. Rabinowitz HK, Diamond JJ, Markham FW, et al.: Critical factors for designing programs to increase the supply and retention of rural primary care physicians. *JAMA* 286:1041, 2001.
37. Smith N: The incidence of severe trauma in small rural hospitals. *J Fam Practice* 25:595, 1987.
38. Stewart RM, Johnson J, Geoghegan K, et al.: Trauma surgery malpractice risk: Perception versus reality. *Ann Surg* 241:969, 2005.
39. Morrisey MA, Ohsfeldt RL, Johnson V, Treat R: Trauma patients: An analysis of rural ambulance trip reports. *J Trauma* 41:741, 1996.
40. Messick WJ, Rutledge R, Meyer AA: The association of advanced life support training and decreased per capita trauma death rates: An analysis of 12,417 trauma deaths. *J Trauma* 33:850, 1992.
41. Brathwaite CEM, Rosko M, McDowell R, et al.: A critical analysis of on-scene helicopter transport on survival in a statewide trauma system. *J Trauma* 45:140, 1998.
42. Diaz MA, Hendey GW, Bivins HG: When is helicopter faster? A comparison of helicopter and ground ambulance transport times. *J Trauma* 58:148, 2005.
43. Gabram SGA, Jacobs LA: The impact of flight systems on access to and quality of care. *Prob Gen Surg* 7:203, 1990.
44. Grossman DC, Hart LG, Rivara FB, et al.: From roadside to bedside: The regionalization of trauma care in a remote rural county. *J Trauma* 38:14, 1995.
45. Cunningham P, Rutledge R, Baker CC, et al.: A comparison of the association of helicopter and ground ambulance transport with the outcome of injury in trauma patients transported from the scene. *J Trauma* 43:940, 1997
46. Urdaneta LF, Miller BK, Ringenberg BJ, et al.: Role of an emergency helicopter transport service in rural trauma. *Arch Surg* 122:992, 1987.
47. Sharar SR, Luna GK, Rice CL, et al.: Air transport following surgical stabilization: An extension of regionalized trauma care. *J Trauma* 28:794, 1988.
48. Wald SL, Shackford SR, Fenwick J: The effect of secondary insults on mortality and long-term disability in a rural region without a trauma system. *J Trauma* 34:377, 1993.
49. Veenema KR, Rodewald LE: Stabilization of rural multiple trauma patients at Level III emergency departments before transfer to a Level I regional trauma center. *Ann Emerg Med* 25:175, 1995.
50. Rutledge R, Shaffer VD, Ridky J: Trauma care reimbursement in rural hospitals: Implications for triage and trauma system design. *J Trauma* 40:1002, 1996.
51. Wenneker WW, Murray DH, Ledwich T: Improved trauma care in a rural hospital after establishing a Level II trauma center. *Am J Surg* 160:655, 1990.
52. Richardson JD: Trauma centers and trauma surgeons: Have we become too specialized? *J Trauma* 48:1, 2000.
53. Richardson JD, Cross T, Lee D, et al.: Impact of Level III verification on trauma admissions and transfer: Comparisons of two rural hospitals. *J Trauma* 42:498, 1997.
54. Sampalis JS, Denis R, Frechette P, et al.: Direct transport to tertiary trauma centers versus transfer from lower level facilities: Impact on mortality and morbidity among patients with major trauma. *J Trauma* 43:288, 1997.
55. Barquist E, Pizzutiello M, Tian L, et al.: Effect of trauma system maturation on mortality rates in patients with blunt injuries in the Finger Lakes region of New York State. *J Trauma* 49:63, 2000.
56. Karsteadt LL, Larsen CL, Farmer PD: Analysis of a rural trauma program using the TRISS methodology: A three-year retrospective study. *J Trauma* 36:395, 1994.
57. Ali J, Adam R, Butler AK, et al.: Trauma outcome improves following the Advanced Trauma Life Support program in an developing country. *J Trauma* 34:890, 1993.
58. Ali J, Adam R, Stedman M, et al.: Advanced Trauma Life Support program increases emergency application of trauma resuscitative procedures in a developing country. *J Trauma* 36:391, 1994.
59. Rogers FB, Shackford SR, Hoyt DB, et al.: Trauma deaths in a mature urban vs. rural trauma system. A comparison. *Arch Surg* 132:376, 1997.
60. Harrington DT, Connolly M, Biffl WL, et al.: Transfer times to definitive care facilities are too long. A consequence of an immature trauma system. *Ann Surg* 241:961, 2005.
61. Cone JB: Tertiary trauma care in a rural state. *Am J Surg* 160:652, 1990.
62. Stabilization and Transport, in *Advanced Trauma Life Support Program for Physicians*, 6th ed. Chicago: American College of Surgeons, 1997.
63. Bitterman RA: Overview of hospital and physician responsibilities mandated by EMTALA, in *Providing Emergency Care under Federal Law EMTALA*. Dallas: American College of Emergency Physicians, 2000, p. 15.
64. ACS statement on managed care and the trauma system. *Bull Am Coll Surg* 80:86, 1995.
65. Gilligan JE, Griggs WM, Jelly MT, et al.: Mobile intensive care services in rural South Australia. *Med J Aust* 171:617, 1999.
66. Hirshberg A, Walden R: Damage control for abdominal trauma. *Surg Clin North Am* 77:813. 1997.
67. Granchi TS, Liscum KR: The logistics of damage control. *Surg Clin North Am* 77:921, 1997.
68. Mattox KL: Introduction, background, and future projections of damage control surgery. *Surg Clin North Am* 77:753, 1997.
69. Kudsk KA, Ivatury RR, Morris JA, Rotondo MF: Symposium: Damage control in the trauma patient. *Contemp Surg* 57:325, 2001.
70. Vargo DJ, Battistella FD: Abbreviated thoracotomy and temporary chest closure: An application of damage control after thoracic trauma. *Arch Surg* 136:21, 2001.
71. Mann NC, Mullins RJ, Hedges JR, et al.: Mortality among seriously injured patients treated in remote rural trauma centers before and after implementation of a statewide trauma system. *Med Care 2001* 39:643, 2001.
72. Head Injury, in *Advanced Trauma Life Support Program for Physicians*, 6th ed. Chicago: American College of Surgeons, 1997.
73. Rinker CF, McMurry FG, Groeneweg VR, Emergency craniotomy in a rural Level III trauma center. *J Trauma* 44:984, 1998.
74. Schecter WP, Peper E, Tuatoo V: Can general surgery improve the outcome of the head-injury victim in rural America? A review of the experience in American Samoa. *Arch Surg* 120:1163, 1985.
75. Cohen JE, Montero A, Israel ZH: Prognosis and clinical relevance of anisocoria-craniotomy latency for epidural hematoma in comatose patients. *J Trauma* 41:120, 1996.
76. Mangus RS, Mann NC, Worrall, et al.: Statewide variation in the treatment of patients hospitalized with spleen injury. *Arch Surg* 134:1378, 1999.
77. Engelhardt S, Hoyt D, Coimbra R, et al.: The 15-year evolution of an urban trauma center: What does the future hold for the trauma surgeon? *J Trauma* 51:633, 2001.
78. Richardson JD, Miller FB: Will future surgeons be interested in trauma care? Results of a resident survey. *J Trauma* 32:229, 1992.
79. Esposito TJ, Maier RV, Rivara FP, et al.: Why surgeons prefer not to care for trauma patients. *Arch Surg* 126:292, 1991.
80. Maniscalco-Theberge ME, Elliott DC: Virtual reality, robotics, and other wizardry in 21st century trauma care. *Surg Clin North Am* 79:1241, 1999.
81. Boulanger B, Kearney P, Ochoa J, et al.: Telemedicine: A solution to the follow up of rural trauma patients? *J Am Coll Surg* 192:447, 2001.
82. Kirkpatrick A, Brenneman F, McCallum A, et al.: Prospective evaluation of the potential role of teleradiology in acute interhospital trauma referrals. *J Trauma* 46:1017, 1999.
83. Aucar J, Granchi T, Liscum K, et al.: Is regionalization of trauma care using telemedicine feasible and desirable? *Am J Surg* 180:535, 2000.
84. Rogers FB, Ricci M, Shackford SR, et al.: The use of telemedicine for real time video consultation between trauma center and community hospital in a rural setting improves early trauma care. *J Trauma* 51:1037, 2001.
85. Buntic RF, Siko PP, Buncke GM, et al.: Using the internet for rapid exchange of photographs and x-ray images to evaluate potential extremity replantation candidates. *J Trauma* 43:342, 1997.
86. Ching-Hila H, Seng-Feng J, Chih-Yuan C, et al.: Teleconsultation with the mobile camera-phone in remote evaluation of replantation potential. *J Trauma* 58:1208, 2005.
87. Mahoney D: Telemedicine program serves rural Vermont. *Surgery News* 1:1,20, 2005.
88. Satava RM, Bowersox JC, Mack M, Krummel TM: Robotic surgery. State of the art and future trends. *Contemp Surg* 57:489, 2001.
89. Satava RM: Emerging technologies for surgery in the 21st century. *Arch Surg* 134:1197, 1999.
90. Marescaux J, Smith M, Folscher D, et al.: Telerobotic laparoscopic cholecystectomy: Initial clinical experience with 25 patients. *Ann Surg* 234:1, 2001.
91. Reichenspurner H, Damiano RJ, Mack M, et al.: Use of the voice-controlled and computer-assisted system ZEUS for endoscopic coronary artery bypass graft. *J Thorac Cardiovasc Surg* 118:11, 1999.
92. Branas CC, ReVelle CS, MacKenzie EJ: To the rescue: Optimally locating trauma hospitals and helicopters. *LDI Issue Brief* 6:1, 2000.
93. Norwood S, Myers MB: Outcomes following injury in a predominantly rural-population-based trauma center. *Arch Surg* 129:800, 1994.

# Commentary ■ ROBERT L. COSCIA

Treatment of patients injured in rural areas presents several unique challenges that are not commonly seen in urban centers. Some of these include delays in recognition or identification, increased distance to care, and weather-related issues. Frequently, first responders are volunteers with BLS or less training. This, coupled with patient arrival at initial receiving hospitals with limited resources and an infrequency of treating severe injuries, may contribute to poor outcomes in rural areas. As noted in this chapter, most trauma in rural environments results from blunt mechanisms such as automobile crashes, falls, or farm-related injuries. The most common causes of fatal injuries are automobile crashes, suicide, homicide, and falls; however, an alarming statistic shows that suicide accounts for 10% of all rural trauma deaths. It is important to recognize that the two greatest problems confronting rural trauma care are access to a trauma system and a lack of resources. Another factor to consider is the limited development of functioning trauma systems in some states in the United States. Less than half of the states have a fully developed functioning trauma system. At least eight states, mostly in the western United States, do not have a designated or verified Level I or II trauma center.

Obviously some of these problems will be difficult to eliminate. The patients sustaining a severe head injury may have little chance of survival regardless of where the injury occurs. Since most traumatic injuries are minor, an emphasis needs to be placed on getting the right patient to the right center at the right time—a concept which has been stated many times. Unnecessary delays in transport may result as a consequence of underequipped facilities which do not have the resources to care for extensive injuries obtaining time-consuming imaging studies rather than arranging for transport. One of the most critical decisions to be made is whether the patient can be treated locally or whether transfer is necessary and this decision must be made in a timely manner.

Trauma outcome is directly related to time to definitive care. Since delays in discovery, retrieval, and transport are the principal causes of death, how can these potentially preventable mortalities and morbidities be addressed? Development of a "true" functioning trauma system by states is a step in the right direction. These questions and others should be a high priority for policy makers. Patients should not die of simple injuries. In this chapter, Charles Rinker has described many issues that patients injured in the rural setting face. While there has been improvement in this area, much work remains to be done to further decrease mortality.

# Initial Assessment and Management

*Christoph R. Kaufmann*

Hospital care of the injured patient begins with initial assessment and management. This first step must be performed aggressively if the patient is to have an uncomplicated hospital course. It may be impossible at a later time for the trauma team to overcome or correct for poor initial assessment and management. Inadequate or delayed care of the trauma patient not only prolongs the hospital course, but can initiate the cycle of organ failure and death. Preplanned, organized, comprehensive, and rapid initial assessment and management must be successful for the patient to be physiologically prepared to survive definitive care of multiple or complex injuries.

Adequate time for the standard history and physical examination does not exist for the severely injured patient. Physicians treating injured patients have long recognized that treatment frequently takes priority over the definitive work-up and that life-saving procedures must be instituted immediately. This realization was the basis for the development of the Advanced Trauma Life Support (ATLS®) course of the American College of Surgeons Committee on Trauma (ACSCOT).[1] ATLS-recommended guidelines have become the "gold standard" for the first hour of hospital care for trauma patients around the world.

ATLS uses the terms *initial assessment and management* for this urgent evaluation and treatment of the trauma victim. The terms *primary survey* and *secondary survey* are used to differentiate between the rapid evaluation and treatment of the immediately life-threatening injuries (*primary survey*) and the more detailed evaluation, diagnosis, and treatment of the occult or nonimmediate threats to life (*secondary survey*). Both the primary survey and the secondary survey are parts of initial assessment and management of the injured patient.

This chapter reviews the systematic approach taught in ATLS. Since 1980, the ACSCOT has developed and continually refined the ATLS course to improve the care of injured patients during this early hospital phase of care. The course includes lectures, surgical and other interactive skills stations, group discussion, testing stations, and a course manual to teach the initial evaluation and management of the patient with multiple injuries. A reliable and systematic approach to the initial assessment and management of the trauma patient improves survival and minimizes disability.[1]

The initial assessment begins with the ABCDEs of the primary survey (airway, breathing, circulation, disability, exposure/environment) performed simultaneously with resuscitation. Reevaluation is continuous and the primary survey may need to be repeated several times throughout the initial assessment of the patient. Following the primary survey and concomitant resuscitation, a secondary survey is performed, which is a head-to-toe history and physical examination. Adjuncts to the secondary survey may include complex diagnostic tests. The secondary survey may also need to be repeated to avoid missing injuries, sometimes referred to as a tertiary survey.[3] The tertiary survey is particularly important in patients with multiple injuries and those taken for emergency operation. Following the primary and secondary survey with concurrent resuscitation, whether performed in the emergency department (ED) or operating room (OR), the patient will require transfer to either another hospital or to an intensive care unit or ward setting. Patient transport needs to be accomplished in a deliberate way.

## PREPARATION

Preparation is critical and must not be overlooked, as it is an integral part of trauma care. The physician must prepare for the arrival of the patient and, ideally, be waiting for the patient in the resuscitation room with all necessary staff and equipment ready.

All physicians providing care for trauma patients must be involved in the planning and preparation for prehospital and hospital trauma care. Protocols must be in place long before the patient is seen to determine what procedures will and will not be performed in the field. One resource in this area is the National Association of Emergency Medical Technicians (EMTs) Prehospital Trauma Life Support (PHTLS) course.[4] Protocols should determine the who, when, how, and where of trauma patient transport. The right patient (who) should be transported at the earliest time that is safe (when), using the ideal available transport method (how), to the right hospital (where), preferably a designated trauma center. Prehospital personnel should obtain as much information as is available and report this information on arrival in the resuscitation room. The history of the incident/mechanism of injury, the environment, and any data regarding prior medical conditions is often important. The prehospital setting is the only place some of these data can be obtained. Interventions performed in the prehospital setting are also important to document.

A triage protocol, created to ensure transport of injured patients to the appropriate hospital, is vital. This triage protocol is applied to determine whether a specific trauma patient needs to be transported to a nearby emergency department or to a designated trauma center. *Resources for Optimal Care of the Injured Patient,* a document from the ACSCOT, explains one method for trauma patient triage.[2] Triage is also important in the face of multiple or mass casualty events. Triage is much more difficult when dealing with a mass casualty event, in which the number or type of casualties overwhelms local resources.[5]

Many decisions should be made prior to patient arrival. Roles of members of the resuscitation team should be planned and defined before the patient arrives. The resuscitation area should be familiar to the team members and must have the proper equipment. Deciding who will be called before the major trauma patient arrives is important as well. The hospital should develop an activation process to ensure that the proper personnel are available and ideally present when a patient with major trauma arrives. These personnel include not only physicians but also specialized hospital personnel including nurses, respiratory therapists, social workers (for family issues), and appropriate radiology technicians (plain film and CT). *Resources for Optimal Care of the Injured Patient 2006* is an excellent document to assist with preparation and planning of the in-hospital phase.[2] For verified trauma centers, it clearly describes which personnel *must* be available at the time of the patient's arrival. The initial resuscitation team ideally would be perfectly matched to the patient's injury severity. This is not possible today because the magnitude of injury and specific injuries cannot be accurately identified until the initial resuscitation is completed. Most trauma centers use a tiered response for evaluation and resuscitation of the trauma patient.[6] A graduated response based on suspected injury severity may vary not only in composition of the team, but also in the location of the resuscitation (ED vs. OR). Preparation must include protection of trauma care personnel from communicable diseases. This involves the use of *universal precautions,* which include hair covers, face masks, eye protection, appropriate gown, shoe covers or leggings, and gloves so that contact with body fluids containing communicable diseases is minimized. As too many trauma patients today arrive in the ED demonstrating aggressive behavior secondary to intoxication from alcohol or other drugs, increased emphasis needs to be placed on team safety. It is often necessary to control these patients through physical or pharmacologic means to protect both the patient and the resuscitation team from harm.

## PRIMARY SURVEY

A rapid primary survey is essential to immediately identify life-threatening situations in the patient with severe injuries or the potential for severe injuries. The primary survey is performed simultaneously with the management of these life-threatening situations as they are identified. If initial interaction reveals that the patient is alert, talking, oriented, and moving all extremities, one can be assured that the patient has an adequate airway, is breathing adequately, that oxygen is being circulated to the brain, and that there is no major neurologic injury. If the initial interaction between the experienced physician and the patient determines that there is no immediate treatment needed, the primary survey is complete within seconds.

The primary survey is a sequence of evaluations. In actual practice, many of the components are being assessed simultaneously, especially when a team is working together efficiently. The evaluation portion of the primary survey consists of the ABCDEs of trauma care which are assessed in order to identify immediately life-threatening conditions. They are:

**A**irway maintenance with cervical spine protection

**B**reathing and ventilation

**C**irculation with hemorrhage control

**D**isability; neurologic status

**E**xposure/**E**nvironment (completely undress the patient and prevent hypothermia)

As the patient is being undressed, adjuncts to the primary survey can be performed, including the following: administering oxygen, applying the electrocardiogram (ECG) and pulse oximetry monitors, starting intravenous crystalloid administration with two large-bore cannulas, drawing blood for initial blood work, and visualizing the entire patient, front and back. The patient should be covered with a warm blanket as soon as possible to avoid hypothermia. Other adjuncts at this point include insertion of a gastric tube and urinary catheter when indicated.

Ideally, the primary survey, its adjuncts, and resuscitation are all taking place simultaneously. Members of the resuscitation team work simultaneously to protect or control the airway, administer oxygen, and make sure that the patient does not aspirate while intravenous lines are started. One team member may provide the definitive airway and breathing for the patient while simultaneously performing a rapid evaluation to see whether injury to the brain or shock from blood loss is the reason for a diminished level of consciousness. At the same time, other team members may be starting intravenous lines, applying monitors, inserting a gastric tube, undressing the patient, or placing a urinary catheter in the bladder (after digital rectal exam).

A patient's response to resuscitative measures is also an important part of the initial assessment. The primary survey and associated therapeutic interventions may need to be repeated several times if the patient does not respond to resuscitation, preventing the physician from proceeding to the secondary survey. Some life-threatening injuries, such as cardiac tamponade, require definitive surgical therapy before even attempting a secondary survey. It may not be possible to complete the entire initial assessment, including both the primary and the secondary survey, until the postoperative period. A single, trained physician is capable of performing the primary survey and initiating appropriate resuscitation. Indeed, the initial assessment is taught, practiced, and tested in this manner during the ATLS course. When more resources are available, a trauma team increases the efficiency and efficacy of the primary survey as well as that of the entire initial assessment and management.

A team leader, preferably a trauma surgeon, should be present during the initial care of the patient. The team leader's task is to ensure an organized effort focused toward returning the patient to a physiologically normal state and making appropriate judgments regarding diagnostic testing, therapeutic interventions, and need for transfer. The management and ultimate outcome of seriously injured patients is improved if board-certified surgeons are immediately available for the early treatment of specific injuries.[7] Trauma patients should be reassessed at regular intervals so that the team can find and treat previously unidentified injuries and monitor the patient's response.

## Airway with Cervical Spine Protection

The highest priority in resuscitation is securing and maintaining the airway because loss of the airway is the most rapidly lethal event. Evaluation of the airway begins by asking the patient a simple question, such as, "What is your name?" A response in a normal voice suggests that the airway is not in immediate jeopardy. A weak voice, breathlessness, hoarseness, or absent response, however, suggests compromise of the airway. Agitation and combativeness may be signs of airway compromise resulting in hypoxia. Some patients with an inadequate airway are misdiagnosed as being intoxicated or having an injury to the brain. Noisy breathing, cyanosis, and use of the accessory muscles of respiration are all strongly suggestive of obstruction of the airway. Common causes of obstruction are the tongue, edematous soft tissues, blood, foreign bodies, teeth, and vomitus. Unconscious and obtunded patients are at particular risk and need to have the airway protected by an endotracheal tube to deliver adequate oxygen, support ventilation, and reduce the risk of aspiration. All adult patients with a Glasgow Coma Scale (GCS) score of 8 or less should have a definitive airway—a cuffed endotracheal tube in the trachea.[1] For children younger than 9 years old, an uncuffed endotracheal tube is preferred because of concern regarding tracheal injury secondary to cuff pressure. Facial trauma is frequently associated with airway problems due to distortion of the anatomy of the upper airway, bleeding, and swelling of soft tissues. Patients with facial burns, particularly those associated with inhalational injuries, are at especially high risk for obstruction of the airway.

Early aggressive airway management with endotracheal intubation will prevent loss of the airway as soft tissue swelling in the neck increases. Other patients at high risk of airway compromise include those with injury to the larynx, hemorrhage into the soft tissues of the neck from penetrating wounds, or penetrating thoracic trauma. Patients who are hoarse or have a weak voice may have a laryngeal fracture or a partial transection of the cervical airway. Intubation of the airway should be approached with extreme caution and by the physician with the most experience in airway management to prevent conversion of a partial airway transection into a complete one. Preparation is the key. The physician must have all necessary or potentially necessary drugs and equipment at the bedside prior to proceeding. Fiberoptic guidance may be helpful in some circumstances.[8]

Rapid sequence intubation (RSI) with the use of paralyzing drugs is a useful method to obtain a definitive airway in patients who are combative, but require tracheal intubation.[9] The use of a short-acting depolarizing agent such as succinylcholine minimizes the duration of paralysis, which is desirable should attempts at intubation fail. Physicians employing RSI should be competent in all techniques of airway management. Additionally, equipment must be readily available to perform a surgical airway (e.g., cricothyroidotomy) if attempts at oral intubation fail. Inability to achieve a definitive airway in a paralyzed patient can be disastrous. As heart rate is the primary determinant of cardiac output in children and because children have a more pronounced vagal response to intubation than adults, atropine should be administered to children prior to RSI.[10]

Special problems are all too frequently encountered in management of the airway. Failure to recognize a partial laryngeal transection can lead to complete loss of the airway if intubation efforts are unsuccessful and/or too vigorous. Patients with suspected laryngeal injury are best intubated in the operating room with all necessary equipment opened and ready for emergency tracheostomy, the surgical airway procedure of choice in the patient with laryngeal injury. Compromise of the airway may be insidious, and loss of the airway may occur several hours after the initial evaluation has been completed. This is especially true for patients with inhalational injury, facial fractures, and laryngeal injury.

Difficulties with ventilation may be confused with airway problems. The patient with a simple pneumothorax who has air hunger and breathlessness may be misdiagnosed as having a compromised airway. If this patient is intubated and provided assisted ventilation (rather than appropriate treatment with a tube thoracostomy), the simple pneumothorax may be converted into a tension pneumothorax, which is immediately life threatening.

Endotracheal tubes, even if positioned correctly at the time of insertion, may get dislodged or malpositioned with patient movement or transport.[11] Frequent reevaluation of the position of the endotracheal tube is essential. Patients who are intubated and transported should be accompanied by individuals who can detect displacement of the endotracheal tube, are capable of intubation or repositioning of the tube, and have the necessary equipment.

After a potential or real problem with the airway is identified, the choice of airway maneuvers is based, in part, on suspicion of an injury to the cervical spine. Any patient who is unconscious, paralyzed, preverbal (younger children), complains of pain in the neck, or has an obvious injury above the level of the clavicles should be assumed to have a fracture of the cervical spine. Such patients (and any polytrauma patient) must have proper immobilization of the neck until radiological studies and physical examination can exclude an injury. A semirigid cervical collar, long backboard, lateral sandbags, and bindings or tape best provide for immobilization of the cervical spine in a neutral position. Immobilization with a semirigid collar alone allows for approximately 50% of normal movement.[12] The use of soft cervical collars should be avoided in the acute trauma setting as the degree of immobilization they provide is minimal, at best.

Diagnostic X-rays of the cervical spine should not delay the performance of emergent airway maneuvers. The emphasis is on protection of the cervical spine and not diagnosis during initial assessment and resuscitation.

Management of airway problems encompasses a spectrum from simple observation to insertion of a surgical airway. The choice in an individual patient depends on the presence of injury or suspected injury to the brain, cervical spine, or face, and the need for an emergent operation for other conditions. The chin lift, jaw thrust, oropharyngeal airway, nasopharyngeal airway, and appropriate use of a large-bore rigid suction device are all maneuvers to relieve simple obstruction.[13] Both the chin lift and the jaw thrust elevate the tongue from the posterior pharynx. The chin lift is performed by placing the fingers of one hand under the anterior mandible and the thumb of the same hand over the lower lip or lower incisors and lifting. The jaw thrust is performed by placing the fingers of both hands behind the angles of the mandible and displacing it forward. Care must be taken with both these techniques to avoid movement of the cervical spine.

An oropharyngeal airway is usually placed using a tongue blade to depress the tongue and inserting the device past the base of the tongue. The airway may be placed in the mouth of the adult upside down and twisted 180° until it is behind the base of the tongue. This insertion technique is not recommended for children because of concern for palatal injury. The nasopharyngeal airway is a soft tube that is lubricated and gently inserted through either nostril into the pharynx. This tube is tolerated by conscious and semiresponsive patients and is less likely to stimulate gagging and vomiting. The nostril with the least resistance to passage should be used in order to prevent injury to the nasal mucosa and epistaxis. Brief, gentle suctioning of saliva, blood, or vomit from the mouth and airway is also useful and may need to be repeated frequently.

The indications for a definitive airway (a cuffed tube in the trachea) include apnea, inability to maintain an airway, need for airway protection, coma, or inability to maintain adequate oxygenation with a face mask. Three methods to obtain a definitive airway are available, including orotracheal intubation, nasotracheal intubation, and a surgical airway (cricothyroidotomy or tracheostomy). Indications for each depend on injury pattern, urgency, lack of success in maintaining the airway with other techniques, as well as the skill set of the physician. Once the tube is in the trachea and the cuff inflated, proper location of the tube must be confirmed. The first step is to listen for breath sounds bilaterally, both anteriorly and in the axillae to confirm tracheal intubation. The finding of epigastric gurgling may diagnose esophageal intubation; however, auscultation alone is not adequate to determine proper or improper placement of the tube.[14] Rapid resolution of hypoxia to normal saturation levels is a good indicator of proper placement of the tube. A more rapid indicator is the use of colorimetric carbon dioxide ($CO_2$) detectors to confirm proper intubation, but these do not provide absolute assurance of *tracheal* intubation. $CO_2$ will be detected with intubation of one mainstem bronchus and, occasionally, $CO_2$ will be detected in gas aspirated from the stomach (but will clear with a half dozen breaths). It is important to remember that $CO_2$ may not be detectable in patients following cardiac arrest, even with proper tube placement. If the patient is spontaneously breathing, nasotracheal intubation with in-line immobilization of the head and neck is sometimes used. Apnea or the possibility of midface fractures preclude use of this technique. Sinusitis can be a major complication if a prolonged period of nasotracheal intubation is required.[15]

The skill and experience of the physician performing the intubation determine which technique is used. With certain airway problems, flexible endoscopy will facilitate successful intubation. Other adjuncts to tracheal intubation include the use of lighted wands and retrograde, wire-guided intubation.[16,17] Laryngeal mask airways (LMA) are adequate for airway management during elective surgical procedures, but as they are not definitive airways, the LMA should be avoided during the initial assessment and resuscitation of the trauma patient. The exception may be the intubating LMA, through which a definitive airway can be placed into the trachea.[18]

A chest X-ray should be performed as soon as is clinically safe in all intubated patients to assess location of the tip of the tube and to recognize and correct intubation of a mainstem bronchus. Clinical reconfirmation of tube location is also necessary each time the patient is moved.

A surgical airway is necessary when there is emergent need for a definitive airway and other intubation methods have failed or are inappropriate (laryngeal fracture or severe facial/pharyngeal trauma). In-line cervical immobilization must be maintained so that hyperextension of the neck is avoided.[19] Surgical cricothyroidotomy is not performed in children less than 12 years of age. Needle cricothyroidotomy with jet insufflation is preferred for temporary oxygenation in children until either endotracheal intubation or tracheostomy can be performed. Jet insufflation is necessary to force oxygen at higher pressure through the catheter. Between insufflation breaths of one second, four-second intervals are necessary to allow $CO_2$ to escape. Over about 45 minutes, the $CO_2$ levels gradually rise to a level mandating insertion of a larger airway.[20] Needle cricothyroidotomy with jet insufflation can be used in adults, as well, but formal cricothyroidotomy is preferred as the cricoid cartilage (the only circular support of the larynx) is less vulnerable to injury in adults.[21]

Surgical cricothyroidotomy has classically been performed with a scalpel and a #11 blade. The larynx and trachea are immobilized securely with one hand while a transverse "stab" incision is made in the cricothyroid membrane in one motion. The handle of the knife blade is then inserted into the defect in the cricothyroid membrane and turned 90° to allow the intake of air. An appropriately sized cuffed endotracheal tube or tracheostomy appliance is then placed through the defect and directed toward the carina.[22] The distance to the carina is short, and intubation of the right mainstem bronchus should be avoided.

A patient wearing a helmet should have it removed when emergency management of the airway is required; otherwise, it may be left in place until injury to the cervical spine has been excluded. A technique that carefully supports the cervical spine in a neutral position must be used and requires two people. One person stands next to the patient and protects the cervical spine by holding the head and face motionless while the other person stands at the head of the patient and springs the helmet open near the ears and removes it without flexing or extending the neck.[23,24] Cutting the helmet is another option.

## Breathing and Ventilation

High-flow delivery of oxygen provides the opportunity for optimal oxygen saturation of hemoglobin. The oxygen saturation is most readily assessed by the use of a pulse oximeter, as the clinical determination of adequate oxygenation is virtually impossible by any other noninvasive means.[25] Two of the factors that affect reliability of the pulse oximeter readings are anemia less than 5 g% and hypothermia less than 30°C (86°F).

Inspection, palpation, percussion, and auscultation are the classic methods employed during the physical examination to detect thoracic problems. Inspection will detect asymmetry in expansion of the chest, flail segments, use of accessory muscles of respiration, contusions, penetrating injuries, open or sucking wounds, distended neck veins, dyspnea, respiratory rate, and restlessness. Palpation may demonstrate tenderness, crepitus, subcutaneous emphysema, tracheal deviation, lack of motion of portions of the chest wall, and bony or cartilaginous deformity. Percussion, although difficult in a noisy trauma room, can identify hyperresonance or dullness. Auscultation may also be difficult because of noise levels, but is a critically important method of examining the chest in the injured patient. In addition to confirming bilateral breath sounds, auscultation is used to identify the following: asymmetric breath sounds as may be seen with pneumothorax or hemothorax, wheezing secondary to reactive airway disease or foreign body in an airway, heart rate and rhythm with potential to identify muffled heart sounds secondary to pericardial fluid, murmurs from possible injury to a heart valve, or abnormal heart sounds such as a gallop which may indicate poor baseline cardiac performance.

Injuries that should be detected during the primary survey include tension pneumothorax, flail chest with pulmonary contusion, open pneumothorax, and massive hemothorax. Massive hemothorax causes derangement of both breathing (hypoventilation) and circulation (hypovolemic shock).

A tension pneumothorax (caused by either blunt or penetrating trauma) develops when air continuously enters the pleural space from the lung, bronchi, trachea, or through the chest wall, cannot escape, and causes the lung to collapse. Eventually, this air under pressure will cause a shift of the mediastinum toward the opposite side, compression of the superior vena cava and inferior vena cava, decreased venous return to the heart, and hypotension. Clinically, a sense of impending death, marked respiratory distress ("air hunger"), deviated trachea, distended neck veins, unilateral absence of breath sounds, cyanosis, and hypotension may be seen. A deviated trachea at the base of the neck is difficult to see or feel and may not be a prominent finding. Distended neck veins may also be undetectable, particularly if hypovolemia from other injuries is present. Because hypotension and distended neck veins are seen in tension pneumothorax and cardiac tamponade, they are sometimes difficult to differentiate. Cardiac tamponade is less common and does not cause mediastinal shift, and breath sounds are usually symmetric. The diagnosis of tension pneumothorax is a clinical one and requires emergent chest decompression with a needle (14-gauge 3 inch catheter-over-needle inserted into the second intercostal space in the midclavicular line). Again, tension pneumothorax is a clinical diagnosis that should never wait for chest X-ray confirmation as this will delay life-saving decompression of the chest. A rush of air escaping through the catheter confirms the diagnosis. This converts the tension pneumothorax into a simple pneumothorax. The absence of a rush of air suggests misdiagnosis or insertion of the needle into the wrong hemithorax. Occasionally, the respiratory distress is so profound that breath sounds are diminished on both sides. If the diagnosis of tension pneumothorax still seems likely, the catheter is left in place and the opposite hemithorax is punctured. If no rush of air occurs, the wrong diagnosis is likely, and cardiac tamponade should be considered. Whether or not the needle confirms the presence of a tension pneumothorax, tube thoracostomy should follow.

Infiltration with a local anesthetic in any responsive patient should be performed prior to insertion of a thoracostomy tube. A large-caliber chest tube in adults (number 32 to 40 French) is placed into the affected hemithorax in the midaxillary line at the level of the nipple. The procedure is accomplished by sharply incising the skin and subcutaneous tissue at the desired interspace. A surgical clamp is then used to penetrate the chest immediately cephalad to a rib to avoid the neurovascular structures on the inferior surface. The clamp is spread to make the chest defect large enough to permit a finger to pass into the chest for inspection. A finger is inserted into the pleural space to identify adhesions or organs to be avoided and to feel the lung. Finally, the thoracostomy tube is inserted through the incision, directing it posteriorly and superiorly. Both blood and air are effectively evacuated in the supine patient when the tube is in a posterosuperior position.[26] Trocars should never be used when placing a chest tube because their use has been associated with damage to the diaphragm, lung, liver, spleen, and even mediastinal structures. After the tube is inserted, it must be secured with a suture. The tube is then connected to an underwater seal drainage system. A subsequent chest X-ray will confirm expansion of the lung, determine the position of the tube, and may identify other injuries.

A flail chest consists of segmental fractures of three or more adjacent ribs, one or more rib fractures with an associated costochondral separation, or fracture of the sternum. This causes an unstable or "floating" segment of the chest wall that moves paradoxically during respiration. A force of injury strong enough to cause a flail chest usually causes an underlying pulmonary contusion. A pneumothorax or hemothorax may be present, as well. An injury to the chest wall of this magnitude is associated with significant pain, and respiratory efficiency is reduced. The treatment of a flail chest is directed toward reversing the hypoventilation (caused by pain) and hypoxia (caused by an associated pulmonary contusion).[27] Careful monitoring of ventilation and oxygenation is required, and intubation and ventilatory support may be indicated in 20 to 40% of patients. An associated hemopneumothorax is treated by insertion of a thoracostomy tube. Control of pain from multiple rib fractures using regional anesthetic techniques such as repeated intercostal nerve blocks or insertion of an epidural catheter is important to improve the respiratory mechanics. Over-resuscitation should be avoided in patients with a pulmonary contusion.

An open pneumothorax or "sucking chest wound" results when a defect in the chest wall exceeds two-thirds the diameter of the trachea. Inspiration draws air into the chest through the chest wound (and into the pleural cavity) rather than into the lungs via the trachea, and hypoxia ensues. When an open pneumothorax is present, prompt closure of the defect with a sterile occlusive dressing will improve ventilation. Three sides of the dressing should be taped to the skin and the fourth side allowed to remain open to create a one-way valve for escape of trapped air. This will prevent conversion to a tension pneumothorax. A chest tube should be placed as soon as it is clinically safe to do so. Intubation and assisted ventilation should be instituted if these methods fail to alleviate the respiratory distress and hypoxia persists (arterial partial pressure of oxygen, $po_2$ <60 mmHg). All defects in the chest wall resulting in an open pneumothorax require surgical closure, usually in the operating room.

A massive hemothorax, defined as >1500 mL of blood in the chest acutely, may be caused by penetrating or blunt trauma.[28] The ipsilateral lung is compressed with diminished or absent breath sounds. Massive hemothorax may also cause hypovolemic shock and(or shifting of the mediastinum. Distention of the neck veins is usually absent because of the massive blood loss.

Massive hemothorax is treated by evacuating blood from the chest by tube thoracostomy and attempting to restore blood volume with crystalloids and blood. Patients with 1500 mL of immediate drainage through the thoracostomy tube will almost always need an emergent or urgent thoracotomy. Thoracotomy is also indicated in patients who continue to drain 200 mL/hour for several hours after the original evacuation.[29] Evacuated blood may be collected in special collection systems, anticoagulated, filtered, and immediately reinfused into the patient.

## Circulation with Hemorrhage Control

***Stop the bleeding!*** After the airway has been secured and the dynamics of breathing are being restored, the status of the circulatory system is addressed next. Shock, defined as inadequate organ perfusion and tissue oxygenation, must be diagnosed and treated. The most common type of shock in the trauma patient is hemorrhagic shock. Cardiogenic shock (cardiac tamponade, tension pneumothorax, or cardiac injury/insufficiency), neurogenic shock (spinal cord injury), and septic shock (usually occurs late) may also occur. In every patient in shock, two large-bore intravenous catheters are inserted into the peripheral veins, and volume restoration is begun by the infusion of warmed fluids.

The most important management principle in treating hemorrhagic shock is to find the source of blood loss and stop the bleeding.[30,31] Hemorrhage from open wounds is treated by direct pressure at the wound site or, if required, at proximal pressure points where arterial inflow can be compressed (e.g., femoral artery at the groin or brachial artery at the elbow). The use of hemostats and other clamps is best reserved for the operating room. Large scalp wounds may be difficult to control with pressure, and rapid suture or staple closure is often necessary to stop the bleeding. Raney clips are another excellent temporary solution for scalp bleeding.[32]

Pulse rate and character, color and temperature of the skin, and mental status are rapidly evaluated to assess perfusion. Blood pressure is determined at the onset of resuscitation and then every 5 to 10 minutes until the initial assessment is complete and the patient's vital signs have stabilized. Later, pulse pressure, central venous pressure, and urinary output are helpful in the assessment of the adequacy of resuscitation.

Many factors cause tachycardia, but, in the trauma patient, tachycardia is always suggestive of hypovolemic shock. A heart rate greater than 120 in adults and 160 in preschool children is assumed to be hemorrhagic shock until proven otherwise. Patients who have pacemakers or who are taking digoxin, beta-blockers, or calcium channel blockers may have a slow pulse rate despite the presence of shock. A strong pulse is obviously associated with a higher cardiac output than a weak, thready pulse, although the presence or absence of palpable pulses is dependent on too many factors to be useful in estimating blood pressure. Catecholamine-induced vasoconstriction of vessels to the skin and muscle is one of the earliest compensatory changes as a response to hypovolemia. It results in pale, cool skin and sweating; therefore, the patient with tachycardia and cool, clammy skin should be considered to be in hypovolemic shock until proven otherwise.

Normal mental function implies adequate cerebral perfusion and probable absence of significant injury to the brain. Conversely, decreased mental function may be from the shock state, from brain injury, or from metabolic causes (e.g., intoxication). The most

important factors in preventing secondary injury to the brain are avoiding hypoxia and hypotension. Mortality and morbidity are doubled in patients with traumatic brain injury who are hypotensive and increased nearly three times if both hypotension and hypoxia are present.[33]

Blood pressure is often misleading in the evaluation and treatment of shock. Up to 30% of the blood volume may be lost before a significant decrease in blood pressure can be measured because of vasoconstriction as compensation for the lost volume. The pulse pressure (the numeric difference between systolic and diastolic pressures) is more sensitive. A decrease in pulse pressure is noted when as little as a 15% blood loss has occurred. When the systolic blood pressure is below 90 mm Hg, a shock state exists in most adolescents and adults.

Cardiogenic shock may be caused by injury to cardiac muscle, perforation of the heart, cardiac disease, or a tension pneumothorax and must be urgently diagnosed and treated. Cardiac tamponade is usually associated with penetrating trauma to the parasternal area, upper abdomen, or (rarely) the neck. Blunt cardiac rupture is rare. Cardiac tamponade causes significant hypotension and early death if diagnosis and intervention are not immediate. Patients with cardiac tamponade usually have a gray deathlike appearance, extreme anxiety, tachycardia, hypotension, distended neck veins, and muffled heart sounds. The hypotension may partially respond to the infusion of fluids but is only temporarily responsive to volume. A needle pericardiocentesis, using a long 16- or 18-gauge needle via the subxiphoid route to aspirate even small amounts of blood, can temporarily relieve the tamponade, but definitive operation is almost always necessary to treat the underlying injury. If the tamponade is unrelieved by pericardiocentesis and the patient is dying, immediate left anterolateral thoracotomy, pericardiotomy, and cardiac repair in the emergency department are appropriate. Median sternotomy is also an excellent incision for emergent access to the heart in more stable patients, particularly in those trauma centers that utilize an operating room for resuscitation of the most severely injured patients.[34] That the patient has not succumbed to the cardiac injury increases the likelihood that the injury is small enough to repair without cardiopulmonary bypass.

Blunt cardiac injury is associated with a direct blow to the anterior chest.[35] Few patients with blunt thoracic trauma have ECG abnormalities, life-threatening arrhythmias, or secondary cardiogenic shock. In the presence of any of these, an emergency echocardiogram is useful to determine the magnitude of the cardiac injury and should be used liberally when cardiac injury or disease is suspected. Treatment of cardiac injury includes monitoring in the surgical intensive care unit, with treatment of arrhythmias or hypotension as indicated.

Neurogenic shock is caused by injury to the spinal cord and is not associated with injuries to the brain. Shock in the presence of injury to the brain is almost always hypovolemic, and the source of hemorrhage must be found and controlled. An exception, preterminal shock, may occur in the presence of a severe injury to the brain that is about to cause the death of the patient. Neurogenic shock due to injury of the spinal cord is associated with the loss of sympathetic tone, vasodilation, and absence of an increased pulse rate. Hypovolemic shock can occur simultaneously, thus the initial treatment of suspected neurogenic shock should be fluid resuscitation. Monitoring of the central venous pressure may be useful to determine appropriate treatment. Lack of tachycardia, or even bradycardia, occurs because injury to the spinal cord leaves unopposed vagal stimulation to the heart. Vasoactive medications have a role in treatment of both neurogenic shock and septic shock.

While septic shock is rarely seen in the early postinjury period, it may be seen in patients arriving at the hospital many hours or days after the trauma incident. Injuries to hollow viscera that have been untreated usually lead to sepsis. Patients with septicemia who are normovolemic have minimal hypotension, wide pulse pressure, and warm skin. Patients with hypovolemia and septic shock present clinically as if in a hypovolemic shock state. Treatment is initially directed toward restoration of volume, and ultimately to surgical control of the source of sepsis.

Two large-bore intravenous catheters should be placed into peripheral veins in all patients with suspected or confirmed serious injuries. Because the diameter and length of the catheter determine flow rate, short large-bore catheters are ideal. In the adult, 14- and 16-gauge plastic cannulas are ideal. The insertion site is usually in the upper extremities unless there is likelihood of a major venous injury to the arm, upper chest, or ipsilateral neck that will interfere with flow of fluids to the central circulation. Frequently, central lines placed into subclavian, internal jugular, or femoral veins are used in urgent resuscitations. These procedures require experience and expertise and should be used with care because of the potential for complications. In difficult situations, venous cutdowns may be required. Cutdowns are usually placed into the greater saphenous vein either at the ankle or the groin or just above the antecubital crease into the basilic or cephalic vein. In the child, the largest catheter that a vein can accommodate should be inserted. The use of percutaneous insertion techniques is preferable to cutdowns because of simplicity and safety. In children less than 6 years of age, an intraosseous needle inserted into the proximal tibia may be appropriate during the initial resuscitation until volume restoration allows direct venous cannulation. Any of these techniques can provide appropriate access, and the choice is primarily based on the clinical circumstance and the skill of the physician. When the intravenous catheter is inserted, blood should be drawn for type and cross-match, baseline hematologic studies, and a pregnancy test for all females of child-bearing age.

Patients with hypovolemic shock are not treated acutely with vasopressors, steroids, or sodium bicarbonate. Improving tissue oxygenation with supplemental oxygen and restoring adequate volume treats the acidosis seen in patients with hypovolemia. The choice of resuscitation fluid depends on the condition of the patient. The use of a warmed balanced salt solution such as Ringer's lactate is considered safe and effective. A bolus of 2 L is given to the adult patient with hypotension, and 20 mL/kg to the child. If a hemodynamically normal state is restored, crystalloids can be continued. If the patient remains unstable, a second bolus is utilized while blood is being obtained. If the patient's vital signs have not returned to normal after two boluses, blood should be administered. If the need is urgent, type-specific blood may be used. When this is not immediately available, low-titer type O-positive blood for men or O-negative blood for women is acceptable. The patient who requires uncrossmatched blood usually needs to be in the operating room.

ED thoracotomy for the patient who arrives in extremis or has a cardiac arrest after suffering penetrating parasternal trauma may be life-saving. Patients with blunt trauma do not benefit from ED thoracotomy if cardiac arrest occurs in the prehospital period.[36]

Only surgeons with the training and expertise necessary to control hemorrhage from the heart, great vessels, and lung should perform this procedure.

## Disability: Neurologic Status

After resuscitation of life-threatening injuries found during the ABCs has begun, a brief baseline neurologic assessment is performed. This should consist of determining the GCS score and examining the pupils for size, symmetry, and reaction to light.[37] Until the patient is hemodynamically normal, a complete and detailed neurologic examination is not likely to be accurate nor is it prudent to perform one during extended resuscitative efforts. Both the GCS score and the pupillary size and reaction are frequently reevaluated. The GCS is the sum of scores for three areas of assessment, including (a) eye opening, (b) verbal response, and (c) best motor response. Pupillary size, symmetry, and reaction to light are important diagnostic tools that aid in determining if there is a lateralizing brain injury. Drugs, an ocular prosthesis, pre-existing pathology, or direct injury to the globe can all affect the pupillary exam.

Frequent reevaluation of the neurologic exam is mandatory to detect changes. The detection of asymmetry in the motor or sensory exam or a deterioration in the GCS score suggests the possibility of a surgical intracranial lesion. The liberal use of CT scanning is advocated for patients with any history, sign, or symptom of trauma to the brain.

## Exposure and Environmental Control

Patients must be completely undressed so that all external injuries are identified, and cutting clothing from the patient to facilitate exposure is necessary when there is severe injury or risk of injury to the spine. Injured patients must be kept warm using warm rooms, warm blankets, warm resuscitation fluids, and warm inspired air to prevent or treat hypothermia. The temperature of the patient should be monitored as early as possible and continuously.[38] A temperature-sensing urinary catheter measuring bladder temperature is ideal. The best way to ensure that the patient maintains his or her body temperature is to stop the bleeding. Efforts to prevent hypothermia and to rewarm the patient are as important as any other part of the primary survey and resuscitation.

## Adjuncts to the Primary Survey

As life-threatening injuries are found during the primary survey, appropriate interventions and resuscitative efforts are instituted concurrently. Resuscitation and the primary survey occur simultaneously.

Following completion of the primary survey and a brief reevaluation, a moment should be taken to ensure that all necessary data have been obtained, are being evaluated, and that the appropriate decisions have been made. During the ABCDEs, the team should have made use of various adjuncts. Completion of the primary survey is the ideal time to review these adjuncts and the information they provide.

Monitoring.   Monitoring begins immediately after arrival of the injured patient. Vital signs, including heart rate, respiratory rate, temperature, and blood pressure are obtained as soon as possible.

Continuous monitoring of cardiac rhythm is mandatory. Arterial blood gases and urinary output should also be measured during the primary survey and resuscitation phases of care. The use of pulse oximetry and end-tidal $CO_2$ monitoring will measure the adequacy of oxygenation and ventilation of the patient. The 12-lead ECG, arterial line, central venous pressure line, and pulmonary artery catheter can all provide helpful information in selected patients. Analysis of vital sign trends may provide an early indication of developing problems.

Catheters and Tubes.    A urinary catheter should be inserted during resuscitation of the severely injured patient unless there is an obvious contraindication. When a male patient has blood at the urethral meatus, a scrotal hematoma, a penile hematoma, or a high-riding prostate on rectal exam, a retrograde urethrogram must be performed prior to insertion of the catheter. When a urethral injury is discovered, catheterization should be avoided and specialty consultation requested. The patient with a urethral injury may require a suprapubic cystostomy. Monitoring the ongoing urinary output volume helps determine the adequacy of volume restoration and organ perfusion. Urine should be tested for the presence of blood or glucose and can be used for drug screening. A gastric tube is often placed during resuscitation to empty the stomach and decrease the risk of aspiration. Children are particularly sensitive to gastric dilatation, and decompression frequently improves their vital signs. Because insertion of the gastric tube may induce vomiting, the resuscitation team must be prepared to rapidly logroll the patient should emesis occur.

An orogastric or nasogastric tube is inserted, depending on the presence or absence of maxillofacial injuries. Patients who have bleeding from the nose, ears, or mouth should be suspected of having a fracture of the cribriform plate, base of the skull, mastoid process, and/or a leak of cerebrospinal fluid. Orogastric intubation is safer in these patients to avoid insertion of an (attempted) nasogastric tube into the brain, a potentially fatal injury.[39] Blood aspirated from a gastric tube is often swallowed blood, but can be from gastroduodenal injury.

X-Rays and other Diagnostic Studies.    Two X-rays should be performed during the primary survey-resuscitation phase in all patients with significant blunt trauma. Findings on the chest X-ray or the pelvic X-ray may prompt a change in the treatment plan. The finding of a wide mediastinum, pneumo- or hemothorax, or pelvic fracture may serve to identify a source of blood loss. Other diagnostic X-rays are usually reserved until the secondary survey, after resuscitative efforts are well underway and the patient's vital signs are returning to normal. In the patient with blunt injury who has persistent or recurrent hypotension, a search for occult hemorrhage will include the Focused Assessment Sonography in Trauma (FAST),[40,41] diagnostic peritoneal lavage (DPL),[42,43] or abdominal CT, depending on the specific clinical circumstances.[44] The unstable patient may be quickly identified to have intra-abdominal hemorrhage using the FAST or DPL and be rapidly transferred to the operating room. The FAST is an ultrasound exam that is done in the resuscitation room, usually by the trauma surgeon, which examines the recesses of the peritoneal cavity for fluid (presumed to be blood in the injured patient). FAST also allows an examination of the pericardial sac (see Chap. 17).[45]

## Decision for Early Transfer

The need to transfer a patient for specialized care is commonly identified during the primary survey and resuscitation phase. If transfer is planned, then any additional therapeutic efforts should be directed toward resuscitation of the patient's vital signs and restoration of cellular perfusion to normal. Additional diagnostic tests prior to transfer only waste the "golden hour". Once it is recognized that the needs of the patient exceed the capabilities and resources of the local facility, preparation should begin for completion of resuscitation efforts, ensuring a safe transport process, and preparing for contingencies that may occur en route. Once the decision to transfer has been made, physician to physician communication is mandatory. A plan must be agreed upon regarding the optimal mode of transport, who will accompany the patient, and what should be accomplished before and during transport.

The ongoing evaluation, reevaluation, monitoring, and resuscitation must continue until the patient safely reaches the destination. While awaiting the ambulance or helicopter, the secondary survey should continue; diagnostic procedures that will delay the transfer should not be performed. During the secondary survey, a complete history, "head-to-toe" examination, laboratory tests, X-ray studies, and special tests (computed tomography [CT] scan, etc.) are performed. The definitive care phase occurs in the receiving hospital ED, operating room, or intensive care unit. Proper management of the patient in the definitive care phase may require surgical specialists (general/trauma/emergency surgeons, orthopaedic surgeons, neurosurgeons, and others).

# SECONDARY SURVEY

The secondary survey is not started until the primary survey is complete, resuscitation has been initiated, reevaluation of the vital signs has been performed, and the patient's vital functions are beginning to return to normal. The secondary survey is the traditional history and physical examination. A complete history is taken (if possible), and the physical examination from "head to toe" is carefully performed. Further X-ray examinations and special studies such as arteriography, computed tomography, and laboratory tests are completed during the secondary survey if not performed earlier. The secondary survey should be organized and efficient so that delays in definitive care do not occur. Some issues from the primary survey may need reevaluation during the secondary survey, and continuous monitoring of vital signs is mandatory. On occasion, the secondary survey is performed after the patient has had a definitive operation to correct problems with the ABCDEs. If a patient was hemodynamically normal or returning toward normal and then becomes unstable, attention is immediately redirected to the ABCs with the primary survey being repeated and necessary interventions performed.

## History

History is an important part of the secondary survey. The history of the injury event may be unavailable if the patient is unconscious, an endotracheal tube has been inserted, response is impaired secondary to alcohol or other drug ingestion, or simply confused. Prehospital personnel should be questioned before they leave, as they are usually aware of the circumstances surrounding the event and the specific mechanism of injury. Fifteen to 30 seconds of silence (but not inactivity) at the time of patient arrival will permit medics the opportunity to present important information that may serve to guide the initial focus of the trauma resuscitation team. The essential historical elements may be described by the mnemonic **AMPLE**.

**A**llergies

**M**edications currently being taken by the patient

**P**ast illness and operations

**L**ast meal

**E**vents and **E**nvironment related to the injury

Most allergic reactions can be avoided if information about drug allergies is known. Not only do medications taken by patients indicate other chronic conditions, but they can alter the patient's physiologic response to shock. Beta-blockers, digitalis, and calcium channel blockers can be associated with inability to increase heart rate; therefore, they may mask hypovolemia. A history of anticonvulsants or nitroglycerin-type drug use should suggest a seizure or a cardiac event as the possible cause of the injury event. The status of tetanus immunization should be determined, if possible.[46] Past illnesses and operations sometimes explain current findings. The timing of the last meal is important for the individual patient with diabetes, because of medication and blood sugar levels, and for all patients because of the potential for vomiting and aspiration.

The events and environmental issues associated with the injury are important to understand. Knowledge of the mechanism of injury provides valuable information related to expected patterns of injury (see Chap. 7). Vehicular crashes, falls, occupational injuries, and recreational injuries commonly cause blunt trauma. Useful information related to vehicular crashes includes the speed, use of restraints (seatbelts and air bags), direction of impact, ejection, deformity of the vehicle, and condition of the steering wheel and windshield. Absence of skid marks, no evidence of braking, or witnessed absence of attempts to avoid a car crash may indicate a primary cardiac event (dysrhythmia or arrest), neurologic event (stroke or seizure), or even a suicide attempt. Specific patterns of injury are frequently associated with the direction of impact. When ejection from the vehicle occurs, injuries to the brain and spine are very common, but many other injuries are likely because of the magnitude of impact this mechanism implies. Car—pedestrian (or car—bicycle/car—motorcycle) collisions often result in a combination of injuries, including fractures of the lower extremity as well as injuries to the brain and torso.

For gunshot wounds, the distance from the weapon to the injured person, mass and velocity of the missile (kinetic energy), and region of the body injured determines the extent of injury. High velocity bullets, such as from M16 or AK47, rifles have the most kinetic energy and the most potential to cause extensive injuries. Close range shotgun injuries can also be devastating. As much information as possible should be obtained from the medics or police regarding weapon types and distances in order to provide optimal care for the patient with a gunshot wound.

Patients with burns may have inhaled smoke and/or other noxious substances. These inhalation exposures may result in compromise of the airway or carbon monoxide poisoning. The environment, open or closed space fire, and substances burned in the fire can all affect the patient. Chemical fires and combustion of plastics may cause particularly serious inhalation injuries. The history is critically important in these cases. Hypothermia is a significant problem even at moderate temperatures if alcohol or other drugs, hemorrhage, wet clothes, and(or inactivity compromise conservation of heat.

Hazardous materials that cause injury to patients may also be harmful to health care providers. Each area or health care system in a community must be aware of the potential hazards from chemicals, toxins, and radiation in their region that may require treatment. The staff in the ED must be prepared and have appropriate antidotes and protective devices immediately available. Today, biological agents should also be considered a risk to the patient and health care team. Universal precautions are mandatory.

## Physical Examination

### Head and Face.
Brisk bleeding from the scalp can be masked by thick hair, and a significant amount of blood may be lost before adequate evaluation is performed. A trauma patient may present in hemorrhagic shock from an isolated scalp wound if the prehospital care providers did not control the bleeding. Occipital scalp lacerations are easily overlooked, especially in the immobilized patient, and a gloved hand for palpation of the scalp will aid in their identification. Cleansing the hair of blood may be necessary for complete scalp examination. If rapid suture, staple, or Raney clip closure of a scalp laceration has been necessary to control bleeding, further assessment, irrigation, debridement, and reclosure can be done during the secondary survey.

Facial lacerations and associated underlying injuries should be carefully examined. Epistaxis from the anterior aspect of the nose can usually be controlled by pressure. When serious bleeding from the posterior nose or nasopharynx is present, temporary nasal packing may be necessary. Occasionally, angiography with embolization may be necessary to control hemorrhage from facial fractures. Once all sites of scalp and facial bleeding are identified and controlled, the eyes are fully examined. Visual acuity, pupillary size and reactivity, direct globe injury, hyphema, foreign bodies (including contact lenses), and extraocular movements are assessed. If the patient is able to read newsprint with each eye independently, serious ocular injury is unlikely. Palpation of all bony prominences for deformity will detect most facial fractures. Facial fine-cut computed tomography can identify bony injuries not apparent on physical exam or other radiographic studies. Hypesthesia inferior to the eye, diplopia, and limitation of ocular motion are associated with "blowout" fractures of the inferior aspect of the orbit. A mid-face fracture is present when a gloved finger placed into the mouth can move the central incisors and palate. Malocclusion of the teeth is seen with either mandibular or maxillary fractures.

Basilar skull fractures are suggested by the presence of bruising around the eyes (raccoon's eyes) or behind the ears (Battle's sign). Hemotympanum and/or disruption of the auditory canal on otoscopic exam are additional findings suggestive of a basilar skull fracture. Cerebrospinal fluid leaking from the ear is confirmatory. The external ear is subject to lacerations that may be complex, and early wound care is necessary to avoid complications and optimize cosmetic appearance. In the absence of compromise of the airway or bleeding, treatment of facial injuries can be delayed without affecting definitive care; a saline-soaked sponge can be placed over these wounds while other injuries are being addressed.

Neurologic Assessment.    A brief neurologic exam, usually confined to examination of the pupils and determination of the GCS score, is performed during the primary survey. The neurologic exam during the secondary survey is a complete one and includes reevaluation of GCS scoring, reassessing the pupils for size and reactivity, and evaluating the function of the cranial nerves, motor and sensory function, coordination, and reflexes. The identification of asymmetry in the neurologic examination is suggestive of a localized intracranial injury that may require operative intervention. CT scanning of the head is appropriate for all patients with abnormalities of the neurologic exam or history of an alteration in level of consciousness at any point since the trauma episode.

Neck.    Any patient who is unconscious, has a neurologic deficit, or has injury above the clavicles has presumptive evidence of an injury to the cervical spine. A complete X-ray series of the cervical spine or cervical CT scan is needed to exclude occult bony injuries. Ligamentous injuries of the cervical spine can be excluded by magnetic resonance imaging (MRI) or flexion-extension plain films (or fluoroscopy).[47] The cervical spine should be protected until radiographic and clinical exams are reviewed by a physician skilled in evaluation of this area.

Neck wounds that penetrate the platysma require careful, detailed investigation; compromise of the airway is a concern. The presence of significant palpable crepitus or subcutaneous emphysema on X-rays of the neck is suggestive of an injury to the airway or esophagus. An expanding hematoma over the carotid artery or jugular vein mandates immediate operation, whereas duplex scanning, arteriography, or CT angiography may evaluate a small stable hematoma or a bruit. Missed injuries in the neck, whether bony, vascular, or digestive tract related may be lethal.

Spine.    Any loss of sensation, paralysis, or weakness in the extremities suggests an injury to the spinal cord. Neurologic findings should be documented. Serial reevaluation is critical because a change in the neurologic examination may be due to an expanding intraspinal or epidural hematoma, and emergency surgical intervention may be required. The entire spine should be X-rayed with CT or plain films in patients with a significant mechanism for spinal injury or patients in whom one spinal fracture has already been found.

Chest.    The chest is re-examined to find occult injuries and reassess the injuries that required treatment during the primary survey and resuscitation. Inspection for contusions and deformity, palpation for crepitus and tenderness, percussion for hyperresonance and tympany, and auscultation for abnormal breath sounds and heart sounds are performed. Shortness of breath, pain, and tenderness to direct palpation or anterior posterior compression suggest rib fractures which can impair ventilation secondary to pain. Should the chest X-ray show an abnormality, special studies may be indicated to make a definitive diagnosis. CT is now able to make many diagnoses that previously required multiple tests. Other special studies may still be necessary to define aortic disruption (transesophageal echocardiogram and(or aortogram), tracheobronchial injuries (bronchoscopy), and esophageal tears (esophagoscopy and contrast studies).

Abdomen.    Any trauma patient in shock must have abdominal injuries excluded. Detecting the presence of blood in the abdomen is more important than identifying a specific anatomic injury. Pain and bleeding from associated rib and pelvic fractures often interfere with the examination of the abdomen. Once the presence of an abdominal injury is suspected or confirmed, a general surgeon must be involved not only to help with diagnosis and resuscitation, but to provide definitive care. The three basic regions of the abdomen are the peritoneal cavity with its intrathoracic component, the retroperitoneum, and the pelvic portion. Because the diaphragm rises as high as the fourth intercostal space, blunt and penetrating trauma to the lower chest may involve abdominal organs. Suspected retroperitoneal injuries require CT scanning to confirm the diagnosis. Historical information from prehospital personnel or the patient can provide clues to the presence of abdominal injury.

The physical examination itself begins with inspection for contusions and penetrating injuries. Both the front and the back of the abdomen, flanks, perineum, and lower chest need to be viewed. Careful log-rolling of the patient must be done to examine the back. The presence or absence of bowel sounds is nonspecific. Percussion may demonstrate tenderness and peritoneal irritation. Abdominal palpation may detect localized or generalized tenderness, masses, voluntary guarding, or involuntary guarding. Clear evidence of intra-abdominal injury (peritonitis or evisceration) will lead to laparotomy. Penetrating injuries to the abdomen must be identified and evaluated by a surgeon early to plan the workup and operative strategy. In some centers, the presence of any peritoneal penetration mandates operation. In others, patients with gunshot wounds are always operated on, but patients with stab wounds and no peritonitis or hypotension are observed. Some surgeons are doing more extensive workups including triple contrast CT (oral, rectal, and intravenous contrast) for possible tangential, flank, or back wounds in stable patients to determine which require operation. Examination of the perineum, rectum, vagina, and external genitalia should be performed as part of the examination of the abdomen.

Contrast studies to define injuries to the urinary tract are occasionally necessary. The retrograde urethrogram has been mentioned above. Cystograms are performed with the catheter in place for patients with gross hematuria and evidence of pelvic trauma. A CT scan is used to evaluate the kidneys.

Pelvic fractures are frequently associated with other abdominal injuries.[48] Hemodynamically unstable patients with pelvic fractures who require a DPL (when FAST is unavailable) should have a supraumbilical approach to avoid entering a pelvic preperitoneal hematoma. Transfusion is necessary in most patients with severe pelvic fractures, especially those fractures that open the pelvis and increase pelvic volume.[49–51] Hemorrhagic shock may be present. Early control of bleeding from fractures of the pelvic ring can sometimes be achieved by binding the pelvis with a bedsheet or commercial sling; these may even be applied in the prehospital setting. Similarly, external fixation of unstable pelvic fractures to control bleeding from the bony fracture site can be considered an adjunct to resuscitation. When these measures fail, arteriography for embolization of arterial bleeding or operation for pelvic packing may be necessary.

When CT scanning is performed, patients with multiple injuries are at risk of deterioration during transport or during the scan itself and must be carefully monitored by experienced personnel. The

CT scan defines specific injuries, particularly to the solid organs in the abdomen. Children especially benefit from this exam, as nonoperative management for injuries to solid organs is so frequently successful in the young. Today, nonoperative management is often used for patients of all ages, but it is important to specifically identify the injuries being observed.

If multiple CT scans are indicated, one trip to the scanning area is the goal. A CT scan of the head is performed first, when indicated, so that the intravenous contrast needed for neck, chest, or abdominal studies can be given after the noncontrast head scan.

### Musculoskeletal and Peripheral Vascular.

All four extremities including the hands and feet should be inspected for gross deformity, swelling, or open injury. Palpation of the extremities for tenderness, crepitus, and abnormal mobility are clues to the presence of fractures. All joints must be assessed for tenderness, swelling, and abnormal mobility. Bones or joints with suspected injury should be immobilized to alleviate pain and prevent further damage.

Assessment of the neurovascular status of the limbs is crucial to detect injuries that might lead to limb loss. Decreased or absent pulses suggest a vascular injury. Asymmetry of the pulse or blood pressure as compared to the opposite extremity is also presumptive evidence of vascular injury. Arterial hemorrhage or an expanding hematoma is an indication for urgent operation. Loss of pulse is also an indication for operation, but a diagnostic arteriogram may be necessary first to delineate the location of injury. Proximity of penetrating injuries or major fractures to large vessels is an indication for repeated physical examinations or further studies, depending on local practice. Liberal use of arteriography (or CT angiography) will identify most vascular injuries.[52] If pulses return with reduction of associated fractures or dislocations, careful serial monitoring may suffice.

A compartment syndrome may develop insidiously, and every patient with an injured extremity should be considered at risk, particularly those with fractures and crush injuries. Pain is the first sign of ischemia and should be aggressively evaluated. The unconscious patient who cannot verbalize the presence of pain is at particular risk because of potential for delay in diagnosis. Frequent reevaluation of the extremity is essential. If there is any suspicion that a compartment syndrome is developing or exists, compartment pressures should be measured or fasciotomy performed. For crush injuries, rhabdomyolysis must be considered. The function of peripheral nerves should also be assessed and recorded as a baseline.

## REEVALUATION

During all phases of trauma care, frequent reevaluation is performed to detect and treat any deterioration in the patient's condition. If there is a sudden deterioration in the condition of the patient, the safest procedure is to immediately begin again at the beginning, with evaluation of the ABCs. Many examples of deterioration of the patient during or after the primary survey have been described. One of the most common scenarios is the patient who presents with a normal neurologic examination and subsequently develops a dilated pupil, decreasing level of consciousness, and contralateral hemiparesis, suggesting an acute epidural hematoma ("talk and die"). Another common occurrence is conversion of a simple pneumothorax to a tension pneumothorax over time. A severe blunt cardiac injury may be associated with abnormal cardiac rhythms that develop during the course of treatment. Cardiac tamponade, particularly that originating from the atrium, may develop slowly and not be evident initially. In summary, a comprehensive secondary survey, including an investigation of all complaints from the patient, soliciting further information on the patient's pre-existing medical conditions, and continuous monitoring of vital signs and response to therapy, would ideally be completed before definitive care or transfer. Completing the secondary survey is not, however, an appropriate reason to delay transfer of the critically injured patient.

## STABILIZATION AND TRANSFER

Most injured patients can be treated in the local hospital. One of the responsibilities of the physician who first treats the trauma patient is to determine whether the patient's needs exceed the capability and available resources of that hospital. In an organized trauma system, transfer agreements are in place to facilitate transfer of injured patients to a trauma center or other designated hospital. In the absence of a formalized system for transfer, physicians who care for the trauma patient should be aware of which hospitals have advanced capabilities for trauma care or surgical critical care in their region. Satisfactory transfers are guided by the principle of "do no further harm." Once the determination has been made that the patient will require transfer to another facility for definitive care, the referring physician should continue to perform those interventions that assist in resuscitation of the patient and ensure patient safety during the transfer. Time should not be spent performing additional diagnostic procedures.

The referring physician must resuscitate the patient to the best of his or her ability using all available local resources. This physician also needs to determine the urgency of the transfer, mode of transportation, and the level of care required during transport. Direct physician-to-physician consultation is essential. Some decisions about how to transport may be shared by the referring and accepting physicians. The accepting physician may suggest additional maneuvers to enhance the safety of the patient during transfer. Usually the referring physician will be able to complete the primary survey, resuscitation, and secondary survey phases of care prior to transport. Sometimes, because of urgency, the secondary survey will be performed after transport.

Occasionally, a patient that requires transfer for subspecialist care (such as neurosurgery) is not hemodynamically stable because of ongoing hemorrhage. If hemodynamic status can be improved by operative intervention (such as splenectomy), at the local hospital, immediate evaluation by the local surgeon is imperative. The decision to transfer the patient prior to or following surgical intervention should be made by a surgeon. One interfacility transfer system has been established in which the accepting trauma surgeon travels by air to the referring hospital for transfer of extremely critical trauma patients. Using this transfer method, the accepting trauma surgeon can assist the referring surgeon in the operating room, if necessary, prior to transporting the patient.[53]

The decision between air and ground transport is based on patient acuity, available resources, weather, distance/time involved, safety, and the skill level of the transport providers. Most accredited air ambulance programs provide committed personnel specially trained in both trauma and critical care.

The transport providers should be given detailed information and a description of any potential unsolved problems. They must have the capability to continue resuscitation efforts, including management of the ABCDEs. All available information should accompany the patient and include the original assessment including history, physical examination, and description of vital signs, treatments, medications administered, fluids or blood received, results of laboratory tests, response to interventions, and status of the patient before arrival at the receiving hospital. X-rays and their interpretations should also accompany the patient to avoid repeating studies, if possible.

Finally, the patient must be appropriately "packaged." The airway must be secured by whatever means necessary. Intubation in transit is difficult. If there is potential for compromise of the airway en route, intubation should be accomplished prior to the transport. Chest tubes should be placed liberally, even for small pneumothoraces, because a pneumothorax can enlarge en route. Control of external bleeding, two large-bore intravenous lines, crystalloids and/or blood infusing, gastric and urinary catheters in place, and continuous cardiac monitoring are all necessary as well. Patients with severe injuries to the brain require a definitive airway, adequate ventilation, oxygenation, and resuscitation from shock prior to transport.

## RECORD KEEPING

Precise record keeping is important for good care and enables appropriate retrospective review for quality improvement. Timed entries on pre-existing forms facilitate both recording and later recovery of data. Numerous types of trauma flow sheets are utilized in individual facilities and systems. A careful review of the patient's initial assessment and management may explain the patient's subsequent clinical course.

## REFERENCES

1. American College of Surgeons Committee on Trauma: *Advanced Trauma Life Support® for Physicians.* Chicago, IL: American College of Surgeons, 2004.
2. American College of Surgeons Committee on Trauma: *Resources for the Optimal Care of the Injured Patient.* Chicago, IL: American College of Surgeons, 1998.
3. Enderson BL, Reath DB, Meadors J, et al.: The tertiary trauma survey: A prospective study of missed injury. *J Trauma* 30:666, 1990.
4. National Association of Emergency Medical Technicians: *Basic and Advanced Prehospital Trauma Life Support.* St. Louis: Mosby, 2003.
5. Borden Institute, *Emergency War Surgery: 3rd United States Revision, Washington, D.C., 2004.*
6. Eastes LS, Norton R, Brand D, et al.: Outcomes of patients using a tiered trauma response protocol. *J Trauma* 50:908, 2001.
7. Rogers FB, Simons R, Hoyt DB, et al.: In-house board-certified surgeons improve outcome for severely injured patients: A comparison of two university centers. *J Trauma* 34:871 (discussion 875), 1993.
8. Baumgartner FS, Ayers B, Theuer C: Danger of false intubation after traumatic tracheal transection. *Ann Thoracic Surg* 63:227, 1997.
9. Bergen JM, Smith DC: A review of etomidate for rapid sequence intubation in the emergency department. *J Emerg Med* 15:221, 1997.
10. Gerardi MJ, Sacchett AD, Cantor RM, et al.: Rapid-sequence intubation of the pediatric patient. *Ann Emerg Med* 28:55, 1996.
11. Mitchell FL, Thal ER, Wolferth CC: American College of Surgeons verification/consultation program: Analysis of unsuccessful verification reviews. J Trauma 37:557, 1994.
12. Cline JR, Scheidel E, Bigsby EF: A comparison of methods of cervical immobilization used in patient extrication and transport. *J Trauma* 25:649, 1985.
13. Guildner CV: Resuscitation-opening the airway. A comparative study of techniques for opening an airway obstructed by the tongue. *J Am Coll Emerg Phys* 5:588, 1976.
14. Knapp S, Kofler J, Stoiser B, et al: The assessment of four different methods to verify tracheal tube placement in the critical care setting. *Anesth Analg* 88:766, 1999.
15. Bell RM, Page GV, Bynoe RP, et al.: Post traumatic sinusitis. *J Trauma* 28:923, 1988.
16. Butler FS, Circilo AA: Retrograde intubation. *Anesth Analg* 39:333, 1960.
17. Sanches TF: Retrograde intubation. *Anesth Clin North Am* 13:439, 1995.
18. Miller GT, Fastrach LMA: EMS discovers the intubating laryngeal mask airway. *J Emerg Med Serv* 27:68, 2002.
19. Majernick TG, Bieniek, Houston JB, et al.: Cervical spine movement during orotracheal intubation. *Ann Emerg Med* 15:417, 1986.
20. Jorden RC, Moore EE, Marx JA, et al.: A comparison of PTV and endotracheal ventilation in an acute trauma model. *J Trauma* 25:978, 1985.
21. Brantigan CO, Grow JB Sr: Cricothyroidotomy: Elective use in respiratory problems requiring tracheotomy. *J Thoracic Cardiovascular Surg* 71:72, 1976.
22. Brofeldt BT, Panacek EA, Richards JR: An easy cricothyroid approach: The rapid four-step technique. *Acad Emer Med* 3:1060, 1996.
23. McSwain NE: Techniques of helmet removal from injured patients. *Bull Am Coll Surg* 66:19, 1981.
24. Meyer RD, Daniel WW: The biomechanics of helmets and helmet removal. *J Trauma* 25:329, 1985.
25. Yeston NS: Noninvasive measurement of blood gases. *Infect Surg* 9:18, 1990.
26. Lewis FR: Initial assessment and resuscitation. *Emerg Med Clin North Am* 2:733, 1984.
27. Richardson JD, Adams L, Flint LM: Selective management of flail chest and pulmonary contusion. *Ann Surgery* 196:481, 1982.
28. Feliciano DV, Rozycki GS: Advances in the diagnosis and treatment of thoracic trauma. *Surg Clin North Am* 79:1417, 1999.
29. Demetriades D, Velhamos GC: Penetrating injuries of the chest: Indications for operation. *Scand J Surg* 91:41, 2002.
30. Bickell WH, Wall MJ, Pepe PE, et al.: Immediate versus delayed fluid resuscitation for hypotensive patients with penetrating torso trauma. *N Engl J Med* 331:1105, 1994.
31. Capone AC, Safar PK, Sterzoski SW, et al.: Uncontrolled hemorrhagic shock outcome model in rats. *Resuscitation* 29:143, 1995.
32. Turnage B, Maull KI: Scalp laceration: An obvious 'occult' cause of shock. *South Med J* 93:265, 2000.
33. Chestnut RM, Marshall LF, Klauber MR, et al.: The role of secondary brain injury in determining outcome from severe head injury. *J Trauma* 34:216, 1993.
34. Rhodes M, Brader A, Lucke J, et al.: Direct transport to the operating room for resuscitation of trauma patients. *J Trauma* 29:907, 1989.
35. Illig KA, Swierzewski MJ, Feliciano DV, et al.: A rational screening and treatment strategy based on the electrocardiogram alone for suspected cardiac contusion. *Am J Surg* 162:537, 1991.
36. Mansour MA, Moore EE, Moore EA, et al.: Exigent postinjury thoracotomy analysis of blunt versus penetrating trauma. *Surg Gynecol Obstet* 175:97, 1992.
37. Jennett B, Teasdale G: Aspects of coma after severe head injury. *Lancet* 1:878, 1977.
38. Gentilello LM: Practical approaches to hypothermia. In Maull KI et al., eds. *Advances in Trauma and Critical Care.* St. Louis: Mosby, 1994, p. 39.
39. Fremstad JD, Martin SH: Lethal complications from insertion of nasogastric tube after severe basilar skull fracture. *J Trauma* 18:820, 1978.
40. Rozycki GS, Oschner MG, Jaffin JH, et al.: Prospective evaluation of surgeons' use of ultrasound in the evaluation of trauma patients. *J Trauma* 41:368 (discussion 567), 1996.
41. Dolich MO, McKenney MG, Varela JE, et al.: 2,576 ultrasounds for blunt abdominal trauma. *J Trauma* 50:108, 2001.
42. McAnena OJ, Marks JA, Moore EE: Peritoneal lavage enzyme determinations following blunt and penetrating abdominal trauma. *J Trauma* 31:1161, 1991.
43. Feliciano DV: Diagnostic modalities in abdominal trauma. Peritoneal lavage, ultrasonography, computerized tomography scanning, and arteriography. *Surg Clin North Am* 71:241, 1991.
44. Liu M, Lee C, Veng F: Prospective comparison of diagnostic peritoneal lavage, computed tomographic scanning, and ultrasonography for the diagnosis of blunt abdominal trauma. *J Trauma* 35:267, 1993.
45. Rozycki GS, Feliciano DV, Ochsner MG, et al.: The role of ultrasound in patients with possible penetrating cardiac wounds: A prospective multicenter study. *J Trauma* 46:542, 1999.
46. Rhee P, Nunley M, Demetriades D, et al.: Tetanus and trauma: A review and recommendations. *J Trauma* 58:1082, 2005.
47. Sees DW, Rodriguez Cruz LR, Flaherty SF, et al.: The use of bedside fluoroscopy to evaluate the cervical spine in obtunded trauma patients. *J Trauma* 45:768, 1998.
48. Burgess AR, Eastridge BJ, Young JWR, et al.: Pelvic ring disruptions: Effective classification system and treatment protocols. *J Trauma* 30:848, 1990.
49. Cryer HM, Miller FB, Evers BM, et al.: Pelvic fracture classification: Correlation with hemorrhage. *J Trauma* 28:973, 1988.

50. Alonso JE, Lee J, Burgess AR, et al.: The management of complex orthopedic injuries. *Surg Clin North Am* 76:879, 1996.
51. Whitbeck MG, Zwally HJ, Burgess AR: Innominosacral dislocation: Mechanism of injury as a predictor of resuscitation requirements, morbidity and mortality. *J Ortho Trauma* 11:82, 1997.
52. O'Gorman RB, Feliciano DV, Bitondo CG, et al.: Emergency center arteriography in the evaluation of suspected peripheral vascular injuries. *Arch Surg* 119: 568, 1984.
53. Long WB, Michaels AJ: Mobile surgical transport team: The first twenty years. Manuscript in preparation. Personal communication.

# Commentary ■ JAMEEL ALI

As outlined in this chapter, the Advanced Trauma Life Support (ATLS®) Program has established the international standard for initial assessment and management of the trauma patient. The underlying basic principle of this approach is to prioritize management based on the degree of life threat. It emphasizes the concept that resuscitation of the trauma patient can be successfully achieved without a definitive diagnosis. The very nature of the traumatic event frequently prevents detailed history taking and assessment of the mechanism of the injury so that a definitive diagnosis is virtually impossible within the short period of time available for resuscitation. One of the main differences between the trauma patient and the elective patient seen in the office or ambulatory setting is that the trauma patient's condition can deteriorate rapidly not allowing sufficient time to establish a firm diagnosis based on detailed physical examination and investigation.

Although the principles of trauma resuscitation are standard, variations in the approach may be warranted depending on the level of clinical expertise and available resources, including physical, medical, and paramedical. In outlining the approach to the multiply injured patient, the ATLS concepts describe a sequential identification and correction of abnormalities during the primary survey following the ABCDE order. In making A or the airway our first priority, it matters not whether the airway is indirectly compromised from a head injury, hypovolemic shock, or directly by structural damage to the airway. The trauma physician needs to correct the airway problem by the recognized airway maneuvers as described in the chapter regardless of the underlying definitive cause of this airway compromise. Although in describing this approach, the ABCDE order of priorities is followed and is entirely appropriate when one physician is managing the multiply injured patient, there are many circumstances where several physicians and nurses may be available allowing simultaneous correction of different components of the ABCDE. For instance, while one physician is assessing and securing the airway another could be establishing intravenous access or stopping external hemorrhage by the application of pressure and splints. When several physicians are available it is critical to ensure that one physician is in charge of the entire resuscitative process—the Team Leader whose responsibility is to ensure adherence to the priorities in the initial assessment.

Successful outcome following management in the hospital setting depends to a large extent on what type of prehospital care the trauma victim receives. Indeed, improvement in prehospital care has been shown to positively affect outcome for the same injury severity among patients admitted with multiple injuries to the referral hospital.[1,2] Simple, prehospital maneuvers aimed at protecting the airway and preventing hypoxic cellular damage, maintaining oxygenation, protection of the spine, and control of hemorrhage can all contribute toward a better outcome of the trauma patient after arrival in the hospital. Regarding hemorrhage control, use of tourniquets in the hospital setting is usually not indicated but in the prehospital setting this can be life-saving provided it is properly applied with the appropriate tension to exceed arterial pressure in the damaged extremity.[3] In this circumstance, the prehospital personnel needs to make a decision of risking loss of limb in order to preserve the life of the trauma patient. Because the approach in the initial assessment allows the physician to identify abnormalities in a sequence based on the degree of life threat, once an abnormality is identified it can be immediately corrected.

Although the ATLS Program originated in North America in the late 1970s, the international promulgation process has resulted in over 50% of the 750,0000 ATLS trained physicians being from outside North America. This means that the approach taught for initial assessment has universal application but while maintaining the overall basic principles there may be differences depending on the local environment.

Following are some of these differences in approach which may be specific for certain environments:

## A. Airway

The combative patient may be impossible to intubate and use of a paralyzing agent may be necessary to secure the airway. Overall, the safest agent, as described, in spite of its limitations, is succinylcholine mainly because of its very short duration of action. If a high level of airway expertise is lacking, inability to secure intubation with a paralyzing agent such as succinylcholine can be followed by mechanical manual ventilation for the brief period of time until the succinylcholine wears off and the patient is able to breathe spontaneously. In many settings where greater level of expertise in airway management is available, intermediate acting paralyzing agents are frequently used because of their more acceptable hemodynamic responses in the trauma patient. In the emergency room setting one must always anticipate the possibility of a difficult airway. Surgical instruments for establishing a surgical airway as well as flexible fiber optic devices should be immediately and readily available.

In the trauma patient, preparation is essential and this requires strategically placed devices such as IV fluids, chest tubes, airway equipment in the ED. Continuous inventory is required on a daily basis to ensure that supplies which have been used are replenished and are ready for the next patient.

## B. Breathing

Traditional teaching recommends needle decompression for the treatment of a tension pneumothorax which is a clinical diagnosis made during the primary survey. The advantages of this maneuver are that it is simple, quick, and safe. This is definitely the preferred approach in the hands of a nonexpert. However, this technique may sometimes not be effective in decompressing a tension pneumothorax because of such problems as kinking of the plastic cannula which is frequently used with the needle decompression. In a sophisticated trauma centre setting where all equipment is in readiness including chest tubes and highly skilled staff, the chest tube may be inserted just as expeditiously and would result in more effective and definitive decompression of the tension pneumothorax than by needle decompression.

With an open pneumothorax the simplest technique is to apply an occlusive dressing as outlined in this chapter. When the defect in the chest wall is very large it may be impossible to provide a secure occlusive dressing and in these circumstances endotracheal intubation and mechanical ventilation is an effective way of maintaining hemodynamics, ventilation, and oxygenation. This technique facilitates stabilization of the patient who can then be taken to the operating room for formal surgical correction of the chest wall defect using more complex procedures.

The area of lung contusion following blunt trauma to the chest can increase with crystalloid infusion and the technique of conservative fluid administration is advised to minimize the enlargement of the contused area and its effect on gas exchange. However, in the trauma patient who is in shock and requires massive fluid infusion, the enlargement of the contusion takes second priority to aggressive fluid resuscitation, mechanical ventilation being instituted to treat the hypoxemia resulting from enlargement of the area of contusion leading to V/Q mismatch.

## C. Circulation

The first choice for vascular access is peripheral large-bore short catheters and, as mentioned, the expertise available often dictates what method is used for vascular access. In many trauma centres, the central route particularly in the neck is the first choice and this has become even more so because of the increased accuracy and safety associated with central venous access under ultrasound guidance.

The type of fluid used in initial resuscitation is usually a balanced salt solution such as Ringer's Lactate or Normal Saline in spite of many studies suggesting possible benefit from hypertonic saline.[4-6] There maybe some advantage in the head-injured patient by using hypertonic saline over isotonic solutions.[7] The demonstrated advantages in the laboratory of hypertonic saline in attenuation of the polymorpho nuclear neutrophil cytotoxicity in hemorrhagic shock have not led to general clinical application. This lack of clinical benefit may be related to the timing of hypertonic fluid resuscitation.[9] Earlier institution of hypertonic fluid resuscitation appears more likely to benefit the patient.[8]

In the laboratory setting and specially designed clinical studies, it has been suggested that in penetrating torso trauma aggressive fluid resuscitation may result in increased bleeding and a worse outcome for the trauma patient.[10-13] However, these studies are based on special circumstances where immediate operating room access and short prehospital time apply. Even in these circumstances the patient with significant head trauma is better served by more aggressive fluid resuscitation in order to prevent secondary brain injury from cerebral hypoperfusion and hypoxia. A reasonable approach would appear to be the maintenance of borderline hypotension by conservative fluid administration in penetrating torso trauma in the absence of traumatic brain injury with the aim of prompt hemorrhage control in the operating room.

In neurogenic shock, the vasodilatation from loss of sympathetic vascular tone results in a relative hypovolemia because of the expanded vascular space for the same circulating blood volume. Thus, the initial management of these patients requires fluid resuscitation. It should be noted that bradycardia may not always be an accompaniment of this type of shock depending on the level of interruption of the sympathetic pathway from the spinal cord. Preservation of the sympathetic nerve supply to the heart would allow an appropriate cardiac response to hypotension in the form of a tachycardia. In resuscitating the patient in neurogenic shock the aim should be to establish normal perfusion recognizing that this can be achieved without necessarily reaching a normal blood pressure. If, in the presence of borderline hypotension, there is adequate cerebral and renal perfusion as evidenced by normal CNS function and urine output then fluid administration purely for the purpose of increasing the blood pressure is not necessary. Under some circumstances it may be necessary to temporarily increase systemic vascular resistance by the administration of alpha agonists when the blood pressure is unacceptably low and associated with signs of hypo perfusion. Indeed, attempts to achieve a normal blood pressure in the patient with neurogenic shock by fluid administration alone may result in pulmonary edema before achieving normalcy of blood pressure. Ideally, fluid administration, particularly in the elderly patient with poor cardiac reserve, should be guided by central hemodynamic pressure monitoring.

The diagnosis of cardiac tamponade has been facilitated greatly by the more liberal use of FAST in the emergency room.[14] This allows the prompt identification of fluid in the pericardial sac. In the presence of chest trauma this is an indication for decompression of the pericardial space. Where the expertise is not immediately available for performing a subxiphoid pericardiotomy, pericardiocentesis, if properly performed, can be life saving.[15] This is only a temporizing measure until the patient can be taken to the operating room for definitive repair of the offending injury. In situations where the operating room is easily accessible and with appropriately trained staff, the preferred route is a subxiphoid pericardiotomy for immediate pericardial decompression followed by open thoracotomy for formal repair of the cardiac wound.

The DPL is still presented as a technique for assessing the abdomen as a source of hemorrhage in the trauma patient. This has application in settings where ultrasound is not immediately available. However, in most trauma centres, FAST has replaced DPL because it is much quicker, safer, and more reliable for identifying intra-abdominal hemorrhage.

## D. Neurologic Disability

The main stay of management of the head-injured patient during the initial assessment is the maintenance of oxygenation and perfusion to prevent secondary brain injury. The effect of hypocapnea in decreasing intracranial pressure is accomplished at the expense of cerebral ischemia and can have deleterious effects on brain function if instituted for prolonged periods of time. Hence, patients with severe head injuries are ventilated to maintain $PCO_2$

very close to normal (approximately 35 mm Hg) and an appropriate inspired oxygen concentration to maintain $O_2$ saturation above 95%.

In centres where neuro surgical expertise is not immediately available and the patient has a rapidly potentially lethal expanding intracranial hematoma, such as an epidural hematoma, it may be appropriate to consider craniotomy by non-neurosurgeons who may be either guided by a neurosurgeon from a distance or who may have had previous limited experience in this technique. Generally, however, these procedures are more optimally performed by an appropriately trained neurosurgeon because the offending clot is often difficult to evacuate without a generous craniotomy.

### E. Exposure and Environment

As previously stated, it is important to completely expose the patient in order to identify all possible injuries. However, the patient must be promptly covered with warm blankets and kept in a warm environment; fluid-warming devices must be immediately available so that fluid administered would be appropriately warmed to protect from hypothermia. This continues to be a major problem particularly when patients are in shock requiring massive volume infusion and the effects of the hypothermia and its consequences are frequently worse than the initiating injury itself.[16–18]

## The Secondary Survey

The secondary survey begins after the patient's hemodynamic, respiratory, and metabolic status has been corrected and represents a more deliberate process of head-to-toe assessment for injuries, which, if left unattended, could produce significant morbidity or even late death. It is frequently not possible to complete the secondary survey for several hours in situations where the patient is taken to the operating room for operative resuscitation which is then considered part of the primary survey. During the primary survey, the attending physician should continuously assess the patient's needs in light of the available resources (physical and personnel) to determine whether the patient should be transferred to a higher level of care. This transfer should be initiated as quickly as possible and should not be delayed in order to obtain imaging and other laboratory test results. In ordering a particular investigation in these circumstances, the principle should be that if the results of the tests would change management of the patient at the original institution then it is appropriate to conduct the tests. Otherwise, these investigations are better left for the referral centre.

In the initial assessment of the trauma patient with a possible spine injury, as mentioned in the chapter, the major goal is spine protection rather than establishing a definitive diagnosis. Imaging is therefore conducted only after the patient's condition has been stabilized. Occasionally, cervical spine X-rays (lateral cervical spine and open mouth odontoid views) may be conducted if this does not interfere with the sequence and conduct of the primary survey and resuscitation of the trauma patient. Plain X-ray films are still mentioned as part of the routine assessment for spine injury. This is primarily because of the variation in environments where patients are managed according to ATLS principles and more sophisticated imaging techniques may not be available. In most major trauma centers, CT assessment of the spine has completely replaced plain X-rays because this gives a more complete and accurate assessment.

---

## SUMMARY

The simple system of dividing the management of the multiply injured patient into the phases of primary survey, secondary survey, and definitive care has uniform applicability and has become the standard for initial assessment and management. Variations in the approach based on local environments such as the level of medical expertise, physical resources, and training may be necessary. However, the underlying basic principle of identifying and treating the life threats in the appropriate sequence and then proceeding to an orderly process of secondary survey provides the safest means of optimizing management of the acutely multiply injured patient.

## References

1. Ali J, Adam R, Butler AK, et al.: Trauma outcome improves following the advanced trauma life support (ATLS) program in a developing country. *J Trauma* 34:890, 1993.
2. Ali J, Adam R, Gana TJ, et al.: Trauma patient outcome after the prehospital trauma life support program. *J Trauma* 42:1018, 1997.
3. Walters TJ, Mabry RL: Use of tourniquets on the battlefield: a consensus panel report. *Mil Med* 170:770, 2005.
4. Angle N, Hoyt DB, Coimbra R, et al.: Hypertonic saline resuscitation diminishes lung injury by suppressing neutrophil activation after hemorrhagic shock. *Shock* 9:164, 1998.
5. Ciesla DJ, Moore EE, Zallen G, et al.: Hypertonic saline attenuation of polymorphonuclear neutrophil cytotoxicity: timing is everything. *J Trauma* 48:388, 2000.
6. Rotstein OD: Novel strategies for immunomodulation after trauma: revisiting by hypertonic saline as a resuscitation strategy for hemorrhagic shock. *J Trauma* 49:580, 2000.
7. Wade CE, Grady JJ, Kramer GC, et al.: Individual patient cohort analysis of the efficacy of hypertonic saline/dextran in patients with traumatic brain injury and hypotension. *J Trauma* 42:S61, 1997.
8. Hashiguchi N, Lum L, Romeril E, et al.: Hypertonic saline resuscitation: efficacy may require early treatment in severely injured patients. *J Trauma* 62:299, 2007.
9. Vassar MJ, Fischer RP, O'Brien PE, et al.: A multicenter trial for resuscitation on injured patients with 7.5% sodium chloride. *Arch Surg* 128:1003, 1993.
10. Bickell WH, Wall MJ Jr, Pepe PE, et al.: Immediate versus delayed fluid resuscitation for hypotensive patients with penetrating torso injuries. *N Eng J Med* 331:1105, 1994.
11. Burris D, Rhee P, Kaufman C, et al.: Controlled resuscitation for uncontrolled hemorrhagic shock. *J Trauma* 46:216, 1999.
12. Capone AC, Safar P, Stezoski W, et al.: Improved outcome with fluid restriction in treatment of uncontrolled hemorrhagic shock. *J Am Coll Surg* 180:49, 1995.
13. Kowalenko T, Stern S, Dronen S, et al.: Improved outcome with hypotensive resuscitation of uncontrolled hemorrhagic shock in a swine model. *J Trauma* 33:349, 1992.
14. Rozycki GS, Feliciano DV, Ochsner MG, et al.: The role of ultrasound in patients with possible penetrating cardiac wounds: a prospective multicenter study. *J Trauma* 46:543, 1999.
15. Breaux EP, Dupont JB Jr, Albert HM, et al.: Cardiac tamponade following penetrating mediastinal injuries: improved survival with early pericardiocentesis. *J Trauma* 19:362, 1979.
16. Patt A, McCroskey BL, Moore EE: Hypothermia induced coagulopathies in trauma. *Surg Clin North Am* 68:775, 1988.
17. Jurkovich GJ, Greiser WB, Luterman A, et al.: Hypothermia in trauma victims: an ominous predictor of survival. *J Trauma* 27:1019, 1987.
18. Gentilello LM, Jurkovich GJ, Maier R, et al.: Is hypothermia in the victim of major trauma protective or harmful? A randomized prospective study. *Ann Surg* 226:439, 1997.

# Airway Control

Eric A. Toschlog ■ Scott G. Sagraves ■ Michael F. Rotondo

## INTRODUCTION

Oxygen is the primary substrate for aerobic metabolism, and failure to deliver cellular oxygen represents the most common cause of mortality following injury and critical illness. Although many trauma patients die secondary to nonsurvivable primary injury to vital organs, a significant number of patients perish secondary to lack of available cellular oxygen. Cellular oxygen consumption is dependent upon adequate oxygen delivery, which in turn is dependent upon hemoglobin concentration, oxygen saturation of arterial hemoglobin, and cardiac output.

### The Priority of the Airway

In the crucial initial management of the injured patient, securing the airway is quite literally the single most important priority; failure to oxygenate and ventilate represents the difference between life and death as well as functionality and disability. Loss of the airway frequently initiates a terminal and irreversible cascade of events. In emergency airway procedures performed outside of the operating room, including the prehospital environment, the incidence of severe hypoxemia preceding cardiac arrest is 90%.[1] Of all prehospital advanced life support (ALS) interventions, successful airway management has been demonstrated to have the most profound effect on outcome, representing a truly life-saving intervention.[2] Correspondingly, airway management in the injured patient represents one of the most important requisite skills for clinicians caring for this population. Not only are hypoxia and hypoventilation common injury-related causes of mortality, they additionally represent one of the most common causes of *preventable* mortality following injury.

The trauma patient represents a unique and exquisite airway challenge, from both anatomic and physiologic perspectives. Any injury or component of airway failure contributing to a reduction of any single component of oxygen delivery can be lethal. Failure of oxygenation and ventilation may be unrelated to craniofacial or thoracic trauma, resulting solely from severe reduction in oxygen delivery secondary to any one of a number of isolated or concurrent shock states. Conversely, reduced oxygen delivery may be secondary to isolated anatomic injury to any structure responsible for oxygenation and ventilation, including the brain and spinal cord. The multisystem trauma patient represents the culmination of interrelated insults to oxygenation and ventilation. Clinicians must rapidly recognize multiple injuries in such patients and prioritize the airway in what may be seemingly multiple conflicting priorities. It is the complexity and stress of the multisystem patient that have mandated the development of a consistent and reproducible approach to the airway useful to clinicians of varying degrees of clinical skill.

### The Foundation of Advanced Trauma Life Support

Assurance of adequate cellular oxygenation and ventilation has retained primacy in algorithms to support critically ill adults and children. They are incorporated as the first and second steps, "Airway" and "Breathing," in the primary patient surveys of Advanced Cardiac, Pediatric Prehospital, Burn, and Trauma Life Support courses. The Advanced Trauma Life Support (ATLS) course emphasizes prevention of hypoxemia through maintenance of an unobstructed airway with adequate ventilation having priority over all other conditions in the trauma patient.[3] "Airway compromise may be sudden and complete, insidious and partial, and progressive and/or recurrent."[3] One of the foundations of ATLS emphasizes that early preventable death after injury is not infrequent, and that preventable death can originate from the following:

Failure to recognize the need for an airway

Inability to establish an airway

Failure to recognize an incorrectly placed airway

Displacement of a previously established airway

Failure to recognize the need for ventilation

Aspiration of gastric contents

The additional steps in the ATLS primary survey—breathing, circulation, disability, and exposure—are not undertaken until the airway has been effectively secured. Following assessment of the airway, further emphasis on oxygenation and ventilation is assured through assessment of breathing. Although the goal of the ATLS course is to provide a basic and fundamental approach to the early management of the injured for providers of all levels of expertise, many principles remain valuable for the most advanced provider. They include the following:

Recognition of the priority of the airway

Recognition of the difficult airway

Basic airway maintenance techniques

Strict attention to immobilization of the cervical spine

Endotracheal intubation as the definitive airway

Inability to intubate the trachea is a clear indication for creating a surgical airway

The importance of a team approach to the airway

## BASIC AIRWAY EQUIPMENT AND PREPARATION

### Introduction

The maintenance of a patent airway and adequate ventilation are the first priorities in managing any injured patient. An open airway supports adequate oxygenation and ventilation, and is the initial step in preventing hypoxemia. The creation of an open airway and maintenance of that open airway, prior to intubation, may be one of the most difficult skills for a healthcare provider to master. Careful attention to the possibility of an injury to the cervical spine, and the protection of normal cervical alignment are mandatory.

### Preparation for Airway Management

Airway management can be a stressful undertaking that is often approached with a degree of trepidation. Successful airway management starts with planning and preparation as a failure to secure an adequate airway has life-threatening consequences. Planning begins by assembling an airway kit or cart containing all the necessary equipment for intubation. The practitioner should take the time to inventory the equipment prior to the intubation. By doing so, the practitioner assures themselves as to the availability and proper working order of the equipment.[4]

Equipment.    The airway cart should consist of drugs, endotracheal tubes, airways, laryngoscopes, airway adjuncts, a variety of syringes and needles, and equipment to establish a surgical airway. This kit/cart should be well marked and placed in an easily accessible and highly visible location.[5,6] The airway kit should contain induction and sedation agents, including etomidate, ketamine, midazolam, barbiturates, fentanyl, and propofol. The cart should also have a variety of paralytic agents including succinylcholine, vecuronium, and rocuronium. Besides these essential medications, adjunctive medications such as lidocaine (both injectable and gel forms) and atropine should also be readily available on the airway

cart. These medications should be in their standard dosing vials and be checked daily and replaced after each use of the airway cart. An oxygen source should also be readily available for preoxygenation needs and during the intubation itself.[5,6]

The mainstay of the airway kit is the endotracheal tube. The airway cart should have a variety of tubes in both cuffed and uncuffed types. If the cart is in a general location where both adult and pediatric patients may need to be intubated, the airway cart should have endotracheal tubes down to a 2.0 internal diameter size as well as a variety of stylet sizes. In addition to the endotracheal tubes, the airway cart should be stocked with both oropharyngeal and nasopharyngeal airways in all sizes to handle infants to adults.

The other key piece of equipment that should be included on the airway cart is the laryngoscope. The cart should contain both Macintosh (curved) and Miller (straight) laryngoscope blades in various sizes. The bulbs should be checked to verify that they have been screwed into the blade securely, and a spare bulb should be available. There should also be at least two handles with well-charged batteries. The practitioner should verify that the blades engage the handle correctly and that the light source is adequate. In addition, the cart should have laryngeal mask airways (LMA) in sizes 1.0–6.0 and an intubating LMA as a rescue airway.[5,6]

Several pieces of additional equipment should be included in the standard airway cart or readily available, and these are listed as follows:[4]

Lighted wand stylet in multiple sizes

Retrograde intubation set

Combitube (Sheridan Catheter Corp., Argyle, NY)

Jet ventilation set

Percutaneous and open cricothyroidotomy sets

$CO_2$ detector

The goal of airway management in the trauma admitting area is to closely simulate the control of the operating room. Once the airway cart has been assembled, key personnel should be summoned to the bedside to work as a team to assure a successful intubation (Fig. 12-1). Novice practitioners should attempt to gain experience on stimulators and in controlled, supervised settings prior to attempting to intubate in a critical situation. In most trauma situations, the intubating team should consist of at least three members including the person intubating, a respiratory therapist, and an additional person to maintain alignment of the cervical spine or to provide the Sellick maneuver on the cricoid cartilage to prevent aspiration. The team may expand if an additional person is needed for surgical airway support. Once the team has been established, a standard preintubation checklist should be reviewed.[4]

### Monitoring and Troubleshooting

*Pulse Oximetry.*    This device measures the amount of arterial oxyhemoglobin saturation ($SpO_2$) and the patient's pulse rate. This device is portable, reliable, easily applied, and is noninvasive. The device measures $SpO_2$ by emitting near red light from one diode, which is specific for oxygenated hemoglobin, while a second diode emits infrared light, which is specific for deoxygenated hemoglobin. Each hemoglobin state absorbs some fraction of the emitted light, thus preventing it from reaching the corresponding sensor. The state that absorbs the most light has the higher percentage of that type of

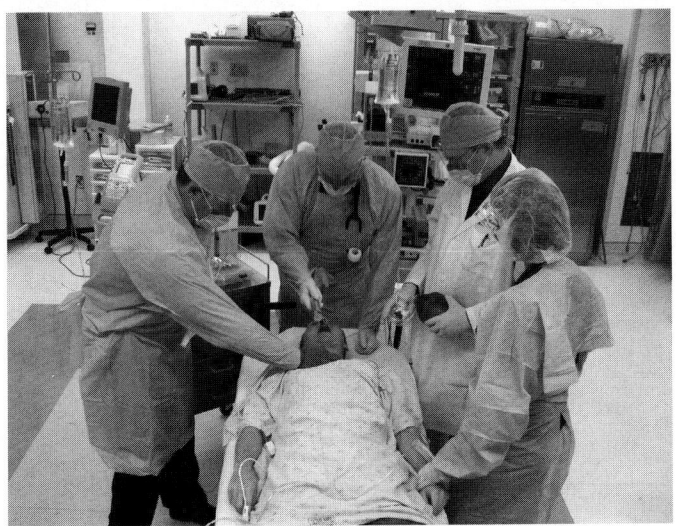

**FIGURE 12-1.** The optimal rapid sequence intubation team comprises (1) the intubating provider at the head of the bed, (2) an assistant to the patient's right to facilitate passage of necessary equipment from the airway cart (to the intubating provider's right) and to provide cricoid cartilage pressure, (3) a provider to administer drugs to the patient's left, and (4) a respiratory therapist to assist with airway maneuvers. Note the presence of full barrier precautions, pulse oximetry, telemetry, colorimetry, and two functioning large bore intravenous catheters.

hemoglobin. The device then computes a ratio of the hemoglobin states and displays it as a number—the $SpO_2$. Although very accurate, the pulse oximeter may display inaccurate readings in the case of carbon monoxide poisoning, high-intensity lighting, hemoglobin abnormalities, a pulseless extremity, or in severe anemia.[7-9] The goal is to maintain an $SpO_2$ greater than 93%.

*Capnography.*     End-tidal carbon dioxide (ETCO2) detectors measure the partial pressure of carbon dioxide in a sample gas. The closer the sample is to end-exhalation, the closer the correlation with arterial PCO2. The patient's PaCO2 is typically 2–5 mmHg higher than the ETCO2. A normal reading in a trauma patient is approximately 30–40 mmHg.[10] Traditionally, an ETCO2 reading is used to confirm placement of the endotracheal tube. The presence of carbon dioxide in the exhaled air strongly suggests correct placement of the endotracheal tube in the trachea in a perfusing patient. The disposable capnometer indicates the presence of carbon dioxide with a color change.[10] The electronic capnometer provides the healthcare provider with a numerical ETCO2 and plots the PaCO2 concentration against time. It is composed of four-part curve, including an ascending portion, a plateau, a descending portion, and a baseline. These portions of the curve are usually distinct, sharp phases of the capnogram. In a disease state, the curves soften and the slope of the curves is less. Additionally, the capnogram can be used to monitor a patient's breathing rhythm and the patient's interaction with the ventilator. Although the use of capnometry as an adjunct to monitor the patient's exhaled carbon dioxide has met some success, conditions such as hypotension, increased intrathoracic pressure, and pulmonary embolus resulting in increased dead space ventilation may decrease the accuracy of the capnometer.[7] Overall, end-tidal carbon dioxide concentration prior to prehospital intubation and 20 minutes thereafter has been demonstrated to correlate with outcome.[11]

The team intubating the patient should have the patient attached to a cardiac monitor, a blood pressure cuff, and an oxygen saturation monitor (Fig. 12-1). An intravenous line of normal saline should be established and flowing properly as well as a second intravenous line in the event that the primary line becomes nonfunctional or there is urgent need for resuscitation. The patient should receive supplemental oxygen via a nonrebreather mask or a bag-valve-mask (BVM) depending upon the patient's inherent respiratory drive. The correct size of endotracheal tube should be brought to the bedside and a correctly sized stylet should be inserted. The endotracheal balloon should be checked for leaks. Once the balloon has been checked, a 10 cc syringe is left attached to the pilot balloon. A suction device with a large catheter tip should be readily available and working properly and be placed near the right side of the patient's head.[7] The laryngoscope blade should be selected, and the handle/blade connection checked for a functional light source. A means to secure the endotracheal tube should be available. Consideration should be made to restraining the patient's hands if the patient is awake. Dentures should be looked for and removed just before intubation, particularly if the patient is being bagged and the dentures allow for a tight mask seal. The patient should be placed into an optimal position for intubation if not contraindicated by a cervical spine injury. This position has the patient's neck slightly flexed and the head slightly extended on an imaginary axis through the patient's ears. Placing a pillow or towel under the patient's occipital region and elevating the head approximately ten centimeters may facilitate this position. An end-tidal carbon dioxide detector should be available once the intubation has been completed to help to confirm placement of the endotracheal tube. Finally, a postintubation chest radiograph should be obtained to confirm appropriate placement of the endotracheal tube. Due diligence with respect to preparation of both personnel and equipment makes for a less stressful intubation and improves the practitioner's chances of successfully intubating the patient.[3]

*Manual Airway Maneuvers.*     Before any airway maneuver can be undertaken, a quick visual inspection of the oropharyngeal cavity should be done. Any foreign or loose material should be swept clear with a gloved finger or removed with suctioning. Blood is often present in the mouth of a trauma patient, and adequate suctioning is essential to maintaining an open airway.[7] Prolonged suctioning should be avoided to eliminate the potential for hypoxemia, while administration of oxygen prior to suctioning may also prevent hypoxemia due to suctioning. The tongue is the number one cause of airway obstruction in the unresponsive patient as it often lacks tone and falls back into the oropharynx. Manual airway maneuvers serve to elevate the tongue out of the hypopharynx.

*Jaw Thrust.*     The patient's cervical spine should be kept in normal alignment. The provider should gasp the sides of the patient's face with fingers 3–5 along the ramus portion of the patient's mandible. The provider's thumb is on the patient's cheek and the index finger on the patient's chin and lower lip. These two fingers can open the patient's lips or serve to seal the mask on a manual ventilator bag. The provider's fingers should form an "E" with their three lower fingers and a "C" with their thumb and index finger. Force is applied to the angle of the mandible forcing the mandible forward and anteriorly, while simultaneously opening the mouth with the index finger on the chin. When done properly, the cervical spine remains in a neutral position, while the elevation of the mandible lifts the tongue out of the oropharynx with minimal movement of the head and cervical spine.[12]

*Chin Lift.* With either a free, gloved hand, or another provider's gloved hand, the provider's thumb is placed into the patient's mouth, the patient's lower incisors and chin are grasped, and the patient's mandible is lifted anteriorly. This maneuver supplements the jaw thrust and works to lift the mandible anteriorly, thus lifting the tongue out of the oropharynx. Combined, the two maneuvers effectively clear the tongue from the hypopharynx; the provider, however, should exercise caution when using these techniques in an awake patient or one with a traumatic brain injury who may attempt to clinch their teeth on the provider's fingers.

*Sellick's Maneuver.* Prevention of gastric aspiration is one of the key components in airway maintenance. Typically, the injured patient has either swallowed large amounts of air into their stomach, or air has been forcibly placed into the stomach during ventilation with a BVM. The use of the Sellick Maneuver, particularly during BVM ventilation, aids in preventing aspiration.

The maneuver is accomplished by applying gentle posterior pressure to the patient's cricoid cartilage. This pressure causes the cricoid cartilage to be displaced posteriorly thus effectively closing off the esophagus. The pressure is applied by a healthcare provider placing their thumb and index anteriorly and laterally onto the cricoid cartilage near the midline of the patient's neck.[10]

## Basic Mechanical Airway Devices

*Oropharyngeal Airway (OPA).* Oropharyngeal and nasopharyngeal devices can be inserted into either the patient's mouth or nose, and both serve to elevate the patient's tongue out of the oropharynx. The OPA is typically a curved, plastic or hard rubber device, which comes in various sizes and has channeling for suction catheters. The device is sized by placing the OPA in the space between the patient's ear and corner of the patient's mouth. A correctly sized OPA will extend from the patient's mouth to the angle of their jaw.

Indications for the use of the OPA include a patient who is unable to maintain their airway or to prevent an intubated patient from biting the endotracheal tube. Advantages for use of the OPA include the following:

1. Prevention of obstruction from the patient's teeth and lips

2. Maintains the airway of a spontaneously breathing unconscious patient

3. Suctioning is easier

4. May serve as a bite block in a patient who is having a seizure

The OPA is contraindicated in a conscious patient as it may stimulate a gag reflex. In addition, it does not isolate the trachea, nor can it be inserted through clenched teeth. It may obstruct the airway if it is improperly placed, and can be dislodged easily.

To place the OPA, the mouth is opened and the OPA is inserted with the curve reversed and the tip pointing toward the roof of the patient's mouth. Using a twisting motion the OPA is rotated into position behind the base of the patient's tongue. Alternatively, a tongue blade can be used to depress the tongue and the OPA placed directly into the oropharynx.[7,8]

*Nasopharyngeal Airway (NPA).* The NPA is a soft rubber or latex uncuffed tube that is designed to conform to the patient's natural nasopharyngeal curvature. It is designed to lift the posterior tongue out of the oropharynx. Like the OPA it is indicated for patients who cannot maintain their own airway. The advantages of the NPA include ease and rapidly of insertion, patient tolerance and comfort, and it can be inserted when the patient's teeth are clenched.

Disadvantages of the NPA include its smaller size and the risk of nasal bleeding during insertion, and the NPA is not used if a basilar skull fracture is suspected.[13–15]

The provider should first size the NPA by determining that the NPA is slightly smaller than the patient's nostril. Next, the distance from the patient's nose to earlobe determines the proper length of the NPA. Once the proper sized NPA is chosen, it is liberally lubricated with lidocaine gel prior to insertion. The right nare is preferentially chosen, as it is typically larger.

Gentle pressure should be applied until the flange rests against the patient's nostril.[7,8] Once the basic mechanical airway has been inserted, the patient will either have supplemental oxygen administered, or the patient will need to have their oxygenation and ventilation assisted with a BVM device.

*Bag-Valve-Mask.* The BVM is a device to assist the provider in oxygenation and ventilation in the apneic or hypoventilating patient. When used properly with an effective mask seal and an open airway, the BVM can deliver tidal volumes approaching 1.5 L and nearly 100% inspired oxygen with an attached oxygen reservoir. The BVM consists of a bag with a volume of 1600 mL. A standard facemask is attached to the bag via a one-way, nonrebreathing valve. A reservoir bag and oxygen source is attached to the opposite end of the bag. Multiple sizes should be available to treat neonatal, infant, children, and adult patients. To effectively use the BVM device, a second provider may be required to establish a properly fitted mask seal while the other provider squeezes the bag. Success in maintaining oxygenation and ventilation can be improved upon by utilizing a basic mechanical airway and proper jaw thrust and chin lift techniques while "bagging" the patient.[7,8] An alternative to the basic mechanical airway is the esophageal tracheal Combitube (Sheridan Catheter Corp., Argyle, NY) to assist the provider with BVM oxygenation and ventilation.

## ASSESSMENT OF THE AIRWAY

The assessment, management, and the securing of an adequate airway should be the most important goal in treating critically injured patients. The difficult airway has been defined as "a clinical situation in which the practitioner experiences difficulty with ventilation, laryngoscopy, or tracheal intubation."[16] In the unstable trauma patient, assessment may be difficult due to the fact that the patient may be hypoxic and may be combative. Additionally, the trauma patient may have direct injury to the face and neck and often has secretions or blood in the oropharynx. Typically, the injured patient has a full stomach, presents fully immobilized with a cervical collar in place, and may not be able to speak or follow commands, thus complicating the assessment of the airway.[17] One single indicator has not been successfully identified to predict the inability to intubate. An attempt at an airway assessment should be done, however, in an effort to prevent the situation where the healthcare provider can neither intubate nor ventilate the patient.[18]

## History

A history of the patient's previous intubations and overall general medical conditions should be obtained if possible. The patient should be interrogated as to their dental health and prosthetic dental devices, any previous difficulty with anesthesia or intubation, sleep apnea, trismus, and their last meal. Additionally, a review of the patient's health with respect to mobility of the cervical spine, including a history of arthritis or ankylosing spondylitis, soft tissue disease of the oropharynx and neck, and, if nasotracheal intubation is a possibility, discussion of previous surgery, clotting disorders, or a history of epistaxis should be undertaken.[14]

## Physical Examination

A general assessment of the oropharynx, nose, maxilla, mandible, and neck should be rapidly undertaken in the acute situation. An assessment of the patient's overall level of consciousness (e.g., Glasgow Coma Score), and the ability of the patient to open their mouth should also be investigated. If possible, have the patient stick out their tongue to allow for evaluation of the size of the tongue. The vocal quality of the patient should be noted during the physical exam, as well. The presence of stridor usually indicates some type of injury to the upper airway. The examination will document the presence of dentures or other prosthetic devices which may need to be removed prior to intubation, but with their removal, may make it difficult to establish or maintain a seal with a BVM device.

## INTUBATION OF THE TRACHEA

The majority of injured patients are able to undergo successful orotracheal intubation. In compliance with recommendations from the ATLS course, the preferred definitive airway is tracheal intubation through the mouth using direct laryngosocopy.[3]

## Guidelines for Emergency Tracheal Intubation

Indications for intubation relate to the three following simple questions.

First, is the patient able to oxygenate and ventilate?

Second, is the patient able to maintain an airway?

Third, will the underlying injury and physiology of the patient lead to a failure to maintain the airway, oxygenate, or ventilate?

The practice management guidelines of The Eastern Association for the Surgery of Trauma (EAST) for tracheal intubation secondary to trauma reveal no Level I data (evidence from randomized, controlled trials) that predict the need for urgent intubation.[19] In the absence of Level I data, the guidelines calls for emergency tracheal intubation in trauma patients exhibiting the following characteristics:

Acute airway obstruction

Hypoventilation

Severe hypoxemia despite supplemental oxygen

Severe cognitive impairment (Glasgow Coma Scale score $\leq$ 8)

Cardiac arrest

Severe hemorrhagic shock

In concurrence with ATLS, the EAST guidelines promulgate the notion that orotracheal intubation utilizing direct laryngoscopy is the procedure of choice for airway control following trauma.[19] In the absence of a flaccid mandible in an obtunded patient, rapid sequence intubation, utilizing neuromuscular paralysis and aspiration precautions via a modified RSI approach, is the technique of choice.

## Anatomy and Technique of Direct Laryngoscopy and Intubation

Success in intubating the injured patient is dependent on a thorough knowledge of the anatomy of the upper airway and a meticulous adherence to proper technique. The vocal cords lie posterior and inferior to the pliable epiglottis, which should be visualized as a constant reference point during laryngoscopy. The posterior-most esophagus may be lifted into view with sufficient elevation of the epiglottis. Positioning of the laryngoscopist and the patient are dependent upon the intubation environment and status of the cervical spine. Since the majority of intubations occur prior to clearance of the cervical spine, immobilization of the head and neck is of highest priority. Emergency medical personnel are often required to intubate while patients are trapped in vehicles, from unusual angles, or in the confines of a helicopter. In the rare instance that the cervical spine is cleared, the patient should be placed in the sniffing position (extension of the head, slight flexion of the lower cervical spine) which optimizes the alignment of the oral, pharyngeal, and laryngeal axes.

Following optimal preparation of equipment and personnel, including selection of drugs for intubation, the laryngoscope is grasped firmly with the left hand. It should be emphasized that the right hand should be kept free for suctioning, manipulation of oral structures, and placement of the endotracheal tube. Selection of a straight versus curved blade has less to do with proven efficacy in a particular scenario than the comfort and proficiency of the laryngoscopist with a particular blade. In general, the straight blade is utilized to pass beneath and directly elevate the epiglottis. The straight blade is inserted visually or nonvisually into the esophagus, with the blade withdrawn slowly under direct visualization to expose the glottic opening. The same technique can be applied with a curved blade of sufficient size, although the curved blade technique typically utilizes insertion of the tip of the blade into the vallecula with anterior traction of the epiglottis, thus exposing the glottic opening. The tongue should be displaced by the blade to the patient's left such that the tongue is not visualized on the right, which may obscure visualization of the epiglottis.

The motion and direction of the laryngoscope in the left hand during laryngoscopy is of critical importance to safe and successful intubation of the trachea. As the blade is withdrawn from the esophagus and the epiglottis and/or vallecula are elevated, the glottic opening should be visualized. The proper technique of laryngoscopy employs upward motion of the laryngoscope in the parallel plane of the handle. A "rocking" motion during which the handle is rotated counterclockwise and posterior should never be used. This posterior circular motion can impart dangerous extension on the cervical spine or fracture or dislodge teeth. In addition, the left elbow should not be placed on the bed or spine board for stabilization. As the blade is positioned to visualize the glottic opening, the right hand can be utilized to employ the B.U.R.P. maneuver if the glottic opening is not readily visible. This technique includes **B**ackward, **U**pward, **R**ightward, **P**ressure on the thyroid cartilage and is distinct from the Sellick maneuver. When the laryngoscopist grasps the endotracheal tube for placement with the right hand, an assistant can continue with Sellick pressure and the BURP maneuver.

## RAPID SEQUENCE INTUBATION

### Overview

Rapid sequence induction intubation (RSI) has become the gold standard for management of the airway in trauma and critical illness. The technique of RSI has been demonstrated to increase success rates for intubation and reduce complications compared to pre-RSI techniques in a variety of emergent settings.[20–27] The benefits of RSI relate to the ability of the technique to mitigate against adverse effects of airway control under duress. RSI benefits include provision of optimal intubating conditions for injured patients, rapid airway control, high success rates, and reduction of pulmonary aspiration. The adaptability of RSI to individual patients renders the technique optimal for airway control in the injured.

First developed to facilitate intubations in the operating room in patients with full stomachs, thereby minimizing risk of aspiration,[28] the technique is now widely utilized by prehospital paramedics,[29,30] emergency medicine physicians,[31] and trauma surgeons, with high reported success rates for intubation.[20,32] Approximately 80% of intubations performed in modern emergency departments utilize RSI, with a 90% success rate by the first intubator.[31] In the technique of RSI, laryngoscopy and intubation are facilitated by use of sedating induction agents and short acting neuromuscular blockade (NMB). Rapid sequence intubation is not without risk, and the decision to employ RSI must be preceded by a risk-benefit analysis based upon proficiency with non-intubating airway maintenance skills, RSI pharmacology, and emergent intubation. Rapid sequence intubation can be divided into five phases: (1) **preparation** of patient and equipment; (2) **preoxygenation**; (3) **premedication**; (4) **paralysis**; and (5) **placement** of the tube.

### Preparation

Although significant injury with physiologic instability may preclude prolonged preparation for RSI, all efforts should be made to allow for individualized assessment of comorbid conditions, airway status, predictors of difficult intubation, and anticipated pharmacologic regimen. Equipment and personnel should be prepared sufficiently to address all ranges of airway compromise, from controlled RSI to emergent surgical intervention. The potentially difficult airway should mandate presence of a difficult airway cart, including adjuncts to orotracheal intubation. Under this circumstance,

preparation of the neck for cricothyroidotomy, including the opening of a surgical instrument tray, may prove invaluable once the RSI sequence is initiated. The selection and sequence of pharmacologic agents should be determined, with all agents available in clearly labeled syringes. As previously noted, two large-bore, functioning intravenous lines are advisable.

A *horizontal approach* to the preparatory phase of RSI is optimal, defined as a concerted effort toward intubation in which multiple personnel with predetermined responsibilities and positions work simultaneously (Fig. 12-1). In this manner, the preoxygenation phase is initiated during preparation. The history, assessment of comorbidities, and prediction of airway difficulty should proceed as positioning occurs, pharmacologic agents are readied, and equipment and the neck are prepared. Attention to detail in the preparation phase of RSI may yield significant benefits once the RSI sequence is initiated.

### Preoxygenation

Although not originally considered an essential component of RSI, preoxygenation is mandatory if the oxygenation, ventilation, and hemodynamic status of the patient permit. The purpose of preoxygenation is to replace the nitrogen-dominant room air occupying the pulmonary functional residual capacity with a 100% oxygen reservoir, such that saturation of arterial hemoglobin ($SaO_2$) is prolonged. This can be accomplished by gently assisting spontaneous respirations with 100% oxygen or simply allowing the patient to breathe 100% oxygen. Forceful BVM ventilation should be assiduously avoided during the intubation sequence, as it may produce unnecessary gastric distention and increase the risk for pulmonary aspiration of gastric contents. Recommendations for the duration of preoxygenation necessary for optimal hemoglobin saturation range from 3 to 5 minutes, recognizing that the effectiveness of preoxygenation is dependent on the physiologic status of the patient as well as age, size, and comorbid conditions. For example, an optimally preoxygenated healthy 70-kg adult will maintain $SaO_2$ over 90% for approximately 8 minutes, an obese adult less than 3 minutes, and a 10-kg child less than 4 minutes.[33] More importantly, the desaturation from 90% $SaO_2$ to 0% occurs much more rapidly than the fall from 100% to 90%. The approximate $PaO_2$ at 90% $SaO_2$ is 60 mm Hg, and this decreases to 27 mm Hg at an $SaO_2$ of 50%. An injured patient with little compensatory reserve can decline from 90% to 0% literally in seconds.

## PHARMACOLOGY OF RAPID SEQUENCE INTUBATION

It is imperative that providers caring for the injured be facile with all pharmacologic agents utilized for RSI, including both barbiturate and nonbarbiturate hypnotics, neuromuscular blocking agents, benzodiazepines, dissociative agents, and opiates (Table 12-1). A "one method fits all" approach is not always applicable,[16] and each patient should be individualized based upon type and mechanism of injury, comorbidities, and potential for adverse events. The majority of trauma patients, however, can be effectively intubated using a generalized pharmacologic regimen.

Clinical predictors of the need for sedation and paralysis have been identified. In data from a prospective study of endotracheal

**TABLE 12-1**

| **Pharmacology of Rapid Sequence Intubation** | | | | |
|---|---|---|---|---|
| AGENT | DOSE | ONSET | DURATION | PRECAUTIONS |
| **Premedication Agents** | | | | |
| Fentanyl | 1.0–4.0 mcg/kg | 30–45 s | 0.5–1.0 h | Chest wall rigidity |
| Midazolam | 0.1–0.3 mg/kg | 2–3 min | 2–3 h | Slow onset |
| Lidocaine | 1.0–1.5 mg/kg | 30–90 s | 10–20 min | Hypotension |
| Esmolol | 2.0 mg/kg | 2–5 min | 9–30 min | Hypotension |
| Vecuronium | 0.01 mg/kg | 90–120 s | 60–75 min | Extended duration |
| **Induction Agents** | | | | |
| Etomidate | 0.05–0.3 mg/kg | 10–60 s | 2–5 min | Adrenal suppression |
| Propofol | 0.5–2.0 mg/kg | 10–50 s | 2–10 min | Hypotension |
| Thiopental | 1.0–3.0 mg/kg | 10–60 s | 5–30 min | Hypotension |
| Methohexital | 1.0–3.0 mg/kg | 30 s | 5–10 min | Hypotension |
| Ketamine | 0.5–2.0 mg/kg | 30–120 s | 5–15 min | Intracranial hypertension |
| **Neuromuscular Blockade** | | | | |
| Succinylcholine | 0.6–2.0 mg/kg | 30–60 s | 5–15 min | Hyperkalemia |
| Rocuronium | 1.0 mg/kg | 45–60 s | 30–60 min | Long duration |

intubation, factors associated with drug-facilitated intubation, defined as intubation facilitated by the use of sedatives or paralytics, included clenched jaw or trismus, declining verbal component of the Glasgow Coma Scale (GCS) score, and use of cervical spine precautions.[34] The vast majority of patients currently undergoing RSI receive both sedative and paralytic agents. Evidence-based principles identified by the airway workgroup of EAST for drugs administered during orotracheal intubation include the following[19]:

Neuromuscular paralysis

Sedation

Regimen which maintains hemodynamic stability

Regimen which minimizes intracranial hypertension

Regimen that prevents vomiting

Regimen that prevents extrusion of intraocular contents

Premedication Agents.    Airway stimulation, including laryngoscopy and placement of an endotracheal tube, results in the *pressor response*, an intense autonomic sympathetic discharge producing tachycardia, hypertension, and increased intracranial pressure.[28,35,36] The degree of airway stimulation, including the number of direct laryngoscopies or attempts at intubation, is proportional to the magnitude of the pressor response. Correspondingly, increased intragastric, intrathoracic, and intracranial pressures may result from a valsalva maneuver, bronchospasm, or coughing. As the foundation of RSI relates to abrogating the untoward effects of airway stimulation, particularly in trauma patients, preinduction agents are routinely utilized to blunt the physiologic response to laryngoscopy and placement of the endotracheal tube. A common mnemonic for the preinduction regimen is **LOAD**, which includes **L**idocaine, **O**piates, **A**tropine, and a **D**efasciculating agent, although atropine is typically utilized in pediatric populations only.

Opioids.    Depth of sedation may correlate with speed of intubation in RSI.[37] The sedative and analgesic effects of opioids may provide benefit to the injured patient prior to induction. A commonly used opioid for RSI in the prehospital and emergency department setting is fentanyl, which at a dose of 5.0 mcg/kg has been shown to be hemodynamically neutral compared to midazolam and thiopental during RSI.[37] Fentanyl effectively blunts airway reactivity[38] and confers the significant added benefit of analgesia in the injured patient.

Benzodiazepines.    Benzodiazepines, a family of gamma aminobutyric acid (GABA) agonists, have been utilized in RSI for sedation. Midazolam is the most widely studied agent, having favorable pharmacokinetics for RSI, including rapid onset and short half-life. Advantages include hemodynamic neutrality and retrograde amnesia, although onset is slower than comparable agents and the intubation reflex is not attenuated.[37] Therefore, it is less commonly used in RSI protocols than opioids.

Antiarrhythmics.    Despite a great deal of controversy regarding the potential benefits of lidocaine during RSI, it is a preinduction agent common to RSI protocols[39] and is advocated in many emergency airway courses. Lidocaine has a number of theoretical beneficial preintubation effects, including abrogation of airway reactivity following placement of the endotracheal tube, the tachycardic response to intubation, and succinylcholine-induced myalgia and fasciculations.[40,41] The two primary potential benefits of use of lidocaine in RSI are to avoid reflex bronchospasm and increased intracranial pressure. The decision to use lidocaine in RSI becomes a potential benefit versus risk analysis. Although definitive data are lacking regarding effects on intracranial pressure, the potential benefits outweigh the negligible side effects of the RSI dose.

Beta-Adrenergic Blockers.    Esmolol has been utilized as a preinduction agent for mitigation of the tachycardic component of the pressor response. In comparison to lidocaine and fentanyl, esmolol has demonstrated superiority in attenuating the pressor response.[42,43] Beneficial pharmacokinetics include rapid onset and short action, but the bradycardic and negative inotropic effects of esmolol may blunt the compensatory response to hemorrhage and the cardiac effects may produce corresponding reductions in cerebral blood flow. Therefore, esmolol should be considered only in controlled circumstances in which hemorrhage and injury to the brain have been definitively excluded.

*Defasciculation Paralytic Agents.*    Succinylcholine, the standard neuromuscular blocking agent utilized for RSI, produces significant myoclonal fasciculations, prompting a rise in intracranial pressure. Therefore, a defasciculating dose of a competitive neuromuscular blocking is administered during RSI. Common defasciculating agents include vecuronium and rocuronium, and, less commonly, pancuronium. Defasciculating doses are administered as 10% of the paralyzing dose, given 3 to 5 minutes prior to administration of succinylcholine. It is unusual for defasciculating doses of neuromuscular blockers to cause apnea. As patient weight is commonly an estimate during RSI following injury, however, preparations to assist with ventilation should be made.

Induction Agents.    The purpose of induction agents in RSI is to induce rapid loss of consciousness to facilitate endotracheal intubation. The perfect induction agent would possess rapid onset and elimination, render the patient unconscious but also amnestic, possess analgesic properties, and have negligible side effects. In injured and critically ill patients, the ideal agent would produce little cardiovascular effects and maintain cerebral perfusion pressure. Regrettably, such an agent does not yet exist. Because many agents produce side effects, including myocardial depression with the potential for hypoperfusion, careful attention should be dedicated to the selection of individual agents, focusing on clinical presentation and patient specific characteristics.

*Etomidate.*    Etomidate is a short acting carboxylated imidazole hypnotic agent frequently utilized for rapid sequence induction. Etomidate possesses ideal characteristics for urgent and emergent RSI in trauma patients, including rapid onset and clearance, reduction in cerebral metabolic rate,[44] and negligible effects on hemodynamics. This favorable pharmacokinetic profile has led to the widespread use of etomidate for RSI in patients with injury to the brain and hemodynamically labile patients. The most significant side effect of etomidate relates to adrenal insufficiency, as it produces a reversible blockade of adrenal 11-beta-hydroxylase. In patients at risk for adrenal insufficiency, including brain injured, mechanically ventilated, and septic populations, etomidate has been independently correlated with reductions in serum cortisol.[45–47] The controversial question relates to whether transient adrenal suppression produces lasting effects on outcome. Further studies are warranted to determine the long-term safety of etomidate for RSI; however, given the multiple favorable characteristics of the drug, etomidate will remain the standard induction agent in most RSI protocols.

*Propofol.*    Propofol is a nonbarbiturate hypnotic agent that rapidly induces deep sedation and significant relaxation of laryngeal musculature.[28] When used for induction, propofol produces intubation conditions equal to thiopental[48] and equal to or superior to etomidate.[49] Propofol should be used with caution in patients with injury to the brain or hemodynamically labile patients due to a consistent hypotensive effect and potential reduction of cerebral blood flow. Therefore, it should be considered an alternative agent in RSI.

*Barbiturates.*    Thiopental is the most commonly used barbiturate for RSI. Like other induction agents used in RSI, thiopental has rapid onset and clearance. In the aeromedical setting, thiopental has been shown equally efficacious to etomidate as an adjunct to RSI.[50] Similarly, in an evaluation of 2380 RSI procedures, patients were more likely to be successfully intubated using thiopental or propofol as compared to etomidate or a benzodiazepine.[49] In addition, thiopental reduces cerebral oxygen consumption and exhibits anticonvulsant effects, rendering it useful in patients with injury to the brain. The significant limitation of thiopental use for RSI in trauma relates to inhibition of the sympathetic response of the central nervous system. Therefore, thiopental reduces myocardial contractility and systemic vascular resistance, and causes hypotension. Therefore, it is best reserved for patients who are euvolemic and normotensive, limiting its application in injured and critically ill patients.

Methohexital is an additional barbiturate that has been used for rapid sequence intubation. It exhibits similar effects to thiopental, although it is significantly more potent and has shorter onset and duration than thiopental. The cerebroprotective and cardiac effects of methohexital are similar to thiopental, confining the agent to the same small subset of potential use. In summary, the barbiturates are effective induction agents, inducing rapid unconsciousness and exhibiting short half-life. The cardiodepressent effects of this class limit utility in injury and critical illness, and etomidate has supplanted the class in many RSI protocols.

*Dissociative Agents.*    Ketamine, a rapid onset dissociative sedative and anesthetic agent, is frequently used for RSI in the pediatric population[51] and in adults with chronic obstructive pulmonary disease.[52] In addition to its sedative effects, ketamine exhibits the beneficial properties of potent analgesia and a partial amnesia. As a sympathomimetic agent, ketamine may induce tachycardia and increase blood pressure. In addition, ketamine induces cerebral vasodilatation, potentially exacerbating intracranial hypertension. Trauma patients with documented or potential injury to the brain should not undergo induction for RSI with ketamine. Given the sympathomimetic properties of ketamine, it is best reserved for patients with proven reactive airway disease and hypovolemia when injury to the brain has been definitively excluded.

## Paralysis

Neuromuscular Blocking Agents.    Pharmacologic paralysis represents an integral component of RSI, facilitating emergent intubation for more than three decades.[53,54] Paralysis of facial musculature facilitates optimal visualization during laryngoscopy, confers total control of the patient, and reduces complications during intubation. Prehospital neuromuscular blockade has been demonstrated to be safe[26,27] and to improve the success of intubation in injured patients undergoing RSI.[55,56] In a recent study of RSI in patients with traumatic brain injury, 72% of prehospital intubations in AIS head $\geq$ 3 were performed using neuromuscular blocking agents, with an unadjusted mortality of 25% versus 37% for those intubated without paralysis.[25] Potential adverse effects should be diligently assessed, particularly with use of succinylcholine. In addition, preparations for rescue techniques must be made prior to administration of a paralytic agent in the event of intubation failure. Because paralytic agents provide no sedative, analgesic, or amnestic effect, it is imperative to combine use of a paralytic agent with an appropriate induction agent.

*Succinylcholine.* Succinylcholine, a depolarizing acetylcholine dimer, acts noncompetitively at the acetylcholine receptor in a biphasic manner to produce muscular paralysis at the motor end plate. Succinylcholine stimulates all muscarinic and nicotinic cholinergic receptors of both parasympathetic and sympathetic systems. Initial brief depolarization results in clinically notable muscular fasciculations, followed by sustained myocyte depolarization. Succinylcholine degradation is dependent on hydrolysis by pseudocholinesterase, and it is resistant to acetylcholinesterase. Due to rapid onset of action and a short half-life, succinylcholine remains the gold standard for RSI in patients not at risk for adverse events. The standardized dose of succinylcholine for RSI is 1.0 mg/kg, although the optimal dose for RSI is under evaluation. Recent data suggest that a smaller dose of 0.5–0.6 mg/kg is sufficient for RSI,[57] facilitating more rapid resumption of spontaneous respiration. Because complete paralysis represents an integral component of RSI, it is better to err toward complete paralysis when dosing in patients not at risk for adverse events. Intramuscular injection of succinylcholine has been described, although the required dose, 4 mg/kg is higher and onset is slower than with intravenous injection.[58] Intramuscular injection should be absolutely reserved for the injured patient in whom a delay associated with intravenous or intraosseous access would be life-threatening.

A clear understanding of the potential adverse effects of succinylcholine is critical to its appropriate use in RSI. Contraindications are primarily related to existing hyperkalemia or conditions which accentuate the hyperkalemic effects of succinylcholine, as it normally produces a 0.5–1.0 mEq/L elevation of serum potassium. Contraindications related to hyperkalemia include a thermal injury greater than 24 hours old,[59] although upregulation of receptors likely does not become clinically relevant until postburn day 5. Therefore, it is safe to use succinylcholine for RSI in most acute burns. It is contraindicated in patients with crush injury or rhabdomyolysis with hyperkalemia,[60] congenital or acquired myopathies, conditions of subacute and chronic upper and motor neuron denervation including paralysis and polyneuropathy of critical illness,[28] a history of malignant hyperthermia and pseudocholinesterase deficiency. In addition, succinylcholine is reported to raise intragastric and intracranial pressure due to muscle fasciculations and may contribute to increased intraocular pressure. It should be used with caution in patients with injury to the brain and penetrating injury to the globe, although the evidence that succinylcholine raises intraocular pressure is anecdotal at best.[61]

*Nondepolarizing Agents.* Nondepolarizing NMBAs, through competitive blockade of acetylcholine transmission at postjunctional, cholinergic nicotinic receptors, provide a paralytic alternative for those injured patients in whom succinylcholine is contraindicated. The aminosteriod compounds, including rocuronium, pancuronium, and vecuronium, represent the commonly used NMBAs for RSI and postintubation paralysis. Nondepolarizing agents for RSI are selected based upon the ability to best approximate the rapid onset and elimination of succinylcholine. The most intensively studied nondepolarizing agent utilized for RSI is rocuronium, which exhibits short onset and intermediate duration of action. In a recent Cochrane Database analysis comparing rocuronium to succinylcholine during RSI, rocuronium use was associated with inferior production of "excellent" intubating conditions, but equal "acceptable" conditions.[62] Similarly, in a recent prospective, randomized comparative trial under emergent conditions, succinylcholine produced more rapid intubation and superior intubating conditions.[63] Despite the reported inferiority compared to succinylcholine, rocuronium has been shown to produce superior intubating conditions in comparison to vecuronium in the prehospital environment.[25] When contraindications to succinylcholine exist, rocuronium produces acceptable intubating conditions and should remain in the RSI armamentarium as an alternative to succinylcholine.

## Cricoid Cartilage Pressure (Sellick's Maneuver)

Most practitioners consider the use of Sellick's maneuver to be an essential part of RSI.[64] Efficacy of Sellick's maneuver requires a force of greater than 40 Newtons, and this pressure has been demonstrated to reduce lower esophageal sphincter pressure by half[65] and make fiberoptic techniques (WuScope™) more difficult.[66] Alternatively, a recent blinded, randomized study of 700 patients undergoing elective anesthesia using direct laryngoscopy reported that the technique did not increase the difficulty of intubation or rate of failure.[67] In use of the Sellick maneuver, proper technique is imperative. In a review of videotaped RSI evaluating deviations from RSI protocol in emergency medicine residents, 45% employed improper use of the technique.[68]

## Confirmation of Placement

The setup and technique of intubation have been described previously. Confirmation of tube placement is critical to the subsequent care of the injured or critically ill patient. The first method to confirm placement is visualization of the endotracheal tube passing through the vocal cords, although this relies on the subjective impression of the operator and is not infallible. Other useful but nonspecific methods include auscultation of breath sounds in both lung fields, visualization of both rise and fall of the chest and condensation in the endotracheal tube with exhalation. The standard confirmatory method for RSI is detection of exhaled carbon dioxide through use of capnography or colorimetric end-tidal devices, which change from purple to yellow in its presence.[69] Capnography is superior to colorimetric detection,[70] although both techniques are quite reliable.[71] The two primary clinical circumstances which may render the colorimetric device inaccurate include false positive detection after esophageal intubation when sufficient carbon dioxide is present in the esophagus and false negative detection during cardiac arrest with undetectable levels of tracheal carbon dioxide. Due to the reliability, portability, and ease of use of colorimetric capnography, the technique represents the mainstay for confirming proper placement of the endotracheal tube after RSI. If color change is not noted within 2 to 3 breaths, improper placement is likely and the endotracheal tube should be replaced. A standardized timeline for RSI is helpful to ensure adherence to proper sequencing and administration of drugs. The timeline utilized for emergent RSI at our institution is displayed in Table 12-2.

**TABLE 12-2**

### How We Do It: Steps and Timing of Rapid Sequence Intubation In A 70 Kilogram Adult

| STEP | TIMING | ACTION |
|------|--------|--------|
| Preparation | Zero–10 min | Prepare equipment |
| | | Assess patient |
| | | Position personnel |
| | | Select drugs |
| Preoxygenation | Zero–5 min | Passive administration of high flow oxygen via bag valve mask |
| Premedication | Zero–2 min | Lidocaine 100 mg IVP |
| | | Vecuronium 1.0 mg IVP |
| | | Etomidate 20 mg IVP |
| Paralysis | Zero | Succinylcholine 100 mg IVP |
| Placement | Zero + 20 s | Sellick's maneuver |
| | Zero + 45 s | Intubation |
| | Zero + 1 min | Tube confirmation |

## Complications and Outcomes after Rapid Sequence Intubation

Success rates for RSI are well established, and a recent international study including a database with over 10,000 intubations noted a success rate exceeding 97% for trauma patients,[72] but complications do occur. Sedative and paralytic agents utilized in RSI place injured patients at risk for cardiovascular collapse, diminution of respiratory effort, pulmonary aspiration, and abrupt loss of the airway. The primary complication of RSI involves airway failure, particularly esophageal intubation. The National Emergency Airway Registry (NEAR) classifies adverse events related to intubation as immediate, technical, and physiologic.[72] Immediate events include witnessed aspiration, airway trauma, and undetected esophageal intubation. Technical events include recognized esophageal intubation and mainstem intubation. Physiologic events, often difficult to separate from underlying patient conditions related to injury, include pneumothorax, dysrrhythmia, and cardiac arrest. Because the most critical adverse event related to RSI is airway failure, practitioners of the technique must be facile with airway rescue maneuvers including cricothyroidotomy in the event of failed intubation.

## ALTERNATIVES AND ADJUNCTS TO ENDOTRACHEAL INTUBATION

### Nasotracheal Intubation

Nasotracheal intubation (NTI) is identified within the ATLS course as an alternative to orotracheal intubation under select circumstances. Any discussion of nasotracheal intubation should begin by noting the two absolute contraindications: apnea, and severe trauma to the midface or suspicion of a basilar skull fracture during which nasotracheal intubation could breach the cranial vault. Relative contraindications include coagulopathy, combativeness, intracranial hypertension, and suspected obstruction of the upper airway. NTI should also be avoided in patients with little

oxygenation or ventilatory reserve due to possible delays incurred with the technique. Because of contraindications, failure rate, and complications, NTI has been nearly supplanted by RSI. The primary indication for NTI relates to the difficult airway. In a spontaneously breathing patient with an anticipated difficult airway and in whom RSI is predicted to fail, NTI can be considered for tracheal intubation.

Following preparation of all necessary equipment, as well as planning an algorithm for procedure failure, the patient is preoxygenated similar to RSI. The nares, nasopharynx, and trachea should be anesthetized. Lidocaine jelly or topical cocaine solution can be instilled into the selected nare, topical anesthetic sprayed into the oropharynx and nasopharynx, and lidocaine solution injected through the cricothyroid membrane. An appropriate size tube should be selected, typically having an internal diameter of 6.0 to 7.5 mm. The tube should be well lubricated and gently inserted into the nare, with the tip directed toward the occiput. When the tube passes into the posterior nasopharynx, it should be directed caudad, and resistance is commonly encountered. The tube should be rotated approximately one-quarter turn toward the opposite nare, and advanced. When the tube advances into the distal nasopharynx, it should be restored to neutral and advanced. When breath sounds are heard through the tube (condensation may be visible), the tube should be advanced carefully but rapidly for approximately 3–5 centimeters. If the tube has entered the trachea, the patient will cough repeatedly, and condensation may be seen. Placement should be confirmed with auscultation of breath sounds and use of an end-tidal carbon dioxide detector. If the esophagus is entered or the tube will not advance, it should be repositioned, and the procedure attempted again, depending upon the condition of the patient.

### Retrograde Intubation

First described by Butler and Cirillo in 1960 as an alternative to conducting unplanned preoperative tracheostomies,[73] retrograde endotracheal intubation (REI) represents another potential adjunctive airway. Variations in the technique exist, but REI usually involves needle cannulation of the trachea through the cricothyroid membrane with passage of a flexible guidewire or epidural catheter into the oropharynx (Fig. 12-2). If a catheter is utilized, it can be affixed to the Murphy's eye of an endotracheal tube, which is pulled in an anterograde fashion into the trachea. When the ET tube is at the cricothyroid membrane, the catheter is cut flush with the skin and removed. More commonly, an ET tube is passed over a flexible guidewire or obturator into the trachea, with the wire removed by transection at the skin and withdrawal through the oropharynx. Current commercial kits include a large bore needle, a flexible guidewire, and a thicker flexible obturator to guide passage of the ET tube.

The cited mean time to intubation utilizing REI has been reported to be from approximately one minute in simulators[74] and cadavers[75] to approximately 3–5 minutes in actual patient scenarios.[76,77] A recent retrospective review of REI over an 8-year period at a Level I trauma center documented use of the technique in only 8 patients (0.5% of intubations), with success and complication rates of 50% and 38%, respectively.[77] Alternatively, a separate review of 24 patients undergoing REI by anesthesiologists identified a success rate of 100%, with 88% intubated on the first

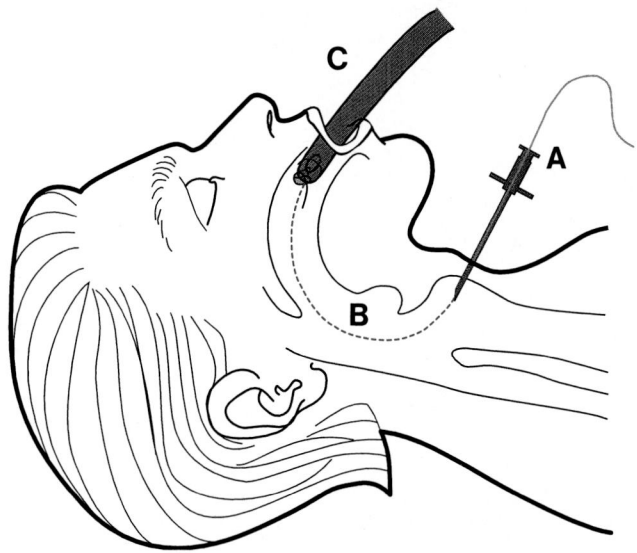

**FIGURE 12-2.** Retrograde intubation. An epidural size 17 Tuahy needle is inserted through the cricothyroid membrane as close to the upper border of the cricoid cardilage as possible and angled cephalad **(A)** An epidural catheter **(B)** is advanced through the vocal cords into the oropharynx and pulled out of the mouth. The epidural needle is withdrawn, and the catheter is tied to the Murphy's eye of a size ID 7- to 8-mm endotracheal tube **(C)**, which is then pulled thorough the vocal cords. Once through or at the vocal cords, the endotracheal tube is pushed into the trachea, and once in position, the epidural catheter can be cut at the skin. Modifications include threading the endotracheal tube or a tube changer over the catheter or a J wire, and railroading the endotracheal tube into the trachea; or feeding the distal end of a J wire through the suction port of a bronchoscope over which an endotracheal tube has been loaded.

attempt.[78] Although infrequently performed with variable results, the technique remains in the practice guidelines for the difficult airway put forth by the American Society of Anesthesiologists Task Force,[79] and commercial kits remain on many difficult airway carts. Given infrequent use and potential complications, REI should be reserved for failure of conventional techniques of intubation.

## Gum Elastic Bougie

The gum elastic bougie (GEB) or Eschmann stylet is a semirigid, malleable endotracheal tube introducer which has been used for airway emergencies in a variety of settings. The 60 cm bougie, which has a diameter of 5 mm, is angled at 40° 3.5 cm from the distal end. During difficult laryngoscopy, when the vocal cords are not well visualized, the GEB is advanced to the level of the epiglottis, with the angled portion directed anteriorly. With further advancement, the tube may enter the trachea, and if successful, a "washboard" effect is palpated, as the bougie tip passes over tracheal rings. An ETT can then be passed over the GEB into the trachea.

If a smooth unobstructed course is encountered, and the GEB passes greater than 40–45 cm, a presumed esophageal intubation has occurred. In a prospective blinded trial in 20 human cadavers, the accuracy of tracheal ring "clicks" for tracheal intubation was assessed.[80] Overall, 93% of tracheal placements were correctly identified, with ring clicks being 95% sensitive for tracheal intubation. In a recent review of 1442 prehospital intubations, the GEB

was utilized in 41 patients.[81] Of the 3% requiring GEB use, intubation was successful in 33 patients (78%).

## Esophageal Tracheal Combitube (ETC)

The ETC is a relatively new device that is primarily used as a rescue airway in the prehospital arena. Although inserted as a single tube, it is essentially a two-tube system with a divider in the distal tube. The device has two balloons, one proximal to occlude the oropharynx and a second balloon distally to occlude either the esophagus or trachea depending upon into which structure the device is placed (Fig. 12-3). The ETC is inserted blindly and commonly into the esophagus. Both balloons are inflated. The longer, blue tube is ventilated first. If sounds are auscultated in the chest and the there are no sounds auscultated over the epigastrium, the ETC is in the esophagus and ventilation should continue through the blue tube. If sounds are heard in the epigastrium, this suggests that the ETC is in the trachea. Ventilation should then be changed to the clear, shorter tube, while not changing the position of the ETC. Indications for its use include the following:

1. Immediate intubation cannot be performed.

2. Unsuccessful endotracheal intubation in a patient requiring an airway.

3. The patient may be entrapped and access to the patient's head is poor.

4. Direct visualization of the larynx cannot be obtained due to secretions.

Contraindications for ETC use include the following:

1. Patients younger than 16 years old

2. Patients less than 5 ft. tall

Potential advantages include ease in insertion, the ability to ventilate through either tube, insertion does not require visualization, and aspiration can be prevented with inflation of the proximal balloon. Disadvantages to ETC use include making endotracheal intubation more difficult as the ETC obscures the trachea, the trachea cannot be directly suctioned with the ETC in place, and it cannot be used in the conscious patient with a gag reflex.[82]

## Supralaryngeal Airways

*Laryngeal Mask Airway.* The laryngeal mask airway (LMA North America, Inc., San Diego) was introduced over 20 years ago by Dr. Archie Brain[83] and has evolved into a viable temporizing rescue maneuver for the difficult airway. The LMA Classic consists of a flexible tube attached to an inflatable cuff that is passed into the hypopharynx and advanced over the larynx (Fig. 12-4). When the cuff is inflated, a seal is created around the glottic aperture, permitting selective ventilation of the trachea. Since introduction of the LMA, a number of incarnations have ensued, each with theorized situation specific advantages. In addition to the Classic, the LMA is available in Unique (disposable Classic), Proseal (added glottic suction lumen), Flexible (wire reinforced for positioning), Fastrach (intubating LMA) and Ctrach (Fastrach with a viewing screen) models (All products LMA North America, Inc., San Diego, CA).

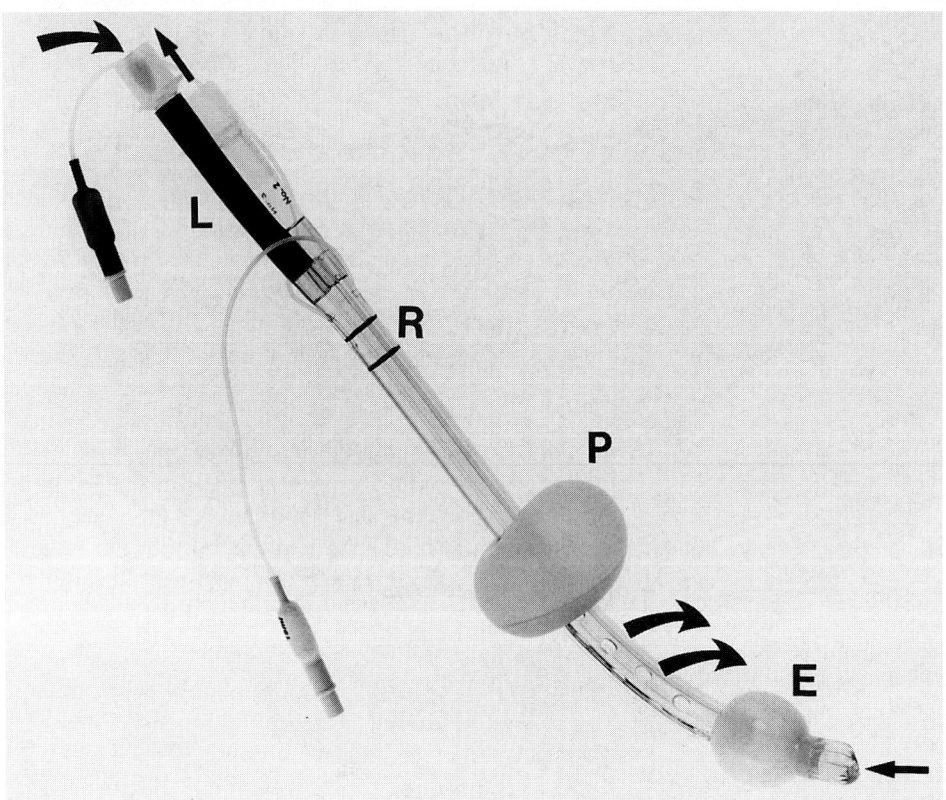

A

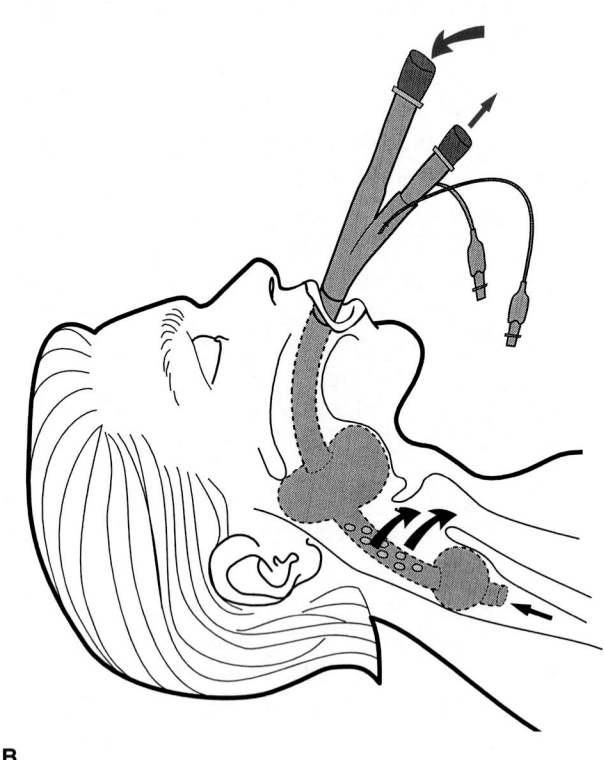

B

**FIGURE 12-3. (A)** Lateral photograph of the Combitube double-lumen tube. **(B)** The Combitube in place for emergency airway control. The tube is inserted blindly by lifting the jaw and tongue upward until the two printed rings (R) are at the teeth. The tip of the tube usually enters the esophagus. The pharyngeal cuff (P) is inflated with 100 mL of air and, when correctly placed, seals off the nasopahrynx and oral cavity. The distal cuff (E) is inflated with 15 mL of air. Ventilation through the longer (blue) connecting tube (L) will inflate the lungs via the eight side holes in the pharyngeal portion of the Combitube (as illustrated). If no breath sounds are heard, ventilation is attempted through the other lumen (the shorter tube) as the distal tube and cuff (E) has probably entered the larynx.

The LMA may be utilized in the difficult airway during resuscitation in an unconscious patient, when intubation skills are lacking or intubation has been unsuccessful. Accordingly, the primary clinical indications for use of the LMA include the following: airway rescue and maintenance in an "unable to intubate, able to ventilate" situation, and as a first line adjunct in an "unable to intubate, unable to ventilate" situation. Under the latter condition, LMA placement should proceed while preparations for cricothyroidotomy are underway. Under such conditions, the LMA may offer temporizing delivery of supplemental oxygen[79] and assist ventilation. The Classic LMA has been successfully placed as an airway adjunct by prehospital personnel,[84] Navy

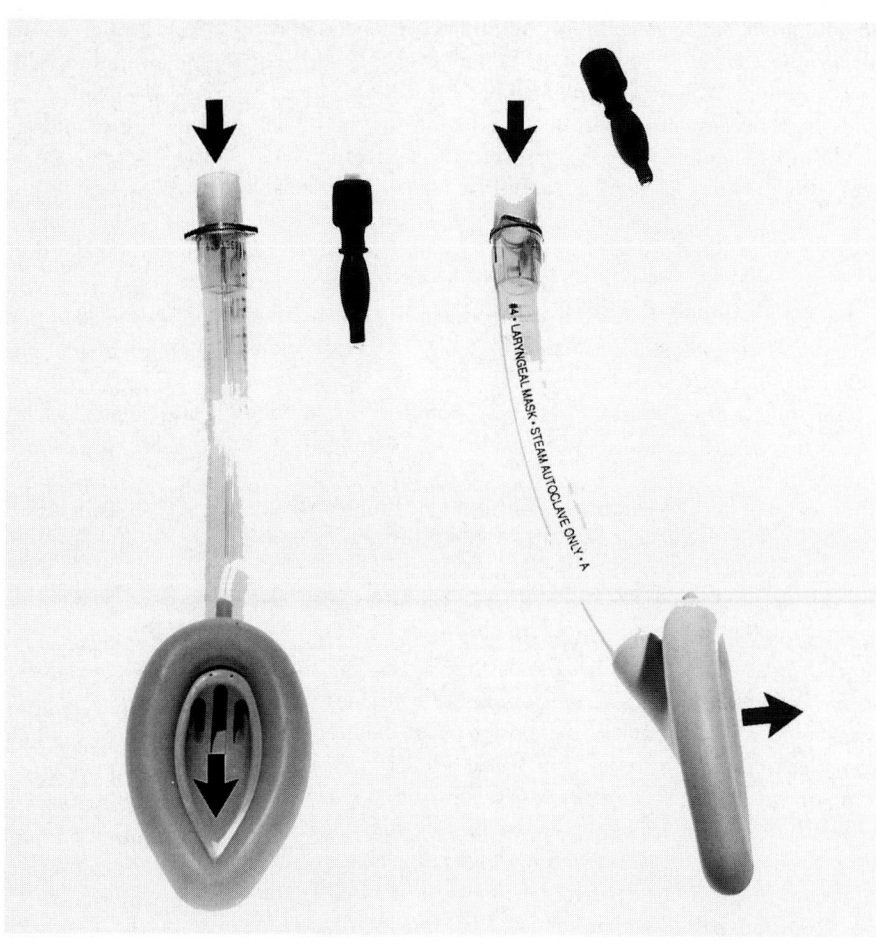

**FIGURE 12-4. (A)** Anterior and lateral photograph of the Bain laryngeal mask airway (LMA). **(B)** The LMA in position. The LMA is inserted blindly with the cuff deflated or partly inflated over the tongue and pushed as far as it will go. The cuff is inflated with 20 to 30 mL of air. When correctly placed, the cuff lies in the pharynx, its tip obstructing the upper esophageal lumen, and the mask interposed between the base of the tongue and the posterior pharyngeal wall to open the airway. Patients can breathe spontaneously through it (when it is used to reduce upper airway obstruction) or can be ventilated via the LMA if apneic.

SEAL corpsmen under fire,[85] emergency medicine physicians, and trauma surgeons.[83] The Proseal modification has an added suction lumen for control of esophageal or gastric secretions. In addition, the design of the cuff permits higher peak airway pressure during positive pressure ventilation. Placement of the Proseal LMA is potentially easier than the conventional LMA under conditions of cervical in-line stabilization,[86] and, in a recent review of its use in 11 episodes of airway rescue, the Proseal was found to have a high level of success.[87]

The LMA Fastrach potentially represents the most important version of the LMA for the difficult airway. It combines the advantages of the Classic LMA with technology that allows facilitation of blind intubation. An epiglottic elevating bar has been incorporated into the distal cuff, combined with a guide channel for the endotracheal tube. Following hypopharyngeal placement, an ETT can be passed blindly into the larynx. In a recent study of prehospital aeromedical intubation during flight, the intubating LMA (ILMA) was shown to be easy to use and facilitated intubation in less than one minute.[88] In addition, in a large review of ILMA use by emergency medicine physicians in 245 patients with difficult airways, including those with injury to the cervical spine, the success rates for blind and fiberoptic intubation through the ILMA were 97% and 100%, respectively.[89] The applicability of the variations in design of the LMA in the trauma and prehospital setting have not been sufficiently studied to assess superiority of one model; however, the Classic, Unique, and intubating LMA may prove to be valuable adjuncts.

Placement of an LMA does not constitute a definitive airway. Contraindications to the use of an LMA exist, and complications have been reported. Use of the LMA should never delay cricothyroidotomy when warranted and expertise exists. Under urgent conditions, the LMA is contraindicated in patients who are not obtunded or deeply sedated. Irritation of the airway induced by insertion in a semiconscious patient may exacerbate injury to the cervical spine and intracranial hypertension. Care should be exercised under conditions of severe craniofacial or pharyngeal trauma so as not to worsen injury. Leakage from around the cuff may occur in patients with fixed reductions in pulmonary compliance secondary to thoracic injury. Reported complications include aspiration, as it does not effectively separate the respiratory and alimentary tracts.[17] Although rare, other reported complications include mucosal trauma, local hematoma, cyanosis of the tongue, dislocation of the arytenoids, and paralysis of the lingual, hypoglossal, or recurrent laryngeal nerves.[90]

Laryngeal Tube Airway.    The laryngeal tube airway (LTA), a relatively new supralaryngeal device, is a variation on the form and function of the combitube, although it is reported to exhibit substantially less resistance on insertion. The LTA is primarily intended as an emergency airway device.[91] The LTA is a single lumen silicon tube with low-pressure oropharyngeal and esophageal cuffs, with the esophageal cuff terminating in a rounded tip. Between the two cuffs lies a ventilation outlet for selective ventilation of the trachea. Four variations of the LTA now exist, with addition of distal suction capabilities representing the newest versions. Literature assessing the role of the LTA in trauma patients is limited. In the anesthesia literature, the LTA has demonstrated equal efficacy in oxygenation and ventilation as compared to the LMA, is easy and safe to place, and permits higher airway pressures during ventilation than the LMA.[92] In a recent review of the existing literature on the LTA, the ease of placement, efficacy of oxygenation and ventilation, higher permissible airway pressure, and potential role in cardiopulmonary resuscitation were reiterated.[93] Due to the positive attributes demonstrated in the scant literature to date, the LTA warrants study in the emergent, difficult airway, particularly in comparison to the combitube.

Cobra Perilaryngeal Airway (CobraPLA).    The CobraPLA (Engineered Medical System, Indianapolis, IN) is a novel supraglottic airway device which has been utilized in "difficult to intubate, difficult

to ventilate" scenarios.[94] The device consists of a flexible ventilation tube with inner diameters ranging from 6.5 mm to 12.5 mm corresponding to five sizes. Similar to the LMA, the distal end of the tube contains an inflatable pharyngeal cuff with inflation volumes ranging from 10 cc in the pediatric size one to 85 cc in the adult size five. The "cobra head" configuration of the flexible distal tip is designed for positioning in the glottic inlet such that the ventilation outlets distal to the cuff selectively ventilate the trachea. The tube is placed blindly until resistance is felt, the cuff is then inflated, and ventilation ensues. The ventilation lumen permits passage of a flexible bronchoscope for confirmation of proper positioning.

The CobraPLA has been studied nearly exclusively in the operating room, where it has proven easy to insert[95] and effective at establishing an airway.[96] In recent studies, the device has been utilized to maintain the airway during percutaneous tracheostomy[97] and to assist with fiberoptic intubation in a child with an unstable cervical spine.[98] Further studies are warranted in prehospital and trauma scenarios.

Cricothyroidotomy.    In this era of constantly evolving gadgetry, the surgical airway remains the mainstay for rapid control of the difficult airway. Cricothyroidotomy is an ancient procedure which, despite having undergone a myriad of incarnations in the past two decades, remains an effective method to secure a compromised airway.

Multiple reviews of surgical cricothyroidotomy in recent years have redemonstrated a success rate of greater than 90% at obtaining an airway,[99–101] including performance by prehospital providers.[102] Cricothyroidotomy may be performed as the first airway maneuver in cases of craniofacial trauma precluding oral or nasotracheal intubation; however, it is more commonly utilized after translaryngeal intubation attempts have failed.[101] In published series, as many as 50% of patients undergoing the procedure are in cardiac arrest.[100] The greatest impediments to cricothyroidotomy are the delayed recognition that it is necessary and subsequent performance of the procedure. Given the duress under which cricothyroidotomy is typically performed, a number of complications, both acute and chronic, have been described. Acute complications include failure of the procedure, pneumothorax, hemorrhage, and misplaced tube, while late complications include tracheal stenosis. In a series of 122 patients undergoing emergency department cricothyroidotomy identified by the EAST workgroup, the complication rate was 28.7%.[19] The single contraindication to cricothyroidotomy is young age. Traditional recommendations suggest needle cricothyroidotomy for children less than 12 years of age, although body size should be taken into account.

## Technique of Cricothyroidotomy

Preparation for any potentially difficult airway should include securing necessary equipment for cricothyroidotomy, and all difficult airway carts should include the necessary instruments. It is important to prepare all participants in the process of obtaining an emergent airway that a cricothyroidotomy may need to be performed. In addition, an evaluation of surface anatomy and sterile preparation of the neck may facilitate the procedure in the event of a failed intubation. The most important instrument for surgical cricothyroidotomy is a scalpel, with many procedures having been performed with little else. Additional instruments may include tissue forceps and a hemostat. Cuffed endotracheal tubes with internal diameters of 5.0 mm to 7.0 mm should be available.

The procedure is initiated under universal precautions with rapid antiseptic preparation of the skin and palpation of the thyroid and cricothyroid cartilages with identification of the position of the cricothyroid membrane just superior to the cricoid cartilage. The trachea and larynx are then stabilized with the nondominant hand, with the thumb and index and long fingers immobilizing the superior cornua of the larynx. Following stabilization, a generous vertical incision is made over the membrane. The pretracheal tissue and fascia anterior to the membrane is rapidly divided with the scalpel, followed by a horizontal incision in the membrane. The index finger of the stabilizing hand may be utilized to palpate the membrane, guiding correct orientation of the incision. Many descriptions of the technique include insertion of the scalpel handle through the incised membrane to dilate the opening; however, given the conditions under which the procedure is typically performed, this technique may lead to inadvertent injury and should be abandoned. The cricoid incision can be dilated with artery forceps, a hemostat, a Trousseau dilator, or digitally. The index finger of the stabilizing hand should be used to maintain control of the cricoidotomy and guide insertion of the tube. Care should be taken to insert the endotracheal tube in a controlled fashion to a depth of approximately 5 cm. Insertion is facilitated by use of a rigid stylet; otherwise, the tube may selectively pass retrograde toward the vocal cords.

It should be emphasized that cricothyroidotomy is a poorly visualized or blind procedure in many instances. The obese neck may render superficial landmarks less than obvious, and transection of branches of the anterior jugular vein or thyroid tissue can lead to significant and unnerving hemorrhage. The stabilizing hand on the larynx may prove invaluable under such circumstances and should not be removed until the airway is secure.

A number of commercial alternatives to traditional surgical cricothyroidotomy have recently been developed in an attempt to expedite the procedure and reduce the degree of expertise required. The devices known as cricothyrotomes typically utilize one of the two techniques to cannulate the trachea, depending on whether a Seldinger technique is utilized. For Seldinger-type kits, the cricothyroid membrane is punctured with a needle, a flexible guidewire is passed, and a tracheostomy tube is passed over a dilator. Alternatively, other kits utilize a tracheostomy tube placed over a puncture device without the intervening placement of a guidewire.

## Needle Cricothyroidotomy

Percutaneous needle cricothyroidotomy with transtracheal jet ventilation is an alternative to traditional surgical cricothyroidotomy. The technique is utilized for temporization of oxygenation and ventilation, primarily in one of two scenarios. First, the technique can be used in adults following failure of tracheal intubation or other temporizing measures, when expertise with surgical cricothyroidotomy is lacking. Alternatively, it is an effective method to temporize the pediatric patient, in whom the algorithm for airway failure calls for a surgical airway.

The skin over the neck should be rapidly sterilized, and the skin anesthetized. The cricothyroid cartilage and membrane should be identified in a similar fashion to surgical cricothyroidotomy.

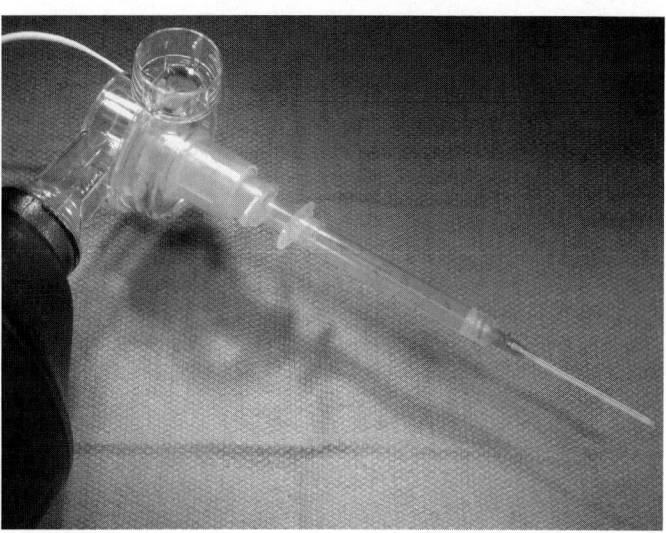

**FIGURE 12-5.** A photograph of a useful set up for needle cricothyroidotomy, consisting of a standard 8 millimeter diameter endotracheal tube adapter, a three cc syringe, and a 14 gauge angiocatheter. The endotracheal tube adapter is removed and inserted into the open end of the three cc syringe (plunger removed). The angiocatheter is affixed to the syringe. A bag-valve-mask is then able to be attached to the adapter, allowing easy ventilation of the patient.

A large-bore catheter (14–16 gauge) is attached to a syringe half filled with saline. The cricothyroid membrane is cannulated in an inferior and caudal direction, at an angle of 30 to 60° from the trachea. The trachea is aspirated, with positioning confirmed by air bubbles visualized in the saline. The needle is removed, and the catheter is then attached to a jet ventilation system using a Luer lock. Alternatively, a 5 mL syringe can be cut and attached directly to oxygen tubing or the tubing can be wedged into the open end of the syringe, then connected to a high-flow 100% oxygen source. An alternative method is to attach a three cc syringe to a 14 gauge catheter with an endotracheal tube adapter inserted into the open end of the syringe (Fig. 12-5). This technique allows direct attachment of the BVM to the syringe. Whatever system is utilized, an aperture should be created such that when occluded, jet insufflation occurs, and, when open, flow may escape. Jet insufflation should proceed at approximately 1 second of flow (inspiration) for every 3 seconds of release (expiration). Because ventilation is not actually occurring, alveolar carbon dioxide rises as the partial pressure of alveolar oxygen declines. A point of emphasis is the temporizing nature of the procedure; life may be sustained for approximately 30 minutes until a definitive airway can be achieved.

## AIRWAY CHALLENGES IN THE INJURED PATIENT

### Maxillofacial Trauma

Patients with craniofacial, maxillofacial, and tracheolaryngeal injuries commonly present with threatened airways. Direct injury to the facial soft tissues and bony skeleton, tongue, and larynx may cause intrinsic and extrinsic obstruction of the airway from edema, hemorrhage, secretions, or loss of bony architecture. In a recent large review of craniomaxillofacial trauma at a Level I trauma center, 16,465 patients sustained injuries to the head, neck, or face over a 12-year period. Many required advanced airway techniques or cricothyroidotomy.[103] Most maxillofacial injuries are secondary to blunt mechanisms and are commonly associated with multisystem injuries, including those to the brain.[104] In penetrating injury, the airway may be no less challenging. In a review of 92 patients with maxillofacial gunshot wounds, 22% presented with a threatened airway, 60% of whom required an emergent surgical airway.[105] Similarly, in a separate 4-year review of 84 patients with maxillofacial gunshot wounds, 21% required an urgent tracheostomy.[106]

Although emergent surgical intervention is often required, many patients with severe injury to bone and soft tissue are able to clear blood and secretions. If the potential for an injury to the spine does not preclude the patient sitting upright, slight forward positioning, suctioning, and calming of the patient frequently allow for forward displacement of bilateral mandibular fractures or macerated soft tissue and maintenance of a precarious but patent airway. Under these conditions, close observation and transport to the operating room may optimize conditions for definitive airway procedures such as an awake tracheostomy or a submental intubation. In the context of massive injury to bone and soft tissue (Fig. 12-6), such as the catastrophic self-inflicted submental gunshot wound, an urgent need for a definitive airway does not necessarily mean that a surgical airway will be necessary. Despite the intimidating appearance of such injuries, many of these patients can undergo orotracheal intubation due to loss of restrictive anatomy. In summary, when maxillofacial trauma is present, the patient's ability to maintain an airway should not be underestimated; however, it is essential not to delay the insertion of a definitive airway when indicated. Orotracheal intubation is the preferred definitive airway, while nasotracheal intubation should be undertaken with extreme caution when the severity of an injury to the mid-face is unclear. If

orotracheal intubation is not plausible or fails, the rescue technique of choice is cricothyroidotomy.

## Laryngotracheal Trauma

The management of laryngotracheal injuries is based foremost upon status of the airway. In the previously mentioned study of craniomaxillofacial trauma over a 12-year period, 0.2% of patients with injuries to the head, neck, or face sustained laryngeal fractures, and 97% of these sustained concomitant maxillofacial trauma.[103] In patients with laryngeal fractures, 74% required advanced airway maneuvers.[103] In another report, 71 patients with laryngotracheal trauma were identified over an eight-year period.[107] Of note, 73% of injuries were penetrating, but patients with a blunt mechanism were more likely to require an emergent airway (79% vs. 46%). The need for an emergency airway was an independent predictor of mortality.[107]

Recognition of either overt or potential injury to the larynx and cervical trachea is critical to subsequent airway planning. Clues to the diagnosis of laryngotracheal injury include marked pain, tenderness and ecchymosis across the anterior neck or larynx, hoarseness or stridor, or the presence of subcutaneous emphysema. Subcutaneous emphysema and crepitance are the chief clinical signs.[108] In a review of 19 patients presenting to a Level I trauma center with injury to the upper aerodigestive tract, 100% had radiographic evidence of subcutaneous emphysema or palpable crepitance, 21% had dysphagia, and 63% had stridor or hoarseness.[109]

Treatment options for this constellation of injures include fiberoptic intubation, orotracheal intubation, and insertion of a surgical airway depending on the acuity of the presentation. In patients who are oxygenating, ventilating, and protecting their airway despite a clinical suspicion of tracheolaryngeal injury, the procedures of choice are fiberoptic laryngoscopy or bronchoscopy to assess integrity of the airway under controlled conditions, with performance of a surgical airway if necessary. If a tracheolaryngeal injury is visualized, an attempt at passage of an endotracheal tube over the scope is appropriate. Under urgent conditions, unless obvious tracheal or laryngeal disruption is evident, orotracheal intubation remains the procedure of choice. If resistance is met, intubation should be aborted and a surgical airway performed corresponding to the suspected level of injury. Temporizing supralaryngeal devices should be avoided in this circumstance, as the potential for worsening subcutaneous emphysema and distortion of anatomy exists. For open wounds in which a tracheal injury is visualized, the trachea may be cannulated directly, with conversion to orotracheal intubation under controlled conditions.

## Trauma to the Cervical Spine

Injury to the cervical spine is common in patients with blunt trauma, and more than half of spine injuries occur in the cervical spine. In patients with an injury above the clavicles, 15% overall and 5% with injury to the brain have a concomitant injury to the cervical spine. The critical need to immobilize and protect the cervical spine in virtually all patients with blunt trauma complicates management of the airway. Fear of injury to the spinal cord by cervical manipulation during laryngoscopy has led to the purely theoretical practice of blind nasotracheal intubation for all patients with multisystem blunt trauma in some centers. Accumulating evidence

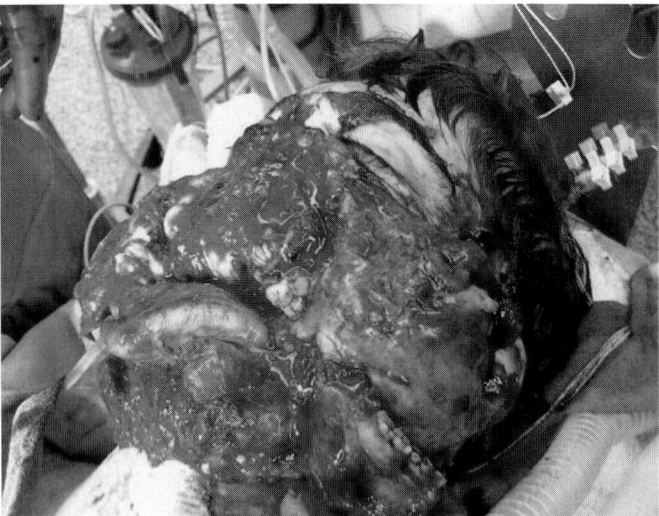

**FIGURE 12-6.** Despite the extreme destructive nature of the maxillofacial injury, orotracheal intubation is the first method to secure a definitive airway. If orotracheal intubation fails and hypoxia ensues, cricothyroidotomy should be performed inferior to the tissue destruction. If the patient is able to oxygenate, an urgent yet controlled tracheostomy in the operating room is an alternative.

suggests that orotracheal intubation, with strict stabilization of the cervical spine, is safe as a standard of care.

A number of studies in the past decade have assessed the effects of various intubation techniques on motion of the cervical spine. The majority have utilized fluoroscopic images in cadavers or in the controlled setting of the operating room.[110–115] Nearly all studies compare cervical motion incurred during direct laryngoscpy with a Macintosh blade versus techniques which utilize either fiberoptic laryngoscopy or devices which facilitate blind intubation. To summarize findings to date, direct laryngoscopy produces more extension at all levels of the cervical spine than the intubating LMA,[113,114] Lightwand (intubating lighted stylet),[111] GlideScope,[111] Bullard laryngoscope,[113] Bonfils fibrescope,[110,113] and fiberoptic laryngoscopy.[112] Nearly all techniques are significantly more time-consuming than direct laryngoscopy, however, and the degree of extension, depending on the cervical level, ranges from 3.5 to 22.5°.[112–113] If sufficient time, equipment, and expertise exist, alternate techniques to direct laryngoscopy may be considered, particularly with the intubating LMA, which has been reasonably well studied in the prehospital environment. Given the emergent nature of most intubations performed in the field and emergency department, constraints of equipment and expertise and the small degree of extension with proper cervical stabilization during direct laryngoscopy, the tried and true method of airway control in the injured patient remains rapid sequence intubation using direct laryngoscopy.

## Thermal Trauma

Multiple scenarios in thermal injury may precipitate compromise of the airway. After thermal injury, airway edema with obstruction has many causes including major nonfacial burns with shock treated with requisite large volumes of crystalloid solutions, circumferential thoracic burns, direct thermal or caustic injury to the lips, tongue or pharynx, and inhalational injury. The Advanced Burn Life Support course, similar to ATLS, emphasizes the primacy of airway in thermal and inhalational injury.[3]

The incidence of smoke inhalation, the most common inhalational injury, is approximately 20% in all patients admitted to Level I burn centers and, in isolation, carries a 5–8% mortality rate.[116] Inhalational injury can affect any of the three distinct areas of the respiratory tract, including the supraglottic, tracheobronchial, and pulmonary parenchymal regions. Inhalation injury is defined as aspiration of superheated gases, steam, hot liquids, or noxious products of incomplete combustion. Inhalational injury causes a number of physiologic derangements including the following: (1) loss of airway patency secondary to mucosal edema; (2) bronchospasm secondary to inhaled irritants; (3) intrapulmonary shunting from small airway occlusion caused by mucosal edema and sloughed endobronchial debris; (4) diminished compliance secondary to alveolar flooding and collapse with mismatching of ventilation and perfusion; (5) pneumonia and tracheobronchitis secondary to loss of ciliary clearance and tracheobronchial epithelium; and (6) respiratory failure secondary to a combination of the above factors.[117] Such physiologic derangements are variable in different populations. The injuries evolve over time and parenchymal lung dysfunction is often minimal for 24 to 72 hours.

Normal oxygenation and chest radiographs do not exclude the diagnosis,[117] and the etiology of early death from smoke inhalation is most commonly compromise of the airway.[118] Recent consensus recommendations from the American Burn Association (ABA) state the following: "Inhalation injury is suspected in the presence of one or more specific points of history (closed space exposure to hot gasses, steam or products of combustion), physical examination (singed vibrissae and carbonaceous sputum), or laboratory findings (elevated carboxyhemoglobin or cyanide level)."[117]

Inhalation injury alone is an ABA criterion for transfer to a burn center.[117] Therefore, the critical maneuvers for the initial care of the patient with a severe thermal and inhalational injury must focus upon oxygenation and protection of the airway prior to and during triage and transfer. The crux of decision-making pertains to establishment of a definitive airway. Because no Level I evidence supporting the diagnosis of inhalational injury exists and the onset of symptoms is variable and frequently insidious, significant clinical suspicion should prompt establishment of a definitive airway.[117] Currently, bronchoscopic examination is the standard definitive diagnostic measure, assessing for the presence of carbonaceous debris and mucosal erythema or ulceration.[117] Although intubation alone is fraught with both early and late sequelae, a window of opportunity may exist for controlled intubation. Subsequent airway edema and rapid pulmonary deterioration can convert a controlled situation into an emergent, difficult airway at an inopportune time during transport. If clinical suspicion is significant or bronchoscopy suggests an inhalational component, clinicians should err on the side of intubation. The Eastern Association for the Surgery of Trauma Management Guidelines Workgroup completed an extensive review of the literature assessing data to suggest need for intubation following inhalational injury. No Level I data (predicated on randomized, controlled trials) were cited; however, consensus of the Committee identified airway obstruction, severe cognitive impairment (GCS score < 8), cutaneous burn exceeding 40% total body surface area, prolonged transport time, and impending airway obstruction (due to moderate to severe facial burn, oropharyngeal burn, and airway injury visualized on endoscopy) as indications for intubation.[19]

Due to efficient cooling capabilities of the upper respiratory tract, thermal injury is usually confined to the upper airways, unless smoke with high water content or steam is inhaled.[119] Significant oropharyngeal or facial burns with mucosal edema do not preclude oral intubation. Attempts at laryngoscopy are warranted, although failure of orotracheal intubation should prompt the insertion of a surgical airway. Circumferential third-degree burns of the chest may impair oxygenation and ventilation secondary to reductions in compliance of the chest wall, pulmonary static compliance, and increased intra-abdominal pressure.[120] Under these circumstances, it is imperative for clinicians to address the airway definitively with endotracheal intubation or rescue maneuvers and to concurrently address the need for escharotomy of the chest wall as expeditiously as possible.

## Traumatic Brain Injury (TBI)

Injury to the brain is the most common, single indication for a definitive airway in patients with blunt trauma. Initial goals focus upon airway protection and maintenance, while sustained goals focus on prevention of secondary injury to the brain through optimization of oxygenation and regulation of carbon dioxide. Airway management is particularly challenging in patients with TBI because of the associated problem of intracranial hypertension. It is well recognized that hypoxia, even a single episode, has deleterious effects on outcome, and uncontrolled hyperventilation, with resultant cerebral vasoconstriction, may worsen outcome, as well.[121] The Brain Trauma Foundation guidelines state that hypoxia, defined as apnea, cyanosis, oxygen saturation < 90%, or partial pressure of arterial oxygen < 60 mm Hg, *must be scrupulously avoided*.[122] In addition to prevention of hypoxia, the avoidance of hypercarbia is of critical importance. Hypercarbia results in cerebral vasodilatation, effectively increasing intracranial blood volume, with resultant elevated intracranial pressure. Early definitive airway control, with the ability to more directly control oxygenation and ventilation, is theoretically appealing, and the recommendation that a GCS score < 8 should prompt intubation remains in the ATLS course.[3] Rapid sequence intubation may help to eliminate prolonged awake intubation attempts and, therefore, the risk of hypercarbia.

Despite the intuitive belief that early intubation may prevent hypoxia or extremes of ventilation, data assessing prehospital intubation in TBI are conflicting. In two recent studies, prehospital use of RSI by paramedics was shown to correlate with poor functional outcome and death in patients with injury to the brain.[123,124] In a study of pediatric airway management, prehospital endotracheal intubation by paramedics was not demonstrated to confer outcome benefit compared to BVM ventilation.[125] Correspondingly, 8% of patients suffered either esophageal intubation or dislodgement of the tube, and 93% died.[125] Conversely, other recent studies have demonstrated an outcome benefit in patients with TBI undergoing RSI, particularly when neuromuscular blocking agents are utilized.[126] In a recent swine model evaluating the effects of various RSI regimens on intracranial pressure, those utilizing paralytic agents produced three-fold increases in peak intracranial pressure as compared to regimens using sedation only.[127] The association between RSI and mortality may have little to do with the procedure itself; rather, preintubation hypoxia and postintubation hyperventilation, may represent the causes of death.[128] In a study of 291 patients with TBI, 144 patients underwent continuous measurement of end-tidal carbon dioxide ($ETCO_2$).[128] Patients with $ETCO_2$ monitoring had a lower incidence of inadvertent severe hyperventilation (defined as partial pressure carbon dioxide < 25 mm Hg), and patients with severe hyperventilation had significantly higher mortality than those without hyperventilation.[128] In further work from the San Diego Paramedic RSI trial, 79% of patients were documented to have $ETCO_2$ values less than 30 mm Hg during RSI or transport, and 59% of patients had levels less than 25 mm Hg.[129]

From existing data, it appears that RSI may be appropriate when clinically indicated in TBI, provided preintubation hypoxia and postintubation extreme hyperventilation are avoided. Of concern, the incidence of hypoxia incurred during RSI may be significant. In a study assessing the frequency of hypoxia (defined as oxygen saturation measured by oximetry < 90%) during RSI performed by paramedics, 57% of patients demonstrated hypoxia lasting a median duration of 160 seconds.[130] The median decrease in oxygen saturation was 22%.[46] In summary, rapid sequence intubation should be undertaken with strict attention to preoxygenation and rate of postintubation ventilation in patients with TBI.

## THE PEDIATRIC AIRWAY

Management of the airway in the critically ill and injured child presents a number of unique challenges which render emergent management less successful by clinicians primarily trained in managing the adult airway.[131] First, anatomy is dependent upon body mass, and knowledge of development-based anatomy is critical to selection of equipment and pharmacology. Second, physiology unique to children, including increased susceptibility to the deleterious effects of hypoxia, may amplify the urgency of the airway. Finally, psychological stress, affecting both the clinician and patient, is inherent in establishing a pediatric airway. In general, principles of airway management for the pediatric population are similar to those in the adult population, but selected fundamental principles do differ.

### Anatomy

As the pediatric cranium comprises a larger relative percentage of body surface and mass and flexes the cervical spine in the supine position, cervical stabilization is critical at all times. Internal differences in the airway at laryngoscopy which have the potential to render the pediatric airway challenging include a larger amount of distensible soft tissue.[132] Children may have significant tonsilar and adenoid tissue as well as a large tongue which collapses into the posterior pharynx, and these have the potential to obstruct laryngoscopy and bleed with instrumentation. Compounded by the fact that the glottic opening of the trachea is at the level of C-1 in infancy and the larynx is more anterior with decreasing age, the angle between the laryngeal orifice and the glottic opening is more acute. Other anatomic variations from adults include a narrower cricoid ring, narrower and shorter trachea, and smaller cricothyroid membrane. As the larynx becomes less anterior with advanced age, the technique of laryngoscopy and intubation more closely approximates that of adults. As a rule, children less than two years of age have high anterior airways while children greater than 8 years of age have an alignment similar to adults. Children aged two through eight have transitional airways with less consistency among individuals.

### Physiology

More rapid onset of hypoxemia in children is related to higher basal oxygen consumption, 6 to 8 mL kg$^{-1}$ min$^{-1}$ in infants versus 3 to 4 mL kg$^{-1}$ min$^{-1}$ in adults. Increased susceptibility to hypoxemia leads to a higher incidence of cardiac arrests due to compromise of the airway than in adults. The higher metabolic rate, compounded by reduced cardiovascular tolerance to hypoxia, accentuates the urgency of establishing an airway in children with hemorrhagic, obstructive or neurogenic shock. In addition, rapid oxygen desaturation in children is coupled to a relative reduction is functional residual capacity.

### Equipment

Anatomic and physiologic attributes of children mandate alterations in airway equipment and drug preparation, as well as anticipated algorithms for management of the difficult airway. The Broselow Pediatric Emergency Tape, although intended as a guide only, is an excellent airway resource for clinicians unfamiliar with standard sizes and doses. The tape includes length-based estimates of kilogram body weight, with corresponding recommendations for drug dosing and equipment sizing. The tape includes recommendations for size of endotracheal tube, insertion length, stylet, suction catheter, laryngoscope, BVM, end-tidal carbon dioxide detector, as well as oral, nasopharyngeal, and laryngeal mask airways.

The BVM apparatus should be selected with attention to both size of facemask, ensuring proper seal, and delivered tidal volume. Although pop-off valves set at 35 to 45 cm of $H_2O$ are often recommended, a higher generated airway pressure may be required to ventilate the injured child, and air may escape from the valve unrecognized. Circular masks often provide a better seal in infants and children. Oral airways, utilized solely in the unconscious child, should be selected from recommendations of the Broselow tape, or by approximating the distance from the angle of the mouth to the angle of the mandible or the tragus of the ear. Correspondingly, the internal diameter of the endotracheal tube is based upon the Broselow tape or formulas, including age/4 + 4, or (16 + age)/4. Uncuffed endotracheal tubes are recommended in younger children, with cuffed tubes employed for children requiring a 5.5 mm internal diameter or greater. Given the short tracheal length in children, intubation of the right mainstem bronchus is a potential complication following endotracheal intubation. In addition to recommendations on the Broselow tape, depth of insertion may be calculated as the internal diameter of the tube multiplied by three. A nasopharyngeal airway is selected based upon the approximate distance from the tip of the nose to the angle of the tragus. The size of end-tidal carbon dioxide measurement also differs with use in children. The pediatric model should be used for children weighing less than 15 kilograms.

## Technique

Although all clinicians caring for injured patients should be facile with the pediatric airway, it is frequently difficult to recall specific differences in drug doses to establish an airway. Again, the Broselow tape may be invaluable when determining appropriate dosing. During rapid sequence intubation, defasciculating doses of nondepolarizing neuromuscular blocking agents are not recommended for children less than 20 kilograms body weight. In addition, it is imperative to remember that children have a higher percentage of extracellular volume than adults, requiring higher dose of succinylcholine (2 mg/kg). Finally, due to the potential for reflex bradycardia during RSI,[133] all children should receive atropine when receiving succinylcholine. This is also true for children less than 5 years of age undergoing any form of manipulation of the airway, although atropine does not universally abrogate bradycardia.[134,135]

Given the unique impact of hypoxia on pediatric physiology, failure to gain definitive control of the airway can be catastrophic. Conversely, the decision to intubate has unique ramifications in children. Failure rates for intubation are extremely variable in children, with higher rates noted in smaller children and infants. In addition, a number of studies have questioned the utility of prehospital intubation in children. The Pediatric Airway Management project, a controlled trial of 830 patients requiring prehospital control of the airway, found no benefit and more complications with prehospital intubation.[125] BVM offers an excellent means to oxygenate and ventilate children. When definitive airway control is necessary, rapid sequence intubation is the technique of choice and is now recommended by pediatric life support courses. When intubation fails, a paucity of data exist to guide clinicians regarding adjuncts to establishing a definitive airway. Surgical cricothyroidotomy is considered a contraindication in infants[136] and small children, due to the size of the cricothyroid membrane, although data are limited. For children less than 8 to 10 years of age, needle cricothyroidotomy should be utilized, although limited data exist regarding the efficacy of this technique.[137] The laryngeal mask airway represents a temporizing alternative to cricothyroidotomy, although it does not represent a definitive airway. Accumulating data suggest that LMA use is feasible and efficacious in children, although the majority of studies are focused in controlled operative settings.[138,139] The utility of the LMA in the injured child under urgent or emergent conditions is not yet validated.

## EMERGENCY AIRWAY ALGORITHMS

Airway algorithms are beneficial as they provide a reproducible structural framework for recognition and response that guides management under complex and stressful situations. Once the need for definitive airway protection has been identified, a concise and logical approach to airway control, based upon situational and patient characteristics, is imperative.

### Definitions

The failed airway and the difficult airway are distinct. The two entities are not unrelated, as the difficult airway frequently leads to the failed airway. To negotiate the sequence of both the failed and difficult airways, an understanding of current definitions is necessary. A failed airway is defined as any clinical scenario in which a patient is unable to oxygenate or ventilate. A failed airway may exist upon presentation secondary to a disease process or after a clinician has initiated any one of a number of airway interventions that have failed to maintain oxygenation or ventilation. Therefore, failure of initial attempts at BMV ventilation, with $SpO_2$ falling below 90%, represents a failed airway. Thus, a failed airway may manifest at any intervention from BVM to tracheal intubation. Some authors have expanded the definition of failed airway to include failure of tracheal intubation after three attempts, despite maintenance of oxygenation and ventilation.

There is no literature-based definition of a difficult airway. In general, the difficult airway refers to any preintubation characteristics, related to injury type or pattern, physiology, anatomy, comorbidities, or skills of the practitioner that predict difficulty with the standard algorithm for orotracheal intubation. In the emergent situation, scant time may be available to use alternatives to orotracheal intubation, such as an awake technique or nasotracheal intubation. Alternatively, an identified difficult airway may be followed by an uneventful progression through the standard RSI technique. In summary, the difficult airway does not always portend a failed airway, nor does the failed airway universally arise from a predicted difficult airway. In the words of one author, "The difficult airway

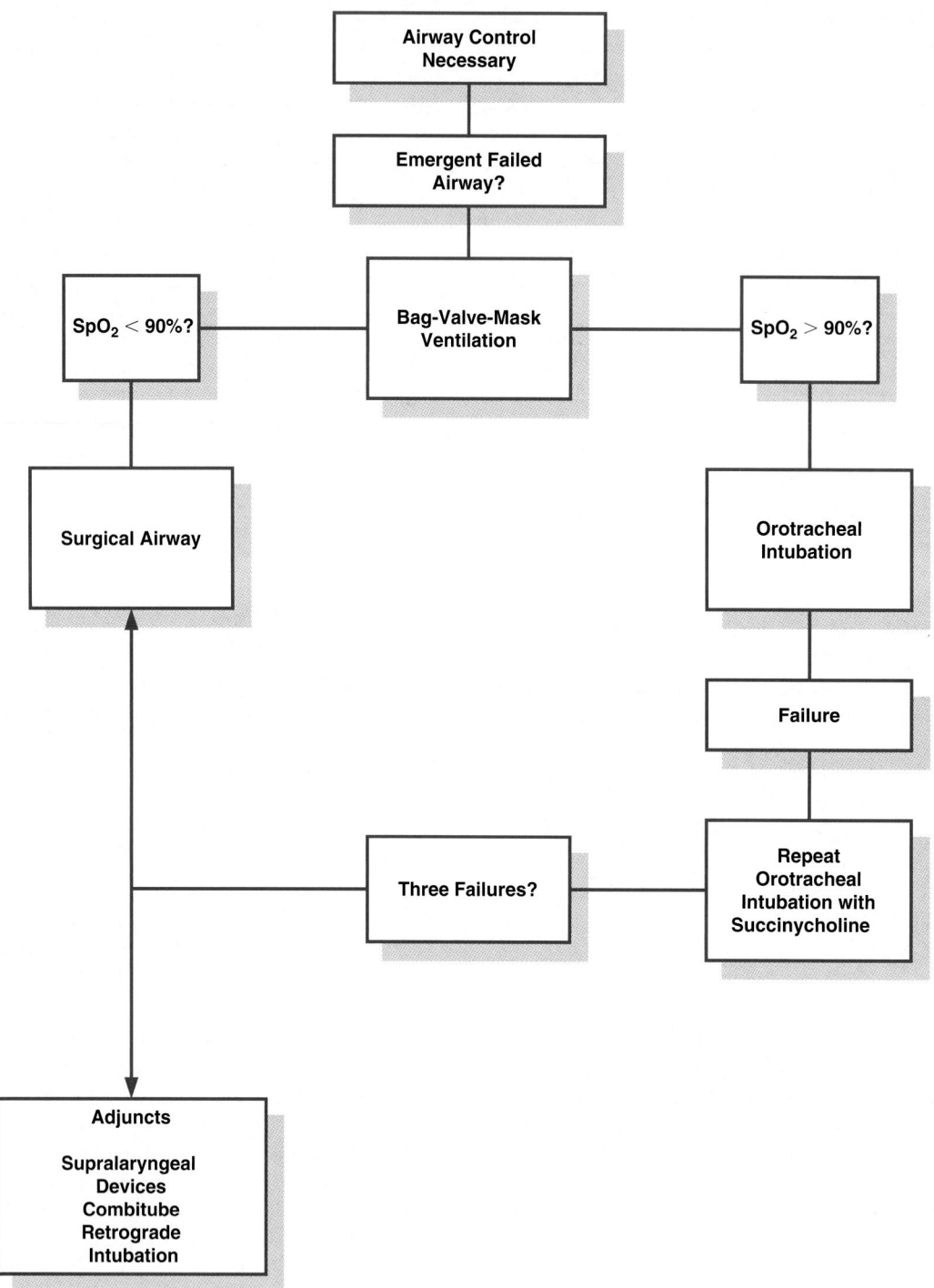

**FIGURE 12-7.** Algorithm for the failed airway.

is something one anticipates, the failed airway is something one experiences."[140]

## Decision Making in the Failed Airway

When airway control is required, the first assessment is determining whether airway failure is present. Patients who are apneic, in extremis, or manifest inability to protect the airway with resultant failure of oxygenation and ventilation, represent airway failure. The first step in airway failure is BVM ventilation while rapid preparations

for tracheal intubation are made (Fig. 12-7). Further management steps are based upon success of BVM.

Airway Failure: Bag-Valve-Mask Ventilation, $SpO_2$ >90%. The effectiveness of BMV ventilation determines the progression to either orotracheal intubation or urgent surgical intervention. If BMV results in successful oxygenation and ventilation, orotracheal intubation (OTI) should be attempted. If OTI is unsuccessful, further treatment always depends on the ability to oxygenate and ventilate the patient with BMV. If at any point the patient cannot be ventilated or develops hypoxia, an emergent surgical airway is necessary. Following an initial failure of OTI, an assessment of reasons for failure should quickly follow. If paralysis is deemed beneficial based upon the status of facial musculature on the first attempt at OTI, succinylcholine should be administered followed by a repeat attempt at OTI. If a second failure occurs, a third attempt should only occur if BVM remains effective and a more experienced clinician is available. If a third failure at OTI occurs, two options exist. First, a surgical airway is always acceptable after three OTI failures and should be the mainstay for a definitive airway at this juncture. If surgical expertise is unavailable, alternate methods of tracheal intubation such as retrograde intubation or the intubating LMA may be considered provided BVM ventilation remains effective. If alternatives fail, temporizing measures to maintain oxygenation and ventilation, including ETC and supralaryngeal airways, should be utilized until surgical expertise is available.

Airway Failure: Bag-Valve-Mask Ventilation, SpO$_2$ <90%. The foundation of this scenario is rapid transition to a definitive surgical airway (Fig. 12-7). If SpO$_2$ cannot be maintained >90% using BMV, emergent transition to a rapid single attempt at orotracheal intubation or a surgical airway should be undertaken. The decision at this point should be based upon available equipment and expertise. If a surgical airway is possible, delay for even a single attempt at tracheal intubation may be lethal. The decision to attempt tracheal intubation should be predicated upon anticipated ease of placement and lack of surgical expertise. If OTI fails and a surgical airway is not possible, alternate methods of tracheal intubation should be avoided, with progression to attempts at temporizing measures to oxygenate and ventilate.

Spontaneous Respirations.    A number of trauma patients are alert and breathing spontaneously, but are not oxygenating or ventilating adequately, hence, they have a failed airway. Under these circumstances, vigorous BMV should be avoided, with supplemental oxygen applied to spontaneous breaths. The patient should be assessed for injuries that might not require intubation, such as a pneumothorax, with oxygen administered in the highest concentration possible. Emergent RSI should follow. If unable to intubate, a surgical airway should be undertaken. In the event that a surgical airway is not possible, temporizing alternatives, including the insertion of a supralaryngeal airway or ETC, should be considered.

## The Difficult Airway

For patients who have need for a definitive airway but do not present with airway failure, there is time to assess and prepare for a potentially difficult airway. In patients who do not meet the criteria for difficult airway, RSI should be employed, with attention to all five phases of RSI, including preparation, drug selection, and preoxygenation (Fig. 12-8). If OTI is unsuccessful after three attempts, a failed airway exists.

Prediction of the Difficult Airway.    As many as 20% of all emergency intubations meet the criteria for a difficult airway. Many indicators of a difficult airway may be subtle or masked in injured patients, further emphasizing the need to prepare for all possible scenarios. Disease states, anatomic variations, and congenital abnormalities may all contribute to the inability to successfully intubate

the trachea. Problematic disease states include those involving the temporomandibular joint disease, arthritis, ankylosing spondylitis, infections, foreign bodies, and malignancy. Anatomic abnormalities include scoliosis, hypoplasia of either the mandible or the maxilla, and cleft lip. Anatomic variations, which can usually be noticed on physical exam, include the short, thick mandible, the fat/thick neck ("bull neck"), narrow opening of the mouth, and a large tongue.[16]

Traditionally, the most commonly used predictive scheme used in anesthesiology is the Mallampati airway classification system. The tenet of this system is that gradations are assigned to an increasingly difficult airway based upon the ability to visualize the structures of the oropharynx.[141] Samsoon and Young modified the Mallampati system and compared the tongue's ability to obscure the oropharynx as a predictor of the difficulty to establish an airway.[82] Both of these systems require a cooperative patient who can follow commands. The "Rule of Threes" was developed to combine the physical characteristics of mouth opening, jaw size, and mandible size (thyromental distance) as a predictor of a difficult airway at the bedside. Simplistically, if three provider finger breaths can be placed between the patient's upper and lower teeth, the hyoid bone and the chin, and the thyroid cartilage and the sternal notch, the provider has a higher success rate in direct laryngoscopy.[8,142]

Equipment and Technique for the Difficult Airway.    In a survey of program directors of training programs in emergency medicine regarding airway adjunct, the frequency of various adjuncts was reported and included the following: cricothyroidotomy kits (95%), fiberoptic scopes (76%), Bougies (70%), LMAs (66%), intubating LMAs (61%), lighted stylets (54%), retrograde intubation kits (49%), Combitube (46%), and esophageal obturator airways (15%). Despite the preparedness, 94% of airways were managed with orotracheal intubation.[143] The standard airway cart should have all potential adjuncts useful in the difficult airway, including fiberoptic devices.

Although difficult airway criteria are common, the majority of difficult airways are managed with RSI, with a low incidence of complications. Therefore, anticipation of a difficult airway, with preparation for alternatives to orotracheal intubation, including insertion of a surgical airway, is critical. The step in RSI which may prove precarious in the patient with a difficult airway and precipitating airway failure is paralysis. Therefore, the single deviation from a standard RSI approach is laryngoscopy without paralysis (Fig. 12-8). In patients not meeting the criteria for airway failure, the pharynx and trachea can be topically anesthetized followed by administration of a sedative agent, typically etomidate. Sedation with a sedative hypnotic agent may be sufficient to allow laryngoscopy, visualization of the vocal cords, and endotracheal intubation. In addition, although laryngoscopy without paralysis may not always allow intubation, the process may identify the airway as amenable to RSI with paralysis. If RSI fails to secure the difficult airway, management proceeds according to a failed airway (Fig. 12-7).

## COMPLICATIONS ASSOCIATED WITH THE EMERGENCY AIRWAY

Complications associated with management of the emergency airway are multiple and common and cause significant morbidity and mortality both during, and subsequent to, airway procedures. For

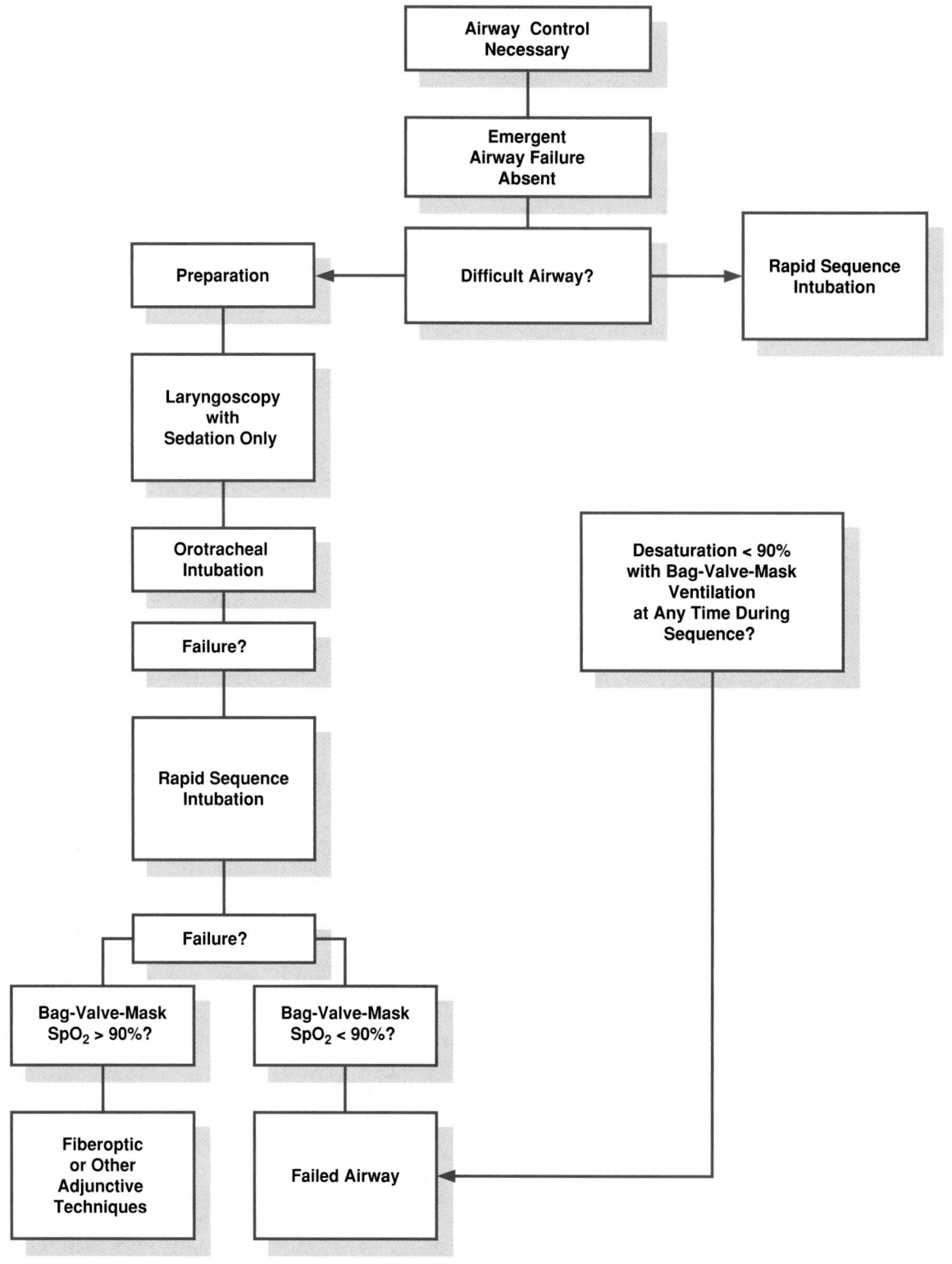

**FIGURE 12-8.** Algorithm for the difficult airway.

intubation, primarily rapid sequence, morbidity increases as the number of attempts at laryngoscopy increases.[144] Complications can be defined as immediate and late relative to attempts at an emergent airway. The most common and ominous immediate complications are failure to intubate, failure to recognize esophageal intubation, and failure to ventilate.[145] Pulmonary aspiration of gastric contents, an immediate complication, imparts both early and late morbidity, secondary to the potential for acute lung injury and pneumonia.

## Failure to Intubate

Rapid sequence orotracheal intubation is the preferred means of airway control in the majority of injured and critically ill patients. Correspondingly, failure to intubate is the most feared complication of emergent airway intervention, initiating the critical pathway of alternate means of oxygenation and ventilation. Published rates of failure of intubation are as varied as the patient populations and environments from which they originate. The majority of recent series report failure rates of emergent intubation as 2% to 13%, including those performed by rural basic emergency medical technicians,[146] single center emergency medicine and anesthesia residents,[147] single and multicenter paramedics,[69,148,34] and emergency medicine and anesthesia attendings.[149] In a recent multicenter prospective trial, the success rate of endotracheal intubation across providers for out-of-hospital intubation was 86.8%.[34] In a comprehensive review of cardiac arrest during 3000 emergent intubations, 60 deaths (2%) were reported, of which only 32% of patients were intubated on the first attempt. Even in patients intubated on the first attempt, over 33% experienced profound hypoxemia.[1] Unrecognized, misplaced intubation represents a potentially lethal subset of failed intubation. Rates of prehospital misplaced intubation, primarily esophageal, reported in the multiple studies evaluating this complication range from 0.4% to 25%, with most documenting rates of less than 10%.[150] In a review of over 1600 intubations by paramedics, only 2% were unrecognized failed intubations, but 57% of the failures were in trauma patients.[69]

## Esophageal Intubation

Esophageal intubation, comprising a subset of intubation failure, can represent a minor or catastrophic complication, depending on time of recognition. Early recognition is facilitated by lack of appropriate color change on colorimetry, desaturation, lack of breath sounds over bilateral lung fields, and auscultation of inspired air over the epigastrium. The incidence of esophageal intubation is unknown, as it is likely underreported if recognition is not delayed. The incidence of unrecognized esophageal intubation ranges from 0% in small series[146,151] to 10%. Under urgent circumstances, this complication contributes to hypoxemia, regurgitation, aspiration, bradycardia, cardiac dysrrhythmias, and cardiac arrest.[144] When esophageal intubation is proven, or suspected, it is imperative to rapidly remove the tube and reintubate.

## Aspiration

Due to the urgent and unplanned nature of airway control in injured and critically ill patients, pulmonary aspiration of gastric contents represents a feared and morbid complication. The untoward effects of aspiration range from obscuration of vocal cords during intubation to death secondary to failed intubation, chemical pneumonitis with acute respiratory distress syndrome, and pneumonia. Studies of emergent airway management have reported the incidence of aspiration to range from 1% to 20%, depending on the patient population and environment.[152] The few studies focusing on the prehospital setting have reported an aspiration incidence of 34% to 39%.[153,154] A recent study, using pepsin assay of tracheal aspirates, identified an aspiration incidence of 22% for urgent intubations in the emergency department compared to 50% in the prehospital environment.[152]

## Pneumonia

Emergency intubation has been identified as a risk factor for pneumonia after trauma, likely related to pulmonary aspiration during the procedure. In a review of 99 patients with early onset ventilator associated pneumonia (VAP), multivariate regression identified emergency intubation and aspiration as factors independently associated with multidrug resistant infections.[155] The incidence of pneumonia is significantly higher after a field versus emergency department airway[156] and has been independently associated with RSI performed by paramedics.[157]

## REFERENCES

1. Mort TC: The incidence and risk factors for cardiac arrest during emergency tracheal intubation: A justification for incorporating the ASA guidelines in the remote location. J Clin Anesth 16:508, 2004.
2. Schmidt U, Frame SB, Nerlich ML, et al.: On-scene helicopter transport of patients with multiple injuries: A comparison of a German and American system. J Trauma 33:548, 1992.
3. Krantz BE: Advanced Trauma Life Support for Doctors, American College of Surgeons, Committee on Trauma, Advanced Trauma Life Support (ATLS) Course. 7th ed., Chicago, IL, 2004.
4. Roberts JR: Clinical Procedures in Emergency Medicine, 4th ed., Philadelphia, PA: Saunders, 2004, p. 71.
5. Kaide CG, Hollingsworth JC, Stafford PW: Current strategies for airway management of the trauma patient. Trauma Reports 4:1, 2003.
6. Kaide CG, Hollingsworth JC, Stafford PW: Current strategies for airway management of the trauma patient, part II: Managing difficult and failed airways. Trauma Reports 4:1, 2003.
7. McSwain NE, Frame S, eds: Pre-Hospital Trauma Life Support (PHTLS), 5th ed. St. Louis, MO: Mosby, 2003, p. 98.
8. Bledsoe BE, Porter RS, Shade BR, eds: Paramedic Emergency Care, 2nd ed.. Brady, NJ: Englewood, 1994, p. 228.
9. Barnes TA, MacDonald D, Nolan J, et al.: Airway devices. Ann Emer Med 37:S145, 2001.
10. Marini JJ, Wheeler AP, eds: Critical Care Medicine-The Essentials, 2nd ed. Baltimore, MD: Williams & Wilkins, 1997, p. 107.
11. Deakin CD, Sado DM, Coats TJ, et al.: Prehospital end-tidaly carbon dioxide concentration and outcome in major trauma. J Trauma 57:65, 2004.
12. Zimmerman JL, ed: Fundamental Critical Care Support (FCCS), 3d ed. Des Plaines, IL: Society of Critical Medicine (SCCM), 2002, p. 2.
13. Hazinski MF, Chameides L, Elling B, et al.: Adjuncts for airway control and ventilation. Circulation 112:IV-51, 2005.
14. Stoneham MD: The nasopharyngeal airway: Assessment of position by fiber optic laryngoscopy. Anesthesia 48:575, 1993.
15. Schade K, Borzotta A, Michaels A: Intracranial malposition of nasopharyngeal airway. J Trauma 49:967, 2000.
16. Blanda M, Gallo U: Emergency airway management. Emerg Med Clin N Am 21:1, 2003.
17. Butler KH, Clyne B: Management of the difficult airway: Alternative airway techniques and adjuncts. Emerg Med Clin N Am 21:259, 2003.
18. Levitan RM, Everett WW, Ochroch EA: Limitations of difficult airway prediction in patients intubated in the emergency department. Ann Emer Med 44:307, 2004.
19. Dunham CM, Barraco RD, Clark DE, et al.: Guidelines for emergency tracheal intubation immediately after traumatic injury. J Trauma 55:162, 2003.
20. Kovacs G, Law JA, Ross J, et al.: Acute airway management in the emergency department by non-anesthesiologists. Can J Anaesth 51:174, 2004.
21. Pearson S: Comparison of intubation attempts and completion times before and after the initiation of a rapid sequence intubation protocol in an air medical transport program. Air Med J 22:28, 2003.
22. Bair AE, Filbin MR, Kulkarni RG, et al.: The failed intubation attempt in the emergency department: Analysis of prevalence, rescue techniques, and personnel. J Emerg Med 23:131, 2002.
23. Jones JH, Weaver CS, Rusyniak DE, et al.: Impact of emergency medicine faculty and an airway protocol on airway management. Acad Emerg Med 9:1452, 2002.
24. Bernard S, Smith K, Foster S, et al.: The use of rapid sequence intubation by ambulance paramedics for patients with severe head injury. Emerg Med 14: 406, 2002.
25. Bulger EM, Copass MK, Maier RV, et al.: An analysis of advanced prehospital airway management. J Emerg Med 23:183, 2002.

26. Zonies DH, Rotondo MF, Sing RF, et al.: The safety of urgent paralysis and intubation (UPI) in the trauma admitting area (TAA): A review of 570 consecutive patients. *J Trauma* 44:431, 1998.
27. Rotondo MF, McGonigal MD, Schwab CW, et al.: Urgent paralysis and intubation of trauma patients: Is it safe? *J Trauma* 34:242, 1993.
28. Reynolds SF, Heffner J: Airway management of the critically ill patient rapid-sequence intubation. *Chest* 127:1397, 2005.
29. Smith CE, Kovach B, Polk JD, et al.: Prehospital tracheal intubating conditions during rapid sequence intubation: Rocuronium versus vecuronium. *Air Med J* 21:26, 2002.
30. Sing RF, Rotondo MF, Zonies DH, et al.: Rapid sequence induction for intubation by an aeromedial transport team: A critical analysis. *Am J Emerg Med* 16:598, 1998.
31. Sagarin MJ, Barton ED, Chng YM: Airway management by US and Canadian emergency medicine residents: A multicenter analysis of more than 6,000 endotracheal intubation attempts. *Ann Emerg Med* 46:328, 2005.
32. Dibble C, Maloba M: Best evidence topic report. Rapid sequence induction in the emergency department by emergency medicine personnel. *Emerg Med J* 23:62, 2006.
33. Walls RM: Rapid sequence intubation. In Walls RM, Murphy MF, Luten RC, Schneider RE, eds. *Manual of Emergency Airway Management*, 2nd ed. Philadelphia: Lippincott, Williams & Wilkins, 2004, p. 24.
34. Wang HE, Kupas DF, Paris PM, et al.: Preliminary experience with a prospective, multi-centered evaluation of out-of-hospital endotracheal intubation. *Resuscitation* 58:49, 2003.
35. Singh S, Smith JE: Cardiovascular changes after the three stages of nasotracheal intubation. *Br J Anaesth* 91:667, 2003.
36. Tong JL, Ashworth DR, Smith JE: Cardiovascular reponses following laryngoscopic assisted, fiberoptic orotracheal intubation. *Anaesthesia* 60:754, 2005.
37. Sivilotti ML, Ducharme J: Randomized, double-blind study on sedatives and hemodynamics during rapid-sequence intubation in the emergency department: The SHRED study. *Ann Emerg Med* 31:313, 1998.
38. Tagaito Y, Isono S, Nishino T: Upper airway reflexes during a combination of propofol and fentanyl anesthesia. *Anesthesiology* 88:1433, 1998.
39. Robinson N, Clancy M: In patients with head injury undergoing rapid sequence intubation, does pretreatment with intravenous lignocaine/lidocaine lead to an improved neurologic outcome? A review of the literature. *Emerg Med J* 18:453, 2001.
40. Lev R, Rosen P: Prophylactic lidocaine use preintubation: A review. *J Emerg Med* 12:499, 1994.
41. Schreiber JW, Lysakowski C, Fuchs-Buder T, et al.: Prevention of succinylcholine-induced fasciculation and myalgia: A meta-analysis of randomized trials. *Anesthesiology* 103:877, 2005.
42. Kindler CH, Schumacher PG, Schneider MC, et al.: Effects of intravenous lidocaine and/or esmolol on hemodynamic responses to laryngoscopy and intubation: A double-blind, controlled trial. *J Clin Anesth* 8:491, 1996.
43. Feng CK, Chan KH, Liu KN, et al.: A comparison of lidocaine, fentanyl, and esmolol for attenuation of cardiovascular response to laryngoscopy and tracheal intubation. *Acta Anaesthesiol Sin* 34:61, 1996.
44. Rodricks MB, Deutschman CS: Emergent airway management: Indications and methods in the face of confounding conditions. *Crit Care Clinics* 16:389, 2000.
45. Cohan P, Wang C, McArthur DL, et al.: Acute secondary adrenal insufficiency after traumatic brain injury: A prospective study. *Crit Care Med* 33:2358, 2005.
46. Malerba G, Romano-Girard F, Cravoisy A, et al.: Risk factors of relative adrenocortical deficiency in intensive care patients needing mechanical ventilation. *Intensive Care Med* 31:388, 2005.
47. Jackson WL Jr: Should we use etomidate as an induction agent for endotracheal intubation in patients with septic shock?: A critical appraisal. *Chest* 127:1031, 2005.
48. El-Orbany MI, Wafai Y, Joseph NJ, et al.: Does the choice of intravenous induction drug affect intubation conditions after a fast-onset neuromuscular blocker? *J Clin Anesth* 15:9, 2003.
49. Sivilotti ML, Filbin MR, Murray HE, et al.: Does the sedative agent facilitate emergency rapid sequence intubation? *Acad Emerg Med*, 10:612, 2003.
50. Sonday CJ, Axelband J, Jacoby J, et al.: Thiopental vs. etomidate for rapid sequence intubation in aeromedicine. *Prehospital Disaster Med* 20:324, 2005.
51. Lee BS, Gausche-Hill M: Pediatric airway management. *CPEM* 2:91, 2001.
52. Marvez E, Weiss SJ, Houry DE, et al.: Predicting adverse outcomes on a diagnosis-based protocol system for rapid sequence intubation. *Am J Emerg Med* 21:23, 2003.
53. Thompson JD, Fish S, Ruiz E: Succinylcholne for endotracheal intubation. *Ann Emerg Med* 11:526, 1982.
54. Brown EM, Krishnaprasad D, Smiler BG: Pancuronium for rapid induction technique for tracheal intubation. *Can Anaesth Soc J* 26:489, 1979.
55. Bozeman WP, Kleiner DM, Huggett V: A comparison of rapid-sequence intubation and etomidate-only intubation in the prehospital air medical setting. *Prehosp Emerg Care* 10:8, 2006.
56. Davis DP, Ochs M, Hoyt DB, et al.: Paramedic administered neuromuscular blockade improves prehospital intubation success in severely head-injured patients. *J Trauma* 54:444, 2003.
57. Naguib M, Samarkandi A, Riad W, et al.: Optimal dose of succinylcholine revisited. *Anesthesiology* 99:1045, 2003.
58. Schuh FT: The neuromuscular blocking action of suxamethonium following intravenous and intramuscular administration. *Int J Clin Pharmacol Ther Toxicol* 20:399, 1982.
59. MacLennan N, Heimbach DM, Cullen BF: Anesthesia for major thermal injury. *Anesthesiology* 89:749, 1998.
60. Gronert GA: Cardiac arrest after succinylcholine: Mortality greater with rhabdomyolysis than receptor upregulation. *Anesthesiology* 94:523, 2001.
61. Vachon CA, Warner DO, Bacon DR: Succinylcholine and the open globe. Tracing the teaching. *Anesthesiology* 99:220, 2003.
62. Perry J, Lee J, Wells G: Rocuronium versus succinylcholine for rapid sequence induction intubation. *Cochrane Database Syst Rev* 1:CD002788, 2003.
63. Sluga M, Ummenhofer W, Studer W, et al.: Rocuronium versus succinylcholine for rapid sequence induction of anesthesia and endotracheal intubation: A prospective, randomized trial in emergent cases. *Anesth Analg* 101:1356, 2005.
64. Morris J, Cook TM: Rapid sequence induction: A national survey of practice. *Anaesthesia* 56:1090, 2001.
65. Tournadre JP, Chassard D, Berrada KR, et al.: Cricoid cartilage pressure decreases lower esophageal sphincter tone. *Anesthesiology* 867, 1997.
66. Smith CE, Boyer D: Cricoid pressure decreases ease of tracheal intubation using fiberoptic laryngoscopy (WuScope System). *Can J Anaesth* 49:614, 2002.
67. Turgeon AF, Nicole PC, Trepanier CA, et al.: Cricoid pressure does not increase the rate of failed intubation by direct laryngoscopy in adults. *Anesthesiology* 102:315, 2005.
68. Olsen JC, Gurr DE, Hughes M: Video analysis of emergency residents performing rapid-sequence intubations. *J Emerg Med* 18:469, 2000.
69. Bair AE, Smith D, Lichty L: Intubation confirmation techniques associated with unrecognized non-tracheal intubations by pre-hospital providers. *J Emerg Med* 28:403, 2005.
70. Puntervoll SA, Soreide E, Jacewicz, Bjelland E: Rapid detection of oesophageal intubation: Take care when using calorimetric capnometry. *Acta Anaesthesiol Scand* 46:455, 2002.
71. Grmec S. Comparison of three different methods to confirm tracheal tube placement in emergency intubation. *Intensive Care Med* 28:701, 2002.
72. Sagarin MJ, Chiang V, Sakles JC, et al.: Rapid sequence intubation for pediatric emergency airway management. *Pediatr Emerg Care* 18:417, 2002.
73. Butler FS, Cirillio AA: Retrograde endotracheal intubation. *Anesth Analg* 39:333, 1960.
74. Van Stralen DW, Rogers M, Perkin RM, et al.: Retrograde intubation training using a mannequin. *Am J Emerg Med* 13:50, 1995.
75. Stern Y, Spitzer T: Retrograde intubation of the trachea. *J Laryngol Otol* 105:746, 1991.
76. Barriot P, Riou B: Retrograde technique for tracheal intubation in trauma patients. *Crit Care Med* 16:712, 1988.
77. Gill M, Madden MJ, Green SM: Retrograde endotracheal intubation: An investigation of indications, complications, and patient outcomes. *Am J Emerg Med* 23:123, 2005.
78. Weksler N, Klein M, Weksler D, et al.: Retrograde tracheal intubation: Beyond fibreoptic endotracheal intubation. *Acta Anaesthesiol Scand* 48:412, 2004.
79. Caplan RA, Benumof JL, Berry FA, et al.: Practice guidelines for management of the difficult airway. An updated report by the American Society of Anesthesiologist Task Force on management of the difficult airway. *Anesthesiology* 98:1269, 2003.
80. Bair AE, Laurin EG, Schmitt BJ: An assessment of a tracheal tube introducer as an endotracheal tube placement confirmation device. *Am J Emerg Med* 23:754, 2005.
81. Jabre P, Combes X, Leroux B, et al.: Use of gum elastic bougie for prehospital difficult intubation. *Am J Emerg Med* 23:552, 2005.
82. Samsoon GLT, Young JRB: Difficult tracheal intubation. *Anaestheia* 42:487, 1987.
83. Matioc AA, Wells JA: The LMA-Unique in a prehospital trauma patient: Interaction with a semirigid cervical collar: A case report. *J Trauma* 521:162, 2002.
84. Martin SE, Ochsner MG, Jarman RH, et al.: Use of the laryngeal mask airway in air transport when intubation fails. *J Trauma* 47:352, 1999.
85. Calkins MD, Robinson TD: Combat trauma airway management: Endotracheal intubation versus laryngeal mask airway versus combitube use by Navy SEAL and Reconnaissance combat corpsmen. *J Trauma* 46:927, 1999.

86. Asai T, Murao K, Shingu K: Efficacy of the ProSeal laryngeal mask airway during manual in-line stabilisation of the neck. *Anaesthesia* 57:918, 2002.

87. Cook TM, Silsby J, Simpson TP: Airway rescue in acute upper airway obstruction using a ProSeal laryngeal mask airway and an Aintree catheter: A review of the ProSeal laryngeal mask airway in the management of the difficult airway. *Anaesthesia* 60:1129, 2005.

88. Swanson ER, Fosnocht DE, Matthews K, et al.: Comparison of the intubating laryngeal mask airway versus laryngoscopy in the Bell 206-L3 EMS helicopter. *Air Med J* 23:36, 2004.

89. Ferson DZ, Rosenblatt WH, Johansen MJ, et al.: Use of the intubating LMA-Fastrach in 254 patients with difficult-to-manage airways. *Anesthesiology* 95:1175, 2001.

90. Chan TV, Grillone G: Vocal cord paralysis after laryngeal mask airway ventilation. *Laryngoscope* 115:1436, 2005.

91. Bein B, Scholz J: Supraglottic airway devices. *Best Pract Res Clin Anaesthesiol* 19:581, 2005.

92. Ocker H, Wenzel V, Schmucker P, et al.: A comparison of the laryngeal tube with the laryngeal mask airway during routine surgical procedures. *Anesth Analg* 95:1094, 2002.

93. Asai T, Shingu K: The laryngeal tube. *Br J Anaesth* 95:729, 2005.

94. Szmuk P, Ezri T, Akca O, et al.: Use of a new supraglottic airway device—the CobraPLA—in a "difficult to intubate/difficult to ventilate" scenario. *Acta Anaesthesiol Scand* 49:421, 2005.

95. Turan A, Kaya G, Koyuncu O, et al.: Comparison of the laryngeal mask (LMA™) and laryngeal tube (LT®) with the new perilaryngeal airway (CobraPLA®) in short surgical procedures. *Eur J Anaesthesiol* 23:234, 2006.

96. Gaitini L, Yanovski B, Somri M, et al.: A comparison between the PLA Cobra and the laryngeal mask airway unique during spontaneous ventilation: A randomized prospective study. *Anesth Analg* 102:631, 2006.

97. Agro F, Carassiti M, Magnani C, et al.: Airway control via the CobraPLA during percutaneous dilational tracheostomy in five patients. *Can J Anaesth* 52:418, 2005.

98. Szmuk P, Ezri T, Narwani A, et al.: Use of CobraPLA as a conduit for intubation in a child with neck instability. *Paediatr Anaesth* 16:217, 2006.

99. Wright MJ, Greenberg DE, Hunt JP, et al.: Surgical cricothyroidotomy in trauma patients. *South Med J* 96:465, 2003.

100. Isaacs JH Jr, Pederson AD: Emergency cricothyroidotomy. *Am Surg* 63:346, 1997.

101. Salvino CK, Dries D, Gamelli R, et al.: Emergency cricothyroidotomy in trauma victims. *J Trauma* 34:503, 1993.

102. Jacobson LE, Gomez GA, Sobieray RJ, et al.: Surgical Cricothyroidotomy in trauma patients: An analysis of its use by paramedics in the field. *J Trauma* 41:15, 1996.

103. Verschueren DS, Bell RB, Bagheri SC, et al.: Management of laryngo-tracheal injuries associated with craniomaxillofacial trauma. *J Oral Maxillofac Surg* 64:203, 2006.

104. Hohorieder M, Hinterhoelzl J, Ulmer H, et al.: Maxillofacial fractures masking traumatic intracranial hemorrhages. *Int J Oral Maxillofac Surg* 33:389, 2004.

105. Tsakiris P, Cleaton-Jones PE, Lownie MA: Airway status in civilian maxillofacial gunshot injuries in Johannesburg, South Africa. *S Afr Med J* 92:803, 2002.

106. Hollier L, Grantcharova EP, Kattash M: Facial gunshot wounds: A 4-year experience. *J Oral Maxillofac Surg* 59:277, 2001.

107. Bhojani RA, Rosenbaum DH, Dikmen E, et al.: Contemporary assessment of laryngotracheal trauma. *J Thorac Cardiovasc Surg* 130:426, 2005.

108. Kuttenberger JJ, Hardt N, Schlegel C: Diagnosis and initial management of laryngotracheal injuries associated with facial fractures. *J Craniomaxillofac Surg* 32:80, 2004.

109. Goudy SL, Miller FB, Bumpous JM: Neck crepitance: Evaluation and management of suspected upper aerodigestive tract injury. *Laryngoscope* 112:791, 2002.

110. Rudolph C, Schneider JP, Wallenborn J, et al.: Movement of the upper cervical spine during laryngoscopy: A comparison of the Bonfils intubation fibrescope and the Macintosh laryngoscope. *Anaesthesia* 60:668, 2005.

111. Turkstra TP, Craen RA, Pelz DM, et al.: Cervical spine motion: A fluoroscopic comparison during intubation with lighted stylet, GlideScope, and Macintosh laryngoscope. *Anesth Analg* 101:910, 2005.

112. Sahin A, Salman MA, Erden IA, et al.: Upper cervical vertebrae movement during intubating laryngeal mask, fibreoptic, and direct laryngoscopy: A video-fluoroscopic study. *Eur J Anaesthesiol* 21:819, 2004.

113. Wahlen BM, Gercek E: Three-dimensional cervical spine movement during intubation using the Macintosh and Bullard laryngoscopes, the bonfils fibrescope and the intubating laryngeal mask airway. *Eur J Anaesthesiol* 21:907, 2004.

114. Waltl B, Melischek M, Schuschnig C, et al.: Tracheal intubation and cervical spine excursion: Direct laryngoscopy vs. intubating laryngeal mask. *Anesthesia* 56:221, 2001.

115. Lennarson PJ, Smith DW, Sawin PD, et al.: Cervical spine motion during intubation: Efficacy of stabilization maneuvers in the setting of complete segmental instability. *J Neurosurg* 94:265, 2001.

116. Rocker GM: Acute respiratory distress syndrome: Different syndromes, different therapies? *Crit Care Med* 29:202, 2001.

117. American Burn Association: Inhalational injury: Diagnosis. *J Am Coll Surg* 196:307, 2003.

118. Miller K, Chang A: Acute inhalational injury. *Emerg Med Clin North Am* 21:533, 2003.

119. Rabinowitz PM, Siegel MD: Acute inhalation injury. *Clin Chest Med* 23:707, 2003.

120. Tsoutsos D, Rodopoulou S, Keramidas E: Early escharotomy as a measure to reduce intraabdominal hypertension in full-thickness burns of the thoracic and abdominal area. *World J Surg* 27:1323, 2003.

121. Davis DP, Dunford JV, Poste JC, et al.: The impact of hypoxia and hyperventilation on outcome after paramedic rapid sequence intubation of severely head-injured patients. *J Trauma* 57:1, 2004.

122. Brain Trauma Foundation. Guidelines for prehospital management of traumatic brain injury. http://www.braintrauma.org. Accessed January 13, 2006.

123. Wang HE, Peitzman AB, Cassidy LD, et al.: Out-of-hospital endotracheal intubation and outcome after traumatic brain injury. *Ann Emerg Med* 44:439, 2004.

124. Davis DP, Hoyt DB, Ochs M: The effect of paramedic rapid sequence intubation on outcome in patients with severe traumatic brain injury. *J Trauma* 54:444, 2003.

125. Gausche M, Lewis RJ, Stratton SJ, et al.: Effect of out-of-hospital pediatric endotracheal intubation on survival and neurological outcome : A controlled clinical trial. *JAMA* 283:783, 2000.

126. Bulger EM, Copass MK, Sabath DR, et al.: The use of neuromuscular blocking agents to facilitate prehospital intubation does not impair outcome after traumatic brain injury. *J Trauma* 58:718, 2005.

127. Bozeman WP, Idris AH: Intracranial pressure changes during rapid sequence intubation: A swine model. *J Trauma* 58:278, 2005.

128. Davis DP, Dunford JV, Ochs M, et al.: The use of quantitative end-tidal capnometry to avoid inadvertent severe hyperventilation in patients with head injury after paramedic rapid sequence intubation. *J Trauma* 56:808, 2004.

129. Davis DP, Heister R, Poste JC, et al.: Ventilation patterns in patients with severe traumatic brain injury following paramedic rapid sequence intubation. *Neurocrit Care* 2:165, 2005.

130. Dunford JV, Davis DP, Ochs M, et al.: Incidence of transient hypoxia and pulse rate reactivity during paramedic rapid sequence intubation. *Ann Emerg Med* 42:721, 2003.

131. Orenstein JB: Prehospital pediatric airway management. *CPEM* 7:31, 2006.

132. Mandell DL: Traumatic emergencies involving the pediatric airway. *CPEM* 6:41, 2005.

133. Sing RF, Reilly PM, Rotondo MF, et al.: Out-of-hospital rapid-sequence induction for intubation in the pediatric patient. *Acad Emerg Med* 3:41, 1996.

134. Zelicof-Paul A, Smith-Lockridge A, Schnadower D, et al.: Controversies in rapid sequence intubation in children. *Curr Opin Pediatr* 17:355, 2005.

135. Fastle RK, Roback MG: Pediatric rapid sequence intubation: Incidence of reflex bradycardia and effects of pretreatment with atropine. *Pediatr Emerg Care* 20:651, 2004.

136. Navsa N, Tossel G, Boon JM: Dimensions of the neonatal cricothyroid membrane—how feasible is a surgical cricothyroidotomy? *Paediatr Anaesth* 15:402, 2005.

137. Peak DA, Roy S: Needle cricothyroidotomy revisited. *Pediatr Emerg Care* 15:224, 1999.

138. Goldman K, Roettger C, Wulf H: Use the ProSeal laryngeal mask airway for pressure-controlled ventilation with and without positive end-expiratory pressure in paediatric patients: A randomized, controlled study. *Br J Anaesth* 95:831, 2005.

139. Bortone L, Ingelmo PM, De Ninno G, et al.: Randomized controlled trial comparing the laryngeal tube and the laryngeal mask in pediatric patients. *Paediatr Anaesth*, 16:251, 2006.

140. Walls RM, Murphy MF, Luten RC, Schneider RE, eds: *Manual of Emergency Airway Management*, 2nd ed. Philadelphia: Lippincott, Williams & Wilkins, 2004, p. 70.

141. Mallampati SR, Gatt SP, Gugino LD, et al.: A clinical sign to predict difficult tracheal intubation. A prospective study. *Can Anaesth Soc J* 32:429, 1985.

142. Watson CB: Prediction of difficult intubation. *Resp Care* 44:777, 1999.

143. Reeder TJ, Brown CK, Norris DL: Managing the difficult airway: A survey of residency directors and a call for change. *J Emerg Med* 28:473, 2005.

144. Mort TC: Emergency tracheal intubation: Complications associated with repeated laryngoscopic attempts. *Anesth Analg* 99:607, 2004.

145. Dorges V: Airway management in emergency situations. *Best Pract Res Clin Anaesthesiol* 19:699, 2005.

146. Pratt JC, Hirshberg AJ: Endotracheal tube placement by EMT-basics in a rural EMS system. *Prehosp Emerg Care* 9:172, 2005.

147. Levitan RM, Rosenblatt B, Meiner EM, et al.: Alternating day emergency medicine and anesthesia resident responsibility for management of the trauma

airway: A study of laryngoscopy performance and intubation success. *Ann Emerg Med* 43:48, 2004.

148. Slagt C, Zondervan A, Patka P: A retrospective analysis of the intubations performed during 5 years of helicopter emergency medical service in Amsterdam. *Air Med J* 23:36, 2004.

149. Mackay CA, Terris J, Coats TJ: Prehospital rapid sequence induction by emergency physicians: Is it safe? *Emerg Med J*, 18:20, 2001.

150. Silvestri S, Ralls GA, Krauss B, et al.: The effectiveness of out-of-hospital use of continuous end-tidal carbon dioxide monitoring on the rate of unrecognized misplaced intubation within a regional emergency medical services system. *Ann Emerg Med* 45:497, 2005.

151. Davis DP, Fisher R, Buono C, et al.: Predictors of intubation success and therapeutic value of paramedic airway management in a large, urban EMS system. *Prehosp Emerg Care* 10:356, 2006.

152. Ufberg JW, Bushra JS, Karras DJ, et al.: Aspiration of gastric contents: Association with prehospital intubation. *Am J Emerg Med* 23:379, 2005.

153. Lockey DJ, Coats T, Parr MJ: Aspiration in severe trauma: A prospective study. *Anaesthesia* 54:1097, 1999.

154. Oswalt JL, Hedges JR, Soifer BE, et al.: Analysis of trauma intubations. *Am J Emerg Med* 10:511, 1992.

155. Akca O, Koltka K, Uzel S, et al.: Risk factors for early-onset, ventilator-associated pneumonia in critical care patients: Selected multiresistant versus nonresistant bacteria. *Anesthesiology* 93:638, 2000.

156. Eckert MJ, Davis KA, Reed RL II, et al.: Urgent airways after trauma: Who get pneumonia? *J Trauma* 57:750, 2004.

157. Davis DP, Stern J, Sise MJ: A follow-up analysis of factors associated with head-injury mortality after paramedic rapid sequence intubation. *J Trauma* 59:486, 2005.

# Commentary ■ RONALD I. GROSS

There are few aspects in the care of the acutely injured patient, short of a traumatic arrest, that cause more angst and trepidation than airway management. Toschlog, Sagraves, and Rotondo captured the very essence of the issue when they stated, "Not only are hypoxia and hypoventilation common injury-related causes of mortality, they additionally represent one of the most common causes of *preventable* mortality following injury." The authors appropriately pointed out that the incidence of severe hypoxia preceding cardiac arrest is 90% in all emergency airway procedures performed outside the operating room, highlighting the urgency that that must be given to the appropriate and immediate management of the airway of the trauma patient.

Throughout the chapter, the authors have emphasized the basic tenet espoused in all of the advanced life support courses (PHTLS, ATLS, PALS, ABLS); airway and breathing must be the primary focus of attention for any health care giver providing life-saving care to the injured patient. Evaluation and resuscitation of the trauma patient begins with airway management, and does not proceed any further until airway and breathing have been insured.

The concept of tracheal intubation is by no means a new one. In fact, the first documented report of tracheal intubation dates back to 1543, and actually refers to a tracheostomy. In his atlas *On the Fabric of the Human Body*, the Renaissance anatomist Anreas Vesalius observed, "Life may, in a manner of speaking, be restored. An opening must be attempted in the trunk of the trachea into which a reed or cane should be put; you will then blow into this so that the lung may rise again."[1] In this chapter, the authors have managed to distill the basic elements of achieving this opening into the trachea (airway control) into an organized and practical approach that can be adapted to all levels of expertise and resource availability.

The success of achieving and maintaining a definitive and protected airway is dependent on many factors, but perhaps the most important step in the process is the recognition that the patient and/or provider is incapable of providing and maintaining a protected airway without intervention. Throughout this chapter, the authors have provided excellent guides to the assessment of the airway, and the concepts, personnel, equipment, and maneuvers necessary to achieve airway control under almost any circumstance.

A successful outcome depends on the operators experience and on having immediate access to all the correct equipment. The importance of advanced preparation and a team approach to airway management have been properly reinforced, and explicit protocols have been provided that serve to highlight the chapter as a valuable resource to even the most experienced of clinicians. For example, the authors' comprehensive and thorough review of the medications commonly used for RSI, including their advantages, disadvantages, and potential complications, as well as the indications for their use, is excellent in its scope, and provides both the novice and expert with useful information that can be applied to the clinical arena with ease.

Endotracheal intubation (ETI) remains the accepted standard as the definitive airway in the injured patient. However, ETI may fail even in the most expert of hands. Fortunately, there are now several "rescue" techniques that are available to ensure our ability to oxygenate and ventilate in the absence of the successful placement of an endotracheal tube. Toshlog et al. have provided the reader with a comprehensive review of the use of the three most useful airway rescue tools that that are becoming commonplace in both the prehospital and the emergency room setting: the CombiTube; the Laryngeal Mask Airway (LMA) and intubating LMA; and the gum elastic bougie (GEB). All three of these tools can be used when laryngoscopic visualization and orotracheal intubation are impaired or impossible, or when intubating skills (or tools) are lacking. The indications, contraindications, and the rationale for the use of each adjunct are clearly presented, leaving the reader with a clear understanding of the alternatives available should intubation be necessary but unsuccessful.

The surgical cricothyroidotomy is most often used after all attempts at orotracheal intubation have failed. While the authors discuss the techniques of percutaneous tracheostomy and retrograde endotracheal intubation, these procedures are, in fact, not indicated in the true emergency situation; as the authors state, "The greatest impediment to cricothyroidotomy is the recognition that it is necessary." The cricothyroidotomy procedure is presented to the reader in a manner that provides even the most inexperienced clinician a vivid verbal picture of the technique, as well as potential complications that need to be anticipated and prevented.

Although management of the potentially difficult airway in the adult trauma resuscitation room can certainly be stressful and anxiety-provoking, management of the difficult pediatric airway in an emergency situation tends to raise the stress on all providers to the highest levels, due not only to the anatomical differences and physical constraints of the pediatric patient, but to the emotional and visceral reactions elicited by the badly injured child. This chapter deals with issues in airway control of the pediatric airway that are rarely dealt with in such a detailed manner in the standard surgical text. As with the adult airway, not all institutions will have all the equipment, nor will all institutions have appropriately trained personnel. This chapter will certainly provide the clinician with the information needed to understand exactly what one would need for equipment and individual training.

As I have been stated previously, every clinician needs to train and be prepared to manage the emergency airway, regardless of where we might find our skills necessary. All the equipment in the world will be to no avail without extensive individual training that provides the clinician with an excellent, instinctual command of the procedural and technical aspects of airway management. While "on-the-job" training has been the way that most of us have trained in the past, I believe that extensive training in the simulated environment is an imperative that we should all impose on ourselves and on our colleagues. That, coupled with a chapter of the superior quality provided in this text, will go a very long way to insure our ability to alleviate pain and suffering while we do no further harm.

## Reference

1. Vesalius A: *de Humani Corporis Fabrica Libris Septum.* Basel: Oporinus, 1543, p. 658

# Management of Shock

*Brian G. Harbrecht* ■ *Raquel M. Forsythe* ■ *Andrew B. Peitzman*

Shock has been defined in a variety of ways over the hundreds of years that man has inflicted injury upon his fellow man. Most trauma surgeons can recognize the patient in fulminant shock, but creating a useful working definition for shock that incorporates all the relevant clinical and pathophysiological features has proven to be more difficult. Gross defined shock as a "rude unhinging of the machinery of life"[1] but his characterization, while accurate, does not fully reflect the significant tissue and cellular changes that occur. Shock is not simply a disturbance of one parameter of homeostasis such as blood pressure. Significant hypoperfusion and impending cellular death may be present despite normal systemic blood pressure, so equating shock with hypotension and cardiovascular collapse is a vast oversimplification. Shock is most precisely defined as a condition of inadequate delivery of the oxygen and nutrients that are necessary for normal tissue and cellular function. The rapid recognition of the patient in shock and the reflexive institution of steps to correct shock is a basic and essential skill for the trauma surgeon. Surgeons caring for injured patients should be prepared to initiate active treatment prior to a definitive diagnosis of the cause of shock and, at times, prior to absolute proof that shock is even present.

The management of the patient in shock has been an integral component of the surgeon's realm of expertise for centuries. The treatment of wounds and injuries can be traced to ancient times, but the understanding of clinical factors associated with shock and essential steps in its management made significant progress only in the late 19th and early 20th centuries. Claude Bernard suggested that an organism attempts to maintain constancy in the internal environment despite external forces that attempt to disrupt the "milieu interie."[2] In the intact animal, the failure of physiologic systems to buffer the organism against these external forces results in what we call the *shock state*. Walter B. Cannon made several significant contributions in the early 20th century to our understanding of shock. He described the "fight or flight response" generated by elevated levels of catecholamines in the bloodstream and introduced the term homeostasis in 1926. Cannon spent two years on the battlefields of Europe and published his classic monograph, *Traumatic Shock,* in 1923. Cannon's observations led him to propose that shock was due to a disturbance of the nervous system which resulted in vasodilatation and hypotension. He proposed that secondary shock with its attendant capillary permeability leak was caused by a "toxic factor" released from the tissue.[3,4] Interestingly, Cannon is also credited with first proposing deliberate hypotension in patients with penetrating wounds of the torso to minimize internal bleeding since "if the pressure is raised before the surgeon is ready to check the bleeding that may take place, blood that is sorely needed may be lost."[5]

Alfred Blalock generated key contributions to our understanding of shock during his time at Vanderbilt. In a series of elegant experiments, Blalock documented that shock after hemorrhage was associated with reduced cardiac output and that hemorrhagic shock was due to volume loss, not a "toxic factor."[6] He also noted, however, that toxins could be important initiators of shock. In 1934, Blalock proposed the following four categories of shock that continue to be utilized today: hypovolemic, vasogenic, cardiogenic, and neurogenic (Table 13-1).[6] Hypovolemic shock, the most common type, results from loss of circulating blood or its components. Therefore, loss of circulating volume may be due to decreased whole blood (hemorrhagic shock), plasma, interstitial fluid, or a combination thereof. Vasogenic shock as seen in sepsis results from decreased resistance to blood flow within capacitance vessels of the circulatory system causing an effective decrease in circulating volume. Neurogenic shock is a form of vasogenic shock in which spinal cord injury (or spinal anesthesia) causes vasodilatation. Cardiogenic shock results from failure of the pump function as may occur with arrhythmias or acute heart failure. Two additional categories of shock have been added to those originally proposed by Blalock. Obstructive shock is present when circulatory flow is mechanically impeded as with pulmonary embolism or a tension pneumothorax. Laboratory experiments and clinical experience

**TABLE 13-1**

| Forms of Shock |
| --- |
| Hypovolemic |
| Cardiogenic |
| Neurogenic |
| Inflammatory (Septic) |
| Obstructive |
| Traumatic |

have also confirmed the appropriateness of Cannon's proposal of traumatic shock as a unique entity. Injuries to soft tissue and fractures of long bones that occur in association with multisystem trauma can produce an upregulation of proinflammatory mediators which can create a state of shock that can often be more complex than simple hemorrhagic shock.

In addition to seminal observations on the clinical syndrome of shock on the battlefield, the early and mid-20th century witnessed important laboratory contributions to our understanding of shock. In 1947, Wiggers developed a model of graded hemorrhagic shock based on the uptake of shed blood into a reservoir to maintain a prescribed level of hypotension.[7] G. Tom Shires performed a series of classical laboratory studies in the 1960s and 1970s that demonstrated that a large extracellular fluid (ECF) deficit occurred in severe hemorrhagic shock that was greater than could be attributed to vascular refilling alone.[8] A triple isotope technique in dogs revealed that this ECF deficit persisted when shed blood or shed blood plus plasma was used in resuscitation. Only the infusion of both shed blood plus lactated Ringer's solution (an ECF mimic) repleted the red blood cell mass, plasma volume, and ECF.[9] The mortality rate after hemorrhage dramatically illustrated the importance of this observation: resuscitation with blood alone (80%), blood plus plasma (70%), and blood plus lactated Ringer's solution (30%).[9] The existence of this ECF deficit was subsequently confirmed in patients.[8] Additional studies by this group demonstrated significant dysfunction of the cellular membrane in prolonged hemorrhagic shock.[10] Depolarization of the cell membrane resulted in an uptake of water and sodium by the cell and loss of potassium in association with the loss of membrane integrity.[10] The depolarization of the cell membrane was proportional to the degree and duration of hypotension. Studies in red blood cells, hepatocytes, and skeletal muscle suggested that an abnormality in membrane active transport (Na-K-ATPase pump) was the basis of the cellular membrane dysfunction.[10] In addition, the uptake of fluid by the intracellular compartment was a major site of fluid sequestration following prolonged hemorrhagic shock. These changes were reversible with appropriate resuscitation. Thus, the importance of fluid resuscitation of severe hemorrhagic shock with isotonic saline or lactated Ringer's solution in addition to red blood cells was confirmed. These studies also emphasized the important cellular effects from what had previously appeared to be a global circulatory phenomenon.

With advances in our understanding of the pathophysiology and treatment of shock, new clinical problems soon became apparent. The Vietnam War provided a clinical laboratory for the rapidly expanding field of shock research. Aggressive fluid resuscitation with red blood cells, plasma, and crystalloid solutions allowed patients who previously would have succumbed to hemorrhagic shock to survive. Renal failure became a less frequent clinical problem, but fulminant

pulmonary failure appeared as an early cause of death after severe hemorrhage. Initially labeled "shock lung" or "DaNang lung," the clinical problem soon became recognized as the Acute Respiratory Distress Syndrome (ARDS). Flooding of the lung with large volumes of crystalloid solution was initially proposed as the primary mechanism of ARDS. Currently, ARDS is seen as a component of the Multiple Organ Dysfunction Syndrome (MODS), a result of the complex upregulation of proinflammatory mediators and mechanisms of the homeostatic response. The concept of MODS will be discussed in a subsequent chapter (see Chap. 68).

Several decades of research utilizing modified Wiggers' models of hemorrhagic shock emphasized the importance of early control of hemorrhage in conjunction with restoration of intravascular volume with red blood cells and crystalloid solutions. Studies over the past decade have extended the observations initially made by Cannon in 1918 on the futility of vigorously resuscitating patients with ongoing bleeding and have challenged traditional thinking on the appropriate endpoints of resuscitation from uncontrolled hemorrhage.[11] The concepts of delayed fluid resuscitation and hypotensive resuscitation are still being debated, fueled by the clinical study by Bickell et al. of patients with penetrating torso trauma.[12] Several essential concepts in the management of shock in the trauma patient, however, have withstood the test of time: (a) early definitive control of the airway must be achieved; (b) delays in control of active hemorrhage increase mortality; (c) poorly corrected hypoperfusion increases morbidity and mortality; i.e., inadequate resuscitation results in avoidable early deaths; and (d) excessive fluid resuscitation may exacerbate problems; i.e., uncontrolled resuscitation is harmful.

This chapter will describe our current understanding of the pathophysiology of shock. The diagnosis and treatment of each category of shock will be presented. It will conclude by reviewing endpoints in resuscitation that can be utilized clinically. The field of shock research is expanding exponentially. Our understanding of the cellular changes initiated by shock, the interaction between integrated cellular and intercellular pathways, the effect of genetics on the host response to shock, and many other aspects of the physiology of shock is increasing daily. The goal of this chapter is to provide a broad overview of the relevant clinical and basic science principles that are important in the management of the patient in shock. The interested reader can use this information as the foundation for more detailed investigation into specific areas of interest.

## PATHOPHYSIOLOGY

### Pathophysiology of Shock

Shock is defined as a state of inadequate tissue perfusion in which the delivery of oxygen to tissues and cells is insufficient to maintain normal aerobic metabolism. This concept implies an imbalance between substrate delivery (supply) and substrate requirements (demand) at the cellular level. A distinction must be made between the sequelae of shock, a total body circulatory disturbance that induces a systemic response, and localized ischemia and reperfusion, which predominantly induces a local response that can subsequently produce downstream effects. Tissue hypoperfusion is associated with a number of cardiovascular and neuroendocrine

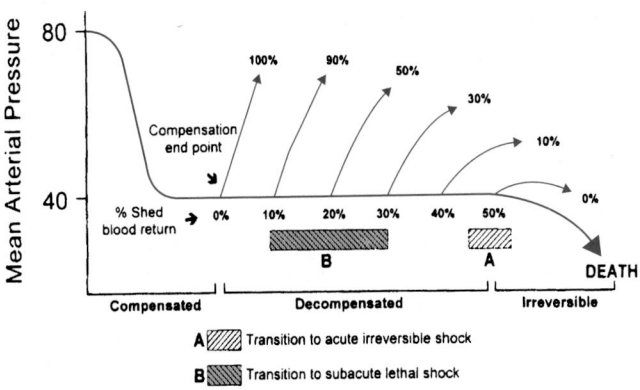

**FIGURE 13-1.** A rodent model of hemorrhagic shock depicting the relation between volume loss, duration of shock, and transition from reversible to fatal, irreversible shock.
*(Reproduced with permission from Peitzman AB, Billiar TR, Harbrecht BG, et al.: Hemorrhagic Shock. Curr Prob Surg 32:974, 1995.)*

responses designed to compensate for and reverse inadequate tissue perfusion. The pathophysiologic sequelae of shock may be due to either the direct effects of inadequate tissue perfusion on cellular and tissue function, or they may be due to the body's adaptive responses producing undesirable consequences. The magnitude of the shock insult and, therefore, the magnitude of the response, varies depending on the depth and duration of shock.[13,14] The consequences of shock may also vary from minimal physiologic disturbance with complete recovery at one end of the spectrum to profound circulatory disturbance, end-organ dysfunction, and death at the other (Fig. 13-1). The accumulating evidence suggests that, while the quantitative nature of the host response to shock may differ between the various etiologies of shock, the qualitative nature of the body's response to shock is similar regardless of the cause of the insult. This response consists, in part, of profound changes in cardiovascular, neuroendocrine, and immunologic function. While these innate mechanisms of host response are discussed separately, they are not independently functioning homeostatic pathways. There is considerable overlap and cross-talk between the various mechanisms of host response induced by shock.

## Afferent Signals

Afferent impulses transmitted from the periphery are processed within the central nervous system (CNS) and activate the reflexive effector responses or efferent impulses that are designed to expand plasma volume, maintain peripheral perfusion and tissue oxygen delivery, and reestablish homeostasis. The afferent impulses that initiate the body's intrinsic adaptive responses converge in the CNS and originate from a variety of sources. The sensation of pain from injured tissue is transmitted via the spinothalamic tracts and activates the hypothalamic-pituitary-adrenal axis.[15] The sensation of pain can also activate the autonomic nervous system (ANS) and increase direct sympathetic stimulation of the adrenal medulla to release catecholamines. Baroreceptors represent an important afferent pathway in initiating adaptive or corrective responses to shock. Volume receptors are present within the atria of the heart and are sensitive to changes in both chamber pressure and wall stretch.[15] They become activated with low-volume hemorrhage or mild

reductions in right atrial pressure. Receptors in the aortic arch and carotid bodies respond to alterations in pressure or stretch of the arterial wall and respond to greater reductions in intravascular volume or changes in pressure. These receptors normally inhibit activation of the ANS. When these baroreceptors are activated, their output is diminished. Thus, there is increased ANS output principally via sympathetic activation at the vasomotor centers of the brainstem, and this produces centrally mediated constriction of peripheral vessels.[15]

Receptors exist in the aorta and carotid bodies that are sensitive to changes in oxygen tension, $H^+$ ion concentration, and $CO_2$ level (chemoreceptors).[16] These receptors also provide afferent stimulation when the circulatory system is disturbed and activate effector response mechanisms. In addition, a variety of protein and nonprotein mediators produced at the site of injury and inflammation act as afferent impulses and induce a host response to shock and trauma. Some of these compounds are components of the host immunologic response to shock and include histamine, cytokines, eicosanoids, endothelins, and others which will be discussed in greater detail both in this chapter and in subsequent chapters.

## EFFERENT SIGNALS

### Cardiovascular Response

Changes in cardiovascular function are intimately tied to the neuroendocrine response to shock and constitute a prominent feature of both the body's adaptive response mechanisms and the clinical presentation of the patient in shock. Stimulation of sympathetic fibers innervating the heart leads to activation of $\beta_1$-adrenergic receptors that increase heart rate and contractility to increase cardiac output.[16] Increased myocardial oxygen consumption occurs as a result of the increased workload. Myocardial oxygen supply must be maintained or myocardial ischemia and dysfunction will develop.

Direct sympathetic stimulation of the peripheral circulation via the activation of $\alpha_1$-adrenergic receptors on arterioles increases vasoconstriction and causes a compensatory increase in systemic vascular resistance and blood pressure. Selective perfusion of tissues due to regional variations in arteriolar resistance from these compensatory mechanisms occurs in shock. Blood is shunted away from organs such as the intestine, kidney, and skin that are less essential to the body's immediate need to correct and respond to shock.[17] Organs such as the brain and heart have autoregulatory mechanisms that attempt to preserve their blood flow despite a global decrease in cardiac output. Direct sympathetic stimulation also induces constriction of venous vessels, decreasing the capacitance of the circulatory system, and accelerating blood return to the central circulation.

Increased sympathetic output increases catecholamine release from the adrenal medulla. Catecholamine levels are increased and peak within 24 to 48 hours of injury before returning to baseline.[16] Most of the epinephrine that circulates systemically is produced by the adrenal medulla, while norepinephrine is derived from synapses of the sympathetic nervous system.[17] Catecholamines also have profound effects on peripheral tissues in ways that support the organism's ability to respond to shock and hypovolemia. Catecholamines stimulate hepatic glycogenolysis and gluconeogenesis to increase the availability of circulating glucose to peripheral tissues, increase glycogenolysis in skeletal muscle, suppress the release of insulin, and increase the release of glucagon.[15] These responses increase the availability of glucose to the tissues that require it for maintenance of essential metabolic activity.

## Neuroendocrine Response

As discussed earlier, a variety of afferent stimuli lead to activation of the hypothalamic-pituitary-adrenal axis that functions as an integral component of the adaptive response of the host following shock. Shock stimulates the hypothalamus to release corticotropin-releasing hormone, which results in the release of adrenocorticotropin hormone (ACTH) by the pituitary. ACTH subsequently stimulates the adrenal cortex to release cortisol. Cortisol acts synergistically with epinephrine and glucagon to induce a catabolic state.[16] Cortisol stimulates gluconeogenesis and insulin resistance, resulting in hyperglycemia. It also induces protein breakdown in muscle cells and lipolysis, which provide substrates for hepatic gluconeogenesis. Cortisol causes retention of sodium and water by the kidney that aids restoration of circulating volume. In the setting of severe hypovolemia, ACTH secretion occurs independently of negative feedback inhibition by cortisol. Absence of appropriate cortisol secretion during critical illness or after traumatic injury has recently been postulated as an underappreciated contributor to ongoing circulatory instability in the intensive care unit.[18-20] The cellular mechanisms that may be involved in states of "relative" or secondary adrenal insufficiency in critically ill and shocky patients have not yet been defined, but presumably are similar to those present in primary adrenal insufficiency.

The pituitary also releases vasopressin or antidiuretic hormone (ADH) in response to hypovolemia, changes in circulating blood volume sensed by baroreceptors and stretch receptors in the left atrium, and increased plasma osmolality detected by hypothalamic osmoreceptors.[15] Epinephrine, angiotensin II, pain, and hyperglycemia enhance the production of ADH. ADH levels remain elevated for about 1 week after the initial insult, depending on the severity and persistence of the hemodynamic abnormalities. ADH acts on the distal tubule and collecting duct of the nephron to increase water permeability, decrease losses of water and sodium, and preserve intravascular volume. Also known as arginine vasopressin, ADH acts as a potent mesenteric vasoconstrictor, shunting circulating blood away from the splanchnic organs during hypovolemia.[21] The intense mesenteric vasoconstriction produced by vasopressin may contribute to intestinal ischemia and predispose to dysfunction of the intestinal mucosal barrier in shock states. Vasopressin also regulates hepatocellular function by increasing hepatic gluconeogenesis and hepatic glycolysis.

The renin-angiotensin system is activated in shock, as well. Decreased perfusion of the renal artery, β-adrenergic stimulation, and increased sodium concentration in the renal tubules cause the release of renin from the juxtaglomerular cells.[16] Renin catalyzes the conversion of angiotensinogen (produced by the liver) to angiotensin I, which is then converted to angiotensin II by angiotensin-converting enzyme (ACE) produced in the lung. While angiotensin I has no significant functional activity, angiotensin II is a potent vasoconstrictor of both splanchnic and peripheral vascular beds and also stimulates the secretion of aldosterone, ACTH, and ADH. Aldosterone, a mineralocorticoid, acts

on the nephron to promote reabsorption of sodium and, as a consequence, water in exchange for potassium and hydrogen ions that are lost in the urine.

## Immunologic and Inflammatory Response

The function of the host's immune system after shock is intimately related to alterations in the production of mediators generally considered part of the body's response to localized inflammation and infection. When these mediators gain access to the systemic circulation, they can induce changes in a number of tissues and organs. Therefore, activation of proinflammatory pathways is an integral component of the host response to shock. While proinflammatory activation is a central feature of septic shock, proinflammatory cytokine production and mediator release also occurs in other forms of shock such as hypovolemic shock.[22-24] As initially proposed by Cannon almost a century ago, inflammatory mediators can be a cause of shock as well as a byproduct of the body's response to shock. As previously discussed, most mediators have a variety of effects due to the redundant and overlapping nature of the host response to injury. Therefore, in addition to regulating immune function in the host, many of these mediators have effects on the cardiovascular system, cellular metabolism, and cellular gene expression. It deserves to be mentioned, however, that many compounds already discussed that have substantial effects on the cardiovascular or neuroendocrine response to shock, such as catecholamines, can also have effects on immune function and the activation of proinflammatory cytokines.[25] Cytokines are small polypeptides and glycoproteins that exert most of their actions in a paracrine fashion and are responsible for fever, leukocytosis, tachycardia, tachypnea, and the upregulation of other cytokines. Their levels are elevated in hemorrhagic, septic, and traumatic shock.[22] The overexpression of certain cytokines is associated with the metabolic and hemodynamic derangements often seen in septic shock or decompensated hypovolemic shock, and cytokine production after shock correlates with the development of the multiple organ dysfunction syndrome.[22-24,26] The immune response to injury and infection is discussed in greater detail in Chap. 67. A brief review of several of the key components of the immune response is provided below.

Tumor necrosis factor-α (TNF-α) is one of the earliest proinflammatory cytokines released by monocytes, macrophages, and T cells in response to injurious stimuli.[27] The classic model of TNF-α production is the injection of bacterial endotoxin in an animal or human subject. Under these controlled conditions, TNF-α levels peak within 90 minutes of the insult and return to baseline within 4 hours. Endotoxin stimulates TNF-α release and may be a primary inducer of cytokines, as in the case of septic shock. TNF-α release may also be a secondary event following the release of bacteria from the intestinal lumen that may occur after hemorrhage and ischemia.[28,29] Also, TNF-α levels are increased after hemorrhagic shock,[30] and TNF-α levels correlate with mortality in animal models of hemorrhage.[31] In human patients, TNF-α, interleukin-6 (IL-6), and IL-8 levels increase during hemorrhagic shock although the magnitude of the increase is less than that seen in septic patients.[32] Once released, TNF-α can cause peripheral vasodilation, activate the release of other cytokines such as IL-1β and IL-6, induce procoagulant activity, and stimulate a wide array of cellular metabolic changes.[27] TNF-α has also been associated with mechanisms of host defense against infection by promoting activation of macrophages and intracellular killing of pathogens.[33] During the stress response, TNF-α contributes to breakdown of muscle protein and cachexia, as well.[27] Despite being linked to tissue injury and dysfunction, TNF-α may be essential in combating bacterial infection since neuralizing TNF-α in infection models using live bacteria (peritonitis, pneumonia) increases mortality.[34–36]

IL-1β has actions that are similar to TNF-α and can cause hemodynamic instability and vasodilation.[27] IL-1β has a very short half-life (6 minutes) and primarily acts locally in a paracrine fashion. IL-1β produces a febrile response by activating prostaglandins in the posterior hypothalamus and causes anorexia by activating the satiety center. This cytokine also augments the secretion of ACTH, glucocorticoids, and β-endorphins.[27] In conjunction with TNF-α, IL-1β can induce the release of other cytokines such as IL-2, IL-4, IL-6, IL-8, granulocyte/macrophage colony-stimulating factor (GM-CSF), and interferon-γ (IFN-γ). IL-2 expression is important for the cell-mediated immune response, and its attenuated expression has been associated with transient immunosuppression of injured patients. IL-6 has consistently been shown to be elevated in animals subjected to hemorrhagic shock or trauma and in patients with major surgery or trauma. And, elevated IL-6 levels correlate with mortality in some forms of shock.[37] IL-6 contributes to neutrophil-mediated injury to the lung after hemorrhagic shock[38] and may play a role in the development of diffuse alveolar damage and ARDS. IL-6 and IL-1β are mediators of the hepatic acute phase response to injury and enhance the expression and/or activity of complement, C-reactive protein, fibrinogen, haptoglobin, amyloid A, and α-antitrypsin. Activation of neutrophils is promoted by IL-6, IL-8, and GM-CSF, and IL-8 also serves as a potent chemoattractant to neutrophils.

The complement cascade is activated by injury and shock and contributes to proinflammatory activation in both animal models and in human patients. Complement consumption can occur after hemorrhagic shock and may contribute to the hypotension and metabolic acidosis observed following resuscitation.[39] The degree of complement activation is proportional to the magnitude of the traumatic injury and may serve as a marker for severity of injury in trauma patients.[40] Patients in septic shock also demonstrate activation of the complement pathway with elevation of the activated complement proteins C3a and C5a.[41] Activation of the complement cascade can contribute to the development of organ dysfunction.[42] Thus, patients with extensive injuries and significant activation of complement may be prone to develop MODS. Activated complement factors C3a, C4a, and C5a are potent mediators of vascular permeability, contraction of smooth muscle cells, release of histamine, synthesis of the by-products of arachidonic acid, and adherence of neutrophils to vascular endothelium. These activated complement factors, known as anaphylatoxins, synergistically induce the release of TNF-α and IL-1β with endotoxin.[43] The development of ARDS and MODS in trauma patients correlates with the intensity of complement activation.[23] In fact, complement and neutrophil activation (as measured by C3a level, C3a/C3 ratio, and neutrophil elastase level) were the most significant parameters to predict death in multiply injured patients in one study.[24]

Activation of neutrophil is one of the early changes induced by the inflammatory response, and neutrophils are the first cells to be recruited to sites of injury and inflammation. These cells are important in the clearance of infectious agents, foreign substances that have penetrated host barrier defenses, and nonviable tissue. Unfortunately, activated neutrophils and their products may also produce cell injury and organ dysfunction. Activated neutrophils generate and release a number of substances such as reactive oxygen species, lipid-peroxidation compounds, proteolytic enzymes (elastase, cathepsin G), and vasoactive mediators (leukotrienes, eicosanoids, and platelet-activating factor, or PAF). Oxygen radicals such as superoxide anion, hydrogen peroxide, and the hydroxyl radical are potent inflammatory molecules that activate peroxidation of lipids, inactivate cellular enzymes, and consume cellular antioxidants (such as glutathione and tocopherol). Intestinal ischemia and reperfusion cause activation of neutrophils and induce neutrophil-mediated organ injury in experimental animal models.[44] In animal models of hemorrhagic shock, activation of neutrophils correlates with irreversibility of shock and mortality,[45] and neutrophil depletion prevents the pathophysiologic sequelae of hemorrhagic and septic shock.[46,47] Human data corroborate the activation of neutrophils in trauma and shock and suggest that neutrophil activation may play a role in the development of MODS after injury.[48] Plasma markers of neutrophil activation such as elastase may correspond to phagocytic activity or correlate with severity of injury.[23] In this context, elastase and other markers of neutrophil activation may predict the development of ARDS and MODS after shock.

Interactions between endothelial cells and leukocytes are important in host defense and the initiation and perpetuation of the inflammatory response in the host. The vascular endothelium regulates blood flow, adherence of leukocytes, and activation of the coagulation cascade. Adhesion molecules such as intercellular adhesion molecules (ICAMs), vascular cell adhesion molecules (VCAMs), and the selectins (E-selectin, P-selectin) are expressed on the surface of endothelial cells and are responsible for the adhesion of leukocytes to the endothelium. The interaction of surface proteins on leukocytes and vascular endothelial cells allows activated neutrophils to marginate into the tissues in order to engulf invading organisms. Unfortunately, the migration of activated neutrophils into tissues can also lead to neutrophil-mediated cytotoxicity, microvascular damage, and tissue injury.[49] This tissue damage may contribute to organ dysfunction after shock.

## Cellular Effects

Depending on the magnitude of the insult and the intrinsic compensatory mechanisms present in different cells, the response at the cellular level may be one of adaptation, dysfunction and injury, or death. The aerobic respiration of the cell, i.e., oxidative phosphorylation by mitochondria, is the pathway most susceptible to inadequate oxygen delivery. As oxygen tension within cells decreases, there is a decrease in oxidative phosphorylation and the generation of adenosine triphosphate (ATP) slows or stops. The loss of ATP, the cellular "energy currency," has widespread effects on cellular function, physiology, and morphology.[50] As oxidative phosphorylation slows, the cells shift to anaerobic glycolysis that generates ATP from the rapid breakdown of cellular glycogen[50,51]; however, anaerobic glycolysis is much less efficient than oxygen-dependent mitochondrial pathways. Under aerobic conditions, pyruvate, the end-product of glycolysis, is fed into the Kreb's cycle for further oxidative metabolism. Under hypoxic conditions, the mitochondrial pathways of oxidative catabolism are impaired and pyruvate is instead converted to lactate. The accumulation of lactic acid and inorganic phosphates is accompanied by a reduction in pH resulting in intracellular metabolic acidosis. As cells become hypoxic and ATP-depleted, other ATP-dependent cell processes are affected such as synthesis of enzymes and structural proteins, repair of DNA damage, and intracellular signal transduction. Tissue hypoperfusion also results in decreased availability of metabolic substrates and the accumulation of metabolic by-products such as oxygen radicals and organic ions that may be toxic to cells.

The consequences of intracellular acidosis on cell function can be quite profound. Decreased intracellular pH can alter the activity of cellular enzymes, lead to changes in cellular gene expression, impair cellular metabolic pathways, and interfere with ion exchange in the cell membrane.[52–54] Acidosis can also lead to changes in cellular calcium ($Ca^{2+}$) metabolism and $Ca^{2+}$-mediated cellular signaling which can, by itself, interfere with the activity of specific enzymes and alter cell function.[52,55] These changes in normal cell function can produce cellular injury or cell death.[56] Changes in both cardiovascular function and immune function in the host can be induced by acidosis,[57,58] although translating these in vitro effects to the physiologic sequelae of shock produced in the intact organism may be difficult.

As cellular ATP is depleted under hypoxic conditions, the activity of the membrane $Na^+,K^+$-ATPase slows and thus the regulation of cellular membrane potential and volume is impaired.[10] $Na^+$ accumulates intracellularly while $K^+$ leaks into the extracellular space. The net gain of intracellular sodium is accompanied by an increase in intracellular water and the development of cellular swelling. This cellular influx of water is associated with a corresponding reduction in extracellular fluid volume.[59] Swelling of the endoplasmic reticulum is the first ultrastructural change seen in hypoxic cell injury. Eventually, swelling of the mitochondria and cells is observed. The changes in cellular membrane potential impair a number of cellular physiologic processes such as myocyte contractility, cell signaling, and the regulation of intracellular $Ca^{2+}$ concentrations. Once intracellular organelles such as lysosomes or cell membranes rupture, the cell will undergo death by necrosis.[60]

Hypoperfusion and hypoxia can induce cell death by apoptosis, as well. Animal models of shock and ischemia/reperfusion have demonstrated apoptotic cell death in lymphocytes, intestinal epithelial cells, and hepatocytes.[61] Apoptosis has also been detected in trauma patients with ischemia and reperfusion injury. Apoptosis of lymphocytes and intestinal epithelial cells occurs within the first 3 hours of injury.[62] Apoptosis in intestinal mucosal cells may compromise barrier function of the intestine and lead to translocation of bacteria and endotoxin into the portal circulation during shock. Also, lymphocyte apoptosis has been hypothesized to contribute to the immune suppression that is observed in trauma patients.

Tissue hypoperfusion and cellular hypoxia result not only in intracellular acidosis but also in systemic metabolic acidosis as metabolic by-products of anaerobic glycolysis exit the cells and gain access to the circulation. In the setting of acidosis, oxygen delivery to the tissues is altered as the oxyhemoglobin dissociation curve is shifted toward the right.[15] The decreased affinity of hemoglobin for oxygen in erythrocytes results in increased tissue $O_2$ release and increased tissue extraction of oxygen. In addition, hypoxia stimulates the production of erythrocyte 2,3-diphosphoglycerate (2,3-DPG), which also contributes to the shift to the right of the oxyhemoglobin dissociation curve and increases $O_2$ availability to the tissues during shock.

Epinephrine and norepinephrine released after shock have a profound impact on cellular metabolism in addition to their effects on vascular tone. Hepatic glycogenolysis, gluconeogenesis, ketogenesis, breakdown of skeletal muscle protein, and lipolysis of adipose tissue are all increased by these catecholamines.[21] Cortisol, glucagon, and ADH also participate in the regulation of catabolism during shock. Epinephrine induces the release of glucagon while inhibiting the release of insulin by pancreatic β-cells. The result is a catabolic state with glucose mobilization, hyperglycemia, protein breakdown, negative nitrogen balance, lipolysis, and insulin resistance during shock and injury.[21,59] The relative underutilization of glucose by peripheral tissues preserves it for the glucose-dependent organs such as the heart and brain. In addition to inducing changes in cellular metabolic pathways, shock also induces changes in cellular gene expression. The deoxyribonucleic acid (DNA) binding activity of a number of nuclear transcription factors is altered by the production of oxygen radicals, nitrogen radicals, or hypoxia that occur at the cellular level in shock.[63] The expression of other gene products including heat shock proteins,[64] vascular endothelial growth factor (VEGF), inducible nitric oxide synthase (iNOS), and cytokines is also increased in shock.[23,30,65] The role these proteins play in the cellular and tissue response to shock continues to be explored.[66,67] Many of these shock-induced gene products, such as cytokines, have the built-in ability to subsequently alter gene expression in specific target cells and tissues.[27] These pathways will be discussed in greater detail elsewhere but they emphasize the complex, integrated, and overlapping nature of the response to shock.

Shock induces profound changes in tissue microcirculation that may contribute to organ function, organ dysfunction, and the systemic sequelae of severe hypoperfusion. These changes have been studied most extensively in the microcirculation of skeletal muscle in models of sepsis and hemorrhage. Whether microcirculatory changes are primarily a result of the development of shock or a pathophysiologic response that promotes tissue injury and organ dysfunction has been difficult to determine. Intuitively, it would seem that both are likely to be true. After hemorrhage, larger arterioles vasoconstrict, most likely due to sympathetic stimulation, while smaller distal arterioles dilate, presumably due to local mechanisms.[68] Flow at the capillary level, however, is heterogeneous with swelling of endothelial cells and the aggregation of leukocytes producing diminished capillary perfusion in some vessels both during shock and following resuscitation.[68–70] Hemorrhage-induced microcirculatory dysfunction also occurs in vascular beds besides skeletal muscle and may contribute to tissue injury and organ dysfunction.[71,72] In sepsis, similar changes in microcirculatory function occur. Regional differences in blood flow can be demonstrated after proinflammatory stimuli, and the microcirculation in many organs is heterogeneous.[73–77] Differences may also be evident depending on whether acute or chronic sepsis models are utilized.[76,77] Aggregation and sludging of neutrophils in the microcirculation can aggravate shock-induced hypoperfusion, induce direct cellular injury via toxic neutrophil-dependent processes such as production of oxygen radicals or release of proteolytic enzymes, and impair cellular metabolism.[78]

The decreases in microcirculatory blood flow and capillary perfusion result in decreased capillary hydrostatic pressure. The changes in hydrostatic pressure promote an influx of fluid from the extravascular or extracellular space into the capillaries in an attempt to increase circulating volume. These changes are associated, however, with additional decrements in the volume of extracellular fluid due to increased cellular swelling. These basic cellular and microcirculatory changes have significant physiologic importance in the ability of the organism to recover from circulatory shock. Resuscitation with volumes of fluid sufficient to restore the extracellular fluid deficit is associated with improved outcome after shock as described earlier.[9]

## Quantifying Cellular Hypoperfusion

Hypoperfused tissues and cells experience what has been called oxygen debt, a concept first proposed by Crowell.[79] The oxygen debt is the deficit in tissue oxygenation over time that occurs during shock. When oxygen delivery ($DO_2$) is limited, oxygen consumption ($VO_2$) may be inadequate to match the metabolic needs of cellular respiration creating a deficit in oxygen at the cellular level. The measurement of oxygen deficit is calculated by taking the difference between the estimated oxygen demand and the actual value obtained for oxygen consumption ($VO_2$). Under normal circumstances, cells can "repay" the oxygen debt during reperfusion. The magnitude of the oxygen debt correlates with the severity and duration of hypoperfusion. In a canine model of hemorrhagic shock, Crowell and Smith demonstrated a direct relation between survival and degree of shock.[80] They determined that a marker of mortality was the inability to repay the oxygen debt. The median lethal dose ($LD_{50}$) occurred at 120 mL/kg of oxygen debt. Dunham et al. showed via regression analysis that the probability of death could be directly correlated to the calculated oxygen debt in a canine model of hemorrhagic shock.[81] Their study demonstrated that the $LD_{50}$ for oxygen debt was similar (113.5 mL/kg) to that found by Crowell in their earlier studies. Dunham et al. were also able to confirm a relation between the rate of accumulation of the oxygen debt and survival. In human patients a relation between oxygen debt and survival has also been shown. In over 250 high-risk surgical patients, the calculated oxygen debt correlated directly with organ failure and mortality.[82] The maximum oxygen debt in nonsurvivors (33.2 L/m²) was greater than that of survivors with organ failure (21.6 L/m²) and survivors without organ failure (9.2 L/m²). In addition, the total duration of oxygen debt and the time required to repay it correlated with outcome in this study. Survivors were able to repay the oxygen debt while the hallmark of nonsurvivors was the inability to repay the oxygen debt. Thus, the magnitude of the oxygen debt, its rate of accumulation, and the time required to correct it may all correlate with survival.

It is difficult to directly measure the oxygen debt in the resuscitation of trauma patients. The easily obtainable parameters of arterial blood pressure, heart rate, urine output, central venous pressure, and pulmonary artery occlusion pressure are poor indicators of the adequacy of tissue perfusion. Therefore, surrogate parameters have been sought to estimate the oxygen debt. Experimental animal studies show that serum lactate and base deficit correlate with oxygen debt.[81] Cardiac output, blood pressure, and shed blood volume were all inferior to the base deficit and lactate in estimating the oxygen debt and in predicting mortality in hemorrhaged animals.[81] Dunham et al. showed a direct correlation between arterial lactate and probability of survival in a model of canine hemorrhage (Fig. 13-2).[81] The $LD_{50}$ for lactate was 12.9 mmol/L in hemorrhaged dogs.

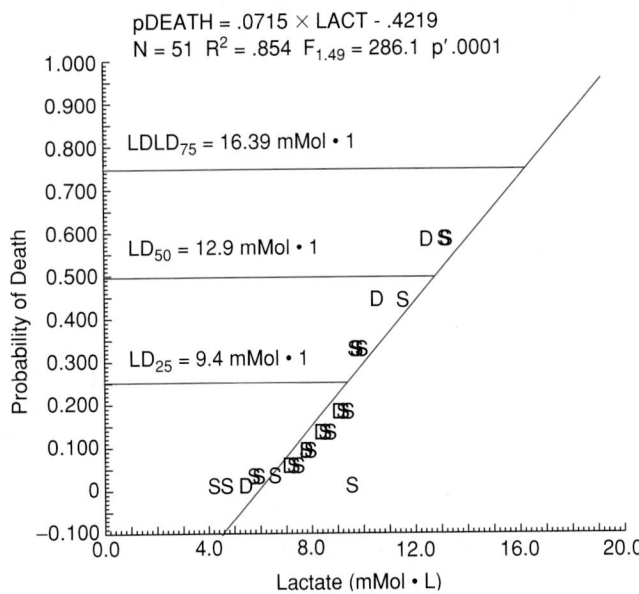

**FIGURE 13-2.** The relation between mortality and serum lactate levels is described by data generated in a canine hemorrhagic shock model. (Reproduced with permission from Dunham CM, Siegel JH, Weireter L, et al.: Oxygen debt and metabolic acidemia or quantitative predictors of mortality and the severity of the ischemic insult in hemorrhagic shock. *Crit Care Med* 19:231, 1991.)

Base deficit is the amount of base in millimoles that is required to titrate 1 L of whole blood to a pH of 7.40 with the blood fully saturated with $O_2$ at 37 °C (98.6 °F) and a $PaCO_2$ of 40 mm Hg. It is usually measured by arterial blood gas analysis using automated devices and has a rapid turnaround time. Good correlation between the base deficit and survival has been shown in patients with shock.[83] At a base deficit of 0 mmol/L there was an 8% mortality, while there was a 95% mortality at a base deficit of 26 mmol/L. The $LD_{50}$ occurred at a base deficit of 11.8 mmol/L (Fig. 13-3).[83] Other clinical parameters such as blood pressure, heart rate, hemoglobin, plasma lactate, and oxygen transport variables were not nearly as accurate as the base deficit in determining the probability of death in these trauma patients. Neither base deficit nor serum lactate, however, is as precise at measuring physiologic stress as the oxygen debt. When compared in a model of hemorrhage and resuscitation, the lactate level decreased more slowly and tended to estimate higher residual oxygen debt while the base deficit decreased more rapidly and tended to estimate lower values of oxygen debt[81]; however, the base deficit appeared to reflect the measured oxygen debt more accurately. As will be discussed more fully later in the chapter (see *Endpoints of Resuscitation of the Trauma Patient*), both lactate and base deficit are useful in the assessment of trauma patients and in the evaluation of the patient's response to resuscitation.

## EVALUATION OF THE TRAUMA PATIENT IN SHOCK

### General Overview

Shock represents a condition of abnormal tissue perfusion. The manifestations of shock may be dramatic, as in the patient with profound hypotension or obvious external sources of blood loss,

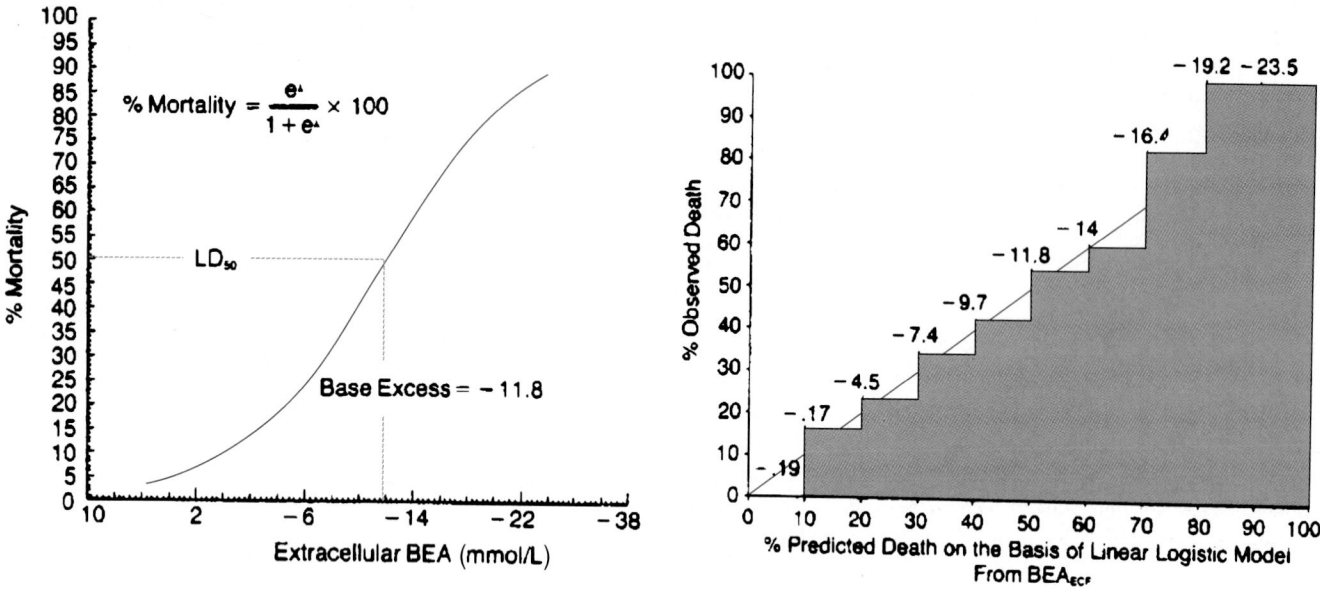

**FIGURE 13-3.** The relation between base deficit (negative base excess) and mortality is depicted for patients who suffered blunt hepatic injury. *(Reproduced with permission from Siegel JH, Rivkind AI, Dalal S, et al.: Early physiologic predictors of injury severity and death in blunt multiple trauma. Arch Surg 125:498, 1990.)*

or findings may be subtle. As with other trauma-induced injuries, the evaluation, diagnosis, and treatment of the trauma patient in shock begins with the ABCs of the primary survey.[84] Advanced shock may produce coma with loss of the ability to maintain and protect the airway, so that endotracheal intubation is necessary. Marked tachypnea may be present as the respiratory system attempts to compensate for metabolic acidosis or in response to generalized anxiety from hypoperfusion of the central nervous system. In the primary survey, the circulation can be rapidly assessed by evaluation of the presence and location of the pulse (central vs. peripheral), its rate, and its character. Absent peripheral pulses (radial, pedal) associated with weak, rapid central pulses (femoral, carotid) denote a profound circulatory disturbance that requires prompt intervention. Associated findings that may be manifestations of abnormal tissue perfusion include cool clammy skin, altered sensorium (confusion, lethargy, coma), and tachycardia. Low urine output, often used as an indicator of hypovolemia, is unlikely to be a useful tool in the initial assessment of the patient in shock in the trauma resuscitation area. The rate of urine formation is difficult to estimate during the initial evaluation of the injured patient and may be confounded by factors such as alcohol consumption. Measurement of blood pressure may be misleading. Compensatory mechanisms to maintain cerebral and coronary perfusion may maintain relatively normal systemic arterial pressure despite significant underperfusion of splanchnic and peripheral tissues. Up to 30% of the blood volume may be lost before significant changes in blood pressure occur.[84] When present, however, hypotension represents a profound circulatory derangement and the failure of compensatory mechanisms and requires immediate attention.

The correction of shock should begin immediately once it is recognized. Treatment generally begins before an etiology for shock is identified. The forms of shock are listed in Table 13-1, but the most common etiology for shock in the trauma patient is hypovolemia from loss of circulating volume (see algorithm Fig. 13-4). Two large-bore intravenous lines (at least 14- or 16-gauge

peripheral or number 7.5 to 8.5 French resuscitation lines) should be inserted and volume resuscitation instituted. The availability of rapid infusion systems in many trauma centers facilitates rapid volume expansion with the delivery rate limited predominantly by the size and length of the intravenous cannula. Warmers to heat the infusate are essential to prevent hypothermia. For patients in profound shock, immediate blood replacement may be necessary. As correction of the shock state is underway, a source/etiology for shock is rapidly sought. Physical examination may indicate potential etiologies (i.e., obvious external hemorrhage, flaccid extremities from spinal cord injury, or penetrating precordial wounds). Rapidly performed radiologic examinations (X-rays of chest and pelvis, diagnostic ultrasound) can provide additional information while the initial resuscitation is being conducted and the response to resuscitation is evaluated. Diagnostic maneuvers that do not directly contribute to the identification and treatment of shock should be deferred until shock has been corrected. Trauma patients can be categorized into three general groups with respect to their response to resuscitative maneuvers (see treatment algorithm Fig. 13-5). Responders are those patients who rapidly correct their shock state with minimal replacement of intravascular volume. These patients often have an intravascular volume loss that is not ongoing, bleeding that has stopped or been tamponaded (multiple extremity fractures), or an etiology for hypoperfusion other than hypovolemia such as neurogenic shock or obstructive shock. Transient responders represent patients who initially improve with resuscitative efforts, but subsequently deteriorate. This group of patients frequently has intracavitary bleeding that requires surgical control. Nonresponders represent those patients who have persistent manifestations of shock despite vigorous resuscitative efforts. These patients are gravely ill and often present *in extremis*. These patients typically have high-volume bleeding from injuries to major vessels or severe injuries to solid organs that require immediate operative control. They will rapidly expire from circulatory collapse or develop the progressive spiral of hypothermia,

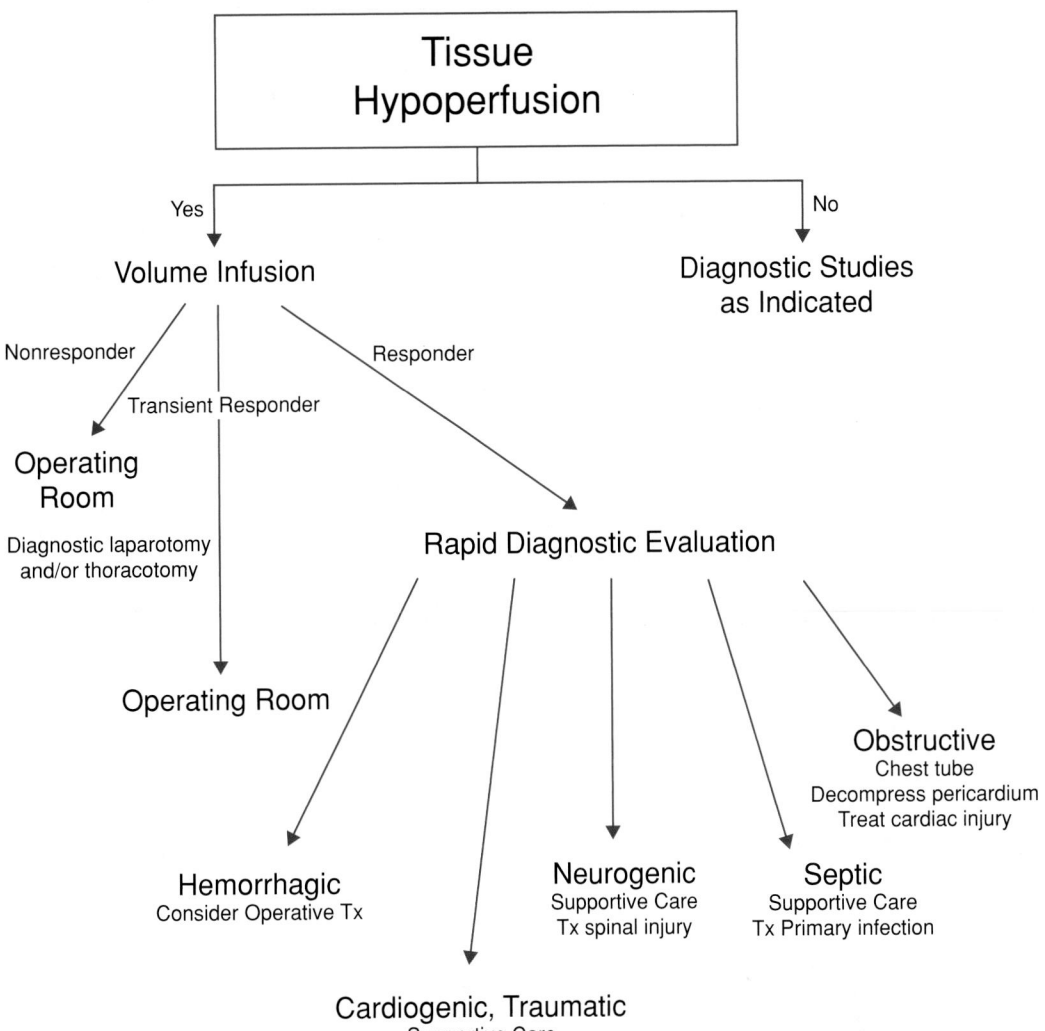

**FIGURE 13-4.** Tissue Hypoperfusion Algorithm. The most common etiology for shock in the trauma patient is Hypovolemia from loss of circulating volume.

coagulopathy, and irreversible shock unless bleeding is rapidly controlled. Patients who have active, ongoing hemorrhage cannot be successfully resuscitated until hemorrhage has been controlled, and rapid identification of patients who require operative intervention is essential.

## FORMS OF SHOCK

### Hemorrhagic and Hypovolemic Shock

As previously noted, the most common cause of shock in the trauma patient is loss of circulating volume from hemorrhage. Acute blood loss causes decreased stimulation of baroreceptors (stretch receptors) in the large arteries resulting in decreased inhibition of vasoconstrictor centers in the brainstem, increased stimulation of chemoreceptors in vasomotor centers, and diminished output from atrial stretch receptors. These changes increase vasoconstriction and peripheral arterial resistance. Hypovolemia also induces sympathetic stimulation leading to the release of epinephrine and norepinephrine, activation of the renin-angiotensin cascade, and increased release of vasopressin. Peripheral vasoconstriction is prominent while lack of sympathetic effects on cerebral and coronary vessels and local autoregulation promote maintenance of blood flow to the heart and brain.[15]

*Diagnosis.* Shock in a trauma patient should be presumed to be due to hemorrhage until proven otherwise. Treatment is instituted as soon as shock is identified, typically before a source of hemorrhage is located.

The clinical and physiologic response to hemorrhage has been classified according to the magnitude of volume loss.[84] Loss of up to 15% of the circulating volume (700 to 750 mL for a 70-kg patient) may produce little in terms of obvious symptoms, while loss of up to 30% of the circulating volume (1.5 L) may result in mild tachycardia, tachypnea, and anxiety. Hypotension, marked tachycardia (pulse >110 to 120 beats/minutes) and confusion may not be evident until more than 30% of the blood volume has been lost, while loss of 40% of circulating volume (2 L) is immediately life-threatening. Thus, there is a fine line between the development of mild symptoms of shock and the presence of life-threatening blood loss. Young, healthy patients with vigorous compensatory mechanisms may tolerate larger volumes of blood loss while manifesting fewer clinical signs. These patients may maintain a near-normal blood pressure until a precipitous cardiovascular collapse occurs. Elderly patients may be taking medications that either promote bleeding (warfarin, aspirin) or mask the compensatory response to hypovolemia (beta blockers). In addition, atherosclerotic vascular disease, diminished cardiac compliance with age, inability to elevate heart rate or cardiac contractility in response to

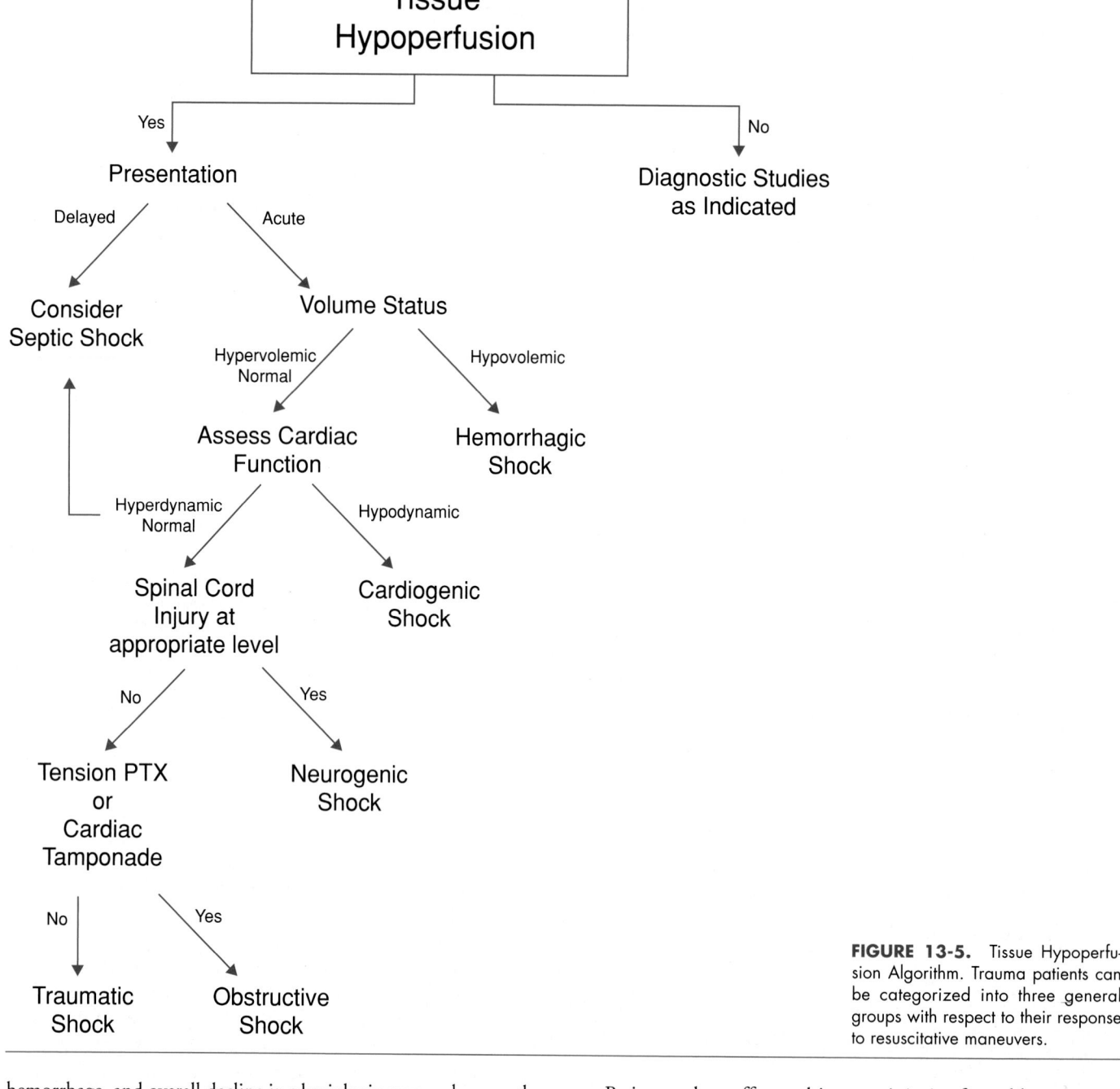

**FIGURE 13-5.** Tissue Hypoperfusion Algorithm. Trauma patients can be categorized into three general groups with respect to their response to resuscitative maneuvers.

hemorrhage, and overall decline in physiologic reserve decrease the ability of the elderly patient to tolerate hemorrhage.[85,86]

Understanding the mechanism of injury of the patient in shock will help direct the evaluation and management. Identifying the source of blood loss in patients with penetrating wounds is relatively simple since potential bleeding sources will be located along the known or suspected path of the wounding agent. Patients with penetrating injuries who are in shock usually require operative intervention. Occasionally, patients in shock from penetrating injuries may have problems that are readily treated by simple maneuvers outside the operating room. Treatment of a tension pneumothorax with insertion of a thoracostomy tube in the emergency department (ED) is one example. Generally speaking, though, shock from penetrating wounds is typically due to ongoing hemorrhage that mandates operative control.

Patients who suffer multisystem injuries from blunt trauma have multiple sources of potential hemorrhage. There are a limited number of sites, however, that can harbor sufficient extravascular blood volume to induce hypoperfusion or hypotension. Prehospital medical reports may confirm a significant blood loss at the scene of an accident, history of massive blood loss from wounds, visible brisk bleeding, or presence of an open wound in proximity to a major vessel. Injuries to major arteries or veins should be suspected when there is ongoing hemorrhage from an open pelvic fracture. Persistent bleeding from uncontrolled small vessels can, over time, precipitate shock if left untreated; however, attributing profound blood loss to these wounds (i.e., scalp lacerations) should be done only after major intracavitary bleeding has been excluded. When major blood loss is not immediately visible, internal (intracavitary) blood loss should be suspected. Intraperitoneal hemorrhage is probably the most common source of blood loss inducing shock. Its presence may be suspected based on physical examination (distended abdomen, abdominal tenderness, visible abdominal wounds) although the sensitivity of the physical exam for detecting substantial abdominal injuries after blunt trauma is unreliable. A large volume of intraperitoneal blood from abdominal injuries may be present before the physical examination is abnormal. Therefore, ultrasound Focused Assessment Sonography in Trauma (FAST) or diagnostic peritoneal lavage is used frequently in the resuscitation area to rapidly identify intraperitoneal blood. In selected patients, diagnostic laparotomy may be indicated. Each pleural cavity can hold 2 to 3 L of blood and can, therefore, also be a site of significant blood loss. Diagnostic and therapeutic tube thoracostomy may be indicated in patients based on clinical findings, clinical suspicion, or evidence of a hemopneumothorax on a chest X-ray or pleural FAST. Major retroperitoneal hemorrhage occurring in association with a pelvic fracture can be diagnosed by pelvic radiography in the resuscitation bay (Fig. 13-6). The pattern of the pelvic fracture may provide clues as to the risk of massive blood loss.[87]

Treatment. The method of treatment will depend on the patient's response to resuscitation, the specific injury or injuries responsible for the blood loss, and consideration of factors such as mechanism of injury, age of the patient, associated injuries, and institutional resources. Patients who fail to respond to initial resuscitative efforts should be assumed to have ongoing active hemorrhage from major vessels (external bleeding, pleural cavity, peritoneal cavity, retroperitoneum, or both thighs) and require prompt operative intervention. Identification of the body cavity harboring active hemorrhage will help focus operative efforts, but since time is of the essence, rapid treatment is essential and

diagnostic laparotomy or thoracotomy may be indicated. The actively bleeding patient cannot be resuscitated until control of ongoing hemorrhage is achieved.

Patients who respond to initial resuscitative efforts but then deteriorate hemodynamically frequently have injuries that require operative intervention. The duration of their response will dictate whether diagnostic maneuvers can be performed to identify the site of bleeding. Usually, however, hemodynamic deterioration denotes ongoing bleeding for which some form of intervention (operation, interventional radiology) is required (Fig. 13-7). As noted above, patients who have lost significant intravascular volume but have their hemorrhage controlled or have no active bleeding will often respond to resuscitative efforts if the depth and duration of shock have been limited.

A subset of patients fails to respond to resuscitative efforts despite adequate control of ongoing hemorrhage. These patients present in the following manner: have ongoing fluid requirements despite adequate control of hemorrhage; have persistent hypotension despite restoration of intravascular volume; often require vasopressor support to maintain their systemic blood pressure; and may exhibit a futile cycle of uncorrectable hypothermia, hypoperfusion, acidosis, and coagulopathy that cannot be interrupted despite maximum therapy. These patients have classically been described to be in decompensated or irreversible shock,[59] and mortality is inevitable once the patient manifests shock in its terminal stages; however, this is always a diagnosis made in retrospect. Hemodynamic decompensation or the paradoxical peripheral vasodilation that occurs with prolonged hemorrhage has been studied in animal models of shock,[13,88] but the mechanisms responsible for its development and the clinical factors that predict its onset in humans with shock have not been elucidated.

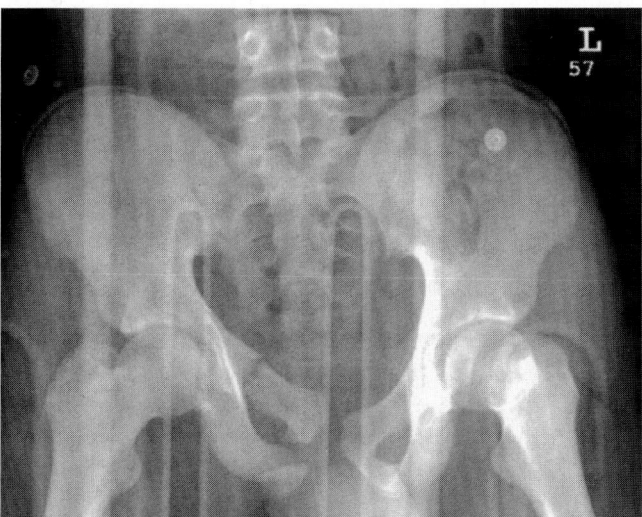
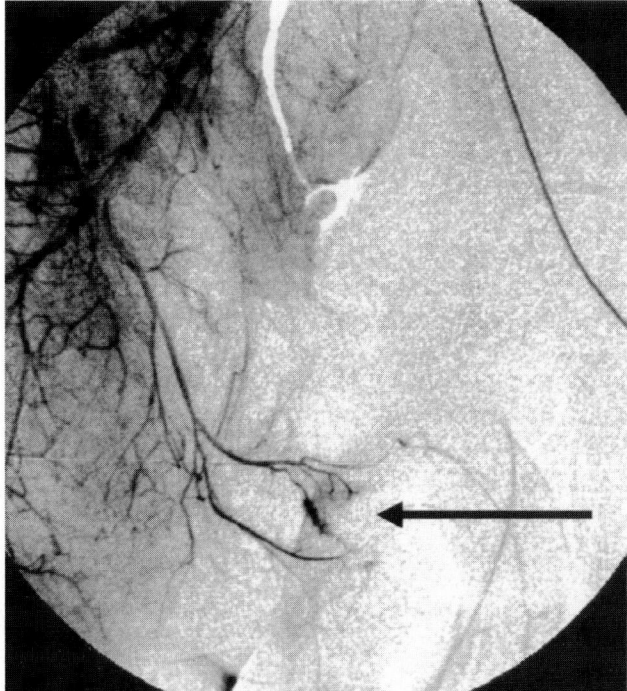

**FIGURE 13-6.** This patient was involved in a motor vehicle crash and presented to the ED in shock. His radiographic evaluation demonstrated a pelvic fracture (**left**). Angiography and coil embolization of a bleeding vessel was required (**right**) to control pelvic hemorrhage.

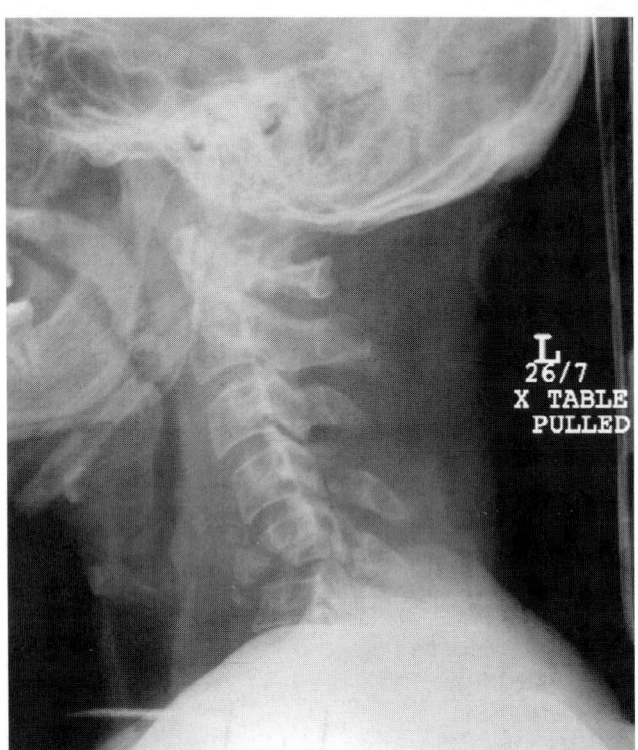
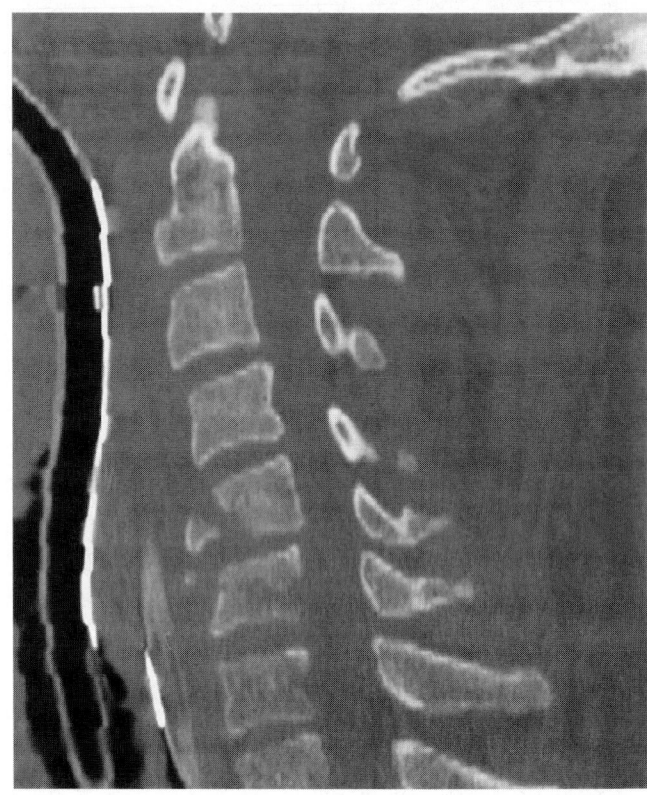

**FIGURE 13-7.**   This patient dove into shallow water and struck his head. He immediately complained of neck pain and presented to the emergency room with brachycardia, hypotension, flaccid lower extremities, and weak upper extremities. His radiographic evaluation demonstrated multiple fractures of the cervical spine, and he required phenylephrine to maintain a systolic blood pressure greater than 90 mm mm Hg.

## Neurogenic Shock

Neurogenic shock refers to diminished tissue perfusion as a result of loss of vasomotor tone to peripheral arterial beds. Loss of vasoconstrictor impulses results in increased vascular capacitance, decreased venous return, and decreased cardiac output. Neurogenic shock is usually due to injuries to the spinal cord from fractures of the cervical or high thoracic vertebrae that disrupt sympathetic regulation of peripheral vascular tone. Occasionally, an injury such as an epidural hematoma impinging on the spinal cord can produce neurogenic shock without an associated vertebral fracture. Penetrating wounds to the spinal cord can produce neurogenic shock, as well. Sympathetic input to the heart that normally increases heart rate and cardiac contractility and input to the adrenal medulla that increases the release of catecholamines can be disrupted by a high injury to the spinal cord, preventing the typical reflex tachycardia that occurs with the relative hypovolemia from increased venous capacitance and loss of vasomotor tone.

Diagnosis.   The classic findings of neurogenic shock consist of decreased blood pressure associated with bradycardia (absence of reflexive tachycardia due to disrupted sympathetic discharge), warm extremities (loss of peripheral vasoconstriction), motor and sensory deficits indicative of an injury to the spinal cord, and radiographic evidence of a fracture in the vertebral column (Fig. 13-7). Determining the presence of neurogenic shock may be difficult, however, since patients with multisystem trauma that includes an injury to the spinal cord often have a traumatic brain injury that may make identification of motor and sensory deficits difficult. Furthermore, associated injuries may cause hypovolemia and

complicate the clinical presentation. In a subset of patients with injuries to the spinal cord from penetrating wounds, most patients with hypotension had blood loss as the etiology (74%) and not a neurogenic cause, and few (7%) had all the classic findings of neurogenic shock.[89] Hypovolemia should be sought and excluded before the diagnosis of neurogenic shock is made.

Treatment.   After the airway is secured and ventilation is adequate, fluid resuscitation and restoration of intravascular volume will often improve systemic blood pressure and perfusion in neurogenic shock. Administration of vasoconstrictors can improve peripheral vascular tone, decrease vascular capacitance, and increase venous return, but should only be considered once hypovolemia is excluded and the diagnosis of neurogenic shock established. Specific treatment for the shock state per se is often brief and the need to administer vasoconstrictors typically lasts only 24 to 48 hours. The duration of the need for vasopressor support for neurogenic shock may correlate with the overall prognosis for improvement in neurologic function.[90] Appropriate rapid restoration of blood pressure and circulatory perfusion may also improve perfusion to the spinal cord, prevent progressive ischemia of the spinal cord, and minimize secondary injury to the spinal cord.[91] Restoration of normal hemodynamics should precede any operative attempts to stabilize the vertebral fracture.

## Cardiogenic Shock

Cardiogenic shock refers to a failure of the circulatory pump leading to diminished forward flow and subsequent tissue hypoxia. Inadequate cardiac function after blunt thoracic trauma can be due to a myocardial contusion, myocardial infarction, or injury to a valve.

As the average age of the population increases, the prevalence of comorbid medical conditions in trauma patients will also increase. Elderly patients with pre-existing intrinsic cardiac disease will be more susceptible to suffering an acute myocardial infarction or significant arrhythmia associated with the stress of injury that can also induce cardiac failure and cardiogenic shock. Diminished cardiac output or contractility in the face of adequate intravascular volume (preload) may lead to underperfused vascular beds and reflexive sympathetic discharge. Increased sympathetic stimulation of the heart, either through direct neural input or from circulating catecholamines, increases heart rate, myocardial contraction, and myocardial oxygen consumption. Patients with fixed, flow-limiting stenoses of the coronary arteries may not be able to increase coronary perfusion to meet the increased myocardial oxygen demands and these lesions, therefore, further increase the risk for myocardial damage.[15] Diminished cardiac output decreases coronary artery blood flow, resulting in a scenario of increased myocardial oxygen demand at a time when myocardial oxygen supply may be limited. Acute heart failure can also result in fluid accumulation in the pulmonary microcirculatory bed, impairing the diffusion of oxygen from the alveolar space and decreasing myocardial oxygen delivery even further.

Diagnosis.   Rapid identification of the patient with pump failure and institution of corrective action are essential in preventing further decreases in cardiac output after such an injury. If increased myocardial oxygen needs cannot be met, there will be progressive and unremitting cardiac dysfunction. Blunt injury to the heart is rarely severe enough to induce pump failure,[92] but manifestations of shock in the setting of a patient at risk should raise one's index of suspicion. Evidence of blunt thoracic injury such as sternal fracture, multiple rib fractures, tenderness or hematomas in the chest wall or precordial area, or a history of a direct precordial impact may heighten one's suspicion and identify a patient at increased risk for a blunt cardiac injury. Elderly patients with known preexisting cardiac disease are at increased risk of suffering injury-related cardiac complications including cardiac failure. Furthermore, elderly patients with intrinsic cardiac disease are at risk to suffer a primary cardiac event that induces syncope, a fall, or loss of control of one's vehicle that then leads to presentation to a trauma center. Defining the frequency of the latter condition may be difficult.

Making the diagnosis of cardiogenic shock involves the identification of cardiac dysfunction or acute heart failure in a susceptible patient. Since patients with blunt cardiac injury typically have multisystem trauma,[93,94] hemorrhagic shock from intra-abdominal bleeding, intrathoracic bleeding, and bleeding from fractures must be excluded. Most instances of blunt cardiac injury are self-limited with no long-term cardiac sequelae. Relatively few patients with blunt cardiac injury will develop dysfunction of the cardiac pump and those who do generally exhibit cardiogenic shock early in their evaluation.[92] Therefore, establishing the diagnosis of blunt cardiac injury is secondary to excluding other etiologies for shock and establishing that significant cardiac dysfunction is present. This typically involves measurement of diminished cardiac output by catheterization of the pulmonary artery or documenting abnormalities of wall motion or other manifestations of cardiac dysfunction by echocardiography.[95–98] Invasive hemodynamic monitoring with a pulmonary artery catheter can reveal diminished cardiac output and elevated pulmonary artery pressures. The pulmonary artery catheter can also guide the response to therapy. Transesophageal echocardiography (TEE) provides excellent views of the pericardium that are not interfered with by subcutaneous air, bandages covering chest wounds, chest tubes, or unfavorable body habitus that may limit evaluation of cardiac function by transthoracic echocardiography (TTE). The rapid evaluation of cardiac function by TEE may be problematic, however, in the presence of severe cervical trauma, maxillofacial trauma, or unstable injuries to the cervical spine that can interfere with placement of the probe. TEE also requires experienced ultrasonographers who may not be rapidly available at all hours. Trauma surgeons are becoming increasingly more experienced in the use of ultrasound as part of the initial resuscitation. While the sensitivity of surgeon-performed ultrasound to diagnose penetrating cardiac wounds may be high,[99,100] the ability of surgeons to effectively evaluate cardiac performance as part of the ultrasound examination for trauma has not been established.

Treatment.   Patients with blunt cardiac injury will often have associated injuries that produce hypovolemia, and expansion of intravascular volume as an initial maneuver can improve perfusion significantly. Hypervolemia, however, can magnify the physiologic derangements produced by cardiac dysfunction and should be avoided. When profound cardiac dysfunction exists, ionotropic support may be indicated to improve cardiac contractility and cardiac performance.[101] Dobutamine stimulates primarily cardiac $\beta_1$ receptors to increase cardiac output, but may also vasodilate peripheral vascular beds, lower total peripheral resistance, and lower systemic blood pressure through effects on $\beta_2$ receptors. Ensuring adequate preload and intravascular volume is, therefore, essential prior to instituting therapy with dobutamine. Dopamine stimulates $\alpha$ receptors (vasoconstriction), $\beta_1$ receptors (cardiac stimulation), and $\beta_2$ receptors (vasodilation) with its effects on $\beta$ receptors predominating at low doses. Epinephrine stimulates $\alpha$ and $\beta$ receptors and may increase cardiac contractility and heart rate, but can also cause intense peripheral vasoconstriction that can further impair cardiac performance. It is important to balance the beneficial effects of improved cardiac performance versus the potential side effects of excessive reflex tachycardia and peripheral vasoconstriction. This will require serial assessment of tissue perfusion including capillary refill, character of peripheral pulses, adequacy of urine output, or improvement in laboratory parameters of resuscitation such as arterial blood pH, base deficit, and lactate.

Patients whose cardiac dysfunction is refractory to cardiotonics may require mechanical circulatory support with an intra-aortic balloon pump.[101] This can be inserted at the bedside in the intensive care unit via the femoral artery through either a cutdown or percutaneous approach. Aggressive circulatory support of patients with cardiac dysfunction from intrinsic cardiac disease has led to more widespread application of these devices and more familiarity with their operation by both physicians and critical care nurses.

Patients who have suffered an acute myocardial infarction following injury should have preservation of existing myocardium and cardiac function as priorities of therapy. This is accomplished by the following: ensuring adequate systemic oxygen delivery and peripheral tissue oxygenation; maintaining adequate preload with judicious volume restoration; minimizing sympathetic discharge through adequate relief of pain; and correcting electrolyte imbalances. The use of anticoagulation or thrombolytic therapy for the management of acute coronary syndromes will depend on associated injuries and the risk of secondary intracavitary or intracranial bleeding. Patients in cardiac failure from an acute myocardial infarction may benefit from pharmacologic or mechanical circulatory support in a manner similar to that of patients with cardiac failure related to blunt cardiac injury. There are additional pharmacologic tools that are useful in patients with cardiac ischemia from intrinsic coronary artery disease. These include the use of beta blockers to control heart rate and myocardial oxygen consumption, nitrates to promote coronary blood flow through vasodilation, and angiotensin-converting enzyme (ACE) inhibitors to reduce ACE-mediated vasoconstriction that increases myocardial work load and oxygen consumption.[102] Selected patients who do not have significant associated injuries may be candidates for coronary angiography and subsequent procedures to improve coronary blood flow such as transluminal angioplasty, coronary artery stents, or urgent coronary artery bypass grafting.

## Septic Shock

Septic shock is a by-product of the body's response to invasive or severe localized infection, typically from bacterial or fungal pathogens. In its attempt to eradicate the pathogens, the reticuloendothelial system elaborates a wide array of protein mediators (cytokines). These mediators enhance effector mechanisms for macrophage- and neutrophil-killing, increase procoagulant activity and fibroblast activity to localize the invaders, and increase microvascular blood flow to enhance delivery of killing forces to the area of invasion. When this response is overly exuberant or becomes systemic rather than localized, manifestations of sepsis may be evident. These findings include enhanced cardiac output, peripheral vasodilation, fever, leukocytosis, and tachycardia.[103,104] Sepsis is an uncommon etiology for shock in the acute presentation of a trauma patient unless there has been a substantial delay between injury and presentation to the ED. Typically, invasive infection in the injured patient occurs days to weeks after injury and is prevalent in the severely injured patient who develops a nosocomial infection in the intensive care unit.

Diagnosis.    Attempts to standardize terminology have led to the establishment of criteria for the diagnosis of sepsis in the hospitalized adult. These criteria include manifestations of the host response to infection (fever, leukocytosis, mental contusion, tachypnea, tachycardia, hypotension, oliguria), as well as identification of an offending organism.[105] Septic shock requires the presence of these conditions associated with evidence of tissue hypoperfusion. Recognizing septic shock in the trauma patient begins with defining high-risk groups as follows: critically ill patients in the intensive care unit where nosocomial infection rates are high; patients who have suffered injuries associated with significant contamination (colorectal wounds with fecal spillage, soft tissue wounds embedded with soil or dirt); patients with injuries that may be associated with persistent devitalized tissue (crush injuries);

patients whose wounds put them at risk from complications (anastomotic disruption, pancreatic leak); or patients with missed injuries (shotgun wounds). The clinical manifestations of septic shock will usually prompt the initiation of treatment before bacteriologic confirmation of an organism or source of active infection is identified. An aggressive search for the source of the infection includes a thorough physical exam, inspection of all wounds, evaluation of intravascular catheters or other foreign bodies, sampling of appropriate body fluids for culture, and adjunctive imaging studies as needed.

Treatment.    Severely obtunded patients may require intubation to protect their airway while patients whose work of breathing is excessive may require intubation and mechanical ventilation to prevent respiratory collapse. Since vasodilation and a decrease in total peripheral resistance may produce hypotension, restoration of circulatory volume with balanced salt solutions is essential. Since the portal of entry of the offending organism and its identity may not be evident until culture data return or imaging studies are completed, empiric antibiotics that cover the most likely pathogens are chosen. Knowing the bacteriologic profile of infectious events in an individual intensive care unit can be obtained from the infection control department and may identify potential responsible organisms. In the trauma patient, intravenous antibiotics will frequently be insufficient to adequately treat the infectious episode. Therefore, drainage of infected fluid collections (Fig. 13-8), removal of infected foreign bodies, and debridement of devitalized tissue are essential to eradicate the infection. This process may require multiple operations. For patients who manifest symptoms of septic shock early in their hospitalization, consideration of the possibility of a missed injury to a hollow viscus should be entertained. Missed abdominal injuries represent a significant source of sepsis and the septic response leading to multiple organ dysfunction syndrome.[106,107] Antibiotics should be tailored to cover the responsible organisms once culture data are available and, if appropriate, the spectrum of coverage narrowed. Long-term empiric use

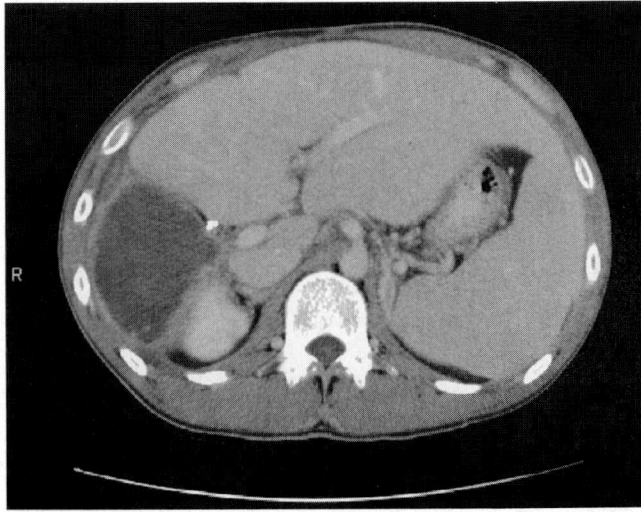

**FIGURE 13-8.**  This patient suffered a gunshot wound to the abdomen and required a laparotomy, hepatorrhapy, and repair of an intestinal injury. He returned to the hospital after discharge with fever, tachycardia, malaise, and abdominal tenderness. This abdominal abscess was treated with percutaneous drainage.

of broad spectrum antibiotics should be minimized to reduce the development of resistant organisms and avoid the potential complications of fungal overgrowth and antibiotic-associated colitis from Clostridium difficile.[108]

Vasopressor therapy may be required as a supportive measure when hypotension is refractory to volume infusion in patients in septic shock. Alpha adrenergic agents promote peripheral vasoconstriction, improve systemic blood pressure, and can be titrated by continuous infusion to target an adequate mean arterial pressure. Unfortunately, high doses of alpha-adrenergic agents can be associated with tachyarrhythmias, ischemia of the midgut, gangrene of the digits, or the development of hyposensitivity requiring increasing doses to achieve the desired goals. As previously noted, vasopressin has been utilized as an adjunct for the treatment of vasodilatory shock in some centers and may be associated with a decreased need for alpha adrenergic agents.[109] High doses of vasopressin should be avoided so as to decrease adverse gastrointestinal and cardiovascular side effects.

Adrenal insufficiency can be a cause of ongoing shock in susceptible individuals as described above, and relative adrenal insufficiency has been suggested to be an underappreciated cause of ongoing hemodynamic instability in critically ill patients.[18–20] This condition has been studied most extensively in patients suffering sepsis, and only preliminary information is available for the role of an inadequate adrenal response in trauma patients. The relative importance of secondary adrenal insufficiency, the best method to diagnose the condition, the proper treatment regimen, and the appropriate duration of therapy continue to be studied.

Strategies for immune modulation have been developed for the treatment of septic shock. These include the use of anti-endotoxin antibodies, anti-cytokine antibodies, cytokine receptor antagonists, immune enhancers, anti-nitric oxide compounds, and oxygen radical scavangers.[110–116] Each of these compounds are designed to alter some aspect of the host immune response to shock. Most of these strategies, however, have failed to demonstrate efficacy in patients despite utility in well-controlled animal experiments. It is unclear whether the failure of these compounds is due to poorly designed clinical trials, inadequate understanding of the interactions of the complex immune response to injury and infection, or animal models of shock that poorly represent human disease. Recent trials have demonstrated the efficacy of activated protein C in improving mortality from sepsis.[117] Subgroup analysis of patients with sepsis, but at low risk of death, did, however, document an increased risk of bleeding complications associated with therapy without a substantial improvement in survival.[118] Sepsis and nosocomial infections in critically ill patients continue to represent significant sources of morbidity and consume substantial health care resources. The magnitude of this problem ensures that investigation into novel therapies for the treatment of sepsis will continue until better agents are identified.

## Obstructive Shock

Hypoperfusion can be due to mechanical obstruction of the circulation impeding venous return to the heart or preventing cardiac filling. The end result of either of these two events is decreased cardiac output leading to decreased peripheral perfusion. Most commonly, mechanical obstruction is due to the presence of a tension pneumothorax or cardiac tamponade. With either condition, there is decreased cardiac output associated with increased central venous pressure.

Diagnosis and Treatment. The manifestations of a tension pneumothorax are a presence of shock in the context of diminished breath sounds over one hemithorax, hyperresonance to percussion, jugular venous distension, and shift of mediastinal structures to the unaffected side. Unfortunately, not all of the clinical manifestations of tension pneumothorax may be evident on physical examination. Hyperresonance may be difficult to appreciate in a noisy resuscitation area. Jugular venous distension and/or tracheal deviation may be obscured by a cervical collar in the multiply injured patient and not seen unless specifically searched for. Furthermore, hypovolemia from concurrent bleeding may diminish central venous pressure and prevent jugular venous distension even when increased pleural or pericardial pressure restrict flow. When a surgeon with skill in interpreting pleural ultrasound is unavailable, empiric treatment with pleural decompression is indicated rather than waiting for an emergent X-ray. When a chest tube cannot be immediately inserted, such as in the prehospital setting, the pleural space can be decompressed with a large caliber needle inserted in the second interspace at the midclavicular line. Immediate return of air and rapid resolution of hypotension suggest strongly that a tension pneumothorax was present. Typical findings on a chest X-ray include deviation of mediastinal structures, depression of the hemidiaphragm, and hypo-opacification with absent lung markings.

Cardiac tamponade results from the accumulation of blood within the pericardial sac and most commonly occurs from penetrating trauma. While precordial wounds are most likely to injure the heart and produce tamponade, any projectile or wounding agent that passes in proximity to the mediastinum can potentially produce tamponade. Blunt rupture of the heart is fortunately rare, but difficult to diagnose unless a FAST exam is performed immediately on all patients at risk. The manifestations of cardiac tamponade may be as catastrophic as total circulatory collapse and cardiac arrest or they may be more subtle. A high index of suspicion is warranted to make a rapid diagnosis. Patients who present with circulatory arrest due to cardiac tamponade from a precordial penetrating wound require emergency pericardial decompression through a left anterolateral thoracotomy, and the indications for this maneuver are discussed in Chap. 15. Cardiac tamponade may also be associated with tachycardia, muffled heart tones, jugular venous distension, and elevated central venous pressure. Absence of these clinical findings, however, may not be sufficient to exclude cardiac injury and cardiac tamponade. Muffled heart tones may be difficult to appreciate in a busy trauma center and jugular venous distension and central venous pressure may be diminished by coexistent bleeding and hypovolemia. Therefore, patients at risk for cardiac tamponade whose hemodynamic status permits should undergo additional diagnostic tests.

Invasive hemodynamic monitoring may support the diagnosis of cardiac tamponade if elevated central venous pressure, pulsus paradoxus (decreased systemic arterial pressure with inspiration), or elevated right atrial and right ventricular pressure by pulmonary artery catheter are present. These hemodynamic profiles suffer from lack of specificity, the time required to obtain them, and their inability to exclude cardiac injury in the absence of tamponade. Chest radiographs may provide information on the possible trajectory of a projectile, but are rarely diagnostic since the acutely filled pericardium distends poorly. Pericardial ultrasound as part of a surgeon-performed FAST examination, either through the subxiphoid or transthoracic approach, is practiced routinely at many trauma centers. Excellent results in detecting pericardial fluid have been reported.[99,100] The yield in identifying pericardial fluid obviously depends on the skill and experience of the ultrasonographer, body habitus of the patient, and absence of wounds that preclude visualization of the pericardium. Standard two-dimensional transthoracic or transesophageal echocardiography to evaluate the pericardium for fluid is typically performed by cardiologists or anesthesiologists skilled at evaluating ventricular function, valvular abnormalities, and integrity of the proximal thoracic aorta. These skilled examiners are usually not immediately available at all hours of the night and waiting for this test may result in inordinate delays. In addition, while both ultrasound techniques may demonstrate the presence of fluid or characteristic findings of tamponade (large volume of pericardial fluid, right atrial collapse, poor distensibility of the right ventricle), they do not exclude cardiac injury per se[119,120] and their utility will be discussed in greater detail in Chap. 16.

Pericardiocentesis to diagnose pericardial blood and potentially relieve tamponade has a long history in the evaluation of the trauma patient. Its inability to evacuate clotted blood and potential to produce cardiac injury make it a poor alternative in most busy trauma centers.

Diagnostic pericardial window represents the most direct method to determine the presence of blood within the pericardium. It can be performed through either the subxiphoid or transdiaphragmatic approach.[121,122] Some authors report performing this technique using local infiltrative anesthesia; however, the ability to achieve satisfactory safety and visualization in the trauma victim who may be intoxicated, in pain, or anxious from hypoperfusion usually mandates the use of general anesthesia. Once the pericardium is opened and tamponade relieved, hemodynamics usually improve dramatically and formal pericardial exploration can be performed. Exposure of the heart can be achieved by extending the incision to a formal sternotomy, performing a left anterolateral thoracotomy, or performing bilateral anterior thoracotomies ("clamshell") as discussed in Chaps. 15 and 25.

## Traumatic Shock

Some authors consider traumatic shock a separate clinical entity.[59] The term is used to represent a combination of several insults after injury that, by themselves, may be insufficient to induce shock, but produce profound hypoperfusion when combined. Hypoperfusion from relatively modest loss of volume can be magnified by the proinflammatory activation that occurs following injury or shock. In addition to ischemia or ischemia/reperfusion, accumulating evidence demonstrates that even simple hemorrhage induces proinflammatory activation and causes many of the cellular changes typically attributed previously only to septic shock.[22,26] Examples of traumatic shock might include small-volume hemorrhage accompanied by injury to soft tissue (femur fracture, crush injury) or any combination of hypovolemic, neurogenic, cardiogenic, and obstructive shock that induces rapidly progressive activation of proinflammatory cytokines. Therapy for this form of shock is focused on correcting the individual elements contributing to its existence. Therapeutic maneuvers include prompt control of hemorrhage, adequate volume

resuscitation to correct oxygen debt, debridement of nonviable tissue, stabilization of bony injuries, and appropriate treatment of soft tissue wounds.

## ENDPOINTS IN RESUSCITATION OF THE TRAUMA PATIENT

The ultimate goal in the treatment of shock from any etiology is to restore tissue perfusion, re-establish normal cellular function, and prevent damage to end-organs. Resuscitation of the trauma patient is complete when aerobic cellular metabolism is restored, tissue acidosis is corrected, and the oxygen debt has been repaid. The difficult question remains how to determine when this has occurred. The ideal standard to measure, or the appropriate endpoint to monitor, to determine when shock has been fully reversed has not yet been determined.

Clinical parameters used to assess the adequacy of resuscitation in the patient with shock include heart rate, blood pressure, and urine output as described in the Advanced Trauma Life Support course. When these parameters are abnormal, the need for ongoing resuscitation is clear. These clinical parameters can normalize, however, despite evidence of persistent abnormalities in tissue perfusion,[123–125] and more objective or sensitive measures that signify the normalization of homeostasis have been sought. Endpoints in resuscitation can be divided into systemic or global parameters, tissue specific parameters, and cellular parameters. In addition to vital signs, other global endpoints include cardiac output, pulmonary artery wedge pressure, oxygen delivery and consumption, lactate level, and base deficit. It is not entirely clear, as will be discussed below, if these parameters represent actual goals to be achieved in resuscitation since some patients will not achieve these goals despite heroic efforts. One could argue that inability to normalize these parameters represents a marker or predictor for poor outcome. Several recent comprehensive reviews on resuscitation of the trauma patient have been published, and the interested reader is directed to these publications for additional details.[126,129] Endpoints are discussed below.

## Oxygen Transport

Correction of the cellular oxygen debt is the goal of resuscitation of the patient in shock. It has been hypothesized that generating supranormal oxygen delivery to optimize oxygen consumption will more rapidly correct the oxygen debt. This finding was supported by studies that demonstrated improved outcome in patients suffering shock or undergoing high-risk surgery when they had elevated cardiac output and oxygen delivery.[130,131] Bishop reported reduced mortality, decreased organ failure, decreased need for mechanical ventilation, and fewer ICU days in trauma patients managed with supranormal oxygen delivery.[132] The results of other studies using supranormal oxygen transport as a goal of therapy, however, have had conflicting results. Several studies report no survival benefit with this approach.[123,133] One complicating factor with studies attempting to optimize oxygen transport is the finding that many "control" patients will spontaneously achieve goal levels of oxygen delivery while many patients in the treatment arm cannot achieve these goals despite maximal therapy.[134,135] It appears that the ability to achieve elevated oxygen delivery after resuscitation identifies patients who have greater physiologic reserve and will have lower mortality than those who do not.[129,136]

Some investigators have suggested that the timing of therapeutic interventions to optimize oxygen transport significantly impacts the results of therapy. In studies where oxygen transport was optimized after the onset of organ dysfunction, there was no improvement in mortality; however, early optimization has been associated with improved survival in selected studies.[127,128,137] Most of these studies have been conducted in patients with sepsis or in mixed surgical populations and their direct relevance to resuscitation after trauma remains to be demonstrated. Another drawback to wide acceptance of oxygen transport-directed therapy is the need for insertion of a pulmonary artery catheter. Pulmonary artery catheters are invasive, associated with a low but definable incidence of complications, and have not been universally shown to improve mortality in critically ill adults.[138,139] Some investigators have suggested that central venous oxygen saturation ($SO_2$) may represent a reasonable approximation of mixed venous $SO_2$ and, thus, be an easier endpoint to monitor for goal-directed therapy.[140,141] The relationship between central and mixed venous $SO_2$, though, has not yet been confirmed in injured patients. Further studies will be required before the role of optimization of oxygen transport in patients suffering from shock will be fully understood.

## Lactate

As previously described lactate dehydrogenase converts pyruvate to lactate during anaerobic metabolism. The lactate is then released into the systemic circulation and measured as an indirect marker of oxygen debt after shock. Several measures of lactate correlate with mortality after traumatic injury including admission lactate, highest serum lactate, and time to normalize lactate.[142,143] In one study, mortality was zero in patients who normalized serum lactate within 24 hours, 22% in those who normalized lactate within 24–48 hours, and 86% in patients who took greater than 48 hours to normalize lactate levels.[144] A number of factors can influence serum lactate level, and these include excessive alcohol intake, cocaine intoxication, ketoacidosis, and hepatic dysfunction. Also, some investigators have found lactate to be imperfect in estimating oxygen debt in patients after shock.[144–146] A recent analysis of over 15,000 trauma admissions revealed higher lactate levels in patients with positive drug and alcohol screens. On the other hand, multiple logistic and linear regression analyses

confirmed lactate and base deficit as independent predictors of mortality, ICU and hospital length of stay.[147] Similar to the concept of increasing oxygen delivery, lactate may be most useful as a predictor of outcome, normalizing in patients with sufficient reserve to respond to resuscitation.

## Arterial Base Deficit

Base deficit can also be used as an estimate of the oxygen debt in patients who have been injured or suffered shock. As noted above, the base deficit is defined as the amount of base in millimoles required to titrate a liter of arterial blood to a normal pH in the presence of normal oxygenation, carbon dioxide, and body temperature. Several studies have correlated the base deficit with survival, development of organ failure, and the need for blood transfusion in trauma patients.[148–152] Base deficit can be stratified into mild (3 to 5), moderate (6 to 14) and severe ($\geq$15); and these strata correlate with resuscitation requirements (Table 13-2) and mortality.[148,149] Of interest, patients with markedly severe base deficits after traumatic injury can have a reasonable survival rate if they can survive the first several hours after injury.[153] Magnitude of the base deficit does not appear to equate to therapeutic futility. In addition, minor abnormalities in base deficit may still be associated with significant injuries.[154] Failure to normalize the base deficit with ongoing resuscitation is associated with greater mortality, increased risk of multiple organ failure, and the potential for ongoing undetected blood loss.[149,155] Factors that can influence base deficit besides metabolic acidosis from shock include hypothermia, alcohol, drugs, and the use of bicarbonate-rich or chloride-rich resuscitation fluids.[156] Nevertheless, base deficit continues to be widely used to stratify severity of illness after injury.[129] Serum bicarbonate has been postulated to reflect base deficit and to be easier to obtain.[157,158] Initial studies appear promising, but whether serum bicarbonate will ultimately replace base deficit in the monitoring of patients in shock will require further study.

## Gastric Tonometry

Tissue-specific endpoints as an index of global tissue perfusion have been proposed as being more predictive of outcome and adequacy of resuscitation and have been used as markers of resuscitation of the splanchnic bed. Gastric tonometry, for example, has been used to assess the adequacy of perfusion of the gastrointestinal tract. The $pCO_2$ in gastric secretions readily

**TABLE 13-2**

| Volume Requirements (Ringer's Lactate and Blood) in Base Deficit Groups[a] | | | | | |
|---|---|---|---|---|---|
| | | **HOURS AFTER ADMISSION** | | | |
| **BASE DEFICIT GROUP** | **N** | **1** | **2** | **4** | **24** |
| Mild (2 to –5) | 70 | 2,966 ± 335 | 4,030 ± 520 | 5,881 ± 817 | 7,475 ± 766 |
| Moderate (–6 to –14) | 110 | 3,893 ± 322 | 7,522 ± 642 | 8,120 ± 718 | 13,007 ± 1,078 |
| Severe (<–15) | 29 | 6,110 ± 589 | 9,800 ± 982 | 10,909 ± 1,435 | 16,396 ± 3,252 |
| | | $p < 0.001$ | $p < 0.001$ | $p < 0.008$ | $p < 0.001$ |

"Values expressed as cc ± SEM.
*(Reproduced with permission form Davis JW, Shackford SR, Mackersie RC, et al: Base deficit as a guide to volume resuscitation. J Trauma 28:1464, 1988.)*

equilibrates with the gastric muscosa, and gastric tonometry converts $pCO_2$ to a measurement of intramucosal pH (pHi) using the Henderson-Hasselbach equation. For gastric tonometry to be accurate, gastric feedings must be withheld and gastric acid should be suppressed. Gastric mucosal pHi after resuscitation and the time to normalize gastric pHi correlate with mortality.[159,160] A recent randomized, prospective study involving 151 trauma patients, however, demonstrated no survival benefit with splanchnic hypoperfusion-directed therapy.[161] Similar to the global parameters discussed so far, the ability of injured patients to normalize gastric pHi may reflect intrinsic ability of a given patient to reestablish homeostasis and respond to resuscitation rather than representing a goal of therapy that will increase survival.[162,163]

## Near-Infrared Spectroscopy

Near-infrared spectroscopy (NIRS) is a noninvasive technique that utilizes the differential absorption properties of hemoglobin to evaluate skeletal muscle oxygenation by emitting light in the near-infrared spectrum (650–1000 nm). Photons from multiple wavelengths are either absorbed or reflected back to the probe and measure tissue oxyhemoglobin levels. In animal models of shock, NIRS has been suggested to be a better predictor of the inability to be successfully resuscitated and subsequent mortality than oxygen transport or lactate.[164] NIRS of tissue oxygen saturation ($StO_2$) in patients being resuscitated after injury correlated with systemic $O_2$ delivery, base deficit and lactate in one study.[165] NIRS has also been shown to identify patients in severe shock and may do so better than base deficit.[166] A multicenter trial to evaluate the role of NIRS in trauma patients in shock and to determine its ability to predict shock-induced multiple organ dysfunction syndrome is currently underway.

## Tissue pH, Oxygen, and Carbon Dioxide Concentration

Measurement of tissue pH, $PO_2$, and $PCO_2$ also hold promise for guiding resuscitation in trauma patients based on many of the same principles as previously discussed for gastric tonometry. Either transcutaneous or percutaneous measurements can be performed, but their current use remains experimental. Sublingual capnometry correlated with gastric tonometry in the resuscitation of critically ill adults in one study and may be a less cumbersome tissue specific parameter to follow.[167] Animal models of hemorrhagic shock and resuscitation suggest that peripheral tissue measurements may adequately reflect those of the splanchnic bed and provide a more readily accessible measure of visceral perfusion.[168–170] Whether these relationships are true for septic shock remains to be demonstrated, and some investigators have identified discrepancies between measurements obtained from different body areas following resuscitation.[171] This technology may be subject to the same limitations discussed above for gastric tonometry and other endpoints of resuscitation. It remains to be proven that resuscitating the injured patient to specific endpoints of visceral perfusion will impact survival in a meaningful way. These technologies remain active areas of investigation in both the animal laboratory and clinical arena.

## REFERENCES

1. Gross SA: *A System of Surgery: Pathologic, Diagnostic, Therapeutic, and Operative.* Philadelphia: Lee & Febiger, 1872.
2. Bernard C: *Lecons sur les Phenomenes de la Vie Communs aux Animaux et Aux Vegetaux.* Paris: JB Ballieve, 1879, p. 4.
3. Cannon WB: *Traumatic Shock.* New York: Appleton, 1923.
4. Chambers NK, Buchman TG: Shock at the millennium. Walter B. Cannon and Alfred Blalock. *Shock* 13:497, 2000.
5. Cannon WB, Frasen J, Cowell EM: The preventative treatment of wound shock. *JAMA* 70:618, 1918.
6. Blalock A: *Principle of Surgical Care, Shock, and Other Problems.* St. Louis: Mosby, 1940.
7. Wiggers CJ: *Experimental hemorrhagic shock, in Physiology of Shock.* New York: Commonwealth, 1950, p. 121.
8. Carrico CJ, Canizaro PC, Shires GT: Fluid resuscitation following injury-rationale for the use of balanced salt solutions. *Crit Care Med* 4:46, 1976.
9. Shires T, Coln D, Carrico J, et al.: Fluid therapy in hemorrhagic shock. *Arch Surg* 88:688, 1964.
10. Peitzman AB, Corbett WA, Shires GT III, et al.: Cellular function in liver and muscle during hemorrhagic shock in primates. *Surg Gynecol Obstet* 161:419, 1985.
11. Bickell WH, Bruttig SP, Millnamow GA, et al.: The detrimental effects of intravenous crystalloid after aortotomy in swine. *Surgery* 110:529, 1991.
12. Bickell WH, Wall MJ, Pepe PE, et al.: Immediate versus delayed resuscitation for hypotensive patients with penetrating torso injuries. *N Engl J Med* 331:1105, 1994.
13. Bond RF, Manley ES Jr, Green HD: Cutaneous and skeletal muscle vascular responses to hemorrhage and irreversible shock. *Am J Physiol* 212:488, 1967.
14. Bereiter DA, Zaid AM, Gann DS: Adrenocorticotropin response to graded blood loss in the cat. *Am J Physiol* 250:E76, 1984.
15. Guyton AC: *Textbook of Medical Physiology.* Philadelphia: Saunders, 1981.
16. Taylor BS, Harbrecht BG: The physiologic response to injury. In Peitzman AB, Rhodes M, Schwab CW, et al. ed: *The Trauma Manual,* 2nd ed. Philadelphia: Lippincott, Williams & Wilkins, 2002, p. 17.
17. Aneman A, Eisenhofer G, Olbe L, et al.: Sympathetic discharge to mesenteric organs and the liver; evidence for substantial mesenteric organ norepinephrine spillover. *J Clin Invest* 97:1640, 1996.
18. Annane D, Sebille V, Charpentier C, et al.: Effect of treatment with low doses of hydrocortisone and fludocortisone on mortality in patients with septic shock. *JAMA* 288:862, 2002.
19. Minneci PC, Deans KJ, Banks SM, et al.: Mita-analysis: The effect of steroids on survival and shock during sepsis depends on the dose. *Ann Intern Med* 14:47, 2004.
20. Cooper MS, Stewart PM: Costicosteroid insufficiency in acutely ill patients. *N Engl J Med* 348:727, 2003.
21. Runciman WB, Skowronski GA: Pathophysiology of haemorrhagic shock. *Anaesth Intens Care* 12:193, 1984.
22. Roumen RM, Hendriks T, van der Ven-Jongekrijg J, et al.: Cytokine patterns in patients after major vascular surgery, hemorrhagic shock, and severe blunt trauma. Relation with subsequent adult respiratory distress syndrome and multiple organ failure. *Ann Surg* 218:769, 1993.
23. Nuytinck JK, Goris JA, Redl H, et al.: Posttraumatic complications and inflammatory mediators. *Arch Surg* 121:886, 1986.
24. Roumen RM, Redl H, Schlag G, et al.: Inflammatory mediators in relation to the development of multiple organ failure in patients after severe blunt trauma. *Crit Care Med* 23:474, 1995.
25. Farmer P, Pugin J: β-adrenergic agonists exert their "anti-inflammatory" effects in monocytic cells through the IκB/NF-κB pathway. *Am J Physiol* 279:L675, 2000.
26. Nast-Kolb D, Waydhas C, Gippner-Steppert C, et al.: Indicators of the posttraumatic inflammatory response correlate with organ failure in patients with multiple injuries. *J Trauma* 42: 446, 1997.
27. Akira S, Hirano T, Taga T, et al.: Biology of multifunctional cytokines; IL-6 and related molecules (IL-1 and TNF). *FASEB J* 4:2860, 1990.
28. Peitzman AB, Udekwu AO, Ochoa J, et al.: Bacterial translocation in trauma patients. *J Trauma* 31:1083, 1991.
29. Rush BF Jr, Redan JA, Flanagan JJ, et al.: Does the bacteremia observed in hemorrhagic shock have clinical significance? *Ann Surg* 210:342, 1989.
30. Rhee P, Waxman K, Clark L, et al.: Tumor necrosis factor and monocytes are released during hemorrhagic shock. *Resuscitation* 25:249, 1993.
31. Jiang J, Bahrami S, Leichtfried G, et al.: Kinetics of endotoxin and tumor necrosis factor appearance in portal and systemic circulation after hemorrhagic shock in rats. *Ann Surg* 221:100, 1995.
32. Endo S, Inada K, Yamada Y, et al.: Plasma endotoxin and cytokine concentrations in patients with hemorrhagic shock. *Crit Care Med* 22:949, 1994.
33. Decker T, Lohmann-Matthes ML, Gifford GE. Cell-associated tumor necrosis factor (TNF) as a killing mechanism of activated cytotoxic macrophages. *J Immunol* 138:957, 1987.

34. Bagby GJ, Plessala KJ, Wilson LA, et al.: Divergent efficacy of antibody to tumor necrosis factor-α in intravascular and peritonitis models of sepsis. *J Infect Dis* 163:83, 1991.

35. Echtenacher B, Falk W, Mannel DN, et al.: Requirement of endogenous tumor necrosis factor/cachetin for recovery from experimental peritonitis. *J Immunol* 145:3762, 1990.

36. van der Poll T, Keogh CV, Burirman WA, et al.: Passive immunization against tumor necrosis factor-alpha impairs host defense during pneumococial pneumonia in mice. *Am J Respir Crit Car Med* 155:603, 1997.

37. Wakefield CH, Barclay GR, Fearon KC, et al.: Proinflammatory mediator activity, endogenous antagonists and the systemic inflammatory response in intra-abdominal sepsis. Scottish Sepsis Intervention Group. *Brit J Surg* 85:818, 1998.

38. Hierholzer C, Kalff JC, Omert L, et al.: Interleukin-6 production in hemorrhagic shock is accompanied by neutrophil recruitment and lung injury. *Am J Physiol* 275:L611, 1998.

39. Younger JG, Sasaki N, Waite MD, et al.: Detrimental effects of complement activation in hemorrhagic shock. *J Appl Physiol* 90:441, 2001.

40. Kapur MM, Jain P, Gidh M: The effect of trauma on serum C3 activation and its correlation with injury severity score in man. *J Trauma* 26:464, 1986.

41. Stove S, Welte T, Wagner TO, et al.: Circulating complement proteins in patients with sepsis or systemic inflammatory response syndrome. *Clin Diagn Lab Immunol* 3:175, 1996.

42. Dehring DJ, Steinberg SM, Wismar BL, et al.: Complement depletion in a porcine model of septic acute respiratory disease. *J Trauma* 27:615, 1987.

43. Cavaillon JM, Fitting C, Haeffner-Cavaillon N: Recombinant C5a enhances interleukin 1 and tumor necrosis factor release by lipopolysaccharide-stimulated monocytes and macrophages. *Eur J Immunol* 20:253, 1990.

44. Moore EE, Moore FA, Franciose RJ, et al.: The postischemic gut serves as a priming bed for circulating neutrophils that provoke multiple organ failure. *J Trauma* 37:881, 1994.

45. Barroso-Aranda J, Schmid-Schonbein GW: Transformation of neutrophils as indicator of irreversibility in hemorrhagic shock. *Am J Physiol* 257:H846, 1989.

46. Vedder NB, Winn RK, Rice CL, et al.: A monoclonal antibody to the adherence-promoting leukocyte glycoprotein, CD18, reduces organ injury and improves survival from hemorrhagic shock and resuscitation in rabbits. *J Clin Invest* 81:939, 1988.

47. Squadrito F, Altavilla D, Canale P, et al.: Contribution of intercellular adhesion molecule 1 (ICAM-1) to the pathogenesis of splanchnic artery occlusion shock in the rat. *Brit J Pharm* 113:912, 1994.

48. Adams JM, Hauser CJ, Livingston DH, et al.: Early trauma polymorphonuclear neutrophil responses to chemokines are associated with development of sepsis, pneumonia, and organ failure. *J Trauma* 51:452, 2001.

49. Marzi I, Bauer C, Hower R, Buhren V: Leukocyte-endothelial cell interactions in the liver after hemorrhagic shock in the rat. *Circ Shock* 40:105, 1993.

50. Chaudry IH: Cellular mechanisms in shock and ischemia and their correction. *Am J Physiol* 245:R117, 1983.

51. Ozawa K: Biological significance of mitochondrial redox potential in shock and multiple organ failure-redox theory. *Prog Clin Biol Res* 11:39, 1983.

52. Stacpoole PW: Lactic acidosis and other mitochondrial disorders. *Metabolism* 46:306, 1997.

53. Bevington A, Brown J, Pratt A, et al.: Impaired glycolysis and protein catabolism induced by acid in L6 rat muscle cells. *Eur J Clin Invest* 28:908, 1998.

54. Lateroza OF, Curthoys NP: Specificity and functional analysis of the pH-responsive element within renal glutaminase mRNA. *Am J Physiol* 278:F970, 2000.

55. Dasso LLT, Buckler KJ, Vaughan-Jones RD: Interactions between hypoxia and hypercapnic acidosis on calcium signaling in carotid body type I cells. *Am J Physiol* 279:L36, 2000.

56. Ding D, Moskovitz SI, Li R, et al.: Acidosis induces necrosis and apoptosis of cultured hippocampal neurons. *Exp Neurol* 162:1, 2000.

57. Simonis G, Marquetant R, Rothele J, et al.: The cardiac adrenergic system in ischaemia; differential role of acidosis and energy depletion. *Cardiovas Res* 38:646, 1998.

58. Lardner A: The effects of extracellular pH on immune function. *J Leukoc Biol* 69:522, 2001.

59. Peitzman AB, Billiar TR, Harbrecht BG, et al.: Hemorrhagic shock. *Curr Prob Surg* 11:925, 1995.

60. Cotran RS, Kumar V, Collins T: Cell pathology I: Cell injury and cell death. In Cotran RS, Kumar V, Collins T, eds: *Robbins Pathologic Basis of Disease.* Philadelphia: Saunders, 1999, p. 5.

61. Xu YX, Ayala A, Monfils B, et al.: Mechanism of intestinal mucosal immune dysfunction following trauma-hemorrhage: Increased apoptosis associated with elevated Fas expression in Peyer's patches. *J Surg Res* 70:55, 1997.

62. Hotchkiss RS, Schmieg RE Jr, Swanson PE, et al.: Rapid onset of intestinal epithelial and lymphocyte apoptotic cell death in patients with trauma and shock. *Crit Care Med* 28:3207, 2000.

63. Sen CK, Packer L: Antioxidant and redox regulation of gene transcription. *FASEB J* 10:709, 1996.

64. Kelly E, Morgan N, Woo ES, et al.: Metallothionein and HSP-72 are induced in the liver by hemorrhagic shock and resuscitation but not by shock alone. *Surgery* 120:403, 1996.

65. Kelly E, Shah NS, Morgan NN, et al.: Physiologic and molecular characterization of the role of nitric oxide in hemorrhagic shock: Evidence that type II nitric oxide synthase does not regulate vascular decompensation. *Shock* 7:157, 1997.

66. Benjamin IJ, Kroger B, Williams RS: Activation of the heat shock transcription factor by hypoxia in mammalian cells. *Proc Natl Acad Sci U S A* 87:6263, 1990.

67. Williams RS, Thomas JA, Fina M, et al.: Human heat shock protein 70 (hsp70) protects murine cells from injury during metabolic stress. *J Clin Invest* 92:503, 1993.

68. Garrison RN, Cryer HM: Role of the microcirculation in skeletal muscle during shock. *Prog Clin Biol Res* 299:43, 1989.

69. Mazzoni MC, Borgstrom P, Intaglutta M, et al.: Lumenal narrowing and endothelial cell swelling in skeletal muscle capillaries during hemorrhagic shock. *Circ Shock* 29:27, 1989.

70. Bagge V, Amundson B, Launitzen C: White blood cell deformability and plugging of skeletal muscle capillaries in hemorrhagic shock. *Acta Physiol Scand* 180:159, 1980.

71. Koo A, Liang IYS: Blood flow in hepatic sinusoids in experimental hemorrhagic shock in the rat. *Microvasc Res* 13:315, 1977.

72. Gosche JR, Garrison RN: Prostaglandins mediate the compensatory responses to hemorrhage in the small intestine of the rat. *J Surg Res* 50:584, 1991.

73. Spain DA, Wilson MA, Bar-Natan MF, et al.: Role of nitric oxide in the small intestinal microcirculation during bacteremia. *Shock* 2:41, 1994.

74. Cryer HM, Garrison RN, Kaebnick HW, et al.: Skeletal microcirculatory responses to hyperdynamic Escherichia coli sepsis in unanesthetized rats. *Arch Surg* 122:86, 1987.

75. Nishida J, McCusky RS, McDonnell D, et al.: Protective role of NO in hepatic microcirculatory dysfunction during endotoxemia. *Am J Physiol* 267:G1135, 1994.

76. Wang P, Zhan M, Rane W, et al.: Differential alterations in microvascular perfusion in various organs during early and late sepsis. *Am J Physiol* 263:G38, 1992.

77. Lang CH, Bagby GJ, Ferguson JI, et al.: Cardiac output and redistribution of organ blood flow in hypermetabolic sepsis. *Am J Physiol* 246:R331, 1984.

78. Amundson B, Jennische E, Haljamae H: Correlate analyses of microcirculatory and cellular metabolic events in skeletal muscle during hemorrhagic shock. *Acta Physiol Scand* 108:147, 1980.

79. Crowell JW: Oxygen debt as the common parameter in irreversible hemorrhagic shock. *Fed Proc* 20:116, 1961.

80. Crowell JW, Smith EE: Oxygen deficit and irreversible hemorrhagic shock. *Am J Physiol* 206:313, 1964.

81. Dunham CM, Siegel JH, Weireter LJ, et al.: Oxygen debt and metabolic acidemia as quantitative predictors of mortality and the severity of the ischemic insult in hemorrhagic shock. *Crit Care Med* 19:231, 1999.

82. Shoemaker WC, Appel PL, Kram HB: Role of oxygen debt in the development of organ failure sepsis, and death in high-risk surgical patients. *Chest* 102:208, 1992.

83. Siegel JH, Rivkind AI, Dalal S, et al.: Early physiologic predictors of injury severity and death in blunt multiple trauma. *Arch Surg* 125:498, 1990.

84. American College of Surgeons Committee on Trauma: *Advanced Trauma Life Support Course Manual.* Chicago: American College of Surgeons, 1997.

85. Osler T, Hales K, Baack B, et al.: Trauma in the elderly. *Am J Surg* 156:537, 1988.

86. Schwab CW, Kauder DR: Trauma in the geriatric patient. *Arch Surg* 127:701, 1992.

87. Cryer HM, Miller FB, Evers BM, et al.: Pelvic fracture classification: Correlation with hemorrhage. *J Trauma* 28:973, 1988.

88. Flint LM, Cryer HM, Simpson CJ, et al.: Microcirculatory norepinephrine constrictor response in hemorrhagic shock. *Surgery* 96:240, 1984.

89. Zipnick RI, Scalea TM, Trooskin SZ, et al.: Hemodynamic responses to penetrating spinal cord injuries. *J Trauma* 35:578, 1993.

90. Wolf L, Wolf A, Belzberg H: Hemodynamic parameters in patients with acute cervical cord trauma: Description, intervention, and prediction of outcome. *Neurosurgery* 33:1007, 1993.

91. Hall ED, Wolf DL: A pharmacological analysis of the pathophysiological mechanisms of post-traumatic spinal cord ischemia. *J Neurosurg* 69:951, 1986.

92. Baxter TB, Moore EE, Moore FA, et al.: A plea for sensible management of myocardial contusion. *Am J Surg* 158:557, 1989.

93. Flancbaum L, Wright J, Siegel JH: Emergency surgery in patients with post-traumatic myocardial contusion. *J Trauma* 26:795, 1986.

94. Ross P, Degutis L, Baker CC: Cardiac contusion: The effect on operative management of the patient with traumatic injuries. *Arch Surg* 124:506, 1989.

95. Simmons TA, Meijborg HW, de la Riviere AB: Traumatic papillary muscle rupture. *Ann Thor Surg* 72:257, 2001.

96. Nekkanti R, Aaluri SR, Nanda NC, et al.: Transesophageal echocardiographic diagnosis of traumatic rupture of the moncoronary cusp of aortic valve. *Echocardiography* 18:189, 2001.

97. Amorim MJ, Almeida J, Santos A, et al.: Atrioventricular septal defect following blunt chest trauma. *Eur J Cardio Thor Surg* 16:679, 1999.

98. Garcia-Fernandez MA, Lopez-Perez JM, Perez-Castellano N, et al.: Role of transesophageal echocardiography in the assessment of patients with blunt chest trauma: Correlation of echocardiographic findings with electrocardiogram and creatine kinase monoclonal antibody measurements. *Am Heart J* 135:476, 1998.

99. Rozycki GS, Feliciano DV, Schmidt JA, et al.: The role of surgeon-performed ultrasound in patients with possible cardiac wounds. *Ann Surg* 223:737, 1996.

100. Rozycki GS, Feliciano DV, Ochsner MG, et al.: The role of ultrasound in patients with possible penetrating cardiac wounds: A prospective multicenter study. *J Trauma* 46:543, 1999.

101. Snow N, Lucas AE, Richardson JD: Intra-aortic balloon counterpulsation for cardiogenic shock from cardiac contusion. *J Trauma* 22:426, 1982.

102. Hennekens CH, Albert CM, Godfried SL, et al.: Adjunctive drug therapy of acute myocardial infarction—evidence from clinical trials. *N Engl J Med* 335:1660, 1996.

103. Fink MP, Heard SO: Laboratory models of sepsis and septic shock. *J Surg Res* 49:186, 1990.

104. Wheeler HP, Bernard GP: Treating patients with severe sepsis. *N Engl J Med* 340:207, 1999.

105. ACCP/SCCM Consensus Conference Committee: Definitions for sepsis and organ failure and guidelines for the use of innovative therapies in sepsis. *Crit Care Med* 20:864, 1992.

106. Enderson BL, Maull KI: Missed injuries: The trauma surgeon's nemesis. *Surg Clin North Am* 71:399, 1991.

107. Davis JW, Hoyt DB, McArdle MS, et al.: An analysis of errors causing morbidity and mortality in a trauma system: A guide for quality improvement. *J Trauma* 32:660, 1992.

108. Dallal RM, Harbrecht BG, Boujoukas AJ, et al.: Fulminant clostridium difficile colitis: An underappreciated and increasing cause of death and complications. *Ann Surg* 235:363, 2002.

109. Luckmen G, Dunser MW, Jochberger S, et al.: Arginine vasopressin in 316 patients with advanced vasodilatory shock. *Crit Care Med* 33:2659, 2005.

110. The HA-1A Sepsis Study Group: Treatment of gram negative bacteremia and septic shock with HA-1A human monoclonal antibody against endotoxin: A randomized, double-blind placebo-controlled trial. *N Engl J Med* 324:429, 1991.

111. Abraham E, Anzueto A, Gutierrez G, et al.: Double-blind randomized trial of monoclonal antibody to human tumor necrosis factor in treatment of septic shock. *Lancet* 351:929, 1998.

112. Fischer CJ Jr, Slotman GJ, Opal SM, et al.: Initial evaluation of human recombinant interleukin-1 receptor antagonist in the treatment of sepsis syndrome: A randomized, open-label, placebo-controlled multicenter trial. *Crit Care Med* 22:12, 1994.

113. Stauback K-H, Schroder J, Stuber F, et al.: Effect of pentoxifylline in severe sepsis: Results of a randomized, double-blind, placebo-controlled study. *Arch Surg* 133:94, 1998.

114. Petros A, Lamb G, Leone A, et al.: Effects of a nitric oxide synthase inhibitor in humans with septic shock. *Cardiovas Res* 28:34, 1994.

115. Grover R, Zaccardelli D, Colice G, et al.: An open-label dose escalation study of the nitric oxide synthase inhibitor $N^G$-monomethyl hydrochloride (546C88) in patients with septic shock. *Crit Care Med* 27:913, 1999.

116. Porter JM, Ivatury RR, Azimuddin K, et al.: Antioxidant therapy in the prevention of organ dysfunction syndrome and infectious complications after trauma: Early results of a prospective randomized study. *Am Surg* 65:478, 1999.

117. Bernard GR, Vincent J-L, Laterre P-F, et al.: Efficacy and safety of recombinant human activated protein C for severe sepsis. *N Engl J Med* 344:699, 2001.

118. Abraham E, Laterre P-F, Gary R, et al.: Drotrecogin alfa (activated) for adults with severe sepsis and a low risk of death. *N Engl J Med* 353:1332, 2005.

119. Bolten JWR, Bynoe RP, Lazar HL, et al.: Two-dimensional echocardiography in the evaluation of penetrating intrapericardial injuries. *Ann Thorac Surg* 56:506, 1993.

120. Freshman SP, Wisner DH, Weber CJ: 2-D echocardiography: Emergent use in the evaluation of penetrating precordial trauma. *J Trauma* 31:902, 1991.

121. Miller FB, Bond SJ, Shumate CR, et al.: Diagnostic pericardial window: A safe alternative to exploratory thoracotomy for suspected heart injuries. *Arch Surg* 122:605, 1987.

122. Garrison RN, Richardson JD, Fry DE: Diagnostic transdiaphragmatic pericardiotomy in thoracoabdominal trauma. *J Trauma* 22:147, 1982.

123. McKinley BA, Kozar RA, Cocanoun CS, et al.: Normal vs supranormal oxygen delivery goals in shock resuscitation: The response is the same. *J Trauma* 53:825, 2002.

124. Abou-Khalil B, Scalea TM, Trooskin SZ, et al.: Hemodynamic responses to shock in young trauma patients: Need for invasive monitoring. *Crit Care Med* 22:633, 1994.

125. Claridge JA, Crabtree TD, Pelletier SJ, et al.: Persistent occult hypoperfusion is associated with a significant increase in infection rate and mortality in major trauma patients. *J Trauma* 48:8, 2000.

126. Moore FA, McKinley BA, Moore EE: The next generation in shock resuscitation. *Lancit* 363:1988, 2004.

127. Kern JW, Shoemaker WC: Meta-analysis of hemodynamics optimization in high-risk patients. *Crit Care Med* 30:1686, 2002.

128. Bilkovski RN, Rivera EP, Horst HM: Targeted resuscitation strategies after injury. *Curr Open Crit Care* 10:529, 2004.

129. Tisherman SA, Barie P, Bokhari F, et al.: Clinical practice guidelines: Endpoints of resuscitation. *J Trauma* 57:898, 2004.

130. Clowes GHA, del Guercio LR: Circulatory response to trauma of surgical operations. *Metabolism* 9:67, 1960.

131. Shoemaker WC, Montgomery ES, Kaplan E, et al.: Physiologic patterns in surviving and nonsurviving shock patients. *Arch Surg* 106:630, 1973.

132. Bishop MH, Shoemaker WC, Appell PL, et al.: Prospective, randomized trial of survivor values of cardiac index, oxygen delivery, and oxygen consumption as resuscitation endpoints in severe trauma. *J Trauma* 38:780, 1995.

133. Velmahos GC, Demetriades D, Shoemaker WC, et al.: Endpoints of resuscitation of critically injured patients: Normal or supranormal? *Ann Surg* 232:409, 2000.

134. Gattinoni L, Brazzi L, Pelosi P, et al.: A trial of goal-oriented hemodynamic therapy in critically ill patients. *N Engl J Med* 333:1025, 1995.

135. Heyland DK, Cook DJ, King D, et al.: Maximizing oxygen delivery in critically ill patients: A methodologic appraisal of the evidence. *Crit Care Med* 24:517, 1996.

136. Durham RM, Neunaber K, Mazuski JE, et al.: The use of oxygen consumption and delivery as endpoints for resuscitation in critically ill patients. *J Trauma* 41:32, 1996.

137. Rivers E, Nguyen B, Havstad S, et al.: Early goal-directed therapy in the treatment of severe sepsis and septic shock. *N Engl J Med* 345:1368, 2001.

138. Chittock DR, Dhingra VK, Ronco JJ, et al.: Severity of illness and risk of death associated with pulmonary artery catheter use. *Crit Care Med* 32:911, 2004.

139. Shah MR, Hasselbad V, Stevenson LW, et al.: Impact of the pulmonary artery catheter in critically ill patients: Meta-analysis of randomized clinical trials. *JAMA* 1664, 2005.

140. Rhodes A, Bennett D: Early goal-directed therapy: An evidence-based review. *Crit Care Med* 32:S448, 2004.

141. Reinhart K, Kuhn HJ, Hartog C, et al.: Continuous central venous and pulmonary artery oxygen saturation monitoring in the critically ill. *Intensive Care Med* 30:1572, 2004.

142. Abramson D, Scalea TM, Hitchcock R, et al.: Lactate clearance and survival following injury. *J Trauma* 35:584, 1993.

143. Manikis P, Jackowski S, Zhang H, et al.: Correlation of serial blood lactate levels to organ failure and mortality after trauma. *Am J Emerg Med* 13:619, 1995.

144. Mikulaschek A, Henry SM, Donovan R, et al.: Serum lactate is not predicted by anion gap or base excess after resuscitation. *J Trauma* 40:218, 1996.

145. James JH, Luchette FA, McCarter FD, et al.: Lactate is an unreliable indicator of tissue hypoxia in injury in sepsis. *Lancet* 354:505, 1999.

146. Gore DC, Jahoor F, Hibbert JM, et al.: Lactic acidosis during sepsis is related to increased pyruvate production, not deficits in tissue oxygen availability. *Ann Surg* 224:97, 1996.

147. Dunne JR, Tracy JK, Scalea TM, et al.: Lactate and base deficit in trauma: Does alcohol or drug use impair their predictive accuracy? *J Trauma* 58:959, 2005.

148. Rutherford EJ, Morris JA Jr, Reed GW, et al.: Base deficit stratifies mortality and determines therapy. *J Trauma* 33:417, 1992.

149. Davis JW, Shackford SR, Mackersie RC, et al.: Base deficit as a guide to volume resuscitation. *J Trauma* 28:1464, 1988.

150. Davis JW, Parks SN, Kaups KL, et al.: Admission base deficit predicts transfusion requirements and risk of complications. *J Trauma* 41:769, 1996.

151. Rixen D, Siegel JH: Metabolic correlates of oxygen debt predicts post trauma early acute respiratory distress syndrome and the related cytokine response. *J Trauma* 49:392, 2000.

152. Eberhard LW, Morakito DJ, Matthay et al.: Initial severity of metabolic acidosis predicts the development of acute lung injury in severely traumatized patients. *Crit Care Med* 28:125, 2000.

153. Tremblay LN, Feliciano DV, Rozycki GS: Are resuscitation and operation justified in injured patients with extreme base deficits (less than -20)? *Am J Surg* 186:597, 2003.

154. Davis JW, Kaups KL: Base deficit in the elderly: A marker of severe injury and death. *J Trauma* 45:873, 1998.

155. Kincaid EH, Miller PR, Meredith JW, et al.: Elevated arterial base deficit in trauma patients: A marker of impaired oxygen utilization. *J Am Coll Surg* 187:384, 1998.

156. Brill SA, Stewart TR, Brundage SI, et al.: Base deficit does not predict mortality when secondary to hyperchloremic acidosis. *Shock* 17:459, 2002.

157. Fitz Sullivan E, Salim A, Demetriades D, et al.: Serum bicarbonate may replace the arterial base deficit in the trauma intensive care unit. *Am J Surg* 190:941, 2005.

158. Eachempati SR, Barie PS, Reed RL: Serum bicarbonate as an endpoint of resuscitation in critically ill patients. *Surg Inf* 4:193, 2003.

159. Maynard N, Bihari D, Beale R, et al.: Assessment of splanchnic oxygenation by gastric tonometry in patients with acute circulatory failure. *JAMA* 270:1203, 1993.

160. Chang MC, Cheatham MC, Nelson LD, et al.: Gastric tonometry supplements information provided by systemic indications of oxygen transport. *J Trauma* 37:448, 1994.

161. The Miami Trauma Clinical Trials Group: Splanchnic hypoperfusion-directed therapies in trauma: A prospective randomized trial. *Am Surg* 71:252, 2005.

162. Gutierrez G, Palizas F, Doglio G, et al.: Gastric intramucosal pH as a therapeutic index of tissue oxygenation in critically ill patients. *Lancet* 339:195, 1992.

163. Gomersall CD, Joynt GM, Freebairn RC, et al.: Resuscitation of critically ill patients based on the results of gastric tonometry. *Crit Care Med* 28:607, 2000.

164. Taylor JH, Mulier KE, Myers DE, et al.: Use of near-infrared spectroscopy in early determination of irreversible hemorrhagic shock. *J Trauma* 58:1119, 2005.

165. McKinley BA, Marvin RG, Cocanour CS, et al.: Tissue hemoglobin $O_2$ saturation during resuscitation of traumatic shock monitored using near infrared spectroscopy. *J Trauma* 48:637, 2000.

166. Crookes BA, Cohn SM, Block S, et al.: Can near-infrared spectroscopy identify the severity of shock in trauma patients? *J Trauma* 58:806, 2005.

167. Marik PE: Sublingual capnography: A clinical validation study. *Chest* 120:923, 2001.

168. Soller BR, Khan T, Favreau J, et al.: Investigation of muscle pH as an indicated of liver pH and injury from hemorrhagic shock. *J Surg Res* 114:195, 2003.

169. Clavijo-Alvarez JA, Sims CA, Pinsky MR, et al.: Monitoring skeletal muscle and subcutaneous acid-based status and oxygenation during hemorrhagic shock and resuscitation. *Shock* 24:270, 2005.

170. Soller BR, Cingo N, Puyana JC, et al.: Simultaneous measurement of tissue pH, venous oxygen saturation and hemoglobin by near infrared spectroscopy. *Shock* 15:106, 2001.

171. Guzman JA, Dikin MJ, Kruse JA: Lingual, splanchnic, and systemic hemodynamics and carbon dioxide tension changes during endotoxic shock and resuscitation. *J Appl Physiol* 98:108, 2005.

# Commentary ■ DENNIS W. ASHLEY

Drs. Harbrecht, Forsythe, and Peitzman have written an excellent overview on shock. They elegantly describe the complex pathophysiology of this disease process as we understand it today followed by a review of each type of shock with the appropriate treatment. The authors note that shock is not just a disturbance in blood pressure but involves inadequate delivery of oxygen to the tissues resulting in an oxygen debt. This may happen despite a relatively normal blood pressure and heart rate. Additionally, inflammatory cytokine production is upregulated with shock and resuscitation and can be associated with multiple organ failure. Even brief periods of hypotension and hypoxia have been shown to have deleterious effects on outcome in traumatic brain injury. Since the magnitude of this oxygen debt and the time required to repay it have correlated with survival in some studies, it appears that quickly diagnosing the patient with shock and performing adequate resuscitation to limit the period of oxygen debt should be the main goal of treatment. In some cases this may require the initiation of aggressive resuscitation before the exact etiology of the shock state is identified.

Regardless of the shock type, initial resuscitation must start with the ABCs of trauma. Despite significant cardiovascular collapse, control of the airway must be accomplished first so that adequate oxygenation can be achieved. This may require immediate intubation and mechanical ventilation in severe cases. The patient's breathing is then examined by auscultation. This should lead to a clinical diagnosis of tension pneumothorax if present and placement of a therapeutic thoracostomy tube. There is no time to obtain a chest radiograph in this scenario. Finally, circulation is addressed by obtaining appropriate venous access, administration of crystalloid and/or blood products, and control of hemorrhage. The authors correctly point out that delay in control of hemorrhage and inadequate resuscitation resulting in prolonged hypotension can result in increased morbidity and mortality. Therefore, patients requiring definitive control of hemorrhage should be moved to the operating room expeditiously avoiding long periods of resuscitation in the emergency room.

All types of shock must be considered in the initial differential diagnosis but the most common type for trauma patients is hemorrhagic or hypovolemic shock. In addition to the four types of classic shock (hemorrhagic, neurogenic, cardiogenic, and septic) the authors describe another type shock that results in obstruction of venous return to the heart.[1] This is obstructive shock and results from a tension pneumothorax or cardiac tamponade. It is imperative that the trauma surgeon quickly differentiate between hemorrhagic and nonhemorrhagic shock as the treatment for each is different. Continued aggressive volume resuscitation for the obstructive shock patient will not resolve the underlying etiology as the patient needs a tube thoracostomy or release of tamponade followed by cardiac repair.

To assist with a rapid diagnosis in the trauma resuscitation bay, I have found it beneficial to simply divide shock into two categories, hemorrhagic and nonhemorrhagic. The hemorrhagic category includes bleeding from any or all of the following sites: (1) chest; (2) abdomen; (3) pelvis; (4) external; and (5) long bones. The etiologies of shock in the nonhemorrhagic category includes: (1) tension pneumothorax; (2) cardiac tamponade; (3) cardiac contusion; (4) myocardial infarction; (5) spinal cord injury (neurogenic); and (6) sepsis (extremely rare in acute trauma). By utilizing clinical examination, ultrasound and limited radiography the trauma surgeon can quickly diagnose the etiology of shock and proceed to the appropriate definitive treatment.

After initiation of resuscitation and control of hemorrhage, the next challenge involves finding the appropriate endpoint of resuscitation. This is difficult as the clinical parameters such as heart rate, blood pressure, and urine output may normalize despite continued tissue hypoperfusion and accumulation of oxygen debt. In addition to clinical parameters, many sophisticated parameters have been used including cardiac output, oxygen delivery, and oxygen consumption obtained from a pulmonary artery catheter. Resuscitation of the patient to achieve supranormal oxygen delivery values as the endpoint of resuscitation initially appeared beneficial in some studies but has not withstood the test of time and is no longer recommended. This should not be confused with the "early goal-directed therapy" described by Rivers. He measured central venous oxygen saturation via a central line and showed a decrease in mortality by optimizing resuscitation within the first six hours of critical illness in the emergency room. Although, the etiology of shock in this study population was sepsis, it seems that early goal directed therapy to decrease the period of oxygen debt would lead to increased survival in trauma patients.

Currently, one of the most common parameters used to define the endpoint of resuscitation is base deficit. This measurement can be obtained from the arterial blood gas and is readily available in the emergency room, operating room, and intensive care unit. It has been correlated with survival and organ failure and is an excellent indicator of appropriate resuscitation if the value is normalizing with continued resuscitation. Although, other factors may cause the base deficit to remain elevated despite adequate resuscitation, failure of the base deficit to correct should be considered inadequate resuscitation until proven otherwise. Regardless of the parameter used to evaluate the "best" endpoint of resuscitation, early identification of shock, control of hemorrhage and early resuscitation to prevent a large oxygen debt should be the goal for all physicians caring for the patient in shock.

## Reference

1. Rivers E, Nguyen B, Havstad S, et al.: Early goal-directed therapy in the treatment of severe sepsis and septic shock. *N Engl J Med* 345:1368, 2001.

# Transfusion, Autotransfusion, and Blood Substitutes

*Scott R. Petersen* ■ *Jordan A. Weinberg*

Transfusion medicine is an integral part of trauma practice. As early as World War I, blood transfusion was used to combat hemorrhagic shock in injured soldiers, and it continues to be the resuscitation fluid of choice for critical hemorrhage. Historically, blood transfusion has been perceived as a low-risk, routine intervention, but more recent recognition of both the infectious and noninfectious complications of blood transfusion has led to greater consideration of its potential benefits and risks in both the elective and emergent settings. Despite this appreciation, the annual number of transfusions continues to increase by approximately 6%.[1] Although the number of units collected is on the rise as well, there is a shrinking margin between blood collections and transfusions, and blood remains a limited resource (Fig. 14-1).[1] In this chapter, the indications for allogenic erythrocyte transfusion, logistics of transfusion, complications of red blood cell transfusion, indications for the administration of other blood products, alternatives to erythrocyte transfusion, and progress in the development of red blood cell substitutes will be discussed.

## INDICATIONS FOR ERYTHROCYTE TRANSFUSION

The initial management of hemorrhagic shock is directed toward achieving cellular perfusion by restoring and maintaining intravascular volume. At some point, however, the clinician must consider the adequacy of oxygen delivery, which is the underlying goal of resuscitation. Although the administration of crystalloid solution can effectively replace the lost volume of blood, it will not augment oxygen delivery. Conversely, the primary purpose of erythrocyte transfusion is to restore oxygen delivery and should not be equated to volume expansion, although it secondarily serves this intention.

In the emergency department, the initial assessment of the patient's hemodynamic status helps determine the need for immediate transfusion, as outlined in the algorithm presented in Fig. 14-2. Patients in mild to moderate hemorrhagic shock (class I and II as

described in the Advanced Trauma Life Support guidelines of the American College of Surgeons) tend to respond well to fluid replacement with crystalloid solutions without the need for immediate blood transfusion.[2] Patients in severe shock (class III and IV), however, have incurred massive blood loss approaching or exceeding 30% of their blood volume, necessitating the empiric transfusion of red blood cells during initial resuscitation to restore both intravascular volume and oxygen delivery.

During the ongoing resuscitation of the trauma patient, including the perioperative period, the need for blood transfusion, or so-called transfusion trigger, is a clinical decision that should be tailored to the individual patient. Prior to the appreciation of the infectious and immunomodulatory risks of transfusion, patients were routinely transfused to maintain hemoglobin and hematocrit levels of 10 g/L and 30%, respectively. The "10/30" rule was introduced by Adams and Lundy based on their clinical experience.[3] Subsequent laboratory studies and clinical reviews offered additional support to this practice.[4,5]

In the 1980s, concern for transmission of human immunodeficiency virus (HIV) and hepatitis by blood transfusion prompted the evaluation of transfusion principles and practices. In 1988, the National Institutes of Health produced a consensus paper stating the following: (a) available evidence did not support the use of a single transfusion criterion such as a critical hemoglobin level; (b) there is no evidence that mild-to-moderate anemia contributes to perioperative morbidity; and (c) clinical judgment should be the basis for decision-making with respect to transfusion.[6] This philosophy encourages a transfusion practice that is patient-specific, based on clinical evaluation and physiologic principles, in addition to the plasma hemoglobin or hematocrit.

The signs and symptoms of anemia include tachycardia, exertional dyspnea, chest pain, pallor, and impaired consciousness. In most patients, anemia is well tolerated and the majority remains asymptomatic until hemoglobin levels are in the range of 6 to 7 g/dL.[7] For trauma patients, the clinical picture is further obscured

## Red Cell Collections and Transfusions (1987–2001)*

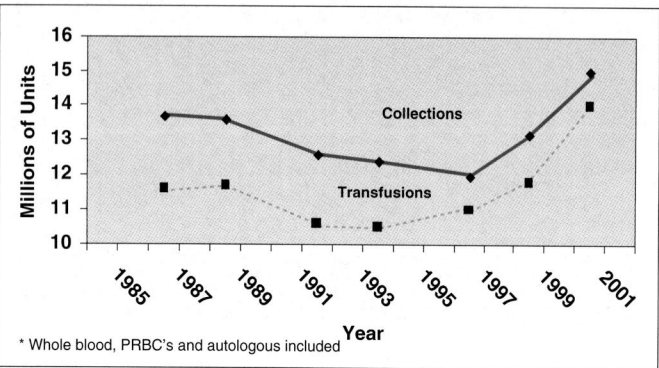

**FIGURE 14-1.** Allogenic whole blood transfusions and collections from 1987 to 2001. Data includes autologus transfusions and was obtained from surveys conducted by the Center for Blood Research. *(Reproduced with permission from National Blood Data Resource Center, Bethesda, MD, 2005.)*

by confounding issues such as injury to the chest, systemic inflammatory response syndrome, and pain, all of which can produce the signs and symptoms described earlier.

Basing the transfusion of red blood cells on physiologic parameters offers the appeal of making the decision to transfuse more responsive to a patient's oxygen requirements at a given time. Many physiologic parameters can be calculated or obtained directly from pulmonary artery catheters, including cardiac index and mixed venous oxygen saturation. With variations on the Fick equation (Table 14-1), one can use these measurements, along with hemoglobin and arterial oxygen saturation, to calculate oxygen delivery, consumption, and extraction ratio. The decision to transfuse can then be made with the rationale of improving these parameters by increasing the hemoglobin level. In practice, however, the use of these parameters to guide transfusion has had mixed success. The effect of blood transfusion on oxygen extraction and consumption has been demonstrated to be limited.[8,9] The role of such physiologic parameters as transfusion triggers has yet to be defined. Also, the

determination of these parameters requires invasive monitoring, which is not indicated for all trauma patients.

A threshold for hemoglobin level has been the historic transfusion trigger as described earlier and continues to be used in clinical practice, although with a higher threshold for transfusion. Surgical experience with patients who are Jehovah's Witnesses has demonstrated that individuals can tolerate hemoglobin levels as low as 6 g/dL without an observed increase in morbidity or mortality.[10] Robertie and Gravlee proposed the following basic transfusion guidelines based on hemoglobin level: (a) 6 g/dL for well-compensated patients without heart disease or postoperative complications; (b) 8 g/dL for patients with stable cardiac disease and less than 300 mL blood loss; and (c) 10 g/dL for older patients and those with postoperative complications who cannot increase cardiac output.[11] Similar "rule of thumb" approaches are in use across North America, whereby the threshold for transfusion is lowered for the more compromised patient. A multicenter, randomized, controlled clinical trial of two transfusion triggers (one restrictive, 7 g/dL, and one liberal, 10 g/dL) for patients in the intensive care unit demonstrated no difference in mortality between groups. In a subsequent subset analysis of those patients with cardiovascular disease, no difference in mortality was noted, with the possible exception of patients with acute myocardial infarction and unstable angina.[12,13] Other studies call into question the rationale of lowering the transfusion threshold based on hemoglobin for more compromised patients.[14] The important association between hemoglobin and blood volume must be recognized. Spence et al. did not identify a difference in outcome in Jehovah's Witnesses undergoing major elective surgery, when patients with preoperative hemoglobins of greater than 10 g/dL were compared to patients with hemoglobins between 6 to 10 g/dL. When intraoperative blood loss exceeded 500 mL in both groups, mortality increased from 0 to 7.4%.[15] In a randomized study in critically ill patients who had been injured, McIntyre et al. demonstrated that a restrictive transfusion strategy (7 g/dL versus 10 g/dL) was safe and used less red cell transfusions with similar mortality rates, incidence of multiple organ dysfunction and length of stay.[16]

In summary, the decision to transfuse erythrocytes must be individualized to the patient. The healthy 30-year-old patient with euvolemia without ongoing blood loss and a hemoglobin of 7 g/dL is less likely to benefit from transfusion than the 70-year-old patient with hypovolemia with ongoing hemorrhage and a hemoglobin of 9 g/dL. It is the clinician's responsibility to combine the available clinical, laboratory, and physiologic data as previously described to make rational decisions on the need for transfusion.

## TABLE 14-1

### Hemodynamic and Oxygen Transport Variables

| VARIABLE | FORMULA |
|---|---|
| Arterial Oxygen Content (mL/dL) | $C_aO_2 = 1.39 \times Hgb + (0.0031 \times P_aO_2)$ |
| Mixed Venous Oxygen content (mL/dL) | $C_vO_2 = S_vO_2 \times 1.39 \times Hgb + (0.0031 \times P_vO_2)$ |
| Cardiac Output (Fick Equation) (L/min) | $CO = VO_2 / (C_aO_2 - C_vO_2) \times 10$ |
| Oxygen Delivery (mL/min) | $DO_2 = CO \times C_aO_2 \times 10$ |
| Oxygen Consumption (mL/min) | $VO_2 = CO (C_aO_2 - C_vO_2) \times 10$ |
| Oxygen Extraction Ratio (Oxygen Utilization Coefficient) | $O_2 \, Ext = DO_2 / VO_2$ |

## BLOOD STORAGE AND PREPARATION

The need to maximize the use of the blood pool and the lack of a demonstrated benefit of whole blood transfusion over component therapy have led to the widespread use of separated components (red blood cells, platelets, plasma, cryoprecipitate) over whole blood. Fresh, warm whole blood is theoretically ideal for use in trauma, replacing both the erythrocyte and plasma contents of shed blood in a balanced fashion, as well as platelets and clotting factors. For practical purposes, since donors of each blood type are not available at a moment's notice, fresh whole blood is rarely

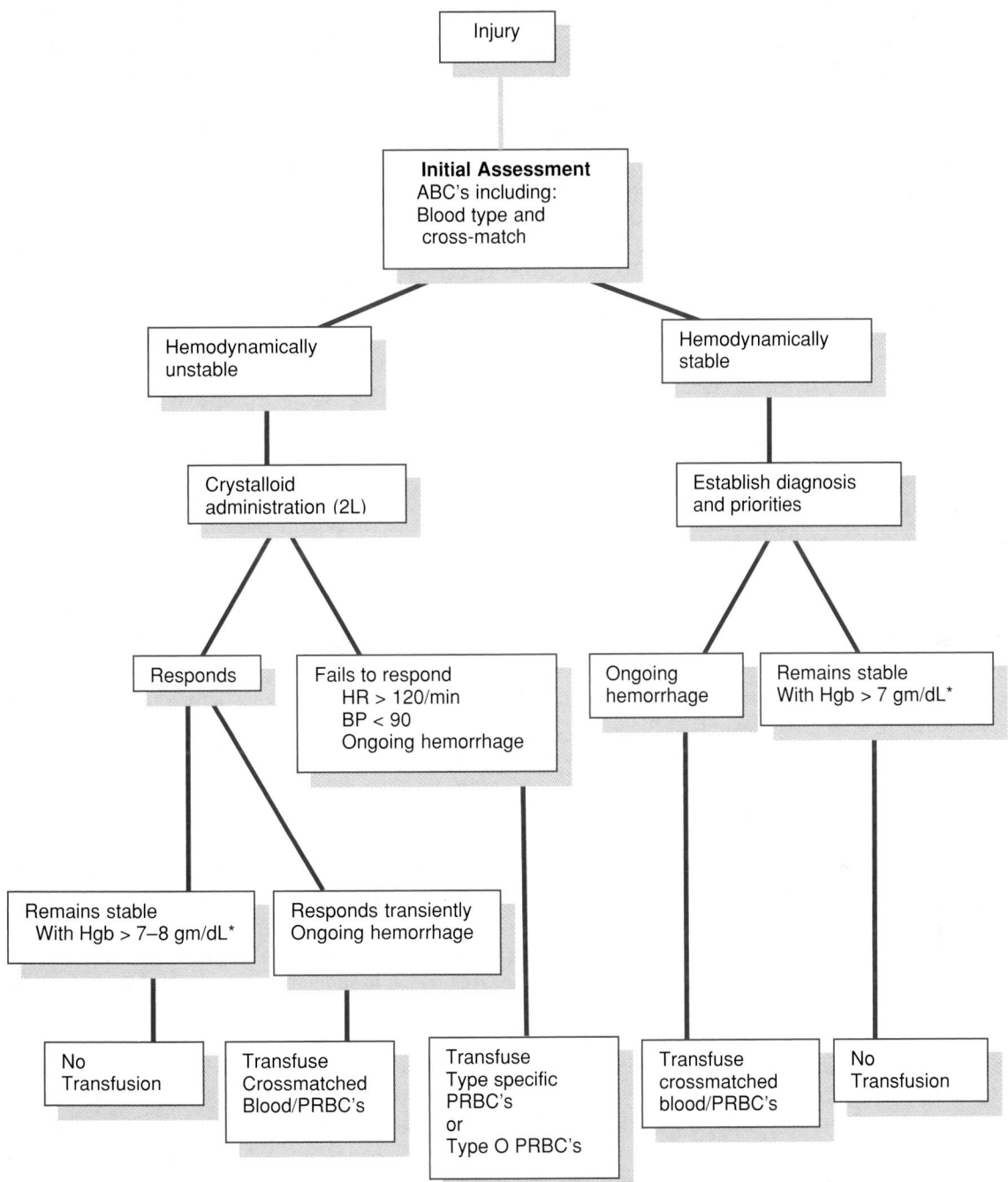

**FIGURE 14-2.** Algorithm for transfusion to restore intravascular volume following injury. (*Hemoglobin of 7 gm/dL reflects usual practice. In less stable patients and those with pre-existing cardiovascular or pulmonary disease, a higher hemoglobin may be desirable.)

available. In addition, the storage process for whole blood inactivates the platelets and much of the clotting efficacy of heat labile factors V and VIII, diminishing the potential advantage of whole blood over component-separated red blood cells. Thus, component therapy is the mainstay of blood banking practice in the United States.

Red blood cells are units of whole blood with most of the plasma removed by differential centrifugation. They are the most frequently administered component, representing nearly 50% of the 29 million U of blood products administered in 2001.[1] The volume of 1 U of red blood cells is between 300 and 350 mL with a hematocrit of 65 to 80%. In the patient with euvolemia without

ongoing hemorrhage, transfusion of 1 U of red blood cells would be expected to raise the hemoglobin level approximately 1 g/dL.[17] It should be noted, however, because of the variability in donor volume withdrawn ("short draw" vs. "large draw"), hemoglobin concentration in a "unit," and difference in the survival of red blood cells depending on the length of storage, the expected incremental rise in hemoglobin concentration following erythrocyte transfusion often does not occur.

Blood is collected into bags containing anticoagulant-preservative solutions. Citrate prevents coagulation by chelating calcium, inhibiting the calcium-dependent steps of the coagulation cascade. Dextrose is added to support the generation of adenosine triphosphate (ATP) by glycolytic pathways. Sodium biphosphate buffers the buildup of lactic acid secondary to glycolysis, while adenine is often added to provide a substrate for ATP synthesis. Despite these measures, there is a progressive degradation of red blood cells during storage. These so-called storage lesions include the depletion of red blood cell 2,3 diphosphoglycerate (2,3-DPG), which increases the affinity of hemoglobin for oxygen, thus diminishing oxygen release to the tissues. Clinically, this degradation has little significance, even in massively transfused recipients.[17] After 24 hours of circulation, transfused red blood cells obtain complete restoration of 2,3-DPG and normal hemoglobin function.

Frozen storage of red blood cells with glycerol allows for preservation times as long as 21 years.[17] The high cost and short shelf life following deglycerolization, however, make this preparation less useful for routine blood storage. It is most often reserved for storage of units with a rare blood type.

## BLOOD TYPES AND CROSS-MATCHING

A blood sample for the purpose of cross-matching should be urgently analyzed for almost all trauma patients, in case blood transfusion becomes necessary during the course of resuscitation. Although blood that has been fully cross-matched is the ideal choice for transfusion, it takes the most time to obtain, so the urgent need for transfusion forces the consideration of other options, including type O (universal donor) and type-specific blood.

Cross-matched blood is tested for compatibility concerning ABO and Rh type, as well as for the presence of known antibodies (including Lewis, Kell, Kidd, MNS, and Duffy). Cross-matched blood should be readily available for the relatively stable trauma patient who may require transfusion during ongoing resuscitation or in the perioperative period.

Type O red blood cells are immediately available without any sort of blood cross-matching, making them appropriate for the patient in extremis who requires emergency transfusion. Type O blood contains no A or B surface antigens and is accepted in type A, B, and AB patients with little risk of transfusion reaction. The administration of large quantities of type O blood, however, can lead to a positive direct Coomb's test or rarely a hemolytic reaction, secondary to the presence of anti-A or anti-B antibodies in the reduced amount of plasma remaining in the donor units. In addition, transfusion of more than four units of type O blood can result in an admixture of blood types, leading to subsequent difficulties in compatibility testing. It is recommended that type-specific blood be transfused as soon as it is available. The administration of type O blood to women of child-bearing age is complicated by the need to avoid Rh sensitization by the administration of Rh-positive blood to an Rh-negative recipient. Type O, Rh-negative blood is often held in reserve for emergent administration to women of child-bearing age.

Type-specific blood is ABO and Rh compatible. It is usually available within ten minutes of receipt of the patient's blood specimen. Type-specific blood transfusion has been demonstrated to be safe during emergency resuscitation.[18–22] Newer techniques for blood typing and cross-matching may obviate the necessity of using type-specific blood, since fully cross-matched units may become more readily available in a shorter period.

Coordination between the trauma team and the hospital transfusion service is essential to an effective system for providing safe and rapid availability of blood. Physicians should be familiar with their hospital's protocols for emergency transfusion, particularly the mechanisms for the release of type O and/or type-specific blood. When confusion arises over requests for blood products, direct communication between the physician and the transfusion service is essential.

## COMPLICATIONS OF BLOOD TRANSFUSION

### Transfusion-Transmitted Diseases

Transfusion-transmitted diseases (TTDs) are the most common cause of late transfusion death. Increased awareness of TTDs, particularly HIV infection, has contributed substantially to the reconsideration of indications for blood transfusion.[23–25] Advances in donor screening have lessened the risk of viral transmission significantly. The current estimated risks of TTDs are listed in Table 14-2. Hepatitis continues to be the most frequent viral infectious complication related to blood transfusion. Transfusion-transmitted HIV infection is a rare event (1 per 1,800,000 units transfused), but it remains a major concern of patients and physicians. Other less common diseases that may be transmitted include human T-cell lymphotrophic virus (HTLV-1 and -2). The incidence of transmission of HTLV-1 is 1 per 250,000 to 1 per 2,000,000 units.[26] Its clinical importance stems from the fact that patients with an HTLV-1 infection have a 4% lifetime risk of developing an associated fatal illness (e.g., T-cell leukemia, tropical spastic paraparesis). West Nile virus emerged as a transfusion-transmitted infection during the 2002 epidemic; however, the rapid adoption of screening processes for this pathogen by blood banks has markedly reduced the risk of transmission.[27]

Cytomegalovirus (CMV) has a high prevalence in the general population, and approximately 50% of blood donors can be expected to be CMV-seropositive.[28] In immunocompetent persons, the infection is most often asymptomatic and remains dormant. In immunosuppressed individuals, however, CMV can cause significant morbidity and mortality. Transfusion of leukocyte-reduced erythrocyte units should be considered for the immune-compromised patient as they effectively prevent the transmission of CMV.[17]

Bacterial contamination of red blood cells occurs rarely, but can cause severe and fatal reactions. Previous reports implicated gram-negative organisms as the most common contaminants,

**TABLE 14-2**

| Infectious Transmission Risks with Blood Transfusion | |
|---|---|
| **AGENT TRANSMITTED** | **ESTIMATED RISK** |
| Bacterial | 1 in 100,000–500,000 |
| Hepatitis B | 1 in 220,000 |
| Hepatitis C | 1 in 1,600,000 |
| HIV | 1 in 1,800,000 |

Adapted from Dellinger EP, Anaya DA. Infectious and immunologic consequences of blood transfusion. *Critical Care* 8(Suppl 2):S18, 2004.

but data from the U.S. Centers for Disease Control and Prevention (CDC) demonstrate that contamination with gram-positive bacteria is actually more common.[29,30] The CDC data suggest a risk of transfusion-transmitted bacterial infection of 1 per 5,000,000 units. Bacterial contamination of platelet products resulting in sepsis has also been described with an estimated risk of 1 per 100,000 units.[30] Clinical signs and symptoms of transfusion-associated sepsis usually begin during the transfusion. When a recipient experiences fever, chills, or unexplained hypotension during or shortly after transfusion, the possibility of bacterial contamination should be entertained. Treatment, including broad-spectrum antibiotics and intravenous fluids, should be initiated immediately after cultures of the recipient's blood are obtained. In addition to cultures from the recipient, the blood bag and filter should be cultured and the transfusion service notified of the event for further investigation. Parasitic contamination causing malaria and Chagas' disease is exceedingly rare, but has been reported, as well.[31]

## Transfusion Reactions

Transfusion reactions can be thought of in two broad categories, namely hemolytic and nonhemolytic. Major hemolytic transfusion reactions are the result of ABO incompatibility, and they are caused by clerical error in which mistakes were made in the identification of blood samples or in the administration of appropriately crossmatched blood to the incorrect patient. The urgent nature of trauma may contribute to human error, as suggested by the fact that more than half of the major reactions in trauma patients occur in the emergency department and the operating room. It is critically important that specimens are appropriately labeled and properly checked prior to administration. Symptoms of a major hemolytic reaction include hemogobinuria, fever, chills, coagulopathy, chest pain, and hypotension. Treatment involves immediate discontinuation of the transfusion and hemodynamic support as necessary.

Delayed hemolytic reactions are caused by non-ABO antigen-antibody incompatibilities. They are often the result of recipient antibodies of the non-ABO system, such as those in the Kidd system. Delayed reactions are frequently unrecognized as complications. Individuals who have had an antibody response to prior transfusion may have undetectable levels of antibody present at the time of subsequent incompatibility testing. Following transfusion, an anamnestic response can develop and mimic autoimmune hemolytic anemia. Typical findings are low-grade hemolysis with an unexplained fall in hemoglobin level 4 to 14 days after transfusion, as well as jaundice, fever, and hemoglobinuria. The diagnosis can be confirmed by repeat compatibility testing in conjunction with a positive direct antiglobulin (Coombs') test. The usual course of delayed hemolytic transfusion reaction is mild and requires no specific therapy; however, in rare cases, such reactions may be severe and fatal.

## Massive Transfusion

Massive blood transfusion is most commonly defined as complete replacement of a patient's blood volume (about 10 units of packed red blood cells in an adult) within a 24-hour period. The clinical consequences of massive transfusion are of both theoretical and genuine concern and include hyperkalemia, hypocalcemia, hypothermia, and coagulopathy.[32-37]

Refractory coagulopathy accounts for the majority of trauma deaths occurring within the first 24 hours of hospitalization.[38-43] Although the causes of coagulopathy are multifactorial, including coagulation abnormalities resembling disseminated intravascular coagulation, excessive fibrinolysis, hypothermia, and acidosis, dilutional coagulopathy as a result of massive infusion of crystalloid solutions and transfusion of packed red blood cells are significant contributors. Under such circumstances, the administration of fresh frozen plasma and/or platelet concentrates is indicated.

Thrombocytopenia is the most common contributor to clotting abnormalities in the setting of massive transfusion.[44] The platelet count should be monitored in trauma patients requiring large volumes of blood transfusion, but the function of the platelets under such circumstances is unpredictable. Thus, while circulating platelet counts of 20,000/$\mu$L and less may be adequate in non-bleeding patients, platelet transfusion is indicated in the early postoperative period following trauma when the platelet count is below 100,000/$\mu$L and there is evidence of ongoing microvascular bleeding. In the face of proven microvascular bleeding, the first dose of platelets may be given before the results of the platelet count are available. Additionally, if there is a history of preexisting platelet dysfunction or if the patient has taken nonsteroidal anti-inflammatory drugs (NSAIDs) and hemostasis is inadequate despite local measures, the administration of platelet concentrates may be indicated regardless of the platelet count.

Platelet concentrates may be extracted from platelet-rich plasma by centrifugation or may be obtained by platelet pheresis to yield $5 \times 10^{10}$ platelets in 50 mL, respectively. The administration of platelet concentrate will raise the circulating platelet count for 6 to 7 days in the absence of a consumptive coagulopathy or platelet specific antibodies in the recipient. $3 \times 10^{11}$ platelets are considered an "adult dose," as this number will provide a rise in platelet count of 30,000 to 60,000/$\mu$L.[17]

The aforementioned dilution of clotting factors mandates the administration of fresh frozen plasma (FFP), as well. FFP is plasma that is stored in a frozen state to maintain shelf life. One unit of FFP typically has a volume of 200 to 250 mL and contains levels of coagulation factors found in fresh whole blood except for factors V and VIII. The level of factor V, however, is still higher than that required for hemostasis, and though the level of factor VIII is less than that in fresh blood, recipient factor VIII levels rarely fall below critical levels during active hemorrhage in the absence of hemophilia.

Although the risk of TTD is low with respect to FFP administration, there have been relative advances in storage and acquisition to lower the risk of TTDs. A solvent (tri-*N*-butylphosphate)/detergent (Triton x-100) solution is a licensed product that effectively eliminates the risk of lipid-envelope virus transmission (such as HIV, hepatitis B, and hepatitis C) when used to treat frozen plasma. This process does not inactivate viruses with nonlipid envelopes, so there is still a potential risk of transmission of parvovirus B19, hepatitis A, and other pathogens. This potential use is of little benefit in the acute trauma setting if the patient has been transfused and exposed with other blood products. Another available product is donor-retested FFP, whereby FFP is stored for 90 days and the donor is retested for TTDs such as HIV to ensure that the donation was not made during the seronegative window period. This procedure is used infrequently in most blood banks.

FFP is indicated to correct abnormalities in the prothrombin time (PT) or international normalized ratio (INR) and activated partial thromboplastin time (aPTT). Generally, 10 to 15 mL/kg of FFP should be initially administered when the PT and/or aPTT is greater than 1.5 times the normal range. Although the need for both FFP and platelets can be anticipated during massive transfusion, the prophylactic administration of these products, based on the number of units of red blood cells administered, has not proven to be effective.[45,46] The challenge is to administer these products in a timely manner, once their need has been documented by laboratory results. To accomplish this goal, coagulation studies and platelet counts can be ordered simultaneously with requests for the preparation of FFP and/or platelets. The preparation time for these components (30 to 45 minutes) is roughly equivalent to the time it takes for the laboratory results to be obtained, and, if abnormalities are detected, they may then be rapidly treated without additional preparation time. If the laboratory results are not available and microvascular bleeding is clinically evident, treatment may begin empirically.

There has been much recent interest in the utility of recombinant activated coagulation factor VII (rFVIIa) in the setting of a coagulopathy resulting from massive transfusion, and, although the product is approved in the United States only for treatment of bleeding associated with hemophilia, significant off-label use has been reported.[47] A recent randomized clinical trial comparing rfVIIa to placebo in the setting of traumatic hemorrhage demonstrated a reduction in RBC transfusion requirements in patients with blunt trauma. No difference in outcomes, however, was observed.[48] Further study and clinical experience are necessary to better define the role of rFVIIa therapy in the setting of traumatic hemorrhage.

The concentration of potassium in a unit of red blood cells is between 5.2 and 6.6 mEq/L and increases with duration of storage. In most cases, the clinical impact of this potassium load is inconsequential. In patients with significant hypothermia, acidosis, and shock, as well as in those with major injury to soft tissue and those with renal insufficiency, significant hyperkalemia can occur. In these situations, electrocardiographic monitoring and frequent measurement of potassium levels should be performed. If there is evidence of potential hyperkalemia and red blood cell transfusion is required, the use of blood within its first week of storage or use of washed red blood cells that have little if any potassium should be considered. Washed red blood cells are units of PRBCs that have been washed with normal saline. The washing process removes approximately 99% of plasma proteins, electrolytes, and antibodies. It is indicated for use in the setting described earlier and may also reduce the incidence of febrile, urticarial, and, possibly, anaphylactic reactions.

Calcium chelation by citrate is the principal means of anticoagulating banked blood, and a significant citrate load is administered during massive transfusion. In patients with hypovolemia and hypothermia and those with hepatic injury or insufficiency, this citrate load can lead to reduced calcium availability. This can result in cardiac effects, including ventricular fibrillation and depression of myocardial contractility. Citrate toxicity can be monitored by measuring ionized calcium levels, with supplemental intravenous calcium given to maintain ionized calcium levels above 3.8 mg/dL.

## Transfusion-Related Acute Lung Injury

Transfusion-related acute lung injury (TRALI) is an acute respiratory distress syndrome observed soon after the administration of red blood cells (within 4 hours). It is characterized by hypoxia secondary to noncardiac pulmonary edema. The estimated frequency of TRALI is 1 in 5000 transfusions.[49] Reactive lipid products from breakdown of donor cells during the storage process have been implicated as a possible causative factor.[50] In the trauma setting, the causes of acute noncardiac pulmonary edema may be multiple, making it difficult to distinguish TRALI from other causes of acute respiratory distress syndrome (ARDS). Clinically, this distinction is not essential, because there is no specific difference in treatment for TRALI versus ARDS.

## Transfusion-Mediated Immunomodulation

The adverse immunosuppressive effect of allogenic blood transfusion has been noted in various clinical settings, including orthopaedics, colorectal surgery, and cardiac surgery.[51–55] In general, the available evidence suggests that exposure to allogenic blood increases the risk of postoperative infection and recurrence of cancer postresection.[56] Most pertinent to the trauma setting, allogenic blood transfusion has been demonstrated to be an independent risk factor for the development of multiple organ failure in injured patients.[57–59] Transfusion has also been demonstrated to be independently associated with ventilator-associated pneumonia, ARDS, and death in trauma patients regardless of injury severity.[60] It is theorized that the leukocytes present in units of red blood cells are mediators of transfusion-related immunomodulation. As the leukocytes die in storage, they release cytotoxic enzymes that can act as proinflammatory mediators. Leukocyte-reduced red blood cell units have been proposed to prevent transfusion-related immunomodulation, but the efficacy of leukoreduction has not been clearly demonstrated.[61] Universal leukoreduction of blood products has become standard blood bank practice in some countries, but the Food and Drug Administration has not advocated this policy for the United States to date. The University Health System Consortium, an alliance of more than 80 academic medical centers, evaluated leukoreduction according to evidence-based medicine guidelines, and concluded that leukoreduced blood components are not indicated to ameliorate the immunomodulatory effects of transfusion as described above.[62] In 1999, 42% of allogenic RBC transfusions in the United States were leukoreduced.[62]

## ALTERNATIVES TO ALLOGENIC ERYTHROCYTE TRANSFUSION

### Autotransfusion

The concern for both allogenic blood conservation and the transmission of TTDs has contributed to an increase in the use of autologous blood transfusion, which accounts for 5 to 10% of blood transfusions at many institutions. The majority of autologous transfusions are performed in association with elective surgery, whereby the patient is able to schedule autologous donation prior to operation. In the trauma setting, autotransfusion typically involves the salvage and reinfusion of shed blood from the hemorrhaging patient. Intraoperative recovery of blood involves the collection of shed blood in suction canisters. The collected blood is then anticoagulated with heparin and washed, yielding red blood cell units containing virtually no plasma or clotting factors. This technique typically requires 20 to 30 minutes, special equipment, and trained personnel. Because the washing process does not completely remove bacteria from the recovered blood, intraoperative autotransfusion should be limited if the operative field is grossly contaminated.[64] Appropriate intravenous antibiotics should be administered simultaneously.

Shed blood may also be collected from drainage tubes, most commonly thoracostomy tubes, anticoagulated with citrate, and directly reinfused through a macroaggregate filter without additional processing. The most notable adverse effect is the development of disseminated intravascular coagulation, which may be the result of reinfusion of activated products of coagulation and fibrinolysis in the shed blood. This complication most often occurs with autotransfusion of greater than 1500 mL, but can be encountered with smaller volumes. Most institutional guidelines limit autotransfusion of citrate-anticoagulated blood to less than 1500 mL and restrict its use to patients in profound shock. The length of time that salvaged blood may remain outside of the patient is uncertain, but the currently recommended limit is 4 to 6 hours.[17]

## Recombinant Erythropoietin

Endogenous erythropoietin, a glycoprotein produced predominately by the kidneys, stimulates the production of red blood cells. Recombinant human erythropoietin, or epoietin alfa, is commonly used to treat anemia associated with renal failure, but it has also been shown to be effective in a variety of clinical settings. Because of the lag between administration of the product and its effect, it is not a useful therapy for acute hemorrhage in the setting of trauma. There may, however, be a role for this therapy for trauma patients with prolonged stays in the intensive care unit. Ongoing anemia in the nonbleeding, critically ill patient has been observed to be of similar character to the anemia of chronic disease. Inappropriately low levels of circulating endogenous erythropoietin have been demonstrated in such patients.[65–67] The administration of epoetin alfa has been demonstrated to raise hematocrit concentrations while reducing the total number of red blood cell transfusions when compared with controls.[68] It is unknown, however, whether this therapy ultimately influences the clinical outcome of such patients, and clinical studies are ongoing.

## Hemoglobin-Based Red Blood Cell Substitutes and Oxygen Carrier Solutions

In recent years, there has been increasing interest and progress in the development of red blood cell substitutes. At the time of writing this chapter, however, no such product is available for human use in North America outside of controlled clinical trials. Scientific efforts have been directed toward the development of various perfluorocarbon emulsions and, alternatively, cell-free hemoglobin solutions to substitute for the oxygen delivery capacity of cellular hemoglobin.

Perfluorocarbons are chemically and biologically inert molecules that are capable of dissolving nonpolar gases including oxygen and carbon dioxide. They must be combined with a surfactant to produce a stable emulsion to be suitable for intravenous administration. Fluosol DA is a perfluorocarbon product that showed initial promise. Multicenter trials failed to demonstrate differences in mortality and morbidity between groups given the perfluorocarbon product and controls given lactated Ringer's solution.[69] It was withdrawn from the market in 1994 as a result of poor product sales. To date, no perfluorocarbon emulsion has been approved for clinical use by the FDA.

Hemoglobin-based oxygen carrier solutions exploit the well-understood ability of hemoglobin to load and unload oxygen in response to local physiologic conditions. The absence of antigenicity in such solutions as well as a relatively long storage life compared with banked blood offer the potential for a versatile, durable red blood cell substitute that could be utilized both in the hospital and in the field. Free, unmodified hemoglobin is rapidly cleared from the circulation and is nephrotoxic, necessitating the development of delivery solutions that can overcome this problem. Such modifications include hemoglobin cross-linking, polymerization of hemoglobin, surface modification of hemoglobin, and encapsulation of hemoglobin in liposomes. Sources of hemoglobin utilized in the current generation of products include outdated human banked blood, bovine hemoglobin, and recombinant hemoglobin. The availability of outdated human red blood cells limits the manufacturing potential of substitutes based on this source. Bovine hemoglobin, although widely available and abundant, carries with it a perceived, but undocumented risk of transmission of prions. Recombinant hemoglobin is limited largely by the economics of large-scale manufacture of such products.

No hemoglobin-based substitute has been approved for use in human medicine in North America, but clinical trials continue. HemAssist, a diaspirin cross-linked hemoglobin solution, was demonstrated in trauma patients to be a significant predictor of worse outcome compared with controls, and, hence, has been withdrawn from further development.[70] PolyHeme, a polymerized human hemoglobin solution, has been demonstrated to be effective in reducing mortality of patients with severe acute anemia compared with historical controls who refused blood transfusion on religious grounds.[71] At the time of writing, Polyheme is being evaluated in a multiinstitutional phase III trial in the prehospital setting, whereby the product is given to severely injured patients in the field and compared with standard prehospital resuscitation with crystalloid solutions. Hemopure, a polymerized bovine hemoglobin solution, has been approved for use in South Africa, and is undergoing evaluation by the FDA. The liposomal encapsulated hemoglobin solutions have not advanced beyond preclinical studies at this time. The major obstacles to development include technical issues with respect to reproducibility of uniformly sized liposomes and the unknown impact of clearance of the by-products by the reticuloendothelial system.

## SUMMARY

The rational use of blood products is essential to the successful management of the critically injured patient. The known metabolic and infectious risks of transfusion must be balanced against the need to augment oxygen delivery during both acute and prolonged resuscitation. As more knowledge is acquired, the guidelines for judicious transfusion will become more clearly defined. In the near future, the inevitable development of red blood cell substitutes will provide an entirely new dimension to the treatment of hemorrhagic shock.

# REFERENCES

1. *National Blood Data Resource Center FAQs.* (n.d.) http://www.aabb.org/About_the_AABB/Nbdrc/faqs.htm. Accessed December 8, 2005

2. Advanced Trauma Life Support: *Faculty Manual,* 7th ed. Chicago, IL: American College of Surgeons, 2004.

3. Adams RC, Lundy JS: Anesthesia in cases of poor surgical risk: Some suggestions for decreasing the risk. *Surg Gynecol Obstet* 74:1011, 1942.

4. Clark JH, Nelson W, Lyons C, et al.: Chronic shock: The problem of reduced blood volume in the chronically ill patient. *Ann Surg* 125:618, 1947.

5. Chapler CK, Carn SM: The physiologic reserve in oxygen carrying capacity: Studies in experiment hemodilution. *Can J Physiol Pharmacol* 64:7, 1986.

6. Perioperative red cell transfusion. *NIH Consensus Development Conference Statement.* Bethesda: National Institutes of Health, 1988, p. 1.

7. McFarland JG: Perioperative blood transfusions: Indications and options. *Chest* 115:113, 1999.

8. Spence RK, Cernaianu AC, Carson J, et al.: Transfusion and surgery. *Curr Probl Surg* 30:1101, 1993.

9. Gramm J, Smith S, Gamelli RL, et al.: Effect of transfusion on oxygen transport in critically ill patients. *Shock* 5:190, 1996.

10. Carson JL, Spence RK, Poses RM, et al.: Severity of anemia and operative mortality and morbidity. *Lancet* 1:727, 1988.

11. Robertie P, Gravlee G: Safe limits of hemodilution and recommendations for erythrocyte transfusion. *Int Anesthesiol Clin* 28:197, 1990.

12. Hebert PC, Wells G, Blajchman MA, et al.: A multicenter, randomized, controlled clinical trial of transfusion requirements in critical care. *N Engl J Med* 340:409, 1999.

13. Hebert PC, Yetisir E, Martin C, et al.: Is a low transfusion threshold safe in critically ill patients with cardiovascular diseases? *Crit Care Med* 29:227, 2001.

14. Carson JL, Duff A, Berlin JA, et al.: Effect of anemia and cardiovascular disease on surgical mortality and morbidity. *Lancet* 348:1055, 1996.

15. Spence RK, Carson JA, Poses R, et al.: Elective surgery without transfusion; influence of preoperative hemoglobin level and blood loss on mortality. *Am J Surg* 159:320, 1990.

16. McIntyre L, Hebert PC, Wells G, et al.: Is a restrictive transfusion strategy safe for resuscitated and critically ill trauma patients? *J Trauma* 57: 563, 2004.

17. Brecher ME, ed: *Technical Manual,* 14th ed. Bethesda, MD: American Association of Blood Banks. 2002.

18. Simon TL, Alverson DC, AuBuchon J, et al.: Practice parameters for the use of red blood cell transfusions. *Arch Pathol Lab Med* 122:130, 1998.

19. Crosby WH: The safety of blood transfusion in treatment of mass casualties. *Milit Med* 117:354, 1955.

20. Barnes A: Transfusions of universal donor and uncrossmatched blood. *Bibl Haematol.* 46:132, 1980.

21. Klein HG, Dodd RY, Dzik WH, et al.: Current status of solvent/detergent-treated frozen plasma. *Transfusion* 38:102, 1998.

22. Gervin AS, Fisher RP: Resuscitation of trauma patients with type specific uncrossmatched blood. *J Trauma* 24:327, 1984.

23. Donahue JG, Munoz A, Ness PM, et al.: The declining risk of post-transfusion hepatitis C virus infection. *N Engl J Med* 327:369, 1992.

24. Seidl S, Kuhnl P: Transmission of diseases by blood transfusion. *World J Surg* 11:30, 1987.

25. Dodd RY: The risk of transfusion-transmitted infection. *N Engl J Med* 327:419, 1992.

26. Goodnough LT, Mrecher ME, Kanter MH, et al.: First of two parts – blood transfusion. *N Engl J Med* 340:438, 1999.

27. Busch MP, Kleinman SH, Nemo GJ: Current and emerging infectious risks of blood transfusions. *JAMA* 289:959, 2003.

28. Weber B, Doerr HW: Diagnosis and epidemiology of transfusion-associated human cytomegalovirus infection: Recent developments. *Infusionsther Transfusme* 21:32, 1994.

29. Red blood cell transfusions contaminated with Yersinia enterocolitica—United States, 1991–1996, and initiation of a national study to detect bacteria-associated transfusion reactions. *MMWR Morb Mortal Wkly Rep* 46:553, 1997.

30. Kuehnert MJ, Roth VR, Haley NR, et al.: Transfusion-transmitted bacterial infection in the United States, 1998 through 2000. *Transfusion* 41:1493, 2001.

31. Dodd RY: Transmission of parasites and bacteria by blood components. *Vox Sang* 78:236, 2000.

32. Valeri CR, Feingold H, Cassidy G, et al.: Hypothermia-induced reversible platelet dysfunction. *Ann Surg* 205:175, 1987.

33. Flancbaum L, Trooskin SZ, Petersen H: Evaluation of blood-warming devices with the apparent thermal clearance. *Ann Emerg Med* 18:355, 1989.

34. Collins JA, Simmons RL, James PM, et al.: Acid-base status of seriously wounded combat casualties: Restoration with stored blood. *Ann Surg* 173:6, 1971.

35. Kahn RC, Jaxcott D, Carlon GC, et al.: Massive blood replacement: Correlation of ionized calcium, citrate and hydrogen ion concentration. *Anesth Analg* 58:274, 1979.

36. Linko K, Saxelin I: Electrolyte and acid-base disturbances caused by blood transfusion. *South Med J* 77:315, 1984.

37. Ferrara A, MacArthur JD, Wright HK, et al.: Hypothermia and acidosis worsen coagulopathy in the patient requiring massive transfusion. *Am J Surg* 160:515, 1990.

38. Burch JM, Ortiz VB, Richardson RJ, et al.: Abbreviated laparotomy and planned reoperation for critically injured patients. *Ann Surg* 215:476, 1992.

39. Cue JI, Cryer HG, Miller FB, et al.: Packing and planned reexploration for hepatic and retroperitoneal hemorrhage: Critical refinements of a useful technique. *J Trauma* 30:1007, 1990.

40. Hoyt DB, Bulger EM, Knudson MM, et al.: Death in the operating room: An analysis of a multicenter experience. *J Trauma* 37:426, 1994.

41. Moore EE: Staged laparotomy for the hypothermia, acidosis, and coagulopathy syndrome. *Am J Surg* 172:405, 1996.

42. Morris JA, Eddy VA, Blimman TA, et al.: The staged celiotomy for trauma: Issues in unpacking and reconstruction. *Ann Surg* 217:576, 1993.

43. Rotondo MF, Schwab CW, McGonigal MD, et al.: Damage control: An approach for improved survival in exsanguinating penetrating abdominal injury. *J Trauma* 35:375, 1993.

44. Moore EE, Dunn E, Brestich DJ, et al.: Platelet abnormalities associated with massive autotransfusion. *J Trauma* 20:1052, 1980.

45. Counts RB, Haisch C, Simon TL, et al.: Hemostasis in massively transfused trauma patients. *Ann Surg* 190:91, 1979.

46. Reed RL, Ciavarella D, Hemibach DM, et al.: Prophylactic platelet administration during massive transfusion. *Ann Surg* 203:40, 1986.

47. Harrison TD, Laskosky J, Jazaeri O, et al.: "Low-dose" recombinant activated factor VII results in less blood and blood product use in traumatic hemorrhage. *J Trauma* 59:150, 2005.

48. Boffard KD, Riou B, Warren B, et al.: Recombinant factor VIIa as adjunctive therapy for bleeding control in severely injured trauma patients: Two parallel randomized, placebo-controlled, double-blind clinical trials. *J Trauma* 59:8, 2005.

49. Popovsky MA, Moore SB: Diagnostic and pathogenic considerations in transfusion-related acute lung injury. *Transfusion* 25:573, 1985.

50. Silliman CC, Paterson AJ, Dickey WO, et al.: The association of biologically active lipids with the development of transfusion-related acute lung injury: A retrospective study. *Transfusion* 37:719, 1997.

51. Carson JL, Duff A, Berlin JA, et al.: Perioperative blood transfusion and post operative mortality. *JAMA* 279:199, 1998.

52. Tatten PI: Transfusion-induced immunosuppression and perioperative infections. *Beitr Infusionsther* 31:52, 1993.

53. Houbiers JG, van de Velde CJ, van de Watering LM, et al.: Transfusion of red cells is associated with increased incidence of bacterial infection after colorectal surgery: A prospective study. *Transfusion* 37:126, 1997.

54. Quintilianai L, Pescini A, Di Girolamo M, et al.: Relationship of blood transfusion, post-operative infections and immunoreactivity in patients undergoing surgery for gastrointestinal cancer. *Haematologica* 82:318, 1997.

55. Van de Watering LMG, Hermans J, Houbiers JGA, et al.: Beneficial effects of leukocyte depletion of transfused blood on postoperative complications in patients undergoing cardiac surgery: A randomized clinical trial. *Circulation* 97:562, 1998.

56. Vamvakas EC: Transfusion-associated cancer recurrence and postoperative infection: Meta-analysis of randomized, controlled clinical trials. *Transfusion* 36:175, 1996.

57. Moore FA, Moore EE, Sauaia A: Blood transfusion. An independent risk factor for postinjury multiple organ failure. *Arch Surg* 132:620, 1997.

58. Sauaia A, Moore FA, Moore EE, et al.: Multiple organ failure can be predicted as early as 12 hours after injury. *J Trauma* 45:291, 1998.

59. Sauaia A, Moore FA, Moore EE, et al.: Early predictors of postinjury multiple organ failure. *Arch Surg* 129:39, 1994.

60. Croce MA, Tolley EA, Claridge JA, et al.: Transfusions result in pulmonary morbidity and death after a moderate degree of injury. *J Trauma* 59:19, 2005.

61. Biffl WL, Moore EE, Offner PJ, et al.: Plasma from aged stored red blood cells delays neutrophil apoptosis and primes for cytotoxicity: Abrogation by poststorage washing but not prestorage leukoreduction. *J Trauma* 50:426, 2001.

62. Ratko TA, Cummings JP, Oberman HA, et al.: Evidence-based recommendations for the use of WBC-reduced cellular blood components. *Transfusion* 41:1310, 2001.

63. Sullivan MT, Wallace EL: Blood collection and transfusion in the United States in 1999. *Transfusion* 45:141, 2005.

64. Napier JA, Bruce M, Chapman J, et al.: Guidelines for autologous transfusion. II. Perioperative haemodilution and cell salvage. *Br J Anaesth* 78:768, 1997.

65. Krafte-Jacobs B, Levetown ML, Bray GL, et al.: Erythropoietin response to critical illness. *Crit Care Med* 22:821, 1994.

66. Rogiers P, Zhang H, Leeman M, et al.: Erythropoietin response is blunted in critically ill patients. *Intensive Care Med* 23:159, 1997.

67. Hobisch-Hagen P, Wiedermann F, Mayr A, et al.: Blunted erythropoietic response to anemia in multiply traumatized patients. *Crit Care Med* 29:743, 2001.
68. Corwin HL, Gettinger A, Pearl RG, et al.: Efficacy of recombinant human erythropoietin in critically ill patients: A randomized controlled trial. *JAMA* 288:2827, 2002.
69. Gould SA, Rosen A, Sehgal K, et al.: Fluosol-DA as a red-cell substitute in acute anemia. *N Engl J Med* 314:1653, 1986.
70. Sloan EP, Koenigsberg M, Gens D, et al.: Diaspirin cross-linked hemoglobin (DCLHb) in the treatment of severe traumatic hemorrhagic shock. A randomized controlled efficacy trial. *JAMA* 282:1857, 1999.
71. Gould SA, Moore EE, Hoyt DB, et al.: The life-sustaining capacity of human polymerized hemoglobin when red cells might be unavailable. *J Am Coll Surg* 195:445, 2002.

## Commentary ■ LENA M. NAPOLITANO

Blood transfusion is a life-saving treatment for trauma patients in hemorrhagic shock. No alternative resuscitative fluids are currently available. In light of this, every effort should be made to conserve blood utilization for the trauma patient with hemorrhage, and alternative strategies for the treatment of anemia in hemodynamically stable euvolemic trauma patients must be considered. Furthermore, rigorous investigation of strategies to promote earlier cessation of traumatic hemorrhage with prompt correction of coagulopathy are vitally important.

Drs. Peterson and Weinberg have provided a comprehensive review of the risks and benefits of blood transfusion in trauma. In most circumstances, other than for the treatment of hemorrhagic shock, the risks of blood transfusion outweigh the benefits. There are a number of potential mechanisms that have been delineated regarding the adverse effects of blood transfusion, including increased storage time of blood, decreased red blood cell deformability resulting in reduced microcirculatory perfusion, increased red blood cell adhesion to vascular endothelial cells, increased inflammatory response, transfusion-associated immunosuppression, and increased free hemoglobin related to hemolysis which results in binding of nitric oxide with subsequent vasoconstriction and pulmonary hypertension.[1–3]

Many of these adverse effects are a result of increased blood storage time. During storage, red blood cells undergo a series of biochemical and biomechanical changes that reduce their survival and function, and collectively are referred to as the "storage lesion." A number of observational studies have raised the possibility that prolonged red blood cell storage adversely affects clinically outcomes.

Most importantly, there is little evidence documenting improved tissue oxygen consumption with the transfusion of red blood cells. Although an increase in hemoglobin concentration is evident after blood transfusion, only 2 of 20 studies have documented a significant increase in tissue oxygen consumption posttransfusion. RBC transfusion is not associated with improvements in clinical outcome in the critically ill and may result in worse outcomes in some patients.

Additionally, transfusion-associated microchimerism, the stable persistence of an allogeneic leukocyte population, has been documented as a common complication of blood transfusion in injured patients. Transfusion-associated microchimerism is present in approximately half of transfused severely injured patients at hospital discharge and is not decreased by leukoreduction. In approximately 10% of patients, the chimerism from a single blood donor may increase in magnitude over months to years, reaching as much as 5% of all circulating leukocytes in a trauma patient. This may have the potential to be pathologic, resulting in either autoimmunity or graft-versus-host disease. The recent use of fresh whole blood for military combat casualties may result in a higher incidence of transfusion-associated microchimerism, and warrants additional study.

Interestingly, blood transfusion has never undergone prospective safety and efficacy testing. The recent data presented in this chapter regarding increased inflammatory response, decreased microcirculation, and lack of increase in tissue oxygen consumption, all point toward potential problems with allogeneic blood transfusion.

The vast majority of blood transfusion in trauma and critical care is administered for the treatment of anemia. A number of recent studies have documented that trauma patients are more likely to be transfused (55% of trauma ICU patients), are transfused at a higher hemoglobin level, and receive more red blood cell units than other critically ill patients. The mean pre-transfusion hemoglobin concentrations in critically ill trauma patients have been documented as 8 to 9 g/dL. Trauma patients are also at highest risk for hospital-acquired infections, and blood transfusion has been confirmed as an independent risk factor for infection, systemic inflammatory response syndrome, and increased mortality. In an effort to decrease such adverse events, immunosuppression and hyperinflammation, all attempts to minimize the use of blood transfusion in trauma patients is warranted.

The pathophysiology of anemia post-injury is related initially to hemodilution and blood loss, but subsequently to an inflammatory state with release of inflammatory cytokines that result in (1) direct inhibition of red blood cell production by the bone marrow, (2) direct inhibition of the erythroid precursor cell response to erythropoietin, (3) inhibition of erythropoietin gene transcription in the renal juxtaglomerular cells, and (4) increased hepcidin expression with indirect limitation of iron availability by hepcidin-induced increase in iron sequenstration in macrophages. Blood transfusion has been documented to further incite an inflammatory response with resultant inflammatory cytokine release, and further impair the normal bone marrow response to anemia after traumatic injury.

It is therefore critically important to weigh the risks and benefits of red blood cell transfusion in trauma patients with anemia who are hemodynamically stable and demonstrate no evidence of ongoing hemorrhage. The optimal hemoglobin in the stable trauma patient postinjury is not known. But based on existing literature, the evidence is sufficient to state that the benefits of blood transfusion exceed the risks when hemoglobin concentrations fall below 7.0 g/dL in this population.

Other strategies to prevent and treat anemia in the stable trauma patient should be implemented. The authors importantly point out that autotransfusion and the use of recombinant erythropoietin are important strategies for the treatment of anemia that are infrequently considered in trauma. Other simple strategies, including reduction of phlebotomy for diagnostic laboratory testing, use of smaller volume diagnostic laboratory sampling tubes, and the use of blood conservation devices to minimize diagnostic phlebotomy blood loss have all been documented to be efficacious. Despite this, less than 20% of ICUs utilize these strategies.

Clearly, future randomized controlled clinical trials in the area of optimal transfusion practice in trauma are needed. Transfusion of the injured patient with stored packed red blood cells requires careful vigilance during the acute resuscitative and recovery phases postinjury. At present, blood transfusion is the only option for treatment of severe hemorrhagic shock. The future of hemoglobin-based oxygen carriers in the treatment of hemorrhagic shock holds great promise. We await the findings of the clinical trials with hemoglobin-based oxygen carriers for early trauma resuscitation. In the interim, we should attempt to conserve blood transfusion for trauma victims with hemorrhagic shock and minimize blood transfusion in the stable anemic trauma patient.

## References

1. Malone DL, Dunne J, Tracy JK, et al.: Blood transfusion, independent of shock severity, is associated with worse outcome in trauma. *J Trauma* 54:898, 2003.
2. Napolitano LM: Cumulative risks of early red blood cell transfusion. *J Trauma* 60:S26, 2006.
3. Napolitano LM, Corwin HL: Efficacy of red blood cell transfusion in the critically ill. *Crit Care Clin* 20:255, 2004.

# Emergency Department Thoracotomy

*C. Clay Cothren* ■ *Ernest E. Moore*

The number of patients arriving at hospitals *in extremis*, rather than expiring in the prehospital setting, has increased due to the maturation of regionalized trauma systems (see Chap. 4). Salvage of individuals with imminent cardiac arrest or those already undergoing cardiopulmonary resuscitation often requires immediate thoracotomy as an integral component of their initial resuscitation in the emergency department (ED). The optimal application of emergency department thoracotomy (EDT) requires a thorough understanding of its physiologic objectives, technical maneuvers, and the cardiovascular and metabolic consequences. This chapter reviews these features and highlights the specific clinical indications, all of which are essential for the appropriate use of this potentially lifesaving yet costly procedure.

## HISTORICAL PERSPECTIVE

Emergent thoracotomy came into use for the treatment of heart wounds and anesthesia-induced cardiac arrest in the late 1800s and early 1900s.[1] The concept of a thoracotomy as a resuscitative measure began with Schiff's promulgation of open cardiac massage in 1874.[1] Block first suggested the potential application of this technique for penetrating chest wounds and heart lacerations in 1882.[2] Following use of the technique in animal models, the first successful suture repair of a cardiac wound in a human was performed at the turn of the century.[3] Subsequently, Igelsbrud described the successful resuscitation of a patient sustaining cardiac arrest during a surgical procedure using emergent thoracotomy with open cardiac massage.[1] The utility of the emergent thoracotomy was beginning to be tested in a wide range of clinical scenarios in the early 1900s.

With improvement in patient resuscitation and an ongoing evaluation of patient outcomes, the indications for emergent thoracotomy shifted. Initially, cardiovascular collapse from medical causes was the most common reason for thoracotomy in the early 1900s. The demonstrated efficacy of closed-chest compression by

Kouwenhoven and colleagues[4] in 1960 and the introduction of external defibrillation in 1965 by Zoll and colleagues[5] virtually eliminated the practice of open-chest resuscitation for medical cardiac arrest. Indications for emergent thoracotomy following trauma also became more limited. In 1943, Blalock and Ravitch advocated the use of pericardiocentesis rather than thoracotomy as the preferred treatment for postinjury cardiac tamponade.[6] In the late 1960s, however, refinements in cardiothoracic surgical techniques reestablished the role of immediate thoracotomy for salvaging patients with life-threatening chest wounds.[7] The use of temporary thoracic aortic occlusion in patients with exsanguinating abdominal hemorrhage further expanded the indications for emergent thoracotomy.[8,9] In the past decade, critical analyses of patient outcomes following postinjury EDT has tempered the unbridled enthusiasm for this technique, allowing a more selective approach with clearly defined indications.[10,11]

## DEFINITIONS

The literature addressing emergency department thoracotomy (EDT) appears confusing, likely due to widely varying terminology. As a result, there is a lack of agreement amongst physicians regarding the specific indications for EDT as well as the definition of "signs of life."[12] In this chapter, EDT refers to a thoracotomy performed in the ED for patients arriving *in extremis*. At times, the term EDT is used interchangeably with the term resuscitative thoracotomy; however, this should not be confused with a thoracotomy that is performed in the operating room (OR) or intensive care unit (ICU) within hours after injury for delayed physiologic deterioration. The value of and indication for EDT for acute resuscitation may also be confusing because of the variety of indices used to characterize the patient's physiologic status prior to thoracotomy. Because there have been a wide range of indications for which EDT has been performed in different trauma centers, comparisons in the literature are difficult. The authors define "no signs of life" as no detectable blood pressure, respiratory or motor effort, cardiac electrical activity, or pupillary activity (i.e., clinical death). Patients with "no vital signs" have no palpable blood pressure, but demonstrate electrical activity, respiratory effort, or pupillary reactivity.

## PHYSIOLOGIC RATIONALE FOR EDT

The primary objectives of EDT are to (a) release pericardial tamponade; (b) control cardiac hemorrhage; (c) control intrathoracic bleeding; (d) evacuate massive air embolism; (e) perform open cardiac massage; and (f) temporarily occlude the descending thoracic aorta. Combined, these objectives attempt to address the primary issue of cardiovascular collapse from mechanical sources or extreme hypovolemia.

### Release Pericardial Tamponade and Control Cardiac Hemorrhage

The highest survival rate following EDT is in patients with penetrating cardiac wounds, especially when associated with pericardial tamponade.[7] Early recognition of cardiac tamponade, prompt pericardial decompression, and control of cardiac hemorrhage are the key components to successful EDT and patient survival following penetrating wounds to the heart (see Chap. 28).[13] The egress of blood from the injured heart, regardless of mechanism, results in tamponade physiology. Rising intrapericardial pressure produces abnormalities in hemodynamic and cardiac perfusion that can be divided into three phases.[14] Initially, increased pericardial pressure restricts ventricular diastolic filling and reduces subendocardial blood flow.[15] Cardiac output under these conditions is maintained by compensatory tachycardia, increased systemic vascular resistance, and elevated central pressure (i.e., ventricular filling pressure). In the intermediate phase of tamponade, rising pericardial pressure further compromises diastolic filling, stroke volume, and coronary perfusion, resulting in diminished cardiac output. Although blood pressure may be maintained deceptively well, subtle signs of shock (e.g., anxiety, diaphoresis, and pallor) become evident. During the final phase of tamponade, compensatory mechanisms fail as the intrapericardial pressure approaches the ventricular filling pressure. Cardiac arrest ensues as profound coronary hypoperfusion occurs.

The classic description of clinical findings, Beck's triad, is rarely observed in the ED; therefore, a high index of suspicion in the at-risk patient sustaining penetrating torso trauma is crucial, with prompt intervention essential. In the first two phases of cardiac tamponade, patients may be aggressively managed with definitive airway control, volume resuscitation to increase preload, and pericardiocentesis. The patient in the third phase of tamponade, with profound hypotension (SBP < 60), should undergo EDT rather than pericardiocentesis as the management for evacuation of pericardial blood.[16,17] Following release of tamponade, the source of tamponade can be directly controlled with appropriate interventions based on the underlying injury (see *Technical Considerations*).

### Control Intrathoracic Hemorrhage

Life-threatening intrathoracic hemorrhage occurs in less than 5% of patients following penetrating injury presenting to the ED, and in even lower percentage of patients sustaining blunt trauma.[18] The most common injuries include penetrating wounds to the pulmonary hilum and great vessels; less commonly seen are torn descending thoracic aortic injuries with frank rupture or penetrating cardiac wounds exsanguinating into the thorax through a traumatic pericardial window. There is a high mortality rate in injuries to the pulmonary or thoracic great-vessel lacerations due to the lack of hemorrhage containment by adjacent tissue tamponade or vessel spasm (see Chaps. 26 and 29). Either hemithorax can rapidly accommodate more than half of a patient's total blood volume before overt physical signs of hemorrhagic shock occur. Therefore, a high clinical suspicion is warranted in patients with penetrating torso trauma, particularly in those with hemodynamic decompensation. Patients with exsanguinating wounds require EDT with rapid control of the source of hemorrhage if they are to be salvaged.

### Perform Open Cardiac Massage

External chest compression provides approximately 20 to 25% of baseline cardiac output, with 10 to 20% of normal cerebral perfusion.[19,20] This degree of vital organ perfusion can provide reasonable salvage rates for 15 minutes, but few normothermic patients survive 30 minutes of closed-chest compression. Moreover, in models of inadequate intravascular volume (hypovolemic shock) or restricted ventricular filling (pericardial tamponade), external chest compression fails to augment arterial pressure or provide adequate systemic perfusion; the associated low diastolic volume and pressure result in inadequate coronary perfusion.[21] Therefore, closed cardiac massage is ineffective for postinjury cardiopulmonary arrest. The only potential to salvage the injured patient with ineffective circulatory status is immediate EDT.

### Achieve Thoracic Aortic Cross Clamping

The rationale for temporary thoracic aortic occlusion in the patient with massive hemorrhage is two-fold. First, in patients with hemorrhagic shock, aortic cross clamping redistributes the patient's limited blood volume to the myocardium and brain.[9] Second, patients sustaining intraabdominal injury may benefit from aortic cross clamping due to reduction in subdiaphragmatic blood loss.[8] Temporary thoracic aortic occlusion augments aortic diastolic and carotid systolic blood pressure, enhancing coronary as well as cerebral perfusion.[22,23] Canine studies have shown that the left ventricular stroke-work index and myocardial contractility increase in response to thoracic aortic occlusion during hypovolemic shock.[24] These improvements in myocardial function occur without an increase in the pulmonary capillary wedge pressure or a significant change in systemic vascular resistance. Thus, improved coronary perfusion resulting from an increased aortic diastolic pressure presumably accounts for the observed enhancement in contractility.[25]

These experimental observations suggest that temporary aortic occlusion is valuable in the patient either with shock due to nonthoracic trauma or in patients with continued shock following the repair of cardiac or other exsanguinating wounds. Indeed, occlusion of the descending thoracic aorta appears to increase the return of spontaneous circulation following cardiopulmonary resuscitation.[26,27] Reports of successful resuscitation using EDT in patients in hemorrhagic shock and even sustaining cardiac arrest following extremity and cervical injuries exist.[28] In these situations, EDT may be a temporizing measure until the patient's circulating blood volume can be replaced by blood product transfusion. However, once the patient's blood volume has been restored, the aortic cross clamp should be removed. Thoracic cross clamping in the normovolemic patient may be deleterious because of increased myocardial oxygen demands resulting from the increased systemic vascular resistance.[29] Careful application of this technique is warranted as there is substantial metabolic cost and a finite risk of paraplegia associated with the procedure.[30–32] However, in carefully selected patients, aortic cross clamping may effectively redistribute the patient's blood volume until external replacement and control of the hemorrhagic source is possible. Typically, complete removal of the aortic cross clamp or replacement of the clamp below the renal vessel should be performed within 30 minutes; the gut's tolerance to normothermic ischemia is 30–45 minutes.

## Evacuate Bronchovenous Air Embolism

Bronchovenous air embolism can be a subtle entity following thoracic trauma, and is likely to be much more common than is recognized.[33–35] The clinical scenario typically involves a patient sustaining penetrating chest injury who precipitously develops profound hypotension or cardiac arrest following endotracheal intubation and positive-pressure ventilation. Traumatic alveolovenous communications produce air emboli that migrate to the coronary arterial systems; any impedance in coronary blood flow causes global myocardial ischemia and resultant shock. The production of air emboli is enhanced by the underlying physiology—there is relatively low intrinsic pulmonary venous pressure due to associated intrathoracic blood loss and high bronchoalveolar pressure from assisted positive pressure ventilation. This combination increases the gradient for air transfer across bronchovenous channels.[36] Although more often observed in penetrating trauma, a similar process may occur in patients with blunt lacerations of the lung parenchyma (see Chap. 26).

Immediate thoracotomy with pulmonary hilar cross clamping prevents further propagation of pulmonary venous air embolism. Thoracotomy with opening of the pericardium also provides access to the cardiac ventricles; with the patient in the Trendelenburg's position (done to trap to air in the apex of the ventricle), needle aspiration is performed to remove air from the cardiac chambers. Additionally, vigorous cardiac massage may promote dissolution of air already present in the coronary arteries.[35] Aspiration of the aortic root is done to alleviate any accumulated air pocket, and direct needle aspiration of the right coronary artery may be attempted.

## CLINICAL RESULTS FOLLOWING EDT

The value of EDT in resuscitation of the patient in profound shock but not yet dead is unquestionable. Its indiscriminate use, however, renders it a low-yield and high-cost procedure.[37–39] In the past three decades there has been a significant clinical shift in the performance of EDT, from a nearly obligatory procedure before declaring any trauma patient to very few patients undergoing EDT. During this swing of the pendulum, several groups have attempted to elucidate the clinical guidelines for EDT. In 1979, we conducted a critical analysis of 146 consecutive patients undergoing EDT and suggested a selected approach to its use in the moribund trauma patient, based on consideration of the following variables: (1) location and mechanism of injury, (2) signs of life at the scene and on admission to the ED, (3) cardiac electrical activity at thoracotomy, (4) systolic blood pressure response to thoracic aortic cross-clamping.[39]

To validate these clinical guidelines, we established a prospective study in which these data were carefully documented in all patients at the time of thoracotomy. In 1982, the first 400 patients were analyzed.[38] A more recent review has summarized the data on 868 patients who have undergone EDT at the Denver Health Medical Center.[40] Of these, 676 (78%) were dead in the ED, 128 (15%) died in the operating room, and 23 (3%) succumbed to multiple organ failure in the surgical intensive care unit. Ultimately, 41 (5%) patients survived, and 34 recovered fully without neurologic sequelae. While this yield may seem low, it is important to emphasize that thoracotomy was done on virtually every trauma patient delivered to the ED. In fact, 624 (72%) were without vital signs in the field, and 708 patients (82%) had no vital signs at the time of presentation to the ED. In contrast, it is equally important to stress that patients without signs of life at the scene but who responded favorably to resuscitation were excluded from this analysis because they did not require EDT; these patients remind the practitioner that prehospital clinical assessments may not always be reliable in triaging these severely injured patients.[43] Indeed, the authors have salvaged a number of individuals sustaining blunt and penetrating trauma who were assessed to have no signs of life at the scene of injury.

The survival rate and percentage of neurologic impairment following EDT varies considerably, due to the heterogeneity of patient populations reported in the literature. As previously discussed, critical determinants of survival include the mechanism and location of injury and the patient's physiologic condition at the time of thoracotomy.[42,43] We have attempted to elucidate the impact of these factors in ascertaining the success rate of EDT by collating data from a number of clinical series reporting on 50 or more patients (Table 15-1). Unfortunately, inconsistencies in patient stratification and a paucity of clinical details limit objective analysis of these data. Although some reviews provide a specific breakdown of the injury mechanism and clinical status of patients presenting to the ED, others combine all injury mechanisms. We believe it is crucial to stratify patients according to the location and mechanism of injury as well as the status of signs of life (i.e., blood pressure, respiratory effort, cardiac electrical activity, and pupillary activity).

The data summarized to date confirms that EDT has the highest survival rate following isolated cardiac injury (Table 15-1). An average of 35% of adult patients presenting in shock, defined as a SBP <70 mm mm Hg, and 20% without vital signs were salvaged after isolated penetrating injury to the heart if EDT was performed. In contrast, only 1–3% of blunt trauma patients undergoing EDT survive, regardless of clinical status on presentation. Following penetrating torso injuries, 14% of patients requiring EDT are salvaged if they are hypotensive with detectable vital signs, whereas 8% of those who have no vital signs but have signs of life at presentation, and 1% of those without signs of life are salvaged. These findings are reiterated by a recent report incorporating all patients undergoing EDT for either blunt or penetrating mechanism from 24 separate studies;[42] survival rates for patients undergoing EDT for penetrating injuries was 8.8% and 1.4% for blunt mechanisms. Additionally,

**TABLE 15-1**

## Outcome Following Emergency Department Thoracotomy in Adults

| INJURY PATTERN | SHOCK | NO VITAL SIGNS | NO SIGNS OF LIFE | TOTAL |
|---|---|---|---|---|
| **Cardiac** | | | | |
| Denver[67] | 3/9 (33%) | 0/7 (0%) | 1/53 (2%) | 4/69 (6%) |
| Detroit[70] | 9/42 (21%) | 3/110 (3%) | | 12/152 (8%) |
| Johannesburg[71] | | | | 13/108 (12%) |
| Los Angeles[66] | 2/5 (40%) | 6/11 (55%) | 2/55 (4%) | 10/71 (14%) |
| New York[69] | 7/20 (35%) | 18/53 (32%) | 0/18 (0%) | 24/91 (26%) |
| San Francisco[10] | 18/37 (49%) | 0/25 (0%) | | 18/63 (29%) |
| Seattle[68] | 4/11 (36%) | 11/47 (23%) | | 15/58 (26%) |
| Overall | 43/124 (35%) | 47/254 (19%) | 4/126 (3%) | 96/612 (16%) |
| **Penetrating** | | | | |
| Denver[15] | 19/78 (24%) | 14/399 (4%) | | 33/477 (7%) |
| Detroit[70] | 9/42 (21%) | 3/110 (3%) | | 12/152 (8%) |
| Houston[73] | 14/156 (9%) | 18/162 (11%) | | 32/318 (10%) |
| Indianapolis[16] | 3/7 (43%) | 1/50 (2%) | 0/80 (0%) | 4/137 (3%) |
| Johannesburg[71] | 31/413 (8%) | 10/149 (7%) | 1/108 (1%) | 42/670 (6%) |
| Los Angeles[66] | 2/5 (40%) | 6/11 (55%) | 2/55 (4%) | 10/71 (14%) |
| New York[75] | 8/32 (25%) | 8/77 (10%) | 0/25 (0%) | 16/134 (12%) |
| Oakland[20] | 8/24 (33%) | | 2/228 (1%) | 10/252 (4%) |
| San Francisco[10] | | | | 32/198 (30%) |
| Seattle[68] | 4/11 (36%) | 11/47 (23%) | | 15/58 (25%) |
| Washington[72] | 7/13 (54%) | 3/47 (6%) | | 10/60 (17%) |
| Overall | 145/1007 (14%) | 100/1252 (8%) | 6/615 (1%) | 283/2986 (10%) |
| **Blunt** | | | | |
| Denver[15] | 4/86 (5%) | 4/311 (1%) | | 8/397 (2%) |
| Houston[73] | 0/42 (0%) | 0/27 (0%) | | 0/69 (0%) |
| Johannesburg[71] | 1/109 (1%) | 0/39 (0%) | 0/28 (0%) | 1/176 (1%) |
| San Francisco[10] | | | | 1/60 (2%) |
| Seattle[18] | | | | 1/88 (1%) |
| Overall | 5/237 (2%) | 4/377 (1%) | 0/28 (0%) | 11/790 (1.4%) |

more patients survive EDT for isolated cardiac wounds (19.4%) followed by stab wounds (16.8%) and gunshot wounds (4.3%).

Although there is a clear role for EDT in the patient presenting in shock but with measurable vital signs, there is disagreement about its use in the patient population undergoing cardiopulmonary resuscitation prior to arrival in the ED. Although there have been multiple reports with low survival rates and dismal outcomes following prehospital CPR, termination of resuscitation in the field should not be performed in all patients.[44] Our most recent evaluation, spanning 26 years of experience, indicates EDT does play a significant role in the critically injured patient undergoing prehospital CPR.[10] The majority of patients arriving in extremis who survived to discharge sustained a stab wound to the torso, consistent with previous reports. Additionally, over 80% of patients were neurologically intact at discharge. We believe this study provides simple, clear guidelines for the use of EDT as a resuscitative measure to ensure that all potentially salvageable patients are included (Table 15-2). All survivors undergoing CPR on arrival to the ED had lost vital signs less than 15 minutes prior to arrival for penetrating mechanisms and less than 5 minutes for blunt mechanisms.

Emerging data indicates the clinical results in the pediatric population mirror that of the adult experience (Table 15-3).

One might expect that children would have a more favorable outcome compared to adults, due to improved results following head injury (see Chap. 46); however, this has not been borne out in multiple studies.[45–49] Beaver and colleagues reported no

**TABLE 15-2**

## Current Indications and Contraindications for EDT

INDICATIONS:

*Salvageable postinjury cardiac arrest:*

Patients sustaining witnessed penetrating thoracic trauma with < 15 min of prehospital CPR

Patients sustaining witnessed penetrating non-thoracic trauma with < 5 min of prehospital CPR.

Patients sustaining witnessed blunt trauma with < 5 min of prehospital CPR

*Persistent severe postinjury hypotension (SBP < 60 mmHg) due to:*

Cardiac tamponade

Hemorrhage–intrathoracic, intraabdominal, extremity, cervical

Air embolism

CONTRAINDICATIONS:

*Penetrating trauma:* CPR > 15 min and no signs of life (pupillary response, respiratory effort, or motor activity)

*Blunt trauma:* CPR > 5 min and no signs of life or asystole

**TABLE 15-3**

**Outcome Following Emergency Department Thoracotomy in Children**

| INJURY PATTERN | SHOCK | NO VITAL SIGNS | NO SIGNS OF LIFE | TOTAL |
|---|---|---|---|---|
| **Penetrating** | | | | |
| Baltimore[46] | | 0/2 (0%) | | 0/2 (0%) |
| Denver[47] | 1/3 (33%) | 1/5 (20%) | 0/28 (0%) | 2/36 (6%) |
| Mobile[49] | 0/1 (0%) | 3/9 (33%) | | 3/10 (30%) |
| Sacramento[48] | 1/4 (25%) | 0/4 (0%) | | 1/8 (13%) |
| Overall | 2/8 (25%) | 4/20 (20%) | 0/28 (0%) | 6/56 (11%) |
| **Blunt** | | | | |
| Baltimore[46] | | 0/15 (0%) | | 0/15 (0%) |
| Denver[47] | 1/11 (9%) | 0/6 (0%) | 0/30 (0%) | 1/47 (2%) |
| Mobile[49] | | 0/5 (0%) | | 0/5 (0%) |
| Sacramento[48] | 0/6 (0%) | 0/9 (0%) | | 0/15 (0%) |
| Overall | 1/17 (6%) | 0/35 (0%) | 0/30 (0%) | 1/82 (1%) |

survivors among 27 patients, from 15 months to 14 years of age, undergoing postinjury EDT at Johns Hopkins Hospital.[46] Powell and coworkers, at the South Alabama Medical Center, described an overall survival of 20% (3 of 15 patients) in patients ranging from 4 to 18 years.[49] In a study at Denver Health Medical Center, encompassing an 11-year experience with 689 consecutive EDT, we identified 83 patients (12%) who were under 18 years old.[47] Survival by injury mechanism was 9% (1 of 11) for stab wounds, 4% (1 of 25) for gunshot wounds, and 2% (1 of 47 patients) for blunt trauma. Among 69 patients presenting to the ED without vital signs, only 1 patient (1%) survived (with a stab wound). This contrasted to a salvage of 2 (14%) among 14 patients with vital signs. The outcome in blunt trauma, the predominant mechanism of lethal injury in children, was disappointing, with only 2% salvage, and no survivors when vital signs were absent. Thus, as in adults, outcome following EDT in the pediatric population is largely determined by injury mechanism and physiologic status on presentation to the ED.

In sum, overall analysis of the available literature indicates that the success of EDT approximates 35% in the patient arriving in shock with a penetrating cardiac wound, and 15% for all penetrating wounds. Patients undergoing CPR upon arrival to the ED should be stratified based upon injury and transport time to determine the utility of EDT. Conversely, patient outcome is relatively poor when EDT is done for blunt trauma; 2% survival in patients in shock and less than 1% survival with no vital signs.

## INDICATIONS FOR EDT

Based on our 26 successive years of EDT prospective analysis, we propose current indications for EDT[10] (Table 15-2). Clearly, the specific application of these guidelines must include consideration of the patient's age, pre-existing disease, signs of life, and mechanism of injury, as well as logistic issues such as the proximity of the ED to the OR, and qualified personnel. Our current decision algorithm for resuscitation of the moribund trauma patient and use of EDT was formulated and implemented as a key clinical pathway in the ED (Fig. 15-1). At the scene, patients *in extremis* without electrical cardiac activity are declared dead. Patients *in extremis* but with electrical cardiac activity are intubated, supported with cardiac compression, and rapidly transported to the ED.

On arrival to the ED, the time from initiation of CPR is recorded; blunt trauma patient with greater than 5 minutes of prehospital CPR and no signs of life are declared while penetrating trauma patients with greater than 15 minutes of prehospital CPR and no signs of life are pronounced. Patients within the time guidelines or those with signs of life trigger ongoing resuscitation and EDT. After performing a generous left anterior thoracotomy and subsequent pericardotomy, the patient's intrinsic cardiac activity is evaluated. Patients in asystole without associated cardiac injury are declared. Patient's with a cardiac wound, tamponade, and associated asystole are aggressively treated; the cardiac wound is repaired first followed by manual cardiac compressions and intracardiac injection of epinephrine. Following several minutes of such treatment and volume resuscitation, one should reassess salvageability, typically defined as the patient's ability to generate a systolic blood pressure > 70 mm Hg.

Patient's with an intrinsic rhythm following EDT should be treated according to underlying pathology. Those with tamponade should undergo cardiac repair, either in the trauma bay or the operating room (see Chap. 28). Control of intrathoracic hemorrhage may entail hilar crossclamping, digital occlusion of the direct injury, or even packing of the apices for subclavian injuries. Treatment of bronchovenous air embolism includes crossclamping of the hilum, putting the patient in Trendelenberg's position, aspirating the left ventricle and aortic root, and massaging the coronaries. Finally, aortic crossclamping is performed to decrease the required effective circulating volume, for either thoracic or abdominal sources of hemorrhage, and facilitate resuscitation. In all of these scenarios, reassessment of the patient following intervention and aggressive resuscitation efforts is performed, with the goal systolic pressure of 70 mm Hg used to define salvageability.

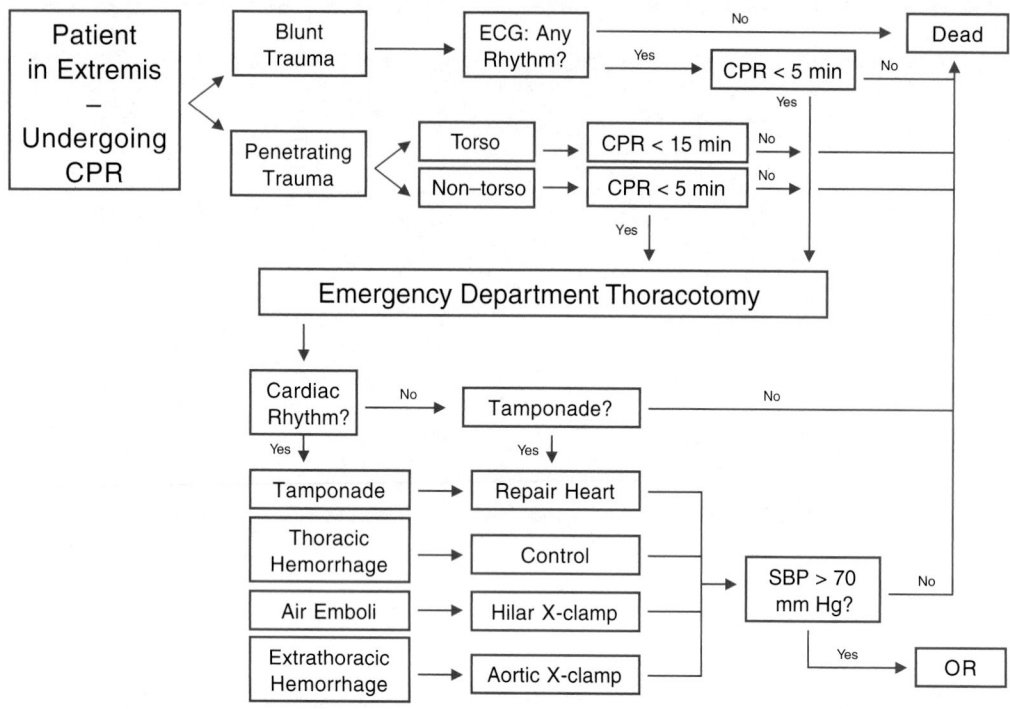

**FIGURE 15-1.** Algorithm directing the use of EDT in the multiply injured trauma patient.

## TECHNICAL DETAILS OF EDT

The optimal benefit of EDT is achieved by a surgeon experienced in the management of intrathoracic injuries. The emergency physician, however, should not hesitate to perform the procedure in the moribund patient with a penetrating chest wound when thoracotomy is the only means of salvage. The technical skills needed to perform the procedure include the ability to perform a rapid thoracotomy, pericardiotomy, cardiorrhaphy, and thoracic aortic cross clamping; familiarity with vascular repair techniques and control of the pulmonary hilum are advantageous. Once life-threatening intrathoracic injuries are controlled or temporized, the major challenge is restoring the patient's hemodynamic integrity and minimizing vital-organ reperfusion injury.

### Thoracic Incision

A left anterolateral thoracotomy incision is preferred for EDT. Advantages of this incision in the critically injured patient include (a) rapid access with simple instruments, (b) the ability to perform this procedure on a patient in the supine position, and (c) easy extension into the right hemithorax, a clamshell thoracotomy, for exposure of both pleural spaces as well as anterior and posterior mediastinal structures. The key resuscitative maneuvers of EDT, namely, pericardiotomy, open cardiac massage, and thoracic aortic cross clamping are readily accomplished via this approach. The initial execution of a clamshell thoracotomy should be done in hypotensive patients with penetrating wounds to the right chest. This provides immediate, direct access to a right-sided pulmonary or vascular injury while still allowing access to the pericardium from the left side for open cardiac massage. Clamshell thoracotomy may also be considered in patients with presumed air embolism, providing access to the cardiac chambers for aspiration, coronary vessels for massage, and bilateral lungs for obliteration of the source.

Preparation for EDT should be performed well ahead of the patient's arrival. Set-up should include a 10-blade scalpel, Finochietto's chest retractor, toothed forceps, curved Mayo's scissors, Satinsky's vascular clamps (large and small), long needle holder, Lebsche's knife and mallet, and internal defibrillator paddles. Sterile suction, skin stapler, and access to a variety of sutures should be available (specifically 2-0 prolene on a CT-1 needle, 2-0 silk ties, and teflon pledgets). Upon patient arrival and determination of the need for EDT, the patient's left arm should be placed above the head to provide unimpeded access to the left chest. The anterolateral thoracotomy is initiated with an incision at the level of the fifth intercostal space (Fig. 15-2). Clinically, this level for incision corresponds to the inferior border of the pectoralis major muscle, just below the patient's nipple. In women, the breast should be retracted superiorly to gain access to this interspace, and the incision is made at the inframammary fold. The incision should start on the right side of the sternum; if sternal transection is required, this saves the time-consuming step of performing an additional skin incision. As the initial incision is carried transversely across the chest, and one passes beneath the nipple, a gentle curve in the incision toward the patient's axilla rather than direct extension to the bed should be performed; this curvature in the skin correlates with the natural curvature of the rib cage. The skin, subcutaneous fat, and chest wall musculature are incised with a knife to expose the ribs and associated intercostal space. Intercostal muscles and the parietal pleura are then divided in one layer with either curved Mayo scissors or sharply with the scalpel; the intercostal muscle should be divided along the superior margin of the rib to avoid the intercostal neurovascular bundle. Chest-wall bleeding is minimal in these patients and should not be a concern at this point in the resuscitation. Once the incision is completed and the chest entered, a standard Finochietto's rib retractor is inserted, with the handle directed inferiorly toward the axilla (Fig. 15-3). Placement of the handle toward the bed rather than the sternum allows extension of

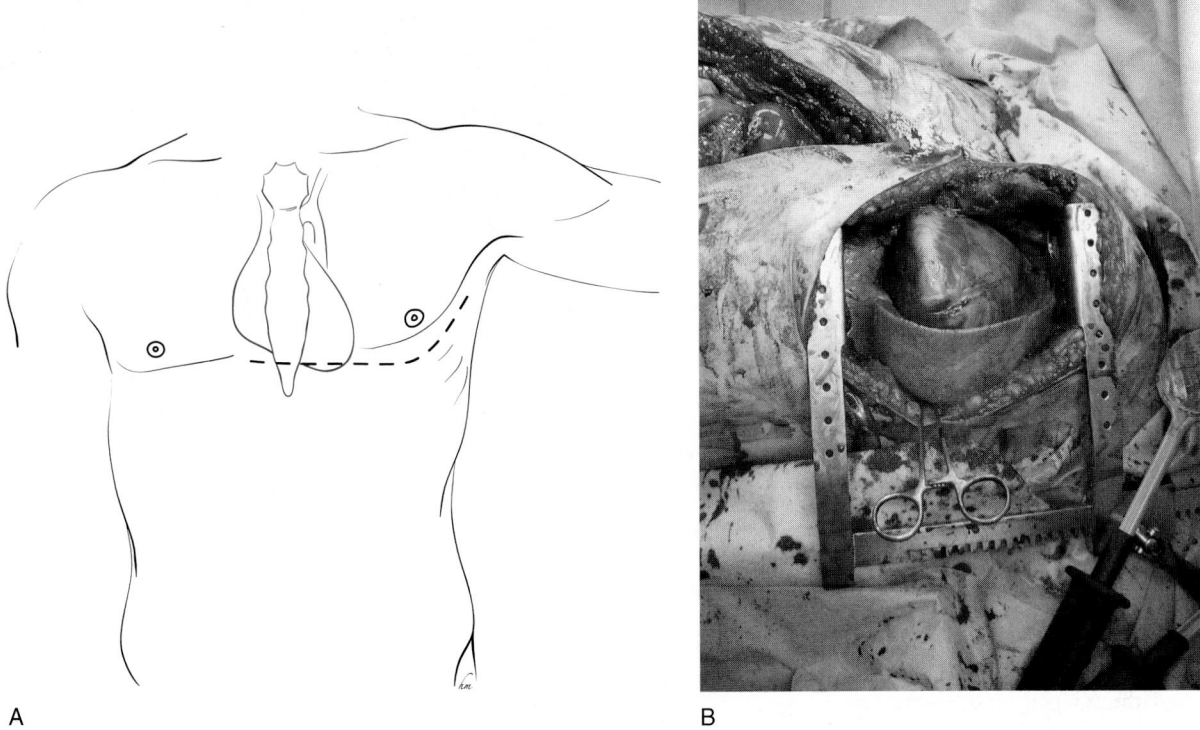

A                                                    B

**FIGURE 15-2.** **(A)&(B):** The thoracotomy incision is performed through the fourth or fifth intercostal space; the incision should start to the right of the sternum, and begin curving into the axilla at the level of the left nipple.

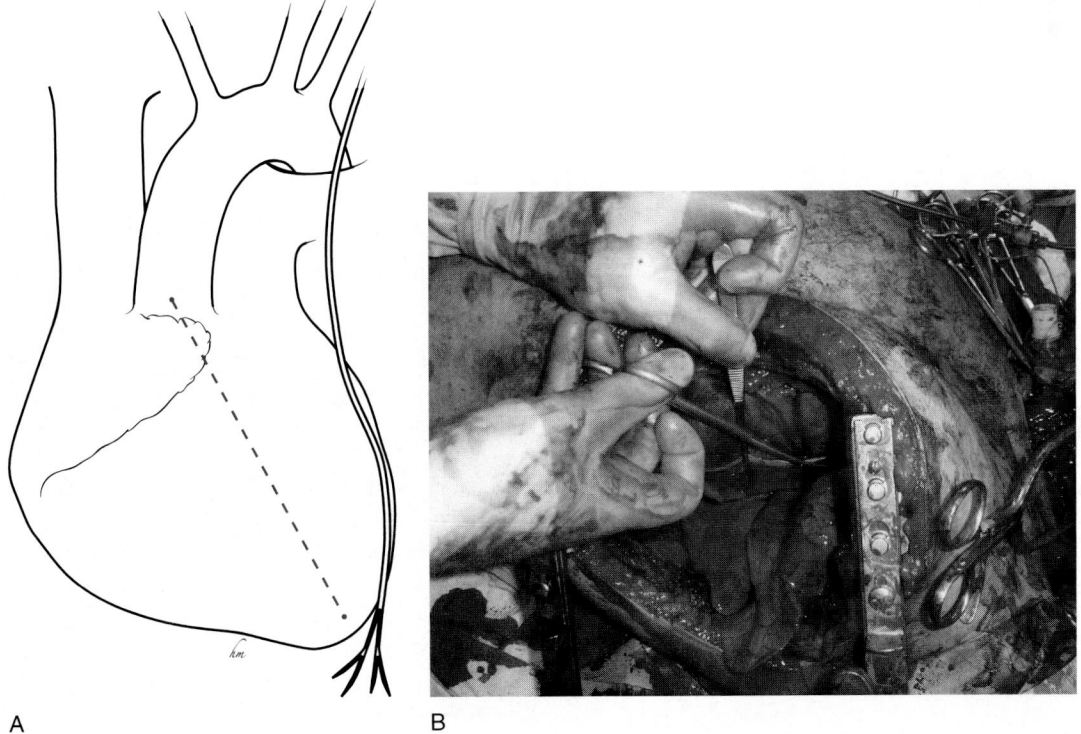

A                                                    B

**FIGURE 15-3.** **(A)&(B):** The Finochietto's rib retractor is placed with the handle directed inferiorly toward the bed. Pericardiotomy is done with toothed pick-ups and curved Mayo scissors; the incision begins at the cardiac apex, anterior to the phrenic nerve, and extends on the anterior surface of the heart toward the great vessels.

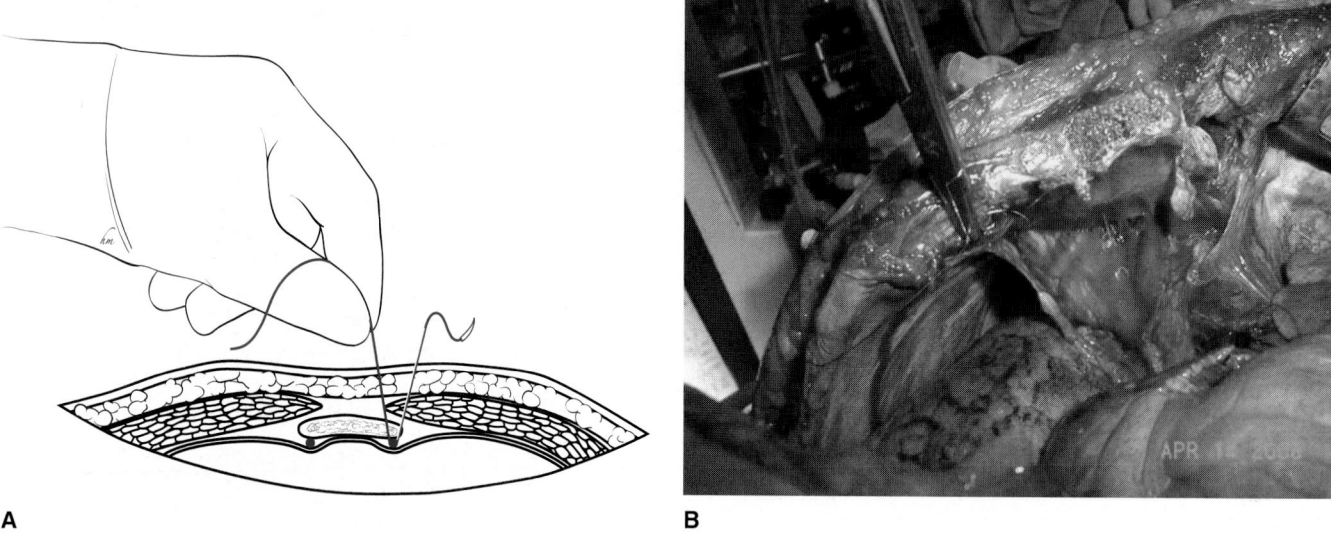

**FIGURE 15-4.** **(A)&(B):** Transverse division of the sternum requires individual ligation of the internal mammary arteries.

the left thoracotomy into a clamshell thoracotomy with crossing of the sternum without replacing the rib retractor.

If the left anterolateral thoracotomy does not provide adequate exposure, several techniques may be employed. The sternum can be transected for additional exposure with a Lebsche's knife; care must be taken to hold the Lebsche's knife firmly against the underside of the sternum when using the mallet to forcefully transect the sternum, or the tip of the instrument may deviate and result in an iatrogenic cardiac injury. If the sternum is divided transversely, the internal mammary vessels must be ligated when perfusion is restored; this may be performed using either a figure of eight suture with 2-0 silk or by clamping the vessel with a tonsil and individually ligating it with a 2-0 silk tie (Fig. 15-4). A concomitant right anterolateral thoracotomy produces a "clamshell" or "butterfly" incision, and achieves wide exposure to both pleural cavities as well as anterior and posterior mediastinal structures (Fig. 15-5). Once

the right pleural space is opened, the rib retractor should be moved to more of a midline position to enhance separation of the chest wall for maximal exposure. When visualization of penetrating wounds in the aortic arch or major branches is needed, the superior sternum is additionally split in the midline.

## Pericardiotomy and Cardiac Hemorrhage Control

The pericardium is incised widely, starting at the cardiac apex and extending toward the sternal notch, anterior and parallel to the phrenic nerve (Fig. 15-3). If the pericardium is not tense with blood it may be picked up at the apex with toothed forceps and sharply opened with scissors. If tense pericardial tamponade exists, a knife or the sharp point of a scissors is often required to initiate the pericardiotomy incision. Blood and blood clots should be completely evacuated from the pericardium. The heart should be delivered from the

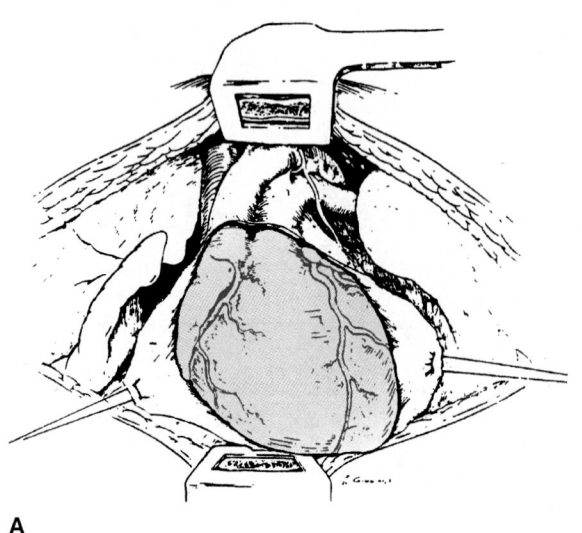

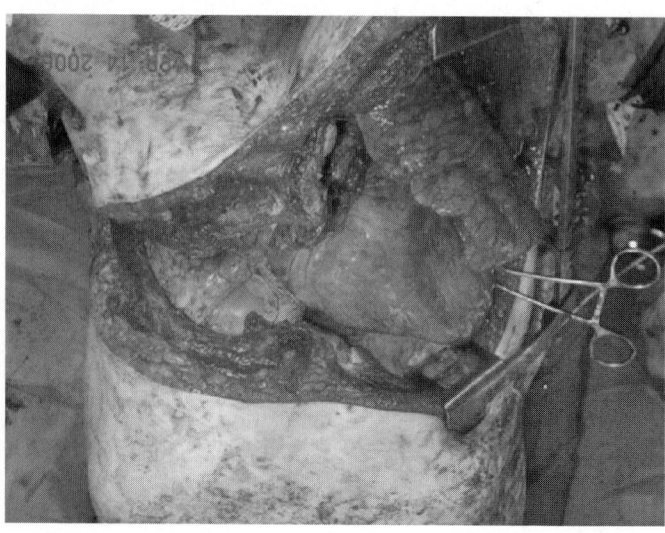

**FIGURE 15-5.** **(A)&(B):** A bilateral anterolateral ("clamshell") thoracotomy provides access to both thoracic cavities including the pulmonary hila, heart, and proximal great vessels.

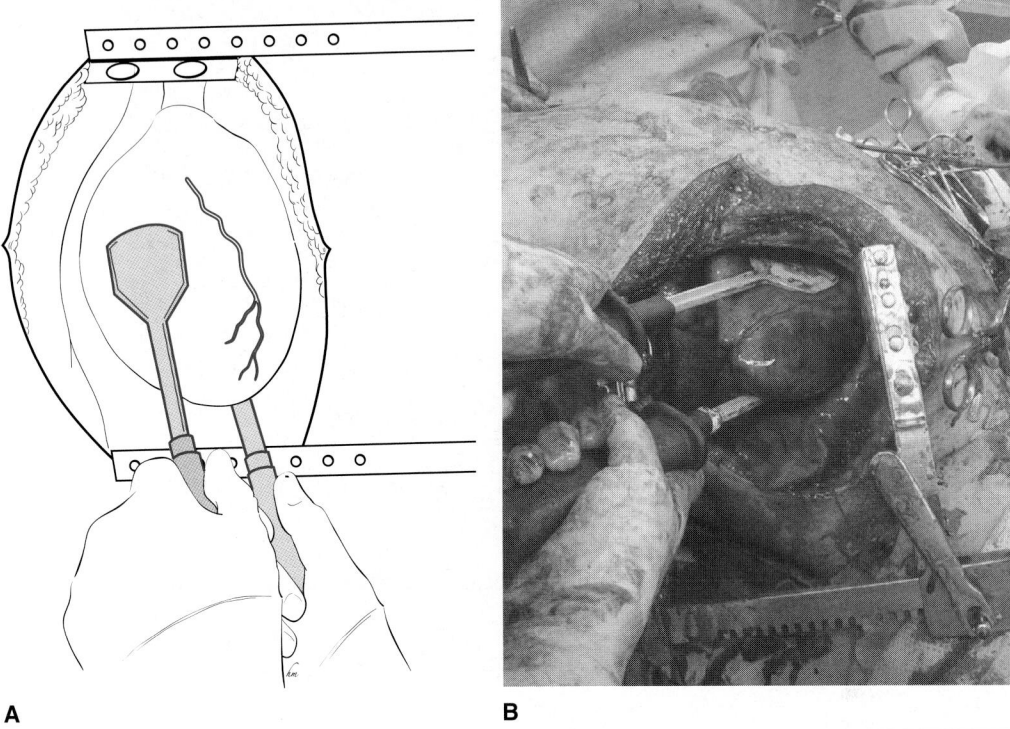

**FIGURE 15-6.** **(A)&(B)**: Internal paddles for defibrillation are positioned on the anterior and posterior aspects of the heart.

**A**                                  **B**

pericardium by placing the right hand through the pericardial incision, encircling the left side of the heart and pulling it into the left chest. This effectively places the left side of the pericardium behind the heart allowing access to the cardiac chambers for repair of cardiac wounds and access for effective open cardiac massage.

Prompt hemorrhage control is paramount for a cardiac injury. In the beating heart, cardiac bleeding sites should be controlled immediately with digital pressure on the surface of the ventricle and partially occluding vascular clamps on the atrium or great vessels. Efforts at definitive cardiorrhaphy may be delayed until initial resuscitative measures have been completed. In the nonbeating heart, cardiac repair is done prior to defibrillation and cardiac massage. Cardiac wounds in the thin walled right ventricle are best repaired with 3-0 nonabsorbable running or horizontal mattress sutures. Buttressing the suture repair with Teflon pledgets is ideal for the thinner right ventricle, but not essential. When suturing a ventricular laceration, care must be taken not to incorporate a coronary vessel into the repair. In these instances, vertical mattress sutures should be used to exclude the coronary and prevent cardiac ischemia. In the more muscular left ventricle, particularly with a linear stab wound, control of bleeding can often be achieved with a skin-stapling device. Low-pressure venous, atrial, and atrial appendage lacerations can be repaired with simple running or pursestring sutures. Posterior cardiac wounds may be particularly treacherous when they require elevation of the heart for their exposure; closure of these wounds is best accomplished in the OR with optimal lighting and equipment. For a destructive wound of the ventricle, or for inaccessible posterior wounds, temporary inflow occlusion of the superior and inferior vena cava may be employed to facilitate repair (see Chap. 29). Use of a foley catheter for temporary occlusion of cardiac injuries has been suggested; in our experience this may inadvertently extend the injury due to traction forces.

## Advanced Cardiac Life Support Interventions Including Cardiac Massage

The restoration of organ and tissue perfusion may be facilitated by a number of interventions.[50] First, a perfusing cardiac rhythm must be established. Early defibrillation for ventricular fibrillation or pulseless ventricular tachycardia has proven benefit, and evidence supports the use of amiodarone (with lidocaine as an alternative) following epinephrine in patients refractory to defibrillation. Magnesium may be beneficial for *torsades de pointes*; other dysrhythmias should be treated according to current guidelines.[50] Internal defibrillation may also be required, with similar indications as closed chest CPR. Familiarity with the internal cardiac paddles and appropriate charging dosages in joules is required (Fig. 15-6). In the event of cardiac arrest, bimanual internal massage of the heart should be instituted promptly (Fig. 15-7). We prefer to do this with a hinged clapping motion of the hands, with the wrists apposed, sequentially closing from palms to fingers. The ventricular compression should proceed from the cardiac apex to the base of the heart. The two-handed technique is strongly recommended, as the one-handed massage technique poses the risk of myocardial perforation with the thumb.

Pharmacologic adjuncts to increase coronary and cerebral perfusion pressure may be needed. The first agent in resuscitation at this juncture is intracardiac epinephrine. Epinephrine should be administered using a specialized syringe, which resembles a spinal needle, directly into the left ventricle. Typically, the heart is lifted up slightly to expose the more posterior left ventricle, and care is taken to avoid the circumflex coronary during injection. Although epinephrine continues to be advocated during resuscitation, there is a growing body of data suggesting that vasopressin may be superior to epinephrine in augmenting cerebral perfusion and other vital organ blood flow.[51] Administration of calcium, while theoretically deleterious

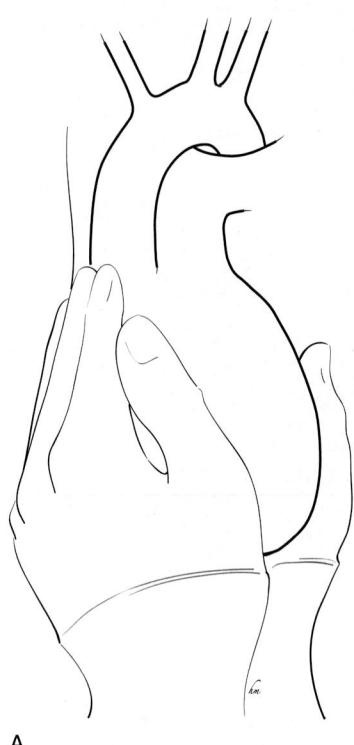

A

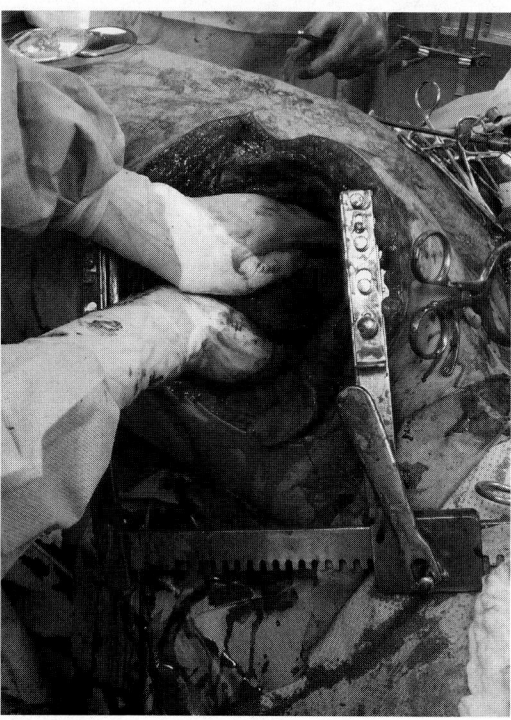

B

**FIGURE 15-7. (A)&(B):** Open cardiac massage is performed with a two-handed hinged technique; the clapping motion sequentially closes the hands from palms to fingers.

during reperfusion injury, increases cardiac contractility, and may be helpful in the setting of hypocalcemia produced by massive transfusion. While metabolic acidosis is common following EDT and resuscitation, the mainstay of therapy is provision of adequate alveolar ventilation and restoration of tissue perfusion. Sodium bicarbonate therapy has not been proven beneficial in facilitating defibrillation, restoring spontaneous circulation, or improving survival. It may be warranted following protracted arrest or resuscitation, because catecholamine receptors may be sensitized.

## Thoracic Aortic Occlusion and Pulmonary Hilar Control

Following thoracotomy and pericardiotomy with evaluation of the heart, the descending thoracic aorta should be occluded to maximize coronary perfusion if hypotension (SBP < 70 mmHg) persists. We prefer to cross-clamp the thoracic aorta inferior to the left pulmonary hilum (Fig. 15-8). Exposure of this area is best provided by elevating the left lung anteriorly and superiorly. Although some advocate taking down the inferior pulmonary ligament to better mobilize the lung, this is unnecessary and risks injury to the inferior pulmonary vein. Dissection of the thoracic aorta is optimally performed under direct vision by incising the mediastinal pleura and bluntly separating the aorta from the esophagus anteriorly and from the prevertebral fascia posteriorly. Care should be taken in dissecting the aorta, and completely encircling it may avulse thoracic and other small vascular branches. Alternatively, if excessive hemorrhage limits direct visualization, which is the more realistic clinical scenario, blunt dissection with one's thumb and fingertips can be done to isolate the descending aorta. Once identified and isolated, the thoracic aorta is occluded with a large Satinsky or DeBakey's vascular clamp. If the aorta cannot be easily isolated from the surrounding tissue, digitally occlude the aorta against the

spine to affect aortic occlusion. Although occlusion of the thoracic aorta is typically performed after pericardiotomy, this may be the first maneuver upon entry into the chest in patients sustaining extrathoracic injury and associated major blood loss.

Control of the pulmonary hilum has two indications. First, if coronary or systemic air embolism is present, further embolism is prevented by placing a vascular clamp across the pulmonary hilum (Fig. 15-9). Associated maneuvers such as vigorous cardiac massage to move air through the coronary arteries and needle aspiration of air from the left ventricular apex and the aortic root are also performed (Fig. 15-10). Second, if the patient has a pulmonary hilar injury or marked hemorrhage from the lung parenchyma, control of the hilum may prevent exsanguination. Hilar control can be performed by a Satinsky's clamp, the pulmonary hilar twist, or temporarily with digital control (see Chaps. 26 and 27).

## COMPLICATIONS AND CONSEQUENCES OF EDT

### Procedural Complications

Technical complications of EDT involve virtually every intrathoracic structure. The list of such misadventures included lacerations of the heart, coronary arteries, aorta, phrenic nerves, esophagus, and lungs, as well as avulsion of aortic branches to components of the mediastinum. Previous thoracotomy virtually assures technical problems from the presence of dense pleural adhesions and is therefore a relative contraindication to EDT. Additional postoperative morbidity among ultimate survivors of EDT includes recurrent chest bleeding, infection of the pericardium, pleural spaces, sternum, and chest wall, and post-pericardiotomy syndrome.

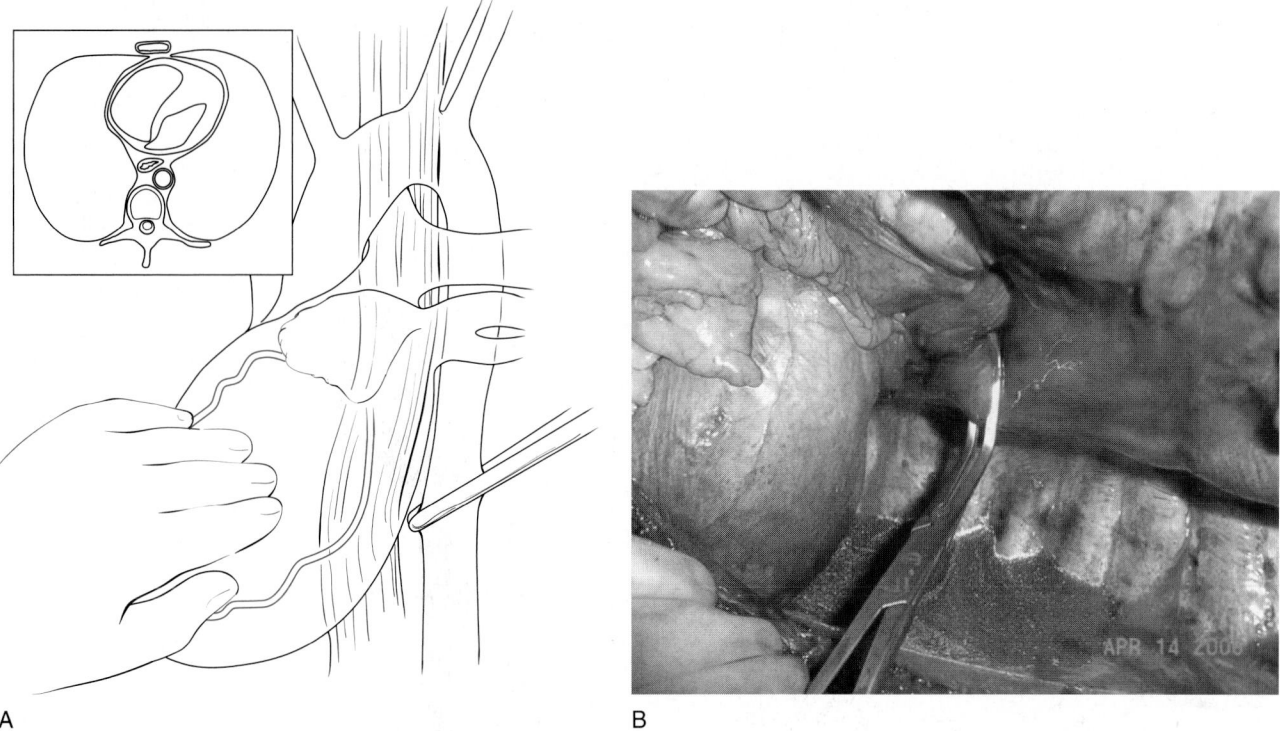

**FIGURE 15-8.** **(A)&(B)**: Aortic crossclamp is applied with the left lung retracted superiorly, below the inferior pulmonary ligament, just above the diaphragm. The flaccid aorta is identified as the first structure encountered on top of the spine when approached from the left chest.

Importantly, there is a finite risk to the health care providers and trauma team performing an EDT.[52] The use of EDT by necessity involves the rapid use of sharp surgical instruments and exposure to the patient's blood. Even during elective procedures in the OR, the contact rate of patient's blood with the surgeon's skin can be as high as 50%, and the contact rate of patients' blood with health care workers' blood as high as 60%. The overall seroprevalence rate of human immunodeficiency virus (HIV) among patients admitted to the ED for trauma is around 4%, but is much higher among the subgroup of patients most likely to require an EDT, e.g., 14% of

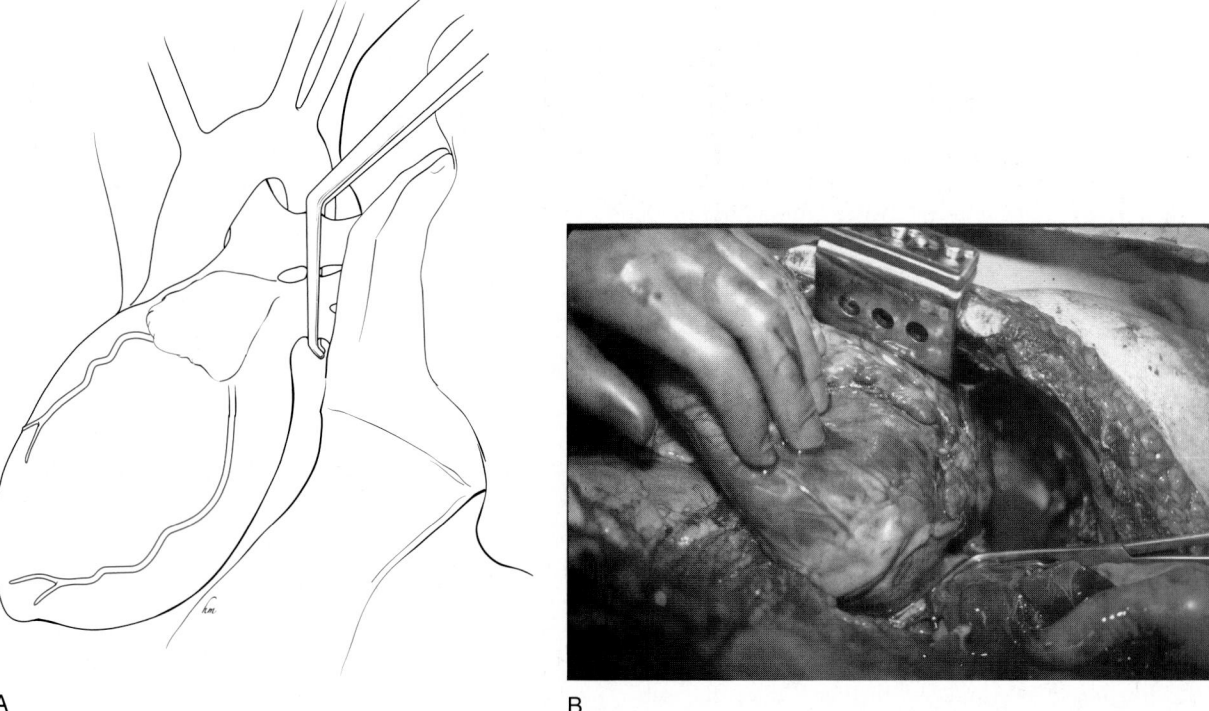

**FIGURE 15-9.** **(A)&(B)**: A Satinsky clamp is used to clamp the pulmonary hilum for hemorrhage control or to prevent further bronchovenous air embolism.

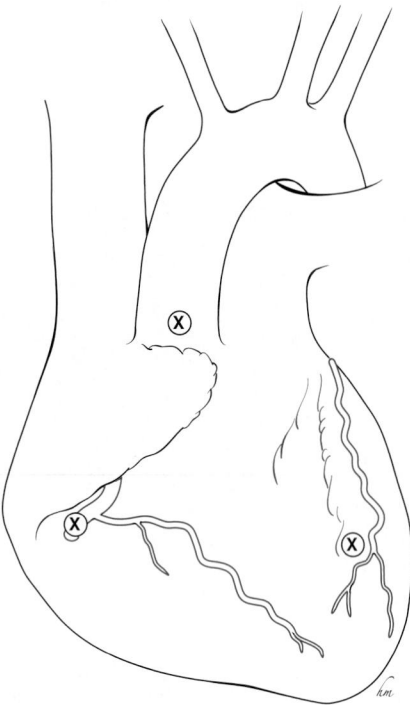

**FIGURE 15-10.** In cases of bronchovenous air embolism, sequential sites of aspiration include the left ventricle (1), the aortic root (2), and the right coronary artery (3).

penetrating trauma victims and nearly 30% of intravenous drug abusers. Caplan et al.[53] found that 26% of acutely injured patients had evidence of exposure to HIV (4%), hepatitis B (20%), or hepatitis C virus (14%); there was no difference in the incidence comparing blunt to penetrating trauma. Thus, the likelihood of a health care worker sustaining exposure to HIV or hepatitis in the ED is substantial. The risk of contagion from exposures to HIV and other blood-borne pathogens can be minimized by the use of appropriate barrier precautions and the selective use of EDT.

## Hemodynamic and Metabolic Consequences of Aortic Cross-Clamping

Aortic cross clamping may be life saving during acute resuscitation, but there is a finite cost to the patient. Occlusion of the aorta results in an increase in blood pressure, but there is an associated 90% reduction in femoral artery systolic blood pressure; in addition, abdominal visceral blood flow decreases to 2 to 8% of baseline values.[31,32] Therefore, cross clamping magnifies the metabolic cost of shock by reducing local blood flow to abdominal viscera even further. This results in tissue acidosis and increased oxygen debt, and may ultimately contribute to post-ischemic multiple organ failure.[32] Additionally, return of aortic flow may not result in normalization of flow to vital organs; in animal models, blood flow to the kidneys remained at 50% of baseline despite a normal cardiac output. The metabolic penalty of aortic cross clamping becomes exponential when the normothermia occlusion time exceeds 30 minutes, both in trauma as well as in elective thoracic aortic procedures.[54–56] Hypoxia of distal organs, white blood cells, and endothelium induces the elaboration, expression, and activation of inflammatory cell adhesion molecules and inflammatory mediators; this systemic inflammatory

response syndrome has been linked to impaired pulmonary function and multiple organ failure[57] (see Chap. 68). Consequently, the aortic clamp should be removed as soon as effective cardiac function and adequate systemic arterial pressure have been achieved.

Removal of aortic occlusion may result in further hemodynamic sequelae.[58] Besides the abrupt reperfusion of the ischemic distal torso and washout of metabolic products and inflammatory mediators associated with aortic declamping, there are direct effects on the cardiopulmonary system. The return of large volumes of blood from the ischemic extremities, with its lower pH, elevated lactate, and other mediators may exert a cardiodepressant activity on myocardial contractility.[59] Overzealous volume loading during aortic occlusion may also result in left ventricular strain, acute atrial and ventricular dilatation and, consequently, precipitous cardiac failure.[32] Following release of aortic occlusion there is impaired left ventricular function, systemic oxygen utilization, and coronary perfusion pressure in the postresuscitation period.[58,60] The transient fall in coronary perfusion may not be clinically relevant in patients with efficient coronary autoregulation; however, in patients with coronary disease or underlying myocardial hypertrophy, this increase in cardiac work may result in clinically critical ischemia.[60]

## OPTIMIZING OXYGEN TRANSPORT FOLLOWING EDT

Following EDT, patients are frequently in a tenuous physiologic state. The combination of direct cardiac injury, ischemic myocardial insult, myocardial depressants, and pulmonary hypertension adversely impact postinjury cardiac function (see Chap. 62). Additionally, aortic occlusion induces profound anaerobic metabolism, secondary lactic academia, and release of other reperfusion-induced mediators. Consequently, once vital signs return, the resuscitation priorities shift to optimizing cardiac function and maximizing oxygen delivery to the tissues. The ultimate goal of resuscitation is adequately tissue oxygen delivery and cellular oxygen consumption (see Chap. 60). Circulating blood-volume status is maintained at the optimal level of cardiac filling in order to optimize cardiac contractility, and the oxygen-carrying capacity of the blood is maximized by keeping the hemoglobin above 7–10 g/dL. If these measures fail to meet resuscitative goals[61] (e.g., oxygen delivery ≥500 mL/min/,[2] resolution of base deficit, or clearance of serum lactate), inotropic agents are added to enhance myocardial function.

## FUTURE CONSIDERATIONS

### Defining Nonsalvageability

As clinicians faced with increasing scrutiny over appropriation of resources, it is critical to identify the patient who has permanent neurologic disability or death. Resuscitative efforts should not be abandoned prematurely in the potentially salvageable patient but field assessment of salvageability is unreliable.[41,62–64] Our clinical pathway attempts to optimize resource utilization, but outcomes must continue to be evaluated, searching for more definitive predictors of neurologic outcome. For example, markers of brain metabolic activity such as increased serum-neuron-specific enolase activity appear to have prognostic significance for irreversible brain damage.[65] Use of more advanced monitoring devices in the ED, together with further elucidation of the characteristics of irreversible shock, may permit a more physiologic prediction of outcome for these critically injured patients in the future.

## Temporary Physiologic Hibernation

A potential adjunct in the care of traumatic arrest is the timely application of hypothermia. Recent randomized studies suggest the use of hypothermia for central nervous system protection after nontraumatic cardiac arrest.[66,67] In these studies, patients randomized to a period of mild to moderate hypothermia (32° to 34°C) after cardiac arrest had improved neurologic outcomes compared to those kept normothermic. This favorable effect was presumably due to a decrease in cerebral metabolic demand during hypothermia. In addition, hypothermia may reduce oxygen radical generation and inflammatory mediator production. By extension, then, if an injured patient in transport could be cooled to a minimal metabolic rate (i.e., suspended animation), one can posit that transfer to definitive care might be possible.[68,69] Application of this principle to the multiply injured or bleeding patient, however, is problematic. Rapid cooling is not currently practical in the field, and there are legitimate concerns about the adverse effects of hypothermia on immune function and effective clot formation. Overall, while some[70] preclinical work supports the application of hypothermia after resuscitation from hemorrhage, other investigators have reached the opposite conclusion.[71]

## Temporary Mechanical Cardiac Support

The concept of temporary mechanical cardiac support for the failing heart following injury is intuitively attractive. Unfortunately, experience with the intra-aortic balloon pump in this scenario has been unrewarding. The advent of centrifugal pumps (Bio-Medicus Pump, Bio-Medicus, Inc., Minneapolis, MN), that allow partial cardiac bypass without systemic anticoagulation, offers another potential means for increasing salvage of the moribund patient. Centrifugal pumps have become the standard approach to the torn descending thoracic aorta in the patient with associated myocardial contusion (see Chap. 29).[72,73] The adjunctive use of extracorporeal membrane oxygenation may also play a critical role in supporting the patient with massive injuries or early multiple organ failure.[74] Finally, hypothermia circulatory arrest may find utility in a broad spectrum of patients with injuries that are considered "irreparable."[75,76]

## REFERENCES

1. Hemreck AS: The history of cardiopulmonary resuscitation. *Am J Surg* 156:430, 1988.
2. Beck CS: Wounds of the heart. *Arch Surg* 13:205, 1926.
3. Blatchford JW III: Ludwig Rehn—The first successful cardiography. *Ann Thorac Surg* 39:492, 1985.
4. Kouwenhoven WB, Jude JR, Knickerbocker GG: Closed-chest cardiac massage. *JAMA* 173:1064, 1960.
5. Zoll PM, Linenthal AJ, Norman LR, et al.: Treatment of unexpected cardiac arrest by external electric stimulation of the heart. *NEJM* 254:541, 1956.
6. Blalock A, Ravitch MM: A consideration of the nonoperative treatment of cardiac tamponade resulting from wounds of the heart. *Surgery* 14:157, 1943.
7. Beall AC Jr, Diethrich EB, Crawford HW, et al.: Surgical management of penetrating cardiac injuries. *Am J Surg* 112:686, 1966.
8. Ledgerwood AM, Kazmers M, Lucas CE: The role of thoracic aortic occlusion for massive hemoperitoneum. *J Trauma* 16:610, 1976.
9. Millikan JS, Moore EE: Outcome of resuscitative thoracotomy and descending aortic occlusion performed in the operating room. *J Trauma* 24:387, 1984.
10. Powell DW, Moore EE, Cothren CC, et al.: Is emergency department resuscitative thoracotomy futile care for the critically injured patient requiring prehospital cardiopulmonary resuscitation? *JACS* 199:211, 2004.
11. ACS-COT Subcommittee on Outcomes: Practice management guidelines for emergency department thoracotomy. *JACS* 193:303, 2001.
12. Miglietta MA, Robb TV, Eachempati SR et al.: Current opinion regarding indications for emergency department thoracotomy. *J Trauma* 51:670, 2001.
13. Breaux EP, Dupont JB Jr, Albert HM, et al.: Cardiac tamponade following penetrating mediastinal injuries: Improved survival with early pericardiocentesis. *J Trauma* 19:461, 1979.
14. Shoemaker WC, Carey JS, Yao ST, et al.: Hemodynamic alterations in acute cardiac tamponade after penetrating injuries to the heart. *Surgery* 67:754, 1970.
15. Wechsler AS, Auerbach BJ, Graham TC, et al.: Distribution of intramyocardial blood flow during pericardial tamponade. *J Thorac Cardiovasc Surg* 68:847, 1974.
16. Mattox KL, Beall AC Jr, Jordon GL Jr, et al.: Cardiorrhaphy in the emergency center. *J Thorac Cardiovasc Surg* 68:886, 1974.
17. Wall MJ Jr, Mattox KL, Chen CD, et al.: Acute management of complex cardiac injuries. *J Trauma* 42:905, 1997.
18. Graham JM, Mattox KL, Beall AC Jr: Penetrating trauma of the lung. *J Trauma* 19:665, 1979.
19. Boczar ME, Howard MA, Rivers EP, et al.: A technique revisited: Hemodynamic comparison of closed- and open-chest cardiac massage during human cardiopulmonary resuscitation. *Crit Care Med* 23:498, 1995.
20. Rubertsson S, Grenvik A, Wiklund L: Blood flow and perfusion pressure during open-chest versus closed-chest cardiopulmonary resuscitation in pigs. *Crit Care Med* 23:715, 1995.
21. Luna GK, Pavlin EG, Kirkman T, et al.: Hemodynamic effects of external cardiac massage in trauma shock. *J Trauma* 29:1430, 1989.
22. Spence PA, Lust RM, Chitwood WR Jr, et al.: Transfemoral balloon aortic occlusion during open cardiopulmonary resuscitation improves myocardial and cerebral blood flow. *J Surg Res* 49:217, 1990.
23. Wesley RC Jr, Morgan DB: Effect of continuous intra-aortic balloon inflation in canine open chest cardiopulmonary resuscitation. *Crit Care Med* 18:630, 1990.
24. Dunn EL, Moore EE, Moore JB: Hemodynamic effects of aortic occlusion during hemorrhagic shock. *Ann Emerg Med* 11:238, 1982.
25. Michel JB, Bardou A, Tedgui A, et al.: Effect of descending thoracic aortic clamping and unclamping on phasic coronary blood flow. *J Surg Res* 36:17, 1984.
26. Gedeborg R, Rubertsson S, Wiklund L: Improved hemodynamics and restoration of spontaneous circulation with constant aortic occlusion during experimental cardiopulmonary resuscitation. *Resuscitation* 40:171, 1999.
27. Rubertsson S, Bircher NG, Alexander H: Effects of intra-aortic balloon occlusion on hemodynamics during, and survival after cardiopulmonary resuscitation in dogs. *Crit Care Med* 25:1003, 1997.
28. Sheppard FR, Cothren CC, Moore EE, et al.: Emergency department resuscitative thoracotomy for non-torso injuries. *Surgery* 139:574, 2006.
29. Kralovich KA, Morris DC, Dereczyk BE, et al.: Hemodynamic effects of aortic occlusion during hemorrhagic shock and cardiac arrest. *J Trauma* 42:1023, 1997.
30. Connery C, Geller E, Dulchavsky S, et al.: Paraparesis following emergency room thoracotomy: Case report. *J Trauma* 30:362, 1990.
31. Mitteldorf C, Poggetti RS, Zanoto A, et al.: Is aortic occlusion advisable in the management of massive hemorrhage? Experimental study in dogs. *Shock* 10:141, 1998.
32. Oyama M, McNamara JJ, Suehiro GT, et al.: The effects of thoracic aortic cross-clamping and declamping on visceral organ blood flow. *Ann Surg* 197:459, 1983.
33. King MW, Aitchison JM, Nel JP: Fatal air embolism following penetrating lung trauma: An autopsy study. *J Trauma* 24:753, 1984.
34. Thomas AN, Stephens BG: Air embolism: A cause of morbidity and death after penetrating chest trauma. *J Trauma* 14:633, 1974.
35. Yee ES, Verrier ED, Thomas AN: Management of air embolism in blunt and penetrating thoracic trauma. *J Thorac Cardiovasc Surg* 85:661, 1983.
36. Graham JM, Beall AC Jr, Mattox KL, et al.: Systemic air embolism following penetrating trauma to the lung. *Chest* 72:449, 1977.

37. Baxter BT, Moore EE, Moore JB, et al.: Emergency department thoracotomy following injury: Critical determinants for patient salvage. *World J Surg* 12:671, 1988.

38. Cogbill TH, Moore EE, Millikan JS, et al.: Rationale for selective application of emergency department thoracotomy in trauma. *J Trauma* 23:453, 1983.

39. Moore EE, Moore JB, Galloway AC, et al.: Postinjury thoracotomy in the emergency department: A critical evaluation. *Surgery* 86:590, 1979.

40. Branney SW, Moore EE, Feldhaus KM, et al.: Critical analysis of two decades of experience with postinjury emergency department thoracotomy in a regional trauma center. *J Trauma* 45:87, 1998.

41. Pickens JJ, Copass MK, Bulger EM: Trauma patients receiving CPR: Predictors of survival. *J Trauma* 58:951, 2005.

42. Rhee PM, Acosta J, Bridgeman A, et al.: Survival after emergency department thoracotomy: Review of published data from the past 25 years. *JACS* 190:288, 2000.

43. Baker CC, Thomas AN, Trunkey DD: The role of emergency room thoracotomy in trauma. *J Trauma* 20:848, 1980.

44. Stockinger ZT, McSwain NE: Additional evidence in support of withholding or terminating cardiopulmonary resuscitation for trauma patients in the field. *JACS* 198:227, 2004.

45. Li G, Tang N, DiScala C, et al.: Cardiopulmonary resuscitation in pediatric trauma patients: Survival and functional outcome. *J Trauma* 47:1, 1999.

46. Beaver BL, Colombani PM, Buck JR: Efficacy of emergency room thoracotomy in pediatric trauma. *J Pediatr Surg* 22:19, 1987.

47. Rothenberg SS, Moore EE, Moore FA, et al.: Emergency department thoracotomy in children: A critical analysis *J Trauma* 29:1322, 1989.

48. Sheikh AA, Culbertson CB: Emergency department thoracotomy in children: Rationale for selective application. *J Trauma* 34:323, 1993.

49. Powell RW, Gill EA, Jurkovich GJ, et al.: Resuscitative thoracotomy in children and adolescents. *Am Surg* 54:1988, 1988.

50. American Heart Association: Guidelines 2000 for cardiopulmonary resuscitation and emergency cardiovascular care. *Circulation* 102:I1, 2000.

51. Nolan JP, de Latorre FJ, Steen PA, et al.: Advanced life support drugs: Do they really work? *Curr Opin Crit Care* 8:212, 2002.

52. Sikka R, Millham FH, Feldman JA: Analysis of occupational exposures associated with emergency department thoracotomy. *J Trauma* 56:867, 2004.

53. Caplan ES, Preas MA, Kerns T, et al.: Seroprevalence of human immunodeficiency virus, hepatitis B virus, hepatitis C virus, and rapid plasma reagin in a trauma population. *J Trauma* 39:533, 1995.

54. Fabian TC, Richardson JD, Croce MA, et al.: Prospective study of blunt aortic injury: Multicenter trial of the American Association for the Surgery of Trauma. *J Trauma* 42:374, 1997.

55. Gharagozloo F, Larson J, Dausmann MJ, et al.: Spinal cord protection during surgical procedures on the descending thoracic and thoracoabdominal aorta. *Chest* 109:799, 1996.

56. Katz NM, Blackstone EH, Kirklin JW, et al.: Incremental risk factors for spinal cord injury following operation for acute traumatic aortic transection. *J Thorac Cardiovasc Surg* 81:669, 1981.

57. Adembri C, Kastamoniti E, Bertolozzi I, et al.: Pulmonary injury follows systemic inflammatory reaction in infrarenal aortic surgery. *Crit Care Med* 32:1170, 2004.

58. Kralovich KA, Morris DC, Dereczyk BE, et al.: Hemodynamic effects of aortic occlusion during hemorrhagic shock and cardiac arrest. *J Trauma* 42:1023, 1997.

59. Perry MO. The hemodynamics of temporary abdominal aortic occlusion. *Ann Surg* 168:193, 1968.

60. Michel JB, Bardou A, Tedgui A, et al.: Effect of descending thoracic aorta clamping and unclamping on phasic coronary blood flow. *J Surg Research* 36:17, 1984.

61. McKinley BA, Kozar RA, Cocanour CS, et al.: Normal versus supranormal oxygen delivery goals in shock resuscitation: the response is the same. *J Trauma* 53:825, 2002.

62. Battistella FD, Nugent W, Owings JT, et al.: Field triage of the pulseless trauma patient. *Arch Surg* 134:742, 1999.

63. Fulton RL, Voigt WJ, Hilakos AS: Confusion surrounding the treatment of traumatic cardiac arrest. *J Am Coll Surg* 181:209, 1995.

64. Stratton SJ, Brickett K, Crammer T: Prehospital pulseless, unconscious penetrating trauma victims: Field assessments associated with survival. *J Trauma* 45:96, 1998.

65. Fogel W, Krieger D, Veith M, et al.: Serum neuron-specific enolase as early predictor of outcome after cardiac arrest. *Crit Care Med* 25:1133, 1997.

66. Bernard SA, Gray TW, Buist MD, et al.: Treatment of comatose survivors of out-of-hospital cardiac arrest with induced hypothermia. *N Engl J Med* 346:557, 2002.

67. The Hypothermia After Cardiac Arrest Study Group: Mild therapeutic hypothermia to improve the neurologic outcome after cardiac arrest. *N Engl J Med* 346:549, 2002.

68. Rhee P, Talon E, Eifert S, et al.: Induced hypothermia during emergency department thoracotomy: An animal model. *J Trauma* 48:439, 2000.

69. Safar P, Tisherman SA, Behringer W, et al.: Suspended animation for delayed resuscitation from prolonged cardiac arrest that is unresuscitatable by standard cardiopulmonary-cerebral resuscitation. *Crit Care Med* 28:N214, 2000.

70. Prueckner S, Safar P, Kenter R, et al.: Mild hypothermia increases survival from severe pressure-controlled hemorrhagic shock in rats. *J Trauma* 50:253, 2001.

71. Mizushima Y, Wang P, Cioffi WG, et al.: Should normothermia be restored and maintained during resuscitation after trauma and hemorrhage? *J Trauma* 48:58, 2000.

72. Read RA, Moore EE, Moore FA, et al.: Partial left heart bypass for thoracic aorta repair: Survival without paraplegia. *Arch Surg* 128:746, 1993.

73. Szwerc MF, Benckart DH, Lin JC, et al.: Recent clinical experience with left heart bypass using a centrifugal pump for repair of traumatic aortic transection. *Ann Surg* 230:484, 1999.

74. Perchinsky MJ, Long WB, Hill JG, et al.: Extracorporeal cardiopulmonary life support with heparin-bonded circuitry in the resuscitation of massively injured trauma patients. *Am J Surg* 169:488, 1995.

75. Chughtai TS, Gilardino MS, Fleiszer DM, et al.: An expanding role for cardiopulmonary bypass in trauma. *Can J Surg* 45:95, 2002.

76. Howells GA, Hernandez DA, Olt SL, et al.: Blunt injury of the ascending aorta and aortic arch: Repair with hypothermic circulatory arrest. *J Trauma* 44:716, 1998.

77. Moreno C, Moore EE, Majure JA, et al.: Pericardial tamponade: A critical determinant for survival following penetrating cardiac wounds. *J Trauma* 26:821, 1986.

78. Tyburski JG, Astra L, Wilson RF, et al.: Factors affecting prognosis with penetrating wounds of the heart. *J Trauma* 48:587, 2000.

79. Velhamos GC, Degiannis E, Souter I, et al.: Outcome of a strict policy on emergency department thoracotomies. *Arch Surg* 130:774, 1995.

80. Asensio JA, Berne JD, Demetriades D, et al.: One hundred five penetrating cardiac injuries: A 2-year prospective evaluation. *J Trauma* 44:1073, 1998.

81. Rohman M, Ivatury RR, Steichen FM, et al.: Emergency room thoracotomy for penetrating cardiac injuries. *J Trauma* 23:570, 1983.

82. Rhee PM, Foy H, Kaufmann C, et al.: Penetrating cardiac injuries: A population-based study. *J Trauma* 45:366, 1998.

83. Durham LA, Richardson RJ, Wall MJ, et al.: Emergency center thoracotomy: Impact of prehospital resuscitation. *J Trauma* 32:775, 1992.

84. Brown SE, Gomez GA, Jacobson LE, et al.: Penetrating chest trauma: Should indications for emergency room thoracotomy be limited? *Am Surg* 62:530, 1996.

85. Ivatury RR, Kazigo J, Rohman M, et al.: "Directed" emergency room thoracotomy: A prognostic prerequisite for survival. *J Trauma* 31:1076, 1991.

85. Mazzorana V, Smith RS, Morabito DJ, et al.: Limited utility of emergency department thoracotomy. *Am Surg* 60:516, 1994.

87. Danne PD, Finelli F, Champion HR: Emergency bay thoracotomy. *J Trauma* 24:796, 1984.

88. Esposito TJ, Jurkovich GJ, Rice CL, et al.: Reappraisal of emergency room thoracotomy in a changing environment. *J Trauma* 31:881, 1991.

# Commentary ■ BRADFORD G. SCOTT

The authors of the chapter should be commended for a thorough review of the subject of emergency department thoracotomy (EDT). A few comments may improve the readers understanding of the topic. The indications for EDT are often expanded when the practitioner meets the patient in extremis. Often the trauma team is waiting patiently in the ED for the arrival of the victim. Anticipation builds expecting a dramatic life saving intervention, the pabulum of productivity for trauma nurses and doctors. When the patient arrives with no signs of life, the energy in the resuscitation area goads the treating team into initiating an

EDT, in the hope of one more dramatic save. Every trauma center has an antidotal story of an extreme survivor from an EDT and this story is handed down to each successive generation which fuels the push for the next attempt. The authors have set out clear guidelines for the indications for EDT. Not so subtle to these guidelines is the need to recognize futility. I would add from our own institutions review of indications for EDT the presence of field intubation with the presence of cardio-pulmonary resuscitation (CPR) extended the window of survivors at 9.4 minutes from nonsurvivors of 4.2 minutes. Therefore, in our practice a nonintubated patient with CPR in progress for greater than 5 minutes has a low probability of survival and EDT is considered with more suspect.[1] Obviously if EDT is restricted to those with better physiology the outcomes will be better.[2] Inversely, if no EDT are ever attempted there will be no survivors in this small group of patients *in extremis.* Invariably when there is a survivor of an EDT, at that week's conference the comment will be made that the patient did not need the procedure, because they clearly survived. Also, when there is a death presented at the same conference a comment will be made that obviously the procedure was futile and therefore not indicated.

EDT should not be entertained wantonly, as this limited success procedure is potentially dangerous to the health care workers. There is no known rate of exposure during EDT, but it was estimated by the authors to approximate elective exposures of 50%. Cost of the procedure should also be considered. It is well established that the procedure itself is costly and the ramifications of producing a neurologically devastated patient drives the overall cost to very high levels.[3] This burden of a nonintact patient is carried by the patient's family and health care system at a high emotional and financial cost. Finally, some institutions have (not so public) protocols to resuscitate every body coming into the trauma center in a hope of (expensively) increasing the potential donor pool for a solid organ transplant program.

Each caregiver should have a clear indication for EDT in their own mind prior to encountering the patient. Emotion of the moment should not sway the decision to embark on this dangerous yet potentially life-saving maneuver.

The technical description of how to perform an EDT is an excellent primer for any practitioner. From our institutional experience a few suggestions might be entertained. A generous incision should be made to start the procedure. If transaction of the sternum is necessary the authors suggest Lebsche's knife, in our practice a few swipes of Gigli's Saw or a strong hand on Mayo scissors can easily achieve the same. The technical point is to transect the sternum at a diagonal, instead of straight across, so that if the patient does survive, reconstruction will be easier to achieve with larger sections of bone for purchase of the sternal wires.

During the repair of cardiac injuries the authors suggest the use of skin staples to control left ventricle injuries. This is possible in simple scratches of the epicardium but in more complex destructive injuries, such as gun shot wounds, it is found not to be useful.[4] If the injury extends into the chamber of the heart the use of skin staples will not temporize the situation and will delay the operator with futile attempts. Skin staples can only be used on the most simple

of wounds. The myocardium is very soft and difficult to repair. When an injury is found in the emergency center the most skilled surgeon available should be the one to attempt repair. Quite often a simple incised wound of the heart can be made worse with failed attempts by an inexperienced operator. Most survivable cardiac injuries can be temporized with digital pressure, while waiting for appropriate personnel. This will allow the treating team to resuscitate the patient to a better physiologic condition. In short, put your finger in the hole that is bleeding, resuscitate the patient, and once the proper personnel and supplies are available, then repair the hole.

The authors of the chapter prefer to clamp the descending thoracic aorta below the pulmonary hilum. At our institution, the teaching has been to clamp the aorta above the pulmonary hilum and just below the left subclavian artery. A single spread in the pleura above the aorta with either Satinsky or DeBakey's clamp will allow a finger to be inserted between the aorta and the spine. The aorta can be pulled away from the spine and esophagus and the clamp placed across the entire aorta. At this anatomic position the aorta is freely mobile and is not tethered to the spine by the investing pleura and intercostal arteries as it is inferior to the pulmonary hilum. Thus, clamping the aorta low in the chest, as the authors suggest, is difficult to dissect away the pleura, risks tearing an intercostal artery and is very difficult to place the clamp across the aorta. Thus the aorta will slip out of the grasp of the clamp as it is filled with resuscitation and increasing pressure. As always for any surgical procedure the operator, based on their thoughts, hands, and experience, should decide which route to take.

At the beginning of the chapter the authors define their discussion to emergency center based thoracotomies and not those performed elsewhere. If an operating theater is available to the trauma team the patient requiring the thoracotomy should be triaged from the street to the suite. Better lights, instruments, and assistance will help optimize the outcome of the patient.[5] Of course, if local concerns such distance to the operating room, staffing, availability, etc. does not allow this to happen the situation in the ED should be optimized prior to arrival. The calling for a surgical technologist from the operating room to the ED to hand instruments greatly facilitates the procedure. Each institution should establish guidelines and protocols for this event to maximize success.

## References

1. Durham LA III, Richardson RJ, Wall MJ Jr, et al.: Emergency center thoracotomy: impact of prehospital resuscitation. *J Trauma* 32:775, 1992.
2. Aihara R, Millham FH, Blansfield J, et al.: Emergency room thoracotomy for penetrating chest injury: effect of an institutional protocol. *J Trauma* 50:1027, 2001.
3. Branney SW, Moore EE, Feldhaus KM, et al.: Critical analysis of two decades of experience with postinjury emergency department thoracotomy in a regional trauma center. *J Trauma* 45:87 (discussion 94), 1998.
4. Macho JR, Markison RE, Schecter WP: Cardiac stapling in the management of penetrating injuries of the heart: rapid control of hemorrhage and decreased risk of personal contamination. *J Trauma* 34:711, (discussion 715), 1993.
5. Blake DP, Gisbert VL, Ney AL, et al.: Survival after emergency department versus operating room thoracotomy for penetrating cardiac injuries. *Am Surg* 58:329, (discussion 332), 1992.

# Diagnostic and Interventional Radiology

*Luana Stanescu* ■ *Ken F. Linnau* ■ *Tom Burdick* ■ *F. A. Mann*

Trauma imaging (TI) serves broad constituencies, including individual and cohorts of patients, their caregivers, healthcare organizations, and society. TI may be used to provide rapid and broad surveys when clinical evaluation is likely to be incomplete or unreliable or used to characterize recognized injuries as part of treatment planning. And, TI may be used to guide observational, surgical, and minimally invasive therapies. This way, TI may inform clinical diagnosis, but it cannot make management decisions.

Specific TI strategies reflect many factors, some of which will be unique to a given clinical setting. Such factors include the proximity of available imaging technology to the resuscitation area, the capabilities of the imaging equipment, the experience and availability of radiology technologists performing emergent imaging procedures, and timely access to expert interpretation and reporting.

The timing of diagnostic imaging ought to reflect the needs of individual patients and the local system. With the exception of image-guided endovascular hemostasis, hemodynamically unstable patients should be resuscitated prior to imaging. In order to enhance efficiency, triage priorities for imaging should be based on the acute needs for information to direct treatment of the patient. Close cooperation and open communication between the trauma team, nurses, imaging technologists, and radiologists is always necessary to optimize any imaging assessment.

One chapter cannot reasonably teach interpretation of diagnostic images. Therefore, we present a general approach to the role of TI in the evaluation of selected clinical scenarios, while pointing out the advantages and disadvantages of a given imaging strategy. As previously noted, our strategies may suit some institutions better than others. Among transferred patients, approximately 90% arrive with prior imaging. It's not uncommon to repeat images performed at initial institutions due to technical deficiencies, including CT slice thickness/interval, reconstruction algorithm, absence of reformations. For this reason, we provide explication of indications and details on radiological technique.

## PRIMARY IMAGING SURVEY: INITIAL IMAGING ASSESSMENT OF BLUNT TRAUMA

### Trauma Series

As part of the secondary survey of victims of blunt trauma, an imaging survey of the chest [supine anteroposterior (AP) chest with 10° of caudal angulation of the central x-ray beam], pelvis (supine AP pelvis), and cervical spine (horizontal-beam cross-table lateral cervical spine obtained with bilateral arm pull) may be performed, if clinical evaluation alone is deemed insufficient (Fig. 16-1).[1] The trauma resuscitation ABCD strategy may be extended to this "trauma series." Verification of the integrity of the airway (and other tubes and lines) should be specifically made on the radiographs of both the chest and lateral cervical spine. Radiographic pulmonary opacities associated with hypoxemia include pulmonary contusions, aspiration pneumonitis, and atelectasis (including collapse due to aspirated dental or foreign debris). Tension pneumo- and hemothorax are typically detected on clinical examination, while clinically occult pneumo- or hemothoraces are commonly shown by chest radiographs as a "deep sulcus" sign and generalized hemithoracic opacity, respectively. Other injuries, such as rupture of the hemidiaphragm, flail chest, pneumopericardium, and pneumo- and hemomediastinum are often diagnosed or suggested by initial conventional radiographic findings. Hemodynamic instability may be due to extraperitoneal hemorrhage from disruption of the pelvic ring. Biomechanically-unstable disruptions of the pelvic ring are almost always shown on AP radiographs and may be associated with injuries to the bladder and urethra. In addition, pelvis radiographs may show hip dislocations, and fractures of the acetabulum and proximal femur.

A technically adequate (C1-T1) lateral radiograph of the cervical spine provides a reasonable "screening" study to identify most

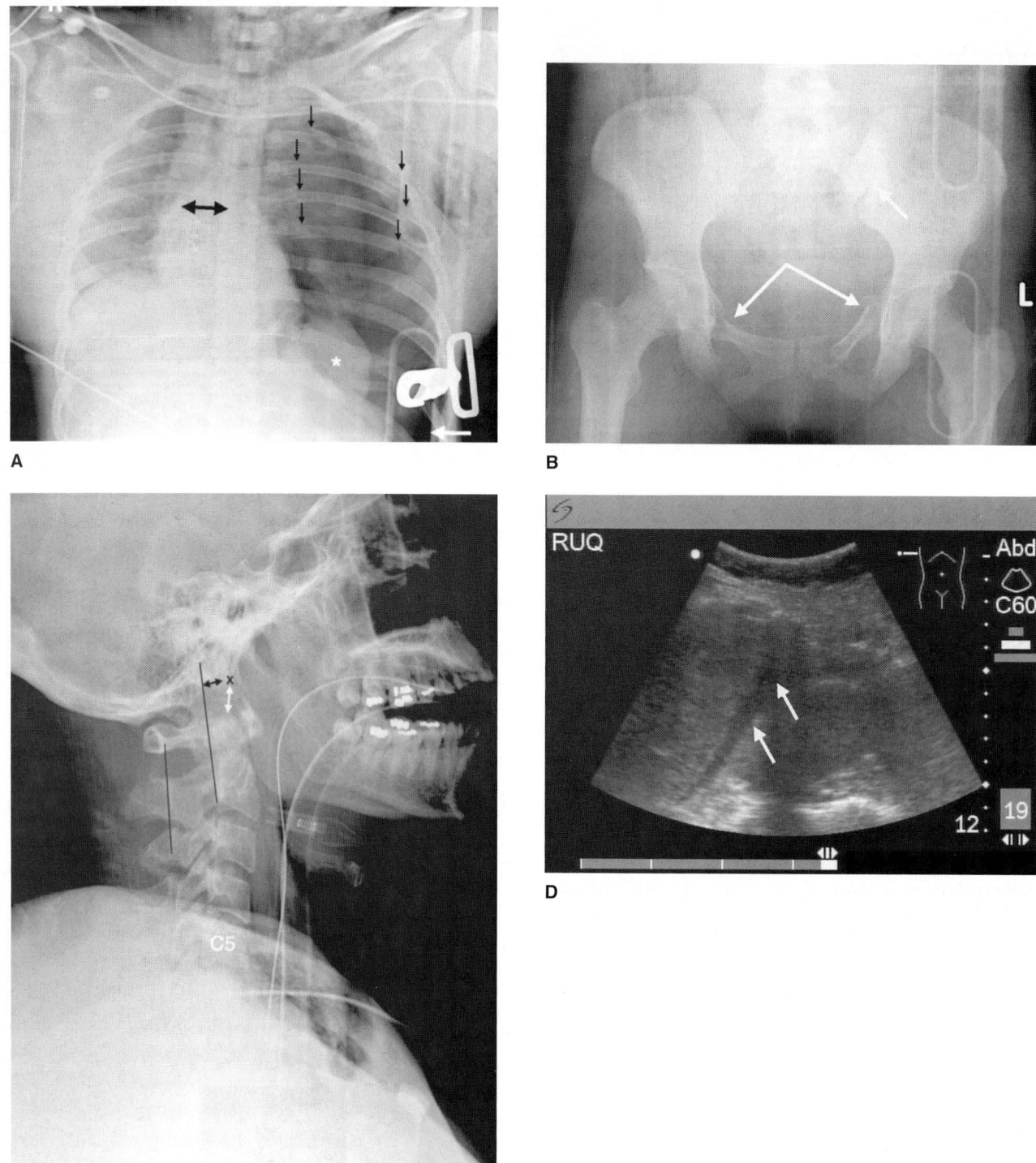

**FIGURE 16-1.** Trauma series. This 27-year-old woman sustained multiple injuries, including splenic rupture, as an unrestrained left rear seat passenger in a high-speed side-impact crash. **(A)** Anteroposterior (AP) recumbent chest radiograph shows hyperexpanded and hyperlucent left hemithorax with "deep sulcus" sign (short white arrow) and rightward mediastinal shift (double-ended arrow) due to left tension pneumothorax. Short black arrows show multiple displaced rib fractures. Asterisk shows irregularity of left hemidiaphragm, which strongly suggests herniation of abdominal contents through left diaphragmatic laceration. **(B)** AP recumbent pelvis radiograph shows lateral-compression-type pelvic ring disruption consisting of bilateral ilio- and ischiopubic ramus fractures (long arrows) and left sacral and sacroiliac joint disruptions (short arrow). **(C)** Cross-table lateral cervical spine radiograph shows interval placement of orogastric tube. Alignment is grossly normal to C5. Careful attention must be given to craniocervical alignment. Dens-basion distance (white double-ended arrow) is normally no greater than 12 mm. Posterior axial line represents cephalad extension of posterior cortex of C2 body (ignoring the dens) and is normally no more than 12 mm posterior or 4 mm anterior to basion (black double-ended arrow). Anterior atlantodens interval is normally no greater than 3 mm in adults and 5 mm in children (8 years and younger). Laminar point of C2 (laminar points are most anterior extent of neural canal margin of lamina) should be within 1.5 mm of line connecting laminar points of C1 and C3. **(D)** Coronal image of right upper quadrant from focused abdominal sonography for trauma (FAST) shows free intraperitoneal fluid in anterior subhepatic (Morison's) space (arrows), compatible with hemoperitoneum.

unstable injuries to the cervical spine. It may provide important information regarding the best technique for airway control and may confirm that spinal shock from a fracture of the cervical spine is the cause of otherwise unexplained hypotension.

## Focused Abdominal Sonography for Trauma (FAST)

FAST is performed as part of the secondary survey in victims of blunt-force torso trauma (Fig. 16-2; see Chap. 17). FAST is a temporally (2–5 minutes) and anatomically limited real-time sonographic examination[2] whose core components include direct sonographic search for free fluid in the pericardial sac, both upper abdominal quadrants and in the intraperitoneal recesses adjacent to the urinary bladder. Scanning is optimally performed in two orthogonal planes (e.g., longitudinal and transverse), and intra-parenchymal and retroperitoneal injuries are generally not sought. FAST may be extended to detect abnormal pleural collections (hemo- and pneumothorax). Commercially available, portable hand-held real-time imaging devices are technically adequate to perform FAST.

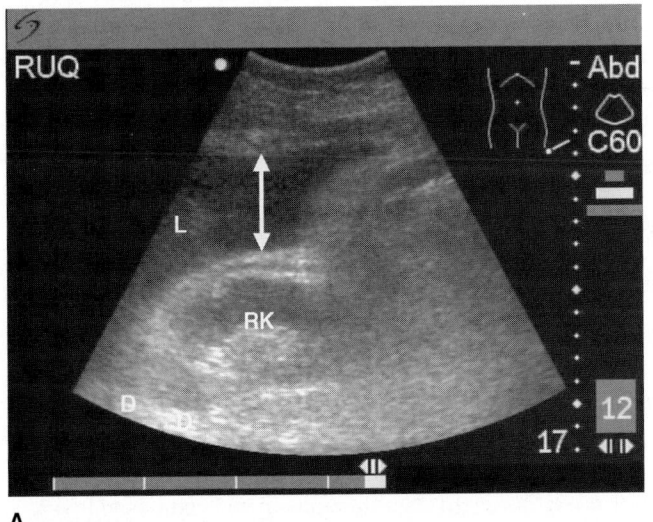

A

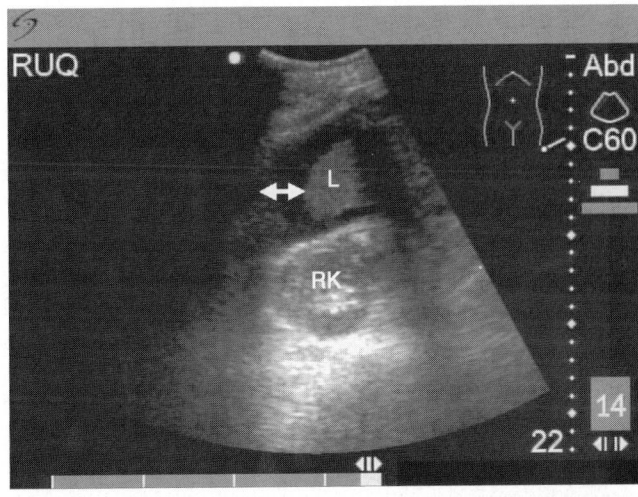

B

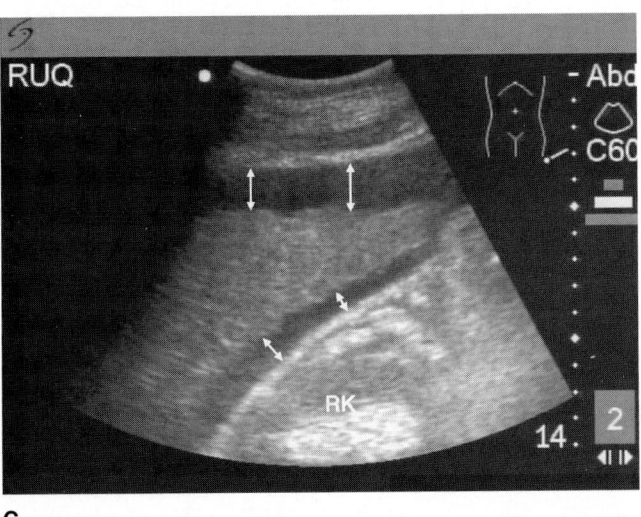

C

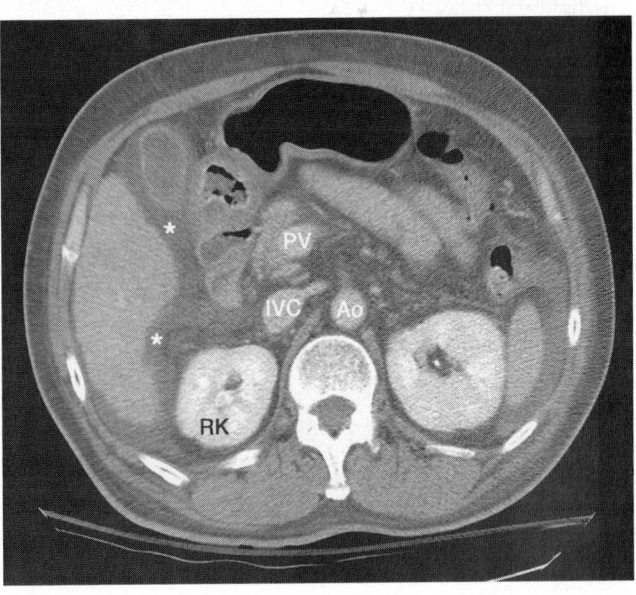

D

**FIGURE 16-2.**    Focused abdominal sonography for trauma (FAST): This 58-year-old alcoholic man was struck by an automobile while crossing a highway. **(A)** Coronal sonogram from right upper quadrant has depth adjusted to show diaphragm (D) and shows free intraperitoneal fluid (double-ended arrow). L, liver; RK, right kidney. **(B)** Transverse sonogram from right upper quadrant shows irregular surface to liver (L) with surrounding fluid (double-ended arrow). RK, right kidney. **(C)** Coronal sonogram of right upper quadrant, adjusted to show Morison's pouch, shows macronodularity of liver margin, consistent with macronodular cirrhosis, surrounded by free intraperitoneal fluid (double-ended arrows). In such situations, differentiation between hemoperitoneum and chronic ascites may be difficult (although uncomplicated ascites usually shows little or no debris, as seen in hemoperitoneum). RK, right kidney. **(D)** Axial image from computed tomography abdomen correlates well with sonography. Free fluid (asterisks) proved to be hemoperitoneum at laparotomy. PV, portal vein; IVC, inferior vena cava with left renal vein insertion; Ao, abdominal aorta at take-off of superior mesenteric artery; RK, right kidney.

FAST is uniformly accurate for the detection of intraperitoneal fluid with volumes >400 cc (i.e., user dependency is very small; at smaller volumes, accuracy varies with user experience).[3–5] Of interest, isolated injuries to the liver and spleen with minimal or no hemoperitoneum represent as many as one-third of solid organ injuries.[6,7] Isolated intraparenchymal lesions with small (<250 mL) or no hemoperitoneum rarely require endovascular or surgical intervention (liver <1%, spleen <5%).[8] False-positive interpretation of FAST can result from improper machine settings (gain), sonolucent perinephric fat (which is rarely sonolucent in both axial and coronal scanning planes), fluid-filled bowel loops, bladder, various types of fluid-filled intra-abdominal cysts, and physiologic or nontraumatic free fluid (ascites). FAST is widely available, inexpensive and noninvasive, uses no ionizing radiation, and can be repeated serially. In the setting of patients admitted with severe hemodynamic compromise or obvious hemorrhagic shock, FAST can establish the abdomen as a source of hemorrhage within a few seconds. An important limitation of FAST is that isolated injuries to the bowel and retroperitoneal injuries are not reliably detected. Therefore, patients who have suffered blunt trauma with clinical presentations suspicious for injury to the bowel (e.g., lap belt sign and associated Chance or flexion-distraction injury to the thoraco-lumbar spine) or hematuria (e.g., gross hematuria in all age groups, microscopic hematuria [>50 red blood cell count per high-power field] in those individuals 16 years old and younger, or in those older with at least one documented episode of hypotension) should undergo diagnostic peritoneal lavage (DPL) and intravenous contrast-enhanced computer tomography (CT) of the abdomen and pelvis, respectively. Hemodynamically stable patients with a positive FAST or DPL (not gross blood) typically have contrast-enhanced CT performed. Further, FAST requires operator training and experience for reliable performance and interpretation. Caveat: a recent Cochrane collaborative systematic review concluded that the current literature does not support use of FAST as a replacement for DPL and CT in blunt abdominal trauma.[9]

## "THE TRAUMA TRAIN" FOR BLUNT POLYTRAUMA

Victims of blunt multiple trauma at our institution are initially imaged in the trauma suite and then triaged based on their hemodynamic status to the operating room, intensive care units, or angiography suite for ongoing resuscitation or remain in the trauma center for completion of secondary and tertiary surveys, including initial imaging. For these patients remaining in the trauma center, the route through radiology at our institution is sometimes referred to as the "trauma train." Typically, this consists of a trip to the CT suite for imaging (e.g., head, neck, chest, abdomen, and pelvis) for the most severely injured. Subsequently, conventional radiographic images of the extremities and spine may be obtained. Less severely injured individuals may take a slightly different route with conventional radiographs preceding CT and directed at abnormalities found by prior imaging or clinical examination. For the purpose of this section, the authors use an order that includes CT of the head, face, soft tissue neck; CT of the chest, abdomen, pelvis, orthopaedic pelvis or acetabulum; imaging of the spine, to include conventional radiographs, CT, flexion-extension radiographs, and magnetic resonance imaging (MRI); angiography, including its role in imaging and guiding therapy for aortic injuries, and embolization of hemorrhage associated with disruption of the pelvic ring; and evaluation of the extremities, focusing on approaches to injuries of long bones and joints, separately.

## Multidetector Computed Tomography (MDCT)

Advent of multidetector(multislice CT scanners (e.g., 2-row, 16-channel, 64-detector) has changed the way CT is used in imaging trauma.[10,11] Multidetector CT scanners, with 16 or more detectors can provide nearly isotropic volume imaging (i.e., equivalent resolution in all three imaging planes), at progressively shorter and shorter scan times. Near-isotropic imaging greatly improves the quality of both two- (multiplanar) and three-dimensional reformations. The rapidity of multidetector helical scanning and enormously improved designs of X-ray tubes allow single-session scanning from cranial vertex to pelvic ischia in less than 90 seconds,[12,13] with two-dimensional and three-dimensional reformations of the thoracic and abdominal aorta, maxillofacial skeleton, cervical and thoracolumbar spines, and orthopaedic pelvis and acetabulae.

The X-ray detector in the new generation CT scanners may be configured to divide the X-ray beam width (i.e., collimation) into two or more thinner channels (slice thickness), the details of which are vendor-specific. For example, an 8-channel multidetector CT scanner may use several different collimation widths (e.g., 10-mm, 5-mm, and 2.5-mm) for the x-ray beam, and several different combinations of the eight potential channels. With x-ray beam collimation set at 10 mm, the slice thicknesses of eight equally sized channels is 1.25 mm. Alternatively, these could be configured to give four 2.5-mm-thick sections. With 5-mm collimation of the x-ray beam, the slice thickness of eight equally sized channels would be approximately 0.63 mm, which could be reconstructed as four 1.25-mm sections.[2] With appropriate anticipation, scanning parameters allow raw axial data to be reconstructed using different thicknesses (e.g., 5-mm-thick slices for abdominal viscera and 2.5-mm-thick slices for CT aortography).

CT terminology can be confusing. Scanning pitch for multidector scanners has been defined by all vendors to be the table speed (in millimeters per second) divided by the x-ray beam collimation (NOT slice thickness). Definition of pitch differed among vendors among older generation multidetector scanners. The volume raw data acquired by CT is "reconstructed" using specialized back-projection algorithms (synonym: kernels) that are optimized to portray different tissue characteristics (e.g., soft tissue versus bone), and may be viewed as cross-sectional "slices" of various thickness made at user-defined intervals (e.g., 2.5 mm thick slices made at 1.25 mm intervals have a 1.25 mm [50%] overlap). Reformations are made from the reconstructed data sets and can be made as 2D (sagittal, coronal, curved-plane) or 3D (volume rendered, maximum intensity projection, etc). For specific imaging protocols, please see the webpage for Harborview Medical Center CT protocols: http://depts.washington.edu/hmcrad/Protocols/H-Radiology-Protocols-Index.htm

MRI safety link: http://mrisafety.com/

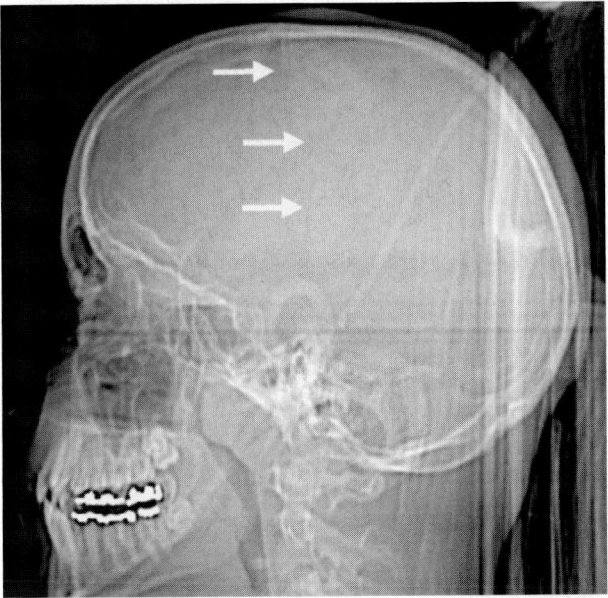

A

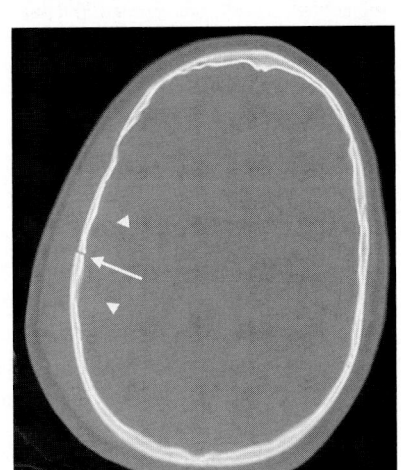

B

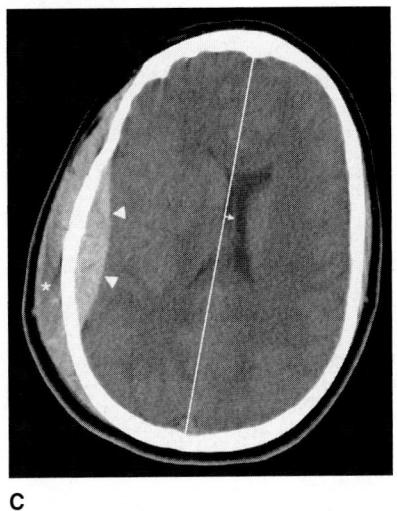

C

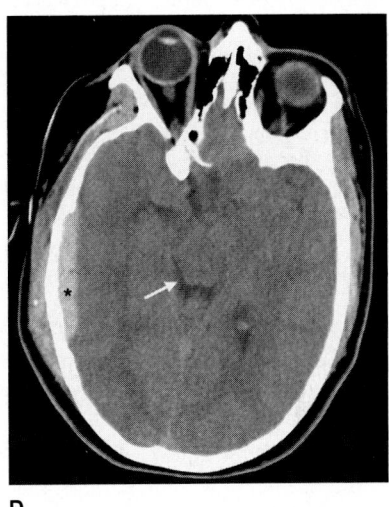

D

**FIGURE 16-3.** Epidural hematoma. Helmetless bicyclist in crash. **(A)** Lateral scout scanogram shows linear lucency compatible with fracture (arrows). **(B)** Axial computed tomography (CT) displayed at bone window shows minimally displaced right parietal skull fracture with overlying subgaleal hematoma. Fracture is marked by white arrow, and barely visible hyperintensity of extra-axial blood collection by arrowheads. **(C)** Axial CT at brain windows shows epidural hematoma (arrowheads), associated midline shift (short arrow), and subgaleal hematoma (asterisk). **(D)** Axial CT at level of the suprasellar cistern, brain windows, shows epidural hematoma (black asterisk), asymmetric widening of perimesencephalic cistern (arrow), which suggests impending uncal herniation.
*(Reproduced with permission from DK Hallam.)*

## Computed Tomography of the Cranium

General Indications.    Axial noncontrast CT scanning remains the reference standard in patients with acute craniocerebral trauma, guiding initial decisions regarding the clinical management.[14,15]

Indications for CT of the cranium include objective evidence of closed injury to the brain, including decreased level of consciousness; cranial or facial deformity; hemotympanum; or evidence for leakage of cerebrospinal fluid (Figs. 16-3, 16-4, and 16-5). Recent studies identified clinical criteria that reliably predict association with significant intracranial injury (ICI) in patients who will require CT head scanning. In pediatric population, significant ICI is extremely unlikely in any child who does not exhibit at least one

of the following high-risk criteria: (1) evidence of significant skull fracture, (2) altered level of alertness, (3) neurologic deficit, (4) persisting vomiting, (5) scalp hematoma, (6) abnormal behavior, or (7) coagulopathy.[16] In the adult population over 65, the same criteria were found to be associated with significant ICI.[17] More generically, minor trauma to the head may lead to surgically important injuries to the brain, and liberal utilization of CT is appropriate among individuals who have sustained "high-risk" mechanisms. Single-photon emission CT (SPECT) may be helpful in initial diagnostic evaluation of patients with mild traumatic brain injury (MTBI), particularly for those with normal CT findings and associated posttraumatic amnesia (PTA), post concussion syndrome (PCS), and loss of consciousness.[18]

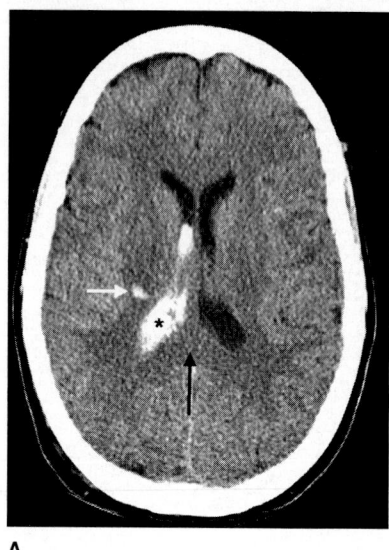
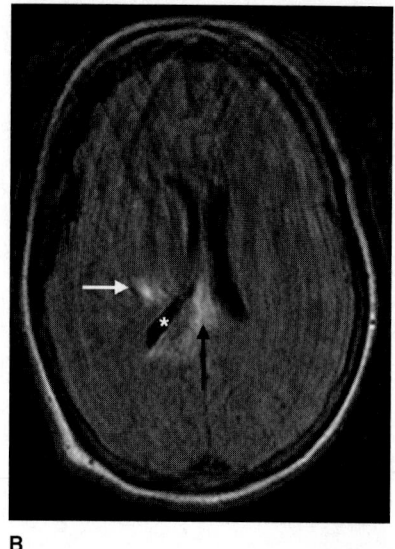
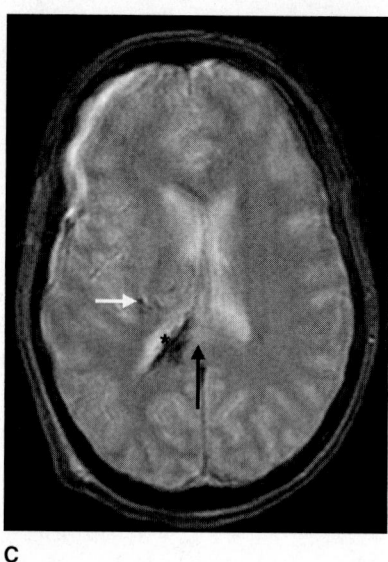

A                              B                              C

**FIGURE 16-4.** Blunt head injury: Diffuse axonal injury. This 48-year-old helmeted female motorcyclist sustained diffuse axonal injury. **(A)** Axial computed tomography (CT) at level of lateral ventricles demonstrates intraventricular hemorrhage (asterisk), "tear" hemorrhage in posterior limb of internal capsule (white arrow). Black arrow notes splenium of corpus callosum, which appeared normal by CT. **(B)** Axial magnetic resonance imaging (MRI) using FLAIR shows clot in right lateral ventricle as extended region of low signal (asterisk), edema associated with tear hemorrhage (white arrow), and splenium of corpus callosum (black arrow) to better advantage. **(C)** MRI gradient recalled echo (GRE) sequence shows low signal intensity of magnetic susceptibility due to hemorrhage in region of posterior horn of internal capsule (white arrow) and in right lateral ventricle (asterisk). Splenium of corpus callosum has region of mildly increased signal intensity compatible with edema (black arrow). In general, the more central findings of diffuse axonal injury, the greater the degree of neurologic disability.
*(Reproduced with permission from WA Cohen.)*

**Examination Prescription.** For helical CT scanners, the authors use a slice thickness of 5 mm in adults and older children and 1.25 mm for infants (<4 years) from the vertex through the skull base. In infants, the authors extend the CT scan down to the base of C2, because injuries to the upper cervical spine are particularly common in this age group. Images are reconstructed using both bone and soft tissue algorithms and viewed at bone windows and two different soft tissue windows ("brain" and "blood"). In general, the axial images are obtained parallel to the cantho-meatal or porion-orbitale (Frankfurt) lines.

**Comment.** CT scanning is highly sensitive for the detection of extra-axial and intra-axial hemorrhage and mass effect, as well as for soft tissue injuries to the globe and paranasal sinuses. In patients with diffuse axonal injury, however, CT may even be normal and discordant between the severity of the clinical brain injury and radiographic findings. On a cautionary note, skull fractures aligned in the plane of scanning may be subtle, and review of the scout views used to plan the CT-head study may act to alert the clinician to such fractures. Except for medicolegal imaging of nonaccidental trauma (child abuse), conventional radiographs of the skull are usually not necessary.[19,20]

## Computed Tomography of the Maxillofacial Skeleton

**General Indications.** Indications include deformity or instability of the maxillofacial structures found by clinical (physical) examination; deformity, opacification, or fracture of the periorbital or paranasal sinus shown on head CT; and clinical evidence for leakage of cerebrospinal fluid (Fig. 16-6). The mnemonic LIPS-N

(lip lacerations, intraoral lacerations, periorbital contusions, subconjunctival hemorrhage, or nasal lacerations) also provides a helpful tool during clinical examination of trauma patients, given the high association between any of LIPS-N lesions and facial fractures.[21] Absence of opacification of a paranasal or periorbital sinus on CT generally excludes surgically important injury to the maxillofacial skeleton.[22]

**Examination Prescription.** Images can be obtained either directly in axial and coronal planes, directly in either axial or coronal plane with reformations in the orthogonal plane, or as reconstruction from a CT of the cranium obtained from an appropriately prescribed study (i.e., 1.00 to 1.25-mm slice thickness). In general, direct acquisition in orthogonal planes at 2.5–3-mm contiguous slice thickness has been the standard of care in outpatient settings. With the evolution of spiral CT, and especially MDCT, 1.0- to 1.25-mm thick sections in the axial plane can be reformatted into 2D reformations orthogonal planes (e.g. coronal, sagittal, oblique sagittal) and 3D reformations, without loss of image quality, accuracy, and without further radiation.

Primary axial images are obtained parallel to the Frankfurt horizontal plane using 1.0- to 1.25-mm slice thickness from above the frontal sinus through the hard palate or maxillary alveolus and are commonly extended to include the mandible to aid surgical planning (Buttress and Facial Subunit Concept)[23,24] especially in children, as fractures of the condyle of the mandible are the most commonly missed maxillofacial fractures in this age group.[25] Reformations in the coronal and sagittal planes should be perfectly orthogonal to the axial images. Reformations in the sagittal plane may be performed either relative to the coronal plane or as sagittal oblique reformations parallel to the optic

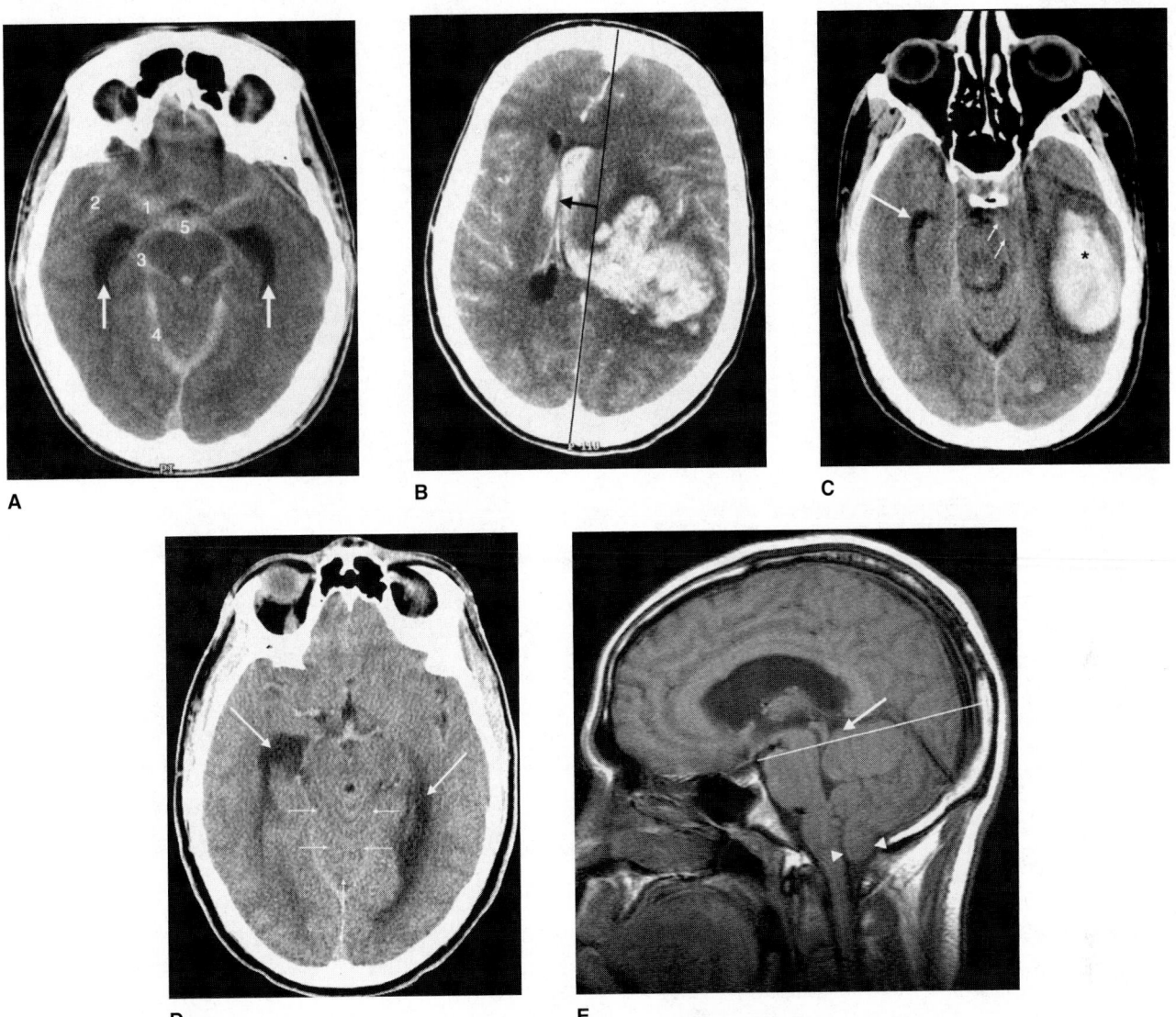

**FIGURE 16-5.**    Patterns of herniation. **(A)**. Axial computed tomography (CT) at level of suprasellar cistern shows extensive subarachnoid hemorrhage extending from lateral aspect of suprasellar cistern (1), into the sylvian fissure (2), circumferentially about brainstem and perimesencephalic cistern (3), along tentorium (4), and interpedunculate cistern of mesencephalon (5). Entrapment of lateral ventricles is shown as dilatation of temporal horns (white arrows). Brainstem appears relatively lucent and heart-shaped, with pointed inferior portion of heart due to "beaking" of mesencephalon due to upward herniation. **(B)** Subfalcine shift. Axial CT, at brain windows, at level of lateral ventricles shows marked rightward subfalcine shift (black arrow), quantified as distance from 3rd ventricle to line connecting anterior and posterior portions of sagittal sinus (which tend not to shift due to their fixed relation to calvarium). Note extensive hemorrhage in left frontal parietal region extending into left ventricle. (*Reproduced with permission from WA Cohen.*) **(C)** Uncal herniation. Axial CT at level of middle cranial fossa shows large left temporal hematoma (black asterisk) associated with left uncal herniation (small white arrows). Enlargement of right temporal horn (large white arrow) is compatible with obstruction to cisternal system. (*Reproduced with permission from AB Baxter.*) **(D)** Combined upward and downward herniation. This is a 38-year-old with posterior leukoencephalopathy due to hypertension. Axial CT at level of suprasellar cistern shows enlargement of lateral ventricles and right temporal horn (long white arrows). Suprasellar cistern is poorly seen. Perimesencephalic cisterns are absent and posterior aspect is beaked, compatible with superior herniation from posterior fossa. Upward herniation is also shown by the cerebellar vermis filling the subtentorial cisternal space (multiple small arrows). (*Reproduced with permission from WA Cohen.*) **(E)** Same patient as in (D) Sagittal T1-weighted magnetic resonance imaging shows tonsillar herniation through the foramen magnum (arrowheads), as well as superior herniation of cerebellum and mesencephalon at level of tentorium (white arrow).

nerve, if evaluating for blow-out fractures of the orbital floor.[26] Images are reconstructed using both soft tissue and bone algorithms and viewed using soft tissue and bone windowing, respectively.

If a 16-detector CT scan is obtained, for example, using 2 cm collimation of the x-ray beam, in which the 20 mm detector array is composed of 16 1.25-mm wide channels, postprocessing allows for separation of the information from each of those channels to create individual 1.25-mm slice thicknesses. Such imaging prescription provides the raw data for reconstruction of the maxillofacial skeleton and soft tissues in various spatial planes without further radiation exposure to the patient.

Comment.    While CT is highly accurate at detecting and characterizing surgically important injuries, it does not show the magnitude of osseous fragmentation found at surgery in

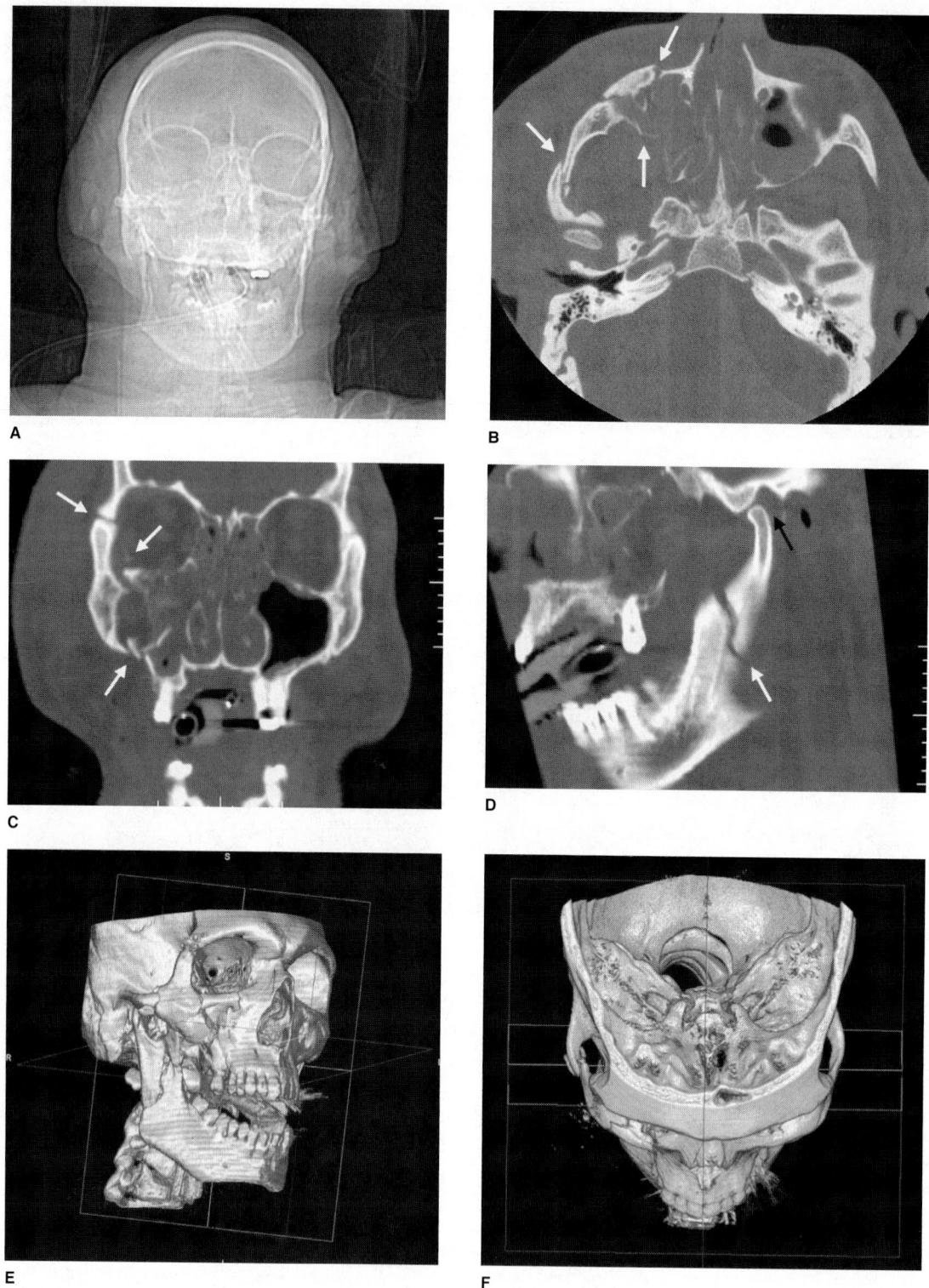

**FIGURE 16-6.** Facial fracture: Zygomaticomaxillary complex (ZMC) fracture. This 54-year-old male sustained a blow to the face in a motorcycle crash. **(A)** Anteroposterior (AP) scanogram shows loss of symmetry to orbital volumes, with elliptoid enlargement of right orbit. Associated indistinctness of orbital floor and lateral maxillary sinus walls is also present. Opacification of right maxillar sinus is shown. **(B)** Axial computed tomography (CT) image at the level of zygomatic arches shows depression and overriding apposition of impacted zygomatic arch fracture (lateral white arrow), segmental comminuted fracture of anterior maxillary wall (anterior arrow), and posterolateral maxillary sinus wall disruption (posterior arrow). Asterisk marks the base of nasofrontal process of maxilla and shows fracture of nasolacrimal duct just posterior to it. Minimal internal rotation of anterior aspect and associated fracture of nasolacrimal duct are not portions of zygomaticomaxillary complex fracture and represent an associated heminasoethmoidal orbital complex fracture. **(C)** Coronal CT reformations shows separation of right frontozygomatic suture (lateral and superior arrow), disruption of orbital floor (white arrow projected over orbit), and lateral maxillary wall (inferior white arrow). **(D)** Sagittal CT reformation shows associated vertical fracture of right ramus of mandible, with anterior subluxation at temporomandibular joint (white and black arrows, respectively). **(E)** Three-dimensional CT reformation gives an overview of complex fracture of zygomaticomaxillary region and right mandibular fracture. It is important to note that spatial resolution is lost with three-dimensional reformations, although spatial comprehension is often improved. **(F)** Three-dimensional CT reformation shows depression of right zygomatic arch and loss of projection of the right zygoma (flat cheek).

complex fractures. Orbital and maxillary fractures should heighten suspicion of more complex fractures. Although their incremental diagnostic value is small, 3D-CT reformation appear to be the best imaging method for the global portrayal of complex maxillofacial injury patterns, such as Le Fort type fractures, providing valuable information of spatial relationship, and being particularly useful in planning the treatment by surgeons.[27–30]

On the other hand, axial and 2D reformations best portray soft tissue complications, interposition of osseous fragments and soft-tissue herniations, and are best for quantifying size of fractures and associated soft-tissue herniation (e.g., orbital floor blow-out fractures).[26,31]

Maxillofacial CT delivers a significant radiation dose to the orbits, and scan extension to include the mandible is associated with clinically meaningful radiation to the soft tissues of the neck (e.g., thyroid), an important consideration in the pediatric population.[32]

## Soft Tissue Injuries of the Neck

General Indications.   Clinical findings for blunt injury to the aerodigestive tract include subcutaneous crepitus, hemoptysis, hoarseness, neck pain, and abrasions or hematomas (e.g., from the shoulder harness of a 3-point restraint; Figs. 16-7 and 16-8). Due to liberal screening, blunt carotid and vertebral injury (BCVI) is now known to be much more common than previously appreciated. Vascular imaging of the neck is warranted in injury patterns associated with a high risk of blunt injury to the carotid and vertebral arteries, including the following: cervical spine fracture (especially involving C1-C3, involving the transverse foramena or extension into foramen magnum), neurologic deficits not

explained by findings at brain imaging, Horner's syndrome, high energy facial fractures (Le Fort II or III), skull base fracture involving foramen lacerum or soft tissue injury in the neck (neck belt sign and "hangings" sufficient to cause central anoxia).[33,34] Catheter angiography is indicated emergently in patients with an expanding cervical hematoma, active extravasation from nose, mouth or ears, or a cervical bruit in individuals younger than 50-years-old.[35] Four-vessel-catheter arteriography and transcranial Doppler studies are useful in the application of endovascular therapy of high-grade BCVI and selection of patients at risk for embolic stroke, respectively.[33,36] Duplex Doppler US sensitivity is inadequately low (38.5%) for directly depicting BCVI, while MDCT, with a sensitivity of 90–100%, allows rapid acquisition of an angiographic assessment without delaying rapid trauma work-up.[37]

In the absence of a pneumothorax, radiographic findings that suggest injury to the aerodigestive tract include parapharyngeal or precervical emphysema. In general, penetrating injuries to zones I and III of the neck are best evaluated with imaging in the hemodynamically stable patient.

Examination Prescription.   Noncontrast MDCT neck (larynx) axial imaging with a slice thickness of 2.5 mm and reconstruction interval of 1.25 mm from the hyoid bone to the sternal notch. Images are reconstructed using both bone and standard (soft tissue) algorithms and portrayed at bone and soft tissue windows, respectively.

CT arteriography of the neck is obtained following a timing bolus performed at the C6 level using 20 mL of contrast at 3 mL/s and a slice thickness of 5 mm. Based on the timing

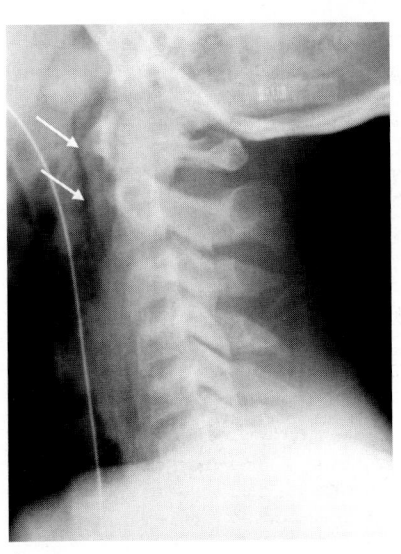 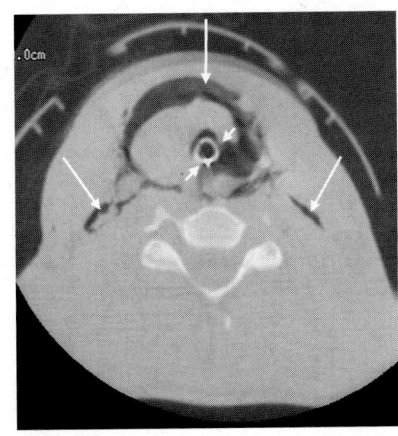 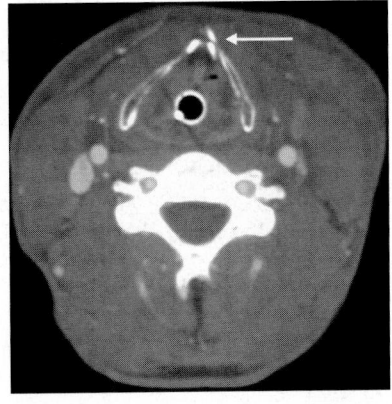

**A**     **B**     **C**

**FIGURE 16-7.**   Soft tissue neck injury. **(A)** This is a 15-year-old male motorcyclist with clothesline injury, causing tracheal and esophageal transection. Lateral view of cervical spine shows extensive subcutaneous emphysema (white arrows). Endotracheal cuff balloon is abnormally large (diameter >3 cm), compatible with either soft tissue injury or abnormal airway. In general, presence of precervical or parapharyngeal emphysema in neck without pneumothorax should raise question of airway or digestive tract injury. **(B)** Axial computed tomography (CT), lung windows. Same patient as in A. Cervical tracheal disruption is shown between two short white arrows at posterior and left side of trachea. Extensive parapharyngeal and precervical emphysema is present (long arrows). **(C)** Axial CT at level of thyroid cartilage, soft tissue windows. This 27-year-old man sustained thyroid cartilage fracture in strangulation. White arrow points to paramedian thyroid cartilage fracture. Thyroid cartilage fractures typically occur within 2 or 3 mm of anterior junction of lamina of thyroid cartilage and are thought to be due to wishbone-like spreading of thyroid cartilage as it is driven on to vertebrae. Overriding apposition of fracture fragments shortens vocal cord on affected side, causing hoarseness and lower voice. Air seen adjacent to cartilage fracture suggests compound injury.

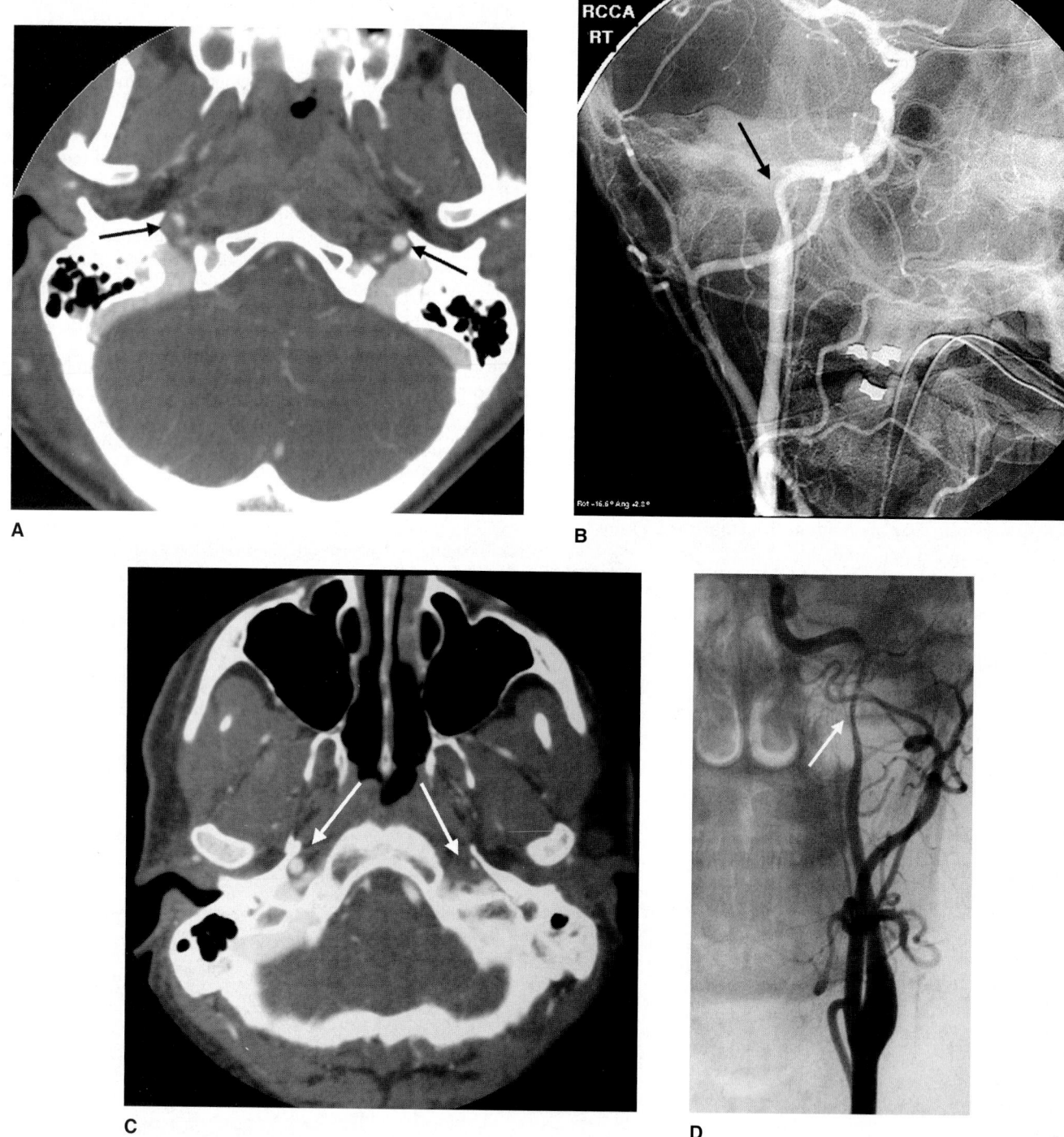

**FIGURE 16-8.** Carotid dissections. **(A)** This 19-year-old female right rear seat passenger sustained injuries in a side-impact crash. Axial image from computed tomography (CT) arteriogram shows asymmetry of the internal carotid arteries (black arrows), with right showing findings suggestive of dissection. Also note abnormal contours to mandibular condyles, compatible with bilateral fractures. *(Reproduced with permission from WA Cohen.)* **(B)** Same patient as in (A). Transorbital oblique view of right internal carotid angiogram shows abrupt luminal narrowing and irregularity (black arrow) compatible with traumatic dissection (Biffl grade 2). **(C)** This is a 36-year-old man with spontaneous left carotid dissection. Axial CT arteriography at level of skull base shows asymmetry between the internal carotids (long arrows), with the left showing a much narrower and slightly eccentric lumen compatible with dissection. *(Reproduced with permission from AB Baxter.)* **(D)** Same patient as in (C). Anteroposterior arteriogram of left common carotid injection shows fusiform narrowing of internal carotid before its entry into skull base (arrow). No extravasation nor intraluminal clot was evident.

bolus, the CT arteriography of the neck is performed using slice thickness at 1.25–2.5 mm and reconstruction interval of 50% of the slice thickness using bone and soft tissue algorithms. Reformations, performed as multiplanar volume reformations

(MPVR) maximum-intensity projections are obtained using 1.25-mm slice thickness at 0.6-mm intervals. Three-dimensional reformations are also obtained using a MPVR maximum-intensity projection.

*Comment.* CT is often most helpful in the evaluation of laryngotracheal injuries when deformed anatomy or extensive hemorrhage makes direct or indirect endoscopy more difficult. Careful search for open injuries (e.g., air adjacent to cartilaginous fractures) guides the need for intervention for debridement and mucosal closure. CT can assist in the grading of laryngotracheal injuries, but tends to understage compared to endoscopy or open exploration. The search should begin in the region of the valleculae epiglottica and extend anteriorly along the larynx and trachea. The most common injuries are those to the thyroid cartilage. Fractures of the thyroid cartilage typically occur within 2 to 3 mm of the anterior crest of the two lateral laminae. Comminuted fractures of the laminae generally reflect higher energy, direct impact injuries to the larynx, and are more commonly associated with thyrocricoid dislocation. Also, CT will demonstrate subluxations and dislocations of the arytenoid cartilage, findings that are more readily appreciated if the patient is well centered. Most tracheal disruptions are in the membranous portion of the trachea and will heal with conservative (e.g., endotracheal tube placed distal to the disruption) therapy. Soft tissue emphysema immediately adjacent to the trachea suggests an injury in this location. Searches for a fracture of a tracheal ring are often fruitless unless the fracture is displaced. Coronal reformations through the trachea may show separation (vertical diastasis between tracheal rings) of the trachea compatible with more serious grades of injury.

Blunt traumatic rupture of the esophagus tends to be in the proximal third, particularly within the cervical portion. Radiographically, this manifests as gas in the soft tissues. A definitive diagnosis may require the administration of contrast or endoscopy. When esophagography is requested, the authors prefer to evaluate with injection through an enteral tube placed into the esophagus to assure adequate distension.

Penetrating injuries of the soft tissues of the neck, particularly gunshot wounds, may be evaluated with CT arteriography.[38] The advantages of direct exploration of isolated penetrating injuries of zone II of the neck in symptomatic patients commonly outweigh having an imaging road map of the injury.

Advances in MDCT technology and PACS monitor viewing improved the diagnostic accuracy of CTA compared to digital subtraction angiography (DSA) in detecting injury to the carotid or vertebral artery.[39] Current generation MDCT with 16 or more channels show essentially all clinically important BCVI, if performed using appropriate thin-section technique following rapid intravenous contrast administration.[35]

## Survey Computed Tomography of the Cervical Spine

*General Indications.* In adult and older children (≥10 years-old), validated clinical prediction rules can reliably determine those trauma victims warranting cervical spine imaging (or not); i.e., National Emergency X-Radiography Utilization Study Group (NEXUS) and the Canadian Cervical Spine Rule. Another clinical prediction rule helps determine which imaging modality is most cost-effective. Specifically, Blackmore et al.[40] developed a clinical prediction rule to determine pre-imaging risk of fracture in select patients about to undergo a helical CT to survey the cervical spine for fracture and soft tissue injuries (Figs. 16-9 to 16-12). For the application of this clinical prediction rule, it is assumed that the patient will already be undergoing CT of the cranium. Any one of three mechanisms of injury or any one of three clinical findings puts the patient at a pretest risk of harboring an injury in the cervical spine of greater than 5%. High-risk mechanisms of injury include a high-speed motor vehicle crash >35 mph or >50 km/h combined impact; motor vehicle crash with a death at the scene; or a fall from a height of >10 ft or >3 m. Clinical parameters signifying increased risk for injury to the cervical spine that are found on a primary patient survey and associated with a high-risk mechanism include a significant closed injury to the brain (or intracranial hemorrhage shown by CT of the cranium); acute neurologic deficits referable to the cervical spine (acute myelopathy or radiculopathy); or either pelvic fracture or multiple extremity fractures. Hanson et al.[41] validated the clinical prediction rule prospectively and showed its application by separating victims of blunt trauma into a high-risk group (12% prevalence of acute cervical spine injuries) and low-risk group (0.2% prevalence of cervical spine injury). In infants (<1 year-old) and younger children (<9 year-old) no validated rule exists. In general, patients with greater severities of injury (ISS >25) have elevated risk of injury to the cervical spine. Conventional radiographs will depict essentially all clinically important fractures and dislocations in patients aged 9 years and younger. CT is NOT useful /indicated in younger children and infants to screen the cervical spine, nor in search for other occult injuries causing neurological deficit.[42,43] CT should be reserved as a staging/treatment planning procedure among patients with a known bony abnormality.

*Examination Prescription.* Axial slices of thickness of 1.25 to 3.0 mm are obtained from the skull base through the T4 vertebral body. Depending on the scanner type (e.g., single vs. multiple detector helical scanners), it may be more temporally efficient to scan from the T4 level to the skull base, which allows for cooling of the x-ray tube and minimizes delays before further scanning of the torso. MDCT's with four or more detector arrays are not as susceptible to tube overheating and scanning can be performed cranio-rostral. Images are typically reconstructed at half the slice-thickness interval for creation of parasagittal and coronal reformations. Reformations are typically contiguous 2.5–3.0 mm thick images and can be reconstructed using either a bone or soft tissue algorithm, but evaluated using bone windows. (Note: At Harborview Medical Center [HMC] we reconstruct with high-resolution bone algorithm.)

Since helical CT produces large numbers of axial images, the review of the examination is substantially facilitated by use of PACS (Picture Archiving and Communication Systems) workstations and the so-called scroll functions. In addition, use of cross-referencing tools on the PACS workstation facilitates identification of specific vertebral levels.

In many ways, the coronal reformations may be reviewed using the same approach as open mouth views of the craniocervical junction and anteroposterior (AP) views of the cervical spine, while reviews of the sagittal reformations are performed with guidelines used for the lateral cervical spine. Particular attention in parasagittal images to alignment at C0-C1 will avoid missing subtle incongruity of the typically perfectly matched C0-C1 joint—a finding suggestive of atlanto-occipital instability.

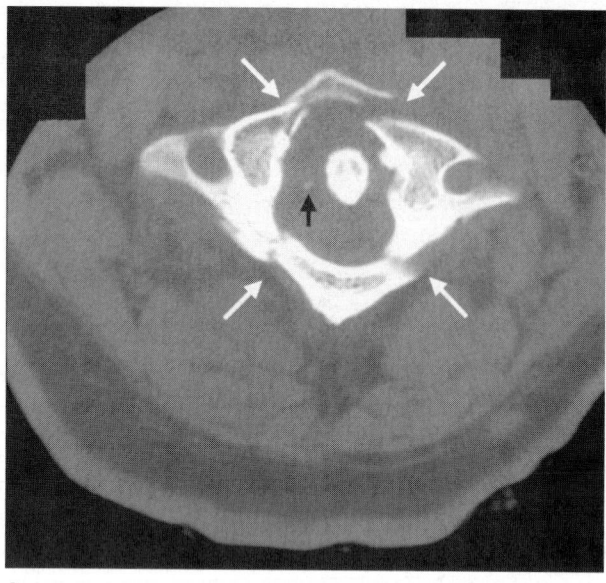

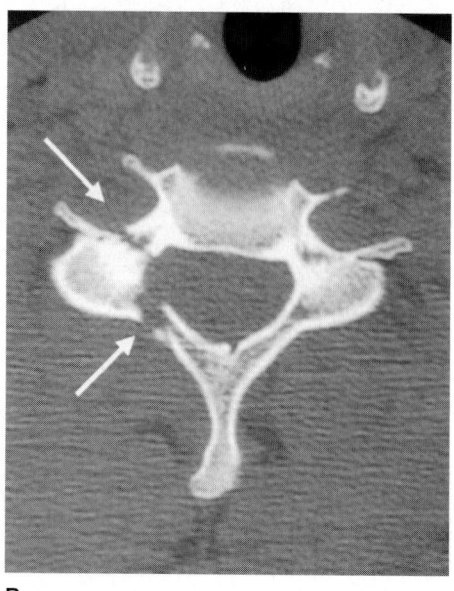

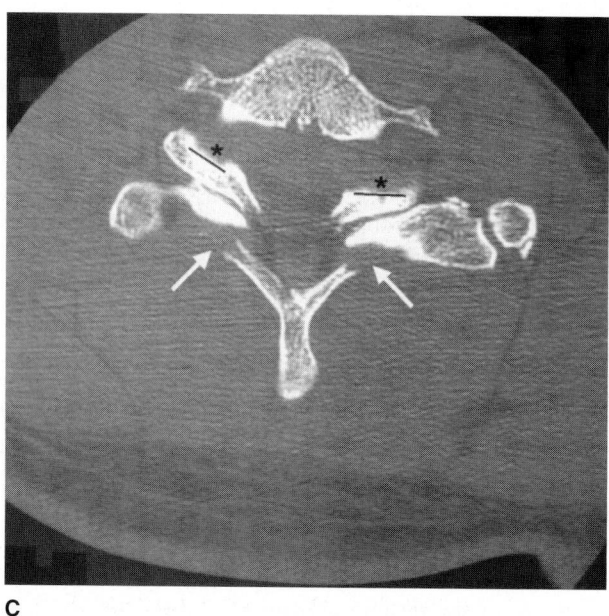

**FIGURE 16-9.** Cervical spine, axial computed tomography (CT) examples of pathology. **(A)** Axial CT at C1. White arrows show a four-part Jefferson burst fracture, with displacement of anterior tubercle on left side. Note increased distance between anterior aspect of dens and anterior tubercle, compatible with disruption of transverse atlantal ligament. Black arrow marks small flake fracture due to type 1 dens fracture (avulsion of dens insertion of right alar ligament). **(B)** C5–C6 pediculaminar fracture shown on axial CT. White arrows mark pedicle and laminar portions of lateral mass fracture. Note lateral mass is slightly laterally displaced, as shown by widening of laminar portion of fracture. *(Reproduced with permission from CC Blackmore.)* **(C)** C7–T1 bilateral facetal dislocation with bilateral C7 laminar fractures is shown on axial CT. White arrows mark bilateral laminar fractures of C7. Asterisks mark empty inferior facets of C7. Superior facets are shown immediately posterior with their curved articular surfaces posterolaterally oriented, best seen on right.
*(Reproduced with permission from W. A. Cohen.)*

Similarly, careful evaluation of sagittal reformations will avoid oversight of "in-plane" (axial plane) fractures, such as type II fractures of the dens and fractures of the horizontal spinous process/lamina. Nonetheless, careful attention to axial images is necessary to detect fractures involving the craniocervical junction,[44] transverse processes (potential vertebral artery injury), margins of vertebral bodies, pedicles, lateral mass, or lamina and spinous processes.

Comment. The sensitivity of this survey CT for acute bony injuries to the cervical spine is above 95% with specificity around 95%. Although CT does not directly show soft tissue injuries to the spine, focal kyphosis, focal lordosis, and widening of the disk space can be used as it is with conventional radiography to suggest associated soft tissue injuries. Some authors purport that clinically important soft tissue injuries causing biomechanical instability are almost always evident on technically

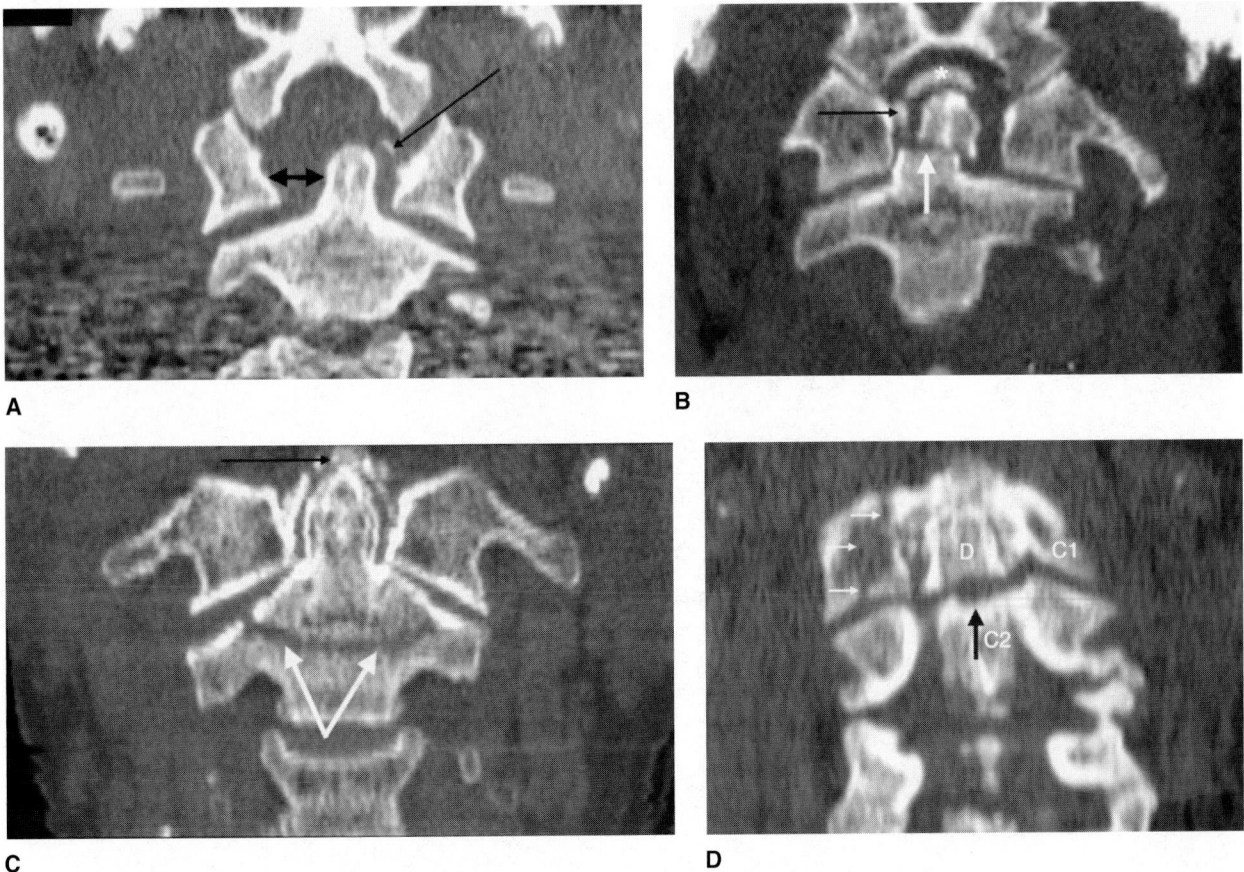

**FIGURE 16-10.** Upper cervical spine, coronal reformations from computed tomography (CT). **(A)** Coronal reformation of craniocervical junction CT shows pathologic widening of right lateral atlantoaxial interval (double-ended arrow), widening of left occipital condyle–C1 lateral mass interval, and bony flake due to left type 1 dens fracture (long arrow). These findings are compatible with variant of atlanto-occipital dissociation. **(B)** Coronal reformation of dedicated axial CT performed at 1-mm intervals of craniocervical junction shows transverse type 2 dens fracture (white arrow). Black arrow marks tubercle on C1 for the insertion of transverse atlantal ligament. Asterisk marks osteophyte at superior margin of C1 portion of anterior atlantodens articulation, a common finding in older patients. **(C)** Coronal reformations from CT survey of cervical spine in patient who sustained high-energy trauma (performed at 2.5-mm slice thickness) shows type 3 dens fracture (white arrows), which is minimally distracted. Black arrow notes osteophyte seen at superior margin of C1 tubercle of the anterior atlantodens articulation. **(D)** Coronal reformations from survey CT of cervical spine focused at craniocervical junction. Black arrow demonstrates displaced type 2 dens fracture. White arrows show a right lateral mass fracture of C1. Intra-articular (lateral mass) fractures of C1 less often have involvement of transverse atlantal ligament compared to Jefferson burst fractures, which are more commonly extra-articular or minimally intra-articular.

---

adequate CTs of the cervical spine (especially on the sagittal and parasagittal reformations).[45]

## Conventional Radiographs of the Spine

General Indications.   Clinical decision rules and expert recommendations[46–49] provide guidelines as to who does not require an image survey of the cervical spine (Figs. 16-13 and 16-16). Basically, oriented asymptomatic individuals without findings at physical examination following trauma do not require subsequent imaging.

Imaging of the thoracic and lumbar spine following blunt trauma injury is indicated when patients present with one or more of the following: (1) signs or symptoms of local injury (pain, tenderness, interspinous step-off); (2) depressed level of consciousness, including intoxication; (3) acute myelopathy or radiculopathy referable to the thoracolumbar spine; (4) major distracting injury, including concomitant injuries to the cervical spine.[50,51]

Examination Prescription.   Cervical spine: Given the differences in the incidence of injury to the cervical spine in children and the differences in their distribution (far more common in the upper cervical spine) relative to adults,[52] the authors only obtain AP and lateral views in infants 0 to 4 years of age; AP, lateral, and open mouth views in children 5 to 9 years of age; and treat individuals 10 years or older as adults. In the adult population, a minimum of three views, and often five or six views, are required to adequately survey the cervical spine. The minimum views include an AP view of the craniocervical junction (open mouth view), an AP view of the subdental cervical spine, and a lateral view of the cervical spine that extends down to the C7–T1 interspace. To supplement these three views, bilateral trauma oblique views and a swimmer's lateral are often used, both of which are intended to give more conclusive views of the lower cervical spine including the cervicothoracic junction. Trauma oblique views are obtained without moving the patient. The imaging cassette is placed on the surface of the table or gurney on which the patient is lying and positioned such that its leading edge is near the patient's midline and its inferior edge is beneath a portion of the patient's shoulder girdle. The x-ray beam is angled at 45° to the plate with the central beam centered

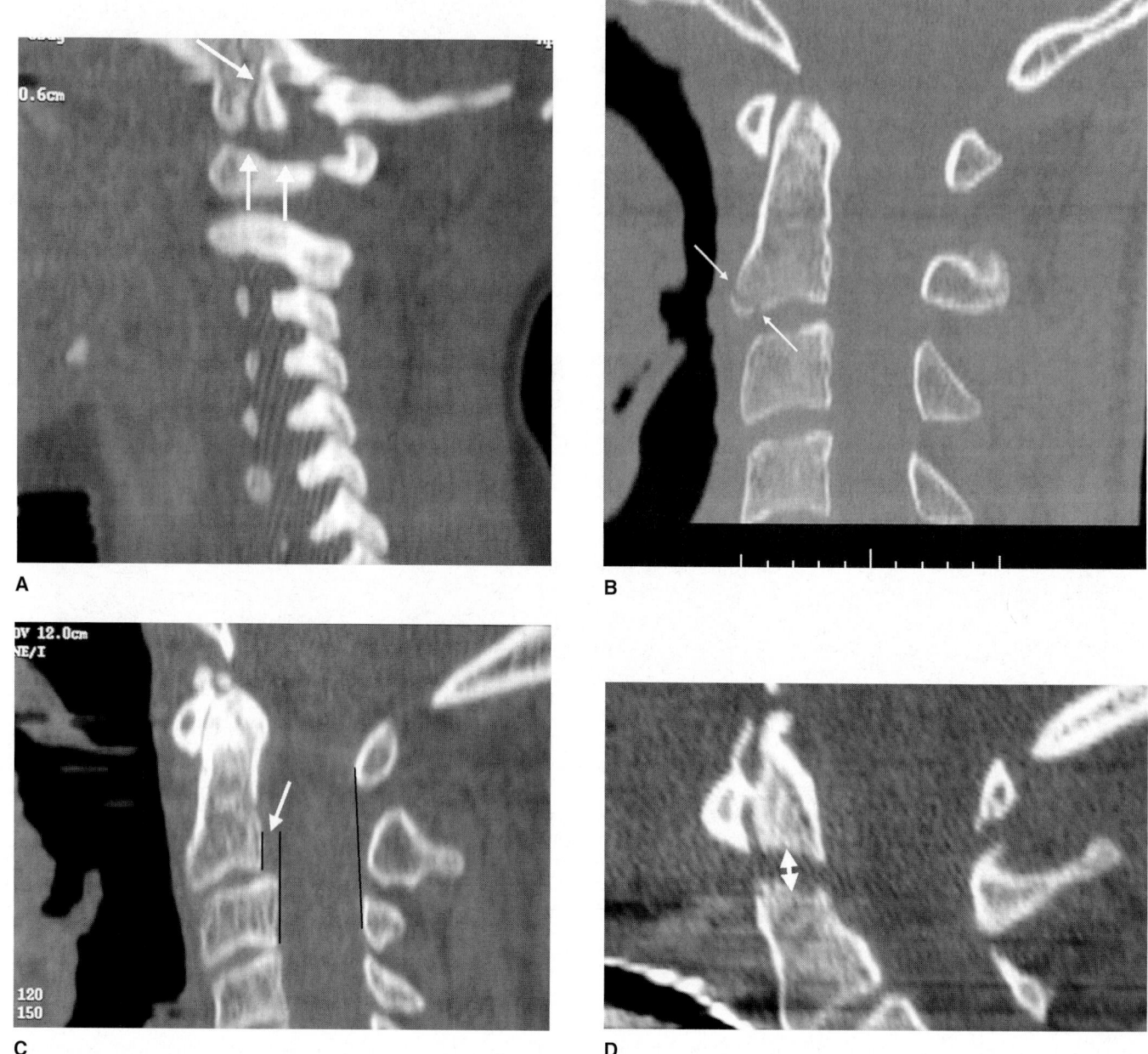

**FIGURE 16-11.**  Upper cervical spine, sagittal reformations from computed tomography (CT). **(A)** Left parasagittal CT reformation. This 3-year-old was run over by a trailer. Arrowheads show superior articular surface of C1 lateral mass, with anterior subluxation of head. The long white arrow shows a vertically and coronally oriented fracture of occipital condyle. **(B)** Midline sagittal reformation shows hyperextension teardrop fracture at C2 (white arrows) in a 20-year-old man. **(C)** Midline sagittal CT reformation shows a combination of anterior subluxation of C2 relative to C3 (white arrow), as well as posterior displacement of lamina of C2 relative to C1–C3 line as manifestation of hyperextension hangman's fracture of C2. **(D)** Sagittal mid-plane CT reformation shows diastasis of type 2 dens fracture (double-ended arrow). Distraction of >3 mm is commonly associated with disruption of anterior and posterior longitudinal ligaments.

on the anterior aspect of the patient's neck, with approximately 10° to 15° of cranial angulation. Trauma oblique projections obtained in this fashion show the posterior elements and the endplates of the vertebral body.

Films of the thoracic and lumbar spine are usually obtained as separate sets of frontal and lateral projections. The upper thoracic spine may require addition of a swimmer's lateral, if one has not been previously obtained as part of a cervical spine series, to show the cervicothoracic junction and upper thoracic

spine. In general, if pathology is identified, the authors recommend "coned" views of the affected vertebral body. This represents more collimated images centered on the level of abnormality.

Comment.    When examinations of the cervical or thoracic spine are technically inadequate, it is almost always due to the inability to adequately visualize the cervicothoracic junction and the upper thoracic spine. Swimmer's laterals are generally

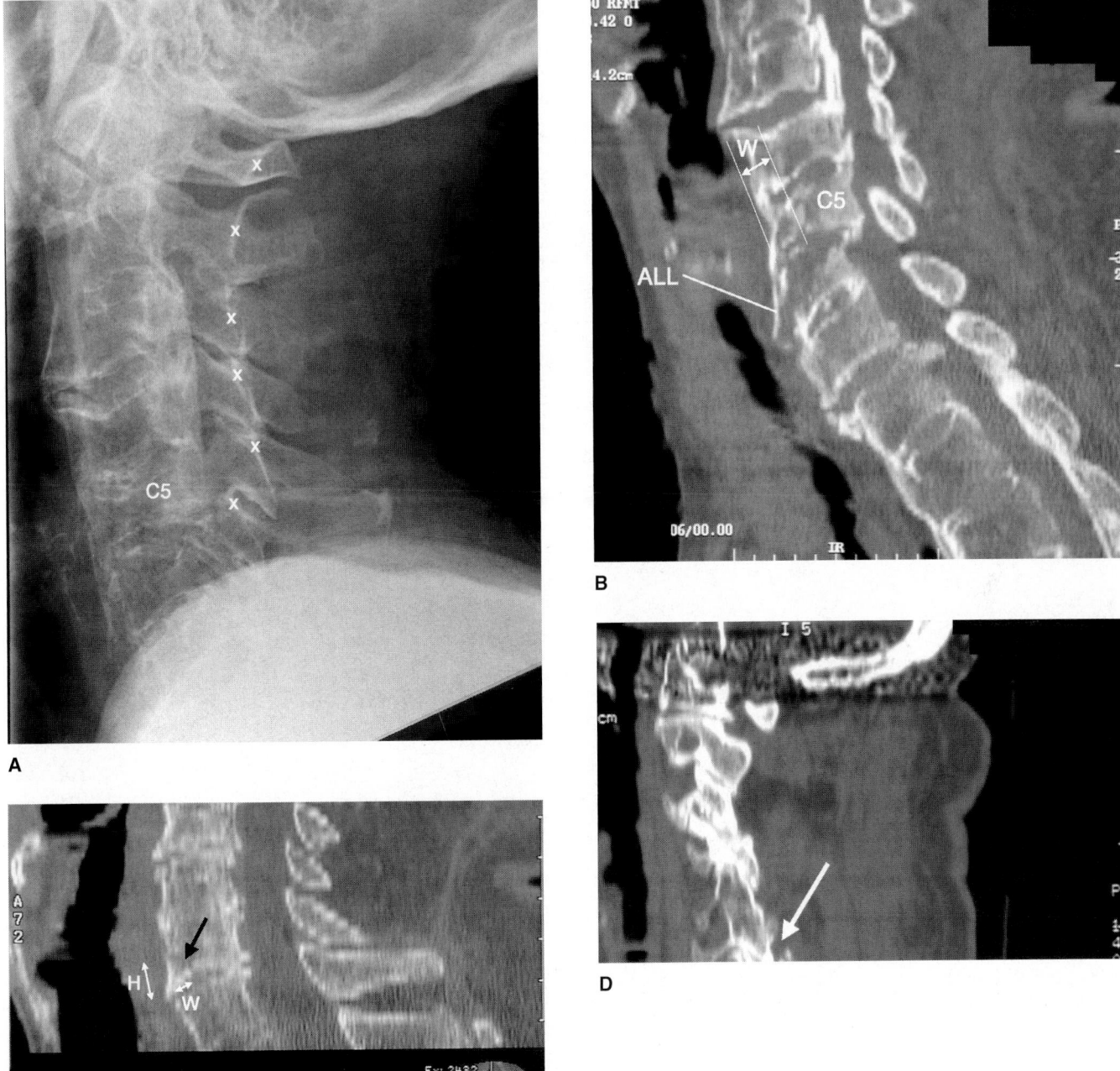

**FIGURE 16-12.** Lower cervical spine, sagittal reformations from computed tomography (CT). **(A)** This 84-year-old woman sustained C5 hyperexten-sion injury in a fall. Lateral cervical spine shows extensive spondylosis but no obvious fracture to vertebral bodies. However, white Xs mark laminar points and show definite retrolisthesis of C5 on C6. Careful attention to laminae, particularly in the elderly, is good practice in detecting translational abnor-malities. **(B)** Same patient as in (A). Sagittal reformation in midline from CT shows complex fracture of C6 with marked neurocanal narrowing at C5 body–C6 laminar level. Disruption of flowing osteophytosis of anterior longitudinal ligament (ALL), seen in diffuse idiopathic skeletal hyperostosis, should be presumed grossly unstable. Extent of anterior, appositional osteophytes is marked by "W" and is fairly typical of diffuse idiopathic skeletal hyperos-tosis. **(C)** Midline sagittal CT reformation shows flexion teardrop fracture of C6 in a 79-year-old man. Mechanistic classification of these fractures is based on relation of height relative to width of avulsed fragment (H and W). Teardrop fracture (black arrow) separates anterior inferior corner of C6 vertebral body from its corpus. In this case, H is greater than W, compatible with hyperflexion injury. In lower cervical spine, hyperextension injuries tend to have greater width than height of their corner fragments and can be either from anteroinferior or anterosuperior corner. Note this relation is different at C2, where hyperextension fragments typically have greater height than width, due to peculiar shape of anteroinferior corner of C2. **(D)** Parasagittal CT refor-mation shows oblique corner fracture through the C7 lateral mass, with anterior and inferior displacement of C6 lateral mass relative to inferior cervical spine (white arrow).

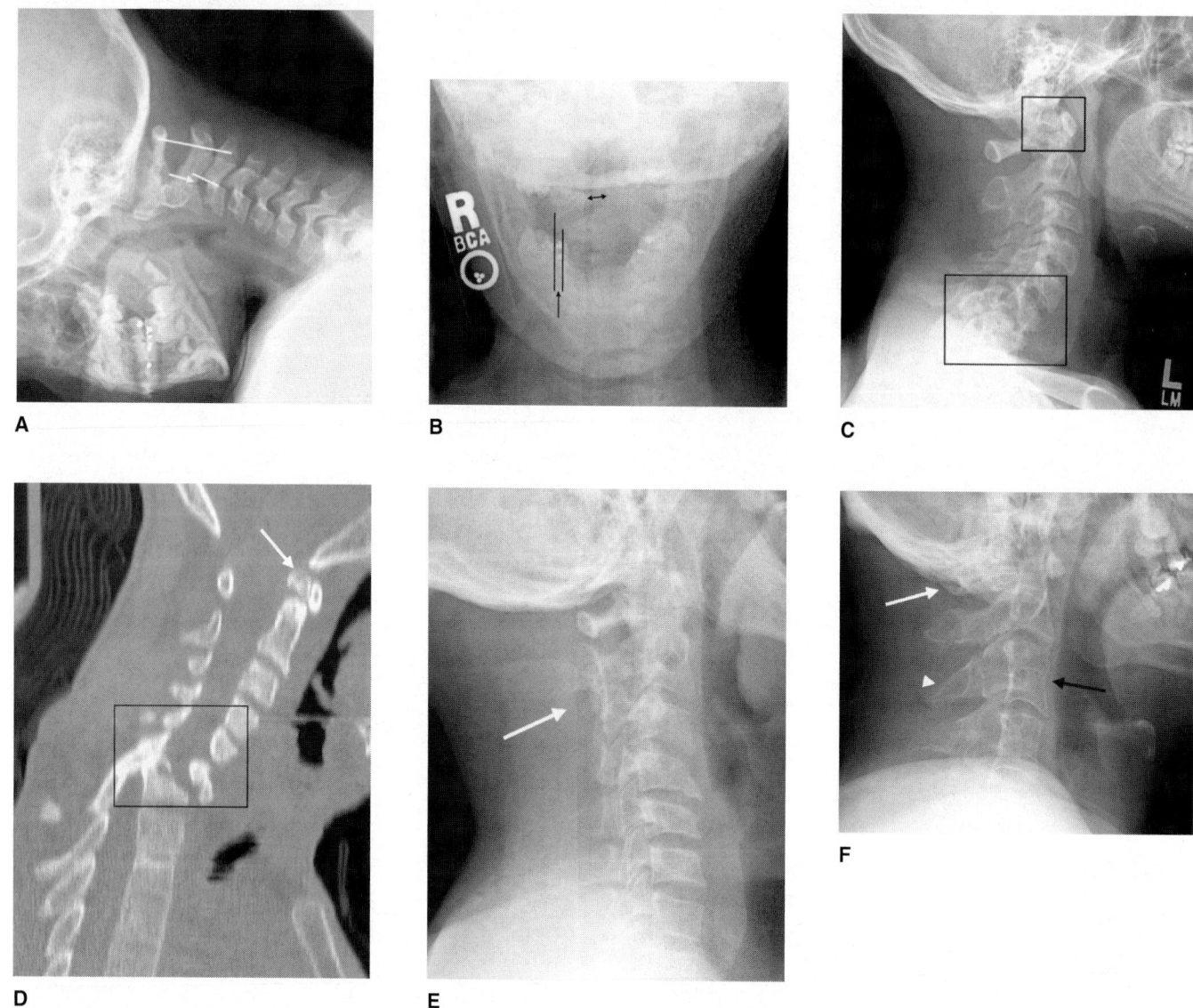

**FIGURE 16-13.** Cervical spine: selected normal variants. **(A)** Pseudosubluxation C2–C3 in 5-year-old struck by an automobile. Lateral cervical spine shows apparent anterolisthesis of C2 on C3 (arrow). This apparent anterolisthesis can be up to 4 mm and be normal *if* C1–C3 spinolaminar line is normal. C1–C3 spinolaminar line is constructed by connecting anteriormost portions of lamina on C1 and C3, and shortest distance to lamina of C2 should be 1.5 mm or less (long white line). Note that approximately 2% of normals, and many young infants, have not fused posterior arch of C1 and spinolaminar line is clinically ambiguous in that setting. **(B)** Pseudospreading of C1. Jefferson fracture is suggested by apparent overhang of lateral mass of C1 relative to C2 (arrow). This is a developmental variant; which is maximal around age of 4 years but may be seen up to puberty. Typically, amount of C1 overhang on C2 does not exceed 2 mm on either side, and the lateral atlantodens intervals (double-ended arrow) remain normal. **(C)** Klippel-Feil syndrome showing os odontoideum (upper square) and complex multilevel developmental kyphosis due to interbody fusion from adjacent hemivertebrae (lower square bracket). While os odontoideum shows well-corticated ossicle, compatible with either developmental anomaly or remote fracture nonunion, lower cervical anomaly is not well evaluated by conventional films alone. **(D)** Same patient as in (C). Sagittal reformation from CT better shows both os odontoideum (arrow) and portions of complex developmental anomaly of lower cervical spine (square bracket). Careful analysis of axil images in conjunction with both coronal and sagittal reformations is necessary to fully understand lower anomaly. No fracture, however, was shown. **(E)** Pseudospreading of interspinous distances (arrow) due to dysplasia of C3–C4 spinous processes in patient with mild platyspondyly and spondylosis. **(F)** Congenital fusion of C1 to occiput (C1 assimilation, occipitalization of C1) is shown by white arrow. Congenital fusion of C3–C4 vertebral bodies is shown as hourglass deformity of fused anterior bodies (black arrow) and fusion of posterior elements (arrowhead). Isolated fusion of posterior elements is almost always developmental or congenital, rather than acquired, and this distinction may be used to determine whether fused segment is acquired or developmental.

obtained with one arm elevated above the head and the other arm in caudal traction. Obviously, when there are fractures of the upper extremity, it may be either difficult or impossible to humanely obtain such studies in a conscious patient. It is possible for experienced observers to substitute carefully evaluated trauma oblique views for swimmer's views; however, most centers

would use CT in a targeted fashion when the conventional radiographs are inadequate to view this area. To reinforce the point, it is necessary to see the top of T1 on the cervical spine and the bottom of C7 on radiographs of the thoracic spine.

One of the common errors made in evaluating the cervical spine is mistaking developmental variations for pathology.

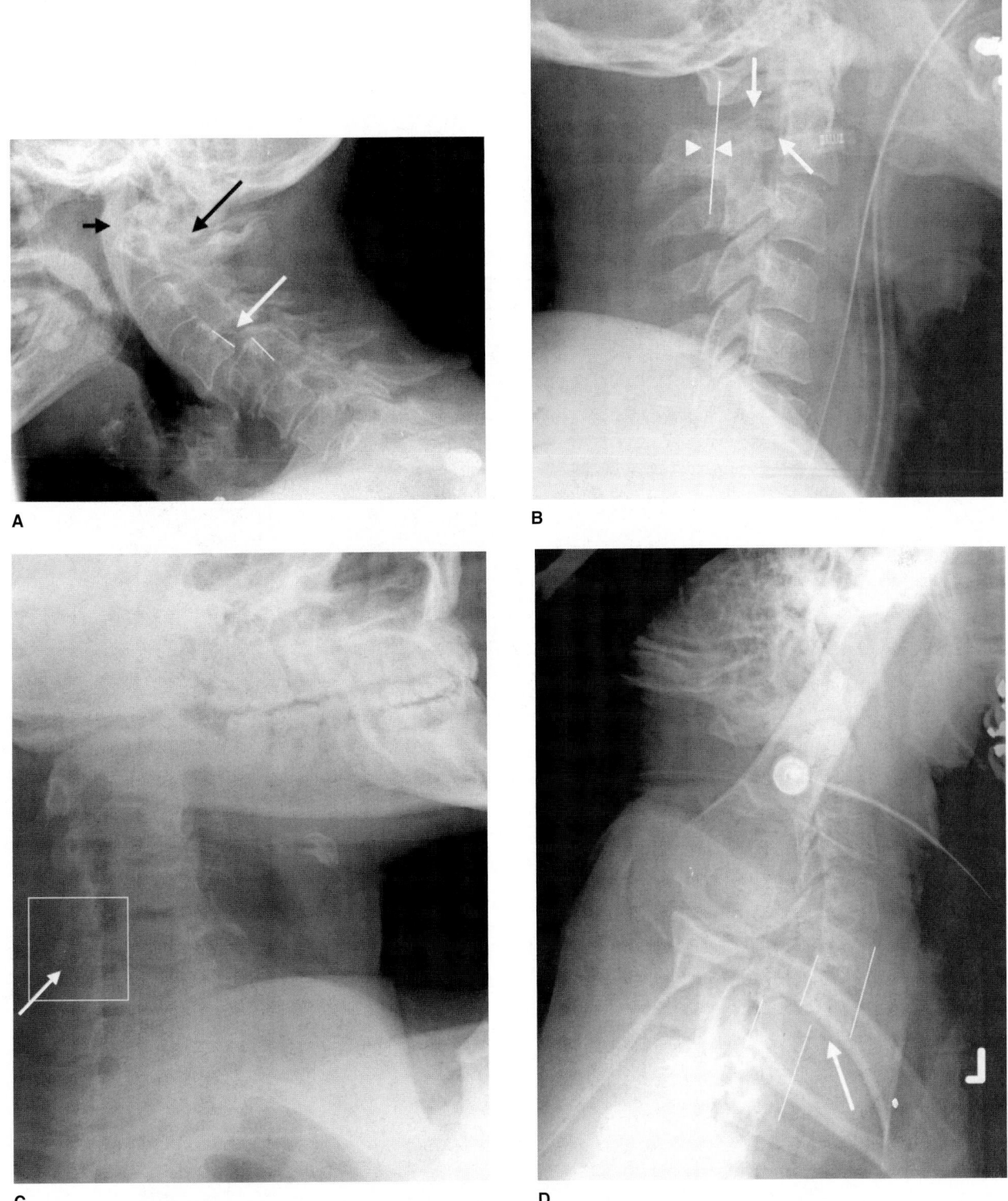

**FIGURE 16-14.** Cervical spine injuries. Conventional radiographic uses. **(A)** This 85-year-old woman fell from her wheelchair at the nursing home. Combined C1 Jefferson fracture and dens fractures and C4–C5 anterior subluxation. Lateral view shows increase in precervical soft tissues anterior to upper cervical spine, with anterior convexity. Short black arrow shows displaced type 2 dens fracture. Long black arrow shows posterior element fractures of C1. While up to 3 mm of anterolisthesis can be attributed to degenerative disk disease if there is concordant degenerate facet disease, in absence of degenerate facet disease anterolisthesis should be considered traumatic (white arrow). **(B)** This 38-year-old man was thrown 70 ft after being struck by racecar traveling at 80 mph. Lateral view of cervical spine shows lucency through pars interarticularis of C2 (arrows) consistent with traumatic bilateral spondylolysis (hangman's fracture). Note also posterior displacement of C2 arch relative to C1 to C3 spinolaminar line (arrowheads). **(C)** This 29-year-old man sustained right C5 lateral mass and pedicle fracture in fall down stairs. Right trauma oblique shows disruption of imbrication of right lamina (white square bracket) and displacement of portion of right lateral mass (arrow). Oblique radiographs are most useful in evaluation of posterior bony structures, but if careful attention is given to anterior body and endplates, particularly with up-angled views of cervicothoracic junction, body fractures and translation may be reliably depicted. **(D)** This 34-year-old man sustained C6–C7 fracture-dislocation while performing karate. Lateral view (swimmer's view) of cervical spine demonstrates approximately 50% anterior translation of C6 on C7 (arrow), compatible with bilateral facet dislocation.

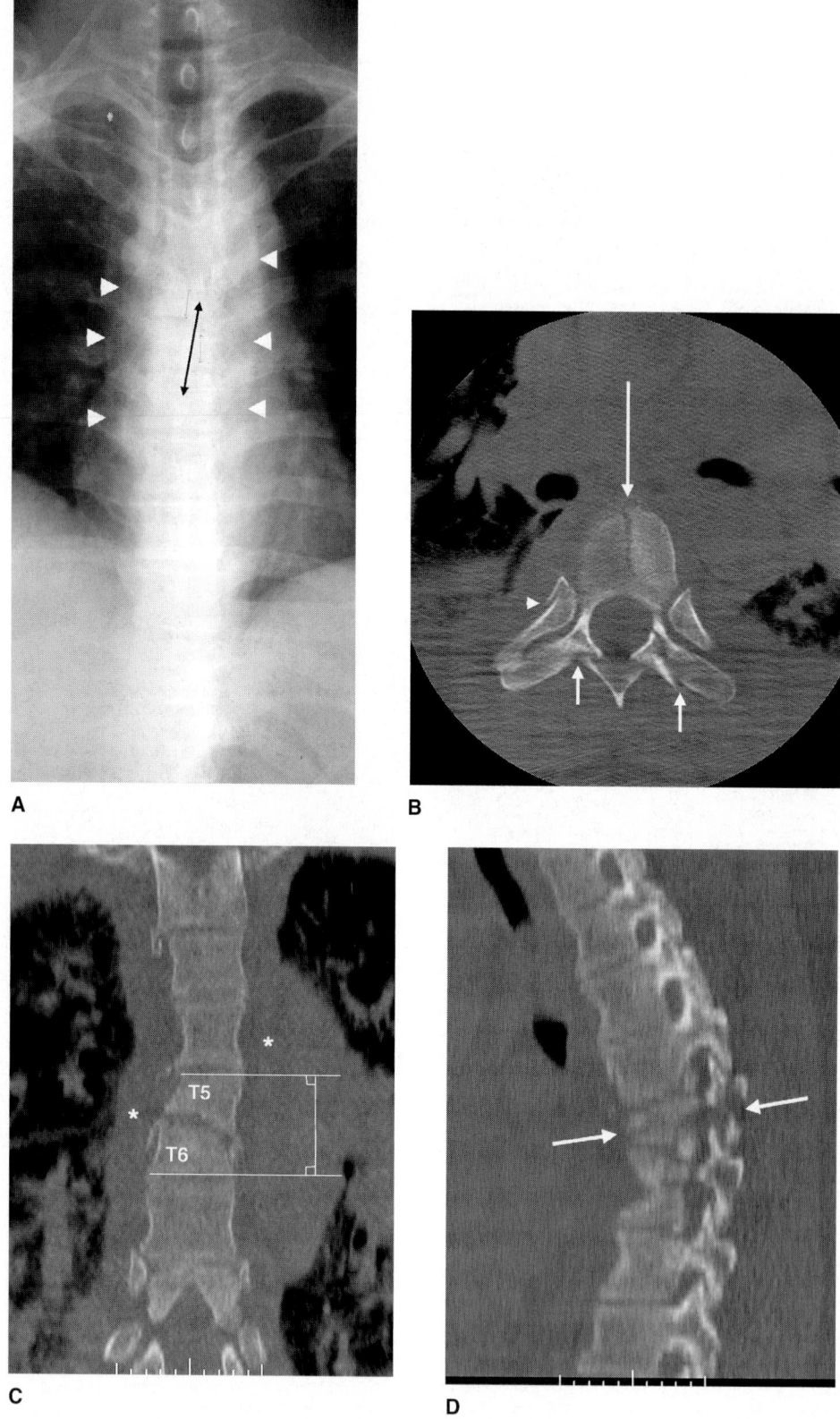

**FIGURE 16-15.** Thoracic spine: T5–T6 flexion-distraction fracture-dislocation. This 39-year-old man was ejected in a high-speed all-terrain-vehicle crash. **(A)** Anteroposterior (AP) radiograph of thoracic spine shows pathologic widening of interspinous distance (double arrow) at T5–T6 level. Large paraspinal hematomas are suggested (arrowheads). Mild left convex scoliosis is present. **(B)** Axial computed tomography (CT) shows compression deformity of anterior column (long arrow) and bilateral posterior element fractures (short arrows). Presence of relatively horizontal (axial) fractures bilaterally of posterior elements or spinous processes is a strong predictor of flexion-distraction injuries. Note associated fracture of T6 rib head (arrowhead). **(C)** Coronal CT reformation shows lateral compression deformities of T5 and T6 vertebral bodies with short local scoliosis, but without loss of overall colinear alignment of thoracic spine. Asterisks show large paraspinal hematomas. **(D)** Sagittal CT reformation shows horizontal plane fracture extending through all columns (arrows), characteristic of flexion-distraction injuries. It is important to recall that these injuries can be at either single level, multiple levels, purely osseous, or mixture of osseous and ligamentous injuries.

*(Reproduced with permission from CC Blackmore.)*

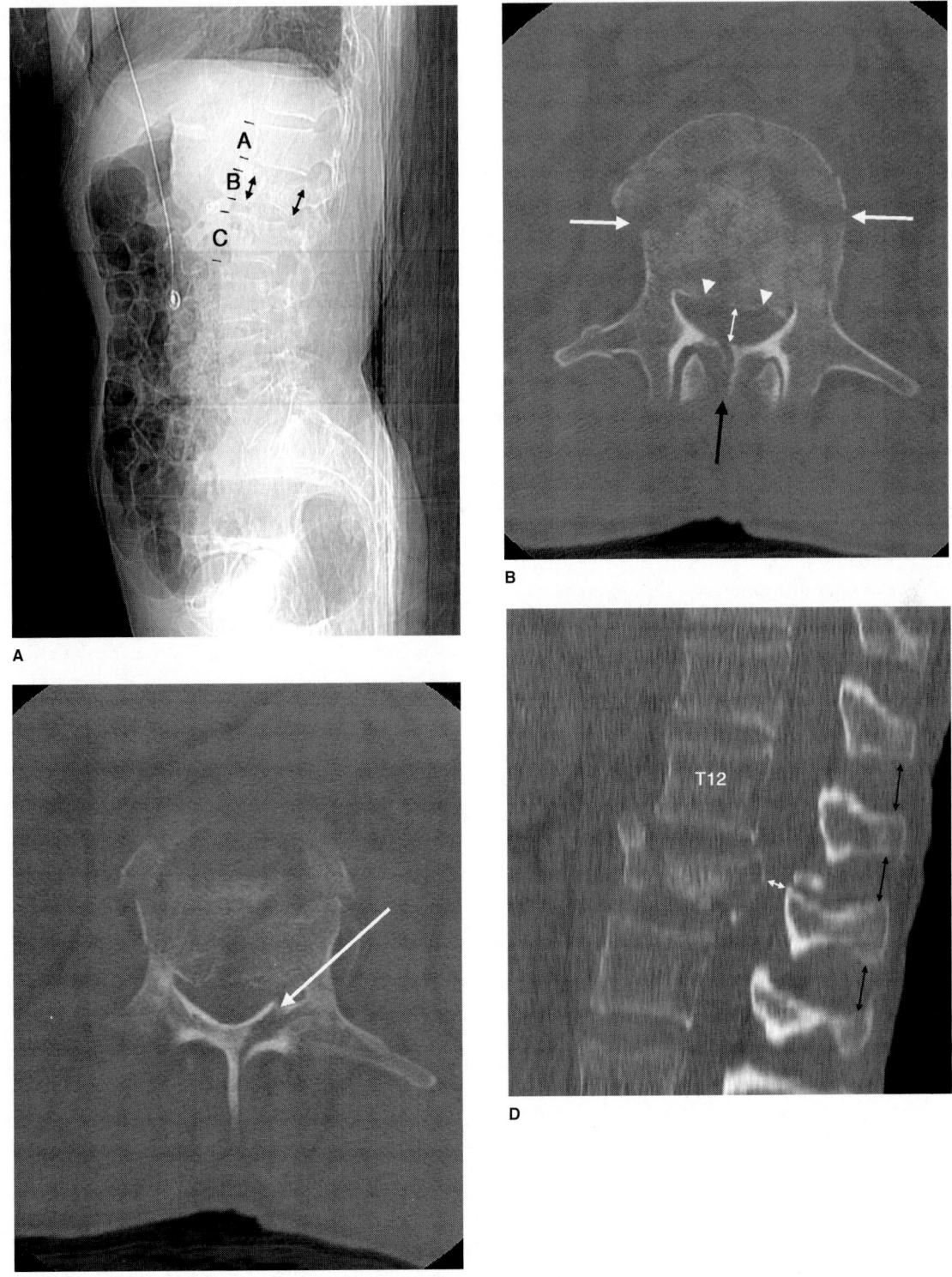

**FIGURE 16-16.** Lumbar spine: three column burst fracture. **(A)** A 64-year-old man fell 12 ft. from a roof. Lateral view of lumbar spine shows loss of both anterior and middle column heights of L1 vertebral body (double-ended arrows). This can be quantified as ratio of B over average of A and C (that is, anterior height of L1 vertebral body divided by average of anterior height of T12 and L2, providing these are normal). Posterior height loss may be similarly quantified. Careful inspection of posterior elements is mandated, where involvement is often best shown on anteroposterior (AP) projection and more readily seen by computed tomography (CT). Careful inspection should include search for superimposed flexion-distraction injury. **(B)** Axial CT of L1 shows coronal plane fracture (white arrows) involving anterior column of L1 vertebral body with retropulsion of superoposterior cortex (middle column, arrowheads). This fragment typically extends down to basivertebral venous complex and is limited by pedicles laterally. Percentage of AP encroachment is calculated as a measurement at level of lamina (double arrow) divided by average canal distance of unaffected vertebral body above and below. Note also "wishbone" fracture at base of spinous processes (black arrow), which may be associated with entrapment of nerve roots and tearing of dura, which may be difficult to see during surgical exploration. **(C)** Axial CT of L1 vertebral body. Long arrow points to displaced left-sided lamina fracture associated with three-column burst fracture. Displaced laminar fractures are also associated with dural tears. **(D)** Sagittal reformation from axial CT shows L1 burst fracture with loss of both anterior and posterior heights and encroachment on neural canal maximal at level of top of lamina (white arrow). Indirect evidence for flexion-distraction injury, such as focal kyphosis or pathologic widening of interspinous distances, is not shown. *(Reproduced with permission from CC Blackmore.)*

Common variations at the craniocervical junction include fusion of C1 to the occiput, which may be partial or complete; failure of fusion or development of the posterior elements of C1; pseudospreading of C1 relative to C2, which may mimic Jefferson burst fractures (most common in the 0- to 4-year age range, but may be seen up through puberty); pseudosubluxation of C2 on C3 in pediatric patients, which can be recognized as normal by a normal C1–C3 spinolaminar line; and os odontoideum (anomalous bone that replaces all or part of the dens axis and is not attached to the atlas).

In the thoracic and lumbar spine, the authors recommend a careful count of the vertebral bodies on the frontal examination to establish the correct levels, based on the number of rib-bearing (thoracic) and non rib-bearing (lumbar) vertebrae. On the lateral, it is important to look at the corners of the vertebral bodies, especially the anterior superior corner, which is affected in approximately 90% of all vertebral body fractures. On the frontal, it is most important to evaluate the adjacent endplates for continuity, the lateral margins of the vertebrae, the posterior elements for pathologic interspinous and interpediculate widening, and horizontal lucencies that would suggest horizontal soft-tissue and/or osseous disruption of a flexion-distraction type injury.

Once an abnormality is identified on conventional radiographs, CT and/or MRI may be used to further characterize the injury for planning of treatment and provide information on the patient's prognosis.

## Computed Tomography of the Thoracolumbar Spine

General Indications.   Among patients undergoing CT of the chest and/or abdomen, review of axial images in bone algorithm and bone windows, sagittal reformations, or lateral and AP scanograms (topograms) may be used in lieu of conventional radiographs to survey the thoracic and lumbar spine.[53] The authors are very liberal in their use of CT for the further evaluation of vertebral body deformities, which are thought to be related to trauma based on conventional radiographs (Figs. 16-15 and 16-16). In addition, patients with high-risk mechanisms and impressive signs or symptoms without abnormal radiographs (e.g., a palpable step-off suggesting disruption of the posterior elements) undergo a thoracolumbar CT to detect occult minimal burst fractures or Chance or flexion-distraction type injuries.

Examination Prescription.   A 2.5- to 3.0-mm axial slice thickness is used to acquire images from two vertebral body levels above an abnormality through two vertebral body levels below. Images are reconstructed using both bone and soft tissue algorithms. Sagittal reformations are made in both algorithms and viewed at bone and soft tissue windows, respectively.

Comment.   In the thoracic or lumbar spine, it is important to have some reference to the scanogram or to the reformations to allow accurate assessment of the vertebral levels imaged. In addition to careful evaluation of the vertebral elements, some attention should be paid to possible injuries to ribs, aorta, sternomanubrial junction, and the kidneys. If flexion-distraction or Chance fractures are detected, careful attention to the aorta, bowel, and retroperitoneal structures, including the ureteropelvic junction, is appropriate.

## Magnetic Resonance Imaging of the Spine

General Indications.   The principal indications for MRI are to characterize soft tissue injuries associated with vertebral body fractures and luxations, and to assess the neural elements (Fig. 16-17). Edema of the spinal cord has a much better prognosis than hemorrhage into the cord, and MRI in the subacute setting can help make this distinction, as well as detect epidural hematomas that may require treatment. Furthermore, evaluations of the disk spaces, ligaments, and facet joints, including the cranio-occipital articulation, are helpful. MRI is indicated in individuals who have no conventional radiographic or CT abnormality, but who have an acute myelopathy or radiculopathy (spinal cord injury without radiographic abnormality, SCIWORA).

The use of MRI is frequently controversial in the setting of dislocation of bilateral or unilateral facets. The local practice is to first reduce the dislocation, with subsequent imaging, but this is a practice that varies from institution to institution. In general, emergent MRI is appropriate when there is an evolving neurologic deficit or neurologic deficits without explanation.

Examination Prescription.   Sagittal and axial T1-weighted and fluid-sensitive sequences (e.g., T2-weighted STIR) are standard. Gradient echo sequences are useful in detecting an artifact of magnetic susceptibility, a finding in the acute and subacute setting that allows more reliable assignment of a fluid collection to being blood. When assessing the transverse atlantal ligament, images should be obtained in the axial plane parallel to Ranawat's line (a line from the anterior most portion of the anterior tubercle of C1 through the most posterior aspect of the posterior arch of C1).

Comment.   MR has been used to "clear" the cervical spine in obtunded or unexaminable patients with otherwise normal imaging (CT or high quality conventional radiographs).[54,55] The absence of abnormal high signal intensity in ligaments and disc effectively excludes biomechanically significant injuries; however, abnormal signal does not imply instability. At this time, MR has not been shown to accurately grade injuries to the posterior longitudinal ligament (PLL) or anterior longitudinal ligament (ALL).

## Flexion and Extension X-Rays of the Cervical Spine

General Indications.   Among individuals who are completely alert and who have normal radiographs and tenderness at the posterior midline, flexion and extension radiographs may be used to assess ligamentous stability (Fig. 16-18). Some centers have recommended the use of passive (guided by the physician) flexion and extension studies using fluoroscopy. While this may be appropriate in very limited circumstances in the hands of physicians of considerable experience, the authors do not advocate this practice at our center and believe that the published data are not sufficiently strong to warrant generalization.

Examination Prescription.   A qualified physician should be in attendance if examination is performed shortly after injury (hours vs. days), and the patient needs to be completely alert and

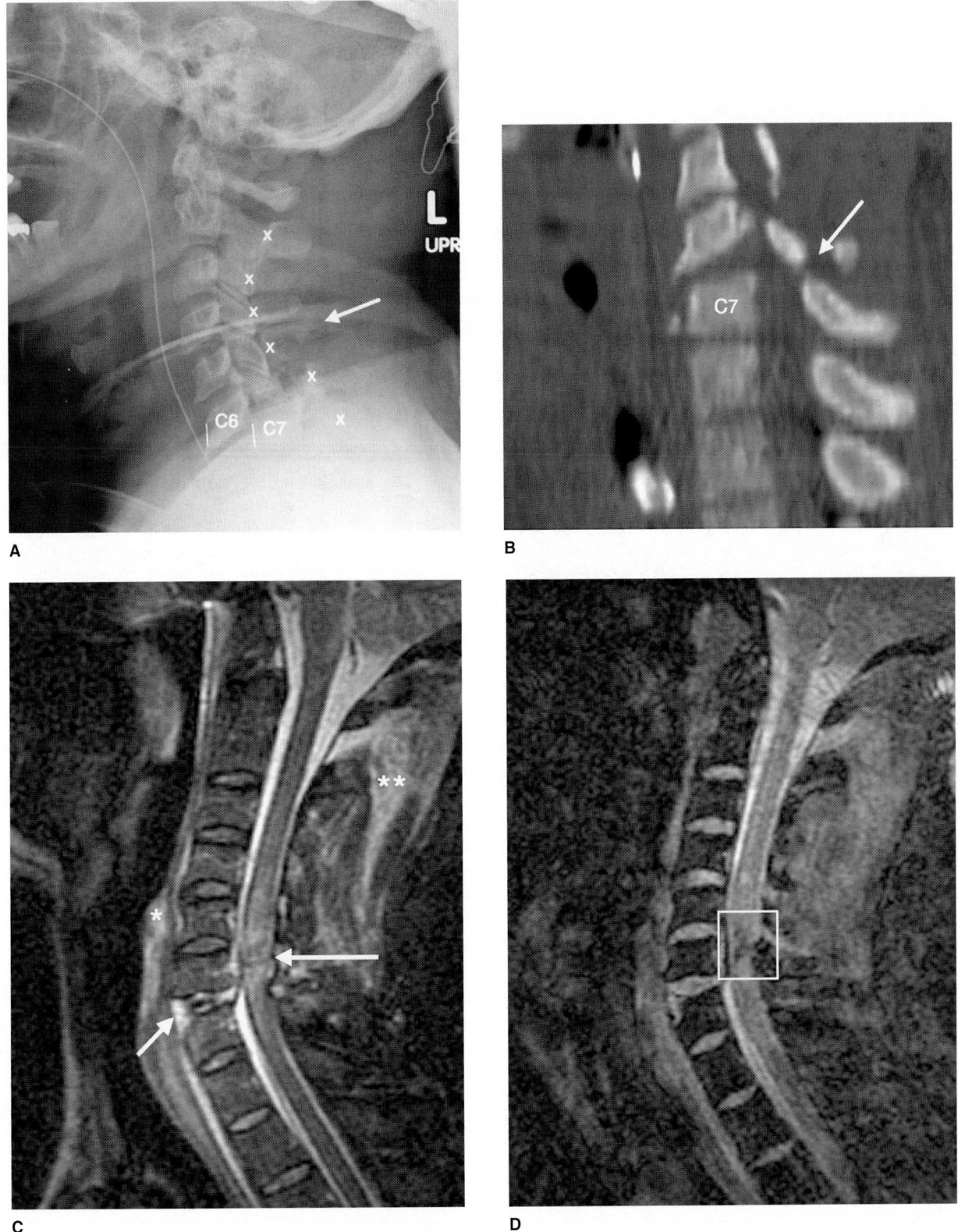

**FIGURE 16-17.** Transmodality correlations: cervical spine. **(A, B)** Lateral conventional radiograph and sagittal reformation from axial computed tomography (CT) of C6–C7 fracture-dislocation, pre- and postreduction, respectively. White Xs mark laminar points and connecting them shows disruption of spinolaminar line at C6–C7. Arrow points to fractures of inferior articular process of C6. **(B)** Same patient as in (A). Sagittal CT reformation shows improved alignment of vertebral bodies but persistent encroachment of neural canal from bony fragments from body and posterior elements (arrow). **(C, D)** Sagittal magnetic resonance imaging performed using short tau inversion recovery (STIR) and gradient recalled echo (GRE) sequences on same patient as shown in Fig. 16-14D following reduction of C6–C7 fracture-dislocation. Single asterisk shows precervical edema and double-asterisk edema in posterior spinal musculature. Long white arrow shows a region of cord swelling with heterogeneous signal, suggesting cord transection at C6 level. Short arrow shows abnormal signal within C6–C7 disk space. GRE sequences show decreased signal at C6 level within centrum of cord compatible with hemorrhage (white square), which portends poorer neurologic prognosis than does edema alone.

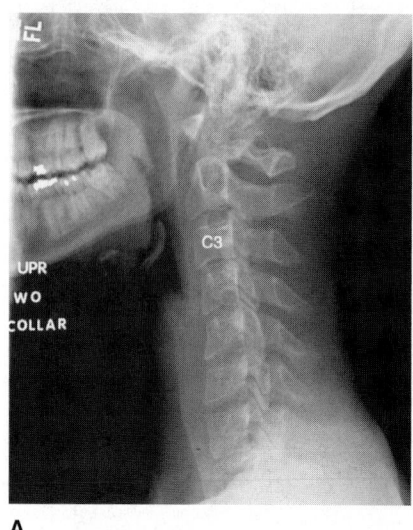 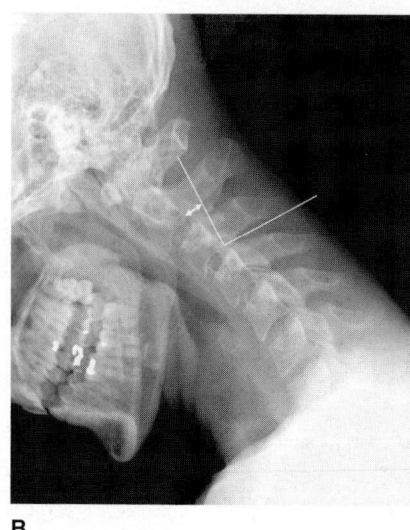 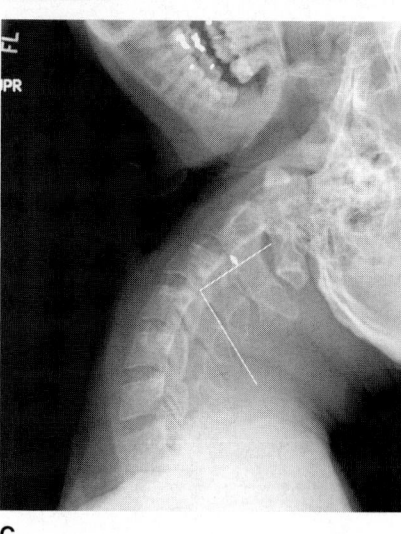

A                                    B                                    C

**FIGURE 16-18.** Flexion-extension radiograph: cervical spine. This 24-year-old male bicyclist was struck by a car from behind. Posterior midline tenderness of upper cervical spine. Dynamic instability at C2–C3. **(A)** Upright lateral out-of-collar radiograph shows loss of usual cervical lordosis without focal kyphosis or translation. Precervical soft tissues are normal. **(B)** Upright lateral flexion radiograph of cervical spine shows no gross interspinous widening or loss of parallelism of facet joint. Reference lines are drawn from posteroinferior corner of C3 to most inferior aspect of C3 spinous process. Perpendicular to that line from posteroinferior corner, a line is used as a reference for translation of C2 relative of C3, as demonstrated by double-arrowed line. **(C)** Upright lateral extension radiograph of cervical spine again shows no gross widening of anterior disk space. Using same reference for translation of C2 on C3, 2.5 mm of difference at C2–C3 disk space is demonstrated between flexion and extension, compatible with partial, dynamic instability.

able to assume an upright posture and precisely follow commands. An initial radiograph is obtained with the patient upright and with the cervical spine in a neutral position. This examination is reviewed by the physician overseeing the examination and, in our center, an emergency radiologist. If this examination is normal, the patient is asked to actively extend to the maximum and a radiograph is obtained. The patient's cervical spine is then returned to a neutral position. This extension radiograph is evaluated in a manner similar to that taken with the cervical spine in a neutral position. If normal, the examination is repeated with maximum effort at flexion and a radiograph is obtained.

**Comment.**    Standards for an adequate examination vary from a range of motion of 30°[46] to 90° (Harborview Medical Center). The authors suggest the larger range of motion, as the test is intended to study the capability of the spine to resist physiologic stresses, and the mean normal range of motion in adults is approximately 90°. If the patient's midline tenderness is in the upper or mid-cervical spine, it is not critical to see the C7–T1 interspace. If the discomfort is in the lower cervical spine or more diffuse, the entire area of abnormality needs to be visualized.

Evaluation of cranio-occipital stability by conventional radiographs is based on detection of translation and distraction between the basion and the cervical spine. In the authors' practice, if the flexion-extension radiographs are abnormal in the acute or subacute setting, MRI is pursued. If the examination does not show an adequate range of motion, the patient's spine is immobilized (hard collar) and the exam is repeated in two weeks (if the patient remains symptomatic).

## Computed Tomography of the Chest

**General Indications.**    Chest CT is generally performed to evaluate adult victims of high-energy blunt trauma (especially those with chest pain, deformity, or hypoxia),[56] with particular attention to the mediastinal contents (Figs. 16-19 to 16-23). Children presenting with hypotension, elevated respiratory rate, abnormal physical examination, depressed consciousness, and femur fractures after blunt trauma are at substantially increased risk for intrathoracic injury.[57] In this setting, CT provides a wealth of information about the lungs, pleural cavities, and chest wall. Indications for evaluating the mediastinum are principally to exclude injury to the intrathoracic aorta and great vessels (sensitivity 97–99%[58]). The role of MDCT in diagnosis of acute traumatic aortic injury has been evolving, and it is believed to be most cost-effective when patients are already undergoing another CT examination (e.g., CT cranium); are at risk for injury to the thoracic aorta because of high-energy mechanism, associated injuries, or age (>50 years old); or have a previously abnormal study (chest x-ray). A decision rule has been proposed by Blackmore et al.,[59] in which individuals with two or more of the following are at high risk for aortic injury: age >50; unrestrained occupant in motor vehicle crash; hypotension; thoracic injury (rib fracture, pneumothorax, pulmonary contusion, or laceration); abdominopelvic injury (fracture of lumbar spine or pelvic ring, injury requiring laparotomy); fractures of appendicular skeleton; or injury to the brain.

**Examination Prescription.**    Axial images are obtained with a slice thickness of 2.5 mm from the thoracic inlet to at least the

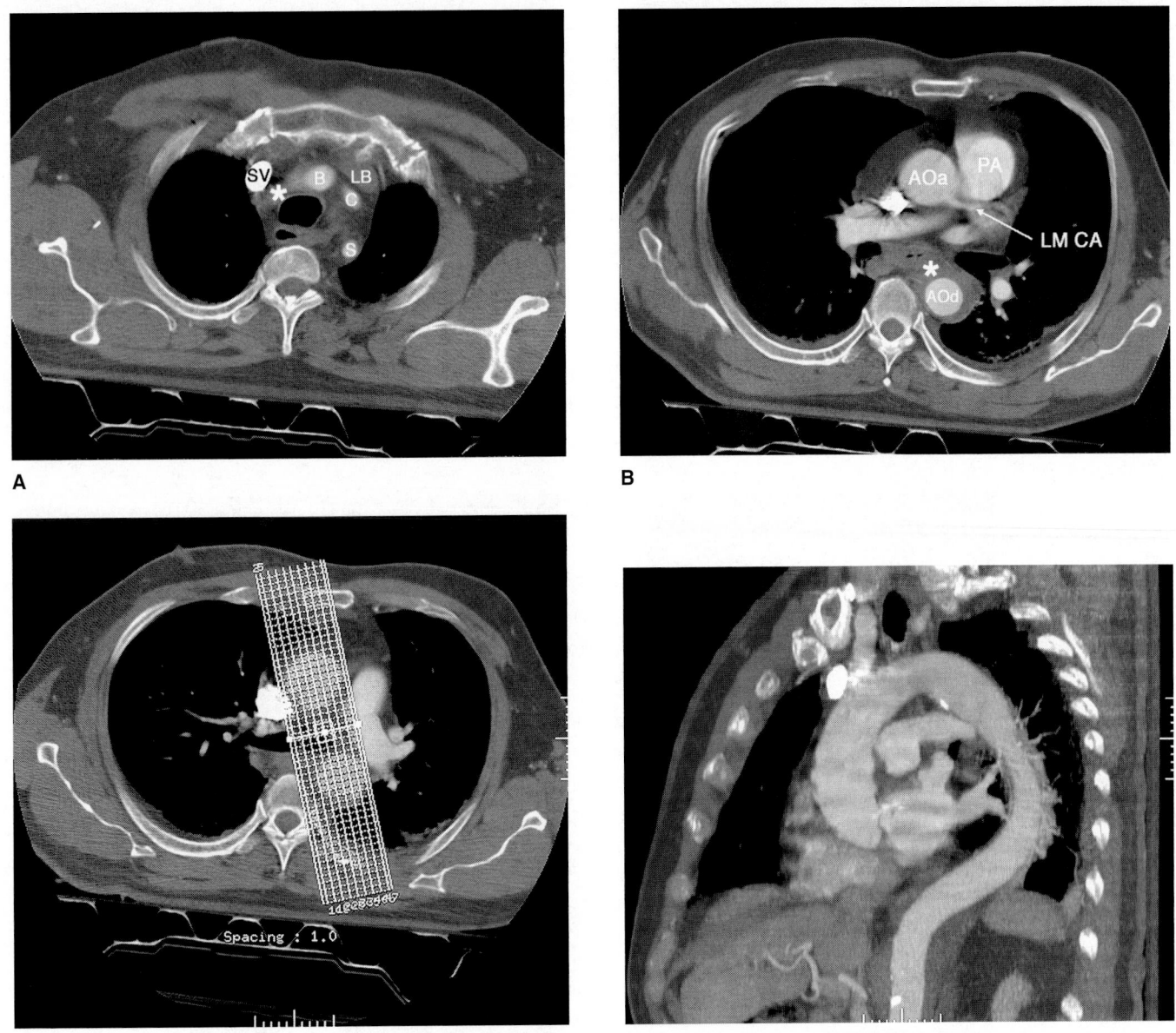

**FIGURE 16-19.** Mediastinal hematoma with normal thoracic aorta. This 68-year-old man sustained multiple injuries in a motor vehicle crash. **(A)** Computed tomography (CT) at level of left brachiocephalic vein (LB). Small amount of hematoma (asterisk) is shown insinuating itself between the superior vena cava (SV) and brachiocephalic artery (B). Left carotid (C) and left subclavian (S) are also shown. **(B)** CT at level of the aortic root, ascending aorta (AOa) is shown giving-off left main coronary artery (LM CA). Mediastinal hematoma is seen in posterior mediastinum (asterisk) with fat plane thinly separating itself from descending aorta (AOd). Right anterolateral rib fracture is present. **(C)** Prescription for multiplanar reformations. Oblique sagittal multiplanar reformations are made at 1-mm intervals and oriented based on source image. **(D)** Oblique sagittal reformation of aorta showed no evidence of pseudoaneurysm or intimal injury. Reformations were made using maximum intensity projection technique, which records the highest value found in volume used for reformation. Thus, intimal calcifications seen in the region of ductus arteriosus and proximal abdominal aorta are seen as density greater than that of intravascular contrast.
*(Reproduced with permission from EJ Stern.)*

aortic bifurcation and through the perineum if there is a known fracture of the pelvic ring. The 2.5-mm images are reconstructed at 1.25-mm intervals for the purposes of developing the multiplanar volume rendered reformations and three-dimensional reformations useful for portraying the anatomy of the aorta and great vessels. Reconstructing the images at 5 mm and 2.5 mm can be used for evaluating the chest and abdomen, and thoracolumbar spine, respectively, at bone and soft tissue algorithms and windows.

In patients unable to receive contrast, noncontrast CT can be effective in detecting a mediastinal hematoma and guiding the patient to evaluations such as transesophageal echocardiography, magnetic resonance angiography, etc.

Comment.   CT is generally the most cost-effective survey study for patients at modest to moderate risk for injury to the thoracic aorta. The role of CT-aortography is evolving and has mostly replaced that previously held by catheter angiography.

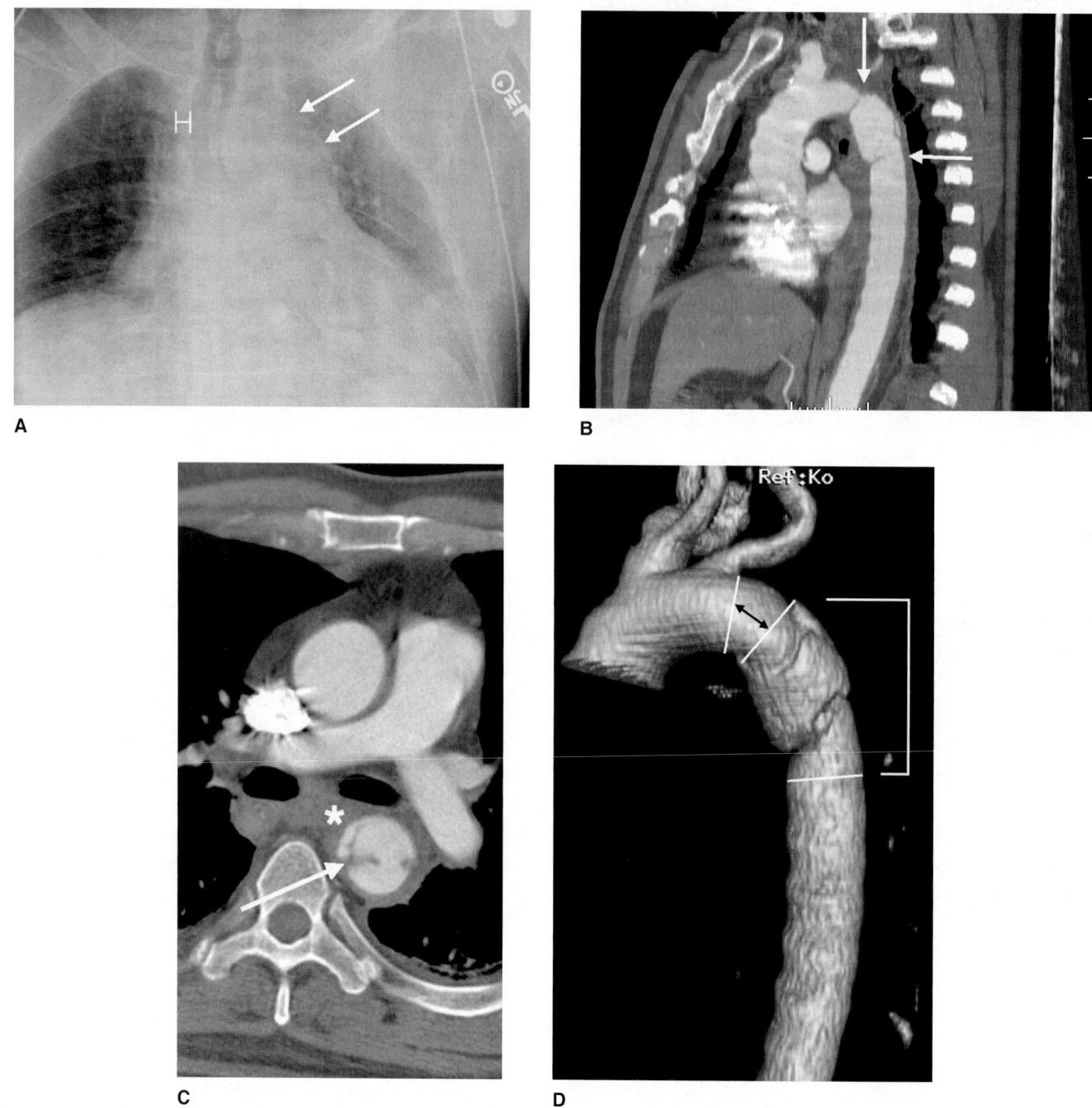

**FIGURE 16-20.** Acute traumatic aortic injury. This 48-year-old man in a motor vehicle crash sustained multiple injuries. **(A)** Anteroposterior (AP) recumbent chest radiograph shows abnormal contour to aortic arch (arrows) and widening of right paratracheal stripe to >4 mm (H). Deviation of left wall of trachea to right of spinous processes of T3 or T4 suggests mediastinal hematoma. **(B)** Oblique sagittal computed tomography (CT) reformation shows pseudoaneurysm and intimal flaps (arrows). Mediastinal hematoma is shown sheathing aorta from brachiocephalic artery take-off into the lower mediastinum. **(C)** Axial images demonstrate mediastinal hematoma (asterisk) obliterating para-aortic fat. Complex intimal flap shown (arrow) as low-density curvilinear structures within contrast of proximal descending aorta. **(D)** Three-dimensional CT reformations can depict relation of intimal injuries to take-off of great vessels, and "cuff" distances should be measured along central axis of the aorta between lines perpendicular to the aortic axis (arrow). Length of intimal and wall injury is shown within white bracket. *(Reproduced with permission from EJ Stern.)*

Findings on CT can be divided into direct and indirect. Direct findings are visualization of pseudoaneurysms, intimal flaps, and pseudocoarctation (due to subadventitial dissection). A mediastinal hematoma, however, is an indirect finding. To suggest an aortic injury, a mediastinal hematoma should be contiguous with the aortic wall and should not be separated from the aorta by a rim of fat. Thus, in very thin patients or in patients with extensive edema and pleural or parenchymal opacification, determination of whether or not a mediastinal hematoma has obliterated juxta-aortic fat can be difficult. Complex atheromatous disease can also make interpretation of the examination difficult, particularly for more subtle injuries.

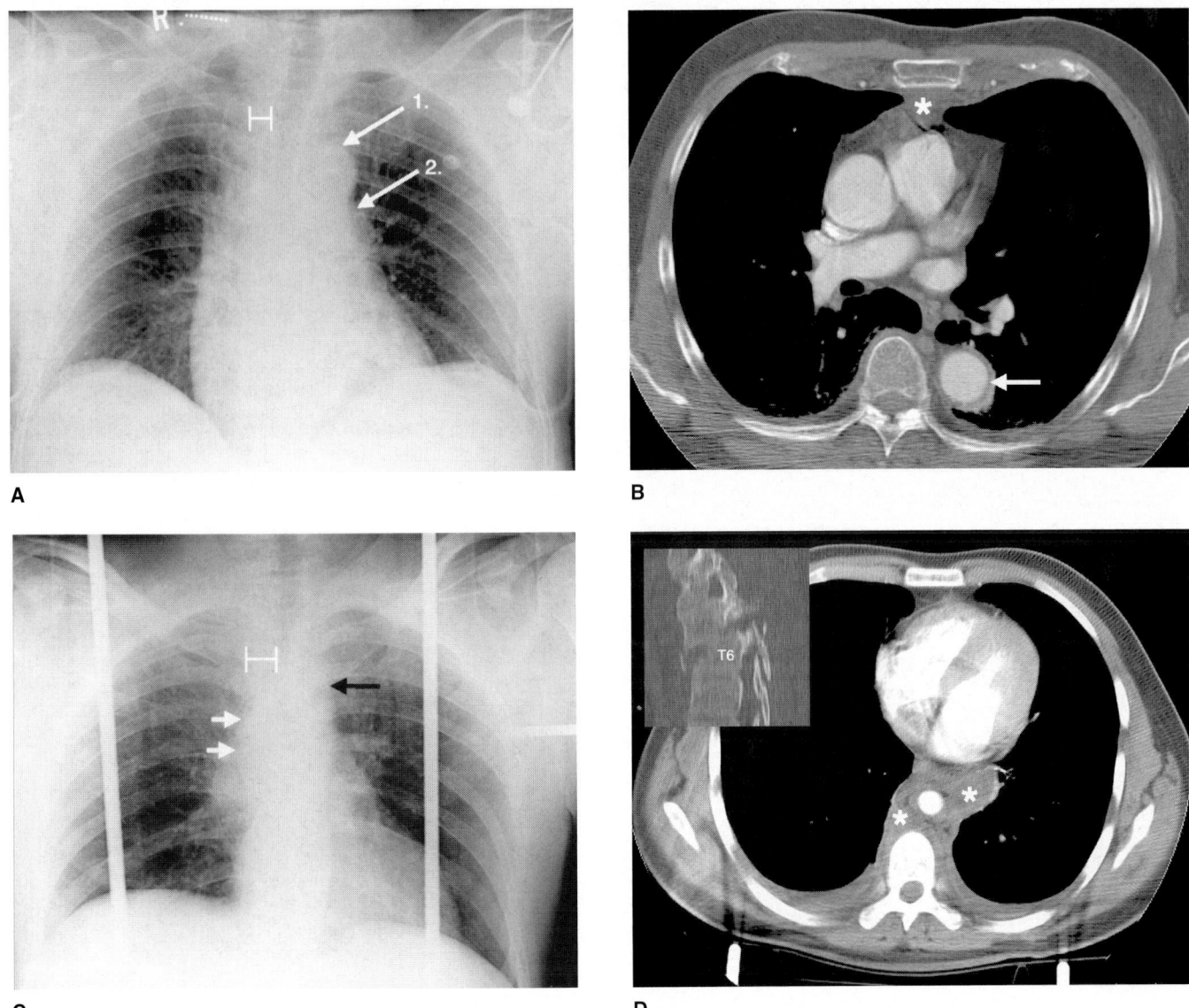

**FIGURE 16-21.** Mediastinal hematoma caused by nonaortic injury. **(A)** This 75-year-old man was injured in high-speed motor vehicle crash with sternal fracture. Anteroposterior (AP) recumbent chest shows widening of right paratracheal stripe (H), with maintenance of normal para-aortic arch and aortopulmonary window (# 1 and 2, respectively). **(B)** Same patient as in (A), axial computed tomography (CT) shows anterior mediastinal hematoma (asterisk). Note maintenance of normal fat surrounding descending aorta (arrow). **(C)** AP chest radiograph performed on 19-year-old unrestrained driver in head-on motor vehicle crash shows multiple injuries, including T6 and left shoulder fractures. Widening of right paratracheal stripe (H), obscuration of aortic arch (black arrow), and abnormal right paraspinal line (white arrows) suggest mediastinal hematoma. In absence of osteophytes, right paratracheal stripes are not typically seen in young adults and their presence locally should direct search for underlying pathology. Left paraspinal line is typically seen due to descending aorta and should not be seen as continuous line between the lower chest and the apex of lung. Continuous left paraspinal line from apex to diaphragm is pathognomonic for mediastinal collection, such as hematoma in setting of trauma. **(D)** Same patient as in (C), axial CT following intravenous contrast shows extensive posterior mediastinal hematoma (asterisks). Partial sparing of para-aortic fat planes and normal appearing aorta suggest nonaortic source for hematoma. Note inset picture showing sagittal plane translational fracture-dislocation of T6.

And, finally, artifacts of the technique, including aortic pulsations and beam hardening due to dense contrast in adjacent venous structures, may make interpretation difficult.

It is particularly important in the presence of an abnormal examination to delineate the anatomy of interest to the trauma surgeon, such as the distance from the most proximal point of injury to the take-off of the left subclavian artery or any anomalous branches. This information is readily provided by CT, particularly with three-dimensional and multiplanar reformations. These capabilities have begun to alter the role of angiography

from its traditional role of diagnosis, staging, and pretreatment planning to one more often used for resolving diagnostic conundrums raised by CT or transesophageal echocardiography, or as part of treatment (e.g., placement of aortic stent grafts).

CT is the most sensitive diagnostic method for detection of acute blood in the pericardium.[60] It is also among the most sensitive methods for detection of injuries to the chest wall, pleural cavities, or lungs. It is less sensitive in the detection of injuries to the hemidiaphragm (sensitivity is 65–70%) or the tracheobronchial

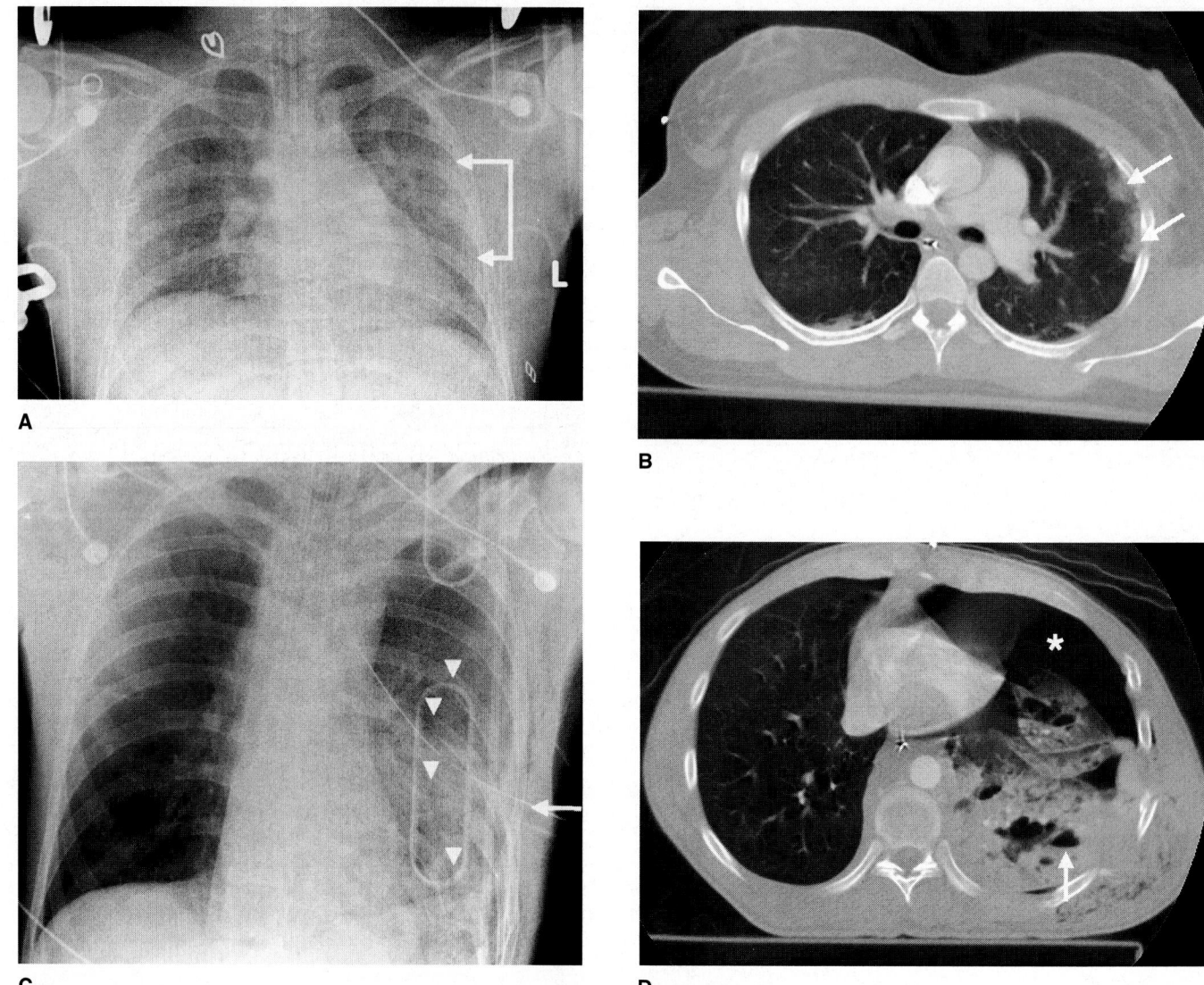

**FIGURE 16-22.**  Pulmonary contusion and laceration due to blunt force injury. **(A)** This 22-year-old woman was in a high-speed motor vehicle crash. Anteroposterior (AP) recumbent chest shows peripheral nonanatomic patchy opacity (bracketed arrows). Pulmonary contusions are typically present by the time patient presents to the hospital and may evolve for 48 to 72 hours. Progression thereafter should be considered a complication, such as pneumonia or adult respiratory distress syndrome. Typically, pulmonary contusions resolve within 1 week. **(B)** Same patient as in (A), contrast-enhanced axial CT shows subpleural location of patchy opacities compatible with contusion (arrows). Atelectasis is seen in right posterior hemithorax. **(C)** This 22-year-old male passenger was involved in a side-impact crash with significant intrusion into passenger compartment. AP recumbent chest shows extensive pulmonary opacities, with mixed lucency seen in left mid-lung (arrow) and multiple displaced rib fractures (arrowheads). Mediastinal contours are also abnormal with obscuration of aortic arch, aortopulmonary window, and widening of right paratracheal stripe. **(D)** Contrast-enhanced axial computed tomography in same patient as (C) shows moderately large anterior pneumothorax (asterisk), dense opacification throughout left lung compatible with contusions, and air-fluid level within cystic structure compatible with lacerations (arrow).

tree. For suspected diaphragmatic injuries, coronal and sagittal multiplanar reformations are useful, as they better display characteristic findings (Fig. 16-24).

## Computed Tomography of Abdomen and Pelvis

### General Indications.

Abdominopelvic CT is one of many adjunctive tests to assist the trauma surgeon in the evaluation of otherwise occult intra-abdominal injury or to aid in characterization of injuries previously detected by other diagnostic tests (e.g., DPL or FAST; Figs. 16-25 to 16-29). Usual indications include abdominal signs (e.g. lap belt sign) or symptoms

(e.g. pain and tenderness) following high-energy trauma. The combination of left costal margin and pleuritic chest pain is an independent predictor of splenic injury and warrants diagnostic evaluation.[61]

Among patients with distracting injuries (e.g., femur or pelvic ring fractures), physical examination may lead to underdiagnosis of surgically important intra-abdominal injuries in up to 15%. In addition, abdominopelvic CT is the principal means of both detection and characterization of renal injuries among adults with gross hematuria, children with microscopic hematuria (>50 red blood cell count per high-power field), or microscopic hematuria among adults who have had one or more episodes of systolic hypotension.

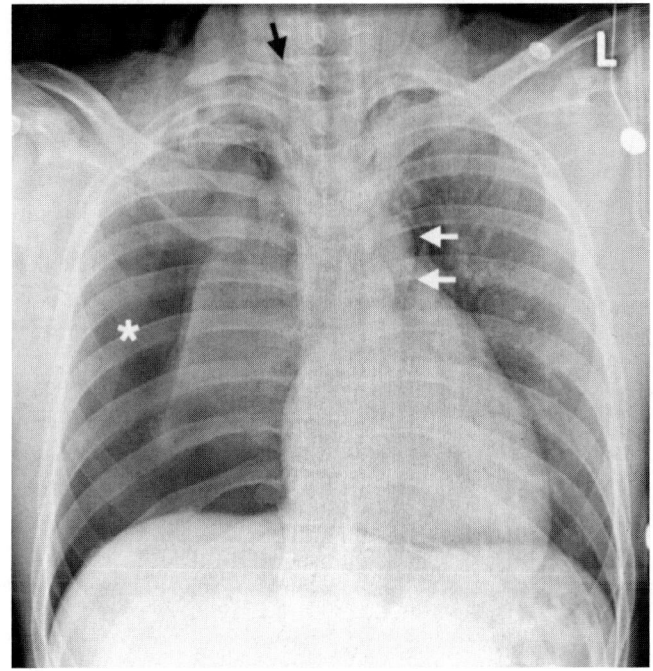

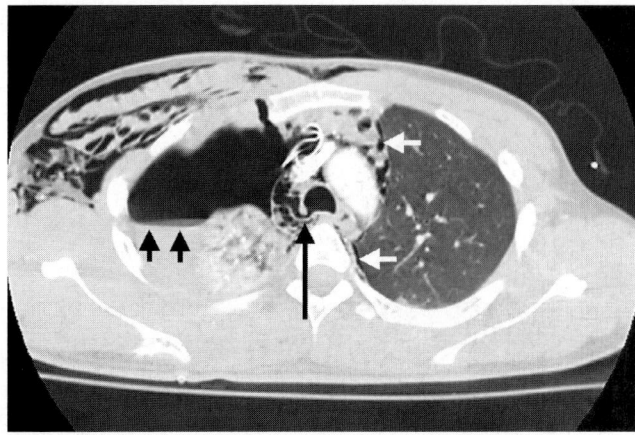

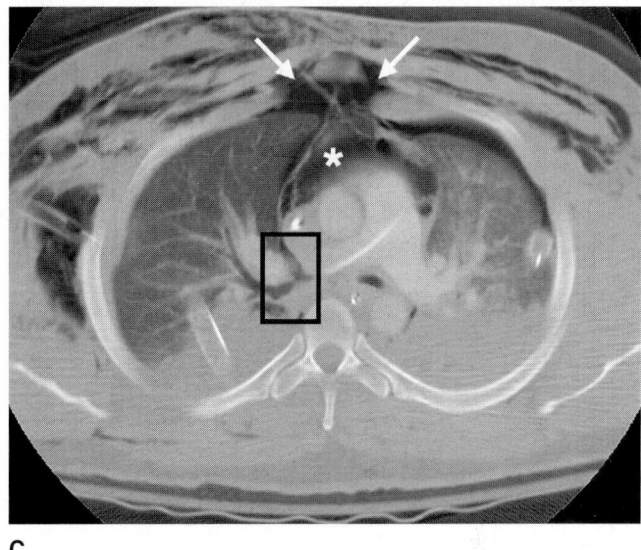

**FIGURE 16-23.** Trachea rupture. **(A)** AP recumbent chest shows large right pneumothorax (asterisk). Pneumomediastinum is shown as lucent lines within posterior mediastinum (white arrows), at base of neck (black arrow), and as "continuous diaphragm sign" projecting over lower thoracic spine. **(B)** Same patient as in (A). Contrast-enhanced axial CT at lung window shows large right hemopneumothorax (black arrows), sternocostal separation on right as air extending adjacent to manubrium, and directly shows tracheal rupture (long black arrow). Pneumomediastinum is shown along left aspect of mediastinum (white arrows). **(C)** This 28-year-old man (different patient) was in a high-speed head-on collision. Right main bronchus injury. Bilateral pneumothoraces, pneumopericardium (asterisk), and bilateral costosternal separation (white arrows) are associated with bilateral pneumothoraces. Focal stenosis of right lower lobe bronchus (black square) is consistent with focal injury.
*(Reproduced with permission from EJ Stern.)*

Indication for CT cystography includes hematuria and fracture of either the pelvic ring or acetabulum or hematuria and free intraperitoneal fluid. In the absence of hematuria, cystography is not necessary.

Examination Prescription.    A "dual-phase" intravenous contrast-enhanced study is used to acquire 5-mm slice thickness from the lower chest to the aortic bifurcation during mid portal venous phase and from the iliac crest through the perineum following a brief delay to avoid "outrunning" the IV bolus and to allow opacification of distal ureters. Images are reconstructed using standard algorithm and viewed at soft tissue and bone windows. In those patients whose arterial or parenchymal phase images demonstrate a renal injury, the authors obtain a series of images through the upper urinary tract following a 10-minute delay using 5-mm slice thickness to detect and quantify extravasation of urine. In addition, for those patients requiring evaluation of the thoracolumbar spine,

chest, and abdominal CT may be reconstructed at 2.5 mm intervals using a bone algorithm, with sagittal reformations, and analysis of the AP and lateral scout views as a substitute for conventional radiographs.

CT cystography typically is performed prior to the administration of intravenous contrast and following the instillation of 100 mL of diluted iodinated contrast. If this shows no extravasation, additional contrast is instilled into the urinary bladder until 40 cm of water pressure is achieved and 2.5-mm axial images are obtained through the bony pelvis. No postdrainage scanning is obtained. Images are reconstructed using a soft tissue algorithm and reviewed at soft tissue and bone windows.

Comment.    The arterial-weighted parenchymal phase images are particularly useful for the detection of extravasation, especially if a pseudoaneurysm or arteriovenous fistula is present.

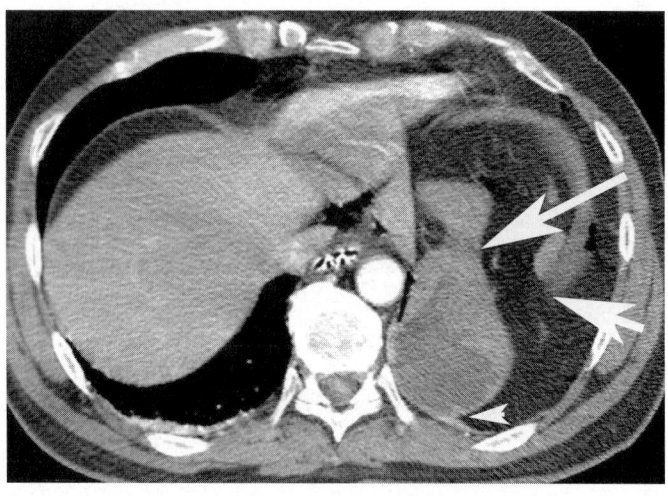
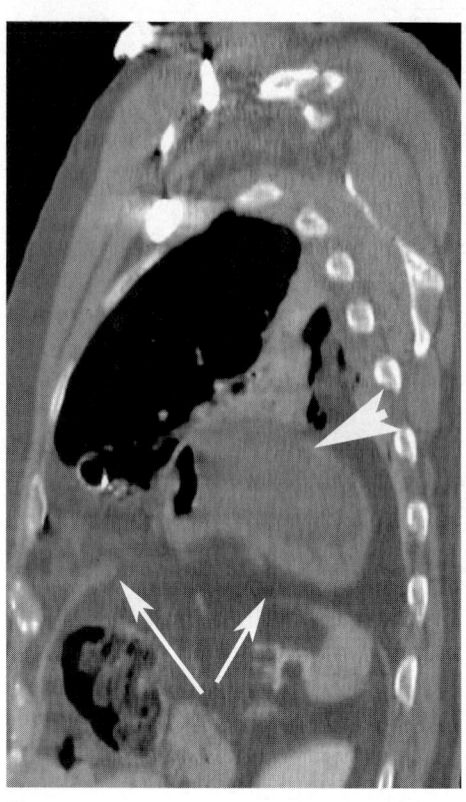

**A**                                              **B**

**FIGURE 16-24.** Diaphragm rupture: 55 year-old man sustained left hemidiaphragm rupture and gastric hernia in high-speed MVC. **(A)** Intravenous contrast enhanced axial CT abdomen shows three of the classic CT findings of traumatic diaphragmatic hernia: (1) Discontinuous diaphragm (short arrow); (2) "Fallen organ" sign, which is present when intra-abdominal viscera (stomach) is abutting the posterior thoracic wall when the scan level is in the upper-third of the liver or spleen) (arrow head); (3)visceral "waist" or "collar sign", where narrowed waist of the herniated intra-abdominal organ is due to compression as it squeezes through the diaphragmatic rupture (long arrow). **(B)** Sagittal reformation from intravenous contrast enhanced CT abdomen shows discontinuous diaphragm (arrows) and stomach herniated above the disrupted diaphragm (arrow head).

Extravasation of venous contrast is seen in 5–10% of victims of high-energy blunt trauma. Splenic hemorrhage is the most commonly appreciated isolated extravasation; however, pelvic ring fractures are most commonly associated with multiple sites of extravasation.[62] The amount of hematoma associated with pelvic ring disruptions directly correlates with the likelihood of an angiographically demonstrable arterial injury (200 cc, 5% arterial injury; more than 500 cc, approx. 50% arterial injury)[63] (Fig. 16-30–16-31). Nonetheless, otherwise unexplained continued hemodynamic instability in patients with blunt pelvic fractures warrant angiographic evaluation, even if the initial CT showed NO extraperitoneal hematoma.[64]

Regarding splenic (Fig. 16-32) and hepatic lacerations, detection of extravasation is a more powerful guide to the need of intervention than is grading of the organ injury. The detection of lacerations that extend to the hepatic veins is of particular importance in the liver, as these have a strong predictive value for failure of nonoperative management when associated with large (>10 cm) hypoperfused regions.[65] Adrenal hemorrhage is relatively common, particularly on the right. In general, it is not of clinical importance unless bilateral, and even then, posttraumatic hypoadrenalism is rare.

CT is relatively insensitive to the detection of isolated injury to the bowel. Findings may include thickened bowel wall, asymmetric mural enhancement, and free fluid not explained by other injuries

(Figs. 16-33–16-34). Nonetheless, when interloop fluid is present, this is very suspicious for transmural injury to the bowel even in the presence of injury to a solid organ and even immediately following DPL. One note of caution regarding free intraperitoneal fluid is that women of child-bearing age have small amounts of fluid (±50 mL) in their pelvis. Patients who have been vigorously resuscitated (especially if they are >24 h from their injury) may have ascites and interloop fluid present due to a capillary leak syndrome. Acute and subacute hemorrhage typically measures 40 to 70 Hounsfield units (H), while urine, bowel contents, and ascites measure closer to water (e.g., 0 to 30 H).

CT performs slightly better at detection of diaphragmatic ruptures than conventional radiography, with sensitivity about 60%. A normal diaphragm contour and no pleural collections or adjacent airspace disease effectively excludes injury to the diaphragm. Caveat: this is not necessarily true in patients receiving positive pressure ventilation. Thus, diaphragmatic elevation following extubation should be viewed as a potential occult injury to the diaphragm. Another pitfall in the search for diaphragmatic injuries is the increasing prevalence of fibrous replacement of diaphragmatic muscle among older (>65 years old) individuals, which may mimic the so-called discontinuous diaphragm sign of a ruptured diaphragm (Note: one should look for adjacent hemorrhage or bulbous retraction to suggest acute injury).[66,67]

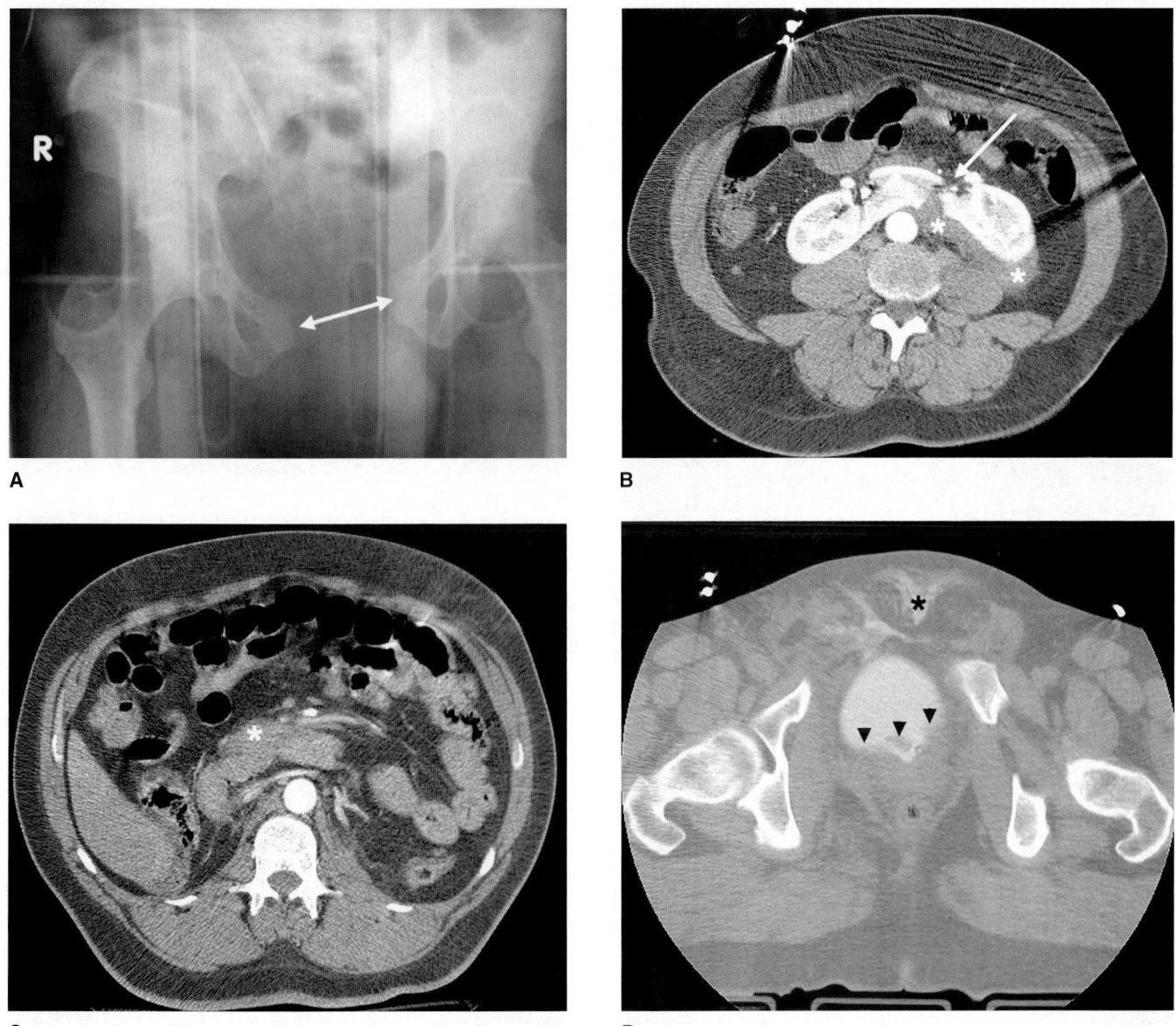

**FIGURE 16-25.** Patterns of injury: central package. This 54-year-old male motorcyclist sustained multiple injuries, including laceration of horseshoe kidney, duodenal contusion, bladder rupture, and anteroposterior (AP) compression fracture of pelvic ring. **(A)** AP radiograph of pelvis. Greater than 2.5 cm diastasis of pubic symphysis is compatible with disruption of sacrospinous, sacrotuberous, and anterior capsular ligaments of sacroiliac joints. Appearance supports AP compression mechanism and is associated with increased risk for intra-abdominal, intrathoracic, and head injuries. **(B)** Axial computed tomography (CT) abdomen at L3–L4 level. White arrow shows median fracture of horseshoe kidney with posterior perinephric hematoma (asterisks). Arterial phase image shows dense opacification of aorta directly posterior to neck of horseshoe kidney and without opacification of the inferior vena cava immediately to its right. Arterial phase images best demonstrate active extravasation and pseudoaneurysms. **(C)** Axial CT at level of third portion of duodenum shows paraduodenal hematoma (asterisk), suggestive of duodenal contusion. **(D)** Axial CT at level of right acetabulum shows widening of symphysis and extraperitoneal bladder laceration as contrast in anterior abdominal wall (asterisk). Posterior wall of bladder is irregular with double densities within urine contrast compatible with hematoma (arrowheads).

## Computed Tomography of the Orthopaedic Pelvis and Acetabulum

**General Indications.** CT is generally indicated for unstable fractures of the pelvic ring, as determined by physical examination or appearances on conventional radiographs (simultaneous anterior and posterior displacement of fractured pelvic ring; Figs. 16-35 to 16-39). Acetabular CT is indicated following reduction of hip dislocations to detect entrapped intra-articular debris and for the evaluation of unstable fractures.

Finally, individuals who sustain bilateral sacral fractures benefit from a sacral CT obtained with coronal imaging of S1-S3 and sagittal reformations.

The general goal of imaging for unstable fractures of the pelvic ring and acetabulum is to aid in surgical planning. CT scans of acetabular fractures are performed for the assessment of fracture types,[68] secondary congruence of the hip (e.g., are the fracture fragments symmetrically oriented about the intact femoral head?), evidence for marginal impaction (e.g., subarticular bone depressed or impacted, and not showing secondary congruence), detection of a

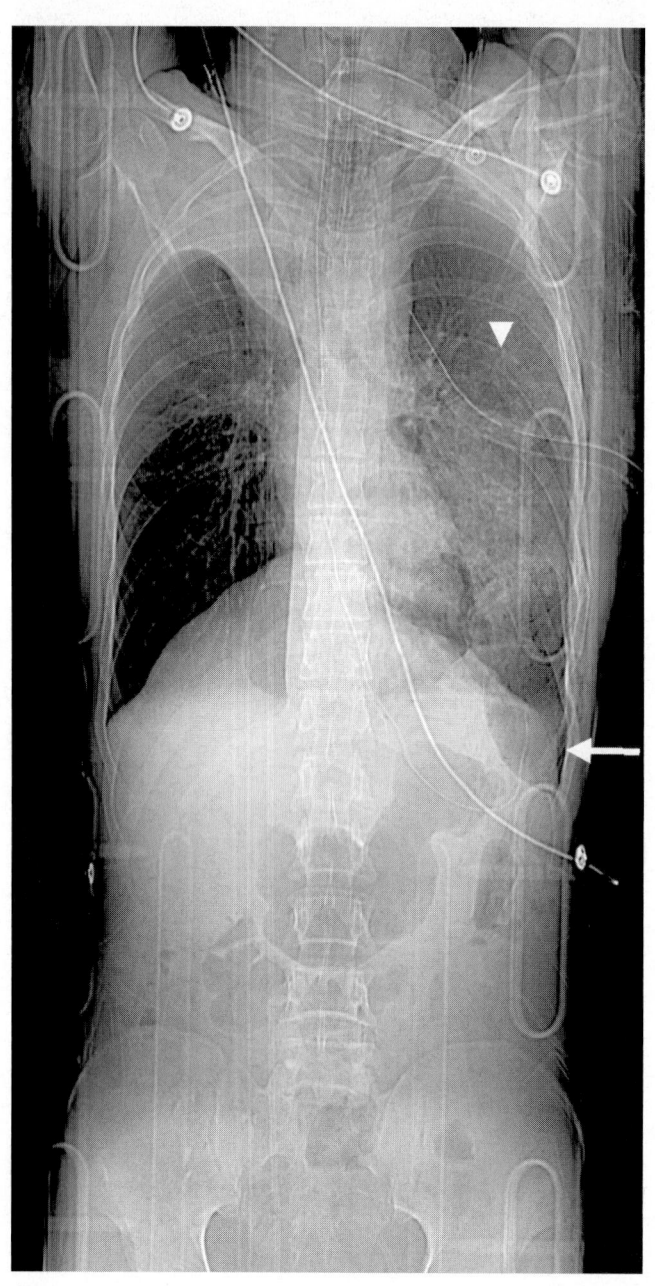

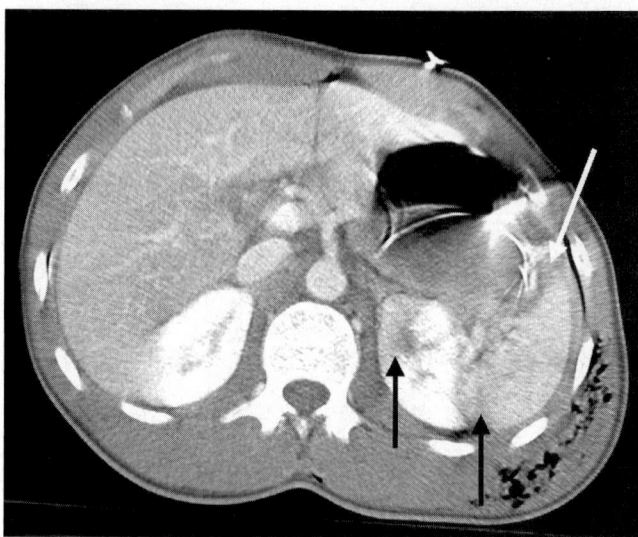

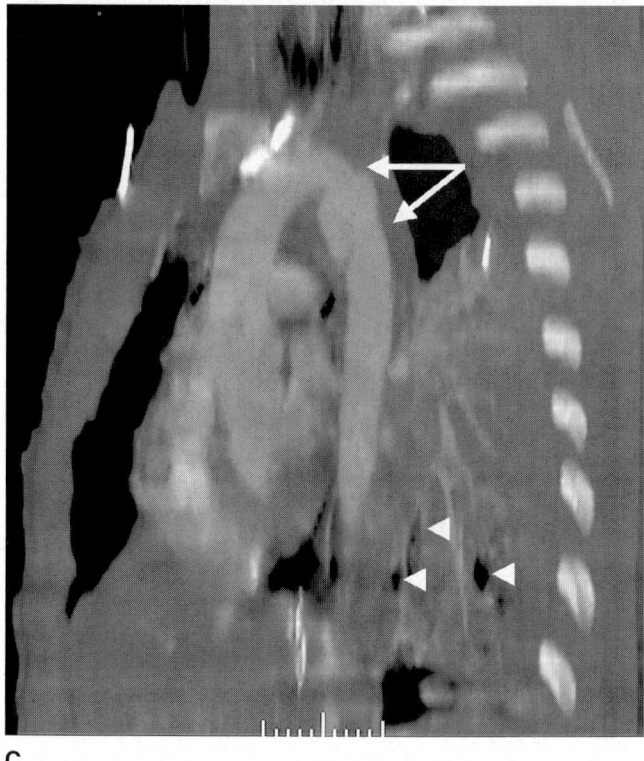

**FIGURE 16-26.** Patterns of injury: left package. This 22-year-old male driver was injured in a side-impact crash with substantial intrusion to driver's side of car. Multiple injuries sustained. **(A)** Anteroposterior (AP) scanogram from computed tomography (CT) of chest, abdomen, and pelvis shows extensive opacity of left mid- and lower lung fields compatible with contusion; a deep sulcus (arrow) at left costophrenic angle compatible with left pneumothorax; and multiple left-sided rib fractures (arrowhead). Patient is intubated, and there is right upper lobe collapse. **(B)** Axial CT of upper abdomen during parenchymal phase shows contusion of anterior portion of left kidney (medial arrow) and splenic laceration with sentinel clot (black and white arrows, respectively). Although rib fractures are not shown on current image, subcutaneous emphysema in left chest wall and distal extent of small pneumothorax are shown. **(C)** Oblique sagittal reformation from CT aortography shows complex segmental intimal injury to proximal descending aorta in the typical location (arrows) and pseudoaneurysm formation due to acute traumatic aortic injury. Air-fluid levels (arrowheads) are compatible with pulmonary lacerations.

fracture of the femoral head, and detecting intra-articular debris. There is approximately a 15% concurrent rate for fractures of the pelvic ring and acetabulum.

Examination Prescription.    CT of the pelvis typically uses a slice thickness of 2.5 to 5 mm in the axial plane from the level of the

L5 transverse processes through the ischia. Images are reconstructed using a bone algorithm and reviewed at bone and soft tissue windows. If using a multidetector CT scanner, 5-mm thicknesses can be obtained by coupling two contiguous 2.5-mm channels and thus allow scanning of the acetabulum without additional radiation. Similarly, 2.5-mm slice thicknesses obtained from

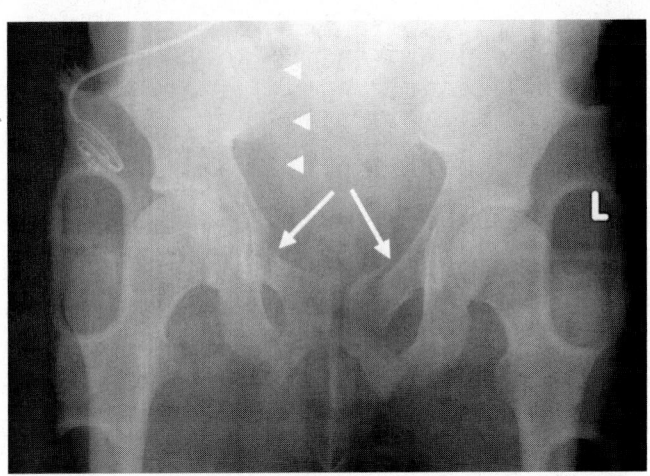

A

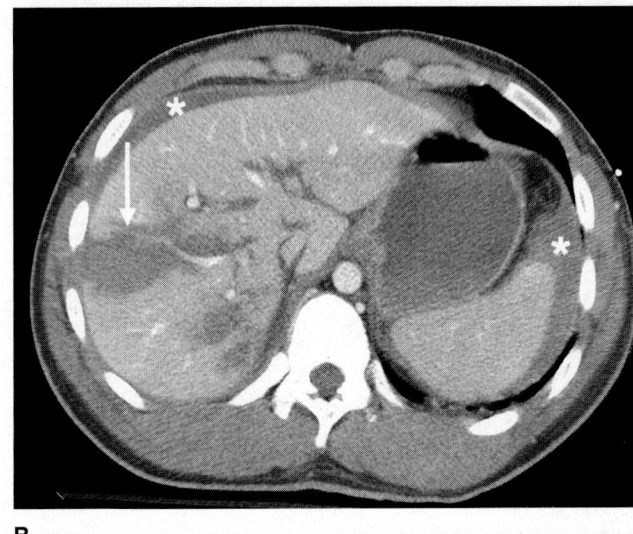

B

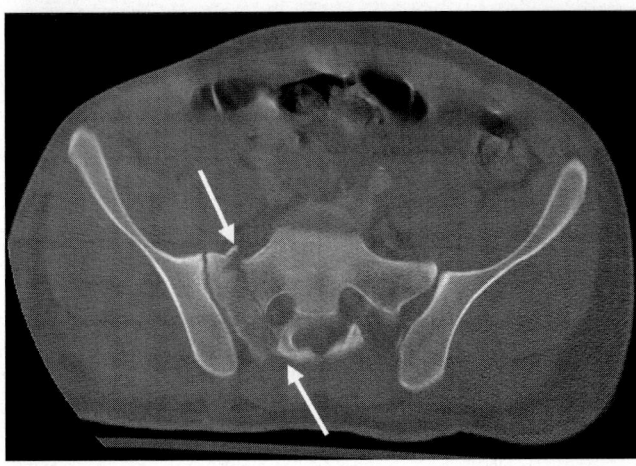

C

**FIGURE 16-27.**  Patterns of injury: Right package. This 22-year-old unrestrained passenger was ejected from car in side-impact high-speed crash. **(A)** Anteroposterior (AP) view of pelvis shows bilateral ilio- and ischiopubic ramus fractures (white arrows) and disruption of right sacral arcuate lines (arrowheads); findings are compatible with lateral compression fracture due to right-lateral impact. **(B)** Axial contrast-enhanced abdominal CT shows free intraperitoneal fluid (asterisks) due to complex ("bear claw") collection of liver lacerations (arrow). **(C)** Axial computed tomography through S1, bone windows, shows through-and-through fracture of S1 ala, which traverses S1 neuroforamina (white arrows). Such through-and-through fractures are typically associated with biomechanical instability.

multidetector scanning may be reconstructed at 1.25-mm intervals when bilateral sacral fractures are present to obtain oblique coronal (in plane of S1-S3 sacral promontory) and sagittal reformations of diagnostic quality.

Acetabular CTs are usually performed using a slice thickness of 2.5 to 3.0 mm in the axial plane through the acetabulae, with 5 mm slick thickness in the remainder of the bony pelvis. If PACS is not available, the authors typically will also reconstruct the affected acetabulum using a display field of view (DFOV) of 10 to 20 cm (a magnification factor of 1.5 to 1.8 X). Occasionally, sagittal and coronal reformations may be helpful in better depicting anatomy.

Comment.    In assessing CT for a disruption of the pelvic ring, it is important to correlate with at least an AP radiograph for the pelvis. A top to bottom, posterior to anterior approach of reviewing images is recommended, such that the authors initiate

their review at the level of L5 looking for avulsions of the transverse processes due to the iliolumbar ligament and the posterior superior iliac spine due to the strong posterior sacroiliac ligaments. The sacroiliac joints are subsequently assessed for their side-to-side symmetry and integrity of their subchondral white lines. The anterior surface of the sacrum is carefully evaluated for "buckle" fractures due to internal rotation of the hemipelvis as seen with the most common fracture mechanism, internal rotation of the hemipelvis due to a lateral impact (lateral compression mechanism). Fractures of the sacrum are assessed relative to the neural canals, particularly at S1 and S2, the neural foramina from S1 through S5, and the origins of the sacrospinous and the sacrotuberous ligaments. Fractures of the ilio- and ischiopubic rami are assessed for their orientation (lateral compression fractures typically show orientation in the axial plane or coronal plane, while AP compression and vertical shear fractures will show orientation in the sagittal plane). The normal

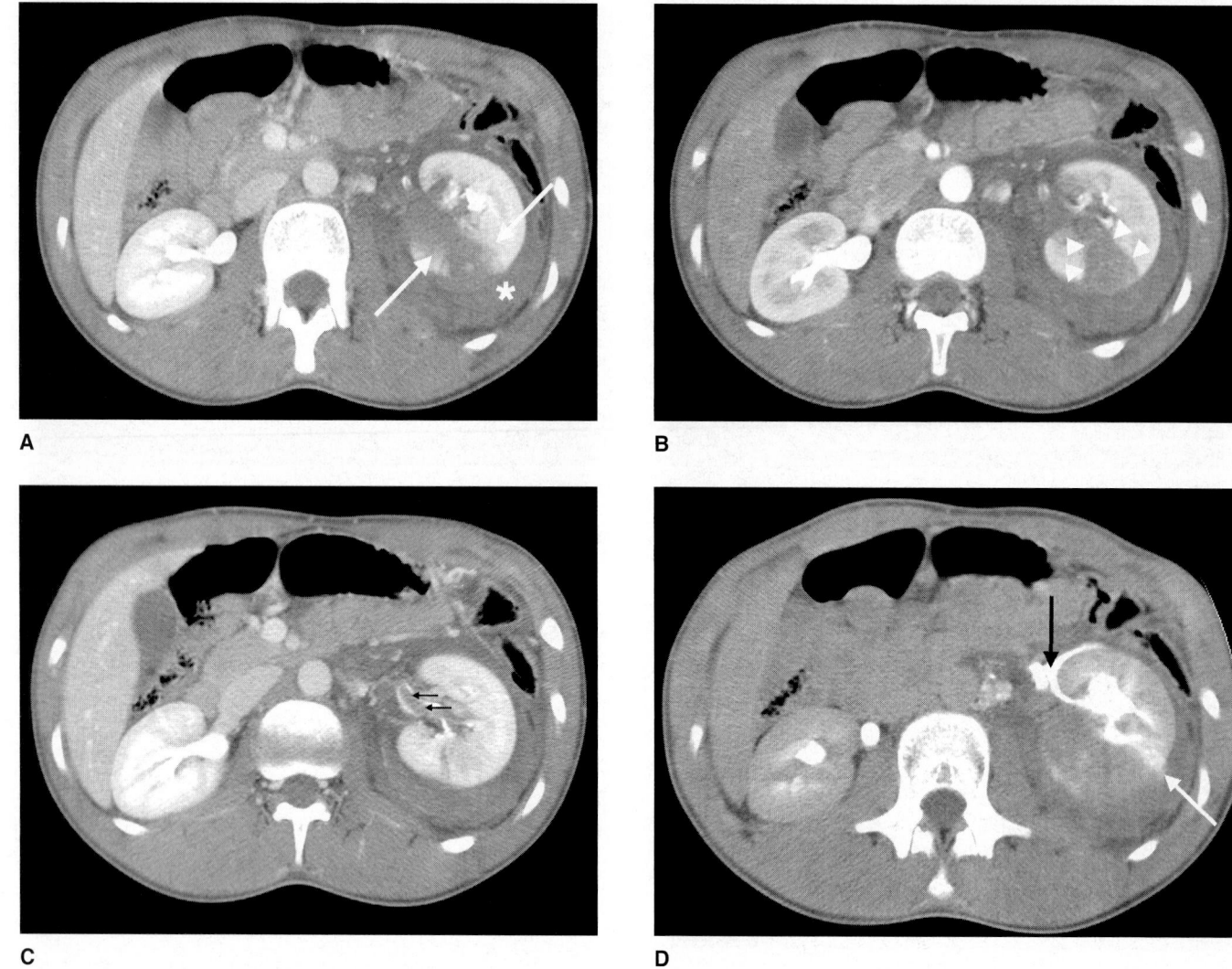

**FIGURE 16-28.**   Grade 4 renal laceration. This 14-year-old sustained an injury in a fall from a dirt bicycle while jumping. **(A)** Contrast-enhanced axial CT scan, soft tissue windows, performed in parenchymal phase shows perinephric hematoma on left (asterisk) adjacent to laceration that extends into renal hilum (arrows). Right kidney shows normal pyelographic phase. Free intra-abdominal fluid is due to grade 3 splenic laceration (not shown). **(B)** Contrast-enhanced axial computed tomography (CT) obtained in arterial phase shows wedge-shaped defect in left kidney compatible with laceration and infarct extending to capsule from renal hilum (arrowheads). **(C)** Contrast-enhanced axial CT at level of kidneys shows thrombus within collecting system (black arrows), perinephric hematoma, and contusion of posterior aspect of kidney, just below laceration seen on image (A). Perinephric hematoma surrounds kidney. **(D)** Following contrast-enhanced CT at level of kidneys, 10-minute delayed images show extravasation of contrast-enhanced urine from anterior and medial pole of kidney into anterior pararenal space (black arrow). Striated nephrogram is present posteriorly (white arrow), compatible with contusion adjacent to laceration.

pubic symphysis is never more than 1 cm in width in normal subjects, regardless of age. When pubic symphysis is traumatically wider than 2.5 cm, disruptions of both sacrospinous and sacrotuberous ligaments are assumed. In the posterior ilium, it is important to look for avulsion fractures of the posterior superior iliac spine, so-called crescent fractures, as these are strongly associated with biomechanically unstable fractures of the pelvic ring in the presence of disruption of the anterior pelvic ring. The axial images give good evaluation of the amount of internal or external rotation, but underestimate the amount of flexion or extension of a hemipelvis relative to the intact pelvis. Furthermore, evaluation of the amount of pelvic hematoma may be helpful in determining the need for angiography for embolization.

Pelvic CT is not a dynamic study, and the assessment of biomechanical instability may be difficult. Certainly, the combination of a crescent fracture from the posterior superior iliac spine

and displaced, anterior pelvic ring fractures will be unstable under anesthesia. The stability of other patterns, however, is not so predictable, even though CT images provide a great deal of anatomic and conceptual (injury pattern) information. Therefore, conventional radiographs are necessary as guides to intraoperative reduction.

Currently, the Letournel and Judet classification system is used to classify acetabular fractures, but it was developed based on conventional radiography. CT typically shows a greater number and complexity of fractures, and not all fractures fit into the Letournel and Judet classification.

Evaluation of the acetabulum with CT is usually accomplished by an initial rapid survey, in which obvious fractures are ignored and the observer completes the general survey. Initiating the search at the anterior surface of the sacrum, evaluating symmetry of the sacroiliac joint, and following along the

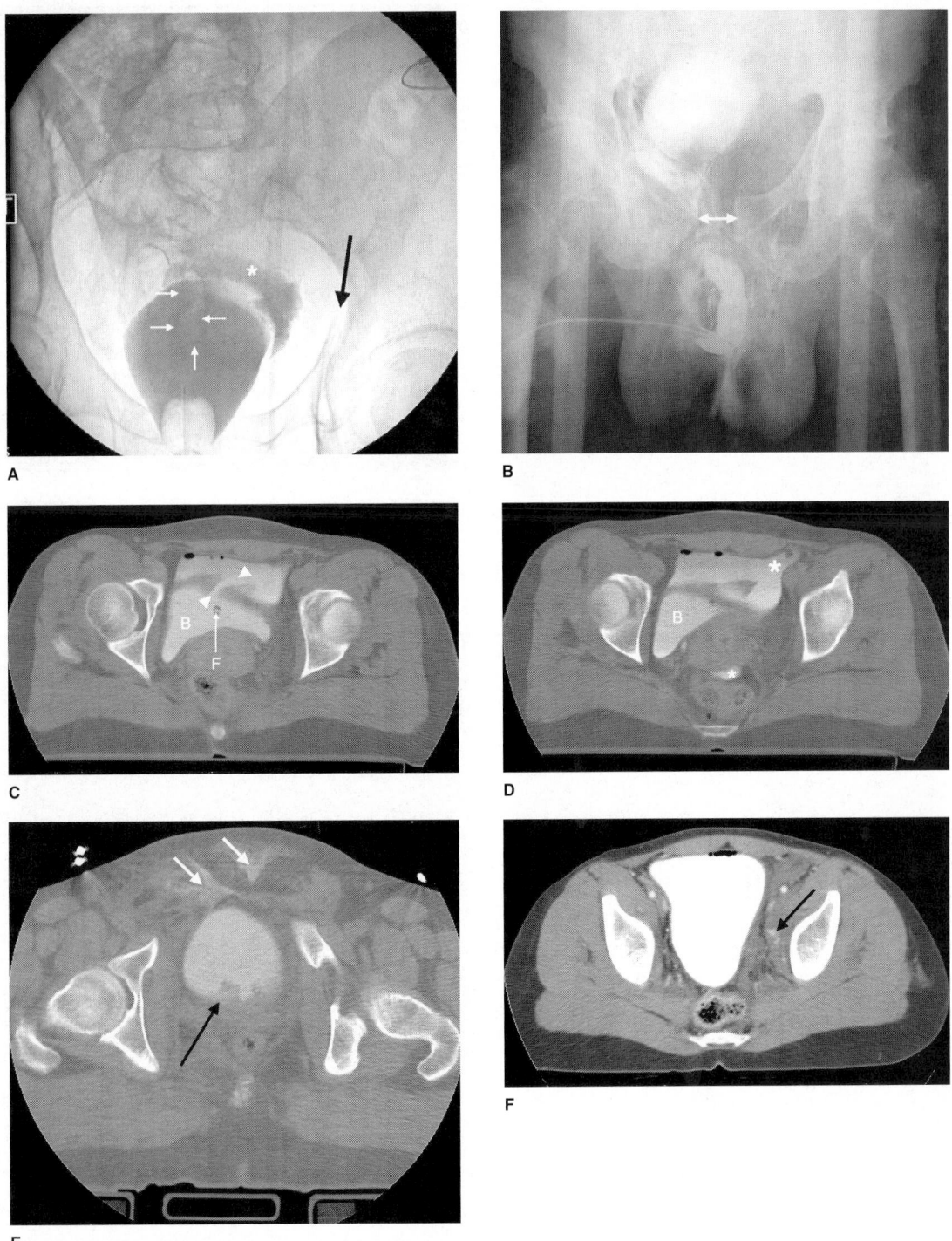

**FIGURE 16-29.** Bladder rupture. **(A)** Anteroposterior (AP) radiograph from conventional cystogram, obtained from 43-year-old female unrestrained passenger in a high-speed motor vehicle crash, shows extraperitoneal extravasation (asterisk), intrabladder clot (multiple arrows), evidence of extraperitoneal bladder hematoma with elevation of the bladder from its base. Note lateral iliopubic ramus fracture (black arrow). **(B)** AP film of pelvis obtained during retrograde urethrogram in 48-year-old man who was crushed by 1000-kg rack shows pubic symphyseal diastasis (double-ended arrow), high-riding bladder, and extensive extravasation of contrast above and below urogenital diaphragm. Bladder contrast came from prior intravenous contrast as part of computed tomography (CT) abdomen. No definite communication of urethra was shown to bladder, and disruption was shown to be transverse to urogenital diaphragm. Suprapubic tube was placed to decompress bladder. **(C)** Axial image from CT cystogram performed on 22-year-old woman involved in head-on motor vehicle crash shows intraperitoneal bladder rupture with extravasation (arrowheads). Tip of Foley catheter (white arrow) is shown centrally in bladder (B). **(D)** Same patient as in (C), slightly cephalad axial section from CT cystogram shows fluid (asterisk) both anterior and posterior to bladder (B) and uterus, respectively. **(E)** Extraperitoneal bladder laceration shown in 54-year-old man injured in motorcycle crash. Axial CT following administration of intravenous contrast shows irregularities along posterior wall of bladder compatible with intraluminal hematoma (black arrow). Note also contrast in anterior abdominal wall from extraperitoneal laceration near the dome of bladder (white arrows). **(F)** Contrast-enhanced CT at level of acetabula shows active extravasation into left iliopsoas and obturator internus muscles (black arrow). Bladder contour was deformed, but wall was intact. *(Reproduced with permission from CC Blackmore.)*

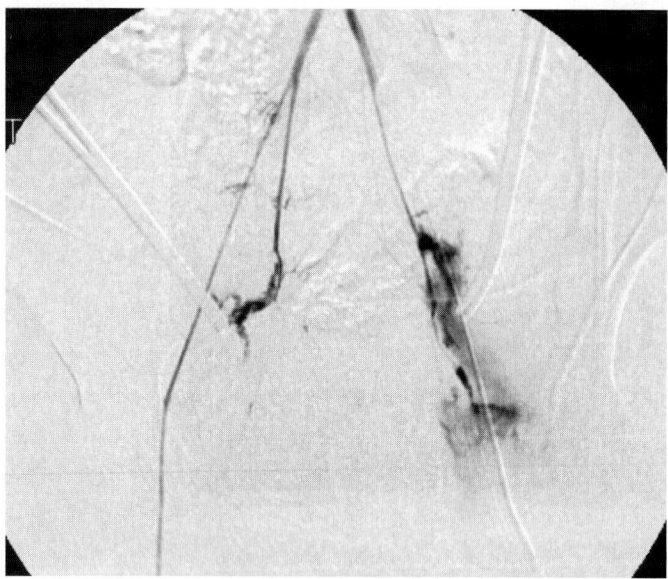

**FIGURE 16-30.**  Fatal bleed from internal iliac arteries: 28-year-old female hit by bus. AP Pelvic digital subtraction angiogram shows exsanguinating hemorrhage from the internal iliac arteries bilaterally. This was treated with placement of a distal aortic occlusion balloon prior to emergent surgery. Note the small size of the iliac arteries due to spasm and profound hypovolemic shock.

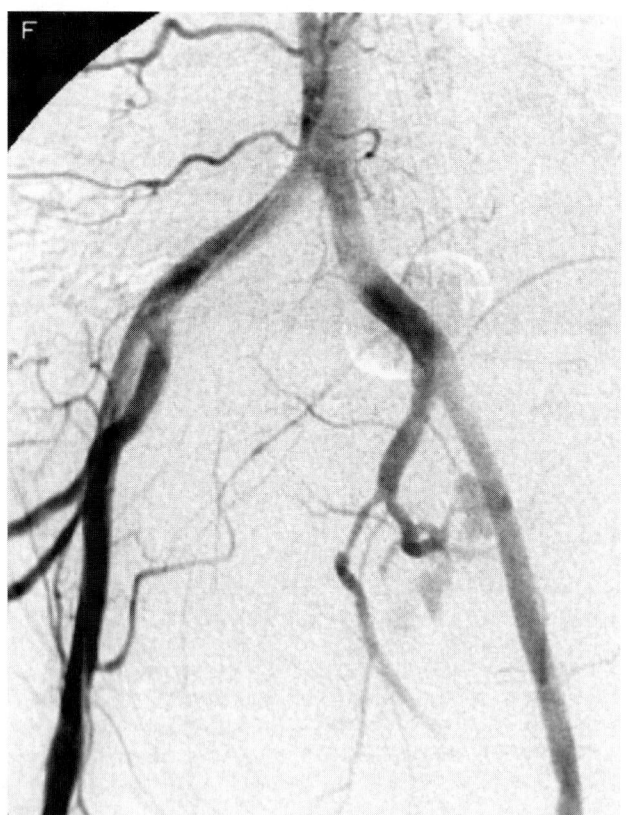

**FIGURE 16-31.**  Left superior gluteal artery bleed. Left Posterior Oblique (LPO) digital subtraction pelvic angiogram in this 56-year-old male post motorcycle accident and pelvic fracture reveals a large active bleed from the left superior gluteal artery. This was treated with selective coil embolization.

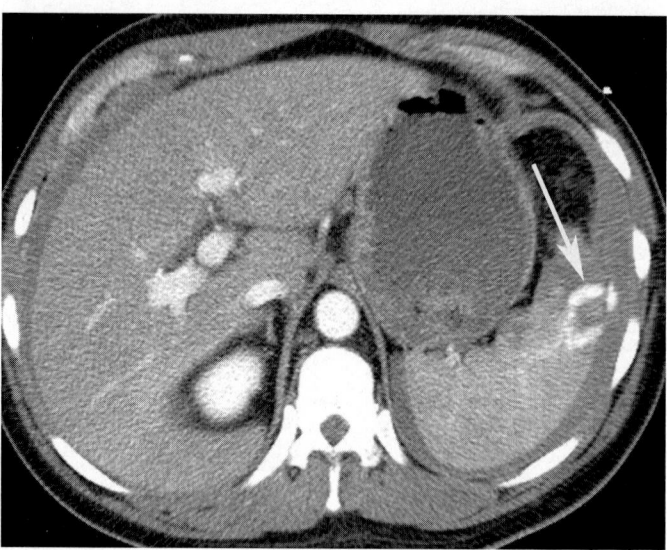

**FIGURE 16-32.**  Splenic laceration and active extravasation: 43-year-old-male post MVC. Contrast enhanced axial CT abdomen shows anterior splenic laceration with active focal extravasation (long arrow).

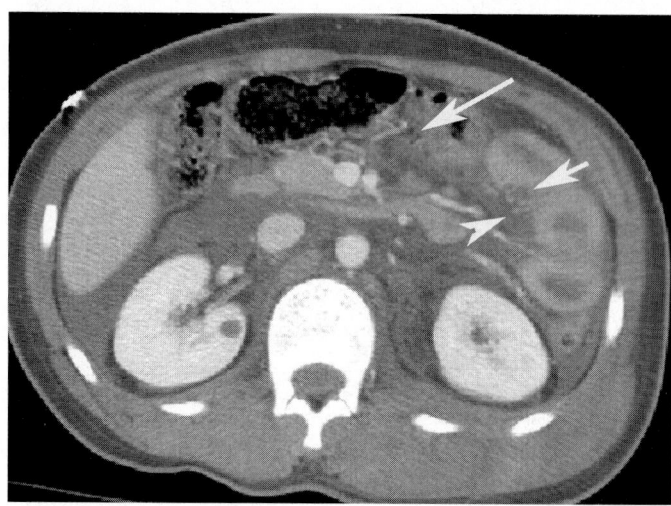

**FIGURE 16-33.**  Small bowel perforation: 14-year-old-boy, unhelmeted bicycle rider hit by car, sustained small bowel perforation. Intravenous contrast enhanced axial CT shows three findings consistent with small bowel (jejunal) injury: (1) Diffusely enhancing and thickened jejunum loops within the left side of the abdomen, with a focal hypoenhancing segment compatible with at least partial transmural injury (short arrow); (2) high-density interloop fluid within the mesentery adjacent to abnormal bowel (arrow head) strongly suggests transmural bowel laceration; (3) small amount of pneumoperitoneum (long arrow) collecting within mesentery. Extra-alimentary air almost always correlates with transmural laceration of bowel.

cortical margin of the sciatic buttress to the tectum provide an anatomic approach that extends from the intact hemipelvis toward the fracture. Assessment of the posterior through anterior walls, the ischium for the posterior column, the pubis and symphysis for evaluation of the anterior column, the iliac wing for superior extension, and the secondary congruence between the femoral head and tectum allows for a more complete recognition of fracture fragments. If fractures involve the acetabulum, the goal is to determine what remains attached to the

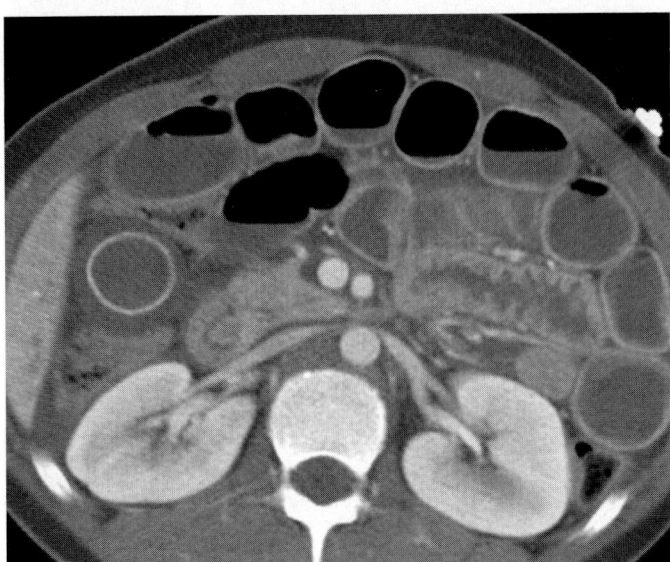

**FIGURE 16-34.** Shock-bowel syndrome: 11-year-old-girl sustained fall from height. Intravenous contrast enhanced axial CT abdomen shows flat (slit-like) IVC, diffusely dilated small bowel loops with thickened and enhancing walls, and extensive mesenteric and retroperitoneal edema. Reduced splanchnic blood flow due to under-resuscitation results in capillary leak and prolonged transit time for intravenous contrast. This constellation of findings is consistent with shock bowel. Also note moderate intraperitoneal fluid from DPL.

intact hemipelvis and describe and characterize the major fracture fragments and their relation to each other and the femoral head.

## APPENDICULAR SKELETON

### Conventional Radiography

General Indications.    Conventional radiography is for evaluation of long bones showing obvious deformity, instability, palpable crepitus, pain, and swelling. For periarticular regions, conventional radiography is indicated for deformity, instability, decreased range of motion, pain, and swelling. The Ottawa ankle and knee clinical prediction rules add considerable precision to specificity.[69–71]

Examination Prescription.    For long bones (Figs. 16-40 and 16-41), two orthogonal views are obtained, including an AP view and lateral projection centered at the midshaft. Projections should include the joint above and the joint below the long bone, or the end of the bone. Periarticular regions (joints) (Figs. 16-42 to 16-50) should have two orthogonal views and one or two oblique views, centered at the midportion of the articulation.

Comment.    Soft tissue swelling is a very helpful radiographic marker for the detection of otherwise occult injuries. Analysis of the long bone should allow assessment of the direction of the force that created the fracture pattern (e.g., twisting injuries result in spiral fractures; bending injuries result in wedge fractures). In general, higher energy injuries tend to be more comminuted and displaced. If there is a mismatch between the apparent amount of comminution and the reported energy of the injury, osteoporosis or otherwise abnormal bone should be suspected. For the appendicular skeleton, description of displacements are relative to the proximal and intact skeleton.

For periarticular regions, luxations or subluxations are suggested by partial or complete loss of congruity of the joint, the appearance of a so-called white line due to overlapping of bones, and disruption of expected alignment of adjacent articulating structures.

Careful attention to soft tissues (e.g., focal swelling, obliteration of normal fat pads, joint effusions) is helpful for subtle or otherwise occult fractures (e.g., elbow, knee, wrist).

### Computed Tomography of Appendicular Joints

General Indications.    CT of appendicular joints (e.g., shoulder, supracondylar femur, tibial plateau, pilon, calcaneus) is indicated for "displaced" intra-articular fractures (e.g., 1 to 2 mm at the wrist or scapula, and glenoid, 5 to 10 mm at the tibial plateau) or unstable fracture patterns (see Figs. 16-42 to 16-50). CT may be very helpful in presurgical planning and in the detection of otherwise occult fractures.

Examination Prescription.    In most patients, CT should be performed after provisional placement of traction or reduction. Slice thicknesses of 0.5 to 1.25 mm in the axial plane may be used in all appendicular joints to acquire raw data and may be reconstructed using bone algorithms. Initial reformations are usually obtained perpendicular to the joint of interest and orthogonal to source data and initial reformation planes. Three-dimensional volume-rendered reformations should be made from reconstructions created using standard (soft tissue) algorithms and variable (user-defined) opaqueness.

Comment.    Use of traction prior to imaging allows ligamentotaxis to indirectly reduce fracture fragments and support indirect assessment of the integrity of soft tissue attachments to major bone fragments. Specifically, bone fragments that do not move or reduce on stretch are presumed to be no longer attached to soft tissue and may require debridement or direct repositioning. In addition, CT facilitates the assessment of intact bone and the integrity of subchondral bone (e.g., need for bone grafting.)

CT for injuries to the scapula allows for the assessment of intra-articular step-offs and displacement of 1 to 2 mm or more and for the determination of stability of shoulder projection (which is determined by an intact clavicle, acromion, basiacromion, and glenoid neck). In addition, function of the supraspinatus and infraspinatus muscles may be disrupted in the presence of scapular spine fractures that are displaced for 10 mm or more.

## CATHETER ANGIOGRAPHY

### Arch Angiography for Acute Blunt-Force Traumatic Aortic Injury [ATAI]

General Indications.    Blackmore[59] has published a clinical prediction rule as an aid to determine which patients should

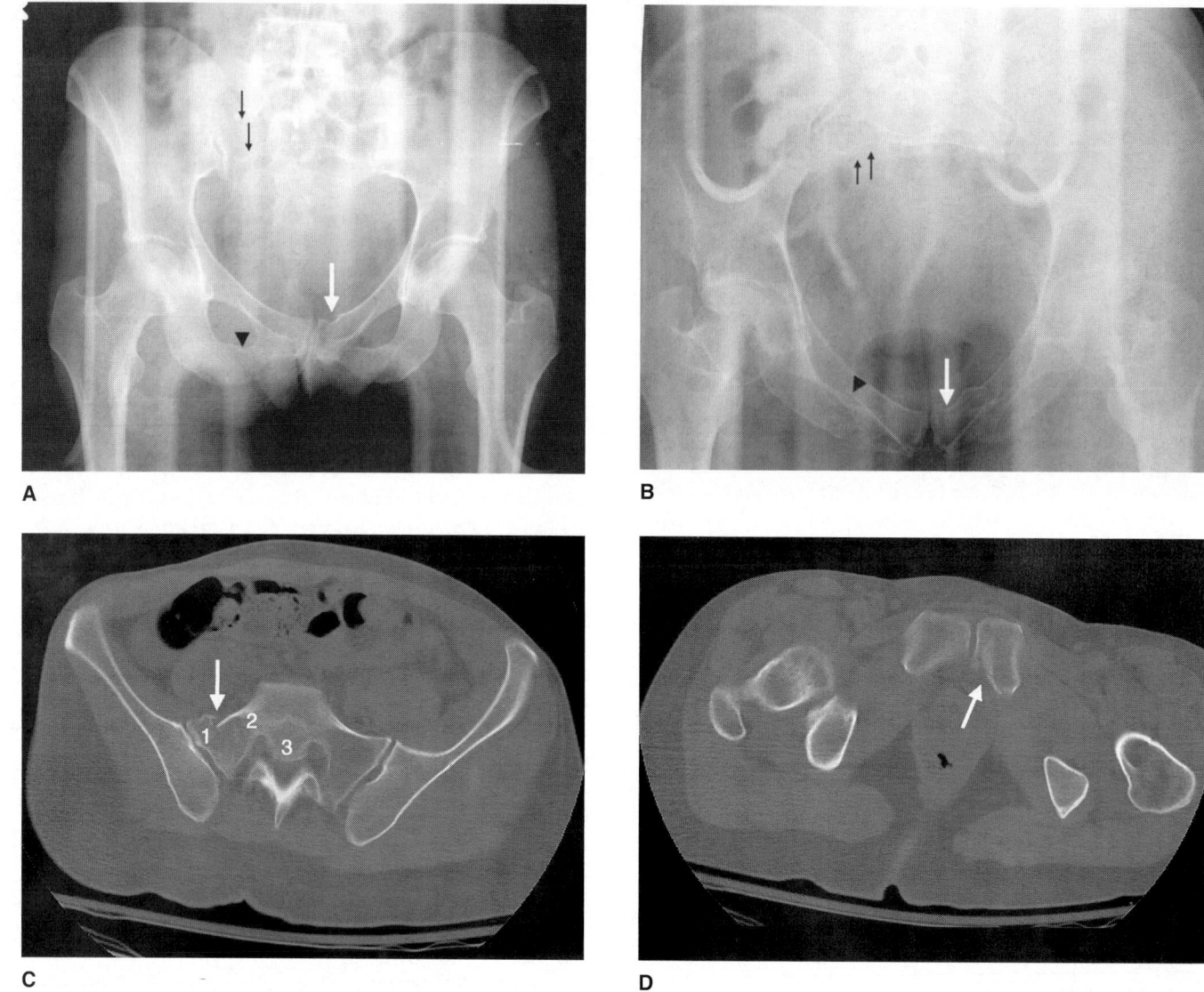

**FIGURE 16-35.**  Pelvic ring fracture: lateral compression type. This 36-year-old unrestrained woman in rollover motor vehicle crash sustained injuries to right upper and lower extremities. **(A)** Anteroposterior (AP) conventional radiograph of pelvis shows disruption of right-sided arcuate lines at S1 and S2 (black arrows), left iliopubic ramus at pubis (white arrow), and right ischial pubic ramus near synchondrotic scar (black arrowhead). **(B)** Inlet view of pelvis better shows the disruption of anterior sacrum at right alae (black arrows), left pubic (white arrow), and right ischial pubic ramus (black arrowhead). Inlet view nicely demonstrates mild internal rotation of right hemipelvis, relative to left. Inlet views are also useful to detect AP displacement. **(C)** Axial computed tomography (CT) shows impacted fracture of right S1 ala, lateral to neuroforamen (arrow). Frequency of injury to sacral nerve roots is greatest when fractures involve neural canal (Denis zone 3), lowest when lateral to the neuroforamen (Denis zone 1), and intermediate when involving neuroforamen (Denis zone 2). **(D)** Axial CT image at superior margin of symphysis pubis demonstrates an impacted fracture of posterior margin of left pubis (arrow).

be screened for ATAI. Usual indications are either direct (pseudoaneurysm Fig. 16-51, intimal flap) or indirect (juxtaaortic hematoma) CT findings, especially if the abnormality involves the ascending aorta. If patients are going directly to angiography for evaluation of pelvic ring disruptions and the mediastinum is not normal by chest radiograph, catheter arch angiography is the preferred "screening" modality; otherwise, CT is preferred modality for patients at >0.5% risk for ATAI.[72] Among selected patients sustaining ATAI who are not operative candidates, endovascular stent grafts have been advocated as either temporizing or definitive therapy.

**Examination Prescription.**  Typically, a 6 French pigtail catheter is guided to the ascending aorta via a femoral arterial

approach. Patients are positioned and imaged in both 35° right anterior oblique (RAO) and left anterior oblique (LAO) projections, using injection rates of approximately 25–30 cc/second for 40–50 cc volume and positioning to include great vessels and diaphragm.

## Hepatic Angiography for Blunt-Force Lacerations

**General Indications.**  Visceral catheter angiography is appropriate for hepatic lacerations (Fig. 16-52), especially those associated with abnormal hemodynamic status, showing active extravasation or vascular abnormalities at contrast-enhanced CT.

**Examination Prescription.**  Selective catheterization of the celiac trunk and superior mesenteric artery (SMA) is diagnostically

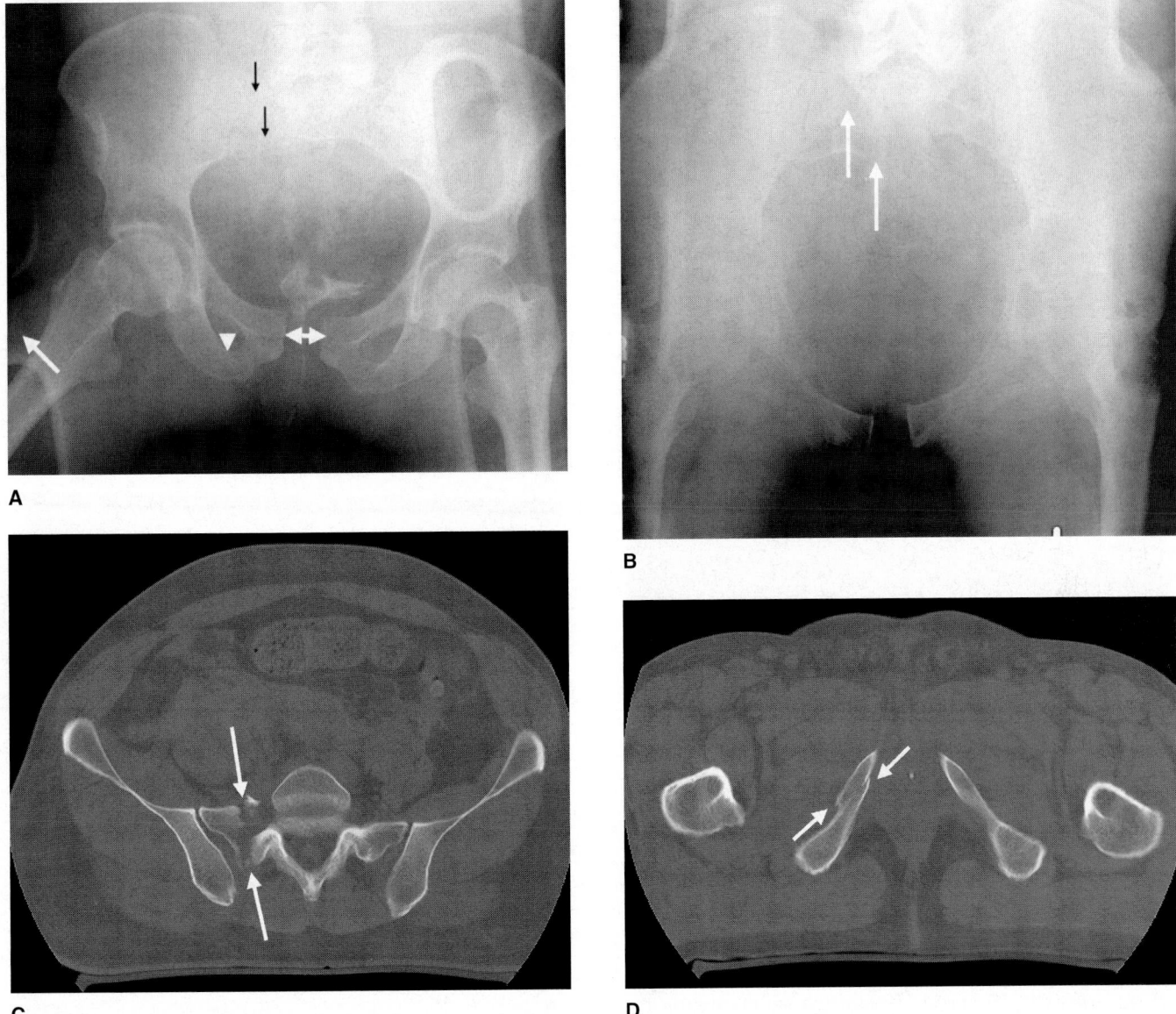

**FIGURE 16-36.** Pelvic ring fracture: anteroposterior (AP) compression type. This 55-year-old male sustained an injury during a 7-m fall onto concrete. **(A)** AP radiograph of pelvis shows symphyseal diastasis (double-ended arrow); right ischiopubic ramus fracture, which is minimally displaced (arrowhead); and disruption of right sacral arcuate lines (black arrows). Right femur is abducted (white arrow), a finding that is common with fractures of femoral shaft. **(B)** Inlet view of pelvis (obtained with 45° angulation caudally) better shows disruption of arcuate lines (white arrows) and again shows pubic symphyseal diastasis. **(C)** Axial CT at the lumbosacral junction shows through-and-through fracture (arrows) of right lateral mass of S1 with 6 mm of lateral and 8 mm of anterior translation. **(D)** Axial CT image at ischial tuberosities shows oblique sagittal fracture through right ischial pubic ramus (white arrows). Orientation of ischial fractures often reflects mechanism injury (sagittal plane fractures due to AP compression or vertical shear; transverse or axial plane fractures due to lateral compression).

essential due to the high rate of hepatic vascular variants, particularly the aberrant replaced right hepatic artery. Imaging should be continued through the late portal venous phase. Embolization of discretely abnormal vessels is typically performed by coils using a coaxial microcatheter technique. Diffusely abnormal parenchymal injury with arterial bleeding may be safely embolized with Gelfoam due to the dual blood supply of the liver (hepatic arterial and portal venous).

## Splenic Arteriography for Blunt-Force Lacerations

*General Indications.*    Similar to the liver, a patient with an abnormal hemodynamic status is a candidate for angiography and embolization when the CT demonstrates active arterial extravasation

or a parenchymal vascular abnormality (arteriovenous fistula versus pseudoaneurysm).

*Examination Prescription.*    Diagnostic angiography of the celiac trunk is followed by selective splenic artery catheterization with a 4 or 5 French catheter. If splenic artery tortuosity permits, and a solitary pseudoaneurysm or focus of extravasation is seen, distal coil embolization at the site of injury is preferred. Diffuse injury is more common and splenic tortuosity often prevents rapid catheterization. In such cases, embolization of the splenic artery proximal to the pancreatic magna branch is advocated by many authors to reduce the arterial pressure head at the injury site (Fig. 16-53). This may also prevent splenic infarction by allowing persistent collateral perfusion through the short gastric and gastroepiploic branches.

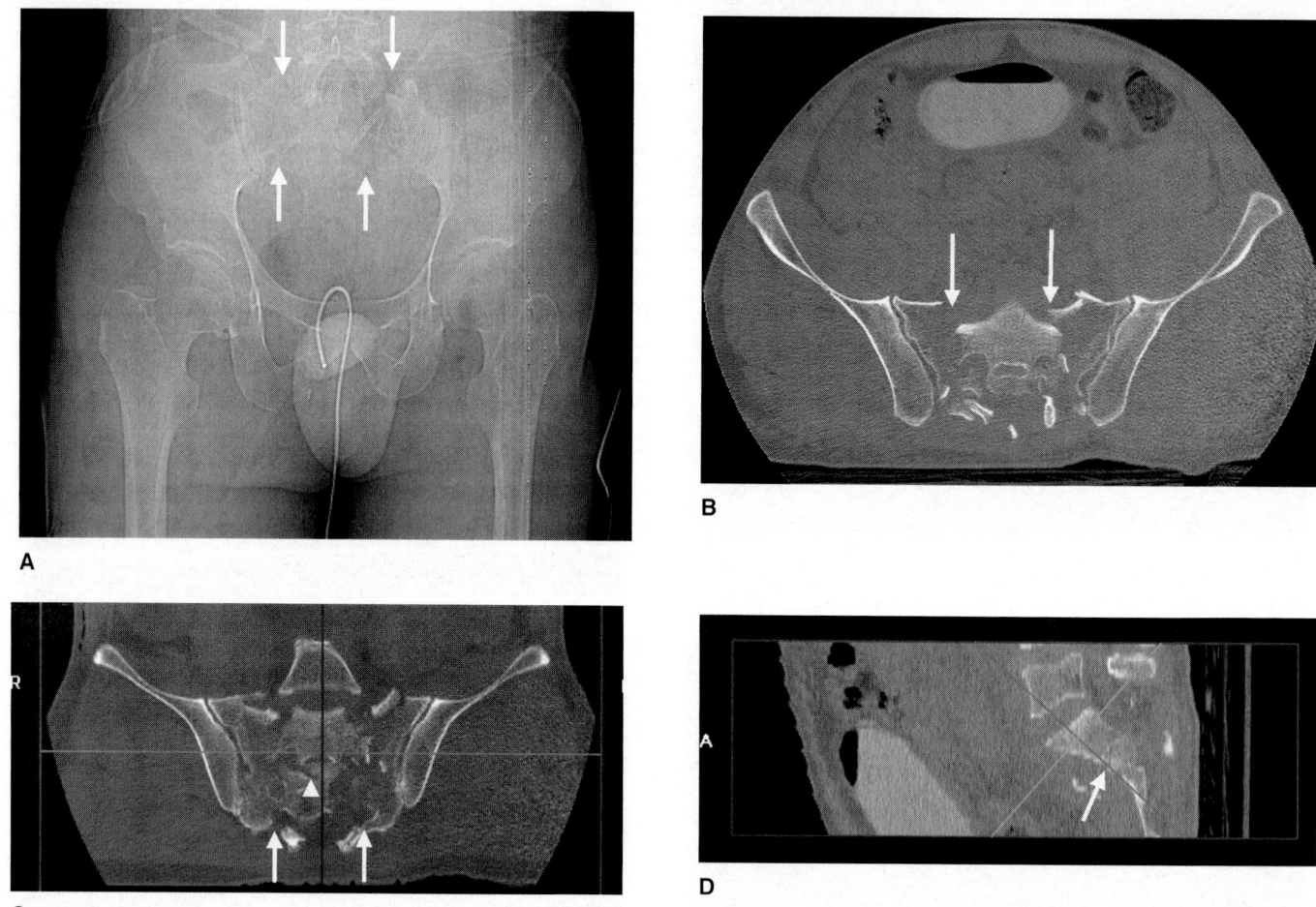

**FIGURE 16-37.** Unstable sacral fracture. An "H"-shaped sacral fracture was sustained in 40-ft fall. This was associated with right calcaneus and T12 compression fractures. **(A)** Anteroposterior (AP) pelvis CT scout shows disruption of arcuate lines bilaterally (arrows). Such finding requires excellent lateral view of sacrum to exclude transverse components of the fracture to create either "H"- or "U"-shaped sacral fractures, which are typically biomechanically unstable. Computed tomography (CT) better evaluates this area and may be performed as direct coronal scan or as coronal reformations of thin-section axial CT. **(B)** Axial CT shows bilateral through-and-through sacral fractures (arrows) that are transforaminal in their course. At this level, no transverse fracture is appreciated. **(C)** Coronal oblique CT reformation shows bilateral lateral mass fractures (arrows), as well as a portion of transverse fracture (arrowhead). **(D)** Sagittal CT reformation shows transverse fracture (arrow).

## Renal Arteriography for Trauma

**General Indications.** Grade I-III renal injuries are usually well tolerated with supportive management, and the surgical trend is toward initial nonoperative management of all injuries that are not associated with hemodynamic instability if the vascular pedicle is intact. Angiography with embolization complements this approach nicely and is recommended for patients with CT evidence of renal injury and hemodynamic instability, ongoing blood loss, or persistent hematuria (Fig. 16-54).

**Examination Prescription.** Aortography is mandatory to assess injury at the origin of the renal artery and to exclude renal parenchymal injury perfused by accessory renal arteries. A selective renal artery angiogram using 4 or 5 French catheter is then performed. Most injuries will require coaxial microcatheter selection and embolization of small branches. Coils are preferred as they can be carefully placed to prevent infarction of adjacent noninjured renal tissue.

## PENETRATING INJURIES

Penetrating injuries are a model for conceptualizing imaging for trauma. Specifically, the course of the penetration and its energy deposition predicts which organs are at risk for surgically important injuries. To estimate the likely injury vector, frontal and lateral radiographs, or at least orthogonal views, with markers at the presumed entrance and exit sites (e.g., bullet injuries) allow a reasonable prediction of the likely course of a penetrating high-energy gunshot or low energy stab wound could take. Low-velocity bullets pass through fascial planes and, despite an appearance suggesting a transvisceral course, may remain entirely superficial. Analysis of any retained missile (e.g., bullet size, deformity, amount of bony comminution) allows an assessment of the composition and energy of the penetrating object.

Fragments of bullets or bone fragments due to impaction by high-energy missiles are independent projectiles with their own potential for injury. In addition to noting injuries to bones and solid organs, it is important to query what important neurovascular structures are in the path of injury.

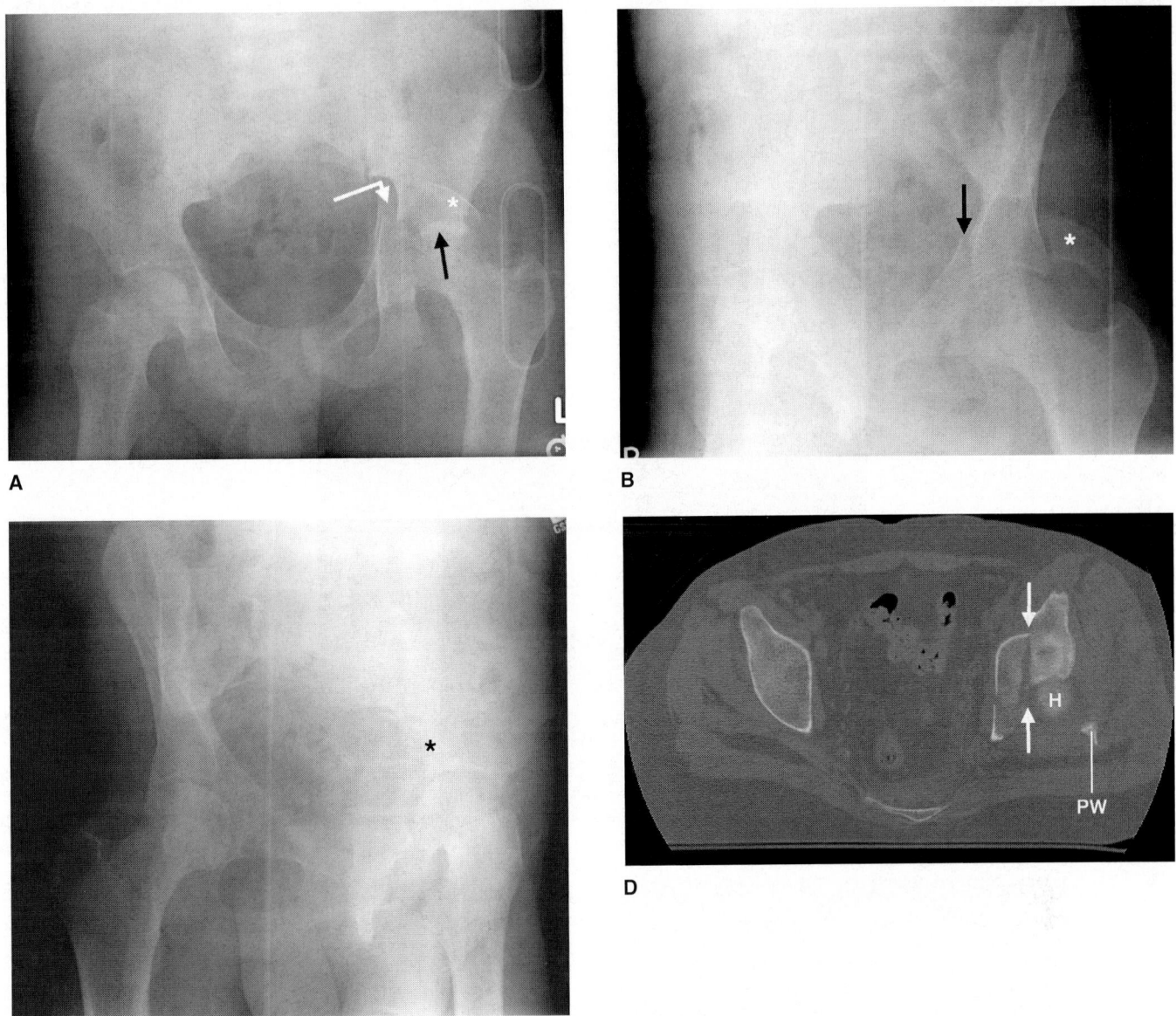

**FIGURE 16-38.** Acetabulum: transverse acetabular fracture with associated posterior wall fracture. This 25-year-old unrestrained male backseat passenger partially ejected in high-speed motor vehicle crash. **(A)** Anteroposterior (AP) view of pelvis shows disruption of iliopectineal and ischiopubic lines adjacent to acetabulum, with medial and proximal displacement of distal fragment (white arrow). Note that no fracture involving obturator foramen is evident, and no supraacetabular extension fracture is shown to suggest a column fracture. Black arrow shows concentric-shaped region of radiodensity due to overlap of tectum and femoral head, characteristic of dislocation. Position of femur in adduction and internal rotation is characteristic for posterior dislocation. Asterisk shows eyebrow-shaped radiopacity of displaced posterior wall fragment. **(B)** Left obturator oblique again shows transverse fracture (black arrow) and posterior wall fragment (asterisk), following relocation of posterior hip dislocation. Careful attention to shape of femoral head allows detection of subtle fractures associated with dislocation. Femoral head fractures may be either shear injuries or impaction fractures (the latter, similar to Hill-Sachs fractures associated with anterior shoulder dislocations). **(C)** Left iliac oblique shows location of posterior wall fragment (asterisk) and better shows transverse fracture course through anterior wall. **(D)** Axial computed tomography (CT) image at level of tectum shows a sagittal plane fracture (arrows) characteristic of transverse fractures of acetabulum. Transverse fractures typically divide acetabulum into superior and lateral moiety, which maintains its connection to the intact hemipelvis, and a medial and inferior moiety in continuity with ischium. In this case, CT was obtained prior to reduction, and femoral head (H) is posterior to tectum (circular radiodensity just anterior to dislocated femoral head). The most inferior portion of posterior wall fracture fragment (PW) is also shown.

Impalements can be from metal, glass, or wood. Wood may be either dried or green, and the latter may be impossible to reliably image by any modality. When retained green wood is possible, a strong clinical suspicion and vigilant clinical follow-up is mandated.

## Conventional Radiographs

**General Indications.** The goal with conventional radiographs is to detect any retained radio-opaque foreign bodies and to determine

the most likely path of injury and, thereby, inspect organs at greatest risk for injury (e.g., intracranial parenchymal injury in gunshot wounds to face, great vessel injury, pneumothorax or hemothorax, spine injury; Figs. 16-55 and 16-56).

**Examination Prescription.** Gunshot wounds, to include shotgun injuries and shrapnel, typically require frontal and lateral, or at least orthogonal projections of the suspected zone of injury after placement of markers at suspected entrance and

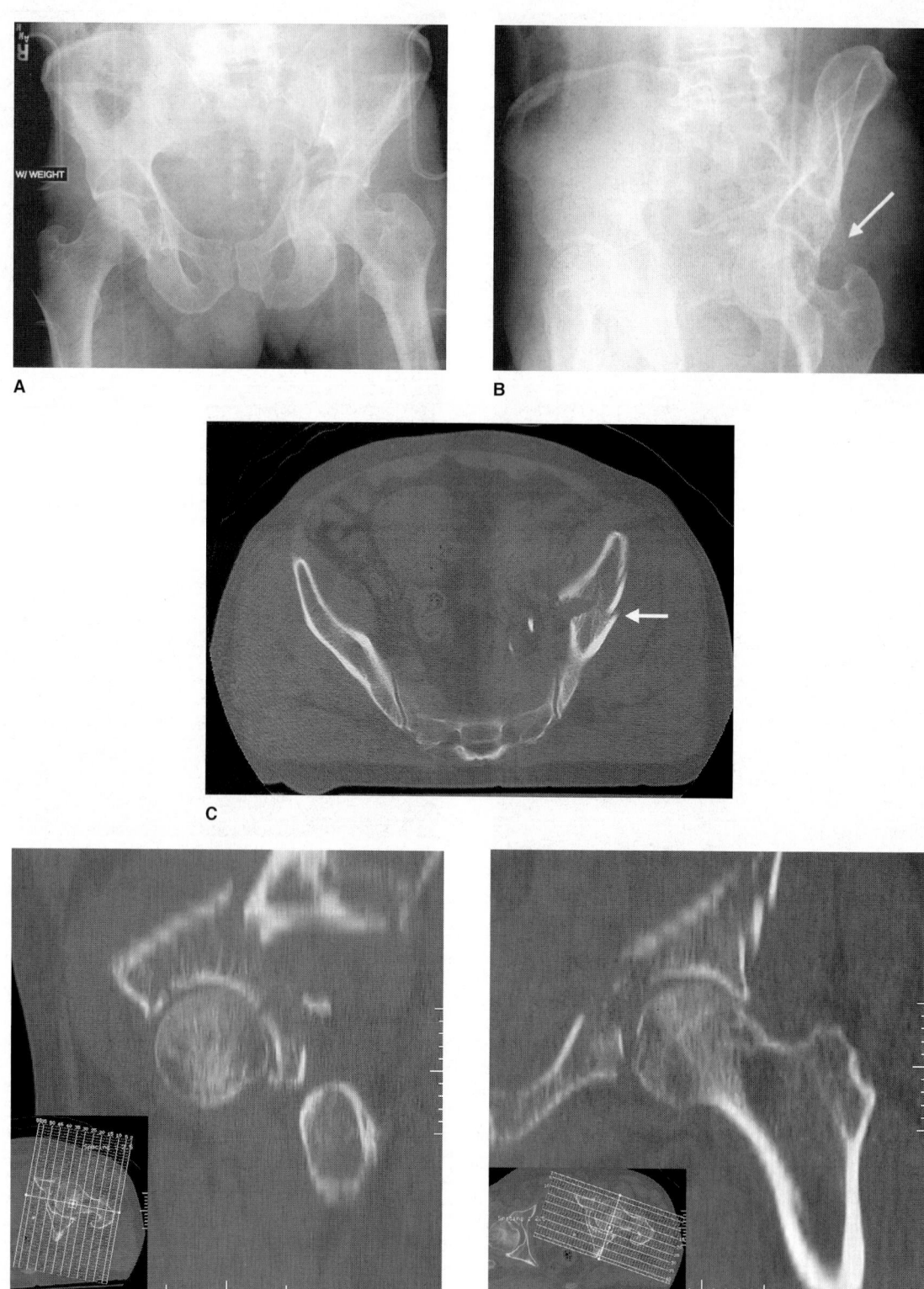

**FIGURE 16-39.**   Acetabulum: both column fractures. This 63-year-old man sustained left acetabular fracture in 12-ft fall onto concrete. **(A)** Anteroposterior (AP) conventional radiograph of pelvis shows disruption of both iliopectineal and ischiopubic line on left, and disruption of left ischiopubic ramus. **(B)** Left obturator oblique view shows so-called spur sign, characteristic of both column fractures. Spur (arrow) represents intact iliac bone connected to sacroiliac joint, exposed due to medial migration of unstable anterior hemipelvis. Judet obliques are named for affected side, such that when obturator foramen is visible en face, image is termed an *obturator oblique,* and when iliac wing is imaged en face with foreshortening of obturator foramen the view is termed *iliac oblique.* Oblique views give best conventional film representation of acetabular anatomy. **(C)** Axial computed tomography (CT) image obtained just above tectum shows comminuted coronal plane fracture of left acetabulum. White arrow marks intact supraacetabular ileum and is piece of bone that accounts for "spur" seen on obturator oblique views of affected hip (B). On CT, column fractures, whether anterior, posterior, or both columns, are typically shown as coronal plane fractures. **(D)** Sagittal CT reformation shows separation of acetabular roof from intact hemipelvis, characteristic of both column acetabular fractures. **(E)** Oblique coronal plane reformation from axial CT shows good secondary congruence between femoral head and free-floating tectum. Disruptions of medial acetabular wall, as well as supra-acetabular wall, are demonstrated.

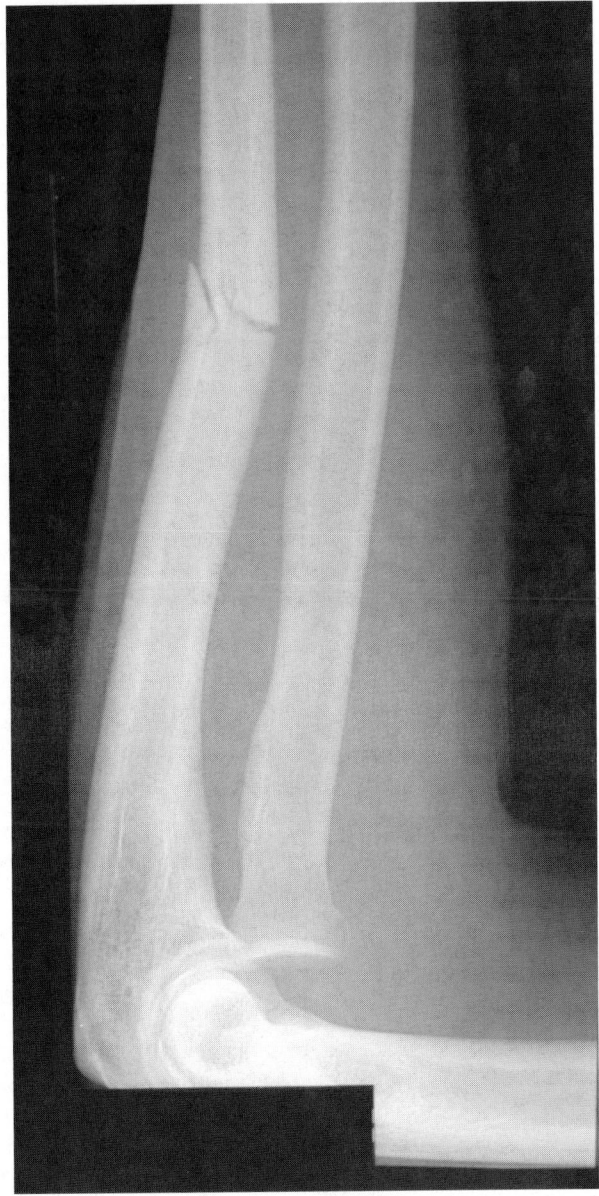

**FIGURE 16-40.** Long-bone fracture: Monteggia. Lateral view of proximal forearm shows anterior convex angulation of midshaft fracture of ulna. Anterior dislocation of radius at radiocapitellar articulation is present. While Monteggia and Galeazzi fractures are well-known long-bone fractures with associated dislocations at adjacent joint, the evaluation of any long-bone fractures should include careful evaluation of adjacent joints. *(Reproduced with permission from CC Blackmore.)*

exit sites. If no definite foreign body is seen where expected (e.g., gunshot wound with only an entrance site), radiographs of the anatomic zone above and below should be obtained to account for deflection or embolization. Cross-table imaging should also look carefully for evidence of free intraperitoneal or intrathoracic air.

For stab wounds and impalements, AP and lateral views are recommended if the object is known or suspected to remain within the patient. Cross-table projections may be helpful to detect free intraperitoneal or intrapleural air. A radiograph with the central ray parallel to the impaling object best shows the pathway of the injuring vector.

General Indications for the Use of Angiography in Penetrating Injury.   Should a single stab or gunshot wound traverse the

mediastinum, a thorough imaging evaluation of the mediastinal contents has historically included a FAST examination, aortography, bronchoscopy, esophagoscopy, and, occasionally, esophagography. With advances in multidetector CT, CT aortography may supplant catheter aortography for transmediastinal gunshot wounds.

A single penetrating or gunshot wound to the appendicular skeleton in the region of an important vascular structure is surgically explored when "hard signs" of a vascular injury are present, as long as the clinical findings do not suggest anomalous underlying anatomy (e.g., absent dorsalis pedis pulse with a stab wound to the posterior lateral calf), and some also use angiography if the ankle-brachial index is <0.9. When there are multiple penetrating injuries (such as might be seen with multiple stab wounds, multiple gunshot wounds, severe bullet fragmentation,

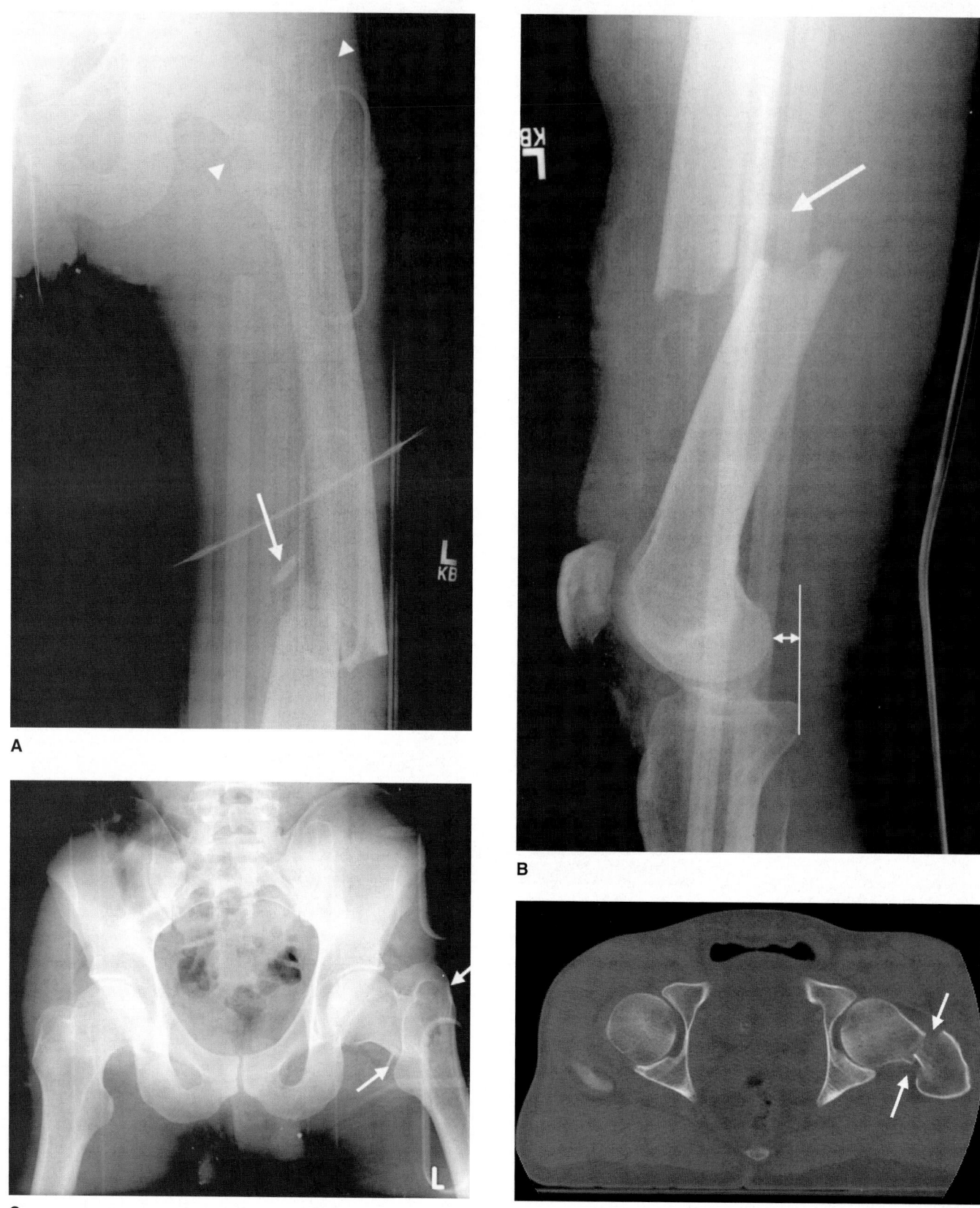

**FIGURE 16-41.** Long-bone fractures: ipsilateral femoral shaft and proximal femur fracture. This 35-year-old driver was in a high-speed head-on motor vehicle crash. **(A)** Wedge fracture of midshaft of femur (arrow) is associated with basicervical fracture of proximal femur (arrowheads). **(B)** White arrow points to displaced wedge fragment at transverse fracture of midshaft. Distal shaft fragment is 100% medially and posteriorly displaced and shows 1 cm of overriding apposition and anterior angulation. These injuries are typically "dashboard" injuries and associated injuries of knee should be specifically sought. Double arrows show apparent posterior translation of tibia relative to distal femur, a finding worrisome for knee dislocation. **(C)** Anteroposterior (AP) view of pelvis better shows basicervical fracture (arrows) but neither pelvic ring nor acetabular pathology. **(D)** Axial CT image at level of acetabula shows basicervical fracture (arrows). Fracture is more vertically oriented than fractures typically seen with falls in the elderly.

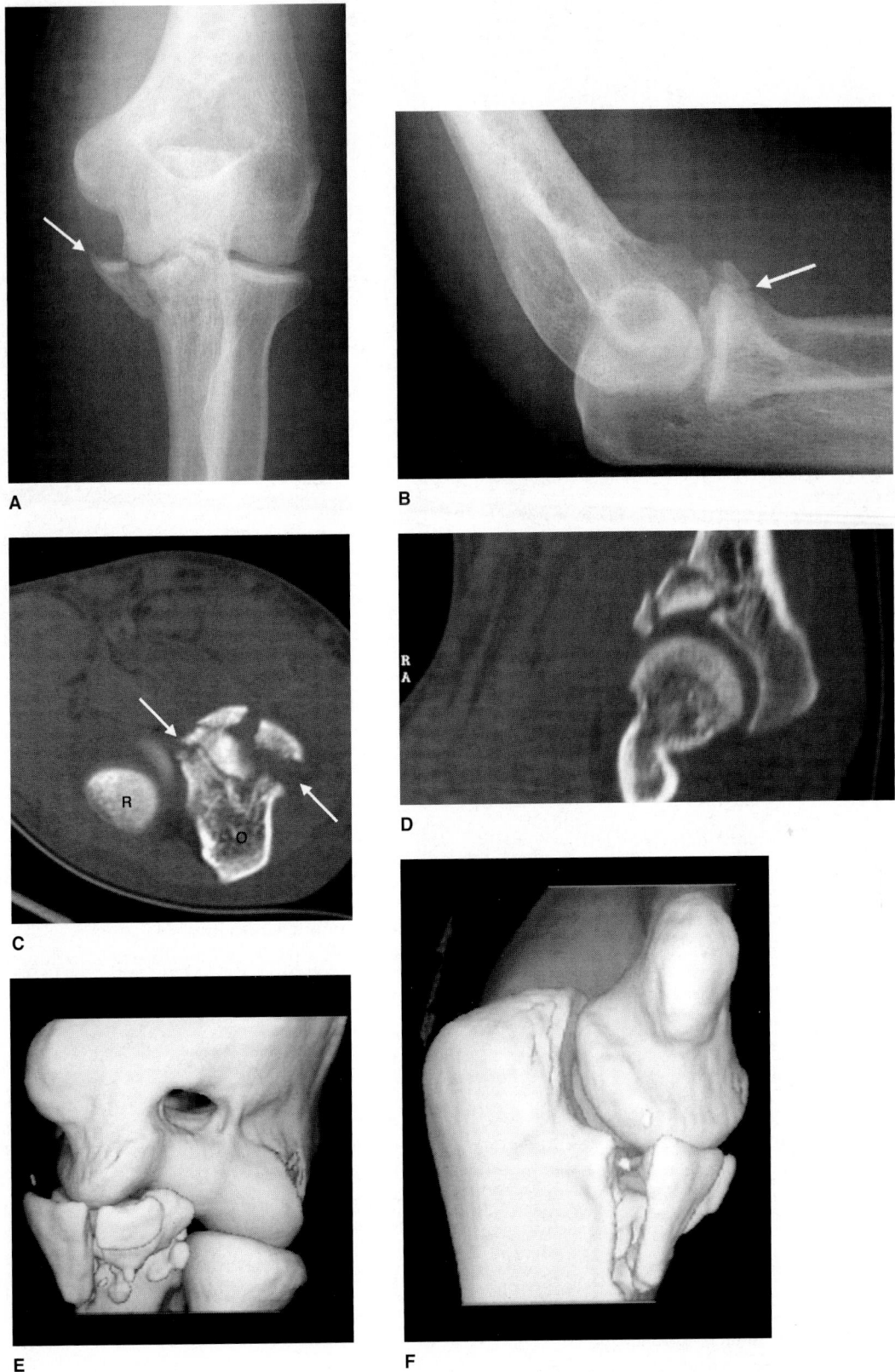

**FIGURE 16-42.** Periarticular fracture: coronoid process fracture of elbow. **(A)** Anteroposterior (AP) radiograph of left elbow shows displaced coronoid process (arrow). Elsewhere, joint appears congruent. **(B)** Lateral view of left elbow shows tip of coronoid process fracture (arrow). Coronoid process fractures can be graded by amount of coronoid process involved, such that larger coronoid process fracture fragments are more likely to result in elbow instability. **(C)** Axial computed tomography (CT) obtained because of mismatch between radiographic and clinical findings of instability shows highly comminuted fracture of coronoid process (arrows). Radial head (R) and olecranon process (O) appear normal. **(D)** Sagittal CT reformation shows nearly all the coronoid process is involved in fracture. Secondary congruence between trochlea and olecranon-coronoid process is fair. **(E, F)** Three-dimensional CT reformations more graphically demonstrate transverse and distal extent and displacement of coronoid process fracture.

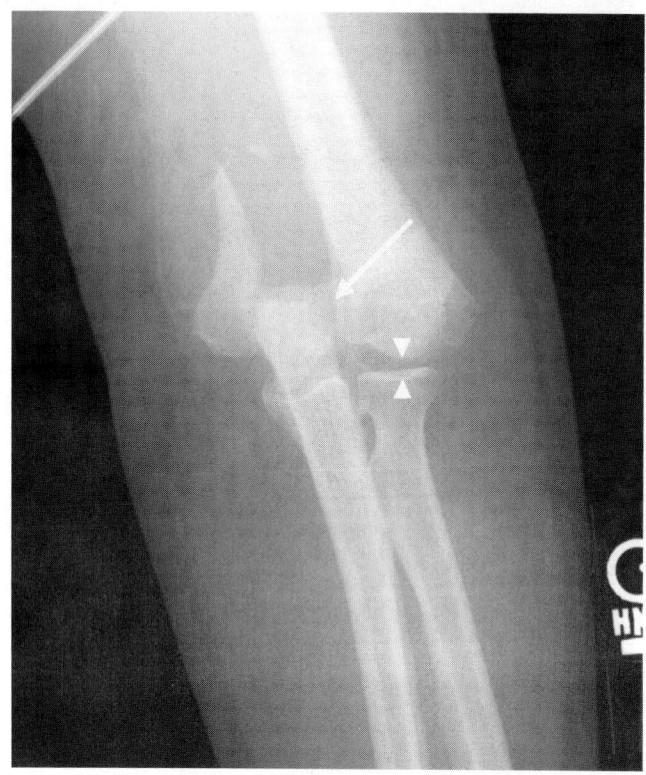
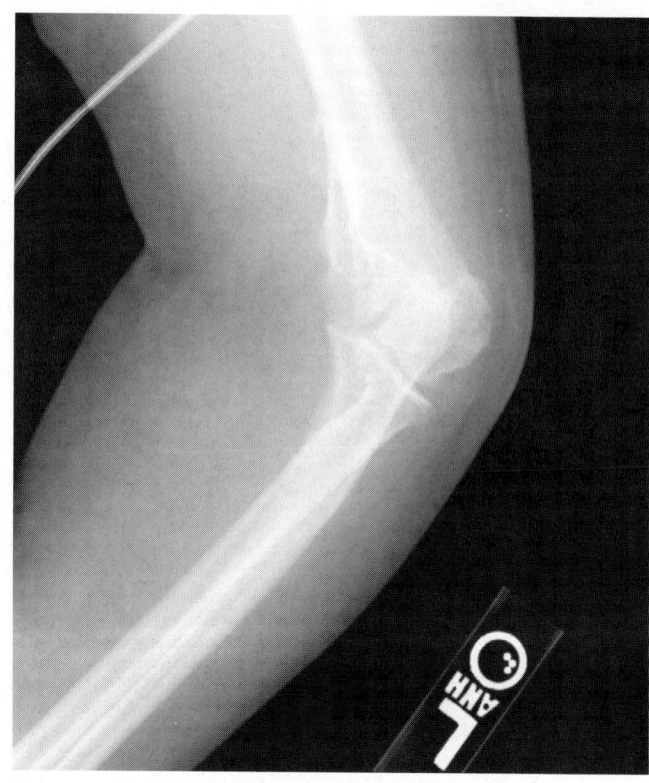

A

B

**FIGURE 16-43.**   Periarticular fractures: supracondylar fracture of distal humerus. This 54-year-old restrained passenger sustained injury in head-on motor vehicle crash at 40 mph. **(A, B)** Anteroposterior (AP) and lateral views of elbow show intra-articular T-type fracture of supracondylar distal humerus (arrow) with subluxation at radiocapitellar articulation (arrowheads). To fully evaluate these fractures, repeat radiographs after placement of traction may be necessary, and these certainly facilitate operative planning.

or shotgun injuries), surgical exploration may be relatively inefficient at fully evaluating the peripheral vascular arterial tree, and diagnostic arteriography is preferable (Fig. 16-57).

Examination Prescription: We typically perform selective external iliac catheterization and obtain digital subtraction angiography to the level of the foot.

## General Indications for the Use of Sonography and CT in Penetrating Injuries

Ultrasound can be quite helpful in localizing foreign bodies with low radiographic contrast, such as wood and glass. Ultrasound relies on the difference in acoustical impedance between soft tissues and the structure reflecting the soundwave back to the transducer. On rare occasions, glass can be oriented such that its reflections do not come back, and multiple different scanning angles toward the expected location of the foreign body are necessary to accurately localize it.

Many centers use vascular ultrasound, in conjunction with physical examination, to evaluate for morphologic (e.g., pseudoaneurysm) or physiologic abnormalities such as an abnormal duplex [pulse] Doppler wave-form or decreased arterial-brachial index to suggest that surgically important peripheral arterial injuries have been sustained.

**Comments on Imaging in Penetrating Injuries.**   Nonoperative management is far less common for injuries penetrating the peritoneum than for blunt injuries; however, MDCT may be used to exclude extraperitoneal involvement, such as use of "triple

contrast" abdominal-pelvic CT (oral, IV, and rectal contrast) in evaluation of penetrating injuries to the back and flank. Some trauma surgeons have advocated use of contrast-enhanced CT to evaluate hemodynamically stable patients with gunshot wounds to the right upper quadrant (liver), although this remains controversial.

CT performed at thin-section (1.0–1.25 mm thickness) with reformations remains the single most reliable preoperative imaging modality to characterize penetrating injuries to the face, head, and neck. Particular attention to the airway and great vessels will minimize overlooking potentially fatal or debilitating injuries. CT can be helpful, beyond recognizing specific organ injuries, by excluding the transperitoneal or transthoracic course of a missile (Figs. 16-58 and 16-59). Particularly with handguns (low-velocity projectiles), bullets will tend to follow the course of least resistance and may track around important visceral compartments by coursing within the superficial fascia. CT nicely demonstrates hemorrhage and edema caused by "crush" or "diepunch" injuries caused by missiles.

## General Indications for Esophagography for Possible Pharyngeal and Esophageal Injuries

As noted earlier, any penetrating injury to the chest or neck that traverses the mediastinum may injure the esophagus, trachea, or aorta. Although less commonly injured in blunt trauma, forceful compression of the thorax can lead to ruptures, most commonly in

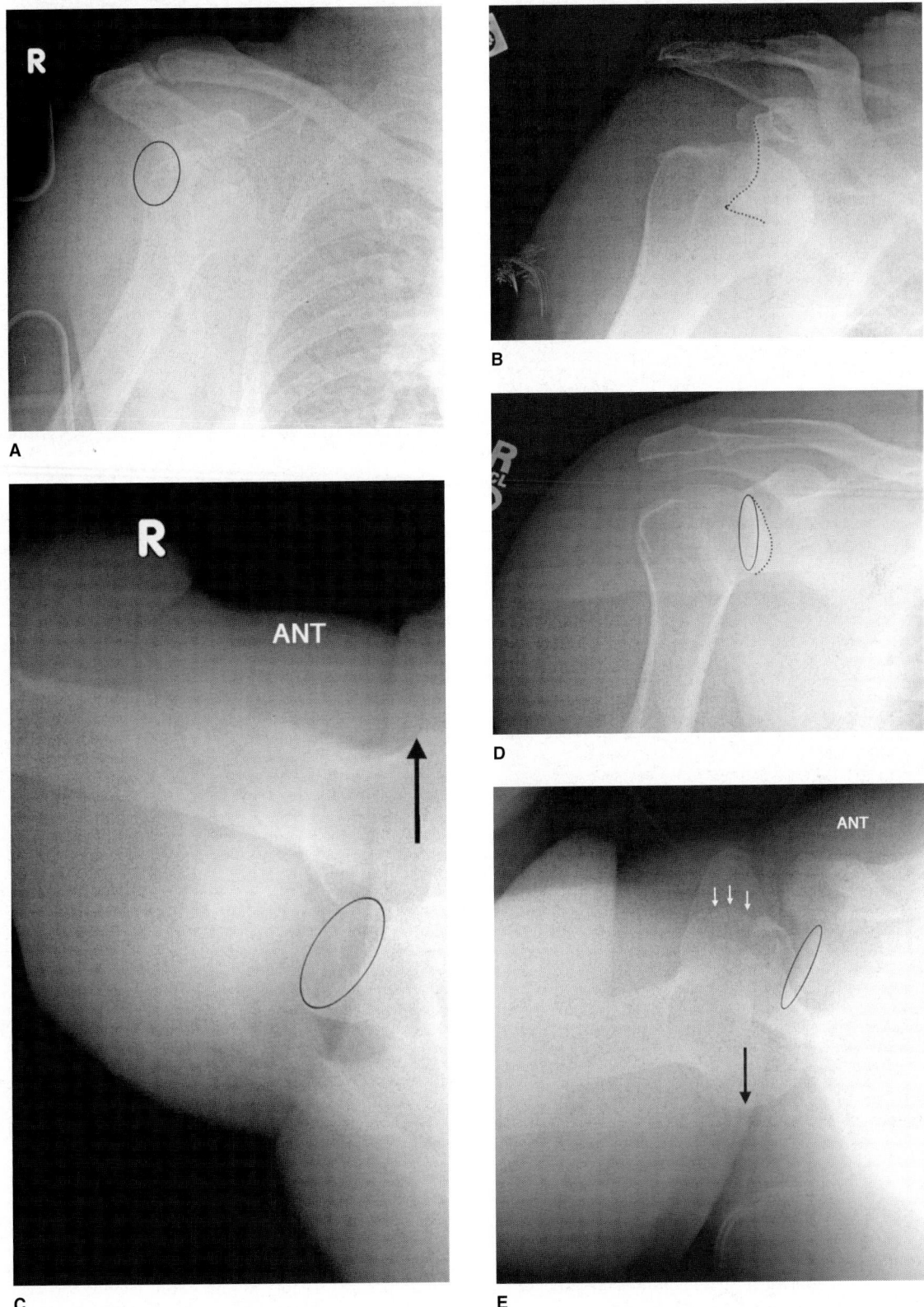

**FIGURE 16-44.**   Periarticular injury: shoulder dislocation. A, B, and C show anterior dislocation sustained by a 52-year-old struck by falling tree on his back. **(A)** shows an anteroposterior (AP) radiograph with medial location of humeral head relative to glenoid (circle). **(B)** shows postero-oblique radiograph of humeral head and glenoid (dotted line). Note that amount of overlap of scapula is less on this posterior oblique view than it is on anterior view (A), characteristic of anterior dislocation. **(C)** shows anterior location of humeral head relative to glenoid (upward pointing arrow and circle, respectively) on axillary lateral view. Axillary laterals are obtained by placing imaging plate on top of patient's shoulder, x-ray tube down by patient's waist with minimal angulation toward patient's spine. **(D)** and **(E)** show posterior dislocation sustained in a 42-year-old man who fell during a seizure. Posterior oblique radiograph (D) shows overlap of glenoid (circle) and medial aspect of humeral head (dotted line). **(E)** is an axillary projection that shows the location of the humeral head posterior to glenoid (oval). Posterior margin of the head is denoted by downward pointing black arrow. Three downward pointing white arrows show impaction on anterior margin of humeral head, so-called trough fracture or reverse Hill-Sachs deformity.

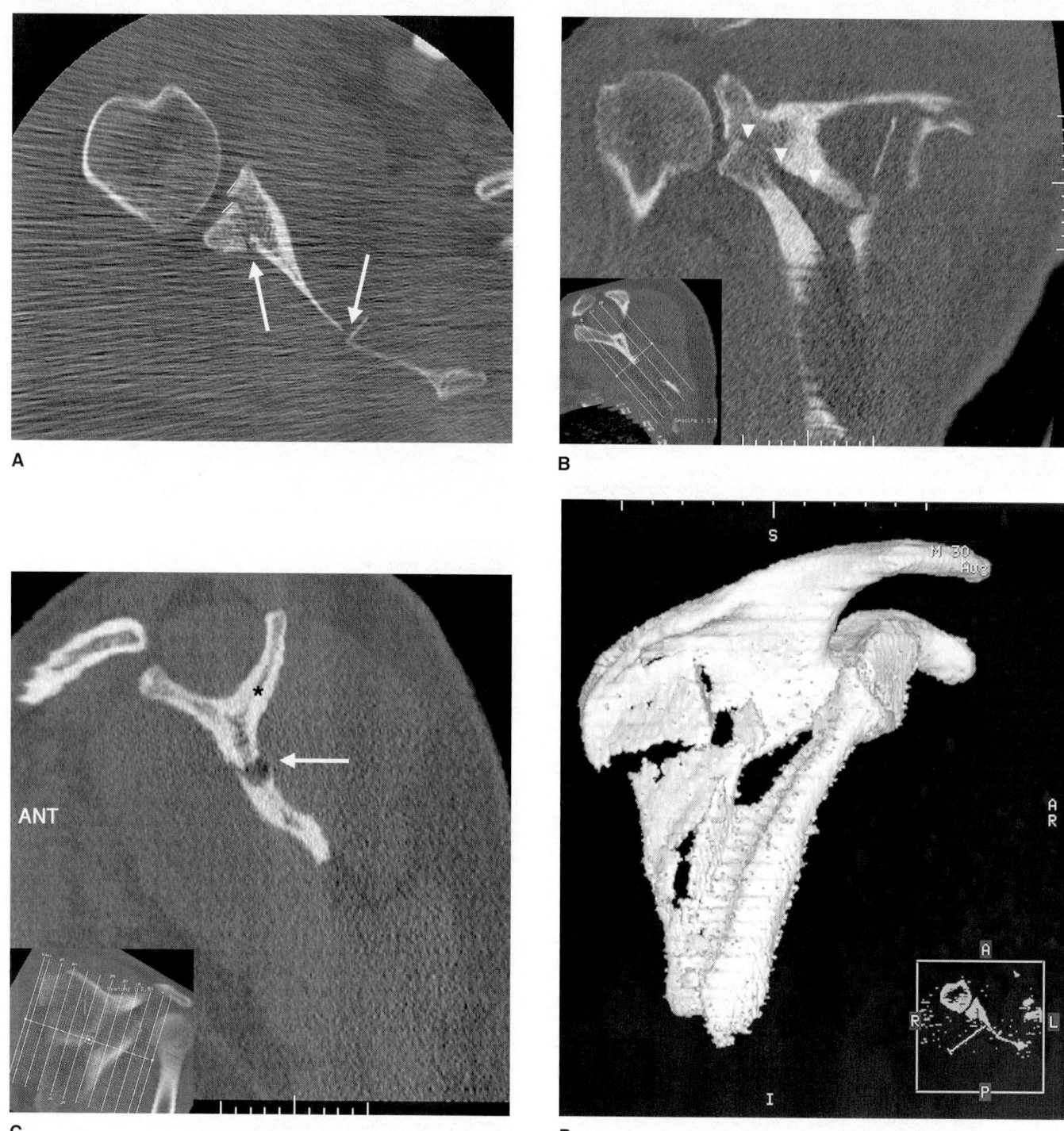

**FIGURE 16-45.** Periarticular fractures: scapular fractures involving the glenoid. This 30-year-old man was involved in high-energy jet-ski accident with intra-articular fracture of the scapular body. **(A)** Axial computed tomography (CT) image through the glenoid (slice thickness 1 mm through glenoid, 3-mm slice thickness elsewhere in the scapular body). Arrows show fractures of glenoid and body. Note 2-mm depressed fragment of posterior glenoid. **(B)** Coronal oblique CT reformation shows upper glenoid attached to coracoid process, basiacromion process, and remaining shoulder girdle. Transverse subspinous fracture is comminuted and extends into glenoid (arrowheads). Inferior and posterior glenoid retains one fragment that is impacted and rotated with intra-articular incongruity of surgical importance. **(C)** Sagittal oblique CT reformation shows transverse subspinous component of comminuted scapula fracture (arrow). Note that spine of scapula (asterisk) is not involved in fracture. **(D)** Three-dimensional CT reformation (posterior view) shows step artifact of thicker sections. Biplane deformity to glenoid articular surface is well shown.

the upper third of the esophagus (as contrasted to those seen in Boerhaave's syndrome which tend to be near the gastroesophageal junction). An injury to the aerodigestive tract in blunt trauma should be suspected when there is a pneumomediastinum or pre-cervical emphysema without evidence for a pneumothorax;

however, the presence of a pneumomediastinum alone is a very nonspecific finding.

**Examination Prescription.** In all but the most cooperative patients, the authors inject water-soluble contrast through a feeding

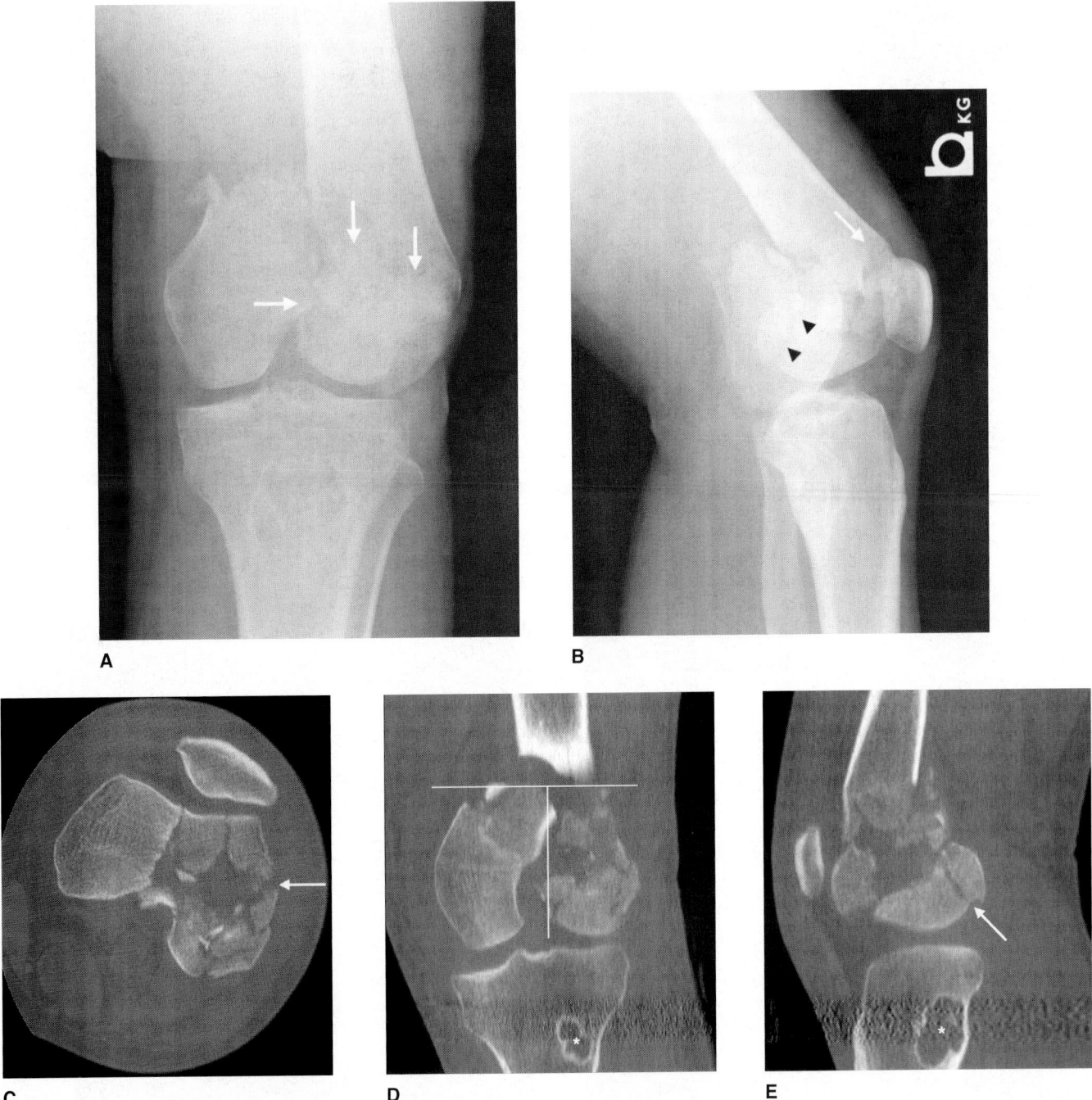

**FIGURE 16-46.** Periarticular fractures: intra-articular supracondylar distal femur fracture. This 20-year-old man was involved in a high-speed motor vehicle crash as a belted driver. **(A)** Anteroposterior (AP) radiograph of knee shows transverse T-type fracture of distal supracondylar femur, with intra-articular extension into intercondylar notch (arrows). **(B)** Lateral radiograph of knee shows transverse supracondylar component (arrow), from which femoral condyles have dissociated. In addition, lateral femoral condyle shows coronal plane, comminuted fracture of posterior aspect of condyle (arrowheads). In up to 40% of intra-articular supracondylar fractures caused by high-energy mechanisms, such coronal plane fractures (Hoffa's fracture) may be overlooked. **(C)** Axial computed tomography (CT) shows a sagittal plane fracture extending into midportion of trochlea of the patellofemoral joint and a comminuted coronal plane fracture of posterior aspect of lateral femoral condyle (arrow). **(D)** Coronal plane reformation from axial CT shows T-type intra-articular fracture with dissociation of medial and lateral femoral condyles (white lines). Asterisk marks developmental variant, nonossifying fibroma. **(E)** Sagittal reformation from axial CT in central portion of lateral knee joint compartment shows coronal plane fracture of posterior femoral condyle (Hoffa's fracture) as marked by arrow. Asterisk notes nonossifying fibroma, a benign developmental variant.

tube or a nasogastric tube to obtain full distention of the esophagus as an essential portion of the evaluation. To initiate the examination, the patient is placed in a 45° left posterior oblique projection with a feeding tube or nasogastric tube positioned at the junction of the middle and distal thirds of the esophagus. To obtain full distention, 50 mL of nonionic, iso-osmolar water-soluble contrast agent is rapidly injected, during which time fluoroscopic cineradiographs are obtained at 2 to 3 frames per second. If no perforation is demonstrated, the nasogastric tube is repositioned at the junction of the proximal and middle thirds, and the procedure repeated. This

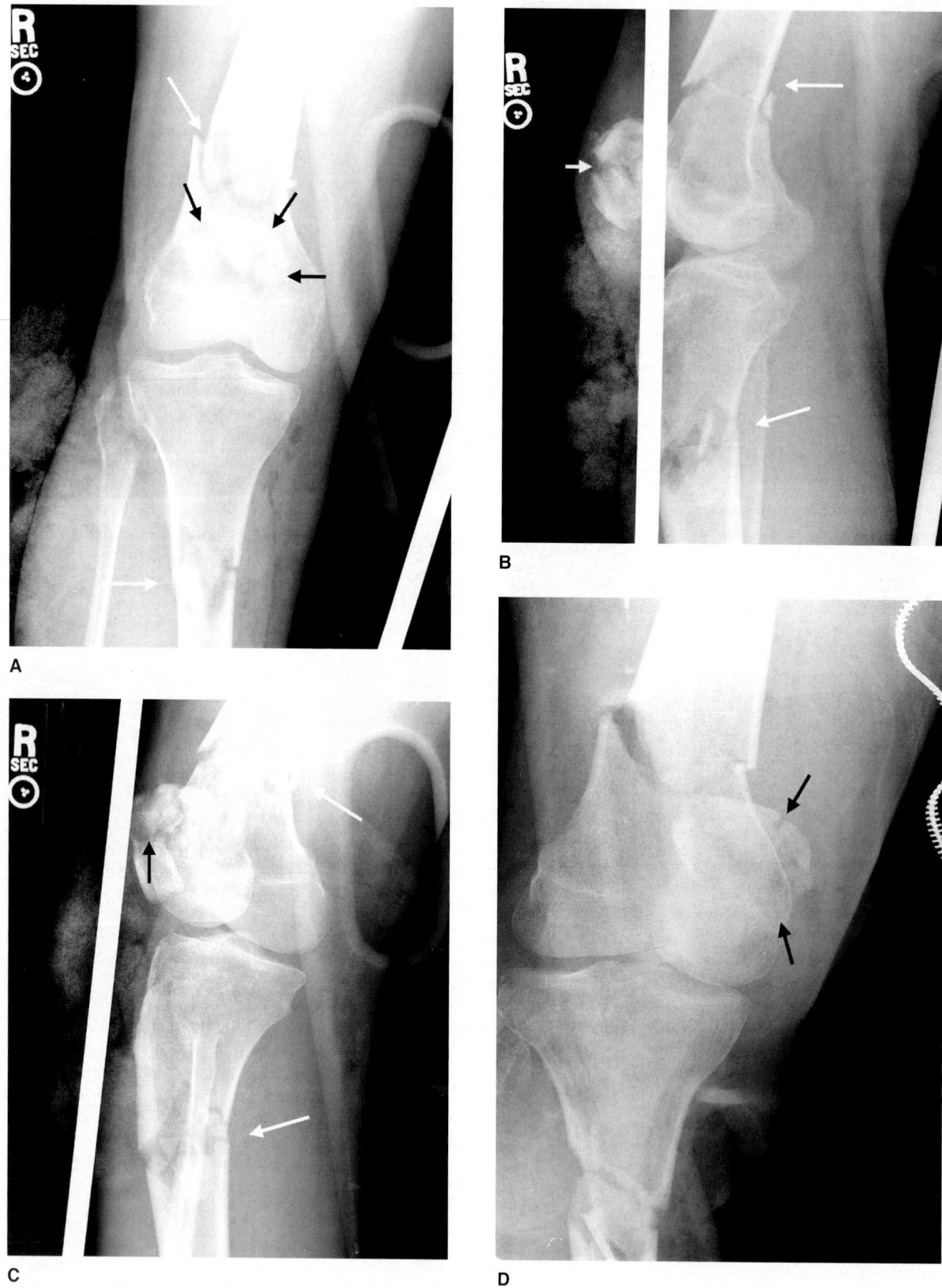

**FIGURE 16-47.**   Periarticular fractures: stellate fracture of patella. This 50-year-old unrestrained rear seat passenger in a motorcycle crash sustained multiple injuries when colliding with a horse trailer at 50 mph. **(A)** Anteroposterior (AP) conventional radiograph shows a so-called floating knee, with associated transverse, extra-articular supracondylar femur fracture and transverse, comminuted proximal tibial diaphyseal fractures (white arrows). Looking through femoral condyles, distracted, stellate fracture of patella is shown (black arrows). **(B)** Lateral conventional radiograph shows floating knee caused by fractures of distal femur and proximal tibia, respectively (white arrows). Transverse component of stellate fracture of patella is marked by anterior short arrow. **(C)** External oblique view of knee better shows stellate pattern and incongruity of articular surface of patella (black arrow). Again shown by white arrows are extra-articular fractures of distal femur and proximal tibia, respectively. **(D)** Conventional radiograph obtained with internal rotation shows stellate fracture of patella (black arrows), as well as comminuted extra-articular fractures of distal femur and proximal tibia (not marked).

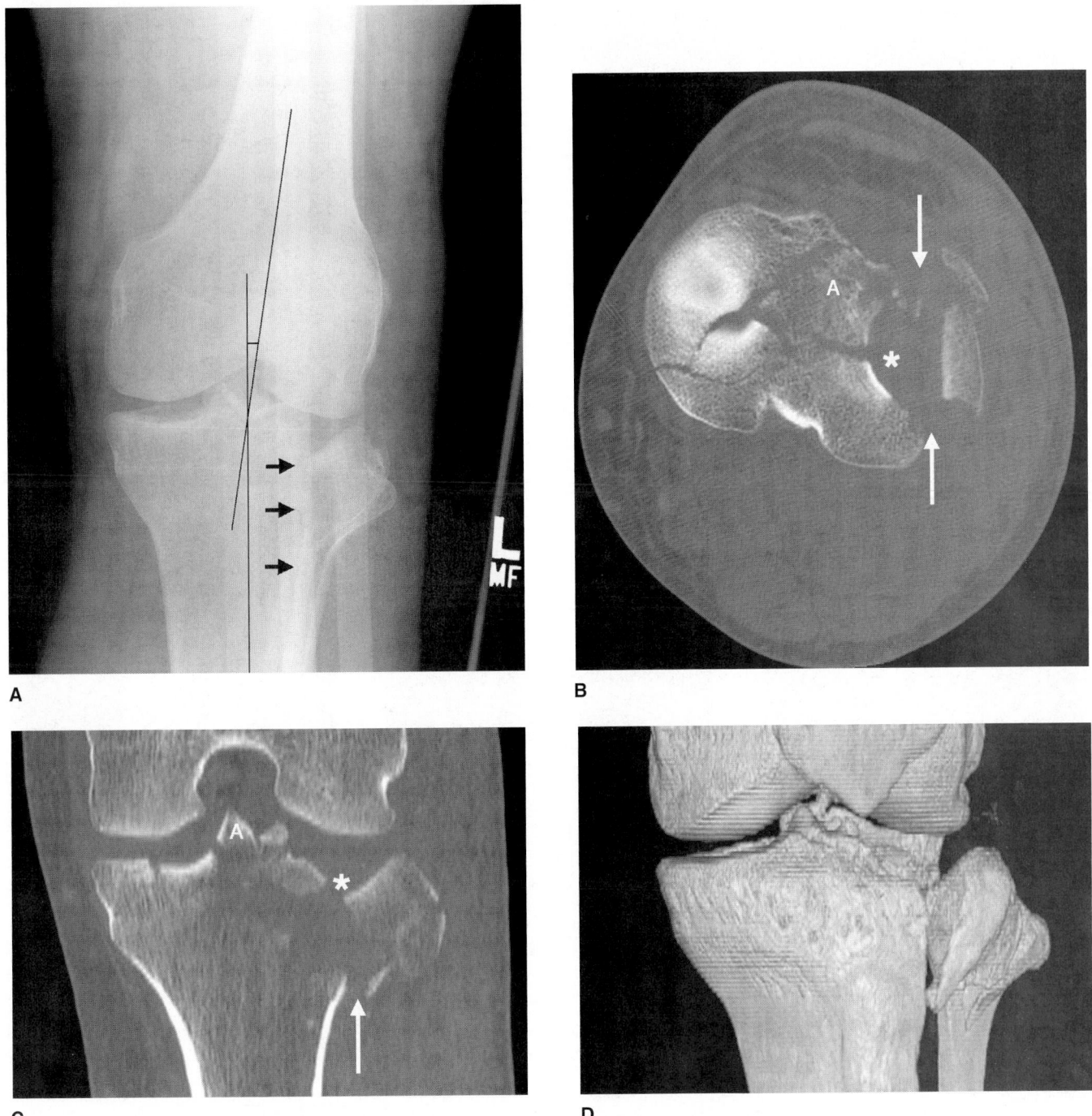

**FIGURE 16-48.** Periarticular fractures: tibial plateau fracture (Schatzker 2). This 46-year-old man fell on the stairs. **(A)** Anteroposterior (AP) radiograph of knee shows valgus angulation due to collapse of lateral femoral condyle into a split depressed fracture of tibial plateau (arrows). **(B)** Axial image from computed tomography (CT) shows depressed left (asterisk) and split (arrows) portions of split depressed fracture. Note extension of comminuted fracture lines into medial tibial plateau across posterior aspect of proximal tibia and into intercondylar eminences, where anterior eminence (A) is minimally displaced. **(C)** Coronal reformation from axial CT shows split (arrow) and depressed (asterisk) portions of Schatzker type 2 fracture. Also note apparent elevation of anterior tibial eminence (A), on which anterior cruciate ligament inserts. Less striking step-off is seen in central portion of medial tibial plateau. **(D)** Three-dimensional CT reformation graphically demonstrates depression and lateral displacement of articular surface and lateral rim of tibial plateau, respectively. Also shown on this view is fracture of proximal fibula.

latter injection typically extends to the hypopharynx. If the first two series are normal, the patient is repositioned into a right posterior oblique position, and the process repeated using "thin barium."

Where pharyngeal perforations are suspected and if the patient is able to swallow, the study is again initiated with nonionic, iso-osmolar water-soluble contrast. Two orthogonal obliques are obtained, the first with the nonionic, water-soluble contrast and the second with thin barium, provided the initial esophagram was normal. In patients who are unable to cooperate, a 25-mL bolus of the nonionic, water-soluble contrast is injected into the hypopharynx (only performed in patients with airway control).

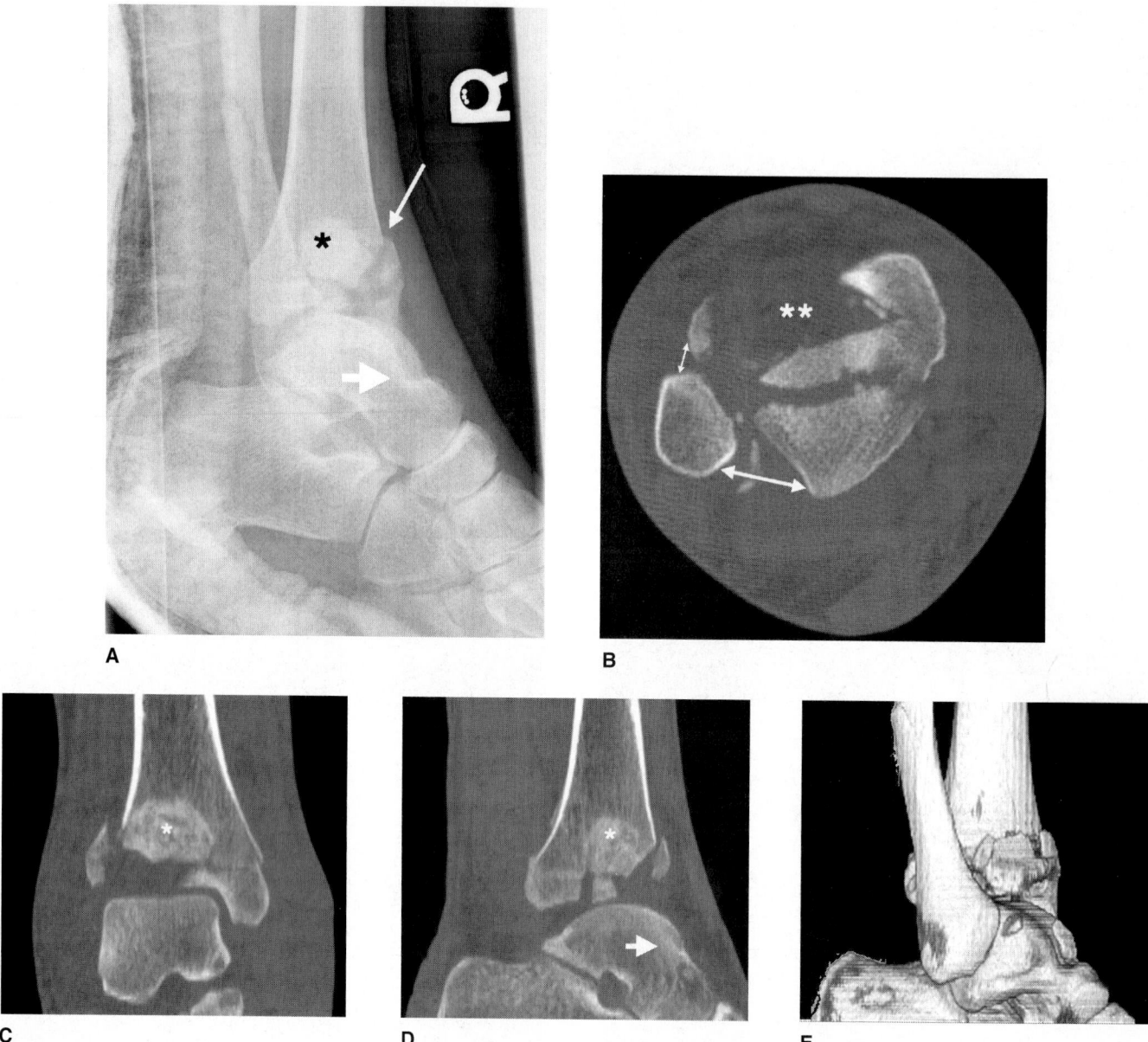

**FIGURE 16-49.** Periarticular fractures: pilon fracture. This 23-year-old male motorcyclist attempted 15-ft jump with dirt bike and sustained fracture during hard landing while standing up on his "pegs." **(A)** Conventional lateral radiograph of ankle shows anterior translation of talus relative to tibia (bold arrow). Comminuted fracture of distal tibial articular surface involving anterior aspect of distal tibia (arrow) shows circular double-density projected over metaphysis of tibia (asterisk), which represents impacted subchondral bone from anterior articular surface of tibia. Also note unmarked distal fibular fracture. **(B)** Axial computed tomography (CT) at level of plafond clearly shows three major components of disruption. Double asterisk marks origin of impacted subchondral articular bone from anterior tibial articular surface. Longer of two double-ended arrows shows displacement of fibula from peroneal groove and implies disruption of posterior inferior tibiofibular ligament. Shorter double-ended arrow shows expected relation between anterior aspect of fibula and anterolateral corner of distal tibia (so-called Chaput fragment). In analysis of these fractures, it is important to determine relations of articular surface to intact distal tibia (the posterior malleolus, in this case) and association between posterior malleolus and distal fibula. **(C)** Coronal reformation from axial CT shows defect in anterolateral aspect of distal tibia. Asterisk notes impacted subchondral bone. **(D)** Sagittal reformation from axial CT again demonstrates anterior translation of talus (bold arrow) relative to the articular surface of intact distal tibia at posterior malleolus. Asterisk marks impacted subchondral bone from anterior plafond. **(E)** Three-dimensional reformation from axial CT, lateral view, well shows comminution of anterior lateral aspect of distal tibia, compatible with hyperdorsiflexion injury.

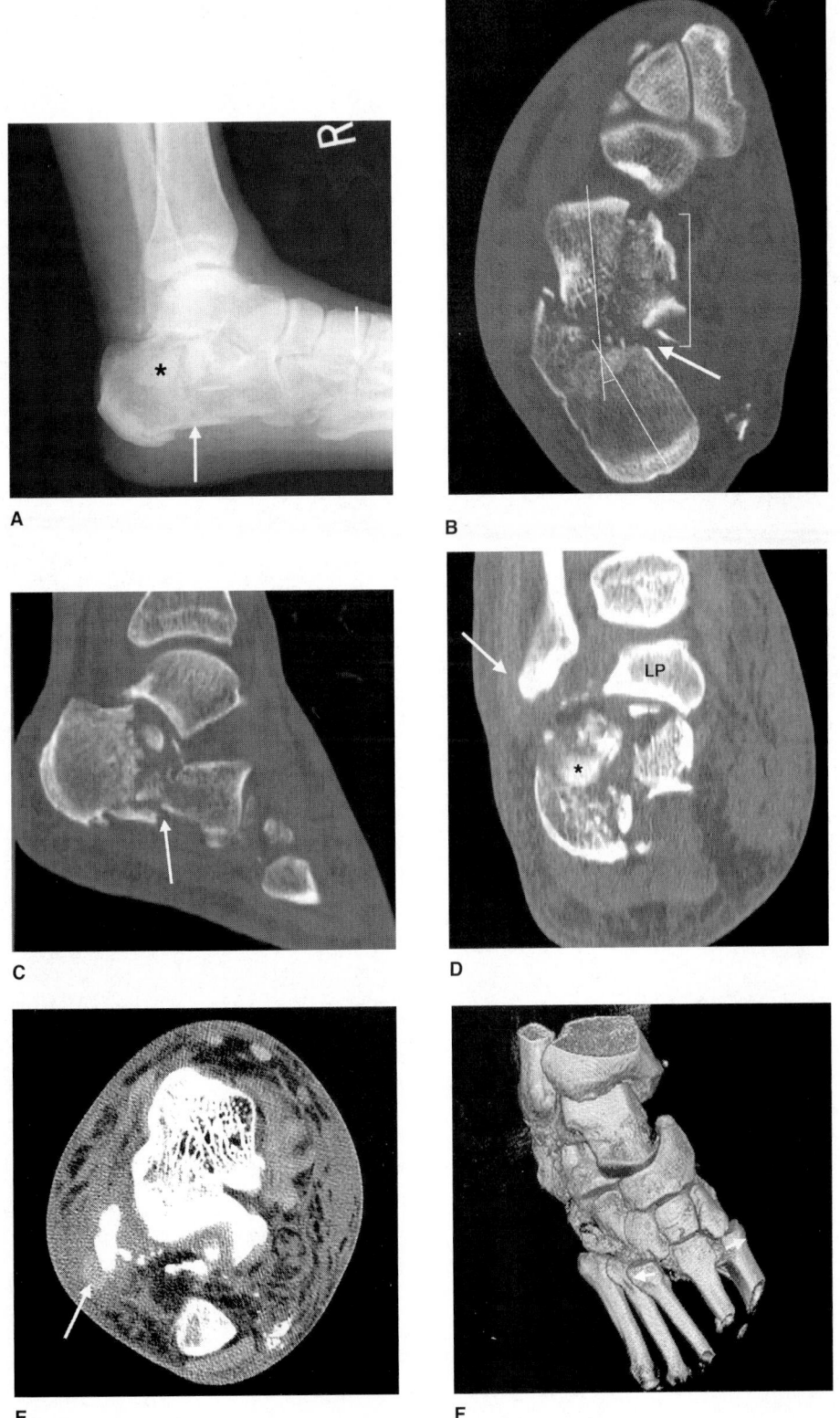

**FIGURE 16-50.** Periarticular fractures: calcaneus and Lisfranc fractures of midfoot. This 51-year-old restrained driver in a high-speed motor vehicle crash sustained multiple extremity and torso injuries. **(A)** Lateral conventional radiograph shows intra-articular fracture of calcaneus (upward pointing arrow denotes primary fracture plane; asterisk shows double density of central lateral fragment of posterior subtalar joint of calcaneus). Downward pointing arrow shows displacement of one of the metatarsal bases with an adjacent cuneiform fracture. **(B)** Axial computed tomography (CT) image at level of base of sustentaculum tali shows varus deformity through primary fracture (arrow). Secondary fracture plane extends toward anterior process (bracket). It is important to note continuity of cortex of medial wall of anterior process, as it influences distal extent of necessary fixation. **(C)** Sagittal reformation from axial CT shows primary fracture plane (upward arrow) with centrolateral fragment rotated dinto its superior extent. **(D)** Coronal reformation shows comminuted fracture of posterior facet of calcaneus due to bursting of body by lateral process (LP) of the talus. Centrolateral fragment is shown by asterisk. White arrow denotes lateral dislocation of peroneal tendons from peroneal groove in posterior fibula. **(E)** Axial CT at level of sinus tarsi, soft tissue window, shows lateral and anterior dislocation of peroneal tendons surrounded by hemorrhage and edema (white arrow). **(F)** Three-dimensional reformation from axial CT, medial oblique projection, shows divergent dislocations of great toe and third to fifth metatarsal bases (arrows).

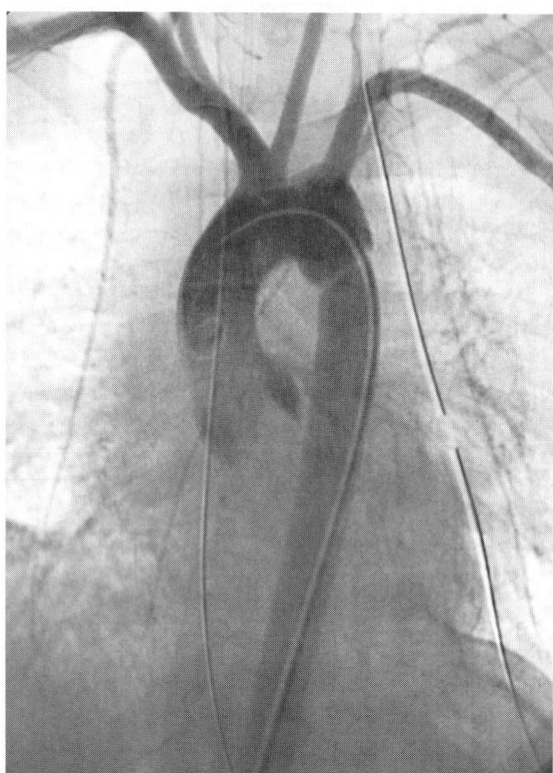

**FIGURE 16-51.** Traumatic aortic pseudoaneurysm. 30 year-old-male following high speed motor vehicle accident. Left Anterior Oblique (LAO) digital subtraction arch aortogram shows traumatic aortic pseudoaneurysm extending proximal to the left subclavian artery. Of note, the aortic size and the distance from the left subclavian artery is important when considering endovascular therapy.

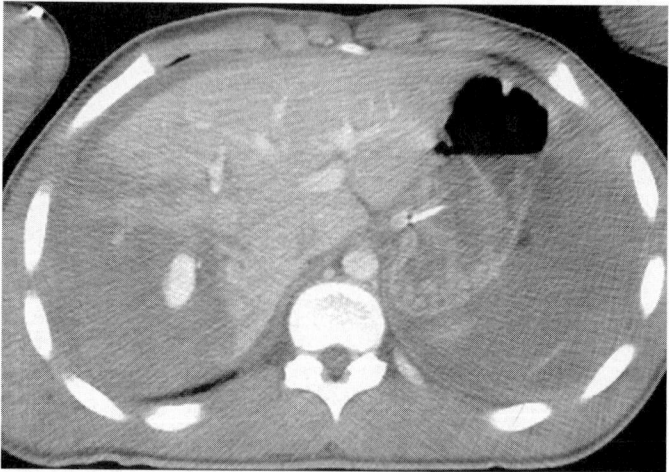

A

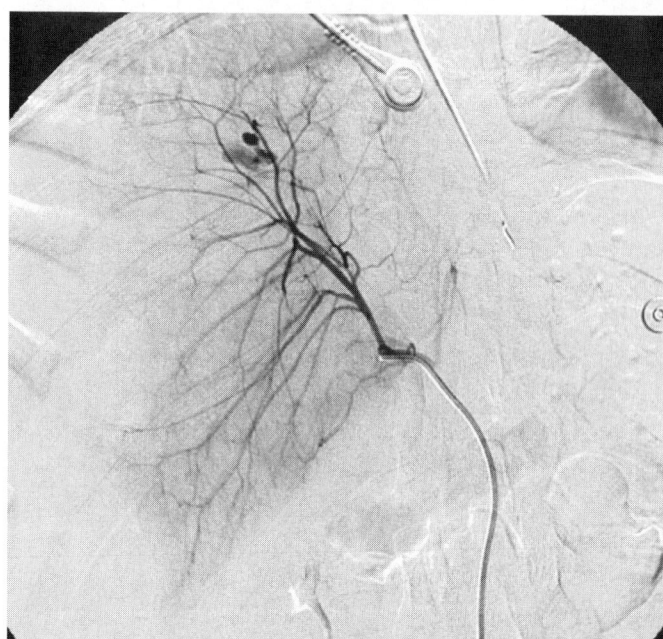

B

**FIGURE 16-52.** Liver laceration. **(A)** Trauma CT of the upper abdomen reveals a grade 5 liver laceration with pseudoaneurysm of the right hepatic lobe in this 18-year-old male status post high-speed MVA. **(B)** Right hepatic angiogram identified the pseudoaneurysm. Note the size of the feeding vessel in relation to the 5 French diagnostic catheter. Selective coil embolization was performed through a microcatheter. When selective catheterization is not possible, the liver is quite tolerant of wide arterial embolization due to the dual blood supply provided by the portal vein.

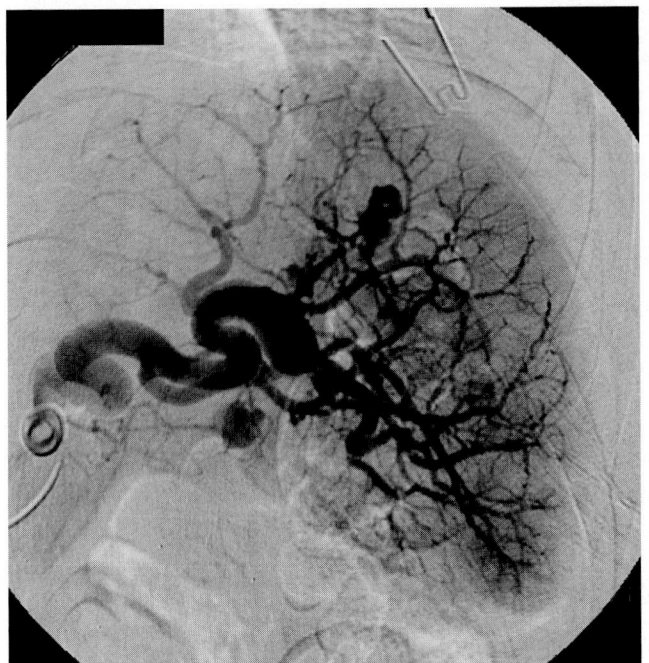

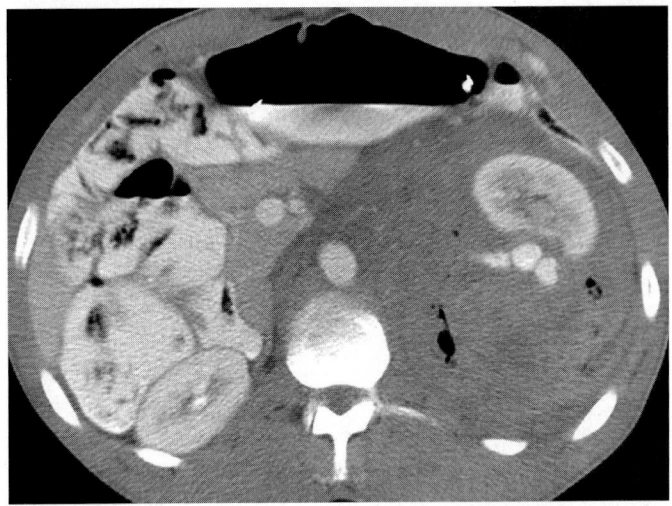

A

B

**FIGURE 16-53.** Splenic traumatic pseudoaneurysms. Digital subtraction angiogram of the splenic artery reveals multiple pseudoaneurysms in this 56-year-old male status post MVA. Selective embolization may not be possible due to splenic artery tortuosity. In such cases proximal splenic artery coil embolization proximal to the pancreatic magna branch is advocated in poor surgical candidates.

**FIGURE 16-54.** Renal laceration. **(A)** Abdominal CT in this 39-year-old male status post stab wound to the flank demonstrates a laceration to the lower pole of left kidney with massive perinephric hematoma and active extravasation. **(B)** Selective left renal arteriogram reveals active extravasation from a lower pole interlobar artery. Selective catheterization for embolization is mandatory as there is little arterial collateralization in the renal parenchyma.

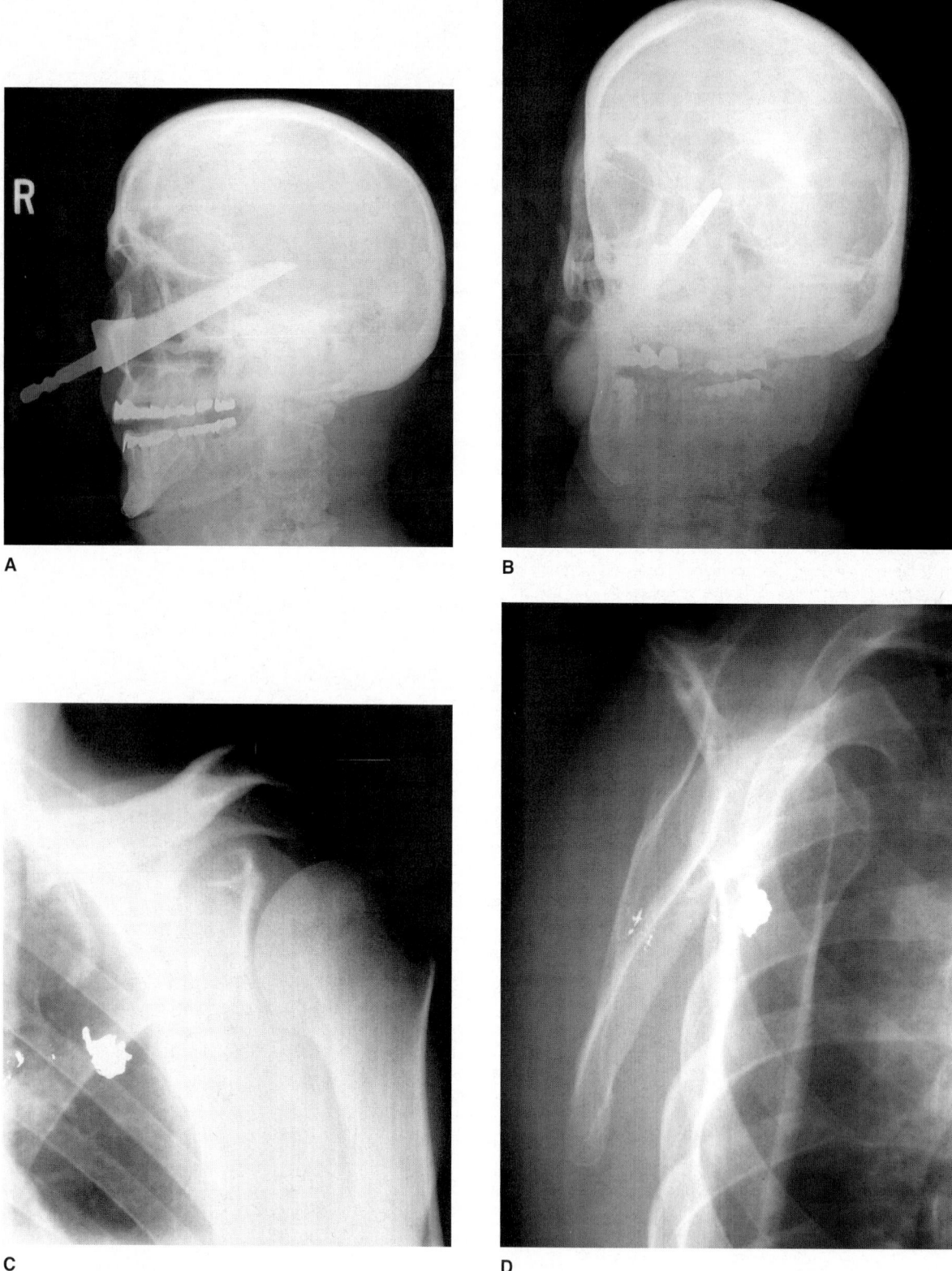

**FIGURE 16-55.**    Penetrating injuries: stab wounds and gunshot wounds. **(A)** Off-lateral projection of skull shows metallic portions of knife projected over anterior face and calvarium. On single view, it is not possible to determine course of knife or location of tip. **(B)** Anteroposterior (AP) radiograph of skull demonstrates tip projecting superior to sphenoid sinus and left of midline. Compared to (A), this location can only be intracranial, and course would appear to be from right maxillary sinus through and across midline structures. Triangulation afforded by orthogonal views allows reasonable estimation of structures at risk in this fatal assault. *(Reproduced with permission from AJ Wilson.)* **(C)** Posterior oblique view of left shoulder shows deformed bullet and adjacent fragment in individual who had been shot in the back. Pulmonary parenchyma appears unremarkable. **(D)** Same patient as in (C), anterior oblique of shoulder shows bullet fragments overlying scapula adjacent to entrance site with deformed bullet lying just inside chest wall. *(Reproduced with permission from AJ Wilson.)*

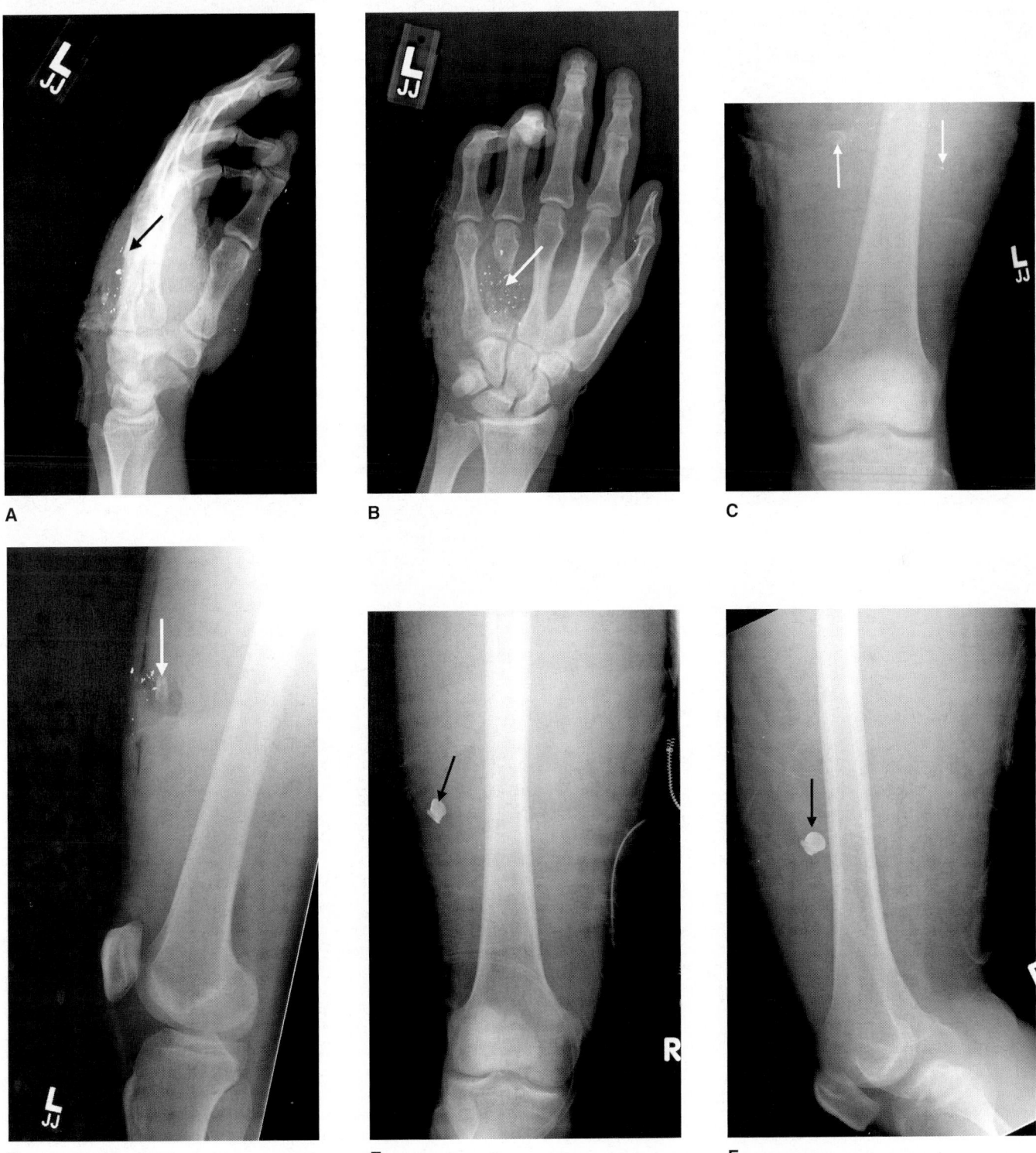

**FIGURE 16-56.** Penetrating injuries: gunshot wound. This 18-year-old male driver sustained unintentional gunshot wound from high-powered rifle fired from a distance of half a mile by firearm enthusiast practicing marksmanship. **(A)** Lateral view of left hand shows dorsal aspect of bony defect over metacarpals (arrow) with overlying metallic bullet debris. **(B)** Anteroposterior (AP) view of left hand shows segmental defect of ring finger metacarpal with many small stippled metallic fragments. **(C)** AP view of left femur shows metallic debris in lateral aspect of thigh (downward pointing arrow) and calcific density along medial aspect (upward pointing white arrow). **(D)** Lateral conventional radiograph demonstrates subcutaneous emphysema and rounded gas lucency in center of which lies tubular portion of bone (downward white arrow). Bone fragment represents ring finger metacarpal shaft embedded in soft tissues of anterior left thigh. **(E, F)** AP and lateral conventional radiographs of right distal thigh show deformed bullet (black arrows) lying in soft tissues of anterior lateral right thigh. Bones appear normal.

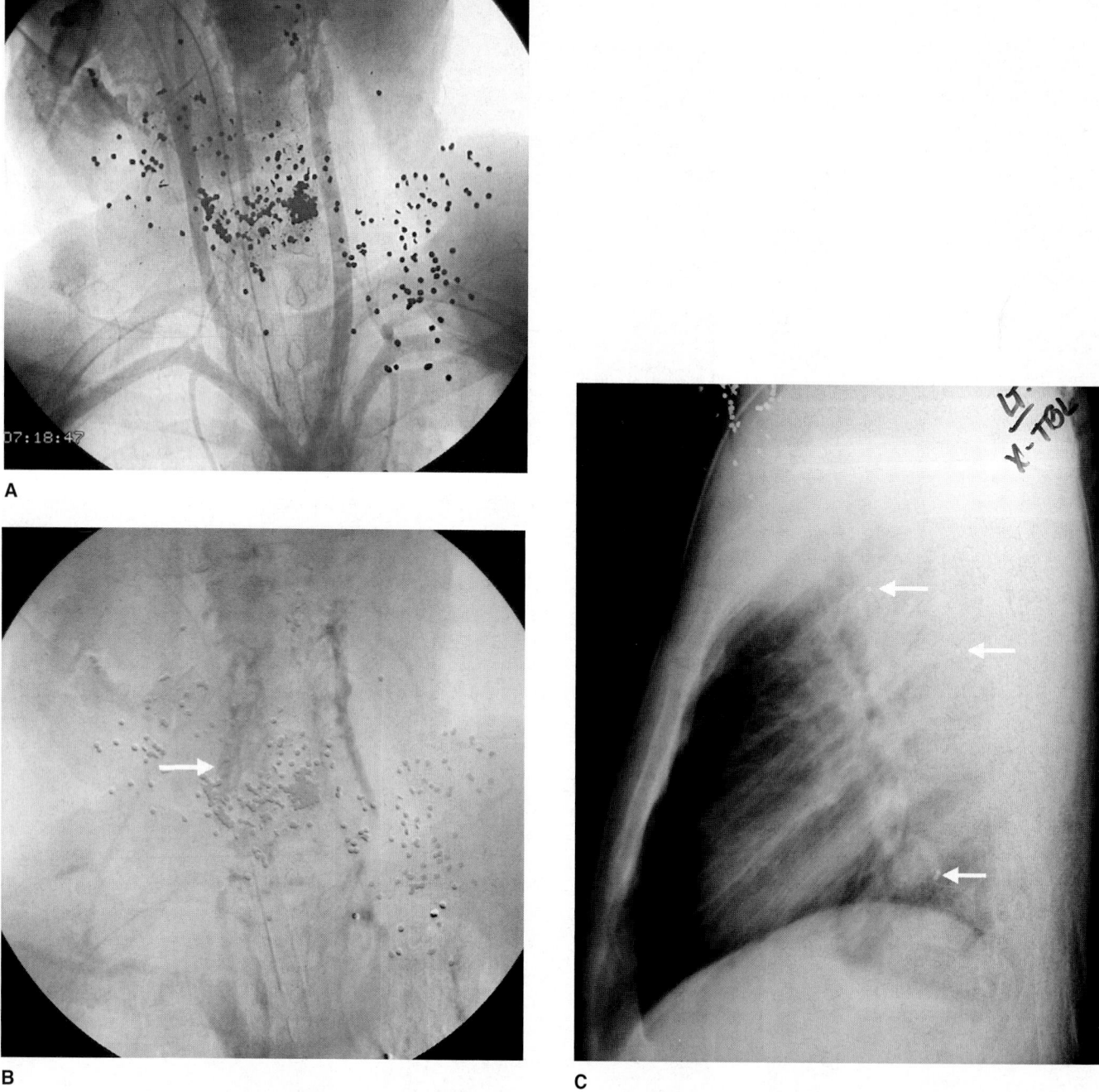

**FIGURE 16-57.**  Penetrating injury: shotgun wound with venous embolization. This 28-year-old man with close range shotgun wound sustained mandibular burst injury, disruption of larynx and right jugular vein, and multiple venous pulmonary pellet emboli. **(A)** Unsubtracted anteroposterior (AP) view from aortic arch angiogram shows wide distribution of many highly deformed shotgun pellets (deformation suggests lead rather than steel shot). In single view, it is not possible to determine location of pellets. Note the destruction of mandible. **(B)** Although no arterial disruption is evident, this venous phase image shows extravasation from partially occluded right jugular vein (white arrow). **(C)** Lateral chest shows multiple pulmonary pellet emboli (white arrows).

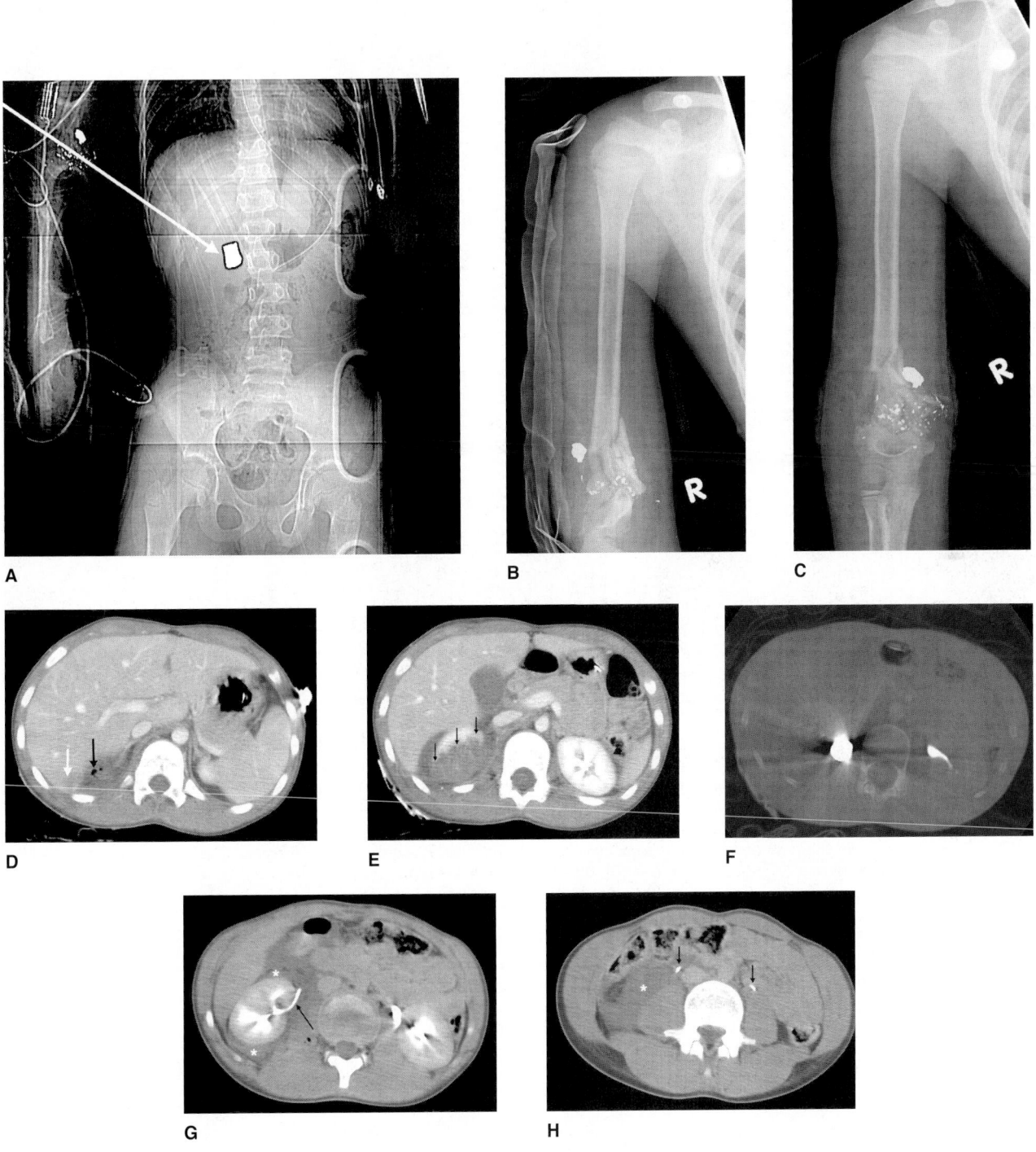

**FIGURE 16-58.** Penetrating injury: multiorgan gunshot wound. An 8-year-old girl shot by brother with 50-caliber muzzle-loading black powder musket. **(A)** Anteroposterior (AP) scanogram from abdominal CT shows large metallic caliber missile overlying right upper quadrant, with debris along its course through right distal humerus (long white arrow). **(B)** Lateral projection of right humerus shows a large fragment posterior to comminuted, intra-articular supracondylar distal humerus fracture. Bullet debris is admixed with multiple fracture shards. **(C)** AP radiograph of right humerus shows windswept appearance of bone, with osseous fragments projecting from lateral entrance site toward medial exit wound. **(D)** Contrast-enhanced axial CT image at level of right adrenal shows air in retroperitoneum (black arrow) surrounded by hematoma and including subtle enlargement of adrenal compatible with focal hematoma. There is inhomogeneous enhancement of posterior rim of liver, consistent with liver contusion (white arrow). Other organs are unremarkable. Metallic density over anterolateral left chest wall is an electrocardiogram electrode. **(E)** Axial image from contrast-enhanced computed tomography (CT), 2.5 cm caudal to D shows right renal laceration (black arrows) and infarction with surrounding hematoma. Small metallic fragment from bullet projects in posterior pararenal space. **(F)** Axial CT image 2 cm caudal to E shows large bullet adjacent to right side of vertebral column. Small amount of contrast is seen in right collecting system and normal amount of contrast in the left. Anteriorly, lucency is gastric antrum with the tip of nasogastric tube. **(G)** Axial CT image at level of right renal hilum from intravenous contrast-enhanced CT with 10-minute delay shows integrity to inferior pole and renal pelvis and proximal ureter (black arrow). Asterisks mark surrounding perinephric hematoma. **(H)** Axial image from contrast-enhanced abdominal CT at L3 level shows retroperitoneal hematoma (asterisk) and psoas enlargement (compatible with psoas hematoma). Continuity of ureters is demonstrated in this 10-minute delayed exam as contrast filling (black arrows).
*(Reproduced with permission from CC Blackmore.)*

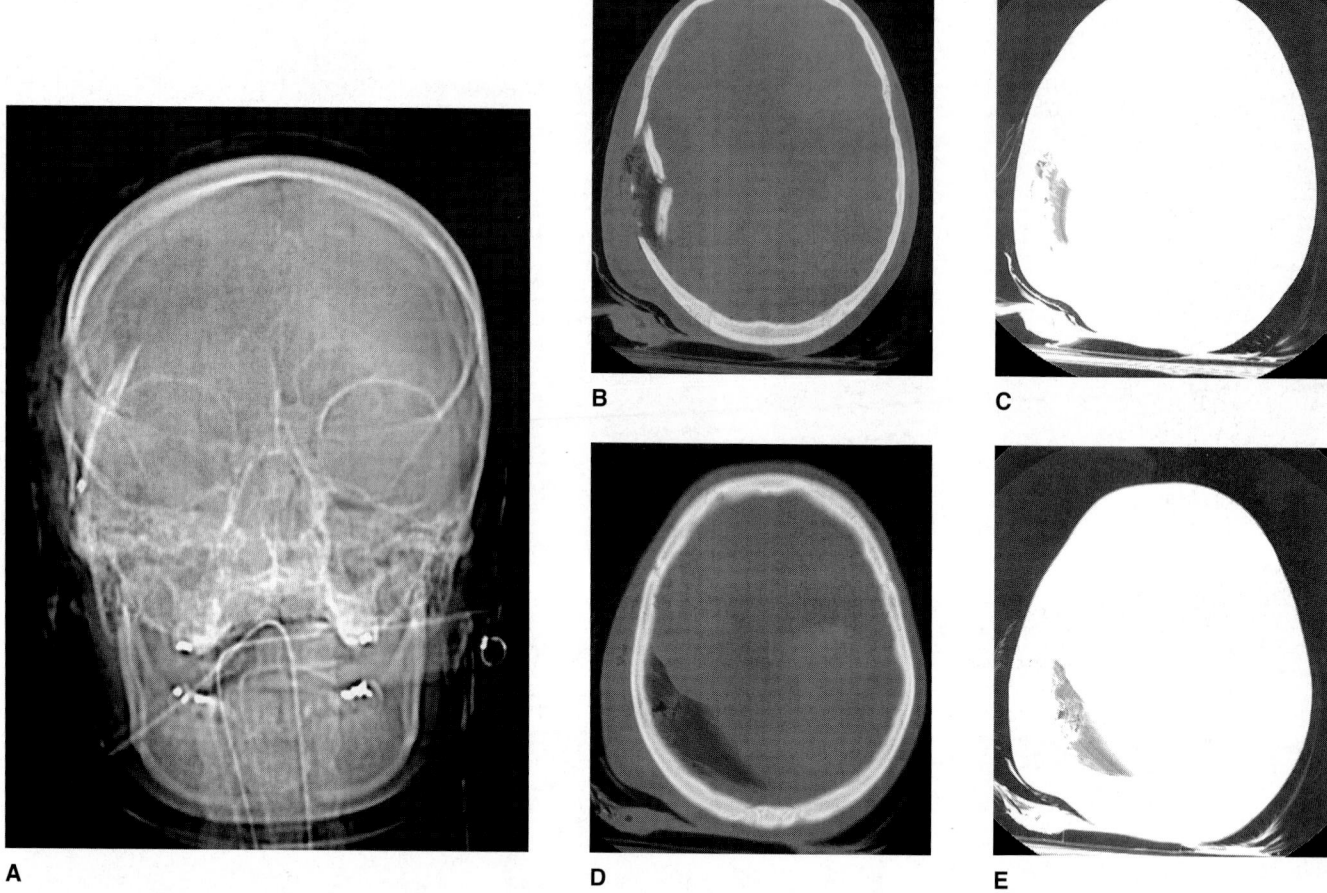

**FIGURE 16-59.** Penetrating injuries: wood impalement. **(A)** Anteroposterior (AP) scanogram from head computed tomography (CT) shows soft tissue irregularity over right parietal region and double-density cephalad to right orbital rim laterally, representing displaced calvarium. **(B)** Axial CT image at level of parietal convexities shows segmental depressed skull fracture with lucencies lateral to it. **(C)** Same image as in (B), but using lung windows, demonstrates air lucency within soft tissue region lateral to depressed skull fracture. Careful inspection demonstrates linear opacities and streaky linear lucencies. **(D)** Axial CT image just above images B and C again shows intracranial flame-shaped lucency, which on careful inspection shows structured linear opacities and included stippled lucencies. **(E)** Same image as in (D), but at lung windows, shows striations characteristic of wood. Wood-formed bodies can be among the most difficult to appreciate by any imaging modality, particularly if they are green wood, they may not be distinguished from the adjacent water-density soft tissues by any standard modality.
*(Reproduced with permission from DK Hallam.)*

## CONCLUSIONS

An effective imaging strategy for victims of trauma requires a commitment from hospitals to provide the necessary physical and personnel resources, organized spatially and procedurally, to allow the accomplished trauma surgeons to lead the trauma team. We have attempted to provide in this chapter an overview of imaging modalities, with their strengths and weaknesses. In order to facilitate high-quality studies, we hoped to guide the expectations of the trauma surgeon for specific imaging techniques. Finally, we have illustrated radiographic findings for many common traumatic conditions.

## REFERENCES

1. Blackwood GA, Blackmore CC, Mann FA, et al.: The importance of trauma series radiographs: Have we forgotten the ABC's? In: *13th Annual Scientific Meeting of the American Society of Emergency Radiology,* 2002.

2. Bushberg JT, Seibert SJ, Leidholdt EMJ, et al.: *The Essential Physics of Medical Imaging,* 2nd ed. Williams and Wilkins: Philadelphia, 2001.
3. Stengel D, Bauwens K, Sehouli J, et al.: Systematic review and meta-analysis of emergency ultrasonography for blunt abdominal trauma. *Br J Surg* 88:901, 2001.
4. Davis DP, Campbell CJ, Poste JC, et al.: The association between operator confidence and accuracy of ultrasonography performed by novice emergency physicians. *J Emerg Med* 29:259, 2005.
5. Branney SW, Wolfe RE, Moore EE, et al.: Quantitative sensitivity of ultrasound in detecting free intraperitoneal fluid. *J Trauma* 39:375, 1995.
6. Chiu WC, Cushing BM, Rodriguez A, et al.: Abdominal injuries without hemoperitoneum: A potential limitation of focused abdominal sonography for trauma (FAST). *J Trauma* 42:617, (discussion 623),, 1997.
7. Poletti PA, Wintermark M, Schnyder P, et al.: Traumatic injuries: Role of imaging in the management of the polytrauma victim (conservative expectation). *Eur Radiol* 12:969, 2002.
8. Ballard RB, Rozycki GS, Knudson MM, et al.: The surgeon's use of ultrasound in the acute setting. *Surg Clin North Am* 78:337, 1998.
9. Stengel D, Bauwens K, Sehouli J, et al.: Emergency ultrasound-based algorithms for diagnosing blunt abdominal trauma. *Cochrane Database Syst Rev* CD004446, 2005.
10. Becker CD, Poletti PA: The trauma concept: The role of MDCT in the diagnosis and management of visceral injuries. *Eur Radiol* 15:D105, 2005.

11. Fang JF, Wong YC, Lin BC, et al.: Usefulness of multidetector computed tomography for the initial assessment of blunt abdominal trauma patients. *World J Surg* 30:176, 2006.

12. Linsenmaier U, Krotz M, Hauser H, et al.: Whole-body computed tomography in polytrauma: Techniques and management. *Eur Radiol* 12:1728, 2002.

13. Novelline RA, Rhea JT, Rao PM, et al.: Helical CT in emergency radiology. *Radiology* 213:321, 1999.

14. Toyama Y, Kobayashi T, Nishiyama Y, et al.: CT for acute stage of closed head injury. *Radiat Med* 23:309, 2005.

15. Parizel PM, Van Goethem JW, Ozsarlak O, et al.: New developments in the neuroradiological diagnosis of craniocerebral trauma. *Eur Radiol* 15:569, 2005.

16. Oman JA, Cooper RJ, Holmes JF, et al.: Performance of a decision rule to predict need for computed tomography among children with blunt head trauma. *Pediatrics* 117:e238, 2006.

17. Mower WR, Hoffman JR, Herbert M, et al.: Developing a decision instrument to guide computed tomographic imaging of blunt head injury patients. *J Trauma* 59:954, 2005.

18. Gowda NK, Agrawal D, Bal C, et al.: Technetium Tc-99m ethyl cysteinate dimer brain single-photon emission CT in mild traumatic brain injury: A prospective study. *AJNR Am J Neuroradiol* 27:447, 2006.

19. de Lacey G, McCabe M, Constant O, et al.: Testing a policy for skull radiography (and admission) following mild head injury. *Br J Radiol* 63:14, 1990.

20. Masters SJ, McClean PM, Arcarese JS, et al.: Skull x-ray examinations after head trauma. Recommendations by a multidisciplinary panel and validation study. *N Engl J Med* 316:84, 1987.

21. Holmgren EP, Dierks EJ, Assael LA, et al.: Facial soft tissue injuries as an aid to ordering a combination head and facial computed tomography in trauma patients. *J Oral Maxillofac Surg* 63:651, 2005.

22. Lambert DM, Mirvis SE, Shanmuganathan K, et al.: Computed tomography exclusion of osseous paranasal sinus injury in blunt trauma patients: The "clear sinus" sign. *J Oral Maxillofac Surg* 55:1207, (discussion 1210), 1997.

23. Manson P: Organization of treatment in panfacial fractures. In: Rein PJ, ed. *Manual of Internal Fixation in the Cranio-Facial Skeleton.* Berlin: Springer Verlag, 1998, p. 95.

24. Stanley R: Maxillofacial trauma. In Cummings CW FJ, Harker LA, et al. eds. *Otolaryngology: Head and Neck Surgery,* 3rd ed. St. Louis: Mosby-Year Book, 1998, p. 453.

25. Schuknecht B, Graetz K: Radiologic assessment of maxillofacial, mandibular, and skull base trauma. *Eur Radiol* 15:560, 2005.

26. Rake PA, Rake SA, Swift JQ, et al.: A single reformatted oblique sagittal view as an adjunct to coronal computed tomography for the evaluation of orbital floor fractures. *J Oral Maxillofac Surg* 62:456, 2004.

27. Dos Santos DT, Costa e Silva AP, Vannier MW, et al.: Validity of multislice computerized tomography for diagnosis of maxillofacial fractures using an independent workstation. *Oral Surg Oral Med Oral Pathol Oral Radiol Endod* 98:715, 2004.

28. Klenk G, Kovacs A: Do we need three-dimensional computed tomography in maxillofacial surgery? *J Craniofac Surg* 15:842, (discussion 850), 2004.

29. Saigal K, Winokur RS, Finden S, et al.: Use of three-dimensional computerized tomography reconstruction in complex facial trauma. *Facial Plast Surg* 21:214, 2005.

30. Chen WJ, Yang YJ, Fang YM, et al.: Identification and classification in le fort type fractures by using 2D and 3D computed tomography. *Chin J Traumatol* 9:59, 2006.

31. Ploder O, Klug C, Voracek M, et al.: Evaluation of computer-based area and volume measurement from coronal computed tomography scans in isolated blowout fractures of the orbital floor. *J Oral Maxillofac Surg* 60:1267, (discussion 1273), 2002.

32. Brenner D, Elliston C, Hall E, Berdon W: Estimated risks of radiation-induced fatal cancer from pediatric CT. *AJR Am J Roentgenol* 176:289, 2001.

33. Biffl WL: Diagnosis of blunt cerebrovascular injuries. *Curr Opin Crit Care* 9:530, 2003.

34. Miller PR, Fabian TC, Croce MA, et al.: Prospective screening for blunt cerebrovascular injuries: Analysis of diagnostic modalities and outcomes. *Ann Surg* 236:386, (discussion 393), 2002.

35. Biffl WL, Egglin T, Benedetto B, et al.: Sixteen-slice computed tomographic angiography is a reliable noninvasive screening test for clinically significant blunt cerebrovascular injuries. *J Trauma* 60:745, (discussion 751), 2006.

36. Cothren CC, Moore EE, Ray CE Jr, et al.: Carotid artery stents for blunt cerebrovascular injury: Risks exceed benefits. *Arch Surg* 140:480, (discussion 485), 2005.

37. Mutze S, Rademacher G, Matthes G, et al.: Blunt cerebrovascular injury in patients with blunt multiple trauma: Diagnostic accuracy of duplex Doppler US and early CT angiography. *Radiology* 237:884, 2005.

38. LeBlang SD, Nunez DB Jr: Noninvasive imaging of cervical vascular injuries. *AJR Am J Roentgenol* 174:1269, 2000.

39. Bub LD, Hollingworth W, Jarvik JG, et al.: Screening for blunt cerebrovascular injury: Evaluating the accuracy of multidetector computed tomographic angiography. *J Trauma* 59:691, 2005.

40. Blackmore CC, Emerson SS, Mann FA, et al.: Cervical spine imaging in patients with trauma: Determination of fracture risk to optimize use. *Radiology* 211:759, 1999.

41. Hanson JA, Blackmore CC, Mann FA, et al.: Cervical spine injury: A clinical decision rule to identify high-risk patients for helical CT screening. *AJR Am J Roentgenol* 174:713, 2000.

42. Adelgais KM, Grossman DC, Langer SG, et al.: Use of helical computed tomography for imaging the pediatric cervical spine. *Acad Emerg Med* 11:228, 2004.

43. Hernandez JA, Chupik C, Swischuk LE: Cervical spine trauma in children under 5 years: Productivity of CT. *Emerg Radiol* 10:176, 2004.

44. Aulino JM, Tutt LK, Kaye JJ, et al.: Occipital condyle fractures: Clinical presentation and imaging findings in 76 patients. *Emerg Radiol* 11:342, 2005.

45. Van Goethem JW, Maes M, Ozsarlak O, et al.: Imaging in spinal trauma. *Eur Radiol* 15:582, 2005.

46. Marion D, Domeier R, Dunham CM, et al.: Determination of cervical spine stability in trauma patients. In *Eastern Association for the Surgery of Trauma (EAST),* 2000.

47. Mower WR, Hoffman JR, Pollack CV Jr, et al.: Use of plain radiography to screen for cervical spine injuries. *Ann Emerg Med* 38:1, 2001.

48. Stiell IG, Wells GA, Vandemheen KL, et al.: The Canadian C-spine rule for radiography in alert and stable trauma patients. *JAMA* 286:1841, 2001.

49. Hoffman JR, Wolfson AB, Todd K, et al.: Selective cervical spine radiography in blunt trauma: Methodology of the National Emergency X-Radiography Utilization Study (NEXUS). *Ann Emerg Med* 32:461, 1998.

50. Holmes JF, Panacek EA, Miller PQ, et al.: Prospective evaluation of criteria for obtaining thoracolumbar radiographs in trauma patients. *J Emerg Med* 24:1, 2003.

51. Hsu JM, Joseph T, Ellis AM: Thoracolumbar fracture in blunt trauma patients: Guidelines for diagnosis and imaging. *Injury* 34:426, 2003.

52. Kuhns L: *Imaging of Spinal Trauma in Children.* BC Decker Inc.: Hamilton, Ontario, 1998.

53. Roos JE, Hilfiker P, Platz A, et al.: MDCT in emergency radiology: Is a standardized chest or abdominal protocol sufficient for evaluation of thoracic and lumbar spine trauma? *AJR Am J Roentgenol* 183:959, 2004.

54. Richards PJ: Cervical spine clearance: A review. *Injury* 36:248, (discussion 270), 2005.

55. Sliker CW, Mirvis SE, Shanmuganathan K: Assessing cervical spine stability in obtunded blunt trauma patients: Review of medical literature. *Radiology* 234:733, 2005.

56. Rodriguez RM, Hendey GW, Marek G, et al.: A pilot study to derive clinical variables for selective chest radiography in blunt trauma patients. *Ann Emerg Med* 47:415, 2006.

57. Holmes JF, Sokolove PE, Brant WE, et al.: A clinical decision rule for identifying children with thoracic injuries after blunt torso trauma. *Ann Emerg Med* 39:492, 2002.

58. Mirvis SE, Shanmuganathan K, Miller BH, et al.: Traumatic aortic injury: Diagnosis with contrast-enhanced thoracic CT–five-year experience at a major trauma center. *Radiology* 200:413, 1996.

59. Blackmore CC, Zweibel A, Mann FA: Determining risk of traumatic aortic injury: How to optimize imaging strategy. *AJR Am J Roentgenol* 174:343, 2000.

60. Omert L, Yeaney WW, Protetch J: Efficacy of thoracic computerized tomography in blunt chest trauma. *Am Surg* 67:660, 2001.

61. Holmes JF, Ngyuen H, Jacoby RC, et al.: Do all patients with left costal margin injuries require radiographic evaluation for intraabdominal injury? *Ann Emerg Med* 46:232, 2005.

62. Ryan MF, Hamilton PA, Chu P, et al.: Active extravasation of arterial contrast agent on post-traumatic abdominal computed tomography. *Can Assoc Radiol J* 55:160, 2004.

63. Sheridan MK, Blackmore CC, Linnau KF, et al.: Can CT predict the source of arterial hemorrhage in patients with pelvic fractures? *Emerg Radiol* 9:188, 2002.

64. Brown CV, Kasotakis G, Wilcox A, et al.: Does pelvic hematoma on admission computed tomography predict active bleeding at angiography for pelvic fracture? *Am Surg* 71:759, 2005.

65. Poletti PA, Mirvis SE, Shanmuganathan K, et al.: CT criteria for management of blunt liver trauma: Correlation with angiographic and surgical findings. *Radiology* 216:418, 2000.

66. Killeen KL, Shanmuganathan K, Mirvis SE: Imaging of traumatic diaphragmatic injuries. *Semin Ultrasound CT MR* 23:184, 2002.

67. Patselas TN, Gallagher EG: The diagnostic dilemma of diaphragm injury. *Am Surg* 68:633, 2002.

68. Hunter JC, Brandser EA, Tran KA: Pelvic and acetabular trauma. *Radiol Clin North Am* 35:559, 1997.

69. Stiell IG, Greenberg GH, McKnight RD, et al.: Decision rules for the use of radiography in acute ankle injuries. Refinement and prospective validation. *JAMA* 269:1127, 1993.

70. Stiell IG, Greenberg GH, Wells GA, et al.: Prospective validation of a decision rule for the use of radiography in acute knee injuries. *JAMA* 275:611, 1996.

71. Stiell IG, Wells GA, Hoag RH, et al.: Implementation of the Ottawa Knee Rule for the use of radiography in acute knee injuries. *JAMA* 278:2075, 1997.

72. Ouwendijk R, Kock MC, Visser K, et al.: Interobserver agreement for the interpretation of contrast-enhanced 3D MR angiography and MDCT angiography in peripheral arterial disease. *AJR Am J Roentgenol* 185:1261, 2005.

# Commentary ■ STUART E. MIRVIS

The chapter on imaging and intervention in blunt and penetrating trauma by Stanescu et al. presents a concise overview of the applications of imaging in trauma. By necessity, this overview must focus on what concepts and imaging strategies are both current and generally well-established. Of course, these imaging applications are a moving target, subject to advances in technology and the influence of greater experience.

The utility of imaging for diagnoses of traumatic injury has made amazingly rapid advances in the last two decades, perhaps faster than some nonimaging specialists are comfortable with. The dramatic advances in computed tomography, magnetic resonance imaging, and bedside sonographic technology have fostered this trend toward increasing utilization of imaging techniques. Also, the development of electronic image review, transmission, and storage has made images available at multiple sites simultaneously and has facilitated communication of critical information.

The goals of the trauma team have always been the same, to make rapid and accurate diagnoses, to institute appropriate and timely treatment, to minimize morbidity and mortality, and to do all of this in a cost and resource efficient manner. I believe that the greater reliance on diagnostic imaging in the trauma setting has contributed very positively toward these efforts.

What are the trends in trauma imaging evolving today and what can be anticipated in the near future? As clearly established in this chapter multi-detector computed tomography (MDCT) has become the principle imaging device in assessing the "stable" trauma victim. Almost all important diagnoses can be established or excluded with this single modality. Increasingly, more body region, including full body surveys, are performed by MDCT. The speed of the study, the greater image resolution, the higher sensitivity to subtle injuries, the capacity to directly detect vascular injury, and the ability to reconstruct images in any plane, volume, or within structures have all contributed to this development.

Concurrent with increased reliance on MDCT, the use of plain radiography in the admission phase of trauma care has declined. It is well recognized that bedside radiography is far less sensitive for diagnosis of spine and thoracic pathology, is often of limited technical quality, is time-consuming, and is relatively expensive. The use of anterior-posterior and lateral thoracic and lumbar radiography has also declined, as it has been established that injuries in these areas are more accurately detected by the "screening CT" of the chest, abdomen, and pelvis, without need for special thin-section dedicated CT imaging. Facial radiographs have virtually disappeared in acute trauma. I expect that the decline in the use of the plain film in initial imaging triage will continue unabated.

Many physicians involved in trauma care may see this as an unfortunate or perhaps dangerous trend. As always, appropriate patient selection is required before imaging outside the immediate confines of the admissions area can proceed. In our practice, MDCT supports confident and rapid exclusion of major injury, permits quick decisions regarding patient disposition, limits hospital stays, keeps beds available, and decreases the total cost of care. In today's litigious environment of health care, the CT scanner has unfortunately often served as the "ultimate second opinion" and is perhaps overutilized in that respect. On the positive side, automatic x-ray dose modulation (real-time dose adjustment as different tissue thicknesses are scanned) is becoming routinely available on new CT units and will decrease patient exposure, in part compensating for the increased use of ionizing radiation.

Each new generation of CT technology has improved our ability to diagnose vascular injury and detect active bleeding. This capacity directs our attention to the most appropriate site for surgical or catheter-directed treatment with concurrent knowledge of the spectrum of the patient's injuries. CT angiography is now well-established in the pelvis, abdomen, and chest wall, and is increasingly used in the neck and extremities leading to a decreasing need for time-consuming, expensive, and labor-intensive diagnostic angiography. Therapy is now the mainstay of interventional radiology in trauma care. As an example, in our center, the combined use of MDCT and angiographic embolization for splenic vascular injury has reduced the need for splenectomy, while achieving an extremely high spleen preservation rate.

MDCT has also shown promise in the assessment of patients sustaining penetrating torso trauma. Historically, most of these patients have been surgically explored, unless the wound was clearly superficial. MDCT can often demonstrate the course of a penetrating object and determine the likelihood of visceral injury. Time and further experience will dictate the future of MDCT for this application.

Other imaging techniques will become more common in management of trauma patients. Perfusion CT will be used increasingly for cerebral trauma to establish regional perfusion, tissue viability, and effects of treatment. Interactive volume-rendered images will be routinely acquired for assessment of complex injuries on increasingly user-friendly workstations that will have the capacity for the treating physicians to manipulate image data in their offices or in the operating room. So-called PACS (picture-archiving, communication, and storage) systems will become more robust, allowing faster movement of images across networks and more image manipulation capability on reviewing stations as opposed to dedicated workstations. Almost certainly, this improvement will facilitate decision making and treatment initiation.

The application of new technologies must occur in well-considered steps using scientific methods to ensure they perform as expected and clearly improve upon what has gone before. The acquisition of diagnostic information, the communication of such information, and its rapid application require direct interaction between bedside physicians and imaging specialist to assure optimal use of imaging technology for maximum patient benefit. Today, the imaging physician can contribute more than ever to the improving care of the trauma patient and must be a fully integrated member of the trauma care team, working and communicating with other team members. "Being there" only in spirit while interpreting images in complete isolated from the clinical circumstances and failing to provide pertinent clinical data to the imaging specialist can minimize the benefits of even the best technology.

# Surgeon-Performed Ultrasound in Trauma and Surgical Critical Care

*Christopher J. Dente* ■ *Grace S. Rozycki*

## INTRODUCTION

For nearly 15 years, surgeons in American trauma centers have successfully performed, interpreted, and taught ultrasound examinations of patients who are injured or critically ill.[1–13] Real-time imaging allows the surgeon to receive instantaneous information about the clinical condition of the patient and, therefore, helps to expedite the patient's management. In many trauma centers, ultrasound machines are owned by surgeons and are part of the standard equipment in the trauma resuscitation area as well as in the intensive care unit (ICU). While diagnostic peritoneal lavage (DPL) and computed tomography (CT) scanning are still valuable diagnostic tests for the detection of intra-abdominal injury in patients, ultrasound is faster, as well as noninvasive and painless.

As an extension of the physical examination, surgeons routinely use ultrasound in the acute setting to determine the presence or absence of fluid in the peritoneal cavity, the pericardium, and the pleural cavities. Additional uses of this modality include the detection of pneumothoraces, sternal fractures, soft tissue infections, common femoral vein thromboses, as well as assistance for such procedures as ultrasound guided thoracentesis, bedside placement of vena caval filters, and placement of intravenous central lines.

The objectives of this chapter include a discussion of the following: (1) select principles of ultrasound physics related to the use of ultrasound in the evaluation of patients who are injured or critically ill; and (2) the components, indications, and pitfalls of these focused ultrasound examinations as used in the acute care setting.

## ULTRASOUND PHYSICS

Ultrasonography is operator dependent and, therefore, an understanding of select principles of ultrasound imaging is necessary so that images may be acquired rapidly, performed precisely, and interpreted correctly. This skill is facilitated by knowledge of some basic principles of physics that enable the surgeon to select the appropriate transducer, optimize resolution of the image, and recognize artifacts. Some basic terms and principles of physics relative to ultrasound imaging in the acute setting are defined in Tables 17-1, 17-2, and 17-3.

In general, an ultrasound system includes the following components: (1) a *transmitter* that controls electrical signals sent to the transducer; (2) a *receiver* or image processor that admits the electrical signal; (3) a *transducer* containing piezoelectric crystals to interconvert electrical and acoustic energy; (4) a *monitor* to display the ultrasound image; and (5) an *image recorder* or printer.[14,15] The ultrasound images that are obtained depend on the orientation of the transducer relative to the structure or organ being imaged. Each transducer has an indicator that directs the orientation of imaging (Fig. 17-1). The orientations or scanning planes are described in Table 17-4 and the projected patient positions on the ultrasound monitor are shown in Fig. 17-2.[16]

Although diagnostic ultrasound uses transducer frequencies ranging from 1 MHz (megahertz = one million cycles per second) to 30 MHz, medical diagnostic imaging most often uses frequencies between 2.5 and 10 MHz (Table 17-5). Accordingly, transducers are chosen on the basis of the depth of the structure or organ to be imaged. High-frequency transducers ($\geq$5 MHz) provide excellent resolution for imaging superficial structures such as an abscess in the soft tissue of an extremity. Lower frequency transducers emit waves that penetrate deeply into the tissue and, therefore, are preferred for visualizing organs such as the liver or spleen.[14,17,18] Caveats of ultrasound imaging relative to physics principles are listed in Table 17-6.

## SURGEON-PERFORMED ULTRASOUND IN TRAUMA

### Fast

Introduction.   Developed for the evaluation of injured patients, the Focused Assessment for the Sonographic Examination of the Trauma Patient (FAST) is a rapid diagnostic examination to assess

**TABLE 17-1**

### Ultrasound Physics Terminology Relevant to Ultrasound Imaging[19]

| TERM | DEFINITION | SIGNIFICANCE |
|------|------------|--------------|
| Ultrasound | High-frequency (>20 kHz) mechanical radiant energy transmitted through a medium | Diagnostic ultrasound: 1–30 MHz<br>Medical diagnostic ultrasound: 2.5–10 MHz |
| Frequency | Number of cycles/sec ($10^6$ cycles/sec = 1 MHz) | Increasing frequency improves resolution<br>Higher frequency transducers (e.g., 7.5 MHz) provide better resolution of tissues |
| Propagation speed | Speed with which wave travels through soft tissue (1540 m/s) Propagation speed (determined by density and stiffness of medium) is greater in solids than in liquids and greater in liquids than in gases. | To image an organ, the ultrasound wave must be emitted from the transducer, travel through a medium (soft tissue or liquid), strike the organ, and bounceback to the transducer. It is the reflected wave that forms the ultrasound image. Ultrasound waves travel better through solids and liquids (molecules are more compact, less interference) than through gas. Therefore, ultra sound waves do not travel well through air-filled structures (e.g., lungs or bowel) These organs are visualized, however, when they are surrounded by fluid which acts as an acoustic window and allows the through transmission of waves. |
| | | The formation of a good ultrasound image depends on two principles of physics: (1) how well sound waves are transmitted through the tissue (acoustic impedance, which equals the density of the material times the speed of sound through the material); and (2) the amount of sound waves reflected once they hit a target organ. A good ultrasound image, therefore, is formed when sound waves travel well through tissues of higher and similar density, such as the liver and kidney. |
| | | In the presence of subcutaneous emphysema, a large impedance mismatch exists because of the difference in densities between the air-filled tissue and the soft tissue (liver). As a result, the waves travel poorly through the air-filled tissue and not enough of them are reflected back to the transducer to form a good image. |
| | | The air filled lung is not normally visualized because the air within the lung reflects the sound waves too strongly and therefore, no image is formed. When a hemothorax or pleural effusion is present, the differences in tissue acoustic impedance between fluid and the lung allow the lung to be visualized |
| Acoustic Impedance | | Acoustic impedance = density of tissue times the speed of sound in tissue (sound velocity) |
| | | The strength of the returning wave depends on difference in density between two organs imaged. Structures of different acoustic impedance (e.g., bile and gallstone) are relatively easy to distinguish from one another. Those of similar acoustic impedance (e.g., spleen and kidney) are more difficult to distinguish, although Gerota's fascia has a higher tissue acoustic impedance (more dense) and, therefore, allows the spleen and kidney to be visualized as two distinct organs. |
| Amplitude | Strength or height of wave | Amplitude and intensity are reduced (attenuated) as waves travel through tissue. The higher the frequency, the more the wave is attenuated. Therefore, higher frequency transducers cannot visualize deep structures well. Increasing the gain setting on the machine enhances the amplitude of the returning or reflected ultrasound waves. If the gain setting is too high, echo amplification is too strong and the image appears too bright. |
| Attenuation | Decrease in amplitude and intensity of wave as it travels through a medium; attenuation is affected by absorption, scattering, and reflection | |
| Absorption | Conversion of sound energy into heat | |
| Scattering | Redirection of wave as it strikes a rough or small boundary | |
| Reflection | Return of wave toward transducer | |
| Artifact | Error in imaging. Features on the ultrasound image that do not have precise correspon-dence to the image being scanned. | Examples include shadowing (gallstones), reverberation (comet tail, metallic fragment), and mirror image (diaphragm as strong reflector) In the normal sagittal ultrasound image of the lower thoracic cavity, the supradiaphragmatic area (lung) appears to have a similar echogenicity to the liver because of a mirror image artifact. This artifact occurs because the diaphragm acts as a strong reflector of the ultrasound waves, sending them back to the transducer and then re-reflecting them again as they return to the interface of the diaphragm and the liver. (It should be recalled that it is the *returning* or *reflected* wave that forms the ultrasound image on the screen). These re-reflected or smaller waves return to the transducer *after* the original reflected waves and, therefore, "create" an image that appears to be deeper than the liver and diaphragm, hence the "mirror image."[20] |

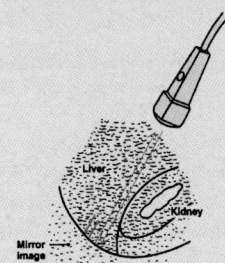

**TABLE 17-2**

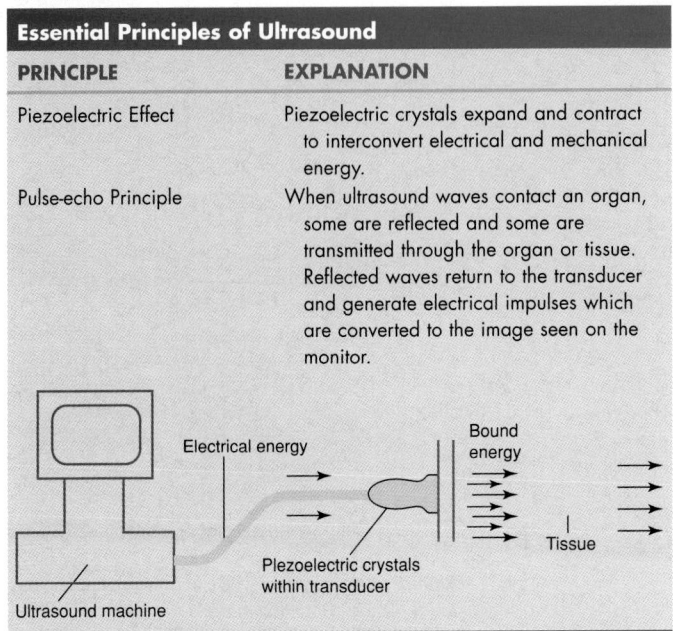

| Essential Principles of Ultrasound | |
| --- | --- |
| **PRINCIPLE** | **EXPLANATION** |
| Piezoelectric Effect | Piezoelectric crystals expand and contract to interconvert electrical and mechanical energy. |
| Pulse-echo Principle | When ultrasound waves contact an organ, some are reflected and some are transmitted through the organ or tissue. Reflected waves return to the transducer and generate electrical impulses which are converted to the image seen on the monitor. |

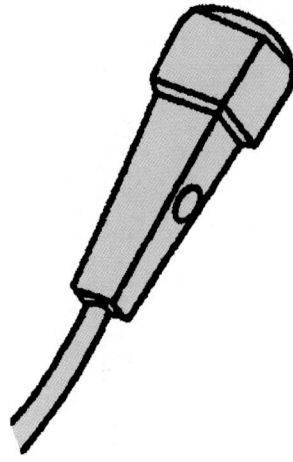

**FIGURE 17-1.** Schematic of multifrequency (2.5 to 5.0 MHz) convex transducer. Dot is an example of an indicator for imaging orientation.

**TABLE 17-3**

| Terminology Used in Interpretation of Ultrasound Images[21] | |
| --- | --- |
| **TERM** | **DEFINITION** |
| Echogenicity | Degree to which tissue echoes the ultrasonic waves (generally reflected in ultrasound image as degree of brightness) |
| Anechoic | Showing no internal echoes, appearing dark or black |
| Isoechoic | Having appearance similar to that of surrounding tissue |
| Hypoechoic | Less echoic or darker than surrounding tissue |
| Hyperechoic | More echoic or brighter than surrounding tissue |

Adapted from Hedrick WR, Hykes L, Starchman DE: Glossary. Anonymous In: Ultrasound physics and instrumentation. 3rd ed. St. Louis: Mosby; 1995. p. 355.

**TABLE 17-4**

| Scanning Planes Used in Ultrasound Imaging[16] | | |
| --- | --- | --- |
| **SCANNING PLANE (FIG. 17-2)** | **DEFINITION** | **TRANSDUCER ORIENTATION** |
| Sagittal | Divides body into right and left sections parallel to long axis | Transducer indicator points toward patient's head |
| Transverse | Divides body into superior and inferior sections perpendicular to long axis | Transducer indicator points toward patient's right side |
| Coronal | Divides body into anterior and posterior sections perpendicular to sagittal and parallel to long axis | Transducer indicator points toward patient's head when imaging exteriorly |

Adapted from Tempkin BB: Scanning Planes and Methods. In Tempkin BB, ed.: Ultrasound Scanning: Principles and Protocols. Philadelphia: W.B. Saunders Company; 1993. p. 7.

patients with potential injuries to the thorax or abdomen. The test sequentially surveys for the presence or absence of fluid in the pericardial sac and in the dependent abdominal regions, including Morison's pouch region in the right upper quadrant (RUQ), the left upper quadrant (LUQ) behind the spleen and between the spleen and kidney, and the pelvis posterior to the bladder. Surgeons can perform the FAST during the primary or secondary survey of the American College of Surgeons Advanced Trauma Life Support[22] algorithm and, although minimal patient preparation is needed, a full urinary bladder is ideal to provide an acoustic window for visualization of blood in the pelvis.

Blood, as any fluid, will accumulate in dependent regions of the abdomen.[23] In the supine position, this corresponds to Morison's pouch, the spleno-renal recess, and above the spleen as well as in the pelvis posterior to the bladder. All these regions may be visualized rapidly and dependably with the FAST. Furthermore, ultrasound is an excellent modality for the detection of intra-abdominal fluid, having been shown to detect ascites in small amounts.[24,25] Although the exact minimum amount of intraperitoneal fluid that can be detected by ultrasound is not known,[26] most authors agree that it is a sensitive modality.

The FAST is performed in a specific sequence for several reasons. The pericardial area is visualized first so that blood within the heart can be used as a standard to set the gain (Table 17-1). Most modern ultrasound machines have presets so that the gain does not need to be reset each time the machine is turned on. Occasionally, if multiple types of examinations are performed with different transducers, the gain should be checked to ensure that intracardiac blood appears anechoic. This maneuver ensures that a hemoperitoneum will also appear anechoic and will be readily detected on the ultrasound image. The *abdominal* part of the FAST begins with a survey of the RUQ which is the location within the peritoneal cavity where blood most often accumulates and is most readily detected with the FAST. Indeed, investigators from four Level I trauma centers examined true positive ultrasound images of 275 patients who sustained either blunt (#220) or penetrating (#55) injuries.[27] They found that regardless of the injured organ (with the exception of those patients who had an isolated perforated viscus), blood was most often identified on the RUQ image of the FAST. This can be a time-saving measure because when hemoperitoneum is identified on the FAST examination of a

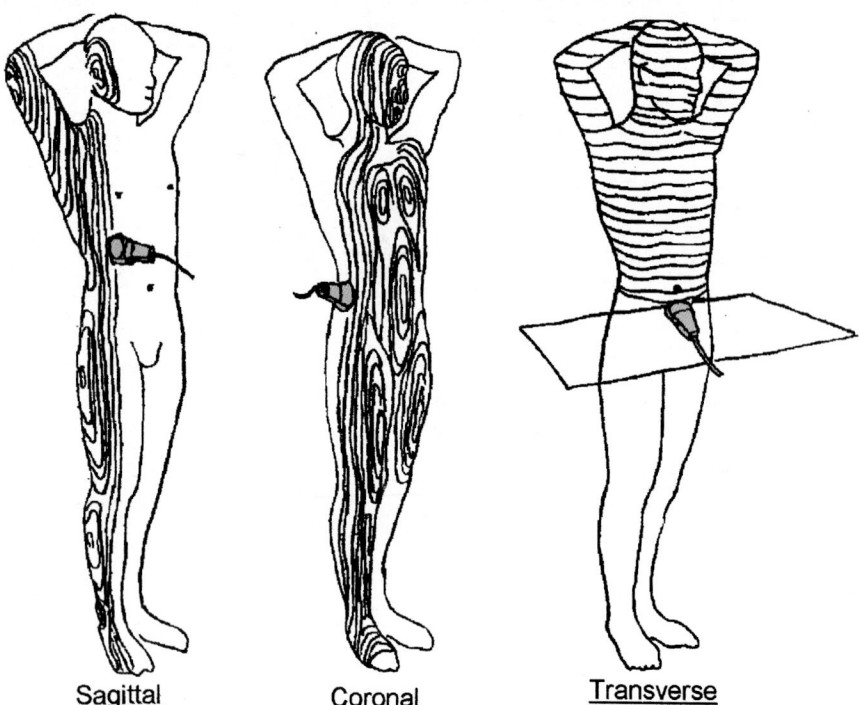

Sagittal          Coronal          Transverse

**FIGURE 17-2.** Scanning planes used in ultrasound imaging.
*(Adapted from Tempkins, BB. Scanning Planes and Methods. Ultrasound Scanning: Principles and Protocols. Philadelphia: WB Saunders Company; 1993.)*

hemodynamically unstable patient, then that image alone, in combination with the patient's clinical picture, is sufficient to justify an immediate abdominal operation.[27] In a stable patient, following the exam of the RUQ, the LUQ and pelvis are visualized as discussed below.

Technique.    Ultrasound transmission gel is applied on four areas of the thoracoabdomen, and the examination is conducted in the following sequence: the pericardial area, RUQ, LUQ, and the pelvis (Fig. 17-3).

A 3.5 MHz convex transducer is oriented for sagittal or longitudinal views and positioned in the subxiphoid region to identify the heart and to examine for blood in the pericardial sac. The normal and abnormal views of the pericardial area are shown in Fig. 17-4. The subxiphoid image is usually not difficult to obtain, but a severe injury to the chest wall, a very narrow subcostal area, subcutaneous emphysema, or morbid obesity can prevent a satisfactory examination.[28] Both of the latter conditions are associated with poor imaging because air and fat reflect the wave too strongly and prevent penetration into the target organ.[14] If the subcostal pericardial image cannot be obtained or is suboptimal, a parasternal ultrasound view of the heart should be performed (Figs. 17-5 and 17-6).

**TABLE 17-5**

| Clinical Applications of Selected Transducer Frequencies | |
|---|---|
| **FREQUENCY** | **APPLICATIONS** |
| 2.5–3.5 MHz | General abdominal |
| 5.0 MHz | Transvaginal |
| | Pediatric abdominal |
| | Testicular |
| 7.5 MHz | Vascular |
| | Soft tissue |
| | Thyroid |

Next, the transducer is placed in the right anterior or mid-axillary line between the 11th and 12th ribs to obtain sagittal images of the liver, kidney, and diaphragm (Fig. 17-7) and determine the presence or absence of blood in Morison's pouch and in the right subphrenic space. Next, attention is turned to the LUQ. With the transducer positioned in the left posterior axillary line between the 10th and 11th ribs, the spleen and left kidney are visualized and the presence or absence of blood between the two organs and in the left subphrenic space is determined (Fig. 17-8). The splenic window is often the most difficult window to adequately visualize and the probe should be placed significantly more posterior (posterior vs. anterior or mid-axillary line) and superior (one to two rib spaces higher) than with the RUQ window.

Finally, the transducer is directed for a transverse view and placed about 4 cm superior to the symphysis pubis. It is swept inferiorly to obtain a coronal view of the full bladder and the pelvis examining for the presence or absence of blood (Fig. 17-9).

Accuracy of the FAST.    Improper technique, inexperience of the examiner, and inappropriate use of ultrasound have long been known to adversely impact the accuracy of ultrasound imaging. More recently, the etiology of injury, the presence of hypotension on admission, and select associated injuries have also been shown to influence the accuracy of this modality.[2,3,8] Failure to consider these factors has led to inaccurate assessments of the accuracy of the FAST by comparing it inappropriately to a CT scan and not recognizing its role in the evaluation of patients with penetrating torso trauma.[29,30] Both false-positive and negative pericardial ultrasound examinations have been reported to occur in the presence of a massive hemothorax or mediastinal blood.[4,8,10,31] Repeating the FAST after the insertion of a tube thoracostomy improves the visualization of the pericardial area and decreases the number of false positive and negative studies. While false studies may occur, a rapid focused ultrasound survey of the subcostal pericardial area is a very

**TABLE 17-6**

**Suggestions to Maximize Accuracy of Ultrasound Imaging**

1. Ultrasound machines should be maintained properly in conjunction with an institution's department of biomedical engineering.
2. To ensure the correct orientation of the patient relative to the monitor, gel should be applied to the edge of the transducer near the indicator line, which is then rubbed with a finger. Motion should occur on the left side of the screen indicating that the transducer is properly oriented.
3. Liberal amounts of gel, as an acoustic coupler, should be used to reduce the amount of reflection.
4. The transducer should be manipulated slowly and with small motions rather than with wide sweeps and pressure should be gentle initially. This is particularly true when imaging superficial structures, as too much pressure will compress the area and distort the image.
5. For bilateral structures, imaging should be performed on the normal side first to have a comparison for the area in question. For example, when trying to assess a deep vein thrombosis in an extremity, inspect the normal extremity first so that you can see the normal compressibility and size of the vessel. This may help distinguish subtle pathologic changes in the abnormal tissue.
6. A nasogastric tube may help decompress the stomach and improve visualization of the spleen and splenorenal recess.
7. A full bladder acts as an acoustic window to the pelvis and if a urinary catheter has already been inserted, temporarily clamping it will allow the bladder to fill and the examination can be repeated.
8. Differentiating artery from vein is generally not difficult with B-Mode ultrasonography, but application of the Doppler mode, compression of the vessel (veins compress much easier than arteries), or having the patient perform the Valsalva maneuver (which dilates venous structures) can help differentiate arterial and venous structures.

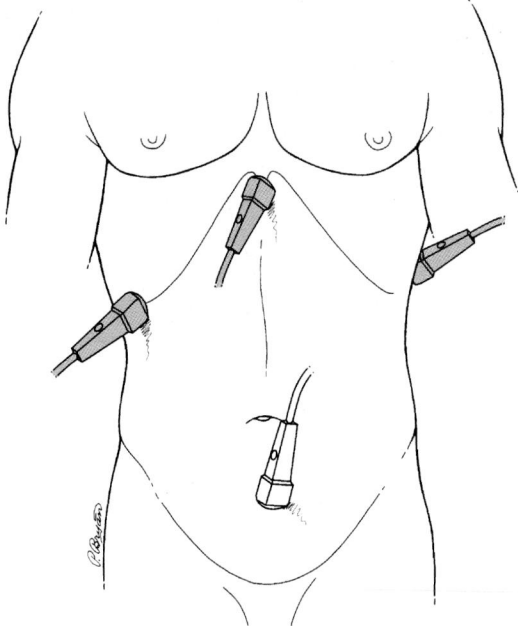

**FIGURE 17-3.** Schematic diagram of transducer positions for FAST: pericardial, right upper quadrant, left upper quadrant, and pelvis.

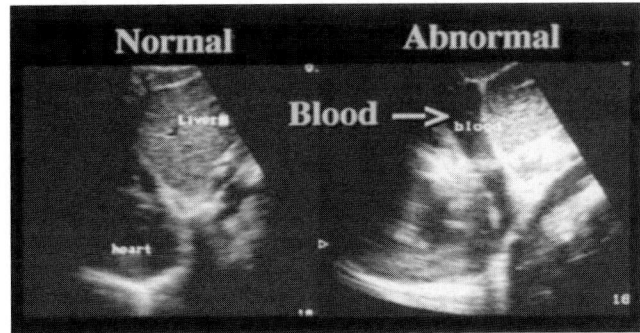

**FIGURE 17-4.** (**Left**) Sagittal view of pericardial area showing pericardium as single echogenic line. (Normal) (**Right**) Sagittal view of pericardial area showing separation of visceral and parietal areas of pericardium with blood (arrow) that appears anechoic.

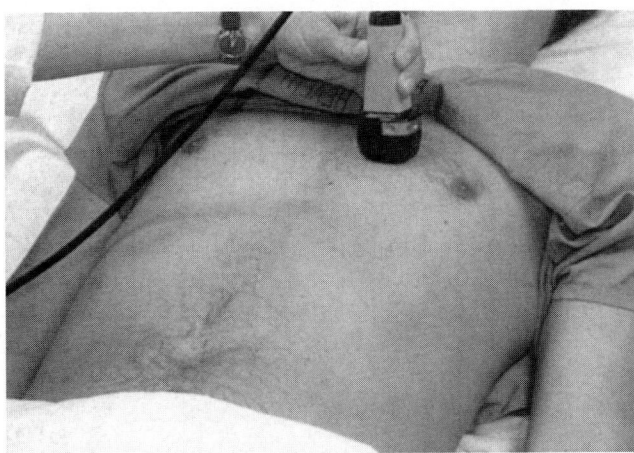

**FIGURE 17-5.** Transducer position for left parasternal view of heart.

decreases the number of false positive and negative studies. While false studies may occur, a rapid focused ultrasound survey of the subcostal pericardial area is a very accurate method to detect hemopericardium in most patients with penetrating wounds in the "cardiac box."[4,10] In a recent large study of patients who sustained either blunt or penetrating injuries, the FAST was 100% sensitive and 99.3% specific for detecting hemopericardium in patients with precordial or transthoracic wounds. Furthermore, the use of pericardial ultrasound has been shown to be especially helpful in the evaluation of patients who have no overt signs of pericardial tamponade. This was highlighted in a study in which 10 of 22 patients with precordial wounds and a hemopericardium on an ultrasound examination had admission systolic blood pressures >110 mm Hg and were relatively asymptomatic. Based on these signs and the lack of symptoms, it is unlikely that the presence of cardiac wounds would have been strongly suspected in these patients and, therefore, this rapid ultrasound examination provided an early diagnosis of hemopericardium before the patients underwent physiologic deterioration.

The FAST is also very accurate when it is used to evaluate hypotensive patients who present with blunt abdominal trauma. In this scenario, ultrasound is so accurate that when the FAST is positive, an immediate operation is justified.[4,8,10,33]

Because the FAST is a focused examination for the detection of blood in dependent areas of the abdomen, its results should not be

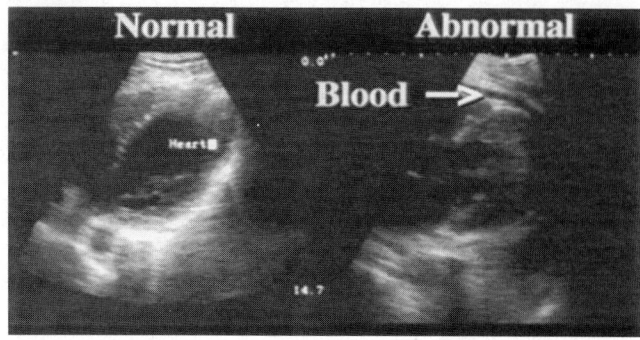

**FIGURE 17-6.** Normal (**Left**) and abnormal (**Right**) heart, parasternal view.

Because the FAST is a focused examination for the detection of blood in dependent areas of the abdomen, its results should not be compared to those of a CT scan because the FAST does not readily identify intraparenchymal or retroperitoneal injuries. Therefore, select hemodynamically stable patients considered to be at high risk for occult intra-abdominal injury should undergo a CT scan of the abdomen regardless of the results of the FAST examination. These patients include those with fractures of the pelvis or thoracolumbar spine, major thoracic trauma (pulmonary contusion, lower rib fractures), and hematuria. These recommendations are based on the results of two studies from Chiu et al. in 1997[34] and Ballard et al. in 1999.[35] Chiu et al. reviewed their data on 772 patients who underwent FAST examinations after sustaining blunt torso injury. Of the 772 patients, 52 had intra-abdominal injury but 15 (15/52 = 29%) of them had no hemoperitoneum on the admitting FAST examination or on the CT scan of the abdomen. In other work conducted by Ballard et al. at Grady Memorial Hospital, an algorithm was developed and tested over a 3.5 year period to identify patients who were at high risk for occult intra-abdominal injuries after sustaining blunt thoracoabdominal trauma.[35] Of the 1490 patients admitted with severe blunt trauma, there were 102 (70 with pelvic fractures, 32 with spine injuries) who were considered to be at high risk for occult intra-abdominal injuries. Although there was only one false negative FAST examination in the 32 patients who had spine

injuries, there were 13 false negatives in those with pelvic fractures. Based on these data, the authors concluded that patients with pelvic fractures should have a CT scan of the abdomen regardless of the result of the FAST examination. Both studies provide guidelines to decrease the number of false-negative FAST studies, but, as with the use of any diagnostic modality, it is important to correlate the results of the test with the patient's clinical picture. Suggested algorithms for the use of FAST are depicted in Figs. 17-10a and 17-10b. Indeed, the FAST exam has been included in recently published evidence-based guidelines for the evaluation of patients with blunt abdominal trauma with reported accuracy rates of 96–98%.[36]

**Quantification of Blood.**    The amount of blood detected on the abdominal CT scan[37] or in the DPL aspirate (or effluent) has been shown to predict the need for operative intervention.[38] Similarly, the quantity of blood that is detected with ultrasound may be predictive of a therapeutic operation.[39,40] Huang et al. developed a scoring system based on the identification of hemoperitoneum in specific areas such as Morison's pouch or the perisplenic space.[39] Each abdominal area was assigned a number from 0 to 3, and the authors found that a total score of ≥3 corresponded to more than 1 liter of hemoperitoneum. This scoring system had a sensitivity of 84% for determining the need for an immediate abdominal operation. Another scoring system developed and prospectively validated by McKenney et al., examined the patient's admission blood pressure, base deficit, and the amount of hemoperitoneum present on the ultrasound examinations of 100 patients.[40] The hemoperitoneum was categorized by its measurement and its distribution in the peritoneal cavity, so that a score of 1 was considered a minimal amount of hemoperitoneum but a score of >3 signified a large hemoperitoneum. Forty-six of the 100 patients had a score >3, and 40 (87%) of them underwent a therapeutic abdominal operation. This scoring system had a sensitivity, specificity, and accuracy of 83%, 87%, and 85%, respectively. The authors concluded that an ultrasound score of >3 is statistically more accurate than a combination of the initial systolic blood pressure and base deficit for determining which patients will undergo a therapeutic abdominal operation. Although the quantification of hemoperitoneum is not exact, it can provide valuable information about the need for an abdominal operation as well as its potential to be therapeutic.

**Recent Advances and Organ Specificity.**    As surgeons have become more facile with ultrasound exams and as technology has

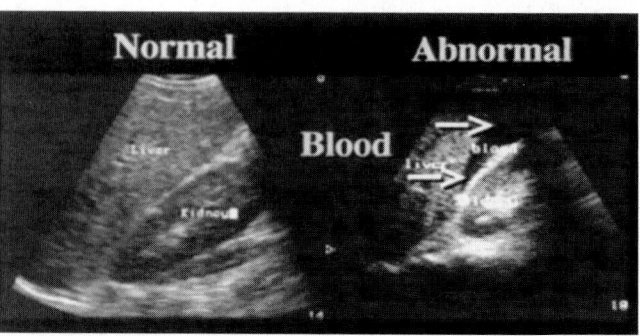

**FIGURE 17-7.**  **(A)** Normal sagittal view of liver, kidney, and diaphragm. Note Gerota's fascia is hyperechoic. **(B)** Abnormal sagittal view of liver, kidney, and diaphragm. Note fluid (blood) in between liver and kidney (arrows).

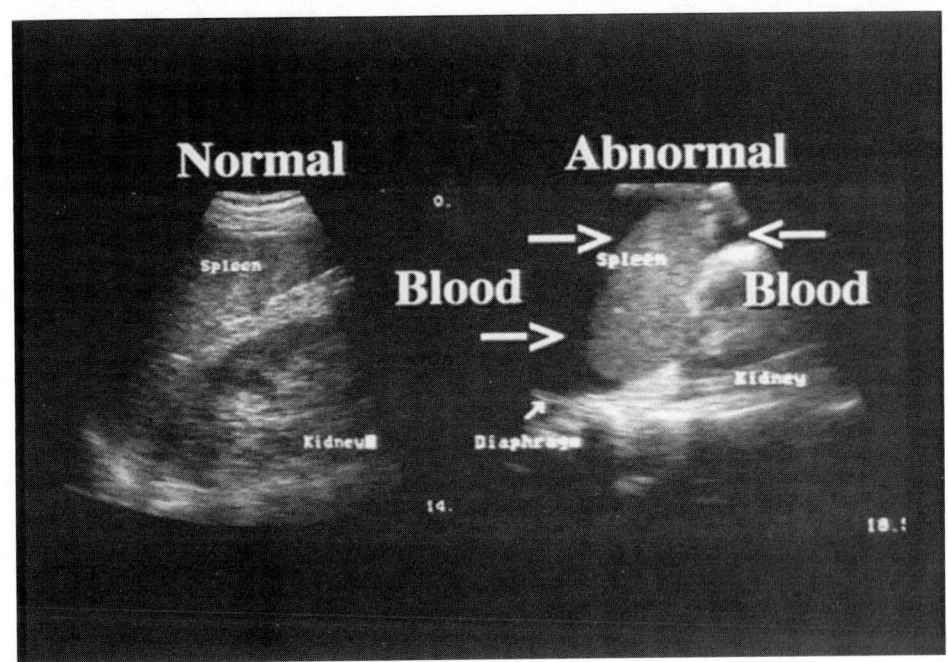

**FIGURE 17-8.** (**Left**) Normal sagittal view of spleen, kidney and diaphragm. (**Right**) Abnormal sagittal view of spleen, kidney, and diaphragm with fluid (blood) in between spleen and kidney and above the spleen in the subphrenic space.

improved, extensions of the FAST exam have been described. Again, it is noted that the standard FAST exam is designed to accurately answer two simple questions: Is there fluid in the peritoneal cavity and is their fluid in the pericardial sac? The use of ultrasound for more complex diagnostic interventions is described below, but these areas are less well studied and beyond the purview of the traditional FAST exam.

A recent prospective, multicenter trial conducted by the Western Trauma Association reported on the use of ultrasound to serially evaluate patients with documented solid organ injuries (SOI) after trauma.[41] The so-called BOAST exam, or the Bedside Organ Assessment with Sonography after Trauma, was performed by a limited number of experienced surgeon-sonographers in 126 patients with 135 SOI in four American trauma centers. This study, performed over nearly two years, was designed to be a more thorough abdominal ultrasound examination with multiple views obtained of each solid organ (kidneys, liver, and spleen). Criteria

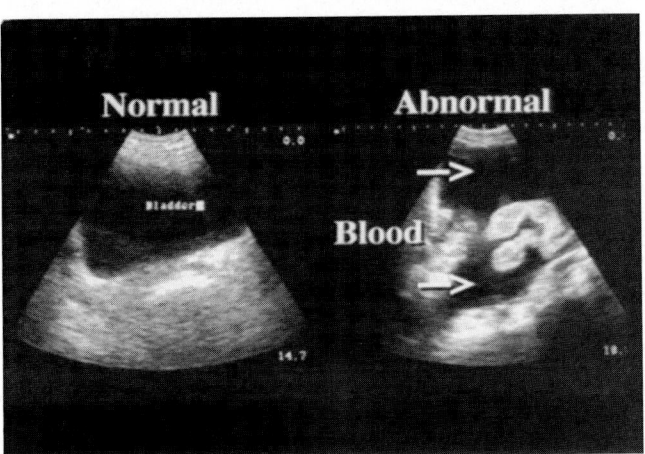

**FIGURE 17-9.** (**Left**) Normal coronal view of full urinary bladder. (**Right**) Abnormal coronal view of full bladder with fluid in pelvis. (Note the bowel floating in fluid).

for enrollment included normal hemodynamics, absence of peritonitis or other need for urgent laparotomy, and lack of excessive blood transfusion in the attending physician's judgment. All patients were victims of blunt trauma with a mean Injury Severity Score (ISS) of nearly 15.

Overall, only 34% of injuries to solid organs were seen with BOAST yielding an error rate of 66%. None of the 34 grade I injuries were identified and only 13 (31%) of the grade II injuries were identified. Sensitivities for grade III and IV injuries ranged from 25 to 75,% and only one grade V injury (to the liver) was examined and positively identified. Eleven patients developed 16 intra-abdominal complications (8 pseudoaneurysms, 4 bilomas, 3 abscesses and 1 necrotic organ), and 13 (81%) were identified by the sonographers. This study emphasizes that ultrasound, in most surgeons' hands, should not be considered a reliable modality for diagnosis and grading of SOI although it may be acceptably accurate in the diagnosis of posttraumatic abdominal complications in patients with SOI managed nonoperatively.

In Europe, preliminary work using Power Doppler ultrasonography to identify specific organ injuries has been published in recent years.[42,43] Many of these exams include the use of a sonographic contrast agent injected peripherally during the scan. In one study, the authors were able to document extravasation of contrast in 20 of 153 patients (13%). Extravasation was seen not only from the spleen, liver, and kidney after trauma, but also in postoperative patients (aortic aneurysm repair, postsplenectomy) and in a patient with a ruptured aortic aneurysm. In 9 of 20 patients, CT scan was performed and all nine confirmed extravasation of contrast. In the 133 patients without extravasation, the absence of active bleeding was inferred by a subsequent CT scan in 82 patients, surgical data in 13 patients, and clinical follow-up in 38 patients, with no cases of active bleeding missed by ultrasound. Thus, the addition of an ultrasonic contrast agent and Power Doppler may be of some benefit in the diagnosis of specific injuries. It should be emphasized, however, that the FAST exam in most American trauma centers is used simply as a screening tool to

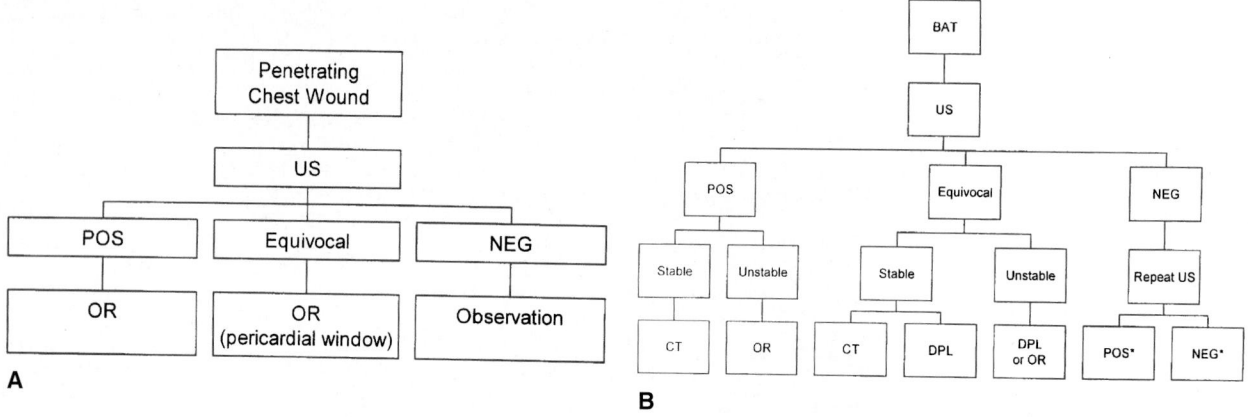

**FIGURE 17-10.**   Algorithm for the use of ultrasound in patients with **(A)** penetrating chest wounds and **(B)** blunt abdominal trauma.

identify the presence or absence of hemoperitoneum or hemopericardium in a trauma patient.

## Traumatic Hemothorax

Introduction.   A focused thoracic ultrasound examination was developed by surgeons to rapidly detect the presence or absence of a traumatic hemothorax in patients during the Advanced Trauma Life Support (ATLS) secondary survey.[9] This focused thoracic ultrasound examination employs the ultrasound physics principles of the mirror image artifact and tissue acoustic impedance as presented in Table 17-1. A test that promptly detects a traumatic effusion or hemothorax is worthwhile because it dramatically shortens the interval from the admission of the patient with hemothorax to the insertion of a thoracostomy tube.

Technique.   The technique for this examination is similar to that used to interrogate the upper quadrants of the abdomen in the FAST and also uses the same type and frequency transducer. In point of fact, it is performed one to two rib spaces higher than the RUQ and LUQ FAST views using the same probe. Ultrasound transmission gel is applied to the right and left lower thoracic areas in the mid to posterior axillary lines between the 9th and 10th intercostal spaces (Fig. 17-11). The transducer is slowly advanced cephalad to identify the hyperechoic diaphragm and to interrogate the supradiaphragmatic space for the presence or absence of fluid (Figs. 17-12a and 17-12b) which appears anechoic. In the positive thoracic ultrasound examination, the hypoechoic lung can be seen "floating" amidst the fluid. The same technique can be used to evaluate a critically ill patient for a pleural effusion as discussed earlier.

Accuracy.   One of the earliest reports on the use of ultrasound for the evaluation of fluid collections in the pleural space was described by Joyner et al. in 1967.[44] Later, Gryminski et al. documented the superiority of ultrasound over standard radiography for the detection of pleural fluid.[45] In that study, they reported that ultrasound detected even small amounts of pleural fluid in 74 (93%) of 80 patients, whereas plain radiography detected pleural fluid in only 66 (83%) of these patients.

Surgeons at Emory University have also examined the accuracy of this examination in 360 patients with blunt and penetrating torso injuries.[9] They compared the time and accuracy of ultrasound

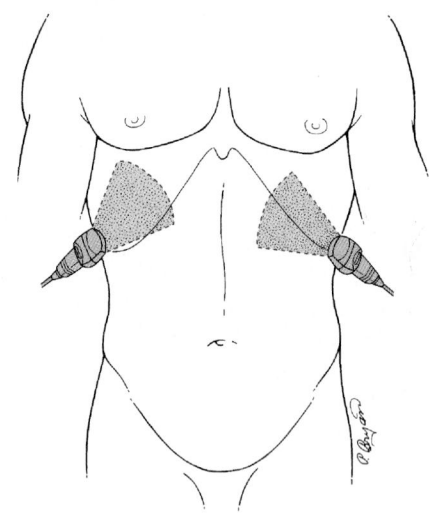

**FIGURE 17-11.**   Transducer positions for thoracic ultrasound examination (detection of hemothorax).

with that of the supine portable chest x-ray and found both to be very similar with 97.4% sensitivity and 99.7% specificity observed for thoracic ultrasound versus 92.5% sensitivity and 99.7% specificity for the portable chest x-ray. Performance times, however, for the thoracic ultrasound examinations were statistically much faster ($p < 0.0001$) than those for the portable chest x-ray. Although it is not recommended that the thoracic ultrasound examination replace the chest x-ray, its use can expedite treatment in many patients and decrease the number of chest radiographs obtained.

## Pneumothorax

Introduction.   The use of ultrasound for the detection of a pneumothorax is not a new diagnostic test, having been reported by several authors.[46–50] This examination is useful to the surgeon to evaluate a patient for a potential pneumothorax in the following circumstances: (1) bulky radiology equipment is not readily available; (2) inordinate delays for obtaining a chest x-ray are anticipated; or (3) numerous injured patients (mass casualty situation) must be rapidly assessed and triaged.[51,52] Although useful in the trauma resuscitation area, surgeons may also find this examination

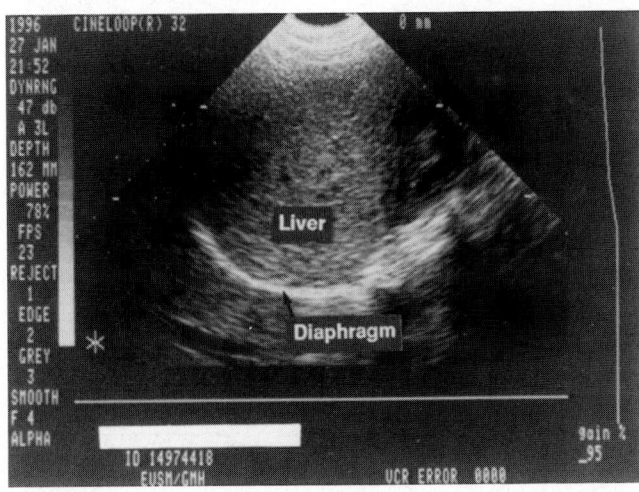

A

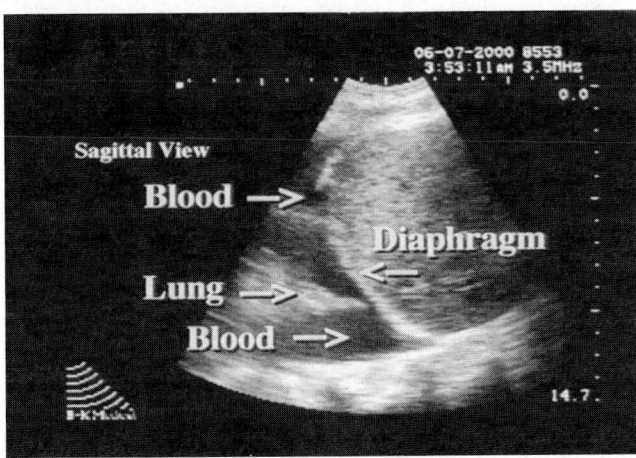

B

**FIGURE 17-12. (A)** Sagittal view of liver, kidney, and diaphragm. Note supradiaphragmatic (lung) area but absence of pleural effusion. **(B)** Sagittal view of right supradiaphragmatic space. The right hemithorax contains fluid (blood) which appears anechoic.

helpful to detect a pneumothorax in a critically ill patient who is on a ventilator, after a thoracentesis procedure, or after discontinuing the suction on an underwater seal device.

Technique.   A 5.0 to 7.5 MHz linear array transducer is used to evaluate a patient for the presence of a pneumothorax. The examination may be performed while the patient is in the erect or the supine position. Ultrasound transmission gel is applied to the right and left upper thoracic areas at about the 3rd to 4th intercostal space in the mid-clavicular line and the presumed unaffected thoracic cavity is examined first. The transducer is oriented for longitudinal imaging, is placed perpendicular to the ribs, and is slowly advanced medially toward the sternum and then laterally toward the anterior axillary line. The normal examination of the thoracic cavity identifies the rib (seen as black on the ultrasound image because it is a refraction artifact), pleural sliding, and a comet-tail artifact (Table 17-1). Pleural sliding is the identification of the visceral and parietal layers of the lung seen as hyperechoic superimposed pleural lines. When a pneumothorax is present, air becomes trapped between the visceral and parietal pleura and does not allow for the transmission of the ultrasound waves. Therefore,

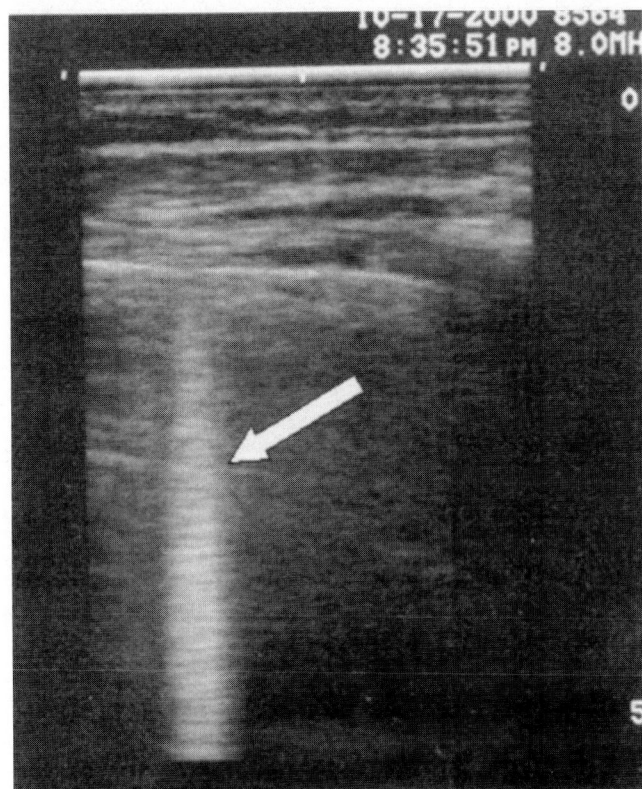

**FIGURE 17-13.** Comet tail artifact (arrow)

the visceral pleura is not imaged and pleural sliding is not observed. The comet tail artifact is generated because of the interaction of two highly reflective opposing interfaces, i.e., air and pleura (Fig. 17-13). When air separates the visceral and parietal pleurae, the comet tail artifact is not visualized. If desired, the examination may be repeated with the transducer oriented for transverse views, with images obtained with the probe parallel to the ribs.

Accuracy.   Several studies have documented excellent sensitivity and specificity of ultrasound for the detection of a pneumothorax.[46,48,49,53] Dulchavsky et al. from Detroit Receiving Hospital/Wayne State University showed that ultrasound can be successfully used by surgeons to detect a pneumothorax in injured patients.[54] Of the 382 patients (364 trauma; 18 spontaneous) evaluated with ultrasound, 39 had pneumothoraces and ultrasound successfully detected 37 of them, yielding a 95% sensitivity. Not unexpectedly, pneumothoraces in two patients could not be detected because of the presence of significant subcutaneous emphysema. The authors recommended that when a portable chest x-ray cannot be readily obtained, the use of this bedside ultrasound examination for the identification of a pneumothorax can expedite the patient's management.

### Sternal Fracture

Introduction.   Fractures of the sternum are visualized on a lateral x-ray view of the chest, but this film may be difficult to obtain in a patient with multiple injuries. For this reason, an ultrasound examination of the sternum can rapidly detect a fracture while the patient is still in the supine position and, therefore, avoid the need to obtain a lateral x-ray.[55]

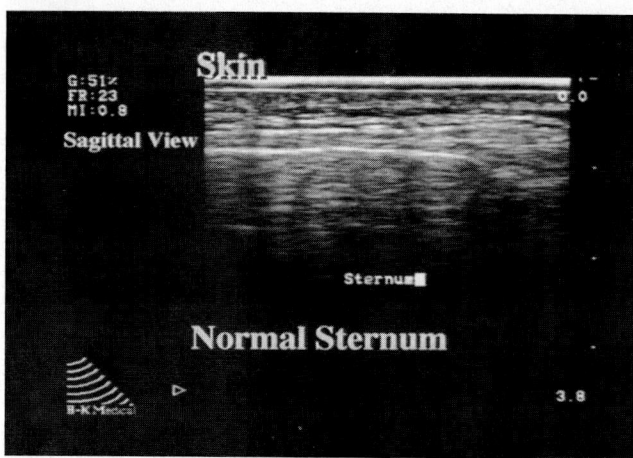

**FIGURE 17-14.** Sagittal view of sternum. Normal findings.

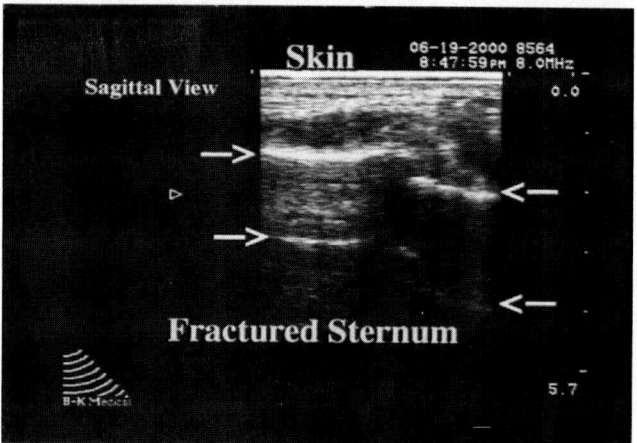

**FIGURE 17-15.** Sagittal view of sternum illustrating fracture (interruption of hyperechoic line).

**Technique.** The ultrasound examination of the sternum is performed using a 5.0 or 8.0 MHz linear array transducer that is oriented for sagittal or longitudinal views. Ultrasound transmission gel is applied over the sternal area while the patient is in the supine position. Beginning at the suprasternal notch, the transducer is slowly advanced in a caudad direction to interrogate the bone for a fracture. The examination is then repeated with the transducer oriented for transverse views. The examination of the intact sternum is shown in Fig. 17-14. A sternal fracture is identified on the ultrasound examination as a disruption of the cortical reflex (Fig. 17-15). Investigators have found that the use of ultrasound for this diagnosis is as accurate (and much more rapid) than a lateral x-ray view of the chest.[55]

## Special Situations

**Ultrasound in the Pregnant Trauma Patient.** Ultrasound would seem to be an ideal method of evaluating a pregnant patient with suspected blunt abdominal trauma as it is portable, noninvasive, and free of ionizing radiation. The ATLS course teaches that unrecognized abdominal trauma is a major problem in the pregnant trauma patient.[22] Concerns over changes in abdominal anatomy

leading to difficulty in obtaining images have not borne out in objective evaluations. Goodwin et al.[56] reported on their eight-year experience with the FAST exam in 127 pregnant patients, including 5 of 6 patients with hemoperitoneum who were found to have fluid on the FAST exam (sensitivity 83%). Of the 120 without abdominal injury, 117 had a true-negative FAST (specificity 98%), with three false-positive exams due to serous intraperitoneal fluid. Furthermore, Brown et al.[57] reported on their experience with a more extensive ultrasound exam in 101 stable, pregnant patients with suspected blunt abdominal trauma. Median gestational age was just over 24 weeks, and these patients underwent an official abdominal ultrasound by a certified technician to include images of the fetus and placenta. The sensitivity was 80% (4 of 5 patients had correct identification of injuries) with one missed placental hematoma that required an emergent cesarean delivery for fetal distress. Injuries identified included one placental abruption, two splenic lacerations, one hepatic laceration, and one renal injury. None of the 96 patients with a negative ultrasound had injuries discovered later in their hospital course (specificity 100%). Thus, it would seem that ultrasound remains a good screening tool for the pregnant patient with blunt abdominal trauma and has the advantages of repeatability and a lack of radiation exposure.

**Ultrasound in Penetrating Trauma.** Ultrasound for the diagnosis of injuries after penetrating trauma has been studied much less extensively than ultrasound used after blunt trauma. Several of the larger, well-known series[4,9,10] have included patients with penetrating trauma and, as stated previously, ultrasound of the pericardium has been shown to be accurate for diagnosis of injury in patients with penetrating injury to the "cardiac box".[9] In a recent study of 32 patients with penetrating anterior chest trauma, ultrasound was used to diagnose 8 pericardial effusions with a reported 100% accuracy (8 true-positive and 24 true-negative exams). Eight other patients were noted to have intraperitoneal fluid and underwent therapeutic exploration including repair of five diaphragmatic injuries, three hepatic lacerations, three splenic lacerations, three gastric injuries, two injuries to the small bowel, and one injury to the adrenal gland. No false-positive or fast-negative examinations of the peritoneum were reported.[58] Other studies have shown that the accuracy of FAST after penetrating trauma is somewhat less with one study reporting a sensitivity for abdominal injury after penetrating trauma as low as 67%.[59]

A recent report by Murphy et al. looked at the utility of ultrasound to diagnose fascial penetration after anterior abdominal stab wounds.[60] In this study, 35 patients underwent ultrasonic evaluation of their anterior abdominal fascia with an 8.0 MHz linear array probe followed by a local wound exploration. While ultrasound had only a 59% sensitivity (13/22 patients), it did have a 100% specificity with no false positive studies. Thus, if fascial penetration is noted on ultrasound, a more invasive wound exploration is probably not needed; however, a negative ultrasound evaluation is clearly less helpful and does not preclude peritoneal penetration.

## Use of Ultrasound in Austere Settings

**Ultrasound on Deployment.** The portability of ultrasound makes it ideal for use in forward settings. Training courses are in place to teach the use of the FAST exam to military surgeons, and handheld ultrasound is now routinely deployed within the British Defence Medical Services.[61] Indeed, in a survey of surgeons reviewing potential preventable casualties in Vietnam, ultrasound was the fourth most commonly mentioned advancement in technology (behind modern ventilators, CT scanners, and modern antibiotics) that may have assisted in better patient salvage.[62]

Although up to 90% of war wounds are penetrating, ultrasound may allow quicker, more accurate triage decisions as patients with penetrating abdominal trauma with no or minimal hemoperitoneum may be transferred to the next echelon where the study may be repeated or additional diagnostic maneuvers undertaken.[63] In a study from the Croatian conflict in 1999, FAST was shown to have a sensitivity of 86%, a specificity of 100% and an accuracy of 97% when applied to 94 casualties evaluated over a 72-hour period. This was comparable to the accuracy achieved by the authors in their civilian experience with FAST in more than 1000 patients over the three years prior to the conflict. In a recent small series,[63] FAST was used with excellent results in a British military hospital in Iraq. Fifteen casualties were evaluated with serial FAST exams, and 14 had negative exams at admission and again at six hours. One patient underwent laparotomy based on trajectory and had no intraperitoneal fluid but two small holes were discovered in the cecum that required repair. The other 13 patients recovered without sequelae. One exam was positive and led to immediate laparotomy in a patient with a grade V liver injury after a motor vehicle collision.

Because ultrasound is portable enough to use in active combat situations, research is ongoing to evaluate the best method to teletransmit images obtained in the field. Several different satellite transmission systems have been evaluated, and high quality images were able to be obtained in the majority of cases; however the balance between the weight of the system and the minimum image quality has still not been completely achieved.[63] It has been noted that images can be transmitted from up to 1500 ft. from the antennae without significant degradation.[64] As technology advances, one would expect imaging systems to continue to become smaller and lighter with improved image quality, making ultrasound even more appealing as a modality for use in the forward setting.

Ultrasound in Space. Many of the same qualities that make ultrasound appealing for use in combat make it equally appealing as a diagnostic modality in space, where an injury might mandate abortion of a multimillion dollar mission. Indeed, ultrasound is one of the only feasible diagnostic modalities on space missions, given the size and weight restrictions. Also, ultrasound examinations are easily taught and images can be relayed with minimal delay to physicians on the ground. ATLS procedures are also feasible in space,[65] and life-saving procedures could be performed based on ultrasound findings.

Ultrasound has been used in space for several decades. Indeed, it has been ultrasound technology that has taught us much about the physiologic effects of microgravity, especially the fluid shifts associated with space travel.[66] As early as 1982, cardiac ultrasound was used to evaluate left ventricular systolic function and cardiac chamber size in cosmonauts. The first American ultrasound system in space was the American flight echograph from Advanced Technology Laboratories (Bothel, WA) which first flew in 1984 and eventually was capable of three-dimensional images using a tilt frame device. Currently, the Human Research Facility aboard the International Space Station (ISS) is equipped with a state-of-the-art Philips HDI 5000 (Philips Medical, Bothel, WA).[66]

Because surface tension and capillary action are the principal physical forces in space, scientists questioned whether images obtained on the standard FAST exam would be useful in microgravity. There are now several published studies of ultrasounds performed on parabolic flights in the NASA Microgravity Research Facility, a KC-135 aircraft. This aircraft can generate 25–30 second intervals of weightlessness using serial parabolic trajectories. A porcine model of intra-abdominal hemorrhage was created on the ground and studied during parabolic flights.[67] Over 2000 ultrasound segments were recorded with 80% of these considered feasible for diagnosis of the presence or absence of abdominal fluid. The sonographers felt the exam was no more difficult than one done on the ground as long as the sonographer and patient were adequately restrained. For the intraperitoneal portion of the exam, a fourth view (the midline "Abdominal Sweep") was added and, with this addition, the FAST exam was able to reliably detect even relatively small amounts of intraperitoneal fluid. The Morison's pouch view remained the most sensitive window for fluid detection.[67] Further study using a similar model revealed that ultrasound can also reliably detect both hemothorax and pneumothorax in microgravity.[68]

Recently, astronauts aboard the ISS performed FAST ultrasounds that were transmitted with a two-second satellite delay to directors on the ground, who were able to provide them with real-time instructions for probe position and system adjustments. Exams were able to be completed in roughly five minutes with adequate images obtained in all views.[69] Astronauts have also been able to perform comprehensive ocular ultrasounds aboard the ISS with the same real-time feedback.[70]

In summary, ultrasound fulfills all the necessary criteria for a diagnostic modality in space. It is sufficiently portable, teletransmittable, teachable, and accurate. It will likely continue to be the only feasible technology to assist with medical diagnoses on space missions in the near future.

## SURGEON-PERFORMED ULTRASOUND IN THE INTENSIVE CARE UNIT

The surgeons' use of ultrasound is particularly applicable to the evaluation of critically ill patients in the intensive care unit for the following reasons: (1) many patients have a depressed mental status making it difficult to elicit pertinent signs of infection; (2) physical examination is hampered by tubes, drains, and monitoring devices; (3) the clinical picture often changes necessitating frequent reassessments; (4) transportation to other areas of the hospital is not without inherent risks[71]; and (5) these patients frequently develop complications, which if diagnosed and treated early, may lessen their morbidity and length of stay in the ICU.[72] Indeed, both diagnostic and therapeutic ultrasound examinations can be performed by the surgeon without disrupting rounds in the ICU. These focused examinations should be performed with a specific purpose and as an extension of the physical examination, *not* as its replacement.[12]

Several retrospective studies have documented the utility of portable ultrasound examinations performed in diverse groups of critically ill patients.[71,73,74] In these studies, evaluation for sepsis of unknown origin, suspected gallbladder pathology, and renal dysfunction were the most common indications for the examinations. Slasky et al. reported their findings on the ultrasound evaluations of 107 patients in the ICU.[74] The sonographic results of their examinations supported the suspected diagnosis in 29 (27%) patients and excluded the initial diagnosis in 78 (73%) patients. There were no false-negative studies in this series. Additionally, 22 of the ultrasound examinations showed unsuspected abnormalities, although only five patients had their management altered based on these findings. In another study, however, Lichtenstein and Axler prospectively performed ultrasound examinations in 150 consecutive patients admitted to the medical ICU.[73] They examined the pleural cavity, abdomen, and the femoral veins of critically ill patients and found that information derived from their sonographic examinations directly contributed to a change in the management of 33 (22%) patients. Other investigators have reported similar results and further suggest that critically ill patients most likely to benefit from a bedside ultrasound examination are those with occult hemorrhage, sepsis of unknown origin,[75] and pleural effusion.[12]

Surgeons most commonly use bedside ultrasound examination for the evaluation of patients in the ICU to detect pleural effusions, intra-abdominal and soft-tissue fluid collections, hemoperitoneum, femoral vein thrombosis, and as a guide for the cannulation of central veins in patients with difficult access. Before introducing specific ultrasound techniques and procedures, some basic principles of interventional ultrasound will be discussed.[76,77] Advantages of interventional ultrasound as used by the surgeon in the ICU include the following: (1) visualization in real-time imaging to allow direct placement of a catheter and confirmation of complete drainage of a fluid collection; (2) performance at the patient's bedside to avoid transport; and (3) ultrasound is safe, minimally invasive, and repeatable, if necessary. Contraindications to the performance of an ultrasound-guided interventional procedure include the lack of a safe pathway, presence of a coagulopathy, and an uncooperative patient.

Larger needles and those that are Teflon coated produce more echogenicity and are easier to visualize with ultrasound.[78] But, when performing a transabdominal procedure, an 18 gauge (or smaller needle) is probably preferred to avoid large injuries to the bowel. Although minor procedures may be done with minimal preparation, basic principles of sterility should be followed for major interventional procedures.

## Soft Tissue Infections

Introduction. Soft tissue infections may be difficult to assess by physical examination because the signs of infection may only be superficial and may not reflect the status of the entire wound. With the ultrasound transducer in hand, the surgeon can assess the presence, depth, and extent of an abscess at the patient's bedside and determine the appropriate treatment. Furthermore, the collection can be localized to ensure its complete drainage, especially if it is loculated. In the postoperative period, wounds can be imaged to examine for hematomas or seromas. Because the fascia can be precisely delineated with ultrasound, a fascial dehiscence (Fig. 17-16) can be diagnosed at an earlier stage.

Foreign bodies can be the cause of recurrent soft tissue infections and, therefore, removal is often recommended. Several

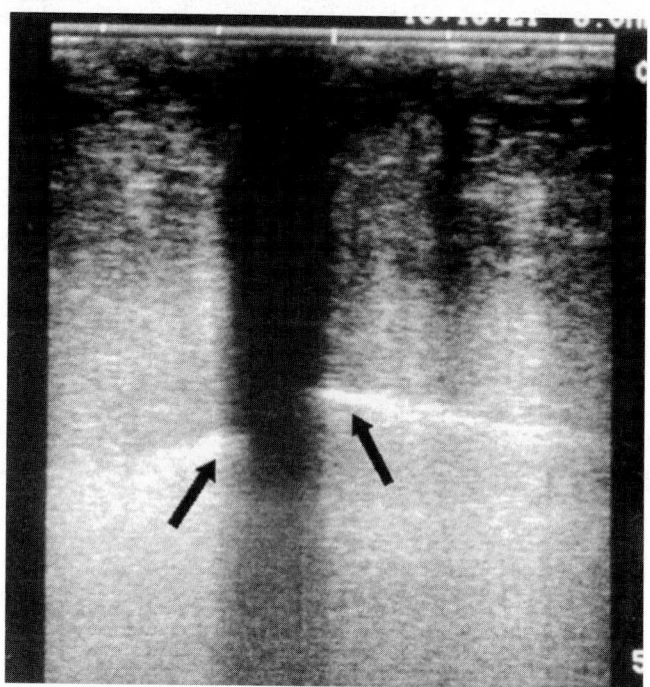

**FIGURE 17-16.** Fascial dehiscence (arrow)

studies have confirmed the value of ultrasound in the detection of radiolucent foreign bodies in human tissue.[20,79,81] In another application, Fry et al. reported the utility of ultrasound in patients with truncal wounds.[79] They showed that ultrasound delineated the subcutaneous and fascial layers, and the authors were able to determine whether the peritoneum or parietal pleura was violated. In their study, this evaluation obviated the need for a local wound exploration.

Technique. The ultrasound examination of soft tissue is performed using a 5.0–8.0 MHz linear array transducer (Table 17-5). The area of inflammation is scanned in both the transverse and longitudinal views to accurately assess the depth and extent of the fluid collection. The depth should be measured so that the appropriate length of the needle is chosen. Once the fluid collection is assessed, an ultrasound-guided needle aspiration may be performed. Aspiration of the collection is performed after the planned point of needle insertion is marked with a felt-tipped pen. The field is prepped and draped, and an 18- or 20-gauge needle attached to a 10cc or 12cc syringe is inserted into the tissue at the marked site. An alternate method involves using real-time ultrasound imaging with sterile transmission gel and a sterile plastic cover for the transducer. The ultrasound transducer is held in the nondominant hand and the area is imaged as the needle is directed into the fluid collection. The advantage of this method is that the surgeon visualizes the active drainage of the entire fluid collection and collapse of the cavity.

## Pleural Effusions

Introduction. The use of ultrasound for the detection of a pleural effusion is similar to that described earlier in this chapter for the detection of a traumatic hemothorax.[12] Although the technique for the focused thoracic ultrasound examination has already been described, the following is the technique used for an ultrasound-guided thoracentesis.

Technique.    The head of the bed is elevated to a 45–60° angle (if the patient's spine is not injured), or the patient may be supine if spinal precautions are needed. A 3.5 or 5.0 MHz convex array transducer is oriented for sagittal views and placed in the midaxillary line at the 6th or 7th intercostal space. The liver (or spleen) and diaphragm are identified, and then the thoracic cavity is interrogated for the presence of pleural fluid. After the fluid is localized, the area adjacent to the transducer is marked using a felt-tipped pen and the chest is prepped and draped. A local anesthetic is injected into the skin near the mark and infiltrated into the underlying subcutaneous tissue and parietal pleura. The pleural space is entered with an 18-gauge needle obtained from a central line kit, and the fluid from the pleural space is aspirated in its entirety. For large effusions, a guidewire is passed through the needle into the pleural cavity using the Seldinger technique. A small skin incision is made around the guidewire and, if necessary, the stiff dilator is passed just through the dermis to allow easy passage of the catheter but minimize the risk of a pneumothorax. A standard central line catheter is placed into the pleural space and a three-way stopcock is connected to the port so that the pleural fluid can be aspirated entirely and collected into a separate container. The central line catheter is removed from the pleural space while applying constant suction with a syringe, and an occlusive dressing is placed over the small incision. Real-time ultrasound imaging can also be used for the detection and aspiration of small or loculated fluid collections because the needle is observed as it enters the collection and collapse of the space confirms that the fluid is entirely removed.

## Intraperitoneal Fluid/Blood

A sudden decrease in a patient's blood pressure or persistent metabolic acidosis despite continued resuscitation is a common indication to reassess the peritoneal cavity as the source of hemorrhage. The FAST examination can be performed as needed at the patient's bedside to exclude hemoperitoneum as a potential source of hypotension. This may be applied to a critically ill patient who has multisystem injuries or one receiving anticoagulation therapy. Ultrasound is also used to evaluate a patient with cirrhosis who has abdominal pain. An ultrasound-guided aspiration of ascites can also be performed, minimizing the risk of injury to the bowel.

## Insertion of a Central Venous Catheter

Introduction.    The placement of a central venous catheter is a commonly performed procedure in critically ill patients. Although surgical residents are generally adept at the insertion of central lines, ultrasound-guided procedures may be helpful when the resident is initially learning the technique or when the patency of a vessel is uncertain. Ultrasound-guided central line insertions are especially useful in patients with anasarca or morbid obesity and for the immobilized patient with a potential injury to the cervical spine.[82,83] In the past decade, several studies have evaluated the use of ultrasound as an aid for central line placement in order to reduce the risk of complications.[83–89] Fry et al. successfully used ultrasound-guided central venous access in 52 patients and, with the

exception of a pneumothorax that occurred in one patient, no other complications were noted.[88] These studies suggested that the use of ultrasound results in a decreased number of cannulation attempts and complications for insertion of subclavian and internal jugular venous catheters. A recent study reported similar excellent results with ultrasound guided percutaneous access of the cephalic vein in the deltopectoral groove.[89]

Technique.    The central veins in the cervical and upper thoracic region are imaged with a 7.5 MHz linear transducer. The skin insertion site may be marked prior to creating a sterile field, or the procedure may be performed with real-time imaging. Cannulation of the subclavian vein is slightly more difficult because of its location beneath the clavicle and, therefore, colorflow duplex and Doppler may be helpful to identify the vein prior to cannulation. Gualtieri et al.[86] suggest identification of the axillary vein and artery just inferior to the lateral aspect of the clavicle. Patency of the vein is determined by its ability to be easily compressed with the ultrasound transducer. The vein is then imaged about two to three centimeters medial to the point of the planned insertion site. The transducer should be held in the nondominant hand and the cannulating needle is followed during real-time imaging as it traverses the soft tissue toward the vein. Once the vein is cannulated, the remainder of the procedure is completed using the standard Seldinger technique.

## Thrombosis of the Common Femoral Vein

Introduction.    Despite the administration of prophylactic agents and routine screening by duplex imaging, deep venous thrombosis (DVT) still occurs in high-risk patients. The characteristics of venous thrombosis as seen on the duplex imaging study include the following: dilation, incompressibility, echogenic material within the lumen, absence or decreased spontaneous flow, and loss of phasic flow with respiration. Although each ultrasound characteristic of a thrombosed vein is important in making the diagnosis of DVT, loss of compressibility of a thrombus-filled vein is the most useful with the other criteria considered supportive of the diagnosis.[90–93]

A focused ultrasound examination of the femoral veins is based on the following principles: (1) most lethal pulmonary emboli originate from the iliofemoral veins[94]; (2) the common femoral artery is identified as a pulsatile vessel lateral to the common femoral vein on B-mode (Brightness-mode) ultrasound and provides a consistent anatomic landmark; (3) B-mode ultrasound can be used to evaluate for incompressibility of the vein, echogenic material (thrombus) within the lumen of the vein, and dilation of the vein; and (4) surgeons are familiar with B-mode ultrasound because it is frequently used to detect hemopericardium, hemoperitoneum, and pleural effusion/traumatic hemothorax in critically ill patients, hence enhancing its practical applicability in this setting.

Technique.    The focused ultrasound examination of the common femoral veins is performed with the patient in the supine position as an extension of the physical examination. A 7.5 MHz linear array transducer is used to examine the common femoral veins according to the following protocol as described by Lensing et al.[90]

1. The transducer is oriented for transverse imaging, and the right common femoral vein and artery are visualized (Fig. 17-17).

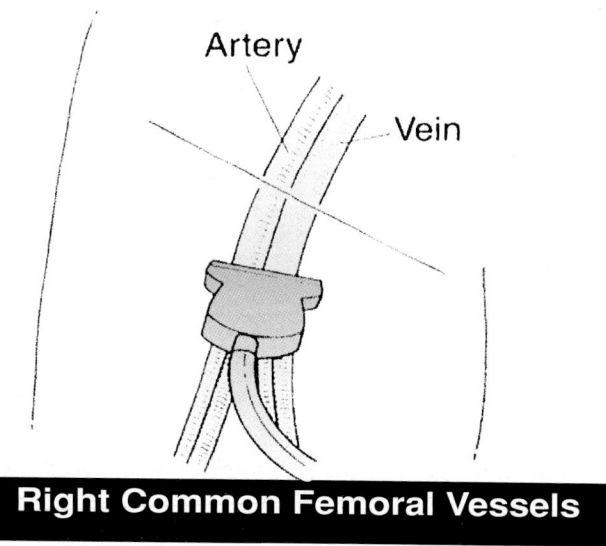

**Right Common Femoral Vessels**

**FIGURE 17-17.** Transducer position for the evaluation of femoral vein.

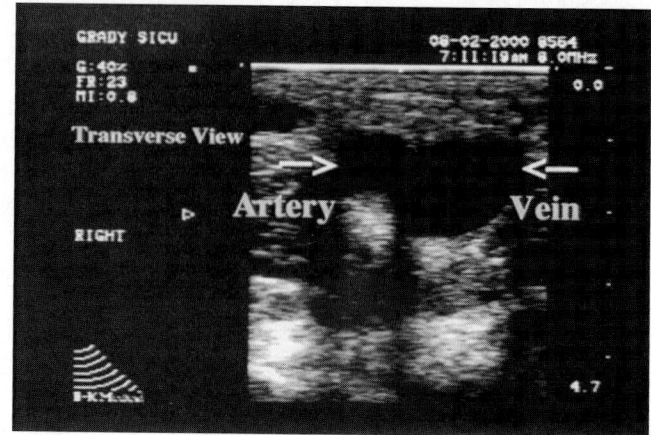

**FIGURE 17-18.** Transverse ultrasound image of right common femoral vein and artery

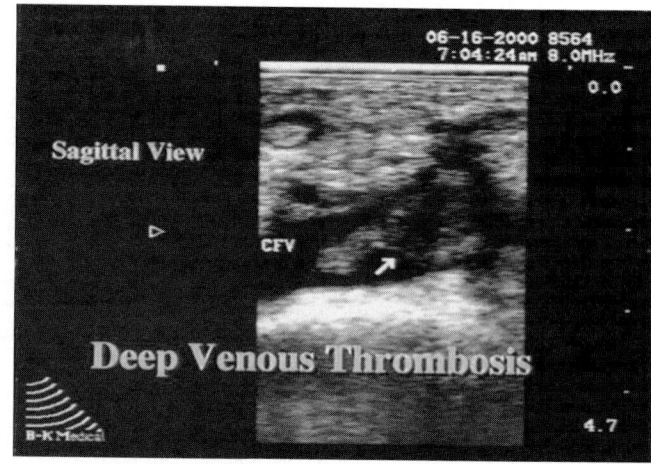

**FIGURE 17-19.** Sagittal ultrasound image of right common femoral vein with thrombus.

2. The vein is examined for the presence or absence of intraluminal echogenicity (consistent with thrombus) (Fig. 17-18) and for ease of compressibility.

3. The transducer is positioned for sagittal images, and a view of the common femoral vein is identified. The vein is inspected for intraluminal thrombus (Fig. 17-19) and adequate compressibility. The diameter of the vein is measured just distal to the saphenofemoral junction.

4. The same examination (1 through 3) is then conducted on the left lower extremity.

A positive study is defined as dilation of the common femoral vein (more than 10% increase) when compared to the same vein in the opposite extremity,[95] incompressibility of the vein, and /or the presence of echogenic foci consistent with an intraluminal thrombus. A negative study is the presence of a normal caliber vein with good compressibility and the absence of an echogenic intraluminal thrombus.

## Insertion of Inferior Vena Caval Filters

*Introduction.*  Because critically ill surgical patients are at significant risk for deep venous thrombosis and because many have contraindications to anticoagulation, therapeutic and prophylactic inferior venal caval filters (IVCF) are being used more and more frequently. Indeed, while the topic is quite controversial, one author recommends prophylactic insertion of an IVCF within 48 hours in critically ill patients who are at high risk for DVT and have a contraindication to anticoagulation.[96]

While many other authors are less apt to be this aggressive, enough critically ill surgical patients require this procedure that a bedside technique for insertion would be ideal. In fact, with improvements in technology and the advent of intravascular ultrasound (IVUS), bedside insertion of IVCF is now possible.

Indeed both trans-abdominal duplex ultrasonography[97,98] as well as intravascular ultrasound[99,100] have been used to insert vena caval filters successfully and safely at the bedside. Ashley et al.[100] reported on their experience with bedside insertion of 29 IVCF using IVUS

in the trauma intensive care unit. All patients were able to have their vena caval diameter measured and renal veins located. All filters were successfully deployed in good position without complication. Follow-up CT scans in 27 of the 29 patients were available which indicated proper placement (in reference to the renal veins) in all 27 patients. A much larger experience with bedside IVCF insertion was recently published with similarly excellent results.[101]

*Technique.*  After preparing the right groin and right thigh, a 9 French introducer sheath is placed in the right common femoral vein using a Seldinger technique. The stiff guidewire is passed into the right atrium. A 10 MHz IVUS catheter is aligned tip-to-tip with the filter deployment sheath. The IVUS catheter is then marked at the level of the deployment sheath hub. The IVUS images of the vena cava from the right atrium to the iliac confluence are obtained. The IVC is measured and a point 1 cm below the lowest renal vein is determined. The reference mark on the IVUS is transferred to the patient's thigh, and the IVUS is removed. The introducer sheath is exchanged for the deployment sheath which is advanced to the correct depth and deployed. A follow-up abdominal x-ray confirms proper position of the filter.

## EDUCATION OF SURGEONS IN ULTRASOUND

Although many approaches have been shown to be effective in teaching these focused ultrasound examinations, surgeons should have a solid understanding of the physics principles of ultrasound imaging as an integral part of that education process. Furthermore, these principles should be emphasized each time the examinations are taught.

The first educational model for how surgeons can learn ultrasound was published by Han et al. from Emory University.[7] Incoming interns took a pretest and then attended a lecture and videotape about the FAST examination. After completion of the ATLS laboratory session, three swine had diagnostic peritoneal lavage catheters reinserted to infuse fluid and produce "positive" ultrasound examinations. Two other fresh swine were "negatives". All five swine were draped similarly to disguise interventions. Incoming interns were tested individually by surgeon sonographers to determine whether the ultrasound image was "positive" or "negative." The interns completed a posttest which showed a statistically significant improvement from the pretest ($p < 0.001$). The authors concluded that incoming interns could learn the essential ultrasound principles of the FAST and that swine are feasible models for learning it.

In another study using pre- and post-testing, Ali et al. showed how a workshop in ultrasound consisting of didactics, videotapes, and hands-on demonstrations improved the ultrasound skills of nonradiologists.[102]

Other paradigms that have been used as educational models include cadavers whose peritoneal cavities were instilled with saline[103] and simulators which had data stored in three-dimensional images.[104] In the latter study, Knudson and Sisley conducted a prospective cohort study involving residents from two university trauma centers. They compared the posttest results between residents trained on a real-time ultrasound simulator versus those trained in a traditional hands-on format. The main outcome measured was the residents' performance on a standardized posttest, which included interpretation of ultrasound cases recorded on videotape. They determined no significant difference between those residents trained on the simulator or those trained on models or patients. From their study, the authors concluded that the use of a simulator is a convenient and objective method of introducing ultrasound to surgery residents.

Another issue is that of the learning curve. One of the best studies to address this issue for the FAST was conducted by Shackford et al. from the University of Vermont.[11] In this study, the authors questioned the recommendations that various numbers of ultrasound examinations should be done under supervision before a surgeon is considered qualified to perform them. The authors calculated the primary and adjusted error rates and then determined the potential clinical utility of the FAST. They found that although the clinician's (nonradiologists) initial error rate was 17%, it fell to 5% after the clinicians performed ten examinations. Additionally, in that study, the authors proposed the following recommendations for credentialing: (1) The process for credentialing of surgeons in the use of ultrasound should occur within the Department of Surgery either by surgeons or a committee composed of surgeons and nonsurgeons which reports to the Chairperson of the Department of Surgery; (2) A formal course with 4 hours of didactic and 4 hours of "hands-on" training is adequate. The curriculum for the performance of ultrasound in trauma, recently developed by the American College of Surgeons, is strongly recommended. (3) Competency for performance of the FAST exam should be determined based on error rate with respect to the prevalence of the target disease in the series. (4) "Control" or repeat scans should be allowed during the proctored experience. (5) After completion of proctoring, an ongoing monitoring process of error rates and causes of indeterminate studies using the Department of Surgery's quality improvement program is essential.[11]

The teaching of surgeon-performed ultrasound is now an integral part of the American College of Surgeons' educational program. Modular courses begin with an ultrasound basics course, which is now available on compact disc. Advanced courses in many topics, including an "Acute/Trauma" module, are taught at the College meetings and across the country each year. A very recent survey of surgeons participating in these courses show that they have been a tremendous success.[105]

Experience with ultrasound is now a mandated part of residency training in general surgery. In a recent published survey, 95% of all residency programs are teaching ultrasonography, either in a didactic or clinic form.[106] FAST, general abdominal, and breast ultrasound were all being taught in both academic and community-based programs. Academic centers additionally reported significant resident experience with IVUS, laparoscopic, and endocrine ultrasound.[106] These data suggest that ultrasound is being incorporated to a larger and larger extent in surgical training programs.

## SUMMARY

As the role of the general surgeon continues to evolve, the surgeon's use of ultrasound will surely influence practice patterns, particularly for the evaluation of patients in the acute setting. With the use of real-time imaging, the surgeon receives "instantaneous" information to augment the physical examination, narrow the differential diagnosis, or initiate an intervention.

The advantages of ultrasound are easily seen in each of the following clinical scenarios. As a *noninvasive* modality, ultrasound can be used to evaluate the injured pregnant patient and simultaneously identify the fetal heart so that its rate can be recorded. For the patient with multiple fractures who is in traction, the *portable* machine is wheeled to the patient's bedside and the FAST is performed without having to move the patient. If hypotension or an unexpected decrease in hematocrit occurs, an ultrasound examination can be easily *repeated* to exclude hemoperitoneum as the source of hypotension. When several patients with penetrating thoracoabdominal injuries present simultaneously to the emergency department, a *rapid* FAST examination with thoracic views can assess for pericardial effusion, massive hemothorax, or hemoperitoneum within seconds. This information helps the surgeon to prioritize resources and triage patients. Finally, ultrasound may be suitable for the initial assessment of the injured child. A recent study showed that ultrasound is an effective tool to screen for hemoperitoneum in the hypotensive pediatric patient.[107] This *painless* noninvasive modality is well accepted by children because it is performed at the bedside and is not intimidating.

As surgeons become more facile with ultrasound, it is anticipated that other uses will develop to further enhance its value for the assessment of patients in the acute setting.

# REFERENCES

1. Tso P, Rodriguez A, Cooper C, et al.: Sonography in blunt abdominal trauma: A preliminary progress report. *J Trauma* 33:39, 1992.
2. Rozycki GS, Ochsner MG, Jaffin JH, et al.: Prospective evaluation of surgeons' use of ultrasound in the evaluation of trauma patients. *J Trauma* 34:516, 1993.
3. Rozycki GS, Ochsner MG, Schmidt JA, et al.: A prospective study of surgeon-performed ultrasound as the primary adjuvant modality for injured patient assessment. *J Trauma* 39:492, 1995.
4. Rozycki GS, Feliciano DV, Schmidt JA, et al.: The role of surgeon-performed ultrasound in patients with possible cardiac wounds. *Ann Surg* 223:737, 1996.
5. McKenney MG, Martin L, Lentz K, et al.: 1000 consecutive ultrasounds for blunt abdominal trauma. *J Trauma* 40:607, 1996.
6. Boulanger BR, McLellan BA, Brenneman FD, et al.: Emergent abdominal sonography as a screening test in a new diagnostic algorithm for blunt trauma. *J Trauma* 40:867, 1996.
7. Han DC, Rozycki GS, Schmidt JA, et al.: Ultrasound training during ATLS: An early start for surgical interns. *J Trauma* 41:208, 1996.
8. Rozycki GS, Ballard RB, Feliciano DV, et al.: Surgeon-performed ultrasound for the assessment of truncal injuries: Lessons learned from 1,540 patients. *Ann Surg* 228:557, 1998.
9. Sisley AC, Rozycki GS, Ballard RB, et al.: Rapid detection of traumatic effusion using surgeon-performed ultrasound. *J Trauma* 44:291, 1998.
10. Rozycki GS, Feliciano DV, Ochsner MG, et al.: The role of ultrasound in patients with possible penetrating cardiac wounds: A prospective multicenter study. *J Trauma* 46:543, 1999.
11. Shackford SR, Rogers FB, Osler TM, et al.: Focused abdominal sonogram for trauma: The learning curve of nonradiologist clinicians in detecting hemoperitoneum. *J Trauma* 46:553, 1999.
12. Rozycki GS, Pennington SD: Surgeon-performed ultrasound in the critical care setting: Its use as an extension of the physical examination to detect pleural effusion. *J Trauma* 50:636, 2001.
13. Dolich M, McKenney MG, Varela J, et al.: 2,576 ultrasounds for blunt abdominal trauma. *J Trauma* 50:108, 2001.
14. Edelman SK, ed: *Understanding Ultrasound Physics, Fundamentals and Exam Review,* 2nd ed. College Station, TX: Tops Printing, Inc, 1997, p. 75.
15. Hedrick WR, Hykes L, Starchman DE: *Ultrasound physics and instrumentation,* 3rd ed. St. Louis: Mosby, 1995, p. 31.
16. Tempkin BB: Scanning Planes and Methods. In Tempkin BB, ed. *Ultrasound Scanning: Principles and Protocols.* Philadelphia: W.B. Saunders Company, 1993, p. 7.
17. Zagzebski JA: Properties of Ultrasound Transducers. In Zagzebski JA, ed. *Essentials of Ultrasound Physics.* St. Louis, Missouri: Mosby-Year Book, Inc, 1996, p. 20.
18. Hedrick WR, Hykes L, Starchman DE: Static Imaging Principles and Instrumentation. In Hedrick WR, Hykes L, Starchman DE, ed. *Ultrasound physics and instrumentation,* 3rd ed. St. Louis: Mosby, 1995, p. 71.
19. Hedrick WR, Hykes L, Starchman DE: Basic ultrasound physics. In Hedrick WR, Hykes L, Starchman DE, ed. *Ultrasound Physics and Instrumentation,* 3rd ed. St. Louis: Mosby, 1995, p. 1.
20. Fornage BD, Schernberg FL: Sonographic diagnosis of foreign bodies of the distal extremities. *AJR* 147:567, 1986.
21. Hedrick WR, Hykes L, Starchman DE: Glossary. Anonymous In *Ultrasound Physics and Instrumentation,* 3rd ed. St. Louis: Mosby, 1995, p. 355.
22. American College of Surgeons Committee on Trauma: *Advanced Trauma Life Support Course for Physicians. Anonymous.* Chicago: American College of Surgeons, 1997.
23. Grant JCB: Abdomen. In Grant JCB, ed. *Grant's Atlas of Anatomy,* 6th ed. Baltimore: Williams & Wilkins, 1972, p. 130.
24. Goldberg BB, Goodman GA, Clearfield HR: Evaluation of ascites by ultrasound. *Radiology* 96:15, 1970.
25. Goldberg BB, Clearfield HR, Goodman GA: Ultrasonic determination of ascites. *Arch Intern Med* 131:217, 1973.
26. Branney SW, Wolfe RE, Moore EE, et al.: Quantitative sensitivity of ultrasound in detecting free intraperitoneal fluid. *J Trauma* 39:375, 1995.
27. Rozycki GS, Ochsner MG, Feliciano DV, et al.: Early detection of hemoperitoneum by ultrasound examination of the right upper quadrant: A multicenter study. *J Trauma* 45:878, 1998.
28. Weyman AE, Feigenbaum H, Dillon JC, et al.: Cross-sectional echocardiography in assessing the severity of valvular aortic stenosis. *Circulation* 52:828, 1975.
29. Pearl WS, Todd KH: Ultrasonography for the initial evaluation of blunt abdominal trauma: A review of prospective trials. *Ann Emerg Med* 27:353, 1996.
30. Mutabagani K, Coley B, Zumberge N, et al.: Preliminary experience with focused abdominal sonography for trauma (FAST) in children: Is it useful? *J Ped Surg* 4:48, 1999.
31. Meyer DM, Jessen ME, Grayburn PA: Use of echocardiography to detect cardiac injury after penetrating thoracic trauma: A prospective study. *J Trauma* 39:902, 1995.
32. Rozycki GS: Ultrasonography: Surgical Applications. In Wilmore DW, Cheung LY, Harkin AH, et al., ed. *Scientific American Surgery.* New York: Scientific American, 1999, p. 1.
33. Wherrett LJ, Boulanger BR, McLellan BA, et al.: Hypotension after blunt abdominal trauma: The role of emergent abdominal sonography in surgical triage. *J Trauma* 41:815, 1996.
34. Chiu WC, Cushing BM, Rodriguez A, et al.: Abdominal injuries without hemoperitoneum: A potential limitation of focused abdominal sonography for trauma (FAST). *J Trauma* 42:617, 1997.
35. Ballard RB, Rozycki GS, Newman PG, et al.: An algorithm to reduce the incidence of false-negative FAST examination in patients at high-risk for occult injury. *J Am Coll Surg* 189:145, 1999.
36. Huff WS, Holevar M, Nagy KK, et al.: Practice Management Guidelines for the Evaluation of Blunt Abdominal Trauma: The EAST Practice Management Guidelines Work Group. *J Trauma* 53:602, 2002.
37. Federle MP, Jeffrey RB Jr: Hemoperitoneum studied by computed tomography. *Radiology* 148:187, 1983.
38. American College of Surgeons Committee on Trauma: *Advanced Trauma Life Support Course for Physicians.* Chicago: American College of Surgeons, 1997.
39. Huang M, Liu M, Wu J, et al.: Ultrasonography for the evaluation of hemoperitoneum during resuscitation: A simple scoring system. *J Trauma* 36:173, 1994.
40. McKenney KL, McKenney MG, Cohn SM, et al.: Hemoperitoneum score helps determine the need for therapeutic laparotomy. *J Trauma* 50:650, 2001.
41. Rozycki GS, Knudson MM, Shackford SR, et al.: Surgeon-Performed Bedside Organ Assessment with Sonography after Trauma (BOAST): A pilot study from the WTA Multicenter Group. *J Trauma* 59:1356, 2005.
42. Nilsson A, Loren I, Nirhov N, et al.: Power Doppler ultrasonography: Alternative to computed tomography in abdominal trauma patients. *J Ultrasound Med* 18: 669, 1999.
43. Catalano O, Sandomenico F, Raso MM, et al.: Real-time, contrast-enhanced sonography: A new tool for detecting active bleeding. *J Trauma* 59:933, 2005.
44. Joyner CR Jr, Herman RJ, Reid JM: Reflected ultrasound in the detection and localization of pleural effusion. *JAMA* 200:399, 1967.
45. Gryminski J, Krakowka P, Lypacewicz G: The diagnosis of pleural effusion by ultrasonic and radiologic techniques. *Chest* 70:33, 1976.
46. Lichtenstein D, Menu Y: A bedside ultrasound sign ruling out pneumothorax in the critically ill. *Chest* 108:1345, 1995.
47. Targhetta R, Bourgeois J, Chavagneux R, et al.: Diagnosis of pneumothorax by ultrasound immediately after ultrasonically guided aspiration biospy. *Chest* 101:855, 1992.
48. Wernecke K, Galanski M, Peters P, et al.: Pneumothorax: Evaluation by ultrasound—preliminary results. *J Thorac Imaging* 2:76, 2000.
49. Goodman T, Traill Z, Phillips A, et al.: Ultrasound detection of pneumothorax. *Clin Radiology* 54:736, 1999.
50. Knudtson JL, Dort JM, Helmer SD, et al.: Surgeon-performed ultrasound for pneumothorax in the trauma suite. *J Trauma* 56: 527, 2004.
51. Dulchavsky SA, Hamilton DR, Diebel LN, et al.: Thoracic ultrasound diagnosis in pneumothorax. *J Trauma* 47:970, 1999.
52. Sarkisian AE, Khondkarian RA, Amirbekian NM, et al.: Sonographic screening of mass casualties for abdominal and renal injuries following the 1988 Armenian earthquake. *J Trauma* 31:247, 1991.
53. Sistrom CL, Reiheld C, Gay S, et al.: Detection and estimation of the volume of pneumothorax using real-time sonography: Efficacy determined by receiver operating characteristic analysis. *AJR* 166:317, 1996.
54. Dulchavsky SA, Schwarz KL, Kirkpatrick A, et al.: Prospective evaluation of thoracic ultrasound in the detection of pneumothorax. *J Trauma* 50:201, 2001.
55. Fenkl R, von Garrel T, Knaepler H: Emergency diagnosis of sternum fracture with ultrasound. *Unfallchirurg* 95:375, 1992.
56. Goodwin H, Holmes JF, Wisner DH: Abdominal ultrasound examination in pregnant blunt trauma patients. *J Trauma* 50:689, 2001.
57. Brown MA, Sirlin CB, Farahmand N, et al.: Screening sonography in pregnant patients with blunt abdominal trauma. *J Ultrasound Med* 24:175, 2005.
58. Tayal VS, Beatty MA, Marx JA, et al.: FAST (Focused Assessment with Sonography in Trauma) accurate for cardiac and intraperitoneal injury in penetrating anterior chest trauma. *J Ultrasound Med* 23:467, 2004.

59. Boulanger BR, Kearney PA, Tsuei B, et al.: The routine use of sonography in penetrating torso injury is beneficial. *J Trauma* 51:320, 2001.

60. Murphy JT, Hall J, Provost D: Fascial ultrasound for evaluation of anterior abdominal stab wound injury. *J Trauma* 59:843, 2005.

61. Brooks AJ, Price V, Simms M: FAST on operational military deployment. *Emerg Med J* 22:263, 2005.

62. Sustic A, Miletic D, Fuckar Z, et al.: Ultrasonography in the evaluation of hemoperitoneum in war casualties. *Mil Med* 164:600, 1999.

63. Strode CA, Rubal BJ, Gerhardt RT, et al.: Satellite and mobile wireless transmission of focused assessment with sonography in trauma. *Acad Emerg Med* 10:1411, 2003.

64. Strode CA, Rubal BJ, Gerhardt RT, et al.: Wireless and satellite transmission of prehospital focused abdominal sonography for trauma. *Prehosp Emerg Care* 7:375, 2003.

65. Campbell MR, Billica RD, Johnston SL, et al.: Performance of advanced trauma life support procedures in microgravity. *Aviat Space Environ Med* 73:907, 2002.

66. Martin DS, South DA, Garcia KM, et al.: Ultrasound in space. *Ultrasound Med Biol* 29:1, 2003.

67. Kirkpatrick AW, Hamilton DR, Nicolaou S, et al.: Focused assessment with sonography for trauma in weightlessness: A feasibility study. *J Am Coll Surg* 196:833, 2003.

68. Hamilton DR, Sargsyan AE, Kirkpatrick AW, et al.: Sonographic detection of pneumothorax and hemothorax in microgravity. *Aviat Space Environ Med* 75:272, 2004.

69. Sargsyan AE, Hamilton DR, Jones JA, et al.: FAST at MACH 20: Clinical ultrasound aboard the international space station. *J Trauma* 58:35, 2005.

70. Chiao L, Sharipov S, Sargsyan AE, et al.: Ocular examination for trauma; clinical ultrasound aboard the International Space Station. *J Trauma* 58:885, 2005.

71. Braxton CC. *The Traveling Intensive Care Unit Patient: Road Trips.* 80 No. 3. Philadelphia, PA: W.B. Saunders, 2000, p. 949.

72. Ballard RB, Rozycki GS, Knudson MM, et al.: The surgeon's use of ultrasound in the acute setting. In Rozycki GS, ed. *Surgeon-Performed Ultrasound.* Philadelphia: W.B. Saunders, 1998, p. 337.

73. Lichtenstein D, Axler O: Intensive use of general ultrasound in the intensive care unit. Prospective study of 150 consecutive patients. *Intensive Care Med* 19:353, 1993.

74. Slasky BS, Auerbach D, Skolnick ML: Value of portable real-time ultrasound in the ICU. *Critical Care Medicine* 11:160, 1983.

75. Lerch MM, Riehl J, Buechsel R, et al.: Bedside ultrasound in decision making for emergency surgery: Its role in medical intensive care patients. *Am J Emerg Med* 10:35, 1992.

76. Staren ED, Torp-Pedersen S: General interventional ultrasound. In Staren ED, ed. *Ultrasound for the Surgeon.* Philadelphia: Lippincott-Raven, 1997, p. 137.

77. Holm HH, Skjoldbye B: Interventional ultrasound. *Ultrasound Med Biol* 22:773, 1996.

78. Staren ED, ed: *Ultrasound for the Surgeon.* Philadelphia: Lippincott-Raven, 1997.

79. Fry WR, Smith RS, Schneider JJ, et al.: Ultrasonographic examination of wound tracts. *Arch Surg* 130:605, 1995.

80. Banerjee B, Das RK: Sonographic detection of foreign bodies of the extremities. *Br J Radiol* 64:107, 1991.

81. Hill R, Conron R, Greissinger P, et al.: Ultrasound for the detection of foreign bodies in human tissue. *Ann Emerg Med* 29:353, 1997.

82. Mansfield PF, Hohn DC, Fornage BD, et al.: Complications and failures of subclavian-vein catheterization. *N Engl J Med* 331:1735, 1994.

83. Gilbert TB, Seneff MG, Becker RB: Facilitation of internal jugular venous cannulation using an audio-guided Doppler ultrasound vascular access device: results from a prospective, dual-center, randomized, crossover clinical study. *Crit Care Med* 23:60, 1995.

84. Mallory DL, McGee WT, Shawker TH, et al.: Ultrasound guidance improves the success rate of internal jugular vein cannulation. A prospective, randomized trial. *Chest* 98:157, 1990.

85. Gratz I, Afshar M, Kidwell P, et al.: Doppler-guided cannulation of the internal jugular vein: A prospective, randomized trial. *J Clin Monit* 10:185, 1994.

86. Gualtieri E, Deppe SA, Sipperly ME, et al.: Subclavian venous catheterization: Greater success rate for less experienced operators using ultrasound guidance. *Crit Care Med* 23:692, 1995.

87. Leger D, Nugent M: Doppler localization of the internal jugular vein facilitates central venous cannulation. *Anesthesiology* 60:481, 1984.

88. Fry WR, Clagett GC, O'Rourke PT: Ultrasound guided central venous access. [Unpublished] 1998.

89. LeDonne J: Percutaneous cephalic vein cannulation (in the Deltopectoral groove), with ultrasound guidance. *J Am Coll Surg* 200:810, 2005.

90. Lensing AW, Prandoni P, Brandjes D, et al.: Detection of deep-vein thrombosis by real-time B-mode ultrasonography. *New Eng J Med* 320:342, 1989.

91. Appleton PT, De Jong TE, Lampmann LE: Deep venous thrombosis of the leg: US Findings. *Radiology* 163:743, 1987.

92. Polak JF, Culter SS, O'Leary DH: Deep veins of the calf: assessment with color Doppler flow imaging. *Radiology* 171:481, 1989.

93. Vogel P, Laing FC, Jeffrey RB Jr, et al.: Deep venous thrombosis of the lower extremity: US evaluation. *Radiology* 163:747, 1987.

94. Wheeler HB, Anderson FA Jr: Can noninvasive tests be used as the basis for treatment of deep vein thrombosis. In Bernstein EF, ed. *Noninvasive Diagnostic Techniques in Vascular Disease*, 3rd. ed. St. Louis: Mosby, 1985, p. 805.

95. Effeney DJ, Friedman MB, Gooding GA: Iliofemoral venous thrombosis: Real-time ultrasound diagnosis, normal criteria, and clinical application. *Radiology* 150:787, 1984.

96. Carlin AM, Tyburski JG, Wilson RF, et al.: Prophylactic and therapeutic inferior vena cava filters to prevent pulmonary emboli in trauma patients. *Arch Surg* 521, 2002.

97. Corriere MA, Passman MA, Guzman RJ, et al.: Comparison of bedside transabdominal duplex ultrasound versus contrast venography for inferior vena cava filter placement: What is the best imaging modality? *Ann Vasc Surg* 19:229, 2005.

98. Conners MS, Becker S, Guzman RJ, et al.: Duplex scan-directed placement of inferior vena cava filters: A five-year institutional experience. *J Vasc Surg* 35:286, 2002.

99. Gamblin TC, Ashley DW, Burch S, et al.: A prospective evaluation of a bedside technique for placement of inferior vena cava filters: Accuracy and limitations of intravascular ultrasound. *Am Surg* 69:382, 2003.

100. Ashley DW, Gamblin TC, McCampbell BL, et al.: Bedside insertion of vena cava filters in the intensive care unit using intravascular ultrasound to locate renal veins. *J Trauma* 57:26, 2004.

101. Passman MA, Dattilo JB, Guzman RJ, et al.: Bedside placement of inferior vena cava filters by using transabdominal duplex ultrasonography and intravascular ultrasound imaging. *J Vasc Surg* 42:1027, 2005.

102. Ali J, Rozycki GS, Campbell JP, et al.: Trauma ultrasound workshop improves physician detection of peritoneal and pericardial fluid. *J Clin Res* 63:275, 1996.

103. Frezza EE, Solis RL, Silich RJ, et al.: Competency-based instruction to improve the surgical resident technique and accuracy of the trauma ultrasound. *Am Surg* 65:884, 1999.

104. Knudson MM, Sisley AC: Training residents using simulation technology: Experience with ultrasound for trauma. *J Trauma* 48:659, 2000.

105. Staren ED, Knudson MM, Rozycki GS, et al.: An evaluation of the American College of Surgeons' ultrasound education program. *Am J Surg* 191:489, 2006.

106. Freitas ML, Frangos SG, Frankel HL: The status of ultrasonography training and use in general surgery residency programs. *J Am Coll Surg* 202:453, 2006.

107. Thourani VH, Pettitt BJ, Schmidt JA, et al.: Validation of surgeon-performed emergency abdominal ultrasound in pediatric trauma patients. *J Pediatr Surg* 33:322, 1998.

# Commentary ■ ALEXANDER L. EASTMAN ■ HEIDI FRANKEL

This chapter by Drs. Dente and Rozycki provides an excellent review of the basic principles that underlie surgeon-performed ultrasound in the trauma and ICU setting. It summarizes succinctly the 15-year experience of American surgeons using this modality as described by the authors and their colleagues at Emory University/Grady Memorial Hospital in Atlanta. Their review of ultrasound physics, techniques, and indications for the sonographic examinations will serve the practicing trauma surgeon and trainee well. The modifications to this edition on the use of ultrasound in penetrating trauma and in special situations as well as in the ICU are also valuable and timely.

Surgeon-performed FAST is a rapid, simple, and fairly accurate bedside study that, when used wisely, provides expedient information in real-time during trauma resuscitation. Through the work of the authors of this chapter and the diligence of organizations like the American College of Surgeons, the use of surgeon-performed ultrasound, specifically FAST, has become a standard part of the evaluation of the injured patient. Moreover, interest and competence in the performance of surgeon-performed FAST have led to use of ultrasound by surgeons in the intensive care unit and in nontrauma settings as well, both for diagnosis and for therapy.

Drs. Dente and Rozycki aptly note that trauma ultrasound is most accurate and helpful in the management of the hypotensive blunt injured patient when *positive* and in those with penetrating injury to the "box" where cardiac damage is possible. On the other hand, the reliability of the *negative* ultrasound of the abdomen has been questioned by many, including our group, prompting reliance on CT scanning for normotensive, hemodynamically stable patients at risk for abdominal injury. For example, we have reported that, in the presence of a significant pelvic fracture, FAST sensitivity is low. Moreover, after several "false-negative" FAST examinations in hypotensive patients, we have experienced an increase in the number of diagnostic peritoneal lavages performed at our institution.

Furthermore, the authors point out that the results of trials extending the indications for abdominal ultrasound in trauma have been disappointing. The Western Trauma Association's multicenter trial on the BOAST examination, or advanced, organ-specific imaging, demonstrated that experienced surgeon-sonographers were unable to identify solid organ injuries the majority of the time. Murphy and colleagues from our institution, and others have shown that ultrasound was far too insensitive for use as an appropriate screening examination for penetrating trauma. Clearly, the appropriate role for FAST is evolving and will continue to do so as technology improves.

On the other hand, there are novel uses for ultrasound in the evaluation of the injured. As technology has improved and simplified with increased portability, ultrasound may be useful in locations remote from the hospital by nonphysician providers. The authors cite examples from the British Defense Medical Services and NASA, although we believe these are only a few of the novel applications for trauma outside of the trauma center or surgical ICU. Several authors have advocated the potential use of ultrasound by paramedics in the field and use by US military medics and corpsman during Operations Iraqi Freedom and Enduring Freedom as a triage tool during mass casualty incidents.

Additionally, as the authors describe, the use of surgeon-performed ultrasound in the surgical intensive care unit has allowed improved, more efficient care of patients. The identification of a pleural effusion, pneumothorax, and deep vein thrombosis now no longer requires a radiologist for definitive diagnosis. As the authors point out, this has dramatically improved efficiency of diagnosis of these complications in the surgical intensive care unit. Furthermore, ultrasound-guided drainage of fluid collections and central line insertion have become the standard of care in many centers. With regards to the placement of central venous catheters, the authors present data on improved efficiency and decreased complications by the use of ultrasound guidance. Several regulatory agencies have suggested that ultrasound-directed central catheter insertion, particularly for those placed in the internal jugular vein, be mandatory. Some have undertaken ultrasound guidance for IVC filter insertion. Others—our group included—have begun to use limited focused echocardiography to assist in resuscitation, particularly as pulmonary artery catheters have fallen into disfavor.

We concur with the belief of the authors and the American College of Surgeons that a successful surgeon-led ultrasound program requires a process of continuous quality assessment and improvement. Ultrasound machines age and transducers may be dropped and mishandled in the hectic trauma resuscitation area. This can result in the acquisition of substandard images and misdiagnosis.

Understanding its role and limitations, surgeon-performed ultrasound will continue to assist in diagnosis and conduct of procedural skills. We look forward to the future, where a health care provider armed with a durable, PDA-sized high-resolution "smart" ultrasound machine can travel from the prehospital setting to the ICU to improve the care of the injured.

## References

1. Friese RS, Malekzadeh S, Shafi S et al.: Abdominal ultrasound (FAST) is an unreliable modality for the detection of hemoperitoneum in patients with pelvic fracture. J Trauma 63:97, 2007.
2. Murphy JT, Hall J, Provost D: Fascial ultrasound for evaluation of anterior stab wound injury. J Trauma 59:843, 2005.

# Anesthesia

*James C. Duke*

Few patients offer greater challenge to the anesthesiologist than the critically injured patient. The acuity of the situation and uncertainty of the extent of injury requires the anesthesiologist to be aggressive, keenly vigilant, and methodical in approach, so that injuries will not be missed or, lamentably, exacerbated. This chapter discusses the risk of anesthesia, anesthetic assessment and concerns, intraoperative monitoring, selection of the appropriate anesthetic and anesthetic agents, and concerns for injury to specific body regions and patient groups.

## ANESTHETIC RISK

Risk associated with the administration of anesthesia was first recognized in the mid-19th century.[1] Adverse perioperative outcomes are often multifactorial and the contribution of anesthesia cannot easily be separated from pre-existing illness, acute injury, and surgery. As pointed out by Keats, "No control study of the hazards of operation without anesthesia, or conversely, anesthesia without operation, will ever be performed. The hazards of anesthesia can therefore never be considered independent of a second procedure."[2] Aitkenhead reviews anesthetic-related injuries from a global perspective.[3]

The most important predictor of death may be severity of comorbid disease. Progression of presenting disease has been estimated in the United Kingdom as contributing to more than two-thirds of preoperative deaths.[4] Assessment of outcomes must also include some accounting for severity of illness. This is particularly true for busy trauma centers. Crude, unadjusted rates of mortality and morbidity may unfairly judge the quality of care of institutions charged with treating the sickest patients (see Chap. 6).

Perioperative death is the most commonly researched assessment of anesthetic risk. Prior to 1979, mortality rates, in which anesthesia either contributed to or was the principal cause of death, were estimated about 1 in 6789.[5] Numerous studies published since 1979 demonstrate remarkable declines in anesthetic-related mortality

and morbidity (Table 18-1). Many of these studies were performed on a national basis. The *British Report of a Confidential Enquiry into Perioperative Deaths* found mortality rates attributable solely to anesthesia of roughly 1:185,000.[6] This study is valuable as it assessed nearly 1 million cases in three large regions of the United Kingdom, and data sent to the confidential enquiry were protected from subpoena. In 1988, Eichorn reviewed the Harvard experience and found only nine deaths or cases of significant central nervous system injury attributable to anesthesia in approximately 1 million patients.[7] With reductions in mortality of this magnitude, further studies would of necessity be enormous and multi-institutional. Advances in computerized database management may make such investigations less burdensome. In view of concerns in the United States regarding confidentiality and liability, any such studies would likely take place in other countries.

Besides death, there have also been substantial reductions in hypoxic central nervous system (CNS) injury, myocardial infarction, pulmonary aspiration, and other significant morbid events. Numerous factors contributing to this decline include improvements in monitoring technology (particularly pulse oximetry and capnography), development of intraoperative monitoring standards, and an exploding interest in anesthesia patient safety and risk management.[8,9] Improvement in anesthetic outcomes is supported by results of the American Society of Anesthesiologists (ASA) closed malpractice claims investigations. Between 1975 and 1990, closed medicolegal claims for death decreased from 41 to 27%, and claims for CNS damage decreased from 15 to 6%. It also appears that participation of anesthesiologists in intraoperative care is of positive benefit, and one can speculate that this would be particularly true for the multiply injured patient.[10]

Although estimating mortality rates are useful, they do not determine mechanisms contributing to patient injury. Critical incident analysis identifies perianesthetic events that may lead to adverse outcomes. A critical incident is a human error or equipment failure that led or may have led (if undiscovered and uncorrected in a timely manner) to an undesirable outcome.[11] Cooper and colleagues grouped anesthetic critical incidents into causal patterns

**TABLE 18-1**

| Representative Anesthetic Mortality Statistics | | | |
|---|---|---|---|
| STUDY | YEARS | ANESTHETICS | MORTALITY RATE |
| Farrow et al.[5] | Pre-1979 | 1,147,362 | 1:6,789 |
| Eichom[7] | 1976–1985 | 757,000 | 1:151,400 |
| Eichom[7] | 1985–1988 | 244,000[a] | No deaths |
| Buck et al.[6] | 1986 | 485,850 | 1:185,000 |

[a]1985 was the year Harvard Standards for Intraoperative Monitoring were instituted.

**TABLE 18-2**

| American Society of Anesthesiologists (ASA) Physical Status Classification | |
|---|---|
| STATUS | DISEASE STATE |
| ASA class I | No organic, physiologic, biochemical, or psychiatric disturbance |
| ASA class II | Mild to moderate systemic disturbance that may or may not be related to the reason for surgery |
| ASA class III | Severe systemic disturbance that may or may not be related to the reason for surgery |
| ASA class IV | Severe systemic disturbance that is life-threatening with or without surgery |
| ASA class V | Moribund patient who has little chance of survival but is submitted to surgery as a last resort |
| Emergency | Any patient in whom an emergency operation is required |

and developed strategies for prevention or detection of the adverse events. Of particular interest is the fact that while 86% of events occurred in healthy patients, only 6% led to significant injury. Errors occurring in more severely ill patients (ASA physical class III or greater) accounted for 43% of significant adverse events (e.g., mortality, cardiac arrest, canceled operative procedure, extended hospital or intensive care unit [ICU] stay). However, they recommend that review of adverse occurrences involve not just an examination of outcomes but of process. Currently such "root cause" analysis has become a routine part of quality review and improvement at all hospitals (see Chap. 6).

Remarkable information concerning anesthetic risk has emerged from the ASA Closed Claims Study, a structured analysis of adverse anesthetic outcomes ongoing since 1985. Records from cases that led to litigation were carefully reviewed to identify factors that contributed to either death or significant morbid events. Though the results are sometimes compelling, limitations of this methodology include lack of comparison groups, probable bias toward adverse outcomes, reliance on partial observers, and the inability to provide numerical estimates of risk (there is a lack of denominator data as only closed medicolegal cases are reviewed). Though some of the results have received peer review publication (respiratory events,[12] neurologic injury,[13] intraoperative awareness[14]), additional information on this project can be obtained through the ASA website (www.asahq.org).

There is a paucity of information available to estimate anesthetic risk in trauma patients per se. Clearly, patients operated upon emergently have greater mortality and morbidity. Tiret and coworkers found a three-fold increase in the rate of complications (death and persistent coma) when any procedure was performed emergently.[15] Cohen found emergency procedures to be independent predictors of mortality (along with advanced age, male gender, increasing ASA status, major or intermediate surgery, and complications within the operating room).[16] Vacanti and colleagues reviewed over 68,000 anesthetics and also found that mortality rates were higher for emergency procedures as well as for more seriously ill patients.[17] However, in neither of these studies was an effort made to distinguish traumatic injuries from other emergencies. Koch, Cohen, and colleagues found that ASA physical status was a powerful predictor of mortality in trauma patients and correlated highly with severity of injuries.[16,18]

## Anesthetic Assessment and Concerns

Initial Assessment.   The thoroughness of the preoperative evaluation is often a function of the acuity of the situation. Paradoxically, the most complicated, gravely injured patient affords the least time for assessment. Such limitations require the anesthesiologist to be aggressive and methodical in assessment and preparation. All severely injured patients should be considered at risk for aspiration, cervical spine and closed-head injury, hypovolemia, alcohol abuse, and potential difficultly to intubate.

If time permits, important prior medical history (possibly taken from family) includes cardiac and pulmonary complaints. Because most anesthetic agents are metabolized and excreted through hepatic and renal mechanisms, knowledge of chronic impairment of these systems may alter the choice or dosage of many anesthetic agents and neuromuscular blocking agents. Although gastroparesis is assumed after any traumatic event, the time since the last meal is also of interest. Current medications, allergies, prior surgeries and associated adverse events, last menstrual cycle, endocrine disease, viral illness such as hepatitis or human immunodeficiency virus (HIV), and substance abuse are also pertinent historical features. Events surrounding the traumatic event may suggest that pre-existing illness was a contributing factor to the accident. Mechanism of injury may alert one to certain injury patterns (see Chap. 7).

The ASA has developed a five-category classification system based on preoperative assessment (Table 18-2).[19] This system separates patients by the estimated severity of systemic diseases. An *E* is added to the numerical value if the patient requires an emergency operation. The classification system does not take into account extremes of age or complexity of the surgical procedure. No other system of classification has achieved such widespread use among anesthesiologists. Though the system was developed to facilitate communication and not as a risk assessment, several investigators have identified higher ASA physical class patients as being at greater risk for pulmonary and cardiac complications as well as death.[17,18,20]

## Physical Assessment

Features of the physical examination of special interest include assessing vital sign trends and response to resuscitative efforts. Maintaining airway patency is a major role for the anesthesiologist as well as the surgical team and devices for definitively establishing an airway are discussed extensively elsewhere (see Chap. 12). Once an airway is established, it is necessary to assess adequacy of ventilation and assist if needed. Respiratory drive may be impaired secondary to head injury or intoxicants, and the mechanical aspects of ventilation may be compromised due to spinal cord, chest wall, or diaphragmatic injury, as well abdominal distention, pulmonary contusion, hemothorax, pneumothorax, and so forth. The adequacy of the circulation should be assessed, noting the relative insensitivity of vital signs in detecting moderate degrees of blood loss (see Chap. 13). The ability to resuscitate a patient with significant blood loss should be ensured; numerous large-gauge intravenous lines should be inserted if previous caregivers have not done so (14- and 16-gauge peripheral cannulae and 9 French central introducers are ideal). Consideration should be given to placing intravenous lines above and below the diaphragm if physical findings suggest major thoracic or upper extremity vascular injury. Intravenous infusions should be warmed, isotonic, and compatible with blood products. Blood should be drawn for type and cross-match, as well as hematology, chemistry (including lactate), and coagulation profiles. Arterial blood gas analysis is invaluable for detecting ventilation perfusion disturbances. A cursory neurologic examination should be undertaken and recorded, noting level of consciousness (Glasgow Coma Scale [GCS]), cervical spine tenderness, and lateralizing defects.

## Airway Management

The injured patient is at risk for a compromised airway for multiple reasons (see Chap. 12). The tongue is the most common cause of an obstructed airway and is readily treated by anterior displacement of the mandible with a jaw thrust and oral airway. Direct trauma to the face may distort or obstruct the airway through disruption of the supporting bony architecture. Bilateral fractures of the mandible are particularly likely to result in loss of airway patency. Blunt trauma to the anterior neck may fracture the larynx or trachea and precipitate subcutaneous emphysema and soft tissue swelling. Penetrating neck injuries may produce hematomas sufficient to obstruct airflow. Hoarseness, stridor, use of accessory respiratory musculature, and paradoxical motions of the chest or abdominal wall suggest some degree of airway obstruction and impending total airway collapse. Cyanosis, pallor, declining pulse oximetry values, and apnea are signs mandating immediate airway intervention.

The basic materials for airway management include bag–valve–mask (BVM, Ambu) devices attached to high-flow oxygen; suction devices; oral and nasopharyngeal airways; laryngoscopes with blades of various lengths and shapes; endotracheal tubes (ETTs) of graduated sizes with stylets; and amnestic, analgesic, and neuromuscular-blocking agents appropriate to the clinical situation. Difficult intubations require the use of such airway adjuncts as gum elastic bougies, light wands, laryngeal mask airways (LMAs), and fiberoptic bronchoscopes. The intubating laryngeal mask airway (Fastrach, LMA North America, San Diego, CA) has led to successful intubations in patients with maxillofacial injuries and where there is difficult tracheal intubation along with difficult mask ventilation.[21,22] Esophageal tracheal combitube (ETC-Sheridan Catheter Corp., Argyle, NY) and transtracheal jet ventilation (TTJV) are additional techniques, that along with the LMA, should be considered bridging maneuvers to definitive airway control. The combitube and LMA are unsatisfactory when laryngeal fractures are present. The Bullard laryngoscope facilitates intubation while maintaining the neck in a neutral position, and now there are laryngoscope handles that transmit the viewed image

to an attached screen and reduce (but not eliminate) the amount of cervical motion associated with intubation (Glidescope, Saturn Biomedical, Burnaby, BC, Canada). Devices to verify end-tidal $CO_2$ and proper endotracheal tube placement are necessary, as the physical examination can be unreliable.[23]

Prior to administration of medications that render the patient unconscious or pharmacologically paralyzed, the likelihood of encountering a difficult airway should be made. A difficult airway is defined as one in which a trained, experienced laryngoscopist experiences difficulty with mask ventilation, tracheal intubation, or both. Difficulty may arise from an injury or to intrinsic anatomic airway variability. The ease of mask ventilation may be thought of as a continuum, ranging from an airway that is patent without intervention to the airway that is impossible to mask-ventilate by even the most experienced practitioners using available airway adjuncts under any conditions (Fig. 18-1).[24] Similarly, ease of intubation by direct laryngoscopy is a continuum from an unremarkable successful first attempt to impossible despite optimum positioning, changes in laryngoscopy blades, and multiple attempts by various experienced laryngoscopists. The difficult extremes of ventilation and intubation result in the "cannot ventilate, cannot intubate" (CVCI) scenario. Recognizing the likelihood and appropriate planning for this situation are of utmost importance. The ASA Task Force on Management of the Difficult Airway has developed an algorithm to assist in CVCI scenarios (Fig. 18-2).[22] Special considerations in trauma include concerns for a full stomach, cervical spine stability, hypovolemia, closed-head injury, and the likelihood that partial airway obstruction portends total airway obstruction.

Ease of intubation is a function of complete laryngoscopic viewing; Cormack and Lehane (Fig. 18-3) described a grading classification.[25] The entire laryngeal aperture is visualized by direct laryngoscopy in grade I; posterior laryngeal anatomy (arytenoid cartilages) at most are visualized in grade II; only the epiglottis is visualized in grade III; and only the soft palate is visualized in grade IV. Grades III and IV are considered difficult intubations. The inability to open the mouth by at least three fingerbreadths and a thyromental distance of less than three fingerbreadths suggests visualization of the glottic aperture upon direct laryngoscopy may not be possible. Short, muscular, or obese necks, prominent incisors or large breasts may make laryngoscopy difficult. Morbidly obese patients are difficult to ventilate and intubate and experience rapid oxygen desaturation due to loss of functional residual capacity.

The size of the tongue relative to the oropharyngeal cavity has been noted to correlate with intubation difficulty. Mallampati and coworkers divided the visual appearance of the oral pharynx into four classes. The structures visualized with each class are as follows: class I—soft palate, uvula, and tonsillar pillars; class II—soft palate and uvula; class III—base of uvula only and soft palate; and class IV—soft palate only (Fig. 18-4).[26] Intubations where the glottis could not be visualized on direct laryngoscopy were found in 35% of patients when only the base of the uvula could be seen; essentially all class IV patients have inadequate glottic exposure. However, this assessment requires the patient to be upright and to fully open the mouth and protrude the tongue, which is often impossible after trauma. Satisfactory laryngoscopic views are less likely to be obtained when cervical spine precautions are employed, as in-line stabilization purposefully limits atlantoaxial extension. Laryngoscopy is also made difficult by rigid (Philadelphia) cervical spine collars.[27]

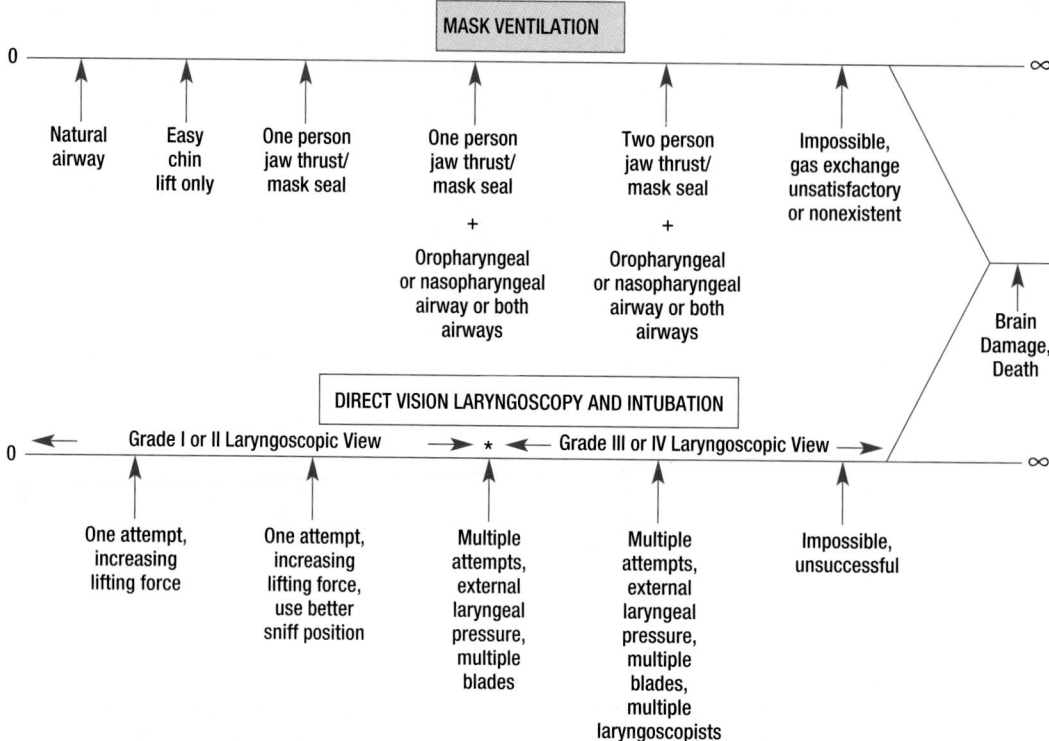

**FIGURE 18-1.**  Definition of difficult airway. Airway refers to either mask ventilation or endotracheal tube (ETT) intubation by direct vision laryngoscope. The degree of difficulty can range from 0 (extremely easy) to infinite (impossible). In between these extremes, there are several well-defined and commonly encountered degrees of difficulty. Laryngoscopic views as described by Cormack and Lehane and intubation also can be described across a continuum. *(Reproduced with permission from Benumof JL. Management of the difficult adult airway. Anesthesiology 75:1088, 1991.)*

**Confirmation of Endotracheal Intubation.**    Standard clinical detection methods, such as noting chest wall movement and auscultation over the lungs and epigastrum, are all associated with significant error. Fiberoptic bronchoscopy is the best means of verification but requires equipment not always available. The most popular and reliable indirect method is confirming exhaled carbon dioxide ($CO_2$). Quantitative analysis is standard in all anesthetizing locations and qualitative $CO_2$ detection using dye indicators is common elsewhere. False-positive detection may occur after ingestion of carbonated beverages and the like, but the effect is transitory. Detection of $CO_2$ may be difficult in severe hypoperfusion states or during cardiac arrest. A self-inflating esophageal detector bulb has been described that is not dependent on $CO_2$ detection and may be of value in such circumstances.[23]

**Extubation and Tube Changing.**    It is sometimes necessary to convert nasal to oral endotracheal tubes or replace small or leaking tubes to facilitate bronchoscopy or weaning from ventilatory support. Tube changing may result in unintentional loss of airway. By using fenestrated endotracheal tube changers, jet ventilation may be instituted if the replacement endotracheal tube is not easily inserted[28] (Fig. 18-5). Should advancing the replacement tube prove unexpectedly difficult once the initial endotracheal tube is withdrawn, the jet stylet can be attached by Luer-Lok connectors to a high-pressure oxygen supply and the patient oxygenated as issues of difficulty are resolved. Jet stylets may induce barotrauma.[29] Jet stylets can also be used during trials of extubation.

The patient can be extubated over the stylet and if the trial fails, the endotracheal tube is reinserted over the indwelling jet stylet.

## Fluid Resuscitation

Chapter 13 covers this topic extensively. It is mentioned here for it is the responsibility of the anesthesia team to manager and monitor the unstable circulatory system of the trauma patient while surgery is taking place. Obviously it will be difficult to fully restore intravascular volume as long as bleeding is ongoing and the patient is experiencing the physiologic changes associated with the shock state. Lactated Ringer's solution is preferable to normal saline because of the hyperchloremic metabolic acidosis which has been associated with excessive use of the latter, and confounds interpretation of the lactic acidosis that invariably occurs with severe hypovolemia.[30] Blood products and blood substitutes are administered predicated upon hemodynamic indicators and serial laboratory examinations.

## Allergic Reactions

Allergic reactions may be difficult to diagnose intraoperatively.[31] For instance, hypotension associated with an allergic reaction would easily be confused with hypovolemia from blood loss. Increased airway resistance associated with an allergic reaction can be confused with increased airway pressures due to endobronchial intubation, mucus plugging, a kinked endotracheal tube, anesthesia machine malfunction, pulmonary contusion,

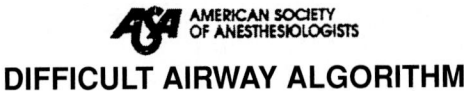

## DIFFICULT AIRWAY ALGORITHM

1.  Assess the likelihood and clinical impact of basic management problems:
    - A. Difficult Ventilation
    - B. Difficult Intubation
    - C. Difficulty with Patient Cooperation or Consent
    - D. Difficult Tracheostomy

2.  Actively pursue opportunities ro deliver supplemental oxygen throughout the process of difficult airway management

3.  Consider the relative merits and feasibility of basic management choices:

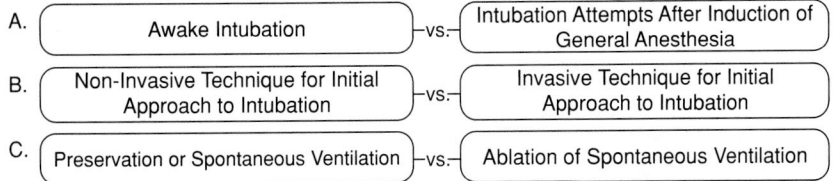

|   | | |
|---|---|---|
| A. | Awake Intubation | -vs- | Intubation Attempts After Induction of General Anesthesia |
| B. | Non-Invasive Technique for Initial Approach to Intubation | -vs- | Invasive Technique for Initial Approach to Intubation |
| C. | Preservation or Spontaneous Ventilation | -vs- | Ablation of Spontaneous Ventilation |

4.  Develop primary and alternative strategies:

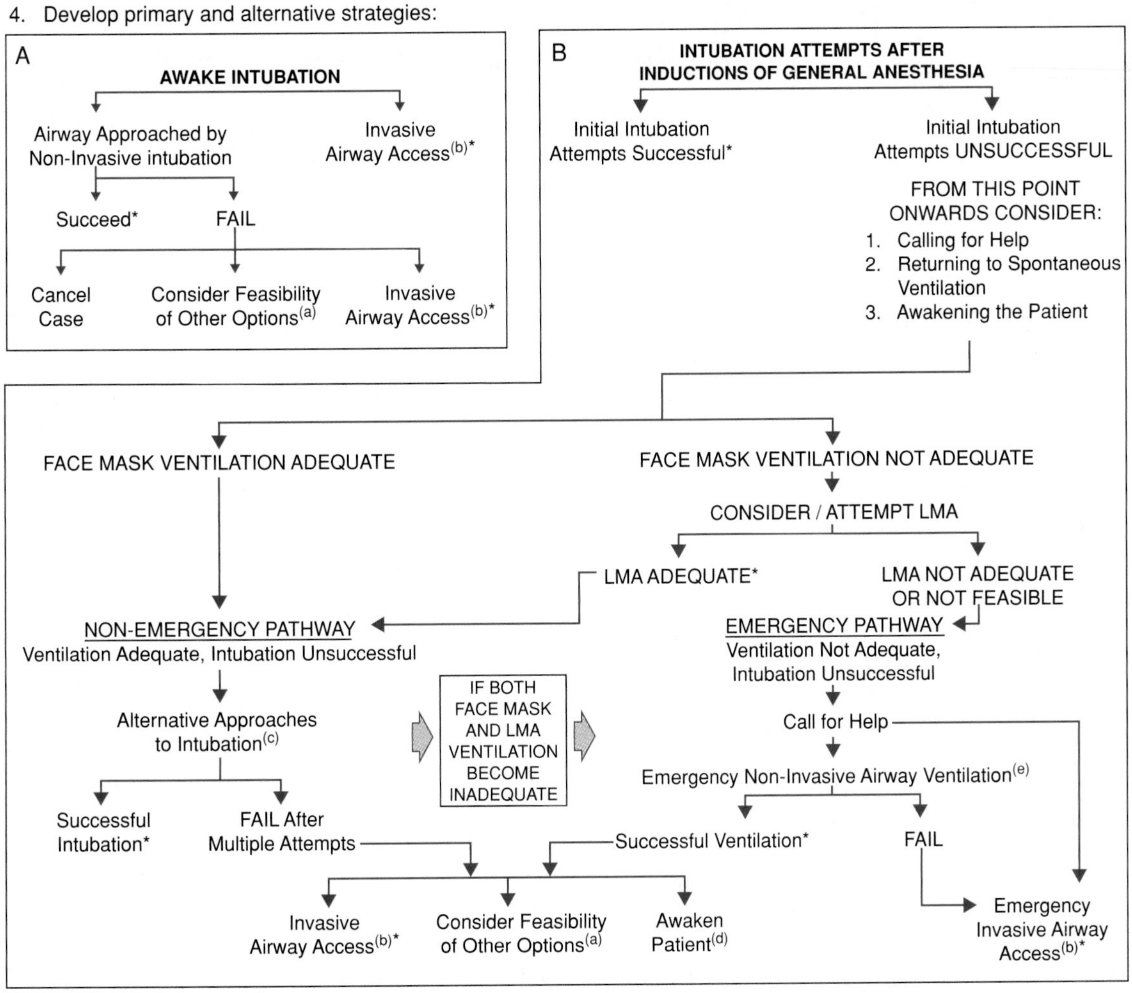

**A**
**AWAKE INTUBATION**

Airway Approached by Non-Invasive intubation | Invasive Airway Access[(b)]*

Succeed* | FAIL

Cancel Case | Consider Feasibility of Other Options[(a)] | Invasive Airway Access[(b)]*

**B**    **INTUBATION ATTEMPTS AFTER INDUCTIONS OF GENERAL ANESTHESIA**

Initial Intubation Attempts Successful* | Initial Intubation Attempts UNSUCCESSFUL

FROM THIS POINT ONWARDS CONSIDER:
1. Calling for Help
2. Returning to Spontaneous Ventilation
3. Awakening the Patient

FACE MASK VENTILATION ADEQUATE | FACE MASK VENTILATION NOT ADEQUATE

CONSIDER / ATTEMPT LMA

LMA ADEQUATE* | LMA NOT ADEQUATE OR NOT FEASIBLE

**NON-EMERGENCY PATHWAY**
Ventilation Adequate, Intubation Unsuccessful | **EMERGENCY PATHWAY**
Ventilation Not Adequate, Intubation Unsuccessful

Alternative Approaches to Intubation[(c)]

IF BOTH FACE MASK AND LMA VENTILATION BECOME INADEQUATE

Call for Help

Emergency Non-Invasive Airway Ventilation[(e)]

Successful Intubation* | FAIL After Multiple Attempts | Successful Ventilation* | FAIL

Invasive Airway Access[(b)]* | Consider Feasibility of Other Options[(a)] | Awaken Patient[(d)] | Emergency Invasive Airway Access[(b)]*

**\* Confirm ventilation, tracheal intubation, or LMA placement with exhaled Co₂**

a. Other options include (but are not limited to): surgery utilizing face mask or LMA anesthesia, local anesthesia infiltration or regional nerve blockade. Pursuit of these options usually implies that mask ventilation will not be problematic. Therefore, these options may be of limited value if this step in the algorithm has been reached via the Emergency Pathway.

b. Invasive airway access includes surgical or percutaneous tracheostomy or cricothyrotomy.

c. Alternative non-invasive approaches to difficult intubation include (but are not limited to): use of different laryngoscope blades, LMA as an intubation conduit (with or without fiberoptic guidance), fiberoptic intubation, intubating stylet or tube changer, light wand, retrograde intubation, and blind oral or nasal intubation.

d. Consider re-preparation of the patient for awake intubation or canceling surgery.

e. Options for emergency non-invasive airway ventilation include (but are not limited to): rigid bronchoscope, esophageal-tracheal combitube ventilation, or transtracheal jet ventilation.

**FIGURE 18-2.** The ASA Difficult Airway Algorithm.
*(Reproduced with permission American Society of Anesthesiologists. Practice guidelines for management of the difficult airway: An updated report. Anesthesiology 98:1269, 2003.)*

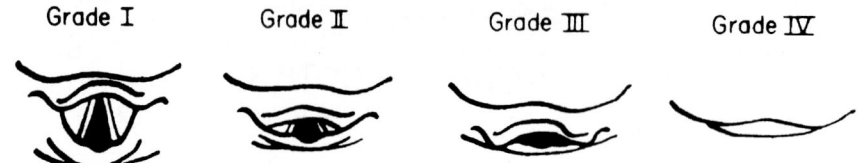

**FIGURE 18-3.** Classification of laryngoscopic views. Correct technique is assumed. The approximate frequencies follow the grade: grade I, 99%; grade II, 1%; grade III, 1 per 2000; grade IV, 1 per 1000. *(Reproduced with permission from Cormack RS, Lehane J. Difficult trachea intubation in obstetrics. Anaesthesia 39:1106, 1984.)*

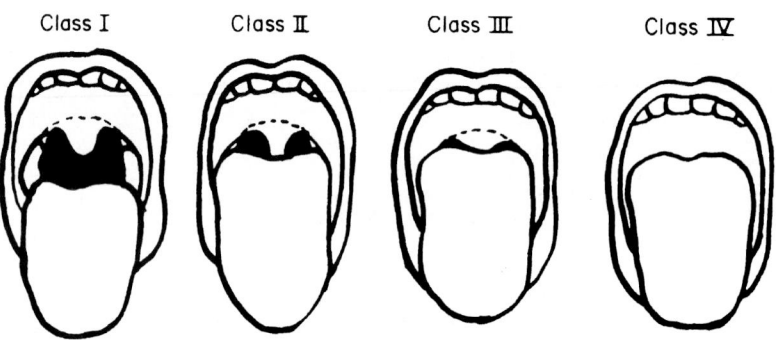

**FIGURE 18-4.** The "Mallampati classification" of the appearance of upper airway structures upon mouth opening. *(Reproduced with permission from Mallampati SR, Gugino LD, Desai SP, et al.: A clinical sign to predict difficult tracheal intubation: A prospective study. Can Anaesth Soc J 32:430, 1985.)*

pulmonary edema, primary reactive airway disease, etc. Because the patient is surgically draped, a rash may be missed. Dark urine may be myoglobinuria or due to a primary urinary tract injury. Tachycardia is nonspecific, and of course, the anesthetized patient cannot vocalize any complaints.

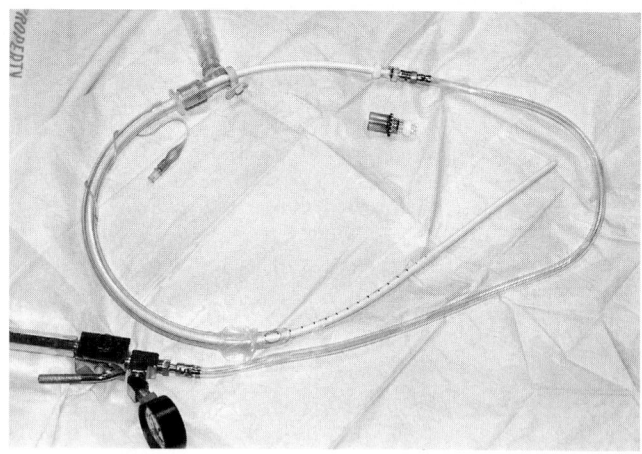

**FIGURE 18-5.** Demonstration of an assembly for jet ventilating through a tube changer. The endotracheal tube is connected to a ventilating circuit. The tube changer is threaded through a rubber adapter, which maintains ventilating circuit integrity. The tube changer is connected to a removable Luer-Lok adapter. A Sanders-type jet ventilator is shown connected via this adapter. The Sanders ventilator would be connected to a wall source of oxygen. The tube changer adapter can be quickly removed, allowing interchange of endotracheal tubes. If the act of tube changing proves difficult, the adapter can be reconnected and the patient temporarily jet ventilated. Also shown is a standard 15-mm adapter fitting for the tube changer, which can be connected to a manual resuscitating bag.

The most common medications used regularly by anesthesiologists that cause an allergic reaction are muscle relaxants, but one should also consider antibiotics administered (e.g., penicillin), as well as colloidal preparations (e.g., dextran), heparin, protamine, and ester-based local anesthetics (procaine, chlorporcaine, benzocaine, tetracaine.) Latex allergy has become increasingly recognized in the perioperative environment.[32] Finally, blood components, particularly packed red blood cells, may cause allergic reactions ranging from the mild to life-threatening. If a blood product is thought to be the cause, the unit responsible for the reaction (if it can be identified) should be returned to the lab, the patient should be retyped and cross-matched, and a blood sample should be sent for diagnostic screening.

Treatment of an allergic reaction includes removing the offending agent, decreasing the concentration of volatile anesthetics (while ensuring amnesia), epinephrine titrated intravenously to the severity of the hypotension, direct bronchodilators, and intravenous antihistamines and steroids. Volume expansion should be aggressive, and 100% oxygen administered.

## Monitoring

Publication of the Harvard Medical School standards for patient monitoring during anesthesia was a sentinel event in the establishment of guidelines for minimal mandatory monitoring in the operating room.[33] These standards were notable for being one of the initial attempts at standardization of care in medicine in general. Notable also was their acceptance; the community of anesthesiologists embraced the standards with little dissension at large. The standards are technically achievable and cost-effective (especially considering the expense of defending adverse outcomes). Eichorn reviewed catastrophic outcomes before and after institution of these standards at the component hospitals of the Harvard Department of Anesthesiology.[7] When reviewing the period before monitor standardization, he determined that 88% of major intraoperative events (death, permanent CNS injury, and cardiac arrest) could have been prevented if minimum monitoring standards had been in effect. No major preventable anesthetic-related injuries were found in over 319,000 anesthetics conducted after institution of the guidelines.

The Harvard standards were the basis for development of the ASA Standards for Basic Intraoperative Monitoring. The current standards mandate continuous presence of an anesthesiologist or anesthetist within the operating room as well as continuous evaluation of oxygenation, ventilation, circulation, and temperature.[34] Pulse oximetry is the standard for estimating patient oxygenation but it also necessary to monitor the delivered concentration of oxygen. Capnometry is clearly the superior means of monitoring ventilation but assessing exhaled volumes is also encouraged. Electrocardiography and blood pressure monitoring are the usual assessments of circulation, assisted by pulse oximetry. It is often unappreciated that electrocardiography may not detect coronary insufficiency if the leads are not placed accurately, particularly the V5 lead, and accurate placement of such leads may prove impossible secondary to the particular surgical needs of injured patients. It should be reinforced that these standards are *minimal* standards, and it is expected that such levels of monitoring will be routinely exceeded, predicated on patient and surgical factors. Invasive monitoring, such as intra-arterial, central venous, and pulmonary arterial catheterization, offer additional diagnostic information in the compromised patient and are regular features in the care of the injured patient (see Chap. 60). It should not go unmentioned that, despite great advances in monitoring technology, inspection of the patient continues to offer diagnostic clues to the astute clinician.

## Pulse Oximetry

Methods of measuring hemoglobin saturation have existed for decades but were bulky and difficult to use, making them impractical in the clinical setting.[35] A significant technical problem was separating the absorption of light by arterial blood from that of tissues, venous, and capillary blood. Rather ingeniously, an engineer discovered that the absorbance of light by arterial blood could be separated from that of other sources by measuring absorbance of the pulsatile component of the signal, thereby arriving at a means of estimating arterial hemoglobin saturation.

Contemporary pulse oximeters measure light absorbance at two wavelengths, visual red (660 nm) and infrared (940 nm). The ratios of pulsatile absorbances at the two wavelengths determine an "R" value. A certain "R" value correlates with an estimated value for hemoglobin saturation ($SpO_2$; Fig. 18-6).

Because pulse oximeters measure absorbance at only two wavelengths, an inaccurate estimate of hemoglobin occurs when more than two hemoglobin species are present. Ordinarily found in measurable concentrations are oxyhemoglobin ($HbO_2$) and reduced hemoglobin (RHB). However, when methemoglobin (MetHb) and carboxyhemoglobin (COHb) are present, spurious $SpO_2$ values may result, and if undiagnosed, may affect the patient adversely. To accurately measure four hemoglobin species, it is necessary to measure absorbance at four wavelengths of light. Co-oximeters have this capability and analysis by co-oximetry is necessary to measure the concentration of all these species simultaneously. Stan-

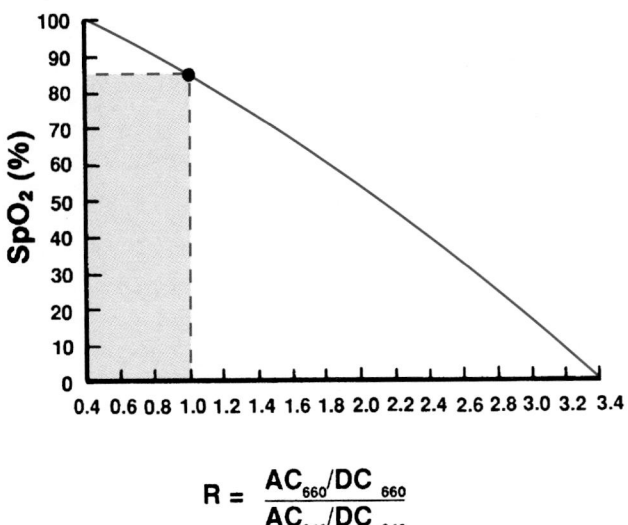

$$R = \frac{AC_{660}/DC_{660}}{AC_{940}/DC_{940}}$$

**FIGURE 18-6.** A typical oximetry calibration curve. Percent saturation estimated by pulse oximetry ($SpO_2$) is estimated by determining the ratio (R) of pulse added red absorbance at 660 nm to the pulse added infrared absorbance at 940 nm.
*(Reproduced with permission from Tremper KK, Barker SJ. Pulse oximetry. Anesthesiology 70:101, 1989. Adapted from JA Pologe. Pulse oximetry: Technical aspects of machine design. In Tremper KK, Barker SJ, eds. International Anesthesiology Clinics, Advances in Oxygen Monitoring. Boston: Little, Brown, 1987, p. 142.)*

dard clinical pulse oximetry will likely have four-wavelength capability in the future.

The impact of methemoglobin on pulse oximetry values occurs due to the coincidental relationship of methemoglobin's extinction coefficients. Extinction coefficients are physical constants of the species dependent only on the wavelength at which they are measured. At the two wavelengths pulse oximeters utilize, the coefficients for methemoglobin are nearly equal. The consequence of this, the "R" value approximates one, correlating with a pulse oximetry value of 85%. Clinically, patients developing methemoglobinemia experience declining pulse oximetry values that level off in the mid-80s. However, it should be noted that true hemoglobin saturation continues to decline (Fig. 18-7).[36] Methemoglobinemia should be considered any time hemoglobin saturation, as estimated by pulse oximetry, correlates poorly with saturation as measured by blood gas analysis. Polymerized hemoglobin red blood cell substitutes contain sufficient methemoglobin to render pulse oximetry inaccurate.[37]

Carbon monoxide binds avidly to hemoglobin, preventing oxygen loading. However, its effect on pulse oximetry is less significant than methemoglobin and its detection requires clinical suspicion prompting blood gas analysis by co-oximetry.

Limitations of pulse oximetry measurement include degradation of signal measurement by ambient light and low signal to noise ratios due to a weak pulse or patient movement. The accuracy of pulse oximeters is +/−2% between 100 and 70% saturation and +/−3% between 70 and 50% saturation. Finally, it is important to remember what pulse oximetry does not measure. Pulse oximetry does not measure oxygen transport or delivery, and does not measure distal perfusion. An anemic patient may have 100% hemoglobin saturation yet have inadequate oxygen to

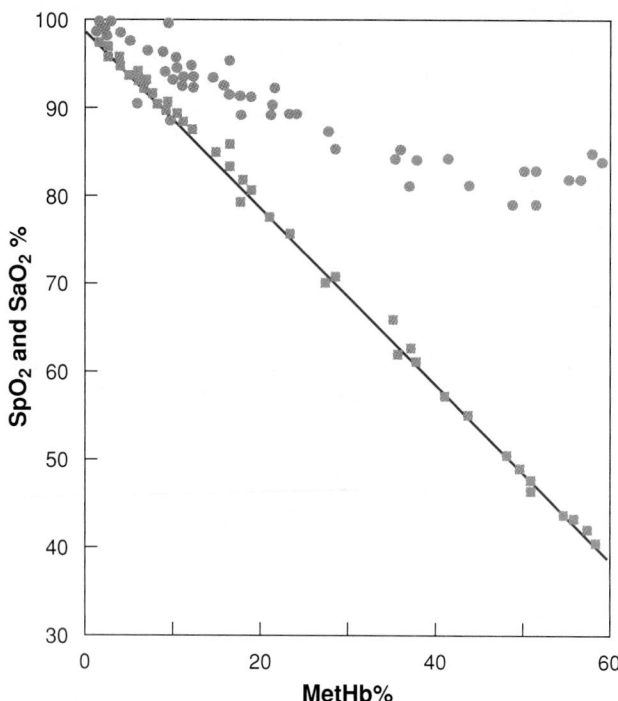

**FIGURE 18-7.** Comparison of pulse oximetry saturation (SpO$_2$—circles) and arterial saturation (SaO$_2$—squares) as methemoglobin (MetHb) concentration increases. Note the SpO$_2$ value levels off in the mid-80s while arterial oxygen saturation continues to decrease as MetHb concentration increases.
*(Reproduced with permission from Barker SJ, Tremper K, Hyatt J. Effects of methemoglobinemia on pulse oximetry and mixed venous oximetry. Anesthesiology 70:113, 1989.)*

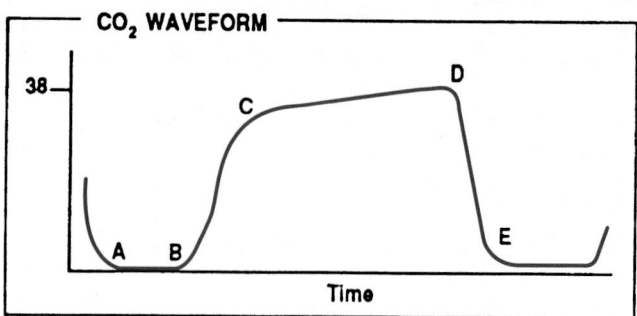

**FIGURE 18-8.** The capnographic waveform. A–B: exhalation of CO$_2$ free gas from dead space; B–C: combination of dead space and alveolar gas; C–D: exhalation of mostly alveolar gas; D: "end-tidal" point (alveolar plateau); D–E: inhalation of CO$_2$ free gas.
*(Reproduced with permission from Advanced Concepts in Capnography. Pleasanton, CA: Nellcor Puritan Bennett, 1988.)*

meet metabolic needs. Furthermore, it will not detect deterioration in oxygenation until arterial partial pressures of oxygen fall below 75 to 80 mm Hg—the point where hemoglobin saturations fall below 100%.

## Capnography

End-tidal CO$_2$ monitoring has been an important factor in reducing anesthesia-related adverse outcomes.[8] Carbon dioxide monitoring is considered the best method of easily verifying correct ETT placement. Capnometers or colorimetric CO$_2$ detectors (Easy Cap II, Nellcor Puritan Bennett, Pleasanton, CA) should be regularly used to establish correct endotracheal intubation. End-tidal CO$_2$ levels have been used to predict outcome of resuscitation.[38]

Within the operating room the rise and fall of expired CO$_2$ is monitored over time (capnography). The important features of the capnographic waveform include contour, baseline level, and rate of rise of CO$_2$. There are four distinct phases (Fig. 18-8). The first phase (A–B) is the initial stage of exhalation, where the gas sampled is dead space gas, free of CO$_2$. At point B, there is mixing of alveolar gas with dead space gas and the CO$_2$ level abruptly rises. The expiratory or alveolar plateau is represented by phase C–D, and the gas sampled is essentially alveolar. Point D is the maximal CO$_2$ level, the best reflection of alveolar CO$_2$, and is known as end-tidal CO$_2$ (ETCO$_2$). Fresh gas is entrained as the patient inspires (phase D–E), and the trace returns to the baseline level of CO$_2$, approximately 0.

Alveolar and arterial carbon dioxide partial pressures (PaCO$_2$) normally differ by only 2 to 3 mm Hg, assuming ventilation and perfusion are matched and there is complete alveolar emptying. However, should there be a maldistribution between ventilation and perfusion, the correlation between ETCO$_2$ and PaCO$_2$ decreases, with ETCO$_2$ being lower. Increased dead space results in an increased gradient; is common in trauma patients; and may be due to shock, air- or thromboembolism, cardiac arrest, chronic lung disease, or lateral decubitus positioning. Shunt has little effect on arterial–alveolar CO$_2$ gradients.

Exponential decreases in CO$_2$ waveforms are significant events, often associated with sudden blood loss or other causes of hypotension. Low cardiac output states, cardiac arrest, or pulmonary embolism may produce this pattern. Gradual decreases in ETCO$_2$ may reflect hypothermia, hypovolemia, decreasing cardiac output, or decreased metabolic activity (e.g., after neuromuscular blockade). A sustained but constant decrease in ETCO$_2$ may be due to hyperventilation or increases in dead space ventilation.

ETCO$_2$ values may rise gradually secondary to hypoventilation, increasing body temperature, increased metabolic activity (e.g., fever, sepsis, and malignant hyperthermia), or exogenous CO$_2$ absorption (laparoscopy). Transient increases in ETCO$_2$ may be noted after intravenous bicarbonate administration, release of extremity tourniquets, or removal of vascular cross-clamps. Obstructive lung disease results in a gradually up-sloping phase B–C.

## Airway Pressure Monitoring

Increasing airway pressures may be related to the anesthesia machine, the anesthesia circuit, the endotracheal tube, or changes within the patient. There may be malfunctions within the anesthesia ventilatory circuit, such as kinks or valve malfunction, or the endotracheal tube may be kinked, obstructed, or has migrated into a main stem bronchus. Patient related events (e.g., abdominal compartment syndrome) may suggest that a change in management is required or that a critical event (such as a tension pneumothorax, bronchospasm, mucus plugging, and the like) is occurring. In regards to patient-related events, it is often valuable to evaluate increasing airway pressures within the context of the changes in capnographic waveforms.

## Intra-arterial Monitoring

Intra-arterial blood pressure monitoring is indicated when blood pressure changes may be rapid and when serial blood analysis is needed, or when noninvasive measurements are inaccurate. Most commonly, the radial artery is cannulated at the wrist, but alternative sites include the ulnar, brachial, axillary, femoral, and dorsal pedal arteries, and preference for these alternative sites are dependent on institutional practices.

Arterial waveforms may be subject to misinterpretation. Arterial monitoring systems (transducer and fluid-filled tubing) may be underdamped, resulting in overestimation of the systolic and underestimation of the diastolic blood pressure. Alternatively, an overdamped system underestimates the systolic and overestimates the diastolic blood pressure. Such artifacts and patently inaccurate values are reduced by use of rigid connecting tubing no more than 120 cm in length, assuring that the tubing is free of kinks, clots, and bubbles, maintaining only one stopcock in the system, maintaining patency through flushing the system, accurate placement of the transducer at the level of the right atrium, and periodic calibration ("zeroing") of the transducer system.

Complications of arterial cannulation include distal ischemia, arterial thrombosis, hematoma formation, catheter site infection, systemic infection, necrosis of the overlying skin, and potential blood loss due to disconnection. The incidence of infection increases with duration of catheterization. The risk of arterial thrombosis increases with duration of catheterization, prolonged shock, and pre-existing peripheral vascular disease.

## Bispectral Index Monitoring

Though intraoperative awareness is estimated to occur in roughly 0.5% of general surgical populations, recall after surgery for major trauma is probably greater. Bogetz and Katz found 11% of trauma patients who received anesthesia intraoperatively and 43% of all patients too unstable to receive anesthesia (at least for a portion of the procedure) experienced intraoperative awareness.[39] Lubke et al. found remarkably different results. In 1999 they reported that none of the 96 patients undergoing surgery for acute trauma experienced recall.[40] Perhaps this difference is explained by improvements in resuscitation. Clearly, low doses of anesthetics are the most frequent cause of awareness.[14] Patient movement does not correlate with awareness, as movement under anesthesia is a spinal-cord-mediated event.[41] Vital signs are poor monitors of awareness.[14] Events known to decrease anesthetic requirements (hypotension, hypothermia, and acute alcohol intoxication) do not decrease the likelihood of awareness. Intraoperative awareness has many manifestations. Possibly the worse is pain, but the sensation of paralysis and auditory stimulation are also encountered and disagreeable. Patients having experienced intraoperative awareness describe this as their worst hospital experience and frequently go on to develop posttraumatic stress disorders.

Intraoperative analysis of raw electroencephalographic (EEG) signals is too difficult to be useful. However, computer processing of certain components of EEG signals (using a mathematical technique called *bispectral analysis,* or *BIS*) has permitted development of a clinically useful monitor of anesthetic effect.[42] BIS monitors (Aspect Medical Systems, Natick, MA) translate EEG signals into dimensionless numbers from 0 to 100, with 0 representing no brain activity and 100 being the awake state. Values less than 40 represent a deep hypnotic state such as may be associated with barbiturate coma. Values between 40 and 60 correlate with unconsciousness and are the target values while under general anesthesia. Light hypnosis is associated with values between 60 and 70, and the probability of recall is small. As patients rise above 70, awareness cannot be ruled out.

During routine anesthesia care, use of BIS technology regularly allows downward titration of anesthetic agents, saving drug costs, and facilitating rapid emergence from anesthesia. Practically speaking, using this technology during the resuscitation of the seriously injured patient may be difficult as the time for correct placement of the monitoring electrodes takes one away from other urgent matters. Additionally, in the current environment it is most unusual for such a patient not to receive some amnestic agent, such as scopolamine or a benzodiazepine. However, BIS technology is being used to monitor depth of sedation within the ICU.[43]

## Temperature Monitoring

Hypothermia is common in the trauma population. The etiologies and physiologic consequences of hypothermia are well reviewed elsewhere (see Chap. 51). A few points relative to thermoregulation in the anesthetic state and intraoperative warming are appropriate.[44]

There are three phases of thermoregulation: afferent sensing, central thermoregulatory integration, and efferent response. Within a narrow range of temperatures (the interthreshold range), no efferent response is triggered by hypothalamic thermoregulatory centers. Above and below certain thresholds, efferent mechanisms activate in an attempt to, respectively, decrease or increase body temperature. Warm responses include active vasodilation and sweating; cold responses include vasoconstriction, nonshivering thermogenesis (found in infants), and shivering. General anesthesia widens the interthreshold range, and body temperature passively changes with existing temperature gradients. The thermoregulatory response is markedly less robust under general anesthesia, and shivering is unavailable as a compensatory mechanism (Fig. 18-9). The vasodilatory effects of volatile anesthetics, increasing heat loss, attenuate vasoconstriction.

Perioperative heat loss is caused by four mechanisms: conduction, convection, radiation, and evaporation. The degree of conductive loss is determined by temperature differences between the patient and adjacent surfaces; unwarmed intravenous fluids and blood products and cold surgical preparation solutions increase conductive loss. Temperature loss to adjacent air is convective in nature and increased by frequent turnover of air within the operating room. Radiant losses are significant when gowned surgeons require a cool room to remain comfortable. Evaporative heat losses occur with the exposure of viscera during surgery.

Strategies for minimizing hypothermia include decreasing cutaneous heat loss by increasing the ambient temperature of the room and limiting further heat loss by use of blankets, plastic bags for wrapping the extremities and head, and active warming devices. Forced air warming devices are especially beneficial and superior to circulating water blankets.[45] Warming of lower extremities during vascular clamping may predispose the patient to thermal injury and should be avoided in this instance. Warm-

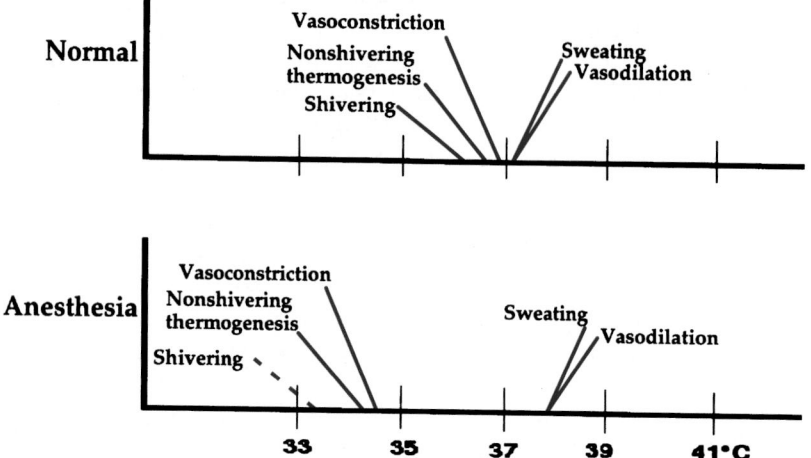

**FIGURE 18-9.** Thresholds for common thermoregulatory responses in awake and anesthetized humans. *(Reproduced with permission from Sessler DI. Monitoring body temperature. In Saidman LJ, Smith NT, eds. Monitoring in Anesthesia, 3rd ed. Boston: Butterworth-Heinemann, 1993, p. 317. Modified from Sessler DI. Temperature Monitoring, in Miller RD, ed. Anesthesia, 3rd ed. New York: Churchill Livingstone, 1990, p. 1217.)*

ing of all intravenous fluids and blood products is essential to avoid further heat loss. Each liter of fluid infused at ambient temperature and each unit of blood transfused at 4°C (39.2°F) decreases body temperature by approximately 0.25°C (0.45°F).[44] Heating of cold, dry gases offers little, as the heat content of gases is very small. Passive humidification via moisture-exchanging filters ("artificial nose") is useful in preventing exposure to cold, dry gases and maintaining normal airway cilial function, though temperature gain is unimpressive. The use of active rewarming is discussed in Chap. 51.

## Monitoring Coagulation

Thromboelastography (TEG) is a near-site monitor of hemostasis. It differs from other tests of coagulation (platelet count, prothrombin time, partial thromboplastin time, fibrinogen levels, and fibrin split products), which measure specific hemostatic lesions, in that it is an integrated in vivo assessment of whole blood coagulation, interaction of the separate coagulation components, and hemostasis overall. TEG results are also responsive to the influence of hypothermia, a common occurrence in massive resuscitation. Given the complex physiologic phenomenon associated with major resuscitative efforts, an integrated measurement of coagulation has benefits.[46,47] Technical aspects and interpretation are discussed further in Chap. 61

## Anesthetic Choices: Advantages and Disadvantages

An anesthetic should be appropriate to the planned procedure and the condition of the patient. Choices include monitored anesthesia care (MAC), regional anesthesia (spinal and epidural anesthesia or sometimes peripheral nerve block), and general anesthesia. During MAC, sedation accompanies peripheral nerve block or local anesthetic infiltration of the surgical site, and suffices only for minor procedures. Recommended local anesthetic doses for infiltration are found in Table 18-3. Regional anesthesia may be appropriate for isolated extremity trauma unless hypovolemia is a consideration. Most assuredly, general anesthesia will be the technique of choice for the majority of injured patients. The following discussion will review advantages and disadvantages of regional and general anesthesia within the context of the injured patient.

To perform spinal or epidural anesthesia, local anesthetic is instilled into the neuraxis, impairing neural conduction. Sympathetic, pain, and motor fibers are blocked in that order, as this is roughly the sequence from small to large nerve fibers, though there is some overlap. Opioids are often administered coincident with the local anesthetic and modulate transmission of painful impulses at the spinal cord level.

Advantages of neuraxial anesthetic techniques include avoiding airway manipulation and intubation, reducing the risk of pulmonary aspiration, and reducing the number of medications administered intraoperatively (anesthetic induction, neuromuscular blockade, and reversal of blockade are avoided). Additionally, mental status can be followed and the physiologic stress response is lessened (Table 18-4). There may be decreased intraoperative blood loss, hastened recovery of bowel function, improved blood flow to extremities, and decreased incidence of deep venous thrombosis (notably in hip fractures).[48] Epidural catheters left in situ postoperatively may be used for postoperative analgesia. Thoracic epidural analgesia is regularly instituted in patients with rib frac-

**TABLE 18-3**

| Maximal Recommended and Typical Doses for Local Anesthetics for Infiltration | | | | | |
|---|---|---|---|---|---|
| | **PLAIN SOLUTION** | | | **EPINEPHRINE-CONTAINING SOLUTION**[a] | |
| **DRUG** | **Concentration (%)** | **Max Dose (mg)** | **Duration (min)** | **Max Dose (mg)** | **Duration (min)** |
| Bupivacaine | 0.25–0.5 | 175 | 120–240 | 225 | 180–420 |
| Chloroprocaine | 1–2 | 800 | 15–30 | 1000 | 30–90 |
| Lidocaine | 0.5–1.0 | 300 | 30–60 | 500 | 120–360 |
| Mepivacaine | 0.5–1.0 | 300 | 45–90 | 500 | 120–360 |

[a]Suggested epinephrine concentration is 1:200,000 (5 μg/mL).

**TABLE 18-4**

**The Advantages and Disadvantages of Regional Anesthesia in the Injured Patient**

**ADVANTAGES OF REGIONAL ANESTHESIA**

Attenuates stress response
Avoids "cannot ventilate, cannot intubate" scenario
Decreased deep venous thrombosis
Decreases intraoperative blood loss in orthopedic trauma
Improved outcome with microvascular surgery
Improves extremity blood flow
May facilitate postoperative pain management
Mental status can be continuously evaluated
Rapid recovery of bowel function
Reduces the risk of pulmonary aspiration

**DISADVANTAGES OF REGIONAL ANESTHESIA**

Cannot address impaired oxygenation and ventilation
Epidural hematoma or abscess
Lose pain as a monitor of evolving injuries
Needle trauma to nerves
Risks of the procedure
Sympathectomy poorly tolerated in hypovolemic patients
Time-consuming
Toxic local anesthetic reaction

tures (see Chap. 26) and has been shown to improve ventilatory function, decrease intubation and mechanical ventilation, and reduce the incidence of pneumonia as well as the duration of ICU stays.[49,50]

A major disadvantage of neuraxial anesthesia is hypotension due to sympathetic blockade, particularly if the patient is hypovolemic. It is always prudent to administer a fluid challenge before performing spinal or epidural anesthesia and avoid the technique when volume status is uncertain. If local anesthetics are inadvertently injected into the circulation, seizures and cardiovascular collapse are a risk. Side effects of epidural infusions include motor blockade, nausea, vomiting, and pruritis. Urinary retention is common, and urinary catheters are usually indicated. Performing regional anesthesia is more time-consuming than initiating general anesthesia, but some time may be made up at case conclusion because anesthetic emergence and extubation are obviated. Anyone requiring physiologic support is not a candidate for regional anesthesia.

A risk when instrumenting the neuraxis is epidural hematoma. Coagulation status should always be assessed prior to considering these procedures. Coagulation disturbances and anticoagulant medications render a patient at risk for this complication and may contraindicate neuraxial techniques. Thrombocytopenia and loss of clotting factors are regular occurrences in the multiply injured patient (see Chap. 61). Additionally, many patients receive low-molecular-weight heparin (LMWH) to prevent deep venous thrombosis. The decision to instrument the neuraxis while on LMWH is complicated. It is believed that twice daily dosing of LMHW contraindicates this procedure. If the patient is on LMWH and antiplatelet drugs, the procedure is likewise contraindicated. In a multiply injured patient, once a day dosing of LMWH and performing neuraxial instrumentation may be safe, though in this setting the risks versus benefits becomes an important consideration.[51,52]

Peripheral nerve blocks can also provide isolated regional anesthesia. They avoid general anesthesia and the sympathectomy of neuraxial techniques, and if catheters are inserted into anatomic sheaths surrounding these nerves (rather than one shot dosing), many days of analgesia may be afforded postoperatively. This may be particularly important for limb reattachments.[53] Disadvantages include confounding subsequent physical exams of that extremity, time required initiating the blocks, and significant failure rate. A thorough knowledge of regional anatomy and regular practice is required for consistent success.

Neuraxial anesthesia and peripheral nerve blocks may mask pain as an important sign for compartment syndromes. While not representing a contraindication, the clinician should be attuned to other symptoms of increasing compartment pressures, including swelling, loss of pulses, etc.

General anesthesia with endotracheal intubation will be the anesthetic course for most injured patients, certainly any undergoing surgery on a body cavity. General anesthesia is appropriate and indicated for any patient undergoing significant fluid resuscitation, requiring hyperventilation or mechanical ventilation for any reason, in the obtunded patient, and in anyone at risk for aspiration or experiencing significant metabolic abnormalities. As opposed to regional anesthesia, general anesthesia can be titrated to the severity of the surgical stimulus. Oxygen may be delivered in high concentration and positive end-expiratory pressure (PEEP) administered. Muscle relaxants may improve operating conditions.

Disadvantages include the necessity to intubate a patient with a potential cervical spine injury. In any patient with an uncleared cervical spine, precautions must be taken to prevent excessive neck motion. The CVCI scenario is a risk, as is pulmonary aspiration. Finally, mental status cannot be followed, and many patients with closed-head injuries will require intraoperative intracranial pressure (ICP) monitoring.

Whether one anesthetic technique is superior to another has been long debated, but in general it appears that there is little difference between well-conducted techniques. The decrease in postoperative deep venous thrombosis thought attributable to epidural analgesia may now be effectively managed with thromboprophylaxis. However there are fewer pulmonary complications if intubation can be avoided, and orthopedic rehabilitation may be improved with the use of regional techniques. But it does appear clear that postoperative pain is a major complication and may slow recovery; hence, effective, multimodal postoperative analgesia is recommended.[54]

## Anesthetic Agents

The anesthetic armamentarium useful in the care of injured patients includes intravenous hypnotics and amnestics, inhalational agents, opioid analgesics, and muscle relaxants. Injudicious use of any of these agents in the trauma victim may result in disastrous respiratory or cardiovascular complications. All anesthetic agents have significant hemodynamic impact, and their therapeutic indices are generally much lower in the trauma patient. Anesthetic induction agents available include etomidate, thiopental, propofol, ketamine, and midazolam, though all may not be appropriate in the hypovolemic patient, at least in usually recommended doses. Amnestic agents include the benzodiazepines

**TABLE 18-5**

### Cardiovascular Effects of Induction Agents

| AGENT | MAP | HR | SVR | CO | CONTRACTILITY | VENODILATION |
|---|---|---|---|---|---|---|
| Etomidate | 0 | 0 | 0 | 0 | 0 | 0 |
| Ketamine[a] | ++ | ++ | + | + | + or − | 0 |
| Midazolam | 0 to − | 0 to + | 0 to − | 0 to − | − | + |
| Propofol | − | + | − | 0 to − | − | + |
| Thiopental | − | + | 0 to − | − | − | + |

CO, cardiac output; HR, heart rate; MAP, mean arterial pressure; SVR, systemic vascular resistance; (+) increases; (0) no effect: (−) decreases.
[a]Ketamine's effect depends on patient's catecholamine levels.

and scopolamine. Opioid analgesics include morphine, hydromorphone, fentanyl and its congeners, sufentanil, alfentanil, and remifentanil. Inhalational agents for maintenance of general anesthesia include isoflurane, desflurane, sevoflurane, and nitrous oxide.

Etomidate is a cardiostable induction agent, having little effect on cardiac contractility or sympathetic function. Hence, etomidate is useful for anesthetic induction of the hemodynamically unstable trauma patient. Hypotension may still occur in the severely hypovolemic patient, so this medication, as all induction agents, should be titrated to effect. Etomidate may be of use in the head-injured patient, for it significantly reduces cerebral blood flow, cerebral oxygen consumption, and ICP while maintaining cerebral perfusion pressure (CPP). A notable side effect is transient inhibition (6 to 8 h) of steroidogenesis. Single bolus administration does not raise concerns for adrenal depression.[55] The cardiovascular effects of induction agents are reviewed in Table 18-5.

Thiopental has long been used for anesthetic induction because of its rapid, reliable hypnotic effect. However, thiopental is a potent cardiovascular depressant due to its negative inotropic effect, impairment of sympathetic activity, and increase in venous capacitance. Some degree of hypotension is seen even in healthy euvolemic patients after standard dosing. These effects are certainly magnified in the hypovolemic trauma victim and severe, refractory hypotension may occur if dosage is not properly adjusted. Pentothal decreases cerebral oxygen consumption and ICP but also decreases CPP. Few would consider it first-line treatment in the injured patient.

Propofol is an intravenous sedative–hypnotic agent used for anesthetic induction in bolus form and maintenance of anesthesia when infused continuously, but its utility in acute injury is limited by cardiovascular depression.[56]

Recently, short-term sedative infusions of large-dose propofol have been noted to result in lactic acidosis, and increases in serum creatinine and rhabdomyolysis that tends to be reversible after discontinuation of the infusion, though deaths have been noted. This entity has been denoted the propofol infusion syndrome (PRIS). Propofol infusions should be considered in the differential diagnosis of refractory lactic acidosis with renal impairment and increasing creatinine kinase.[57]

Ketamine is a rapid-acting IV anesthetic agent that produces a functional and electrophysiologic dissociation between the cortex and limbic system, producing analgesia and in larger doses, unconsciousness.[56] A state of catalepsy is attained where the eyes remain open in a slow, nystagmic gaze, yet intense analgesia and amnesia

is produced. Varying degrees of hypertonus and purposeful movements may be noted. Ketamine's sympathomimetic effects support blood pressure and heart rate, making it a desirable induction agent in trauma, but it also has direct myocardial depressant effects, and cardiovascular depression may occur in catecholamine-depleted patients. Other side effects include increased ICP and cerebral blood flow, contraindicating its use in head-injured patients. Ketamine increases myocardial oxygen demand, produces copious airway secretions, and may be associated with emergence delirium, usually in adults.

Benzodiazepines produce anxiolysis and amnesia and though rarely used as such in trauma patients, may induce anesthesia in high doses. Benzodiazepines in and of themselves are cardiostable and maintain respirations, though this is dose-dependent. However, they may act synergistically with opioids or volatile anesthetics, resulting in hypotension and apnea. Midazolam, diazepam, and lorazepam are available as IV preparations, but midazolam is popular in the operating room as it is nonirritating on injection.[58] Midazolam has a short elimination half-life when given in bolus form, but its effect may be prolonged when administered by continuous infusion.[59] Midazolam is useful for awake intubations. If necessary, benzodiazepine effect may be reversed by the competitive antagonist flumazenil. Profoundly hypovolemic trauma patients are sometimes administered scopolamine to minimize recall, though this may be less reliable than benzodiazepines.

Commonly used opioids within the operating room include morphine, hydromorphone, fentanyl, and its congeners, sufentanil, alfentanil, and remifentanil. There are numerous opioid receptors but the principal analgesic receptor is the mu receptor. Supraspinal opioid receptors have also been identified but their role in analgesia appears to be complex and is as yet ill defined. Clearly, the principal analgesic action takes place within the spinal cord. The substantia gelatinosa is dense with opioid receptors and application of opioids to this area produces dense analgesia. Opioids fundamentally modify and inhibit nociceptive signals from peripheral nerves by inhibiting release of the mediator of pain, substance P, as well as acting as neurotransmitters themselves.

Opioids in and of themselves are cardiostable agents, though factors such as volume status, associated medications, and ventricular function may modify cardiostability. The more agents administered, the more likely such stability will be lost. They reduce the magnitude of surgery-induced stress response. Opioids are respiratory depressants, decreasing both the hypercarbic and hypoxic drive to breathe. They decrease gastrointestinal motility and are legendary for promoting nausea and vomiting.

Morphine and fentanyl are regularly administered with local anesthetics during neuraxial techniques. Morphine, hydromorphone, and fentanyl are used postoperatively with patient-controlled analgesia. Alfentanil and remifentanil are notable as their rapid onset of action may be used to blunt brief but highly stimulating noxious stimuli. Remifentanil is unique amongst opioids as it undergoes ester hydrolysis within blood and tissue, rather than hepatic metabolism characterized by other opioids. It is the first "ultrashort-" acting opioid and is administered by infusion. As its effect terminates precipitously, the clinician must provide other means of analgesia whenever postprocedural pain is anticipated.[60]

Opioids should not be spared in acute settings out of concern for promoting dependency. To the contrary, good pain control returns individuals to a functional status more rapidly. Lack of adequate analgesia promotes a maladaptive stress response, results in sympathetic stimulation resulting in hypertension and tachycardia, delays ambulation, may increase the incidence of chronic pain syndromes, and does not support positive patient–physician interactions. Similarly, adequate analgesia should not be denied to substance-abusing individuals.

Opioids have pharmacologic antagonists, the most frequently used being naloxone, a pure mu-receptor antagonist. Respiratory depression may be reversed but analgesia dissipates as well. Injudicious use may result in sympathetic storm, pulmonary edema, and an out-of-control patient. Under some circumstances it may be prudent to support ventilations rather than reverse opioid effect. At any rate, naloxone should be slowly titrated to effect.

The most common inhaled halogenated anesthetics include isoflurane, desflurane, and sevoflurane. These agents are titratable and produce unconsciousness, amnesia, analgesia, and a degree of muscle relaxation. Though their mechanism of action is incompletely understood, volatile anesthetics impair ion transport in CNS tissues through lipid membrane interactions. They are all vasodilators and have cardiac depressant effects in larger doses. They increase cerebral blood flow while decreasing cerebral oxygen consumption. Desflurane is the most insoluble; its effects diminish rapidly upon discontinuance. Isoflurane and desflurane are metabolized to only a small degree and are principally eliminated by the lungs. When sevoflurane is metabolized, fluoride (a potential nephrotoxin) is produced.[61] But due to its extreme insolubility, it is rapidly excreted from the lungs, metabolism is minimal, and serum fluoride levels rapidly diminish. Postoperative renal dysfunction has not been a problem.

Nitrous oxide is a potent analgesic but insufficiently potent to induce unconsciousness when used as a sole agent. It is insoluble like desflurane, but because it is administered in high concentration (50 to 60%), it achieves higher serum levels. It is contraindicated in the trauma patient because, due to its insolubility, it will diffuse into air-filled spaces, such as an untreated pneumothorax or pneumocephalus, and will expand an air embolus.[62,63]

## Neuromuscular Blocking Agents

Neuromuscular blockers (NMBs) relax skeletal muscle, facilitating endotracheal intubation, mechanical ventilation, and surgical exposure. Understanding the action of NMBs requires an appreciation of normal neuromuscular transmission. The neuromuscular junction (NMJ) is the synapse found between neuron and muscle. An action potential propagating down a neuron will initiate release of acetylcholine from the distal neuron. Acetylcholine diffuses across the synapse and binds to its receptor on the muscle membrane, resulting in depolarization. A muscle action potential is produced when sufficient acetylcholine receptors are bound and depolarization spreads across the full length of the muscle membrane, resulting in actin-myosin interaction and muscular contraction.

NMBs can be classified as depolarizing or nondepolarizing, depending on their effect at the NMJ. The only depolarizing agent available is succinylcholine (Sch), an agonist at the NMJ. The initial binding of Sch produces random and disorganized muscular contraction, known as fasciculations. Sch is not metabolized within the synaptic area and must diffuse away to be metabolized, explaining its duration of effect.

Due to its rapid onset of action (approximately 45 seconds) and short duration of action (5 to 8 minutes), Sch is primarily used to facilitate tracheal intubation under emergent circumstances (see Chap. 12). When used in conjunction with induction agents, this process of rapidly securing the airway is known as "rapid sequence induction." This technique is regularly performed in trauma patients to minimize the risk of pulmonary aspiration of gastric contents. Table 18-6 suggests doses of commonly used relaxants to facilitate endotracheal intubation.

There are numerous risks inherent in the administration of Sch. Anoxic injury and death may occur if the patient cannot be ventilated or intubated. Succinylcholine may cause arrhythmias, rhabdomyolysis, and masseter muscle spasm (complicating attempts at intubation); it is a trigger for malignant hyperthermia in susceptible individuals and may increase intracranial and intraocular pressure. Though Sch normally causes an insignificant, transient rise in the serum potassium levels (0.5 to 1.0 mEq/L), patients having sustained major trauma, burns, spinal cord injuries, or major crush injuries are susceptible to profound potassium efflux from skeletal muscle.[64] These patients have upregulated acetylcholine receptors, which are responsible for the exaggerated hyperkalemic response, and cardiac arrest is a risk after Sch administration.[65]

Nondepolarizing relaxants are true competitive antagonists, and the degree of neuromuscular blockade achieved is a balance between the amount of acetylcholine and nondepolarizing relaxant available at the NMJ. Small amounts of NMB may be found at the NMJ, yet no deficits in transmission are detected because the number of available junctional receptors far exceeds the number needed to produce the excitation–contraction response, demonstrating the tremendous reserve in neuromuscular transmission.

The nondepolarizing agents are divided into two groups based on chemical structure: the aminosteroid compounds (vecuronium, rocuronium, and pancuronium), and the benzylisoquinoline group

## TABLE 18-6

### Suggested Doses of Muscle Relaxants for Rapid Intubation

| DRUG | INTUBATING Dose (mg/kg) | INTUBATION Time (sec) | FULL Recovery[a] (min) |
|---|---|---|---|
| Atracurium | 0.6–0.8 | 90 | 60–90 |
| Mivacurium | 0.16–0.3 | 90 | 40–60 |
| Pancuronium | 0.15–0.2 | 90 | 210–270 |
| Rocuronium | 0.9–01.2 | 60 | 60–160 |
| Succinylcholine | 0.7–1.5 | 60 | 12–15 |
| Vecuronium | 0.07–0.15 | 90 | 75–120 |

[a]Full recovery is considered return of twitch height of 95% of control.

(atracurium, cisatracurium, and mivacurium). These agents are also classified by their duration of action.

Rapid-onset, short-acting, nondepolarizing NMBs may be used in lieu of Sch as long as the airway is believed to be manageable. Mivacurium has a relatively short duration of action. When administered in a dose sufficient to result in total paralysis within 2 minutes, essentially complete return of motor function can be expected in 20 to 25 minutes due to its rapid hydrolysis by plasma cholinesterase.[66] Rocuronium has also been used effectively in place of Sch. However, when administered in doses to achieve rapid onset, recovery takes about 35 minutes, considered intermediate in duration. Vecuronium and the atracurium compounds are of intermediate duration, workhorses within the operating room, and are administered as infusions in the ICU. Pancuronium is a long-acting muscle relaxant.

Cardiovascular stability can be a concern for the nondepolarizing NMBs. Many in the benzylisoquinoline group produce histamine release with associated bronchospasm and hypotension, especially if administered rapidly or in large doses. Pancuronium produces vagolysis, resulting in tachycardia, though the impact on already tachycardic trauma patients appears minimal. With the exception of the atracurium compounds, which break down spontaneously, the effect of nondepolarizing relaxants may be prolonged in the presence of hepatic and renal dysfunction.

## Monitoring Neuromuscular Blockade

As respiratory insufficiency due to prolonged neuromuscular blockade is an event with significant yet preventable morbidity, monitoring neuromuscular transmission while administering NMBs is essential. Neuromuscular monitoring involves electrically stimulating a peripheral nerve and assessing the response of a corresponding muscle. Two silver–silver chloride electrodes are placed over the nerve and a visual and tactile observation of muscular contraction, called a twitch, is made. Often the ulnar nerve at the elbow or wrist is stimulated and the response of the adductor pollicis assessed. Alternatively, the facial nerve may be stimulated, resulting in contraction of the orbicularis oculi. Any peripheral nerve may be stimulated if one of its innervated muscles can be isolated enough to quantify its contraction. The usual current applied is about 60 to 80 mA. Patterns of response estimate depth of blockade and discriminate between depolarizing and nondepolarizing relaxants.

Single-twitch stimulation offers little diagnostic information to the clinician and has been supplanted by train-of-four (TOF) stimulation. Four stimuli at the rate of 2 Hz are applied, and the number of twitches, as well as the ratio of intensity of the fourth twitch relative to the first, is determined, defining the train-of-four ratio. As blockade deepens, successive twitches fade, and then disappear (Fig. 18-10). The fewer the twitches noted, the deeper the blockade.

A 50-Hz tetanic stimulus is a sensitive monitor of residual neuromuscular blockade. While a patient may have recovered a full TOF, the muscular contraction after tetanic stimulation may fade, indicating residual blockade. A patient with full return of TOF but fade on tetanus has 70% of receptors blocked. A patient without tetanic fade has roughly 50% of receptors blocked. An important point, nerve stimulation only quantifies deep levels of neuromuscular blockade (>50%). Further termination of relaxant effect and recovery of function can only be assessed by clinical means, such as demonstrating sustained head lift, hand grip, and generating an inspiratory force of greater than −40 cm H$_2$O.

Practically speaking, while it is common to incur deep blockade with intubating doses of NMBs, if long-acting relaxants are avoided, some pattern of electrical stimulation should return soon. Subsequently, whether in the operating room or ICU, doses and dosing intervals should be sufficiently circumspect so that the depth of blockade can always be monitored by electrical stimulation.

As long as serum levels of muscle relaxants are not substantial, acetylcholinesterase inhibitors can antagonize nondepolarizing relaxants. These medications interfere with breakdown of acetylcholine by acetylcholinesterase. An undesirable side effect of acetylcholinesterase inhibition is bradycardia due to stimulation of cardiac muscarinic cholinergic receptors. Anticholinergics such as glycopyrrolate or atropine are administered prior to the acetylcholinesterase inhibitors to prevent this.

Common causes of prolonged relaxant effect include hepatic or renal failure, electrolyte abnormalities, hypothermia, concurrent medications, and acidosis. Prolonged relaxant administration in critically ill patients has unique complications as discussed in Chap. 60.

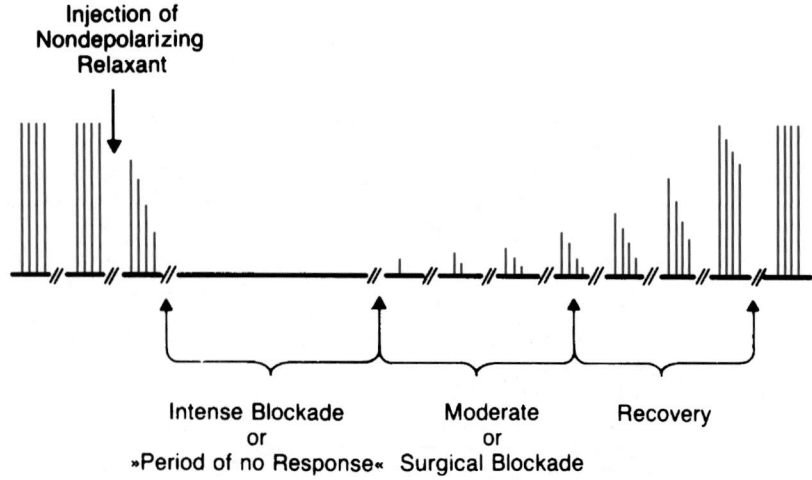

**Injection of Nondepolarizing Relaxant**

Intense Blockade or
»Period of no Response«

Moderate or
Surgical Blockade

Recovery

**FIGURE 18-10.** Changes in response to train-of-four stimulation during nondepolarizing neuromuscular blockade.
*(Reproduced with permission from Viby-Mogensen J. Neuromuscular monitoring. In Miller RD, ed: Anesthesia, 4th ed. New York: Churchill Livingstone, 1994, p. 1357.)*

The great majority of agents used in general anesthesia have been discussed. The majority of anesthetic procedures will use an induction agent to establish, and a volatile anesthetic to maintain, a state of unconsciousness or hypnosis. Noxious stimuli will be blunted by opioids; immobility and operating conditions will be facilitated by muscle relaxants. This represents what is commonly known as "balanced anesthesia." While one or two agents in large doses may conceivably achieve the necessary results, they may do so at the cost of cardiovascular instability, prolonged emergence, and other toxic manifestations. Using multiple agents with specific actions but in smaller doses permits anesthesia to be safely administered to most patients.

## ANESTHETIC CONCERNS AFTER INJURY TO SPECIFIC BODY REGIONS AND SPECIAL PATIENT GROUPS

### Traumatic Brain Injury

Little medical intervention is available to temporize the immediate effects of kinetic and mechanical forces on intracranial neuronal and vascular structures, the so-called primary brain injury. However, there is substantial evidence suggesting that ischemic secondary brain injury is deleterious (see Chap. 20).[67] Cerebral blood flow is lowest in the hours following the injury.[68] One-third of patients, even if normotensive, have ischemic levels of cerebral blood flow (CBF).[69] Autoregulation, the ability to maintain a constant blood flow over a range of perfusion pressures, may be lost, at least regionally, and CBF changes passively with perfusion pressure.[70] Maintaining cerebral oxygenation and perfusion in anyone having traumatic brain injury is fundamental.

Issues of concern include airway management, cervical protection, control of ICP, and choice of IV fluids and appropriate anesthetic agents. When faced with a head-injured patient requiring intubation, care should be taken to prevent further elevation of ICP while protecting the cervical spine. Thiopental and etomidate decrease cerebral metabolic activity, CBF, cerebral blood volume, and ICP. Neuromuscular blockade is appropriate to prevent coughing, or "bucking," which substantially increases ICP. Though theoretically unattractive, Sch has not been shown to result in clinically relevant increases in ICP.[71] Lidocaine (1.5 mg/kg 90 second before intubation) blunts the autonomic response to intubation, as does esmolol, administered in 10-mg boluses.

Though hyperventilation has been a mainstay in the treatment of elevated ICP, its benefit has undergone critical reexamination because of the potential for rendering the brain ischemic (see Chap. 20). Hyperventilation decreases cerebral perfusion at a time when CBF is likely reduced. Current guidelines recommend that prophylactic hyperventilation be avoided. However, hyperventilation may be necessary for brief periods when suctioning is planned, when there is acute neurologic deterioration, or when ICP fails to respond to other measures, such as sedation, paralysis, cerebrospinal fluid drainage, osmotic diuresis, head-up positioning, modest hypothermia, and barbiturate coma. Brief periods of hyperventilation are not associated with changes in cerebrospinal bicarbonate. If the patient has received chronic hyperventilation, weaning should be carried out with attention given to changes in ICP.

Intraoperative ICP monitoring should be used widely in patients with closed-head injury when other surgical procedures are planned[67] and serial neurologic exams become impossible.

Dextrose-free isotonic crystalloid solutions are the treatment of choice to maintain intravascular volume and CPP (see Chap. 20). Conventional volume resuscitation does not increase ICP. Isotonic crystalloids have superior osmotic effects while colloid solutions, though hyperoncotic, do not. Dextrose is converted to lactate within the cells, producing intracellular acidosis. Hyperglycemia is associated with poor outcomes in traumatic brain injury.[72] Hypotonic crystalloids should be avoided because the free water in these solutions contributes to total brain water. Hypertonic solutions decrease brain water and are occasionally used to lower ICP.

Ideally, anesthetic agents should decrease cerebral oxygen consumption ($CMRO_2$), maintain CPP, and not increase ICP. Barbiturates, benzodiazepines, propofol, and etomidate decrease $CMRO_2$ and CBF. However, barbiturates, benzodiazepines, and propofol decrease peripheral resistance and, when associated with hypovolemia, are likely to result in reductions in CPP. Etomidate is the IV anesthetic of choice when increased ICP is associated with hypovolemia because of its cardiovascular stability. Ketamine increases $CMRO_2$ and CBF, in turn increasing ICP. Despite maintaining systemic perfusion it is contraindicated in head injury. The cerebrovascular effects of induction agents are reviewed in Table 18-7.

The volatile anesthetics have remarkably different effects on CBF and $CMRO_2$. Though $CMRO_2$ decreases, CBF increases as volatile anesthetics are cerebral vasodilators. Isoflurane is the weakest vasodilator and is the volatile anesthetic of choice in neurotrauma. In impending brainstem herniation, any volatile anesthetic is contraindicated.

### Spinal Cord Injury

Though spinal cord injury is relatively uncommon, such injuries are devastating, resulting in profound life-long disability. Little can be offered to such patients in the way of improvement. However, as in head injuries, prevention of secondary injuries through spinal stabilization, careful airway control, hemodynamic support, and recognition and treatment of associated injuries are important therapeutic goals (see Chap. 24).

Immobilization of the spine is essential in all injured patients. Secondary injury will occur in 2–10% of such patients but is related principally to the initial injuries, hypotension, and hyoxemia.

**TABLE 18-7**

| Cerebrovascular Effects of Induction Agents | | | | |
|---|---|---|---|---|
| AGENT | CBF | ICP | CPP | CMRO$_2$ |
| Etomidate | − | − | 0 | − |
| Ketamine | ++ | + | + | + |
| Midazolam | − | − | − | − |
| Propofol | − | − | − | − |
| Thiopental | − | − | − | − |

CBF, cerebral blood flow; CPP, cerebral perfusion pressure; CMRO$_2$, cerebral metabolic oxygen rate; ICP, intracranial pressure; (+) increases; (0) no effect; (−) decreases.

All forms of airway control, including chin lift, jaw thrust, and oral and nasopharyngeal airway insertion, result in some cervical spine motion, though immobilization may mitigate this somewhat. Direct laryngoscopy, even with in-line spine stabilization, results in cervical motion, especially at atlanto-occipital and atlantoaxial levels. There is much less motion at lower cervical levels. Straight and curved laryngoscope blades do not differ substantially in the motion they produce, though the Bullard laryngoscope causes less head and cervical spine extension than does conventional laryngoscopy.[73] Fiberoptic bronchoscopy is considered by some to be the preferred method of securing the airway in patients with potential cervical spine injuries. However, the overall experience using a standard laryngoscope is satisfactory and no particular recommendation can be made based on outcome data.

Some degree of neurogenic shock should be expected with injuries above the T6 level. However, hypotension in cord-injured patients is most likely due to other injures. Catecholamine surges may produce pulmonary vascular damage, resulting in neurogenic pulmonary edema. There may be some element of myocardial dysfunction. If moderate fluid resuscitation does not result in hemodynamic improvement, a pulmonary artery catheter may provide valuable data (see Chap. 60). Fluid administration should be limited to pulmonary artery diastolic pressures of approximately 18 mm Hg.[74] Spinal cord injuries cephalad to midthoracic levels interrupt sympathetic cardioaccelerator fibers, resulting in bradycardia. If accompanied by hypotension, administration of atropine is indicated. Occasionally, infusion of vasopressors such as phenylephrine is needed to support blood pressure. Anesthetic agents should be titrated carefully, as drug-associated cardiovascular depression cannot be compensated for by increases in sympathetic tone. Doses of 30 to 50% of normal are likely to be sufficient. Succinylcholine may be administered in the first 24-hour period after cord injury but avoided thereafter to avoid the potential for life-threatening hyperkalemia.

Sympathetic tone eventually returns postinjury and sympathetic responses to stimuli distal to the injury may be exaggerated. Despite a loss of sensation, any surgical procedure or distention of a hollow viscus below the injury may produce life-threatening hypertension, termed *autonomic hyperreflexia*. Exaggerated reactions manifest as the patient moves into the period of spastic paralysis (4 to 8 weeks postinjury) and beyond. The more distal the stimulus, the more exaggerated the reaction. Urologic procedures or fecal disimpaction, common procedures in chronic cord patients, are examples. All procedures on chronic cord-injured patients require some anesthetic to prevent or attenuate autonomic hyperreflexia. Neuraxial and inhalational anesthetics are usually satisfactory though occasionally vasodilators such as nitroprusside are necessary to control hypertension.

## Highlights in Trauma-Perioperative Visual Loss Associated with Spine Surgery

Postoperative visual loss (POVL) is a devastating postoperative complication. While it has been reported following cardiopulmonary bypass (CPB), hip arthroplasty, abdominal procedures, craniotomies, and procedures on the head and neck, an increasing association with prone spine surgery has been noted over the last decade.

Overall, POVL is relatively infrequent, about 0.2% of spine surgeries. The most common etiology of blindness is ischemic optic neuropathy, and may be subclassified as either anterior or posterior ischemic optic neuropathy (AION, PION).

Patient-related risk factors include preoperative anemia and factors suggesting vascular disease, such as chronic hypertension, smoking, diabetes mellitus, carotid artery disease, etc. Procedure-related risk factors include prone or head-down procedures, surgical durations greater than 6.5 hours, blood loss exceeding about 45% of intravascular volume, and hypotension (MAP 40% below baseline). Other associated factors may be hypoxia, hemodilution, facial edema, and increases in intraocular pressure (IOP).

Ischemic optic neuropathy should be suspected if a patient complains of painless visual loss during the first postoperative week and may be first notice upon awakening from sleep, when IOP is highest. Urgent ophthalmologic consultation should be sought to comprehensively examine the patient, establish the diagnosis, and to recommend further evaluation and therapy. The most common prognosis is little return of visual function. Though the prognosis tends to be poor, prompt treatment may be the patient's only chance at recovering vision.

Strategies to avoid ION include avoiding external pressure on the eye. However, POVL has been noted in patients when supine and when prone but in Mayfield pins. In truth, compression upon the eyes is a rare intraoperative event. Perhaps more beneficial is maintaining acceptable blood pressure and hematocrit, particularly in high-risk patients.

At the current level of knowledge, it is believed there is a certain subset of patients having spine surgery in the prone position who are at increased risk for POVL. Who these patients are is as yet poorly understood. It is likely these high-risk patients are chronically hypertensive and likely have other risk factors for vascular disease, as has been discussed. The trend toward ever-decreasing hematocrit transfusion triggers may not be as prudent as previously supposed since a low hematocrit in the presence of other factors appears to put these patients at risk for visual loss. Additionally, while not absolutely contraindicated, the appropriate use of induced hypotension and hemodilution during prone spine procedures ought to be carefully considered when patients have risk factors for POVL. Finally, patients who may need both anterior and posterior instrumentation, and who are high risk, might be best managed with staged procedures, though the validity of this strategy is as yet unproven.[75]

## Thoracic Injury

For this broad topic, the reader is referred to Chaps., 25, 26, and 27. The following discussion will be limited to airway management during distal airway repairs, single-lung ventilation, air embolism, and cardiac tamponade.

Large airway injuries usually occur within 2.5 cm of the carina and are usually immediately recognizable; distal bronchial injuries are more difficult to identify (see Chap. 27). Physical features that may be associated with these injuries include respiratory distress, subcutaneous or mediastinal air, hemoptysis, pneumothorax, and persistent large air leak after tube thoracostomy. Delay in diagnosis may result in bronchopleural fistula, empyema, and mediastinitis.

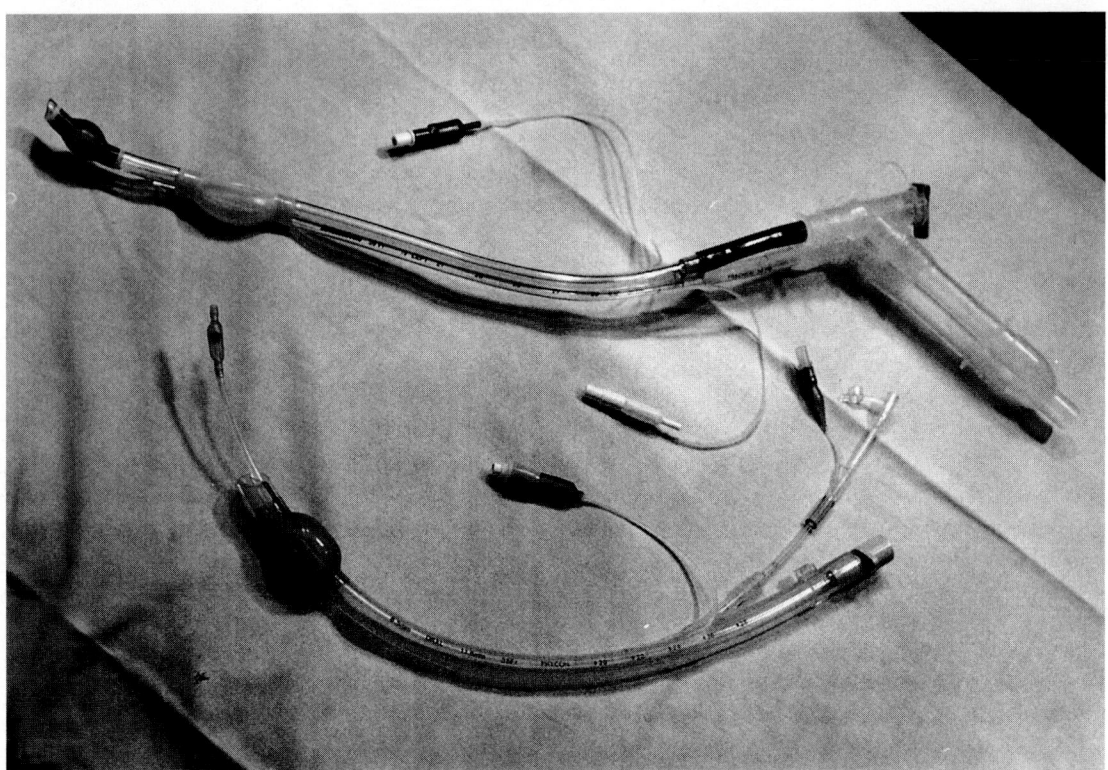

**FIGURE 18-11.** A left-sided double-lumen endotracheal tube (Sher-I-Bronch Endobronchial Tube, Kendall Health Care Products, Mansfield, MA) and bronchial blocking tube (Univent, Fuji Systems Corporation, Tokyo, Japan) are demonstrated. All cuffs are inflated. The bronchial blocker is extended. Each double-lumen endotracheal tube has two inflatable cuffs.

Lung Isolation. Any injury near the carina is likely to require lung isolation and single-lung ventilation. A single-lumen ETT might be inserted into the uninvolved main stem bronchus. Other options include inserting a double-lumen ETT or using a bronchial blocker. A fiberoptic bronchoscope is essential for any option chosen.

Double-lumen endotracheal tubes (DLET) are available in 35, 37, 39, and 41 French external diameters (Fig. 18-11). These tubes possess tracheal and bronchial ventilating channels and isolation is achieved by inflating the respective low-pressure cuffs. Unless precluded by the injury, a left bronchial DLET is preferred as right bronchial tubes often obstruct the right upper lobe bronchus. A major disadvantage of a DLET is that they must be exchanged for single-lumen endotracheal tubes at case conclusion unless differential lung ventilation is planned. Patients having major fluid resuscitations may be too edematous to perform this exchange safely.

An alternative to avoid the risk of airway loss at case conclusion would be to insert a bronchial blocker. The Univent tube (Fuji Systems Corp., Tokyo, Japan) has a balloon-tipped hollow stylet contained within the wall of the single-lumen ETT. Under endoscopic guidance, this stylet can be inserted into a main stem bronchus and inflated, isolating the lung (Fig. 18-12). A disadvantage of any

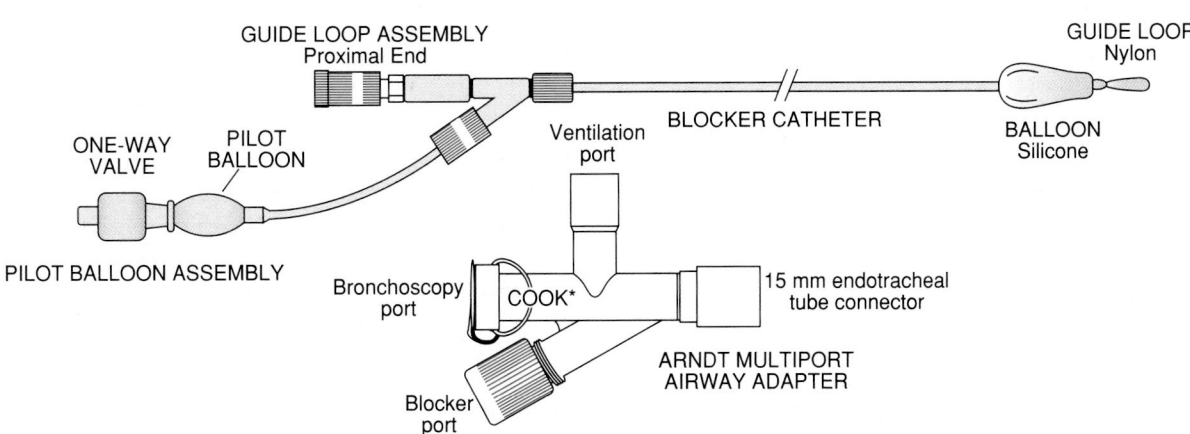

**FIGURE 18-12.** The Arndt bronchial blocker. Note the nylon snare that threads over the bronchoscope. The multiport airway adapter is also pictured. *(Reproduced with permission from Cook Critical Care, Bloomington, IN.)*

blocker, suctioning of the collapsed lung during the surgical procedure cannot be undertaken without resulting in reinflation. Additionally, lung deflation can sometimes be a problem and a solution is to disconnect the airway circuit, allow the lungs to passively collapse, then inflate the bronchial balloon. A contused or noncompliant lung may still not collapse well.

The Arndt endobronchial blocker (Cook Critical Care, Bloomington, IN) is inserted through a conventional single-lumen ETT (Fig. 18-12).[76] A multiport airway adapter is attached to the proximal ETT connector. The ventilating circuit remains connected and continues to ventilate the patient. A fiberoptic bronchoscope is inserted through a second arm of the adapter. The blocker is inserted through a third arm and has a snare that is passed around the bronchoscope. The bronchoscope is threaded into a main stem bronchus, the blocker is advanced, the bronchoscope is withdrawn slightly to confirm optimal blocker positioning, the blocker's cuff is inflated, and the lungs are isolated. This may be the optimal method of obtaining lung separation when postoperative ventilation is planned.

Single-Lung Ventilation.    The patient in lateral decubitus position with an open chest is likely to have considerable ventilation–perfusion (V/Q) imbalances due to injury as well as single-lung ventilation. There is greater ventilation and less perfusion to the nondependent lung, and greater perfusion but less ventilation to the dependent lung. Gravity influences blood flow distribution while the open chest, diaphragmatic paralysis, and weight of the mediastinum and abdominal contents on the dependent lung favor ventilation of the nondependent lung. To facilitate optimal V/Q matching, the following practices are suggested: maintain two-lung ventilation as long as possible; begin one-lung ventilation with tidal volumes of 7–10 mL/kg; adjust respiratory rate to maintain normocarbia (use an FiO$_2$ of 1.0); and utilize frequent blood gas analysis to monitor the effectiveness of initial ventilatory strategies.[85] PEEP to the dependent lung may be incrementally added but should not exceed 10 cmH$_2$O. Occasionally, continuous positive airway pressure (CPAP) to the nondependent lung may be applied. Low levels (5 to 10 cmH$_2$O) will inflate nondependent alveoli slightly, allowing for some gas exchange while not impairing surgical progress. Occasionally, high-frequency ventilation is necessary. Advantages include minimizing gas leakage from the bronchial tear while limiting airway pressures. The challenges of one-lung ventilation in adults and pediatrics has been recently reviewed.[77,78]

Air Embolism.    Penetrating lung injuries may result in systemic air entrainment via bronchovenous or alveolocapillary fistulas. Increased airway pressures associated with loss of pulmonary compliance as well as reduced venous pressure increases the likelihood of air embolism. Frothy, sanguineous secretions emanating from injured lung surfaces should make one wary of systemic air embolization. Air may be observed within coronary arteries. Systemic air embolism should be suspected whenever unexpected signs of CNS or myocardial ischemia and precipitous cardiovascular collapse occur in the appropriate clinical context (see Chap. 27). When treating patients at risk, minimize inspiratory airway pressure, avoid PEEP, and administer small tidal volumes.

Cardiac Tamponade.    Cardiac tamponade should be suspected with blunt or penetrating trauma to the chest or upper abdomen (see Chap. 28). The clinical and hemodynamic findings may be subtle and the dramatic physical findings associated with associated traumatic injuries may divert attention from these subtle findings. Clinical acumen is paramount.

An acutely distended pericardium is noncompliant. As pericardial pressure reaches right atrial pressure, cardiac filling diminishes. Only through preload augmentation can cardiac output be maintained. But as pericardial pressure reaches right ventricular diastolic pressure, acute cardiac decompensation ensues.

Anesthetic agents should be administered with the greatest of caution in untreated acute tamponade. Insertion of invasive monitors is useful but only if the patient is hemodynamically stable. It is often advisable to perform pericardiocentesis or subxiphoid pericardial drainage under local anesthesia before anesthetic induction. Intravenous fluid augmentation is usually necessary. Once pericardial drainage has occurred, general anesthesia can be cautiously induced, and ketamine is recommended due to its sympathomimetic effects, though direct myocardial depression has been described.[79] Once the patient is intubated, high airway pressures and PEEP should be avoided as both may impair venous return to the heart. Tachycardia is a compensatory mechanism and should not be overtreated. Vagally-mediated bradycardia due to pericardial distention requires atropine. Contractility is ordinarily intact and inotropes are rarely beneficial. Vasodilator therapy may be catastrophic in the hypovolemic patient.

## Abdominal Injury

Anesthesiologists and surgeons alike have similar concerns for patients experiencing intra-abdominal injuries; these are well reviewed in Chaps. 30 and 41. The abdominal compartment syndrome (ACS) is regularly encountered and challenges the anesthesiologist as cardiac output declines and ventilation is impaired (see Chap. 41).[80] Prompt recognition is important as the treatment, surgical decompression, is usually straightforward. However, low cardiac output may be associated with elevated pulmonary arterial occlusion pressure, suggesting cardiac failure, calling into question optimal fluid management. A porcine model has elegantly demonstrated the impact of increased intra-abdominal pressure (IAP) on intrathoracic pressures and invasive monitor interpretation.[81] When IAP was increased to 25 mm Hg, cardiac index significantly decreased. Measured pleural, pulmonary arterial, and occlusion pressures increased linearly with IAP. The declines in cardiac index resolved with further volume expansion despite hemodynamic indices that suggested satisfactory intravascular filling. The increases in pleural pressure were transmitted to the intravascular compartment, elevating the measured occlusion pressure (the sum of the left atrial diastolic pressure and pleural pressure), but the transmural occlusion pressure (the difference between the measured occlusion and pleural pressure) actually decreased with increasing IAP. A trial of volume expansion is usually indicated when pathologic IAP is suspected despite seemingly normal intravascular status as assessed by invasive hemodynamic monitors.

## Orthopedic Injury

Orthopedic injuries consume a remarkable portion of operating time in busy trauma centers. Life-threatening orthopedic injuries include exsanguination from complex pelvic or long-bone fractures and fat embolism syndrome but associated injuries are the major determinants of outcome.[82] Guidelines have recently been published describing optimal management of pelvic fractures in the multiply injured patient (see Chaps. 43 and 44).[83,84]

Many orthopedic procedures require nonsupine positioning. Care should always be taken to ensure ventilation is not compromised. Positioning should ensure adequate diaphragmatic excursion and thoracic expansion without producing excessive airway pressure. All extremities should be placed in positions of comfort, preventing torsion or pressure on neurovascular bundles, particularly the brachial plexus. The eyes, nose, ears, genitals, and breasts should be protected.

Tourniquets are often used to improve operative visualization and limit blood loss. When maintained in an inflated state for excessive durations or at excessive pressures, tourniquets may result in injury to underlying nerves, blood vessels, and muscle. Recommendations for inflation pressures are 100 mm Hg above systolic pressures for thigh cuffs and 50 mm Hg above systolic pressures for upper-extremity cuffs.[85]

Compartment syndromes associated with severe musculoskeletal trauma or vascular injury may produce permanent disability from permanent nerve injury, myonecrosis, and loss of extremity function and may occur pre-, intra-, or postoperatively (see Chap. 43). Acute renal failure may affect overall outcome. A principal sign of compartment syndrome (besides loss of pulses in a pale, cool extremity) is pain out of proportion to the injury, but patients may have a disordered perception of pain postoperatively. Excessive requests for analgesics should alert one to the possibility of this complication. Administration of local anesthetics may also rob the clinician of this valuable clinical sign.

Although up to 90% of long-bone fractures have some degree of fat embolism associated with them, only 3 to 4% progress to the fat embolism syndrome (FES).[86] Up to 10% of patients with multiple long-bone fractures may develop FES (see Chap. 63). The lungs, CNS, and skin are the major affected organ systems. Independent of pre-existing lung injury, FES should be considered whenever alveolar–arterial oxygen gradients deteriorate in conjunction with loss of pulmonary compliance and CNS deterioration (confusion, delirium, seizures, coma, etc.). Intraoperatively, patients may become hypotensive and intolerant of general anesthesia, and pressor agents may become necessary. If clinically important fat embolization is suspected, it is advisable to terminate the procedure as quickly as is possible and temporary stabilization may be appropriate. Pulmonary arterial catheterization is often necessary to optimize the hemodynamic profile, especially if failure of right side of the heart is suspected. Echocardiography may be of value in estimating chamber filling. Treatment of pulmonary dysfunction is supportive.

Myoglobinuria often follows crush injuries and compartment syndromes and may be recognized intraoperatively by the appearance of dark urine. Obstruction of renal tubules may ensue if untreated, followed by acute renal failure (see Chap. 65). Intraoperative management includes optimizing hemodynamics to improve renal blood flow and promoting diuresis to clear renal tubules. Loop and osmotic diuretics enhance urine output at the risk of decreasing intravascular volume.

## Geriatric Patients

The trauma mortality rate is greatest in geriatric patients compared to any other age group (see Chap. 47). Older patients are more prone to injury due to decreased cognitive ability and are less able to tolerate traumatic insults due to comorbidities and a lack of physiologic reserve. Myocardial contractility is impaired, there is decreased sensitivity to catecholamines, decreased pulmonary function, increased intracranial space due to brain atrophy (rendering them prone to intracranial hemorrhage), decreased hepatic and renal function, and impaired immunity and thermoregulation.[87] Invasive monitoring is necessary to optimize perfusion in the severely injured. They are also likely to have altered drug distribution due to obesity and hypoalbuminemia and enhanced sensitivity to any medication. Induction agents, opioids, benzodiazepines, muscle relaxants, and volatile anesthetics all have accentuated effects and dose reduction is prudent.

## Obstetric Patients

Trauma during pregnancy does not increase mortality to the mother compared to nonpregnant patients but the outcome of the pregnancy may be affected, especially if there is maternal death, severe maternal injury, the presence of severe maternal abdominal injury, and hemorrhagic shock.[88] The presence of pelvic fractures, and persistent hypoxemia may also increase the incidence of fetal death, which ordinarily presents soon after hospital admission (see Chap. 40).

The increased plasma volume of pregnancy results in a functional anemia and confuses interpretation of the hematocrit. Pregnancy is a vasodilated state, and the natural alteration in vital signs may confound their interpretation. All pregnant patients should be considered to have full stomachs and impaired gastroesophageal sphincter tone and are at increased risk for aspiration. Pregnancy is also an edematous state, and endotracheal intubation may be difficult. Functional residual capacity is decreased by 20% due to the weight of the gravid uterus upon the diaphragm, and oxygen consumption increases by an equal amount. Rapid oxygen desaturation is likely at onset of anesthesia and neuromuscular blockade. The weight of the uterus upon the abdominal aorta and inferior vena cava often impairs blood flow to the uterus and venous return to the thorax. Left uterine displacement is necessary and is achieved by placing a wedge under the right hip.

The fetus is the second patient and monitoring of fetal heart tones and uterine activity is recommended (see Chap. 40). During radiographic procedures, the fetus should be shielded whenever possible. Maternal hyperventilation left-shifts the oxyhemoglobin curve, increasing the maternal affinity for oxygen, decreasing oxygen release to the fetus. Alpha-adrenergic agonists may decrease uterine blood flow.

In general, aggressive resuscitation of the mother is the best management for the fetus. Loss of fetal heart rate variability is common in hyperadrenergic states and often seen after injury but is also a sign of uterine rupture and abruption. Abruption complicates 20% of major injuries. Loss of fetal tones also suggests uterine rupture or loss of uterine perfusion, and immediate abdominal delivery should be considered.

Fetal monitoring should continue after any surgical procedure addressing traumatic injuries to detect premature labor as well as impaired fetal oxygenation. Postoperative opioid administration may mask onset of premature labor but the benefits of analgesia should never be denied. A previable or dead fetus shifts concern back to the mother.

**TABLE 18-8**

## Safety of Drugs and Drug Classes Frequently Used in Trauma Patients Based on FDA Classification of Drug Safety in Pregnancy

| CATEGORY A AND B | CATEGORY C | CATEGORY D AND X |
|---|---|---|
| Amphotericin | Acyclovir | ACE inhibitors |
| Cephalosporins | Albuterol | Angiotensin receptor antagonists |
| Cimetidine | Aminoglycosides | Coumadin |
| Clindamycin | Atropine | Salicylates |
| Glycopyrrolate | Bretylium | Tetracycline |
| Insulin | Benzodiazepines | Toradol |
| Lidocaine | Beta blockers | |
| Magnesium sulfate | Bupivicaine | |
| Methyldopa | Catecholamines | |
| Naloxone | Dantrolene | |
| Opioids | Digoxin | |
| Penicillins | Haloperidol | |
| Propofol | Flumazenil | |
| Ranitidine | Fluconazole | |
| Terbutaline | Furosemide | |
| | Heparin | |
| | Hydralazine | |
| | Labetalol | |
| | Metronidazole | |
| | Midazolam | |
| | Muscle relaxants | |
| | Nifedipine | |
| | Nitroglycerine | |
| | Nitroprusside | |
| | Phenytoin | |
| | Prednisone | |
| | Procainamide | |
| | Thiopental | |
| | Vancomycin | |

*Modified and updated from Lapinsky SE, Kruczynsiki K, Slutsky AS: Critical care in the pregnant patient. Am J Respir Cnt Care Med 152:427–455, 1995.*
Category A and B drugs have not demonstrated fetal risk in human and/or animal studies. Category C drugs have demonstrated adverse effects in animal studies and the risk and benefits should be weighed before administering these drugs. Category D and X drugs have demonstrated adverse human fetal effects.

The hormonal changes of pregnancy increase the potency of a given dose of volatile anesthetic by 25 to 40%. The potency of neuraxial local anesthetics increases by 30%. All lipid soluble drugs reach the fetus. The teratogenic potential of all drugs should be considered (Table 18-8).

## Pediatric Patients

Upper airway obstruction is common and oxygen desaturation occurs quickly due to increased oxygen consumption relative to size (see Chap. 46). Intubation should occur early in any child who is cyanotic, unconscious, combative, or if the airway is in imminent risk of compromise. However, the pediatric airway differs from the adult in that the tongue is large relative to the oral cavity, the epiglottis is floppy, and the larynx is at a higher cervical level; thus intubation may be difficult. Always maintain cervical spine precautions as children have a high incidence of ligamentous cervical injuries inapparent on routine cervical radiographs (see Chap. 24). The cricoid cartilage is the point of greatest airway narrowing, and

an endotracheal tube may cross the vocal cords without difficulty then encounter resistance. Once intubated, vigorous ventilation should be avoided to reduce the risk of barotrauma. The chest wall is compliant, and there may be a lack of physical signs despite significant intrathoracic injury; rib fractures suggest severe injury.

Vital signs change with age and blood pressure and heart rate may be difficult to interpret, so it is important to look for signs of decreased perfusion such as loss of peripheral pulses and impaired capillary refill. Bradycardia is an ominous sign and suggests hypoxia or significant hypovolemia. Isotonic crystalloid solutions should be administered in 20 mL/kg boluses. Insufficient hemodynamic response after two to three crystalloid boluses should prompt administration of packed red blood cells in 10 mL/kg boluses. Saphenous venous cutdowns or tibial intraosseus infusions may be necessary to achieve adequate venous access (see Chap. 46). Heat loss is rapid and aggressive efforts to reestablish normal body temperature should be made since vasoconstriction will markedly impair distal perfusion. Volatile and intravenous anesthetics should be titrated carefully, anticipating a decreased volume of distribution and enhanced effect.

## The Burned Patient

An "ABC" approach to the burned patient is important (see Chap. 50). While respiratory distress may not be an initial presenting complaint, the significant fluid resuscitation and subsequent extracellular fluid expansion (usually observed with 30% total burns or greater) is likely to result in airway compromise. Hence, in anticipation of later problems, endotracheal intubation should be accomplished early. An index of suspicion for pulmonary injury (burns occurring in closed spaces, in industrial settings, etc.) is necessary and may be supported by physical features such as soot on the face, singed facial hair, mucous erythema or swelling, and wheezing or other signs of respiratory distress. Of note, carbon monoxide poisoning cannot be detected with standard two wavelength pulse oximetry and arterial blood gases as measured by co-oximetry will be required to detect carbon monoxide. Topical silver nitrate may increase serum methemoglobin levels. As previously mentioned, major fluid resuscitation (usually with Ringer's lactate and by formula) is necessary to maintain functional intravascular volume. Intravenous access may be problematic. Circumferential injuries require urgent escharotomies to maintain circulation or chest expansion. Electrical injuries may produce cardiac injury and electrocardiographic abnormalities.

Burn patients have lost temperature regulation with loss of skin integrity. Burn units and operating rooms must be maintained at a temperature uncomfortable to care providers so as not to render patients hypothermic. Loss of thermoregulatory control during general anesthesia only exacerbates this potential.

Standard anesthetic monitoring may be difficult. Electrocardiographic leads may need to be stapled onto whatever skin site is reasonable. Noninvasive blood pressure monitoring may be difficult as well, and direct arterial pressure monitoring is often employed. All vascular catheters must be inserted under strict aseptic conditions and changed according to institutional protocol.

Major burns lead to a proliferation of extrajunctional neuromuscular receptors, and these patients are at risk for life-threatening hyperkalemia after Sch administration, though the first 24 hours postburn phase is considered safe for Sch use. As these patients are extremely catabolic, anesthetic needs (assuming intravascular volume is adequate) are often increased, though hypoalbuminemia may increase the free fraction of many drugs. These patients are also resistant to nondepolarizing neuromuscular blockers. Their analgesic requirements can be enormous in comparison to other patient groups. Administration of blood products is virtually guaranteed during operative management of burns. Patient comorbidities have an impact on overall burn outcome and should be taken into consideration when planning an anesthetic as well.

## The Obese Patient

The obese and morbidly obese patient creates numerous anesthetic challenges. They may be difficult to mask ventilate and intubate, and they experience rapid oxygen desaturation when anesthetized and paralyzed because frequently they have alveolar collapse during tidal respiration. The triad of difficult ventilation, difficult intubation, and rapid oxygen desaturation creates a situation where the likelihood of a hypoxic brain injury is increased, and obese patients probably have an increased incidence of emergently created surgical airways. They also have an increased incidence of gastroparesis, predisposing them to pulmonary aspiration of gastric contents.

Blood pressure cuffs fit poorly, obtaining suitable electrocardiographic monitoring may be difficult, and inserting invasive monitoring lines is likewise challenging. Airway pressures are frequently excessive. Determining the correct dose of all medications is challenging as medications are based on an accurate assessment of lean body weight.

Obese patients have metabolic abnormalities as well, most notably diabetes mellitus, which often is insulin-dependent. They are often hypertensive and have coronary artery disease. They may have restrictive lung disease, be chronically hypoxemic and hypercarbic, and in the extreme, are associated with pulmonary hypertension and right heart failure.[89] Deep venous thrombosis is also an increased risk.

Obese patients sustaining blunt injuries have more complications (including multiple organ failure, acute respiratory distress syndrome, myocardial infarction, and renal failure), require vasopressor support more often, have more ventilator days, fail extubation more frequently, and require longer hospital stays.[90] Obesity itself is independently associated with increased mortality.[91]

## REFERENCES

1. Snow J: *On Chloroform and Other Anesthetics.* London: John Churchill, 1858.
2. Keats AS: What do we know about anesthetic mortality? *Anesthesiology* 50:387, 1979.
3. Aitkenhead AR: Injuries associated with anaesthesia. A global perspective. *Br J Anaesth* 95:95, 2005.
4. Spence AA: The lessons of CEPOD. *Br J Anaesth* 60:753, 1988.
5. Farrow SC, Fowkes FGR, Lunn JN, et al.: Epidemiology in anesthesia. II. Factors affecting mortality in hospital. *Br J Anaesth* 54:811, 1982.
6. Buck N, Devlin HB, Lunn JN: *Report of a confidential enquiry into perioperative deaths.* London: Kings Fund. Nuffield Provincial Hospitals Trust, 1987.
7. Eichorn JH: Prevention of intraoperative anesthesia accidents and related severe injury through safety monitoring. *Anesthesiology* 70:572, 1989.
8. Lee LA, Domino KB: The Closed Claims Project. Has it influenced anesthetic practice and outcome? *Anesthesiol Clin N Amer* 20:485, 2002.
9. Caplan RA, Posner KL, Ward RJ, et al.: Adverse respiratory events in anesthesia: A closed claims analysis. *Anesthesiology* 72:828, 1990.
10. Silber JH, Kennedy SK, Even-Shoshan O: Anesthesiologist direction and patient outcomes. *Anesthesiology* 93:152, 2000.
11. Cooper JB, Newbower RS, Kitz RJ: An analysis of major errors and equipment failures in anesthesia management: Considerations for prevention and detection. *Anesthesiology* 60:34, 1984.
12. Caplan RA, Posner KL, Ward RJ, et al.: Adverse respiratory events in anesthesia: A closed claims analysis. *Anesthesiology* 72:828, 1990.
13. Cheney FW, Domino KB, Caplan RA, et al.: Nerve injury associated with anesthesia: A closed claims analysis. *Anesthesiology* 90:1062, 1999.
14. Domino KB, Posner KL, Caplan RA, et al.: Awareness during anesthesia: A closed claims analysis. *Anesthesiology* 90:1053, 1999.
15. Tiret L, Desmonts JM, Hatton F, et al.: Complications associated with anaesthesia—A prospective survey in France. *Can Anaesth Soc J* 33:336, 1986.
16. Cohen MM, Duncan PG, Tate RB: Does anesthesia contribute to operative mortality? *JAMA* 260:2859, 1988.
17. Vacanti CJ, van Houten RJ, Hill RC: A statistical analysis of the relationship of physical status to postoperative mortality in 68,388 cases. *Anesth Analg* 49:564, 1970.
18. Koch JP, McLellan BA, Wortzman D, et al.: Is the ASA physical status classification adequate in predicting mortality in blunt trauma? *Anesthesiology* 67:A482, 1987.
19. American Society of Anesthesiologists: New classification of physical status. *Anesthesiology* 24:111, 1963.
20. Wolters U, Wolf T, Stützer H, et al.: ASA classification and perioperative variables as predictors of postoperative outcome. *Br J Anaesth* 77:217, 1996.
21. Parmet JL, Colonna-Romano P, Horrow JC, et al.: The laryngeal mask airway reliably provides rescue ventilation in cases of unanticipated difficult tracheal intubtion along with difficult mask ventilation. *Anesth Analg* 87:661, 1998.
22. American Society of Anesthesiologists: Practice guidelines for management of the difficult airway: An updated report. *Anesthesiology* 98:1269, 2003.
23. Salem MR: Verification of endotracheal tube position. *Anesth Clin N Amer* 19:813, 2001.
24. Benumof JL: Management of the difficult airway with special emphasis on awake tracheal intubation. *Anesthesiology* 75:1087, 1991.
25. Cormack RS, Lehane J: Difficult tracheal intubation in obstetrics. *Anaesthesia* 39:1105, 1984.
26. Mallampati SR, Gugino LD, Desai SP, et al.: A clinical sign of predictable difficult tracheal intubation: A prospective study. *Can Anaesth Soc J* 32:429, 1985.
27. Pennant JH, Pace NA, Gajraj NM: Role of the laryngeal mask airway in the immobile cervical spine. *J Clin Anesth* 5:226, 1993.
28. Bedger RC, Chang JL: A jet-stylet endotracheal catheter for difficult airway management. *Anesthesiology* 66:221, 1987.
29. Benumof JL: Airway exchange catheters: Simple concept, potentially great danger. *Anesthesiology* 91:342, 1999.
30. Ho AM, Karmakar MK, Contardi LH et al.: Excessive use of normal saline in managing traumatized patients in shock: A preventable contributor to acidosis. *J Trauma* 51:173, 2001.
31. Laxenaire MC, Mertes PM: Anaphylaxis during anaesthesia. Results of a two-year survey in France. *Br J Anaest* 87:549, 2001.
32. Hepner DL, Castells MC: Latex allergy: An update. *Anesth Analg* 96:1219, 2003.
33. Eichorn JH, Cooper JB, Cullen BF, et al.: Standards for patient monitoring during anesthesia at Harvard Medical School. *JAMA* 256:1017, 1986.
34. American Society of Anesthesiologists: Standards for basic intraoperative monitoring, in *ASA Standards, Guidelines, and Statements.* American Society of Anesthesiologists, 1986, amended 2005.
35. Aoyagi T: Pulse oximetry: Its invention, theory, and future. *J Anesth* 17:259, 2003.
36. Barker SJ, Tremper KK, Hyatt J: Effects of methemoglobinemia on pulse oximetry and mixed venous oximetry. *Anesthesiology* 70:112, 1989.
37. Gould SA, Moore EE, Hoyt DB: The first randomized trial of human polymerized hemoglobin as a blood substitute in acute trauma and emergent surgery. *J Am Coll Surg* 187:113, 1998.
38. Levine RL, Wayne MA, Miller CC: End-tidal carbon dioxide and outcome of out-of-hospital cardiac arrest. *N Engl J Med* 337:301, 1997.
39. Bogetz MS, Katz JA: Recall of surgery for major trauma. *Anesthesiology* 61:6, 1984.
40. Lubke GH, Kersens C, Phaf H, et al.: Dependence of explicit and implicit memory on hypnotic state in trauma patients. *Anesthesiology* 90:670, 1999.
41. Eger EI, Koblin DD, Harris RA, et al.: Hypothesis: Inhaled anesthetics produce immobility and amnesia by different mechanism at different sites. *Anesth Analg* 84:915, 1997.
42. American Society of Anesthesiologists Task Force on Intraoperative Awareness: Practice advisory for intraoperative awareness and brain function monitoring. *Anesthesiology* 104:847, 2006.
43. DeDeyne C, Struys M, Decruyenaere J, et al.: Use of continuous bispectral EEG monitoring to assess depth of sedation in ICU patients. *Intens Care Med* 24:1294, 1998.
44. Sessler DI: Complications and treatment of mild hypothermia. *Anesthesiology* 95:531, 2001.

45. Kurz A, Kurz M, Poeschl G, et al.: Forced-air warming maintains intraoperative normothermia better than circulating-water mattresses. *Anesth Analg* 77:89, 1993.
46. Whitten CW, Greilich PE: Thromboelastography: Past, present and future. *Anesthesiology* 92:1223, 2000.
47. Kaufmann CR, Dwyer KM, Crews JD: Usefulness of Thromboelastography in assessment of trauma patient coagulation. *J Trauma* 42:716, 1997.
48. Liu S, Carpenter RL, Neal JM: Epidural anesthesia and analgesia: Their role in postoperative outcome. *Anesthesiology* 82:1474, 1995.
49. Bulger EM, Edwards T, Klotz P, et al.: Epidural analgesia improves outcome after multiple rib fractures. *Surgery* 136:426, 2004.
50. Karmakar MK, Ho AM: Acute pain management of patients with multiple rib fractures. *J Trauma* 54:615, 2003.
51. Horlocker TT, Wedel DJ, Benzon H et al.: Regional anesthesia in the anticoagulated patient: Defining the risks (the second ASRA Consensus Conference on Neuraxial Anesthesia and Anticoagulation). *Reg Anesth Pain Med* 28:172, 2003.
52. Horlocker TT, Wedel DJ: Spinal and epidural blockade and perioperative low molecular weight heparin: Smooth sailing on the Titanic (comment). *Anesth Analg* 86:1153, 1998.
53. Kurt E, Ozturk S, Isik S et al.: Continuous brachial plexus blockade for digital replantations and toe-to-hand transfers. *Ann Plast Surg* 54:24, 2005.
54. Bonnet F, Marret E: Influence of anesthetic and analgesic techniques on outcome after surgery. *Br J Anaesth* 95:52, 2005.
55. Absalom A, Pledger D, Kong A: Adrenocortical function in critically ill patients 24 hours after a single dose of etomidate. *Anaesthesia* 54:861, 1999.
56. Sneyd JR: Recent advances in intravenous anaesthesia. *Br J Anaesth* 93:725, 2004.
57. Liolios A, Guerit J-M, Scholtes J-L: Propofol infusion syndrome associated with short-term large-dose infusion during surgical anesthesia in an adult. *Anesth Analg* 100:1804, 2005.
58. Nordt SP, Clark RF: Midazolam: A review of therapeutic uses and toxicity. *J Emerg Med* 15:357, 1997.
59. Young CC, Prielipp RC: Benzodiazepines in the intensive care unit. *Crit Care Clinics* 17:843, 2001.
60. Egan TD: Remifentanil pharmacokinetics and pharmacodynamics. A preliminary appraisal. *Clin Pharmacokinet* 29:80, 1995.
61. Mazze RI, Jamison RL: Low flow sevoflurane: Is it safe? *Anesthesiology* 86:1225, 1997.
62. Kaur S, Cortiella J, Vacanti CA: Diffusion of nitrous oxide into the pleural cavity. *Br J Anaesth* 87:894, 2001.
63. Souders JE: Pulmonary air embolism. *J Clin Monit Comput* 16:375, 2000.
64. Martyn JA, Richtsfeld M: Succinylcholine-induced hyperkalemia in acquired pathologic states: Etiologic factors and molecular mechanisms. *Anesthesiology* 104:158, 2006.
65. Martyn JAJ, White DA, Gronert GA: Up and down regulation of skeletal muscle acetylcholine receptors. *Anesthesiology* 76:822, 1992.
66. Caldwell JE: New skeletal muscle relaxants. *Int Anesth Clinics* 33:39, 1995.
67. Meagher RJ, Narayan RK: The triage and acute management of severe head injury. *Clin Neurosurg* 46:127, 2000.
68. Marion DW, Darby J, Yonas H: Acute regional cerebral blood flow changes caused by severe head injuries. *J Neurosurg* 74:407, 1991.
69. Bouma GJ, Muizelaar JP, Stringer WA, et al.: Ultra-early evaluation of regional cerebral blood flow in severely head-injured patients using xenon-enhanced computerized tomography. *J Neurosurg* 77:360, 1992.
70. Brain Trauma Foundation. The American Association of Neurological Surgeons, Joint Section on Neurotrauma and Critical Care: Use of mannitol. *J Neurotrauma* 17:521, 2000.
71. Kovarik WD, Mayberg TS, Lam AM, et al.: Succinylcholine does not change ICP, cerebral blood flow velocity or the electroencephalogram in patients with neurologic injury. *Anesth Analg* 78:469, 1994.
72. Jeremitsky E, Omert LA, Dunham CM, et al.: The impact of hyperglycemia on patients with severe brain injury. *J Trauma* 58:47, 2005.
73. Crosby ET: Airway management in adults after cervical spine trauma. *Anesthesiology* 104:1293, 2006.
74. Mackenzie CF, Shin B, Krishnaprasad D, et al.: Assessment of cardiac and respiratory function during surgery on patientswith acute paraplegia. *J Neurosurg* 62:843, 1985.
75. ASA Task Force on Perioperative Blindness: Practice advisory for perioperative visual loss associated with spine surgery. *Anesthesiology* 104:1319, 2006.
76. Arndt GA, Kranner PW, Rusy DA, et al.: Single-lung ventilation in a critically ill patient using a fiberoptically directed wire-guided endobronchial blocker. *Anesthesiology* 90:1484, 1999.
77. Campos JH: Current techniques for perioperative lung isolation in adults. *Anesthesiology* 97:1295, 2002.
78. Mirzabeigi E, Johnson C, Ternian A: One-lung anesthesia update. *Semin Cardiothorac Vasc Anesth* 9:213, 2005. 79. Weiskopf RB, Bogez MS, Roizen MF, et al.: Cardiovascular and metabolic sequelae of inducing anesthesia with ketamine or thiopental in hypovolemic swine. *Anesthesiology* 60:214, 1984.
80. Sugrue M: Abdominal compartment syndrome. *Curr Opin Crit Care* 11:333, 2005.
81. Ridings PC, Bloomfield GL, Blocher CR: Cardiopulmonary effects of raised intra-abdominal pressure before and after intravascular volume expansion. *J Trauma* 39:1071, 1995.
82. Dente CJ, Feliciano DV, Rozycki GS, et al.: The outcome of open pelvic fractures in the modern era. *Am J Surg* 190:830, 2005.
83. Heetveld MJ, Harris I, Schlaphoff G: Hemodynamically unstable pelvic fractures: Recent care and new guidelines. *World J Surg* 28:904, 2004.
84. Dunham CM, Bosse MJ, Clancy TV, et al.: Practice management guidelines for the optimal timing of long-bone fracture stabilization in polytrauma patients: The EAST practice management guidelines work group. *J Trauma* 50:958, 2001.
85. Pedowitz RA: Tourniquet-induced neuromuscular injury. A recent review of rabbit and clinical experiments. *Acta Orthop Scand* 245:1, 1991.
86. Parisi DM, Koval K, Egol K: Fat embolism syndrome. *Amer J Orthop* 31:507, 2002.
87. Johnson C, Ashley SA: Perioperative care of patients with shock and multiple trauma. In Lake CL, Rice LJ, Sperry RJ, eds. *Advances in Anesthesia*. St. Louis: Mosby, 2001, p. 262.
88. Shah AJ, Kilcline BA: Trauma in Pregnancy. *Emerg Med Clin North Am* 21:615, 2003.
89. Abir F, Bell R: Assessment and management of the obese patient. *Crit Care Med* 32:S87, 2004.
90. Brown CV, Neville AL, Rhee P, et al.: The impact of obesity on the outcomes of 1,153 critically injured blunt trauma patients. *J Trauma* 59:1048, 2005.
91. AL, Brown CVR, Weng J, et al.: Obesity is an independent risk factor of mortality in severely injured blunt trauma patients. *Arch Surg* 139:983, 2004.

# Commentary ■ SALLY RATY

Dr. Duke has provided the nonanesthesiologist with a well-organized, thorough text outlining the concerns confronting the anesthesiologist when faced with caring for a traumatized patient. In this edition of *Trauma*, Dr. Duke has included updated descriptions and explanations of a wide range of anesthetic concepts, considerations, medications, and techniques, the knowledge of which is essential to the successful trauma surgeon. His addition of five new sections focused on allergic reaction, airway pressure, intra-arterial, and coagulation monitoring, and postoperative vision loss are important anesthesia related issues for all surgical

patients, not just for the traumatically injured patient. In acknowledgement of the increasing numbers of obese patients, Duke wisely adds a special section regarding the care of the traumatized obese patient. The author correctly emphasizes, the anesthesiologist faced with caring for the critically injured patient is often unable to obtain important medical history from the patient. Early preoperative inclusion of the anesthesiologist in patient care, preferably in the emergency center for a critically injured patient, can provide the anesthesiologist with crucial information about the patient that would otherwise be unobtainable. Undoubtedly, some of the information relevant to the safe conduct of anesthesia will be routinely asked by the attending surgeon and the emergency center staff. However, it is unrealistic to expect a nonanesthesiologist to focus on all of the issues that are of particular importance to the anesthesiologist. The skilled anesthesiologist will begin formulating a plan for the traumatized patient immediately. Clearly, the earlier an anesthesiologist can evaluate the patient, the more comprehensive and well planned the anesthetic is likely to be. While the surgeons are physically caring for the patient in the emergency center, the informed anesthesiologist can brief the operating room personnel on the condition of the patient, call in additional personnel if needed, confer with the blood bank, lab, and radiology on the likely need of services, delegate responsibility to the anesthesia team, and organize other ongoing cases. There is clearly no advantage to the patient if the anesthesiologist is surprised by his/her arrival in the operating room.

The author's inclusion of extensive discussions on the mechanism and limitations of neuromuscular monitoring, pulse oximetry, BIS, capnography, and intra-arterial monitoring are relevant for every surgeon, not just those who specialize in the care of traumatized patients.

For the initial emergent procedure, most trauma patients are placed in the supine position with both arms extended. Every effort should be made to protect pressure points from injury. If the patient requires fluoroscopy near the pelvic region, care must be taken to protect his/her gonads from excessive radiation exposure.

Finally, the importance of communication between the surgeon and the anesthesiologist cannot be overstated. Communication between the surgery team and the anesthesia team should begin at the earliest possible moment. As soon as the emergency response services in the region notify the hospital of the imminent arrival of a trauma patient, all caregivers likely to be involved in the patient's care should be notified. It is only with early notification that available resources can be appropriately allocated. An air of cooperation and assistance among everyone helping to care for a seriously injured patient is absolutely essential.

Despite the best efforts and plans of a trauma team, there will occasionally be a catastrophic event during the care of a patient. Mostly commonly, this catastrophe is the loss of a patient who is "supposed to" survive. Such an event can be truly devastating to the care team. Debriefing after such a loss has enormous value. The goal of the debriefing, facilitated by someone skilled in the process, is to review the events leading up to the catastrophe, to review what went wrong and what went right, to brainstorm for solutions to implement the "next time" while avoiding blaming and finger pointing.

# Infection

*Philip S. Barie* ■ *Soumitra R. Eachempati* ■ *Fredric M. Pieracci*

The incidence of infection following traumatic injury is approximately 25%.[1] Although most trauma-related deaths occur from either exsanguination or massive injury to the central nervous system within 24 hours of injury, the leading cause of later posttraumatic death is infection, usually manifesting as multiple organ dysfunction syndrome[2,3] (Table 19-1). Trauma patients are at high risk of infection for many reasons, including the host immunosuppressive response to injury[4]; direct inoculation of wounds by clothing, dirt, or debris; inadequate infection control practice under emergency conditions; blood transfusions; and poor control of blood sugar.[5] In some respects, the epidemiology of infection following trauma differs from that in other critically ill surgical patients, with trauma patients being more likely to become infected (Table 19-2) and also to develop infection earlier after admission.

Infections following injury occur in the injured tissue itself (or an incision made to treat the injury) or as nosocomial infections, such as pneumonia or catheter-related blood stream infection (CR-BSI) (Table 19-2).[6] Unfortunately, nosocomial infections are collectively as common as infections of the injured tissues themselves.[6] Among the nosocomial infections, pleuro-pulmonary infections (e.g., pneumonia, empyema) are more common than CR-BSIs,[7–9] which in turn are more common than urinary tract infections. This review will examine the factors that contribute to the markedly increased risk of infection after trauma, consider what can be done to reduce the risk of infection, and how best to diagnose and treat infection when it occurs.

## HOST FACTORS

The host is defined by genotype, expressed phenotypically as various characteristic traits. The host immune response is highly conserved across mammalian species. Traumatic injury, by definition a breach of a natural epithelial barrier (e.g., skin, respiratory, and digestive tract mucosa) creates a portal by which tissue invasion by pathogens may occur. Innate immunity provides continuous surveillance in the interstitial spaces just beneath the natural epithelial barriers against tissue invasion by foreign antigens. Potential pathogens are ubiquitous in the environment, but although colonization of epithelial surfaces occurs even in healthy hosts, invasion is relatively uncommon. Injury also stimulates a repair response (inflammation), which may cause a wide-ranging counter-productive augmentation of the inflammatory response that is destructive to the host.

The stress hormone phenotype that characterizes the "fight or flight" response augments cardiovascular function through the autonomic nervous system, enhances glycogenolysis, mobilizes peripheral lean tissue and fat for gluconeogenesis, enhances coagulation to stanch hemorrhage, and stimulates a pro-inflammatory cytokine response to begin the process of tissue repair (Table 19-3).[10] Humoral and cellular immunity are depressed in large part by the actions of cortisol (Tables 19-4 and 19-5).[4,10]

Older age (generally age ≥65 years) is a definite risk factor for increased mortality from trauma,[11] which appears to be related directly to the depression of immunity and the increased rate of nosocomial infection that afflicts older patients. Hyperglycemia is increasingly recognized as a risk factor for infection (Tables 19-6 and 19-7), and it is well documented that hyperglycemia induces immune cell dysfunction. Even transitory hyperglycemia has been associated with an increased risk of surgical site infection[12–15] and nosocomial infection that translates into increased mortality after trauma[5] and sepsis.[16,17] The effects of the stress response (increased cortisol secretion, decreased insulin secretion, peripheral insulin resistance) make hyperglycemia a risk for diabetic and nondiabetic patients alike.

Profound hypocholesterolemia occurs rapidly during critical surgical illness,[18] possibly as part of a cytokine-induced negative acute-phase response that downregulates the synthesis of lipoproteins important for the trafficking of endotoxins. Hypocholesterolemia increases the risk of both surgical site and nosocomial infections[19] and may also be an independent predictor of mortality.[20]

## TABLE 19-1

| Temporal Relationships of Trauma Deaths to Causation | | | |
|---|---|---|---|
| | ACUTE | EARLY | LATE |
| | (<24 H) | (24 H–7 D) | (>7 D) |
| Central nervous system | 40% | 64% | 39% |
| Exsanguination | 55% | 9% | 0 |
| Multiple organ dysfunction syndrome | <1% | 18% | 61% |

Adapted from: Asensio JA, Stewart BM, Murray J, et al.: Penetrating cardiac injuries. Surg Clin North Am 76:685, 1996.

## TABLE 19-3

| Overview of the "Stress Response" to Injury |
|---|
| Activation of the sympathetic nervous system |
| Activation of hypophyseal-pituitary-adrenal axis |
| Peripheral insulin resistance |
| Production of pro-and anti-inflammatory cytokines |
| Acute-phase changes of hepatic protein synthesis |
| Recruitment and activation of neutrophils, monocyte/macrophages, and lymphocytes |
| Upregulation of pro-coagulant activity |

## Genetic Predisposition to Sepsis

It is possible, but unproved, that gender may make a difference in outcome following injury. In vitro and animal studies indicate clearly that androgens are immunosuppressive, and that male animals have higher mortality after both trauma and sepsis,[21,22] however, human studies are conflicting on this issue. Offner et al. found male gender to be an independent risk factor for the development of infection following severe injury (Injury Severity Score [ISS] <15, odds ratio [OR] 1.58),[23] but there was no difference in mortality. A large, population-based study demonstrated higher mortality among males with the acute respiratory distress syndrome (ARDS).[24] In contrast, population-based studies by Gannon et al.[25] and Angus et al.[26] cast doubt on the clinical importance of the laboratory observations of gender-based differences. Gannon et al.[25] found no gender-based difference of mortality among 18,892 trauma patients; of interest, male patients were more likely to develop pneumonia, but female patients were more likely to succumb.[25] Angus et al.[26] were unable to detect any adverse outcome among females from sepsis in a nationwide population-based study.

## Genomics of Trauma and Sepsis (see Chap. 57)

Modern high-throughput, multiplexed assays allow the molecular characterization of pathophysiologic conditions. Whereas most genes have hundreds of nucleotides in sequence, only a relatively short sequence is needed for precise identification of each. Glass slide "chips" have been designed to exploit this finding by affixing minute quantities of vast numbers (i.e., many thousands) of short, gene-specific probe nucleotides in an array called a *DNA microarray*. Messenger RNA can be isolated from cells or tissues and labeled to produce complementary nucleotides (cDNA or cRNA), that, when incubated with the microarray, will bind by conventional base pairing. With a scanner and the aid of computational biomedicine, the label signal intensity (mRNA abundance) may be calculated. By comparing various samples used for derivation of mRNA, the mRNA abundance can be compared, generating an expression profile, called the *transcriptome*, for the cell or tissue of interest; however, it is estimated that fewer than one-half of changes in mRNA are translated into changes at the protein level. Proteomic analysis may thus be more valuable for characterization, but unlike nucleotides, amino acids are more difficult to characterize,

## TABLE 19-2

| Rates of Healthcare-Associated Pneumonia and Catheter-Related Blood Stream Infection Among Various ICU Types. National Nosocomial Infection Surveillance System, U.S. Centers for Disease Control and Prevention | | | | |
|---|---|---|---|---|
| ICU TYPE | CVC USE | CR-BSI RATE (Mean/ Median) | TT USE | VAP RATE (Mean/ Median) |
| Medical | 0.52 | 5.0/3.9 | 0.46 | 4.9/3.7 |
| Pediatric | 0.46 | 6.6/5.2 | 0.39 | 2.9/2.3 |
| Surgical | 0.61 | 4.6/3.4 | 0.44 | 9.3/8.3 |
| Cardiovascular | 0.79 | 2.7/1.8 | 0.43 | 7.2/6.3 |
| Neurosurgical | 0.48 | 4.6/3.1 | 0.39 | 11.2/6.2 |
| Trauma | 0.61 | 7.4/5.2 | 0.56 | 15.2/11.4 |

CVC Use: Number of days of catheter placement/1000 patient-days in ICU.

CR-BSI: Catheter-related blood stream infection.

TT Use: Number of days of indwelling endotracheal tube or tracheostomy/1000 patient-days in ICU.

VAP: Ventilator-associated pneumonia.

Infection rates are indexed per 1000 patient-days.

Data available at www.cdc.gov, and are in the public domain

Adapted from: National Nosocomial Infections Surveillance (NNIS) System report, data summary from January 1992–June 2004, issued October 2004. Am J Infect Control 232:470, 2004.

## TABLE 19-4

| Principal Hormonal Responses to Surgical Stress | | |
|---|---|---|
| ENDOCRINE GLAND | HORMONES | CHANGE IN SECRETION |
| Anterior pituitary | | |
| | ACTH | Increased |
| | Growth hormone | Increased |
| | TSH | Variable |
| | FSH/LH | Variable |
| Posterior pituitary | | |
| | AVP | Increased |
| Adrenal cortex | | |
| | Cortisol | Increased |
| | Aldosterone | Increased |
| Pancreas | | |
| | Insulin | Decreased |
| | Glucagon | Increased |
| Thyroid | | |
| | Thyroxine | Decreased |
| | Triiodothyronine | Decreased |

ACTH, adrenocorticotropic hormone; AVP, arginine vasopressin; FSH, follicle-stimulating hormone; LH, luteinizing hormone; TSH, thyroid-stimulating hormone.

## TABLE 19-5

### Immune Dysfunction after Trauma

**Specific Immunity**
- Lymphopenia
- Helper: Suppressor T-cell ratio <1
- Downregulated:
  - T, B cell proliferation
  - NK cell activity
  - IL-2 receptor expression
  - IL-4, -10 production
  - HLA-DR expression
  - DTH skin test response

**Nonspecific Immunity**
- Monocytosis
- Upregulated:
  - Acute-phase proteins
  - TNFα, IL-6 production
  - Eicosanoid production
- Downregulated:
  - Neutrophil function

NK: Natural killer cell, IL: Interleukin, HLA: Human leukocyte antigen.
DTH: Delayed topical hypersensitivity, TNF: Tumor necrosis factor.

## TABLE 19-7

### Glucose Dyshomeostasis during Stress and Effects on Cellular Immunity

**Effects of Stress Response Upon Carbohydrate Metabolism**
Enhanced peripheral glucose uptake/utilization
Hyperlactatemia
Increased gluconeogenesis
Depressed glycogenolysis
Peripheral insulin resistance

**Effects of Hyperglycemia Upon Immune Cell Function**
Decreased respiratory burst of alveolar macrophages
Decreased insulin-stimulated chemokinesis
Glucose-induced protein kinase C activation
Increased adherence
Increased adhesion molecule generation
Spontaneous activation of neutrophils

largely because of their biochemical heterogeneity and post-translational modification. As a result, the development of "protein chips" has lagged.

Such techniques have been used to further the understanding of host predisposition and response to sepsis and may enable the development of more effective diagnosis and therapy.[27,28] Reduced T-cell proliferation has been confirmed after severe injury, along with increased cell surface receptors of negative signaling receptors.[29] Therefore, application of cell separation, genome-wide expression, and cell-specific pathway analyses can be used to characterize alterations in human disease for earlier identification and intervention.

In infection, genomic variability may correlate with disease susceptibility. *Single nucleotide polymorphisms* (SNPs), single point-mutations in the nucleotide structures of genes related to inflammation (e.g., tumor necrosis factor-alpha, interleukins–1, –6, and –8), the anti-inflammatory response (e.g., interleukin–10, interleukin–1 receptor antagonist), the innate immune response response

(e.g., Toll-like receptor 4), and the coagulation system (e.g., factor V, plasminogen activator inhibitor-1) have been identified and associated with predisposition to sepsis and provide important insights into the pathogenesis of sepsis-induced organ dysfunction.[30] Complex genetic heterogeneity in the immune response and predisposition to infection, as well as its severity and related mortality, make conclusions difficult to draw, especially in that many reported associations have been made in small populations of patients. The impact of allelic variants in multiple genes on clinical outcomes makes it unlikely that a single SNP will be identifiable in an individual patient to characterize risk or outcome. When multiple SNPs act together in the presence of infection, the disease pheotype associated with a specific outcome, such as increased risk of death, may become apparent using new analytical tools. A recently developed genome-wide SNP genotyping assay may facilitate the identification of genotypes associated with specific clinical outcomes.[31]

## Interactions Between the Host and Therapy

The risk of infection may exist as the result of injury itself, resuscitation, or definitive care. Hypothermia may occur as the result of exposure, large-volume infusion of unwarmed fluids or blood products, or evaporative losses during intracavitary surgery, especially if more than one body cavity has been opened. Hypothermia causes peripheral and cutaneous vasoconstriction in an attempt to preserve core heat. Vasoconstriction decreases microcirculatory blood flow, which may also be disrupted by hypovolemia, the inflammatory response, activation of coagulation, and the decreased deformability of transfused red blood cells.[32] Also, hypothermia increases mortality after multiple trauma.[33]

Tissue hypoxia after trauma may result from injury to the facial bones, airways, lungs, or chest wall; inability to secure the airway; massive blood loss; cardiovascular instability; disruption of the microcirculation; or ARDS. Tissue hypoxia may predispose to surgical site infection (SSI),[34] and administration of supplemental oxygen ($F_IO_2$, 0.8) has reduced the risk of SSI after elective surgery in two randomized, prospective studies (reviewed in ref. 35).

The manner of resuscitation may influence outcome. Fluids are necessary to restore hemodynamics and microcirculatory perfusion, but the quantity and type of fluid that should be administered is

## TABLE 19-6

### Medical Conditions Known to Increase the Risk of Infection

Extremes of age
Malnutrition
Obesity
Diabetes mellitus
Prior site irradiation
Hypothermia
Hypoxemia
Remote infection
Corticosteroid therapy
Recent operation, especially of the chest or abdomen
Chronic inflammation
Hypocholesterolemia

still debated. Crystalloid fluids remain preferable to colloids, being less expensive with results that are at least equivalent.[36] Early, small-volume resuscitation with hypertonic saline (HTS, 7.5% NaCl) is gaining interest, not only because of early restoration of hemodynamics, but also because HTS may attenuate the pro-inflammatory response.[37] Functionally, resuscitation of the immune system may be crucial, as evidenced by observations that a persistent systemic inflammatory response after injury is associated with an increased risk of nosocomial infection and death.[38]

Blood transfusion can be lifesaving after trauma, but an increased risk of infection is clearly recognized following transfusion of trauma patients. Transfusions are believed to exert immunosuppressive effects through presentation of leukocyte antigens and the induction of a shift to the T-helper 2 (immunosuppressive) phenotype; however, the mechanism remains somewhat controversial because transfusion of leukocyte-depleted red blood cell concentrates does not reduce the risk of infection.[39] In a landmark study, Nichols et al.[40] identified risk factors for infection after penetrating abdominal trauma by multivariate analysis of data from patients who received prophylactic antibiotics. Although factors such as four or more organs injured (odds ratio [OR] 10.5, 95% confidence interval [CI] 2.4–46.9), left colon injury (OR 5.7, 95% CI 2.2–14.3), and shock (OR 3.6, 95% CI 1.4–8.9) were predictors of infection,[40] the risk of infection increased significantly by 5% for each unit of blood transfused. In a retrospective multicenter multivariate analysis of 5366 patients (incidence of infection, 15%), Agarwal et al.[41] identified the number of blood transfusions to be the most powerful predictor of infection following trauma, both overall and after stratification for severity of injury (Table 19-8).[41] Claridge et al. identified an exponential relationship between transfusion risk and infection risk among trauma patients, detectable with even one unit of transfusion and becoming a virtual certainty after more than 15 units of transfused blood (RR 1.084, 95% CI 1.028–1.142).[42] Hill et al. have estimated by meta-analysis the risk of infection related to blood transfusion to be increased for trauma patients by more than five-fold (OR 5.26, 95% CI 5.03–5.43).[43] This increased risk for infection by transfusion has also been identified for critically ill patients in general,[44] and for CR-BSI[45] and ventilator-associated pneumonia (VAP)[46] specifically.

Banked blood is affected by a "storage lesion" characterized by loss of membrane 2–3 diphosphoglycerate and adenosine triphosphate, leading to loss of membrane deformability.[47] As a result, erythrocytes cannot deform as they must to transit the microcirculation, causing disruption of nutrient blood flow and impairment of oxygen offloading. Consequently, blood transfusion does not increase oxygen consumption for critically ill patients with sepsis[48] and, in fact, may actually increase the risk of organ dysfunction.[49] The storage lesion becomes fully manifest after about 14 days of storage; therefore, transfusion of older blood is an independent risk factor for the development of infection.[50] Unfortunately, no alternative to blood yet exists, but it is safe to be more conservative in the administration of red blood cell concentrates, especially for stable patients in the ICU.[51]

## PREVENTION

No single method of prevention is universally effective, thus a number of prevention methods are used. Even if all available modalities are utilized for every patient and executed perfectly, infection may still occur. Traumatic wounds must be cleansed thoroughly and debrided as needed to remove devitalized tissue. Surgical incisions must be handled gently, inspected daily, and dressed if necessary using aseptic technique. Drains and catheters must be avoided if possible and removed as soon as possible if needed. Prophylactic and therapeutic antibiotics should be used sparingly so as to decrease the development of antibiotic-resistant pathogens.

### Reducing the Risk of Infection

Infection control is often sacrificed under the often-chaotic conditions of trauma resuscitation, but this is not necessary (see below). Endotracheal tubes should be kept sterile until the moment of intubation. Central venous catheters inserted under suboptimal conditions (i.e., lack of cap, mask, sterile gown, or sterile gloves for the operator, lack of a full-bed drape for the patient) must be removed and replaced (if necessary) by a new puncture at a new site as soon as the patient's condition permits. Detailed evidence-based guidelines for the prevention of infection have been developed by the Centers for Disease Control and Prevention (CDC).[52,53] Evidence-based guidelines for the prevention of ventilator-associated pneumonia have been published, as well.[54,55]

Control of Blood Sugar.    Hyperglycemia is deleterious to host immune function as it impairs function of neutrophils and mononuclear phagocytes and may also reflect the catabolism and insulin resistance associated with the surgical stress response. Poor control of blood glucose in the perioperative period increases the risk of infection and worsens outcome from sepsis. Diabetic patients undergoing cardiopulmonary bypass surgery have a higher risk of infection of both the sternal incision and the vein harvest incisions on the lower extremities.[56] Moderate hyperglycemia (>200 mg/dL) at any time on the first postoperative day increases the risk of SSI fourfold after cardiac[57] and noncardiac surgery.[58] The infusion of insulin to keep blood glucose concentrations <110 mg/dL was associated with a 40% decrease in mortality among critically ill postoperative patients, who also had fewer nosocomial infections and less organ dysfunction in one study.[59] Meta-analysis of 35 existing trials indicates that the risk of mortality is decreased significantly (RR 0.85, 95% CI 0.75–0.97) by tight glucose control, especially so for critically ill surgical patients (RR 0.58, 95% CI, 0.22–0.62), regardless of whether the patients had

**TABLE 19-8**

| Blood Transfusion and the Risk of Infection (%) | | | | |
|---|---|---|---|---|
| **INJURY SEVERITY SCORE** | **UNITS TRANSFUSED** | | | |
| | **0** | **1–2** | **3–7** | **>8** |
| 1–10 | 7 | 24 | 34 | 73 |
| 11–24 | 10 | 24 | 31 | 45 |
| >25 | 37 | 54 | 37 | 59 |
| **Overall** | **9** | **27** | **34** | **57** |

Adapted from: Agarwal N, Murphy JG, Cayten CG, et al.: WM:Blood transfusion increases the risk of infection after trauma. Arch Surg 128:171, 1993.

diabetes mellitus (RR 0.71, 95% CI 0.54–0.93) or stress-induced hyperglycemia (RR 0.73, 95% CI 0.58–0.90).[60]

Nutritional support is also essential, considering that trauma patients are catabolic and that restoration of anabolic conditions requires the provision of calories and nitrogen far in excess of basal requirements of 25–30 kcal and 1 g nitrogen/kg/day. In the midst of the stress response, it may be challenging to provide sufficient calories and protein while also preventing hyperglycemia. Parenteral nutrition appears to convey no advantage over not feeding the patient at all,[61] perhaps because of the inherent infectious morbidity of central intravenous feeding (i.e, the risk of CR-BSI) and hyperglycemia. In contrast, early enteral feeding (within the first 48 hours and, perhaps, immediately if the gut is functional), is unquestionably beneficial, with the possible exception of preventing pneumonia prevention (see below). Marik and Zaloga[62] found that the risk of infection was reduced by 55% (OR 0.45, 95% CI 0.30–0.66) and that total hospital stay was reduced by a mean of 2.2 days (95% CI 0.81–3.63 days) in a meta-analysis of 15 randomized trials of early enteral feeding following surgery, trauma, or burns.

Infection Control.    Hand hygiene is the single most effective means to reduce the spread of infection, yet, whenever studied, it is invariably found to be underutilized. To be effective, hand cleansing with soap and water requires a minimum of 30–45 seconds. Alcohol gel hand cleansers are as effective as soap and water, compliance with use is higher, and,when used, the prevalence of multi-drug-resistant (MDR) bacteria is reduced.[63] Universal precautions (i.e., cap, mask, gown, gloves, and protective eyewear) must be observed whenever there is a risk of splashing of body fluids (at all times in the trauma bay and the operating room, and commonly in the ICU).

The source of most pathogenic bacteria is the patient's endogenous flora. Skin surfaces, artificial airways, gut lumen, wounds, catheters, and inanimate surfaces within the patient's room (e.g., bed rails, computer terminals) may all become colonized. Any break in natural epithelial barriers (e.g., incisions, percutaneous catheters, airway or urinary catheters) creates a portal of entry for invasion of a host by pathogens. The fecal-oral route is the most common manner by which pathogens reach the portal, but healthcare workers definitely can facilitate the transmission of pathogens around a unit. Whether infection develops subsequently is determined by complex interactions among host defenses, pathogen, and therapy. Many organisms that cause infection following injury are inherently avirulent (e.g., *Candida, Enterococcus, Pseudomonas*).

Contact isolation is an important part of infection control and should be used selectively to prevent the spread of pathogens such as methicillin-resistant *S. aureus* (MRSA), vancomycin-resistant enterococci (VRE), or MDR gram-negative bacilli. Contact isolation may decrease the amount of time that caregivers have direct patient contact, however, because the process of donning protective garb is time-consuming. By guarding against this phenomenon, an appropriate balance can be struck between attention and protection.

## Catheter Care

Optimal catheter care includes avoidance of use when unnecessary, appropriate skin cleansing and barrier protection during insertion, proper catheter selection, proper dressing of indwelling catheters, and removal as soon as possible when no longer needed. The benefit of the information gained by catheterization must always be weighed against the risk of infection.

Almost any indwelling catheter carries a risk of infection, but nontunnelled central venous catheters (and pulmonary artery catheters) pose the highest risk, including local site infections and CR-BSIs. Other catheters that pose increased infection risk include intercostal thoracostomy catheters (if inserted as an emergency procedure), ventriculostomy catheters for monitoring of intracranial pressure, and urinary bladder catheters. Each day of endotracheal intubation and mechanical ventilation increases the risk of pneumonia, and it is controversial whether tracheostomy decreases that risk. In terms of preventing infection, abdominal drains are superfluous.

Whenever possible, chlorhexidine (which is bactericidal, viricidal, and fungicidal) should be used for skin preparation for insertion of vascular catheters. Chlorhexidine is superior to povidone-iodine solution for skin preparation prior to central venous catheter insertion.[64] If povidone-iodine solution is used, it must be allowed to dry, as it is not bactericidal when wet. Full barrier precautions (i.e., cap, mask, sterile gown, sterile gloves, eye protection, and a large field drape) are mandatory for all bedside catheterization procedures[53] except for insertion of arterial and bladder catheters, for which sterile gloves and a sterile field suffice. Any time a central venous catheter is inserted under less than ideal conditions it must be removed (and replaced at a different site if still needed) as soon as permitted by the patient's hemodynamic status, but no more than 24 hours after insertion. A single dose of a first-generation cephalosporin (e.g., cefazolin), but no more, may prevent some infections following emergency insertion of thoracostomy tubes or ventriculostomies, but is not indicated for vascular or bladder catheterizations. Topical antiseptics placed postprocedure at the insertion site are of no benefit in preventing infection for any type of indwelling catheter.

Dressings must be maintained clean, dry, and intact.[65] Maintaining integrity of dressings may be no small accomplishment when the patient is agitated or the body surface is irregular (e.g., the neck [internal jugular vein catheterization] as opposed to the chest wall [subclavian vein catheterization]). A simple gauze dressing may be best, because occlusive transparent dressings can accumulate moisture that is a growth medium for residual skin flora that can recolonize the skin within a few hours. Marking the dressing clearly with the date and time of each change is simple, effective, and mandatory. Dressing carts should not be brought from patient to patient, and sufficient supplies should be kept in each patient's room. The possibility for inanimate objects (e.g., stethoscopes, scissors) to be transmission vectors if not cleansed thoroughly after contact with each patient must be borne in mind, as well. Finally, dedicated catheter care teams reduce the risk of CR-BSI substantially.

The choice of catheter may play a role in decreasing the risk of infection related to endotracheal tubes, central venous catheters, and urinary catheters. Continuous aspiration of subglottic secretions (CASS), via an endotracheal tube with an extra lumen that opens to the airway just above the balloon, facilitates the aspiration of secretions that accumulate below the vocal cords but above the endotracheal tube balloon. This is an area that cannot be reached by routine suctioning. The incidence of VAP is decreased by one-half by CASS.[66] Silver-impregnated endotracheal tubes are effective in reducing colonization of the airway, but whether the incidence of VAP is reduced is not yet known.[67] Antibiotic- (e.g., minocycline/rifampin) or antiseptic-coated central venous catheters (e.g, chlorhexidine/silver sulfadiazine) are effective in reducing the incidence of catheter-related blood stream infection,[68] especially in high-prevalence units; of interest, the catheters coated with minocycline/rifampin appear to be more effective. Urinary bladder catheters coated with ionic silver reduce the incidence of catheter-related bacterial cystitis by a similar amount.[69]

Every indwelling catheter must be evaluated daily for its continued utility and removed immediately when no longer needed. Protocolized ventilator weaning facilitated by daily cessation of sedation and trials of spontaneous breathing allow earlier endotracheal extubation and decrease the risk of VAP.[70] An even better strategy may be avoidance of catheterization entirely. Some episodes of respiratory failure can be managed with noninvasive positive-pressure ventilation delivered by mask (e.g., continuous positive airway pressure [CPAP]).[71] Improved resuscitation techniques and noninvasive monitoring techniques have decreased the utilization of pulmonary artery flotation catheters, which pose an especially high risk of infection.[72] Most drains do not decrease the risk of infection; in fact, the risk is probably increased[73] because the catheters hold open a portal for invasion by bacteria. Other than for hepatic or pancreatic injuries, abdominal drains are seldom useful as noted previously.

## Antibiotic Prophylaxis

The general principles of antibiotic prophylaxis apply to trauma care as well. Prophylactic antibiotics are used to prevent infection of a wound or surgical site. Prolonged antibiotic prophylaxis does not prevent deep space/intracavitary surgical site infections nor nosocomial infections, but rather selects for more-resistant pathogens when infection does develop.[73] These will occur at an increased rate after prolonged prophylaxis.[74] The antibiotic chosen should be safe and narrowly efficacious against the pathogens of concern (e.g., gram-positive cocci for skin/soft tissue wounds, aerobic and anaerobic gram-negative bacilli for penetrating abdominal trauma with suspected hollow viscus injury). Preoperative antibiotic prophylaxis is given so that tissue concentration is maximized at the time of incision and maintained for the duration of the operation.[75]

The principles of antibiotic pharmacokinetics (PK) must be adhered to (see below), but several circumstances complicate the administration of prophylactic antibiotics after trauma. Vasoconstriction may cause poor tissue penetration of the antibiotic. Ongoing blood loss may cause ongoing antibiotic loss, especially if the antibiotic is highly protein-bound and slow to distribute to tissues. Tissue edema will increase for the first 48–72 hours after injury, changing the volume of distribution ($V_d$) of many antibiotics unpredictably. Dosing may have to be higher to ensure an adequate tissue concentration with increased $V_d$. On the other hand, fluid administration and tissue edema, combined with the effects of the negative acute-phase response, result in hypoalbuminemia. Hypoalbuminemia, in turn, reduces protein binding, increasing free drug concentrations of highly protein-bound drugs.

Some are of the opinion that trauma patients need higher doses of antibiotics for prophylaxis. The answer is unclear, and data are scant. Most PK studies of antibiotic prophylaxis of trauma are dated and examine the use of aminoglycosides, which are seldom used for prophylaxis anymore. Those early studies did suggest that higher doses of aminoglycosides were warranted for prophylaxis,[76] but the modern relevance of those studies is questionable. One contemporary study shows that cefoxitin 1 g is sufficient for prophylaxis after penetrating abdominal trauma.[77]

Reasonably definitive dosing recommendations can be made for cases of penetrating abdominal trauma, which has been well studied. Evidence-based guidelines of the Eastern Association for the Surgery of Trauma (EAST)[78] recommend only a single dose of antibiotic (i.e., second-generation cephalosporin) when there is not an injury to a hollow viscus. Unfortunately, supplies of second-generation cephalosporins are now uncertain. Whether a comparably safe and efficacious choice for single-agent antibiotic prophylaxis of penetrating abdominal trauma will be identified will require prospective investigation. Recognized risk factors for infection following hollow viscus injury include preoperative shock, injury to the colon, the number of injured abdominal organs, injury to the central nervous system, and blood transfusion.[77] When a hollow viscus injury is present, antibiotic prophylaxis should be continued for only 24 hours (longer courses are nonbeneficial and may be harmful, even in the presence of colon injury).[79] It is uncertain whether higher doses should be administered in the presence of shock.[78]

The risk of infection following soft tissue injury is reasonably well defined, but not the duration of prophylaxis. In a retrospective review of 1436 wounds, 1054 of which were abdominal and 382 were in an extremity, Weigelt found the incidence of infection among 331 clean wounds to be 3.2%,[80] whereas 10.5% of 855 clean-contaminated wounds and 24.8% of contaminated wounds became infected. Similarly, a prospective study of 5521 traumatic lacerations repaired in the emergency department (ED) identified an overall rate of infection of 3.5%.[81] The risk factors for the development of infection of repaired minor lacerations were diabetes mellitus (OR 6.9, 95% confidence interval [CI] 1.7–26.4), presence of a foreign body (OR 2.6, 95% CI 1.3–5.2), wound width (per mm) (OR 1.05, 95% CI 1.02–1.08, and age (per year) (OR 1.01, 95% CI 1.00–1.30). Lacerations of the head and neck were significantly less likely to become infected (OR 0.28, 95% CI 0.18–0.45). Although identification of an individual patient as high risk may prompt consideration of antibiotic prophylaxis of a clean wound, antibiotics are probably not necessary for clean lacerations in the extremities that are repaired promptly, according to one prospective, randomized trial.[82] On the other hand, a meta-analysis of eight randomized, placebo-controlled trials of penicillin or macrolide prophylaxis of dog bite wounds showed an infection rate of 16% in control patients, and significant reductions after antibiotic prophylaxis overall (OR 0.56, 95% CI 0.38–0.82), especially for wounds of the hand (OR 0.23, 95% CI 0.05–0.95).[83] The appropriate duration of antibiotic administration was not clearly answered in this study. Human bites, which are much more likely than dog bites to be inoculated with pathogens, should receive empiric therapeutic antibiotics for presumed infection.

Antibiotic prophylaxis of other injuries is less well supported by data. For closed long-bone fractures, a single dose of antibiotic reduced the risk of infection (surgical site infection, urinary tract infection, respiratory tract infection) by 60% (OR 0.40, 95% CI 0.24–0.67) in one trial, but no advantage was conferred by additional doses.[84] Likewise, a single dose of antibiotics was equivalent to five days of prophylaxis for Grade I/II open tibial fractures in a randomized, double-blind trial.[85] Unfortunately, data are lacking

**TABLE 19-9**

## Summary of Evidence-Based Recommendations for Antibiotic Prophylaxis of Open Fractures

**Eastern Association for the Surgery of Trauma[87]**

*Level I:*

Preoperative antibiotic prophylaxis for coverage of gram-positive organisms should be begun for patients with open fractures as soon as possible after injury. For Grade III fractures, additional coverage for gram-negative organisms should be given.

High-dose penicillin should be added when there is a concern for fecal/clostridial contamination, such as in farm-related injuries.

*Level II:*

Antibiotics should be discontinued 24 h after wound closure for Grade I and II fractures.

Antibiotics should be continued for Grade III fractures for only 72 h after injury, or not more than 24 h after soft tissue coverage of the wound is achieved, whichever occurs first.

**Surgical Infection Society[88]**

*Level I:*

No prophylactic antibiotics are required for open fractures resulting from low-velocity civilian gunshot wounds that do not require open reduction and internal fixation.

Administration of a first-generation cephalosporin (or similar agent active against gram-positive bacteria) for 24–48 h perioperatively is safe and effective prophylactic choice for patients with Grade I open fractures.

*Level II:*

Administration of a first-generation cephalosporin (or similar agent active against gram-positive bacteria) for 48 h perioperatively is safe and effective prophylactic choice for patients with Grade II and III open extremity fractures.

*Level III:*

A single broad-spectrum agent given pre-operatively and extended for 48 h post-operatively is safe and effective prophylactic option for patients with Grade II and III open fractures.

**Other recommendations:**

There are insufficient data to:

Conclude that antibiotics directed specifically against gram-negative bacteria are beneficial routinely as prophylaxis in any open fracture.

Conclude that pediatric patients require different antibiotic regimens than adult patients.

Conclude that prophylactic penicillin should be administered routinely to patients receiving other indicated prophylaxis for open fractures with *Clostridium*-prone wounds

Recommend routine placement of antibiotic beads in any open fracture

Recommend that antibiotic therapy be based on routine wound cultures obtained either at presentation or during subsequent operative procedures.

---

regarding appropriate prophylaxis of Grade III open extremity fractures, where the risk of both soft tissue infections and osteomyelitis may be increased. The current standard regimen of 72 hours of cefazolin plus gentamicin is based on retrospective data from the 1970s, and the one contemporary prospective study to examine the issue[86] is underpowered for these high-risk injuries. The EAST guidelines[87] (Table 19-9) acknowledge the weakness of the data, providing only a Level II recommendation to cover open grade I–II fractures for 24 hours and open grade III fractures for 72 hours, or for 24 hours after wound closure, whichever comes first. The Surgical Infection Society (SIS) guidelines for antibiotic prophylaxis of open fractures reviewed a nearly identical group of studies. Using a more rigorous methodology, they reached conclusions that are even more circumspect about the value of prophylaxis of open fractures for more than 24 hours or with an agent of broader spectrum than a first-generation cephalosporin[88] (Table 19-9).

There are almost no data to inform the clinician regarding antibiotic prophylaxis of thoracic trauma. The pathogenesis of pneumonia is seldom related directly to the injury to the lung; therefore, the infection that is to be prevented is empyema, which has such a low incidence that scientific study is difficult. Antibiotic prophylaxis of tube thoracostomy for trauma with 24 hours of a first-generation cephalosporin has been recommended by EAST, but only as a Level III recommendation.[89]

There are also few data regarding antibiotic prophylaxis of traumatic brain injury. Among 215 patients with intracranial pressure monitors, the infection rate of 7.5% was not reduced by prophylaxis. The major risk factors for infection included the presence of a cerebrospinal fluid (CSF) leak (OR 6.3, 95% CI 1.5–27.4), serial device placement (OR 4.9, 95% CI 1.7–13.8), and duration of monitoring greater than five days (OR 4.4, 95% CI 1.3–11.9).[90] In a meta-analysis of 12 studies of 1241 patients with basilar skull fracture,[91] 58% of whom received antibiotic prophylaxis, antibiotics did not prevent meningitis overall (OR 1.15, 95% CI 0.68–1.94), among patients with a CSF leak (OR 1.34, 95 CI 0.75–2.41), or among pediatric patients (OR 1.04, 95% 0.07–14.90).

## VACCINATION OF INJURED PATIENTS

Nearly any antigen can be prepared for use as a vaccine. The difficulties are in identifying protective antigens and persuading the immune system to respond correctly to them. Over the last 200 years, success has been achieved in controlling major infectious diseases predominantly by vaccinating with attenuated living or inactivated organisms, inactivated toxoids, and bacterial capsular polysaccharides. There are limited data on the current use of vaccines after injury. The utility of rabies and tetanus vaccines after injury is poorly documented.[92,93] Recent evidence-based recommendations of the SIS provide some clarity[94] (Table 19-10).

**TABLE 19-10**

## Surgical Infection Society Evidence-Based Recommendations for Vaccination of Injured Patients

### Rabies

*Pre-exposure Prophylaxis*

Vaccination should be provided to persons at risk (laboratory workers, diagnosticians, veterinarians and their staffs, animal control officers, rabies researchers, and some travelers to areas where rabies is prevalent (Grade A))

*Post-exposure Prophylaxis*

A five-dose regimen is recommended. Five one-milliliter doses of vaccine are given intramuscularly (deltoid muscle) on days 0, 3, 7, 14, and 28 in conjunction with a single dose of human rabies immune globulin (HRIG) 20 IU/kg infiltrated into the wound on day 0. Any remaining HRIG should be administered IM at a site distant from the vaccine site (Grade D)

### Anthrax

*Pre-exposure Prophylaxis*

Vaccination may be indicated for veterinarians and other high-risk persons handling potentially infected animals in areas with a high incidence of anthrax. Routine vaccination of emergency first-responders, federal responders, medical practitioners, and private citizens is not recommended (Grade B)

*Post-exposure Prophylaxis*

Administration of the vaccine and antibiotics against *B. anthracis* is recommended following an aerosol exposure to spores. Post-exposure vaccination should be administered as three injections of vaccine, beginning as soon as possible, at 0, 2, and 4 weeks (Grade E)

### Tetanus

*Prophylaxis of Acute Wound*

Administration of tetanus immune globulin (HTIG) 250 IU is recommended only for patients with tetanus-prone wounds who have never completed a primary immunization series. The HTIG should be given at a site different from the tetanus toxoid to avoid interaction (Grade B)

For small children, the routine dose of HTIG may be calculated by body weight (4 IU/kg). However, it may be advisable to administer the entire 250 IU, because theoretically, the same amount of toxin will be produced in a child's as in an adult's body (Grade B)

If a patient with an acute soft tissue injury has not been immunized previously, a tetanus toxoid booster is required. The patient must have followup to complete the series. If the patient has been immunized previously, a booster dose is given if the last dose was more than five years previously (for a tetanus-prone wound) or more than 10 years previously (for a non-tetanus-prone wound). Patients with a contraindication to tetanus toxoid must be managed with HTIG alone (Grade B)

*Immunization of High-risk Persons*

The elderly, HIV-infected, or otherwise immunocompromised patient may not respond adequately to vaccination alone. More liberal use of HTIG may be warranted for these patients, regardless of primary immunization status. More frequent dosing of tetanus toxoid may help to sustain adequate antibody titers (Grade E)

Intravenous drug users may present with complaints unrelated to acute wounds. However, their drug use should be considered a risk factor that requires consideration of tetanus prophylaxis (Grade E)

### Vaccination After Splenectomy

The 23-valent polysaccharide pneumococcal vaccine is recommended for persons 2 to 64 years of age who have functional or anatomic asplenia (Grade D)

High-risk individuals should be considered for vaccination with *Haemophilus influenzae* type b conjugate vaccine (Grade D)

Asplenic patients should receive meningococcal vaccine (Grade D)

*Timing and Redosing*

For patients undergoing elective splenectomy, vaccination should be performed at least two weeks before surgery to maximize the antibody response against T-cell-dependent immunogens (Grade C)

Patients who undergo emergency splenectomy should receive immunizations 14 days postoperatively (Grade D)

A single revaccination with the 23-valent polysaccharide pneumococcal vaccine should be given at least five years after the first dose. No further dosing is recommended routinely (Grade D). There is currently no recommendation to revaccinate for *H. influenzae* type b or meningococcus

*Vaccination of Children Younger than Five Years*

The 7-valent pneumococcal conjugate vaccine is recommended for all children 24 to 59 months of age who are at high risk for invasive pneumococcal infection. High-risk children include those with sickle cell disease and other types of functional or anatomic asplenia

For high-risk children 24 to 59 months of age who have received no previous dose of either the 23-valent or the 7-valent pneumococcal polysaccharide vaccine, two doses of the 7-valent conjugate vaccine are recommended, to be given at an interval of six to eight weeks, followed by a single injection of the 23-valent vaccine no less than six to eight weeks after the last dose of the 7-valent vaccine. An additional dose of 23-valent vaccine is recommended three to five years after the last dose (Grade D)

High-risk children 24 to 59 months of age should also receive vaccination against meninococcus and *H. influenzae* type b (Grade D)

Antibiotic prophylaxis is recommended for all children with sickle cell disease and functional or anatomic asplenia, regardless of whether they have received pneumococcal immunization (Grade B)

Oral penicillin V potassium is recommended in a dose of 125 mg twice a day, until three years of age and in a dose of 250 mg twice a day after three years of age. Children who have not experienced invasive pneumococcal infection and have received recommended pneumococcal immunizations may discontinue penicillin *prophylaxis after five years of age* (Grade B)

Adapted from: Howdieshell TR, Heffernan D, Dipiro JT; Therapeutic Agents Committee of the Surgical Infection Society: Surgical infection society guidelines for vaccination after traumatic injury. Surg Infect 7:275, 2006.

## Rabies

Rabies virus is transmitted in the saliva of infected animals. The infection is widespread in some species and, occasionally, is transmitted to human beings. Over the last 50 years, the incidence of rabies has declined, and human rabies infection is rare in the United States, even though animal bites are encountered frequently. Dog bites alone account for more than 300,000 ED visits annually, with total costs of more than $100 million.[95]

Rabies is almost invariably fatal in the absence of specialized treatment, but is preventable with proper measures, including postexposure prophylaxis, to the point that only 32 cases of human rabies were diagnosed in the United States between 1980 and 1998.[96]

### Postexposure Prophylaxis.

Bites from bats (which can be so small as to go unnoticed) and high-risk wild carnivores such as raccoons, skunks, foxes, bobcats, and coyotes warrant consideration of immediate postexposure prophylaxis. In the case of direct contact with a bat (even in the same room), a bite injury should be considered unless the exposed person can be reasonably certain that one did not occur. An apparently healthy domesticated dog, cat, or ferret that bites a person should be confined and observed, unvaccinated, for ten days. Management of animals kept as pets other than dogs, cats, and ferrets depends on the species, the circumstances of the bite, the local rabies epidemiology, and the biting animal's history, health status, and potential for exposure to rabies, even if vaccinated recently (vaccination of animals is not invariably successful). If the animal is confirmed to have rabies, postexposure prophylaxis should be completed, whereas if the test results are negative within 24–48 hours, postexposure prophylaxis can cease. If testing will take longer, prophylaxis should be started, pending the results of testing.[97]

Rabies postexposure prophylaxis consists of three primary elements including wound care, infiltration of human rabies immune globulin (HRIG), and administration of the vaccine. Immediate, thorough washing of all bite wounds and scratches with soap and water is perhaps the most effective measure for preventing rabies.

The Advisory Committee on Immunization Practices (ACIP) of the CDC recommends a five-dose regimen for postexposure prophylaxis. Five 1-mL doses of Imovax® rabies vaccine are given intramuscularly (I.M.) in the deltoid muscle on days 0, 3, 7, 14, and 28 in conjunction with a single dose of HRIG 20 IU/kg on day 0. As much as possible of the dose of HRIG should be infiltrated into the wound. Any remaining volume should be administered IM at a site distant from the site of vaccination.[98]

## Anthrax

Anthrax is caused by *Bacillus anthracis*, a gram-positive, spore-forming bacillus capable of infecting human and animal hosts. Several factors affect the destructive capabilities of anthrax as a biological weapon. Spores can be spread easily by airborne dissemination, but the anthrax particles can be damaged by an explosion.[99] Particle size also affects virulence and infective potential. When a particle is larger than 5–10 micrometers, infectivity may decrease substantially, as the 8000 to 10,000 spores necessary for infection may not be inhaled. One- to two-micrometer spores are highly lethal, but the creation of stable spores smaller than five micrometers has

not been reported outside state-sponsored laboratories.[99] Also, the concentration of the powder affects its pathogenicity. The most concentrated anthrax known has as many as one trillion spores per gram. Lastly, clumping of spores limits widespread dissemination, but admixture with silica and treatment to offset the electrostatic charge of the particles allows maximum dispersal. Anthrax spores that are smaller than five micrometers, treated to prevent clumping, and then concentrated are referred to as "weapons-grade" anthrax.

### Postexposure Prophylaxis.

Postexposure vaccination should be administered as follows: three injections of vaccine (which is only available routinely to the military), one as soon as possible and the others at two and four weeks. Postexposure prophylaxis with the vaccine and antibiotics against *B. anthracis* are recommended following an aerosol exposure to spores.[100] The ACIP recommends at least a 30-day course of ciprofloxacin or doxycycline postexposure for persons who have been vaccinated partially or fully. Antibiotics should be administered at least until the third vaccine dose is given.[101] Although the shortened vaccine regimen has been effective postexposure when coadministered with antibiotics, the duration of protection from vaccination is not known. Because human-to-human transmission has not been documented, contacts and friends do not need prophylaxis unless they also were exposed to the aerosol.[100]

## Tetanus

Since 1975, fewer than 100 cases of tetanus have been reported annually in the United States and, for the past ten years, the number has averaged less than 50 per year.[101] Because the primary tetanus toxoid (TT) series used for universal immunization of children and the military induces excellent immune memory, booster doses reliably result in a brisk anamnestic antibody response, even when intervals of 20 years or more have elapsed since the last dose. In more than 20 years of CDC data, no deaths have been reported from tetanus among individuals who have been fully immunized at any time.[102]

### Tetanus Prophylaxis of the Acute Wound.

Many characteristics of wounds encountered in the ED render them non-tetanus-prone including those that are recent and linear with sharp edges, well vascularized, and not obviously contaminated or infected. All other wounds are considered tetanus-prone, particularly those resulting from blunt trauma and bites and those that are grossly contaminated or infected. The CDC recommends human tetanus immune globulin (HTIG) 250 IU given at a site separate from the tetanus toxoid (TT) 0.5 mL I.M. to avoid interaction between the two and only for patients with tetanus-prone wounds who have never completed a primary immunization series. In small children, the routine dose of HTIG may be calculated by the body weight (4 IU/kg). It may, however, be advisable to administer the entire 250 IU regardless of the child's size, because theoretically, the same amount of toxin will be produced in a child's as in an adult's body by the infecting organism.

If a patient has not completed a primary immunization series, a tetanus booster is required, and the patient will need follow-up to complete the series. If the patient has had primary immunization, a booster is given if the last dose was more than five years previously with a tetanus-prone wound or more than 10 years previously with a non-tetanus-prone wound. Patients with a contraindication to TT must be managed with HTIG alone.

### Immunization in High-risk Groups.

Patients from certain high-risk groups require special attention, including elderly patients, individuals with human immunodeficiency virus (HIV) infection, and intravenous drug users (IVDUs), as standard prophylaxis may not provide sufficient protection from tetanus. If prophylaxis is indicated, more liberal use of HTIG may be warranted to ensure protection against tetanus, regardless of primary immunization status. More frequent dosing of TT may help sustain antibody concentrations in the protective range, but official guidelines do not endorse such an approach. HTIG and TT are safe, however, whereas the morbidity and mortality associated with acute tetanus are considerable.[103] Intravenous drug users are a burgeoning group at high risk for tetanus. They accounted for 18% of all cases of tetanus between 1995 and 1997 but only 2.1–4.5% of the cases seen between 1982 and 1994.[102] Factors that place IVDUs at risk include low rates of immunization, contaminated drugs, repeated injection wounds under dirty conditions, and formation of skin abscesses and chronic ulcers, which provide ideal conditions for tetanus development.[102]

## Post-Splenectomy Vaccination

### Overwhelming Post-Splenectomy Infection (OPSI).

Overwhelming post-splenectomy infection is a fulminant, life-threatening condition that may occur even years after splenectomy. The precise incidence of OPSI remains controversial. Published estimates vary because of different definitions of disease, duration of follow-up, stratification for age, indication for splenectomy, and underlying disease.[104]

The risk of post-splenectomy sepsis is highest in children, especially those under two years of age. There are, however, reported cases 20 to 40 years after splenectomy.[105] A collective critical review of the literature on OPSI from 1952 to 1987 estimated the incidence in children under 16 years of age at 4.4% with a mortality rate of 2.2%. The corresponding figures for adults were 0.9% and 0.8%. The incidence of sepsis after splenectomy caused by trauma was 15.7% in infants and 10.4% in children younger than 5 years.[106] Splenectomy performed for a hematologic disorder such as thalassemia, hereditary spherocytosis, or lymphoma carries a higher risk than splenectomy performed as a result of trauma. A potential contributor to the lower rate of infection after splenectomy for trauma is the frequent existence of splenic implants or accessory spleens.[107]

The time since splenectomy is also an important risk factor. Several studies have shown that 50–70% of admissions to the hospital for serious infections occur within the first two years. In splenectomized young children, 80% of OPSI cases occur within this time[108]; however, some degree of risk persists indefinitely. There are individual cases of OPSI reported more than 40 years after splenectomy[104]; also, 33% of post-splenectomy pneumococcal infections and 42% of OPSI occur more than five years post-splenectomy.

Most OPSIs are caused by encapsulated bacteria. Pneumococcal infections account for approximately 50–90% of reported cases, with a mortality rate as high as 60%. *Haemophilus influenzae* type b,

*Neisseria meningitidis,* and Group A *Streptococcus* account for an additional 25% of infections. *Haemophilus* infections are particularly important in children. Others are Group B streptococci, *Enterococcus* spp., *Bacteroides* spp., and *Pseudomonas aeruginosa.*

### Evidence-Based Recommendations.

The ACIP recommends the use of the 23-valent polysaccharide pneumococcal vaccine for persons 2 to 64 years of age who have functional or anatomic asplenia.[109] Because the true incidence of OPSI is unknown, the efficacy of vaccination cannot be ascertained precisely. True vaccine failures are uncommon.[110] Vaccination against *H. influenzae* type b should also be considered using the conjugate vaccine.[111] Meningococcal vaccination will not eliminate risk because the vaccine does not protect against serotype B and because protection against serogroups C and Y is only partial.[112] Nevertheless, those at risk for the disease (including asplenic patients) should be vaccinated.

### Timing.

The timing of immunization after emergency splenectomy for trauma is debated, with conflicting data supporting a variety of recommendations. Part of the problem has stemmed from studies using antibody assays, which may be misleading. Extensive studies in Denmark led to the establishment in 1991 of national guidelines for vaccination and revaccination of splenectomized children and adults.[113] The Danish guidelines recommend that patients undergoing urgent or otherwise unplanned splenectomy be immunized no less than 14 days postoperatively. Waiting two weeks before vaccinating carries the risk of forgetting to vaccinate, but solid data suggest that the antibody response is suboptimal when patients are vaccinated less than 14 days post-splenectomy.[114] Delaying vaccination beyond 14 days did not appear to improve the immune response.

### Revaccination.

The literature documents a variety of revaccination practices. The CDC suggests a single booster dose for those older than two years of age who are at high risk for serious pneumococcal infection and those most likely to have a rapid decline in antibody titers, which includes those with either functional or anatomic asplenia. A single revaccination should be given at least five years after the first dose, with further dosing not recommended routinely. Currenlty, there is no recommendation to revaccinate for either *H. influenzae* type b or meningococcus.[109]

The 7-valent pneumococcal conjugate vaccine (PCV7) is recommended for all children 24–59 months of age who are at high risk for invasive pneumococcal infection, including those with functional or anatomic asplenia.[115] For high-risk children 24–59 months of age who have not received either the 23-valent pneumococcal polysaccharide vaccine or the PCV7, two doses of PCV7 should be given at an interval of six to eight weeks, followed by a single dose of the 23-valent vaccine no less than six to eight weeks after the last dose of PCV7. An additional dose of the 23-valent vaccine is recommended three to five years after the last dose.[115] This age group should also receive vaccination against meningococcus and *H. influenzae* type b. Antibiotic prophylaxis with oral penicillin V potassium 125 mg BID until three years of age and 250 mg BID thereafter is recommended for all children with functional or anatomic asplenia until adulthood, regardless of immunization status.

# MICROBIOLOGY

## Principles of Resistance

In general, bacteria develop resistance to antibiotics by one or more of four different mechanisms.[116–120] Cell wall permeability to antibiotics is decreased by changes in porin channels (especially important for gram-negative bacteria with complex cell walls, affecting aminoglycosides, β-lactam drugs, sulfonamides, tetracyclines, and possibly quinolones). Production of specific antibiotic-inactivating enzymes by either plasmid-mediated or chromosomally-mediated mechanisms affects aminoglycosides, β-lactam drugs, and macrolides. Alteration of the antibiotic binding target in the cell wall affects β-lactam drugs and vancomycin, whereas alteration of target enzymes can affect β-lactam drugs, sulfonamides, and quinolones. Binding to the bacterial ribosome (e.g., aminoglycosides, macrolides, lincosamides, streptogramins, tetracyclines) is susceptible to alteration of the ribosomal receptor. Intracellular antibiotics may be extruded actively by efflux pumps in the cell membrane in the case of macrolides, lincosamines, streptogramins, quinolones, and tetracyclines.

Gram-Positive Cocci.   Gram-positive cocci collectively are the most common causes of infection following injury, having superceded gram-negative bacilli more than 20 years ago. Infections that are most likely caused by gram-positive cocci include those after neurosurgery (e.g., ventriculitis from intracranial pressure monitoring catheters), sinusitis, CR-BSI, device/implant-associated infections, and complicated skin/skin structure infections (cSSSI). Respiratory tract and urinary tract infections may also be caused by gram-positive cocci. Most important among the gram-positive pathogens is *S. aureus*. More than 60% of hospital-acquired isolates of *S. aureus* are MRSA[6]; the incidence of resistance is approaching that among community-acquired strains (CA-MRSA). Staphylococcal resistance to vancomycin is reported but fortunately remains rare and is induced only after prolonged exposure to vancomycin among very debilitated patients (e.g., dialysis patients). *Staphylococcus aureus* is a major pathogen in sinusitis, CR-BSI, cSSSI, and pneumonia. *Staphylococcus epidermidis* is almost invariably resistant to methicillin (MRSE, 85%) and is the major pathogen in CR-BSI and infections associated with device/implants. *Enterococcus* spp. can cause cSSSI, CR-BSI, and infections of the urinary tract. About 30% of enterococci are VRE, but the pattern is species-specific (*E. faecium*, 70% VRE; *E. faecalis* 3%).[6] The incidence of VRE has plateaued, but VRE poses a threat only to debilitated patients after prolonged hospitalization. Fecal colonization with VRE usually precedes invasive infection and cannot be eradicated pharmacologically. Risk factors for VRE acquisition include prolonged hospitalization, re-admission to the ICU, and therapy with vancomycin or third-generation cephalosporins.

Because of the high prevalence of MRSA, vancomycin remains the most-prescribed antibiotic for infection caused by resistant gram-positive cocci, despite poor tissue penetration and the risk of toxicity. Alternatives for therapy[121] include linezolid, tigecycline, daptomycin (but NOT for pneumonia),[122] and quinupristin/dalfopristin (used seldom because of multiple toxicities).

Gram-Negative Bacilli.   Gram-negative bacilli are less common as pathogens after injury, but are important in the pathogenesis of cSSSI (e.g., infected traumatic wound), lower respiratory tract infection, and intra-abdominal infection. Although Enterobacteriaceae such as *E. coli* or *Klebsiella* spp. predominate in intra-abdominal infection, *Pseudomonas aeruginosa* is the second most common ICU pathogen overall and the bacterium most closely associated with death from VAP. *Pseudomonas aeruginosa* can infect virtually any tissue, including synovium and vitreous humor. *Pseudomonas aeruginosa* bacteremia can cause or complicate pneumonia, and other metastatic infections can follow. Antimicrobial resistance is a major, growing problem with *P. aeruginosa*, *Acinetobacter* spp., and *Klebsiella* spp., and increasing among Enterobacteriaceae other than *Klebsiella*.

Cephalosporin resistance among Enterobacteriaceae is often the result of induction of chromosomal β-lactamases after prolonged or repeated antibiotic exposure. Extended-spectrum cephalosporins are rendered ineffective when the bacteria mutate (or are selected clonally) to produce constitutively a β-lactamase that is normally an inducible enzyme. Although resistance to cephalosporins can occur by several mechanisms, chromosomally-mediated extended-spectrum β-lactamase (ESBL) production has been related to use of third-generation cephalosporins. The induction of an ESBL in *Klebsiella* by ceftazidime was first reported 20 years ago, and more than 120 genetic mutations have now been identified in various Enterobacteriaceae, with more identified continuously. Affected bacteria develop resistance rapidly not only to all cephalosporins, but also to entire other classes of β-lactam antibiotics. Restricted ceftazidime use is justifiable in institutions grappling with an ESBL-producing bacterium, and resistance rates decline when use is restricted.[123] Carbapenems and aminoglycosides generally retain useful microbicidal activity against ESBL-producing strains, but ESBL-producing strains can cause fatal infections because of delayed recognition and consequent delayed empiric antimicrobial therapy. Unfortunately, routine susceptibility testing does not detect ESBL-producing strains; therefore, heightened clinical suspicion must be followed by confirmatory laboratory testing of the suspicious organism.[124]

Resistance problems among gram-negative bacteria are not limited to cephalosporins. Metalloproteinases and carbapenemases threaten the utility of carbapenems to treat infections caused by *Klebsiella*, *Pseudomonas*, and *Acinetobacter*.[125,126] The fastest-growing resistance problem for gram-negative bacilli in the United States is quinolone resistance, particularly against *Pseudomonas*.[125] Quinolone resistance is chromosomally-mediated for the most part, primarily by changes in the target sites (DNA gyrase or topoisomerase IV) for the antibiotic. Changes in permeability or efflux may sometimes cause resistance to quinolones as well. Resistance to the quinolone class may develop rapidly if a less-than-maximally effective drug or dose is chosen for initial therapy, so a highly-active agent given in adequate dosage is essential for empiric therapy with quinolones. Unfortunately, even as the problem of antibiotic resistance among gram-negative bacilli proliferates, few new antimicrobial agents are being developed to meet this clinical need.

Fungi and Yeast.   Most fungi and yeast are avirulent opportunistic pathogens that pose no threat to healthy patients. Such infections should also be rare in the "typical" injured patient, who is usually not profoundly immunosuppressed (i.e., cancer chemotherapy with neutropenia, bone marrow transplant, or nonrenal solid organ transplant); however, fungal infections are associated with antibiotic overuse, suppression of host flora, and overgrowth of commensal flora. The most common health care-acquired fungal infections are caused by *Candida* spp., which are part of gut flora in approximately one-quarter of patients.

Some experts believe that high-risk patients (including those who require intensive antibiotic therapy) should be treated prophylactically with an azole antifungal agent (e.g., fluconazole) to prevent invasive infection, which can be lethal.[126] Although *Candida* colonization does precede invasive infection, the utility of antifungal prophylaxis requires confirmation. Widespread prescribing of fluconazole has led to resistant *Candida* spp. that are normally fluconazole-susceptible (e.g., *C. albicans, C. tropicalis*).[127] Empiric antifungal coverage as part of empiric antimicrobial therapy is probably unnecessary in centers with a low incidence of such infections, but must address the possibility of resistant *Candida* if administered. Empiric therapy choices include conventional amphotericin B, lipid formulations of amphotericin B, or an echinocandin. Conventional amphotericin B is seldom used any more because of substantial toxicity (e.g., febrile reactions, hypokalemia, renal insufficiency). The lipid formulations mitigate the toxicity, but at high cost. Echinocandins have broad activity against yeast and fungi including *Candida* spp. and *Aspergillus* sp. and are a logical, if expensive, choice for empiric therapy, but data are scant. Comparative studies suggest that the triazole voriconazole may be more effective than amphotericin B for invasive aspergillosis.[128] Fluconazole should be reserved for organisms that are likely to be fluconazole-susceptible (e.g., *C. albicans*) (many centers do not perform fungal susceptibility testing).

## PRINCIPLES OF ANTIBIOTIC THERAPY

Antimicrobial therapy is a mainstay of the treatment of infections, but widespread overuse and misuse of antibiotics have led to an alarming increase in MDR pathogens. New agents may allow shorter courses of therapy and prophylaxis, which are desirable for cost savings and control of microbial flora. To provide effective therapy with no toxicity requires an understanding of the principles of *pharmacokinetics* (PK).

### Pharmacokinetic Principles

Pharmacokinetics is collectively the principles of drug absorption, distribution, and metabolism.[129] For any medication, the dose-response relationship is influenced by dose, dosing interval, and route of administration. Drug concentrations in plasma and tissue are influenced by absorption, distribution, and elimination, which in turn depend on drug metabolism and excretion. Plasma and tissue concentrations may or may not correlate, depending on tissue penetration. Relationships between local drug concentration and effect are defined by *pharmacodynamic* (PD) principles (see below).[130]

Basic concepts of PK include *bioavailability*, the percentage of drug dose that reaches the systemic circulation. Bioavailability is 100% after intravenous (I.V.) administration, but is affected by absorption, intestinal transit time, and the degree of hepatic metabolism after oral administration. *Half-life* ($T_{1/2}$), the time required for the drug concentration to reduce by one-half, reflects

both clearance and *volume of distribution* $(V_D)$[124] and is useful to estimate for interpretation of data on drug concentration. The proportionality constant $V_D$, a derived parameter of no particular physiologic significance that is independent of a drug's clearance or $T_{1/2}$, is useful for estimating the plasma drug concentration achievable from a given dose. Volume of distribution varies substantially due to pathophysiology. A reduced $V_D$ causes a higher plasma drug concentration for a given dose, whereas fluid overload and hypoalbuminemia (which decrease drug binding) increase $V_D$, making dosing more complex.

*Clearance* refers to the volume of liquid from which drug is eliminated completely per unit of time, whether by tissue distribution, metabolism, or elimination. A knowledge of drug clearance is important for determining the dose of drug necessary to maintain a steady-state concentration. Drug elimination may be by metabolism, excretion, or dialysis. Most drugs are metabolized by the liver to polar compounds for eventual renal excretion, which may occur by filtration or either active or passive transport. The degree of filtration is determined by molecular size and charge and by the number of functional nephrons. In general, if less than or equal to 40% of administered drug or its active metabolites is eliminated unchanged in the urine, decreased renal function will require a dosage adjustment.

### Pharmacodynamic Principles

Pharmacodynamics are unique for antibiotic therapy, because drug-patient, drug-microbe, and microbe-patient interactions must be accounted for[130] In contrast to most drug treatment, the key drug interaction is not with the host, but with the microbe. Microbial physiology, inoculum size, microbial growth phase, mechanisms of resistance, micro-environmental factors such as local pH at the site of infection, and the host's response are important factors. Because of microbial resistance, mere administration of a drug may not be microbicidal.

Antibiotic PD parameters determined by laboratory analysis include the *minimal inhibitory concentration* (MIC), the lowest serum drug concentration that inhibits bacterial growth ($MIC_{90}$ refers to 90% inhibition); however, some antibiotics may suppress bacterial growth at subinhibitory concentrations (*postantibiotic effect* [PAE]). Appreciable PAE can be observed with aminoglycosides and fluoroquinolones for gram-negative bacteria, and with some β-lactam drugs (notably carbapenems) against *S. aureus*. MIC testing may not, however, detect resistant bacterial subpopulations within the inoculum (e.g., "heteroresistance" of *S. aureus*).[131,132] Moreover, in vitro results may be irrelevant if bacteria are inhibited only by drug concentrations that cannot be achieved clinically.

Sophisticated analytic strategies utilitze both PK and PD, for example, by determination of the peak serum concentration: MIC ratio, the duration of time that plasma concentration remains above the MIC, and the area of the plasma concentration-time curve above the MIC (the *area under the curve*, or AUC).[133] Accordingly, aminoglycosides have been characterized as having concentration-dependent killing,[134,135] whereas β-lactam agents exhibit efficacy determined by time above the MIC.[136] For β-lactam antibiotics with short $T_{1/2}$, it may be efficacious to administer by continuous infusion.[137,138] Some agents (e.g., fluoroquinolones) exhibit both properties; i.e., bacterial killing increases as drug concentration increases up to a saturation point, after which the effect becomes concentration-independent.

## Empiric Antibiotic Therapy

Empiric antibiotic therapy must be administered carefully. Injudicious therapy could result in undertreatment of established infection or unnecessary therapy when the patient has only inflammation or bacterial colonization. Inappropriate therapy (e.g., delay, therapy misdirected against usual pathogens, failure to treat MDR pathogens) leads unequivocally to increased mortality.[139–142]

Strategies have been promulgated to optimize the administration of antibiotics, including reliance upon physician prescribing patterns, computerized decision support,[143] administration by protocol,[144–148] and formulary restriction programs. Owing to the increasing prevalence of MDR pathogens, it is crucial for initial empiric antibiotic therapy to be targeted appropriately, administered in sufficient dosage to assure bacterial killing, narrowed in spectrum (de-escalation)[149] as soon as possible based on microbiology data and clinical response, and continued only as long as necessary. Appropriate antibiotic prescribing not only optimizes patient care, but supports infection control practice and preserves microbial ecology.[150,151]

The decision to treat the patient may need to be made before definitive information is available, considering the likelihood of infection, its source, and whether delay will be detrimental. Outcomes of serious infections are improved if antibiotics are started promptly. On the other hand, only about 50% of fever episodes in hospitalized patients are caused by infection[152] (Table 19-11). Many causes of the systemic inflammatory response syndrome (SIRS) are not due to infection (e.g., aspiration pneumonitis, burns, trauma, pancreatitis), although they may be complicated later by infection.[153] Multiple organ dysfunction syndrome (MODS) may progress even after an infectious precipitant has been controlled, due to a dysregulated host response.[154] The patient's environment must also be considered (e.g., recent hospitalization or antibiotic treatment, the presence of MDR pathogens in the unit, and any recent positive cultures).

**TABLE 19-11**

| Nosocomial Infections in the Intensive Care Unit |
| --- |
| **Common** |
| Pneumonia |
| Catheter-related infection |
| Intraabdominal (in surgical units) |
| Urinary tract |
| Skin/soft tissue |
| Decubitus ulcer |
| Surgical site infection |
| **Uncommon** |
| Sinusitis |
| Empyema |
| Endocarditis |
| Endophthalmitis |
| Parotitis |
| Suppurative phlebitis |

**TABLE 19-12**

| Factors Influencing Antibiotic Choice |
| --- |
| Activity against known/suspected pathogens |
| Disease believed responsible |
| Distinguish infection from colonization |
| Narrow-spectrum coverage most desirable |
| Antimicrobial resistance patterns |
| Patient-specific factors |
| Severity of illness |
| Age |
| Immunosuppression |
| Organ dysfunction |
| Allergy |
| Institutional guidelines/restrictions |

Choice of Antibiotic.  Antibiotic choice is based on several interrelated factors (Table 19-12). Paramount is activity against identified or likely (for empiric therapy) pathogens, presuming infecting and colonizing organisms can be distinguished, and that narrow-spectrum coverage is always desired. Estimation of likely pathogens depends on the disease process believed responsible; whether the infection is community-, health care-, or hospital-acquired; and whether MDR organisms are present. Local knowledge of antimicrobial resistance patterns is essential, even at the unit-specific level. Patient-specific factors of importance include age, debility, immunosuppression, intrinsic organ function, prior allergy or other adverse reaction, and recent antibiotic therapy. Institutional factors of importance include guidelines that may specify a particular therapy, formulary availability of specific agents, outbreaks of infections casued by MDR pathogens, and antibiotic control programs.

Numerous agents are available for therapy (Table 19-13).[121,155,156] Agents may be chosen based on spectrum, whether broad or targeted (e.g., antipseudomonal, antianaerobic), in addition to the above factors. If a nosocomial gram-positive pathogen is suspected (e.g., wound or surgical site infection, CR-BSI, prosthetic device infection, pneumonia) and MRSA is endemic, then empiric vancomycin (or linezolid) is appropriate. Some authorities recommend dual-agent therapy for serious Pseudomonas infections (i.e., an antipseudomonal (β-lactam drug plus an aminoglycoside), but evidence of efficacy is lacking.[157] It is important to use at least two antibiotics for empiric therapy of any infection that may be caused by either a gram-positive or -negative infection (e.g., nosocomial pneumonia).[158]

## Antifungal Prophylaxis and Therapy

The incidence of invasive fungal infections is increasing among critically ill surgical patients. Several conditions are predictors for invasive fungal infection complicating critical illness, including length of stay in the intensive care unit, altered immune responsiveness, and the number of medical devices placed. Neutropenia, diabetes mellitus, new-onset hemodialysis, total parenteral nutrition, broad-spectrum antibiotic administration, bladder catheterization, azotemia, diarrhea, and corticosteroid therapy are also associated with invasive fungal infections.[126,159]

The recovery of Candida spp. from multiple sites of colonization (without symptoms) has been linked to a high likelihood of

## TABLE 19-13

### Antibacterial Agents for Empiric Use

**Antipseudomonal**
Piperacillin-tazobactam
Cefepime, ceftazidime
Imipenem, meropenem
? Ciprofloxacin, levofloxacin (depending on local susceptibility patterns)
Aminoglycoside

**Targeted-Spectrum**
*Gram-positive*
Glycopeptide
Lipopeptide (not for known/suspected pneumonia)
Oxazolidinone

*Gram-negative*
Third-generation cephalosporin (not ceftriaxone)
Monobactam

*Anti-anaerobic*
Metronidazole

*Broad-spectrum*
Piperacillin-tazobactam
Carbapenems
Fluoroquinolones
Tigecycline (plus an anti-pseudoomonal agent)

*Anti-anaerobic*
Metronidazole
Carbapenems
Beta-lactam/beta-lactamase combination agents
Tigecycline

invasive candidiasis (the *colonization index*).[159] Risk factors for *Candida* colonization include prior use of antibiotics or a bacterial infection prior to ICU admission, a prolonged stay in the ICU, and multiple gastrointestinal operations. The source of the pathogen is often the patient's own gastrointestinal tract. Some data suggest that antifungal prophylaxis for colonized, nonneutropenic critically ill surgical patients can decrease the risk of invasive candidiasis,[126,160] whereas data strongly suggest that antifungal prophylaxis with fluconazole leads to resistance of previously susceptible fungi.[127,161] Table 19-14 presents a list of selected antifungal agents and susceptibility to *Candida* spp.[162]

*Duration of Therapy.*    The endpoint of therapy is largely undefined, in part because quality data are few.[149,163,164] If cultures are

negative, empiric antibiotic therapy should be stopped in most cases. Unnecessary antibiotic therapy in the absence of infection clearly increases the risk of MDR infection, therefore, therapy beyond 48–72 hours with negative cultures usually is unjustifiable. The morbidity of antibiotic therapy includes the following: allergic reactions; development of nosocomial superinfections, (e.g., fungal, enterococcal, and *Clostridium difficile*-related infections)[165–167]; organ toxicity; promotion of antibiotic resistance; reduced yield from subsequent cultures; and induced vitamin K deficiency with a coagulopathy or accentuation of warfarin effect.

If bona fide evidence of infection is evident, then treatment is continued as indicated clinically. Many infections can be treated with therapy lasting five days or less. Every decision to start antibiotics must be accompanied by a decision regarding the duration of therapy.[149] A reason to continue therapy beyond the predetermined endpoint must be compelling. Bacterial killing is rapid in response to effective agents, but the host response may not subside immediately. Therefore, the clinical response of the patient should not be the sole determinant for continuation of therapy. If a patient still has SIRS at the predetermined end of therapy, it is more useful to stop therapy and obtain new cultures to look for persistent or new infection, resistant pathogens, and noninfectious causes of SIRS. There is seldom justification to continue antibacterial therapy for more than 7–10 days. Examples of bacterial infections that require more than 14 days of therapy include tuberculosis of any site, endocarditis, osteomyelitis, and selected cases of brain abscess, liver abscess, lung abscess, postoperative meningitis, and endophthalmitis.

## Choosing and Administering Antibiotics

Antibiotic selection pressure is the major factor in the emergence of MDR pathogens, but there are other risk identified factors (Table 19-15), including increasing severity of illness, immunosuppression owing to illness (e.g., cancer, trauma) or therapy (e.g., antineoplastic therapy, transplant immunosuppression, glucocorticoid therapy), and invasive procedures. Ineffective infection control practice is a major issue in healthcare facilities, and hand washing is the single most effective deterrent of infection. Antibiotic selection is obiviously crucial to maximize the antibacterial effect while minimizing both toxicity and the potential for development of resistance.

**Cell Wall-Active Agents: Beta-lactam Antibiotics.**    The β-lactam antibiotic group consists of penicillins, cephalosporins, monobactams, and carbapenems. Within this group, several agents have been

## TABLE 19-14

### Usual Susceptibilities of *Candida* Species to Selected Antifungal Agents

| CANDIDA SPECIES | FLUCONAZOLE | ITRACONAZOLE | VORICONAZOLE | AMPHOTERICIN B | CASPOFUNGIN |
|---|---|---|---|---|---|
| C. albicans | S | S | S | S | S |
| C. tropicalis | S | S | S | S | S |
| C. parapsilosis | S | S | S | S | S to I (?R) |
| C, glabrata | S-DD to R | S-DD to R | S to I | S to I | S |
| C. krusei | R | S-DD to R | S to I | S to I | S |
| C. lusitaniae | S | S | S | S to R | S |

S = Susceptible.

S-DD = Susceptible-dose dependent (increased MIC may be overcome by higher dosing–e.g. 12 mg/kg/day fluconazole).

I = Intermediate.

R = Resistant.

**TABLE 19-15**

**Factors Contributing to Antibiotic Resistance**

Increased severity of illness
Severely immunocompromised
Invasive devices and procedures
Resistant organisms in the community
Ineffective infection control and compliance
Inappropriate antibiotic usage

combined with β-lactamase inhibitors to broaden the spectrum and increase the efficacy of the drugs. Several subgroups of antibiotics are recognized within the group, notably several "generations" of cephalosporins and penicillinase-resistant penicillins.

Penicillins. Penicillin is useful against most strains of *Streptococcus*, except for penicilin-resistant *S. pneumoniae* (PRSP, up to 40% of isolates). Penicillins retain little or no activity against most gram-negative bacteria, but those that are susceptible to penicillins include *Neisseria meninigidis* (highly-resistant strains exist), some strains of *Proteus mirabilis*, and *Pasturella multocida*. Penicillins are also effective against all *Clostridium* spp. other than *C. difficile*.

The primary use of penicillinase-resistant semisynthetic penicillins (e.g., methicillin, nafcillin, oxacillin) is for therapy for sensitive strains of staphylococci, against which they are highly bactericidal. These drugs are the treatment of choice for infections caused by susceptible isolates of *S. aureus*, but hospitalized patients should not be treated empirically with these agents, because of the high prevalence of MRSA, MR- *S. epidermidis* (MRSE), and VRE.[6]

Combination with a β-lactamase inhibitor (e.g., sulbactam, tazobactam, clavulanic acid) enhances the effectiveness of the parent β-lactam agent (piperacillin > ticarcillin > ampicillin), and to a lesser extent the inhibitor (tazobactam > sulbactam ~ clavulanic acid). The spectrum of activity varies within the class, and the treating clinician needs to be familiar with each of the drugs. All β-lactamase inhibitor combination drugs are effective against streptococci and methicillin-sensitive strains of *S. aureus* and widely effective against anaerobes (except for *C. difficile*). Piperacillin–tazobactam has the widest spectrum of activity against gram-negative bacteria and the most potency among β-lactam drugs against *P. aeruginosa*. Although ampicillin–sulbactam is unreliable against *E. coli* and *Klebsiella* (resistance rate ~50%), it has useful activity against *Acinetobacter* spp. because of sulbactam.[168]

Cephalosporins. More than 20 antibiotics comprise the class and are placed within four broad "generations." "First-generation" agents retain useful activity against gram-positive organisms, whereas "second-generation" agents generally lose that activity in favor of antianaerobic activity. "Third-generation" agents have enhanced activity against gram-negative bacilli (some have specific antipseudomonal activity), but most are ineffective against gram-positive cocci and none against anaerobes. Cefepime, the "fourth-generation" cephalosporin available in the United States, has useful antipseudomonal activity and has regained activity against most gram-positive cocci, but not MRSA. None of the cephalosporins are useful against enterococci. The heterogeneity of spectrum, especially among third-generation agents, requires broad familiarity with all of these drugs.

First-Generation Cephalosporins. First-generation cephalosporins (cefadroxil, cefazolin, cephalexin, cephalothin, cephapirin, and cephradine) are useful to treat community-acquired gram-negative infections caused by *E. coli* and *Klebsiella* spp., but not nosocomial pathogens. Parenteral first-generation cephalosporins still have a major role in surgical prophylaxis. First-generation agents are the most active cephalosporins against staphylococci (not MRSA) and streptococci.

Second-Generation Cephalosporins. Second-generation cephalosporins are useful to the trauma surgeon, but they are in short supply. These agents include cefaclor, cefamandole, cefmetazole, cefonicid, cefotetan, cefoxitin (technically a cephamycin), and cefuroxime. These drugs retain activity against aerobic and anaerobic streptococci, but lose some activity against methicillin-sensitive staphylococci. Activity against gram-negative bacilli is intermediate between that of the first- and third-generation agents. In general, there is activity against the *Enterobacteriaceae* except for *Enterobacter* spp., but no activity against *Acinetobacter*, *Pseudomonas*, or *Stenotrophomonas*. Cefmetazole, cefotetan, and cefoxitin have some activity against anaerobic gram-negative bacilli, including *B. fragilis*, but not to the extent of β-lactamase combination drugs, carbapenems, or metronidazole.

Third-Generation Cephalosporins. Third-generation cephalosporins include cefoperazone, cefotaxime, ceftazidime, and ceftriaxone, among others. They possess a modestly extended spectrum of activity against gram-negative bacilli, but not against gram-positive bacteria (except for ceftriaxone) or anaerobic bacteria. Third-generation cephalosporins, particularly ceftazidime, have been associated with the induction of ESBLs among many of the *Enterobacteriaceae*.[169] Activity is reliable only against non-ESBL producing species of *Enterobacteriaceae* including *Enterobacter, Citrobacter, Providencia*, and *Morganella*. Activity is no longer reliable for empiric use against nonfermenting gram-negative bacilli (e.g., *Acinetobacter* spp., *P. aeruginosa*, *S. maltophilia*).

Fourth-Generation Cephalosporins. The gram-negative spectrum of cefepime is more broad than that of the third-generation cephalosporins (antipseudomonal activity exceeds that of ceftazidime), whereas the anti-gram-positive activity is comparable to that of a first-generation cephalosporin. The potential for induction of ESBL production appears to be less. Similar to the carbapenems, cefepime appears to be intrinsically more resistant to hydrolysis by β-lactamases, but cefepime has variable activity against ESBL-producing bacteria.[170]

Monobactams. The single agent of this class, aztreonam, has activity against gram-negative bacilli that is similar to the third-generation cephalosporins, with no activity against either gram-positive organisms or anaerobes. Aztreonam is not a potent inducer of β-lactamases. Resistance to aztreonam is widespread, but the drug may be useful for directed therapy against known susceptible strains and may be used safely for penicillin-allergic patients because the incidence of cross-reactivity is low.

Carbapenems. Imipenem-cilastatin, meropenem, and ertapenem are available for clinical use in the United States. Imipenem-cilastatin and meropenem have the widest antibacterial spectrum of any antibiotics, with excellent activity against aerobic and anaerobic streptococci, methicillin-sensitive staphylococci, and virtually all gram-negative bacilli except *Legionella*, *P. cepacia*, and *S. maltophilia*.[171,172] Activity against the *Enterobacteriaceae* exceeds that of all antibiotics with the possible exceptions of piperacillin-tazobactam and cefepime, and activity of meropenem against *P. aeruginosa* is approached only by that of amikacin. All carbapenems are superlative antianaerobic agents. Ertapenem is not useful against *Pseudomonas* spp., *Acinetobacter* spp., *Enterobacter* spp., or MRSA, but its long half-life and substantial PAE permit once-daily dosing.[173] Ertapenem is highly active against ESBL-producing *Enterobacteriaceae*.

### Cell Wall Active Agents: Lipoglycopeptides.

Vancomycin, a soluble lipoglycopeptide, is rapidly bactericidal, but only on dividing organisms. A PAE persists for about two hours. Unfortunately, tissue penetration of vancomycin is generally poor, which limits its effectiveness. Both *S. aureus* and *S. epidermidis* are susceptible to vancomycin, although MICs for *S. aureus* are increasing, requiring higher doses for effect.[174] *Streptococcus pyogenes*, group B streptococci, *S. pneumoniae* (including PRSP), and *C. difficile* are also susceptible. Most strains of *E. faecalis* are inhibited (but not killed) by attainable concentrations, but *E. faecium* is predominantly VRE.

It is important for the public health that widespread inappropriate usage of vancomycin should be curtailed (Table 19-16). Bona fide indications include serious infections caused by MRSA/MRSE, gram-positive infections in patients with serious penicillin allergy, and enteral therapy for *C. difficile*-associated disease (CDAD) in patients who have failed or are intolerant of metronidazole. Parenteral vancomycin (a dose of 15 mg/kg is now recommended) must be infused over at least one hour.

### Cell Wall Active Agents: Cyclic Lipopeptides.

Daptomycin has potent, rapid bactericidal activity against most gram-positive organisms. The mechanism of action is novel, causing rapid membrane depolarization, potassium ion efflux, arrest of DNA, RNA, and protein synthesis, and cell death. Daptomycin exhibits concentration-dependent killing, has a long half-life (8 hours), and demonstrates a prolonged PAE, up to 6.8 hours.[175]

---

#### TABLE 19-16

**Situations in Which the Use of Vancomycin is Discouraged**

Routine surgical prophylaxis in the absence of life-threatening allergy to beta-lactam antibiotics

Empiric therapy of febrile neutropenia in the absence of evidence for a gram-positive infection

Continued empiric use when microbiologic data suggest a reasonable alternative

Systemic or local (i.e., catheter flush) prophylaxis of indwelling vascular catheters

Selective decontamination of the digestive tract

Eradication of colonization of methicillin-resistant staphylococci

Primary treatment of antibiotic-associated colitis due to *Clostridium difficile*

Routine prophylaxis for patients on hemodialysis or continuous ambulatory peritoneal dialysis

Use for topical irrigation or application

---

A dose of 4 mg/kg once daily is recommended for complicated skin/skin structure infections (6 mg/kg/day for bacteremia). Renal excretion requires increasing the dosing interval to 48 hours when creatinine clearance <30 mL/min. No antagonistic drug interactions have been observed. Daptomycin must not be used for the treatment of pneumonia or empiric therapy when pneumonia is in the differential diagnosis, even when caused by a susceptible organism, because daptomycin penetrates lung tissue poorly and is also inactivated by pulmonary surfactant.[176]

### Protein Synthesis Inhibitors.

Several classes of antibiotics, despite dissimilar structure and divergent spectra of activity, exert their antibacterial effects via binding to bacterial ribosomes, inhibiting protein synthesis. Because clindamycin, streptogramins, and macrolides have little utility for therapy of trauma patients, further mention is omitted.

### Aminoglycosides.

Once disdained as toxic and superceded by newer antibiotics, aminoglycoside use is ironically resurgent owing to the epidemic of infections caused by MDR pathogens. Aminoglycosides bind to the bacterial 30S ribosomal subunit. With the exception of better activity against gram-positive cocci possessed by gentamicin, the spectrum of activity for the various agents is nearly identical. Differences among the agents are based upon toxicity and local resistance patterns. Gentamicin, tobramycin, and amikacin are still used frequently. Nevertheless, potential toxicity is real, and aminoglycosides are seldom first-line therapy, except in a synergistic combination to treat a serious *Pseudomonas* infection, enterococcal endocarditis, or an infection caused by a MDR gram-negative bacillus. As second-line therapy, aminoglycosides are active against the *Enterobacteriaceae*, but there is less activity against *Acinetobacter*, and limited activity against *P. cepacia*, *Aeromonas* spp., and *S. maltophilia*.

Aminoglycosides kill bacteria most effectively with a concentration peak: MIC >12; therefore, a loading dose is necessary and serum drug concentration monitoring is often performed.[7] Synergistic therapy with a β-lactam agent is theoretically effective because β-lactam-induced cell wall damage enhances intracellular penetration of the aminoglycoside, but evidence of improved clinical outcomes is lacking.[157] Serious infections require 5 mg/kg/day of gentamicin or tobramycin after a 2 mg/kg loading dose or 15 mg/kg day of amikacin after a loading dose of 7.5 mg/kg. Clearance and $V_D$ are variable and unpredictable in critically ill patients, and higher doses are sometimes necessary (e.g., burn patients). High doses (e.g., gentamicin 7 mg/kg/day, amikacin 20 mg/kg/day) administered as a single daily dose can obviate these problems in selected patients.[134] Marked dosage reductions are necessary in renal failure, but the drugs are dialyzed and a maintenance dose should be given after each hemodialysis treatment.

### Tetracyclines.

Tetracyclines bind irreversibly to the 30S ribosomal subunit, but, unlike aminoglycosides, they are bacteriostatic agents. Widespread resistance limits their utility in the hospital setting (with two exceptions, doxycycline and tigecycline). Tetracyclines are active against anaerobes, and *Actinomyces* can be treated successfully. Doxycycline and tigecycline are active against *B. fragilis*. All tetracyclines are contraindicated in pregnancy and for children under the age of eight years owing to dental toxicity. Tigecycline is a novel glycylcycline derived from minocycline,[177] with broad-spectrum activity againse many MDR gram-positive and –negative bacteria with the exception of *P. aeruginosa*. Tigecycline has notable activity against MDR *Acinetobacter* spp. and excellent activity against MDR gram-positive cocci without exception.

**Oxazolidinones.** Oxazolidinones bind to the ribosomal 50S subunit, preventing complexing with the 30S subunit.[178] Assembly of a functional initiation complex for protein synthesis is blocked, and this prevents translation of mRNA. This mode of action differs from other inhibitors such as chloramphenicol, macrolides, lincosamides, and tetracyclines, which permit mRNA translation but then inhibit peptide elongation. The first marketed oxazolidinone, linezolid, prevents the synthesis of staphylococcal and streptococcal virulence factors (e.g., coagulase, hemolysins, protein A), but is bacteriostatic. With minor exceptions, gram-negative bacteria are oxazolidinone-resistant, because oxazolidinones are excreted by efflux pumps. Linezolid is equally active against MSSA and MRSA, vancomycin-susceptible enterococci and VRE, and against susceptible and PRSP pneumococci. Most gram-negative bacteria are resistant, but *Bacteroides* spp. are susceptible. Linezolid exhibits excellent tissue penetration, and requires no dosage reduction in renal insufficiency.

### Drugs that Disrupt Nucleic Acids

**Quinolones.** Quinolones inhibit DNA gyrase, which folds DNA into a superhelix in preparation for replication. The fluoroquinolones exhibit broad-spectrum activity and excellent oral absorption and bioavailability, but are prone to develop resistance rapidly. Agents with both parenteral and oral formulations include ciprofloxacin, levofloxacin, and moxifloxacin (which has some anti-anaerobic activity). Quinolones are most active against enteric gram-negative bacteria, particularly the *Enterobacteriaceae* and *Haemophilus* spp. There is activity against *P. aeruginosa*, *S. maltophilia*, and gram-negative cocci. Activity against gram-positive cocci is variable, being least for ciprofloxacin and best for the so-called "respiratory quinolones" (e.g., moxifloxacin). Ciprofloxacin is most active against *P. aeruginosa*. Unfortunately, rampant overuse of fluoroquinolones is rapidly causing resistance that may severely limit the future usefulness of these agents.[125,179] Fluoroquinolone use has been associated with the emergence of resistant *P. aeruginosa*[48] and MRSA.[180]

### Cytotoxic Antibiotics

**Metronidazole.** Metronidazole is active against nearly all anaerobic pathogens and many protozoa that are human parasites. Metronidazole has potent bactericidal activity, including activity against *B. fragilis*, *Prevotella* spp., *Clostridium* spp. (including *C. difficile*), and anaerobic cocci, although it is ineffective in actinomycosis. Resistance is rare and of negligible clinical significance. Metronidazole causes DNA damage after intracellular reduction of the nitro group of the drug. Acting as a preferential electron acceptor, it is reduced by low-redox-potential electron transport proteins, decreasing the intracellular concentration of the unchanged drug and maintaining a transmembrane gradient that favors uptake of additional drug. The drug thus penetrates nearly all tissues well, including neural tissue, making it effective for deep-seated infections even against bacteria that are not multiplying rapidly. Absorption after oral or rectal administration is rapid and nearly complete. The $T_{1/2}$ of metronidazole is eight hours, owing to an active hydroxy metabolite. Increasingly, intravenous metronidazole is administered every 8–12 hours in recognition of the active metabolite, but once-daily dosing is possible.[181] No dosage reduction is required for renal insufficiency, but the drug is dialyzed effectively and administration should be timed to follow dialysis if twice-daily dosing is used. Pharmacokinetics in patients with hepatic insufficiency suggest a dosage reduction of 50% with marked impairment.

**Trimethoprim-Sulfamethoxazole (TMP-SMX).** Sulfonamides exert bacteriostatic activity by interfering with bacterial folic acid synthesis necessary for DNA synthesis. Resistance is widespread, and use is limited. The addition of sulfamethoxazole to trimethoprim, which prevents the conversion of dihydrofolic acid to tetrahydrofolic acid by the action of dihydrofolate reductase (downstream from the action of sulfonamides), accentuates the bactericidal activity of trimethoprim.

The combination of TMP-SMX is active against *S. aureus*, *S. pyogenes*, *S. pneumoniae*, *E. coli*, *P. mirabilis*, *Salmonella* and *Shigella* spp., *Yersinia enterocolitica*, *S. maltophilia*, *L. monocytogenes*, and *Pneumocystis carinii*. It is the treatment of choice for infections caused by *S. maltophilia* and outpatient treatment of skin infections caused by CA-MRSA.

### Antibiotic Toxicities

**Beta-lactam Allergy.** Allergic reaction, although less common than generally believed, is the most common toxicity of β-lactam antibiotics. The incidence is approximately 7–40/1000 treatment courses of penicillin.[182] Reactions of four distinct types are recognized. Immediate hypersensitivity reactions occur via interaction with preformed β-lactam-specific IgE antibodies bound to mast cells or circulating basophils. Cytotoxic antibody reactions occur when β-lactam-specific IgG (usually) or IgM antibodies bind to antigen-fixed red blood cells or renal interstitial cells, resulting in complement-dependent cell lysis. Complement-independent toxicity (e.g., leukopenia, thrombocytopenia, hemolytic anemia, interstitial nephritis) may result from binding cell membranes of neutrophils or macrophages. Immune complex (Arthus) reactions occur when circulating antigen-antibody (IgG, IgM) complexes fix complement and lodge in various tissue sites, causing serum sickness-like reactions and a possible drug fever. The onset of these reactions is usually 7–14 days after therapy has begun, even if drug has already been stopped. Certain reactions do not fall under these classifications, including pruritis, maculopapular reactions, erythema multiforme, erythema nodosum, photosensitivity, and exfoliative dermatitis.

The immunochemistry of penicillin reactions is well defined. Penicillin binds tissue proteins to produce multivalent hapten-protein complexes necessary for induction of immunity. The most common hapten form of penicillin in vivo is the penicilloyl derivative, which is called the major determinant. Accelerated (1–72 hour) and late reactions are usually in response to the major determinant. Small quantities of other minor determinants may be formed by metabolic activity and induce a variable response. Anaphylactic reactions are usually in response to a minor determinant.

Parenteral therapy causes more clinical allergic reactions as a dose-dependent function. Most serious reactions occur in patients with no history of penicillin allergy, simply because a history of penicillin allergy is sought commonly and reported by 5–20% of patients (far in excess of the true incidence). Patients with a prior reaction have a four- to six-fold increased risk of another reaction compared to the general population; however, this risk decreases with time, from 80–90% skin test reactivity at two months to 20% reactivity at ten years. The risk of cross-reactivity between penicillins and carbapenems and cephalosporins is 5–10%, being highest for first-generation cephalosporins.[183] There is negligible cross-reactivity to monobactams.

Nephrotoxicity.    Aminoglycosides differ little as potential nephrotoxins. Aminoglycosides do not provoke inflammation, thus allergic reactions do not occur. Aminoglycoside toxicity relates both to ischemia and toxicity to the renal proximal tubular cell (PTC).[184] Ischemia is prominent owing to afferent arteriolar vasoconstriction. Aminoglycoside binding to the brush border membrane of the PTC leads to enzymuria, excretion of calcium and magnesium, and internalization by pinocytosis. The phosphatidyl inositol "middle messenger" system is perturbed, with membrane damage, excretion of membrane phospholipids, perinuclear localization of drug, disturbed protein synthesis, and impaired mitochondrial respiration. Ultimately, there is necrosis of the PTC, reduction of the glomerular filtration rate (GFR), and decreased creatinine clearance. Postulated mechanisms of reduced GFR include release of vasoconstrictive hormones, trans-epithelial back-leak of toxins, obstruction by necrotic cellular debris, or a change in glomerular fenestrae and the ultrafiltration coefficient. Injury is usually nonoliguric and reversible, and progression to dialysis dependence is rare. The risk of nephrotoxicity is increased by frequent dosing, older age, sodium and volume depletion, acidemia, hypokalemia, hypomagnesemia, coexistent hepatic disease, and other nephrotoxins, but ameliorated by single-daily-dose therapy.

Vancomycin nephrotoxicity is less common than previously believed. Multiple courses of therapy, administration of very high doses (dosage reductions are necessary in renal insufficiency), and concurrent administration of an aminoglycoside are known risk factors for toxicity.

Ototoxicity.    Aminoglycosides cause cochlear or vestibular toxicity that is usually irreversible and may develop after cessation of therapy.[185] Repeated exposures create a cumulative risk. Most patients develop either cochlear toxicity or a vestibular lesion, but not both. Cochlear toxicity can be a subtle diagnosis to make, because baseline audiograms are seldom available, and formal screening programs are seldom undertaken. Few patients complain of hearing loss, yet when sought, the incidence of cochlear toxicity may be more than 60%. Clinical hearing loss may occur in 5–15% of patients. Amikacin is less ototoxic than gentamicin, and tobramycin is intermediate in toxicity. Risk factors include duration of treatment, high serum drug concentrations, a large cumulative dose, concomitant ototoxic drug therapy (e.g., vancomycin, furosemide), hypovolemia, and renal or hepatic disease. There is no correlation with nephrotoxicity.

The target of vestibular toxicity is the type I hair cell of the summit of the ampullar cristae. The true incidence of vestibular toxicity is estimated to be 5%. Patients can suffer considerable injury before becoming symptomatic, owing to the compensatory contribution of visual and proprioceptive cues (therefore, symptoms may be worse at night). Complaints of nausea, vomiting, and vertigo are most common, and patients may exhibit nystagmus.

Ototoxicity caused directly by vancomycin is accepted as fact, but poorly documented in the literature. Hearing loss attributed to vancomycin is better described as neurotoxicity, manifesting as auditory nerve damage, tinnitus, and loss of acuity for high-frequency tones. Synergistic injury is possible with coadministration of other ototoxic drugs, especially aminoglycosides and furosemide.

Quinolone Toxicity.    Quinolones are generally well tolerated, but adverse effects increase with higher doses and prolonged therapy. Gastrointestinal side effects are common (up to 13%), but mild. Adverse effects on the central nervous system are also common (up to 7%). Headache and dizziness predominate, followed by insomnia and mood alteration, while hallucinations, delirium, and seizures are rare. Allergic and skin reactions occur in up to 2% of patients. Phototoxicity after exposure to ultraviolet A light (sunlight is sufficient exposure) occurs in some patients. While anaphylactoid reactions are rare, arthopathy and tendinitis, reversible bone marrow depression, leukopenia, and hemolytic anemia have been reported. Rare but important is prolongation of the electrocardiogram QT interval, which may precipitate the dangerous ventricular dysrhythmia *torsades de pointes*.[186]

## Avoiding Toxicity: Adjustment of Antibiotic Therapy

Hepatic Insufficiency.    The liver metabolizes and eliminates drugs that are too lipophilic for renal excretion. The cytochromes $P_{450}$ (a gene superfamily of more than 300 different enzymes) oxidize lipophilic compounds to water-soluble products. Other enzymes convert drugs or metabolites by conjugating them with sugars, amino acids, sulfate, or acetate to facilitate biliary or renal excretion, whereas enzymes such as esterases and hydrolases act by other distinct mechanisms. Many of these functions are disrupted when hepatic function is impaired, especially oxidative metabolism.

Drug dosing in hepatic insufficiency is complicated by insensitive clinical assessments of function and changing metabolism as the degree of impairment fluctuates (e.g., resolving cholestasis). Changes in renal function with progressive hepatic impairment add considerable complexity, especially with concomitant ascites. Adverse drug reactions are more frequent with cirrhosis than with other forms of hepatic disease.

The effect of hepatic disease on drug disposition is difficult to predict in individual patients as none of the usual tests of hepatic function can be used to guide dosage.[187] Generally, a dosage reduction of up to 25% of the usual dose is considered if hepatic metabolism is 40% or less and renal function is normal (Table 19-17). Greater dosage reductions (up to 50%) are advisable if the drug is administered chronically, there is a narrow therapeutic index, protein binding is significantly reduced, or the drug is excreted renally but renal function is severely impaired.

## TABLE 19-17

### Antimicrobials Requiring Dosage Reduction in Hepatic Disease

Aztreonam
Cefoperazone
Chloramphenicol
Clindamycin
Erythromycin
Isoniazid
Metronidazole
Nafcillin
Quinupristin/dalfopristin
Rifampin
Tigecycline

**Renal Insufficiency.** Renal drug elimination depends on the GFR, tubular secretion, and reabsorption, any of which may be decreased with renal dysfunction. Renal failure may affect hepatic as well as renal drug metabolism. Drugs whose hepatic metabolism is likely to be disrupted in renal failure include aztreonam, cefotaxime, and imipenem-cilastatin (Tables 19-18 and 19-19). Renal failure can change $V_D$ due to fluid overload or hypoproteinemia. Antimicrobials known to have increased $V_D$ in renal failure include aminoglycosides, cefazolin, cefoxitin, and vancomycin, while methicillin will have decreased $V_D$ in renal failure.

Accurate estimates of renal function are important in patients with mild-to-moderate renal dysfunction, because the clearance of many drugs by dialysis actually makes management easier. Factors influencing drug clearance by hemofiltration include molecular size, aqueous solubility, plasma protein binding, equilibration kinetics between plasma and tissue, and the apparent $V_D$.[188,189] New high-flux polysulfone dialysis membranes can clear molecules up to 5kD efficiently (the molecular weight of vancomycin is 1.486 kD). Patients may need to be redosed during or after dialysis; also, during continuous renal replacement therapy, the estimated creatinine clearance is ~15 mL/min in addition to the patient's intrinsic clearance.[188,189] Cefoperazone, ceftriaxone, doxycycline, linezolid, methicillin/nafcillin/oxacillin, metronidazole, and tigecycline are among the antimicrobial agents that do not require dosage reduction in renal failure.

## TABLE 19-18

### Dosage Reductions for Selected Antimicrobials in Renal Insufficiency

| DRUG (USUAL DOSE) | DOSE FOR $C_{Cr}{}^a$ (10–50 mL/m) | DOSE FOR $C_{Cr}{}^a$ (<10 mL/m) | DIALYZED?[b] |
|---|---|---|---|
| **Aminoglycosides** | Individualize | Individualize | Yes |
| Ampicillin (1–2 g q4h) | 0.5–1 g q6h | 0.5–1 g q12h | Yes |
| Aztreonam (1 g q8h) | 0.5 g q8h | 0.5 g q12h | HD only |
| Cefamandole (1–2 g q6h) | 1–2 g q8–12h | 1–2 g q8–24h | HD/CRRT |
| Cefazolin (1 g q8h) | 1 g q12–24h | 1 g q48h | HD only |
| Cefepime (2 g q12h) | 1 g q12h | 1 g q24h | Yes |
| Cefotaxime (1 g q 6h) | 1 g q8–12h | 1 g q24h | HD only |
| Cefotetan (1 g q12h) | 1 g q24h | 0.5–1g q24h | No |
| Cefoxitin (1–2 g q6h) | 1–2 g q8–12h | 1–2 g q24h | HD/CRRT |
| Ceftazidime (1 g q8h) | 1 g q24h | 1 g q48h | Yes |
| Ceftizoxime (1 g q8h) | 1 g q12–24h | 1 g q48h | HD only |
| Ciprofloxacin (0.4 g q8–12h) | 0.4 g q8h | 0.4 g q16h | No |
| Imipenem/cilastatin (0.5 g q6h) | 0.25–0.5 g q6–8h | 0.25–0.5 g q12h | HD only |
| Levofloxacin (0.5–0.75 g q12h) | 0.5g q24h | 0.5 g q248h | CRRT only |
| Piperacillin (2–4 g q4h) | 2–4 g q6h | 2–3 g q8h | HD/CRRT |
| Vancomycin (1 g q12h) | Individualize | Individualize | High-flux HD only |

[a]Formula for estimation of creatinine clearance [$C_{Cr}$]:

$$C_{Cr} \text{ [mL/min]} = \frac{140\text{-age} \times (1.00 \text{ [male]} \ 0.85 \text{ [female]}) \times \text{weight [kg]}}{\text{Serum Cr concentration [mg/dL]} \times 72}$$

[b]Dialysis by hemodialysis (HD), peritoneal dialysis (PD), or continuous renal replacement therapy (CRRT).

**TABLE 19-19**

| Dosing of Selected Parenteral Antibiotics in Dialysis Patients | |
|---|---|
| Amikacin | 2.5–3.75 mg/kg |
| Ampicillin | 1 g |
| Azlocillin | 3 g |
| Aztreonam | 0.125 g |
| Cefamandole | 0.5–1 g |
| Cefepime | 0.5 g |
| Cefoxitin | 1 g |
| Ceftazidime | 1 g |
| Ceftizoxime | 1–3 g |
| Cefuroxime | 0.75 g |
| Chloramphenicol | 1 g |
| Gentamicin | 1.0–1.7 mg/kg |
| Imipenem/cilastatin | 0.25–0.5 g |
| Meropenem | 0.5 g |
| Mezlocillin | 2–3 g |
| Netilmicin | 2 mg/kg |
| Piperacillin | 2 g |
| Piperacillin/tazobactam | 2.25 g |
| Ticarcillin | 3 g |
| Ticarcillin/clavulanic acid | 3.1 g |
| Tobramycin | 1.0–1.7 mg/kg |
| Trimethoprim/sulfamethoxazole | 5 mg/kg trimethoprim |
| Vancomycin | 0.5 g if using polysulfone dialysis membrane otherwise no supplement |

**TABLE 19-20**

| Risk Factors for Ventilator-Associated Pneumonia |
|---|
| Age ≥60 y |
| Acute respiratory distress syndrome |
| Chronic obstructive pulmonary disease or other underlying pulmonary disorder |
| Coma or impaired consciousness |
| Serum albumin <2.2 g/dL |
| Burns, trauma |
| Blood transfusion |
| Organ failure |
| Supine position |
| Large-volume gastric aspiration |
| Sinusitis |
| Immunosuppression |

## SPECIFIC NOSOCOMIAL INFECTIONS

### Pneumonia

Trauma patients are particularly susceptible to pneumonia, particularly if they require mechanical ventilation. Ventilator-associated pneumonia (VAP), defined as pneumonia occurring at some point after endotracheal intubation, is the most common infection in the intensive care unit (ICU) among trauma patients. Unfortunately, VAP is partially iatrogenic, and nonspecific diagnostic criteria, indiscriminate use of antibiotics, and unclear therapeutic endpoints have all contributed to increased episodes of VAP caused by MDR pathogens. In turn, MDR pathogens increase the likelihood of inadequate initial antimicrobial therapy, which exerts further selection pressure for these pathogens, and results in higher mortality. Several evidence-based strategies can prevent VAP and promote effective diagnosis and therapy.

Distinction is made between early-onset VAP (occurring <5 days after intubation) and late-onset VAP (occurring ≥5 days after intubation). Early-onset VAP, to which trauma patients are particularly prone, is often a result of aspiration of gastric contents and is usually caused by antibiotic-sensitive bacteria such as methicillin-sensitive *S. aureus*, *S. pneumoniae*, and *H. influenzae*.[190–192] Conversely, patients with late-onset VAP are at increased risk for infection with MDR pathogens (e.g., MRSA, *P. aeruginosa*, or *Acinetobacter* spp.).

The incidence of VAP depends upon the diagnostic criteria utilized and varies in published reports. Clinical criteria alone overestimate the incidence of VAP as compared with either microbiologic or histologic data.[193,194] A systematic review of 89 studies of VAP among mechanically-ventilated patients[195] reported a pooled incidence of VAP of 22.8% (95% CI 18.8–26.9%). The National Nosocomial Infection Surveillance (NNIS) system reported recently that VAP occurred at a rate of 4.9 cases per 1000 ventilator days in medical ICUs and 9.3 per 1000 ventilator days in surgical ICUs[6] (Table 19-2). The risk for trauma patients, especially those with traumatic brain injury, is especially high. The incidence of VAP increases with the duration of mechanical ventilation at a rate of 3% per day during the first five days, 2% per day during days 5–10, and 1% per day after that.[196]

Risk factors for VAP are summarized in Table 19-20. The risk of VAP increases 6–20 fold in mechanically-ventilated patients,[197,198] and VAP is especially common in patients with ARDS, owing to prolonged mechanical ventilation and impaired host defenses in the local airway.[199–201]

It is controversial whether VAP increases mortality.[202] The crude mortality rate of VAP is reported to be between 9–27%.[192,203–206] Attribution of mortality to VAP is problematic, as there often is no single, identifiable cause of death due to critical illness, or VAP may be a marker of generalized host immunosuppression. Moreover, mortality may be due in fact to inappropriate initial empiric therapy.[207] Meta-analysis of pooled matched-cohort studies of patients with VAP no indicate that the risk of death is doubled (Odds ratio [OR] 2.03, 95% CI 1.16–3.56, $p=0.03$).[195]

Pathogenesis. Both impaired host defenses and oropharyngeal colonization by pathogens predispose critically ill and mechanically ventilated patient to VAP. Normal airway host defenses, such as the epiglottis, vocal cords, cough reflex, and ciliated epithelium and mucus of the upper airways are either bypassed or rendered ineffective during intubation. Bacteria may enter the lower respiratory tract via aspiration through the endotracheal tube (bacterial colonies in the glycocalyx biofilm that coats the lumen of artificial airway devices are impervious to antibiotics), migration around it (particularly with cuff "leak"), or, rarely, by hematogenous spread from remote infections.

Currently, the most common pathogens isolated from patients with VAP are MRSA (15%), *P. aeruginosa* (14%), *Enterobacter* spp. (3%), *E. coli* (3%), and *Acinetobacter* spp. (2%),[5,23] often by MDR

**TABLE 19-21**

**Rank Order of Key Pathogens in ICU Infections (by Incidence)**

| | BLOODSTREAM INFECTION | URINARY TRACT INFECTION | PNEUMONIA |
|---|---|---|---|
| Gram-positive | 1: Coag-neg staphylococci | 1: Enterococcus | 1: S. aureus |
| | 2: Enterococcus | 2: Coag-neg staphylococci | |
| | 3: S. aureus | 3: S. aureus | |
| Gram-negative | 1: Enterobacter | 1: E. coli | 1: P. aeruginosa |
| | 2: P. aeruginosa | 2: P. aeruginosa | 2: Enterobacter |
| | 3: K. pneumoniae | 3: K. pneumoniae | 3: K. pneumoniae |
| | 4: E. coli | 4: Enterobacter | 4: E. coli |

pathogens (Table 19-21). Infection with MRSA is particularly common in patients with diabetes mellitus and after traumatic brain injury.[208–210] *Pseudomonas aeruginosa* is increasingly common with an MDR phenotype, especially to both fluoroquinolones[211] and third-generation cephalosporins.

Anaerobic bacteria are isolated infrequently from patients with VAP.[212] Isolation of fungi (e.g., *Candida* spp., *A. fumigatus*) from endotracheal aspirates is common, but almost always represents colonization when the host is immunocompetent.[213–216] When fungi are isolated from two or more normally-sterile sites (e.g., urine and lower respiratory tract) in an immunocompromised patient, systemic antifungal therapy should be considered.

Prevention.    Prevention of VAP requires a thorough understanding of modifiable risk factors (Table 19-22). Strict infection control, including hand hygiene with alcohol-based hand disinfectants, gowning, and gloving, minimizes person-to-person transmission of pathogens and is paramount to deterring all ICU infections.[217–218] Prevention of VAP begins with instituting endotracheal intubation only when necessary and minimizing the duration of mechanical ventilation. Non-invasive, positive-pressure ventilation (NIPPV) should be considered in lieu of intubation, as management of respiratory failure with NIPPV leads to a lower incidence of VAP.[219]

**TABLE 19-22**

**Strategies to Prevent Ventilator-Associated Pneumonia**

| STRATEGY | RECOMMENDED | INSUFFICIENT EVIDENCE |
|---|---|---|
| Universal infection control precautions | + | |
| Orotracheal intubation | + | |
| Maintenance of endotracheal cuff pressure >20 cmH₂O | + | |
| Continuous aspiration of subglottic secretions | + | |
| Semirecumbent positioning | + | |
| Postpyloric feeding | | + |
| Postponement of enteral feeding for at least 48 hours following intubation | + | |
| Selective decontamination of the digestive tract | | + |
| Topical antiseptics | | + |
| Transfusion restriction | + | |
| Antibiotic cycling | | + |

Evidence-based strategies to decrease the duration of mechanical ventilation include daily interruption of sedation,[220] standardized weaning protocols, and adequate ICU staffing.[221]

If endotracheal intubation is required, the orotracheal route is preferred to nasotracheal intubation as it decreases the risk of VAP by as much as one-half.[222] Nasotracheal intubation is strongly associated with the development of nosocomial sinusitis,[223] which often precedes and is caused by the same pathogen that subsequently causes VAP.

After intubation, most VAP preventive measures decrease the risk of aspiration. Both maintenance of endotracheal cuff pressure >20 cmH₂O[224] and continuous aspiration of subglottic secretions via a specialized multilumen endotracheal tube reduce the incidence of VAP significantly (see above). Semirecumbent positioning (30°–45° head-up) is also protective as compared to supine positioning, especially during enteral feeding.[225]

Compared to postpyloric feeding, intragastric feeding increases both gastroesophageal reflux and aspiration.[226] A meta-analysis of 11 randomized trials reported a RR of 0.77 (95% CI 0.60–1.00, $p = 0.05$) for VAP with postpyloric as compared to gastric feedings.[227] Pro-motility agents such as erythromycin may facilitate safe intragastric feeding should this route be used.[228] Early enteral feedings may increase the risk of VAP. Shorr et al. reported that enteral nutrition begun ≤48 hours after the initiation of mechanical ventilation was independently associated with the development of VAP (OR 2.65, 95% CI 1.93–3.63, $p <0.0001$).[46]

Pharmacologic strategies to minimize the risk of aspiration include selective use of prophylaxis for stress gastritis and selective decontamination of the digestive tract (SDD) with either topical or systemic antibiotics or antiseptics. Many clinical trials have reported a significant decrease in the incidence of VAP, but methodology has often been questionable,[229] studies have taken place in ICUs in which MDR pathogens were rare, and an increased number of infections caused by MDR bacteria have been observed in the SSD groups. For these reasons, use of SDD is currently not recommended for the routine prevention of VAP. Alternatively, studies of oropharyngeal decontamination with topical chlorhexidine have provided conflicting evidence of efficacy,[230,231] and further research is needed.

Prophylaxis against stress gastritis is a known risk factor for VAP,[232] and its use should be reserved for patients at high risk for gastrointestinal mucosal hemorrhage (e.g., mechanical ventilation >2 days, intracranial hemorrhage, coagulopathy, glucocorticoid therapy). Results of randomized trials comparing histamine type-2 antagonists, sucralfate, and antacids are conflicting for prevention of VAP.

Ample data document the relationship between blood transfusion and infection risk in surgical, trauma, and critically ill patients (see above). Shorr et al. found red blood cell transfusion to be an independent risk factor for VAP (OR 1.89, 95% CI 1.33–2.68, $p = 0.0004$).[46] Early et al. documented a 90% decreased incidence of VAP in a surgical ICU following implementation of a management protocol for anemia that resulted in fewer blood transfusions.[232]

Diagnosis.   The diagnosis of VAP requires a determination that the patient has pneumonia and the etiologic pathogen. Poor specificity is problematic in the diagnosis of VAP because it not only exposes patients to unnecessary risk from overtreatment with antibiotics, but also increases selection pressure and, thus, the emergence of MDR bacteria.[149] Conversely, inadequate initial therapy in patients with VAP (poor sensitivity) is associated with increased mortality that cannot be reduced by subsequent changes in antibiotics.[233]

Historically, the diagnosis of VAP requires one or more of the following: fever, leukocytosis or leukopenia, purulent sputum, hypoxemia, or a new or evolving infiltrate on a chest x-ray (CXR). Several noninfectious respiratory disease processes may mimic these nonspecific signs including congestive heart failure, atelectasis, pulmonary thromboembolism, pulmonary hemorrhage, and ARDS, making clinical criteria alone unreliable. The presence of a new infiltrate on CXR, along with two of the three aforementioned criteria, was only 69% sensitive and 75% specific for VAP as compared to postmortem histology.[234] Several subsequent reports have confirmed the low specificity of clinical acumen in the diagnosis of VAP,[235] and clinically-diagnosed VAP is confirmed microbiologically in fewer than 50% of cases.[236]

The Clinical Pulmonary Infection Score (CPIS) incorporates clinical, radiographic, and microbiologic criteria (i.e., temperature, leukocyte count, CXR infiltrates, appearance and volume of tracheal secretions, $P_aO_2:F_IO_2$, culture and gram stain of tracheal aspirate (0–2 points each) to yield a maximum CPIS score of 12 points.[237] A CPIS of >6 points indicates a high probability of VAP; however, the specificity of CPIS is no better than clinical acumen alone when compared to cultures of the lower respiratory tract obtained via bronchoscopic bronchoalveolar lavage (BAL) or protected specimen brush (PSB).[238–240] Of interest, the negative predictive value of a gram stain showing no organisms in a clinically stable patient approaches 100%.[241]

Because of the low specificity of traditional diagnostic criteria for VAP, cultures of the lower respiratory tract prior to the institution of antibiotics are mandatory in order to minimize false-negative results. The method of specimen collection (invasive vs. noninvasive) and the method of specimen analysis (semi-quantitative vs. quantitative) are debated continously. Noninvasive techniques include endotracheal suction aspiration (EAs), blinded plugged telescoping catheter (PTC), blinded PSB, and mini-BAL. Endotracheal aspirates are less specific due to an increased likelihood of contamination by oropharyngeal flora reflecting colonization rather than infection.

Invasive techniques (BAL or PSB) collect samples using fiberoptic bronchoscopy and allow for direct visualization of the airways. These are, of course, more expensive and resource-intensive than noninvasive techniques. Furthermore, although bronchoscopy is generally well-tolerated, arterial desaturation may persist for up to 24 hours after the procedure, possibly due to alveolar flooding

caused by residual lavage fluid; however, this desaturation has not been correlated with poorer outcomes.[242]

Irrespective of the method of collection, respiratory tract cultures may be analyzed using either semi-quantitative or quantitative microbiology. The crucial issue is distinction of colonization from infection.[243] Whereas semi-quantitative microbiology reports growth in ordinal categories (e.g., light, moderate, or heavy), quantitative microbiology reports growth in terms of colony forming units (CFUs)/mL of aliquot. In the latter case, a threshold value is selected to distinguish colonization from infection. Commonly used thresholds are $10^3$ CFU/mL for PSB, $10^4$ CFU/mL for BAL, and $10^5$ CFU/mL for EA. Any threshold should be lowered by one order of magnitude if antibiotics have been changed recently or started prior to acquisition of the sample.[244]

Endotracheal aspirates have an inferior specificity when compared to either blinded PTC or bronchoscopic BAL or PSB. Two systematic reviews, one of bronchoscopic BAL[242] and one of blinded invasive techniques,[245] reported similar test characteristics for the two techniques, but methodologic variability is rampant. Bronchoscopic techniques are more specific than blinded techniques, and both techniques are superior to EAs.

The largest randomized, controlled trial for the diagnosis of VAP compared an invasive, quantitative approach with a noninvasive, semi-quantitative approach.[194] A total of 413 patients suspected of VAP were randomized to evaluation with either bronchoscopic BAL or PSB with quantitative cultures or "clinical" management consisting of semi-quantitative analysis of EAs. Antibiotic therapy was discontinued in clinically stable patients with negative cultures, regardless of study arm. Compared to the clinical strategy, patients in the invasive group demonstrated decreased 14-day mortality (16% vs. 25%, $p = 0.02$), less antibiotic use (11.9 vs. 7.7 antibiotic-free days), decreased sepsis-related organ failure, and decreased 28-day mortality after adjustment for severity of illness. The clinical strategy also resulted in more and broader-spectrum antibiotic therapy compared to the invasive strategy and increased emergence of fungi. It is unclear whether these improved outcomes resulted from the use of an invasive vs. a noninvasive sample acquisition strategy or quantitative vs. semi-quantitative microbiology.

Shorr et al. performed a meta-analysis of randomized trials that compare outcomes of patients with VAP managed with invasive vs. noninvasive sampling when both samples were cultured quantitatively.[246] Although the pooled OR suggested a survival advantage to the invasive approach (OR = 0.62), the result was not significant ($p = 0.62$); however, patients in the invasive group were more likely to undergo changes in antimicrobial regimen.

Samples obtained via bronchoscopic BAL or PSB and then analyzed quantitatively have the highest specificity in diagnosing VAP. Data reporting outcomes in patients managed with an invasive vs. a "clinical" strategy are conflicting, although the largest such trial showed a significant survival advantage for the invasive/quantitative approach. Patients so managed are also more likely to undergo antibiotic changes, which may be the real value of quantitative analysis of specimens obtained invasively.

Therapy.   Neither the decision to initiate antimicrobial therapy nor the choice of agents requires interpretation of cultures as this information will not become available for 48–72 hours. Rather, the decision is based on clinical suspicion and microscopic examination

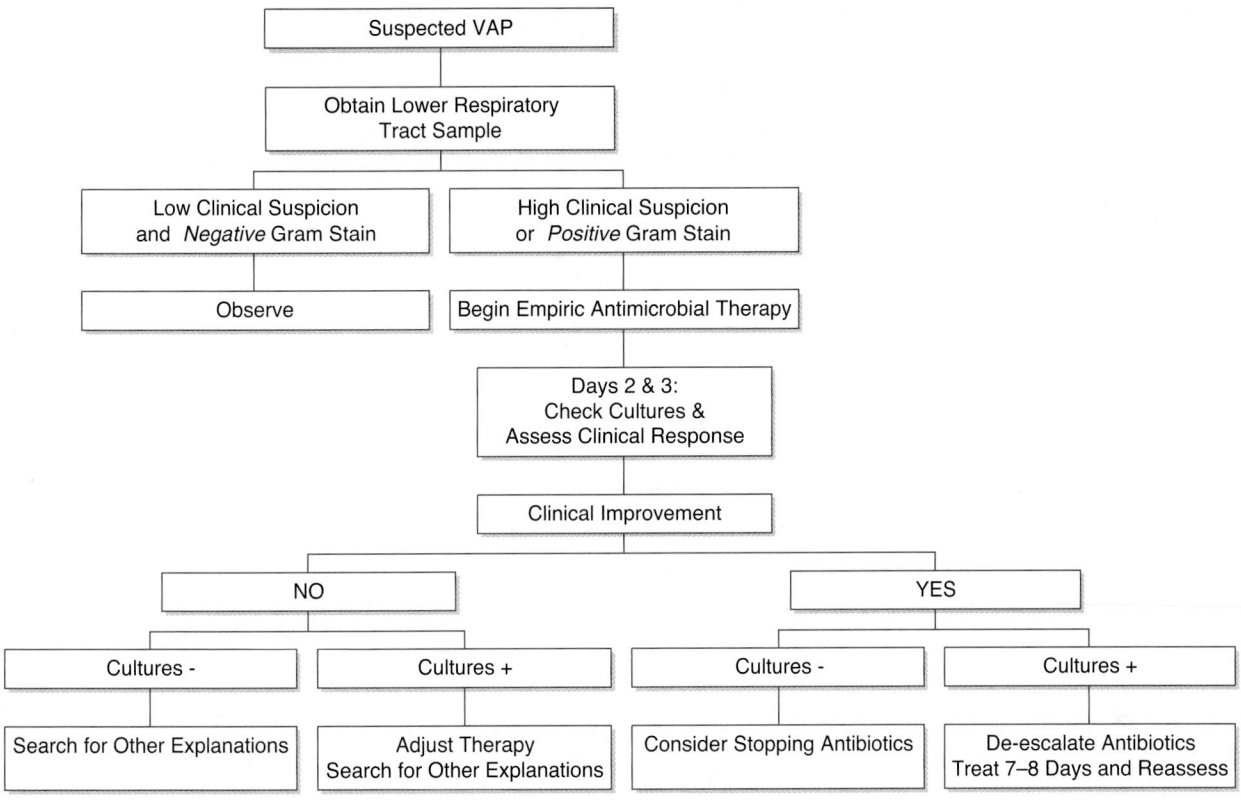

VAP; ventilator-associated pneumonia.

**FIGURE 19-1.** Ventilator-associated pneumonia management algorithm.

of gram-stained sputum (Fig. 19-1). Furthermore, choice of agent is based on both individual patient risk factors for infection with MDR organisms and data from institutional antibiograms (Tables 19-12, 19-21, and 19-23). Antimicrobial therapy may be withheld safely if (1) the gram-stain reveals no organisms and (2) the patient has no signs of severe sepsis.[246,247] Clinical signs of infection with a negative sputum gram stain suggest either an extrapulmonary source of infection or sterile inflammation.

Patients with microorganisms on gram stain or clinical instability should receive empiric therapy for VAP pending the results of cultures. The primary concern is the administration of "adequate therapy," defined as one antimicrobial agent to which the pathogen is sensitive, in the correct dose, via the correct route

of administration, and in a timely manner. A second crucial aspect of VAP therapy involves serial re-evaluation and interpretation of initial microbiology so that (1) therapy may be discontinued if no organism is isolated and the patient has not deteriorated clinically; (2) therapy is de-escalated to treat only the specific etiologic pathogen; and (30 an endpoint of therapy may be identified in prospect and adhered to.

Ample data detail the increased mortality associated with inadequate initial antimicrobial therapy of VAP. Iregui et al.[247] showed that delayed therapy (defined as initial antibiotic treatment administered $\geq$24 hours after meeting diagnostic criteria for VAP) was associated with increased mortality (OR 7.68, 95% CI 4.50–13.09, $p < 0.001$). Similarly, Kollef et al. reported that inadequate initial antimicrobial therapy of gram-negative infections is a risk factor for mortality (OR 4.22, 95% CI 3.57–4.98, $p < 0.001$).[207] Alvarez-Lerma et al. demonstrated that attributable mortality from VAP was lower among patients who received initial appropriate antibiotic treatment (16.2% vs. 24.7%; $p = 0.03$).[233]

Choice of initial antimicrobial therapy depends not only on patient risk factors, but also local (ideally, unit-specific) microbiologic data (Fig. 19-2), which increases the likelihood that appropriate empiric therapy will be prescribed.[248] In general, therapy for patients at risk for infection with a MDR organism should provide coverage against MRSA, *P. aeruginosa*, *Acinetobacter* spp., and ESBL-producing *Klebsiella* spp. (Table 19-23). At least two drugs are usually required, one effective against MRSA (e.g., vancomycin,

**TABLE 19-23**

**Risk Factors for Ventilator-Associated Pneumonia (VAP) with Multidrug-Resistant Organisms**

Late-onset VAP
Antibiotics within previous 90 d
Hospitalization within previous 90 d
Current hospitalization >5 d
Admission from a long-term care/hemodialysis facility
High frequency of antibiotic resistance in the community
Immunosuppressive disease or therapy

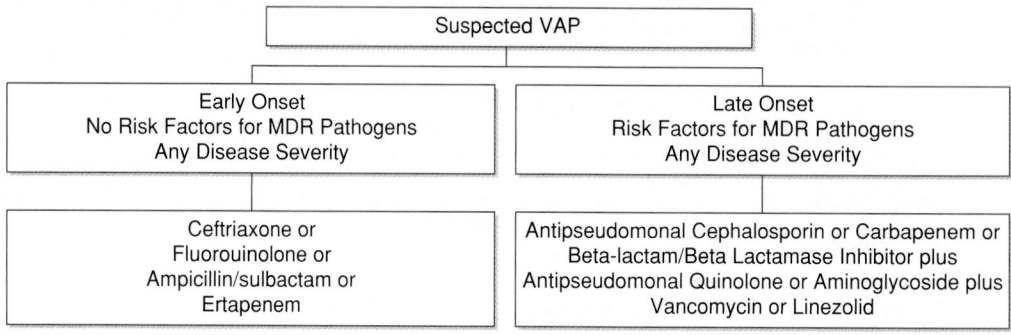

FIGURE 19-2. Algorithm for selection of initial antimicrobial therapy in suspected ventilator-associated pneumonia.

linezolid) and one effective against MDR gram-negative bacilli, particularly *P. aeruginosa* (e.g., piperacillin-tazobactam, meropenem). Patients with early-onset VAP and none of the aforementioned risk factors may be treated with narrow-spectrum therapy as outlined in Fig. 19-2.

Initial antimicrobial therapy for VAP should be given parenterally. Enteral therapy may be considered if patients respond adequately to intravenous therapy, gut function is normal, and the oral antibiotics have equal bioavailability.[249] The use of adjunctive aerosolized aminoglycoside therapy eradicates bacteria but does not affect mortality.[250]

Inadequate dosing of antibiotics leads to the emergence of MDR bacteria and is associated with poorer outcomes in VAP. Appropriate initial dosing of vancomycin (15 mg/kg q12h), aminoglycosides (gentamicin, tobramycin 7 mg/kg daily; amikacin 20 mg/kg daily) and fluoroquinolones (levofloxacin 750 mg daily, ciprofloxacin 400 mg q8h) is paramount to achieving adequate therapy (all doses assume normal renal function). Abundant data now document an association between fluoroquinolone use and the emergence of VAP caused by MDR pathogens, particularly *Pseudomonas*[251–253] and MRSA.[254] Fluoroquinolone use in the treatment of VAP should be judicious, based on regular updates of unit-specific antibiograms.

Whereas multidrug empiric therapy is necessary to treat patients with suspected VAP until culture results become available, combination therapy of a specific pathogen (e.g., "double-coverage" of *Pseudomonas*) is unlikely to provide benefit and may worsen outcomes. Neither in vitro nor in vivo synergy of such combination therapy has been demonstrated consistently. A meta-analysis of all trials of β-lactam monotherapy versus β-lactam-aminoglycoside combination therapy for immunocompetent patients with sepsis, including 64 trials and 7586 patients, found no difference in either mortality (RR 0.90, 95% CI 0.77–1.06) or the development of resistance.[157] In fact, clinical failure was more common with combination therapy.

The goal of empiric therapy is to initiate a combination of antibiotics likely to cover all pathogens, followed by tailored therapy if possible. Ideal treatment of suspected VAP thus involves

both an initial period of perfect sensitivity followed by a period of perfect specificity, based on microbiology results. Thus, no patient with VAP is untreated, and no patient without VAP is treated after microbiologic data are available.

Following initiation of therapy for suspected VAP, cultures of the lower respiratory tract may reveal either (1) no or insignificant growth (below the predetermined threshold value); (2) significant (above threshold) growth of a pathogen sensitive to a narrow-spectrum agent; or (3) significant growth of a pathogen sensitive only to a broad-spectrum agent. Regarding the first scenario, antimicrobial therapy may be discontinued safely if the patient has not deteriorated clinically.[246,255] In the second scenario, therapy is de-escalated to a narrow-spectrum agent active against the pathogen. In the last scenario, the initial broad-spectrum agent active against the pathogen is continued.

Once pathogen-specific therapy has been initiated, its duration must be determined with the goal of avoiding prolonged and unnecessary administration. Resolution of clinical and radiographic parameters takes longer than the eradication of infection.[158] Vidaur et al. found that improved oxygenation and normothermia occurred within three days in VAP patients without ARDS.[239] Dennesen et al. observed a clinical response to therapy (e.g., normalization of temperature, WBC count, arterial oxygen saturation, and decreased bacterial count in sputum) within six days of therapy of VAP.[256]

A randomized, multicenter trial of 401 patients (VAP proved by bronchoscopy and quantitative microbiology) assigned subjects to receive either eight or 14 days of antibiotic therapy.[164] All patients received adequate empiric therapy, and patients in the eight-day therapy group were stable at that time. Patients treated for eight days had equivalent mortality, duration of mechanical ventilation, and recurrence of infection despite significantly more antibiotic-free days. Recurrent infections were less likely to be caused by MDR pathogens in patients treated for eight days; however, patients with VAP caused by nonfermenting gram-negative bacilli (e.g., *Pseudomonas, Acinetobacter, Stenotrophomonas*) were more likely to develop recurrent pneumonia if treated for eight days only. Thus, an eight-day course of initially appropriate antimicrobial therapy appears safe and effective provided that the patient is stable and the pathogen is not a nonfermenting gram-negative bacillus.

In select patients, a shorter course of therapy may be effective for therapy of VAP. Singh et al. randomized patients with suspected VAP and a CPIS score ≤6 points to receive either standard therapy (physician discretion) versus ciprofloxacin monotherapy, with re-evaluation at day three and discontinuation of antibiotics if the CPIS remained ≤6.[257] If the CPIS remained ≤6 at the day-three evaluation, antibiotics were continued in 96% (24/25) of the standard therapy group, but for none in the experimental therapy group ($p = 0.0001$). Mortality did not differ despite a shorter duration ($p = 0.0001$) and lower cost ($p = 0.003$) of antimicrobial therapy in the short-course arm.

Patients who do not respond to appropriate therapy for VAP pose a dilemma.[255] Inadequate therapy, misdiagnosis, or a pneumonia-related complication (e.g., empyema or lung abscess) must be considered. A diagnostic evaluation should be repeated, including repeat quantitative sputum cultures (using a lower diagnostic threshold when interpreting quantitative microbiology given recent antibiotic exposure) and consideration of broadened coverage until new data become available.

## Catheter-Related Blood Stream Infection

Trauma patients often require reliable large-bore central venous access (e.g., femoral, internal jugular, or subclavian vein), and these catheters are prone to local infection at the insertion site and blood stream infection. Strict adherence to infection control[44] and proper insertion technique is crucial for prevention,[258] because trauma patients are at particularly high risk (Table 19-1). When placed under elective (controlled) circumstances, optimal insertion technique includes chlorhexidine skin preparation (not povidone-iodine),[50] draping the entire bed into the sterile field, and donning a cap, a mask, and sterile gown and gloves.[44] If technique is breached, the risk of infection increases exponentially. The catheter should be removed and replaced (if still needed) at a different site using strict asepsis and antisepsis as soon as the patient's condition permits, but certainly within 24 hours. Infection risk for femoral vein catheters is highest, and lowest for catheters placed via the subclavian route.[51] Peripheral vein catheters, peripherally-placed central catheters (PICC), and tunneled central venous catheters (e.g., Hickman, Broviac) pose less risk of infection than percutaneous central venous catheters.[51] Information campaigns, educational initiatives,[259] and strict adherence to insertion protocols are all effective to decrease the risk of CR-BSI. Antibiotic- and antiseptic-coated catheters are controversial, but may help decrease the risk of infection in units that have a high rate of infection.[54]

Catheter infection is diagnosed by isolation of >15 CFU from the subcutaneous 2-cm segment of catheter by the semi-quantitative roll-plate technique. The diagnosis of CR-BSI is confirmed when isolates from blood and the cultured catheter are identical. Blood culture collection technique is crucial. Povidone–iodine skin preparation solution must be allowed to dry on the patient and the rubber stopper of the collection bottle before the specimen is collected. A minimum of two blood cultures (not two bottles from one culture set) must be inoculated. Blood should be collected from two separate peripheral venipunctures whenever possible. When peripheral venous access is poor, it is permissible to collect one set of cultures (two bottles) from a central venous catheter.

Each bottle should be inoculated with a minimum volume of 10 mL blood (from adults).

New automated blood culture incubation/detection systems allow rapid identification of bacteria by turbidimetric assay (often within 24 hours). The presence of antibiotics in blood interferes little with isolation of the pathogen, although it remains true that blood (and, indeed, all specimens for culture) should be collected before antibiotics are begun. If fungal infection is suspected, several days of incubation may be required.

The pathogens of CR-BSI are predominantly gram-positive cocci, most commonly MRSE, MRSA, and enterococci. Unfortunately, MRSE is both the most common cause of CR-BSI and the most common cause of false-positive blood cultures because of contamination during the collection process. Most authorities consider the isolation of MRSE from a single blood culture to be a contaminant and do not treat the patient who does not have indwelling hardware that might become infected secondarily (e.g., prosthetic joint or heart valve). Gram-negative bacillary pathogens are less common (but seldom are contaminants), and fungal CR-BSI are unusual in trauma patients.

Treatment is by removal of the catheter (for peripheral or percutaneous central venous catheters) and parenteral antibiotics, at least initially. It is unclear whether a positive catheter culture requires therapy beyond removal of the catheter, absent local signs of infection or a true-positive blood culture. Catheter-related blood stream infections caused by S. aureus probably require at least two weeks of therapy, although some authorities argue for a longer course (4–6 weeks) because of the risk of metastatic infection (e.g., pneumonia, endocarditis). Vancomycin or linezolid may be chosen for MRSA CR-BSI (or MRSE when treatment is indicated), with daptomycin as an alternative. Therapy for enterococcal or gram-negative CR-BSI is dictated by bacterial susceptibility, with no clear consensus as to duration of therapy. Beyond removal of the catheter, treatment of fungal CR-BSI is controversial. Some authorities recommend removal of the catheter as sole therapy, whereas others recommend at least two weeks of systemic antifungal therapy.

## Peritonitis

The peritonitis that is associated commonly with a perforated viscus is called secondary peritonitis. In the trauma setting, secondary peritonitis may follow penetrating injury to the intestine that is not recognized or treated promptly (>12-hour delay). Other causes include dehiscence of a bowel anastomosis with leakage of succus entericus or development of an intra-abdominal abscess. Secondary peritonitis is polymicrobial, with anaerobic gram-negative bacilli (e.g., B. fragilis) predominating, and E. coli and Klebsiella spp. isolated commonly. Any of a number of antibiotic regimens of appropriate spectrum may be prescribed. Enterococci, Pseudomonas, and other bacteria may be isolated, but do not require specific therapy if the patient is otherwise healthy (e.g., not immunocompromised) and responding to therapy as prescribed.

When secondary peritonitis develops in a hospitalized patient as a complication of disease or therapy, the flora (Table 19-24) are more likely to reflect MDR pathogens encountered in the hospital[260–262] and outcomes are worsened if empiric therapy is not appropriate. For example, enterococci, Enterobacter, and Pseudomonas are more prevalent, whereas E. coli and Klebsiella are less common. Antibiotic therapy must be adjusted accordingly, and surgical

**TABLE 19-24**

**Flora in Different Types of Intra-Abdominal Infection**

| PRIMARY (MONOMICROBIAL) | SECONDARY (POLYMICROBIAL) | TERTIARY (POLYMICROBIAL) |
|---|---|---|
| E. coli | B. fragilis group | S. epidermidis |
| Klebsiella spp. | Other anaerobes | Enterococci |
| S. pneumoniae | E. coli | P. aeruginosa |
| Enterococci | Klebsiella spp. | Candida spp. |
| Anaerobes rare | Other enterics | Enterococci |

source control must be achieved. Failure of two source control procedures with persistent intra-abdominal collections is referred to as *tertiary peritonitis*. Tertiary peritonitis is also characterized by complete failure of intra-abdominal host defenses.[263] There is controversy as to whether tertiary peritonitis is a true invasive infection, or rather peritoneal colonization with incompetent local host defenses. This impacts on whether antibiotics should be prescribed and, if so, for how long. Bacteria isolated in tertiary peritonitis are avirulent opportunists such as MRSE, enterococci, *Pseudomonas*, and *C. albicans*, supporting the hypothesis of incompetent host defense. Some authorities recommend management with an open-abdomen technique, so that peritoneal toilet can be provided manually (at the bedside in some cases) under sedation or anesthesia, until local host defenses recover. There may be no alternative to open-abdomen management if the infection extends to involve the abdominal wall, and extensive debridement is required.

### *Clostridium difficile*-Associated Disease

*Clostridium difficile*-associated disease (CDAD), formerly pseudomembranous colitis, develops because antibiotic therapy disrupts the balance of colonic flora and allows the selection and overgrowth of *C. difficile*, which is present in the fecal flora of about 3% of normal hosts. Any antibiotic can induce this selection pressure, even when given appropriately as single-dose surgical prophylaxis, although clindamycin, third-generation cephalosporins, and fluoroquinolones are the most common causes. Paradoxically, even antibiotics used to treat CDAD (e.g., metronidazole) have been associated with CDAD.

*Clostridium difficile*-associated disease is unquestionably a nosocomial infection. Spores can persist on inanimate surfaces for prolonged periods, and pathogens can be transmitted from patient-to-patient by contaminated equipment (e.g., bedpans, rectal thermometers) or on the hands of healthcare workers. The alcohol gel that is used increasingly for hand disinfection is not active against spores of *C. difficile*; therefore, hand washing with soap and water is necessary when caring for an infected patient or during outbreaks.

The clinical spectrum of CDAD is wide, ranging from asymptomatic (8% of affected patients do not have diarrhea) to life-threatening transmural pan-colitis with perforation and severe sepsis or septic shock. The typical patient will have fever, abdominal distention, copious diarrhea, and leukocytosis. Hemorrhage from the colon is rare and, if observed, should prompt an alternative diagnosis. Diagnosis is by assay for the enterotoxins in a fresh stool specimen. This has largely supplanted colonoscopy because up to 50% of patients do not have the "characteristic" colonic mucosal pseudomembranes (hence, the change is nomenclature, as well).

Treatment of patients with mild cases consists of withdrawal of the putative offending antibiotic; oral antibiotic therapy is often prescribed but may or may not be necessary. Patients with severe cases may require parenteral metronidazole or oral or enteral vancomycin (by gavage or enema, if ileus precludes oral therapy) as parenteral vancomycin is ineffective.[156–158] Some patients with severe disease may require a total abdominal colectomy. The prevalence of severe disease has increased markedly with the emergence of a new strain of *C. difficile*. The new strain has undergone a mutation of a gene that suppresses toxin production, such that far more toxin is elaborated, resulting in clinically severe disease.[156–158] More of these patients will require surgery, but it remains to be determined whether or how antibiotic therapy should be modified to combat this dangerous bacterium.

### Sinusitis

Nosocomial sinusitis is a dangerous, closed-space infection that is increasing in incidence, but difficult to diagnose and controversial as to its actual incidence and importance.[264] Patients with transnasal intubation (particularly nasotracheal intubation, after seven days of which the incidence is one-third) and maxillofacial trauma are at particular risk. Purulent or foul-smelling nasal discharge is an obvious clue to the diagnosis. As it is not always present, sinusitis must be sought radiographically by computed tomography of the facial bones to identify sinus mucosal thickening or opacification. Because the process is often occult, the more the diagnosis is sought, the more often it will be confirmed.

Sinusitis should be suspected in any patient with sepsis, particularly if initial cultures (e.g., blood, sputum, urine, indwelling vascular catheters) are unrevealing. If sinusitis is suspected, the diagnosis is confirmed by a maxillary antral tap, lavage, and culture using aseptic technique. Gram-positive cocci, gram-negative bacilli (including *P. aeruginosa*), and fungi (incidence, 8%) are possible pathogens, so initial therapy should be based on local susceptibility patterns. Most antibiotics achieve adequate tissue penetration. The optimal duration of therapy is unknown, so the patient's clinical response is monitored. Refractory cases may require repetitive lavage of the sinus or a formal drainage procedure.

Sinusitis is a predisposing factor for VAP and may be a source of pathogens in the lower respiratory tract. There is an 85% concordance between pathogens of sinusitis and pneumonia in patients who develop VAP subsequently, lending credence to the hypothesis that purulent sinus drainage inoculates the lower airway.

### Decubitus Ulcer

Decubitus ulcer is another source of occult or overt infection. Patients are at substantially increased risk with prolonged bed rest (>7 days),[265] which may be mitigated by specialized bedding. Neither vasopressor therapy nor poor nutrition has been substantiated as an additional risk factor. Morbid obesity is a clear risk factor, given that routine turning and positioning of such patients is a formidable undertaking. Most decubitus ulcers form in the presacral area, but can form where unremitting pressure is placed upon tissue. For example, if the position of the endotracheal tube at the lips is not changed periodically, ulceration may occur at the corner of the mouth. Also, occipital decubitus have been reported from ill-fitting cervical collars when used in obtunded or comatose patients or when "clearance" of the cervical spine is delayed.

When evaluating a patient for occult infection, the skin must be inspected systematically for decubitus ulcers. Deep (Stage III-involving subcutaneous fat; Stage IV-involving fascia, muscle, or bone) ulcers may require debridement or systemic antibiotic therapy. In rare cases, a decubitus ulcer may transform into a life-threatening necrotizing soft tissue infection.

# REFERENCES

1. Stillwell M, Caplan ES: The septic multiple-trauma patient. *Infect Dis Clin North Am* 3:155, 1989.
2. Barie PS, Hydo LJ: Epidemiology of multiple organ dysfunction syndrome in critical surgical illness. *Surg Infect* 1:173, 2000.
3. Asensio JA, Stewart BM, Murray J, et al.: Penetrating cardiac injuries. *Surg Clin North Am* 76:685, 1996.
4. Napolitano LM, Faist E, Wichmann MW, et al.: Immune dysfunction in trauma. *Surg Clin North Am* 79:1385, 1999.
5. Yendamuri S, Fulda GJ, Tinkoff GH: Admission serum glucose as a prognostic indicator in trauma. *J Trauma* 55:33, 2003.
6. National Nosocomial Infections Surveillance (NNIS) System report, data summary from January 1992–June 2004, issued October 2004. *Am J Infect Control* 232:470, 2004.
7. Dente CJ, Tyburski J, Wilson RF, et al.: Ostomy as a risk factor for posttraumatic infection in penetrating colonic injuries: Univariate and multivariate analyses. *J Trauma* 49:628, 2000.
8. Papia G, McLellan BA, El-Helou P, et al.: Infection in hospitalized trauma patients: Incidence, risk factors, and complications. *J Trauma* 47:923, 1999.
9. Wallace WC, Cinat M, Gornick WB, et al.: Nosocomial infections in the surgical intensive care unit: A difference between trauma and surgical patients. *Am Surg* 65:987, 1999.
10. Desborough JP: The stress response to trauma and surgery. *Br J Anaesth* 85:109, 2000.
11. Gardner EM, Murasko DM: Age-related changes in Type 1 and Type 2 cytokine production in humans. *Biogerontology* 32:281, 2002.
12. Latham R, Lancaster AD, Covington JF, et al.: The association of diabetes and glucose control with surgical-site infections among cardiothoracic surgery patients. *Infect Control Hosp Epidemiol* 22:607, 2001.
13. Cheadle WG: Risk factors for surgical site infection. *Surg Infect* 7:S7, 2006.
14. Zerr KJ, Furnary AP, Grunkemeier GL, et al.: Glucose control lowers the risk of wound infection in diabetics after open heart operations. *Ann Thorac Surg* 63:356, 1997.
15. Pomposelli JJ, Baxter JK III, Babineau TJ, et al.: Early postoperative glucose control predicts nosocomial infection rate in diabetic patients. *JPEN J Parenter Enteral Nutr* 22:77, 1998.
16. van den Berghe G, Wouters P, Weekers F, et al.: Intensive insulin therapy in the critically ill patients. *N Engl J Med* 345:1359, 2001.
17. Pittas AG, Siegel RD, Lau J: Insulin therapy for critically ill hospitalized patients: A meta-analysis of randomized controlled trials. *Arch Intern Med* 164:2005, 2004.
18. Gordon BR, Parker TS, Levine DM, et al.: Relationship of hypolipidemia to cytokine concentrations and outcomes in critically ill surgical patients. *Crit Care Med* 29:1563, 2001.
19. Delgado-Rodriguez M, Medina-Cuadros M, Gomez-Ortega A, et al.: Cholesterol and serum albumin levels as predictors of cross infection, death, and length of hospital stay. *Arch Surg* 137:805, 2002.
20. Bonville DA, Parker TS, Levine DM, et al.: The relationships of hypocholesterolemia to cytokine concentrations and mortality in critically ill surgical patients with systemic inflammatory response syndrome. *Surg Infect* 5:39, 2004.
21. Wichmann MW, Zellweger R, DeMaso CM, et al.: Enhanced immune responses in females, as opposed to decreased responses in males following haemorrhagic shock and resuscitation. *Cytokine* 8:853, 1996.
22. Diodato MD, Knoferl MW, Schwacha MG, et al.: Gender differences in the inflammatory response and survival following haemorrhage and subsequent sepsis. *Cytokine* 14:162, 2001.
23. Offner PJ, Moore EE, Biffl WL: Male gender is a risk factor for major infections after surgery. *Arch Surg* 134:935, 1999.
24. Moss M, Mannino DM: Race and gender differences in acute respiratory distress syndrome deaths in the United States: An analysis of multiple-cause mortality data (1979–1996). *Crit Care Med* 30:1679, 2002.
25. Gannon CJ, Napolitano LM, Pasquale M, et al.: A statewide population-based study of gender differences in trauma: Validation of a prior single-institution study. *J Am Coll Surg* 195:11, 2002.
26. Angus DC, Linde-Zwirble WT, Lidicker J, et al.: Epidemiology of severe sepsis in the United States: Analysis of incidence, outcome, and associated costs of care. *Crit Care Med* 29:1303, 2001.
27. McDunn JE, Chung TP, Laramie JM, et al.: Physiologic genomics. *Surgery* 139:133, 2006.
28. Cobb JP, O'Keefe GE: Injury research in the genomic era. *Lancet* 363:2076, 2004.
29. Laudanski K, Miller-Graziano C, Xiao W, et al.: Cell-specific expression and pathway analyses reveal alterations in trauma-related human T cell and monocyte populations. *Proc Natl Acad Sci U S A* 103:15564, 2006.
30. Arcaroli J, Fessler MB, Abraham E: Genetic polymorphisms and sepsis. *Shock* 24:300, 2005.
31. Gunderson KL, Steemers FJ, Lee G, et al.: A genome-wide scalable SNP genotyping assay using microarray technology. *Nat Genet* 37:549, 2005.
32. Machiedo GW, Powell RJ, Rush BF Jr, et al.: The incidence of decreased red blood cell deformability in sepsis and the association with oxygen free radical damage and multiple-system organ failure. *Arch Surg* 124:1386, 1989.
33. Danks RR: Triangle of death. How hypothermia, acidosis and coagulopathy can adversely impact trauma patients. *J Emerg Med Serv* 27:61, 2002.
34. Ives CL, Harrison DK, Stansby GS: Tissue oxygen saturation, measured by near-infrared spectroscopy, and its relationship to surgical-site infections. *Br J Surg* 94:87, 2007.
35. Dellinger EP: Roles of temperature and oxygenation in prevention of surgical site infection. *Surg Infect* 7:S27, 2006.
36. Human albumin administration in critically ill patients: Systematic review of randomised controlled trials. Cochrane Injuries Group Albumin Reviewers. *BMJ* 317:235, 1998.
37. Rotstein OD: Novel strategies for immunomodulation after trauma: Revisiting hypertonic saline as a resuscitation strategy for hemorrhagic shock. *J Trauma* 49:580, 2000.
38. Bochicchio GV, Napolitano LM, Joshi M, et al.: Persistent systemic inflammatory response syndrome is predictive of nosocomial infection in trauma. *J Trauma* 53:245, 2002.
39. Nathens AB, Nester TA, Rubenfeld GA, et al.: The effects of leukoreduced blood transfusion on infection risk following injury: A randomized controlled trial. *Shock* 26:342, 2006.
40. Nichols RL, Smith JW, Klein DB, et al.: Risk of infection after penetrating abdominal trauma. *N Engl J Med* 311:1065, 1984.
41. Agarwal N, Murphy JG, Cayten CG, et al.: Blood transfusion increases the risk of infection after trauma. *Arch Surg* 128:171, 1993.
42. Claridge JA, Sawyer RG, Schulman AM, et al.: Blood transfusions correlate with infections in trauma patients in a dose-dependent manner. *Am Surg* 68:566, 2002.
43. Hill GE, Frawley WH, Griffith KE, et al.: Allogeneic blood transfusion increases the risk of postoperative blood infection: A meta-analysis. *J Trauma* 54:908, 2003.
44. Taylor RW, O'Brien J, Trottier SJ, et al.: Red blood cell transfusions and nosocomial infections in critically ill patients. *Crit Care Med* 34:2302, 2006.
45. Shorr AF, Jackson WL, Kelly KM, et al.: Transfusion practice and blood stream infections in critically ill patients. *Chest* 127:1722, 2005.
46. Shorr AF, Duh MS, Kelly KM, et al. (CRIT study Group): Red blood cell transfusion and ventilator-associated pneumonia: A potential link? *Crit Care Med* 32:666, 2004.
47. Scharte M, Fink MP: Red blood cell physiology in critical illness. *Crit Care Med* 31:S651, 2003.
48. Fernandes CJ Jr, Akamine N, De Marco FV, et al.: Red blood cell transfusion does not increase oxygen consumption in critically ill septic patients. *Crit Care* 5:362, 2001.
49. Moore FA, Moore EE, Sauaia A: Blood transfusion. An independent risk factor for postinjury multiple organ failure. *Arch Surg* 132:620, 1997.
50. Offner PJ, Moore EE, Biffl WL, et al.: Increased rate of infection associated with transfusion of old blood after severe injury. *Arch Surg* 137:711, 2002.
51. Hebert PC, Wells G, Blajchman MA, et al.: A multicenter, randomized, controlled clinical trial of transfusion requirements in critical care. Transfusion Requirements in Critical Care Investigators, Canadian Critical Care Trials Group. *N Engl J Med* 340:409, 1999.
52. Mangram AJ, Horan TC, Pearson ML, et al.: Guideline for prevention of surgical site infection, 1999. Hospital Infection Control Practices Advisory Committee. *Infect Control Hosp Epidemiol* 20:250, 1999.
53. O'Grady NP, Alexander M, Dellinger EP, et al.: Guidelines for the prevention of intravascular catheter-related infections. Centers for Disease Control and Prevention. *MMWR Recomm Rep* 51:1, 2002.
54. Minei JP, Nathens AB, West M, et al.: Inflammation and the host response to injury large scale collaborative research program investigators. Inflammation

and the host response to injury, a large-scale collaborative project: Patient-oriented research core-standard operating procedures for clinical care. II. Guidelines for prevention, diagnosis and treatment of ventilator-associated pneumonia (VAP) in the trauma patient. *J Trauma* 60:1106, 2006.

55. Kollef MH: The prevention of ventilator-associated pneumonia. *N Engl J Med* 340:627, 1999.
56. Latham R, Lancaster AD, Covington JF, et al.: The association of diabetes and glucose control with surgical-site infections among cardiothoracic surgery patients. *Infect Control Hosp Epidemiol* 22:607, 2001.
57. Zerr KJ, Furnary AP, Grunkemeier GL, et al.: Glucose control lowers the risk of wound infection in diabetics after open heart operations. *Ann Thorac Surg* 63:356, 1997.
58. Pomposelli JJ, Baxter JK III, Babineau TJ, et al.: Early postoperative glucose control predicts nosocomial infection rate in diabetic patients. *JPEN J Parenter Enteral Nutr* 22:77, 1998.
59. van den Berghe G, Wouters P, Weekers F, et al.: Intensive insulin therapy in the critically ill patients. *N Engl J Med* 345:1359, 2001.
60. Pittas AG, Siegel RD, Lau J: Insulin therapy for critically ill hospitalized patients: A meta-analysis of randomized controlled trials. *Arch Intern Med* 164:2005, 2004.
61. Heyland DK, MacDonald S, Keefe L, et al.: Total parenteral nutrition in the critically ill patient: A meta-analysis. *JAMA* 280:2013, 1998.
62. Marik PE, Zaloga GP: Early enteral nutrition in acutely ill patients: A systematic review. *Crit Care Med* 29:2264, 2001.
63. Trick WE, Vernon MG, Welbel SF, et al.: Chicago Antimicrobial Resistance Project. Multicenter intervention program to increase adherence to hand hygiene recommendations and glove use and to reduce the incidence of antimicrobial resistance. *Infect Control Hosp Epidemiol* 28:42, 2007.
64. Chaiyakunapruk N, Veenstra DL, Lipsky BA, et al.: Chlorhexidine compared with povidone-iodine solution for vascular catheter-site care: A meta-analysis. *Ann Intern Med* 136:792, 2002.
65. McGee DC, Gould MK: Preventing complications of central venous catheterization. *N Engl J Med* 348:1123, 2003.
66. Collard HR, Saint S, Matthay MA: Prevention of ventilator-associated Pneumonia: An evidence-based systematic review. *Ann Intern Med* 138:494, 2003.
67. Rello J, Kollef M, Diaz E, et al.: Reduced burden of bacterial airway colonization with a novel silver-coated endotracheal tube in a randomized multiple-center feasibility study. *Crit Care Med* 34:2766, 2006.
68. Hanna HA, Raad II, Hackett B, et al.: M.D. Anderson Catheter Study Group. Antibiotic-impregnated catheters associated with significant decrease in nosocomial and multidrug-resistant bacteremias in critically ill patients. *Chest* 124:1030, 2003.
69. Johnson JR, Kuskowski MA, Wilt TJ: Systematic review: Antimicrobial urinary catheters to prevent catheter-associated urinary tract infection in hospitalized patients. *Ann Intern Med* 144:116, 2006.
70. Ely EW, Baker AM, Dunagan DP, et al.: Effect on the duration of mechanical ventilation of identifying patients capable of breathing spontaneously. *N Engl J Med* 335:1864, 1996.
71. Esteban A, Frutos-Vivar F, Ferguson ND, et al.: Noninvasive positive-pressure ventilation for respiratory failure after extubation. *N Engl J Med* 350:2452, 2004.
72. Shah MR, Hasselblad V, Stevenson LW, et al.: Impact of the pulmonary artery catheter in critically ill patients: Meta-analysis of randomized controlled trials. *JAMA* 294:1664, 2005.
73. Manian FA, Meyer PL, Setzer J, et al.: Surgical site infections associated with methicillin-resistant Staphylococcus aureus: Do postoperative factors play a role? *Clin Infect Dis* 36:863, 2003.
74. Velmahos GC, Toutouzas KG, Sarkisyan G, et al.: Severe trauma is not an excuse for prolonged antibiotic prophylaxis. *Arch Surg* 137:537, 2002.
75. Bratzler DW, Houck PM, Richards C, et al.: Use of antimicrobial prophylaxis for major surgery: Baseline results from the National Surgical Infection Prevention Project. *Arch Surg* 140:174, 2005.
76. Reed RL II, Ericcson CD, Wu A, et al.: The pharmacokinetics of prophylactic antibiotics in trauma. *J Trauma* 32:21, 1992.
77. Bozorgzadeh A, Pizzi WF, Barie PS, et al.: The duration of antibiotic administration in penetrating abdominal trauma. *Am J Surg* 177:125, 1999.
78. Luchette FA, Borzotta AP, Croce MA, et al.: Practice management guidelines for prophylactic abtibiotic use in penetrating abdominal trauma: The EAST practice management guidelines work group. *J Trauma* 48:508, 2000.
79. Delgado G Jr, Barletta JF, Kanji S, et al.: Characteristics of prophylactic antibiotic strategies after penetrating abdominal trauma at a level I urban trauma center: A comparison with the EAST guidelines. *J Trauma* 53:673, 2002.
80. Weigelt JA: Risk of wound infections in trauma patients. *Am J Surg* 150:782, 1985.
81. Hollander JE, Singer AJ, Valentine SM, et al.: Risk factors for infection in patients with traumatic lacerations. *Acad Emerg Med* 8:716, 2001.
82. Cassell OC, Ion L: Are antibiotics necessary in the surgical management of upper limb lacerations? *Br J Plast Surg* 50:523, 1997.
83. Cummings P: Antibiotics to prevent infection in patients with dog bite wounds: A meta-analysis of randomized trials. *Ann Emerg Med* 23:535, 1994.
84. Gillespie WJ, Walenkamp G: Antibiotic prophylaxis for surgery for proximal femoral and other closed long bone fractures. *Cochrane Database Syst Rev* 1:CD000244, 2001.
85. Carsenti-Etesse H, Doyon F, Desplaces N, et al.: Epidemiology of bacterial infection during management of open leg fractures. *Eur J Clin Microbiol Infect Dis* 18:315, 1999.
86. Dellinger EP: Antibiotic prophylaxis in trauma: Penetrating abdominal injuries and open fractures. *Rev Infect Dis* 13:847, 1991.
87. http://www.east.org/tpg.html. Accessed November 13, 2002.
88. Hauser CJ, Adams CA Jr, Eachempati SR, Council of the Surgical Infection Society: Surgical Infection Society guideline: Prophylactic antibiotic use in open fractures: An evidence-based guideline. *Surg Infect* 7:379, 2006.
89. Luchette FA, Barie PS, Oswanski MF, et al.: Practice management guidelines for prophylactic antibiotic use in tube thoracostomy for traumatic hemopneumothorax. The EAST Practice Management Guidelines Workgroup. Eastern Association for the Surgery of Trauma. *J Trauma* 48:753, 2000.
90. Rebuck JA, Murry KR, Rhoney DH, et al.: Infection related to intracranial pressure monitors in adults: Analysis of risk factors and antibiotic prophylaxis. *J Neurol Neurosurg Psych* 69:381, 2000.
91. Villalobos T, Arango C, Kubilis P, et al.: Antibiotic prophylaxis after basilar skull fractures: A meta-analysis. *Clin Infect Dis* 27:364, 1998.
92. Moran GJ, Talan DA, Mower W, et al.: Appropriateness of rabies postexposure prophylaxis treatment for animal exposures. *JAMA* 284:1001, 2000.
93. Gergen PJ, McQuinllan GM, Kiely M, et al.: A population-based serologic survey of immunity to tetanus in the United States. *N Engl J Med* 332:761, 1995.
94. Howdieshell TR, Heffernan D, Dipiro JT: Therapeutic Agents Committee of the Surgical Infection Society: Surgical infection society guidelines for vaccination after traumatic injury. *Surg Infect* 7:275, 2006.
95. Weiss HB, Friedman DI, Coben JH: Incidence of dog bite injuries treated in emergency departments. *JAMA* 279:51, 1998.
96. Noah DL: Epidemiology of human rabies in the United States, 1980 to 1986. *Ann Intern Med* 128:922, 1998.
97. Human Rabies Prevention–United States, 1999: Recommendations of the Immunization Practices Advisory Committee (ACIP). *MMWR Morb Mortal Wkly Rep* 48:1, 1999.
98. Rupprecht CE, Gibbons RV: Prophylaxis against rabies. *N Engl J Med* 351:2626, 2004.
99. Modlin JF: Advisory Committee on Immunization Practices. Use of anthrax vaccine in the United States. *MMWR Morb Mortal Wkly Rep* 49:1, 2000.
100. Wassilak SGF, Orenstein WA, Sutter RW: Tetanus toxoid. In Plotkin SA, Orenstein WA, eds. *Vaccines*, 4th ed. Philadelphia: WB Saunders, 2004, p. 745.
101. Centers for Disease Control and Prevention: Tetanus surveillance–United States, 1995–1997. CDC Surveillance Summaries. *MMWR Morb Mortal Wkly Rep* 47:1, 1998.
102. Hsu SS, Groleau G: Tetanus in the emergency department: A current review. *J Emerg Med* 20:357, 2002.
103. Brigden ML, Pattullo AL: Prevention and management of overwhelming postsplenectomy infection—An update. *Crit Care Med* 27:836, 1999.
104. Lortan JE: Management of asplenic patients. *Br J Haematol* 84:566, 1993.
105. Holdsworth RJ, Irvin AD, Cushierr A: Postsplenectomy sepsis and mortality rate: Actual versus perceived risk. *Br J Surg* 78:1031, 1991.
106. Weintraub LR: Splenectomy: Who, when, and why? *Hosp Pract* 29:27, 1994.
107. Shaw JHF, Print CG: Postsplenectomy sepsis. *Br J Surg* 76:1074, 1989.
108. Prevention of pneumococcal disease: Recommendations of the Advisory Committee on Immunization Practices (ACIP). *MMWR Morb Mortal Wkly Rep* 46:12, 1997.
109. Butler JC, Breiman RF, Campbell JF, et al.: Pneumococcal polysaccharide vaccine efficacy: An evaluation of current recommendations. *JAMA* 270:1826, 1993.
110. Recommendations of the Advisory Committee on Immunization Practices (ACIP): Use of vaccines and immune globulins in persons with altered immunocompetence. *MMWR Morb Mortal Wkly Rep* 42:1, 1993.
111. Prevention and control of meningococcal disease: Recommendations of the Advisory Committee on Immunization Practices (ACIP). *MMWR Morb Mortal Wkly Rep* 49:1, 1999.
112. Pedersen FK, Nielsen JL, Andersen V, et al.: Proposal for the prevention of fulminant infection after splenectomy. *Ugeskr Laeger* 144:1453, 1992.
113. Shatz DV, Schinsky MF, Pais LB, et al.: Immune responses of splenectomized trauma patients to the 23-valent pneumococcal polysaccharide vaccine at 1 versus 7 versus 14 days after splenectomy. *J Trauma* 44:760, 1998.
114. Giebink GS, Le CT, Schiffman G: Decline of serum antibody in splenectomized children after vaccination with pneumococcal capsular polysaccharides. *J Pediatr* 105:576, 1984.

115. American Academy of Pediatrics, Committee on Infectious Disease. Policy statement: Recommendations for the prevention of pneumococcal infections, including the use of pneumococcal conjugate vaccine, pneumococcal polysaccharide vaccine, and antibiotic prophylaxis. *Pediatrics* 106:362, 2000.

116. Bradley JS, Guidos R, Baragona S, et al.: Anti-infective research and development–problems, challenges, and solutions. *Lancet Infect Dis* 7:68, 2007.

117. Champney WS: The other target for ribosomal antibiotics: Inhibition of bacterial ribosomal subunit formation. *Infect Disord Drug Targets* 6:377, 2006.

118. Harbottle H, Thakur S, Zhao S, et al.: Genetics of antimicrobial resistance. *Anim Biotechnol* 17:111, 2006.

119. Navon-Venezia S, Ben-Ami R, Carmeli Y: Update on Pseudomonas aeruginosa and Acinetobacter baumannii infections in the healthcare setting. *Curr Opin Infect Dis* 18:306, 2005.

120. Paterson DL: Resistance in gram-negative bacteria: Enterobacteriaceae. *Am J Infect Control* 34:S20, 2006.

121. Giamarellou H: Treatment options for multidrug-resistant bacteria. *Expert Rev Anti Infect Ther* 4:601, 2006.

122. Paterson DL: Clinical experience with recently approved antibiotics. *Curr Opin Pharmacol* 6:486, 2006.

123. Rice LB: Successful interventions for gram-negative resistance to extended-spectrum beta-lactam antiobiotics. *Pharmacotherapy* 19:120S, 1999.

124. Hope R, Potz NA, Warner M, et al.: Efficacy of practised screening methods for detection of cephalosporin-resistant Enterobacteriaceae. *J Antimicrob Chemother* 59:110, 2007.

125. Neuhauser MM, Weinstein RA, Rydman R, et al.: Antibiotic resistance among gram-negative bacilli in US intensive care units: Implications for fluoroquinolone use. *JAMA* 289:885, 2003.

126. Eggimann P, Pittet D: Postoperative fungal infections. *Surg Infect* 7:S53, 2006.

127. Brion LP, Uko SE, Goldman DL: Risk of resistance associated with fluconazole prophylaxis: Systematic review. *J Infect* 54:521, 2007.

128. Patterson TF: Treatment of invasive aspergillosis: Polyenes, echinocandins, or azoles? *Med Mycol* 44:357, 2006.

129. Fry DE: The importance of antibiotic pharmacokinetics in critical illness. *Am J Surg* 172:20S, 1996.

130. DiPiro JT, Edmiston CE, Bohnen JMA: Pharmacodynamics of antimicrobial therapy in surgery. *Am J Surg* 171:615, 1996.

131. Naimi TS, LeDell KH, Como-Sabetti K, et al.: Comparison of community- and health care-associated methicillin-resistant Staphylococcus aureus infection. *JAMA* 290:2976, 2004.

132. Anstead GM, Owens AD: Recent advances in the treatment of infections due to resistant Staphylococcus aureus. *Curr Opin Infect Dis* 17:549, 2004.

133. Schentag JJ, Gilliland KK, Paladino JA: What have we learned from pharmacokinetic and pharmacodynamic theories? *Clin Infect Dis* 32:S39, 2001.

134. Nicolau DP, Freeman CD, Belliveau PP, et al.: Experience with a once-daily aminoglycoside program administered to 2,184 adult patients. *Antimicrob Agents Chemother* 39:650, 1995.

135. Kashuba AD, Bertino JS Jr, Nafziger AN: Dosing of aminoglycosides to rapidly attain pharmacodynamic goals and hasten therapeutic response by using individualized pharmacokinetic monitoring of patients with pneumonia caused by gram-negative organisms. *Antimicrob Agents Chemother* 42:1842, 1998.

136. Thomas JK, Forrest A, Bhavnani SM, et al.: Pharmacodynamic evaluation of factors associated with the development of bacterial resistance in acutely ill patients during therapy. *Antimicrob Agents Chemother* 42:521, 1998.

137. Benko AS, Cappelletty DM, Kruse JA, et al.: Continuous infusion versus intermittent administration of ceftazidime in critically ill patients with suspected Gram-negative infections. *Antimicrob Agents Chemother* 40:691, 1996.

138. Lau WK, Mercer D, Itani KM, et al.: Randomized, open-label, comparative study of piperacillin-tazobactam administered by continuous infusion versus intermittent infusion for treatment of hospitalized patients with complicated intra-abdominal infection. *Antimicrob Agents Chemother* 50:3556, 2006.

139. Kollef MH, Ward S, Sherman G, et al.: Inadequate treatment of nosocomial infections is associated with certain empiric antibiotic choices. *Crit Care Med* 28:3456, 2000.

140. Alvarez-Lerma F: Modification of empiric antibiotic treatment in patients with pneumonia acquired in the intensive care unit: ICU-Acquired Pneumonia Study Group. *Intensive Care Med* 22:387, 1996.

141. Iregui M, Ward S, Sherman G, et al.: Clinical importance of delays in the initiation of appropriate antibiotic treatment for ventilator-associated pneumonia. *Chest* 122:262, 2002.

142. Garnacho-Montero J, Garcia-Garmendia JL, Barrero-Almodovar A, et al.: Impact of adequate empirical antibiotic therapy on the outcome of patients admitted to the intensive care unit with sepsis. *Crit Care Med* 31:2742, 2003.

143. Evans RS, Pestotnik SL, Classen DC, et al.: A computer-assisted management program for antibiotics and other antiinfective agents. *N Engl J Med* 338:232, 1998.

144. Kollef MH, Vlasnik J, Sharpless L, et al.: Scheduled rotation of antibiotic classes: A strategy to decrease the incidence of ventilator-associated pneumonia due to antibiotic-resistant gram-negative bacteria. *Am J Respir Crit Care Med* 156:1040, 1997.

145. Gruson D, Hilbert G, Vargas F, et al.: Strategy of antibiotic rotation: Long term effect on incidence and susceptibilities of gram-negative bacilli responsible for ventilator-associated pneumonia. *Crit Care Med* 31:1908, 2003.

146. Raymond DP, Pelletier SJ, Crabtree TD, et al.: Impact of a rotating empiric antibiotic schedule on infectious mortality in an intensive care unit. *Crit Care Med* 29:1101, 2001.

147. van Loon HJ, Vriens MR, Fluit AC, et al.: Antibiotic rotation and development of gram-negative antibiotic resistance. *Am J Respir Crit Care Med* 171:480, 2005.

148. Kollef MH: Is antibiotic cycling the answer to preventing the mergence of bacterial resistance in the intensive care unit? *Clin Infect Dis* 43:S82, 2006.

149. Niederman MS: Appropriate use of antimicrobial agents: Challenges and strategies for improvement. *Crit Care Med* 31:608, 2003.

150. Kollef MH, Micek ST: Strategies to prevent antimicrobial resistance in the intensive care unit. *Crit Care Med* 33:1845, 2005.

151. LeDell K, Muto CA, Jarvis WR, et al.: SHEA guideline for preventing nosocomial transmission of multidrug-resistant strains of Staphylococcus aureus and Enterococcus. *Infect Control Hosp Epidemiol* 24:639, 2003.

152. Talmor M, Hydo L, Barie PS: Relationship of systemic inflammatory response syndrome (SIRS) to organ dysfunction, length of stay, and mortality in critical surgical illness: Effect of intensive care unit resuscitation. *Arch Surg* 134:81, 1999.

153. Barie PS, Hydo LJ: Epidemiology of multiple organ dysfunction syndrome in critical surgical illness. *Surg Infect* 1:173, 2000.

154. Barie PS, Hydo LJ, Eachempati SR: Characteristics and consequences of fever complicating critical surgical illness. *Surg Infect* 5:145, 2004.

155. Bosso JA: The antimicrobial armamentarium: Evaluating current and future treatment options. *Pharmacotherapy* 25:55S, 2005.

156. Padmanabhan RA, Larosa SP, Tomecki KJ: What's new in antibiotics? *Dermatol Clin* 23:301, 2005.

157. Paul M, Benuri-Silbiger I, Soares-Weiser K, et al.: Beta-lactam monotherapy versus beta-lactam-aminoglycoside combination therapy for sepsis in immunocompetent patients: Systematic review and meta-analysis of randomized trials. *BMJ* 328:668, 2004.

158. American Thoracic Society: Guidelines for the management of adults with hospital-acquired, ventilator-associated, and healthcare-associated pneumonia. *Am J Resp Crit Care Med* 171:388, 2005.

159. Pittet D, Monod M, Suter PM, et al.: Candida colonization and subsequent infections in critically ill surgical patients. *Ann Surg* 220:751, 1994.

160. Lipsett PA: Surgical critical care: Fungal infections in surgical patients. *Crit Care Med* 34:S215, 2006.

161. Gleason TG, May AK, Caparelli D, et al.: Emerging evidence of selection of fluconazole-tolerant fungi in surgical intensive care units. *Arch Surg* 132:1197, 1997.

162. Pappas PG, Rex JH, Sobel JD, et al.: Infectious Diseases Society of America. Guidelines for treatment of candidiasis. *Clin Infect Dis* 38:161, 2004.

163. Dellinger EP: Duration of antibiotic treatment in surgical infections of the abdomen. Undesired effects of antibiotics and future studies. *Eur J Surg* 576:29, 1996.

164. Chastre J, Wolff M, Fagon JY, et al.: Comparison of 15 vs. 8 days of antibiotic therapy for ventilator-associated pneumonia in adults: A randomized trial. *JAMA* 290:2588, 2003.

165. Bartlett JG, Perl TM: The new Clostridium difficile. What does it mean? *N Engl J Med* 343:2503, 2005.

166. Loo V, Poirier L, Miller MA, et al.: A predominantly clonal multi-institutional outbreak of Clostridium difficile-associated diarrhea with high morbidity and mortality. *N Engl J Med* 353:2442, 2005.

167. McDonald LC, Kilgore GE, Thompson A, et al.: An epidemic, toxin gene-variant strain of Clostridium difficile. *N Engl J Med* 353:2433, 2005.

168. Ferrara AM: Potentially multidrug-resistant non-fermentative Gram-negative pathogens causing nosocomial pneumonia. *Int J Antimicrob Agents* 27:183, 2006.

169. McGowan JE Jr: Resistance in nonfermenting gram-negative bacteria: Multidrug resistance to the maximum. *Am J Med* 119:S29, 2006.

170. Labombardi VJ, Rojtman A, Tran K: Use of cefepime for the treatment of infections caused by extended spectrum beta-lactamase-producing Klebsiella pneumoniae and Escherichia coli. *Diagn Microbiol Infect Dis* 56:313, 2006.

171. Rodloff AC, Goldstein EJ, Torres A: Two decades of imipenem therapy. *J Antimicrob Chemother* 58:916, 2006.

172. Edwards SJ, Emmas CE, Campbell HE: Systematic review comparing meropenem with imipenem plus cilastatin in the treatment of severe infections. *Curr Med Res Opin* 21:785, 2005.

173. Zhanel GG, Johanson C, Embil JM, et al.: Ertapenem: Review of a new carbapenem. *Expert Rev Anti Infect Ther* 31:23, 2005.

174. Jones RN: Microbiological features of vancomycin in the 21st century: Minimum inhibitory concentration creep, bactericidal/static activity, and applied breakpoints to predict clinical outcomes or detect resistant strains. *Clin Infect Dis* 42:S13, 2006.

175. Lee SY, Fan HW, Kuti JL, et al.: Update on daptomycin: The first approved lipopeptide antibiotic. *Expert Opin Pharmacother* 7:1381, 2006.

176. Silverman JA, Mortin LI, Vanpraagh AD, et al.: Inhibition of daptomycin by pulmonary surfactant: In vitro modeling and clinical impact. *J Infect Dis* 191:2149, 2005.

177. Stein GE, Craig WA: Tigecycline: A critical analysis. *Clin Infect Dis* 43:518, 2006.

178. Wilcox MH: Update on linezolid: The first oxazolidinone antibiotic. *Expert Opin Pharmacother* 6:2315, 2005.

179. Nseir S, Di Pompeo C, Soubrier S, et al.: First-generation fluoroquinolone use and subsequent emergence of multiple drug-resistant bacteria in the intensive care unit. *Crit Care Med* 33:283, 2005.

180. Charbonneau P, Parienti JJ, Thibon P, et al.: Fluoroquinolone use and methicillin-resistant Staphylococcus aureus isolation rates in hospitalized patients: A quasi experimental study. *Clin Infect Dis* 42:778, 2006.

181. Sprandel KA, Drusano GL, Hecht DW, et al.: Population pharmacokinetic modeling and Monte Carlo simulation of varying doses of intravenous metronidazole. *Diagn Microbiol Infect Dis* 55:303, 2006.

182. Demoly P, Romano A: Update on beta-lactam allergy diagnosis. *Curr Allergy Asthma Rep* 5:9, 2005.

183. Madaan A, Li JT: Cephalosporin allergy. *Immunol Allergy Clin North Am* 24:463, 2004.

184. De Broe ME, Giuliano RA, Verpooten GA: Aminoglycoside nephrotoxicity: Mechanism and prevention. *Adv Exp Med Biol* 252:233, 1989.

185. Bates DE: Aminoglycoside ototoxicity. *Drugs Today* 39:277, 2003.

186. Owens RC Jr, Ambrose PG: Antimicrobial safety: Focus on fluoroquinolones. *Clin Infect Dis* 41:S144, 2005.

187. Roberts JA, Lipman J: Antibacterial dosing in intensive care: Pharmacokinetics, degree of disease and pharmacodynamics of sepsis. *Clin Pharmacokinet* 45:755, 2006.

188. Pinder M, Bellomo R, Lipman J: Pharmacological principles of antibiotic prescription in the critically ill. *Anaesth Intensive Care* 30:134, 2002.

189. Trotman RL, Williamson JC, Shoemaker DM, et al.: Antibiotic dosing in critically ill adult patients receiving continuous renal replacement therapy. *Clin Infect Dis* 41:1159, 2005.

190. Kollef MH, Shorr A, Tabak YP, et al.: Epidemiology and outcomes of healthcare-associated pneumonia. *Chest* 128:3854, 2005.

191. Guidelines for the management of adults with hospital-acquired, ventilator-associated, and healthcare-associated pneumonia. *Am J Respir Crit Care Med* 171:388, 2005.

192. Vincent JL, Bihari DJ, Suter PM, et al.: The prevalence of nosocomial infection in intensive care units in Europe: Results of the European Prevalence of Infection in Intensive Care (EPIC) study. *JAMA* 274:639, 1995.

193. Rello J, Ollendorf DA, Oster G, et al.: Epidemiology and outcomes of ventilator-associated pneumonia in a large US database. *Chest* 122:2115, 2002.

194. Fagon JY, Chastre J, Wolff M, et al.: Invasive and noninvasive strategies for management of suspected ventilator-associated pneumonia. A randomized trial. *Ann Intern Med* 132:621, 2000.

195. Safdar N, Dezfulian C, Collard HR, et al.: Clinical and economic consequences of ventilator-associated pneumonia: A systematic review. *Crit Care Med* 33:2184, 2005.

196. Cook DJ, Walter SD, Cook RJ, et al.: Incidence and risk factors for ventilator-associated pneumonia in critically ill patients. *Ann Intern Med* 129:433, 1998.

197. Celis R, Torres A, Gatell JM, et al.: Nosocomial pneumonia: A multivariate analysis of risk and prognosis. *Chest* 93:318, 1988.

198. Torres A, Aznar R, Gatell JM, et al.: Incidence, risk, and prognosis factors of nosocomial pneumonia in mechanically ventilated patients. *Am Rev Respir Dis* 142:523, 1990.

199. Chastre J, Trouillet JL, Vuagnat A, et al.: Nosocomial pneumonia in patients with acute respiratory distress syndrome. *Am J Respir Crit Care Med* 157:1165, 1998.

200. Delclaux C, Roupie E, Blot F, et al.: Lower respiratory tract colonization and infection during severe acute respiratory distress syndrome: Incidence and diagnosis. *Am J Respir Crit Care Med* 156:1092, 1997.

201. Markowicz P, Wolff M, Djedaini K, et al.: Multicenter prospective study of ventilator-associated pneumonia during acute respiratory distress syndrome. Incidence, prognosis, and risk factors. ARDS Study Group. *Am J Respir Crit Care Med* 161:1942, 2000.

202. Barie PS: Importance, morbidity, and mortality of pneumonia in the surgical intensive care unit. *Am J Surg* 197:S2, 2000.

203. Haley RW, Hooton TM, Culver DH, et al.: Nosocomial infections in US hospitals, 1975–1976: Estimated frequency by selected characteristics of patients. *Am J Med* 70:947, 1981.

204. Pennington JE: Nosocomial respiratory infection. In Mandell GL, Douglas RG Jr, Bennet JE, eds. *Principles and practice of infectious diseases*. St. Louis: Churchill Livingstone, 1990, p. 2199.

205. Centers for Disease Control and Prevention: Monitoring hospital acquired infections to promote patient safety: United States, 1990–1999. *MMWR Morb Mortal Wkly Rep* 49:149, 2000.

206. Kollef MH, Morrow LE, Niederman MS, et al.: Clinical characteristics and treatment patterns among patients with ventilator-associated pneumonia. *Chest* 129:1210, 2006.

207. Kollef MH, Ward S, Sherman G, et al.: Inadequate treatment of nosocomial infections is associated with certain empiric antibiotic choices. *Crit Care Med* 28:3456, 2000.

208. Richards, MJ, Edwards, JR, Culver, DH, et al.: Nosocomial infections in medical intensive care units in the United States: National Nosocomial Infections Surveillance System. *Crit Care Med* 27:887, 1999.392

209. Lowy FD: Staphylococcus infections. *New Engl J Med* 320:520, 1998.

210. Fridkin SK: Increasing prevalence of antimicrobial resistance in intensive care units. *Crit Care Med* 29:N64, 2001.

211. Scheld WM: Maintaining fluoroquinolone class efficacy: Review of influencing factors. *Emerg Infect Dis* 9:1, 2003.

212. Marik PE, Careau P: The role of anaerobes in patients with ventilator-associated pneumonia and aspiration pneumonia: A prospective study. *Chest* 115:178, 1999.

213. El-Ebiary M, Torres A, Fabregas N, et al.: Significance of the isolation of Candida species from respiratory samples in critically ill, non-neutropenic patients. *Am J Respir Crit Care Med* 156:583, 1997.

214. Krasinski K, Holzman RS, Hanna B, et al.: Nosocomial fungal infection during hospital renovation. *Infect Control* 6:278, 1985.

215. Lentino JR, Rosenkranz MA, Michaels JA, et al.: A retrospective review of airborne disease secondary to road construction and contaminated air conditioners *Am J Epidemiol* 116:430, 1982.

216. Loo VG, Bertrand C, Dixon C, et al.: Control of construction-associated nosocomial aspergillosis in an antiquated hematology unit. *Infect Control Hosp Epidemiol* 17:360, 1996.

217. Girou E, Loyeau S, Legrand P, et al.: Efficacy of hand rubbing with alcohol based solution versus standard hand washing with antiseptic soap: Randomized clinical trial. *BMJ* 325:362, 2002.

218. Pittet D, Hugonnet S, Harbarth S, et al.: Effectiveness of a hospital-wide programme to improve compliance with hand hygiene. *Lancet* 356:1307, 2000.

219. Girou E, Brun-Buisson C, Taille S, et al.: Secular trends in nosocomial infections and mortality associated with noninvasive ventilation in patients with exacerbations of COPD and pulmonary edema. *JAMA* 290:2985, 2003.

220. Kress J, Pohlman A, O'Connor M, et al.: Daily interruption of sedative infusions in critically ill patients undergoing mechanical ventilation. *New Engl J Med* 342:1471, 2000.

221. Marelich GP, Murin S, Battistella F, et al.: Protocol weaning of mechanical ventilation in medical and surgical patients by respiratory care practitioners and nurses: Effect on weaning time and incidence of ventilator-associated pneumonia. *Chest* 118:459, 2000.

222. Holzapfel L, Chevret S, Madinier G, et al.: Influence of long-term oro-or nasotracheal intubation on nosocomial maxillary sinusitis and pneumonia: Results of a prospective, randomized trial. *Crit Care Med* 21:1132, 1993.

223. Rouby JJ, Laurent P, Gosnach M, et al.: Risk factors and clinical relevance of nosocomial maxillary sinusitis in the critically ill. *Am J Respir Crit Care Med* 150:776, 1994.

224. Cook D, De Jonghe B, Brochard L, et al.: Influence of airway management on ventilator-associated pneumonia: Evidence from randomized trials. *JAMA* 279:781, 1998.

225. Drakulovic MB, Torres A, Bauer TT, et al.: Supine body position as a risk factor for nosocomial pneumonia in mechanically ventilated patients: A randomised trial. *Lancet* 354:1851, 1999.

226. Heyland DK, Drover J, MacDonald S, et al.: Effect of postpyloric feeding on gastroesophageal regurgitation and pulmonary microaspiration: Results of a randomized controlled trial. *Crit Care Med* 29:1495, 2001.

227. Heyland DK, Dhaliwal R, Drover JW, et al.: Canadian clinical practice guidelines for nutrition support in mechanically ventilated, critically ill adult patients. *JPEN J Parent Enteral Nutr* 27:355, 2003.

228. Berne JD, Norwood SH, McAuley CE, et al.: Erythromycin reduces delayed gastric emptying in critically ill trauma patients: A randomized, controlled trial. *J Trauma* 53:422, 2002.

229. van Nieuwenhoven CA, Buskens E, van Tiel FH, et al.: Relationship between methodological trial quality and the effects of selective digestive decontamination on pneumonia and mortality in critically ill patients. *JAMA* 286:335, 2001.

230. DeRiso AJ, Ladowski JS, Dillon TA, et al.: Chlorhexidine gluconate 0.12% oral rinse reduces the incidence of total nosocomial respiratory infection and nonprophylactic systemic antibiotic use in patients undergoing heart surgery. *Chest* 109:1556, 1996.

231. Fourrier F, Dubois D, Pronnier, P, et al.: Effect of gingival and dental plaque antiseptic decontamination on nosocomial infections acquired in the intensive care unit: A double-blind placebo-controlled multicenter study. *Crit Care Med* 33:1728, 2005.

232. Bonten MJ, Gaillard CA, de Leeuw PW, et al.: Role of colonization of the upper intestinal tract in the pathogenesis of ventilator-associated pneumonia. *Clin Infect Dis* 24:309, 1997.

233. Alvarez-Lerma F: Modification of empiric antibiotic treatment in patients with pneumonia acquired in the intensive care unit: ICU-Acquired Pneumonia Study Group. *Intensive Care Med* 22:387, 1996.

234. Fabregas N, Ewig S, Torres A, et al.: Clinical diagnosis of ventilatory associated pneumonia revisitited: Comparative value using immediate post-mortum lung biopsies. *Thorax* 54:867, 1999.

235. Fagon JY, Chastre J, Hance AJ, et al.: Evaluation of clinical judgment in the identification and treatment of nosocomial pneumonia in ventilated patients. *Chest* 103:547, 1993.

236. Rodriguez de Castro F, Sole-Violan J, Aranda Leon A, et al.: Do quantitative cultures of protected brush specimens modify the initial empirical therapy in ventilated patients with suspected pneumonia? *Eur Respir J* 9:37, 1996.

237. Pugin J, Auckenthaler R, Mili N, et al.: Diagnosis of ventilator-associated pneumonia by bacteriologic analysis of bronchoscopic and nonbronchoscopic "blind" bronchoalveloar lavage fluid. *Am Rev Respir Dis* 143:1121, 1991.

238. Fartoukh M, Maitre B, Honore S, et al.: Diagnosing pneumonia during mechanical ventilation: The clinical pulmonary infection score revisited. *Am J Respir Crit Care Med* 168:173, 2003.

239. Luyt CE, Chastre J, Fagon J,et al.: Value of the clinical pulmonary infection score for the identification and management of ventilator-associated pneumonia. *Intensive Care Med* 30:844, 2004.

240. Veinstein A, Brun-Buisson C, Derrode N, et al.: Validation of an algorithm based on direct examination of specimens in suspected ventilator-associated pneumonia. *Intensive Care Med* 32:676, 2006.

241. Blot FB, Raynard B, Chachaty E, et al.: Value of gram stain examination of lower respiratory tract secretions for early diagnosis of nosocomial pneumonia. *Am J Respir Crit Care Med* 162:1731, 2000.

242. Torres A, Mustafa E: Bronchoscopic BAL in the diagnosis of ventilator-associated pneumonia. *Chest* 117:198, 2000.

243. Niederman MS: Gram-negative colonization of the respiratory tract: Pathogenesis and clinical consequences. *Semin Respir Infect* 5:173, 1990.

244. Vidaur L, Gualis B, Rodriquez A, et al.: Clinical resolution in patients with suspicion of VAP: A cohort study comparing patients with and without ARDS. *Crit Care Med* 33:1248, 2005.

245. Campbell GD: Blinded invasive diagnostic procedures in ventilator-associated pneumonia. *Chest* 117:207S, 2000.

246. Shorr AF, Sherner JH, Jackson WL, et al.: Invasive approaches to the diagnosis of ventilator-associated pneumonia: A meta-analysis. *Crit Care Med* 33:46, 2005.

247. Iregui M, Ward S, Sherman G, et al.: Clinical importance of delays in the initiation of appropriate antibiotic treatment for ventilator-associated pneumonia. *Chest* 122:262, 2002.

248. Rello J, Sa-Borges M, Correa H, et al.: Variations in etiology of ventilator-associated pneumonia across four treatment Sites. Implications for antimicrobial prescribing practices. *Am J Respir Crit Care Med* 160:608, 1999.

249. Paladino JA: Pharmacoeconomic comparison of sequential IV/oral ciprofloxacin versus ceftazidime in the treatment of nosocomial pneumonia. *Can J Hosp Pharm* 48:276, 1995.

250. Brown RB, Kruse JA, Counts GW, et al.: Endotracheal Tobramycin Study Group. Double-blind study of endotracheal tobramycin in the treatment of gram-negative bacterial pneumonia. *Antimicrob Agents Chemother* 34:269, 1990.

251. Nsier S, Pompeo C, Soubrier S, et al.: First-generation fluoroquinolone use and subsequent emergence of multiple drug-resistant bacteria in the intensive care unit. *Crit Care Med* 33:283, 2005.

252. Trouillet J, Vuagnat A, Combes A, et al.: Pseudomonas aeruginosa ventilator-associated pneumonia: Comparison of episodes due to piperacillin-resistant versus piperacillin-susceptible organisms. *Clin Infect Dis* 34:1047, 2002.

253. Daniel F, Sahm D, Critchley I, Kelly L, et al.: Evaluation of current activities of fluoroquinolones against gram-negative bacilli using centralized in vitro testing and electronic surveillance. *Antimicrob Agents Chemother* 45:267, 2001.

254. McDougall C, Powell JP, Johnson CK, et al.: Hospital and community fluoroquinolones use and resistance in Staphylococcus aureus and Escherichia coli in 17 US hospitals. *Clin Infect Dis* 41:435, 2005.

255. Kollef MH, Kollef KE: Antibiotic utilization and outcomes for patients with clinically suspected VAP and negative quantitative BAL cultures results. *Chest* 128:2706-, 2005.

256. Dennesen PJ, van der Ven AJ, Kessels AG, et al.: Resolution of infectious parameters after antimicrobial therapy in patients with ventilator-associated pneumonia. *Am J Respir Crit Care Med* 163:1371, 2001.

257. Singh N, Rogers P, Atwood CW, et al.: Short-course empiric antibiotic therapy for patients with pulmonary infiltrates in the intensive care unit. *Am J Respir Crit Care Med* 162:505, 2000.

258. Rizzo M: Striving to eliminate catheter-related bloodstream infections: A literature review of evidence-based strategies. *Semin Anesth* 24:214, 2005.

259. Coopersmith CM, Rebmann TL, Zack JE, et al.: Effect of an education campaign on decreasing catheter-related bloodstream infections in the surgical intensive care unit. *Crit Care Med* 30:59, 2002.

260. Montravers P, Gauzit R, Muller C, et al.: Emergence of antibiotic-resistant bacteria in cases of peritonitis after intraabdominal surgery affects the efficacy of empirical antimicrobial therapy. *Clin Infect Dis* 23:486, 1996.

261. Sitges-Serra A, Lopez MJ, Girvent M, et al.: Postoperative enterococcl infection after treatment of complicated intra-abdominal sepsis. *Br J Surg* 361, 2002.

262. Roehrborn A, Thomas L, Potreck O, et al.: The microbiology of postoperative peritonitis. *Clin Infect Dis* 33:1513, 2001.

263. Bujik SE, Bruining HA: Future directions in the management of tertiary peritonitis. *Intensive Care Med* 28:1024, 2002.

264. Talmor M, Li P, Barie PS: Acute paranasal sinusitis: Guidelines for prevention, disgnosis, and treatment. *Clin Infect Dis* 25:1441, 1997.

265. Eachempati SR, Hydo LJ, Barie PS: Factors influencing the development of decubitus ulcers in critically ill patients. *Crit Care Med* 29:1678, 2001.

# Commentary ■ MARK A. MALANGONI

Barie and his colleagues correctly emphasize that infectious complications and their consequences are responsible for the majority of deaths from trauma that are not due to the immediate and early effects of injury. They outline important preventive measures that are critical for trauma surgeons to understand and practice. These principles are simple and well-proven. When applied appropriately they help avoid infection and its attendant risks.

The use of perioperative antimicrobial prophylaxis for patients undergoing emergent operation for trauma is a simple concept. It involves administering the right drug at the right dose to the patient at the right time. A simple way to remember which agents are appropriate for traumatic abdominal injury is to use cefazolin for patients with blunt abdominal trauma and a second-generation cephalosporin (cefoxitin, cefotetan) for those with penetrating injury. Recent problems with the availability of second generation cephalosporins or the presence of an allergy to penicillins or cephalosporins require the use of alternative agents.

Prospective, randomized clinical trials of perioperative antimicrobial prophylaxis for abdominal trauma have demonstrated no benefit to continuing antibiotics beyond 24 hours after operation. Exceptions to this rule include the presence of significant soft tissue contamination or compromised viability usually as a result of blast effect, in which case a repeat exploration within 48 hours is indicated. An adequate antibiotic dose should be used and higher doses should be given to patients who weigh more than 80 kg. Antibiotics should be redosed every three to four half-lives and for every six units of blood loss.

With the more frequent use of damage control laparotomy, a question has arisen as to whether prophylaxis should be continued between operations. There are no peer-reviewed data concerning this particular situation. I recommend that antimicrobial prophylaxis should be given before each operation and stopped between operations.

Ventilator-associated pneumonia (VAP) is the nosocomial infection with the highest attributable mortality. Conflict continues as to how VAP should be appropriately diagnosed. As a general rule, endotracheal sputum cultures are most accurate when obtained immediately after intubation (or tracheostomy), when the likelihood of obtaining a sample from the lower respiratory tract is optimal. When the diagnosis of VAP is questionable, broncho-alveolar lavage (BAL) has been demonstrated to be more specific for diagnosis. If BAL is used to establish the diagnosis of VAP, the clinician should commit to stopping empiric antibiotics in the face of a negative result. The use of broad spectrum empiric therapy should always be reassessed when culture and sensitivity results are available and agents with a narrower spectrum chosen when appropriate. The authors present some logical algorithms, which serve as a good basis for clinical care.

Catheter-related blood stream infections are best treated by catheter removal and a short course of antimicrobial therapy (3–5 days). Many patients who develop these infections are also susceptible to the development of an associated bacteremia. For infections due to *Staphylococcus aureus* bacteremia, I favor a four to six week course of therapy because of the potential devastating effects of persistent staphylococcal infection.

Methicillin resistant *S. aureus* (MRSA) has become commonplace in most healthcare institutions and in the general community. When infection with MRSA is suspected, vancomycin should be used as a first line agent. It is important to review the antimicrobial sensitivity results of cultures since the injudicious vancomycin use has been associated with the proliferation of vancomycin-resistant enterococci and *S. aureus* strains that are only intermediately sensitive to vancomycin. Trimethoprim-sulfamethoxazole is a useful alternative to vancomycin in these situations and it can be given orally.

Abdominal CT has been the mainstay for the diagnosis of intraabdominal infections. Percutaneous drainage is often useful to achieve source control in this situation but is less effective than operation for patients who have multiple or multilocular abscesses, necrotic tissue or debris contained within the abscess cavity, or when an enterocutaneous fistula is present. The accuracy of CT is suboptimal until about one week following the time of contamination. Once a negative scan is obtained, there is little value to repeated CT scans to work up fever in the absence of abdominal signs and symptoms.

Urinary tract infection is not mentioned in the chapter. A recent study from our institution has demonstrated that urinary tract infection is an infrequent cause for fever or nosocomial infection among seriously injured patients.[1] It is most important however that urinary tract infection be considered in patients who have had injury to the upper or lower urinary tract.

Posttraumatic meningitis is an uncommon disorder but can be fatal if unrecognized. Risk factors include the presence of open skull fractures, pneumencephalus, and the prolonged presence of ventriculostomy or intracranial pressure monitor. Treatment should consist of vancomycin and meropenem until cultures have returned. Even with rapid diagnosis and treatment, mortality is high.

It is important for the trauma surgeon and surgical critical care specialist to develop expertise in the proper treatment of patients with infection. Understanding the principles of infection prevention is also important. Tracking infectious complications is a valuable quality indicator and should be done routinely. The continued proliferation of antibiotic-resistant organisms can be minimized by the judicious use of antibiotics.

## Reference

1. Golob JF, Sando MJ, Phipps WR, et al: Fever and leukocytosis in critically ill trama patients: it's not the urine. Presented at Surgical Infection Society meeting. *Surg Infect* 8:277, 2007.

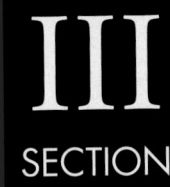

III
SECTION

# MANAGEMENT OF SPECIFIC INJURIES

# The Brain

*Peter Letarte*

## INTRODUCTION

In the United States each year 1.4 million people sustain a traumatic brain injury (TBI) of some kind; 1.1 million present to an Emergency Room and are treated and released; 235.000 are hospitalized and 50,000 die,[1] while each year 80,000 to 90,000 patients suffer permanent disability from their injury.[1]

The cumulative burden of this epidemic is estimated to be 5.3 million Americans, that is, 2% of the population living with TBI-related disability. The annual economic burden from this TBI population was estimated to be $37.8 billion in 1985, with $4.5 billion in direct expenditure for hospital care, extended care, and other medical care and services; $20.6 billion in injury-related work loss and disability; and $12.7 billion in lost income from premature death.[2]

## ETIOLOGY

The cause, natural history, and consequence of TBI vary with age and demographics.

The largest cause of all TBI in the United States is falls which accounted for 28% of all such injuries; motor vehicle-traffic accidents accounted for 20%, while assault, including with a firearm, accounted for 11% of TBI.[1]

Motor vehicle-traffic related incidents, however, are the largest source of death and hospitalization from TBI; they account for 25% of annual hospitalizations that survive and 34% of annual deaths from TBI. Falls accounted for 21% of the hospitalizations and 13% of the deaths, while assault accounted for 6% of the hospitalizations and 13% of the deaths.[1]

If suicides are included in the firearm TBI rate and TBI death rate, then firearms become the largest source of TBI death.

## PATHOLOGY

### Cerebral Injury

Introduction.   From prehistoric times, man appears to have appreciated the significance of brain swelling in cerebral injury and the potential benefits of relieving that swelling. Archeologist tell us that throughout human evolution and in multiple and widespread locations, trephination was practiced.

During the Enlightenment, physicians were aware that draining fluid and blood compressing the brain could be beneficial. They understood that delayed loss of consciousness could result from compressive mass lesions of the brain and by the 1700s they had described the pathologic findings, the clinical syndromes and thus the significance of increased intracranial pressure.

In 1793, Alexander Monroe proposed the ideas that would become the "Kellie-Monroe" doctrine which states that the brain is essentially incompressible, that the intracranial space was completely closed and that all of the volume within the calvarium is occupied by brain, blood, and cerebral spinal fluid.

The clinical findings associated with increased intracranial pressure, slowed pulse, deep snoring and varying respirations, vomiting, headache, and declining mental status were described in the 19th century.

The measurement of elevated subarachnoid pressure was introduced in 1891 by Quincke who soon after proposed the therapeutic reduction of intracranial pressure (ICP) via repeated lumbar taps as a treatment for head injury.

Thus, by the early 20th century it was understood that mass effect, either from edema or blood, and the consequences of the closed intracranial space were central to the understanding and treatment of cerebral injury.

## Mass Effect

Edema.   Historically, cerebral edema was thought to be tightly related to cerebral blood flow. Increased brain mass from autoregulatory dysfunction was recognized quite early. Such increase in brain mass is today referred to as vasogenic edema. Vasogenic edema is the result of loss of cerebral autoregulation and the subsequent cerebral vasodilatation.

With the advent of more sophisticated histologic and biochemical techniques, it became apparent that increased brain mass also came from swelling of the neurons and glial cells themselves. This is referred to as cytotoxic edema. Cytotoxic edema is the result of loss of energy stores within the cells, resulting in cellular swelling.

## Intracranial Hematomas and Contusions

The most important acute source of mass effect after trauma is hemorrhage.

Subdural Hematomas.   The most common traumatic mass lesion is the subdural hematoma which occurs in approximately 20% to 40% of severely head-injured patients. This lesion originates in the space between the dura and arachnoidal meningeal layer on the surface of the brain and is a result of injury to the bridging veins and the brain parenchyma beneath it. As it layers on the surface of the brain it forms a crescent shape (Fig. 20-1).

The morbidity of subdural hematomas is due to the rapid onset of mass effect as well as injury to the brain parenchyma beneath the subdural.

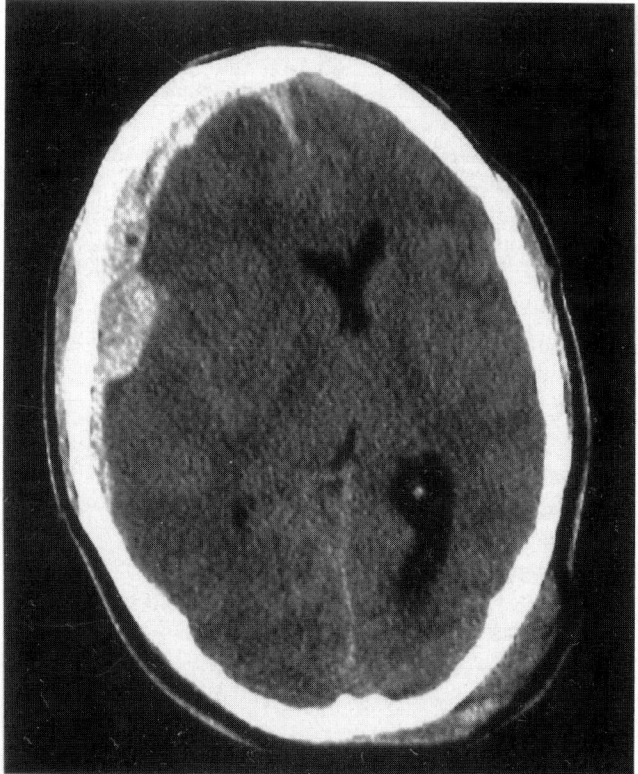

**FIGURE 20-1.**  Computed tomography scan showing large right acute subdural hematoma with marked shift of midline to the left.

Epidural Hematomas.   The injury from epidural hematomas is more likely due to isolated mass effect. The dura adheres to the inner table of the skull like a laminate. The epidural space, the space between the dura, and the inner table is therefore a potential space, created only when something peels the dura off of the inner table. For this reason, epidural hematomas have a lens shape, formed as the blood peels the dura back, creating a pocket of blood trapped between the inner table and the dura (Fig. 20-2).

Epidural hematomas are caused by lacerations of the middle meningeal artery caused by fractures in the temporal bone, which is extremely thin and susceptible to fracture.

Epidural hematomas can also be caused by lacerations to the dural sinuses or fractures through the diploic spaces, causing venous bleeding into the epidural space.

These hematomas most often occur at the locations of the dural sinuses, in the low parieto occipital region and along the convexity.

Epidural hematomas are more the result of skull injury than of brain injury, although brain injury can certainly occur with them. Their morbidity and mortality is to a large extent due to mass effect from the clot and the ensuing herniation that can occur if left unchecked. Rapid identification and removal of epidural hematomas is therefore essential.

In pre-imaging days, a lucid interval was felt to be diagnostic for epidural hematomas.

In fact, only about 1/3 of patients with epidural hematomas actually experience this "lucid interval" and it may also occur with other intracranial bleeds, making it an alarming but nonspecific finding.

Intracerebral Hematomas/Contusions.   Damage to the brain itself may produce an intracerebral hematoma or cerebral contusions. Cerebral contusions are relatively common, occurring in about 20% to 30% of severe brain injuries but occurring in a significant percentage of moderate head injuries as well. Although these injuries are typically the result of blunt trauma, they may also occur from penetrating trauma such as a gunshot wounds to the brain. In blunt trauma, cerebral contusions may be numerous. Cerebral contusions are the result of a complex pattern of transmission and reflection of forces within the intracranial space. As a result, contusions often occur in locations remote from the site of impact, often on the opposite side of the brain, the familiar "contracoup" injury.

Cerebral contusions often take 12–24 hours to appear on CT scans and so a patient with a cerebral contusion may have an initially normal head CT. The only clue to its presence will be a depressed Glasgow Coma Score (GCS), with many patients with contusions presenting as moderate head injuries with GCS 9–13.

Contusions consist of areas of bruised tissue in which the blood-brain barrier has lost its integrity, creating a heterogeneous region of injured cerebral parenchyma mixed with extravasated blood (Fig. 20-3). As contusions evolve after injury they not only become more apparent on head computed tomography (CT), they also can cause increased mass effect through cerebral edema in the injured brain, hemorrhage from injured smaller blood vessels, or they may coalesce to form intracranial hemorrhages (Fig. 20-4). Moderate head injuries can deteriorate to severe head injuries in about 10% of cases[3] and contusions and hematomas that are initially small may progressively enlarge and lead to rapid worsening, even in previously awake and alert patients who have sustained apparently moderate head injuries.

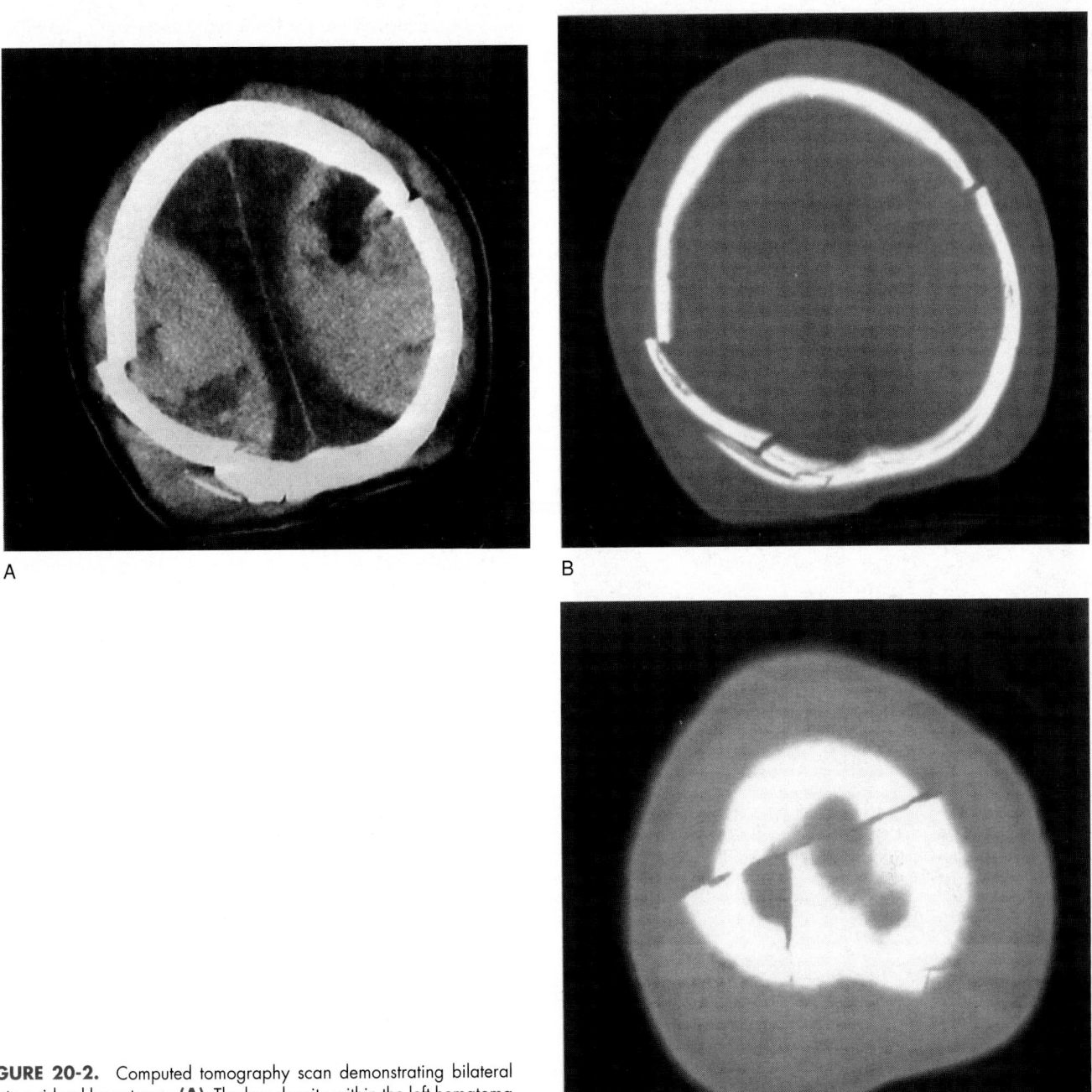

**FIGURE 20-2.** Computed tomography scan demonstrating bilateral acute epidural hematomas (**A**). The low density within the left hematoma (i.e., on the right side of the picture) represents hyperacute blood that has not yet formed a solid clot (**B**). Bone settings reveal detail of accompanying bilateral skull fractures that meet at the vertex (**C**).

Contusions most commonly occur in the frontal and anterior temporal lobes. During sudden rotation of the head, these regions impact upon the rough surface of the underlying skull base.

It should be remembered that many or even all of these types of lesions can occur concurrently.

## Secondary Injury

Secondary injury is the brain injury that occurs as a consequence of the primary event, or primary injury. It is not immediately incurred but rather is a result of pathological processes set in motion at the time of the injury. Its importance is that these processes can potentially be interrupted, thereby limiting the consequences of injury. While little can be done for the damage incurred at the time of initial injury, a great deal can be done to treat traumatic brain injury by limiting secondary injury.

While expanding intracranial masses act as secondary injury mechanisms, traditionally the term has been identified with hypoxia and hypotension. Before routine imaging of brain injury became available, brain trauma management focused on decompression of mass effect and management of ICP. By 1977, when routine CT scanning of brain injury became available, it became clear that not all bad outcome from head injury was due to mass effect. This lead to articles by, among others, Rose and Miller describing the impact of hypoxia and hypotension on outcome from head injury.[4,5] These insults became the traditional secondary injury mechanisms. With the advent of sophisticated cellular and biochemical techniques, it became clear that inadequate blood flow

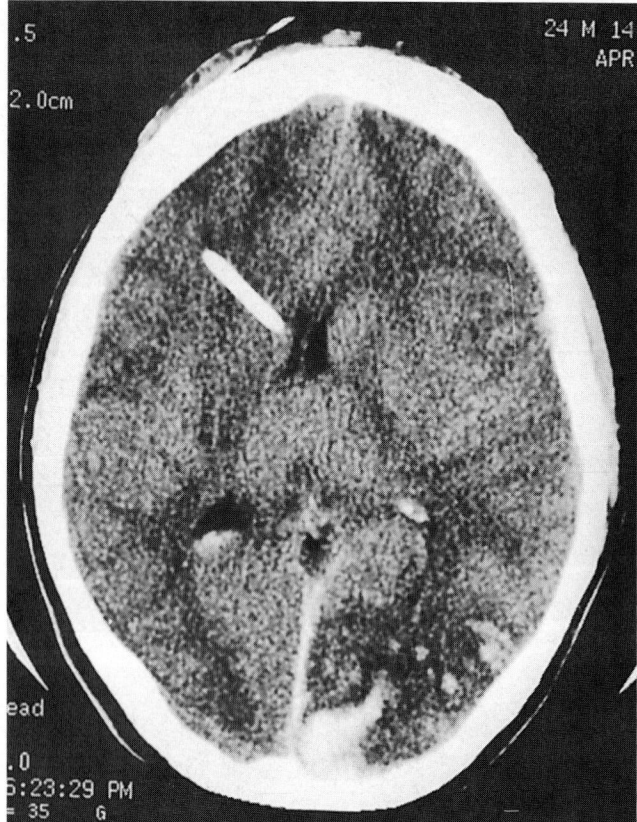

**FIGURE 20-3.** Computed tomography scan demonstrating large left occipital contusion. Although this location is atypical for cerebral contusions, the heterogeneous pattern of alternating high and low densities is classic. A right frontal ventriculostomy is also present. Considerable mass effect is evident. This patient eventually required surgical evacuation of the contusion to bring intracranial pressure under control.

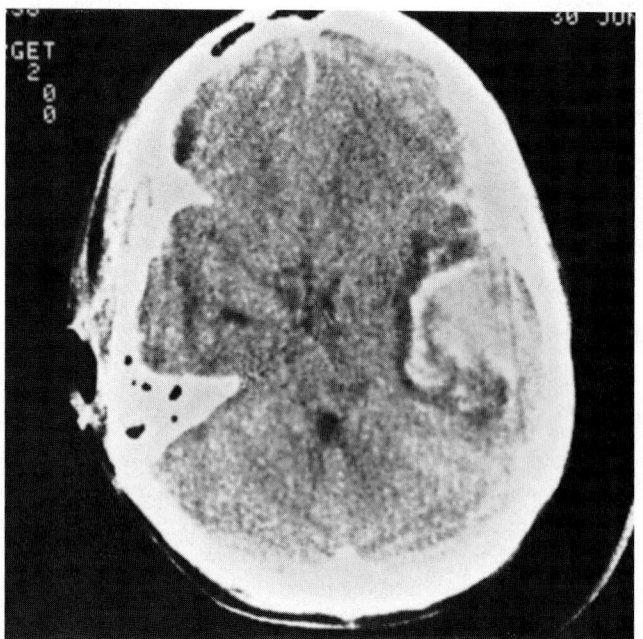

**FIGURE 20-4.** Computed tomography scan showing large left posterior temporal intracerebral hematoma with surrounding edema. Considerable mass effect is present.

and substrate delivery to the brain could also result in severe exacerbation of neurological injury if not promptly addressed.

Thus, there are currently three identified mechanisms for secondary injury, mass effect, hypoxia, and ischemia.

Ischemia.   It has been known for sometime that brain ischemia is common in head injury. Evidence of ischemia is found in 90% of the patients who die of TBI and many of the survivors have evidence of ischemic injury.[6] In the National Trauma Brain Injury data bank, the two most significant predictors of poor outcome from TBI were time spent with an ICP > 20 and an SBP < 90 mm Hg. In fact, a single episode of an SBP < 90 mm Hg can lead to a poorer outcome.[7] Several studies have confirmed from an epidemiologic viewpoint the profound impact that SBP < 90 mm Hg has on the outcome from TBI. Cerebral ischemia is one of the two major sources of secondary injury and is to be avoided.

Hypoxia.   One of the most critical substrates delivered to the injured brain by the circulation is oxygen. Irreversible brain damage can occur within only four  to six minutes of cerebral anoxia.

The injured brain appears to be even less tolerant of hypoxia than the normal brain.

Studies have also demonstrated a significant impact of a $pO_2 <$ 60 mm Hg on TBI victims.[7–9] In addition, a significant number of the victims of TBI are not adequately resuscitated in the field.[9] Several studies have demonstrated that significant numbers of TBI victims present with low or inadequate $pO_2$ or $O_2$ saturations.[10] The emphasis on prehospital airway management and oxygen delivery for brain injured patients has, in part, been the result of these studies.

Elegant work with brain tissue oxygen monitors has demonstrated the impact of hemorrhagic shock on oxygen delivery to the brain. Limiting hypotension is a key component in assuring that the brain receives an adequate supply of oxygen during the postinjury phase.[11]

## Diffuse Lesions

As opposed to focal lesions, diffuse lesions are injuries to the entire brain. The mildest form is the concussion; a far more severe form is diffuse axonal injury.

Mild Head Injury.   Mild head injury is usually defined using the Glasgow Coma Score, that is, a GCS 14–15. A related but separate definition is that of concussion. Concussion has traditionally been defined as an alteration in consciousness without findings on imaging, usually CT. Recently, this definition has been refined. The hallmarks of concussion are now known to be any confusional episode or antigrade amnesia occurring after head trauma. Confusion and amnesia can occur immediately or several minutes after the event. Loss of consciousness is not required to make a diagnosis of concussion. Amnesia is the hallmark of concussion.[12,13]

Other features can be presenting findings after concussion and several are commonly missed by inexperienced providers. These include a vacant stare (befuddled facial expression), delayed verbal and motor responses (slow to answer questions or follow instructions), confusion and inability to focus attention (easily distracted and unable to follow through with normal activities), disorientation (walking in the wrong direction, unaware of time, date, place), slurred or incoherent speech (making disjointed or incomprehensible statements), gross observable incoordination (stumbling, inability to walk tandem(straight line), emotions out of proportion to circumstances (distraught, crying for no apparent reason), memory deficits (exhibited by repeatedly asking the same question that has already been answered, or inability to memorize and recall three of three words or three of three objects in five minutes) and any period of loss of consciousness (paralytic coma, unresponsiveness to arousal).[12,13]

Depending on how it is administered, the GCS may or may not identify patients with confusion or amnesia. Because of this, it is possible to have clinical findings of concussion and a GCS of 15. Tests for the hallmarks of concussion, amnesia, and confusion, are available but are not currently routinely used in most emergency departments (ED).[14]

Diffuse Axonal Injury.    Despite the rapid evacuation of mass lesions, many patients remain vegetative or severely disabled for long periods of time after injury. Other patients may suffer profound neurologic deficits despite initial CT scans that are relatively unimpressive. A common cause of these deficits is diffuse axonal injury (DAI). During sudden rotation of the head, mechanical forces acting on long axonal cylinders may cause certain axons to experience stresses and for some structural failure. While immediate traumatic axotomy does occur, a large part of the disruption occurs later. Most of the axons that will ultimately be damaged are in continuity immediately after injury. Within 5–15 minutes of injury the structure of the axon starts to be disrupted followed by a functional change in the microtubules. Within two to six hours hours, the neurofilaments start to compact and the neurofilament side arms collapse. At the same time calpain, a calcium activated protease, is activated. It is only four hours to *days* later that the calpain finishes its work, the neurofilament is destroyed, and axotomy occurs. Presumably, if axonal disconnection disrupts a sufficient number of pathways within the brain, profound deficits may result. At present, there are no effective treatments for DAI. If, however, an axon is injured but not severed, then providing the optimal internal milieu for healing may allow it to recover, whereas secondary insults may seal its fate.

## Vascular Injuries

Subarachnoid Hemorrhage.    Subarachnoid hemorrhage (SAH) is quite common after trauma; in fact, the most common cause of subarachnoid hemorrhage is trauma. Because the blood from such a hemorrhage is spread diffusely, it does not cause mass effect, hence does not pose an immediate threat to the patients. However, the diffuse layer of blood may predispose these patients to cerebral vasospasm, although the clinical significance of this remains to be worked out.

Posttraumatic subarachnoid hemorrhage does, however, act as a marker for the severity of injury. Patients with subarachnoid hemorrhage have an increased chance of other space occupying lesions. The chances of these patients developing cerebral contusions increases by 63–77% and 44% of patients with tSAH will develop subdural hematomas. In addition, patients with subarachnoid hemorrhage have increased risk of elevated ICP and intraventricular

hemorrhage. The positive predictive value of tSAH (more than a 1 cm thickness of blood or blood in the suprasellar or ambient cisterns) for a poor outcome is 72–78%. In the Trauma Coma Data Bank the presence of traumatic SAH doubled the incidence of death in brain-injured patients.[15]

Intraventricular Hemorrhage.    Intraventricular hemorrhage may also be seen after TBI. Its main significance is as an indicator of the severity of trauma. Blood in the ventricular system may also predispose the patient to posttraumatic hydrocephalus.

## EMERGENCY DEPARTMENT MANAGEMENT

A solid appreciation for the profound impact of secondary injury on the outcome from TBI creates the basis for understanding the initial priorities in its resuscitation.

### Airway

Epidemiology has demonstrated that patients who are allowed oxygen saturations < 90% have poorer outcomes. Work with brain tissue monitors has demonstrated that hypoxic insults are additive. This means that multiple brief hypoxic insults add up to a total time of hypoxic insult. Studies have shown that a total of 30 minutes of hypoxia time can result in significantly poorer outcomes.[16,17]

It would seem then that limiting such small insults via a well secured airway would be best for the brain-injured patient. For this reason, orotracheal intubation has been advocated as part of prehospital care for all patients with a GCS < 9. Interestingly, when the impact of prehospital intubation on patients with severe head injuries was studied, patients who were intubated actually did worse.[18,19] The reasons for this are still being discovered but several observations can be made. First, it appears that delay in achieving intubation must be weighed against the quality of the intubation, that is, the skill of the provider performing the intubation. In large urban centers with low transport times, the most skilled intubation may be available in the ED. Injured patients in such settings can be rapidly transported to the ED where they can then receive a prompt and skilled intubation. Conversely, patients in remote or rural settings may have to wait hours prior to arriving at the ED. The outcome for these patients may be best served by field intubation allowing a secure airway throughout the prolonged transport. Further research will be needed to better define these issues. For now, it appears that every effort must be made to assure meticulous cerebral oxygenation in the prehospital and ED phases of care. In deciding how best to achieve this goal, the issue of time to definitive airway versus the skill of the available providers must be balanced in each practice setting.

### Breathing

Once the airway is secured, the patient must be ventilated appropriately. The studies demonstrating poorer outcomes for patients intubated in the field have suggested that another source of the increased morbidity is inadvertent hyperventilation.[20] Patients presenting to EDs with lower $pCO_2$ appear to have poorer outcomes.[18,21] Various strategies have been proposed to address this issue. The Guidelines for the Prehospital Management of Traumatic Brain Injury published by the Brain Trauma Foundation have suggested standardized ventilation rates which can be taught to providers.[22] Others have suggested the use of capnography to monitor end-tidal $pCO_2$. Unfortunately, most protocols utilizing capnography assume a stabile relationship between end-tidal $CO_2$ and serum $pCO_2$ which in fact does not exist, especially in the physiologically fluid and dynamic environment of prehospital and ED care.[23–28] Early data is beginning to emerge suggesting that there are meaningful end-tidal $CO_2$ thresholds below which outcome appears to be affected but more work needs to be done to make this a meaningful tool in the early management of postinjury hyperventilation.[29,30]

There should be no confusion that hyperventilation in the presence of signs of herniation is appropriate. In the prehospital or ED environments, before intracranial pressure monitoring has been instituted, patients who manifest clinical signs of herniation such as a unilaterally dilated pupil, an asymmetric motor examination, or declining GCS should be hyperventilated in an attempt to blunt the impact of herniation. However, prophylactic or inadvertent hyperventilation should be avoided.

Similarly, all measures need to be taken to assure adequate oxygenation and serum oxygen saturations. The first ventilatory priority is always adequate oxygenation.

## Circulation

As noted above, even a single episode of systolic blood pressure below 90 mm Hg can result in poor outcomes for the victims of TBI.[7,8] For this reason, victims of traumatic brain injury require vigorous resuscitation of their systolic blood pressure to greater than 90 mm Hg. Ninety millimeters of mercury has traditionally been the threshold used in studies of outcome after head injury. Its basis lies in historical precedent and it may be that sharp changes in mortality are actually observed at a different threshold.

There is a trend in trauma surgery to set lower resuscitation thresholds and to limit crystalloid resuscitation, especially in penetrating trauma, to prevent exacerbation of physiologically staunched severe bleeding and to prevent dilution of oxygen carrying capacity. Both of these concerns argue that lower systolic blood pressure resuscitation end points may be appropriate. Without denying the validity of either argument, the fact remains that epidemiologically, TBI patients with systolic blood pressure less than 90 mm Hg have poorer outcomes. While further research is needed to determine if another cut off might make more sense from a physiological, mortality, or outcome point of view, for now the data supports resuscitation of patients with suspected brain injury to 90 mm Hg and all efforts should be expended to assure that patient's systolic blood pressures are kept at this level.

## Neurologic Assessment

Pupillary Response.    Pupillary asymmetry, the clinical manifestation of temporal lobe herniation, has high diagnostic and prognostic utility.

Pupillary asymmetry is defined as a difference of >1 mm between pupils. A dilated pupil is >4 mm. A fixed pupil shows no response to bright light. Pupillary asymmetry and its duration should be carefully documented.

Hypotension, hypoxia, and direct orbital trauma are common causes of pupillary dilation. Hypoxia and hypotension should be corrected as herniation is being excluded as the cause for pupillary dilatation. Orbital trauma can be excluded using a swinging light test which assesses the direct and consensual response of each pupil.

Fixed and dilated pupils are a grave prognostic sign and require and emergent response.[31]

## Glasgow Coma Score

Description of GCS.    An important part of the primary survey is to obtain an accurate GCS. The GCS[32] is critical in classifying the severity of head injury and determining its subsequent management (Table 20-1). Patients with a GCS of 14–15 are classified as having mild head injury, they have a 2% chance of elevated intracranial pressure, a 2% chance of any lesion on CT, and <0.1% chance of that lesion being surgically significant. Moderate head injuries have a GCS of 9–13, a 20% chance of elevated ICP, and an approximately 10% chance of having a lesion on CT scan. Severe head injuries need to be intubated and have an approximately 50% chance of having elevated ICP. Severely head-injured patients with a normal head CT do not need ICP monitoring unless they are in a high-risk group defined as having two of the following three characteristics, age >40, a history of hypotension (SBP < 90), or unilateral or bilateral motor posturing. Severe head injuries have a GCS of 3–8.[32–34]

Confounding Factors.    Unfortunately, in as many as 44% of patients a full GCS cannot be obtained, especially early in the course of care. The accuracy of the GCS in predicting outcome relies on the patient being well resuscitated. Patients who are hypoxic, hypotensive, hypothermic, or hypoglycemic have depressed mental status due to a poor environment for the brain and not due to brain pathology. These conditions should be corrected prior to relying on the GCS for management decisions. Similarly, the common use of paralytics and sedatives in rapid sequence intubation introduces confounding factors which must clear prior to relying on the GCS.

The principal uses of the GCS are to allow uniform communication among providers concerning the patient's level of consciousness. Unfortunately, it is possible for different hospitals or departments within hospitals to apply the criteria differently. In addition, the fact that the scoring of patients who are intubated and can not be tested for a verbal score or patients with periorbital edema and can not be tested for eye opening is not uniform throughout institutions or systems is problematic.

**TABLE 20-1**

**Glasgow Coma Scale**

| SCORE | MOTOR | VERBAL | EYE OPENING |
|---|---|---|---|
| 6 | Obeys commands | — | — |
| 5 | Localizes stimulus | Oriented | — |
| 4 | Withdraws from stimulus | Confused | Spontaneously |
| 3 | Flexes arm | Words/phrases | To voice |
| 2 | Extends arm | Makes sounds | To pain |
| 1 | No response | No response | Remain closed |

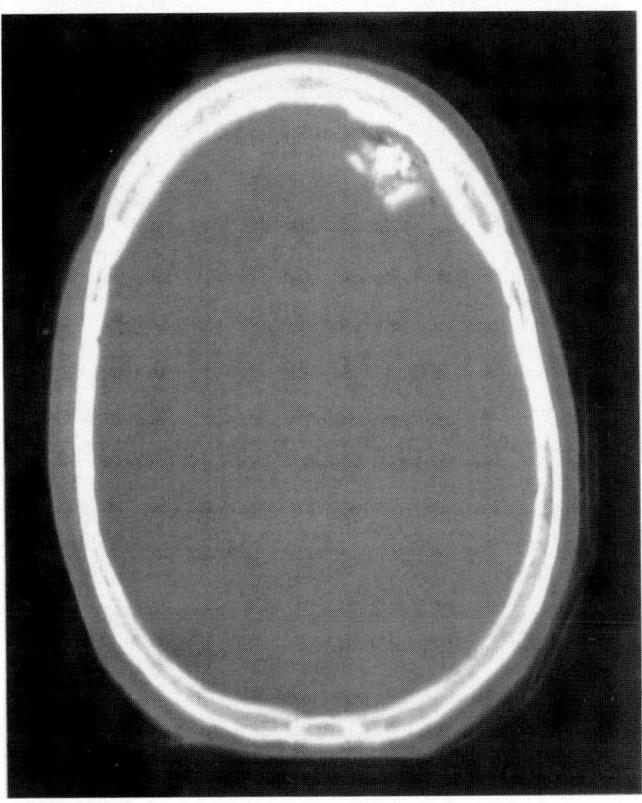
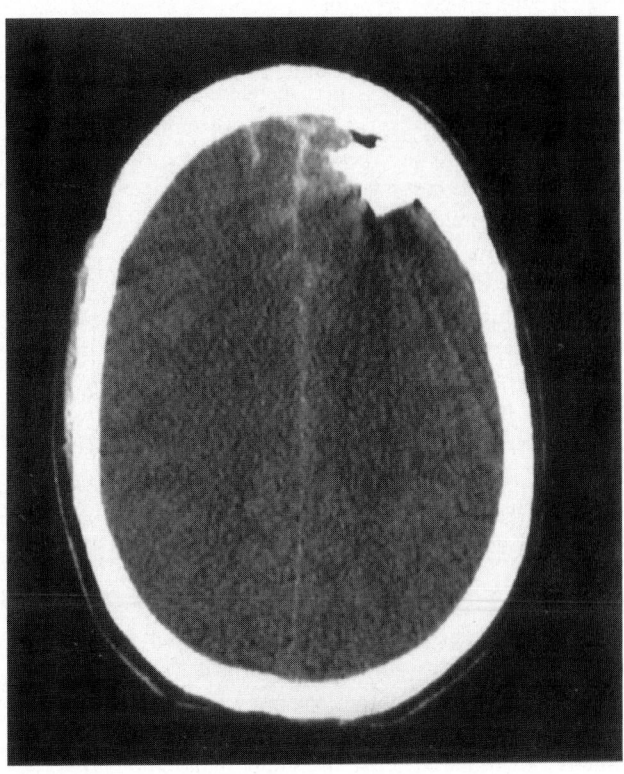

**FIGURE 20-5.** Bony **(A)** and soft tissue **(B)** views of computed tomography scan showing indriven bone fragments from a gunshot wound to the head. The patient was neurologically normal.

## Penetrating Injuries

Penetrating injuries to the head, particularly gunshot wounds to the head can carry as high as 90% mortality. Decisions on who should be resuscitated can often be particularly difficult.

Important factors to assess in making this decision are the age of the patient, the circumstance of the injury, and the caliber of weapon. In addition, it is useful to classify PBI into tangential, penetrating, or perforating injuries. Tangential injury occurs when the bullet glances off of the skull, sometimes driving bone into the brain (Fig. 20-5). Tangential injuries have a lower mortality rate.[35] A penetrating injury occurs when the projectile enters the calvarium, often driving bone before it into the brain, but remains lodged within the calvarium. A perforating injury occurs when the projectile also exits the brain, creating a tract completely across the head. Traditional PBI teaching has been that injuries which cross the midline are the most lethal and some Class III data supports this.[35,36]

Victims of penetrating head trauma who present with a GCS of 3–5 have only a small chance of an acceptable outcome. At the same time several studies have shown a reasonable prognosis for patients with PBI and GCS 13–15.[35,37–39] It should be remembered that these assumptions are based on postresuscitation GCS.

Patients with a depressed respiratory rate or hypotension on presentation after penetrating trauma are likely near death and are at greater risk for a poorer outcome.

Abnormalities in coagulation studies also may be a marker for poor outcome in PBI. A single abnormal PT or PTT is associated with 80% mortality, as opposed to a 7.4% mortality for patients without such an abnormality.[40]

## EMERGENCY RADIOLOGIC STUDIES

### Cervical Spine Films

All patients sustaining traumatic brain injury should have their cervical spines cleared according to accepted protocols. Details on imaging modalities and techniques for clearing the cervical spine are covered in Chap. 24.

### Computed Tomography of the Head

The introduction of routine computed tomography revolutionized the treatment of head injury. It provided the capacity to immediately and easily identify life-threatening space occupying lesions to most EDs in the country.

*Who Should Get a CT?.* Since the overwhelming majority of head injuries which present every day are mild and insignificant, multiple organizations have released guidelines on which brain injury patients should undergo CT scanning, in an effort to limit the unnecessary utilization of this modality. The summary of these guidelines is that it is not necessary to obtain a head CT in patients who have no loss of consciousness and are neurologically normal. Problems arise, however, in defining what is meant by "neurologically normal." All guidelines define this as the absence of posttraumatic amnesia (PTA), confusion, or impaired alertness.[41–43] Some of these features may be present with a GCS of 15, depending on the method used for obtaining the GCS. While tests for PTA and screening tests for mild head injury are available, they are not in wide use in emergency rooms today and their utility in this busy environment is questionable.[14] It is therefore difficult to reliably identify and document patients who may not require CT scanning. While it is possible to omit CT scanning in some patients, in most cases, it appears to be cost effective and safer to triage head injury patients, including mild head injury patients, with CT.

Timing of CT.    CT scanning should be obtained as early as is safely possible in the patient's care. Patients should be adequately resuscitated prior to being taken to the CT scanner.[43] In many urban trauma centers, CT scans can often be obtained within minutes of arrival in the ED, indeed within minutes of the injury. These "ultra early" CT scans can be obtained prior to significant accumulation of intracranial blood or swelling. Note should be made of patients who receive "ultra early" scanning and subsequently decline in mental status. Such patients may warrant repeat scanning.

Features on CT.    The focus of the CT examination is to identify intracranial hematomas, which are described elsewhere in this chapter. There are several other features of the scan which are important.

Compression of the basal cisterns is important to note. Basal cistern effacement is the anatomic correlate for progressing temporal lobe herniation. Effaced or compressed basal cisterns are a warning, absent basal cisterns a grim marker of well-advanced herniation.

Midline shift is also important, its use as a criteria for removal of various hematomas is discussed elsewhere. It is important to note that midline shift is caused not only by hematomas, but also by subfalcine herniation and cerebral edema.

Traumatic subarachnoid blood is, in fact, the most common cause of subarachnoid hemorrhage. Its significance has been previously described.

CT scanning also allows good imaging of the skull and skull base. Many fractures can be identified on CT. Particular attention should be paid to skull fractures in "ultra early" scans, since they may portend delayed development of a hematoma.[15]

Penetrating Head Injury.    In penetrating head injury, perforating lesions carry a higher mortality; these lesions can be seen on CT. One exception worth noting is bilateral frontal lobe involvement. Kaufman noted a mortality rate of 12% in this group and good outcomes in 30%, considerably better than the outcomes for bihemispheric lesions in general.[44] Conversely, if the tract is further posterior in the brain, more critical structures will be damaged. Such a posterior tract is likely to traverse the ventricles and ventricular penetration by the tract has been shown to have a strong association with increased mortality.[37,40,45]

## Skull Films

Skull films have a long history in the management of head injury. Features such as fractures, intracranial air, or a shift of the pineal gland from the midline have traditionally been associated with a higher incidence of intracranial pathology. The presence of a linear fracture of the skull vault has been reported to increase the likelihood of intracranial pathology 400-fold.[46]

In the post CT era, however, direct imaging of this intracranial pathology is readily and quickly available in most EDs. Acquiring skull films in many cases introduces needless delay.

In settings with limited or no availability of CT scanning, skull films remain useful for identifying patients at high risk for intracranial pathology. In addition, in penetrating trauma and for the treatment of some skull fractures, skull films can provide useful additional information on the morphology of the injury, supplementing the acutely obtained CT.[43]

## Cerebral Angiography

Until it was supplanted by CT scanning, angiography was the method of choice for detecting intracranial lesions by their displacement of cerebral vessels. Currently, angiography is used only occasionally in cases of acute head injury, primarily in those situations in which vascular injury is suspected. During the first few days after resuscitation and stabilization, angiography should be considered to evaluate for pseudoaneurysms and other vascular lesions in patients with gunshot wounds and other penetrating injuries. In addition, patients with relatively normal cranial imaging who present with or develop neurological deficits should have angiography considered to rule out vertebral or carotid injury and dissection.

## Air Ventriculography

It may not be possible in multiply injured patients who must be taken immediately to the operating room because of hemodynamic instability to obtain a head CT. In such cases, it is possible for the neurosurgeon to perform an air ventriculogram while the general or thoracic surgeons evaluate the patient or perform an operation.[47] After 5 to 10 mL of cerebrospinal fluid (CSF) have been drained and replaced with air, a portable anteroposterior skull film is obtained to ascertain the presence of midline shift. A shift of 5 mm or more suggests a possible mass lesion that may require immediate evacuation. In these cases, a craniotomy may be performed concurrently with the abdominal or thoracic procedure.

## MRI

Magnetic resonance imaging (MRI) has no role in the emergency evaluation of a head-injured patient. Reasons for this include the time required to obtain images, the limited access to a patient in the magnet, the incompatibility of magnetic fields with much of the metallic resuscitative equipment used in the emergency setting, and the inferiority of MRI to CT for visualizing acute hemorrhage and bony pathology. However, for the subacute or chronic phases after injury, MRI is more sensitive than CT in detecting subtle or diffuse injuries that may have prognostic significance.

# SURGICAL MANAGEMENT

## Removal of Mass Lesions

Calculation of Clot Volume.    In the post-imaging era, most decisions on when to remove clot or mass effect are based on appearance on CT. Some criteria on how large a clot should be removed refer to clot volume, not clot dimensions such as width or length. Many CT imaging programs can calculate clot volume but this may not be routinely available at many institutions for a variety of reasons.

In the absence of a formal calculation, clot volume can be estimated by the following formula. On a CT scan with 10 mm slices, identify the slice on which the clot has the largest area. This will be slice 1. Measure the largest diameter, designate this value as A. Measure the length of the axis 90° from A on the same slice and designate this B. On the remaining CT slices on which the clot is visible, compare the size of the clot on each slice to slice 1. If the clot size is >75% of the size of the clot on slice 1, assign the slice a value of 1. If it is 25–75% of the area, assign it a value of 0.5. If it is <25%, assign it a value of 0. Total the assigned points for the remaining slices and designate this value C. Clot volume can be estimated by the value $(A*B*C)/2$.[48]

### Acute Epidural Hematoma.
All epidural hematomas with a volume $> 30$ cm$^2$ need to be evacuated, regardless of the patient's GCS. The criteria for nonoperative management are a volume on CT $< 30$ cm$^2$, a thickness of $<15$ mm and midline shift $< 0.5$ mm in a patient with a GCS $> 8$, and no focal deficit. All of these criteria should be met for the patient to be managed nonoperatively.[49]

Patients with an acute epidural hematoma, anisocoria, and a GCS $<9$ should undergo craniotomy as soon as possible, regardless of the size of the hematoma.[49]

No recommendation on the method of evacuation is made but guideline authors mention that craniotomy allows a more complete removal.[49]

### Acute Subdural Hematomas.
For subdural hematomas, those with a thickness greater than 10 mm or a midline shift greater than 5 mm should be evacuated regardless of the patient's GCS. A patient with an acute subdural hematoma that is less than 10 mm thick and midline shift less than 5 mm but who has fixed and dilated or asymmetric pupils, an ICP $> 20$ mm Hg, or a decline in GCS of two or more points from the time of injury to hospital admission should also have their hematoma removed. Patients with acute subdural hematomas also need to have their clots removed as soon as possible.[50] Subdural hematomas should be removed using craniotomy. All patients with a GCS $< 9$ and an acute subdural hematoma should be monitored with an ICP monitor.[50]

### Parenchymal Lesions.
Parencymal lesions consist of interparenchymal clots and contusions. Their management has always been less clearly defined than the management of epidural and subdural hematomas.

Focal parenchymal lesions should be removed in three circumstances. Any patient with a parenchymal mass lesion and signs of progressive neurological deterioration due to the lesion, medically refractory intracranial hypertension, or signs of mass effect on CT scan should be treated operatively. Any patient with any lesion greater than 50 cm$^3$ in volume should be treated operatively. Patients with GCS scores of 6 to 8 with frontal or temporal contusions greater than 20 cm$^3$ in volume with midline shift of at least 5 mm and/or cisternal compression on CT scan should be treated

operatively.[51] Craniotomy with evacuation of mass lesion is recommended for these patients.[51]

Patients with parenchymal mass lesions who do not show evidence for neurological compromise, have controlled ICP, and no significant signs of mass effect on CT scan may be managed nonoperatively with intensive monitoring and serial imaging.[51]

### Posterior Fossa Lesions.
Posterior Fossa lesions are particularly dangerous. These lesions often do not manifest their mass effect by mental status change but rather by vital sign changes. These changes are often subtle and missed, with the ensuing tonsillar herniation then presenting as cardiopulmonary collapse.

Patients with mass effect on CT scan or with neurological dysfunction or deterioration referable to the lesion should undergo operative intervention. Mass effect on CT scan is defined as distortion, dislocation, or obliteration of the fourth ventricle; compression or loss of visualization of the basal cisterns, or the presence of obstructive hydrocephalus. The operation should take place as soon as possible. The most commonly performed procedure is a suboccipital craniectomy.[52]

Patients with lesions and no significant mass effect on CT scan and without signs of neurological dysfunction may be managed by close observation and serial imaging.[52]

## Surgical Management of Diffuse Brain Swelling-Decompressive Craniectomy

As with many emerging techniques, the term decompressive craniectomy has been used by authors to refer to several different operations. A wide hemispheric craniectomy and bifrontal craniectomy with several different methods of dural opening have all been described.[53–55]

The quandary in decompressive craniectomy is its use in treating isolated diffuse cerebral swelling. Decompressive craniectomy may be done incidental to a craniotomy for removal of clot but the decision making in this case is driven by the need to remove the clot. The more difficult problem is the decision and timing of surgery where the only indication is diffuse cerebral swelling.

Currently, it is felt that decompressive craniectomy should not be a "last ditch" salvage procedure, rather it should be a deliberate part of the treatment protocol which is aggressively invoked early in the patient's care when lower tier therapies fail. Expert guidelines suggest that for patients with diffuse cerebral swelling, bifrontal decompressive craniectomy within 48 hours of injury is a treatment option. These patients should have diffuse, medically refractory posttraumatic cerebral edema and resultant intracranial hypertension.[51] In addition to bifrontal decompressive craniectomy other decompressive procedures, including subtemporal decompression, temporal lobectomy, and hemispheric decompressive craniectomy, are treatment options for patients with refractory intracranial hypertension and diffuse parenchymal injury with clinical and radiographic evidence for impending transtentorial herniation.[51]

## Depressed Skull Fractures

Patients with open (compound) depressed cranial fractures should undergo operative intervention to prevent infection and decompress the brain if clinical or radiographic evidence of dural penetration, significant intracranial hematoma, bone depression greater than 1 cm, frontal sinus involvement, gross cosmetic deformity, wound infection, pneumocephalus, or gross wound contamination is present. Nonoperative management is appropriate for patients without any of these findings.

Elevation of the fracture and debridement of the skull, scalp, and brain followed by closure of the dura is the surgical method of choice. Replacement of the bone at the time of surgery is appropriate, although the risk of infection must be considered when one is replacing bone fragments associated with an open wound. However, such replacement can be safe if thorough irrigation and debridement have been utilized. Antibiotics can be started on all patients with open (compound) depressed fractures.[56] Early operation is recommended to reduce the incidence of infection.

Closed (simple) depressed cranial fractures that are less than the width of the skull deep may be treated non operatively.[56]

In children, ping-pong fractures, or large depressions on the convexity of the skull reminiscent of the depressions commonly seen on old ping-pong (table tennis) balls, sometimes require elevation if the depression is deeper than the thickness of the skull. These fractures may be elevated by simply drilling an adjacent burr hole, carefully sliding a stout instrument underneath the fracture, and levering the fragments outward.

Fractures at the base of the skull which involve the frontal sinuses or ethmoid sinuses are more complex to manage and often require a collaborative approach with otolaryngology, plastics or oromaxillofacial surgery.

Operative decision making for frontal sinus fractures can be difficult. Some advocate surgical exploration for anyone with a fracture in the posterior wall of the sinus. Others recommend surgery only if it is displaced, still others use evidence of dural tear as criteria for surgical intervention. The goals for this surgery, however, are the same as for all depressed fractures with the added goals of repair of the sinuses, prevention of mucoceles in the sinus, and the sealing and reconstruction of the floor of the frontal fossa.

## Penetrating Injuries

The goals of surgery for the victim of PBI are to remove mass effect, control bleeding, control infection, to prevent CSF leak, and to close the scalp. Although advocated in the past, aggressive removal of all bone and bullet fragments are no longer goals for this surgery.[57-61]

Retained bullet and bone fragments do not have a large impact on the post-PBI infection rates but CSF leakage does.[58,60] Tight dural closure is a mainstay of surgery for PBI. Scalp lacerations which result from PBI are often complex. Scalp incisions for PBI operations should be planned to allow for complex scalp repair at the end of the case.

## Cerebrovascular Injury

Patients who present with potential arterial hemorrhage from mouth, nose, ears, or wounds, expanding cervical hematomas, cervical bruit in patients less than 50 years old, or incongruous lateralizing neurologic deficit not explained by CT, or other findings should have carotid dissection considered in their diagnosis. In addition, trauma patients who present with evidence of cerebral

infarction should have carotid as well as vertebral artery injury considered in the diagnosis, although like contusion, infarction does not present on CT for 12–24 hours after the infarction. Patients suspected of harboring a carotid injury should undergo angiography on an emergent basis if they are otherwise stable. Coordination of the appropriate management for both the vascular and intracranial injuries requires a well-coordinated multispecialty approach. More details on the management of carotid and vertebral injuries are available in Chap. 23.

## Emergency Burr Holes

In patients with signs strongly suggestive of a rapidly expanding intracranial hematoma, such as a witnessed sudden loss of consciousness and a rapidly enlarging pupil, it may be best to proceed directly with surgery or even with burr holes drilled in the ED. The problems surrounding emergency burr holes concern localization of the lesion and efficacy of the evacuation. With a CT scan to localize the lesion, the localization concern is addressed. Without such localization, significant time can be spent placing multiple holes searching for the lesion. Secondly, gelatinous fresh clots can have only a fraction of their volume removed through burr holes. In most cases, decompression will not occur until a complete craniotomy is performed. Patients are best served by rapid transport to facilities able to perform the complete craniotomy. Emergency burr holes are best reserved for those who will absolutely not survive this process.[62]

# INTENSIVE CARE UNIT MANAGEMENT

## Neurologic Management

Intracranial Pressure.    At the turn of the century the critical lumbar puncture pressure threshold for the surgical treatment of head injury was 20 cm of water.[63]

Early workers used cutoffs ranging from 20–30 mm Hg as the intraventricular pressure threshold for the treatment of intracranial pressure.[34,47,64,65] Analyzing data from the NTCB, Marmarou found 20 mm Hg to be the critical cut off identified by regression analysis.[66] Current guidelines recommend keeping the ICP below 20–25 mm Hg water.[67]

The intraventricular catheter had been in use since the 19th century but it was its coupling with the strip chart recorder to allow continuous ICP monitoring that made it the measurement device of choice for ICP. This radical innovation was introduced by Guillamie and Jenny in 1954 and put into clinical use by Lundberg in 1959.[68-70]

Placement of an intraventricular catheter, however, requires a certain level of skill and practice. Placement can not always be achieved. They can require a high level of maintenance and they carry an approximately 2% infection rate.

For these reasons, over the years there has been a steady effort to create a more reliable, less invasive, and easier to use ICP measurement device. Subarachnoid wicks and epidural sensors have all been tried. Currently, fiber optic based intraparencymal or intraventricular devices, in addition to plain intraventricular catheters are used to measure ICP. The intraparenchymal sensor is easier to place and probably has a lower infection rate than an intraventricular catheter. It does not, however, allow CSF drainage for immediate ICP management, which is a significant disadvantage. Coupling it with an intraventricular drain, however, overcomes this disadvantage.

Although requiring a more complex skill set to institute and maintain, external ventricular drainage via an intraventricular catheter offers the gold standard for ICP measurement and immediate treatment for ICP elevations.

Hyperosmolar Therapy.    Hyperosmolar therapies reduce ICP by two distinct mechanisms. The commonly appreciated mechanism is via the establishment of an osmolar gradient across the blood brain barrier, with the gradient favoring the flow of water out of the brain and into the circulation. This mechanism is estimated to require 15–30 minutes to act and can last 90 minutes to six hours.[71]

Osmolar agents, however, can act in a much shorter time frame via a second mechanism. These agents also improve the rheology of the blood via plasma expansion, reduced hematocrit, and reduced blood viscosity resulting in more efficient cerebral blood flow. This increased efficiency means that at any given CPP, the cerebrovascular resistance will be higher, the cerebral blood volume will be lower, ICP will therefore be lower while cerebral blood flow remains unaltered.[72] Mannitol and hypertonic saline are believed to utilize both these mechanisms.[73]

Mannitol.    Mannitol has long been accepted as an effective tool for reducing intracranial pressure.[74–78] Numerous mechanistic laboratory studies support this conclusion. Its impact on outcome has never, however, been directly demonstrated via a Class I trial testing mannitol against placebo.

There is a commonly held belief that mannitol administration can cause or exacerbate hypotension in the early resuscitation of trauma victims. There is Class III data that infusion of mannitol at rates of 0.2–0.8 g/kg/min can lead to transient drops in blood pressure.[79–81] From these observations, a recommended rate of no higher than 0.1 g/kg/min or 1 g/kg delivered over 10 minutes or more is recommended.[72] Careful monitoring of urine output with aggressive replacement of this fluid loss is also recommended to prevent hypotension associated with the use of mannitol.

Mannitol can be given in response to an elevated ICP or as a continuous drip in a more prophylactic fashion. Class II data have found bolus administration to be more effective and some Class III data have found no difference between the two modes of delivery.[74,76,82–85]

Mannitol and other osmotics are known to be able to briefly open the blood brain barrier. Furthermore, at rates of administration which exceed the rate of excretion of mannitol, mannitol can accumulate in the extracellular space. These factors lead to the accumulation of mannitol in extracellular spaces and a reverse osmotic gradient which can lead to a "rebound effect" or movement of water into the brain. Class III data suggests that this effect is more likely with continuous infusion of mannitol, as opposed to bolus administration.[86,87]

Class II and Class III data have shown that doses of 0.25–1.0 g/kg of mannitol may be needed to achieve a reduction in ICP. This required dose varies from patient to patient and even may vary from time to time in the same patient.[76,87,88]

Hypertonic Saline.    Hypertonic saline offers an attractive alternative to mannitol as a therapy for elevated intracranial pressure. Its ability to reduce elevated ICP has been demonstrated with Class II and III data in the ICU and in the operating room.[89–92]

Hypertonic saline has been used in two very different ways in the resuscitation of trauma victims. In addition to being proposed as a hyperosmolar agent for the management of elevated ICP, it is also advocated as a low volume resuscitation fluid. While the qualities that make it useful both as a low volume resuscitation fluid and as a brain-targeted therapy are related, its efficacy in one role does not guarantee its efficacy in the other. Each therapeutic endpoint must be analyzed independently.

There is no consensus on what is meant by "hypertonic saline." Concentrations of 3%, 7.2%, 7.5%, 10%, and 23.4% have all been used and described in the literature. There is no consensus on a standard concentration for reduction of ICP.[89–91,93]

In addition, hypertonic saline is described in the literature as being administered in a variety of different ways. The goals and endpoints in each of these studies are different.

In some studies, hypertonic saline is given as an infusion, the goal of which is to elevate serum sodium to 155–160 mEq/L, although some investigators have gone as high as 180 mEq/L. This elevated serum sodium is thought to help stabilize ICP and reduce the therapeutic intensity required to manage elevated ICP.[94,95]

Another way to use hypertonic saline is as a bolus in an attempt to achieve an immediate reduction in ICP. This method takes advantage of the rapid rheologic improvement and improved cerebral blood flow which, like mannitol, hypertonic saline can create.

Multiple animal studies and several human studies have demonstrated that hypertonic saline, as a bolus, can reduce ICP in a monitored environment such as the operating room or ICU where ICP monitoring is present.[96–98] Comparison of these studies is difficult since they do not use the same concentrations or protocols. No study has demonstrated an effect on clinical indicators of herniation such as pupillary widening or posturing.

One Class I study looked at the impact of prehospital hypertonic saline on neurological outcome. In this study, hypertonic saline did not demonstrate any advantage over normal saline on neurological outcome when given as a prehospital resuscitation fluid.[99] Based on this data, hypertonic saline is not yet a mainstream treatment for elevated ICP.

Albumin.    Albumin has several theoretical properties that make it attractive as a resuscitation fluid. Its purported ability to rapidly expand intravascular volume with lower infusion volumes while limiting cerebral edema by augmenting intravascular oncotic pressure make it attractive as a neuroresuscitation fluid.

For years, the relative benefits of colloid resuscitation, such as albumin versus crystalloid resuscitation for trauma have been debated and studied.[100,101] Several meta-analysis have failed to demonstrate any clear advantage to albumin resuscitation. One analysis actually found a higher mortality rate for patients resuscitated with albumin.[102] While a subsequent randomized prospective clinical trial of albumin versus crystalloid failed to confirm this increased mortality, it also did not find any advantage to albumin resuscitation.[103] Since albumin is more costly, in the absence of definitive data demonstrating a clear advantage to its use, its use as a resuscitation and neuroresuscitation fluid has declined.[101,104]

It continues to be used, however, among many neuroscience clinicians. Within this group, albumin, in addition to its previously mentioned properties, is valued as a hemodilutant, improving cerebral microcirculation and reducing thrombus formation in ischemic brain.[105]

In addition, some clinicians, feel that the blood brain barrier, created in large part by the unique cerebrovascular endothelium, creates a special environment for albumin's oncotic action. "Lund Therapy" relies heavily on this notion. Lund therapy is described as a third alternative to either ICP-centered or CPP-centered management. In Lund therapy, CPP is kept to the minimum necessary to keep the brain perfused, often at a level of 50 mm Hg. Cerebral edema is controlled by increasing the oncotic pressure on the vascular side of the blood brain barrier through the use of albumin. In theory, by minimizing the hydrostatic pressure driving fluid into the cerebral interstitial space (CPP) and by decreasing the oncotic drive out of the vascular space by infusing albumin, cerebral edema can be minimized and ICP will be better controlled.[106]

Ongoing work attempting to validate these ideas has led to a great deal of interesting work about the action of albumin in the environment of the blood–brain barrier.[106]

In addition, animal experimental work has explored albumin's reported properties as an antioxidant, its laudatory influence on the vascular endothelium, its antiedema effects, and its positive effects on metabolism in brain injury. Such work has demonstrated decreased infarction size with albumin use in animal stroke models.[107]

Although there are significant concerns about albumin's potential to sequester fluid in the cerebral interstitial space and even data suggesting that patients with TBI may do worse with albumin resuscitation, its theoretical potential as a neuroresuscitation fluid remains.[103] While the currently available data does not demonstrate this potential, work on albumin as a neuroresuscitation fluid is likely to continue for the foreseeable future.

### Hyperventilation.

The observation that respiratory rate can impact cerebral blood flow and swelling dates to the 19th century. A large body of work on the effects of respiration on cerebral blood flow was done in the early 20th century.

Lundberg was aware of this work when he performed his first clinical observations of continuous ICP monitoring. Since he was the first to report on a large series of continuously ICP monitored patients, Lundberg was also the first to report on the impact of hyperventilation on the ICP. He pointed out that hyperventilation did not always work to reduce ICP and expressed concern over its ability to precipitate cerebral ischemia.[108]

Thus from its introduction, it was understood that hyperventilation was potentially useful for reducing intracranial pressure but also posed the threat of cerebral ischemia.

A debate on the risks and benefits of its use started almost immediately. Current thinking about hyperventilation can be traced to Raichle's work in the 1970s, which demonstrated that hyperventilation reduced cerebral swelling but also reduced cerebral blood flow. He also pointed out that prolonged hyperventilation had not been shown to be beneficial to patients.[109]

The only study of hyperventilation's impact on outcome demonstrated that at 12 months there was no difference between patients who were hyperventilated and those who were not. However, at 3 and 6 months, patients who were hyperventilated did worse.[110]

This outcome data, combined with a growing body of data concerning the low blood flow and near ischemic conditions found in newly injured brains, led to an increasing concern about hyperventilation's ischemic potential.[111–113] In the 1990s, published guidelines discouraged hyperventilation except in the presence of impending herniation, as manifest by elevated ICP or clinical signs of herniation. This position has remained the therapeutic recommendation since. Hyperventilation is an acceptable modality in the presence of impending herniation for short periods of time or in the presence of elevated ICP refractory to sedation, paralysis, CSF drainage, or osmotic diuresis.[114]

### Barbiturate Therapy.

Barbiturate therapy or barbiturate "coma" can be used as a third-tier therapy for elevated ICP when other more standard therapies have failed. It has been demonstrated be effective in reducing ICP.[115]

Barbiturate therapy also carries with it a high morbidity.[116] Barbiturates affect the function of not only the brain but also the heart and kidneys, among other organs. Significant declines in the functioning of both of these organ systems can occur during therapy. For this reason, barbiturate coma should not be initiated if the victim of malignant ICP is also hemodynamically unstable. Patients should be carefully monitored to assure maintenance of hemodymanic stability during therapy.

### Propofol.

Propofol is commonly used as a sedative in TBI.[117] While it is convenient and can be reversed quickly during the first few days of use, there is little data that it useful for ICP control. Propofol has been associated with myocardial death in children and this complication is also possible in adults. Propofol infusion syndrome can present with hyperkalemia, hepatomegaly, lipemia, metabolic acidosis, myocardial failure, and rhabdomyolysis.[118–120] The possibility of this complication must be considered when propofol is used in doses greater than 5 mg/kg/hour or for more than 48 hous.[121]

### Hypothermia.

It has long been suspected that cooling the brain would have a protective effect and limit injury. Anecdotal observations of phenomenon such as brain survival after prolonged immersion and near-drowning in very cold water have led providers to assume that the cold provides some protective effect.

Hypothermia has been shown to reduce elevated intracranial pressure.[122–125] There is also some clinical data which demonstrates that hypothermia has a beneficial effect on the outcome from TBI.[122,126,127]

The National Acute Brain Injury Study: Hypothermia (NABISH) study was a large randomized prospective clinical trial designed to demonstrate this beneficial effect for hypothermia on the outcome from TBI. It failed to achieve that.[128]

Although the NABISH study failed to demonstrate the efficacy of hypothermia, many still believe that it has potential value as a therapy. Both the analysis of the factors which confounded the NABISH study and other research leave room for this opinion.

Therapeutic hypothermia for TBI is considered to be the rapid reduction and maintenance of a core body temperature to 32–35°C for 48 hours or less. The decision to induce the hypothermia must be made almost immediately upon presentation and the patient must have the hypothermia induced and reach target temperature within 60 or perhaps even 30 minutes of presentation.[129] The therapy has no demonstrated efficacy as a third-tier therapy that could be considered for use several days into treatment as other therapies fail.[129]

Hypothermia is a complex therapy which should only be performed at centers that are willing to make the substantial commitment to doing it correctly. It appears that marginal or inept application of this therapy at best will do no good and at worst will harm the patients.

It has been shown that hyperthermia results in a poorer outcome from TBI.[130] Efforts to prevent excessive temperatures in the victims of TBI are appropriate.

Cerebral Perfusion Pressure.   Cerebral perfusion pressure (CPP) is the difference between the mean arterial pressure and the intracranial pressure (CPP = MAP-ICP). The role of CPP in TBI is complex and our understanding of it is incomplete and controversial. Establishing what the correct CPP should be is therefore difficult.

There are actually many reasons cited to maintain an adequate CPP.[131] The most common is to reduce the incidence of secondary insults to the injured brain. This approach focuses on inadvertent hypotension to the brain and reduces the number of secondary insults, i.e., the number of hypotensive episodes.

A second reason to maintain adequate CPP is to assure that the brain is functioning within the autoregulatory limits. Autoregulation uses cerebral vasodilation to maintain constant cerebral blood flow in the face of varying CPP. For autoregulation to function, the CPP must be above a certain threshold. In injured brains, this threshold may rise. Maintaining the CPP above the autoregulatory threshold allows substrate delivery to be maintained via efficient flow rather than large volume. As cerebral vasoconstriction is allowed to work, cerebral blood volume (CBV) falls. The endpoint for this approach is to assure that the autoregulatory threshold is met.

The third way to evaluate the effectiveness of CPP is to look at its effect on oxygen delivery to the brain, the PbrO$_2$. In these studies, above a certain CPP threshold, PbrO$_2$ is no longer dependent on CPP. In most studies this threshold is 60 mm Hg, in one it is 70 mm Hg. One caveat to this approach to CPP management is the issue of regional ischemia. In the injured brain, there can be selected regions that lose autoregulation and will require higher CPP than the noninjured areas of the brain.[132,133] Guiding therapy based on average CPP for the whole brain will result in suboptimal perfusion and treatment for these areas of injury. Patients with areas of regional ischemia may require higher CPP.[134]

A fourth school of thought, the advocates of the previously discussed Lund Therapy, believe that elevated CPP increases transcapillary hydrostatic pressure, increasing cerebral edema, and mass effect. While not advocating the old practice of keeping TBI patients dry, this group believes that once the goals of adequate cerebral perfusion are met, that is, meeting the autoregulatory threshold and preventing hypotensive episodes, further increases in CPP are detrimental.[135]

Robertson et al. examined some of these issues in a study published in 1999. In this Class I study, patients were randomized to either a CBF targeted therapy or an ICP targeted therapy.[136]

In the ICP treatment group, standard ICP control strategies were used, MAP > 70, CPP > 50. Hyperventilation, with its subsequent ischemic effects, was included in the techniques being used to control ICP.

In the CBF group, much more aggressive CBF management was utilized with MAP > 90, CPP > 70 and, while elevated ICP was controlled, hyperventilation was not used as a modality.[136]

The study showed that CBF focused therapy was more successful in meeting some of the surrogate markers of adequate CBF. The incidence of SjvO$_2$ desaturation was 50.6% in the ICP focused group and 30% in the CBF focused group. The median length of time the CPP was < 60 mm Hg in the ICP targeted group was 13 hours, it was 4 hours in the CBF targeted group. The total length of time the SjvO$_2$ was low for the ICP targeted group was 58.9 hours and 7.8 hours for the CBF targeted group.

While CBF targeted therapy in this study demonstrated considerable improvement in many surrogate markers for CPP success, the study failed to show any improvement in outcome for CBF directed therapy over ICP focused therapy. Further, the study showed that patients with CPP of 70 mm Hg had a higher incidence of ARDS.[136]

Multiple studies have looked at outcomes when CPP is maintained at 70 mm Hg, none has convincingly demonstrated improved outcomes.[134] Oxygen delivery studies have demonstrated that over a CPP of 60 mm Hg, little improvement in cerebral oxygen delivery is achieved by higher levels, with the important exception of patients with regional ischemia. Patients whose CPP is kept at 70 mm Hg appear to have a higher incidence of ARDS. While the advocates of Lund therapy would recommend a CPP of 50 mm Hg, there is not enough data to make this a widely accepted approach. The current synthesis of this data appears to be that of Robertson which is that, except in cases of regional ischemia, a CPP of 60 mm Hg is adequate and no benefit and some harm may come from elevating CPP to 70 mm Hg.[134]

Optimum Hemoglobin and Hematocrit.   The impact of hypoxia and hypotension on TBI has been previously discussed. Each is assumed to impair oxygen delivery to the injured brain and cerebral oxygen delivery is assumed to be the underlying factor which must be maintained. Crucial to adequate oxygen delivery is the hemoglobin content of the blood and so it is assumed that the victims of neurotrauma must have adequate hemoglobin levels.

Equally critical, however, is the effect of blood viscosity on cerebral blood flow, especially in the cerebral microcirculation. Good data suggests that as hematocrit decreases, cerebral blood flow increases.[137]

Estimates of the hematocrit needed to optimize cerebral blood flow based on Poiseuille's law arrived at an optimum hematocrit between 30 and 35%. Later work which took into account the non-Newtonian characteristics of blood flow, especially in the microcirculation, brought this value into question.[138]

More importantly, there is little data on the appropriate hematocrit to optimize cerebral oxygen delivery. The point at which the benefit of increased cerebral blood flow from hemodilution outweighs the resulting decline in blood oxygen carrying capacity is not known. Thomas et al. found that a drop in hematocrit from 49.3 to 42.6% resulted in a 50% increase in cerebral blood flow while oxygen carrying capacity was calculated to fall by only 13%.[139] Lee et al. found in a canine cerebral infarction model that a hematocrit of 30% resulted in the smallest infarction size.[140] Morimoto in a rabbit model found that brain tissue oxygenation declined immediately upon the institution of hemodilution in spite of increasing cerebral blood flow.[141] Other data however, implies that lower hematocrits result in poorer outcomes for patients with various neurological conditions.

The optimum hemoglobin and hematocrit is probably the result of many factors including the integrity of cerebral autoregulation and the metabolic status of the brain. The traditional goals of a hematocrit of 30–35% and a hemoglobin of 10 mg/dl appear to be the best current recommendations.

Advanced Cerebral Monitoring.   Oxygen delivery to the brain is traditionally monitored via pulseoxymetery. Knowing that blood oxygen saturation is >90%, however, is a long way from knowing anything about oxygen delivery to the brain.

**AVO$_2$:** Several methods for measuring oxygen delivery to the brain are available. One method is to measure the arterial–venous oxygen difference across the brain. This value is difference in the oxygen content of the blood entering the cranial vault and the content of the blood leaving the cranial vault. The oxygen content of the blood leaving the cranial vault is measured by placing a sensor or sampling catheter high in the jugular vein.

This "utilized oxygen content" is known as the AVO$_2$ difference. A metabolically active brain will require more oxygen and more delivery of oxygen than a quiet brain. The brain will be injured when this demand is not met. The AVO$_2$ difference helps assess this balance.

**SjvO$_2$:** Estimates of the adequacy of oxygen delivery to the brain can also be made by simply measuring the saturation of blood leaving the brain in the jugular bulb, the SjvO$_2$. Most patients have saturations of 55–69% in the blood leaving the brain.

SjvO$_2$ appears to adequately reflect the status of oxygen delivery to the brain. While it has never been shown that maintaining SjvO$_2$ in the normal range improves outcome, multiple studies have shown that patients with increased numbers of episodes of SjvO$_2$ desaturation <50% have worse outcomes.[142–146]

**PbtO$_2$:** A more direct approach is to measure cerebral tissue oxygen tension. This can be measured via cerebral tissue oxygen monitoring. Normal cerebral tissue oxygen pressures, PbrO$_2$, are approximately 32 mm Hg. Studies have shown that patients whose PbrO$_2$ is allowed to dip to 15 or lower have poorer outcomes.[146–148]

It appears that active management of cerebral oxygen delivery has the potential to improve outcomes from TBI. Applying technologies that allow the SjvO$_2$ to be kept above 50% and the PbrO$_2$ above 15 mm Hg is now a reasonable option to pursue in the management of TBI (Table 20-2).

Investigational Compounds.   Numerous experimental advances have occurred in the area of pharmacologic intervention for TBI. Therapies to combat the effects of excitotoxicity and free radicals have been explored. Despite encouraging preclinical results, clinical trials using various therapeutic agents for TBI have so far been disappointing. In some cases, the treatment and control groups were not comparable despite attempts at accurate randomization. In other trials, the outcome measures may not have been sufficiently sensitive to detect the beneficial effects of an intervention. These results emphasize the difficulty of orchestrating multicenter trials for diseases as complex as TBI.

**TABLE 20-2**

**Techniques of Monitoring Cerebral Metabolism**

| PHYSIOLOGIC PARAMETER | MONITOR | GLOBAL OR REGIONAL MONITOR? | CRITICAL VALUE |
|---|---|---|---|
| Intracranial pressure (ICP) | Ventriculostomy | Global | ICP > 20 mm Hg |
| | Intraparenchymal catheter | | |
| Cerebral blood flow (CBF) | Xenon-enhanced CT scan | Both | Ischemic threshold: 18 mL/ |
| | Nitrous oxide clearance | Global | 100 g/min |
| | PET (positron emission tomography) scan | Both | |
| | SPECT (single photon emission computed tomography) scan | Both | |
| | Thermal diffusion probe | Regional | |
| | Laser Doppler probe | Regional | |
| | Transcranial Doppler sonogram | Regional | Normal values vary for different arteries |
| Brain parenchymal oxygen tension (Pbto$_2$) | Intraparenchymal Po$_2$ catheter | Regional | Poto$_2$ < 15 mm Hg?[b] |
| Jugular venous oxygen saturation (Sjvo$_2$) | Jugular bulb oximetric catheter | Global | Saturation < 50% |
| Cerebral perfusion pressure (CPP)[a] | Arterial blood pressure and ICP monitors | Global | CPP < 60 mm Hg?[b] |
| Arterial oxygen saturation | Pulse oximeter | Global | <90%? |

[a]CPP is mean arterial pressure (MAP) minus ICP.
[b]Reference 52.

## Penetrating Injury

PBI can lead to delayed posttraumatic cerebral aneurysms. Between 3 and 33% of all victims of PBI may have a posttraumatic aneurysm.[149,150] Such aneurysms can develop as late as two weeks after the injury and an early negative cerebral angiogram does not exclude an aneurysm later in the patient's course. Any patient who develops delayed or unexplained subarachnoid hemorrhage or other delayed bleeding should be suspected of harboring a posttraumatic aneurysm and should undergo cerebral angiography.

Half of all CSF leaks may occur at sites remote from the entry or exit sites in PBI. These CSF leaks will not be apparent at surgery and will manifest after surgery. 72% of these leaks will appear within two weeks of surgery and 44% will seal spontaneously.[151]

Current infection rates for PBI in a military setting are 4–11%. Current civilian rates are at 1–5%.[152] Half (55%) of all intracranial infections occur within three weeks of the injury and 90% occur within six weeks.[152] Factors affecting infection risk are CSF leaks, air sinus wounds, and wound dehiscence. Because of the high infection rates with this injury, long-term antibiotics are commonly used.

In PBI, 30–50% of victims develop posttraumatic epilepsy (PTE).[57,153] This is slightly higher than the estimates of 4–42% for nonpenetrating TBI.[154–156] Early seizures in the TBI literature are defined as seizures in the first seven days after injury, when the vast majority of early seizures occur.[156] Current guidelines for antiepileptic therapy after PBI are the same as after TBI.[157]

The risk of PTE after PBI appears to decline with time. While 18% of victims may not have their first seizure until five or more years after the injury, 80% will have their first seizure within two years of the injury, and 95% of patients will remain seizure-free if they remain seizure-free for three years following injury.[57,153] Followed out to 15 years, 50% of patients who do develop PTE will stop having seizures.[57]

## Systemic Management

The management of systemic parameters in head-injured patients is similar to the management of other trauma patients. Cardiovascular, pulmonary, renal, and other organ systems must be watched closely and supported as necessary with the goal of preventing secondary cerebral insults. There are some unique aspects of critical care management for brain-injured patients which should be highlighted.

### Hypoglycemia and Hyperglycemia.
The impact of decreased glucose delivery to the injured brain and the brains utilization of glucose after injury are less studied areas of TBI. After head injury, cerebral glucose metabolism can be deranged in complex ways. Some compelling evidence indicates that glucose metabolism and therefore, cerebral glucose need actually goes up after severe head injury, threatening a mismatch between glucose delivery and utilization.[158–160]

On the other hand, good clinical and laboratory data in stroke patients shows that patients whose serum glucose is allowed to be elevated for protracted periods in the ICU may have larger areas of infarction and less effective resuscitation of salvageable brain. Limited studies have seemed to indicate that these same factors apply after head injury. Prolonged elevations in blood glucose levels in patients with TBI have been associated with poorer neurologic outcome.

Both elevations (hyperglycemia) and decreases (hypoglycemia) in blood sugar can jeopardize ischemic brain tissue. The disastrous impact of significant hypoglycemia on the nervous system, during injury and at other times is well known. In the absence of glucose, ischemic neurons can be permanently damaged. However, it is also true that prolonged serum glucose of >150 and perhaps >200 mg/dl may be harmful to the injured brain and should be avoided.[161,162]

### Steroids.
Although steroids were commonly administered to head-injured patients in the past to try to improve outcome or reduce ICP, multiple studies have failed to show any benefit to mortality or outcome for steroid administration. The largest study to date, the CRASH trial, was terminated early after accrual of 10,008 patients when analysis showed a significant increase risk of death for the head injury population receiving steroids.[163] There is currently no known benefit to administering steroids to brain-injured patients for the purpose of neuroprotection or ICP control.

### Anticonvulsants.
Current guidelines for antiepileptic therapy after TBI distinguish between two uses for antiepileptic drugs; postinjury treatment, and prophylaxis. Antiepileptic drugs do appear to be effective in treating an established posttraumatic seizure disorder and in preventing immediate postinjury seizures in the first week after injury. They do not appear to be effective in reducing the incidence of posttraumatic epilepsy. Maintenance of TBI victims on prophylactic doses of anticonvulsant medications beyond the first week of therapy does not appear to reduce the incidence of posttraumatic seizures. The recommendation for TBI is to treat the patient with anticonvulsants for seven days and then discontinue the medication, only restarting it if seizures develop.[157]

# PREVENTION AND MANAGEMENT OF COMPLICATIONS

## Coagulopathy

The frequent occurrence of coagulopathies in head-injured patients is widely known. One investigation of head-injured children found a 71% incidence of abnormal clotting tests and a 32% incidence of the disseminated intravascular coagulation and fibrinolysis (DICF) syndrome.[164]

Unlike most critically injured trauma patients, who tend to have low plasma antithrombin (AT) activity, those with closed head injury tend to have supranormal plasma AT activity, perhaps explaining in part the frequent occurrence of coagulopathy after TBI.[165] DICF is often associated with the development of potentially dangerous delayed or recurrent intracranial hematomas in head-injured patients and can cause expansion of otherwise small hematomas and contusions.[166]

In addition, the increasing use of anticoagulants in treating various cardiac, vascular, and neurological conditions has resulted in an increasing older population of patients with iatrogenic coagulopathy. These patients are also at risk for expansion of seemingly insignificant clots into life-threatening masses. Special caution should be observed if the initial CT scan is a "hyperacute" scan, that is, one obtained very soon after the precipitating trauma.

Fresh-frozen plasma is a commonly used and effective empiric treatment for these conditions. Unfortunately, reduction of an elevated INR to acceptable levels for surgery can sometimes take several hours. The decision to operate in the face of significantly elevated INR can easily lead to surgical disaster. Recombinant Factor VIIa offers a potential solution to this dilemma, with the ability to rapidly reverse an elevated INR and allow almost immediate surgery.[167,168] This use of Factor VIIa is currently an off-label indication and further work is needed to assure the safety and efficacy of this drug in the treatment of the victims of TBI.[169]

## Thromboembolic Events

Head-injured patients are at increased risk of deep venous thrombosis (DVT) and pulmonary embolism (PE). In a large series of trauma patients, 4.3% of those with head injury were diagnosed with DVT, which was half as common in patients without neurologic injury.[170]

Neurosurgeons are concerned about potentially catastrophic postoperative hemorrhagic complications and prefer DVT prophylaxis techniques which avoid compromise of the clotting cascade.

Pneumatic compression stockings are one such technique. In several clinical series of patients with various types of neurosurgical disease, such devices were associated with an incidence of DVT of 1.7 to 2.3% and PE of 1.5 to 1.8%.[171,172] These results have not been uniformly demonstrated by all studies but pneumatic stockings are a mainstay of DVT prophylaxis.

Experience with low-molecular-weight heparin used in conjunction with pneumatic compression suggests that this regimen is even more effective than pneumatic compression alone in general neurosurgery patients[171] and is safe and effective in trauma patients (including those with head injury).[173]

Treatment of thromboembolic events in head-injured patients must weigh the dangers of PE with the risk of bleeding. There is scant data relating the risk of bleeding to time after injury. Anticoagulation may be deferred from 72 hours to as long as 6 weeks after injury in an attempt to prevent recurrent bleeding, depending on local custom.

Thromboembolic events within this window are usually best treated by insertion of an inferior vena cava filter (IVCF). Prophylactic use of IVCFs in all high-risk patients is controversial.

## Fat Embolism

Fat embolism syndrome (FES) is most commonly associated with long-bone fractures. Emboli of fat particles from the bone marrow can disseminate widely and, in the most severe cases, produce multiple organ failure both from a direct embolic effect and from activation of inflammatory cascades.[174]

Although the majority of cases are mild or subclinical, FES can cause dramatic worsening of neurologic status, including confusion, disorientation, seizures, and lethargy. More ominous neurologic changes have been reported, including those mimicking intracranial hypertension or enlargement of intracranial mass lesions. The classical triad of symptoms is acute respiratory failure, global neurologic dysfunction, and a petechial rash, but not all patients exhibit all these features. Acute respiratory failure may be the only symptom in over one-half of all cases.

The diagnosis is difficult and is often made on clinical grounds. Diagnostic confusion may occur if the combination of acute respiratory failure and arterial blood gases showing hypoxemia and hyperventilation are interpreted as signs of pulmonary embolism. A chest x-ray showing diffuse fluffy infiltrates may be more suggestive of FES. It has been suggested that the diagnosis of FES may be made if >5% of cells in washings from bronchoalveolar lavage stain positive for neutral fat with oil red O.[175]

## WHERE AND BY WHOM SHOULD PATIENTS BE MANAGED

Neurotrauma care is complex, highly specialized care. Assuring universal access to complex, highly specialized care has always been problematic. Traditional analysis of this problem has yielded two paradigms for addressing it. The first is to make the care widely available by investing widely in training and equipment to make the capability available at the point where patients access care.

Alternatively, the small numbers of patients requiring complex care can be concentrated at specialty centers. This allows adequate case loads to maintain competence among the staff and concentrates resources on a more cost-effective manner. The drawbacks to this approach are that the services are often maintained at some distance from some of the served population and are not readily available at the point of presentation for care. This necessitates efficient transportation and communication systems to get patients to the appropriate level of care.

The trauma systems in the United States were the result of a decision to take the later approach, concentrating the 11% of trauma victims having major trauma at advanced specialty centers.[176–178]

There has been significant recent concern on the part of the trauma community about access to neurotrauma care. As with complex trauma, most neurotrauma patients do not require complex neurotrauma care but those that do, require a sophisticated system.

Once again, the choice will be dispersing care, creating low level neurotrauma capabilities at all trauma centers by training non-neurosurgeons to provide neurotrauma care or consolidating care at specialty neurotrauma centers.

Assuring timely access to high quality neurotrauma services for the majority of the United States population is a daunting challenge that must be met. Deciding between the center of excellence or the dispersed care approaches involves powerful financial and political factors. Different solutions will probably be applied in different parts of the country. It is hoped that the dedication and experience which created the trauma systems of the United States can now be applied to providing high-quality and universal neurotrauma care to its population.

## OUTCOME

### Disability

Of the patients who survive to reach the ED, 80% have mild injuries. Moderate and severe injuries each account for 10% of the total. Survivors of TBI are often left with varying degrees of

**TABLE 20-3**

**Glasgow Outcome Scale**

| SCORE | CATEGORY | DESCRIPTION |
|---|---|---|
| 5 | Good recovery (GR) | Able to live and work independently despite minor disabilities |
| 4 | Moderate disability (MD) | Able to live independently despite disabilities; can use public transportation, work with assistance/supervision, etc |
| 3 | Severe disability (SD) | Conscious but dependent upon others for self-care; often institutionalized |
| 2 | Persistent vegetative state (PVS) | Not conscious, but may appear "awake" |
| 1 | Death (D) | Self-explanatory |

disability, which occur in roughly 10% of mild, 50 to 67% of moderate, and > 95% of severe closed TBI survivors.[179] The most widely used tool for assessing outcome after TBI is the GCS[180] (Table 20-3).

Outcome can be defined in many different ways. While patient survival may be considered a good outcome by the healthcare team, the significant attendant disability might make the same outcome a poor one to the family or patient. Being clear on how outcome and good outcome is to be defined is critical when discussing outcome prediction.

Similarly, disabilities are relative. The same impairment might be disastrous to one patient and a minor nuisance to another. An example would be the impact of a loss of the ability to calculate, which would be a major disability to an accountant but minor nuisance to a gardener.

Epidemiologic and financial data tell only part of the story, however. The psychological and social sequelae of TBI are tremendous. Many patients experience significant depression from loss of independence, social withdrawal, decreased earning power, which is often permanent and substantial (if not complete), and loss of economic status. Family members commonly experience anger and depression from the upheaval in their lives caused by the injury.

## Outcome Prediction

Many prediction models have been developed over the years. Different indicators of outcome have different significance and different precedence depending on the population to which they are applied. A grim prognostic indicator in the elderly might have much less dire implications for a younger patient. As a result, generalization of findings from a specific population and prediction model to the general population is often inappropriate.[181,182] Care needs to be used when applying prediction models in everyday practice.

Although very good and very bad outcomes can usually be predicted with a high degree of confidence early after injury, it is much harder to prognosticate about patients in intermediate categories. Studies have shown that even with the diligent application of known indicators, physicians tend to overestimate the likelihood of poor outcome and underestimate the likelihood of good outcome early in the care of head-injured patients. In one study, physician's predictive accuracy was only 56%.[183] This "false

pessimism" phenomenon takes on greater significance when combined with work demonstrating that providers will alter their care based on these predictions, increasing the use of therapies considered beneficial for those thought to have a good outcome, and decreasing it for those felt not to have a good prognosis.[184] Care should therefore be exerted when offering predictions or withholding care of the brain-injured patient early in the course of their treatment.

## BRAIN DEATH AND ORGAN DONATION

The diagnosis of brain death is made when there is no clinical evidence of neurological function in a patient whose core temperature is greater than 32.8°C, whose mental status is not impacted by sedating or paralyzing medications, who is completely resuscitated with a systolic blood pressure >90 mm Hg and whose oxygen saturations are >90%.[185]

The absence of neurological function must be scrupulously established and documented. Most errors in declaring brain death are the result of poorly performed neurological examinations. Nationally recognized standards for examination can be found in the references.[185]

Many clinical protocols and some state statutes also require that brain death be confirmed by further neurological tests, an ancillary test such as radio nucleotide cerebral blood flow studies or EEG.[185]

The physiologic definition of brain death described above is the one commonly used in the United States. Various hospitals and systems will have differing methods for declaring brain death and the states have varying legal statute on who may declare death and brain death and how it is to be declared. Those interested should ask within their local system.

What must be emphasized, however, is that brain death is not the same as a hopeless prognosis. Brain death is a physiologic event where the brain dies while the heart and lungs are still functioning through artificial support. In contrast, a hopeless prognosis is a medical judgment that a good outcome is not possible from the current injuries. This distinction is often blurred by health care providers, with the resulting confusion resulting in a loss of credibility on the part of the healthcare system.

This credibility is critical because the victims of TBI that progresses to brain death provide an important source of organs for transplantation. In 1999, TBI was the cause of brain death for more than 40% of individuals from whom organs were procured, with the majority of organs coming from those between 18 and 49 years of age. Despite the presence of a fatal brain injury, an individual's heart, lungs, liver, kidneys, pancreas, and corneas may benefit others with chronic illnesses. Enlisting the trust and support of the public in obtaining these organs is critical to assuring their availability to those who so desperately need them. To gain this trust, the family members of the victims of TBI first need to be sure that the resuscitation of the injured brain has been the first priority of the treating team and second, when that resuscitation has failed, they need to clearly understand the issues surrounding physiologic brain death versus a futile situation. A clear understanding of these issues empowers families to make good decisions for themselves and their loved one, decisions that they can live with as they gain more information in the aftermath of the event. Blurring or confusing these issues erodes the trust of the family and the credibility of the healthcare and organ procurement communities. While the task of approaching families for permission for donation is increasingly being performed by representatives of organ procurement networks, it essential for all members of the patient's care team to be informed and involved in these matters.

# REFERENCES

1. Langlois JA, Rutland-Brown W, Thomas KE: Traumatic brain injury in the United States: *Emergency Department Visits, Hospitalizations, and Deaths.* Centers for Disease Control and Prevention, National Center for Injury Prevention and Control, 2004.
2. Thurman DJ, Alverson C, Browne D, et al.: Traumatic brain injury in the United States: a report to Congress, Atlanta: Centers for Disease Control and Prevention, National Center for Injury Prevention and Control, 1999.
3. Rimel RW, Giordani B, Barth JT: Moderate head injury: Completing the clinical spectrum of brain trauma. *Neurosurgery* 11:344, 1982.
4. Rose J, Valtonen S, Jennett B: Avoidable factors contributing to death after head injury. *BMJ* 2:615, 1977.
5. Miller JD, Sweet RC, Narayan R, et al.: Early insults to the injured brain. *JAMA* 240:439, 1978.
6. Graham DI, Ford I, Adama JH, et al.: Ischeaemic brain damage is still common in fatal non-missle head injury. *J Neurol Neurosurg Psychiatry* 52:346, 1989.
7. Marmarou A, Anderson RL, Ward JL, et al.: Impact of ICP instability and hypotension on outcome in patients with severe head trauma. *J Neurosurg* 75:S59, 1991.
8. Chestnut RM, Marshall LF, Klauber MR, et al.: The role of secondary brain injury in determining outcome from severe head injury. *J Trauma* 34:216, 1993.
9. Stochetti N, Furlan A, Volta F: Hypoxemia and arterial hypotension at the accident scene in head injury. *J Trauma* 40:764, 1996.
10. Silverston P: Pulse oximetry at the roadside: A study of pulse oximetry in immediate care. *BMJ* 298:711, 1989.
11. Manley GT, Pitts LH, Morabito D, et al.: Brain tissue oxygenation during hemorrhagic shock, resuscitation, and alterations in ventilation. *J Trauma-Inj Inf Crit Care* 46:261, 1999.
12. Practice parameter: The management of concussion in sports (summary statement). Report of the Quality Standards Subcommittee. *Neurology* 48:581, 1997.
13. Kelly JP, Rosenberg JH: Diagnosis and management of concussion in sports. *Neurology* 48:575, 1997.
14. McCrea M, Kelly JP, Kluge J, et al.: Standardized assessment of concussion in football players. *Neurology* 48:586, 1997.
15. CT Scan Features. *Management and Prognosis of Severe Traumatic Brain Injury.* New York: Brain Trauma Foundation, 2000, p. 65.
16. Bardt TF, Unterberg AW, Kiening KL, et al.: Multimodal cerebral monitoring in comatose head-injured patients. *Acta Neurochir* 140:357, 1998.
17. Bardt TF, Unterberg AW, Hartl R, et al.: Monitoring of brain tissue $PO_2$ in traumatic brain injury: Effect of cerebral hypoxia on outcome. *Acta Neurochir Suppl* 71:153, 1998.
18. Davis DP, Dunford JV, Poste JC, et al.: The impact of hypoxia and hyperventilation on outcome after paramedic rapid sequence intubation of severely head-injured patients. *J Trauma* 57:1, 2004.
19. Davis DP, Hoyt DB, Ochs M, et al.: The effect of paramedic rapid sequence intubation on outcome in patients with severe traumatic brain injury. *J Trauma* 54:444, 2003.
20. Lal D, Weiland S, Newton M, et al.: Prehospital hyperventilation after brain injury: A prospective analysis of prehospital and early hospital hyperventilation of the brain-injured patient. *Prehospital Disaster Med* 18:20, 2003.
21. Davis DP, Stern J, Sise MJ, et al.: A follow-up analysis of factors associated with head-injury mortality after paramedic rapid sequence intubation. *J Trauma* 59:486, 2005.
22. Treatment: Airway, Ventilation and Oxygenation. In: Brain Trauma Foundation, ed. *Guidelines for Prehospital Management of Traumatic Brain Injury.* New York: Brain Trauma Foundation, 2000.
23. Christensen MA, Bloom J, Sutton KR: Comparing arterial and end-tidal carbon dioxide values in hyperventilated neurosurgical patients. *Am J Crit Care* 4:116, 1995.
24. Grenier B, Verchere E, Mesli A, et al.: Capnography monitoring during neurosurgery: Reliability in relation to various intraoperative positions. *Anesth Analg* 88:43, 1999.
25. Isert P: Control of carbon dioxide levels during neuroanaesthesia: Current practice and an appraisal of our reliance upon capnography. *Anaesth Intensive Care* 22:435, 1994.
26. Kerr ME, Rudy EB, Weber BB, et al.: Effect of short-duration hyperventilation during endotracheal suctioning on intracranial pressure in severe head-injured adults. *Nurs Res.* 46:195, 1997.
27. Mackersie RC, Karagianes TG: Use of end-tidal carbon dioxide tension for monitoring induced hypocapnia in head-injured patients. *Crit Care Med* 18:764, 1990.
28. Russell GB, Graybeal JM: Reliability of the arterial to end-tidal carbon dioxide gradient in mechanically ventilated patients with multisystem trauma. *J Trauma* 36:317, 1994.
29. Davis DP, Dunford JV, Poste JC, et al.: The impact of hypoxia and hyperventilation on outcome after paramedic rapid sequence intubation of severely head-injured patients. *J Trauma* 57:1, 2004.
30. Davis DP, Stern J, Sise MJ, et al.: A follow-up analysis of factors associated with head-injury mortality after paramedic rapid sequence intubation. *J Trauma* 59:486, 2005.
31. Pupillary Diameter and Light Reflex. *Management and Prognosis of Severe Traumatic Brain Injury.* New York: Brain Trauma Foundation, 2000.
32. Teasdale G, Jennett B: Assessment of coma and impaired consciousness: A practical scale. *Lancet* 2:81, 1974.
33. Narayan RK, Greenberg RP, Miller JD: Improved confidence of outcome prediction in severe head injury: A comparative analysis of the clinical examination, multimodality evoked potentials, CT scanning, and intracranial pressure. *J Neurosurg* 54:751, 1981.
34. Narayan RK, Kishore PR, Becker DP: Intracranial Pressure: To monitor or not to monitor? A review of our experience with severe head injury. *J Neurosurg* 56:650, 1982.
35. Arabi B: Surgical outcome in 435 patients who sustained missile head wounds during the Iran-Iraq War. *Neurosurgery* 27:692, 1990.
36. Part 2: Prognosis in penetrating brain injury. *J Trauma* 51:S44, 2001.
37. Brandvold B, Levi L, Feinsod M, et al.: Penetrating craniocerebral injuries in the Israeli involvement in the Lebanese conflict, 1982–1985. Analysis of a less aggressive surgical approach. *J Neurosurg* 72:15, 1990.
38. Grahm TW, Williams FC Jr, Harrington T, et al.: Civilian gunshot wounds to the head: A prospective study. *Neurosurgery* 27:696, 1990.
39. Kaufman HH, Makela ME, Lee KF, et al.: Gunshot wounds to the head: A perspective. *Neurosurgery* 18:689, 1986.
40. Shaffrey ME, Polin RS, Phillips CD, et al.: Classification of civilian craniocerebral gunshot wounds: A multivariate analysis predictive of mortality. *J Neurotrauma* 9:S279, 1992.
41. The management of minor closed head injury in children. Committee on Quality Improvement, American Academy of Pediatrics. Commission on Clinical Policies and Research, American Academy of Family Physicians. *Pediatrics* 104:1407, 1999.
42. The East Practice Management Guidelines Work Group: Practice Management Guidelines for the Management of Mild Traumatic Brain Injury. Eastern Association for the Surgery of Trauma. Eastern Association for the Surgery of Trauma, 2001.
43. ACR Appropriateness Criteria Expert Panel on Neurologic Imaging: *Head Trauma.* American College of Radiology, 2006. http://www.acr.org/s_acr/
44. Kaufman HH, Levy ML, Stone JL, et al.: Patients with Glasgow Coma Scale scores 3, 4, 5 after gunshot wounds to the brain. *Neurosurg Clin N Am* 6:701, 1995.
45. Clark WC, Muhlbauer MS, Watridge CB, et al.: Analysis of 76 civilian craniocerebral gunshot wounds. *J Neurosurg* 65:9, 1986.
46. Jennett B., Teasdale G: Early assessment of the head-injured patient. *Management of Head Injuries.* Philadelphia: FA Davis Company, 1981.
47. Becker DP, Miller JD, Ward JD, et al.: The outcome from severe head injury with early diagnosis and intensive management *J Neurosurg* 47:491, 1977.
48. Kothari RU, Brott T, Broderick JP, et al.: The ABCs of measuring intracerebral hemorrhage volumes *Stroke* 27:1304, 1996.
49. Bullock MR, Chesnut R, Ghajar J, et al.: Surgical Management of acute epidural hematomas. *Neurosurgery* 58:S2, 2006.
50. Bullock MR, Chesnut R, Ghajar J, et al.: Surgical Management of Acute Subdural Hematomas. *Neurosurgery* 58:S2, 2006.
51. Bullock MR, Chesnut R, Ghajar J, et al.: Surgical management of traumatic parenchymal lesions. *Neurosurgery* 58:S25, 2006.
52. Bullock MR, Chesnut R, Ghajar J, et al.: Surgical management of posterior fossa mass lesions. *Neurosurgery* 58:S47, 2006.
53. Aarabi B, Hesdorffer DC, Ahn ES, et al.: Outcome following decompressive craniectomy for malignant swelling due to severe head injury. *J Neurosurg* 104:469, 2006.
54. Hejazi N, Witzmann A, Fae P: Unilateral decompressive craniectomy for children with severe brain injury. Report of seven cases and review of the relevant literature. *Eur J Pediatr* 161:99, 2002.
55. Polin RS, Shaffrey ME, Bogaev CA, et al.: Decompressive bifrontal craniectomy in the treatment of severe refractory posttraumatic cerebral edema. *Neurosurgery* 41:84, 1997.

56. Bullock MR, Chesnut R, Ghajar J, et al.: Surgical management of depressed cranial fractures. *Neurosurgery* 58:S56, 2006.

57. Salazar AM, Jabbari B, Vance SC, et al.: Epilepsy after penetrating head injury. I. Clinical correlates: A report of the Vietnam Head Injury Study. *Neurology* 35:1406, 1985.

58. Carey ME, Young HF, Rish BL, et al.: Follow-up study of 103 American soldiers who sustained a brain wound in Vietnam. *J Neurosurg* 41:542, 1974.

59. Chaudhri KA, Choudhury AR, al Moutaery KR, et al.: Penetrating craniocerebral shrapnel injuries during "Operation Desert Storm": Early results of a conservative surgical treatment. *Acta Neurochir (Wien)* 126:120, 1994.

60. Gonul E, Baysefer A, Kahraman S, et al.: Causes of infections and management results in penetrating craniocerebral injuries. *Neurosurg Rev* 20:177, 1997.

61. Hammon WM: Analysis of 2187 consecutive penetrating wounds of the brain from Vietnam. *J Neurosurg* 34:127, 1971.

62. Wester K: Decompressive surgery for "pure" epidural hematomas: Does neurosurgical expertise improve the outcome? *Neurosurgery* 44:495, 1999.

63. Langfitt TW: Increased intracranial pressure. *Clin Neurosurg* 16:436, 1969.

64. Saul TG, Ducker TB: Effect of intracranial pressure monitoring and aggressive treatment on mortality in severe head injury. *J Neurosurg* 56:498, 1982.

65. Marshall LF, Smith RW, Shapiro HM: The outcome with aggressive treatment in severe head injuries. Part I: The significance of intracranial pressure monitoring. *J Neurosurg* 50:20, 1979.

66. Marmarou A, Anderson RL, Ward JD: Impact of ICP instability and hypotension on outcome in patients with severe head trauma. *J Neurosurg* 75:S159, 1991.

67. *Intracranial Pressure Treatment Threshold. Management and Prognosis of Severe Traumatic Brain Injury.* New York: Brain Trauma Foundation, 2000, p. 71.

68. Guillaume J, Janny P: Continuous intracranial manometry; physiopathologic and clinical significance of the method. *Presse Medicale* 59:953, 1951.

69. Guillaume J, Janny P: Continuous intracranial manometry; importance of the method and first results. *Revue Neurologique* 84:131, 1951.

70. Lundberg N: Continuous recording and control of ventricular fluid pressure in neurosurgical practice. *Acta Psychiatr Scand* 36:1, 1960.

71. Barry KG, Berman AR: Mannitol infusion. III: The acute effect of the intravenous infusion of mannitol on blood and plasma volumes. *N Engl J Med* 264:1085, 1961.

72. Schrot RJ, Muizelaar JP: Is there a "best" way to give Mannitol? In: Valadka AB, Andrews BT, eds. *Neurotrauma.* New York: Thieme, 2005, p. 142.

73. *Management and Prognosis of Severe Traumatic Brain Injury,* 2nd ed. New York: Brain Trauma Foundation, 2000.

74. Becker DP, Vries JK: The alleviation of increased intracranial pressure by the chronic administration of osmotic agents. In Brock M, Dietz H, eds. *Intracranial Pressure.* Berlin: Springer, 1972, p. 309.

75. Eisenberg HM, Frankowski RF, Contant CF: High-dose barbiturate control of elevated intracranial pressure in patients with severe head injury. *J Neurosurg* 69:15, 1988.

76. James HE: Methodology for the control of intracranial pressure with hypertonic mannitol. *Acta Neurochir (Wein)* 51:161, 1980.

77. Schwartz ML, Tator CH, Rowed DW: The University of Toronto Head Injury Treatment Study: A prospective, randomized comparison of pentobarbitol and mannitol. *J Neurol Sci* 11:434, 1984.

78. Smith HP, Kelly DL Jr, McWhorter JM, et al.: Comparison of mannitol regimens in patients with severe head injury undergoing intracranial monitoring. *J Neurosurg* 65:820, 1986.

79. Cote CJ, Greenhow DE, Marshall BE: The hypotensive response to rapid intravenous administration of hypertonic solutions in man and in the rabbit. *Anesthesiology* 50:30, 1979.

80. Domaingue CM, Nye DH: Hypotensive effect of mannitol administered rapidly. *Anaesth Intensive Care* 13:134, 1985.

81. Ravussin P, Archer DP, Tyler JL: Effects of rapid mannitol infusion on cerebral blood volume. A positron emission tomography study in dogs and man. *J Neurosurg* 64:104, 1986.

82. Smith HP, Kelly DL, McWorter JM, et al.: Comparison of mannitol regimens in patients with severe head injury undergoing intracranial monitoring. *J Neurosurg* 65:820, 1986.

83. Marshall LF, Smith RW, Rausher LA: Mannitol dose requirements in brain-injured patients. *J Neurosurg* 48:169, 1978.

84. Muizelaar JP, Lutz HA III, Becker DP: Effect of mannitol on ICP and CBF and correlation with pressure autoregulation in severely head-injured patients. *J Neurosurg* 61:700, 1984.

85. Unterberg AW, Kiening KL, Hartl R, et al.: Multimodal monitoring in patients with head injury: Evaluation of the effects of treatment on cerebral oxygenation. *J Trauma-Inj Infect Crit Care* 42:S32, 1997.

86. Kaufmann AM, Cardoso ER: Aggravation of vasogenic cerebral edema by multiple-dose mannitol. *J Neurosurg* 77:584, 1992.

87. McGraw CP, Alexander E, Howard G: Effect of dose and dose schedule on the response of intracranial pressure to mannitol. *Surg Neurol* 10:127, 1978.

88. Marshall LF, SMith RW, Rauscher LA, et al.: Mannitol dose requirements in brain-injured patients. *J Neurosurg* 48:169, 1978.

89. Gemma M, Cozzi S, Tommasino C: 7.5% hypertonic saline versus 20% mannitol during elective neurosurgical supratentorial proceedures. *J Neurosurg Anesthesiol* 9:329, 1997.

90. Munar F, Ferrer AM, de Nadal M: Cerebral hemodynamic effects of 7.2% hypertonic saline in patients with head injury and raised intracranial pressure. *J Neurotrauma* 17:41, 2000.

91. DeVivo P, Del Gaudio A, Ciritella P: Hypertonic saline solution: A safe alternative to mannitol 18% in neurosurgery. *Minerva Anestesiol* 67:603, 2001.

92. Peterson B, Khanna S, Fisher B et al.: Prolonged hypernatremia controls elevated intracranial pressure in head-injured pediatric patients. *Crit Care Med* 28:1136, 2000.

93. Suarez JI, Qureshi AI, Bhardwaj A: Treatment of refractory intracranial hypertension with 23.4% saline. *Crit Care Med* 26:1118, 1998.

94. Peterson B, Khanna S, Fisher B, et al.: Prolonged hypernatremia controls elevated intracranial pressure in head-injured pediatric patients. *Crit Care Med* 28:1136, 2000.

95. Qureshi AI, Wilson DA, Traystman RJ: Treatment of elevated intracranial pressure in experimental intracerebral hemorrhage: Comparison between mannitol and hypertonic saline. *Neurosurg* 44:1055, 1999.

96. Doyle JA, Davis DP, Hoyt DB: The use of hypertonic saline in the treatment of traumatic brain injury. *J Trauma* 50:367, 2001.

97. Schatzmann C, Heissler HE, Konig K, et al.: Treatment of elevated intracranial pressure by infusions of 10% saline in severely head injured patients. *Acta Neurochir Suppl* 71:31, 1998.

98. Shackford SR: Effect of small-volume resuscitation on intracranial pressure and related cerebral variables. *J Trauma* 42:S48, 1997.

99. Cooper DJ, Myles PS, McDermott FT: Prehospital hypertonic saline resuscitation of patients with hypotension and severe traumatic brain injury: A randomized controlled trial. *JAMA* 291:1350, 2004.

100. Moore FA, McKinley BA, Moore EE: The next generation in shock resuscitation. *Lancet* 363:1988, 2004.

101. Devlin JW, Barletta JF: Albumin for fluid resuscitation: Implications of the Saline versus Albumin Fluid Evaluation. *Am J Health Syst Pharm* 62:637, 2005.

102. Human albumin administration in critically ill patients: Systematic review of randomised controlled trials. Cochrane Injuries Group Albumin Reviewers. *BMJ* 317:235, 1998.

103. Finfer S, Bellomo R, Boyce N, et al.: A comparison of albumin and saline for fluid resuscitation in the intensive care unit. *N Engl J Med* 350:2247, 2004.

104. Tanzi M, Gardner M, Megellas M, et al.: Evaluation of the appropriate use of albumin in adult and pediatric patients. *Am J Health Syst Pharm* 60:1330, 2003.

105. Sundt TM Jr, Waltz AG: Hemodilution and anticoagulation. Effects on the microvasculature and microcirculation of the cerebral cortex after arterial occlusion. *Neurology* 17:230, 1967.

106. Grande PO, Asgeirsson B, Nordstrom CH: Volume-targeted therapy of increased intracranial pressure: The Lund concept unifies surgical and non-surgical treatments. *Acta Anaesthesiol Scand* 46:929, 2002.

107. Belayev L, Liu Y, Zhao W, et al.: Human albumin therapy of acute ischemic stroke: Marked neuroprotective efficacy at moderate doses and with a broad therapeutic window. *Stroke* 32:553, 2001.

108. Lundberg N, Kjallquist A, Bien C: Reduction of increased intracranial pressure by hyperventilation. A therapeutic aid in neurological surgery. *Acta Psychiatr Scand* 34:1, 1959.

109. Raichle ME, Plum F: Hyperventilation and cerebral blood flow. *Stroke* 3:566, 1972.

110. Muizelaar JP, Marmarou A, Ward JD, et al.: Adverse effects of prolonged hyperventilation in patients with severe head injury: A randomized clinical trial. *J Neurosurg* 75:731, 1991.

111. Bouma GJ, Muizelaar JP, Choi SC, et al.: Cerebral circulation and metabolism after severe traumatic brain injury: The elusive role of ischemia. *J Neurosurg* 75:685, 1991.

112. Bouma GJ, Levasseur JE, Muizelaar JP, et al.: Description of a closed window technique for in vivo study of the feline basilar artery. *Stroke* 22:522, 1991.

113. Jaggi JL, Obrist WD, Gennarelli TA, et al.: Relationship of early cerebral blood flow and metabolism to outcome in acute head injury. *J Neurosurg* 72:176, 1990.

114. *Hyperventilation, in Management and Prognosis of Severe Traumatic Brain Injury.* New York: Brain Trauma Foundation, 2000, p. 101.

115. Eisenberg HM, Frankowski RF, Contant CF, et al.: High-dose barbiturate control of elevated intracranial pressure in patients with severe head injury. *J Neurosurg* 69:15, 1988.

116. Ward JD, Becker DP, Miller JD, et al.: Failure of prophylactic barbiturate coma in the treatment of severe head injury. *J Neurosurg* 62:383, 1985.

117. Kelly DF, Goodale DB, Williams J, et al.: Propofol in the treatment of moderate and severe head injury: A randomized, prospective double-blinded pilot trial. *J Neurosurg* 90:1042, 1999.

118. Cremer OL, Moons KG, Bouman EA, et al.: Long-term propofol infusion and cardiac failure in adult head-injured patients. *Lancet* 357:117, 2001.

119. Cannon ML, Glazier SS, Bauman LA: Metabolic acidosis, rhabdomyolysis, and cardiovascular collapse after prolonged propofol infusion. *J Neurosurg* 95:1053, 2001.

120. Kelly DF: Propofol-infusion syndrome. *J Neurosurg* 95:925, 2001.

121. Kang TM: Propofol infusion syndrome in critically ill patients. *AnnPharmacother* 36:1453, 2002.

122. Marion DW, Penrod LE, Kelsey SF, et al.: Treatment of traumatic brain injury with moderate hypothermia. *N Engl J Med* 336:540, 1997.

123. Shiozaki T, Sugimoto H, Taneda M, et al.: Effect of mild hypothermia on uncontrollable intracranial hypertension after severe head injury. *J Neurosurg* 79:363, 1993.

124. Shiozaki T, Sugimoto H, Taneda M, et al.: Selection of severely head injured patients for mild hypothermia therapy. *J Neurosurg* 89:206, 1998.

125. Shiozaki T, Hayakata T, Taneda M, et al.: A multicenter prospective randomized controlled trial of the efficacy of mild hypothermia for severely head injured patients with low intracranial pressure. Mild Hypothermia Study Group in Japan. *J Neurosurg* 94:50, 2001.

126. Marion DW, Obrist WD, Carlier PM, et al.: The use of moderate therapeutic hypothermia for patients with severe head injuries: A preliminary report. *J Neurosurg* 79:354, 1993.

127. Zhi D, Zhang S, Lin X: Study on therapeutic mechanism and clinical effect of mild hypothermia in patients with severe head injury. *Surg Neurol* 59:381, 2003.

128. Clifton GL, Miller ER, Choi SC, et al.: Lack of effect of induction of hypothermia after acute brain injury. *N Engl J Med* 344:556, 2001.

129. Markgraf CG, Clifton GL, Moody MR: Treatment window for hypothermia in brain injury. *J Neurosurg* 95:979, 2001.

130. Diringer MN, Reaven NL, Funk SE, et al.: Elevated body temperature independently contributes to increased length of stay in neurologic intensive care unit patients. *Crit Care Med* 32:1489, 2004.

131. Robertson CS: Management of cerebral perfusion pressure after traumatic brain injury. *Anesthesiology* 95:1513, 2001.

132. Marion DW, Darby J, Yonas H: Acute regional cerebral blood flow changes caused by severe head injuries. *J Neurosurg* 74:407, 1991.

133. McLaughlin MR, Marion DW: Cerebral blood flow and vasoresponsivity within and around cerebral contusions. *J Neurosurg* 85:871, 1996.

134. Hlatky R, Robertson C: Does Raising Cerebral Perfusion Pressure Help Head Injured Patients? In Valadka AB, Andrews BT, eds. *Neurotrauma*. New York: Thieme, 2005, p. 75.

135. Eker C, Asgeirsson B, Grande PO, et al.: Improved outcome after severe head injury with a new therapy based on principles for brain volume regulation and preserved microcirculation. *Crit Care Med* 26:1881, 1998.

136. Robertson CS, Valadka AB, Hannay HJ, et al.: Prevention of secondary ischemic insults after severe head injury. *Crit Care Med* 27:2086, 1999.

137. Heros RC, Korosue K: Hemodilution for cerebral ischemia. *Stroke* 20:423, 1989.

138. Harel D, Ullman JS: What is the Optimal Hematocrit and Hemoglobin for Head-Injured Patients? In Valadka AB, Andrews BT, eds. *Neurotrauma*. New York: Thieme, 2005.

139. Thomas DJ, Marshall J, Russell RW, et al.: Effect of haematocrit on cerebral blood-flow in man. *Lancet* 2:941, 1977.

140. Lee SH, Heros RC, Mullan JC, et al.: Optimum degree of hemodilution for brain protection in a canine model of focal cerebral ischemia. *J Neurosurg* 80:469, 1994.

141. Morimoto Y, Mathru M, Martinez-Tica JF, et al.: Effects of profound anemia on brain tissue oxygen tension, carbon dioxide tension, and pH in rabbits. *J Neurosurg Anesthesiol* 13:33, 2001.

142. Robertson CS, Narayan RK, Gokaslan ZL, et al.: Cerebral arteriovenous oxygen difference as an estimate of cerebral blood flow in comatose patients.. *J Neurosurg* 70:222, 1989.

143. Obrist WD, Langfitt TW, Jaggi JL, et al.: Cerebral blood flow and metabolism in comatose patients with acute head injury. Relationship to intracranial hypertension. *J Neurosurg* 61:241, 1984.

144. Robertson C: Desaturation episodes after severe head injury: Influence on outcome. *Acta Neurochir Suppl (Wien)* 59:98, 1993.

145. Gopinath SP, Robertson CS, Contant CF, et al.: Jugular venous desaturation and outcome after head injury. *J Neurol Neurosurg Psychiatry* 57:717, 1994.

146. Gopinath SP, Valadka AB, Uzura M, et al.: Comparison of jugular venous oxygen saturation and brain tissue Po2 as monitors of cerebral ischemia after head injury. *Crit Care Med* 27:2337, 1999.

147. Kiening KL, Hartl R, Unterberg AW, et al.: Brain tissue pO2-monitoring in comatose patients: Implications for therapy. *Neurol Res* 19:233, 1997.

148. Stiefel MF, Spiotta A, Gracias VH, et al.: Reduced mortality rate in patients with severe traumatic brain injury treated with brain tissue oxygen monitoring. *J Neurosurg* 103:805, 2005.

149. Aarabi B: Traumatic aneurysms of brain due to high velocity missile head wounds. *Neurosurg* 22:1056, 1988.

150. Aarabi B: Management of traumatic aneurysms caused by high-velocity missile head wounds. *Neurosurg Clin N Am* 6:775, 1995.

151. Meirowsky AM, Caveness WF, Dillon JD, et al.: Cerebrospinal fluid fistulas complicating missile wounds of the brain. *J Neurosurg* 54:44, 1981.

152. Antibiotic prophylaxis for penetrating brain injury. *J Trauma* 51:S34, 2001.

153. Caveness WF, Meirowsky AM, Rish BL, et al.: The nature of posttraumatic epilepsy. *J Neurosurg* 50:545, 1979.

154. Antiseizure prophylaxis for penetrating brain injury. *J Trauma* 51:S41, 2001.

155. Annegers JF, Hauser WA, Coan SP, et al.: A population-based study of seizures after traumatic brain injuries. *N Engl J Med* 338:20, 1998.

156. Temkin NR, Dikmen SS, Wilensky AJ, et al.: A randomized, double-blind study of phenytoin for the prevention of post-traumatic seizures. *N Engl J Med* 323:497, 1990.

157. Bullock R, Chesnut RM, Clifton G, et al.: Guidelines for the management of severe head injury. Brain Trauma Foundation. *Eur J Emerg Med* 3:109, 1996.

158. Caron MJ, Hovda DA, Mazziotta JC, et al.: The structural and metabolic anatomy of traumatic brain injury in humans: A computerized tomography and positron emission tomography analysis. *J Neurotrauma* 10:S58, 1993.

159. Caron MJ, Mazziotta JC, Hovda DA, et al.: Quantification of cerebral glucose metabolism in brain injured humans utilizing positron emission tomography. *J Cereb Blood Flow Metab* 13:S379, 1993.

160. Caron MJ: PET(SPECT Imaging in Head Injury. In: Narayan RK, Wilberger JE, Povlishock JT, eds. *Neurotrauma*. New York: McGraw-Hill, 1996, 163.

161. Lam AM, Winn HR, Cullen BF, et al.: Hyperglycemia and neurological outcome in patients with head injury. *J Neurosurg* 75:545, 1991.

162. Young B, Ott L, Dempsey R, et al.: Relationship between admission hyperglycemia and neurologic outcome of severely brain-injured patients. *Ann Surg* 210:466, 1989.

163. Roberts I, Yates D, Sandercock P, et al.: Effect of intravenous corticosteroids on death within 14 days in 10008 adults with clinically significant head injury (MRC CRASH trial): Randomised placebo-controlled trial. *Lancet* 364:1321, 2004.

164. Miner ME, Kaufman HH, Graham SH, et al.: Disseminated intravascular coagulation fibrinolytic syndrome following head injury in children: Frequency and prognostic implications. *J Pediatr* 100:687, 1982.

165. Owings JT, Bagley M, Gosselin R, et al.: Effect of critical injury on plasma antithrombin activity: Low antithrombin levels are associated with thromboembolic complications. *J Trauma* 41:396, 1996.

166. Kaufman HH, Moake JL, Olson JD, et al.: Delayed and recurrent intracranial hematomas related to disseminated intravascular clotting and fibrinolysis in head injury. *Neurosurgery* 7:445, 1980.

167. Boffard KD, Riou B, Warren B, et al.: Recombinant factor VIIa as adjunctive therapy for bleeding control in severely injured trauma patients: Two parallel randomized, placebo-controlled, double-blind clinical trials. *J Trauma* 59:8, 2005.

168. Mayer SA, Brun NC, Begtrup K, et al.: Recombinant activated factor VII for acute intracerebral hemorrhage. *N Engl J Med* 352:777, 2005.

169. O'Connell KA, Wood JJ, Wise RP, et al.: Thromboembolic adverse events after use of recombinant human coagulation factor VIIa. *JAMA* 295:293, 2006.

170. Dennis JW, Menawat S, Von Thron J, et al.: Efficacy of deep venous thrombosis prophylaxis in trauma patients and identification of high-risk groups. *J Trauma* 35:132, 1993.

171. Frim DM, Barker FG, Poletti CE, et al.: Postoperative low-dose heparin decreases thromboembolic complications in neurosurgical patients. *Neurosurgery* 30:830, 1992.

172. Black PM, Baker MF, Snook CP: Experience with external pneumatic calf compression in neurology and neurosurgery. *Neurosurgery* 18:440, 1986.

173. Knudson MM, Morabito D, Paiement GD, et al.: Use of low molecular weight heparin in preventing thromboembolism in trauma patients. *J Trauma* 41:446, 1996.

174. Shier MR, Wilson RF: Fat embolism syndrome: Traumatic coagulopathy with respiratory distress. *Surgery Annual* 12:139, 1980.

175. Chastre J, Fagon JY, Soler P et al.: Bronchoalveolar lavage for rapid diagnosis of the fat embolism syndrome in trauma patients.[see comment]. *Annals of Inter Med* 113:583, 1990.

176. Nathens AB, Jurkovich GJ, MacKenzie EJ et al.: A resource-based assessment of trauma care in the United States. *J Trauma* 56:173, 2004.

177. Mullins RJ, Mann NC: Introduction to the Academic Symposium to Evaluate Evidence Regarding the Efficacy of Trauma Systems. *J Trauma* 47:S3, 1999.

178. Mullins RJ. A historical perspective of trauma system development in the United States. *J Trauma* 47:S8, 1999.

179. Kraus JF: Epidemiology of head injury. In Cooper PR, ed. *Head Injury*. Baltimore: Williams & Wilkins, 1993, p. 1.
180. Jennett B, Bond M: Assessment of outcome after severe brain damage. *Lancet* 1:480, 1975.
181. *Early Indicators of Prognosis in Severe Traumatic Brain Injury. Management and Prognosis of Severe Traumatic Brain Injury.* New York: Brain Trauma Foundation, 2000, p. 1.
182. Choi SC, Muizelaar JP, Barnes TY et al.: Prediction tree for severely head-injured patients. *J Neurosurg* 75:251, 1991.
183. Kaufmann MA, Buchmann B, Scheidegger D et al.: Severe head injury: Should expected outcome influence resuscitation and first-day decisions? *Resuscitation* 23:199, 1992.
184. Murray LS, Teasdale GM, Murray GD, et al.: Does prediction of outcome alter patient management? *Lancet* 341:1487, 1993.
185. Guidelines for the determination of death. Report of the medical consultants on the diagnosis of death to the President's Commission for the Study of Ethical Problems in Medicine and Biomedical and Behavioral Research. *JAMA* 246:2184, 1981.

# Commentary ■ JACK WILBERGER

The quality of acute care provided to victims of TBI has a significant impact on their survival and functional outcome. In the United States, most studies show that the mortality rate from severe TBI has declined by at least 50% during the last four–five decades due in large part to improved trauma systems, emergency medical systems, and ICU critical care. Additionally, our enhanced understanding of the pathophysiology of secondary brain injury and the increasing availability of multimodality monitoring to detect and prevent or ameliorate the deleterious effects of secondary injury are further improving outcomes.

This chapter provides a comprehensive overview of our current state of knowledge and reviews available evidence-based guidelines on the medical and surgical treatment of severe TBI. There are, however, several areas that deserve amplification or clarification.

## POSTTRAUMATIC SUBARACHNOID HEMORRHAGE

The authors correctly point out that SAH is a very frequent occurrence after severe TBI.

Indeed, it is seen in over 50% of these patients. It has been recently been elucidated that the incidence of vasospasm in this setting is over 40%, most commonly manifesting on postinjury day two. Thus, transcranial doppler monitoring should be considered in this context in an attempt to monitor and treat significant alterations in cerebrovascular resistance and flow. Alternatively, cerebral blood flow monitoring would provide a more sensitive means of detecting vasospasm, however its availability is quite limited at this time.

Irrespective of monitoring capabilities, posttraumatic vasospasm should be considered in any severe TBI patient with CT evidence of SAH who clinically deteriorates or in whom ICP is difficult to control—especially in the first several days after injury.

The treatment of symptomatic posttraumatic vasospasm can be problematic in the severe TBI patient. The calcium channel blocker nimodipine has proven effective in ameliorating vasospasm from other causes. However, its use can be associated with significant hypotension which must be avoided in this setting. Hypervolemic therapy may also be helpful, but possibly contraindicated in patients with large contusions or ICP control issues. Thus, early

use of interventional therapies such as angioplasty may be the best approach for these patients.

## SURGICAL TREATMENT

There are a number of dogmatic statements regarding the indications for surgical intervention in severe TBI patients with mass lesions. The reader must recognize that the majority of these statements are taken from the recently published Guidelines for the Surgical Management of Traumatic Brain Injury.[1] Every recommendation made in this evidence-based review is at the level of an option. It is of unclear clinical certainty, based on available literature, whether the interventions recommended positively affect outcome. Readers with a particular interest in this area are thus encouraged to review the original Guidelines.

## DECOMPRESSIVE CRANIECTOMY

Based on a recent survey, decompressive craniectomy—either in conjunction with evacuation of a mass lesion or as a stand-alone procedure—is being almost as frequently performed as is ICP monitoring. While there are a number of anecdoctal reports, retrospective reviews and at least one meta-analysis, information is still lacking on its effectiveness or lack thereof. It is however reasonably clear that if decompressive craniectomy is going to be done that the decompression must be extensive and the timing early. There is now an active randomized, controlled clinical trial on decompressive craniectomy after severe TBI, the results of which should be available by 2008.

## GERIATRIC TBI

While not addressed in this chapter, head injury in patients over 65 years of age is being seen with increasing frequency. While a predominant mechanism is same height falls, the injuries are often severe and fatalities are high.

An additional problem in this population is concomitant antiplatelet, anticoagulatant prescription. Even seemingly trivial injuries, with minimal or no initial neurologic or CT findings may result in rapid deterioration, resulting in a recent proliferation of recommendations for the management of this specific patient population. A reasonable approach in the anticoagulated patient with a supratherapeutic INR is to correct the INR to therapeutic levels with Vitamin K and fresh frozen plasma and follow clinically and with repeat CT. If the CT is abnormal, the INR should be corrected to normal and the patient followed closely with frequent clinical and appropriate CT monitoring.

Currently, there is tremendous interest and pressure to use recombinant factor VII (rVIIa) in this setting. While rVIIa will rapidly correct the INR, it must be remembered that its effect is short-lived and it does not replenish the other Vitamin K- dependent clotting factors.

## THE FUTURE

Unfortunately, as noted in this chapter, in spite of dozens of clinical trials involving tens of thousands of severe TBI patients, we have failed to find a pharmacologic treatment to halt the biochemical secondary injury cascade. We, however, have come to realize not only the significant pathophysiologic heterogeneity amongst seemingly similar injuries but also that the operant pathophysiology may be different at different times in the same patient. This provides the opportunity to better target currently available treatments and subsequent clinical trials. Just as importantly we are beginning to understand that genetics plays a key role in susceptibility, response, and recovery from TBI. For example, individuals with the APOe gene appear predisposed to TBI and have worse outcomes.

Hopefully when this chapter is next revised, our understanding of these key issues will have exponentially increased and outcomes from severe TBI dramatically improved.

## Reference

1. *Neurosurgery* 58:S2-1, 2006.

# Injury to the Eye

*Geoffrey Broocker* ■ *Maria E. Aaron* ■ *Joung Y. Kim*

## HISTORICAL PERSPECTIVE

Among the many causes of blindness, trauma has long been one of the major causes of visual loss.[1] Technical advances and developments in medical and surgical expertise have greatly improved visual outcomes in patients with injuries to the eye. Understanding the timing of microsurgical techniques for the anterior segment and vitreoretinal area, intraocular viscoelastic materials, improved imaging modalities, ocular and orbital implants, and plastic surgical techniques have all played major roles in preserving sight and maintaining acceptable patient appearances following significant injuries to the eye. The importance of prevention through protective eyewear and awareness cannot be overemphasized.

## EPIDEMIOLOGY OF EYE INJURIES

As with all areas of trauma, interest in the epidemiology of eye injuries has grown over the past two decades. This is due to an increased awareness of the significant impact ocular injuries have on long-term disability and the economics of health care. Besides case series and isolated studies of prevalence, national and international centers created to help track injuries to the eye have provided important data. In particular, the United States Eye Injury Register (USEIR), National Electronic Injury Surveillance System, National Institute for Occupational Safety and Health, National Athletic Injury/Illness Reporting System, and the National Hospital Discharge Survey play important roles in helping to define rates and the relative risks of injuries to the eye in the United States. Worldwide, roughly 500,000 injuries to the eye leading to monocular blindness occur annually, and eye injuries are the second leading cause of visual impairment following cataracts (which are reversible).[2] In the United States, it is estimated that there are 2.5 million new eye injuries each year, and 40,000 to 60,000 of these patients suffer trauma-related blindness.[3,4] The cumulative lifetime prevalence for eye injuries in the United States is approximately 143.6 per 1000 people.[5] The National Institute for Occupational Safety and Health estimates that there are at least 650,000 work-related eye injuries each year. Based on information provided by Prevent Blindness America for the year 2000, the total cost of disabling eye injuries in the workplace in the United States, including medical expenses, lost wages, administrative costs, and production slowdowns, was $3.9 billion.[3,4] If all types of eye injuries (e.g., assaults, injuries at home, automobile accidents, sports-related injuries, and nondisabling injuries) are included, the annual cost is much higher.

As one of the largest case series of its kind representing 39 states, information reported by the USEIR provides valuable insight into eye injuries across the United States. Between 1988 and 1998 the USEIR reported on 8952 severe injuries to the eye, and the types of data gleaned from these injuries are consistent with information gathered from other sources. The major findings from the USEIR address severe vision-threatening injuries. The average age of the injured patient was 29, and 58% of patients were less than 30 years old. The vast majority of these patients were male, and the relative rate of injuries for men was approximately five times that for women. Blunt and sharp injuries were the most common causes (48%). Frequently implicated blunt objects include rocks, fists, baseballs, and lumber. Sharp objects were likely to be sticks, knives, scissors, screwdrivers, and nails. Vehicle crashes, gunshots, BB injuries, fireworks, and falls were also highly represented. Most injuries (40%) occurred at home, while industrial settings, streets and highways, and sporting activities accounted for roughly 14% each. Approximately 20% of injuries were work related. Anatomically, the cornea was involved in 52% of injuries, the retina in 46%, and the sclera in 31%. Posterior ocular injuries carried a worse visual prognosis. Only 4% of these injuries were bilateral, with gunshot wounds and motor vehicle crashes the most common causes. Approximately 3% of patients were wearing some form of eye protection when injured.[6,7]

Other studies show a higher prevalence of eye injuries in non-whites and in patients with lower levels of education. Additionally, patients under the influence of alcohol are at higher risk for eye trauma.[2,3,8,9] A surveillance study of eye injuries in military personnel on active duty during 1998 showed that approximately 1% were treated for eye injuries, and the demographic data for these injuries are similar to information obtained from studies of civilian populations.[10] With regard to children, eye trauma is the leading cause of noncongenital unilateral visual loss.[11] Prevent Blindness America estimates that 35% of eye injuries occur in individuals less than 17 years of age, though these rates may actually be higher.[4] The American Academy of Pediatrics reported that 66% of all eye injuries occur in individuals less than 16 years of age, and that boys are four times more likely to be injured than girls.[11] Studies of urban eye trauma have revealed a preponderance of injuries to the left eye in assaults and a 10% rate of bilateral injuries.[8,9,10] Sports-related eye injuries have also been well studied. Basketball has the highest rate of eye injuries in organized and recreational sports (20%). Baseball is second overall and is highest for participants between the ages of 5 and 14; it also tends to have the most severe injuries.[13–16] Hockey has shown drastic reductions in the rates of eye injuries with the implementation of effective face shields, but racquet sports continue to account for high rates of sports-related injuries to the eye.[14,16]

## FUNCTION AND ANATOMY

The function of the eye is primarily to give sight. The eyelids and orbit have structural and protective importance and secondary importance in cosmesis. Familiarity with external and internal ocular anatomy and orbital and eyelid structure is paramount to evaluating and managing injuries to the eye. A detailed review of ocular and orbital anatomy is outside the scope of this chapter. Briefly, the eye resides in the orbital cavity and rests within orbital fat. The eyelids close reflexively when objects approach rapidly, and both the upper and lower lid are complex structures endowed with fibrous tarsal plates for further eye protection. The wall of the eye is composed of the cornea anteriorly, the choroid, retina, and sclera posteriorly. The cornea is optically clear, while the sclera is white and makes up the remainder of the external wall of the eye. The limbus is the region of the eye where the sclera and cornea meet, and the sclera is covered anteriorly by conjunctiva. The eye is divided anatomically into the anterior and posterior segments. The anterior segment of the eye includes the cornea, anterior chamber (space between cornea and iris), the iris, and the lens of the eye. The anterior chamber is filled with aqueous fluid. Zonular fibrils hold the lens (just behind the iris) in place by securing it to the ciliary body. The ciliary body produces the aqueous fluid and lies peripherally at the junction between the anterior and posterior segments. The posterior segment includes the vitreous cavity filled with clear vitreous gel and then the retina and choroid that rest internally on the posterior two-thirds of the sclera. The macula is the center portion of the retina and provides fine visual acuity (the fovea is the center of the macula and gives the most discriminating 20/20 vision). The optic nerve (cranial nerve II) consists of 1 million retinal ganglion fibers. It exits the globe at the optic disk and traverses the posterior orbit until it enters the optic foramen. It then travels through the optic canal before forming the optic chiasm where branches depart for the midbrain as well as the optic

tracts and radiations toward the occipital cortex. Cranial nerve III innervates the medial, superior, and inferior recti muscles, the inferior oblique extraocular muscle, and the lid levator muscle; it also constricts the pupil. Cranial nerve IV innervates the superior oblique muscle, and cranial nerve V provides sensation to the eye through the ciliary nerves. Cranial nerve VI innervates the lateral rectus muscle, while cranial nerve VII closes the eye by constricting the orbicularis muscle. The six extraocular muscles originate on the bony orbit and insert on the globe and provide ocular motility. The orbital space is formed on each side from the frontal, ethmoid, lacrimal, maxillary, palatine, sphenoid, and zygomatic bones and is closely related to the paranasal sinuses (usual sources for orbital cellulitis).

## CLASSIFICATION OF OCULAR TRAUMA

It is important for all physicians to be able to communicate clearly with each other when describing ocular injuries. It is also important to have consistent terminology for accurate reporting and interpretation of data regarding injuries to the eye. In response to this need, the Birmingham Eye Trauma Terminology system was established (Table 21-1). Figure 21-1 shows how injuries to the globe should be classified and described. The descriptions of soft tissue injuries and orbital fractures are generally more straightforward and can accompany the description of injury to the globe or stand-alone.[17,18]

**TABLE 21-1**

### Ocular Trauma Terminology

**Eyewall**

Sclera and cornea

**Closed-Globe Injury**

The sclera and/or cornea have not been violated full-thickness.

A contusion of the globe (associated with hyphema, and varying degrees of internal tissue tears, disorganization/dislocation); also corneal abrasion (only corneal epithelial injury), or partial thickness (cornea/sclera) injury.

**Open-Globe Injury**

Full-thickness wound to the eyewall (cornea and/or sclera).

The internal ocular structures (iris, lens, ciliary body, vitreous, choroid, retina) may be uninvolved, damaged, or prolapsed out of the eye.

**Rupture**

An open eyewall from the impact of a blunt object with enough force to cause the intraocular pressure to exceed the tensile strength of the eyewall at its weakest points (often the sclera at the rectus muscle insertions and the corneoscleral limbus). Tissue herniation is frequent.

**Laceration**

An open eyewall usually caused by a sharp object. The wound is at the impact site.

**Penetrating Injury**

Usually a sharp object with a single eyewall wound site. There is no exit wound.

Intraocular foreign body (IOFB)

A retained intraocular object from a penetrating injury.

**Perforating Injury**

Two eyewall lacerations (an entry and exit wound), usually caused by the same sharp or high-velocity object.

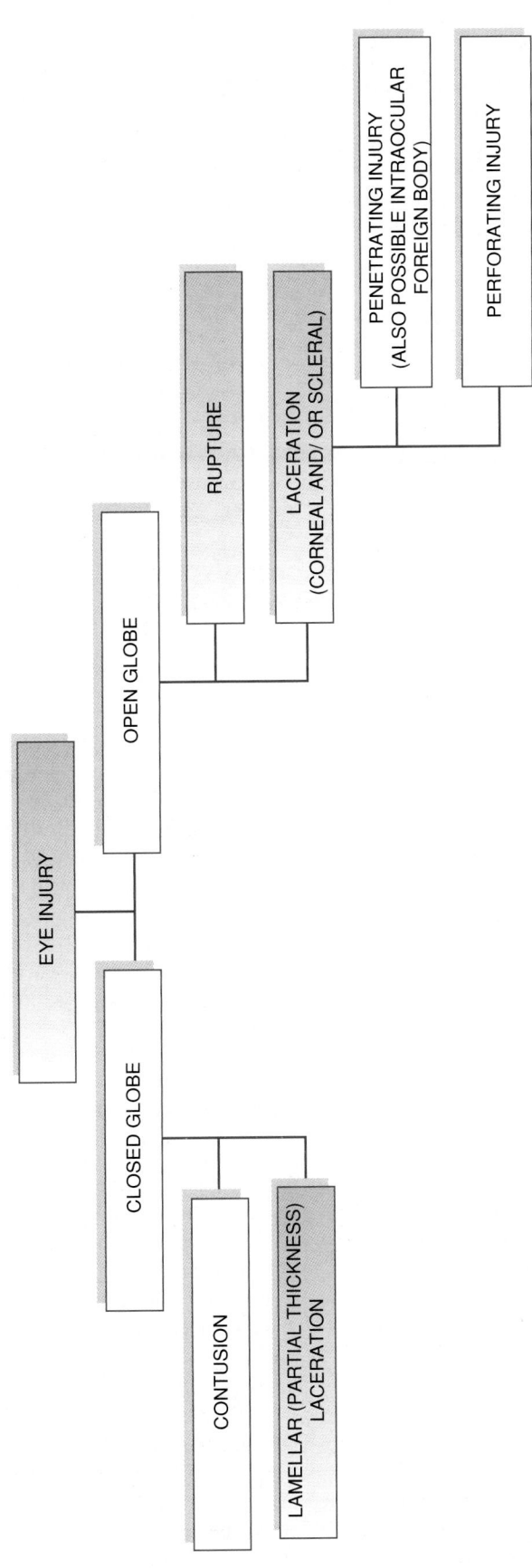

**FIGURE 21-1.** Schematic diagram illustrating terminology of ocular trauma.

## INITIAL EVALUATION

Many patients presenting to the trauma center with severe ocular injuries will have other associated trauma such as to the head and neck. Often, facial and skull fractures, tissue disruption, and hemorrhage associated with these injuries may delay recognition or evaluation of ocular damage. In potentially severe or life-threatening trauma, ophthalmic evaluation and intervention are appropriately delayed. Early integration of the ophthalmologist into the treatment plan for the injured patient is desirable. Not only may further damage to the globe be avoided and emergency treatment instituted, but additional surgical procedures and anesthetic exposures can be minimized.

The initial evaluation of injuries to the eye must be cautious, thorough, and expedient. Recognition of potentially sight-threatening disorders is of the highest priority, and prevention of secondary injury is equally important. The examining physician should always remain cognizant of the possibility for occult rupture of the globe, an intraocular foreign body, or injury to the optic nerve as these conditions can be overlooked in some settings. In particular, there is significant medicolegal risk associated with missed intraocular foreign bodies. Identifying other types of injuries to the eye and orbit is important in making appropriate referrals and decisions on management.[19]

## HISTORY

When a history can be obtained, there are several key pieces of information that need to be ascertained. A detailed description of the exact mechanism of injury is necessary. For example, a patient with any type of ocular complaint after hammering metal on metal (sharp, high velocity) defines a situation where an intraocular foreign body should be highly suspected. Even if the eye is quiet and the patient has good vision, facial x-rays and dilated fundoscopy are warranted. Likewise, blunt trauma, with significant impact velocity (e.g., fists, hockey pucks), points toward possible occult rupture of the globe and/or orbital fracture. Additionally, information about the offending object needs to be elicited, as shattered glass, a BB, or an airbag injury all point to different types of severe injuries. Knowing the origins of contaminating materials such as a tree branch or a dirty nail increases the probability of identifying serious infectious complications.

Injured patients may be unconscious, combative, or under the influence of alcohol or other substances. Force should not be used to open the lids in combative patients, because this may facilitate extrusion of ocular contents when an open globe is the injury. Occasionally, there will be witnesses, friends, or family members who can give helpful information with regard to the mechanism of injury, immediate postinjury complaints, and past medical history. Other times, an examination is all that is possible, and even that is often difficult. There is one occasion where treatment needs to begin immediately and that is chemical injury to the eye. Ocular irrigation should take precedence, and a history and examination should be temporarily deferred. Information about the chemical itself should be obtained concurrently with ocular lavage.

Another related question is whether the patient wears glasses or contacts, and, if so, were contacts on the eyes at the time of injury? Whether protective eyewear was worn should also be documented as it may be important later for medicolegal reasons.

Following the description of the injury, it is important to inquire about the quality of a patient's vision immediately after the event. Sometimes swelling of the lid, progressive corneal edema, and intraocular hemorrhage (hyphema, vitreous hemorrhage) can limit testing for visual acuity. The status of immediate postinjury vision can help direct work-up and referrals and offer prognostic information. Other visual symptoms also need to be addressed. Photopsia and the sudden onset of floaters points to vitreoretinal pathology, whereas double vision points to motility abnormalities, orbital injury, or even neurological involvement. Laterality, pain, and discharge are also relevant.

A patient's past ocular history and family ocular history should be reviewed. A history of corneal scarring, glaucoma, amblyopia, diabetic retinopathy, or optic neuropathy have implications for the physical examination and management. Information about previous ocular surgery is extremely pertinent. A prior radial keratotomy or recent LASIK (laser in situ keratomileusis) can increase the risk for corneal complications of trauma. Importantly, a history of corneal transplantation, glaucoma surgery, or cataract surgery warns the examiner to carefully evaluate incision sites as they tend to be more likely to rupture in trauma to the globe.

A brief review of a patient's past medical history is also necessary. Diabetes mellitus, hypertension, and thyroid disease can have significant ocular complications that may be manifest on examination and be unrelated to trauma. Hemoglobinopathies, especially sickle cell disease, can complicate injuries to the eye (hyphema implications). The possibility of pregnancy needs to be considered since it can affect decision-making, especially in the first trimester. Current medications and drug allergies should also be recorded. Anticoagulant therapy (including aspirin and other NSAIDs) can complicate surgery. Allergies to medications can affect treatment decisions. When necessary, tetanus status should also be established. The entire history can often be accomplished in just a few minutes and plays an invaluable role in subsequent management of the patient.[20–22]

## PHYSICAL EXAMINATION

Trauma patients can present some of the most challenging circumstances for ocular examination. With understanding and practice, examiners who are not ophthalmologists can develop the skill and facility to carry out a meaningful ocular examination. Often, lid swelling and pain severely hamper attempts to view the eye itself. A topical anesthetic such as proparacaine is often necessary but, on occasion, systemic analgesics or even a facial nerve block can facilitate opening of the lid. After gentle application of topical anesthesia, a Demarres retractor, a lid speculum, or two large paper clips bent under at the ends in a U-shape with a hemostat can also assist with retraction of the lid and thus enable an initial ocular assessment. Fig. 21-2 demonstrates schematically an algorithmic approach for examiners who are not ophthalmologists when assessing orbital injuries. If a rupture of the globe is confirmed or highly likely, the examination should cease, a Fox shield (no patch) should

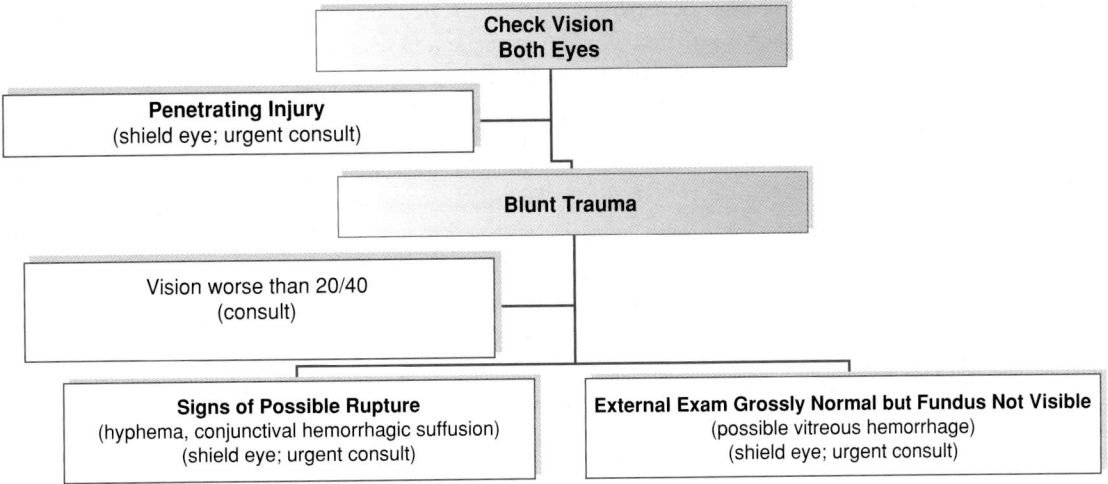

**FIGURE 21-2.** Schematic diagram illustrating steps in determining level of urgency for ophthalmic consultation by nonophthalmic examiners.

be placed over the eye, and an ophthalmologist consulted emergently. In patients with severe injuries or those with an altered mental status, it is often possible to perform only parts of the eye examination initially. When assessing the status of the eye and visual system, ocular vital signs are used as a template for evaluation and examination. These vital signs include the visual acuity, the pupils, the intraocular pressure, the ocular position/motility, and the visual fields by confrontation.[23] The measurement of visual acuity and testing for a relative afferent papillary defect at the initial examination should be performed in all injured eyes because of their relative prognostic significance.[24]

## VISUAL ACUITY

The most important (and often overlooked) part of the ocular examination is the testing of visual acuity which should precede a more sophisticated evaluation of the eye. After stabilization of the patient, visual acuity should be recorded accurately as it has significant prognostic importance. Subsequent administration of analgesics, sedatives, or anesthesia may render vision testing very difficult, if not impossible. Each eye must be evaluated independently. An ocular occluder or patch can be used to cover one eye at a time. Vision should be tested at a distance with correction (glasses), if available. With reduced vision tested, or glasses not available, rechecking the vision through a pinhole (which minimizes the impact of refractive error on visual acuity) placed in front of an eye is appropriate. Usually, it is not possible to test distance vision in the emergency setting. A near card can give a reasonable assessment of vision. The card or even a magazine, newspaper, package label, or identification badge (indicate in the medical record what is used and at what distance) should be held at 14 inches from the patient. If a patient is unable to see letters, numbers, or words during acuity testing, vision should be measured as counting fingers (at the farthest distance a patient responds correctly), hand motions, light perception (i.e., with or without projection, reporting accurately the direction from where the light is shined), or no light perception. When evaluating an eye for light perception, it is important to completely block all light from

entering the other eye (e.g., tape with eye patch). It should be noted that patients with reduced mental status or dense intraocular hemorrhage may not perceive light. Sometimes serial measurements of visual acuity need to be performed during the course of an acute injury, as in patients with an evolving retrobulbar hematoma or injury to the optic nerve.

## Pupils

Like the visual acuity, examination of the pupil is extremely important for the assessment of an ocular injury. Pupils can assist in demonstrating injury to the anterior visual pathways (predominantly the optic nerve, but retina and optic chiasm may be involved). If possible, it is best to test pupillary reactions in trauma patients prior to the administration of systemic medications that may affect pupillary function (e.g., narcotics, anticholinergic/cholinergic drugs). Examination of the pupil consists of measuring the size and shape of the pupil in ambient light, shining a bright light in the eye and watching the pupil constrict, and then taking away the light and observing the pupil size return to that seen in ambient light. Again, each eye is tested individually. An examiner must become proficient with the swinging flashlight test. This test is the best method for diagnosing a relative afferent pupillary deficit (RAPD or Marcus-Gunn pupil). Both pupils should constrict equally to light and maintain that constriction as a light source is moved smoothly but quickly from one eye to the other. Dilation of one pupil when the light is shining in it points toward an RAPD in that eye. An RAPD can be diagnosed in the setting of trauma to the iris by observing the uninjured pupil during the swinging flashlight test. This maneuver is called testing for a reverse RAPD and also relies on the consensual pupillary response to light. During the test, if the uninjured eye paradoxically dilates when the flashlight is shined into the injured eye, an RAPD can be diagnosed in the injured eye. RAPDs are typically graded on a scale of 1 to 4, with 1 being mild and 4 severe. Injuries to the optic nerve such as avulsions, transections, traumatic contusions, and large retinal detachments usually demonstrate a marked RAPD.

Pathologic processes, such as tears to the sphincter of the iris and root and palsies of cranial nerve III, can cause anisocoria or irregularities of the pupil, so pupil size and shape must be carefully documented. "Peaking" of the pupil is commonly associated with anterior penetrating injuries or scleral ruptures complicated by uveal (iris) incarceration.

## Orbit and Eyelids

The eyelids are often swollen and frequently covered with dried blood after injures to the eye and face. The periorbital skin should be cleaned gently but thoroughly with gauze 4 × 4's and normal saline to allow for proper assessment of the lid, face, and orbit. Cleaning frequently uncovers facial and lid lacerations that were not originally apparent. Lid lacerations may be full-thickness or partial-thickness. Lacerations that involve the lid margin and/or nasal ends of the eyelids (where the puncta of the lacrimal canaliculi originate) require triaging to the ophthalmologist. This will allow for proper evaluation of the lacrimal drainage system and the issue of protecting the posterior lid margins from sutures that might damage the ocular surface. The external examination needs to identify periorbital foreign bodies, ecchymoses, and/or crepitus (subcutaneous or orbital air). The presence of enophthalmos (sunken), exophthalmos (proptosis), or other forms of orbital dystopia should also be noted. Frequently, the patient will complain of vertical diplopia and have restriction of upgaze. Additionally, if a fracture of the orbital floor is suspected, infraorbital sensation should be tested gently with a cotton applicator and compared from one side to the other. Infraorbital hypesthesia is frequently associated with fractures of the orbital floor (blowout fracture), where the maxillary division of the fifth cranial nerve runs. Ptosis should also be documented. Another important aspect of eyelid inspection is eversion of the lids. Superficial foreign bodies have a tendency to embed themselves on the inner surface of the upper lids (superior tarsal sulcus). As the eyelid blinks, these foreign bodies will rub against the cornea, causing track like abrasions. Eyelid eversion is accomplished with an applicator stick resting horizontally against the upper portion of the upper lid. While having the patient look down, the examiner pulls on the lashes outward and upward to expose the palpebral conjunctiva for inspection.

## Extraocular Motility

Determination of the function of extraocular muscles is essential in all patients who complain of binocular diplopia or have a suspected fracture of the orbital wall. Cranial nerve palsies, direct muscle trauma or incarceration, hemorrhage, edema, and orbital foreign bodies/infection may all cause disturbances of the extraocular muscles. It should be noted that if a ruptured globe is suspected, the motility exam should be performed cautiously as vigorous contraction of the extraocular muscles may facilitate extrusion of intraocular contents. Extraocular motility is assessed by asking a patient to look in the cardinal positions of gaze as follows: up, down, right, left, up and right, down and right, up and left, and down and left. Deficits in motility and diplopia should be noted. Forced duction testing can differentiate between restriction of an extraocular muscle or paresis. The eye should be anesthetized by soaking a cotton swab with topical proparacaine and holding it at a convenient place just posterior to the limbus. A 0.3-mm forceps can then grasp the eye at that location and pull the eye in the direction of the movement

deficit. Care should be taken so as not to inadvertently abrade the epithelium of the cornea. If the eye moves easily in the direction of the deficit, the test is negative and there is no restrictive component, so a paretic muscle is likely. If the eye does not move in that direction at all, the test is positive and muscle entrapment may be possible. Swelling of orbital tissue can often cause dysfunction of ocular movements with findings similar to that of muscle restriction. A short interval of observation can help discern the difference. Orbital computed tomography (CT) is a valuable adjunct in these settings.

## Confrontational Visual Fields

A patient's visual field can be assessed rapidly at the bedside, and this evaluation can play a role in evaluating retinal detachments (often a horizontal defect) and intracranial pathology (obeying the vertical midline). One eye is tested while the other eye is completely covered. The examiner (who can be a control) moves one or two of his own fingers from the far periphery toward the center of a patient's visual axis, from up, down, right, and left in sequence. The patient should report the correct number of fingers when they become visible.

## Measurement of Intraocular Pressure

The Tonopen (Medtronic Ophthalmics, Jacksonville, FL) is a versatile and valuable instrument in the setting of trauma to the eye. It is handheld, easy to use, and provides fairly accurate measurements of intraocular pressure. A low intraocular pressure often supports a diagnosis of a ruptured globe, and high pressures can be seen in hyphemas, retrobulbar hemorrhages, and edema of the orbital lid. Pressures above normal (20 to 22 mm Hg) should be followed, and, generally, those above 30 mm Hg should initiate urgent ophthalmic consultation. Because evaluation of intraocular pressure is difficult in the setting of trauma, it may be hazardous for non-ophthalmologists to assess this vital sign if the globe might be open (facilitating extrusion of ocular contents).

## Evaluation of the Globe

It is critical to assess whether the globe is ruptured. Clues to rupture include brown uveal tissue (iris or ciliary body) visible on the surface or protruding through a laceration with a teardrop or eccentrically "peaked" pupil. The anterior chamber may be deeper (posterior rupture) or shallower (anterior rupture) along with a hyphema. A suffused subconjunctival hemorrhage (bulging hematoma) may be indicative of a scleral rupture (and/or orbital fractures). If rupture or laceration is then suspected, no further ocular exam is necessary, and the eye should be covered with a protective shield (Fox) as previously noted to prevent potential extrusion of intraocular contents by external pressure.

## Slit-Lamp Examination

A slit-lamp is the preferred method for examining the eye. If the patient is mobile or can sit safely, a slit lamp should be employed. If that is not possible, a careful inspection of the globe with the naked eye and penlight or a direct ophthalmoscope will suffice.

The sclera and conjunctiva should be examined for the presence of partial- or full-thickness lacerations and epithelial defects. Subconjunctival hemorrhage, a dramatic yet common finding, is significant in the setting of trauma only if the history suggests possible rupture or laceration (e.g., high velocity) and other predictors of rupture are present. Examination of the normal cornea should reveal it to be crystal clear and smooth in contour. Any irregularity of the corneal light reflex suggests the presence of a corneal abrasion or deeper injury. Fluorescein staining should be used to confirm such an injury. Fluorescein stains areas of the cornea and conjunctiva that have been denuded of epithelium. The tip of a fluorescein strip should be wetted and touched to the conjunctiva in the inferior cul-de-sac. By blinking, the patient disperses the fluorescein in the precorneal tear film, coating the entire cornea. Using a penlight with a cobalt blue filter, the area of green fluorescence corresponding to any abrasion can easily be seen and may also be seen with a white light, alone. In addition, due to the pH difference between the aqueous humor and the tear film, one may see a dark stream of aqueous in the green fluorescein if there is a leaking corneal laceration.

The depth and contents of the anterior chamber should then be examined. Both excessively shallow or deep anterior chambers when compared to the other eye may suggest possible rupture of the globe. A hyphema is often subtle in appearance, but indicative of severe injury to the anterior segment of the eye. Inspection of the lens should reveal it to be clear and centered immediately behind the pupil. Traumatic subluxation of the lens is often manifest as a dark "crescent moon" in the center of the pupil and complicates fundoscopy significantly.

The value of the direct ophthalmoscope should not be discounted in emergent settings. This powerful and easily transportable instrument can provide magnified views of the conjunctiva, sclera, cornea, and lens. There is often a blue filter to assist with fluorescein evaluations. Additionally, confirming the presence of a red reflex is reassuring.

## Examination of the Fundus

An injured eye needs to have a dilated fundus examination. If there are neurosurgical concerns, communication with the neurosurgical service should be obtained prior to dilating a patient's eyes. Neurosurgeons frequently monitor pupillary function in the setting of trauma to the brain and elevated intracranial pressure. Regardless, pharmacologic dilation of the pupils should be recorded in the medical record, and the patient's nurse should be informed verbally. Phenylephrine 2.5% and tropicamide 1%, one drop each in both eyes, is generally sufficient to produce adequate mydriasis (for 4–6 hours). Indirect ophthalmoscopy is the "gold standard" for a retinal evaluation, but this technique is generally performed only by ophthalmologists as it requires significant training to master. A direct ophthalmoscope, however, can be a very effective tool for examining the ocular fundus through a dilated pupil. The presence or absence of a red reflex should be noted. A decreased or absent red reflex suggests a media opacity (hyphema or vitreous hemorrhage), cataract, or large retinal detachment. Attention should be placed on the optic disk, vessels, and macula (peripheral retinal exam is performed by indirect ophthalmoscopy). Intravitreal, retinal, and subretinal hemorrhages can be identified. Disk edema and retinal injuries can also be noted with this technique. An attempt to ascertain further fundoscopic detail should be made, as the initial examining physician may have the only view of the fundus prior to a delayed hemorrhage or development of a traumatic cataract. Barring a severe traumatic optic neuropathy, however, a normal fundus examination can be very reassuring to patient and family.

## ANCILLARY STUDIES

### Radiologic Assessment

CT of the orbits with 1.0–1.5 mm axial cuts is the radiologic study of choice in the acute setting of trauma to the globe and orbit. Although it may no longer be necessary to primarily request axials and direct coronal studies at institutions with state-of-the-art scanners (because digitally reconstructed coronal images are of high quality), it still may be best to order "axials and coronals of the orbits" generically. Direct coronal images can be difficult to obtain acutely in the patient with injuries to the head and neck, so reconstructed images will be necessary. CT images can give valuable information about the integrity of the globe, presence of intraocular hemorrhage, and intraocular foreign bodies. The orbital CT is also ideal for assessing orbital fractures, retrobulbar hemorrhage, orbital foreign bodies, and optic nerve injuries. In the event CT is not available, plain film radiographs (e.g., Water's views) can be helpful and cost-effective to help rule out foreign bodies and provide preliminary information on orbital fractures. An orbital CT should be requested in the setting of a ruptured globe, disturbance of the ocular motility, possible ocular or orbital foreign body, or when the history and examination suggest the presence of orbital fractures, open globe, or an orbital hematoma. The study should always be reviewed with a radiologist. Contrast CT and MRI are generally not indicated in the setting of acute orbital trauma.[24]

MRI is contraindicated if there is the possibility of a metallic foreign body, due to high flux magnetic fields causing movement of the foreign body inside the eye.

### Ultrasonography

B-scan ultrasonography is an important adjunct when hemorrhage or a cataract prevents visualization of the ocular fundus. The study is generally performed by ophthalmologists and ophthalmic technicians capable of performing the procedure. It takes some level of expertise to be able to differentiate between intraocular hemorrhage, fibrin membranes, and a retinal detachment. Ocular ultrasound can also be useful in the assessment of intraocular and orbital foreign bodies.

## COUNSELING THE PATIENT WITH AN INJURY TO THE EYE

Blindness is one of the most feared disabilities, and sudden eye injuries can create significant emotional distress. Goals of counseling are to comfort, to inform, and to obtain consent for treatments. As a general rule, it is best to explain to the patient who has suffered a severe injury to the eye that it is difficult to predict outcomes at this time. It is also important to make the patient and family aware that multiple operations may be required and that it may take months before a final outcome is known. Similar guidelines apply to patients who have suffered disfiguring orbital or facial trauma. This type of preliminary communication can help to prevent anger toward and disappointment with the physician later. Likewise, examination of the noninjured eye and reassurance to the family if it is normal can also help ease these difficult encounters.[25] It is very important for the patient and family to understand that certain ocular injuries may occasionally benefit from a delay in repair and may require the use of corticosteroids to reduce the incidence of intraocular hemorrhage and improve outcomes.[26]

## TRANSPORTING THE PATIENT WITH AN INJURY TO THE EYE

Frequently, patients with severe injuries must be transferred to another medical facility for definitive management. Trauma patients should have an ophthalmic examination prior to transfer. In the setting of a suspected open globe, a shield needs to be placed over that eye. If a metal shield is unavailable, the bottom half of a Dixie or styrofoam cup should be taped over the injured eye. Pain medicines and antiemetics should be administered as needed. Patients with orbital or intraocular foreign bodies should be stabilized until they can be removed in a controlled surgical setting. Patients with injured eyes who need to be transported by air should receive supplemental oxygen to decrease retinal vasodilation and rises in intraocular pressure associated with hypoxia. Gauze soaked in sterile normal saline should be placed next to injured tissues to prevent dessication of the surface especially with an exposed globe. Ointments should not be used if the globe might be open, and the patient's head should be elevated.[27]

## SPECIFIC INJURIES AND THEIR MANAGEMENT

It is important to understand that many of the injuries described in the following sections can coexist in the same patient.

## CHEMICAL INJURY

A chemical injury to the eye is an ophthalmic emergency.

Chemical burns represent 7.7 to 18% of ocular trauma.[28,29] Both acids and alkalis are capable of causing significant damage to the eye, but alkalis tend to cause the more severe injury. The severity of a chemical burn is primarily dependent on the pH of the chemical itself.[28] Alkalis penetrate ocular tissues rapidly through saponification of cell membranes, resulting in liquefactive necrosis of all ocular structures contacted. The degradative process is augmented and prolonged by hydroxylation of collagen fibers and the neutrophilic release of various proteases and collagenases. These may result in corneal opacification or melting,

cataract formation, severe glaucoma, generalized ocular ischemia, and necrosis of ocular contents.[30]

With only a few exceptions (e.g., hydrofluoric acid), acids and other nonalkalis (e.g., organics) do not cause nearly the degree of ocular damage as do alkali exposures. Acids cause a coagulative necrosis with protein precipitation within the tissues, thus limiting the depth of chemical penetration into the eye. As a result of the poor penetration of acids, fewer deep corneal and intraocular complications develop. Potential severe complications of acid and nonalkali exposures include superficial conjunctival and corneal scarring and vascularization, glaucoma, and uveitis.

Immediate irrigation should begin in the field with tap water, saline, lactated Ringer's, or any commercially available irrigant with a neutral pH, and then continue in the emergency department (ED) for a minimum of 30 minutes for significant exposures. Topical anesthesia can facilitate the process. The nature of the offending material should be identified as the pH of the solution, duration of contact, and volume of exposure are major determinants of the severity of chemical injuries to the eye. During irrigation, the lids should be held open and the stream of irrigating fluid directed into the superior and inferior conjunctival fornices in an attempt to wash away any particulate matter. If the cornea is intact, irrigation with either a Morgan or Mediflow lens or the Morgan Mortlex lens (Mortram, Inc., Missoula, MT) is desirable. An irrigating lens should not be used if a deep corneal injury or foreign body is suspected. The fornices should be swept with moistened swabs in order to loosen and dislodge any retained particulate matter. An ophthalmologist should be called immediately unless the injury is clearly the result of an organic, innocuous compound (e.g., alcohol) and the damage sustained is no more than a mild corneal abrasion. Irrigation should continue until the pH of the tear lake remains neutral (7.4) at least five minutes after cessation of active infusion of irrigant.

Following sufficient irrigation, the acute treatment of severe chemical burns is directed at reducing ocular inflammation and ischemia and toward detection and treatment of complications. This involves the judicious use of topical steroids, topical antibiotics, cycloplegics, and anticollagenolytic agents such as doxycycline,[31] n-acetylcysteine, and topical or oral ascorbate.[32,33] Surgical treatments in the acute phase may include amniotic membrane transplantation to reduce inflammation of the ocular surface, promote epithelial healing, and reduce formation of a symblepharon.[34–36] Emergent corneal transplantation may be required if the patient develops a corneal perforation.

Chemical burns to the cornea are classified as grade 1–4.[37] Conjunctival hyperemia and corneal clarity (grades 1 and 2) are good prognostic indicators, while corneal clouding and limbal ischemia (grades 3 and 4) portend worse prognoses. Outcomes for significant alkali injuries are poor (Fig. 21-3). In general, the patient with a severe chemical injury will require prolonged and expert follow-up care. Long-term management may involve multiple operations on the anterior segment. These may include reconstruction of the conjunctival fornicies, transplantation of limbal stem cells,[38] cataract surgery, and corneal transplantation to replace a permanently scarred and opaque cornea. It is important to remember, however, that the outcome in such patients is often determined by the expediency with which the initial treatment is given. Any

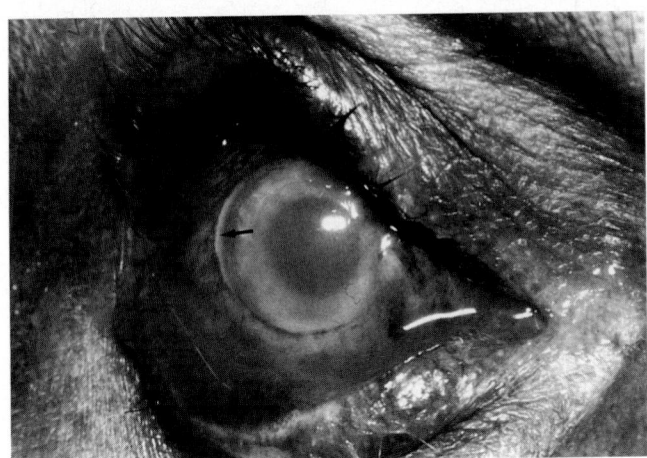

**FIGURE 21-3.** A severe alkalai burn. Note the diffusely hazy cornea and limbal whitening (arrow). Indicative of ocular ischemia. *(Reproduced with permission from David Palay, MD.)*

injury greater than a mild chemical exposure should involve emergent ophthalmologic consultation.

## CORNEAL ABRASION

Corneal epithelial abrasions frequently occur as isolated events but can accompany more severe injuries to the eye. Among the many causes of abrasions, the presence of a contact lens increases the risk of infectious complications.

The cornea is a transparent tissue, which is approximately 0.5 mm in thickness. It is covered with a thin layer of epithelium overlying a basement membrane. The epithelium protects the corneal stroma against infection and, along with the precorneal tear film, acts as the principal refracting surface of the eye. Beneath the corneal epithelium lies a dense plexus of corneal sensory nerves. Therefore, if the epithelium is removed, these sensory nerve endings become exposed, resulting in severe pain.

Based on an appropriate history and diagnostic findings (corneal fluorescein uptake), a corneal abrasion can be treated in the ED. The traditional treatment of non-contact lens related, traumatic corneal abrasions has involved the instillation of a cycloplegic agent (e.g., homatropine 5%) and antibiotic ointment followed by the placement of a pressure patch to securely close the eye.[39] Several studies have now shown that the use of a pressure patch does not increase the healing rate nor decrease the pain associated with a corneal abrasion in both adults[40–42] and children.[43] One study that prospectively compared patching versus no patching of non-contact lens related, traumatic corneal abrasions showed significantly faster healing of abrasions when cycloplegic and antibiotic ointments are used alone without patching of the eye.[44] Therefore, routine patching is not indicated. The addition of a topical nonsteroidal agent (e.g., ketorolac or diclofenac) to the regimen may increase patient comfort[45] and decrease the need for oral analgesia.[46] For larger abrasions, the placement of a therapeutic bandage contact lens by an eye care professional may also improve the patient's comfort allowing a quicker return to normal daily activities.[47,48] Follow-up should include daily re-examination of the eye (depending on abrasion size

and circumstances of injury) to monitor the healing of the defect and to evaluate for signs of infection. In general, a clean, noninfected corneal abrasion will heal completely in two to three days, and long-term visual loss is uncommon.

Non-contact lens related traumatic corneal abrasions may be treated adequately with instillation of a topical cycloplegic agent (e.g., 5% homatropine) and topical antibiotic ointment (erythromycin or bacitracin/polymixin B ophthalmic ointment) three times per day until the lesion is healed. Larger abrasions may require firm patching and are followed daily until they resolve. The corneal epithelium regenerates rapidly, and patients usually do well. A corneal infiltrate (stromal opacity) associated with an abrasion may be a sign of infection and needs to be referred urgently to an ophthalmologist.

## CORNEAL FOREIGN BODY

Small corneal foreign bodies are frequently encountered in the ED (Fig. 21-4). In the majority of patients, corneal foreign bodies are very superficially embedded and easily visible on slit-lamp examination. Following careful examination to rule out a penetrating injury (in conjunction with fluorescein to aid in diagnosis), the examiner may attempt removal of the foreign body. After the instillation of a topical anesthetic, a moistened, sterile cotton swab may be rolled across the cornea or gentle irrigation with balanced salt solution is performed in an attempt to loosen and remove a superficial foreign body. If this is unsuccessful, ophthalmic consultation should be obtained as more deeply embedded foreign bodies may require removal at the slit lamp with a foreign body spud or 25-gauge needle. In addition, the upper lid should be everted to ensure that no additional particles are present. Following removal of the foreign body, the eye should be treated for the residual corneal abrasion (as noted previously). Linear "ice track" abrasions (seen on fluorescein staining) on the upper cornea should alert the physician to evert the upper lid to ensure that there are no other foreign bodies present. After removal of a foreign body, topical antibiotic and cycloplegic medicines are utilized in the same manner as with other corneal abrasions.

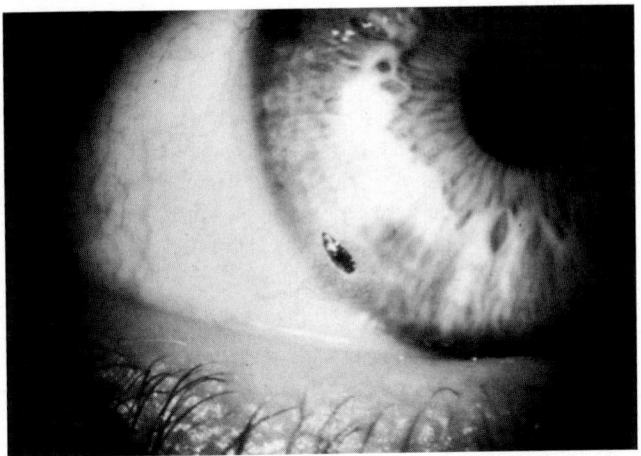

**FIGURE 21-4.** A superficially embedded corneal foreign body. *(Reproduced with permission from David Palay, MD.)*

## SUBCONJUNCTIVAL HEMORRHAGE AND CONJUNCTIVAL LACERATION

Although they are dramatic in appearance and often prompt patients to seek urgent medical attention, subconjunctival hemorrhages are most often benign. Exceptions include a history of blunt or high-velocity trauma that may present with significant subconjunctival hematomas (hemorrhagic suffusion) and chemosis. Typically, they are associated with Valsalva maneuvers or minor trauma (eye rubbing), but may arise spontaneously in the setting of severe hypertension and bleeding diatheses. Clinically, subconjunctival hemorrhages appear as a flat, bright red area noted on the bulbar conjunctiva. Visual acuity is not affected, and the hemorrhage will resolve spontaneously in about two weeks or less.

Isolated conjunctival lacerations generally do not need to be repaired unless they are large or over the insertion of a rectus muscle. It may be difficult to determine if the laceration involves the sclera, and, thus, ophthalmic consultation may be required. Scleral penetration is associated with vitreous hemorrhage, which may be noted clinically on exam, as well as decreased visual acuity.

## BLUNT OCULAR TRAUMA

Severe concussive injury to the globe and orbit can produce damage to almost every ocular tissue.[49] A concussive force striking the eye, such as a fist or steering wheel, pushes the globe further back into the orbit. If the eye is deeply set in the orbit, the orbital rim may absorb much of the impact. Generally, however, the globe is compressed, with a shortening of the anteroposterior dimension and a compensatory increase in the circumference at the equator.[50] This in turn can produce damage to the soft lining tissues of the globe (choroid, iris, ciliary body, retinal pigment epithelium, and retina), which are subjected to stretching vectors, in addition to causing fractures of the thin medial orbital wall and floor (blowout fractures). In a review of 727 patients with generalized blunt trauma, Holt and associates noted ocular injury in 67% of cases, 18% of which were deemed serious injury.[51] Of eyes that have sustained contusion injury, fewer than 50% will regain reading vision (better than or equal to 20/40).

Scleral rupture following severe blunt trauma may be difficult to clinically detect because intraocular or subconjunctival hemorrhage may obscure visualization of a wound. Some predictors of scleral rupture include an abnormally deep or shallow anterior chamber, lowered intraocular pressure, severe ocular hemorrhage (intraocular or periocular), and media opacity preventing a view of the fundus.[52] When a ruptured globe is suspected, further ocular manipulation should be avoided as previously noted. Immediate treatment includes a Fox shield or other rigid device (such as a styrofoam cup) placed over the eye, analgesics (no aspirin products), and antiemetics administered as needed until ophthalmologic consultation is obtained. Eye pads are contraindicated and may cause further damage.

## OPEN GLOBE

An open globe requires emergency ophthalmologic consultation. Open globe injuries include rupture, penetrating injuries (entry wound only), lacerations, intraocular foreign bodies, and perforating injuries (entry and exit wounds). Details regarding the differentiation between these entities are described earlier in the section *Classification of Ocular Trauma*. The diagnosis of an open eye is sometimes obvious. The eye is misshapen, and uveal (pigmented structures including the iris, ciliary body, and choroid) tissue is prolapsing out of an anterior scleral or corneal wound (Fig. 21-5). Sometimes an obvious foreign body is still in the eye when the patient arrives at the ED or a laceration can be easily noted at the slit lamp. Frequently, however, the injury is occult, and diagnostic acumen is required to identify these injuries. Ruptures can be associated with a low, normal, or even high intraocular pressure. Very sharp small foreign bodies can enter the eye through small wounds that are difficult to visualize, even for expert examiners. Thus, the history plays an invaluable role in the work-up of these severe injuries. Signs of occult rupture on examination include decreased vision, chemosis (clear fluid elevation of the conjunctiva), areas of dense subconjunctival hemorrhage, a shallow or a deepened anterior chamber, and dense vitreous hemorrhage. These and other irregularities of the globe *may* be noted on CT studies, as well. If an open globe is suspected, further evaluation should be suspended, and a metal shield placed over the eye as noted above. The administration of prophylactic broad spectrum intravenous antibiotics (e.g., ceftazidime and vancomycin)[53] should occur in timing with surgical intervention. The initial physician should, however, treat pain and nausea, give tetanus toxoid if indicated, order the patient to be NPO ("nil per os", English equivalent, "nothing by mouth"), and obtain an orbital CT scan. Surgical exploration and wound repair should be performed within 6 to 24 hours. Goals of primary repair are to reform the integrity of the globe while maintaining the normal anatomic architecture of the eye as much as possible. Intraocular foreign bodies are common in open eye injuries and should be removed at the time of primary repair.[54–56] Depending on visibility and other circumstances, procedures such as extraction of the lens, vitrectomy, or scleral buckling can be undertaken primarily or delayed secondarily to help reduce the risk of further complications. These secondary surgical procedures are often necessary for corneal scarring, cataract, vitreous hemorrhage, retinal detachment, and/or glaucoma.

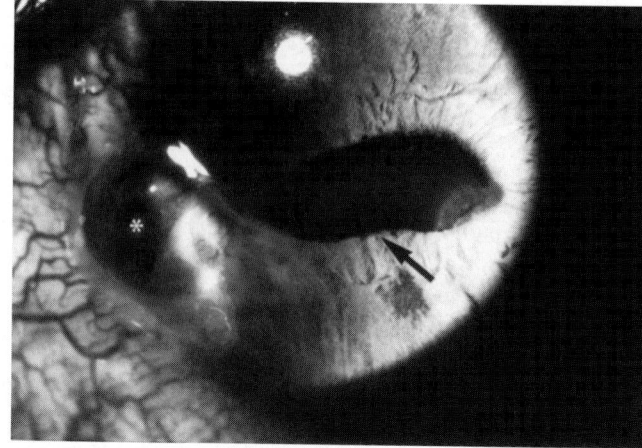

**FIGURE 21-5.**  A ruptured globe with herniation of iris and ciliary body (asterisk) through a corneal laceration. Note the irregular, "peaked" pupil (arrow).
*(Reproduced with permission from David Palay, MD.)*

The prognosis for open-eye injuries is variable. Lacerations have better outcomes than ruptures, but this may be related to total size of the wound.[57] Anterior injuries tend to fare better than those more posterior, and eyes with initial visual acuity better than 20/200 have a far better prognosis than those presenting with a vision of light perception only or worse.[25,58] Severe retinal scarring (proliferative vitreoretinopathy) can complicate these injuries and is a major cause of poor visual results. Perforating injuries also have poor prognoses as the offending object can frequently involve the macula while intraocular BBs carry a high risk for eventual enucleation.[54,56] Even severe injuries should be considered for repair as there exists a chance for some visual function in all but the most severe injuries. Additionally, if an enucleation is eventually indicated, it can be psychologically advantageous for the patient to wait a short time as opposed to having the eye removed primarily.

## ENDOPHTHALMITIS

Traumatic endophthalmitis occurs in 2.8 to 7.4% of patients with penetrating injuries and is frequently caused by organisms of high virulence.[59,60] Prophylactic systemic and topical antibiotics are part of the routine management of open eyes to reduce the risk of this severe complication.[53] There has been a recent tendency to use third or fourth generation fluoroquinolones with good ocular penetration (levofloxacin or gatifloxacin) orally after surgery, limiting inpatient stay and demonstrating cost-effectiveness.

The risk for traumatic endophthalmitis is highest in patients with intraocular foreign bodies, injuries occurring in rural settings, injuries to the crystalline lens, and delays in presentation. Prophylactic intravitreal injection of antibiotics (ceftazidime and vancomycin) is sometimes administered to eyes with these risk factors.[54,60] In severe trauma it can be challenging to diagnose infectious endophthalmitis as a sterile hypopyon and significant inflammatory debris are not uncommon findings. Suspicion must remain high, however, and culturing anterior chamber and vitreous fluid (and possibly a vitreous biopsy specimen) plays an integral role in the evaluation of these eyes. In addition to antibiotic therapy, treatment can include core vitrectomy, close follow-up, and serial cultures. Prognosis can be poor in these cases, especially when highly virulent organisms such as *Bacillus cereus* are present.[54,60]

## CLOSED GLOBE

Closed globe injuries can also be associated with severe visual loss, and many intraocular structures can be injured simultaneously.

### Lamellar Laceration

Partial-thickness lacerations of the cornea are occasionally seen with an injury from a sharp object. These wounds should be evaluated closely to ensure there is no full-thickness component. Surgical repair is generally not indicated.

### Traumatic Iritis

Blunt trauma may result in injury to the iris and ciliary body, which subsequently causes inflammatory signs in the anterior chamber. Following even mild blunt injury to the globe, a patient will often describe eye pain, photophobia, and mild blurry vision. Symptoms are often delayed and typically begin 24 to 48 hours following injury. Examination reveals a red eye (perilimbal injection), a small, poorly reactive pupil, and an inflammatory reaction in the anterior chamber (seen on slit lamp exam as cell and flare). Treatment includes topical cycloplegia (homatropine 5% two or three times daily) to reduce photophobia and often anti-inflammatory medications (prednisolone acetate 1% suspension, four times a day). The condition should resolve within a few days to a week and requires an ophthalmologic follow-up visit to ensure that no other serious intraocular injury is present.

### Hyphema

*Hyphema* is defined as blood in the anterior chamber of the eye. Hyphemas can range from microscopic findings seen only under slit-lamp illumination to total, or "eight ball," hyphemas.

The overall treatment strategy for management of hyphemas is directed at reducing the chance for secondary hemorrhage (rebleed) and lowering intraocular pressure. Rebleeding into the anterior chamber usually occurs within three to five days. Metal-shield protection and bedrest with ambulation are essential mainstays of management. Even with such measures, rebleeds occur in 10 to 30% of cases and significantly complicate the management and worsen the overall prognosis of patients with hyphema.[61] Hyphemas tend to layer when a patient is upright and can be measured (percent of layered blood within the anterior chamber) and followed serially. Hyphemas are usually caused by tears in the anterior face of the ciliary body, the iris root, or pupillary margin.[62] Small hyphemas usually clear in less then a week without sequelae as the blood cells pass through the trabecular meshwork of the anterior chamber into the venous system. Larger hyphemas carry a higher risk of vision-threatening complications. The major risks associated with a hyphema are severe elevations of intraocular pressure causing damage to the optic nerve or bloodstaining of the cornea. Treatment includes topical cycloplegics and steroids, bed rest with elevation of the head of the bed to 30° to help the hyphema layer, and a protective shield to minimize the risk of secondary blunt injury to the eye. Intraocular pressure needs to be serially measured, and ocular antihypertensives are generally administered for pressures that reach greater than 25 mm Hg. Aspirin, nonsteroidal antiinflammatory medicines, and antiplatelet and anticoagulant agents should be discontinued if possible to reduce the risk of rebleeding. Some ophthalmologists recommend antifibrinolytic agents (aminocaproic or transexamic acid) or oral steroids to reduce the risk of rebleeding in select patient groups. Surgical removal of the clot is indicated when the intraocular pressure cannot be controlled medically, when early corneal blood-staining develops, and for large persistent hyphemas. Some patients may require earlier intervention depending on pre-existing conditions. African-American patients (and rarely other ethnic groups) with a hyphema require special attention. These patients need urgent screening for sickle cell disease (and trait), and hemoglobin electrophoresis should also be considered. The reason for this urgency is that the red blood cells of affected patients can sickle in the hypoxic environment of the anterior chamber and create more difficulty in their clearance with subsequent elevations of intraocular pressure (with even small bleeds).

Due to sickling in the capillaries of the head of the optic nerve, these pressure elevations facilitate damage to the optic nerve. Therefore, surgical intervention is indicated earlier for control of intraocular pressure in sickle-screen-positive patients. Use of carbonic anhydrase inhibitors is somewhat controversial in these patients due to their potential to aggravate sickling via their tendency to create metabolic acidosis. Approximately 75% of patients overall who develop a hyphema have a visual outcome of 20/50 or better. Patients with a hyphema need a detailed ocular examination one month postinjury and yearly follow-up as these patients have an increased lifetime risk for glaucoma in the injured eye.[62–64]

## Injury to the Lens

Injuries to the lens from trauma may be manifested as cataracts and subluxation or dislocation of the lens. Trauma is the most common cause of unilateral cataracts in young individuals. Various causes include direct penetrating injury to the lens, blunt trauma, electrical shock, and ionizing radiation. Small, focal disruptions of the lens capsule may be well tolerated and result in small segmental opacities that do not significantly affect vision. If cataracts develop over weeks to months, they can cause severe visual defects. Modern techniques to remove cataracts yield exceptional results as long as the cornea, macula, and optic nerve are healthy. When patients who have had previous cataract surgery with placement of an intraocular lens suffer eye injuries, dislocation of the intraocular lens can occur.

The lens is suspended behind the iris by zonular fibers that attach to the ciliary body. With blunt trauma, the zonules may break, resulting in a subluxed (partially dislocated) or completely dislocated lens. The edge of a dislocated lens may be visible following dilation of the pupil, while a totally dislocated lens may be seen in the anterior chamber or posteriorly on the retina. A sign of dehiscence of the lens zonules may be seen at the slit-lamp as a shimmering of the iris with rapid eye movements. This is termed *iridodonesis*. Dilated slit-lamp examination aids in making this diagnosis, although CT images can also reveal lens dislocation. Mild subluxation of the lens can be compatible with good uncorrected vision, while more significant subluxations and posterior dislocations can occasionally be tolerated with spectacle correction. If treatment is needed, it is not emergent unless an anteriorly dislocated lens is causing endothelial damage on the cornea or obstructing aqueous outflow through the pupil, causing acute angle-closure glaucoma. Significant direct damage to the lens, especially when associated with ocular inflammation, endothelial damage to the cornea, or an elevated intraocular pressure, usually requires a lens extraction procedure for visual rehabilitation.[64] This procedure can be performed primarily or secondarily depending on the severity of the injury, the surgeon's preference (visibility), and other related factors.

## Vitreous Hemorrhage

A vitreous hemorrhage can range from only small amounts of blood peripherally to dense hemorrhage precluding visualization of the ocular fundus. It can occur in both open and closed globe injuries. There are many potential sources of bleeding, including the ciliary body, retinal or choroidal vessels, a wound in the wall of the eye, or even the optic nerve. B-scan ultrasonography is performed in dense hemorrhages to evaluate the eye for the presence of a retinal detachment and foreign bodies. Vitrectomy is generally indicated within two weeks for open eye injuries and, if the hemorrhage does not clear spontaneously, in closed globe injuries.[54] Unilateral or bilateral vitreous hemorrhages can also be seen after traumatic subarachnoid bleeds, which is a condition called Terson's syndrome.

## Choroidal Rupture

A concussive force will deform the globe and stretch ocular tissue. This mechanism can sometimes result in a rupture of the choroid, the vascular layer of the internal wall of the eye. Such ruptures are generally found in a pattern concentric to the optic disk and are often associated with varying amounts of subretinal hemorrhage. When these ruptures extend directly under the fovea, they cause significant loss of acuity. There is no surgical method to repair choroidal ruptures, and management consists of observation and caring for the other eye injuries. When these injuries are associated with significant amounts of subfoveal hemorrhage, some practitioners advocate pneumatic displacement of the hemorrhage by injecting an expansile gas into the eye and positioning the patient to force the blood away from the center of vision. Late complications of choroidal rupture include subretinal neovascular membranes that can lead to further visual loss. Laser therapy or subretinal surgical techniques can be effective methods for treating patients with these subretinal neovascular membranes.[54,64]

# INJURIES TO THE RETINA

While many retinal injuries have a good visual outcome, even the most advanced surgical techniques cannot prevent blindness in all patients.

## Commotio Retinae

*Commotio retinae* is also known as Berlin's edema and refers to a retinal contusion. It is thought that concussive injury causes a shearing within the highly ordered photoreceptor cell layer of the retina. The retina appears whitened when viewed with an ophthalmoscope. This condition can be associated with a decrease in visual acuity, but generally resolves after two to four weeks with excellent visual outcomes. Late complications of *commotio retinae* include atrophy of the fovea and underlying pigment epithelium of the retina, formation of a hole in the macula, and visual distortion.[54,64,65]

## Retinitis Sclopeteria

*Retinitis sclopeteria* is a result of direct external trauma to the wall of the eye generally associated with a high-velocity contusive mechanism. The choroid and retina underlying the site of injury retract and necrose leaving a view of bare sclera in the peripheral or posterior fundus. Even though these injuries tear the retina, treatment is generally not necessary because the inflammation associated with the injury causes enough chorioretinal adhesion to prevent subsequent detachment. This injury is consistent with good vision as long as the macula and optic nerve are spared.[54,64]

## Traumatic Macular Hole

A traumatic macular hole can develop after blunt trauma either immediately due to vitreoretinal traction at the fovea or later as retinal macular edema resolves. Without treatment visual acuity can range from 20/80 to 20/400, but vitrectomy surgery may lead to better visual outcomes.[64,65]

## Retinal Breaks and Retinal Detachments

Following injuries to the globe, several forms of retinal breaks (tears) can occur. These breaks can lead to retinal detachment and require early identification and appropriate management. A thorough examination of the peripheral retina is indicated in all patients suffering significant injuries to the eye. This examination must be delayed in some cases (i.e., corneal laceration, hyphema) to avoid placing external pressure to the globe, but it should be performed when safe. Retinal dialyses (disinsertions) are one of the most common causes of retinal detachment after severe blunt trauma and can occur in isolation or be associated with avulsions of the base of the vitreous or other injuries.[65] Giant retinal tears and smaller horseshoe tears can result from trauma-induced vitreoretinal traction. These lesions also carry significant risk for detachments. Early identification can allow for successful prophylactic treatment with laser retinopexy or cryotherapy. Symptoms of a retinal break include photopsia (peripheral flashing lights) and seeing a sudden new onset of floaters. A retinal detachment will cause peripheral visual loss (curtains coming across the vision) that eventually affects central vision. Retinal detachments can be caused by tractional membranes associated with proliferative vitreoretinopathy, as well. Retinal detachments need surgical intervention and usually require scleral buckling and/or vitrectomy procedures.

## Purtscher's Retinopathy

A retinopathy with multiple focal areas of superficial retinal whitening in both eyes has been well described after trauma to the head, fractures of long bones, compression of the chest, and childbirth. This condition, called Purtscher's retinopathy, may be caused by arterial leukoemboli following complement activation. There is no treatment, and visual acuity function may return to normal or be diminished.[64,65]

## Sympathetic Ophthalmia

Sympathetic ophthalmia is one of the most feared complications of severe eye trauma because it affects the patient's only remaining eye. It is estimated to occur in 0.2 to 0.5% of severe nonsurgical eye wounds and is presumed to be an autoimmune inflammatory response generated toward ocular antigens (these antigens are usually sheltered from the immune system). The condition consists of a posterior *granulomatous uveitis*, and its onset can be from days to years after the inciting traumatic event. Clinical presentation is an insidious or acute anterior uveitis with mutton-fat keratic precipitates.

The posterior segment manifests moderate to severe vitritis, usually accompanied by multiple yellowish-white choroidal lesions. Treatment of sympathetic ophthalmia consists of systemic anti-inflammatory agents such as high-dose oral corticosteroids. If the inflammation cannot be controlled with steriods, alternate immunosuppressive agents may be necessary. The role of enucleation of the injured eye after the diagnosis of sympathetic ophthalmia remains controversial.[54,67] Visual prognosis is reasonably good with prompt wound repair and appropriate immunomodulatory therapy.[66]

## INJURY TO CRANIAL NERVES

Any of the cranial nerves coursing through the orbit (II, III, IV, V, and VI) may be injured during trauma to the head, orbit, or eye (see Chap. 20).

### Direct Injury to the Optic Nerve

Direct injuries to the optic nerve are caused by deep and sharp penetrating orbital trauma, compression on the nerve by bone fragments or foreign bodies in the orbit, or by a hematoma in the nerve sheath. Trauma to the optic nerve should be suspected when visual loss is associated with an obvious relative afferent pupillary defect. When a reversible cause can be clearly identified radiographically, surgical decompression may be indicated. Generally, these procedures are performed by ophthalmologists with subspecialty training in orbital surgery or by neurosurgeons. Avulsion of the optic nerve results in monocular blindness.

### Traumatic Optic Neuropathy

Traumatic optic neuropathy occurs after indirect injury to the optic nerve. Anterior injuries from a sudden forceful rotation of the globe are those where the damage is manifest in the intraorbital portions of the nerve and there is edema or hemorrhage of the optic disk. Posterior injuries tend to involve traumatic shearing forces that are transmitted to the nerve through the optic canal where it is tightly bound and immobile.

The diagnosis is confirmed when a relative afferent pupillary deficit shows no other sufficient ocular cause for that finding. Visual acuity is affected in varying degrees. The mainstay of current treatment guidelines is urgent high-dose intravenous methylprednisolone followed by a steroid taper, while transethmoidal surgical decompression of the optic nerve may be indicated in some patients. Outcomes are variable and can be difficult to predict, but severe visual loss is not an uncommon result.[68,69] Optic disk pallor becomes prominent approximately four weeks after significant injuries to the optic nerve.

### Cranial Nerve Palsies

Palsies of ocular motor nerves present with acquired strabismus, dysfunction of extraocular motility, and subsequent diplopia. Injuries of cranial nerve III can also be associated with ptosis and pupillary dilation. Recovery generally occurs, but may not begin for weeks to months and may demonstrate aberrant regeneration.

If disturbances of ocular motility persist for six or more months, strabismus surgery can be considered. It is obviously important to differentiate orbital from intracranial origins for cranial nerve palsies.

## ORBITAL INJURIES

An orbital CT scan is integral to the management of patients with possible injuries to the orbit. When a foreign body is present in the orbit, it should be removed if this can be done with limited morbidity. Small inert posterior orbital foreign bodies (such as a BB) can be left in place if they are not causing visual or functional problems because there is risk to exploring the posterior orbit.[70] An acute traumatic carotid-cavernous sinus fistula is generally high flow, and neuroradiologic or neurosurgical consultation and intervention are usually required (see Chap. 16). Extraocular muscles can develop hematomas, be lacerated/avulsed, and subsequently develop restrictive fibrosis in the setting of orbital trauma.

### Retrobulbar Hemorrhage

A retrobulbar hemorrhage presents with pain, proptosis, and hemorrhagic suffusion (bloody chemosis). Visual acuity, pupillary function, and intraocular pressure should be monitored, and a CT scan of the orbit is obtained to confirm the diagnosis. Lateral canthotomy and, if necessary, cantholysis (upper and lower) are indicated emergently to decompress the orbit and allow the globe to displace anteriorly when pupillary function demonstrates neuroretinal compromise (e.g., retinal artery pulsations) or if intraocular pressure cannot be lowered medically. When the above abnormalities are clearly noted, this canthotomy procedure need not wait for CT results.[71,72] Close postprocedure follow-up is warranted.

### Orbital Blow-Out Fracture

Orbital fractures are common in patients with severe facial and orbital trauma. These fractures can be multiple, usually involving either the medial or inferior orbital walls, often sparing the orbital rim, and may involve other facial structures as well. They are classically the result of blunt injury to the orbit by a mass larger than the diameter of the bony orbital rim. Such forces cause an acute increase in intraorbital pressure, and subsequent decompression occurs most easily through the very thin orbital floor or medially located lamina papyracea (hydraulic theory). Herniation of periorbital fat and/or extraocular muscle into the maxillary sinus or, less commonly, the ethmoid sinus may complicate a blowout fracture. Diplopia may result from muscle entrapment and/or contusion or dysfunction of a cranial nerve. Signs suggestive of an orbital blowout fracture include subconjunctival hematoma, periorbital ecchymosis, crepitus, orbital emphysema, enophthalmos, restrictive or paretic extraocular muscle function, and hypesthesia in the distribution of the infraorbital nerve (cheek).

The diagnosis of orbital fractures is largely based on radiographic evaluation of the orbits. While plain films can delineate most orbital fractures quite well, high-resolution CT is the modality of choice. Both axial and coronal slices less than or equal to 1.0-mm thickness through the entire orbit, optic canal, and cavernous sinus are recommended for optimal evaluation. Bone windows are especially useful to detect the more subtle fractures.

Indications for surgical repair with an orbital implant can include enophthalmos greater than 2 mm, diplopia in primary or inferior (reading) gaze, a fracture greater than 50% of the orbital floor, and entrapment of an extraocular muscle. Because surgical complications can be significant, the decision to operate should be made carefully. Significant intraocular injury should be considered first.[73] Because most patients have significant soft-tissue swelling concurrent with an orbital wall fracture, most ophthalmic surgeons advocate observation for a minimum of seven days, during which time most of the swelling will resolve. Immediate surgery may be indicated for severe orbital apex fractures, fractures associated with leaks of cerebrospinal fluid, the presence of a nonresolving oculocardiac reflex, and early enophthalmos or hypoglobus with facial asymmetry. In children, isolated floor fractures are often "trap door" in nature with significant muscle entrapment and are often associated with persistent nausea and vomiting. Studies have shown good outcomes with early (<3 days postinjury) surgery with prompt resolution of diplopia, nausea, vomiting, and bradycardia. Indications for delayed (one to two weeks postinjury) surgical repair of an isolated orbital wall fracture include the following: persistent diplopia in primary gaze associated with positive forced ductions and evidence of prolapsed orbital soft tissue on CT imaging; enophthalmos greater than 2 mm; and large fractures with greater than 50% disruption of the orbital floor which may lead to late enophthalmos or hypoglobus. Surgical correction delayed beyond two weeks may be associated with less desirable outcomes. Oral steroids and antibiotics have been used in some centers.[71,72,74] These considerations for treatment should be influenced by the presence of prior sinus disease or possible involvement of the cranial vault.

## LACERATIONS OF THE EYELID

Lid lacerations can be divided into three groups including nonmarginal, those involving the lid margin, and those involving the canalicular system. Superficial nonmarginal lacerations of the lid can be closed primarily without subspecialty consultation (unless there is prolapse of fat). Lacerations of the margin of the lid require special attention to ensure proper realignment and closure (Figs. 21-6 and 21-7). Lacerations of the margin of the lid medial to the puncta will involve the canaliculus and should be closed in the operating room with a microscope. The distal and proximal ends of the canaliculus are identified, the lacrimal drainage system is stented with silicone tubing to maintain patency for the initial postrepair period, the canalicular epithelium is reapproximated with 7-0 vicryl suture, and the laceration is then closed.[74,75] Failure

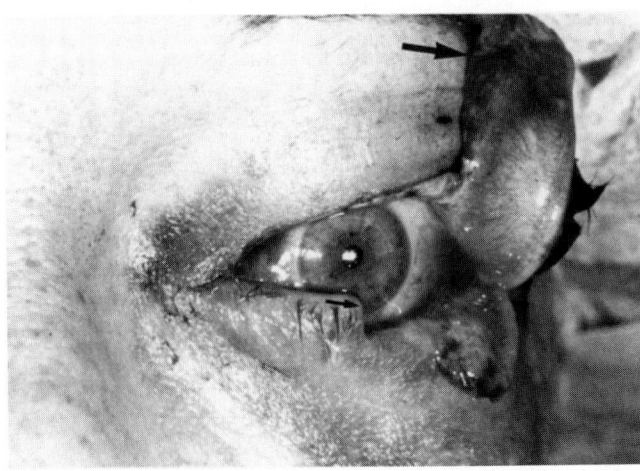

**FIGURE 21-6.** Lacerations of both the upper and lower eyelids (large arrow and small arrow, respectively). Note the large, temporally based flap of upper eyelid (large arrow), indicating probable medial canthal injury as well.
*(Reproduced with permission from Ted Wojno, MD.)*

to diagnose and repair canalicular lacerations can lead to an abnormal overflow of tears down the cheek (epiphora).

## PEDIATRIC TRAUMA

In the pediatric population there are several special situations with regard to ophthalmic trauma. Birth, especially forceps deliveries, can be associated with periorbital edema, lacerations of the lid, corneal damage, and retinal hemorrhages. Fortunately, these injuries tend to resolve spontaneously, but damage to the cornea can lead to corneal astigmatism. Therefore, ophthalmologic consultation is indicated after complicated deliveries. Shaken baby syndrome is a well-described entity in which intracranial and retinal hemorrhages are often seen with no other external signs of trauma. It is generally seen in children less than two years of age and may lead to severe cognitive and visual impairment or death. Retinal hemorrhages resolve fairly quickly, but other retinal or optic nerve complications may cause visual loss. Finally, it is important to be aware of the risk of amblyopia in any child less than 8 years of age with an injury to the eye. Ophthalmologic consultation and close follow-up is indicated in any child suffering an ocular injury.[11,76]

## INJURY PREVENTION

Education of the lay public is necessary to reduce the risk of injury to the eye at home, at work, and in recreational activities (see Chap. 3). Polycarbonate lenses with frames appropriate to the proposed activity meets a general standard for reasonable protective eyewear.[2] Most severe injuries to the eye occur in patients who were not wearing appropriate eye protection.[6,16] Legislation controlling the use of fireworks and BB guns would also decrease the incidence of serious injuries to the eye.

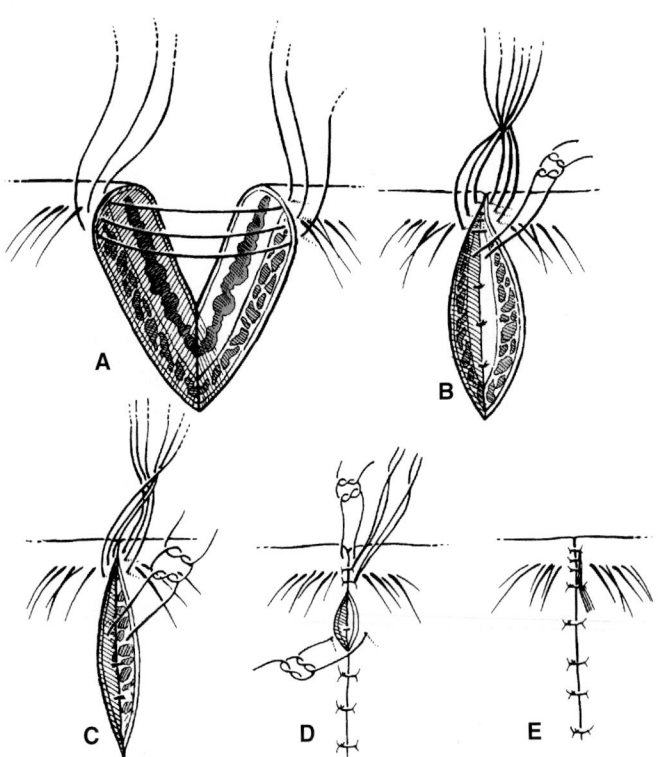

**FIGURE 21-7.** Repair of full-thickness eyelid laceration. **(A)** A 6-0 silk suture is placed through the gray line and on either side of the lash line. Together these are used for traction. **(B)** The tarsoconjunctiva is approximated with 6-0 Vicryl, avoiding a full-thickness bite. **(C)** The orbicular muscle is approximated with 6-0 plain catgut. **(D)** The skin is closed with interrupted 6-0 silk or 6-0 plain catgut. **(E)** The margin sutures are tied and brought forward and tied to one of the skin sutures.
*A-E (With permission from Leone CR: Plastic surgery. In Spaeth GL, ed. Ophthalmic Surgery: Principles and Practice. Philadelphia: W.B. Saunders, 1990, pp. 534–535.)*

Likewise, manufacturers must continually attempt to improve the design of their products and associated safety features. For example, laminated windshields and airbags have had positive impact in reducing the severity of eye injuries associated with motor vehicle crashes.[77–79] The trade-off, of course, is that ocular injuries can be caused by these same airbags.[80,81] As a final note, monocular patients should be advised to always wear eye protection with polycarbonate lenses.

## ACKNOWLEDGMENT

The authors would like to thank David M. Kleinman MD, for his original contributions to this manuscript.

## REFERENCES

1. Alfaro DV, Egan CA, Kellicut DC, et al.: Surgical management of the eye: Modern history 1900-present. In: Alfaro DV, Liggett PE , eds. *Vitreoretinal Surgery of the Injured Eye.* Philadelphia: Lippincott-Raven, 1999, p. 1.
2. Congdon NG, Schein OD: The epidemiology of ocular trauma: A preventable ocular emergency. In MacCumber MW, ed. *Management of Ocular Injuries and Emergencies.* New York: Lippincott-Raven, 1998, p. 9.
3. Kuhn F, Mester V, Douglas C, et al.: Epidemiology and socioeconomic impact of ocular trauma. In Alfaro DV, Liggett PE, eds. *Vitreoretinal Surgery of the Injured Eye.* Philadelphia: Lippincott-Raven, 1999, p. 17.

4. Prevent Blindness America: The scope of the eye injury problem. 2001. http://preventblindness.org/vpus/vp.html.

5. Katz J, Tielsch JM: Lifetime prevalence of ocular injuries from the Baltimore eye survey. *Arch Ophthalmol* 111:1564, 1993.

6. May DR, Kuhn FP, Morris RE, et al.: The epidemiology of serious eye injuries from the United States Eye Injury Registry. *Graefe's Arch Clin Exp Ophthalmol* 238:153, 2000.

7. Xiang H, Stallones L, Guanmin C, et al.: Work-related eye injuries treated in hospital emergency departments in the U.S. *Am J Ind Med* 48:57, 2005.

8. Hemady RK: Ocular injuries from violence treated at an inner-city hospital. *J Trauma* 37:5, 1994.

9. Sastry SM, Paul BK, Bain L, et al.: Ocular trauma among major trauma victims in a regional trauma center. *J Trauma* 34: 223, 1993.

10. Andreotti G, Lange JL, Brundage JF: The nature, incidence and impact of eye injuries among US military personnel. *Arch Ophthalmol* 119:1693, 2001.

11. Coody D, Banks J, Yetman R, et al.: Eye Trauma in children: Epidemiology, management, and prevention. *J Pediatr Health Care* 11:182, 1997.

12. Zagelbaum BM, Tostanoski JR, Kerner DJ, et al.: Urban eye trauma: A one-year prospective study. *Ophthalmology* 100:851, 1993.

13. Starkey C, Zagelbaum BM: Basketball. In: Zagelbaum BM, ed. *Sports Ophthalmology*. Cambridge: Blackwell Science, 1996, p. 43.

14. Napier SM, Baker RS, Sanford DG, et al.: Eye injuries in athletics and recreation. *Surv Ophthalmol* 41:229, 1996.

15. Zagelbaum BM: Baseball. In: Zagelbaum BM, ed. *Sports Ophthalmology*. Cambridge: Blackwell Science, 1996, p. 23.

16. United States Eye Injury Registry: *Selected Data 1988–2001*. Birmingham, 2001.

17. Kuhn F, Morris R, Witherspoon CD: Classification of ocular trauma: The Birmingham Eye Trauma Terminology. In: Alfaro III DV, Liggett PE, eds. *Vitreoretinal Surgery of the Injured Eye*. Philadelphia: Lippincott-Raven, 1999, p. 17.

18. Kuhn F, Morris R, Witherspoon D, et al.: A standard classification of ocular trauma. *Ophthalmology* 103:240, 1996.

19. Harlan JB Jr, Pieramici DJ: Evaluation of patients with ocular trauma. *Ophthalmol Clin North Am* 15:153, 2002.

20. Juang PS, Rosen P: Ocular examination techniques for the emergency department. *J Emerg Med* 15:793, 1997.

21. Congdon NG, MaCumber MW: Ocular evaluation. In: MacCumber MW, ed. *Management of Ocular Injuries and Emergencies*. New York: Lippincott-Raven, 1998, p. 29.

22. Weisman RA, Savino PJ: Management of patients with facial trauma and associated ocular/orbital injuries. *Otolaryngol Clin North Am* 24:37, 1991.

23. Broocker G: The Ophthalmic Examination. In: Harwood-Nuss A, Wolfson AB, eds. *The Clinical Practice of Emergency Medicine*, 3rd ed. Philadelphia: Lippincott Williams & Wilkins, 2001, p. 42.

24. Joseph DP, DiBernardo C, Miller NR: Radiographic and echographic imaging studies. In: MacCumber MW, ed. *Management of Ocular Injuries and Emergencies*. New York: Lippincott-Raven, 1998, p. 55.

25. Morris R, Kuhn F, Witherspoon CD: Counseling of the trauma victim and the family. In: Alfaro DV, Liggett PE, eds. *Vitreoretinal Surgery of the Injured Eye*. Philadelphia: Lippincott-Raven, 1999, p. 25.

26. Kuhn F, Slezakb Z: Damage control surgery in ocular traumatology. *Injury* 35:690, 2004.

27. Hamill MB: Clinical evaluation. In: Shingleton BJ, Hersh PS, Kenyon KR, eds. *Eye Trauma*. St. Louis: Mosby-Year Book, 1991, p. 22.

28. Pfister RR: Chemical injuries of the eye. *Ophthalmology* 90:1246, 1983.

29. Liggett P: Ocular trauma in an urban population. *Ophthalmology* 97:581, 1989.

30. Cangadhar DV, Kenyon KR, Wagoner MD: The surgical management of chemical ocular injuries: Present and future strategies. *Int Ophthalmol Clin* 35:63, 1995.

31. Ralph RA: Tetracyclines and the treatment of corneal stromal ulceration: A review. *Cornea* 19:274, 2000.

32. Reim M, Redbrake C, Schrage N: Chemical and thermal injuries of the eyes. Surgical and medical treatment based on clinical and pathophysiological findings. *Arch Soc Esp Oftalmol* 76:79, 2001.

33. Brodovsky SC, McCarty CA, et al.: Management of alkali burns: An 11-year retrospective review. *Ophthalmology* 107:1829, 2000.

34. Meller D, Pires RT, Mack RJ, et al.: Amniotic membrane transplantation for acute chemical or thermal burns. *Ophthalmology* 107:980, 2000.

35. Kobayashi A, Shirao Y, Yoshita T, et al.: Temporary amniotic membrane patching for acute chemical burns. *Eye* 17:149, 2003.

36. Arora R, Mehta D, Jain V: Amniotic membrane transplantation in acute chemical burns. *Eye* 19:273, 2005.

37. Roper-Hall MJ: Thermal and chemical burns of the eye. *Trans Ophthalmol Soc UK* 85:631, 1965.

38. Kenyon KR, Tseng SC: Limbal autograft transplantation for ocular surface disorders. *Ophthalmology* 96:709 (discussion 722), 1989.

39. Sabri K, Pandit JC, et al.: National survey of corneal abrasion treatment. *Eye* 12:278, 1998.

40. Patterson J, Fetzer D, Krall J, et al.: Eye patch treatment for the pain of corneal abrasion. *South Med J* 89:227, 1996.

41. Hart A, White S, Conboy P, et al.: The management of corneal abrasions in accident and emergency. *Injury* 28:527, 1997.

42. Arbour JD, Brunette I, Boisjoly HM, et al.: Should we patch corneal erosions? *Arch Ophthalmol* 115:313, 1997.

43. Michael JG, Hug D, Dowd MD: Management of corneal abrasion in children: A randomized clinical trial. *Ann Emerg Med* 40:67, 2002.

44. Kaiser PK: A comparison of pressure patching versus no patching from corneal abrasions due to trauma or foreign body removal. *Ophthalmology* 102:1936, 1995.

45. Kaiser PK, Pineda R: A study of topical nonsteroidal anti-inflammatory drops and no pressure patching in the treatment of corneal abrasions. Corneal Abrasion Patching Study Group. *Ophthalmology* 104:1353, 1997.

46. Goyal R, Shankar J, Fone DL, et al.: Randomized controlled trial of ketorolac in the management of corneal abrasions. *Acta Ophthalmol Scand* 79:177, 2001.

47. Salz JJ, Reader AL, Schwartz LJ, et al.: Treatment of corneal abrasions with soft contact lenses and topical diclofenac. *J Refract Corneal Surg* 10:640, 1994.

48. Donnenfeld ED, Selkin BA, Perry HD, et al.: Controlled evaluation of a bandage contact lens and a topical nonsteroidal anti-inflammatory drug treating traumatic abrasions. *Ophthalmology* 102:979, 1995.

49. Joseph E, Zak R, Smith S, et al.: Predictors of blinding or serious eye injury in blunt trauma. *J Trauma* 33:19, 1992.

50. Delori F, Pomerantzeff O, Cox MS, et al.: Deformation of the globe under high-speed impact: Its relation to contusion injuries. *Invest Ophthalmol Vis Sci* 8:290, 1969.

51. Holt JE, Holt GR, Blodgett JM, et al.: Ocular injuries sustained during blunt facial trauma. *Ophthalmology* 90:14, 1983.

52. Kylstra JA, Lamkin JC, Runyan DK, et al.: Clinical predictors of scleral rupture after blunt ocular trauma. *Am J Ophthalmol* 115:530, 1993.

53. Alfaro DV: Intravenous antibiotics in open-globe injuries. In: Alfaro DV, Liggett PE, eds. *Vitreoretinal Surgery of the Injured Eye*. Philadelphia: Lippincott-Raven, 1999, p. 65.

54. Aaberg TM Jr, Sternberg PS Jr: Trauma: Principles and techniques of treatment. In: Wilkinson CP, ed. *Retina*, 3rd ed. St. Louis: Mosby, 2001, p. 2400.

55. Navon SE: Management of the ruptured globe. *Int Ophthalmol Clin* 35:71, 1995.

56. McCabe CM, Mieler WF, Postel EA: Surgical management of intraocular foreign bodies. In: Alfaro DV, Liggett PE, eds. *Vitreoretinal Surgery of the Injured Eye*. New York: Lippincott-Raven, 1999.

57. Pieramici DJ, MacCumber MW, Humayun MU, et al.: Open-globe Injury. Update on types of injuries and visual results. *Ophthalmology* 103:1798, 1996.

58. Edwards MG, Pieramici DJ, Fekrat S, et al.: Corneoscleral lacerations and ruptures. In: MacCumber MW, ed. *Management of Ocular Injuries and Emergencies*. New York: Lippincott-Raven, 1998, p. 207.

59. Merbs SL, Abrams LS, Campochiaro PA: Endophthalmitis. In: MacCumber MW, ed. *Management of Ocular Injuries and Emergencies*. New York: Lippincott-Raven, 1998, p. 275.

60. Alfaro DV, Pastor JC, Meredith T: Posttraumatic endophthalmitis. In: Alfaro DV, Liggett PE, eds. *Vitreoretinal Surgery of the Injured Eye*. Philadelphia: Lippincott-Raven, 1999, p. 339.

61. Thomas MA, Parrish RK II, Feuer WJ, et al.: Rebleeding after traumatic hyphema. *Arch Ophthalmol* 104:206, 1986.

62. Berrios RR, Dreyer EB: Traumatic hyphema. *Int Ophthalmol Clin* 35:93, 1995.

63. Raja SC, Goldberg MF: Injuries of the anterior segment. In: MacCumber MW, ed. *Management of Ocular Injuries and Emergencies*. New York: Lippincott-Raven, 1998, p. 227.

64. King LP, Hudson SJ: Closed-globe trauma. In: Alfaro DV, Liggett PE, eds. *Vitreoretinal Surgery of the Injured Eye*. Philadelphia: Lippincott-Raven, 1999, p. 29.

65. Dugel PU, Ober RR: Posterior segment manifestations of closed-globe contusion injury. In: Wilkinson CP, ed. *Retina*, 3rd ed. St. Louis: Mosby, 2001, p. 2386.

66. Damiro FM, Kiss S, et al.: Sympathetic ophthalmia, *Semin Ophthalmol* 20:191, 2005.

67. Power WJ, Foster CS: Update on sympathetic ophthalmia. *Int Ophthalmol Clin* 35:127, 1995.

68. Warner JE, Lessell S: Traumatic optic neuropathy. *Int Ophthalmol Clin* 35:57, 1995.

69. Levin LA, Beck RW, Joseph MP, et al.: The treatment of traumatic optic neuropathy: The international optic nerve trauma study. *Ophthalmology* 106:1268, 1999.

70. Dunya IM, Rubin PA, Shore JW: Penetrating orbital trauma. *Int Ophthalmol Clin* 35:25, 1995.

71. Bains RA, Rubin PA: Blunt orbital trauma. *Int Ophthalmol Clin* 35:37, 1995.

72. Kerrison JB, Iwamoto MA, Merbs SL, et al.: Orbital trauma. In: MacCumber MW, ed. *Management of Ocular Injuries and Emergencies*. New York: Lippincott-Raven, 1998, p. 107.

73. Cook T: Ocular and periocular injuries from orbital fractures. *J Am Coll Surg* 195:831, 2002.

74. Leone C: Periorbital trauma. *Int Ophthalmol Clin* 35:1, 1995.
75. Leone CR: Plastic surgery. In: Spaeth GL, ed. *Ophthalmic Surgery: Principals and Practice.* Philadelphia: Saunders, 1990, p. 534.
76. Fard AK, Repka MX: Special issues in pediatric ocular trauma. In: MacCumber MW, ed. *Management of Ocular Injuries and Emergencies.* New York: Lippincott-Raven, 1998, p. 39.
77. Linden JA, Renner GS: Trauma to the globe. *Emerg Med Clin North Am* 13:581, 1995.
78. Duma SM, Rath AL, Jernigan MV, et al.: The effects of depowered airbags on eye injuries in frontal automobile crashes. *Am J Emerg Med* 23:13, 2005.
79. Lehto KS, Sulander PO, Tervo TM: Do motor vehicle airbags increase risk of ocular injuries in adults? *Ophthalmology* 110:1082, 2003.
80. Mieler WF: Ocular Injuries: Is it possible to further limit the occurrence? *Arch Ophthalmol* 119:1712, 2001.
81. Kuhn F, Pieramici DJ: *Ocular Trauma: Principles and Practice.* New York: Thieme, 2002.

# Commentary ■ TERRY KIM

Drs. Broocker, Aaron, and Kim provide a very comprehensive, well-written, and well-referenced chapter on the topic of eye trauma. This chapter starts with an interesting and useful introduction on the epidemiology of eye injuries, providing surprising statistics on the incidence, cost, and etiology. After an overview of the function and anatomy of the eye and adnexa, the authors provide a classification schema of ocular trauma, followed by important pearls in the initial evaluation and history-taking of these patients. One major recommendation they make here is the early involvement of an ophthalmologist in the treatment plan, in order to avoid further eye damage, facilitate an emergency treatment plan, and minimize unnecessary tests or procedures. They also emphasize the importance of obtaining information on prior surgical procedures. (i.e., corneal transplantation, cataract surgery, LASIK, etc.), as this can warn the examiner about potential rupture sites after trauma.

The authors then proceed to provide detailed and well-organized instruction on the physical examination of these patients, all the way from measuring visual acuity to examining the fundus. Very useful pearls on examination tips in these trauma patients are provided along the way. A section on ancillary studies (i.e., CT scans, ultrasonography, etc.) provides practical updates on what tests to order and how these tests can help assess these eye injuries. The chapter concludes with a section devoted to the evaluation and management of specific eye injuries that are commonly encountered in the emergency room: chemical injuries, corneal abrasions, corneal foreign bodies, conjunctival lacerations, blunt traumas, open/closed globe injuries, and a host of other traumatic injuries involving the optic nerve, orbit, and eyelids.

In summary, this chapter provides one of the most comprehensive reviews on the subject of eye trauma. The authors are to be commended for providing an up-to-date and practical resource that will be a must for any medical provider in need of information on this topic.

# Face

Robert M. Kellman ■ Matthew L. Rontal

## INTRODUCTION

Facial structures participate in essential functions of human life, including respiration, mastication, deglutition, vision, and the expression of both verbal and nonverbal communication. Indeed, the face is the focal point of human social interaction.[1] Thus, to restore facial form and function is to restore much of a patient's opportunity to live a normal life.

Facial and craniofacial injuries range from simple soft-tissue lacerations to penetrating trauma that may also involve the brain above or the neck below, to high-speed, blunt force injuries that result in panfacial fractures and soft-tissue destruction as well as involvement of multiple organ systems. In order to effectively manage facial trauma, the surgeon must understand the various tissues of the face, the possible mechanisms of trauma to these tissue elements, and the diagnosis and management of resulting facial injuries. Management also requires an understanding of the possible import of these injuries in the most emergent setting, the means of early diagnosis and treatment during the acute and subacute periods, and the management of possible secondary complications.

Thus, the care of the facial trauma patient in the emergency room and trauma bay will be covered first. Then, the anatomy, evaluation, and management of injuries to the soft tissue, visceral, and bony components of the face will be covered in detail. Finally, the management of secondary deformities and complications will be discussed. In this manner, not only is a broad discussion of facial trauma achieved, but the reader is also made aware of the place occupied by facial trauma within the Advanced Trauma Life Support (ATLS) evaluation (see Chap. 11) and subsequent management.

## EMERGENCY DEPARTMENT CARE

### Primary Survey

Care of facial trauma in the emergent setting, as in the management of any trauma, is initially focused on the "ABCs." The adequacy of airway, breathing, and circulation are determined, and the appropriate ATLS algorithms are instituted. In addition to airway and circulation or bleeding issues, the cervical spine must be appropriately managed in the setting of facial trauma.

Airway.   Injuries to the upper aerodigestive tract and craniofacial skeleton may result in airway obstruction from tissue trauma and edema, foreign debris, or bleeding. The natural mechanisms of airway protection rely on functioning oropharyngeal structures supported by an intact facial skeleton. Soft-tissue injuries in the mouth and pharynx as well as facial skeletal trauma may render the tongue and pharynx ineffective at maintaining an open airway. Severe facial injuries may also present with coincident injury to the neuraxis or neck. An injury to the brain may result in central loss of the mechanisms of airway protection, and cervical trauma may produce laryngeal or lower airway obstruction or disruption.

Airway compromise may be rapidly lethal and is assessed first. Vital signs, including pulse oximetry, are ascertained and the ability to move air through the upper respiratory tract is assessed. The reader is cautioned that significant airway obstruction, even impending loss of the airway, may be accompanied by normal or near-normal oximetry. The Glasgow Coma Scale (GCS) is used to rapidly understand the presence of any neurologic impairment that may portend centrally based loss of the ability to protect the airway. The presence of laryngeal injury or tracheal deviation is determined by inspection and palpation. Subcutaneous emphysema may suggest pharyngeal, laryngeal, or tracheal disruption. Stridor (stereotypical high-pitched sounds of breathing through a partially obstructed airway) suggests airway narrowing and possible impending obstruction, and stertor (variable inspiratory or expiratory sounds usually resulting from poorly managed airway secretions) may suggest an inability to manage secretions. If time permits, flexible fiberoptic nasopharyngolaryngoscopy allows rapid and definitive evaluation of the potentially compromised hypopharyngeal and laryngeal airway.

Foreign material may be finger-swept, and blood and secretions are suctioned from the oral cavity and pharynx. A "jaw thrust," even in the setting of mandibular trauma, and bag-valve mask (BVM) assistance may temporize an airway, especially in the setting of injury to the brain or spinal cord. The compromised airway can then be secured via rapid sequence orotracheal or nasotracheal intubation. Orotracheal intubation is preferred in the setting of possible midface fractures.[2,3] Through the nose, intubation of the disrupted skull base is possible, albeit unlikely, and the midface may be further injured. If intubation proves impossible, the airway should be accessed through an emergent tracheotomy or cricothyrotomy.

Bleeding.   After management of the airway, any brisk bleeding should be controlled. The face is very well vascularized, and soft-tissue injuries may result in profuse hemorrhage. In particular, the scalp bleeds profusely because large vessels are located near the surface and because the tissue is relatively inelastic.[4] Intraoral and pharyngeal bleeding may involve injury to the carotid artery, internal jugular vein, or their branches and may result in compromise of the airway. After securing the airway, the throat may be packed in order to control pharyngeal bleeding, the source of which may be difficult to determine during initial management. Injuries to the carotid artery and/or jugular vein may also occur with coincident trauma to the neck. A neck hematoma may threaten the airway via extrinsic compression. Bullet wounds involving the parapharyngeal and retropharyngeal spaces, the nasopharynx, and the infratemporal fossa carry the risk of injury to the internal carotid artery, and emergent angiography may be indicated. Massive, high-energy wounds to the face may present with massive bleeding. Direct pressure and pressure dressings are applied. Naimer et al. have described a pressure dressing secured to the face with a clear synthetic full-face wrap after airway diversion through a tracheostomy or cricothyrotomy.[5]

Cervical Spine.   Facial injuries may also be associated with trauma to the cervical spine and brain. In order to minimize further damage, any patient with suspected injury to the cervical spine should be immobilized on a backboard with a rigid cervical collar until definitive evaluation can be completed.[2] Most notably, cervical spine precautions are maintained during intubation or emergent tracheotomy by maintaining a neutral position of the head via in-line traction and minimal extension such that at least the supraglottis may be visualized.

Finally, assessment of the patient's level of consciousness and neurologic function is summarized by the GCS. Up to 15 points are allocated based on a patient's motor, verbal, and eye-opening performance. Computed tomography (CT) scan of the head and brain and neurosurgical consultation are indicated with a GCS <14.[2,3]

## Secondary Survey

With the airway, breathing, hemodynamics, and cervical spine stabilized, the remainder of the trauma survey is undertaken. Injuries that continue to pose an impending threat to the patient's life are identified and addressed. At this time, facial and craniomaxillofacial injuries are also identified. The location and severity of wounds are determined, as is the involvement of skin and soft tissue, facial bones, and viscera. The need for imaging should also be determined since radiographic studies are often readily available in the emergency department. Since the multitrauma patient will undergo CT examination of other anatomic regions, radiographic evaluation of craniofacial injuries can be expedited. During this time, the input of consultants who care for craniofacial and associated wounds is sought. This may include otolaryngology/facial plastic surgery, plastic surgery, oral and maxillofacial surgery, ophthalmology, and neurosurgery.

## NORMAL ANATOMY

In order to make an accurate assessment of craniofacial injuries and to effect an adequate reconstruction, an understanding of the normal anatomy is required. While a complete discussion of craniofacial anatomy is well beyond the scope of this chapter, key anatomic points will be highlighted to the extent that they are encountered in the care of facial trauma.

## Soft Tissue

The scalp covers the entire cranial vault and extends over the upper face. It consists of five layers including, skin, subcutaneous fat, galea aponeurosis (including the frontalis muscle in the forehead), loose areolar tissue, and periosteum of the skull known as the pericranium. Lateral to the temporal lines, the galea gives way to a fibrofatty fascial plane known as the temporoparietal fascia, which is contiguous inferiorly with the superficial muscular aponeurotic system of the face. In the inferior aspect of the temporal scalp, the temporal branch of the facial nerve travels in the deep aspect of the loose areolar tissue on the superficial surface of temporalis investing fascia, to innervate the frontalis muscle (Fig. 22-1). The supratrochlear and supraorbital neurovascular bundles travel sagitally in the substance of the frontal scalp. These structures emanate from notches or foramina in the medial and midpupillary superior orbital rims and penetrate the frontalis muscle 2 cm (supratrochlear) to 4 cm (supraorbital) above the superior orbital rim.[6,7] Therefore, subperiosteal dissection of the 3–4 cm above the supraorbital rims ensures protection of these structures until they are encountered at the orbital rim itself.

The eyelid is a trilamellar structure (Fig. 22-2). The anterior lamella consists of skin and the sphincteric orbicularis muscle and the posterior lamella consists of the conjunctiva. The tarsal plates comprise the middle layer, and they are attached at their transverse extents to the medial and lateral orbital rims by the medial and lateral canthal tendons, respectively. The orbital septum separates the peripheral aspects of the orbicularis from the deep periorbital fat. In the upper lid, the superior orbital septum is contiguous with a levator aponeurosis which connects the levator muscles to the anterior face of the tarsus. The inferior orbital septum inserts directly on the

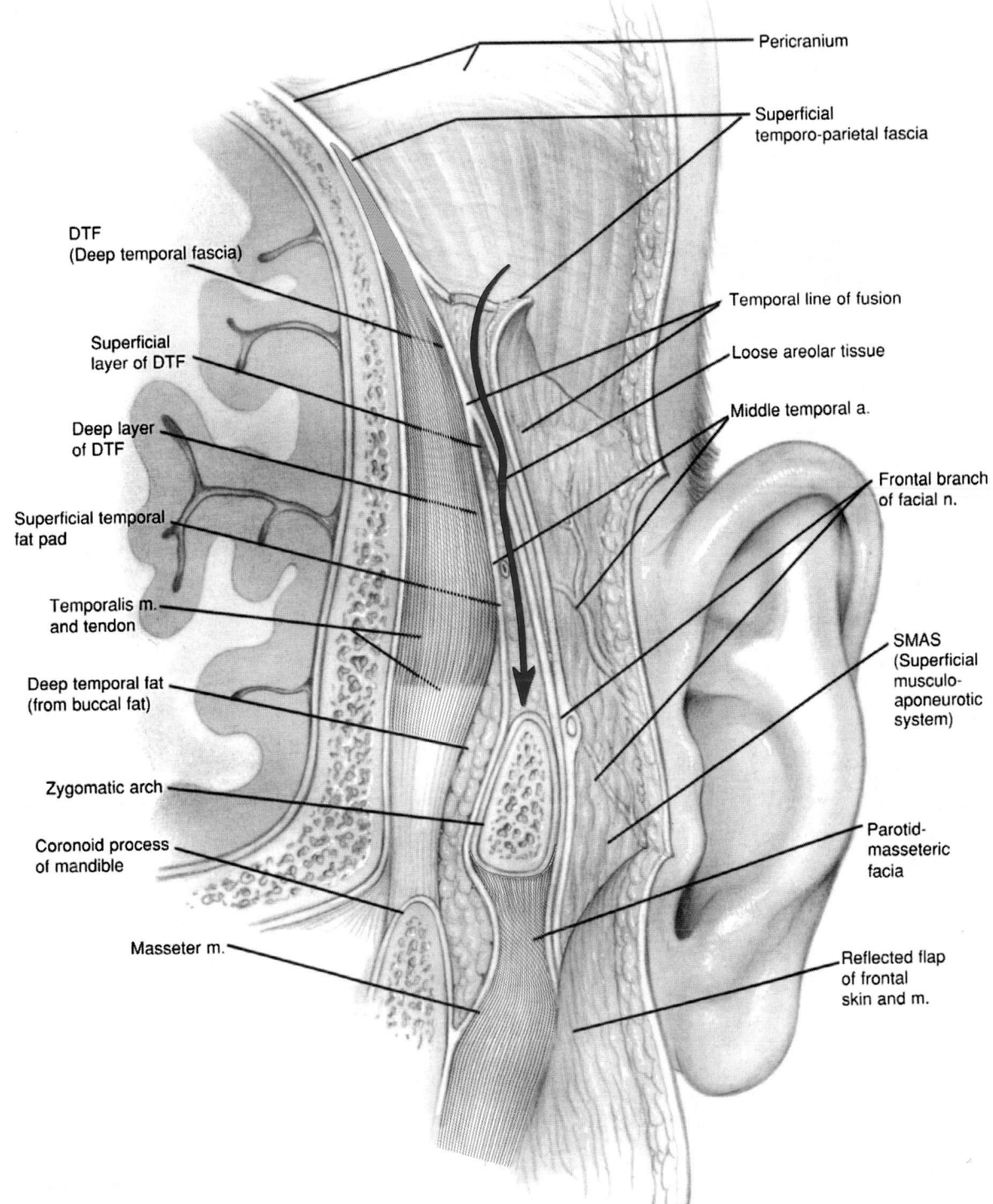

Pericranium

Superficial
temporo-parietal fascia

DTF
(Deep temporal fascia)

Temporal line of fusion

Superficial
layer of DTF

Loose areolar tissue

Deep layer
of DTF

Middle temporal a.

Superficial temporal
fat pad

Frontal branch
of facial n.

Temporalis m.
and tendon

SMAS
(Superficial
musculo-
aponeurotic
system)

Deep temporal fat
(from buccal fat)

Zygomatic arch

Parotid-
masseteric
facia

Coronoid process
of mandible

Masseter m.

Reflected flap
of frontal
skin and m.

**FIGURE 22-1.** The fascial planes of the temporal scalp and underlying temporalis muscle. The frontal branch of the facial nerve located on or within the superficial layer of deep temporalis fascia.
*(Reproduced with permission from Kellman RM, Marentette LJ. Atlas of Craniomaxillofacial Fixation. New York, Raven Press, 1995, p. 97.)*

inferior margin of the inferior tarsus. Levator and depressor muscles insert on the superior and inferior margins of the upper and lower lid tarsal plates, respectively, and open the eyelids upon stimulation by the third cranial nerve. The orbicularis closes the lids and is innervated by the eye branch of the temporal branch of the facial nerve. The conjunctiva, or posterior lamella, covers the inner surface of the lid and extends over the anterior aspect of the globe itself.

The medial canthal tendon is derived from the pretarsal and preseptal portions of the orbicularis oculi muscle, which divide at their medial extent into anterior and posterior slips. The anterior and posterior components of each muscle then fuse, forming the common anterior and posterior limbs of the medial canthal tendon (MCT). These insert on the anterior and posterior lacrimal crest, respectively. A third slip of the tendon also attaches more superiorly.

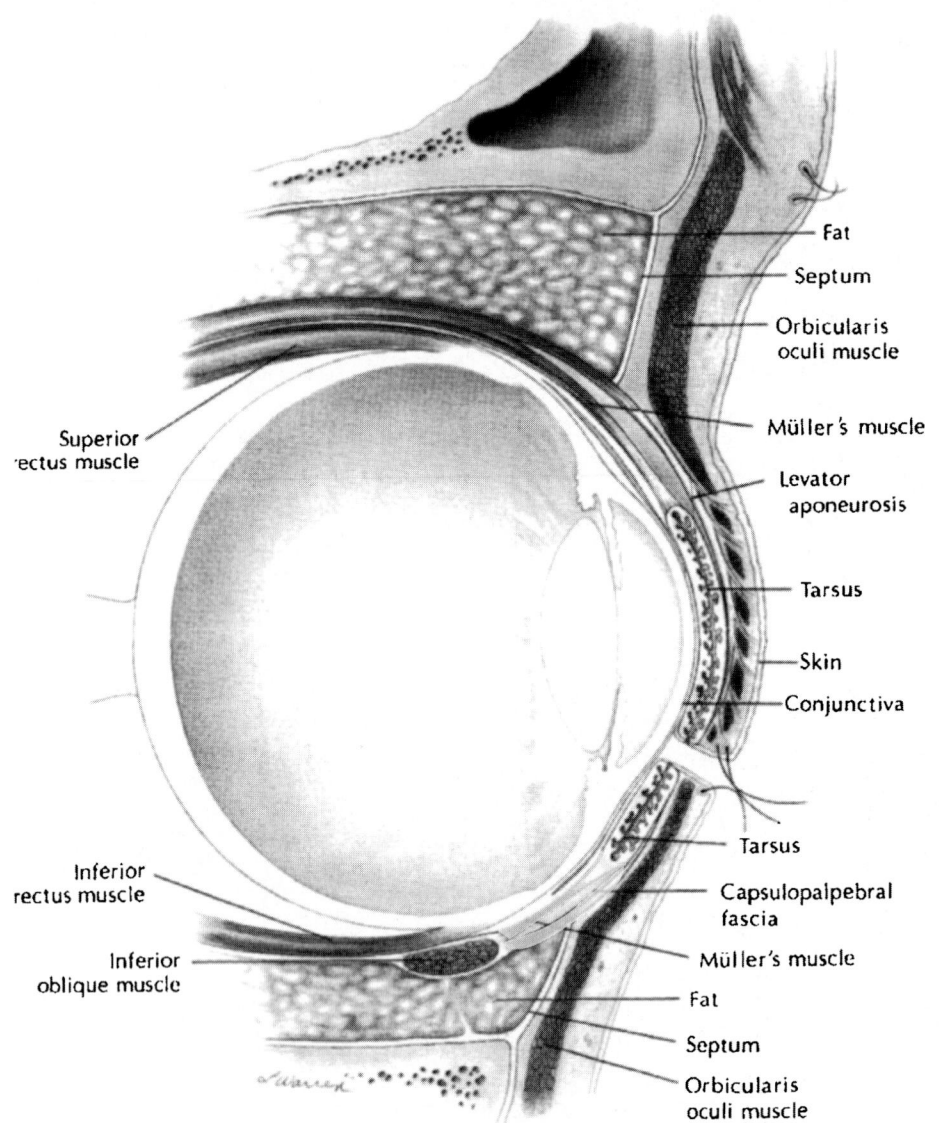

Fat

Septum

Orbicularis
oculi muscle

Müller's muscle

Levator
aponeurosis

Tarsus

Skin

Conjunctiva

Superior
rectus muscle

Tarsus

Capsulopalpebral
fascia

Müller's muscle

Fat

Septum

Orbicularis
oculi muscle

Inferior
rectus muscle

Inferior
oblique muscle

**FIGURE 22-2.** Cross section of eyelids and
schematized globe.
*(Reproduced with permission from Wobig J. Eyelid Anatomy. In: Putterman AM, ed. Cosmetic Oculoplastic Surgery, 2nd ed. Philadelphia: W.B. Saunders, p. 73, 1993.)*

Together, these structures surround the lacrimal sac within the lacrimal fossa. Tears enter the lacrimal cannaliculi through the punctcae of the upper and lower lids and flow into the lacrimal sac. With blinking, the components of the MCT squeeze the sac and force tears into the nasolacrimal duct. Zide et al. showed that the vector of the medial canthal tendon attachment is tangential to the medial aspect of the eyelids and that the vector of reconstruction is best directed just posterior and superior to the attachment of the anterior limb[8] (Fig. 22-3).

Fascial extensions from the upper and lower tarsal plates as well as the levator aponeurosis coalesce to form the superior and inferior limbs of the lateral canthal tendon. These limbs fuse laterally, creating a common tendon, and insert on a prominence of the lateral orbital wall called Whitnall's tubercle. The tubercle is usually located 2 mm posterior to the lateral orbital rim and 9 mm inferior to the zygomaticofrontal suture.

The external ear, or auricle, emanates superiorly, posteriorly, and inferiorly in an oblique lateral fashion from an external canal in the temporal bone. Normally, it projects 15–25° from the parasagittal plane. The cartilaginous framework defines ridges and hollows covered by perichondrium and skin with no subcutaneous fat. The innermost component is a conchal bowl divided into a superior and inferior portion by the root of the helix. The helix is the outermost fold and is supported in its superior two-thirds by cartilage. The inferior third consists only of a roll of skin. The antihelical fold is interposed between the helix and the concha and bifurcates in its superior third creating a triangular fossa in the interval between its superior and inferior crus. The anterior aspect of the concha and the external auditory canal is protected by a projection of cartilage known as the tragus.

The nose consists of nine aesthetic subunits and comprises a bony and cartilaginous framework with an overlying skin-soft tissue envelope. In the upper and middle third, these subunits include the midline dorsum and paired sidewalls. The dorsum is normally a straight projection from the nasofrontal junction supported in its superior half by the bony nasal pyramid and in its lower half by the cartilaginous septum and upper lateral cartilages. The subunits of the lower third include the midline tip, and columella, as well as the paired lateral sidewalls, soft triangles or facets, and alae. Only the facets contain no cartilage. The modern understanding of nasal architecture states that the lower third is analogous to a tripod consisting of the septum and the paired lower lateral cartilages.[9]

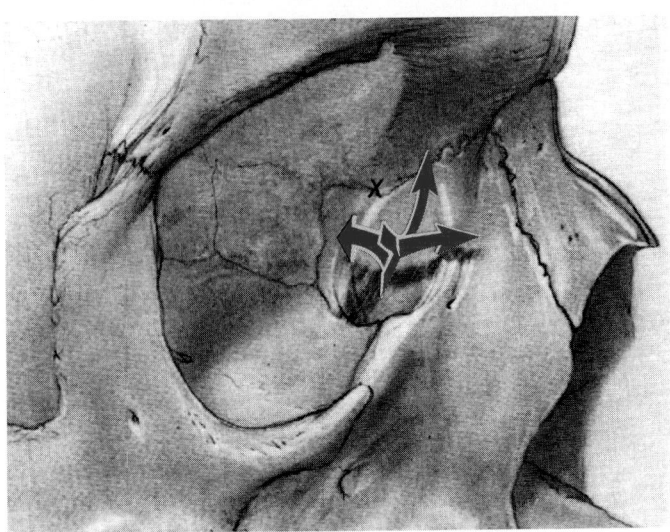

**FIGURE 22-3.** The components of the medial canthal tendon are represented by arrows. The resultant vector is best reconstructed by placing the tendon or a canthopexy stitch in a posterior-superior position, at the point X.
*(Reproduced with permission from Rodriguez L, Zide B. Reconstruction of the Medial Canthus. Clinics in Plastic Surgery 15:257, 1988.)*

Like the eyelids, the lips consist of a sphincteric orbicularis muscle (the orbicularis oris), adjunctive levator and depressor muscles, and tendonous support in the form of the modiolus. The modiolus is a tendonous meeting point of the orbicularis fibers and the depressors and levators of the oral commisure. Loss of muscular attachment to the modiolus or of the modiolus itself may result in rounding of the commisure and oral incompetence. The lip margins consist of vermillion, a thin non-keratinizing squamous epithelium overlying rich capillary beds. The junction of the vermillion and lip skin is called the white roll, and the junction of vermillion and mucosa is known as the wet line. The philtrum is found in the central aspect of the upper lip, extending vertically from the columella to the vermillion. The medial aspect is depressed and bounded by lateral philtral ridges that end inferiorly at two elevated points of the vermillion that form the handle of the "Cupid's bow."

The cheeks comprise the lateral aspect of the face, extending from its medial boundaries, the nasofacial sulcus and the melolabial groove, to its posterior boundary, the preauricular crease, and superiorly from the lower eyelid and temple to the inferior margin of the mandible. The key aesthetic point of the cheek is the malar prominence, discussed below. Most of the muscles of the facial expression live within a fibrofatty fascial layer of the cheek known as the superficial muscular aponeurotic system (SMAS). The SMAS lies superficial to the fascia over the parotid gland and the masseter muscle and is the key layer of lift and strength in the modern rhytidectomy.

## Visceral

The deep aspect of the cheek contains the parotid gland and facial nerve. The parotid gland gives bulk to the posterior cheek. It extends anteriorly from the external auditory canal to the posterior border of the masseter and from the zygomatic arch superiorly to just below the angle of the mandible. The parotid duct coalesces and exits from the midportion of the anterior aspect of the gland. It crosses the lateral surface of the masseter and enters the mouth through an orifice in the buccal mucosa lateral to the second maxillary

molar. The duct is intimately associated with the buccal branches of the facial nerve.

The facial nerve exits the stylomastoid foramen of the temporal bone medial to the styloid and lateral to the transverse process of the first cervical vertebral body and immediately enters the posterior aspect of the parotid gland. The nerve almost immediately divides into a superior and inferior division and then ramifies further creating five divisions: the frontal, the zygomatic, the buccal, the marginal mandibular, and the cervical. The frontal branch is the most superficial as it crosses the midpoint of the zygomatic arch. The zygomatic branch travels inferior to the zygomatic arch until it inserts on the deep surface of the upper and lower aspect of the orbicularis oculi. The buccal division consists of multiple anastomotic branches that course over the masseter muscle to innervate the nasal muscles as well as the levator muscles of facial expression. The inferior buccal branches eventually terminate in the upper lip portion of the orbicularis oris and the levator muscles of facial expression. The marginal mandibular branch loops over the antegonial notch of the mandible into the neck before returning to the face and terminating in the depressor anguli oris and lower aspect of the orbicularis. The cervical branch innervates the platysma muscle, itself contiguous with the SMAS and the temporoparietal fascia.

Sensory innervation of the face is supplied by the divisions of the fifth cranial nerve. The supraorbital and supratrochlear nerves serve the upper face, and the mental nerves innervate the lower lip and chin. The infraorbital nerve is the terminal extent of the second division of the fifth nerve and innervates the skin of the medial cheek, lateral nose, and upper lip. Its course extends from the foramen rotundum into the infraorbital fissure and canal, from which it exits through the infraorbital foramen. The foramen is found in the face of the maxilla 1 cm below the infraorbital rim in the midpupillary line. Prior to entering the inferior orbital groove, the second division of the trigeminal nerve divides, sending branches inferiorly in the walls of the maxillary antrum to the maxillary dentition.

The contents of the orbit include the globe, the extraocular muscles, the terminal branches of the second, third, fourth, and sixth cranial nerves, as well as terminal branches of the internal carotid arterial system. Notably, the anterior and posterior ethmoid arteries branch from the ophthalmic artery and traverse the medial orbital wall at the level of the frontoethmoid suture. They then course intracranially over the superior surface of the cribriform plate and terminate in the nasal cavity.

## Bony

The cranial vault, or neurocranium, extends superiorly and posteriorly from the bones of the basi- and viscerocranium. The upper face (the forehead) is supported by the paired, broad, flat frontal bones that articulate inferiorly with the nasal bone and frontal process of the maxilla medially and with the frontal process of the zygoma laterally. Posterior to the lateral orbital rims, the frontal bone articulates with the greater wing of the sphenoid. Inferiorly, the frontal bone is thickened over the orbits, creating the orbital bar, and at its inferior midline aspect, the diploic layer is replaced by a broad, pyramidal air-containing space with a narrow floor. This frontal sinus communicates with the nasal passage through the paired nasofrontal ducts that penetrate the sinus floor medially.

Intersinus septae are oriented vertically in roughly the parasagittal plane, but only partially separate frontal sinus cavities.

The midface comprises the paired maxillae, zygomas, and nasal bones. It articulates deeply with the orbital walls and ethmoid structures. Thickened regions of these structures comprise the medial, lateral, and posterior "vertical buttresses" as well as the "horizontal beams"—lines of thickened cortical bone that withstand greater loads than the intervening regions of thin, weak bone (Fig. 22-4). This lattice-like arrangement of the midface is suspended from the orbital bar and is projected from the skull base via its articulations with the ethmoid, pterygoid, and temporal bones. The vertical buttresses resist the forces of mastication and include the paired nasomaxillary (medial), zygomaticomaxillary (ZM) (lateral), and pterygomaxillary (posterior) struts. The zygomaticomaxillary is the strongest of these structures, extending from the maxillary alveolus above the first molar, across the ZM suture and the zygomaticofrontal (ZF) suture in the lateral orbital rim to the suprorbital bar. The nasomaxillary buttress ascends from the canine fossa into the lateral wall of the piriform aperture and the medial orbital wall. The pterygomaxillary buttress comprises thickened bone at the junction of the posterior maxillary sinus and the take-off of the pterygoid plates.

The horizontal stabilizers of the vertical struts are less robust and include the maxillary alveolar bone, the infraorbital rims, and the supraorbital rims (frontal bone). In addition, the orientation of medial and lateral pterygoid plates provides horizontal stabilization for the posterior buttress.

In the central midface, the infraorbital rims are connected across the midline by the bony nasal pyramid, and the medial orbits abut the ethmoid complex. The paired nasal bones project anteriorly from the ascending or frontal processes of the maxillae and articulate above with the supraorbital bar and below with the cartilaginous septum and upper lateral cartilages. Although the nasal bones connect the relatively thick inferior orbital rims and glabella, they are thin and impart little strength to the central midface. The ethmoid complex contributes little strength to the central midface, owing to the paper-thin nature of most of its components. The ethmoid bone consists of paired cassettes of air cells connected by a horizontal cribriform plate (the medial anterior fossa floor, transmitting the fibers of the first cranial nerve) and separated vertically by the perpendicular plate and the crista gali. Together, the nasal bones and ethmoid compex create a weak central midfacial skeleton that is dependent on the remainder of the craniofacial skeleton to produce the anterior projection of the nose and the appropriate attachment of the medial canthal tendons.[10]

The ethmoid also contributes the paper-thin lamina papyracea to the medial wall of the orbit. Anterior to the lamina, the medial orbital wall consists of the thick lacrimal bone which houses the lacrimal sac in a depression (the lacrimal fossa) between the raised anterior and posterior lacrimal crests and the segments of the medial canthal tendon. At the anterior-most aspect of the medial orbit is the ascending process of the maxilla. The frontal bone forms the roof of the orbit and articulates with the lamina papyracea before extending medially as the roof of the ethmoid air

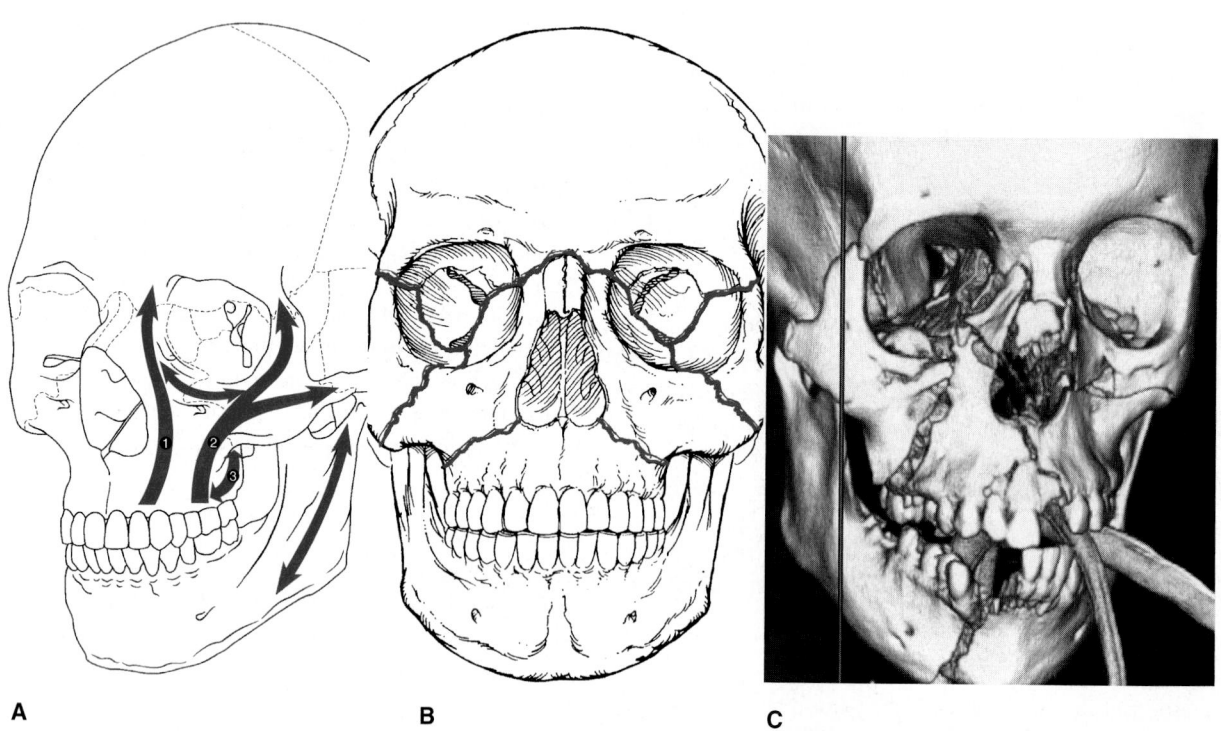

**A**                    **B**                    **C**

**FIGURE 22-4.** **(A)** Classic medial (1), lateral (2), and posterior (3) vertical maxillary buttresses and the infraorbital horizontal buttress. **(B)** Lines of the classic LeFort fractures of the midface. **(C)** Comminuted midface fractures, including right LeFort III, bilateral Le Fort II, and left Le Fort I fractures as well as frontal sinus, orbital, and palatal fractures, demonstrating the complex pathology commonly resulting from high-speed blunt force trauma.
*(A) (Reproduced with permission from Forrest CR, Pillips JH, Prein J. Craniofacial Fractures, Le Fort I-III Fractures. In: Prein J, ed. Manual of Internal Fixation in the Cranio-Facial Skeleton. Berlin Heidelberg: Springer-Verlag, 1998, p. 109.)*
*(B) (Reproduced with permission from Ducic Y, Hamlar DD. Fractures of the Midface. Facial Plast Surg Clin North Am. 6:471, 1998.)*

cells. The lateral orbital wall consists of the greater wing of the sphenoid and the zygoma anteriorly. The orbital floor is predominately formed by the orbital plate of the maxilla, although the zygoma contributes on the lateral side. Vertical processes of the palatine bones also contribute to the medial orbital walls. Posteriorly, the orbital plate of the maxilla sweeps medially and superiorly to meet the lamina papyracea. The orbital roof and floor are mostly concave anteriorly and house the globe, but the floor is convex antero-medially. Thus, an antero-medial fracture that eliminates this convexity will significantly enlarge the orbital volume and result in enophthalmos.

The zygoma is the keystone structure of the midfacial buttress system. The infraorbital rim and lateral buttress intersect in the body of the zygoma. Thus, the zygoma and maxilla in this region are considered together as a zygomaticomaxillary complex (ZMC). The components of the ZMC are commonly referred to as a "tripod," although in reality all five articulations between the zygoma and the adjacent facial skeleton support the malar eminence. These include not only the zygomaticomaxillary (ZM) suture, the zygomaticofrontal (ZF) suture, and the inferior orbital rim, but also the zygomatic arch, and the zygomaticosphenoid (ZS) suture in the infero-lateral orbital wall. These components support a key aesthetic landmark, the malar projection, which can be understood as two arcs intersecting at the zygoma: a vertical arc comprises the ZM buttress and the lateral orbital rim (the ZF suture), and a horizontal arc comprises the infraorbital rim and the zygomatic arch[11] (Fig. 22-5).

The lower facial skeleton is dominated by the mandible. The mandibular alveolus is the arch of tooth-bearing bone that extends anteriorly from the angle. The alveolar bone is supported inferiorly by the symphyseal, paraysmphyseal, and body portions of the mandibular arch, which is thicker along its inferior border. Anteroinferiorly, the symphyseal and parasymphyseal bone projects slightly anteriorly, creating the skeletal basis of the chin. The mandibular arch projects anteriorly from the angle, and posterosuperiorly, the flat, roughly sagitally oriented rami extend vertically to their articulation with the temporal bone at the temporomandibular joint (TMJ). The superior extent of the ramus ends in the coronoid process anteriorly, the condylar process posteriorly, and an intervening sigmoid notch. Along the anterosuperior surface of the angle, the transition from ramus to alveolus is marked by an oblique ridge of bone called the oblique line. The inferior alveolar neurovascular triad enters the lingual surface of ramus at its midportion and then travels inferiorly and anteriorly in the substance of the body. Before exiting the mental foramen below the first or second premolar, the inferior alveolar nerve ramifies to each tooth providing afferent sensory information. After exiting the mental foramen, the mental nerve provides sensation to the lower lip and chin.

## EVALUATION

An understanding of the pathophysiology of facial trauma informs the clinical and radiographic evaluation of facial injuries.

### Soft Tissue

Soft-tissue injuries are generally obvious on initial physical exam; however, all soft-tissue wounds must be accurately evaluated and documented. After adequate local anesthesia, wounds should be carefully probed and examined. The surgeon is interested in the location, longitudinal extent, and depth of a wound, as well as the loss of tissue, the quality of residual tissue, and the involvement of skeletal and visceral structures. The ability to reconstruct soft tissue wounds is dependent on the degree of soft-tissue loss.[12–14] After high-energy soft tissue wounding resulting from avulsion or ballistic energy, a zone of lost tissue is surrounded by a zone of injured tissue. In the days following an injury, tissue necrosis will continue to evolve within the zone of injured tissue.[12–14]

Close-range versus distant gunshot wounds are differentiated based on the amount of energy imparted to a wound. Most non-shotgun ballistic wounds occur from a distance and are, therefore,

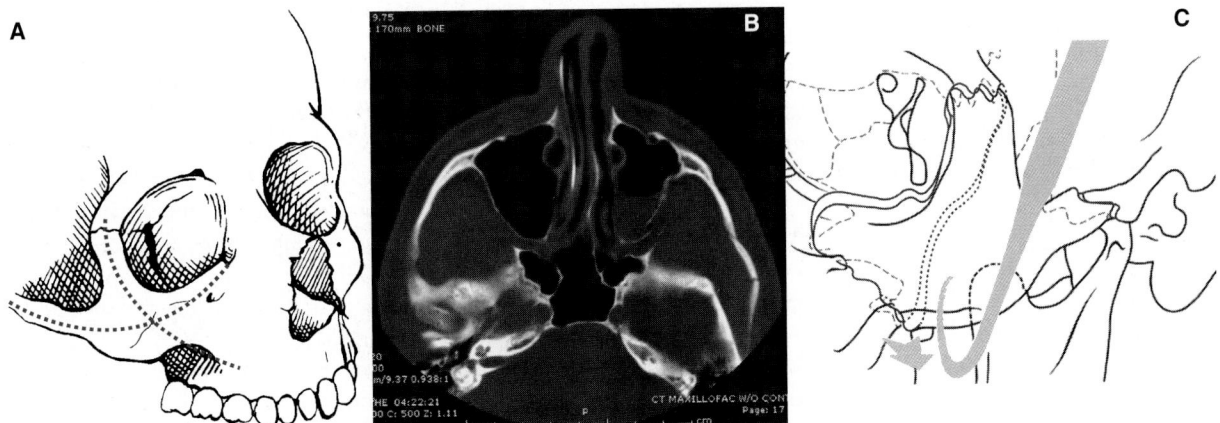

**FIGURE 22-5.** **(A)** The vertical and horizontal arcs created by the zygomaticomaxillary complex. **(B)** Axial CT image of left zygomaticomaxillary fracture demonstrates loss of malar projection. **(C)** Schematic illustration of use of the bone hook to mobilize the zygomaticomaxillary complex.
(A) (Reproduced with permission from American Medical Association. *Archives of Otolaryngology – Head and Neck Surgery, Citation* 115:1459, 1989.)
(C) (Reproduced with permission from Markowitz BL, Manson PN. Craniofacial Fractures, Zygomatic Complex Fractures. In: Prein J, ed. *Manual of Internal Fixation in the Cranio-Facial Skeleton.* Berlin: Springer-Verlag, 1998, p. 133.)

low velocity (less than 1200 ft/second).[14] They usually cause limited loss of soft tissue and localized injury to the craniofacial skeleton. They are treated similar to blunt wounds with overlying soft tissue lacerations and are classified by the path of the bullet.[14] Close-range ballistic wounds, in contrast, may cause massive loss of soft tissue and bone, a limiting factor in the likelihood for successful reconstruction[12–14]; they can be classified according to the region of tissue loss. Shotgun wounds are commonly inflicted from close range and impart energy to an even wider field of tissue. Suicide attempts represent the most common shotgun wounds, and these usually direct energy to the lower face and midface from below.[12–14]

Skin does not respond to blunt trauma randomly. Lee et al. determined that blunt trauma results in repeatable patterns of soft tissue wounding.[15] In a study of blunt wounds to cadaver heads, they found that in approximately 80% of wounds the skin broke along cleavage planes as previously defined by others. These cleavage planes resemble the relaxed skin tension lines along which wrinkles occur (cleavage lines originally described by Langer), and are likely related to the orientation of collagen fibers and elastic bundles within the dermis.[15] Lee et al. also proposed a complex method of documenting soft-tissue wounds so that future study may be improved.[16] However, this has not been widely adopted.

## Visceral

Vital visceral structures are housed within and around the face. High-energy mechanism, deep soft-tissue wounds, craniofacial fractures, and multiorgan trauma suggest the possibility of an intracranial injury. The neurologic exam should be repeated and a head CT should be obtained routinely. Ophthalmologic examination of acuity, afferent pupillary defects, and extraocular motion should be performed and repeated, and injury to the lacrimal drainage system must be considered as well. The loss of facial sensation may suggest the depth or extent of injury. Facial paralysis must be identified, given that primary facial nerve anastamosis should be attempted during primary repair of a facial wound. Wounds to the cheek or submental region that injure the salivary glands or ducts should be identified.

## Bony

Most often, craniofacial fractures occur along well-recognized lines of weakness in the midfacial skeleton and in repeated patterns in the mandible. Clinical evaluation is directed by knowledge of these typical fractures.

Upper Face.    Upper facial fractures usually involve the frontal sinus. A laceration of the forehead skin and depression of the forehead suggest a possible fracture of the anterior table of the frontal sinus. The presence of an anterior table fracture associated with mental status changes or CSF rhinorrhea should alert the surgeon to possible posterior table involvement, a dural tear, or a traumatic brain injury.

Midface.    The lattice system of medial and lateral buttresses usually prevents random fractures through the midface.[17] Instead, the midface most commonly fractures along the classic weak lines described

by Rene LeFort in 1901, although variations in the pattern and in the combination of LeFort fractures are the rule[11,18] (Fig. 22-4). A Le Fort I fracture usually results from horizontal or downward force applied to the anterior alveolus. The fracture line crosses the medial, lateral, and posterior buttresses in their inferior aspect as well as the antral walls, piriform aperture, and septum. This separates the maxillary alveolus and palate from the upper midface. In the upper midface, the level, pattern, and combination of Le Fort II and III fractures depend less on the point of impact than on the vector of impact relative to the Frankfort Horizontal.[17] Horizontal impact of the upper midface usually results in Le Fort II fracture line, which crosses from the nasal dorsum, ascending process of the maxilla, and lacrimal bones into the orbit. In the orbit, the fracture line descends through the floor and infraorbital rim, into the anterior and lateral antral walls and through the pterygoid plates. This separates a pyramidal central midfacial and alveolar segment from the zygomas and pterygoid plates. In contrast, downward, oblique impact separates the facial skeleton from the skull base ("craniofacial disjuncture") via fractures across the nasofrontal suture, the lacrimal and ethmoid bones, and into the orbital floor. At the inferior orbital groove, the fracture trifurcates, extending across the ZF suture, the zygomatic arch, and the pterygoid plates.

Clinical examination of the vertical and horizontal buttresses involves inspection and palpation. Massive soft-tissue injury suggests underlying facial fractures, although massive edema may obscure the exam. Mobility of the midface relative to the skull base suggests a Le Fort fracture. Le Fort fractures can be differentiated based upon the axial level of mobility, signs of orbital wall fractures (discussed below), and evidence of central midface fractures such as loss of nasal pyramid projection and telecanthus. Palatal fractures in the sagittal plane are suggested by palatal lacerations, widening of the dental arch, and abrupt changes in the vertical level of dentition. Step-off deformities of the infraorbital rims may be palpated. The upper midface fractures classically cause the face to recede posteroinferiorly, creating a flat or "dish-face" appearance. This commonly results in early posterior contact and anterior open-bite. Le Fort III fractures, especially in isolation, are relatively rare.[19]

The lateral application of force to the malar prominence most commonly results in fractures of the ZMC, although a high-speed blow to the malar eminence may transmit force to the vertical buttresses. Fractures free the zygoma from its articulations, collapsing the horizontal and vertical arcs. The masseter rotates the zygomatic body inferiorly. The zygomatic arch fracture (as with the Le Fort III fracture) disrupts the relationship of the zygoma to the temporal bone, reducing the anterior projection of the zygoma.[10,11,17,18,20] Displacement at the inferior orbital rim reduces lateral projection. The result is loss of the anterior, lateral, and vertical position of the malar eminence. Despite varying degrees of edema, malar flattening is evident from the vertex or basal perspective.[19]

Fractures of the weak, central compartment of the midface result in characteristic naso-orbital ethmoid (NOE) injuries. The sine-quo-non of the NOE fracture is telecanthus. Disruption of the bony attachment of the medial canthi can be determined through inspection and palpation. The nasal root will appear broad and the canthus will appear rounded and lateralized. The central bony fragments may be easily mobilized, and the canthal tendons may give easily with gentle lateral tugging. The canthi should be no further apart than the alar base of the nose and should be roughly one half of the interpupillary

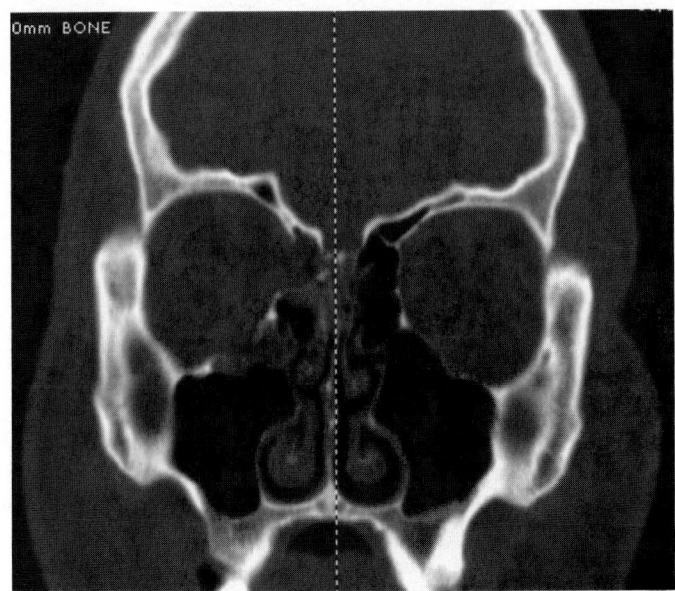

**FIGURE 22-6.** Coronal CT image of orbital blowout fracture with disruption of the orbital floor and medial orbital wall. Entrapment of the medial rectus muscle is also seen.

distance. In general, an intercanthal distance of greater than 35 mm is suggestive of telecanthus, and greater than 45 mm is usually definitive.[21,22] Care must be taken to measure with calipers directly applied to the medial extent of the canthus, touching bone if possible. Soft tissue edema can produce the illusion of telecanthus. CSF rhinorrhea may result from disruption of the cribriform plate of the ethmoid bone or the roof of the ethmoid air cells. Ocular and orbital findings should also alert the surgeon to possible NOE injury.

Orbit.   If force is transmitted through the midface articulations with the orbit, orbital wall and floor fractures may result (Fig. 22-6). Isolated orbital blowout fractures (fractures of the orbital walls without associated fractures through the orbital rims) occur when blunt force is applied directly to the orbital contents and transmitted to the walls. Intraorbital volume is increased, the orbital soft tissues take on a spherical rather than conical shape,[11] and the

globe recedes posteriorly (known as "enophthalmos"). Diplopia is readily recognized by the patient. Enophthalmos is often evident on the basal or vertex view of the patient, although orbital and periorbital edema may fill the enlarged orbital volume, temporarily preventing recession of the globe. Orbital wall fractures may also result in herniation and entrapment, most commonly of the inferior or medial rectus muscle, restricting extraocular movements. Chemosis, scleral injection, periorbital ecchymosis, and diplopia suggest orbital fractures.

Mandible.   Mandibular fractures also occur in stereotypical patterns relating to the point of impact and the amount of energy imparted. The weakest points of the mandible include the subcondylar region, the angle, and the parasymphsyseal regions. The presence of a third molar or a wisdom tooth weakens the angle, and the canine tooth root and mental foramen compromise the parasymphysis. Not surprisingly, these sites are the most common points of fracture, regardless of the point of impact. Energy may be absorbed at the point of impact or, if it does not exceed the strain capacity of that point, may be transmitted to distant, weaker points of the bone where fractures may occur. Thus, lower velocity impact at the symphysis may be transmitted such that a parasymphyseal fracture or bilateral subcondylar fractures may occur. In contrast, a high-energy impact at the symphysis may result in immediate, local fracture of the symphysis as well as bilateral angle or subcondylar fractures. Similarly, a low-velocity blow to the body or parasymphysis will result in a nondisplaced fracture at the point of impact and a contralateral angle or subcondylar fracture. A high-energy blow to the body may result in massive comminution at the point of impact if the force is not transmitted so that no distant fractures occur.

Clinical evaluation can be directed by knowledge of the mechanism of injury. In addition, gingival lacerations, ecchymoses, and bleeding are signs of underlying fracture. Malocclusion, facial asymmetry, stepoff deformities of the dental arch, mobility of the arch with palpation (performed gently), pain, trismus (restricted mandibular movement) are obvious indications for radiographic imaging (Fig. 22-7).

Radiographic Evaluation.   CT scanning has essentially replaced plain film radiography for evaluation of craniofacial fractures.

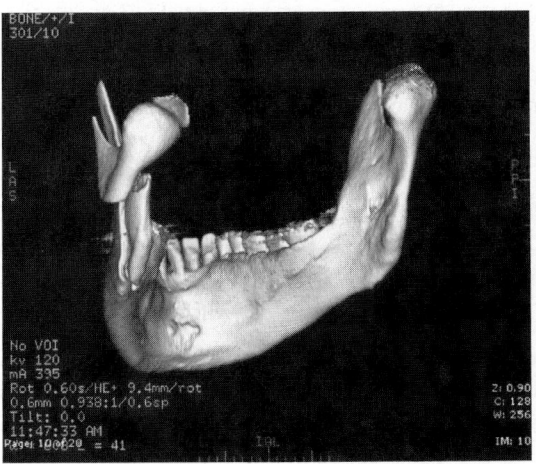

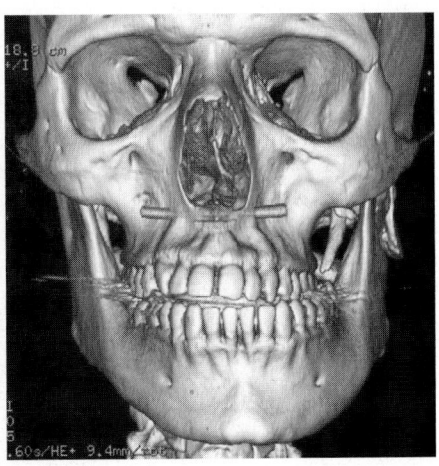

**FIGURE 22-7.** **(A)** Three-dimensional CT scan of the mandible demonstrates the ease with which the special orientation of the segments of this subcondylar and ramus fracture are visualized. **(B)** Three-dimensional CT scan of the same patient with mandible in situ. Evident are the cross bite and anterior open bite as well the facial asymmetry that results from vertical shortening of the left ramus.

A                                      B

Studies have shown that CT evaluation of the mandible will reveal fractures not visible on plain and panoramic radiographs,[23] and only horizontal subcondylar fractures may prove difficult to identify on CT images. Here, the panoramic radiograph still proves useful, although panorex images will not clearly demonstrate midline symphyseal fractures and may not be feasible during the management of a trauma. As mentioned, most polytrauma patients with any sign of facial injury may undergo maxillofacial CT during the initial workup. It has been determined that specific soft tissue injuries including lip lacerations, intraoral lacerations, periorbital contusion, subconjunctival hemorrhage, and nasal laceration are statistically correlated with the presence of facial fractures in trauma patients undergoing head CT. Perhaps the most siginificant advancement in imaging is the three-dimensional (3D) reconstruction of axial CT sections (see Chap. 16). Three-dimensional CT images can be rotated 180 or 360° on a variable axis and clearly reveal fracture lines as well as the relations of small bony fragments (Fig. 22-7). With multiple complex fractures, 3D images facilitate surgical planning; however, it must kept in mind that the computer algorithms that create the 3D images do create some inaccuracies, so that careful analysis of directly obtained CT images remains essential.[24,25]

## MANAGEMENT

### Soft Tissue

Low-Energy Wounds.   Careful written and photographic documentation of injuries and their repair may be useful in counseling patients and in interacting with the legal system, which may be necessary. Such documentation should not delay the administration of narcotic analgesia if needed. Most soft-tissue wounds are then managed at the bedside using local anesthesia. When possible, the sequence of nerve block, followed by field block, and then local infiltration may reduce the discomfort of the injection and reduce the volume of anesthetic required.[26]

After local anesthesia is achieved, wounds are debrided and cleansed. Contamination and foreign material are sources of deep tissue infection which further destroys tissue via reduced partial pressure of oxygen and collagenolysis,[27] spoils attempts at reconstruction, and causes systemic illness. In addition, granules of foreign material embedded in the skin can cause permanent tattooing.[4] Embedded foreign material, identified both visually and radiographically, is, therefore, carefully picked away or scrubbed clear. Some foreign bodies, such as glass particles, are not readily evident radiographically and are only found with painstaking inspection of the wound. Local application of antibiotic solutions (e.g., hydrogen peroxide) is not helpful and may cause further tissue damage.[4,27] Copious saline irrigation is commonly performed, although one group found that irrigation does not significantly reduce the risk of infection or improve the cosmetic outcome in facial wounds that are superficial, minimally contaminated, and less than six hours old.[28] They suggest that irrigation may damage tissue and that such wounds are amenable to cleansing with saline and gauze.

Debridement is limited to frankly necrotic soft tissue. Given the abundant vascularity of the face, tissue that appears compromised,

but not necrotic, is likely to survive.[4,27] Abraded tissue will demonstrate abnormal texture and color relative to the depth of abrasion; however, unless the area of abrasion is small and can be easily excised, it is best to allow the abrasion to heal and to consider secondary scar revision in the future. Similarly, jagged wound edges should not be trimmed, but rather re-approximated and revised secondarily. The broken line may actually prove advantageous, preventing scar contracture and providing better camouflage than straight-line closures.[4,26,27]

The following general principles may then be applied to the closure of soft tissue wounds of the face. First, with adequate debridement and irrigation, the robust vascularity of the face supports primary closure of almost all facial wounds. With proper antimicrobial therapy, the incidence of secondary infection is low, even in the setting of bite wounds less than 24 hours old. Closure of facial wounds by secondary intention typically results in unacceptable scars. Second, wounds should be closed in a layered fashion. Mucosa is closed with interrupted absorbable sutures, while muscle should be reapproximated with braided, absorbable suture. Failure to reapproximate muscular layers can result in loss of function and facial deformity, as well as depressed and excessively wide scars. Skin closure is accomplished with interrupted absorbable polyglycan 4-0 dermal stitches (except in the thin skin of the nose, eyelids, and ear) followed by 5-0, or 6-0 monofilament sutures in the epidermis. In small children, where suture removal presents an additional challenge, 6-0 fast absorbing gut may be used. Every attempt is made to achieve eversion of wound edges. Where tissue is lost via avulsion, undermining the skin up to 2–4 cm from the wound edge will often allow primary closure. Undermining is usually accomplished in the subcutaneous plane, although the forehead and scalp are undermined in the subgaleal plane, and nasal skin is undermined in the submuscular plane. In larger avulsions, local or regional flaps may be needed. Alternatively, a skin graft can be used in the acute setting, and definitive closure can be achieved in the future when the full range of reconstructive techniques may be more available.[26] Facial sutures should be removed early, often at four to five days and certainly within one week, in order to prevent "railroad track" scars.

The reconstruction of specialized soft-tissue structures of the face requires attention. In a schematized sense, the lips and eyelids share a common anatomic construction, as do the nose and ear. The lips and eyelids comprise sphincteric orbicularis muscle, adjunctive levator and depressor muscles, and tendinous supporting structures located at their transverse margins. (The eyelids possess the additional features of an indwelling tarsal plate and fascial septum.) The nose and ears are distinguished by soft tissue envelopes supported by an underlying cartilaginous framework. Based on these anatomic similarities, distinct principles guide the repair of the lips and eyelids and the repair of the nose and ears.

Lips.   The mucosa, the orbicularis, and the skin are closed in discrete layers. The primary aim is reapproximation of the white roll and the vermillion margin, as well as the wet line and the orbicularis. Great care is taken to precisely reapproximate the vermillion-cutaneous junction, since the slightest mismatch is easily observed, and the white roll can be surprisingly difficult to visualize when obscured by injury and by blanching caused by epinephrine. Thus, the authors commonly begin lip closures with a single interrupted skin suture at the vermillion-cutaneous border followed by a muscular stitch that also contributes to precise alignment. Next, the mucosa is closed with interrupted absorbable sutures. The remainder of the muscle and skin is then closed. Several muscular sutures are required, not only to reconstitute the oral sphincter, but to prevent notching and segmental depression resulting from an underlying muscle diastasis.

Multiple algorithms exist for the reconstruction of full thickness lip defects.[29] Primary closure can be accomplished for defects of less than half of a lip. Local flaps are utilized in defects of up to two-thirds of the lip, and free flap reconstruction is useful in defects of the entire lip. These efforts are rarely employed in the acute phase. The philtral ridges are especially difficult to reconstruct. When defective, an Abbe flap (a pedicled lip-switch procedure) provides the appearance of a discrete filtral subunit in the midline.[30] The extended Abbe flap can be used to reconstruct lip defects that include portions of the medial cheek or columella.[30] A sharp and competent angle at the commisure is also difficult to reconstitute. Reattachment of oral and facial muscles to the modiolus is key to this reconstruction. Although a full commissuroplasty may not be possible in the acute setting, primary reconstitution of the modiolus should be attempted. Contracture of disconnected muscles impedes secondary commisuroplasty.

Eyelids.    Similar to lip repair, eyelid closure involves layered closure of the lamellae, as well as careful reconstruction of the lateral supporting structures, in this case the canthal tendons. Thus, the tarsus is reapproximated with interrupted absorbable 6-0 stitches; however, the levator aponeurosis must be repaired such that lid ptosis is prevented. The grey line is reapproximated with 6-0 silk suture. The conjunctiva may be closed with interrupted sutures, although often this is not necessary. Finally, the skin and orbicularis may be closed as a single flap.

The canthal tendons must be repaired if torn or if displaced from the orbital rims. The crura of the lateral tendon are reapproximated, and the stump of the common lateral canthal tendon is sewn either to the periosteum or to a drill-hole in the lateral rim. If the periosteum is used, consideration should be given to a slightly superior repositioning given that some relaxation will occur postoperatively. Failure to reposition the lateral canthus will result in a rounded, sad appearing eye and ectropion. Note that there is a common misperception that the lateral canthus attaches more superiorly than the medial canthus; however, recent analyses have revealed that these attachments are actually along a horizontal line.[31] Repair of the medial canthal tendon is covered below in a discussion of nasal orbital ethmoid complex fractures.

With medial lid and medial canthal injuries, the lacrimal drainage system may be damaged, resulting in epiphora. After probing and cannulation of the punctum, lacerations may be repaired over a silastic stent. The stent is brought out through the end of the nasolacrimal duct in the inferior meatus of the nose and is left in place until inflammation subsides, typically three to six months. In all cases, significant disruption of the lower lid may indicate the need for a temporary Frost stitch to prevent lid retraction during healing. This consists of a stitch through the lower lid margin, which is taped to the forehead keeping the lower lid on mild tension.

Nose.    The principles of augmentive rhinoplasty[9] and of nasal reconstruction of skin cancer defects[32] are utilized in repairing soft-tissue trauma of the nose. Superficial lacerations can often be closed primarily. The relatively inelastic nasal skin is, however, prone to scar contracture, trapdoor deformity, and scar depression. Therefore, wound edges are everted via submuscular undermining, deep sutures that reapproximate wound margins, and skin closure with vertical mattress sutures. Small areas ($<1$ cm) of skin loss located in concavities of the nasal surface (such as the nasofacial or alar facial sulci) can be left to granulate, as these tend to heal nicely by secondary intention.[32] If necessary, the underlying cartilaginous framewok is reconstructed. Lacerated lateral cartilages should be reapproximated with interrupted 4-0 polydioxanone sutures. The alar rims, especially in the soft triangles, are especially prone to notching as a result of scar contracture. Here, eversion of wound edges is essential, and skin is supported with underlying cartilage batten grafts harvested from the septum or auricular conchae.

In the case of significant loss of soft tissue, multiple nasal skin flaps, cartilage grafts, and composite grafts from the ear can be employed for partial thickness reconstruction,[32] but are beyond the scope of this chapter. In general, full thickness defects require three-layer repair of the nasal mucosal lining, the cartilaginous framework, and the overlying skin envelope. Commonly, pedicled septal or turbinate mucosa flaps are used to line a defect. Auricular or septal cartilage is fashioned into grafts that batten the lower lateral cartilages, open the internal valves and buttress the dorsum, or augment the dorsum and tip. Interpolated, two-stage forehead or cheek flaps then provide external cover.

The septum must be examined. The septal cartilage is fed through its mucoperichondrium and is devascularized when the mucuperichondrium is raised by a hematoma. Devitalization and resorption of the caritlagenous septum can occur within days to weeks and, over time, this will result in a saddle-nose deformity which may require extensive reconstruction. Hematomas are therefore aspirated or drained via incision and drainage. A quilting stitch or a nasal pack is placed in order to coapt the cartilage and mucoperichondrium and to prevent reaccumulation.

Ear.    As with the nose, ear skin is inelastic and supported by a cartilaginous framework. Lacerations of skin and cartilage must be meticulously repaired. Auricular cartilage is directly repaired and/or the anterior and posterior perichondrium are reapproximated, and, where the cartilaginous support is absent, supporting cartilaginous grafts may be introduced and wound edges everted in order to prevent notching. Analogous to the septal hematoma, an auricular hematoma separates the skin from the underlying cartilage and must be evacuated. The cartilagenous architecture may become severely distorted as a result of devascularization, the development of organized scar between skin and cartilage, or infection. A hematoma may be removed through needle aspiration or a small stab incision, and a bolster is then sewn to the ear.

Significant tissue loss requires grafting of cartilage, often taken from the contralateral concha, and soft tissue coverage. For large defects, pedicled, staged soft tissue flaps provide coverage. Postauricular skin flaps cover the helix and antihelix well, and the temporoparietal fascial flap covered by a skin graft is useful for larger defects.

For complete or near-complete avulsion, primary reattchment of the auricle, two-stage postauricular skin flap coverage of the auricle, and microvascular reanastomosis have been reported. If the amputated segment is available, simply sewing the avulsed segment into place is unlikely to succeed, even with the use of hyperbaric oxygen therapy. Most authors support removal of skin and perichondrium from the avulsed cartilage, reapproximation of the avulsed cartilage to the intact auricular cartilage, and implantation of the exposed, reconnected cartilage in a postauricular skin pocket within six hours. The second stage is performed after a period of approximately three months. The postauricular skin is incised posterior to the embedded cartilage and is raised with that cartilage from the surface of the mastoid. The posterior surface of the auricle is skin grafted and the postauricular region is closed via a local flap, skin grafted, or left to granulate. Delay of the second-stage flap elevation may be useful in order to ensure that the raised postauricular skin may survive on its anterior attachments. Microvascular anastomosis has proven successful, but requires prompt action and appropriate expertise for anastomosis of 1mm vessels.

## Visceral

Injuries to the cheek involving deep tissue must be explored for possible trauma to the parotid gland and duct. Laceration of the gland itself is often not reparable, although an attempt at closure of the parotidomasseteric fascia may be made. Injury to the parotid gland may result in a salivary-cutaneous fistula or sialocele.

It is particularly important to assess for a possible injury to Stenson's duct. Treatment options for ductal injuries include primary anastomosis, creation of an oral fistula, ductal ligation, and conservative nonoperative measures. Primary anastomosis is best suited to injuries of the proximal ⅔ of the duct. Upon exploration of the wound, lacerated ends of the duct are identified and cannulated with a lacrimal probe. An angiocatheter or silastic stent is then inserted from the ductal orifice in the mouth into both the distal segment, across the open interval, and then into proximal segment. The duct is then anastomosed under magnification, and the stent is left in place for up to two weeks. If the ductal segments cannot be coapted without tension, autologous vein may be interposed.[33,34]

When injuries are located in the distal third of the duct or when they involve tissue loss such that reanastomosis is not possible, the proximal segment may be diverted to a new, more proximal orifice created in the cheek. A new orifice is opened through the buccinator and buccal mucosa, and the end of the duct is sewn to the buccal mucosa. No stent is required. Ductal ligation may be necessary when both primary anastomosis and ductal diversion prove impossible, as occurs with severe tissue loss. In this case, the proximal duct may be ligated. The gland will at first swell and become painful, but will eventually atrophy. In this situation, antisialogogues are useful to reduce salivary output and pain.

Alternatively, conservative management is supported by some authors.[35–37] Gland and ductal injuries have been managed successfully through salivary suppression and expectant management of sialoceles or cutaneous fistulas as they arise.

Salivary cutaneous fistula and sialoceles may result from injury to the gland, an unrecognized ductal laceration, or intentionally conservative management of parotid injury. Sialoceles should be aspirated in serial fashion. Fluid can be assayed for amylase in order to confirm its nature. Reaccumulation of the sialocele and persistence of the salivary fistula is reduced by the application of a pressure dressing, which may encourage atrophy of the gland. In addition, parotid output should be suppressed by antisialogogues. Antisialogogues include anticholinergics and may be administered via oral or transdermal routes.[38] Recently, the use of botulinum toxin A (Botox A) in the treatment of traumatic sialocele and salivary fistula has been reported.[39] More radical means of reducing parotid output include tympanic neurectomy, parotidectomy, and low-dose radiotherapy,[40] although these modalities carry significant risk of complications.

Injury to facial nerve branches often accompanies injury to the parotid gland. If evidence of paralysis in one or more regions of the seventh nerve is found on physical exam, an attempt at primary microsurgical reanastomosis should be made at the time of initial wound repair. If necessary, the nerve is mobilized such that segments may be coapted without tension. The epineurium is then reapproximated under magnification with interrupted 8-0 or 10-0 sutures.[4] If a tension free anastomosis is not possible, a cable graft may be used to span the open interval. Recovery after reanastomosis may be prolonged for up to 24 months.[41] If permanent paralysis is encountered, techniques for static and active facial reanimation may be employed secondarily.[42–44] Eyelid paralysis should be managed conservatively with lubricants and artificial tears, and a gold weight can be placed to aid in upper lid closure, since this can be removed if function of the facial nerve returns. At night, a moisture chamber or eyelid tape should be applied in order to prevent corneal dessication until a secondary lid procedure can be performed.[45]

## Facial Skeleton

**Soft Tissue Approaches.** If facial lacerations exist, they may provide adequate exposure with minimal extension. Otherwise, the principles of soft tissue approaches include minimizing (and avoiding) incisions in facial skin and protecting neurovascular structures while achieving maximal exposure.

The coronal approach exposes the entire upper face down to the nasal bones as well as the anterior calvarium, lateral orbital rims, and zygomas.[46,47] The scalp is incised in serpentine, geometric, or gently curved (Soutar) fashion from the root of the auricular helix on one side to the other. A scalp flap is raised anteriorly in either the subgaleal or subperiosteal plane between the temporal lines. If a pericranial flap will be harvested, the subgaleal plane is often followed, leaving a healthy layer of loose areolar tissue down on the pericranium. Alternatively, the pericranium can be raised with the scalp and harvested from the scalp flap secondarily.

Extreme care is required not to disrupt the temporal branches of the facial nerve. Lateral to the temporal lines, dissection is carried forward and inferior just over the fascia of the temporalis muscle until the temporal line of fusion is encountered. Below this line, the temporalis fascia divides in the sagittal plane, and the temporalis fat pad can be seen through the superficial layer of temporalis fascia. The authors recommend opening the superficial fascia over the temporalis fat pad and carrying the superficial fascial layer forward with the scalp flap, thus protecting the frontalis branch (Fig. 22-1 and 22-8A). Alternatively, hugging this layer during elevation will generally avoid nerve injury. The pericranium is then raised and dissection is carried forward to the superior and lateral orbital rims and inferiorly to the zygomatic arches. Dissection is carried into the orbit, protecting the supratrochlear and supraorbital neurovascular bundles. The lacrimal apparatus is freed from the lacrimal fossa, and the orbital contents are allowed to drop forward slightly out of the orbits themselves. The anterior ethmoid arteries are clipped or cauterized and divided.

If unilateral exposure is needed, an extended hemi-coronal flap can be raised on one side only. Similarly, dissection down to the zygomatic arches can be avoided if no management of the arches is required. Still, the dissection is always carried over the temporalis muscle, simply to allow adequate rotation of the anterior flap.

Scalp closure is achieved in layers. A wide scar is prevented by taking particular care to reapproximate the galea, the most robust and inelastic layer. The skin may be sutured or stapled, and drains may be placed if no connection with the subarachnoid space exists, although they are not essential.

Exposure of the midface is obtained through a sublabial or midface degloving approach (Fig. 22-8B). When combined with a coronal approach, tissue of the entire upper two-thirds of the face is raised in continuity. After an incision in the superior oral vestibule is made perpendicular to mucosa and then deepened perpendicular to bone, a subperiosteal dissection over the face of the maxilla is performed. The infraorbital nerve is usually easily identified and protected, even when fracture lines traverse its foramen. Transversely, the exposure extends from the lateral aspect of the zygomatic process of the maxilla to the nasal bones. Superiorly, dissection is carried over the inferior orbital rim and the inferior aspect of the medial and lateral orbital rims. The approach is tailored to the clinical situation so as to minimize subperiosteal dissection.

Conversely, even greater midface exposure is obtained, particularly of the frontal processes of the maxillae by converting a bilateral sublabial approach to a midface degloving approach.[48] Subperiosteal dissection is extended into the floor of the piriform aperture and into the nose. The nasal vestibule is incised circumferentially, connecting the nasal floor, membranous septum and intercartilagenous region. Thus, the lower one-third of the nose is raised with the entire bilateral soft tissue envelope of the midface. Increased exposure of the bony nasal pyramid and superior aspect of the medial buttresses as well as access to the nasal passages is achieved. Mucosal incisions are closed with interrupted 2-0 or 3-0 absorbable suture such as chromic gut or polyglycan, and the alar base is narrowed with polyglycan suture.[48] The lateral crurae of the upper and lower lateral cartilages are reapproximated in order to prevent internal valve collapse, and the alar bases are brought together with a muscular-layer stitch, thereby avoiding ptosis of the tip and broadening of the alar base.[48] Similarly, the midface soft tissue is resuspended in order to prevent secondary ptosis. This is a particularly important aspect of closure, since neglecting this resuspension can result in significant droop of the midface.

The orbits are directly approached through modified brow and blepharoplasty incisions.[46,48] The brow incision provides direct access to the superior and lateral orbital rims when reconstructive efforts do not otherwise mandate a coronal approach. The incision is placed just above or just below the hairline of the brow, beveling in line with the hair follicles. The superior and lateral orbicularis is split in line with its fibers, and soft tissue over the orbital rims is divided. A layered closure with good eversion of wound edges via vertical mattress sutures is essential. While this incision has been advocated for years, many surgeons have abandoned it in favor of the upper lid blepharoplasty incision.[46]

Blepharoplasty incisions provide the best direct exposure of the orbital floor and inferior, medial, and lateral rims.[48] In the upper lid, an incision in the lateral aspect of the lid fold may be extended into a relaxed skin tension line in the crow's foot area. A preseptal flap of skin and orbicularis is undermined and then deepened to a subperiosteal plane over the lateral rim in the region of the zygomaticofrontal suture. In the inferior lid, a subciliary skin incision can provide access to the inferior rim and floor, but it does produce a facial scar (albeit fine) and does carry greater risk of lid retraction than does an approach through the conjunctiva. The transconjunctival approach may include a lateral canthotomy (sectioning the common lateral canthal tendon) and cantholysis (lysis of the inferior tendinous limb). In this case, it is initiated with the lateral incision and canthotomy, and then the conjunctiva is incised with a high-temperature cautery at the inferior border of the tarsal plate. Otherwise, only the conjunctival incision is used. The surgeon develops either a pre- or post-septal plane (often, with trauma, the septum is torn, obviating the distinction) and carries the dissection to the inferior rim (Fig. 22-8C). Subsequent subperiosteal exposure of the orbital floor requires care in protecting the inferior rectus muscle. Injury to the muscle can result in scarring, restriction of gaze, and diplopia. The medial extent of the incision is generally in the region of the lacrimal punctum, although the approach can be extended medially into the caruncle, affording excellent exposure of the medial orbit and ascending process of the maxilla. In closing, the surgeon repairs the canthotomy and reattaches the common tendon to the periosteum of the lateral orbital rim or to a small drill hole created in the rim itself. The conjunctiva may be left open or is closed with a 6-0 running fast absorbing gut suture.

The inferior oral vestibular approach exposes the mandibular symphysis and body. Again, an adequate mucosal cuff for closure is maintained below the gingival; however, care is taken not to place the incision too low so that the mental nerves are not inadvertently injured. Subperiosteal dissection exposes the mental nerves and the anterior two-thirds of the mandible. Closure is water-tight and, as with the midface, the soft tissue of the mentum must be resuspended from the skeleton—often from the midline aspect of a plate or to a hole drilled in the bone. An incision along the length of the anterior border of the ramus, carried into the retromolar trigone and just inferior to the crowns of the posterior molars is used to expose the ramus, including the coronoid process, the sigmoid notch, and the condylar neck. This ramus approach combined with a transbuccal stab incision is usually adequate for reduction of a subcondylar, ramus, or angle fracture.

Occasionally, the ramus and angle are approached through an external skin incision. A submandibular incision may be used or extended to include a parotidectomy incision. This is placed in the inferior aspect of the preauricular crease and is deepened posterior to the posterior inferior aspect of the parotid gland until the inferior ramus is identified. Subperiosteal dissection exposes the ramus, condyle, and temporomandibular joint. Particular care is taken to first approach the inferior, posterior aspect of the ramus so as to avoid the main trunk and branches of the facial nerve. Mandibular fractures are difficult to expose externally and may require a submental incision connected via a Z-plasty to a submandibular incision.

Fundamentals of Rigid Fixation. Skeletal support for the soft tissue and visceral structures of the face must be reconstituted. The surgeon reduces and fixates fractured skeletal elements in order to restore proper form and function and to optimize bony

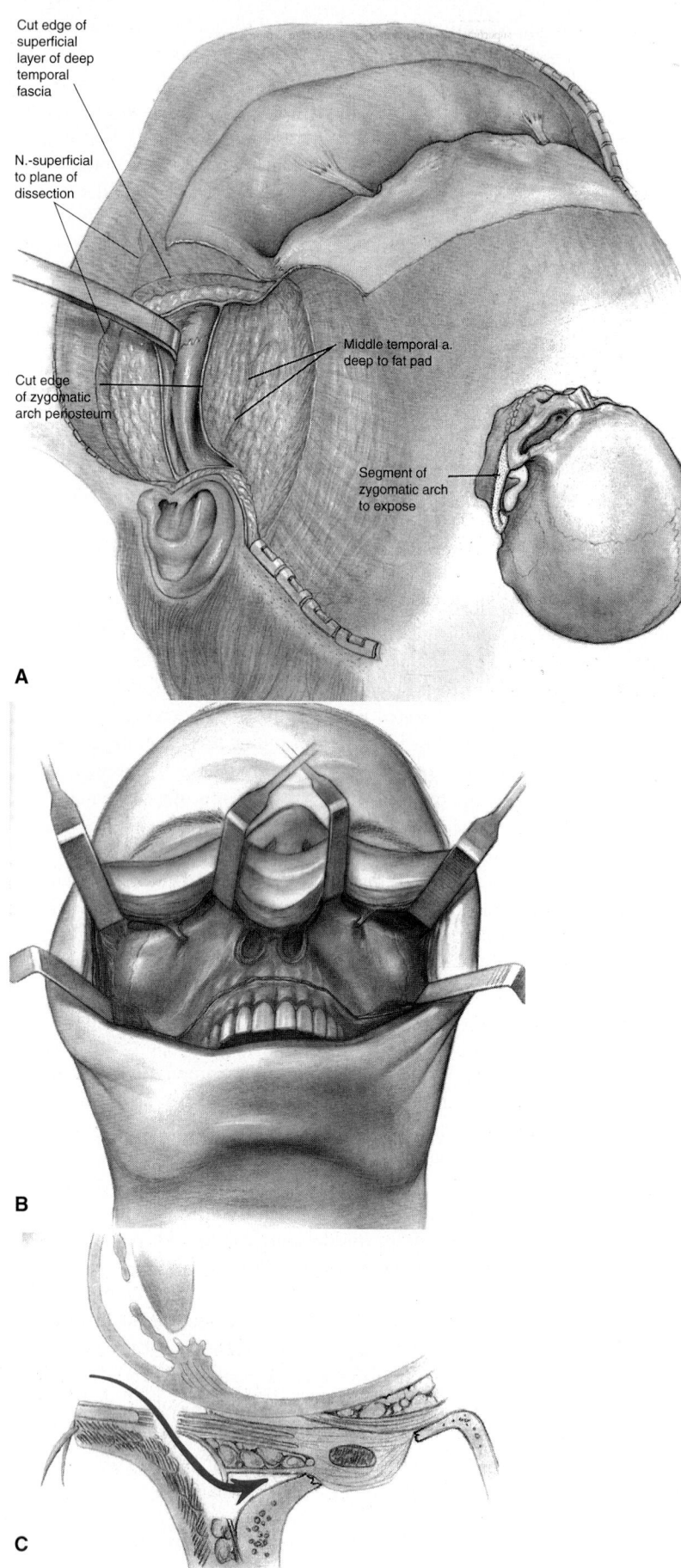

Cut edge of
superficial
layer of deep
temporal
fascia

N.-superficial
to plane of
dissection

Cut edge
of zygomatic
arch periosteum

Middle temporal a.
deep to fat pad

Segment of
zygomatic arch
to expose

A

B

C

**FIGURE 22-8.** Surgical approaches. **(A)** The left half of a coronal approach. The plane of dissection is carried deep to the superficial layer of deep temporal fascia thereby protecting the facial nerve. **(B)** The transconjunctival approach with the preseptal plane of dissection demonstrated. **(C)** The midface degloving approach combines bilateral sublabial approaches and circumferential incisions in the nasal vestibule, permitting access to nearly the entire midface.
*(Reproduced with permission from Kellman RM, Marentette LJ. Atlas of Craniomaxillofacial Fixation. New York, Raven Press, 1995, p. 98, 113, 116.)*

healing.[18,46,49–51] Interfragmentary motion prevents the formation of the delicate vascular support of growing bone, thereby preventing osteoblastic bone formation and the development of a stable population of osteocytes. Rigid fixation not only maintains alignment of bone segments, but also eliminates motion in the fracture gap.[18,49] Lack of adequate fixation increases the chance of device failure and nonunion as well as wound infection and osteomyelitis.[46,50,51]

Fixation has evolved such that currently available strategies include maxillomandibular fixation (MMF, wire fixation of arch bars to the maxillary and mandibular dental or skeletal elements and to each other), interosseous wiring, rigid fixation with compression plates or lag screws, and semi-rigid fixation with miniplates. MMF, with and without interosseous wiring, was the mainstay of primary facial fracture management for most of the 20th century. It is still useful in aligning fracture segments for plating and in some mandibular fractures. Interosseous wiring was employed extensively in the 1950s and 1960s until the advent of rigid fixation, introduced in the early 1970s by Spiessl in Switzerland and Luhr in Germany utilizing compression plating, and in France by Soujeris, Michelet, and Champy who advocated miniplate fixation.[28,52]

Plate and screw fixation now represent the primary means of interosseous fixation. Fixation is achieved only when screws tightly apply a well-adapted plate to apposed bony segments in a manner that overcomes the dynamic forces of distraction. The plate provides immobilization and strong, rigid splinting. Multiple plating strategies have been developed. Compression plates take advantage of eccentric, ramped screw holes that force the turning screw to slide down the shoulders of the screw hole[46] (Fig. 22-9). This applies force axially across a fracture line. Fracture segments are pressed together, friction between fragments is increased, and rigid fixation results, so long as the plates have been applied in a biomechanically advantaged position. Recently however, compression plates have fallen out of favor, not because they are ineffective, but as a result of comparably high success rates with the technically easier and more tolerant miniplate approaches. Compression plates are generally bulkier and more difficult to bend, so that malocclusion is more likely if extreme precision is not achieved. Furthermore, there is concern that fixation of larger plates to the surface of a bone may compromise periosteal blood supply and induce cortical resorption. In addition, compression requires bicortical screw placement, which is limited to the inferior aspect of the mandible by the presence of tooth roots and the inferior alveolar canal, making it more difficult to overcome biomechanical disadvantages of placement. The sliding action of compression across an overlapping or oblique fracture will cause fracture segments to override inappropriately.[46,51]

Instead, smaller, thinner, lower-profile miniplates are increasingly utilized. Miniplate screws are placed only through the outer cortex, and compression is not applied. The lack of compression results in less frictional force between fracture segments, achieving only a "semirigid fixation." This implies some micromovement at the fracture line. This was originally thought by some to be a disadvantage that would lead to failure; however, miniplate technology reliably achieves complete healing with comparable success rates, albeit via a combination of direct (primary) and indirect (secondary) intention, including some minimal callus formation.[53] Three-dimensional miniplates are fashioned in geometric patterns and offer increased resistance to torsion relative to straight-line plates, though they nonetheless represent a form of miniplate (noncompression) fixation.

The newer "locking plates" add a margin of safety by fixing the screw heads to the plate itself. The heads of locking screws thread-lock to a "locking plate" which stabilizes the screws in 3-D space. This is similar to the function of an external fixator and requires less precision in adapting the plate.[54] Like compression plates, locking plates are thicker than miniplates, but they tend to minimize contact with underlying bone, reducing potential devascularization of the periosteum.

Compression fixation is also achieved with lag screws—either alone or in combination with a plate (Fig. 22-10). Lag screws are inserted into a hole in the proximal segment that is over-drilled so that the hole is wider than the screw, and the hole in the distal segment is drilled so that the screw threads will engage. Engaging and tightening the screw then draws the bone segments together. Lag screws may only be placed across fractures that overlap or run obliquely to the surface of a bone and in suitable bone stock. Such fractures occur most commonly in the mandibular symphysis where the curvature creates the equivalent of an overlap and at the angle, where the change of direction of the bone allows lag screw placement.[18,46,49] Lag screws can similarly be used in selected overlapping midface fractures[55] and when fixing bone grafts to underlying bone.

In general, screw placement requires precision in drilling, tapping, and tightening. Except in the case of lag screws, drill bits, taps, and screws are inserted at 90° to the bone surface and with minimum wobble such that the screw hole is not enlarged. Screw holes are also enlarged when the bony walls resorb as a result of overheating and osteocyte necrosis. Therefore, screw holes are drilled at low speeds (<1000 RPM) with constant cool irrigation. Recently, self-tapping and self-drilling monocortical screws have become increasingly popular.

Titanium is currently the metal of choice for nearly all metal craniofacial plates. Titanium does not corrode and does not interfere with imaging based on ionizing radiation. In addition, it demonstrates "pseudobiological" activity in bonding with host tissue.[46,51] Specifically, the hydroxyl moiety of titanium dioxide interacts with organic ligands and the space between metal and bone is obliterated at the atomic level.[49] This effect, termed "osseointegration," is variable and can be enhanced by chemical modification of the implant surface.[46,56–59] Bioabsorbable plates are also available and are discussed in greater detail below.

Mandibular Repair.   The goals of treatment are restoration of form, manifested by normal occlusion, and restoration of function, or the capacity to bear the load of mastication. While many fractures could heal solely through the application of MMF, there is increased risk of malunion due to less dependability of maintenance of position and increased risk of nonunion due to lack of adequate stabilization; therefore, most fractures are treated with open reduction and internal fixation (ORIF) so that healing is accelerated and patient comfort and safety are improved.[18,46,51] Potential adverse sequelae in the temporomandibular joint (TMJ) and masticatory muscles resulting from prolonged immobility are also avoided, though it remains unclear that this is a result of MMF. Note however, that all techniques begin with realignment of fracture segments and that MMF remains an excellent method of achieving and maintaining realignment through stabilization of occlusion.[23] Thus, maxillofacial repair is often started with application of arch bars and wires. Moreover,

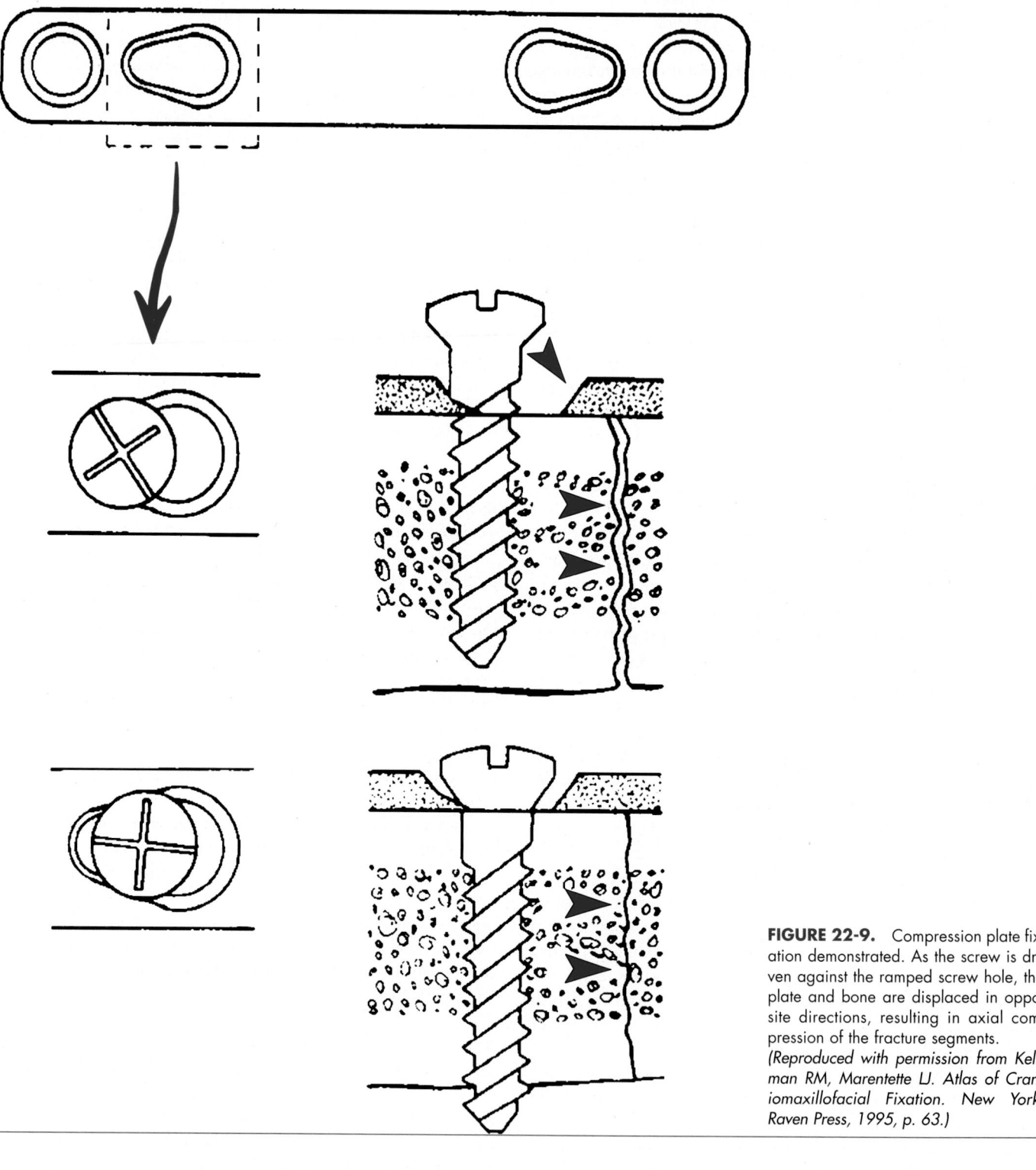

**FIGURE 22-9.** Compression plate fixation demonstrated. As the screw is driven against the ramped screw hole, the plate and bone are displaced in opposite directions, resulting in axial compression of the fracture segments. *(Reproduced with permission from Kellman RM, Marentette LJ. Atlas of Craniomaxillofacial Fixation. New York, Raven Press, 1995, p. 63.)*

arch bars are often desirable in the postoperative period in case training elastics are required for further adjustment of the muscles to maintain occlusion. It should be noted, however, that MMF will not overcome rigid fixation of the bones in a suboptimal position. In the absence of adequate dentition, the patient's dentures may be wired into position and MMF may be achieved via circummandibular and transnasal wires or MMF screws.

Once fractures have been realigned, they are then plated. Repair of mandibular fractures requires understanding of the biomechanics

so that distracting forces acting on the fragments can be overcome. While the fundamental screw and plating techniques have been reviewed, the physiologic basis for fixation in the mandible is founded on an understanding of the forces acting on the fractured segments.[18,46,53,60–62] Thus, the fixation strategy is chosen based on the site, orientation, and severity of the fracture.

Older studies schematized the mandible as two beams or an arch, cantilevered at the angle and suspended from the TMJ.[53] Classically, bite forces are thought to cause strain, classified as bending (tension, however, experience a greater degree of torsion than bending or shearing, bending predominates across fractures of the body, and shearing forces are greatest in the angle.

In direct response to these forces, Champy et al. proposed "ideal lines" of osteosynthesis, along which miniplates should be placed[63] (Fig. 22-12). With tension at the superior border and compressive forces at the inferior border of symphysis, parasymphsysis, and body fractures, Champy demonstrated the mechanical advantage of placing a "tension band" across the superior border. For fractures of the symphysis and parasymphysis, Champy proposed a second plate, placed inferiorly. Thus, the tension band resists bending and both plates in combination resist torsion.

Multiple combinations of strategies for fixation fulfill the need for a tension band and an inferior border fixator. In the dentulous patient, a well-applied arch bar may serve as a tension band; however, any evidence that an arch bar will not remain well fixed, such as the lack of adequate dentition, suggests that the tension band function should be fulfilled by a plate or lag screw. A tension band at the superior border and a compression plate may be used in combination. Recently, compression plating has given way in most cases to semi-rigid miniplate fixation[23] and to locking plate fixation.[54,64,65] Thus, most commonly, two miniplates comprise the tension band and the inferior border plate. Alternatively, two lag screws or a single 3-D miniplate plate will account for the tension-band and inferior fixation elements.

Champy's technique also dictates that in the body, the predominance of bending forces and the lack of significant rotational force suggest that a fracture may be stabilized by a single, superiorly-placed plate. In the angle, one plate, fixed along the oblique line, will resist the predominant shearing force, though several groups have demonstrated better outcomes when two miniplates are fixed at the angle.

In reality, however, the bite forces applied to the mandible are far more complex than those suggested in the simplified model, and they depend on the site of the fracture, the position at which a bite force is applied, and the presence of comminution and

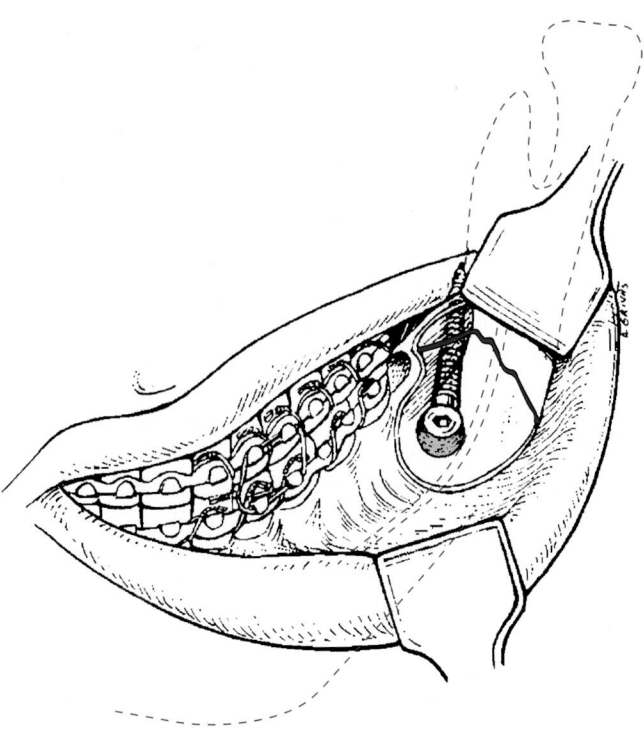

**FIGURE 22-10.** Lag screw fixation of a manibular angle fracture through an inferior oral vestibular approach. Note that the proximal segment is overdrilled and that a countersink is created in its cortical surface. *(Reproduced with permission from Kellman RM, Marentette LJ. Atlas of Craniomaxillofacial Fixation. New York: Raven Press, 1995, p. 238.)*

or the spreading of fracture segments, at the superior border and compression at the inferior border), torsion (rotational movement of segments relative to each other), and shearing (translation of segments relative to each other) (Fig. 22-11). In general, fractures of the symphysis, parasymphsysis, body, and angle all experience some tension at the superior border. The symphysis and parasymphysis,

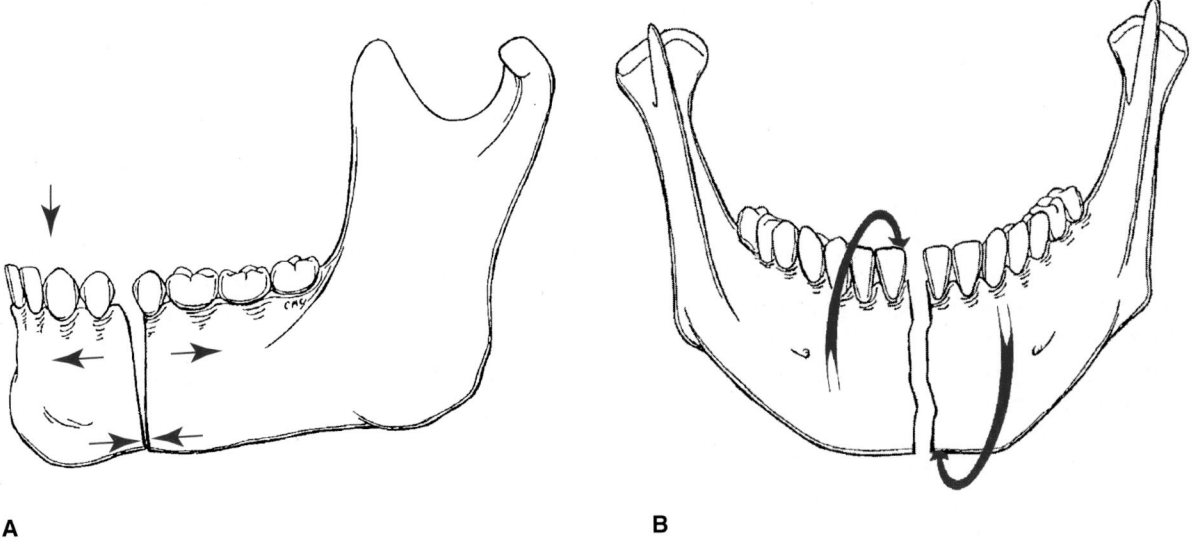

**A**                                                                                      **B**

**FIGURE 22-11.** **(A)** Bending forces in the mandibular body resulting from downward force applied to the anterior mandible. This causes at the superior border and at the inferior border. **(B)** Torsional forces predominate at the symphysis. *(Reproduced with permission from Kellman RM, Marentette LJ. Atlas of Craniomaxillofacial Fixation. New York: Raven Press, 1995, p. 40, 41.)*

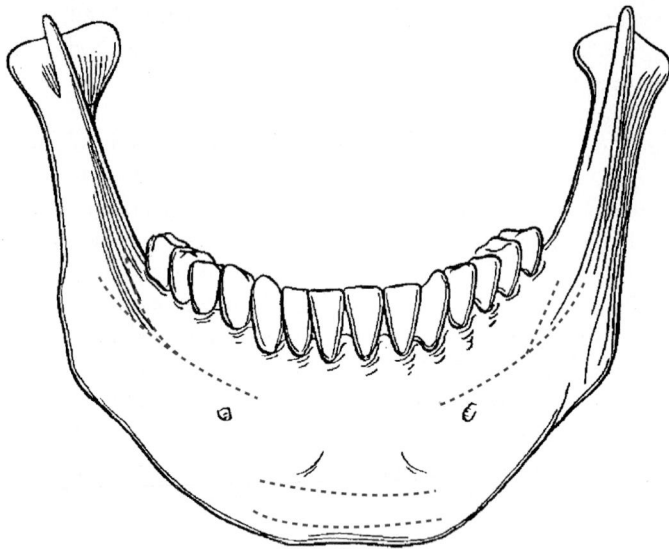

**FIGURE 22-12.** Dotted lines represent "Champy's Ideal Line of Osteosynthesis" as defined by Professor Maxime Champy. Miniplate fixation along these lines counteracts the predominant forces acting in each region. *(Reproduced with permission from Kellman RM, Marentette LJ. Atlas of Craniomaxillofacial Fixation. New York: Raven Press, 1995, p. 43.)*

multiple fractures. Increasingly sophisticated techniques, including computer modeling, demonstrate the differential loads borne by discrete areas of the mandible relative to the placement of fracture lines and bite force.[53,54,60–62,66–73] Notably, bite force is also relative to the postoperative compliance of the patient. Thus, while Champy's technique is certainly adequate for almost all situations in the symphysis and parasymphysis, it may be best considered the minimum treatment required in the body and angle. Simple fractures in the body with minimal displacement in compliant patients may fare well with Champy's technique, and many surgeons now agree that simple angle fractures do not require a heavy compression plate.[23] Yet, the authors suggest that a body or angle fracture of any complexity (including the presence of comminution or other fractures) requires that the superior tension band or oblique line plate should be complemented by a second miniplate.[74] In the angle, this may be placed on the buccal surface of the oblique line or at inferior aspect of the angle. Haug et al. demonstrated that multiple techniques for providing a second line of stability to a fracture of the angle, including miniplates, bicortical compression plates, and lag screws, produce similar biomechanical results.[75]

Management of condylar and subcondylar fractures remains a focus of debate. While it is widely agreed that fractures of the condyle and the subcondylar region may cause a significant disturbance of masticatory movement, the patient's ability to adapt to such a disturbance may be great.[76] Thus, debate continues over the role of ORIF versus closed treatment without surgical reduction. The heart of this debate concerns the most appropriate measures of outcomes. Closed reduction and the use of arch bars and training elastics may result in what some consider reasonable occlusion, fracture alignment, and masticatory function. This result is achieved, however, at the expense of physiologic adaptation, including altered kinematics of the jaw while chewing[77] and possible foreshortening of the mandible on the fractured side. This may produce significant facial asymmetry at rest and with mouth

opening.[76,78,79] Moreover, some patients may not be capable of adaptation, and altered jaw movement may result in chronic pain or trismus.[76,77]

Surgical reduction has been shown to improve alignment of fracture segments and prevent foreshortening of the mandible,[79–81] although the external approach carries some risk of injury to the facial nerve and scarring. An intraoral approach assisted by an endoscope with or without a right-angle drill and a right-angle screw driver has been shown to reduce the risk of injury to the facial nerve and to eliminate facial scarring while effecting excellent results in selected patients[79,82] (Fig. 22-13). In general, isolated, unilateral subcondylar fractures with minimal displacement and fractures in patients who refuse open reduction are treated with placement of an arch bar and training elastics. Otherwise, the authors perform an endoscope-assisted reduction and internal fixation with rare conversion to an external approach. Exact indications for open and endoscopic open repair continue to evolve with technology and surgical experience.[78,79] The obvious limitation is in acquiring the requisite training in endoscopic surgery. The reader is referred to the literature for a complete description of the endoscopic technique.[79]

Miniplate fixation does have limitations. When a segment of mandible is severely injured by comminution or bone loss, miniplate fixation cannot provide adequate stability. A mandibular reconstruction plate is fixated to adequate proximal and distal bone stock incorporating the comminuted fragments between.[18,46,65] Comminuted fragments may be fixed to one another with miniplates or wires or lagged to the reconstruction plate. Although the size of a reconstruction plate mandates its placement at the less advantageous inferior border, the bulk also enables the bar to provide resistance against both bending and torsion.[46] At least three screws are placed into solid bone on each side of the comminuted area, and additional screws contribute to the safety and stability of the repair. Reconstruction plates, however, can be difficult to use. Even the slightest malocclusion will be rigidly maintained by a reconstruction plate, and, in placing screws, bone segments are drawn to the stiff, heavy plate rather than vice versa. In addition, Haug et al. showed that any offset between bone and plate reduces the plate's effectiveness.[54] Thus, not only is bending a heavy reconstruction plate more difficult than bending a miniplate, greater precision in adapting reconstruction plates is required.

In contrast, locking reconstruction plates retain the advantage of load-bearing strength (i.e., strong enough to replace the load-bearing burden of the damaged bone) while mitigating the difficulty in adapting a heavier plate.[18,65] The end point of screw placement in a locking plate is the screw head thread-locking to the screw hole rather than the plate contacting bone. Thus, there is less risk of bone segments being drawn out of position to the surface of the plate. In addition, the compression of a heavy reconstruction plate to a surface of bone may result in mild cortical bone resorption. The consequent offset may reduce fixation[54,65]; however, since locking plates impart stability to a fracture through the screws themselves, less contact with the bone surface results in less periosteal injury. Moreover, a minor offset of a locking plate does not result in loss of position.[54]

**Midface.**    The forces acting across midface fractures are far less than those found in mandibular fractures. Occlusal forces impart only compressive forces to the medial and lateral buttress, and the

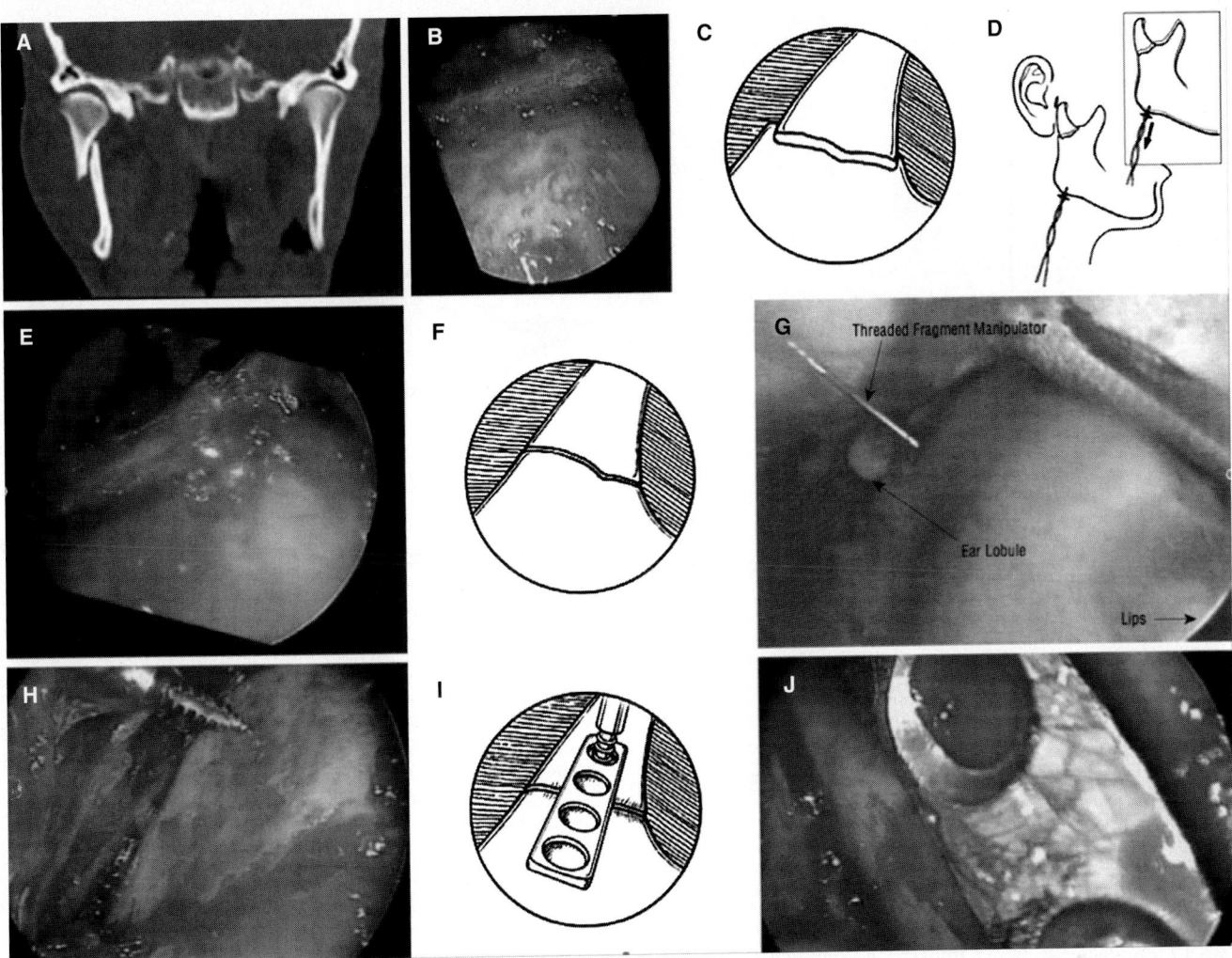

**FIGURE 22-13.** Endoscopic subcondylar fracture repair. **(A)** Frame of a coronal computed tomographic scan demonstrating a right subcondylar fracture with lateral overlap of the proximal fragment. **(B)** Lateral overlap of the proximal fragment as seen through the endoscope. **(C)** Artist's depiction of B. **(D)** Wire through the angle of the mandible. Inset, Inferior traction on the distal fragment allows the proximal fragment to fall into a reduced position. **(E)** Proximal fragment falling into place as inferior traction is applied. **(F)** Artist's depiction of E. **(G)** Threaded fragment manipulator being passed through the right cheek. **(H)** The manipulator in position over the proximal fragment. **(I)** Artist's depiction of the manipulator passing through the proximal plate hole into the proximal bone fragment. **(J)** Endoscopic view of the reduced fracture after plate placement is complete. *(Reproduced with permission from Kellman RM. Endoscopically assisted repair of subcondylar fractures of the mandible: An evolving technique. Arch Facial Plast Surg 5:244, 2003.)*

masseter muscle imparts only mild to moderate amounts of shearing and rotation to a fractured zygoma.[46] Thus, repair considerations focus less on the fixation strategy than on the realignment of skeletal elements such that the buttresses are restored and soft tissue and visceral structures are properly supported. In general, single miniplate fixation of buttresses and microplate fixation of intervening segments are sufficient.

Repair of lower midface or Le Fort I fractures involves exposure of the bones, disimpaction of the midface, realignment of fracture segments, and plating of the vertical buttresses. Primary principles are the restoration of occlusion and vertical facial height.[19] After sublabial exposure of the midface, fractures are evaluated. Significant comminution and open bite deformities (after mandibular height and continuity have been re-established) suggest midface intrusion. Rowe forceps, inserted into the nose and mouth, allow the surgeon to grasp the nasal and oral surfaces of the palate and disimpact the inferior aspect of the maxillae (Fig. 22-14). The palate is first mobilized in a downward movement, and then proper repositioning usually requires anterior and superior movement. The disimpacted position of the palate is secured with MMF while miniplates are adapted and fixated to the medial and lateral buttresses. Thus, an intact or restored mandible is often needed to stabilize the maxilla in proper occlusion prior to plating. Pre-bent L- or Y-shaped plates are particularly useful in spanning a fracture line and finding enough bone stock on the alveolar aspect of the fracture for plating (Fig. 22-15). The posterior buttress is inaccessible, and, therefore, it is not plated. MMF is then released, unless adequate fixation is not achieved or adjunctive procedures such as bone grafting for the treatment of severe injuries is required.

Comminution complicates repair by eliminating reference points that determine the proper position of fracture segments and by reducing the potential for stable fixation. Comminution resulting in fracture gaps in the buttresses of less than 5 mm[18] to 7.5 mm[19] can be spanned by a miniplate alone. Larger gaps, however, should be spanned by bone grafts from the calvarium, rib, or iliac crest.[19,46,83] Comminuted fragments of the face of the maxillary

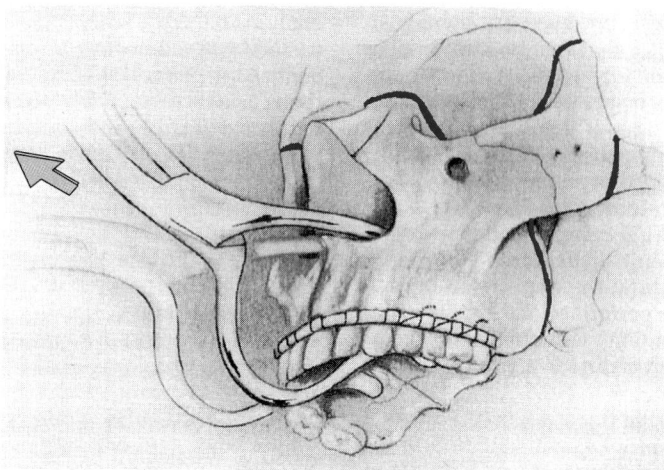

**FIGURE 22-14.** Disimpaction of the midface with Rowe forceps. (Reproduced with permission from Ducic Y, Hamlar DD. Fractures of the Midface. Facial Plast Surg Clin North Am 6:478, 1998.)

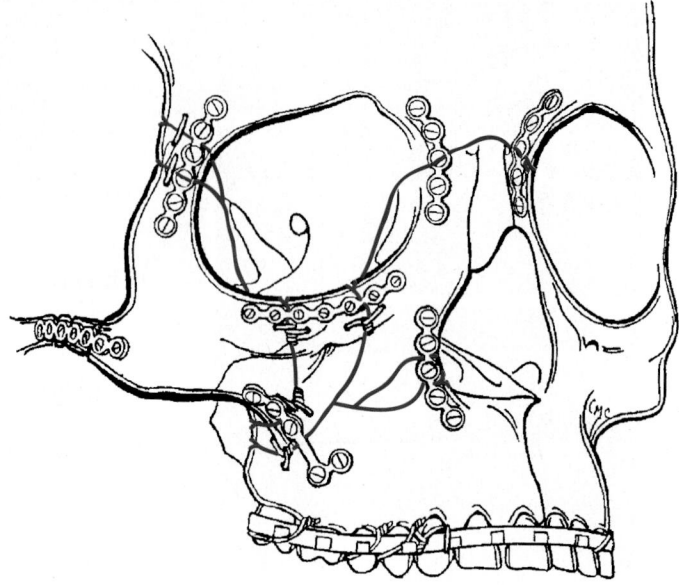

**FIGURE 22-15.** Repair of complex midfacial fractures including multi-level Le Fort with zygomatic fractures. The presence of Le Fort fractures demands that intermaxillary fixation be used to reestablish and maintain occlusion during the repair. Comminuted segments have been approximated with wire suture. Projection from the skull base is re-established through reduction and fixation of the zygomatic arch and the nasal root. The orbital rims and then the medial and lateral buttresses are then reconstituted. (Reproduced with permission from Kellman RM, Marentette LJ. Atlas of Craniomaxillofacial Fixation. New York: Raven Press, 1995, p. 292.)

sinus intervening between medial and lateral buttresses are often fixed to microplates that span across any combination of vertical buttresses, inferior orbital rims, and alveolus. This prevents contraction of soft tissue into the sinus. In the presence of severe comminution such that facial projection and height cannot be determined based on the patient's anatomy, known concepts of ideal facial dimensions (e.g., incisal show, vertical facial thirds) are utilized.[18,19]

Upper midface fractures include buttress fractures in the Le Fort II and III pattern, as well as fractures through the orbital walls and zygomatic articulations. The maxillary vestibular approach is again utilized to approach the upper midface in combination with the transconjuntival approach to the orbital rims and floor. Like Le Fort I fractures, Le Fort II fractures often involve impaction of the midface relative to the skull base. Thus, Rowe forceps are again needed to disimpact the midface, which is then locked into position using MMF. It is important to rotate the midface downward prior to disimpaction, to avoid potential damage or disruption of the anterior skull base. Any free segments of buttresses are reduced and the buttresses are plated (Fig. 22-15). Occasionally, segments may be temporarily held in position with interosseous wires in order to simplify reduction. Comminution of the maxillary face can be repaired via microplate fixation of bone fragments in order to prevent soft tissue prolapse into the antrum. The orbital floor is explored and repaired as described below.

Unlike LeFort I and II fractures, the face of the maxilla is uninvolved in an isolated LeFort III fracture. Therefore, nearly the entire fracture can be accessed through the coronal approach to the orbital rims, the nasal pyramid, and the zygoma. The midface is disimpacted, fixed below in MMF, and plated at the ZF suture and zygomatic arch (Fig. 22-15).[18,46] Lastly, the orbital floors are explored and repaired through the transconjunctival or subciliary approach. In reality, pure Le Fort III fractures are almost never seen in clinical experience, and we generally name fractures by the most severe component, adding descriptive information about intervening fractures.

The midface may also transmit force to the deeper skeletal elements of the orbit. Therefore, after the lateral buttress and orbital rims are approached and repaired, the orbital walls, especially the

floor, are explored. The same exploration is required with isolated orbital blowout fractures. Dissection through the transconjunctival approach is carried from the inferior and lateral rims onto the floor. The periorbita is freed from bony fragments along the floor, the orbital contents are elevated from the maxillary sinus, and the floor is examined. Visualization of the posterior orbital floor may be impeded by herniated orbital soft tissue. Defects in the floor of less than 1cm can generally be observed.[19] Any larger defect is reconstructed in order to prevent enlargement of orbital volume and consequent enophthalmos or entrapment of the medial rectus. A profusion of materials and techniques for repair of the orbital floor have been described, nearly all with reasonable success. The authors suggest that calvarial bone grafts plated anteriorly to the orbital rim offer time-tested success[18,19,46] and resist resorption and extrusion (Fig. 22-16). Alternatively, alloplast material such as Medpore or nylon sheeting may be laid across a defect. Even larger defects may require additional support with titanium mesh embedded within or covered with a smooth surface such as Medpore or nylon sheeting. Orbital fractures resulting from zygomatic complex injuries are discussed below.

Most recently, endoscopic repair of the orbital floor has been described. The floor is approached through the maxillary vestibular incision and an anterior maxillotomy. This approach avoids possible complications of eyelid incisions and may afford better visualization of the posterior orbital floor.[84] The orbital contents are reduced and the floor is grafted.

Le Fort II and III fractures also imply disruption of the nasal pyramid. The medial buttress is plated superiorly, reestablishing the frontal process of the maxilla and the medial orbital rim. A strong tendency for posterior rotation of the lower facial skeleton,

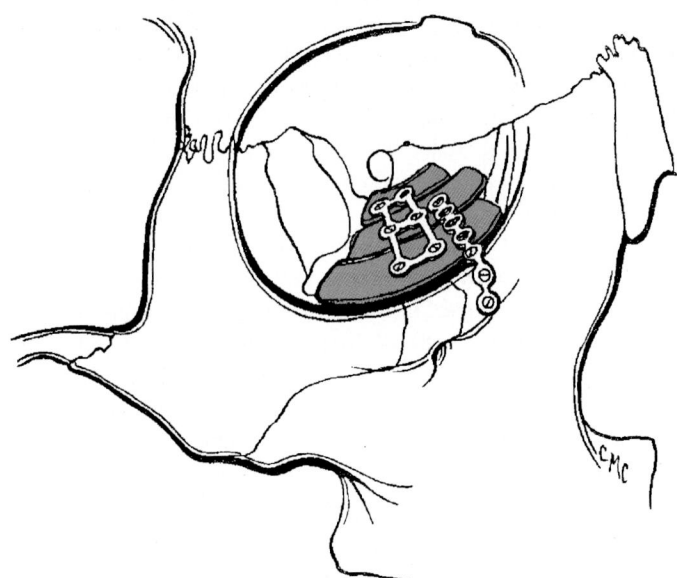

**FIGURE 22-16.** Orbital floor repair using autogenous bone graft. The graft is fixed to the inferior orbital rim. Multiple pieces may be plated or wired together in order to account for defects with complex shapes. *(Reproduced with permission from Kellman RM, Marentette LJ. Atlas of Craniomaxillofacial Fixation. New York: Raven Press, 1995, p. 293.)*

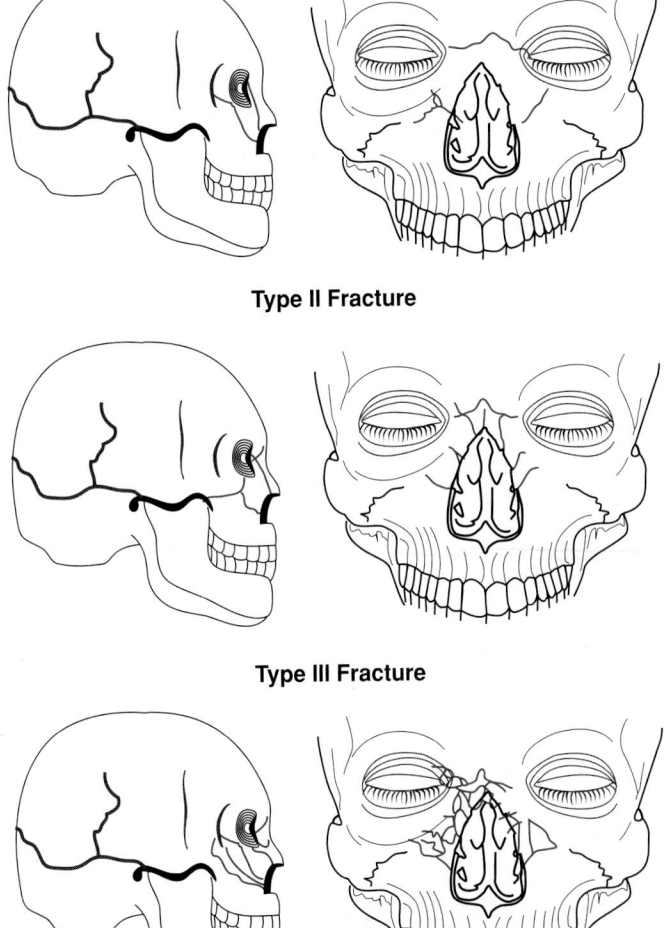

**FIGURE 22-17.** Naso-orbito-ethmoid fracture classification.

hinged at the nasal root, is an indication for plating nasal fractures, and stabilizing the nasal root to the frontal bone[18,46] (Fig. 22-15). Defects in the nasal dorsum may be closed with a free bone graft cantilevered from the glabella.[46]

Rarely are LeFort III fractures encountered in the absence of some disruption of the ethmoid bone, medial orbital walls, and thus, the attachments of the medial canthal ligaments. As previously described, naso-orbito-ethmoid (NOE) fractures result in telacanthus. For the purpose of repair, NOE fractures are categorized as types I, II, and III, depending on the severity of disruption of the medial canthal ligaments (Fig. 22-17). Type I injuries result in a large, undisturbed central fragment. Displacement of such a fragment should be reduced and plated at its superior and inferior aspects separately. Stripping the periosteum of this central fragment in order to place a single plate from frontal bone to lower medial buttress is not recommended, since this may unnecessarily release the medial canthal tendon.[10]

Type II fractures involve comminution of the central fragment without avulsion of the medial canthal ligament from at least a fragment of the lacrimal bone. If the comminution is minimal, telacanthus is repaired through microplate fixation of fracture segments. With greater comminution, microplate fixation should be augmented by transnasal fixation of the medial canthi with 28 gauge wire or 2-0 permanent suture.[46,85] A posterior-superior vector of fixation is achieved, since anterior placement of the wire will result in lateral rotation of central fragment and postoperative telacanthus[85] (Fig. 22-3). If fragments interfere with transnasal fixation, detachment of the ligaments may be performed prior to fixation.

Type III injuries involve severe comminution of the NOE complex and avulsion of the medial canthus. In this case, the stumps of the canthi are approximated with a wire or permanent suture that crosses the nasal septum. Again, the suture is given a posterior and

superior vector and slight overcorrection is achieved in order to prevent postoperative telacanthus. Comminuted fragments are microplated or free bone grafts are used to span any gap between the medial buttress and the frontal bone.[86] Often severe NOE injuries involve the lacrimal system, which should be probed and stented, as discussed above.

Zygoma fractures may be isolated to the arch or may involve the entire "zygomaticomaxillary complex" (ZMC) or "tripod." Simple, nondisplaced fractures of the arch may be treated with observation. Displacement, however, may result in impingement of the temporalis muscle and dimpling of the cheek and should be reduced. Classically, this is accomplished via an external, Gilles incision in the temporal hair tuft through which the fracture is reduced with a small elevator. An external splint such as a finger splint may be sutured percutaneously to the arch. Any complex arch fracture and any fracture resulting in noticeable reduction of malar projection is approached more widely, reduced, and fixed with a mini- or microplates as needed. The amount of exposure and selection of incisions is dependent upon the severity of the fractures and the degree of displacement and comminution. Comminution is overcome by plating multiple fragments by bone grafting long gaps.

Most ZMC fractures require open reduction and internal fixation. Nondisplaced fractures may be observed and, since many displaced fractures result only in cosmetic rather than functional deficits, patients may decline surgical repair. The central principle of repair is fracture realignment and fixation to reestablish the malar prominence. The anterior and lateral projection is restored with reconstruction of the horizontal arc, and the vertical height of the eminence is reset with reconstruction of the vertical arc. While not all components of the ZMC are plated, they each play a role in ensuring proper reduction. The ZF suture provides the best indication of facial height. The continuity of the ZM suture and infraorbital rim are easily visualized and reestablished, barring significant comminution. The continuity of the zygomatic arch determines proper anterior malar projection. Although the ZS suture may be overlooked, it often provides the key information in determing final ZMC reduction. In addition, malalignment of the ZS articulation can result in a significant step-off in the lateral orbital floor and change in the orbital volume.

The sublabial, transconjunctival and blepharoplasty approaches are useful in approaching the buttresses and orbital rims, and arch fractures are exposed through the coronal approach. Disimpaction of the ZMC is usually accomplished through anterolateral traction applied with large bone hook placed just behind the take-off of the zygomatic arch. Often, this traction is maintained by an assistant until key fracture lines can be plated. The ZM, ZF, and infraorbital rim all provide adequate cortical bone stock for plating, though the infraorbital rim is plated less frequently. Two-point fixation is usually adequate unless the complexity of the fracture reduces its stability or the zygomatic arch is significantly disrupted. The ZF suture provides an ideal point of temporary wire fixation around which the ZMC may be pivoted into final reduction. This wire fixation may be left in place if two-point fixation is obtained at the

ZM suture and infraorbital rim. Otherwise, the wire can be removed and a miniplate applied. The arch can be repaired as detailed above. Care should be taken to achieve the proper length of the arch, recognizing that the midsection arch is actually flat.[18–20,46] Relatively stable fractures may be repaired with a simple ZM plate and, in rare cases, no fixation is needed.

Upper facial fractures consist of either anterior cranial vault fractures, beyond the scope of this chapter, or frontal sinus fractures. Frontal sinus fractures may be isolated, but often occur in the setting of upper midface fractures including Lefort II and III and NOE injuries (Fig. 22-18). Multiple algorithms for the evaluation and repair of the frontal sinus injuries are described.[11,86,87] The principles of treatment include reestablishing an aesthetic anterior wall, ensuring the function of the frontal sinus should it be preserved, and safe management of a possible leak of cerebrospinal fluid (CSF). Despite minor variations, the authors agree that the following distinctions determine the treatment needed to achieve those principles:

1. Site of fracture—anterior versus posterior table
2. Degree of fracture displacement in either the anterior or posterior wall
3. The presence of fractures through the nasofrontal duct (NFD)
4. The presence of possible CSF leak

Nondisplaced fractures of the anterior table can be observed. Anterior table fractures with significant depression or displacement should be repaired for cosmetic reasons, though the patient may opt for observation, utilizing delayed repair if a significant cosmetic deformity develops. Nondisplaced fractures of the posterior wall can also be observed. Classically, displacement of posterior table fractures greater than the width of the posterior table itself has been used as an indication for exploration. The fear is communication between the frontal sinus and the intracranial compartment with

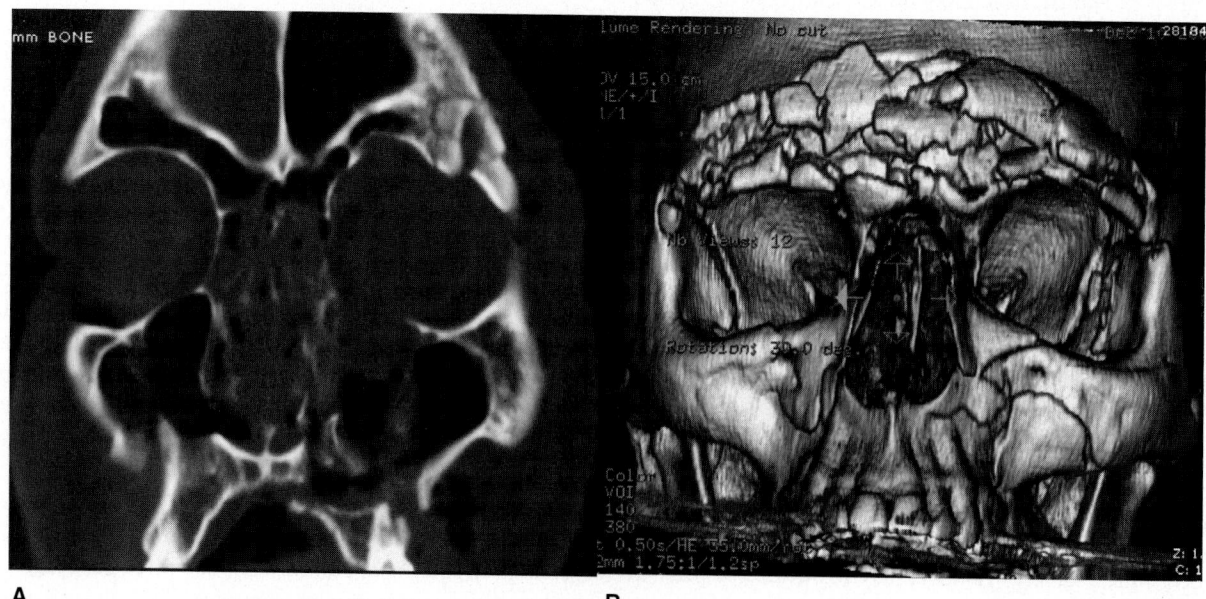

A                                    B

**FIGURE 22-18.**   Variation in severe panfacial fractures. **(A)** Coronal CT demonstrating left Le Fort III, frontal sinus, NOE, and bilateral Le Fort I fractures as well as a split palate. **(B)** Three-dimensional CT demonstrating severely comminuted frontal sinus, bilateral Le Fort III, left Le Fort II, NOE, and bilateral high Le Fort I fractures. Both injuries resulted from high-speed motor vehicle accidents.

increased risk of dural tear, CSF leak, and meningitis.[11,86,87] In reality, any displacement suggests these risks, though obviously, increasing severity of a posterior table fracture including the presence of CSF leak mandates increasingly aggressive treatment. Fractures that traverse the floor of the sinus, especially medially, are likely to produce dysfunction of the NFD. Possible sequelae include frontal sinusitis, mucocele, and mucopyocele. Thus, involvement of the NFD in anterior or posterior table fractures requires more aggressive management. Minimal or questionable fractures through the sinus floor or posterior table can be further assessed via endoscopy for the presence of CSF leak or obstruction of the NFD.

Management options include observation, observation with medical management including antibiotic coverage, open reduction and internal fixation, sinus and duct obliteration, and sinus cranialization with duct obliteration. The frontal sinus may be approached through lacerations in the forehead skin. Otherwise, the coronal approach is utilized. Brow incisions create forehead numbness and unsightly scars and are no longer advocated. Displaced anterior table fractures can be reduced with small bone hooks and microplated, given the lack of forces acting on the upper face. Comminuted fragments can be removed, plated on a back table and reimplanted. Camouflage can be achieved using grafts or implants. Posterior table fractures are often explored through a fractured anterior table. Again, reduction can be achieved with careful use of small bone hooks. If the anterior table is not fractured, an osteoplastic flap of the anterior table can be raised with the use of a template cut from a Caldwell plain x-ray of the frontal sinus taken at 6 ft. away from the patient. Through the osteoplastic flap, posterior table repair, sinus and duct obliteration, and sinus cranialization with duct obliteration can be accomplished. Sinus and duct obliteration involves complete removal of all sinus mucosa (preventing mucocele formation), reduction of the intersinus septae and the filling of air-containing spaces with bone chips, abdominal fat graft, or a pedicled pericranial flap. Hydroxyappetite cement is not recommended for this purpose. Finally, cranialization can also be accomplished through the subcranial approach.

In reality, upper face and midface fractures most commonly occur in combination as the result of high-speed motor vehicle accidents and may also present with lower facial injuries (Fig. 22-18). Although such "pan-facial" fractures represent daunting challenges to the surgeon, the authors and others espouse a "subunit" approach, by which complex fractures are repaired, sequentially resulting in less complex fractures.[10,46] For instance, when LeFort II and III fractures and a ZMC fracture are encountered together, repairing the lateral orbital rims leaves a residual LeFort II fracture and a zygomatic arch fracture, each of which is handled as isolated subunits. The question then remains as to how to organize the repair effort. Classical approaches have been described as either 'outside-in' or 'inside out'; i.e., from the periphery toward the center or vice-versa. The authors use somewhat of a combined approach, first stabilizing the occlusion and then proceeding from the periphery toward the center ('outside-in'). The central midface is the most dependent portion of the craniofacial skeleton, providing the least in terms of native strength. Facial height and projection is, therefore, established through reconstitution of the mandible and the maxillary alveolus below and the cranial vault and upper midface above. The zygomatic arches relate the upper midface to the cranial base posteriorly. The vertical and horizontal buttresses are then reconstituted, and the upper and lower halves of the craniofacial skeleton are thus linked. The central midface is addressed last, repairing telecanthus and restoring projection of the nasal root.[10,18,46]

Proper reduction of the mandibular arch is key.[18] If the mandible is incompletely reduced and then used to set the midfacial width and projection via occlusal relationships, a wide and insufficiently projected midface results. Furthermore, a split palate combined with a fracture of the mandibular symphysis make this extremely difficult to repair. Buccal version of the posterior mandibular dentition and a resulting open bite deformity should alert the surgeon to a splayed dental arch. Bilateral pressure on the mandibular angles during repair of the symphysis will help reduce splaying. Direct repair of the palate will also help. Subcondylar fractures of the mandible should also be opened and repaired. Offering an alternative view, Gruss et al. suggest that first setting the midface projection, dependent on the full length of the zygomatic arch rather than the mandible, may prevent insufficient restoration of facial projection.[20]

Finally, fractures of the frontal sinus and the upper midface, especially the NOE complex, may well result in disruption of the anterior skull base. Severely comminuted fractures of the frontal sinus, suspected dural lacerations, or impingement on the optic nerve suggest fractures of the anterior skull base. In this case, the authors perform a subcranial approach to the anterior skull base. This involves temporary removal of the nasoglabellar complex and a variable extent of the superior orbital rims and frontal calvarium.[88] The reader is referred to the literature for an in-depth review of the subcranial technique.[88-90] The approach affords superior exposure of the frontal lobe dura, and anterior skull base with minimal retraction of the brain.[88-90] The medial canthi are also directly exposed, simplifying telecanthus repair.[88]

## MASSIVE WOUNDS

High-energy insults resulting in massive full-thickness wounds to the face deserve particular attention. These include both high-speed motor vehicular trauma and close-range gunshot injuries. Management of such wounds is complex; however, primary principles and treatment approaches that maximize success have been be identified (Fig. 22-19).[12-14,91,92] All authors agree that blast wounds to the face require immediate stabilization of remaining skeletal elements, especially the mandible and midfacial buttresses, and closure of overlying soft tissue. Delay results in severe retraction of soft tissue and devitalization of the underlying skeleton. Large bony defects should be spanned by reconstruction plates in the mandible or by miniplates and bone grafts in the midface and cranial vault. Debridement in the zone of injury is repeated over the first several days until further tissue loss is not encountered. Early reconstruction utilizing local and regional tissue provides an aesthetic outcome far superior to that obtained by delayed secondary repair including free tissue transfer.[12-14,92] Where free tissue transfer is needed, one should expect that more than one flap will be needed. Finally, Clark et al. suggest that lack of lining tissue in the oral cavity and sinuses is an underappreciated cause of infection and failure of bone grafting.[14]

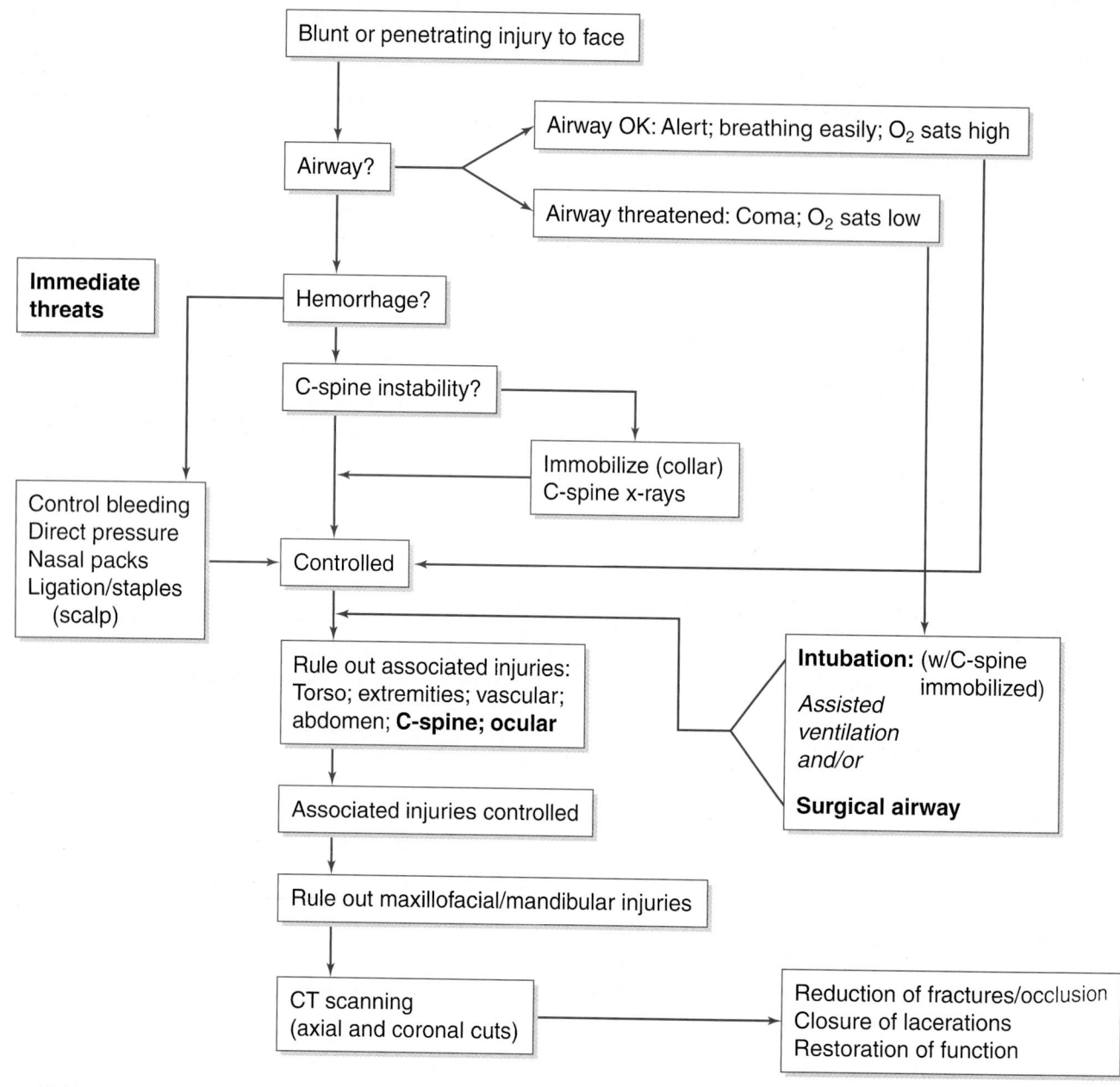

**FIGURE 22-19.**  An approach to maxillofacial and mandibular injury.

## COMPLICATIONS

Complications may result from injuries that are beyond our capability to repair, from the vagaries of an individual's healing, or from the surgeon's failure to adhere to known principles of repair.

### Soft Tissue

Although scars may be minimized, their presence following lacerations is inevitable. Wound healing is directed by a cascade of cytokines that bring about three overlapping stages of repair, including inflammation, proliferation, and remodeling.[93] Hypertrophic and keloid scarring are produced by excessive and disorganized collagen deposition during the proliferative stage. While hypertrophic scars are wide, they are contained within the margins of a wound. Keloids, on the other hand, extend beyond the margins of a wound, may take months to grow, are more likely to recur following excision, and most commonly occur in darker skin and at the earlobe (as well as the back and chest). Minimizing surgical manipulation and preventing infection will reduce inflammation. Beveling scalp incisions parallel to the hair follicles and placing facial incisions (when they cannot be avoided) within relaxed skin tension lines also minimizes the appearance of scars.

Scar contracture from fibroblasts peaks during the third week of wound healing.[29] Scar contracture over fracture sites may frustrate fracture reduction and accentuate facial deformity. Thus, early repair of the underlying craniofacial skeleton is critical, and delay beyond two weeks is detrimental. Localized scar contracture in critical sites of the face results in unacceptable cosmetic results and loss of function. Notching is immediately noticeable in the helical rim of the auricle and in the alar margins and soft triangles of the nose.

Scar in the region of the oral commisure may result in loss of the commissural angle and oral incompetence. In the eyelid, scarring may result in loss of the normal canthal angles and lid retraction. Eyelid injuries may also result in lid defects, ectropion, entropion, trichiasis, blepheraptosis, or telecanthus.

## Visceral

Complications involving the visceral structures of the face may be devastating. These include traumatic brain injury, loss of vision, and facial palsy. It has been suggested that certain attributes of facial architecture may serve to minimize force transmission to vital structures; however, injury to the brain is common with facial fractures and increases with the severity of the fracture and with fractures of the upper face and upper midface. Moreover, no difference in the severity of injury to the brain has been found in patients with facial fractures compared to those without. Facial fractures are, in fact, a marker for suspected injury to the brain.[94–98]

Facial palsy has a devastating impact on the quality of life. Proximal facial nerve injuries (resulting from facial injuries or temporal bone fractures) result in a completely flaccid hemi-face. Inability to close the eye may lead to exposure keratopathy, and oral incompetence may be frustrating and embarrassing. Distal facial nerve injuries result in more localized loss of function, depending upon the branches affected.

## Bony

Complications of bony injuries include nonunion (failure of bony healing), malunion (successful bony healing of malpositioned segments), and infection. In the mandible, this may result from failure to choose the appropriate fixation strategy or technical failure in applying fixation. Infection and nonunion in a properly fixated fracture line is rare.[65,74] Malunion most commonly results in malocclusion. Common and avoidable mistakes include failure to properly adapt compression or reconstruction plates and failure to recognize an improperly positioned mandible during plating. Care is taken to ensure that the mandibular condyle is well seated in the glenoid fossa (centric relation) and that maximal intercuspation of teeth (centric occlusion) is maintained. Also, the mandibular arch may remain splayed along the lingual surface, despite the appearance of reduction on the labial surface. The authors routinely avoid lingual splaying of the mandibular arch via application of digital pressure to the gonial angles while fixating a reduced fracture.

Malocclusion may also result from complications of midface repair. Relapse of midface retrusion may result in early posterior contact of molars and anterior open bite. This may be avoided by maintaining MMF in the early postoperative period in the setting of complex midface LeFort fractures.[10,18] Several authors remark on the importance of reestablishing the native relationship of the midface to the skull base through the zygomatic arch.[10,20,46] Inadequate reduction of the arch, especially in failing to reestablish the length of the straight midsection of the arch, will reduce the anterior projection of the ZMC and midface. Midface retrusion may also relapse after LeFort II and III repair if the nasal root is not fixated to the glabella.[10,11,17,18,46] As mentioned above, inadequate repair of midface fractures involving the orbit may result in

enophalmos, diplopia, gaze restriction, or facial asymmetry. Lastly, a mucocele may form in the ethmoid labyrinth secondary to NOE fractures with subsequent scarring and obstruction of ethmoid outflow.

A mucocele in the frontal sinus may form in the setting of residual mucosal elements in an obliterated frontal sinus or obstruction of the nasofrontal ducts. Failure in repair or healing of posterior table fractures may result in leakage of cerebrospinal fluid into the sinus and nasal cavity. Communication between the intracranial compartment and frontal sinus may also set up an ascending infection in the form of an epidural abscess or meningitis.

# SECONDARY REPAIR

## Scar Tissue

Scar revision may take the form of medical or surgical intervention. The injection of corticosteroids reduces fibroblast chemotaxis and collagen deposition. Dermabrasion and laser resurfacing reduce raised scars and address erythema of the scar. Surgical scar revision techniques include scar excision, Z-plasty, W-plasty, and asymmetric geometric broken line closure. Scar excision is usually performed in a fusiform fashion, necessarily resulting in a longer scar, although the goal is decreased width of the scar. Key principles include absence of tension, eversion of wound edges, and serial excision when necessary. Serial excision allows excision of large scars where adequate lack of tension is not initially possible. Through multiple excisions over many weeks or months, the surrounding skin may be stretched such that a low-tension or tension-free closure is achieved. The scar may also be moved over time into hairline or an aesthetic subunit boundary.

Z-plasty is a versatile technique that involves the conversion of a linear scar into opposing triangular flaps oriented obliquely to the original scar.[26,99] The flaps are incised, undermined, and transposed, and the skin is then closed. This results in lengthening and reorientation of the scar, dependent on the angle at which limbs of the Z-plasty are cut relative to the originial scar. Compound Z-plasty techniques are applied to longer scars. Contracted scars can be lengthened and re-oriented to lay within relaxed skin tension lines. Moreover, recurrent scar contracture is inhibited by the interruption of the straight-line closure.

W-plasty and asymmetric geometric broken line techniques further advance scar excision through the creation of an irregular wound margin.[26] After a scar is removed, wound edges are incised in a running W pattern or in other random geometric shapes. The eye does not as easily perceive the broken line, and wound contraction across the broken line is inhibited.

A complete discussion of specific secondary corrections of eyelid,[100,101] nasal,[32,102] and lip[102] deformities is beyond the scope of this chapter. The reader is referred to the literature.

## Visceral

A facial palsy is best addressed through primary reanastomosis or cable graft of the facial nerve, if possible. If this is not possible, secondary procedures are directed either at restoring neurologic input to the facial musculature or resuspending the facial soft tissues in a dynamic or static manner. Currently accepted strategies for restoring facial function when distal branches are preserved include hypoglossal-facial anastomosis, cross-facial grafting, and microneurovascular free muscle transfer. Although muscular tone is often improved, no procedure is known to achieve normal facial movement and dyskinesis is common.

Hypoglossal-facial anastomosis provides an ample stock of neurons, but carries the disadvantage of ipsilateral loss of tongue function and loss of emotional movement of facial muscles. Tone is often restored, and a volitional smile is accomplished when the patient performs a tongue movement. Alternatively, a hypoglossal nerve (CN XII)– facial nerve (CN VII) jump graft may preserve ipislateral tongue function, although less stimulation of the seventh nerve is achieved. The cross-facial graft connects buccal branches of an intact facial nerve to divisions of the severed nerve. It provides facial tone and the chance for emotional input to the injured hemiface; however, a small stock of neurons is engrafted compared to the hypoglossal procedures. Several authors support a combination of CNXII-CNVII jump grafting, such that innervation to the mimetic muscles is preserved (the so-called "baby-sitting procedure") prior to cross-facial grafting or a free neuromuscular transfer.[103–107]

Facial slings and adjunctive procedures may be used to suspend lax tissue of a paralyzed face, either in combination with nerve anastomosis procedures or where those procedures are refused or contraindicated. A portion of the temporalis muscle may be freed from its bed, transposed over the zygoma, and connected to the lateral canthus or oral commisure. The deep temporal nerves are protected, producing a dynamic sling. The temporal defect may be filled with a temporoparietal fascial flap or allograft implant. A static sling may be fashioned from fascia lata or an allograft such as acellular dermis and suspended from the zygomatic arch. A brow lift and face lift are often useful in improving laxity of the face and ptosis of the brow. A gold weight implant may be inserted over the tarsus of the upper eyelid in order to achieve passive eyelid closure. Correction of lower lid paralytic ectropion and oral incompetence may be obtained through wedge excisions from the eyelids and lips, respectively.

## Bony

Secondary corrections of the craniofacial skeleton are undertaken in order to address unacceptable facial asymmetry, orbital complications, or malocclusion. Malocclusion is usually obvious to the patient, manifesting as a lack of intercuspation, open bite, or discomfort with chewing, especially in the temporomandibular joint. Patient history, physical examination, cephalometric study, 3-D CT scan, and dental models comprise a full evaluation of the problem and assist in planning corrective measures. If a malocclusion is minor and if skeletal relationships are acceptable or discrepancies minor, then the patient may be managed through nonsurgical orthodontic techniques. Orthodontics may also be necessary in "setting up" a skeletal correction.

Skeletal corrections are accomplished via a number of well-studied craniofacial osteotomies. The soft-tissue approaches for these osteotomies are the same as those described above. The osteotomies themselves maintain adequate vascular support to the skeletal elements and facilitate horizontal, vertical, and angular

movements of the jaws. Through a LeFort I osteotomy, the maxillary alveolus is advanced or retruded, with or without superior impaction or down-grafting. The mandible may be split in a sagittal fashion at the angle, in a vertical oblique manner through the ramus, or less commonly in an inverted 'L' pattern through the inferior and anterior aspects of the ramus. Set back, advancement, and angular adjustment of the projection of the mandibular arch from the ramus are possible. Malunion of the midface also requires osteotomies of the affected subunits in order to achieve repositioning.

Finally, orbital fractures may require secondary correction. Failure to recognize enophthalmos, late development of enophthalmos, and inadequate reconstruction lead to the need for secondary or delayed correction. Blowout fractures should be differentiated from orbitozygomatic, LeFort, and central midace fractures that involve both the orbital rims and walls because the required correction is far greater if the midface is involved. Rim position can affect globe position and, therefore, orbital wall repair should not be attempted without correction of a malunion of the rims.[108] A complete ophthalmologic exam will also differentiate dipopia due to enophthalmos from dysfunction of eye muscle, which may require surgery in addition to bony repair of the orbit. Soft-tissue approaches to the orbit and repair of fractures are accomplished secondarily just as in primary repair. As in primary repair, both the anterior and posterior orbital floor must be repaired.

## THE CUTTING EDGE AND BEYOND

The principles of minimizing facial incisions, reducing any unneeded impact of plating, and improving the management of massive tissue loss are driving advances in craniofacial repair. Endoscopic management of orbital floor and subcondylar fractures have already been mentioned; however, the endoscope is increasingly utilized throughout the craniofacial skeleton. Indeed, the frontal sinus, the medial orbital walls, and the zygomatic arch may be accessed endoscopically, transnasally, or through minimal incisions and repaired.[109–112] Orthognathic osteotomies may be performed through limited incisions using endoscopic assistance. This science will continue to develop with the continued desire on part of patients and surgeons alike for minimally-invasive approaches. The addition of computer-guided technologies to minimally invasive techniques will further advance the ability to perform these procedures through less invasive approaches.

Semirigid fixation in the craniofacial skeleton may be accomplished with bioabsorbable plates. These plates consist of polymers of lactic acid or glycolic acid and are known to retain strength for up to three months and to completely absorb over several months thereafter. Their use is gaining wide acceptance in pediatric craniofacial surgery where metallic plates may migrate during or interfere with facial growth. Most recently, fiber-reinforced bioabsorbable materials have demonstrated sufficient strength even for mandibular repair.[66,68,69]

Finally, tissue engineering represents a nascent but promising field with applications in repairing defects of the face and craniofacial skeleton. The use of cells, cytokines, genetic material, and biocompatible materials to regenerate normal skeletal and soft tissues in the exact conformation of lost tissue and under the direction of the recipient's own physiology is currently moving from the bench to the realm of clinical research. Regeneration of bone and cartilage through gene therapy techniques is already possible in the laboratory[113] and, recently, Kopp et al. described the clinical application of engineered skin in burn patients.[114,115] These approaches hold the promise of minimizing and perhaps someday even eliminating the devastating effects of tissue loss and scarring.

## HIGHLIGHTS OF CARE

### Repair of Complex of Facial Fractures

1. Work from stable to unstable

2. Reduce complex fractures to increasingly simpler patterns by treating individual components in progression.

3. Re-establish projection of the face from the skull base

    (a) Utilize occlusal relationships so that mandibular height and projection guide the reduction and correction midface deformities.

    (b) Re-establish anterior projection by correctly reducing the zygomatic arch.

4. Ensure that the mandibular arch is properly reduced, especially in the setting of a symphyseal or parasymphyseal fracture and a split palate.

    (a) Bimanual pressure applied the gonial angles will reduce splaying of the lingual cortex.

5. Utilize wire suture at key fracture lines in order to partially stabilize fracture segments to facilitate definitive fracture reduction.

### Treatment of Massive Wounds

1. Early reduction of facial fractures

    (a) Prevent soft tissue contracture over an inadequately treated facial skeleton

    (b) Consider bone grafting in severely comminuted or lost skeletal segments

2. Serial debridement within the evolving zone of necrosis

3. Early reconstruction of soft tissue defects

## REFERENCES

1. Holt G: Acute Soft Tissue Injuries. In: I. Papel, ed. *Facial Plastic and Reconstructive Surgery.*. New York, NY: Theime, 2002, p. 689.
2. Trauma TACoSCo: *Advanced Trauma Life Support for Doctors.* 2nd ed. Vol. 1. Chicago, IL: American College of Surgeons, 1999.
3. Rosen P: *Emergency Medicine: Concepts and Clinical Practice.* 4th ed. St. Louis: Mosby, 1998.
4. Hoffmann J: Management of facial soft-tissue injuries. *Facial Plast Surg Clin North Am* 6:407, 1998.
5. Naimer SA, Nash M, Niv A, et al.: Control of massive bleeding from facial gunshot wound with a compact elastic adhesive compression dressing. *Am J Emerg Med* 22:586, 2004.
6. Potparic Z, Fukuta K, Colen LB, et al.: Galeo-pericranial flaps in the forehead: A study of blood supply and volumes. *Br J Plast Surg* 49:519, 1996.
7. Fukuta K, Potparic Z, Sugihara T, et al.: A cadaver investigation of the blood supply of the galeal frontalis flap. *Plast Reconstr Surg* 94:794, 1994.
8. Rodriquez RL, Zide BM: Reconstruction of the medial canthus. *Clin Plast Surg* 15:255, 1988.
9. Johnson CM, Toriumi DM: *Open Structure Rhinoplasty.* Philadelphia: W.B. Saunders, 1990, p. 516.
10. Manson PN, Clark N, Robertson B, et al.: Subunit principles in midface fractures: The importance of sagittal buttresses, soft-tissue reductions, and sequencing treatment of segmental fractures. *Plast Reconstr Surg* 103:1287, 1999, quiz 1307.
11. Stanley R: Maxillofacial Trauma. In: Cummings, CEA, ed. *Otolaryngology–Head & Neck Surgery.* St. Louis: Mosby, 1998, p. 453.
12. Motamedi MH: Primary management of maxillofacial hard and soft tissue gunshot and shrapnel injuries. *J Oral Maxillofac Surg* 61:1390, 2003.
13. Alper M, Totan S, Cankayali R, et al.: Gunshot wounds of the face in attempted suicide patients. *J Oral Maxillofac Surg* 56:930, (discussion 933), 1998.
14. Clark N, Birely B, Manson PN, et al.: High-energy ballistic and avulsive facial injuries: Classification, patterns, and an algorithm for primary reconstruction. *Plast Reconstr Surg* 98:583, 1996.
15. Lee RH, Gamble WB, Mayer MH, et al.: Patterns of facial laceration from blunt trauma. *Plast Reconstr Surg* 99:1544, 1997.
16. Lee RH, et al.: The MCFONTZL classification system for soft-tissue injuries to the face. *Plast Reconstr Surg* 103:1150, 1999.
17. Stanley R, Nowack G: Midfacial fractures: Importance of angle of impact to horizontal craniofacial buttresses. *Otolaryngol Head Neck Surgery* 93, 1985.
18. Prein J, Assael LA: Arbeitsgemeinschaft feur Osteosynthesefragen, *Manual of Internal Fixation in the Cranio-Facial Skeleton: Techniques Recommended by the AO/ASIF-Maxillofacial Group.* Berlin, New York: Springer, 1998, p. 227.
19. Ducic Y, Hamler D: Fractures of the midface. *Facial Plast Surg Clin North Am* 6:467, 1998.
20. Gruss JS, Van Wyek L, Phillips JH, et al.: The importance of the zygomatic arch in complex midfacial fracture repair and correction of posttraumatic orbitozygomatic deformities. *Plast Reconstr Surg* 85:878, 1990.
21. Vora NM, Fedok FG: Management of the central nasal support complex in naso-orbital ethmoid fractures. *Facial Plast Surg* 16:181, 2000.
22. Stranc MF: Primary treatment of naso-ethmoid injuries with increased intercanthal distance. *Br J Plast Surg* 23:8, 1970.
23. Gear AJ, Apasova E, Schmitz JP, et al.: Treatment modalities for mandibular angle fractures. *J Oral Maxillofac Surg* 63:655, 2005.
24. Levy FE, Smith RW, Odland RM, et al.: Monocortical miniplate fixation of mandibular angle fractures. *Arch Otolaryngol Head Neck Surg* 117:149, 1991.
25. Levy RA, Rosenbaum AE, Kellman RM, et al.: Assessing whether the plane of section on CT affects accuracy in demonstrating facial fractures in 3-D reconstruction when using a dried skull. *AJNR Am J Neuroradiol* 12:861, 1991.
26. Davidson T: Lacerations and Scar. In: Cummings CEA, ed. *Revision in Otolaryngology - Head and Neck Surgery.*, St. Louis, MO: Mosby, 1998, p. 431.
27. Leach J: Proper handling of soft tissue in the acute phase. *Facial Plast Surg* 17:227, 2001.
28. Hollander JE, Richman PB, Werblud M, et al.: Irrigation in facial and scalp lacerations: Does it alter outcome? *Ann Emerg Med* 31:73, 1998.
29. Baker SR, Swanson NA: *Local Flaps in Facial Reconstruction.* St. Louis: Mosby, 1995, p. 606.
30. Naficy S, Baker SR: The extended Abbe flap in the reconstruction of complex midfacial defects. *Arch Facial Plast Surg* 2:141, 2000.
31. Rosenstein T, Talebzadeh N, Pogrel MA: Anatomy of the lateral canthal tendon. *Oral Surg Oral Med Oral Pathol Oral Radiol Endod* 89:24, 2000.
32. Baker SR, Naficy S: *Principles of Nasal Reconstruction.* St. Louis: Mosby,, 2002, p. 301.
33. Chudakov O, Ludchik T: Microsurgical repair of Stensen's & Wharton's ducts with autogenous venous grafts. An experimental study on dogs. *Int J Oral Maxillofac Surg* 28:70, 1999.
34. Heymans O, Nelissen X, Medot M, et al.: Microsurgical repair of Stensen's duct using an interposition vein graft. *J Reconstr Microsurg* 15:105, (discussion 107), 1999.
35. Lewis G, Knottenbelt JD: Parotid duct injury: Is immediate surgical repair necessary? *Injury* 22:407, 1991.
36. Parekh D, Glezerson G, Stewart M, et al.: Post-traumatic parotid fistulae and sialoceles. A prospective study of conservative management in 51 cases. *Ann Surg* 209:105, 1989.
37. Landau R, Stewart M: Conservative management of post-traumatic parotid fistulae and sialoceles: A prospective study. *Br J Surg* 72:42, 1985.
38. Lapid O, Kreiger Y, Sagi A: Transdermal scopolamine use for post-rhytidectomy sialocele. *Aesthetic Plast Surg* 28:24, 2004.
39. Vargas H, Galati LT, Parnes SM: A pilot study evaluating the treatment of postparotidectomy sialoceles with botulinum toxin type A. *Arch Otolaryngol Head Neck Surg* 126:421, 2000.
40. Cavanaugh K, Park A: Postparotidectomy fistula: A different treatment for an old problem. *Int J Pediatr Otorhinolaryngol* 47:265, 1999.

41. Malik TH, Kelly G, Ahmed A, et al.: A comparison of surgical techniques used in dynamic reanimation of the paralyzed face. *Otol Neurotol* 26:284, 2005.

42. Alex JC, Nguyen DB: Multivectored suture suspension: A minimally invasive technique for reanimation of the paralyzed face. *Arch Facial Plast Surg* 6:197, 2004.

43. Sherris DA: Refinement in reanimation of the lower face. *Arch Facial Plast Surg* 6:49, 2004.

44. Takushima A, Harii K, Asato H, et al.: Neurovascular free-muscle transfer for the treatment of established facial paralysis following ablative surgery in the parotid region. *Plast Reconstr Surg* 113:1563, 2004.

45. Levine R: *Care of the Eye in Facial Paralysis.* In: Brackman D, Shelton C, Arriaga M, eds. *Otologic Surgery.* Philadelphia, PA: W.B. Saunders Company, 2001, p. 611.

46. Kellman RM, Marentette LJ: *Atlas of Craniomaxillofacial Fixation.* New York: Raven Press, 1995, p. 337.

47. Frodel JL, Marentette LJ: The coronal approach. Anatomic and technical considerations and morbidity. *Arch Otolaryngol Head Neck Surg* 119:201, 1993, discussion 140.

48. Ellis E, Zide MF: *Surgical Approaches to the Facial Skeleton.* 2nd ed. Philadelphia: Lippincott Williams & Wilkins, 2006.

49. Greenberg AM, Prein J: *Craniomaxillofacial Reconstructive and Corrective Bone Surgery: Principles of Internal Fixation Using AO/ASIF Technique.* New York: Springer, 2002, p. 784.

50. Kellman RM, Tatum SA: Internal fixation of maxillofacial fractures: Indications and current implant technologies and materials. *Facial Plast Surg* 14:3, 1998.

51. Kellman R: Clinical applications of bone plating systems to facial fractures. In: Papel I, ed. *Facial Plastic and Reconstructive Surgery.* New York, NY: Thieme Medical Publishers, Inc., 2002, p. 720.

52. Spiessl B: Rigid internal fixation of fractures of the lower jaw. *Reconstr Surg Traumatol* 13:124, 1972.

53. Winzenburg SaIM: Mandible Fractures. *Facial Plast Surg Clin North Am* 6:445, 1998.

54. Haug RH, Street CC, Goltz M: Does plate adaptation affect stability? A biomechanical comparison of locking and nonlocking plates. *J Oral Maxillofac Surg* 60:1319, 2002.

55. Frodel JL Jr, Marentette LJ: Lag screw fixation in the upper craniomaxillofacial skeleton. *Arch Otolaryngol Head Neck Surg* 119:297, 1993.

56. Cooley DR, Van Dellen AF, Burgess JO, et al.: The advantages of coated titanium implants prepared by radiofrequency sputtering from hydroxyapatite. *J Prosthet Dent* 67:93, 1992.

57. Buser D, Broggini N, Wieland M, et al.: Enhanced bone apposition to a chemically modified SLA titanium surface. *J Dent Res* 83:529, 2004.

58. Steinemann SG: Titanium—the material of choice? *Periodontol* 17:7, 2000, 1998.

59. Listgarten MA, Buser D, Steinemann SG, et al.: Light and transmission electron microscopy of the intact interfaces between non-submerged titanium-coated epoxy resin implants and bone or gingiva. *J Dent Res* 71:364, 1992.

60. Tams J, Otten B, van Loon JP, et al.: A computer study of fracture mobility and strain on biodegradable plates used for fixation of mandibular fractures. *J Oral Maxillofac Surg* 57:973, (discussion 981), 1999.

61. Tams J, van Loon JP, Otten E, et al.: A three-dimensional study of bending and torsion moments for different fracture sites in the mandible: An in vitro study. *Int J Oral Maxillofac Surg* 26:383, 1997.

62. Tams J, van Loon JP, Rozema FR, et al.: A three-dimensional study of loads across the fracture for different fracture sites of the mandible. *Br J Oral Maxillofac Surg* 34:400, 1996.

63. Champy M, Lodde JP, Schmitt R, et al.: Mandibular osteosynthesis by miniature screwed plates via a buccal approach. *J Maxillofac Surg* 6:14, 1978.

64. Herford AS, Ellis E III: Use of a locking reconstruction bone plate/screw system for mandibular surgery. *J Oral Maxillofac Surg* 56:1261, 1998.

65. Ellis E III, Graham J: Use of a 2.0-mm locking plate/screw system for mandibular fracture surgery. *J Oral Maxillofac Surg* 60:642, (discussion 645), 2002.

66. Yerit KC, Enislidis G, Schopper C, et al.: Fixation of mandibular fractures with biodegradable plates and screws. *Oral Surg Oral Med Oral Pathol Oral Radiol Endod* 94:294, 2002.

67. Enislidis G, Yerit K, Witter G, et al.: Self-reinforced biodegradable plates and screws for fixation of zygomatic fractures. *J Craniomaxillofac Surg* 33:95, 2005.

68. Yerit KC, Hainich S, Turhani D, et al.: Stability of biodegradable implants in treatment of mandibular fractures. *Plast Reconstr Surg* 115:1863, 2005.

69. Yerit KC, Hainich S, Enislidis G, et al.: Biodegradable fixation of mandibular fractures in children: Stability and early results. *Oral Surg Oral Med Oral Pathol Oral Radiol Endod,* 100:17, 2005.

70. Gerlach KL, Schwarz A: Bite forces in patients after treatment of mandibular angle fractures with miniplate osteosynthesis according to Champy. *Int J Oral Maxillofac Surg* 31:345, 2002.

71. Wagner A, Krach W, Schicho K, et al.: A 3-dimensional finite-element analysis investigating the biomechanical behavior of the mandible and plate osteosynthesis in cases of fractures of the condylar process. *Oral Surg Oral Med Oral Pathol Oral Radiol Endod* 94:678, 2002.

72. Tams J, van Loon JP, Otten B, et al.: A computer study of biodegradable plates for internal fixation of mandibular angle fractures. *J Oral Maxillofac Surg* 59:404, (discussion 407), 2001.

73. Haug RH: The effects of screw number and length on two methods of tension band plating. *J Oral Maxillofac Surg* 51:159, 1993.

74. Fox AJ, Kellman RM: Mandibular angle fractures: Two-miniplate fixation and complications. *Arch Facial Plast Surg* 5:464, 2003.

75. Haug RH, Fattahi TT, Goltz M: A biomechanical evaluation of mandibular angle fracture plating techniques. *J Oral Maxillofac Surg* 59:1199, 2001.

76. Ellis E, Throckmorton GS: Treatment of mandibular condylar process fractures: Biological considerations. *J Oral Maxillofac Surg* 63:115, 2005.

77. Throckmorton GS, Ellis E III, Hayasaki H: Jaw kinematics during mastication after unilateral fractures of the mandibular condylar process. *Am J Orthod Dentofacial Orthop* 124:695, 2003.

78. Miloro M: Considerations in subcondylar fracture management. *Arch Otolaryngol Head Neck Surg* 130:1231, 2004.

79. Kellman RM: Endoscopically assisted repair of subcondylar fractures of the mandible: An evolving technique. *Arch Facial Plast Surg* 5:244, 2003.

80. Raveh J: Closed mind to an open technique. *J Oral Maxillofac Surg* 47:773, 1989.

81. Iizuka T, Ladrach K, Geering AH, et al.: Open reduction without fixation of dislocated condylar process fractures: Long-term clinical and radiologic analysis. *J Oral Maxillofac Surg* 56:553, (discussion 561), 1998.

82. Schon R, Gutwald R, Schramm A, et al.: Endoscopy-assisted open treatment of condylar fractures of the mandible: Extraoral vs intraoral approach. *Int J Oral Maxillofac Surg* 31:237, 2002.

83. Phillips JH, Forrest CR, Gruss JS: Current concepts in the use of bone grafts in facial fractures. Basic science considerations. *Clin Plast Surg* 19:41, 1992.

84. Farwell DG, Strong EB: Endoscopic repair of orbital floor fractures. *Facial Plast Surg Clin North Am* 14:11, 2006.

85. Markowitz BL, Manson PN, Sargent L, et al.: Management of the medial canthal tendon in nasoethmoid orbital fractures: The importance of the central fragment in classification and treatment. *Plast Reconstr Surg* 87:843, 1991.

86. Strong E, Sykes J: *Frontal Sinus and Nasoorbitoethmoid Complex Fractures.* In: Papel I, ed. *Facial Plastic and Reconstructive Surgery.* New York, NY: Thieme Medical Publishers, 2002, p. 747.

87. Yavuzer R, Sari A, Kelly CP, et al.: Management of frontal sinus fractures. *Plast Reconstr Surg* 115:79e, (discussion 94e), 2005.

88. Kellman R: Use of the Subcranial Approach in Maxillofacial Trauma. *Facial Plast Surg Clin North Am* 6:507, 1998.

89. Kienstra MA, Van Loveren H: Anterior skull base fractures. *Facial Plast Surg* 21:180, 2005.

90. Fliss DM, Zucker G, Cohen T, et al.: The subcranial approach for the treatment of cerebrospinal fluid rhinorrhea: A report of 10 cases. *J Oral Maxillofac Surg* 59:1171, 2001.

91. Taher AA: Management of weapon injuries to the craniofacial skeleton. *J Craniofac Surg* 9:371, 1998.

92. Yuksel F, Celikoz B, Ergun O, et al.: Management of maxillofacial problems in self-inflicted rifle wounds. *Ann Plast Surg* 53:111, 2004.

93. Chen MA, Davidson TM: Scar management: Prevention and treatment strategies. *Curr Opin Otolaryngol Head Neck Surg* 13:242, 2005.

94. Gentry LR: Facial trauma and associated brain damage. *Radiol Clin North Am* 27:435, 1989.

95. Keenan HT, Brundage SI, Thompson DC, et al.: Does the face protect the brain? A case-control study of traumatic brain injury and facial fractures. *Arch Surg* 134:14, 1999.

96. Carlin CB, Ruff G, Mansfeld CP, et al.: Facial fractures and related injuries: A ten-year retrospective analysis. *J Craniomaxillofac Trauma* 4:44, (discussion 43), 1998.

97. Martin RC II, Spain DA, Richardson JD: Do facial fractures protect the brain or are they a marker for severe head injury? *Am Surg* 68:477, 2002.

98. Kraus JF, Rice TM, Peek-Asa C, et al.: Facial trauma and the risk of intracranial injury in motorcycle crashes. *Ann Emerg Med* 41:18, 2003.

99. Frodel J, Wang T: Z-plasty. In: Baker S, Swanson N, eds. *Local Flaps in Facial Reconstruction.* St. Louis, MO: Mosby, 1995, p. 131.

100. Patel B, Flaharty P, Anderson R: Reconstruction of the eyelids. In: Baker S, Swanson N, eds. *Local Flaps in Facial Reconstruction.* St. Louis, MO: Mosby, 1995, p. 275.

101. Bersani T, Courchesne M: Post-traumatic eyelid deformities. *Facial Plast Surg Clin North Am* 6:511, 1998.

102. Gregory R: *Reconstruction of the Lip.* In: Baker S, Swanson N, eds. *Local Flaps in Facial Reconstruction.* St. Louis, MO: Mosby, 1995.

103. Kalantarian B, et al.: Gains and losses of the XII-VII component of the "baby-sitter" procedure: A morphometric analysis. *J Reconstr Microsurg* 14:459, 1998.

104. Mersa B, Tiangco DA, Terzis JK: Efficacy of the "baby-sitter" procedure after prolonged denervation. *J Reconstr Microsurg* 16:27, 2000.

105. Terzis JK, Kalantarian B: Microsurgical strategies in 74 patients for restoration of dynamic depressor muscle mechanism: A neglected target in facial reanimation. *Plast Reconstr Surg* 105:1917, (discussion 1932). 2000.
106. Guelinckx PJ, Sinsel NK: Muscle transplantation for reconstruction of a smile after facial paralysis past, present, and future. *Microsurgery* 17:391, 1996.
107. Yoleri L, et al.: Cross-facial nerve grafting as an adjunct to hypoglossal-facial nerve crossover in reanimation of early facial paralysis: Clinical and electrophysiological evaluation. *Ann Plast Surg* 46:301, 2001.
108. Kellman RM, Bersani TA: Delayed and secondary repair of posttraumatic enophthalmos and orbital deformities. *Facial Plast Surg Clin North Am* 10:311, 2002.
109. Strong EB, Kellman RM: Endoscopic repair of anterior table-frontal sinus fractures. *Facial Plast Surg Clin North Am* 14:25, 2006.
110. Shumrick KA: Endoscopic management of frontal sinus fractures. *Facial Plast Surg Clin North Am* 14:31, 2006.
111. Rhee JS, Chen CT: Endoscopic approach to medial orbital wall fractures. *Facial Plast Surg Clin North Am* 14:17, 2006.
112. Czerwinski M, Lee C: The rationale and technique of endoscopic approach to the zygomatic arch in facial trauma. *Facial Plast Surg Clin North Am*, 14:37, 2006.
113. Nussenbaum B, Rutherford RB, Krebsbach PH: Bone regeneration in cranial defects previously treated with radiation. *Laryngoscope* 115:1170, 2005.
114. Kopp J, Jeschke MG, Bach AD, et al.: Applied tissue engineering in the closure of severe burns and chronic wounds using cultured human autologous keratinocytes in a natural fibrin matrix. *Cell Tissue Bank* 5:89, 2004.
115. Horch RE, Kopp J, Kneser U, et al.: Tissue engineering of cultured skin substitutes. *J Cell Mol Med* 9:592, 2005.

# Commentary ■ VINCENT J. PERCIACCANTE ■ SAM E. FARISH

The chapter on facial trauma by Kellman and Rontal is extremely well organized. In the introduction the authors outline the material they will present and go from care of the facial trauma patient in the emergency room and trauma bay to the anatomy, evaluation, and management of facial injuries. They subdivide their discussions into the soft tissue, visceral, and bony components of the face. They emphasize that early management is dictated by the magnitude of facial injuries in the most emergent setting. Early diagnosis and treatment during the acute and subacute periods and management of secondary complications are also well described. The presentation of such a broad discussion of the subject of facial trauma is a credit to their knowledge of the subject, but also a bit of a problem to the intended audience of this text. What a trauma surgeon needs to know about facial trauma can be summed up in far fewer pages than the authors chose to use. Surgical approaches, fixation modalities, and reconstruction procedures are elegantly presented by the authors but the details presented tend to blunt the important take-home messages about facial trauma for trauma center personnel.

We agree with the authors that the reader of this text should be made aware of the place occupied by facial trauma within the ATLS evaluation and subsequent management. Evaluation and initial management of facial injury is part of the ATLS secondary survey except when these injuries involve compromise to the airway or severe hemorrhage. Potential airway compromise is the biggest threat to the well being of the facial trauma patient. The authors covered most airway topics quite well. Markedly displaced, bilateral mandible fractures can result in a flail mandible that allows the contents of the oral cavity to fall back on the posterior pharyngeal wall. Simply pulling the segment forward with the hand or a towel clip can frequently relieve the obstruction and allow for less urgency in securing an airway by intubation or surgery. Well-placed "bridle wires" can fix such flail segments in dentate patients and serve as a temporary measure to lessen the need for emergent airway intervention. Severely displaced maxillary fractures may also cause airway compromise.

Bleeding, most frequently, is not a major problem with facial injuries, but can be a major issue with severe injuries. When it is, good lighting and suction are essential for identification of the bleeders and their management by ligation or well-placed pressure.

The value of pressure in facial bleeding cannot be overemphasized and the author's reference to pressure wrap techniques utilized in Isreal[1] is very interesting. Posterior nasal packing with a Foley catheter under anterior traction and anterior nasal packing with nasal "rhino-rockets" must also be emphasized. If bleeding associated with facial injuries that cannot be readily controlled with the above measures or is known to be from inaccessible skull base sources then angiography and targeted embolization cannot be delayed.

Since cervical spine injuries frequently accompany facial injuries, protection of the neck is essential until it can be cleared clinically and/or radiographically. The maintenance of in-line cervical support can hinder some manipulations needed in diagnosis and management of facial trauma, but with care these can be overcome. The chapter on neck injuries in this text details the evaluation and emergent management of these injuries quite well.

If the airway is secured and bleeding is adequately managed, most of the implications of facial trauma are under immediate control and the diagnostic goals can be addressed when all other life-threatening injuries are addressed. It is at this point that the discipline which will treat the facial injuries should be involved. In some instances, when the patient is being fast tracked to the OR for the treatment of life-threatening injuries, those that manage facial trauma may be of valuable service for placement of temporary fixation, definitive or temporary closure of extensive laceration as well as airway assistance for anesthesia. The basic facial examination, including palpitation for crepitance and mobility of facial skeletal components, inspection for malocclusion and step deformities, examination of ocular function and cranial nerve examination is a critical element of evaluation.

The panorex radiograph is widely available at trauma centers and is a most valuable film, whose importance in mandible fracture diagnosis and treatment planning cannot be diminished. A reverse Townes view of the skull can also be an important plain film for the diagnosis of mandibular condyle fractures. We agree that CT is the most important radiologic modality. There should be standard protocols in trauma centers where the elements needed (cut size, reconstruction potentials, etc.) that constitute a routine facial bones CT are clearly specified. This saves repeat examinations as most trauma patients will get CT of other anatomic regions as the authors pointed out. We agree that 3-D reformatted images of the facial bones are a very valuable treatment planning and teaching tool. We do not think the inaccuracies, noted by the authors demean their importance, in mid-face trauma in particular, especially when viewed in different penetrations.

From personal experience, we feel that the fact that the authors made no reference to facial trauma as a marker for intimate partner violence or the role in recognition of possible child abuse associated with facial trauma is a notable oversight. We also would like to point out to the trauma community that a facial injury severity scale has been developed as a research tool, by Bagheri et al.[2] in Portland. Tools such as this will make research data on facial trauma easier to collate and broaden our ability to improve our management and assess outcomes.

As regards the surgical techniques for facial fractures presented in perhaps too much detail by the authors, their emphasis of the need for open reduction of mandibular condyle fractures is currently not well supported by the literature and endoscopic open reduction of condylar fractures is not commonly practiced in but a few centers. Though open reduction with internal fixation for these injuries is important and performed frequently in our institution, it is not necessarily the definitive standard of care. Additionally, the term "closed-reduction", when referring to mandibular condylar and subcondylar fractures, is, in our opinion a misnomer and the term "closed-treatment" is more appropriate. Variance of opinion on treatment is far beyond the scope of this text, but we feel these points were worthy of comment.

## References

1. Naimer SA, Nash M et al.: Control of massive bleeding from facial gunshot wound with a compact elastic adhesive compression dressing. *Am J Emerg Med* 22:586, 2004.
2. Bagheri SC, Dierks EJ et al.: Application of a facial injury severity scale in craniomaxilofacial trauma. *J Oral Maxillofac Surg* 64:408, 2006.

# Management of Acute Neck Injuries

*L.D. Britt* ■ *Leonard J. Weireter, Jr.* ■ *Frederic J. Cole, Jr.*

## INTRODUCTION

The neck has been a source of tremendous interest in the trauma surgical literature for several hundred years. The high density of vital structures, in a relatively small and unprotected anatomic region, makes an adult or child vulnerable to potentially fatal injuries. Unfortunately, critical injuries of the neck are not always apparent during the initial assessment and failure to recognize aerodigestive and major vascular or neurologic injuries to the neck can substantially increase morbidity and mortality. Airway compromise resulting from laryngotracheal injuries, along with sustained hemorrhage from injuries to the major vessels, are the main contributing factors in the mortality of neck injuries. However, the debate about the proper treatment of neck trauma has persisted for centuries.

## ANATOMY OF THE NECK

Knowledge of the surface landmarks of the neck is imperative for optimal evaluation and management of neck injuries. The defining borders of the neck encompass the area between the lower margin of the mandible and the superior nuchal line of the occipital bone and the suprasternal notch and the upper border of the clavicle.

Palpable structures (Figs. 23-1 and 23-2) from the upper to lower border of the neck include the symphysis menti, which is where the two halves of the body of the mandible unite in the midline. The submental triangle, located between the symphysis menti and the body of the hyoid bone, is bounded inferiorly by the hyoid bone and anteriorly by the midline of the neck. Laterally, it is bounded by the anterior belly of the digastric muscle. The mylohyoid muscle forms the floor. The body of the hyoid bone lies opposite the third cervical vertebra. The area between the hyoid bone and the thyroid cartilage is the thyrohyoid membrane. The notched upper border of the thyroid cartilage is at the level of the cervical vertebra. The cricothyroid ligament or membrane occupies the space between the cricoid cartilage and the thyroid cartilage. The cricoid cartilage lies at the level of the sixth cervical vertebra and the junction of the pharynx with the esophagus. The interval between the cricoid cartilage and the first tracheal ring is filled by the cricotracheal ligament. The isthmus of the thyroid gland is at the level of the second, third, and fourth tracheal rings. The suprasternal notch can be palpated between the clavicular heads and lies opposite the lower border of the body of the second thoracic vertebra. The structures that can be palpated in the midline posteriorly are the following: the external occipital protuberance, the nuchae groove and the seventh cervical vertebra (the first spinous process that can be palpated for the cervical spines 1–6 are covered by the ligamentum nuchae). The sternocleidomastoid muscle can be palpated from sternum and clavicle to the mastoid process. The sternocleidomastoid muscle is the landmark that divides the neck into anterior and posterior triangles. The borders of the anterior triangle are the body of the mandible, the sternocleidomastoid muscle, and the midline. The posterior triangle is bounded by the sternocleidomastoid muscle anteriorly, the border of the trapezius muscle posteriorly, along with the clavicle inferiorly.

The platysma, a thin muscular sheet, is enclosed by the superficial fascia. Its origin is from the deep fascia that covers the upper part of the pectoralis major and deltoid muscles and it inserts into the lower margin of the body of the mandible. It is the anatomic landmark that is often cited when determining whether a penetrating neck wound is superficial or deep. The potential for injury to a vital structure exists when this structure is penetrated.

Traditionally, wounds to the neck have been grouped into three separate zones, with most surgical discussions centering on the anatomy of the anterior triangles which encompass the area

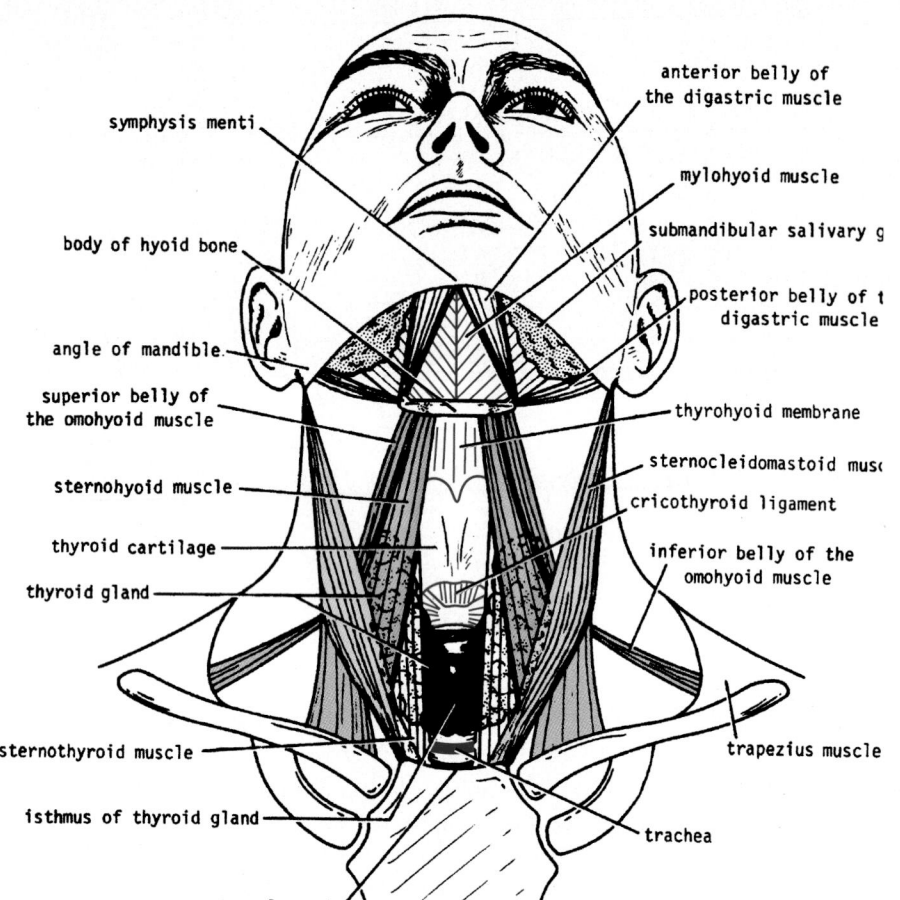

symphysis menti

body of hyoid bone

angle of mandible

superior belly of
the omohyoid muscle

sternohyoid muscle

thyroid cartilage

thyroid gland

sternothyroid muscle

isthmus of thyroid gland

anterior belly of
the digastric muscle

mylohyoid muscle

submandibular salivary g

posterior belly of t
digastric muscle

thyrohyoid membrane

sternocleidomastoid musc

cricothyroid ligament

inferior belly of the
omohyoid muscle

trapezius muscle

trachea

**FIGURE 23-1.**  Surface anatomy of the neck from the front view.
*(Reprinted with permission from Snell RS. Clinical Anatomy for Medical Students. Boston: Little, Brown, 1973, p. 616.)*

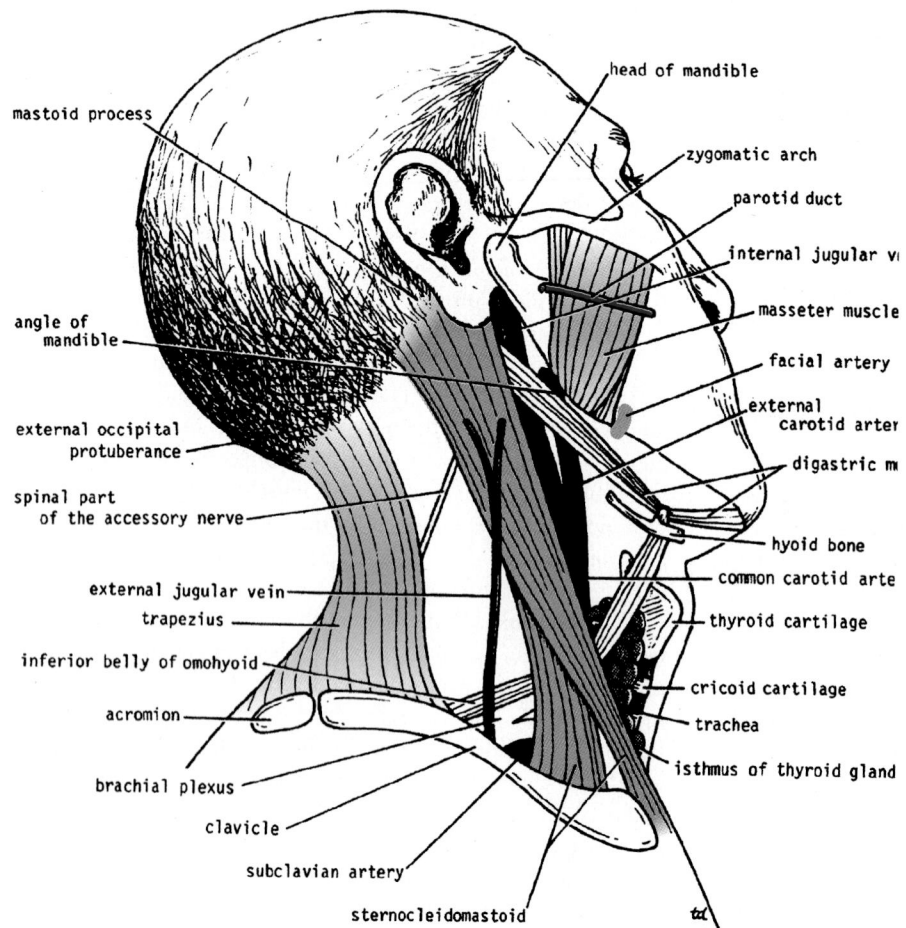

mastoid process

angle of
mandible

external occipital
protuberance

spinal part
of the accessory nerve

external jugular vein

trapezius

inferior belly of omohyoid

acromion

brachial plexus

clavicle

subclavian artery

sternocleidomastoid

head of mandible

zygomatic arch

parotid duct

internal jugular v

masseter muscle

facial artery

external
carotid arter

digastric m

hyoid bone

common carotid arte

thyroid cartilage

cricoid cartilage

trachea

isthmus of thyroid gland

**FIGURE 23-2.**  Surface anatomy of the neck from the lateral aspect.
*(Reprinted with permission from Snell RS. Clinical Anatomy for Medical Students. Boston: Little, Brown, 1973, p. 616.)*

A

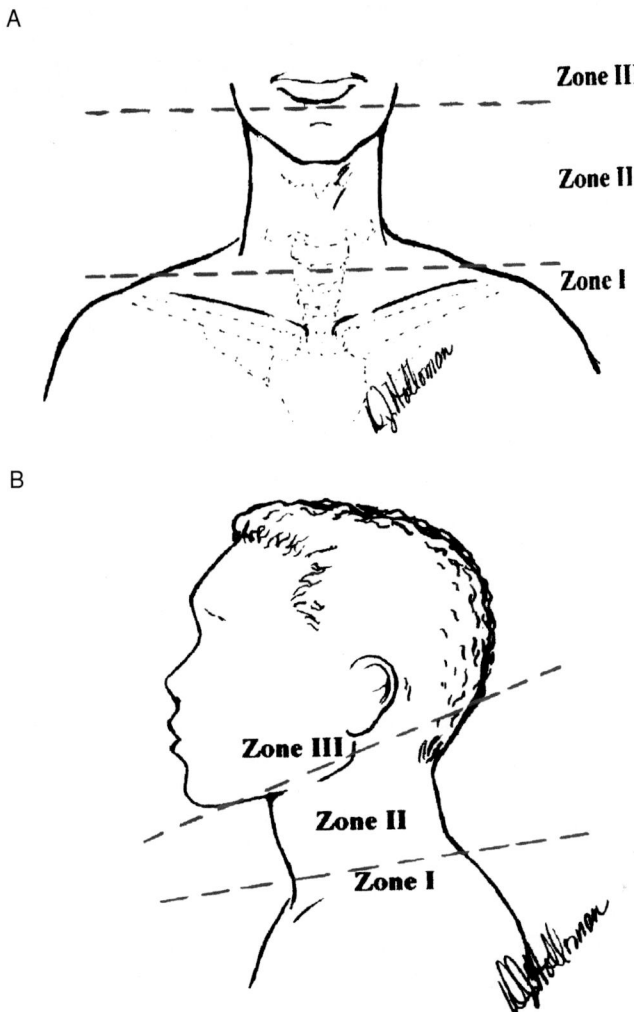

Zone III

Zone II

Zone I

B

Zone III

Zone II

Zone I

**FIGURE 23-3.** Anatomic zones of the neck. **(A)** Anterior view. **(B)** Lateral view.

between the left and right sternocleidomastoid muscles. These three "anatomic" zones of the neck provide an important guideline in the management of penetrating neck injuries (Fig. 23-3). Zone I is that horizontal area between the clavicles and the cricoid cartilage that encompasses the thoracic outlet vasculature, along with the vertebral and proximal carotid arteries, the lung, trachea, esophagus, spinal cord, thoracic duct, and major cervical nerve trunks. Zone II is that area between the cricoid cartilage and the angle of the mandible. The jugular veins, vertebral and common carotid arteries, and external and internal branches of the carotid are located in this zone. The trachea, esophagus, spinal cord, and larynx also traverse this area. Zone III, the most cephalad area, lies between the angle of the mandible and the base of the skull. The pharynx is located in this zone, along with the jugular veins, vertebral arteries, and the distal internal carotid arteries. Unlike Zones I and III that are bounded by bony structures, the central neck area (Zone II) can be accessed more expeditiously should an injury necessitate operative intervention. Zone I could possibly require a clavicle resection or median sternotomy, while exposure of Zone III might necessitate disarticulation of the mandible or resection of the base of the skull.

## INITIAL EVALUATION

In all cases, the first step in management is securing an adequate airway. The essential principles of the initial assessment in the Advanced Trauma Life Support (ATLS) are just as applicable with neck trauma as with any other injury.[1] The ATLS-directed primary survey, with its mandatory emphasis on the ABCs (airway, breathing, circulation), resuscitative efforts, and secondary survey are all imperative in the optimal management of major injuries of the neck. A definitive airway, preferably a translaryngeal endotracheal intubation, should be performed for establishment of a secure airway if there are doubts about a secure airway. In the event a translaryngeal airway cannot be established in an emergency setting, a surgical airway should be the next option. For most situations, a cricothyroidotomy should be the surgical airway of choice. However, on the rare occasion, expeditious intubation of a tracheostomy site that has been created by a neck injury may be an immediate life-saving procedure. Depending on the object and the trajectory of the sharp object or missile, pleural space entry is a possibility with penetrating neck injury.

Life-threatening complications, such as pneumo/hemothorax or a tension pneumothorax, can be associated with penetrating or blunt neck injuries, necessitating prompt recognition and pleural space decompression. Circulatory assessment and stabilization are required after appropriate airway and ventilatory management. Significant bleeding at the wound site should be managed by, preferably, direct pressure application. At no time should blind clamping, tourniquet, or pressure dressing be applied. With a team approach, these life-saving measures can all be done simultaneously.

For hemodynamically stable patients, who have undergone the primary survey and the necessary resuscitative measures, a complete history and thorough physical examination should be performed during the secondary survey. Pertinent history should include the mechanism and time of injury, whether or not loss of consciousness occurred, and whether there was significant blood loss at the scene. If the patient cannot be questioned, this and other vital information should be obtained from the prehospital personnel, family members, or persons at the injury scene.

## INJURY MANAGEMENT

The majority of penetrating trauma is a result of stabbings and gunshot injuries. High velocity injuries, (>2,500 feet/second), such as high-powered rifles, often generate a missile velocity which has 60 times more energy generated than handguns that are associated with substantially lower missile velocities. Tissue destruction is related to the energy of the projectile by the formula $k = 1/2 \ mv^2$ ($k$ = kinetic energy $3m$ = mass, and $v$ = velocity). The energy produced increases four-fold as the velocity doubles. The impact of shotgun blasts, which generate multiple low-velocity projectiles, depends on several factors including the weapon–victim range, weapon type, choke setting, and the type of shot (birdshot or buckshot).[2,3] However, at close range, a shotgun blast wound is a high velocity-type injury. Although there were isolated single case reports of surgical intervention for penetrating injuries prior to and during World War I, nonoperative management was the standard approach to penetrating neck wounds, with an associated high mortality.[4] Almost a decade after World Ward II, Fogelman and Steward reported on the first large civilian series on penetrating neck injuries.[5] With 86 total injuries in 100 patients, the authors advocated mandatory exploration of all deep penetrating wounds after reporting a significant difference in the mortality rates of immediate mandatory exploration (6%) versus delayed or expectant management (35%). This policy of routine neck exploration for Zone II penetrating wounds was broadly accepted.[6,7] However, a selective management approach evolved because of the high rate of negative exploration.[8–10] Shirkeg et al. reported one of the first studies to advocate returning to a policy of selective management of penetrating neck injuries to avoid the increased rate of nontherapeutic exploration.[11]

With respect to the general management approach in penetrating neck trauma, it should always be resource and institution dependent. For example, with the transfer of a patient with a penetrating Zone II injury not being an option, the surgeon managing the patient should consider mandatory exploration if the medical facility has limited capabilities. Although the policy of mandatory exploration for all central neck (Zone II) penetrating injuries was developed after World War II and during the Korean conflict, it was subsequently challenged by others because of the high nontherapeutic exploration rate.[11] Noyes et al. demonstrated no cost benefit to selective management of penetrating Zone II injuries as compared to mandatory exploration.[12] Several authors have advocated that selective management of penetrating neck injuries should be done to avoid unnecessary and potential morbidity.[13–15] The recommendation for selective management is influenced by the "zone" of penetration. Unless the patient has profound hemodynamic stability, a more selective approach is taken for both Zone I and III because of the difficulty in examining and operatively exposing the areas. For example, a median sternotomy or an anterolateral thoracic approach may be required to optimally manage a vascular injury in Zone I, while operative exposure for a Zone III penetrating injury might necessitate disarticulation of the mandible, resection of the angle of the mandible, resection of the styloid, or other maneuver. Obvious signs and symptoms (the so-called "hard findings") suggestive of major vascular or aerodigestive injuries require urgent operative intervention (Table 23-1). More subtle signs ("soft") necessitate a diagnostic workup (Table 23-2). The main controversy continues to center around those patients who present hemodynamically stable, with a Zone II penetrating neck wound and no signs or symptoms suggestive of a major injury to a vital structure.[16] Both mandatory and selective management of penetrating injuries in this zone have been challenged. Because of the relatively low yield of these approaches, a more expectant or observational approach has been advocated when there are no signs

## TABLE 23-1

### "Hard Findings" a Vascular or Aero-Digestive Injury

Airway compromise
Shock or active bleeding
Pulsatile hematomas
Extensive subcutaneous emphysema

## TABLE 23-2

### "Soft Findings" a Vascular or Aero-Digestive Injury

Dysphagia
Voice Change
Hemoptysis
Wide Mediastinum

of major injury to a vital structure. Hall et al. recommended nonoperative management for penetrating Zone II injuries in children.[17] Twenty-four children had penetrating injuries through the platysma in the Zone II region of the neck. Their morbidity of 21% was all secondary to neurologic injury. For the adult population, Atteberry et al. emphasized that physical examination alone is a safe and accurate method for evaluation of vascular injuries in penetrating Zone II neck trauma.[18] Demetriades et al. demonstrated in a prospective study that in patients who are hemodynamically stable with no clinical signs of vascular injuries, nonoperative management is safe.[19] The authors highlighted a negative predictive value of 100%. Intuitively it would seem that gunshot wounds to the neck, particularly transcervical, should prompt operative exploration; however, mandatory exploration of gunshot wounds to the neck has a high rate of negative and nontherapeutic operative interventions. In another study by Demetriades and colleagues, only 21% of transcervical gunshot wounds required a therapeutic operation. The authors emphasized that the majority of all transcervical gunshot wounds can be managed nonoperatively.[20] Caution must be exercised with expectant management. An occult esophageal injury can result from a penetrating neck injury, even without sign and symptoms. However, Vassiliu et al. reported that in 76 patients with aerodigestive injuries, each had suspicious signs and symptoms on admission.[21] Also, Ngakane et al. highlighted no mortality with the nonoperative approach for penetrating esophageal injuries when there was no gross spillage demonstrated.[22] A proposed treatment algorithm for penetrating neck injuries is highlighted in Fig. 23-4. All patients who are hemodynamically unstable from a penetrating neck wound should be explored. Also, high-velocity injuries to the neck dictate operative intervention. Management guidelines for blunt trauma to the neck is depicted in Fig. 23-5. Although the proposed algorithm is a helpful guideline for the treatment of penetrating neck injuries, the specific management paradigm depends on the resources of the institution and the capabilities of the surgeon.

If surgical intervention is required, the exposure options most commonly used to achieve optimal visualization of injuries are depicted in Fig. 23-6. Operative exposure of Zone I injuries may necessitate a supraclavicular incision, with removal of the head of the clavicle or a "trapdoor" approach that requires a supraclavicular incision and a median sternotomy along with an anterolateral incision. For Zone III injuries, optimal operative exposure may necessitate cephalad extension of an incision at the anterior border of the sternocleidomastoid muscle with the possibility of needing a disarticulation or partial resection of the mandible. Also, a limited craniotomy might be necessary in order to achieve the best exposure. Unlike Zone I and III neck wounds, operative exposure of the vital aerodigestive and vascular structure in Zone II can be easily done through either a standard vertical neck incision along the anterior border of the

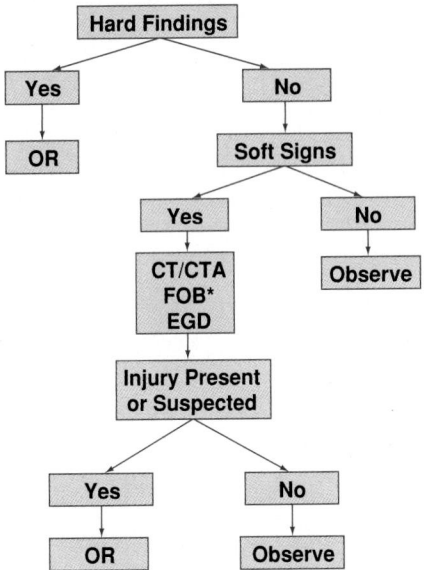

**FIGURE 23-4.** Management algorithm for penetrating neck injuries.* Fiberoptic Bronchoscopy.

sternocleidomastoid muscle or a transverse collar incision. The advantage of the latter is that this type of exposure provides access to both sides of the neck.

## Aero-Digestive Injury

Simultaneous injuries of the airway and digestive tract are not uncommon due to the close proximity of the trachea and esophagus in the neck. Aero-digestive tract injuries are seen in 10% of penetrating injuries.[23] As highlighted above, optimal airway management is paramount. In a patient who requires urgent airway management, the translaryngeal endotracheal approach is still the best option, particularly when it is performed by skilled practitioners.[24,25] The role of the surgical airway should always be considered when approaching any patient who might have a difficult airway for conventional management. However, an expert with emergency airway management should make an attempt at rapid sequence translaryngeal endotracheal intubation. The surgical airway of choice in a true emergency setting is a cricothyroidotomy. A tracheostomy should only be considered in the adult when there

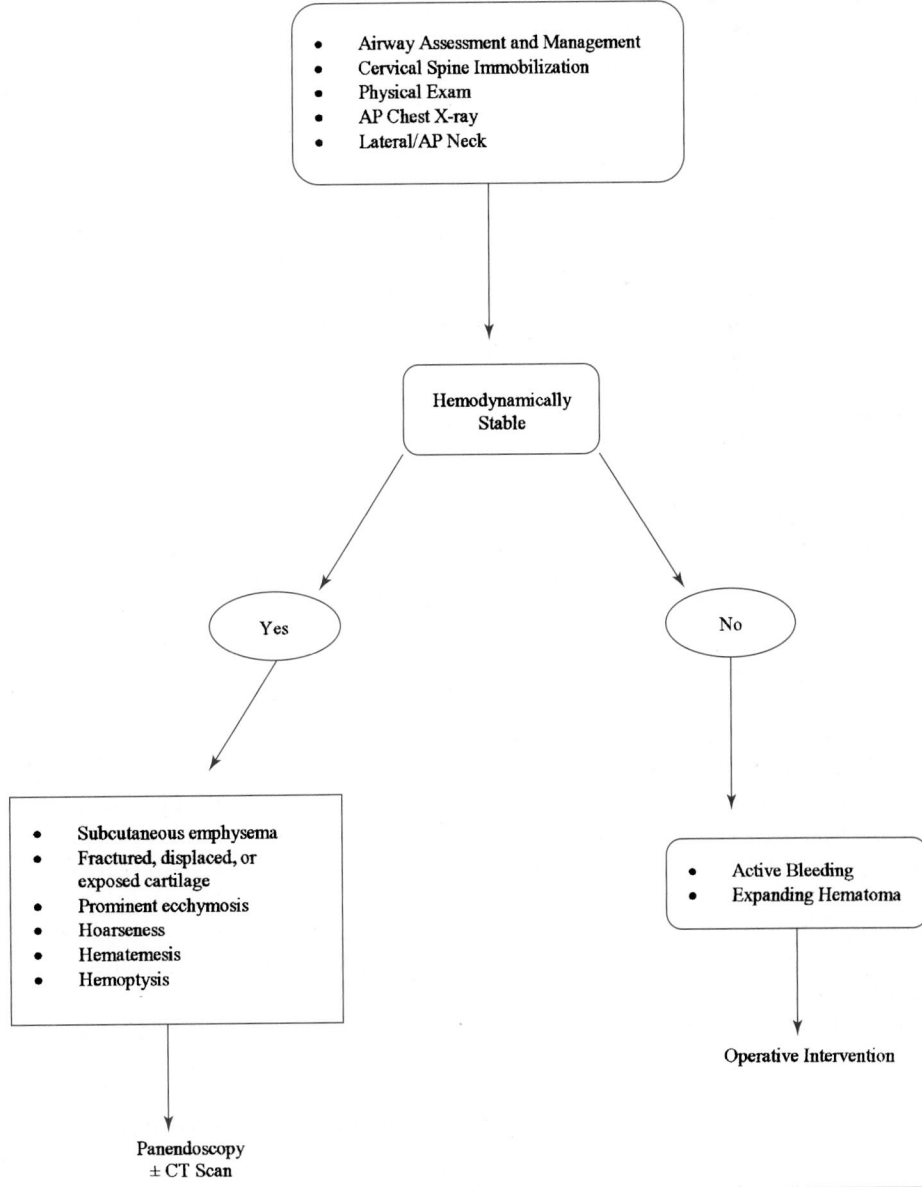

**FIGURE 23-5.** Management algorithm for blunt neck injuries.

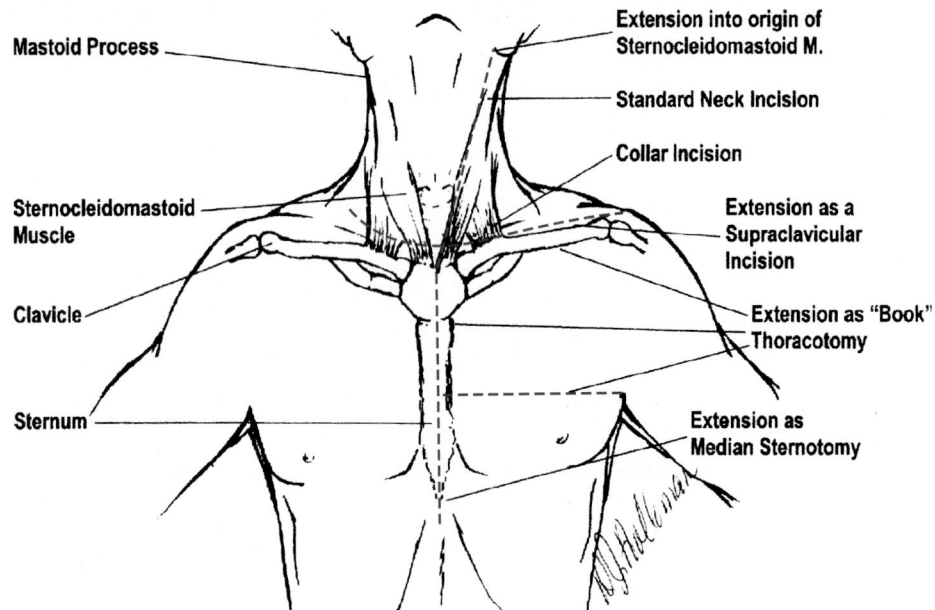

Mastoid Process

Sternocleidomastoid Muscle

Clavicle

Sternum

Extension into origin of Sternocleidomastoid M.

Standard Neck Incision

Collar Incision

Extension as a Supraclavicular Incision

Extension as "Book" Thoracotomy

Extension as Median Sternotomy

**FIGURE 23-6.** Incisions for operative exposure of penetrating neck injuries.

is an urgent need for an airway in a patient who you suspect might have a partial laryngo-tracheal separation. Even in that setting, an attempt should be made, if possible, by an airway expert to perform a careful translaryngeal endotracheal intubation.

After achieving airway control and if a selective management approach is chosen, the available modalities include flexible fiberoptic laryngoscopy, flexible esophagoscopy, flexible bronchoscopy, and contrast esophography. Using a water-soluble contrast agent and multiple views of the esophagus, extravasation can be safely excluded. The 85% sensitivity and specificity of this study can be increased to near 100% by the addition of esophagoscopy.[26] Increased experience with flexible fiberoptic scopes and enhanced technology have led to less dependence on the use of both studies as more emphasis is placed on the use of endoscopy. Visualization of the proximal 3–5 centimeters of the cervical esophagus immediately inferior to the cricopharyngeal constrictor is critical for this area can be past easily on scope insertion and withdrawal unless specifically inspected.

While direct laryngoscopy should be used to determine if there is a laryngeal injury, fiberoptic bronchoscopy is used for detection of a tracheal or bronchial injury. Alternatively, CT scan of the neck may identify injuries that require further investigation or operative intervention.

Laryngotracheal injuries can occur in both penetrating and blunt neck trauma. The presenting signs and symptoms include stridor, acute respiratory distress, cervical tenderness, and subcutaneous emphysema. The preferred method of evaluating possible injuries to the larynx and trachea is by the combined use of direct laryngoscopy and bronchoscopy. Concomitant injuries are frequent; therefore, diagnostic evaluation of possible arterial and esophageal injuries is imperative.

The classification of acute trauma to the larynx includes supraglottic, glottic, and subglottic injuries. Although some injuries involve all three levels, isolated supraglottic injuries usually result in a depression of the superior notch of the thyroid cartilage. Invariably, a vertical thyroid fracture is present. Rupture of the thyroepiglottic ligament is a common associated injury. This results in retraction of the epiglottis and herniation of soft tissue of the pre-epiglottic space into the laryngeal line. Glottic injuries typically

result in a fracture of the thyroid cartilage and comminution and blunting of the thyroid notch. The thyroarytenoid muscles are ruptured with tears extending into the true vocal cords, ventricular bands and aryepiglottic folds. Subglottic usually involve the lower thyroid and cricoid cartilage. If there is no fracture of the cricoid cartilage, symptoms may be minimal or consist of coughing with hemoptysis, and cervical emphysema. Cricotracheal separation with inferior retraction of the transected trachea can result from a transverse blow to the neck just below the cricoid cartilage. Subglottic injuries often cause rapid compromise of the airway necessitating emergency surgical management.[27]

Complete cricotracheal separation resulting from blunt trauma to the neck is uncommon. Optimal management includes primary end-to-end anastomosis. If the attending surgeon is unprepared for this type of definitive repair or if the operative conditions are not conducive to optimal management, a temporary tracheotomy should be performed as a life-saving measure and a first-stage procedure. Although the hemodynamic status of the patient will often dictate the operative approach, early definitive repair should be the goal for there is higher incidence of structure formation at the anastomotic site with delayed repair.[28] Tracheal injuries can usually be primarily repaired in a one-layer fashion with a three or four polyglycolic suture. Interposition of vascularized tissue such as omohyoid or sternocleidomastoid muscles is essential when there is an associated esophageal and/or arterial injury. This operative maneuver can lessen the chance of tracheoesophageal or tracheoarterial fistula development. When there is a severe laryngotracheal injury, tracheostomy should be performed. Table 23-3 highlights the recommended principles of management of acute laryngotracheal trauma as advocated by Mathisen and Grillo.[29] In addition to fistula development, other complications include possible erosion of arteries by drains, development of a laryngotracheal stenosis, and ongoing sepsis with associated mediastinitis. Timely diagnosis, early intervention, and appropriate surgical management should minimize these complications. Stents have been advocated for severe injury to the cartilaginous framework of the larynx.

The majority of esophageal injuries are a result of penetrating trauma. Penetrating injuries to the esophagus were rarely reported

**TABLE 23-3**

**Principles of Management of Acute Laryngotracheal Trauma**

Proper airway management
Evaluation of associated injuries
Avoid searching for recurrent laryngeal nerves
Separation of tracheal and esophageal suture lines
Conservation of viable trachea
Avoid tracheostomy through the repair
Flexion of the neck postoperatively to reduce tension

prior to World War II. This was probably because many of the victims died from associated vascular injuries prior to receiving any evaluation of a possible esophageal wound. Jemerin reported significant reduction in the mortality rate from esophageal wounds when the operative approach included drainage of the injury.[30] Barrett reported the first successful suture repair of the esophagus.[31] Delays in the diagnosis and management of penetrating esophageal injuries correlate with increased morbidity and mortality, with the greatest mortality occurring when there is an injury to the thoracic and abdominal esophagus. Optimal management of cervical esophageal injuries include early recognition, nonoperative means to establish an airway, meticulous debridements, two-layer closure of the esophageal wound, closed-suction drainage, and postoperative esophagography before drain removal.[32] For large esophageal wounds that cannot be primarily closed, or if there is a significant delay in diagnosis with significant contamination, the operative approach would be to establish a controlled fistula with catheter drainage or construct an esophagostomy. A necessary adjunctive measure is to initiate total parenteral nutrition or establish a feeding jejunostomy. Penetrating hypopharyngeal wounds can be safely managed conservatively. With isolated wounds, this selective management would include a nasogastric tube for feeding and a seven-day course of parenteral antibiotics.

## Vascular Injury

Although venous injuries can contribute to morbidity and mortality in neck trauma, a carotid artery injury is the most challenging. Over the centuries, management of carotid artery injuries has been documented. In 1552, the French surgeon, Ambroise Pare, ligated both the common carotid artery and the jugular vein of a soldier who was injured in a duel.[33] Fortunately, the soldier survived the injury; however, the patient subsequently developed an aphasia and hemiplegia. Over two centuries later, Fleming reported a successful outcome after ligating a lacerated common carotid artery.[34] Injury to the carotid artery comprises 5% of all arterial injuries.[35] Although motor vehicles crashes account for most of the blunt carotid injuries, penetrating trauma is the main mechanism of injury to the carotid artery, with gunshot wounds accounting for approximately half of the injuries.[36-39] Diagnosis of this injury can be challenging, for patients are frequently neurologically intact. Radiologic evaluation is, therefore, essential to the identification and localization of carotid injuries. Angiography continues to be the "gold standard" diagnostic procedure in the evaluation of vascular trauma.

Scalfani reported on a study of proximity angiograms and notes that physical examination had a sensitivity of 61% and a specificity

of 80%.[40] He argued that not incorporating proximity angiography in the evaluation of penetrating neck injuries was premature. However, Menawat who reported on a series of 110 patients with penetrating neck injuries,[41] only one patient had an injury not predicted by physical examination findings. Nine arterial injuries were treated nonoperatively without sequelae.

Azuaje's series of penetrating neck injuries demonstrated a sensitivity and negative predictive value of 100% for physical examination in detecting surgically significant vascular injuries.[42] When considering injuries detected by angiography, physical examination showed a sensitivity of 93% and a negative predictive value of 97%. No patient in this series with a negative physical examination required a vascular repair regardless of the zone of injury.

Referring specifically to Zone III wounds, Ferguson reports a series of 72 patients with penetrating wounds.[43] The absence of "hard signs" reliably excluded surgically significant injuries. Sixty percent of the patients with "hard signs" of injury were explored. Only one patient in this group had no identifiable injury. The remainder of the patients with "hard signs" of injury underwent emergent angiography with endovascular angiographic treatment. The authors recommended that Zone III injuries with "hard signs" of vascular injury should undergo angiography as they maybe amenable to endovascular intervention.

Mazolewski performed a prospective evaluation of 14 stable patients with penetrating Zone II injuries.[44] All patients underwent thorough physical examination, infusion CT scan, and operative exploration. Three of the 14 patients had five injuries. These patients had a high probability for injury based on the computed tomography (CT) scan findings. Although a small sample size, the CT scan had a sensitivity of 100%, specificity of 91%, positive predictive value of 75%, and a negative predictive value of 100%. The authors felt that the CT scan should play a pivotal role in the evaluation of neck injuries. Gracias conducted a retrospective series of 23 patients evaluated by CT scan for penetrating neck trauma that spanned all three zones.[45] All the patients lacked "hard signs" of vascular or aero-digestive injury. Thirteen patients had the trajectory of injury remote from important structures identified and no further evaluation carried out. There were no adverse events.

Gonzalez reported on a prospective study of CT in patients with Zone II penetrating wounds without "hard signs" of injury necessitating immediate exploration.[46] The authors concluded that CT added little to the information obtained by physical examination with Zone II injuries.

Hollingsworth conducted a meta-analysis of computed tomographic angiography (CTA) for detection of carotid and vertebral lesions of either atherosclerotic or traumatic origin.[47] It was concluded that there was insufficient high-quality data to comment on the sensitivity or specificity of CTA for trauma.

Woo studied patients with Zone II penetrating wounds who underwent CTA as a diagnostic test.[48] They reported that with increase utilization of CTA and enhanced staff experience, there was an associated decrease in the number of negative neck explorations. The authors highlighted that with this imaging that wound tracts could be visualized and potentially dictate the use of other diagnostic studies.

The role of angiography continues to evolve. Currently, it does not appear to be superior to a through physical examination. Angiography has been advocated for Zone I injuries at the base of the neck because injury in the thoracic outlet would be difficult to diagnose and control. Eddy conducted a multi-institutional retrospective study surveying patients over ten years.[49] Exactly 138 patients were studied and 28 arterial injuries were found. However, the group concluded that in the presence of a normal physical examination and a normal chest radiograph, angiographic study may not be needed. Gasparri confirmed this finding after conducting a retrospective review of 100 patients.[50] All patients with "hard signs" of vascular injury were taken for expeditious surgical exploration. Eighty one patients without "hard signs" of injury underwent angiography. Eleven occult injuries are discovered. When a normal physical examination and a normal chest radiograph are combined they have a sensitivity of 100%, a specificity of 80%, a positive predictive value of 40%, and a negative predictive value of 100%. The group concluded that proximity alone does not mandate angiography.

However, other diagnostic modalities have proven to be less expensive and less invasive. Bok and Peter demonstrated the efficacy of magnetic resonance angiography (MRA) in blunt trauma patients.[51] They emphasized that in addition to identifying the injured vessel, MRA could possibly delineate specific injury patterns to the brain. Munera et al. demonstrated that CTA had a sensitivity of 90% and a specificity of 100%.[52] They highlighted that this diagnostic modality compared favorably with traditional angiography, with the main advantage being the ability to avoid selective arterial cannulation. However, the disadvantages included the requirement for large amounts of contrast and the increased dependence on the skill of the operator. Fry et al. advocated duplex scanning for the diagnosis of carotid artery injuries.[53] They compared this method to angiography and reported no false positives or negatives. There was a cost savings of $1,252 per case. Management of common internal carotid artery injury should be managed by restoration of cerebral blood flow, whenever possible.[54-57] Weaver et al. concluded that neurologic outcome and survival were not compromised or worsened by restoration of arterial blood flow.[56] Ledgerwood et al. recommended carotid artery repair, if technically possible in all patients who are not comatose and have stable vital signs.[58]

When a carotid artery injury is found, there are several therapeutic options. Observation or expectant management is advocated for patients who are comatose as a result of either a penetrating or blunt injury to the carotid artery.[36,59] There is no advantage to revascularization or ligation, although Liekweg and Greenfield emphasized that coma is the single most important factor in determining the indication for repair versus ligation of the carotid artery.[60] Carotid artery ligation is an option for those patients presenting with uncontrollable hemorrhage and when placement of a temporary shunt is technically impossible to achieve. In the neurologically intact patient, the carotid injury should be repaired. Anticoagulation has been advocated for some carotid injuries when there are no existing contraindications to heparinization. Cogbill reported a benefit to anticoagulation, particularly with carotid dissections.[61] Fabian et al. found anticoagulation effective with all blunt injuries to the carotid and small intimal flap injuries resulting from penetrating trauma.[62] Although the open surgical approach is the "gold standard" when an operative procedure is required, the role of minimally invasive management is evolving as a viable option. At our institution, Duane et al. demonstrated the efficacy of endovascular stenting.[63] Biffl et al. recommended that stent utilization be complemented by full heparinization to decrease the rate of stent occlusions.[64] Bejjani et al. treated three patients with traumatic carotid dissections (one penetrating and two blunt) with endovascular stents.[65] All these patients had symptoms leading to diagnosis, and were symptomatically improved postprocedure. There were no procedure-related complications. Brandt and her colleagues retrospectively identified six patients with blunt injuries who were treated with stents. There were no deaths or procedure-related complications. There were no occlusions, stenoses, or stent malfunctions in follow-up from one month to two years.[66] Diaz-Daza et al. retrospectively identified eight patients with traumatic lesions of the carotid and/or vertebral arteries. Four patients had penetrating mechanisms of injury (three GSW's and one stab). There were a total of 17 lesions in the eight patients including pseudoaneurysms, fistulas, and extravasation. Treatments included deployment of coils, Polyvinyl alcohol, gelfoam, and stents. There were no procedure-related complications reported. Six of the 8 remained stable or improved at varying intervals of follow-up. Two patients experienced interval development of new small pseudoaneurysms which did not require further intervention.[67] Joo et al. reported 10 patients with traumatic carotid injuries, nine victims of blunt mechanisms, and one stab wound.[68] The majority were symptomatic leading to a variety of imaging studies. Half of the lesions were carotid cavernous fistulas, and the remainder were pseudoaneurysms. Treatments included balloon embolizations in three patients, stenting in six patients, some with concomitant embolizations, and one patient underwent embolization with platinum coils and glue. All 10 patients had successful treatment of their traumatic lesions with preservation of the parent artery. Five had resolution of their antecedent symptoms, three had gradual improvement of antecedent weakness, and two had stability of symptoms with no new neurological symptoms. Such intervention remains controversial.

Located in the posterior triangle of the neck and deep to the bony and fascial compartments through its course, the vertebral artery is the first branch of the subclavian artery. It takes a cephalad course and enters the foramina in the transverse process of the sixth cervical vertebrae. This proximal section is considered the first part of the artery. The second portion includes the course of the artery as it continues within the bony vertebral foramina. The third and fourth part of the vertebral artery is beyond the first cervical vertebrae (Fig. 23-7).[69] Injury to the vertebral artery is infrequent because of its protected location. In the trauma setting, the majority of vertebral artery injuries are diagnosed in Zone I and are often associated with injuries to the subclavian and internal jugular veins. Unilateral vertebral artery occlusion rarely results in a neurologic deficit if the contralateral vertebral artery is normal and the posterior inferior cerebellar artery is preserved.[70] Even though the majority of vertebral artery injuries can be managed nonoperatively, operative intervention can be life-saving in some situations. Operative intervention should be reserved for injuries that have active hemorrhage or large pseudoaneurysms and arteriovenous fistulas which cannot be successfully embolized. Fortunately, vertebral artery injuries requiring aggressive management can be done in the interventional radiology suite where angiographic embolization can be definitive management. McConnell and Trunkey emphasized that if a detailed angiogram is available and demonstrates that the remaining vertebral artery is hypoplastic, operative repair of the injured vertebral artery should be performed instead of ligation.[71] Reid and Weigelt reported on one of the largest series of vertebral

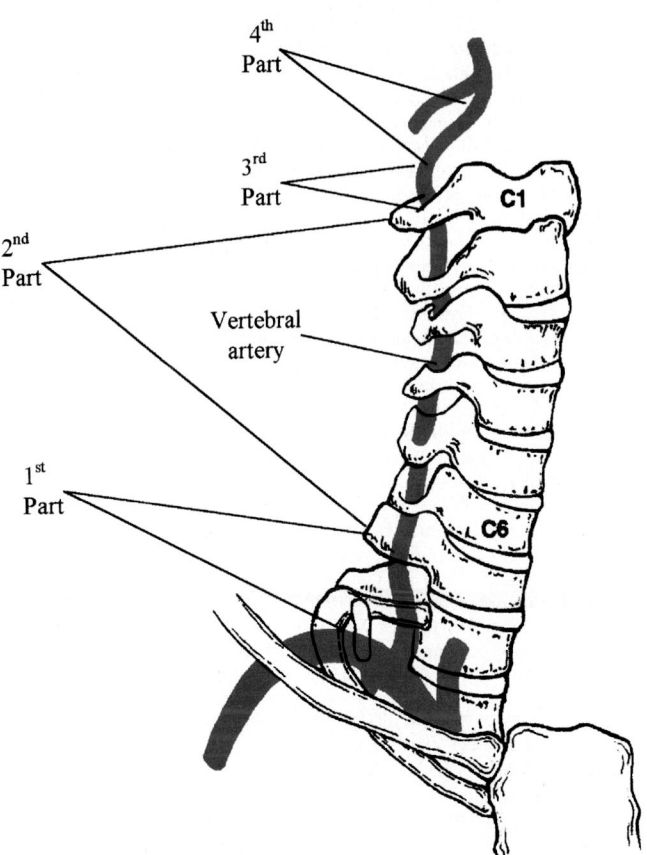

**FIGURE 23-7.** Line drawing of vertebral artery demonstrating anatomic relation to the cervical spine. C1, first cervical vertebra; C6, sixth cervical vertebra.
*(Reproduced with permission from Blickenstaff KL, Weaver FA, Yellin AE, et al.: Trends in the management of traumatic vertebral artery injuries. Amer J surg 158:104, 1989.)*

artery injuries consisting of 43 cases over a ten-year period.[72] Of the 43 patients who sustained this injury, 38 had a normal Glasgow Coma Scale Score, and no patient presented with vertebrobasilar neurologic signs. The majority of patients were hemodynamically stable on admission. However, there were seven patients who presented in shock, with the vertebral artery as the sole bleeding site in five of these patients.

In the shock state, any venous injury should be managed by expeditious ligation. Injuries to the internal jugular vein are important and can account for significant external bleeding and hematoma development. As a result of extrinsic compression, the airway can become severely compromised. If at all possible, an injury to the internal jugular vein should be repaired by, preferably, a lateral venorrhaphy, although patch venoplasty and segmental resection with primary anastomosis are acceptable procedures if the patient is hemodynamically stable. Irrespective of the type of repair, subsequent thrombosis is common. Ligation is the option of choice if repair is difficult or adds too much time to the operation of critically injured patients. The external jugular vein, if injured, can be ligated without adverse sequelae. Massive air emboli can result from major venous injuries. Van Ieperen reported that 11 patients died from air emboli after sustaining penetrating neck injuries.[73] A high index of suspicion needs to be maintained to diagnose this complication. As in the case with all neck injuries, the possibility of a cervical spine injury should always be considered. Approximately 10% of penetrating cervical trauma victims have an

associated spinal cord or brachial plexus injury. In spinal cord injuries above the fourth cervical vertebra, there is significant mortality. Bracken and colleagues have advocated the use of methylprednisolone and naloxone in the treatment of acute blunt spinal cord injury of patients when there is spinal cord trauma within eight hours.[74] Such a management protocol has not been shown to be advantageous for penetrating cord injuries.

## SUMMARY

Penetrating and blunt neck wounds still present serious challenges in diagnosis and management. Astute physical examination with attention to the overt findings of vascular and aero-digestive injury ("hard signs") appears to be the most efficient approach to evaluation of penetrating neck injuries. Injuries resulting from blunt trauma require a high index of suspicion for a possible occult injury. The complexity of injuries to the neck in both penetrating and blunt trauma, along with steadily advancing technology, often requires changes in diagnostic and management paradigms. Although the open operative approach for definitive repair has and continues to be a major thrust in the definitive management of neck injuries in the severely compromised patient, the emerging role of expectant management and surgical alternatives, such as endovascular stenting of carotid injuries, needs to continue to be carefully employed in the management of certain neck injuries. The caveat that must continue to be stated is that having the occasional success with a certain novel approach does not make it an acceptable protocol. Outcome analysis remains the best method to determine which specific management approach is appropriate.

## REFERENCES

1. American College of Surgeons Advanced Trauma Life Support for Doctors: *Instructor Course Manual.* Chicago, IL, 1997, p. 21.
2. Ordog GJ, Albin D, Wasserberger J, et al.: Shotgun "birdshot" wounds to the neck. *J Trauma* 28:491, 1998.
3. Ordog GJ: Penetrating neck trauma. *J Trauma* 27:543, 1987.
4. Mocquot P: Plaies des gros vaisseaus du cou. *Rev de Chir* 52:241, 1917.
5. Fogelman MJ, Stewart RD: Penetrating wounds of the neck. *Am J Surg* 91:581, 1956.
6. Ashworth C, Williams LF, Bynre JJ: Penetrating wounds of the neck: Reemphasis of the need for prompt exploration. *Am J Surg* 121:387, 1971.
7. Lee C, May M, Sapote B, et al.: Penetrating wounds of the neck: Selective management. A study of 100 cases. *Trans Am Acad Opthm Oto* 75:496, 1971.
8. Cabasares HV: Selective surgical management of penetrating neck trauma: 15 year experience in a community hospital. *AM Surg* 48:355, 1982.
9. Cohen ES, Breaux CW, Johnson PN, et al.: Penetrating neck injuries: Experience with selective exploration. *South Med J* 80:26, 1987.
10. Dunbar LL, Adkins RB, Waterhouse G: Penetrating injuries to the neck: Selective management. *Am Surg* 50:198, 1984.
11. Shirkeg AL, Beall AC, DeBakey ME: Surgical management of penetrating wounds of the neck. *Arch Surg* 86:96, 1983.
12. Noyes LD, McSwain NE, Markowitz IP: Panendoscopy with arteriography versus mandatory exploration of penetrating wounds of the neck. *Ann Surg* 204:21, 1986.
13. Gerst PH, Sharma SK, Sharma PK: Selective management of penetrating neck trauma. *Am Surg* 56:553, 1990.
14. Stroud HW, Yarbrough DR III: Penetrating neck wounds. *Am J Surg* 140:323, 1980.
15. Ayuyao AM, Kaledzi YL, Parsa MH, et al.: Penetrating wounds: Mandatory vs. selective exploration. *Am Surg* 202:563, 1985.
16. Britt LD, Riblet JL: Penetrating neck trauma. In: Cameron JL, ed. *Current Surgical Therapy,* 6th ed. St. Louis: Mosby, 1998, p. 1000.
17. Hall JR, Reyes HM, Meller JL: Penetrating zone II neck injuries in children. *J Trauma* 31:1614, 1991.

18. Atteberry LR, Dennis JW, Menawatt SS, et al.: Physical examination alone is safe and accurate for evaluation of vascular injuries in penetrating zone II neck trauma. *J Am Coll Surg* 179:657, 1994.
19. Demetriades D, Theodorou D, Cornwell E, et al.: Evaluation of penetrating injuries of the neck: Prospective study of 223 patients. *World J Surg* 21:41, 1997.
20. Demetriades D, Theodorou D, Cornwell E, et al.: Transcervical gunshot injuries: Mandatory operation is not necessary: *J Trauma* 40:758,1996.
21. Vassiliu P, Baker J, Henderson S, et al.: Aerodigestive injuries of the neck. *Am Surg* 67:75, 2001.
22. Ngakane II, Muckart DJ, Luvuno FM: Penetrating visceral injuries of the neck: Results of a conservative management policy. *Br J Surg* 77:908, 1990.
23. Ascensio JA, Valenziano CP, Falcone RE, et al.: Management of penetrating neck injuries: The controversy surrounding zone II injuries. *Surg Clin North Am* 71:267, 1991.
24. Mandavia DP, Qualls S, Rokos I: Emergency airway management in penetrating neck injury. *Ann Emer Med* 35:221, 2000.
25. Shearer VA, Giesecke AH: Airway management for patients with penetrating neck trauma: a retrospective study. *Anesth Analg* 77:1135, 1993.
26. Weigelt JA, Thal ER, Snyder WH, et al.: Diagnosis of penetrating cervical esophageal injuries. *Am J Surg* 154:619, 1987.
27. Brandenburg JH: Management of acute blunt laryngeal injuries. *Otolaryngology Clin North Am* 12:741, 1979.
28. Ashbaugh DG, Gordon JH: Traumatic avulsion of the trachea associated with cricoid fracture. *J Thor Cardiovasc Surg* 69:800, 1975.
29. Mathisen DJ, Grillo H: Laryngotracheal trauma. *Ann Thoracic Surg* 43:254, 1987.
30. Jemerin EE: Results of treatment of perforation of the esophagus. *Ann Surg* 128:971, 1948.
31. Barrett NR: Report of a case of spontaneous perforation of the esophagus successfully treated by operation. *Br J Surg* 35:216, 1947.
32. Winter RP, Weigelt JA: Cervical esophageal trauma: Incidence and cause of esophagel fistulas. *Arch Surg* 125:849, 1990.
33. Watson WL, Silverstone SM: Ligature of the common carotid artery in cancer of head and neck. *Ann Surg* 109:1, 1939.
34. Fleming D: Case of rupture of the carotid artery: The wounds of several of its branches successfully treated by tying the common trunk of the carotid itself. *Med Chir J Rev* 3:2, 1817.
35. Ward RE: Injury to the cervical cerebral vessels. In: Blaisdell FW, Trunkey DD, eds. *Trauma Management*, Vol III: Cervicothoracic Trauma. New York: Thieme, 1986, p. 262.
36. Kraus RR, Bergstein JM, DeBord JR: Diagnosis, treatment and outcomes of blunt carotid arterial injuries. *Am J Surg* 178:190, 1999.
37. Berne JD, Norwood SH, McAuley CE, et al.: The high morbidity of blunt cerebrovascular injury in an unscreened population: More evidence of the need for mandatory screening protocols. *J Am Coll Surg* 192:314, 2001.
38. Timberlake GA, Rice JC, Kersten MD, et al.: Penetrating injury to the carotid artery: A reappraisal of management. *Am Surg* 55:154, 1989.
39. Padberg FT, Hobson RW, Yeager RA, et al.: Penetrating carotid arterial trauma. *Am Surg* 50:277, 1984.
40. Scalfani SJ, Cavaliere G, Atwew N, et al.: The Role of Angiography in penetrating neck trauma. *J Trauma* 31:557, 1991.
41. Menawat SS, Dennis JW, Laneve LM: Are arteriograms necessary in penetrating zone I neck injuries? *J Vasc Surg* 16:397, 1992.
42. Azuaje RE, Jacobson LE, Glover J, et al.: Reliability of physical examination as a predictor of vascular injury after penetrating neck injury. *Am Surg* 69:804, 2003.
43. Ferguson E, Dennis JW, Frykberg ER: Redefining the role of arterial imaging in the management of penetrating zone 3 neck injuries. *Vascular* 13:158, 2005.
44. Mazolewski PJ, Curry JD, Browder T, et al.: Computer tomographic scanning can be used for surgical decision making in Zone II penetrating neck injuries. *J Trauma* 51:315, 2001.
45. Gracias VH, Reilly PM, Philpot J, et al.: Computed Tomography in the Evaluation of Penetrating Neck Trauma. *Arch Surg* 136:1231, 2001.
46. Gonzalez RP, Falimirski M, Holevar MR, et al.: Penetrating zone II neck injury: Does dynamic computed tomographic scan contribute to the diagnostic

47. Hollingworth W, Nathens AB, Kanne JP, et al.: The diagnostic accuracy of computed tomographic angiography for traumatic or atherosclerotic lesions of the carotid and vertebral arteries: A systematic review. *Eur J Radiol* 48:88, 2003.
48. Woo K, Magner DP, Wilson MT, et al.: CT Angiography in penetrating neck trauma reduces the need for operative neck exploration. *Am Surg* 71:754, 2005.
49. Eddy VA: Is routine Arteriography mandatory for penetrating injury to Zone I of the neck? Penetrating Injury Study Group. *J Trauma* 48:208, 2000.
50. Gasparri MG, Lorelli DR, Kralovich KA, et al.: Physical examination plus chest radiography in penetrating peri-clavicular trauma: The appropriate trigger for angiography. *J Trauma* 49:1029, 2000.
51. Bok AP, Peter JC: Carotid and vertebral artery occlusion after blunt cervical injury: The role of MR angiography in early diagnosis. *J Trauma* 40:968, 1996.
52. Munera F, Soto JA, Palacio D, et al.: Diagnosis of arterial injuries caused by penetrating trauma to the neck: Comparison of helical CT angiography and conventional angiography. *Radiology* 216:356, 2000.
53. Fry WR, Dort JA, Smith RS, et al.: Duplex scanning replaces arteriography and operative exploration in the diagnosis of potential cervical vascular injury. *Am J Surg* 168:693, 1994.
54. Meyer JP, Walsh J, Barrett J, et al.: Analysis of eighteen recent cases of penetrating injuries to the common and internal carotid arteries. *Am J Surg* 156:96, 1988.
55. Ledgerwood AA, Mullins RJ, Lucas C: Primary repair vs. ligation for carotid artery injuries. *Arch Surg* 115:488, 1980.
56. Weaver FA, Yellin AE, Wagner WH, et al.: The role of arterial reconstruction in penetrating carotid injury. *Arch Surg* 123:1106, 1988.
57. Unger SW, Tucker WS, Mrdeza MA, et al.: Carotid arterial trauma. *Surgery* 87:477, 1980.
58. Ledgerwood AM, Mullins RJ, Lucas CE: Primary repair vs. ligation for carotid injuries. *Arch Surg* 115:488, 1980.
59. Fabian TC, George SM, Croce MA, et al.: Carotid artery trauma: Management based on mechanism of injury. *J Trauma* 30:953, 1990.
60. Liekweg WG, Greenfield LJ: Management of penetrating carotid arterial injury. *Ann Surg* 188:582, 1978.
61. Cogbill TH, Moore EE, Meissner M, et al.: The spectrum of blunt injury to the carotid artery: A multicenter perspective. *J Trauma* 37:473, 1994.
62. Fabian TC, Patton JH, Croce MA, et al.: Blunt carotid injury: Importance of early diagnosis and anticoagulation therapy. *Ann Surg* 223:513, 1996.
63. Duane TM, Parker F, Stokes GR, et al.: Endovascular carotid stenting after trauma. *J Trauma* 52:149, 2002.
64. Biffl WL, Moore EE, Offmer PJ, et al.: Blunt carotid arterial injuries: Implications of a new grading scale. *J Trauma* 47:845, 1999.
65. Bejjani GK, Monsein LH, Laird JR, et al.: Treatment of symptomatic cervical carotid dissections with endovascular stents. *Neurosurg* 44:755, 1999.
66. Brandt M, Kazanjian S, Wahl WW: The utility of endovascular stents in the treatment of blunt arterial injuries. *J Trauma* 51:901, 2001.
67. Diaz-Daza O, Arraiza FJ, Barkley JM: Endovascular therapy of traumatic vascular lesions of the head and neck. *Cardiovasc Intervent Radiol* 26:213, 2003.
68. Joo JY, Ahn JY, Chung YS, et al.: Therapeutic endovascular treatments for traumatic carotid artery injuries. *J Trauma* 58:1159, 2005.
69. Blickenstaff KL, Weaver FA, Yellin AE, et al.: Trends in the management of traumatic vertebral artery injury. *Am J Surg* 158:101, 1989.
70. Golueke P, Sclafani S, Phillips T, et al.: Vertebral artery injury: Diagnosis and management. *J Trauma* 27:856, 1987.
71. McConnell DB, Trunkey DD: Management of penetrating trauma to the neck. *Adv Surg* 27:97, 1994.
72. Reid JD, Weigelt JA: Forty-three cases of vertebral artery trauma. *J Trauma* 28:1007, 1988.
73. Van Ieperen L: Venous air embolism as a cause of death—a method of investigation. *S Afr Med J* 63:442, 1983.
74. Bracken MB, Shepard MJ, Collins WF: A randomized, controlled trial of methylprednisolone or naloxone in the treatment of acute spinal cord injury. Results of the Second National Acute Spinal Cord Injury Study. *N Eng J Med* 322:1405, 1990.

# Commentary ■ ALI SALIM

The neck is a small anatomical area with a dense concentration of numerous vital structures. The diagnosis and management of injuries to this area remain challenging and at times, controversial. Dr. Britt and colleagues have provided an excellent review addressing these complexities. There are a number of points that are worth emphasizing.

As mentioned throughout the chapter, the physical exam is the most efficient approach in evaluating the neck with respect to penetrating trauma. The exam should be systematic and specifically directed at signs or symptoms of airway, vascular, pharyngoesophageal, spinal cord, and other nerve injuries. A detailed exam, preferably according to a written protocol, will identify injuries that need to be addressed. Patients with "hard" signs of vascular or aerodigestive injuries should be taken promptly to the operating room. Patients with minimal symptoms or "soft" signs are selected to undergo further evaluation and observation. Following this approach will prevent unnecessary neck exploration. Only about 17% of gunshot wounds (21% for transcervical wounds), and 10% of stab wounds to the neck require a therapeutic operation.[1,2]

For patients with "soft" signs of injury, selecting the most appropriate investigation depends on the mechanism, clinical status of the patient, and the resources of the hospital. Helical CT has become the initial diagnostic test of choice in hemodynamically stable patients with no indication for exploration. It provides valuable information regarding missile trajectory, the site and nature of spinal fractures, and any involvement of the spinal cord. It has now become the test of choice in evaluating vascular structures. Evaluation of the aerodigestive tract involves endoscopy and contrast imaging studies.

Because of the risk of airway compromise, prompt diagnosis and intervention for laryngotracheal injuries is necessary. The only "hard" sign for injury is air bubbling through a penetrating wound. Minor blunt and small penetrating wounds may be managed conservatively. Early definitive repair is the goal for the majority of injuries. Tracheostomy is used only in patients with extensive tracheal injuries.

Pharyngoesophageal injuries are not immediately life threatening. Ensuring an adequate airway is always the first and most urgent priority. Since there are no "hard" signs diagnostic of pharyngoesophageal injuries, a high index of suspicion is warranted. Small penetrating injuries to the pharynx can safely be managed nonoperatively. All injuries to the cervical esophagus should be repaired in a timely fashion. Early repair is associated with a reduction in septic complications and leaks.

Penetrating carotid injuries usually result from low-velocity gunshot wounds and stab wounds. Minor injuries such as small intimal defects and pseudoaneurysms can be managed nonoperatively. All other injuries require surgical repair. As the authors noted, controversy exists regarding the management of patients with established coma or dense contralateral neurologic deficits. The best chance for any neurologic recovery is urgent revascularization. However, patients with prolonged coma (> 4 hours) have an extremely poor prognosis regardless of treatment and revascularization may worsen cerebral edema and intracranial hypertension. Penetrating vertebral artery injuries are much less common. Often, the artery is thrombosed at presentation and no intervention is necessary. Active bleeding requires angiographic or operative intervention. Significant advances in imaging quality with CT angiography have increased the diagnosis of blunt carotid and vertebral artery injuries. The majority of injuries are not amenable to surgical intervention and are managed with endovascular treatment and/or prolonged anticoagulation.

Brachial plexus and other nerve injuries resulting from blunt and penetrating trauma are often overlooked. They are usually associated with other vascular injuries. Injuries are diagnosed by physical exam and confirmed with the use of magnetic resonance imaging. Prognosis depends on the mechanism of injury, with blunt and gunshot injuries having the worse prognosis.

As the authors have noted, there have been significant advances in the evaluation and management of injuries to the neck. Selective nonoperative management has become more commonplace. A careful and systematic physical exam will identify significant injuries that require attention. The shift from invasive angiography to less invasive CT angiography and noninvasive color flow duplex has been an important change in the evaluation of vascular injuries. The advancement of interventional radiology has altered the management of certain vascular injuries, avoiding the need for complex surgery in many patients.

## References

1. Demetriades D, Theodorou D, Cornwell EE, et al.: Evaluation of penetrating injuries of the neck: Prospective study of 223 patients. *World J Surg* 21:41, 1997.
2. Demetriades D, Theodorou D, Cornwell E, et al.: Transcervical gunshot injuries: mandatory operation is not necessary. *J Trauma* 40:758, 1995.

# Injury to the Vertebrae and Spinal Cord

*Ronald W. Lindsey* ■ *Zbigniew Gugala* ■ *Spiros G. Pneumaticos*

## INTRODUCTION

Injuries to the spine are common and when associated with a neurologic compromise they can be most devastating to the patient. Among all trauma victims, the incidence of spinal injury is approximately 4.3% in the cervical spine and 6.3% in the thoracolumbar spine with spinal cord injury occurring in approximately 1.3%.[1–4] This seemingly small incidence of spine injury is offset by the prevalence of morbidity and mortality associated with these injuries. A significant number of spinal injuries occurs in polytraumatized patients[5] (Fig. 24-1) and further complicates the management of these patients (Table 24-1). Understandably, spine injury represents a major cause of permanent disability and death among trauma patients.

The risk for spinal injury can vary depending on the patient's age and the anatomic region injured. Cervical spine injuries have a bimodal prevalence based on the age, involving either the young (age 15–45 years) or elderly (age 65–85 years)[6] (Fig. 24-2); in the thoracolumbar spine, a single patient age group is typically affected (age 50–80 years)[1] (Fig. 24-3). Although modern medicine has improved our care of spine injuries, the types of patients affected may influence the incidence of morbidity and mortality. Traditionally, spine injuries had occurred in a young and active patient population; however, the recent trend has been toward these injuries occurring in elderly patients due to longer life expectancies, a more active elderly population, and the inherent risks which accompany increasing age such as osteoporosis.

Although the incidence of females sustaining spinal injury has increased in recent years, males continue to comprise approximately 70% of all spine injury patients. The most common mechanism of injury is a motor vehicle accident, followed by falls, act of violence (gunshots, stab wounds), and sport activities.[1] In urban regions assaults and gunshot injury have surpassed sports and occasionally even falls as the principle mechanism of spinal injury.

Spine injuries usually occur in the most mobile spinal segments: the cervical spine, and the thoracolumbar spine. In the cervical spine 25% of all injuries occur in the upper cervical spine (Oc–C2), while 75% occur in the subaxial region (C3–C7). Multiple level spine injuries have been estimated to occur in 4 to 20% of all cases. In the thoracolumbar spine the anatomic distribution of injury is most common around the thoracolumbar junction with L1 accounting for 16% of all injuries. Approximately, 5 to 20% of patients with thoracolumbar spine injuries have noncontiguous fractures.

The annual incidence of spinal cord injury in the United States (excluding lethal cases) is approximately 40 cases per million population and results in 11,000 new cases each year.[7] Spinal cord injury occurs in approximately 1.3% of all spine fractures, and most commonly occurs in the cervical spine (55%), followed by the thoracic spine (30%), and the lumbar spine (15%) (Fig. 24-4). Approximately 40% of all spinal cord injuries present as complete lesions, and the associated mortality rate following spinal cord injury can approach 16 times that for other injuries.[8] In the United States, 4000 patients with spinal cord injury (SCI) die annually before reaching the hospital, and another 1000 patients die during their hospitalization.

The prevalence of individuals with SCI is estimated to average 755 (range 679–870) per million USA population.[7] The increasing prevalence of SCI patients is the direct result of the recent advances in the management of SCI patients that improve their life expectancy. The median time of survival for patients who sustained SCI at the age 25–34 has been predicated to be 38 years postinjury, with 43% surviving for at least 40 years.[9]

The social and economic impact of SCI not only affects the patient and his family, but the entire society. The economic burden of SCI in the United States is estimated at $9.7 billion per year.[10] Life-time costs for a paraplegic patient at age 35 years are estimated to be $500,000, and for a quadriplegic at age 27 years more than $1,000,000.[10] The additional social costs of SCI include divorce

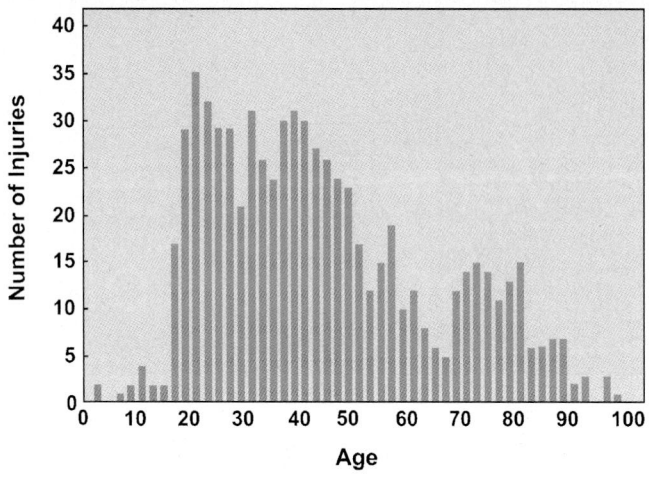

**FIGURE 24-1.** Prevalence of cervical spine injury by age. *(Reproduced with permission from Lowery DW, Wald MM, Browne BJ, et al.: Epidemiology of cervical spine injury victims. Annals of Emergency Medicine, 38:12–16, 2001.)*

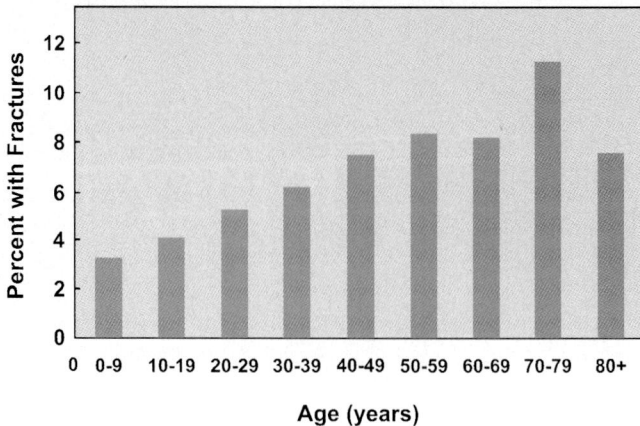

**FIGURE 24-2.** Prevalance of thoracolumbar spine injury by age. *(Reproduced with permission from Holmes J, Miller P, Panacek E, Lin S, et al.: Epidemiology of thoracolumbar spine injury in blunt trauma. Academic Emergency Medicine 8:866–872, 2001.)*

**TABLE 24-1**

| Associated Trauma with Spinal Cord Injury | |
| --- | --- |
| **INJURY TYPE** | **OCCURRENCE (%)** |
| No Additional Injury | 55.8 |
| Fractures of the Trunk | 17.2 |
| Long Bone Fractures | 13.9 |
| Head and Face Trauma | 13.8 |
| Pneumothorax and Chest Injury | 8.8 |
| Abdominal Injury | 8.6 |

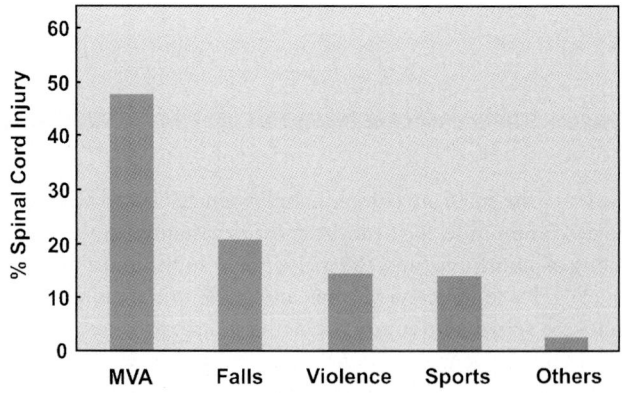

**FIGURE 24-3.** Etiology of spinal cord injury as a result of spinal trauma. *(Reproduced with permission from Holmes J, Miller P, Panacek E, et al.: Epidemiology of thoracolumbar spine injury in blunt trauma. Academic Emergency Medicine 8:866–872, 2001.)*

and separation in more than 50% of victims and less than 1% subsequently will marry.

Traditionally, injuries of the spine have been treated nonoperatively. Over the past century, numerous surgical techniques have been described, implants and instrumentations have been devised, and surgical indications have been better defined facilitating the operative management of these injuries. Optimal management must consider early patient mobilization, the maintenance of acceptable spinal alignment and stability, the influence of associated injuries, and the risks and severity of complications associated with each treatment modality.

The basic principles of spine injury management consist of the following: (1) to avoid the progression of neurologic deficit, and when deficit is present to enhance its resolution; (2) to reduce unacceptable spinal deformity or malalignment to facilitate neurologic decompression and eventually permit an acceptable functional range; (3) to maintain spinal alignment within a functional range throughout the course of treatment; and (4) to achieve healing of the spine in a functional alignment sufficient to permit return of physiologic loads through the spine.

Spine injury represents a common, potentially devastating portion of the trauma patient population. Proper initial emergency center management, early detection, and appropriate treatment can minimize many of the complications associated with these injuries, and maximize their potential for recovery

## ANATOMY AND KINEMATICS OF VERTEBRAL COLUMN

### Pertinent Anatomy

The vertebral column forms the axial skeleton of the body and extends from the base of the skull to the coccyx. Among 33 vertebrae, 24 are movable (7 cervical, 12 thoracic, and 5 lumbar), whereas five sacral and four coccygeal vertebrae are fused forming the sacrum and the coccyx. The adjacent movable vertebrae form articulations via intervening intervertebral discs and facets. The spine is curved in sagittal plane exhibiting lordosis in the cervical, kyphosis in the thoracic, and lordosis in the lumbar segments.

Anatomical distinctions of the vertebrae differentiate the cervical spine into upper (C1–C2) and lower (subaxial) (C3–C7) regions. The C1–C2 along with the occiput form complex, highly specialized articulations. The atlas (C1) consists of a ring formed by the anterior and posterior arches and two lateral masses.

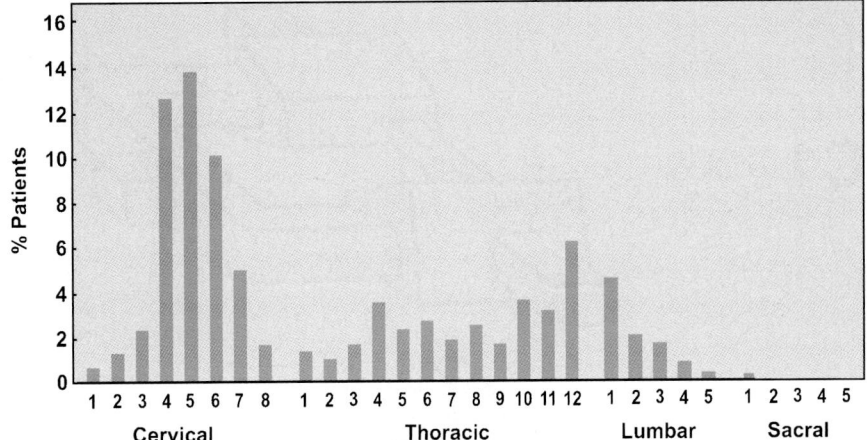

**FIGURE 24-4.** Distribution of the level of spinal injury with neurologic deficit.
*(Reproduced with permission from Stover SL, Fine PR (eds). Spinal Cord Injury: The Facts and Figures. Birmingham, The National Spinal Cord Injury Statistical Center, University of Alabama, 1986, p. 36.)*

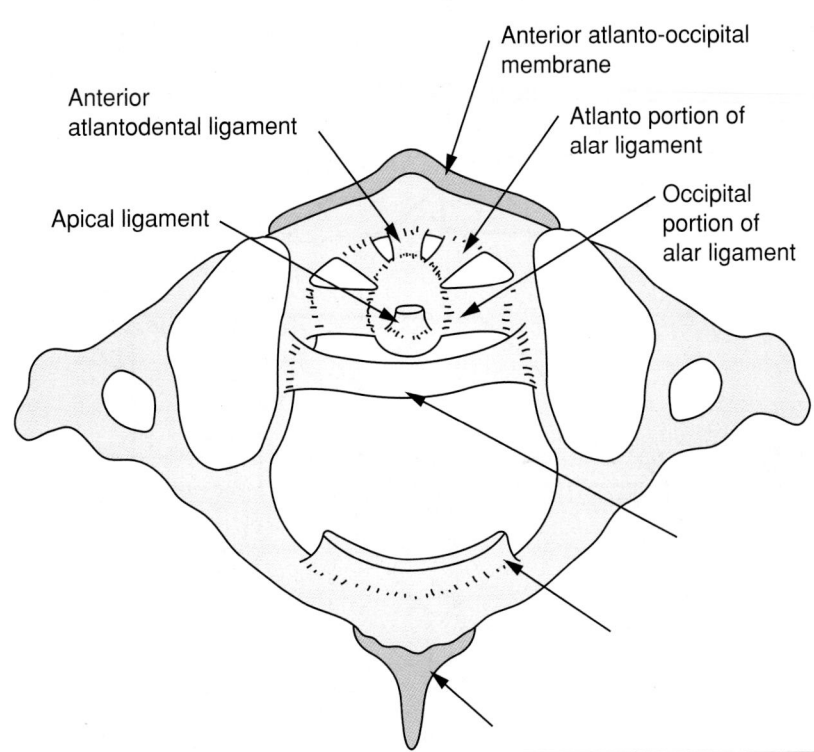

**FIGURE 24-5.** Axial anatomy of the atlas and its stabilizing ligaments.
*(Reproduced with permission from Dvorak J, Panjabi MM. Functional anatomy of the alar ligaments. Spine 12:183, 1987.)*

C1 articulates with occipital condyles, dens and facets of C2 (Fig. 24-5). A distinctive feature of the axis (C2) includes the odontoid process that forms joints with the anterior arch of C1 and the transverse ligament. The pedicles of C2 run obliquely in the sagittal plane connecting thereby anteriorly located facets of C1 with posteriorly located facets of C3 (Fig. 24-6). The remaining C3–C7 vertebrae are more uniform. The bodies of these vertebrae articulate via the intervertebral discs; the lateral aspects of the vertebral body have the uncinate processes forming with the adjacent vertebra joints of Luschka. Facet joints are arranged like shingles at 45° in coronal plane angulation.

Thoracic vertebrae differ from the cervical in having thin pedicles, large transverse processes, and long spinous processes. The thoracic spine forms a rigid column because of its attachments to the rib cage. The facets of thoracic vertebrae are angulated 20° in the coronal plane. At the thoracolumbar junction, the facet joints change gradually from the coronal to more sagittal angulations.

The subsequent lumbar spine is composed with largest five vertebrae (L1–L5) forming lordotic curve. The relatively large bodies, wide and short pedicles, and absence of the costal facets distinguish the lumbar vertebrae from the cervical and thoracic regions. The lumbar facets are oriented at 45° of sagittal angulation. L5 is the largest of all vertebrae and is associated with the prominence of the lumbosacral angle.

## Spine Kinematics

The spine comprises a complex, segmented mechanical structure that provides support, protects the neural elements, and allows erect posture and body movement. The basic unit in spinal kinesiology is the motion segment. The motion unit includes two adjacent vertebral bodies, intervening disc, the facet joints, and connecting ligamentous structures. The coupling nature of motion occurring at the given segment is a consequence of the anatomic

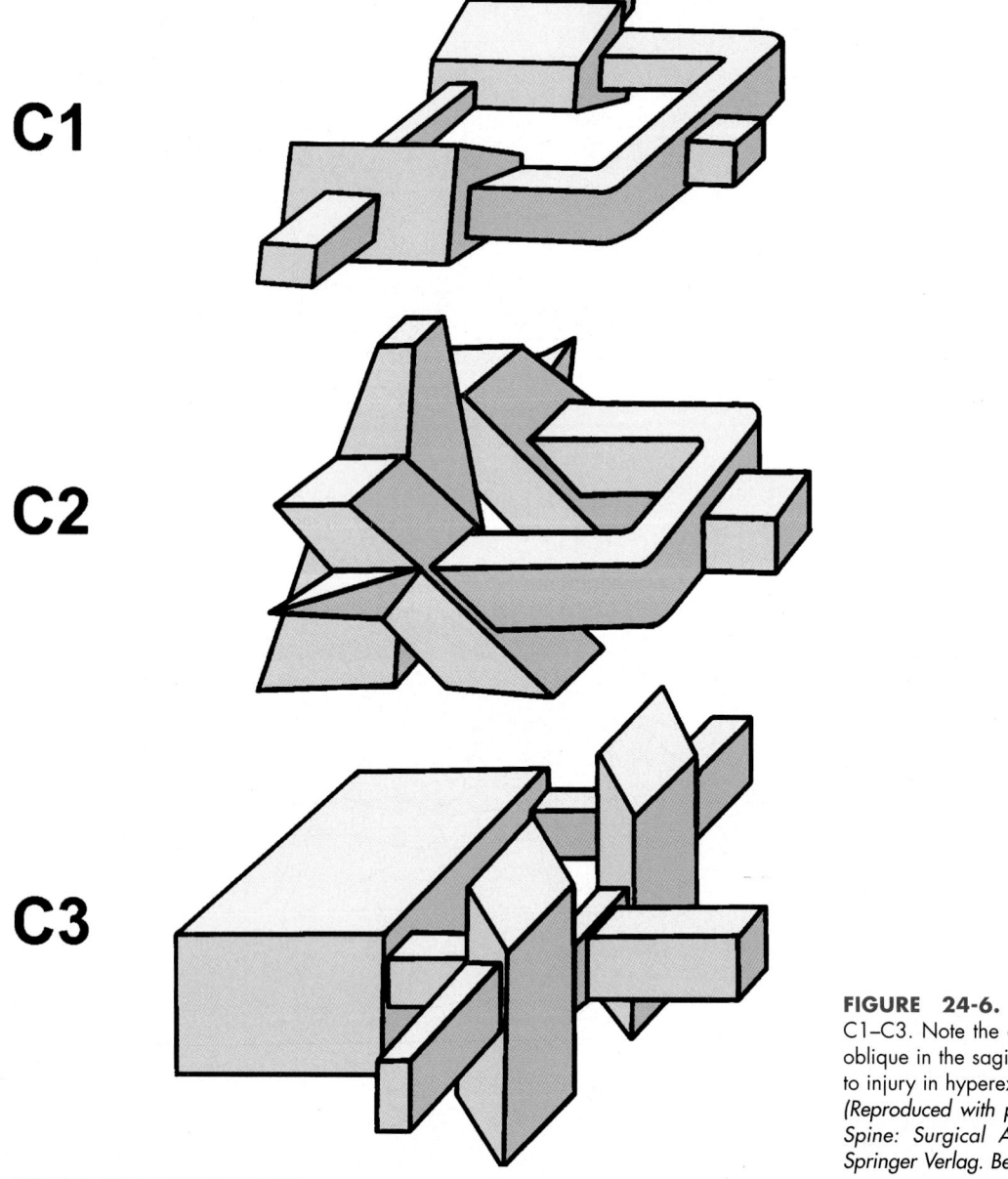

C1

C2

C3

**FIGURE 24-6.** Anatomical relationships between C1–C3. Note the orientation of the pedicle of the axis is oblique in the sagittal plane thereby making it susceptible to injury in hyperextension (hangman's fracture).
*(Reproduced with permission from Louis R. Surgery of the Spine: Surgical Anatomy and Operative Approaches. Springer Verlag. Berlin, 1982, p. 57.)*

configurations.[11] Spinal motion segments are responsible for maintaining spinal stability while permitting its flexibility In addition to providing support and weight-bearing, the spine protects neurologic structures.

Spinal ligaments and discs serve as restraints for the movable osseous structures of the vertebral column. In the upper cervix, the odontoid process is stabilized by the alar, transverse, and apical ligaments. Stabilizers of the entire cervical spine can be grouped in anterior and posterior columns.[12] Intervertebral discs along with the anterior and posterior longitudinal ligaments are stabilizers of anterior column, while the main posterior stabilizers include facet capsules, ligamenta flava, interspinal, supraspinal ligaments, and ligamentum nuchae (Fig. 24-7). The thoracolumbar spine, ligamentous stabilizers are divided into three columns (Fig. 24-8). The anterior column includes the anterior longitudinal ligament, the anterior portion of the annulus, and the anterior half of the vertebral body. The middle column consists of the posterior longitudinal ligament, posterior portion of the annulus, and posterior portion of the vertebral body. The posterior bony arch made up of the pedicles, facets, laminae, and

posterior ligamentous complex comprises the posterior column. The three-column model is useful in understanding the mechanism of injury and diagnosing spinal instability.

The most of axial rotation of the head and some flexion and lateral bending occur in the upper cervical spine. At the occiput and C1 major movement include flexion-extension and lateral bending, whereas at the atlantoaxial articulation 50% of the head rotation takes places. The motion of the upper cervical spine is limited by the alar ligaments. The cruciate ligaments restrict potentially dangerous anterior translation during flexion, while sill torsion around the dens. The apical ligament has negligible effect of restricting motion between occiput and C2.

The anatomical features of the lower cervical spine are adapted to flexion-extension as a primary motion of this region. The presence of intervertebral disc and the orientation of the facets joint support the axial loads and limit the rotation. The lateral bending in this region is coupled with an axial rotation to the same side. The motion segments of the upper cervical spine stabilize with anterior and posterior longitudinal ligaments.

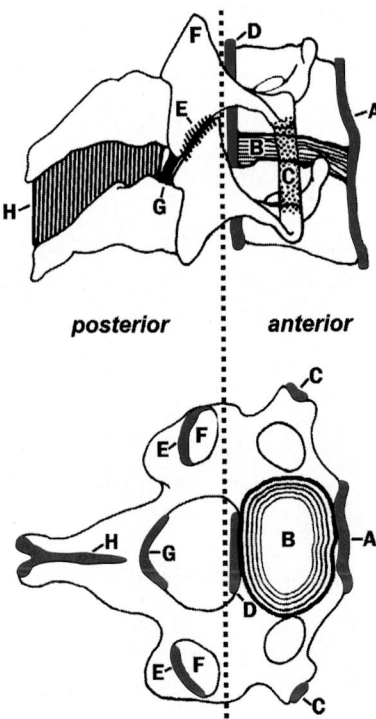

**FIGURE 24-7.** The stabilizing elements of the subaxial cervical spine can be grouped into anterior and posterior columns. A, anterior longitudinal ligament; B, intervertebral disc; C, intertransverse ligament; D, posterior longitudinal ligament; E, capsular ligament; F, facet joint; G, ligamentum flavum; H, interspinous ligament.
*(Reproduced with permission from White AA., et al. Biomechanical analysis of clinical stability in the cervical spine. Clin Orthop 109:85–96, 1975.)*

The thoracic region is the most rigid segment of the vertebral column due to the stabilizing effects of the rib cage and sternum. The motion allowed in the thoracic spine include rotation and to small extent flexion-extension and lateral bending. The peculiar kinematics of thoracolumbar junction is a consequence of the transition between rigid thoracic spine and flexible lumbar segment. Disrupting the anterior column decreases the load-carrying capacity of the thoracolumbar junction decreased by 30%; whereas ablating the anterior and middle columns can decrease its load-carrying capacity by 70%. The posterior column alone participates in the load-carrying capacity by only 25%; whereas together with middle column 65% of load can be shared. The annulus is the major rotatory stabilizer of the spine. By ablating the annulus, the rotatory stability of the thoracolumbar junction was diminished by 80%, while ablation of the facets decreased the rotatory stability by only 20%.

## ANATOMY AND PHYSIOLOGY OF THE SPINAL CORD

The spinal cord and its meninges represent a caudal continuation of the brain, extending from the foramen magnum through the spinal canal to T12–L1 where it terminates as the conus medullaris. A cluster of lumbosacral nerve roots below conus medullaris forms cauda equina (Fig. 24-9). At each intervertebral space, the ventral and dorsal roots join to form a nerve root that exits the spinal canal through the neural foramen. The spinal cord and intraspinous portions of the nerve roots are contained in a dura

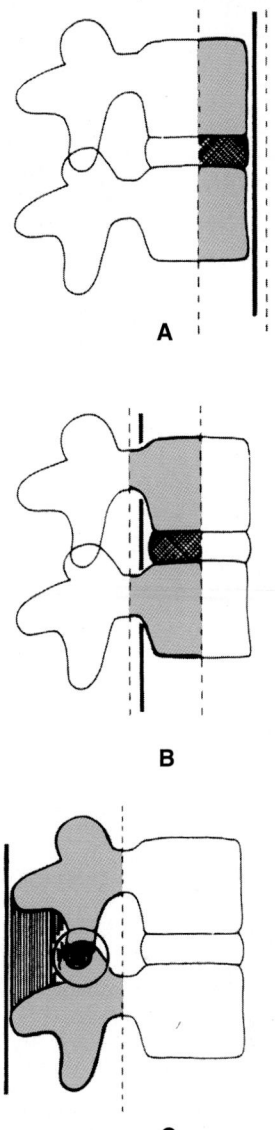

**FIGURE 24-8.** The three-column theory of the thoracolumbar spine distinguishes between the anterior (**A**), middle (**B**) and posterior columns (**C**). *(Reproduced with permission from Denis F. The three-column spine and its significance in the classification of acute thoracolumbar spinal injuries. Spine 8:817–831, 1983).*

mater (Fig. 24-10). Between the cord and the dura is the subarachnoid space, which contains the cerebrospinal fluid that completely surrounds the spinal cord and acts as a shock absorber. This fluid circulates from the subarachnoid space in the brain to communicate with the subarachnoid space around the spinal cord.

At the level of C1, the spinal cord occupies 33% of the canal with remaining space distributed equally between dens and cushioning fat (Fig. 24-11). In the lower cervical and thoracic spine, spinal cord filled the canal in about 50%. The remainder of the canal is filled with cerebrospinal fluid, epidural fat, and dura matter. The spinal cord has a variable diameter with enlargement of the cervical and lumbar regions to supply the nerve roots of the brachial and lumbosacral plexuses. In contrast to spinal cord in the cervical and thoracic regions, cauda equina is biomechanically less susceptible to injury due to the relatively larger spinal canal size in that region and higher flexibility. Furthermore, the nerves of cauda equina comprise the lower motor neuron axons,

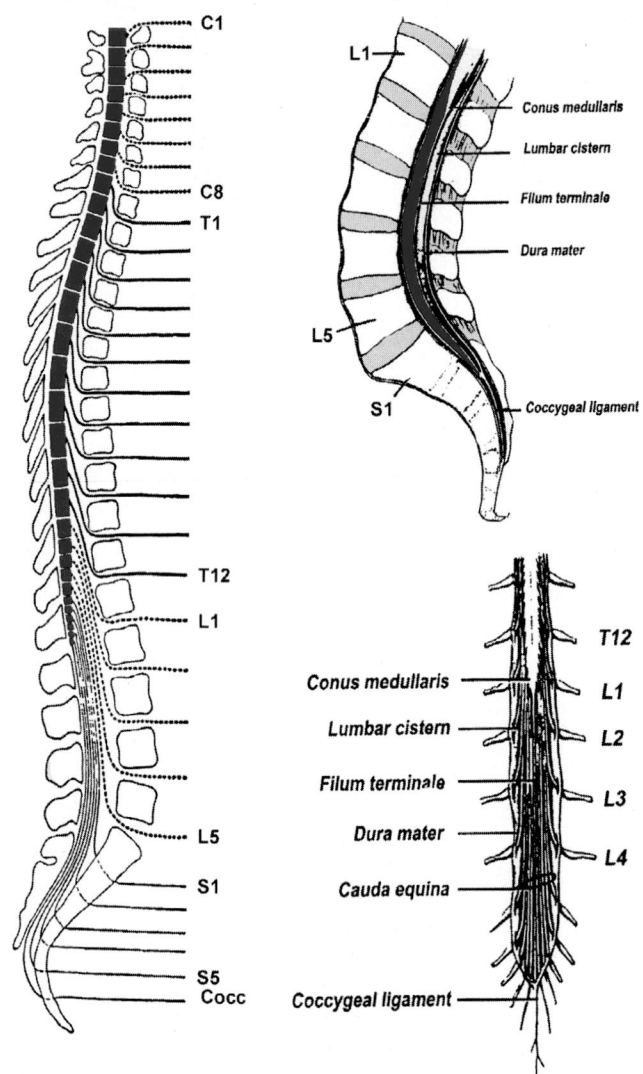

FIGURE 24-9.    The general anatomy and alignment of the spine and its neural elements.

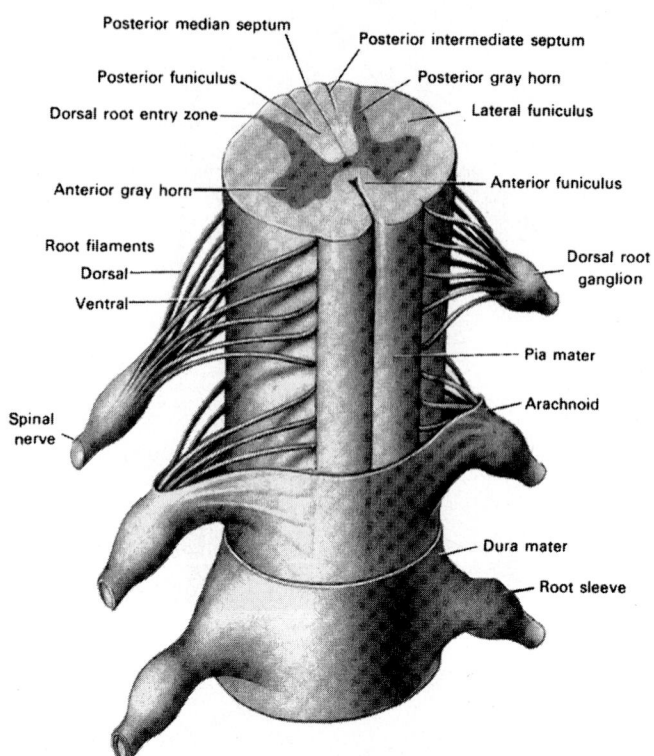

FIGURE 24-10.    Anatomy of the spinal cord and its nerve roots.

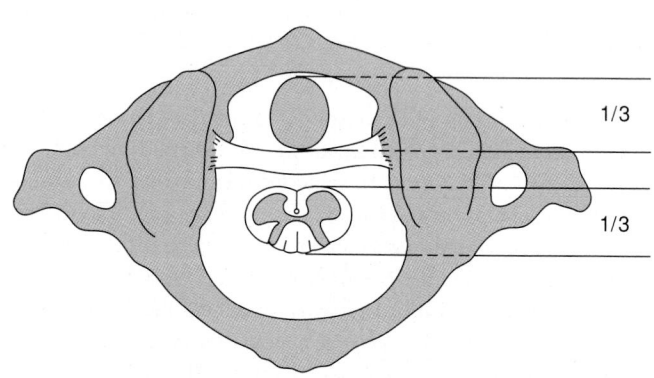

FIGURE 24-11.    Steel's rule of thirds which refers to the space occupied by the dens and the cord within the ring of the atlas.

which are more physiologically resilient to trauma than the upper motor neuron.

The spinal cord cross-sectional anatomy consists of centrally located gray matter with white matter located at the periphery (Fig. 24-12). The gray matter contains primarily neurons and unmyelinated axons. The anterior horns of the gray matter include somatic *lower motor neurons* that innervate the muscles of the neck, trunk, and the extremities; the posterior horns include neurons synapsing with afferent sensory axons; while the intermediate horns contains the preganglionic autonomic sympathetic neurons between T1–L3 and parasympathetic between S2–S4. The white matter contains myelinated axons forming ascending and descending spinal tracts. Although the spatial relationships of gray and white matter remain consistent throughout the entire length of the cord, their proportions change based on the level. The white matter comprises proportionally more of the cervical cross-sectional area than in more caudal segments due to the accumulation of the ascending tracts of the bellow located segments. Throughout the cord segments, the gray matter is enlarged in the cervical and lumbar levels due to accumulation of motor neurons innervating the upper and lower extremities. The *upper motor neurons* originate in the

cerebral cortex or brain stem, mostly crossing to the opposite side they descend as lateral and anterior corticospinal (pyramidal) tract to synapse with the lower motor neurons in the anterior horns of the gray matter (Fig. 24-13).

Spinal cord plays a crucial role in receiving and transmitting somatic and visceral sensory information to the brain as well as transmitting and modulating signals to the body's motor and autonomic effectors (Fig. 24-14). The ascending sensory input originates from the somatic or visceral receptors, and via axons is transmitted to neurons located in the dorsal root ganglia. Next, the sensory afferent axons enter the posterior horns of the gray matter and travel cephalad in different areas of the spinal cord, depending on the type of sensation. Pain and temperature sensation immediately cross to the opposite side of the cord and ascend in the lateral spinothalamic tract (Fig. 24-15). Touch also crosses immediately and ascends

**Posterior**

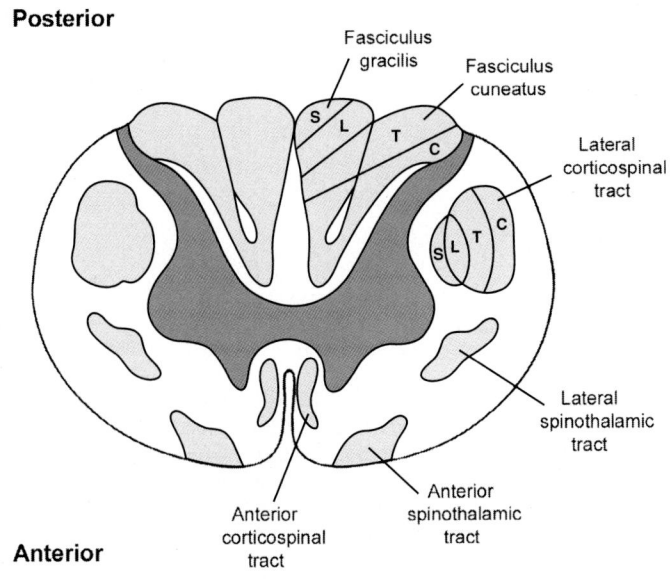

**Anterior**

**FIGURE 24-12.** Cross-sectional anatomy of the subaxial cervical spinal cord.

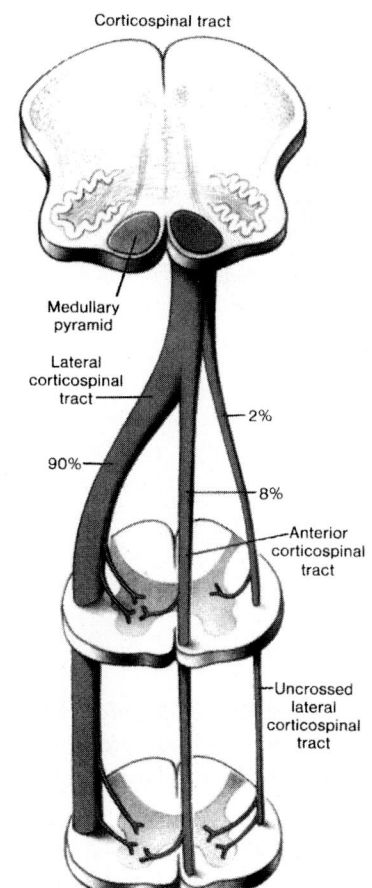

**FIGURE 24-13.** Distribution of the axons within the pyramidal tract.

in a diffuse manner, but primarily in the anterior spinothalamic tract. Proprioception and vibratory sensation ascend in the fibers of the posterior column and cross in the brain stem. The posterior columns are also structured topologically. The fasciculus gracilis

(lower extremities) is medial to the fasciculus cuneatus (upper extremities).

Depending on whether upper or lower motor neuron function is deficient different symptoms occur. The upper motor neuron injury produces spastic paralysis which also includes symptoms of inability for voluntary movement, increased deep tendon reflexes, loss of superficial reflexes, and positive Babinski sign. The damage of the anterior horns of the spinal cord gray matter constitute the lower motor neuron injury with symptoms like flaccid parlay which also includes inability for voluntary movement, loss of all reflexes, and atrophy of muscles. The injured spinal cord typically produces symptoms of the lower motor neuron injury at the level of the injured segment and the upper motor neuron symptoms to all segments bellow. Spinal cord also integrates and modulates body reflexes. The bulbocavernosus reflex is a simple sensory-motor pathway that functions autonomically without involvement of the ascending or descending spinal tract. If the level of the reflex arc is both physiologically and anatomically intact, the reflex will function despite cephalad dysfunctional spinal cord. Return of the bulbocavernosus reflex is sign of termination of the spinal shock following spinal cord injury.

## ACUTE INJURY TO VERTEBRAL COLUMN

### Spinal Instability as a Result of Trauma

Biomechanically spinal instability can refer to an abnormal response to applied loads, and can be characterized by motion in spinal segments beyond the normal constraints. Clinical instability refers to as the loss of the ability of the spine to maintain its pattern of the displacement of its elements under physiologic loads which can lead to subsequent damage or irritation to the spinal cord, its nerve roots, or can cause incapacitating deformity or pain.[13] This clinical definition takes into account neurologic as well as mechanical instability. In practice, spine fractures associated with neurologic injury are by definition unstable, except for those injuries secondary to penetrating trauma (i.e., gunshot, stabbing).

Spinal instability occurs when the anatomic elements of the motion segment or its supportive structures are disrupted, so that loads that are normally tolerated result in excessive or abnormal spinal motions, displacements, or strains, causing the development of progressive deformities. Recognition of spinal instability posttrauma is crucial to preventing injury to neural structures, late spinal deformity, and pain. In order to facilitate the diagnosis of the instability a checklist using point systems have been devised for each region of the vertebral column (Tables 24-2–24-4).

Division of the spine into columns has been used to estimate the potential for instability[14] (Fig. 24-8). A two-column model in which components posterior to the posterior longitudinal ligament are separated from the anterior components suggests that complete column injury results in instability.[12] A three-column model suggests that in the thoracolumbar spine, injury involving two or three columns produces instability[15,16] (Table 24-5). Biomechanical studies and clinical observations suggest that a loss of 50% of vertebral body height or angulation of the thoracolumbar spine

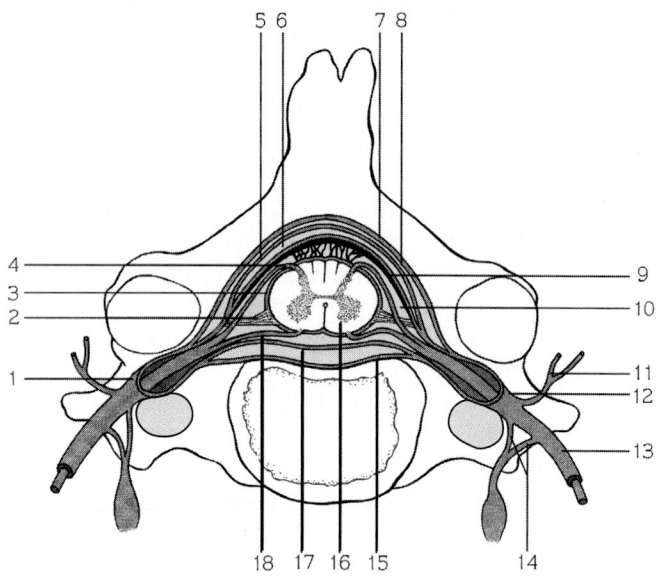

1 Spinal ganglion
2 Dentate ligament
3 Pia mater
4 Dorsal root of spinal n.
5 Dura mater
6 Subdural space
7 Periosteum
8 Epidural space
9 Arachnoid membrane
10 Subarachnoid space
11 Dorsal ramus
12 Spinal n.
13 Ventral ramus of spinal n.
14 Ramus communicans
15 Periosteum
16 Medulla spinalis
17 Dura mater
18 Ventral root of spinal n.

**FIGURE 24-14.** Anatomical relations of the neural and bony structures of the spine. (Reproduced with permission from An HS, Simpson JM, eds. Surgery of the Cervical Spine. Baltimore: Lippincott Williams & Wilkins. 1994, p. 21.)

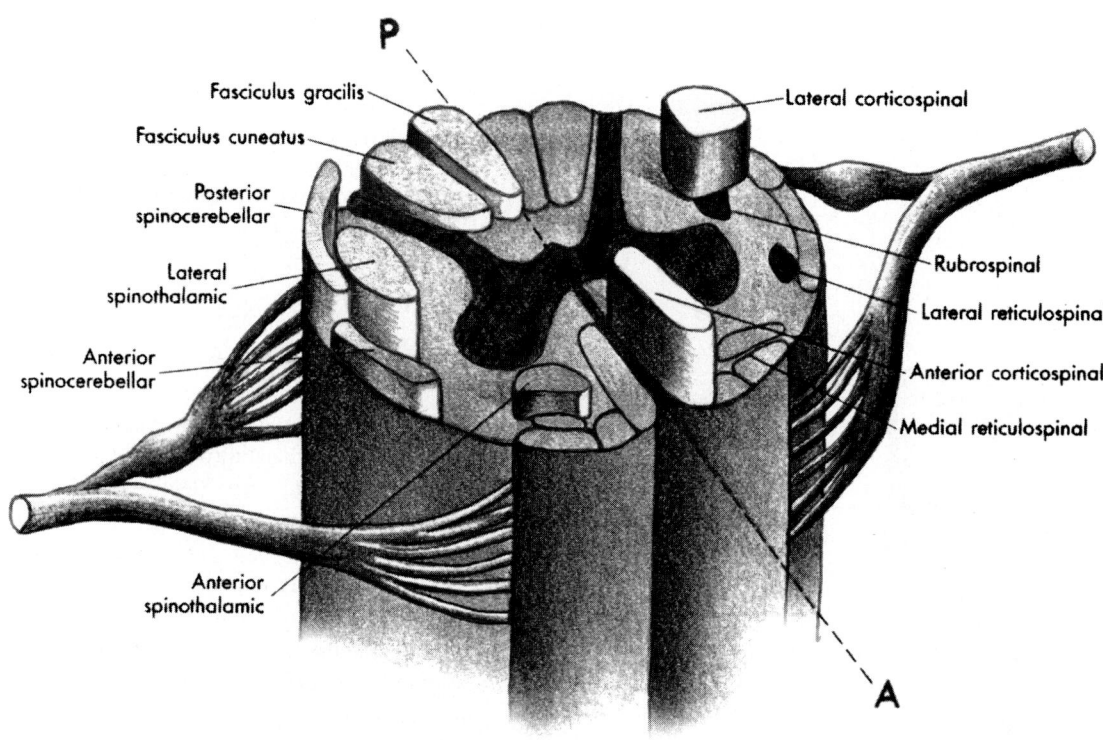

**FIGURE 24-15.** The major ascending and descending tracts of the spinal cord.

greater than 20° renders the spinal segment unstable. Under these conditions compression and burst fractures should be considered unstable. Clinical studies demonstrate that biomechanical instability occurs when at least two contiguous columns of the three spinal columns fail.

According to the magnitude and direction of injuring forces, five major types of spinal trauma mechanisms can be distinguished. They can produce varying degree of spinal instability:

1. *Flexion-compression.* Excessive flexion or biomechanical incompetence of the vertebral body (i.e., osteoporosis) typically results in the simple wedge fracture that involves the anterior portion of the vertebral body. The pivot point in this injury is located in the middle column; therefore this column is typically spared in compression fracture. Severe types of compression fractures can also occur as a result in disruption of posterior stabilizing elements, rendering the injury unstable. Combined flexion and compression and also flexion teardrop fracture which is very unstable injury involving all three spinal columns.

2. *Axial compression.* Axially applied load results in burst fractures that causes failure of anterior and middle spinal columns. The magnitude of the injuring force determines injury severity manifesting by fracture comminution, degree of retropulsion (spinal canal compromise) with concomitant neurologic deficit, and the residual deformity (loss of body height). Axial compression of the axis can cause Jefferson fracture as a burst fracture equivalent.

3. *Flexion-distraction.* The combination of flexion and distraction load with the pivot point located anteriorly causes significant

## TABLE 24-2

### Checklist for the Diagnosis of Clinical Instability of the Lower Cervical Spine (Total ≥ 5 Points = Unstable)

| ELEMENT | | POINTS |
|---|---|---|
| Anterior elements destroyed or unable to function | | 2 |
| Posterior elements destroyed or unable to function | | 2 |
| Radiographic criteria | Total | 4 |
|    A. Sagittal displacement >3.5 mm | 2 | |
|    B. Relative sagittal angulation >11° | 2 | |
| Positive stretch test | | 2 |
| Spinal cord injury | | 2 |
| Nerve root Injury | | 1 |
| Abnormal disc narrowing | | 1 |
| Dangerous loading anticipated | | 1 |

Adapted from: White, A.A.; Southwick, W.O.; Panjabi, M.M. Clinical instability in the lower cervical spine. Spine 1:15-27, 1976.

## TABLE 24-3

### Checklist for the Diagnosis of Clinical Instability of the Thoracic and Thoracolumbar Spine (Total ≥ 5 Points = Unstable)

| ELEMENT | | POINTS |
|---|---|---|
| Anterior elements destroyed or unable to function | | 2 |
| Posterior elements destroyed or unable to function | | 2 |
| Radiographic criteria | Total | 4 |
|    A. Sagittal displacement >2.5 mm | 2 | |
|    B. Relative sagittal angulation >5° | 2 | |
| Spinal cord or cauda equina damage | | 2 |
| Disruption of costovertebral articulations | | 1 |
| Dangerous loading anticipated | | 2 |

Adapted from: White, A.A.; Penjabi, M.M. Clinical Biomechanics of the Spine. Philadelphia, JB Lippincott, 1978, pp.236-251.

## TABLE 24-4

### Checklist for the Diagnosis of Clinical Instability of the Lumbosacral Spine (Total ≥ 5 Points = Unstable)

| ELEMENT | | POINTS |
|---|---|---|
| Anterior elements destroyed or unable to function | | 2 |
| Posterior elements destroyed or unable to function | | 2 |
| Radiographic criteria | Total | 4 |
| A. Flexion-extension radiographs: | | |
|    1. Sagittal translation | >4.5 mm or 15% | 2 |
|    2. Sagittal rotation | >15° at L1–L2, L2–L3, L3–L4 | 2 |
| | >20° at L4–L5 | 2 |
| | >25° at L5–S1 | 2 |
| B. Resting radiographs | | |
|    1. Sagittal displacement | >4.5 mm or 15% | 2 |
|    2. Relative sagittal angulation | >22° | 2 |
| Cauda equina damage | | 3 |
| Dangerous loading anticipated | | 1 |

Adapted from: White, A.A.; Penjabi, M.M. Clinical Biomechanics of the Spine. Philadelphia, JB Lippincott, 1978, pp.236-251.

7. *Avulsion.* Typical examples of avulsion fractures include type I odontoid fracture, clay-shovelers fracture of C7, or extension "teardrop" fracture.

## ACUTE SPINAL CORD INJURY

Spinal cord injury usually results from a mechanical stress or impact that occurs at the time of the trauma. The degree of cord damage depends on the nature and dynamics of the traumatic force and on the level at which the spine and cord are injured. Based on the nature and extent of mechanism of injury, the acute lesions of the spinal cord can be identified as:

1. *Direct space-occupying lesions* that result in a focal injury to the neural elements at the site of impact. These lesions created high forces concentrated at small area of the cord and can occur due to spine fractures, dislocation, disc herniation, or direct penetrating trauma. Typically the site of the injury can be localized using imaging studies.

2. *Direct non-occupying lesions* which result from stretching, shearing, or compressive forces applied to spinal cord via bony-ligamentous components of the spine. This occurs when the impact causes a comparatively small load distributed over large area of the cord. The injuries in this group present more diffuse patterns of neurologic deficit;

3. *Secondary injuries* due to disruption of blood supply to spinal cord or passage of the cerebrospinal fluid.

In general, the cord lesion is rarely confined to the point of impact to the spine, but may spread away over several segments. This is due to both primary and secondary traumatic changes.

Due to the anatomic and biomechanical conditions of the spine, the cervical region and thoracolumbar junction are the most frequent sites of traumatic damage. Cervical spine injuries are particularly devastating and occasionally lethal. About 60% of acute fatal cervical injuries are associated with traumatic craniocerebral lesions. They often involve the upper cervical cord, while fracture-dislocations and subluxations of the cervical spine are most

disruption of the posterior stabilizing elements, with the extension to the middle and anterior column. This very unstable injury can occur through bony and/or ligamentous components of the spinal motion segment (Chance fracture).

4. *Hyperextension.* These injuries result in disruption of anterior and middle columns in tension and commonly are often accompanied by subluxation or dislocation, when translation or rotation component is present. Typical examples include traumatic spondylolisthesis of C2 (hangmen's fracture), and extension "teardrop" fracture. These injuries are typically unstable due due to the disruption of the stabilizing ligamentous apparatus and injury to the disc.

5. *Rotation.* Flexion and extension injuries that include significant rotation component often result in subluxation, dislocations, and fracture-dislocations of the spinal facets. Rotational injuries often have a translational component and are very unstable. Bilateral facet dislocation typically produces very unstable three-column injury.

6. *Shear.* The spinal translation is a component of majority of spinal fractures and/or ligamentous disruptions. Shear mechanism of the spinal injury produces failure of all the three columns and is often associated with facet dislocation.

**TABLE 24-5**

### Modes of Failure of the Spine Using the Three-Column Stability Model

| FRACTURE TYPE | COLUMN | | |
| --- | --- | --- | --- |
| | Anterior | Middle | Posterior |
| Simple Compression | Compression | None | None |
| Severe Compression | Compression | None | Distraction |
| Burst | Compression | Compression | None |
| Flexion-Distraction | None/Compression/Distraction | Distraction | Distraction |
| Fracture-Dislocation | Compression/Rotation/Shear | Distraction/Rotation | Distraction/Rotation |

Adopted from: Denis F. The three column spine and its significance in the classification of acute thoracolumbar spinal injuries. Spine 8: 817, 1983.

common at the level of the C5–C6 vertebrae. Thoracic fractures are less common than cervical, and in these the lower thoracic levels are more likely to be involved. Low thoracic injuries are typically caused by crushing or extreme flexion of the spine in falls or road or mining accidents. Upper thoracic spine trauma may show second-level injury. Lesions of the lumbar spine can damage the conus or compress the cauda equina.

## Morphological Changes following Spinal Cord Injury

According to their relationship to the site of injury and to the presumed pathogenesis, the pathologic changes are separated into *main damage,* situated at the level of or adjacent to the site of injury, representing the local consequence of physical trauma; *neighboring lesions,* occurring in the areas adjacent to the main damage, including hemorrhages, ischemic or hemorrhagic necroses, edema; and remote lesions as result of deprived circulation.

The region within the spinal cord which is most susceptible to direct injury is the gray matter located within the central substance. This is due to higher metabolic rate of the gray matter, and the presence of its repair mechanisms (neurons) within the site of injury. This is in contrast to the white matter where the neuronal cell bodies are at a remote site.[17]

Depending on the period of survival, the pathologic lesions can be categorized as early or acute, intermediate, and late changes, the character and chronological consequences. It has been implied that, except for petechial hemorrhage, the human spinal cord may show no significant macroscopic or histopathologic changes until 6–24 hours after trauma. Therefore, there is a considerable latent period between the moment of injury and the necrosis in the traumatized area of the spinal cord. This has been confirmed in several trauma models.[18]

## Functional Changes following Spinal Cord Injury

Concomitantly with the primary mechanical injury that causes direct tissue insult to the spinal cord secondary events are triggered which are detrimental to neural tissue function. Although structural damage of neural tissue is irreversible, the prompt ablation of persistent direct cord compression and justifies the immediate surgical to arrest progressive neurologic compromise. Current recognition, identification, and prevention of secondary spinal cord injury mechanisms has been the major premise for early pharmacological intervention in spinal cord injury.

The initial traumatic impacts typically results in compression and contusion of the spinal cord, and with mechanical damage to

nerve cells, axonal tracts, and blood vessels. Complete transection of the spinal cord following blunt trauma is rare. As a response to the mechanical insult, hemorrhage, edema, and ischemia, rapidly follow extending to contiguous areas in the neural tissue. Persistent pressure on the cord by space occupying bone, ligaments, or disc can potentiate mechanical damage to the cord after the primary injury. The mechanical injury to the neural tissue triggers the secondary events which comprise a complex cascade of biochemical and cellular processes. Although exact mechanism of secondary spinal cord damage is not well understood, various functional hypotheses are proposed.

After the initial hemorrhage, inflammation proceeds in the central gray matter of the cord. On a systemic level, autonomic nervous system dysfunction, hypotension, and bradycardia (neurogenic shock) contribute to impaired spinal cord perfusion, which further increases the ischemia. Experimental studies in animal models of spinal cord injury have shown an increase of products of anoxic metabolism in neural tissue. Although there are number of theories emphasize certain events the pathophysiology of secondary injury, the synergistic effect of these events most likely take places.[19]

The neurotransmitters theory suggests that excitatory amino acid, derivatives glutamate and aspartate, increase 6-fold the baseline levels[20] yielding concentrations detrimental to neurons within one hour after injury.[21] Experimentally-induced neurologic dysfunction can occur when the cord is exposed to excitatory amino acids,[22,23] whereas pretreatment with these amino acid antagonists can reduce the extent of functional deficit.[23,24] The free-radical theory suggests that free radicals accumulate in the injured neural tissue and damage lipids and proteins the cell membrane as well as nucleic acids. The inability to maintain the integrity of cell membrane is responsible for death of neurons due to uncontrolled influx of ions and unbalanced osmotic pressure. The calcium ion theory implicates the influx of extracellular calcium ions into nerve cells in the propagation of secondary injury. Intracellular accumulation of calcium with efflux of potassium has been observed after experimental spinal cord injury.[25] Excess of calcium ions activate phospholipases, proteases, and phosphatases which in turn lead to interruption of mitochondrial activity and disruption of the cell membrane. Initial neuronal swelling is related to sodium influx, whereas subsequent neuronal disintegration results from calcium influx.[26] Both competitive and noncompetitive calcium channel blockers have been demonstrated experimentally to reduce secondary neurologic injury.[22,27–29]

Another theory postulates the involvement of the endogenous opioid such as peptides, dynorphin, endorphin, and enkephalins may be involved in the producing secondary effects of spinal cord injury.[27] This is substantiated by the fact that graded time-dependent injuries can be related to dynorphin,[30,31] while application of opiate antagonists such as naloxone improved neurologic recovery in experimental models of spinal cord injury.[32] In the inflammation theory, increased activity of cyclo- and lipoxygenase results in accumulation of inflammatory mediators (i.e., prostaglandins, leukotrienes, platelet-activating factor, serotonin) producing secondary neuronal damage.[33,34] More specifically, the increasing imbalance between levels of thromboxane or prostacyclin was observed soon after experimental spinal cord injury.[34,35] The effect of inflammatory mediator seemed to be potentiated in anoxic conditions with a diminished tissue perfusion.[36]

## Novel Neuroprotective and Therapeutic Interventions

The concept of neuroprotection has been recently coined to characterize all of the measures utilized to attenuate the extent of spinal cord injury and possibly at support the dormant reparative potential of the neural tissue. Neuroprotective interventions are based on the premise that neurologic outcome can be improved by the elimination of secondary injuring mechanisms and the ability of the damaged neural tissue to recover functionally. Although several neuroprotective interventions have proven efficacious in animal spinal cord injury models, demonstrating efficient neuroprotection in humans has been exceedingly difficult.

The early institution of high-dose steroids currently remains the standard clinical neuroprotective intervention in the acute phase of spinal cord injury. Steroids effectively limit the cellular and molecular events of the injury-induced inflammation, and, thereby, decreases the extent of secondary effects on the neural tissue.[33,37] The clinical role of anti-inflammatory steroids has been extensively tested in spinal cord injury and, although all the present theories seem to have merit on a scientific basis, the clinical results have not been successful in limiting secondary injury. Methylprednisolone is currently the only pharmacologic substance whose ability to limit the extent of secondary neural injury has been prospectively validated.[38] Conversely, other agents such as GM1 ganglioside, naloxone, thyreotropin-releasing hormone, nimodipine, triliazad mesylate have proven promising in animals, but have not demonstrated sufficient efficacy in clinical trails.[39,40]

Presently, several new, promising neuroprotective agents are being investigated and these include minocycline, erythropoietin, neurotrophic growth factors, and cellular therapies. Minocycline, a tetracycline derivative, exhibits its neuroprotective properties by inhibiting matrix metalloproteinases, microglial activation (both present during neuroinflammation), and preventing cell apoptosis.[41] The administration of minocycline shortly after an experimentally-induced spinal cord injury increased axonal sparing, reduced the apoptotic demise of oligodendrocytes, diminished axonal death, and culminated in improved locomotor and behavioral outcomes in animals.[42] Erythropoietin, a hormone produced primarily by the kidney in response to hypoxia, has proven to be especially capable of minimizing spinal cord injury in ischemic models based on aortic occlusion. Erythropoietin prevented motoneuron apoptosis spinal cord injury in animals, and thereby promoted their motor

functional recovery.[43] Interestingly, erythropoietin reduced lipid peroxidation at the site of injury to a greater extent than methylprednisolone at the doses recommended per Second National Acute Spinal Cord Injury Study (NASCII).[44]

Recently, there have been a renewed interest in applying neurotrophic factors, growth factors, cytokines, and various forms of cell therapies in the treatment of SCI. Neurite outgrowth at the site of injury can be inhibited by myelin and myelin-associated protein (MAG), and the protein called Nogo. The application of brain- and glial-derived neurotrophic factors (BDNF and GDNF) has been shown to favorably alter the injury environment. Both, BDNF and GDNF increase the levels of cyclic adenosine monophosphate (cAMP) in neurons and thereby promote the axonal regeneration over long distances relevant for functional recovery of the spinal cord.[45] The application of specific Nogo receptor blockers has been promising as evidenced by its facilitation of axonal sprouting and enhanced functional recovery in rats.[46] Among other noggin, several types of bone morphogenetic proteins (BMPs), and interleukin 6 (IL-6) are being actively investigated to elucidate their roles in triggering reparative cascades in the injured spinal cord.[40]

The necrosis and apoptosis of cells in the injured spinal cord as evidenced by the presence of cystic cavity at the injury site intuitively postulate this cellular be replenished. Cellular therapies aim to deliver committed or uncommitted cells locally to the injury site, thereby restoring functionally competent cellular environment of the injured cord. The primary cell types used in this approach include Schwann cells and olfactory ensheathing cells, and uncommitted stems cells. Schwann cells have been recognized as the key cellular constituent of peripheral nerve regeneration. Several studies demonstrated that transected spinal cord can be morphologically bridged when by Schwann cells are delivered.[47,48] Schwann cells function as chaperons by guiding the sprouting axons.[48] Olfactory ensheathing cells are distinct glial cells that guide the growing axons and play a crucial role in the renewal of sensory neurons within the olfactory epithelium. Unlike Schwann cells, olfactory ensheathing cells have demonstrated the unique ability to extend across glial scar within the transected cord.[49] The transplantation of olfactory ensheathing cells into a completely transected spinal cord facilitates the long-distance regeneration of corticospinal, noradrenergic, and serotonergic fibers which culminate in significant functional recovery.[50,51] Prompted by these results, many spinal cord injury centers have initiated human trials which focus on the application of putative OECs for spinal cord injury patients.

Uncommitted bone marrow mesenchymal and hematopoetic cells are particularly promising for spinal cord repair due to their apparent ability to trans-differentiate into neurons and glia without cell fusion.[52] These cells have a great appeal because they can be easily procured, expanded in culture, and delivered intravenously. Preclinical studies have supported the feasibility of this approach, and have confirmed the ability of intravenously administered mesenchymal stem cells to target regions of intraspinal cavitation.[53–55]

Experimental animal models of spinal cord injury have generated a number of promising experimental neuroprotective interventions, but have also exposed the overwhelming complexity of the neurobiological challenges. Major progress has occurred in the field of cellular replacement therapies; neural tissue transplantation, initially considered as only a powerful experimental tool for central nervous system

(CNS) injury and disease, has become a major focus in translational spinal cord injury neurobiology. A greater understanding of this technology will be necessary for the further development of the optimal therapeutic approaches to the injured spinal cord.

## NEUROLOGICAL PATTERNS OF SPINAL CORD INJURY

All spinal cord lesions can be broadly classified as neurologically complete or incomplete using Frankel score (Table 24-6) or the American Spinal Injury Association Scale (ASIA), (ASIA Standards 1989) (Fig. 24-16). A patient with a complete cord injury has no motor or sensory function caudal to the level of the injury. In order to designate the spinal injury as neurologically incomplete or complete, the spinal cord must recover from spinal shock. Return of spinal reflexes, mainly bulbocavernosus reflex confirms the resolution of the spinal shock, which typically last up to 48 hours postinjury. Beyond this point, if there is no sensory or motor recovery, the injury is pronounced as complete and no further significant neurologic improvement can be expected.[56] The severity of the

**TABLE 24-6**

| Frankel Classification of Spinal Cord Injury | |
|---|---|
| **FRANKEL TYPE** | **DEFICIT** |
| A | Complete, no sensory, no motor function |
| B | Preserved sensory function, no motor function |
| C | Useless motor function |
| D | Useful motor function |
| E | Normal sensory and motor function |

*Adopted from: Frankel HL, Hancock DO, Hyslop G, et al. The value of postural reduction in initial management of closed injuries of the spine with paraplegia and tetraplegia. Paraplegia 7:179, 1970.*

complete spinal cord injury is inversely proportional to the anatomic levels of the injured segment.

Among incomplete spinal cord injuries, four distinct patterns can be identified which demonstrate specific neurologic deficits (Fig. 24-17). These spinal cord syndromes are characterized by variable loss of motor and sensory function, are associated with specific injuries of the spine, and present a different prognosis for neurologic recovery.

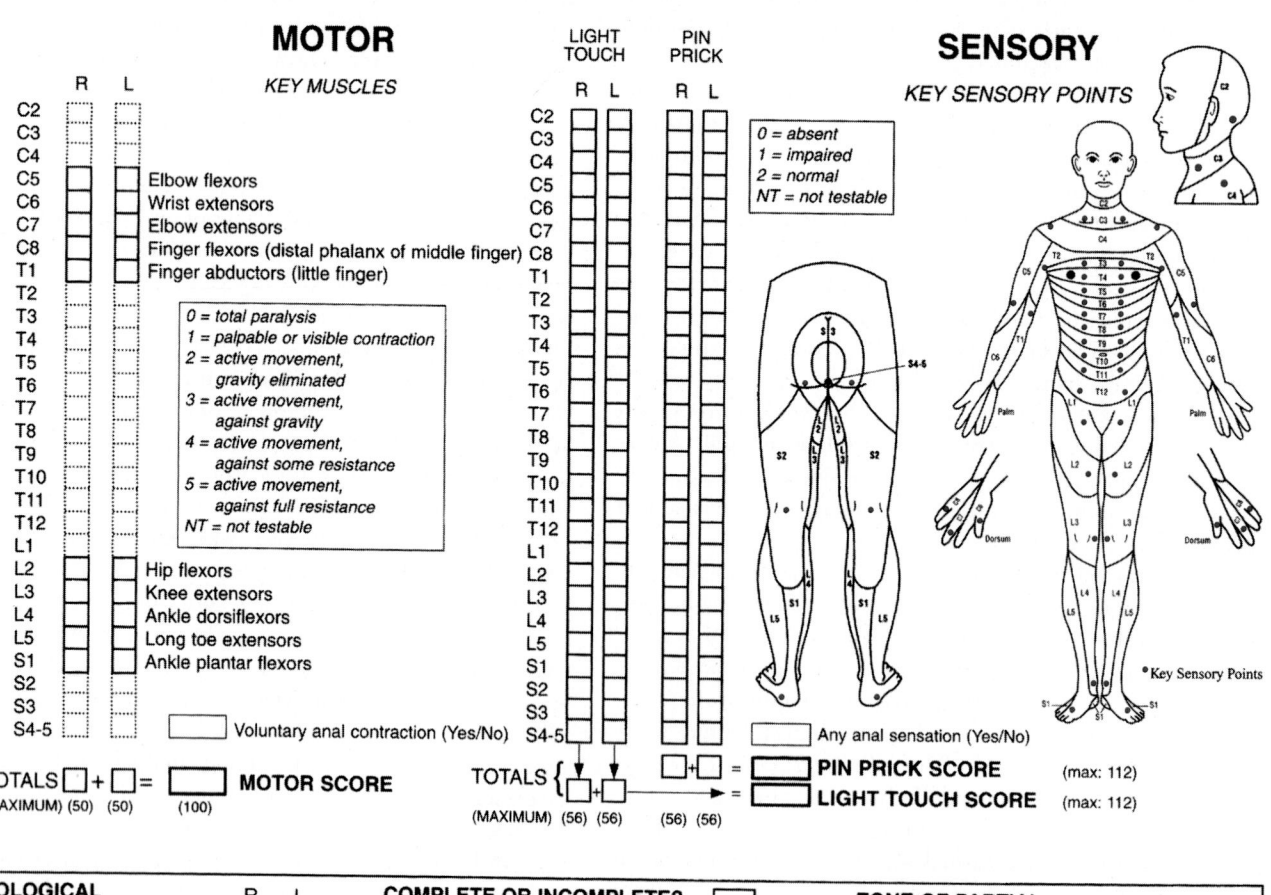

**FIGURE 24-16.** The ASIA classification of neurologic deficit following spine injury.

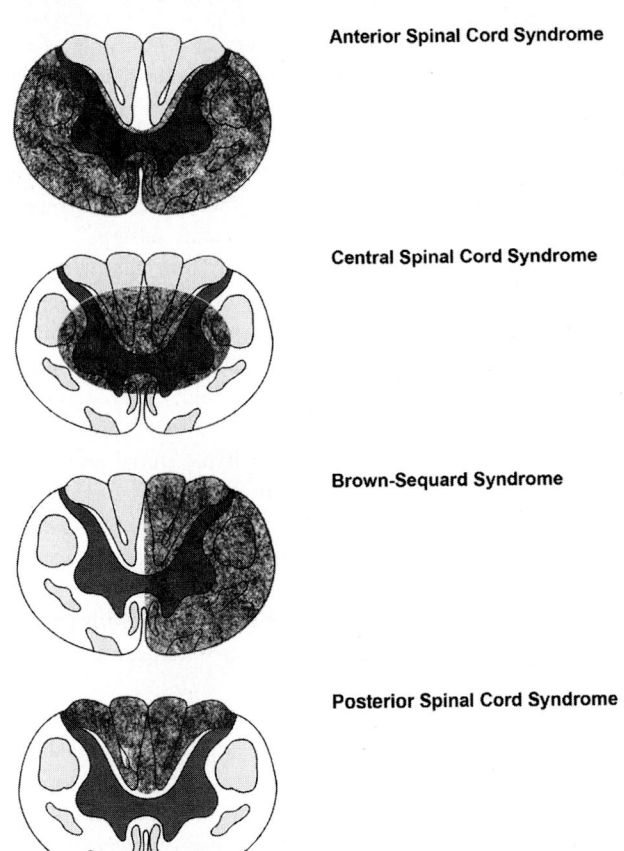

Anterior Spinal Cord Syndrome

Central Spinal Cord Syndrome

Brown-Sequard Syndrome

Posterior Spinal Cord Syndrome

**FIGURE 24-17.** The most common patterns of spinal cord injury.

## Anterior Cord Syndrome

The anterior cord syndrome is characterized by injury to the anterior two-thirds of the cord, on the opposite site of spine injury. The mechanism of injury is usually a compression or flexion type which causes subsequent vascular injury. Clinically, patients present with complete loss of motor function, sharp pain, and temperature below the level of injury, but retain proprioception and the ability to sense vibration and deep pressure. The prognosis for recovery is poor, with minimal chance of return of meaningful function.[57]

## Central Cord Syndrome

The central cord syndrome is common and typically results from a hyperextension injury in an older patient with a preexisting cervical spondylosis. The injury involves the central portion of the cord. Clinically, the upper extremities present with more sensory/motor deficit than the lower extremities, due to the more peripheral positioning of the lower extremity axons within the spinal cord tracts. The recovery from this type of injury is fair, with some patients regaining the ability to walk, with limited return of upper extremity function.[56]

## Brown-Sequard Syndrome

This syndrome results from hemitransection of the spinal cord with unilateral damage to the corticospinal and spinothalamic tracts, with subsequent loss of ipsilateral motor and dorsal column function, and contralateral pain and temperature sensation. Substantial recovery may be expected from this syndrome.[58]

## Posterior Cord Syndrome

This syndrome is rare and involves the dorsal column with subsequent loss of proprioception and vibration, while motor function is preserved. The prognosis is generally good, although many patients experience difficulty walking due to deficit in proprioceptive sensation.

## Cervical Root Syndrome

This represents an isolated nerve root that causes a deficit in sensation and the lower motor neuron. This injury is typically associated with acute disc herniation or a dislocation of the facet joint.

## Conus Medullaris Syndrome

The conus medullaris is located at the level of the T11–L1 intervertebral space. Injury of conus medullaris can produce mixed upper and lower motor neuron symptoms. Isolated injury to the conus may result in loss of bowel and bladder control (no sacral sparing). The prognosis for recovery is poor.

## Cauda Equina Syndrome

The cauda equina extends from L1 to L5 and is composed entirely from lumbar and sacral nerve roots. Injury to this region will resemble a peripheral nerve injury demonstrating lower motor injury symptoms. The physical findings are variable motor and sensory loss. Patients may present with bladder and bowel dysfunction. The prognosis for motor recovery is good. Surgical treatment in this area of the spine may produce the best results.

# INJURY DIAGNOSIS AND ACUTE MANAGEMENT

## Clearing of the Cervical Spine

In the trauma setting, cervical spine clearance is defined as reliably ruling out the presence of cervical injury in a patient when cervical injury is not present.[59] Contrary to the common misconception, the purpose of cervical clearance is not to detect, classify, and/or determine the appropriate treatment for cervical injury; clearance simply establishes that a cervical spine injury does not exist. Cervical clearance always requires a thorough clinical evaluation, while adjunctive imaging is warranted only as indicated. Although it is preferable that the cervical spine be cleared as early as feasible, the major emphasis of the clearance process major emphasis is its accuracy and not the speed at which it is accomplished.

The primary objective of cervical spine clearance is to improve both the efficiency and accuracy of the entire trauma assessment process. When the cervical spine can be cleared, neck immobilization precautions can be discontinued, additional cervical spine diagnostic or therapeutic modalities are not warranted, and the evaluating physicians can focus on the other areas of the patient's assessment. However, there are some patients who cannot be safely cleared in the acute setting and when this occurs, cervical spine precautions must be maintained and efforts to establish the presence or absence of cervical spine injury must continue.

A comprehensive clinical examination is essential in achieving cervical spine clearance, and this requires that the patient is alert, orient, and cooperative. Therefore, the clinician's initial objective should be to determine the patient's level of consciousness based on the Glasgow Coma Scale (GCS) which consists of six varying levels of alertness ranging from full orientation through deep coma (Table 24-7). An alert patient (GCS >14) can provide a valid history and a creditable physical examination, and corroborate the data obtained from all other diagnostic modalities. Even when cervical imaging appears normal, injury cannot be conclusively excluded unless the patient is able to contribute to the process.

The clinician's ability to perform a reliable clinical examination constitutes the basis by which patients can be divided into one of three cervical spine clearance groups[59] (Fig. 24-18): Group I — patients who can be cleared of cervical spine injury by clinical examination alone without diagnostic imaging; Group II — patients who can be cleared only when clinical examination is supported by negative diagnostic imaging, or Group III — patients upon whom a reliable clinical examination is not feasible at presentation and are not candidates for cervical spine clearance, even if adjunctive imaging is negative.[59]

*Group I:* Patients that meet all of the five following criteria: (1) full alertness; (2) no intoxication; (3) no midline tenderness; (4) no focal neurological deficit; and (5) no distracting painful injury. A randomized, prospective study[60,61] by the NEXUS group of 34,069 patients demonstrated that significant cervical spine injury could be reliably excluded by physical examination alone. The reliability of cervical spine clearance by physical examination of the alert patient has also been corroborated by other studies.[62–65] These studies have demonstrated that many trauma patients are alert on presentation to a medical facility and, thereby, can potentially be clinically cleared. Successfully cleared patients do not require further diagnostic measures, and cervical spine precautions can be discontinued.

*Group II:* Fully oriented and alert patients who demonstrate symptoms of neck pain, tenderness, neurologic deficit, decreased mobility on physical examination require additional diagnostic assessment to effectively clear the cervical spine. This group also includes patients with a distracting injury or past history of cervical spine pathology. Additional diagnostic studies typically consist of three-view radiography (AP, lateral, open-mouth odontoid) and may require adjunctive CT or MRI.[59] Voluntary lateral flexion-extension radiography is indicated only after symptomatic treatment has failed over a brief period of time (typically two weeks), and is not generally recommended in the acute setting.

An alert patient who presents with partial or complete neurologic deficit is assumed to have a spine injury, and thereby requires imaging. Whether the deficit is due to spinal cord, spinal root, or peripheral nerve injury, an exhaustive diagnostic effort must be made to rule out spine instability and/or injury. Throughout this process, the physician must strictly adhere to all precautionary spine immobilization techniques, even if the initial examination suggests a complete neurologic deficit. Plain radiography and/or sophisticated imaging are always indicated to diagnose and categorize the injury. Prophylactic modalities such as high-dose steroids administration, when indicated, must be instituted emergently. Serial examinations are warranted for the patients with partial or complete neurologic deficit to document neurologic progression or improvement.

*Group III:* In the obtunded trauma patients, strict adherence to basic principles of cervical spine external support and/or stabilizing precautions is recommended. Imaging, to detect but not to definitively exclude injury, is always required in these patients. Imaging should begin with the standard three-view plain radiography series, and advance on computerized tomography or magnetic resonance imaging as indicated. If cervical spine imaging is positive, this should be addressed in accordance with the standard of care for that particular injury. If the cervical spine imaging is negative, the prudent physician is obliged to maintain all neck precautions until the patient becomes more alert and receptive to supplemental clinical assessment. Although some reports[66–69] suggest that negative sophisticated imaging (CT and/or magnetic resonance imaging [MRI]) may adequately clear the cervical spine of these patients, the present authors submit that definitive clearance cannot be reliably established until the patient is alert and a valid physical examination can be performed.

The effectiveness of cervical spine clearance is greatly facilitated when trauma patients are assigned to one of these three clinical groups. Although the usual clinical objective of detecting injury can be difficult, its proficient exclusion can be an even greater challenge. Cervical spine imaging, which is more sensitive for injury detection than it is specific for its exclusion, does not substitute for a thorough clinical evaluation in establishing clearance. Moreover, the effectiveness of cervical spine imaging in clearance of cervical spine is enhanced when it is combined with a valid clinical assessment.

## Imaging

A thorough radiographic evaluation must follow appropriate initial clinical examination according to the Advanced Trauma Life Support (ATLS) protocol[70] in patients with suspected spinal column injury. Noncontiguous multilevel spinal injuries have been reported in 4.5 to 16.7% of all spine trauma cases.[71–73] Proper imaging will identify these injuries and avoid delay in diagnosis and treatment. The initial cervical spine radiographic evaluation consists of a cross table lateral view (CTLV), which can depict 70 to 79% of all injuries (Fig. 24-19). The lateral film must

**TABLE 24-7**

| Glasgow Coma Scale | | |
|---|---|---|
| **FEATURE** | **RESPONSE** | **SCORE** |
| Eye opening | Spontaneous | 4 |
| | To speech | 3 |
| | To pain | 2 |
| | None | 1 |
| Verbal response | Oriented | 5 |
| | Confused conversation | 4 |
| | Words inappropriate | 3 |
| | Sounds incomprehensible | 2 |
| | None | 1 |
| Best motor response | Obeys commands | 6 |
| | Localizes pain | 5 |
| | Flexion normal | 4 |
| | Flexion abnormal | 3 |
| | Extended | 2 |
| | None | 1 |
| Total Coma Score | | 3–15 |

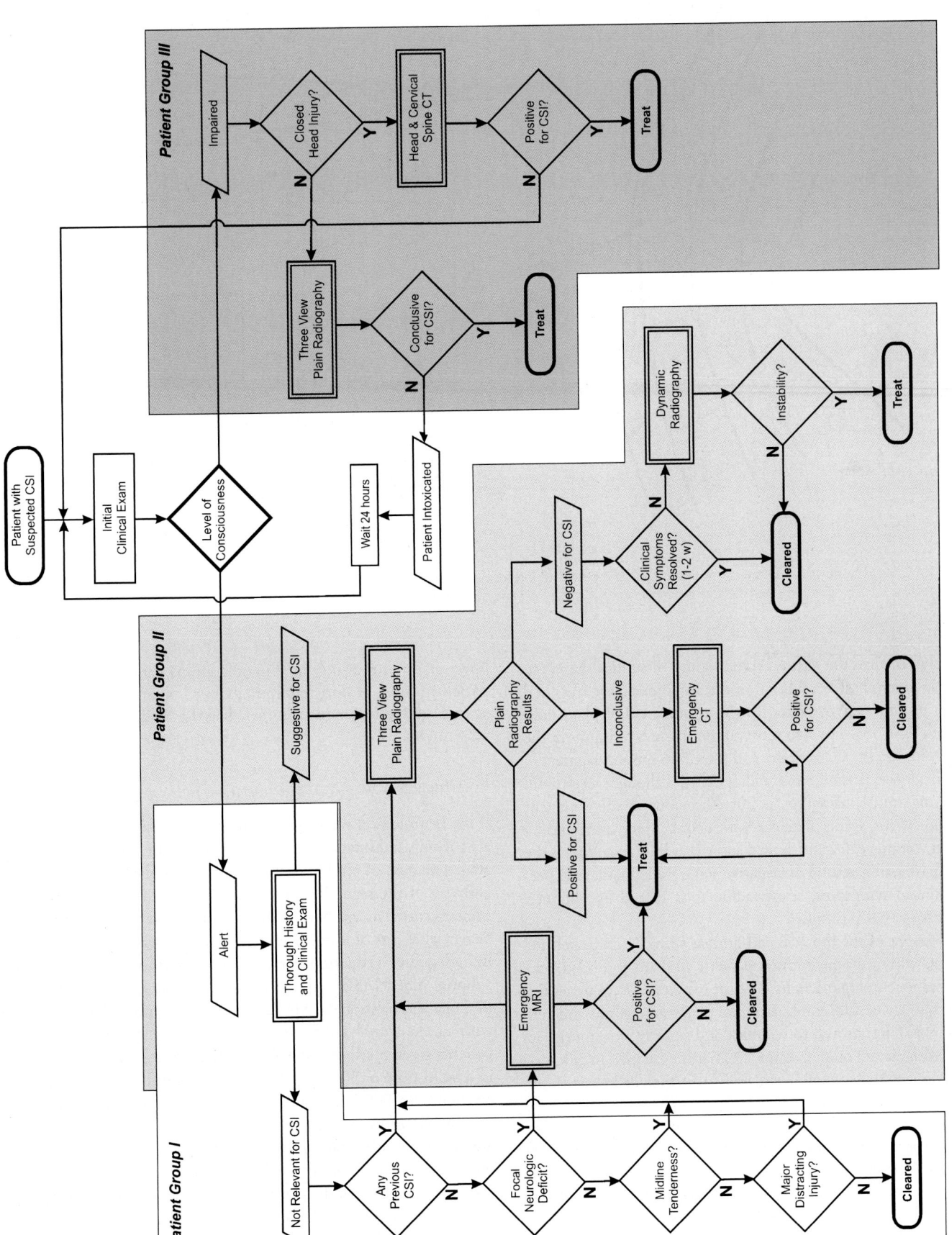

**FIGURE 24-18.** A comprehensive algorithm for clearing of the cervical spine. (Reproduced with permission from Lindsey RW, Gugala Z. Clearing of the Cervical Spine. In The Cervical Spine Research Society Editorial Committee: Clark CL, et al. The Cervical Spine. 4th ed. Philadelphia: Lippincott Williams & Wilkins, 2005, p. 375.)

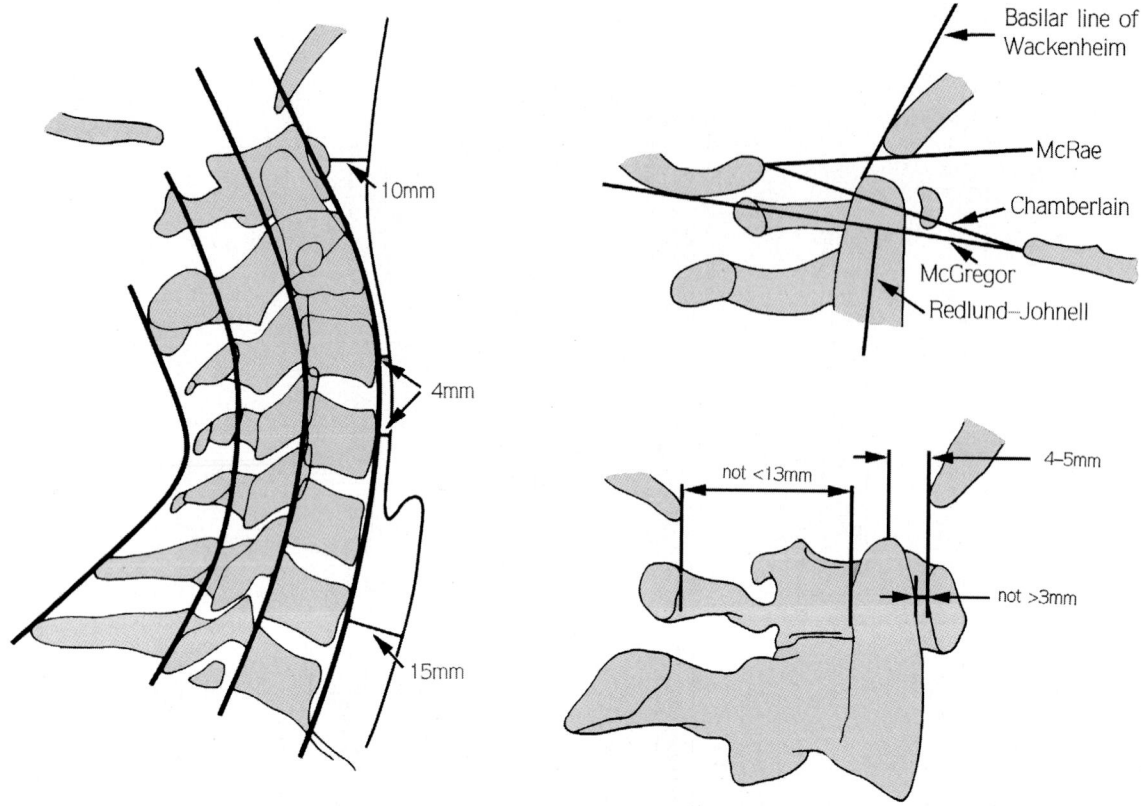

**FIGURE 24-19.**  The normal anatomical relationships on the normal lateral plain radiography.

adequately visualize the entire cervical spine including the cervicothoracic junction. The addition of the anteroposterior (AP) and the open mouth view increases the diagnostic yield of plain radiographs to 90–95%. The two most common areas of injury in the cervical spine are the C2 vertebra and the C5–6 motion segment.[74]

The flexion-extension stress radiography, although very useful in detecting spinal instability, is not efficacious in the emergent evaluation of the spine. Patients with acute injury are typically unable to voluntary flex and extend spine in a full range due to the muscle spasm. In a setting of negative static radiographs and persistent clinical symptoms, stress radiographs should be obtained two to three weeks postinjury.[75]

Radiographs of the thoracic and lumbar spine are indicated for all patients with multiple injuries, patients who are obtunded, and patients with neurologic deficits. The use of spiral CT improves the imaging sensitivity. The combination of plain radiographs and cervical spiral CT has proved to be quick and sensitive for injuries in patients with altered mental status.[76] CT scans are used to enhance visualization of transitional areas, and to further delineate suspicious areas on plain films.[77]

Acute CT is indicated in all cases when inadequate or inconclusive radiographic images are obtained in face of present clinical symptoms. All patients with impaired neurological status following blunt head trauma, should undergo emergent CT of the head which can be extended to include the cervical spine. Emergent MRI scanning is indicated in all patients with neurologic deficit, discordant levels of skeletal and neurologic injury, and worsening neurologic status. MRI may also be useful in detecting posterior ligamentous injury despite negative plain radiographs. MRI,

however, is not routinely used in polytrauma patients because these patients often require equipment (i.e., ventilators, extremity splints, and intravenous pumps) that the magnetic field cannot accommodate.

## Pharmacologic Management

If the neurological symptoms attributable to the spinal cord injury are present, pharmacologic treatment should be immediately initiated. The goal of pharmacology is to prevent and/or interrupt the pathway of the secondary injury mechanisms associated with the primary cord damage. Several clinical studies have demonstrated the beneficial effects of immediate steroid administration when utilized in adequate reduction and immobilization of the spinal column. The NASCIS-II[78] evaluated the efficacy of methylprednisolone and naloxone in a placebo-controlled study of 487 patients with acute spinal cord injury. This study demonstrated that patients given methylprednisolone within eight hours of the injury in a bolus dose of 30 mg/kg followed by an infusion of 5.4 mg/kg per hour for 23 hours had better recovery of the neurologic function at six weeks, six months, and one year following the injury. There were no statistically significant differences in the mortality and the morbidity of the patients receiving methylprednisolone compared to the placebo group. Patients with acute spinal cord injury should optimally receive methylprednisolone within three hours of the injury for a period of 24 hours.[79] Patients with methylprednisolone therapy initiated between three and eight hours from the time of injury, should continue this regimen for 48 hours. Based on these clinical trials, methylprednisolone is widely used in the treatment of acute spinal cord injury and is considered by many as the standard of care.

However, NASCIS have been controversial. It has been suggested that these studies do not provide sufficient clinical evidence to support the use of this treatment in acute injury. Furthermore, a number of concerns exist regarding the potential risks of this intervention.[80] Despite these issues, methylprednisolone remains one of the few neuroprotective agents available. It is currently suggested that methylprednisolone be recommended at the level of a guideline (Class II evidence) for acute nonpenetrating spinal cord injury within eight hours of trauma.[39,81]

## Immediate Spinal Immobilization

Once injury to the spinal column has been identified, the involved spinal segment must be stabilized. In the cervical spine initial immobilization may be achieved with the use of tongs or halo ring traction. Application of cervical tongs is simple, and can easily be achieved quickly by one person in the emergency room. In contrast, halo application is more demanding, often requiring at least two people, and generally requires more time. The advantage of halo, however, is that can provide stabilization in three planes. Regardless of the method of immobilization, it is preferable to use tongs or halo made out of materials compatible with CT and/or MRI.

Cervical fractures and dislocations are considered for reduction in the acute setting by means of axial traction. The goals of traction include reduction of the deformity, indirect decompression of the traumatized neural elements, and provisional stability of the spine. Traction should be initiated as soon as deformity is noted on the radiographs. The urgency of the reduction is based on experimental studies of spinal cord injuries which suggest a window of six to eight hours during which decompression may reverse neurologic deficits.[82,83] Some controversy exists about whether pretraction MRI is warranted to determine the presence of intervertebral disc herniation prior to traction.[84] More recently, in a retrospective study to determine the risk of neurological deterioration following early closed reduction of cervical spine injuries, the authors concluded that disc herniation and disruption can occur following all types of traumatic cervical fracture subluxations. However, the incidence of neurological deterioration following closed reduction in these patients was rare, and early closed reduction in patients presenting with significant motor deficits without prior MRI was deemed reasonable.

After application of tongs, cervical traction may begin under the lose supervision of a physician with repeated monitoring of the patient's neurologic status. Serial lateral radiographs must be obtained after the addition of extra load to avoid overdistraction. Generally, traction weight is added incrementally, with approximately 10 lbs for the occiput and an additional 5 lbs for each vertebra to the injury level. The maximum amount of weight that can safely be applied is not clearly defined. Regardless of the outcome of closed reduction, it is imperative that the maximum traction weight is reduced to 10 to 15 lbs once monitored reduction process has been terminated.

Immobilization in the thoracolumbar spine may initially be achieved by bed rest and log-rolling the patient. Additionally, these injuries may be stabilized with the use of a rigid brace, which in many instances may also be the definitive treatment.

## NONOPERATIVE MANAGEMENT OF SPINE INJURIES

The nonoperative management of spine fractures usually consists of immobilization that is well tolerated, permits timely mobilization, and permits healing of the injury in a timely fashion. The success of nonoperative treatment modality is dependent first upon proper patient selection, and secondarily upon the physician's understanding of the principles of nonoperative spine trauma management. Most acute injuries to the spine are managed nonsurgically. In treating spine trauma, the term nonsurgical treatment is not synonymous with the conservative management. Most fractures of the cervical spine do not require surgery. Nonsurgical management is typically most appropriate for stable injuries without neurologic deficit. Most bony injuries have the potential to heal with orthotic immobilization; healing of ligamentous injuries is unpredictable and most likely involves surgery.

### Cervical Traction

Cervical traction is often indicated in the management of cervical spine injury to reduce cervical spine deformity, indirectly decompress traumatized neural elements, and provide cervical spine stability. The utilization of traction is essential in the management of cervical spine trauma due to the ease of its application and low morbidity when applied properly.

Cervical traction should be initiated with 10 to 15 lb to avoid overdistraction, and gradually increased following radiographic assessment. Cervical traction can be applied through a head halter, tongs, or a halo ring. The head halter attaches to the head at the chin and the occiput, and only small amounts of weight (up to 20 lb) can be applied safely. The limitations of head halter traction are its poor fixation to the skull, and its ability to control only axial compression through longitudinal distraction. Additionally, even acceptable weights over a prolonged period of time can cause chin or occiput pressure decubiti.

Traction tongs achieve fixation into the bony skull through special pins with a pointed tip that abruptly flares out. This design allows for fixation into the outer cortical table of the skull but prevents inner cortex penetration, while distributing the pressure of pin insertion on the outer table over the entire width of the pin. In tongs these pins are placed below the cranial brim or the widest diameter of the skull, just anterior and superior to the earlobe. Pins must be positioned posterior to the temporalis muscle, which can become symptomatic due to either the thin bone in this region, or from muscle irritation with mastication. The pins are oriented in the tongs at 180° from each other, and tightened to 6 to 8 in-lb torque. Usually these pins require repeat tightening within 24 hours to maintain the applied load. If the pins loosen again, they can be retightened; if loosening continues to recur, the pins should be replaced. Tongs, like head halters, control motion in a single plane through the application of longitudinal traction. Tongs are associated with a greater incidence of loosening than halo rings, due to their ability to resist motion in only one plane. Tongs are ideally indicated, when the need for longitudinal traction is temporary, or the patient has to remain bedridden.

The halo apparatus was introduced by Nickel et al.[85] and its effectiveness in stabilizing the cervical spine was later demonstrated by Perry.[86] Halo ring immobilization achieves better skeletal fixation due to its multipin circumferential application, and is, therefore, able to withstand higher loads for a longer period of time. Additionally, the halo ring can resist multiplane motion, and following fixation to a body cast or plastic vest, allows for upright mobilization, while maintaining spine stability. The halo can be applied with local or general anesthesia; the ring is positioned below the crown of the skull similar to tongs, and the pins are inserted with approximately 6 to 8 inch-lb of torque. Pins should ideally be placed in the hairline for cosmesis and, as with tongs, pin fixation must not involve the temporal region. The halo ring can be adapted to either a cast or a fitted vest with metal upright struts. The cast or vest must be well fitted to the iliac crest to prevent vertical toggle of the apparatus. Despite adequate fit, the halo vest does not guarantee complete spine stabilization, especially when the patient is upright.

Once tongs or a halo ring has been applied, cervical traction can begin with approximately 10 to 15 lb, and immediately evaluated by lateral radiographs. The traction weight can then be increased by 5 to 10 lb increments with subsequent serial lateral radiographs obtained at approximately 10 to 15 minute intervals after each weight application. The patient must be completely relaxed, and analgesia or muscle relaxants are often required to relieve muscle spasms or tension. At higher weights (40 to 50 lb) a 30 to 60 minute interval should be permitted before the load is increased. The head of the bed should be elevated to provide body and weight resistance to the traction, and the shoulder portion should be depressed to optimize visualization of the cervicothoracic region.

The maximum amount of weight that can be safely applied for closed traction reduction of the cervical spine is controversial. Crutchfield[87] recommended a maximum of 5 lb per level of cervical injury, beginning with 10 lb for the head. This would limit the weight applied to a C5–6 facet up to 35 lb. It has also been suggested that a slow, gradual increase in traction weight will affect spinal reduction at a lower total traction load.[88] Others[89] have supported the more rapid incremental increase in load, applying weights up to 150 lb without any adverse effects. Typically, the maximum weight tolerated is limited by the skeletal fixation utilized, and for cranial tongs this limit is up to 100 lb.

Most cervical spine injuries can be reduced with only longitudinal traction, but small changes in the vector of traction (i.e., slightly more flexion or more extension) is necessary in some cases. Spinal manipulation can be hazardous, and is, therefore, controversial. Evans[90] recommended manual manipulation with the patient under general anesthesia. Lee et al.[89] compared traction to manipulation under anesthesia, and it was deemed that traction alone was preferable. Cotler et al.[91] recommended that gentle manipulation in combination with traction could be of benefit in the alert patients. Whether the patient is awake and alert, or under general anesthesia, manual manipulation as a means of achieving cervical spine reduction is rarely advocated. If manipulation is warranted, it is best performed as an open surgical procedure; otherwise longitudinal traction is preferred for closed reduction.

## Spinal Orthotics

Nonsurgical treatment of spine trauma involves immobilization of the spinal segment with an orthosis. Spinal orthoses are external devices that can restrict the motion of the spine by acting indirectly to reinforce the intervening soft tissue. Despite the heterogeneity of designs, the theoretical functions of all spinal braces are analogous, and include restriction of spinal movement, maintenance of spinal alignment, reduction of pain, and support of the trunk musculature. Spinal braces also act psychologically as proprioceptive reminders for the patient to restrict the spinal motion. The immobilizing effectiveness of spine braces is dependent on the mobility and anatomical features of the spine to be stabilized; injury biomechanics; length and rigidity of the orthosis; thickness of the intervening soft tissues; and patient's compliance with the orthosis. Although spinal braces are generally applied to stabilize a specific motion segment, their immobilization properties typically affect the entire spinal region (i.e., cervical, thoracic, or lumbar).

Cervical spine bracing is particularly challenging due to the wide range of normal spinal motion in extent, direction, and variation of movements. Due to the inability of the vital structures in the neck to withstand prolonged compression, cervical braces utilize the cranium and thorax as fixation points. Cervical orthoses can be used as a definitive treatment for some spinal injuries or as temporary immobilizers for postinjury transport or during the early hospital diagnostic process. These braces can generally be divided into two basic types: cervical orthoses (COs), and high- and low cervicothoracic orthoses (CTOs) (Fig. 24-20).

COs include both soft and rigid cervical collars. The former are basically foam cylinders that encircle the neck (Fig. 24-20A). The mechanical function of soft collars is negligible, and their immobilizing effectiveness relates to the psychological effect of the orthosis wearing. Soft collars are indicated for mild cervical sprains, or to provide postoperative comfort following stable internal fixation.

High-thoracic CTOs have molded occipital-mandibular supports which extend to the upper the thorax, typically not lower than the level of the sternal notch anteriorly, and the T3 spinous process posteriorly (Fig. 24-20B). Typical appliance in this group includes the Philadelphia collar, the Miami J brace, NecLoc collar, the Newport/Aspen collar, the Stifneck collar, the Malibu brace, and the Nebraska collar, among others. Biomechanical differences, however, exist even among the various high CTO designs. The comparative effectiveness of the various COs and CTOs in restriction of total cervical motion are presented in Table 24-8. The immobilizing properties of selected COs and CTOs for specific cervical motion segments are depicted in Table 24-9.[92]

Low-thoracic CTO, similarly to high-thoracic CTOs, attach to the cranium at the occiput and mandible but they extend to the lower thorax below the sternum notch and T3 spinous process (Fig. 24-20C). Commonly employed low CTOs include the Sternal-Occipital-Mandibular Immobilizer (SOMI), the Yale brace, four-poster brace, and the Minerva-type orthoses. All of these braces provide better fixation to the head and trunk than high CTOs and, thereby, constitute the most effective of all cervical braces. The major difference between high- and low-thoracic CTOs is the ability of the latter to provide better control of spinal rotation and sagittal motion in mid- and lower cervical spine.

The thoracic spine is unique among spinal regions in terms of its inherent rigidity and location between highly mobile adjacent cervical and lumber segments. The mid-spine location of the thoracic segments makes this region particularly amendable to bracing. Furthermore, the presence of the rib cage, sternum, and shoulder girdle act as additional stabilizers. However, achieving significant restriction of movement in the unstable thoracic spine can be difficult due to the continuous breathing movements. Also

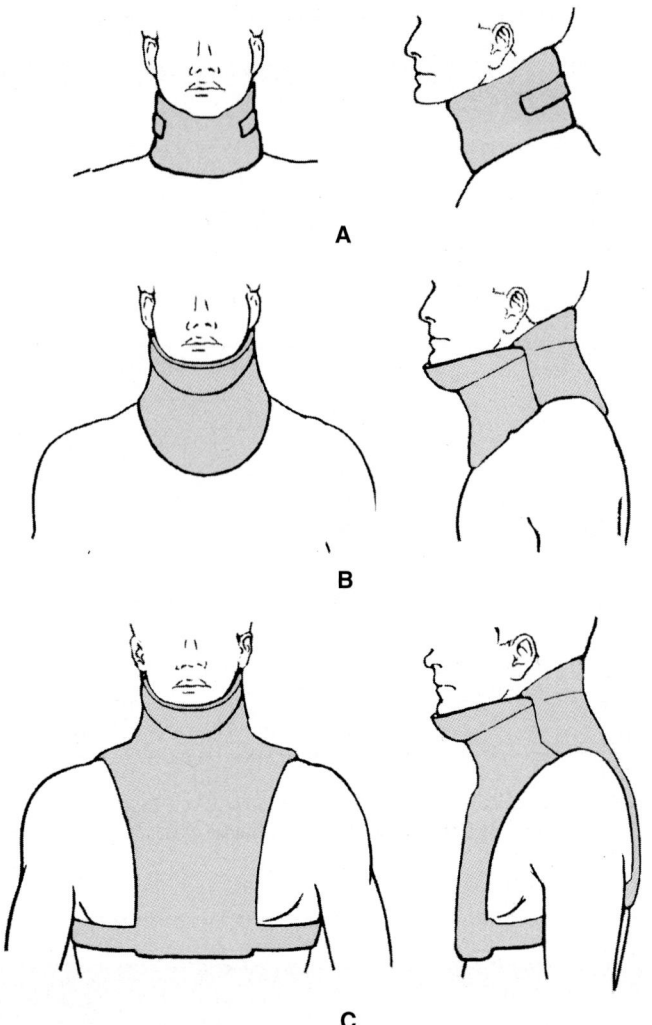

**FIGURE 24-20.** Basic types of cervical orthoses. **(A)** Cervical collars, **(B)** high thoracic, **(C)** and low thoracic braces. *(Reproduced with permission from Sypert GW. External spinal orthotics. Neurosurgery 20:642–649, 1987.)*

rotation, the principal motion of the thoracic spine, is much more difficult to control than flexion and extension. Therefore, thoracic spinal bracing is indicated only for acute spine trauma or postoperative support, and is rarely effective for degenerative disorders.

The lumbar spine, particularly its lower segments, is difficult to brace due to the limited caudal fixation points and its physiologic hypermobility. Typically, adequate stabilization requires that the brace extends as much as four or five vertebra levels proximal and distal to the unstable segment.[93] Even when the brace includes a hip spica component, hip flexion is not adequately controlled resulting in inadequate lumbar protection.[94]

The goal of thoracolumbar bracing is to support the spine by limiting overall trunk motion, decreasing muscular activity, increasing the intraabdominal pressure, reducing spinal loads, and limiting spinal motion. Current available orthoses include lumbosacral corsets, Jewett braces, and full-contact custom-molded orthoses. The selection of the appropriate orthotic is dependent on the type of injury, the extent of spinal stability, the associated injuries, body habitus, and the patient's age.[95,96]

## SURGICAL MANAGEMENT OF SPINE INJURY

The surgical management of spine fractures requires a thorough knowledge of the anatomic and biomechanical characteristics of the injury. Injury classification schemes have been devised to assist the clinician with the injury diagnosis, indications for surgical intervention, and prognosis.

### Spine Injury Classification

Cervical spine fractures and dislocations were most comprehensively classified by Allen and Ferguson.[97] In this system the injury patterns are described according to the position of the neck at the time of the injury and the direction of the injuring force. The six common patterns of cervical injuries include: flexion-compression, vertical compression, compression-extension, distraction-extension, and lateral flexion injuries (Fig. 24-21). Each injury pattern is graded in terms of the degree of injury to the involved motion segment and a higher stage denotes a more complex injury.

The management of thoracolumbar fractures has improved due to imaging techniques such as CT and MRI that better delineate fracture patterns, neural canal compromise, and ultimately spinal instability. A number of classification systems have been developed to determine spine stability. Holdsworth[98] introduced the concept of columns dividing the thoracolumbar spine into two columns. The anterior column consisted of the anterior longitudinal ligament, vertebral body, intervertebral disc, and the posterior longitudinal ligament. The posterior column consisted of the remaining osteo-ligamentous structures. According to Holdsworth's model, instability occurs when both columns have been compromised.

Denis[14–16] developed the three-column classification system and according to this model, spinal instability occurs when two of the three columns are injured. Panjabi et al.[99] tested ex vivo cadaveric burst fracture model and validated the three-column theory. In this study the middle column proved to be the principal determinant of thoracolumbar spine stability.

Gertzbein[100] modified a classification of thoracic and lumbar fractures initially described by Magerl et al.[101] that provided a simple description of fracture patterns based on the mechanism of the injury and the injury severity (Fig. 24-22). Type A injuries are caused by compression forces; Type B injuries by distraction forces; and Type C injuries by rotation-translation forces. In Gertzbein's system, the more complex types are more unstable and more likely to warrant surgical treatment.

### Spinal Stability

Classification systems provide a descriptive analysis of various fracture patterns, and the extent to which these injuries reflect spine stability remains controversial. In the cervical spine, clinical instability is determined by translation in excess of 3.5 mm, or angulation greater than 11° compared to adjacent segments.[13] Checklists exist to determine clinical instability in the cervical (Table 24-2), thoracolumbar (Table 24-3), as well as the lumbar and lumbosacral spine (Table 24-4). These checklists incorporate the pertinent clinical and radiographic parameters that determine spinal instability.[102,103]

**TABLE 24-8**

**Comparison of Total Cervical Motion Restricted by Various Cervical Orthoses**

| ORTHOSIS | MOTION RESTRICTED [%] | | | | |
|---|---|---|---|---|---|
| | Combined Flexion-Extension | Flexion | Extension | Lateral Bending | Axial Rotation |
| **CO** | | | | | |
| Soft Collar[1-3] | 26 | 23 | 20 | 8 | 7 |
| **High-Thoracic CTO** | | | | | |
| Philadelphia[1-5] | 70 | 74 | 59 | 34 | 56 |
| Miami J[5] | 73 | 85 | 75 | 51 | 65 |
| NecLoc[3-5] | 80 | 86 | 78 | 60 | 73 |
| Newport/Aspen[5,6] | 62 | 59 | 64 | 31 | 38 |
| Stifneck[5,7] | 70 | 73 | 63 | 50 | 57 |
| Malibu[8] | - | 86 | 82 | 55 | 74 |
| Nebraska[9] | 87 | 74 | 60 | 75 | 91 |
| **Low-Thoracic CTO** | | | | | |
| SOMI[1,2] | 72 | 93 | 42 | 34 | 66 |
| Yale[2] | 86 | - | - | 61 | 76 |
| Four Poster[1] | 79 | 89 | 82 | 54 | 73 |
| Minerva[10] | 79 | 78 | 78 | 51 | 88 |
| LMCO[9] | 83 | 68 | 66 | 50 | 60 |
| **Halo-Vest[2]** | 96 | - | - | 99 | 96 |

SOMI (Sternal Occipital Mandibular Immobilizer); LMCO (Lehrman-Minerva Cervical Orthosis).

[1]Johnson RM et al. JBJS 59A:332-339, 1977; [2]Johnson RM et al. JBJS 59A:332, 1977; [3]Kufman WA et al. Orthot Posthet 39, 1986; [4]Rosen PB et al. Ann Emerg Med 21, 1992; [5]Askins V et al. Spine 22, 1997; [6]Hughes SJ. J Trauma 45, 1998; [7]Graziano A et al. Ann Emerg Med 16, 1987; [8]Lunsford TR et al. J Prosthet Orthot 6, 1994; [9]Alberts LR et al. J Orthop Trauma 12, 1998; [10]Sharpe KP et al. Spine 20, 1995.

**TABLE 24-9**

**Recommended Orthosis for Selected Cervical Injuries**

| INJURY | MOTION SEGMENT AFFECTED | PLANE OF INSTABILITY | RECOMMENDED ORTHOSIS |
|---|---|---|---|
| Ring C1 (Jefferson's Fracture) | | | |
| Stable | Occ–C1 | All | Yale brace |
| Unstable | Occ–C2 | All | Halo-Vest |
| Odontoid Fracture (Types II and III) | C1–C2 | All | Halo-Vest |
| Atlantoaxial Instability | C1–C2 | Flexion | SOMI |
| Hangman's Fracture | | | |
| Stable | C2–C3 | Flexion | SOMI |
| Unstable | C2–C3 | All | Halo-Vest |
| Mid-cervical Flexion Injuries | C3–C5 | Flexion | Yale brace, SOMI |
| Low-cervical Flexion Injuries | C5-T1 | Flexion | Yale brace, SOMI, Four poster brace |
| Mid-cervical Extension Injuries | C3–C5 | Extension | Halo |
| Low-cervical Flexion Injuries | C5-T1 | Extension | Yale brace, Four Poster Brace |

## Goals of Surgical Management

The majority of the spine fractures can be treated nonoperatively. Only injuries that are unstable, with or without neurologic involvement, require surgical treatment. Surgical objectives include the correction of spine alignment; the restoration and maintenance of spine stability; and the decompression of compromised neural elements.

The initial objective of spine trauma surgery is the reduction of spine deformity to a functionally acceptable alignment. The choice of spinal instrumentation is dependent upon its ability to reduce a fracture and maintain stability according to the deforming forces. For example, using distraction instrumentation for a flexion-distraction type of fracture will further destabilize the spine. By contrast, the application of extension-compression posterior instrumentation will correct and stabilize this deformity.

The next goal of surgery is to restore the spinal stability. Modern anterior and posterior surgical fixation devices provide better stabilization and compromise a minimum number of motion segments. The final goal of spinal trauma surgery is the decompression of the neural elements to permit maximum functional recovery. The injury type and the time to surgical intervention determine

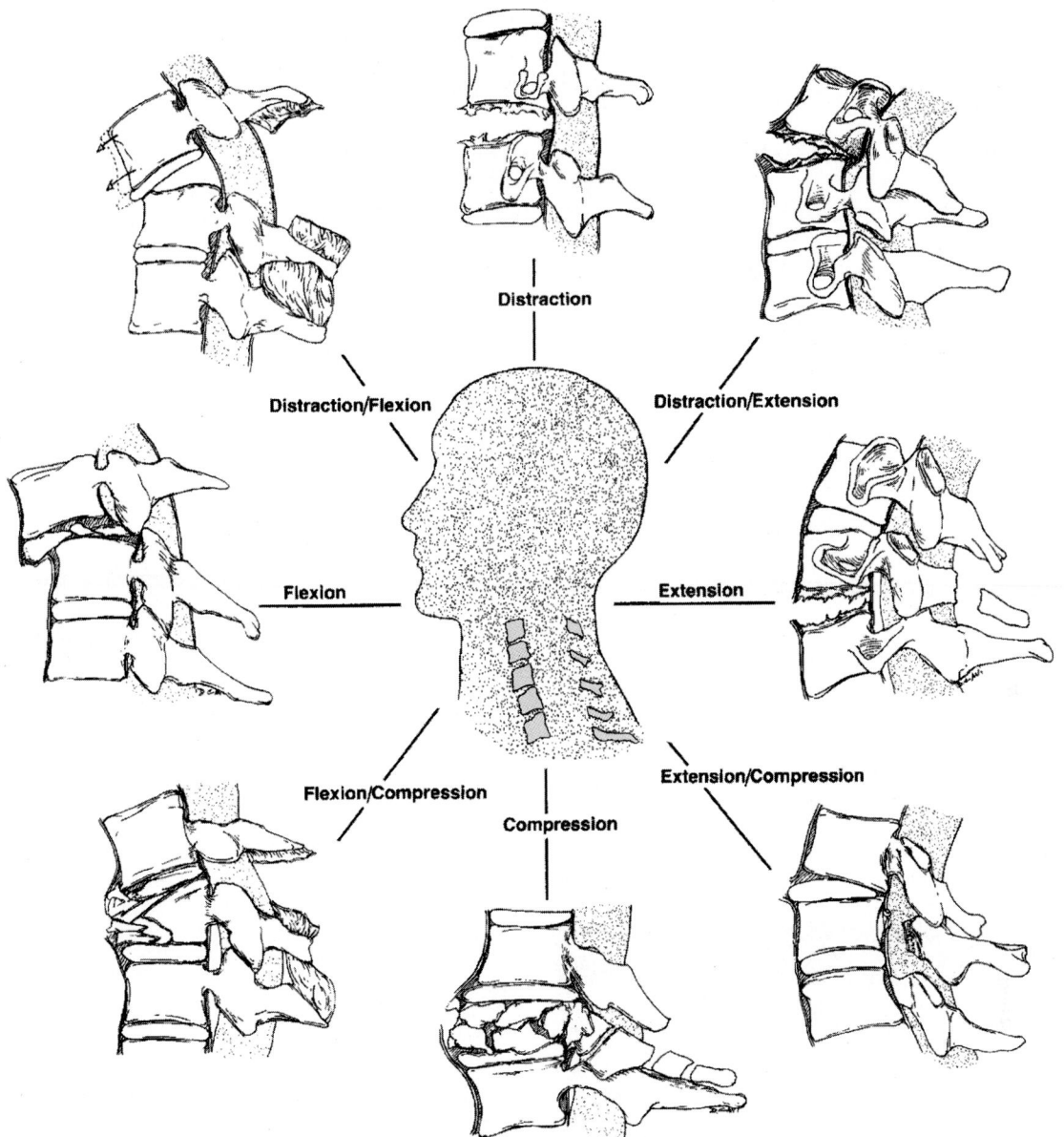

**FIGURE 24-21.**    Patterns of subaxial cervical spine injury based on the injury mechanism.
*(Reproduced with permission from McAfee P. Cervical spine trauma. In Frymoyer, JW, (ed) Adult Spine, New York: Raven Press, 1991, p. 1080.)*

the most appropriate type of decompression. Neural decompression can be performed anteriorly, posterolaterally transpedicularly, and/or indirectly. In the thoracolumbar spine, indirect decompression, as a result of posterior instrumentation to restore spinal alignment, is very effective in patients undergoing surgery within 48 to 72 hours.[104] By applying distraction through posterior instrumentation indirect reduction is achieved through ligamentotaxis.

The literature suggests that the results of anterior direct versus the posterior indirect spinal canal decompression are similar for patients with incomplete neurologic deficits.[105–108] Posterior indirect reduction technique currently constitutes the most frequently utilized method of treatment for the majority of thoracolumbar spine fractures. The absolute indications for anterior decompression would include the neurologically incomplete patient with greater than 50% canal compromise, greater than 72 hours postinjury, following a failed attempt at posterior reduction, or significant loss of anterior and middle column (vertebral body) support despite posterior reduction.

## Timing of Surgery

The optimal timing of surgery following spinal injury is controversial. Some physicians insist that surgery be performed as soon as possible, while others advocate a delay of surgery to allow for the resolution of posttraumatic swelling. The absolute indications for immediate surgery are progressive neurologic deterioration and spine fracture-dislocations associated with incomplete or no neurologic deficit.[109]

The expedient stabilization and mobilization of spinal injury patients has reduced the incidence of complications such as the adult respiratory distress syndrome and deep venous thrombosis.[110,111] In the absence of neurologic deficit, it is reasonable to delay surgery to facilitate surgical planning, and allow for spinal cord and nerve root edema to resolve. Furthermore, hematoma organization occurs at about 48 hours after the injury and decreases intraoperative blood loss.[112] Excessive delay of surgery

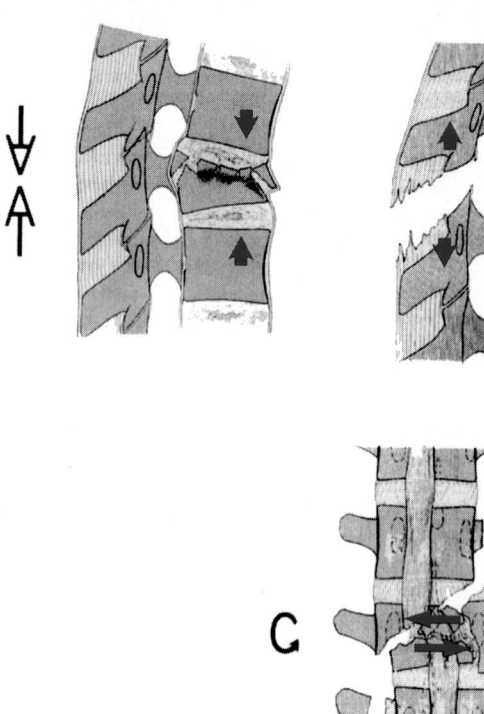

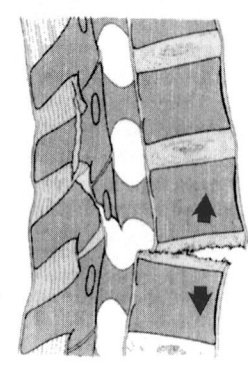

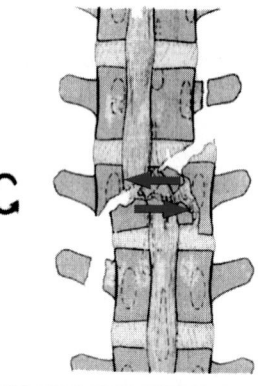

**FIGURE 24-22.** The classification of the thoracolumbar fractures based on the injury mechanism. Compression injuries **(A)**; distraction injuries **(B)**, and rotational injuries **(C)**. *(Reproduced with permission from Magerl F, Aebi M, Gertzbein SD, Harms J, Nazarian S. A comprehensive classification of thoracic and lumbar injuries. Eur Spine J 3:184-201, 1994.)*

**TABLE 24-10**

**Effect of Surgical Timing for Patients Spine Fracture and ISS Greater than 18**

| | TIMING OF STABILIZATION | |
|---|---|---|
| | Early (<48 h) | Late (>48 h) |
| Patients (n) | 16 | 46 |
| GCS | 14 | 13 |
| AISS-Head | 1 | 3 |
| AISS-Chest | 2 | 2 |
| Ventilator Days | 1.0 | 11.0 |
| ICU Days | 3.9 | 14.0 |
| Hospital Days | 11.0 | 26.0 |
| Average Costs | $26,250 | $54,130 |

Abbreviations: ISS, Injury Severity Score; GCS, Glasgow Coma Scale; AISS, Abbreviated Injury Severity Score; ICU, Intensive Care Unit.

may adversely affect the clinician's ability to reduce the fracture and achieve canal clearance. Reports have shown that optimum canal clearance is most effective if surgery is ideally performed within four days, and certainly no later than seven to ten days from the time of injury.[104,113,114]

Management of the polytrauma patient with an associated spinal injury is a particularly difficult problem. In several studies examining the effects of early versus late stabilization of spinal fractures in polytrauma patients surgery performed within 72 hours on patients with injuries severity score (ISS) greater than 18 consistently and significantly decreased morbidity and hospital stay without significant differences in the rate of preoperative complications[115–117] (Table 24-10).

## SPECIFIC SPINAL INJURY CHARACTERISTICS

### Injuries of the Occipito-Cervical Articulation

Occipital cervical injuries are rare and usually fatal. These injuries consist of subluxations or dislocations and can include fractures of occipital condyles. Occipital-cervical injuries can be detected by lateral X-ray using the Power's ratio (Fig. 24-23). These injuries are classified as Type I (anterior displacement of the occiput on the atlas), Type II (longitudinal facet distraction injury with diastases of the occiput from the atlas), and Type III (posterior displacement of the occiput on the atlas)[118] (Fig. 24-24). Type I and III injuries require minimal traction (5 lb) in either slight extension or flexion respectively to reduce; in Type II injuries alignment is generally acceptable and distraction is strictly contraindicated. Initial treatment consists of traction, which should be limited to 5 lb only due to the extremely unstable nature of the injury. Reduction is achieved by either extension or flexion of the occiput in combination with light traction. Definitive nonoperative treatment requires initial traction for three months followed by mobilization within to a halo-vest for three months if alignment can be maintained. Typically, however, these injuries are extremely unstable and require surgical stabilization and fusion.

### Fractures of the Atlas

Fractures of the atlas rarely involve neurologic deficit but cause pain and compromise neck mobility. Atlas fractures can consist of bone disruption without instability, or bone, and ligament injuries with subsequent displacement of the lateral mass articulation.

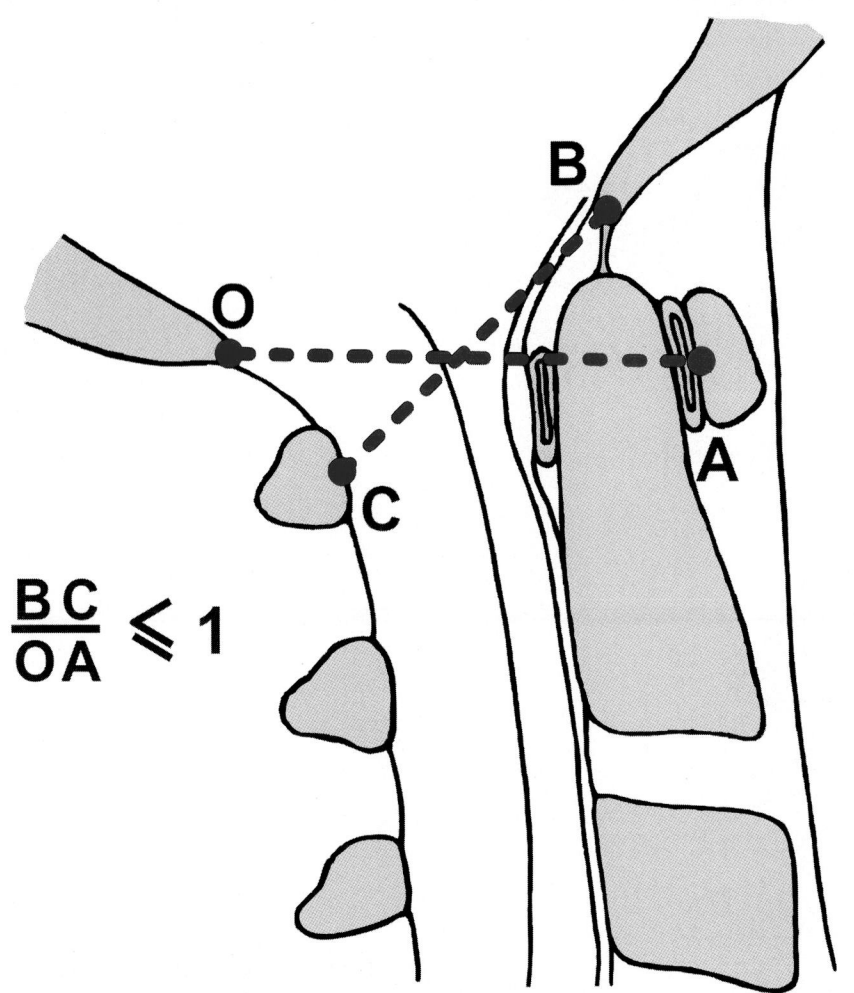

$$\frac{BC}{OA} \leqslant 1$$

**FIGURE 24-23.** The sagittal view of the normal craniocervical junction depicting the Powers ratio (**B**, basion; **O**, opision; **A**, anterior arch of the C2; **C**, posterior arch of C2).

The five distinct fracture patterns include the posterior arch fracture (the most common), the lateral mass fracture, the four-part burst fracture (Jefferson fracture), the horizontal fracture of the anterior arch of C1, and the transverse process fracture of the atlas (unilateral or bilateral) (Fig. 24-25). Stable fractures with an intact transverse ligament and simple posterior arch fraction can be treated with a brace. Unstable, displaced fractures in which the transverse ligament is disrupted require traction initially to reduce the displaced lateral masses and then can be placed in a halo-vest.[119] Atlas fractures with significant displacement can require traction for up to six to eight weeks before a halo vest can be applied. Surgery is usually not required acutely, but reserve for those patients who develop a delayed or nonunion.

## Atlanto-Axial Joint Injuries

Atlantoaxial subluxation occurs when the transverse ligament is disrupted and the ring of C1 remains intact (Fig. 24-26). In addition to being extremely unstable, this injury has a high risk for neurologic deficit. Traction is an appropriate initially only to achieve reduction. Definitive treatment consists of a posterior cervical fusion of C1–C2. Rotary subluxation of C1–C2 clinically presents with the patient's head in fixed rotation. This subluxation will usually reduce with traction and requires only brace support. Surgery for rotatory subluxation is warranted if an open reduction is necessary and, in these patients, a surgical fusion is also indicated.

## Fractures of the Odontoid

Odontoid fractures can be visualized on lateral X-rays, but are best seen on the open mouth views. Odontoid fractures have been classified by Anderson and D'Alonzo according to the anatomical level of the fracture (Fig. 24-27).[120] Type I fractures consist of apical ligament avulsion injuries which are essentially stable and require limited, if any, external support. Type III fractures extend below the waist of the odontoid into the body of C2 and usually result in uneventful bony union. To ensure adequate dens alignment, these injuries are optimally immobilized in a halo vest as other cervical orthoses are associated with up to a 15% incidence of nonunion.[121] Type II odontoid injuries occur at the waist of the odontoid, require anatomic reduction of both translation and angulation, and maintenance of fracture stability, if healing is to occur nonoperatively. Therefore, after an adequate reduction has been achieved, a halo vest is essential for a favorable outcome. In these fractures, as little as 10° of angulation, or 5 mm displacement has been correlated with a greater incidence of fracture nonunion or malunion.[121] Type III fractures of the waist (junction of the dens and body) can be treated with either a halo or preferentially surgical stabilization, especially if they are displaced.

## Traumatic Spondylolisthesis of the Axis

C2 pedicle or pars interarticularis fracture (hangman's fracture) rarely involves neurologic injury, and can be detected on lateral

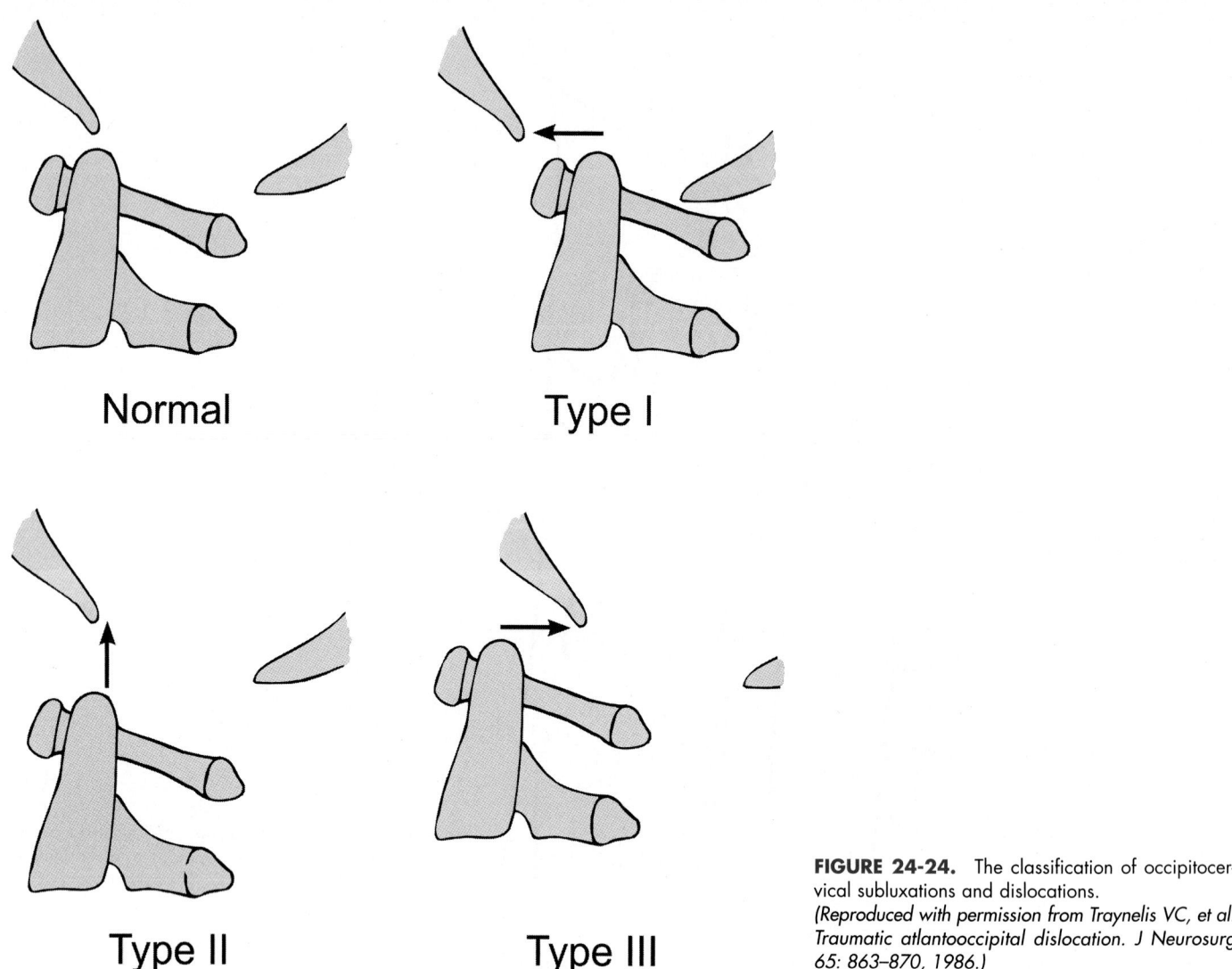

**Normal**

**Type I**

**Type II**

**Type III**

**FIGURE 24-24.** The classification of occipitocervical subluxations and dislocations.
*(Reproduced with permission from Traynelis VC, et al. Traumatic atlantooccipital dislocation. J Neurosurg 65: 863–870, 1986.)*

X-rays. These injuries have been classified by Levine and Edwards (Fig. 24-28)[122] based on the extent of fracture displacement and angulation. The treatment is dependent on the extent of associated disc and ligament injury.[122] In the minimally displaced fracture (Type I), a soft collar is sufficient treatment. In fractures with severe angulation (greater 11°) are without translation (Type IIA) treatment consists of a halo vest with the neck extended. In fractures with greater 11° angulation or 6 mm of translation (Type II) halo mobilization head, neck extension reduction is appropriate. Type IIA fractures are extremely unstable and should never be subjected to traction/distraction. Treatment should consist of extension-reduction with a halo. A surgical fusion is indicated for II or IIA injuries if reduction cannot be maintained. C2 pars fractures with facet dislocation (Type III) are common and nonoperative management is ineffective due to the disrupted continuity between the C2 body and the posterior elements. Surgery is absolutely indicated to achieve reduction and establish stability.

## Injuries of the Subaxial Cervical Spine (C3–C7)

Subaxial cervical injuries can consist of fractures, dislocations, subluxation, or a combination of these injuries. The diagnosis can usually be made with lateral or oblique cervical radiographs; displaced

segments may reduce spine positioning and require stress views to delineate. Subaxial cervical spine instability has been described by White et al.,[123] and is based on the extent of segmental angular or translation (Fig. 24-29).[124] Unilateral or bilateral facet subluxations or dislocations and/or fractures are variations of the same injury pattern. As unilateral or bilateral facets injuries progress from subluxation to perched facets, or to dislocation, the extent of cervical spine malalignment provides a good indication of the degree of disruption of the facet capsule and/or posterior ligaments. Neurologic deficit can present as root irritation and radiculopathy with unilateral facet injuries while the cord compromises frequently occurs with bilateral injuries. Both unilateral and bilateral facet disruptions should be initially treated with closed traction. Following reduction, unilateral injuries can be managed in a brace with halo immobilization if reduction can be maintained. If the facet is locked in a dislocated position, open reduction and fusion is indicated. Bilateral facet injuries are grossly unstable and require surgical fusion.

## Compression Fractures

Compression fracture consists of wedging of the anterior position of the vertebral of body with the posterior body and spinal canal

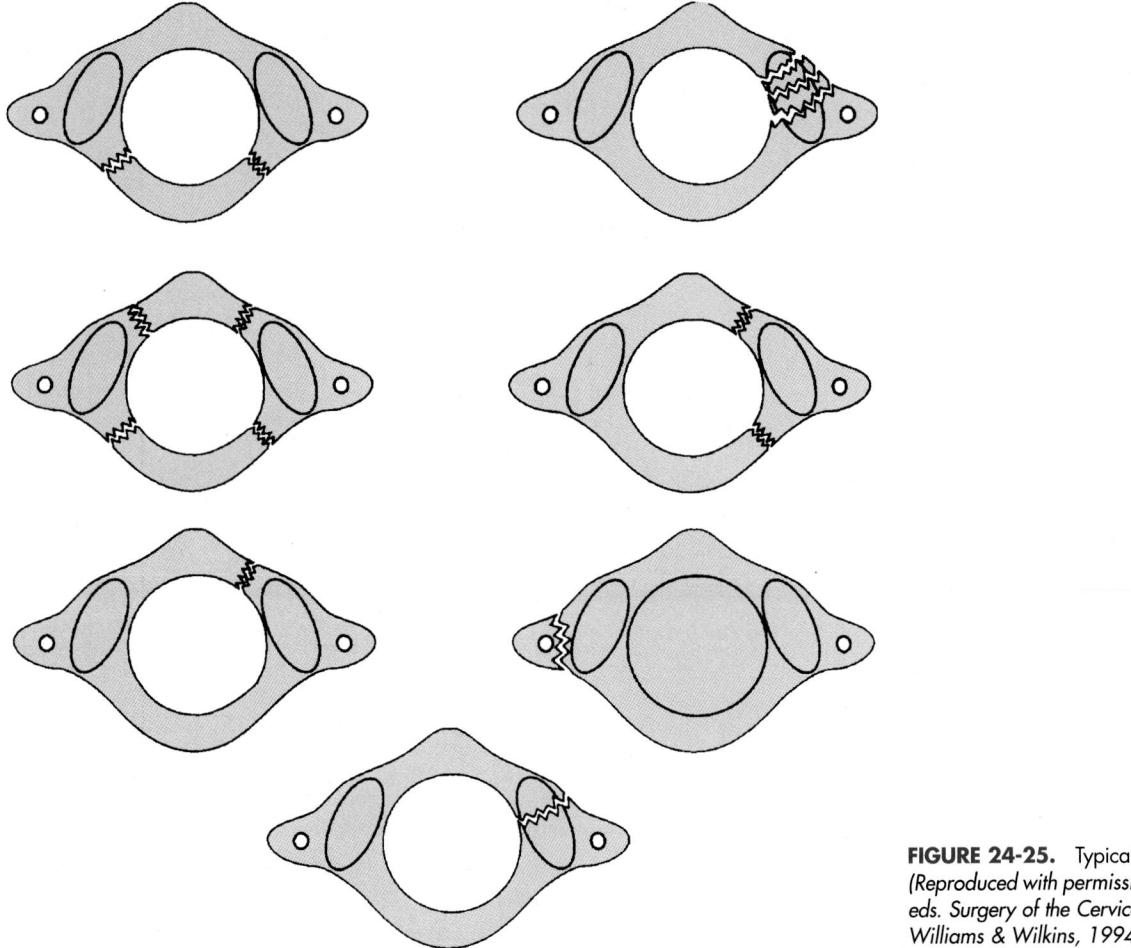

**FIGURE 24-25.** Typical fracture patterns of the atlas. (Reproduced with permission from An HS, Simpson JM, eds. Surgery of the Cervical Spine. Baltimore: Lippincott Williams & Wilkins, 1994, p. 235.)

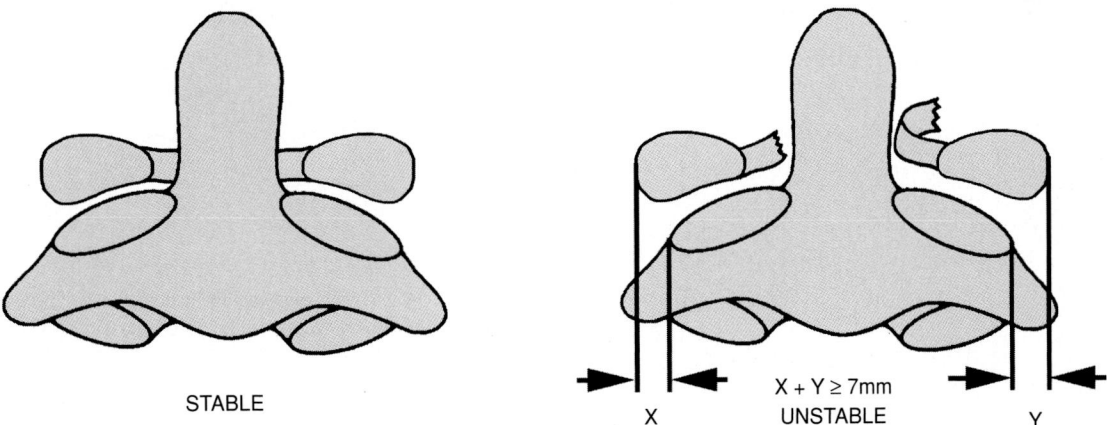

STABLE

X + Y ≥ 7mm

X    UNSTABLE    Y

**FIGURE 24-26.** Disruption of the transverse ligament results in the lateral displacement of the lateral masses of C1 making the C1–C2 articulation unstable.

remaining intact (Fig. 24-30). This injury is visualized on lateral x-ray and does not typically involve neurologic compromise. If angulation is less than 11° or wedge compression is less 25% of the anterior vertebral body height or translation less than 2.5 mm, brace immobilization is sufficient. When the anterior body compression fracture exceeds 50%, flexion-distraction occurs and is associated with posterior ligamentous disruption. When these injuries also include disc disruption, cervical collar or halo vest immobilization alone are plagued by progression of fracture

collapse and increasing loss of alignment.[125–127] The inherent instability of this form of compression injury requires surgical stabilization and fusion.

## Burst Fractures

Burst fractures occur as a result of a large axial load applied to the cervical spine in straight position (Fig. 24-31). Burst fractures are characterized by disruption of the anterior and middle columns of

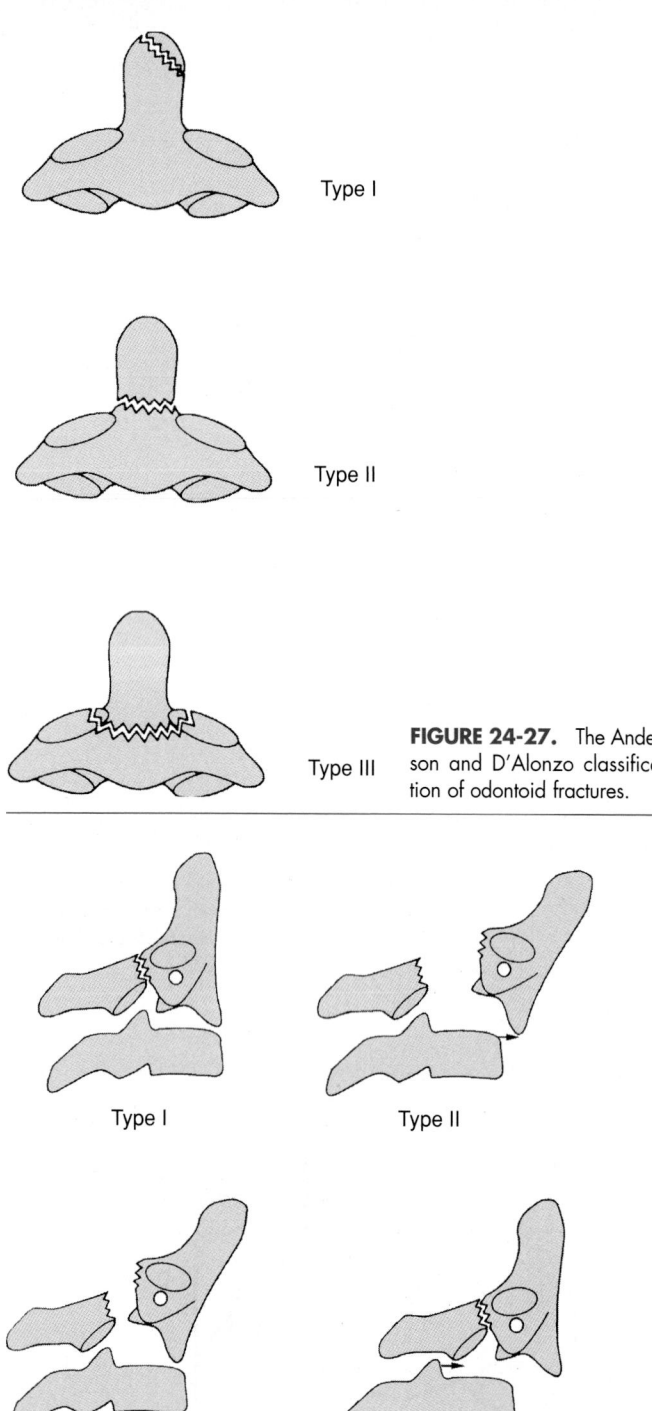

**FIGURE 24-27.** The Anderson and D'Alonzo classification of odontoid fractures.

Type I

Type II

Type III

Type I

Type II

Type IIA

Type III

**FIGURE 24-28.** The Levine and Edwards classification of traumatic spondylolisthesis of the axis (hangman's fracture).

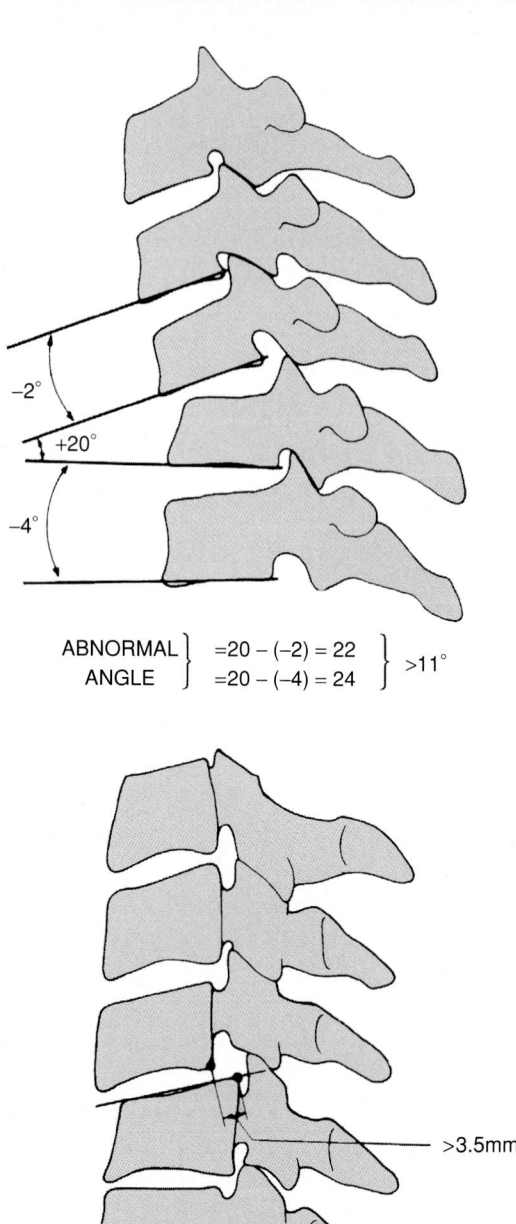

ABNORMAL } =20 − (−2) = 22 } >11°
ANGLE    } =20 − (−4) = 24 }

>3.5mm

**FIGURE 24-29.** The angular and translational displacement measurements used to determine instability in the subaxial spine.

## Other Fractures

Common cervical spine fractures include: flexion teardrop fractures, lateral mass fracture, extension teardrop fractures, and injuries to the posterior bony and/or ligamentous fractures. Among these injuries, the flexion teardrop fracture (Fig. 24-32) is among the most devastating injuries of the cervical spine. The injury results from the flexion–compression mechanisms, involves all three columns and have very high incidence of the neurologic compromise. Extension teardrop fracture is a stable avulsion injury involving only anterior spinal column (Fig. 24-33). Lateral mass fractures are often complicated with subluxation or dislocation of the facets (Fig. 24-34). These injuries warrant acute reduction. Posterior bony or ligamentous injuries (lamina fractures, clay-shoveler fracture) are typically stable injuries restricted to the posterior column

the spine with some degree of canal compromise. Appropriate treatment is determined by the presence of neurologic deficit, degree of malalignment, and the extent of instability. If there is no neurologic deficit and alignment is acceptable, a halo and dressed application is justified as long as fracture alignment can be maintained. If reduction cannot be achieved or maintained, surgery for anterior decompression and fusion is indicated. If combined anterior and posterior longitudinal ligament injury occurs, surgical stabilization is required.

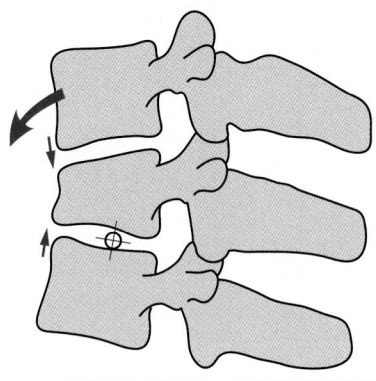

**FIGURE 24-30.** A simple compression fracture involves the anterior column of the spine.

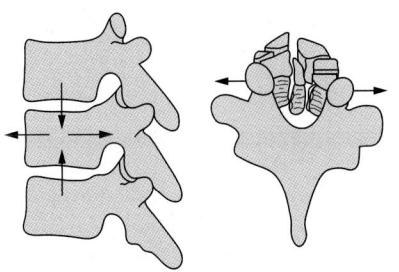

**FIGURE 24-31.** A burst fracture is the result of axial compression, and involves the anterior and middle spinal columns.

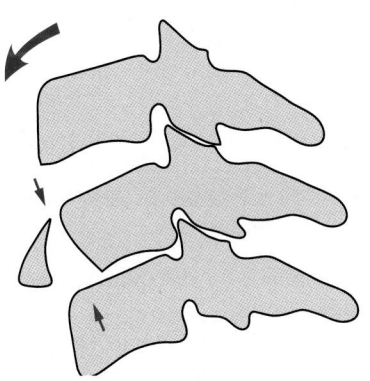

**FIGURE 24-32.** A flexion-compression teardrop fracture involves multiple cervical columns, is extremely unstable, and has a high incidence of neurologic deficit.

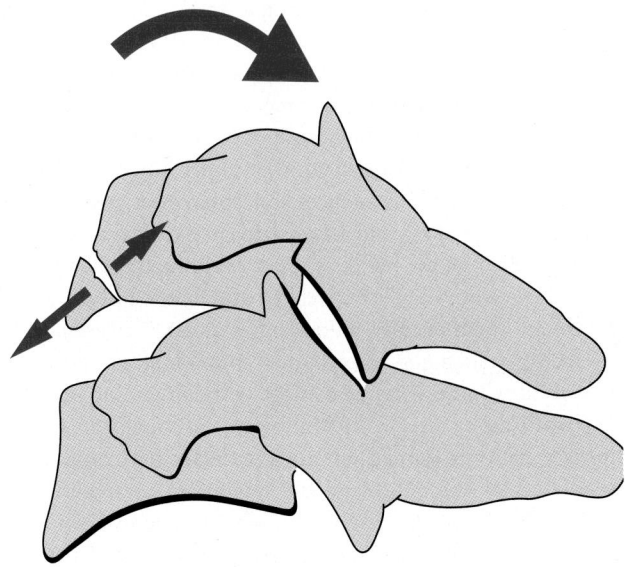

**FIGURE 24-33.** An extension teardrop fracture is an avulsion of the anterior inferior portion of the vertebral body and is a stable injury.

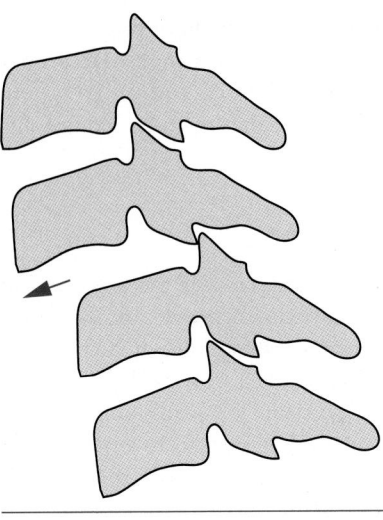

**FIGURE 24-34.** Bilateral dislocation of the cervical facet joints is an unstable injury which is associated with translational malalignment of the spine.

of the spine. Treatment for all the above-mentioned fractures is either conservative or operative depending on the injury stability, ability to achieve reduction by traction, and neurological involvement.

## Injuries of the Thoracic Spine

The thoracic spine is inherently stable due to the rigid structural configuration of the spine, sternum, and rib cage. Injuries to this region usually result from a high-energy insult. Associated injuries occur in approximately 75% of all thoracic spine injuries, and can include rib fractures, pulmonary contusions, or pneumothorices, cardiac contusions, or vascular injuries. Although stable injuries rarely involve neurologic compromise, profound neurologic deficit typically occurs in the more unstable fractures.[128] This high risk for complete neurologic injury is due to the small size of the neural canal, the tenuous arterial blood supply to the thoracic cord, and the energy required to inflict injury. Stable thoracic spine fractures with intact neurologic status can usually be treated nonoperatively in a brace. These fractures often consist of compression or burst fractures without significant flexion, rotation, or translation. Unstable thoracic spine fractures usually have associated neurologic deficit and/or present with excessive flexion, rotation, or translation.

## Injuries of the Thoracolumbar Spine

Thoracolumbar spine fractures are second only to cervical spine injuries in frequency of occurrence. Due to its increase mobility compared to the adjacent thoracic spine and sacrum, this region is highly susceptible to injury. Thoracolumbar spine consists of compression fractures, burst fractures, flexion-distraction injuries, and fracture dislocation. The criteria for thoracolumbar spine posttraumatic stability was described by White and Panjabi[124] (Table 24-3), and defined as a spine that was able to maintain anatomic relationships between vertebra, when subjected to physiologic loads.[102,124]

Compression fractures are the most frequent of all thoracolumbar spine fractures and present with a decreased anterior vertebral body height without disruption of the posterior body or spinal cord. Stable compression fractures present with less than 50% anterior body height diminution, less than 30°

angulation, and can be treated in a brace without progression of deformity. Unstable compression fractures demonstrate greater than 50% anterior body height collapsed and/or greater in 30° angulation. The unstable compression fractures require surgical stabilization.

## Burst Fractures

Burst fractures consist of bony destruction of the anterior and posterior vertebral body, and have an increased risk for spinal cord compromise with subsequent neurologic deficit. Stable burst fractures present with less than 50% decrease in body height, less than 25° of angulation, and less than 50% canal compromise. Stable burst fractures can be treated and/or an orthosis but require close follow-up to insure that the spinal alignment is maintained. Unstable burst fractures occur with greater than 50% of body height diminution, greater than 25° of angulation, greater than 50° of compromise, and/or present with neurologic deficit. Unstable burst fractures need surgery to realign and stabilize the fracture. If the neuro-elements are not decompressed with indirect, reduction methods, desired decompression of the spinal cord is indicated.

## Flexion-Distraction Injuries

Flexion distraction injuries involve a combination of bone and ligaments disruption of the anterior and posterior spine without loss of body height (Fig. 24-35). Care must be taken to avoid all traction/distraction maneuvers during the initial stabilization of this injury. Closed reduction and bracing is appropriate in those injuries involving bone with less than 30° angulation. Surgical reduction and fixation is indicated for flexion distraction injuries which involved primarily ligaments or disc, demonstrates more than 30° angulation.

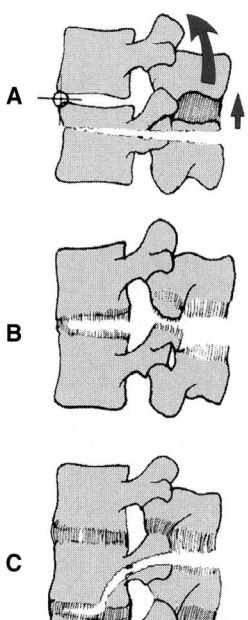

**FIGURE 24-35.** A flexion-distraction injury (Chance fracture) is an unstable injury that can occur through bone (**A**), ligaments (**B**), or both of these structures (**C**).

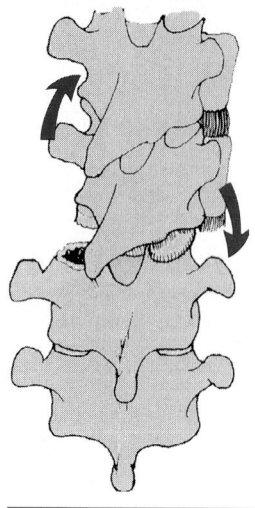

**FIGURE 24-36.** Rotational spinal injuries involve all three columns, are extremely unstable, and are associated with a high incidence of neurologic deficit.

## Fracture-Dislocations

Fracture-dislocations are extremely unstable injuries, which consist of various components of rotation, flexion, and translation (Fig. 24-36). These injuries result in an approximately two-thirds of cases in neurologic deficit of which half are complete lesions. Nonoperative treatment is rarely appropriate. Neurologically, incomplete injuries benefit from early posterior reduction by surgical decompression and stabilization. Neurologically, complete or intact patients will require surgical stabilization to facilitate early mobilization and rehabilitation.

## GUNSHOT INJURY TO THE SPINE

The incidence of civilian gunshot injuries to the spine has been steadily increasing and in many urban areas is presently the second leading cause of spinal cord injury.[129] In the urban setting, gunshot injury (GSI) to the spine has become especially prevalent. Currently, a missile injury counts for 13% of all spinal injuries and is third only to falls and motor vehicle accidents.

Likewise, according to the National Spinal Cord Injury Data Research Center, between 1973 through 1982, 13% of cord injuries resulted from gunshot wounds. However, since 1990, gunshot injuries to the spine have reported incidence of 25% and has become the second leading cause of cord injury.[129]

The wounding capacity of a gunshot injury or its kinetic energy is directly proportional to its mass and, to an even greater extend, its velocity ($E = \frac{1}{2} mv^2$). The tissue damage is related to the energy that is dissipated by the bullet as it passes through the body. Low-velocity (low-energy) bullets travel at 1000 ft/second or less, while high-velocity (high-energy) bullets travel at 2000 ft/second.[130] In low-velocity, civilian gunshot wounds from a bullet or a fragment of a projectile can cause tissue damage without coming into direct contact with the tissue. As the bullet passes through soft tissues, a temporary cavity is formed due to soft tissues stretching. A concussive effect of the bullet and the cavitations creates the tissue damage, which correlates with the kinetic energy. Neurologic injury can occur not only from direct contact, but if the bullet passes within close proximity to the spinal cord.[121,131] Usually, civilian GSI to the spine must transverse or remain inside the spinal canal to neurologic deficit.

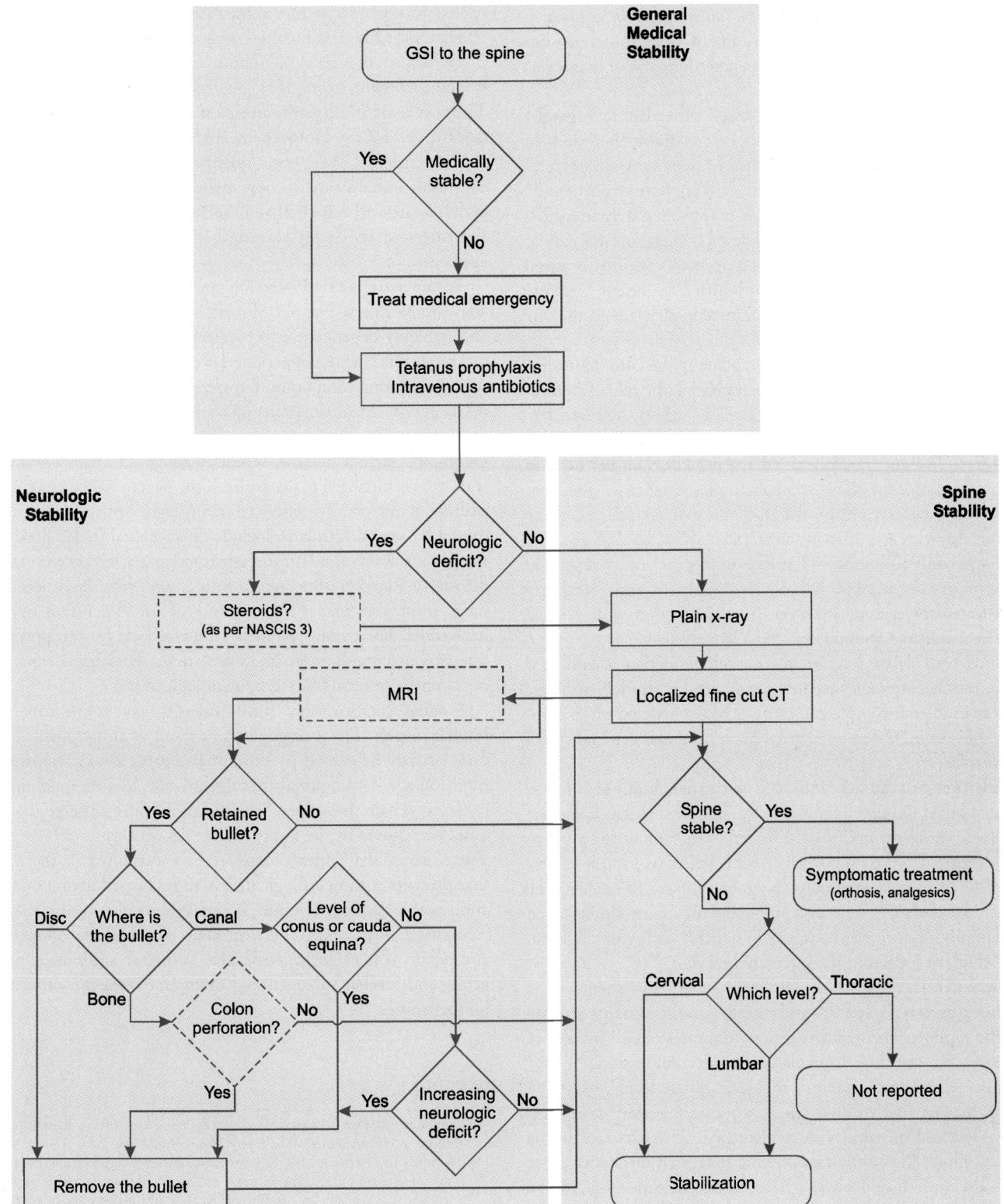

**FIGURE 24-37.** A comprehensive algorithm for the management of gunshot injuries to the spine.
*(Reproduced with permission from Lindsey, RW and Gugala Z. Spinal cord injury as a result of ballistic trauma. In: Chapman, JR, ed. Spine: State of the Art Reviews. Vol. 13(3) Spinal Cord Injuries. Hanley & Belfus Inc, 1999.)*

All gunshot wounds to the spine should be evaluated according to a routine management algorithm (Fig. 24-37). A patient's general medical condition should be addressed and stabilized prior to focusing on the spine. A detailed neurologic examination should be performed to determine a neurologic condition according to the Frankel Score[112] or the ASIA Scale (ASIA Standards 1989). Gunshot injuries to the neck mandate routine angiography and panendoscopy. Due to the potential increase in morbidity, surgical expiration of the wound track is not recommended for civilian GSI unless there is evidence of expanding hematoma or vascular disruption.[132] Thoracic spine gunshot injuries may be associated with pulmonary or cardiac injuries, and lumbar spine gunshot injuries may involve abdominal viscera genitourinary, or major vascular injury.

The spine should be routinely accessed with plain radiography and CT to localize the level of injury and establish the extent of bony disruption.[133] MRI is contraindicated due to the artifacts created by the missile fragment as well as their ferromagnetism.[134] Dynamic flexion-extension stress radiographs are rarely indicated in the acute setting, but can be considered in alert, or in a patient with suspected instability. Although spine instability is often thought to be preserved with gunshot injuries, the recent literature has suggested that stability is not guaranteed, especially in the cervical spine.[135]

Although the benefits of steroid for acute spinal cord injury due to indirect trauma have been well documented, the role of steroids following GSI to the spine is less clear. The authors, however, recommend methylprednisolone in a 30 mg per kilogram bolus followed by a 24-hour infusion of 5.4 mg per kilogram per hour in patients with gunshot injury-related neurologic deficits.[78] The benefits of prophylactic antibiotics and the management of spine gunshot injuries are also unclear. Usually several days of a broad-spectrum antibiotic will suffice unless the injury results in the perforation of a hollow viscous. In these cases, antibiotics may be indicated for one or two weeks in combination with surgical debridement of the fracture site.[132,135–141]

Spinal cord decompression for neurologic deficit is indicated only in the face of progressive neurologic deterioration. Neurologic recovery in these incomplete lesions is also limited and often complicated by an increased incidence of infection and cerebral spinal fluid fistula.[142]

Bullet removal is rarely indicated with spine gunshot injuries. Retained bullet or bone fragment in the spinal canal may cause late neurologic problems and should be removed should those symptoms develop.[143,144] As previously noted, bullet removal is preferable if the missile has perforated large bowel prior to entering the spine.[136] Lead toxicity is rarely a problem with retained bullets, and can typically occur if the missile is in contact with synovial fluid, spinal fluid, or lodged in the intervertebral disc.[145–148]

The potential for spinal instability following low energy spine gunshot injuries is low[149] and these patient usually require orthotic support. The majority of reported cases of GSI instability are estrogenic resulting from ill-advised decompression.[138,141,142] Recently, Isiklar and Lindsey[135] reported on late spinal instability among patients with spinal gunshot injuries treated nonoperatively. Of the all instability cases identified, 75% occurred in the cervical spine. Therefore, the potential for spinal instability exists with GSI and should always be considered, especially in the cervical spine.

## COMPLICATIONS

Complications of the spine trauma treatment have frequently been reported. Most complications are the result of failure to understand the patient's altered spinal biomechanics, selection of the treatment, improper surgical technique, or choice of instrumentation.[150] Failure to achieve and maintain an adequate reduction can be related to the severity of the fracture, the quality of the patient's bone, and technical difficulties with the surgery.

Failure of the instrumentation can be assigned to improper implant selection or implant construct for a specific spinal injury. The choice of an implant, and its mode of application, is always determined by the biomechanical stability of the segment to be instrumented.[151] Poor bone quality or poor fixation technique can result in hardware dislodgement construct to failure. Finally, all hardware will eventually fail in the presence of pseudarthrosis, regardless of its design, strength, or the manner in which is applied.

Postoperative wound infections are also a common complication after spine surgery. The risk of infection ranges between 1 and 6%, and is highly dependent on expedient surgery, meticulous surgical technique, and the use of perioperative prophylactic antibiotics. The most devastating complication in spine trauma surgery is neurologic deterioration. Most situations of neurologic decompensation result from inadequate decompression of the neural structures. When an incomplete deficit persists, repeat imaging (i.e., myelogram, CT scan, etc.) is indicated to determine if the patient would benefit from additional surgery. Postoperative neurologic deterioration may be caused by several factors to include direct neural injury during the surgery from manipulation, instrumentation, or correction of a deformity. Rapid postoperative deterioration when the patient is initially improved may be the result of an expanding epidural hematoma. The treating physician must be alert for this potentially catastrophic complication, and evacuate the hematoma emergently to minimize residual long-term neurologic deficit.

Finally, cerebrospinal fluid leakage may complicate spine trauma surgery. The leakage can be a result of an iatrogenic laceration, or may be caused by the initial injury. When cerebrospinal fluid leakage is recognized intraoperatively, an attempt should be made to repair the injury. Cerebrospinal fluid leakage due to a dural tear caused by the injury is a special concern in spine trauma. Therefore, a high index of suspicion is warranted in the patient that presents with neurologic deficit and a burst fracture in association with a laminar fracture. If the cerebrospinal fluid leakage is recognized postoperatively, treatment may include re-operation and repair of the leak in the lumbar spine, or antibiotics, recumbency and lumbar subarachnoid drains for both the cervical and lumbar spine.

## REFERENCES

1. Holmes J, Miller P, Panacek E, et al.: Epidemiology of thoracolumbar spine injury in blunt trauma. *Acad Emerg Med* 8:866, 2001.
2. Samuels LE, Kerstein MD: Routine radiologic evaluation of the thoracolumbar spine in blunt trauma patients; a reappraisal. *J Trauma* 34:85, 1993.
3. Cooper C, Dunham DC, Rodriquez A: Falls and major injuries are risk factors for thoracolumbar injuries: Cognitive impairment and multiple injuries impede the detection of back pain and tenderness. *J Trauma* 38:692, 1995.
4. Frankel HL, Rozycki GS, Ochsner GM, et al.: Indications for obtaining surveillance thoracic and lumbar spine radiographs. *J Trauma* 37:673, 1994.
5. Stover SL, Fine PR, eds.: *Spinal Cord Injury: The Facts and Figures.* Birmingham, The National Spinal Cord Injury Statistical Center, University of Alabama, 1968, p. 15.
6. Lowery DW, Wald MM, Browne BJ, et al.: Epidemiology of cervical spine injury victims. *Annals of Emergency Medicine* 38:12, 2001.
7. National Spinal Cord Injury Statistical Center (NSCISC): *The 2005 Annual Statistical Report for the Model Spinal Cord Injury Care Systems.* Birmingham AL, 2005.
8. DeVivo MJ, Stover SL, Black KJ: Prognostic factors for 12-year survival after spinal cord injury. *Arch Phys Med Rehab* 73:156, 1992.

9. McColl MA, Walker J, Stirling P, et al.: Expectations of life and health among spinal cord injured adults. *Spinal Cord* 35:818, 1997.

10. Berkowitz M, O'Leary P, Kruse D, et al.: *Spinal Cord Injury: An Analysis of Medical and Social Costs.* New York: Demos Medical Publishing, Inc., 1998.

11. White AA, Panjabi MM: *Clinical Biomechanics of the Spine,* 2nd ed. Philadelphia: JB Lippincott, 1990.

12. Panjabi MM, White AA, Johnson RM: Cervical spine mechanics as a function of transection of components. *J Biomech* 8:327, 1975.

13. White AA, Johnson RM, Panjabi MM, et al.: Biomechanical analysis of clinical stability in the cervical spine. *Clin Orthop* 109:85, 1975.

14. Denis F: The three column spine and its significance in the classification of acute thoracolumbar spinal injuries. *Spine* 8:817, 1983.

15. Denis F: The three-column spine and its significance in the classification of acute thoracolumbar injuries. *Spine* 8:817, 1984.

16. Denis F: Spinal instability as defined by the three-column spine concept in acute spinal trauma. *Clin Orthop* 189:65, 1984.

17. Geisler FH: GM-1 ganglioside and motor recovery following human spinal cord injury. *J Emerg Med* 11:49, 1993.

18. Jellinger K: Pathology of spinal cord trauma. In Errico TJ, Bauer RD, Waugh T, eds. *Spinal Trauma.* Baltimore, BD: Lippincott, 1990, p. 455.

19. Hall ED, Springer JE: Neuroprotection and acute spinal cord injury: A reappraisal. *NeuroRx* 1:80, 2004.

20. Panter SC, Yum SW, Faden AI: Alteration in extracellular amino acids after traumatic spinal cord injury. *Ann Neurol* 27:96, 1990.

21. Liu D, Thangnipon W, McAdoo DJ: Excitatory amino acids rise to toxic levels upon impact injury to the rat spinal cord. *Brain Res* 547:344, 1991.

22. Takeda H, Caiozzo VJ, Gardner VO: A functional in vitro model for studying the cellular and molecular basis of spinal cord injury. *Spine* 18:1125, 1993.

23. Wrathall JR, Teng YD, Choiniere D, et al.: Evidence that local non-NMDA receptors contribute to functional deficits in contusive spinal cord injury. *Brain Res* 586:140, 1992.

24. Liu D, McAdoo DJ: Methylprednisolone reduces excitatory amino acid release following experimental spinal cord injury. *Brain Res* 609:293, 1993.

25. Young W, Koren I: Potassium and calcium changes in injured spinal cords. *Brain Res* 365:42, 1986.

26. Choi DW: Ionic dependence of glutamate neurotoxicity. *J Neurosci* 7:369, 1987.

27. Gentile NT, McIntosh TK: Antagonists of excitatory amino acids and endogenous opioid peptides in the treatment of experimental central nervous system injury. *Ann Emerg Med* 22:1028, 1993.

28. Faden AI, Simon RP: A potential role for excitotoxins in the pathophysiology of spinal cord injury. *Ann Neurol* 23:623, 1988.

29. Gomez-Pinilla F, Tram H, Cotman CW, et al.: Neuroprotective effect of MK-801 and U-50488H after contusive spinal cord injury. *Exp Neurol* 104:118, 1989.

30. Faden AI, Jacobs TP: Dynorphin induces partially reversible paraplegia in the rat. *Eur J Pharmacol* 91:321, 1983.

31. Faden AI, Molineaux CJ, Rosenberg JG, et al.: Endogenous opioid immunoreactivity in rat spinal cord following traumatic injury. *Ann Neurol* 17:386, 1985.

32. Faden AI, Jacobs TP, Holaday JW: Opiate antagonism improves neurologic recovery after spinal injury. *Science* 211:493, 1981.

33. Anderson DK, Hall ED: Pathophysiology of spinal cord trauma. *Ann Emerg Med* 22:987, 1993.

34. Hsu CY, Halushka PV, Hogan EL, et al.: Alteration of thromboxane and prostacyclin levels in experimental spinal cord injury. *Neurology* 35:1003, 1985.

35. Hsu CY, Halushka PS, Spicer KM, et al.: Temporal profile of thromboxane–prostacyclin imbalance in experimental spinal cord injury. *J Neurol Sci* 83:55, 1988.

36. Tempel GE, Martin HF: The beneficial effects of a thromboxane receptor antagonist on spinal cord perfusion following experimental cord injury. *J Neurol Sci* 109:162, 1992.

37. Hall ED: Lipid antioxidants in acute central nervous system injury. *Ann Emerg Med* 22:1022, 1993.

38. Bracken MB: Steroids for acute spinal cord injury. *Cochrane Database Syst Rev* Issue 2. Art. No. CD001046, 2002.

39. Lammertse DP: Update on pharmaceutical trials in acute spinal cord injury. *J Spinal Cord Med* 27:319, 2004.

40. Kwon BK, Fisher CG, Dvorak MF, et al.: Strategies to promote neural repair and regeneration after spinal cord injury. *Spine* 30:S3, 2005.

41. Zemke D, Majid A: The potential of minocycline for neuroprotection in human neurologic disease. *Clin Neuropharmacol* 27:293, 2004.

42. Stirling DP, Khodarahmi K, Liu J, et al.: Minocycline treatment reduces delayed oligodendrocyte death, attenuates axonal dieback, and improves functional outcome after spinal cord injury. *J Neurosci* 24:2182, 2004.

43. Gorio A, Gokmen N, Erbayraktar S, et al.: Recombinant human erythropoietin counteracts secondary injury and markedly enhances neurological recovery from experimental spinal cord trauma. *Proc Natl Acad Sci USA* 99:9450, 2002.

44. Kaptanoglu E, Solaroglu I, Okutan O, et al.: Erythropoietin exerts neuroprotection after acute spinal cord injury in rats: Effect on lipid peroxidation and early ultrastructural findings. *Neurosurg Rev* 27:113, 2004.

45. Qiu J, Cai D, Dai H, et al.: Spinal axon regeneration induced by elevation of cyclic AMP. *Neuron* 34:895, 2002.

46. Li S, Liu BP, Budel S, et al.: Blockade of Nogo-66, myelin-associated glycoprotein, and oligodendrocyte myelin glycoprotein by soluble Nogo-66 receptor promotes axonal sprouting and recovery after spinal injury. *J Neurosci* 24:10511, 2004.

47. Cheng H, Cao Y, Olson L: Spinal cord repair in adult paraplegic rats: Partial restoration of hind limb function. *Science* 273:510, 1996.

48. Oudega M, Xu XM: Schwann cell transplantation for repair of the adult spinal cord. *J Neurotrauma* 23:453, 2006.

49. Ruitenberg MJ, Vukovic J, Sarich J, et al.: Olfactory ensheathing cells: Characteristics, genetic engineering, and therapeutic potential. *J Neurotrauma* 23:468, 2006.

50. Ramon-Cueto A, Cordero MI, Santos-Benito FF, et al.: Functional recovery of paraplegic rats and motor axon regeneration in their spinal cords by olfactory ensheathing glia. *Neuron* 25:425, 2000.

51. Barnett SC, Riddell JS: Olfactory ensheathing cells (OECs) and the treatment of CNS injury: Advantages and possible caveats. *J Anat* 204:57, 2004.

52. Camargo FD, Chambers SM, Goodell MA: Stem cell plasticity from transdifferentiation to macrophage fusion. *Cell Prolif* 37:55, 2004.

53. Lee J, Kuroda S, Shichinohe H, et al.: Migration and differentiation of nuclear fluorescence-labeled bone marrow stromal cells after transplantation into cerebral infarct and spinal cord injury in mice. *Neuropathology* 23:169, 2003.

54. Hofstetter CP, Schwarz EJ, Hess D, et al.: Marrow stromal cells form guiding strands in the injured spinal cord and promote recovery. *Proc Natl Acad Sci USA* 99:2199, 2002.

55. Sykova E, Jendelova P, Glogarova K, et al.: Bone marrow stromal cells – a promising tool for therapy of brain and spinal cord injury. *Exp Neurol* 187:220, 2004.

56. Bosch A, Stauffer ES, Nickel VL: Incomplete traumatic quadriplegia: A ten-year review. *JAMA* 216:473, 1971.

57. Stauffer ES: Neurologic recovery following injuries to the cervical spinal cord and nerve roots. *Spine* 9:532, 1984.

58. Little JN, Halar E: Temporal course of motor recovery after Brown-Sequard spinal cord injuries. *Paraplegia* 23:39, 1985.

59. Lindsey RW, Gugala Z: Clearing of the Cervical Spine. In The Cervical Spine Research Society Editorial Committee: Clark CR, Benzel EC, Currier BR, eds. *The Cervical Spine* 4th ed. Lippincott Williams & Wilkins, 2005, pp. 375–386.

60. Hoffman JR, Wolfson AB, Todd K, et al.: Selective cervical spine radiography in blunt trauma: Methodology of the national Emergency X-Radiography Utilization Study (NEXUS). *Ann Emerg Med* 32:461, 1998.

61. Hoffman JR, Mower WR, Wolfson AB, et al.: Validity of a set of clinical criteria to rule out injury to the cervical spine in patients with blunt trauma. National Emergency X-Radiography Utilization Study Group. *N Engl J Med* 343:94, 2000.

62. Fischer RP: Cervical radiographic evaluation of alert patients following blunt trauma. *Ann Emerg Med* 13:905, 1984.

63. Bachulis BL, Long WB, Hynes GD, et al.: Clinical indications for cervical spine radiographs in the traumatized patient. *Am J Surg* 153:473, 1987.

64. Diliberti T, Lindsey RW: Evaluation of the cervical spine in the emergency setting: Who does not need an X-ray? *Orthopedics* 15:179, 1992.

65. Lindsey RW, Diliberti TC, Doherty BJ, et al.: Efficacy of radiographic evaluation of the cervical spine in emergency situations. *South Med J* 86:1253, 1993.

66. Stassen NA, Williams VA, Gestring ML, et al.: Magnetic resonance imaging in combination with helical computed tomography provides a safe and efficient method of cervical spine clearance in the obtunded trauma patient. *J Trauma* 60:171, 2006.

67. Widder S, Doig C, Burrowes P, et al.: Prospective evaluation of computed tomographic scanning for the spinal clearance of obtunded trauma patients: Preliminary results. *J Trauma* 56:1179, 2004.

68. Harris MB, Kronlage SC, Carboni PA, et al.: Evaluation of the cervical spine in the polytrauma patient. *Spine* 25:2884, 2000.

69. D'Alise MD, Benzel EC, Hart BL: Magnetic resonance imaging evaluation of the cervical spine in the comatose or obtunded trauma patient. *J Neurosurg* 91:54, 1999.

70. (ATLS) American College of Surgeons Committee on Trauma: Spine and Spinal Cord Trauma. In: *Advanced Trauma Life Support for Doctors. The Student Manual.* 7th ed. Chicago: First Impression Publishing, 2004, p. 177.

71. Calenoff L, Chessare JW, Rogers LF, et al.: Multiple level spinal injuries: Importance of early recognition. *AJR Am J Roentgenol* 130:665, 1978.

72. Henderson RL, Reid DC, Saboe LA: Multiple noncontiguous spine fractures. *Spine* 16:128, 1991.

73. Vaccaro AR, Jacoby SM: Thoracolumbar fractures and dislocations. *OKU* 2:263, 2002.

74. Ryan MD, Henderson JJ: The epidemiology of fractures and fracture-dislocations of the cervical spine. *Injury* 23:38, 1992.

75. Herkowitz HN, Rothman RH: Subacute instability of the cervical spine. *Spine* 9:348, 1984.

76. Schenarts PJ, Diaz J, Kaiser C, et al.: Prospective comparison of admission computed tomographic scan and plain films of the upper cervical spine in trauma patients with altered mental status. *J Trauma* 51:663, 2001.

77. Berne JD, Velmahos GC, El-Tawil Q, et al.: Value of complete cervical helical computed tomographic scanning in identifying cervical spine injury in the unevaluable blunt trauma patient with multiple injuries: A prospective study. *J Trauma* 48:988, 2000.

78. Bracken MB, Shepard MJ, Collins WF, et al.: A randomised, controlled trial of methylprednisolone or naloxone in treatment of acute spinal cord injury: Results of the Second National Acute Spinal Cord Injury Study. *N Eng J Med* 322:1405, 1990.

79. Bracken MB, Shepard MJ, Holford TR, et al.: Spinal Cord Injury Randomized Controlled Trial. National Acute Spinal Cord Injury Study. *JAMA* 277:1597, 1997.

80. Hurlbert RJ: Methylprednisolone for acute spinal cord injury: An inappropriate standard of care. *J Neurosurg* 93:1, 2000.

81. Fehlings MG: Summary statement: The use of methylprednisolone in acute spinal cord injury. *Spine* 15:S55, 2001.

82. Delamarter RB, Sherman JE, Carr JB: Cauda equina syndrome: Neurologic recovery following immediate, early, or late decompression. *Spine* 16:1022, 1991.

83. Delamarter RB, Sherman J, Carr JB: Pathophysiology of spinal cord injury. Recovery after immediate and delayed decompression. *J Bone Joint Surg* 77A:1042, 1995.

84. Eismont FJ, Arena MJ, Green BA: Extrusion of an intervertebral disc associated with traumatic subluxation or dislocation of cervical facets. Case report. *J Bone Joint Surg* 73A:1555, 1991.

85. Nickel VL, Perry J, Garrett A, et al.: The halo. A spinal skeletal traction fixation device. *J Bone Joint Surg* 50A:1400, 1968.

86. Perry J: The halo in spinal abnormalities: Practical factors and avoidance of complications. *Orthop Clin North Am* 3:69, 1972.

87. Crutchfield WG: Skeletal traction in treatment of injuries to the cervical spine. *J Am Med Assoc* 1:29, 1954.

88. Miller LS, Cotler HB, De Lucia FA, et al.: Biomechanical analysis of cervical distraction. *Spine* 12:831, 1987.

89. Lee AS, MacLean JCB, Newton DA: Rapid traction for reduction of cervical spine dislocations. *J Bone Joint Surg* 76B:352, 1994.

90. Evans DK: Reduction of cervical dislocations. *J Bone Joint Surg* 43B:552, 1961.

91. Cotler HB, Miller LS, DeLucia FA, et al.: Closed reduction of cervical spine dislocations. *Clin Orthop* 214:185, 1987.

92. Johnson RM, Owen JR, Hart DL, et al.: Cervical orthoses: A guide for their selection and use. *Clin Orthop* 154:34, 1981.

93. Benzel EC: Spinal orthosis. In Benzel EC, ed. *Biomechanics of Spinal Stabilization*. New York: McGraw-Hill, 1995, p. 247.

94. Axelsson P, Johnsson R, Strömqvist B: Lumbar orthosis with unilateral hip immobilization. *Spine* 18:876, 1993.

95. Anderson PA: Nonsurgical treatment of patients with thoracolumbar fractures. *Instr Course Lect* 44:57, 1995.

96. Sypert GW: External spinal orthotics. *Neurosurgery* 20:642, 1987.

97. Allen BL, Ferguson RL, Lehmann TR, et al.: A mechanistic classification of closed, indirect fractures and dislocations of the lower cervical spine. *Spine* 7:1, 1982.

98. Holdsworth F: Fractures, dislolcations, and fracture-dislocations of the spine. *J Bone Joint Surg* 52A:1534, 1970.

99. Panjabi MM, Oxland TR, Kifune M, et al.: Validity of the three-column theory of thoracolumbar fractures: A biomechanic investigation. *Spine* 20:1122, 1995.

100. Gertzbein SD: Spine update. Classification of thoracic and lumbar fractures. *Spine* 19:626, 1994.

101. Magerl F, Aebi M, Gertzbein SD, et al.: A comprehensive classification of thoracic and lumbar injuries. *Eur Spine J* 3:184, 1994.

102. Panjabi MM, Hausfeld JN, White AA: A biomechanical study of the ligamentous stability of the thoracic spine in men. *Acta Orthop Scand* 52:315, 1981.

103. Posner I, White AA, Edwards WT, et al.: A biomechanical analysis of clinical stability of the lumbar and lumbosacral spine. *Spine* 7:374, 1982.

104. Gertzbein SD, Crowe PJ, Fazl M, et al.: Canal clearance in burst fractures using the AO internal fixator. *Spine* 17:558, 1992.

105. Chapman JR, Anderson PA: Thoracolumbar spine fractures with neurologic deficit. *Orthop Clin North Am* 25:595, 1994.

106. Hu SS, Capen DA, Rimoldi RL, et al.: The effect of surgical decompression on neurologic outcome after lumbar fracture. *Clin Orthop* 288:166, 1993.

107. Lemons VR, Wagner FC, Montesano PX: Management of thoracolumbar fractures with accompanying neurological injury. *Neurosurgery* 30:667, 1992.

108. Mumford J, Weinstein JN, Spratt KF, et al.: Thoracolumbar burst fractures: The clinical efficacy and outcome of nonoperative management. *Spine* 18:955, 1993.

109. Bohlman HH: Surgical management of cervical spine fractures and dislocations. *Instr Course Lect* 34:163, 1985.

110. Brazinksi M, Yoo JU: Review of pulmonary complications associated with early versus late stabilization of thoracic and lumbar fractures. *Proc 12th Annual Meeting of the Orthopedic Trauma Association*, 1996.

111. Fellrath RF, Hanley EN: Multitrauma and thoracolumbar fractures. *Semin Spine Surg* 7:103, 1995.

112. Frankel HL, Hancock DO, Hyslop G, et al.: The value of postural reduction in initial management of closed injuries of the spine with paraplegia and tetraplegia. *Paraplegia* 7:179, 1969.

113. Edwards CC, Levine AM: Early rodsleeve stabilization of the injured thoracic and lumbar spine. *Orthop Clin North Am* 17:121, 1986.

114. Willen J, Lindahl S, Irstam L, et al.: Unstable thoracolumbar fractures: A study by CT and conventional roentgenology of the reduction effect of Harrington instrumentation. *Spine* 9:215, 1984.

115. Schiegel J, Bayley J, Yuan H, et al.: Timing of surgical decompression and fixation of acute spinal fractures. *J Orthop Trauma* 10:323, 1996.

116. Campagnolo DI, Esquieres RE, Kopacz KJ: Effect of stabilization on length of stay and medical complications following spinal cord injury. *J Spinal Cord Med* 20:331, 1997.

117. McLain RF, Benson DR: Urgent surgical stabilization of spinal fractures in polytrauma patients. *Spine* 24:1646, 1999.

118. Traynelis VC, Marano GD, Dunker RO, et al.: Traumatic atlantooccipital dislocation. *J Neurosurg* 65:863, 1986.

119. Spence KF, Decker S, Sell KW: Bursting atlantal fracture associated with rupture of the transverse ligament. *J Bone Joint Surg* 52A:543, 1970.

120. Anderson LD, D'Alonso RT: Fractures of the odontoid process of the axis. *J Bone Joint Surg* 56A:1663, 1974.

121. Clark RA Jr: Analysis of wounds involving the lumbosacral canal in the Korean War. In Meirowsky A, ed. *Neurological Surgery of Trauma*. Washington D.C.: Office of the Surgeon General, 1965, p. 337.

122. Levine AM, Edwards CC: The management of traumatic spondylolisthesis of the axis. *J Bone Joint Surg* 67:217, 1985.

123. White AA, Southwick WO, Panjabi MM: Clinical instability of the lower cervical spine. *Spine* 1:85, 1976.

124. White AA, Panjabi MM: *Clinical Biomechanics of the Spine*. Philadephia: JB Lippincott, 1978, p. 236.

125. Cooper PR, Maravilla KR, Sklar FH, et al.: Halo immobilization of cervical spine fractures. *J Neurosurg* 50:603, 1979.

126. Cheshire DJE: The stability of the cervical spine following the conservative treatment of fractures and fracture-dislocations. *Paraplegia* 7:193, 1969.

127. Waters RL, Adkins RH, Nelson R, et al.: Cervical spinal cord trauma: Evaluation and nonoperative treatment with halo-vest immobilization. *Contemp Orthop* 14:35, 1987.

128. Meyer PR: Fractures of the thoracic spine. In Meyer PR, ed. *Surgery of Spine Trauma*. Oxford: Churchill Livingstone, 1989, p. 525, 717.

129. Yoshida GM, Garland D, Waters RL: Gunshot wounds to the spine. *Orthop Clin North Am* 26:109, 1995.

130. Johnson A: Principles of wound ballistics. *Emerg Nurse* 6:12, 1998.

131. Demuth WE: Bullet velocity as applied to military rifle wounding capacity. *J Trauma* 9:27, 1969.

132. Golueke P, Sclafari S, Phillips T, et al.: Vertebral artery injury diagnosis and management. *J Trauma* 27:856, 1987.

133. Plumney TF, Kilocyne RF, Mack LA: Computed tomography in evaluation of gunshot wounds of the spine. *J Comput Assist Tomogr* 7:310, 1983.

134. Teitelbaum GP, Yee CA, Van Horn DD, et al.: Metallic ballistic fragments: MR imaging safety and artifacts. *Radiology* 175:855, 1990.

135. Isiklar ZU, Lindsey RW: Low velocity civilian gunshot wounds of the spine. *Orthopedics* 20:967, 1997.

136. Romanick PC, Smith TK, Kopariky DR, et al.: Injection about the spine associated with low velocity injury to the abdomen. *J Bone Joint Surg* 67A:1195, 1985.

137. Roffl RP, Waters RL, Adkins RH: Gunshot wounds to the spine associated with a perforated viscus. *Spine* 14:808, 1989.

138. Kupcha PC, An HC, Cotler JM: Gunshot wounds to the cervical spine. *Spine* 15:1058, 1990.

139. Waters RL, Adkins RH: The effects of removal of bullet fragments retained in the spinal canal: A collaborative study by the National Spinal Cord Injury Model Systems. *Spine* 16:934, 1991.

140. Venger B, Simpson R, Narayan R: Neurosurgical intervention in penetrating spinal trauma associated with visceral injuries. *J Neurosurg* 70:514, 1989.

141. Heiden JS, Weiss MH, Rosenbery AW, et al.: Penetrating gunshot wounds of the cervical spinal cord in civilians: Review of 38 cases. *J Neurosurg* 42:575, 1975.

142. Stauffer ES, Wood RW, Kelly EG: Gunshot wounds of the spine: The effects of laminectomy. *J Bone Joint Surg* 61A:389, 1979.

143. Arasil E, Tascioglu AO: Spontaneous migration of an intracranial bullet to the cervical spinal canal causing Lhermitte's sign: A case report. *J Neurosurg* 56:158, 1982.

144. Conway JE, Crofford TW, Terry AF, et al.: Cauda equina syndrome occurring nine years after a gunshot injury to the spine. *J Bone Joint Surg* 75A:760, 1993.

145. Dillman RO, Crumb CK, Lidsky MJ: Lead poisoning from a gunshot wound. Report of a case and review of the literature. *Am J Med* 66:509, 1979.

146. Grogan DP, Bucholz RW: Acute lead intoxication from a bullet in an intervertebral disc space: A case report. *J Bone Joint Surg* 63A:1180, 1981.

147. Leonard MH: Solution of the lead by synovial fluid. *Clin Orthop* 64:255, 1969.

148. Linden MA, Manton WI, Stewart RM, et al.: Lead poisoning from retained bullets. Pathogenesis, diagnosis and management. *Ann Surg* 195:305, 1969.

149. Waters RL, Hu SS: Penetrating injuries of the spinal canal. Stab and gunshot injuries. In: Frymoyer JW, ed. *The adult spine.* Vol. 1. New York: Raven Press, 1991, p. 815.

150. Taylor BA, Albert TJ: Complications of adult thoracolumbar surgery. *OKU* 2:449, 2002.

151. McAfee PC, Bohlman HH, Yuan HA: Anterior decompression of traumatic thoracolumbar fractures with incomplete neurological deficit using a retroperitoneal approach. *J Bone Joint Surg* 67A:89, 1985.

# Commentary ■ LISA K. CANNADA

The authors should be commended for an excellent job on their chapter. It is often the trauma doctors who are the first physicians evaluating a trauma patient with a spinal cord injury. The explanation of acute spinal cord injury and the changes which occur in the spinal cord was especially thorough. As the chapter describes, there are a number of mediators which may be detrimental in compounding the insult to the spine. By understanding the various possible mechanical and physiological means of insult to the spinal cord, the trauma surgeons can then fully appreciate the need to prevent further injury to the spinal cord and facilitate the early institution of any interventions which may be important to improve one's outcome.

One of the common pharmacologic treatments is the high-dose steroid protocol. As much as this has been accepted as the universal protocol, it is important to realize that the benefits gained have been limited to cervical spine injuries caused by blunt trauma. The patients who have gunshot wounds to the spine show an increased infection rate if, in fact, the steroid protocol is used. The steroid protocol would not be significantly beneficial in thoracic or lumbar spine lesions.

An exciting area of research is the use of mesenchymal stem cells to target regions of the spinal cord which are injured. In addition, the authors mention the application of olfactory sheathing cells (OEC) as a treatment for spinal cord injury patients. These novel agents have the ability to target the injured region and may also assist in nerve regeneration for significant injury to the spinal cord. Perhaps the exciting research which is going on now might not have been occurring without the increased awareness of spinal cord injury and its devastating effects.

A topic of big interest is cervical spine clearance. The authors, using the protocols described by Lindsey, have divided patients into three different groups and discussed a protocol regarding spine clearance for each group. In patients who are alert and able to participate in the evaluation, a protocol to clear the spine and/or to evaluate the spine for further injury is much easier to follow; the dilemma is clearance of the obtunded trauma patient. The authors recommend that the spine should not be cleared until the patient is alert, and evaluation and physical examination can be performed. However, there are patients who linger on for days and weeks in an obtunded state, and there is enough literature that supports a combination of studies (including radiographs, helical CT

scan, and MRI) to exclude cervical spine injury be used. In a patient who is unable to participate in the exam, a combination including all three modalities would be prudent. What is interesting is at major trauma centers, cervical spine radiographs are not a routine part of spine clearance protocol at this time. If follow-up patients and any patient with a spine fracture cannot get CT scans at every clinical visit, the use of routine radiographs of the injured spine region is still necessary.

The authors have discussed variable treatment recommendations for the different types of injuries including cervical, thoracic, and lumbar trauma. With thoracolumbar fractures the literature clearly does not demonstrate operative treatment providing superior results. In addition, in thoracolumbar burst fractures multiple studies have been completed comparing anterior versus posterior fusion in terms of treatment and complications. Overall, it is important to realize that in a patient without a neurologic deficit, nonoperative treatment may provide just as good, if not better, results with less complications than operative treatment. In choosing an anterior versus a posterior approach, the surgeon treating the patient must consider stability of the injury, neurologic compromise, and ability to provide restoration of alignment and appropriate stabilization to make the operation a success.

The authors commented on an increasing number of fractures occurring in the elderly. The elderly with even simple compression fractures may benefit from increased use of more recent interventions. A vertebral fracture whether due to osteoporosis or trauma can cause significant pain and possibly neurologic deficits in the patient. Vertebroplasty involves a percutaneous technique in which bone cement is injected into the vertebral body. Bone tamps or instrumentation can be used prior to the injection of cement to create a void in the vertebral body. The technique is known as balloon vertebroplasty or kyphoplasty. These procedures are not without risk and there are case reports of this throughout the literature. However, the use of kyphoplasty or vertebroplasty by itself and/or in conjunction with short segment instrumentation and/or fusion provides an attractive alternative with good results for thoracic and lumbar fractures.

The authors emphasize that there is increasing incident of gunshot wounds and spine fractures. A recently published article discussed the role of debridement and antibiotics in gunshot wounds to the spine. The article concluded there was a significantly high rate of spine and wound infections with transgastrointestinal gunshots wound to the spine. Although much further research is needed in this context, there is no specific protocol for intravenous antibiotic therapy in the setting of transgastrointestinal gunshot wounds to the spine. In general, gunshot wounds to the cervical spine region are often thought to have a higher infection rate and may warrant antibiotics due to the proximity of the esophagus.

The authors did not specifically address one of the biggest risks in patients with spine fractures and spinal cord injury, that is, DVT prophylaxis. It is important that DVT prophylaxis be initiated early. With advances in interventional radiology to include a removable filter that represents another treatment option open for the patient. It is the teamwork between the trauma surgeons and the treating spine surgeons with consideration of the patient's injuries and risks, that an optimal protocol be initiated as soon as possible with the minimum of mechanical compression and begin chemical prophylaxis and/or placement of a removable filter pending the specific spine injury and surgical intervention which may be planned.

There has been an increased awareness of posttraumatic stress disorder and depression after trauma. Recent studies have reported the occurrence in up to 50% of trauma patients. It is important that the physician who sees the patient in follow-up ask the patient questions regarding their feelings of depression and/or posttraumatic stress and refer them to the proper health professional for treatment. The authors did provide a great insight into some of the social impact following spinal cord injury including the high divorce rate and marriage rate of less than 1% of patients who have spinal cord injury. It is important that we as health care professionals are aware of this and the mental complications which can occur following spine trauma in addition to the physical complications. In this way we can better serve the patient and assist in the recovery.

# Indications for and Techniques of Thoracotomy

*Matthew J. Wall, Jr.* ■ *Joseph Huh* ■ *Kenneth L. Mattox*

## BACKGROUND

Thoracic injury is responsible for approximately 16,000 deaths per year in the United States.[1] Immediate deaths from blunt thoracic trauma are often secondary to a major disruption of the heart or thoracic aorta. Deaths within three hours of injury due to thoracic trauma are often secondary to cardiac tamponade, aortic disruption, or continued hemorrhage. Later deaths from blunt thoracic injuries occur in the intensive care unit due to multiorgan failure and systemic inflammatory response syndrome, respiratory complications, infection, and, occasionally, unrecognized injuries. While the massive cardiovascular injuries are the most spectacular, the most common thoracic injury is chest wall contusion or rib fracture.[1]

Furthermore, approximately 85% of patients with thoracic injuries that require intervention can be treated with tube thoracostomy, observation, and pain control. Adjuncts to this regimen include respiratory support, intercostal blocks, and epidural anesthesia. Thus, only 10 to 15% of patients with significant thoracic injury require formal thoracotomy. The decision process regarding thoracotomy can thus require significant judgment.

## EVOLUTION

One of the earliest citations of thoracic injury is a report of penetrating trauma to the sternum noted in the *Edwin Smith Surgical Papyrus,* approximately 3000 BC. likely authored by Imhotep, the builder of the step pyramid.[2] Open chest injuries during the time of the Romans were considered fatal injuries. Galen reported attempting to treat gladiators who sustained chest injuries with open packing. Perrier recommended closing chest wounds three to five days postinjury. In North America, the first written thoracic operative record appeared in the diary of Cabeza de Vaca in 1635.

This account described the operative removal of an arrowhead from the chest wall of an Indian.[3] The mortality from chest wounds in military campaigns was 28.5% in the Crimean War (1853–1856), 27.8% in the American Civil War (1861–1865), 24.1% in World War I (1914–1918), only improving to 5.4% by the second World War (1939–1945).[4]

It was not until World War II that guidelines were established for treating thoracic trauma. The development of endotracheal intubation resulted in the ability to manage open thoracotomy as well as treat patients with respiratory insufficiency. The understanding and treatment of posttraumatic respiratory insufficiency advanced dramatically during the Vietnam War. While trauma care often advances during wartime, it is significant that the majority of wartime injuries that survive to treatment are extremity injuries and not truncal. In the civilian sector, there are higher ratios of truncal-to-extremity wounds. In contemporary mobile society, high-speed vehicular accidents have contributed to the increasing incidence of blunt thoracic trauma.

With the redesign of automobile interiors and the addition of passenger restraints such as airbags, it is anticipated that the incidence of thoracic injury may change. However, injury profiles specifically related to these restraint devices (such as seat belt signs and airbag sequelae) are emerging. Patients with thoracic vascular injuries that previously were dead at the scene may now survive transport to the hospital.

## CLINICAL APPROACH/PHILOSOPHY

The evaluation and management of patients with thoracic injuries can be philosophically different depending on mechanism, timing, and associated injuries. For patients with blunt injuries to the chest, the history can be illuminating. For vehicular trauma, conferring with emergency medical services (EMS) providers to determine the mechanism of injury, condition of the vehicle, amount of intrusion, direction of impact on the vehicle, presence of rollover, difficult extrication, and other injuries or deaths in the vehicle (all signs of significant injury transfer) can give clues to initiate further studies. While the majority of penetrating trauma to the chest can be managed with tube thoracostomy, the evaluation and management of patients with mediastinal traverse is evolving. In the past, it was felt that all required operation. However, because of the lower-than-expected incidence of significant injuries, and the recognition that many are not true "mediastinal traverse," there have been recommendations for evaluation with endoscopy, arteriography, and observation.[5] The multicenter helical computed tomography (CT) scans are providing resolution capable of demonstrating trajectories, which can then guide further decisions regarding workup or operation. Few patients not *in extremis* now undergo empiric thoracotomy for mediastinal traverse.

Emergency center thoracotomy philosophically has been reserved for patients who suffer penetrating trauma, are hemodynamically unstable, but have signs of life. The patients who benefit most from emergency center thoracotomy are those with penetrating injury to the chest that have short transport times and who have undergone prehospital endotracheal intubation.[6] While endotracheal intubation allows maximal oxygenation of the available red cells, overventilation may further drop venous return in these markedly hypovolemic patients. Survivable injuries are usually limited to a single organ system that can be readily controlled. Emergency center thoracotomy for blunt trauma has had very limited success. Blunt trauma more often causes multiorgan injury that can involve multiple cavities. Emergency center thoracotomy for injuries outside the thoracic cavity also has a much lower yield. Due to constraints and limited resources, while many continue to be aggressive with the use of thoracotomy in the emergency center, most centers have become increasingly selective of which patients are brought to the operating room. Thus, some suggest that patients that are unable to sustain a blood pressure greater than 70 mmHg after thoracotomy in the emergency center should not be brought to the operating room. Thus, patient care decisions must be individualized.[7]

Thoracoabdominal injuries can cause significant judgmental pitfalls. These are daunting injuries, which, when an empiric exploration is required, often result in an initial exploration into the wrong cavity. The signs of an injury outside the explored cavity are often noted first by the anesthesiologist during the case. Subtle findings, such as unexplained deterioration in the patient's hemodynamic status, or an increase in ventilatory pressures, might cause one to consider an injury in a cavity that has not yet been explored.[8]

It is common to treat the initial penetrating thoracoabdominal injury with tube thoracostomy. If the chest tube output is noted to be minimal, the operative approach focuses on the abdomen. Unfortunately, chest tube output can be notoriously unreliable and give a false sense of security. New imaging modalities such as using ultrasound to evaluate for hemopericardium or hemothorax may assist in decision making. Thus, thoracoabdominal injuries require judgment and a significant amount of flexibility.

There has been significant work in termination of resuscitation for medical cardiac arrest.[9] As experience is gained, particularly in population-based studies, there is recognition of injuries that are fatal. When these are able to be identified, eliminating the need for transport by EMS, then resources can be preserved. It must be remembered, however, that with advances in both EMS and resuscitation, some previously fatal injuries are now being successfully managed. Thus, it is important that a label of futility does not result in a self-fulfilling prophecy. One must be careful to allow clinical judgment to intervene in these cases.

With the advent of multiple specialties caring for the trauma patient, credentialing has become a significant issue. The guiding principle is that the most qualified individual available to evaluate a patient or perform a procedure should be the responsible individual. Trauma is clearly a surgical disease. A hospital system committed to trauma should ensure that surgeons comfortable in the management of injured patients are readily available to care for significantly injured patients. Without the surgeon, access to procedures to manage life-threatening injuries and their complications will be limited. Alternatively, tube thoracostomy is a more basic, potentially life-saving procedure that may impact a high number of patients. Nonsurgeons who place chest tubes must be appropriately trained and experienced; otherwise, the complication rate increases. These issues must be examined locally on a system-by-system basis using the performance improvement approach.

## INITIAL EVALUATION AND TREATMENT

Patients with thoracic trauma can be evaluated via the standard Advanced Trauma Life Support (ATLS) protocols.[10] The primary survey in the ATLS course concentrates on life-threatening mechanical problems related to the chest and the airway. The patient's presentation should be discussed with the EMS personnel, as they can provide important details relating to the scene of injury. The patient is carefully examined for all penetrating injuries, and attempts should be made to reconstruct the path of a missile or sharp object. A significant pitfall, however, is that missiles may not always travel in straight lines. The chest is inspected and auscultated to assess for the absence of breath sounds, deviation of the trachea, subcutaneous emphysema, and elevation of the jugular venous pulsations. X-rays should not be required to detect tension pneumothorax. The presence of hematomas, particularly at the thoracic outlet, should arouse suspicion for a thoracic vascular injury. Scars from previous tube thoracostomies or chest incisions may herald a patient with significant fibrosis from a previous thoracic procedure that would make a second operation or placement of a tube thoracostomy much more difficult. Even in the unoperated chest, 15% of patients have a symphysis of the pleura. Thus, it is recommended that after spreading the intracostal muscles the pleura should not be entered with a clamp or a trocar, but with the surgeon's finger.

The chest x-ray remains a fundamental imaging modality in the evaluation of the patient with chest trauma. All wounds should be identified with radiopaque markers to assist in assessing injury patterns. Many recommended that the initial chest x-ray be taken with the patient sitting erect. With a significantly injured patient, this is often impractical, and many now routinely assess the patient with supine films. In addition, in the multiply injured patient in whom there is concern for a cervical, thoracic, or lumbar spine fracture, having the patient sit up may not be feasible.

The chest x-ray is evaluated for the position of the tracheobronchial tree, the lung parenchyma, the mediastinal silhouette, the silhouette of the vascular structures and aortic knob, and the pleural cavities. Specifically, the presence of hemopneumothorax, pneumomediastinum, rib fractures, spinal or other skeletal fractures, foreign bodies, positions of various tubes, and great vessel injuries should be sought if possible.

The most common therapeutic activity in treating a patient with chest trauma is observation with judicious fluid administration to prevent overhydration. With both penetrating and blunt injury to the chest, the contused lung parenchyma absorbs excess fluid. As described by Trinkle and associates over three decades ago, one of the key elements in managing these patients is to limit, if possible, fluid administration to below 1 liter/day.[11] For penetrating truncal trauma, even with hypotension, survival has been shown to be increased when crystalloid resuscitation has been delayed until operation.[12] Some vascular injuries may clot when the blood pressure drops. Patients often autoresuscitate by shifting fluid from the interstitial space. Iatrogenic elevation of blood pressure may dislodge this tenuous clot and increase bleeding. Delay in resuscitation may be difficult in patients with multiple injuries.

## TUBE THORACOSTOMY

Tube thoracostomy is one of the most underrated procedures performed in the patient with chest injury. It is the only invasive procedure that 85% of the patients with penetrating chest trauma will require. One pitfall with tube thoracostomy relates to the use of trocar chest tubes, which contain a sharp metal rod that can produce injury to both upper abdominal and intrathoracic organs. These tubes characteristically are smaller in diameter, and their use may result in an unevacuated clotted hemothorax and the need for a subsequent thoracotomy. As mentioned earlier, many have some element of pleural symphysis, blind insertion of a trocar chest tube often results in lung injury with subsequent air leak. In adolescents and adults, the chest tube should be at least 36 French or larger and have at least four to six distal holes in the tube. During placement, it is important to assure that the tube is in the pleural cavity, as many tubes are misplaced. There are a number of devices designed to collect shed blood from the chest tube. These range from custom-made multiple bottle systems to expensive plastic commercial devices with in-line autotransfusion attachments. Regardless of the system, the physician should understand the three-chamber concept of the collection device, as up to 30% of chest tubes in any hospital are connected incorrectly.

The majority of these systems have a suction control chamber or device. The amount of suction applied to the chest tube is approximately 20 cm of negative pressure. "High" suction can be temporarily accomplished by stripping the chest tubes or occluding the airvent port on the pressure regulator of the collection device. This should be used judiciously, because high suction in a patient with significant air leak can completely evacuate the patient's tidal volume. If a patient's arterial saturation decreases and the physician is unable to ventilate the patient because of a large air leak, the patient should be removed from suction and left to water seal. The patient may then be taken to the operating room for definitive repair. There is seldom an indication in trauma to clamp a chest tube, because a patient with a significant air leak may rapidly develop an iatrogenic tension pneumothorax.

Chest tube removal, although a simple procedure, can result in significant complications. The decision for chest tube removal is based on several factors including the likelihood of a lung injury, the absence of an air leak, the trend in the amount of fluid removed from the chest, as well as the surgeon's determination of the functionality of the tube. Examining the water seal chamber for fluctuation with respiration can give an indication of whether the tube continues to be functional. After a pulmonary resection or with a lung injury in which there has been a significant air leak, a trial of water seal may be helpful in avoiding replacement of a tube. In many patients who have sustained an open pneumothorax with low likelihood of pulmonary parenchymal injury, a trial of water seal may only extend their hospitalization. The incidence of pneumothorax after chest tube removal can be a performance improvement indicator in some trauma systems.

## ACUTE INDICATIONS FOR THORACOTOMY

Thoracotomy may be indicated for acute or chronic conditions (Tables 25-1, 25-2). Indications for thoracotomy in acute thoracic injury are based on historical and physical findings, clues noted on radiographic studies, and the clinical course of the patient. One clinical presentation, pericardial tamponade, is recognized by the classic physical findings of hypotension, narrow pulse pressure, and muffled heart sounds. These findings combined with proximity are appropriate indications for operation. Unfortunately, from a practical standpoint, the presentation is often not definitive. Pulsus paradoxus or simply the loss of the radial pulse when the patient takes a deep breath may be suggestive of tamponade. The demonstration of hemopericardium by surgeon-directed ultrasound has made the diagnosis of tamponade much more straightforward. Acute or hypovolemic cardiac arrest in the patient with penetrating trauma to the chest suggests the need for resuscitative thoracotomy. A rare indication for acute thoracotomy in a patient that has sustained blunt trauma is herniation of the heart through a defect in the pericardium. These patients can present after a lateral deceleration with acute deterioration after positional changes.[13] Widening of the upper mediastinum on routine chest film is suggestive of vascular injury to the thoracic outlet, which can be confirmed by angiography, if possible, to plan incisions and the operative

**TABLE 25-1**

### Acute Indications for Thoracotomy

Acute hemodynamic deterioration and cardiac arrest in the trauma center[7]
Patients with penetrating truncal trauma (resuscitative thoracotomy)[44]
Cardiac tamponade
Ultrasound demonstration of hemopericardium[43]
Vascular injury at the thoracic outlet[45]
Massive air leak from the chest tube[46]
Suspected cardiac herniation[13]
Endoscopic or radiographic demonstration of tracheal or bronchial injury[47,48]
Radiographic evidence of great vessel injury[49,50]
Significant missile embolism to the heart or pulmonary artery[51]
Traumatic thoracotomy (loss of chest wall substance)
True mediastinal traverse with penetrating object
Transcardiac placement of inferior vena caval shunt for hepatic vascular wounds[52]

**TABLE 25-2**

**Nonacute Indications for Thoracotomy**

Nonevacuated clotted hemothorax[19]
Chronic (or neglected) posttraumatic empyema
Chronic traumatic diaphragmatic hernia
Traumatic cardiac septal or valvular lesions[21]
Chronic traumatic thoracic aortic pseudoaneurysms[20]
Nonclosing thoracic duct fistula
Missed tracheal or bronchial injury
Infected intrapulmonary hematoma (traumatic lung abscess)
Tracheoesophageal fistula
Innominate artery and tracheal fistula
Traumatic arterial venous fistula

approach. Traumatic thoracotomy may be produced by high-velocity missiles, blast injury, or massive blunt trauma. The presence of cervical, mediastinal, and pleural air may be a significant clue to an injury to intrathoracic structures. This may be determined by physical examination or on chest x-ray. "Massive" air leaks via tube thoracostomy are also indicative of major injury to the airway. Tracheal, bronchial, and esophageal injuries are diagnosed by endoscopy or contrast studies and require thoracotomy for repair and prevention of postinjury complications such as abscess.

Blunt great-vessel injury, particularly to the descending thoracic aorta, can be highly lethal, and angiography continues to be the diagnostic procedure of choice for diagnosis.[14] Computed tomography (CT) and transesophageal echocardiography have limitations but may have selected indications in multiply injured patients to assist in triage. The high-resolution multidetector CT is increasingly used for the screening of patients with blunt aortic injury, due to the ability to resolve subtle injuries as well as the short scan time. This has become an extremely controversial modality. The newer scanners often have resolution showing findings not previously seen and thus may be oversensitive. The most important factor is probably the local experience with each of these modalities. As this evolves, each hospital's trauma quality assurance system can track the efficacy of each of these modalities for a particular system.

A common indication for acute thoracotomy is based on the amount of bleeding from the chest tube. The threshold for the amount of blood evacuated by the tube has recently been increased from an immediate output of 1 to 1.5 liter as being sufficient indication for thoracotomy. However, the trend is probably more important. Many patients arrive well after injury, and if a large amount of blood is evacuated, the lung is reexpanded, and no further output occurs, the patient can be observed for continuing bleeding or recurrence of hemothorax. If bleeding persists with a steady trend of over 250 ml/h, thoracotomy is often indicated. Many advocate routine exploration anytime when 1500 cc is obtained.[15]

As discussed earlier, stable patients with potential mediastinal traverse are managed with endoscopy/arteriography or with CT to define wound track, followed by directed examinations or imaging. However, the limitations of each of these diagnostic modalities must be remembered.[5] Missile emboli can be an extremely confusing presentation, again emphasizing the inability to draw straight lines from injury to the final resting place of the projectile. Missile embolus can occur from the venous circulation to the lung. This often requires removal, usually by interventional techniques, unless it is small (i.e., less than the size of a BB). It can occur on the left

side of the heart to the aorta and the major branches such as the carotid and iliac arteries. The authors have also seen the transseptal embolus of missiles that enter the right side of the circulation, cross the cardiac septum, and embolize systemically. Careful examination of all peripheral pulses, for example, can lead to the diagnosis of missile embolus to the iliac arteries with an absent femoral pulse or to the innominate, subclavian, or carotid arteries with absent radial or carotid pulses.[16]

Infrequently, a thoracic incision can be made to treat an abdominal injury, such as for transcardiac placement of an inferior vena caval shunt for retrohepatic vena cava injury or for proximal control of a supraceliac aortic injury.[17,18] Often however, other approaches such as packing or medial visceral rotation are available to avoid the morbidity of entering a second, uninjured cavity. Hybrid procedures combining open surgery, intravascular occlusion balloons, and intravascular stent/grafts may eliminate the need for thoracic incisions from vascular control.

Nonacute conditions related to previous trauma that may require thoracotomy are often secondary to unrecognized or incompletely treated acute injuries.[19,20] Examples include clotted hemothorax; empyema; trapped lung; posttraumatic chronic aortic pseudoaneurysms; stenosis from a bronchial injury; septal and valvular cardiac lesions; and nonhealing bronchopleural fistula. Injuries to the bronchial tree are often difficult to diagnose and commonly present as poststenotic atelectasis weeks after the original injury. Intracardiac injuries in patients that survive to the hospital are a special subset. The majority of intracardiac injuries are recognized in the ICU after an emergent operation to control bleeding from an injury to the heart. Even if recognized acutely, it is usually appropriate to stage the repair of these intracardiac injuries. In a review of 711 heart injuries, it was extremely rare to require acute cardiopulmonary bypass in these patients.[21] It may be that many of these patients self-triage in that they die on the scene of massive intracardiac injuries and the patients that survive to hospital are a special subset.

Historically, the most common chronic postinjury condition that leads to operation is an unevacuated clotted hemothorax. For management, there may be little difference between video-assisted evacuation of a clotted hemothorax and a small, muscle-sparing thoracotomy in which the ribs are spread only enough to permit admission of the tonsil suction or the surgeon's hand.

In the past, thoracoabdominal injury was cited during World War II as an indication for thoracotomy. Today, thoracoabdominal wounds are more commonly an indication for laparotomy but not necessarily formal thoracotomy. Unfortunately, the algorithms for chest injury and the algorithms for abdominal injury are often difficult to integrate. In over half the cases the wrong cavity is entered initially. One of the keys to managing these injuries intraoperatively is communication with the anesthesiologist, who may notice unexplained hemodynamic instability. There is a four times greater chance of a missed injury or complication when one of the other cavities contains the only injuries.[8] Thus, in patients with both thoracic and abdominal wounding, extremely close surveillance, flexibility, and increased sensitivity to potential injuries is essential (Table 25-3).

Several clinical conditions that have soft indications for thoracotomy for which treatment should be individualized include flail chest or fractured sternum,[22] fibrothorax, posttraumatic pulmonary embolism, and selected vascular injuries for proximal vascular control. (Figs. 25-1 and 25-2)

**TABLE 25-3**

**Pitfalls in the Care of Thoracoabdominal Injuries[8]**

Wrong cavity initially entered
Reliance on low chest tube output (clotted tube)
Inadequate communication with anesthesiologist
Bleeding from liver through diaphragm into chest
Need for vigilance and flexibility

## OPERATIVE ISSUES

### Incisions

The approach chosen for an unstable trauma patient who requires an empiric operation for chest injury is often an educated guess suggested by the anticipated injuries. For the abdomen, the midline laparotomy is the utility incision in trauma. However, there are many incisions available for thoracic trauma. These include anterolateral thoracotomy, transsternal anterolateral thoracotomy, posterolateral thoracotomy, "book incision" (anterolateral thoracotomy, partial upper sternotomy to a supraclavicular extension), and median sternotomy (Fig. 25-3). The left anterolateral thoracotomy is the utility incision for resuscitation under circumstances of acute deterioration or cardiac arrest.[23] This incision allows exposure for opening the pericardium, open cardiac massage, clamping of the descending thoracic aorta, and treatment of a large percentage of cardiac and left lung injuries. Pitfalls associated with the performance of emergent left anterolateral thoracotomy include making the incision too small initially, not following the interspace with the incision (Fig. 25-4), injury to the aorta, the intercostal arteries or the esophagus during aortic clamping, and injury to the phrenic nerve when opening the pericardium. Injury to the right side of the heart often requires transsternal extension for full visualization and repair (Fig. 25-5). The right anterolateral incision alone provides limited exposure to the heart and is used primarily for anticipated injuries to the right lung and chest wall. The azygous venous

system is posterior in the chest. These can be difficult injuries to visualize through anterior incisions, and carry mortality similar to vena cava injuries. They may be suggested by venous bleeding from a posterior location.[24] While many routinely place a right chest tube during performance of an EC thoracotomy, a simpler way to assess for hemothorax/pneumothorax is to pass a hand into the right pleural cavity anterior to the pericardium. These incisions often have to be made in a rapid fashion. At the completion of the procedure, the internal mammary arteries and intercostals should be examined and ligated to prevent delayed bleeding. Unfortunately, due to the rapidity of exposure and closure, delayed bleeding is not uncommon as these vessels are often in spasm at the time of operation.

The left posterolateral thoracotomy incision provides excellent exposure of the posterior mediastinum, left lung, hilum, and descending thoracic aorta. This incision provides access to the heart for cardiac massage and management of lateral and posterior cardiac injuries, as well as good exposure of the proximal left subclavian artery with some access to the proximal left common carotid artery.[25] Unfortunately, anterior cardiac injuries and injuries that extend to the right can be difficult to manage.

A right posterolateral thoracotomy incision provides good exposure for managing pulmonary, tracheal, and mid-esophageal injuries. Although this incision provides some exposure of the heart for management of right atrial and some left atrial injuries, this exposure is suboptimal for the management of cardiac injuries. This incision also provides exposure to the superior and inferior venae cavae and the azygous vein. Its primary use, however, is for pulmonary, esophageal, or tracheal injuries. The interspace entered is chosen to be centered on the area of interest.

The "book" or "trap door" incision is seldom used but can be considered for exposure of left-sided thoracic outlet injuries. It has the advantage of providing exposure of a long segment of the left common carotid and left subclavian artery. The anterolateral thoracotomy component of this incision can be made above or below the breast, and attention must be paid to the internal mammary artery. Lebschke's knife or a sternal saw may be used to make the sternal osteotomy. The sternocleidomastoid muscle may be cut to

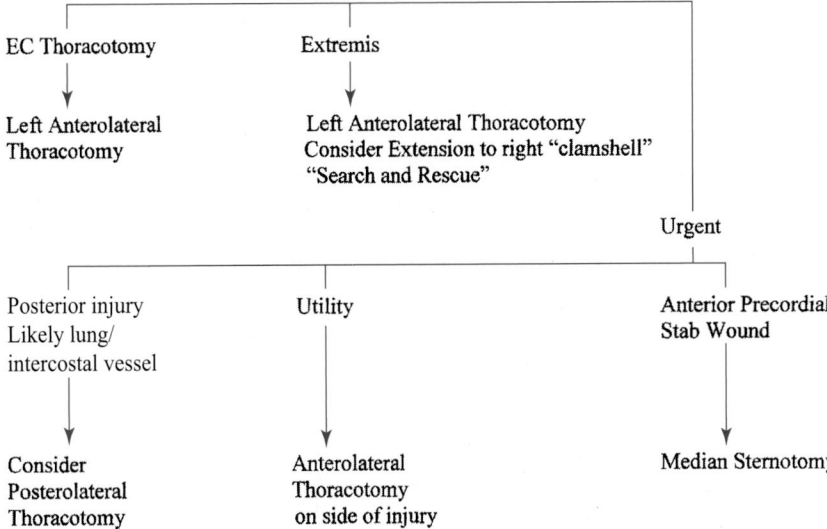

INCISION ALGORITHM

**FIGURE 25-1.** Incision algorithm.

SPECIFIC INJURIES

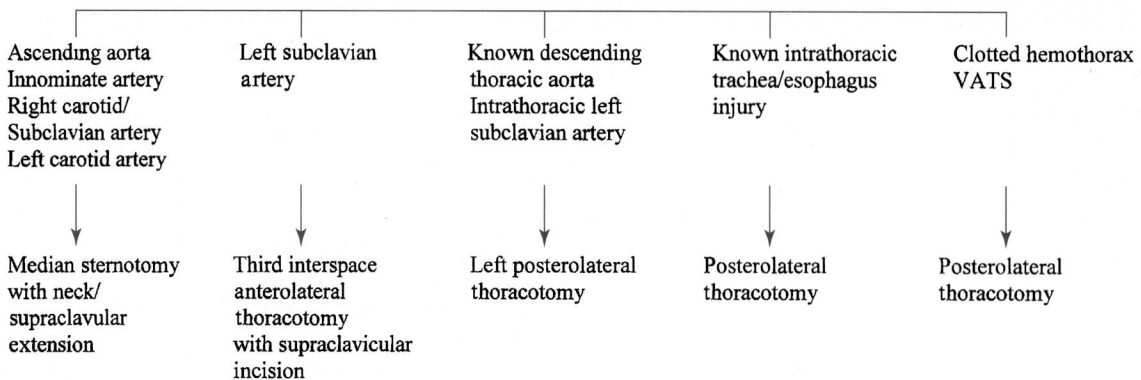

| Ascending aorta<br>Innominate artery<br>Right carotid/<br>Subclavian artery<br>Left carotid artery | Left subclavian<br>artery | Known descending<br>thoracic aorta<br>Intrathoracic left<br>subclavian artery | Known intrathoracic<br>trachea/esophagus<br>injury | Clotted hemothorax<br>VATS |
|---|---|---|---|---|
| ↓ | ↓ | ↓ | ↓ | ↓ |
| Median sternotomy<br>with neck/<br>supraclavular<br>extension | Third interspace<br>anterolateral<br>thoracotomy<br>with supraclavicular<br>incision | Left posterolateral<br>thoracotomy | Posterolateral<br>thoracotomy | Posterolateral<br>thoracotomy |

**FIGURE 25-2.** Specific injuries algorithm.

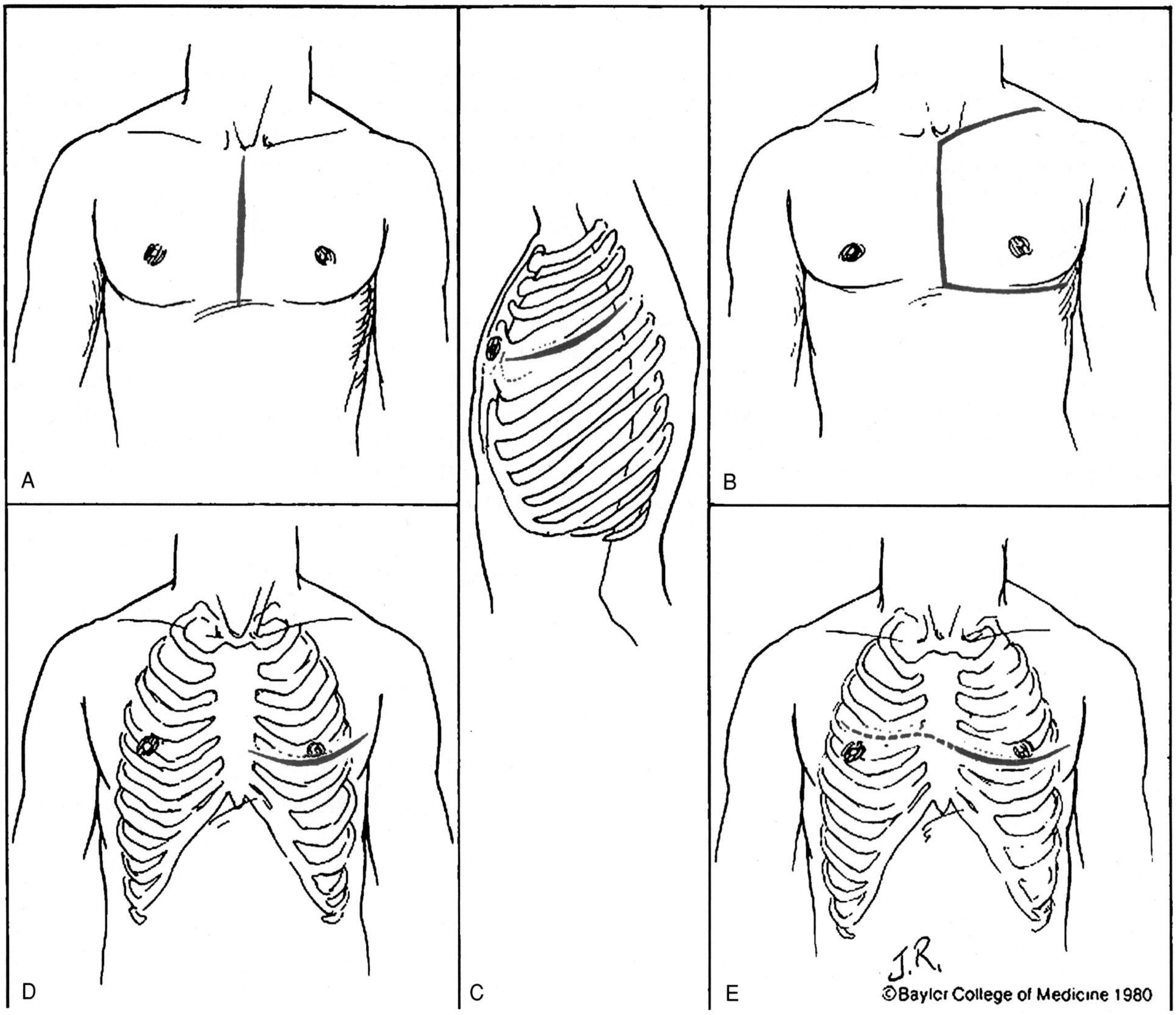

**FIGURE 25-3.** Thoracic incisions for trauma include **(A)** median sternotomy, **(B)** book thoracotomy, **(C)** posterolateral thoracotomy, **(D)** anterolateral thoracotomy, and **(E)** extension of an anterolateral thoracotomy across the sternum. *(Reproduced with permission from Baylor College of Medicine.)*

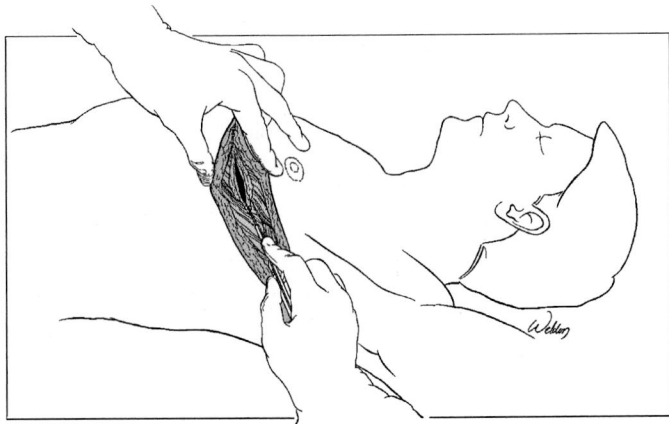

**FIGURE 25-4.** The emergent left anterolateral thoracotomy incision should follow the intercostal space.
*(Reproduced with permission from Baylor College of Medicine.)*

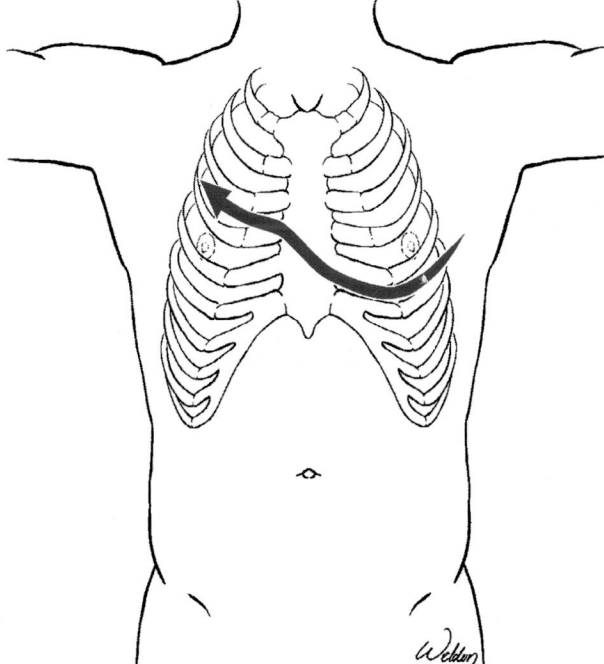

**FIGURE 25-5.** When extending a left anterolateral thoracotomy to the right, the incision should track superiorly to avoid a low interspace incision on the right.
*(Reproduced with permission from Baylor College of Medicine.)*

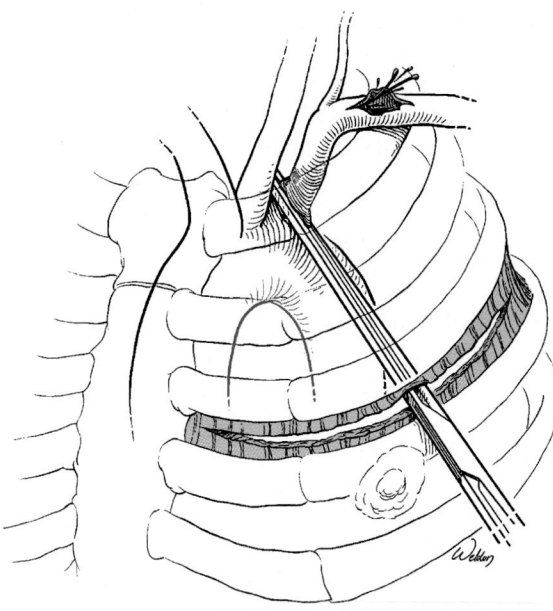

**FIGURE 25-6.** Proximal control of a left subclavian artery is obtained via a third interspace anterolateral thoracotomy. Definitive repair is then performed through a separate supraclavicular incision.
*(Reproduced with permission from Baylor College of Medicine.)*

trauma. It provides excellent exposure for isolated anterior cardiac and great-vessel injuries but provides no access to the esophagus and posterior thorax. In addition, it is very difficult to clamp the descending thoracic aorta via this approach. Therefore, it is recommended primarily for anticipated isolated anterior cardiac injuries, where there is no need to repair injuries to other organ systems. The median sternotomy incision is also useful for injury to anterior mediastinal structures such as the ascending aorta, innominate artery, and left common carotid artery. Further exposure can be obtained with extension into either the supraclavicular area or the neck.

The subxiphoid pericardiotomy is an abdominal approach to a suspected cardiac wound that provides less than ideal exposure. With increasing use of the focused abdominal sonogram for trauma (FAST) to exclude tamponade, this procedure is rarely indicated. Much more useful is pericardiotomy during laparotomy in the operating room. This can be helpful intraoperatively to investigate unexplained hypotension secondary to undiagnosed tamponade.

facilitate exposure, but care should be taken to avoid injury to the phrenic nerve, which is located on the anterior border of the scalenus anterior muscle. Difficulties with the book incision include stretch of the brachial plexus and upper posterior costal junctions, which can result in long-term neurologic and upper back pain syndromes that can be quite disabling. This pain simulates causalgia and may require extensive rehabilitation or later sympathectomy for pain control. Thus, this incision is used only when necessary for control and repair. The current approach for the management of left subclavian artery injuries is to gain proximal control via anterolateral thoracotomy in the left third interspace combined with a separate clavicular incision for definitive repair. (Fig. 25-6) The standard median sternotomy incision, while the most common elective cardiac incision, has limited usefulness in

## PATIENT POSITIONING

The most common operative position for the patient with injury to the chest is supine with both arms out on arm boards. The patient is prepped from the chin to the knees or ankles. Positioning and operative preparation thus permit vascular access at multiple sites, as well as allow harvest of a conduit for repair of small-vessel injuries. For posterolateral thoracotomy, the patient is placed in the decubitus position, with the appropriate side accessible. The hips are often rotated back somewhat to permit access to the abdomen if needed for sudden deterioration and suspected intraabdominal injury. Unfortunately, these "half way" positions often are not optimal for any injury, and it may be best to control life-threatening problems via an anterior incision, close perhaps with a damage control closure, then turn and reprepare the patient. If the patient is placed in the decubitus position, care should be taken not to place central venous lines in the down side, as pneumothorax from the line intraoperatively can result in collapse of the opposite lung, inability to ventilate the patient, and intraoperative death.

## DAMAGE CONTROL

Damage control in the abdomen has consisted of limiting the operative procedure to acutely control injuries, usually vascular, that are imminently lethal, followed by planned reoperation after the patient's condition has stabilized.[26] Damage control approaches in the chest include pulmonary tractotomy with selective vascular ligation to avoid formal resection[27] (Fig. 25-7), en masse resection of a lobe of the lung with the stapling device,[28] pulmonary hilar twist[29] (Fig. 25-8), packing of the limits of the chest, placement of intravascular shunts, massive drainage of esophageal injuries, stapling of heart injuries, and rapid closure techniques. Towel clip closures or vacuum closures of the abdomen work well because the midline is devoid of significant vascular structures. Many of the thoracotomy incisions involve cutting large muscles that continue to bleed. Thus, en masse closure with a single large suture may be a more efficacious closure technique. Thus, rather than planned reoperation, damage control techniques in the chest are philosophically a simpler procedure to accomplish hemostasis in a more rapid manner.[30]

## OTHER CONSIDERATIONS

### Digital Thoracotomy

Valuable information may be obtained by a digital exploration through the chest tube site prior to chest tube placement, particularly

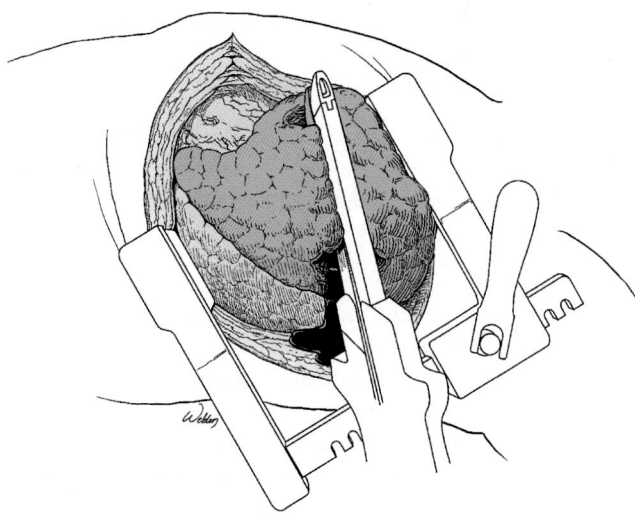

**FIGURE 25-7.** Pulmonary tractotomy with selective vascular ligation can be used for deep penetrating injuries to the lung as a damage control technique to avoid formal lung resection.
*(Reproduced with permission from Baylor College of Medicine.)*

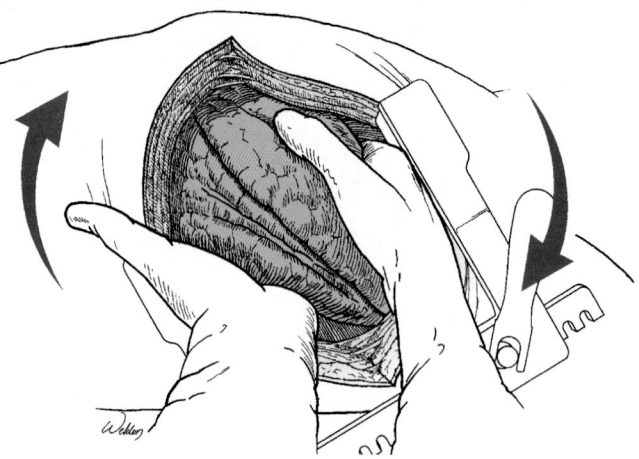

**Figure 25-8.** Pulmonary hilar twist can be used to rapidly achieve hilar control for significant injuries of the lung. After dividing the inferior pulmonary ligament, the entire lung is rotated 180°. This wraps the hilar vessels around the bronchus, providing vascular control and preventing systemic air embolis.
*(Reproduced with permission from Baylor College of Medicine.)*

for the left side of the chest. After spreading the intercostal muscles, the pleural space is entered by the surgeon's finger rather than by a sharp instrument or trocar. Digital exploration of the pleural space is performed to examine for the conditions noted in Table 25-4, which, if present, indicate the need for further diagnostic and therapeutic measures.

Technically, the incision for the chest tube can be oriented to access the area of concern. These intrathoracic structures should be palpated routinely with any chest tube insertion as pathologic findings are often subtle. The chest tube is then placed.

### Thoracoscopy

Thoracoscopy has been used to remove clotted blood, evaluate the diaphragm, look for hemopericardium, remove foreign bodies, control chest wall and mammary artery bleeding, and examine for hemomediastinum or hematomas around the great vessels.[31–34] If the clotted hemothorax is evacuated early, it can often be removed thoracoscopically or via a small incision by performing a muscle sparing thoracotomy through the auscultatory triangle. Either approach works well. Thoracoscopy has a theoretical advantage that it does not spread the ribs and thus results in less postoperative pain. However, the small muscle sparing thoracotomies are often simpler and are equally well tolerated. Significant differences of postoperative length of stay are difficult to demonstrate.[31] The video systems technically make the procedure much more user-friendly for the entire operative team. Unfortunately, thoracoscopy requires differential lung ventilation, increases intraoperative costs,

| **TABLE 25-4** |
| --- |
| **Positive Findings During Digital Thoracotomy** |
| Tense, ballotable pericardium without cardiac pulsation, suggesting hemo pericardium |
| Pleural symphysis from previous trauma or disease |
| Palpable holes in the pericardium or diaphragm |
| Palpable abdominal organs herniated through a tear in the diaphragm |

and does not clearly result in shorter hospital stays. Thoracoscopy has had its greatest application in chest trauma for early evacuation of clotted hemothorax.

## EXTRACORPOREAL SUPPORT DEVICES

There continues to be significant interest in the use of external cardiopulmonary support devices for trauma patients, particularly those with thoracic injuries. There are pneumatic, mechanical, and hand-driven devices to perform external cardiac massage. Although they are very popular with the EMS, there are very few reports of survivors with these devices. We have found no single trauma patient with truncal injuries who has survived as a result of the use of one of these devices. The intraaortic balloon pump has been used after elective cardiac surgery to support the failing heart. It has been used in a small number of patients with posttraumatic myocardial dysfunction, heart failure, or congestive heart failure, and has been considered to be lifesaving in certain instances.[35] Unfortunately, many trauma patients have tachycardia and significant dysrhythmias such that the intra-aortic balloon pump is unable to track their rhythm and provide adequate counterpulsation. Also, patients with low systemic vascular resistance get little augmentation during counterpulsation. The intraaortic balloon pump is most efficacious in posttraumatic cardiac failure caused by direct cardiac injury such as an unrevascularizable coronary artery injury or bridge support of an exacerbation of pre-existing congestive heart failure. More applications in trauma for similar devices are anticipated.

Cardiopulmonary bypass may be indicated for proximal coronary artery injuries, posttraumatic massive pulmonary embolism, acute valvular and septal lesions that are hemodynamically unstable, and myocardial or ascending aortic rupture.[36] Reports of heparin-bonded circuits and heparinless cardiopulmonary bypass resulted in a few survivors with massive trauma. However, this approach requires a significant commitment of resources per patient and is extremely expensive. Acute cardiopulmonary bypass is commonly reserved for the high proximal left anterior descending coronary artery lesions, ascending aortic and arch injuries, or refractory intracardiac injuries.[21]

The centrifugal pump can be used to augment flow without the need for total body heparinization. These are most commonly used for left heart bypass for operations on the descending thoracic aorta. It may also be used to bypass retrohepatic vena caval injuries and portal venous injuries to avoid the problems of passive shunts. This technology has also been applied to hypothermic patients for rewarming and in the treatment of severe adult respiratory distress syndrome.[37]

## EVOLVING IMAGING ISSUES

### Angiography

Angiography in the patient with penetrating injuries to the chest is most useful to visualize the brachiocephalic vessels. As the incisions for proximal control and repair are different for each injury, angiography, if the patient's status permits, significantly aids in planning the operation. Angiography for penetrating trauma to the aorta itself has significant pitfalls. The large column of contrast agent in the aorta allows small, subtle injuries to be missed. If angiography is to be used for a patient with a potential penetrating aortic injury, a view tangential to the anticipated missile path should be obtained so that small pseudoaneurysms may be visualized.

Angiography continues to be the "gold standard" for the evaluation of blunt injury to the aorta.[14] It allows visualization of the entire thoracic aorta, multiple injuries, and multiple veins. It defines arch vessel congenital anomalies that are common and can significantly affect conduct of the operation.

### Computed Tomography

Many centers now use a multidetector CT scan for the initial evaluation of blunt injury to the thoracic aorta. These scanners require much shorter scan times in the unstable patient. In addition, the higher resolution available may suggest an injury or small intimal flap. Furthermore, three-dimensional reconstructions eventually may allow visualization equivalent to aortography. The development of small portable CT scanners may allow their use in the intensive care unit. Fabian and coworkers showed promising results and suggested more work was needed in this area.[14] Currently however, few surgeons would operate based on CT scan alone, and angiography is still the standard confirmatory test. As experience is gained with the algorithms for 3D reconstruction, CT scan may become increasingly important.

When evaluating the aorta, it is philosophically helpful to distinguish screening examinations from diagnostic and planning examinations. Classically, patients would be screened with history, physical examination, and plain chest x-ray-then the diagnosis made with aortography. Other examinations such as CT scan or transesophageal echocardiography have been incorporated into the screening process. Aortography, however, is still currently the diagnostic and planning examination in most centers prior to repair. Thus, it is helpful to remember that the screening examinations have much different objectives and limitations than the diagnostic and planning investigations such as aortography.

### Transesophageal Echocardiography

Transesophageal echocardiography (TEE) continues to be championed by many for evaluation of the descending thoracic aorta.[38-40] It is also useful for evaluating cardiac function and traumatic intracardiac lesions. It is a modality noted to be very technician- or operator-dependent. During evaluation of the aorta, even with multiplane technology, there are blind areas due to the tracheal air column such as the aortic arch and innominate junction. TEE may be useful as a screening test, particularly in the hands of surgeons who are skilled in its use. This might apply to the patient already in the operating room during laparotomy or to an unstable patient in the intensive care unit who would not tolerate being moved to the arteriogram suite. It may also be useful to follow a patient with a questionable aortogram. As many patients already undergo CT with the multidetector technology, TEE seems to lately be less often utilized.

### Surgeon-Performed Ultrasound

The surgeon-performed ultrasound exam of the pericardium and peritoneal cavity has been a significant advance in the care of the trauma patient.[41–43] The initial view is a subxiphoid window visualizing the liver, heart, and pericardium and is anticipated to become the standard of care for diagnosing pericardial tamponade. In many centers the abdominal component of the FAST examination has been abandoned, leaving the pericardial view as the most useful. By avoiding the use of ionizing radiation, this test can also be repeated as many times as needed to follow a patient. It is most useful when positive, and local experience varies. The FAST exam can be used prior to laparotomy for thoracoabdominal trauma, thus virtually eliminating the need for subxiphoid pericardiotomy and pericardiocentesis. Like all examinations, it is important to recognize the local experience with this modality.

## SUMMARY

Thoracic injury accounts for significant morbidity and mortality in the trauma patient. The majority of thoracic injuries can be managed conservatively or with tube thoracostomy alone; however, the more unstable presentations require significant diagnostic and therapeutic decisions. Managing the thoracoabdominal injury is a pitfall for which no specific integrated algorithm currently exists. The choice of incision is guided by clinical judgment, road maps provided by imaging, or the surgeon's best guess of the anticipated pathology. New technology, such as extracorporeal support devices, thoracoscopy, multidetector CT, portable CT, and ultrasound technology, may affect the approach to the patient with thoracic injuries. Limitation of fluid resuscitation while managing penetrating thoracic injuries may decrease mortality and postoperative complications.

## REFERENCES

1. LoCicero J, Mattox KL: Epidemiology of chest trauma. *Surg Clin North Am* 69:15, 1989.
2. Breasted JH: *The Edwin Smith Surgical Papyrus,* vol. 1. Chicago: University of Chicago Press, 1930.
3. Sparkman RS, Nixon PI, Croswait RW, et al. In: Sparkman RS, ed. *The Texas Surgical Society: The First Fifty Years.* Dallas: Texas Surgical Society, 1965, p. 3.
4. Berry FB: Historical note. In: Coates JB, ed. *Surgery in World War II, Thoracic Surgery.* Washington, DC: Office of the Surgeon General, Department of the Army, 1963, vol. 1, p. 3.
5. Richardson JD, Flint LM, Snow NJU, et al.: Management of transmediastinal gunshot wounds. *Surgery* 90:671, 1981.
6. Durham LA, Richardson R, Wall MJ Jr, et al.: Emergency center thoracotomy: Impact of prehospital resuscitation. *J Trauma* 32:775, 1992.
7. Working Group, Ad Hoc Subcommittee on Outcomes, American College of Surgeons Committee on Trauma: Practice management guidelines for emergency department thoracotomy. *J Amer Coll Surg* 193:303, 2001.
8. Hirshberg A, Mattox KL, Wall MJ Jr: Double jeopardy: Thoracoabdominal injuries requiring surgery in both chest and abdomen. *J Trauma* 39:1, 1995.
9. Bonnin MJ, Pepe PE, Kimball KT, et al.: Distinct criteria for termination of resuscitation in the out-of-hospital setting. *JAMA* 270:1457, 1993.
10. American College of Surgeons Committee on Trauma: *Advanced Trauma Life Support Manual.* Chicago, IL: American College of Surgeons, 1997.
11. Trinkle JK, Furman RW, Hiushaw MA, et al.: Pulmonary contusion: Pathogenesis and effect of various resuscitative measures. *Ann Thorac Surg* 16:568, 1973.
12. Bickel WH, Wall MJ, Pepe PE, et al.: Immediate versus delayed fluid resuscitation for hypotensive patients with penetrating torso injuries. *N Engl J Med* 331:1105, 1994.
13. Wall MJ Jr, Mattox KL, Wolf DA: The cardiac pendulum: Blunt rupture of the pericardium with strangulation of the heart. *J Trauma* 59:136, 2005.
14. Fabian TC, Richardson JD, Croce MA, et al.: Prospective study of blunt aortic injury: Multicenter trial of the American Association for the Surgery of Trauma. *J Trauma* 42:374, 1997.
15. Karmy-Jones R, Jukovich GJ, Shatz D, et al.: Urgent thoracotomy for hemorrhage following trauma: A multicenter study. *Arch Surg* 136:513, 2001.
16. Mattox KL, Beall AC Jr, Ennix CC, et al.: Intravascular migratory bullets. *Am J Surg* 137:192, 1979.
17. Burch JM, Feliciano DV, Mattox KL: The atriocaval shunt. Facts and fiction. *Ann Surg* 207:555, 1988.
18. Ledgerwood AM, Kazmers M, Lucas CE: The role of thoracic aortic occlusion for massive hemoperitoneum. *J Trauma* 16:610, 1976.
19. Coselli JS, Mattox KL, Beall AC Jr: Reevaluation of early evacuation of clotted hemothorax. *Am J Surg* 148:786, 1984.
20. McCollum CH, Graham JM, Noon GP, et al.: Chronic traumatic aneurysms of the thoracic aorta: An analysis of 50 patients. *J Trauma* 19:248, 1979.
21. Wall MJ Jr, Mattox KL, Chen C, et al.: Acute management of complex cardiac injuries. *J Trauma* 42:905, 1997.
22. Moore BP: Operative stabilization of nonpenetrating chest injuries. *J Thorac Cardiovasc Surg* 70:619, 1975.
23. Feliciano DV, Mattox KL: Indications, technique, and pitfalls of emergency center thoracotomy. *Surg Rounds* 4:32, 1981.
24. Wall MJ Jr, Mattox KL, DeBakey ME: Injuries to the azygous venous system. *J Trauma* 60:357, 2006.
25. Schaff HV, Brawley RK: The operative management of penetrating vascular injuries of the thoracic outlet. *Surgery* 82:1822, 1977.
26. Rotondo MF, Schwab CW, McGonigal MD, et al.: Damage control: An approach for improved survival in exsanguinating penetrating abdominal injury. *J Trauma* 35:375, 1993.
27. Wall MJ Jr, Villavicencio RT, Miller CC, et al.: Pulmonary tractotomy as an abbreviated thoracotomy technique. *J Trauma* 45:1015, 1998.
28. Huh J, Wall MJ Jr, Estrera AL, et al.: Surgical management of traumatic pulmonary injury. *Amer J Surg* 186:620, 2003.
29. Wilson A, Wall MJ Jr, Maxson RT, et al.: Pulmonary hilum twist as damage control procedure for severe lung injury. *Am J Surg* 186:49, 2003.
30. Wall MJ Jr, Soltero E: Damage control for thoracic injuries. *Surg Clin North Am* 77:863, 1997.
31. Mancini M, Smith LM, Nein A, et al.: Early evacuation of clotted blood in hemothorax using thoracoscopy: Case reports. *J Trauma* 34:144, 1993.
32. Branco JMJ: Thoracoscopy as a method of exploration in penetrating injuries of the thorax. *Dis Chest* 12:330, 1946.
33. Senno A: Thoracoscopy with the fiberoptic bronchoscope. *J Thorac Cardiovasc Surg* 67:606, 1974.
34. Jones JW, Kitahama A, Webb WR, et al.: Emergency thoracoscopy: A logical approach to chest trauma management. *J Trauma* 21:280, 1981.
35. Snow N, Lucas A, Richardson D: Intra-aortic balloon counter-pulsation for cardiogenic shock from cardiac contusion. *J Trauma* 22:426, 1982.
36. Mattox KL, Beall AC: Resuscitation of the moribund patient using portable cardiopulmonary bypass. *Ann Thorac Surg* 22:436, 1976.
37. Anderson HL, Shapiro MB, Delius RE, et al.: Extracorporeal life support for respiratory failure after multiple trauma. *J Trauma* 37:266, 1994.
38. Kearney PA, Smith DW, Johnson SB, et al.: Use of transesophageal echocardiography in the evaluation of traumatic aortic injury. *J Trauma* 34:696, 1993.
39. Hiatt JR, Yeatman LA, Child JS: The value of echocardiography in blunt chest trauma. *J Trauma* 28:914, 1988.
40. Fernandez LG, Lain KY, Messersmith RN, et al.: Trans-esophageal echocardiography for diagnosing aortic injury. A case report and summary of current imaging techniques. *J Trauma* 36:877, 1994.
41. Hauenstein KH, Wimmer B, Billmann P, et al.: The role of sonography in blunt abdominal trauma. *Radiology* 22:106, 1982.
42. Tso P, Rodriguez A, Cooper C, et al.: Sonography in blunt abdominal trauma: A preliminary progress report. *J Trauma* 33:39, 1992.
43. Rozycki GS, Ochsner MG, Jaffin JH, et al.: Prospective evaluation of surgeons' use of ultrasound in the evaluation of trauma patients. *J Trauma* 34:516, 1993.
44. Washington B, Wilson RF, Steiger Z, et al.: Emergency thoracotomy: A four year review. *Ann Thorac Surg* 40:188, 1985.
45. Bricker DL, Noon GP, Beall AC Jr, et al.: Vascular injuries of the thoracic outlet. *J Trauma* 10:1, 1970.
46. Grover FL, Ellestad C, Arom KV, et al.: Diagnosis and management of major tracheobronchial injuries. *Ann Thorac Surg* 28:384, 1979.
47. Kirsh MM, Orringer MB, Behrendt DM, et al.: Management of tracheobronchial disruptions secondary to blunt trauma. *Ann Thorac Surg* 22:93, 1976.
48. Defore WW, Mattox KL, Hansen HA, et al.: Surgical management of penetrating injuries of the esophagus. *Am J Surg* 134:734, 1977.
49. Reul GJ, Beall AC Jr, Jordan GL Jr, et al.: The early operative management of injuries to the great vessels. *Surgery* 74:862, 1973.
50. Mattox KL, Pickard LR, Allen MK, et al.: Suspecting thoracic aortic transection. *J Am Coll Emerg Phys* 7:12, 1978.
51. Mattox KL, Beall AC Jr, Ennix CL, et al.: Intravascular migratory bullets. *Am J Surg* 137:192, 1979.
52. Yellin AE, Chaffee CB, Donovan JD: Vascular isolation in treatment of juxtahepatic venous injuries. *Arch Surg* 102:506, 1971.

# Commentary ■ RICARDO FERRADA

Trauma to the chest is quite common in Cali, Colombia, South America. Most of our patients arrive with penetrating trauma, and majority due to gunshot wounds. The following comments are on what we have learned with this specific type of trauma, and what we do in routine practice.

Once inside the thoracic cavity, the surgeon must perform several maneuvers almost simultaneously, however, the first one is crucial in our opinion: *The assessment of endotracheal tube position.* If the patient arrives in agonal condition, the correct position of the endotracheal tube is a crucial step taking one or two seconds, by verifying the movements of the lungs with the anesthesiologist's insufflations. Even in experienced hands, fatal esophageal intubation is possible. In this particular situation, the anesthesiologist has no time to verify the correct position of the tube, which among others, is usually made by auscultation of the thorax. Auscultation is not possible in this setting due to the speed of the maneuvers and because at the same time the surgeons are preparing the area with iodine. Esophageal intubation results in severe hypoxemia, and due to the patient's previously agonal condition, irreversible cardiac arrest follows.

As the authors point out, the type of incision is very important. A correctly-chosen incision can make the procedure easier, however an error at this point can result in catastrophic consequences. Before the thoracotomy is made, the surgeon does not know what structure is compromised. Many of these patients have injuries to many structures, which must be treated at this time or at least controlled. Accordingly, the majority of the patients require an incision that allows easy exploration of the entire cavity and access for repair to the potentially injured structures. For these reasons, the incision used most often is the left submammary anterolateral because it can be made with basic instruments, it is very fast and it allows management of most of the thoracic viscera, including the heart.

The incision on the skin is made 1 cm below the nipple in males, and in females below the breast by mobilizing the gland cephalad in order to avoid cutting through breast tissue. In both, the thoracic cavity is accessed through the fourth or fifth space, and by cutting the upper cartilage with the edge of the knife up.

Thoracotomy through the third space for proximal control on the left side has been suggested. This incision is not only of no use in bleeding trauma patients, but is also troublesome. On the third space the pectoral muscle is bulky and thick, and as a consequence, the access is laborious, takes a lot of time, and the exposure is extremely limited. As already noted, in injured and unstable patients the access has to be fast and easy and the exposure wide.

During a two-year period, we performed 242 urgent thoracotomies at the University Hospital in Cali, Colombia. During this period, use of the open-book incision was not necessary.

When the hemorrhage is exsanguinating, the aorta must be occluded, which is an easy maneuver. However, unless the surgeon is very experienced, it is wiser to use fingers rather than a clamp at this moment. Clamping without direct inspection can result in injury to the esophagus or to the small branches of the aorta. The surgeon should not plan to palpate the aorta for this purpose, since it is empty. Instead, the fingers are placed against the vertebral bodies as a temporary occlusion. Once the aorta has been identified, the assistant must be asked to do the clamping. This frees the surgeon to perform other maneuvers, but more importantly, avoids tremors in his hands resulting from the effort. In these cases, it is very important that the surgeon remain mentally and physically calm.

The initial occlusion is made with the fingers. However, the hands inside the thoracic cavity prevent intrathoracic visualization of injuries and repair. For this reason, the next step is to apply a vascular clamp on the aorta. For this purpose, the pleura must be opened in order to put the clamp under direct view. The clamp is applied laterally, not transversely, to avoid iatrogenic injuries to the esophagus and aortic branches.

Myocardial suture. After pericardial tamponade is released, hemodynamic status improves but tachycardia usually persists. It is wiser not to suture the myocardium at this time because of increased difficulty. Instead, a finger should be placed on the wound, thus avoiding blood loss, and the surgeon should then wait for a few minutes until the cardiac rhythm becomes normal. Besides the intravenous (IV) fluids, the anesthesiologist can help to lower the frequency, which makes the suture much easier to manage.

Most of these patients are young, and interrupted simple sutures without pledgets are well tolerated. However, since patients older than 50 and/or with previous hypertension have friable myocardium, Teflon or pericardium felt pads are used. In the latter group of patients, all caution should be taken to avoid myocardial tearing by following the heart movements. Nonabsorbable suture such as silk or tycron is used, with a nontraumatic needle. Polypropylene can also be used, but the authors' preference is the former because it has no memory and consequently the knots are faster and safer. It is much easier to use two needle holders: one for the surgeon and the other for the assistant, who receives the needle at the moment of suturing.

One problem not found in the articles on the subject is heart dilatation during the procedure. An increase must be assumed to be acute cardiac failure and the surgeon must perform a manual massage. In our experience, other techniques, like clamping the caval veins, lead to cardiac arrest. If after anterolateral submammary thoracotomy the heart is significantly larger than the pericardial sac, a prosthetic material can be used to enlarge the sac. We have used IV fluids in the same way (and guided by the same concepts) as for management of abdominal compartment syndrome If available, a polytetrafluoroethylene (PTFE) or Dacron prosthesis may be used, with the advantage that a return to the operating room may not be necessary.

Transmediastinal stable patients are uncommon but controversial. For years we have performed multislice CT scan in these particular cases and have found that this diagnostic approach is cost-effective, and with no false negative or false positive result so far.

## References

1. Ferrada R, Garcia AF: Torso Penetrating Trauma. *Advances in Trauma and Critical Care* 8:85, 1993.
2. Ferrada R: Trauma Cardíaco. Manejo Operatorio. *Rev Col Cirugía* 16:5, 2001.
3. Ferrada R, Mejia W: Toracotomia de Resuscitacion. *S Am J Thorac Surg* 7:64, 2001.
4. Ferrada R, Rivera D, Ramos LG: *Emergency and Resuscitative Thoracotomy. Patient Management Problems in Trauma.* ACS Committee on Trauma, BC Decker, 2004.

# Chest Wall and Lung

*David H. Livingston* ■ *Carl J. Hauser*

Thoracic injuries are common following both penetrating and blunt trauma and it has been estimated that chest injuries are responsible for 20 to 25% of all trauma deaths. Chest injuries are also common in multiply injured patients and are a major contributing factor in the development of subsequent organ failure.

## CHEST TRAUMA IN HISTORY

Despite the potentially lethal nature of many chest injuries, evidence exists that early man both sustained and survived blunt and penetrating chest trauma. A Neanderthal skeleton unearthed in Shanidar Cave, in Iraq, showed evidence of a healing of a penetrating wound across the left ninth rib. A second skeleton at that site revealed multiple healed rib fractures.[1] Thoracic injuries continued to be an important focus during the early history of trauma care. The Edwin Smith Papyrus, written at the time of the Great Pyramid, circa 3000 BC, gave explicit instructions as to the management of a wide variety of chest injuries. These included "wounds in the breast," "diseased (infected) wounds in the breast," "breaks in the ribs of the breast," "dislocation in the ribs of the breast," and both "breaks" and "dislocations in the collar-bone".[2] Of special interest, the author showed considerable clinical judgment in draining infections with a "fire-drill," in the avoidance of occlusive dressings for wounds that were draining pus, and in declining to treat self-limited conditions such as isolated simple rib fractures. In fact, eight of the 43 cases discussed concerned chest injuries, suggesting that even at that time, chest injuries accounted for 20–25% of all trauma. In classical Greek times, Pythagoras states that Euphorbus died of a chest wound in the battle over the body of Patroclus, and Hippocrates recognized that if empyemas were not drained the patient would die. In the 19th century, there was controversy over whether Hippocrates' approach was correct, because opening the chest could cause asphyxia if the lung collapsed. Also, occasionally clear fluid would be found which would then "putrefy." Thus in 1835, when Napoleon's personal physician Dupuytren developed an empyema, he stated that "he would rather die at the hands of God than of surgeons" and refused surgery. Twelve days later he got his wish! Trousseau finally established trocar drainage as the definitive treatment for empyema.

In modern trauma care, the approach to thoracic injuries typically depends upon the mechanism (penetrating vs. blunt), severity (life threatening vs. stable), and the location of injury (chest wall vs. pleura vs. lung). While these somewhat arbitrary divisions can provide a useful mechanism to describe the injuries and their proper management, they should not give the reader the impression that injury to the chest is truly compartmentalized; such is not the case. This chapter does examine specific chest injuries, but it also attempts to outline a global approach and a continuum of care for the trauma patient with chest injuries. We begin with the initial evaluation and management, proceed with diagnosis and treatment management of thoracic injuries, and conclude with important ward and critical care aspects of these patients.

## HISTORY AND PHYSICAL EXAMINATION IN CHEST TRAUMA

Speed is of the essence in the management of all major or unstable trauma patients. Thus, by necessity the history and physical examination should be kept to the bare essentials in the more critical injuries, whereas they may be more detailed in lesser injuries. The Advanced Trauma Life Support (ATLS) approach[3] to management of major trauma stresses the simultaneous diagnosis and management of conditions that can kill the patient rapidly by asphyxia or circulatory arrest. Many of these conditions are chest injuries. Thus the physical examination of the chest is performed during the ATLS "Primary Survey," and optimally it will be fully integrated into the resuscitation of the patient.

## History

Wherever patients can give a history this should be sought, and patients with chest injuries will typically complain of chest pain and shortness of breath, and may point to their pathology. Patients with a major chest injury however, will usually be unable to give a useful history. Whenever available therefore, a "field history" should be obtained from the prehospital providers (or occasionally from the patient) as the patient is transferred off of the stretcher. Whether the patient has a penetrating or blunt mechanism of injury is a key initial concern. Subsequently, in blunt injuries, a history of the type of impact, of vehicular intrusion, entrapment or ejection may give important clues as to the degree of energy transfer. In penetrating injuries, any available descriptions as to the weapons used, the number or direction of the shots fired, of the size of knife, or of the caliber of the gun used may yield important early clues as to the likelihood of subsequent deterioration. Field vital signs, transport times, and records of fluids administered to the patient prior to or in transport should be reviewed and documented, since they give vital clues as to patient's stability. In situations where patients are transferred from another hospital, the care of the patient at the referring institution and any available radiographs should be carefully reviewed and documented. Other significant historical details can often be inferred from physical examination, such as the presence of operative scars.

## Physical Examination

### General inspection of the patient.

The key to effective trauma management is to minimize the time to definitive treatment of life-threatening conditions. The initial physical examination in chest trauma is therefore focused and abbreviated. After assessment of the airway, the patient is completely uncovered and rapidly inspected while the vital signs are assessed. Frank hypotension or tachycardia, or the presence of ashen or cyanotic skin color suggests shock. In the presence of a known or suspected thoracic injury, shock must be assumed to be from an intra-thoracic source. If not already endotracheally intubated, such patients should undergo rapid sequence intubation and control of the airway[4] prior to any further diagnostic evaluation. Presumptive chest tube placement on limited evidence will often be indicated and may be life-saving in this subset of patients. Patients with parasternal penetrating wounds who insist on sitting bolt upright or who show agitation, confusion, or air hunger have a very high likelihood of pericardial tamponade. Diaphoresis is also a common presentation of low-flow states such as tamponade, and all such signs commonly precede the development of hypotension in young trauma patients with tamponade. Distension of the neck veins may suggest either tension pneumothorax or pericardial tamponade, but this sign is often unreliable, and may occur when patients grunt or bear down against a closed glottis (Valsalva) due to pain. Similarly, the absence of neck vein distension does not exclude either pericardial tamponade or tension pneumothorax, especially in hypovolemic patients. Although tracheal deviation is also frequently cited as a sign of tension pneumothorax, in practice it is rarely if ever seen, even in patients with mediastinal deviation on chest x-ray (Fig. 26-1).

The inspection of the chest per se should also be rapid. Intercostal and supraclavicular retractions may suggest airway obstruction. The chest wall should also be seen to rise symmetrically. The

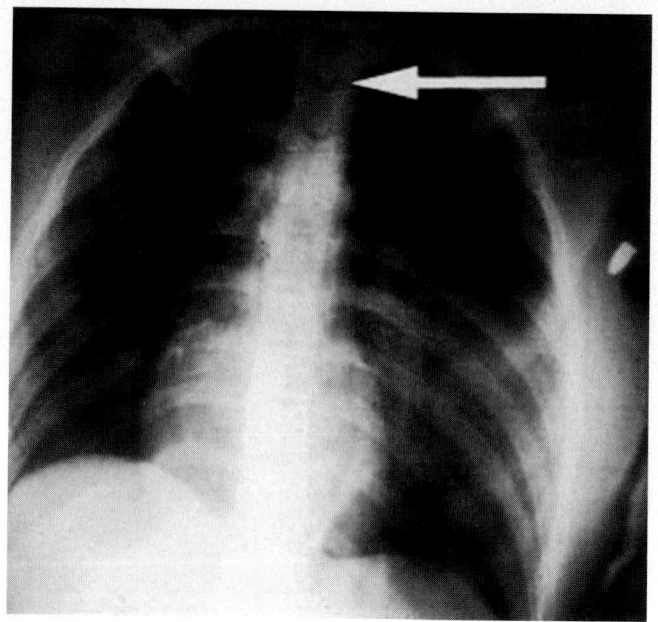

**FIGURE 26-1.** Tension pneumothorax showing normal tracheal positioning in the neck (arrow) despite the presence of a mediastinal shift.

number and distribution of wounds should be evaluated. Abrasions, sucking chest wounds, subcutaneous emphysema, crepitus, and unstable "flail" segments of the chest wall should be noted. Occasionally, information as to the course of a penetrating wound may be suggested. However, the time spent evaluating what are essentially forensic considerations may delay attention to more physiologically important processes, and this should be avoided. Moreover, experienced examiners come to recognize that assumptions as to trajectory based on inspection of the wounds often turn out to be incorrect.

Remember, it is crucial to examine the patient's back (Fig. 26-2). In blunt trauma this requires "logrolling" the patient, noting that airway security and ventilation must be assured first. In penetrating injuries however, the risk of vertebral instability is remote.[5] Thus, formal "logrolling precautions" may represent more of an impediment to rapid diagnosis of a potentially lethal injury than any protection against spinal cord injury. Good clinical judgment is the best guide as to whether such precautions will be required or not.

## Palpation

Palpation of the chest is both rapid and informative in chest trauma, but unfortunately it is often overlooked. Mobile segments of chest wall and sternum can often be palpated even when not visible on inspection. It is often helpful in spontaneously breathing patients to place both hands on the two hemithoraces and palpate the symmetry of chest wall motion. Crepitance is a common finding in chest trauma. The examiner should distinguish between the finer crepitance of subcutaneous emphysema and the coarse crepitations felt with movement of broken ribs. In cooperative patients, the presence and location of pain on lateral and anterior-posterior (AP) chest compression may help in localizing chest wall trauma. Point tenderness is rarely noted in multiple trauma where patients have significant distracting injuries or an altered level of consciousness, but it may be very helpful in localizing lesser injuries such as isolated rib fractures and costochondral injuries.

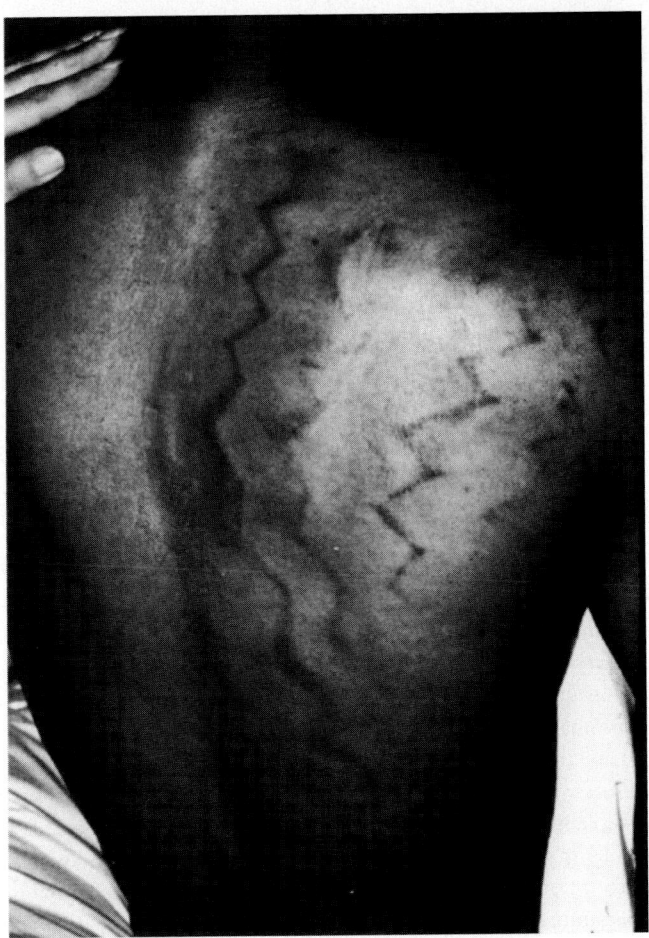

**FIGURE 26-2.** Significant trauma to the back that would be concealed without rolling the patient to ensure a compete physical examination.

## Auscultation and Percussion

Accurate, rapid auscultation of the chest maintains a central role in the modern management of chest injuries. In practice, however, auscultation of the chest is always suboptimal in trauma. This is especially so in the setting of multiple trauma in the busy trauma-room setting. In essence, auscultation of the chest in trauma has very poor sensitivity but a high specificity. During the initial management of chest trauma, the examiner should therefore simply focus on the presence and symmetry of air entry. An abnormal examination (i.e., absent or asymmetric breath sounds) will then have a high specificity for life threatening pathology and will often lead to an intervention. In the unstable patient such interventions will often be immediate (e.g., manipulation of the endotracheal tube or placement of a chest tube) and the effect of the intervention should be checked by the normalization of breath sounds on repeated examination. Absence or markedly diminished breath sounds *does not* mandate diagnostic tests such as chest x-rays (CXR) but often indicate immediate intervention, and CXR is often contraindicated in unstable patients. Findings of untreated high-grade pathology, such as large hemo- or pneumothoraces on CXR are evidence of the failure of physical diagnosis. Conversely, a negative auscutatory examination (i.e., symmetric breath sounds) is frequent in the presence of early intra-thoracic pathology. Thus, normal breath sounds should never be assumed to confirm the absence of significant intrathoracic injury and small, asymptomatic

hemo- or pneumothoraces will be assessed radiologically prior to selection of management options. Patients who are *in extremis* with suspected chest injury will on occasion warrant empiric placement of bilateral chest tubes on the basis of their hemodynamic presentation alone.

As with auscultation, the thoracic percussion note can often be difficult to hear in crowded, noisy environments although it may sometimes be possible to sense an enhanced or dulled percussion note digitally. Again, though, a clearly positive finding suggests advanced pathology and rapid intervention rather than diagnostic dalliances. Heart sounds are also poorly heard in the trauma bay environment, and specific physical signs such as Beck's triad for tamponade and Hamman's sign for mediastinal air are rarely if ever found. Thus, detailed auscutation of heart sounds in trauma is seldom productive.

## DIAGNOSTIC RADIOLOGY IN CHEST TRAUMA

### Overview

Radiology plays a central role in the management of chest trauma, and every trauma surgeon needs to be facile in the rapid interpretation of the suboptimal, supine, AP CXR. In addition, though, emerging technologies for imaging the chest are in rapid evolution. These may hold enormous promise for improving diagnostic accuracy in chest trauma, but their integration into the care of chest trauma must be approached with great caution. The potentially rapidly lethal nature of chest trauma creates a conundrum: over-reliance on imaging techniques, or an insistence on levels of diagnostic accuracy that can only be achieved at the expense of time delays can easily lead to death.

Radiological tests in acute chest trauma should therefore always be aimed at functional and practical ends. Each available imaging modality, traditional or novel, needs to be directed toward very specific ends within the context of specific types of clinical injury. Films destined to end up in "teaching files" such as large tension pneumothoraces with mediastinal shift and depression of the diaphragm, are often films that should never have been taken. Similarly, fast helical computed tomography (CT) may detect pericardial fluid very well, but patients suspected of a traumatic hemopericardium may deteriorate rapidly and should never be placed in a CT scanner. In patients demonstrating marginal hemodynamic stability, any time spent obtaining CT scans for any purpose imposes some risk of deterioration and death. These risks should only be accepted after careful weighing of the potential benefits of the test. Moreover, such patients may be better managed by empiric interventions with or without rapid bedside tests such as focused ultrasonography (US) depending on their level of hemodynamic stability and the clinical level of suspicion for an injury.

Thus, in the early management of chest trauma, the exquisitely accurate diagnostic studies now available may be less appropriate than rapidly obtained studies performed at the bedside which, while less accurate, yield working diagnoses that can be used to protect the patient from acute deterioration. In effect, often the more spectacular an x-ray is, the less likely it is that it was indicated; and impressive appearing x-rays may often suggest poor clinical skills.

After potential immediate causes of respiratory and hemodynamic deterioration are excluded or treated, it may be safe and highly productive to investigate the patient's injuries in detail using advanced imaging modalities. It is clear, though, that the role of advanced imaging in acute trauma is in rapid evolution. As imaging technologies become more portable they may be brought to the patient's bedside more readily. Moreover, as imaging becomes more rapid and accurate, the risks of delay in management during evaluation will diminish and the diagnostic benefits obtained may justify new patient care algorithms. Thus new imaging technologies will always have to justify their integration into the management of chest trauma in the context of the nature of the problems they seek to address, as well as in the context of the system- and operator-specific advantages and limitations of those technologies.

## Traditional X-Rays

At present, the AP CXR performed in the trauma receiving area is the single most valuable diagnostic study in the management of chest trauma (Fig. 26-3). The CXR is performed early in the ATLS secondary survey. It must be accepted that the CXR is taken under adverse conditions in trauma and so is both less sensitive and specific than classic standing postero-anterior and lateral chest films taken in a dedicated radiology suite. Backboards are of variable x-ray compatibility, and x-ray incompatible boards should be changed when patients are logrolled to examine the back. The trauma CXR is also often done using portable x-ray equipment. It may be a suboptimal projection, and can be limited in penetration, especially in obese or muscular individuals. Nonetheless, the AP portable CXR still diagnoses or excludes a wide variety of immediately life-threatening pathology. In major chest trauma, therefore, the CXR is

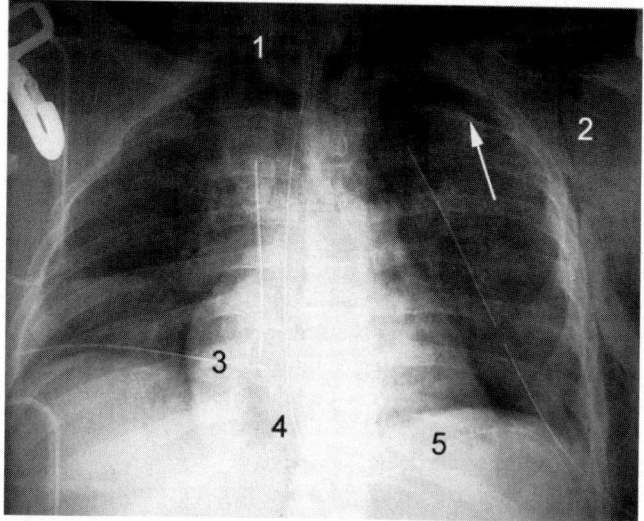

**FIGURE 26-3.** The importance of the screening AP CXR in the care of the patient with severe chest trauma is exemplified by many findings on this radiograph. The endotracheal tube inserted in the field is too high and needs to be advanced (1). A persistent pneumothorax (white arrow) and subcutaneous emphysema is present (2) despite the apparent good position of an emergent left chest tube. The right-sided chest tube is kinked at the last hole (3). There is gross displacement of the left sided ribs from their vertebral bodies (4) and a suspicion of a thoracic spine injury at T9-10. There are also posterior fractures of the left 9th and 10th ribs (5). Lastly, to facilitate further x-rays, the metallic clasp in the upper left needs to be removed from the board and returned to EMS.

always obtained and must be carefully reviewed in the trauma receiving area prior to any transport of the patient to any other area. In stable or minor injuries it may be possible to sit patients up to improve the CXR. Direct digital and computerized radiology systems now allow CXR images to be enhanced and manipulated. This may help to overcome some of the inherent shortcomings of these films.

The trauma CXR is evaluated first for evidence of pulmonary and pleural pathology. Radiological evaluation of the status of the lungs and pleura should be seen as an extension of the "Airway, Breathing and Circulation" (ABC) phases of the ATLS Primary Survey. The position of the endotracheal tube if present is noted, as is the expansion of the lungs. The presence of pneumo- or hemo-thoraces should be noted, and this information will help guide the patient's ventilatory and circulatory management. Pulmonary infiltrates suggesting contusions or aspiration are noted, and will help guide management of gas exchange. The mediastinum is next evaluated for widening, blurring of the aortic knob, apical "capping," or displacement of the left mainstem bronchus or nasogastric tube. Any of these may suggest an injury of the mediastinal great vessels and the potential for hemorrhage. The diaphragms are then evaluated for evidence of direct injury or elevation due to abdominal pathology.

Last, the ribs, clavicles, scapulae, and humerus are evaluated for fractures. Alignment of the thoracic and upper lumbar vertebrae should also be checked, recognizing that only the grossest vertebral pathology will be seen. Fractures provide important clues as to the degree of energy transfer to the thorax, and thus the potential for other, unrecognized injuries. Any indicated specific radiographs of the thoracic bony structures should be deferred until the patient has a stable airway, respiratory, and cardiovascular status. Bone films have no bearing on the acute care of the patient, and an inappropriate focus on them will often delay the recognition and care of truly life-threatening injuries. Scapular films are occasionally required for orthopedic purposes, but dedicated clavicle or sternal films are rarely needed. The thoracic spine should always be imaged prior to mobilizing blunt truncal trauma patients if physical examination cannot exclude instability of the axial spine. In patients with penetrating injuries however, thoracic spine stability is not an issue.[5] Rib fractures that appear on the initial screening CXR provides clear evidence of thoracic and torso trauma and the number of fractures have been associated with morbidity and mortality. Rib fractures that cannot be seen on a CXR will have little effect on the acute care of patients with low-energy trauma and thus dedicated "rib series" films as are often done in ambulatory patients are of little medical value and should be relegated to radiology museums. If documentation is truly needed, such patients can be evaluated with a low radiation noncontrasted CT. Occasionally fractures of the sternum may be symptomatic, and if needed, these can be evaluated either with computed tomograms or with lateral sternal films in an elective fashion.

## Contrast Studies

Traditional contrast studies are rarely obtained in chest trauma patients and are used most commonly in situations where there is concern for perforation of the esophagus. This is a very uncommon concern in blunt trauma, but it is occasionally necessary to evaluate esophageal integrity in otherwise stable patients with penetrating injuries that cross the mediastinum. Since water-soluble contrast studies miss approximately 15% of leaks seen on barium studies[6] and have significant potential for pulmonary toxicity in the event of aspiration,[7,8] barium is clearly the contrast agent of choice for this indication. There is no clear consensus, however, as to whether esophagography as opposed to esophagoscopy or direct operation should be the mainstay of diagnosis of esophageal injury.[9–11] Currently, computed tomography is widely used as a screening study to triage patients with gunshot wounds at high risk for traversing the mediastinum into those that do and do not require further evaluation.[12,13]

## Computed Tomography (CT)

Computed tomography of the chest using modern multidetector helical CT scanners machines has now begun an integral part of the evaluation and treatment of patients sustaining high energy torso trauma. Older studies prior to the development of helical CT suggested that while the CXR detected rib fractures better than CT, CT was much more sensitive for pneumothoraces, fluid collections, and infiltrates. CT was also much more specific than CXR for aortic injury. Nonetheless, in that patient cohort, the chest CT findings uncommonly led to changes in management. More recent studies by Omert[14] reported that CT discovers unsuspected injuries in about two-thirds of major trauma patients who have evidence of chest injury on their initial CXR. More importantly, when the CXR was abnormal the new CT findings resulted in significant management changes 20% of the time. In the patient described in Fig. 26-4, the pneumothorax on the chest CT was the only positive finding and resulted in the patient's admission to the hospital rather than discharge from the trauma receiving area. In patients with a high-energy mechanism of injury but a normal CXR, CT found new pathology in 39% of the cases, but those findings only led to changes in therapy in 5% of cases. Exadaktylos found significant pathology on CT even in patients with an ostensibly "normal" CXR.[15] Guerrero–Lopez found that chest CT changed initial management 30% of the time and was far more sensitive to the presence of spine injuries than plain films.[16] Greiser[17] noted an even higher rate of CT-based management changes than that reported by Omert.[14]

The application of rapid, multidetector helical CTs to the global diagnosis of high energy truncal trauma has led to a multitude of advances in the management of chest injuries.[18] CT of the thoracic spine is now considered the "gold standard" for identifying the extent of vertebral body injuries as well as the degree of involvement of the posterior elements.[16,18,19] CT is also especially helpful in excluding vertebral injuries at the cervico-thoracic junction, which is otherwise notoriously difficult to image.

Chest CT has also been shown to aid in the evaluation of pulmonary contusions by determining their extent and by possibly allowing early prediction of respiratory deterioration.[20] Widening of the mediastinum may suggest aortic injury, but this finding is nonspecific and CXR evaluation of the mediastinum is often difficult and error-prone.[21] High-quality chest CTs allow us to limit application of aortography with its risk and expense, to evaluation of patients with known or likely aortic injuries.[22–25] Several groups have also now shown that CT can be used effectively to triage hemodynamically stable patients with suspected transmediastinal penetration into groups that may be observed, or may benefit by selective management based upon the risk of injury to specific organs[12,26] (Fig. 26-5). There is now no question that chest CT has proven enormously beneficial in trauma. Nonetheless, appropriate concerns exist that its advantages must be balanced against potential increased costs, increased intravenous contrast exposure, and especially the need to avoid delays in the treatment of patients who may become unstable. In our experience, most of these concerns are unwarranted, since truncal CTs markedly expedite the diagnostic work-up of major blunt trauma patients[19]. It should also be recognized that fast multidetector helical scanners now allow complete

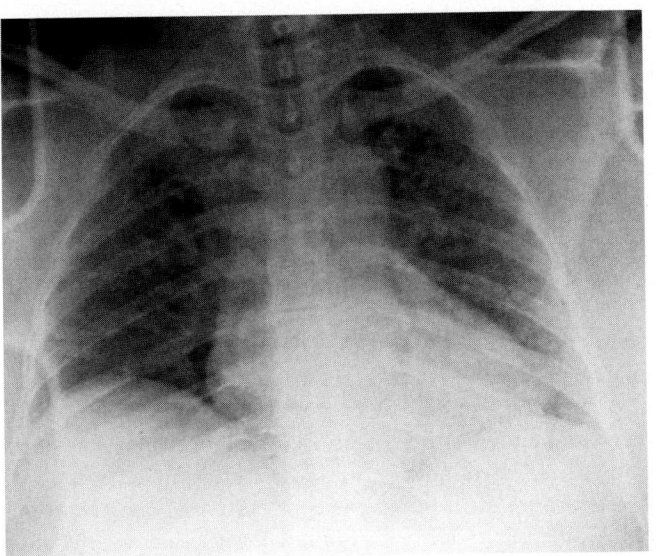

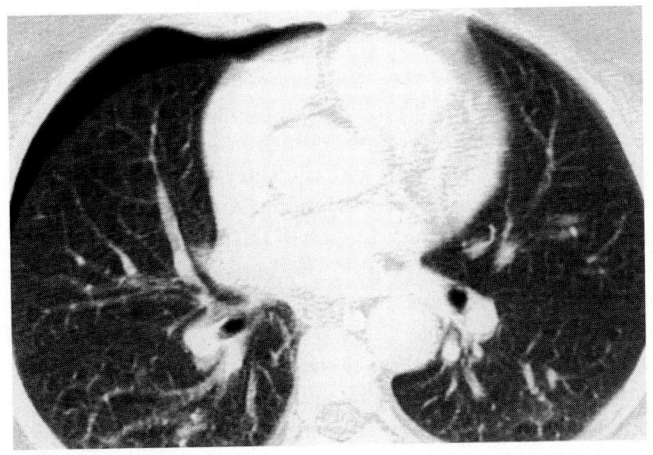

**A**                    **B**

**FIGURE 26-4.** CXR (**A**) of a 54-year-old patient involved in a MVC. The CT (**B**) disclosed an unsuspected pneumothorax, for which the patient was admitted and observed. Six hours later the follow-up CXR demonstrated that the pneumothorax was now visible and had increased in size. The patient was treated with a tube thoracostomy.

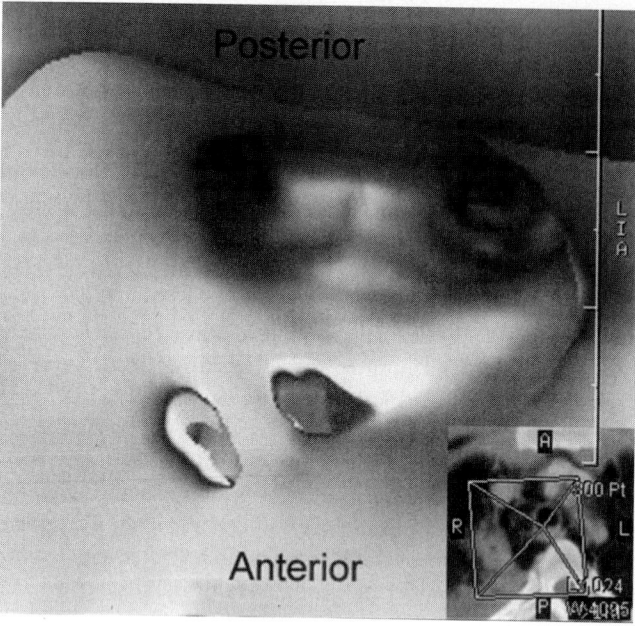

**FIGURE 26-5.** Virtual tracheoscopy using a multidetector CT for a transmediastinal GSW that demonstrated a tracheal injury. The anterior and posterior directions are "reversed" on the CT reconstruction. The injury could not be visualized by bronchoscopy even after the endotracheal tube was pulled back. A through and through injury of the trachea was found above the level of the azygous vein high in the chest.

integration of chest CT protocols with abdominal CT protocols currently used in the management of blunt truncal trauma. We now use focused offline reformatting of the original high-density data routinely to image injuries selectively on the basis of their appearance on the initial CT screen. Thus, definitive diagnosis of lesions found on screening CT can often be achieved without returning sick and often ventilator-dependent patients to the Radiology Department. We expect that with careful study, further appropriate clinical adaptations of emerging helical CT technology to trauma of the chest will be developed.

## Ultrasonography

Ultrasonography, and especially surgeon-performed focused sonography, now plays an important role in the diagnosis of intra-abdominal hemorrhage. An important by-product of that trend has been the application of ultrasound to the diagnosis of traumatic conditions of the chest. Sonography has rapidly become the gold standard for rapid diagnosis of traumatic pericardial fluid collections. A smaller number of reports now extend the use of sonography to evaluation of the pleural spaces. Sonography has inherent limitations for imaging of the pleural spaces because sound waves are reflected rather than transmitted by bone and air. Thus, these uses have been slower to develop. On the other hand, sonography is inexpensive and typically more rapid than conventional radiology, so its use in chest trauma would potentially be advantageous. Recent reports do suggest that sonography can be used to diagnose pneumothoraces and hemothoraces.[27–29] Thus with advances in ultrasound technology and further experience in its application, sonography may play an increasing important role in the early management of chest trauma.

## TRAUMA TO THE CHEST WALL

Direct injuries to the chest wall are common problem in clinical trauma. The most common causes of chest wall injuries and rib fractures in adults are motor vehicle crashes (MVC), falls, and blows to the chest with blunt objects. It is important to recall that rib fractures in infants and younger children occur almost exclusively in the setting of child abuse. In older pediatric populations, motor vehicles versus pedestrian accidents become the predominant mechanism of injury.

Injuries of the chest wall may vary enormously in severity depending upon the clinical circumstances where they are seen. In routine emergency room settings, chest trauma may be incurred as a result of a low-energy impact, and be relatively minor. In such cases, care is symptomatic only, and even plain chest radiography or rib series may be of little or no value.[30] On the other hand, chest injuries sustained by patients treated in trauma centers following high energy trauma from motor vehicle crashes are typically severe and are often life-threatening. Ziegler noted that in a population of over 7000 patients seen in a trauma center, 10% had rib fractures. Of the patients with rib fractures, 94% had associated injuries and 12% died. One-half required operations or admission to the intensive care unit (ICU), one-third developed pulmonary complications, and one-third were discharged to an extended care facility.[31]

Rib fractures are normally the hallmark of significant blunt chest trauma, and increasing numbers of rib fractures are related to increasing morbidity and mortality. The presence of greater than three rib fractures on CXR in adults is a marker for associated solid visceral trauma and mortality, and thus has been used as a marker for trauma center transfer.[32] In hemodynamically stable patients, the presence of blunt chest trauma has also been shown to double the rate of intra-abdominal injuries detected by abdominal CT.[33] Rib fractures are less common in children due to the resilience of their bony chest wall. Thus, children may suffer major intrathoracic injury without rib fractures and the presence of any rib fracture in a child should be considered a marker for severe injury.[34] The presence of acute rib fractures in a young child whose mechanism of injury is unclear or the finding of rib fractures of varying ages should also serve as an indicator for potential child abuse.[35,36] Conversely, elderly patients with brittle bones will occasionally have little in the way of intrathoracic injury despite extensive rib fractures.[37]

## Outcomes

Most deaths after chest wall injuries are the result of associated trauma, but severe chest wall trauma alone can be an independent cause of death. Death due to chest wall trauma per se is typically related to respiratory failure, and so is dependent upon the other conditions that predispose to SIRS, respiratory failure, and MOF. Associated injuries, Injury Severity Score (ISS), and increasing numbers of blood transfusions can be shown to increase the morbidity and mortality attributable to chest wall trauma.[38,39] Historically, the association of radiologically visible pulmonary contusion on CXR with flail chest more than doubles the mortality of either condition seen independently[40] and associated flail chest makes patients with pulmonary contusion far more likely to require mechanical ventilation.[41] But in the era of CT diagnosis, it remains to be seen what the importance of CT-only pulmonary contusion will be. Future experience will tell how to apply the historical data to the new paradigm.

The need for ventilatory support, increased ICU days and overall length of stay, pneumonia, and mortality are clearly higher in elderly rib fracture patients than in younger patients.[42] Other studies suggest that such complications and mortality tend to be concentrated mostly in the subset of elderly patients with pre-existing cardiopulmonary diseases.[43] Similarly, the mortality of the subset of patients with flail chest is found to increase with age.[44]

## Initial Clinical Approach to Chest Wall Trauma

The structured ATLS approach to trauma guides the early approach to chest wall injuries. Initial diagnostic efforts are aimed at finding and treating lesions that impair gas exchange and circulation. Major chest wall trauma is associated with blunt pulmonary trauma, and disturbances in pulmonary compliance and gas exchange after pulmonary injury occur in the absence of visible pulmonary contusions. Nonetheless, such alterations take time to develop, so early deterioration of gas exchange should not be assumed to be due to pulmonary parenchymal pathology. Airway compromise, pneumothoraces, aspiration, and sucking chest wounds are more likely causes and should be sought. Abnormal vital signs or acidosis should raise the suspicion of associated bleeding injuries in the chest and abdomen. After all these conditions have been stabilized, a thorough examination of the chest wall and a simple AP CXR will reveal the majority of significant chest wall injuries. The location and number of rib fractures should be noted, but although rib fractures in specific areas have often been said to be associated with specific injuries, most of these associations have proved loose or nonexistent. In particular, injuries of the first rib are now known not to require angiography to exclude blunt aortic injury. Thus, the presence of multiple rib fractures or any other evidence of high-energy trauma to the chest should alert the examiner to the possibility of multiple visceral injuries.[33,45] Patients should be managed with that possibility in mind rather than allowing the location of the rib fractures to focus, and therefore limit diagnostic efforts.

## Management of Chest Wall Injuries

Injuries of the bony thorax per se can be viewed as leading to four common and important sequelae: (1) pain, (2) hemorrhage, (3) mechanical chest wall instability, and (4) chest wall defects. To differing extents, these can contribute directly or indirectly to pulmonary gas-exchange dysfunction, hemodynamic instability, and pneumonia, and thus all can be important contributors to the morbidity and mortality of multisystem injuries.

## Chest Wall Pain

Pain is often the single most important consideration in the management of stable nonbleeding chest wall injuries. These injuries have no direct, immediate effect on chest wall stability or pulmonary function, but they may have significant delayed morbidity. It is widely believed that immobility of the chest wall due to "splinting" from pain is a major contributor to the occurrence of pneumonia after rib fractures. This has never been proven in any

scientific fashion and our recent studies suggest that the onset of pneumonia in the trauma patients in general reflect the evolution of innate immune function.[46] Nonetheless, pain management is a crucial contribution to patient care in general, and failure of pulmonary toilet with retention of secretions can contribute substantially to pulmonary dysfunction and the development of pneumonia. Thus, chest wall pain should be treated with appropriate analgesic regimens. These are discussed in the section on pain management. There is no scientific support for the use of approaches such as chest taping or strapping to relieve pain.

Clearly, the ability to clear secretions is diminished by chest wall pain and immobilization, but a wide variety of other systemic influences are now thought to be involved in the etiology of posttraumatic pneumonia. The most important of these are associated shock and other soft-tissue trauma,[47] which probably act via modulation of immune function.[48] Elderly patients are also more likely to develop pneumonia.[42] Whenever safe, management without endotracheal intubation is associated with lower rates of pneumonia in prospective studies.[49] All of these other influences however, are likely to act synergistically with the direct chest wall injury. Thus, in selected patients where pain impedes adequate respiratory function, aggressive pain management should be a primary consideration. This is discussed at length below.

## Chest Wall Hemorrhage

Chest wall bleeding associated with rib fractures typically presents as a hemothorax. Traumatic hemothoraces typically require chest tube drainage, but may require thoracotomy for control. The management of hemothorax is discussed later. If the parietal pleura remains intact however, chest wall bleeding tends to be contained and self-limited. Such contained bleeding may present as an extrapleural hematoma. Traumatic extrapleural hematoma is found in about 7% of cases of major chest trauma. It is almost uniformly associated with rib fractures, and about half the time it is associated with a hemothorax.[50] Our experience is that it is often seen as a residual pleural-based density after drainage of a hemothorax, but it is not itself amenable to chest tube drainage. The frequency with which chest wall bleeding is diagnosed depends on how hard it is sought. The 7% figure quoted above probably represents that subset of contained chest wall hemorrhages that accumulate laterally, and thus can be seen on AP radiographs. Many more at other locations are seen on CT.[51] Most interstitial chest wall bleeding is asymptomatic, but on occasion it may be a primary cause of continued unexplained blood loss in patients with multiple trauma. Contained chest wall bleeding rarely requires intervention, but documenting its presence occasionally allays concerns for bleeding at other sites as well as concern for other intrathoracic processes on AP CXR. On rare occasions we have used CT angiography of the chest to localize a contrast extravasation "blush" (Fig. 26-6). Treatment options in stable patients include expectant management or angiography and embolization.[52] We have not seen truly interstitial chest wall bleeding be rapid enough to warrant operation, but such injuries may be partially decompressed into the pleura and present as an associated hemothorax. Also, reports of delayed hemorrhage and death do exist.[53] As with any hematoma, the possibility of secondary infection by hematogenous seeding or by direct extension from a pneumonia must be considered. These possibilities should be kept in mind when searching for a source of unexplained fever.

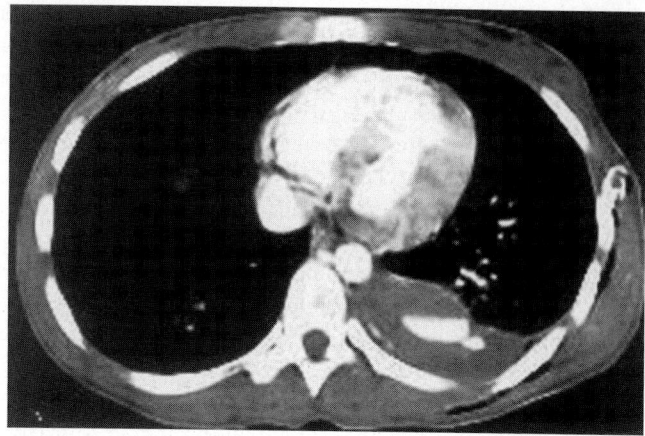

**FIGURE 26-6.** Chest CT demonstrating an extrapleural hematoma with an obvious contrast blush.

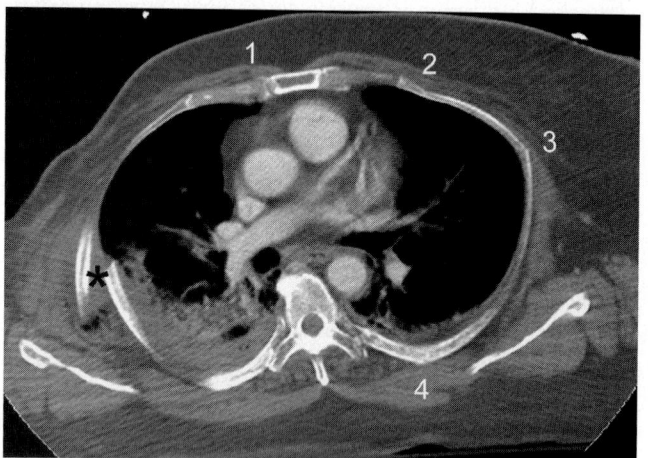

**FIGURE 26-7.** Multiple right-sided rib fractures. During spontaneous respiration, the patient had a clinical flail, but contiguous and left-sided fractures cannot be found on the chest radiograph. In fact, many of the other fractures occurred at the costosternal junction (see Fig. 26-8). Note the suggestion of the pulmonary contusion as well as a subpulmonic pneumothorax.

## Chest Wall Instability and Flail Chest

Chest wall instability is a common occurrence in the presence of multiple rib fractures. Typically, three or more contiguous ribs must be fractured segmentally in order to create a flail segment (Fig. 26-7). Flail segments are most common in the anterior and antero-lateral chest, and are more common in the mid to lower than the upper chest wall. This distribution is probably related to the fact that the anterior and lateral segments of the chest wall are more commonly injured and the thicker overlying chest wall structures in other areas both protect the ribs and limits their paradoxical movement if fractured. Similarly, in our experience flail segments are more common (or perhaps more commonly noted) in thinner, older, and less heavily muscled patients. The paradoxical movement of the flail segment is caused by negative intrapleural pressure generated during inspiration.[54] Thus flail segments are only seen in spontaneously ventilating patients, or those who can generate a negative inspiratory force while on ventilatory support. Subtle flail segments will often be appreciated best by palpation of the chest during spontaneous ventilation.

Although CXR will often demonstrate the classic picture of multiple segmental fractures, it is not uncommon for one or both

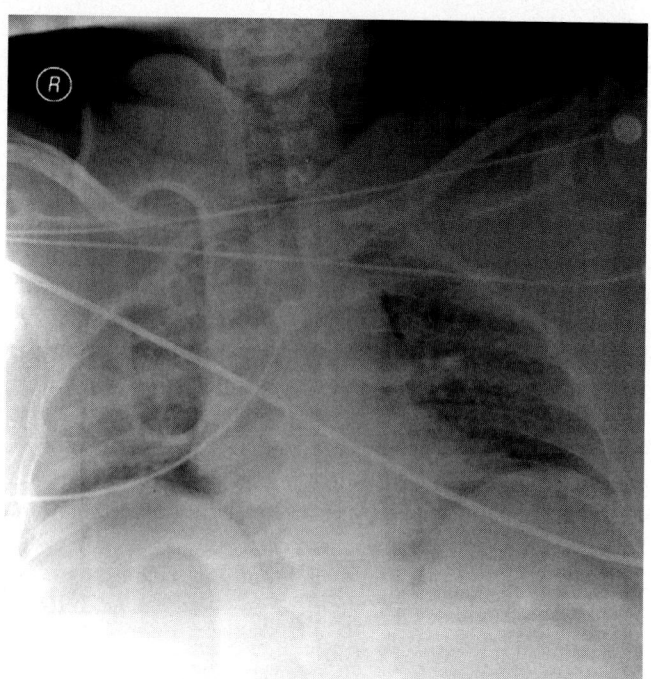

**FIGURE 26-8.** CT of the same patient in Fig. 26-7. In addition to the obvious displaced right-sided rib fractures that was seen on the initial CXR (*), an additional four rib fractures (numbered 1–4) can be observed. When this patient began breathing spontaneously off mechanical ventilation, she had evidence of bilateral flail chest which would be predicted from the CT scan.

ends of a flail segment to be composed of costochondral fractures which will not be seen on plain x-rays. While they may be seen on CT, we would emphasize that the diagnosis of flail chest is clinical and not radiological. On occasion, the potential for a flail segment will only be suspected on the basis of CT findings in an intubated, ventilated patient (Fig. 26-8). However diagnosed, the presence of a flail segment may impact weaning from ventilatory support. Occasionally, the entire anterior chest wall may move paradoxically as a flail. Typically, this will be associated with bilateral fractures in the anterior axillary lines or bilateral fractures of the costochondral cartilages, best seen of chest CT. Such patients may appear to have a "flail sternum." The physiological implications of flail chest injuries, however, are fairly constant and show no constant relationship to the location of the unstable segment.

Instability of the chest wall due to mobile fracture segments has traditionally been thought critical to the pathogenesis of abnormal gas exchange after trauma. Paradoxical flail segment motion was previously thought to allow to-and-fro gas movement ("pendelluft") in the airways during spontaneous respiration. Although this simplistic concept was attractive when initially proposed and large flail segments clearly do make ventilation inefficient, direct applications of the pendelluft concept to clinical chest wall instability are erroneous. Physiologically, the rebreathing of airway gas will create a dead-space (VD/VT) abnormality. In practice, an elevated shunt fraction (QS/QT) and hypoxemia are the hallmarks of respiratory failure after blunt chest trauma, and after trauma in general. Moreover, pendelluft is routinely observed in acute lung injury without chest wall instability, most likely due to the heterogeneous viscoelastic properties of the injured lung itself.[55]

In fact, flail chest does impose additional work of breathing, but respiratory failure after chest wall injury is almost never due to the mechanical ventilatory dysfunction imposed by the chest wall injury itself. In great measure, it is caused by the underlying pulmonary contusion.[56] Pulmonary contusion almost universally accompanies flail chest. Pulmonary contusion decreases pulmonary compliance and increases QS/QT. The flail chest causes both chest wall pain and inefficient mechanical ventilation. Thus these two injuries each contribute to hypoventilation, and together lead to ventilatory failure. Hypoventilation along with pain and thus impaired coughing will also contribute to atelectasis and mucus plugging. These factors contribute directly to shunting and thus hypoxemia. The loss of chest wall expansion under a flail segment directly decreases functional residual capacity and contributes to hypoxemia.[57] Taken together, the complex interplay of physiologic disturbances after chest wall trauma suggests that flail chest and pulmonary contusion are best considered as a single syndrome characterized by (1) inefficient ventilation and increased work of breathing which lead to ventilatory failure, and (2) a complex of chest wall and parenchymal pathology that leads to intra-pulmonary shunting and impaired oxygen transport. The management of flail chest-pulmonary contusion is thus one of the most important and challenging aspects of trauma care. The critical care of flail chest-pulmonary contusion, including possible operative options, is therefore considered separately.

## Chest Wall Defects

All chest wall defects can prevent spontaneous ventilation and thus lead to rapid death from asphyxia. Sucking chest wounds occur most commonly after penetrating injuries that are large enough to allow rapid equilibration of pleural and atmospheric pressures. This prevents lung inflation and alveolar ventilation. The classic teaching is that such wounds are dressed with occlusive petrolatum gauze taped on three sides to allow gas exit from the pleural space only. This approach may be useful in the field setting, but we believe it has no place in definitive care. In all but the most rudimentary medical care settings, such wounds should be treated with a chest tube placed through a clean site. The primary wound can be treated temporarily with an occlusive dressing or simple skin closure. Temporary closure is followed by definitive wound closure in the operating room. It should also be recognized that the majority of major chest wall injuries will require endotracheal intubation, and that once positive pressure ventilation is instituted, temporary chest wall closure is not necessary for respiration.

In fact, true chest wall defects with significant tissue loss are quite rare. They may occur occasionally due to penetrating injuries like close range shotgun blasts, or after impalements. Major chest wall defects due to high-energy blunt trauma are clinical novelties since most die before reaching medical attention. In the case of large defects, occlusive dressings are of no value. All such wounds mandate endotracheal intubation and positive pressure ventilation. After control of the airway and establishing ventilation, control of bleeding from the chest wall and from associated injuries should be the major focus of operative interventions. The chest wall bleeding in major defects is often life-threatening. Typically, emergency thoracotomy is needed and operative control of bleeding may be very difficult (Fig. 26-9). Abbreviated operation with packing may sometimes be the safest course. It is common to see some degree of disruption of the chest wall at thoracotomies performed for hemorrhage after major blunt trauma. Posttraumatic lung hernias are

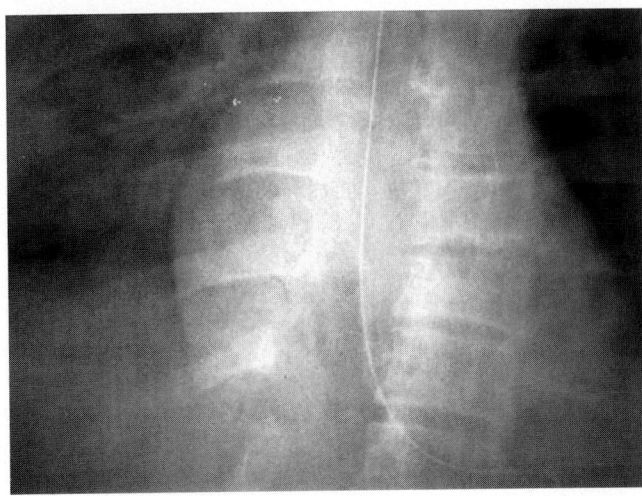

**FIGURE 26-9.** Close-up of CXR from Fig. 26-3 demonstrating a massive degree of displacement of the costo-vertebral joints. The patient required an urgent thoracotomy for bleeding. The operative findings included a huge defect in the posterior chest wall down to the overlying skin that required packing with eight large laparotomy pads.

another rare finding which may represent a more chronic presentation of this same process.[58]

The definitive closure of chest wall defects often requires tissue-transfer procedures, but such lengthy operations should never be considered in the initial care of a gravely ill patient. Rather, modern principles of damage control should be applied. Temporary closures can be achieved using any available skin or prosthetic materials until such time as the patient is physiologically fit and will tolerate definitive repair. Chronic deformities of the chest wall have also been reported after trauma. The cases reported have all been those treated surgically, but the denominator of asymptomatic chest wall deformities after trauma is completely unknown. In all likelihood the vast majority of posttraumatic chest wall deformities are minor and never come to clinical attention.

# OTHER INJURIES TO THE CHEST WALL

## Scapular Fractures

Due to its location and structure, fractures of the scapula are uncommon. Considerable direct force is therefore required to cause a scapular fracture, and associated injuries are common. Thus, a scapula fracture, especially when present on the initial CXR, should serve as an indication that the patient has sustained severe chest trauma. In that group of blunt trauma patients the incidence of scapular fractures has been reported to be about 1% with over 80% of patients having associated injuries. As with other types of fractures, the use of modern CT technology has revealed considerably more nondisplaced scapula fractures than previously reported.[59] The increasing number of scapular fractures does not negate the previous reported data as the potential severity of these injuries, rather the astute clinician must alter their practice pattern based upon additional information gleaned from new technology. Recognition of a scapular fracture should prompt careful examination for thoracic, neurologic, vascular, and abdominal injury in addition to orthopedic consultation. Clinical signs of scapular fracture include local pain, tenderness, swelling, and crepitus. Although many scapular fractures are visible on an initial chest radiograph, they are often obscured or overlooked on initial evaluation of the CXR.[60] Present imaging includes CT scanning to determine any extension into the shoulder joint. Initial management is analgesia and immobilization followed by progressive physical therapy. Scapular fractures only occasionally require reconstruction.

## Scapulothoracic Dissociation

Scapulothoracic dissociation is a dramatic but rare injury secondary to severe blunt trauma to the shoulder girdle. A spectrum of injuries can involve the musculoskeletal, vascular, and neurologic structures of the shoulder girdle. In a collected review of 58 cases, Damschen and coworkers reported complete brachial plexus injury in 81% of patients and partial injury in 13%.[61] Disruption of the subclavian or axillary artery occurred in 88% of patients, and in our experience may be a rare cause of occult but life-threatening hemorrhage into the chest wall Associated thoracic, craniocerebral, and spinal injuries are frequent. The management of these patients' complex injuries will depend upon the severity of injury. Nonetheless, the nearly uniform presence of severe neurologic deficits almost always results in an extremely poor functional outcome. The surgeon should carefully consider the high likelihood of a poor result before embarking upon long and potentially life-threatening vascular and soft tissue reconstructions that may salvage a useless or flail extremity that will ultimately require amputation.

## Clavicular Fractures

In contrast to scapular and sternal fractures, fractures of the clavicle commonly occur as isolated injuries. Clavicle fractures are also found in association with other thoracic and extra-thoracic trauma. The majority (80%) of fractures of this S-shaped bone occur in the middle third, following a fall or blow with lateral force applied to the shoulder.

Clinical signs of clavicular fracture are tenderness, crepitus, and palpable deformity. The ipsilateral shoulder may be positioned inferiorly and medially if the fracture is displaced. Most fractures are visible on the AP CXR. The initial management should consist of immobilization with a figure-of-eight dressing or shoulder immobilizer. This has been shown to be superior to operative fixation.[62] Although nonunion of a clavicle fracture may occur in up to 20% of patients it is not uniformly associated with a worse functional outcome with regard to strength or range of motion. A poor cosmetic appearance and disfiguring prominence can occur in patients with and without union. Late thoracic outlet syndrome with neurovascular compression from exuberant callus formation or a pseudoarthrosis has also been reported.[63] Nonunion of the clavicle can result in pain, cosmetic deformity, or thoracic outlet compression and severely symptomatic patients have been managed most successfully by open reduction and fixation.[64]

## Sternal Fractures

Sternal fractures are another uncommon injury following blunt chest trauma. The classic mechanism of injury continues to be a direct impact of the sternum of an unrestrained driver against the steering column of an automobile involved in a deceleration crash. It remains to be seen if the widespread availability of airbags will have an impact upon the frequency of these fractures. Occasionally sternal fractures are seen following a fall or other direct impact on the chest. The majority of sternal fractures involve the upper or mid-portion of the bone.[65] Sternal fractures following motor vehicle crashes are associated with other significant thoracic and extrathoracic injuries in 50 to 60% of patients.[65] Hence similar to scapular fractures, sternal fractures should be regarded as a hallmark of severe multiple injuries until proven otherwise. These include rib fractures in 40% of patients, long-bone fractures in 25%, and head injuries in 18%. Cardiac arrythmias may occur, but the association between sternal fractures and blunt myocardial injury has proved inconstant.

The clinical manifestations of sternal fracture per se include anterior chest pain, tenderness, ecchymosis, swelling, and a palpable deformity and motion of the fracture fragments upon respiration. The initial treatment of patients with sternal fractures should focus on the associated injuries. A baseline ECG should be obtained, especially in patients over age 40. Most patients like this with significant anterior chest trauma will have transient right ventricular dysfunction but the need for ongoing cardiac monitoring is based upon the associated injuries and underlying cardiac status rather than the sternal fracture. Patients with isolated sternal fractures and a normal emergency department evaluation do not require hospital admission.[66–68] Specific management of the sternal fracture consists of analgesics and the avoidance of motion. Occasionally open reduction and internal fixation of sternal fractures is indicated for patients with severe pain and grossly displaced fractures.

## PNEUMOTHORAX

Pneumothorax is one of the most common injuries sustained in major trauma, with a reported prevalence over 20% in patients arriving alive to trauma centers.[69] A pneumothorax is defined as a collection of air in the pleural space. There are three subtypes of pneumothoraces: simple, open, and tension. A simple pneumothorax is merely a collection of air trapped in the pleural space. The most common cause of pneumothorax is egress of air from an injury of the lung into the pleural space. Open pneumothoraces occurs when wounds of the chest wall allow air to enter the pleural space from the outside. A tension pneumothorax occurs when air collects in the pleural space under pressures exceeding atmospheric pressure. This pressure will then be transmitted to the mediastinum and can result in a shift of the heart and great vessels away from the side of the pneumothorax (Fig. 26-1). As with most injuries, the pathogenesis of the pneumothorax will vary in blunt and penetrating mechanisms. Pneumothoraces following blunt trauma may occur through several mechanisms: (1) a sudden increase in intrathoracic pressure may rupture alveoli resulting in an air leak, (2) rib fractures may be displaced inward and lacerate the lung itself, (3) deceleration injuries may tear the lung, causing an air leak, and (4) blunt forces may directly crush and disrupt alveoli. In contrast, the etiology of pneumothoraces following penetrating trauma is almost always from the direct laceration of lung parenchyma.

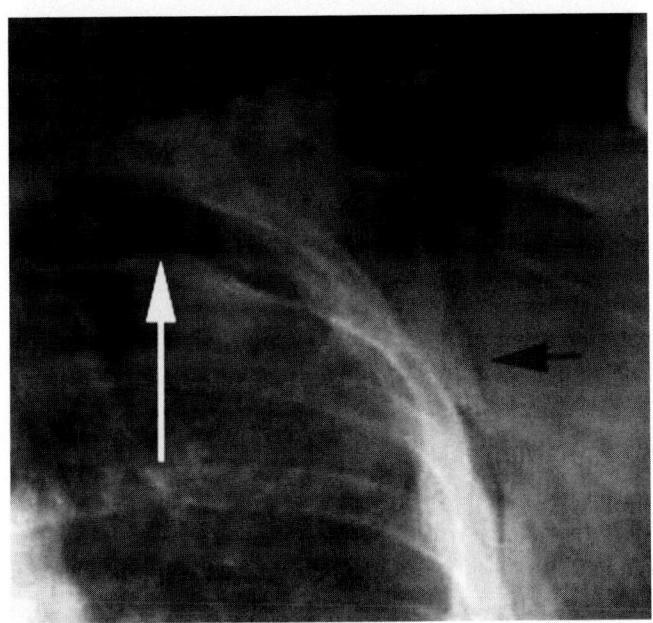

**FIGURE 26-10.** A CXR demonstrating a pneumothorax (white arrow) and overlying subcutaneous emphysema (black arrow), which can be seen tracking up to the neck. The lack of a tube thoracostomy indicates that the diagnosis of this pneumothorax was unfortunately made by this CXR instead of by the obvious physical exam findings.

The definitive diagnosis of pneumothorax is made by CXR although it can often be suspected from physical examination. The finding of subcutaneous emphysema following either blunt or penetrating trauma is indicative of an underlying pneumothorax (Fig. 26-10). While decreased breath sounds are a useful finding when present, the relatively high ambient noise in most trauma resuscitation bays and the fact that breath sounds are often well transmitted from the other lung make this finding less than universal, and our experience is that breath sounds may be present even in face of a substantial pneumothorax. An open wound on the chest wall with obvious escape of air makes the diagnosis of an open pneumothorax readily apparent.

As stated, the diagnosis of a pneumothorax is most commonly made using portable AP CXR. Recently though, ultrasound has also been shown to be of value in the diagnosis of pneumothoraces and hemothoraces pneumothorax.[27,70,71] This is especially true in those anterior pneumothoraces which are poorly seen on the supine AP chest radiograph. It has been suggested that examination of both hemithoraces should be part of the focused abdominal sonogram for trauma (FAST). The ultrasound diagnosis of pneumothorax can be made by visualizing the pleura between echogenic rib windows and observing for the characteristics signs of pneumothorax.[27,71] In a prospective evaluation of 382 patients sustaining blunt and penetrating trauma, ultrasound diagnosed 37 of 39 pneumothoraces seen on the AP CXR. Two pneumothoraces could not be diagnosed due to the presence of subcutaneous emphysema, but the combination of physical examination and ultrasound therefore correctly identified all patients. Although these reports are interesting, it remains to be seen if routine ultrasound may prove to be a more accurate "stethoscope" in the rapid diagnosis of pneumothorax.

Often, estimates of the size of pneumothoraces are used in attempts to predict their clinical significance. This is done by describing the distance from the collapsed lung edge to the chest wall as a percentage of the total size of the hemi-thorax. As abdominal CT scanning became more commonplace in the evaluation of stable patients following blunt trauma, it became apparent that many blunt trauma patients have significant anterior pneumothoraces that are not seen on plain chest radiographs (Fig. 26-4). The rate of missed pneumothoraces on the supine AP CXR has been estimated at 20–35%. In fact, the inability of the plain AP CXR to render a truly three-dimensional picture of the thoracic space makes commonly used "percentage" descriptions of pneumothoraces highly inaccurate and of little value. Clinically, these limitations of plain radiographs explain why so many pneumothoraces that seem fairly innocuous on chest radiography may actually cause significant shortness of breath. It also helps in understanding why a seemingly small amount of pleural fluid on CXR may result in a large fluid output through a chest tube. Thus, the individual patient's symptoms and physiologic responses are far more important than the apparent size of a pneumothorax on CXR, and should dictate the urgency of their treatment. Experienced providers have also seen patients with complete collapse of a lung who are not short of breath and who have normal blood gasses at rest. In contrast, other patients may have severe dyspnea and hypoxia with much more modest collapse. In retrospect, it is likely that some of the patients in the latter group would have had large pneumothoraces if subjected to a CT of the chest.

This conundrum brings up a recent controversy in the diagnosis and management of pneumothorax, namely, the appropriate management of patients whose pneumothorax is only visible on a CT examination of the chest and/or abdomen. The reported incidence of these occult pneumothoraces is between 2–8% of all blunt trauma victims.[72,73] While the detection of occult pneumothorax is increasing, the optimal management of these patients remains to be defined. In a retrospective study, the size of the occult pneumothorax was correlated with placement of a tube thoracostomy, and tube thoracostomy was suggested for all pneumothoraces greater than 5×80 mm.[74] In addition, these authors suggested that two or more rib fractures also predicted the need for a tube thoracostomy. Enderson and colleagues prospectively documented that eight of 15 patients with occult pneumothoraces on positive pressure ventilation required tube thoracostomy, and three of these patients developed tension pneumothorces. The authors recommended that all occult pneumothoraces in patients requiring positive pressure ventilation be treated with tube thoracostomy.[75] Conversely, in a prospective study of 44 similar patients, Brasel et al. found that neither size nor positive pressure ventilation correlated with the development of a clinically significant pneumothorax that required tube thoracostomy.[76] Thus from the available literature, it appears that approximately 20% of patients with occult pnuemothoraces will require tube thoracostomy, but that these pneumothoraces need to be treated in the context of the whole patient. Patients with multiple injuries, hemorrhagic shock, or a traumatic brain injury may not tolerate the small but very real chance of their pneumothorax increasing in size. Similarly, patients who will require emergent operative treatment by subspecialty services such as orthopaedics or neurosurgery may not be observed for progression of their pneumothorax as reliably as patients who are being managed in a trauma intensive care unit. In such scenarios we believe the risk–benefit ratio falls on the side of treating patients with a chest tube. In cases where it is thought that observation can be safely elected, follow-up radiographs should be performed at 6 and 24 hours after diagnosis to ensure that the pneumothorax has not progressed.

The treatment of pnuemothorax in the field is usually limited to the management of open and tension pneumothoraces. Open wounds should be covered with an occlusive dressing taped on three sides. This creates a flap-valve type dressing which lets air escape from, but not enter the space. The advisability of field decompression of tension pneumothoraces remains controversial. In the United States, needle aspiration is the standard first-line treatment for a suspected tension pneumothorax. In other countries where physicians are utilized as part of the prehospital teams, a high degree of success has been reported with the placement of field tube throracostomies.[77,78] There is no doubt that prompt recognition and rapid decompression of a tension pneumothorax can be a life-saving maneuver. The problem with field decompression is achieving a balance between making the correct diagnosis and instituting early treatment, and avoiding the small but measurable rate of iatrogenic injures and unnecessary tube thoracostomies that result from empiric field decompression.[79] The proper technique for emergent chest decompression is to place a 14-gauge IV catheter in the mid-clavicular line 1–2 fingerbreadths below the clavicle. This will place the needle in the second or third intercostal space. Over the past decade, manufacturers have made their intravenous catheters shorter and the old style 3-inch catheters may not be available. One should recognize that in muscular or obese individuals, even a 3-inch catheter, properly placed, still might not reach the pleural space.

The standard treatment for a traumatic pneumothorax, from either blunt or penetraing trauma, found on the screening AP CXR is tube thoracostomy to allow re-expansion of the lung. In our opinion, attempts at removal of air by needle aspiration should not be undertaken as a primary therapy, and may be especially dangerous in patients with multiple injuries. If a tension pneumothorax is suspected, it should be treated urgently. In patients manifesting any distress, desaturation, or hemodynamic instability, this is typically done *without* radiologic confirmation. Conversely, in stable patients suspected of having a simple pneumothorax, we will obtain a confirmatory chest radiograph prior to chest tube insertion. The acquisition of a CXR has several advantages: (1) it confirms the diagnosis and occasionally prevents unnecessary chest tube placement; (2) it sometimes demonstrates unexpected abnormalities, such as diaphragmatic rupture, that might lead to catastrophic complications of chest tube placement (Fig. 26-11); and (3) it may demonstrate other findings that would change the size or location of tube placement, such as a large associated hemothorax or a chest wall hematoma. Similar to the discussion of occult pneumothoraces discovered on CT above, select patients who are stable from a hemodynamic and respiratory standpoint, and who have what appears to be a small pneumothorax on CXR, may be observed. We routinely obtain follow-up radiographs at 6 and 24 hours after diagnosis to ensure that the pneumothorax has not progressed. Patients may be placed on supplemental oxygen to enhance reabsorption of the pneumothorax, but it is unlikely that very high inspired oxygen tensions (i.e.,>60%) will have any more effect than supplemental $O_2$ given by nasal prongs.[80] Another option is the placement of a "pigtail" catheter into the pleural space by Seldinger technique. This approach may be

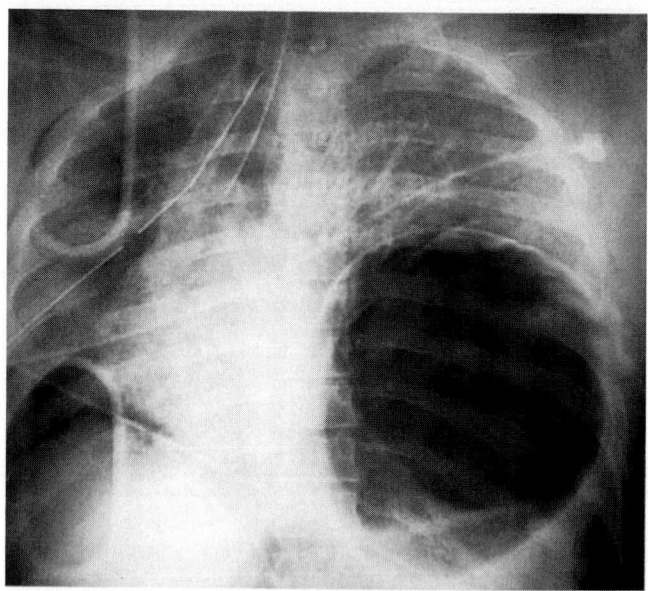

**FIGURE 26-11.** CXR demonstrating a large gastric bubble through a diaphragmatic rupture. The patient was intubated in the field and a chest tube was placed on the right for decreased breath sounds and subcutaneous air. Chest tube placement on the left side was avoided by this CXR.

curative for selected simple pneumothoraces without entailing the risks and discomfort of a traditional tube thoracostomy. Hemodynamically stable patients with penetrating chest trauma without evidence of a pneumothorax on their initial CXR undergo a follow-up film at 6 hours. If that film is normal they may be discharged from the emergency department.

## Tube Thoracostomy

The placement and management of a tube thoracostomy is basic to the care of patients with chest trauma. The standard placement for a chest tube is in the midaxillary line in the fifth to sixth intercostal space. The reasoning behind this location is two-fold. First, this location is usually safely above the diaphragm. Second, it is the area is with the thinnest chest wall musculature, thus allowing for a more rapid and less painful tube insertion than if it were to be positioned more anterior or posterior.

Appropriate positioning of the patient will aid in the placement of a tube thoracostomy cannot be minimized. In patients that are supine on a long spine board who require emergent tube placement, the ipsilateral arm should be raised and placed behind the patient's head whenever possible. This further "opens" the space between the latisimus dorsi and pectoralis musculature and allows a better window for insertion. In women, care should be taken to move the breast medially to avoid placing the chest tube through the lateral portion of the breast tissue. In patients who sustain penetrating trauma or those whose spine has been cleared, elevating the hemithorax 15–20° markedly increases the ease of insertion and the ability to position the tube.

The area chosen should be cleansed with an antiseptic solution and anesthetized. We routinely utilize 10 cc of 1% lidocaine and infiltrate all layers of the chest wall including the rib surface and the intercostal muscles and pleura. A useful trick to prolong the anesthesia associated with chest tube insertion especially in the presence of rib fractures is to mix the lidociaine with bipuvicaine essentially providing a rib block for the patient. This should be done without concern about entering the pleural space, since a chest tube is being placed. In patients whose hemodynamic and respiratory status is sufficient, conscious sedation with morphine and midazolam may be used to supplement the local anesthesia. In addition, where time permits placement of intercostals blocks (with bipuvicaine) posterior to the proposed insertion site can make insertion and early management less painful. It is also our experience that the ease of placing the chest tube is directly related to discomfort of the patient. In part, this is because patients will forcefully contract their chest wall muscles due to pain, and drastically narrow their intercostal spaces.

Some standard texts recommend placing the skin incision one to two rib spaces below the proposed intercostal insertion site of the tube. This is meant to create a subcutaneous tunnel in order to help seal the tube track, but we believe that this maneuver is generally unnecessary. It is also more easily performed in the operating room or in patients who are sedated and mechanically ventilated than in awake patients. Last, such tunnels have in fact been shown not to affect the rate of development of recurrent pneumothoraces following chest tube removal.[81]

Our practice is to make a 2 cm incision over the rib immediately below the interspace chosen for tube insertion. Dissection should proceed directly down to the rib using the knife. The superior border of the rib is identified to avoid injury to the inferiorly located intercostal vessels, and the pleural space is entered. While the use of a Kelly or Pean clamp to enter the pleura is often recommended, we often prefer to continue with the knife, and to enter the pleural space sharply, immediately over the rib. This technique is particularly helpful in heavily muscled individuals. After entering the pleura, a finger should always be inserted through the opening and the pleural space explored. This will confirm that the entry has been made into the pleural cavity rather than into the lung or the abdominal cavity. Also, the lung and diaphragm should be palpated and the presence or absence of adhesions from the lung to the chest wall should be determined. These maneuvers are especially important in patients who may have a ruptured diaphragm, or who may have had previous chest surgery or pulmonary infections. We condemn the blind placement of chest tubes using a trocar technique, since the risk of placing the tube into the lung or the abdomen, resulting in a trauma patient shish-ka-bob is significant. Once entry into the pleural space is confirmed digitally, the chest tube can be placed safely through the incision, over the rib, and into the pleural space. The appropriate size of the tubes to be used is also a subject of some debate. Classically, trauma patients received a large bore (38–40 French) chest tube regardless of their diagnosis. It is clear now that in patients who only have a pneumothorax, a small-bore tube (20–22 French or even a "pigtail" catheter) will suffice. Large-bore tubes may be more difficult to place between the rib spaces of smaller patients and may result in significantly increased pain secondary to intercostal nerve irritation. Last, the difference in cross sectional diameter between a 38–40 French tube and our preferred size (32–34 French) is really quite small. Moreover, while liquid blood will drain well from either size tube, clotted blood will not drain from either. In a patient with only a pneumothorax, the tube can often be directed superiorly and anteriorly. If an associated hemothorax is present, a larger tube (32–34 French) should be placed and the tube advanced in a more posterior and superior direction.

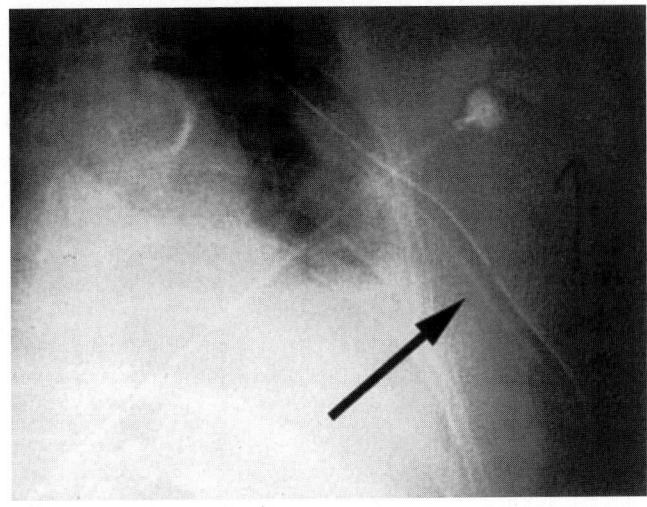

**FIGURE 26-12.** The last hole of the chest tube is seen outside the chest wall (arrow).

Attention should be paid to the "last hole" in the chest tube to ensure that it is located within the pleural space (Fig. 26-12). If time permits, holding the tube against the patient's thorax to gauge the mark where the tube will exit the chest wall can be useful. A tube that is placed too far into the chest will often kink at the last hole. This frequently causes the tube to occlude or malfunction. Theoretically, the pleural space is (initially) continuous, and can be drained completely by a single tube. In practice however, when tubes are placed in a dependent position optimal for fluid evacuation, pneumothoraces may not be evacuated as well. Similarly, more superiorly placed "air tubes" may be suboptimal for fluid removal. Thus, whenever a single chest tube is used, its placement always represents a compromise between optimal fluid and optimal air drainage. With large hemothoraces, and particularly in the presence of displaced rib fractures, we often use two chest tubes, a smaller one placed superiorly for the removal of air and a larger tube placed inferior and posterior for the removal of fluid.

Following placement, tubes are generally connected to an underwater seal with negative suction. A negative pressure of 20 cm $H_2O$ is helpful in promoting drainage. Rapid re-expansion of the lung should not be attempted in situations where the lung has been collapsed for several days (this is unusual in blunt trauma), since it may lead to "re-expansion pulmonary edema." The rapid re-expansion of the lung that occurs with treatment of a major pneumothorax can cause considerable pain as the pleura stretches. In the case of an isolated pneumothorax therefore, it may be worthwhile to allow the patient to breathe deeply and cough gently in order to gradually expand the lung before applying suction. This approach to care is inappropriate in the unstable or multiple-injury situation, but it will diminish pain and alleviate fear of the thoracostomy tube, particularly among adolescents and children, when time and stability allow. The tube should be well secured to the skin of the chest wall, and a sterile dressing should be applied at the point of tube entry.

It is important to obtain a chest x-ray immediately after placement of the tube. This will help confirm proper placement of the tube and aid in evaluating for complete evacuation of fluid and air from the pleural space. If intrapleural fluid still seems to be present, a second chest tube should be placed. The inability to evacuate blood from the pleural space completely is one of the indications for early surgical intervention in cases of chest injury. The complete evacuation of air and blood from the pleural space is important for complete expansion of the lung. This will help decrease bleeding and air leaks from the lung as well as decreasing the risk of subsequent empyema.

Daily chest x-rays help to provide evidence of the effective elimination of air and fluid from the pleural space. The chest tube is left in place until there is no air leak from the lung and less than 100 to 150 mL of fluid drainage per 24 hours. In a randomized prospective study, Martino and colleagues found that a 6–8 hour trial of water seal was superior to no water seal in decreasing the incidence of recurrent pneumothorax following tube removal.[81]

The use of antibiotic prophylaxis for the placement of chest tubes has been studied extensively. Nonetheless, the literature is very problematic and the issue remains highly controversial. Opinion is clearly divided among those who believe[82] and those who do not believe[83] in their use. It is our present practice not to use prophylactic antibiotics when we place tube thoracostomies. We believe that the *chest-tube-specific* infectious complication rates (predominantly of empyema) are much more directly related to adequacy of drainage of the pleural space, and to the degree of injury and shock present than to the use of antibiotics. Moreover, the risks of indiscriminant antibiotic use in trauma patients are very real. If one feels the urge to use prophylactic antibiotics, we strongly recommend that only a single dose of a first generation cephalosporin be given prior to the incision, as has been shown to be the appropriate mode of administration in virtually every other type of prophylactic antibiotic use.

Although tube thoracostomy insertion can be a life-saving procedure and is often relatively straightforward, its performance should not be taken lightly since the reported overall complication rates approach 25%.[84] Important factors in determining complication rates included the urgency of placement, the location of tube placement, and the level of operator experience. Complication rates are also significantly dependent on the training of the provider. One study found complication rates of 33% in tubes placed by prehospital personnel, 13% in tubes placed by emergency department physicians, and 6% in tubes placed by surgeons.[85] Thus, it is clear that surgeons should be actively involved in educating nonsurgeons as to the proper technique of chest tube insertion and the recognition of complications. In a study utilizing CT scanning, chest tube malposition was observed in 26% of patients.[86]

While we would like to believe that our placement of a tube thoracostomy is always ideal, it should be understood that placement is a "blind" procedure, which is often done under less than ideal conditions. Thus, the finding of several studies that successful placement is related to experience should come as no surprise. The high incidence of chest tube malposition contributes to the inability to evacuate the pleural space as well as to the persistence of air leaks. Also, early CT scanning can be helpful in patients where there are questions as to either the adequacy of the pleural drainage or the etiology of a persistent air leak. Carillo and colleagues using thoracoscopy reported a high rate of air leaks that required surgical intervention.[87] Even if chest tubes have been placed correctly, they should not lead to a false sense of security about the occurrence of a tension pneumothorax (Fig. 26-13). Fibrin plugs may occlude tubes that have been in place for a few days

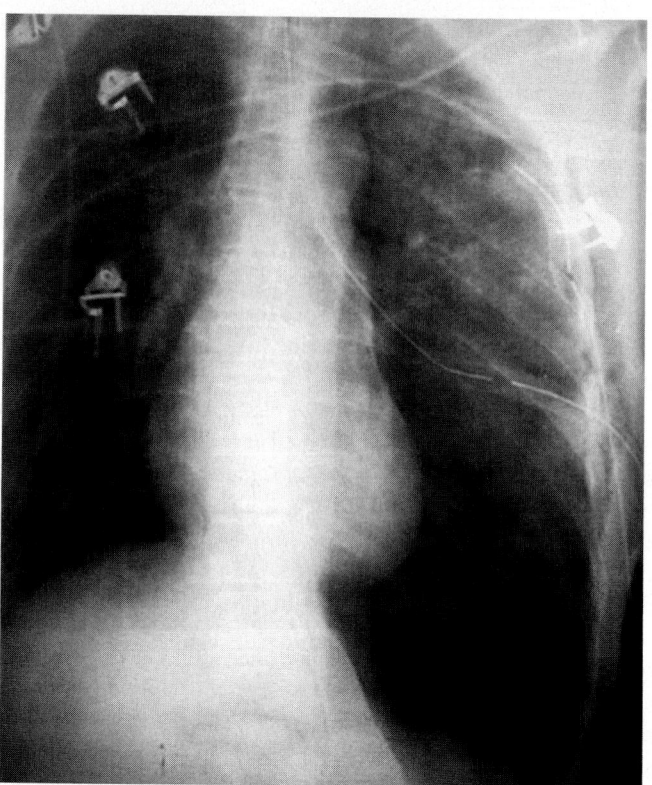

**FIGURE 26-13.** A tension pneumothorax developed despite the presence of two chest tubes.

and allow a pneumothoraces to develop in a delayed fashion. Thus, any patient with a chest tube in place who shows signs of respiratory deterioration (either hypoxia or diminishing compliance) should be suspected of having a recurrent pneumothorax and be evaluated accordingly.

Whenever a new air leak is discovered or the chest tube fails to re-expand the lung, several potential causes should be considered. All connections from the tube to the suction canisters need to be checked. The last hole of the tube needs to be checked to see that it has not migrated out of the chest cavity. This is a frequent cause of air leak, but it is an unusual cause of large pneumothoraces. Immediately after placement, a tube can be "prepped" and advanced a small distance, but as the skin entry site becomes colonized this will become unwise. Malposition of the tube in the major fissure can also result in failure to expand the lung and inadvertent placement of the tube into the pulmonary parenchyma is not uncommon as a cause of continuing air leaks. In our experience, chest CT has proved invaluable in diagnosing such events, and if intraparenchymal placement is found, the tube should be removed and another tube placed at a new site. It is also common for chest tubes to become occluded over time and such tubes can often be removed without the need for replacement, since they were nonfunctional in any case.

## HEMOTHORAX

A hemothorax is defined as the presence of blood in the pleural space. The blood can come from any number of sources. Thoracic sources include the lung parenchyma, the chest wall including the

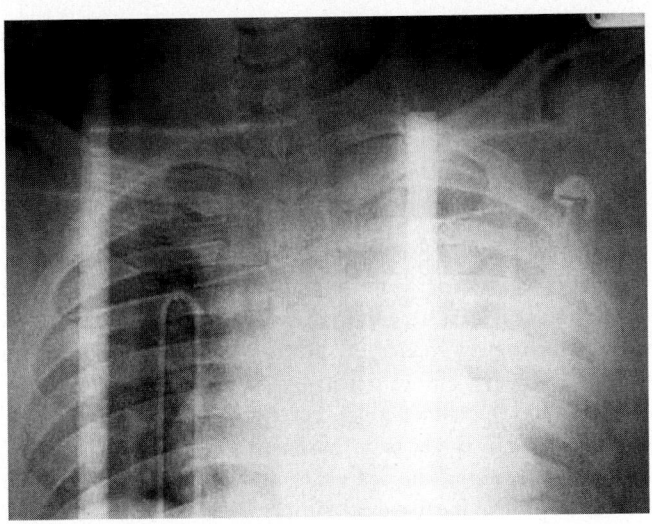

**FIGURE 26-14.**  CXR demonstrating large hemothorax.

intercostal or internal mammary arteries, or the heart and great vessels. Hemothoraces can also arise from intra-abdominal organs, especially the liver and spleen, in the setting of diaphragmatic laceration. In unstable patients following blunt or penetrating trauma, the diagnosis of hemothorax is usually suspected on the basis of physical examination, and confirmed by the insertion of a chest tube. A massive hemothorax is defined as the presence of (1 L of blood in the pleural space and is typically associated with systemic signs of shock and hypoperfusion (Fig. 26-14). In hemodynamically stable patients, the diagnosis of hemothorax is more commonly made on CXR. It has been estimated that 200 to 300 mL of blood must be present in the pleural space before a hemothorax can be detected on standard chest x-rays. In most patients with penetrating trauma, the initial CXR can be taken in an upright position. This will increase the sensitivity of the study for both hemo- and pneumothoraces. Following blunt trauma however, there is almost always concern regarding the stability of the vertebral column and thus the initial CXR is usually taken with the patient supine on a long spine board. In these circumstances, fluid will layer posteriorly and a significant hemothorax may be visible only as a slight increase in opacification (or "haziness") of the affected hemithorax. In stable patients, the diagnosis of posterior fluid collections may also be made on the most cephalad cuts of a CT scan of the abdomen. CT scans can also be quite useful acutely in discriminating pleural fluid collections that require drainage from parenchymal densities, such as pulmonary contusions. Our current experience is that CT scans can be very useful in the management of stable penetrating chest trauma, but that they should never be used until patient stability is assured.

As with pneumothoraces, the major goal in the treatment of hemothoraces is to evacuate the pleural space completely. Expansion of the lung will appose the parietal and visceral pleura. This decreases bleeding from the lung and other low-pressure sources, and in most cases results in definitive control of bleeding. Overall, thoracotomy to control bleeding is required in less than 10% of all chest trauma patients. This percentage is somewhat higher in victims of penetrating trauma and lower in patients sustaining blunt trauma.[88–90] Once the chest tube has been placed, a CXR should be obtained immediately. This will confirm the position of the tube and show whether the blood has been completely evacuated from the pleural cavity. If

the pleural space still appears to contain blood, a second chest tube should be placed. Recall that early opacification of the hemithorax on chest radiograph may also represent a pulmonary contusion, hematoma, infiltrates from aspiration, or collapse due to intubation of one of the main-stem bronchi. Thus, it may be difficult to exclude the presence of residual pleural blood, especially in blunt trauma patients.[91] In such cases, chest CT of the stable patient may help resolve the dilemma and avoid unnecessary placement of a second chest tube or urgent thoracotomy. If an acute hemothorax cannot be adequately drained by chest tubes, it is probably clotted. Clotted hemothoraces typically require operative drainage to allow expansion of the lung and resolution of bleeding. Moreover, it is impossible to ascertain the rate of ongoing bleeding in the presence of a clotted hemothorax. This makes any observation extremely hazardous. Traditionally, operative drainage has been accomplished by a thoracotomy, but video assisted thoracoscopic surgery (VATS) may also be possible in selected stable patients to remove residual undrained blood and to determine if there is any ongoing bleeding.

A common and unanswered question asked on rounds with residents and students is, How much blood can be safely left in the pleural space? Clearly, chest tubes cannot evacuate every last drop of blood from the pleura. On the other hand, numerous studies have shown that failure to drain the pleural space adequately is associated with the later development of empyemas. This paradox appears to be related to systemic and local inflammatory responses. In experimental studies, dogs with either simple hemothoraces or minor injuries to the lung itself were able to clear their pleural space of blood promptly. In contrast, animals that had pleural or systemic inflammatory conditions did not.[92] Thus the injured lung and chest wall set up an inflammatory milieu. Sterile pleural fluid samples from trauma patients are rich in a wide variety of inflammatory mediators.[93] These can activate some neutrophil functions, while simultaneously suppressing vital anti-infective functions such as phagocytosis.[46,94] Thus, the inflammation which accompanies clinical trauma can alter both how the pleural cavity will handle retained blood as well how it will respond to whatever microbial innoculum may reach it. Moreover, it is a common clinical experience for patients to defervesce after drainage of a suspected empyema that proves sterile on culture. Such findings may reflect a clinical response to the removal of inflammatory products from a mature sterile hemothorax rather than any failure of microbiologic culture techniques. In our experience, bile in the pleural space from patients with penetrating thoracoabdominal injuries involving the liver will also result in an intense pleural reaction. In the absence of any hard data to the contrary, we continue to advocate aggressive drainage of the pleural space and diversion of the bile away from the chest as completely as possible. This may require peri-hepatic drainage, repair of the diaphragm, and decompression of the biliary tree as well as pleural drainage.

Immediate removal of more than a liter of blood from the pleural cavity should alert one to the potential need for urgent thoracotomy. However, patients who remain stable, have minimal or no further drainage of blood from the chest tube, have a CXR that demonstrates complete evacuation of the pleural space, and have no other indication for an operation can be admitted to a monitored bed and be observed. Occasionally such patients may present to medical care in a delayed fashion, and the large amount of drainage may reflect a slow accumulation of blood in the pleural space rather than rapid active bleeding.

Persistent bleeding from the chest tube is another indication for thoracotomy. As with the expectant management of other conditions with continuing hemorrhage, at some point continuing blood loss becomes a disease in and of itself, and the risks of transfusion and coagulopathy begin to outweigh the risks of operation. The general guidelines used to indicate thoracotomy are a continuing chest tube output of between 500–1000 mL over a defined period of time, e.g., 200 mL/hr for four hours. Patients whose chest tube outputs begin to increase may also require early operation. An important pitfall in the management of these patients is the failure to adhere to the agreed upon algorithm for operative intervention at a set amount of bleeding. The temptation to allow "just one more hour" to pass or "just another 200 mL of blood" to bleed increases, rather than decreases the morbidity and mortality of thoracic bleeding.[95] Last, close observation should also include repeat CXR to insure that a clotted hemothorax is not developing and is not the reason that the chest tube output is slowing down.

Considering the cost and risks of blood transfusion, we also strongly advocate the collection and auto-transfusion of chest tube output from any moderate-to-large hemothorax. Since the majority of blood loss often occurs immediately after placement of a chest tube, the collection apparatus should be available in the emergency department and used whenever there is suspicion that a large acute hemothorax may be drained. Ideally, such systems should be able to be adapted to the existing collection device used, rather than being a totally separate system. This may allow the use of auto-transfusion even in situations where one did not expect a large hemothorax. Our experience has also been that the auto-transfusion of blood from chest tubes diminishes the coagulopathy and inflammatory response to injury that is often seen in these patients.

## VIDEO-ASSISTED THORACOSCOPIC SURGERY (VATS) IN TRAUMA

Experience and facility with VATS has made it an important part of the operative skills of surgeons taking care of trauma patients. VATS can be useful in the diagnostic evaluation and repair of small injuries of the diaphragm, assessment of continued hemorrhage or air leaks, and control of bleeding from intercostal vessels, but its main advantage is in the evacuation of retained pleural clot.[87,96–100] Optimally, VATS requires the patients to be placed in the lateral decubitus position. Inability to tolerate the lateral decubitus position is therefore a relative contraindication to VATS. Also, while VATS may occasionally be possible using single lumen endotracheal tubes, a double-lumen tube that allows deflation of the involved lung facilitates it greatly, and is almost always required. The inability to pass a double lumen tube or concerns about changing/replacing the single lumen tube for a double lumen tube can sometimes be managed by advancing the indwelling single lumen tube into the mainstem bronchus on the unaffected side. This maneuver is most easily accomplished when attempting to thoracoscope the left pleural space.

In most patients a chest tube will already be present, and the thoracoscope can be inserted through the existing chest tube site after removal of the tube. If not, our preference is to place the scope in the fifth intercostal space in the anterior axillary line. This allows

excellent visualization of the posterior and inferior portion of the pleural space where blood clot is most likely to accumulate. Using small incisions that allow the placement of standard as well as thoracoscopic instruments into the chest, the clot can be broken up and evacuated. Using the large thoracoscopic suction or a high-pressure pulse irrigation device can be of assistance in breaking up and evacuating the clot.

The ability of VATS to successfully evacuate the pleural space is in great measure related to the timing of the procedure. In general, procedures performed after a week are more difficult and have a much lesser chance of success.[98–100] Also, in some cases where VATS alone cannot evacuate the pleural space, combining VATS with open techniques has proven successful. In these cases, a mini-thoracotomy can be performed using minimal or no spreading of the ribs. Traditional thoracic instruments are used and the video-thoracoscope can be used to supplement direct vision. This approach may avoid some of the short and long-term morbidity associated with traditional thoracotomies.

## LUNG INJURIES

Blunt and penetrating trauma result in markedly different types of lung injury. Penetrating injuries cause lung lacerations directly, with resultant hemopneumothoraces. Lung injuries following blunt trauma are less common and most often due to displaced rib fractures. In both cases, insertion of a tube thoracostomy and evacuation of the pleural space are the initial treatment, and will usually control hemorrhage and air leaks from the peripheral lung. In older series, of patients undergoing thoracotomy following penetrating trauma, only about 20% of patients required a resective procedure to control hemorrhage from lung injuries.[88,89] In a recent multicenter review from five Level I trauma centers, however, Kharmy-Jones reported that 40% of patients who required a thoracotomy following penetrating trauma and 17% of those requiring a thoracotomy following blunt trauma required some form of lung resection.[101] Many possible reasons exist for this apparent increase in the rate of lung resection. It may reflect an increased sophistication of the weaponry used (e.g., a greater rate of high caliber gunshot wounds vs. a prior predominance of low-velocity gunshot wounds and stab sounds). Alternatively, there may be a selection bias in that more severely injured patients are now presenting to Level I trauma centers in locations with mature trauma systems, or that operative indications have become more stringent. Nonetheless, most lung lacerations following penetrating trauma can be handled by pulmonary tractotomy or stapled nonanatomic resections.[101]

When performing a thoracotomy for lung hemorrhage there can often be a great temptation to clamp the lung entry and exit wounds immediately to halt the bleeding. It should be recognized that this does little to stop the actual bleeding. It does stop bleeding into the pleural cavity, but unfortunately that maneuver often simply results in the hemorrhage being directed into the lung parynchema. More dangerous still, the blood can be forced into the tracheo-bronchial tree. Communication with anesthesia is essential to warn them of the possibility of significant endobronchial bleeding. Blood suffusing the alveoli can result in profound hypoxemia and be extremely difficult to evacuate. For these

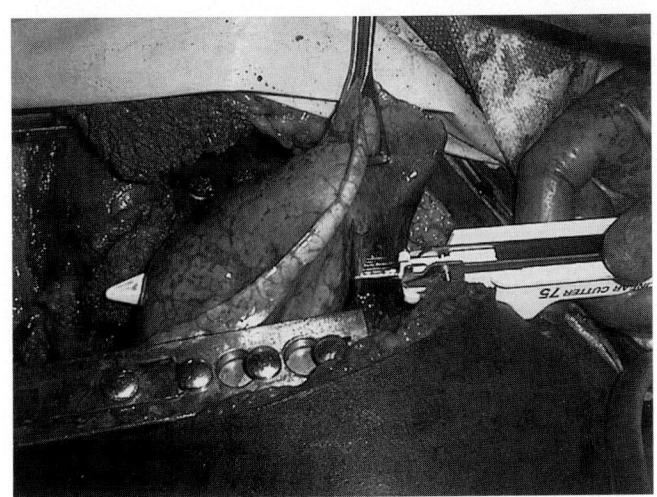

**FIGURE 26-15.** Intraoperative photograph of a pulmonary tractotomy. The linear stapler is placed through the gunshot wound tract.

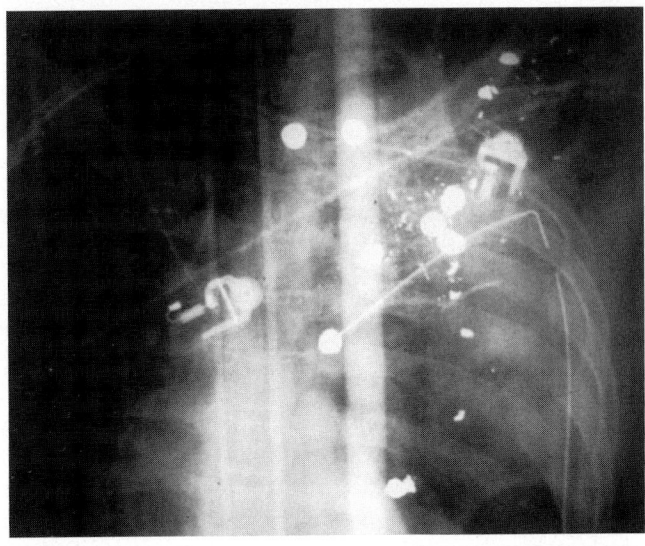

**FIGURE 26-16.** Close-range shotgun wound to the left upper chest wall. This devastating injury required left upper lobectomy to control hemorrhage.

reasons, the practice of simply oversewing penetrating lung injuries should be used with caution. In contrast, pulmonary tractotomy preserves lung parenchyma as well as simultaneously controlling both bleeding and air leakage.[102,103] The principle of this operation is to open the knife or gunshot wound tract using a linear stapler (Fig. 26-15). This exposes the inner portion of the tract. Large individual vessels are suture-ligated. Our preference is then to control residual minor hemorrhage and air leaks using a running #3-0 polypropylene suture on a long needle to oversew the entire injury tract at right angles to the staple line. Using this type of needle allows one to span the distance needed easily. Compressing the lung edges with a lung clamp can also be helpful in areas where the lung is thick. Alternatively, if the geometry of the injury allows, the edge may be stapled.

In more extensive injuries, anatomic lobectomies may be required to control hemorrhage. In our experience this occurs most often with close-range shotgun or high-velocity gunshot wounds. These can easily result in a cavitating injury that involves an entire lobe (Fig. 26-16). But in addition, severe parenchymal lung injuries requiring resection can be seen in a significant percentage of patients requiring thoracotomy for blunt trauma.[101] Some central injuries may result in a proximal bronchial injury that will require lobectomy to close the air leak. Anatomic lobectomy has been associated with an increased mortality compared to nonanatomic resection or tractotomy, but this may be due to an increase in the incidence of shock, in the percentage of patients sustaining more extensive injuries, or in patients sustaining blunt rather than penetrating trauma. Those patients requiring lobectomy for bronchial injury have a better outcome than patients requiring lobectomy for hemorrhage.[104]

The need for pneumonectomy following penetrating trauma is thankfully rare, since it is associated with reported mortality rates ranging from 50 to 100%.[88,101,104,105] The combination of hemorrhagic shock and the sudden increase in pulmonary vascular resistance that accompanies pneumonectomy can result in sudden and often irreversible right heart failure, which can lead rapidly to cardiac arrest.[106] But another possible reason for the dismal results reported with pneumonectomy is that the procedure is often performed late and in desperation after lesser options have failed. Such

patients may therefore represent a subgroup that has suffered extensive blood loss, and in which prolonged shock is present. Our impression is that when lobar resections and pneumonectomies seem inevitable, they probably should be carried out expeditiously to prevent ongoing blood loss. In appropriately chosen patients this may still lead to significant salvage rates.[101,107] Also, because of the otherwise lethal nature of these injuries, we and others have attempted to apply damage control techniques to their management.[108] Temporary control of hemorrhage using a Satinsky clamp or a hilar snare[109] or even simply torsing the lung on its hilar pedicle to affect a "physiologic pneumonectomy" with the idea of returning to the operating room for the formal anatomic resection if the patient can be successfully resuscitated may be an attractive alternative under extreme conditions.

The majority of injuries to the lung following blunt trauma consist of contusions and hematomas. Contusions are common whether or not there is an associated injury to the chest wall.[110] Pulmonary contusions may not be apparent on the initial chest radiograph but may still manifest themselves physiologically as a decreased arterial oxygen saturation. Lesions not visible on a screening AP CXR are frequently seen on a CT scan. Similar to the classic picture of bronchopneumonia, the lung contusions may begin to "blossom" and become visible on the CXR several hours after admission. Some may not however, and it is still unclear what the natural history of "CT-only" pulmonary contusions is. Contusions are usually irregular, and have ill-defined edges that do not follow segmental anatomy. The role of fluid therapy in the progression and treatment of pulmonary contusions remain controversial, and will be discussed further in the section on critical care. Uncomplicated pulmonary contusions will often improve and disappear within three to four days following injury unless a secondary insult occurs.

Whereas pulmonary contusions may contain hemorrhagic areas with some intra-alveolar hemorrhage, a pulmonary hematoma represents a true, space-occupying blood clot within the parenchyma of the lung. These lesions are usually apparent on the initial CXR, and while they may initially be thought to represent early pulmonary contusions, they signify a much greater degree of damage to the lung, and are far slower to resolve. On physical examination, such patients may often have bloody secretions or frank hemoptysis.

## THE CRITICAL CARE OF CHEST TRAUMA

Pulmonary failure is the single greatest cause of ICU morbidity and is a significant contributor to mortality after trauma.[111] The root causes of impaired gas exchange after chest injuries are typically multifactorial and therefore especially difficult to diagnose and treat. A wide variety of diagnostic and therapeutic approaches have been tried. Over the past 20 years these have included the use of steroids, prostanoids, surfactant, biologic response modifiers, fluid restriction, fluid "optimization," chest wall fracture fixation, open lung biopsies, prone positioning, oscillating beds, ECMO, partial liquid ventilation, use of inhaled nitric oxide, and a wide variety of ventilation schemes. The lack of rigorous scientific validation of the efficacy of any of these approaches attests to the difficulties in treating and even in studying these conditions. Yet, the mortality of respiratory failure after trauma has noticeably decreased.[112] Thus in the aggregate, modern approaches to the care and support of major chest injuries do seem to have improved their prognosis.

## CAUSES OF PULMONARY DYSFUNCTION AFTER CHEST TRAUMA

### Pulmonary Contusion

The most consistent source of pulmonary dysfunction after chest trauma is a direct injury, or pulmonary contusion. Pulmonary contusions alter pulmonary ventilation-perfusion (V/Q) matching and thus cause arterial hypoxemia. The underlying pathophysiology is complex, involving pathologic vasomotion, airway collapse, and immunologic attack on the alveolar-capillary membrane. Microvascular endothelial cells are in fact, directly activated by percussion trauma, although this effect is much better described in the central nervous system (CNS) than in the lung.[113] This process is poorly understood in general, however. Consequently, the management of pulmonary contusion is almost entirely supportive. In less severe cases, supplemental oxygen can be given by mask to prevent arterial desaturation. Continuous positive airway pressure (CPAP) delivered by a tight-fitting mask has been used to improve oxygenation further, but the natural history of pulmonary contusion is a gradual worsening over the first few days. Moreover, CPAP can predispose to gastric distention and aspiration, especially in trauma patients who may be obtunded or receiving narcotics. Thus in our experience, the use of CPAP as a "hedge" to avoid endotracheal intubation in major chest trauma patients is almost always unwise, being both doomed to failure in most cases and risking significant complications. Since endotracheal intubation will be required in most patients with significant contusions, prophylactic intubation prior to deterioration should be considered early and is often warranted. Once the patient is

intubated, measures that increase mean airway pressure should be used early to improve oxygenation. These may include positive end expiratory pressure (PEEP) or the reversal of normal inspiratory/expiratory(I/E) time relationships by any one of several ventilator strategies. The physiologic effects of the pulmonary contusion itself typically resolve over about a week.

### Pulmonary Infections

Up to half the patients with significant chest injuries will develop pneumonia during their hospital course.[114,115] The accurate diagnosis of pneumonia is important since the inappropriate use of antibiotics will enhance colonization and infection of the patient with more resistant organisms. Yet the diagnosis and management of pulmonary infection is especially difficult in the face of chest trauma. All patients with major chest injuries have an abnormal CXR and abnormal oxygenation. Moreover, the systemic inflammatory responses to injury are at present, essentially indistinguishable from those seen in infections. Thus, although the diagnosis of pneumonia may be clear on occasion, most commonly it is very difficult to make after chest injury. Our practice therefore has been to supplement clinical diagnosis with liberal use of bronchoscopic alveolar lavage[116] in the diagnosis of pneumonia. This approach is clearly imperfect, and will have a substantial false positive and false negative rate. Nonetheless, we find that it has helped us a great deal to limit and focus antibiotic use.

Pneumonia early after chest injury is most commonly caused by Gram-positive, community-acquired organisms like *S. aureus, streptococci,* and *H. influenza*. After two to four days, the airway becomes colonized with hospital-acquired flora like enteric gram negatives and *pseudomonas sp.* This transition is hastened by the inappropriate and prolonged use of empiric antibiotics[117] administered in the hope of preventing infections at other injured sites. Similarly, once diagnosed, pulmonary infections should be treated with as narrow an antibiotic regimen as possible, recognizing that many infections will prove to be polymicrobial and some will require multidrug therapy. Aggressive endobronchial toilet is often required. This may entail tracheostomy and repeated bronchoscopy.

### Inflammatory Lung Injury

In many cases, the deterioration of pulmonary function after chest trauma will be related as much or more to the systemic inflammatory effects of injury as to the local injury. The early acute lung injury (ALI) and more advanced adult respiratory distress syndrome (ARDS) observed following shock and trauma are widely believed to result from pathologic neutrophil (PMN)–endothelial cell (EC) interactions. These injure pulmonary capillary endothelial membranes, leading to interstitial and alveolar edema. The net results are diminished pulmonary compliance and diffusion capacity.

The diagnosis of ALI/ARDS is based upon empiric criteria. X-ray changes are generally diffuse and there should be no evidence of left ventricular failure, but in chest trauma patients coexisting pathology often make the published criteria for ARDS less than uniformly applicable. In effect, ARDS is a diagnosis of exclusion and, in reality all major trauma patients probably have some ALI/ARDS component to their pulmonary dysfunction.

The goals of therapy are therefore to minimize the patient's exposure to those factors that are known or thought to cause, prolong or exacerbate ALI/ARDS. Theoretically, the avoidance of shock and prolonged periods of incomplete resuscitation may be preventive, but these problems can seldom be controlled. Considerable data also suggests that patients with chest injuries may be at special risk for pulmonary deterioration after fracture fixation.[118] Some of these occurrences may therefore be avoidable. Our studies suggest that ALI after fracture fixation may result when inflammatory fracture hematoma fluids are mobilized into the circulation.[119] Such fluids can activate PMN,[120] and PMN activation at a time period when EC are activated[121] will enhance their capacity to attack the lung. Blood loss, imprecise resuscitation, and transfusion with banked blood during other surgical procedures may also be important contributors to a "second hit" at the time of fracture management, and may help precipitate ARDS. Since the inflammatory mediator content of fractures peaks two to three days after injury;[119] in the multiply injured patient with a chest injury we favor a "resuscitative orthopedics" approach to the timing of long-bone fracture fixation. Needed wound cleansing and temporary stabilization are performed early in a damage control fashion. In critically ill patients, however, we prefer to delay definitive fracture fixation until the end of the first week, or when the patient has improving pulmonary function.

The treatment of acute ARDS itself is supportive at present. No intervention or pharmaceutical agent has proven of significant value in treating posttraumatic ARDS. Several small series[122,123] have suggested that the late fibroproliferative stage of ARDS may respond in some measure to corticosteroids, but considering the dangers of steroids, we await prospective data before using them routinely.

## Extravascular Lung Water

Historically, the avoidance of fluid overload and of sequestration of extravascular lung water was a cornerstone of the management of chest injuries.[124] The current recognition that SIRS related to systemic hypoperfusion causes immune lung injury[125,126] must modify that concern. Our approach to fluid management in the patient with chest injures is therefore primarily aimed at insuring circulatory adequacy and "euvolemia." Shock and resuscitation by any regimen leads to a relative expansion of extravascular water, but the highly effective pulmonary lymphatic pumps tend to spare the lung from interstitial fluid accumulation.[127,128] Patients with coexisting cardiac, renal, or hepatic diseases however, will show a greater tendency to accumulate symptomatic excess interstitial lung water with resuscitation. Unfortunately, since the alternative in this group is inadequate resuscitation and prolonged tissue hypoperfusion, extravascular fluid sequestration must often be accepted. Such patients will often require inotropic, diuretic, or oncotic support during their course. Pleural effusions will be common and will often require drainage in patients with marginal pulmonary function. Last, it is common for all trauma patients to mobilize sodium and water from cellular and interstitial spaces as they improve. Such fluid shifts are often predictable and their early management may lessen their clinical impact on the patient.

## Endobronchial Secretions

The accumulation of bronchial secretions is an important problem in the chest trauma patient. Excessive secretions may lead to lobar collapse, hypoxemia, diminished compliance, and postobstructive airway infections. Gross aspiration at the time of injury as well as the continuing micro-aspiration that accompanies endotracheal intubation will both increase secretions, and lead to their colonization with oropharyngeal flora. Blood may accumulate in the airway and form bronchial casts. Nonintubated patients may retain secretions due to pain and impaired cough. Thus, the most important early management strategy in spontaneously ventilating patients will often be the institution of good pain control.

Intubated patients cannot cough and are completely dependent upon suctioning for airway toilet. Mucolytic agents such as n-acetylcysteine may be helpful if secretions are thick, but should be accompanied by a bronchodilator. Overly prolonged therapy may cause bronchorrhea. Chest physiotherapy may be helpful, but the percussion of injured ribs should be avoided. Often, the clearance of tenacious secretions in intubated patients will require therapeutic bronchoscopy.

## MANAGEMENT OF PULMONARY DYSFUNCTION AFTER CHEST TRAUMA

Because of the complex pathology described above, management of respiratory dysfunction in the chest trauma patient can be very complex. In such patients it is often useful to consider ventilatory management of $CO_2$ exchange separately from the treatment of impaired oxygen transport.

### Ventilation

The ventilation of chest trauma patients may differ from that of other patients in several respects. Only patients with rather mild chest trauma and an absence of associated injuries can be safely managed without endotracheal intubation and mechanical ventilation. Intubated patients with lesser degrees of injury will require some support of air exchange, but whenever possible should be allowed to use their muscles of respiration to the fullest extent possible. We find that the use of the pressure support ventilation (PSV) mode is highly satisfactory for such moderate support of spontaneously breathing patients. The major exception to the use of PSV in our spontaneously ventilating patients is the presence of a clinically significant flail chest. Early after flail chest, even the modest negative pressures needed to trigger the ventilator cycle may destabilize the chest wall.[54] Patients can find such instability very painful, and fracture segment motion may delay spontaneous stabilization. We therefore often prefer to use a volume controlled mode such as SIMV initially, with a minute ventilation sufficient to raise arterial pH to slightly >7.40. A slight alkalosis will suppress spontaneous ventilation without the need for excessive sedation. Flail chest segments generally tend to stabilize over about a week, although patients with thicker chest walls often appear to stabilize more quickly. At that time, patients can be allowed to breathe spontaneously using a PSV mode to support their work of breathing. We institute PSV at a pressure equal to the peak inspiratory pressure minus the end expiratory pressure ("PIP–PEEP") noted in the SIMV mode at the prior tidal volume. This insures a comfortable transition for the patient. The patient can then be weaned by progressively lowering their pressure support.

After major chest trauma however, both pulmonary contusion and ARDS can cause the pulmonary parenchyma to be noncompliant. Stiff lungs often require relatively high airway pressures to sustain "traditional" tidal volumes of 10–15 mL/kg. High airway pressures ($\geq$35 cm $H_2O$) however, predispose to ventilator induced lung injury.[129] Thus the use of lower tidal volumes ($\leq$6 ml/kg) has been shown to improve outcomes.[130] Maintaining a "normal" $PaCO_2$ is not needed and "permissive" hypercapnia is often useful in chest trauma.[131,132] Acidosis can be controlled using buffers if the pH falls below $\geq$7.25, but we have found this is rarely necessary. Concurrent acid loads, such as from excess chloride in NaCl, should be avoided. All patients treated this way require paralysis and sedation both because of the air hunger associated with respiratory acidosis, and to lower their oxygen consumption and $CO_2$ production. Similarly, excess $CO_2$ production due to excessive calorie intake and other metabolic sources must be avoided.

In some patients, lowering inspiratory flow rates will also help decrease airway pressures. Limiting airway pressure may be especially important in the event of traumatic or postoperative broncho-pleural fistulas, and a variety of ventilator modes can be used to achieve these conditions. Chest trauma patients with an abrupt change in compliance should always be suspected of either a pneumothorax requiring drainage, or mucus plugging requiring suctioning or bronchoscopy.

## Oxygenation

All patients with major chest trauma will have some degree of hypoxemia for the reasons described above. Whereas this may be managed initially by increasing $FIO_2$, prolonged high $FIO_2$ is in itself deleterious to the lung both because of oxygen free-radical generation and absorptive atelectasis due to the absence of nitrogen. The longer-term management of hypoxemia therefore entails raising mean airway pressures by the use of PEEP and plateau or "reverse I/E" ventilation. These modes increase either the time spent in inhalation or the end-expiratory pressure. Such interventions are designed to recruit alveoli as well as to diminish alveolar and interstitial water, and thus to diminish intrapulmonary shunting. The degree of reversal of I/E time will only be limited by the need to excrete $CO_2$. As noted above, the maintenance of "normal" $PaCO_2$ is not a requirement. Right ventricular preload must be maintained in order to compensate for the decreased venous return seen when using high PEEP.[133]

A multitude of unproven therapies have been used in profoundly hypoxemic patients. Such patients have been treated with rotating or oscillating beds, differential lung ventilation, inhaled nitric oxide, partial liquid ventilation, hypertonic saline, red blood cell transfusions, or inotropic support to raise mixed venous oxygen saturation, and other modalities. All may have some effect and may "buy some time" for the primary process to abate in occasional patients. None has been prospectively validated.

## TRACHEOSTOMY IN CHEST TRAUMA

As noted above, tracheostomy can be an important tool to optimize ventilation in severe pulmonary failure. It is also a key adjunct in pulmonary toilet, which can be a life-threatening problem for chest trauma patients with copious, bloody, or thick secretions. Thus, tracheostomy is seen as a treatment for respiratory failure as well as for weaning patients from support, rather than as a marker for the failure of therapy. Tracheostomy is frequently needed in chest trauma patients who deteriorate, but whenever considered, it should be performed early. In fact, as patients' requirements for ventilatory and oxygenation support increase, tracheostomy itself becomes increasingly dangerous. Thus, the clinician should always be looking for a "window" when it has become clear that a tracheostomy is likely to be needed, but still before it becomes unsafe to perform. Early problems with clearing secretions or dependence on a small ($<$8 mm) endotracheal tube placed during prehospital care should suggest prompt conversion to tracheostomy.

In critically ill chest trauma patients, we prefer to perform tracheostomies in the ICU. This approach will avoid the substantial intrinsic risks of deterioration in transport. Occasionally, there may be concern for the proximity of a tracheostomy to a sternotomy incision. In such cases, using a dilatational technique can allow for more cephalad placement of the tracheostomy. Also, where required, an elective cricothyrotomy can be a useful alternative to tracheostomy placement.

## CHEST WALL STABILIZTION

Although it is clear that most flail chest injuries can be managed by selective intubation and mechanical ventilation,[123] there has been recurring interest in the operative management of flail chest.[134–137] Unfortunately, the evidence supporting the concept that stabilization of rib fractures is useful in major chest trauma continues to be scanty with many of the papers being case reports that are testimonial in nature. The few reported series are retrospective over long periods of time and comprise highly selected patients where those with the most severe pulmonary dysfunction have not typically been considered surgical candidates. In stratifying patients with flail chests with and without significant pulmonary contusions, Voggenreiter found that operative chest wall stabilization provided no benefit in patients with pulmonary contusion. However, chest wall fixation did permit earlier extubation and a shortened length of stay in the subgroup of patients that had respiratory insufficiency without pulmonary contusions.[137] These data support the conclusion that whereas fixation does stabilize flail segments, the major physiologic deficit in chest trauma patients requiring mechanical ventilation is usually their underlying pulmonary contusions and ALI/ARDS. In the one randomized prospective series in the literature, Takana et al. randomized patients five days after injury to operative stabilization or continuing nonoperative management.[137] Despite waiting five days after injury, the operative group required less ventilatory support and had fewer infections.

Thus, at present our conclusion is that operative chest wall stabilization will not benefit the vast majority of patients with flail chest and significant pulmonary contusions. In patients undergoing thoracotomy for other indications, fixation of adjacent rib sections using wires or small plates will provide markedly improved chest wall stability and should be done at the time of closure as it adds no additional physiologic cost to the patient. In patients with flail chest injuries that do not require endotracheal intubation, operative fixation will clearly provide no benefit. In the subset of patients requiring intubation with physiologically important pulmonary contusions, operative fixation of the flail segment cannot be recommended on the basis of available data.

# PAIN CONTROL IN CHEST TRAUMA

Adequate pain control is among one of the most important aspects of managing patients with chest injuries.[138] The failure to provide sufficient analgesia in this setting has been shown to result in hypoventilation, retained secretions, increased atalectasis and lobar collapse, pneumonia, and respiratory failure.[139] In addition, inadequate pain control has been shown to perpetuate the stress response to injury[140] and may have a negative impact on posttraumatic immune function.[141] In patients who are mechanically ventilated, the failure to provide adequate pain control will hamper their ability to be weaned and extubated.

Traditionally, the pharmacological approach to pain management in chest injury has consisted of the use of narcotics with or without regional anesthesia. Recently however, more powerful nonsteroidal anti-inflammatory drugs (NSAID) such as ketorolac have proven effective in relieving pain from mild to moderate injuries.[142]

## Narcotics

Parenteral narcotics remain the standard method of pain control in the majority of trauma patients. Narcotic preparations can be given orally, intramuscularly, or intravenously. But whereas intramuscular administration has been the standard for decades, we strongly advise against this route of administration since it is both painful to the patient and results in unreliable absorption of the narcotic. With the exception of meperdine (Demerol), however, which narcotic is used is less important than ensuring that an adequate dose is administered.[143] The doses of narcotics required for pain control will vary greatly depending upon previous or current narcotic use, age, extent of injury, and other factors that may alter the patient's perception of and reaction to pain. Thus, narcotic analgesics must be monitored for and titrated to effect.

The use of visual pain scales in combination with physical examination and performance on incentive spirometry can be very effective in determining the adequacy of pain control.[144,145] Our present approach is to begin most awake patients on a patient controlled analgesia (PCA) regimen using morphine or fentanyl. Later, patients are transitioned to long-acting narcotic preparations such as oxycontin or MS-contin with the use of oxycodone for breakthrough pain. At this time, we may add a NSAID to further reduce inflammation and improve analgesia. It should be remembered that in the narcotic-addicted patient or patients who have received narcotic infusions for a prolonged period, one may have to use "extraordinary" doses of morphine to achieve adequate analgesia. In such cases, the addition of methadone may be useful to provide a baseline level of narcotic effect without excessive sedation. Last, it is important to avoid narcotic-induced constipation. This can result in severe abdominal pain, nausea, and vomiting in patients requiring long-term opioids.

## Regional Anesthesia

Rib blocks using a mixture of 1–2% lidocaine with 0.25% bipuvicaine have been used to decrease the pain of rib fractures. This simple technique involves the administration of 2–3 mL of the anesthetic mixture to the inferior rib margin several centimeters posterior to the site of the rib fracture. To obtain optimal analgesia, one intercostals nerve above and one below the fractured rib should be blocked. Intercostal blocks may last for up to six hours and can be repeated. The limitations of the technique are that the pain control is short-lived and that it can only be used for patients with mid or lower rib fractures. Last, in our experience the results vary widely and the risks of pneumothorax in patients without a chest tube are real.[146]

Intrapleural administration of local anesthetics has also been used following chest trauma. This technique has been questioned by some groups and embraced by others.[147–149] Its utility has usually been limited to those patients who have chest tubes in place to allow for repetitive administrations, but some groups have suggested the placement of small subpleural or paravertebral catheters for this purpose.[150,151]

Epidural analgesia/anesthesia is the delivery mode that has been shown to have the greatest impact on pulmonary mechanics following moderate to severe chest trauma, especially in those patients with bilateral injuries.[152,153] There are several different combinations of local anesthetics and narcotics which can be used. In our institution, the most common combination is fentanyl with bipuvicaine. Hypotension may result from an epidural block. Thus, if the blood pressure either cannot be corrected with vascular expansion, or if the infusion of volume is undesirable, the local anesthetic can be omitted. But such combination therapy can be advantageous because it works via two different mechanisms of action. Opioids modulate pre- and postsysnaptic nerve transmission in dorsal horn neurons by effects on their specific receptors. Local anesthetics work by blocking sodium channels. Thus the analgesic effects of the two classes of drug are synergistic. Moreover, the potential for side effects is lessened in combination therapy since the doses of each drug used can be lower than the amount used if either were administered alone.

Epidural analgesia does have significant practical drawbacks, however. The many specific complications of epidural narcotics and local anesthetics include ileus, pruritis, and urinary retention as well as transient hypotension. The use of epidural catheters per se also requires that the spine be documented to be free of injury. In severely injured patients this can sometimes be impossible to accomplish for several days. In addition, the concomitant use of low molecular weight heparin (LMWH) in patients with an epidural catheter has been implicated in the development of spinal epidural hematomas with resultant neurologic deficits. This complication resulted in an FDA Public Health Advisory in 1997. Thus, if an epidural catheter is to be placed the patient should not have received LMWH for at least 24 hours or subcutaneous standard heparin for at least 12 hours. Last, epidural catheters can only be left in place safely for 7–10 days because of the possibility of epidural abscess formation. Thus, it is strongly recommended that epidural catheters not be placed in mechanically ventilated patients until they are ready to be weaned.

Mackersie demonstrated that the use of epidural fentanyl alone was safe and was associated with significant improvements in vital capacity and in maximum negative inspiratory force.[154] Eighty-five percent of the patients in that study experienced good relief of pain with this technique alone and required no supplemental parenteral narcotics. In a subsequent randomized prospective study it was found that while both methods improved visual analog pain scores, epidural fentanyl improved ventialory mechanics significantly better than intravenous fentanyl. Intravenous narcotics were associated with increases in $PaCO_2$ and decreases in $PaO_2$ that were not observed in the epidural group. These data have been replicated by numerous other investigators. Most recently, in a randomized prospective trial, Bulger et al. reported a 2-fold increase in the number of ventilator days for the opioid group versus patient receiving epidural analgesia.[155] Most importantly, they also point out that the ability to provide epidural analgesia is limited in the trauma population due to the presence of exclusion criteria in over 50%. Thus, we believe that the use of epidural analgesia, when feasible, is of considerable benefit to patients following severe chest injury, as it has been strongly associated with a decrease in the rate of nosocomial pneumonia and a shorter duration of mechanical ventilation.

## COMPLICATIONS AND OTHER CONDITIONS

### Empyema

Posttraumatic bacterial empyema continues to be a significant source of morbidity and mortality following severe chest trauma.[156] The etiologies of posttraumatic empyema are multifactorial and include (1) iatrogenic infection of the pleural space after tube thoracostomy for hemothorax or pneumothorax; (2) direct contamination of the pleural space resulting from penetrating injuries; (3) secondary infection of the pleural space secondary to an intra-abdominal injury associated with diaphragmatic disruption; (4) secondary infection of a clotted hemothorax; and (5) parapneumonic empyema secondary to posttraumatic pneumonia, pulmonary contusion, or ARDS.[157,158]

The specific organisms that cause posttraumatic empyema will vary greatly depending upon which mechanism was responsible for the empyema. Direct contamination as a result of a chest tube insertion almost always results in a gram-positive infection, most commonly with *Staphyloccus aureus* and *Streptococcus* species.[159,160] Pneumonic processes may result in secondary pleural contamination with a variety of organisms, but often involve gram-negative or mixed pathogens. The specific agents will depend on the prevailing bacteriology of nosocomial pneumonia in the institution. Similarly, secondary infection of the pleural space from hematogenous or contiguous sources will usually result in either a gram-negative or a mixed infection.

The reported incidence of empyema varies widely, with published rates from 0 to 18%.[83,159–161] Examination of the data suggests that these wide variations can be attributed to (1) the retrospective nature of the studies, (2) which patients were included in the denominator group at risk (blunt trauma vs. penetrating trauma; all patients with a chest tube vs. selected groups etc.), and (3) whether the fluid collection needed to be "culture positive." This is important, since many clinical "empyemas" in blunt trauma patients are in fact "culture negative."[158] Our experience is that

sterile pleural collections are also rich in inflammatory mediators.[93] Thus they may have clinical systemic effects indistinguishable from those of infected collections. We believe that a reasonable estimate of the true empyema rate in major trauma patients is about 5%. With advances in trauma and critical care that have resulted in increasing survival of severely injured patients, it is possible that the incidence of this complication may be increasing. The *sine qua non* for the development of an empyema is an inadequately drained pleural space fluid collection.[159–162] Other risk factors include the mechanism of injury, the location of chest tube placement, the presence of pulmonary contusion or pneumonia, and the number of chest tubes. However, it will be recognized that all these factors are themselves dependent variables, which are related to the severity of either regional chest injury, or to the degree of systemic injury and shock.

A pleural collection or empyema should be suspected in any patient with chest trauma who has unexplained fever, leukocytosis, or respiratory failure. In our experience, the majority of patients in whom the issue arises are critically ill, and are in the trauma ICU. In this group, the AP CXR is of little or no use in the delineation of pleural collections. Early and liberal use of CT scanning has proved invaluable in identifying loculated fluid collections and pleural peels that have not been apparent on plain chest radiographs (Fig. 26-17). Moreover, the CT may guide therapy.[158,163] The early use of CT scanning can also prevent delays in diagnosis. Such delays may both prolong the patient's illness and also result in the need for more extensive surgical procedures should operative management of the empyema prove necessary.

Current treatment options for empyema include (1) chest tube or CT-guided drainage, (2) chest tube drainage with intrapleural fibrinolytic therapy, (3) VATS, and (4) open thoracotomy and decortication. Classically, empyemas proceed through several phases. They begin as exudative effusions, changing over time into loculated effusions, and finally into organized empyemas. The pleural fluid becomes progressively more viscous as these stages proceed. This process may occur quite rapidly in major trauma patients due to the high degree of tissue damage present and to the concentrations of activated mediators that are present in the pleural space. These factors also underscore the need for rapid diagnosis and treatment.

Chest tube or CT-guided tube drainage is often quite effective in the early phases and typically should be attempted as a primary treatment. The presence of a visible peel on the chest CT scan has been associated with a high rate of failure of chest tube drainage. These patients are probably better served by proceeding directly to a VATS or to an open thoracotomy. Fibrinolytics have been used successfully by some groups, but the benefit of this approach as compared to chest tube drainage alone or to VATS is unknown.[163] With its increasing use, there have been reports of VATS being highly successful in treating established empyemas.[100] In distinction, our experience has been that it is very difficult to enter the chest in these cases, and it has often proved impossible to obtain enough maneuvering room to begin to successfully decorticate the pleural space thoracoscopically. This is in contrast to our experience with early retained hemothoraces.[98] We recognize that the success of the procedure may be directly related to the patience one has to perform it. Conversely, other groups may be reporting on early patients that we might have

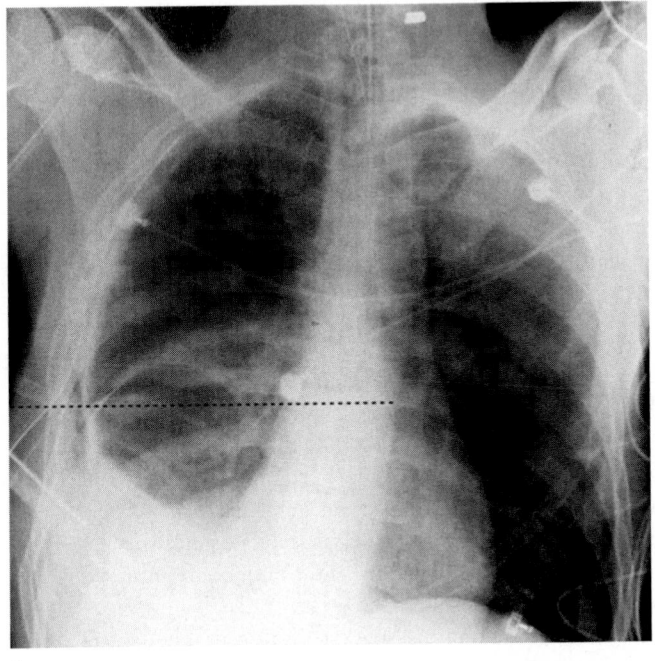

A

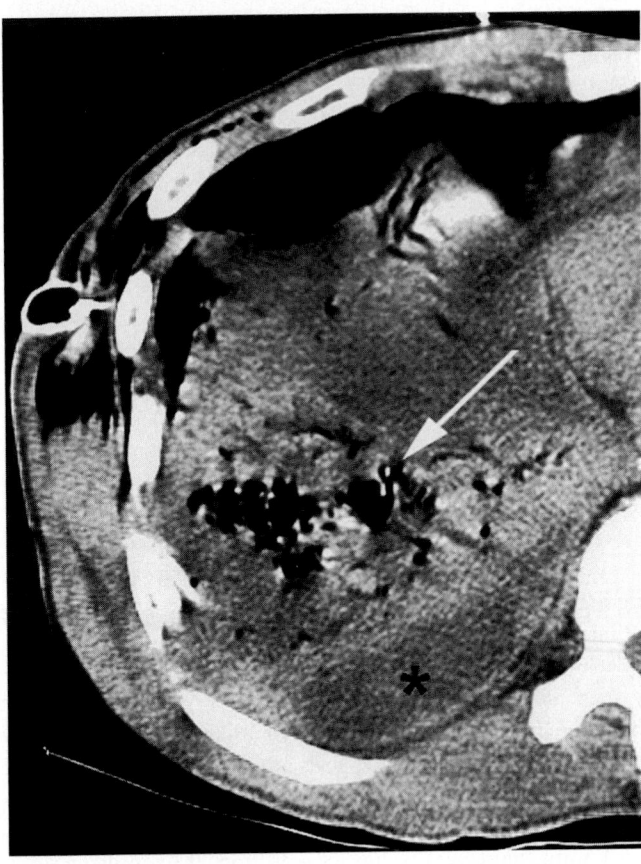

B

**FIGURE 26-17.** Plain CXR (**A**) and corresponding Chest CT (**B**) demonstrating the superiority of CT to diagnose complex thoracic pathology. The dotted line of the CXR marks that level of the CT slice. The CXR show loss of volume on the right, the presence of a chest tube, and moderate haziness in the right lower lobe. The chest CT, however, shows an undetected loculated pneumothorax despite the chest tube (which enters the chest more superiorly), significant right lower lobe consolidation and pneumonia (arrow), and the presence of an empyema (*) with a surrounding inflammatory rind. The patient underwent thoracotomy and decortication.

classified as a retained hemothorax. In either case, our experience is that in sick trauma patients with a well-established infective process, an open thoracotomy and deocortication is often the most expedient approach.

Following decortication it is not uncommon for the CXR to look worse in the first few days than it did preoperatively. If good drainage has been established, however, the patient will begin to improve clinically even though the CXR lags behind the clinical course. Vigorous pulmonary toilet must be used to keep the lung expanded after thoracotomy. It is not uncommon to have an increase in purulent secretions that must be suctioned after the release of an entrapped lung. Culture-specific antibiotics should be used for organisms cultured from the pleura or sputum.

## Pneumatocele

Posttraumatic cysts or pneumatoceles are uncommon following chest trauma although CT scanning has made it easier to diagnose this condition. Airway disruption can lead to the development of an air collection within the lung parenchyma that does not connect with the pleural space. We have observed this condition with increased frequency in the subset of patients with

severe chest trauma who have required prolonged and intensive ventilatory support (Fig. 26-18). Most of these lesions do not require specific treatment and will resolve following successful weaning for the ventilator. If these lesions are large or continue to expand, or if they become secondarily infected, CT guided percutaneous drainage can be very effective in draining and collapsing

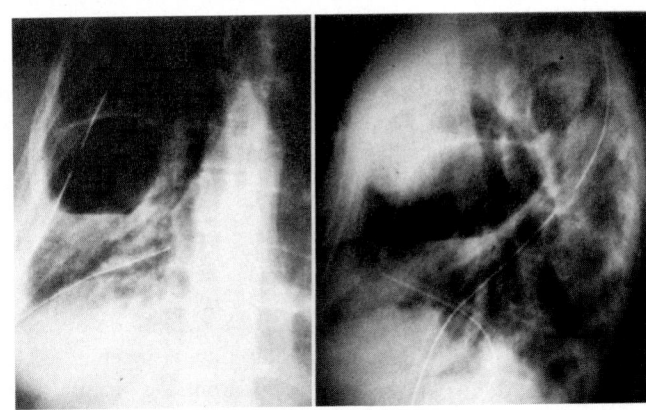

**FIGURE 26-18.** PA and lateral CXR of a large pneumatocele following a severe crush injury to the right lung.

the cyst. Concern for injury to the lung here is unfounded, and our experience is that this approach treats rather than causes air leaks.

## Persistent Air Leaks and Bronchopleural Fistula

Air leaks are very common following chest trauma, but they seldom require any treatment other than tube thoracostomy. The presence of a large air leak soon after injury mandates urgent bronchoscopy to rule out tracheo-bronchial injury. Air leaks may also be observed if the lung fails to re-expand due to chest tube malposition or large pulmonary lacerations. Small air leaks can be exacerbated by respiratory failure requiring mechanical ventilation, especially at high tidal volumes or high airway pressures.

The treatment of a persistent air leak also requires bronchoscopy to ensure that a bronchial injury has not occurred. Once this has been excluded, complete lung expansion becomes the cornerstone of therapy. CT scanning may be needed to assure that the lung is fully expanded. If bronchoscopy does not disclose a proximal injury, other causes of air leakage should be excluded, including leaks within the chest-tube system itself. In patients undergoing mechanical ventilation with high PEEP or other advanced modalities, it is not uncommon for air leaks to persist for many days or weeks. The therapeutic goals in this group are to minimize peak airway pressures to the extent possible while maintaining oxygenation, with the realization that the air leaks will not stop completely until the patient begins to wean from the ventilator. Since it decreases the anatomic dead space, tracheostomy will often markedly lower the peak airway pressures required to achieve satisfactory gas exchange. In hemodynamically stable patients who have a prolonged air leak, thoracoscopic approaches have been helpful in some situations.[87]

## Traumatic Asphyxia

Traumatic asphyxia is a rare syndrome of craniocervical cyanosis and edema, petechiae, and subconjunctival hemorrhage which results from a severe crush injury to the thorax by a very heavy object that remains in place. A common scenario in our experience is the person who is working under his car when it falls on his chest. The pathophysiology of traumatic asphyxia involves two elements: a direct increase in thoracic and superior vena cava pressure from the crush injury combined with closure of the glottis which further exacerbates the increase in central venous pressure. The syndrome is easily recognized and the treatment is similar to any patient with severe chest injury and hypoxemia. Outcome is related to the degree of hypoxemia and extent of anoxic neurologic injury. Such patients may need to be evaluated and treated for posthypoxic cerebral edema.

## Chylothorax

Chylothorax following chest trauma is an uncommon event.[164] The vast majority (80%) of chylothoraces are iatrogenic, resulting either from operative procedures or from the percutaneous placement of central venous catheters. Nonetheless blunt injuries, especially those to the vertebral bodies, as well as penetrating wounds can lacerate the thoracic duct. The effusion resulting from this usually presents within ten days after the injury, although on occasion it may present weeks to months later. The diagnosis is made from the milky appearance of the fluid and from the presence of fat that can be stained with Sudan III.

The principles of treatment for chylothorax involve decreasing the production of chyle and the establishment of chest tube drainage. Re-expansion of the lung can help in closing the fistula responsible for the condition. Controversy exits as to how long to continue with conservative therapy before going to surgical correction. It is likely that the early use of VATS to ligate the injured thoracic duct will be shown to be the optimal therapy.

## DISABLILTY FOLLOWING CHEST TRAUMA

As the sophistication of trauma care has increased, so has our ability to successfully treat victims of severe chest trauma and respiratory failure. A significant question arises as to how these patients function months and years following discharge from the trauma center. Patients with penetrating chest trauma who do not require pulmonary resection generally have little ongoing disability once their condition has stabilized and their pain subsided. The disability following blunt pulmonary injury, however, may be much more severe.

The relevant literature suggests quite variable degrees of disability following major chest injuries. The contradictory findings of various studies may in part be due to differences in study design or to bias in patient selection. Landerscaper and colleagues noted significant pulmonary disability following flail-chest injury, and found that a significant proportion of their patients remained breathless for several years following injury.[165] Others found that while there was some degree of measurable pulmonary dysfunction compared to expected values, the objective findings did not correlate with the subjective symptoms reported.[166,167] A limitation of all but one of these studies was that they only measured pulmonary function at one time point following injury. In a group of patients followed sequentially after severe chest trauma, Livingston and Richardson[168] demonstrated that pulmonary recovery continued for up to 18 months following injuries when measured by standard spirometric tests. In that study, all patients who were employed prior to injury returned to work. Subjective complaints were few and did not correlate with the results on spirometry. The two patients that had the most subjective and objective disability were both over 60 years of age, although other older patients appear to recover well. No patient in that study was an "olympic athlete," and it remains possible that patients who have been very athletic, or are required to perform significant aerobic activities may experience sufficient impairment to prevent them from returning to their prior level of activity. Thus, while we do not wish to underemphasize the importance of subjective complaints following lung injury, the available data cannot correlate objective data with symptoms. The outlook for the survivors of severe chest trauma remains generally good, and suggests the importance of caregivers maintaining a positive outlook, and encouraging such patients to return to work and to their preinjury levels of activity after their acute illness has resolved.

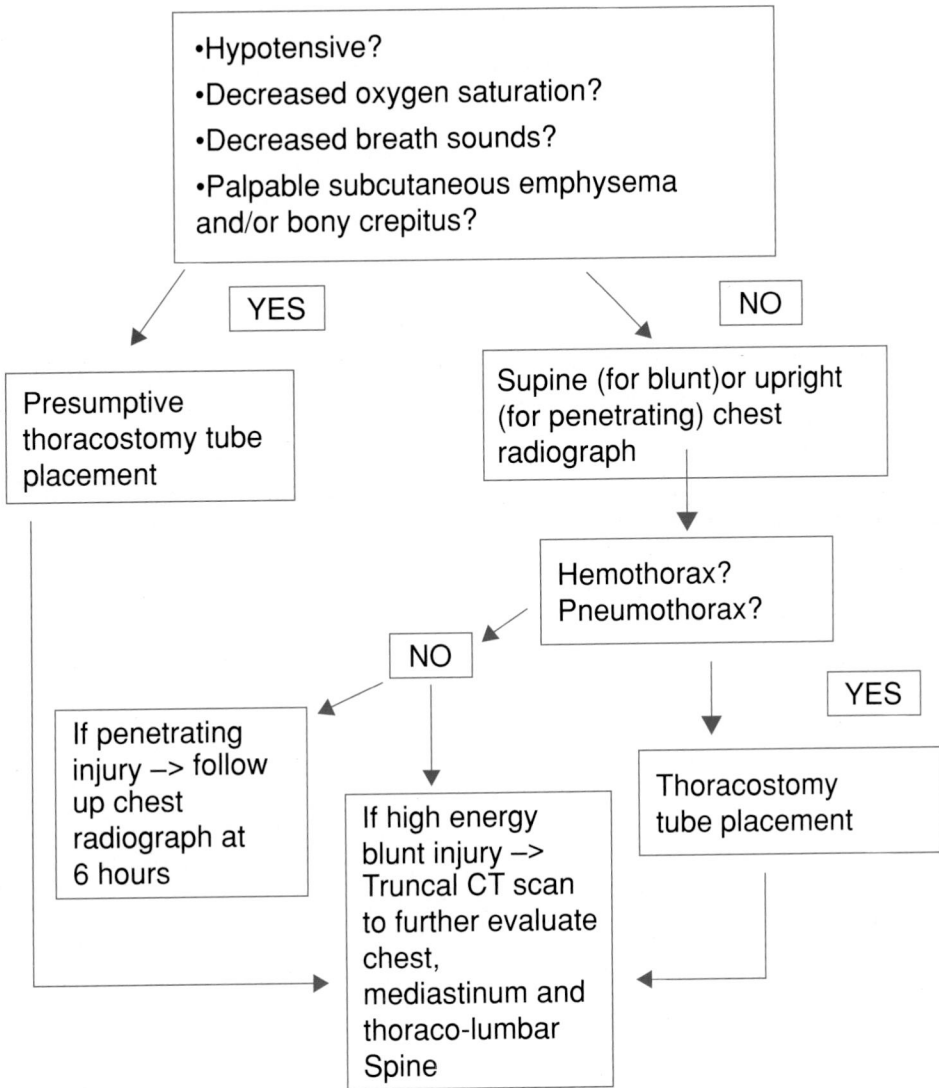

SUSPECTED CHEST TRAUMA

- Hypotensive?
- Decreased oxygen saturation?
- Decreased breath sounds?
- Palpable subcutaneous emphysema and/or bony crepitus?

YES → Presumptive thoracostomy tube placement

NO → Supine (for blunt) or upright (for penetrating) chest radiograph

Hemothorax? Pneumothorax?

NO

If penetrating injury –> follow up chest radiograph at 6 hours

YES → Thoracostomy tube placement

If high energy blunt injury –> Truncal CT scan to further evaluate chest, mediastinum and thoraco-lumbar Spine

# REFERENCES

1. Trinkaus E, Zimmerman M: Trauma among the Shanidar Neandertals. *Am J Phys Anthropol* 57:61, 1982.
2. Breasted J: *The Edwin Smith Surgical Papyrus.* Chicago: Chicago University Press, 1980.
3. American College of Surgeons Committee on Trauma. *Advanced Trauma Life Support.* 6th ed. Chicago: 1997.
4. Livingston D, Lavery R, Mosenthal M, et al.: Rapid sequence intubation (RSI) of the trauma patient: A safe and justified procedure. *J Trauma* (submitted).
5. Cornwell ER, Chang D, Bonar J, et al.: Thoracolumbar immobilization for trauma patients with torso gunshot wounds: Is it necessary? *Arch Surg* 136:324, 2001.
6. Tanomkiat W, Galassi W: Barium sulfate as contrast medium for evaluation of postoperative anastomotic leaks. *Acta Radiol* 41:482, 2000.
7. Bellasfar G, Duchene P, Le Mee J, et al.: Pulmonary complications after gastrografin inhalation during radiographic control of esophageal anastomosis. *Ann Fr Anesth Reanim* 5:533, 1986.
8. Fan ST, Lau WY, Yip WC, et al.: Limitations and dangers of gastrografin swallow after esophageal and upper gastric operations. *Am J Surg* 155:495, 1988.
9. Popovsky J, Lee YC, Berk JL: Gunshot wounds of the esophagus. *J Thorac Cardiovasc Surg* 72:609, 1976.
10. Pass LJ, LeNarz LA, Schreiber JT, et al.: Management of esophageal gunshot wounds. *Ann Thorac Surg* 44:253, 1987.
11. Asensio JA, Chahwan S, Forno W, et al.: Penetrating esophageal injuries: Multicenter study of the American Association for the Surgery of Trauma. *J Trauma* 50:289, 2001.
12. Hanpeter DE, Demetriades D, Asensio JA, et al.: Helical computed tomographic scan in the evaluation of mediastinal gunshot wounds. *J Trauma* 49:689, 2000.
13. Stassen NA, Lukan JK, Spain DA, et al.: Reevaluation of diagnostic procedures for transmediastinal gunshot wounds. *J Trauma* 53:635, 2002.
14. Omert L, Yeaney WW, Protetch J: Efficacy of thoracic computerized tomography in blunt chest trauma. *Am Surg* 67:660, 2001.
15. Exadaktylos AK, Sclabas G, Schmid SW, et al.: Do we really need routine computed tomographic scanning in the primary evaluation of blunt chest trauma in patients with "normal" chest radiograph? *J Trauma* 51:1173, 2001.
16. Guerrero-Lopez F, Vazquez-Mata G, Alcazar-Romero PP, et al.: Evaluation of the utility of computed tomography in the initial assessment of the critical care patient with chest trauma. *Crit Care Med* 28:1370, 2000.
17. Grieser T, Buhne KH, Hauser H, et al.: Significance of findings of chest X-rays and thoracic CT routinely performed at the emergency unit: 102 patients with multiple trauma. A prospective study. *Rofo Fortschr Geb Rontgenstr Neuen Bildgeb Verfahr* 173:44, 2001.
18. Gavelli G, Canini R, Bertaccini P, et al.: Traumatic injuries: Imaging of thoracic injuries. *Eur Radiol* 12:1273, 2002.
19. Hauser CJ, Visvikis G, Hinrichs C, et al.: Prospective validation of computed tomographic screening of the thoracolumbar spine in trauma. *J Trauma* 55:228, 2003.
20. Miller PR, Croce MA, Bee TK, et al.: ARDS after pulmonary contusion: Accurate measurement of contusion volume identifies high-risk patients. *J Trauma* 51:223, 2001.
21. Gleeson CE, Spedding RL, Harding LA, et al.: The mediastinum–is it wide? *Emerg Med J* 18:183, 2001.

22. Melton SM, Kerby JD, McGiffin D, et al.: The evolution of chest computed tomography for the definitive diagnosis of blunt aortic injury: A single-center experience. *J Trauma* 56:243, 2004.

23. Parker MS, Matheson TL, Rao AV, et al.: Making the transition: The role of helical CT in the evaluation of potentially acute thoracic aortic injuries. *AJR Am J Roentgenol* 176:1267, 2001.

24. Downing SW, Sperling JS, Mirvis SE, et al.: Experience with spiral computed tomography as the sole diagnostic method for traumatic aortic rupture. *Ann Thorac Surg* 72:495, 2001.

25. Pate JW, Gavant ML, Weiman DS, et al.: Traumatic rupture of the aortic isthmus: Program of selective management. *World J Surg* 23:59, 1999.

26. Stassen NA, Lukan X, Spain DA, et al.: Re-evaluation of diagnostic procedures for transmediastinal gunshot wounds. *J Trauma* 2001.

27. Dulchavsky SA, Schwarz KL, Kirkpatrick AW, et al.: Prospective evaluation of thoracic ultrasound in the detection of pneumothorax. *J Trauma* 50:201, 2001.

28. Rozycki GS, Feliciano DV, Davis TP: Ultrasound as used in thoracoabdominal trauma. *Surg Clin North Am* 78:295, 1998.

29. Rozycki GS, Ballard RB, Feliciano DV, et al.: Surgeon-performed ultrasound for the assessment of truncal injuries: Lessons learned from 1540 patients. *Ann Surg* 228:557, 1998.

30. Dubinsky I, Low A: Non-life-threatening blunt chest trauma: Appropriate investigation and treatment. *Am J Emerg Med* 15:240, 1997.

31. Ziegler DW, Agarwal NN: The morbidity and mortality of rib fractures. *J Trauma* 37:975, 1994.

32. Lee RB, Bass SM, Morris JA Jr, et al.: Three or more rib fractures as an indicator for transfer to a Level I trauma center: A population-based study. *J Trauma* 30:689, 1990.

33. Livingston D, Lavery R, Passannante M, et al.: Admission or observation is not necessary after a negative abdominal computed tomographic scan in patients with suspected blunt abdominal trauma: Results of a prospective, multi-institutional trial. *J Trauma* 44:273, 1998.

34. Garcia VF, Gotschall CS, Eichelberger MR, et al.: Rib fractures in children: A marker of severe trauma. *J Trauma* 30:695, 1990.

35. Bulloch B, Schubert CJ, Brophy PD, et al.: Cause and clinical characteristics of rib fractures in infants. *Pediatrics* 105:E48, 2000.

36. Cadzow SP, Armstrong KL: Rib fractures in infants: Red alert! The clinical features, investigations and child protection outcomes. *J Paediatr Child Health* 36:322, 2000.

37. Cameron P, Dziukas L, Hadj A, et al.: Rib fractures in major trauma. *Aust N Z J Surg* 66:530, 1996.

38. Freedland M, Wilson RF, Bender JS, et al.: The management of flail chest injury: Factors affecting outcome. *J Trauma* 30:1460, 1990.

39. Gaillard M, Herve C, Mandin L, et al.: Mortality prognostic factors in chest injury. *J Trauma* 30:93, 1990.

40. Clark GC, Schecter WP, Trunkey DD: Variables affecting outcome in blunt chest trauma: Flail chest vs. pulmonary contusion. *J Trauma* 28:298, 1988.

41. Johnson JA, Cogbill TH, Winga ER: Determinants of outcome after pulmonary contusion. *J Trauma* 26:695, 1986.

42. Bulger EM, Arneson MA, Mock CN, et al.: Rib fractures in the elderly. *J Trauma* 48:1040, 2000.

43. Stawicki SP, Grossman MD, Hoey BA, et al.: Rib fractures in the elderly: A marker of injury severity. *J Am Geriatr Soc* 52:805, 2004.

44. Albaugh G, Kann B, Puc MM, et al.: Age-adjusted outcomes in traumatic flail chest injuries in the elderly. *Am Surg* 66:978, 2000.

45. Poole GV Jr, Myers RT: Morbidity and mortality rates in major blunt trauma to the upper chest. *Ann Surg* 193:70, 1981.

46. Tarlowe MH, Hauser CJ: Prospective study of neutrophil chemokine responses in trauma patients at risk for pneumonia. *Am J Resp Crit Care Med* 171:753, 2005.

47. Croce MA, Fabian TC, Waddle-Smith L, et al.: Identification of early predictors for post-traumatic pneumonia. *Am Surg* 67:105, 2001.

48. Adams JM, Hauser CJ, Livingston DH, et al.: Early trauma PMN responses to chemokines are associated with development of sepsis, pneumonia and organ failure. *J Trauma* 51:452, 2001.

49. Bolliger CT, Van Eeden SF: Treatment of multiple rib fractures. Randomized controlled trial comparing ventilatory with nonventilatory management. *Chest* 97:943, 1990.

50. Rashid MA, Wikstrom T, Ortenwall P: Nomenclature, classification, and significance of traumatic extrapleural hematoma. *J Trauma* 49:286, 2000.

51. Toombs BD, Sandler CM, Lester RG: Computed tomography of chest trauma. *Radiology* 140:733, 1981.

52. Carrillo EH, Heniford BT, Senler SO, et al.: Embolization therapy as an alternative to thoracotomy in vascular injuries of the chest wall. *Am Surg* 64:1142, 1998.

53. Reiter C, Denk W: Delayed epipleural hematoma as a fatal complication following blunt chest injury. *Wien Klin Wochenschr* 97:535, 1985.

54. Cappello M, Legrand A, De Troyer A: Determinants of rib motion in flail chest. *Am J Respir Crit Care Med* 159:886, 1999.

55. Pelosi P, Cereda M, Foti G, et al.: Alterations of lung and chest wall mechanics in patients with acute lung injury: Effects of positive end-expiratory pressure. *Am J Respir Crit Care Med* 152:531, 1995.

56. Craven KD, Oppenheimer L, Wood LD: Effects of contusion and flail chest on pulmonary perfusion and oxygen exchange. *J Appl Physiol* 47:729, 1979.

57. Gyhra A, Torres P, Pino J, et al.: Experimental flail chest: Ventilatory function with fixation of flail segment in internal and external position. *J Trauma* 40:977, 1996.

58. Busch T, Sirbu H, Aleksic I, et al.: Incarcerated postraumatic intercostal lung hernia. Case report and review of the literature. *J Cardiovasc Surg (Torino)* 40:901, 1999.

59. Haapamaki VV, Kiuru MJ, Koskinen SK: Multidetector CT in shoulder fractures. *Emerg Radiol* 11:89, 2004.

60. Harris R, Harris JJ: The prevalence and significance of missed scapular fractures in blunt chest trauma. *AJR Am J Roentgenol* 151:747, 1988.

61. Damschen D, Cogbill T, Siegel M: Scapulothoracic dissociation caused by blunt trauma. *J Trauma* 42:537, 1997.

62. Grassi F, Tajana M, D'Angelo F: Management of midclavicular fractures: Comparison between nonoperative treatment and open intramedullary fixation in 80 patients. *J Trauma* 50:1096, 2001.

63. Connolly J, Dehne R: Nonunion of the clavicle and thoracic outlet syndrome. *J Trauma* 19:1127, 1989.

64. Ebraheim N, Mekhail A, Darwich M: Open reduction and internal fixation with bone grafting of clavicular nonunion. *J Trauma* 42:701, 1997.

65. Buckman R, Trooskin S, Flancbaum L, et al.: The significance of stable patients with sternal fractures. *Surg Gynecol Obstet* 164:261, 1987.

66. Hills M, Delprado A, Deane S: Sternal fractures: Associated injuries and management. *J Trauma* 35:55, 1993.

67. Jackson M, Walker W: Isolated sternal fracture: A benign injury? *Injury* 23:535, 1992.

68. Chiu W, D'Amelio L, Hammond J: Sternal fractures in blunt chest trauma: A practical algorithm for management. *Am J Emerg Med* 15:252, 1997.

69. Di Bartolomeo S, Sanson G, Nardi G, et al.: A population-based study on pneumothorax in severely traumatized patients. *J Trauma* 51:677, 2001.

70. Goodman T, Traill Z, Phillips A, et al.: Ultrasound detection of pneumothorax. *Clin Radiol* 54:736, 1999.

71. Lichtenstein DA, Meziere G, Lascols N, et al.: Ultrasound diagnosis of occult pneumothorax. *Crit Care Med* 33:1231, 2005.

72. Neff M, Monk JJ, Peters K, et al.: Detection of occult pneumothoraces on abdominal computed tomographic scans in trauma patients. *J Trauma* 49:281, 2000.

73. Rhea J, Novelline R, Lawrason J, et al.: The frequency and significance of thoracic injuries detected on abdominal CT scans of multiple trauma patients. *J Trauma* 29:502, 1989.

74. Garramone RJ, Jacobs L, Sahdev P: An objective method to measure and manage occult pneumothorax. *Surg Gynecol Obstet* 173:257, 1991.

75. Enderson BL, Abdalla R, Frame SB, et al.: Tube thoracostomy for occult pneumothorax: A prospective randomized study of its use. *J Trauma* 35:726, 1993.

76. Brasel K, Stafford R, Weigelt J, et al.: Treatment of occult pneumothoraces from blunt trauma. *J Trauma* 46:987, 1999.

77. Schmidt U, Stalp M, Gerich T, et al.: Chest tube decompression of blunt chest injuries by physicians in the field: Effectiveness and complications. *J Trauma* 44:98, 1998.

78. Coats T, Wilson A, Xeropotamous N: Pre-hospital management of patients with severe thoracic injury. *Injury* 26:581, 1995.

79. Eckstein M, Suyehara D: Needle thoracostomy in the prehospital setting. *Prehosp Emerg Care* 2:132, 1998.

80. England G, Hill R, Timberlake G, et al.: Resolution of experimental pneumothorax in rabbits by graded oxygen therapy. *J Trauma* 45:333, 1998.

81. Martino K, Merrit S, Boyakye K, et al.: Prospective randomized trial of thoracostomy removal algorithms. *J Trauma* 46:369, 1999.

82. Wilson R, Nichols R: The EAST Practice Management Guidelines for Prophylactic Antibiotic use in Tube Thoracostomy for Traumatic Hemopneumothorax: A commentary. *J Trauma* 48:758, 2000.

83. Luchette F, Barrie P, Oswanski M, et al.: Practice Management Guidelines for Prophylactic Antibiotic Use in Tube Thoracostomy for Traumatic Hemopneumothorax: The EAST Practice Management Guidelines Work Group. Eastern Association for Trauma. *J Trauma* 48:753, 2000.

84. Chan L, Reilly K, Henderson C, et al.: Complication rates of tube thoracostomy. *Am J Emerg Med* 15:368, 1997.

85. Etoch S, Bar-Natan M, Miller F, et al.: Tube thoracostomy. Factors related to complications. *Arch Surg* 130:521, 1995.

86. Baldt M, Bankier A, Germann P, et al.: Complications after emergency tube thoracostomy: Assessment with CT. *Radiology* 195:539, 1995.

87. Carrillo E, Schmacht D, Gable D, et al.: Thoracoscopy in the management of posttraumatic persistent pneumothorax. *J Am Coll Surg* 186:636, 1998.

88. Thompson D, Rowlands B, Walker W, et al.: Urgent thoracotomy for pulmonary or tracheobronchial injury. *J Trauma* 28:276, 1988.

89. Borlase B, Metcalf R, Moore E, et al.: Penetrating wounds to the anterior chest. Analysis of thoracotomy and laparotomy. *Am J Surg* 152:649, 1986.

90. Feliciano D: The diagnostic and therapeutic approach to chest trauma. *Semin Thorac Cardiovasc Surg* 4:156, 1992.

91. Velmahos GC, Demetriades D, Chan L, et al.: Predicting the need for thoracoscopic evacuation of residual traumatic hemothorax: Chest radiograph is insufficient. *J Trauma* 46:65, 1999.

92. Condon R: Spontaneous resolution of experimental clotted hemothorax. *Surg Gynecol Obstet* 126:505, 1968.

93. Adams JM, Hauser CJ, Livingston DH, et al.: The immunomodulatory effects of damage control abdominal packing on local and systemic neutrophil activity. *J Trauma* 50:792, 2001.

94. Adams JM, Hauser CJ, Livingston DH, et al.: *Damage Control Abdominal Packing Causes Prolonged Suppression of Neutrophil IL-8 Responses and Phagocytosis.* Surgical Forum, Vol. 51. Chicago, IL: American College of Surgeons, 2000, p. 178.

95. Karmy-Jones R, Jurkovich G, Nathens A, et al.: Timing of urgent thoracotomy for hemorrhage after trauma: A multicenter study. *Arch Surg* 136:513, 2001.

96. Ochsner M, Rozycki G, Lucente F, et al.: Prospective evaluation of thoracoscopy for diagnosing diaphragmatic injury in thoracoabdominal trauma: A preliminary report. *J Trauma* 34:704, 1993.

97. Lowdermilk G, Naunheim K: Thoracoscopic evaluation and treatment of thoracic trauma. *Surg Clin North Am* 80:1535, 2000.

98. Abolhoda A, Livingston DH, Donahoo JS, et al.: Diagnostic and therapeutic video assisted thoracic surgery (VATS) following chest trauma. *Eur J Cardiothorac Surg* 12:356, 1997.

99. Heniford BT, Carrillo EH, Spain DA, et al.: The role of thoracoscopy in the management of retained thoracic collections after trauma. *Ann Thorac Surg* 63:940, 1997.

100. Scherer L, Battistella F, Owings J, et al.: Video-assisted thoracic surgery in the treatment of posttraumatic empyema. *Arch Surg* 133:637, 1998.

101. Karmy-Jones R, Jurkovich G, Shatz D, et al.: Management of Traumatic Lung Injury: A Western Trauma Association Multicenter Review. *J Trauma* 51:1049, 2001.

102. Wall MJ Jr, Villavicencio RT, Miller CC III, et al.: Pulmonary tractotomy as an abbreviated thoracotomy technique. *J Trauma* 45:1015, 1998.

103. Velmahos G, Baker C, Demetriades D, et al.: Lung-sparing surgery after penetrating trauma using tractotomy, partial lobectomy, and pneumonorrhaphy. *Arch Surg* 134:186, 1999.

104. Jones W, Mavroudis C, Richardson J, et al.: Management of tracheobronchial disruption resulting from blunt trauma. *Surgery* 95:319, 1984.

105. Bowling R, Mavroudis C, Richardson J, et al.: Emergency pneumonectomy for penetrating and blunt trauma. *Am Surg* 51:136, 1985.

106. Cryer H, Mavroudis C, Yu J, et al.: Shock, transfusion, and pneumonectomy. Death is due to right heart failure and increased pulmonary vascular resistance. *Ann Surg* 212:197, 1990.

107. Tominaga G, Waxman K, Scannell G, et al.: Emergency thoracotomy with lung resection following trauma. *Am Surg* 59:834, 1993.

108. Wall MJ, Soltero E: Damage control for thoracic injuries. *Surg Clin North Am* 77:863, 1997.

109. Powell R, Redan J, Swan K: The hilar snare, and improved technique for securing rapid vascular control of the pulmonary hilum. *J Trauma* 30:208, 1990.

110. Shorr RM, Crittenden M, Indeck M, et al.: Blunt thoracic trauma. Analysis of 515 patients. *Ann Surg* 206:200, 1987.

111. Sauaia A, Moore FA, Moore EE, et al.: Pneumonia: Cause or symptom of postinjury multiple organ failure? *Am J Surg* 166:606, 1993.

112. Nast-Kolb D, Aufmkolk M, Rucholtz S, et al.: Multiple organ failure still a major cause of morbidity but not mortality in blunt multiple trauma. *J Trauma* 51:835, 2001.

113. Gourin CG, Shackford SR: Links Influence of percussion trauma on expression of intercellular adhesion molecule-1 (ICAM-1) by human cerebral microvascular endothelium. *J Trauma* 41:129, 1996

114. Livingston DH: Prevention of ventilator-associated pneumonia. *Am J Surg* 179:12S, 2000.

115. Deitch EA, Livingston DH, Hauser CJ: Septic complications in the trauma patient. *New Horizons* 7:158, 1999.

116. Croce MA, Fabian TC, Schurr MJ, et al.: Using bronchoalveolar lavage to distinguish nosocomial pneumonia from systemic inflammatory response syndrome: A prospective analysis. *J Trauma* 39:1134, 1995.

117. Ewig S, Torres A, El-Ebiary M, et al.: Bacterial colonization patterns in mechanically ventilated patients with traumatic and medical head injury. Incidence, risk factors, and association with ventilator-associated pneumonia. *Am J Respir Crit Care Med* 159:188, 1999.

118. Pape H-C, Auf'm Kolk M, Paffrath T, et al.: Primary intramedullary femur fixation in multiple trauma patients with associated lung contusion-A cause of posttraumatic ARDS. *J Trauma* 33:540, 1993.

119. Hauser CJ, Zhou X, Joshi P, et al.: The immune microenvironment of human fracture/soft-tissue hematomas and its relationship to systemic immunity. *J Trauma* 42:895, 1997.

120. Hauser CJ, Desai N, Fekete Z, et al.: Priming of neutrophil $[Ca^{2+}]i$ signaling and oxidative burst by human fracture fluids. *J Trauma* 47:854, 1999.

121. Moss M, Gillespie MK, Ackerson L, et al.: Endothelial cell activity varies in patients at risk for the adult respiratory distress syndrome. *Crit Care Med* 24:1782, 1996.

122. Biffl WL, Moore FA, Moore EE, et al.: Are corticosteroids salvage therapy for refractory acute respiratory distress syndrome? *Am J Surg* 170:591, 1995.

123. Meduri GU, Belenchia JM, Estes RJ, et al.: Fibroproliferative phase of ARDS. Clinical findings and effects of corticosteroids. *Chest* 100:943, 1991.

124. Richardson JD, Adams L, Flint LM: Selective management of flail chest and pulmonary contusion. *Ann Surg* 196:481, 1982.

125. Magnotti LJ, Upperman JS, Xu DZ, et al.: Gut-derived mesenteric lymph but not portal blood increases endothelial cell permeability and promotes lung injury after hemorrhagic shock. *Ann Surg* 228:518, 1998.

126. Zallen G, Moore EE, Johnson JL, et al.: Posthemorrhagic shock mesenteric lymph primes circulating neutrophils and provokes lung injury. *J Surg Res* 83:83, 1999.

127. Erdmann AJ III, Vaughan TR Jr, Brigham KL, et al.: Effect of increased vascular pressure on lung fluid balance in unanesthetized sheep. *Circ Res* 37:271, 1975.

128. Drake RE, Weiss D, Gabel JC: Active lymphatic pumping and sheep lung lymph flow. *J Appl Physiol* 71:99, 1991.

129. Slutsky AS: Lung injury caused by mechanical ventilation. *Chest* 116:9S, 1999.

130. ARDS-Network: Ventilation with lower tidal volumes as compared with traditional tidal volumes for acute lung injury and the acute respiratory distress syndrome. The Acute Respiratory Distress Syndrome Network. *N Engl J Med* 342:1301, 2000.

131. Eisner MD, Thompson T, Hudson LD, et al.: Efficacy of low tidal volume ventilation in patients with different clinical risk factors for acute lung injury and the acute respiratory distress syndrome. *Am J Respir Crit Care Med* 164:231, 2001.

132. Bigatello LM, Patroniti N, Sangalli F: Permissive hypercapnia. *Curr Opin Crit Care* 7:34, 2001.

133. Dhainaut JF, Brunet F: Right ventricular performance in adult respiratory distress syndrome. *Eur Respir J Suppl* 11:490s, 1990.

134. Lardinois D, Krueger T, Dusmet M, et al.: Pulmonary function testing after operative stabilisation of the chest wall for flail chest. *Eur J Cardiothorac Surg* 20:496, 2001.

135. Ahmed Z, Mohyuddin Z: Management of flail chest injury: Internal fixation versus endotracheal intubation and ventilation. *J Thorac Cardiovasc Surg* 110:1676, 1995.

136. Voggenreiter G, Neudeck F, Aufmkolk M, et al.: Operative chest wall stabilization in flail chest—outcomes of patients with or without pulmonary contusion. *J Am Coll Surg* 187:130, 1998.

137. Tanaka H, Yukioka T, Yamaguti Y,et al.: Surgical stabilization of internal pneumatic stabilization? A prospective randomized study of management of severe flail chest patients. *J Trauma* 52:727, 2002.

138. Hedderich R, Ness T: Analgesia for trauma and burns. *Crit Care Clin* 15:167, 1999.

139. Desai P: Pain management and pulmonary dysfunction. *Crit Care Clin* 15:151, 1999.

140. Rady MY, Kirkman E, Cranley J, et al.: Nociceptive somatic nerve stimulation and skeletal muscle injury modify systemic hemodynamics and oxygen transport and utilization after resuscitation from hemorrhage. *Crit Care Med* 24:623, 1996.

141. Yokoyama M, Itano Y, Mizobuchi S, et al.: The effects of epidural block on the distribution of lymphocyte subsets and natural-killer cell activity in patients with and without pain. *Anesth Analg* 92:463, 2001.

142. Rainer TH, Jacobs P, Ng YC, et al.: Cost effectiveness analysis of intravenous ketorolac and morphine for treating pain after limb injury: Double blind randomised controlled trial. *BMJ* 321:1247, 2000.

143. Clark RF, Wei EM, Anderson PO: Meperidine: Therapeutic use and toxicity. *J Emerg Med* 13:797, 1995.

144. Gallagher EJ, Liebman M, Bijur PE: Prospective validation of clinically important changes in pain severity measured on a visual analog scale. *Ann Emerg Med* 38:633, 2001.

145. Myles PS, Troedel S, Boquest M, et al.: The pain visual analog scale: Is it linear or nonlinear? *Anesth Analg* 89:1517, 1999.

146. Shanti CM, Carlin AM, Tyburski JG: Incidence of pneumothorax from intercostal nerve block for analgesia in rib fractures. *J Trauma* 51:536, 2001.

147. Short K, Scheeres D, Mlakar J, et al.: Evaluation of intrapleural analgesia in the management of blunt traumatic chest wall pain: A clinical trial. *Am Surg* 62:488, 1996.

148. Gabram SG, Schwartz RJ, Jacobs LM, et al.: Clinical management of blunt trauma patients with unilateral rib fractures: A randomized trial. *World J Surg* 19:388, 1995.

149. Knottenbelt JD, James MF, Bloomfield M: Intrapleural bupivacaine analgesia in chest trauma: A randomized double-blind controlled trial. *Injury* 22:114, 1991.

150. Haenel JB, Moore FA, Moore EE, et al.: Extrapleural bupivacaine for amelioration of multiple rib fracture pain. *J Trauma* 38:22, 1995.

151. Barron DJ, Tolan MJ, Lea RE: A randomized controlled trial of continuous extra-pleural analgesia post-thoracotomy: Efficacy and choice of local anaesthetic. *Eur J Anaesthesiol* 16:236, 1999.

152. Mackersie RC, Karagianes TG, Hoyt DB, et al.: Prospective evaluation of epidural and intravenous administration of fentanyl for pain control and restoration of ventilatory function following multiple rib fractures. *J Trauma* 31:443, 1991.

153. Mandabach MG: Intrathecal and epidural analgesia. *Crit Care Clin* 15:105, 1999.

154. Mackersie RC, Shackford SR, Hoyt DB, et al.: Continuous epidural fentanyl analgesia: Ventilatory function improvement with routine use in treatment of blunt chest injury. *J Trauma* 27:1207, 1987.

155. Bulger EM, Edwards T, Klotz P, et al.: Epidural analgesia improves outcome after multiple rib fractures. *Surgery* 136:426, 2004.

156. Walker W, Kapelanski D, Weiland A, et al.: Patterns of infection and mortality in thoracic trauma. *Ann Surg* 201:752, 1985.

157. Arom K, Grover F, Richardson J, et al.: Posttraumatic empyema. *Ann Thorac Surg* 23:254, 1977.

158. Watkins J, Spain D, Richardson J, et al.: Empyema and restrictive pleural processes after blunt trauma: An under-recognized cause of respiratory failure. *Am Surg* 66:210, 2000.

159. Aguilar M, Battistella F, Owings J, et al.: Posttraumatic empyema. Risk factor analysis. *Arch Surg* 132:647, 1997.

160. Eddy AC, Luna GK, Copass M: Empyema thoracis in patients undergoing emergent closed tube thoracostomy for thoracic trauma. *Am J Surg* 157:494, 1989.

161. Mandal A, Thadepalli H, Mandal A, et al.: Posttraumatic empyema thoracis: A 24-year experience at a major trauma center. *J Trauma* 43:764, 1997.

162. Helling TS, Gyles NR III, Eisenstein CL, et al.: Complications following blunt and penetrating injuries in 216 victims of chest trauma requiring tube thoracostomy. *J Trauma* 29:1367, 1989.

163. de Souza A, Offner P, Moore E, et al.: Optimal management of complicated empyema. *Am J Surg* 180:507, 2000.

164. Merrigan B, Winter D, O'Sullivan G: Chylothorax. *Br J Surg* 84:15, 1997.

165. Landercasper J, Cogbill T, Lindesmith L: Long-term disability after flail chest injury. *J Trauma* 24:410, 1984.

166. Davidson I, Bargh W, Cruickshank A, et al.: Crush injuries of the chest. A follow-up study of patients treated in an artificial ventilation unit. *Thorax* 24:563, 1969.

167. Svennevig J, Vaage J, Westheim A, et al.: Late sequelae of lung contusion. *Injury* 20:253, 1989.

168. Livingston D, Richardson J: Pulmonary disability after severe blunt chest trauma. *J Trauma* 30:562, 1990.

# *Commentary* ■ KENNETH L. MATTOX

The authors of this chapter aptly noted that injuries to the chest wall and lungs account for the majority of chest injuries. They reemphasized the value of the traditional physical examination and chest X-ray. The statement that "the anteroposterior chest X-ray, preformed in the trauma receiving area is the single most valuable diagnostic study in the management of chest trauma" would be supported by most surgeons caring for trauma patients. The authors then cite the benefits in other imaging modalities in evaluating subtle fractures and pulmonary contusion.

With the advent of advanced CT chest scanning, "occult" pneumothoraces have been increasingly discovered. As the authors point out, up to 20% of occult pneumothoraces will require treatment; however, they do not have any strong suggestions or guidelines for which can be managed conservatively. Therefore, the authors recommend that any occult pneumothorax discovered on CT of an ICU patient be treated with a tube thoracostomy.

The single largest section of this chapter is devoted to the technical aspects of tube thoracostomy, management, and associated complications. Those involved in the care of patients with chest trauma outside the continuum of care in the surgical intensive care unit often assume that tube thoracostomy is a simple, rather benign procedure and with straightforward and simple algorithmic principles of management. The authors report that 25% of patients with tube thoracostomy will have a problem or complication. This section of the chapter is especially helpful in attempting to "troubleshoot" a chest tube problem.

One area that requires some reinforcement focuses CLAMPING of chest tubes. Nontrauma, non-thoracic surgeons have often clamped chest tubes as a "test" to determine if the chest tube can be removed. Clamping a chest tube to preserve acute hemothorax blood while autotransfusion equipment is being set up is supportable. However, no class I or II evidence data exist to support clamping of chest tubes for any other reason. Clamping of chest tubes also has a number of inherent dangers, such as contributing to a tension pneumothorax, empyema, and other complications. The historic urban legend of clamping chest tubes prior to their removal cannot be supported.

One subject of recurring interest is that of operative fixation of chest wall bony fractures. The authors stipulate that the data to support this practice is "scanty." There is some meager suggestive evidence that operative chest wall stabilization allows earlier extubation of the patient. Certainly, the vast majority of patients with rib fractures will not benefit from this procedure.

The issue of pain control is of considerable interest to all physicians caring for patient with chest wall injury. The various modalities of chest wall pain control are cited, and the advantages of regional epidural anesthesia are well documented.

The common complications following chest wall and lung injury are listed and adequately covered. One uncommon but troublesome complication is biliary-bronchial fistula, which is typified in a patient with liver, diaphragm, and lung injury, coughing up bile stained material, and usually has had some bouts of postinjury pneumonia. Treatment is most often accomplished by lower lobectomy and diaphragmatic closure.

# Esophagus, Trachea, and Bronchus

*Riyad Karmy-Jones* ■ *Douglas E. Wood* ■ *Gregory J. Jurkovich*

## TRACHEA AND BRONCHUS

*Highlights in Management*

- The initial priority is airway stabilization, which may require flexible or rigid bronchoscopy
- Penetrating injury predominantly affects the cervical trachea, blunt the distal trachea and carina
- Diagnosis should be suspected in patients with significant air-leak, subcutaneous emphysema, and/or pneumothorax despite tube thoracostomy
- The diagnosis can be missed, resulting in airway stricture, parenchymal necrosis, and/or late onset "asthma"
- The upper half of the trachea is best exposed via a collar cervical incision, the distal half in most cases by a right 4th intercostals posterolateral thoracotomy
- Operative repair involves precise debridement of devitalized tissue, but in most cases simple reconstruction with absorbable interrupted sutures suffices.

Tracheobronchial injury is uncommon but can be immediately life threatening. The immediate sequelae can include death from asphyxiation, whereas lack of recognition or incorrect management may result in life-threatening or disabling airway stricture. Penetrating injuries can occur with any laceration to the neck or from projectile injuries to the neck or chest. Blunt injuries can occur from a variety of direct and indirect trauma. Laryngotracheal injuries are sometimes classified together, but in this discussion they are separated from laryngeal trauma, including laryngotracheal separation, which is discussed elsewhere.

## INCIDENCE

The true incidence of tracheal and bronchial rupture is difficult to establish but has been estimated that only 0.5% of all patients with multiple injuries managed in modern trauma centers suffer from tracheobronchial injury.[1] This estimate is crude, however, because virtually all studies of airway trauma combine penetrating and blunt causes and do not publish a denominator of cervical and thoracic injuries with which to calculate the true incidence of airway involvement.

Penetrating neck injuries have a 3–6% incidence of cervical tracheal injury.[2] Less than 1% (4/666) of patients admitted with penetrating chest trauma had tracheal injury in a series published from the Ben Taub Hospital in Houston.[3] Based on an annual incidence at major trauma centers of three to four cases of penetrating tracheal trauma per year, it appears that the incidence of penetrating tracheobronchial trauma constitutes 1–2% of thoracic trauma admissions.[2,4–6]

Bertelsen and Howitz provided perhaps the best information regarding tracheobronchial injuries in blunt trauma.[7] The authors reviewed 1178 autopsy reports of patients dying of blunt trauma and found an incidence of tracheobronchial injury of 2.8%, with over 80% of these patients dying instantly of airway or associated injuries and the rest dying within two hours of reaching the hospital. Kemmerer and associates in 1961 reported an incidence of tracheobronchial rupture of under 1% in a study of nearly 600 traffic fatalities.[8] Thirty years later, Symbas and colleagues reviewed 20 years of English language literature, spanning from 1970 to 1990, that reported airway injury secondary to blunt trauma.[4] In this time frame, 47 articles described 183 patients, with six patients added in the 20-year period from the Grady Memorial Hospital experience in Atlanta. Unfortunately, these data do not provide a meaningful denominator on which to calculate the incidence of airway injury in blunt chest trauma.

There is an apparent increase in the incidence of patients with airway injuries reaching the emergency department alive, which may occur as a result of improved prehospital care and development of specialized regional trauma units.[9] However, this is difficult to establish, given the inherent inaccuracies in the historical and current data regarding airway injuries. De La Rocha and Kayler reported an incidence of tracheobronchial injuries of 1.8% in 327 patients who were discharged from a centralized trauma unit, whereas another series reported an incidence of 0.5% in a series of 2000 patients requiring an intensive care unit admission for multiple trauma.[10,11]

The best consolidation of these data shows an incidence of tracheobronchial injury occurring in 0.5–2% of individuals sustaining blunt trauma, including blunt trauma to the neck. More than 80% of tracheobronchial injuries from blunt trauma are located within 2.5 cm of the carina.[9] Most injuries related to blunt trauma involve the intrathoracic trachea and mainstem bronchi, with only 4% of these injuries reported in the cervical trachea.[4] In this review, 22% of the blunt airway injuries involved the distal thoracic trachea; 27%, the right mainstem bronchus; and 17%, the left proximal mainstem bronchus. Eight percent were complex injuries involving the trachea and mainstem bronchi, and 16% involved the lobar orifices.[4] The rate of tracheobronchial injury from penetrating thoracic trauma is also 0.5–2%, but, in contrast, penetrating cervical injuries involve the airway 3–8% of the time. Penetrating injuries predominantly involve the cervical trachea, with only 25% of the penetrating injuries involving the intrathoracic airways.[2]

## MECHANISM

Most tracheobronchial injuries result from blunt or penetrating trauma, although iatrogenic injuries and less common causes such as strangulation, burns, or caustic injury occasionally result in airway injury. Most penetrating trauma is due to stab wounds or gunshot wounds and only uncommonly may occur from impalement or slash injuries. Nearly all stab injuries of the trachea are cervical in origin, owing to the deep location of the intrathoracic trachea. Knife injuries produce a tearing or shearing effect, resulting in perforation, linear laceration, through and through injuries, or transsection.[2]

Gunshot wounds are a more common cause of penetrating airway injury and can affect any portion of the cervical or intrathoracic airways. However, cervical injuries are still more common, being the site of injury in 75–80% of penetrating tracheal trauma overall.[2] This may be, in part, because more distal penetrating injuries of the trachea may have associated fatal injuries of the heart or great vessels, and such patients never arrive at the trauma center for evaluation and management. Knowledge of the missile trajectory based on history and the entrance and exit wounds is very helpful in predicting the path of the bullet and subsequent structures at risk for injury. However, this can be unpredictable, with bullet paths frequently altered by impact with bone or other dense tissue. Therefore, a high index of suspicion for airway injury must be maintained in all cervical and upper thoracic gunshot wounds. Gunshot wounds produce a crush injury and wound cavity that varies depending on the muzzle velocity, the caliber, and the type of ammunition, with the greatest damage being produced by high-velocity rifles firing hollow-point ammunition. These injuries produce much greater cavitation and soft tissue destruction than do relatively low-velocity injuries from handguns.

Blunt injuries of the cervical trachea most commonly result from direct trauma or from sudden hyperextension. Direct cervical trauma produces a crush injury of the trachea, because it may be impinged on by the rigid vertebral bodies. This has classically been described as a "dashboard" injury because unrestrained automobile passengers may hyperextend the neck during head-on collisions, striking the neck on the steering wheel or dashboard and producing a crush injury of the larynx or cervical trachea.[12] However, even the restrained passenger may incur a laryngeal or cervical tracheal injury when a high-riding shoulder harness applies a compressive and rotational force to the neck on front-impact automobile injuries.[13] Clothesline injuries may produce similar direct crushing trauma but with the force concentrated across a very narrow band. Other injuries may occur with rapid hyperextension, producing a traction and distraction injury that most commonly results in laryngotracheal separation. Hyperextension injuries most commonly occur in automobile crashes but can occur in any other situations in which forced rapid cervical hyperextension occurs.

The exact mechanism of intrathoracic tracheobronchial disruption from blunt trauma is unknown but, as discussed, 80% of these injuries occur within 2.5 cm of the carina.[14] Kirsch and associates proposed three potential mechanisms for the cause of blunt intrathoracic tracheobronchial injuries.[15] First, they noted that sudden, forceful anteroposterior compression of the thoracic cage is the most common type of injury associated with tracheobronchial disruption. They postulated that this produces a decrease in the anteroposterior diameter with subsequent widening of the transverse diameter. Because the lung remains in contact with the chest wall because of negative intrapleural pressure, lateral motion pulls the two lungs apart, producing traction on the trachea at the carina. Airway disruption occurs if this lateral force exceeds tracheobronchial elasticity. A second mechanism may be due to airway rupture as a consequence of high airway pressures. Compression of the lung, trachea, and major bronchi between the sternum and vertebral column during blunt trauma produces a sudden increase in intratracheal airway pressure; and in a patient with a closed glottis at the moment of impact, rupture can occur when the intraluminal pressure exceeds the elasticity of the membranous trachea and bronchi.[16] Rupture in these circumstances occurs most commonly at the junction of the membranous and cartilaginous airway or between cartilaginous rings. The third potential mechanism may be due to a rapid deceleration injury, producing shear forces at points of relative airway fixation such as the cricoid cartilage and the carina, similar to the mechanism of traumatic injuries of the thoracic aorta.

## ASSOCIATED INJURIES

Because of the adjacent cervical and intrathoracic structures, penetrating airway trauma frequently is associated with other major injuries in the body region affected. Blunt trauma is often associated with multiple injuries involving not only chest, but abdomen, head, and orthopedic.[17] Cervical trauma of the airway frequently involves the esophagus, the recurrent laryngeal nerves, the cervical spine and spinal cord, the larynx, and the carotid arteries and jugular veins. Intrathoracic penetrating trauma may involve the esophagus, left recurrent laryngeal nerve, and spinal cord, but it can also involve any of the great vessels, including the ascending arch and descending aorta and the pulmonary arteries, and may involve any of the four heart chambers or the lung parenchyma. Obviously, concomitant great vessel and cardiac injury from penetrating trauma is frequently fatal and may lead to exsanguination or asphyxiation on blood in the airway before presentation in a trauma unit. These associated injuries are common and frequently determine the ultimate outcome in terms of the patient's survival and morbidity.

In a series of 100 penetrating tracheobronchial injuries reported by Kelly and colleagues in patients with a primary airway injury in the cervical trachea, 28% of the patients had an associated esophageal injury, 24% had a hemopneumothorax, 13% had a major vascular injury, 8% had a recurrent laryngeal nerve injury, and 3% had a spinal cord injury.[18] In contrast, primary injuries of the intrathoracic trachea were associated with an incidence of esophageal injury of 11%; hemopneumothorax, 32%; a major vascular injury, 18%; cardiac injury, 5%; spinal cord injury, 7%; and intra-abdominal injuries, 18%.[18] Several other series have shown an overall incidence of associated major injuries with penetrating tracheobronchial trauma to be in the range of 50–80%, most of these being esophageal and vascular injuries, followed by spinal cord, pulmonary, and intra-abdominal injuries.[4–6,19,20]

Because of the magnitude of blunt trauma necessary to produce an airway injury, associated injuries are also common in this group and may be the primary determinant in patient outcome. Any other structure or organ system may be involved as in any multiple trauma patient. Head, facial, and cervical spine injuries are frequent and important predictors of mortality and morbidity. Blunt intra-abdominal, intrathoracic, and skeletal trauma also occur frequently, as well as specific injuries to the esophagus and great vessels that are adjacent to the major airways. Major associated injuries are present in 40–100% of patients suffering blunt airway trauma and are dominated by orthopedic injuries in most patients, with a third to half of the patients having concomitant facial trauma, pulmonary contusions, or intra-abdominal injuries. Ten percent to 20% of the patients have major closed-head injuries, and approximately 10% have associated spinal cord injuries.[17,20] In one series, a very high incidence was reported of recurrent nerve injury associated with blunt airway trauma as evidenced by vocal cord dysfunction without evidence of direct laryngeal injury.[21] In this series, 49% of patients had recurrent nerve injuries and two-thirds of these had bilateral recurrent nerve palsy. In this same series, a 21% incidence of esophageal perforation was reported, clearly suggesting the need for high index of suspicion for associated esophageal injuries, even in the setting of blunt trauma. A high percentage of cervical crush injuries producing tracheal disruption may have associated laryngeal injuries that require careful assessment by an otolaryngologist during the primary assessment phase and before treatment decisions are made regarding repair of the tracheal injury.

Associated injuries are extremely common with both blunt and penetrating trauma of the airway and may be the major determinants of both short-term mortality and long-term morbidity. Knowledge of the relational anatomy, mechanism of injury, and incidence of related injuries helps define a prompt but thorough algorithm for diagnosing or excluding important injuries that require immediate or urgent management. Consideration of the known or potentially associated injuries becomes a critical factor in later choices of the surgical approach for addressing the airway injury.

## DIAGNOSIS

Accurate diagnosis of tracheobronchial injury requires an understanding of the mechanism of injury and a high index of suspicion when these mechanisms or common associated injuries are present (Fig. 27-1). Airway injuries become the first priority in trauma, and because of their acuity and critical importance in stabilizing the patient, initial steps in management may precede simultaneously with the diagnosis of airway pathology and associated injuries. Dyspnea and respiratory distress are frequent symptoms, occurring in 76–100% of patients.[18,20,21] The other common symptom is hoarseness or dysphonia, which occurred in 46% of the patients in a series published by Reece and Shatney.[21]

The most common signs of airway injury reported in most series were subcutaneous emphysema (35–85%), pneumothorax (20–50%), and hemoptysis (14–25%).[18,20–23] Air escaping from a penetrating wound in the neck is a pathognomonic sign of airway laceration and occurs in approximately 60% of patients with cervical penetrating trauma to the trachea,[5] cervical air leak that ceases after intubation confirms the diagnosis.

The most useful initial diagnostic studies are those obtained routinely in the initial trauma survey (i.e., chest and cervical spine radiographs). Deep cervical emphysema and pneumomediastinum will be seen in 60% and pneumothorax occurs in 70% of patients with tracheobronchial injuries.[23,24] The cervical spine or chest radiograph may also show a disruption of the tracheal or bronchial air column on careful examination. Overdistention of the endotracheal tube balloon cuff or displacement of the endotracheal tube may give additional radiologic signs of airway injury.[24] Complete transsection of a mainstem bronchus may result in the classic signs of atelectasis, "absent hilum," or a collapsing of the lung away from the hilus toward the diaphragm, known as the "falling lung sign of Kumpe."[25–27] A persistent pneumothorax with large air leak from a well-placed chest tube should increase the suspicion of intrathoracic tracheal or bronchial injury. With the chest tube on suction, the patient may experience more respiratory difficulties, and this finding is almost invariably associated with bronchial disruption.[28]

Although neck and upper chest computed tomography (CT) scan has become critical to the accurate diagnosis of traumatic laryngeal injuries, the role in more distal tracheobronchial injuries is not well established.[12] Commonly, a chest CT may be obtained as a part of the trauma workup and is extremely valuable in detecting the presence of a mediastinal hematoma or the possibility of associated injuries of the great vessels. The CT scan may show mediastinal air, disruption of the tracheobronchial air column, deviation of the airway, or the specific site of airway disruption. Although not specifically indicated for the workup of suggested acute tracheobronchial trauma, preoperative CT can be useful in assessing associated laryngeal injuries or other unsuspected chest injuries that should be dealt with at the time of surgical exploration. CT is contraindicated in the hemodynamically unstable trauma patient or the patient with an unstable airway. A negative CT scan does not obviate the need for bronchoscopy or other diagnostic studies. CT bronchography, or virtual bronchoscopy, may be helpful in some cases.[29] Our experience suggests that this is best when a CT is done for other reasons, and there is suspicion of injury rather performing CT primarily with the view of obtaining a CT bronchogram.

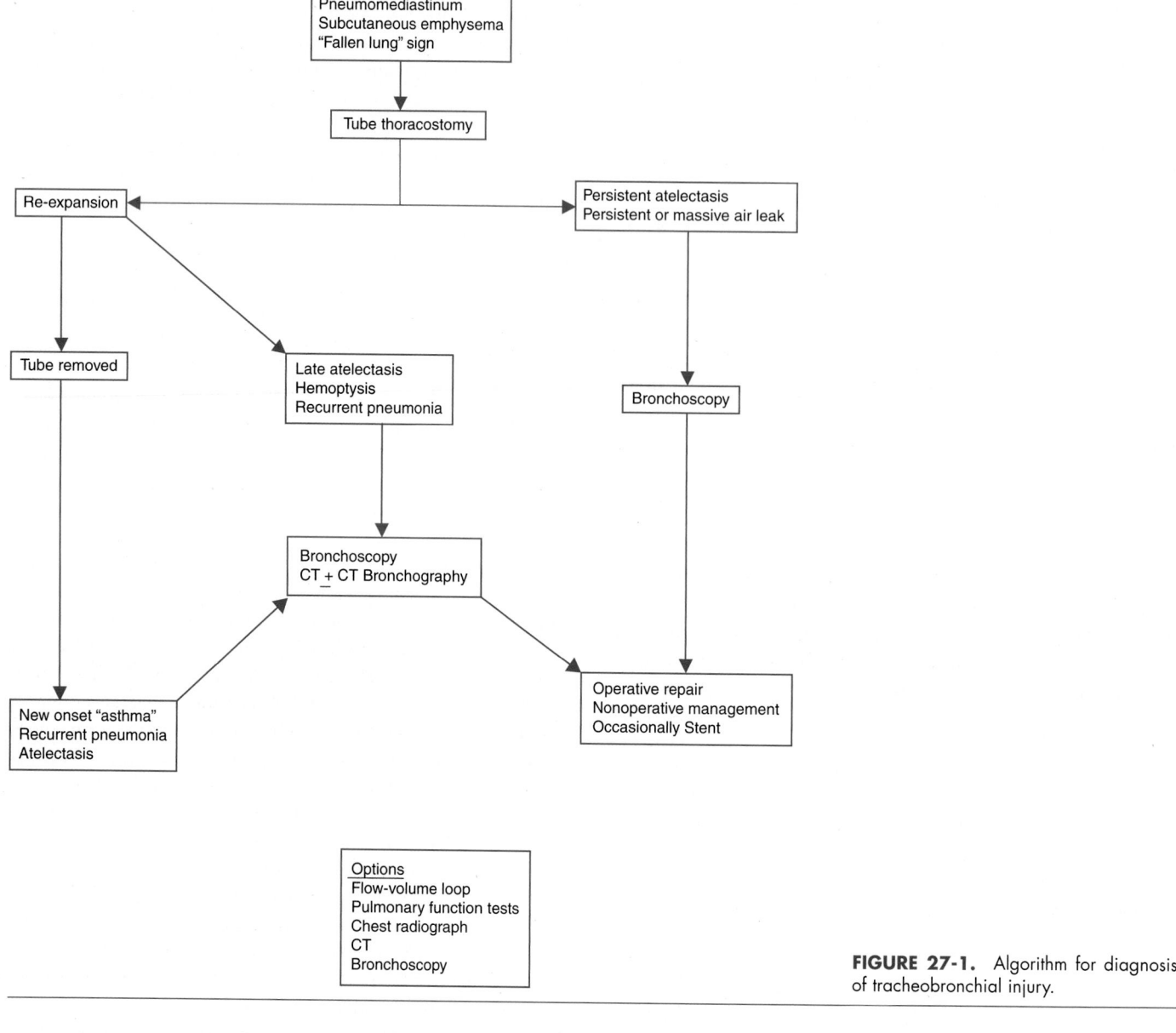

**FIGURE 27-1.** Algorithm for diagnosis of tracheobronchial injury.

Other imaging of suspected associated injuries is performed as indicated. Because of the common association of esophageal injuries, particularly after penetrating trauma, a contrast esophagogram is often necessary. Esophageal injuries may be distant from the airway injuries because of the distortion of tissues on traumatic impact.[30] Angiography of the aortic arch or cervical vessels is performed for penetrating injuries in a stable patient or in a blunt chest trauma patient when the chest radiograph or CT raises the suspicion for great vessel injury.

If the initial diagnosis of airway injury is missed, granulation tissue and stricture of the trachea or bronchus will develop within the first one to four weeks and in the majority of cases lead to symptoms, signs, and radiologic findings of pneumonia, bronchiectasis, atelectasis, and abscess.[9,31] Stridor and dyspnea are the common signs of late tracheal stenosis, whereas wheezing and postobstructive pneumonia are the common presentations of bronchial stenosis. Chest radiography and CT have been useful in the delayed setting and may directly reveal the site of stenosis and the secondary consequences of airway narrowing.

Bronchoscopy provides the single definitive diagnostic study in a patient with suspected airway injury. Direct or fiberoptic laryngoscopy is an important part of the endoscopic study in patients with cervical trauma and should be performed with the assistance of an experienced otolaryngologist when laryngeal injuries are suggested. Careful examination of the tracheobronchial tree with the fiberoptic bronchoscope will allow determination of the site and extent of injury. Bronchoscopy is the only study that can reliably exclude central airway trauma, although minor lacerations may occasionally be missed. The advantages of fiberoptic bronchoscopy are that it can be performed quickly and easily, even in the setting of concomitant head and neck injuries or cervical spine trauma. If bronchoscopy is being performed for a suspected airway injury in an intubated patient, it is important to carefully withdraw the endotracheal tube during endoscopy to avoid missing proximal tracheal injuries.

Bronchoscopy may also prove critical to the initial management of the patient with an injured airway. The flexible bronchoscope can be used as a guide to help intubate across a lacerated or transsected trachea or to intubate selectively into a mainstem bronchus. With this in mind, many major trauma units have now made the presence of a fiberoptic bronchoscope an integral part of their trauma suite equipment to help provide assistance for the establishment of an airway and quick evaluation of potential airway injuries.[9] Rigid bronchoscopy is rarely needed and, in fact, has the potential of exacerbating or extending the airway injury and is contraindicated in cervical spine trauma. However, skilled intubation with a ventilating bronchoscope may be life-saving in cases in which tracheal transsection and displacement does not allow identification or intubation of the distal segment with the fiberoptic bronchoscope. In these cases, the rigid bronchoscope may help realign the displaced airway and allow establishment of emergency ventilation before subsequent surgical repair. In most such cases, proceeding directly to open surgical control of the airway is most expedient and appropriate, as discussed later.

## Management

Airway Management.    The initial and most important priority in acute tracheobronchial injury is to secure a satisfactory airway. Patients with respiratory distress and the clinical suspicion of an airway injury should be intubated immediately, preferably with the guidance of a flexible bronchoscope, as described earlier. Fiberoptic intubation provides several advantages. First, it does not require neck extension for direct laryngoscopy and so can be performed while stabilization of the cervical spine is maintained before the exclusion of cervical spine injuries. Second, fiberoptic intubation can be easily performed in the awake, spontaneously ventilating patient. This prevents the need for sedation and paralysis, which is contraindicated in the patient with an unstable airway, until a satisfactory airway can be established. Sedation and paralysis is also contraindicated during the immediate evaluation and stabilization of an injured patient who requires several simultaneous assessments and hemodynamic stabilization. Third, flexible bronchoscopy can act as an obturator for the endotracheal tube and direct the tube past an area of injury under direct vision, allowing accurate placement into the distal trachea or either mainstem bronchus as necessary. Lastly, immediate bronchoscopy by an experienced endoscopist allows early evaluation of the location and extent of airway injury. This provides the best early information about the indications and approach for airway repair, allowing this to be calculated into the priority list of possible interventions for the multiply injured patient.

In published reports, the incidence of upper airway obstruction or severe distress that requires immediate intubation is variable and dependent on the degree of injuries and the criteria used. Flynn and associates reported eight of 22 patients (36%) requiring an immediate airway and three of these patients requiring an emergency tracheostomy or cricothyroidotomy. A series by Gussack and colleagues revealed 92% of patients requiring an emergency airway, 73% of these being successfully managed by orotracheal intubation, and three emergently intubated through an open neck wound.[1] Edwards and associates and Rossbach and Johnson reported that approximately 60% of their patients required prompt control of the airway.[20,32] In Rossbach and Johnson's series, 74% of the patients requiring emergency intubation were successfully managed by orotracheal intubation alone, whereas 10% required

intubation with fiberoptic guidance, 10% were intubated through an open neck wound, and only one patient (5%) required an emergent surgical airway through tracheostomy or cricothyroidotomy.[20] In the series reported by Edwards and coworkers, approximately 60% of the emergency airways were managed by nasotracheal or orotracheal intubation, and the other 40% required tracheostomy.[32] Important points are raised concerning the three patients in this series who were initially stable but experienced sudden deterioration secondary to the airway injury while they were being evaluated for multiple injuries. Two patients with a transsected cervical trachea required emergency tracheostomy with intubation of the distal tracheal segment through the tracheostomy incision. In one patient, an attempted emergency cricothyroidotomy produced a significant laryngeal injury that necessitated subsequent delayed repair.[32] A high index of suspicion and prompt securing of the injured airway are paramount to both the initial resuscitation and the ultimate outcome.

Patients with air emanating from a penetrating cervical injury may be intubated through the neck injury directly into the tracheal lumen. This technique has been utilized in approximately 25% of airway trauma in reports that include penetrating cervical injuries.[1,20,23,32] However, attempts at oral intubation or blind intubation through a cervical wound may be futile and can either precipitate total obstruction or allow the progressive loss of an unstable airway if repeated attempts are unsuccessful. Although intubation guided by a flexible bronchoscope may solve most of these difficulties, delay in obtaining a bronchoscope or successfully traversing the injury may also cause complete obstruction, with the tragic loss of a salvageable patient. In cases in which airway injury is suspected, preparation for immediate tracheostomy must be made simultaneously with the attempts at intubation. In cases of severe maxillofacial trauma, immediate tracheostomy is the procedure of choice for airway control. Cricothyroidotomy is rarely useful in tracheobronchial trauma because the injury lies distal to the insertion point of the tracheostomy tube, which is placed blindly and with no additional accuracy over oral or nasotracheal intubation alone. If a tracheostomy is performed, the tracheostomy tube should be placed through the area of injury if possible to prevent extension of the tracheal injury by the tracheal stoma. A transsected cervical trachea may retract into the mediastinum; in these cases it is best found by inserting a finger into the mediastinum anterior to the esophagus, locating the distal trachea by palpation, and grasping the clamp to allow retraction into the cervical wound and distal intubation.[33]

Management of the airway for injuries of the distal trachea, the carina, and the proximal mainstem bronchi can be extremely challenging. Use of double-lumen tubes should be avoided because of their rigidity and size, which increases the possibility of injury extension. In these cases, a long endotracheal tube should be positioned beyond the injury or into the appropriate mainstem bronchus to provide single-lung ventilation. This can best be performed with the aid of the flexible bronchoscope serving as a guide and to confirm the final position. In almost all cases, standard ventilation can be initiated once distal airway control is ensured. In cases of distal injuries of the left mainstem bronchus, the bronchus intermedius, or lobar orifices, a bronchial blocker placed proximal to the injury under endoscopic guidance provides another alternative for stabilizing the airway and allowing ventilation.

## STABILIZATION AND PRIORITIZATION OF ASSOCIATED INJURIES

Establishment of a stable airway and assurance of ventilation are the first two priorities of any resuscitation. Once the airway is secured, the priority shifts to circulation, with the recognition, stabilization, and resuscitation of cardiovascular injuries. Neurologic, intrathoracic and intra-abdominal, vascular, and orthopedic injuries are identified during the primary and secondary trauma surveys. A patient with multiple injuries frequently has several simultaneous, competing priorities for the sequencing of and approach to operative procedures. Fortunately, intubation distal to the injury or into the unaffected proximal mainstem bronchus usually allows adequate oxygenation and ventilation for emergency management of associated life-threatening injuries. The sequence of operative procedures must be individualized, but establishment of effective ventilation allows the initial priority to be given to the management of life- or organ-threatening injuries. Subdural hematomas, intra-abdominal bleeding, or major cardiovascular injuries should usually be repaired before definitive repair of the tracheobronchial injury.

## ANESTHETIC MANAGEMENT

Close cooperation between the anesthesiologist and the surgeon is critical to the successful management of a tracheobronchial injury. In cases in which the airway has not already been established, the anesthesiologist may provide invaluable assistance in airway control and selective intubation. The choice and timing of anesthetic agents and muscle relaxants, the type of endotracheal tubes used, and the mode of intraoperative ventilation require close communication between the anesthesiologist and surgeon for planning of an efficient and effective operative strategy. If a bronchoscopy has not already been performed, it is necessary at the initiation of the procedure to define the location and extent of injury and to guide the surgeon regarding the operative approach and intended repair. This is best performed with a standard diagnostic bronchoscope through a large single-lumen endotracheal tube. In cases of mainstem bronchial or lobar injuries, a contralateral double-lumen endotracheal tube is preferred for the ease of isolated single-lung ventilation. However, in all other injuries involving the trachea or carina, a long, single-lumen tube can traverse and be seated distal to the injury and is preferred because it is less bulky and easier to guide past the torn airway without injury extension.

High-frequency jet ventilation provides an effective option for ventilation with relatively low airway pressures. Its main advantage is during airway reconstruction, because it can be delivered through a small catheter with less bulk and rigidity, allowing easier placement of sutures or approximation of the newly reconstructed airway without tension. However, in most cases, it is usually easiest to perform standard ventilation through the oral endotracheal tube or through a sterile endotracheal tube inserted through the operative field into the transsected airway. This does not require additional equipment or experience and has the added advantage of a cuffed tube preventing aspiration of blood into the distal airway and less aerosolization of blood around the surgical team.

Cardiopulmonary bypass is virtually never necessary for the intraoperative management of isolated airway injuries. Associated injuries of the heart or great vessels may require cardiopulmonary bypass (CPB). In cases in which CPB is already being used, it may facilitate a concomitant tracheobronchial repair. However, CPB after major trauma can exacerbate intracerebral or intra-abdominal hemorrhage and potentiate the systemic inflammatory response that produces adult respiratory distress syndrome, with a very high subsequent mortality. In simple injuries, standard ventilation is straightforward, precluding consideration of CPB. In complex injuries, or those in which associated trauma makes ventilation difficult, the anticoagulation and added trauma of CPB probably results in exacerbation of bleeding and the systemic inflammatory response more than it helps in allowing airway repair.

Virtually all patients with isolated tracheobronchial injuries can be easily extubated at the end of the operative procedure and should be managed by the anesthesiologist with this in mind. Patients who require postoperative ventilation because of their associated injuries should finish the procedure with a large-bore, single-lumen endotracheal tube to allow good pulmonary toilet and fiberoptic bronchoscopy if necessary. If possible, this should be placed with the balloon cuff distal to the area of tracheal repair in proximal injuries or should lie proximal and away from the repair for carinal and mainstem bronchial injuries. Major laryngeal or maxillofacial injuries with the anticipated need for prolonged ventilation are indications for placement of a tracheostomy at the completion of the tracheobronchial repair. This tracheostomy should not be placed through the tracheal repair, which will lead to a contamination of the suture line with subsequent dehiscence or stenosis.[33]

## NONOPERATIVE MANAGEMENT

On occasion, injuries will be found that do not require operative repair. These include small injuries, primarily mucosal, which are not associated with significant ongoing air leak or distal obstruction. These lesions typically should be smaller than one-third of the entire circumference and not be associated with tissue devitalization. These injuries still require follow-up as late stricture and related complications can occur. One very unusual presentation is the patient who has experienced a partial mucosal "blow out" in which there is no discreet mucosal rupture but endoscopically there is a "patulous" nature of the membrane. This can, especially if there is associated inflammation, result in a "ball-valve," which leads to progressive obstruction and/or air trapping distally that prompts interval operative repair.[22,23]

## SURGICAL MANAGEMENT

Management is determined by location, extent of injury, and associated injuries (Fig. 27-2). The proximal one-half to two-thirds of the trachea is best approached through a low cervical collar incision that also provides excellent exposure to vascular or esophageal injuries in the neck. Creating a "T" incision over the manubrium and splitting the manubrium down to the second interspace opens the thoracic inlet and provides a broader exposure to the middle

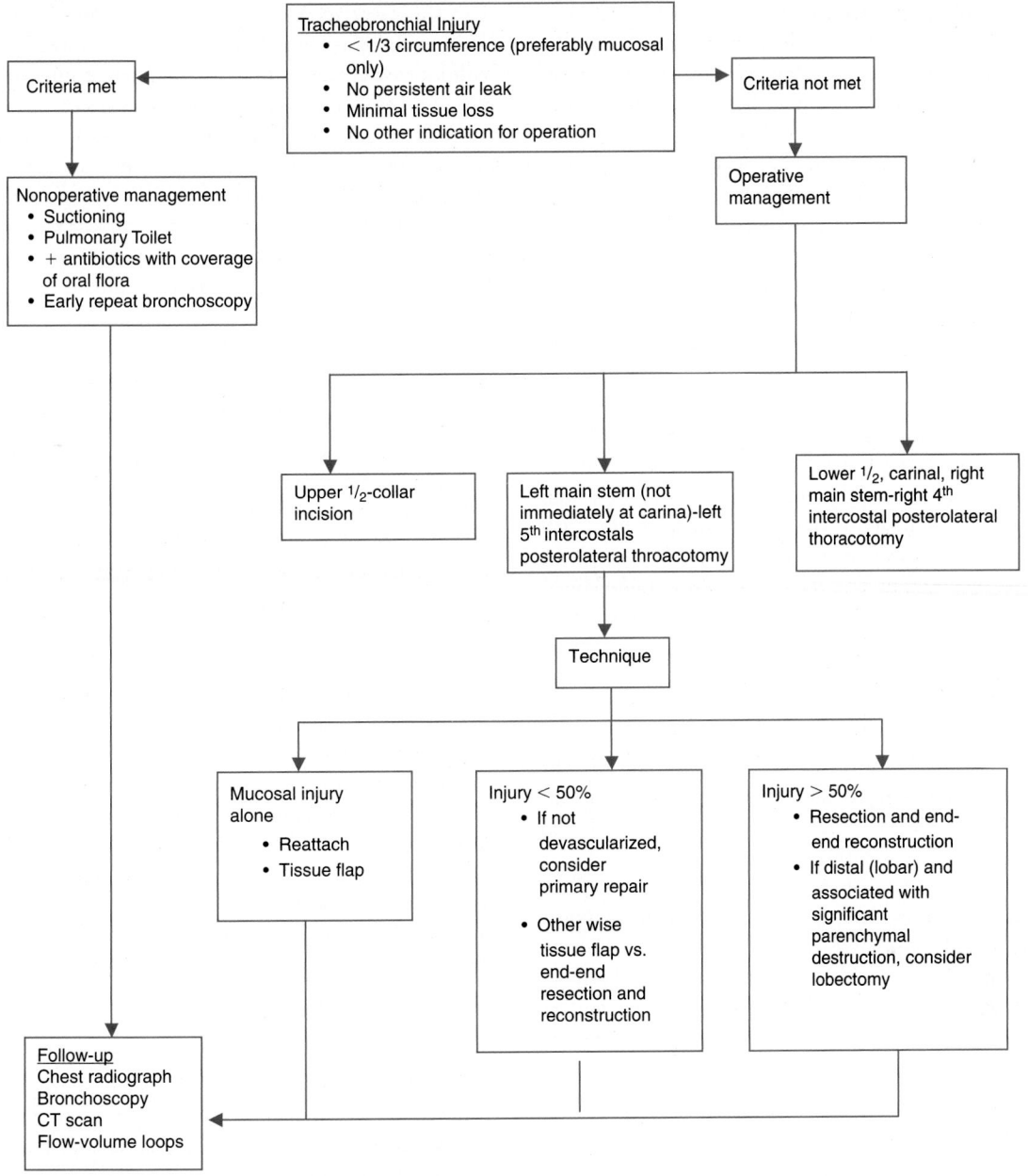

**FIGURE 27-2.** Algorithm for management of tracheobronchial injury.

third of the trachea as well as proximal control of the innominate artery or veins. A full median sternotomy does not provide significant additional airway exposure except in specific circumstances, which are discussed later. The distal third of the trachea, the carina, and the right mainstem bronchus are most easily approached through a right thoracotomy, which also provides good exposure to the azygous vein, superior vena cava, and right atrium, as well as all of the intrathoracic esophagus. Injuries of the left mainstem bronchus are most easily approached through a left thoracotomy, which also provides good exposure to the distal portion of the aortic arch, the descending thoracic aorta, and the proximal left subclavian artery. However, exposure to the proximal left mainstem, the carina, the distal trachea, or the right mainstem is extremely difficult through a left thoracotomy, owing to the overlying aortic arch. Adequate proximal exposure may be gained by mobilization of the arch with retraction cephalad laterally and division of the ligamentum arteriosum.

These approaches may not be adequate for the management of potential associated injuries. Because of the proximity of the heart and great vessels anterior to the distal trachea, the carina, and the proximal mainstem bronchi, penetrating injuries to the chest are likely to have associated life-threatening cardiovascular injuries. A median sternotomy will often be performed to provide optimal access to the heart or great vessels but provides far less satisfactory exposure to the trachea, carina, and bronchi than did respective thoracotomies as described earlier. However, it is possible to obtain exposure to the anterior airway in the vicinity of the carina to allow anterior repair or limited primary resection and reconstruction. This requires mobilization of the superior vena cava with reflection to the right, retraction of the ascending aorta to the left, and longitudinal division of the posterior pericardium cephalad to the right pulmonary artery and caudal to the innominate vein. Unfortunately, this does not provide any exposure to the posterior airway where blunt injuries frequently occur. It also does not provide adequate exposure for repair of concomitant esophageal injuries. A bilateral thoracosternotomy or "clamshell" incision through the fourth interspace provides good exposure to both hemithoraces and the anterior mediastinum and may be a considered as an approach because of associated injuries. However, this approach provides little additional airway exposure or airway advantages over those incisions previously described.

Simple, clean lacerations without airway devascularization can be repaired primarily with simple interrupted absorbable sutures. We prefer 4-0 Vicryl (Ethicon, Cincinnati, OH), although others have successfully utilized permanent and absorbable monofilament. In cases in which there is significant tracheobronchial damage, all devitalized tissue should be débrided, with care taken to preserve as much viable airway as possible. In these cases, a circumferential resection and end-to-end anastomosis is almost always preferable to partial wedge resections of traumatized airway with attempted primary repair. The principles of airway resection and reconstruction are similar for tracheal, carinal, or bronchial injuries, although the anatomy of reconstruction is unique to the surgical exposure, the location, and the extent of resection. This is particularly true when a portion of the carina must be resected or reconstructed, because a large variety of techniques may be necessary to achieve reconstruction in this area.[34] Dissection of the airway is limited to the region to be resected to preserve tracheobronchial blood supply to the area of anastomosis. Precise placement of interrupted absorbable suture allows an airtight anastomosis, correction of size discrepancy between the distal and proximal airway, and minimal anastomotic granulations if the anastomosis is brought together without tension.

In most patients, up to half of the trachea can be resected and primarily reconstructed so that the most significant tracheal injuries should be able to allow primary resection and reconstruction without difficulty. Both mainstem bronchi can be completely resected with primary reconstruction without tension in all cases. Extensive injuries of the carina are more problematic and should be repaired rather than resected if at all possible. Only 3 to 4 cm of airway involving the carina can be resected and allowed for primary reconstruction. A variety of tracheobronchial release maneuvers have been used to allow a tension-free anastomosis. For most limited tracheal resections, blunt development of the anterior avascular pretracheal plane combined with neck flexion is all that is necessary. For more extensive proximal tracheal resections, a suprahyoid laryngeal release can provide 1-2 cm of additional proximal mobilization. For resections of the mainstem bronchi or carina, division of the pericardium around the inferior aspect of the hilum provides an additional 1-2 cm of distal airway mobilization.[35]

Associated injuries of the esophagus should be repaired in two layers. When working through an anterior cervical exposure, the esophagus may be best exposed by complete tracheal transsection through the area of planned tracheal repair. A vascularized flap of muscle or soft tissue should be interposed between the tracheal and esophageal repairs to minimize the risk of postoperative tracheoesophageal fistula. Intrathoracic tracheobronchial suture lines are also preferably wrapped with pedicled pericardial fat, intercostal muscle, or pleura to separate the airway anastomosis from overlying blood vessels. In cases in which a portion of the trachea or carina has been resected and reconstructed, much of the airway mobility is provided by neck flexion. This position is maintained in the postoperative period by placement of a "guardian suture" between the chin and the sternum. As discussed earlier, patients with isolated airway injuries are routinely extubated in the operating room, even after complex reconstructions.

In those cases in which the diagnosis has been missed, and patients develop persistent atelectasis, pneumonia, and/or mediastinitis, management is determined by parenchymal viability. If extensive lung necrosis has occurred, management would include resection. If not, attempts at airway reconstruction, or in specific cases, temporizing stenting, may be possible.[9,31]

## POSTOPERATIVE MANAGEMENT

Careful airway observation is maintained in the early postoperative period. Aggressive pulmonary toilet, including the liberal use of bedside bronchoscopy, is important because these patients may have difficulty clearing secretions past their anastomosis or area of airway repair. Patients who have an associated vocal cord paralysis may have even more difficulty with pulmonary toilet owing to their inability to produce an effective cough. These patients may benefit from a commercially available minitracheostomy (Minitrach II, Portex, Keene, NH), which is placed through their cricothyroid membrane to allow direct tracheal suctioning. Some patients with tracheal resection may have problems with postoperative aspiration because of difficulty in elevating the larynx during deglutition. This is more profound in the patients with associated recurrent nerve injuries or in those who have had a suprahyoid laryngeal release. The remainder of the postoperative management is similar to the routine care after other neck operations or thoracotomy for pulmonary resection. In the trauma setting, management of the associated injuries and their complications may dominate the care of the patient. For the ventilated patient, care should be taken to position the endotracheal balloon distal or proximal to the tracheal suture line and minimize airway pressures in cases where the endotracheal tube lies above the airway anastomosis by necessity. These patients should be managed at the lowest possible airway pressures that provide satisfactory oxygenation and ventilation and extubated as soon as their other injuries will allow. Bronchoscopy should usually be performed seven to ten days after tracheobronchial repair or before discharge to ensure satisfactory healing without granulation tissue or the early development of anastomotic stenosis.

## COMPLICATIONS

The complications of tracheobronchial repair are similar to those of airway resection and reconstruction and consist mostly of anastomotic problems. Anastomotic dehiscence or restenosis occurs in 5–6% of patients after tracheal reconstruction.[36] All patients should have baseline flow volume loops, even if managed nonoperatively, as rarely patients may present later in life with "asthma" which really reflects a stricture. Initial management involves securing the airway, usually with an endoluminal or tracheal T-tube until healing is complete and the perioperative inflammation has subsided. Most of these patients can be managed with subsequent airway resection and reconstruction three to six months after the original repair, if necessary.[37,38] Other options may include serial dilation and stenting. Anastomotic dehiscence is life-threatening if this results in fistula formation to the innominate artery or esophagus. Tracheal/innominate artery fistula is rare but frequently fatal and requires immediate operation for division of the innominate artery and interposition of healthy tissue between the airway and great vessels. Tracheoesophageal fistula can usually be managed initially by establishing gastric drainage, enteral nutrition, and treatment of pneumonia. When the patient is stable and no longer requires ventilatory support, the tracheoesophageal fistula can be divided, with the esophageal and tracheal defects resected or repaired and healthy soft tissue interposed between the adjacent suture lines. If vocal cord paralysis is permanent, it can usually be palliated by vocal cord lateralization or medialization procedures.

## LATE MANAGEMENT

Patients may incur delayed treatment after tracheobronchial trauma for three reasons. First, the initial injury may have been subtle and initially missed in the early or intermediate trauma management. Second, severe associated injuries may have prevented early definitive management of recognized airway injury. Third, initial attempts at repair may fail, resulting in dehiscence or late stenosis.

In any of these scenarios, the sequelae are similar. Although the airway may be partially or completely disrupted at the time of initial injury, it may be held together by strong peritracheal connective tissue, allowing an airway to be established and ventilation to be maintained. However, as the primary injury or secondary dehiscence heals, granulation tissue and scar contracture result, with subsequent stricture formation that usually develops one to four weeks after injury. Taskinen and associates reported nine patients with blunt tracheobronchial rupture, five of whom had operations purposely delayed from 9 to 89 days because of complete lung expansion with suction drainage.[39] However, in all five patients, dyspnea later developed, with bronchoscopy revealing obstruction and granulation tissue at the site of airway injury. Each of these patients required subsequent airway resection with primary reconstruction.

These patients may initially have dyspnea on exertion but may also have wheezing, stridor, cough, difficulty in clearing secretions, or recurrent respiratory infections. Any of these symptoms with a history of trauma or prolonged intubation should raise the suspicion of a late airway stenosis, which should be diagnosed or excluded by bronchoscopy. A 50% reduction in the cross-sectional area of the trachea usually results in dyspnea only with significant exertion, whereas narrowing of the lumen to less than 25% usually produces dyspnea and stridor at rest. Patients may be reasonably compensated in spite of significant stenosis but can have acute life-threatening deterioration with a minor amount of airway edema or secretions. A high index of suspicion in these patients is critical to their subsequent workup and timely diagnosis.[9]

Once recognized, critical airway stenosis can be evaluated and initially stabilized by bronchoscopy and dilatation.[40] However, the appropriate, definitive management of most of these patients is subsequent tracheal or bronchial resection with primary reconstruction as for benign airway strictures from other causes. Except in cases of distal lung destruction by chronic infection, re-establishment of ventilation to lung parenchyma can be expected to restore significant function, even years after the injury. There may be little or no apparent function by preoperative perfusion scanning; this is likely due to reflexive pulmonary vasoconstriction and is reversible on resumption of ventilation to the lung parenchyma. Airway reconstruction should always be considered first in these instances, with pulmonary resection reserved for patients with unreconstructable lesions or those with destroyed parenchyma from chronic infection or bronchiectasis.

## RESULTS

Injury to the trachea and proximal bronchi is lethal, with more than 75% of patients with blunt tracheobronchial trauma dying before arrival to the emergency department.[7] There are no known series of autopsy studies of penetrating tracheobronchial trauma to give us a similar prehospital mortality denominator. However, in both instances, death is most likely due to associated injuries rather than to the tracheobronchial injury itself.

In patients operated on for penetrating injuries, the mortality is 6–18%.[5,6] Of 17 survivors of penetrating tracheal trauma, 88% had a good result, apparently without symptoms.[6] One of 17 patients had permanent hoarseness from concomitant recurrent nerve injury and a second patient required a permanent tracheostomy because of complications and failed reconstruction of a combined tracheal and esophageal injury. In Rossbach's series of 32 patients with penetrating (59%) and blunt (41%) tracheobronchial trauma, 78% of patients required postoperative mechanical ventilation. In patients with a penetrating injury, this ranged from one to three days with a mean of two days, and in patients with blunt injury, intubation ranged from three to nine days with a mean of five days. The average length of intensive care unit stay was four days for patients with penetrating trauma and nine days for patients with blunt injury, whereas the mean hospitalization was 15 days and 17 days for penetrating and blunt injuries, respectively.[20] Nineteen percent of patients in this series sustained postoperative complications but 93% of patients were ultimately asymptomatic and returned to preinjury function. Only one of 32 patients (3%) had a symptomatic late stenosis after repair of complex avulsion injury. The mortality rate in this series was 6% and was related to multiple injuries in the setting of blunt trauma. Results from other series show a mortality of 10–25% for patients undergoing repair of tracheobronchial injury in the setting of penetrating or blunt trauma with associated injuries.[4,23,32]

Patients with early definitive airway repair had a long-term good result in over 90% of patients, with poor airway-related outcomes generally being due to associated recurrent nerve injury or failed initial tracheobronchial repair.[1,21] However, in the series by Reece and Shatney, good results were only obtained in 67% of patients who had tracheal repair over a stent or with a tracheostomy, leaving the authors to conclude that primary early repair provides the best long-term outcomes. In many series, the ultimate prognosis after airway injury is dependent on the associated injuries, particularly closed-head injuries. Thirteen percent of the patients in a series published by Angood and associates were left in a vegetative state in spite of excellent functional airways after definitive tracheobronchial repair.[10]

## Traumatic Esophageal Perforation

### Highlights in Management

- Signs and symptoms are nonspecific, thus a high degree of suspicion is required to make the diagnosis

- Most injuries require simple repair

- All repairs should be buttressed by local tissue

- Outcome is critically affected by a delay in diagnosis

- The management of caustic injuries is determined by initial esophagoscopy which ideally should be within 24 hours of injury

- The role of corticosteroids remain debatable

- Patients with peritonitis or obvious mediastinitis require urgent exploration

- Alkali injuries result in full thickness coagulation necrosis while acid injuries tend to be more often superficial

Diagnosis, management, and outcome are critically affected by etiology, location, and duration between event and intervention. In trauma, there is a tendency for the diagnosis to be made in a delayed fashion.[41] There has been a trend of moving away from "time-based" therapy, with injuries diagnosed >24 hours after injury being managed by "exclusion-diversion" to therapy based on an understanding of the clinical stability of the patient, underlying esophageal pathology, and quality of the mediastinal tissues, with an emphasis on primary repair, usually with some form of tissue buttressing.

## INCIDENCE AND MECHANISM

Overall, esophageal injuries are present in less than 1% of patients admitted following traumatic injury.[42] The most common traumatic injury occurs following penetrating neck injury, accounting for >80% of all traumatic perforations.[41] However, only 0.5–7% of penetrating neck injuries are associated with esophageal involvement.[42,43] This number increases to as much as 12% if one considers cervical explorations for penetrating injuries that violate the platysma.[44,45] Although penetrating trauma is rarely associated with intra-thoracic esophageal injury, it is not unheard of. Cornwell and associates noted a 0.7% incidence among 1961 patients admitted following thoracic gunshot wounds.[46] Transmediastinal gunshot wounds, involving "low-velocity" missiles that course close to the spine, can result in tough and through injuries. Stab wounds to the abdomen, particularly through the back, rarely are associated with intra-abdominal esophageal perforation. Injuries to these areas due to high-velocity gunshot wounds usually are fatal and are diagnosed postmortem. Depending on the prevalence of mechanisms seen, gunshot wounds account for 43–95% and stab wounds 7–57% of esophageal injuries.[47–49] Blunt trauma leads to esophageal perforation in <0.1% of cases, the majority in the cervical area caused by a sudden blow to the anterior hyper-extended neck.[50] Other mechanisms described include blast injury (particularly compressed air) and acute gastric compression resulting in complex lower third intra-thoracic esophageal tears, analogous to Boerhaave's syndrome.[42]

## DIAGNOSIS

The majority of traumatic esophageal injuries are discovered because the mechanism of injury suggests the possibility. Signs and symptoms clearly are related to location and mechanism. The diagnosis can be suggested or obscured by the presence of associated injuries (Table 27-1). Penetrating cervical injuries were diagnosed on clinical grounds in 68% of patients in the series reported by Meyer and coworkers, while Weigelt and colleagues reported that 50% of patients following stab wounds, and 100% following gunshot wounds, presented with signs or symptoms suggestive of esophageal injury.[44,45] However, they may present in a more occult fashion.[41] Initial presentation of cervical perforations may be simply hoarseness, spiting up blood, subcutaneous air, and/or anterior tracheal deviation. Untreated, fever, erythema, swelling, increasing credits, and airway distress, and finally frank abscess formation occurs. Infection often spreads along the precervical plane to involve upper mediastinal structures leading to signs and symptoms of mediastinitis. Patients who present with Zone II injuries that are associated with penetration of the platysma should be considered at risk for esophageal injury. Whether or not, in the asymptomatic patient without evidence of injury, mandatory exploration should be performed as opposed to the combination of swallow, endoscope, and angiography is still being debated. Rarely, ethylene or brilliant blue dye given orally will confirm the injury. Intra-thoracic injuries may be clinically silent or be obscured until mediastinitis and empyema result in unrelenting septic shock. Pleural fluid that is foul smelling, associated with pH <6.0 or with elevated amylase, should raise the possibility.[51] Sub diaphragmatic injuries present with abdominal tenderness, referred shoulder tip pain, and ultimately, in over 50% of cases, peritonitis and sepsis.[50]

Because, in many cases, symptoms are obscure and nonspecific, particularly with respect to the intra-thoracic esophagus, a great deal of reliance is placed on suspicion based on mechanism and imaging studies. Conventional radiographs may demonstrate

**TABLE 27-1**

| Incidence of Various Injuries Associated with Esophageal Trauma | |
| --- | --- |
| SITE | PERCENTAGE OF TIME INJURED |
| Carotid | 4–25 |
| Diaphragm | 9–20 |
| Great vessels | 5–10 |
| Heart | 10 |
| Lung | 5–37 |
| Major venous | 8–17 |
| Spinal cord | 8–16 |
| Thoracic duct | 4–5 |
| Thyroid | 5–18 |
| Trachea | 15–64 |
| Vascular | 26–43 |
| Vocal cord or recurrent nerve | 5–10 |

*Sources: Armstrong et al.,[55] Attar et al.,[47] Defoire et al.,[67] Fetterman et al.,[68] Flynn et al.,[48] Glatterer et al.,[69] Ngakane et al.,[70] Richardson and Tobin,[54] Sheely et al.,[43] Weiman et al.,[49] Winter and Weigelt,[71] Yugueros et al.[72]*

*(From: Riley RD, Miller PR, Meredith JW: Injury to the esophagous, trachea and bronchus. In Moore EE, Feliciano DV, Mattox KL, eds, Trauma (5th ed.), New York: McGraw-Hill, 2004, pp. 539–553.[42])*

**TABLE 27-2**

**Diagnostic Evaluation of Suspected Esophageal Injuries**

|  | REFERENCE | SENSITIVITY (%) | SPECIFICITY (%) | ACCURACY (%) |
|---|---|---|---|---|
| Clinical presentation | Weigelt et al.[45] | 80 | 64 | 72 |
| Contrast esophagography | Noyes et al.[73] | 80 | 94 | 90 |
|  | Armstrong et al. (C)[55] | 62 | – | – |
|  | Weigelt et al.[45] | 89 | 100 | 94 |
|  | White and Morris[74] | 100 | 95 | 95 |
|  | Sheely et al. (C)[43] | 48 | – | – |
| Rigid esophagoscopy | Armstrong et al.[55] | 100 | – | – |
|  | Weigelt et al.[45] | 89 | 95 | 94 |
|  | Noyes et al. (C)[73] | 67 | 89 | 86 |
| Flexible esophagoscopy | Weigelt et al.[45] | 37 | 99 | 94 |
|  | Flowers et al.[75] | 100 | 96 | 97 |
|  | White and Morris (C)[74] | 67 | 67 | 82 |
|  | White and Morris (T)[74] | 100 | 100 | 100 |

C, cervical; T, thoracic; others are combined sites or unspecified.

(From: Riley RD, Miller PR, Meredith JW: Injury to the esophagus, trachea, and bronchus. In Moore EE, Feliciano DV, Mattox KL, eds, Trauma (5th ed.), New York: McGraw-Hill, 2004, pp. 539–553.[42])

subcutaneous emphysema, hydropneumothorax, hydropneumomediastinum, or free abdominal air depending on location of perforation and duration of injury. Occasionally, a nasogastric tube will be noted to be lying extra-esophageal. Gastrograffin swallows are favored by radiologists who fear barium contamination. However, gastrograffin can miss up to 15% of perforations and therefore, if negative, should be followed by barium. We prefer to use "thin" barium as the initial study. The advantage of a contrast study is that it will confirm location of leak, which side of the esophagus the leak predominantly tends to, as well as determine if this is significant stricture or other pathology that needs to be addressed. Overall, the false negative rate using combined gastrograffin-tin barium is as high as 10%.[50] CT scan may demonstrate contrast and/or air in the surrounding mediastinum, reveal pleural effusions, and can be used to follow up. In addition, in stable patients, computed tomography (CT) angiography can obviate the need for routine bronchoscopy, esophagoscopy, angiography, and esophageal swallow in all patients with transmediastinal gunshot wounds by defining the tract of the missile. More selective evaluation can then be performed.[52]

Esophagoscopy and contrast studies are complimentary in the trauma setting (Table 27-2).[41] Esophagoscopy can miss 15–40% of traumatic injuries, but when combined with contrast studies the sensitivity approaches 100%. Flexible and rigid esophagoscopy are both acceptable in the trauma setting. Flexible endoscopy tends to be less sensitive for detecting injuries in the most proximal cervical esophagus, as blind passage of the scope through the cricopharyngeus tends to miss the most proximal 2–4 cm. Rigid esophagoscopy is limited by the need for anesthesia and the requirement that the patient's neck be cleared for flexion.

## MANAGEMENT

Basic principles include control of leak, debridement and drainage of all areas of suppuration, nutritional support (with emphasis on gastric and/or jejunostomy tubes), and early use of broad spectrum antibiotics. The vast majority of traumatic perforations require operative therapy, and the majority of cases should be approached

with the intention of performing primary repair.[51] However, the presence of significant underlying esophageal pathology, extreme inflammation of tissues, and/or degree of shock may mandate other approaches.

The cervical esophagus can be explored via a collar incision, which is particularly useful if bilateral injuries are present. Unilateral penetrating injuries, particularly stab wounds, can be explored by a "carotid" incision, but one should be prepared to "T" the incision as needed for exposure. The upper two-thirds of the thoracic esophagus is best exposed via a right posterolateral thoracotomy, the level determined by the need for repair of other structures, or by the level of injury. The thoracic esophagus at or below the inferior pulmonary vein is best exposed by a 7th or 8th intercostals left posterolateral approach. If in doubt, the simplest rule is to operate on the side of the leak, although bilateral approaches may be required in cases where there has been a delay in diagnosis leading to bilateral empyema. The majority of injuries can be repaired primarily. Additional protection can be achieved by buttressing the repair.[53] In the cervical area, the sternocleidomastoid or other strap muscles can be mobilized as an onlay patch, particularly if there has been associated carotid or tracheal injury, to prevent the risk of late fistula formation. In the chest, intercostal muscle flap can be laid on to the repair. It may not be advisable to circumferentially wrap the esophagus as late calcification can result in an unyielding extrinsic stricture. Other options include diaphragm, pericardium, and/or pericardial fat pad flaps. Latissimus dorsi, rhomboid, and other muscle flaps have been described for complex long tears.[54] In the abdomen, omentum, a fundoplication or Thal (gastric tube) patches are options.

Primary repair should still be considered even in the setting where diagnosis has been delayed for >24 hours.[51,53] The limiting factors in these circumstances are tissue quality and patient stability. In fact, in a field of moderate inflammation, repair with tissue flaps (either as primary method or to reinforce primary repair) may be even more effective. The "Grillo" pleural flap appears to be particularly effective when there is pleural inflammation.[51,53] It is critical, however, one attempts to deal with the delayed perforation, that a thorough decortication is performed to allow full lung expansion. Some authors feel that if the tissue is tenuous, primary repair can still be performed if either a diversion (cervical fistula or drainage with T-tube) or exclusion (absorbable suture or staples at E-G junction) is performed to "protect" the repair.[50]

Occasionally in the cervical or thoracic esophagus, through and tough wounds are significant enough that primary repair would lead to critical narrowing. Short (1–2 cm) circumferential resection and end-to-end anastamosis can be performed for penetrating traumatic injuries in the neck or chest. When the tear or perforation is very large, resection can be performed in an expeditious manner. A long cervical esophagostomy can be brought out onto the anterior chest wall below the clavicle.[50] This has the advantages of being more comfortable for the patient and maximizing the length of residual esophagus for later reconstruction. In stable patients, immediate reconstruction can be considered.

Drainage is best suited for the management of late-diagnosed cervical perforations.[41,50] The precervical plane needs to be drained and a closed suction drain placed. Open drainage will usually be successful, but strictures can occur late and based on the experience with cervical leaks after gastroesophagectomy, early dilation may be helpful. Drainage of complex thoracic aortic perforation that either because of size of injury, inadequate tissue and/or patient instability, are not candidates for primary repair or resection, is best achieved with a tracheal T-tube, into which a 28 Fr. chest tube can be intussuscepted. At least two other chest tubes should be placed nearby. This creates a controlled fistula that, once the patient recovers, can be downsized by removing the T-tube via esophagoscopy and then slowly changing the chest tube to smaller and smaller caliber tubes. This should only take a minute or two longer than is required to simply place chest tubes and is ideally utilized in patients who are in septic shock. Simple drainage with chest tube is associated with nearly 70% mortality. On the other hand, in hemodynamically unstable patients, with other injuries, simple drainage with or without stapling or ligating the esophagus above and below the injury, may be needed simply to "get the patient of the table."[41,50]

## COMPLICATIONS

Traumatic esophageal injuries carry mortality rates ranging from 0 to 19%.[41] Stab wounds clearly have a lower mortality rate than gunshot wounds which can be associated with significant devitalization and associated injuries. Complications of esophageal resection or repair are the same following trauma as for any other cause and include leak, fistula, and stricture. Armstrong and associates described a leak rate of 20% when traumatic cervical injuries were repaired within 12 hours, but 100% when greater than 24 hours.[55] The approach to managing leaks are varied, and also depend on location, patient physiology, size of the leak, and degree of surrounding tissue plane involvement. Small cervical leaks can be managed by open drainage. Small thoracic leaks without gross empyema or mediastinitis can be occasionally managed by radiologically placed drains. A mid-esophageal leak may also be controlled by temporizing, retrievable, esophageal stent. As the degree of contamination and sepsis increases, so should the aggressiveness of the operation. In the most severe cases, esophagectomy with diversion, T-tube drainage (with a tracheal T-tube in the defect with chest tube to provide drainage attached), or esophageal exclusion described for complicated iatrogenic or spontaneous rupture may be required. In general,

### TABLE 27-3

**Endoscopic Grading of Caustic Injury**

| DEGREE OF INJURY | DEPTH | ENDOSCOPIC FINDINGS |
|---|---|---|
| Grade I | Mucosal | Superficial hyperemia and friability |
| Grade II | Partial | Mucoasl sloughing, friability |
| • A | Thickness | superficial ulcers, psuedomembranes |
| • B | Patchy | Circumferential |
|  | Circumferential | • deep |
|  |  | • ulceration |
| Grade III | Full thickness | Eschar |
|  |  | • gray |
|  |  | • black |
|  |  | Ulcers |
|  |  | • transmural |
|  |  | • necrosis |

(From: Paidas, CN: Caustic burns of the esophagus. In Yang SC, Cameron DE, eds. Current therapy of thoracic and cardiovascular surgery. Philadelphia: Mosby, 2004, pp. 98–101.[57])

we feel that in the setting of severe esophageal disruption, either acutely or if there has been a delay in diagnoisis, esophagectomy is favoured over complex diversion approaches.[56]

## Caustic Injuries

Although the incidence appears to have been significantly reduced owing to increased awareness and change in formulation, the leading etiologies of caustic injury remain accidental ingestion in children less than five years of age, and suicide attempts in adults.[57] The most common offending agent remains liquid alkaline household cleaners.

The extent and severity of injury depend upon the nature of the material (Table 27-3). Patients often present with severe oral and neck pain, increasing dysphagia, and respiratory distress requiring emergent airway control. Severe retrosternal pain, crepitus, and/or peritoneal findings imply esophageal and/or gastric perforation. Of note, up to 20% of children present without any symptoms, at least half of whom go on to develop complications requiring treatment.[57] In the absence of symptoms, observation for 24 hours to make sure that oral liquids can be tolerated, is usually sufficient. Patients with oral lesions should undergo early esophagoscopy within 24 hours. Other indications include stridor, drooling, vomiting, and/or intended ingestion. In the absence of obvious perforation, management is directed by endoscopic grading of injury (Fig. 27-3). Transesophageal ultrasound does not appear to add information that would change the management based on visual inspection by esophagoscopy.[58]

In patients with grade IIB and III lesions, but without obvious perforation, contrast studies may be performed to confirm absence of leak. Patients with persistent acidosis, increasing coagulaopathy, peritoneal findings, or pneumomediastinum should be explored. Alkali injuries, because of the full thickness coagulation necrosis, are often associated with significant abdominal organ destruction in addition to gastric necrosis, including pancreas, small bowel, and colon.[59] Acid ingestion may be limited to stomach, as pyloric spasm often protects the small bowel. However, if it is extensive gastric injury, a careful inspection of the esophagus is required.[57] Esphagectomy in the acute setting can be performed transhiatally, with long

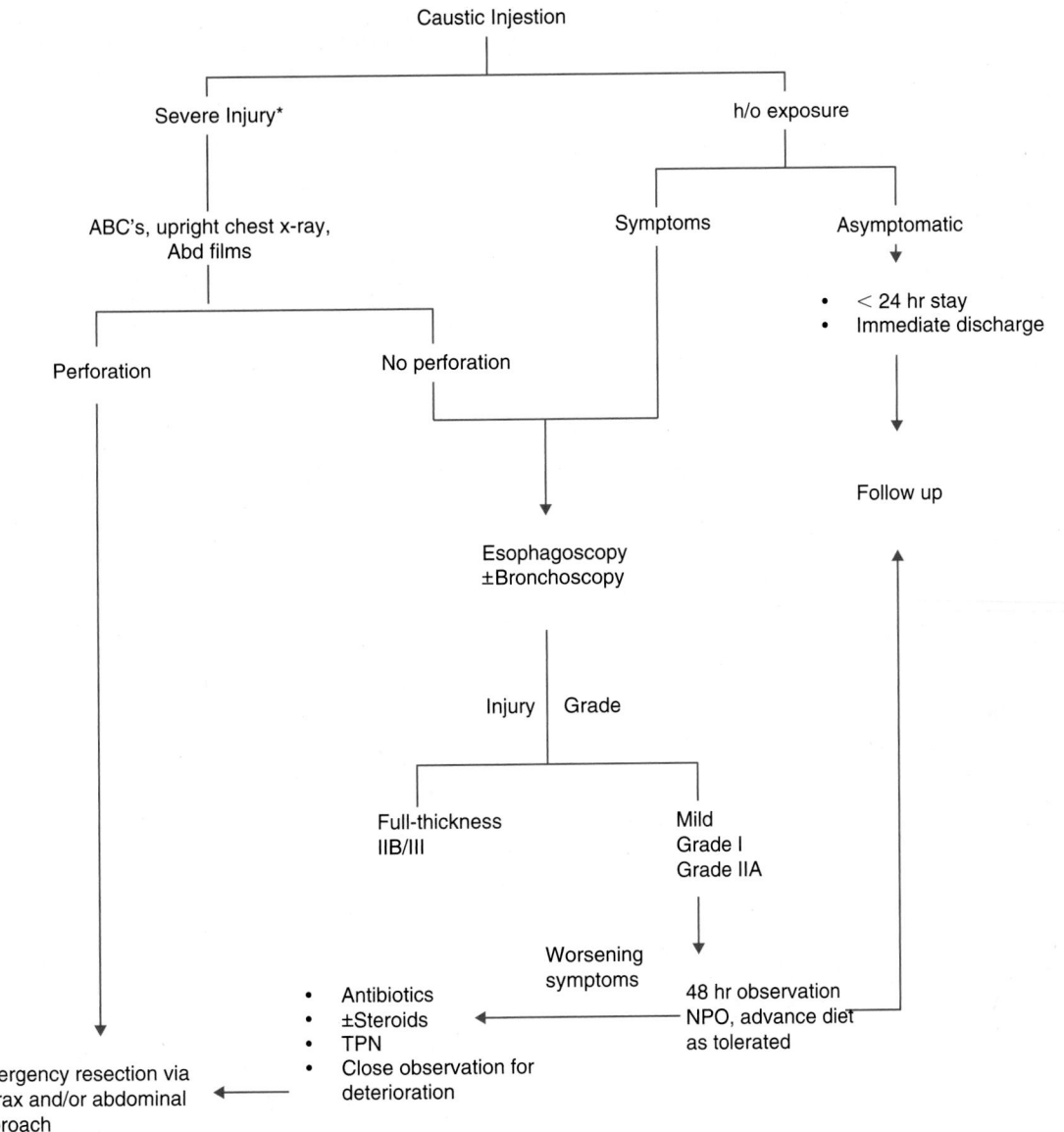

**FIGURE 27-3.** Algorithm for acute management of caustic injestion.
*Severe injury = respiratory compromise, neck crepitus, severe epigastric or retrosternal pain, unkown corrosive, or intentional injestion.
(From: Paidas, C.N. Caustic burns of the esophagous, In Yang SC, Cameron DE, eds. Current therapy of thoracic and cardiovascular surgery. Philadelphia: Mosby, 2004, pp. 98–101. Reproduced with permission.[57])

cervical ostomy and mediastinal drainage both from the neck and abdomen. Feeding jejunostomy should also be performed.

The management of patients with grade IIB or III injuries that do not require immediate operation is varied. In brief, antibiotics and NPO with parenteral feeding forms the cornerstone of therapy. Some groups advocate early corticosteroid use to reduce stricture formation, although this is not uniformly accepted.[57,60] Circumferential injuries have been managed by open gastrostomy and passage of a string through the nares for later dilitations.[57] On the other hand, some groups try and avoid any foreign objects in the esophagous, using delayed contrast studies to predict the need for dilatation.[61] Ultimately, patients usually require prolonged repetitive dilitations. Reconstruction may be required, either of the entire esophagus or a short segment, utilizing jejunal grafts, colon interposition or gastric flaps, or pull-ups (depending on extent of injury). When operated in a delayed fashion, there is usually extensive mediastinal scarring that

makes even open thoracocotomy approaches difficult. In patients who do not under go resection, surveillance for the development of cancer is required for the remainder of their lives.

## Tracheoesophageal Fistula

Tracheoesophageal fistula usually arises as a complication of resection. As noted previously, buttressing tracheal repair or resection with sternocleidomastoid or other available muscle flaps does appear to reduce the risk of this complication.[62] "Primary" tracheoesophageal fistula can occur from penetrating injury either immediately from dual penetration, or in a delayed fashion as necrosis or blast trauma affects surrounding tissues. Tracheoesophageal fistula can rarely occur after crush injury to the extended neck or compression injury just at or proximal to the carina.[63–65] The incidence following blunt trauma is as little as 0.001%.[66] In one review of 61 cases, the predominant mechanism was air-bag or steering wheel injuries, and the most common site was just above the carina.[66] This has led to the hypothesis that simultaneous compression of the trachea and esophagus between the sternum and vertebral column results in contusion or frank injury to the anterior esophagous and membranous trachea. The latter heals but progressive necrosis of the former results in delayed fistulization ten or more days after injury. The diagnosis is suggested by new-onset cough or pneumonia after swallowing or evidence of aspiration of tube feeds. Operative treatment is associated with mortality of 10–15% while nonoperative treatement carries mortality rates as high as 80%, although this may reflect more severe underlying lung dysfunction, sepsis etc.[65]

In general, operative repair through a right fourth intercostals posterolateral thoracotomy with tracheal resection and esophageal repair with viable tissue (e.g., omentum) or gastric pull-up is performed. If severe pneumonia or adult respiratory distress syndrome precludes operative repair, gastric decompression (nasogastric tube and/or gastrostomy), feeding jejunostomy tube, and temporization are appropriate. If significant air-leak into the esophagus complicates ventilator management, the endotracheal tube may be advanced. If, however, this is not possible or there is concern that prolonged cuff or tube pressure will exacerbate the fistula, then earlier repair should be undertaken.

# REFERENCES

1. Gussack GS, Jurkovich GJ, Luterman A: Laryngotracheal trauma: a protocol approach to a rare injury. *Laryngoscope* 96:660, 1986.
2. Lee RB: Traumatic injury of the cervicothoracic trachea and major bronchi. *Chest Surg Clin N Am* 7:285, 1997.
3. Graham JM, Mattox KL, Beall AC Jr: Penetrating trauma of the lung. *J Trauma* 19:665, 1979.
4. Symbas PN, Justicz AG, Ricketts RR: Rupture of the airways from blunt trauma: treatment of complex injuries. *Ann Thorac Surg* 54:177, 1992.
5. Symbas PN, Hatcher CR, Jr, Vlasis SE: Bullet wounds of the trachea. *J Thorac Cardiovasc Surg* 83:235, 1982.
6. Symbas PN, Hatcher CR Jr, Boehm GA: Acute penetrating tracheal trauma. *Ann Thorac Surg* 22:473, 1976.
7. Bertelsen S, Howitz P: Injuries of the trachea and bronchi. *Thorax* 27:188, 1972.
8. Kemmerer WT, Eckert WG, Gathright JB, et al.: Patterns of thoracic injuries in fatal traffic accidents. *J Trauma* 1:595, 1961.
9. Karmy-Jones R, Jurkovich GJ: Blunt chest trauma. *Curr Probl Surg* 41:211, 2004.
10. Angood PB, Attia EL, Brown RA, et al.: Extrinsic civilian trauma to the larynx and cervical trachea–important predictors of long-term morbidity. *J Trauma* 26:869, 1986.
11. de la Rocha AG, Kayler D: Traumatic rupture of the tracheobronchial tree. *Can J Surg* 28:68, 1985.
12. Lupetin AR: Computed tomographic evaluation of laryngotracheal trauma. *Curr Probl Diagn Radiol* 26:185, 1997.
13. Guertler AT: Blunt laryngeal trauma associated with shoulder harness use. *Ann Emerg Med* 17:838, 1988.
14. Lynn RB, Iyengar K: Traumatic rupture of the bronchus. *Chest* 61:81, 1972.
15. Kirsh MM, Orringer MB, Behrendt DM, et al.: Management of tracheobronchial disruption secondary to nonpenetrating trauma. *Ann Thorac Surg* 22:93, 1976.
16. Martin de Nicolas JL, Gamez AP, Cruz F, et al.: Long tracheobronchial and esophageal rupture after blunt chest trauma: injury by airway bursting. *Ann Thorac Surg* 62:269, 1996.
17. Ramzy AI, Rodriguez A, Turney SZ: Management of major tracheobronchial ruptures in patients with multiple system trauma. *J Trauma* 28:1353, 1988.
18. Kelly JP, Webb WR, Moulder PV, et al.: Management of airway trauma. I: Tracheobronchial injuries. *Ann Thorac Surg* 40:551, 1985.
19. Grover FL, Ellestad C, Arom KV, et al.: Diagnosis and management of major tracheobronchial injuries. *Ann Thorac Surg* 28:384, 1979.
20. Rossbach MM, Johnson SB, Gomez MA, et al.: Management of major tracheobronchial injuries: a 28-year experience. *Ann Thorac Surg* 65:182, 1998.
21. Reece GP, Shatney CH: Blunt injuries of the cervical trachea: review of 51 patients. *South Med J* 81:1542, 1988.
22. Baumgartner F, Sheppard B, de Virgilio C, et al.: Tracheal and main bronchial disruptions after blunt chest trauma: presentation and management. *Ann Thorac Surg* 50:569, 1990.
23. Flynn AE, Thomas AN, Schecter WP: Acute tracheobronchial injury. *J Trauma* 29:1326, 1989.
24. Stark P: Imaging of tracheobronchial injuries. *J Thorac Imaging* 10:206, 1995.
25. Endress C, Guyot DR, Engels JA: The "fallen lung with absent hilum" signs of complete bronchial transection. *Ann Emerg Med* 20:317, 1991.
26. Kumpe DA, Oh KS, Wyman SM: A characteristic pulmonary finding in unilateral complete bronchial transection. *Am J Roentgenol Radium Ther Nucl Med* 110:704, 1970.
27. Wintermark M, Schnyder P, Wicky S: Blunt traumatic rupture of a mainstem bronchus: spiral CT demonstration of the "fallen lung" sign. *Eur Radiol* 11:409, 2001.
28. Deslauriers J, Beaulieu M, Archambault G, et al.: Diagnosis and long-term follow-up of major bronchial disruptions due to nonpenetrating trauma. *Ann Thorac Surg* 33:32, 1982.
29. Jones CM, Athanasiou T: Is virtual bronchoscopy an efficient diagnostic tool for the thoracic surgeon? *Ann Thorac Surg* 79:365, 2005.
30. Minard G, Kudsk KA, Croce MA, et al.: Laryngotracheal trauma. *Am Surg* 58:181, 1992.
31. Velly JF, Martigne C, Moreau JM, et al.: Post traumatic tracheobronchial lesions. A follow-up study of 47 cases. *Eur J Cardiothorac Surg* 5:352, 1991.
32. Edwards WH Jr, Morris JA, Jr, DeLozier JB III et al.: Airway injuries. The first priority in trauma. *Am Surg* 53:192, 1987.
33. Mathisen DJ, Grillo H: Laryngotracheal trauma. *Ann Thorac Surg* 43:254, 1987.
34. Mitchell JD, Mathisen DJ, Wright CD, et al.: Clinical experience with carinal resection. *J Thorac Cardiovasc Surg* 117:39, 1999; discussion 52–3.
35. Heitmiller RF: Tracheal release maneuvers. *Chest Surg Clin N Am* 13:201, 2003.
36. Grillo HC, Zannini P, Michelassi F: Complications of tracheal reconstruction. Incidence, treatment, and prevention. *J Thorac Cardiovasc Surg* 91:322, 1986.
37. Wright CD, Grillo HC, Wain JC, et al.: Anastomotic complications after tracheal resection: prognostic factors and management. *J Thorac Cardiovasc Surg* 128:731, 2004.
38. Donahue DM, Grillo HC, Wain JC, et al.: Reoperative tracheal resection and reconstruction for unsuccessful repair of postintubation stenosis. *J Thorac Cardiovasc Surg* 114:934, 1997; discussion 938.
39. Taskinen SO, Salo JA, Halttunen PE, et al.: Tracheobronchial rupture due to blunt chest trauma: a follow-up study. *Ann Thorac Surg* 48:846, 1989.
40. Stephens KEJ, Wood DE: Bronchoscopic management of central airway obstruction. *J Thorac Cardiovasc Surg* 119:473, 2000.
41. Asensio JA, Chahwan S, Forno W, et al.: Penetrating esophageal injuries: multicenter study of the American Association for the Surgery of Trauma. *J Trauma* 50:289, 2001.
42. Riley RD, Miller PR, Meredith JW: Injury to the esophagous, trachea and bronchus. In Moore EE, Feliciano DV, Mattox KL, eds. *Trauma*. New York: McGraw-Hill, 2004, p. 539.
43. Sheely CH II, Mattox KL, Beall AC Jr, et al.: Penetrating wounds of the cervical esophagus. *Am J Surg* 130:707, 1975.
44. Meyer JP, Barrett JA, Schuler JJ, et al.: Mandatory vs selective exploration for penetrating neck trauma. A prospective assessment. *Arch Surg* 122:592, 1987.
45. Weigelt JA, Thal ER, Snyder WH III, et al.: Diagnosis of penetrating cervical esophageal injuries. *Am J Surg* 154:619, 1987.
46. Cornwell EE III, Kennedy F, Ayad IA, et al.: Transmediastinal gunshot wounds. A reconsideration of the role of aortography. *Arch Surg* 131:949, (discussion 952), 1996.
47. Attar S, Hankins JR, Suter CM, et al.: Esophageal perforation: A therapeutic challenge. *Ann Thorac Surg* 50:45, (discussion 50), 1990.
48. Flynn AE, Verrier ED, Way LW, et al.: Esophageal perforation. *Arch Surg* 124:1211, (discussion 1214), 1989.
49. Weiman DS, Walker WA, Brosnan KM, et al.: Noniatrogenic esophageal trauma. *Ann Thorac Surg* 59:845, (discussion 849), 1995.
50. Kao L, Karmy-Jones R: Esophageal injury and perforation. In Stern E, ed. *Thoracic trauma and critical care*. Boston: Kluwer Medical Publishers, 2002, p. 209.
51. Whyte RI, Iannettoni MD, Orringer MB: Intrathoracic esophageal perforation. The merit of primary repair. *J Thorac Cardiovasc Surg* 109:140, (discussion 144), 1995.
52. Grossman MD, May AK, Schwab CW, et al.: Determining anatomic injury with computed tomography in selected torso gunshot wounds. *J Trauma* 45:446, 1998.
53. Gouge TH, Depan HJ, Spencer FC: Experience with the Grillo pleural wrap procedure in 18 patients with perforation of the thoracic esophagus. *Ann Surg* 209:612, (discussion 617), 1989.
54. Richardson JD, Tobin GR: Closure of esophageal defects with muscle flaps. *Arch Surg* 129:541, (discussion 547), 1994.
55. Armstrong WB, Detar TR, Stanley RB: Diagnosis and management of external penetrating cervical esophageal injuries. *Ann Otol Rhinol Laryngol* 103:863, 1994.
56. Salo JA, Isolauri JO, Heikkila LJ, et al.: Management of delayed esophageal perforation with mediastinal sepsis. Esophagectomy or primary repair? *J Thorac Cardiovasc Surg* 106:1088, 1993.

57. Paidas CN: Caustic burns of the esophagus. In Yang CS, Cameron DE, eds. *Current therapy in thoracic and cardiovascular surgery.* Philadelphia: Mosby, 2004, p. 98.

58. Chiu HM, Lin JT, Huang SP, et al.: Prediction of bleeding and stricture formation after corrosive ingestion by EUS concurrent with upper endoscopy. *Gastrointest Endosc* 60:827, 2004.

59. Cattan P, Munoz-Bongrand N, Berney T, et al.: Extensive abdominal surgery after caustic ingestion. *Ann Surg* 231:519, 2000.

60. Boukthir S, Fetni I, Mrad SM, et al.: High doses of steroids in the management of caustic esophageal burns in children. *Arch Pediatr* 11:13, 2004.

61. Baskin D, Urganci N, Abbasoglu L, et al.: A standardised protocol for the acute management of corrosive ingestion in children. *Pediatr Surg Int* 20:824, 2004.

62. Losken A, Rozycki GS, Feliciano DV: The use of the sternocleidomastoid muscle flap in combined injuries to the esophagus and carotid artery or trachea. *J Trauma* 49:815, 2000.

63. Braun RA, Goldware RR, Flores LM: Cervical tracheal transsection with esophageal fistula. *Arch Otolaryngol* 96:67, 1972.

64. Chapman ND, Braun RA: The management of traumatic tracheo-esophageal fistula caused by blunt chest trauma. *Arch Surg* 100:681, 1970.

65. Sebastian MW, Wolfe WG: Traumatic thoracic fistulas. *Chest Surg Clin N Am* 7:385, 1997.

66. Reed WJ, Doyle SE, Aprahamian C: Tracheoesophageal fistula after blunt chest trauma. *Ann Thorac Surg* 59:1251, 1995.

67. Defore WW Jr, Mattox KL, Hansen HA, et al.: Surgical management of penetrating injuries of the esophagus. *Am J Surg* 134:734, 1977.

68. Fetterman BL, Shindo ML, Stanley RB Jr, et al.: Management of traumatic hypopharyngeal injuries. *Laryngoscope* 105:8, 1995.

69. Glatterer MS Jr, Toon RS, Ellestad C, et al.: Management of blunt and penetrating external esophageal trauma. *J Trauma* 25:784, 1985.

70. Ngakane H, Muckart DJ, Luvuno FM: Penetrating visceral injuries of the neck: results of a conservative management policy. *Br J Surg* 77:908, 1990.

71. Winter RP, Weigelt JA: Cervical esophageal trauma. Incidence and cause of esophageal fistulas. *Arch Surg* 125:849, 1990; discussion 851.

72. Yugueros P, Sarmiento JM, Garcia AF, et al.: Conservative management of penetrating hypopharyngeal wounds. *J Trauma* 40:267, 1996.

73. Noyes LD, McSwain NE Jr, Markowitz IP: Panendoscopy with arteriography versus mandatory exploration of penetrating wounds of the neck. *Ann Surg* 204:21, 1986.

74. White RK, Morris DM: Diagnosis and management of esophageal perforations. *Am Surg* 58:112, 1992.

75. Flowers JL, Graham SM, Ugarte MA, et al.: Flexible endoscopy for the diagnosis of esophageal trauma. *J Trauma* 40:261, 1996; discussion 265.

# Commentary ■ J. WAYNE MEREDITH

Drs. Karmy-Jones, Wood, and Jurkovich have contributed a review of the epidemiology, diagnosis, and management of the injuries to the esophagus, trachea, and bronchus which is excellent, thorough, well organized, and thoughtful. These injuries are life-threatening, difficult to manage, and occur frequently enough to be commonly considered and rarely enough to be uncommonly encountered by any given practitioner. They may occur in the neck, thorax, or upper abdomen and require a great breadth and depth of understanding of cardiopulmonary physiology, anatomy, surgical technique, judgment, and skill.

These authors have combined a superb and extensive review of the literature with a thoughtful analysis of that review combined with a practical approach from a wealth of institutional experience to provide valuable insights for the reader on this important topic.

The authors provide an excellent discussion of the role of the CT scanning in the management of these injuries. CT scans have dramatically changed the flow of diagnosis in injured patients, as well as in many areas changed the management of injuries. The authors provide a good discussion of the role of CT scanning and correctly emphasize the point that a CT scan is not appropriate when the patient is either hemodynamically unstable or the patient's airway is unstable.

Furthermore, it is worth repeating that a "negative CT scan does not completely exclude the need for bronchoscopy or other tests" and that "bronchoscopy is the only study that can reliably exclude central airway trauma."

Management of tracheal injuries typically pose challenges in airway management and the authors have deftly and pragmatically described the importance of preplanning the management of the airway during each step of the operation, excellent communication between the anesthesia team and the operating team, and the importance of flexibility in intraoperative options. These include on-field endotracheal tubes and anesthesia circuits, the use of bronchial blockers to exclude one side or the other, the appropriate use of double lumen tubes, and the important observation that these tubes, though hypothetically attractive, in practical terms are often too stiff to use for main stem bronchial injuries.

One of the most difficult areas to expose appropriately for repair is the proximal left main stem bronchus. Approaching from a left thoracotomy the aorta and great vessels impair access proximally and from the right thoracotomy the lung may fall away making it difficult to manage the airway or get good exposure of the airway segment distal to the injury. The authors recommend primarily a left-sided approach to the entire left main stem bronchus. I would add the observation that often the very proximal left main stem bronchus and usually the proximal left main stem when combined with a carinal injury is, I believe, most easily approached through a right thoracotomy. Clearly, however, associated injuries rather than the site of airway injuries dictate which thorax should be opened.

Like the discussion on airway injuries in this chapter, the discussion on esophageal injuries is comprehensive, thoughtful, and practical. Several points are worth re-emphasizing. The diagnosis of esophageal injury can be challenging. It is best done with a combination of esophagoscopy and contrast studies. The basic management principles of leak control, debridement, drainage, and reinforcement with viable tissue are well described. The authors propose the controversial position, with which I agree, that in the setting of severe esophageal disruption, either acutely or if there has been a delay in diagnosis, esophagectomy is favored over complex diversion approaches. This strategy avoids multiple failed diversions and drainage attempts and prolonged bouts of uncontrolled sepsis, and provides an opportunity for the patient to have an early recovery and a subsequent planned, careful reconstruction. The authors also describe well the management of caustic ingestion of the esophagus. The management is profoundly influenced by the injuring agent; acids producing a more superficial injury and alkalines producing a deeper injury when in liquid form may result in full-thickness gastric or even gastrointestinal injuries.

In summary, these authors have provided a superb, well-organized, comprehensive, and practical treatise on the management of tracheal, bronchial, and esophageal injuries.

# Trauma to the Heart

*Juan A. Asensio* ■ *Luis M. García-Núñez* ■ *Patrizio Petrone*

## INTRODUCTION

The heart is a vital, unique, and amazing organ and constant in its function. It is romantic in its very reason for existing. No other organ has inspired so many poets, musicians, and writers to create poems, beautiful rhythms, and enchanting novels. Injury to the heart will be approached in this chapter from two major perspectives: penetrating injuries and blunt injuries.

## PENETRATING CARDIAC INJURY

### Historical Perspective

The earliest description of a cardiac injury is found in the *Iliad*[1] which describes the death of Sarpedon from impalement with a lance.[2] The Edwin Smith Surgical Papyrus describes penetrating wounds of the chest.[3,4] Hippocrates,[5] Ovid,[6] Celsus,[7] Pliny,[8] Aristotle,[9] and Galen[10] stated that all wounds of the heart were deadly. Paulus Aegineta[11] described the venting of a pericardial tamponade, while Fallopius[12] made observations describing the difference between wounds of the right and left ventricles.

Ambroise Paré,[13,14] described two cases of penetrating cardiac injuries, while both Fabricius[15] and Boerhaave[16] described the futility in the management of these injuries. However, Hollerius[17] first advanced the idea that wounds of the heart could heal. Wolf,[18] in 1642, was first to describe a healed wound of the heart, while Senac,[19] in 1749, concluded that all wounds of the heart were serious, although some wounds might heal and not be fatal. Morgagni,[20] in 1761, described the effects of compression on the heart secondary to hemopericardium.

Larrey[21,22] is credited with pioneering the technique for pericardial window. Jobert,[23] in 1839, correlated the lifespan of a cardiac wound with the quantity of blood lost. Purple,[24] in 1850,

compiled a total of 42 cardiac injury cases, while Fischer,[25] in 1868, collected 452 cases from the literature and reported a 10% survival rate. Billroth, in 1875[26] and 1883,[27] proclaimed his resistance to any attempt at cardiac injury repair, although he did suture the heart.[26–28] Roberts,[29] in 1881, suggested the possibility that cardiac injuries could be sutured; he, however, did not attempt to do so. Block,[30] in 1882, created cardiac wounds in a rabbit model and was successful in achieving repair. These concepts were soon questioned by Riedenger,[31] who in 1888 stated that any suggestion of suturing a wound of the heart, although made in all seriousness, should scarcely deserve notice. Similarly, Paget,[32] in 1896, clearly stated that surgery of the heart had probably reached limits set by nature to all surgery. Del Vecchio,[33] however, was not deterred, as he demonstrated cardiac injury healing after suturing the heart in a canine model.

In 1895, Cappelen[34] from Norway repaired a 2 cm left ventricular laceration including ligation of a large branch of the distal left anterior descending coronary artery. The patient survived for three days, but later succumbed to sepsis. At autopsy the cause of death was found to be septic pericarditis from diplococci. This was followed by Farina[35] in Italy also in 1896, who also attempted to repair a left ventricular wound; however, both patients succumbed. In 1896, Rehn[36] in Germany was successful in repairing a wound of the right ventricle sustained in a fencing duel. Duval[37] described the median sternotomy incision, while in the United States Hill,[38] in 1902, was the first surgeon to successfully repair a left ventricular injury. Both Dalton[39] in St. Louis (1891) and Williams[40] in Chicago (1893) successfully sutured pericardial lacerations.

In 1906, Spangaro[41] described the left anterolateral thoracotomy incision, while in 1907 Sauerbruch[42] described a method for controlling hemorrhage from a wound of the heart. Matas[43] warned of the dangers of rapidly relieving a pericardial tamponade resulting in exsanguinating hemorrhage. In 1909, Peck[44] was the first to describe a successful repair of a stab wound of the right atrium and reported 11 patients, while in 1912 Pool[45] collected additional cardiac injury cases and concluded that "the treatment of heart wounds should be surgical." Smith[46] developed a comprehensive plan for cardiac injury management and for the first time pointed out the dangers of dysrhythmias occurring during cardiac manipulation. In 1926, Beck[4] described the physiology of cardiac tamponade. Borchardt[47] provided evidence of the rarity of Beck's Triad. In 1928 Schoenfeld[48] and in 1939 Bigger[49] reported their collective experiences in the management of penetrating cardiac injuries.

In 1942, Beck[50] astutely pointed to the necessity of sparing ligation of coronary arteries in wounds adjacent to these structures and described the technique of placing mattress sutures under the bed of the coronary arteries. In 1942, Turner[51] reviewed the experience with cardiac injury management during World War I and addressed the need for emergency treatment. In the same year, Griswold[52] refined the techniques in the management of cardiac injuries and recommended that every large General Hospital should have available a sterile set of instruments plus an available operating room 24 hours a day.

In 1943, Blalock and Ravitch[53] described a stepwise approach to the management of cardiac injures in the European theatre of war recommending first pericardiocentesis followed by cardiorrhaphy after recurrence of pericardial hemorrhage. In 1944, Elkin[54–56] recommended the administration of intravenous infusions prior to operation and pointed to the beneficial effects of increasing blood volume and thus cardiac output, while in 1946, Harken[57] described techniques to remove foreign bodies adjacent to the heart and major blood vessels. Beall[58–61] was first to describe the technique of emergency department (ED) thoracotomy and along with Cooley[60] reported the benefits of cardiopulmonary bypass in the management of selected intracardiac injuries. Meanwhile, Mattox[62–64] refined and protocolized ED thoracotomy and cardiorrhaphy including emergency cardiopulmonary bypass.

## Incidence

The true incidence of penetrating cardiac injuries is difficult to determine from the literature. In 1983, Feliciano[65] described a one-year experience consisting of 48 cardiac injuries at Ben Taub Hospital in Houston in a very busy urban trauma center. In 1989, Mattox[66] described a 30-year experience from the same institution with 4459 patients, reporting 539 cardiac injuries which translates to 18 cardiac injuries per year. Asensio[67,68] reported two prospective consecutive series reporting a total of 165 cardiac injuries in a three-year period or 55 cardiac injuries per year accounting for 1.38% of all of the trauma admissions to LA County/USC Medical Center in Los Angeles. Asensio[69] looked at the National Trauma Data Bank (NTDB) of the American College of Surgeons (ACS), consisting of 1,310,720 patients, which identified a total of 2016 patients sustaining penetrating cardiac injuries and calculated the national incidence of 0.16%. Thus, penetrating cardiac injures are uncommon and are usually seen only in busy urban trauma centers.

## Etiology

In the civilian arena, penetrating cardiac injuries are usually caused by gunshot wounds (GSW), stab wounds (SW), and rarely by shotgun wounds, ice picks, and iatrogenic instrumentation.[70] Asensio,[69] in a recent review of the NTDB of the ACS consisting of 2016 patients, found that 63% of all reported cardiac injuries in America are caused by gunshot wounds, 36% are caused by stab wounds, while shotgun and impalement injuries accounted for approximately 1% of these injures. Rarely, fractured ribs may impale and/or lacerate the heart. In the military arena, Rich[71] reported 96 cardiac injuries from the Vietnam conflict. The majority of these patients sustained injuries from fragments of grenades or shrapnel while a few of these patients were impaled by flechettes. This series describes very few gunshot wounds most likely because American soldiers sustaining missile injuries from high-velocity automatic rifles did not survive medical evacuation extraction to reach an operating room.

## Clinical Presentation

Beck's Triad—muffled heart tones, jugular venous distention, and hypotension—describes the classical presentation of a patient with pericardial tamponade.[4,70] Kussmaul's sign, described as jugular venous distention upon inspiration, is another classic sign attributed to pericardial tamponade. In reality, the presence of Beck's Triad and Kussmal's signs represent the exception rather than the rule.[4,47,70] It is estimated that Beck's Triad is only present in approximately 10% of patients.[70] In general, penetrating cardiac injuries can be extremely deceptive in their presentation. Patients may present with injuries directly located over the precordium, while others sustain cardiac injuries from extra-precordial penetration. Most stab wounds generally penetrate the heart if located in the precordium, whereas gunshot wounds can injure the heart from both precordial and extra-precordial locations.[70] Hirschberg and Mattox[72] described a series of patients presenting with thoracoabdominal injures in which 82 patients sustained 21 associated cardiac injuries for an incidence of 26%. Asensio,[73] in a series of 73 patients undergoing both thoracotomy and laparotomy for thoracoabdominal injuries, reported 32 patients which incurred penetrating cardiac injuries for an incidence of 44%.

The clinical presentation of penetrating cardiac injuries may range from complete hemodynamic stability to cardiopulmonary arrest; in fact, some penetrating cardiac injuries can be very deceptive in their presentation.[70,74] Some patients with penetrating precordial injuries are resistant to lying down, signaling with their restlessness the presence of a pericardial tamponade. The clinical presentation of penetrating cardiac injuries may also be related to factors including the wounding mechanism, the length of time elapsed prior to arrival at a trauma center; the extent of the injury, which if sufficiently large in terms of myocardial destruction will invariably lead to exsanguinating hemorrhage into the left hemithoracic cavity. Patients that lose between 40% and 50% of intravascular blood volume develop cardiopulmonary arrest. The muscular nature of the left ventricle and to a lesser extent that of the right ventricle may seal penetrating injuries and prevent exsanguinating hemorrhage allowing these patients to arrive with some signs of life.[70,74]

The most unique presentation of a penetrating cardiac injury is pericardial tamponade. The tough fibrous nature, lack of elasticity, and noncompliance of this structure translates to acute rise in intrapericardial pressure when blood is acutely lost into the pericardium, leading to compression of the thin wall of the right ventricle impairing its ability to accept the returning blood volume, resulting in a concomitant decrease in left ventricular filling, and ejection fraction. This results in a drastic decrease in cardiac output (CO) and stroke volume (SV). The impaired ability to generate both right and left ventricular ejection fractions increases cardiac work and myocardial wall tension. This results in an increase in myocardial volume of oxygen consumption ($MVO_2$) which cannot be met, leading to myocardial hypoxemia and lactic acidosis.[70,74]

The pericardium is able to accommodate gradual quantities of blood, provided that the rate of hemorrhage is slow and does not cause acute rises in intrapericardial pressures exceeding the right ventricle and subsequently the left ventricle's ability to fill. This explains why a subset of patients presenting with pericardial tamponade are hemodynamically stable even with relatively large volumes of fluid in the pericardial cavity, whereas patients in whom blood losses into the pericardium have accumulated rapidly will develop with hemodynamic instability from smaller volumes of blood in the pericardial cavity.[67,68,70,74]

Pericardial tamponade can have both deleterious and protective effects. Its deleterious effects can lead to a rapid rise in pericardial pressure and cardiopulmonary arrest, whereas its protective effect will limit extrapericardial hemorrhage into the left hemithoracic cavity preventing exsanguinating hemorrhage. This allows selected patients to reach a trauma center alive, albeit with varying degrees of hemodynamic instability.[67,68] Moreno,[75] in a retrospective study consisting of 100 patients presenting with penetrating cardiac injuries, reported 77 patients that presented with pericardial tamponade and a 31% survival rate. He concluded that for patients presenting with pericardial tamponade the survival rate was much higher — 73% versus 11%, a survival advantage regardless of the wounding agent. When stratified to cardiac chambers injured, Moreno[75] reported a 79% survival rate in favor of patients presenting with right-side chamber injuries versus 28% for those sustaining left-side chamber injuries. The authors concluded by suggesting that pericardial tamponade may be an even more influential factor than presenting vital signs in determining outcomes. However, Buckman[76] and Asensio[67] in prospective studies could not identify pericardial tamponade as a critical independent factor in survival. Although there is significant differences between these four studies,[67,68,75,76] there appears to be a period of time in which pericardial tamponade has a protective effect allowing selected patients to reach trauma centers with varying signs of life to undergo definitive surgical procedures. What remains undefined is the actual period of time after which the protective effect of pericardial tamponade is lost and when exactly this transition occurs causing its adverse effect on cardiac function.[67,68]

## Diagnosis

Physical Examination. Clearly any patient with a penetrating injury to the precordium or a thoracoabdominal injury should be suspected as having a cardiac injury. Jugular venous distention occurs from multifactorial causes such as pain, presence of a pneumo or hemopneumothorax, straining due to pain elicited during physical examination as well as a pericardial tamponade, or rarely a pneumopericardium.[70]

Frequently these patients present with associated pneumohemothoraces and decreased breath sounds in the ipsilateral hemithoracic cavity. The detection of muffled heart sounds in a busy and noisy trauma center is often difficult. Occasionally, patients presenting with precordial injuries are restless and refuse to lie down; this may be a subtle indicator suggesting the presence of hemopericardium and/or impending pericardial tamponade. The most dramatic presentation for a patient sustaining a penetrating cardiac injury is, of course, cardiopulmonary arrest. Although pericardiocentesis has been advocated in the past as a diagnostic tool to detect the presence of blood in the pericardium, it is only mentioned to note that it currently has no role in establishing the diagnosis of cardiac injuries.

Subxiphoid Pericardial Window. The original technique of pericardial window was described by Larrey[21,22,70] in the 1800s. It is remarkable that only small variations in the original technique have been added to this procedure. This technique, although occasionally employed in patients with penetrating precordial injury, has seen a marked diminution in its role during recent times due to the advent of two-dimensional echocardiography.[77] Nevertheless, it is a technique that is still employed in many countries that do not have access to ultrasound equipment.

Trinkle,[78] in 1974, published a series of 45 patients comparing patients undergoing pericardiocentesis versus subxiphoid pericardial window and recommended its use under local anesthesia in the operating room. Subsequently, in 1977, Arom[79] published a series of 50 patients and proved the reliability of this procedure. This paper described the modern version of the technique and recommended it as the technique of choice at that time, to evaluate patients with potential cardiac injuries. In 1979, Trinkle[80] clearly established pericardial window, as the technique of choice for the evaluation of cardiac injuries based on a series of 101 patients and recommended abandoning the use of pericardiocentesis. Garrison,[81] in a series of 60 patients with combined thoracoabdominal injuries, described and refined the technique of diagnostic transdiaphragmatic pericardial window, recommending it as a safe and rapid method for the evaluation of patients with injuries in proximity to the heart undergoing laparotomy. In this paper he also outlined the indications of this technique for patients developing unexplained hypotension during abdominal exploration.[81]

Miller,[82] Brewster,[83] and Duncan[84] further confirmed the accuracy of this technique, while Andrade-Alegre and Mon[85] described its use in resource-poor countries when no two-dimensional echocardiography is available.

Two-Dimensional Echocardiography. Echocardiography has become a "gold standard" in the evaluation of patients with penetrating thoracic injury. Major benefits of echocardiography include being noninvasive, rapid, accurate, and its ability to be repeated at any time. Most importantly, it is also painless.[70] In 1965, Feigenbaum,[86–88] Moss,[89] and Goldberg[90] first began to define echocardiography as a valuable technique for the diagnosis of pericardial fluid. Horowitz,[91] in 1974, defined the limits of sensitivity and specificity of this technique and concluded that a minimum of 50 mL of pericardial fluid is necessary before echocardiography can demonstrate an effusion. Weiss[92] and Miller[93] then applied two-dimensional echocardiography to establish the diagnosis of blunt cardiac injury such as myocardial contusions. Choo[94] suggested the use of this technique for evaluating penetrating cardiac injuries while Lopez,[95] in a canine model, studied the echocardiographic characteristics of hemopericardium with or without thrombus formation; concluding that hemopericardium could be identified by two-dimensional echocardiography and differentiated from other types of pericardial effusions of lower acoustic density.

Both Hasset[96] and Robison[97] used two-dimensional echocardiography to locate foreign bodies within the heart and concluded that missiles embedded within the wall of the myocardium could be observed, versus those located within the cardiac chambers which should be removed. DePriest[98] and Freshman[99] also used two-dimensional echocardiography emergently in the evaluation of patients with penetrating precordial injuries while Jimenez[100] prospectively compared hemodynamically stable patients admitted with penetrating chest injuries; 73 underwent two-dimensional echocardiography followed by subxiphoid pericardial window. There were 64 negative and nine positive windows. In this study, echocardiography was found to have a 96% accuracy, 97% specificity, and a 90% sensitivity in detecting penetrating cardiac injury. Only one patient had a false negative finding in this study. From these findings, the authors proposed that bedside two-dimensional echocardiography become the procedure of choice for the diagnosis of penetrating cardiac injuries in patients with stable vital signs that have sustained penetrating thoracic injuries in proximity to the heart.[100] Similar findings were confirmed by both Plummer[101] and Aaland.[102]

Meyer[103] prospectively evaluated 105 hemodynamically patients sustaining thoracic injuries for the presence of cardiac injuries. All patients underwent two-dimensional echocardiography followed by subxiphoid pericardial windows. For the entire group, as a technique, the subxiphoid window revealed a sensitivity of 100%, a specificity and accuracy of 92% versus echocardiography, with a reported sensitivity of 56%, specificity of 93%, and accuracy of 90%. However, when the subxiphoid pericardial window was compared with echocardiography in patients without associated pneumo or hemothorax, parameters such as sensitivity 100% versus 100%, specificity 89% versus 91%, and accuracy 90% versus 91% were comparable. From these results the author concluded that echocardiography has significant limitations in identifying cardiac injuries in patients with associated hemothoraces; however, for patients without an associated pneumo or hemothorax, echocardiography missed no significant injuries and is recommended as a reliable diagnostic technique.[103]

The sonography has assumed a prominent role in the evaluation of all trauma patients, it has also assumed the preeminent role for the evaluation of penetrating cardiac injuries.[70] Rozycki,[104] in a multicenter study consisting of 209 patients admitted with precordial and/or transthoracic wounds, utilized sonography to evaluate for the presence of cardiac injuries, 21 patients had true positive examinations, all of whom were confirmed as having cardiac injuries. In this study, sonography had a 100% sensitivity and a 97.3% specificity in detecting pericardial fluid. Rozycki,[105] in another multicenter study including five trauma centers, evaluated 261 patients with sonography for the presence of pericardial fluid. In this study, 29 patients (11%) had true positive examinations, whereas 225 (86%) had a true negative evaluation. Seven patients (3%) had false-positive examinations and none had false-negative examinations resulting in a sensitivity of 100%, specificity of 96.9%, and accuracy of 97.3%. The authors reported a mean time from ultrasound to surgical intervention of $12.1 \pm 5$ minutes. Data from these two studies[104,105] conclusively supports the role of sonography as the initial investigative tool for the evaluation of patients

with penetrating cardiac injuries, given its accuracy and ease of performance. Other techniques such as transesophageal echocardiography (TEE) have no role in the immediate evaluation sustaining penetrating precordial injuries.[70]

## Minimally Invasive Methods

Thoracoscopy.    Although technically thoracoscopy may be utilized to evaluate the pericardium as well as perform a pericardial window, it has not been employed widely in the United States. Morales,[106] in a series of 100 patients that underwent thoracoscopy and thoracoscopic pericardial window, reported a 31% incidence of positive windows describing a technique that was both accurate and well tolerated without any complications. The authors recommend this technique to be used in patients also requiring evacuation of a retained hemothorax. In our opinion, thoracoscopic pericardial window has no role in the acute evaluation of penetrating cardiac injuries.

Laparoscopy.    Similarly, laparoscopy has been used to detect peritoneal violation in patients sustaining penetrating abdominal trauma. It has been utilized to evaluate patients with thoracoabdominal injuries to evaluate presence of diaphragmatic or solid organ injuries. During laparoscopy the pericardium can also be evaluated. Zantut[107] and Porter[108] have reported performing laparoscopic pericardial windows. Although this technique can be used, it is the opinion of the authors that it has no role in the acute evaluation of penetrating cardiac injuries.

## Management

Prehospital.    Emergency medical systems (EMS) providing rapid transport to trauma centers have allowed patients with penetrating cardiac injuries an opportunity to undergo life-saving surgical procedures. Perhaps in no other injury is rapid transport of such paramount importance. Field stabilization of patients with penetrating cardiac injuries should consist of intubation. Under no circumstances EMS personnel should delay transport in attempting to establish intravenous lines. Insertion of intravenous lines should be carried out only during transport. Immediate notification should mobilize the trauma team.[70]

Gervin,[109] in an analysis of factors influencing the outcome of patients with penetrating cardiac injuries, reported 23 patients with cardiopulmonary arrest, 13 of whom were deemed to be potentially salvageable. These patients were stratified into two groups: the first group was immediately transported and arrived within nine minutes at the trauma center. Five of six patients survived. The second group of patients underwent field stabilization lasting greater than 25 minutes, and all succumbed. On the basis of this data, Gervin[109] suggested that prompt transport to trauma centers without attempts at field resuscitation increases the survival in patients with penetrating cardiac injuries. Similarly, Mattox[110] found no survivors when they analyzed 100 patients that had received external cardiac compression for more than three minutes in the prehospital period.

Lorenz[111] associated survival with the physiologic state of patients in the field and upon arrival in the ED, utilizing systolic blood pressures of less than 60 mm Hg as a predictive factor. Durham,[112] in a series consisting of 207 patients arriving at a trauma center, concluded that a period of prehospital cardiopulmonary resuscitation of less than five minutes is a significant predictor of outcome in surviving patients. In this series, they determined that the average time of prehospital CPR for survivors was 5.1 minutes versus a period of 9.1 minutes for nonsurvivors. Durham[112] linked prehospital endotracheal intubation with both tolerance and prolongation of successful cardiopulmonary resuscitation. Ivatury[113] also reported that prompt transport to a trauma center without field stabilization yielded better survival rates after penetrating cardiac injuries.

Millham,[114] in an analysis of 3845 patients subjected to ED thoracotomy of which 2,253 were performed for penetrating chest injuries, correlated the presence of vital signs upon arrival in the ED and recommended that patients with chest wounds without vital signs in the field or upon hospital arrival be excluded from this technique. These studies[109,112–114] strongly support and advocate for the need of immediate transport of patients with penetrating thoracic injuries to a trauma center, with the only predictors of outcome being the achievement of an airway via endotracheal intubation. Endotracheal intubation has been proven to increase both duration and tolerance of cardiopulmonary resuscitation administered for a period of less than five minutes. The return of organized cardiac electrical activity will provide the best opportunity at survival for these patients.

Emergency Department. All patients with potential penetrating cardiac injuries should undergo rapid initial assessment and resuscitation following Advanced Trauma Life Support (ATLS) protocols.[115] Patients will usually self-stratify into those that are hemodynamically stable and may be subject to more detailed evaluation, those that are hemodynamically unstable but will respond to fluid resuscitation and allow for rapid transport to the operating room (OR), and those that present in cardiopulmonary arrest and will necessitate life-saving surgical interventions such as ED thoracotomy. Patients can be initially and rapidly evaluated with sonography, chest x-ray, and optionally an electrocardiogram (EKG). Volume resuscitation with an appropriate fluid and O- or typespecific blood should be initiated. An arterial blood gas to determine initial pH and base deficit and lactic acid level should also be obtained. However, a significant majority of these patients will arrive in extremis requiring life-saving interventions.[67,68,70,74]

ED thoracotomy is a surgical procedure of great value if undertaken following strict indications for its performance and a special chapter of this textbook has addressed this procedure (Chap.15). Wide disparity in the reporting of outcomes exist in the literature ranging from 0 to 72%.[62,63,116–118] Asensio, Wall, and others,[119] in an extensive analysis of the literature generated practice management guidelines for ED thoracotomy. They analyzed 42 series totaling 1165 patients with penetrating cardiac injuries and reported 363 patients that survived yielding a survival rate of 31.1%.[58,63,65–69,75,78,80–109,113,116,117,120–152] Forty of these 42 series were retrospective. Asensio,[77] in a prospective one-year study whose inclusion criteria was cardiopulmonary arrest secondary to traumatic injury, reported 215 patients subjected to ED thoracotomy. One hundred and sixty-seven (78%) patients incurred penetrating injuries with 142 (66%) sustaining gunshot

wounds, 21 (10%) stab wounds, and four (2%) shotgun wounds. The mean injury severity score (ISS) for these patients was 42 and the mean cardiovascular respiratory score (CVRS) 1. Mean duration of CPR was 12 minutes. In the ED, 162 patients (75%) succumbed, while 53 (25%) were able to reach the OR, with an overall survival rate of six patients (3%). Of the 215 patients, 62 (29%) sustained penetrating cardiac injures. The only survivors in this series were six (10%) of the 62 patients with penetrating cardiac injuries; this remains, thus far, the only prospective study in the literature. Asensio,[67] in a prospective one-year pilot study consisting of 60 patients with penetrating cardiac injuries, reported a 16% survival rate. Tyburski,[152] in a 17-year series reporting 302 patients, admitted with penetrating cardiac injuries stratified these patients into four categories according to the location of their cardiopulmonary arrest. A total of 152 patients required ED thoracotomy, 43 arrested at the scene of which none survived, 63 arrested in the ambulance and three survived, 27 arrested in the ED and five survived while 15 deteriorated in the ED with four survivors. Twelve of the 152 patients (8%) survived to leave the hospital.

Asensio[69] recently reviewed data from the National Trauma Data Bank (NTD) on penetrating cardiac injuries. Out of 1,310,720 patients, 2016 were identified with penetrating cardiac injuries, 830 (41%) underwent ED thoracotomy and 47 (6%) survived (Table 28-1).

## Techniques for Cardiac Injury Repair

Incisions. Two main incisions are used in the management of penetrating cardiac injuries: median sternotomy and anterolateral thoracotomy.[67,68,70,74,77] Median sternotomy described by Duval[37] is an acceptable incision for patients admitted with penetrating precordial injuries that arrive with some degree of hemodynamic instability and may either undergo preoperative investigation with sonography and/or chest x-ray and patients thought to harbor occult cardiac injuries. The left anterolateral thoracotomy is the incision of choice in the management of patients that arrive in extremis. This incision is used in the ED for resuscitative purposes.[67,68,70,74,77]

The left anterolateral thoracotomy described by Spangaro[41] can also be extended across the sternum as bilateral anterolateral thoracotomies, if it is determined during the resuscitative period that the patient's injury extends into the right hemithoracic cavity. Extension into bilateral anterolateral thoracotomies is also the incision of choice for patients that are hemodynamically unstable after incurring mediastinal traversing injuries. This incision allows full exposure of the anterior mediastinum and pericardium as well as both hemithoracic cavities. Upon transection of the sternum both internal mammary arteries are also transected and must be ligated after restoration of perfusion pressure. Uncontrolled, they can serve as a significant source of blood loss. This is a frequent pitfall during the institution of damage control; as trauma surgeons may forget to ligate these vessels prompting return to the OR. For patients that sustain thoracoabdominal injuries, the left anterolateral thoracotomy is also the incision of choice if patients deteriorate in the OR while undergoing a laparotomy.[67,68,70,74,77,153]

**TABLE 28-1**

### Emergency Department Thoracotomy for Cardiac Injuries

| AUTHOR AND YEAR | TYPE OF STUDY | SURVIVORS/ PENETRATING TRAUMA | SURVIVORS/ TOTAL NUMBER OF EDT |
|---|---|---|---|
| Boyd and Strieder 1965[120] | R | 0/0 | 17/25 |
| Beall 1966[58] | R | 3/16 | 42/197 |
| Sauer 1967[121] | R | 12/0 | 12/13 |
| Sugg 1968[122] | R | 0/0 | 63/459 |
| Yao 1968[123] | R | 0/0 | 61/80 |
| Steichen 1971[124] | R | 7/21 | 35/58 |
| Beall 1971[59] | R | 29/52 | 42/66 |
| Borja 1971[125] | R | 0/0 | 24/145 |
| Carrasquilla 1972[126] | R | 8/30 | 20/245 |
| Beall 1972[127] | R | 0/0 | 67/269 |
| Bolanowski 1973[128] | R | 0/0 | 33/44 |
| Trinkle 1974[78] | R | 0/0 | 38/45 |
| Mattox 1974[63] | R | 25/37 | 31/62 |
| Harvey 1975[129] | R | 0/0 | 22/28 |
| Symbas 1976[130] | R | 0/0 | 50/98 |
| Beach 1976[131] | R | 0/4 | 26/34 |
| Asfaw 1977[132] | R | 0/0 | 277/323 |
| Sherman 1978[133] | R | 32/41 | 31/92 |
| Trinkle 1979[80] | R | 0/0 | 89/100 |
| Evans 1979[134] | R | 0/4 | 29/46 |
| Breaux 1979[135] | R | 39/44 | 78/197 |
| Mandal 1979[136] | R | 0/38 | 26/55 |
| Gervin 1982[109] | R | 4/21 | 4/21 |
| Demetriades 1983[137] | R | 2/16 | 40/125 |
| Demetriades 1984[138] | R | 1/11 | 0/45 |
| Tavares 1984[117] | R | 21/37 | 64 |
| Feliciano 1984[65] | R | 5/15 | 2/3 |
| Mattox 1985[64] | R | 50/119 | 204 |
| Demetriades 1986[139] | R | 1/18 | 70 |
| Moreno 1985[75] | R | 4/69 | 100 |
| Ivatury 1987[113] | R | 28/91 | – |
| Jebara 1989[140] | R | 4/17 | – |
| Attar 1991[141] | R | 21/55 | – |
| Knott-Craig 1992[142] | R | 5/13 | – |
| Buchman 1992[143] | R | 1/2 | 23 |
| Benyan 1992[144] | R | 1/13 | – |
| Macho 1993[116] | R | 12/24 | – |
| Mitchell 1993[145] | R | 7/47 | – |
| Kaplan 1993[146] | R | 2/23 | |
| Henderson 1994[147] | R | 6/122 | 215 |
| Coimbra 1995[148] | R | 0/20 | |
| Arreola-Risa 1995[149] | R | 11/40 | |
| Karmy-Jones 1997[150] | R | 3/6 | 16 |
| Rhee 1998[151] | R | 15/58 | 41/96 |
| Asensio 1998[67] | P | 6/37 | 6/37 |
| Asensio 1998[68] | P | 10/71 | 10/71 |
| Tyburski 2000[152] | R | 12/152 | 12/152 |
| Asensio (NTDB)[69] | R | 47/830 | 47/830 |

*Note:* There were no survivors of blunt trauma.

EDT, emergency department thoracotomy; P, prospective; R, retrospective.

**Adjunct Maneuvers.** In 1907, Sauerbuch[42] described controlling blood flow by compression of the base of the heart. This maneuver is difficult to perform via a left anterolateral thoracotomy. Total inflow occlusion to the heart is accomplished by cross clamping both the superior (SVC) and inferior vena cava (IVC) in their intrapericardial location to arrest total blood flow to the heart.

The clamp must be placed carefully and sometimes at an angle so as to totally occlude the intrapericardial IVC.[70,77]

Total inflow occlusion of the heart is indicated for the management of injuries in the lateral-most aspect of the right atrium and/or the superior or inferior atriocaval junction. Total inflow occlusion will lead to immediate emptying of the heart and allow the injury to be visualized and thus repaired. Frequently this procedure results in cardiac arrest. The safe period for this maneuver is unknown, although a one to three minute range is often quoted in the literature as the period of time after which clamps must be released. As the clamps are released, venous return fills the right-sided cardiac chambers and forward cardiac pumping motion may begin, but more often than not, the heart will fibrillate requiring immediate direct defibrillation along with pharmacologic manipulation.[70,77]

Cross-clamping of the pulmonary hilum is another valuable maneuver indicated for the management of associated pulmonary injuries, particularly those that present with hilar central hematomas and/or active bleeding. This maneuver arrests bleeding from the lung and prevents systemic air emboli from reaching the systemic circulation. However, one of its negative effects is responsible for significantly increasing the afterload of the right ventricle, as half of the pulmonary circulation is no longer available for perfusion. Sequential declamping of the hilum is carried out as expediently as possible along with a direct approach by stapled pulmonary tractotomy.[70,74]

Grabowski[154] described a maneuver to facilitate exposure of posterior cardiac wounds by placing a Satinsky clamp at the right ventricular angle, which is formed at the acute anteroinferior margin of the right ventricle as it reflects on the right diaphragm by grasping a small portion of the right ventricle. He recommends this maneuver to elevate the heart out of the pericardium to repair posterior injures.

Maneuvers such as venting either the right or left ventricle post cardiorrhaphy are recommended to provide an avenue of egress for air emboli trapped in these chambers. This is usually accomplished by placing 16-gauge intravenous catheters. Theoretically, air should eject out of the repair chambers thus reducing venous or systemic air emboli.

At times a trauma surgeon will need to elevate the heart out of the pericardium in order to repair certain injuries. Rapid and injudicious manipulation of the heart will often result in complex dysrhythmias that might include ventricular fibrillation and even arrest. If hemorrhage can be digitally controlled, gradual elevation of the heart by placing multiple laparotomy packs will allow better tolerance of this maneuver while decreasing the chances for the development of dysrhythmias.[70,74]

Waterworth[155] reported a case in which the Octopus IV Mechanical Cardiac Stabilizer was utilized on a 20-year-old patient that sustained a two cm stab wound in the right ventricular outflow tract approximately one cm below the pulmonary valve. According to the author, this area was difficult to suture without causing further tearing due to tachycardia sustained by the patient and the fragile nature of this area. After control of hemorrhage by direct pressure, the Octopus IV Mechanical Cardiac Stabilizer was placed providing for immobility to this area of the heart and this facilitating repair.

### Repair of Atrial Injuries.

Right atrial injuries can usually be controlled by placement of a Satinsky partial occlusion vascular clamp (Fig. 28-1). Control of the wound will allow the trauma surgeon to perform cardiorrhaphy. We recommend utilizing 2-0 or 3-0 polypropylene monofilament sutures on an MH needle either in a running or in an interrupted fashion. It is important to visualize both sides of the atrial injury particularly those caused by missiles.

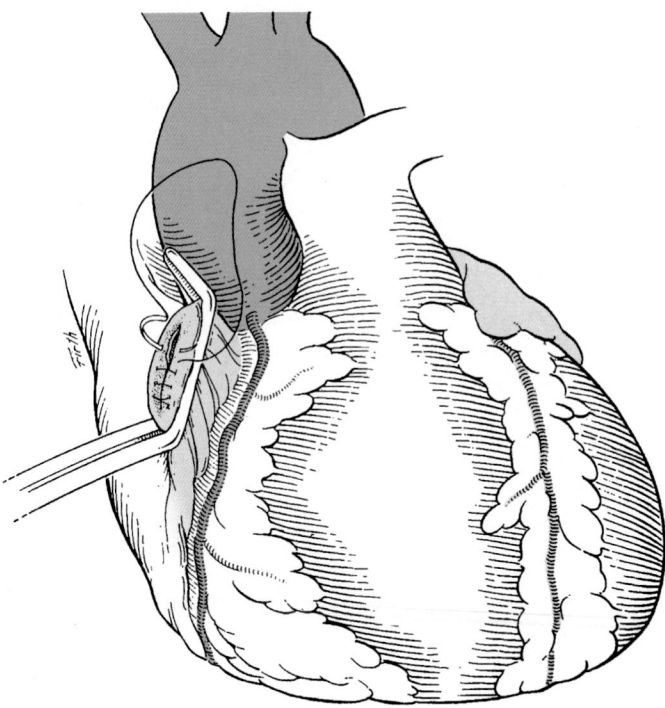

**FIGURE 28-1.** Satinsky partial occlusion clamp applied for right atrial repair.
*(Reproduced with permission from Juan A. Asensio, MD, FACS, FCCM and Demetrios Demetriades, MD, PhD, FACS.)*

The trauma surgeon must be aware that the atria have fairly thin walls and demand gentleness during cardiorrhaphy; as they can easily tear and enlarge the original injury. The use of pledgets are not recommended for the management of these injuries.[70,74]

### Repair of Ventricular Injuries.

Ventricular injuries usually cause significant hemorrhage. They should be occluded digitally while simultaneously repaired by either simple interrupted or horizontal mattress sutures of Halsted. Ventricular cardiorrhaphy can also be accomplished with a running monofilament suture of 2-0 polypropylene. Some surgeons prefer 3-0 or 4-0 polypropylene suture. Performing cardiorrhaphy for ventricular stab wounds is usually less challenging than for gunshot wounds. Missile injuries often produce some degree of blast effect which causes myocardial fibers to retract. Frequently, missile injuries that have been successfully sutured and controlled enlarge, as the damaged myocardium retracts and becomes more friable. Frequently these injuries require multiple sutures to control significant hemorrhage. In this scenario, bioprosthetic materials such as Teflon strips and/or pledgets are used by some surgeons to buttress the suture line (Figs. 28-2 and 28-3). This is usually performed by fashioning a Teflon strip that may measure anywhere from one to five centimeters. This strip is held by two straight hemostats held by an assistant. Simultaneously, the trauma surgeon may then place double-armed 2-0 polypropylene monofilament sutures, first through the strip and then through both sides of the injury. A second strip is then held similarly so that the trauma surgeon then places both needles through the second Teflon strip. The sutures are then gently tied against the Teflon strip and/or pledgets,

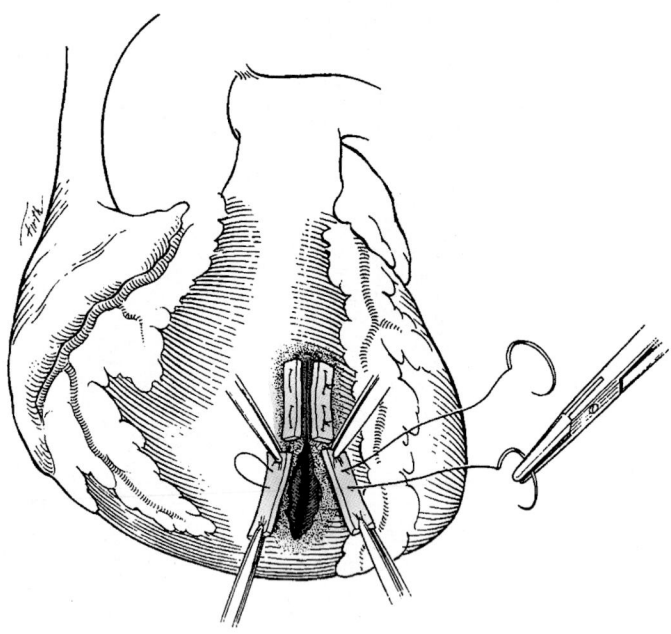

**FIGURE 28-2.** Method for repairing a complex left ventricular injury utilizing Teflon strips.
*(Reproduced with permission from Juan A. Asensio, MD, FACS, FCCM and Demetrios Demetriades, MD, PhD, FACS.)*

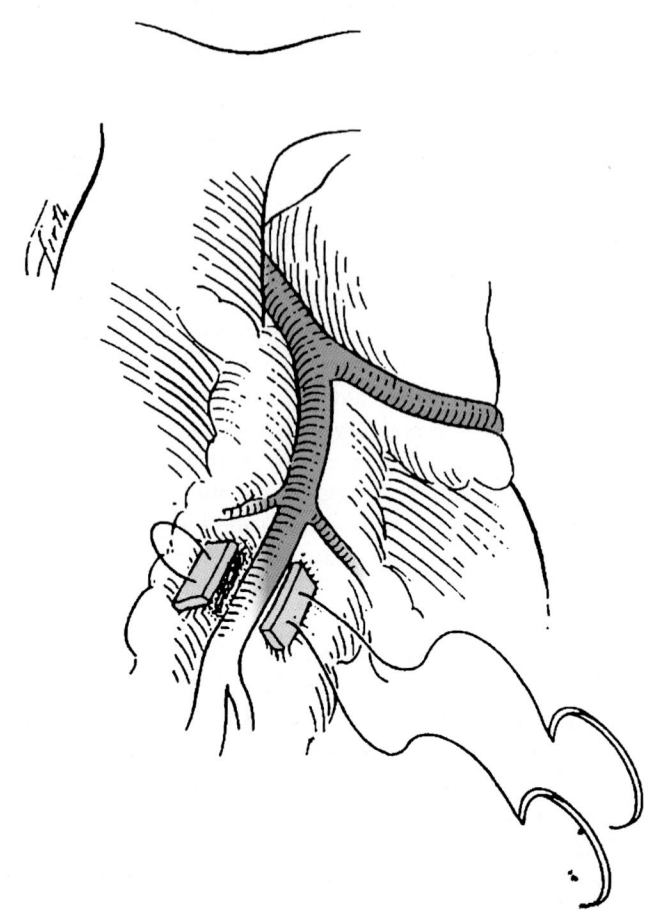

**FIGURE 28-4.** Technique depicting placement of sutures under the coronary artery bed. We recommend 2-0 polypropylene monofilament suture on a MH needle.
*(Reproduced with permission from Juan A. Asensio, MD, FACS, FCCM and Demetrios Demetriades, MD, PhD, FACS.)*

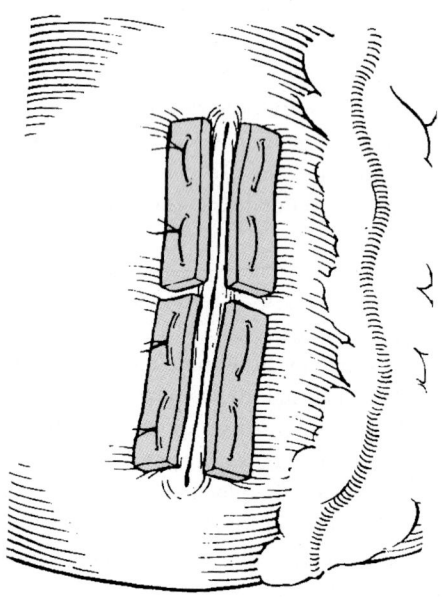

**FIGURE 28-3.** Sutures tied against the Teflon strips to buttress suture line.

which will buttress and reinforce the suture line. This maneuver must be repeated until total control of ventricular hemorrhage is achieved. Alternatively, one may use commercially made fibrin sealants.[70,74]

Coronary Artery Injuries.    The repair of cardiac injuries adjacent to coronary arteries can be very challenging. Injudicious and/or inappropriate placement of sutures during cardiorrhaphy may narrow and/or occlude a coronary artery or one of its branches (Fig. 28-4). Sutures should be placed underneath the bed of the coronary artery. Injuries to the proximal segment of a

coronary artery will usually require revascularization. Lacerations of the distal segment of the coronary artery, particularly in the distal most third of the vessel, are managed by ligation.[70,74,157-159]

Complex and Combined Injuries.    Complex and combined cardiac injuries can be defined as a penetrating cardiac injury plus associated neck, thoracic, thoracic-vascular, abdominal, abdominal vascular, or peripheral vascular injuries. These injuries are quite challenging to manage. Priority should be given early to the injury causing the greatest blood loss or threatening the patient's life.[70,74,160-165]

Wall and Mattox[156] described 60 patients with complex cardiac injuries, which they defined as those beyond lacerations of the myocardium. They described these injuries as those with concomitant coronary artery injuries, cardiac valvular injuries, intracardiac fistulas, and other unusual injuries. In this series, they described 39 coronary artery injuries, two valvular injuries, and 14 intracardiac fistulas including ventriculoseptal defects, atrioseptal defects (ASD), and another ten injuries, which they considered unusual ranging from ventricular false aneurysms to coronary sinus injuries, and two patients who developed missile emboli to the heart. These types of injuries can also be considered complex and combined injuries.

**TABLE 28-2**

### Anatomic Location of Injuries

| AUTHOR | YEAR | SPAN (Years) | NO. OF PATIENTS | CARDIAC CHAMBERS (#/%) | | | | Multiple Chambers | ASSOCIATED CORONARY ARTERIES |
|---|---|---|---|---|---|---|---|---|---|
| | | | | RV | LV | RA | LA | | |
| Ivatury[157] | 1981 | 20 | 228 | 90 (39.4%) | 44 (19.2%) | 15 (6.5%) | 6 (2.6%) | 38 (16.6%) Location NR 20 (8.8%) | 11 (4.8%) |
| Buckman[76] | 1993 | 2.25 | 66 | Single Chamber 42 (63.6%) | | | | 24 (36.3%) | NR |
| Henderson[147] | 1994 | 6 | 251 | 96 (38.2%) | 98 (39.8%) | 57 (22.7%) | 31 (12.3%) | 101 (40.2%) | NR |
| Arreola[149] | 1998 | 7 | 55 | 29 (52%) | 17 (30%) | 7 (12%) | 2 (3%) | 11 (20%) | 1 (1.5%) |
| Wall[156] | 1997 | 20 | 711 | 284 (40%) | 284 (40%) | 171 (24%) | 21 (3%) | 14 (1.9%) | 39 (5.4%) |
| Asensio[67] | 1998 | 1 | 60 | 40 (66.6%) | 15 (25%) | 11 (18.3%) | 3 (5%) | NR | 5 (8.3%) |
| Asensio[68] | 1998 | 2 | 105 | 39 (37.1%) | 26 (24.7%) | 8 (7.6%) | 5 (4.7%) | 23 (21.9%) | 9 (8.5%) |
| Tyburski[152] | 2000 | 17 | 302 | 121 (40%) | 75 (24.8%) | 17 (5.6%) | 6 (1.9%) | 83 (27.4%) | NR |
| Totals | | | 1778 | 699 | 559 | 328 | 74 | 314 | 65 |

NR, Not reported.

## Anatomic Location of Injury

A great deal of variability exists in the literature when it comes to reporting the breakdown of cardiac injuries by chambers (Table 28-2). Ventricular injuries occur with an incidence ranging from 37% to 67% of all cardiac injuries, whereas left ventricular injuries occur with an incidence ranging from 19% to 40%. Right atrial injuries appear to occur with greater frequency ranging from 5% to 20%, whereas the left atrium, the most recessed chamber of the heart, is injured between 2% and 12% of the times.[67,68,76,147,149,152,156,157]

Wall and Mattox[156] reported a 40% incidence of both right and left ventricular injuries in their series of 711 patients. Tyburski[152] reported a 40% incidence of right ventricular injuries and a 25% incidence of left ventricular injuries in 302 patients. Multiple-chamber injuries occur with a frequency ranging from 2% to 36%. With the highest reported incidence of multiple-chamber injuries reported by Henderson (40%)[147] and Buckman (36%).[76] Associated coronary artery injuries occur infrequently with the largest experience in the literature reported by Wall and Mattox[156] consisting of 39 associated coronary arterial injuries (5%) in their series of 711 patients. In both prospective studies of Asensio,[67,68] the incidence of coronary artery injuries remained stable at 8%.

## Associated Injuries

Stab wounds are generally isolated and usually only involve one chamber due to their precordial penetration; however, missile injuries may injure the heart either from precordial as well as extra precordial locations and thus have a greater propensity for causing multiple chamber and associated injuries. Buckman[76] reported that of the 23 (50%) of their 46 patients sustaining penetrating gunshot wounds of the heart, 23 (50%) had associated injuries to the pulmonary hilum, great vessels, and solid abdominal viscera in comparison to only four (20%) of the 20 patients that sustained stab wounds.

Henderson,[147] in a series of 251 patients, reported that associated injuries were present in most of his patients stating that the majority were minor injuries involving the skin, soft tissues, or the musculoskeletal system, but that potentially lethal associated injuries involving the abdominal viscera, lung, abdominal vasculature, and thoracic vascular structures were also relatively common.

Asensio,[67] in a one-year prospective study of 60 patients, reported 13 associated intrathoracic vessel injuries which included three patients each with aortic, pulmonary artery, and superior vena caval injuries, respectively. In addition, 19 patients sustained pulmonary injuries and one intrathoracic esophageal injury. A total of 19 patients sustained associated intraabdominal injuries. Asensio,[68] in a two-year prospective study of 105 patients, reported 21 (20%) associated intrathoracic major vessel injuries that included seven aortic injuries, four superior vena caval injuries, three pulmonary venous, two pulmonary arterial injuries, and five other associated vessels. In addition, 47 (45%) patients sustained associated pulmonary injuries and two (2%) intrathoracic esophageal injuries. Forty-five (43%) patients sustained associated abdominal injuries, which included 19 (18%) with hollow viscous injuries, 16 (15%) with solid organ injuries, and 10 (9%) with associated abdominal vascular injuries. Nine other patients (9%) sustained injuries to the extremities and back, respectively, while six (6%) sustained associated head and neck injuries.

## Prognostic Factors

The American Association for the Surgery of Trauma (AAST) and its Organ Injury Scaling (OIS)[158] committee have developed a cardiac injury scale to uniformly describe cardiac injuries (Table 28-3). This scale has been available since 1994, and few studies have correlated cardiac injury grade with mortality. Asensio,[67] in a one-year prospective pilot study of 60 patients followed by a two-year prospective study of 105 patients, correlated AAST-OIS for cardiac injuries with mortality, demonstrating 99 (94%) of the 105 patients incurred injury grades IV–VI injuries. Mortality progressively increased with injury grade. Grade IV injuries incurred a mortality of 56%, grade V 76%, and grade VI 91%, respectively. Further work is necessary to confirm their findings and all cardiac injuries should be graded according to this scale.[67,68,70,74]

**TABLE 28-3**

| American Association for the Surgery of Trauma (AAST) Organ Injury Scaling (OIS): Heart Injury Scale | |
|---|---|
| GRADE[a] | INJURY DESCRIPTION |
| I | Blunt cardiac injury with minor electrocardiographic abnormality (nonspecific T- or T-wave changes, premature atrial or ventricular contraction, or persistent sinus tachycardia) |
| | Blunt or penetrating pericardial wound without cardiac injury, cardiac tamponade or cardiac herniation |
| II | Blunt cardiac injury with heart block (right or left bundle branch, left anterior fascicular, or atrioventricular) or ischemic changes (ST depression or T-wave inversion) without cardiac failure |
| | Penetrating tangential myocardial wound up to, but not extending through, endocardium, without tamponade. |
| III | Blunt cardiac injury with sustained (≥5 beats /min) or multifocal ventricular contractions |
| | Blunt or penetrating cardiac injury with septal rupture, pulmonary or tricuspid valvular incompetence, papillary muscle dysfunction, or distal coronary arterial occlusion without cardiac failure |
| | Blunt pericardial laceration with cardiac herniation |
| | Blunt cardiac injury with cardiac failure |
| | Penetrating tangential myocardial wound up to, but not extending through, endocardium, with tamponade |
| IV | Blunt or penetrating cardiac injury with septal rupture, pulmonary or tricuspid valvular incompetence, papillary muscle dysfunction, or distal coronary arterial occlusion producing cardiac failure |
| | Blunt or penetrating cardiac injury with aortic or mitral valve incompetence |
| | Blunt or penetrating cardiac injury of the right ventricle, right atrium, or left atrium |
| V | Blunt or penetrating cardiac injury with proximal coronary arterial occlusion |
| | Blunt or penetrating left ventricular perforation |
| | Stellate wound with <50% tissue loss of the right ventricle, right atrium, or left atrium |
| VI | Blunt avulsion of the heart; penetrating wound producing >50% tissue loss of a chamber |

[a]Advance one grade for multiple penetrating wounds to a single chamber or multiple chamber involvement.

(From: Moore EE, Malangoni MA, Cogbill TH, et al.: Organ injury scaling IV: Thoracic, vascular, lung, cardiac, and diaphragm. J Trauma 36:229, 1994.)

Prognostic factors such as mechanism of injury, the presence or absence of physiologic parameters at the scene of the traumatic incident, during transport, and upon arrival such as the presence of pupillary response, spontaneous ventilation, presence of a carotid pulse, presence of a measurable blood pressure, presence of a sinus rhythm, any extremity movement, need for intubation and cardiopulmonary resuscitation as well as scene times greater than ten minutes are also significant risk factors.[67,68,76,109] The presence of cardiopulmonary arrest upon arrival is a poor predictor of outcome.[65,66,113,147,152,160]

Moreno and Moore[75] confirmed the presence of a pericardial tamponade as a positive prognostic factor for survival; however, this could not be independently confirmed by Buckman,[76] Mattox,[66] and Ivatury.[157] Asensio[67,68] and Buckman[76] have also validated the presence of significant associated injuries, such as coronary and major blood vessel injuries as well as multiple chamber injuries which are significant as poor predictors of outcome. Buckman[76] also defined the absence of an organized rhythm upon opening the pericardium as a significantly poor predictor of outcome. Stepwise, logistic regression analysis identified gunshot wounds, exsanguination, and restoration of blood pressure to be the single most important predictors of both mortality and survival for these patients.

## BLUNT CARDIAC INJURY

### Historical Perspective

The first unquestionable case of myocardial contusion was reported in 1764 by Akenside.[166] He treated a 14-year-old boy struck

between the ribs by plate. The patient died six months after the blow. At autopsy, an area of necrosis of the left ventricle was found extending nearly but not completely through the heart wall. The first recorded case of blunt cardiac chamber rupture was reported in 1679 by Borch.[167,168] He described an eight-year-old boy that fell and bruised his chest, whose chief complaint was pain in the chest and abdomen. During a period of four months the child became anemic and subsequently died. An autopsy report revealed a right atrial injury with clot formation. From 1676 to 1868, only 27 cases of blunt traumatic cardiac injuries were reported in the literature.[169] In 1868, Fischer[25] published an impressive description of 76 cases describing 69 traumatic ruptures of the heart and seven myocardial contusions. In 1932, Kissane[170] reported a 15% incidence of blunt cardiac injury. In 1936, Glendy[171] reported a single case of nonpenetrating wound of a heart and reviewed 7600 autopsies at the Massachusetts General Hospital but could not identify any other cases of blunt cardiac trauma. In 1940, Leinoff[172] reported 15 unselected consecutive cases of fatal automobile accidents of which eight (16%) revealed macroscopic evidence of cardiac injury.

Bright and Beck[173] analyzed 168 patients, in which death occurred in 157 and of those 157 blunt cardiac rupture occurred in 152. From this review, as well as from their own clinical and experimental work on animals, they showed that enormous force is required to rupture the heart and also pointed that severe and lesser forces may produce an entire range of cardiac trauma in which recovery is generally the rule and rupture is the exception. As part of their animal studies they established the pathologic diagnosis of myocardial contusion in an autopsy series as well as experimentally in a canine model in which they described interstitial hemorrhage and muscle necrosis.

In 1958, Parmley[174] reviewed 207,548 autopsy cases from the Armed Forces Institute of Pathology (AFIP) and described 546 patients with nonpenetrating traumatic injury to the heart reporting an incidence of 0.1%. In this hallmark study, the authors reported 353 cases of cardiac chamber rupture, 273 isolated and 80 associated with combined aortic ruptures. The breakdown per chamber included 66 ruptured right ventricles, 59 ruptured left ventricles, 41 ruptured right, and 26 left atria. One hundred and six patients sustained multiple-chamber injuries.

## Mechanism, Pathophysiology, and Incidence

Since Bright and Beck[173,175] established the pathologic diagnosis of myocardial contusion and focused attention on nonpenetrating trauma to the heart, establishing a firm definition for what blunt cardiac injury is has remained somewhat elusive. This entity was for quite some time known as myocardial contusion and has even been described as myocardial concussion. The exact definition of blunt cardiac injury has remained difficult to pinpoint because it is not really one entity but rather a spectrum of entities.

Blunt cardiac injury (BCI) can range from a mild myocardial contusion to frank cardiac chamber rupture including the rare entity of *comotio cordis* described as sudden cardiac arrest from a sternal blow, leading to cardiogenic shock. Blunt cardiac injuries may occur secondary to compression, deceleration, blast, and direct forces applied to the chest or transmitted increases in intravascular abdominal pressures associated with compression of the abdominal contents. In fact, any mechanism that delivers kinetic energy to the heart may cause injury. High-speed motor vehicular collisions, causing crushing injuries to the thoracic cage or objects of great weight falling directly on to the sternum or thoracic cage will directly compress the heart against the vertebral column causing blunt cardiac injury. Similarly, accidental falls from great heights as well as blast injuries can also cause blunt cardiac injuries. Iatrogenic blunt cardiac injuries have also been reported during closed cardiopulmonary resuscitation.

Risk factors for blunt cardiac injuries include any mechanism that may result in any significant force applied to the thoracic cage that is transmitted to the heart. Direct impacts in high-speed motor vehicular collisions exceeding greater than 20 miles per hour as well as bending of the steering wheel are well-known risk factors for these injuries. The true incidence of blunt cardiac injuries remains difficult to estimate from the literature.[176]

## Clinical Presentation

Blunt cardiac injury encompasses an entire spectrum of different processes; therefore clinical presentation for patients sustaining blunt cardiac injury may range from complete hemodynamic instability to cardiopulmonary arrest. Similarly, these patients may also present with the classical syndrome of pericardial tamponade. Symptoms consistent but not necessarily specific for blunt cardiac injury include tenderness and pain over the anterior chest wall. Chest pain experienced by some of these patients and its distribution may be indistinguishable from the classical pain of myocardial infarction. Physical findings may include pain and tenderness over the anterior chest wall, contusion, ecchymosis, anterior rib fractures, and even a central flail chest.[176]

**Diagnosis.** Diagnostic modalities for blunt cardiac injury include chest x-rays, EKGs, Holter monitoring, measurement of cardiac enzymes, trans-thoracic (TTE) and trans-esophageal (TEE) echocardiography, and nuclear medicine scans including Radionuclide Angiography (RNA), thallium 201, single photon emission computed tomography (SPECT), and multiple-gated image acquisition scans (MUGA).[176] Chest x-rays are routinely obtained in all trauma patients, they may detect the presence of fractured ribs and flail chest and rarely may reveal a globular-shaped cardiac silhouette; however, findings associated with severe blunt chest trauma such as multiple fractured ribs or flail chest are often missed on plain films and are visualized with greater detail with computed tomography (CT). EKG were one of the first modalities utilized for the diagnosis of blunt cardiac injury. EKG has been traditionally used to screen patients and detect conduction disturbances. However, there is no pathonogmonic finding that can reliably establish the diagnosis of blunt cardiac injury.[176]

According to Tenzer,[177] EKG is an unreliable tool to establish the diagnosis of blunt cardiac injuries because it reflects abnormalities of the left ventricle and not of the right ventricle which, given its more anterior location, is the chamber more frequently affected by blunt cardiac injury. Electrocardiographic abnormalities detected by EKG may range from sinus tachycardia, the most commonly encountered arrhythmia to supraventricular arrhythmias such as atrial flutter (AF) and atrial fibrillation (AF), ventricular tachycardia (VT), premature ventricular contractions (PVCs), ventricular fibrillation (VF), right bundle branch block (RBB) followed by first-degree heart block, right bundle branch block with hemiblock and third-degree heart block as well as T-wave and ST-segment abnormalities.[176,177] All these findings may occur in patients sustaining blunt cardiac injury although presence of many of these conduction abnormalities is uncommon. Right bundle branch block (RBB) or any type of block in the presence of blunt thoracic trauma, particularly when associated with direct sternal impacts, should raise the suspicion that further investigation is needed to detect blunt cardiac injury in these patients.

EKG still continues to be used as a simple screening test for patients suspected of harboring blunt cardiac injury. The presence of a normal EKG in a hemodynamically stable patient warrants no further investigation. Currently, the authors utilize EKG as a screening tool and will proceed to institute further investigation only in the presence of significant electrical disturbances.[178]

**Cardiac Enzymes and Troponin.** The measurement of creatine phosphokinase (CPK) or creatine kinase (CK) with measurement of the myocardial band (MB) was for a time utilized to establish the diagnosis of blunt cardiac injury. Frazee[179] utilized measurements of CPK-MB as part of their diagnosis of both "cardiac contusion" and "cardiac concussion." Tenzer[177] reported the utilization of CPK and the measurements as sensitive tests to diagnose myocardial contusion. However, studies by Hossack,[180] Potkin,[181] Kettunen,[182] Anderson,[183] Cachecho,[184] and Biffl[185] contradict these findings and have proven that measurement of these enzymes does not establish nor correlate with the presence of blunt cardiac injury.

More specific measurements of contractile proteins of different muscle types including troponin (cTn) have emerged as diagnostic tools to diagnose blunt cardiac injury as both troponin T and I belong to a group of proteins of the contractile apparatus that are unique to cardiac muscle. Katus,[186,187] in 1989, used a new assay to demonstrate a new elevated level of cardiac troponins (TcTnT) in patients that suffered myocardial infarction and extrapolated its use for the detection of blunt cardiac injury. Similarly, Adams[188,189] also used measurements of troponin I (cTnI) to detect blunt cardiac injury.

Fulda[190] prospectively evaluated 71 patients with thoracic wall injuries utilizing signal-averaged EKG, serum troponin T levels, standard EKG, and CPK-MB measurements. Patients were monitored electrocardiographically and by serial measurements of troponin-T and CPK-MB fractions. Two-dimensional echocardiography (TTE) was performed for patients with abnormal CPK-MB levels. Upon admission, 17 of their 71 patients (24%) had normal sinus rhythm and 13 (18%) had a clinically significant finding. The repeat EKG was abnormal in 50 patients and in 26, the findings were clinically significant. In the 17 patients with a normal initial EKG, seven (41%) developed a clinically significant abnormality and six required interventions for the findings detected on EKG. Eleven of 71 patients (16%) had positive troponin T, 5 of 71 (7%) had positive CPK-MB, 15 of 71 (21%) had positive signal averaged EKG and four of 13 had positive echocardiograms. Only the initial EKG abnormalities and an elevated troponin T levels greater than 0.20 m/L were the only variables found to predict clinically significant electrocardiographic events.

Fulda[190] reported that the sensitivity and specificity of troponin–T in predicting clinically significant abnormalities was 27 and 91%, respectively. From the findings of this study, the authors concluded that the best predictors for the development of significant electrocardiographic changes are an abnormality detected in the initial EKG as well as an elevated serum troponin T level recommending that both of these tests be obtained to diagnose blunt cardiac injury.

Salim[191] investigated the role of serum cardiac troponin I and EKG to identify patients at risk for the development of cardiac complications after blunt cardiac trauma. In this prospective 115-patient study, the authors utilized the previously described tests to identify patients at risk for significant blunt cardiac injury defined as cardiogenic shock, arrhythmias requiring treatment, or structural cardiac abnormalities directly related to blunt cardiac trauma. All patients were evaluated with EKG upon admission which was repeated at an eight-hour interval. Cardiac troponin I was obtained at admission and also at four and eight hours. TTE were obtained when clinically indicated. Nineteen patients (16.5%) had significant blunt cardiac injuries. In 18 of the 19, symptoms were present within 24 hours. Of the 115 patients, 58 (50%) had abnormal EKGs and 27 (23.5%) had increased cTnI; cTnI had positive predictive values of 28% and 48% and negative predictive values of 95% and 93%, respectively. However, when both tests were abnormal (positive) or normal (negative) the positive and negative predictive values increased to 62% and 100%, respectively. From these data the authors concluded that the combination of EKG and troponin I reliably identified the presence or absence of significant and blunt cardiac injuries. They recommended that patients with an abnormal EKG and an abnormal troponin I level require close monitoring for at least 24 hours and recommended that patients with normal admission EKG and troponin I levels can be safely discharged in the absence of other injuries.

Bertinchant,[192] however, evaluated the incidence, clinical significance, and prognostic value for both troponin I and troponin T elevations in hemodynamically stable patients to exclude suspected blunt cardiac injury and concluded that both cTnI and cTn-T had low sensitivity and predictive values in diagnosing cardiac contusions and did not represent an improved method to diagnose blunt cardiac injuries. Currently, the authors recommend an admission EKG as well as serial troponin levels for patients suspected of blunt cardiac injury followed by TTE if clinically significant arrhythmias are present.

**Two-Dimensional Transthoracic and Transesophageal Echocardiography.** The use of TTE has been extensively used as diagnostic modality for the evaluation of patients with suspected blunt cardiac injury. Patients are selected for evaluation by this modality after abnormal EKG and abnormal cardiac enzymes and troponin level measurements are detected. TTE evaluates segmental wall abnormalities or valvular dysfunction.[176] However, although useful, it has not been shown to correlate with complications or eventual outcome in BCI, and whereas it may detect and identify structural defects and abnormalities with wall motion it is limited by chest wall edema, traumatic structural abnormalities such as fractured ribs and flail chest but most importantly it cannot detect the electrical instability that is a hallmark for blunt cardiac injury. Transesophageal echocardiography (TEE) has been shown to be a useful adjunct to evaluate patients with blunt cardiac injury as it is more versatile in its ability to detect blunt cardiac injury. In the hands of skilled operators, blunt periaortic hematomas and other mediastinal injuries can also be detected. However, it is an invasive procedure which is operator-dependent and not always available around the clock.[185,193–197]

**Radionuclide Scans.** A number of different radionuclide scans have been utilized in the past for the diagnosis of blunt cardiac injury. They include technetium-99m pyrophosphate, thallium 201, single photon emission computed tomography (SPECT), and multiple-gated acquisition scans (MUGA). The respective radioactive substances used in this scans bind injured or infarcted areas of the myocardium to detect blunt cardiac injury and ischemia. None of these scans were sufficiently sensitive or specific to reliably establish the diagnosis of blunt cardiac injury and have been abandoned.[176]

## Spectrum of Blunt Cardiac Injury

Clinically, blunt cardiac injury can be divided into two types: acute and subacute. The acute type is usually the catastrophic injury that causes death immediately or rapidly if surgical intervention is not instituted. These injuries include cardiac chamber rupture with acute pericardial tamponade, combined chamber and pericardial rupture with hemorrhage into the pleural cavity, and acute myocardial injury with cardiogenic shock. Subacute cardiac injury may not lead to immediate death but does impact cardiac hemodynamics while placing the patient at risk for the development of significant arrhythmias and hemodynamic complications. Subacute injuries include myocardial contusion, subacute pericardial tamponade, myocardial infarction, valvular injury, intracardiac shunts, mural thrombi, and of course, arrhythmias.

**Pericardial Injury.** Blunt rupture of the pericardium occurs from direct, high-energy impact or from transmitted sudden and acute increases of intrabdominal pressure. Most pericardial injuries whether single or multiple can occur after blunt injury, many are associated with extensive cardiac injuries; however, they may also occur as isolated injuries. Classical but rare physical findings include the Bruit de Moulin described as the sound of a splashing mill wheel by Bricheteau[196] in 1844 and again, by Morell-Lavallee[196] in 1864, as secondary to either a pneumo or hemopericardium. The pericardium may rupture on the diaphragmatic or pleural surfaces usually parallel to the left phrenic nerve. In Fulda's[197] study, 22 patients were reported with pericardial tears, 14 (64%) had left pericardial tears parallel to the phrenic nerve, four (18%) diaphragmatic, and two had right side and mediastinal tears (9%) each. In addition, the heart may eviscerate into the abdominal cavity, in rare cases it can cause torsion of the great vessels acutely. Such an extensive injury requires immediate surgical intervention via a laparotomy to replace the herniated heart back in the pericardial sac. In his series, Parmley[174] reported that if pericardial laceration occurs as an isolated injury, it is usually of no consequence unless complicated by hemorrhage from a lacerated pericardiophrenic artery. Parmley[174] also reported 71 pericardial ruptures present in association with patients that incurred isolated atrial or ventricular rupture.

The clinical presentation of patients sustaining blunt pericardial rupture can range from hemodynamic instability to cardiopulmonary arrest secondary torsion of the heart or great vessels or associated blunt cardiac chamber rupture. Patients should be investigated with a chest x-ray that may reveal displacement of the cardiac silhouette, pneumopericardium, or an abnormal gas pattern secondary to herniated hollow viscera. If hemodynamically stable, the patients may be investigated with sonography and EKG. Diagnosis can also be confirmed via a subxyphoid pericardial window which will reveal a hemopericardium. This should then be followed by median sternotomy. For patients sustaining pericardial tears with or without cardiac herniation, the pericardium may be repaired utilizing simple interrupted sutures of 2-0 polyprolene.[70]

### Valvular, Papillary Muscle/Chordae Tendineae, and Septal Injury.

Blunt cardiac injury may rarely cause valvular injuries. Valves may be ruptured secondary to direct transmission of energy to the sternum. The most frequently injured valves include the aortic, followed by the mitral. The classic signs associated with valvular dysfunction may not be immediately recognized due to the presence of more obvious life-threatening injuries. Hypovolemia and diminished cardiac output may further obscure the extent of valvular damage until cardiac output (CO) can be restored. Important clinical findings include the presence of new cardiac murmurs, thrills, or loud musical murmurs. Similarly, acute left ventricular dysfunction with cardiogenic shock and associated pulmonary edema are important clinical findings. Symptoms of valvular incompetence should immediately prompt further diagnostic studies based on the clinical status of the patient.

Rapid displacement of blood secondary to crushing or compressive forces applied to the thoracic cage during ventricular diastole may lacerate cardiac valve leaflets, papillary muscles, or chordae tendinea leading to valvular insufficiency. From this mechanism, the aortic valve is most frequently injured. The valve cusp most frequently damaged is either the left coronary or the noncoronary aortic leaflet. Injuries to the mitral valve may also occur via the same mechanism during the period of maximum diastolic filling.

Similarly, any sudden increase in intraaortic pressure may lead to laceration or leaflet rupture and can also result in stretching and hematoma formation within the papillary muscle. Sudden alterations in papillary muscle anatomy will render it dysfunctional and may cause valvular insufficiency. Acute severe left ventricular failure with associated increases in pulmonary capillary wedge pressures (PCWP) along with decreases in Cardiac Output (CO)/Cardiac Index (CI) along left ventricular stroke work index (LVSWI) signal the presence of valvular injury, chordae tendinea, or papillary muscle dysfunction.

Fulda,[197] in a study of 59 patients that sustained blunt cardiac injury, reported no valvular injuries. Perchinsky[198] in a series of 27 patients also failed to report a single case of valvular injury. Parmley[174] in a series of 546 autopsied patients reported four patients with aortic valve ruptures of which two had congenitally bicuspid valves. In addition, he reported eight patients with ruptures of the mitral and tricuspid each, one patient with a pulmonary valvular rupture and one that had combined mitral and tricuspid valvular injuries.

Septal ruptures are also uncommon. In 1847, Hewett[199] first described the rupture of the intraventricular septum caused by blunt trauma. In 1935, Bright and Beck[173] described 11 patients with septal rupture in a series of 152 patients that sustained fatal cardiac injury. In 1953, Guilfoil[200] reported the first patient in which a septal defect was diagnosed with cardiac catheterization.

### Blunt Coronary Artery Injury.

Blunt coronary artery injuries are extremely rare. Direct impacts may cause acute coronary thrombosis and may result in intimal disruption caused by significant application of blunt energy to the chest. Blunt coronary artery injuries are usually associated with severe myocardial contusions generally along the distribution of the left anterior descending coronary artery (LAD). In rare cases, the right coronary artery (RCA) may also rupture. The clinical presentation of these patients cannot be distinguished from acute myocardial infarction. The LAD is the most frequently injured vessel as it lies beneath the sternum; however, the RCA is also vulnerable, usually within two centimeters of its origin. The RCA can also be damaged directly by torsion of the heart with displacement of the myocardium caudally while the left can be damaged by a stretch injury usually in the proximal portion of this vessel. Long-term sequelae of these injuries may lead to the development of a ventricular aneurysm with its potential complications such as rupture, ventricular failure, production of emboli, or malignant arrhythmias.[174]

### Cardiac Chamber Rupture.

Blunt cardiac rupture is relatively uncommon.[197,198,201–203] Only a small number of patients sustaining these injuries survive to reach the hospital. Blunt chamber rupture is often the immediate cause of death at the scene of motor vehicular collisions and is frequently found in autopsy findings. Similarly, delayed rupture of the heart may occur when an area of contused myocardium undergoes necrosis and subsequently ruptures causing pericardial tamponade and immediate death. Several mechanisms for blunt cardiac rupture have been postulated[197] which include: direct precordial impacts, hydraulic effect from retrograde transmission of force through the abdomen into the venous system causing rapid rises of venous pressure transmitted to the heart particularly the atria, compression, acceleration or deceleration injuries leading to tears of the heart at its attachment to the great thoracic vessels, blast effects, and concussive blows thought to be fatal secondary to the production of malignant arrhythmias.

Bright and Beck[174] reported 152 patients sustaining cardiac rupture and reviewed the literature reporting the first case of a left atrial injury reported by Berard in 1826. They also collected 30 cases of blunt ruptures of cardiac chambers from 1826–1926. Parmley,[174] in a study of 207,546 autopsy cases, described 546 patients with nonpenetrating injury to the heart and described 66 right ventricular, 59 left ventricular injuries, 41 right atrial and 26 left atrial injuries. Some of these injuries combined with aortic ruptures.

According to Martin,[204] Mayfield,[205] and Shorr,[206] the incidence of blunt cardiac rupture among hospital trauma admissions ranges from 0.5% to 2%. Calhoon[201] estimates a higher incidence— 4–5% of blunt cardiac chamber injuries. Santavirta[207] reported 40,169 nonsurvivors of traffic collisions in Finland of which 75 patients had blunt ruptures of the heart for an incidence of 1.33%. Fulda[197] reported 59 patients with blunt cardiac chamber rupture out of 16,000 blunt trauma patients admitted to their center for an incidence of 0.37%. Türk,[203] in a study of 6264 autopsies, reported 33 patients with blunt cardiac injuries sustained by fatal falls from great heights for an incidence of 0.53%.

DesForges,[208] in 1954, reported the first successful repair of a cardiac chamber rupture following blunt trauma on a patient that sustained a 4 cm longitudinal tear in the right atrium secondary to severe chest trauma from a motor vehicular collision nine hours prior to admission.

Blunt cardiac chamber rupture usually presents with persistent hypotension and/or pericardial tamponade. Similarly, patients may present in cardiopulmonary arrest secondary to exsanguinating hemorrhage. These patients should be rapidly evaluated by sonography to detect pericardial fluid. For those who are hemodynamically stable, subxyphoid pericardial window remains an option to confirm the results of sonography; however, for those that present cardiopulmonary arrest, ED thoracotomy may be their only chance at survival albeit these patients have a dismal prognosis.

There are few series in the literature that report blunt cardiac chamber ruptures.[197,198,201–203] Many include pericardial ruptures as well as epicardial/endocardial tears and myocardial hematomas. Extracting data from these series is challenging given the lack of uniformity in the data reported. A review of five contemporary series in the literature reporting blunt cardiac chamber ruptures describes 139 patients of which 33 were reported by Türk[203] in an autopsy series. From this review of the literature it appears that atrial injuries are more common than ventricular injuries. The most frequently injured cardiac chambers are the right atrium followed by the right ventricle. Left-sided chamber injuries occur with a smaller frequency. Several patients have been reported with multiple-chamber injuries; however, none survived. The overall survival rate is difficult to determine from the data contained in this series. Calhoon,[201] in 1986, reported ten patients of which seven survived; Brathwaite[202] reported 32 patients of which the only survivors were six that arrived with vital signs in the trauma center.

## Myocardial Contusion

Out of all of the blunt cardiac injuries the least important and more difficult to define is myocardial contusion/concussion. The definition of myocardial contusion has evolved over several decades of discussion amongst trauma surgeons. This diagnosis is more often established out of proportion to its incidence, severity, and clinical relevance. Mattox, et al.,[209] in an editorial, strongly suggested that the terms of myocardial contusion and concussion be eliminated in favor of a more reasonable definition for this entity and proposed that they be defined as blunt cardiac injury either with cardiac failure, with the presence of complex arrhythmia, and those patients admitted with blunt cardiac injury with minor EKG or enzyme abnormality. On the basis of their observations, they recommended that asymptomatic patients with anterior chest wall injuries should not be admitted into a surgical intensive care unit (SICU) for continuous electrocardiographic monitoring, serial determination of CPK-MB enzyme levels, or be subjected to further cardiac imaging.

Civetta[210] concluded that significant cardiac events are uncommon in young patients with chest trauma and pointed that initial EKG abnormalities are better indicators of cardiac complications in critically injured patients. He also noted that cardiac morbidity is uncommon in young stable patients with initial EKG abnormalities and suggested that when cardiac abnormalities do occur they need to be treated with or without a diagnosis of myocardial contusion. In the absence of these abnormalities, a diagnosis of myocardial contusion is without clinical significance.

Pasquale and Fabian[211] generated the Eastern Association for the Surgery of Trauma (EAST) practice management guidelines to screen for blunt cardiac injury. The reported incidence of blunt cardiac injury, formerly called myocardial contusion, depends on the modality and criteria used to establish a diagnosis and ranges from 8 to 71% in patients that sustain blunt chest trauma; however, the true incidence remains unknown because there is no diagnostic "gold standard" for diagnosis. The lack of such a standard leads to confusion in establishing the diagnosis as well as interpreting the literature. Moreover, it becomes important to identify a population at risk for the complications of blunt cardiac injury and at the same time identify a cost-effective mechanism to either include or exclude these patients. After a thorough review of the literature, Pasquale and Fabian identified well-conducted primary studies or reviews involving the identification of blunt cardiac injury. On the basis of this review of the literature, EAST generated three recommendations:

### Level I

1. An admission EKG should be performed for all patients in whom there is suspected BCI.

### Level II

1. If the admission EKG results are abnormal (arrhythmia, ST changes, ischemia, heart block, unexplained ST), the patient should be admitted for continuous EKG monitoring for 24–48 hours. Conversely, if the admission EKG results are normal, the risk of having a BCI that requires treatment is insignificant, and the pursuit of diagnosis should be terminated.

2. If the patient is hemodynamically unstable, an imaging study (echocardiogram) should be obtained. If an optimal transthoracic echocardiogram (TTE) cannot be performed, then the patient should have a transesophageal echocardiogram (TEE).

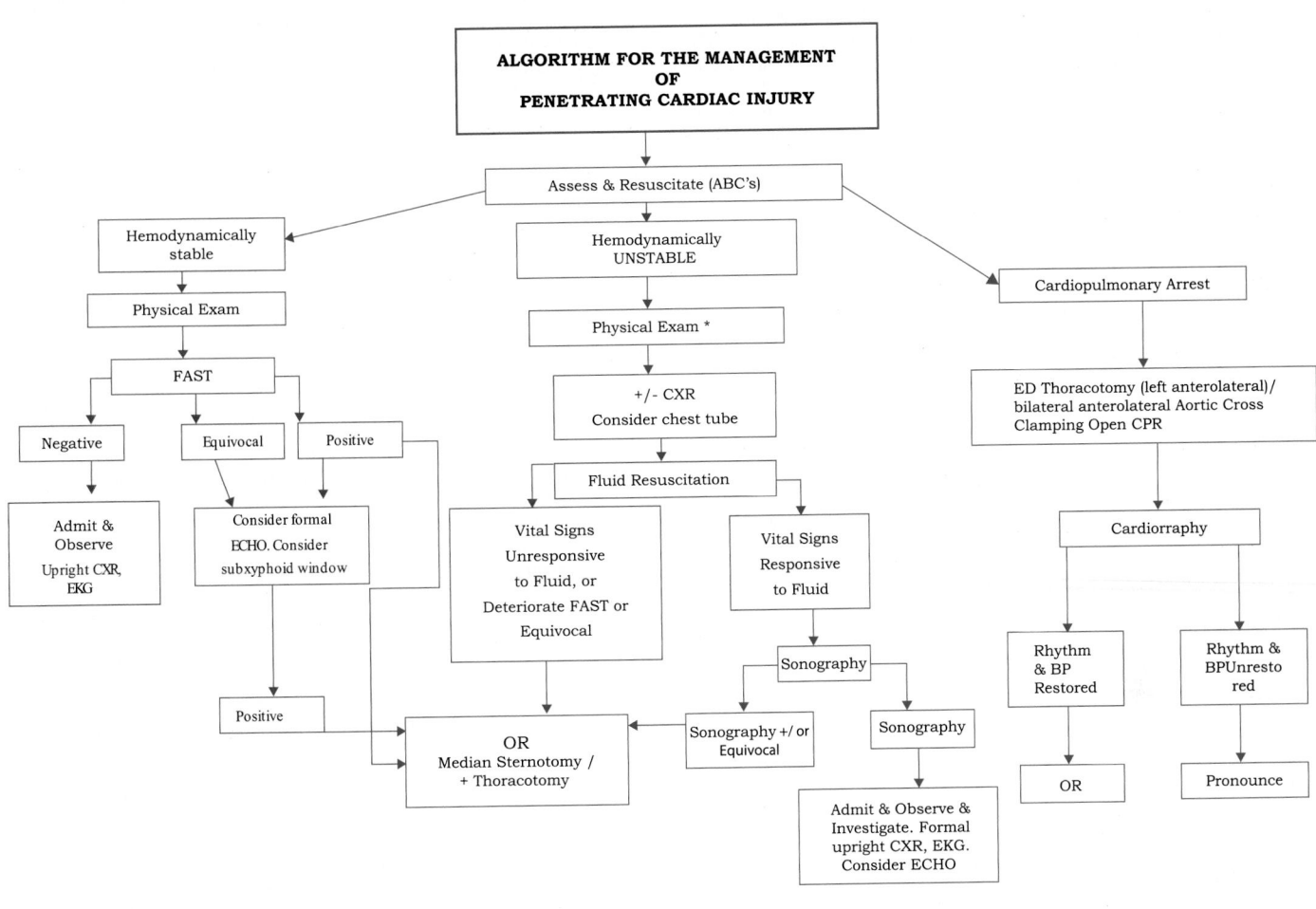

**FIGURE 28-5.** Algorithm for the management of penetrating cardiac injury.

3. Nuclear medicine studies add little compared with echocardiography and, thus, are not useful if an echocardiogram has been performed.

*Level III*

1. Elderly patients with known cardiac disease, unstable patients, and those with an abnormal admission EKG can be safely operated on provided that they are approximately monitored. Consideration should be given to placement of a pulmonary artery catheter in such cases.

2. The presence of a sternal fracture does not predict the presence of BCI and, thus, does not necessarily indicate that monitoring should be performed.

3. Neither creatine phosphokinase with isoenzyme analysis nor measurement of circulating cardiac troponin T are useful in predicting which patients have or will have complications related to BCI.

(see Fig. 28-5)

## CONCLUSIONS

Cardiac injuries remain both challenging and fascinating entities. Only with serious scientific inquiry based on prospective collection and analysis of data can we extend the frontiers in the management of these critical injuries, much like Cappelen, Farina, and Rehn did over 100 years ago.

## REFERENCES

1. Homer: *The Iliad*, Vol XIII, line 442. New York: McMillan & Co, 1922, p. 259. Translated by Lang, Leaf and Myers.
2. Homer: *The Iliad*, Vol XVI, lines 588–625. London: George Bell & Sons, 1904, p. 299. Translated by Alexander Pope.
3. Breasted JH: *The Edwin Smith Papyrus*, Vol 1. Chicago: The University of Chicago Press, 1930.
4. Beck CS: Wounds of the heart: The technique of suture. *Arch Surg* 13:205, 1926.
5. Hippocrates: The genuine works of Hippocrates, Vol 2, Aphorism 18. New York: William Wood and Co, 1886, p. 252. Translated by Francis Adams.
6. Ovid (43 BC–AD 17): Epistolae ex ponto. Lib I, Epist III, lines 21–22. As quoted by Beck CS. Wounds of the heart: The technique of suture. *Arch Surg* 13:205, 1926.
7. Celsus (15th century AD): Medicinae Libri Octo, Lib V, Chap 26 L. Targae, Ludguni Batavorum, 1791, p. 307. Translated by S and J Luchtmans. As quoted by Beck CS. Wounds of the heart: The technique of suture. *Arch Surg* 13:205, 1926.
8. Pliny the Elder (AD 23–79): Historia naturalis, Lib XI, Chap. 37, Vol 3, p. 65. London, Bostock & Riley, 1855. Translated HG Bohr. As quoted by Beck CS. Wounds of the heart: The technique of suture. *Arch Surg* 13:205, 1926.
9. Aristotle (384–322 BC): The Partibus Animalium. Lib III. Chap 4: Opera Edidit Academia Regia Borrusca, Vol 3, 328. As quoted by Beck CS: Wounds of the heart: The technique of suture. *Arch Surg* 13:205, 1926.
10. Galen (AD 130–200): Medicorun Graecorum Opera, Vol VIII, Lipsiae Prostat in officina Libraria Car. Cuoblochii 1824, De Locis Affectis. Edited by Kuhn DC: Tome VIII, Lib V, Chap 2, 304. As quoted by Beck CS. Wounds of the heart: The technique of suture. *Arch surg* 13:225, 1926.

11. Paulus Aegineta (AD 625–690): The seven books of Lib VI, sect 88, Vol 2, p. 421, 1846. Syndenham Society. Translated by Francis Adams. As quoted by Beck CS. Wounds of the heart: The technique of suture. *Arch Surg* 13:205, 1926.

12. Fallopius (AD 1523–1562): Opera omnia tractatus de vulneribus in genere, 1600, Chap 10, p. 163. As quoted by Beck CS. Wounds of the heart: The technique of suture. *Arch Surg* 13:225, 1926.

13. Pare A (AD 1509–1590): The workes of that Famous Chirurgion Ambroise Pare. Translated by T. Johnson. London T, Cates & Co, 1634. As quoted by Beck CS. Wounds of the heart: The technique of suture. *Arch Surg* 13:205, 1926.

14. Pare A: The Apologii and Treatise of Ambroise Pare (Concerning the voyages made into divers places with many of his writings on surgery). Keynes G, ed. Chicago: University of Chicago Press, 1952, p.27.

15. Fabricius ab Aquadependente (AD 1637–1619): Opera Chirurgica, Chap 21. Patavii, 1666, p. 144. As quoted by Beck CS. Wounds of the heart: The technique of suture. *Arch Surg* 13:225, 1926.

16. Boerhaave (1668–1738): De vulnere in Genere. Aphorismi de Cognoscendis et. Curandis Morbis, Aphorism 170, 43. As quoted by Beck CS: Wounds of the heart: The technique of suture. *Arch Surg* 13:205, 1926.

17. Hollerius J: Communis aphorismi allegati. Quoted from Fischer G. Die Wunden des Herzeus und des Herzbeutels. Arch Klin Chir 9:571, 1868. As quoted by Beck CS. Wounds of the heart: The technique of suture. *Arch Surg* 13:225, 1926.

18. Wolf I: Cited by Fischer G. Die Wunden des Herzens und des Herzbentels. *Arch Klin Chir* 9:571, 1868.

19. Senac JB: Traite de la structure du Coeur, de son action, et de ses maladies. Vol 2, p. 366. Paris: Breasson, 1749. As quoted by Beck CS. Wounds of the heart: The technique of suture. *Arch Surg* 13:205, 1926.

20. Morgagni JB: De sedibus et causes morborum. Lipsiae sumptibus Leopoldii Vossii, 1829. As quoted by Beck CS. Wounds of the heart: The technique of suture. *Arch Surg* 13:205, 1926.

21. Larrey DJ: Memoires de chirurgie militaire. *Bull Sci Med* 6:284, 1810.

22. Larrey DJ: Memoires de chirurgie militaire. *Chirurgie* 2:303, 1829.

23. Jobert JA: Reflexions sur les places penetrantes du Coeur. *Arch Gen Med* 6:1, 1839.

24. Purple SS: Statistical observations on wounds of the heart, and on their relations to forensic medicine with a table of fourty-two recorded cases. *NY Med* 14:411, 1855.

25. Fischer G: Die Wunden des Herzens und des Hertzbeutels. *Arch Klin Chir* 9:571, 1968.

26. Billroth T: Quoted by Jeger E: Die Chirurgie der Blutgefasse und des Herzens, Berlin, A Hirschwald, 1913, p. 295. As quoted as Beck CS: Wounds of the heart: The technique of suture. *Arch Surg* 13:205, 1926.

27. Billroth T: Cited by Richardson RG, ed. *The scalpel and the Heart.* New York: Scribner, 1970, p. 27.

28. Billroth T: Offenes Schreibner and Herr der Wittelshofer uver die erste mil gustingen susgange ausgefuhrte pylorectomie. *Wiener Med Wochensch* 31:161, 1881.

29. Robert JB: The surgery of the pericardium. *Ann Anat Surg* 4:247, 1881.

30. Block MH: Verhandlunge der Deutchsen Gesselhoff fur Chirurgie. Elfren Congress, Berlin, part I, p. 108, 1882. As quoted by Beck CS: wounds of the heart: The technique of suture. *Arch Surg* 13:205, 1926.

31. Riedinger KV: Verletzungen und Chirurgische Krankheiten des Thorax und seines Inhaltes, Sttutgart, Ferdinand, Enke, 1888, part 42, p. 189. As quoted by Beck CS. Wounds of the heart: The technique of suture. *Arch Surg* 13:205, 1926.

32. Paget S: Surgery of the Chest. Bristol: John Wright & Co, 1896, p. 122.

33. Del Vecchio S: Sutura del cuore. Napoli, Reforma Med, 1985, p. xi, 38. As quoted by Beck CS. Wounds of the Heart: The technique of suture. *Arch Surg* 13:205, 1926.

34. Cappelen A: Vinia cordis, suture of hjertet. Norsk. Mag. F. Laegy; Kristiania, 4, R; xi, 285, 1896. As quoted by Beck CS. Wounds of the heart: The technique of suture. *Arch Surg* 13:205, 1926.

35. Farina G: Discussion. *Centralbl Chir* 23:1224, 1896. As quoted by Beck CS. Wounds of the heart: The technique of suture. Arch Surg 13:225, 1926.

36. Rehn L: Ueber penetrerende herzwunden und herznaht. *Arch Klin Chir* 55:315, 1897.

37. Duval P: Le incision median thoraco-laparotomie. *Bull Mem Soc Chir Paris* 33:15, 1907. As quoted by Ballana C. Bradshaw Lecture: The surgery of the heart. *Lancet* CXCVIII: 73, 1920.

38. Hill LL: A report of case of successful suturing of the heart, and table of 37 other cases of suturing by different operators with various terminations and conclusions drawn. *Med Record* 62:846, 1902. As quoted by Beck CS. Wounds of the heart: The technique of suture. *Arch Surg* 13:205, 1926.

39. Dalton HC: Report of a case of stab wound of the pericardium terminating in recovery after resection of a rib and suture of the pericardium. *Ann Surg* 21:147, 1895.

40. Williams DH: Stab wounds of the heart and pericardium. Recovery – patient alive three years afterward. *Med Rec* 51:437, 1897.

41. Spangaro S: Sulla tecnica da seguire negli interventi chirurgici per ferrite del cuore e su di un nuovo processo di toracotomia. *Clin Chir* 14:227, 1906. As quoted by Beck CS. Wounds of the heart: The technique of suture. *Arch Surg* 13:205, 1926.

42. Sauerbruch F: Uber die Verwendbarkeit der pneumatischen Kammer fur die Herzschirurgie. *Central Chir* 34:44, 1907.

43. Matas R: Surgery of the vascular system. In Keen WW, Da Costa JC, eds. *Surgery, its principles and practice.* Philadelphia: WB Saunders, 1909, p.5.

44. Peck CH: The operative treatment of heart wounds. *Ann Surg* 50:100, 1909.

45. Pool EH: Treatment of heart wounds. *Ann Surg* 55:485, 1912.

46. Smith WR: Cardiorraphy in acute injuries. *Ann Surg* 78:696, 1923.

47. Borchardt E: Sammlung Klin. Leipzig, Vortrage, 1906. N. f. Chir 102–127, p 297 (Nos. 411, 412; Chir 113, 114). As quoted by Peck CH. The operative treatment of heart wounds. *Ann Surg* 50:100, 1909.

48. Schoenfeld H: Heart injuries with suture. *Ann Surg* 87:823, 1928.

49. Bigger IA: Heart wounds: A report of seventeen patients operated upon in the medical College of Virginia Hospitals and discussion of the treatment and prognosis. *J Thorac Surg* 8:239, 1939.

50. Beck C: Further observations on stab wounds of the heart. *Ann Surg* 115:698, 1942.

51. Turner GG: Gunshot wounds of the heart. In Pingh WS, ed. *War medicine,* A Symposium. London: Podolsky Edward, 1942 .

52. Griswold A, Maguire CH: Penetrating wounds of the heart and pericardium. *Surg Gynecol Obstet* 74:406, 1942.

53. Blalock A, Ravitch MM: A consideration of the non operative treatment of cardiac tamponade resulting from wounds of the heart. *Surgery* 157, 1943.

54. Elkin DC: The diagnosis and treatment of cardiac trauma. *Ann Surg* 114:169, 1941.

55. Elkin DC: Wounds of the heart. *Ann Surg* 120:817, 1941.

56. Elkin DC, Campbell RE: Cardiac tamponade: treatment by aspiration. *Ann Surg* 623, 1941.

57. Harken DE: Foreign bodies in, and in relation to the thoracic blood vessels and heart. *Surg Gynecol Obstet* 14;117, 1946.

58. Beall AC, Dietrich EB, Crawford HW: Surgical management of penetrating cardiac injuries. *Am J Surg* 112:686, 1966.

59. Beall AC, Gasior RM, Bricker DL:Gunshot wounds of the heart. Changing patterns of surgical management. *Ann Thorac Surg* 11:523, 1971.

60. Beall AC, Morris GC, Cooley DA: Temporary cardiopulmonary bypass in the management of penetrating wounds of the heart. *Surgery* 52:330, 1962.

61. Beall AC, Oschner JL, Morris GC, et al.: Penetrating wounds of the heart. *J Trauma* 1:195, 1961.

62. Mattox KL, Espada R, Beall AC, et al.: Performing thoracotomy in the emergency center. *J Am Coll Emerg Phys* 3:13, 1974.

63. Mattox KL, Beall AC, Jordan GL, et al.: Cardiorraphy in the emergency center. *J Am Coll Emerg Phys* 68:886, 1974.

64. Mattox KL, Limacher MC, Feliciano DR, et al.: Cardiac evaluation following heart injury. *J Trauma* 25:758, 1985.

65. Feliciano DV, Bitondo CG, Mattox KL, et al.: Civilian trauma in 1980's. A 1-year experience with 456 vascular and cardiac injuries. *Ann Surg* 199:717, 1984.

66. Mattox KL, Feliciano DV, Burch J, et al.: Five thousand seven hundred sixty cardiovascular injuries in 4459 patients. Epidemiologic evolution 1958 to 1987. *Ann Surg* 210:698, 1989.

67. Asensio JA, Murray J, Demetriades D, et al.: Penetrating cardiac injuries: Prospective one year preliminary report; an analysis of variables predicting outcome. *J Am Coll Surg* 186:24, 1998.

68. Asensio JA, Berne JD, Demetriades D, et al.: One hundred and five penetrating cardiac injuries. A two year prospective evaluation. *J Trauma* 44:1073, 1998.

69. Asensio JA, García-Núñez LM, Petrone P, et al.: Penetrating cardiac injuries in America – Predictors of outcome in 2016 patients from the National Trauma Data Bank. In preparation.

70. Asensio JA, Stewart BM, Murray JA, et al.: Penetrating cardiac injuries. *Surg Clin North Am* 76:685, 1996.

71. Rich NM, Spencer FC: Wounds of the heart. In Rich NM, Spencer FC, eds. *Vascular trauma.* Philadelphia, PA: WB Saunders, 1978, p. 384.

72. Hirshberg A, Wall MJ, Allen MK, et al.: Double jeopardy: Thoracoabdominal injuries requiring surgical intervention in both chest and abdomen. *J Trauma* 39:225, 1995.

73. Asensio JA, Arroyo H Jr, Veloz W, et al.: Penetrating thoracoabdominal injuries: Ongoing dilema – Which cavity and when?. *World J Surg* 26:539, 2002.

74. Asensio JA, Petrone P, Costa D, et al.: An evidenced-based critical appraisal of emergency department thoracotomy. *Evidence-Based Surgery* 1:11, 2003.

75. Moreno C, Moore EE, Majure JA, et al.: Pericardial tamponade. A critical determinant for survival following penetrating cardiac wounds. *J Trauma* 26:821, 1986.

76. Buckman RF, Badellino MM, Mauro LH, et al.: Penetrating cardiac wounds: Prospective study of factors influencing initial resuscitation. *J Trauma* 34:717, 1993.

77. Asensio JA, Hanpeter D, Demetriades D, et al.: The futility of the liberal utilization of emergency department thoracotomy. A prospective study. Proceedings of the American Association for the Surgery of Trauma, 58th Annual Meeting, Baltimore, MD, 1998, p. 210.

78. Trinkle JK, Marcos J, Grover FL, et al.: Management of the wounded heart. *Ann Thorac Surg* 17:231, 1974.

79. Arom KV, Richardson JD, Webb G, et al.: Subxiphoid pericardial window in patients with suspected traumatic pericardial tamponade. *Ann Thorac Surg* 23:545, 1977.

80. Trinkle JK, Toon R, Franz JL, et al.: Affairs of the wounded heart: Penetrating cardiac wounds. *J Trauma* 19:467, 1978.

81. Garrison RN, Richardson JD, Fry DE: Diagnostic transdiaphragmatic pericardiotomy in thoracoabdominal trauma. *J Trauma* 22:147, 1982.

82. Miller FA, Bond SJ, Shumate CR, et al.: Diagnostic pericardial window: A safe alternative to exploratory thoracotomy for suspected heart injuries. *Arch Surg* 122:605, 1987.

83. Brewster SA, Thirlby RC, Snyder WH: Subxiphoid pericardial window and penetrating cardiac trauma. *Arch Surg* 123:937, 1988.

84. Duncan A, Scalea TM, Sclafani S, et al.: Evaluation of occult cardiac injuries using subxiphoid pericardial window. *J Trauma* 29:955, 1989.

85. Andrade-Alegre R, Mon L: Subxiphoid pericardial window in the diagnosis of penetrating cardiac trauma. *Ann Thorac Surg* 58:1139, 1994.

86. Feigenbaum H: *Echocardiography.* Philadelphia: Lea and Febiger, 1972, p. 141.

87. Feigenbaum H, Waldhausen JA, Hyde LP: Ultrasonic diagnosis of pericardial effusion. *JAMA* 191:107, 1965.

88. Feigenbaum H, Zaky A, Waldhausen JA: Use of ultrasound in the diagnosis of pericardial effusion. *Ann Intern Med* 65:443, 1966.

89. Moss AJ, Bruhn F: The echocardiogram. An ultrasound technique for the detection of pericardial effusion. *N Eng J Med* 274:380, 1996.

90. Goldberg BB, Ostrium BJ, Isard JJ: Ultrasonic determination of pericardial effusion. *JAMA* 202:103, 1967.

91. Horowitz MS, Schultz CS, Stinson EB, et al.: Sensitivity and specificity of echocardiographic diagnosis of pericardial effusion. *Circulation* 50:239, 1974.

92. Weiis JL, Bernardine HB, Hutchins GM, et al.: Two-dimensional echocardiography recognition of myocardial injury in man: comparison with postmortem studies. *Circulation* 63:401, 1981.

93. Miller FA, Seward JB, Gersh BJ, et al.: Two-dimensional echocardiographic findings in cardiac trauma. *Am J Cardiol* 50:1022, 1982.

94. Choo MH, Chia BL, Chia FK, et al.: Penetrating cardiac injuries evaluated by two-dimensional echocardiography. *Am Heart J* 108:417, 1984.

95. Lopez J, Garcia MA, Coma I, et al.: Identification of blood in the pericardial cavity in dogs by two-dimensional echocardiography. *Am J Cardiol* 53:1194, 1984.

96. Hassett A, Moran J, Sabiston DC, et al.: Utility of echocardiography in the management of patients with penetrating missile wounds of the heart. *Am J Cardiol* 7:1151, 1987.

97. Robison RJ, Brown JW, Caldwell R, et al.: Management of asymptomatic intracardiac missiles using echocardiography. *J Trauma* 28:1402, 1988.

98. DePriest W, Barish R, Almquist T, et al.: Echocardiographic diagnosis of acute pericardial effusion in penetrating chest trauma. *Am J Emerg Med* 6:21, 1988.

99. Freshman SP, Wisner D, Weber CJ: 2-D echocardiography: emergent use in the evaluation of precordial trauma. *J Trauma* 31:902, 1991.

100. Jimenez E, Martin M, Krukenkamp I, et al.: Subxiphoid pericardiotomy versus echocardiography: A prospective evaluation of the diagnosis of occult penetrating cardiac injury. *Surgery* 108:676, 1990.

101. Plummer D, Burnette D, Asinger R, et al.: Emergency department echocardiography improves outcome in penetrating cardiac injury. *Ann Emerg Med* 21:709, 1992.

102. Aaland M, Bryan FC, Sherman R: Two-dimensional echocardiogram in hemodynamically stable victims of penetrating precordial trauma. *Am Surg* 60:412, 1994.

103. Meyer D, Jessen M, Grayburn P: Use of echocardiography to detect occult cardiac injury after penetrating thoracic trauma: A prospective study. *J Trauma* 39:902, 1995.

104. Rozycki GS, Schmidt JA, Oschner MG, et al.: The role of surgeon-performed ultrasound in patients with possible penetrating cardiac wounds: A prospective multicenter study. *J Trauma* 45:190, 1998.

105. Rozycki GS, Feliciano DV, Oschner MG, et al.: The role of ultrasound in patients with posible penetrating cardiac wounds: A prospective multicenter study. *J Trauma* 46:543, 1999.

106. Morales CH, Salinas CM, Henao CA, et al.: Thoracoscopic pericardial window and penetrating cardiac trauma. *J Trauma* 42:273, 1997.

107. Zantut FL, Ivatury RR, Smith RS, et al.: Diagnostic and therapeutic laparoscopy in penetrating trauma: A multicenter experience. *J Trauma* 42:825, 1997.

108. Porter JM, Ivatury RR: The role of laparoscopy in penetrating trauma. *Semin Laparosc Surg* 3:156, 1996.

109. Gervin AS, Fischer RP: The importance of prompt transport in salvage of patients with penetrating heart wounds. *J Trauma* 22:443, 1982.

110. Mattox KL, Feliciano DV: Role of external cardiac compression in truncal trauma. J Trauma 22:934, 1982.

111. Lorenz PH, Steinmetz B, Lieberman J, et al.: Emergency thoracotomy: Survival correlates with physiologic status. *J Trauma* 32:780, 1992.

112. Durham LA, Richardson RJ, Wall MJ, et al.: Emergency center thoracotomy: impact of prehospital resuscitation. *J Trauma* 32:775, 1992.

113. Ivatury RR, Nallathambi MN, Roberge RJ, et al.: Penetrating thoracic injuries. Stabilization vs. prompt transport. *J Trauma* 27:1066, 1987.

114. Millham F, Grindlinger G: Survival determinants in patients undergoing emergency room thoracotomy for penetrating chest injury. J Trauma 34:332, 1993.

115. *Advanced Trauma Life Support Manual.* Chicago, Illinois: Committee on Trauma – American College of Surgeons. 7th ed. 2005.

116. Macho JR, Markinson RE, Schecter WP: Cardiac stapling in the management of penetrating injuries of the heart: Rapid control of hemorrhage and decreased risk of personal contamination. *J Trauma* 34:711, 1993.

117. Tavares S, Hankins JR, Moulton AL, et al.: Management of penetrating cardiac injuries: The role of emergency thoracotomy. *Ann Thorac Surg* 38:183, 1984.

118. Schwab CW, Adcock OT, Max MH: Emergency department thoracotomy (EDT): A 26-month experience using an "agonal" protocol. *Am Surg* 52:20, 1986.

119. Asensio JA, Wall MJ Jr, Minei J, et al.: Working Group, Ad Hoc Subcommittee on Outcomes, American College of Surgeons – Committee on Trauma. Practice management guidelines for emergency department thoracotomy. *J Am Coll Surg* 193:303, 2001.

120. Boyd TF, Strieder JW: Immediate surgery for traumatic heart disease. *J Thorac Cardiovasc Surg* 50:305, 1965.

121. Sauer PE, Murdock CE: Immediate surgery for cardiac and great vessel wounds. *Arch Surg* 95:7, 1967.

122. Sugg WL, Rea WJ, Ecker RR, et al.: Penetrating wounds of the heart. *J Thorac Cardiovasc Surg* 56:530, 1968.

123. Yao ST, Vanecko RM, Printen K, et al.: Penetrating wounds of the heart: A review of 80 cases. *Ann Surg* 168:67, 1968.

124. Steichen FM, Dargan EL, Efron G, et al.: A graded approach to the management of penetrating wounds of the heart. *Arch Surg* 103:574, 1971.

125. Borja AR, Randsell HT: Treatment of penetrating gunshot wounds of the chest. *Am J Surg* 122:81, 1971.

126. Carrasquilla C, Wilson RF, Walt AJ, et al.: Gunshot wounds of the heart. *Ann Thorac Surg* 13:208, 1972.

127. Beall AC, Patrick TD, Ikles JE, et al.: Penetrating wounds of the heart: Changing patterns of surgical management. *J Trauma* 12:468, 1972.

128. Bolanowski PS, Swaminathan AP, Neville WE: Aggressive surgical management of penetrating cardiac injuries. *J Thorac Cardiovasc Surg* 66:52, 1973.

129. Harvey JC, Pacifico AD: Primary operative management method of choice for stab wound to the heart. *South Med* 68:149, 1975.

130. Symbas PN, Harlaftis N, Waldo WJ: Penetrating cardiac wounds: A comparison of different therapeutic methods. *Ann Surg* 183:377, 1976.

131. Beach PM, Bognolo D, Hutchinson JE: Penetrating cardiac trauma. Experience with thirty four patients in a hospital without cardiopulmonary bypass capability. *Am J Surg* 131:411, 1976.

132. Asfaw I, Arbulu A: Penetrating wounds of the pericardium and heart. *Surg Clin North Am* 57:37, 1977.

133. Sherman MM, Saini UK, Yardoz MD, et al.: Management of penetrating cardiac wounds. *Am J Surg* 135:553, 1978.

134. Evans J, Gray LA, Payner A, et al.: Principles for the management of penetrating cardiac wounds. *Ann Surg* 189:777, 1979.

135. Breaux EP, Dupont JB, Albert HM, et al.: Cardiac tamponade following penetrating mediastinal injuries: Improved survival with early pericardiocentesis. *J Trauma* 19:461, 1979.

136. Mandal AK, Awariefe SO, Oparah SS: Experience in the management of 50 consecutive penetrating wounds of the heart. *Br J Surg* 66:565, 1979.

137. Demetriades D, Vander Veen BW: Penetrating injuries of the heart: Experience over two years in South Africa. *J Trauma* 23:1034, 1983.

138. Demetriades D: Cardiac penetrating injuries: Personal experience of 45 cases. *Br J Surg* 71:95, 1984.

139. Demetriades D: Cardiac wounds. Experience with 70 patients. *Ann Surg* 203:315, 1986.

140. Jebara VA, Saade B: Penetrating wounds to the heart: A wartime experience. *Ann Thorac Surg* 47:250, 1989.

141. Attar S, Suter CM, Hankins JR, et al.: Penetrating cardiac injuries. *Ann Thorac Surg* 51:711, 1991.

142. Knott-Craig CJ, Dalton RP, Rossouw GJ, et al.: Penetrating cardiac trauma: Management strategy based on 129 surgical emergencies over 2 years. *Ann Thorac Surg* 53:1006, 1992.

143. Buchman TG, Phillips J, Menker JB: Recognition, resuscitation and management of patients with penetrating cardiac injuries. *Surg Gynecol Obstet* 174:205, 1992.
144. Benyan AKZ, Al-A'Ragy HH: The pattern of penetrating cardiac trauma on Basrah province: Personal experience with seventy-two cases in a hospital without cardiopulmonary bypass facility. *Int Surg* 77:111, 1992.
145. Mitchell ME, Muakkassa FF, Poole GV, et al.: Surgical approach of choice for penetrating cardiac wounds. *J Trauma* 34:17, 1993.
146. Kaplan AJ, Norcross ED, Crawford FA: Predictors of mortality in penetrating cardiac injury. *Am Surg* 59:338, 1993.
147. Henderson VJ, Smith SR, Fry WR, et al.: Cardiac injuries: Analysis of an unselected series of 251 cases. *J Trauma* 36:341, 1994.
148. Coimbra R, Pinto MCC, Razuk A, et al.: Penetrating cardiac wounds: Predictive value of trauma indices and the necessity of terminology standardization. *Am Surg* 61:448, 1995.
149. Arreola-Risa C, Rhee P, Boyle EM, et al.: Factors influencing outcome in stab wounds of the heart. *Am J Surg* 169:553, 1995.
150. Karmy-Jones R, Van Wijngaarden MH, Talwar MK, et al.: Penetrating cardiac injuries. *Injury* 28:57, 1997.
151. Rhee PM, Foy H, Kaufman C, et al.: Penetrating cardiac injuries: A population based study. *J Trauma* 45:366, 1998.
152. Tyburski JG, Astra L, Wilson RF, et al.: Factors affecting prognosis with penetrating wounds of the heart. *J Trauma* 48:587, 2000.
153. Trinkle JK: Penetrating heart wounds: Difficulty in evaluating clinical series. *Ann Thorac Surg* 38:181, 1994.
154. Grabowski MW, Buckman RF, Goldberg A, et al.: Clamp control of the right ventricle angle to facilitate exposure and repair of cardiac wounds. *Am J Surg* 170:399, 1995.
155. Waterworth PD, Musleh G, Greenhalgh D, et al.: Innovative use of Octopus IV Stabilizer in cardiac trauma. *Ann Thorac Surg* 80:1108, 2005.
156. Wall MJ Jr, Mattox KL, Chen C, et al.: Acute management of complex cardiac injuries. *J Trauma* 42:905, 1997.
157. Ivatury RR, Rohman M, Steichen FM, et al.: Penetrating cardiac injuries: Twenty year experience. *Am Surg* 53:310, 1987.
158. Moore EE, Malangoni MA, Cogbill TH, et al.: Organ injury scaling IV: Thoracic, vascular, lung, cardiac and diaphragm. *J Trauma* 36:299, 1994.
159. Espada R, Wisennand HH, Mattox KL, et al.: Surgical management of penetrating injuries to the coronary arteries. *Surgery* 78:755, 1875.
160. Ivatury RR, Shah PM, et al.: Emergency Room Thoracotomy for the resuscitation of patients with "fatal" penetrating injuries of the heart. *Ann Thorac Surg* 32:377, 1981.
161. Bodai BI, Smith P, Ward RE, et al.: Emergency thoracotomy in the management of trauma: A review. *JAMA* 249:1981, 1983.
162. Rohman M, Ivatury R, Steichen F, et al.: Emergency room thoracotomy for penetrating cardiac injuries. *J Trauma* 23:570, 1983.
163. Thourani VH, Feliciano DV, Cooper WA, et al.: Penetrating cardiac trauma at an urban trauma center: A 22-year perspective. *Am Surg* 65:811, 1999.
164. Gonzalez RP, Luterman A: Reviewer summary of "Rhee PM, Foy H, Kaufman C, et al.: Penetrating cardiac injuries: A population based study. *J Trauma* 45:366, 1998." *Current Surgery* 58:173, 2001.
165. Gonzalez RP, Luterman A: Reviewer summary of "Thourani VH, Feliciano DV, Cooper WA, et al.: Penetrating cardiac trauma at an urban trauma center: A 22-year perspective. *Am Surg* 65:811, 1999." *Current Surgery* 58:177, 2001.
166. Akenside M: An account of a blow upon the heart and its effects. *Philosophical Transact* 53:353, 1764.
167. Osborn LR: Findings in 262 fatal accidents. *Lancet* 2:277, 1943.
168. Urbach J: Die Verletzungen des Herzens durch stumple Gewalt. Beitr. *Ger Med* 4:653, 1940.
169. Warburg E: *Traumatic Heart Lesions.* 1st ed. Humphrey Milford, London: Oxford University Press, 1938.
170. Kissane RW: Non-penetrating cardiac injury. *Circulation* 6:109, 1952.
171. Glendy RE, White PD: Non penetrating wound of the heart. Rupture of the papillary muscle and contusion of heart resulting from external violence: Case report. *Am Heart J* 11:366, 1936.
172. Leinoff HD: Direct non-penetrating injuries of the heart. *Ann Int Med* 14:653, 1940.
173. Bright EF, Beck CS: Non penetrating wounds of the heart: A clinical and experimental study. *Am Heart J* 10:293, 1935.
174. Parmley LF, Manion WC, Mattingly TW: Non penetrating traumatic injury of the heart. *Circulation* 18:371, 1958.
175. Beck CS: Contusions of the heart. *JAMA* 104:109, 1935.
176. Newman PG, Feliciano DV: Blunt cardiac Injury. *New Horizons* 7:26, 1999.
177. Tenzer ML: The spectrum of myocardial contusion: A review. *J Trauma* 25:620, 1985.
178. Sutherland GR, Calvin JE, Driedger AA, et al.: Anatomic and cardiopulmonary responses to trauma with associated blunt chest injury. *J Trauma* 21:1, 1981.
179. Frazee RC, Mucha P Jr, Farnell MB, et al.: Objective evaluation of blunt cardiac trauma. *J Trauma* 226:510, 1986.
180. Hossack KF, Moreno CA, Van Way CW, et al.: Frequency of cardiac contusion in nonpenetrating chest injury. *Am J Cardiol* 61:391, 1988.
181. Potkin RT, Werner JA, Trobaugh GB, et al.: Evaluation of noninvasive tests of cardiac damage in suspected cardiac contusion. *Circulation* 66:625, 1982.
182. Kettunen P: Cardiac damage after blunt chest trauma, diagnosed using CK-MB enzyme and electrocardiogram. *Int J Cardiol* 6:355, 1984.
183. Anderson AE, Doyt DB: Cardiac trauma: An experimental model of isolated myocardial contusion. *J Trauma* 15:237, 1975.
184. Cachecho R, Grindlinger GA, Lee VW: The clinical significance of myocardial contusion. *J Trauma* 33:68, 1992.
185. Biffl WL, Moore FA, Moore EE, et al.: Cardiac enzymes are irrelevant in the patient with suspected myocardial contusion. *Am J Surg* 169:523, 1994.
186. Katus HA, Remppis A, Diederich KW, et al.: Serum concentration changes of cardiac troponin T in patients with acute myocardial infarction. *J Mol Cell Cardiol* 21:1349, 1989.
187. Katus HA, Remppis A, Neumann FJ, et al.: Diagnostic efficiency of troponin T measurements in acute myocardial infarction. *Circulation* 83:902, 1991.
188. Adams JE III, Bodor GS, Davilla-Roman VG, et al.: Cardiac troponin I. A marker with high specificity for cardiac injury. *Circulation* 88:101, 1988.
189. Adams JE III, Davila-Roman VG, Bassey PQ, et al.: Improved detection of cardiac contusion with cardiac troponin I. *Am Heart J* 131:308, 1996.
190. Fulda GJ, Giberson F, Hailstone D, et al.: An evaluation of serum troponin T and signal averaged electrocardiography in predicting electrocardiographic abnormalities after blunt chest trauma. *J Trauma* 43:304, 1997.
191. Salim A, Velmahos GC, Jindal A, et al.: Clinically significant blunt cardiac trauma. Role of serum troponin levels combined with electrocardiographic findings. *J Trauma* 50:237, 2001.
192. Bertinchant JP, Polge A, Mohty D, et al.: Evaluation of incidence, clinical significance, and prognostic value of circulating cardiac troponin I and T elevation in hemodynamically stable patients with suspected myocardial contusion after blunt chest trauma. *J Trauma* 48:924, 2000.
193. Hiatt JR, Yeatman LA Jr, Child JS: The value of echocardiography in blunt chest trauma. *J Trauma* 28:914, 1988.
194. Reid CL, Kawanishi DT, Rahimtoola SH, et al.: Chest trauma: Evaluation by two-dimensional echocardiography. *Am Heart J* 971, 1987.
195. King MR, Mucha P Jr, Seward JB, et al.: Cardiac contusion: A new diagnostic approach utilizing two-dimensional echocardiography. *J Trauma* 23:610, 1983.
196. Dubrow TJ, Mihalka J, Eisenhauer DM, et al.: Myocardial contusion in the stable patient: What level of care is appropriate?. *Surgery* 106:267, 1989.
197. Fulda G, Brathwaite CEM, Rodriguez A, et al.: Blunt traumatic rupture of the heart and pericardium: A ten-year experience (1979–1989). *J Trauma* 31:167, 1991.
198. Perchinsky MJ, Long WB, Hill JG: Blunt cardiac rupture. The Emanuel Trauma Center Experience. *Arch Surg* 130:852, 1995.
199. Hewett P: Rupture of the heart and large vessels: The result of injuries. *Lond Med Gaz* 1:870, 1847.
200. Guilfoil P, Doyle JT: Traumatic cardiac septal defect: Report of case in which diagnosis is established by cardiac catheterization. *J Thorac Surg* 25:510, 1953.
201. Calhoon JH, Hoffmann TH, Trinkle K, et al.: Management of blunt rupture of the heart. *J Trauma* 26:495, 1986.
202. Brathwaite CEM, Rodriguez A, Turney SZ, et al.: Blunt traumatic cardiac rupture. *Ann Surg* 212:701, 1990.
203. Türk EE, Tsokos M: Blunt cardiac trauma caused by fatal falls from height: An autopsy-based assessment of the injury pattern. *J Trauma* 57:301, 2004.
204. Martin TD, Flynn JC, Rowlands BJ: Blunt cardiac rupture. *J Trauma* 24:287, 1984.
205. Mayfield W, Hurley EJ: Blunt cardiac trauma. *Am J Surg* 148:162, 1984.
206. Shorr RM, Crittenden M, et al.: Blunt thoracic trauma. *Ann Surg* 206:200, 1987.
207. Santavirta S, Arajarvi E: Ruptures of the heart in seatbelt wearers. *J Trauma* 32:275, 1992.
208. DesForges O, Ridder WP, Lenoci RJ: Successful suture of ruptured myocardium after nonpenetrating injury. *N Eng J Med* 25:567, 1955.
209. Mattox KL, Flint LM, Carrico CJ, et al.: Blunt cardiac injury (Editorial). *J Trauma* 33:649, 1992.
210. Civetta J (discussion of Cachecho R, Grindlinger GA, Lee VW). The clinical significance of myocardial contusion. *J Trauma* 38:68, 1992.
211. Pasquale M, Fabian TC, EAST Ad Hoc Committee on Practice Management Guideline Development. Practice management guidelines for trauma from the Eastern Association for the Surgery of Trauma. *J Trauma* 44:941, 1998.

# Commentary ■ RAUL COIMBRA

Penetrating cardiac injuries remain a formidable challenge to trauma surgeons. In civilian practice, most cardiac injuries are caused either by stab or low-velocity handguns.

Cardiac wounds account for approximately 10% of all deaths following assaults with firearms.[1] Most patients sustaining penetrating injury to the heart die before hospital admission. However, with the development of better prehospital services and shorter transport times, patients that in the past would have died otherwise, are reaching the hospital alive but in critical clinical condition.

The mortality rate following penetrating cardiac wounds varies from 8.5% to 81.3%.[2–4] This variability is likely related to heterogeneity in patient's clinical condition upon admission and lack of standardization of clinical classification as it pertains to study inclusion criteria.

Causes of death are multifactorial, and include, but are not limited to, the mechanism of injury, hemodynamic status upon admission, location and the number of injuries in the heart, presence of associated injuries, promptness of diagnosis and management, and presence of cardiac tamponade.

The issue of the diagnosis of pericardial tamponade and whether or not pericardial tamponade saves lives is an important one. Early diagnosis of pericardial tamponade is important to prevent myocardial ischemia and death due to poor filling pressures and consequently, low cardiac output. Beck's Triad has been considered the hallmark of pericardial tamponade. In cardiac trauma it is the exception rather than the rule.

We tend to forget things that we do not see everyday. With the overall decrease in penetrating mechanisms, the challenge is to avoid missing the diagnosis of blood in the pericardium. Therefore, a high index of suspicion is necessary for timely diagnosis and management of pericardial tamponade and heart injury. The first step is to consider that all patients presenting with a penetrating injury to the chest, upper back, and thoraco-abdominal region have sustained a cardiac injury until proven otherwise. The second step is to objectively rule it out with sonography preferentially, or with pericardial window if sonography is not available. Rationalizing that a patient sustaining a penetrating injury to the chest, who was stable or transiently hypotensive, without a significant hemothorax or pneumothorax, does not need further investigation of the pericardial sac will only delay diagnosis and will certainly affect the outcome.

When diagnosed before decompensation occurs, pericardial tamponade is thought to be life-saving. However, as described in this chapter, not all studies found pericardial tamponade to be a predictor of survival. A possible explanation to these differences may be due to the lack of studies determining the exact moment after which the beneficial tamponade effect becomes deleterious and compromised cardiac function.

Although most centers have sonography available, trauma surgeons should know how to perform a pericardial window. A trans-diaphragmatic pericardial window becomes important in the patient with multiple penetrating wounds who becomes or remains unstable after bleeding has been controlled during an exploratory laparotomy.

Rapid diagnosis and treatment is of utmost importance in the outcome of patients with cardiac wounds. The utility of an operating room resuscitation protocol has been documented by our group in San Diego.[5] We have recently also demonstrated that resuscitation in the operating room positively affects survival of patients with abdominal aortic injuries, suggesting that shortening the time from admission to operative bleeding control is critical in decreasing mortality.[6]

The impact of time from admission to operation on mortality has been well documented. In one study, 67% of the patients where brought to the operating room within 30 minutes after admission, 22% within 6 hours, and 11% after 6 hours. The mortality rate comparing those operated on within 30 minutes and after 30 minutes was 38% and 72%, respectively.[7]

Since the study published by Bickell et al.,[8] there has been increased awareness about the concept of "popping the clot" with aggressive fluid resuscitation. This is perhaps an area in which improvements could be made. There is no debate that agonal patients or those in extremis require vigorous fluid resuscitation and immediate operation. On the other hand, infusing two liters of crystalloid solution in stable or slightly hypotensive patients with penetrating chest wounds who do not have significant pneumothorax or hemothorax on chest x-ray before fluid in the pericardium is ruled out is dangerous and may precipitate sudden decompensation and death.

The surgical principles in the management of cardiac wounds were clearly described in this chapter. The routine use of pledgets is a matter of personal preference. We have used pledgets selectively but we always use mattress U stitches instead of simple suture. One additional adjunct maneuver may be of utility in the management of posterior heart wounds. We have applied a figure-of-eight Prolene stitch to the apex of the heart leaving both arms of the Prolene suture long enough so to apply some degree of traction and superior displacement of the heart. This strategy avoids the dangerous and excessive angulation of the major vessels as one tries to "flip" the heart over to look at its posterior aspect, allowing the surgeon to inspect the posterior heart without using his/her hands and without excessive movement.

The problems with the diagnosis and initial management of patients with suspected blunt cardiac injuries were well presented by Asensio Garcia-Núñez, and Petrone in the present chapter. The most frequent arrhythmia seen in these patients is sinus tachycardia. In our opinion, the most challenging issue is to decide when and for how long one has to be monitored when the initial EKG reveals sinus tachycardia. In face of the right mechanism of injury, measurement of serum troponin levels is the next step. If the patient remains tachycardic after the initial resuscitation and troponin levels are elevated we routinely monitor the cardiac rhythm for at least 12 hours.

# References

1. Ivatury RR: Injury to the heart. In Feliciano DV, Moore EE, Mattox, KL, eds. *Trauma*. 3rd ed. Connecticut: Appleton & Lange, 1996, p. 409.

2. Asensio JA, Berne JD, Demetriades D, et al.: One hundred five penetrating cardiac injury: A 2-year prospective evaluation. *J Trauma* 44:1073, 1998.

3. Asensio JA, Murray J, Demetriades D, et al.: Penetrating cardiac injuries: A prospective study of variables predicting outcomes. *J Am Coll Surg* 186:24, 1998.

4. Coimbra R, Pinto MCC, Razuk A, et al.: Penetrating cardiac wounds: Predictive value of trauma indices and the necessity of terminology standardization. *Am Surg* 61:448, 1995.

5. Steele JT, Hoyt DB, Simons RK, et al.: Is operating room resuscitation a way to save time? *Am J Surg* 174:683, 1997.

6. Deree J, Shenvi E, Fortlage D, et al.: Patient factors and operating room resuscitation predict mortality in traumatic abdominal aortic injury. A 20-year analysis. *J Vasc Surg* 45:493, 2007.

7. Campbell NC, Thomson SR, Muckart DJJ, et al.: Review of 1198 cases of penetrating cardiac trauma. *Br J Surg* 84:1737, 1997.

8. Bickell WH, Wall MJ, Pepe PE, et al.: Immediate versus delayed fluid resuscitation for hypotensive patients with penetrating torso injuries. *N Engl J Med* 331:1105, 1994.

# Thoracic Great Vessel Injury

*Kenneth L. Mattox* ■ *Matthew J. Wall, Jr.* ■ *Scott Lemaire*

Injuries to the thoracic great vessels—the aorta and its brachio-cephalic branches, the pulmonary arteries and veins, the superior and intrathoracic inferior vena cava, and the innominate and azygos veins—occur following both blunt and penetrating trauma. Exsanguinating hemorrhage, the primary acute manifestation, also occurs in the chronic setting when the injured great vessel forms a fistula involving an adjacent structure or when a posttraumatic aneurysm or pseudoaneurysm ruptures.

Vesalius, in 1557, reported a patient who died of a ruptured aorta after being thrown from a horse.[1] Dfhanelidze[2] repaired a puncture wound of the ascending aorta in 1922. Thirty years later, Bahnson[3] reported an aneurysmorrhaphy for a patient with a chronic posttraumatic thoracic aortic aneurysm. DeBakey and Cooley successfully resected a posttraumatic thoracic aneurysm and replaced the aorta with a graft in 1954. As reported by Passaro in 1959, the first successful primary repair of an acute traumatic thoracic aortic injury was accomplished in 1958 by Klassen.

Our current knowledge regarding the treatment of injured thoracic great vessels has been derived primarily from experience with civilian injuries. Since Rich and Spencers' 1978 review of the fewer than 20 successful repairs reported in the English literature, great vessel injuries have been repaired with increasing frequency, a phenomenon that has paralleled the development of techniques for elective surgery of the thoracic aorta and its major branches.

The following issues have dominated the publications and presentation relating to thoracic great vessel injury since the last edition of this book:

- Better understanding of SCREENING methods versus DIAGNOSIS of acute thoracic great vessel injury

- Focus on priorities relating to concomitant injury versus the thoracic great vessel injury

- Support for purposeful delay in treatment of stable patients

- Continuing interest in the evaluation of intraluminal stented grafts as a therapeutic option and cautions relating to routine use.

A detailed description of thoracic vascular anatomy is beyond the purpose of this chapter. However, a detailed understanding of normal and variant anatomy and structural relationships is mandatory for the surgeon and any one who is a consultant to the surgeon in the evaluation of imaging studies. Venous anomalies are infrequent with the most common being absence of the left innominate vein and persistent left superior vena cava. Thoracic aortic arch anomalies are relatively common and only diagnosed with accuracy by thoracic aortography (Table 29-1). Knowledge of such anomalies is essential in open and catheter based therapies.

## ETIOLOGY AND PATHOPHYSIOLOGY

More than 90% of thoracic great vessel injuries are due to penetrating trauma: gunshot, shrapnel, and stab wounds or therapeutic misadventures.[4] Iatrogenic lacerations of various thoracic great vessels, including the arch of the aorta, are frequently reported complications of percutaneous central venous catheter placement. The percutaneous placement of "trocar" chest tubes has caused injuries to the intercostal arteries and major pulmonary and mediastinal vessels. Intra-aortic counter pulsation balloons can produce injury to the thoracic aorta. During emergency center resuscitative thoracotomy, the aorta may be injured during cross clamping if a crushing (nonvascular) clamp is used. Over inflation of the Swan-Ganz balloon has produced iatrogenic injuries to pulmonary artery branches with resultant fatal hemoptysis; therefore, once a linear relationship has been established between the pulmonary artery diastolic pressure and the pulmonary capillary wedge pressure, further "wedging" is an unnecessary and dangerous practice. Self-expanding metal stents have recently produced perforations of the aorta and innominate artery following placement into the esophagus and trachea, respectively.[5]

The great vessels particularly susceptible to injury from blunt trauma include the innominate artery, pulmonary veins, vena cava, and, most commonly, the thoracic aortic.[6,7] Aortic injuries have

**TABLE 29-1**

### Thoracic Aortic Anomalies

Common origin of innominate and left carotid arteries ("bovine arch")
Ductus diverticulum
Persistent left ductus arterioisus
Aorto-pulmonary window
Takeoff of the right subclavian artery from the descending thoracic aorta
Dextroposition of the thoracic aorta
Coarctation of thoracic aorta
Origin of left vertebral artery off the aortic arch
Pseudocoarction of the thoracic aorta ("kinked aorta")
Double aortic arch
Right ductus arteriosus
Persistent truncus arteriosus
Cervical aortic arch (persistent complete third aortic arch)
Absence of the internal carotid artery
Cardio-aortic fistula

caused or contributed to 10–15% of deaths following motor vehicle accidents for nearly 50 years. These injuries usually involve the proximal descending aorta (54–65% of cases), but often involve other segments—i.e., the ascending aorta or transverse aortic arch (10–14%) and the mid- or distal descending thoracic aorta (12%) or multiple sites (13–18%). The postulated mechanisms of blunt great vessel injury include (1) shear forces caused by relative mobility of a portion of the vessel adjacent to a fixed portion, (2) compression of the vessel between bony structures, and (3) profound intraluminal hypertension during the severe traumatic event. The atrial attachments of the pulmonary veins and vena cava and the fixation of the descending thoracic aorta at the ligamentum arteriosum and diaphragm enhance their susceptibility to blunt rupture by the first mechanism. At its origin, the innominate artery may be "pinched" between the sternum and the vertebrae during anterior sternal impact.

Blunt aortic injuries may be partial thickness—histologically similar to the initial tear in aortic dissection—but most commonly full thickness and therefore equivalent to a ruptured aortic aneurysm that is contained by surrounding tissues. The histopathological similarities between aortic injuries and nontraumatic aortic catastrophes mandate that similar therapeutic approaches be employed. Therefore, in hemodynamically stable patients, the concepts of permissive hypovolemia and aggressive minimization of $dP/dT$—which are widely accepted in the treatment of aortic dissection and aneurysm rupture—should be considered in patients with blunt aortic injuries. In opposition to patients with aortic intimal disease where the adventitia is the restraining barrier, with blunt injury to the descending thoracic aorta, it is the intact parietal pleura (not the aventitia) that contains the hematoma and precludes a massive hemothorax.

True traumatic aortic dissection, with a longitudinal separation of the media extending along the length of the aorta, is extremely rare.[8] The use of the term "dissection" in the setting of aortic trauma should be equally rare, being used only in appropriate cases. Similarly, the terms "aortic transection" and "blunt aortic rupture" should be used only when describing specific injuries, i.e., full thickness lacerations involving either the entire or partial circumference, respectively.

Increasingly, patients with thoracic great vessel injury have associated head, abdominal, and extremity injury. Often preexisting medical conditions are present, such as diabetes, hypertension, coronary artery disease, or cirrhosis. Often patients who present themselves are on a large variety of medication, often aspirin, coumadin, or Plavix. These interfere with the clotting mechanism and adaptations in treatment must be made.

## PATIENT CLASSIFICATION

Three distinctly different groups of patients with thoracic aortic trauma exist (Table 29-2). The epidemiology of aortic injury is changing, due to rapid accident notification and emergency medical system (EMS) transport. The mortality statistics reveal that those whose cause of death is exsanguinating hemorrhage almost all die within the first 0–2 hours of injury. Those who die in the emergency department, operating room, or intensive care unit (ICU) within two to four hours of injury often have extensive multisystem injury with hemorrhage often being from sites other than the thoracic aorta. Hemodynamically stable patients who are subsequently found to have aortic injury, but who die, most often have central nervous system injury as the cause of their injury. It is this later group in whom the diagnosis is made by the trauma team, and therefore amenable to appropriate screening, diagnostic, and therapeutic considerations.

## INITIAL EVALUATION

### Prehospital Management

Interventions often performed by paramedics during transport include judicious intravenous fluid administration and endotracheal intubation when indicated.[9] Military Anti-Shock Trousers (MAST) application in patients with thoracic great vessel injuries statistically increases the chance of death in both adult and pediatric populations.[10–11] The MAST elevate blood pressure by increasing afterload and are equivalent to placing a cross-clamp distal to the potential injury—a clearly counterproductive maneuver. Similarly,

**TABLE 29-2**

### Groups of Patients with Thoracic Aortic Injury

| GROUP | DESCRIPTION | TIME TO DIAGNOSIS | LOCATION OF DEATH | MORTALILTY | CAUSE OF DEATH |
|---|---|---|---|---|---|
| 1 | Dead/dying at scene | <60 min | Scene/EMS | 100% | Bleeding |
| 2 | Unstable during transport | 1–6 h | EMS/EC | >96% | Multisystem trauma |
| 3 | Stable | 4–18 h | ICU | 5–30% | CNS injury |

in patients with acute thoracic great vessel injuries, excessive fluid resuscitation with the goal of increasing blood pressure to normal or supernormal levels increases the incidence of mortality, ARDS, and other postoperative complications.[12]

## Emergency Center Evaluation

History.    In cases of penetrating thoracic trauma, information regarding the length of a knife, the firearm type and number of rounds fired, and the patient's distance from the firearm—although not always reliable—is important to obtain from the patient or accompanying persons.

Although the head-on automobile collision is often considered the typical mechanism for blunt aortic injury, recent epidemiological data reveal that up to 50% of cases occur following side-impact collisions. Blunt aortic injuries have also been reported following equestrian accidents, blast injuries, auto-pedestrian accidents, crush injuries, and falls from heights of 30 ft or more.[13]

In addition to information involving the mechanism of injury, the emergency transport personnel can provide medical information important in evaluating the potential for a thoracic great vessel injury, such as the amount of hemorrhage at the accident scene, any history of intermittent paralysis following the accident, and hemodynamic instability during transport.

Physical Examination.    Upon arrival to the emergency center, each patient is given a rapid, thorough examination. External signs of penetrating or blunt trauma are noted. With an intrapericardial vascular injury, the classic signs of pericardial tamponade (distended neck veins, pulsus paradoxus, muffled heart sounds, elevated central venous pressure) may be present. Clinical findings associated with thoracic great vessel injury include:

1. Hypotension
2. Upper extremity hypertension
3. Unequal blood pressures or pulses in the extremities (upper extremity from innominate or subclavian injury, or lower extremity from pseudocoarctation syndrome)
4. External evidence of major chest trauma (e.g., steering wheel imprint on chest)
5. Expanding hematoma at the thoracic outlet
6. Intrascapular murmur
7. Palpable fracture of the sternum
8. Palpable fracture of the thoracic spine
9. Left flail chest

Chest Radiography.    Upon arrival, a supine antero-posterior 36-inch chest radiograph should be performed, ideally in the emergency center and not in a distant radiologic suite. Emergency physicians, radiologists, and surgeons should develop diagnostic experience viewing supine portable chest x-rays as many trauma patients are hemodynamically unstable or have suspected spinal injuries, making an "upright" 72-inch posterior-anterior chest radiograph unsafe. In many cases of great vessel injury, the radiologic findings are sufficient to warrant immediate arteriography or direct transport to the operating room.

For penetrating injuries, it is important to place radiopaque markers to identify the entrance and exit sites. Radiographic findings which suggest penetrating thoracic great vessel injury include:

1. Large hemothorax
2. Foreign bodies (bullets or shrapnel) or their trajectories in proximity to the great vessels
3. A foreign body out of focus with respect to the remaining radiograph, which may indicate its intracardiac location (Fig. 29-1)
4. A trajectory with a confusing course, which may indicate a migrating intravascular bullet (Fig. 29-2)
5. "Missing" missile in a patient with a gunshot wound to the chest, suggesting distal embolization in the arterial tree.

Several radiographic findings have been associated with blunt injuries of the descending thoracic aorta (Table 29-3). The most reliable of these signs is the loss of the aortic knob contour, creating a "funny looking mediastinum." Mediastinal widening at the thoracic outlet and leftward tracheal deviation are suggestive of innominate artery injury. These signs are secondary to a mediastinal hematoma, which is an indirect sign of thoracic great vessel injury. The presence of any of these signs is a positive screening test and not a diagnosis.

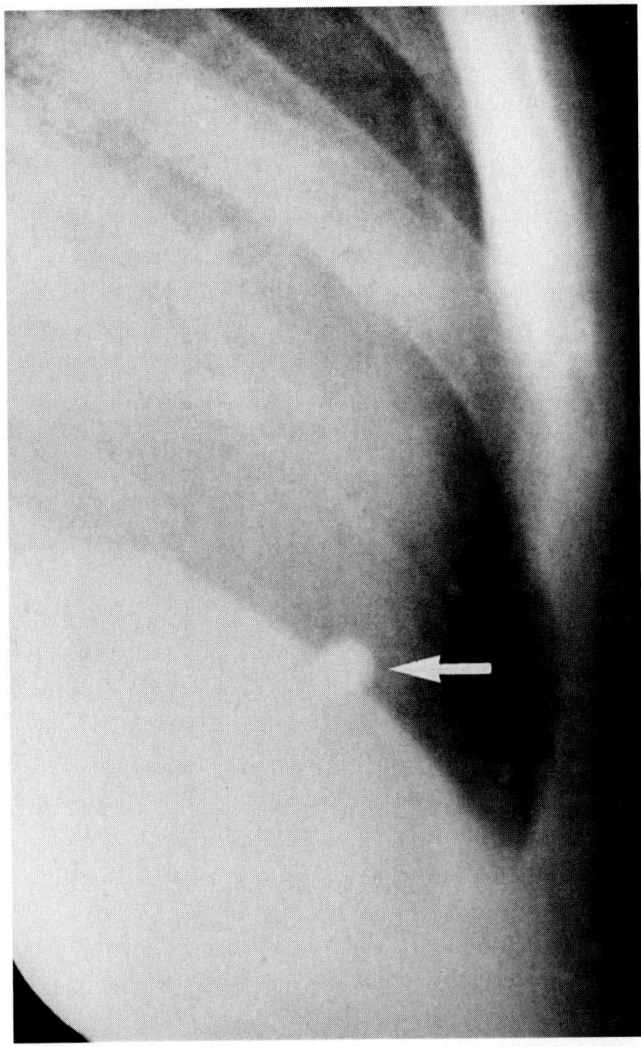

**FIGURE 29-1.** Lateral chest x-ray demonstrating an "out of focus" bullet over the cardiac silhouette. The bullet was lodged in the wall of the right ventricle.

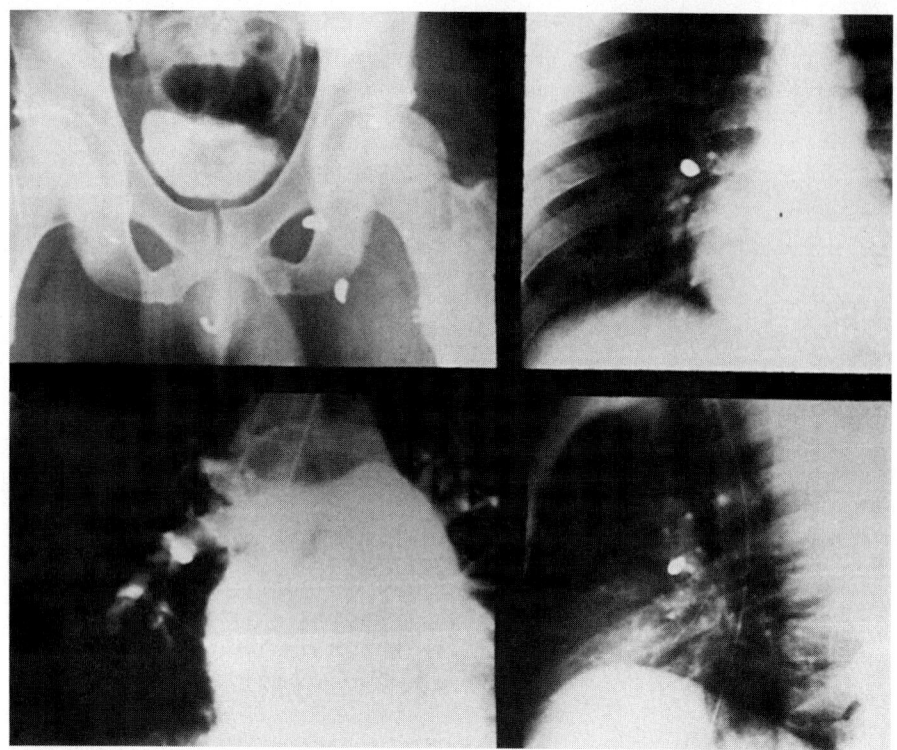

**FIGURE 29-2.** Series of x-rays demonstrating the entrance site of a bullet in the left groin. The bullet embolized to the right pulmonary artery, as confirmed by arteriography.

Missile wounds which appear to traverse the mediastinum create concern regarding injury to the heart, esophagus, trachea, spinal cord, or major vasculature. Should cardiac or vascular injury occur, tamponade or major hemorrhage is usually obvious. A spiral computed tomography (CT) has been proposed to demonstrate missile trajectory and aid the surgeon in a decision regarding thoracotomy or endoscopy.

### TABLE 29-3

**Radiographic Clues That Should Prompt Suspicion of a Thoracic Great Vessel Injury**

**Fractures**
- Sternum
- Scapula
- Multiple left ribs
- Clavicle in multisystem injured patients
- (?) First rib

**Mediastinal Clues**
- Obliteration of aortic knob contour (Fig. 29-3)
- Widening of the mediastinum >8 cm (Fig. 29-4)
- Depression of the left mainstem bronchus >140° from trachea
- Loss of perivertebral pleural stripe
- Calcium layering at aortic knob
- "Funny-looking" mediastinum
- Deviation of nasogastric tube in the esophagus (Fig. 29-5)
- Lateral displacement of the trachea

**Lateral Chest X-ray**
- Anterior displacement of the trachea
- Loss of the aortic/pulmonary window

**Other Findings**
- Apical pleural hematoma
- Massive left hemothorax
- Obvious blunt injury to the diaphragm

## Initial Treatment and Screening

**Emergency Center Thoracotomy.** Emergency center thoracotomy in patients presenting with signs of life and hemodynamic collapse (Chap. 15) may reveal injuries to major thoracic vessels. These injuries require temporizing maneuvers which gain rapid control of bleeding, allowing resuscitation, and subsequent transfer to the operating room for definitive repair.[14] Subclavian vessel injuries, for example, can be controlled by packing or clamping at the thoracic apex or inserting large balloon catheters. Major hemorrhage from the pulmonary hilum can be temporally managed by cross-clamping the entire hilum proximally or twisting the lung 180° after releasing the inferior pulmonary ligament.

**Tube Thoracotomy.** When the chest radiograph indicates a significant hemothorax, the chest tube should be connected to a repository for autotransfusion. An initial "rush" of a large volume of blood (>1500 mL) or significant ongoing hemorrhage (>200 to 250 mL per hour) may indicate great vessel injury, and are considered indications for urgent thoracotomy (Chap. 25).

**Intravenous Access and Fluid Administration.** Currently, unless a patient is in extremis, large bore intravenous portals are avoided, until the time of an operation. If a subclavian venous catheter is required in a patient with a suspected subclavian vascular injury, the contralateral side should be used for cannulation.

The treatment of severe shock should include blood transfusion. However, rapid infusions of excessive volumes of either blood or crystalloid solutions prior to operation may increase the blood pressure to a point that a protective soft perivascular clot is "blown-out" and fatal exsanguinating hemorrhage ensues. The principles of permitting moderate hypotension (systolic blood pressure of 60 to 90 mmHg) and limiting fluid administration until achieving operative control of bleeding are cornerstones in the management of rupturing abdominal aortic aneurysms and *must* equally apply to acute thoracic great vessel injury. Aggressive preoperative fluid resuscitation increases postoperative respiratory complications and may contribute to an increased mortality when compared to fluid restriction.[12] With both penetrating and blunt chest trauma, associated pulmonary contusions are common and provide additional rationale for limiting the infusion of preoperative crystalloid solutions.

### Beta-blockade.

The pharmacologic reduction of $dP/dT$ has remained a critical component of the treatment of aortic dissection since its original description by Wheat et al. in 1965.[15] Based on the histopathologic similarity between aortic dissection and blunt aortic injury, this principle was first applied to $dP/dT$ reduction to patients with the latter condition in 1970. Subsequent reports have described using beta-blockers in hemodynamically stable patients who had proven blunt aortic injuries but required a delay in definitive operative treatment.[16,17] Some centers routinely begin beta-blocker therapy as soon as an aortic injury is suspected—prior to obtaining diagnostic studies—to reduce the risk of fatal rupture during the interval between presentation and confirmation of the diagnosis. While retrospective studies suggest that it is safe, no prospective studies have demonstrated either the safety or efficacy of such treatment.

### "Screening" CT Scan for Thoracic Vascular Injury.

Spiral CT scan of the chest is recommended by many radiologists as a screening test for mediastinal hematoma usually associated with aortic injury.[13–29] In addition, various other aortic wall and intraluminal findings suggest aortic injury on the spiral CT scan. Very often, the initial chest x-ray has already demonstrated findings suggestive of mediastinal hematoma. Some clinicians require the additional screening CT scan to substantiate a request for a diagnostic arteriogram. Although a few surgeons and radiologists have developed a "skill" and comfort level in performing an operation based on the screening CT findings alone, most surgeons require the arteriographic roadmap to determine the specific injury and any unexpected vascular anomalies. Even when radiologists and surgeons have utilized CT scans as a diagnostic test, this test is limited to injuries of the proximal descending thoracic aorta.

If a mediastinal hematoma is visualized on CT, formal aortography is still obtained to specifically determine the site(s) of the injury(s) and to identify any vascular anomalies that require modifications in the operative approach. Because surgeons are very reticent to operate on a major thoracic vascular injury on the basis of conventional CT scan alone, in most instances this test is merely an expensive duplication of the initial chest x-ray and delays aortography.[13–29] Decision trees can be constructed to aid the surgeon is reaching a diagnosis and treating a patient with aortic injury (Fig. 29-3). Three-dimensional reconstruction of the high-resolution data sets adds very little to the knowledge base. Transesophageal echocardiography and intravascular ultrasound have added little in the screening or diagnosis of thoracic aortic injury.[30] Magnetic resonance angiography (MRI) can generate similarly detailed information; however, its application in these potentially unstable trauma patients is not currently practical.

## Diagnostic Studies

### Catheter Arteriography.

In penetrating thoracic trauma, catheter angiography is indicated for suspected aortic, innominate, carotid, or subclavian arterial injuries. Different thoracic incisions are required for proximal and distal control of each of these vessels.

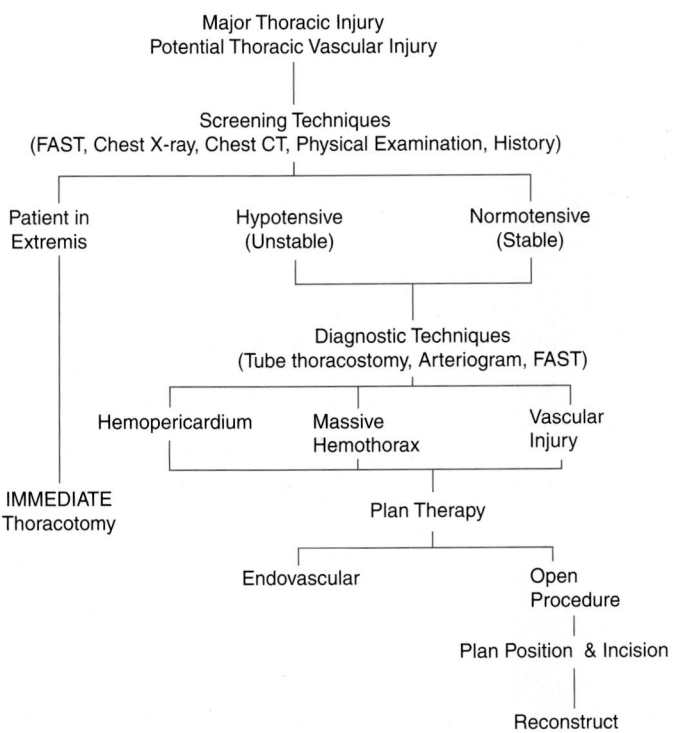

**FIGURE 29-3A.** Algorithm for an approach to patients with suspected thoracic vascular injury.

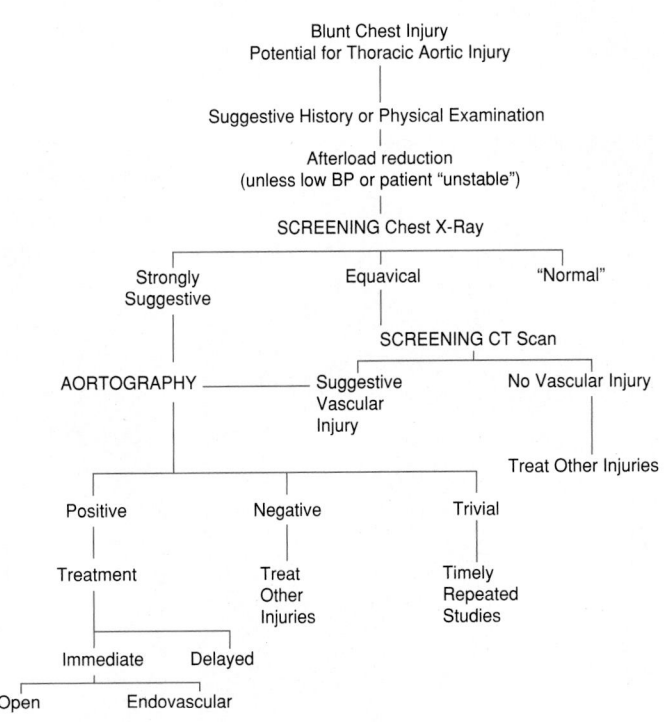

**FIGURE 29-3B.** Algorithm for the evaluation and treatment of a patient suspected of having a blunt injury to the thoracic aorta.

Arteriography, therefore, is essential for localizing the injury and planning the appropriate incision. Proximity of a missile trajectory to the brachiocephalic vessels, even without any physical findings of vascular injury, is an indication for arteriography. Although aortography may also be useful in hemodynamically stable patients with suspected penetrating aortic injuries, its limitations in this setting must be recognized. A "negative" aortogram may convey a false sense of security if the laceration has temporarily "sealed off" or if the column of aortic contrast overlies a small area of extravasation (Fig. 29-4). Therefore, an effort must be made to obtain views tangential to possible injuries (Figs. 29-5 and 29-6).

Following blunt trauma, the potential for thoracic great vessel injury—and, therefore, the need to proceed with aortography—is determined based on (1) the mechanism of injury, (2) physical examination, (3) the standard chest radiograph, or (4) a screening CT scan. As each of these factors has inherent limitations, all must be considered in concert. Traumatic aortic ruptures following seemingly innocuous mechanisms—including low-speed automobile crashes (<10 mph.) with airbag deployment and intrascapular back blows used to dislodge an esophageal foreign body—have been reported. Additionally, 50% of patients with thoracic vascular injuries from blunt trauma present without any external physical signs of injury, and 7% of patients with blunt injury to the aorta and brachiocephalic arteries have a normal appearing mediastinum on admission chest radiography.

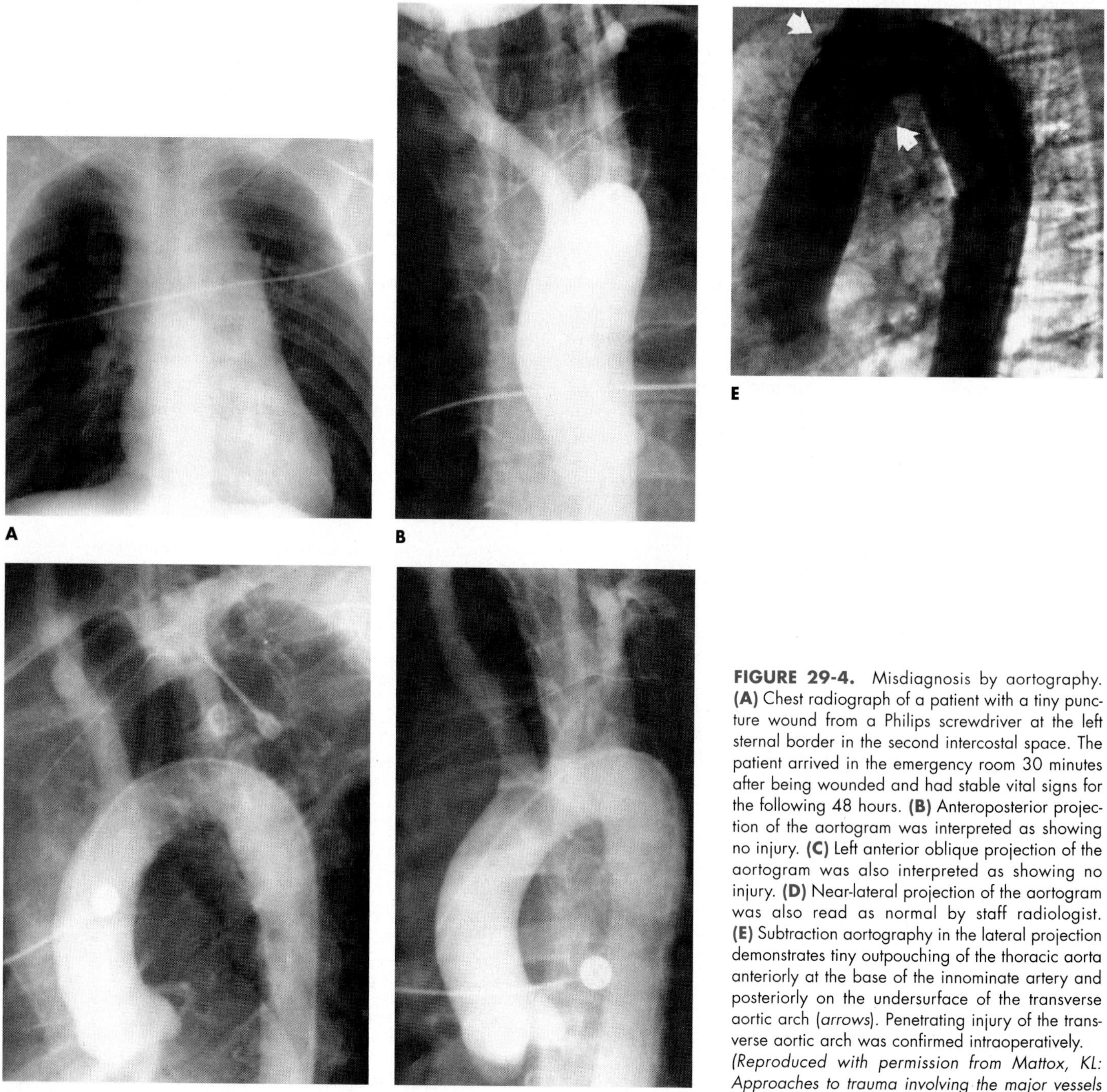

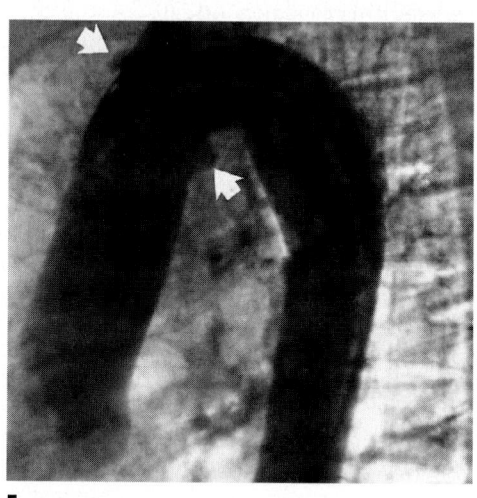

**FIGURE 29-4.** Misdiagnosis by aortography. **(A)** Chest radiograph of a patient with a tiny puncture wound from a Philips screwdriver at the left sternal border in the second intercostal space. The patient arrived in the emergency room 30 minutes after being wounded and had stable vital signs for the following 48 hours. **(B)** Anteroposterior projection of the aortogram was interpreted as showing no injury. **(C)** Left anterior oblique projection of the aortogram was also interpreted as showing no injury. **(D)** Near-lateral projection of the aortogram was also read as normal by staff radiologist. **(E)** Subtraction aortography in the lateral projection demonstrates tiny outpouching of the thoracic aorta anteriorly at the base of the innominate artery and posteriorly on the undersurface of the transverse aortic arch (arrows). Penetrating injury of the transverse aortic arch was confirmed intraoperatively. *(Reproduced with permission from Mattox, KL: Approaches to trauma involving the major vessels of the thorax. Surg Clin North Am 69: 83, 1989.)*

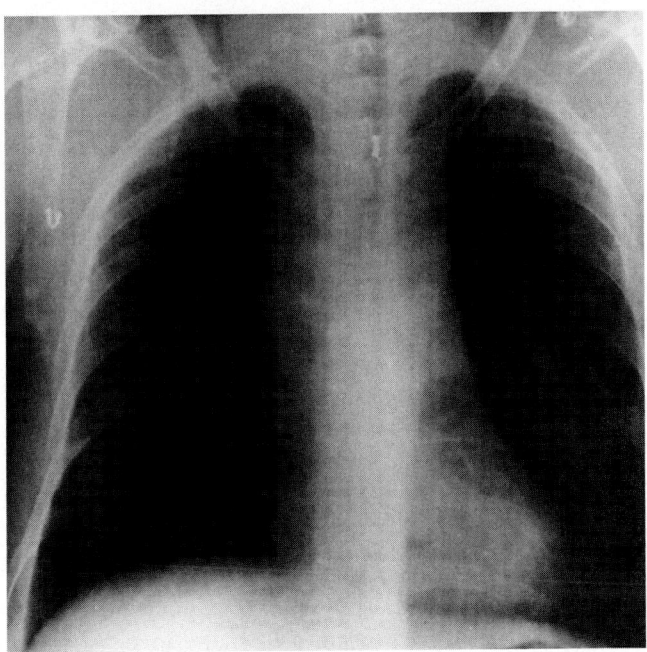

**FIGURE 29-5.** Plain chest x-ray of a patient with a penetrating wound of the ascending aorta.

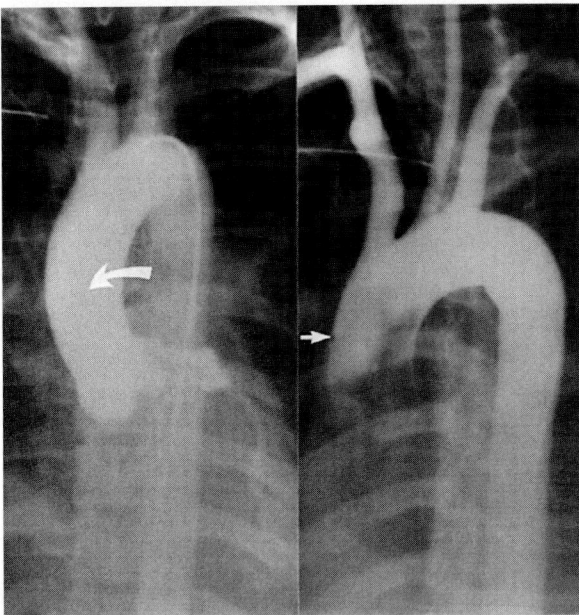

**FIGURE 29-6.** Aortogram of the patient in Fig. 28-7 demonstrating no apparent injury in the anteroposterior projection, but revealing a defect in the anterior aortic wall on the left anterior oblique projection (*arrows*).

*Thoracoscopy.* Thoracoscopy has been used selectively in the past in patients with penetrating thoracic trauma to inspect the mediastinum, pericardial sac, chest wall, diaphragm, and lung. CT scanning has replaced thoracoscopy to evaluate trajectory in patients with suspected mediastinal traverse.

## TREATMENT OPTIONS

### Nonoperative Management

Nonoperative management of blunt aortic injuries should be considered in patients who are unlikely to benefit from an immediate repair:

1. Severe head injury
2. Risk factors for infection
   - major burns
   - sepsis
   - heavily contaminated wounds
3. Severe multisystem trauma with hemodynamic instability and/or poor physiologic reserve

In such instances, nonoperative management is actually a purposeful delay in operation which attempts to achieve physiologic optimization and improve the outcome of repair.[16] Nonoperative management has also been used successfully in cases of "nonthreatening" aortic lesions, e.g., minor intimal defects and small pseudoaneurysms. Close observation without operation is similarly reasonable for small intimal flaps involving the brachiocephalic arteries in asymptomatic patients, as many such lesions will heal spontaneously.

Although apparent minor vascular injuries may resolve or stabilize, their long-term natural history remains uncertain.

Life-threatening complications of great vessel injuries—including rupture and fistulization with severe hemorrhage—occurring more than 20 years after injury are not uncommon.[13] Therefore, careful follow-up, including serial imaging studies, is a critical component of nonoperative management. Avoiding hypertension and use of beta-blocking agents are also recommended when patients with aortic injuries are treated nonoperatively.

### Endovascular Stenting

From a technical standpoint, a chronic posttraumatic false aneurysm of the descending thoracic aorta should be the most logical location for a successful placement of an aortic endograft. Beginning in the late 1990s, single case reports and small series of thoracic endografting for acute transections of the proximal descending thoracic aorta were reported. These were often custom devices using aortic or iliac artery extenders.[31–34] Not infrequently the left subclavian artery was occluded by the endograft, with subsequent left carotid-subclavian bypass in some cases. Iatrogenic injury to the access site of the femoral or iliac artery was occasionally reported. No reports exist for repair of thoracic aortic injury other than the proximal descending thoracic aorta.

In the United States only one commercial device has been approved by the Food and Drug Administration. The approved size range for this device is 26–40 mm in diameter, with 23–24 mm being the recommended diameter for the 26 mm graft. The average diameter of the thoracic aorta among patients with aortic tears is 19.3 cm. The manufacturers allow for 17% oversizing. With greater oversizing, compression and enfolding have been occasionally reported. Over 85% of descending thoracic aortic tears are less than 1 cm. from the orifice of the subclavian artery. A seating distance on either side of the pathology of 2 cm is recommended. Engineering challenges still exist regarding the existing approved thoracic aortic endografts when used in young trauma patients.

**TABLE 29-4**

| Comparison of Open Versus Endovascular Treatment of Blunt Thoracic Aortic Injury | | |
|---|---|---|
| | **OPEN OPERATIONS** | **ENDOVASCULAR STENT GRAFTS** |
| Mortality | 0–55% | 0–12% |
| Average mortality | 13% | 3.8% |
| Paraplegia | 0–20% | 0% |
| Average paraplegia | 10% | 1 out of 239 cases |
| Complications: | ARDS | LSCA occlusion |
| | CNS problems | Graft compression |
| | Nseurologic | Entry site problems |

*ARDS, Adult respiratory distress syndrome; CNS, central nervous system; LSCA, left subclavian artery.*

Using a variety of approved and customized endografts, 239 patients have been reported to have been treated for blunt injury to the proximal descending thoracic aorta (Table 29-4).[35] Many other small series or single case reports exist. Among the 239 cases there were nine deaths (3.8%), and one paraplegia (<0.5%). Even with potential selection bias, the lower mortality and almost nonexistent paraplegia rate makes consideration for endovascular repair very compelling. Yet to be answered are the engineering challenges of graft compression and enfolding as well as available smaller sizes and improved delivery systems. The long-term fate of the endograft as the aorta dilates with age is yet unanswered.

## Surgical Repair

Indications for urgent transfer to the operating room for thoracotomy include hemodynamic instability, significant hemorrhage from chest tubes, and radiographic evidence of a rapidly expanding mediastinal hematoma (Fig. 29-7).

### Preoperative Considerations.

Whenever possible, patients and their families must be made aware of the potential for neurologic complications—paraplegia, stroke, and brachial plexus injuries—following surgical reconstruction of thoracic great vessels. Careful documentation of preoperative neurologic status is critical. With any suspicion of vascular injury, prophylactic antibiotics are administered preoperatively. In hemodynamically stable patients, fluid administration is limited until vascular control is achieved in the operating room. An autotransfusion device should be prepared. During the induction of anesthesia, wide swings in blood pressure must be avoided; while profound hypotension is clearly undesirable, hypertensive episodes can have equally catastrophic consequences.

The operative approach to great vessel injury depends on both the overall patient assessment and the specific injury. The initial steps of patient positioning and incision selection (Table 29-5) are particularly important in surgery for great vessel injuries, as adequate exposure is mandatory for proximal and distal control. Prepping and draping of the patient should provide access from the neck to the knees to allow management of all contingencies. For the hypotensive patient with an undiagnosed injury, the mainstay of thoracic trauma surgery is the left anterolateral thoracotomy with the patient in the supine position. In stable patients, preoperative arteriography may dictate an operative approach by another incision.

Appropriate graft materials should be available. While the failure mode of an infected prosthetic graft is a pseudoaneurysm, a saphenous vein graft is a devitalized collagen tube susceptible to bacterial collagenase, which may cause graft dissolution with acute rupture and uncontrolled hemorrhage. Therefore, for vessels larger than 5 mm, a prosthetic graft is the conduit of choice, especially in potentially contaminated wounds. However, due to patency considerations, a saphenous vein graft may need to be used when smaller grafts are required. For fragile vessels, such as the subclavian artery and the aorta in young people, a soft knitted Dacron graft is useful. Antibiotic irrigation of the graft material may help prevent subsequent infection.

### Damage Control.

Patients with severely compromised physiologic reserve often require damage control injury management to achieve survival. The two approaches to thoracic damage control are (1) definitive repair of injuries using quick and simple techniques that restore survivable physiology during a single operation and (2) abbreviated thoracotomy that restores survivable physiology and requires a planned reoperation for definitive repairs.[14] Severe hilar vascular injuries can be quickly controlled by performing a pneumonectomy using stapling devices. Temporary vessel ligation or placement of intravascular shunts can control bleeding until subsequent correction of acidosis, hypothermia, and coagulopathy allows the patient to be returned to the operating room. En mass closure of a thoracotomy is more hemostatic than towel-clip closure. A "Bogotá bag" can be used as a temporary closure of a median sternotomy in cases with associated cardiac dysfunction.

## ARTERIAL INJURIES

### Ascending Aorta.

Patients with blunt ascending aortic injuries rarely survive transportation to the hospital. Operative repair usually requires use of total cardiopulmonary bypass and insertion of a Dacron graft.[36]

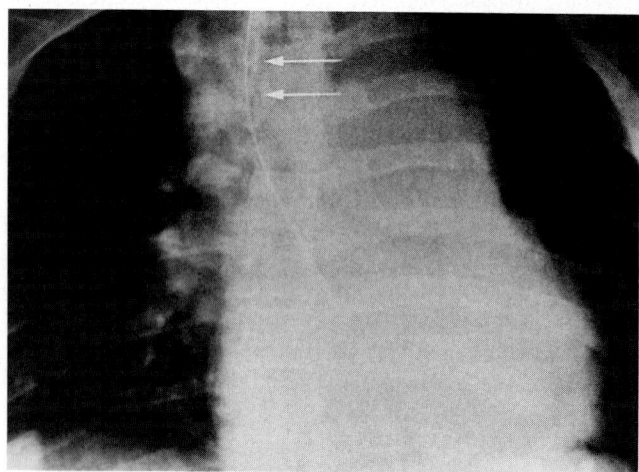

**FIGURE 29-7.** Plain chest x-ray in a patient with a blunt injury to the descending thoracic aorta. Note the rightward deviation of both the trachea and nasogastric tube in the esophagus.

**TABLE 29-5**

**Recommended Incisions for Thoracic Great Vessel Injuries**

| INJURED VESSEL | INCISION |
|---|---|
| Uncertain injury (hemodynamically unstable) | Left anterolateral thoracotomy |
| | ± transverse sternotomy |
| | ± right anterolateral thoracotomy (clamshell) |
| Ascending aorta | Median sternotomy |
| Transverse aortic arch | Median sternotomy |
| | ± neck extension |
| Descending thoracic aorta | Left posterolateral thoracotomy (4th intercostal space) |
| Innominate artery | Median sternotomy with right cervical extension |
| Right subclavian artery or vein | Median sternotomy with right cervical extension |
| Left common carotid artery | Median sternotomy with left cervical extension |
| Left subclavian artery or vein | Left anterolateral thoracotomy (3rd or 4th intercostal space) with separate left supraclavicular incision ± connecting vertical sternotomy ("book" thoracotomy) |
| Pulmonary artery | |
| Main/intrapericardial | Median sternotomy |
| Right or left hilar | Ipsilateral posterolateral thoracotomy |
| Pulmonary vein | Ipsilateral posterolateral thoracotomy |
| Innominate vein | Median sternotomy |
| Intrathoracic vena cava | Median sternotomy |

Penetrating injuries involving the ascending aorta are uncommon (Figs. 29-5 and 29-6). Survival rates approach 50% for patients having stable vital signs on arrival at a trauma center.[37] Although primary repair of anterior lacerations can be accomplished without adjuncts, cardiopulmonary bypass may be required if there is an additional posterior injury. The possibility of a peripheral bullet embolus must always be considered in these patients.

Transverse Aortic Arch. When approaching an injury to the transverse aortic arch, extension of the median sternotomy to the neck is important to obtain complete exposure of the arch and brachiocephalic branches. If necessary, exposure can be further enhanced by division of the innominate vein. When hemorrhage limits exposure, the use of balloon tamponade is useful as a temporary measure. Simple lacerations may be repaired by lateral aortorrhaphy. With difficult lesions, such as posterior lacerations or those with concomitant pulmonary artery injuries, cardiopulmonary bypass is recommended. As with injuries to the ascending thoracic aorta, survival rates approaching 50% are possible.[7,37]

Innominate Artery. Median sternotomy is employed for management of innominate artery injuries. A right cervical extension can be used when necessary. Blunt injuries typically involve the proximal innominate artery (Figs. 29-8 and 29-9) and therefore actually represent aortic injuries and require obtaining proximal control at the transverse aortic arch. In contrast, penetrating trauma injures of the innominate artery may occur throughout its course. Exposure is enhanced by division of the innominate vein.

In selected patients with only partial tears, a running lateral arteriorrhaphy using 4-0 polypropylene suture is occasionally possible. More often, injuries to the innominate artery require repair via the bypass exclusion technique (Fig. 29-10).[38] Bypass grafting is performed from the ascending aorta to the distal innominate artery (immediately proximal to the bifurcation of the subclavian and right carotid arteries) using a Dacron tube graft. The area of injury is avoided until the areas for bypass insertion are exposed. A vascular

clamp is placed proximal to the bifurcation of the innominate artery to allow collateral flow to the brain via the right subclavian and carotid arteries. Neither hypothermia, systemic anticoagulation, nor shunting is required. After the bypass is completed, the area of hematoma is entered, and the injury identified (usually at the origin of the innominate artery) and repaired. If concomitantly injured or previously divided, the innominate vein may be ligated

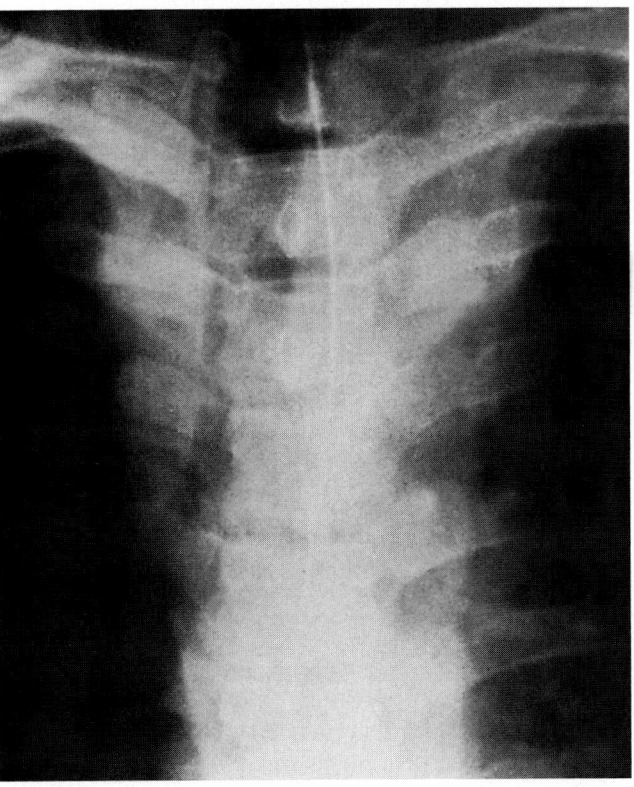

**FIGURE 29-8.** Plain chest x-ray of a patient with a blunt injury of the innominate artery. Note that the hematoma is at the thoracic outlet rather than the aortic isthmus.

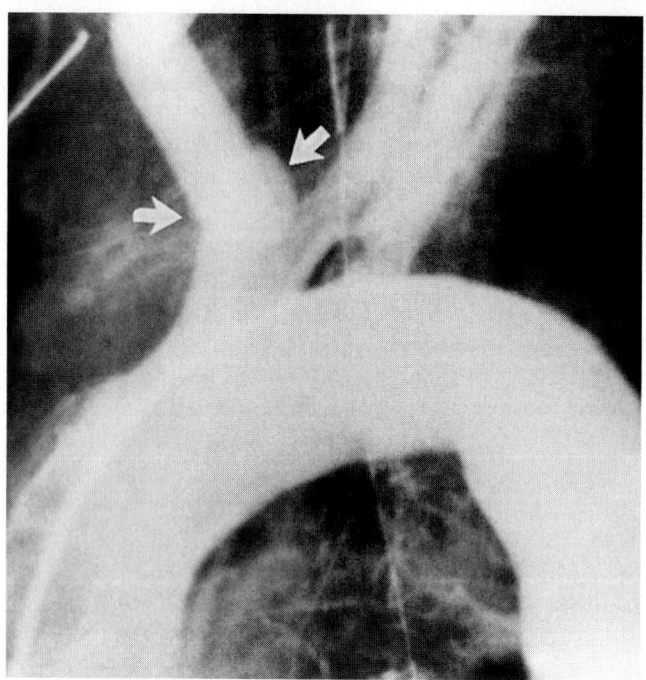

**FIGURE 29-9.** Aortogram of the patient in Fig. 28-1 demonstrating the tear involving the proximal innominate artery.

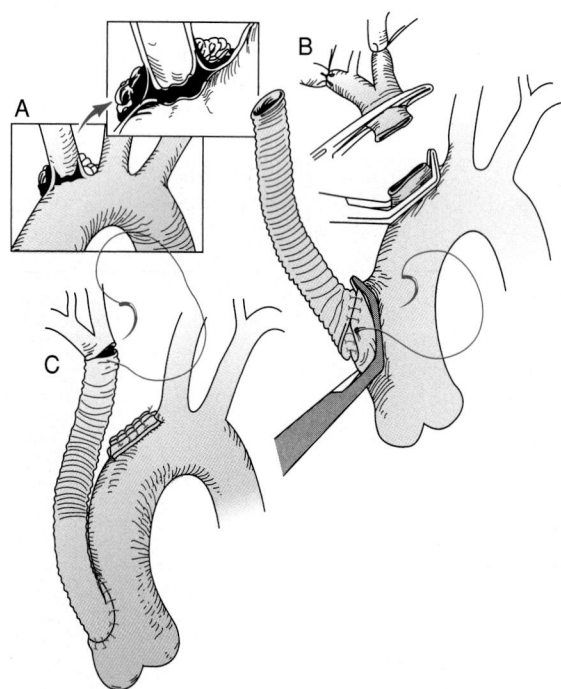

**FIGURE 29-10.** Drawing depicting the bypass exclusion technique employed in patients with innominate artery injuries. (*Copyright © Baylor College of Medicine, 1981.*)

with impunity. If the vein remains intact, a pedicled pericardial flap can be positioned between the vein and overlying graft to prevent erosion.

The treatment of an iatrogenic tracheal-innominate artery fistula deserves special consideration. These fistulae are usually caused by the concave surface of a low riding tracheostomy tube eroding

into the innominate artery. Sentinel bleeding through or around the tracheostomy tube should not be misinterpreted as "trachitis." Arteriography during a "stable interval" is generally not helpful in pinpointing a precise diagnosis; instead, the possibility of a tracheal-innominate fistula should be evaluated via bronchoscopy in the operating room. With massive bleeding, control must be achieved by performing orotracheal intubation, removing the tracheostomy tube, and directly tamponading the bleeding digitally through the tracheotomy during immediate transport to the operating room. Through a median sternotomy with a right neck extension, the innominate artery is ligated at its origin from the aorta and distally just before the division into the carotid and subclavian arteries. Despite a greater than 25% chance of neurologic complications, no attempt should be made at revascularization, since delayed graft infection with its dreaded complications inevitably occurs.

Descending Thoracic Aorta.    Prehospital mortality is 85% for patients with blunt injury to the descending thoracic aorta.[39] In patients who arrive at a hospital alive, the majority of blunt aortic injuries are located at the isthmus (Fig. 29-11). Patients presenting with an injury in the mid-descending thoracic aorta or distally, near the diaphragm, are far less common (Fig. 29-12). Multiple blunt aortic injuries are rare, but may occur.

Injury to the descending thoracic aorta is often accompanied by other organ injuries. If the patient has a stable thoracic hematoma and concomitant abdominal injury, laparotomy should be the initial

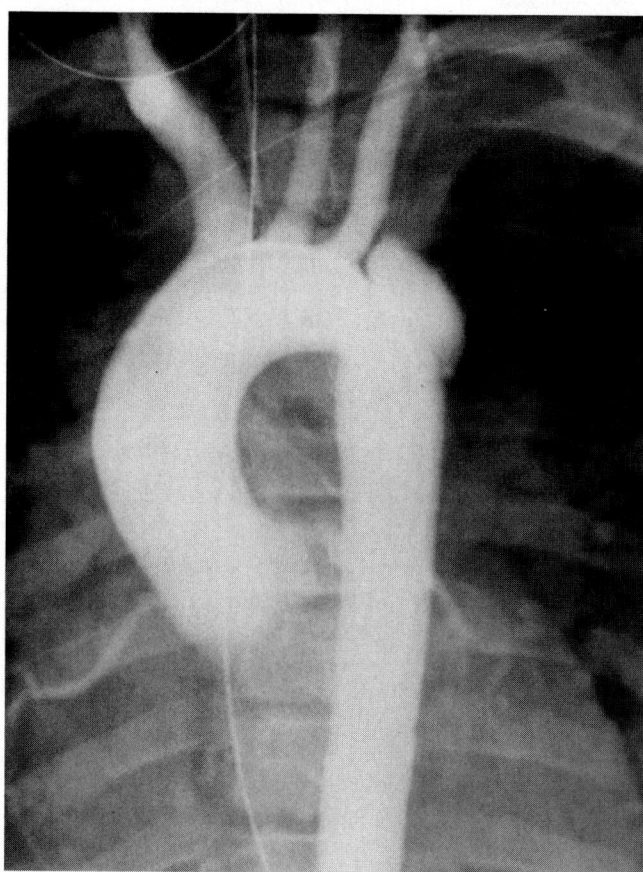

**FIGURE 29-11.** Aortogram demonstrating the classic intimal tear and traumatic pseudoaneurysm of the descending thoracic aorta.

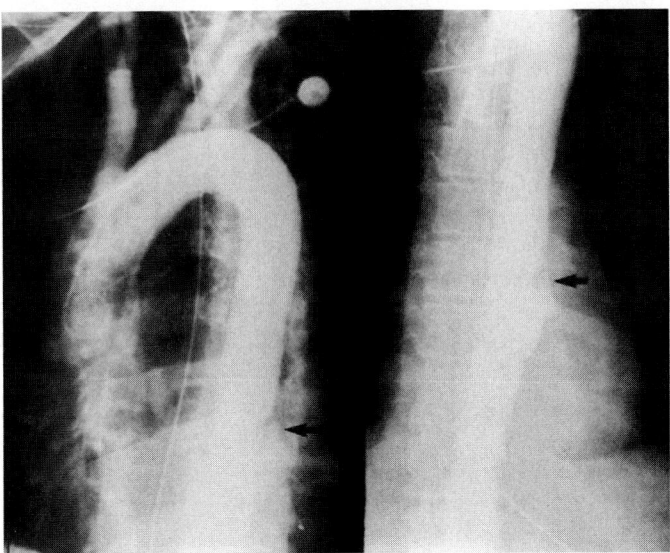

**FIGURE 29-12.** Aortogram in a patient with blunt chest trauma demonstrating an intimal tear of the descending thoracic aorta at the diaphragm.

procedure. For the patient with a rapidly expanding hematoma (Fig. 29-7), however, repair of the thoracic injury should be the primary therapeutic goal.

Numerous surgical procedures for managing injuries of descending thoracic aorta have been described. Although "wrapping" or insertion of stainless steel wire for treatment of traumatic aneurysms should be historic curiosities only, the authors have seen cases treated in this manner during the last 25 years. Exclusion and bypass grafting, as recommended for treatment of innominate artery injuries, has little utility in the descending thoracic aorta.

The current standard technique of repair involves *clamping and direct reconstruction* (Table 29-6). Three commonly employed adjuncts to this approach are (1) pharmacological agents, (2) temporary, passive bypass shunts, and (3) pump assisted atrio-femoral bypass. In the latter approach, two options exist: traditional pump bypass, which requires heparin, and use of centrifugal (heparinless) pump circuits. All three of these adjunctive approaches to the clamp-and-repair principle should be in the armamentarium of the surgeon, who must choose the approach most appropriate to the specific clinical situation.

**TABLE 29-6**

| Current Therapeutic Approaches to the Management of Thoracic Aortic Injuries |
| --- |
| 1. Surgical (clamp and direct reconstruction with or without an interposition graft) |
|    (a) Pharmacological control of proximal hypertension |
|    (b) Passive bypass shunts |
|    (c) Pump-assisted bypass |
|       (1) Traditional cardiopulmonary bypass (with total body heparinization) |
|       (2) Atrio-femoral bypass using centrifugal pump (without heparinization) |
| 2. Nonoperative and/or purposeful delay of operation (with pharmacological treatment and close radiologic surveillance) |
| 3. Endovascular stenting (under investigation) |

Injury to the descending thoracic aorta is approached via a posterolateral thoracotomy through the fourth intercostal space. The injury usually originates at the medial aspect of the aorta at the level of the ligamentum arteriosum; however, one must take care to avoid missing a second injury (usually at the level of the diaphragm).

The initial objective is proximal control, therefore, the transverse aortic arch is exposed, and umbilical tapes are passed around the arch between the left carotid and subclavian arteries. Similarly, the subclavian artery is encircled with umbilical tape. Care must be taken to avoid injuring the left recurrent laryngeal nerve. If it is suspected that the tear extends to the aortic arch or ascending aorta, cardiopulmonary bypass should be available in the operating room. If the patient has had previous coronary artery bypass surgery with use of the left internal mammary artery as a conduit, repair may require profound hypothermic circulatory arrest to eliminate the need to clamp the left subclavian artery.

Vascular clamps are applied to three locations: proximal aorta, distal aorta, and left subclavian artery. Close communication between anesthesiologist and surgeon is essential to maintain stability of hemodynamic parameters before, during, and after clamping. The use of vasodilators (nitroprusside) prevents cardiac strain during clamping. The hematoma is entered and back bleeding from intercostal arteries is controlled. Care is taken to avoid indiscriminate ligation of intercostal vessels; only those required for adequate repair of the aorta should be ligated. The proximal and distal ends of the aorta are completely transected and dissected away from the esophagus; this maneuver allows full-thickness suturing while minimizing the risk of a secondary aortoesophageal fistula. The injury is then repaired by either end-to-end anastomosis or graft interposition. Graft interposition is utilized in more than 85% of reported cases. Prior to clamp removal, large volumes of fluid (colloid and crystalloid) are administered to avoid clamp release hypotension.

For patients undergoing repair of blunt descending thoracic aortic injury, the reported mortality ranges from 0 to 55% (average 13%).[35,40] As expected in these victims of major blunt trauma, the mortality is primarily associated with multisystem trauma, and is ultimately due to head injury, infection, respiratory insufficiency, and renal insufficiency.

The most feared complication of great vessel injury is paraplegia. Utilization of protective adjuncts when repairing descending thoracic aortic injuries remains a topic of considerable debate. There have been proponents of the use of passive shunts and cardiopulmonary bypass, with and without heparinization. The mortality rate with the use of routine cardiopulmonary bypass is probably secondary to the massive cerebral, abdominal, or fracture site hemorrhage that occurs in these victims of multisystem trauma. Recent experience using centrifugal pumps without heparinization has provided an attractive alternative for those who wish to use controlled flow bypass without systemic anticoagulation. The use of bypass systems, however, is not without complications. In the trauma patient, difficulty inserting cannulae may occur due to patient position, the presence of periaortic hematoma, and time constraints imposed by an expanding, pulsatile, uncontrolled hematoma. Intraoperative and postoperative complications include bleeding at the cannulation sites and false aneurysm formation.

Use of simple clamp-and-repair for injuries to the descending thoracic aorta (without the use of systemic anticoagulation or shunts) is a technique that continues to be used with excellent results. Since 1985, review of the literature demonstrates that the simple clamp-repair technique results in the virtually the same statistical incidence of paraplegia as heparin-bonded shunts and use of repair on a variety of pumps. Sweeney[17] reported using simple clamp-repair in 75 patients, only one of whom developed postoperative paraplegia.

Ultimately, the determinants of postoperative paraplegia are multifactorial (Table 29-7); therefore the precise causes cannot be precisely identified in an individual patient. Paraplegia has been associated with perioperative hypotension, injury or ligation of the intercostal arteries, and duration of clamp occlusion during repair.[41] However, there are reports of patients surviving surgery without paraplegia despite having long segments of aorta replaced and ligation of multiple intercostal arteries. The length of cross-clamp time does not *directly* correlate with occurrence of paraplegia. A cross-clamp time under 30 minutes has been argued to provide a safe margin against paraplegia, and shunting techniques have been recommended when longer cross-clamp times are necessary.[41] The use of a shunt, however, does not offer protection for the area of the spinal cord supplied by the arteries between the clamps. Furthermore, patients requiring longer clamp time or interposition grafts have more extensive injuries than those requiring shorter clamp times or end-to-end anastomoses. Thus, it is likely that an increased incidence of paraplegia associated with longer clamp times is secondary to more extensive disruption of intercostal arteries and other flow to the anterior spinal artery caused by the original injury.

Various monitoring techniques are available to assess the effect of aortic occlusion on the spinal cord, including the measurement of somatosensory- and motor-evoked potentials. Although correlation appears to exist between loss of somatosensory-evoked potentials, duration of loss of conduction, and postoperative paraplegia, the use of this modality is not common to all trauma centers, the interpretation of results is still being debated, and actual positive applicability requires further delineation.

Regardless of the technique used, paraplegia occurs in approximately 10% of these patients (range 0–22%).[35,40] No prospective, randomized trial has identified the superiority of any single method. Therefore, the choice of operative technique does not infer legal liability when paraplegia occurs.

Even with potential selection bias in favor or endografts, the low mortality and almost nonexistent paraplegia rate, the use of endografting is very compelling. The reported complications of graft migration, enfolding, compression, occlusion of the subclavian artery, and problems at the entry site are all technical and engineering challenges which will soon be solved by commercial devices. Currently, thoracic aortic endograft insertion should probably be only performed on strict prospective evaluation protocols (Table 29-4).

Subclavian Artery.    Subclavian vascular injuries can involve any combination of the following regions: intrathoracic, thoracic outlet, cervical (zone 1), and upper extremity. Preoperative arteriography allows for planning appropriate incision(s) to obtain adequate exposure and control.

A cervical extension of the median sternotomy is employed for exposure of right-sided subclavian injuries. For left subclavian artery injuries, proximal control is obtained through an anterolateral

**TABLE 29-7**

| Possible Contributing Factors Related to the Multifactorial Development of Paraplegia Following Operations for Thoracic Great Vessel Injury | |
|---|---|
| Injury Factors | Direct segmental artery injury |
| | Direct radicular artery injury |
| | Direct spinal artery injury |
| | Spinal cord contusion/concussion |
| | Spinal canal compartment syndrome |
| | Severity of aortic injury |
| | Specific anatomic location of aortic injury |
| Patient Factors | Location of arteri radicularis magma (?) |
| | Continuity of anterior spinal artery |
| | Caliber of individual segmental radicular arteries |
| | Congenital narrowing of spinal canal |
| | (?) Increased blood alcohol levels |
| | Total perispinal collateral blood supply |
| Operative Factors | Required occlusion of segmental arteries |
| | Pharmacological agents required |
| | (?) Declamping hypotension |
| | (?) Required cross clamp times (in combination with anatomic and injury factors cited in this table) |
| | Length of required interposition grafting or required exclusion |
| | (?) Level of systolic (or mean) proximal aortic blood pressure |
| | (?) Level of distal aortic mean blood pressure |
| | (?) "Flow" in the aorta distal to clamp |
| Postoperative Factors | Progressive swelling of the spinal cord |
| | Spinal canal compartment syndrome |
| | Delayed or secondary occlusion of injured or contused segmental, radicular, or spinal arteries |
| | Pharmacological induced spasm of spinal cord nutrient arteries |

thoracotomy (above the nipple, second or third intercostal space), while a separate supraclavicular incision provides distal control. Although these incisions can be connected to create a formal "book" thoracotomy, this results in a high incidence of postoperative "causalgia" type neurologic complications and its use should be limited to highly selected left-sided subclavian artery injuries.

In obtaining exposure, it is imperative to avoid injuring the phrenic nerve (anterior to the scalenus antics muscle). In subclavian vascular trauma, a high associated rate of brachial plexus injury is seen; thus, documentation of preoperative neurologic status is important. Intraoperative iatrogenic injury to the brachial plexus must also be avoided.

In most instances, repair requires either lateral arteriorrhaphy or graft interposition. It is unusual that an end-to-end anastomosis can be employed. Associated injuries to the lung should be managed with stapled wedge resection or pulmonary tractotomy.[42] One pitfall in subclavian injuries is failure to anticipate the exposure necessary for proximal control. When approaching the subclavian artery via the deltopectoral groove without proximal control, exsanguination may occur. Resection of the clavicle may aid in proximal control. Combination supra- and infraclavicular incisions may be used to avoid the morbidity of clavicular resection. A mortality rate of 4.7% for patients with subclavian artery injuries has been reported, but death is often due to associated injuries.

### Left Carotid Artery.

The operative approach for injuries of the left carotid artery mirrors that used for an innominate artery injury: a median sternotomy with a left cervical extension added when necessary. As with other great vessel injuries, neither shunts nor pumps are employed. With transection at the left carotid origin, bypass graft repair is preferred over end-to-end anastomosis.

### Pulmonary Artery.

The intrapericardial pulmonary arteries are approached via median sternotomy. Minimal dissection is needed to expose the main and proximal left pulmonary arteries.[43] Exposure of the intrapericardial right pulmonary artery is achieved by dissecting between the superior vena cava and ascending aorta. Although anterior injuries can be repaired primarily without adjuncts, repair of a posterior injury usually requires cardiopulmonary bypass. Mortality rates for injury to the central pulmonary arteries or veins are greater than 70%.[4]

Distal pulmonary artery injuries present with massive hemothorax and are repaired through an ipsilateral posterolateral thoracotomy. When there is a major hilar injury, rapid pneumonectomy may be a life-saving maneuver. The use of a large tamponading balloon catheter may control exsanguinating hemorrhage.

### Internal Mammary Artery.

The internal mammary artery in a young patient is capable of flows in excess of 300 mL/min. Injuries to this artery can produce extensive hemothorax or even pericardial tamponade, simulating a cardiac injury. Such injuries are usually serendipitously discovered at the time of thoracotomy for suspected great vessel or heart injury.

### Intercostal Arteries.

Persistent hemothorax can be caused by simple lacerations of the intercostal arteries. Because of difficulty in exposure, precise ligature can be difficult. At times, control must be achieved by circumferential ligatures around the rib on either side of the intercostal vessel injury.

## Venous Injuries

### Thoracic Vena Cava.

Isolated injury to the suprahepatic or superior vena cava is infrequently reported. Injury at either location has a high incidence of associated organ trauma and carries a mortality rate greater than 60%. Intrathoracic inferior vena cava injury produces hemopericardium and cardiac tamponade. Exposure of the thoracic inferior vena cava is extremely difficult unless the patient is placed on total cardiopulmonary bypass with the inferior cannula inserted via the groin in the abdominal inferior vena cava. Repair is enhanced by a right atriotomy and intracaval balloon occlusion to prevent air entering the cannula and massive blood return to the heart except via the hepatic veins. Repair is achieved from inside the cava via the right atrium. Superior vena cava injuries are repaired by lateral venorrhaphy. At times, an intracaval shunt is necessary.[44] For complex injuries a PTFE patch or Dacron interposition tube graft can be used safely and is more expedient than the time-consuming construction of saphenous vein panel grafts.

### Pulmonary Veins.

Injury to the pulmonary veins is difficult to manage through an anterior incision. With major hemorrhage, temporary occlusion of the entire hilum may be necessary. If a pulmonary vein must be ligated, the appropriate lobe needs to be resected. Pulmonary vein injuries are often associated with concomitant injuries to the heart, pulmonary artery, aorta, and esophagus.

### Subclavian Veins.

The operative exposure of the subclavian veins parallels that described for subclavian artery injuries: median sternotomy with cervical extension for right-sided injuries and left anterolateral thoracotomy with a separate supraclavicular incision for left-sided injuries. In most instances, repair requires either lateral venorrhaphy or ligation.

### Azygos Vein.

The azygos vein is not usually classified as a thoracic great vessel, but because of its size and high flow, azygos vein injuries must be considered potentially fatal.[45] Penetrating wounds of the thoracic outlet can produce combinations of injuries involving the azygos vein, innominate artery, trachea or bronchus, and superior vena cava. These complex injuries have a very high mortality rate, and are particularly difficult to control if approached through a median sternotomy. Combined incisions and approaches are frequently needed for successful repair. When injured, the azygous vein is best managed by suture ligature of both sides of the injury. Concomitant injury to the esophagus and bronchus should be considered and ruled out.[46]

## Special Problems

### Mediastinal Traverse Injuries.

Because injuries from both stab and gunshot wounds that traverse the mediastinum are classically felt to have a high probability of injury to the thoracic great vessels and other critical structures, mandatory exploration has been advocated in the past. The evaluation of stable patients using less invasive means—combined aortography, bronchoscopy, echocardiography, and esophagoscopy—has been described. A thoracic spiral CT scan will often show the bullet trajectory and guide a need for surgery or additional diagnostic tests.

Thoracic Duct Injury.   Injuries to the thoracic great vessels may be complicated by concomitant thoracic duct injury, which, if unrecognized, may produce devastating morbidity due to marked nutritional depletion.[47] Diagnosed by chylous material draining from the chest tube, this condition is usually treated medically. Continued chest tube drainage, coupled with a diet devoid of long chain fatty acids, usually result in spontaneous closure in less than one month. Prolonged hyper alimentation beyond three weeks has not consistently resulted in spontaneous closure of thoracic duct fistula. If thoracotomy is required, a heavy fatty meal to increase the chylous flow and facilitate identification of the fistula is given to the patient a few hours before surgery. The fistula is simply ligated with fine monofilament suture (6-0).

Systemic Air Embolism.   A fistula between a pulmonary vein and bronchiole due to a penetrating lung injury results in systemic air embolism. The fistula allows air bubbles enter the left heart and embolize to the systemic circulation, including the coronary and cerebral arteries (Fig. 29-13). Intrabronchial pressure above 60 torr increases the incidence of this complication.[48] Manifestations include seizures and cardiac arrest. Resuscitation requires thoracotomy, clamping of the pulmonary hilum to prevent further air embolization, and aspiration of air from the left ventricle and ascending aorta. Cardiopulmonary bypass can be considered; however, very few survivors have been reported.

Foreign Body Embolism.   Because of their central location, the thoracic great vessels may serve as both an entry site and final resting place for intravascular bullet emboli.[49–51] These migratory foreign bodies present a diagnostic and therapeutic dilemma. As the result of intravascular embolization, bullets may produce infection, ischemia, or injury to organs distant from the site of trauma.

Bullets and catheters can embolize to the pulmonary vasculature; 25% of migratory bullets finally lodge in the pulmonary arteries (Fig. 29-2).[49–51] Although small fragments, such as those the size of a BB, can probably be left in place without causing problems, catheter emboli and larger bullet emboli should be removed to prevent pulmonary thrombosis, sepsis, or other complications.[107]

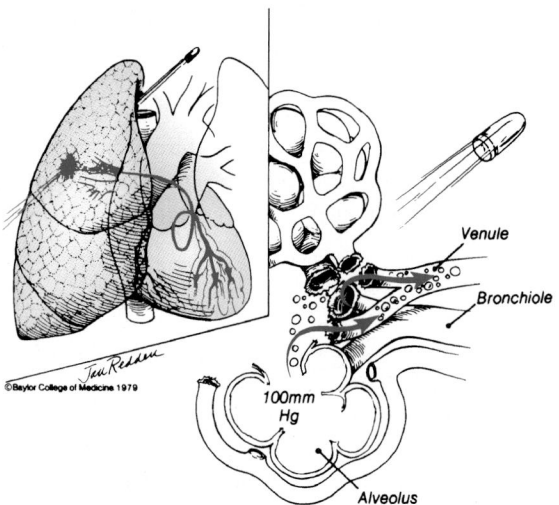

**FIGURE 29-13.** Drawing depicting the mechanism of systemic air embolism following a penetrating lung injury. (*Copyright © Baylor College of Medicine, 1979.*)

Percutaneous retrieval of the foreign body using transvenous catheters and fluoroscopic guidance may obviate the need for thoracotomy.

## Postoperative Management

A significant portion of the in-hospital mortality associated with great vessel injury is secondary to the nature of the multisystem trauma in this group of patients. The operating surgeon is best qualified to direct the patient's postoperative management. Careful hemodynamic monitoring, with avoidance of both hypertension and hypotension, is critical. While urinary output is a generally a good indicator of cardiac function, for the patient with massive injuries, Swan-Ganz monitoring is often necessary to optimize hemodynamic parameters and manage fluids, pressors, and vasodilators.

Various pulmonary problems—including atelectasis, respiratory insufficiency, pneumonia, and adult respiratory distress syndrome—represent the primary postoperative complications in this group of patients. The presence of pulmonary contusions and the potential for development of adult respiratory distress syndrome mandate that fluid administration be carefully monitored. Positive end-expiratory pressure should be provided to hemodynamically stable intubated patients in order to minimize atelectasis. Patient mobility is imperative, and adequate medication for pain relief results in fewer pulmonary complications. For the management of pain related to a thoracotomy or multiple rib fractures, postoperative thoracic epidural anesthesia should be considered in stable patients without spinal injuries; alternatively, intercostal nerve blocks can be performed intraoperatively and repeated in the ICU.

Postoperative hemorrhage may be due to a technical problem, but is often the result of coagulopathy related to hypothermia, acidosis, and massive blood transfusion. Coagulation studies must be carefully monitored and corrected with administration of appropriate blood products. Blood draining via chest tubes can be collected and autotransfused.

The presence of a prosthetic vascular graft requires special attention aimed at avoiding bacteremia. During the initial resuscitation of these critically injured patients, various intravascular lines are often rapidly placed at the expense of strict sterile technique; all such lines should be replaced after the patient has stabilized in the ICU. Antibiotic therapy should be continued into the postoperative period until potential sources of infection are eliminated. Patients are counseled regarding the necessity of antibiotic prophylaxis during invasive procedures, including dental manipulations.

Most late complications are related to infections or sequelae from other injuries. Long-term complications specifically related to the vascular repair—including stenosis, thrombosis, arteriovenous fistula, graft infection, and pseudoaneurysm formation—are uncommon.

## REFERENCES

1. Versalius A: In Beonetus T, ed. *Sepulchretaum sive Anataomia Practica ex Cad a veribus Morbo.* Geneva, 1700.
2. Dfhanelidze II: Manuscript, Petrograd, 1922, cited by Lilienthal H in *Thoracic Surgery: The Surgical Treatment of Thoracic Diseases.* Philadelphia: Saunders, 1926, p. 489.
3. Bahnson HT: Definitive treatment of saccular aneurysms of the aorta with excision of sac and aortic suture. *Surg Gynecol Obstet* 96:383, 1953.
4. Matttox KL, Feliciano DV, Beall AC, Jr, et al.: Five thousand seven hundred sixty cardiovascular injuries in 4459 patients epidemiologic evolution 1958—1988. *Ann Surg* 209:698, 1989.

5. Alfaro J, Varela G, De-Miguel E, de Nicilas M: Successful management of a tracheo-innominate artery fistula following placement of a wire self-explandable tracheal Gianturco stent. *Eur J Cardio-Thorac Surg* 7:615, 1993.

6. Horton TG, Cohn SM, Heid MP, et al.: Identification of trauma patients at risk of thoracic aortic tear by mechanism of injury. *J Trauma* 48:1008, 2000.

7. Katyal D, McLellan BA, Brenneman FD, et al.: Lateral impact motor vehicle collisions; significant cause of blunt traumatic rupture of the thoracic aorta. *J Trauma* 42: 769, 1997.

8. Rogers FB, Osler TM, Shackford SR: Aortic dissection after trauma: Case report and review of the literature. *J Trauma* 41:906, 1996.

9. Mattox KL: Prehospital management of thoracic injury. *Surg Clin North Am* 69:21, 1989.

10. Mattox KL, Bickell W, Pepe P, et al.: Prospective MAST study in 911 patients. *J Trauma* 29:1104, 1989.

11. Mattox KL, Feliciano DV: Role of external cardiac compression in truncal trauma. *J Trauma* 22:934, 1982.

12. Bickell WH, Wall MJ, Pepe PE, et al.: Immediate versus delayed fluid resuscitation for hypotensive patients with penetrating torso injuries. *New Engl J Med* 331:1105, 1994.

13. McCollum CH, Graham JM, Noon GP, et al.: Chronic traumatic aneurysms of the thoracic aorta: an analysis of 50 patients. *J Trauma* 19:248, 1979.

14. Wall MJ, Jr., Soltero E: Damage control for thoracic injuries. *Surgery Clinics of North America* 77:863, 1997.

15. Wheat MW, Jr., Palmer RF, Bartley TD, et al.: Treatment of dissecting aneurysm of the aorta without surgery. *J Thorac Cardiovasc Surg* 50:364, 1965.

16. Fisher RG, Oria RA, Mattox KL, et al.: Conservative management if aortic lacerations due to blunt trauma. *J Trauma* 30:1562, 1990.

17. Sweeney MS, Young DJ, Frazier OH, et al.: Traumatic aortic transections: eight-year experience with the "clamp-sew" technique. *Ann Thorac Surg* 64:384, 1997.

18. Batra P, Bigoni B, Manning J, et al.: Pitfalls in the diagnosis of thoracic aortic dissection at CT angiography. *Radiographics* 20:309, 2002.

19. Brink JA, Wang G, McFarland EG: Optimal section spacing in single-detector helical CT. *Radiology* 214:575, 2000.

20. Demetriades D, Gomez H, Velmahos GC, et al.: Routine helical computed tomographic evaluation of the mediastinum in high-risk blunt trauma patients. *Arch Surg* 133:1084, 1998.

21. Durham RM, Zuckerman D, Wolverson M, et al.: CT as a screening exam in patients with suspected blunt aortic injury. *Ann Surg* 220:699, 1994.

22. Dyer DS, Moore EE, Ilke DN, et al.: Thoracic aortic injury: how predictive is mechanism and is chest computed tomography a reliable screening tool? A prospective study in 1561 patients. *J Trauma* 48:673, 2000.

23. Gedebou TM, Mengesha YM, Fortune JB, et al.: Traumatic aortic rupture: The role of spiral computed tomography in diagnosis. *Contemp Surg* 54:92, 1999.

24. Gotway MB: Helical CT evaluation of the thoracic aorta. *Applied Radiology* 2000:7, 2000.

25. Malhotra AK, Fabian TC, Croce MA, et al.: Minimal aortic injury: a lesion associated with advancing diagnostic techniques. *J Trauma* 51:1042, 2001.

26. Mattox KL: Editorial Comment. *J Trauma* 51:1172, 2001.

27. Nagy, K, Fabian T, Rodman G, et al.: Guidelines for the diagnosis and management of blunt aortic injury: an EAST Practice Management Guidelines Work Group. *J Trauma* 48:1128, 2000.

28. Voggenreiter G, Aufmkolk M, Majetscak M, et al.: Efficiency of chest computed tomography in critical ill patients with multiple traumas. *Crit Care Med* 28:1033, 2000.

29. Buckner BA, DiBardino DJ, Cumbie TC, et al.: Critical evaluation of chest computed tomography scans for blunt descending thoracic aortic injury. *Ann Thorac Surg* 81:1339, 2006.

30. Vignon P, Ostyn E, Francois B, et al.: Limitations of transesophageal echocardiography for the diagnosis of traumatic injuries to aortic branches. *J Trauma* 42:960, 1997.

31. Lin P, Lumsden A: Traumatic thoracic aortic injury. *Endovascular Today* 5:58, 2006.

32. Pratesi C, Dorigo W, Troisi N, Pratesi et al.: Acute traumatic rupture of the descending thoracic aorta: Endovascular treatment. *Am J Surg* 192:291, 2006.

33. Tehrani HY, Peterson BG, Katariya K, et al.: Endovascular repair of thoracic aortic tears. *Ann Thorac Surg* 82:873, 2006.

34. Weiman DS, Gurbuz AT, Gursky A, et al.: Comparison of spinal cord protection utilizing left atrial-femoral with femoral-femoral bypass in patients with traumatic rupture of the aortic isthmus. *World J Surgery* 30:1638, 2006.

35. Mattox KL, Whigham C, Fisher RG, et al.: Blunt Trauma to the Thoracic Aorta: Current Challenges. In Lumsden AB, Lin PH, Chen C, Parodi, eds. *Advanced Endovascular Therapy of Aortic Disease.* London: Blackwell Publishing

36. J.Reyes LH, Rubio PA, Korampai FL, et al.: Successful treatment of transection of aortic arch and innominate artery. *Ann Thorac Surg* 19:468, 1975.

37. Pate JW, Cole FH, Walker WA et al.: Penetrating injuries of the aortic arch and its branches. *Ann Thorac Surg* 55:586, 1993.

38. Johnston RH, Jr, Wall MJ, Mattox KL: Innominate artery trauma: a thirty-year experience. *J Vasc Surg* 17:134, 1993.

39. Parmley LF, Mattingly TW, Marian WC, et al.: Nonpenetrating traumatic injury of the aorta. *Circulation* 17:1086, 1958.

40. von Oppell UO, Dunne TT, De Groot MK, et al.: Traumatic aortic rupture: Twenty-year metaanalysis of mortality and risk of paraplegia. *Ann Thorac Surg* 58:585, 1994.

41. Mattox KL: Fact and fiction about management of aortic transection (editorial). *Ann Thorac Surg* 48:1, 1989.

42. Wall MJ, Hirshberg A, Mattox KL: Pulmonary tractotomy with selective vascular ligation for penetrating injuries to the lung. *Am J Surg* 168:1, 1994.

43. Clements RH, Wagmeister LS, Carraway RP: Blunt intrapericardial rupture of the pulmonary artery in a surviving patient. *Ann Thorac Surg* 64:258, 1997.

44. DeBakey ME, Simeone FA: Battle injuries of arteries in World War II: an analysis of 2,471 cases. *Ann Surg* 123:534, 1946.

45. Sydder CL, Eyer SK: Blunt chest trauma with transection of the azygous vein: case report. *J Trauma* 29:889, 1989.

46. Wall MJ Jr., Mattox KL, DeBakey ME: Injuries to the azygous venous system. *J Trauma* 60:357, 2006.

47. Dulchavsky SA, Ledgerwood AM, Lucas CE: Management of chylothorax after blunt chest trauma. *J Trauma* 28:1400, 1988.

48. Graham JM, Beall AC, Jr, Mattox KL, et al.: Systemic air embolism following penetrating trauma to the lung. *Chest* 72:449, 1977.

49. Mattox KL, Beall AC, Jr, Ennix CL, et al.: Intravascular migratory bullets. *Am J Surg* 137:192, 1979.

50. Van Way CW, III: Intrathoracic and intravascular migratory foreign bodies. *Surg Clin North Am* 69:25, 1989.

51. Symbas PN, Symbas PJ: Missiles in the cardiovascular system. *Chest Surg Clin North Am* 7:343, 1997.

# Commentary ■ AURELIO RODRIGUEZ

The veracity and excellence of this comprehensive review is based on the great experience of the authors and even though some of the concepts could be considered biased, I largely agree with the overall content of the chapter. New issues have emerged since the last publication such as new diagnostic methodologies, treatment prioritization when concomitant injuries exist, delayed treatment in stable patients, and the increasing use of intra luminal stents and grafts. All these areas are masterfully addressed in this review.

## ETIOLOGY AND PATHOPHYSIOLOGY

In addition to the well-known, penetrating, and blunt etiology of the great vessels injuries, the authors elegantly describe other causes usually not addressed in regular medical publications such as those arising iatrogenically from percutaneous central venous placement, trocar chest tubes, intraoartic counter pulsation balloons, and the indiscriminate use of Swanz Ganz catheter balloon inflation, etc.[1]

In regard to the pathogenesis of blunt traumatic aortic injury, the authors describe a provocative and interesting mechanism: the profound increase of intraluminal pressure in the vessel as a cause of the injury. One of the points which I strongly agree with is that the term "aortic dissection" is used very frequently in an inappropriate fashion, mostly by our radiologist colleagues. I also concur that the increase in the elderly population (over 65) in this country, represents a challenge for the clinician assessing patients with preexisting diseases or on anticoagulants (Coumadin, Plavix, Warfarin, Clopidogrel) and a concomitant great vessel injury.

## PATIENT CLASSIFICATION

The new classification by the authors of great vessel injuries, based on the fact that the epidemiology of these lesions is changing due to the rapid EMS transportation and new therapeutic and diagnostic modalities, is very useful.

## INITIAL EVALUATION AND MANAGEMENT

The mechanisms of injury in blunt traumatic aortic injury are discussed, emphasizing the new revelation that 50% of cases occur following side-impact collisions.

## PHYSICAL EXAMINATION

We continue stating that the initial presentation of patients in the emergency suite can be deceiving. Furthermore, many patients can be hemodynamically stable for long periods of time. We continue utilizing Clark's recommendations in regard to signs that predict imminent exsanguination: Hemothorax greater than 500 mL, pseudocoarctation, and left supraclavicular hematoma.[2]

## CHEST RADIOGRAPH

A review by Mirvis and colleagues stated that the correlation between "wide mediastinum" and aortic rupture is inaccurate. We studied the aortic knob, the descending thoracic aorta, and the paraspinal line, with a negative predictive value of these combined parameters of 99%. Nevertheless, we agree that the chest radiograph is a good screening modality.

## COMPUTED TOMOGRAPHY

This is an area of controversy. However, the new advances in computerized tomography are clearly demonstrating the accuracy of this modality, not only in screening for aortic injuries, but also in diagnosing them correctly.[3,4]

I strongly believe, based on my experience, that more cardiothoracic surgeons in the world are using CT scanning as the definitive diagnostic test before going to the operating suite. I agree with the authors that the concept is evolving. Most modern trauma centers are using chest–abdominal–pelvic CT scans almost routinely in blunt trauma patients due to the limitations of the chest x-ray supine films and the lack of resident manpower (due to the 80 hours working rules). Consequently, to have to wait in the middle of the night for the angiographic team could, in my view, be dangerous.

## EMERGENCY DEPARTMENT THORACOTOMY

In blunt trauma, this is generally futile in cases of thoracic aortic disruption. In my experience at my previous institution, no patient survived in these circumstances. In penetrating trauma, the survivability depends on the experience and expedience of the operator.

## ANGIOGRAPHY

We agree with the authors that in penetrating trauma of the great vessels in the presence of hemodynamically stable patients, this procedure is helpful, not only to localize the injury, but to better plan the surgical approach. In blunt trauma, arteriography seems to be relegated to a secondary role due to the sophistication of CT and the preference by an increasing number of surgeons to take the patient to the operating room based only on the CT findings. Nevertheless, we concur that if there is a doubtful diagnosis, angiographic evaluation could be necessary.

## TRANSESOPHAGEAL ECHOCARDIOGRAPHY

The advantage of TEE is that it allows a relatively expeditious evaluation of the great vessels even with concomitant abdominal exploration. Its limitations are the lack of accuracy in the evaluation of the ascending aorta and arch of the aorta. It could be very useful in the work up of morbidly obese patients, where weight prohibits performing CT and angiography. In Allegheny General Hospital, TEE is used routinely in the assessment of blunt aortic trauma with such great success that on several occasions it is the only test performed before going to the operating room. To the best of my knowledge this singular experience has not been repeated in many places.[5]

## THORACOSCOPY

This modality is in the frontiers of the evaluation of the great vessels, mediastinum, etc. However, other procedures such as CT scan or magnetic resonance angiography are less invasive and risky.

## TREATMENT

### Nonoperative Management

The authors present several indications for nonoperative management of blunt thoracic aortic injuries. However, they also describe cases of "nonthreatening" aortic lesions, e.g., minor intraluminal defects and small psuedoaneurysms or small internal flaps of the brachiocephalic vessels. I am not aware of respectable series reporting these "nonthreatening" lesions. We all have anecdotal cases of these "nonthreatening" lesions, but I am not ready to recommend the nonoperative management since this is a very subjective decision.

### ENDOVASCULAR STENTING

This novel approach is revolutionizing the management of these "nightmare injuries" for the cardiothoracic trauma surgeons, despite the present limitation and shortcomings such as in the take-off of the left subclavian, etc. The over 200 cases described by the authors is, in my view, only the "tip of the iceberg." I strongly believe that in the near future, most of the blunt thoracic aortic injuries will be taken care of successfully by the angiographer cardiac surgeon team.

### SURGICAL REPAIR

The description of the operative and perioperative management is masterfully presented by the authors. We all are aware that blunt injuries of the ascending aorta are associated with a high mortality rate. In cases of penetrating trauma, the outcome is more promising.

### TRACHEOINNOMINATE ARTERY INJURY

This lethal injury can occur also iatrogenically when performing tracheostomy. Two scenarios are possible:

1. Intermittent trachoestomy bleeding. In this case, the sequence of treatment should be as follows:
   - Bronchoscopy in the operating room or ICU, with the operating room on standby
   - Immediate surgery of a fistula is identified in the anterior wall
2. Massive bleeding from the trachoestomy tube. In this case, the sequence of treatment should be as follows:
   - Hyperinflation of the tracheostomy balloon
   - Introduction of the right index finger in the tracheostomy wound, compressing the innominate artery between the anterior wall and the sternum.
   - Maintaining finger pressure until a median sternotomy can be done at bedside or the operating room, if the patient's condition allows.

We prefer to oversew the proximal and distal stumps with 3-0 Prolene and do not place an interposition graft (in cases of tracheo-innominate artery fistula).[6]

## ADJUNCTS

- The preoperative use of double lumen Endotracheal tubes facilitate the surgical visualization of the injury.
- Several modalities have been used to prevent paraplegia such as the intraoperative use of somatosensory and motor evoked potentials, centrifugal Vortex pumps etc., without improvement in outcome. We believe that the best way to prevent postoperative paraplegia is to avoid perioperative hypotension.

## DAMAGE CONTROL

Patients severely compromised by the injury should be candidates for this modality. Temporary plastic devices have been used to close the chest.

## SUBCLAVIAN ARTERY INJURY

Angiography definitely helps (if the patient is hemodynamically stable) to plan the surgical approach. If the lesion is behind the scalene muscles or lateral to them, only a supraclavicular incision should be necessary. If the lesion is medial to the scalene muscles, a mid-sternotomy plus a supraclavicular incision is appropriate. We agree with the authors and we do not recommend a "trap door incision." We find that this offers no advantage.

## PULMONARY ARTERY INJURIES AND VENOUS INJURIES

These are described very comprehensively, particularly the intrapericardial approach of the pulmonary artery.

## MEDIASTINAL TRANSVERSE INJURIES

The advances in computerized tomography imaging will eventually displace, in my opinion, standard angiography, pericardial window, bronchoscopy, esophagoscopy.

## THORACIC DUCT INJURIES

Improvements of video thoracoscopy (VATS) technology will help the clinician identify and ligate the thoracic duct in a more expeditious and less invasive fashion.

## SUMMARY

Computerized tomographic angiography is replacing the use of arteriography for the diagnosis of blunt and penetrating thoracic injuries as well as in the assessment of transmediastinal injuries. This near-simple new technology avoids the use of multiple diagnostic procedures. Finally, in the future, the use of stents and nonoperative management will considerably modify the "traditional landscape" in the approach and management of great vessel injuries.

## References

1. Rodriguez A, Elliott D: Blunt traumatic rupture of the thoracic aorta. *Adv Trauma Crit Care* 8:145, 1993.
2. Clark DE, Zeigher MA, Wallace KL, et al.: Blunt aortic trauma: Signs of high risk. *J Trauma* 30:701, 1990.
3. Mirvis SE, Bidwell K, Buddemeyer EU, et al.: Value of chest radiography in excluding traumatic aortic rupture. *Radiology* 163:487, 1987.
4. Mirvis SE, Shanmuganathan K, Buell J, et al.: Use of spinal computed tomography for the assessment of blunt trauma patients with potential aortic injury. *J Trauma* 45:922, 1998
5. Rodriguez A, Elliott D: Blunt thoracic vascular injury. *Vascular Trauma* 269, 2004.
6. Leonard DJ, Rodriguez A: tracheoinnominate artery fistula. In Turney SZ, Rodriguez A, Cowley RA, eds: *Management of Cardiothoracic Trauma*. Baltimore: Williams & Wilkins, 1990, p. 373.

# Indications for and Techniques of Laparotomy

*Demetrios Demetriades* ■ *George C. Velmahos*

## HISTORY

The word laparotomy derives from the Greek words "lapara," which refers to the soft part of the abdomen and "tome," which means incision. The word celiotomy is synonymous and derives from the Greek words "celia," which means abdomen, and "tome," which means "incision."

The history of the first laparotomies for abdominal trauma cannot be traced accurately. Celsus in his writings in the 1st century AD discussed abdominal trauma. The Greek physician Galen (AD 130–200), physician to the gladiators and later personal physician of emperor Marcus Aurelius, had significant experience in penetrating trauma and is known to have performed abdominal wall and intestinal suturing. Significant progress in the management of penetrating abdominal injuries was made with the discovery of chloroform by Simpson in 1847 and introduction of general anesthesia. The American Surgical Association in 1887 recommended exploration of civilian penetrating abdominal wounds. At the beginning of World War I there was a policy not to explore abdominal wounds. Due to the extremely high mortality in 1915, however, a protocol of exploration of all penetrating abdominal wounds was adopted. Although the mortality decreased significantly, it still remained higher than 50% until the availability of blood transfusion. In the next few decades a policy of mandatory laparotomy for all civilian and military penetrating abdominal injuries remained the standard of care. This concept was challenged in the 1960s and 1970s when a policy of selective nonoperative management was gradually introduced and has become an acceptable and widespread practice.

## INJURY GRADING SYSTEMS

### Global Abdominal Grading Systems

The purpose of grading systems is to provide physicians with a relatively simple numerical method for ranking, describing, and comparing injuries. A grading system makes comparisons between various diagnostic or therapeutic modalities more accurate and meaningful and is essential in the development of prognostic models. The severity of injury in the abdomen as a whole is most commonly graded by two systems, the abdominal Abbreviated Injury Scale (AIS) score and the Penetrating Abdominal Trauma Index (PATI). Both systems are purely anatomical which means that no physiologic parameters are included.

*The Abdominal Injury Scale (see Chap.5):* The AIS was developed by the Association for the Advancement of Automotive Medicine and was initially designed to facilitate the coding of blunt trauma. The newer and expanded editions cover penetrating trauma as well. The AIS is a consensus-derived system, which classifies individual organ injuries by body region on a 6-point ordinal severity scale ranging from AIS 1 (minor) to AIS 6 (lethal). The abdomen is one of six body regions assessed and receives an AIS score based on the most severely injured intra-abdominal organ. By adding the squares of the three highest AIS scores from the six body regions, the Injury Severity Score (ISS) is derived and represents an estimation of the severity of the entire trauma. A major limitation of the AIS is the failure to reflect the combined effects of multiple injuries within the same body region. For example, a patient with a major liver laceration will receive an abdominal AIS score of 4. Another patient with the same liver laceration but also lacerations to the head of the pancreas, renal collecting system, small bowel, and colon, may receive the same AIS score of 4, although this patient clearly has a more severe abdominal injury and higher likelihood for adverse outcomes. For this and other reasons, the AIS and ISS may not provide accurate estimations for certain types of injuries and lead to misclassification of the probability for survival.[1] Such misclassifications may have major implications when comparing research results or the performance of different trauma centers. To account for these problems, modifications of the ISS system, such as the new ISS (NISS) have been proposed.[2] The NISS is calculated by adding the squares of AIS of the three most severe organ injuries regardless of body region. By this method, one single body region can contribute more than one AIS in the calculation of NISS. For example, a patient with a spleen AIS of 4, liver AIS of 4, pancreas AIS of 4, lung AIS of 3, and humerus AIS of 2 received an ISS of $4^2+3^2+2^2=29$ but an NISS of $4^2+4^2+4^2=48$. Although it has been suggested that NISS is a more accurate predictor of outcome,[3] the experience with the use of this system is limited.

*The Penetrating Abdominal Trauma Index:* The PATI score was initially described for penetrating injuries. Each intra-abdominal organ is assigned a risk factor and an estimate of the injury severity. The sum of the individual organ scores comprises the final PATI. A score of 25 seems to discriminate adequately between severe and mild injuries. Patients with PATI scores of 25 and above have a postoperative morbidity of 50% compared to 5% in patients with PATI scores below 25.[3] The inventors of PATI revised the system ten years later. The new Abdominal Trauma Index (ATI) required a re-adjustment in the relative rank order of six of the 15 organ systems described (duodenum, major vascular, kidney, extrahepatic biliary, small bowel, stomach) to enhance the prediction of intra-abdominal sepsis. Major vascular injuries presented the greatest risk and small bowel injuries the lowest risk for intra-abdominal infections. The risk of intra-abdominal sepsis increased exponentially with ATI scores greater than 25. The PATI has been extensively used in many studies to describe high-risk groups of patients and remains a good prognostic factor of final outcome.[4]

## INITIAL EVALUATION

### General Principles

The physician evaluating the abdomen should answer two questions: (a) Is there an intra-abdominal injury and (b) does this injury require operative repair? While addressing these issues, two principles should not be violated: (a) the ABCs should be adequately assessed before focusing on the abdomen and (b) clinical examination should be the most important element of the evaluation. Clinical examination can determine the need for emergent exploration following abdominal trauma by the presence of one or both of two signs: (a) peritonitis and (b) hemodynamic instability. In the absence of these two signs, there is time for more detailed investigations.

### Clinical Examination

Despite the technological advances, which undoubtedly add greatly to the ability to evaluate the abdomen, clinical examination remains of paramount importance. Hemodynamic stability (or instability) is a term, which is widely used but insufficiently understood. At the initial stage, the hemodynamic status is usually assessed by crude methods, such as blood pressure, heart rate, and urine output monitoring, serum hemoglobin measurement, and evaluation of the skin and capillary refill (see Chap. 11). Although such information is very important, one needs to remember the limitations of using these measurements to assess hemodynamic stability. Hypotension may occur in the presence of spinal cord injury without blood loss. Hypertension may occur even in the

presence of blood loss due to increased intracranial pressure and a Cushing's reflex. A blood pressure of 110 mm Hg may be normal for a 25-year-old man, abnormally high for a six-month old baby, and profusely low for a 70-year-old hypertensive woman. The heart rate can be high for causes unrelated to bleeding, such as pain or anxiety. On the other hand, a normal or low heart rate cannot exclude bleeding, particularly in patients with high spinal cord injuries, chronic cocaine intoxication, or beta-blocker medication. Paradoxical bradycardia occurs in up to 29% of hypotensive trauma patients.[5] For these reasons a more precise description of the hemodynamic status of the patient is highly desirable. Pulmonary artery catheterization is not logistically feasible in most acute trauma areas. Now, noninvasive technology allows continuous monitoring of the cardiac output, stroke volume, and transcutaneous oxygen tension.[6] These portable devices can be connected to the patient by simple self-adhesive patches, like EKG leads, and provide hemodynamic and oxygen tissue perfusion monitoring even during the very early posttraumatic stages.[7] In summary, hemodynamic instability is a valid reason for laparotomy as long as the physician recognizes the limitations of vital signs and incorporates additional elements in the decision-making to increase its accuracy.

Diffuse abdominal tenderness is the other major indicator of the need for laparotomy. It is important to distinguish between superficial soft tissue tenderness, such as caused by a stab wound or a seatbelt, and deep tenderness caused by a true abdominal organ injury. In the presence of penetrating injuries, it is the tenderness on deep palpation away from the wound site that denotes internal injuries. A significant part of the trauma population is simply nonevaluable because of associated head injuries, spinal cord injuries, or intoxication. Such patients receive the most benefit from additional studies. Intoxication, unless profound, should not be a reason to avoid clinical examination. Most patients with mild or moderate intoxication will manifest abdominal tenderness on careful evaluation, if intra-abdominal structures are injured and the reliability of clinical examination is not impaired.[8,9]

### Ultrasonography (see Chap. 17)

The focused abdominal sonography for trauma (FAST) emerged recently as an important tool in the initial diagnosis of intra-abdominal injuries. Performed by surgeons or emergency room physicians, FAST has shown an excellent sensitivity in identifying intra-abdominal fluid.[10] Because of its ease of use, repeatability, and avoidance of radiation exposure it has rapidly become an essential part of the initial evaluation. In the presence of multiple intraperitoneal injuries, blood is most often found by FAST in the right upper quadrant.[10] Although the sensitivity of FAST ranges between 90% and 100% in most studies, the possibility of publication bias (i.e., good results are reported, bad results are shelved) still exists. Furthermore, specific injuries, such as small bowel trauma[10] or patient subgroups, such as pediatric patients,[11] may be associated with a high incidence of false negative results. The role of FAST in the evaluation of abdominal trauma should be based mainly on the individual center's experience and not on the experience from other centers. In spite of the apparent limitations of this operator-dependant technique, ultrasonography is a useful adjunct to the initial evaluation of the abdomen, when considered into the context of the entire clinical picture, as formed by detailed physical examination and other tests. At this point, it seems that the most significant contribution of the FAST examination is in the detection of intra-abdominal fluid in the hemodynamically unstable and clinically unevaluable blunt trauma victim. These patients should be immediately taken to the operating room for abdominal exploration. Negative FAST exams do not preclude the need for further evaluation of the abdomen by other imaging modalities, most commonly computed tomography (CT).

## Diagnostic Peritoneal Lavage

DPL Technique.    The open technique for DPL consists of a small (2–5 cm) incision below the umbilicus and dissection of the subcutaneous tissue to the fascia. In the presence of pelvic fractures or advanced pregnancy, the incision is made above the umbilicus to avoid entering into an anterior pelvic hematoma or injuring the enlarged uterus. The fascia and peritoneum are opened sharply under direct vision. A catheter is inserted through the opening and directed toward the pelvis.

The percutaneous technique is done in a Seldinger fashion by making a small 0.5-cm incision below (or above) the umbilicus. A needle is inserted through the fascia in a controlled fashion until a "give" is felt after penetration of the peritoneum. A syringe containing fluid may be used to confirm intraperitoneal placement of the needle by unobstructed fluid flow into the abdomen. The syringe is disconnected and a guidewire is fed through the needle. The needle is removed over the guidewire and after a dilator dilates the tract, a catheter is inserted with a direction toward the pelvis and the guidewire is removed. If gross aspiration of the catheter yields no gross blood, one liter of warm normal saline (in children 10–15 mL/kg) is infused into the peritoneal cavity. The fluid is then siphoned back into the empty container which is lowered to below the level of the patient. A specimen of the recovered fluid is then examined macroscopically, microscopically, and biochemically. The retrieval of gross blood or blood-stained fluid with a count of more than 100,000 red blood cells/mm$^3$ constitutes a positive exam for blunt abdominal injuries.[12] The red blood cell count which constitutes a positive DPL for penetrating abdominal injuries is controversial. If the count is kept at >100,000 cells/mm,$^3$ there are no false positives but there is an unacceptably high incidence of false negative results of 11%.[13] The false negative rate decreases to 1%, if the count is considered abnormal at the 10,000 cells/mm$^3$ but the false positive rate increases to 14%. Besides the red blood cell count, a white blood cell count and other elements, such as amylase, alkaline phosphatase, bilirubin, etc. have been used to detect intra-abdominal organ injury. The standard white blood cell count criterion of >500 cells/mm$^3$ used for blunt trauma is not as accurate in penetrating injuries. Of 11 patients lavaged within four hours after injury and a white blood cell count higher than 500 cells/mm,$^3$ nine had no injuries.[14] On the other hand, 15 of 25 patients lavaged at a mean of six to seven hours of an abdominal stab wound and found to have more than 500 white blood cells/mm,$^3$ had a false positive result.[15] A lavage amylase of more than 19 IU/L and lavage alkaline phosphatase of more than 2 IU/L have been also proposed as useful measures to detect hollow visceral injuries. However, of 13 patients with stab wounds or gunshot wounds and proven abdominal organ injuries, only six had amylase levels higher than 19 and only three had alkaline phosphatase higher than two.[16]

The major advantage of DPL is a sensitivity rate higher than 95% for identifying intraperitoneal hemorrhage.[12] However, because the technique is invasive and fails to identify the source of bleeding and the need for operative repair, DPL is used with decreasing frequency over the years. For hemodynamically stable patients, CT provides more accurate information about the quantity of intra-abdominal fluid and the specific abdominal organ injuries. For hemodynamically unstable patients, ultrasonography is a faster, easier, and less invasive test but is operator-dependent and of unknown value in penetrating trauma. Therefore, DPL in today's health care environment is used predominantly when CT or FAST are not available, if there is not sufficient expertise to make decisions based on the FAST results, or if the FAST results are negative but there is no other source to account for the hemodynamic instability.[17] Additionally, DPL can be used to distinguish blood from other type of fluids, not caused by trauma, such as ascites. DPL can be performed by an open or percutaneous technique with similar accuracy and safety but the percutaneous technique is much faster.[18]

In the authors' institutions, the percutaneous technique without infusion of fluid is used in most cases, proceeding only to a diagnostic peritoneal aspiration (DPA) instead of a full lavage. If the patient is hemodynamically unstable due to intra-abdominal bleeding, gross blood should be retrieved upon insertion of the catheter (Fig. 30-1). If no gross blood is detected, the source of hemodynamic instability is elsewhere, and there is no reason to compromise the interpretation of potential CT-imaging by the presence of iatrogenically infused intra-abdominal fluid.

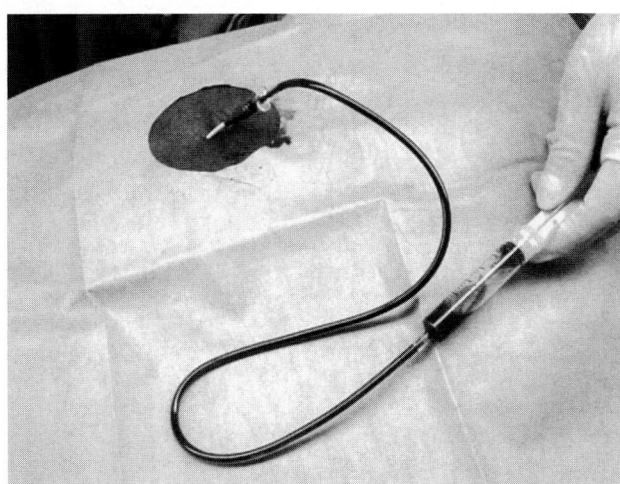

**FIGURE 30-1.** Diagnostic Peritoneal Aspirate (DPA). The catheter is inserted with the closed technique into the peritoneal cavity and directed toward the pelvis. The presence or absence of gross blood on aspiration determines a positive or negative DPA. DPA is very useful in hemodynamically unstable multitrauma patients when the trauma ultrasound is questionable and a quick identification of the source of hypotension is essential.

## Abdominal Computed Tomography (see Chap. 16)

Abdominal CT is becoming the test of preference for evaluating the abdomen of patients with blunt abdominal trauma who are hemodynamically stable and complain of abdominal tenderness or are unevaluable. It allows estimation of the amount of intra-abdominal fluid and accurate imaging of solid parenchymal injuries in most patients.[19] Abdominal CT plays a major role in the decision to manage the injured spleen, liver, or kidney nonoperatively (see Chaps. 32, 33, 39). Although old studies, which for the most part did not use helical technology, challenged the predictive power of organ injury grade on the outcome of nonoperative management, newer studies[20] have shown that the CT-derived organ injury grading is accurate and closely related to the likelihood of success or failure of nonoperative management. As the use of abdominal CT in blunt trauma is increasing, it is important to recognize its limitations. First, CT has limitations in detecting hollow visceral and mesenteric injuries[21,22] (see Chap. 34). This diagnosis is usually suspected on the basis of indirect signs, such as free fluid in the absence of solid visceral injury, pneumoperitoneum, mesenteric fat streaking, bowel wall thickening, or extravasation of luminal contrast.[23,24] Free fluid is the most frequently found and associated with significant hollow visceral or mesenteric injury in 30% to 94% of the patients.[24,25] Based on this incidence, many authors would recommend routine laparotomy in the presence of this sign. The presence of another of the above signs in addition to fluid of unexplained origin increases the likelihood of significant bowel or mesenteric injury to 80% or higher and should almost always prompt surgical exploration. It has been suggested that in children the presence of unexplained fluid on abdominal CT should not always be an indication for laparotomy because the incidence of significant intra-abdominal injuries is only 3%.[26] Another limitation of the CT relates to the possibility of missing superficial lacerations to solid organs. In most occasions, these lacerations are not clinically important and do not require surgical repair.

Abdominal CT is done with administration of intravenous and oral contrast in order to optimize the visualization of the organs. However, oral contrast administration is time-consuming (because at least 30 minutes are required for the contrast to outline the small bowel) and potentially dangerous (because of the risk of aspiration). In a prospective randomized trial of 199 patients who received oral contrast during abdominal CT and 195 patients without oral contrast, Stafford et al.[27] failed to find any differences in the detection of small bowel injury between the two groups. Similarly, in a study of 101 pediatric patients, Shankar et al.[22] concluded that the omission of oral contrast was not associated with delay in the diagnosis of intestinal injury. Our policy is to administer oral contrast provided it does not delay an emergency scanning. Oral contrast certainly has a valuable role in the evaluation of suspected duodenal injuries. The role of abdominal CT has been recently expanded in the evaluation of patients with abdominal gunshot wounds, selected for nonoperative management.[28,29] The CT scan may show the direction of a bullet tract and thus help in selecting patients who may be managed nonoperatively (Fig. 30-2). Also, it may show the site, size, and presence of active bleeding or false aneurysms in solid organ injuries. As abdominal CT is used more and more frequently, it becomes essential to monitor the possibly inappropriate use of technology. CT scanners at the front door of emergency rooms and portable CT scanners are being

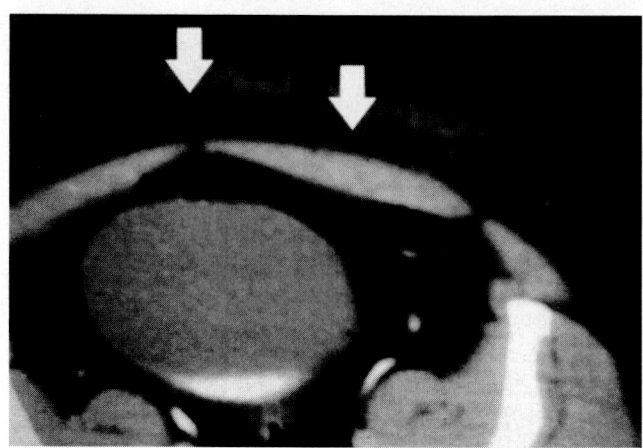

**FIGURE 30-2.** CT scan of the abdomen following a gunshot wound. The bullet tract (*arrows*) is outside the peritoneal cavity. This patient does not need laparotomy.

introduced.[30] Some remain skeptical about the ever-diminishing value of clinical examination and the training of a whole new generation of surgeons who are dependent on CT to diagnose abdominal pathology. On the other hand, there is no doubt that diagnostic accuracy and avoidance of unnecessary operations is related to the ability to image the abdomen accurately. Whether we like it or not, abdominal CT has become an indispensable tool in the evaluation of abdominal trauma. Predictably, the future will make the relation of trauma and CT even greater.

## Rigid Sigmoidoscopy

The value of rigid sigmoidoscopy is significant when it comes to evaluating the extraperitoneal rectum (see Chap. 36) Injuries to this part of the intestinal tract may not produce symptoms initially and escape diagnosis until septic complications prompt further investigation. Classically, gunshot wounds to the gluteal regions, particularly if the trajectory crosses the midline, have the potential of producing initially asymptomatic extraperitoneal rectal injuries. Rectal examination may be helpful but is often unreliable. Rigid sigmoidoscopy reveals intraluminal blood or the exact injury.[31,32] In a series of 30 patients with extraperitoneal rectal injuries, 21 were evaluated by sigmoidoscopy and blood was found in all of them.[32] It is important that air insufflation is kept to a minimum in order to avoid fecal spillage in patients with perforation. The inability to identify the precise site of injury sigmoidoscoppically is not uncommon in unprepared bowel. Therefore, if blood is found in the rectum by sigmoidoscopy, the patient should be treated as if an injury exists. When rigid sigmoidoscopy identifies the exact level of injury, this information serves to plan the appropriate operation, i.e., transanal repair or transabdominal repair with or without diversion.

Patients with pelvic gunshot wounds who are taken to the operating room can be placed in a mild lithotomy position. Then, rigid sigmoidoscopy could be done before or during the operation, if there are doubts about extraperitoneal rectal injuries. Lower-rectal injuries with small surrounding hematomas may not be obvious by looking through the open peritoneal cavity. Opening the peritoneal reflection following an abdominal operation for repair of hollow visceral injuries exposes one more body area to infection and is associated with complications related to dissection of nerves and vessels.

Intra-operative rigid sigmoidoscopy may help in making the decision of opening or leaving undisturbed the peritoneal reflection.

## Diagnostic Laparoscopy

Despite the constantly increasing applications of laparoscopic surgery, trauma has not yet been a fertile field for laparoscopy. The acuity of most trauma patients requiring an operation does not allow the time required to set up and use of laparoscopic equipment. On the other hand, patients who do not need an operation can be followed clinically or imaged by CT without the need for interventional diagnostic techniques. The major limitations of diagnostic laparoscopy in trauma are related to the inability to "run" the bowel, diagnose retroperitoneal injuries, expose adequately deep-lying organs and estimate accurately the quantity of hemoperitoneum.[33] Studies have shown that close to half of the existing injuries can be missed by laparoscopy.[33] On the other hand, diagnostic laparoscopy has an excellent sensitivity and specificity (>95%) when used as a screening tool to establish the presence of peritoneal violation, hemoperitoneum, or enteric content spillage.[33] However, findings such as peritoneal penetration or hemoperitoneum are not always associated with a therapeutic laparotomy and therefore, the information provided by laparoscopy is of questionable use.

At this point, there is only one clear-cut indication for diagnostic laparoscopy and relates to penetrating left thoracoabdominal trauma. In 42% of patients with such injuries, the diaphragm is involved (50% for gunshot wounds, 32% for stab wounds).[34] Many of these patients do not have other injuries requiring a laparotomy. Additionally, imaging tests, such as CT, contrast swallow or enema, or plain radiographs after insertion of a nasogastric tube, are inaccurate in diagnosing small, uncomplicated diaphragmatic penetrations. Direct visualization of the diaphragm by laparoscopy remains the only reliable method to identify these injuries. In a prospective study, Murray et al.[35] evaluated laparoscopically 110 patients with left thoracoabdominal penetrating injuries and no indication for laparotomy, and found an incidence of 24% of occult diaphragmatic injuries. This incidence was similar in anterior, lateral, and posterior injuries. Many patients had a completely normal chest radiograph. The conclusion of the study was that all patients with penetrating trauma to the left lower chest and without an indication for laparotomy should undergo laparoscopic evaluation of the left hemidiaphragm to exclude an occult injury regardless of the presence or absence of associated clinical or radiographic findings.

Although it is suspected that the incidence of occult injuries will be similar to the right hemidiaphragm, the "buttressing effect" of the liver makes their identification less important. Anecdotally, we have seen patients with right visceral herniation after right anterior thoracoabdominal wounds. Therefore, it might be necessary to perform laparoscopy in anterior wounds of the right lower chest. Posterior wounds are very unlikely to produce visceral herniation with the liver lying between the diaphragm and the remaining of abdominal contents. However, there is a risk of bronchobiliary fistula formation in the presence of a liver injury and an unrepaired diaphragmatic defect.

Bedside laparoscopy with or without gas insufflation has been proposed as a convenient screening tool at the emergency department or intensive care unit. The authors' experience with a few cases has been unsatisfactory because of poor visual field and patient discomfort.

## INDICATIONS FOR LAPAROTOMY

The trauma patient often presents a diagnostic puzzle. Incomplete data in the emergency room, unevaluable patients, and multiple injuries may complicate the decision to operate or observe the patient. Delaying laparotomy is associated with serious morbidity. On the other hand, negative laparotomies are not without significant consequences for the patients.[36] The full appreciation of the patient's picture, taking into account all available information provided by clinical examination, radiographic findings, and laboratory tests is more useful than the adherence to rigid protocols that prevent individualization. Understanding basic rules that govern trauma decision-making allows the establishment of policies, regarding the decision to operate, which make good clinical sense and are applicable to the majority of patients. The advent of trauma ultrasonography, increasing use of CT, and successful application of nonoperative techniques have drastically changed the therapeutic algorithms over the last years, including the indications for operation. However, the two signs, which remain absolute indications for laparotomy following penetrating or blunt abdominal trauma are peritonitis and hemodynamic instability. In the presence of either of these two findings the patient should be taken to the operating room without delay. A third indication relates to the inability to examine the patient reliably after a penetrating injury. Patients with significant associated head injuries, spinal cord injuries, severe intoxication, or other injuries requiring emergent operation (such as open long-bone fractures) are included in this group. Although most of these patients are managed safer by routine operation, some discretion is allowed based on hemodynamic stability, time expected to pass until the patient is fully evaluable, and the ability for close observation and additional tests.

## Penetrating Trauma

Stab Wounds.    Over the last 30 years, it became clear that stab wounds to the abdomen can be managed selectively based predominantly on clinical examination. Shaftan in 1960[37] and Nance et al. in 1969[38] were among the first ones to depart from the old policy of routine exploration for all abdominal stab wounds. Following these studies, Demetriades and Rabinowitz[39] reported a prospective study of 651 patients with stab wounds to the anterior abdomen treated with a policy of selective nonoperative management based mainly on serial physical examinations. Half of these patients were successfully managed without a laparotomy. Only 11 (1.6%) patients who were initially observed, required a laparotomy later, and there was no mortality among them. The accuracy of the initial physical examination was 93.9% (false-negative initial exam 3.2%, false-negative exam 2.9%). In a similar study, Shorr et al.[40] found that only 32% of 330 patients with abdominal stab wounds had a therapeutic laparotomy and an additional 14% a nontherapeutic laparotomy. The remaining 53% were discharged without an operation.

Stab wounds to the back result in significant injuries requiring surgical repair in only about 15% of patients. In a South African prospective study of 230 stab wounds to the back the selection of treatment was based predominantly on physical examination; 85% of these patients were successfully managed nonoperatively. The diagnosis was delayed in five patients (2.2%) with no serious

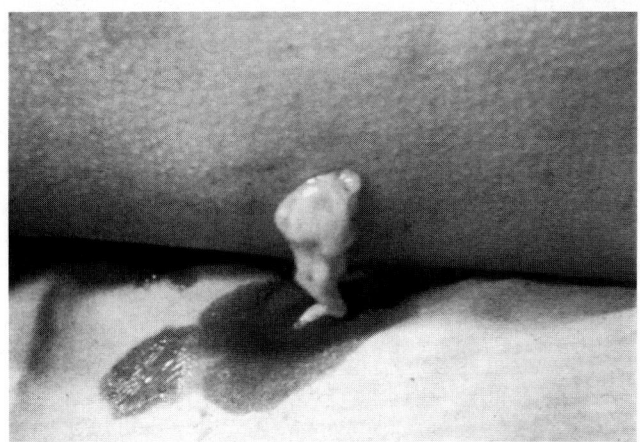

**FIGURE 30-3.** Omental evisceration following a stab wound to the abdomen. In the absence of peritoneal symptoms some authors recommend nonoperative management. Such policy should be considered in centers with 24-hour in-house staffing by trauma surgeons.

consequences. The overall accuracy of the initial physical examination was 95.2% (false-positive 2.6%, false-negative 2.2%).[41]

Indications for laparotomy such as peritoneal penetration, omental evisceration (Fig. 30-3), free air on abdominal radiographs, or blood on abdominal paracentesis are debated. Some investigators report an association of 69% of such findings with significant intra-abdominal injuries, even in the absence of generalized abdominal tenderness.[42] Others have found no such association and continue to use selective management and avoid routine operation in these patients.[39] Such policy should be considered only in centers with experience and appropriate in-house staffing by trauma surgeons.

The role of diagnostic tests in the decision to operate on abdominal stab wounds is limited. DPL has major limitations and very few centers use this modality for this type of trauma. Trauma ultrasonography is reported to have a specificity of 94% but a sensitivity of only 46%.[43] Helical CT may be of value but has not yet been formally studied in stab wounds as it has in gunshot wounds. Laparoscopy is inadequate to diagnose small bowel or retroperitoneal organ injury.[33] The "stabbogram" and local wound exploration are techniques rarely practiced in trauma centers. However, there are occasions in which additional tests are appropriate. For example, in patients with suspected liver injuries or hematuria or blood per rectum as their only symptoms, CT or rigid sigmoidoscopy should be strongly considered.[44,45]

In summary, a careful initial physical examination followed by serial examinations remain the most important tool to set the indications for laparotomy after abdominal stab wounds. Although symptom-directed additional tests may be useful in individual cases, in most patients the decision to operate or not should be based on serial physical exams and close hemodynamic monitoring.

Gunshot Wounds.    Although selective management is considered as the standard of care for stab wounds, abdominal gunshot wounds are treated by routine laparotomy in most trauma centers. The mere presence of a gunshot wound to the abdomen with potential violation of the peritoneum equals a laparotomy. The main reasons cited for this approach are four: (1) There is a high incidence of intra-abdominal organ injury, which approaches 90%, (2) many centers have limited experience with gunshot wounds, (3) negative laparotomy is not particularly morbid, and (4) physical examination is unreliable. There is overwhelming evidence that the two latter statements are not true. Nontherapeutic laparotomy is associated with morbidity ranging

from 12% to 40% and prolongation of hospital stay.[46] Physical examination is reliable for stab wounds and blunt trauma, even in the presence of mild and moderate intoxication,[39] so, some authors suggest, there is no reason to consider it unreliable for gunshot wounds. Therefore, the debate about routine exploration versus selective management of abdominal gunshot wounds is centered around the two former reasons. With regard to the first reason, it is unknown why there are discrepancies among different studies reporting on the incidence of significant intra-abdominal injuries following a gunshot wound to the abdomen. Incidences of 89% to 94% have been presented by some authors,[47–49] whereas others have found much lower incidences, ranging from 68% to 75%.[8,9,50–53] It is possible that the former group of authors have included injuries, which did not require operative repair, or that the latter group of authors have included many probable superficial gunshot wounds. Also, some of the studies with a high incidence refer to injuries with proven peritoneal violation.[49] The authors' group has shown that approximately one-third of the patients with gunshot wounds to the anterior abdomen[9] and two-thirds with gunshot wounds to the back[8] have no significant intra-abdominal injuries and can be safely managed nonoperatively. In a prospective study of 309 patients with abdominal gunshot wounds included over a 16-month period, 34% of the patients were initially selected for nonoperative management and 30% were finally discharged without an operation.[9] In a similar prospective study of 203 patients with gunshot wounds to the back, collected over 12 months, 69% were initially observed and 66% discharged without a laparotomy.[8] The summarized experience from the authors' center with 1856 patients with anterior (1405 patients) or posterior (451 patients) abdominal gunshot wounds over an eight-year period revealed that there was no significant abdominal injury in 47% of the patients (39% with anterior and 74% with posterior gunshot wounds).[54] Eighty patients (4%) developed findings during observation and required a delayed laparotomy. Only five (0.3%) patients suffered complications potentially related to the delay in laparotomy, which were managed successfully. The rate of nontherapeutic laparotomy was 9%. In these three studies, superficial gunshot wounds were excluded. Based on these observations, it seems that there is a sizable portion of patients with abdominal gunshot wounds without significant intra-abdominal organ injury requiring surgical intervention. Selected patients with isolated gunshot wounds to solid organs (liver, spleen, kidney) who are hemodynamically stable and have no peritoneal signs, may be managed nonoperatively (Fig. 30-4). In a study

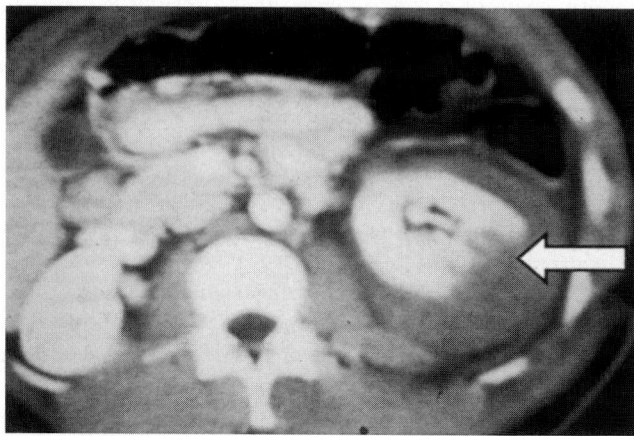

**FIGURE 30-4.** Gunshot wound to the left kidney. The patient was hemodynamically stable and had no signs of peritonitis. He was successfully managed nonoperatively.

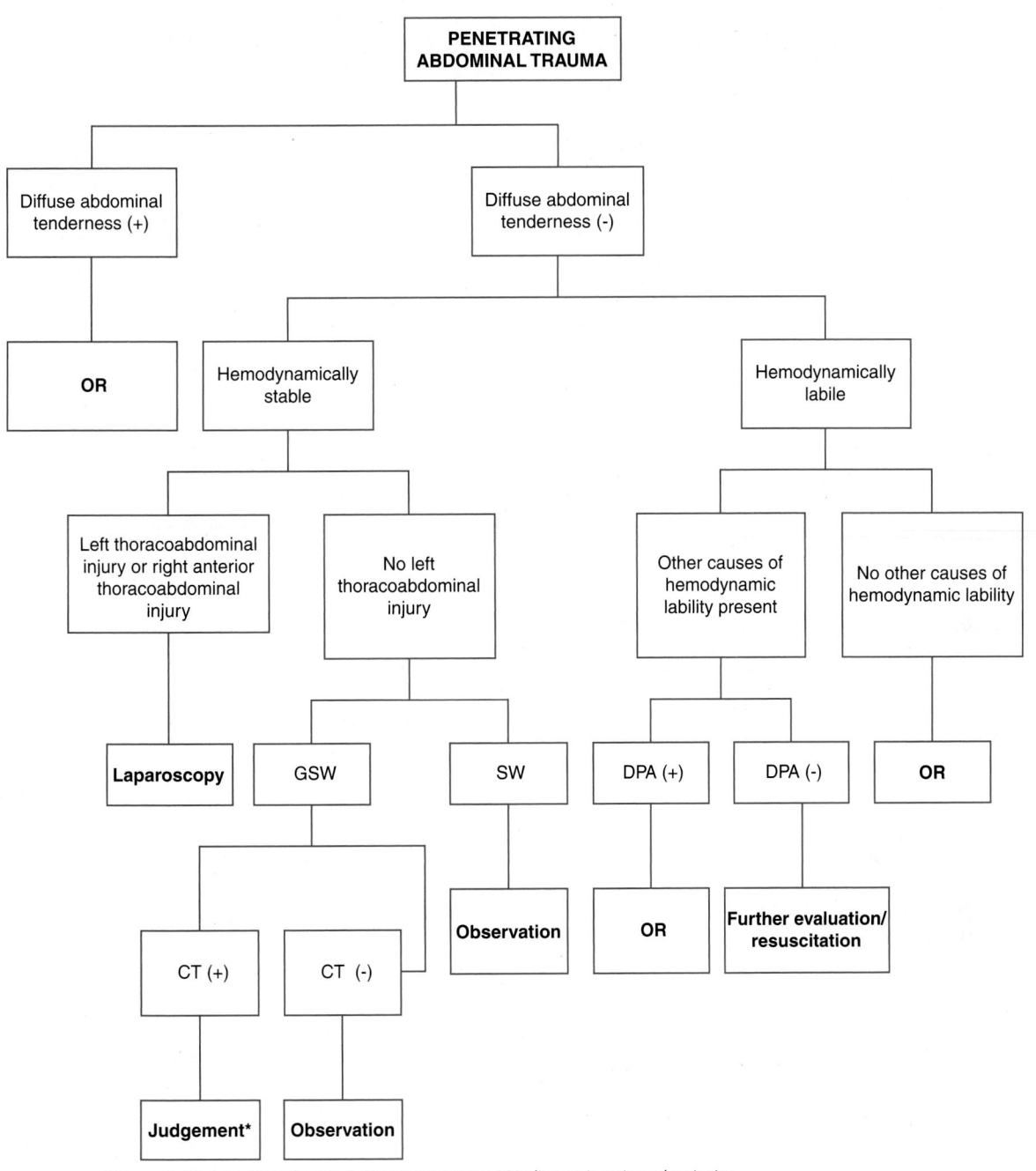

GSW: gunshot wound, SW: stab wound, OR: operating room, DPA: diagnostic peritoneal aspiration

*Judgement = operation or nonoperative management according to CT findings

**FIGURE 30-5.** Algorithm for the management of penetrating abdominal trauma.

of 152 patients with gunshot injuries to the liver, 7% of all cases or 21% of cases with isolated liver injury were successfully managed nonoperatively.[55]

The remaining issue has to do with practicing selective management in trauma centers with a low volume of penetrating trauma or inadequate resources to provide 24-hour in-house coverage. The inability to do serial physical examinations by physicians with reasonable experience in this type of injuries prohibits the practice of selective management. It may be safer for small trauma centers with limited exposure to gunshot wound victims to retain a policy of routine laparotomy. The remaining centers should use for gunshot wounds the same indications of laparotomy that are established for stab wounds.

Recently, CT has also been used as an adjunct to clinical examination in order to determine the bullet trajectory and its relationship to vital structures in patients selected for nonoperative management.[55] (Fig. 30-2) In isolated solid organ injuries which may be considered for nonoperative management, CT scan can demonstrate the site and size of the lesion and identify any false aneurysm or evidence of active bleeding. A practical algorithm for penetrating abdominal trauma is presented in Fig. 30-5. Note that, in contrast with other similar algorithms, the primary decision point relates to the findings of physical examination. The need to investigate the left hemidiaphragm in asymptomatic patients with left thoracoabdominal injuries is highlighted.

## Blunt Trauma

Blunt trauma is managed differently than penetrating trauma. Peritonitis is still a reason for immediate transport to the operating room. However, in contrast with penetrating trauma, hemodynamic instability after blunt multitrauma is not an automatic indication for laparotomy, if there is no confirmation that it is caused by intra-abdominal organ injuries. If hemodynamic instability is caused by pelvic retroperitoneal bleeding, long-bone fractures, blunt myocardial contusion, spinal cord injury, or intrathoracic trauma, an unnecessary laparotomy may be profoundly detrimental. Along the same lines, unevaluable blunt trauma patients need further diagnostic work-up before a decision for laparotomy is made. The presence of a "sealbelt mark" sign is associated with an incidence of about 20% of intraabdominal injuries. These patients should be evaluated very carefully and the threshold for laparotomy should be low (Fig. 30-6).

Besides clinical examination, plain films, and routine laboratory tests, immediate investigation of the abdominal cavity in the emergency room is done by ultrasongraphy or DPL. As increasing experience is gained by trauma ultrasonography, DPL is becoming less frequently used. Positive ultrasonography for intra-abdominal fluid in the presence of hemodynamic instability equals emergent laparotomy. Negative ultrasonography in the presence of hemodynamic instability of unknown origin should be followed up by diagnostic peritoneal aspiration (DPA). If the DPA is positive, the patient should be taken to the operating room. As described above, a full lavage is unnecessary, if the purpose of the test is to evaluate the presence of major intraperitoneal bleeding causing hemodynamic instability. Patients who are hemodynamically stable but unevaluable or with equivocal abdominal exam should be evaluated by CT scan.

CT provides crucial information for the need of laparotomy. It is more sensitive than ultrasound, equally sensitive to DPL, and more specific than both. Basically, there are three types of injuries that can be identified by CT scan: solid visceral, gastrointestinal tract, and a third category, broadly defined as "other", including the mesentery, bladder, and diaphragm. CT is very accurate in detecting solid visceral injuries for the most part but less accurate in the two latter types of injuries.[21] Splenic, hepatic, and renal injuries are characterized adequately by CT. Although superficial

lacerations to these organs can be missed, the majority of injuries are adequately visualized. Pancreatic injuries (see Chap. 35), particularly early after admission, can be missed by CT. Helical technology has dramatically improved the ability of CT to identify most solid visceral injuries of clinical significance. In the absence of hemodynamic instability or peritonitis, CT-diagnosed injuries to the liver, spleen, or kidney can be managed nonoperatively. Overall, approximately one-half of blunt injuries to the spleen and two-thirds to the liver can be managed nonoperatively (see Chaps. 32,33). The success rate of nonoperative management ranges from 70% to over 90%.[56] However, it needs to be mentioned that in most series reporting high success rates of nonoperative management, the injuries to the spleen or liver were low-grade; high-grade injuries were transferred directly to the operating room. Although the grade of injury by itself should not be a deterrent for nonoperative management, it should increase the vigilance of clinical follow-up. Nonoperative management of grade III or higher splenic injuries, requiring more than two units of blood transfusion, is very likely to fail; the threshold for intervention should be low in such cases.[57] Similarly, patients showing a contrast "blush" on CT should have a laparotomy or angiographic embolization.[58]

The diagnostic ability of CT for blunt duodenal, small bowel, and colonic injuries is debatable. The most common finding in these cases is unexplained free fluid. If all patients with this finding are operated on, all hollow visceral injuries will be found but the incidence of unnecessary laparotomy will be high because only 30%–50% of such patients have a clinically significant injury.[23,24] On the other hand, avoiding to act immediately on unexplained free fluid may cause complications related to diagnostic and therapeutic delays in those patients who have significant injuries. Careful clinical examination and information from laboratory tests, including serial arterial blood gases or DPL enzymes, should be integrated in the decision-making process.

CT is a poor test for diagnosing diaphragmatic perforation in the absence of abdominal visceral herniation (see Chap. 31). If this injury is suspected, laparoscopy is the ideal test. Mesenteric injuries can also be easily missed. CT findings related to mesenteric injury include unexplained free fluid, mesenteric stranding, or intravenous contrast extravasation. CT-cystography by injecting contrast through the Foley catheter into the bladder has essentially the same diagnostic accuracy as conventional contrast cystography in detecting bladder injuries (see Chap. 39).

CT has become an integral part of the decision-making on the need for laparotomy. However, the value of clinical examination still remains undisputed. The indications for laparotomy should be placed after a full appreciation of the clinical condition of the patient is being made. Even in the age of technological advancements, clinical examination should be the primary tool determining the need of operation or observation. The variation of practices in the management of blunt trauma is great. A practical algorithm that would cover most blunt trauma patients is shown in Fig. 30-7.

## Combined Head and Abdominal Trauma

The evaluation and management of abdominal trauma in patients with significant head injuries pose four major challenges. (a) Reliable clinical examination, which is the cornerstone of abdominal evaluation, may not be possible because of depressed level of consciousness. (b) The timing of CT evaluation of the head in a

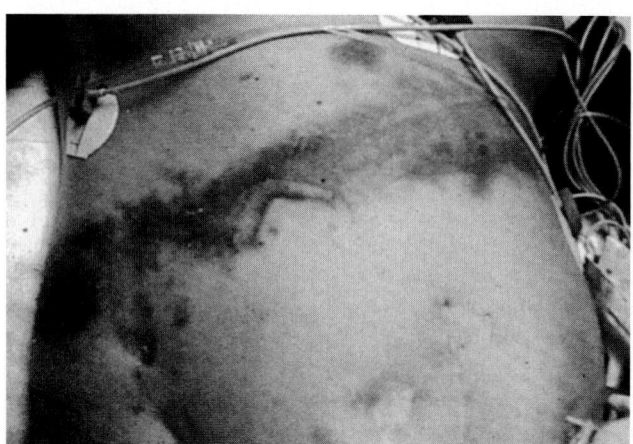

**FIGURE 30-6.** "Seatbelt mark" sign is associated with an incidence of about 20% of intraabdominal injuries.

**Blunt Abdominal Trauma**

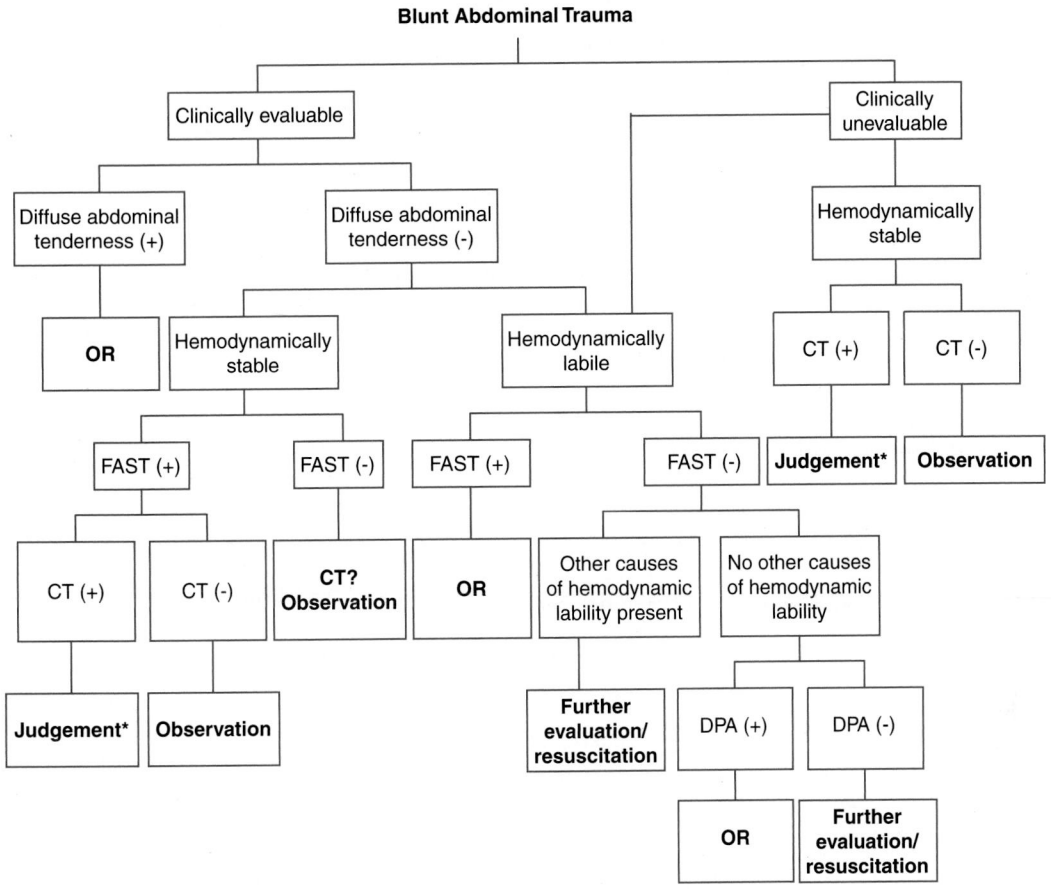

OR: operating room, DPA: diagnostic peritoneal aspiration, CT: computed tomography,
FAST: focused abdominal sonography for trauma
*Judgement: operation or nonoperative management according to CT findings
**CT is desirable as soon as the patient becomes hemodynamically stable

**FIGURE 30-7.** Algorithm for the management of blunt abdominal trauma.

patient requiring an emergency laparotomy may be a difficult decision. (c) Severe head trauma may pose major problems in the nonoperative management of solid organ injuries. (d) Finally, major
intraabdominal injuries with significant blood loss may aggravate
any secondary brain damage.

The incidence of severe abdominal injuries in patients with
major head trauma is fairly low. In a trauma registry review in the
authors' trauma center, 3664 patients with severe head trauma
(AIS≥3), there were 209 (5.7%) cases with severe abdominal
trauma (AIS≥3). Solid organ injuries (minor or major) were found
in 271 (7.4%) and hollow viscus perforation in 61 (1.7%) of
patients. In a prospective study of 2415 patients with severe blunt
trauma to the head and Glasgow Coma Scale (GCS) ≤8, routine
abdominal CT scan revealed injuries in 13.4% of cases. The incidence
of intestinal injury was 3.6%. In a study of 90 patients with severe
blunt head trauma (GCS<8) undergoing routine abdominal
CT scan, Taylor[59] reported an incidence of 27.8% of intra-abdominal injuries. In the group of 392 patients with GCS ≥8 the incidence of intra-abdominal injuries was 17.8%

## Investigations

The selection and timing of abdominal investigations should be
made on the basis of the hemodynamic condition of the patient
along the lines recommended in the algorithm in Fig. 30-7. In

patients requiring an emergency laparotomy the timing of CT scan
evaluation of the head, i.e., before or after laparotomy, should be
determined by the neurological findings and hemodynamic condition of the patient. In general, only few blunt multitrauma patients
require craniectomy (see Chap. 20). In a study of 734 hypotensive
blunt trauma patients, Thomason et al.[60] reported an incidence of
21% of emergency laparotomies. Although 40% of cases had severe
head trauma (AIS≥3), only 2.5% required emergency craniotomy.
In another retrospective analysis of 212 hypotensive blunt multitrauma patients, Winchell et al.[61] reported an overall incidence of
general surgical operations in 19% and craniotomies in 8%. The
incidence of craniotomies increased to 19% in patients with
GCS <8. The study suggested that a preoperative head CT scan is
desirable and safe in hypotensive patients responding to initial
resuscitation.[61] In general, control of significant intra-abdominal
bleeding has priority over CT scan evaluation of the head. Practical algorithms addressing the issue of timing of laparotomy or CT
of the head are shown in Fig. 30-8.

## Nonoperative Management of Solid Organ Injuries in the Presence of Associated Head Injuries

Severe head injuries are often associated with disseminated intravascular coagulopathy. This complication may aggravate any bleeding
from associated solid organ injuries. In the past, associated severe

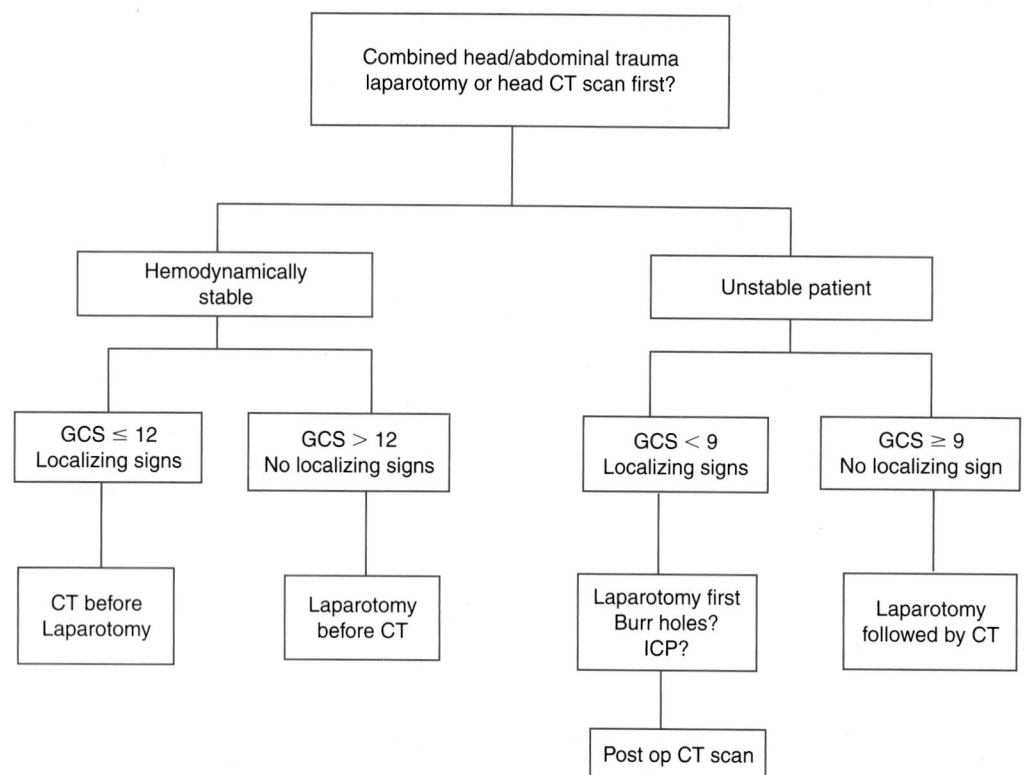

**FIGURE 30-8.** Algorithm for the management of combined head/abdominal trauma.

head trauma was considered as a contraindication for nonoperative management of liver or splenic injury (see Chaps. 32,33). However, subsequent studies have demonstrated that nonoperative management in the presence of neurotrauma is safe and the failure rate is similar to that in patients with no associated head trauma.[62,63] If a nonoperative approach is selected, the patient should be monitored closely and any coagulation problems should be corrected early and aggressively. The threshold for operative intervention should be lower than in patients with no associated head trauma, because of the risk of secondary brain damage in cases with hypovolemic shock. More details on these issues are discussed in Chaps. 32 and 33.

## ANTIBIOTIC PROPHYLAXIS

Antibiotic prophylaxis should be given preferably before the incision is made (see Chap. 19). For many years, second or third generation cephalosporins have been the prophylactic antibiotics of choice in abdominal trauma. More recent studies suggested that cephalosporins might not provide optimal antimicrobial coverage. Weigelt et al.[64] in a prospective randomized study of 595 patients with penetrating abdominal injuries, reported that ampicillin/sulbactam was associated with a significantly lower incidence of wound sepsis than cephalosporin. The study attributed this difference to the anti-enterococal coverage of ampicillin/sulbactam. In another multicenter prospective nonrandomized study of 297 patients with penetrating destructive colon injuries requiring resection, combination antibiotics or ampicillin/sulbactam were associated with a lower rate of abdominal septic complications than cephalosporins.[65]

The duration of antibiotic prophylaxis has been a matter of controversy. There is now good evidence that 24-hour prophylaxis is at least as good as prolonged prophylaxis (three to five days), even in the presence of significant risk factors such as colon injuries, high abdominal trauma index (ATI), and multiple blood transfusions. In a prospective randomized study which included 63 patients with penetrating colon injuries with an associated ATI $\geq 25$ or blood transfusions $\geq 6$ units or delay of operation $\geq 6$ hours, Cornwell et al.[66] reported an incidence of abdominal septic complications of 19% in the 24-hour prophylaxis group and 38% in the five-day prophylaxis group ($p=$ NS). When the patients of this study were combined with similar patients from another study by Fabian et al.,[67] the results were similar. The overall incidence of septic complications was 19% in the 24-hour prophylaxis group and 33% in the five-day prophylaxis group ($p=0.13$).

## OPERATIVE MANAGEMENT

### General Preparation

Warming blankets should always be used on all trauma patients in order to reduce the effects of hypothermia. Leg compression devices are recommended for deep venous prophylaxis, although there is no scientific evidence on their efficacy in the operating room. The operating room nurses and anesthesiology staff should be fully prepared before the patient arrives. In severely injured patients time is of critical importance and even a few minutes delay may have a significant effect on the outcome.

In the unstable patient, skin preparation and induction of anesthesia should proceed simultaneously because induction of anesthesia often results in rapid hemodynamic decompensation. In hemodynamically stable patients with isolated abdominal trauma the skin preparation should include the area between the nipples and the mid-thighs. In patients with thoracoabdominal injuries or hemodynamic instability the skin preparation should include the chest and the thighs, in case a thoracotomy or a saphenous vein graft becomes necessary.

## Incision

A midline laparotomy is the standard incision for trauma, although a transverse incision is acceptable in pediatric cases. The length of the incision should be individualized and should allow adequate exposure. The old dogma that a laparotomy incision for trauma should be one from the xiphoid to the pubic symphysis is not acceptable any more. Depending on the operative findings and the body habitus of the patient the initial incision may be extended upward or downward.

In complex posterior liver or retrohepatic venous injuries the exposure through the midline laparotomy may be improved by adding a midline sternotomy or a right anterolateral thoracotomy. A right subcostal incision is preferred by some surgeons as an alternative to the right thoracotomy. The choice of sternotomy or right thoracotomy or right subcostal incision is a matter of surgeons' preference. However, if an atriocaval shunt is considered, the median sternotomy provides the best option (see Chap. 32)

In patients with distal iliac vessel injuries, vascular exposure through the midline laparotomy may be difficult, especially in males with a narrow pelvis. In these cases the surgical exposure can significantly be improved by extending the lower part of the wound by means of an oblique lower quadrant incision or a separate vertical incision over the inguinal ligament.

The incision can be performed with a scalpel or with cautery. Earlier concerns about tissue damage and possibly impaired healing and infection with the use of cautery have been shown to be unfounded. In a prospective randomized study of 100 patients undergoing elective laparotomy, Kearns et al.[68] showed that cautery incision was associated with significantly less blood loss than the scalpel incision, while the incidence of wound sepsis was similar in both groups.

In the hemodynamically unstable patient the abdominal cavity should be entered as fast as possible and no time should be wasted for meticulous control of subcutaneous small bleeders. Compression with a large gauze achieves spontaneous hemostasis while the surgeon deals with the more urgent issues. The easiest site to enter the peritoneum is the area above the umbilicus, where the linea alba is wide. Patients with previous laparotomy scars may pose special challenges due to the presence of adhesions and the risks of iatrogenic enterotomies or deserosalization of the bowel. The problem is further complicated in the hemodynamically unstable patient where a rapid entry into the peritoneal cavity is necessary. In these patients, whenever possible the peritoneum should be entered through a site proximal or distal to the previous scar, which is usually free from adhesions.

## Abdominal Exploration

Upon entering the peritoneal cavity the surgeon has two urgent priorities: temporary control of any active bleeding followed by temporary control of any intestinal spillage. Bleeding control is usually achieved by tight packing of the suspected source of bleeding. In many cases the source of hemorrhage is known because of a preoperative CT scan or highly suspected from the site of a stab wound, the direction of a bullet tract, or sometimes the clinical signs in blunt trauma. In these cases the surgeon should pack the suspected area and then remove all intraperitoneal blood by a combination of suctioning and manual scooping out. The next step is temporary control of any gastrointestinal spillage by applying tissue clamps. After temporary control of bleeding and gastrointestinal content spillage have been achieved, the abdominal packs should carefully be removed one by one, and the source of bleeding and extent of organ injury are assessed.

In cases with suspected associated cardiac trauma the pericardium can be explored trans-abdominally through a transdiaphragmatic pericardial window. This can be easily achieved by grasping the diaphragm with two tissue clamps and incising it with scissors and cautery. Meticulous hemostasis is essential in order to avoid false positive results. If the pericardium contains blood a median sternotomy is performed, otherwise the pericardial window is closed with a suture.

After definitive control of bleeding has been achieved the next step is the definitive management of any gastrointestinal injuries. The whole gastrointestinal tract, from the stomach to the intraperitoneal rectum, should be evaluated before any definitive procedure is performed. Detailed knowledge of the extent of the gastrointestinal injuries may alter the management, i.e., bowel resection may be a better option than repair of multiple bowel perforations.

The final step is to identify and manage other occult intraabdominal injuries, such as pancreaticoduodenal or other retroperitoneal injuries. In the appropriate cases the lesser sac is opened by dividing the gastrocolic ligament, and the pancreas and the posterior wall of the stomach are examined (see Chap. 35).

## Intraabdominal Hematomas

The intraoperative approach to any intraabdominal hematomas depends on the mechanism of injury (blunt or penetrating), and the site and size of the hematoma. For practical purposes the retroperitoneal hematomas are classified into three zones: Zone I which includes the midline area between the aortic hiatus of the diaphragm and the sacral promontory, Zone II which includes the left and right perirenal areas, and Zone III which includes all pelvic hematomas (Fig. 30-9).

As a general rule, routine exploration in blunt trauma should be considered only for pancreaticoduodenal hematomas. Stable retroperitoneal, pelvic or retrohepatic hematomas should be left undisturbed. Similarly, stable mesenteric hematomas, including those around the superior mesenteric artery, should not be explored routinely. Although many authors recommend routine exploration of all hematomas at the root of the mesentery in order to exclude injuries to the superior mesenteric artery, the authors believe that it is a difficult and potentially dangerous approach. Exploration should be considered only if the hematoma is expanding or the bowel appears ischemic. In all other cases the superior mesenteric artery should be evaluated postoperatively by means of color flow doppler and, if necessary, angiographically. Similarly, stable Zone II (perirenal) or Zone III (pelvic) hematomas due to blunt trauma should be left undisturbed, unless there is evidence of major vascular injury, such as an absent femoral pulse or preoperative diagnosis of renal artery injury.

In penetrating trauma, as a general rule, all hematomas in all three zones should be explored. Often, underneath a small

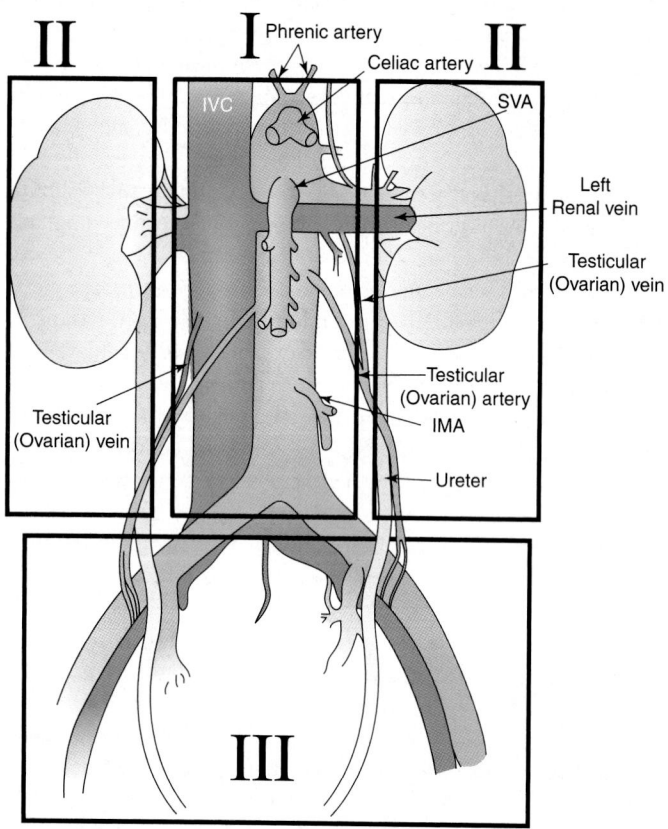

**FIGURE 30-9.** Classification of retroperitoneal hematomas: Zone I, includes the midline area between the aortic hiatus and the sacral promontory; Zone II includes the two perirenal areas; Zone III includes all pelvic hematomas.

hematoma there is an underlying vascular injury or hollow viscus perforation. The only exception to this rule is a stable retrohepatic hematoma, because exploration is technically difficult and dangerous with potentially lethal consequences. The management of perirenal hematomas following penetrating trauma is a matter of controversy. Although most authors advocate routine exploration, it is the authors' experience that stable hematomas away from the hilum, are best left undisturbed. In a study of 52 patients with gunshot wounds to the kidney, the perirenal hematoma was successfully not explored in 20 (38%). No kidneys were lost and no complications occurred as a result of this policy.[69]

## Damage Control

Damage control procedures such as packing of complex liver injuries or difficult bleeding from the retroperitoneum or the pelvis or temporary shunting of vital arteries, should be contemplated early and before the patient becomes severely coagulopathic, hypothermic, and acidotic (see Chap. 41). Stapling of the bowel as part of the damage control strategy should not be considered lightly, because of the possible effects of creating a complete bowel obstruction. There are concerns that this obstruction may aggravate any bowel distention, possibly contribute to bacterial translocation, and sometimes cause bowel necrosis proximal to the stapled end. Although the usual plan is to return the patient to the operating room within 24 hours to reestablish the continuity of the

bowel, often this is not possible because of persistent coagulopathy, the need of high doses of vasopressors, and severe respiratory failure. Detailed description of damage control techniques is presented in Chap. 41.

## Abdominal Drains

The role of abdominal drains following trauma is much debated. There is convincing evidence that the use of sump drains is associated with increased risk of sepsis.[70] However, the use of closed suction drains does not increase the risk of intra-abdominal complications, and there is evidence that in major injuries of either the liver or pancreas they reduce the risk of infection. In a prospective, randomized study of 482 liver injuries, Fabian et al.[70] reported an incidence of perihepatic abscess of 6.7% in patients without drain, 3.5% with closed suction drain, and 13% with sump drains.

Closed-suction drains may be needed to monitor intra-abdominal bleeding or in patients with high-risk hollow viscus repairs. The authors believe that in trauma drains should be used liberally in areas with even minor oozing, especially in the presence of an associated hollow viscus perforation. Undrained blood in the presence of peritoneal contamination may create a favorable environment for intra-abdominal sepsis. Closed drains should also be placed in areas packed as part of damage control, for many reasons. Firstly, it is important to monitor the effectiveness of the packing and, if necessary, return the patient to the operating room for re-exploration or consider angiographic intervention. Secondly, the presence of drains can help explain the source of deteriorating hemoglobin levels, especially in the presence of other severe extraabdominal injuries, such as pelvic or long-bone fractures. Thirdly, the presence of drains may prevent the development of abdominal compartment syndrome, which may occur even when the abdominal wall has been closed with prosthetic material. However, drains may occlude and this may create a false sense of security.

## Abdominal Closure

The abdominal fascia is closed with continuous nonabsorbable sutures provided there is no significant tension. Retention sutures have no role, at least during the initial laparotomy. They are painful and often cause intolerable pain and local complications[71] and they do not reduce the incidence of incisional hernias. Retention sutures may have a role in subsequent laparotomies in the presence of fasciitis precluding standard fascial closure.

The management of the skin wound in the presence of extensive enteric contamination or colon perforation is controversial. In a prospective study of 100 patients with gunshot wounds to the colon who had primary closure of the skin wound, the incidence of wounds sepsis was 11%.[72] However, in another prospective, randomized study from the authors' center, the incidence of wound sepsis in the group of 26 patients with colon injuries and skin wound closure was 65% as compared to 36% in the group of 22 patients managed with open skin wound. The role of primary skin closure over subcutaneous drains is not clear and needs further evaluation.

In the presence of bowel edema or major retroperitoneal hematoma, abdominal wall closure is often not possible or may result in abdominal compartment syndrome. In patients managed with damage-control laparotomy, primary closure of the abdomen should be avoided because of the high incidence of abdominal compartment syndrome. Offner et al.[73] reported an incidence of 80% of compartment syndrome after primary fascial closure in this group of patients. Various methods have been used for temporary abdominal wall closure and these are reviewed in Chap. 41.

## NONTHERAPEUTIC LAPAROTOMIES

The incidence of nontherapeutic laparotomies for trauma varies from 1.7% to 38% and depends on the experience and policies of the individual trauma center. Leppaniemi et al.[74] reported an incidence 37% of negative laparotomies in a series of 459 patients with stab wounds undergoing mandatory laparotomy. Renz et al.[36] in a prospective study of 938 patients undergoing laparotomy for blunt or penetrating abdominal trauma reported 27.1% unnecessary laparotomies. In a prospective study of 651 stab wounds to the abdomen there was an incidence of 3.8% of unnecessary operations.[39] More recent prospective studies by the authors reported unnecessary laparotomies in 10% of 291 patients with gunshot wounds to the anterior abdomen and 3.2% in 188 patients with gunshot wounds to the back.[8,9] The incidence of nontherapeutic laparotomies, for blunt abdominal trauma is similar to that in penetrating trauma and is about 20%.[75]

Although some authors reported a morbidity associated with unnecessary laparotomies as low as 3%,[76] most other studies have shown much higher complication rates. Hasaniya et al.[77] in a study of 222 unnecessary laparotomies reported an incidence of 8.6% of early complications directly related to the laparotomy or anesthesia. Leppaniemi et al.[74] in a review of 172 negative laparotomies following stab wounds to the abdomen, reported an incidence of 17% in patients with no associated extra-abdominal injuries. Renz et al.[36] in a prospective analysis of 254 patients with nontherapeutic laparotomies following trauma reported a complication rate of 25.9% in patients with no associated extraabdominal injuries. In the subgroup of 81 patients with no associated injuries and no peritoneal or retroperitoneal violation, the complication rate was 19.7%. The collective complication rate in 572 nontherapeutic laparotomies for penetrating trauma is 15.6%[8,9,39,41,52,74,75] (Table 30-1).

Respiratory complications (atelectasis or pneumonia), followed by prolonged paralytic ileus, surgical wound infection, and small bowel obstruction are by far the most common complications.[36,74,78]

The incidence of late complications associated with an unnecessary laparotomy is not well documented because of poor follow up. Leppaniemi et al.[74] followed up 102 patients for an average of 57 months (range 1–212 months) and reported an incidence of 5% of incisional hernias. Morrison et al.[79] reviewed the records of 80 patients who belonged to a health maintenance organization and reported no significant late complications, at a mean of $36 \pm 2$ months after a negative or nontherapeutic operation. Weigelt et al.[80] reported a late complication rate of 2.4% with a mean follow-up of 57 months (range 1–164 months). The study found that the incidence of small bowel obstruction in patients with visceral mobilization was higher than in patients without mobilization (5% vs 1.5%).

The costs associated with an unnecessary laparotomy are significant. Renz[36] found that the mean length of hospital stay for patients with a completely negative laparotomy and no associated injuries was 4.7 days. Patients with complications had a mean hospital length of stay of nine days. In another study, the mean hospital charges in successfully observed patients with abdominal gunshot wounds was $8595 and in patients with nontherapeutic laparotomies was $18,123.[9]

## MISSED ABDOMINAL INJURIES

The benefits of successful nonoperative management of abdominal trauma should be weighted against the consequences of missed injuries and delayed treatment. The reported incidence

**TABLE 30-1**

| Incidence and Complication Rates of Nontherapeutic Laparotomies in Penetrating Trauma | | | | |
| --- | --- | --- | --- | --- |
| REFERENCE | MECHANISM OF INJURY | NUMBER OF POINTS | NUMBER OF NONTHERAPEUTIC LAPAROTOMIES | MORBIDITY OF NONTHERAPEUTIC LAPAROTOMIES |
| 8 | GSW (back) | 188 | 6 (3.2%) | Not reported |
| 9 | GSW (Anterior abdomen) | 291 | 29 (10%) | 8 (27.6%) |
| 39 | SW | 651 | 25 (3.8%) | Not reported |
| 41 | SW back | 230 | 5 (2.2%) | Not reported |
| 52 | GSW | 146 | 6 (4.1%) | Not reported |
| 74 | SW | 459 | 172 (37%) | 36 (21%) |
| 76 | GSW | 162 | 13 (8%) | 0 |
| 77 | GSW | 817 | 101 (12.4%) | 22 (22%) |
| 78 | GSW/SW | 240 | 35 (14.6%) | 4 |
| 105 | GSW/SW | 1015 | 222 (21.9%) | 19 (8.6%) |
| Overall | | 4199 | 614 (14.6) | 89/572 (15.6%) |

**TABLE 30-2**

| | | PATIENTS | | COMPLICATION |
|---|---|---|---|---|
| | | SELECTED FOR | PATIENTS | IN PATIENTS |
| | TYPE OF | NONOPERATIVE | WITH DELAYED | WITH DELAYED |
| REFERENCE | INJURY | MANAGEMENT | DIAGNOSIS | DIAGNOSIS |
| 1 | GSW abdomen | 41 | 7 | 2 (wound sepsis) |
| 8 | GSW back | 130 | 0 | 0 |
| 9 | GSW anterior Abdomen | 106 | 5 | 2 (one abscess, one ARDS) |
| 39 | SW-anterior Abdomen | 306 | 9 | 2 (wound sepsis) |
| 41 | SW–back | 145 | 4 | 1 (pancreatic fistula) |
| Total | | 728 | 25 (3.4%) | 7 (28%) |

Table title: Delayed Diagnosis in Patients with Penetrating Abdominal Trauma Selected for Nonoperative Management (Prospective Studies)

of delayed diagnosis in patients with penetrating abdominal injuries selected for nonoperative management is about 3.4% (Table 30-2). The morbidity in this group of patients is acceptable and not higher than the rest of patients. Similar findings have been reported in blunt abdominal injuries.[81] It is possible that patients with delayed diagnosis and no clinical signs of peritonitis on admission have small and confined hollow viscus perforations or slow-bleeding solid organ injuries and delay of treatment by a few hours does not result in excessive morbidity. The mainstay of selective nonoperative management is close continuous monitoring and immediate operation with the first signs of peritonitis. The delay beyond which the morbidity increases has not been defined. Although some authors suggest six hours or up to 12 hours, the existing data do not confirm this. It is possible that in patients with excessive peritoneal contamination even a few hours delay may be associated with significant morbidity. On the other hand, in patients with small perforations and confined contamination, longer delays may be tolerated without increased morbidity.

# REFERENCES

1. Cornwell EE III, Velmahos GC, Berne TV, et al.: Lethal abdominal gunshot wounds at a Level I trauma center: Analysis of TRISS (Revised Trauma Score and Injury Severity Score) fallouts. *J Am Coll Surg* 187:123, 1998.
2. Balogh Z, Offner P, Moore EE, et al.: NISS predicts postinjury organ failure better than the ISS. *J Trauma* 48:624, 2000.
3. Moore EE, Dunn EL, Moore JB, et al.: Penetrating abdominal trauma index. *J Trauma* 21:439, 1981.
4. Sikic N, Korac Z, Krajacic I, et al.: War abdominal trauma: Usefulness of Penetrating Abdominal Trauma Index, Injury Severity Score, and number of abdominal organs injured. *Milit Med* 166:226, 2001.
5. Demetriades D, Chan LS, Bhasin P, et al.: Relative bradycardia in patients with traumatic hypotension. *J Trauma* 45:534, 1998.
6. Shoemaker WC, Belzberg H, Wo CCJ, et al.: Multicenter study of noninvasive monitoring systems as alternatives to invasive monitoring of acutely ill emergency patients. *Chest* 114:1643, 1998.
7. Velmahos GC, Wo CCJ, Demetriades D, et al.: Early continuous noninvasive hemodynamic monitoring after severe blunt trauma. *Injury* 30:209, 1999.
8. Velmahos GC, Demetriades D, Foianini E, et al.: A selective approach to the management of gunshot wounds of the back. *Am J Surg* 174:342, 1997.
9. Demetriades D, Velmahos GC, Cornwell EE III, et al.: Selective nonoperative management of gunshot wounds of the anterior abdomen. *Arch Surg* 132:178, 1997.
10. Rozycki GS, Ballard RB, Feliciano D, et al.: Surgeon-performed ultrasound for the assessment of truncal injuries: Lessons learned from 1540 patients. *Ann Surg* 228:557, 1998.
11. Patel JC, Tepas JJ: The efficacy of Focused Abdominal Sonography for Trauma (FAST) as a screening tool in the assessment of injured children. *J Pediat Surg* 34:44, 1999.
12. Root HD, Hauser CW, McKinley CR, et al.: Diagnostic peritoneal lavage. *Surgery* 57:633, 1965.
13. Merlotti GJ, Marcet E, Sheaff CM, et al.: Use of peritoneal lavage to evaluate abdominal penetration. *J Trauma* 25:228, 1985.
14. D'Amelio LF, Rhodes M: A reassessment of the peritoneal lavage leukocyte count in blunt abdominal trauma. *J Trauma* 30:1291, 1990.
15. Feliciano DV, Bitonod-Dyer CG: Vagaries of the lavage white blood cell count in evaluating abdominal stab wounds. *Am J Surg* 168:680, 1994.
16. McAnena OJ, Marx JA, Moore EE: Contributions of peritoneal lavage enzyme determinations to the management of isolated hollow visceral abdominal injuries. *Ann Emerg Med* 20:834, 1991.
17. Davis JR, Morrison AL, Perkins SE, et al.: Ultrasound: Impact on diagnostic peritoneal lavage, abdominal computed tomography, and resident training. *Am Surg* 65:555, 1999.
18. Velmahos GC, Demetriades D, Stewart M, et al.: Open versus closed diagnostic peritoneal lavage: A comparison on safety, rapidity, efficacy. *J R Coll Surg Edinb* 43:235, 1998.
19. Ochsner MG, Knudson MM, Pachter HL, et al.: Significance of minimal or no intraperitoneal fluid visible on CT scan associated with blunt liver and splenic injuries: A multicenter analysis. *J Trauma* 49:505, 2000.
20. Starnes S, Klein P, Magagna L, et al.: Computed tomographic grading is useful in the selection of patients for nonoperative management of blunt injury to the spleen. *Am Surg* 64:743, 1998.
21. Frick EJ Jr, Pasquale MD, Cipolle MD, et al.: Small bowel and mesenteric injuries in blunt trauma. *J Trauma* 46:920, 1999.
22. Shankar KR, Lloyd DA, Kitteringham L, et al.: Oral contrast with computed tomography in the evaluation of blunt abdominal trauma in children. *Br J Surg* 86:1073, 1999.
23. Brody JM, Leighton DB, Murphy BL, et al.: CT of blunt trauma bowel and mesenteric injury: Typical findings and pitfalls in diagnosis. *Radiographics* 20:1525, 2000.
24. Malhotra AK, Fabian TC, Katsis SB, et al.: Blunt bowel and mesenteric injuries: The role of screening computed tomography. *J Trauma* 48:991, 2000.
25. Cunningham MA, Tyroch AH, Kaups KL, et al.: Does free fluid on abdominal computed tomographic scan after blunt trauma require laparotomy? *J Trauma* 44:599, 1998.
26. Beierle EA, Chen MK, Whalen TV, et al.: Free fluid on abdominal computed tomography scan after blunt trauma does not mandate exploratory laparotomy in children. *J Ped Surg* 35:990, 2000.
27. Stafford RE, McGonigal MD, Weigelt JA, et al.: Oral contrast solution and computed tomography for blunt abdominal trauma: A randomized study. *Arch Surg* 134:622, 1999.
28. Grossman MD, May AK, Schwab CW, et al.: Determining anatomic injury with computed tomography in selected torso gunshot wounds. *J Trauma* 45:446, 1998.
29. Ginzburg E, Carrillo EH, Kopelman T, et al.: The role of computed tomography in selective management of gunshot wounds to the abdomen and flank. *J Trauma* 45:1005, 1998.
30. McCunn M, Mirvis S, Reynolds N, et al.: Physician utilization of a portable computed tomography scanner in the intensive care unit. *Crit Care Med* 28:3808, 2000.
31. Velmahos GC, Demetriades D, Cornwell EE III, et al.: Gunshot wounds to the buttocks: Predicting the need for operation. *Dis Colon Rec* 40:307, 1997.
32. Velmahos GC, Gomez H, Falabella A, et al.: Operative management of civilian rectal gunshot wounds: Simpler is better. *World J Surg* 24:114, 2000.
33. Villavicencio RT, Aucar JA: Analysis of laparoscopy in trauma. *J Am Coll Surg* 189:11, 1999.

34. Murray JA, Demetriades D, Cornwell EE, III, et al.: Penetrating left thoracoabdominal trauma: The incidence and clinical presentation of diaphragm injuries. *J Trauma* 43:624, 1997.

35. Murray JA, Demetriades D, Asensio J, et al.: Occult injuries to the diaphragm: Prospective evaluation of laparoscopy in penetrating injuries to the left lower chest. *J Am Coll Surg* 187:626, 1998.

36. Renz BM, Feliciano DV: Unnecessary laparotomies for trauma: A prospective study of morbidity. *J Trauma* 38:350, 1995.

37. Shaftan GW: Indications for operation in abdominal trauma. *Am J Surg* 99:657, 1960.

38. Nance FC, Wennar MH, Johnson LW, et al.: Surgical judgement in the management of penetrating wounds of the abdomen: Experience in 2212 patients. *Ann Surg* 179:639, 1974.

39. Demetriades D, Rabinowitz B: Indications for operation in abdominal stab wounds. *Ann Surg* 205:129, 1987.

40. Shorr RM, Gottlieb MM, Webb K, et al.: Selective management of abdominal stab wounds. *Arch Surg* 123:1141, 1988.

41. Demetriades D, Rabinowitz B, Sofianos C, et al.: The management of penetrating injuries of the back. A prospective study of 230 patients. *Ann Surg* 207:72, 1988.

42. Granson MA, Donovan AJ: Abdominal stab wound with omental evisceration. *Arch Surg* 118:57, 1983.

43. Udobi KF, Rodriguez A, Chiu WC, et al.: Role of ultrasonography in penetrating abdominal trauma: A prospective clinical study. *J Trauma* 50:475, 2001.

44. Velmahos GC, Demetriades D, Cornwell EE III, et al.: Selective management of renal gunshot wounds. *Br J Surg* 85:1121, 1998.

45. Velmahos GC, Gomez H, Falabella A, et al.: Operative management of rectal gunshot wounds. *World J Surg* 24:114, 2000.

46. Shah R, Max MH, Flint LM Jr, et al.: Negative laparotomy: Mortality and morbidity among 100 patients. *Am Surg* 44:150, 1978.

47. McCarthy MC, Lowdermilk GA, Canal DF, et al.: Prediction of injury caused by penetrating wounds to the abdomen, flank, and back. *Arch Surg* 126: 962, 1991.

48. Henderson VJ, Organ CH Jr, Smith RS: Negative trauma celiotomy. *Am Surg* 59:365, 1993.

49. Moore EE, Moore JB, Van Duzer-Moore S, et al.: Mandatory exploration for gunshot wounds penetrating the abdomen. *Am J Surg* 140:847, 1980.

50. Lowe RJ, Salietta JD, Read DR, et al.: Should laparotomy be mandatory or selective in gunshot wounds of the abdomen? *J Trauma* 17:544, 1977.

51. Muckart DT, Abdool AT, King B: Selective conservative management of abdominal gunshot wounds: A prospective study. *Br J Surg* 77:652, 1990.

52. Demetriades D, Charalambides D, Lakhoo M, et al.: Gunshot wounds of the abdomen: Role of selective management. *Br J Surg* 78:220, 1991.

53. Velmahos GC, Demetriades D, Cornwell EE III: Transpelvic gunshot wounds: Routine laparotomy or selective management? *World J Surg* 22:1034, 1998.

54. Velmahos GC, Demetriades D, Toutouzas KG, et al.: Selective non-operative management in 1,856 patients with abdominal gunshot wounds: Should routine laparotomy still be the standard of care? *Ann Surg* 234:395, 2001.

55. Demetriades D, Gomez H, Chahwan S, et al.: Gunshot injuries to the liver. The role of selective nonoperative management. *J Am Coll Surg* 188:343, 1999.

56. Pachter HL, Hofstetter SR: The current status of nonoperative management of adult blunt hepatic injuries. *Am J Surg* 169:442, 1995.

57. Velmahos GC, Chan LS, Kamel E, et al.: Nonoperative management of splenic injuries: Have we gone too far? *Arch Surg* 135:674, 2000.

58. Schurr MJ, Fabian TC, Tavant M, et al.: Management of blunt splenic trauma: Computed tomographic contrast blush predicts failure of nonoperative management. *J Trauma* 39:507, 1995.

59. Taylor GA, Eich MR: Abdominal CT in children with neurological impairment following blunt trauma. Abdominal CT in comatose children. *Ann Surg* 210:229, 1989.

60. Thomason M, Messick J, Rutledge R, et al.: Head CT scanning versus urgent exploration in the hypotensive blunt trauma patient. *J Trauma* 35:492, 1993.

61. Winchell RJ, Hoyt DB, Simons RK: Use of computed tomography of the head in the hypotensive blunt-trauma patient. *Ann Emerg Med* 25:737, 1995.

62. Shapiro MB, Nance ML, Schiller HJ, et al.: Nonoperative management of solid abdominal organ injuries from blunt trauma: Impact of neurological impairment. *Am Surg* 67:793, 2001.

63. Keller MS, Sartorelli KH, Vane DW: Associated head injury should not prevent nonoperative management of spleen or liver injury in children. *J Trauma* 41:471, 1996.

64. Weigelt JA, Easley SM, Thal ER, et al.: Abdominal surgical wound infection is lower with improved perioperative enterococcus and bacteroides therapy. *J Trauma* 34:579, 1993.

65. Demetriades D, Murray JA, Chan L, et al.: Penetrating colon injuries requiring resection: Diversion or primary anastomosis? An AAST prospective multicenter study. *J Trauma* 50:765, 2001.

66. Cornwell EE, Dougherty WR, Berne TV, et al.: Duration of antibiotic prophylaxis in high-risk patients with penetrating abdominal trauma: A prospective randomized trial. *J Gastrointest Surg* 3:648, 1999.

67. Fabian TC, Croce MA, Payne LW, et al.: Duration of antibiotic therapy for penetrating abdominal trauma: A prospective trial. *Surgery* 112:788, 1992.

68. Kearns SR, Connoly EM, McNally S, et al.: Randomized clinical trial of diathermy versus scalpel incision in elective midline laparotomy. *Br J Surg* 88:41, 2001.

69. Velmahos GC, Demetriades D, Cornwell EE, et al.: Selective management of renal gunshot wounds. *Br J Surg* 85:1121, 1998.

70. Fabian TC, Croce MA, Stanford GG, et al.: Factors affecting morbidity following hepatic trauma. A prospective analysis of 2182 injuries. *Ann Surg* 213:540, 1995.

71. Rink AD, Goldschmidt D, Dietrich J, et al.: Negative side-effects of retention sutures for abdominal wound closure. A prospective randomized study. *Eur J Surg* 166:932, 2000.

72. Demetriades D, Charalambides D, Lakhoo M, et al.: Gunshot wounds of the abdomen: Role of selective conservative management. *Br J Surg* 78:220, 1991.

73. Offner PJ, DeZuza AL, Moore EE, et al.: Avoidance of abdominal compartment syndrome in damage-control laparotomy after trauma. *Arch Surg* 136:676, 2001.

74. Leppaniemi A, Salo J, Haapiainen R: Complications of negative laparotomy for truncal stab wounds. *J Trauma* 38:54, 1995.

75. Sosa JL, Baker M, Puente I, et al.: Negative laparotomy in abdominal gunshot wounds: Potential impact of laparoscopy. *J Trauma* 38:194, 1995.

76. Moore EE, Moore JB, van Duzer-Moore S, et al.: Mandatory laparotomy for gunshot wounds penetrating the abdomen. *Am J Surg* 140:847, 1980.

77. Hasaniya N, Demetriades D, Stephen A, et al.: Early morbidity and mortality of non-therapeutic operations for penetrating trauma. *Am Surg* 60:1, 1994.

78. Demetriades D, Vanderbossche P, Ritz M, et al.: Non-therapeutic operations for penetrating trauma: Early morbidity and mortality. *Br J Surg* 80:860, 1993.

79. Morrison JE, Wisner DH, Bodai BI: Complications after negative laparotomy for trauma: Long-term follow-up in a health maintenance organization. *J Trauma* 41:509, 1996.

80. Weigelt JA, Kingman RG: Complications of negative laparotomy for trauma. *Am J Surg* 156:544, 1988.

81. Bensard DP, Beaver BL, Berner GE, et al.: Small bowel injury in children after blunt abdominal trauma: Is diagnostic delay important? *J Trauma* 41: 476, 1996.

# Commentary ■ C. CLAY COTHREN

The authors have presented a nicely structured, methodical review of the broad topic of trauma laparotomy. As they sagely illustrate, there is not a cookie-cutter approach that incorporates all trauma patients or their injuries. Care for each injured patient requires experienced clinical evaluation, time-honed judgment, and individualized treatment. Residents and junior attendings are

often reminded of the value of experience in the trauma bay when a misstep in management occurs. Hence, to present a unified approach to abdominal trauma and the indications for laparotomy is challenging at best.

Drs. Demetriades and Velmahos make some critical points that I think are worth reiterating. First, the ABCs and the clinical exam are the most important elements in the evaluation of a trauma patient. In the current diagnostic era, it does seem as if computed tomographic (CT) scanning has replaced clinical examination. CT scanning should continue to be seen as an adjunct to the initial evaluation of the patient rather than a component of the primary survey. The presence of peritonitis or hemodynamic instability due to abdominal trauma are indications for emergent laparotomy, and an intervening CT scan merely puts the patient's life at risk—do not forget the mantra, "Death Begins in Radiology."

Second, the use of Focused Abdominal Sonography for Trauma (FAST) should be based on an individual institution's daily experience. In high volume centers with physicians trained in its use, FAST plays a critical role in the evaluation of the injured patient. Patients with a positive FAST examination and hemodynamic instability are rapidly transported to the operating room while stable patients undergo CT scanning for delineation of injuries. Although negative FAST exams typically permit patient observation, do not assume that a negative FAST in an unstable patient is reliable. Patients with hypotension due to abdominal injuries may initially have a negative FAST study, particularly since greater than 300–400 cc of blood within the abdominal cavity is needed before a fluid stripe in Morrison's pouch is evident. With fluid resuscitation and an increase in the patient's blood pressure, bleeding from solid organ injuries or mesenteric rents result in a positive FAST. Therefore, repeat FAST examination in the unstable patient is imperative. Moreover, persistent unexplained hemodynamic embarrassment despite a negative FAST mandates a diagnostic peritoneal aspiration (DPA) to exclude the abdomen as the source of hemorrhagic shock.

Third, despite the ubiquity of CT scanning and its indispensable role in managing blunt solid organ injuries, CT has limitations. As the authors nicely illustrate, CT scan is not reliable for diagnosing hollow visceral or mesenteric injuries. Common subtle findings on CT scan suggestive of such injuries include free fluid without solid organ injury, mesenteric streaking or "haziness", and bowel thickening. The difficulty in diagnosing bowel injuries again reminds the clinician of the importance of clinical examination. Patients with worsening pain, developing peritonitis, hyperpyrexia, unresolving tachycardia, and increasing levels of serum white blood cells (WBC) or amylase warrant consideration for operative exploration. The clinical conundrum of unexaminable patients proves challenging. The most common indication for laparotomy in these patients, particularly those with severe head injuries, is free fluid identified on CT scan without associated solid organ injury. Another diagnostic option in these patients, other than laparotomy, would be diagnostic peritoneal lavage (DPL) to determine enzyme and WBC counts.

Fourth, the utility of laparoscopy for trauma is limited. The majority of trauma explorations are emergent in nature, and hence preclude its use. Moreover, full examination of the bowel for small injuries, particularly in patients with stab wounds who can have punctuate holes in the small intestine, is limited with laparoscopic evaluation. Laparoscopy therefore tends to be limited to two clear uses: (1) determination of peritoneal violation in patients with anterior abdominal penetrating wounds (used in some centers rather than either wound exploration/DPL or CT scanning or clinical observation) and (2) evaluation of the left hemi-diaphragm following

selected cases of thoracoabdominal stab wounds. Laparoscopic visualization of the left diaphragm is suggested for patients with left thoracoabdominal stab wounds to rule out occult injury. Although the authors maintain that all patients not undergoing laparotomy should undergo laparoscopy in this clinical scenario, further stratification of patients is possible. Patients undergoing DPL with a red blood cell (RBC) count less than 1,000 cells/mm$^3$ can be managed expectantly.

With respect to penetrating trauma, our experience and management in Denver is different compared to that expounded by the authors. Patients sustaining stab wounds are evaluated based upon location of injury; those with flank or back wounds undergo triple-contrast CT scanning while those with anterior abdominal stab wounds undergo local wound exploration and diagnostic peritoneal lavage (LWE/DPL). Of note, LWE is not the digital "stab-bogram" occasionally observed in the trauma bay. LWE is performed under sterile condition and local anesthesia, often with sharp enlargement of the wound, to enable direct visual confirmation of the depth of penetration. In patients with a positive LWE, defined as penetration of the anterior rectus sheath or oblique fascia, we perform DPL. In our experience, the diagnostic evaluation of LWE/DPL results in over one-thord of patients being discharged from the Emergency Department without further expensive testing or hospital stay. An additional third of patients are monitored for 12–24 hours in our observation unit following DPL to ensure no complications have occurred. The final third undergo laparotomy based upon clinical evaluation and DPL results. The authors' bias toward serial examination and close monitoring to determine the need for laparotomy is their institution's favored approach. Other institutions opt for CT evaluation of all stable patients with any stab wound to the torso. Perhaps the currently ongoing multicenter trial by the Western Trauma Association will shed some light upon this muddled area of diagnostic investigation.

Regarding the authors' interest in nonoperative management for gunshot wounds, this is a highly controversial topic. Some centers with 24-hour in-house experienced trauma surgeons may elect this practice pattern. However, in the vast majority of facilities, patients with gunshot wounds violating the peritoneum should undergo urgent laparotomy with few exceptions. Patients with isolated high right upper quadrant gunshot wounds *may be* one of the exceptions. If a nonoperative strategy is employed, patients should undergo CT scanning to determine that the bullet tract is visualized throughout and isolated to the liver parenchyma. Admission to the intensive care unit to monitor for hemorrhage as well as a missed gallbladder or hollow viscus injury is critical. The other possible exception to emergent laparotomy following gunshot wounds is in obese patients. Patients with generous subcutaneous fat and a benign abdominal exam may be considered for CT scanning to determine if the tract of the bullet remains extraperitoneal; if diagnosis remains in question, laparoscopy may be performed.

Laparotomy for trauma, as noted by the authors, is a highly individualized decision based upon clinical evaluation and diagnostic adjuncts. Multiple tools exist within the surgeon's armamentarium, including FAST, DPA/DPL, imaging, and laparoscopy, to facilitate diagnosis and management of the trauma patient. Appropriate and timely intervention will limit the number of nontherapeutic laparotomies and their attendant morbidity.

# Injury to the Diaphragm

*James W. Davis* ■ *Babak Eghbalieh*

## INTRODUCTION

The diaphragm is an arched muscle dividing the thorax and the abdomen. Injuries to the diaphragm have been a diagnostic dilemma for surgeons for years. Even though there are early descriptions of postinjury diaphragmatic hernia dating back as far as 400 years,[1] the recognition and management of diaphragmatic injuries remains a challenge. Despite recent advances in diagnostic medical technology, injuries to the diaphragm remain elusive in some cases and complex algorithms have been devised to determine the presence of diaphragm injuries.

Further, once identified, there is some debate as well over whether or not all diaphragm injuries require repair. Clearly, large wounds with obvious herniation of abdominal content to the thorax are not diagnostic or treatment dilemmas. However, small injuries on the right where the liver is unlikely to herniate through have been subject to some debate. The objectives of this chapter are to familiarize the reader with the anatomy and physiology of the diaphragm, to review the incidence of diaphragmatic injury, and provide an approach to the diagnosis, surgical management, and treatment.

## HISTORICAL PERSPECTIVE

The entity of posttraumatic herniation of the stomach was first described by Sennertus.[1] Similarly, Ambrose Paré described the consequences of diaphragmatic injuries in both penetrating and blunt trauma in a series of autopsies.[2] The first case of diaphragmatic injury, described by Paré[3] in 1579, was that of a French artillery captain who sustained a gunshot wound of the left chest eight months earlier, and who subsequently developed colonic obstruction from which he succumbed. Blunt rupture of the diaphragm with gastric incarceration was also described by Paré.[3,4]

Petit[5] was first to differentiate between acquired and congenital diaphragmatic hernias. In 1769, Morgagni[6] published a monograph on the subject of diaphragmatic hernia in which he described the different types of hernias occurring through natural diaphragmatic openings. Bowditch,[7] in 1853, was the first to establish the antemortem diagnosis of a traumatic diaphragmatic hernia and collected 88 cases reported in the literature.

In 1879, Bardenhewer[8] performed a proximal diverting colostomy in a patient who subsequently succumbed and was proven at autopsy to have herniation and strangulation of the colon. In 1886, Riolfi[9] successfully repaired a diaphragmatic laceration with omental herniation. Naumann,[10] in 1888, successfully repaired a traumatic diaphragmatic hernia in which the stomach had herniated into the left chest. In 1899, Walker[11] repaired a lacerated diaphragm in a patient who had been struck by a falling tree. The modern era of diagnosis and treatment of diaphragmatic hernias can be traced to the classical review of 378 cases from the surgical literature by Hedblom,[12] in 1925.

## ANATOMY AND PHYSIOLOGY

### Anatomy

The diaphragm is a dome-shaped partition between the chest above and the abdominal cavity below. Its muscle fibers curve up circumferentially from attachments at the sternum, lower ribs, and posteriorly from periostial attachments (Fig. 31-1). The periostial attachments are from the first through the third lumbar vertebral bodies. The lateral insertion attaches to the internal surfaces of the lower ribs, extending from the sixth rib anteriorly to the twelfth rib posteriorly. The muscle fibers curve up and converge to form the central tendon which acts as the site of insertion for the diaphragm. The

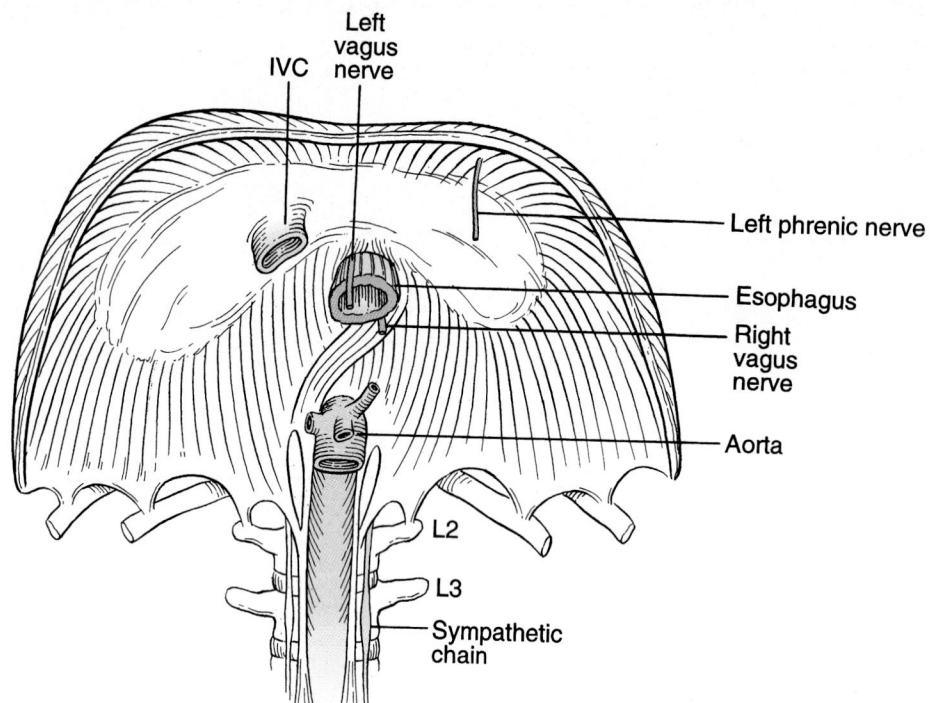

**FIGURE 31-1.** View of the diaphragm, showing the central tendon and the different structures transmitted via each of the apertures. The position of the vagi as they enter the abdominal cavity through the esophageal hiatus is shown.

central tendon has no bony attachments. The diaphragm is interrupted by three major openings: the vena cava, esophageal, and aortic apertures. The aperture for the cava originates at the eighth thoracic vertebral level, the esophageal at the tenth, and the aortic at the twelfth. The aorta, thoracic duct, and the azygous vein all course through the aortic hiatus. The esophagus and the right and left vagus nerves course through the esophageal hiatus and the vena cava is the only structure coursing through the caval hiatus (Fig. 31-2).

The crura of the diaphragm are long, tapering bundles that are muscular above and tendinous below. The right crus arises from the lateral aspect of the border of the upper three lumbar vertebrae and the intervertebral disks while the left crus arises from the upper two lumbar vertebrae. The medial fibers of the two crura decussate in front of the abdominal aorta; the fibers of the right crus encircle

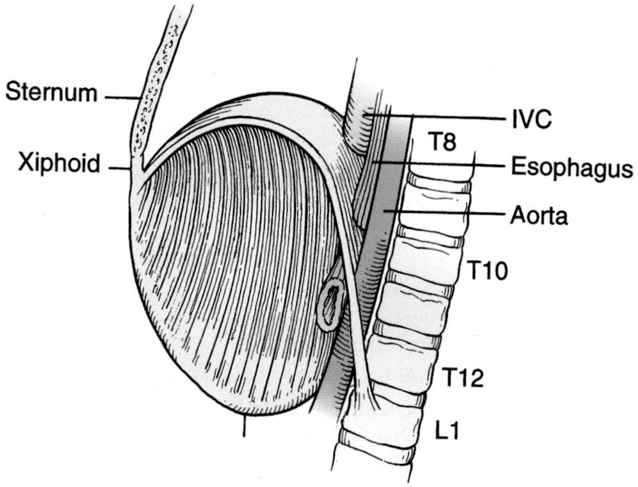

**FIGURE 31-2.** Side view of the diaphragm, showing its dome shape and anterior and posterior areas of attachment: the xiphisternal junction and the lumbar vertebral bodies. The level of the origin of each of the major apertures of the diaphragm are shown.

the esophagus. Both crura ascend forward and reach the posterior border of the central tendon.[13] Understanding this anatomy allows the trauma surgeon to rapidly locate and compress the abdominal aorta during episodes of hypotension and exsanguinating abdominal hemorrhage (see Chap. 37).

Blood supply to the diaphragm arises superiorly from vessels accompanying the phrenic nerve (pericardiophrenic arteries) and inferiorly from branches of the abdominal aorta, such as the phrenic arteries and multiple branches from the intercostal vessels.[13] The diaphragm is a relatively privileged organ. It is relatively resistant to hypoxemia with contractility and oxygen consumption being maintained by compensatory increases in diaphragmatic blood flow and oxygen extraction even at $PaO_2$ levels as low as 30 mmHg.[14]

The diaphragm is innervated by the phrenic nerves. These nerves arise from the third through the fifth cervical roots, with the greatest contribution to diaphragmatic innervation from the fourth cervical root. The phrenic nerves course anteriorly on the medial border of the anterior scalene muscle and traverse the thoracic cavity, traveling along the posterior mediastinum on the pericardial surface. The phrenic nerves typically divide into branches, at or 1 to 2 cm immediately above the level of the diaphragm (Fig. 31-3). The right and left hemidiaphragms are innervated separately by their respective phrenic nerves. Each branch divides into four major rami: a sternal (anterior), anterolateral, posterolateral, and crural (posterior) ramus. The resulting pattern is best described as a double "handcuff," with the anterolateral and posterolateral branches being the main components skirting circumferentially and laterally to the dome of the diaphragm.[15] Irritation of the diaphragm is perceived by the patient in the supraclavicular area (Kehr's sign).

## Physiologic Aspects of Diaphragmatic Function and Injury

The diaphragm is the main respiratory muscle of the body, with inspiratory and expiratory functions. The contraction of the

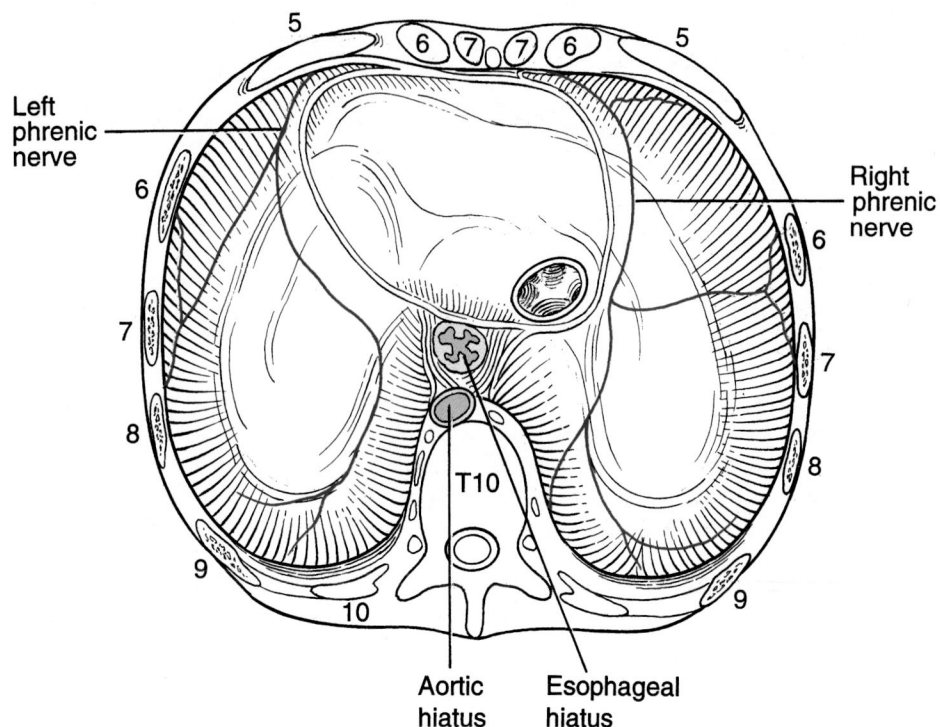

**FIGURE 31-3.** Anatomic distribution and branching pattern of the phrenic nerves. The diaphragm may be detached along its lateral insertions, 2 cm from the costal margin, without damaging the phrenic nerves.

diaphragm flattens the muscle and increases the size of the thoracic cavity, dynamically generating a tidal volume. The generation of a normal tidal volume produces a 3- to 5-cm motion of the diaphragm in each direction, with inferior displacement during inhalation and superior displacement during exhalation. During exhalation, the right hemidiaphragm rises anteriorly to the level of the fourth intercostal space, and the left hemidiaphragm rises to the fifth intercostal space. Posteriorly, both hemidiaphragms rise to about the eighth intercostal space.

Changes in lung volume have a direct effect on diaphragmatic muscle fibers and their function. The transdiaphragmatic pressure obtained with stimulation of the phrenic nerve decreases almost linearly with lung volume.

A relationship also exists between the diaphragm and the musculature of the abdominal wall. These muscles also have both inspiratory and expiratory function. For example, during expiration, they contract pushing the diaphragm superiorly. Marchand[16] demonstrated that there is a normal pattern of fluctuation in the intraperitoneal pressure during quiet respiration, which ranges from +2 to +10 cm $H_2O$, while the corresponding intrapleural pressure fluctuates from −5 to −10 cm $H_2O$. With the body in the supine position, the gradient between abdomen and pleura fluctuates from +7 to +20 cm $H_2O$. With maximal inspiration, this gradient may exceed +100 cm $H_2O$. These physiologic factors have been implicated in the creation of diaphragmatic injury. It has been postulated that sudden and abrupt increases in the pleuroperitoneal pressure gradient, which can occur with the acute transfer of kinetic energy to the domes of the diaphragm (as is the case with severe abdominal trauma), will lead to diaphragmatic disruption. In the presence of a laceration, perforation, or rupture of the diaphragm, the pressure gradient between abdomen and pleura will encourage transdiaphragmatic migration and herniation of intra-abdominal viscera.[17]

Diaphragmatic disruption can cause both hemodynamic and respiratory derangements. Transdiaphragmatic migration of abdominal viscera can restrict ventricular filling and diminish ventricular end-diastolic volumes, effectively reducing the ejection fraction and cardiac output (see Chap. 62). The displaced viscera that migrate into the chest cavity compromise ventilation in that lung and may eventually compromise ventilation in the contralateral lung with subsequent mediastinal shift.

The gastrointestinal system can also suffer acute and chronic sequelae from such disruption. The blood supply of the herniated viscera can be compromised leading to ischemia, necrosis, and perforation with subsequent contamination of the thoracic cavity (see Chap. 64). Gastrointestinal ulceration and hemorrhage have been described as sequelae of chronic herniation.

There are physiologic factors that may prevent diaphragmatic healing. These factors include the continued dynamic movement of the diaphragm and the interplay between the negative intrathoracic and positive intra-abdominal pressures, which fluctuate drastically with coughing, exertion, and other stresses and strains.[18] Additionally, omental migration may act to occlude a diaphragmatic laceration, and separate the transected diaphragmatic muscle fibers, preventing their union and interfering with the healing process.[19]

## Incidence of Diaphragmatic Injuries

Diaphragmatic injuries are infrequent, even in busy trauma centers. The true incidence of diaphragmatic injuries is hard to estimate because of missed and delayed diagnosis. The incidence of diaphragmatic injuries (blunt and penetrating) reported in the literature ranged from 0.8% to 8% of all abdominal injuries.[20] A query to the National Trauma Data Base (NTDB) (952,242 patients from 565 trauma centers, during the years 2000 to 2004) revealed an overall incidence of 0.63% ($n$=6,038); 35% from blunt trauma

**TABLE 31-1**

**Diaphragmatic Injury. NTDB Data from 565 Hospitals from Year 2000 to 2004. This Involved 70% of All Level I, 53% of All Level II, 15% of All Level III, and 48% of All Level IV, V, and Unspecified Trauma Centers That have Reported Their Registry to the NTDB**

| MECHANISM | NUMBER OF PATIENTS | % OF TOTAL TDI | TOTAL NTDB PATIENTS | % OF TOTAL NTDB |
|---|---|---|---|---|
| Blunt | 2093 | 34.7 | 811,531 | 0.26 |
| Penetrating | 3929 | 65.0 | 111,102 | 3.54 |
| Burn | – | – | 12,604 | – |
| Not specified | 16 | 0.3 | 17,005 | – |
| Total | 6038 | 100 | 952,242 | 0.634 |

TDI = Traumatic Diaphragm Injury; NTDB = National Trauma Data Base.

and 65% from penetrating diaphragmatic injuries (Table 31-1).[21] The frequency of penetrating injury may still be greater. In one prospective study, all patients admitted with left-sided penetrating thoraco-abdominal trauma were evaluated by laparoscopy, and 26 of 110 (24%) patients had diaphragmatic injury.[22]

## MECHANISMS OF INJURY

### Overview

The dynamic motion of the muscular diaphragm protects this structure from casual injury (see Chap. 7). Blunt injury is associated with significant transfer of kinetic energy.[23] Up to 90% of diaphragmatic ruptures from blunt trauma occur in young men after motor vehicle accidents.[20] Penetrating trauma occurs most commonly from injury in the thoraco-abdominal region (in the area of diaphragmatic traverse). Less commonly, iatrogenic injuries result from surgical misadventures (see Chap. 30).

### Associated Injuries

The diaphragm is rarely injured alone. Its anatomic location, the close relationship to adjacent intrathoracic and intra-abdominal

organs, and the severity of the trauma account for associated injuries in 52% to 100% of patients with diaphragmatic tears.[24] Certain patterns of associated injuries occur, depending on the mechanism of diaphragmatic injury.

Blunt trauma generally produces a significant number of associated intra- and extra-abdominal injuries. The traumatic forces translate into profound and sudden changes in intra-abdominal pressure, which are then transmitted to the domes of the diaphragm, causing or contributing to diaphragmatic rupture. In the NTDB, diaphragm injuries occurred in conjunction with liver injuries in 48%, splenic injury in 35%, bowel injury in 34%, kidney injury in 16%, pelvic fractures 14%, closed head injury 11%, and spinal cord injury in 4%. Thoracic injuries associated with diaphragm tear include rib fractures (28%), hemo or pneumothorax (47%), and thoracic aortic injury (4%) (Table 31-2).[21]

A larger number of associated injuries are typical penetrating trauma. Demetriades et al.[25] reported associated intra-abdominal injuries in 75% of patients sustaining penetrating injuries to the diaphragm. In a series of 165 patients with diaphragmatic injuries, an average of two associated injuries in patients sustaining stab wounds and three associated injuries in patients sustaining gunshot wounds was noted. This series reported a 50% incidence of associated hepatic injuries, a 26% incidence of gastric injuries, and a 12% to 18% incidence of pulmonary, colonic, splenic, and renal injuries.[26]

**TABLE 31-2**

**Diaphragmatic Injury Associated with Other Organ Injuries. NTDB Data from 565 Hospitals from Year 2000 to 2004. This Involved 70% of All Level I, 53% of All Level II, 15% of All Level III, and 48% of All Level IV, V, and Unspecified Trauma Centers That have Reported Their Registry to the NTDB**

| DIAPHRAGMATIC INJURY AND ASSOCIATED INJURY | NUMBER OF PATIENTS | % OF TOTAL TDI | TOTAL NTDB PATIENTS | % OF TOTAL NTDB |
|---|---|---|---|---|
| Liver | 2872 | 48 | | 0.30 |
| Hemo/Pneumothorax | 2824 | 47 | | 0.30 |
| Spleen | 2084 | 35 | | 0.22 |
| Rib Fractures | 1671 | 28 | | 0.18 |
| Bowel | 1377 | 23 | | 0.14 |
| Extremity | 1047 | 17 | | 0.11 |
| Kidney | 945 | 16 | | 0.10 |
| Pelvic | 840 | 14 | | 0.09 |
| Head Injury | 657 | 11 | | 0.07 |
| Spinal Cord | 242 | 4 | | 0.03 |
| Aortic Injury | 247 | 4 | | 0.03 |
| Total | 6038 | | 952,242 | 0.634 |

TDI = Traumatic Diaphragm Injury; NTDB = National Trauma Data Base.

## Anatomic Location of Injury

Desforges et al.[27] has postulated that diaphragmatic injuries result from the transmission of force through the abdominal viscera to the diaphragm, resulting in rupture. This would explain the more frequent involvement of the left hemidiaphragm, which is unprotected, as compared to the right. The energy from the force applied to the abdomen or flank should be distributed equally in all directions throughout the abdominal visceral contents. This force is distributed to the peritoneal cavity and the left hemidiaphragm, buffered only by the less bulky stomach, spleen, and kidney, which tends to rupture with greater frequency when enough pressure is applied. Bekassy et al.[28] harvested ten diaphragms from cadavers within the first 24 hours of death. Both the right and left hemidiaphragms were mounted separately in a pressure chamber; pressures were progressively increased until rupture of the hemidiaphragm occurred. Although it appeared that the right hemidiaphragm required consistently higher pressures to rupture, the data did not reach statistical significance. The investigators concluded that the right hemidiaphragm appears to be more resistant to applied pressures than does the left, and also suggested that the liver plays a protective role in preventing injuries to the right hemidiaphragm. Other studies have demonstrated that injury to the left hemidiaphragm occurs three times more frequently than does injury to the right after blunt trauma.[24,29,30] Bilateral diaphragmatic injuries and extension of tears into the central tendon are uncommon. They are reported in 2% to 6% of patients with diaphragmatic injury.[24,31]

## Diagnosis (Fig. 31-4)

The diagnosis of diaphragmatic injury may be straightforward, but frequently presents a challenge. Information about the mechanism of injury should be obtained from prehospital care personnel (see Chap. 7). The history obtained after blunt trauma can raise the index of suspicion for diaphragmatic injury. In patients involved in motor vehicle crashes, information about the velocity and direction of impact, the severity of vehicular damage, the presence of passenger-compartment intrusion, the presence or absence of deformity of the steering wheel, and whether extrication was employed to retrieve the victim can indicate the severity of the accident.

Falls from heights or direct impacts on the thoraco-abdominal area from vehicles, from auto–pedestrian incidents, or a history of crush injury should also alert the trauma surgeon to the possibility of an underlying diaphragmatic injury. Blunt trauma generally produces no external signs that are pathognomonic for diaphragm injury.

In contrast, penetrating trauma in the thoracoabdominal area immediately alerts the trauma surgeon to the possibility of diaphragmatic injury. The anterior thoracoabdominal area is defined as the area bounded by the nipples superiorly and the costal margin inferiorly. The lateral portion of the thoracoabdominal area is defined superiorly by a line drawn from the anterior axillary line at the level of the nipples posteriorly to the tip of the scapula and inferiorly to the costal margin. The posterior thoracoabdominal area is defined anteriorly by a line at the level of the tips of the scapula and inferiorly by a line beginning at the posterior axillary line at the level of the inferior most ribs. In general, the same incidence of penetrating injuries is found in the anterior, lateral, and posterior thoracoabdominal area.[22]

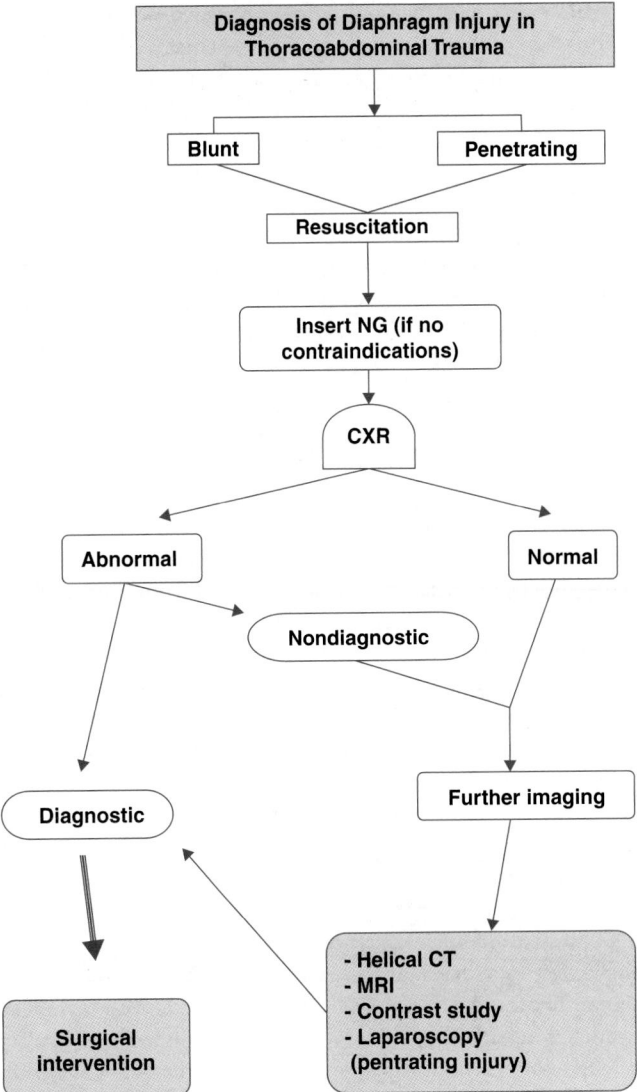

**FIGURE 31-4.** Algorithm for diagnosis of diaphragm injury.

The clinical picture of patients sustaining diaphragmatic injury from thoracoabdominal trauma encompasses the entire spectrum of acuity. Presentations may range from hemodynamic stability with few or no physical findings[22] to shock[51] and massive destruction of the thoraco-abdominal area, as is usually the case with close-range shotgun injuries.

The presenting symptoms in cases of diaphragmatic hernia can be described as thoracic or abdominal. Thoracic symptomatology is generally related to the volume of the pleural space occupied by the displaced intra-abdominal viscera, and whether gastric dilatation is present. Dyspnea, orthopnea, and chest pain are the primary symptoms experienced. Pain may be diaphragmatic, and be referred to the shoulder area (Kehr's sign), or may be related to chest wall injury or pleural violation. In the instance of progressive gastric dilatation with obstruction, respiratory distress may become extreme as the lung collapses, producing symptoms resembling those of tension pneumothorax, whereas abdominal symptoms may range from mild and localized to diffuse with severe abdominal pain.

Physical findings can also be described as thoracic or abdominal. Thoracic signs include decreased breath sounds, or even bowel sounds on chest auscultation, dullness to percussion of the chest, crepitus from rib fractures, and paradoxical chest wall motion from a flail chest. Abdominal signs may include a scaphoid abdomen from displaced viscera, localized or severe and diffuse abdominal tenderness, with guarding and rebound.

## Diagnostic Tests

The initial approach to the diagnosis of a diaphragmatic injury includes portable chest radiograph (CXR). Normal or nonspecific CXRs are seen in 20% to 50% of patients with diaphragmatic injury on initial evaluation. The diagnostic accuracy of the initial CXR for diaphragmatic injury is reported as 27% to 62% for left-sided injuries but only 17% of right-sided injuries.[22,24,31,50]

The initial chest radiograph may reveal the gastric or colonic bubble in the left chest. Occasionally, in acute ruptures of the left hemidiaphragm, nasogastric tubes placed during the resuscitative phase are found coiled in the left hemithoracic cavity (Fig. 31-5). Other findings may include an elevated diaphragm, fractured ribs with or without displacement, flail segments, and/or sternal fractures. Rarely, the liver can be visualized in the right hemithoracic cavity. Other occasional radiographic findings are curvilinear shadows and air-fluid levels consistent with other hollow viscera, such as the colon or small bowel (Fig. 31-6).

On the initial radiograph, diaphragmatic rupture may be confused with atelectasis of the lower lobe that elevates the stomach and hemidiaphragm, hemothorax, pneumothorax, gastric dilatation, pulmonary contusion, intra-abdominal fluid, traumatic pneumatocele, and total or partial eventration of the diaphragm.[33,34]

Contrast studies have been proven useful in cases in which the initial chest x-ray has failed to yield a diagnosis of diaphragmatic injury. The vast majority of such studies will be done to investigate chronic, long-standing herniation of intra-abdominal viscera, although they have also proven valuable in the acute situation.

Clearly, the patient must be hemodynamically stable in order to undergo these studies. An upper gastrointestinal series will often delineate the presence of the stomach within the left hemithoracic cavity. A barium enema, as either a single-column or a double-contrast study, will also outline a herniated colon within the thoracic cavity (Fig. 31-7).[35]

The focused abdominal sonography for trauma (FAST) has emerged as an accurate technique for evaluation of trauma patients (see Chap. 17). There have been some reports describing ultrasound findings of diaphragm injury including disrupted or nonvisualized diaphragm, and herniation of liver or bowel loops through the diaphragmatic defect.[36,37]

Conventional computed tomography (CT) scans have a reported sensitivity of 14–61% and specificity of 76–99% in diagnosing diaphragmatic rupture[20] (Fig. 31-6). This variability reflects limitations of the relatively thick axial slices (10 mm) with patient and respiratory motion and poor quality reconstructions.

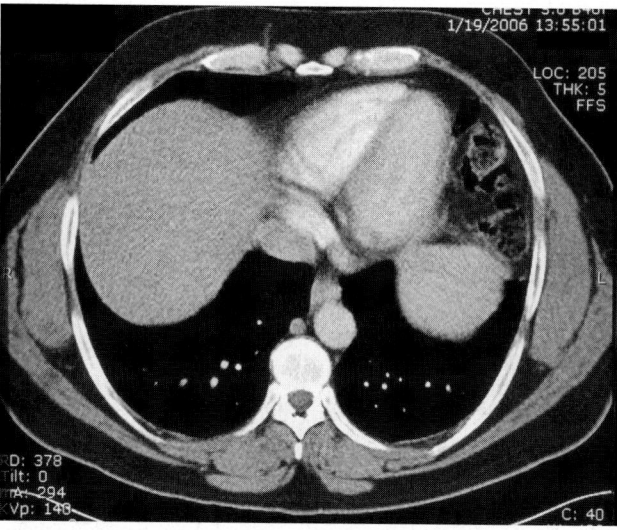

A

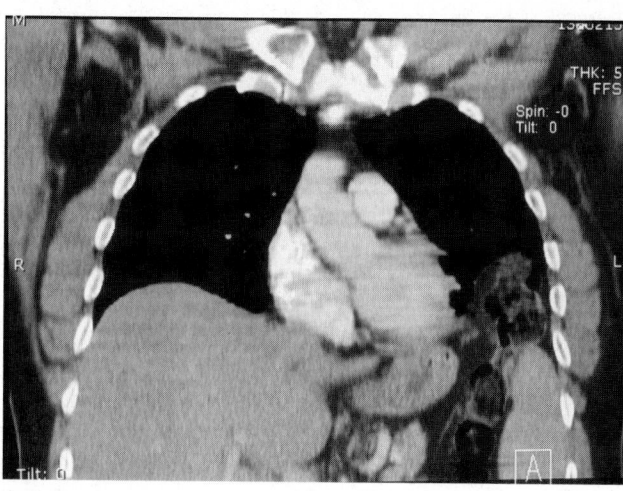

B

**FIGURE 31-6.** Helical CT scan of a patient with a history of left-upper-quadrant discomfort, left chest pain and occasional difficulty in breathing secondary to a stab wound below the left nipple at anterior axillary line. A small gastric bubble as well a part of the left splenic flexure of the colon is seen within the left hemithoracic cavity next to the heart. **(A)** Sagittal view, **(B)** Coronal reconstruction.

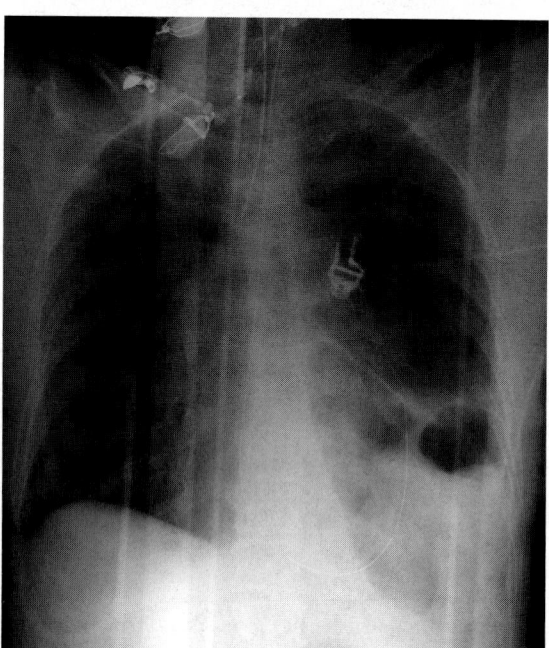

**FIGURE 31-5.** A coiled nasogastric tube within the left hemithoracic cavity is pathognomonic for a rupture of the left hemidiaphragm.

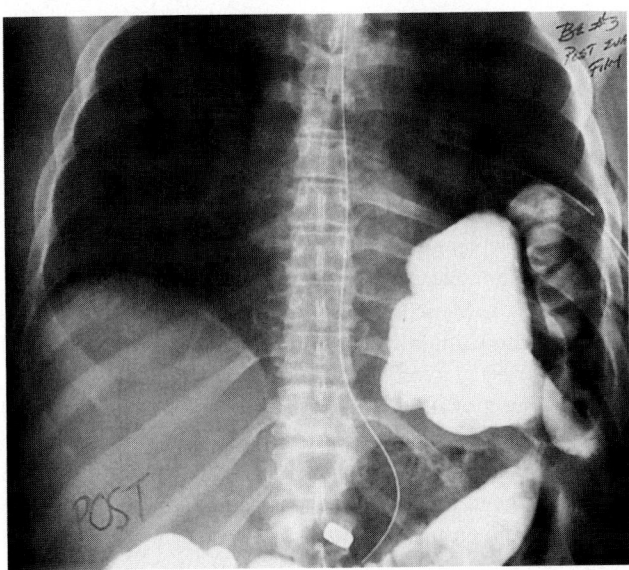

**FIGURE 31-7.** Barium enema reveals the left transverse and splenic flexure of the colon within the left hemithoracic cavity following an old gunshot wound.

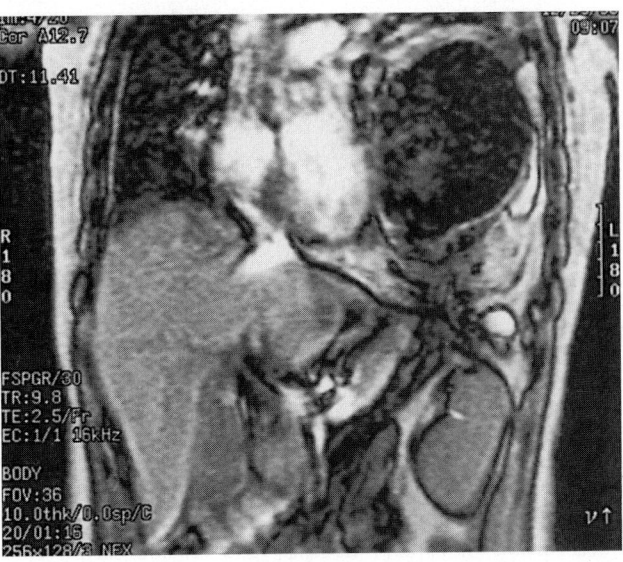

**FIGURE 31-8.** MRI reveals incarceration of the stomach within the left hemidiaphragm through a small defect. The stomach is seen compressing the left lung and displacing the heart.

Advanced helical CT scanners, which provide greater diagnostic accuracy, have been reported to have positive and negative predictive values and accuracy in diagnosing diaphragmatic injury of 80–100%.[38,39] In one series, the multidetector-row CT was found to be useful in the diagnosis of right hemidiaphragm injury.[40]

The use of magnetic resonance imaging (MRI) to diagnose diaphragmatic rupture has been reported (Fig. 31-8). Shanmuganathan et al.[41] confirmed diaphragmatic injury in 44% of patients who were evaluated by MRI after blunt trauma. MRI may become more utilized in the diagnosis of diaphragmatic injuries in the future.

Since its introduction in 1965 by Root et al.,[42] diagnostic peritoneal lavage (DPL) was a mainstay of abdominal evaluation. However, today it has mostly been replaced by the FAST exam and the use of helical CT. The reliability of DPL is overall poor in evaluation of diaphragmatic injury, but may be diagnostic if lavage fluid flows out from the tube thoracostomy. DPL is used currently as a diagnostic technique for diaphragmatic injury only following penetrating wounds (see Chap. 30).

Minimally invasive technology (laparoscopy and thoracoscopy) has been established as an effective means of evaluating the diaphragm for injury. Ivatury and associates[43] reported experience with laparoscopy in a series of 100 hemodynamically stable patients with penetrating abdominal trauma, 60 of which had sustained wounds in the thoracoabdominal area or upper abdominal quadrants, and identified 17 diaphragmatic lacerations. They concluded that the diagnostic accuracy of laparoscopy was excellent for hemoperitoneum, solid-organ injuries, and diaphragmatic lacerations and validated laparoscopy as an excellent tool for evaluating the diaphragm in thoracoabdominal injuries.

A prospective study to evaluate penetrating left thoracoabdominal injury utilized laparoscopy with the aim to determine the incidence of diaphragmatic injuries in penetrating left thoracoabdominal trauma.[44] In this study, 119 consecutive patients sustaining penetrating left thoracoabdominal injury were evaluated with clinical examination, chest radiography, and laparoscopy. Of these patients, 107 were fully evaluated, 50 required emergent laparotomy, and 57 underwent laparoscopy. The overall incidence of diaphragmatic injuries was 42% (59% incidence from gunshot wounds and a 32% incidence for stab wounds). Among the group of patients with diaphragmatic injuries, 31% had no abdominal tenderness, 40% had a normal chest x-ray, and only 49% had an associated hemopneumothorax. Fifteen (26%) of the patients undergoing laparoscopy had occult diaphragmatic injuries. This study concluded that the incidence of diaphragmatic injuries in association with penetrating left thoracoabdominal trauma is high and that clinical and radiographic findings are unreliable at detecting occult diaphragmatic injuries. Laparoscopy proved to be accurate for detecting these injuries among patients who have no other indications for laparotomy. In a prospective study of 34 hemodynamically normal, asymptomatic patients with thoracoabdominal penetrating injuries, all patients underwent diagnostic laparoscopy to evaluate the diaphragm for the presence of injury, followed by a confirmatory laparotomy or video-assisted thoracoscopy.[45] Specificity, sensitivity, and negative predictive value were 100%, 87.5%, and 96.8%, respectively. It was concluded that laparoscopy alone is sufficient to exclude diaphragmatic injury in asymptomatic, hemodynamically normal patients with penetrating thoracoabdominal injury.

Ochsner et al.[46] reported the use of video-thoracoscopy to diagnose diaphragmatic injuries in a series of 14 patients. This technique successfully identified all injuries that were subsequently confirmed by laparoscopy and exploratory laparotomy, although video-thoracoscopy is less frequently used than laparoscopy.

## SURGICAL STRATEGIES IN THE MANAGEMENT OF DIAPHRAGMATIC INJURIES

The surgical care of diaphragmatic injuries, and the operative strategies employed for their definitive management, may be divided into injuries requiring management in their acute phase

**TABLE 31-3**

| | |
|---|---|
| **Adapted from American Association for the Surgery of Trauma-Organ Injury Scale for Diaphragmatic Injuries** | |

| GRADE | INJURY DESCRIPTION |
|---|---|
| I | Contusion |
| II | Laceration ≤2 cm |
| III | Laceration 2–10 cm |
| IV | Laceration >10 cm with tissue loss ≤25 cm² |
| V | Laceration with tissue loss >25 cm² |

and those requiring management in their chronic phase. Additionally, diaphragmatic injuries may be classified using the American Association for the Surgery of Trauma-Organ Injury Scale (AAST-OIS) for diaphragmatic injuries47 (Table 31-3). Using this scale to classify all diaphragmatic injuries allows for standardization of description of injury and has value as a descriptive and research tool.

## Acute Phase (Fig. 31-9)

Once a patient has been resuscitated, a more focused assessment begins. In patients suspected of having diaphragmatic injury, meticulous attention must be paid to the insertion of a nasogastric tube. The tube should not be forced, as herniation of the stomach into the left hemithoracic cavity may distort the esophagogastric junction therefore producing an iatrogenic laceration of the esophagus, stomach, or both. If the tube cannot be passed easily, it is recommended that it be left in the distal esophagus and suction applied to help with the evacuation of swallowed air. Likewise, added caution must be taken when placing a thoracostomy tube if herniated viscera are located by digital exploration prior to placement

of a chest tube. If a chest x-ray has been obtained and suspicious shadows are located in either thoracic cavity, caution must be exercised in chest insertion.

Proven or suspected diaphragmatic injury, coupled with the classic findings of intra-abdominal injury mandates immediate exploratory laparotomy. Most, if not all, acute diaphragmatic injuries can be approached through a midline laparotomy incision. The basic principles of trauma surgery, including control of exsanguinating hemorrhage and gastrointestinal spillage, should be closely followed. Meticulous exploration of the abdominal cavity and retroperitoneum will avoid missed injuries (see Chap. 30). After this has been accomplished, attention should be shifted to a thorough inspection and visualization of the diaphragm. The right hemidiaphragm is best inspected after transection of the falciform ligament and downward traction of the liver. The left hemidiaphragm can be inspected by applying gentle downward retraction of the spleen and greater curvature of the stomach. The central tendon of the diaphragm should also be examined, along with the esophageal hiatus.

All herniated viscera must be carefully reduced and relocated to their original positions within the abdominal cavity (Fig. 31-10). All injuries of the diaphragm should be repaired. It is necessary to carefully debride the edges of a laceration if devitalized tissue is found, as may happen with high-velocity missiles or close-range shotgun wounds. The edges of the diaphragmatic laceration should be grasped with Allis' clamps. The laceration is then spread apart to inspect the chest cavity. This allows for evaluation for ongoing hemorrhage from within the thoracic cavity, as well as to determine the degree of contamination between the abdominal and thoracic cavities. Blood and any enteric contamination should be evacuated from the chest. If there has been significant enteric spillage within the chest, irrigation should be performed.

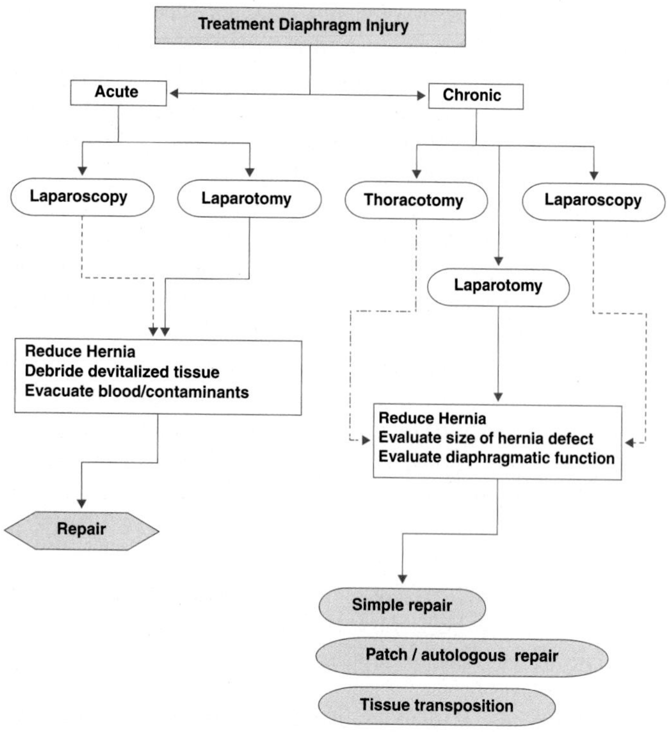

**FIGURE 31-9.** Algorithm for treatment of diaphragm injury, acute vs. chronic.

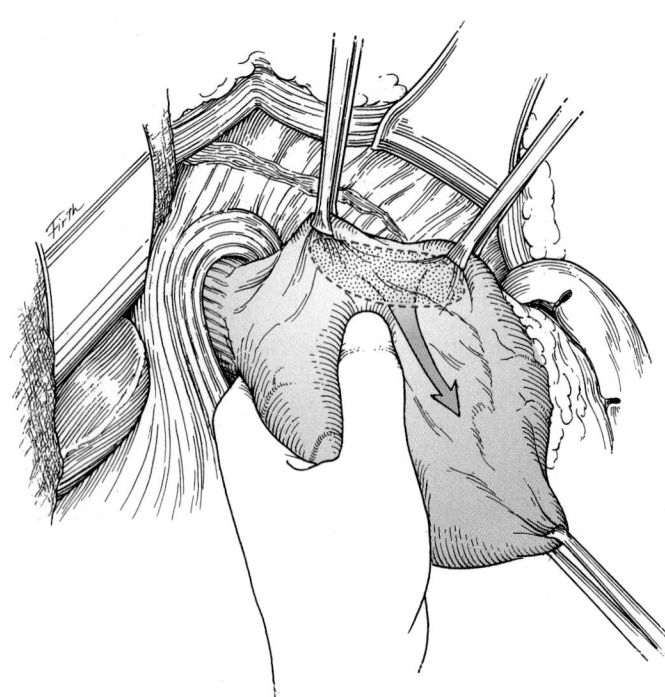

**FIGURE 31-10.** Abdominal approach used to reduce a gastric herniation.

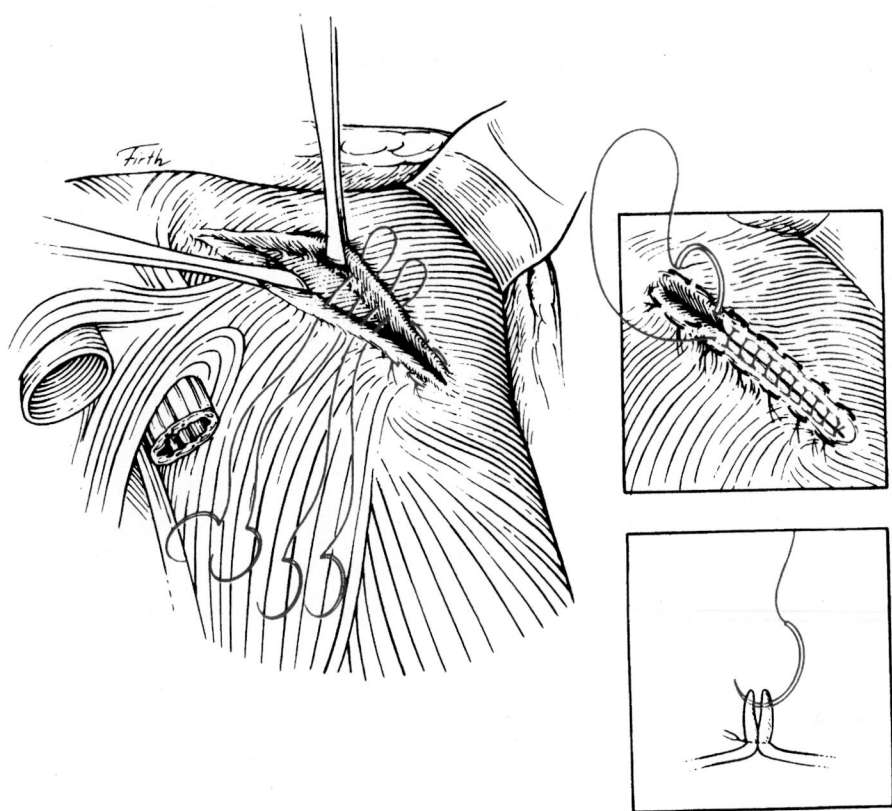

**FIGURE 31-11.** Complex lacerations greater than 5 cm long may require a running suture for reinforcement. One may use 0 or 1 monofilament sutures of nonabsorbable material (polypropylene) or absorbable suture. An alternative means of repairing diaphragmatic injuries involves a continuous running suture. *(Reproduced with permission from Juan A. Asensio, MD, FACS, FCCM and Demetrios Demetriades, MD, PhD, FACS.)*

The management of "cross-contamination" between the peritoneal and pleural cavities has not been studied extensively. A combined thoracotomy and laparotomy approach to enable full visualization has been recommended, although this is controversial. Zellweger et al.[48] studied the management of patients with penetrating thoracoabdominal trauma involving diaphragm laceration and biliary-gastroenteric contamination into the thoracic cavity. They concluded that use of laparotomy and transdiaphragmatic washout of the pleural cavity to remove contamination was effective and simplified the surgical treatment.

Diaphragmatic lacerations may be repaired with a variety of suture material and technique. Interrupted or horizontal mattress suture are commonly used, but some surgeons advocate running, suture repair (Fig. 31-11). Some surgeons prefer 0 or 1 monofilament sutures of nonabsorbable material (polypropylene), but absorbable suture may be used as well.[32] In cases of laceration through the central tendon in which the inferior aspect of the heart is exposed, meticulous attention is given to the placement of the sutures to prevent inadvertent punctures or lacerations of the myocardium (see Chap. 28). At completion of the repair, the integrity of the suture line may be tested by increasing intrathoracic pressure with the administration of large tidal volumes and assessment of diaphragmatic motion. This maneuver is repeated with the field flooded with sterile saline to determine if there is escape of air or pleural fluid through the suture line.

A diaphragmatic injury diagnosed by laparoscopy in the absence of other injuries mandating laparotomy or thoracotomy can be repaired with this approach. This requires that the trauma surgeon be skillful in laparoscopic suturing. Alternatively, they may also be repaired with staples.[22,44]

Evacuation of the air and blood within the chest may be accomplished by placing a tube thoracostomy. The chest tube is classically placed in the fifth intercostal space in the midclavicular line, but may be placed lower under direct observation. Alternatively, with small diaphragmatic injuries, a catheter may be inserted through the laceration and placed to suction. After all the repair sutures are placed, the catheter is quickly withdrawn as the last suture is being tied.

Repair of acute diaphragmatic injuries can be approached via thoracotomy. However, almost all the injuries requiring surgical repair associated with diaphragmatic injury are intra-abdominal and a thorough exploration of the abdominal cavity is mandatory.

Massive diaphragmatic destruction, such as that caused by thoracoabdominal shotgun injuries, merits special mention. Bender and Lucas[49] described the immediate reconstruction of the chest wall following this type of injury by detachment of the affected hemidiaphragm anteriorly, laterally, and posteriorly, thus effectively translocating to a position above the full-thickness chest wall defect and converting the defect functionally into an abdominal wall defect (Fig. 31-12). The diaphragm is then resutured to the muscle of a higher intercostal space, while the abdominal wall defect is managed with local wound care in anticipation of further reconstruction with either split-thickness skin grafts or myocutaneous flaps at a later date (Fig. 31-13). Another technique involves the utilization of prosthetic nonabsorbable mesh material to reconstruct the diaphragm (Fig. 31-14); however, utilization of this material in the presence of contamination in either the thoracic or abdominal cavity poses a risk of infection to the patient.

## CHRONIC PHASE

Patients who initially sustain small, undetected, diaphragmatic lacerations may remain asymptomatic or may experience a progressive increase in visceral herniation of all, or a portion of, a hollow

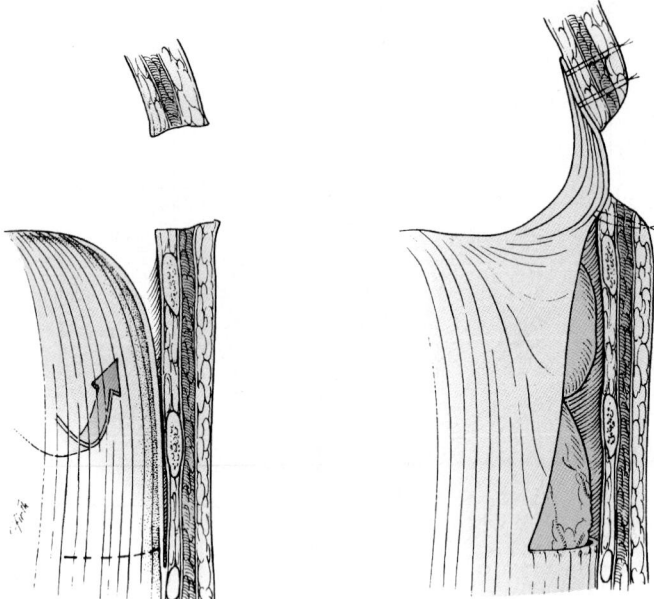

**FIGURE 31-12.** Immediate reconstruction of the chest wall following destructive types of injury may be accomplished by detaching the affected hemidiaphragm anteriorly, laterally, and posteriorly. The diaphragm is then resutured to the muscle of a higher intercostal space, thus effectively translocating it to a position above the full-thickness chest wall defect and converting such a defect functionally into an abdominal wall defect. The abdominal wall defect is then managed with local wound care in anticipation of further reconstruction with either split-thickness skin grafts or myocutaneous flaps at a later date.
*(Reproduced with permission from Juan A. Asensio, MD, FACS, FCCM and Demetrios Demetriades, MD, PhD, FACS.)*

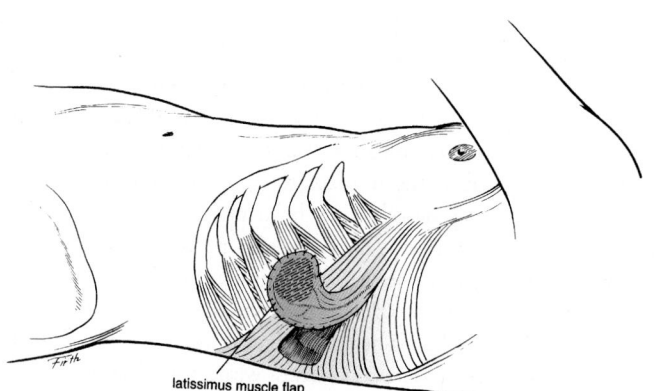

latissimus muscle flap

**FIGURE 31-13.** At times, muscle flaps are necessary to cover thoracoabdominal wall defects. Partial rotational flap of the latissimus dorsi covering a thoracoabdominal wall defect may also be used to reconstruct complex injuries of the chest wall and diaphragm.
*(Reproduced with permission from Juan A. Asensio, MD, FACS, FCCM and Demetrios Demetriades, MD, PhD, FACS.)*

viscus. Some of these injuries are diagnosed years later on routine chest radiograph or on evaluation from a more recent traumatic episode. Some chronic herniations will lead to symptoms and signs of obstruction, and even strangulation.

Miller et al.[50] cautioned about missed diaphragmatic injuries at laparotomy. Feliciano et al.[51] reported 16 patients that experienced delay in diagnosis of diaphragmatic injuries secondary to penetrating

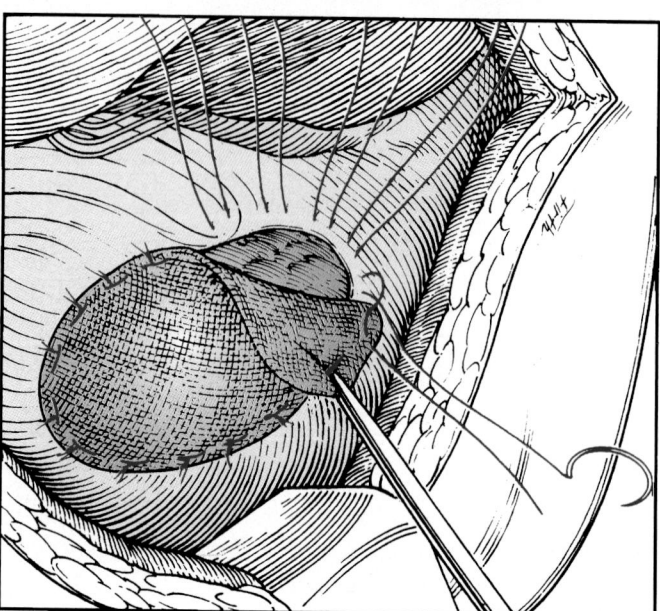

**FIGURE 31-14.** Patients in whom the initial diaphragmatic injury goes undiagnosed may present with large diaphragmatic defects. In general, as time progresses, this defect tends to enlarge due to the constant motion of the diaphragm and negative intrathoracic pressure. It is recommended to attempt a primary repair of the diaphragm, if the diaphragm is mobile. In cases in which the gap cannot be bridged, prosthetic materials, such as the mesh will be necessary.
*(Reproduced with permission from Juan A. Asensio, MD, FACS, FCCM and Demetrios Demetriades, MD, PhD, FACS.)*

trauma. Three of these patients had diaphragmatic injuries missed at the time of laparotomy. Fifteen of the 16 patients had left hemidiaphragmatic involvement, suggesting that the delay in diagnosis of diaphragmatic injury after penetrating trauma most commonly occurs when the left hemidiaphragm is involved.

Delay in repairing a diaphragmatic rupture may increase morbidity and mortality. The diaphragm as a muscle is quick to retract and atrophies, with the result that tissue that could easily be approximated on the day of injury may never be approximated after retraction and atrophy have taken place. Caution is also important with regard to adhesions, which tend to become hazardous during late repairs, as well as the quality of the diaphragmatic tissues in regions of atrophy, which is invariably poor and subject to higher rates of suture line dehiscence once repaired.

The use of nonabsorbable prosthetic meshes (Marlex, Dacron, or Prolene) has been recommended as adjuncts to repair and/or substitute in cases of chronic injury.[52] Edington et al.[53] recommended the use of autologous tissue as the material of choice for reconstruction and described a procedure for reconstructing a functional hemidiaphragm with the use of omentum and a latissimus dorsi flap.

The surgical approach to both acute and chronic diaphragmatic injuries has been a subject of debate.[53–60] For diaphragmatic injuries that are diagnosed on a delayed basis, thoracotomy appears to be a safe approach, and in some cases will facilitate the tedious dissection required to separate herniated intra-abdominal viscera from intrathoracic organs. A significant number of authors, however, recommend the abdominal approach even for chronic injuries.[60]

## Mortality

Mortality from diaphragmatic injuries is generally due to associated injuries. The NTDB reports 1497 deaths of 6038 patients with diaphragm injury (25%). Wieneck et al.[46] reported a series of 165 patients in which 22 of the 43 patients presenting with systolic blood pressures below 70 mm Hg or four or more associated injuries died. Risk factors of a systolic blood pressure below 70 mm Hg, shock lasting longer than 30 minutes, and blood loss exceeding 10 units, with four or more associated injuries invariably predicted a poor outcome.

## Morbidity

Morbidity incurred in diaphragmatic injuries can be subdivided into those directly related to the injury or surgical procedure employed to repair the injury, and that related to the underlying trauma and associated injuries. Morbidity in the first case includes suture-line dehiscence, failure of diaphragmatic repair, hemidiaphragmatic paralysis secondary to iatrogenic phrenic nerve injuries, respiratory insufficiency, empyema, and subphrenic abscess, which are generally manifested during the acute injury period. Whereas strangulation and perforation of herniated intra-abdominal viscera and recurrent bowel obstruction are classified as late morbidity.

The complication rate with diaphragmatic injury has ranged from 30% to 68%.[26,32,54] Atelectasis was seen in 11–68%, with pneumonia and pleural effusions reported in 10–23%. Sepsis, multiorgan system failure, hepatic abscess, and empyema occurred in 2–10%. When complication rates were compared in blunt versus penetrating diaphragmatic injury, the patients with blunt trauma experienced a majority of complications, with an incidence of 60%, as opposed to those with penetrating trauma, who experienced a 40% complication rate.[55] Most of the morbidity figures reported in these studies[26,54,55] is clearly the result of the large number of associated injuries present in association with diaphragmatic injuries.

---

# SPECIAL SITUATIONS

## Strangulated Diaphragmatic Hernias

Gastrointestinal incarceration and strangulation have been recognized as among the most serious complications of diaphragmatic hernias. Sullivan[56] reported 53 cases of obstruction and strangulation in diaphragmatic hernias caused by penetrating injuries and noted that 80% of the cases occurred within the first three years after injury (range 19 hours to 33 years). The etiologic factor in the majority of the cases was a previous stab wound, with gunshot wounds and iatrogenic injury implicated much less frequently. The most common organ herniated was the colon, followed very closely by the stomach. The omentum was found to have herniated in 40% of cases, and the small intestine was found intra-thoracically in only 10% of cases. A mortality rate of 20% has been reported for late incarceration and 40% to 57% for strangulation of traumatic diaphragmatic hernias. The severity of these complications reinforces the importance of making the diagnosis and intervening.[16,56–60]

## Acute Intrapericardial Herniations

Ruptures of the central tendon of the diaphragm involving the pericardium are rare. Most are caused by combined blunt trauma to the chest and abdomen; however, isolated trauma to either one of the cavities can also cause this entity. Coincident rupture of the pericardium into the left and the right pleural space has occurred, as has herniation of the heart inferiorly into the peritoneal cavity. Van Loenhout et al.[61] reported 58 cases of traumatic intrapericardial diaphragmatic hernia collected from the literature. The majority of these patients presented after motor vehicle accidents with cardiopulmonary or abdominal symptoms. Chest x-rays, contrast studies, CT scans, and echocardiography were helpful in establishing the diagnoses. There was a high incidence of associated injuries, including musculoskeletal injuries that occurred predominantly on the left side of the body. The organs most frequently involved in pericardial herniation were the transverse colon, stomach, omentum, liver, and small bowel. Exploratory laparotomy is recommended as the preferred approach for the acute repair of these injuries.

## REFERENCES

1. Sennertus RC (cited by Reed): Diaphragmatic hernia produced by a penetrating wound. *Edinburgh Med Surg J* 53:104, 1840.
2. Paré A: *Oeuvres Completes d'Ambroise Paré*. In Malgaigne JF, ed. *accompangnees de notes historiques et critiques et precedes d'une introduction sur l'origine et les progress de la chirurgie en Occident du Vie au XVIe siecle*. Paris: Bailliere, 1840, vol 11, p. 94.
3. Hamby WB: *The Case Reports and Autopsy Records of Ambroise Paré*. Springfield, IL: Thomas, 1960, p. 50.
4. Paré A: *The Apologii and Treatise of Ambroise Paré, Containing the Voyages Made into Diverse Places with Many of His Writings upon Surgery*. In Keynes G, ed. Chicago: University of Chicago Press, 1952, p. 205.
5. Allison PR: The diaphragm. *Surgery of the Chest*, 2nd ed. Philadelphia: Saunders, 1969, p. 243.
6. Morgagni GB: *Seats and Causes of Diseases*. Monograph on Hernia of the Diaphragm, London: Zellts, 1769, p. 54.
7. Bowditch HI: Diaphragmatic hernia. *Buffalo Med J* 9:1, 1853.
8. Bardenhewer E: Ein von hernia diaphragmatica. *Berl Klin Wochenschr* 16:195, 1879.
9. Riolfi: Bull. Della Soc. Lancisiana degli ospedali di Roma. *Zantralbl Chir* 1893, p 873. As cited by Hedblom CA: Diaphragmatic hernia. A study of three hundred and seventy-eight cases in which operation was performed. *JAMA* 85:947, 1925.
10. Naumann G: Hernia diaphragmatica, laparotomie. DöD as cited by Lauenstein C. *Zentralbl Chir* 15:894, 1888.
11. Walker EW: Strangulated hernia through a traumatic rupture of the diaphragm. Laparotomy: Recovery. *Trans Am Surg Assoc* 18:246, 1900.
12. Hedblom CA: Diaphragmatic hernia: A study of three hundred and seventy-eight cases in which operation was performed. *JAMA* 85:947, 1925.
13. Thorek P: Diaphragm. *Anatomy in Surgery*, 2nd ed. Philadelphia: JB Lippincott, 1962, p. 266.
14. Bark H, Sypinski G, Bundy R, et al.: The effect of hypoxia on diaphragm blood flow, oxygen uptake and contractility. *Am Rev Respir Dis* 138:1535, 1988.
15. Merendino KA, Johnson RJ, Skinner HH, et al.: The intradiaphragmatic distribution of the phrenic nerve with particular reference to the placement of diaphragmatic incisions and controlled segmental paralysis. *Surgery* 39:189, 1956.
16. Marchand P: A study of the forces productive of gastroesophageal regurgitation and herniation through the diaphragmatic hiatus. *Thorax* 12:189, 1957.
17. Hood RM: Traumatic diaphragmatic hernia. *Ann Thorac Surg* 12:311, 1971.
18. Schneider CF: Traumatic diaphragmatic hernia. *Am J Surg* 91:290, 1956.
19. Carter BN, Giuseffi J: Traumatic diaphragmatic hernia. *Am J Roentgenol* 65:56, 1951.
20. Iochum S, Ludig T, Frederic W, et al.: *Radiographics* 22: S103, (discussion S116), 2002.
21. National Trauma Data Base® (NTDB). American College of Surgeons, years 2000 to 2004.
22. Murray JA, Demetriades D, Asensio JA, et al.: Occult injuries to the diaphragm: Prospective evaluation of laparoscopy in penetrating injuries to the lower left chest. *JACS* 187:626, 1998.

23. Kearney PA, Rouhana SW, Burney RE: Blunt rupture of the diaphragm: Mechanism, diagnosis and treatment. *Ann Emerg Med* 18:1326, 1989.
24. Shanmuganathan K, Killeen K, Mirvis SE, et al.: Imaging of diaphragmatic injuries. *J Thorac Imaging* 15:104, 2000.
25. Demetriades D, Kakoyiannis S, Parekh D, et al.: Penetrating injuries of the diaphragm. *Br J Surg* 75:824, 1988.
26. Wiencek RG, Wilson RF, Steiger Z: Acute injuries of the diaphragm: An analysis of 165 cases. *J Thorac Cardiovasc Surg* 92:989, 1986.
27. Desforges G, Strieder JW, Lynch JP, et al.: Traumatic rupture of the diaphragm. *J Thorac Surg* 34:779, 1957.
28. Bekassy SM, Dave KS, Wooler GH, et al.: "Spontaneous" and traumatic rupture of the diaphragm: Long-term results. *Ann Surg* 177:320, 1973.
29. Bergin D, Ennis R, Keogh C, et al.: The "dependent viscera" sign in CT diagnosis of blunt traumatic diaphragmatic rupture. *AJR Am J Roentgenol* 177:1137, 2001.
30. Boulanger BR, Milzman DP, Rosati C, et al.: A comparison of right and left blunt traumatic diaphragmatic rupture. *J Trauma* 35:255, 1993.
31. Bergin D, Ennis R, Keogh C, et al.: The "dependent viscera" sign in CT diagnosis of blunt traumatic diaphragmatic rupture. AJR *Am J Roentgenol* 177:1137, 2001.
32. Beal SL, McKennan M: Blunt diaphragmatic rupture: A morbid injury. *Arch Surg* 123:828, 1988.
33. Hood RM: Injuries involving the diaphragm. In Hood RM, Boyd AD, Culliford AT, eds. *Thoracic Trauma.* Philadelphia: Saunders, 1989, p. 267.
34. Mirvis SE, Shanmuganathan K: Trauma radiology: part II. Diagnostic imaging of thoracic trauma: review and update. *J Intensive Care Med* 9:179, 1994.
35. Payne JH, Yellin AE: Traumatic diaphragmatic hernia. *Arch Surg* 117:18, 1982.
36. Blaivas M, Brannam L, Hawkins M, et al.: Bedside emergency ultrasonographic diagnosis of diaphragmatic rupture in blunt abdominal trauma. *Am J Emerg Med* 22:601, 2004.
37. Kim HH, Shin YR, Kim KJ, et al.: Blunt traumatic rupture of the diaphragm: Sonographic diagnosis. *J Ultrasound Med* 16:593, 1997.
38. Larici AR, Gotway MB, Litt HI, et al.: Helical CT with sagittal and coronal reconstructions: accuracy for detection of diaphragmatic injury. *Am J Radiology* 179:451, 2002.
39. Nchimi A, Szapiro D, Ghaye B, et al.: Helical CT of blunt diaphragmatic rupture. *Am J Radiology* 184:24, 2005.
40. Rees O, Mirvis SE, Shanmuganathan K: Multidetector-row CT of right hemidiaphragmatic rupture caused by blunt trauma: a review of 12 cases. *Clinical Rad* 60:1280, 2005.
41. Shanmuganathan K, Mirvis SE, White CS, et al.: MR imaging evaluation of hemidiaphragms in acute blunt trauma: Experience with 16 patients. *AJR Am J Roentgenol* 167:397, 1996.
42. Root HD, Hauser CW, McKinley CR, et al.: Diagnostic peritoneal lavage. *Surgery* 57:633, 1965.
43. Ivatury RR, Simon RJ, Stahl WM: A critical evaluation of laparoscopy in penetrating abdominal trauma. *J Trauma* 34:822, 1993.
44. Murray JA, Demetriades D, Cornwell EE, et al.: Penetrating left thoracoabdominal trauma: The incidence and clinical presentation of diaphragm injuries. *J Trauma* 43:824, 1997.
45. Friese RS, Coln CE, Gentilello LM: Laparoscopy is sufficient to exclude occult diaphragm injury after penetrating abdominal trauma. *J Trauma* 58:789, 2005.
46. Ochsner MG, Rozycki GS, Lucente F, et al.: Prospective evaluation of thoracoscopy for diagnosing diaphragmatic injury in thoracoabdominal trauma: A preliminary report. *J Trauma* 34:704, 1993.
47. Moore EE, Malangoni MA, Cogbill T, et al.: Organ injury scaling. IV: Thoracic, vascular, lung, cardiac and diaphragm. *J Trauma* 36:299, 1994.
48. Zellweger R, Navsaria PH, Hess F, et al.: Trans-diaphragmatic pleural lavage in penetrating thoracoabdominal trauma. *Br Jr of Surg* 91:1619, 2004.
49. Bender JS, Lucas CE: Management of close-range shotgun injuries to the chest by diaphragmatic transposition: Case reports. *J Trauma* 30:1581, 1990.
50. Miller L, Bennett EV, Root HD, et al.: Management of penetrating and blunt diaphragmatic injury. *J Trauma* 24:403, 1984.
51. Feliciano DV, Cruse PA, Mattox KL, et al.: Delayed diagnosis of injuries to the diaphragm after penetrating wounds. *J Trauma* 28:1135, 1988.
52. Fallazadeh H, Mays ET: Description of the diaphragm by blunt trauma: New dimensions of diagnosis. *Am Surg* 41:337, 1975.
53. Edington HD, Evans S, Sindelar WF: Reconstruction of a functional hemidiaphragm with use of omentum and latissimus dorsi flaps. *Surgery* 105:442, 1989.
54. Chen JC, Wilson SE: Diaphragmatic injuries: Recognition and management in sixty-two patients. *Am Surg* 57:810, 1991.
55. Meyers BF, McCabe CJ: Traumatic diaphragmatic hernia. *Ann Surg* 218:783, 1993.
56. Sullivan RE: Strangulation and obstruction in diaphragmatic hernia due to direct trauma. *J Thorac Cardiovasc Surg* 52:725, 1966.
57. Pomerantz M, Rodgers BM, Sabiston DC Jr: Traumatic diaphragmatic hernia. *Surgery* 64:529, 1968.
58. Skinner EF, Carr D, Duncan JT, et al.: Strangulated diaphragmatic hernia. *J Thorac Cardiovasc Surg* 36:102, 1958.
59. Hoffman E: Strangulated diaphragmatic hernia. *Thorax* 23:541, 1968.
60. Saber WL, Moore EE, Hopeman AR, et al.: Delayed presentation of traumatic diaphragmatic hernia. *J Emerg Med* 4:1, 1986.
61. van Loenhout RMM, Schiphorst TJM, Wittens CHA, et al.: Traumatic intrapericardial diaphragmatic hernia. *J Trauma* 26:271, 1986.

# Commentary ■ MICHAEL L. HAWKINS

This is a well-written review on diaphragmatic injuries with an extensive and up-to-date bibliography. The authors have correctly pointed out that identifying these injuries expeditiously remains problematic in spite of the advances in diagnostic technology with resulting potential for serious morbidity and delayed treatment. The authors provide a brief history of milestones in the recognition and treatment of diaphragmatic injuries which will be of interest to some readers. More significantly, there is a detailed description of the anatomy and physiology of the diaphragm which is important for those who will manage these injuries. The overall incidence of 0.63% as reported from a query of over 950,000 trauma patients in the NTDB must be viewed critically as these data reflect a wide range of trauma severity and undoubtedly grossly underrepresent patients with a delayed diagnosis. Many series report the incidence of diaphragmatic rupture in those patients with significant thoracoabdominal trauma to be in the 5 to 8% range. The authors clearly emphasize that associated injuries are very common, some even report up to a 100% incidence, though the severity of these other injuries varies widely. While there are no pathognomonic external signs, the presence of upper abdominal contusions (such as from an improperly placed lap belt or reflecting a direct blow to this area) should raise one's suspicion in patients suffering blunt trauma. Likewise, diaphragmatic injury must always be considered in patients with lower thoracic/upper abdominal penetrating wounds. In the acute phase, signs and symptoms, if present, generally result from the associated injuries. Diagnosis is easy if there is herniation of the stomach, as shown in Fig.31-5; however, plain films may not be diagnostic in the presence of pulmonary contusion or hemothorax or misinterpreted as diaphragmatic eventration. Ultrasonography, including the FAST exam, may show abnormal diaphragmatic excursion (if the patient is breathing spontaneously) or an abnormal splenic/renal relationship. Multislice CT, especially with sagittal reconstructions, has been shown to be highly reliable in some centers. Although MRI may clearly show visceral herniation through the diaphragm, it has a limited role in the acute setting with current equipment. It is important to keep in mind that herniation of abdominal viscera may not occur while the patient is on positive pressure ventilation with subsequent delay in diagnosis and treatment of a diaphragmatic laceration. Both laparoscopy and thoracoscopy have been touted by some as highly reliable for identifying this injury though either approach is dependent upon the skill and thoroughness of the operator. If diagnostic laparoscopy is employed, one must be aware of the potential for developing a tension pneumothorax during creation of the pneumoperitoneum and be prepared to rapidly decompress the pleural space. While some lacerations may be repaired via the laparoscope or thoracoscope, associated injuries often require an open procedure. The importance of a thorough inspection of the diaphragms, whether approached by an open procedure or by minimally invasive techniques, cannot be overemphasized. There are several series reporting missed injuries, even in experienced hands, following laparotomy. Although a variety of techniques and suture material has been shown to be effective, I prefer nonabsorbable suture, taking large bites to include both the peritoneal and parietal pleural membranes. I close small lacerations using horizontal mattress sutures but use simple running closure for longer lacerations. I do not use pledgets as I believe they are unnecessary additional foreign material. The vast majority of acute injuries can be closed primarily though significant tissue loss, such as a shotgun wound, may require prosthetic material. The surgical repair for chronic diaphragmatic injuries is usually transthoracic and may be challenging due to adhesions, intestinal strangulation, and atrophy or retraction of the diaphragm. Prosthetic mesh, transposition of the diaphragmatic thoracic wall attachments, and/or autogenous tissue flaps may be required. The increasing management of both penetrating and blunt abdominal trauma, including patients with known splenic and/or liver lacerations, nonoperatively may result in a higher incidence of late presentations of diaphragmatic injuries in the future. Physicians who will manage trauma patients must be aware of the anatomy of the diaphragm and the findings, diagnostic difficulties, and treatment options for diaphragmatic injuries. These authors have provided a thorough and easily readable discussion on this topic.

# Liver and Biliary Tract

*Timothy C. Fabian* ■ *Tiffany K. Bee*

## INTRODUCTION

Liver injury occurs in approximately 5% of all trauma admissions.[1] The liver's size and anatomic location, directly under the right costal margin, make it the most susceptible organ for injury in blunt trauma and a frequently involved organ in penetrating trauma. The management of liver injury has evolved greatly over the last decade. There have been many technical advances in medicine, which now allow us to better diagnose and treat liver injuries both operatively and nonoperatively. However, the most severe liver parenchymal and venous injuries as well as those involving the portal triad continue to challenge even the most adept trauma or hepatobiliary surgeon and often lead to death. Therefore, despite our progress in liver injury management, many avenues for improvement remain to be explored.

## HISTORY

Liver injury management has been described in many of the early surgical textbooks. The severity of hepatic injury was emphasized by Edler in 1887. He suggested that if a wound to the liver caused hemorrhage and proved fatal, it would do so within 24 hours.[2] Interestingly, we consider nonoperative management of hepatic injury a modern approach. However, a 1905 surgical text states, "If the evidences of a rupture of the liver, such as the signs of shock and hemorrhage.... the continuous increase in pain, due to progressive abdominal distention, and muscular rigidity, are absent, no operative intervention can be considered."[3] Mortality from liver injury was very high in these early years. Benjamin Tilton reported on 25 liver injuries at New York hospital and found a 62.5% mortality in those operated on for hepatic "rupture," 33% mortality in stab wounds, and 28.5% mortality in cases of gunshot wounds.[4]

J. Hogarth Pringle wrote a landmark paper examining the management of severe liver injury in 1908.[5] Although many authors previous to this paper had described suturing methods of liver parenchyma as well as gauze packing into the liver laceration, Pringle described a maneuver of occluding the porta hepatis with the surgeon's fingers and thus decreasing the amount of hemorrhage from a severely injured liver. This procedure continues to be a useful tool in the management of liver trauma.

During World War II, new ideas in the management of severe liver injury surfaced. Madding et al. used the principles of early laparotomy, drainage procedures, advances in anesthetic and aseptic care, as well as transfusion technology to improve mortality to 27.7%.[6] The techniques of hemorrhage control adopted at that time incorporated parenchymal reapproximation with large blunt liver needles, resection, and direct vessel ligation. These methods prevailed until approximately ten years ago. Trends in management have now led to an emphasis on nonoperative treatment for those patients who remain hemodynamically stable and liver packing with damage control for those who are unstable.

## ANATOMY

Comprehensive knowledge of hepatic anatomy is essential to the proper management of traumatic liver injuries. The understanding of the ligamentous attachments, parenchyma, and intra and extra-parenchymal vascularity of the liver is key to the effective application of methods for control and repair in liver injuries (Fig. 32-1).

### Lobes

Cantlie first described the lobar anatomy in 1898. The liver is divided into two lobes by a 75° angle traversing from the gallbladder fossa posteriorly to the left side of the inferior vena cava. This is the so-called line of Cantlie. Therefore, the left lobe includes the hepatic tissue to the left of the falciform ligament along with the quadrate and caudate lobes. The right lobe consists of the remaining parenchyma.

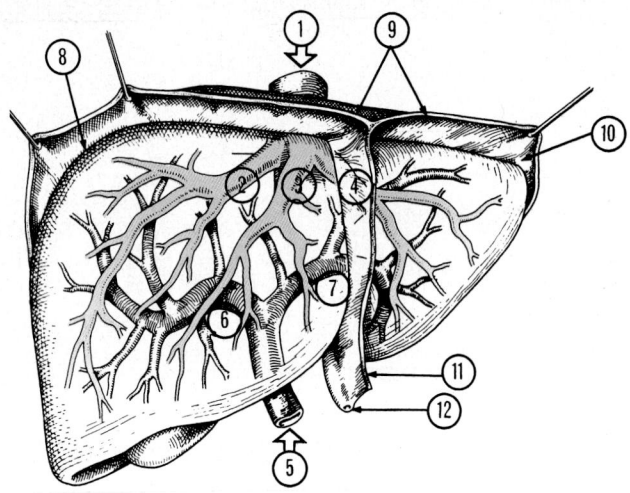

**FIGURE 32-1.** Surgical anatomy of the liver: (1) inferior vena cava; (2) right hepatic vein; (3) middle hepatic vein; (4) left hepatic vein; (5) portal vein; (6) right branch portal vein; (7) left branch portal vein; (8) right triangular ligament; (9) coronary ligament; (10) left triangular ligament; (11) falciform ligament; (12) ligamentum teres.

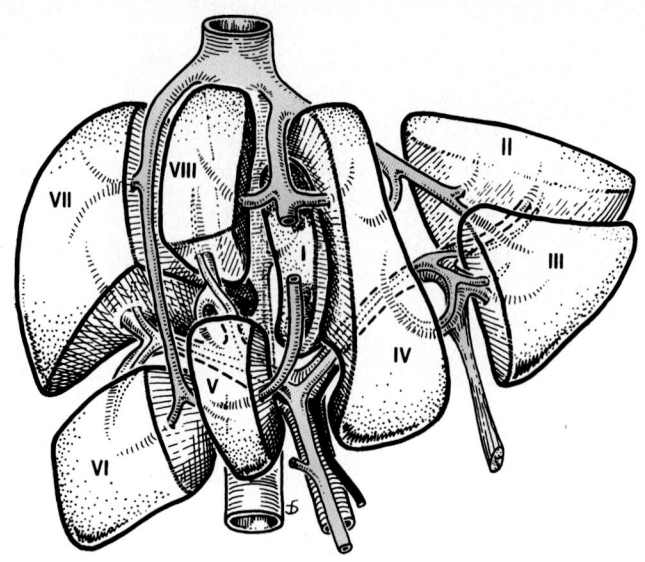

**FIGURE 32-2.** Functional division of the liver, according to Couinaud's nomenclature.
*(Reproduced with permission from Blumgart LH (ed): Surgery of the Liver and Biliary Tract. New York, Churchill Livingstone, 1988.)*

## Functional Anatomy

The functional anatomy of the liver separates the liver into segments pertinent to resection. In 1953, Couinaud provided the basis of modern resection planes by dividing the liver based on the distribution of the hepatic veins and glissonian pedicles. The right hepatic vein traverses between the right posterolateral (VI and VII) and right anteromedial (V and VIII) segments. On the left, the left hepatic vein delineates the anterior (III and IV) and posterior (II) segments. The caudate lobe (I) drains directly into the inferior vena cava (Fig. 32-2).

## Hepatic Artery

The common hepatic artery branches from the celiac artery. This provides about 25% of the hepatic blood flow and 50% of hepatic oxygenation. The artery then branches into the gastroduodenal, right gastric, and proper hepatic. The proper hepatic is found in the porta hepatis usually to the left of the common bile duct and anterior to the portal vein. At the hilum of the liver, the artery bifurcates into a right (the longer branch) and a left hepatic artery. There are a number of anatomic variances. The most frequent (11%) is the aberrant superior mesenteric origin of the right hepatic artery traversing behind the duodenum. Other variants include a left hepatic artery origin from the left gastric artery (8%) and the left and right hepatic arteries arising from a superior mesenteric artery origin (9%). With these multiple variants, great care must be taken when controlling the traumatic hemorrhage.

**Hepatic Veins.** The hepatic veins develop from within the hepatocytes' central lobar veins. The superior, middle, and inferior vein branches originating from the right lobe form the right hepatic vein. The middle hepatic vein derives from the two veins arising from segments IV and V and frequently includes a branch from the posterior portion of segment VIII. In 90% of patients the middle hepatic vein joins the left hepatic vein just before draining into the inferior vena cava. The left hepatic vein is more

variable in its segmental origin. Most important is the posterior positioning of the vein when dissecting the left coronary ligament; great caution must be used in this area to avoid inadvertent injury.

The retrohepatic vena cava is about 8 to 10 cm in length. It receives the blood of the hepatic veins and also multiple small direct hepatic vessels. Exposure to this area can be very difficult, especially when an injury and accompanying hemorrhage make visualization very difficult.

**Portal Vein.** The portal vein is formed from the confluence of the splenic and superior mesenteric veins directly behind the pancreatic head. The portal vein provides about 75% of hepatic blood flow and 50% of hepatic oxygen. The portal vein lies posteriorly to the hepatic artery and bile ducts as it ascends toward the liver. At the parenchyma, the portal vein divides into a short right and longer left extrahepatic branch.

**Ligaments.** When operating on the liver it is crucial to understand the ligamentous attachments. The coronary ligaments attach the diaphragm to the parietal surface of the liver. The triangular ligaments are at the lateral extensions of the right and left coronary ligaments. The falciform ligament with the underlying ligamentum teres attaches to the anterior peritoneal cavity. The medial portion of the coronary ligaments is where the hepatic veins traverse and therefore dissection in this area must be done with caution.

## LIVER INJURY INCIDENCE AND CLASSIFICATION

Liver injury occurs in approximately 5% of all trauma admissions. Since the liver is the largest intra-abdominal organ it is not surprising that the liver is the most commonly injured solid organ in blunt and penetrating injury. Data from the author's institution over the past five years illustrates the frequency of liver injury compared to other abdominal solid organ injury (Table 32-1). Motor

**TABLE 32-1**

| Trauma Admissions, (N = 21,873) | | | | |
|---|---|---|---|---|
| | **MECHANISM OF INJURY** | | | |
| **ORGAN** | **Blunt** | **Penetrating** | **TOTAL** | **% TOTAL** |
| Liver | 938 | 334 | 1272 | 32 |
| Spleen | 903 | 73 | 976 | 25 |
| Kidney | 260 | 122 | 382 | 10 |
| Pancreas | 45 | 54 | 99 | 3 |
| Stomach | 15 | 158 | 173 | 4 |
| Small bowel/ duodenum | 126 | 418 | 544 | 14 |
| Colon/rectum | 92 | 365 | 457 | 12 |
| Total | 2379 | 1524 | 3903 | 100 |

vehicle collision is by far the most common etiology for a blunt liver injury. This is followed by pedestrian/car collisions, falls, assaults, and motorcycle crashes. Liver injury in penetrating trauma is also frequent, ranging from 13% to 35% of penetrating admissions, and is dependent on the weapon utilized.

Uniform classification of liver injury is essential to compare the efficacy of management techniques (Fig. 32-3). The American Association for the Surgery of Trauma established a detailed classification system that has been widely utilized[7] (Table 32-2). This classification provides for uniform comparisons of both nonoperative and operatively managed hepatic injury.

## INITIAL MANAGEMENT

Care for the patient with possible liver injury should proceed by the tenants of Advanced Trauma Life Support (ATLS). Of utmost importance is the initial evaluation, including attention to airway, breathing, and circulation (see Chap. 11).

Decreased sensorium, significant chest or facial injuries, or profound shock may require rapid intubation, chest tube insertion, infusion line placement, or occasionally thoracotomy, (see Chap. 15), all of which may take precedence over possible internal injury. After primary survey has been successfully performed, attention can then focus on the details of resuscitation.

Resuscitation strategies are evolving in the care of trauma patients (see Chap. 13). The prospect of permissive hypotension in trauma patients was examined by Bickell et al. in 1994.[8] They revealed that patients with penetrating torso injuries had an improved survival with delayed resuscitation that began in the operating room. This study has launched many other studies of permissive hypotension in both penetrating and blunt injury. Not all studies have revealed improved mortality.[9] It must also be stressed that hypotension may be deleterious to the severely head injured patient (see Chap. 20) or elderly trauma patient.

Physical exam of the patient remains a critical component of the initial evaluation. However, physical exam of a trauma patient may indeed miss significant internal injury. A study by Olsen et al. found that trauma patients with a "benign" physical exam had a 43%

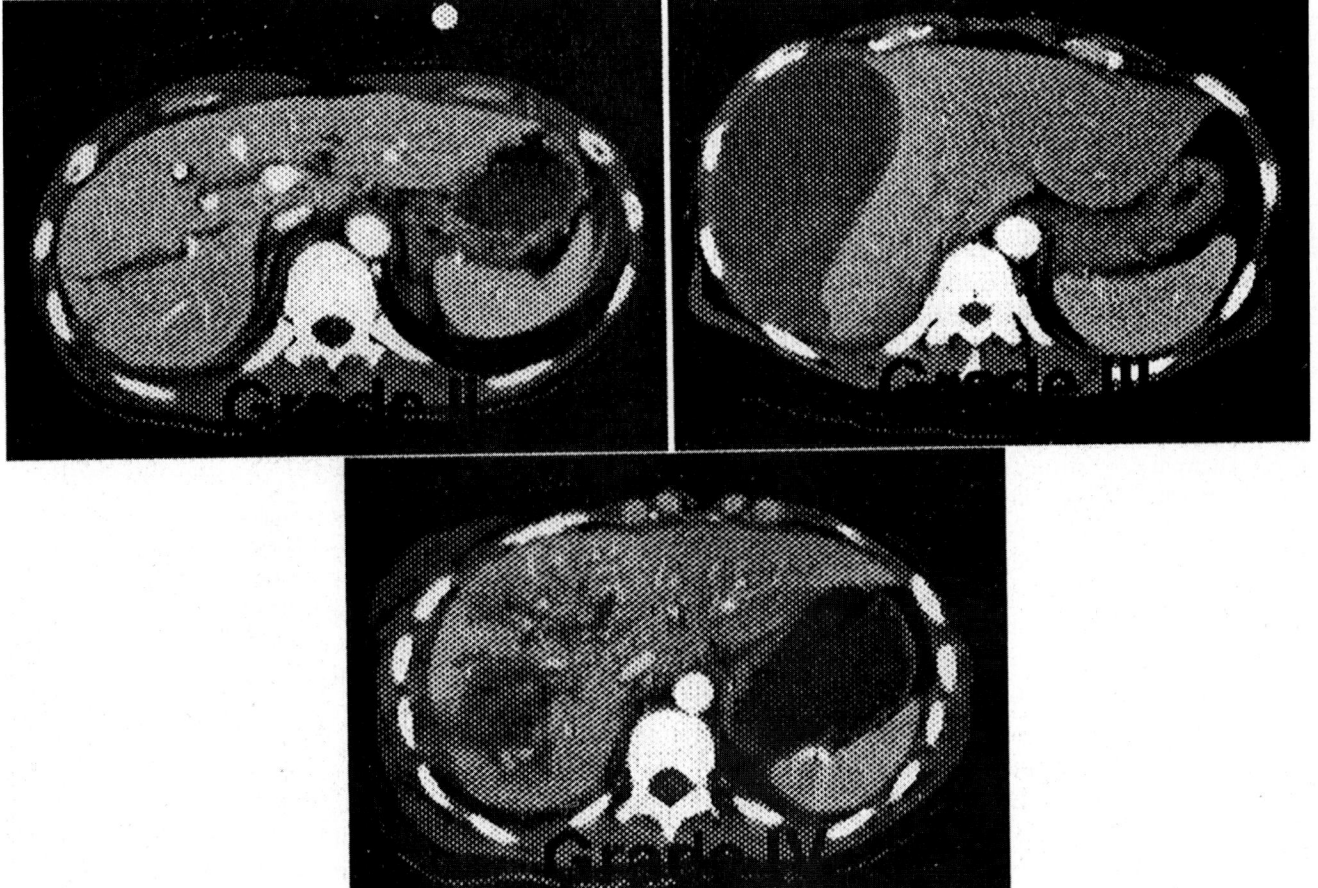

**FIGURE 32-3.** Hepatic injury grading is important to compare outcome.

**TABLE 32-2**

## Liver Injury Scale (1994 Revision)

| GRADE[a] | | INJURY DESCRIPTION | ICD-9[b] | AIS90[c] |
|---|---|---|---|---|
| I | Hematoma | Subcapsualr, nonexpanding <10 cm surface area | 864.01 864.11 | 2 |
| | Laceration | Capsuler tear, nonbleeding. <1 cm parenchymal depth | 864.02 864.12 | 2 |
| II | Hematoma | Subcapsular, nonexpanding, 10 to 50% surface area; intraparenchymal nonexpanding <10 in diameter | 864.01 864.11 | 2 |
| | Laceration | Capsular tear, active bleeding; 1–3 cm parenchymal depth. <10 cm in length | 864.03 864.13 | 2 |
| III | Hematoma | Subcapsular, >50% surface area or expanding; ruptured subcapsular hematoma with active bleeding; intraparenchymal hematoma >10 cm or expanding | | 3 |
| | Laceration | >3cm parenchymal depth | 864.04 864.14 | 3 |
| IV | Hematoma | Ruptured intraparenchymal hematoma with active bleeding | | 4 |
| | Laceration | Parenchymal disruption involving 25 to 75% of hepatic lobe or 1–3 Couinaud's segments within a single lobe | 864.04 864.14 | 4 |
| V | Laceration | Parenchymal disruption involving >75% of hepatic lobe or >3 Couinaud's segments within a single lobe | | 5 |
| | Vascular | Juxtahepatic venous injuries (i.e., retrohepatic vena cava/central major hepatic veins) | | 5 |
| VI | Vascular | Hepatic avulsion | | 6 |

[a]Advance one grade for multiple injuries, up to grade III.
[b]International Classification of Diseases. 9th Revision.
[c]Abbreviated Injury Scale. 1990.

incidence of significant intra-abdominal injury.[10] Therefore, it is justified that patients with benign physical exams are further evaluated either by serial exams or radiologic methods. Plain radiographs may give clues to possible liver injury if lower right rib fractures, hemothorax, or a ruptured diaphragm are diagnosed. Although nonoperative management has become routine, a patient exhibiting clear peritoneal signs and instability requires immediate celiotomy (see Chap. 30).

Important but often overlooked points include keeping the patient warmed and collecting appropriate laboratory data. Hypothermia and its detrimental effects to coagulation and cardiac rhythm can be avoided by setting the trauma room temperature above 80°F (26.6°C) and quickly placing the patient under warmed blankets. Also, warmed IV fluids, air-warmed blankets, and if needed, peritoneal lavage with warmed saline can all prevent hypothermia (see Chap. 51). Appropriate laboratory data should include, type and cross, hematocrit, coagulation profile, amylase, and base deficit. Abnormalities can alert the clinician to possible internal injury and its severity.

## DIAGNOSIS OF LIVER INJURY

### Hemodynamically Unstable Patient

After primary survey and resuscitation have been initiated, the patient may still be hemodynamically unstable. In these cases it is necessary to immediately determine the possible causes of the continued shock state. This can be difficult in patients with multiple injuries involving many organ systems.

Intra-abdominal injury can be an obvious cause of instability if physical exam reveals peritoneal signs, penetrating injury, or increasing distention. More often, a rapid diagnostic modality must be employed. The two most pertinent modalities for these situations are diagnostic peritoneal lavage (DPL) and focused abdominal sonography for trauma (FAST).

### Diagnostic Peritoneal Lavage

DPL is a very accurate method for determining the presence of intraperitoneal blood. Many reports have replicated the work of Root et al. that indicated up to a 98% accuracy of determining the presence of intra-abdominal blood.[11] DPL is rapid and safe if performed with the semiopen or open technique. It remains a very useful tool in those patients who have altered sensorium and remain hemodynamically unstable. A positive DPL is defined as a gross aspiration of 10 mL of blood or greater than 100000 RBC/mm$^3$ in at least 300 mL of irrigant. A finding of gross blood in an unstable patient leads to immediate operative intervention. A DPL can also be examined for WBC, particulate matter, bile, creatinine, and amylase in the more stable patient with possible intestinal or pancreatic injury. DPL does have limitations. It is not useful in determining the origin of the bloody aspirate and can actually be too sensitive since it is positive with minimal hemoperitoneum. Also, it does not evaluate retroperitoneal injury. Therefore, though it has its place in rapid determination of hemoperitoneum and subsequent immediate operative intervention, DPL has been replaced in most trauma centers by ultrasound and in more stable patients, by computed tomography (CT) scanning.

## Focused Abdominal Sonography for Trauma

The FAST exam has superseded DPL in many institutions for the determination of hemoperitoneum in the unstable bluntly injured patient (see Chap.17). Surgeons have become very adept and familiar with this diagnostic modality. Richards et al. reported a 98% sensitivity of ultrasound for hemoperitoneum in grade III and higher liver injury.[12] However, they were not able to identify the anatomical location of the hepatic parenchymal injury in 67% of these severely damaged livers. A study comparing experienced ultrasonographers with less experienced examiners in Japan revealed a sensitivity of 87.5% for hepatic injuries in the experienced group compared to 46.2% in the less experienced group. Differentiation of hepatic injury type and location was up to 80% in the expert group but much less in the less experienced group.[13] A multi-institutional study by Rozycki et al. concluded that the RUQ area is the most common site of hemoperitoneum accumulation in blunt abdominal trauma.[14] This information was reiterated in another study that discovered that the "two most common patterns of fluid accumulation after hepatic injuries were the RUQ only and the RUQ and lower recesses."[15] However, if the initial exam of the RUQ is negative, it is recommended that the pericardial, LUQ, and pelvic areas also be examined. The FAST exam is about 97% sensitive when one liter of peritoneal fluid is present, but the examiner can rarely see volumes less than 400 mL with current technology.[16] FAST exam is very beneficial in those unstable patients in whom the diagnosis of hemoperitoneum requires emergent surgery.

## Hemodynamically Stable Patient

Ultrasound and CT scanning are the mainstays of diagnosing hepatic injury in the hemodynamically stable but bluntly injured patient. Once the primary and secondary surveys have been completed the patient at risk for intra-abdominal injury should undergo further radiologic evaluation for definitive diagnosis (see Chap. 16).

## FAST

FAST examination, as mentioned above, has proven to be a very good diagnostic tool in the evaluation of the blunt trauma patient. Some centers are using ultrasound for definitive diagnosis of intra-abdominal injury. Most examiners though, are unable to distinguish between different grades of hepatic injury by ultrasound.[12] Also, the source of free fluid in the peritoneal cavity is difficult to discern by ultrasound alone, especially if multiple injuries are present. A FAST exam has been reported to have a sensitivity as high as 83.3% and specificity of 99.7%.[17] With these relatively low false negative rates some institutions are observing patients with negative FAST and not proceeding with CT scanning. However, Chiu et al. in 1997 reported a 29% incidence of abdominal injury following negative initial FAST.[18]

They reported confounding clinical factors including contusion, pain, pelvic fracture, and lower rib fractures that were present in many of the false negative patients. Also, 27% of these negative FAST patients underwent laporotomy for undetected splenic injury. A follow-up FAST exam was not performed on these patients prior to surgery and given the time for further hemoperitoneal fluid development these scans may now have been positive. Serial ultrasound exams are now used in many trauma centers if the initial scan is negative. Patients with pelvic ring-type fractures should undergo CT scan even if a negative FAST has been performed due to the more frequent occult injuries in these patients.[19]

Contrast-enhanced sonography is beginning to show some promise in the detection of significant liver injury. Contrast-enhanced ultrasound uses intravenously injected micro bubbles containing gases other than air to produce the "contrasted" images. Though a study by Terrier et al. revealed that contrast-enhanced sonography missed 18% of solid organ injuries, it was able to detect vascular liver and spleen injuries.[20] Another study described the ability of this modality to detect active extravasation from solid organs.[21] With these advancements, patients may be subject to less risk from radiation or CT contrast. Also, this could be done at bedside instead of transporting a critical patient to a radiology suite. Overall, ultrasound is an excellent tool for the diagnosis of significant hepatic injury in the blunt trauma patient. However, in many instances further investigation may be appropriate.

FAST also has an expanding role in penetrating abdominal trauma with an institutional series sensitivity of 46% and specificity of 94% in penetrating injury.[22] Therefore concluding that FAST can be used to triage patients more directly to surgery. However the limitations of FAST in penetrating trauma are significant. In a patient with a possible tangential wound, the question is often if the peritoneum has been penetrated. A finding of fluid in Morison's pouch confirms penetration and will result in immediate surgical intervention. A negative fluid accumulation, however, does not definitively rule out penetration. These results have been validated.[23] Two interesting studies have demonstrated that fascial penetration can be verified by ultrasound examinaton.[24,25] Again, the sensitivity of this modality is low but the specificity is high. Ultrasound may be a good screening tool for finding fascial penetration and a positive result could alleviate the patient of a painful bedside wound exploration and also contribute to operative decision-making. Future study in this area may develop greater uses for ultrasound in select penetrating injuries.

## CT Scanning

The advent of CT scanning and advances in that technology have resulted in tremendous changes in the management of liver injury. Since the first use of CT to diagnose intra-abdominal injury in the early 1980s, CT has become a routine part of the management of trauma patients.[26] One recent study revealed that the specificity of the clinical examination with bedside radiologic investigations of plain x-ray and sonography in addition to laboratory values is not sufficient to preclude the blunt trauma patient from obtaining a CT scan for definitive diagnosis of injury.[27] The advent of the helical CT scan has improved resolution as well as increased the speed of a head to pelvis scan to less

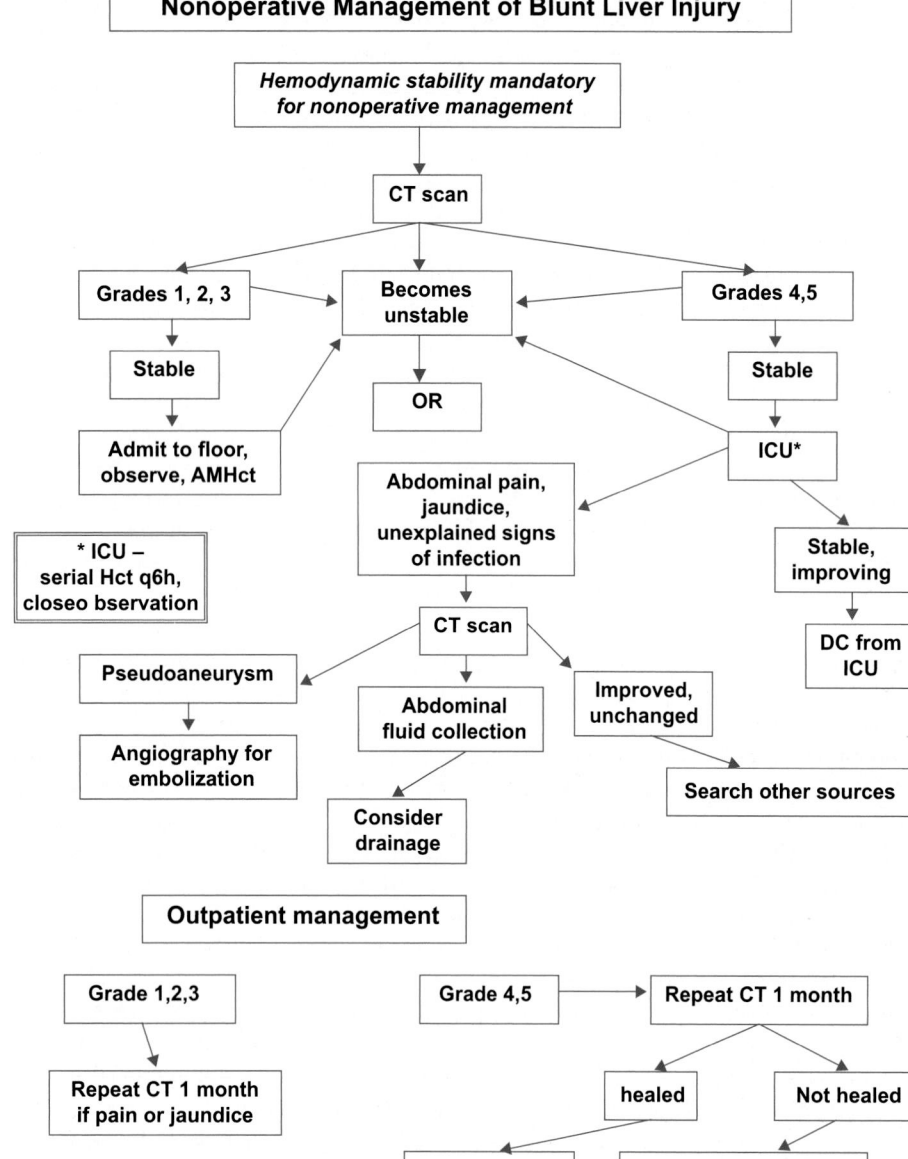

**Nonoperative Management of Blunt Liver Injury**

*Hemodynamic stability mandatory for nonoperative management*

CT scan

Grades 1, 2, 3 — Becomes unstable — Grades 4,5

Stable    OR    Stable

Admit to floor, observe, AMHct

Abdominal pain, jaundice, unexplained signs of infection

ICU*

Stable, improving

* ICU – serial Hct q6h, closeo bservation

CT scan

DC from ICU

Pseudoaneurysm

Abdominal fluid collection

Improved, unchanged

Angiography for embolization

Search other sources

Consider drainage

**Outpatient management**

Grade 1,2,3

Grade 4,5 → Repeat CT 1 month

Repeat CT 1 month if pain or jaundice

healed    Not healed

Ad lib activity    Light duty–repeat CT 1 month until healed

**FIGURE 32-4.** Algorithm for nonoperative management of blunt liver injury.

than ten minutes. Trauma surgeons now use CT scans for diagnosis and for management decisions in liver injuries. Being able to grade the extent of injury and to follow an existing injury can determine if nonoperative management is possible and successful (Fig. 32-4).

CT scanning is also being used in penetrating injury. Triple contrast CT in back and flank wounds has been shown to have good sensitivity; however, the sensitivity for diaphragmatic and small bowel injury is poor.[28] Therefore, a minor hepatic laceration can be evaluated and nonoperatively managed with CT guidance but continued frequent abdominal exam must also accompany this algorithm.

## Laparoscopy

Laparoscopy has been successfully used to diagnose peritoneal penetration of penetrating trauma, thus saving the patient from a nontherapeutic exploratory laparotomy.[29] Repair of hepatic injury

found at laparoscopy has also been reported.[30] In carefully selected patients, laparoscopy can be advantageous in the diagnosis and repair of hepatic injury.

## MANAGEMENT OF LIVER TRAUMA

Anatomic relationships are key to understanding the management of liver trauma. Blunt hepatic injury traverses almost exclusively along the segments of the liver. This most likely occurs due to the strength of the fibrous covering around the portal triad preventing injury from transecting these structures. However, the hepatic veins do not have a similar fibrous structure and therefore, having less resistance, are the primary structures injured in blunt trauma. Penetrating trauma, on the other hand, involves both venous and arterial injury with direct transection of any structure in the trajectory. Those anatomic principles are key to understanding the rationale for making decisions in the management of liver trauma.

## Hemodynamically Stable Patient with Blunt Injury (see Fig. 32-4)

Nonoperative treatment of the hemodynamically stable patient with blunt injury has become the standard of care in most trauma centers. Prior to the 1990s many centers based the decision to operate on grade of injury, hemoperitoneum, possible missed injury, or bile duct injury. Nonoperative therapy became more prevalent in the pediatric population and soon, by the mid 1980s and early 1990s, reports of nonoperatively managed adult liver trauma patients surfaced.[31-33] It was found that concomitant abdominal injuries were not being discovered at laparatomy and many nontherapeutic laparotomies were being performed. Most (up to 80%) liver injuries have stopped bleeding by the time of laparotomy.[34] Additionally, bile radical injuries did not result in abdominal infection and had sealed spontaneously or were able to be successfully managed without operative intervention. In 1995, Croce et al. published a prospective trial of nonoperative management of liver injury.[35] In this study patients with all grades and volumes of hemoperitoneum were evaluated against operative controls. They found that they were able to successfully manage 89% of hemodynamically stable patients without celiotomy. Most blunt liver injuries produce hepatic venous injuries that are low pressure (3–5 cm $H_2O$). Hence, hemorrhage usually stops once a clot forms on the area of disruption. Successful nonoperative therapy resulted in lower transfusion requirements, abdominal infections, and hospital lengths of stay.

Approximately 85% of patients with blunt liver trauma are stable. Once stability has been established, the patient must be carefully analyzed for the appropriateness of nonoperative care. The patient cannot exhibit signs of peritonitis and must continue to be hemodynamically stable without a significant transfusion requirement. The authors are generally comfortable in nonoperatively managing a stable patient with three to five units of blood in their abdomen. A contrast-enhanced helical CT scan should be obtained to evaluate injury grade, amount of hemoperitoneum, evidence for enteric injury, active extravasation of contrast, and presence of pseudoaneurysm (Fig. 32-5).

High-grade injury, large hemoperitoneum, contrast extravasation, and pseudoaneurysm are not contraindications for nonoperative management; however, these patients are at higher risk for

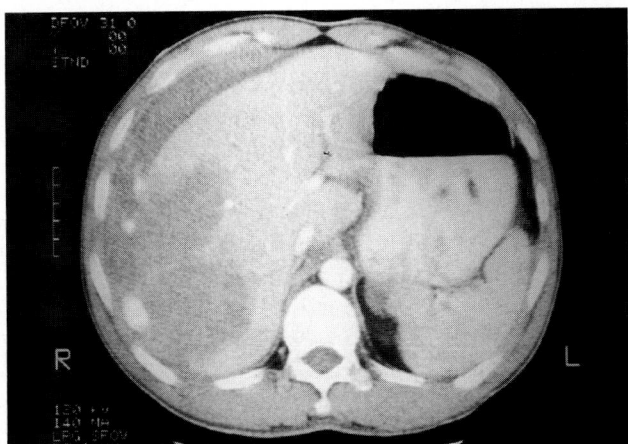

**FIGURE 32-5.** CT scan demonstrating a "contrast blush," indicative of active arterial bleeding in a patient with a grade IV blunt hepatic injury.

nonoperative failure and may need a multimodality approach to stabilize their nonoperative injury. Stable patients with high-grade injury may be observed. However, Malhotra et al. noted that 14% of grade IV and 22.6% of grade V injuries fail nonoperative management, which was substantially higher than the 3–7.5% failure rate of more minor injuries.[36] That same article reports large hemoperitoneum (blood around liver, pericolic gutter, and in the pelvis by CT) as a significant factor in failure of nonoperative management but that it could not predict which patients would ultimately fail nonoperative management. Richardson et al. speculated that many experienced trauma surgeons have taken stable but high-grade injury patients to the operating room only to find that "manipulation of venous injuries resulted in massive hemorrhage that resulted in the patient's death."[37] They concluded that non-surgical treatment has a "positive impact on survival."

A CT finding of contrast blush or extravasation has previously meant that patients were not candidates for nonoperative therapy. However, with the assistance of interventional radiology, some patients may be candidates for embolization and nonoperative treatment. Successful embolization of hepatic arterial injury in patients who are hemodynamically stable but with CT scans demonstrating intrahepatic contrast pooling was reported in 1996.[38] Choosing the appropriate patient for embolization can be a challenge. Fang et al. described 15 patients who exhibited contrast pooling or extravasation on CT scan.[39] They found that all patients that had extravasation and pooling of contrast material in the peritoneal cavity became hemodynamically unstable and required laparotomy. None of these six patients became unstable though only two patients received angiography. If angiography and embolization could have been utilized in the patients with hemoperitoneum and intraparenchymal contrast pooling, they may have had a better nonoperative outcome. Another interesting study looked at 11 patients with hepatic injury and CT evidence of contrast extravasation who were stable "only with continuous resuscitation."[40] These patients were evaluated by hepatic angiography and seven patients were successfully treated with hepatic embolization. The other four patients had no active extravasation seen by angiography and became hemodynamically stable not requiring surgery. These studies constitute a small fraction of hepatic trauma that relates to the guiding principle in liver injury management: Most blunt liver trauma results in venous injury. Therefore, arterial extravasation with blunt liver injury is uncommon. However, many centers are anecdotally noting excellent results with multimodality care and further prospective studies on this issue are currently ongoing.

## Complications of Nonoperative Blunt Hepatic Injury Management

Most patients with blunt nonoperative liver injuries heal without complication. Follow-up CT scans generally show resolution of severe injuries within four months and about 15% show complete resolution at hospital discharge.[35] However, complications can arise and management requires the surgeon to be prepared to deal with the possible adverse outcomes.[41] A retrospective multi-institutional study included 553 patients with grade III-V injury.[42] Of these patients, 12.6% developed hepatic complications that included bleeding, biliary problem, abdominal compartment syndrome, and infection. Significant coagulopathy and grade V injury were found to be predictors of complication. Therefore, with current nonoperative management strategies, complications must be dealt with appropriately.

Bile Leaks.    One of the more frequent complications is bile leakage. Bilomas or bile leak can occur in 3 to 20% of nonoperatively managed patients.[35] Evidence of bile leak by hepatobiliary hydroxy iminodiacetic acid (HIDA) scan does not mandate intervention. In fact, of the 14 patients found to have HIDA evidence of bile leak in a 1995 study, only one patient became symptomatic and required percutaneous drainage.[1] Abnormal liver function tests, abdominal distention, and intolerance to feeding may all indicate a bile leak. CT scan evaluation with drainage percutaneously usually remedies the problem completely. However, large bile leaks can develop. Laparotomy in these cases was often the procedure of choice in past years. The goal of laparotomy was to drain the peritoneal cavity, localize the leak with possible repair or ligation, and to drain the area. Currently, many authors have described management of bile peritonitis or large leaks not responsive to percutaneous drainage using percutaneous drainage techniques with endoscopic retrograde cholangiography (ERC). In some instances, actual stenting of the ductal injury can be accomplished. It has also been demonstrated that sphincterotomy can decrease the biliary pressure and allow healing of the bile leak.[43] Griffen et al. have reported success with a combined laparoscopic and ERC approach. They described patients with biliary ascites taken to operating room for laparoscopic bile drainage and placement of drain near injury site with postoperative ERC and bile duct stenting. They report no septic complications and healing of the substantial biliary leaks.[44] The authors have rarely experienced a persistent bile leak in the nonoperatively managed patient. Bile leaks or bilomas are drained percutaneously, sometimes for up to four to six weeks, and they nearly always resolved without ERC or other decompressive maneuvers.

Abscess.    Perihepatic abscesses have also been uncommonly encountered with nonoperative management. The patient may exhibit signs of sepsis, abnormal liver function tests, abdominal pain, or food intolerance. Abscesses, like biliary collections, can often be managed by CT-guided drainage catheters. However, if the patient fails to improve with drainage and antibiotics, wide surgical drainage should be performed. This may involve merely incision and adequate drainage of the cavity or it may involve extensive debridement of the hepatic parenchyma.

Hemorrhage.    Delayed hemorrhage after nonoperative management is a feared complication. Gates presented a review of the subject in 1994 and suggested an overall incidence of delayed hematoma rupture of 0–14%.[45] The 14% figure is well above current reports. He discussed 13 publications and determined that 69% of these delayed hemorrhage cases could have been successfully treated nonsurgically. Using the same criteria that was originally utilized to manage these patients nonoperatively, namely, hemodynamic stability without ongoing blood loss, patients with delayed hemorrhage can undergo hepatic angiographic embolization and observation with success. Therefore, it seems that delayed hemorrhage is actually a rare and manageable complication.

Devascularization.    Disruption of vascular inflow to a hepatic segment following trauma can lead to necrosis of that segment of liver. The consequences of necrosis may include elevation of liver transaminases, coagulopathy, bile leaks, abdominal pain, feeding intolerance, respiratory compromise, renal failure, and sepsis.[46] Many studies suggest that patients with significant necrosis undergo hepatic resection before complications arise.[47,48] Devascularization can be identified by CT scan. The devascularization can be differentiated from intraparenchymal hemorrhage when follow-up CT scans reveal segments of liver that remain devascularized or have air within the devascularized area.[46] Devascularization can also occur following angiographic embolization and the clinician must be aware of this possibility as well.

Hemobilia.    Hemobilia can occur after blunt hepatic injury. In 1871, Quincke described the triad of right upper quadrant pain, jaundice, and upper GI bleeding that indicated hemobilia. This triad may not be evident in the trauma patients with hemobilia.[49] In a 1994 study, three patients developed hemobilia with massive upper gastrointestinal hemorrhage following blunt hepatic injury.[50] The authors concluded that hepatic artery pseudoaneurysm with hemobilia is predisposed by bile leak and that angiographic embolization was appropriate for patients without sepsis and with small cavities. However, formal hepatic resection or drainage, after angiographic vascular control, may be necessary for septic patients or those with large cavities. Hemobilia is much less common with the prevalence of nonoperative management. With operative interventions of the past including large parenchymal suturing and vessel ligation, communications between vessels and bile ducts often occurred iatrogenically. Now that nonoperative care is practiced, we rarely see hemobilia.

Unusual Complications.    Large subcapsular hematomas have been described to elevate intraparenchymal pressures high enough to cause segmental portal hypertension and hepatofugal flow.[51] This "compartment syndrome of the liver" was described in a patient managed nonoperatively whose decreasing hematocrit and increasing liver function tests promoted angiographic examination revealing the hepatofugal flow in the right portal vein. After operative drainage of the tense hematoma the patient did well with reversal of flow and viability of the right lobe liver tissue. This type of compressive complication has also been described causing a Budd-Chiari syndrome when hematoma results in intrahepatic vena cava compression or hepatic venous obstruction.[52]

## Follow-Up CT Scanning of Blunt Hepatic Injury

Definitive data on the value of follow-up CT scanning of blunt hepatic injury is not available. Recent published reports suggest postobservation CT scans on those with more severe (grade III–V) injuries. Cuff et al. reported that of the 31 patients who received follow-up CT scans three to eight days postinjury, only three patients' scans affected future management.[53] Additionally, the three scans that affected management were obtained due to a change in clinical picture and not merely routine. A 1996 report similarly concluded that follow-up CT did not change decision making in those with grade I–III injury.[54] The author's institution concluded from their follow-up of 530 patients, including 89 grade IV or V, that follow-up CT scans are not indicated as part of the nonoperative management of blunt liver injuries.[55] Follow-up CT scans are indicated only for those patients who develop signs or symptoms suggestive of hepatic abnormality. By scanning only those with clinical suspicion there is a small inherent risk of missing unsuspected, possibly deleterious pseudoaneurysms that may result in delayed hemorrhage and require embolization. If a patient has had a follow-up CT that reveals significant healing, a postdischarge scan is not necessary. However, if significant healing has not occurred or if the patient had a grade IV or V injury, our practice is to obtain a postdischarge scan at four to six weeks after the injury.

## Resumption of Activity

No steadfast rules apply to activity resumption in patients with uncomplicated hospital courses following blunt hepatic injury. The practice of keeping a patient from activity for four months has been commonly employed. This practice most likely resulted from the observation that most hepatic injury seems to have resolved by CT in four months. A contrary approach to this practice can be based on some interesting animal studies. Dulchavsky et al. found in animal studies that hepatic wound burst strength at three weeks was as great or greater than uninjured hepatic parenchyma.[56] This is most likely a result of fibrosis throughout the injured parenchyma and Glisson's capsule. Therefore, activity can be resumed about one month after injury if a follow-up CT (in grade III–V) has shown significant healing.

## Hemodynamically Stable Patient with Penetrating Injury

### Nonoperative Management of Penetrating Injury.
Few penetrating injuries to the abdomen are managed nonoperatively (see Chap. 30). Peritoneal penetration has mandated operative exploration for many years. However, some trauma centers have adopted selective nonoperative management of knife stab wounds to the right upper quadrant. The work of Nance and Cohn in 1969 supported this nonoperative care in patients with stab sounds who were hemodynamically stable and had no evidence of peritoneal irritation.[57] Since then, reports of successful nonoperative management of gunshot wounds have been published. Renz and Feliciano prospectively treated 13 patients with right thoracoabdominal gunshot wounds (GSW) nonoperatively.[58] The rationale behind this management is that these wounds of small caliper weapons may have injury to diaphragm and liver only, sparing any intestinal injury. The authors stressed the importance of serial abdominal exams and contrast CT scanning in their successful nonoperative management of penetrating injury. Other center experience has concurred with this selective nonoperative management.[59] The criteria for nonoperative management includes those patients who are hemodynamically stable, have no peritoneal signs, do not require acute blood transfusion, and are not mentally impaired. These patients then undergo contrast-enhanced CT scan to rule out other abdominal injury or hepatic vascular injury. Serial abdominal exams as well as close hemodynamic monitoring are also implemented. Of 16 patients reported, one required embolization for active bleeding seen on CT and five required delayed operation for decreasing hematocrit or worsening abdominal exam. CT scanning of these patients is required for their management. Triple-contrast CT of 86 abdominal gunshot wounds, as reported by Shanmuganathan, had a sensitivity and specificity of 97% and 98%, respectively.[60] Velmahos and Demetrios do not use triple-contrast

at their center. They report a sensitivity and specificity of 90.5% and 96%, respectively in diagnosing intra-abdominal organ injuries requiring surgical intervention.[61]

All trauma surgeons do not accept nonoperative management of GSW. Missed or deliberate nonrepair of small diaphragmatic lesions may lead to long-term adverse sequelae, not only of diaphragmatic herniation but also to possible biliopleural fistula. Late intervention for other missed injury (e.g., duodenal injury) may also lead to substantial morbidity. Nonoperative management of RUQ penetrating trauma must be performed under the care of a center which not only has the capability of close continuous monitoring but also CT radiology accessibility and immediate operating room availability.

## Operative Management of Patients with Minor Liver Injury

The decision for operative intervention of incidental liver injury may develop due to laparotomy for penetrating injury, patient instability, or concomitant internal injury. The incision of choice is the midline incision in a trauma patient (see Chap. 30). Not only will the operating surgeon be able to gain access to the hepatic region but the entire peritoneal cavity will also be able to be inspected and manipulated. Upon opening the peritoneal cavity, attention should first be focused on stopping uncontrolled hemorrhage. Laparotomy pads should be used to clear the peritoneal cavity of clot. In minor liver injury, the bleeding from the liver can initially be managed with packing of the hemorrhagic area. Before dealing with a minor liver injury, the remainder of the peritoneal cavity should be inspected for injury, including bowel injury, solid visceral injury, Kocherization of the duodenum, and investigation into the lesser sac. Many minor liver injuries do not require operative fixation and nonbleeding wounds should not be probed or otherwise manipulated. Small wounds of the liver parenchyma with minimal bleeding may be able to be controlled with electrocautery or argon beam coagulation. Small to moderate bleeding cavities may first be inspected for any obvious bleeding vessels that can be ligated. Next, packing a tongue of omentum, with its vascular supply intact, into the wound and securing it into place, halts most moderate bleeding. Stone and Lamb first described this technique in 1975.[62] Wrapping a column of absorbable gelatin sponge with oxidized regenerated cellulose makes another beneficial device (Fig. 32-6). This is then inserted like a plug into deeper bleeding cavities. Omentum is often then brought up into the wound and secured to increase hemostasis. These maneuvers are very successful in the management of minor liver injury.

## Operative Management of Patients with Major Liver Injury

### Initial Management.
Patients with major hepatic trauma often present with hemodynamic instability and are therefore taken urgently to the operating room. As in minor injury the most optimal incision for expected major liver injury is the midline incision. Once the peritoneum is entered in these patients, a large amount of blood may be evacuated, which decreases the natural tamponade of a large hemoperitoneum. Adequate resuscitation is the key at this

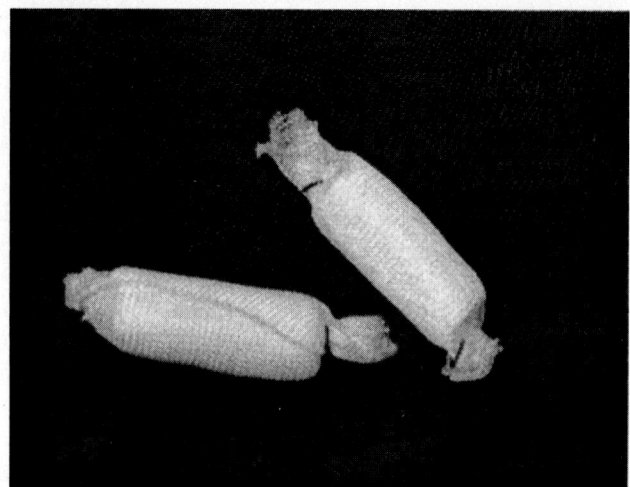

**FIGURE 32-6.** Hepatic injury plugs may be useful for tamponading deep parenchymal wounds.

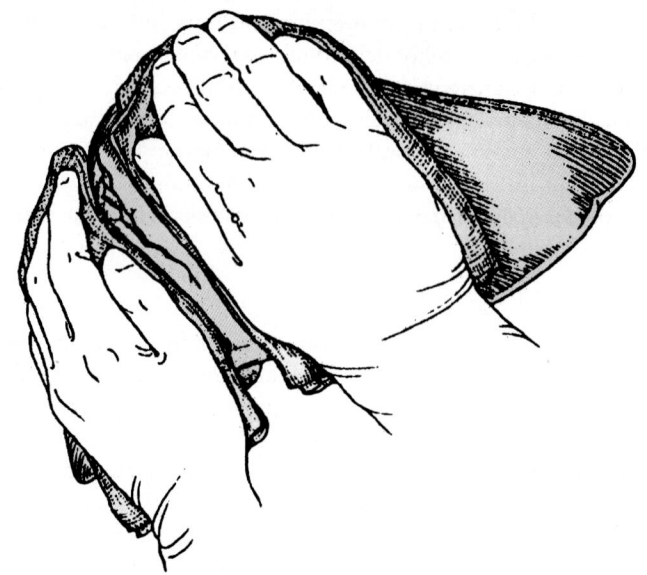

**FIGURE 32-7.** Manual compression of major liver injury.

time. Manual compression of obvious injury will decrease bleeding (Fig. 32-7). It is imperative that the anesthesia team is allowed to catch up with fluid loss prior to proceeding. Fluids should be warmed and coagulopathy corrected. Often these patients will require fresh frozen plasma, platelets, and cryoprecipitate (see Chap. 61). Factor VIIa has been suggested in severe coagulopathy and is undergoing clinical trials as to its effectiveness in traumatic situations. Once the patient has been adequately resuscitated a more thorough exam of the peritoneal cavity must be completed. If indeed the bleeding source is localized to the liver and bleeding continues after manual compression is released, then the portal triad should be identified and a Pringle maneuver performed (Fig. 32-8).

Much controversy has evolved around the normothermic ischemic time produced by the use of the Pringle maneuver. Many authors have advocated clamping for 20 minutes and then allowing reperfusion for five minutes.[63,64] This practice has not been proven to be beneficial in traumatic liver injury. Multiple studies have emerged indicating that longer portal triad occlusion can be accomplished with similar results. In one study describing the management of 1000 cases of hepatic trauma, the Pringle maneuver was utilized for between 30 to 60 minutes in many of the high-grade injuries without adverse sequella.[65] Pachter et al. managed 81 patients with the assistance of the Pringle maneuver for up to 75 minutes without any apparent morbidity from the procedure.[33] Therefore, it seems that longer normothermic ischemic time can be used without added morbidity in the severely injured liver.

The Pringle maneuver often does not control all bleeding. It will control the inflow bleeding from the hepatic artery and portal vein but not the retrograde bleeding from the vena cava and hepatic veins.

## Hemostatic Maneuvers for Severe Parenchymal Injury

Packing.   Perihepatic packing has become the most widely used and successful method for management of severe liver injury. Laparotomy pads are packed around the liver thus compressing the wound between the anterior chest wall, diaphragm, and retroperitoneum. This "damage control" laparotomy provides hemostasis while the patient is able to be hemodynamically optimized in the intensive care unit (ICU) as well as providing pressure on the

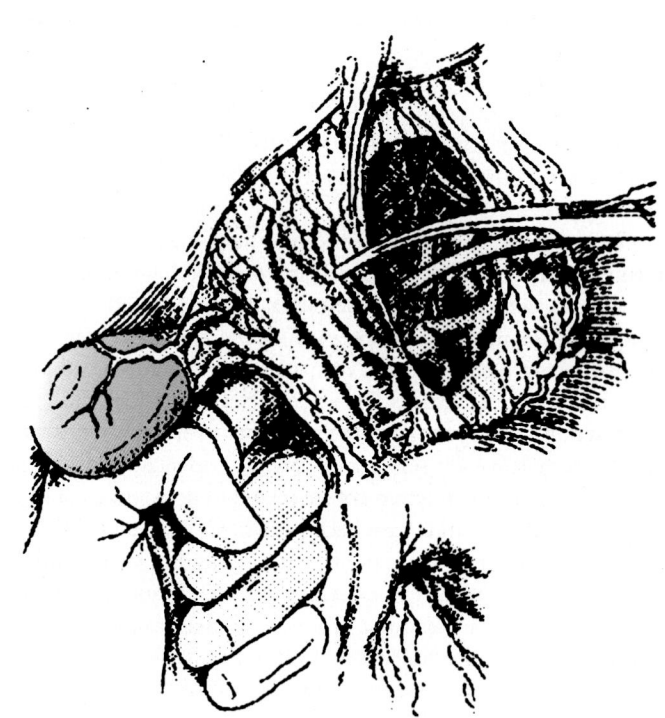

**FIGURE 32-8.** The Pringle maneuver controls arterial and portal vein hemorrhage from the liver. Any hemorrhage that continues must come from the hepatic veins.
*(Reproduced with permission from Burch JM, et al.: Injuries to the Liver, Biliary Tract, Spleen, and Diaphragm. In Wilmore DW, ed. ACSs Surgery: Principles & Practice. New York: WebMD Corporation, 2002.)*

wound to achieve hemostasis. Beal reported an 86% survival rate in 35 patients in whom perihepatic packing was used.[66] In order to provide the tamponade necessary for effective packing, the surgeon must mobilize the liver by taking down the right and left triangular, coronary, and falciform ligaments. If, however, there is obvious hematoma in a ligament this area should not be entered. Hematoma in the ligament may indicate a vena caval or hepatic vein injury and mobilization may lead to rapid exsanguination.

The decision to pack must be made early in the exploration, in order to provide the best chances for patient survival.[67] Indeed, early packing is associated with the increased survival of liver trauma patients. Richardson et al. found that the death rate associated with packing significantly decreased after 1989 and was linked to less packing time, as was demonstrated by a decrease in the average blood loss despite the equal severity of injury.[37] One of the difficulties with packing comes with removal. Often, the bare liver area that has become hemostatic is now adherent to the packs. Pulling off the packs can then cause further bleeding. Different solutions to this problem have been described from wetting the gauze with saline upon removal to a more innovative technique described by Feliciano and Pachter.[68] They suggest placing a nonadherent plastic drape directly on top of the hepatic surface and then placing the laparotomy pads above this plastic interface. An important issue regarding abdominal packing is abdominal closure. These patients will undoubtedly require significant resuscitation. Abdominal compartment syndrome diagnosed with elevated bladder pressure (above 25 mm Hg), increasing peak airway pressures, decreased urine output, and abdominal distention can be a life-threatening consequence of this resuscitation (see Chap. 41). Abdominal compartment syndrome can be avoided in these patients by leaving the fascia and skin edges open and placing a temporary closure device over the open abdomen.

Packing is often useful in blunt, venous injury but cannot be expected to provide hemostasis in major arterial injury. Major arterial injury is often seen with penetrating trauma and therefore packing in penetrating bleeding may not be successful.

The timing of packing removal continues to be the subject of debate. Correction of coagulopathy, acidosis, and hypothermia can almost always be accomplished within 24 to 48 hours of packing. Intra-abdominal sepsis is a risk of prolonged packing. Krige et al. found that packs that remained for more than three days had an 83% incidence of developing perihepatic sepsis whereas those left less than three days had a 27% chance of sepsis.[69] A 1986 report found a 10.2% sepsis rate for patients who had packs removed within 24 to 48 hours along with complete clot evacuation and debridement of devitalized tissue.[70] Caruso and associates advocate the removal of packs at 36 to 72 hours because they have experienced a higher rate of repacking for recurrent hemorrhage in the group of patients who had their packs removed earlier.[67] Overall, it seems that pack removal prior to 72 hours, effective residual peritoneal clot evacuation, and excision of devitalized tissue will provide the optimal circumstance for minimizing perihepatic sepsis.

Direct Suture. Grade III and IV liver lacerations often do not respond to the more topical procedures listed for minor injury control. One of the oldest reported techniques to control deep parenchymal bleeding is direct suturing of the tissue with large, blunt-tipped 0-chromic suture. Utilizing a large blunt needle with 0 suture prevents the suture from tearing through Glisson's capsule when tying. The stitches can be continuous or if a deeper laceration is encountered, a mattress configuration is preferred. This technique is most appropriate for lacerations less than 3 cm in depth. It is best to avoid the direct suture approach as blind passage of these large blunt needles may injure bile ducts and vascular structures thereby leading to possible intrahepatic hematomas or hemobilia.

Finger Fracture. More severe parenchymal laceration may involve larger branches of the hepatic artery or portal system and will not respond to the attempted tamponade with large parenchymal suturing. In these cases some clinicians prefer the technique of finger fracture (Fig. 32-9).[33] The utilization of this technique involves careful extension of the laceration using finger fracture until bleeding vessels can be identified and then controlled with clips, ligation or direct repair. This technique can lead to extensive additional parenchymal bleeding while searching for the initially damaged vasculature.

Omental Packing. Omental packing has been used successfully on its own as well as in conjunction with finger fracturing. Omental packing fills the potential dead space with viable tissue that also is a source of macrophage activity. Stone's original work was reinforced by Fabian and Stone when they managed to stop the venous hemorrhage of severe parenchymal laceration in 95% of patients with an 8% mortality.[62,71] The technical aspects of this process include first mobilizing the greater omentum from the transverse mesocolon in the avascular plain. Next, the omentum is mobilized from the greater curvature preserving the usually right gastroepiploic vascular pedicle (Fig. 32-10). The tongue of omentum is then placed into the injury defect. The ability to achieve hemorrhage cessation with this method reiterates that most hepatic bleeding is venous. Tamponade with viable omental packing is superior to most of the direct techniques of hemorrhage control.

Penetrating Tract. Penetrating tracts through the hepatic tissue provide another challenge for the surgeon. Often these are of great depth and length, therefore making visualization of the entire injury impossible. Management of these injuries has included the packing of omentum into the tract for hemostasis. Also, devices such as the rolled cellulose-covered gelatin sponge can be inserted into the tract for hemostasis. Pogetti et al. advocate the use of balloon tamponade of the tract.[72] A Penrose drain is placed over a hollow, endperforated tube and tied on both ends. The balloon is then placed into the tract and inflated with a contrast agent (Fig. 32-11). If successful tamponade has been achieved the balloon is left in the abdomen and removed 24–48 hours later at a second laparotomy. A similar technique using a Foley balloon has been described.[73] A size-16 Foley is inserted into the tract and inflated. If there is continued active bleeding, the catheter is moved back or forward and inflated again. If bleeding continues through the catheter but not out of tract, the balloon is proximal to the bleeder and needs to be repositioned deeper. If the bleeding continues from the tract orifice, then the balloon must be repositioned further out of the tract. Once the catheter is positioned, drains are placed in the area. The drains and catheter are brought out through the skin. The Foley can be removed after deflation produces no further signs of bleeding in three to four days or at the time of the next planned reexploration.

Deep, small diameter penetrating injury may continue to bleed from the depths of the wound. In these instances finger fracture of a significant liver segment may be necessary. Another alternative, considering institutional availability may be angioembolization for these lesions.

Fibrin Sealants. Fibrin sealants have been a topic of much interest. Fibrin glue combines fibrinogen with thrombin, calcium chloride, and aprotinin to form a stable clot.[74] However, difficulties have been found with the use of fibrin glue. Time required to prepare the

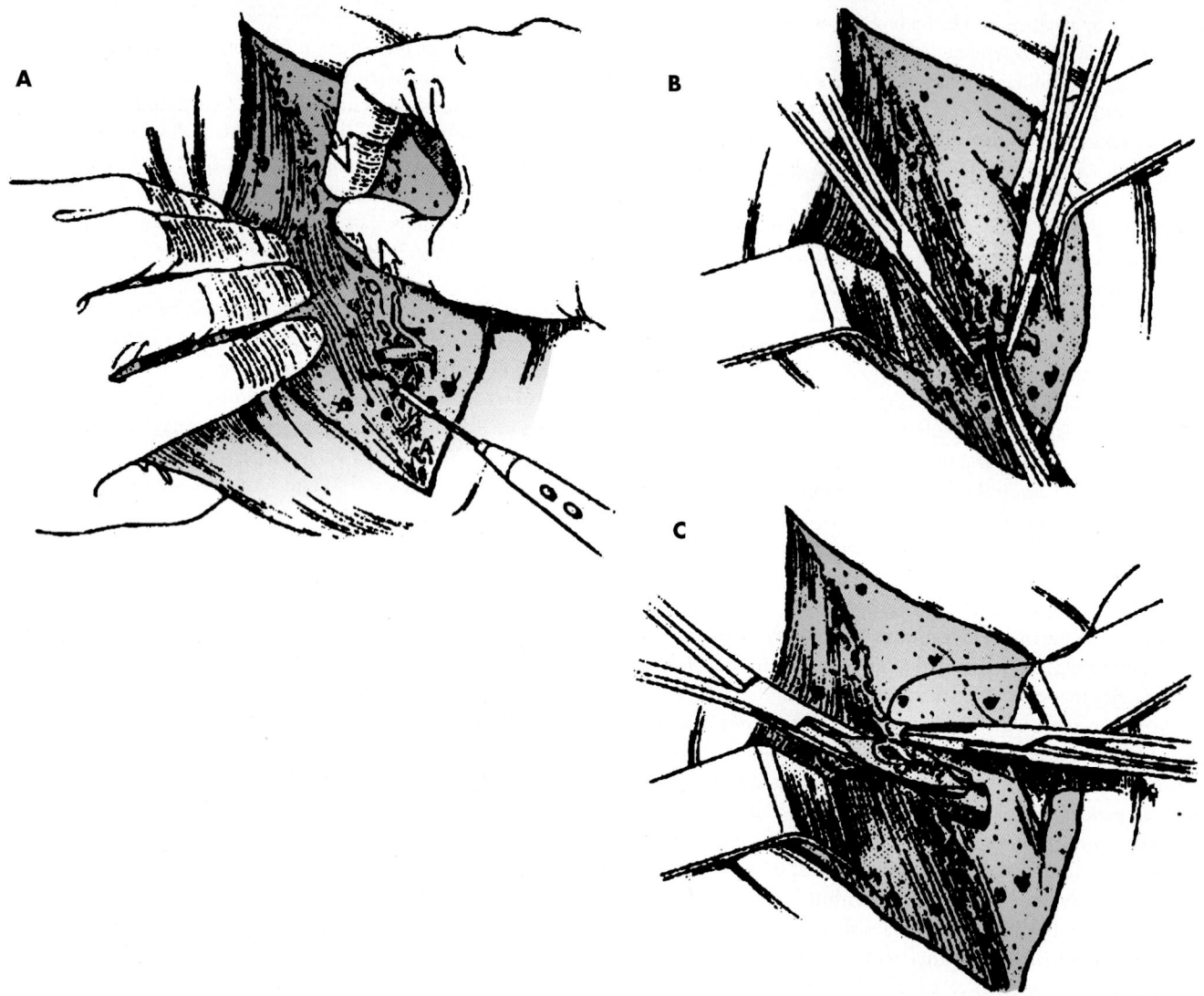

**FIGURE 32-9.** Hepatotomy with selective ligation is an important technique for controlling hemorrhage from deep (usually penetrating) lacerations. This technique includes finger fracture to extend the length and depth of the wound (**A**), division of vessels or ducts encountered (**B**), and repair of any injuries to major veins (**C**).
*(Reproduced with permission from Burch JM, et al.: Injuries to the Liver, Biliary Tract, Spleen, and Diaphragm. In Wilmore DW, ed. ACSs Surgery: Principles & Practice. New York: WebMD Corporation, 2002.)*

glue, inability of the glue to stick to a bleeding surface and hypotension with injection have lead to minimal human use of the preparation. However, swine models using a purified glue thought to cause less hypotension, have shown a decrease in blood loss in complex injury.[75] Other animal studies have used fibrin sealant dressings with good result.[76] This material is made from fibrinogen and thrombin dried on an absorbable mesh. It was found to improve hemorrhage control of grade V liver injury in swine. Human study with these materials is sparse. Fibrin materials may have a future in some aspects of the management of parenchymal bleeding. There is also the possibility of using fibrin products for the more minor diffuse bleeding that occurs after major hemorrhage control has been obtained in trauma patients who are cold and coagulopathic. Promising fibrin sealants are currently undergoing clinical trial.

Other Hemostatic Devices.   The Modified Rapid Deployment Hemostat has been studied in trauma patients with severe liver injury. This device is made of a 1cm layer of acetylated poly-*N*-acetyl glucosamine bonded to a 4 × 4 inch gauze pad. Though the exact mechanism is not yet known, the device was used in nine blunt hepatic injured patients who were acidotic, coagulopathic, and hemodynamically unstable. After applying the bandage in direct contact with the bleeding vessel and applying direct pressure the bleeding ceased or subsided greatly.[77]

The Liver Bag has also been reported. The falciform, coronary, and triangular ligaments are divided in order to mobilize the liver. A radiographic cassette bag is used to completely enclose the liver within the bag. Umbilical tape was then used to snitch the opening of the bag around the porta hepatis. The liver bleeding is thus contained and tamponaded. The patient then returned three days later for successful removal.[78]

These and many other devices are currently being developed to help with the management of severe liver trauma.

Resection.   Anatomic resections for severe hepatic trauma were often performed in the late 1960s and early 1970s. However, the

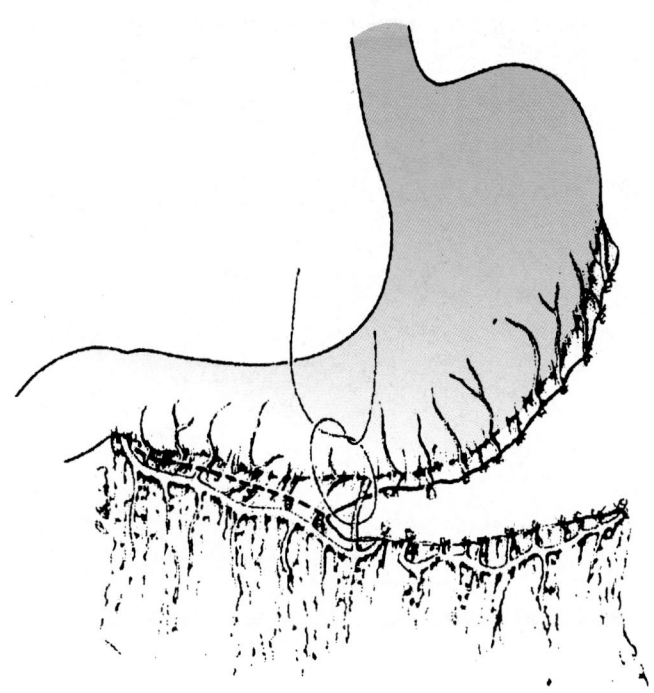

**FIGURE 32-10.** Omental mobilization employed for liver packing.

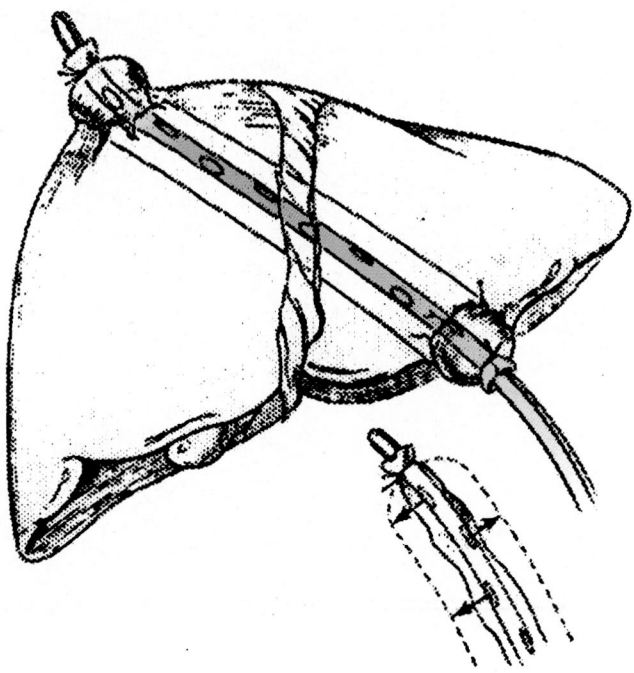

**FIGURE 32-11.** A hand-made balloon from a Robinson catheter and a Penrose drain may effectively control hemorrhage from a transhepatic penetrating wound.[72]
*(Reproduced with permission from Burch JM, et al.: Injuries to the Liver, Biliary Tract, Spleen, and Diaphragm. In Wilmore DW, ed. ACSs Surgery: Principles & Practice. New York: WebMD Corporation, 2002.)*

80% survival reported by McClelland and Shires has not been experienced in other reports.[79] In fact, most series surmise that when anatomic resection is performed for massive bleeding, the mortality is prohibitively high. It has been stated that major lobar resection may be necessary in 10% of liver injury but more than half of these have a mortal wound.[66] Another report from Australia and Hong Kong gave the results of resection in 37 patients with major liver injury.[80] This article suggests that better resectional results occur when trained hepatobiliary surgeons perform the resection. However, the results are less than compelling when actual injury grade, the low number of resections during first laparotomy, and morbidity are taken into account. Better results have been reported by Peitzman et al.[81] They report on 47 patients who underwent hepatic resection during their initial operation with a morbidity of 25% and a mortality of 17.8%. Successful outcome by crushing the injured liver segment between two aortic clamps has also been reported.[82] The hemostatic clamps are left in place and 36 hours later the patient is brought back to the operating room where the now necrotic segment is easily removed and the liver edge oversewn. Anatomic resection may have a place in a large devitalized liver portion when the injury has basically performed the resection already or if the injury is focused to a single anatomic lobe. Otherwise, lobar resection is not commonly or successfully being performed in the acute hemodynamically unstable patient.

Hepatic Artery Ligation. Hepatic arterial ligation can be a useful maneuver either in the operating room or with the aid of angiography. Complete selective hepatic artery ligation is used in only about 1% of patients with severe hepatic trauma.[37] If a patient has a noticeable decrease in bleeding after the Pringle maneuver has been performed, hepatic artery ligation should be considered. Such instances occur in a scenario with a knife wound or small caliper missle wound with continued deep parenchymal bleeding. When the portal vein remains patent, the chance for severe hepatic dysfunction after hepatic artery ligation is minimal.[83] However, with patients who have undergone significant hypoperfusion due to traumatic shock, hepatic artery ligation may produce enough further ischemia to produce necrosis or sepsis.[84] A recent report of hepatic failure following hepatic artery embolization resulted in the patient receiving an urgent liver transplant.[85]

Currently, most centers are advocating a multimodality approach to hepatic arterial bleeding. The role of interventional radiology has gained significant importance in the role of bleeding control after packing. Sclafani et al. in 1984 reported on the successful selective arterial embolization of severely injured liver parenchyma after packing.[86] Angiography has become an important step in the management algorithm for severe liver injury. One report stated that an approach for high-grade liver injury includes "immediate surgery for control of life-threatening hemorrhage, the use of complex surgical techniques to address these injuries, the institution of early hepatic packing and immediate postoperative hepatic angiography and angioembolization." In this report of 22 patients that had sustained grade IV and V injury, 15 underwent angiographic embolization (10 had been previously packed). All of these procedures were successful in arresting the continued bleeding.[87] Therefore, it can not be overemphasized that the care for severe hepatic parenchymal injury requires not only operative skill, but also the judgment to determine the time for packing and collaboration with interventional radiology specialists (Fig. 32-12).

Hepatic Transplantation. Hepatic transplantation has been successfully reported. This is assuredly a drastic approach to traumatic

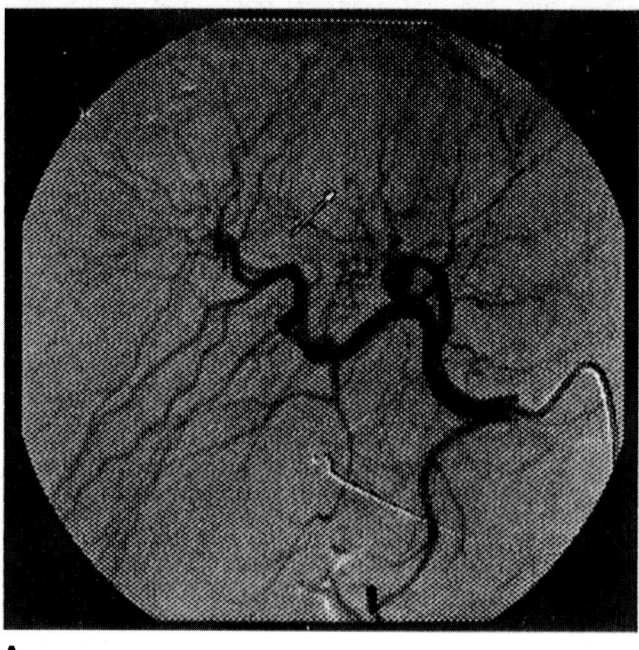
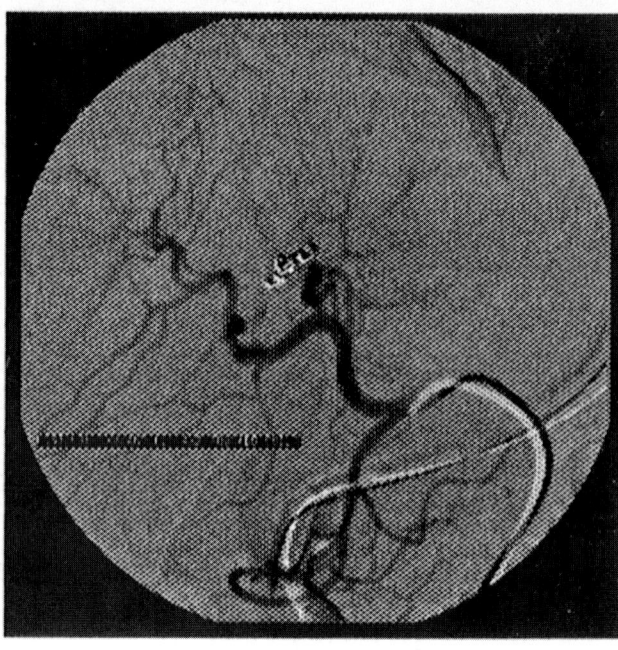

**FIGURE 32-12.** **(A)** Hepatic pseudoaneurysm. **(B)** Coiled hepatic pseudoaneurysm.

injury and is an alternative for very few patients. The patient must have an overall excellent chance of survival with minimal concomitant injury especially other intra-abdominal or neurologic injury. Also, if a trauma patient requires a transplant it must be completed immediately, waiting for a donor organ to arrive is not an option. A case from Philadelphia describes a young patient, initially hemodynamically stable who became unstable and at laparotomy was found to have avulsed her portal vein and proper hepatic artery.[88] The portal vein was reconstructed with vein graft, however, it thrombosed. They were able to correct her coagulation defect and obtain a donor liver within eight hours, whereby she underwent successful transplantation. This case presents the requirements for possible transplantation as the patient had a single liver injury, no neurologic compromise, hemodynamic stability, corrected coagulopathy, and the ability to obtain a donor organ within 36 hours of an anhepatic state.

## Retrohepatic Vena Cava/Hepatic Vein Injury

Severe hepatic trauma can injure the vena cava anywhere along its extraparenchymal course. Also, damage to the hepatic veins can be extra- or intraparenchymal. Life-threatening bleeding from these injuries occurs if the supporting structures, mainly the suspensory ligaments, diaphragm, or liver parenchyma are disrupted. Therefore, the exposure of a major venous injury may release the tamponade and result in free bleeding and exsanguination. As Buckman et al. outlined, there are three main strategies described to deal with these mortal injuries. The first is to directly repair the venous injury with or without vascular isolation. The second is with a lobar resection. The third is by using a strategy of tamponade and containment of the venous bleeding.[89]

## Direct Venous Repair

Direct venous repair without shunting has been advocated by Pachter and Feliciano. They describe occlusion of the portal triad

for a significant time, mobilization of the liver with medial rotation, and efficient finger fracture to the site of injury.[90] With these methods he reported a 43% (6/14) survival. Similar results of a 50% survival have been published by Chen and coworkers.[91]

Various shunting maneuvers have been attempted for complete vascular control of the liver. The atriocaval shunt was first introduced by Schrock et al. in 1968[92] (Fig. 32-13). The goal is to shunt the blood from the infrahepatic vena cava, bypassing the retrohepatic cava, and directing flow into the atria. This, along with the Pringle maneuver, is theoretically used to create a bloodless field. Unfortunately, of the approximately 200 cases published using atriocaval shunting, only at best 10–30% survive their injury.[37] The caveats of this maneuver include the need to plan for the procedure essentially before proceeding with the operation. All the equipment must be ready and a thorocoabdominal exposure is necessary. Shunting a patient cannot be successfully accomplished if the patient has already had major blood loss, become coagulopathic, and has inadequate operative incisional exposure. Shunting, in general, is not often used at present. The patients who require shunting often have catastrophic injury in which time is of the essence. Therefore, more often these patients are packed urgently and brought to angiography for embolization for any hope of true survival.

Other shunting procedures have been utilized as well. Pilcher et al., in 1977, reported on a balloon shunt introduced through the saphenofemoral junction.[93] This occlusive method has had some anecdotal success and avoids emergent thoracotomy without destruction of the surrounding ligamentous tamponade.[94] The multi-institutional trial results in 1988 however did not show any survival benefit of the balloon shunt versus the atriocaval shunt.[95] Venovenous bypass has been used in some institutions as well.[96] Again this method requires considerable planning but obviates the hemodynamic instability of caval occlusion and ligamentous disruption. Direct clamping techniques have also been used in a small number of patients. Carrillo et al. had success with vascular clamps placed upon hepatic vein injured ends, filling the laceration with

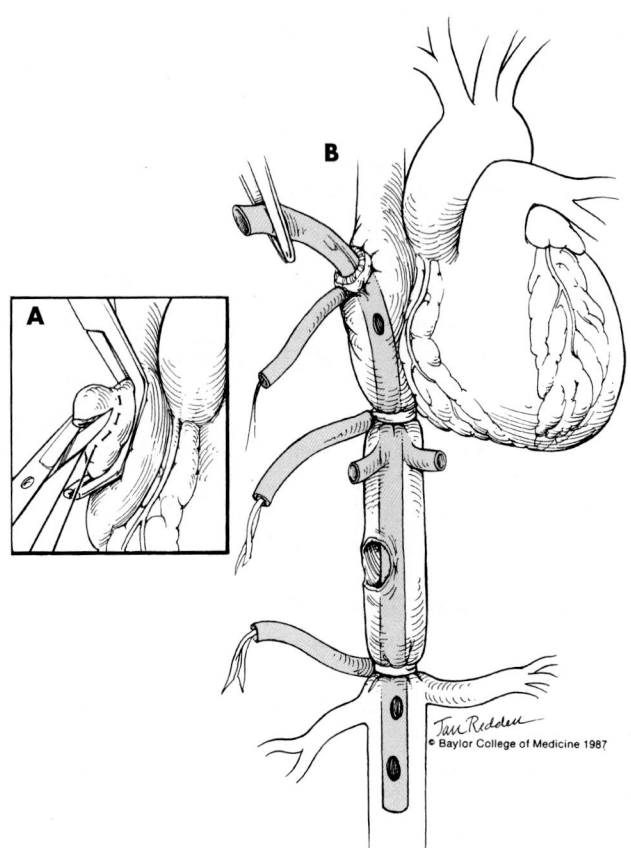

**FIGURE 32–13.** **(A)** A hole is cut in the right atrial appendage above a 2-0 silk purse-string suture. A Satinsky clamp maintains vascular control. **(B)** Final position of No. 36 chest tube acting as an atriocaval shunt. Note the extra hole cut in the chest tube at the level of the right atrium. All holes in the chest tube are outside the umbilical tapes, thereby forcing blood from the lower half of the body and the kidneys through the shunt. *(Reproduced with permission from Feliciano DV, Pachter HL: Hepatic trauma revisited. Curr Probl Surg 26:499, 1989.)*

viable omentum, and packing with planned reoperation.[97] In general, direct approaches to vein repair are difficult and can often result in a profuse uncontrolled bleeding situation, especially since even the most veteran surgeon has little experience in these uncommon injuries.

## Anatomic Resection

As mentioned earlier, anatomic resection has resulted in a high mortality when carried out for traumatic bleeding. In certain circumstances when the dissection has already been done by the injury itself, resection for debridement may be indicated. However, current data does not promote anatomic resection for major venous injury.

## Vena Cava Stenting

Endoluminal stent-grafts are now available for many uses. Reports of using the fenestrated graft in blunt trauma have been reported.[98] The graft used by Watarida was homemade and stayed patent at the 16-month follow-up. More successful reports of commercially available fenestrated grafts used in retrohepatic vena caval injuries are surfacing. These grafts are being placed both after "damage control" laparotomy and also prior to laparotomy when the lesion is

seen on CT.[99,100] Though these grafting procedures are not yet commonplace a significant future for their use is apparent.

## Tamponade with Containment

With the high mortality of direct venous repair and anatomic resection evident, the focus on severe vascular injury management has shifted to methods of tamponading and containing venous injury in addition to embolization of arterial bleeding. Many of the methods utilized for severe parenchymal injury are also effective for large venous injury. In Memphis, the mortality of patients with juxtahepatic venous injuries who were treated with omental packing was a low 20.5%.[101] Another article emphasizing packing included 14 patients with hepatic vein injury, six patients with retrohepatic vena caval injury with an overall mortality of only 14%.[66] Cue et al. depict four patients with retrohepatic vena cava, hepatic vein injury, or both who underwent initial packing and survived.[102] Although packing and resuscitation can lead to abdominal compartment syndrome if care to keep the abdomen open is not addressed, there are no major venous thrombosis cited in the literature when packing maneuvers are used.

At this time it seems that the most successful method of managing severe retrohepatic or hepatic venous injury is by using tamponade and containment. Direct repair of damaged vessels continues to have a very high morbidity even in the most experienced hands. Resection also has shown itself to be a morbid alternative with the survival data primarily being in the hands of experienced hepatobiliary surgeons in somewhat stable patients. Overall, the best approach to severe liver injury includes (a) expedient recognition and operative intervention of unstable hemorrhaging patients, (b) mobilization of the liver ligaments not directly involved with hematoma to better visualize the injury, (c) placement of a viable omental tongue into parenchymal defects, (d) rapid determination of the need for gauze packing when direct surgical maneuvers fail, and (e) angiographic embolization of hepatic arterial injured branches when ongoing hemorrhage or CT blush is seen.

## Drains

Hepatic drains began to be placed shortly after World War II when it was noted that there seemed to be an increase in the incidence of sepsis when collections of bile and blood developed in the perihepatic region after liver trauma. However, in 1978, Fischer et al. found evidence that the Penrose drains most commonly used to drain these collections actually increased the rate of infection in grade I and II liver injury.[103] Higher-grade injury and wounds with obvious bile leakage have been routinely drained.

The use of closed-suction drains has clearly been proven to be superior over Penrose drain use in a number of publications. A 1991 study reported a perihepatic abscess rate of 6.7% with no drain, 3.5% with closed suction, and 13% with penrose drainage.[101] A study from Charity Hospital found an abscess rate of 1.8% in those with no drainage, 0% abscess rate in those with closed suction, and 8.3% abscess rate in those with open drains.[104] Examination of these figures, however, indicates no significant difference in abscess rate between the no drainage group versus the closed-suction cohort. Indeed, in a review of 161 significant liver injuries, 78 patients underwent closed-suction drainage and 83 were left without a drain.[105] The injury grade, blood loss, shock severity, and associated injuries were similar in the two groups. There was no difference in mortality, abscess formation, or biliary fistula between the two groups. Thereby, the study concluded that drainage should be done only in those injuries with obvious bile leaks noted at the time of laparotomy. This viewpoint is reiterated in a 1988 article which states that the presence of hypotension and multiple transfusions are more predictive of abscess formation than drain placement.[104] With the current use of interventional radiology techniques, routine drainage has become less of an issue. Most centers will treat patients expectantly and only place drains in patients with obvious bile leaks. If indeed a collection or abscess develops, many can be dealt with by percutaneous tube placement under radiologic guidance.

## Complications of Operative Management

### Bleeding.
Postoperative hemorrhage is not a common occurrence. Most series quote a 2–7% hemorrhagic complication rate.[68,95] Falling serial hematocrits, increasing abdominal distention, and episodes of hypotension or tachycardia mark continued bleeding. The inability to operatively control the bleeding is often confounded by hypothermia and coagulopathy. In the past these patients were urgently returned to the operating room after correction of their coagulopathy and rewarming. Currently, after resuscitation these patients are often able to be managed with angiographic localization of the bleeding source and embolization. Of course, unstable patients do need operative intervention and may in fact need reexploration of previously packed areas in order to specifically identify the bleeding source. The areas of bleeding must then be addressed by utilizing the previously discussed maneuvers of severe injury control.

### Hemobilia.
Immediate attention should be given to a patient who develops a significant upper gastrointestinal bleed following liver repair. Many times this is the only symptom that can point to the development of hemobilia. The often mentioned signs and symptoms of hemobilia — jaundice, right upper quadrant pain, and falling hematocrit — are common occurrences in most patients after severe liver injury and therefore make the diagnosis of hemobilia difficult. The incidence of hemobilia ranges anywhere from 0.3% to 1.2%.[50,106] The presentation may be days to weeks postinjury. Upper endoscopy and bleeding scans are generally unable to locate the source of bleeding. Angiography will frequently delineate a pseudoaneurysm and accomplish embolization of the damaged vessel.[107,108] Operative debridement and drainage may be necessary is a large cavity has formed or sepsis is apparent.[50]

### Bilhemia.
Biliovenous fistulas have also been described by Clemens and Wittrin in the literature but are quite rare.[109] This entity occurs as the bilious venous blood dissolves in the bloodstream and is carried directly to the right heart. Therefore, one sees a patient with a drastically rising bilirubin with relatively normal liver function tests. Glaser et al. discussed three cases of bilhemia, which were identified by endoscopic retrograde cholangiography (ERC).[110] The management of these cases involved a left hemihepatectomy in the first, spontaneous resolution in one, and controlled biliary fistula in the last. Another method of control included placement of a constant suction T-tube with subsequent resolution.[111] Although spontaneous resolution has occurred, this entity can have a high mortality if left unaddressed.

### Biliary Fistulae.
Biliary fistulae are one of the complications that a surgeon is likely to encounter. Biliary fistula can account for up to 22.5% of traumatic liver management complications.[87] Overall biliary fistulae seem to occur in about 4 to 6% of patients who undergo operative management of severe liver injury.[112,113] Some bile duct injuries are obvious intraoperatively with significant bile staining and a visible disrupted bile duct. Many persistent fistulae may, however, manifest from smaller radicals, which retract into the liver parenchyma and are not visualized. Operative drain placement is advocated in liver injury with obvious bile staining. It is common for liver injuries to have transient early postoperative serosanguinous, bilious drainage. Bilious drainage of at least 50mL per day that continues after two weeks is considered a biliary fistula.[95] Also, persistent earlier drainage of over 300 to 400mL of bile a day should be cause for further evaluation.

The diagnosis of a biliary injury can be done by a fistulogram if a drain is in place, HIDA scan (though not anatomically exact), or ERC. Major left or right bile duct injury often requires further intervention for closure. In the past the surgical approach was recommended with resection or Roux-en-Y procedures predominating. More recently, nonoperative approaches have proven successful. Percutaneous stenting of injuries and drainage of biloma collections has been utilized.[114] Also, many reports are surfacing of management using ERC sphincterotomy with stenting and percutaneous drainage of biloma. A recent study described five patients with intrahepatic bile duct injuries.[115] The injuries included left main hepatic duct, right second-order bile duct, and more peripheral lesions. All were successfully managed nonoperatively. Repeat ERC of these patients led them to conclude that "therapeutic ERC and percutaneous interventional radiology can both treat the complication of the ductal injury and allow healing of the ductal disruption." Confirmation of healing of major ductal injury after ERC stenting and percutaneous drainage has been documented.[87] For bile fistulae that do not involve a main bile duct, drainage alone will provide adequate treatment and other maneuvers are rarely necessary.

### Other Fistulae Problems.
Thoracobiliary fistulae are also encountered with traumatic liver injury. Though it is a rare complication, identification and management can prevent morbidity of progression to bronchobiliary fistula. Many of these injuries occur after thorocoabdominal penetrating injury. Often the patient does well initially with resolution of hemothorax, no evidence of jaundice, and stabilization of liver injury only to become significantly tachypneic a week or more later. One report described the treatment of a thoracobiliary fistula with chest tube drainage and ERC.[116] One patient returning for routine follow-up was operatively managed with thoracic and abdominal drains and diagnosed from an abnormal chest x-ray and subsequent CT.[117] Rothberg et al. promote operative intervention in order to evaluate for significant diaphragmatic injury, liver necrosis, or lung necrosis with possible bronchial involvement.

Penetrating injury can potentially provide a means for many severe fistula communications. Pleurocaval fistula may result from thorocoabdominal injury. This fistula may be the source of life-threatening air embolism.[118] Arterioportal fistula are associated with initial hemorrhage and subsequent portal hypertension.[119] One case report described a gunshot wound which formed a left hepatic artery to portal vein fistula. This fistula was able to be successfully managed by interventional radiology embolization.

## Traumatic Portal Triad/Extrahepatic Biliary Tract Injury

**Overview.** Extrahepatic biliary and portal triad injuries make up only about 0.07–0.21% of all trauma admissions at Level I trauma centers.[120,121] Though these injuries are rare, their evaluation and management prove difficult. Technical problems including continued hemorrhage, adjacent organ injury, and small duct size can prove insurmountable. A timely diagnosis and treatment method may prove to be the survival difference in patients with these severe injuries. In a Seattle paper, 38% were a result of blunt mechanisms, similar to the 31% with blunt mechanism quoted in a 1995 multi-institutional trial.[120,121] Injury to this area carries an overall 50% mortality, with vascular injury (portal vein or hepatic artery) being the most morbid. When examining those with both portal vein and hepatic artery injury the mortality is 99%. It is evident that the management of these injuries is a significant challenge. Most street weapons are now high caliber and medium to high velocity. These weapons usually do not result in simple, single injury. Instead, multiple injuries to the liver, porta, vena cava, and surrounding viscera most often occur. Not only are these portal triad injuries difficult to manage, but the specific injury cannot be identified preoperatively and, therefore, intraoperative decision-making is crucial.

### Injury Types and Diagnostics

**Gallbladder.** Gallbladder injury accounts for up to 66% of extrahepatic biliary tract injury.[120] Injury can be from either blunt or penetrating mechanisms. Blunt injury often involves avulsion, either partial or complete, contusion, or perforation. Penetrating injury has been seen involving everything from the body of the gallbladder down to the cystic duct. A review from 1995 warned that 100% of 22 cases of blunt gallbladder injuries were associated with other intraabdominal trauma; however, this is not uniformly reported and isolated gallbladder injury is encountered.[122] Therefore, though a patient may present with an isolated gallbladder injury, the surgeon must carefully rule out further intraabdominal trauma. A trauma patient may also manifest a gallbladder injury as a result of a significant contusion. Blood in the gallbladder can cause stasis and blockage of the cystic duct, which may present as acute cholecystitis.[123]

Gallbladder injury has been successfully evaluated by CT (Fig. 32-14). The findings of an ill-defined contour of the wall, collapse of the lumen, or intraluminal hemorrhage highly suggest blunt gallbladder injury.[124] Patients may also present with bile peritonitis and right upper quadrant pain. Ultrasound examination in gallbladder injury has not been formally evaluated but intuitively should provide useful information about this injury. Despite these diagnostic methods, the diagnosis of gallbladder injury is most often secured at laparotomy.

**Portal Vein.** A very high mortality is found in those with portal vein injury. Much of the mortality is caused by exsanguination even before attempted repair.[120] Of the 99 patients with portal triad structure injury, evaluated in a 1995 multi-institutional study, 55% included a portal vein injury. The location of the injury is most often within the hepatoduodenal ligament (Fig. 32-15). Portal vein injury also carries about a 70% risk of concomitant major vascular injury.[125]

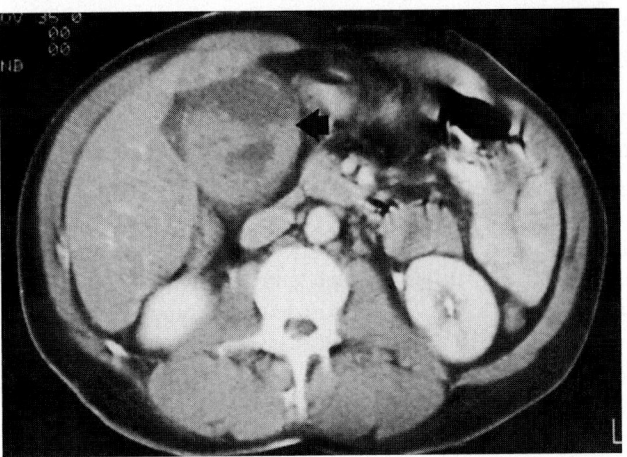

**FIGURE 32-14.** CT scan revealing a distended gallbladder filled with blood (dark arrow) in a patient with blunt abdominal trauma and virtually no peritoneal signs.

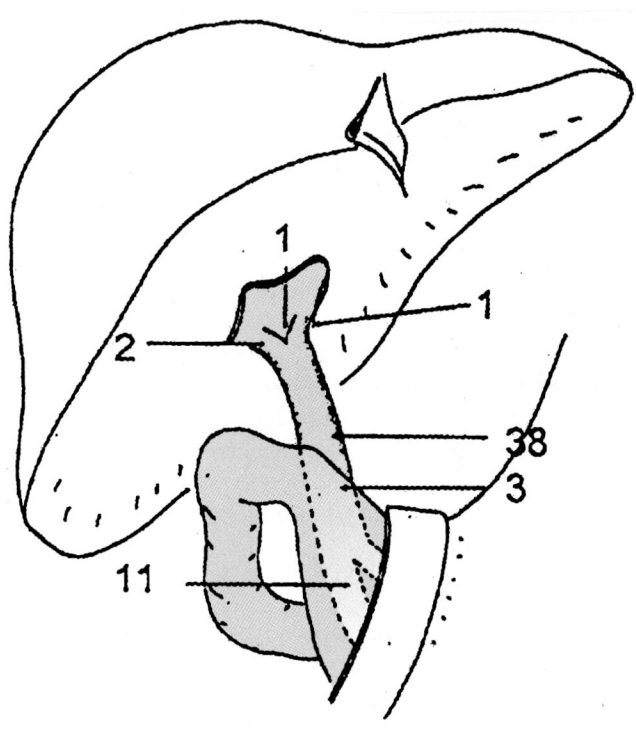

**FIGURE 32-15.** Anatomic location of 56 portal vein injuries in 55 patients. One patient had a penetrating injury to both the main body of the portal vein and the confluence of the mesenteric and vein. *(Reproduced with Permission from Jurkovich GJ, Hoyt DB, Moore FA, et al.: Portal triad injuries-a multicenter study. J Trauma 39:426, 1995.)*

Most patients with significant portal vein injury present in hemorrhagic shock. These patients obviously require immediate exploration. However, a few patients with smaller portal vein injury may respond to initial resuscitation. CT scan evaluation may exhibit periportal fluid or liver injury suspicious for portal involvement.

**Hepatic Artery.** Blunt hepatic artery injury in the porta hepatis is very rare due to its muscular tunica media and meandering course from the celiac axis giving it better strength and more flexibility.[126,127] Blunt injury does occur more frequently near the parenchyma.[120] Penetrating injury to the porta hepatis does, in contrast, occasionally involves the hepatic artery and usually will have a concomitant injured structure in the vicinity.

Most patients with hepatic artery injury arrive in severe shock and are taken urgently to the operating room. There have been, however, late presentations with pseudoaneurysm, thrombosis, or arteriovenous fistula seen on angiography or CT.[121]

Bile Duct.    Bile duct injury is most often encountered in penetrating injury.[120] Blunt ductal injury is most likely to happen where the bile duct is fixed to its surroundings, e.g., the pancreaticoduodenal junction.[128] In a multi-institutional trial it was found that blunt injuries were predominately a complete transaction, whereas penetrating injuries were partial 75% of the time.[120]

Extrahepatic bile duct injuries are evident in two distinct settings: first, at the time of laparotomy for a patient in shock with other severe liver, vascular, pancreatic, or duodenum injury; second, in a late presentation often more than 24 hours and up to six weeks after the original injury time. The patients with late presentation may develop jaundice, abdominal distention and pain, intolerance to enteral feeding, fever, or worsening base deficit dueto bilious ascitis or infection.[121]

Evaluation of the stable patient with CT scan or ultrasound in the acute setting will not be able to differentiate abdominal blood with biliary leak. There may be some indication of pancreatic head fullness, duodenal thickening, or portal edema but these are nonspecific findings. In the presence of bile staining during an operative procedure and no obvious injury, a cholangiogram through the gallbladder can be helpful.[128] DPL has also shown a lack of specificity for biliary injury as duodenal, small bowel, and liver injuries may produce bile.[129] Also, the small amount of bile maybe obscured by the presence of blood in the peritoneum with the DPL. Late presenters of bile duct injury can not be recognized until symptoms are apparent. At that time CT, ultrasound, or ERC can be used to visualize bile collections and localize injury.[130]

## Management of Portal Triad/Extrahepatic Biliary Injuries

General Considerations.    Patients with portal triad and extrahepatic biliary injuries usually arrive in shock. Therefore, the tenets described for major liver injury apply to portal injury as well. A midline incision should be made. Evacuation of blood clots and hemoperitoneum with urgent packing of the bleeding portions should be completed. The patient should be resuscitated and coagulopathy correction initiated by the anesthesia team. Hematoma or bleeding around or within the hepatoduodenal ligament or severe parenchymal injury leading to the porta hepatis should raise suspicion of a portal triad injury. Bile staining should also be fully investigated as 12% of bile duct injury may be missed at the initial operation.[128] The Pringle maneuver may be helpful in decreasing the inflow to a portal injury. In order to obtain adequate examination and exposure for repair, a wide Catell maneuver should be performed, which includes mobilizing the ascending and hepatic flexure areas of the colon, thus exposing the duodenum completely to the head of the pancreas and inferior vena cava.

Gallbladder.    Isolated gallbladder injury is most often managed with open cholecystectomy. However, there have been reports of laparoscopic cholecystectomy in penetrating trauma.[131] This procedure should be done with great reserve since many gallbladder injuries are associated with other intra-abdominal injury both in penetrating and blunt trauma. Though the laparoscope can give a good superficial exam of the peritoneal cavity, visualization of the duodenum, pancreas, and porta is in most hands not sufficient. Minor gallbladder contusions can often be managed nonoperatively.[132] This may lead to cholecystitis or delayed rupture if hematoma is present. Historically, it had been suggested that simple lacerations should undergo cholecystorraphy with absorbable suture.[133] Cholecystorraphy, however, remains a rare procedure, as small gallbladder lacerations are rarely encountered and cholecystectomy is able to be rapidly performed. Cholecystectomy should also be performed on all patients with injury to the cystic duct or right hepatic artery that would eliminate the blood supply to the gallbladder.

Portal Vein.    Initial control of portal vein injury is often by manual decompression or pressure packs. A Pringle maneuver may also control the inflow.[134] If the injury is in the midportion of the hepatoduodenal ligament, clamps may be able to be placed above and below to control both inflow and outflow.[120] The retropancreatic portion of the portal vein can best be visualized with division of the pancreas followed by a distal pancreatectomy once the repair is made.[126]

If the site of hemorrhage can be ascertained and controlled, lateral venorrhaphy has produced the best survival data.[120,121] Obviously these injuries are of lesser severity if control is at all possible. Many other options have been presented in the literature including saphenous vein or polytetrafluoro ethylene (PTFE) interposition grafts, end-to-end primary repairs, and portal caval shunting either directly above the injury or creating superior mesenteric to splenic vein shunts.[135] These procedures may have been successful for anecdotal cases, but have not shown large series success.

In the face of exsanguination, portal vein ligation may be performed. Child first validated the survivability of portal vein ligation in 1954.[136] He was able to show that after portal vein ligation there is a transient rise in portal pressure and drop in systemic pressure until adequate collaterals develop. He stated that these collaterals were adequate in up to 80% of humans. Massive fluid sequestration results after portal vein ligation. These patients require massive resuscitation and will also exhibit bowel edema leading to abdominal compartment syndrome if the abdomen is not left open. Even with adequate resuscitation, the mortality of portal vein ligation is very high. Angiography, duplex ultrasound, and intraoperative pressure measurement months after ligation have documented the resolution of portal hypertension.[137–139] A second-look laparotomy after portal vein ligation has been advocated to assure bowel viability.[138,139] Actual experience with portal vein ligation has shown great variance in survival. In the 1995 multi-institutional report, 90% of patients with portal vein ligation did not survive.[120] However, a study by Stone et al. noted a significantly improved survival of 80%.[137] This survival was obtained by initiating the ligation of the portal vein immediately upon the discovery that lateral venorrhaphy could not be easily accomplished. The high survival of these patients relies again on the principles of damage control with rapid accurate decisions and resuscitation producing a higher survival than long operative repairs with exsanguination.

**Hepatic Artery.** Manual compression or the use of the Pringle maneuver most often obtains control of hemorrhage from the hepatic artery. Isolated hepatic artery injury can be managed by primary repair, but in the case of massive hemorrhage or multiple associated injuries (as is most often the case with today's weaponry) ligation is often prudent. Primary repair and interposition grafts of vein or PTFE have been documented. Hepatic artery ligation can be accomplished safely. Mays reported that hepatic arteries were not "end arteries" and often collaterals reestablished flow.[140] Multiple studies have supported the use of ligation of the hepatic artery, especially when portal flow remains intact.[141,142] The portal system can take over the 25% of blood flow that arose from the hepatic arterial circulation. Reports of liver necrosis or abscess formation, however, continue to indicate a need for caution with ligation. Lucas and Ledgerwood reported a patient with complete hepatic necrosis and death after a hepatic artery ligation with an intact portal system.[143] This patient was in severe shock and also had ligation of his gastroduodenal artery. This continues to reinforce the need for evaluation of evidence of hepatic ischemia after hepatic artery ligation, especially for the patient in shock. The surgeon must also remember to perform a cholecystectomy in those patients in whom the right hepatic blood flow has been disrupted.

**Bile Duct.** Bile duct injury should be addressed after hemorrhage has been controlled. In the patient who remains in shock and coagulopathic, packing and placement of a Jackson-Pratt drain in the area of biliary injury is adequate until reexploration is performed. In the somewhat more stable patient who is becoming coagulopathic, a small T-tube placed in the injured duct will provide adequate drainage until a formal repair can be accomplished.[144] With a partial transection of a right or left hepatic duct, insertion of a small T-tube into the common hepatic duct with a long limb traversing the partially transected area even without suturing, may provide enough support for full healing.[145]

For the stable patient definitive repair is preferred at the first operation. Four broad categories of biliary duct injury have been described: (a) avulsion of cystic duct or small laceration, (b) transection without loss of tissue, (c) extensive defect in the wall, and (d) segmental loss of ductal tissue.[145]

Avulsions and small lacerations in the duct can be repaired primarily with 6-0 polyglycolic suture making sure not to narrow the lumen. A T-tube with a limb under the repair can be used; however, this may be difficult to insert in a patient with a normally small duct. The techniques used to place a T-tube may also devascularize an already compromised duct. Therefore, the author will not place a T-tube in primary repair. For avulsions in which primary repair may narrow the lumen a piece of the cystic duct or proximal gallbladder wall can be used for the repair.[146]

Penetrating injury very occasionally results in a transection of the bile duct without significant tissue loss. In these instances an end-to-end anastomosis can be performed. One must be sure to perform minimal dissection around the duct or the lacerated ends in order to maintain adequate blood supply for healing. Tension on the anastomosis will most certainly lead to stricture. Ivatury et al. reported a 55% stricture rate in the end-to-end anastomosis which then required enteric conversion.[147] Similarly, Stewart and Way had initial success in 67% of patients initially managed with Roux-en-Y for complete laceration following laparoscopic cholecystectomy with failure in all lacerations treated with end-to-end anastomosis.[148]

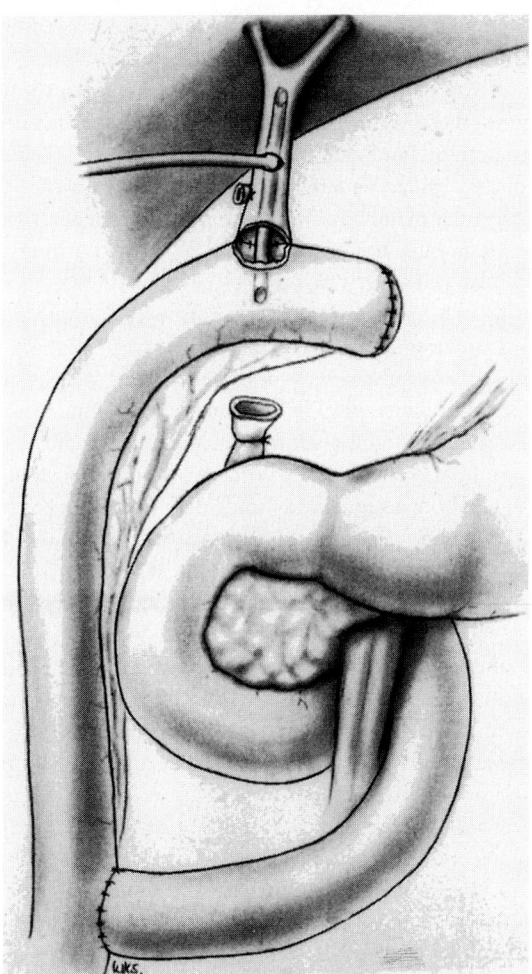

**FIGURE 32-16.** Roux-en-Y choledochojejunostomy. Anastomosis is performed in a one-layer fashion. The T-tube is brought out through a separate proximal stab wound. The gallbladder has been removed.

Extensive wall defects and segmental tissue loss require biliary enteric anastomosis (Fig. 32-16). In the past many methods of "patching" were attempted. Saphenous vein grafts have had difficulties with shrinking and fibrosis, which then required stenting.[149] Prosthetic patches and jejunal mucosal patches have also been tried with anecdotal success only.[150]

Deciding which type of biliary enteric anastomosis to perform depends on the injury location, access, and size. Roux-en-Y hepaticojejunostomy with cholecystectomy and T-tube drainage is the most utilized approach to complex injury. The retrocolic Roux limb is at least 40 cm long and can be brought up to the common hepatic duct or even to the hilar plate similar to the Kasai procedure. An avulsion of the hepatic ducts at the bifurcation can be managed by suturing the ducts together medially before the end-to-side hepatodochojejunostomy.[151] If the distal common duct is not found due to its retraction behind the pancreas, drainage of the area may be all that is necessary.[129] Roux-en-Y choledochojejunostomy with cholecystectomy and T-tube drainage is also useful for the management of common bile duct injury. However, the vascularity in this anastomosis is crucial and any sign of common bile duct vascular injury would lead the surgeon to construct an anastomosis closer to the common hepatic duct. Cholecystojejunostomy and ligation of the very distal common bile duct is a possibility if intraoperative cholangiography reveals a patent cystic duct. This is a viable option especially in patients with small caliper ducts or instability.

Blunt distal hepatic duct injury is rare. However, the surgical treatment of these injuries must be individualized to each situation. Both the right and left hepatic duct injuries have been reported.[152,153] Biliary-enteric anastomosis are sometimes possible right at the hilar plate; however, if the repair is difficult, ligation of a left or right duct has been reported to lead to atrophy of the involved lobe, not biliary cirrhosis.[154]

Stenting in biliary anastomosis is a controversial topic. Surgeons in favor of stenting report that stenting allows for decompression, when edema posttrauma may be significant, as well as allowing access for cholangiography. T-tubes must exit the duct outside of the repair area or stricture will result. Enteric stents are not necessary and some surgeons feel comfortable without their use, stating that a foreign body in an already small duct may promote stricture or obstruction[155] Morbidity data can not support a definitive answer for or against stenting and therefore a stent must be used at the discretion of the surgeon, taking each situation separately.

When ampullary or intrapancreatic bile duct injury is discovered, a pancreaticoduodenectomy may be appropriate if duodenal and pancreatic injury is also seen. An isolated ampullary primary repair or reimplantation may be possible. The author has repaired an ampullary injury by performing a transduodenal sphincteroplasty and primary repair of the ductal injury. Hepatic resection is necessary only in the case of combination injury to the liver parenchyma and hepatic duct traversing that segment.[145]

The major complications associated with biliary duct injury are fistula and stricture. A fistula may be able to be nonoperatively managed with drainage. Persistent fistula may require reexploration. Strictures may present with recurrent cholangitis or biliary cirrhosis. Stenting by endoscopists has become frequent; however, long-term results are not conclusive. A recent publication used an aggressive technique of placing an increasing number of stents until complete disappearance of the biliary stricture occurred. Though they did have a complication rate of 9% their mean duration of treatment was 12 months with a 48.8 month stricture free interval posttreatment thus far.[156] Conversely, Johns Hopkins reported their experience with operative management of all postoperative bile duct strictures and had a 98% success rate.[157]

## REFERENCES

1. Croce MA, Fabian TC, Menke PG: Nonoperative management of blunt hepatic trauma is the treatment of choice for hemodynamically stable patients. *Ann Surg* 221:744, 1995.
2. Edler. *Archiv f Klin Chir Bd* XXXIV, 1887.
3. Moynihan BG: *Abdominal Operations*. Philidelphia: W.B. Saunders, 1905, p. 473.
4. Tilton B: *Ann Surg* Jan 1905, p. 27.
5. Pringle JH: Notes on the arrest of hepatic hemorrhage due to trauma. *Ann Surg* 48:541, 1908.
6. Madding GF, Lawrence KB, et al.: Forward surgery of the severely injured. *Second Aux Surg Group* 1:307, 1942.
6a. Couinaud C: Les enveloppes vasculo-biliares de foie ou capsule de Glisson; leur interet dans la chirurgie vesiculaire, les resections hepatiqes et l'abord du hile du foie. *Lyon Chir* 49:589, 1954.
7. Moore EE, Cogbill TH, Jurkovitch GJ, et al.: Organ injury scaling-spleen, liver (1994 revision). *J Trauma* 38:323, 1995.
8. Bickell WH, Wall MJ, Pepe PE, et al.: Immediate versus delayed resuscitation for hypotensive patients with penetrating torso injuries. *N Engl J Med* 331:1105, 1994.
9. Dutton RP, Mackenzie CF, Scalea TM: Hypotensive resuscitation during active hemorrhage: impact on in-hospital mortality. *J Trauma* 52:1141, 2002.
10. Olsen WR, Redman HC, Hildreth DH: Quantitative peritoneal lavage in blunt abdominal trauma. *Arch Surg* 104:536, 1972.
11. Root HD, Hauser CW, McKinley CR, et al.: Diagnostic peritoneal lavage. *Surgery* 57:633, 1965.
12. Richards JR, McGahan JP, Pali MJ, et al.: Sonographic detection of blunt hepatic trauma: hemoperitoneum and parenchymal patterns of injury. *J Trauma* 47:1092, 1999.
13. Sato M, Yoshii H: Reevaluation of ultrasonography for solid-organ injury in blunt abdominal trauma. *J Ultrasound Med* 23:1583, 2004.
14. Rozycki GS, Ochsner MG, Feliciano DV, et al.: Early detection of hemoperitoneum by ultrasound examination of the right upper quadrant: A multicenter study. *J Trauma* 45:878, 1998.
15. Sirlin CB, Casola G, Brown MA, et al.: Patterns of fluid accumulation on screening ultrasonography for blunt abdominal trauma. *J Ultrasound Med* 20:351, 2001.
16. Branney SW, Moore EE, Cantrill SV, et al.: Ultrasound based key clinical pathway reduces the use of hospital resources for the evaluation of blunt abdominal trauma. *J Trauma* 42:1086, 1997.
17. Rozycki GS, Ballard RB, Feliciano DV, et al.: Surgeon-performed ultrasound for the assessment of truncal injuries: lessons learned from 1540 patients. *Ann Surg* 228:557, 1998.
18. Chiu WC, Cushing BM, Rodriguez A, et al.: Abdominal injuries without hemoperitoneum: a potential limitation of focused abdominal sonography for trauma. *J Trauma* 42:617, 1997.
19. Ballard RB, Rozycki GS, Newman PG, et al.: An algorithm to reduce the incidence of false-negative FAST examinations in patients at high risk for occult injury. Focused Assessment for the Sonographic Examination of the Trauma patient. *J Am Coll Surg* 189:145, 1999.
20. Poletti PA, Platon A, Becker CD, et al.: Blunt abdominal trauma: does the use of a second-generation sonographic contrast agent help to detect solid organ injuries? *Am J Roentgenol* 183:1293, 2004.
21. Catalano O, Sandomenico F, Raso MM, et al.: Real-time, contrast-enhanced sonography: a new tool for detecting active bleeding. *J Trauma* 59:933, 2005.
22. Udobe KF, Rodriguez A, Chiu WC, et al.: Role of ultrasonography in penetrating abdominal trauma: a prospective clinical study. *J Trauma* 50:475, 2001.
23. Soffer D, McKenney MG, Cohn S, et al.: A prospective evaluation of ultrasonography for the diagnosis of penetrating torso injury. *J Trauma* 56:953, 2004.
24. Murphy JT, Hall J, Provost D: Fascial ultrasound for evaluation of anterior abdominal stab wound injury. *J Trauma* 59:843, 2005.
25. Bokhari F, Nagy K, Roberts R, et al.: The ultrasound screen for penetrating truncal trauma. *Am Surg* 70:316, 2004.
26. Federle MP, Goldberg HI, Kaiser JA, et al.: Evaluation of abdominal trauma by computed tomography. *Radiology* 138:637, 1981.
27. Poletti PA, Mirvis SE, Shanmuganathan K, et al.: Blunt abdominal trauma patients: can organ injury be excluded without performing computed tomography? *J Trauma* 57:1072, 2004.
28. Phillips T, Sclafani SJ, Goldstein A, et al.: Use of the contrast-enhanced CT enema in the management of penetrating trauma to the flank and back. *J Trauma* 26:593, 1986.
29. Fabian TC, Croce MA, Stewart RM, et al.: A prospective analysis of diagnostic laparoscopy in trauma. *Ann Surg* 217:557, 1993.
30. Zantut LF, Ivatury RR, Smith RS, et al.: Diagnostic and therapeutic laparoscopy for penetrating abdominal trauma: a multicenter experience. *J Trauma* 42:825, 1997.
31. Farnell MB, Spencer MP, Thompson E, et al.: Nonoperative management of blunt hepatic trauma in adults. *Surgery* 104:748, 1988.
32. Federico JA, Horner WR, Clark DE, et al.: Blunt hepatic trauma: nonoperative management in adults. *Arch Surg* 125:905, 1990.
33. Pachter HL, Spencer FC, Hofstetter SR, et al.: Significant trends in the treatment of hepatic trauma: experience with 411 injuries. *Ann Surg* 215:492,1992.
34. Meredith JW, Ditesheim JA, Stonehouse S, et al.: Computed tomography and diagnostic peritoneal lavage: complementary roles in blunt trauma. *Am Surg* 58:44, 1992.
35. Croce MA, Fabian TC, Menke PG, et al.: Nonoperative management of blunt hepatic trauma is the treatment of choice for hemodynamically stable patients. Results of a prospective trial. *Ann Surg* 221:744, 1995.
36. Malhotra AK, Fabian TC, Croce MA, et al.: Blunt hepatic injury: a paradigm shift from operative to nonoperative management in the 1990s. *Ann Surg* 231:804, 2000.
37. Richardson JD, Franklin GA, Lukan JK, et al.: Evolution in the management of hepatic trauma: a 25-year perspective. *Ann Surg* 232:324, 2000.
38. Pachter HL, Knudson MM, Esrig B, et al.: Status of nonoperative management of blunt hepatic injuries in 1995: a multicenter experience with 404 patients. *J Trauma* 40:31, 1996.
39. Fang JF, Chen RJ, Wong YC, et al.: Classification and treatment of pooling of contrast material on computed tomographic scan of blunt hepatic trauma. *J Trauma* 49:1083, 2000.

40. Ciraulo DL, Luk S, Palter M, et al.: Selective hepatic arterial embolization of grade IV and V blunt hepatic injuries: an extension of resuscitation in the non-operative management of traumatic hepatic injuries. *J Trauma* 45:353, 1998.

41. Kozar RA, Moore JB, Niles SE, et al.: Complications of nonoperative management of high-grade blunt hepatic injuries. *J Trauma* 59:1066, 2005.

42. Kozar RA, Moore FA, Cothren CC, et al.: Hepatic-related morbidity associated with nonoperative management of complex blunt hepatic injuries: AAST multicenter trial. Atlanta, Georgia: *Sixty-Fourth Meeting of the American Association for the Surgery of Trauma*, 2005.

43. Marks, JM, Ponsky JL, Shillingstad RB, et al.: Biliary stenting is more effective than sphincterotomy in the resolution of biliary leaks. *Surg Endosc* 12:291, 1998.

44. Griffen M, Ochoa J, Boulanger BR: A minimally invasive approach to bile peritonitis after blunt liver injury. *Am Surg* 66:309, 2000.

45. Gates, JD: Delayed hemorrhage with free rupture complicating the nonsurgical management of blunt hepatic trauma: a case report and review of the literature. *J Trauma* 36:572, 1994.

46. Anderson IB, Al Saghier M, Kneteman NM, et al.: Liver trauma: management of devascularization injuries. *J Trauma* 57:1099, 2004.

47. Strong RW, Lynch SV, Wall DR, et al.: Anatomic resection for severe liver trauma. *Surgery* 123:251, 1998.

48. Smadja C, Traynor O, Blumgart LH: Delayed hepatic resection for major liver injury. *Br J Surg* 69:361, 1982.

49. Pollack CV: Hemobilia presenting as lower gastrointestinal hemorrhage without pain or jaundice: a case report. *J Miss State Med Assoc* 31:1, 1990.

50. Croce MA, Fabian TC, Spiers JP, et al.: Traumatic hepatic artery pseudoaneurysm with hemobilia. *Am J Surg* 168:235, 1994.

51. Pearl LB, Trunkey DD: Compartment syndrome of the liver. *J Trauma* 47:796, 1999.

52. Markert DJ, Shanmuganathan K, Mirvis SE, et al.: Budd Chiari syndrome resulting from intrahepatic IVC compression secondary to blunt hepatic trauma. *Clin Radiol* 52:384, 1997.

53. Cuff RF, Cogbill TH, Lambert PJ: Nonoperative management of blunt liver trauma: the value of follow-up abdominal computed tomography scans. *Am Surg* 66:332, 2000.

54. Ciraulo DL, Nikkanen HE, Palter M, et al.: Clinical analysis of the utility of repeat computed tomographic scan before discharge in blunt hepatic injury. *J Trauma* 41:821, 1996.

55. Cox JC, Fabian TC, Maish GO III, et al.: Routine follow-up imaging is unnecessary in the management of blunt hepatic injury. *J Trauma* 59:1175, 2005.

56. Dulchavsky SA, Lucas CE, Ledgerwood AM, et al.: Efficacy of liver wound healing by secondary intent. *J Trauma* 30:44, 1990.

57. Nance FC, Cohn I: Surgical judgement in the management of stab wounds of the abdomen: a retrospective and prospective analysis based on a study of 600 stabbed patients. *Ann Surg* 170:569, 1969.

58. Renz RM, Feliciano DV: Gunshot wounds to the liver. A prospective study of selective nonoperative management. *J Med Assoc GA* 84:275, 1995.

59. Demetriades D, Gomez H, Chahwan S, et al.: Gunshot injuries to the liver: The role of selective nonoperative management. *J Am Coll Surg* 188:343, 1998.

60. Shanmuganathan K, Mirvis SE, Chiu WC, et al.: Penetrating torso trauma: triple-contrast helical CT in peritoneal violation and organ injury: a prospective study in 200 patients. *Radiology* 231:775, 2004.

61. Velmahos GC, Constantinou C, Tillou A, et al.: Abdominal computed tomographic scan for patients with gunshot wounds to the abdomen selected for nonoperative management. *J Trauma* 59:1155, 2005.

62. Stone HH, Lamb JM: Use of pedicled omentum as an autogenous pack for control of hemorrhage in major injuries of the liver. *Surg Gyn & Obstet* 141:92, 1975.

63. Sheldon G, Rutledge R: Hepatic trauma. *Adv Surg* 22:179, 1989.

64. Man K, Fan ST, Ng IO, et al.: Prospective evaluation of Pringle maneuver in hepatectomy for liver tumors by a randomized study. *Ann Surg* 226:704, 1997.

65. Feliciano DV, Mattox KL, Jordan GL, et al.: Management of 1000 consecutive cases of hepatic trauma (1979–1984). *Ann Surg* 204:438, 1986.

66. Beal SL: Fatal hepatic hemorrhage: an unresolved problem in the management of complex liver injuries. *J Trauma* 30:163, 1990.

67. Caruso SM, Battistella FD, Owings JT, et al.: Perihepatic packing of major liver injuries. *Arch Surg* 134:958, 1999.

68. Feliciano DV, Pachter HL: Hepatic trauma revisited. *Curr Prob Surg* 26:453, 1989.

69. Krige JE, Bornman PC, Terblanche J: Therapeutic perihepatic packing in complex liver trauma. *Br J Surg* 79:43, 1992.

70. Feliciano DV, Mattox KL, Birch JM: Packing for control of hepatic hemorrhage: 58 consecutive patients. *J Trauma* 26:738, 1986.

71. Fabian TC, Stone HH: Arrest of severe liver hemorrhage by an omental pack. *South Med J* 73:1487, 1980.

72. Poggetti RS, Moore EE, Moore FA, et al.: Balloon tamponade for bilobar transfixing hepatic gunshot wounds. *J Trauma* 33:694, 1992.

73. Demetriades, D: Balloon tamponade for bleeding control in penetrating liver injuries. *J Trauma* 44:538, 1998.

74. Kram HB, Reuben BI, Fleming AW, et al.: Use of fibrin glue in hepatic trauma. *J Trauma* 28:1195, 1988.

75. Cohn SM, Cross JH, Ivy ME, et al.: Fibrin glue terminates massive bleeding after complex hepatic injury. *J Trauma* 45:666, 1998.

76. Holcomb JB, Pusateri AE, Harris RA, et al.: Effect of dry fibrin sealant dressings versus gauze packing on blood loss in grade V liver injuries in resuscitated swine. *J Trauma* 46:49, 1999.

77. King DR, Cohn SM, Proctor KG, et al.: Modified rapid deployment hemostat bandage terminates bleeding in coagulopathic patients with severe visceral injuries. *J Trauma* 57:756, 2004.

78. Sattler S, Gentilello LM: The liver bag: report of a new technique for treating severe, exsanguinating hepatic injuries. *J Trauma* 57:884, 2004.

79. McClelland RN, Shires T: Management of liver trauma in 259 consecutive patients. *Ann Surg* 161:248, 1965.

80. Strong RW, Lynch SV, Wall DR, et al.: Anatomic resection for severe liver trauma. *Surgery* 123:251, 1998.

81. Polanco P, Leon S, Pineda J, et al.: Hepatic resection in the management of complex injury to the liver. Atlanta, Georgia: *Sixty-Fourth Meeting of the American Association for the Surgery of Trauma*, 2005.

82. Ginzburg E, Klein Y, Sutherland M, et al.: Prolonged clamping of the liver parenchyma: a salvage maneuver in exsanguinating liver injury. *J Trauma* 56:922, 2004.

83. Aaron WS, Fulton RL, Mays ET: Selective ligation of the hepatic artery for trauma of the liver. *Surg Gynecol Obstet* 141:187, 1975.

84. Lucas CE, Ledgerwood AM: Liver necrosis following hepatic artery transection due to trauma. *Arch Surg* 113:1107, 1978.

85. Anderson IB, Kortbeek JB, Al-Saghier M, et al.: Liver transplantation in severe hepatic trauma after hepatic artery embolization. *J Trauma* 58:848, 2005.

86. Scalfani SJ, Shaftan GW, McAuley J, et al.: Inteventional radiology in the management of hepatic trauma. *J Trauma* 24:256, 1984.

87. Asensio JA, Demetriades D, Chahwan S, et al.: Approach to the management of complex hepatic injuries. *J Trauma* 48:66, 2000.

88. Angstadt J, Jarrell B, Moritz M, et al.: Surgical management of severe liver trauma: a role for liver transplantation. *J Trauma* 29:606, 1989.

89. Buckman RF, Miraliakbari R, Badellino MM: Juxtahepatic venous injuries: a critical review of reported management strategies. *J Trauma* 48:978, 2000.

90. Pachter HL, Feliciano DV: Complex hepatic trauma. *Surg Clin North Am* 76:763, 1996.

91. Chen RJ, Fang JF, Lin BC, et al.: Surgical management of juxtahepatic venous injuries in blunt hepatic trauma. *J Trauma* 38:886, 1995.

92. Schrock T, Blaisdell W, Mathewson C: Management of blunt trauma to the liver and hepatic veins. *Arch Surg* 96:698, 1968.

93. Pilcher DB, Harman PK, Moore EE: Retrohepatic vena cava balloon shunt introduced via the sapheno-femoral junction. *J Trauma* 17:837, 1977.

94. McAnena OJ, Moore EE, Moore FA: Insertion of a retrohepatic vena cava balloon shunt through the saphenofemoral junction. *Am J Surg* 158:463, 1989.

95. Cogbill TH, Moore EE, Jurkovich GJ, et al.: Severe hepatic trauma: a multicenter experience with 1,335 liver injuries. *J Trauma* 28:1433, 1988.

96. Baumgartner F, Scudamore C, Nair C, et al.: Venoveno bypass for major hepatic and caval trauma. *J Trauma* 39:671, 1995.

97. Carrillo EH, Spain DA, Miller FB, et al.: Intrahepatic vascular clamping in complex hepatic vein injuries. *J Trauma* 43:131, 1997.

98. Watarida S, Nishi T, Furukawa A, et al.: Fenestrated stent-graft for traumatic juxtahepatic inferior vena cava injury. *J Endovasc Ther* 9:134, 2002.

99. Castelli P, Caronno R, Piffaretti G, et al.: Emergency endovascular repair for traumatic injury of the inferior vena cava. *Eur J Cardiothorac Surg* 28:906, 2005.

100. Erzurum VZ, Shoup M, Borge M, et al.: Inferior vena cava endograft to control surgically inaccessible hemorrhage. *J Vasc Surg* 38:1437, 2003.

101. Fabian TC, Croce MA, Stanford GG, et al.: Factors affecting morbidity following hepatic trauma. A prospective analysis of 482 injuries. *Ann Surg* 213:540, 1991.

102. Cue JI, Cryer HG, Miller FB, et al.: Packing and planned reexploration for hepatic and retrperitoneal hemorrhage: critical refinements of a useful technique. *J Trauma* 30:1007, 1990.

103. Fischer RP, Beverlin BC, Engrav LH: Diagnostic peritoneal lavage: Fourteen years and 2586 patients later. *Am J Surg* 136:701, 1978.

104. Noyes LD, Doyle DJ, McSwain NE: Septic complications associated with the use of peritoneal drains in liver trauma. *J Trauma* 28:337, 1988.

105. Mullins RJ, Stone HH, Dunlop WE, et al.: Hepatic trauma: evaluation of routine drainage. *South Med J* 78:259, 1985.

106. Walt AJ, Wilson RF: *Management of trauma: pitfalls and practice.* Philadelphia. Lea and Febiger. 1975. P. 348.

107. Cyret P, Baumer R, Roche A: Hepatic hemobilia of traumatic or iatrogenic origin. Recent advances of diagnosis and therapy. Review of the literature from 1976–1981. *World J Surg* 8:2, 1984.

108. Heimbach OM, Ferguson GS, Harley JD: Treatment of traumatic hemobilia with angiographic embolization. *J Trauma* 18:221, 1978.

109. Clemens M, Wittrin G: *Bilhamie und hamobilie nach reitunfall.* Vortrag 166. Hamburg: Tagung Nordwestdeutscher Chirurgen, 1975.

110. Glaser K, Wetscher G, Pointner R, et al.: Traumatic bilhemia. *Surgery* 116:24, 1994.

111. Enneker C, Berens JP: Schwerste Leberruptur mit lebervenenabriss und massive bilhamie. *Chirurg* 49:311, 1978.

112. Hollands MJ, Little JM: Post-traumatic bile fistulae. *J Trauma* 31:117, 1991.

113. Howdieshell TR, Purvis J, Bates WB, et al.: Biloma and biliary fistula following hepatorraphy for liver trauma: incidence, natural history, and management. *Am Surg* 61:165, 1995.

114. Dick R, Gilliams A, Dooley JS, et al.: Stainless steel mesh stents for biliary stricture. *J Intervent Rad* 4:95, 1989.

115. D'Amours SK, Simons RK, Scudamore DH, et al.: Major intrahepatic bile duct injuries detected after laparotomy: selective nonoperative management. *J Trauma* 50:480, 2001.

116. Sheik-Gafoor MH, Singh B, Moodley J: Traumatic thoracobiliary fistula: report of a case successfully managed conservatively, with an overview of current diagnostic and therapeutic options. *J Trauma* 45:819, 1998.

117. Rothberg ML, Kilngman RR, Peetz D, et al.: Traumatic thoracobiliary fistula. *Ann Thorac Surg* 57:472, 1994.

118. Danetz JS, Yelon JA, Fields CE, et al.: Traumatic pleurocaval fistula: potential source of air embolism. *J Trauma* 50:551, 2001.

119. Eastridge BJ, Minei JP: Intrahepatic arterioportal fistula after hepatic gunshot wound: a case report and review of the literature. *J Trauma* 43:523, 1997.

120. Jurkovich GJ, Hoyt DB, Moore FA, et al.: Portal triad injuries-a multicenter study. *J Trauma* 39:426, 1995.

121. Dawson DL, Johansen KH, Jurkovich GJ: Injuries to the portal triad. *Am J Surg* 161:545, 1991.

122. Sharma O: Blunt gallbladder injuries: presentation of twenty-two cases with review of the literature. *J Trauma* 39:576, 1995.

123. Wilson RF, Walt AJ: *Management of Trauma Pitfalls and Practice.* 2nd ed. Baltimore, Willliams and Wilkins. 1996 p.476.

124. Erb RE, Mirvis SE, Shanmuganathan K: Gallbladder injury secondary to blunt trauma: CT findings. *J Comput Assist Tomogr* 18:778, 1994.

125. McFadden D, Lawelor B, Ali I: Portal vein injury. *Can J Surg* 30:91, 1987.

126. Sheldon G, Lim R, Yee E, et al.: Management of injuries to the porta hepatis. *Ann Surg* 202:539, 1985.

127. Busuttil R, Ketaham A, Cerise E, et al.: Management of blunt and penetrating injuries to the porta hepatis. *Ann Surg* 191:641, 1980.

128. Michelassi F, Ranson J: Bile duct disruption by blunt trauma. *J Trauma* 25:454, 1985.

129. Bourque M, Spigland N, Bensoussan A, et al.: Isolated complete transection of the common bile duct due to blunt trauma in a child, and review of the literature. *J Pediatr Surg* 24:1068, 1989.

130. Jones KB, Thomas E: Traumatic rupture of the hepatic duct demonstrated by endoscopic retrograde cholangiography. *J Trauma* 25:448, 1985.

131. Velez SE, Llaryora RG, Lerda FA: Laparoscopic cholecystectomy in penetrating trauma. *J Laparoendosc Adv Surg Tech A* 9:291, 1999.

132. Soderstrom CA, Maika K, DuPriest RW: Gallbladder injuries resulting from blunt abdominal trauma. *Ann Surg* 193:60, 1981.

133. Smith SW, Hastings TN: Traumatic rupture of the gallbladder. *Ann Surg* 139:521, 1954.

134. Graham JM, Mattox KL, Beall AC: Portal venous system injuries. *J Trauma* 18:419, 1978.

135. Fish JC: Reconstruction of the portal vein. Case reports and literature review. *Am J Surg* 32:472, 1966.

136. Child CG: *The hepatic circulation and portal hypertension.* Philadelphia: WB Saunders, 1954, p. 171.

137. Stone HH, Fabian TC, Turkelson M: Wounds of the portal venous system. *World J Surg* 6:335, 1982.

138. Pachter H, Drager S, Godfrey N, et al.: Traumatic injuries to the portal vein. The role of acute ligation. *Ann Surg* 189:383, 1979.

139. Ivatury R, Nallathambi M, Lankin D, et al.: Portal vein injuries. Noninvasive follow-up of venorrhaphy. *Ann Surg* 206:733, 1987.

140. Mays ET: Observations and management after hepatic artery ligation. *Surg Gynecol Obstet* 124:801, 1967.

141. Aaron WS, Fulton RL, Mays ET: Selective ligation of the hepatic artery for trauma of the liver. *Surg Gynecol Obstet* 141:187, 1975.

142. Walt AJ: The mythology of hepatic trauma-or Babel revisited. *Am J Surg* 135:12, 1978.

143. Lucas C, Ledgerwood A: Liver necrosis following hepatic artery transection due to trauma. *Arch Surg* 113:1107, 1978.

144. Pachter HL, Liang HG, Hofstetter SR: Liver and biliary tract trauma. *Trauma.* 2nd ed. Norwalk, Connecticut: Appleton and Lange, 1991, p.441.

145. Feliciano DV: Biliary injuries as a result of blunt and penetrating trauma. *Surg Clin N Amer* 74:897, 1994.

146. Sandblom P, Tabrizian M, Rigo M, et al.: Repair of common bile duct defects using the gallbladder or cystic duct as a pedicled graft. *Surg Gynecol Obstet* 140:425, 1975.

147. Ivatury RR, Rohman M, Nallathambi M, et al.: The morbidity of injuries of the extrahepatic biliary system. *J Trauma* 25:967, 1985.

148. Stewart L, Way L: Bile duct injuries during laparoscopic cholecystectomy: Factors that influence the results of treatment. *Proceedings of the Pacific Coast Surgical Association*, Seattle, Washington, Feb. 19–21, 1995.

149. Monk JS, Church JS, Agarwal N: Repair of a traumatic noncircumferential hepatic bile duct defect using a vein patch: case report. *J Trauma* 31:1555, 1991.

150. Thomas JP, Metropol HJ, Myers RT: Teflon patch graft for reconstruction of the extrahepatic bile ducts. *Ann Surg* 160:967, 1964.

151. Voyles GR, Blumgart LH: A technique for the construction of high biliary-enteric anastomoses. *Surg Gynecol Obstet* 154:885, 1982.

152. Rodriguez-Montes JA, Rojo E, Martin LG: Complications following repair of extrahepatic bile duct injuries after blunt abdominal trauma. *World J Surg* 25:1313, 2001.

153. Eid A, Almogy G, Pikarsky, et al.: Conservative treatment of a traumatic tear of the left hepatic duct: case report. *J Trauma* 41:912, 1996.

154. Dawson DL, Jurkovich GJ: Hepatic duct disruption from blunt abdominal trauma: case report and literature review. *J Trauma* 31:1698, 1991.

155. Innes J, Ferrara J, Carey L: Biliary reconstruction without transanastamotic stent. *Am Surg* 54:27, 1988.

156. Costa magna G, Pandolfi M, Mutignani M, et al.: Long-term results of endoscopic management of postoperative bile duct strictures with increasing numbers of stents. *Gastrointest Endosc* 54:162, 2001

157. Lillemoe KD, Meltoon GB, Cameron JL, et al.: Postoperative bile duct strictures: management and outcome in the 1990s. *Ann Surg* 232:430, 2000.

# Commentary ■ H. LEON PACHTER

The *Trauma* textbook regarded as the "Bible" for those interested in the field, continues to provide readers with a level of excellence, first conceived by the founding editors, and closely adhered to in all of the subsequent editions. The sixth edition is no exception. Any trauma surgeon or resident will find the chapter on hepatic trauma thorough, complete, and a remarkable reference source of what to do when confronted with any given clinical situation. The chapter excels from "diagnostics" to "therapeutics."

The recognition that FAST continues to play a vital role in the initial evaluation of patients sustaining blunt abdominal trauma has led to its incorporation in the core curriculum training of surgical residents. FAST becomes particularly important in the unstable patient who has sustained multiple trauma and the need to prioritize treatment becomes of paramount importance. As the authors noted, while FAST can determine with a high degree of accuracy the presence of a hemoperitoneum in patients with hepatic injuries, it cannot, however, reliably determine the precise anatomical location of the injury. Additionally, in the patient sustaining blunt abdominal trauma, multiple solid, and/or hollow viscus injuries may have occurred, and the FAST examination, for the most part cannot distinguish the source of free intraperitoneal fluid.

On the flip side, with the relatively low false negative rate with a FAST exam some centers have elected to forgo CT scanning. If such an approach is undertaken it would be prudent to both observe the patient and have them undergo serial ultrasound examinations before discharge as incidences of abdominal injuries following a negative initial FAST have been reported to be as high as 29%.

The role of FAST in penetrating trauma while currently being investigated has serious limitations and is, at best, considered in an evolutionary phase.

In the stable patient, CT scanning, "pound for pound" provides the most complete overall assessment of the peritoneum, retroperitoneum, thorax, and boney structures. For hepatic injuries, particularly those where nonoperative management is contemplated, CT scan serves to determine whether other injuries are present that would preclude nonoperative management; provides prognostic data by determining grade of injury, and the presence or absence of a "contrast blush." The latter two would point to the probability of an unsuccessful outcome without the institution of adjunctive therapeutic maneuvers.

Nonoperative management has stood the test of time, and continues to prove to be applicable in 80–85% of all patients sustaining blunt hepatic injuries with a success rate of 90–95%. The criteria for inclusion are well known with hemodynamic stability being of paramount importance. While grade of injury does not preclude nonoperative management, several studies have documented significant complication and failure rates with grades IV and V injuries. The issue of where hemodymanically stable patients should be observed has always been the subject of controversy, but Fig.32-4 provides the most thorough to date algorithmic approach to the nonoperative management of blunt liver injury and should be followed in detail.

While a three unit liver related bleed from a blunt injury may be acceptable, I am, as opposed to the authors, uncomfortable with five units of blood in the peritoneal cavity. If stable, such patients require additional diagnostic and probably therapeutic maneuvers even in face of the absence of a "contrast blush" on the initial CT scan. The presence of a "contrast blush" is indicative of ongoing hemorrhage and demands prompt attention, even in the face of hemodynamic stability as downward fluctuation in blood pressure can occur instantaneously, suddenly, and without warning. One caveat about "contrast blush." The trauma surgeon must emphasize to the radiologist that it is of paramount importance that the "arterial" phase of the study be properly visualized. The "arterial" phase occurs about 25 seconds after contrast injection, and if not seen at that time, the contrast gets diluted out in the venous phase (approximately 75 seconds from injection) and a "contrast blush," if present may be missed.

The complications associated with nonoperative management, not the failure rate which requires operative intervention, can almost always be managed by an experienced interventional radiologist or by endoscopic or minimally invasive techniques or a combination of all of the above. Bleeding appears to be the most common complication, but operative intervention to arrest such hemorrhage, as the authors point out, when one considers the total number of cases managed nonoperatively is approximately 1%.

The issue of nonoperative management of penetrating gunshot wounds in stable patients particularly when it pertains to the right upper thoraco-abdominal region remains controversial even when applied to a very select patient cohort. As the authors noted, most

trauma centers, but not all, would opt, under these circumstances, for operative intervention. Nevertheless, when the question of peritoneal "penetration" arises as does the possibility of a "blast" effect due to a gunshot wound, diagnostic laparoscopy is warranted. This approach has become firmly established in: (1) assessing peritoneal penetration, and (2) allowing for adequate evaluation of the bowel.

For complex hepatic injuries requiring immediate operative intervention, the sixth edition provides the reader with a series of operative strategies that any surgeon, without the appropriate experience, would do well to familiarize themselves with. The concept of proactive maneuvers, to prevent hypothermia from setting in cannot be overemphasized. In the operating room manual compression of the injury allows for proper fluid resuscitation, and correction of lethal acidosis. Coagulation abnormalities often occur in the presence of systemic hypothermia and frequently tip the balance between life and death. Moreover, if bleeding is excessive, consideration should be given to the use of recombinant Factor VIIa. Factor VIIa bypasses the intrinsic cascade, shortens the time to clot formation by inducing a thrombin burst and fibrin clots at the site of vascular injury. That most complex hepatic injuries often require a multidisciplinary approach, a concept emphatically emphasized in the fifth edition, has firmly been established as the standard of care in 2007. As the number of exposures to operative complex hepatic injuries, grades IV and V, decreases it becomes essential that surgeons familiarize themselves a priori with ten critical "multidisciplinary" steps as outlined in the chapter. They are: (1) the Pringle maneuver, (2) finger fracture of the liver, (3) occlusion of hepatic parenchymal bleeding with large blunt nosed 0-Chromic hepatic sutures, (4) omental Packing, (5) nonanatomic and anatomic resection, (6) damage control laparotomy, (7) angioembolization, (8) vascular endostents, (9) ERCP, sphincterotomy, and endostenting, and (10) interventional radiologic techniques When bleeding persists, "damage control" with peri-hepatic packing should be instituted early and before an irreversible coagulopathy has set in. This simple, yet highly effective maneuver has resulted in increased survival in circumstances where death was all but inevitable. The sixth edition offers the reader helpful hints as to how to place the packing appropriately and the guidelines for its removal.

The sections devoted to hepatic resection and role of transplantation are relevant and current. The latter approach is markedly limited by the unpredictability of getting a donor and the complications that ensue when the recipient remains in a prolonged an-hepatic state. I would submit, however, that there is a role for hepatic resection, provided the availability of a trained hepato-biliary or transplant surgeon. When such expertise is readily available, mortality rates are acceptable and negate historical figures which were prohibitive, to say the least.

Additionally, adjunctive maneuvers, such as employing tampons of absorbable gelatin sponges wrapped with oxidized cellulose and the "Poggetti" balloon tamponade catheter, the modified rapid deployment hemostat, and the use of fibrin sealants are thoroughly depicted, discussed, and when appropriately used, helpful.

Juxtahepatic venous injuries, unfortunately, continue to carry a prohibitive mortality irrespective of virtually any approach attempted to salvage the patient. What is painfully clear is that shunting procedures should be abandoned, and direct repair and resection, at present, are rarely successful. Instead, tamponade with containment should be the preferred treatment modality if the patient has any chance for survival. But, this is "old hat." What is new and exciting and preliminarily has shown great potential is the use of fenestrated graft stents. Properly deployed, these stents can occlude the retrohepatic caval injury while maintaining patency of the hepatic and renal veins.

Finally, the issue "to drain or not to drain" remains the question perhaps dating back to Elizabethan times. The author suggests that "most centers" treat patients expectantly except in those instances where there is an obvious bile leak. They in turn rely heavily on the interventional radiologists to drain and collections usually when the patient becomes septic. Despite adequate debridement and even in the face of nondetectable bile leak at the time of surgery, both abscesses and bilomas can occur particularly in complex hepatic injuries. As "closed suction" drains when used appropriately and removed expeditiously result in almost half the abscess rate when compared to no drains, it would seem prudent to employ them before the onset of sepsis. Drains, in themselves, do not prevent abscesses, bleeding, or bilomas, but can attenuate these processes or make the surgeon aware of their presence at an earlier date. Percutaneous intervention can then be undertaken lessening the risk of severe sepsis or the initiation of the SIRS syndrome as a "second hit" phenomenon.

# Injury to the Spleen

*Robert C. Jacoby* ■ *David H. Wisner*

Splenic injuries are important because they are fairly common and can be deadly. The spleen is listed, along with the liver, as either the first or second most commonly injured solid viscus in the abdomen. Because splenic injuries have a tendency to demonstrate themselves clinically more often than do hepatic injuries, splenic injury was listed as the most commonly injured intra-abdominal solid viscus prior to the advent of computed tomography (CT) scanning. After the advent of CT scanning and our ability to better diagnose clinically silent intra-abdominal injuries, it became apparent that the liver is also commonly injured and some series listed hepatic injuries as more common than splenic injuries. Although the relative incidence of splenic and liver injuries is interesting from an epidemiologic point of view, from a clinical point of view the important point to remember is that the spleen is one of the more common solid abdominal viscera injured and is a frequent site of clinically significant injury.

During the last 50 years, there has been increasing interest in the notion that not all splenic injuries require splenectomy. Our understanding of splenic injury has increased markedly and the management of splenic injury has evolved. Although that evolution has steadily moved us away from routine aggressive operative management, it is important to always keep in mind that splenic injuries can be deadly and that patients with splenic injury can bleed to death.

## HISTORICAL PERSPECTIVE

The spleen has been subject to injury for as long as man has suffered trauma. In ancient India, where malaria was endemic and, as a consequence, large and fragile spleens were commonplace, intentional injury of the spleen was a method of assassination (personal communication by F. William Blaisdell, MD, Sacramento, CA, 1985). Paid assassins called *thuggee* carried out their mission by delivering a blow to the left upper quadrant of the intended victim. They thereby hoped to cause splenic rupture, for which there was no treatment at that time. If the rupture were severe enough, the

victim would bleed to death. As we know from our current imaging capabilities and splenic injury management philosophy, the thuggee must have been frustrated on occasion by the lack of success of their attempted assassinations.

The spleen was felt by the ancient Greeks and Romans to play a significant role in human physiology. Aristotle thought that the spleen was on the left side of the body as a counterweight to the right-sided liver.[1] He believed that the spleen was important in drawing off "residual humors" from the stomach. The close relation of the stomach and spleen and the presence of the short gastric vessels so important in present-day splenic mobilization likely encouraged this belief. The spleen was also felt to "hinder a man's running," and Pliny reportedly claimed that "professed runners in the race that bee troubled with the splene, have a devise to burne and waste it with a hot yron."[2] The exceptional speed of giraffes was felt to be related to the erroneous belief that giraffes were asplenic. Early references to removal of the spleen to increase speed make it apparent that it has long been known that the spleen is not absolutely necessary to sustain life. Paracelsus believed that the spleen could be removed and rejected the notion that it was important for the storage of "black bile."[3]

In 1738, John Ferguson of Scotland removed a portion of the spleen through an open wound in the left side (Fig. 33-1).[3] Once the era of abdominal surgery had begun, it was discovered that the spleen could be removed with what seemed like relative impunity. William Mayo reported in 1910 that "the internal secretion of the spleen is not important, as splenectomy does not produce serious results."[4] Although some suggested that the spleen was important in some way for immune function and for the removal of senescent red blood cells, it was not felt that these functions were of great importance. This resulted in a philosophy until several decades ago in which any traumatic splenic injury, no matter how trivial, was treated with splenectomy.[3,4] Even small iatrogenic injuries occurring during elective surgery were treated with splenic removal.

There were some early thoughts that the spleen plays a role in combating infection, but it only has been in the last half-century that our understanding of the role of the spleen in immune function has

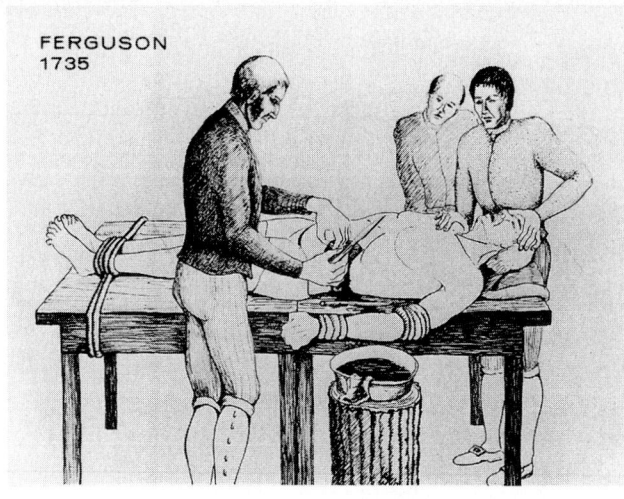

**FIGURE 33-1.** A depiction of the partial splenectomy done by John Ferguson of Scotland and reported in 1738. The operation actually had been done some years earlier.
*(Reproduced with permission from Hiatt JR, Phillips EH, Morgenstern L, eds.: Surgical Diseases of the Spleen, New York: Springer-Verlag, 1997, p. 6.)*

developed.[5–7] The initial impetus to more closely examine the immunologic role of the spleen was based on the observation that neonates and infants who required splenectomy for hematologic disease suffered otherwise inexplicably high rates of postoperative mortality from overwhelming infection. Pneumonia and meningitis secondary to pneumococcus and other encapsulated organisms were particularly common. The dramatic consequences of splenectomy in this very specific group of patients led to the investigation of the effects of splenectomy in pediatric trauma patients. Although the evidence for severe immunologic consequences of splenectomy in this group was less convincing than in pediatric patients with hematologic disease, there was a strong inference that splenectomy for trauma would lead to an increased rate of overwhelming sepsis, just as occurred after splenectomy for hematologic disease.[10] Cases of overwhelmingly postsplenectomy sepsis in adults who had undergone splenectomy for trauma were also then reported.[8,9]

Several other developments that paralleled our increased understanding of the importance of the spleen for immune function were the development of improved abdominal imaging capability and increasing questions about the safety of the blood supply. The advent of CT scanning of the abdomen and its continued improvement in quality markedly increased our ability to diagnose splenic injury nonoperatively, and it became apparent that clinically silent splenic injuries could occur. Nonoperative management was not new. What was new was the fact that we were now able to diagnose splenic injury and nonoperatively manage it in a calculated and chosen way. Concerns about the safety of stored blood transfusion with respect to hepatitis and human immunodeficiency virus led to increasing questions about transfusions for patients with splenic injury.

## SPLENIC FUNCTION

The spleen is important physiologically in several different ways.[10] Histologically, the spleen is divided into what has been termed *red pulp* and *white pulp*. The red pulp is a series of large passageways that filter old red blood cells and also catch bacteria. Filtering of senescent erythrocytes is important in removing poorly functioning red blood cells from the bloodstream and keeping the hematocrit and blood viscosity within a normal range. The capture of bacteria in the filters of the red pulp allows the antigens of the bacterial walls to be presented to the lymphocytes in the adjacent white pulp. The white pulp, as inferred earlier, is filled largely with lymphocytes located such that they can be exposed to antigens either on microorganisms or circulating freely in the circulation. Lymphocyte exposure to antigens results in the production of immunoglobulins,[10,11] the most common of which is IgM. Other potentially important functions of the white pulp are the production of opsonins such as tuftsin and properdin and complement activation in response to appropriate stimuli.

All these functions of the spleen are, of course, lost after splenectomy. Collections of lymph tissue are also found in the liver, thymus, intestinal tract, and skin and these areas may take over some of the functions of the spleen after splenectomy. In addition, accessory spleens are quite common and some of the necessary functions of the spleen could conceivably be carried out by residual splenic tissue left behind in the form of accessory splenic tissue, but the removal of the spleen results in loss of most filtering and immune production functions. How serious these losses are to normal function is a matter of debate. The loss of the filtering function of senescent red blood cells seems to be tolerated reasonably well. Although certain kinds of senescent red blood cells in the bloodstream are more pronounced after splenectomy, the normal production and removal of red blood cells seems, for the most part, to continue. The loss of splenic function has been the subject of a great deal of investigation. A study of isolated splenic injuries revealed an early postinjury infection rate of 9% in postsplenectomy patients as opposed to a rate of only 2% in patients successfully managed nonoperatively. There is also evidence of an increased incidence of overwhelming sepsis after splenectomy for trauma but the precise incidence of such overwhelming infections, especially in adults, is so low that it is difficult to quantify.[12]

The possibility that small accessory spleens might provide residual splenic function raises the question of how much splenic mass is necessary for the filtering and immune functions of the spleen. This is a question of more than academic importance, in that a variety of techniques have been described for partial splenectomy or autotransplantation of the spleen after splenectomy.[13–15] The exact amount of spleen to reimplant after splenectomy or leave behind after partial splenectomy is dependent on the minimum amount of splenic tissue necessary for normal function. How much spleen is necessary for normal function is not precisely known but has been conjectured to be between 30 and 50%.[16]

## SPLENIC ANATOMY

The spleen develops initially as a bulge on the left side of the dorsal mesogastrium and begins a gradual leftward migration to the left upper quadrant. The spleen changes in relative size during maturation. In children, it is large because it is necessary for both reticuloendothelial function and red blood cell production. As the child's bone marrow matures, the spleen becomes relatively less important and diminishes in size relative to the rest of the body. There are also some important differences between pediatric and

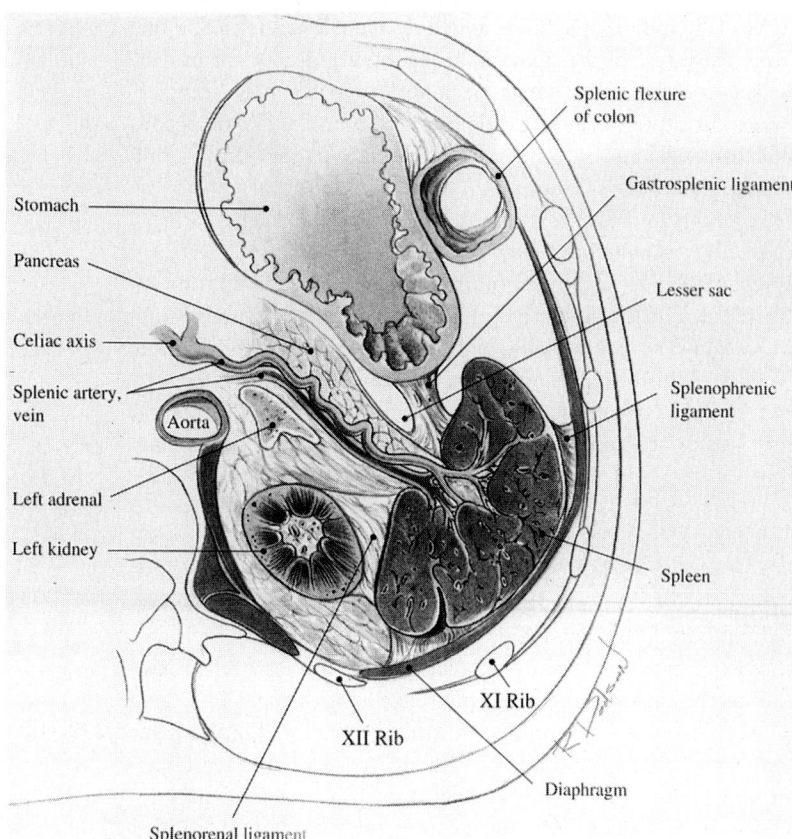

**FIGURE 33-2.** The spleen is located quite posteriorly in the left upper quadrant and is attached to surrounding structures by a variety of ligaments.
*(Reproduced with permission from Carrico CJ, Thal ER, Weigelt JA, eds.: Operative Trauma Management: An Atlas. Copyright 1998, Appleton & Lange, p. 157.)*

adult spleens with respect to the splenic capsule and the consistency of the splenic parenchyma. The capsule in children is relatively thicker than it is in adults, and there is also some evidence that the parenchyma is firmer in consistency in children than it is in adults. These two differences have implications for the success of nonoperative management. A thicker capsule and tougher parenchymal consistency imply that pediatric spleens are more likely to survive an insult without major bleeding and the need for operative intervention, part of the explanation for why children are more often candidates for nonoperative management than are adults and why nonoperative management tends to be somewhat more successful in children than it is in adults.

The normal adult spleen ranges in size from 100 to 250 g. A number of disease processes, however, can change both the size and consistency of the spleen. Malaria and its effects on the spleen with respect to enlargement and changes in consistency have already been referred to earlier. Hematologic diseases such as lymphoma and leukemia can also change both the size and consistency of the spleen and make it more susceptible to damage. Other more common diseases such as mononucleosis make the spleen more vulnerable to injury. An equally important and prevalent pathology that can increase splenic vulnerability is portal hypertension. Usually such portal hypertension is secondary to cirrhosis of the liver and when it is present the spleen can become both enlarged and less firm in consistency.

It is perhaps not intuitive from the anteroposterior views depicted in anatomy textbooks, but the spleen is normally located quite posteriorly in the upper abdomen (Fig. 33-2). It is covered by the peritoneum except at the hilum. The relation of the spleen to surrounding structures and relevant ligamentous attachments is as follows: posteriorly and laterally the spleen is related to the left

hemidiaphragm and the left posterior and posterolateral lower ribs. The lateral aspect of the spleen is attached to the posterior and lateral abdominal wall and the left hemidiaphragm (splenophrenic ligament) with a variable number of attachments; these require division during mobilization of the spleen. The extent of these attachments is quite variable. Minimal attachments result in a fairly mobile spleen; thick attachments, when present, require sharp dissection. The lateral attachments tend to be smaller and less extensive in children than in adults. That the spleen lies adjacent to the posterior ribs on the left side emphasizes the fact that left posterior rib fractures should increase the index of suspicion for underlying splenic injury. Because of the close relation of the spleen to the diaphragm, simultaneous injuries to the two structures are not uncommon (see Chap. 31). After penetrating trauma, a knife or bullet during its course can obviously injure both the left hemidiaphragm and the spleen. The diaphragm can also be injured in blunt trauma, and the spleen, either injured or uninjured, can herniate through a diaphragmatic defect into the left pleural space. The diaphragm should always be closely inspected during surgery for splenic injury.

Posteriorly, the spleen is related to the left iliopsoas muscle and the left adrenal gland. The left adrenal gland is usually fairly small and has a characteristic yellow–gold color. It tends to be related to the posterior aspect of the superior portion of the spleen and should be protected when seen during splenic mobilization.

Posteriorly and medially, the spleen is related to the body and tail of the pancreas. The relation of the spleen and pancreas are of importance during splenic mobilization, and it is very helpful to mobilize the tail and body of the pancreas along with the spleen when elevating the spleen out of the left upper quadrant; including the tail and body of the pancreas increases the extent to which the spleen can be mobilized.

Medially and to some extent anteriorly, the spleen is related to the greater curvature of the stomach. This relation is important in that the spleen can receive a variable amount of blood supply from the greater curvature via short gastric branches from the left gastroepiploic artery. The short gastric vessels require division during full mobilization of the spleen.

Posteriorly and inferiorly, the spleen is related to the left kidney. There are attachments between the spleen and left kidney (splenorenal ligament) that require division during mobilization of the spleen. The left kidney is an important landmark in mobilizing the spleen; it generally should be left in place while mobilizing the spleen and tail of the pancreas from lateral to medial. There are exceptions to leaving the kidney in place, most notably if the kidney also has been injured or if mobilization of the spleen is being done to provide exposure to the aorta from the left side (see Chap. 37).

Finally, the spleen is related inferiorly to the distal transverse colon and splenic flexure. The lower pole of the spleen is attached to the colon (splenocolic ligament), and these attachments require division during splenic mobilization.

The spleen receives its arterial blood supply from the celiac axis. One of the major branches of the celiac axis, the splenic artery, courses along the superior aspect of the body and tail of the pancreas toward the splenic hilum. Although generally located along the upper border of the body and tail of the pancreas, its course can be somewhat variable. The splenic artery also is commonly quite tortuous. It divides into a variable number of branches to supply segmentally the spleen. Both the number of branches and the site at which the branching occurs are quite variable (Fig. 33-3). This variability is of surgical significance in that there is no absolute and dependable number of splenic artery branches that require division during splenectomy or segmental resection of the spleen. Most commonly, a number of separate splenic artery branches are ligated during splenectomy rather than a single ligation of the main splenic artery. It is possible to find the splenic artery along the superior margin of the body and tail of the pancreas if necessary, and sometimes it is helpful to ligate the artery at that location even after hilar branches have been ligated if the surgeon is interested in extra security and hemostasis.

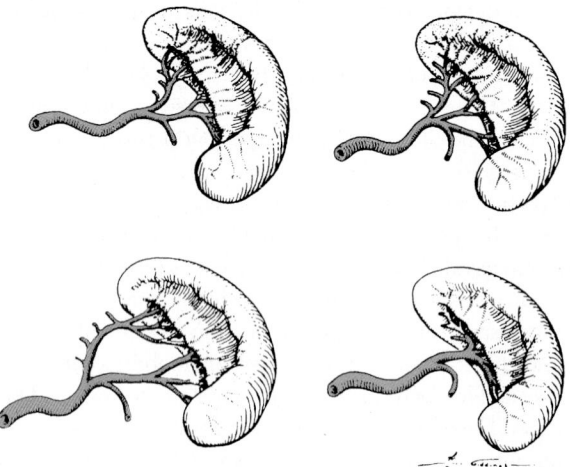

**FIGURE 33-3.** The arterial blood supply to the spleen can be quite variable. The most common configuration consists of two extraparenchymal divisions of the splenic artery (upper left figure).

The other sources of arterial blood supply for the spleen are the short gastric vessels that connect the left gastroepiploic artery and the splenic circulation along the greater curvature of the stomach. There are an average of four to six short gastric arteries. As implied by their name, these branches off the greater curvature are generally fairly short and are easily injured during mobilization of the spleen.

The venous drainage of the spleen, like the arterial inflow, is also via two routes. The splenic vein drains the spleen via a number of branches that coalesce to form a single large vein that courses along the posterior aspect of the body and tail of the pancreas to its confluence with the superior mesenteric vein. Like venous anatomy elsewhere in the body, the splenic vein location, size, and branches can be quite variable. The other route of splenic venous drainage is via short gastric veins that course adjacent to the short gastric arteries. They drain into the left gastroepiploic vein during its course along the greater curvature of the stomach.

## PATHOPHYSIOLOGY OF INJURY

Bleeding should always be the initial concern in patients with splenic injury, as patients with splenic injury can bleed to death. Although nonoperative management is often appropriate after splenic injury, in many instances patients with splenic injury still need emergency surgery to stop the bleeding. In a large multi-institutional survey, approximately 45% of splenic injury patients required emergency surgery.[17] A recent prospective study revealed that 33% of even isolated blunt splenic injuries require immediate operation and a further 23% in that study treated with initial nonoperative management required operation, for an overall 56% operative rate for isolated blunt splenic injury.[18] Overall operative rates vary depending on setting, with higher operative rates for rural and nonteaching hospitals.[19] The rate also varies when comparing large multi-institutional series with single institutional series. Regardless of the setting, however, it is clear that rapid operative intervention is sometimes necessary. This is particularly true when patients have coagulopathy either from preinjury anticoagulation or as a consequence of their injury.

Bleeding can also be a problem on a delayed basis.[20,21] The concept of "delayed rupture" of the spleen is in some ways a misnomer. The initial notion that the spleen could bleed on a delayed basis dates back to an era before abdominal CT scanning. In that era, it was observed that some patients who had suffered a traumatic injury did not manifest overt bleeding from their spleen for a number of days or sometimes even weeks or months after the traumatic event. With the advent of abdominal CT scanning, it became apparent that these were probably cases of "delayed bleeding" rather than of delayed rupture. The distinction between these two entities is more than academic. If "delayed rupture" of the spleen can occur without much evidence of preexisting injury, CT scanning of the abdomen shortly after injury would be negative. In this case, there would be no good way to screen patients and make sure that they were not at risk for delayed splenic bleeding. In contrast, if what used to be called *delayed rupture* is actually just *delayed bleeding*, early diagnosis of the presence of the splenic injury should allow us to tailor our management such that the risk of the delayed bleeding is minimized.

Penetrating injuries to the spleen are most commonly managed operatively, often because of concerns about associated intraperitoneal injuries. Concerns about injury to the diaphragm from the knife or bullet is also a common rationale for operative intervention in patients with penetrating injury to the spleen. Operative intervention, of course, does not mandate splenectomy after penetrating injury any more than it does after blunt injury although the risk of major arterial disruption after penetrating trauma is somewhat higher than after blunt trauma. Attempts at splenic salvage are sometimes appropriate after penetrating splenic injury, especially if the grade of injury is low and associated injuries are not particularly severe.

## INITIAL EVALUATION AND MANAGEMENT

As with any other trauma patient, the initial management of the patient with splenic injury should follow the airway, breathing, and circulation (ABCs) of trauma resuscitation (see Chap.11). A particularly important general comment relative to initial resuscitation is that it is important to recognize refractory shock early and treat it with an appropriate operative response (see Chap. 13). There are some aspects of the initial evaluation, with respect to the spleen, that deserve special mention.

*Highlights for Management:*

1. The possibility of an additional intra-abdominal injury in patients with splenic injury seen on CT scanning should be kept in mind. Bowel injury is of particular concern.

2. While operating on patients with splenic injury, it is important to look for associated injuries, particularly to the left hemidiaphragm and the pancreas.

3. Always mobilize the tail of the pancreas medially with the spleen to optimally expose the splenic hilum and minimize risk to the spleen and pancreas.

4. Despite the fact that nonoperative management of splenic injury is a commonly successful strategy, patients can still bleed to death from splenic injury and a significant percentage of patients still require surgical intervention and splenectomy.

Elements of the history may be helpful in the diagnosis of splenic injury and mechanism of injury is important. In patients injured in a motor vehicle crash, the position of the patient in the car can be of some importance in diagnosing splenic injury. Victims located on the left side of the car (drivers and left rear passengers) are perhaps slightly more susceptible to splenic injury because the left side of their torso abuts the left side of the car. This does not mean, however, that victims in other locations in a vehicle are not also at risk. For patients who have suffered penetrating injury, the type and nature of the weapon is important. When possible, it is helpful to know the caliber of the gun or the length of the knife (see Chap. 7).

In the initial history taking, it is important to note any previous operations the patient has undergone. Of particular importance are any operations that may have resulted in splenectomy (i.e., previous operations for hematologic disease or abdominal trauma). Any pre-existing conditions that might predispose the spleen to enlargement or other abnormality should also be ascertained if possible.

The patient or significant others should be asked also about the presence of liver disease, ongoing anticoagulation, or a recent history of aspirin or nonsteroidal anti-inflammatory drugs.

On physical examination, it is important to determine if the patient has left rib pain or tenderness. Left lower ribs are particularly important in that they overlie the spleen, especially posteriorly. Approximately 14% of patients with left lower rib tenderness will have a splenic injury. Even with left lower rib tenderness as their only indication of possible abdominal injury, 3% of patients will have a splenic injury.[22] In children, the plasticity of the chest wall allows for severe underlying injury to the spleen without the presence of overlying rib fractures. Such a phenomenon is also possible in adults but is less common than it is in children.

The absence of significant physical examination evidence of left lower rib fractures does not preclude the presence of an underlying splenic injury and in some cases may not be related to an altered level of consciousness from associated head injury or intoxication. In the elderly in particular, rib fractures may not manifest in a fashion similar to that seen in younger patients. Patients over the age of 55 may not describe lower rib pain and may not have particularly noteworthy findings on physical examination in spite of severe chest wall trauma and an underlying splenic injury.

Another physical examination finding that is occasionally helpful in the presence of splenic injury is the presence of Kehr's sign. Kehr's sign is the symptom of pain near the tip of the left shoulder secondary to pathology below the left hemidiaphragm. There is minimal shoulder tenderness and the patient typically does not hurt upon range of motion of the left arm and shoulder unless there is an associated musculoskeletal injury. Kehr's sign after splenic injury is the result of irritation of the diaphragm by subphrenic blood. The innervation of the left hemidiaphragm comes from cervical roots 3, 4, and 5, the same cervical roots that innervate the tip of the shoulder. Referred pain from the diaphragmatic irritation thereby causes left shoulder pain. Although it is relatively uncommon, the presence of Kehr's sign shortly after trauma should increase the index of suspicion for splenic injury.

The physical examination of the abdomen sometimes demonstrates localized tenderness in the left upper quadrant or generalized abdominal tenderness, but not all patients with splenic injury will reliably manifest peritoneal or other findings on physical examination. Ecchymoses or abrasions in the left upper quadrant may also be present. The unreliability of the physical examination of the abdomen is obvious in patients with altered mental status. Physical exam findings may also be absent, however, in patients with normal mentation. As a consequence, imaging of the abdomen in hemodynamically stable patients has become an important element of diagnosis and management (see Chap. 30).

The usual initial laboratory studies should be done as in any other trauma patient. There are no laboratory studies specific to patients with splenic injury, although a hematocrit and typing and crossmatching of blood are useful initial laboratory tests. Coagulation studies may be warranted if there is reason to believe that patients are coagulopathic. As with all other early posttraumatic bleeding, bleeding from a splenic injury in the early postinjury period will not always manifest itself as a marked drop in hematocrit. An extremely low hematocrit on arrival of the patient in the resuscitation room, however, especially if the transport has been short and prehospital fluid resuscitation has been minimal, should alert the surgeon to the possibility of severe ongoing hemorrhage (see Chap. 11).

Plain x-rays generally are not helpful in the diagnosis of splenic injury. Left hemidiaphragm ruptures are sometimes apparent on an initial chest x-ray and can suggest an associated splenic injury. A severe pelvic fracture on an anteroposterior pelvic film can sometimes be of importance in subsequent decision-making about how to manage splenic injuries; the presence of simultaneous splenic and severe pelvic injuries often will dictate the removal of the spleen (see Chap. 38). When penetrating trauma is the mechanism of injury, an initial chest x-ray is important in ruling out associated thoracic injury and, in the case of gunshot wounds, helping to determine the path of bullets and the location of retained bullets or bullet fragments.

## IMAGING AND DIAGNOSTIC PERITONEAL LAVAGE

Diagnostic peritoneal lavage (DPL), once a mainstay diagnostic technique after abdominal trauma, is much less frequently used now. Its role as an initial diagnostic maneuver to dictate subsequent testing or operative intervention has been supplanted in many institutions by both ultrasonography and CT scanning of the abdomen (see Chap. 30). Peritoneal lavage remains useful when ultrasonography is not available, however, in that it is a quick way of determining whether or not a hemodynamically unstable patient is bleeding intraperitoneally. Although DPL is not specific for splenic injury, splenic injuries with ongoing bleeding result in positive peritoneal lavage most of the time and lavage can prompt timely operative intervention. When there is an associated diaphragmatic injury, however, diagnostic peritoneal lavage may not yield positive results. Because the instilled fluid may be retained in the pleural space, a diaphragmatic injury should be considered when the DPL yields little or no return of fluid.

Ultrasound of the abdomen for free fluid, the so-called FAST exam, is being used increasingly as a means of diagnosing hemoperitoneum in blunt trauma patients (see Chap. 17). Like DPL, it is most useful in unstable patients. Also, as with peritoneal lavage, the ability of ultrasound to determine exactly what is bleeding in the peritoneal cavity is limited. Small injuries and subcapsular hematomas of the spleen can also be missed by ultrasonography if they do not result in significant hemoperitoneum. There have been attempts to use ultrasound not only to diagnose intraperitoneal fluid but also to diagnose specific injuries such as splenic injuries. Such attempts have met with limited success. It is possible that with improving technology our ability to diagnose specific injuries will improve. As of today, however, the most common method of using FAST exams is for detection of intraperitoneal fluid and as a determinant of the need for either further imaging of the abdomen or for emergency surgery.

CT of the abdomen is the dominant means of nonoperative diagnosis of splenic injury. Patients are sent either directly for abdominal CT scanning after initial resuscitation or are screened by abdominal ultrasonography as reasonable candidates for subsequent CT. When abdominal CT scanning is done, intravenous contrast is quite helpful in diagnosis; oral contrast is much less helpful and does not increase the sensitivity of CT for splenic injury detection.

The findings of splenic injury on CT scan are variable (Fig. 33-4). Hematomas and parenchymal disruption generally show up as hypodense areas. Free fluid can be seen either around the spleen or

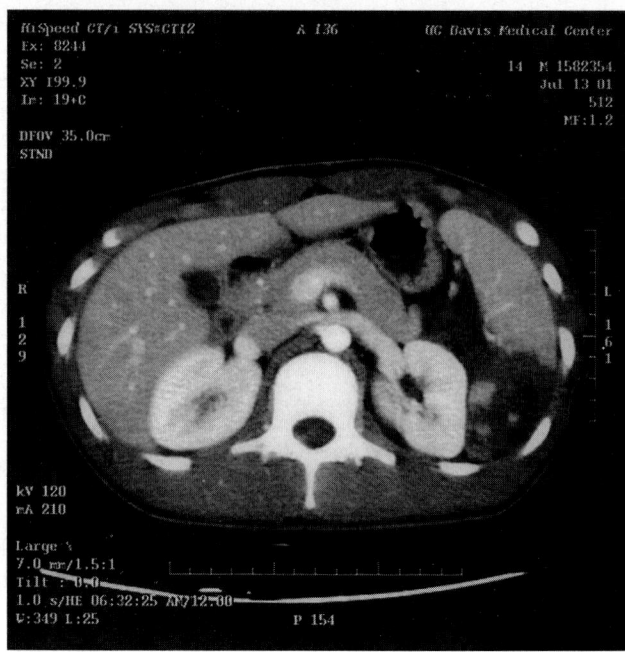

**FIGURE 33-4.** Computed tomographic findings in a patient with a ruptured spleen. The posterior splenic parenchyma is disrupted, and there is some surrounding blood and hematoma. There is also the suggestion of a splenic "blush" in the disrupted parenchyma.

throughout the peritoneal and pelvic spaces. It is particularly important to look in the pelvis, as this is the most dependent portion of the peritoneal cavity in patients who are supine. Other locations where fluid frequently accumulates after splenic injury are Morison's pouch and the paracolic gutters. When a large amount of fluid is present in the peritoneal cavity, it can sometimes be seen between loops of small bowel as well as in the subphrenic spaces.

When looking at CT scans of patients with splenic injury, it is also important to look at the adjacent left kidney and the distal portions of the pancreas. Injury to the spleen implies a blow to the left upper quadrant that can also injure the adjacent organs. The diagnosis of a pancreatic injury is particularly important in that this can significantly affect the patient's subsequent course and prognosis. It is also important to remember that the presence of free fluid is not in all cases solely related to bleeding from a visible splenic injury. One of the pitfalls of CT diagnosis is that free fluid in the peritoneal cavity or in the pelvis may be attributed to a splenic injury when in fact the fluid is secondary to both a splenic injury and an associated mesenteric or bowel injury.

A CT finding in the spleen that has received some attention is the presence in the disrupted splenic parenchyma of a "blush," or hyperdense area with a concentration of contrast in it. When seen, a blush is thought to represent ongoing bleeding with active extravasation of contrast. There is increasingly convincing evidence that the presence of a blush correlates with an increased likelihood of arterial injury. The arterial injury may result in continued or delayed bleeding. Contained hematomas may form psuedoaneurysms. These arterial injuries need further assessment with either angiography or repeat CT scanning.

In addition to the above findings, incidental findings are occasionally seen on CT. Incidental findings in the spleen are rare, with the most common being cysts and granulomas. Primary cysts are parasitic (rare in the United States), congenital, or neoplastic.

Secondary cysts (those without an epithelial lining) may result from trauma or infarction.

A number of scoring systems have been devised to describe the degree of splenic injury seen on CT scanning.[23–28] Some of these scoring systems will be described in further detail later. It is important to remember, however, that there is not a particularly strong correlation between the grade of splenic injury seen on CT scanning and the grade of splenic injury seen at the time of surgery in those patients who require operative intervention. It is also important to remember that the CT grade of splenic injury and a patient's subsequent clinical course are only roughly correlated.

Magnetic resonance imaging (MRI) has also been used sporadically in the diagnosis of splenic injury (see Chap.16). The images obtained are sometimes quite impressive but, given that CT scanning has both a very high sensitivity and specificity for the presence of splenic injury (especially when newer generation multidetector scanners are used), MRI so far has not proven an obvious improvement. Furthermore, MRI is usually less available than is CT scanning, especially after hours. The logistical difficulties inherent in trying to obtain magnetic resonance images in a badly injured patient who requires close monitoring and possibly even mechanical ventilation make MRI even less helpful as a means of splenic injury diagnosis. Continued improvements in MRI and our increasing ability to use it even for very sick patients could conceivably increase the role of MRI in the diagnosis of splenic injury in the future.

Radioisotope scintigraphy has also been used in the diagnosis of splenic injury. Most of the use of radioisotope scintigraphy occurred before the advent of widespread availability of CT scanning, and it is largely of historical interest at this point. Angiography is another test that historically has been used to diagnose splenic injury, and there are even some old reports of the use of angiography for therapy in the case of splenic injury. The description of the blush sign of the spleen seen on CT scanning has revitalized our interest in angiography as a therapeutic maneuver in stable patients with splenic injury.

Laparoscopy has also been tried as a means of diagnosing splenic injury but has not played a major role in the diagnosis or management of the injured spleen. For blunt trauma patients, laparoscopy is not a diagnostic improvement over CT scanning. For penetrating trauma, laparoscopy often misses associated bowel injuries but may have some usefulness in diagnosis and treatment of adjacent injuries to the left hemidiaphragm (see Chap. 30).

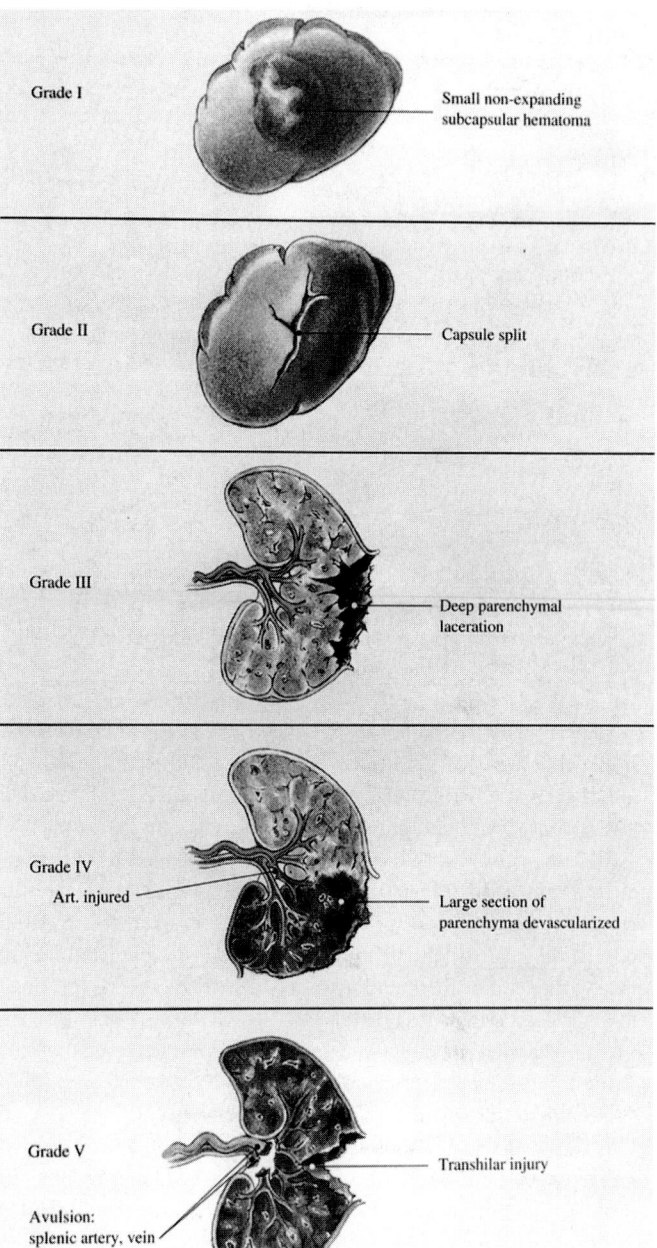

**FIGURE 33-5.** Diagrammatic representation of the splenic organ injury scaling system of the American Association for the Surgery of Trauma. *(Reproduced with permission from Carrico CJ, Thal ER, Weigelt JA, eds.: Operative Trauma Management: An Atlas. Copyright 1998, Appleton & Lange, p. 163.)*

## SPLENIC INJURY GRADING SYSTEMS

A number of different grading systems have been devised to quantify the degree of injury in patients with ruptured spleens.[23–29] These systems have been created based both on the computed tomographic appearance of ruptured spleens as well as the intraoperative appearance of the spleen. Early grading systems included descriptions of the amount of bleeding into the peritoneal cavity as well as attempts to quantify the degree of capsular and parenchymal disruption. The best known splenic grading system is the one created by the American Association for the Surgery of Trauma (AAST) (Fig. 33-5; Table 33-1).[23] As with all of the AAST grading systems, it uses a scale of between 0 and 5.

The CT and intraoperative appearances of a splenic injury are often different from one another. Some of these differences might be because of evolution of the injury between the time of CT scanning and operation, but it is also likely that CT scanning is imperfect in describing the pathologic anatomy of a splenic rupture. Splenic injury scores based on CT scans can both overestimate and underestimate the degree of splenic injury seen at surgery. It is possible to have a CT appearance of fairly trivial injury but at surgery find significant splenic disruption. Conversely, it is possible to see what looks like a major disruption of the spleen on CT scanning and not see the same kind of severity of injury at surgery. In general, the CT scan and associated scores tend, if anything, to

## TABLE 33-1

### The Splenic Organ in Jury Scaling System of the American Association for the Surgery of Trauma, 1994 Revision

| GRADE[a] | | INJURY DESCRIPTION |
|---|---|---|
| I | Hematoma | Subcapsular, <10% surface area |
| | Laceration | Capsular tear, <1 cm parenchymal depth |
| II | Hematoma | Subcapsular, 10–50% surface area, <5 cm In diameter |
| | Laceration | 1–3 cm parenchymal depth that does not involve a trabecular vessel |
| III | Hematoma | Subcapsular, >50% surface area or expanding; ruptured subcapsular or parenchymal hematoma Intraparenchymal hematoma >5 cm or expanding |
| | Laceration | >3 cm parenchymal depth or involving trabecular vessels |
| IV | Laceration | Laceration involving segmental or hilar vessels producing major devascularization (>25% of spleen) |
| V | Laceration | Completely shattered spleen |
| | Vascular | Hilar vascular injury which devascularizes spleen |

[a]Advance one grade for multiple injuries up to grade III.

underestimate the degree of splenic injury compared to what is seen at surgery.[28] Additionally, interrater and intrarater agreement with respect to CT grading of splenic injury is only fair.[30]

An important point about CT-based grading systems is that the patient's subsequent clinical course does not correlate exactly with the degree of injury seen on CT. Although there is a rough correlation between the grade of splenic injury seen on CT scanning and the frequency of operative intervention, exceptions are common. It is possible to have what looks like a fairly trivial injury on CT scan turn out to require delayed operative intervention. In contrast, severe, looking splenic injuries on CT scan quite often follow a benign postinjury course and are successfully managed nonoperatively.

Probably the major usefulness of splenic organ injury grading, especially when the AAST Organ Injury Scale is used, is to allow for objective standardization of terminology and to insure that individual injuries are described in precise terms understandable to others. Standardized organ injury scaling is also useful in research and in describing populations of splenic injury patients. To some extent, they have also been useful in dictating treatment algorithms (Fig.33-6).

## NONOPERATIVE MANAGEMENT

Nonoperative management of splenic injury has become steadily more common over time. Although approximately 40% of patients with splenic injury will require immediate operative intervention, nonoperative management is reasonable for hemodynamically stable patients.[17,18,31]

## PATIENT SELECTION

Appropriate patient selection is the most important element of nonoperative management. Although it is certainly true that nonoperative management is possible in a large number of patients

with splenic injury, emergency surgery is still sometimes necessary to stop life-threatening hemorrhage. Determining which patients require emergency surgery and which can be initially managed nonoperatively is sometimes quite difficult, although hemodynamic status, age, grade of splenic injury, quantity of hemoperitoneum, and associated injuries have been shown to roughly correlate with the success or failure of nonoperative management.[32] Making the right decision is critically important and, as part of the decision-making process, it should never be forgotten that patients with splenic injury can bleed to death.

Of paramount importance in the determination of the appropriateness of nonoperative management is the hemodynamic stability of the patient. *Hemodynamic stability* can be a somewhat illusory concept and one for which there is no consensus definition, but hypotension (systolic blood pressure <90 mm Hg in an adult) is generally considered to be worthy of concern. Prehospital or emergency department hypotension is worrisome, and a high index of suspicion for ongoing hemorrhage should be maintained when either is present. Patients who have been hemodynamically unstable in the prehospital phase and remain hemodynamically unstable during their initial emergency department stay are, in most instances, inappropriate candidates for abdominal CT scanning. They require either a direct trip to the operating room (OR) or, more commonly, abdominal ultrasonography or DPL to help guide the initial decision-making process (see Chap. 30).

Assuming hemodynamic stability, the other important prerequisite for consideration of nonoperative management is the patient's abdominal examination. In patients who are awake and alert and can cooperate with a physical exam and provide feedback, it is important that they should not have diffuse, persistent peritonitis. Although patients with splenic injury often will have abdominal findings secondary to intraperitoneal blood and localized pain and tenderness in the left upper quadrant are quite common, obvious diffuse peritoneal signs can be a sign of intestinal injury and warrants abdominal exploration. If a patient with splenic injury is sent for CT scanning and subsequent nonoperative management, it is important to continue to follow the physical examination. If the exam worsens, the possibility of a blunt intestinal injury should be increasingly considered. The most common CT finding in patients with blunt intestinal injury is free fluid in the peritoneal cavity. In patients with splenic injury, the free fluid can be mistakenly attributed solely to the splenic injury, and the presence of an associated bowel injury can be missed; the physical examination becomes of even greater importance in such circumstances.

The success rates of nonoperative management of splenic injury are truly impressive in many of the published series. Reported success rates for nonoperative management are 95% or higher for pediatric patients and approximately 80% or higher in adults.[29,33–43] These high success rates can be misleading, however, in that they apply only to the group of patients in whom nonoperative management was chosen rather than all patients with splenic injury. When immediate splenectomy patients are included, the overall splenic salvage rates tend to be at best around 50–60% in adult patients. It is also important to remember that these series generally do not include patients in whom the initial impetus was for nonoperative management but in whom emergency surgery was necessary when the patient got into trouble either in the emergency department or upon viewing the CT scanner. The published

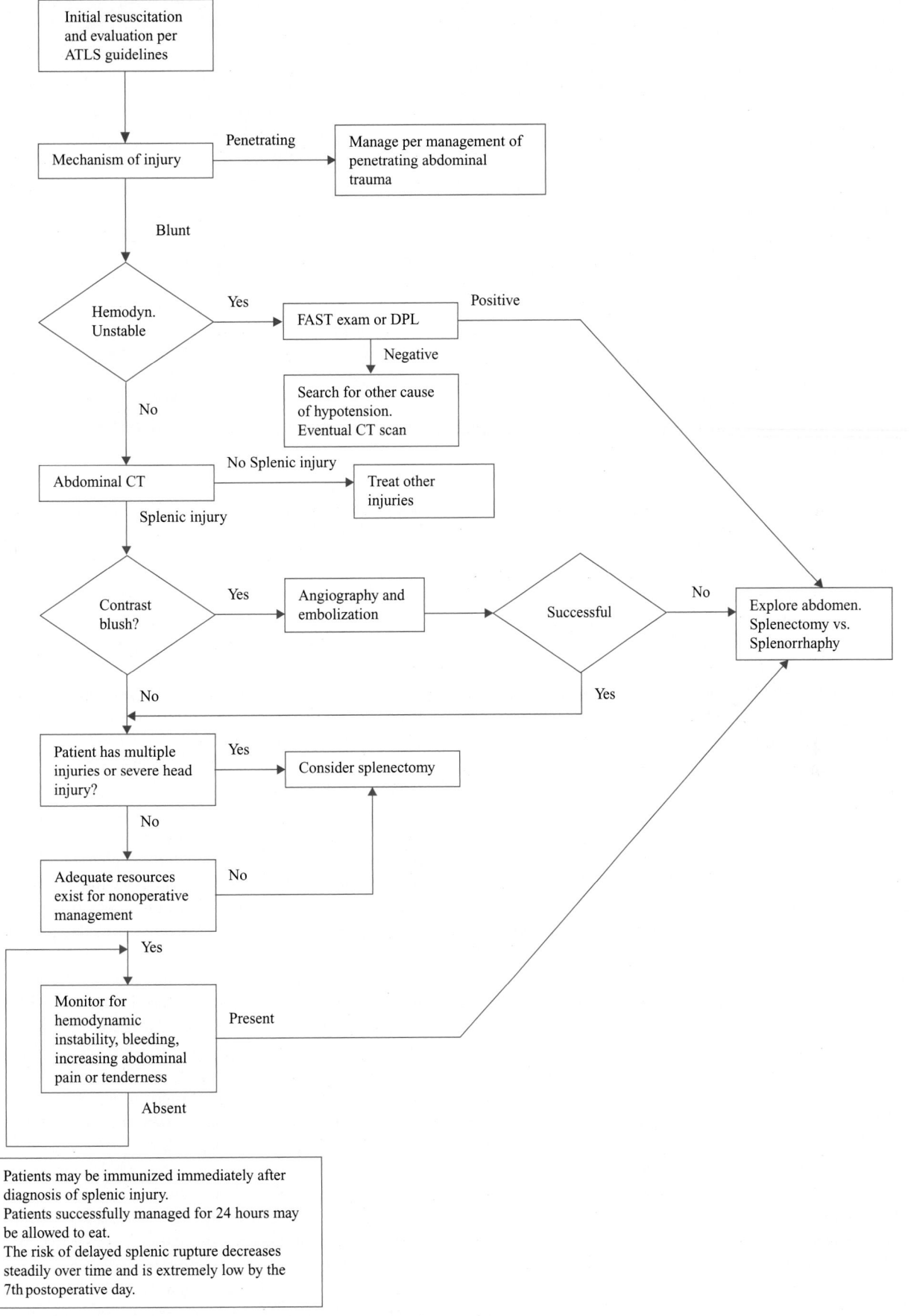

**FIGURE 33-6.** Algorithm for the diagnosis and management of splenetic injury.

series of nonoperatively managed spleens generally include only patients who were stable enough to undergo CT scanning of the abdomen and in whom the CT scan showed a ruptured spleen. It could be argued that this is a select group. Patients who become unstable either before or during the scan and were taken emergently to surgery are usually not counted as patients who underwent "nonoperative" management. In fact, these patients generally when they are reported at all are placed into the "operative" group rather than into the "failed nonoperative" group. This group is admittedly small but is important. It should never be assumed that all splenic injuries can be managed nonoperatively; some patients need to go directly from the resuscitation room to the OR without first having had a CT scan of their ruptured spleen. Finally, the literature on the success of nonoperative management of splenic injury should be interpreted with the awareness that publication bias tends to favor series in which success rates are high.

Other important considerations beyond hemodynamic stability and abdominal findings in the determination of the appropriateness of nonoperative management have to do with the medical environment and some specific characteristics of the patient. Nonoperative management should only be undertaken if it will be possible to closely follow the patient. If close inpatient follow-up is simply not possible, abdominal exploration may be appropriate. Similarly, if rapid mobilization of the OR and quick operative intervention in the case of ongoing or delayed bleeding is not possible, operative intervention may be appropriate. Finally, the patient's circumstances after discharge occasionally may be important in the decision-making process. For patients who are to be discharged to a location extremely far away from medical care, the consequences of delayed bleeding are somewhat greater in that they may not be close enough to operative intervention. In such circumstances, an otherwise reasonable candidate for nonoperative management might undergo operative intervention.

For patients who are stable enough to undergo CT scanning and in whom a ruptured spleen is seen, nonoperative management is reasonable if they continue to remain stable. In addition to vital signs, one of the other commonly followed parameters in such patients is the hematocrit.[44] A common practice is to determine a cut-off value below which the hematocrit will not be allowed to fall. If the hematocrit drops to that level or below, operative intervention is undertaken. Such an approach works best if there are no associated injuries; when associated injuries are present, it can be quite difficult to know if the spleen is continuing to bleed or if the fall in hematocrit is secondary to bleeding from other injuries.

In general, there is consensus that hemodynamically stable patients without obvious or progressive peritoneal signs who can be followed closely are reasonable nonoperative management candidates. There is some debate, however, about certain subgroups of patients and their appropriateness for nonoperative management.

Pediatric patients are generally excellent candidates for nonoperative management. Because of the trauma mechanisms suffered by pediatric patients as opposed to adult patients, children are more likely to have isolated splenic injuries. The relative thickness of the splenic capsule is also greater in children, perhaps conferring more structural integrity to the spleen. The spleen in children is more likely to fracture parallel to the splenic arterial blood supply rather than transverse to it[45] (Fig. 33-7). This orientation of splenic injury tends to decrease the amount of blood loss from the splenic parenchyma. Children are also more likely to have excellent

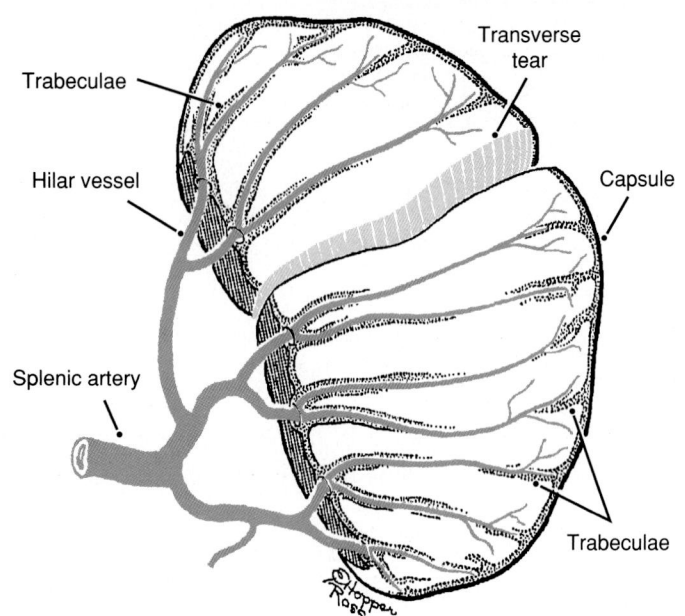

**FIGURE 33-7.** Diagrammatic representation of a transverse laceration relative to the splenic vasculature in a pediatric patient. *(Reproduced with permission from Upadhyaya P: Splenic Trauma in Children. J Am Coll Surg 126:781, 1968.)*

physiologic reserve and minimal pre-existing disease. Finally, the risks of splenectomy with respect to immunologic consequences are thought to be greater in children, especially young children, than they are in adults.[5–8]

There is some evidence that older patients might have a worse prognosis with respect to nonoperative management than do younger patients, and several series have reported that patients older than 55 are less likely to be managed successfully nonoperatively.[46–48] Other series examining the question of the threshold at 55 years of age and nonoperative management suggest the success of nonoperative management is no different in this group than it is in younger patients.[48–50] Although the evidence in this area is somewhat conflicting, one finding from a large multicenter study is that older patients are more likely to fail nonoperative management.[17]

The presence of severe associated injuries, particularly head injury, has been suggested as another relative contraindication to nonoperative management of splenic injury.[47] As has already been pointed out, following the hematocrit in a patient with severe associated injuries can be problematic. Furthermore, there are concerns about the effects of ongoing or delayed splenic bleeding on the prognosis of a severe head injury (see Chap. 20). While these factors do not mandate operative intervention in all patients who fall into these groups they should lower the threshold for operative intervention on an individual basis.[51–53]

There is little uniformity about what constitutes a "failed" attempt at nonoperative management. Different surgeons and different institutions have set different criteria for operative intervention, and much of the decision-making is subjective. As has already been pointed out, there is no perfect relation between the severity of injuries seen on CT scanning and a patient's subsequent success or failure of nonoperative management. Some of this discrepancy is probably related to the imperfect nature of the scoring systems and a lack of sensitivity of CT scanning. It is also likely that some of the differences are in the approach and thresholds for operative intervention. In some instances, concern about a "bad-looking" spleen on a CT scan might prompt more aggressive and quicker surgical intervention and make failed nonoperative management of severe splenic injuries a self-fulfilling prophecy.

An objective finding on CT scan that shows promise as a prognostic sign with respect to nonoperative management is that of a blush in the injured splenic parenchyma.[54–56] Such a blush is thought to represent ongoing bleeding when it is seen shortly after injury and a pseudoaneurysm when seen on later scans. There is evidence that when such a finding is present, the chances of subsequent successful nonoperative management are markedly diminished. A contrast blush seen on initial CT scan should be evaluated with angiography and treated with embolization if ongoing bleeding is present. Contrast blush is associated with a higher need for operative intervention (67% vs. 6% in adults 22% vs. 4% in children).[57,58] This approach seems reasonable as angiography with splenic embolization has improved nonoperative success rates in patients managed nonoperatively. The most dramatic improvement is seen in patients with higher-grade splenic injuries. Available data suggest an improvement in nonoperative success rates from 67% to 83% in grade IV injuries and from 25% to 83% in grade V injuries.[59] A somewhat more extreme approach is to have all patients with splenic injury, with or without a blush, undergo early angiography and embolization as necessary.[60] Most centers do not treat splenic injury in this way because the number of nontherapeutic angiograms with such an approach would be extremely high.

## PATIENT MANAGEMENT

After nonoperative management has been selected, the initial resuscitation should be continued and other diagnostic and therapeutic procedures carried out as necessary. There is little scientific evidence to dictate the specifics of how nonoperative management of splenic injury should be done, and most recommendations are simply matters of common sense and opinion.[45] Most patients should be admitted to an intensive care unit setting for their initial nonoperative management, including those with grade II or above splenic injuries and patients with multiple associated injuries that make following serial hematocrit levels and physical examinations difficult. Exceptions to the intensive care unit admonition are patients who have small, grade I splenic injuries. Even these patients should be initially admitted to an intensive care unit if follow-up in a ward setting will be unreliable.

During initial management patients should be kept with nothing by mouth in case they require rapid operative intervention, most likely necessary in the early postinjury period.[61] Nasogastric suction is not necessary unless needed for other reasons. Whether patients should be kept at bed rest or not is somewhat controversial. Although there are some theoretical reasons why bed rest might be a good idea, there is little empirical evidence that it makes a difference. Early mobilization is generally beneficial for trauma patients and should in general be the practice in patients with splenic injury. Bed rest should only be maintained for a day or two unless there are other reasons for requiring immobility.

Patients should be followed closely hemodynamically and with serial physical examinations. The urine output should be monitored. Serial hematocrits should be obtained and compared with each other as well as with the admission hematocrit. As has been mentioned, changes in hematocrit can be influenced by bleeding from associated injuries as well as by bleeding from a splenic injury; this is important to take into account while following patients. Many surgeons follow the practice of picking a specific hematocrit as a cut-off point below which they will not allow the patient to go without operative intervention. This cut-off point will obviously be influenced by the presence of associated injuries.

Vaccines for meningococcal, streptococcal, and hemophilus infection prevention should be given while the patient is observed nonoperatively. There are some theoretical reasons to believe that the vaccinations are more effective if given while the spleen is still in situ. It is therefore preferable to vaccinate patients who are managed nonoperatively early in their course rather than waiting to vaccinate them after they have required splenectomy. The evidence to support such a practice is somewhat contradictory, and it is very difficult to study the effectiveness of vaccination timing in splenectomy patients because the incidence of overwhelming postsplenectomy sepsis is so low.

How long a patient should remain in the intensive care unit is not clearly defined. Most centers keep patients with splenic injury in the intensive care unit for 24 to 72 hours and then transfer them to a ward bed if they have been stable and other injuries permit. It is also generally at this point that patients are allowed to eat unless other injuries preclude oral intake.

How long a patient should be kept in the hospital is also poorly defined, and there is quite a variety of practice in this regard. There is no strong evidence supporting any particular approach, but a large multi-institutional study showed that most failures of nonoperative management occur within the first six to eight days after injury.[61] Our institutional approach is to keep patients in the hospital for an arbitrary seven days. This approach has obvious financial and insurance implications but will pick up most of the delayed bleeds while the patient is still an inpatient. How long to keep the patient also depends to some extent on the nature of the splenic injury. Clearly, trivial injuries can be safely discharged earlier than more severe injuries. In many circumstances, associated injuries dictate the length of hospitalization more than does the splenic injury. Sometimes it is also important to pay attention to where the patient lives and how close he or she will be to medical attention when deciding about timing of discharge. Patients who live far away and far from medical attention may need to be kept longer.

Deep venous thrombosis prophylaxis can be somewhat difficult in patients with splenic injury who are being followed nonoperatively (see Chap. 61). Sequential compression devices on the lower extremities are always reasonable and should be used routinely. Pharmacologic prophylaxis is more problematic because of concerns about bleeding from the spleen. Early mobilization is important in minimizing thromboembolic complications. After 24–48 hours of successful nonoperative management, it is reasonable, if necessary, to begin deep venous thrombosis prophylaxis in the form of either adjusted-dose heparin or low-molecular-weight heparin. If associated injuries require it, warfarin prophylaxis is also reasonable, beginning approximately one week after injury. It is important to point out that these recommendations are based primarily on common sense rather than on solid data. The rate of clinically significant thromboembolic events in patients with splenic injury and the rate of failure of nonoperative management in anticoagulated patients are both quite low, making prospective study of the risks and benefits of anticoagulation prophylaxis in this patient population difficult to do in a prospective fashion.

The issue of follow-up CT scans in patients with nonoperatively managed splenic injuries is also controversial.[28,62–66] Most series indicate that either they are not necessary or that the frequency with which they alter management is extremely low. A variety of different suggestions have been made in the literature about follow-up CT scans, ranging from no follow-ups at all to follow-ups at frequent intervals. A middle course is taken by some surgeons who only study the spleen with a follow-up CT scan when they are contemplating allowing patients to return to contact sports or other activities that are high risk for spleen injury. The author's institutional policy is to study only patients who have persistent abdominal signs and symptoms after a week of observation. On occasion such patients have developed pseudoaneurysms of the spleen, even if the initial CT scan did not demonstrate a blush. It is difficult to know exactly what the natural history of these pseudoaneurysms would be if left untreated, but they can be impressive in appearance and are amenable to angiographic embolization.

When patients are discharged, they should be counseled not to engage in contact sports or other activities where they might suffer a blow to the torso. The best length of time to maintain this admonition is unknown, but typical recommendations range from two to six months. There is experimental evidence that most injured spleens have not recovered their normal integrity and strength until at least six to eight weeks postinjury,[66] so the recommendation to avoid contact sports for two to six months seems reasonable. Other than with respect to contact sports, there are no major restrictions for patients who have undergone successful nonoperative management.

## OPERATIVE MANAGEMENT

In general, preoperative antibiotics should be given but do not need to be continued in the postoperative period unless dictated by associated injuries (see Chap. 30). Gastric decompression with a nasogastric or orogastric tube is important to decrease the volume of the stomach and allow for easier visualization and mobilization of the spleen. It is important to remember to tell the anesthesiologists not only to place a nasogastric or orogastric tube if one has not already been placed but also to remind them that the tube should be kept on continuous suction.

A midline incision is the best incision for splenic injury surgery as well as most trauma operations on the abdomen. It is versatile, can be extended easily both superiorly and inferiorly, and is also the quickest incision if speed of intervention is important. For operations on an injured spleen, it is often helpful to extend the incision superiorly and to the left of the xiphoid process. This maneuver improves exposure of the left upper quadrant, particularly in large patients and those with a narrow costal angle.

Left upper quadrant transverse incisions occasionally have been suggested for isolated splenic injury. Such an incision should rarely be used. In the case of early operative intervention after injury, a midline incision is preferable because it is more versatile, is quicker, and is more likely to be able to allow the surgeon to deal with a variety of different intra-abdominal findings. If the patient has failed nonoperative management, it is important to

rule out occult-associated injuries, and this is best done through the midline. Even in patients who have failed nonoperative management on a delayed basis and patients in whom it is very unlikely that there is associated occult injury, rapid entry into the abdomen is often important and is best accomplished through a midline incision. One situation in which a left subcostal approach may be the incision of choice is when the patient is morbidly obese and preoperative CT scanning has indicated isolated splenic injury only.

As with all trauma celiotomies, it is important to rapidly examine all four quadrants of the abdomen in patients who are grossly unstable hemodynamically. The upper quadrants should be packed. This initial investigation of the abdomen should not be definitive and should be used only for a quick look at all four quadrants and for packing. Definitive management of any injuries found should not be attempted until the entire abdomen has been investigated. While the quadrants are being inspected, it is helpful to look for clotting. Clotting tends to localize to the site of injury, whereas defibrinated blood will spread diffusely in the abdomen. Clotted blood will therefore often indicate the site of an injury and is helpful in determining where to direct definitive management efforts after the abdomen has been packed.

After the upper abdomen has been packed, it should be inspected in a serial fashion with initial emphasis on areas demonstrating the clot during the initial packing maneuver. In patients who are thought to have an isolated splenic injury based on initial imaging or failed nonoperative management, direct attention can be turned sooner to the left upper quadrant. If viscera other than the spleen seem to be more badly injured and are bleeding more profusely than the spleen, the spleen should necessarily take second priority and be left packed until it is appropriate to attend to it. In comparison, a quick splenectomy is often a wise early move in a patient with multiple serious injuries in that it rapidly eliminates the spleen as a source of ongoing blood loss.

Once attention has been directed to the left upper quadrant, all the structures in that quadrant should be inspected (Fig. 33-2). There should be an initial look at the greater curvature of the stomach and the left hemidiaphragm. The left hemidiaphragm also should be reinspected once the spleen is mobilized if mobilization is necessary. Inspection of the hemidiaphragm is of obvious importance in penetrating trauma patients but is also very important in blunt trauma patients so that an injury is not missed, including iatrogenic injuries that could have been made during splenic mobilization. If the left hemidiaphragm is ruptured in a blunt trauma patient and the spleen is in the left side of the chest, it should be pulled down into the abdomen through the defect. The left lobe of the liver and left kidney should also be inspected as should the tail of the pancreas. If the spleen is to be mobilized, inspection of the tail of the pancreas is easier after mobilization has been accomplished.

The anterior and anterolateral surfaces of the spleen can sometimes be seen fairly easily through the midline incision prior to any splenic mobilization, particularly if the patient is thin and there is a wide costal margin. If the patient is heavy and/or the costal margin is narrow, adequate inspection without some splenic mobilization may be very difficult. If the left upper quadrant is adequately inspected and there is no evidence of any bleeding or splenic injury, the spleen does not require mobilization. If it is known that there is a small splenic injury, but splenic injury is not the primary reason for abdominal exploration or the spleen does not seem to be bleeding at the time of exploration, splenic mobilization is not always necessary. Mobilization of the spleen certainly provides better visualization of any injuries present but is associated with the risk of worsening or "stirring up" the splenic injury. Determining whether or not to mobilize the spleen is a judgment call, but if in doubt, the best thing to do is to mobilize the spleen so that the full extent of injury is elucidated and the spleen can be repaired or removed as necessary. It is important to be as gentle as possible during mobilization of the spleen so that the splenic injury is not worsened.

Splenic mobilization should be done in a stepwise fashion, and a stepwise approach helps in providing adequate mobilization while minimizing the chance of increased injury. Proper mobilization also allows for better visualization of the left kidney, the left hemidiaphragm, and the posterior aspects of the body and tail of the pancreas. The sequence of splenic mobilization is also important in that it allows for splenic salvage and splenorrhaphy up until the final step of hilar ligation.

In mobilizing the spleen, it is important to remember how posteriorly it is situated (Fig. 33-2). It is also important to remember that there is a great deal of variability in the length of the different ligaments around the spleen and therefore in how mobile the spleen is before any dissection is done. If mobilization is done correctly, even spleens with fairly short surrounding ligaments and spleens in obese patients can be mobilized to a level at or above the anterior abdominal wall.

The first step in mobilization of the spleen is to cut the lateral attachments of the spleen, the splenophrenic and splenorenal ligaments (Fig. 33-8). This step should be started with sharp dissection and can then be continued with a combination of blunt dissection and further sharp dissection. The dissection should be taken up to near the level of the esophageal hiatus so that all the lateral and superior attachments are cut. Cutting the lateral attachments is sometimes facilitated by putting a finger or clamp underneath them and then sharply developing the underlying plane. In large patients and in those with a spleen that is very posterior, it may be necessary to do some of the sharp dissection by feel.

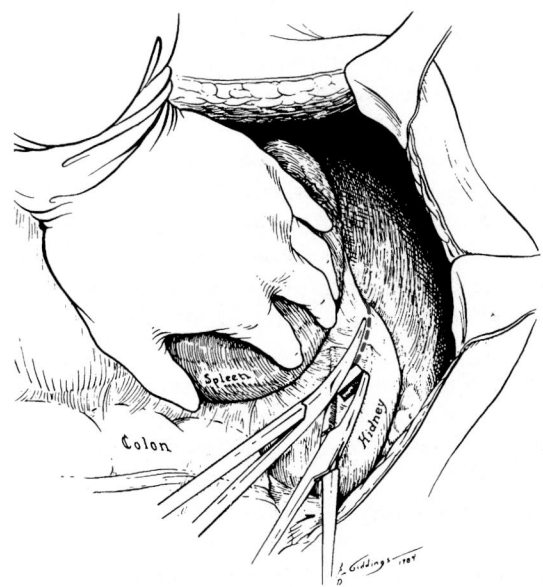

**FIGURE 33-8.** Mobilization of the spleen is begun by early division of its lateral attachments.

After the lateral attachments have been divided, the next step is to mobilize the spleen and tail of the pancreas as a unit from lateral to medial. One of the easier ways to do this is to place the back of the fingernails of the right hand underneath the spleen and tail of the pancreas so that they are adjacent to the underlying left kidney. The kidney can be palpated easily because it is quite hard and provides an excellent landmark for the proper plane of dissection. A common error is to try to mobilize the spleen alone without the adjacent pancreas. Not mobilizing the pancreas with the spleen is easy to do if the surgeon is not posterior enough and is not in the plane between the tail of pancreas and kidney. If the tail of the pancreas is not mobilized with the spleen, the degree of splenic mobilization possible is much more limited and it is also more difficult to avoid injury to the spleen or tail of the pancreas. The splenic hilum can be damaged from behind as the surgeon's fingers attempt mobilization from lateral to medial. The pancreas is more difficult to see if it is not mobilized with the spleen and can be damaged during hilar clamping if the spleen is to be removed. The pancreas is quite variable in length and therefore requires varying degrees of mobilization. In patients with a very short pancreas, very little pancreas, if any, requires mobilization to adequately mobilize the spleen. Conversely, if the pancreas is fairly long, a great deal of its body and tail will require mobilization in order to bring the spleen anteriorly and to the midline.

After the spleen and pancreas have been mobilized as a unit, it is generally apparent that the next constraining attachments of the spleen are the short gastric vessels. Because of the dual blood supply of the spleen through its hilum and also through the short gastric vessels, it is possible to divide the short gastric vessels without compromising splenic viability. The best way to divide the short gastric vessels is to have an assistant elevate the spleen and tail of the pancreas into the operative field and then to securely clamp the vessels starting proximally on the greater curvature of the stomach. The short gastric vessels should always be clamped and tied. They can be small and difficult to see, and it is tempting to simply divide the loose tissue between the spleen and stomach with the scissors or electrocautery. This should not be done, as the short gastric vessels can then bleed either immediately or on a delayed basis. The short gastric vessels, as the name implies, are short. It is therefore not uncommon to be concerned about a clamp on the gastric portion of a short gastric vessel having included a small portion of stomach. In such cases, the tie on the short gastric vessels and nubbin of stomach can necrose the stomach, leading to a delayed gastric leak. This concern can be addressed by oversewing the short gastric tie on the stomach side with a series of Lembert sutures in the seromuscular layer of the stomach.

The final step necessary for full mobilization of the spleen is division of the splenocolic ligamentous attachments between the lower pole of the spleen and the distal transverse colon and splenic flexure. Obvious vessels in these ligamentous attachments should be divided between clamps. During division of both the short gastric vessels and the splenocolic ligament, bleeding from the spleen can be controlled using digital compression of the hilum. If the patient is exsanguinating and the bleeding is massive, occasionally a clamp can be placed on the hilum during the later steps of mobilization. Mass clamping should only be done in extreme circumstances because it increases the chances of injury to the tail of the pancreas; digital compression is preferred.

After the spleen has been fully mobilized, it is possible to inspect it in its entirety. It is also possible to examine the posterior aspect of the body and tail of the pancreas. It is helpful after mobilization to pack the splenic fossa to tamponade any minor bleeding and also to help keep the spleen and distal pancreas elevated into the field. During this packing maneuver, the left adrenal gland can be inspected and the left hemidiaphragm reexamined.

What to do with the spleen after it has been mobilized is a matter of judgment. Factors that figure into the decision about what to do include the degree of splenic injury as well as the overall condition of the patient and the presence of any other intra-abdominal injuries. Obviously, if the spleen is not injured at all, it should be left in place. Similarly, if there is a trivial injury to the spleen and it is not bleeding, the spleen can be simply returned to the left upper quadrant and no further therapy is necessary. If there is a grade I injury of the spleen that is bleeding minimally or not bleeding at all, hemostatic agents can be used to stop the bleeding or forestall any future bleeding. A variety of hemostatic agents are available. These include microfibrillar collagen, gelatin sponge, and fibrin glue. Whichever agent is chosen, the bleeding from the spleen should have ceased by the time the patient is closed.

If the injury is more severe (grades II and III) and the patient's overall condition is not too serious, splenorrhaphy can be done.[68–70] Splenorrhaphy has become somewhat less common with the increasing popularity of nonoperative management. Because we are no longer operating as much on the spleen, especially for lower grades of splenic injury, the number of splenic injuries found at surgical intervention that are amenable to splenorrhaphy has decreased, as has our experience with splenorrhaphy. The simplest version of splenorrhaphy has already been described earlier and is the placement of topical agents. Electrocautery of the spleen is only rarely helpful and has met with limited success. Argon beam coagulators have shown promise in animal models of splenic injury[71,72] and may be helpful for hemostasis, especially of parenchyma that has been denuded of splenic capsule. The spleen can also be sutured, especially when there is an intact capsule, but it does not hold sutures particularly well and it is advisable therefore to use pledget materials to bolster the repair. Several different methods for suturing the spleen have been described, and use of monofilament suture has some advantages in that it is less likely to cause injury while being placed through the splenic parenchyma. The repair sutures should not be pulled too tight. The splenic parenchyma is fairly soft even in the presence of an intact capsule, and it is easy to cinch the suture so tightly that the parenchyma is further disrupted.

Partial splenectomy also has been described and is possible because of the segmental nature of the splenic blood supply. A pole or even half of the spleen can be removed and the remaining spleen will survive provided that its hilar blood supply is left intact. One method of performing partial splenectomy is to ligate the blood supply to the damaged portion of the spleen and then observe the spleen for its demarcation into viable and nonviable portions. The damaged nonviable portion is removed, and the resultant cut splenic parenchyma is made hemostatic with the use of either sutures or mesh wrapping.

Wrapping of either all or part of an injured spleen with absorbable mesh has also been used on occasion. These techniques are moderately time-consuming but reported success rates are high, in part, because of careful patient selection. Such an approach should be reserved for highly selected cases of isolated splenic injury in extremely stable patients.

If the abdomen has been explored, splenectomy should be done in patients who are unstable or who have serious associated injuries. It should also generally be done for the highest grades of splenic injury (grades IV to V) if operative management has been chosen. Bleeding from the splenic parenchyma can be temporarily controlled with digital pressure on the hilum while the spleen has been mobilized; mass clamping of the hilum should be reserved for extremely tenuous cases in that it increases the risk of damage to the adjacent pancreatic tail. If the decision has been made to remove the spleen, this is best done with serial dissection and division of the hilar structures. Suture ligation should be used for large vessels and it is important to ligate arterial and venous branches separately to avoid creation of arteriovenous fistulae. As mentioned in the section *Splenic Anatomy*, usually a number of different splenic artery and vein branches must be divided to complete hilar division (Fig. 33-7). During the course of this dissection, it is not uncommon to encounter accessory spleens, as the most common location for accessory splenic tissue is in the hilum. If accessory spleens are encountered, they should be left in place if possible.

A special circumstance is the patient who has failed nonoperative management. The majority of these patients undergo splenectomy rather than splenorrhaphy.[42,43,45] There are several reasons for the high splenectomy rate in patients who undergo operation after failed nonoperative management. The spleen is somewhat softer after a period of nonoperative management than it was before injury. Both splenic mobilization and splenorrhaphy are therefore more difficult. It is also likely that failed nonoperative splenic injuries are worse than injuries that do not fail nonoperative management. Probably as important as any other factor is that the surgeon operating on a spleen that has failed nonoperative management has already decided that the spleen is a problem and is psychologically prepared for splenectomy at the time of operation. The worst-case scenario for such a surgeon is to perform splenorrhaphy after nonoperative management and have it fail, in which case the patient would require yet another trip to the OR.

As has been mentioned earlier, it is helpful to pack the splenic bed during the latter stages of splenic mobilization and during splenectomy. After the spleen has been removed, the packs in the left upper quadrant should be removed and the splenic fossa reexamined. Inspection of the splenic fossa is facilitated by using a rolled up laparotomy pad. The laparotomy pad is placed deep in the splenic fossa and then rolled by the surgeon's fingers up toward the cut vessels at the splenic hilum. During the course of this inspection, it is important to spread out the laparotomy pad and the greater curvature of the stomach as much as possible to get a good look at the stumps of the short gastric vessels. In addition to looking at the greater curvature, the splenic bed should also be checked for bleeding from the edges of the divided splenic attachments.

Autotransplantation of splenic tissue that has been removed is a controversial topic. It is practiced routinely by some surgeons while other surgeons never autotransplant. Splenic tissue has a remarkable ability to survive in ectopic locations even without a clearly identifiable blood supply. Greater or lesser degrees of spontaneous splenosis after splenectomy for trauma is quite common and patients with splenosis demonstrate some degree of splenic function after splenectomy.[73] The observation that accidentally seeded pieces of splenic tissue could survive and function led to the logical suggestion that portions of the spleen could be intentionally

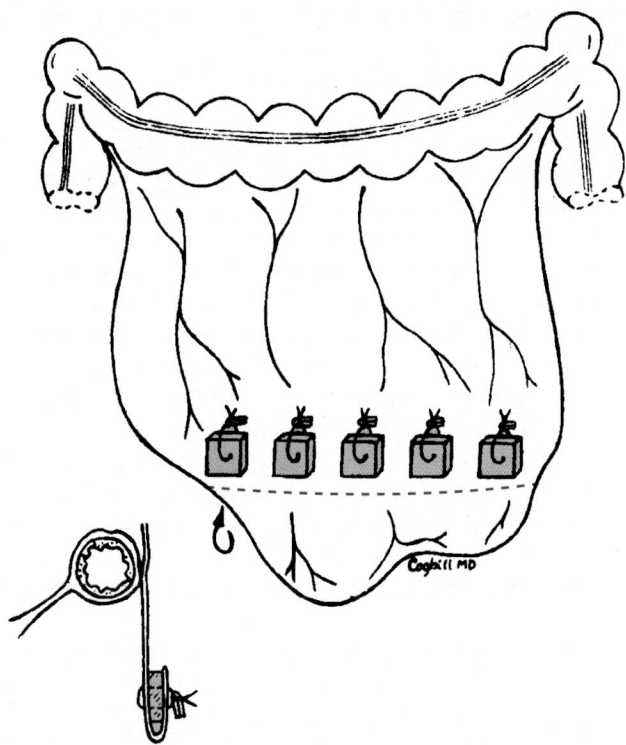

**FIGURE 33-9.** One described method for autotransplantation of splenic tissue is to place small pieces of the spleen into multiple pouches in the greater omentum. *(Reproduced with permission from Millikan JS, Moore EE, Moore GE, et al.: Alternatives to splenectomy in adults after trauma: Repair, partial resection, and reimplantation of splenic tissue. Am J Surg 144:711, 1982.)*

autotransplanted to ectopic sites after splenectomy. Several different methods for autotransplantation of the spleen have been described (Fig. 33-9).[13-15,71-77] One of the more common is to cut the spleen into pieces and place the pieces in omental pouches. Studies of autotransplantation in both animals and humans have demonstrated that some of the splenic tissue survives and has some level of function.[78-80] Whether or not enough of it survives in an adequately functioning form to provide adequate protection against postsplenectomy sepsis is still an open question.[81] Reports of overwhelming infection after autotransplantation suggest that autotransplantation is not universally successful in restoring normal immune function.[82]

Drains should not be routinely placed after either splenectomy or splenorrhaphy as they may actually increase the rate of postoperative complications. Drainage is reasonable if there is associated pancreatic injury or an associated renal injury if there is concern about postoperative urine leak.

## COMPLICATIONS OF SPLENIC INJURY AND MANAGEMENT

### Nonoperative Management

The most common complication of nonoperative management of the spleen is continued bleeding. Many cases of the bleeding are probably just persistent bleeding that never stopped after the original injury. In these circumstances, there is hemodynamic instability or a progressive drop in hematocrit during the first 24 to 48 hours after injury. Although about 60 to 70% of the failures of nonoperative management occur early after admission, many occur on a delayed basis and approximately 10% of the failures occur more than one week after injury.[61]

Early failures of nonoperative management can be determined by closely following the patient's hemodynamic status, hematocrit, and physical examination. In many cases, a drop in hematocrit will be gradual and steady but will ultimately dictate the need for surgical intervention. In other cases, especially those in which the bleeding is delayed, bleeding can occur rather suddenly and be fairly dramatic. If rapid surgical intervention is not done in such cases, the patient is at risk for exsanguination. The pathophysiology of persistent bleeding after splenic injury and early failure of nonoperative management is fairly easy to understand. The pathophysiology of the more delayed bleeds is less obvious, and there are several hypotheses for why nonoperative management can fail on a delayed basis. One hypothesis relating to subcapsular hematomas of the spleen is that as the blood in the subcapsular hematoma breaks down, the increased osmotic forces pull water into the hematoma. A similar pathophysiology has been described as an explanation for the increase in size of subdural hematomas. As the subcapsular hematoma increases in size, it is at an ever-increasing risk for rupture. Another hypothesis for delayed bleeding from splenic injury is the concept of "remodeling" of the clot in the splenic parenchyma. This hypothesis is based on the observation that the clot undergoes revision and degradation over time. It is possible that as this remodeling process occurs, the initial hemostasis of the splenic injury is lost. The observation that splenic injury can result in intraparenchymal pseudoaneurysms raises the possibility that delayed bleeding could also be the result of pseudoaneurysm rupture.[67-69] Finally, it is simply possible that the damaged spleen, highly vulnerable to further injury, suffers what would otherwise be a minor second blow and starts to bleed again. The "failure" rate for nonoperative management varies from surgeon to surgeon and from institution to institution. The variability of these rates is due in part to the lack of a standardized definition of failure. Some surgeons and institutions have a low threshold for operative intervention after an attempt at nonoperative management, and some have a very high threshold. Interestingly, when studied prospectively with specific definitions for who will be initially managed nonoperatively and who will be deemed a failure of nonoperative management, the success rate for nonoperative management is considerably lower than that seen in retrospective studies.[18] When nonoperative management has failed and the patient requires operative intervention, splenectomy is most often the appropriate maneuver unless there is minimal concern about subsequent bleeding.[61] Another potential complication of nonoperative management of splenic injuries is that an associated intra-abdominal injury that requires operative intervention will be missed.[83-85] This is most commonly a problem for missed injuries of the bowel and pancreas. Bowel injury is particularly troublesome, as often free fluid is the only finding of blunt intestinal injury seen on CT of the abdomen. When splenic injury is present, it is easy to attribute the free fluid to the spleen. If patients are good candidates for nonoperative management of their splenic injury, it is possible to miss the bowel injury and delay needed abdominal exploration. Pancreatic injuries are occasionally missed on initial CT scanning done shortly after injury and can result in serious morbidity or even mortality if not treated in an expeditious fashion (see Chap. 35). The proximity of the tail of the pancreas to the spleen makes the combination of injuries to the two organs a possibility. The frequency with which serious associated injuries are present in patients who are good candidates for nonoperative management is fairly low, at most in the 5–10% range, but the possibility of an injury to either the bowel or the pancreas should always be kept in mind when the decision is made to treat a splenic injury nonoperatively. The physical examination of the abdomen will be helpful in raising the suspicion of a missed injury to either the bowel or the pancreas. DPL, pancreatic enzymes, and repeat abdominal CT scanning can also be helpful in pointing to the possibility of bowel and pancreatic injuries (see Chap. 30).

Failure of nonoperative management is not without negative consequences. In a recent multicenter study of failed nonoperatively managed splenic injuries, approximately 13% of the patients who had failed nonoperative management died, with most of the deaths related to either splenic hemorrhage or other intra-abdominal injuries that were missed. A significant number of the cases of failed nonoperative management could be traced to an inappropriate initial decision to proceed with nonoperative management in hemodynamically unstable patients and/or misinterpretation of diagnostic imaging studies.[86] A possible way of minimizing complications after nonoperative management is to obtain follow-up CT scans of the abdomen. A number of series have pointed out that the yield from such CT scans is extremely low and the patient can simply be followed clinically, whereas other studies have shown that in a small percentage of patients, follow-up CT scans demonstrate pathology serious enough to require intervention.[65,66] The most commonly discovered pathology in such patients are pseudoaneurysms, the detection of which is of therapeutic importance because they are amenable to angiographic embolization (Fig. 33-8). The natural history of such pseudoaneurysms seen on a delayed basis is not known, but, as an extension of what we know about blushes and pseudoaneurysms seen in the early postinjury period, there is reason to be concerned about an increased risk of bleeding in such patients. Splenic cysts and abscesses are other pathologic entities sometimes seen on a follow-up CT scan.[21,86] Cysts often are not apparent until a number of months after injury and are at risk for rupture with further trauma. There is a growing consensus that a series of CT scans in the early postinjury period (within the first several days) is not necessary. The question of whether follow-up CT scans are helpful a week or two after injury or several months after injury is still an open question. As mentioned earlier, CT scans done one or two weeks after injury sometimes reveal a blush in the splenic parenchyma indicative of a pseudoaneurysm.[54,55] Such patients can undergo angiographic embolization of their pseudoaneurysms and presumably will be less likely to bleed on a delayed basis. Routine CT scans done several months after injury are generally not indicated if the patient is doing well clinically, although a reasonable circumstance in which some physicians use them is for patients who desire to return to contact sports or some other activity that would put the spleen at risk.

There are no other complications specific to nonoperative management of the spleen, but pulmonary complications are always possible, especially if there are associated rib fractures. The importance of adequate pain control in such patients is critical (see Chap. 26). Epidural analgesia is quite effective in alleviating chest wall pain, especially if the epidural catheter is placed in a thoracic position. Associated pleural effusions are also possible in patients who are managed nonoperatively, either as a sympathetic effusion because of blood and clot beneath the left hemidiaphragm or as a result of intrathoracic bleeding from fractured ribs.

Deep venous thrombosis is another potential complication after nonoperative management of splenic injury (see Chap. 61). Potentially nonoperatively managed patients are particularly at risk because of the dangers of early postinjury anticoagulation, although there is no firm evidence that the rate of thromboembolic complications is higher in patients with nonoperatively managed splenic injuries. When patients who are being managed nonoperatively develop deep venous thrombosis or pulmonary embolism, it can be difficult to decide what to do. Anticoagulation of the patient puts the spleen at risk, but placement of a caval filter also has its associated problems. Such patients should be managed on a case-by-case basis. Fortunately, these cases are rare in that most clinically obvious thromboembolic problems will not manifest themselves until after the major risk of bleeding from a nonoperatively managed spleen has passed.

Patients who are managed nonoperatively often receive blood products, either because of their splenic injury or because of associated injuries, and there are risks associated with transfusion (see Chap. 14). There is the small risk of blood incompatibility and a mismatch complication. There are also risks of blood-borne diseases, particularly hepatitis. The risk of hepatitis C was at one time a particularly important consideration in the management of splenic injury and was used as an argument for early surgical intervention in an attempt to avoid blood transfusion.[87] Improved methods of Hepatitis C and human immunodeficiency virus testing have made the blood supply safer. Even in the absence of major concerns about disease transmission, however, blood transfusion is not without significant drawbacks. Growing evidence indicates significant immunological effects of transfusion, especially in critically ill and injured patients, so transfusion should be avoided when possible.[88–91]

## POSTOPERATIVE COMPLICATIONS

As with any surgical procedure, there is a risk of bleeding after splenectomy or splenorrhaphy. The risk of bleeding from the splenic parenchyma after splenorrhaphy is obvious. When the spleen has been fully mobilized for splenorrhaphy, there is also a risk of bleeding from the splenic bed or more commonly from the cut short gastric vessels. Postoperative bleeding after splenectomy can be from the splenic bed, the short gastric vessels, or the splenic hilum. As after any operative procedure, it is important to closely follow the patient and to reexplore if postoperative bleeding is suspected. Patients with multiple associated injuries and coagulopathy generally should have undergone splenectomy rather than splenorrhaphy. In these patients, the coagulopathy should be treated, but the possibility of surgical bleeding in the postoperative period should always be entertained when the patient is not doing well.

Gastric distention is also a risk after splenic operations, and gastric decompression is reasonable for a short period of time after either splenectomy or splenorrhaphy. When the short gastric vessels have been cut and ligated, gastric distention can result in loss of a tie on the gastric end of a short gastric vessel and resultant bleeding. Even though this danger may be more theoretical than real, a short period of gastric decompression is probably reasonable.

Necrosis of a portion of the greater curvature of the stomach has also been described, most commonly related to inclusion of a portion of the gastric wall in the ties placed on the gastric side of the cut short gastric vessels (see Chap. 34). The resultant gastric leak contaminates the abdomen, in particular the left upper quadrant, and can lead to abscess formation.

Pancreatic injury is another possible postoperative complication (see Chap. 35). Such injuries can be related either to the original trauma or to iatrogenic injury to the pancreas during mobilization or removal of the spleen. Such pancreatic injuries will manifest as an increase in pancreatic enzymes, poor resolution of the patient's ileus, and a generalized inflammatory state. The diagnosis is made from a combination of clinical and CT findings.

The very rare complication of arteriovenous fistula in the ligated hilum of the spleen has also been described as a risk of splenectomy. The best way to avoid such a complication is to individually ligate as many of the hilar vessels as possible and to avoid mass ligation of the hilar structures if at all possible. A measured approach to hilar ligation is also helpful in avoiding injury to the pancreas.

Thrombocytosis is less common after splenectomy for trauma than it is after splenectomy for other diseases. There is no solid evidence that splenectomy for trauma increases the risk of thromboembolic complications. Deep venous thrombosis prophylaxis should be a standard measure in all trauma patients and should cover whatever theoretical risks might be associated with the transient postsplenectomy thrombocytosis (see Chap. 61).

There is some evidence that postoperative complications in the early postoperative period are more common after splenectomy than they are in patients who do not have their spleens removed.[43,92,93] Evidence is conflicting, however, and a difficulty in reviewing the literature on the subject is that it is hard to standardize the severity of injury in patients who have undergone splenectomy as compared to patients who have not undergone splenectomy. Some of the series that have suggested an increased risk of complications after splenectomy have examined postsplenectomy patients who were sicker than control nonsplenectomized patients. Efforts to establish that there is a higher risk of pulmonary and infectious complications after splenectomy have proven difficult. The most common pulmonary complications are those related to rib fractures and critical illness. Pain control is extremely important when there is associated chest wall trauma, as is good pulmonary hygiene. Pneumonia is relatively common after trauma and laparotomy and whether the incidence of postoperative pneumonia is increased after splenectomy is as yet unclear.

## OVERWHELMING POSTSPLENECTOMY SEPSIS

The first experimental evidence supporting the possibility that the spleen is of immunologic importance dates to 1919, but splenectomy remained the treatment of choice for both iatrogenic and traumatic splenic injuries until just several decades ago. In the early 1950s, it was noticed that neonates with hematologic disease who required splenectomy had a very high subsequent risk of serious infection.[5,6] These infections were often severe and the mortality rate was high. It became clear that an asplenic state in neonates

with hematologic disease was a risk factor for overwhelming infection. From this observation, it was a logical next step to investigate the risk of overwhelming infection in both children and adults who had undergone splenectomy for trauma.[94–97] Several studies suggested that the rate of overwhelming sepsis after splenectomy is increased when compared with a control population of patients who have not had their spleens removed. The actual rate at which overwhelming sepsis in asplenic patients occurs is unknown, but one estimate is a 0.026 lifetime risk for adults and a 0.052 lifetime risk for children,[87] and all the estimates of risk tend to be very low. Not all studies have documented an increased risk of overwhelming, life-threatening sepsis after splenectomy for trauma,[41,98,99] and the risk of bleeding should always be weighed against the risk of overwhelming sepsis when considering the most appropriate treatment of an individual patient with splenic injury. Determining the exact risk of overwhelming postsplenectomy sepsis is problematic because it is so low that good epidemiologic studies of the question are very difficult.

When infection does occur in the asplenic state, encapsulated organisms are the most common microorganisms involved. Pneumococcus and meningococcus are the most common pathogens and pneumonia and meningitis are the most common infections.[7] Because of the inference that overwhelming sepsis is more common after splenectomy, vaccines for pneumococcus and meningococcus as well as several other organisms are recommended for splenectomized patients.[99] There is empiric evidence in both animals and humans that the use of vaccines results in an antibody response, but because the incidence of overwhelming sepsis after splenectomy is so low, it is difficult to prove that the vaccines actually have an impact on postsplenectomy infection and mortality. Nonetheless, they have become the standard of care in patients who have had splenectomy. There are theoretical reasons for giving the vaccines early in the course of patients who are managed nonoperatively so that their immune response to the vaccine will be optimal. In patients who have undergone splenectomy, the exact timing of vaccination is somewhat controversial.[101–102] There are theoretical reasons to wait a few days to vaccinate until the patient has had a chance to get over the initial immunosuppression associated with major injury, but the evidence supporting such a delay is mixed. As with the question of the overall effectiveness of vaccines in preventing postsplenectomy sepsis, study of the optimal timing of vaccination is hampered by the low incidence of overwhelming infection after splenectomy for trauma. Probably the most important thing about vaccination after splenectomy is to remember to vaccinate the patient before hospital discharge. Whether or not patients should be revaccinated and when such revaccination should be done remain open questions. One recommendation based on longitudinal antibody studies in a general group of patients (not just trauma postsplenectomy patients) is for revaccination every six years.

Another measure that has been suggested for postsplenectomy patients is the continuous administration of antibiotics or the provision of a supply of antibiotics to splenectomy patients to be taken at the first sign of infection. When such measures have been tried, studies of patients' compliance with the antibiotic regimen have been discouraging.[103] The exact role of antibiotics in postsplenectomy patients is difficult to ascertain for the same reason that the effectiveness of the vaccines is difficult to prove: The incidence of overwhelming sepsis is quite low, and it is therefore difficult to prove the efficacy of any prophylactic maneuver.

# REFERENCES

1. Aristotle: *Parts of Animals* [Peck AL, trans]. London: Heinemann, 1955, p. 261.
2. Krumbhaar EB: The history of extirpation of the spleen. *New York Med J* 6:232, 1915.
3. Morgenstern L: A history of splenectomy. In Hiatt JR, Phillips EH, Morgenstern L, eds. *Surgical Diseases of the Spleen*. New York, Springer, 1997.
4. Mayo WJ: Principles underlying surgery of the spleen. *JAMA* 54:14, 1910.
5. King H, Shumacker HB: Splenic studies: I. Susceptibility to infection after splenectomy performed in infancy. *Ann Surg* 136:239, 1952.
6. Smith CH, Erlandson M, Schulman I, et al.: Hazard of severe infections in splenectomized infants and children. *J Dis Child* 92:507, 1956.
7. Singer DB: Postsplenectomy sepsis. *Perspect Pediatr Pathol* 1:285, 1970.
8. Sherman R: Perspectives in management of trauma to the spleen: 1979 presidential address, American Association for the Surgery of Trauma. *J Trauma* 20:1, 1980.
9. Robinette CD, Fraumeni JF Jr: Splenectomy and subsequent mortality in veterans of the 1939–45 war. *Lancet* 2: 127, 1977.
10. Lynch AM, Kapila R: Overwhelming postsplenectomy infection. *Infect Dis Clin North Am* 10:693, 1996.
11. Shatz DV, Romero-Steiner S, Elie CM, et al.: Antibody responses in post-splenectomy trauma patients receiving the 23-valent pneumococcal polysac-charide vaccine at 14 versus 28 days postoperatively. *J Trauma* 53:1037, 2002.
12. Malangoni MA, Dillon LD, Klamer TW, et al.: Factors influencing the risk of early and late serious infection in adults after splenectomy for trauma. *Surgery* 96:775, 1984.
13. Moore FA, Moore EE, Moore GE, et al.: Risk of splenic salvage after trauma. Analysis of 200 adults. *Am J Surg* 148:800, 1984.
14. Millikan JS, Moore EE, Moore GE, et al.: Alternatives to splenectomy in adults after trauma. Repair, partial resection, and reimplantation of splenic tissue. *Am J Surg* 144:711, 1982.
15. Patel J, Williams JS, Shmigel B: Preservation of splenic function by auto-transplantation of traumatized spleen in man. *Surgery* 90:683, 1981.
16. Van Wyck DB, Wotte MH, Witte CL, et al.: Critical splenic mass for survival from experimental pneumococcemia. *J Surg Res* 28:14, 1980.
17. Harbrecht BG, Peitzman AB, Rivera L, et al.: Contribution of age and gen-der to outcome of blunt splenic injury in adults: Multicenter study of the east-ern association for the surgery of trauma. *J Trauma* 51:887, 2001.
18. Velmahos GC, Toutouzas KG, Radin R, et al.: Nonoperative treatment of blunt injury to solid abdominal organs: A prospective study. *Arch Surg* 138:844, 2003.
19. Todd SR, Arthur M, Newgard C, et al.: Hospital factors associated with splenectomy for splenic injury: A national perspective. *J Trauma* 57:1065, 2004.
20. Kluger Y, Paul DB, Raves JJ, et al.: Delayed rupture of the spleen—myths, facts, and their importance: Case reports and literature review. *J Trauma* 36:568, 1994.
21. Cocanour CS, Moore FA, Ware DN, et al.: Delayed complications of nonop-erative management of blunt adult splenic trauma. *Arch Surg* 133:619, 1998.
22. Holmes JF, Nguyen H, Jacoby RC, et al.: Do All Patients with Left Costal Margin Injuries Require Radiographic Evaluation for Intra-Abdominal Injury? *Ann Emerg Med*, In Press.
23. Moore EE, Cogbill TH, Jurkovich GJ, et al.: Organ injury scaling: Spleen and liver (1994 revision). *J Trauma* 38:323, 1995.
24. Umlas S-L, Cronan JJ: Splenic trauma: Can CT grading systems enable pre-diction of successful nonsurgical treatment? *Radiology* 178:481, 1991.
25. Buntain WL, Gould HR, Maull KI: Predictability of splenic salvage by com-puted tomography. *J Trauma* 28:24, 1988.
26. Resciniti A, Fink MP, Raptopoulos V, et al.: Nonoperative treatment of adult splenic trauma: Development of a computed tomographic scoring system that detects appropriate candidates for expectant management. *J Trauma* 128:828, 1988.
27. Mirvis SE, Whitley NO, Gens DR: Blunt splenic trauma in adults: CT-based clas-sification and correlation with prognosis and treatment. *Radiology* 171:33, 1989.
28. Shapiro MJ, Krausz C, Durham RM, et al.: Overuse of splenic scoring and computed tomographic scans. *J Trauma* 47:651, 1999.
29. Nix JA, Costanza M, Daley BJ, et al.: Outcome of the current management of splenic injuries. *J Trauma* 50:835, 2001.
30. Barquist ES, Pizano LR, Feuer W, et al.: Inter- and intrarater reliability in computed axial tomographic grading of splenic injury: Why so many grading scales? *J Trauma* 56:334, 2004.
31. Alonso M, Brathwaite C, Garcia V, et al.: Practice management guidelines for the nonoperative management of blunt injury to the liver and spleen. *East Practice Management Guidelines*, 2003: p. 1. 32. Peitzman AB, Heil B, Rivera L, et al.: Blunt splenic injury in adults: Multi-institutional study of the east-ern association for the surgery of trauma. *J Trauma* 49:177, 2000.
33. Dent D, Alsabrook G, Erickson BA, et al.: Blunt splenic injuries: High non-operative management rate can be achieved with selective embolization. *J Trauma* 56:1063, 2004.
34. Muehrcke DD, Kim SH, McCabe CJ: Pediatric splenic trauma: Predicting the success of nonoperative therapy. *Am J Emerg Med* 5:109, 1987.
35. Pearl RH, Wesson DE, Spence LJ, et al.: Splenic injury: A 5-year update with improved results and changing criteria for conservative management. *J Pediatr Surg* 24:428, 1989.
36. Lynch JM, Ford H, Gardner MJ, et al.: Is early discharge following isolated splenic injury in the hemodynamically stable child possible? *J Pediatr Surg* 28:1403, 1993.
37. Haller JA Jr, Papa P, Drugas G, et al.: Nonoperative management of solid organ injuries in children. Is it safe? *Ann Surg* 219:625. 1994.
38. Morse MA, Garcia VF: Selective nonoperative management of pediatric blunt splenic trauma: Risk for missed associated injuries. *J Pediatr Surg* 29:23, 1994.
39. Schwartz MZ, Kangah R: Splenic injury in children after blunt trauma: Blood transfusion requirements and length of hospitalization for laparotomy versus observation. *J Pediatr Surg* 29:596, 1994.
40. Coburn MC, Pfeifer J, DeLuca FG: Nonoperative management of splenic and hepatic trauma in the multiply injured pediatric and adolescent patient. *Arch Surg* 130:332, 1995.
41. Malangoni MA, Cue JI, Fallat ME, et al.: Evaluation of splenic injury by com-puted tomography and its impact on treatment. *Ann Surg* 211:592, 1990.
42. Oller B, Armengol M, Camps I, et al.: Nonoperative management of splenic injuries. *Am Surg* 57:409, 1991.
43. Schweizer W, Bölen L, Dennison A, et al.: Prospective study in adults of splenic preservation after traumatic rupture. *Br J Surg* 79:1330, 1992.
44. Velmahos GC, Chan LS, Kamel E, et al.: Nonoperative management of splenic injuries: Have we gone too far? *Arch Surg* 135:674, 2000.
45. Upadhyaya P, Simpson JS: Splenic trauma in children. *J Am Coll Surg* 126:781, 1968.
46. Smith JS, Wengrovitz MA, DeLong BS: Prospective validation of criteria, including age, for safe, nonsurgical management of the ruptured spleen. *J Trauma* 33:363, 1992.
47. Smith JS Jr, Cooney RN, Mucha P Jr: Nonoperative management of the rup-tured spleen: A revalidation of criteria. *Surgery* 120:745, 1996.
48. Godley CD, Warren RL, Sheridan RL, et al.: Nonoperative management of blunt splenic injury in adults: Age over 55 years as a powerful indicator for failure. *J Am Coll Surg* 183:133, 1996.
49. Cocanour CS, Moore FA, Ware DN, et al.: Age should not be a considera-tion for nonoperative management of blunt splenic injury. *J Trauma* 48:606, 2000.
50. Barone JE, Burns G, Svehlak SA, et al.: Management of blunt splenic trauma in patients older than 55 years. *J Trauma* 46:87, 1999.
51. Archer LP, Rogers FB, Shackford SR: Selective nonoperative management of liver and spleen injuries in neurologically impaired adult patients. *Arch Surg* 131:309, 1996.
52. Sartorelli KH, Frumiento C, Rogers FB, et al.: Nonoperative management of hepatic, splenic, and renal injuries in adults with multiple injuries. *J Trauma* 49:56, 2000.
53. Gaunt WT, McCarthy MC, Lambert CS, et al.: Traditional criteria for obser-vation of splenic trauma should be challenged. *Am Surg* 65:689, 1999.
54. Schurr MJ, Fabian TC, Gavant M, et al.: Management of blunt splenic trauma: Computed tomographic contrast blush predicts failure of nonopera-tive management. *J Trauma* 39:507, 1995.
55. Davis KA, Fabian TC, Croce MA, et al.: Improved success in nonoperative management of blunt splenic injuries: Embolization of splenic artery pseudoaneurysms. *J Trauma* 44:1008, 1998.
56. Omert LA, Salyer D, Dunham CM, et al.: Implications of the "contrast blush" finding on computed tomographic scan of the spleen in trauma. *J Trauma* 51:272, 2001.
57. Schurr MJ, Fabian TC, Gavant M, et al.: Management of blunt splenic trauma: Computed tomographic contrast blush predicts failure of nonopera-tive management. *J Trauma* 39:507, 1995.
58. Nwomeh BC, Nadler AP, Meza MP, et al.: Contrast extravasation predicts the need for operative intervention in children with blunt splenic trauma. *J Trauma* 56:537, 2004.
59. Haan JM, Bochicchio GV, Kramer N, et al.: Nonoperative management of blunt splenic injury: A 5-year experience. *J Trauma* 58:492, 2005.
60. Sclafani SJ, Shaftan GW, Scalea TM, et al.: Nonoperative salvage of computed tomography-diagnosed splenic injuries: Utilization of angiography for triage and embolization for hemostasis. *J Trauma* 39:818, 1995.
61. Peitzman AB, Heil B, Rivera L, et al.: Blunt splenic injury in adults: Multi-institutional study of the eastern association for the surgery of trauma. *J Trauma* 49:177, 2000.
62. Uecker J, Pickett C, Dunn E: The role of follow-up radiographic studies in nonoperative management of spleen trauma. *Am Surg* 67:22, 2001.
63. Lawson DE, Jacobson JA, Spizarny DL, et al.: Splenic trauma: Value of follow-up CT. *Radiology* 194:97, 1995.
64. Federle MP: Splenic trauma: Is follow-up CT of value? *Radiology* 194:23, 1995.

65. Allins A, Ho T, Nguyen TH, et al.: Limited value of routine followup CT scans in nonoperative management of blunt liver and splenic injuries. *Am Surg* 62:883, 1996.

66. Thaemert BC, Cogbill TH, Lambert PJ: Nonoperative management of splenic injury: Are follow-up computed tomographic scans of any value: *J Trauma* 43:748, 1997.

67. Dulchavsky SA, Lucas CE, Ledgerwood AM, et al.: Wound healing of the injured spleen with and without splenorrhaphy. *J Trauma* 27:1155, 1987.

68. Cogbill TH, Moore EE, Jurkovich GJ, et al.: Nonoperative management of blunt splenic trauma: A multicenter experience. *J Trauma* 29:1312, 1989.

69. Feliciano DV, Spjut-Patrinely V, Burch JM, et al.: Splenorrhaphy. The alternative. *Ann Surg* 211:569, 1990.

70. Morgenstern L, Shapiro SJ: Techniques of splenic conservation. *Arch Surg* 114:449, 1979.

71. Go PM, Goodman GR, Bruhn EW, et al.: The argon beam coagulator provides rapid hemostasis of experimental hepatic and splenic hemorrhage in anticoagulated dogs. *J Trauma* 31:1294, 1991.

72. Dunham CM, Cornwell EE III, Militello P: The role of the Argon Beam Coagulator in splenic salvage. *Surg Gynecol Obstet* 173:179, 1991.

73. Pearson HA, Johnston D, Smith KA, et al.: The born-again spleen. Return of splenic function after splenectomy for trauma. *N Engl J Med* 298:1389, 1978.

74. Nielsen JL, Sakso P, Sorensen FH, et al.: Demonstration of splenic functions following splenectomy and autologous spleen implantation. *Acta Chir Scand* 150:469, 1984.

75. Mizrahi S, Bickel A, Haj M, et al.: Posttraumatic autotransplantation of spleen tissue. *Arch Surg* 124:863, 1989.

76. Velcek FT, Jongco B, Shaftan GW, et al.: Posttraumatic splenic replantation in children. *J Pediatr Surg* 17:879, 1982.

77. Nicholson S, Hutchinson GH, Hawkins T, et al.: Successful splenosis following autologous splenic implantation. *J R Coll Surg Edinb* 31:67, 1986.

78. Leemans R, Manson W, Snijder JA, et al.: Immune response capacity after human splenic autotransplantation: Restoration of response to individual pneumococcal vaccine subtypes. *Ann Surg* 229:279, 1999.

79. Leemans R, Harms G, Rijkers GT, et al.: Spleen autotransplantation provides restoration of functional splenic lymphoid compartments and improves the humoral immune response to pneumococcal polysaccharide vaccine. *Clin Exp Immunol* 117:596, 1999.

80. Traub A, Gieink GS, Smith C, et al.: Splenic reticuloendothelial function after splenectomy, spleen repair and spleen autotransplantation. *N Engl J Med* 317:1559, 1987.

81. Zhao B, Moore WM, Lamb LS Jr, et al.: Pneumococcal clearance function of the intact autotransplanted spleen. *Arch Surg* 130:946, 1995.

82. Moore GE, Stevens RE, Moore EE, et al.: Failure of splenic implants to protect against fatal postsplenectomy infection. *Am J Surg* 146:413, 1983.

83. Buckman RF Jr, Piano G, Dunham CM, et al.: Major bowel and diaphragmatic injuries associated with blunt spleen or liver rupture. *J Trauma* 28:1317, 1988.

84. Nance ML, Peden GW, Shapiro MB, et al.: Solid viscus injury predicts major hollow viscus injury in blunt abdominal trauma. *J Trauma* 43:618, 1997.

85. Traub AC, Perry JF Jr: Injuries associated with splenic trauma. *J Trauma* 21:840, 1981.

86. Peitzman AB, Harbrecht BG, Rivera L, et al.: Failure of observation of blunt splenic injury in adults: Variability in practice and adverse consequences. *J Am Coll Surg* 201:179, 2005.

87. Luna GK, Delinger EP: Nonoperative observation therapy for splenic injuries: A safe therapeutic option? *Am J Surg* 153:462, 1987.

88. Moore FA, Moore EE, Sauaia A: Blood transfusion. An independent risk factor for postinjury multiple organ failure. *Arch Surg* 132:620, 1997.

89. Taylor RW, Manganaro L, O'Brien J, et al.: Impact of allogenic packed red blood cell transfusion on nosocomial infection rates in the critically ill patient. *Crit Care Med* 30:2249, 2002.

90. Malone DL, Dunne J, Tracy JK, et al.: Blood transfusion, independent of shock severity, is associated with worse outcome in trauma. *J Trauma* 54:898, 2003.

91. Robinson WP III, Ahn J, Stiffler A, et al.: Blood transfusion is an independent predictor of increased mortality in nonoperatively managed blunt hepatic and splenic injuries. *J Trauma* 58:437, 2005.

92. Willis BK, Deitch EA, McDonald JC: The influence of trauma to the spleen on postoperative complications and mortality. *J Trauma* 26:1073, 1986.

93. Wahlby L, Domellof L: Splenectomy after blunt abdominal trauma. A retrospective study of 413 children. *Acta Chir Scand* 147:131, 1981.

94. Pimpl W, Dapunt O, Kaindl H, et al.: Incidence of septic and thromboembolic-related deaths after splenectomy in adults. *Br J Surg* 76:517, 1989.

95. Sekikawa T, Shatney CH: Septic sequelae after splenectomy for trauma in adults. *Am J Surg* 145:667, 1983.

96. Gopal V, Bisno AL: Fulminant pneumococcal infections in "normal" asplenic hosts. *Arch Intern Med* 137:1526, 1977.

97. Green JB, Shackford SR, Sise MJ, et al.: Late septic complications in adults following splenectomy for trauma: A prospective analysis in 144 patients. *J Trauma* 26:999, 1986.

98. Pringle KC, Rowley D, Burrington JD: Immunologic response in splenectomized and partially splenectomized rats. *J Pediatr Surg* 15:531, 1980.

99. Schwartz PE, Sterioff S, Mucha P, et al.: Postsplenectomy sepsis and mortality in adults. *JAMA* 248:2279, 1982.

100. Hutchison BG, Oxman AD, Shannon HS, et al.: Clinical effectiveness of pneumococcal vaccine. Meta-analysis. *Can Fam Physician* 45:2381, 1999.

101. Schreiber MA, Pusateri AE, Veit BC, et al.: Timing of vaccination does not affect antibody response or survival after pneumococcal challenge in splenectomized rats. *J Trauma* 45:692, 1998.

102. Caplan ES, Boltansky H, Synder MJ, et al.: Response of traumatized splenectomized patients to immediate vaccination with polyvalent pneumococcal vaccine. *J Trauma* 23:801, 1983.

103. Waghorn DJ, Mayon-White RT: A study of 42 episodes of overwhelming postsplenectomy infection: Is current guidance for asplenic individuals being followed? *J Infect* 35:289, 1997.

# Commentary ■ JOSEPH P. MINEI

This chapter on injuries to the spleen by Jacoby and Wisner not only gives the reader a comprehensive review of the literature, but is also written by trauma surgeons who impart their extensive experience in dealing with these injuries. It is a must-read for young trauma surgeons as well as those who have spent their share of nights on trauma call in the hospital.

The management of splenic injuries challenges the diagnostic and decision-making skills of the surgeon. Understanding when an injured patient must be in the operating room (OR) for control of surgical bleeding, and when the patient can be closely and safely observed with nonoperative techniques requires modern technical (multislice CT scanners) and monitoring (ICU care) equipment so that sound surgical judgment can be exercised. Jacoby and Wisner repeatedly and appropriately stress that the patient with ongoing

bleeding due to splenic injury should be in the OR for definitive therapy. This is a fundamental concept that is too often overlooked with devastating consequences. Nonoperative management of splenic injuries should not attempt to stretch the envelope. All hemodynamically abnormal patients with a known or suspected splenic injury should be taken to the OR for splenorrhaphy or splenectomy as appropriate. Further, Jacoby and Wisner suggest a limit to transfusion in the nonoperative management of hemodynamically stable patients. I would go one step further as to suggest that in the adult patient with *any* need for transfusion, strong consideration should be made for immediate operative intervention. This approach is supported by recent data that suggests that any transfusion is associated with a higher mortality in this group of patients. The concept of earlier definitive operation prior to transfusion addresses a number of conditions. By operating prior to transfusion need, the patient is potentially freed from transfusion related viral and bacterial transmission as well as the immunosuppression associated with transfusion. Additionally, by operating before transfusion is required decreases the need to treat coagulopathy associated with greater blood loss and red blood cell replacement without other component therapy. Splenic salvage is more likely with earlier surgery. Finally, Jacoby and Wisner put into perspective the very low risk of developing postsplenectomy sepsis particularly in adults. Thus, even if splenectomy is required, postsplenectomy sepsis is a rare event. Many surgeons must have seen a patient bleed to death because of a poor decision to attempt nonoperative therapy of a solid organ injury. Most surgeons never see or hear of a case of postsplenectomy sepsis.

The pendulum of care in the management of splenic injury is approaching equilibrium. We have progressed through the spectrum of operating on most injuries with its inherent complications and nontherapeutic procedures, to pushing the limits of nonoperative therapy to the point of dire consequences. The correct approach is somewhere in between. I believe by adhering to the principles espoused in this chapter by Jacoby and Wisner, the reader will have a firmer understanding of knowing when to operate immediately and when to safely observe with a nonoperative management protocol. Most importantly, if the reader can come away with a clear plan when to abandon nonoperative management before it is too late, then injured patients will be the real beneficiaries from this writing.

# Stomach and Small Bowel

*Lawrence N. Diebel*

## INTRODUCTION

Injuries to the stomach and small bowel are common in penetrating abdominal trauma.

The incidence of gastrointestinal injury following gunshot wounds that penetrate the peritoneal cavity is over 80%. Thus, exploratory laparotomy is warranted on virtually all gunshot wounds that penetrate the peritoneal cavity. The incidence of hollow viscus injury secondary to stab wounds which have penetrated the peritoneal cavity is much less, which in most series is about 30%. Thus, a selective approach to operative exploration has been advocated following stab wounds.

Blunt injuries to the stomach and small bowel are much less common than penetrating injury, but collectively compromise the third most common type of blunt abdominal injury. The increasing use of computed tomography (CT) for diagnostic evaluation of the patient with blunt abdominal trauma and selective nonoperative management of solid organ injuries have contributed to some of the difficulties and controversies in the management of hollow viscus injuries following blunt trauma.[1] In contradistinction to some of the diagnostic difficulties with stomach and small bowel injuries, operative repair of stomach and small bowel injuries is relatively straightforward. The key to the successful management of stomach and small bowel injuries is prompt recognition and treatment, thus decreasing the likelihood of abdominal septic complications and subsequent late death.[2]

## HISTORICAL PERSPECTIVE

Intestinal injuries were reported early in the medical literature (see Chap. 1). Small bowel perforation from blunt trauma was first recognized by Aristotle.[3] Hippocrates was the first to report intestinal perforation from penetrating abdominal trauma. In 1275, Guillaume de Salicet described the successful suture repair of a tangential intestinal wound. Reports of attempted surgical repair of gastric and intestinal wounds appeared in the literature with heightened interest and controversy during the American Civil War, the Spanish–American War, the Russo–Japanese War, and other military conflicts. However, the dismal results of surgical intervention led to abandonment of laparotomy even with obvious intestinal injury during these military campaigns.[4]

By the late 19th century, improved surgical techniques led to renewed interest in laparotomy and repair of penetrating abdominal injuries. Theodore Kocher was the first surgeon to report successful repair of a gunshot wound of the stomach. In 1901, President William McKinley, shot in the abdomen by an assassin, underwent expeditious transport and surgical repair of several gastric wounds, although it was still a controversial technique. However, a wound to the pancreas was overlooked and McKinley died eight days later.

The routine use of exploratory laparotomy for suspected intestinal injury was not observed until late in World War I. A laparotomy for intestinal perforation at the start of World War I carried a mortality rate of 75–80%, almost equal to the mortality rate of nonoperative management.

In World War II, prompt evacuation, improvements in anesthesia, and better understanding and treatment of shock led to mortality rates of 13.9% for jejunal or ileal injuries and 36.3% if multiple injuries were present.[5] Further improvements in mortality were noted during the Korean War and Vietnam conflicts. Lessons learned from the collective military experience were quickly adopted by nonmilitary surgeons. The military term "damage control" has been adopted by civilian and now military surgeons for the surgical approach to patients with profound shock and significant traumatic injuries.

Patients with gastrointestinal injuries under these circumstances may benefit from a staged operative approach for abdominal injuries. Simple repairs or temporizing measures aimed at controlling ongoing peritoneal contamination by gastrointestinal injuries are performed at the initial operation. Definitive repair for more complex gastrointestinal injuries is undertaken at a later operation after hemodynamic stabilization.

Nonetheless, prompt recognition and repair of injuries are responsible for the low morbidity and mortality from isolated gastric and small bowel injuries. Associated injuries contribute significantly to morbidity and mortality in patients with gastric and small bowl injuries.

## ANATOMY AND PHYSIOLOGY

The stomach generally occupies the left upper quadrant of the abdomen. The nondistended stomach, especially in a supine individual, is located largely in the intrathoracic abdomen where it is offered some protection by the lower chest wall. The position of the stomach can be quite variable and in the erect individual may

extend into the lower abdomen, particularly when distended with food or liquid. The stomach is fixed on its lesser curvature by the gastrohepatic ligament, cephally by the gastrophrenic ligament, and distally by the retroperitoneal duodenum. The greater curvature of the stomach is loosely bound to the transverse colon via the greater omentum and to the spleen by the gastrosplenic ligament. The stomach enjoys a rich blood supply from the left and right gastric arteries, the left and right gastroepiploic arteries, and the short gastric arteries (Fig. 34-1). Venous drainage follows the arterial supply to the stomach for the most part.

The normal stomach is relatively free of bacteria and other microorganisms because of the low intraluminal pH.[6] However, up to $10^3$ organisms per mL of species including lactobacilli, aerobic streptococci, and even Candida may be isolated. Low gastric acidity due to $H_2$-receptor blockade or now proton pump inhibitors lead to increased bacterial concentrations in the stomach and proximal gastrointestinal tract, increasing the risk of peritoneal

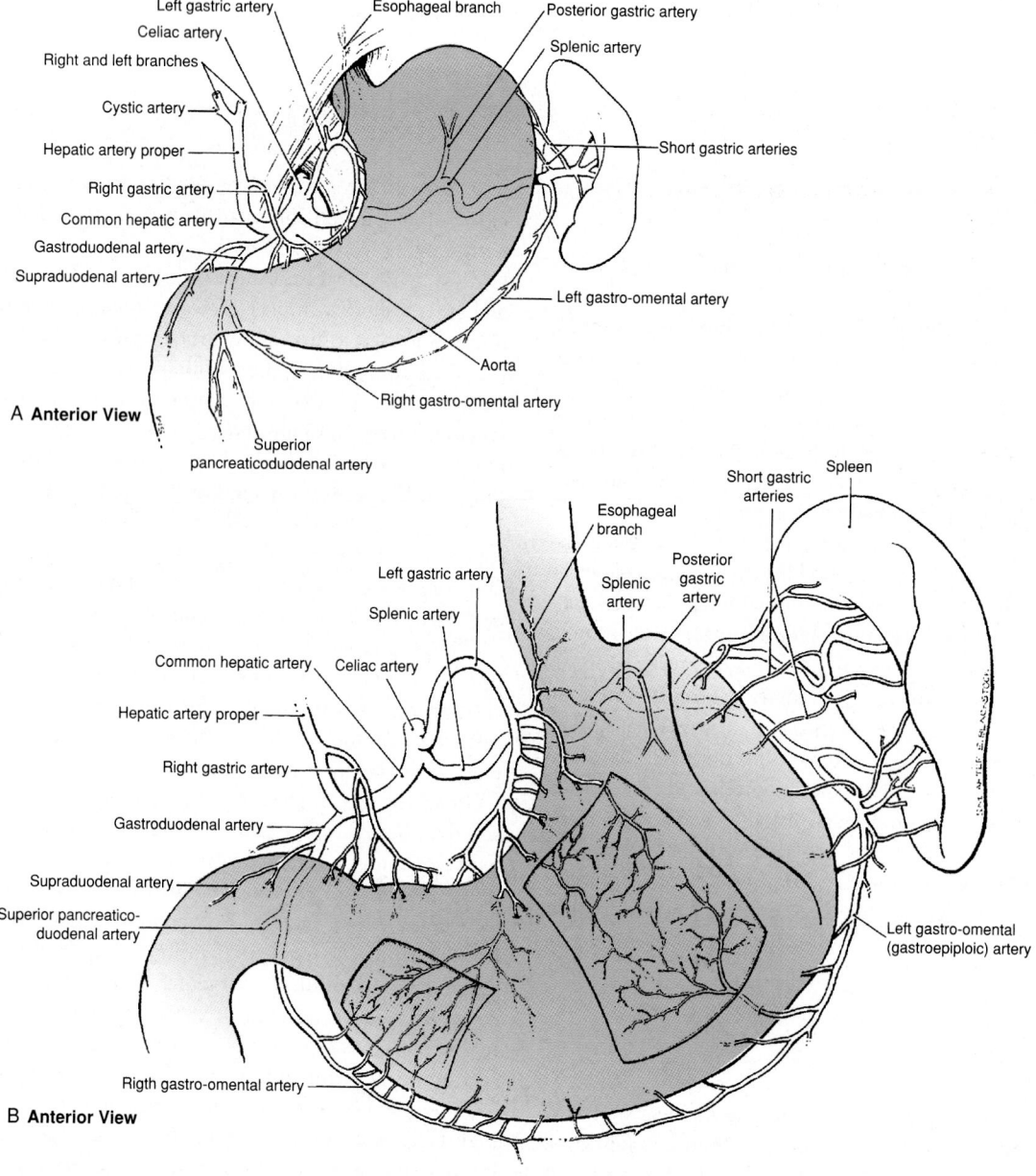

**FIGURE 34-1.**  Blood supply to the stomach. An anomalous left hepatic artery can arise as a branch of the left gastric artery. This should be looked for when doing gastric resections.

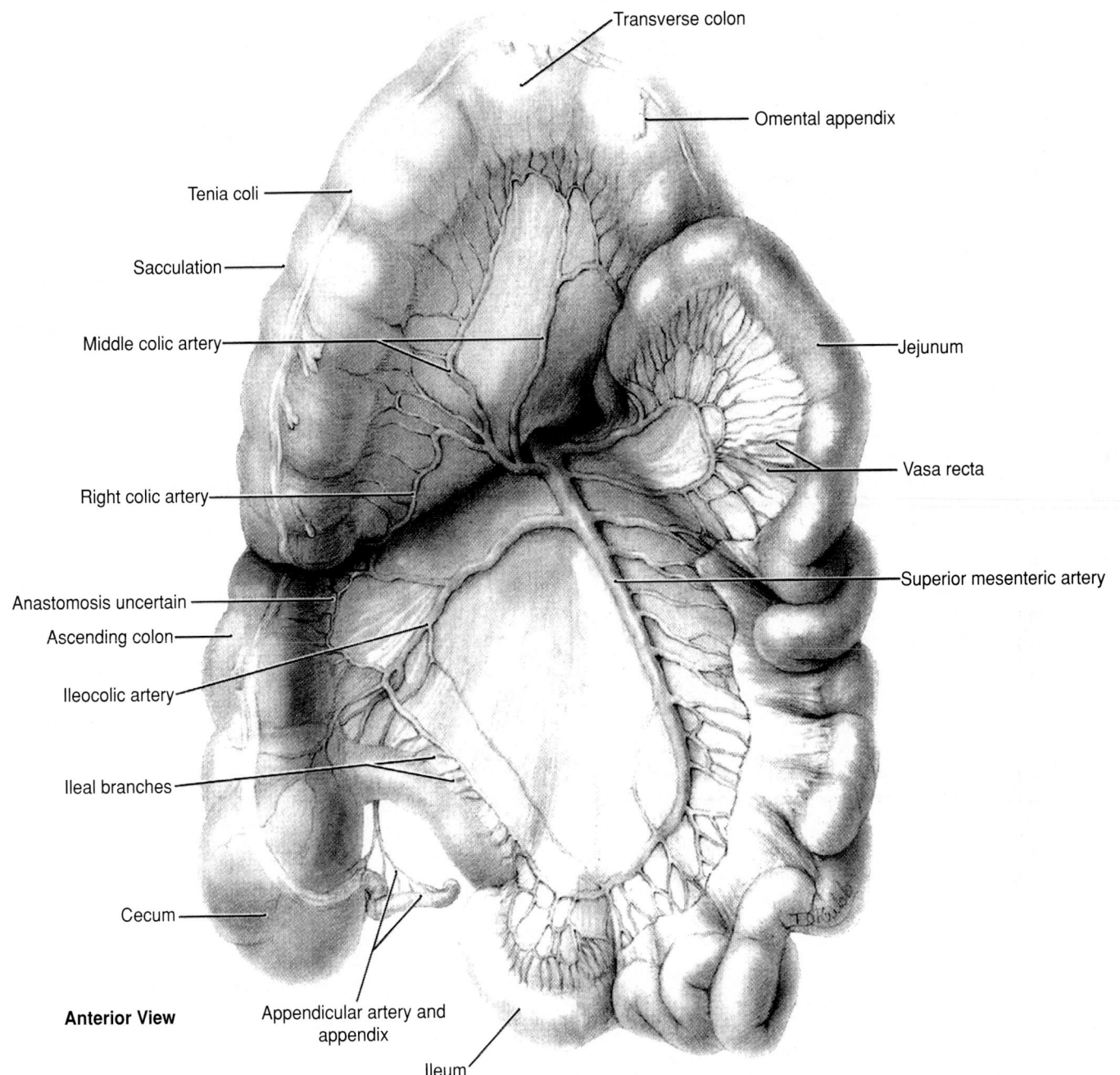

Transverse colon

Omental appendix

Tenia coli

Sacculation

Middle colic artery

Jejunum

Vasa recta

Right colic artery

Anastomosis uncertain

Ascending colon

Ileocolic artery

Superior mesenteric artery

Ileal branches

Cecum

**Anterior View**

Appendicular artery and appendix

Ileum

**FIGURE 34-2.** Blood supply to the small bowel. Multiple branches to the jejunem and ileum originate directly from the superior mesenteric artery. The distal ileum is supplied via the ileocolic artery.

contamination with gastric perforation.[7] Undigested food may also harbor bacteria and increase risk of intraabdominal infection following spillage into the peritoneal cavity.

The small bowel distal to the ligament of Trietz is approximately 5–6 m in length in the adult. Protected anteriorly only by the abdominal wall musculature and occupying most of the true abdominal cavity, the small intestine is anatomically vulnerable to injury.

The small intestine is suspended from the posterior abdominal wall by its mesentery, the base of which extends from the duodenal jejunal flexure, superior to inferior and left to right to the level of the right sacroiliac joint. The arterial supply to the small bowel is provided by the superior mesentery artery (SMA), which emerges from under the pancreas and then courses anterior to the uncinate

process of the pancreas to enter the root of the mesentery. The blood supply to the small bowel comes from the left side of the SMA via intestinal arteries (Fig. 34-2). The jejunal and ileal branches vary in number and supply all but the terminal part of the ileum. This is supplied by branches from the ileocolic artery. Numerous intestinal arcades form within the mesentery to assure excellent collateral blood supply to the small intestine. Venous return from the small intestine follows the arterial supply: the superior mesenteric vein joins the inferior mesenteric vein and splenic vein to form the portal vein.

Although no clear distinction exists, the first 40% or so of the bowel is jejunum and the remainder is the ileum (Fig. 34-3). The jejunum has a larger diameter and thicker folds than the ileum.

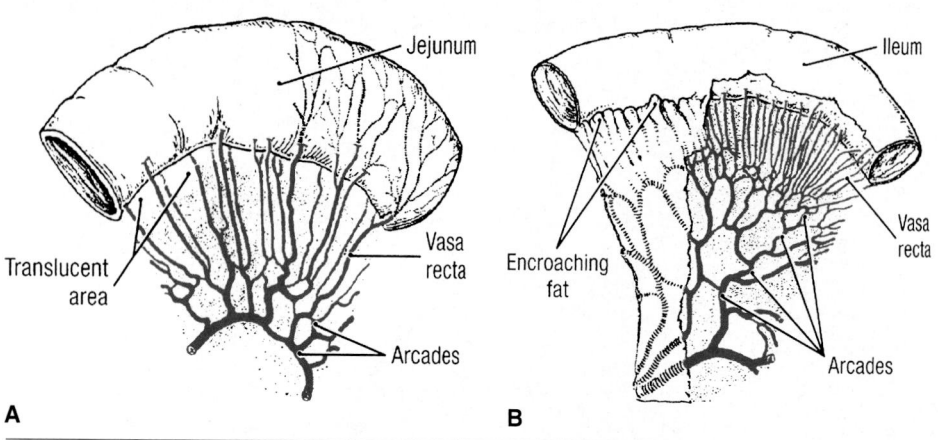

**FIGURE 34-3.** The jejunum and ileum can be distinguished from one another by differences in luminal diameter, number of arterial arcades, and the presence or absence of fat encroaching on the gut wall.

The mesentery of the jejunum contains only a single arcade, whereas more than two or three sets of vascular arcades are present in the ileum. Mesenteric fat is also more prominent in the ileum than in the jejunum. However, these distinctions between jejunum and ileum are of clinical importance only when a significant amount of bowel is to be resected. The ileum is also the site responsible for vitamin $B_{12}$ absorption and the enterohepatic recirculation of bile salts.

The luminal content of the proximal small bowel is of neutral pH and is relatively sterile, containing few bacteria. Most studies of the small bowel microflora have demonstrated increasing bacterial counts with distance away from the pylorus.[8] The proximal small bowel flora resembles the gastric flora. The jejunum and proximal ileum contain gram-positive and gram-negative organisms at $10^4$ to $10^5$ cfu/mL. The bacterial concentration is the distal ileum rises to $10^5$ to $10^8$ in the ileum. There is also a higher number of anerobic species in the ileum. This increase in bacterial load in the ileum is thought to contribute to an increased risk of infection with full thickness injury in the distal small bowel versus the proximal small bowel.

## Mechanism of Injury/Pathophysiology

Contusions, intramural hematomas, full thickness perforations, and mesenteric avulsions of the stomach and small bowel have all been reported to occur following blunt abdominal trauma. Blunt rupture of the stomach is rare. In the East Association for the Surgery of Trauma (EAST) blunt hollow viscus injury multi-institutional trial, the incidence of stomach injuries was 4.3% of a total of 2632 patients identified with any hollow viscus injury. Twelve percent of the 34 gastrointestinal perforations operated on by Ulman et al.[9] were in the stomach. Most blunt gastric injuries are related to pedestrian motor vehicle or high-speed motor vehicle crashes. In adults, most gastric perforations involve the lesser curvature.

Small bowel perforation secondary to blunt abdominal trauma is uncommon, but thought to be increasing in incidence. Localized blows to the abdomen such as the kick of a horse has been replaced by motor vehicle crashes as the most important mechanism of injury. Falls and bicycle accidents resulting in the handlebars striking the abdominal wall are less common causes for blunt intestinal rupture. Mechanisms postulated for injury to the intestine to occur include:

(1) crushing of bowel against the spine, (2) sudden deceleration sheering of the bowel from its mesentery of a fixed point by sudden deceleration, and (3) bursting of a "pseudo closed" loop of bowel owing to sudden increase in intraluminal pressure.[10,11] More recently, Cripps and Cooper have demonstrated experimentally the potential for small intestinal injury in high-velocity, low-momentum impacts which do not greatly compress the abdominal cavity.[12] Earlier series had described proximal jejunum and distal ileum as sites more prone to injury due to their relative immobility. More recent reports have not shown this to be the case, as midjunal perforations have been increasingly reported.[13]

Gastric perforations caused by blunt forces are often large and intraperitoneal contamination is usually significant. Peritoneal signs are usually obvious leading to early surgical intervention. Associated injuries are often severe because of the degree of force necessary to produce a gastric blowout. This accounts for the higher mortality rates for patients with blunt gastric rupture versus patients with other hollow viscus injuries.

Small bowel injury secondary to blunt trauma although uncommon is increasing in frequency due to high-speed motor vehicle crashes as well as mandatory seat belt laws and increasing compliance with the use of passenger restraints. The impact of air bag deployment is not completely known. Use of passenger restraints do save lives but contribute to a higher incidence of certain injuries including bowel perforations.[14] This association has been seen with both lap belts as well as three–point lap and shoulder harness restraints. Anderson and colleagues reported a 4.38-fold increased risk of small bowel injuries with lap/shoulder restraint use and a more than tenfold increased risk with lap belts alone compared to no restraint use.[15]

Injuries due to lap and lap/shoulder restraints encompass a constellation of injuries related to these restraint devices. The "seat belt" syndrome or complex is characterized by injuries to the small bowel, Chance-type lumbar fractures, and occasionally injuries to the stomach or colon. The presence of ecchymoses of the abdominal wall coinciding with the position of lap belt has been referred to as the "seat belt sign" (Fig. 34-4). Chandler et al. reported 112 patients involved in motor vehicle crashes. Sixty percent of patients were wearing a seat belt, and the remainder were unrestrained.[16] There was no difference in the overall incidence of abdominal injury between belted and unbelted patients (15% vs. 10%, respectively). However, the incidence of small bowel perforation was significantly increased in patients with a seat belt versus no belt (6% vs. 2.2%, respectively). The presence of a seat belt sign was associated with an even greater likelihood of abdominal injuries and small bowel perforation (64% and 21%, respectively).

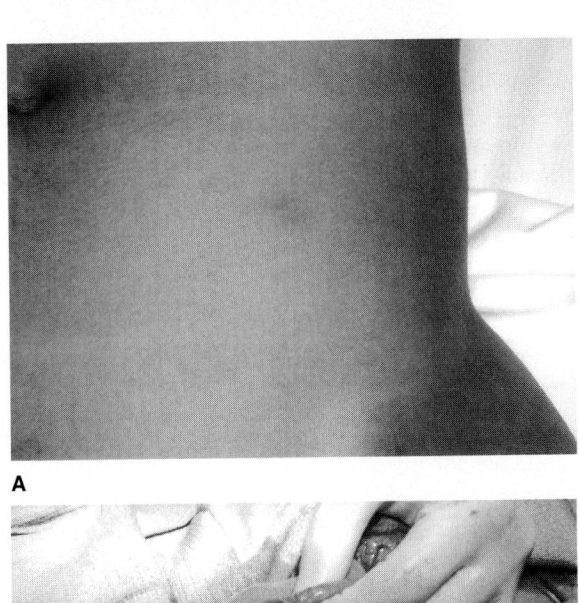

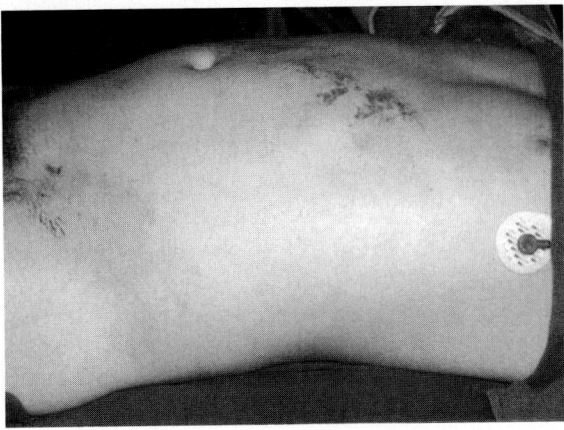

A

B

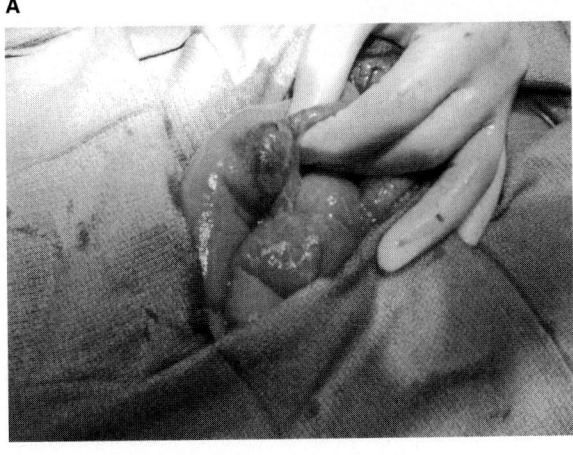

C

**FIGURE 34-4.** Patients with blunt intestinal injury sometimes have ecchymoses of the abdominal wall caused by restraint devices. The findings may be relatively subtle (**A**) or more severe (**B**). The presence of such ecchymoses does not always signify underlying blunt intestinal injury. By the same token, many patients with blunt intestinal injury do not have abdominal wall ecchymoses. The patient in (A) had a grade II injury while a grade IV injury occurred the patient in (B). (**C**) Grade II bowel injury in patient (A).

**FIGURE 34-5.** Some injuries to the lumbar spine are commonly caused by seat belts, and are frequently accompanied by associated blunt intestinal injury. Transversely oriented fractures through bone (**A**) are also sometimes known as Chance fractures. The mechanism of injury responsible for such fractures can cause soft-tissue disruption and dislocation in the same orientation as seen with Chance fracture (**B**).

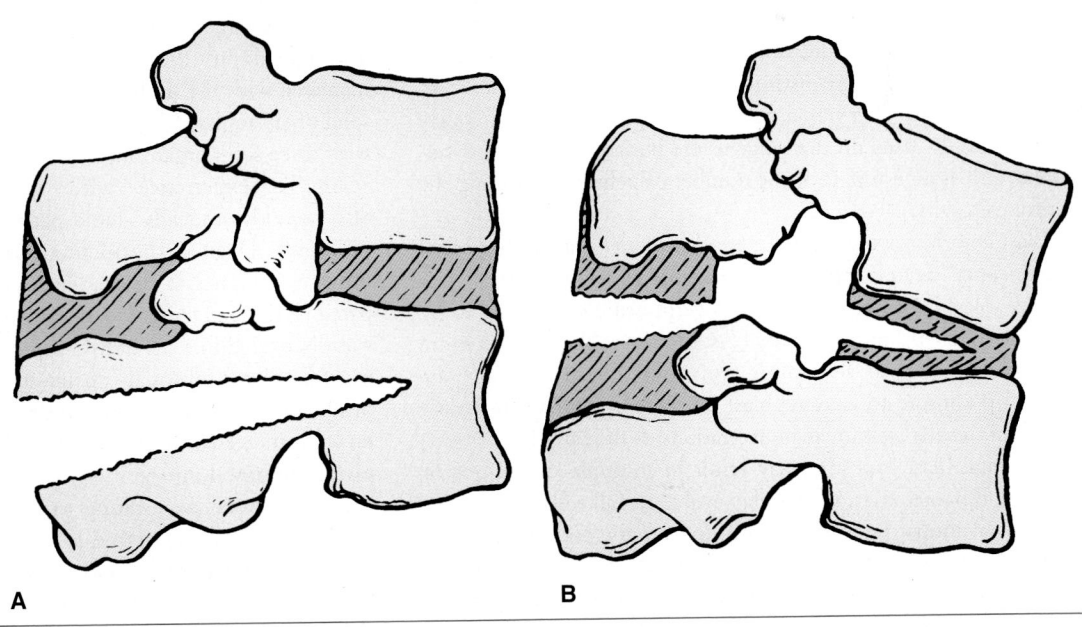

A

B

More recently in the EAST multi-institutional study, the seat belt sign was associated with a 4.7% increase in relative risk of small bowel perforation in patients following motor vehicle crashes.[17] The second highest relative risk of small bowel perforation was the use of a seat belt without evidence of an abdominal seat belt mark (2.4% increase in relative risk). Small bowel injuries noted with the use of seat belt use include small bowel transections (usually in the proximal jejunum) as a manifestation of a deceleration injury, sheering or crushing injuries usually involving the

terminal ileum and associated mesentery, and (blowout) perforations on the antimesenteric aspect of the bowel. This latter injury is felt to be due to an acute sudden increase in intraluminal pressure in a functionally closed loop of bowel.

The association of a Chance-type fracture of the lumbar spine as a predictor of hollow viscus injury is variably reported in the literature (Fig. 34-5). Anderson et al. reported 62.5% of 16 patients with Chance-type fractures had hollow viscus injuries.[15] Nine perforations occurred in the small bowel, the remainder were in the colon. However, in the EAST multi-institutional trial with small bowel perforations there was no difference in incidence of Chance-type fracture in perforating or nonperforating small bowel injury patient groups versus patients without small bowel injury.[18] The incidence of bowel perforations was quite low in all groups, and ranged between 2% and 3% of patients.

In about 20% of patients with blunt intestinal perforations no other injuries are present. Other patients have significant extra abdominal injuries with blunt injury as their sole intraabdominal injury. Approximately 25% of patients with blunt intestinal injury have more than one injury requiring surgical intervention.[19] Thus, in patients undergoing laparotomy for blunt intestinal rupture a complete evaluation for other injuries and a thorough laparotomy are mandated.

On rare occasions, patients may return to the hospital several days or weeks after blunt abdominal trauma with signs and symptoms of bowel obstruction. Contrast-enhanced CT of the abdomen performed at this time usually shows a thickened bowel loop, and narrowing of the lumen. This finding is due to intestinal stenosis resulting from mesenteric vascular injury. The stenosis is felt to be due to infarction resulting from the mesenteric injury rather than a direct injury to the intestine.[20]

Penetrating injuries to the stomach and small intestine are often more obvious. The anatomic location and space occupied by these organs make them the prime target following injury due to knives, gunshot wounds, shotgun wounds, and other piercing instruments. Of those with peritoneal penetration only 30% of patients with knife wounds have significant injuries requiring operation whereas over 80% of patients who suffer gunshot wounds have injuries requiring surgical repair. Thus, most institutions employ selective observation of patients with knife wounds even with peritoneal penetration. The decision for operation is based on clinical signs of peritonitis. Many institutions apply a selective approach to shotgun wounds.[21] For nonclose range shotgun wounds, operative intervention is based on the range of the blast and pellet distribution as well as an estimate of the number of pellets penetrating the peritoneal cavity.

Blast injuries to the GI tract are the result of a "multidimensional injury" as four separate mechanisms may play a role.[22] The primary blast injury results from an overpressure wave induced by the blast itself. Although primary blast injuries to the GI tract more commonly occur in the colon, the small bowel may also be affected. Exposure to extreme blast overpressure (which is invariably fatal) results in immediate lacerations of the bowel.

Nonfatal blast exposure may result in multiple contusions or intramural hematomas, which may evolve to full thickness injury. The initial injury involves the mucosa–submucosa of the bowel wall; the presence of serosal injury is evidence of a transmural lesion at high risk of perforation. Because of the nature of this injury, there may be delay of one or two days, and rarely up to 14 days before clinical symptoms occur. The overall incidence of bowel perforation is low (0.1–1.2%) but is increased with explosive amount, or when the victim is close to the center of the explosion or in an enclosed area.

Secondary blast injuries are caused by projectiles from the explosion that causes perforating injury to the victim. Tertiary blast injuries are the result of the generation of "blast winds" which propel the victim into rigid objects causing blunt injury. Quaternary injuries are the result of fire and heat generated by the explosion.

Most injuries seen clinically are due to secondary or tertiary blast effects. Patients with penetrating torso injury or involving > 4 body areas are at high risk for intra-peritoneal injury.[23] In the presence of peritoneal signs, the decision to perform surgery is easily made. Because bowel perforation may be delayed, careful observation is critical, even with negative initial image studies or diagnostic peritoneal lavage results.

## DIAGNOSIS

An accurate history of the traumatic event can help determine the potential for intraabdominal injuries. In patients with a knife wound of the left thoracoabdominal region, diaphragmatic and gastric injuries are a primary concern. The small bowel is at risk of perforation following virtually any penetrating injury that violates the peritoneum. Evisceration of abdominal contents after abdominal stab wound is associated with significant intraabdominal organ injury in 75% of patients even with no overt clinical signs that would mandate laparotomy.[24] Certain patterns of blunt abdominal injury should alert the clinician as the probability of gastric and small bowel perforations. Thus, a low threshold for laparotomy is appropriate in this setting. These include the use of seat belts, handle bar injury, and blows to the abdomen such as being kicked by a horse or other large animal. An improperly applied Heimlich maneuver has been reported to cause gastric perforations.[25]

The incidence of small bowel injury in patients diagnosed with solid organ injuries by CT is variable. Nance et al., in a review of 3089 patients with solid organ injury from the Pennsylvania Trauma Systems Foundation, found 296 patients who had a hollow viscus injury (9.6%).[26] The frequency of hollow viscus injury increased with the number of solid organs injured: 7.3% with one solid organ injury, 15.4% with two solid organ injuries, and 34.4% with three solid organs injured. More recently, Miller reviewed the Memphis experience with nonoperative management of 803 hemodynamically stable patients with blunt liver or spleen injuries.[27] Overall, the incidence of associated intraabdominal injury was higher in the patients with liver injury at 5% as compared to 1.7% of patients with isolated splenic injury. Bowel injury was discovered in 11% of liver injury patients and no patients with isolated splenic injury. It is believed that the blunt force capable of producing liver injuries or multiple solid organs places the small bowel at increased risk for perforation and should elicit clinical suspicion for bowel injury.

Patients with penetrating gastric injuries usually present with significant peritoneal signs due to the peritoneal irritation from the intraperitoneal leakage of the low pH content of the stomach. Bloody nasogastric aspirate or free air demonstrated on an upright chest x-ray may be indicative of gastric injury but neither is completely sensitive nor specific for the presence of gastric injury.

In patients with obvious peritoneal penetration, clinical findings following penetrating trauma to the small intestine may be minimal at first. This is because the luminal content of the small bowel has an almost neutral pH and is relatively sterile. Intestinal spill may also be relatively small, limiting the initial inflammatory response.

In the EAST multi-institutional trial of blunt small bowel injury 1.2% of 227,972 blunt trauma admits were found to have a hollow viscus injury.[28] The incidence of hollow viscus injury was 3.1% in patients undergoing a workup for possible blunt abdominal injury. Exactly 72.5% of patients with perforating small bowel injury had abdominal tenderness; however, only 33.5% had peritoneal signs.[18] Nonetheless, a careful physical exam by an experienced surgeon may discern the likelihood of intestinal perforation. In patients with a seat belt sign on the abdominal wall, tenderness or guarding away from the seat belt should heighten the concern for the possibility of perforated small bowel injuries. Perforations of the stomach and small bowel are recognized by signs of peritoneal irritation: tenderness with guarding and rebound. Sensitivity of clinical examination to identify patients in need of operation exceeds 95% for stab wounds and gunshot wounds. In other studies, clinical examination of the abdomen has been shown to be unreliable in approximately 50% of blunt abdominal trauma patients.[29,30] Significant limitations include patients with head injury and altered level of consciousness, intoxication due to drugs or alcohol, and spinal cord injury. The variable effect of hemoperitoneum from associated solid organ injuries and the presence of distracting injuries (e.g., pelvic fracture) in the multi-injured patients may also limit the clinical reliability of the findings on physical exam.

Laboratory studies including hematocrit, WBC, and serum amylase are not useful in the initial evaluation of patients with gastric and small intestinal injuries.[18] In patients managed nonoperatively with solid organ injury or in patients with penetrating injuries undergoing serial clinical exams, unexplained tachycardia, hypotension, leucocytosis, an increase in serum amylase, or the development of a metabolic acidosis should arise suspicion of a missed hollow viscus injury.

A variety of diagnostic tests have been used to further evaluate the abdomen following blunt and penetrating injuries (see Chaps.16,17). Diagnostic peritoneal lavage (DPL) is very sensitive in detecting intraperitoneal injury but is now infrequently used. The most common peritoneal lavage finding with bowel injuries is gross blood.[18] However, this may be due to associated solid organ or mesenteric injuries.

Peritoneal lavage with blood cell count has been used to diagnose hollow viscus injury. However, Jacobs et al. found that a lavage white blood cell count >500/mm$^3$ as the sole positive lavage criteria to be a nonspecific indicator of intestinal perforation.[31] It was suggested that sequential determinations of DPL and WBC may be useful in the diagnosis of intestinal perforation. This may be particularly useful in multisystem trauma patients undergoing lengthy extraabdominal surgical procedures where the DPL catheter can be left in place and repeat DPL performed.

Diagnostic peritoneal lavage amylase and alkaline phosphatase levels may also be useful in identifying hollow viscus injuries. Jaffin et al. found an alkaline phosphate level >10 IU in the DPL effluent to have a specificity of 99.8% and a sensitivity of 94.7% in detecting small bowel and colonic injury.[32] McAnena and colleagues used lavage amylase >20 IU/L and lavage alkaline phosphatase levels ≥3 IU/L as predictors of hollow viscus injuries following blunt penetrating trauma.[33] These values had a sensitivity of 54%, specificity of 48%, and a positive predictive value of 88% for significant abdominal injury.

The ability of DPL to detect hollow viscus perforation in the presence of hemoperitoneum secondary to solid organ injury may be improved by adjusting the positive criteria for WBC. Otomo and colleagues proposed a "positive" WBC criteria of WBC ≥RBC/150 when peritoneal lavage was positive for hemoperitoneum.[34] These criteria had a sensitivity of 96.6% and a specificity of 99.4% for intestinal injury when performed more than three hours after injury. Fang et al. used a "cell count ratio" in diagnosing hollow viscus perforation.[35] The cell count ratio was defined as the ratio between white blood cell count and red blood cell count in the lavage fluid divided by the ratio of the same parameters in the peripheral blood. A cell count ratio of ≥1 predicted hollow viscus perforation with a specificity of 97% and a sensitivity of 100% when performed before 1.5 and 5 hours from the time of injury. The "lag time" between intestinal perforation and peritoneal white cell response was felt to account for the reliability of the "corrected" peritoneal lavage white blood cell counts calculated in these later two studies to detect hollow viscus perforations.

The focused assessment by sonography for trauma (FAST) has been a widely used test in the initial evaluation of suspected abdominal trauma. This is not as sensitive as DPL or CT in detecting stomach or small bowel injuries. This is most likely because of the relative inability of the FAST exam to pick up small amounts of free fluid typically found with isolated hollow viscus perforations. Rozycki and colleagues reported on 1540 patients (1227 with blunt injuries, 313 with penetrating injuries) who had FAST examinations performed as part of their initial assessment following injury.[36] The sensitivity and specificity for detecting hemoperitoneum was 83.7% and 99.7%, respectively. However, there were 16 blunt abdominal trauma patients with false-negative ultrasound results. Three of these patients were subsequently found to have significant small bowel injuries. As an isolated finding, an additional patient had small bowel perforation and a ruptured bladder. Bowel injuries have been also missed by FAST examinations in patients with pelvic ring fractures.[37] Detection of actual bowel injuries by FAST is unreliable.

CT scan is the most commonly used diagnostic modality in evaluating the abdomen in hemodynamically stable blunt trauma victims. It is occasionally used in evaluating hemodynamically stable patients with penetrating injuries particularly to the back and flank areas. Findings suspicious for blunt bowel/mesenteric injuries on CT include unexplained intraperitoneal fluid, pneumoperitoneum, bowel wall thickening, mesenteric fat streaking, mesenteric hematoma, and extravasation of either luminal or vascular contrast (Figs. 34-6 and 34-7).[38,39]

It is apparent that when blunt small bowel perforation is present, abdominal CT is usually abnormal. Butela and colleagues did a logistic regression analysis on 54 patients with bowel/mesenteric injuries diagnosed by helial CT.[40] Relevant predictors of bowel injury were mesenteric infiltration, bowel wall thickening, and free intraperitoneal air. Free peritoneal fluid, abnormal bowel wall enhancement, and ileus were less effective predictors. Malhatra et al. reviewed the Presley Regional Trauma Center experience with screening helial CT evaluation of blunt bowel and mesenteric injuries.[41] One hundred of 8112 scans were suspicious of blunt bowel/mesenteric injuries. There were 53 patients with bowel/mesentery injuries (true-positive) and 47 that did not (false-positive). There were seven patients with false-negative scans. Four of these patients were subsequently found to have small bowel perforations and three had mesenteric injuries. The most common findings in both true-positive and false-positive groups was unexplained intraperitoneal fluid present in 74%–79% of scans,

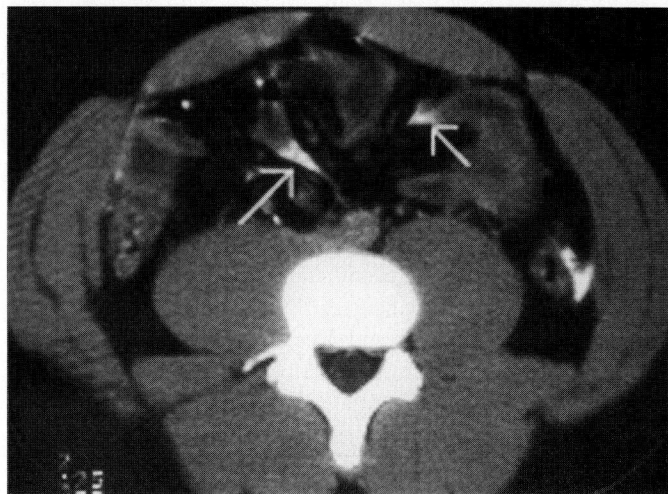

**FIGURE 34-6.** This CT was obtained a few hours after injury. The findings were highly suspicious of oral contrast extravasation (arrows). The patient was found to have rupture of the small intestine at surgery.

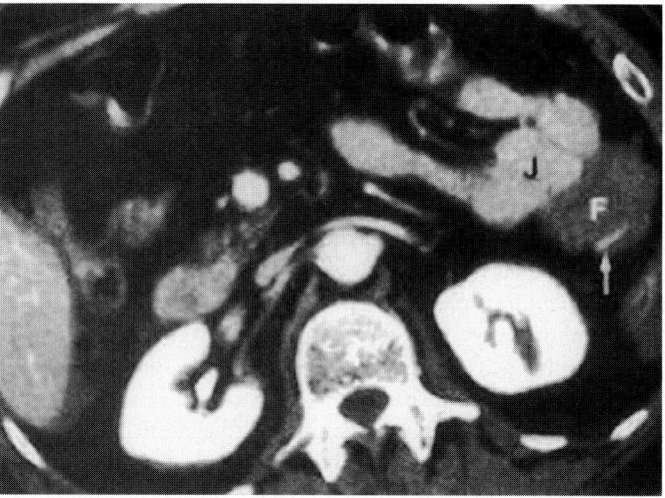

**FIGURE 34-7.** This CT was done shortly after injury. Multiple abnormalities are noted including thickened bowel and free fluid (arrows). However, a large amount of free air is the most notable finding. At operation a midjejunal perforation was found.

respectively. Pneumoperitoneum and bowel wall thickening were much more common in true-positive scans. Multiple findings suspicious for bowel/mesenteric injury were seen in 57% of the true-positive scans but in only 17% of false-positive scans. The overall sensitivity and specificity of CT for bowel/mesenteric injury were 88.3% and 99.4%, respectively. The positive and negative predictor values were 53.0% and 99.9%, respectively.

Malhatra et al. suggested that hemodynamically stable blunt trauma patients undergo exploratory laparotomy if the contrast-enhanced helial CT had multiple abnormal findings suggestive of bowel or mesenteric injury.[41] If a single abnormal finding was noted on the CT, the next step advised was DPL to rule out bowel/mesenteric injury.

The excellent results from Memphis with screening helial CT to detect blunt bowel and mesenteric injuries may not be realistically obtained in centers with smaller trauma volumes and less expertise in interpreting CT findings suggestive of hollow viscus injury. The EAST multi-institutional trial in diagnosing blunt small bowel injury included 1420 patients over two years (1988–1989) from 95 trauma centers.[42] A logistic regression model was used to predict the presence of any small bowel injury or perforating small bowel injury using 25 individual CT findings per patient. The models failed to yield any clinically useful set of discriminators. The most common finding was intraperitoneal free fluid, noted in 68.8% of patients. Of those with free fluid, 29% had perforating small bowel injuries. Free fluid without solid organ injury was associated with a 38.4% incidence of perforating small bowel injury. In an earlier multi-institutional study, 90 of 2299 patients had isolated free fluid on CT and only seven of these patients (8%) had a blunt intestinal injury.[43] A previous large prospective multi-institutional trial has suggested that admission or observation is not necessary after a negative abdominal CT in patients with suspected blunt trauma.[44] Of note, 12.2% of patients diagnosed with small bowel perforations in the EAST trial had a completely normal CT.[42] It would therefore seem prudent to continue a conservative approach at most institutions in this instance. If associated injuries do not mandate admission, a short period of observation may still be warranted, particularly if abdominal tenderness is present or if the patient is obtunded by drugs or alcohol.[45] The time-honored trial of diet when the patient's condition is normalized may be appropriate.

Diagnostic laparoscopy is occasionally helpful in avoiding laparotomy in hemodynamically stable patients with penetrating thoracoabdominal trauma.[46,47] Indications include penetrating left thoracoabdominal trauma with suspected diaphragmatic injuries. On some occasions small diaphragmatic tears and even gastric perforations may be repaired using laparoscopic techniques.[48] Penetrating injuries to the anterior right thoracoabdominal area and tangential gunshot wounds to the abdomen may also be evaluated laparoscopically. Indications for diagnostic laparoscopy are less certain for patients with blunt intestinal trauma. Most feel there is no advantage to diagnostic laparoscopy versus CT and/or DPL.[49]

The major limitation cited with diagnostic laparoscopy is in the relative inability to detect hollow viscus perforations.[50,51] Expertise in advanced laparoscopic surgical techniques is undoubtedly helpful in reliably excluding bowel injuries. Proper selection of sites for port placement is paramount for effective laparoscopic evaluation for bowel injury.[47] This includes initial placement of the laparoscope through a 10 mm port 4 cm above the umbilicus, a second port in the midline suprapubically and a third port in a paramedian position at the level of the umbilicus. Following inspection for blood or bile, the laparoscope is placed in the suprapubic port and the bowel run from the ligament of Treitz to the cecum with atraumatic graspers. In patients found to have intestinal perforation, it is safest to convert to a laparotomy to properly address the bowel injury as well as any additional injuries that may be present. Nonetheless, missed intestinal injuries continue to be a major limitation with laparoscopic evaluation of patients with suspected intra-abdominal injuries.

## OPERATIVE MANAGEMENT

After the initial evaluation and resuscitation of the injured patient, patients with suspected or recognized injury to the stomach or small bowel should undergo immediate operation. Under most circumstances the abdomen should be explored through a midline

**TABLE 34-1**

**Stomach Injury**

| GRADE[a] | DESCRIPTION OF INJURY | AIS-90 |
|---|---|---|
| I | Contusion or hematoma | 2 |
| | Partial thickness laceration | 2 |
| II | Laceration in GE junction or pylorus < 2 cm | 3 |
| | In proximal one-third of stomach < 5 cm | 3 |
| | In distal two-thirds of stomach < 10 cm | 3 |
| III | Laceration > 2 cm in GE junction or pylorus | 3 |
| | In proximal one-third of stomach ≥ 5 cm | 3 |
| | In distal two-thirds of stomach ≥ 10 cm | 3 |
| IV | Tissue loss or devascularization < two-thirds of stomach | 4 |
| | Tissue loss or devascularization > two-thirds of stomach | 4 |

[a]Advance one grade for multiple lesions up to grade III.

*GE, gastroesophageal.*

**TABLE 34-2**

**Small Bowel Injury Scale**

| GRADE[a] | TYPE OF INJURY | DESCRIPTION OF INJURY | AIS-90 |
|---|---|---|---|
| I | Hematoma | Contusion or hematoma without devascularization | 2 |
| | Laceration | Partial thickness, no perforation | 2 |
| II | Laceration | Laceration < 50% of circumference | 3 |
| III | Laceration | Laceration ≥ 50% of circumference without transection | 3 |
| IV | Laceration | Transection of the small bowel | 4 |
| V | Laceration | Transection of the small bowel with segmental tissue loss | 4 |
| | Vascular | Devascularized segment | 4 |

[a]Advance one grade for multiple injuries up to grade III.

*AIS, Abbreviated Injury Score.*

incision. Paraxyphoid extension is useful in the exposure of upper stomach or esophageal wounds. In patients with large abdominal wall defects from close range gunshot wounds, the abdominal wall defect may be used for access to the peritoneal cavity. Usually, debridement with further surgical extension of the abdominal wall defect is necessary. Occasionally, stable patients with large defects and eviscerated bowel or omentum due to stab wounds may be explored through a surgical extension of the abdominal wall defect.

After the initial control of significant hemorrhage, contamination from the GI tract is then addressed. In patients with ongoing hemorrhage temporized by packing, gastric and bowel perforations can be rapidly controlled by placing an atraumatic clamp such as a Babcock clamp on the perforated viscus. Alternatively, these perforations may be controlled by a running closure of the perforation(s) with Vicryl or Dexon suture. This is particularly effective if there is significant bleeding from the lacerated stomach/intestine or adjacent mesentery. All injuries identified are then repaired as the next step.

It is useful to grade stomach and small intestinal injuries according to their severity (Tables 34-1 and 34-2). In the patient who is hemodynamically stable, definitive repair of these injuries is relatively straightforward and based on their severity grade.

## Stomach Injuries

Mobilization of the stomach is essential for detection of gastric injuries. Exposure is generally easier if the stomach is decompressed first by a properly placed nasogastric tube. A bloody nasogastric return may be indicative of a gastric injury. Certain areas of the stomach are more difficult to assess: the gastroesophageal junction, high in the gastric fundus, the lesser curvature, and the posterior wall. Division of the left triangular ligament and mobilization of the lateral segment of the left lobe are helpful in exposing the gastroesophageal junction. A Bookwalter or Omni trac retractor can greatly facilitate this exposure. In the hemodynamically stable patient, the reverse Trendelberg position can aid in exposure of this area and allow better visualization of associated diaphragmatic injuries.

If the gastrohepatic ligament is divided, care must be taken to avoid injury to the vagus nerve or its branches or the occasional anomalous left hepatic artery. To visualize high in the gastric fundus, the short gastric vessels should be divided and ligated. Overzealous traction in this area may cause a tear of these vessels

or of the splenic capsule leading to troublesome bleeding. The posterior wall of the stomach may be inspected by opening the avascular portion of the gastrocolic ligament along the greater curvature of the stomach (Fig. 34-8). This may be extended up to the short gastric vessels to visualize areas high in the fundus if necessary. It is better to enter this space in the upper or mid portion of the greater curvature of the stomach to avoid making a rent in the transverse mesocolon and possibly causing injury to middle colic artery.

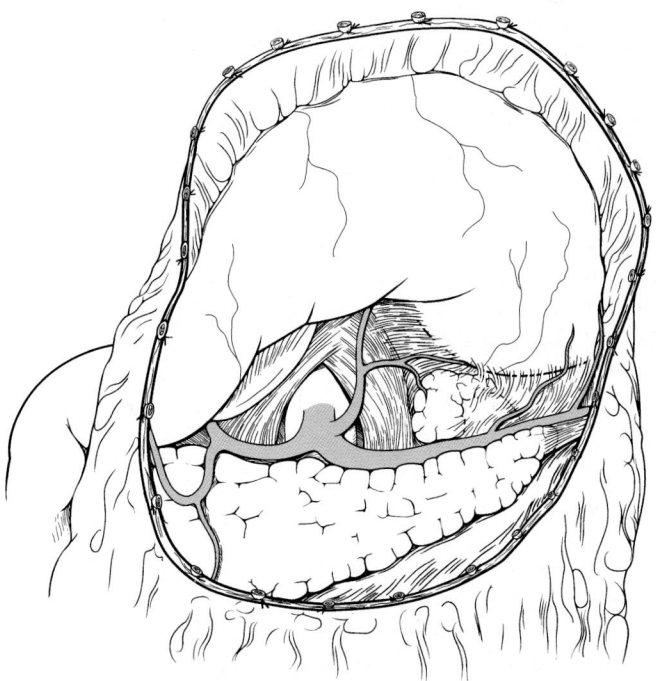

**FIGURE 34-8.** The posterior wall of the stomach, as well as the anterior surface of the pancreas, can be approached by dividing the gastrocolic ligament and lifting the stomach superiorly.

When an anterior hole in the stomach is found, a diligent search for a second hole must be undertaken. This is usually relatively straightforward. However, there are several areas which can hide injuries and should be carefully inspected. These include the greater and lesser curvature of the stomach, the proximal posterior gastric wall, and fundus as well as the posterior cardia. If a suspicion still exists after the search for a second hole comes up empty, a useful diagnostic adjunct is to have the anesthesiologist insufflate the stomach with air through the nasogastric tube. With the stomach submerged in saline, a telltale leakage of bubbles localizes any missed injury. Rarely, it may be necessary to enlarge the known injury so as to inspect the stomach from the inside in search of another injury to the stomach. A tangential wound to the stomach and bowel can occur but this is a diagnosis of exclusion.

Gastric injuries thus identified are treated according to their severity. (Table 34-1) Most intramural hematomas (grades I and II) are repaired with interruptible silk Lembert suture closure after evacuation of the hematoma and hemostasis are obtained. Small grade I and II perforations can be closed primarily in one or two layers. Because the stomach is quite vascular and often bleeds profusely, we prefer a two-layer closure after hemostasis is achieved. A running locked absorbable suture should be used for the inner layer, and interrupted seromuscular sutures of 3.0 or 4.0 silk should be used for the outer layer.

Large (grade III) injuries near the greater curvature can be closed by the same technique or by the use of a GIA stapler. Care must be taken to avoid stenosis in the gastroesophageal and pyloric area. A pyloric wound may be converted to a pyloroplasty to avoid possible stenosis in this area. Extensive wounds (grade IV) may be so destructive that either a proximal or distal gastrectomy is required. Reconstruction with either a Billroth I or II anastomosis is dictated by the presence or absence of an associated duodenal injury. In rare cases, a total gastrectomy and a Roux-en-Y esophojejunostomy is necessary for severe injuries (grade V).

If a diaphragm injury occurs in association with a gastric perforation, contamination of pleural cavity with gastric contents can be problematic. Under most circumstances it is sufficient to clear the pleural space through the diaphragmatic rent following closure of the gastric perforation. It may be necessary to enlarge the diaphragmatic injury to achieve complete evacuation of the pleural contamination. The powered irrigation system used in laproscopic surgery may be an ideal method to clear the pleural cavity prior to chest tube insertion and closure of the diaphragm. Occasionally, the contamination may be so severe, particularly if operation is delayed, that a separate thoracotomy to provide adequate drainage of the pleural space if necessary. Thoracoscopic evacuation of the gastric contamination of the pleural space followed by chest tube placement is another option.

## Small Bowel Injuries

Examination of the small intestine for injury is achieved by evisceration of the small bowel to the right and careful inspection of its entire length. The small bowel is examined loop by loop; no injuries are definitively repaired until the entire bowel is inspected. The decision to resect versus repair bowel is made only after careful assessment of the proximity of bowel perforations and the adequacy of the blood supply to the bowel in question. Mesenteric hematomas adjacent to the bowel wall following penetrating injury

should be carefully opened and the mesenteric aspect of the bowel inspected for injury. Other small nonexpanding mesenteric hematomas should be reassessed at intervals throughout the operative procedure to assure their stability.

If significant bleeding from the mesentery is encountered it should be controlled directly by either placing clamps on the ends of the bleeding vessels followed by suture ligature or by the accurate placement of sutures in a figure-of-eight fashion. Mesenteric defects are closed later. Bleeding at the root of the mesentery requires extra caution in obtaining hemostasis because of the concern for compromising the blood supply to the bowel. Exposure and repair of proximal jejunal injuries may be facilitated by taking down the ligament of Trietz. The inferior mesenteric vein is at risk with injuries in this area. Occasionally, division of this vein is necessary for exposure and repair of bowel injuries near the ligament of Trietz.

Treatment of small bowel injury depends on its grade (Table 34-2).

Obvious serosal tears should be closed with interrupted silk Lembert sutures. Small serosal tears may be left alone if one is certain as to the depth of the intestinal wound. A grade I intramural hematoma can be safely inverted with 3-0 or 4-0 silk seromuscular sutures.

Full-thickness small bowel perforations including less than 50% of the circumference (grade II) are repaired by careful debridement and primary closure (Fig. 34-9). The preferred method is to use a two-layer closure with a continuous Vicryl or Dexon suture for the inner layer and interrupted silk sutures for the outer layer. Alternatively, a single layer closure with a running or interrupted suture can be used. A transverse closure is preferable because it assures the widest luminal opening. A transverse closure without tension may not always be possible, however, particularly with long lacerations along the antimesenteric border of bowel. A longitudinal single layer closure may be preferable in this incidence. Alternatively, a GIA stapler may be placed through the injury and a stapled resection and anastomosis performed (Figs. 34-10 and 34-11).[52] Adjacent through and through wounds of the bowel are joined transversely using electrocautery and closed as a single defect. Multiple grade II injuries can usually be closed individually (Fig. 34-8). Small bowel resection for multiple perforations is not recommended unless resection and anastomosis would take less time than closing the perforations individually and the amount of bowel sacrificed is minimal.

Concerns about the mesenteric circulation and residual luminal diameter dictate the treatment of grade III and IV injuries. Injuries to more than 50% of the small bowel circumference should usually be resected because of the high likelihood of luminal narrowing with primary closure (Fig. 34-12). However, grade III wounds that are oriented transversely or in the relative large proximal to mid jejunum may be primarily repaired provided that an adequate lumen (at least 30% of the circumference) is maintained.

Complete transection of the bowel (grade IV) is treated by resection of the injured bowel and its adjacent blood supply followed by anastomosis (Fig. 34-13). Grade V injuries involve small bowel transections with segmental tissue loss or segmental devascularization and requires resection with anastomosis. (Fig. 34-14).

There remains some controversy as to the safety of stapled versus handsewn anstomoses for traumatic bowel injuries.[53–56] Most of the available data is from retrospective studies with only one prospective study (Table 34-3). There are no controlled clinical

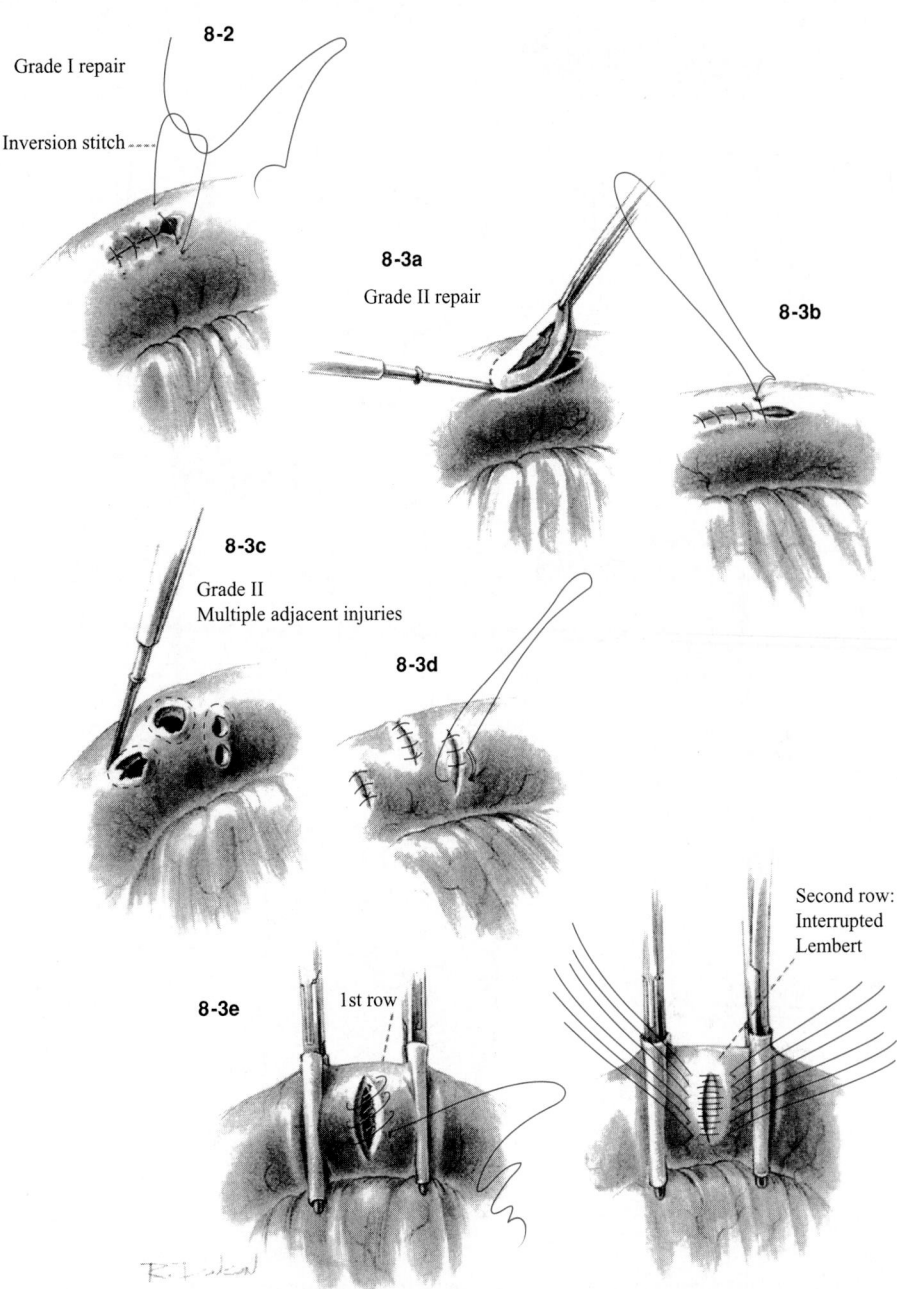

**FIGURE 34-9.** Treatment of grade I and II small bowel injuries. Grade I injuries are treated by inversion with seromuscular sutures. Grade II injuries are treated by careful debridement and primary closure. Either a one or two layer closure may be used. Adjacent through and through perforations are treated as a single defect by dividing the bridge of tissue separating them with electrocautery.

trials comparing techniques for intestinal anastomosis following trauma. However, it is now the general consensus that the complication rate is similar for stapled and handsewn anastomoses.

A hand-sewn anastomosis is the tried and true method to reestablish GI continuity. Techniques include a single layer or two-layered anastomosis. Burch and colleagues conducted a prospective randomized study comparing a single layer anastomosis with 3-0 polypropolene versus a two-layer anastomosis with running absorbable suture for the inner layer and 3-0 silk Lembert for the outer layer.[57] One hundred twenty five patients were enrolled in the study of which only 31 were trauma patients. No differences in anastomotic leaks or intraabdominal abscess between the two groups were noted. Other groups have reported favorable results with a single-layer running absorbable suture technique for traumatic small bowel injuries.[58] If a stapled anastomosis is performed, care should be taken if the enterotomy created for the GIA stapler is closed with a TA stapling device (Fig. 34-11). Regardless of the

technique used, intestinal anastomotic healing is dependent on a good blood supply, a tension-free suture or staple line, an adequate lumen, a water-tight closure, and no distal obstruction.[59] The most appropriate factor in selecting the timing and technique of bowel anastomoses remains sound surgical judgment.

There are several important tenets regarding intestinal anastomoses in the trauma setting. First, the surgeon should rely on techniques that he or she is most experienced with. Secondly, markedly edematous or thickened bowel should be handsewn or one of the newer staplers with a longer staple length should be used. Third, certain circumstances make any anastomosis at risk for complications. These include shock with massive fluid and blood administration, associated pancreatic injury, and the development of an abdominal compartment syndrome.[53,55,56,60]

Patients who incur significant bleeding during laparotomy may develop progressive acidosis, hypothermia, and coagulopathy. These patients should have bleeding controlled or temporized by packing

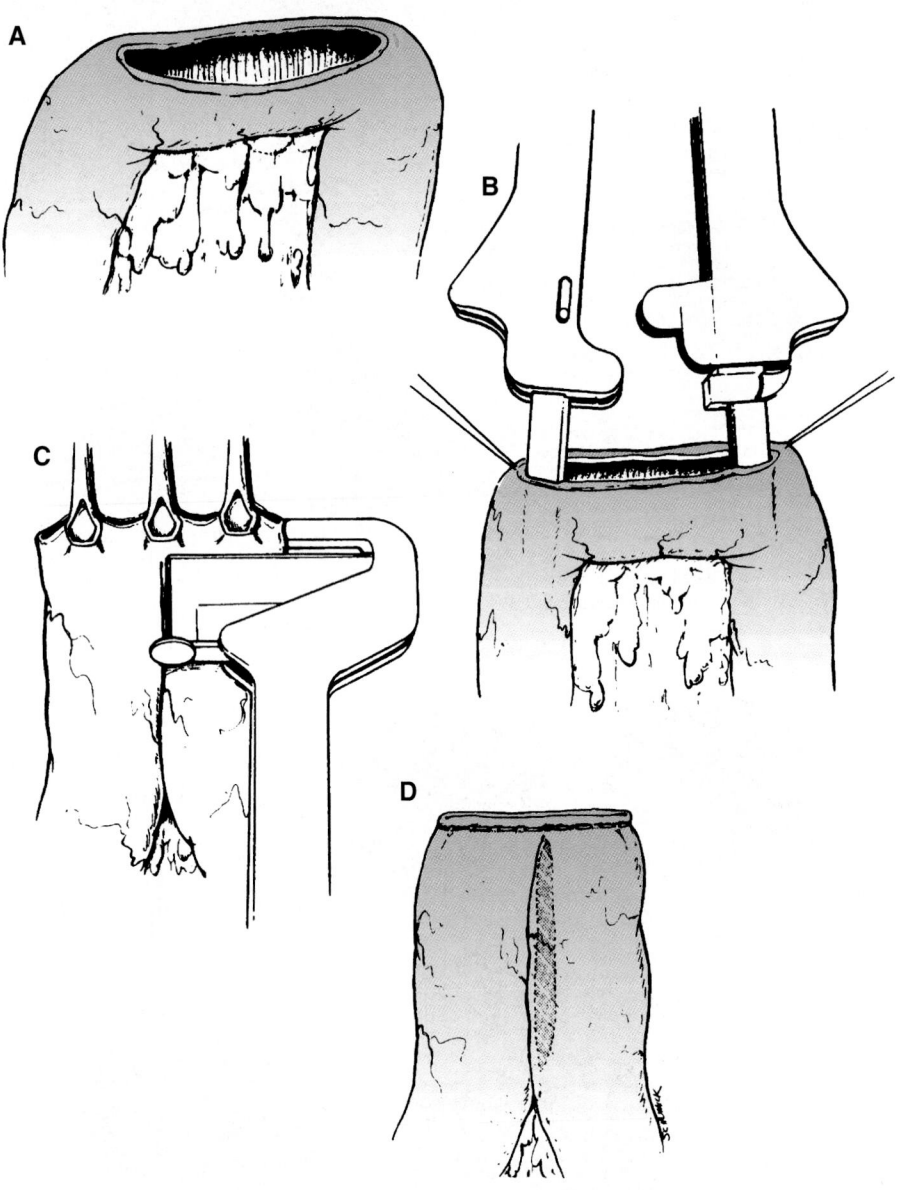

**FIGURE 34-10.** Long lacerations along the antimesenteric aspect of the small bowel may be treated with resection and anastomosis, using GIA and TA staplers.

and undergo further resuscitation before definitive repairs are performed. GI tract injuries should be managed by simple repairs if amenable. More severe bowel injuries may be controlled by stapling of the bowel proximally and distally with resection of the injured part of the bowel.[61] Anastomosis is performed in the operating room 24–48 hours later when the patient has been stabilized.

Bowel resection with anastomosis does not appear to place the anastomosis at risk of breakdown in the patient with an open abdomen.[62] Protection of the bowel anastomosis with omental covering, gental handling of the bowel on reoperation, and early facial closure are advised to prevent intestinal fistula formation.[63,64] Anastomosis at a larger stage is facilated by a decrease in bowel edema which may be significantly less at this time. Additionally, it allows reevaluation of bowel of questionable viability.

Extensive destruction of the small bowel or its mesentery (grade V) necessitates resection and anastomosis. Treatment of isolated mesenteric injuries without bowel perforation is dependent on the viability of the bowel. Resection is required for devascularized bowel. If the involved bowel segment is short and there is doubt about the viability of the bowel, resection should be performed.

Proximal injuries to the mesenteric blood vessels may result in large segments of questionable bowel viability. Clinical judgment about bowel viability has under the best circumstances only a 65% predictive value. Adjunctive techniques to access bowel viability such as intravenous fluorescein and bowel inspection using a Wood's lamp, Doppler flow studies, and bowel surface oximetry may be useful. However, it is usually wiser to terminate the procedure, provide temporary abdominal closure and perform a second look procedure in 24 hours after the patient is rewarmed and perfusion deficits corrected before deciding to perform an extensive bowel resection. Performing resection at this later time may allow preservation of bowel that was of questionable viability at the first operation. With massive bowel resections, it is important to note the location and length of the segment of the resected bowel and to measure the length of the remaining bowel. Preserving as much of the ileum as clinically possible and the ileocecal value if feasible may obviate the complications related to extensive bowel resections.

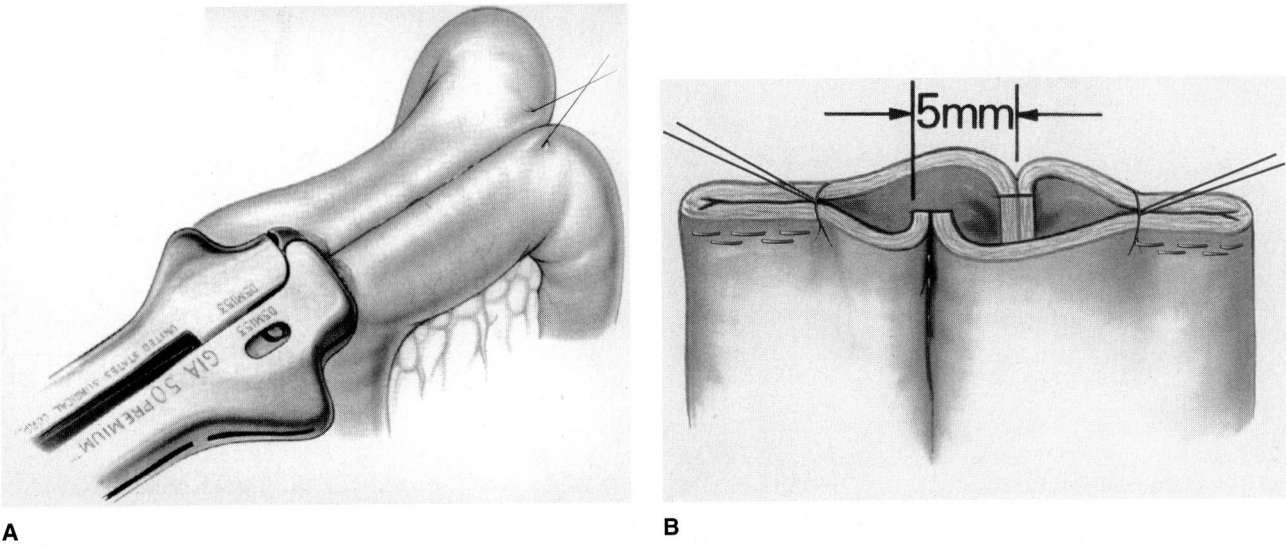

**A**

**B**

**FIGURE 34-11.**    When using a TA stapler to close the defect created for the GIA stapler, it is important to offset staple lines which may create ischemia to the tissues and potentiate an anastomotic leak.

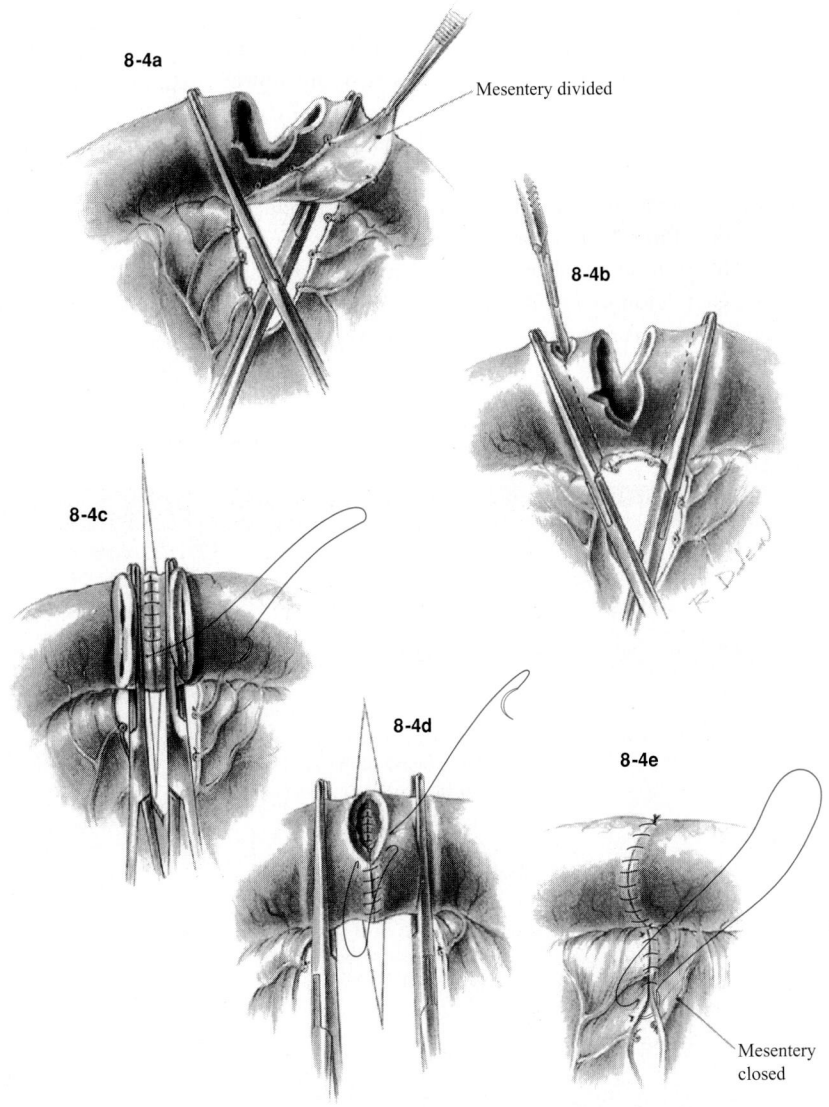

**FIGURE 34-12.**    Grade III small bowel injuries are usually treated by resection and anastomoses. Proximal small bowel injuries or transversely oriented wounds may on occasion be primarily repaired.

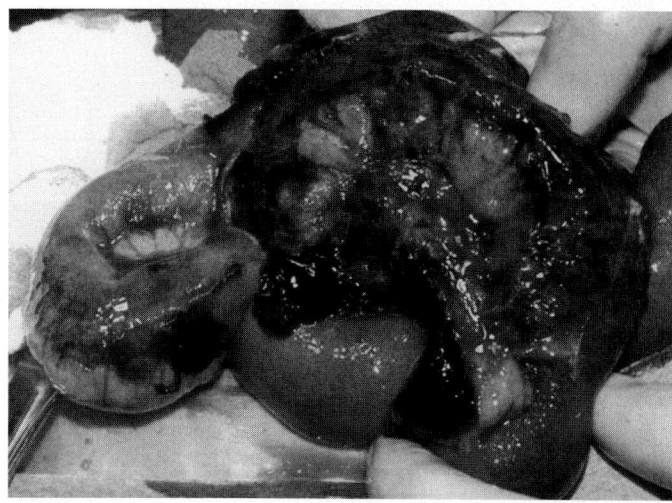

**FIGURE 34-13.** Treatment at grade IV small bowel injuries requires resection of the injured bowel and its adjacent blood supply. Anastomosis may be performed using either suture or stapling techniques.

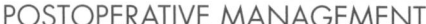

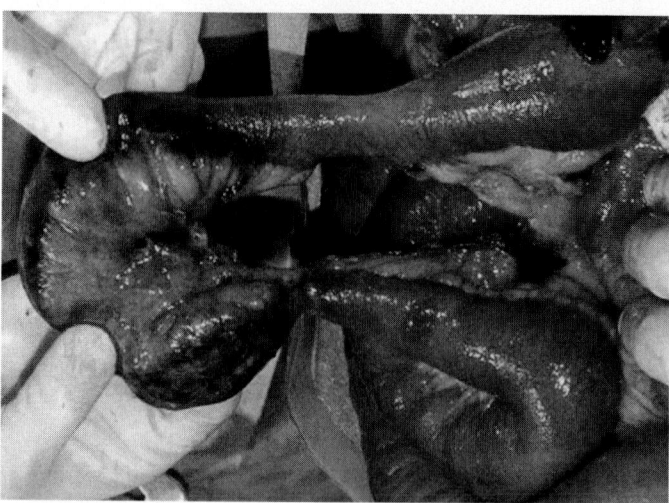

**FIGURE 34-14.** Isolated mesenteric injury: Mesenteric injuries can be caused by both blunt and penetrating mechanisms. If the blood supply is disrupted enough to lead to questions about the viability of a short segment of small intestine, that segment should be resected.

## POSTOPERATIVE MANAGEMENT

The postoperative care of patients with gastric and small bowel injuries is usually relatively straightforward. When complications do arise they are more often related to associated injuries or to delays in the operative management of the stomach and bowel injuries. Antibiotics are limited to a 24-hour course, usually of a single agent such as cefoxitin or ampicillin–sulbactam.[65] However, appropriate dosing may be problematic in patients undergoing massive volume resuscitation with crystalloid and blood products.

The advisability of routine nasogastric decompression following procedures involving an intestinal anastomosis is still controversial, despite prospective randomized controlled trials finding no advantage to this practice.[66–69] A meta-analysis of selective versus routine nasogastric decompression after elective laparotomy was conducted

by Cheatham et al. on 3964 patients from 26 published trials.[67] Routine nasogastric decompression was not supported by this meta-analysis of the literature. However, these studies did not involve trauma patients. The potential impact of other clinically important variables including the presence of multiple associated injuries, hemorrhagic shock, and postresuscitation bowel edema as well as an impaired sensorium from head injuries or drugs and alcohol may make nasogastric decompression the more prudent choice. It is our practice to continue nasogastric decompression, which was initiated during the initial resuscitation, until ileus resolves. In patients in whom a jejunostomy is placed at laparotomy, it is also useful to decompress the stomach and monitor gastric outputs as jejunal enteral feeds are initiated. Jejunal feeding may increase gastric output significantly which may lead to pulmonary aspiration in these patients.[70]

### TABLE 34-3

#### Small Bowel Injury: Hand-Sewn Versus Stapled Anastomoses

| AUTHOR (Year) | NUMBER OF PATIENTS | BOWEL INJURED | TYPE OF SMALL BOWEL ANASTOMOSES | | RESULTS AND COMMENTS |
|---|---|---|---|---|---|
| | | | Hand-Sewn | Stapled | |
| Brundage[53] (1999) | 84 | Small Bowel (101) and Colon (17) | 60 | 58 | Retrospective single institutional study. Stapled anastomoses had significant increase in anastomotic leak requiring reoperation |
| Witzke[54] (2000) | 257 | Small bowel only; but included primary repair (131) and resection/anastomoses (144) | 34 | 110 | Retrospective single institution study showed no difference in rate of intra-abdominal abscess, fistula, a anastomotic leak or postoperative bowel obstruction |
| Brundage[55] (2001) | 199 | Both small bowel (224) and colonic anastomoses (61) | 84 | 140 | Retrospective study from 5 five Level I trauma centers. Higher leak rate and overall complication rate for stapled anastomoses |
| Kirkpatrick[56] (2003) | 227 | Small bowel only; both primary repair (104) and resection with anastomoses (123) | 24 | 52 | Retrospective study from two institutions. No differences in anastomotic complication as related to technique used. Increased anastomotic complications associated with pancreatoduodeno injury, or if done as part of a damage control procedure. Forty-seven anastomoses were done using suture/ staples in a combined technique |

In uncomplicated cases involving stomach or small bowel injuries there is no evidence to support routine nutritional support of patients who were well-nourished preinjury. On the other hand in critically ill or injured patients it is prudent to start nutritional support early before hypermetabolism or sepsis intervenes.[71] Available clinical evidence suggests that moderately to severely injured patients (ISS >16 <25) should have enteral feedings started between 24 and 48 hours postinjury.[71-73] Those with more severe injuries are more likely to have intolerance to enteral feedings.

There is convincing evidence in the literature that patients with blunt and penetrating injuries sustain fewer septic complications when fed enterally as opposed to parenterally.[73] However, total parenteral nutrition should be started by day 7 in severely injured patients who do not tolerate enteral feeding or fail to tolerate at least 50% of their goal rate of enteral feedings. Enteral feeding should start only when patients are completely resuscitated due to the risk of intolerance to the enteral feeds or to the possibility of the development of nonocclusive bowel necrosis.[74,75] There does not appear to be a clear advantage to postpyloric enteral feeding versus gastric feeding in trauma patients. Thus, with few exceptions (severe closed head injury, or severe pancreatic duodenal injury) surgical feeding jejunostomy (with the exception of a needle catheter jejunostomy) should not be routinely performed at the initial laparotomy. Further, bowel edema may make this simple procedure a far greater challenge than necessary. If patients do not tolerate intragastric feeds, it is far simpler to place a nasojejunal tube endoscopically at a later time.

There are a number of studies of patients randomized to enteral support with diets supplemented with Omega-3 fatty acids, arginine, nucleotides, and glutamine to attempt to enhance immunological responses.[76,77] These immune-enhancing formulas may be indicated in the most severely injured patients (ISS >20, ATI >25) when given in conjunction with early and adequate protein/calorie support.

There is some concern for initiating enteral feeds in the early (less than 24–48 hours) postinjury period. It is well known that gastrointestinal motility is adversely impaired following abdominal surgery. Bowel perforation requiring repair or resection and anastomosis is another confounding variable. Postoperative ileus (POI), an inevitable consequence of any laporatomy, may not only hamper attempts at enteral feeding, but also the timely recovery of the patient.[78] There are multiple pathogenic mechanisms responsible for POI.[79] Neural reflexes seem to be the most important, compounded by inflammatory mediators and the administration of opioids for pain control. Conventional treatments of POI include nasogastric suction, early ambulation, implementation of early enteral feeding, and the use of prokinetic drugs. Although nasogastric decompression and early ambulation are time-honored therapies for postoperative ileus, neither method has ever been scientifically proven to speed the resolution of POI.[79,80] Early enteral feeding most likely only has a modest affect on the resolution of POI, even though it is usually tolerated following injury. Enteral feeding tolerance is best achieved using a standardized protocol for initiating feeds and criteria for advancing the rate of infusion.[81]

Metoclopramide and Cisapride were the most commonly used prokinetic agents described in the management of POI.[82] Metoclopramide, however, has no demonstrable effect in relieving postoperative ileus. It is usually administered in a futile attempt to improve GI motility when nothing else is working. Cisapride has shown some positive results for the treatment of postoperative ileus, but was withdrawn from the market because of adverse

cardiovascular effects. Erythromycin, a motilin receptor agonist, also has limited efficacy in resolving postoperative ileus.[83] Sham feeding in the form of gum chewing has been reported to be a helpful method in limiting the duration of POI.[84]

A number of studies have shown that the duration of POI is influenced by the postoperative use of opioids.[85] Opioids sparing analgesic regimens including the use of epideral anesthesia and the adjunctive use of NSAIDS may obviate some of the undesirable side-effects of opioid analgesia. Three main classes of opioid receptors have been identified. The u2 receptors subtype when activated results in respiratory depression and reduced gastrointestinal motility. In this regard, there has been recent interest in the use of the peripherally selective opioid antagonists alivopan and naltrexone to improve postoperative GI motility.[85] However, as these drugs are started prior to surgery, their use appears limited in the trauma setting. As several mechanisms are causally related to the development of postoperative ileus, the multi-modality approach for the treatment of POI will likely be most efficacious.

Complications directly related to gastric and small injuries include intraabdominal septic complications and anastomotic disruption. An intraabdominal septic complication most often presents as an intraabdominal abscess. Anastomotic failures may present as peritonitis and/or the development of an external fistula. Infections complications following gastric injury are most common following blunt trauma and if there is an associated colon injury.[86-89] In these patients, ongoing fever and leukocytosis should mandate diagnostic imaging of both the chest and abdomen to look for foci of infection to drain.

The most important etiologic factor directly relating stomach or small bowel injuries to intraabdominal abscess formation is delayed recognition and surgical treatment. Canty et al. suggested a delay of up to 24 hours after blunt intestinal trauma did not increase mortality or morbidity.[90] A delay in definitive repair over 24 hours was directly associated with increased morbidity but not mortality. Determination of small bowel injury in children is often difficult based on clinical findings and may contribute to delays in operative intervention.[91] Bensard and colleagues reported on the effect of delay in surgical treatment of nine children with small bowel injuries.[92] Six children were operated on 36 ± 16 hours after admission yet had an uneventful recovery. The small numbers of patients in these two studies do not provide convincing evidence as to the potential for harm to the patient with these diagnostic delays. Fang and colleagues retrospectively reviewed 111 consecutive blunt trauma patients with bowel injuries from a single institution.[93] Delays in surgery for more than 24 hours did not significantly increase the mortality compared to when operations were performed within four hours of injury. However, intestinal-related complications including sepsis, wound infection, anastomotic failures, and intraabdominal abscess formation increased dramatically.

Fakhry et al. published a multicenter experience in 198 patients with blunt small bowel injuries.[94] There were 21 deaths (10.6% of total) with nine of these deaths attributable to delay in operation for small bowel injury. In patients in whom small bowel injury was the major injury, the incidence of mortality increased with time to operative intervention. Mortality rates were 2% if the patient was operated on within eight hours, 9.1% if operated between 8–16 hours, 16.7% if operated on between 16 and 24 hours, and 30.8% if operated on more than 24 hours after injury ($p = 0.009$). The incidence of bowel-related complications, especially intraabdominal abscess formation also increased significantly with time to operative intervention. Based on the available literature it seems advisable to determine the need for operation within eight hours of injury and anticipate complications should operative intervention occur at a later time.

Bleeding complications after gastric or small bowel trauma may present as bleeding into the peritoneal cavity or into the bowel lumen. Bleeding from the short gastric vessels or from a torn splenic capsule is a common iatrogenic source of bleeding in this area. Bleeding from the mesentery or lesser curvature of the stomach may not be apparent intraoperatively in the hypotensive patient. This may only become clinically apparent when the patient normalizes his/her blood pressure; continued bleeding postoperatively then manifests as hypotension and a falling hematocrit.[95] After the patient is resuscitated/stabilized, it is necessary to reoperate. Suture line bleeding can be troublesome and may manifest as bloody nasogastric secretions. Endoscopic hemostatic techniques may be carefully employed in this setting, particularly if the bleeding is from the stomach.

Anastomotic failure may present as a contained leak, diffuse fecal peritonitis, or as an enterocutaneous fistula.[96,97] Therapeutic options include medical care only if there is a tiny radiographically evident but clinically insignificant leak. Reoperation is necessary with primary repair and drainage for a small leak discovered early postoperatively if there is minimal peritonitis in the otherwise stable patient. Percutaneous drainage is useful for a symptomatic leak presenting in a delayed fashion as an intraabdominal abcess. If there is complete disruption of an anastomoses with widespread peritoneal contamination, it is advisable to consider a proximal diverting enterostomy.

Anastomotic leaks diagnosed in the immediate postoperative period may be surgically approached as the relevant tissue planes are amenable to surgical dissection. After 10 or 14 days, the inflammatory process makes dissection of bowel extremely difficult. In this case proximal diversion and/or controlled external drainage of the leak may be safer.

There are three phases in the management of an enterocutaneous fistula.[96] The first phase is diagnosis or recognition of the problem. Usually this is quite obvious with either enteric content coming from the wound or postoperative sepsis and a leak defined by imaging studies. The next stage (phase 2) involves stabilization of the patient and radiographic investigation. Stabilization includes correction of fluid and electrolyte deficits and the treatment of sepsis. External loss of intestinal fluids rich in electrolytes, minerals, and protein lead to electrolyte imbalance and malnutrition.

Identification of the fistula site and/or measurement of the electrolyte composition of the fistula effluent are sometimes helpful for fluid replacement (Table 34-4). However, in most cases normal saline with 10–20 milliequivalents of potassium is a suitable fluid to use for the initial intravenous fluid replacement. Patients with enterocutaneous fistula may also develop significant magnesium deficits which should be corrected.

Fistulas are classified as high output (>500 mL per day), moderate output (200–500 mL per day), or low output (<200 mL per day). This may be important to classify fistulas in this manner as it may allow anticipation of the method for nutritional support, and may be useful in predicting the likelihood of spontaneous closure and mortality.[96]

Control of sepsis may include image guided or surgical drainage of intra-abdominal abscesses identified by CT. Empiric antibiotic

**TABLE 34-4**

**Composition and Volume of Gastrointestinal Secretions**

| TYPE | VOLUME (mL/DAY) | NA (mEq/L) | K (mEq/L) | CL (mEq/L) | HCO₃ (mEq/L) |
|---|---|---|---|---|---|
| Salivary | 1500 | 10 | 26 | 15 | 50 |
| Stomach | 1500 | 60–100 | 10 | 100 | 0 |
| Duodenum | 2000 | 130 | 5 | 90 | 0–10 |
| Illeum | 3000 | 140 | 5 | 100 | 15–30 |
| Pancreas | 800 | 140 | 5 | 75 | 70–115 |
| Bile | 800 | 145 | 5 | 100 | 15–35 |

should be started in septic patients and modified after relevant culture data is obtained. The presence of an enterocutanous fistula without clinical signs of sepsis does not warrant antibiotic therapy.

The provision adequate of nutritional support is paramount in the stabilization phase. These patients are usually hypercatabolic and generally require 25 to 32 calories per kilogram per day in total calories with a calorie to nitrogen ratio of 150:1 and a protein intake of at least 1.5 grams per kilogram per day. Total parental nutrition has long been recognized to be an important factor in the management of enterocutaneous fistula. Recent reports have advocated that the provision of at least some of the caloric requirement should be by the enteral route.[96] This may be helpful for its "trophic" affects on the intestine as well as allowing easier management in the outpatient setting. In patients with diversion of the proximal small bowel as an ostomy, reinfusion of the succus entericus into the distal GI tract may be helpful as well.[98]

Adjuncts to control fistula drainage include nasogastric drainage, and acid suppression with H2 receptor antagonists or protein pump inhibitors. Administration of somatostatin and its analog octreotide have an inconsistent effect on fistula output and time to fistula closure. Futhermore, the use of these agents do not increase the rate of nonoperative closure of fistulas.[96]

Protecting the integrity of the skin surrounding the fistulas will improve the quality of the surrounding tissues and decrease infectious complications. Low output fistulas are usually managed with conventional measures. High output fistulas or fistula(s) in the patient with an open abdomen may benefit by the use of the vacuum assisted closure (VAC) system. These may be applied over the entire wound with the fistula or as a VAC dressing with openings for stoma pouches of the fistula openings.[99–101] The main benefit of the use of the VAC system for enterocutaneous fistula appears to be improved wound care before definitive surgery.

Spontaneous closure of enterocutaneous fistulas in patients provided adequate nutritional support and free of sepsis usually occurs within four to six weeks. Unfortunately, spontaneous closure occurs only in about 30% of trauma patients.[97] Definitive surgery (phase 3) in a patient with a persistent enterocutaneous fistula is usually delayed four to six months following the initial operation. Options include resection and reanastomoses of the involved bowel segments or oversewing or wedge resection of the fistula. Recurrence of an enterocutaneous fistulae is related to the method of surgical closure. In a study by Lynch and collegues, oversewing or wedge resection of the enterocutaneous fistula was associated with 36% recurrence rate, while resection with reanastomoses has a 16% recurrence rate.[102]

Differentiating mechanical small bowel obstruction in the early postoperative period from prolonged postoperative ileus can de daunting. Renz and Feliciano reported a 4.3% incidence of prolonged ileus and a 2.4% incidence of small bowel obstruction in 254 patients who had unnecessary laparotomies for trauma.[103] Tortella and colleagues reported an overall incidence of early small bowel obstruction in 7.4% in 298 patients who had a laparotomy for penetrating abdominal trauma.[104]

Patients with small or large bowel injuries were at the greatest risk with a 10.8% incidence of bowel obstruction. However, traumatic bowel injuries do not appear to increase the risk of postoperative bowel obstruction. In a retrospective cohort study, Beck et al. found that 14.3% of patients developed obstructions and 2.8% required adhesiolysis for obstructions following elective colorectal and general surgery.[105]

It has been advised to continue nasogastric suction for 10 to 14 days after laparotomy before considering reoperation for suspected small bowel obstruction.[106] However, it is prudent to obtain a CT scan with oral/IV contrast at an earlier time to look for fluid collections and/or intraabdominal abscesses. CT guided drainage of these processes often leads to return of bowel function and thus avoidance of re-laparotomy. Additionally, CT may contribute significantly to differentiating adhesive small bowel obstruction from ileus and lead to earlier operative intervention.[107] CT may also disclose radiographic findings suspicious for bowel strangulation or volvulus before the appearance of clinical symptoms.

In patients reoperated for postoperative bowel obstruction or in patients who later require elective reestablishment of GI continuity, it may be prudent to attempt to minimize adhesion formation. Both bioresorbable physical barriers and various sprayable polymers are either available or under development in an attempt to reduce adhesions.[108] Sephrafilm®, a hyaluronic acid and carboxymethylcellouse bioresorbable membrane is the most common antiadhesive barrier used in general surgery. It is applied to potentially adhesiogenic tissues before closure of the abdomen. It adheres to moist tissue surfaces and is cleared from the body within 28 days of implantation. Initial clinical studies were promising. A more recent multi-center trial by Fazio et al. compared Sephrafilm® application versus no treatment in 1701 patients who underwent intestinal resections. Although the overall bowel obstruction rate was unchanged, there was a significant reduction in the number of patients requiring reoperation for bowel obstruction.[109] Sephrafilm is, however, somewhat cumbersome to use, especially with distended bowel already complicating abdominal wound closure in the trauma setting. There are a number of other membrane barriers under investigation as well.

Sprayable polymers are another antiadhesive modality.[110] A variety of fibrin glue preparations have been used to limit adhesion formation and several other polymers are under investigation.[111] There is concern that any of these substances may act as a foreign body and promote the development of an intraabdominal abscess or other septic complication. This is especially true with bowel injury and concomitant peritoneal contamination.[112]

Resection of significant amounts of small bowel may lead to problems with malabsorption. In general, jejunal resections are better tolerated than ileal resections. Removal of significant portions of the jejunum may lead to lactose intolerance; however, this is usually self-limited. Resection of the distal ileum often leads to vitamin B12 deficiency as well as bile salt deficiencies, and subsequent fat malabsorption. Ileal resection also removes the "ileal breaking mechanism" which may cause decreased transit time throughout

the gut. This may result in profuse diarrhea and significant fluid and electrolyte imbalances. The ileocecal valve also has an important role as it acts to decrease the volume of stool by slowing intestinal transit time.

The short bowel syndrome occurs following intestinal resection which results in inadequate small bowel absorptive surface.[113] Signs and symptoms of short bowel syndrome include diarrhea, metabolic acidosis, deficiencies of calcium, magnesium and zinc, vitamin B12 and iron deficiency, fat soluble vitamin deficiencies, malabsorption of carbohydrate, fat and protein, gastric acid hypersecretion, the formation of cholesterol gallstones and renal oxalate stones, as well as significant dehydration. Previously the short bowel syndrome was defined as a loss of 50% or more of the small bowel. More recently the short bowel syndrome has been defined as the malabsorption problems that occur in adults who have less than 200 cm of jejunal-ileum remaining. Trauma currently accounts for 8% of all adult patients with the short bowel syndrome.[114]

The chronology of the short bowel syndrome follows three phases: (1) the acute phase involving the initial resection and perioperative care, (2) the subacute phase associated with initial enteral feeding and bowel compensation, and (3) the chronic phase characterized by problems of malabsorption, diarrhea, parenteral nutrition, and a variety of nutritional maladies.[115]

The acute phase occurs during the immediate postoperative weeks and may last 1–3 months. This phase is marked by poor absorption of almost all macro- and micronutrients. Ostomies, if present, may have outputs exceeding five liters per day during the first few days after massive bowel resection. Aggressive intravenous fluid and electrolyte replacement is necessary to prevent life-threatening dehydration and electrolyte imbalances. The primary route of nutrition is parenteral; however, enteral feeding should be slowly initiated later in this phase.[115]

Intestinal adaptation occurs during the subacute phase and enhances bowel absorption. This adaptive process in humans occurs over a period of months to years and is due to dilation of the remaining bowel coupled with improved cell-transport function and prolonged intestinal transit time. Intestinal adaptation may be mediated by growth factors and nutrients including human growth hormone, insulin-like growth factor, epidermal growth factor, transforming growth factor α, and glucagon-like peptides.[116] Nutrients including glutamine and fatty acids may also act as growth factors in intestinal adaptation.

Enteral feeding to provide intraluminal nutrients to maintain gut mass is necessary for the adaptation response to occur. Thus, enteral nutrition remains the primary therapy in maximizing luminal nutrient absorption in the intestinal remnant. In a recent study the use of growth hormone, glutamine, and nutrients to facilitate bowel adaptation led to a significant reduction in the number of TPN-dependent adults with short bowel syndrome.[117] A variety of surgical techniques to slow transit time and/or increase bowel length have met with limited success in the treatment of short bowel syndrome.[118] Restoring the colonic remnant to the GI tract may be helpful as the colon takes on an absorptive function by deriving energy from short chain fatty acids and prolonging transit time, particularly if the ileocecal valve is intact. However, at least 3 ft. of small intestine is required to prevent diarrhea and perianal complications. Other procedures include surgical tapering of dilated dysfunctional intestinal segments and intestinal lengthening procedures. The serial transverse enteroplasty (STEP) procedure is a recent advance as an intestinal lengthening procedure.[118]

Intestinal transplantation is reserved as a last alternative for patients unable to compensate and adapt following intestinal resection. Intestinal transplantation may also be offered to patients who require TPN to maintain body mass and have limited or no remaining venous access for parenteral nutrition, or parenteral nutrition related liver disease. Trauma patients seem to have equivalent long-term survival rates as compared to nontrauma patients following intestinal transplantation.[119]

# REFERENCES

1. Brownstein MR, Bunting T, Meyer AA, et al.: Diagnosis and management of blunt small bowel injury: A survey of the membership of the American Association for the Surgery of Trauma. *J Trauma* 48:402, 2000.
2. Wisner DH, Chun Y, Blaisdell FW: Blunt intestinal injury. Keys to diagnosis and management. *Arch Surg* 125:1319, 1990.
3. Loria Fl: Historical aspects of penetrating wounds of the abdomen. *Int Abstr Surg* 87:521, 1948.
4. Bailey, H (ed): *Surgery of modern warfare.* Vol II 3rd ed. Baltimore: Williams and Williams, 1944.
5. Surgery in World War II, Vol II, General Surgery. Office of the Surgeon General, Department of the Army, Washington D.C., 1955.
6. Finegold SM, Sutter VL, Mathisen GE: Normal indegnous intestinal flora. In Hentges DJ, ed. *Human intestinal microflora in health and disease.* New York: Academic Press, 1983, p.3.
7. Howden CW, Hunt RH: Relationship between gastric secretion and infection. *Gut* 28:96, 1987.
8. Simon GL, Gorbach SL: Intestinal flora in health and disease. *Gastroenterology* 86:177, 1987.
9. Ulman I, Avanoglu A, Ozcan C, et al.: Gastrointestinal perforations in children: A continuing challenge to nonoperative treatment of blunt abdominal trauma. *J Trauma* 41:110, 1996.
10. Talton DS, Craig MH, Hauser, CJ, et al.: Major gastroenteric injuries from blunt trauma. *Am Surg* 61:69, 1995.
11. Guarino J, Hassett JM, Luchette FA: Small bowel injuries: Mechanisms, patterns, and outcome. *J Trauma* 39:1076, 1995.
12. Cripps NP, Cooper GJ: Intestinal injury mechanisms after blunt abdominal impact. *Ann R Coll Surg Engl* 79:115, 1997.
13. Dauterive AH, Flancbaum L, Cox EF: Blunt intestinal trauma. *Ann Surg* 201:198, 1984.
14. Appleby JP, Nagy AG: Abdominal injuries associated with the use of seatbelts. *Am J of Surg* 157:457, 1989.
15. Anderson PA, Rivara FP, Maier RV, et al.: The epidemiology of seatbelt-associated injuries. *J Trauma* 31:60,1991.
16. Chandler CF, Lane JS, Waxman KS: Seatbelt sign following blunt trauma is associated with increased incidence of abdominal injury. *Am Surg* 10:885, 1997.
17. Watts D, Fakhry S, Scalea T, et al.: Blunt hollow viscus injury (HVI) and small bowel injury (SBI): Prevalence, mortality, and morbidity results from a large multi-institutional study. *J Trauma* 51:1233, (abstract) 2001.
18. Fakhry S, Watts D, Daley B, et al.: Current diagnostic approaches lack sensitivity in the diagnosis of perforating blunt small bowel injury (SBI): Findings from a large multi-institutional trial. *J Trauma* 51:1232, (abstract) 2001.
19. Hackam DJ, Ali J, Jastaniah SS: Effects of other intra-abdominal injuries on the diagnosis, management, and outcome of small bowel trauma. *J Trauma* 49:606, 2000.
20. Tsushima Y, Yamada S, Aoki J,et al.: Ischaemic ileal stenosis following blunt abdominal trauma and demonstrated by CT. *Br J Rad* 74:277, 2001.
21. Flint LM, Cryer HM, Howard PA, et al.: Approaches to the management of shotgun injuries. *J Trauma* 24:415, 1984.
22. Singer P, Cohen JD, et al.: Conventional terrorism and critical care. *Crit Care Med* 33(1 Suppl): S61, 2005.
23. Almogy G, Mintz Y, et al.: Suicide bombing attacks: Can external signs predict internal injuries? *Ann Surg* 243:541, 2006.
24. Nagy K, Roberts R, et al.: Evisceration after abdominal stab wounds: Is laperotomy required? *J Trauma* 47:622, 1999.
25. Dupre MW, Silva E, Brotman S: Traumatic rupture of the stomach secondary to Heimlich Maneuver. *Am J Emerg Med* 11:611, 1993.
26. Nance ML, Peden GW, Shapiro MB, et al.: Solid viscus injury predicts major hollow viscus injury in blunt abdominal trauma. *J Trauma* 43:618, 1997.
27. Miller PR, Croce MA, Bee TK, et al.: Associated injuries in blunt solid organ trauma: Implications for missed injury in non-operative management. *J Trauma* 51:1225, 2001.
28. Watts D, Fakhry S, Scalea T, et al.: Blunt hollow viscus injury (HVI) and small bowel injury (SBI): Prevalence, mortality, and morbidity; Results from a large multi-institutional study. *J Trauma* 51:1232, (abstract) 2001.
29. Pikoulis E, Delis S, Psalidas N, et al.: Presentation of blunt small intestinal and mesenteric injuries. *Ann R Coll Surg Engl* 82:103, 2000.
30. Kemmeter PR, Senagore AJ, Smith D, et al.: Dilemmas in the diagnosis of blunt enteric trauma. *Am Surg* 64:750, 1998.
31. Jacobs DG, Angus L, Rodriguez A, et al.: Peritoneal lavage white count: A reassessment. *J Trauma* 30:607, 1990.
32. Jaffin JH, Ochsner G, Cole FJ, et al.: Alkaline phosphatase levels in diagnostic peritoneal lavage fluid as a predictor of hollow visceral injury. *J Trauma* 34:829, 1993.
33. McAnena OJ, Marx JA, Moore EE: Peritoneal lavage enzyme determinations following blunt and penetrating abdominal trauma. *J Trauma* 31:1161, 1991.
34. Otomo Y, Henmi H, Mashiko K, et al.: New diagnostic peritoneal lavage criteria for diagnosis of intestinal injury. *J Trauma* 44:991, 1998.
35. Fang JF, Chen RJ, Lin BC: Cell count ratio: New criterion of diagnostic peritoneal lavage for detection of hollow organ perforation. *J Trauma* 45:540, 1998.
36. Rozycki, GS, Ballard RB, Feliciano DV, et al.: Surgeon-performed ultrasound for the assessment of truncal injuries. *Ann Surg* 228:557, 1998.
37. Ballard RB, Rozycki GS, Newman PG, et al.: An algorithm to reduce the incidence of false-negative FAST examinations in patients at high risk for occult injury. *J Am Coll Surg* 189:145, 1999.
38. Malhatra AK, Fabian TC, Katsis SB, et al.: Blunt bowel and mesenteric injuries: the role of screening computed tomography. *J Trauma* 48:991, 2000.
39. Nghiem HV, Jeffrey RB, Mindelzun RE: CT of blunt trauma to the bowel and mesentery. Seminars in ultrasound, CT, and MRI. 16:82, 1995.
40. Butela ST, Federle MP, Chang PJ, et al.: Performance of CT in detection of bowel injury. *AJR* 176:129, 2001.
41. Hamilton P, Rizoli S, McLellan B, et al.: Significance of intra-abdominal extraluminal air detected by CT scan in blunt abdominal trauma. *J Trauma* 39:331, 1995.
42. Fakhry S,Watts D, Clancy K, et al.: Diagnosing blunt small bowel injury (SBI): an analysis of the clinical utility of computerized tomography (CT) scan from a large multi-institutional trial. *J Trauma* 51:1232 (abstract), 2001.
43. Livingston DH, Lavery RF, Passannante MR, et al.: Free fluid on abdominal computed tomography without solid organ injury after blunt abdominal injury does not mandate celiostomy. *Am J Surg* 182:6, 2001.
44. Livingston DH, Lavery RF, Passannante MR, et al.: Admission or observation is not necessary after a negative abdominal computed tomography scan in patients with suspected blunt abdominal trauma: Results of a prospective, multi-institutional trial. *J Trauma* 44:273, 1998.
45. Hagiwara A, Yukioka T, Satou M, et al.: Early diagnosis of small intestine rupture from blunt abdominal trauma using computed tomography: Significance of the streaky density within the mesentery. *J Trauma* 38:630, 1995.
46. Poole GV, Thomae KR, Hauser CJ: Laparoscopy in trauma. *Surg Clin North Am* 76:547, 1996.
47. Zantut LF, Ivatury RR, Smith RS, et al.: Diagnostic and therapeutic laparoscopy for penetrating abdominal trauma: A multicenter experience. *J Trauma* 42:825, 1997.
48. Smith RS, Fry WR, Morabito DJ, et al.: Therapeutic laparoscopy in trauma. Am J Surg 170:632, 1995.
49. Fabian TC, Croce MA, Steward RM, et al.: A prospective analysis of diagnostic laparoscopy in trauma. *Ann Surg* 217:557, 1993.
50. Guth AA, Pachter HL: Laparoscopy for penetrating thoracoabdominal trauma: Pitfalls and promises. *JSLS* 2:123, 1998.
51. Elliott DC, Rodriguez A, Moncure M, et al.: The accuracy of diagnostic laparoscopy in trauma patients: A prospective, controlled study. *Int Surg* 83:294, 1998.
52. Townsend MC, Pelias ME: Technique for rapid closure of traumatic small intestine perforations with resection. *Am J Surg* 164:171, 1992.
53. Brundage SI, Jurkovich GJ, Hoyt DB, et al.: Stapled versus sutured gastrointestinal anastomoses in the trauma patient. *J Trauma* 3:500, 1999.
54. Witzke JD, Kraatz JJ, Morken JM, et al.: Stapled versus hand sewn anastomosis in patients with small bowel injury: a changing perspective. *J Trauma* 49:660, 2000.
55. Brundage SI, Jurkovich GJ, Hoyt DB, et al.: Stapled versus sutured gastrointestinal anastomoses in the trauma patient: A multicenter trial. *J Trauma* 51:1054, 2001.
56. Kirkpatrick AW, Baxter KA, Simons RK, et al: Intra-abdominal complications after surgical repair of small bowel injuries: an international review. *J Trauma* 3:399, 2003.

57. Burch JM, Franciose RJ, Moore EE, et al.: Single-layer continuous versus two-layer interrupted intestinal anastomosis: A prospective randomized trial. *Ann Surg* 231:832, 2000.

58. Padilla H, Ferrada R: Trauma gastrico. *Panam J Trauma* 3:117, 1992.

59. Pickleman J, Watson W, Cunningham J, et al.: The failed gastrointestinal anastomosis: An inevitable catastrophe. *J Am Coll Surg* 188:473, 1999.

60. Brundage S, Kirilcuk N, et al.: Complications associated with small bowel resections: Concurrent injuries are more relevant to morbidity than method of Gastrointestinal Anastomosis. *J Trauma* 60:249 abstract, 2006.

61. Carillo C, Fogler RJ, Shaftan GW: Delayed gastrointestinal reconstruction following massive abdominal trauma. *J Trauma* 34:233, 1993.

62. Chavarria-Aguilar M, Cockerham WT, et al.: Management of destructive bowel injury in the open abdomen. *J Trauma* 56:560, 2004.

63. Miller RS, Morris JA, Jr, et al.: Complications after 344 damage-control open celiotomies. *J Trauma* 59:1365, (discussion 1371), 2005. Scott BG, Welsh FJ, et al.: Early aggressive closure of the open abdomen. *J Trauma* 60:17, 2006.

64. Scott BG, Welsh FJ, et al.: Early aggressive closure of the open abdomen. *J Trauma* 60:17, 2006.

65 Dellinger EP: Antibiotic prophylaxis in trauma: Penetrating abdominal injuries and open fractures. *Review of Infectious Diseases* 13:S847, 1991.

66. Cunningham J, Temple WJ, Langevin JM, et al.: A prospective randomized trial of routine postoperative nasogastric decompression in patients with bowel anastomosis. *Can J Surg* 35:629, 1992.

67. Cheatham ML, Chapman WC, Key SP, et al.: A meta-analysis of selective versus routine nasogastric decompression after elective laparotomy. *Ann Surg* 221:469, 1995.

68. Nathan BN, Pain JA: Nasogastric suction after elective abdominal surgery: A randomized study. *Ann R Coll Surg Engl* 73:291, 1991.

69. MacRae HM, Fischer JD, Yakimets WW: Routine omission of nasogastric intubation after gastrointestinal surgery. *Can J Surg* 35:625, 1992.

70. Chendrasekhar A: Jejunal feeding in the absence of reflux increases nasogastric output in critically ill trauma patients. *Am Surg* 62:887, 1996.

71. Moore FA, Feliciano DV, Andrassay RJ: Early enteral feeding, compared with parenteral, reduces postoperative septic complications: The results of a meta-analysis. *Ann Surg* 216:172, 1992.

72. Moore FA, Moore EE, Jones TN: Benefits of immediate jejunostomy feeding after major abdominal trauma–A prospective randomized study. *J Trauma* 26:874, 1986.

73. Moore FA, Moore EE, et al.: TEN vs. TPN following major abdominal trauma–Reduced septic morbidity. *J Trauma* 29:916, 1989.

74. Montejo JC: Enteral nutrition-related gastrointestinal complications in critically ill patients: A multicenter study. *Crit Care Med* 27:1447, 1999.

75. Marvin RG, McKinley BA, McQuiggan M, et al.: Nonocclusive bowel necrosis occurring in critically ill trauma patients receiving enteral nutrition manifests no reliable clinical signs for early detection. *Am J Surg* 179:7, 2000.

76. Kudsk KA, Minard G, Croce MA, et al.: A randomized trial of isonitrogenous enteral diets after severe trauma: An immune-enhancing diet reduces septic complications. *Ann Surg* 224:531, 1996.

77. Weinmann A, Bastian L, Bischoff WE, et al.: Influence of arginine, omega-3 fatty acids and nucleotide-supplemented enteral support on systemic inflammatory response syndrome and multiple organ failure in patients after severe trauma. *Nutrition* 14:165, 1998.

78. Kehlet H, Holte K: Review of postoperative ileus. *Am J Surg* 182:3S, 2001.

79. Luckey A, Livingston E, et al.: Mechanisms and treatment of postoperative ileus. *Arch Surg* 138:206, 2003.

80. Waldhausen JHT, Schirmer BD: The effect of ambulation on recovery from postoperative ileus. *Ann Surg* 212:671, 1990.

81. Kozar RA, McQuiggan MM, Moore EE, et al.: Postinjury enteral tolerance is reliably achieved by a standardized protocol. *J Surg Res* 104:70, 2002.

82. Bungard TJ, Kale-Pradhay PB: Prokinetic agents to the treatment of postoperative ileus in adults: A review of the literature. *Pharmacotherapy* 19:2116, 1999.

83. Tack J, Peeters J: What comes after macrolides and other motilin stimulants? *Gut* 49:317, 2001.

84. Hirayama I, Suzuki M, et al.: Gum-chewing stimulates bowel motility after surgery for colorectal cancer. *Hepatogastroenterology* 53:206, 2006.

85. Wolff BG, Michelassi F, et al.: Alvimopan, a novel, peripherally acting mu opioid antagonist: results of a multicenter, randomized, double-blind, placebo-controlled, phase III trial of major abdominal surgery and postoperative ileus. *Ann Surg* 240:728, (discussion 734), 2004.

86. Bruscagin V, Coimbra R, et al.: Blunt gastric injury. A multicentre experience. *Injury* 32:761, 2001.

87. Coimbra R, Pinto MC, et al.: Factors related to the occurrence of postoperative complications following penetrating gastric injuries. *Injury* 26:463, 1995.

88. Croce MA, Fabian TC, et al.: Impact of stomach and colon injuries on intra-abdominal abscess and the synergistic effect of hemorrhage and associated injury. *J Trauma* 45:649, 1998.

89. O'Neill PA, Kirton OC, et al.: Analysis of 162 colon injuries in patients with penetrating abdominal trauma: Concomitant stomach injury results in a higher rate of infection. *J Trauma* 56:304, (discussion 312), 2004.

90. Canty TG, Brown C: Injuries of the gastrointestinal tract from blunt trauma in children: A 12-year experience at a designated pediatric trauma center. *J Trauma* 46:234, 1999.

91. Albanese CT, Meza MP, Gardner MJ, et al.: Is computed tomography a useful adjunct to the clinical examination for the diagnosis of pediatric gastrointestinal perforation from blunt abdominal trauma in children? *J Trauma* 40:417, 1996.

92. Bensard DD, Beaver BL, Besner GE, et al.: Small bowel injury in children after blunt abdominal trauma: Is diagnostic delay important? *J Trauma* 41:476, 1996.

93. Fang JF, Chen RJ, Lin BC, et al.: Small bowel perforation: Is urgent surgery necessary? *J Trauma* 47:515, 1999.

94. Fakhry SM, Brownstein M, Watts DD, et al.: Relatively short diagnostic delays (< 8 hours) produce morbidity and mortality in blunt small bowel injury: An analysis of time to operative intervention in 198 patients from a multicenter experience. *J Trauma* 48:408, 2000.

95. Hishberg A, Wall MJ, Ramchandani MK, et al.: Reoperation for bleeding in trauma. *Arch Surg* 128:1163, 1993.

96. Evenson AR, Fischer JE: Current management of enterocutaneous fistula. *J Gastrointest Surg* 10:455, 2006.

97. Buechter KJ, Leonovicz D, et al.: Enterocutaneous fistulas following laparotomy for trauma. *Am Surg* 57:354, 1991.

98. Calicis B, Parc Y, et al.: Treatment of postoperative peritonitis of small-bowel origin with continuous enteral nutrition and succus entericus reinfusion. *Arch Surg* 137:296, 2002.

99. Alvarez AA, Maxwell GL, et al.: Vacuum-assisted closure for cutaneous gastrointestinal fistula management. *Gynecol Oncol* 80:413, 2001.

100. Goverman J, Yelon JA, et al.: The "Fistula VAC," a technique for management of enterocutaneous fistulae arising within the open abdomen: Report of 5 cases. *J Trauma* 60:428, (discussion 431), 2006.

101. Cro C, George KJ, et al.: Vacuum assisted closure system in the management of enterocutaneous fistulae. *Postgrad Med J* 78:364, 2002.

102. Lynch AC, Delaney CP, et al.: Clinical outcome and factors predictive of recurrence after enterocutaneous fistula surgery. *Ann Surg* 240:825, 2004.

103. Renz BM, Feliciano DV: Unnecessary laparotomies for trauma: A prospective study of morbidity. *J Trauma* 38:350, 1995.

104. Tortella BJ, Lavery RF, Chandrakantan A, et al.: Incidence and risk factors for early small bowel obstruction after celiostomy for penetrating abdominal trauma. *Am Surg* 61:956, 1995.

105. Beck DE, Opelka FG, et al.: Incidence of small-bowel obstruction and adhesiolysis after open colorectal and general surgery. *Dis Colon Rectum* 42:241, 1999.

106. Pickleman J, Lee RM: The management of patients with suspected early postoperative small bowel obstruction. *Ann Surg* 210:216, 1989.

107. Donckier V, Closset J, Gansbeker DV, et al.: Contribution of computed tomography to decision making in the management of adhesive small bowel obstruction. *Br J Surg* 85:1071, 1998.

108. Becker JM, Stucchi AF: Intra-abdominal adhesion prevention: Are we getting any closer? *Ann Surg* 240:202, 2004.

109. Fazio VW, Cohen Z, et al.: Reduction in adhesive small-bowel obstruction by Seprafilm adhesion barrier after intestinal resection. *Dis Colon Rectum* 49:1, 2006.

110. WaxmFan BP: Adhesives and adhesions: intestinal surgery on a sticky wicket! *ANZ J Surg* 74:1037, 2004.

111. Spotnitz WD: Commercial fibrin sealants in surgical care. *Am J Surg* 182:8S, 2001.

112. Tang CL, Jayne DG, et al.: A randomized controlled trial of 0.5% ferric hyaluronate gel (Intergel) in the prevention of adhesions following abdominal surgery. *Ann Surg* 243:449, 2006.

113. Wilmore DW, Robinson MK: Short bowel syndrome. *World J Surg* 24:1486, 2000.

114. Dabney A, Thompson J, et al.: Short bowel syndrome after trauma. *Am J Surg* 188:792, 2004.

115. Sundaram A, Koutkia P, Apovian CM: Nutritional management of short bowel syndrome in adults. *J Clin Gastroenterol* 34:207, 2002.

116. Ray EC, Avissar NE, Sax HC: Growth factor regulation of enterocyte nutrient transport during intestinal adaptation. *Am J Surg* 183:361, 2002.

117. Byrne TA, Morrissey TB, et al.: Growth hormone, glutamine, and a modified diet enhance nutrient absorption in patients with severe short bowel syndrome. *JPEN J Parenter Enteral Nutr* 19:296, 1995.

118. Thompson JS: Surgical rehabilitation of intestine in short bowel syndrome. *Surgery* 135:465, 2004.

119. Nishida S, Hadjis NS, et al.: Intestinal and multivisceral transplantation after abdominal trauma. *J Trauma* 56:323, 2004.

# Commentary ■ RONALD M. JOU ■ SUSAN I. BRUNDAGE

Dr. Diebel has given us a comprehensive and scholarly description of the evaluation and management of stomach and small bowel injuries, and there is little to add by way of detail. However, there are a few points that are worth highlighting.

The history of abdominal trauma provides an interesting perspective and important insights. An other noteworthy military manuscript was: Ogilvie WH. "Abdominal Wounds in the Western Desert." *Surg Gynecol Obstet.* 1944.[1] Of note, the mortality rate for a negative exploratory laparotomy was 23.8% while small bowel injury alone treated by resection and anastomosis carried a 42.8% mortality rate. The statistics reported are startling when compared to today's operative expected morbidity and mortality rates in both civilian and military situations. This historical knowledge imparts weighty perspective. The revealing statistics and the entertaining writing of Ogilvie's is truly a must read for anyone interested in the history of abdominal wounds.

A detailed discussion of various diagnostic tests and an impressive collection of the data behind these maneuvers are provided. Interestingly, there have been times when a physical examination was considered unreliable at best for evaluating abdominal trauma. At other times, the physical examination by a skilled and experienced surgeon has been rediscovered as the most important test for diagnosing abdominal injuries. Likewise, the enthusiasm for laparotomy in trauma has waxed and waned between being totally abandoned in some settings while being mandatory in others. These dilemmas are underscored by the discussion of stomach and small bowel injuries where diagnosis is often difficult and the consequences of missed injuries are significant.

The chapter provides an extensive review of the literature regarding DPL. Given the emergence of the usefulness of the FAST exam and the ubiquity of CT scanners, one could argue that the DPL is now obsolete in most settings. The DPL does have its current utility but that is found in the form of the DPA, or Diagnostic Peritoneal Aspirate. Although widely accepted, it is difficult to find a description of DPA in the literature. Velmahos et al have published an excellent description regarding *the decreasing role of diagnostic peritoneal paracentesis, and the elimination of diagnostic peritoneal lavage (DPL) in favor of aspiration only* and algorithm reflecting the evolution from DPL to DPA.[2]

Mention of the problematic thoracoabdominal "box" is warranted. Recognition that penetrating injuries to the chest which are below the nipple line might result in intra-abdominal injuries is a common pitfall that needs to be emphasized. Although this is a common discussion topic in busy trauma centers, it is difficult to find published acknowledgement of this hazard. Our South African colleagues have provided the best description of this conundrum. "Knowledge of the various regions of the abdominal cavity is vital in penetrating injuries….The diaphragm position at the time of penetrating injuries determines whether thoracoabdominal injuries are intrathoracic only, combined diaphragm and abdominal, or diaphragm and abdominal injuries only. Special

investigations commonly miss hollow visceral injuries, so careful clinical examination is of greater importance than ultrasound or computerized tomography scanning."[3]

As non-operative management of blunt solid organ injuries becomes more common and the incidence of laparotomy for the solid organ injury decreases, there are fewer opportunities to diagnose associated stomach and small bowel injuries that would have been identified during exploration. Therefore, the members of the trauma team must be vigilant in maintaining a high index of suspicion in considering patients for laparotomy.

Once injuries of the stomach and small bowel are recognized, procedures for repair are relatively straightforward. Gastric and small bowel injuries are unlikely to be immediately life threatening. The chapter does emphasize that the elaborateness of the indicated procedures as well as clinical outcomes are dependent primarily on the presence and severity of concomitant injuries such as those of the duodenum or colon. In this context, isolated injuries of the stomach and small bowel may not be particularly complex, but missed injuries do result in significant morbidity and mortality.

The postoperative complications section of the chapter is extremely informative with an excellent discussion of management of post operative fistulas and short gut syndrome. Although briefly mentioned, Dr. Wilmore's contributions to treatment of short gut syndrome are especially noteworthy and the body of literature reflecting his work with this challenging entity should be emphasized.

Lastly, while Dr. Diebel provides an excellent review of the association of the "seatbelt sign" with intra-abdominal injuries and Chance fractures, it is against the tenets of good trauma care not to cite the benefits of prevention. Given the high association of seatbelt signs with intra-abdominal injuries and the potential misuse of the data as an excuse not to "buckle up", we would be remiss not to emphasize the concomitant reduction in mortality associated with restraint use. One must keep the following data foremost in mind while reading the section on the association of intra-abdominal injuries and restraint systems. "Air bag deployment reduced mortality 63%, while lap-shoulder belt use reduced mortality 72%. Combined air bag and seat belt use reduced mortality by more than 80% (OR = 0.18, 95% CI: 0.13, 0.25) confirming the independent effect of air bags and seat belts in reducing mortality."[4] One must balance the risk/benefit ratio of death versus the potential for a relatively straightforward and surgically correctable abdominal injury and enthusiastically promote use of seatbelts.

## References

1. Ogilvie W. Abdominal Wounds in the Western Desert. *Surg Gynecol Obstet.* 1944.
2. Velmahos GC, Toutouzas K, Radin R, et al. High success with nonoperative management of blunt hepatic trauma: the liver is a sturdy organ. *Arch Surg.* 138:475, 2003.
3. Bautz P. The trauma patient: critical decision making. When to explore the abdomen. A South African perspective. *Trauma.* 2:35, 2000.
4. Crandall CS, Olson LM, Sklar DP. Mortality reduction with air bag and seat belt use in head-on passenger car collisions. *Am J Epidemiol.* 153:219, 2001.

# Duodenum and Pancreas

*Jeffry L. Kashuk* ■ *Jon M. Burch*

## INTRODUCTION

Despite implementation of damage control surgery and improved imaging techniques, injuries to the duodenum and pancreas are a continuing challenge, with morbidity and mortality rates changing little over the past 25 years (Tables 35-1 to 35-4). The deep, retroperitoneal location of these organs affords an element of protection from injury but also contributes to the imperfections of diagnostic imaging. Furthermore, most busy trauma centers have only a modest experience with these injuries. These factors mandate that a high index of suspicion must be maintained when confronted with potential trauma to the duodenal-pancreatic axis. In most situations, injuries to the duodenum can be managed satisfactorily with simple repair, and more complicated techniques can be reserved for less frequent destructive injuries. Similarly, many injuries to the pancreas can be managed by observation or closed suction drainage. Complex techniques should be reserved for substantial organ devitalization or duct transection. Paradoxically, the well-protected retroperitoneal location of the duodenum and pancreas may lead to delay in diagnosis, missed injuries, and increased morbidity and mortality. In the setting of a severely injured patient with associated shock, hypothermia, acidosis, and coagulopathy, damage control techniques should be employed (see Chap. 41) for management of hemorrhage and enteric leak, allowing time for the patient's physiological condition to improve. Definitive resection and reconstruction may then be later performed in a staged procedure.

## HISTORY

Most early reports of duodenal and pancreatic injuries are isolated autopsy observations following blunt or penetrating injury. The first acknowledged literature report of pancreatic trauma was described by Travers in 1827.[17] Mickulicz-Radicki[18] identified only 45 cases in the literature 76 years later. Of note, 72% of operated patients survived, a success rate that rivals modern day results. Many of the recommendations suggested in this early series still hold true today: thorough midline exploration, hemostasis, and drainage. In a report by Stern in 1930, 62 patients with pancreatic injuries had a mortality of 52%.[19] Of interest, his recommendation of abdominal puncture for evaluation of trauma to the abdomen may have been a forerunner to modern day diagnostic peritoneal lavage (DPL), as described by Root et al.[20] Scattered case reports of injuries to the pancreas have been reported from wartime experiences dating back to the American Civil War. The first report of five patients included one survivor.[21] A similar experience was reported from World War I, and in World War II only 62 cases of pancreatic trauma were reported (2% of abdominal injuries) with a 56% mortality.[22] Only nine cases of pancreatic injury were reported from the Korean War (22% mortality).[23] Although much sentinel work in trauma was done during the Vietnam war, virtually no reports of pancreatic or duodenal injuries are available except for a single report of two cases of pancreaticoduodenectomy.[24]

Complications of pancreatic trauma became apparent in the earliest reports and have continued through the years. The first report of a pancreatic fistula after isolated pancreatic injury in a surviving patient is attributed to Korte in 1905.[25] Pancreatic pseudocyst was first recognized by Kulenkampff in 1882,[26] and later reported by Moynihan in 1926.[27] Whipple first described pancreaticoduodenectomy in 1935, and later reported the associated complications of hemorrhage, fistula, duodenal leak, and peritonitis.[28]

The first successful surgical repair of a duodenal rupture was reported by Herczel in 1896.[29] Summers, in 1904, recognized the difficulty of diagnosis of a retroperitoneal perforation of the duodenum from a gunshot wound, and may have been the first to describe the potential application of the pyloric exclusion procedure.[30] The earliest reported series of duodenal injuries was reported by Berry in 1909 from 10 London hospitals.[31] There were 24 patients, and all died. The first known patient surviving a duodenal injury is attributed to Godwin in 1905, mentioned in the same report. Another report of survivors was published by Miller

**TABLE 35-1**

### Duodenal Trauma: Mortality by Mechanism of Injury

| AUTHOR | YEAR | TOTAL PATIENTS, N (PENETRATE/ BLUNT) | STAB DIED/TOTAL (% MORTALITY) | GUNSHOT DIED/TOTAL (% MORTALITY) | SHOTGUN DIED/TOTAL (% MORTALITY) | ALL PENETRATING | ALL BLUNT |
|---|---|---|---|---|---|---|---|
| Lucas and Ledgerwood[1] | 1975 | 36 (all blunt) | — | — | — | — | 7/36 |
| Vaughan et al.[2] | 1977 | 175 (152/23) | 2/18 11% | 13/124 11% | 3/10 30% | 18/152 12% | 6/23 26% |
| Stone and Fabian[3] | 1979 | 321 (294/27) | 0/31 0% | 26/239 (11%) | 11/24 46% | 37/294 12.5% | 4/27 15% |
| Flint et al.[4] | 1980 | 75[a] (56/19) | 0/5 (0%) | 0/51 (0%) | — | 11/56 20% | 2/19 11% |
| Ivatury et al.[5] | 1985 | 100 (all penetrating) | 6/30 (20%) | 19/70 (27%) | — | 25/100 25% | — |
| Cogbill et al.[6] | 1990 | 164 (102/62) | 2/31 (6.5%) | 20/66 (30%) | 39118 (40%) | 24/102 (23.5%) | 22798 10% |
| Totals | | 969 (779/190) | 12/134 | 91/550 | 16/39 | 130/779 | 33/190 |
| Mean % Mortality | | | 9% | 17% | 41% | 17% | 17% |

[a]Mortality by specific mechanism not stated in this report.

**TABLE 35-2**

### Duodenal Trauma: Timing and Etiology of Mortality

| AUTHOR | YEAR | TOTAL N (PENETRATING/BLUNT TRAUMA) | OVERALL MORTALITY N (%) | ACUTE MORTALITY: HEMORRHAGE OR ASSOCIATED INJURIES (% TOTAL DEATHS) | DELAYED: SEPSIS/MSOF (% TOTAL DEATHS) | DUODENAL MORTALITY (% DELAYEDDEATHS) |
|---|---|---|---|---|---|---|
| Vaughan et al.[2] | 1977 | 75[a] (64/11) | 14 (19%) | 6 (43%) | 6 (43%) | Not stated |
| Stone and Fabian[3] | 1979 | 321 (294/27) | 41 (13%) | 25 (61%) | 16 (39%) | 5/16 (31%) |
| Flint et al.[4] | 1980 | 75 (56/19) | 14 (19%) | 5 (36%) | 9 (64%) | 4/9 (44%) |
| Snyder et al.[7] | 1980 | 247[b] (180/48) | 43 (17%) | 19 (44%) | 24 (56%) | 9/24 (38%) |
| Martin et al.[8] | 1983 | 128[a] (109/19) | 28 (22%) | 11 (39%) | 14 (50%) | 2/14 (14%) |
| Levison et al.[9] | 1984 | 93 (74/19) | 17 (18%) | 9 (53%) | 8 (47%) | 4/8 (50%) |
| Ivatury et al.[5] | 1985 | 100 (all penetrating) | 25 (25%) | 16 (64%) | 8 (32%) | |
| Shorr et al.[10] | 1987 | 115[c] (94/11) | 14 (12%) | 10 (71%) | 4 (29%) | 2/4 (50%) |
| Cuddington et al.[11] | 1990 | 42 (16/26) | 6 (14%) | 2 (33%) | 3 (50%) | 3/3 (100%) |
| Cogbill et al.[6] | 1990 | 164 (102/62) | 30 (18%) | 25 (83%) | 5 (17%) | 2/5 (40%) |
| Total N (% mortality) | | 1360 | 232 | 128 (9%) | 97 (7%) | 31 (2%) |
| Mean % Mortality | | 1089/342 | 17% | 55% of deaths | 42% of deaths | 37% of late deaths |

[a]Includes only patients undergoing pyloric exclusion with combined duodenal repair.
[b]Mechanism not stated for 19 patients who died within 72 h of injury.
[c]Mechanism not stated for 10 patients who died within 24 h of injury.
Abbreviation: MSOF, multiple-organ system failure.

**TABLE 35-3**

**Pancreatic Trauma: Mortality by Mechanism of Injury**

| AUTHOR | YEAR | TOTAL PATIENTS, N (PENETRATING/ BLUNT) | STAB (%) MORTALITY (TOTAL N) | GUNSHOT (%) MORTALITY (TOTAL N) | SHOTGUN (%) MORTALITY (TOTAL N) | ALL PENETRATING | ALL BLUNT |
|---|---|---|---|---|---|---|---|
| Graham et al.[12] | 1978[a] | 308 (231/77) | 2.8% (1/36) | 15.4% (28/182) | 46% (6/13) | 15.2% | 16.9% |
| Stone et al.[11] | 1981 | 283 (224/59) | 6% (2/32) | 10.6% (19/180) | 66.6% (8/12) | 13% | 17% |
| Jones[13] | 1985 | 500 (362/138) | 5% (4/76) | 22% (55/252) | 56% (19/34) | 22% | 19% |
| Ivatury et al.[5] | 1990 | 103 (all penetrating) | 22% (7/32) | 28% (20/71) | — | 32%[b] | — |
| Cogbill et al.[14] | 1991 | 74 (40/34) | 0% (0/11) | 3.7% (1/27) | 50% (1/2) | 3% | 21% |
| Totals/average | | 1268 (960/308) | 7.5% (14/187) | 17% (123/712) | 56% (34/61) | 18% (171/960) | 18% (56/308) |

[a]Includes only patients treated between 1968 and 1977 in this report.
[b]Includes six patients with unspecified mechanism of injury dying in the late postoperative period.

**TABLE 35-4**

**Pancreatic Trauma: Etiology of Mortality**

| STUDY | YEAR | TOTAL NO. | OVERALL MORTALITY N (%) | HEMORRHAGE OR ASSOCIATED INJURIES (% OF DEATHS) | SEPSIS/MOF (% OF DEATHS) | OTHER |
|---|---|---|---|---|---|---|
| Wilson and Moorehead[15] | 1967 | 84 | 30 (35.7%) | 15 (50%) | 15 (50%) | — |
| Werschky and Jordan | 1968 | 140 | 43 (30.7%) | 19 (44%) | 20 (47%) | 4 |
| Heitsch et al. | 1976 | 100 | 33 (33%) | 16 (48%) | 14 (42%) | 3 |
| Graham et al.[12] | 1978 | 448 | 73 (16.3%) | 47 (64%) | 14 (19%) | 12 |
| Stone et al.[11] | 1981 | 283 | 39 (13.8%) | 19 (49%) | 16 (41%) | 4 |
| Jones[13] | 1985 | 500 | 104 (21%) | 68[a] (65%) | 11 (11%) | 25 |
| Ivatury et al.[5] | 1990 | 103 | 33 (32%) | 27 (82%) | 6 (18%) | — |
| Cogbill et al.[14] | 1991 | 74 | 9 (12%) | 3 (33%) | 5 (56%) | 1 |
| Patton et al[16] | 1997 | 134 | 17 (13%) | 11 (65%) | 4 | 2 |
| Total N (% mortality) | | 1866 | 381 (20.5%) | 225 (12%) | 101 (6%) | 51 (3%) |
| Mean % | | | | 59% of all deaths | 58% of deaths | 13% of deaths |

[a]Includes unspecified number of patients dying within 48 h of admission from head injury.
Abbreviation: MOF, multiple-organ failure.

in 1916.[32] Cave, in a World War II experience, recorded 118 cases of duodenal injuries with a mortality of 57%, which is still the single largest military series of duodenal injuries.[33] Only 17 cases were reported from the Korean War, with a mortality of 22%.[34] Although many of the recommendations suggested in historical series still hold true today, including thorough midline exploration, hemostasis, and drainage of pancreatic injuries, a paradigm shift from nonoperative observation to aggressive surgical treatment has occurred in the modern era of the urban trauma center. Improved anesthesia, shock resuscitation, wound care, and surgical techniques have contributed to better outcomes.

## Recent Historical Trends

Despite continuing urban violence and motor vehicle collisions, pancreatic and duodenal trauma remains uncommon, and no one center has extensive experience. Several reports estimate a frequency of 7–10% of celiotomies for all types of abdominal trauma.[1,9,35] In a large series of blunt trauma patients statewide in

Pennsylvania, only a 0.2% incidence of blunt duodenal injury was reported.[36]

A survey of several large series over the past three decades demonstrates a mortality rate of 17 to 20%, irrespective of mechanism of injury (see Tables 35-1 to 35-4).

Similar to other experiences in trauma, most patients who die from a pancreatic or duodenal injury do so within the first 48 hours from exsanguinating hemorrhage in the setting of multiple associated injuries, namely, vascular, liver, or spleen. (Tables 35-2, 35-4, and 35-5) A recent series of combined pancreatoduodenal injuries[37] emphasized the continuing challenge of this group. Of 240 patients presenting with pancreatic or duodenal injuries, 33 (14%) had combined injury and almost 50% had associated vascular injuries. One third presented in extremis and underwent damage control laparotomy with an 18% mortality and 36% complication rate. The importance of associated vascular injury in duodenal trauma was emphasized in a recent report by Huerta et al.[38] In their series, vascular injury with associated acidosis was a dominant risk factor for mortality.

## TABLE 35-5

### Associated Organ Injuries in 1031 Patients with Pancreatic Wounds

| | TOTAL | |
|---|---|---|
| ORGAN INJURED | No. | % |
| Liver | 483 | 46.8 |
| Stomach | 436 | 42.3 |
| Major arteries and veins | 426 | 41.3 |
| Spleen | 289 | 28.0 |
| Kidney | 241 | 23.4 |
| Duodenum | 199 | 19.3 |
| Colon | 175 | 17.0 |
| Small bowel | 151 | 14.6 |
| Common bile duct | 35 | 3.4 |
| Galbladder | 15 | 1.4 |

Sources: Stone H, Fabian TBS, et al.: Experiences in the management of pancreatic trauma. J Trauma 21:257, 1981; Jones R: Management of pancreatic trauma. Am J Surg 150:696, 1985; and Graham K, Mattox KL, Vaughan G, et al.: Combined pancreatoduodenal injuries. J Trauma 19:340, 1979.

The proximity of the pancreatic-duodenal axis to other vital structures makes isolated injuries distinctly uncommon. (Figs. 35-1 and 35-2) Balasegaram et al.[39] reported a 2.5% mortality rate with one associated injury, with progressive increase in mortality with up to four associated injuries (29.6%). In all series, less than 10% of patients with pancreatic or duodenal trauma will present with a single isolated injury. Multiple series document an average of 3.5 to 4.1 associated injuries per patient.[7,9,11,12,15,35,40–44]

Late deaths in cases of pancreatic and duodenal trauma are most often ascribed to sepsis and multiple-system organ failure (Chap. 68). Numerous reports have shown that over one third of late deaths (1–2 weeks post injury) are due to complications related to the original pancreatic or duodenal injury, underscoring the importance of early and prompt diagnosis.[7,10,13,45,46] Infection most commonly results from either complications of repair(resection or

delayed diagnosis of injury with subsequent peritonitis. Almost one third of patients who survived the first 48 hours developed a complication related to their initial injury.[10,13,16]

Delayed presentation and subsequent late diagnosis of injury in this patient group is disastrous and directly correlates with significantly increased morbidity and mortality in multiple series.[1,7,39,40,47–49]

Tables 35-2 and 35-4 represent a summary of the largest series of timing versus mortality in these injuries, underscoring the importance of prompt diagnosis and a diligent search for associated injuries in this group of patients.

## ANATOMY AND PHYSIOLOGY

Anatomically, the duodenum and pancreas are intimately associated with vital structures in a deep and narrow region. (Fig. 35-1) The duodenum, named from the Latin "duodeni", meaning "twelve each" refers to the 12 fingerbreadths in length or 30 cm extending from the pyloric ring to the ligament of Treitz. Classically the duodenum is divided into four portions: superior or first, descending or second, transverse or third, and ascending or fourth portion.[50,51] The first portion of the duodenum extends from the pylorus to the common bile duct anteriorly and the gastroduodenal artery posteriorly. The second portion extends from the common bile duct and the gastroduodenal artery to the ampulla of Vater. Of significance, this portion is entirely retroperitoneal. The third portion extends from the ampulla of Vater to the mesenteric vessels which descend anteriorly over the junction of the third and fourth portions. The fourth portion extends from the vessels described to the region where the duodenum emerges from the retroperitoneum to join the jejunum just to the left of the second lumbar vertebra, at the ligament of Treitz. The duodenum is almost entirely a retroperitoneal structure, with the exception of the anterior half circumference of the first portion of the duodenum and the most distal part of the fourth portion of the duodenum. The first portion, distal region of the third portion, and the fourth portion

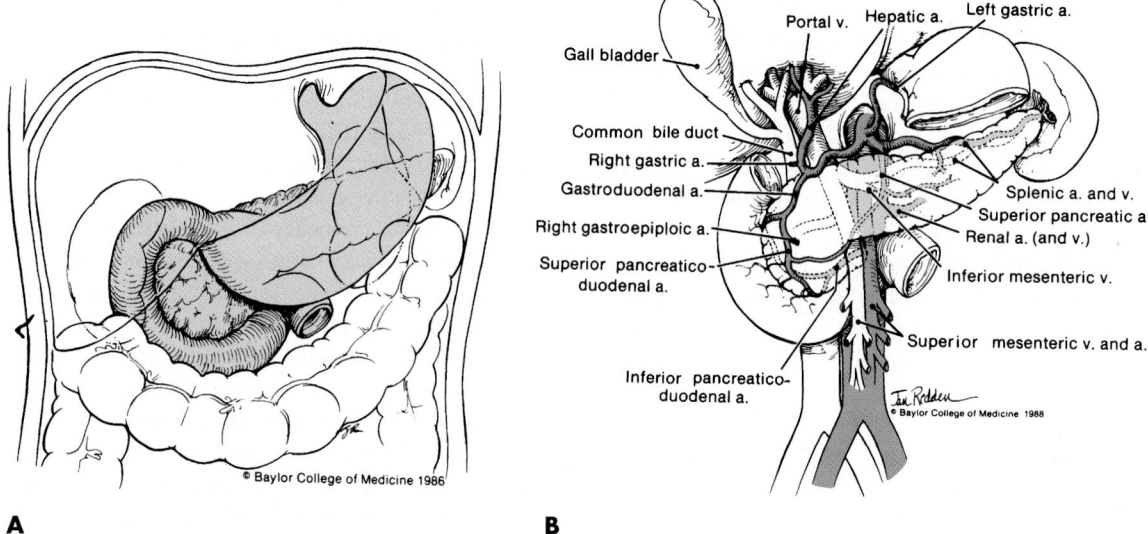

**A**                                          **B**

**FIGURE 35-1.**  Anatomic relation of the pancreas and duodenum, emphasizing the proximity of major associated structures. **(A)** Relation to adjacent organs. **(B)** Important vascular structures in close proximity to the pancreas and duodenum.

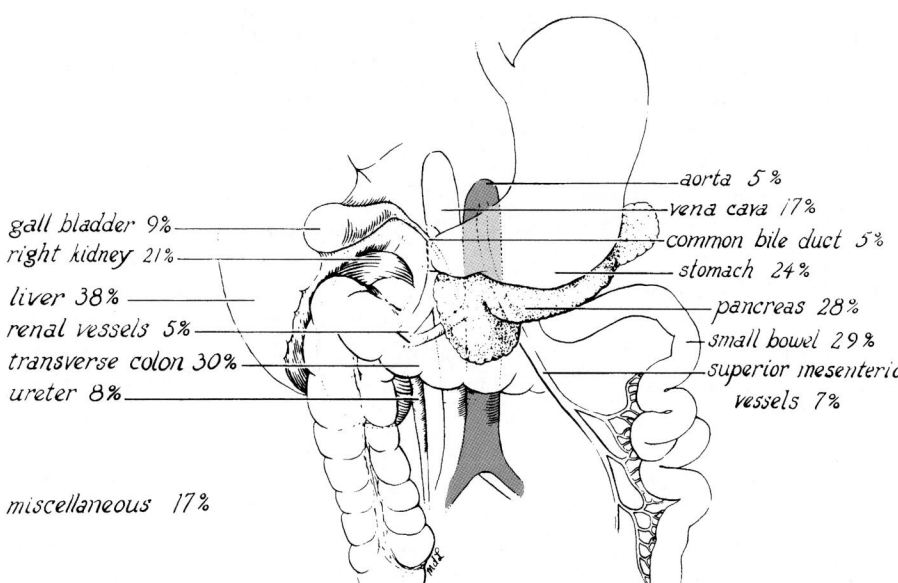

gall bladder 9%
right kidney 21%

liver 38%
renal vessels 5%
transverse colon 30%
ureter 8%

aorta 5%
vena cava 17%
common bile duct 5%
stomach 24%
pancreas 28%
small bowel 29%
superior mesenteric vessels 7%

miscellaneous 17%

**FIGURE 35-2.** Drawing showing the incidence of injuries to nearby organs and vessels in patients with duodenal wounds. *(Reproduced with permission from Morton JR, Jordan GL Jr: Traumatic duodenal injuries: Review of 131 cases. J Trauma 8:127, 1968.)*

of the duodenum lie virtually in their entirety directly over the vertebral column. The psoas muscles, aorta, inferior vena cava, and right kidney complete the posterior boundaries of the duodenum. The liver borders the first and second portions of the duodenum anteriorly, and the fourth portion of the duodenum is bounded by the hepatic flexure of the colon, right transverse colon, mesocolon, and stomach. The gallbladder is positioned medially, and the head of the pancreas is intimately associated within the C loop, or second portion.

The pancreas is divided into the head, contained within the within the C loop, the neck which is the narrowest portion overlying the mesenteric vessels, the body, which is rather triangular in cross section and which extends to the left across the vertebral column, and the tail. The vertebral column may act as a fulcrum causing transection in blunt trauma. The root of the transverse mesocolon crosses the head anteriorly. Posteriorly, the head is separated from the body by the pancreatic incisure, where the superior mesenteric vessels lie. A part of the head, the uncinate process, extends to the left behind the superior mesenteric vessels. The body of the pancreas extends laterally and has superior, anterior, and inferior margins. The base of the transverse mesocolon is attached at the anterior margin, is covered with peritoneum and forms the posterior wall of the omental bursa. The inferior surface is covered with peritoneum from the posterior mesocolon onto the body wall. The body of the pancreas posteriorly rests on the aorta. The tail of the pancreas lies in front of the left kidney, in intimate proximity to the splenic flexure of the colon, often abutting the spleen via the lienorenal ligament. The splenic artery runs along the upper border of the gland, often crossing in front of the tail. The splenic vein lies in a groove behind the body and tail, usually on the inferior edge of the pancreas.

The blood supply of the pancreas and duodenum comes from the gastroduodenal, splenic and superior mesenteric arteries. There are numerous collateral vessels throughout the pancreas which protects it from ischemia, but also contribute to vigorous bleeding following injury. The second portion of the duodenum has a unique blood supply which originates from both the gastroduodenal artery and the inferior pancreatoduodenal artery, a branch of the superior

mesenteric artery. Both of these vessels divide into anterior and posterior branches which are located on the edge of the head of the pancreas and anastomose with each other anteriorly and posteriorly. The second portion of the duodenum receives radial branches from these vessels which comprise its only blood supply. Because the pancreato-duodenal vessels are located on the surface of the head of the pancreas, portions may be resected without causing necrosis of the second portion of the duodenum. If all of the pancreatoduodenal vessels are injured by trauma, a pancreatoduodenectomy will be necessary.

In addition to the blood supply to the head of the gland, the pancreas also receives collateral circulation from the splenic and superior mesenteric arteries through vessels that enter the body and tail of the gland directly. The third portion of the duodenum receives its blood supply from the notorious short mesentery of the superior mesenteric artery.

While the arterial and venous supply as described is relatively constant, variations do exist and should be kept in mind during surgical exploration in this region. Origin of the common hepatic artery (5%) and a replaced right hepatic artery (15–20%) from the superior mesenteric artery are among the most frequent anomalous findings.[51,52] In other instances, the right hepatic may arise from the aorta, gastroduodenal, or even left hepatic artery. In 4% of the population, the entire common or proper hepatic artery is aberrant, arising from the superior mesenteric, the aorta, or the left gastric. In addition, if the bifurcation of the proper hepatic artery is low, the right hepatic may lie in front of the common bile duct or cross in front of it as well as the cystic duct.

Surgeons dealing with injuries to the duodenum and pancreas should be particularly well versed with the anatomic positions of the pancreatic and common bile ducts.[53] After its exit from the liver and cystic branch, the common bile duct extends from above to behind the first part of the duodenum, continuing downward on the posterior surface of the head of the pancreas where it is overlapped by lobules of pancreas obscuring its identification. In this region, the duct curves to the right, and joins with the main pancreatic duct of Wirsung prior to entering the posteromedial wall of the second part of the duodenum as the ampulla of Vater. The main pancreatic duct usually traverses the entire length of the gland and is located posteriorly slightly above a line halfway between the superior and inferior edges of the pancreas. The accessory duct of Santorini typically branches out from the main duct near the neck and empties separately into the duodenum about 2.5 cm proximal to the duodenal papilla. The common bile duct and main pancreatic duct may rarely enter the duodenum through separate openings, precluding intraoperative pancreatography via the gallbladder.

Partially digested chyle from the stomach and the proteolytic and lipolytic secretions of the biliary tract and pancreas mix in the duodenum. The powerful digestive enzymes commonly found in this location include lipase, trypsin, amylase, elastase, and peptidases. Approximately 10 L of fluid from the stomach, bile duct, and pancreas passes through the duodenum in a day.[54] Under normal conditions, the small intestine absorbs more than 80% of this fluid, but following injury, this high volume and enzymatically charged flow accounts for the disastrous consequences of a lateral duodenal fistula and associated derangements in water and electrolyte homeostasis.

The duodenum has several key roles in vitamin and mineral absorption as well as food processing. Vitamin B12 malabsorption may result from extensive duodenal resection. R protein is hydrolyzed by pancreatic enzymes in the duodenum to allow free cobalamin (B12) to bind to gastric parietal cell-derived intrinsic factor.[55]

The duodenum is the main site for transcellular transport of calcium. A key step in transport is mediated by calbindin, a calcium binding protein produced by enterocytes. Regulation of calbindin synthesis appears to be the main mechanism facilitating vitamin D regulated calcium absorption.[55]

The pancreas consists histologically of both endocrine and exocrine cells. The endocrine cells are distributed throughout the substance of the gland, and the a-, b-, and d- islet cells produce glucagon, insulin, and gastrin, respectively. The secretion of insulin and glucagon are responsive to blood glucose levels. Islet cell concentration is thought to be greater in the tail than the body and head of the gland, although it is generally held that approximately 10% of the gland remaining after resection may maintain normal hormonal balance.[56] Both duct and acinar cells of the pancreas secrete between 500–800 mL per day of clear, alkaline, isosmotic fluid. In addition, the acinar cells produce amylase, proteases, and lipases. Pancreatic amylase is secreted in its active form and serves to hydrolyze starch and glycogen to glucose, maltose, maltotriose, and dextrins. Proteolytic enzymes produced by these cells include trypsinogen, which is converted to trypsin in the duodenal mucosa by enterokinase. Pancreatic lipase is secreted in an active form and hydrolyzes triglycerides to monoglycerides and fatty acids. The acinar and duct cells also secrete the water and electrolytes found in pancreatic juice.

Bicarbonate secretion is directly related to the rate of pancreatic secretion and chloride secretion varies inversely with bicarbonate secretion so that the sum total of both remains constant. The hormone secretin, released from the duodenal mucosa, is the major stimulant for bicarbonate secretion, and serves to buffer the acidic fluid entering the duodenum from the stomach. Both endocrine and exocrine pancreatic functions are interdependent. Somatostatin, pancreatic polypeptides, and glucagons are all believed to have a role in inhibition of exocrine secretion. When pancreatic exocrine function is reduced to less than 10%, diarrhea and steatorrhea develop.[57]

## Diagnosis

The approach to patients with pancreatic and duodenal injuries starts with routine evaluation of the trauma patient as described in the Advanced Trauma Life Support (ATLS) manual (see Chap. 11). Approximately 75% of reported duodenal injuries are the result of penetrating trauma, and the injury will be discovered during exploration (see Chap. 30). The hemodynamically unstable patient requires little preoperative evaluation other than expeditious transport to the operating room. Prior to exploration in patients with gunshot wounds, chest, abdomen, and pelvis plain films are valuable (see Chap. 16). Blood typing is performed in anticipation of potential transfusion, and antibiotics are administered. Stable patients with stab wounds undergo focused abdominal sonography for trauma (FAST) exam (see Chap. 17). Grossly positive results require operative exploration. Equivocal tests in the stable patient require further evaluation via local wound exploration, DPL or CT. Unlike blunt trauma, CT findings of free fluid in penetrating injury should be suspect for hollow viscus perforation and undergo exploration. Stable patients with negative FAST, or negative CT require observation and repeat examination over 12–24 hours if their local wound exploration is positive.

Diagnosis of blunt injuries in hemodynamically stable patients is more challenging. Missed injuries result in significant morbidity and mortality.[58] A common mechanism in both duodenum and pancreatic injuries is deceleration with blunt force to the epigastrium resulting in crush injuries from opposition of the anterior abdominal wall with the spinal column. There may be a paucity of physical findings. Patients may have persistent abdominal pain and tenderness,[1,47,59–61] but these findings may be obscured by associated chest, abdominal, or pelvic trauma. Fortunately, isolated duodenal injuries are rare; and when missed on initial evaluation the patient will often develop peritonitis or systemic shock within 48 hours of injury. Initial plain films are of limited use in the diagnosis of blunt pancreatic or duodenal injuries. In blunt trauma, traditional signs such as retroperitoneal air, obliteration of the right psoas shadow, and mild spine scoliosis are often subtle or absent.[62] The FAST exam is useful for identifying hemoperitoneum in hemodynamically unstable patients and will allow for prompt transfer to the operating room (see Chap. 17). In patients with equivocal exam, a high index of suspicion should prompt consideration of DPL. In the stable patient with suspicion of intraabdominal injury, CT scanning is indicated.[63–65] Abdominal CT scans have a reported sensitivity and specificity of around 80% in diagnosing retroperitoneal injury to the duodenum or pancreas, although accuracy is dependent on the qualifications of those reading the scan, the time from injury, and the quality of the scanner.[51,63,64,66,67] Positive findings in duodenal perforation include extraluminal gas or contrast, or fat stranding with loss of sharp tissue planes, but false negative studies occur (Fig. 35-3). Equivocal studies may require repeat CT scanning followed immediately with contrast duodenography first using water soluble contrast and then barium.[68] Although this test has a high specificity (98%), sensitivity is poor. Several series suggest that even with careful inspection and technique to detect subtle findings of duodenal injury, the diagnosis can be elusive.[58] Such subtle

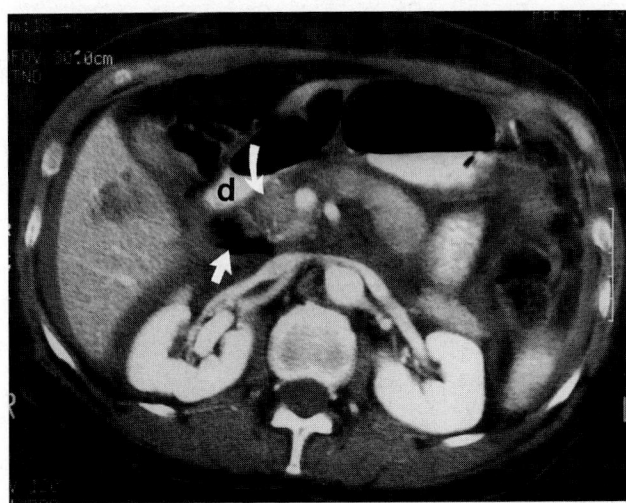

**FIGURE 35-3.** Computed tomography (CT) finding of retroperitoneal duodenal perforation. CT scan shows poor definition of the structures in the region of the head of the pancreas (curved arrow) and diminished enhancement of the head compared to the body. A collection of extraluminal, retroperitoneal gas (straight arrow) lies immediately posterior to the second portion of the duodenum (d), consistent with a duodenal perforation. This patient is also depicted in Fig. 35-4.
*(From Smith DR, Stanley RJ, Rue LW III: Delayed diagnosis of pancreatic transection after blunt abdominal trauma. J Trauma 40:1009, 1996.)*

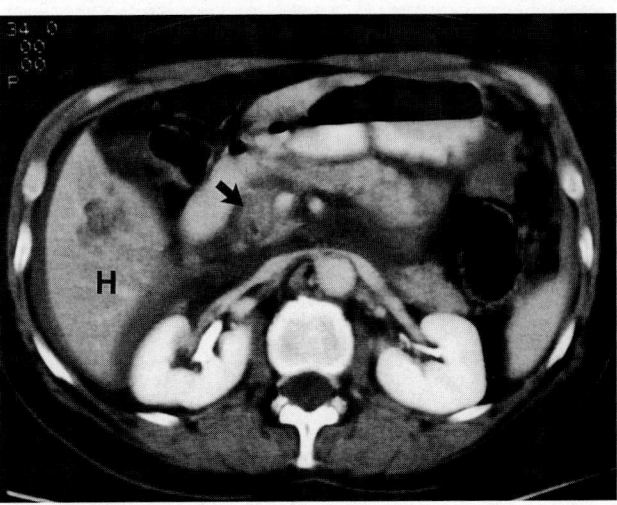

**FIGURE 35-4.** Computed tomography scan of pancreas, demonstrating subtle early signs of injury, including irregularity of the neck of the pancreas (arrow), peripancreatic fluid, and intrahepatic hematoma (H).
*(From Smith DR, Stanley RJ, Rue LW III: Delayed diagnosis of pancreatic transection after blunt abdominal trauma. J Trauma 40:1009, 1996.)*

findings noted in a patient with high risk mechanism of injury may warrant operative exploration.

Preoperative identification of isolated blunt pancreatic injury is also difficult. Blunt pancreatic injuries occur when a high energy crushing force is applied to the upper abdomen. In adults, the majority of injuries result from motor vehicle collisions, often from impact with the steering wheel; whereas in children, the classic presentation is a direct blow to the epigastrium from a bicycle handlebar.[69] CT evaluation of the injured pancreas may be normal, particularly when performed soon after injury.[63] In some patients, small peri-pancreatic collections with inactive pancreatic enzymes may be asymptomatic (Fig. 35-4). Such injuries may

become symptomatic when pancreatic secretions are activated by enteral leak from an associated small bowel injury. Other findings include transection, sometimes in association with fracture of the first lumbar vertebrae, hemorrhage in the area, or peripancreatic fluid or phlegmon when presentation is delayed (Fig. 35-5).[70,71] In a patient with persistent abdominal pain, fever, or elevated amylase, CT scan should be repeated if initially negative. Although a serum amylase is usually performed in patients sustaining blunt abdominal trauma, a single elevated result may not be useful. A persistently increased or rising level, however, mandates further evaluation.[72–76] Table 35-6 outlines the major reports dealing with amylase determination in patients with pancreatic trauma.

The chief determinate of morbidity and mortality in pancreatic injury is the structural integrity of the pancreatic duct. The importance of the status of the duct was first recognized and documented

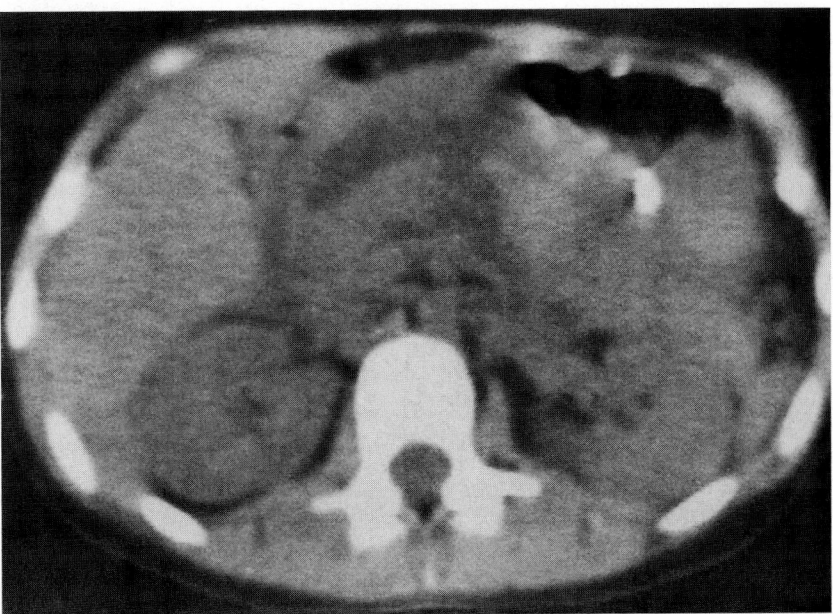

**FIGURE 35-5.** CT scan of pancreas, demonstrating midbody transection from a direct epigastric blow.

**TABLE 35-6**

## Summary of Reports on Hyperamylasemia and Pancreatic Trauma

| AUTHOR | MECHA-NISM | NO. WITH AMYLASE MEASURED | NO. WITH AMYLASE POSITIVE | PAN-CREATIC INJURY | TRUE-POSITIVE AMYLASE | FALSE-NEGATIVE AMYLASE | SENSI-TIVITY | SPECI-FICITY | ACCU-RACY | POSITIVE PREDICTIVE VALUE | NEGATIVE PREDICTIVE VALUE |
|---|---|---|---|---|---|---|---|---|---|---|---|
| White and Benfield 1972 | Penetrating | 33 | 3 (9%) | 33 | 3 | 30 | 9% | 0% | 9% | 100% | 0% |
| White and Benfield, 1972 | Blunt | 25 | 12 (48%) | 25 | 12 | 13 | 48% | 0% | 48% | 100% | 0% |
| Olsent,[91] 1973 | Blunt | 179 | 36 (20%) | 4 | 3 | 1 | 75% | 81% | 81% | 8% | 99% |
| Moretz et al.,[90] 1975 | Blunt | 51 | 23 (45%) | 5 | 3 | 2 | 60% | 56% | 57% | 13% | 93% |
| Bouwman et al.,[94] 1984 | Blunt | 61 | 23 (38%) | 3 | 2 | 1 | 67% | 64% | 64% | 9% | 93% |
| Takishima et al.,[92] 1997 | Blunt | 73 | 61% | 73 | 61 | 12 | 84% | 0% | 84% | 100% | 0% |

by Baker et al. in 1962.[77] Evaluation of duct integrity can be accomplished in stable patients via endoscopic retrograde cholangiopancreatography (ERCP). This technique is particularly valuable in the trauma patient in whom there may be subtle changes on CT, and chemical evidence of pancreatitis but without overt clinical findings mandating laparotomy.[78–81] In such cases, observation may be justified if a duct disruption can be excluded. Another technique that may be useful in a stable patient is magnetic resonance (MR) pancreatography.[82] Verification of ductal injury will require laparotomy in most cases. Although isolated cases of ERCP placed stents as the sole treatment for duct injury have been reported, current evidence suggests that this technique should be reserved for select patients with minimal duct disruption.[83–85]

In patients who require laparotomy, evaluation of pancreatic injury demands consideration of potential duct injury after prioritization of the principles of trauma surgery. Upper or central retroperitoneal hematomas, air, or bile staining require thorough exposure. Other indications of pancreatic injury intraoperatively include peripancreatic fluid collections, subcapsular hematomas, localized hemorrhage, parenchymal disruption, pancreatic fluid leak, and fat necrosis.

Intraoperative evaluation of the duodenum requires thorough evaluation of the anterior and retroperitoneal surfaces from the pylorus to the mesenteric vessels, as well as inspection of the fourth portion of the duodenum to the left of the vessels. To completely evaluate the remaining head, body, and tail of the pancreas, further maneuvers are required. Since the duodenum and pancreas are intimately associated, both structures may be simultaneously evaluated with a Kocher maneuver to the midline with coincident mobilization and medial rotation of the hepatic flexure of the colon. This provides exposure of the anterior and posterior surfaces of the second and third portions of the duodenum as well as further evaluation of the head and uncinate process. The remaining fourth portion of the duodenum requires dividing the ligament of Treitz, taking care to avoid injury to the

superior mesenteric vein. This will allow reflection of the duodenum from left to right. The body and tail of the pancreas are examined by division of the gastrocolic ligament and reflection of the stomach cephalad. Insertion of a curved retractor in the lesser sac allows full inspection of the anterior surface of the pancreas from the head to tail and from superior to inferior surfaces. With this technique, the splenic artery can be exposed along the superior border of the gland and the splenic vein along the inferior margin. In cases of active hemorrhage in the region of the neck of the pancreas suspected to originate from the juncture of the portal vein behind the pancreas, the pancreas should be divided without hesitation. A stapling device will allow for rapid exposure of the injured vessel and hemorrhage control of the pancreas. The discovery of injury to the anterior surface of the pancreas requires assessment of the status of the main pancreatic duct. Further exposure of the posterior surface of the pancreas is accomplished by division of the retroperitoneal attachments along the inferior border of the pancreas and retraction of the pancreas cephalad. Additional mobilization of the spleen and reflection of the spleen and tail of the pancreas from the left to the midline is a useful technique for further evaluation of the remaining areas of the pancreas (see Chap. 30). Most injuries sustained in penetrating trauma will be discovered with direct exploration. Occasionally, however, the integrity of the pancreatic duct remains in doubt. In these situations, it is crucial to attempt to identify a potential injury. To evaluate potential common duct injury, our approach has been to first squeeze the gallbladder to look for bile extravasation. Our next step is contrast infusion into the gallbladder with temporary clamping of the common bile duct above the cystic duct junction (Fig. 35-6). If none is seen, a duodenotomy can be performed for identification and cannulation of the papilla. Evaluation of the main pancreatic duct is performed via cannulation with a blunt tipped probe from the ampulla (Fig. 35-7). If the probe is seen in the wound, the diagnosis is confirmed. Alternatively, intraoperative pancreatography may be performed with

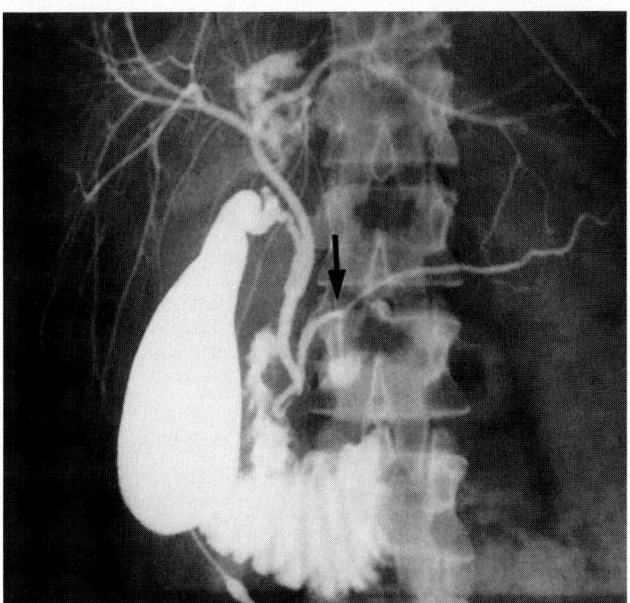

**FIGURE 35-6.** Intraoperative cholangiogram obtained via duodenotomy and direct cannulation of the ampulla. Overly forceful injection resulted in contrast extravasation into the pancreatic head. Also note a distal pancreatic duct injury with contrast extravasation near the laparotomy pad marker.

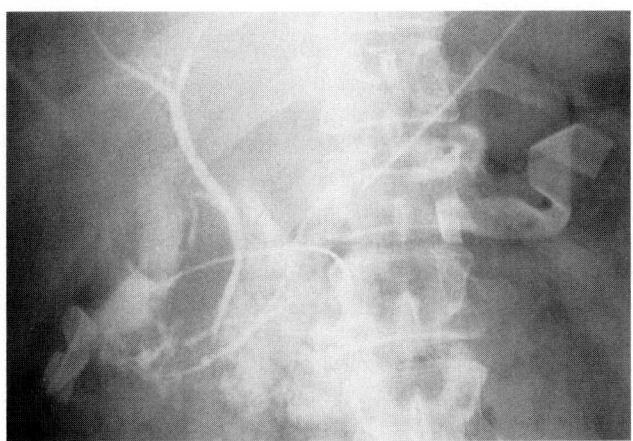

**FIGURE 35-7.** Intraoperative cholangiopancreatogram obtained via the gallbladder. Complete pancreatogram is obtained, depicting proximal pancreatic duct injury and extravasation of contrast.

2–3 cc of water soluble contrast material with very low pressure under fluoroscopic observation (Fig. 35-8). Injuries to the major duct occur in perhaps 15% of pancreatic trauma and are generally the result of penetrating wounds.[12,86] Berni et al. demonstrated that intraoperative pancreatography and accurate determination of the status of the duct resulted in a significant decrease in complications from 55% to 15%.[87] Others have recommended intraoperative pancreatography via transecting the tail of the pancreas and cannulation of the distal duct. This technique has had inconsistent results in most centers, hence transecting the pancreas to perform these evaluations appears ill advised. Finally, intraoperative ERCP is a useful technique which we have employed on a number of occasions with excellent results. One must remember to place a bowel clamp on the distal

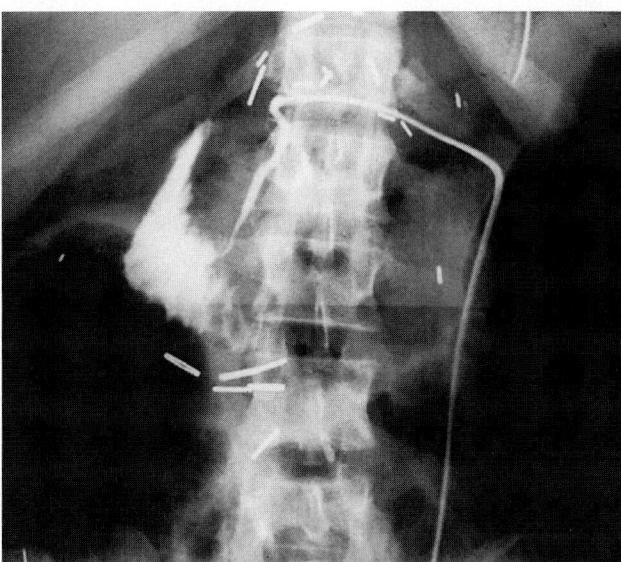

**FIGURE 35-8.** Intraoperative proximal pancreatogram obtained via an injured mid-body pancreatic duct. Normal residual proximal duct is confirmed prior to performing distal pancreatectomy.

portion of the duodenum to avoid air transmission to the gallbladder. Others have reported satisfactory results with this procedure.[88–92] Unfortunately, mobilization of the team to perform ERCP during an emergency exploration may be difficult.

## Decision Making and Treatment Options (see Algorithm I, Fig. 35-9)

Duodenum.    Treatment and decision making is perhaps best reviewed via stratification by organ injury scoring. The current classification system most commonly used is the American Association for the Surgery of Trauma (AAST) Organ Injury Scale (OIS). (Table 35-7) Injuries are graded on a I to V scale in ascending order of severity. In a collective review of 164 duodenal injuries from eight institutions, this management scheme was found to allow satisfactory management of the spectrum of injuries encountered with minimal morbidity and mortality.[93] Of note, this scale adds associated pancreatic injury as a major morbidity cofactor in duodenal injury.

## Grade I and II

Duodenal hematomas (grade I) are commonly identified during exploration[94] but are more often suspected by clinical presentation with gastric outlet obstruction with or without bilious emesis typically on the third postinjury day[95] (Fig. 35-10). This lesion is more common in children (see Chap. 46) but also occur in adults. One report suggested a high frequency in child abuse.[96] Obstruction develops as fluid is sequestered into a hyperosmotic hematoma. If there are no other indications for laparotomy, treatment generally consists of IV hydration and nasogastric tube suction.[95,97] Most duodenal hematomas in children will resolve spontaneously within seven to ten days with such a treatment regimen.[94] If they fail to resolve, repeat CT scan should be done to reevaluate the obstructive process. Operative approaches for evacuation of the hematoma include

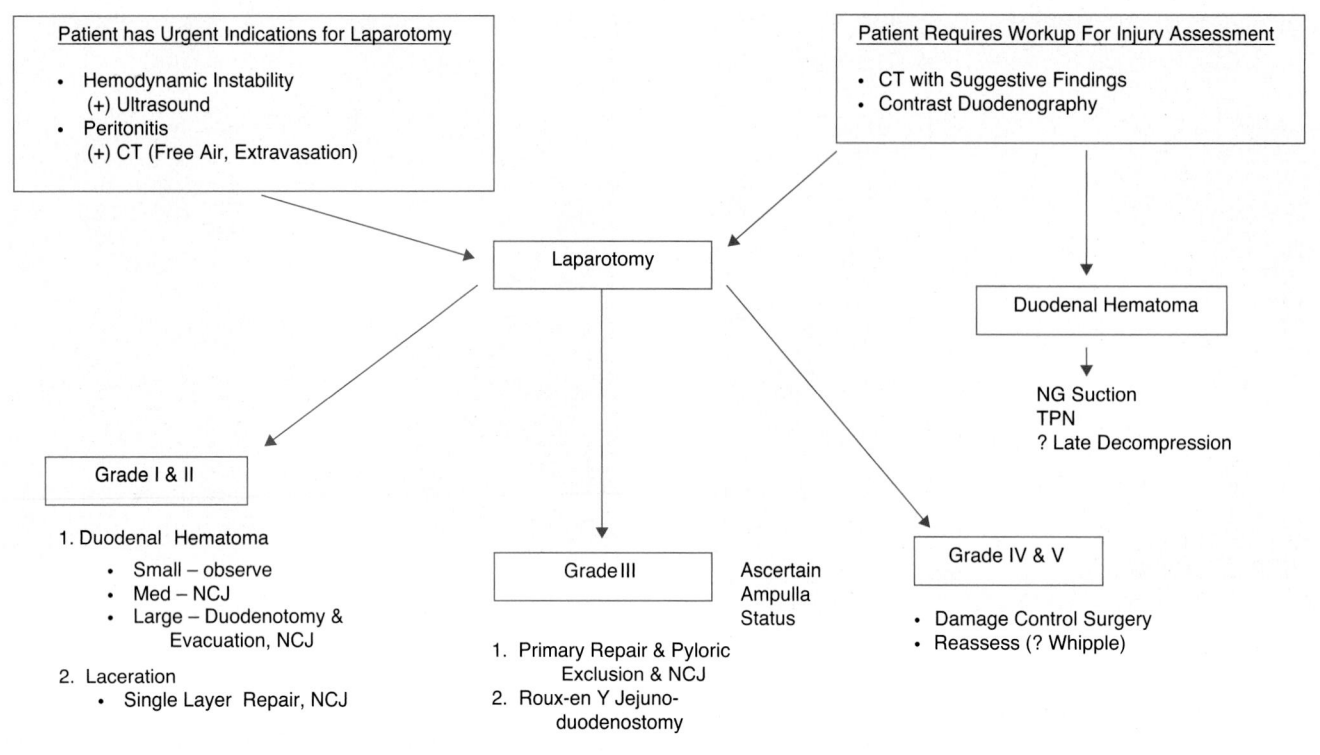

**FIGURE 35-9.** Algorithm I. Algorithm for duodenum injury.

open or laparoscopic drainage procedures. At exploration, the pancreas and duodenum must be thoroughly mobilized and examined. Duodenal stricture or occult perforation or unsuspected injury to the head of the pancreas should be sought, which occur in up to 20% of patients in this group.[95,97] Injuries can range from small serosal staining to obstructing masses. Treatment in this situation is controversial. Opening of the hematoma at the time of initial operation is condoned by some authors, who favor tube decompression of the stomach and distal tube jejunostomy for postoperative enteral nutrition while the hematoma resolves. With patience, almost all hematomas resolve in this setting, and opening of the duodenum risks conversion of a closed to open injury.[95,97] Our group favors a selective approach. We treat small hematomas with minimal luminal compromise with nasogastric suction and distal feeding tube jejunostomy, reserving incision and evacuation for larger hematomas with mass effect and luminal compromise. In such situations, we perform meticulous hemostasis with closure of duodenum with running absorbable closure.

Approximately 75% of duodenal lacerations occur as a result of penetrating trauma.[4,98,99] Exploratory laparotomy is performed via a midline incision. As described previously, standard trauma principles are employed for control of hemorrhage and enteric leaks. Exposure of the pancreas and duodenum is initiated with performance of the Kocher maneuver which allows for evaluation of the head of the pancreas as well as the C loop. The distal common bile duct and third portion of the duodenum are exposed by dissection of the overlying peritoneal attachments and fascia. By detaching the hepatic flexure of the colon from the second portion of the duodenum, evaluation of potential injury to the mesenteric vessels may be assessed. Full medial rotation of the right colon, cecum, and terminal ileum will allow complete evaluation of associated hepatic or vascular injuries in the right upper and middle abdomen. The distal common bile duct and third portion of the duodenum are exposed by dissection of the overlying peritoneal attachments and fascia. Incision in the right side of the root of the transverse colon will allow reflection of the small bowel superiorly for further exposure of the third part of the duodenum. After evaluation of the head of the pancreas, the neck, body, and tail are examined by opening the gastrocolic omentum from the left to the right. Adhesions to the stomach are taken down and the inferior border of the pancreas is visualized by incising the anterior reflection of the transverse mesocolon. Any evidence of

**TABLE 35-7**

**Duodenal Organ Injury Scale: American Association for the Surgery of Trauma**

| GRADE | | INJURY DESCRIPTION |
|---|---|---|
| I | Hematoma | Involving single portion of duodenum |
| | Laceration | Partial thickness, no perforation |
| II | Hematoma | Involving more than one portion |
| | Laceration | Disruption <50% of circumference |
| III | Laceration | Disruption 50 to 75% circumference of D2 |
| | | Disruption 50 to 100% circumference of D1, D3, D4 |
| IV | Laceration | Disruption >75% circumference of D2 |
| | | Involving ampulla or distal common bile duct |
| V | Laceration | Massive disruption of duodenopancreatic complex |
| | Vascular | Devascularization of duodenum |

*Adapted with permission from Moore EE, Cogbill T, Malangoni M, et al.: Organ injury scaling II: Pancreas, duodenum, small bowel, colon, and rectum. J Trauma 30:1427, 1990.*

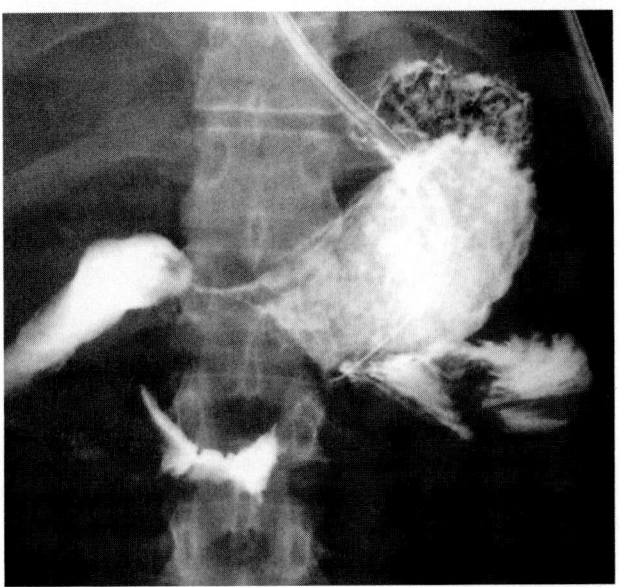
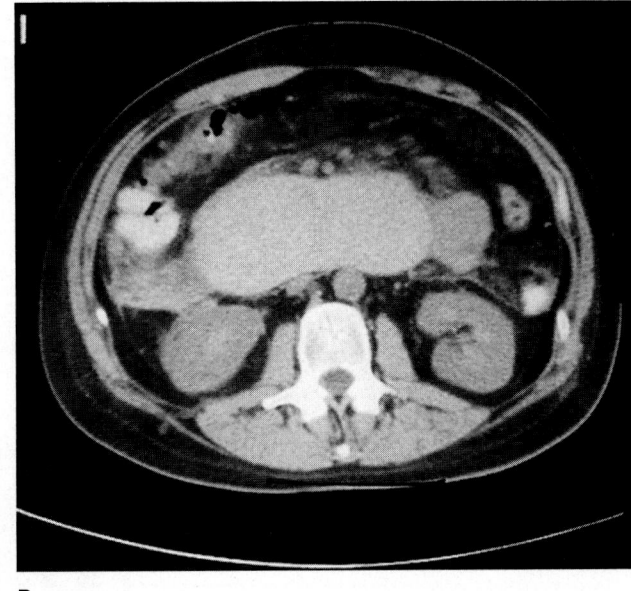

**FIGURE 35-10.** Diagnosing duodenal hematoma in a 30-year-old male. **(A)** Upper gastrointestinal radiograph showing narrowing of the second and third portions of the duodenum. **(B)** Computed tomography scan in the same patient, showing a giant hematoma of the transverse portion of the duodenum.

blood, bile, or air in the retroperitoneum requires thorough exploration. Simple duodenal lacerations with limited injury or minimal tissue destruction often result from either stab wounds or small caliber gunshot wounds. The vast majority can be safely repaired primarily with a meticulous single layer closure if adequate blood supply is ensured.[100] Duodenotomies can be repaired with running or interrupted sutures. We prefer a monofilament repair. Avoidance of tension is paramount. Repair in the direction in which the injury is formed is generally recommended. While earlier reports advocated transverse repair of select longitudinal injuries to minimize luminal compromise, current use of single layer monofilament closure has eliminated this concern in most cases.[6,101] In rare situations of laceration to the pancreatic side of the duodenum, mobilization may not be possible for repair. In such situations, we have performed an antimesenteric duodenotomy with repair of the injury from the inside.

## Grade III

About 20% of injuries (grade III–V) will require more complex procedures.[100,102,103]

If lacerations are judged too extensive for primary repair after mobilization and debridement, primary end-to-end duodeno-duodenostomy may be performed after mobilization of the segments involved without tension. Such a repair is rarely feasible in the second and third portions of the duodenum due to the intimate attachments to the pancreas which preclude obtaining any additional length for tension-free approximation. In this area, careful identification of the ampulla of Vater is essential to avoid injury at the time of repair. Snyder et al.[7] have identified factors that determine whether a duodenal wound can be safely primarily repaired. Table 35-8 outlines determinants of duodenal injury severity from that study, in which five factors were used to differentiate mild from severe injury that would necessitate more complex procedures.

Our policy, when confronted with a patient with a mild duodenal injury but with associated pancreatic injury, has been to perform the pyloric exclusion procedure as described by Vaughn and Jordan[2] (Fig. 35-11). This procedure is simpler than the original diverticulization techniques described by Berne and Donovan.[104] Gastrotomy along the greater curve of the stomach adjacent to the pylorus is used to access the pylorus from the inside. The pylorus is oversewn with nonabsorbable monofilament suture and gastrojejunostomy is created with a loop of jejunum to the gastrotomy on the greater curve. We are careful to use a long jejunal limb to prevent reflux of enteric contents to the duodenum. This procedure diverts the gastrointestinal stream away from the duodenal repair. If a fistula develops, it is a functional end duodenal fistula, which is usually easier to manage than a

**TABLE 35-8**

| Determinants of Duodenal Injury Severity | | |
|---|---|---|
| | **MILD** | **SEVERE** |
| Determinants of Injury Severity | | |
| Agent | Stab | Blunt or missile |
| Size | <75% wall | >75% wall |
| Duodenal location | 3rd, 4th | 1st, 2nd |
| Injury to repair interval | <24 h | >24 h |
| Adjacent injury | No CBD | CBD |
| Outcome | | |
| Mortality (%) | 6% | 16% |
| Duodenal mortality (%) | 0% | 6% |
| Duodenal morbidity (%) | 6% | 14% |
| CBD, common bile duct | | |

Adapted with permission from Snyder W, Weigelt J, Watkins W, et al.: The surgical management of duodenal trauma. Arch Surg 115:428, 1980. Copyright 1980. American Medical Association.

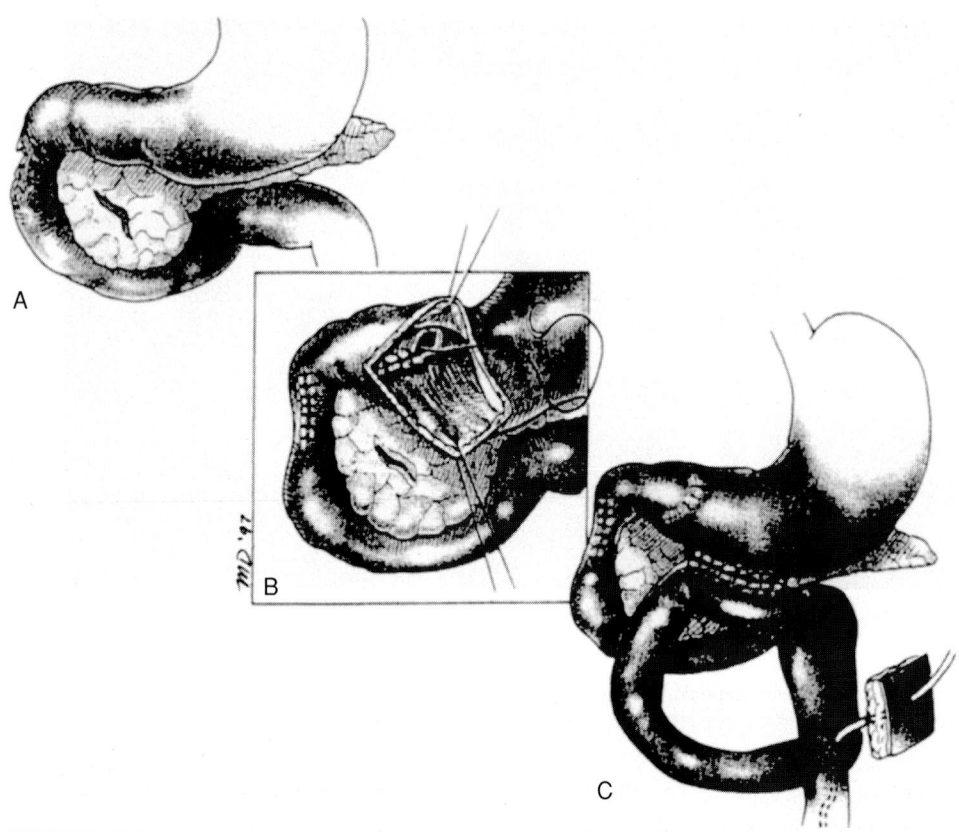

FIGURE 35-11.    **(A)** Pyloric exclusion is used to treat combined injuries of the duodenum and the head of the pancreas, as well as isolated duodenal injuries when the duodenal repair is less than optimal. **(B)** The pylorus is oversewn through a gastrotomy. The gastrotomy will subsequently be used to create a gastrojejunostomy. **(C)** These authors frequently employ needle-catheter jejunostomy tube feedings for these patients.
*(Reproduced with Permission from Brunicardi FC, et al. Schwartz's Principles of Surgery, 8th ed. McGraw-Hill, Inc., 2005. Fig. 6-53, p. 169.)*

higher output lateral fistula. Our policy has been to add needle catheter jejunostomy[105] in this setting to ensure a route for enteral nutrition, and we have found this to be a safer method than standard jejunostomy.[106] Even in the setting of an end fistula, the patient will often tolerate an oral diet after 10–14 days. The pylorus usually opens within 6–12 weeks; therefore vagotomy is not usually performed. This procedure may also be employed as a protective adjunct for a tenuous duodenal repair. Other techniques that have been described include omental patch or jejunal patch with a loop of jejunum, although such procedures are unproven.[5,101] Although there are no randomized prospective studies to prove the benefit of any type of gastric diversion and drainage in severe injuries, several reports do support the use of pyloric exclusion and gastrojejunostomy in selected cases.[8,100,103]

A historical alternative to pyloric exclusion and gastric diversion was advocated by Stone and Fabian,[3] and Hasson[107] using lateral tube duodenostomy and retrograde jejunostomy. Duodenal perforation with extensive surrounding tissue damage usually occurs with large caliber gunshot wounds. If the patient is hemodynamically unstable, these injuries will require appropriate debridement, stapling, drainage, and subsequent reconstruction. If primary repair results in a narrowed, potentially stenotic lumen, then resection and anastomosis will likely fail. In such situations, we have performed Roux-en-Y limb reconstruction with a loop of jejunum passed through the transverse mesocolon to create an end-to-side jejuno-duodenostomy (Fig. 35-12). Although, jejunal mucosal patches and interposition grafts based on a vascular pedicle of the jejunal mesentery have been described[101] we have rarely found a use for these techniques. Injuries to the second portion of the duodenum distal to the

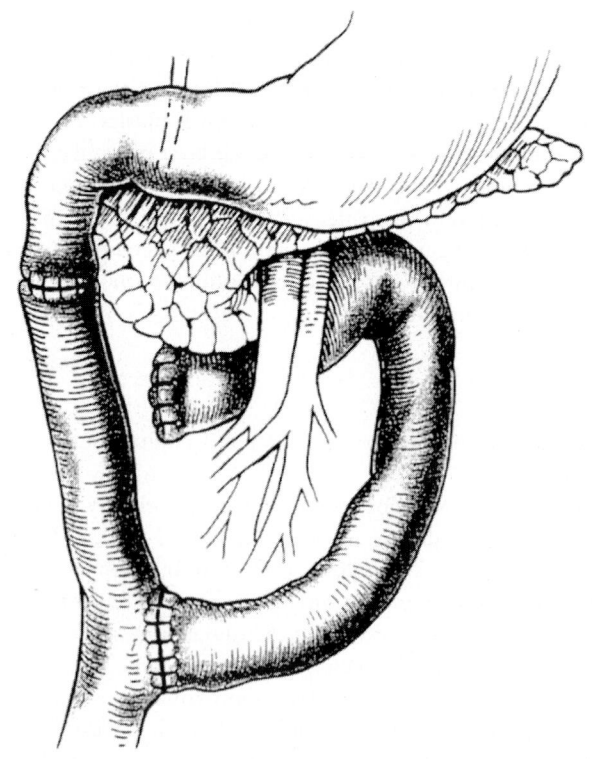

FIGURE 35-12.    Roux-en-Y duodenojejunostomy is used to treat duodenal injuries between the papilla of Vater and superior mesenteric vessel when tissue loss precludes primary repair.
*(Reproduced with Permission from Brunicardi FC et al. Schwartz's Principles of Surgery, 8th ed. McGraw-Hill, Inc., 2005. Fig. 6-52, p. 168.)*

ampulla can be repaired with division of the duodenum and end to end duodenojejunostomy using a roux limb passed through the transverse mesocolon. In these situations, the distal duodenal stump is oversewn and a distal jejuno-jejunostomy is created for intestinal continuity. In injuries to the third and fourth portion of the duodenum, repair may by compromised by the short mesentery causing difficulty in mobilization leading to ischemia. Resection and anastomosis in this setting is associated with a high rate of fistula formation. We have preferred resection and duodeno–jejunostomy to the right of the mesenteric vessels in this setting.

## Grade IV and V (see Section on Combined Duodenal–Pancreatic Injuries)

These injuries involve massive disruption or devascularization of the second portion of the duodenum with avulsion of the ampulla of Vater or distal common bile duct. After hemostasis and debridement via damage control techniques (see Chap. 41) staged reconstruction may be performed. In essence, such a procedure should be considered as a last resort in situations where the injury complex has already accomplished the dissection.

Pancreas (see Algorithm II, Fig. 35-13). The AAST committee on Organ Injury Scaling has issued guidelines for the treatment and categorization of pancreatic injuries (Table 35-9). This evolved from a number of published classification systems that have been devised to describe these injuries.[44,86,93,108] This guideline emphasizes that the chief factor determining morbidity and mortality in pancreatic trauma is the structural integrity of the main pancreatic duct, and the location of injury with regard to the mesenteric vessels.

## Grade I and II

The vast majority of parenchymal injuries and contusions with an intact duct can be treated with surgical hemostasis and drainage.[42]

Capsular tears that are not bleeding are not repaired and may be simply drained with closed suction catheters.[109] Unnecessary attempts at repair of lacerations without evidence of ductal disruption (grade III) or tissue loss can result in late pseudocyst formation, whereas the vast majority of controlled, minor pancreatic fistulae are self-limited and easily managed with soft closed suction drains (Jackson Pratt). We liberally employ catheter drainage, since many minor appearing injuries will drain for several days. If the amylase concentrations in the drain is less than that of serum the drains are usually removed within a few days. If amylase levels are elevated, we continue drainage until there is no further evidence of pancreatic leak. As prolonged gastric ileus is common with even minor pancreatic injuries, we often employ distal enteral access with needle catheter jejunostomy in such cases. Since the composition of most standard tube feeding increases the pancreatic effluent volume and amylase concentration, lower fat and higher pH (4.5) elemental diets are less stimulating to the pancreas and are particularly well suited for use in needle catheter jejunostomies.[110–112]

## Grade III

Pancreatic ductal injuries (grade III–IV) always require treatment to prevent pancreatic ascites or major fistula. Most ductal injuries can

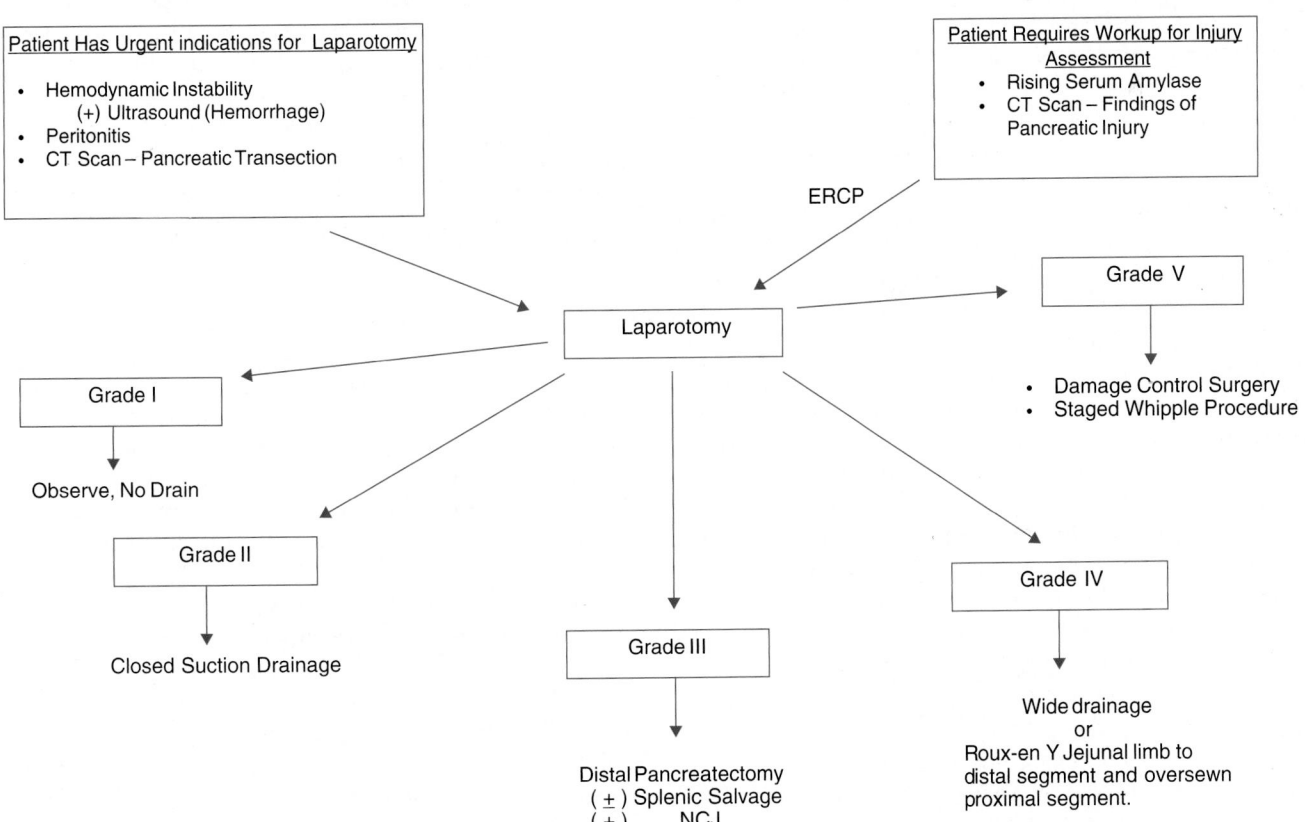

**FIGURE 35-13.** Algorithm II. Algorithm for pancreatic trauma.

## TABLE 35-9

**Pancreatic Organ Injury Scale: American Association for the Surgery of Trauma**

| GRADE[a] | | INJURY DESCRIPTION[b] |
|---|---|---|
| I | Hematoma | Minor contusion without duct injury |
| | Laceration | Superficial laceration without duct injury |
| II | Hematoma | Major contusion without duct injury or tissue loss |
| | Laceration | Major laceration without duct injury or tissue loss |
| III | Laceration | Distal transection or parenchymal injury with duct injury |
| IV | Laceration | Proximal (to right of superior mesenteric vein) transection or parenchymal injury |
| V | Laceration | Massive disruption of pancreatic head |

[a]Advance one grade for multiple injuries to the same organ.

[b]Based on most accurate assessment at autopsy, laparotomy, or radiologic study.

(Modified with permission from Moore EE, Cogbill T, Malangoni M, et al.: Organ injury scaling II: Pancreas, duodenum, small bowel, colon, and rectum. J Trauma 30:1427, 1990.)

be identified by either preoperative studies in the stable patient or intraoperatively at exploration as previously described. The anatomic division between the head and body of the pancreas is located near the point where the superior mesenteric vessels pass behind the neck of the pancreas. This anatomic division will provide an estimated 50% of pancreatic tissue and serves as an anatomic marker of the left and right of the gland.[113,114] Management decisions are based upon the anatomic location of the duct and parenchymal injury (proximal vs. distal). Ductal injuries at or distal to the neck often occurs in blunt trauma, and are treated definitively with distal pancreatectomy.[115–118] In the vast majority of patients, distal resection should leave no concern for later pancreatic endocrine or exocrine function. If there is any concern for injury to the duct proximally in this setting (grade IV), a proximal pancreatogram can be performed through the end of the transected duct. In our experience, such situations are rarely encountered. The pancreas is divided at the injury location, and the proximal stump is closed, often with a stapling devise. We prefer using a TA type with a 4.8 mm stapler to avoid excessively crushing the gland.[118] Alternatively, the parenchyma can be closed with mattress sutures placed in a full thickness non-crushing technique with nonabsorbable sutures. In young trauma patients, the pancreatic duct is small but can be usually identified with loops. If identified, it should be individually ligated at the time of pancreatic division.[115] While some authors have suggested Roux-en-Y pancreaticojejunostomy drainage for the proximal resected pancreas, we do not believe this is warranted. In the hemodynamically stable patient, the distal pancreatectomy can often be performed without splenectomy.[119,120] Every effort should be made to establish enteral access at the time of initial celiotomy in virtually all patients with grade III or more severe injuries to avoid the use of parenteral nutrition, with its attendant risks and complications.[115,121,122]

## Grade IV

Trauma to the right of the vessels and pancreatic head represent the most challenging of pancreatic injuries. Careful assessment of the remaining pancreatic tissue and consideration of future function should be weighed when contemplating an extended distal pancreatectomy.[116] Prior to embarking on such a procedure, one must carefully assess the status of the pancreatic duct and common bile duct. Options for evaluation intraoperatively include duodenotomy and pancreatography,[87] although in most situations, local inspection and exploration of the injury can adequately determine ductal continuity.[123] If ductal status cannot be determined, we have favored wide external drainage and postoperative ERCP evaluation of the duct with stenting if possible.[83,124] Resection of greater than 85% of the pancreas may be associated with a significant risk of pancreatic insufficiency.[77,125] Occasionally, proximal duct injuries (to the right of the vessels) may be treated with extended distal pancreatectomy only when the ampulla is intact and at least 20% of the pancreas will remain. In the rare situation where resection will result in less than 20% of pancreatic tissue intact, the pancreas should be divided, the proximal segment closed, and the distal portion preserved with drainage into a Roux-en-Y pancreaticojejunostomy. This procedure was used in only two (0.5%) of a total of 399 patients in a review of the four largest recent reports of pancreatic trauma published since 1990.[14,16,126,127] Current trends emphasize the effectiveness of closed suction drainage alone even for extensive proximal gland injuries.[16] However, the effectiveness of this technique with major ductal injury remains to be established.

**Combined Pancreatic and Duodenal Injuries.** Combined pancreatic and duodenal injuries are quite common given their intimate anatomic relationship. Such injuries are more common following penetrating trauma. The presence of both injuries significantly increases the complication rates, with morbidity and mortality from combined pancreatic and duodenal injury exceeding 30%, twice that observed in either injury alone. Therefore, combined injuries deserve special attention.[37,49,103,115,128–130] Simple duodenal injuries with limited surrounding tissue loss in combination with pancreatic injuries where the duct is intact can be treated with primary duodenal repair and drainage.[98,100,101] In this situation the risk of duodenal suture line dehiscence is increased and we liberally employ the pyloric exclusion procedure as an adjunct. Consideration of suture line protection with this technique is especially warranted when the pancreatic duct integrity is suspect.

## Grade V

Although rarely warranted, recent experience with staged damage control techniques (see Chap. 41) document that for devastating injury to the head of the pancreas, pancreatoduodenectomy can be performed with success similar to cancer procedures.[131–134] Other indications for this procedure include confirmed transection of both the intrapancreatic bile duct and proximal main pancreatic duct, or avulsion of the ampulla of Vater from the duodenum with complete destruction of the second portion of the duodenum. Evaluation requires cholangiography, usually via the gall bladder, to document continuity or lack thereof between the bile duct and duodenum. Evaluation of the ampulla and common bile duct may be performed through the injury site in some cases. Recent published series of pancreatic trauma suggest a frequency of 3% for pancreatoduodenectomy following trauma.[49,123,132,135] In an occasional patient, late complications of recurrent sepsis with abscess or continued fistula may mandate extirpation.[133]

In sum, patients with extensive trauma to the pancreas and duodenum should be approached individually. Such injuries almost always occur in the face of associated vascular or other organ injuries, and aggressive debridement and reconstruction should be delayed in the unstable coagulopathic patient (see Chap. 41) On occasion, an injury initially judged nonsalvageable in this setting will appear more favorable upon reevaluation the next day.

## Nonoperative Management

With the growth of nonoperative algorithms in the pediatric population, controversy has evolved with regard to the management of blunt pancreatic injury. Several reports[136–139] have documented successful treatment with nonoperative schemes which include complete bowel rest, nutritional support, and serial CT scanning with observation. The success of this technique is undoubtedly related to the fact that major duct injury is very rare in children, with an incidence of 0.12% in one series.[138] Although most successfully treated cases have involved grade I or II injuries, others have reported satisfactory treatment of ductal disruption with ERCP and stenting, including isolated cases in the adult population.[85] Complications such as pancreatic necrosis or pseudocyst formation have been treated with percutaneous drainage and laparotomy has been reserved for selected cases.

We believe that the risk of missed injury and associated morbidity and mortality does not justify nonoperative therapy in most cases. Our policy has been to approach these patients similar to the adult population, with particular effort to preservation of the spleen if distal pancreatectomy is performed[140] (see Chap. 46).

## Complications of Pancreatic and Duodenal Trauma

Although damage control techniques to control associated vascular injuries are essential for survival in the hemorrhagic phase, late septic complications directly related to the pancreatic or duodenal injury occur in up to 40% of patients.[16,60,108,116,141,142] As previously mentioned, the presence of combined pancreatic and duodenal injury doubles the risk of a complication in the postoperative period. The risk of complications can be predicted by the injury grade on the AAST scale, as well as the presence of associated bowel injury.[143] A recent report estimated that up to half of postoperative complications can be avoided with thorough evaluation of the pancreas and determination of the status of the main pancreatic duct.[87] When duct injury is recognized, most complications can be recognized, treated, and will usually be self limited. Unrecognized injuries and complications of duodenal repair or pancreatic duct injury may lead to persistent or recurring sepsis and multiple organ dysfunction syndrome (MODS) (see Chap. 68) which is responsible for nearly 30% of deaths resulting from duodenal and pancreatic trauma. Table 35-10 lists complications seen in 118 patients surviving initial hemorrhage in pancreatoduodenal trauma. Of note, almost 20% involved organ dysfunction/failure.

## Hemorrhage

Exsanguination is the most common cause of early death associated with pancreatic and duodenal injuries. Early use of damage control maneuvers is therefore necessary for successful management. Damage control techniques such as packing of hemorrhage and stapling or drainage of succus leaks will allow for deferred debridement and reconstruction (see Chap. 41). Correction of

**TABLE 35-10**

**Complications of Pancreatoduodenal Wounds in 99 of 118 Patients Surviving More Than 48 h**

| COMPLICATION | NO. |
|---|---|
| Pancreatic fistula | 27 |
| Abscess | 11 |
| Duodenocutaneous fistula | 7 |
| Respiratory failure | 7 |
| Renal failure | 6 |
| Small-bowel fistula | 4 |
| Biliary fistula | 3 |
| Pulmonary embolism | 2 |
| Pancreatic abscess | 2 |
| Gastric fistula | 1 |
| Ureteral fistula | 1 |
| Wound dehiscence | 1 |
| Stomal ulcer | 1 |
| Hemorrhage | 1 |
| Intestinal obstruction | 1 |

coagulopathy (see Chap. 61) hypothermia (see Chap. 51) and optimization of oxygen delivery (see Chap. 60) may be life saving, followed by definitive operative treatment upon return to the operating room.[144] In our experience, this can usually be accomplished within 24–36 hours.

## Recurrent (Secondary) Hemorrhage

Postoperative hemorrhage is a common concern after laparotomy for pancreatic and duodenal injuries, especially given the extent of associated injuries which can be a source of bleeding. Approximately 10% of patients after pancreatic and duodenal trauma will sustain some degree of hemorrhage. Transfusion therapy should be guided by evaluation of the patient's status with attention to oxygen delivery. As in a patient presenting with initial trauma, it is important to resuscitate the patient with efforts to correct associated acidosis, coagulopathy, and hypothermia prior to embarking on a reexploration. On occasion, angiography in this setting may identify the bleeding point for treatment with embolization. Other causes of postoperative hemorrhage late in the treatment course include progressive pancreatic necrosis or intra-abdominal infection/abscess.[130,145] Frequent CT scan evaluation of pancreatic necrosis with aspiration and culture will predict the need for subsequent invasive radiological intervention and drainage. In our experience, many of these patients can be spared complicated and difficult reoperation with these techniques. A rare complication of hemorrhagic pancreatitis which may be indistinguishable from postoperative hemorrhage has been reported with a mortality in excess of 80%.[12,13]

## Pancreatic Fistula

Pancreatic fistula is a significant complication, with an incidence of 7–20% in pancreatic injury and higher in combined injuries.[11,46,141] A pancreatic fistula may be diagnosed in a patient with a measurable drain output with an amylase level greater than three times the serum level.[146] A minor pancreatic fistula is defined as output less than 200 mL/d, and most will resolve within two weeks of injury if adequate drainage without obstruction is established. High output lateral fistulae are rare (greater than 700 mL /d). They are severe management challenges, and many will require long periods of drainage, nutritional support, or late surgical intervention.[12–14,16,112] Stoma therapists can offer creative solutions for skin protection in these patients. ERCP is a useful technique for investigating fistulae that fail to resolve after approximately two weeks.[85] Given the frequency of such complications, surgical foresight in placing enteral access is wise to support a patient with postoperative fistula and may avoid the use of parenteral nutrition and its associated complications. The somatostatin analogue octreotide has shown some promise in treating patients with prolonged high output fistulae; however, the principles of drainage, infection control, and evaluation of obstruction or stricture remain the cornerstones of therapy.[147–151] It has been shown to decrease the volume of fistulae drainage, but does not decrease the duration of the fistulae or increase the rate of spontaneous closure. In a recent multicenter review of distal pancreatectomy for trauma, the postoperative fistula rate was 14% and most (89%) closed within 6–8 weeks. Persistent pancreatic fistulae with associated residual pancreatic sequestrum may require extirpation or other individualized treatment depending on the location of the duct injury. Of note, a recent review of posttraumatic biliary and pancreatic fistulae from a large service showed that pancreatic fistulae had the longest hospitalization and cost of care. No patient in this series died, and only two of 19 required late reoperation for complications related to the fistulae.[152]

## Duodenal Fistula and Stricture

Duodenal fistula results from failure of surgical repair due to suture line dehiscence, sometimes with distal duodenal obstruction from stricture or adhesions. Patients with duodenal obstruction in the postoperative period should be evaluated with CT scan to rule out extrinsic compression from associated phlegmon or abscess. Avoidance of tension at the time of duodenal repair is essential to avoid subsequent stricture formation. With careful attention to these principles, duodenal stricture is rare. The incidence of duodenal fistula in several collated series averaged 7%.[98] As previously discussed, in our group we liberally employ the pyloric exclusion procedure of Vaughn[2] in duodenal injuries. If a duodenal stricture or obstruction occurs, drainage is protected via the gastroenterostomy which allows healing of the duodenal injury and resolution of associated obstruction if present. If a fistula develops, the protective pyloric exclusion results in a less morbid end versus side fistula. In our experience, in this setting, most such fistulae heal within six to eight weeks. We believe that forethought in placement of a needle catheter jejunostomy at the time of pyloric exclusion is essential and allows for enteral access during this period.

## Abdominal Abscess

Abscess formation should be considered in patients who develop a septic picture seven to ten days after major pancreatic and duodenal injury. The best predictors of postoperative peri-pancreatic collections are inadequate debridement or drainage during the initial operative evaluations.[12–14,16]

Diagnostic evaluation via CT will often allow percutaneous decompression and evacuation of collections. Reexploration in this setting carries significant morbidity and mortality and should be avoided whenever possible. Often patients will require several drainage procedures, with repeat CT scanning to evaluate and follow new collections that may develop. Other patients may develop MODS often heralded by respiratory failure (see Chap. 68). Patients who develop such septic complications carry a mortality rate approaching 40%[123,153] (see Tables 35-2, 35-4).

## Pancreatic Pseudocyst and Pancreatitis

Occasionally, pseudocyst formation is the presenting symptom of missed blunt pancreatic trauma. The true incidence is unknown, although a number of cases have been reported.[46] Early pseudocyst formation may be indistinguishable from abscess and percutaneous needle aspiration by invasive radiology may be helpful.[154,155] A recent case report[156] of endoscopic ultrasound guided transgastric stenting of a posttraumatic pseudocyst suggests that this technique may be useful when the cyst is in approximation to the stomach.

In other pseudocyst cases, ERCP will serve to evaluate the continuity of the pancreatic duct. If the duct is intact, percutaneous drainage will often successfully resolve the problem. Late treatment of duct injury with endoscopic stenting[83] has been described, with no long-term results available.

Transient elevation of the serum amylase is common in patients after laparotomy for pancreatic trauma, although acute pancreatitis with clinical abdominal pain is probably less frequent.[11,14,129,157] CT should be performed to rule out associated abscess, pseudocyst, or other complications. If the diagnosis is confirmed, treatment includes nasogastric suction, bowel rest, and nutritional support. Elemental enteral formulas appear to be tolerated well and should be employed with avoidance of TPN and its associated complications. Most cases will resolve spontaneously.

## Pancreatic Insufficiency

With careful attention to injury patterns as described, both exocrine and endocrine insufficiency should be rare after pancreatic trauma. In studies of distal pancreatic resections, only one case of diet controlled hyperglycemia was documented in a patient undergoing a resection in excess of 80% of the gland.[39,125] This assumes normal function of the remaining 10–20% pancreatic tissue. In contrast, patients with chronic pancreatitis and abnormal function had a high incidence of diabetes when undergoing resection of much less than 80% of the gland.[158] In the trauma scenario, it may be assumed that any resection distal to the mesenteric vessels will preserve adequate pancreas for normal function. In a recent multicenter series no instances of exocrine insufficiency were noted after distal pancreatic resections.[14]

## REFERENCES

1. Lucas C, Ledgerwood A: Factors influencing outcome after blunt duodenal injury. *J Trauma* 15:839, 1975.
2. Vaughan G III, Frazier O, Graham D, et al.: The use of pyloric exclusion in the management of severe duodenal injuries. *Am J Surg* 134:785, 1977.
3. Stone H, Fabian T: Management of duodenal wounds. *J Trauma* 19:334, 1979.
4. Flint L Jr, McCoy M, Richardson J, et al.: Duodenal injury: Analysis of common misconceptions in diagnosis and treatment. *Ann Surg* 191:697, 1980.
5. Ivatury RR, Nallathambi M, Gaudino J, et al.: Penetrating duodenal injuries: An analysis of 100 consecutive cases. *Ann Surg* 202:154, 1985.
6. Cogbill T, Moore E, Feliciano D, et al.: Conservative management of duodenal trauma: A multicenter perspective. *J Trauma* 30:1469, 1990.

7. Snyder W, Weigelt J, Watkins W, et al.: The surgical management of duodenal trauma. *Arch Surg* 115:422, 1980.

8. Martin T, Feliciano D, Mattox K, et al.: Severe duodenal injuries: Treatment with pyloric exclusion and gastrojejunostomy. *Arch Surg* 118:631, 1983.

9. Levinson MA, Peterson SR, Sheldon GF, et al.: Duodenal trauma: Experience of a trauma center. *J Trauma* 24:475, 1982.

10. Shorr R, Greaney G, Donovan A: Injuries of the duodenum. *Am J Surg* 154:93, 1987.

11. Stone H, Fabian T, Satiani B, et al.: Experiences in the management of pancreatic trauma. *J Trauma* 21:257, 1981.

12. Graham J, Mattox K, Jordan G: Traumatic injuries of the pancreas. *Am J Surg* 136:744, 1978.

13. Jones R: Management of pancreatic trauma. *Am J Surg* 150:698, 1985.

14. Cogbill T, Moore E, Morris J Jr, et al.: Distal pancreatectomy for trauma: A multicenter experience. *J Trauma* 31:1600, 1991.

15. Wilson R, Moorehead R: Current management of trauma to the pancreas. *Br J Surg* 78:1196, 1991.

16. Patton J Jr, Lyden S, Croce M, et al.: Pancreatic trauma: A simplified management guideline. *J Trauma* 43:234, 1997.

17. Travers B: Rupture of the pancreas. *Lancet* 12:384, 1827.

18. Mickulicz-Radicki JV: Surgery of the pancreas. *Ann Surg* 38:1, 1903.

19. Stern E: Traumatic injuries to the pancreas. *Am J Surg* 8:58, 1930.

20. Root HD, Keizer PJ, Perry JF Jr: Peritoneal trauma, experimental and clinical studies. *Surg* 62:679, 1967.

21. Otis G: The medical and surgical history of the war of the rebellion. In Otis G, ed. *Surgical History*. vol II, part II, Washington DC: Government Printing Office, 1876.

22. Poole H: Wounds of the pancreas. In Coates JJ, DeBakey M, eds. *Surgery in World War II: General Surgery*. vol II. Washington DC: Office of Surgeon General, 1955.

23. Culotta R, Howard J, Jordan GJ: Traumatic injuries to the pancreas. *Surgery* 40:320, 1956.

24. Halgrimson GG, Trimble C, Gale S,et al.: Panreaticoduodenectomy for traumatic lesions. *Am J Surg* 118:877, 1969.

25. Korte W: (Quoted by Robson AWM, Cambridge PJ) in *The Pancreas: Its Surgery and Pathology*. Philadelphia: Saunders, 1907.

26. Kulenkampff D: Ein fall von pancreas-fistel. *Berl Klin Wochenschr* 19:102, 1882.

27. Moynihan B: *Abdominal Operations*. vol II. Philadelphia: Saunders, 1926.

28. Whipple A: Observations on radical surgery for lesions of the pancreas. *Surg Gynecol Obstet* 82:623, 1946.

29. Herczel. Cit. Nach. Jahresber Hildebrands, 1896:691 Cited by Meerwein.

30. Summers JJ: The treatment of posterior perforations of the fixed portions of the duodenum. *Ann Surg* 39:727, 1904.

31. Berry J, Giuseppi P: Traumatic rupture of the intestine, with a case of recovery after operation and an analysis of the 132 cases that have occurred in ten London hospitals during the last fifteen years. *Proc R Soc Med Surg* Sec 1, 1909.

32. Miller R: Retroperitoneal rupture of the duodenum by blunt force. *Ann Surg* 64:550, 1916.

33. Sako Y, Artz P, Howard JM, et al.: A survey of evacuation and mortality in a forward surgical hospital. *Surgery* 37:602, 1955.

34. Cave W: Wounds of the duodenum (118 casualties). In Coates JJ, DeBakey M, eds. *Surgery in World War II: General Surgery*. vol II. Washington DC: Office of Surgeon General; 1955.

35. Kelly G, Norton L, Moore G, et al.: The continuing challenge of duodenal injuries. *J Trauma* 18:160, 1978.

36. Ballard R, Badellino M, Eynon C, et al.: Blunt duodenal rupture: A 6-year statewide experience (discussion 233). *J Trauma* 43:229; 1997.

37. Lopez,PP, Benjamin R, Cockburn M, et al.: Recent trends in the management of combined pancreatoduodenal injuries. *Am Surg* 71:847, 2005.

38. Huerta S, Bui T, Porral D, et al.: Predictors of morbidity and mortality in patients with traumatic duodenal injuries. *Am Surg* 71:763, 2005.

39. Balasegaram M: Surgical management of pancreatic trauma. *Curr Probl Surg* 16:1, 1979.

40. Cuddington G, Rusnak C, Cameron R, et al.: Management of duodenal injuries. *Can J Surg* 33:41, 1990.

41. Sukul K, Lont H, Johannes E: Management of pancreatic injuries. *Hepatogastroenterology* 39:447, 1992.

42. Nowak M, Baringer D, Ponsky J: Pancreatic injuries: Effectiveness of debridement and drainage for nontransecting injuries. *Am Surg* 52:599, 1986.

43. Vargish T, Urdaneta LF, Cram AE, et al.: Duodenal injuries in the rural setting. *Am Surg* 49:211, 1982.

44. Sorensen V, Obeid F, Horst H, et al.: Penetrating pancreatic injuries. *Am Surg* 52:354, 1986.

45. Anderson C, Connors J, Mejia D, et al.: Drainage methods in the treatment of pancreatic injuries. *Surg Gyn Obstet* 138:587, 1974.

46. Kudsk K, Temizer D, Ellison E, et al.: Post-traumatic pancreatic sequestrum: Recognition and treatment. *J Trauma* 26:320, 1986.

47. Roman E, Silva Y, Lucas C: Management of blunt doudenal injury. *Surg Gynecol Obstet* 132:7, 1971.

48. Glancy K: Review of pancreatic trauma. *West J Med* 151:45, 1989.

49. Graham J, Mattox K, Vaughan G III, et al.: Combined pancreatoduodenal injuries. *J Trauma* 19:340, 1979.

50. Edwards E, Malone P, MacArthur J: *Operative Anatomy of Abdomen and Pelvis*. Philadelphia: Lea & Febiger, 1975.

51. Sherck J, Oakes D: Intestinal injuries missed by computed tomography. *J Trauma* 30:1, 1990.

52. Quinlan R: Anatomy, embryology, and physiology of the pancreas. In Shackelford R, Zuidema G, eds. *Surgery of the Alimentary Tract*. Philadelphia: Saunders, 1983, p. 3.

53. Rienhoff WJ, Pickrell K: Variations in terminations of the common bile and main pancreatic ducts. *Arch Surg* 51:205, 1945.

54. Anatomy and Physiology of the Duodenum. In Schackelford R, Zuidema G, eds. *Surgery of the Alimentary Tract*. Philadelphia: Saunders, 1981, p. 38.

55. Rolfs A, Ediger MA: Intestinal metal ion absorption: An update. *Curr Opin Gastroenterol* 17:177, 2001.

56. Yellin A, Vecchione T, Donovan A: Distal pancreatectomy for pancreatic trauma. *Am J Surg* 124:135, 1972.

57. DiMagno EP, Go VL, Summerskill WHJ: Relations between pancreatic enzyme outputs and malabsorption in severe pancreatic insufficiency. *N Engl J Med* 288:813, 1973.

58. Allen G, Moore F, Cox C Jr, et al.: Delayed diagnosis of blunt duodenal injury: An avoidable complication. *J Am Coll Surg* 187:393, 1998.

59. Carr N, Cairns S, Lees W, et al.: Late complications of pancreatic trauma. *Br J Surg* 76:1244, 1989.

60. Leppaniemi A, Haapiainen R, Kiviluoto T, et al.: Pancreatic trauma: Acute and late manifestations. *Br J Surg* 75:165, 1988.

61. Gholson C, Sittig K, Favrot D, et al.: Chronic abdominal pain as the initial manifestation of pancreatic injury due to remote blunt trauma of the abdomen. *South Med J* 87:902, 1994.

62. Cook D, Walsh J, Vick C, et al.: Upper abdominal trauma: Pitfalls in CT diagnosis. *Radiology* 159:65, 1986.

63. Jeffrey R, Federle M, Creass R: Computed tomography of pancreatic trauma. *Radiology* 147:491, 1983.

64. Peitzman A, Makaroun M, Slasky B, et al.: Prospective study of computed tomography in initial management of blunt abdominal trauma. *J Trauma* 26:585, 1986.

65. Lane M, Mindelzun R, Jeffrey R: Diagnosis of pancreatic injury after blunt abdominal trauma. *Semin Ultrasound CT MR* 17:177, 1996.

66. Kunin J, Korobkin M, Ellis J, et al.: Duodenal injuries caused by blunt abdominal trauma: Value of CT in differentiating perforation from hematoma. *Am J Roentgenol* 160:221, 1993.

67. Mirvis S, Gens D, Shanmuganathan K: Rupture of the bowel after blunt abdominal trauma: Diagnosis with CT. *Am J Roentgenol* 159:1217, 1992.

68. Timaran CH, Daley BJ, Enderson BL: Role of duodenography in the diagnosis of blunt duodenal injuries. *J Trauma* 51:648, 2001.

69. Arkovitz MS, Johnson N, Garcia VF: Pancreatic trauma in children: Mechanisms of injury. *J Trauma* 42:49, 1997.

70. Horst H, Bivins B: Pancreatic transection. A concept of evolving injury. *Arch Surg* 124:1093, 1989.

71. Smith D, Stanley R, Rue L: Delayed diagnosis of pancreatic transection after blunt abdominal trauma. *J Trauma* 40:1009, 1996.

72. Moretz J III, Campbell D, Parker D, et al.: Significance of serum amylase level in evaluating pancreatic trauma. *Am J Surg* 150:698, 1975.

73. Olsen W: The serum amylase in blunt abdominal trauma. *J Trauma* 13:200, 1973.

74. Takishima T, Sugimoto K, Hirata M, et al.: Serum amylase level on admission in the diagnosis of blunt injury to the pancreas: Its significance and limitations. *Ann Surg* 226:70, 1997.

75. Liu K, Atten M, Lichtor T, et al.: Serum amylase and lipase elevation is associated with intracranial events. *Am Surg* 67:215 (discussion 219), 2001.

76. Bouwman D, Weaver D, Walt A: Serum amylase and its isoenzymes: A clarification of their implication in trauma. *J Trauma* 24:573, 1984.

77. Baker R, Dippel W, Freeark R: The surgical significance of trauma to the pancreas. *Trans Western Durg Assoc* 70:361, 1962.

78. Vallon A, Lees W, Cotton P: Grey-scale ultrasonography and endoscopic pancreatography after pancreatic trauma. *Br J Surg* 66:169, 1979.

79. Harrell D, Vitale G, Larson O: Selective role for endoscopic retrograde cholangiopancreatography in abdominal trauma. *Surg Endosc* 12:400, 1998.

80. Belohlavek D, Merkle P, Probst M: Identification of traumatic rupture of the pancreatic duct by endoscopic retrograde pancreatography. *Gastrointest Endosc* 24:255, 1978.

81. Whittwell A, Gomez G, Byers P, et al.: Blunt pancreatic trauma: Prospective evaluation of early endoscopic retrograde pancreatography. *South Med J* 82:586, 1989.

82. Soto J, Alvarez O, Munera F, et al.: Traumatic disruption of the pancreatic duct: Diagnosis with MR pancreatography. *AJR Am J Roentgenol* 176:175, 2001.

83. Kozarek R, Ball T, Patterson D, et al.: Endoscopic transpapillary therapy for disrupted pancreatic duct and peripancreatic fluid collections. *Gastroenterology* 100:1362, 1991.

84. Barkin J, Ferstenberg R, Panullo W, et al.: Endoscopic retrograde cholangiopancreatography in patients with injury to the pancreas. *Gastrointest Endosc* 34:102, 1988.

85. Kim H, Dong KL, Whoi K II, et al.: The role of endoscopic retrograde pancreatography in the treatment of traumatic pancreatic duct injury. *Gastrointest Endosc* 54:49, 2001.

86. Lucas C: Diagnosis and treatment of pancreatic and duodenal injury. *Surg Clin North Am* 57:49, 1977.

87. Berni D, Bandyk D, Oreskovich M, et al.: Role of intraoperative pancreatography in patients with injury to the pancreas. *Am J Surg* 143:602, 1982.

88. Sugawa C, Lucas C: The case for preoperative and intraoperative ERCP in pancreatic trauma (Editorial). *Gastrointest Endosc* 34:145, 1988.

89. Laraja R, Lobbato V, Cassaro S, et al.: Intraoperative endoscopic retrograde cholangiopancreatography (ERCP) in penetrating trauma of the pancreas. *J Trauma* 26:1146, 1986.

90. Bozymski E, Orlando R, Holt J: Traumatic disruption of the pancreatic duct demonstrated by endoscopic retrograde pancreatography. *J Trauma* 21:244, 1981.

91. Taxier M, Sivak M Jr, Cooperman A, et al.: Endoscopic retrograde pancreatography in the evaluation of trauma to the pancreas. *Surg Gyn Obstet* 150:65, 1980.

92. Kopelman D, Suissa A, Klein Y, et al.: Pancreatic duct injury: Intraoperative endoscopic transpancreatic drainage of parapancreatic abscess. *J Trauma* 44:555, 1998.

93. Moore E, Cogbill T, Malangoni M, et al.: Organ injury scaling II: Pancreas, duodenum, small bowel, colon, and rectum. *J Trauma* 30:1427, 1990.

94. Jewett T, Caldarola V, Karp M, et al.: Intramural hematoma of the duodenum. *Arch Surg* 123:54, 1988.

95. Touloukian R: Protocol for the nonoperative treatment of obstructing intramural duodenal hematoma. *Am J Surg* 145:330, 1983.

96. Wooley M, Mahour G, Sloan T: Duodenal hematoma in infancy and childhood. *Am J Surg* 136:8, 1978.

97. Czyrko C, Weltz C, Markowitz R, et al.: Blunt abdominal trauma resulting in intestinal obstruction: When to operate? *J Trauma* 30:1567, 1990.

98. Asensio J, Feliciano D, Britt L, et al.: Management of duodenal injuries. *Curr Probl Surg* 11:1021, 1993.

99. McKenney M, Nir I, Levi D, et al.: Evaluation of minor penetrating duodenal injuries. *Am Surg* 62:952, 1996.

100. Kashuk J, Moore E, Cogbill T: Management of the intermediate severity duodenal injury. *Surgery* 92:758, 1982.

101. McInnis W, Aust J, Cruz A, et al.: Traumatic injuries of the duodenum: A comparison of primary closure and the jejunal patch. *J Trauma* 15:847, 1975.

102. Cone JB, Eidt JF: Delayed diagnosis of duodenal rupture. *Am J Surg* 168:676 (discussion 678), 1994.

103. Buck J, Sorensen V, Fath J, et al.: Severe pancreatico-duodenal injuries: The effectiveness of pyloric exclusion with vagotomy. *Am Surg* 58:557 (discussion 561), 1992.

104. Berne C, Donovan A, White E, et al.: Duodenal "diverticulization" for duodenal and pancreatic injury. *Am J Surg* 127:503, 1974.

105. Moore EE, Dunn El, Jones TN: Immediate jejunostomy feeding: Its use after major abdominal trauma. *Arch Surg* 116: 681, 1981.

106. Holmes J IV, Brundage S, Yuen P, et al.: Complications of surgical feeding jejunostomy in trauma patients. *J Trauma* 47:1009, 1999.

107. Hasson J, Stern D, Moss G: Penetrating duodenal trauma. *J Trauma* 24:471, 1984.

108. Jurkovich G, Carrico C: Management of pancreatic injuries. *Surg Clin N Am* 70:575, 1990.

109. Fabian T, Kudsk K, Croce M, et al.: Superiority of closed suction drainage for pancreatic trauma: A randomized prospective study. *Ann Surg* 211:724, 1990.

110. Neviackas J, Kerstein M: Pancreatic enzyme response with an elemental diet. *Surg, Gyn & Obst* 142:71, 1976.

111. McArdle AH, Echave W, Brown RA, et al.: Effect of elemental diet on pancreatic secretion. *Am J Surg* 128:690, 1974.

112. Kellum JM, Holland GF, McNeill P: Traumatic pancreatic cutaneous fistula: Comparison of enteral and panrenteral feedings. *J Trauma* 28:700, 1988.

113. Innes J, Carey L: Normal pancreatic dimensions in the adult human. *Am J Surg* 167:261, 1994.

114. Wittingen J, Frey C: Islet concentration in the head, body, tail and uncinate process of the pancreas. *Ann Surg* 179:412, 1974.

115. Cogbill T, Moore E, Kashuk J: Changing trends in the management of pancreatic trauma. *Arch Surg* 117:722, 1982.

116. Jones W, Finkelstein J, Barie P: Managing pancreatic trauma. *Infect in Surgery* March:29, 1990.

117. Fitzgibbons T, Yellin A, Maruyama M, et al.: Management of the transected pancreas following distal pancreatectomy. *Surg Gyn Obstet* 154:225, 1982.

118. Andersen D, Bolman R III, Moylan J Jr: Management of penetrating pancreatic injuries: Subtotal pancreatectomy using the auto suture stapler. *J Trauma* 20:347, 1980.

119. Pachter H, Hofstetter S, Liang H, et al.: Traumatic injuries to the pancreas: The role of distal pancreatectomy with splenic preservations. *J Trauma* 29:1352, 1989.

120. Schein M, Freinkel W, E'Egidio A: Splenic conservation in distal pancreatic injury: Stay away from the hilum! *J Trauma* 31:431, 1991.

121. Kellum J, Holland G, McNeill P: Traumatic pancreatic cutaneous fistula: Comparison of enteral and parenteral feedings. *J Trauma* 28:700, 1988.

122. Kudsk K, Croce M, Fabian T, et al.: Enteral versus parenteral feeding: Effects on septic morbidity after blunt and penetrating abdominal trauma. *Ann Surg* 215:503, 1991.

123. Feliciano D, Martin T, Cruse P, et al.: Management of combined pancreatoduodenal injuries. *Ann Surg* 205:673, 1987.

124. Huckfeldt R, Agee C, Nichols W, et al.: Nonoperative treatment of traumatic pancreatic duct disruption using endoscopically placed stent. *J Trauma* 41:143, 1996.

125. Dragstedt L: Some physiologic problems in surgery of the pancreas. *Ann Surg* 118:576, 1943.

126. Ivatury R, Nallathambi M, Rao P, et al.: Penetrating pancreatic injuries. Analysis of 103 consecutive cases. *Am Surg* 56:90, 1990.

127. Wisner DH, Wold RL, Frey CF: Diagnosis and treatment of pancreatic injuries. An analysis of management principles. *Arch Surg* 125:1109, 1990.

128. Asensio J, Demetriades D, Berne J, et al.: A unified approach to the surgical exposure of pancreatic and duodenal injuries. *Am J Surg* 174:54, 1997.

129. Moore J, Moore E: Changing trends in the management of combined pancreatoduodenal injuries. *World J Surg* 8:791, 1984.

130. Campbell R, Kennedy T: The management of pancreatic and pancreaticoduodenal injuries. *Br J Surg* 67:845, 1980.

131. Oreskovich M, Carrico C: Pancreaticoduodenectomy for trauma: A viable option? *Am J Surg* 147:618, 1984.

132. Delcore R, Stauffer J, Thomas J, et al.: The role of pancreatogastrostomy following pancreatoduodenectomy for trauma. *J Trauma* 37:395, 1994.

133. Heimansohn D, Canal D, McCarthy M, et al.: The role of pancreaticoduodenectomy in the management of traumatic injuries to the pancreas and duodenum. *Am Surg* 56:511, 1990.

134. McKone T, Bursch L, Scholten D: Pancreaticoduodenectomy for trauma: A life saving procedure. *Am Surg* 54:361, 1988.

135. Lowe R, Saletta J, Moss G: Pancreatoduodenectomy for penetrating pancreatic trauma. *J Trauma* 17:732, 1997.

136. Shilyansky J, Sena L, Kreller M, et al.: Nonoperative management of pancreatic injuries in children. *J Pediatr Surg* 33:343, 1998.

137. Wales PW, Shuckett B, Kim PC: Long-term outcome after nonoperative management of complete traumatic pancreatic transection in children. *J Pediatr Surg* 36:823, 2001.

138. Canty TG Sr, Weinman D: Management of major pancreatic duct injuries in children. *J Trauma* 50:1001, 2001.

139. Kouchi K, Tanabe M, Yoshida H, et al.: Nonoperative management of blunt pancreatic injury in childhood. *J Pediatr Surg* 34:1736, 1999.

140. Meier D, Coln C, Hicks B, et al.: Early operation in children with pancreas transection. *J Pediatr Surg* 36:341, 2001.

141. Sims E, Mandal A, Schlater T, et al.: Factors affecting outcome in pancreatic trauma. *J Trauma* 24:125, 1984.

142. Smego DR, Richardson JD, Flint LM: Determinants of outcome in pancreatic trauma. *J Trauma* 25:771, 1985.

143. Kao LS, Bulger EM, Parks DL, et al.: Predictors of morbidity after traumatic pancreatic injury. *J Trauma* 55:898, 2003.

144. Carrillo C, Fogler RJ, Shaftan GW: Delayed gastrointestinal reconstruction following massive abdominal trauma. *J Trauma* 34:233, 1993.

145. Akhrass R, Yaffe M, Brandt C, et al.: Pancreatic trauma: A ten-year multi-institutional experience. *Am Surg* 63:598, 1997.

146. Bassi C, Dervenis C, Bultirini G, et al.: Post-operative Pancreatic fistula – and international study group (IS6PF) definition. *Surgery* 138:8, 2005.

147. Martineau P, Shwed JA, Denis R: Is octreotide a new hope for enterocutaneous and external pancreatic fistulas closure? *Am J Surg* 172:386, 1996.

148. Amirata E, Livingston DH, Elcavage J: Octreotide acetate decreases pancreatic complications after pancreatic trauma. *Am J Surg* 168:345, 1994.

149. Nwariaku F, Terracina A, Mileski W, et al.: Is octreotide beneficial following pancreatic injury? *Am J Surg* 170:582, 1995.

150. Berberat PO, Friess H, Büchler M, et al.: The role of octreotide in the sprevention of complications following pancreatic resection. *Digestion* 60 (suppl 2):15, 1999.

151. Seidner D, Speerhas R, Trexler K: Can octreotide be added to parenteral nutrition solutions? *Nutr Clin Prac* 13:84, 1998.

152. Vassiliu P, Toutouzas KG, Velahos GC: A prospective study of post-traumatic biliary and pancreatic fistuli. The role of expectant management. *Injury* 35:223, 2004.

153. Wynn M, Hill D, Miller D, et al.: Management of pancreatic and duodenal trauma. *Am J Surg* 150:327, 1985.
154. Bass J, Di Lorenzo M, Desjardins J, et al.: Blunt pancreatic injuries in children: The role of percutaneous external drainage in the treatment of pancreatic pseudocysts. *J Pediatr Surg* 23:721, 1988.
155. Burnweit C, Wesson D, Stringer D, et al.: Percutaneous drainage of traumatic pancreatic pseudocysts in children. *J Trauma* 30:1273, 1990.
156. Rout S, Rahman SH, Sheridan MB: Endoscopic ultrasound guided transgastric stenting of traumatic pancreatic pseudocyst. *JOP* 7:423, 2006.
157. Holland AJA, Davey R, Sparnon A, et al.: Traumatic pancreatitis: Long-term review of initial non-operative management in children. *J Paediatr Child Health* 35:78, 1999.
158. Hutchins RR, Hart RS, Pacifico M, et al.: Long term results of distal pancreatectomy for chronic pancreatitis in 90 patients. *Ann Surg* 236:612, 2002.
159. Bradley EL III, Young PR Jr, Chang MC, et al.: Diagnosis and initial management of blunt pancreatic trauma: Guidelines from a multi-institutional review. *Ann Surg* 227:861, 1998.

# Commentary ■ EDDY H. CARRILLO

This chapter by Drs. Kashuk and Burch reflects their personal experience and their recommendations are supported by the reputation of their institution and by a careful and thorough review from the contemporary literature. They describe the technical details of the surgical management and potential complications of those injuries in a well-written and illustrated chapter. Since most decisions regarding the management of injuries to the pancreatic–duodenal complex are made based upon anatomical findings, it is refreshing to read such an extensive review of the anatomy and physiology.

If the principles of surgical exploration are closely followed, after penetrating trauma, the diagnosis of pancreatic and duodenal injuries should be straightforward. In our unit, we emphasize that if there are any of the "3 Bs" (bile, blood, or bubbles) in or around the pancreas, duodenum, or base of the mesentery at the ligament of Treitz, a thorough exploration of the area should be performed. The same philosophical principle applies to those patients with penetrating proximity wounds and with lower thoracic or upper lumbar fractures. In patients with persistent abdominal pain, fever, and elevated amylase the abdominal CT should be repeated. My preference is to obtain a dedicated pancreatic–duodenal CT that entails the following: (1) intravenous and oral contrast (diatriozate meglumine and diatriozate sodium, MD Gastroview®. Mallinckrodt, Hazelwood, MO); (2) instillation of the oral contrast through a nasogastric tube 15 minutes before the actual test is performed to optimize visualization of the duodenum; and (3) fine cuts (1–2 mm) through the pancreatic-duodenal complex.

Because of the anatomical location of the pancreatic-duodenal complex and its proximity to other organs, including vital vascular structures, isolated injuries are rare and a high morbidity and mortality is common. Much emphasis is placed in the potential morbidity and mortality of duodenal and pancreatic injuries, the overall mortality remains between 16% and 20% and a complication rate of around 30%. As the author's emphasize, "delayed presentation or late diagnosis of the injury in this patient population is disastrous and directly correlates with significantly increased morbidity and mortality." The pancreas or duodenum are directly responsible for less than 2% of all these deaths with associated injuries being responsible for the majority of fatalities. Unrecognized injuries and complications related to the pancreatic-duodenal repairs may lead to persistent or recurring sepsis and MODS which is responsible for nearly 30% of deaths resulting from duodenal and pancreatic trauma.

Pancreatic fistulas are usually harmless unless associated with enteric contents or a high output (more than 200 mL/d). Duodenal fistulas can be more challenging to care for. If sound surgical principles were followed during the initial surgical treatment, most patients will develop end duodenal fistulas, which are better tolerated and easier to manage than lateral duodenal fistulas. In our unit, we follow the SNAP principle (Skin protection, Nutritional support, Abscess drainage/control, Patience) for the treatment of pancreatic or duodenal fistulas with a consistent success rate within a six to eight week period.

The philosophical principles for duodenal and pancreatic injuries should include the following tenets: (1) the overall decision making depends on the severity of the injury, involvement of associated organs, and condition of the patient; (2) less treatment is probably best treatment; (3) most duodenal injuries can be treated by primary repair and most injuries to the pancreas can be managed by observation or closed suction drainage; (4) resection and diversion is indicated only for grade IV and grade V duodenal injuries and pyloric exclusion is probably a better option than duodenal "diverticulization"; (5) pancreatic-duodenal resections should used only in those patients with extensive injuries to the pancreatic-duodenal complex with involvement of the biliary system. The principles of abbreviated laparotomy and planned reoperation should be used in critically ill patients with multiple injuries and associated physiologic derangement, as is usually the case with most patients with complex pancreatic-duodenal injuries.

# Colon and Rectum

*George C. Velmahos*

## HISTORY

The colon is the second most frequently injured organ, next to the small bowel, after penetrating abdominal trauma but is involved in less than 5% of blunt abdominal trauma patients.[1,2] The management of colon injuries has followed a remarkable 360° course that started with primary repair as the procedure of choice, shifted toward colonic diversion, and returned recently to primary repair.

During the World War I era antibiotics did not exist, prehospital times were long, emergent care was underdeveloped, and antisepsis was poor at best. Mortality from colon injuries approached 60%.[3] Primary repair was favored over colostomy, although both techniques were associated with excessive death rates for today's standards.[4,5] Gradual improvements in general surgical care produced new knowledge about the nature and outcome of these injuries. By World War II the pendulum shifted, as Ogilvie described his experience in treating such wounds in the Western desert and recommended colostomy for all military colon injuries.[6] The Office of the Surgeon General of the United States issued a mandate for colostomy[7] and opened the way for establishing it as the standard of care for the next four decades. Ironically, the evidence that supported these conclusions was questionable, as the overall mortality after colon injury in Ogilvie's seminal paper was high (53%) and not different between the primary repair and colostomy groups. It would take over four decades for modern trauma surgeons to understand the differences between high-velocity military wounds and civilian injuries and try to change the unproven surgical dogma of mandatory colostomy. Although reports from Tulane in the 1950s[8] and 1960s[9] reported improved results by using primary repair, colostomy remained the predominant method of managing colon trauma across the country. It would not be before the late 1970s that the seminal reports from Gerogia[10] and then South Africa[11] seriously challenged the concept of mandatory colostomy use and eventually, followed by multiple other studies, succeeded to overturn the dogma.

## MECHANISMS OF INJURY

### Penetrating

Penetrating injuries of the colon are caused by direct perforation from bullets or sharp objects. On rare occasions, the blast effect of a high-velocity missile may create contusion, ischemia, and even perforation of the colon wall without direct contact. Extraperitoneal gunshot wounds have been described to result in colon injury due to such blast effect.[12,13]

### Blunt

During blunt trauma the colon can be injured in one of the three ways: (a) creation of a closed loop with acute increase in intraluminal pressures and blowout (Fig. 36-1), (b) shearing forces causing tears at sites of transition from a relatively immobile segment to a mobile segment (e.g., splenic flexure, rectosigmoid junction), mesocolic avulsions usually coexist, (c) pure mesocolic avulsion which although not associated with immediate colonic perforation, may lead to devascularization, wall necrosis, and late perforation.

### Iatrogenic/Self-inflicted

Perforations of the colon from colonoscopy, sexual activity, or swallowed objects have populated the literature as unusual case reports.[14–16]

## DIAGNOSIS

### Clinical Examination

It is frequently suggested that clinical examination is unreliable in the trauma patient. In general, this is not true (see Chap. 11)!

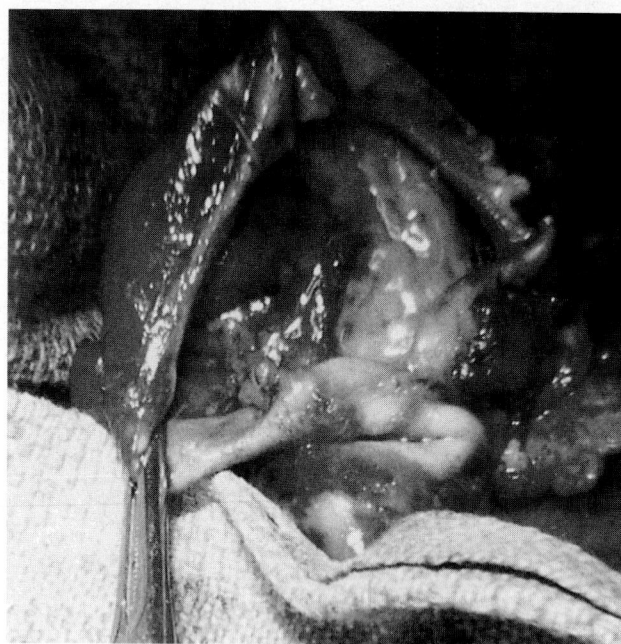

**FIGURE 36-1.** Blowout disruption of the sigmoid colon caused by a motor vehicle accident. (*Courtesy: David V. Feliciano, MD*)

Although neurologically impaired trauma patients cannot be examined reliably, most pitfalls of diagnosis occur due to unfocused and incomplete examinations and not due to an innate ability of the trauma patient to confuse the astute clinician. The argument of unreliable clinical examination was the basis for routine laparotomies after gunshot wounds to the abdomen until large studies proved that selective management based on repeat clinical examination is safe, cost-effective, and reduces the rate of nontherapeutic laparotomies.[17–19] Retroperitoneal perforations of the colon, usually produced by penetrating injuries of the back may take longer (up to 24 hours) to manifest with abdominal tenderness and signs of infection. Such patients may have been initially managed

nonoperatively but such delays in diagnosis are usually not associated with complications or the need for colostomy.[17,19]

Focused assessment with sonography for trauma (FAST) has now become a standard adjunct to the initial clinical examination of almost all trauma patients.[20] However, its value for the specific diagnosis of colon injuries is very low, since such injuries may be associated with very little free abdominal fluid but a substantial amount of intra- and extraluminal gas that obscures the ultrasonographic image (see Chap. 17). FAST can be done according to institutional policies of trauma patient evaluation but not with the purpose or hope of discovering colon injuries, particularly from penetrating trauma.[21]

**Computed Tomography.** Helical computed tomography (CT) has revolutionized the way we practice medicine (see Chap. 16). The ubiquitous fast-speed multidetector CT scanner is now being used for most patients with suspected abdominal trauma. Findings such as extraluminal air, rectal contrast extravasation, thickened colonic wall, and mesocolic stranding are suggestive of colon injury, with the former two being more specific findings than the latter two.[22] Triple-contrast CT (oral, intravenous, rectal) has been adopted by many centers as a sensitive method of detecting intestinal injury, especially after penetrating trauma.[23,24] Triple-contrast administration as a routine policy is cumbersome, unnecessary, and potentially harmful. It has been shown in multiple studies, including a prospective randomized one, that the addition of oral contrast delays time to CT scanning does not increase the sensitivity of detecting hollow visceral injuries.[25–27] Similarly, rectal contrast offers little or no benefit.[28] It is hard to imagine that air will not leak before the contrast material does from a colon perforation; it is similarly hard to imagine that a patient with free air following abdominal trauma would not be explored—given the appropriate clinical presentation—unless contrast material leaks too. However, in a few specific cases rectal contrast may be useful and could be considered.

Single contrast CT (only intravenous) is being increasingly used. The sensitivity and specificity is over 90% and 96%.[28,29] It has been argued that a negative CT allows safe discharge of patients from the emergency department (ED).[30] However, the reliance on CT over clinical examination is of concern. False positive CT findings can lead to nontherapeutic laparotomies (Figs. 36-2A, 36-2B and 36-3A, 36-3B). Clinical examination

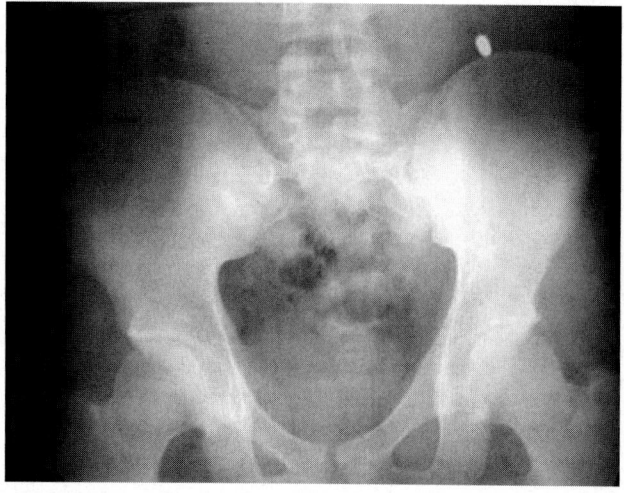

**A**

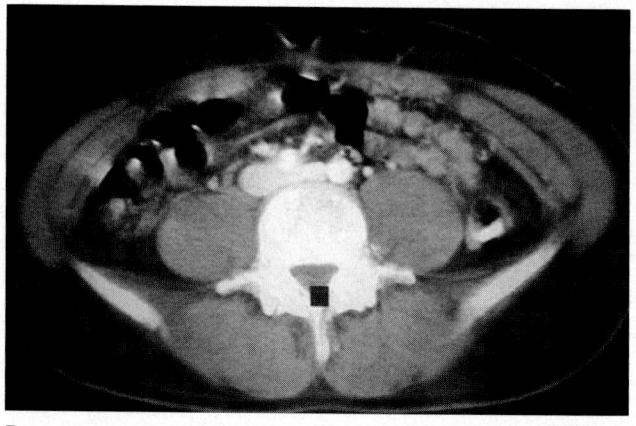

**B**

**FIGURE 36-2.** **(A)** Retained bullet after a gunshot wound to the back. The patient was asymptomatic. **(B)** A CT scan showed the bullet lodged in the wall of the descending colon. Following this, the patient underwent a laparotomy. The bullet was lodged in the mesocolon, adjacent to the wall but not through it. The laparotomy was unnecessary.

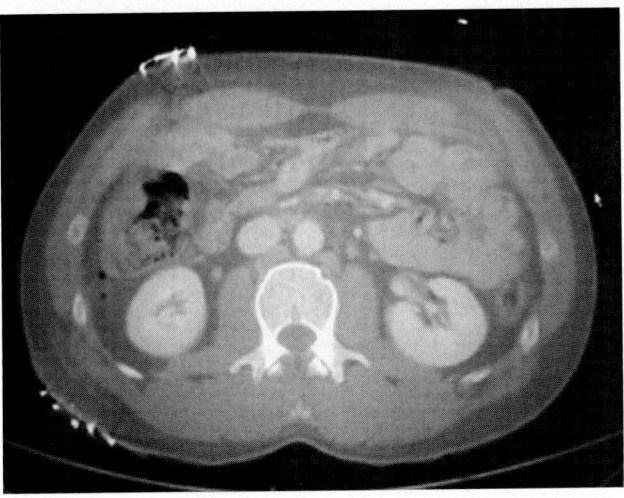

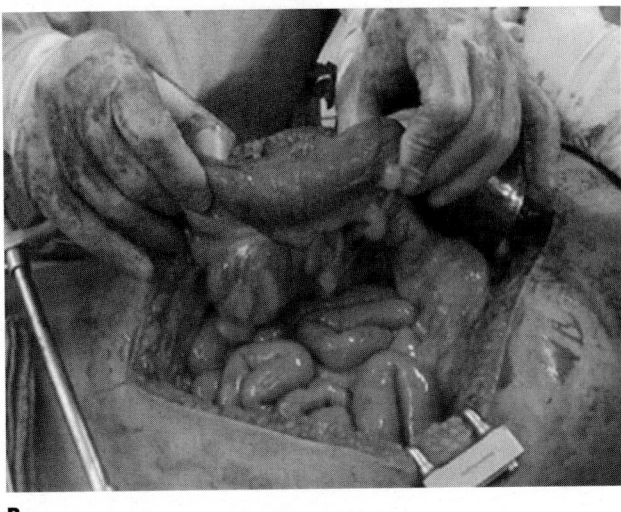

**A**
**B**

**FIGURE 36-3.** **(A)** A CT scan shows extraluminal air following a transabdominal gunshot wound (entry and exit sites marked on skin). The patient complained of mild abdominal tenderness. In the absence of a CT scan this patient would have been observed. **(B)** An exploratory laparotomy revealed an intact colon. The operation was unnecessary.

should remain the mainstay of diagnosis and CT can serve as an adjunct and not the primary method of evaluation.

## Laparoscopy

Diagnostic laparoscopy is struggling to find its appropriate place in trauma.[31] Except for the diagnosis of diaphragmatic injuries,[32] there are a few scenarios in which diagnosis by laparoscopy makes sense. For example, a patient with no abdominal symptoms who has small amounts of free air next to his colon following a gunshot wound to the flank may be a candidate for laparoscopy. Although expert laparoscopists can easily mobilize viscera and access all spaces, reports suggest that retroperitoneal injuries (exactly those that would not cause immediate symptoms and would need to be discovered by laparoscopy) may be missed. In a multicenter study[33] the incidence of negative laparotomy after laparoscopy was 25% and the incidence of additional bowel injuries found on laparotomy but not diagnosed by laparoscopy was 10%. These results, coupled with the risks of general anesthesia and abdominal intervention, indicate that laparoscopy is not yet the diagnostic procedure of choice in colon trauma.

**Intraoperative Diagnosis.** The trauma laparotomy offers a unique opportunity for a systematic and standardized exploration of the abdominal cavity. Attention should be drawn to areas of hematoma, discoloration, or contusion of the colon or mesocolon. Such areas may harbor small contained perforations that are temporarily sealed and may leak later (Figs. 36-4 and 36-5). Such areas should be carefully explored.

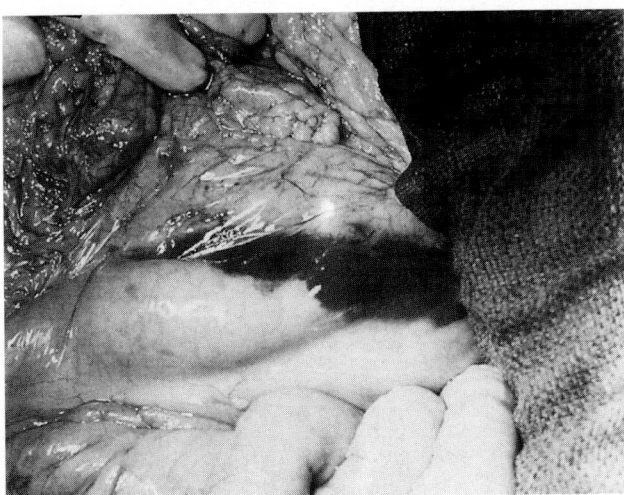

**FIGURE 36-4.** Hematomas such as this, which involves the antimesenteric portion of the transverse colon must be explored in order not to miss colonic injuries.

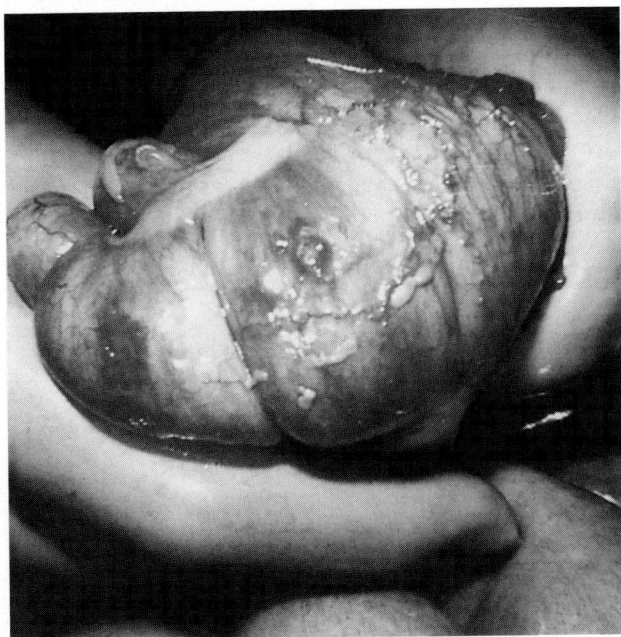

**FIGURE 36-5.** Method for the identification of small perforations by manually increasing the intraluminal pressure. A tiny perforation caused by a shotgun pellet can barely be seen in the center of the colon in this photograph.

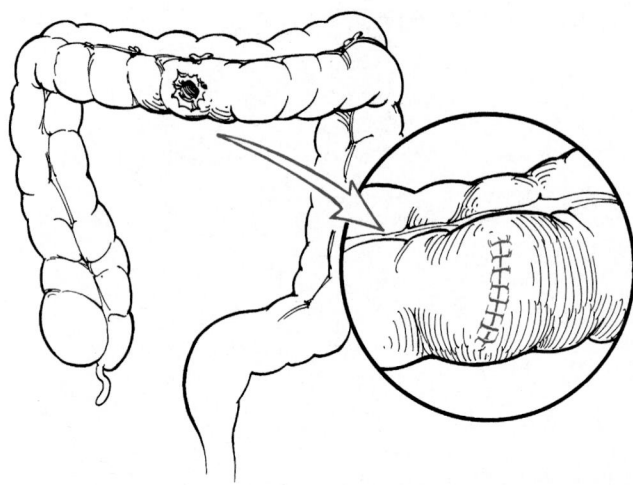

-FIGURE 36-6. Single layer suture repair of colon perforations is successfully employed for the majority of colon injuries encountered in urban environments.
(Reproduced with permission from Baylor College of Medicine.)

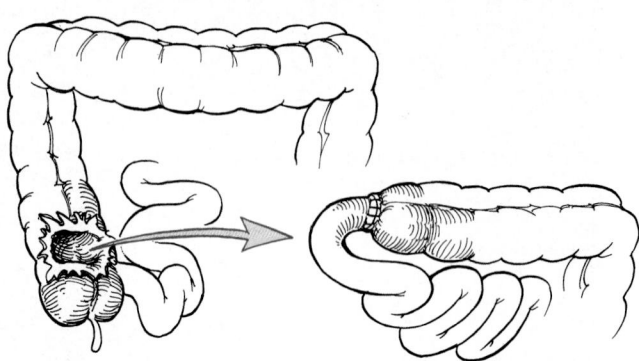

FIGURE 36-7. Resection and ileocolostomy is ideally suited for injuries that require resection proximal to the middle colic artery.
(Reproduced with permission from Baylor College of Medicine.)

## TREATMENT

### Primary Repair Versus Colostomy

The debate of primary repair (PR) versus diverting colostomy (DC) is not completely settled although the pendulum has shifted significantly in favor of PR. From an era of exclusive colostomy, the trauma community moved to the cautious use of PR in the absence of contra-indications, such as shock, extensive fecal contamination, multiple associated injuries, significant blood loss and blood transfusions, prolonged delays from injury to operation, distracting colon injury, and left colon injury.[34] And as experience and confidence was established with PR (Figs. 36-6 and 36-7), more of these subgroups were eventually managed without a DC. A meta-analysis of six prospective randomized trials concludes that the published evidence favors PR as a safer choice of treatment than DC for penetrating colon injuries (Table 36-1).[35] The first prospective randomized study was produced in 1979 by Stone and Fabian.[10] The authors excluded nearly half of patients with colon injury because they had any of the above perceived contraindications for PR. Among the remaining patients, PR was shown to be associated with fewer complications than DC. The second prospective randomized study was done in 1991 by Chappius et al.[36] and

included all patients regardless of high-risk criteria. No difference was found in complications between PR and DC. Only 11 patients were included who had PR after colon resection. The third study was by Falcone et al.[37] in 1992 on a small sample of 20 patients similarly showed no differences between PR and DC. The fourth study by Sasaki et al.[38] in 1995 was again in unselected patients and found a higher incidence of total and colon-related complications in the DC group. This study included only 12 patients with resection and PR. Gonzalez et al.[39] published the fifth study in 2000. They did not use exclusionary criteria and found similar complication rates between PR and DC. Five patients with resection and PR were included. Finally, in 2002, Kawendo et al.[40] published the sixth and largest study and the only one that was done out of the United States. Like in the previous studies, the PR group was not found to be at higher risk for postoperative morbidity and mortality compared to the DC group.

Although it seems clear from the above articles that PR is appropriate for the majority of colon injuries, a gap still exists in the management of distracting colon injuries, defined as those requiring resection. If subjected to PR, such injuries require a 360° anastomosis and therefore may increase the likelihood for failure due to the sheer extent of the anastomotic line. Additionally, there may be vascular impairment, as significant mesocolic trauma is almost always present. Finally, the presence of a distracting colon injury is an indicator of the high general severity of injury, which may affect unfavorably the healing of a fresh anastomotic line. For all these reasons, reluctance for PR in distracting colon injuries was widespread among American[41] and Canadian[42] surgeons who participated in a

**TABLE 36-1**

### Prospective Randomized Studies Comparing Colostomy and Primary Repair

| | | REPAIR | | | COLOSTOMY | | |
|---|---|---|---|---|---|---|---|
| AUTHOR | YEAR | No. of Patients | Fistula | Abscess | No. of Patients | Fistula | Abscess |
| Stone and Fabian | 1979 | 67 | 1 | Not stated | 72 | 1 | Not stated |
| Chappius et al. | 1991 | 26 | 0 | 3 | 28 | 0 | 4 |
| Falcone et al. | 1992 | 9 | 0 | 1 | 11 | 0 | 1 |
| Sasaki et al. | 1995 | 43 | 0 | 1 | 28 | 0 | 5 |
| Gonzalez et al. | 2000 | 56 | 0 | 7 | 53 | 1 | 8 |
| Kamwendo et al. | 2002 | 120 | 2 | Not stated | 118 | 2 | Not stated |

survey of the method for colon repair. Overall, 98% of American and 96% of Canadian chose PR in at least one of the multiple scenarios of colon injury presented in the survey. However, less than half of the American and less than one-forth of the Canadian surgeons considered PR when the scenario included a distracting colon injury.

After a retrospective analysis of 140 patients with severe colon injuries requiring resection[43] showed no difference in abdominal septic complications between PR and DC, a multicenter prospective noncontrolled study was sponsored by the American Association for the Surgery of Trauma to examine the issue.[44] In this study, Demetriades et al. included 297 patients from 19 centers, the largest experience to date on severe colon injuries. Colon-related abdominal complications occurred in 22% of 197 patients managed with PR and 27% of 100 patients managed with DC ($p = 0.373$). In risk-adjusted multivariate analysis the choice of colon repair did not influence outcome. The authors concluded that PR is safe for all colon injuries regardless of perceived risk factors.

Given the lack of a substantial demonstrable benefit of DC, the social implications and poor quality of life associated with it, and the significant risk of the additional operation to reestablish bowel continuity, I agree with these conclusions and practice PR almost exclusively. Only local anatomical conditions (extremely edematous bowel or obviously compromised vascular supply) would factor in a decision to perform DC in the unlikely case. The need for an open abdomen only enforces my preference for PR because a colostomy will increase the risk of infection and make reversal at a later stage significantly challenging (Fig. 36-8).

## Handsewn Versus Stapled Anastomosis

A meta-analysis of 1233 patients from nine prospective randomized studies examined mortality, overall dehiscence, clinical anastomotic dehiscence, radiological anastomotic dehiscence, stricture, anastomotic hemorrhage, reoperation, and wound infection between the 622 patients who were treated with stapled and the

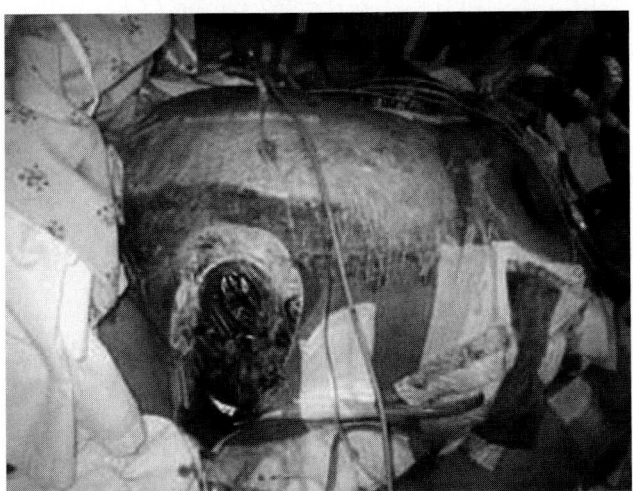

**FIGURE 36-8.**  Open abdomen after damage control operation. Note the colostomy. After multiple operations to reconstruct the abdominal wall, a final operation was undertaken to restore bowel continuity. The anastomosis leaked and the patient required removal of the previously placed mesh to address the problem. To date he is still with a large ventral hernia.

611 with manual anastomosis.[45] The patients were mostly elective surgical patients with cancer or inflammatory bowel disease. The meta-analysis failed to detect any differences in any of the outcomes. Experimental studies have shown that the bursting strength of human colon is similar between stapled and handsewn anastomosis.[46]

A retrospective single-center review[47] of 84 trauma patients with anastomoses throughout the gastrointestinal tract suggested that stapled repairs may be associated with a higher rate of anastomotic leaks and prompted a multicenter retrospective study sponsored by the Western Trauma Association.[48] In this study from 2001 a total of 199 patients with 289 anastomoses of the small and large bowel were identified, 175 had stapled and 114 handsewn procedures. Seven of the stapled and none of the handsewn leaked ($p = 0.04$). Similarly, 19 stapled and four handsewn were associated with intra-abdominal abscess ($p = 0.04$). The authors recommended caution in deciding to staple a bowel anastomosis for trauma. Their reasoning was that staples are made for elective surgery and not edematous bowel, a common occurrence following severe injury and fluid resuscitation. In that study a total of 61 colon anastomoses were included (29 sutured, 32 stapled), and there was inherent bias in favor of stapling the most severe colon injuries. Three of the study's seven anastomotic dehiscences occurred in colon anastomoses; all three were stapled.

The only study that examines exclusively colon injuries and the use of staples versus sutures is based on the population of the previously mentioned multicenter American Association for the Surgery of Trauma trial of PR versus DC. Upon analyzing the patients from this study who underwent PR, Demetriades et al.[49] found the incidence of anastomotic leak to be 6.3% in the stapled group and 7.8% in the handsewn group ($p = 0.69$) and the total colon-related abdominal complications rate to be 22.7% and 20.3%, respectively ($p = 0.3$). The authors concluded that the method of anastomosis does not affect the incidence of abdominal complications and the choice between staples and sutures should be the surgeon's preference.

Obviously, no level 1 recommendations can be made from this data, even if the largest study on colon injuries does not find differences between staples and sutures. It seems safe to assume that for the majority of patients with colon injury, the choice between staples and sutures should be based on convenience, cost, and training rather than expected outcomes. In a minority of patients with anatomical reasons, such as profound bowel edema, stapling may be less than ideal. The thickest staples for the gastrointestinal tract in most commercially available staplers are 4 mm high when open, 2.5 mm high when closed, and 4 mm wide. It can be easily understood how such a stapler would not incorporate the entire thickness of an edematous bowel wall but again, it is not known if a partial thickness capture would lead to an increased incidence of anastomotic leak.

*One- Versus Two-Layer Anastomosis.*  This issue is being researched in trauma and nontrauma patients. A number of reports[50–52] have consistently concluded that a running one-layer anastomosis is at least as safe as a two-layer one. In 2000, Burch et al.[53] published a prospective randomized trial of one versus two layers (Fig. 36-9). Among the different type of patients, 19 trauma patients were included in the one-layer group and 12 in the two-layer. There were 19 and 27 ileocolostomies and colocolostomies,

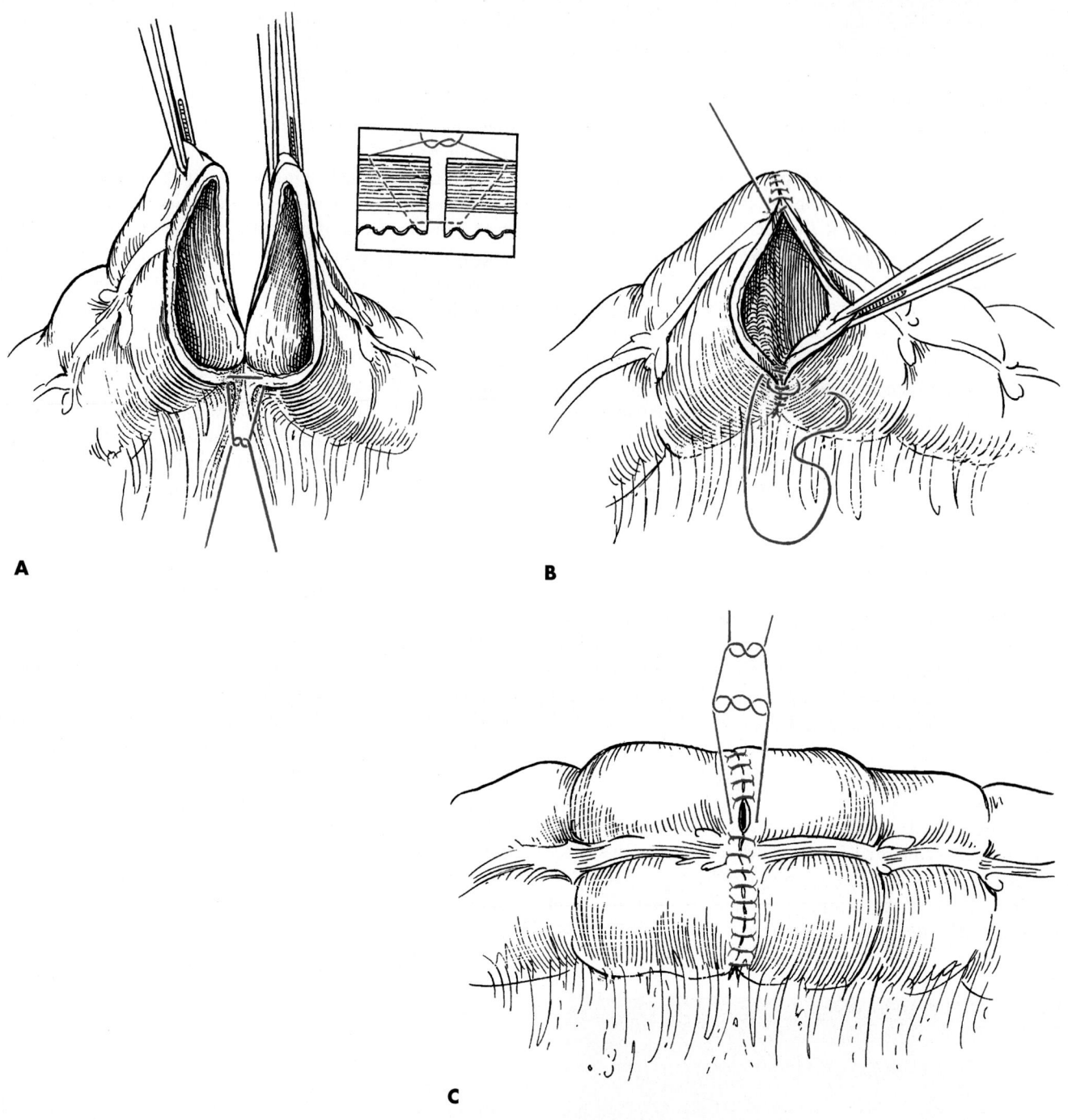

**FIGURE 36-9.** Single-layer running monofilament suture anastomosis after a distructing injury to the colon requiring resection. The anastomosis is faster and probably safer than the traditional two-layer repair. **(A)** Anastomosis begins at the mesenteric border. **(B)** The sutures are placed 3–4 mm from the edge of the bowel and advance 3–4 mm with each stitch. **(C)** The double-needle suture is tied at the antimesenteric border.

respectively, in the one-layer group and 27 and 21 in the two-layer group. There was no difference in anastomotic leaks between the two techniques but the one-layer anastomosis was faster by ten minutes and the patients subjected to this technique were discharged from the hospital by an average of two days earlier than the two-layer group. The authors hypothesized that the earlier discharge was due to a wider lumen and less edema at the anastomotic site, resulting in faster resumption of bowel activity in the one-layer group.

Numerous modifications of the technique for performing an anastomosis have been and will be reported. Even if layers, type of suture material, and running versus interrupted sutures will continue to be debated, the reality is that surgeon's preference will remain the single most important factor to decide how to do it. Adhering to the principles of a well-vascularized, tension-free, adequately-sealed anastomotic line is more important than the number, type, and layers of sutures. Overall, a one-layer running repair is very safe, fast, convenient, and easy to teach.

**End Versus Loop Colostomy.**    Another point of controversy is the type of colostomy in the infrequent case that one is needed. Almost never is a colostomy for trauma permanent. So, minimizing

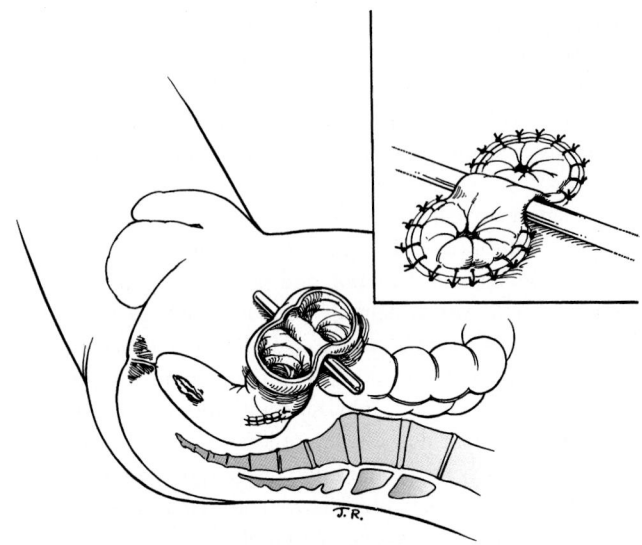

**FIGURE 36-10.** A properly conducted loop colostomy. Note that the spur of the colostomy is supported well above the skin. *(Reproduced with permission from Baylor College of Medicine.)*

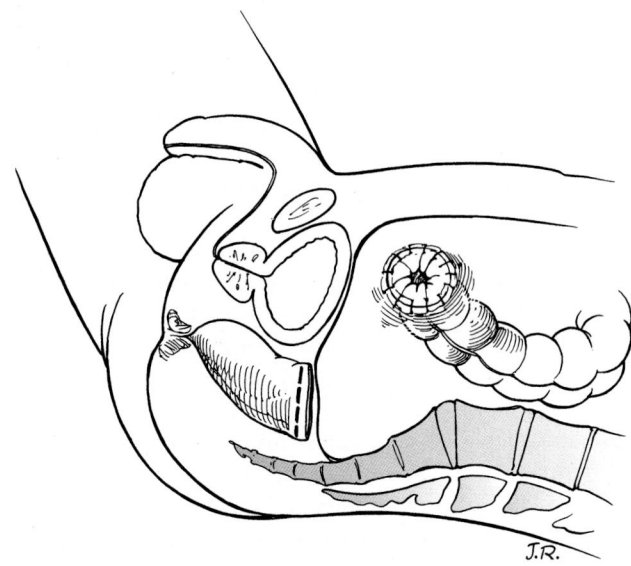

**FIGURE 36-12.** Hartmann's procedure with an end colostomy and a rectal pouch. Reconstituion of bowel continuity will require a full laparotomy and extensive dissection. *(Reproduced with permission from Baylor College of Medicine.)*

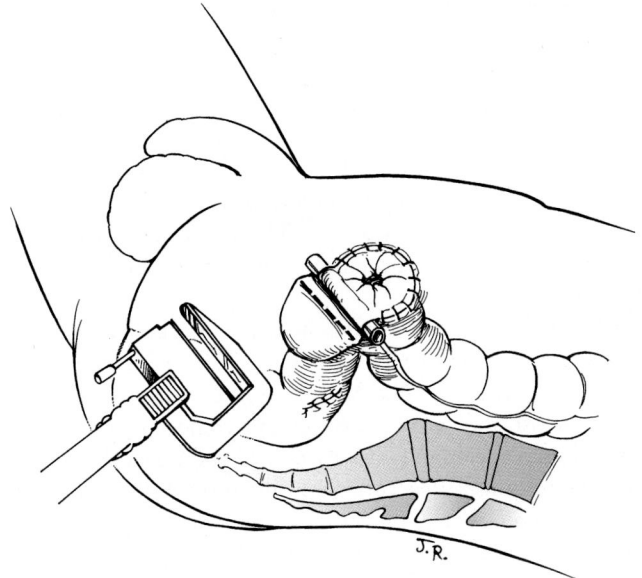

**FIGURE 36-11.** The use of a linear stapler for definitive fecal diversion. *(Reproduced with permission from Baylor College of Medicine.)*

the morbidity of the operation for reconnection is essential.[54,55] According to this principle a loop—but totally diverting—colostomy should be preferred whenever possible (Fig. 36-10). Complete diversion can be achieved by stapling, suturing, or tying off the distal lumen of the loop (Fig. 36-11). An end colostomy with a Hartman's pouch is an alternative method to manage a colon injury following resection (Fig. 36-12).

Drainage Versus No Drainage.   Three meta-analyses on the issue of draining a colonic anastomosis have been published.[56–58] All three conclude that routine drainage is unnecessary. Unfortunately, the studies included in these systematic reviews address predominantly or exclusively elective colon surgery patients.

Therefore, the applicability of this data to trauma is unknown. No studies to my knowledge have examined the need of draining posttraumatic colorectal anastomoses. In trauma, there is usually frank spillage of fecal material in the peritoneal cavity, and the traditional aggressive washout with copious amounts of normal saline takes place at the end of the procedure. Drains are usually placed to facilitate drainage of residual—and by definition infected—fluid that is not suctioned, as well as new fluid that accumulates during resuscitation. I usually drain the peritoneal cavity under such circumstances but remove the drains after 24–48 hours. In this capacity the drain is used to remove early infected fluid for a short postoperative period rather than protect the anastomosis over 5–10 days.

Damage Control.   The concept of controlling the acute problem (bleeding and infection), leaving the abdomen open, and providing definitive repair in a later operation has been well established over the last decade and applies well in severe colon injuries.[59] Although the tenets and technique of damage control will be addressed in a dedicated chapter, a few points specific to colon injuries need to be mentioned. Contamination from a colon wound can be managed by stapling or simply tying off the transected ends after resecting the injured part. Anastomosis or colostomy are not necessary in the first operation. There is concern that if the bowel continuity is not immediately reconstituted, bowel edema will become worse and reanastomosis placed at peril (D. Demetriades, personal communication). In experienced hands a one-layer anastomosis takes eight to ten minutes[53] and therefore, the patient could have bowel continuity restored without major operative delays. However, most damage control advocates seem to feel comfortable with leaving the bowel stapled for one to three days, particularly given the fact that in such severe injuries postoperative colon ileus and lack of forward peristalsis is to be expected. My personal preference is to do a fast stapled or one-layer running anastomosis in the majority of cases during the first operation. Leaving the abdomen open would be an additional—rather than deterring—factor to pursue PR and not DC. Placing a DC in a patient with open abdomen is an invitation to infection throughout the first hospitalization and a formidable challenge when the time comes for colostomy closure.

Open versus Closed Skin Wound.   Although there is literature to suggest that infected abdominal wounds after colon surgery should be left open, there is a paucity of evidence related specifically to trauma. Two articles that are over 20 years old report very different infections rates following primary closure of the skin after colon trauma, 2.7%[60] and 56%.[61] Two more recent studies from South Africa reported significantly lower wound infection rates after routine primary skin wound closure. Demetriades et al.[62] found an 11% incidence of wound infection among 100 prospectively collected patients with colon gunshot wounds and Velmahos et al.[63] a similar 11.6% among 223 retrospectively reviewed colon gunshot wound patients. A retrospective review from the same investigators but in the United States showed an incidence of 26% of 146 colonic resections for trauma.[43] It is obvious that different populations and different medical systems are associated with different wound infection rates.

A prospective randomized study was designed to resolve the wide discrepancies in wound infection rates after primary skin closure in colon trauma. Velmahos et al.[64] introduced strict definitions of wound infection and found an incidence of 65% after primary skin wound closure and 36% when the wound was left open to heal by secondary intent. Wound infection was an independent predictor of wound dehiscence and necrotizing soft tissue infection. Following these results, the majority of wounds were left open in the authors' center. If a skin wound is closed after an operation for colon trauma, it must be followed closely and opened liberally with any suspicion for infection. Delayed primary closure may be of benefit but has not been scientifically studied in this type of patients.

Prophylactic Antibiotics.   Infection remains one of the greatest risk for victims of colon injury, ranging from 10% to 70% depending on the severity of injury.[34,43,44,65,66] Intra-abdominal infections occur in one of every four to one of every six patients and carry attributable mortality.[43,44,67] The issues of appropriate type, timing, and dose of prophylactic antibiotics are still debated (see Chap. 19). For the most part, single broad-spectrum antibiotic agents provide adequate coverage. Second-generation cephalosporins, ampicillin/sulbactam, or piperacillin have been used with success and proven to be at least as effective as combinations of multiple agents.[67–69] Only one study has recently found single antibiotic coverage to be inferior to multiple antibiotic regimens.[44] Whether this is a result of the use of a particular dose of a particular antibiotic, a reflection of the specific subpopulation of this study (severe colon injuries), or a true and reproducible finding remains to be seen.

Cumulative evidence from many studies proves the lack of need for longer prophylaxis than 24 hours.[70–73] Even high-risk patients do not benefit from protracted antibiotic courses. Two prospective randomized trials[71,72] of one versus five days of prophylactic antibiotics in patients with high Penetrating Abdominal Trauma Index scores (≥25) and colon injuries show similar rates of intra-abdominal

infections. In fact, when the populations from both studies were combined,[71] the intra-abdominal infection rate for the 58 patients of the one-day group was 19% and for the 61 patients of the five-day group 33% ($p = 0.13$). It is also possible that longer durations of antibiotic prophylaxis increase the incidence of resistant infections.[67]

Although many patients are served well by the standard antibiotic doses, appropriate dosing in severely injured patients with increased volumes of distribution and rates of drug metabolism or excretion is unknown. A hemodynamically stable patient with an isolated colon stab wound and a critically injured hemodynamically unstable patient with multiple intra-abdominal injuries may receive the same dose of prophylactic antibiotics. The inadequacy of standard antibiotic doses in severe illness is established[74,75] but practices have barely changed. In that light, studies showing certain prophylactic antibiotics administered at standard doses to be equally effective, may reflect equal lack of effect. This is an area in dire need of pertinent research.

Retained Bullets After Colonic Perforation.   Against conventional wisdom the evidence suggests that removal of bullets that traversed the colon is not necessary for the purpose of preventing infection. An experimental study[76] quantified bacterial contamination of steel fragments fired through porcine colon. The bacterial counts decreased drastically along the length of the track and were considerably high only in the first centimeter. The study concluded that wound track excision or bullet removal is not warranted. Similarly, bullets lodged in the spine following a trajectory through the colon did not cause osteomyelitis, meningitis, or disc space infection.[77,78] The tissue trauma caused by attempts to localize and remove a bullet may cause more harm than benefit.

Besides the risk of infection, one needs to consider the unusual complications of bullet migration, embolization, and lead poisoning.[79] For example, a bullet that is lodged next to the aorta may present a risk for vascular erosion and could be considered for removal if an operation is already needed and under the appropriate circumstances. Patients with retained bullets should be informed about it. The presence of a bullet is not prohibitive for future magnetic resonance imaging (MRI), for as long as the ferromagnetic properties of the projectile are pretested by MRI.[80] Each case should be individualized but in general, routine removal of bullets is unnecessary.

# INJURIES OF THE RECTUM

## Mechanism of Injury

The majority of rectal injuries result from penetrating trauma. Pelvic gunshot wounds should always be suspected to have trajectories through the intra- or extaperitoneal rectum.[81] Gluteal gunshot wounds and stabbings may also produce rectal injury.[82,83] Blunt trauma is an unusual cause of rectal perforation. Lower rectal injuries may occur with open pelvic fractures (Fig. 36-13).[84] Foreign bodies and sexual practices are also a cause of rectal perforation.[85]

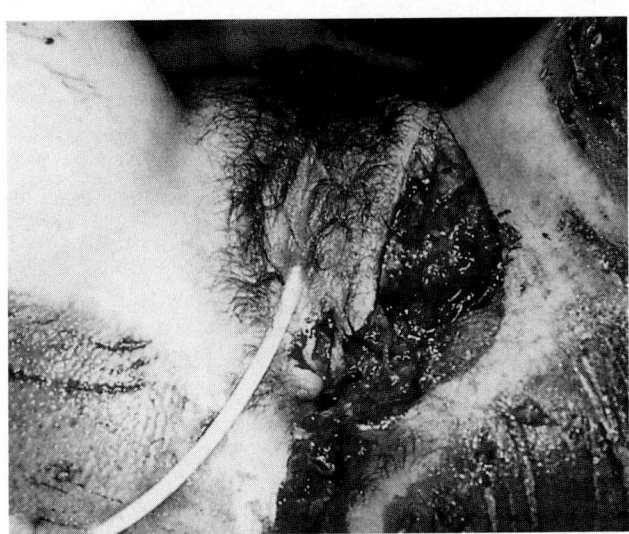

**FIGURE 36-13.** This perineal laceration was caused by a motor vehicle accident. The annal sphincters were completely transected and the tear extends several centimeters up the rectum.

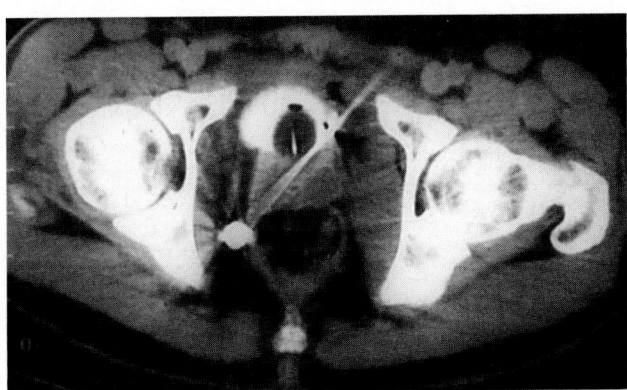

**FIGURE 36-14.** Bullet lodged next to the rectum. No signs of perforation on sigmoidoscopy. The patient was managed without an operation successfully.

## DIAGNOSIS

Clinical Examination.    Injuries to the anterior and lateral walls of the upper two-thirds of the rectum will most likely cause intraperitoneal perforation with symptoms related to peritonitis. However, posterior wall perforations of the upper two-thirds as well as perforations of the lower-third are extraperitoneal and may not cause immediate symptomatology. Clinical examination of these injuries requires a high index of suspicion for rectal perforation, a mental reconstruction of the trajectory, and a careful digital examination to reveal intraluminal blood or palpate a mucosal abnormality.

Radiographic Imaging.    Reconstruction of the bullet trajectory can also be achieved by plain pelvic films after marking the skin hole(s) with a paperclip(s) but even more by helical CT (Fig. 36-14). CT has essentially substituted plain films and should be routinely requested for suspected rectal perforation.[28] When reconstructing a bullet trajectory, it needs to be remembered that a straight line between an entry and an exit or a lodged missile does not always represent the accurate traveled path. Bullets may travel in unpredictable directions depending on missile characteristics, tissue density, and reflection by different anatomical structures. The use of rectal contrast is particularly helpful, whether for plain films or CT.

Sigmoidoscopy.    Rigid sigmoidoscopy is an essential diagnostic tool and should be used if the rectal examination or CT scan are suggestive but ambiguous. It should also be used as the first step following general anesthesia in a hemodynamically stable patient who is being operated for presumed rectal injury in order to help locate the injury precisely and plan the operative strategy. Frequently, sigmoidoscopy will reveal nothing more than intraluminal blood. In the presence of unprepared bowel and a high rectal injury, visualizing the perforation may not be easy. Intraluminal blood should be a reason for operation, as it implies a full-thickness injury after penetrating trauma.

Finally, sigmoidoscopy can be therapeutic by allowing transanal repair of low rectal injuries or removal of foreign bodies.

## TREATMENT

Colostomy, Washout, Presacral Drainage.    The triad of a diverting colostomy, rectal washout, and presacral drainage has defined the operative management of rectal injuries for many years.[86,87] One by one the elements of this triad succumb to new scientific evidence doubting their need. Rectal washout was dispelled as an important part of rectal injury management and even considered to be harmful, as it may force intraluminal contents through a perforation of an unprepared rectum.[87–89] The preoccupation with a completely clean bowel in order to do surgery[90] or allow rectal healing has been shown to carry no scientific weight.

Presacral drainage was advocated as the most reliable method of draining a rectal injury below the peritoneal reflection (Fig. 36-15). This is far from true. Due to dense tissues surrounding the lower rectum, a presacral drain is likely to not be placed exactly next to the injury, particularly if the anterior rather than posterior rectal wall is injured. The discomfort associated with its location, poor functionality, and potential harm during placement negate the alleged benefits. A prospective randomized trial[91] of 48 patients with penetrating rectal injury, 25 randomized to presacral drainage and 23 to no drainage, showed two rectum-related infectious complications in the drainage group and one in the nondrainage group. The study concluded the presacral drainage has no effect on infectious complications associated with rectal injuries.

As opposed to rectal washout and presacral drainage, diverting colostomy remains widely used for rectal injuries. In a retrospective study[92] from the Los Angeles County and University of Southern California group comparing different techniques of extraperitonel rectal gunshot wounds, patients who were treated by a colostomy without rectal repair had the same incidence of complications with patients who had repair of the injury and colostomy. One rectal fistula developed in each one of the groups. The authors concluded that diverting colostomy appears to be safe

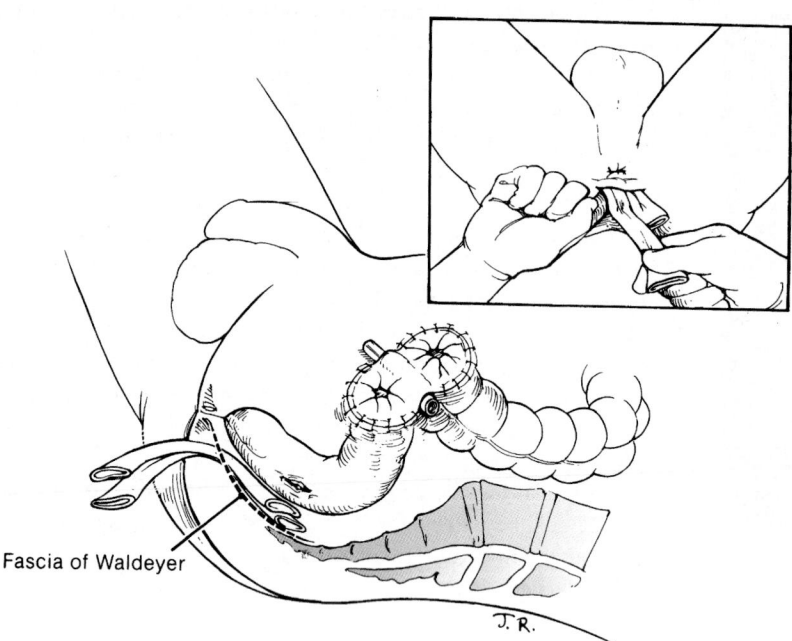

Fascia of Waldeyer

J. R.

**FIGURE 36-15.** Placement of presacral drainage anterior to the Waldeyer's fascia. The membrane is particularly tough below the coccyx and often requires incision with sharp instruments before the drains can be placed. Presacral drains are rarely used any more.
*(Reproduced with permission from Baylor College of Medicine.)*

as the sole method of treatment of most civilian extraperitoneal rectal gunshot wounds. Similarly, a prospective study from South Africa[93] confirmed that a laparoscopically created diverting colostomy was safe as the only treatment for extraperitoneal gunshot wounds. No pelvic sepsis occurred in this study as a result of unrepaired rectal injuries.

**Primary Repair.**   Intraperitoneal rectal injuries can be managed like the rest of colon injuries, that is, with primary repair.[94] However, primary repair without a colostomy has not yet been established for extraperitoneal rectal injuries. The lack of serosal coverage and the difficulty in accessing the low rectal area through a transperitoneal approach are routinely cited reasons for adding colostomy as a safeguard of a challenging repair. If the anatomical planes around the rectum are not disturbed by the extensive dissection of transperitoneal access, primary repair without colostomy may be safe through the anus. Transanal primary repairs have been reported with success.[95,96] Again, the difference between transanal and transperitoneal repair is that in the former the surrounding tissues remain adhered to the rectum, preventing in this way anastomotic breakdown, collection of fluid among dissected planes, and interruption of vascular supply to the injured potion.

   The low frequency of extraperitoneal rectal injuries prevents gaining a large experience by any single group of surgeons. Colostomy is still likely to be used as an integral part of the surgical treatment of this injury, although primary repair is expected to gain increasing acceptance as it happened for the rest of the colon.

## COLOSTOMY CLOSURE

### Timing

Colostomy closure usually takes place three to six months after the initial operation, although the timing of it is debated. While

some authors have extrapolated data from the nontrauma literature and insist on such a long interval between colostomy and its closure, others claim that shorter intervals of one to two months produce the lowest incidence of complications.[97–101] Furthermore, one prospective noncontrolled[102] and two prospective randomized studies[103,104] have shown that same admission colostomy closure, performed within 7–14 days after the first operation is safe and cost-effective. Although same admission closure is not appropriate for all patients, appropriately selected subgroups without other severe injuries or major postoperative complications can be benefited by having the colostomy closed shortly after it was performed. The majority of even unrepaired rectal injuries is well-healed within an average of 7–10 days and therefore same admission colostomy closure seems feasible and safe.

### Technique

The type of colostomy defines the need for access through a local incision or a full laparotomy. Loop and double-barrel colostomies can be easily reconstructed by an incision at the colostomy site that allows debridement of the colostomy edges and closure in one layer. Hartman's procedures with a mucous fistula next to the colostomy also allow local access. Although the majority of such patients will be operated on under general anesthesia, the use of local anesthesia has been described.[105] However, among 14 patients (12 with loop colostomies and two with end colostomies and a mucous fistula) the incidence of serious postoperative complications was unusually high (43%, three anastomotic leaks, two wound infections, one bowel obstruction). It is unclear if the use of local anesthesia, creating suboptimal operative conditions, contributed to these complications.

   In the presence of a Hartman's procedure without a mucous fistula, reopening the midline laparotomy wound under general anesthesia is necessary. Laparoscopic-assisted techniques with or without pneumoperitoneum have been used with success to minimize the operative trauma of the second operation.[106,107] The benefits seems to be higher for Hartman's closures, since loop colostomies can be performed through local incisions in short times with minimal trauma.

## Outcomes

Colostomy closure is associated with significant risk. In an analysis of 40 trauma patients who had their 28 loop and 12 end colostomies closed in an average of 8 months after injury, we found an incidence of intra- and postoperative complications was 30%.[108] Major postoperative complications included a fecal fistula managed non-operatively, a stricture at the anastomotic site requiring reoperation, and two small bowel obstructions, one managed non-operatively and one requiring operative lysis of adhesions. Interestingly, colostomy closures after colon injury had higher morbidity than those after rectal injury.

Similar outcomes have been reported in other studies that have found morbidity rates of 24%,[101] 35%,[109] 32%,[110] and 27%.[111] Although most complications are relatively minor and include wound infections and easily manageable nonabdominal infections, serious complications such as anastomotic breakdowns or intra-abdominal abscesses are not rare, and even mortality has been reported up to 2%.[109,110,112] Preoperative factors and particularly diabetes, cardiac disease, and renal disease increase the risk for complications.[110] Young and otherwise healthy trauma patients should have a low risk but the risk cannot be completely ruled out. Morbidity associated with colostomy closure should be considered additional evidence for performing primary repair of colon injuries.

## COLON INJURY SEVERITY SCALES

The Organ Injury Scaling Committee of the American Association for the Surgery of Trauma produced a grading system to allow reliable and reproducible report of colon and rectal injuries (Tables 36-2 and 36-3).[113]

**TABLE 36-2**

### AAST Colon Injury Scale

| GRADE[a] | | INJURY DESCRIPTION | ICD-9[b] | AIS-90[c] |
|---|---|---|---|---|
| I | Hematoma | Contusion or hematoma without devascularization | 863.40–863.44 | 2 |
| | Laceration | Partial thickness, no perforation | 863.40–863.44 | 2 |
| II | Laceration | Laceration ≤50% of circumference | 863.50–863.54 | 3 |
| III | Laceration | Laceration >50% of circumference | 863.50–863.54 | |
| IV | Laceration | Transection of the colon | 863.50–863.54 | 4 |
| V | Laceration | Transection of the colon with segmental tissue loss | 863.50–863.54 | 4 |

ICD-9:4, .51=ascending; 42, .52=transverse; 43, .53=descending; .44, .54 = rectum.

[a]Advance on grade for multiple injuries, up to Grade III.

[b]International Classification of Diseases, 9th Revision.

[c]Abbreviated Injury Scale, 1990.

(Reproduced with permission from Moore EE, Cogbill TH, Malangoni MA, et al: Organ injury, scaling II: Pancreas, duodenum, small bowel, colon, and rectum. J Trauma 30:1427, 1990.)

**TABLE 36-3**

### AAST Rectal Organ Injury Scale

| GRADE[a] | | INJURY DESCRIPTION[b] | ICD-9[c] | AIS-90[d] |
|---|---|---|---|---|
| I | Hematoma | Contusion or hematoma without devascularization | 863.45 | 2 |
| | Laceration | Partial-thickness laceration | 863.45 | 2 |
| II | Laceration | Laceration ≤50% of circumference | 863.55 | 3 |
| III | Laceration | Laceration >50% of circumference | 863.55 | 4 |
| IV | Laceration | Full-thickness laceration with extension into the perineum | 863.55 | 5 |
| V | Vascular | Devascularized segment | 863.55 | 5 |

[a]Advance on grade for multiple injuries to same organ.

[b]Based on the most accurate assessment at autopsy, laparotomy, or radiologic study.

[c]International Classification of Diseases, 9th Revision.

[d]Abbreviated Injury Scale, 1990.

(Reproduced with permission from Moore EE, Shackford SR, Pachter HL, et al: Organ injury scaling—Spleen, liver and kidney. J Trauma 29:1664, 1989.)

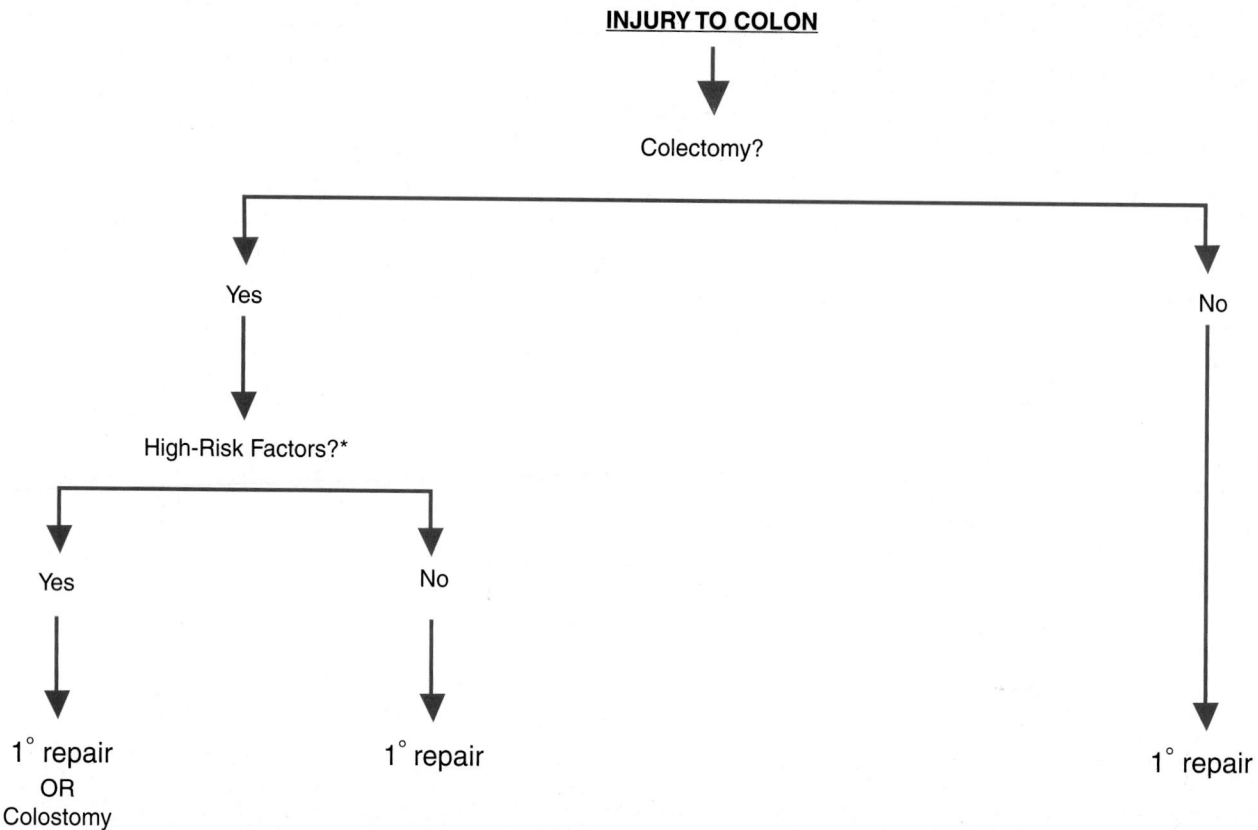

**INJURY TO COLON**

Colectomy?

Yes

High-Risk Factors?*

Yes

1° repair
OR
Colostomy

No

1° repair

No

1° repair

*Damage-control operation, blood transfusion over 6 units, multiple associated abdominal injuries, severe bowel edema, suboptimal vascular supply to resected margins

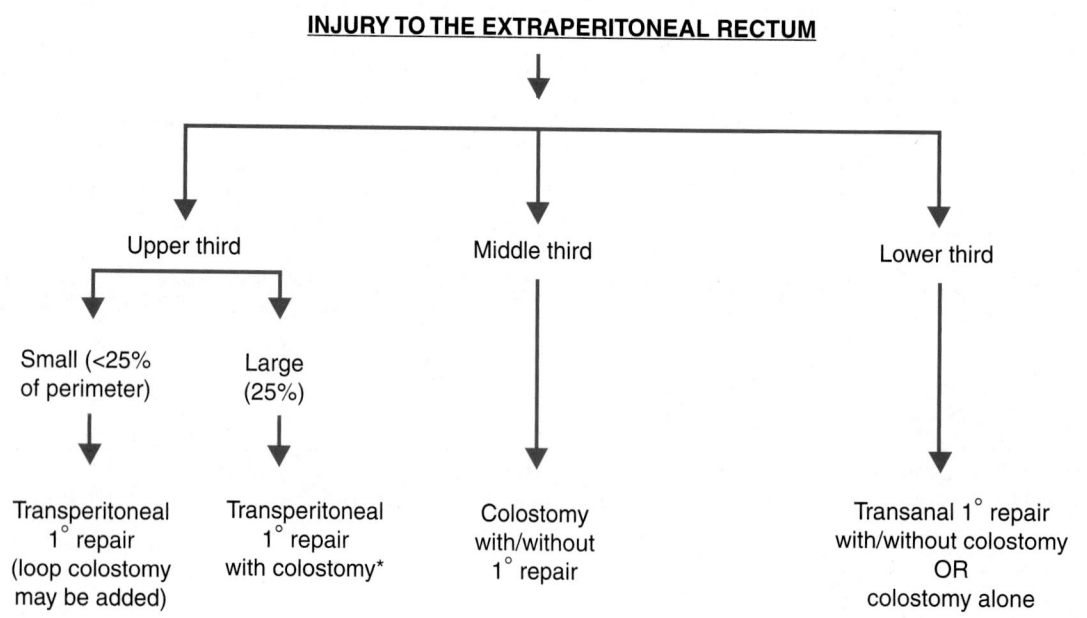

**INJURY TO THE EXTRAPERITONEAL RECTUM**

Upper third

Small (<25% of perimeter)

Transperitoneal 1° repair (loop colostomy may be added)

Large (25%)

Transperitoneal 1° repair with colostomy*

Middle third

Colostomy with/without 1° repair

Lower third

Transanal 1° repair with/without colostomy OR colostomy alone

*On selected cases colostomy alone (without 1° repair) may be adequate

Notes:
1. A loop colostomy is preferred over an end colostomy, whenever possible.
2. Rectal washout and presacral drainage are unnecessary in most cases.

# REFERENCES

1. Burch JM: Injury to the colon and Rectum. In Feliciano DV, Mattox KL, Moore EE, eds. *Trauma.* New York, NY: McGraw-Hill Medical, 2003, p. 763.
2. Williams MD, Watts D, Fakhry S: Colon injury after blunt abdominal trauma: results of the EAST Multi-Institutional Hollow Viscus Injury Study. *J Trauma* 55:906, 2003.
3. Wallace C: A study of 1,200 cases of gunshot wounds of the abdomen. *Br Med J* 4:619, 1916.
4. Fraser J, Drummond H: Three hundred perforating wounds of the abdomen. *Br Med J* x:321, 1917.
5. Gordon-Taylor G, Lond MS: Discussion on the diagnosis and treatment of injuries of the intestines. *Br Med J* 2:639, 1921.
6. Ogilvie WH: Abdominal wounds in the Western desert. *Surg Gynecol Obstet* 78:225, 1944.
7. Office of the Surgeon General. Circular Letter No. 178. October 23, 1943.
8. Woodhall JP, Ochsner A: The management of perforating injuries of the colon and rectum in civilian practice. *Surgery* 29:305, 1951.
9. Isaacson JE, Buck RL, Kahle HR: Changing concepts of treatment of traumatic injuries of the colon. *Dis Colon Rectum* 4:811, 1961.
10. Stone HH, Fabian TC: Management of perforating colon trauma: randomization between primary closure and exteriorization. *Ann Surg* 190:430, 1979.
11. Demetriades D, Rabinowitz B, Sofianos C, et al.: The management of colon injuries by primary repair or colostomy. *Br J Surg* 72:881, 1985.
12. Sharma OP, Oswanksi MF, White PW: Injuries to the colon from blast effect of penetrating extra-peritoneal thoracoabdominal trauma. *Injury* 35: 320, 2004.
13. Stankovich N, Petrovic M, Drinkovic N, et al.: Colon and rectal war injuries. *J Trauma* 40:S183, 1996.
14. Agalar F, Daphan C, Sayek I, et al.: Clinical presentation and management of iatrogenic colon perforations. *Am J Surg* 177:442, 1999.
15. Mana F, De Vogelaere K, Urban D: Iatrogenic perforation of the colon during diagnostic colonoscopy: Endoscopic treatment with clips. *Gastrointest Endosc* 54:258, 2001.
16. Matsuhita M, Takakuwa H, Nishio A: Endoscopic removal techniques and clipping closure for chicken bones wedged transversely in the colon. *Dis Colon Rect* 44:749, 2001.
17. Velmahos GC, Demetriades D, Toutouzas KG, et al.: Selective nonoperative management in 1,856 patients with abdominal gunshot wounds: Should routine laparotomy still be the standard of care? *Ann Surg* 234:395, 2001.
18. Demetriades D, Velmahos G, Cornwell E, et al.: Selective nonoperative management of gunshot wounds of the anterior abdomen. *Arch Surg* 132: 178, 1997.
19. Velmahos GC, Demetriades D, Foianini E, et al.: A selective approach to the management of gunshot wounds to the back. *Am J Surg* 174:342, 1997.
20. Rozycki GS, Newman PG: Surgeon-performed ultrasound for the assessment of abdominal injuries. *Advances in Surgery* 33:243, 1999.
21. Miller MT, Pasquale MD, Bromberg WJ, et al.: Not so FAST. *J Trauma* 54: 52, 2003.
22. Stern E (ed). *Trauma Radiology Companion.* Philadelphia, PA: Lippincott-Raven, 1997, p. 200.
23. Chiu WC, Shanmuganathan K, Mirvis SE, et al.: Determining the need for laparotomy in penetrating torso trauma: A prospective study using triple-contrast enhanced abdominopelvic computed tomography. *J Trauma* 51: 860, 2001.
24. Boyle EM Jr, Maier RV, Salazar JD, et al.: Diagnosis of injuries after stab wounds to the back and flank. *J Trauma* 42:260, 1997.
25. Stafford RE, McGonigal MD, Weigelt JA, et al.: Oral contrast solution and computed tomography for blunt abdominal trauma: A randomized study. *Arch Surg* 134:622, 1999.
26. Tsang BD, Panacek EA, Brant WE, et al.: Effect of oral contrast administration for abdominal computed tomography in the evaluation of acute blunt trauma. *Ann Emerg Med* 30:7, 1997.
27. Allen TL, Mueller MT, Bonk RT, et al.: Computed tomographic scanning without oral contrast solution for blunt bowel and mesenteric injuries in abdominal trauma. *J Trauma* 56:314, 2004.
28. Velmahos GC, Constantinou C, Tillou A, et al.: Abdominal computed tomographic scan for patients with gunshot wounds to the abdomen selected for nonoperative management. *J Trauma* 59:1155, 2005.
29. Ginzburg E, Carillo EH, Kopelman T, et al.: The role of computed tomography in selective management of gunshot wounds to the abdomen and flank. *J Trauma* 45:1005, 1998.
30. Grossman MD, May AK, Schwab CW, et al.: Determining anatomic injury with computed tomography in selected torso gunshot wounds. *J Trauma* 45:446, 1998.
31. Degiannis E, Bowley DM, Smith MD: Minimally invasive surgery in trauma: Technology looking for an application. *Injury* 35:474, 2004.
32. Murray JA, Demetriades D, Asensio JA, et al.: Occult injuries to the diaphragm: Prospective evaluation of laparoscopy in penetrating injuries to the left lower chest. *J Am Coll Surg* 187:626, 1998.
33. Zantut LF, Ivatury RR, Smith RS, et al.: Diagnostic and therapeutic laparoscopy for penetrating abdominal trauma: A multicenter experience. *J Trauma* 42:825, 1997.
34. Maxwell RA, Fabian TC: Current management of colon trauma. *World J Surg* 27:632, 2003.
35. Nelson R, Singer M: Primary repair for penetrating colon injuries. *Cochrane Database of Systematic Reviews* 3:CD002247, 2003.
36. Chappuis CW, Frey DJ, Dietzen CD, et al.: Management of penetrating colon injuries: A prospective randomized trial. *Ann Surg* 213:492, 1991.
37. Falcone RE, Wanamaker SR, Santanello SA, et al.: Colorectal trauma: Primary repair or anastomosis with intracolonic bypass vs. ostomy. *Dis Colon Rec* 35:957, 1992.
38. Sasaki LS, Allaben RD, Golwala R, et al.: Primary repair of colon injuries: A prospective randomized trial. *J Trauma* 39:895, 1995.
39. Gonzalez RP, Merlotti GJ, Holevar MR: Colostomy in penetrating colon injury: Is it necessary? *J Trauma* 41:271, 1996.
40. Kamwendo NY, Modivba MC, Matlala NS, et al.: Randomized clinical trial to determine if delay from time of penetrating colonic injury precludes primary repair. *Br J Surg* 89:993, 2002.
41. Eshraghi N, Mullins RJ, Mayberry JC, et al.: Surveyed opinion of American trauma surgeons in management of colon injuries. *J Trauma* 44:93, 1998.
42. Pezim ME, Vestrup JA: Canadian attitudes toward use of primary repair in management of colon trauma. A survey of 317 members of the Canadian Association of General Surgeons. *Dis Colon Rectum* 39:40, 1996.
43. Murray JA, Demetriades D, Colson M, et al.: Colonic resection in trauma: Colostomy versus anastomosis. *J Trauma* 46:250, 1999.
44. Demetriades D, Murray JA, Chan LC, et al.: Penetrating colon injuries requiring resection: Diversion or primary anastomosis? An AAST prospective multicenter study. *J Trauma* 50:765, 2001.
45. Lustosa SA, Matos D, Atallah AN, et al.: Stapled versus handsewn methods for colorectal anastomosis surgery. *Cochrane Database of Systematic Reviews* 3:CD003144, 2001.
46. Schwab R, Wessendorf S, Gutcke A, et al.: Early bursting strength of human colon anastomoses – an in vitro study comparing current anastomotic techniques. *Langenbecks Arch Surg* 386:507, 2002.
47. Brundage SI, Jurkovich GJ, Grossman DC, et al.: Stapled versus sutured gastrointestinal anastomoses in the trauma patient. *J Trauma* 47:500, 1999.
48. Brundage SI, Jurkovich GJ, Hoyt DB, et al.: Stapled versus sutured gastrointestinal anastomoses in the trauma patient: A multicenter trial. *J Trauma* 51:1054, 2001.
49. Demetriades D, Murray JA, Chan LS, et al.: Handsewn versus stapled anastomosis in penetrating colon injuries requiring resection: A multicenter study. *J Trauma* 52:117, 2002.
50. Mann B, Kleinschmidt S, Stremmel W: Prospective study of hand-suture anastomosis after colorectal resection. *Br J Surg* 83:29, 1996.
51. Law WL, Bailey HR, Max E, et al.: Single-layer continuous colon and rectal anastomosis using monofilament absorbable suture (Maxon): Study of 500 cases. *Dis Colon Rectum* 42:736, 1999.
52. Ceraldi CM, Rypins EB, Monahan M, et al.: Comparison of continuous single layer polypropylene anastomosis with double layer and stapled anastomoses in elective colon resections. *Am Surg* 59:168, 1993.
53. Burch JM, Franciose RJ, Moore EE, et al.: Single-layer continuous versus two-layer interrupted intestinal anastomosis: A prospective randomized trial. *Ann Surg* 321:832, 2000.
54. Madiba TE, Mahomva O, Haffejee AA: Does type of colostomy influence outcome of colostomy closure? *S Afr J Surg* 36:57, 1998.
55. Berne JD, Velmahos GC, Chan LS, et al.: The high morbidity of colostomy closure after trauma: Further support for the primary repair of colon injuries. *Surgery* 123:157, 1998.
56. Urbach DR, Kennedy ED, Cohen MM: Colon and rectal anastomoses do not require routine drainage: a systematic review and meta-analysis. *Ann Surg* 229:174, 1999.
57. Jesus EC, Karlicek A, Matos D, et al.: Prophylactic anastomotic drainage for colorectal surgery. *Cochrane Database for Systematic Reviews* 4:CD002100, 2004.
58. Petrowsky H, Demartines N, Rousson V, et al.: Evidence-based value of prophylactic drainage in gastrointestinal surgery: A systematic review and meta-analyses. *Ann Surg* 240:1074, 2004.
59. Shapiro MB, Jenkins DH, Schwab CW, et al.: Damage control: Collective review. *J Trauma* 49:969, 2000.
60. Adkins RB, Zirkle PK, Waterhouse G: Penetrating colon trauma. *J Trauma* 24:491, 1984.
61. Voyles CR, Flint LM, Jr: Wound management after trauma to the colon. *South Med J* 70:1067, 1977.

62. Demetriades D, Charalambides D, Pantanowitz D: Gunshot wounds of the colon: Role of primary repair. *Ann R Coll Surg Engl* 74:381, 1992.

`63. Velmahos GC, Souter I, Degiannis E, et al.: Primary repair for colonic gunshot wounds. *Aust N Z J Surg* 66:344, 1996.

64. Velmahos GC, Vassiliu P, Demetriades D, et al.: Wound management after colon injury: Open or closed? A prospective randomized study. *Am Surg* 68:795, 2002.

65. Fabian TC: Infection in penetrating abdominal trauma: risk factors and preventive antibiotics. *Am Surg* 68:29, 2002.

66. Bozorgzadeh A, Pizzi WF, Barie PS, et al.: The duration of antibiotic administration in penetrating abdominal trauma. *Am J Surg* 177:125, 1999.

67. Velmahos GC, Toutouzas KG, Sarkisyan G, et al.: Severe trauma is not an excuse for prolonged antibiotic prophylaxis. *Arch Surg* 137:537, 2002.

68. Heseltine PN, Berne TV, Yellin AE, et al.: The efficacy of cefoxitin versus clindamycin/gentamycin in surgically treated stab wounds of the bowel. *J Trauma* 26:241, 1986.

69. Sims EH, Lou MA, Williams SW, et al.: Piperacillin monotherapy compared with methornidazole and gentamicn combination in penetrating abdominal trauma. *J Trauma* 34:205, 1993.

70. Cayten CG, Fabian TC, Garcia VF, et al.: Patient management guidelines for penetrating colon injury. Eastern Association of the Surgery of Trauma; Trauma Practice Guidelines, 1998, http://www.east.org.

71. Cornwell EE III, Dougherty WR, Berne TV, et al.: Duration of antibiotic prophylaxis in high-risk patients with penetrating abdominal trauma: a prospective randomized trial. *J Gastroint Surg* 3:648, 1999.

72. Fabian TC, Croce MA, Payne LW, et al.: Duration of antibiotic therapy for penetrating abdominal trauma: a prospective trial. *Surgery* 112:788, 1992.

73. Dellinger EP, Wertz MJ, Lennard ES, et al.: Efficacy of short-course antibiotic prophylaxis after penetrating intestinal injury. *Arch Surg* 121:23, 1986.

74. Belzberg H, Zhu J, Cornwell EE III, et al.: Imipenem levels are not predictable in the critically ill patient. *J Trauma* 56:11, 2004.

75. Oparooji EC, Siram S, Shoheiber O, et al.: Appropriateness of a 4 mg/kg gentamicin or tobramycin loading dose in post-operative septic shock patients. *J Clin Pharmacy Therapeutics* 23:185, 1998.

76. Edwards DP, Brown D, Watkins PE: Should colon-penetrating small missiles be removed? An experimental study of retrocolic wound tracks. *J Invest Surg* 12:25, 1999.

77. Velmahos GC, Demetriades D: Gunshot wounds of the spine: Should retained bullets be removed to prevent infection? *Ann Roy Coll Surg Eng* 76:85, 1994.

78. Kumar A, Wood GW II, Whittle AP: Low-velocity gunshot injuries of the spine with abdominal viscus trauma. *J Orthop Trauma* 12:514, 1998.

79. Scuderi GJ, Vaccaro AR, Fitzenry LN, et al.: Long-term clinical manifestations of retained bullet fragments within the intervertebral disk space. *J Spin Disorders & Techniques* 17:108, 2004.

80. Hess U, Harms J, Schneider A, et al.: Assessment of gunshot bullet injuries with the use of magnetic resonance imaging. *J Trauma* 49:704, 2000.

81. Velmahos GC, Demetriades D, Cornwell EE III: Transpelvic gunshot wounds: Routine laparotomy or selective management. *World J Surg* 22:1034, 1998.

82. Susmalian S, Ezri T, Elis M, et al.: Gluteal stab wounds is a frequent and potentially dangerous injury. *Injury* 36:148, 2005.

83. Velmahos GC, Demetriades D, Cornwell EE III, et al.: Gunshot wounds to the buttocks: Predicting the need for operation. *Dis Col Rect* 40:307, 1997.

84. Pell M, Flynn WJ Jr, Seibel RW: Is colostomy always necessary in the treatment of open pelvic fractures? *J Trauma* 45:371, 1998.

85. Cohen CE, Giles A, Nelson M: Sexual trauma associated with fisting and recreational drugs. *Sex Transm Infect* 80:469, 2004.

86. Burch JM, Feliciano DV, Mattox KL: Colostomy and drainage for civilian rectal injuries: Is that all? *Ann Surg* 209:600, 1989.

87. Thomas DD, Levison MA, Dykstra BJ, et al.: Management of rectal injuries. Dogma versus ptiracce. *Am Surg* 56:507, 1990.

88. Trunkey DA, Hays RJ, Shires GT: Management of rectal trauma. *J Trauma* 13:411, 1973.

89. Ivatury RR, Licata J, Gunduz Y, et al.: Management options in penetrating rectal injuries. *Am Surg* 57:50, 1991.

90. Zmora O, Mahanja A, Bar-Zakai B, et al.: Colon and rectal surgery without mechanical bowel preparation: A randomized prospective trial. *Ann Surg* 237:363, 2003.

91. Gonzalez RP, Falimirski ME, Holevar MR: The role of presacral drainage in the management of penetrating rectal injuries. *J Trauma* 45:656, 1998.

92. Velmahos GC, Gomez H, Falabella A, et al.: Operative management of civilian rectal gunshot wounds: Simpler is better. *World J Surg* 24:114, 2000.

93. Navsaria PH, Shaw JM, Sellweger R, et al.: Diagnostic laparoscopy and diverting sigmoid loop colostomy in the management of civilian extraperitoneal rectal gunshot injuries. *Br J Surg* 91:460, 2004.

94. McGrath V, Fabian TC, Croce MA, et al.: Rectal trauma: Management based on anatomic distinctions. *Am Surg* 64:1136, 1998.

95. Machado GR, Bojalian MO, Reeves ME: Transanal endoscopic repair of rectal anastomotic defect. *Arch Surg* 140:1219, 2005.

96. Ameh EA: Anorectal injuries in children. *Pediatric Surg International* 16:388, 2000.

97. Machiedo GW, Casey KF, Blackwook JM: Colostomy closure following trauma. *Surg Gynecol Obstet* 151:58, 1980.

98. Thal ER, Yeary EC: The morbidity of colostomy closure following colon trauma. *J Trauma* 20:287, 1980.

99. Pachter HL, Hoballah JJ, Corcoran TA, et al.: The morbidity and financial impact of colostomy closure in trauma patients. *J Trauma* 30:1510, 1990.

100. Mealy K, O'Broin E, Donohue J, et al.: Reversible colostomy-what is the outcome? *Dis Colon Rectum* 39:1227, 1996.

101. Sola JE, Bender JS, Buchman TG: Morbidity and timing of colostomy closure in trauma patients. *Injury* 24:438, 1993.

102. Renz BM, Feliciano DV, Sherman R: Same admission colostomy closure (SACC). A new approach to rectal wounds: A prospective study. *Ann Surg* 218:279, 1993.

103. Velmahos GC, Degiannis E, Wells M, et al.: Early closure of colostomies in trauma patients: A prospective randomized trial. *Surgery* 118:815, 1995.

104. Khalid MS, Moeen S, Khan AW, et al.: Same admission colostomy closure: A prospective, randomized study in selected patient groups. *Surgeon J Roy Coll Surg Edin Ireland* 3:11, 2005.

105. Cantele H, Mendez A, Leyba J: Colostomy closure using local anesthesia. *Surgery Today* 31:678, 2001.

106. Rosen MJ, Cobb WS, Kercher KW, et al.: Laparoscopic restoration of intestinal continuity after Hartmann's procedure. *Am J Surg* 189:670, 2005.

107. Bossotti M, Bona A, Borroni R, et al.: Gasless laparoscopic-assisted ileostomy or colostomy closure using an abdominal wall-lifting device. *Surg Endosc* 15:597, 2001.

108. Berne JD, Velmahos GC, Chan LS, et al.: The high morbidity of colostomy closure after trauma: Further support for the primary repair of colon injuries. *Surgery* 123:157, 1998.

109. Mealy K, O'Broin E, Donohue J, et al.: Reversible colostomy-what is the outcome? *Dis Colon Rectum* 39:1227, 1996.

110. Ghorra SG, Rzeczycki TP, Natarajan R, et al.: Colostomy closure: Impact of preoperative risk factors on morbidity. *Am Surg* 65:266, 1999.

111. Riesener KP, Lehnen W, Hofer M, et al.: Morbidity of ileostomy and colostomy closure: Impact of surgical technique and perioperative treatment. *World J Surg* 21:103, 1997.

112. Chandramouli B, Srinivasan K, Jagdish S, et al.: Morbidity and mortality of colostomy and its closure in children. *J Ped Surg* 39:596, 2004.

113. Moore EE, Cogbill TH, Malangoni MA, et al.: Organ injury scaling II: Pancreas, duodenum, small bowel, colon, and rectum. *J Trauma* 30:1427, 1990.

# Commentary ■ KATHRYN M. TCHORZ

The management of colonic and rectal injuries has been the subject of considerable change over the past three decades. The author of this chapter, an experienced urban trauma surgeon, presents an up-to-date and evidence-based surgical perspective on management of today's blunt and penetrating civilian injuries. One of the major points highlighted by the author is the critical impor-

tance of clinical examination. Albeit brief and focused at times, it is the thoughtful attention to the clinical examination that enables prudent surgical care. I am in full agreement with the author's statement that clinical examination of the abdomen is reliable in most trauma patients. However, I have significant reservations about potential delay in the treatment of retroperitoneal colon injuries.

The author contends that there is no morbidity in delay; however, his paper on this topic had no cases of delayed retroperitoneal colonic injuries. Even small bowel injuries have significant morbidity and mortality when the diagnosis is delayed. The liberal use of abdominal CT scanning or other diagnostic modalities as required to properly identify abdominal injuries is valuable, but the global mindset of discounting the reliability of a physician's clinical examination may often delay optimal intervention.

Another major point presented in this chapter regarding the management of penetrating colon injuries is the preference for primary colon repair over colostomy, which was previously a standard practice and covered much of the chapter in the previous edition of this trauma text. It is rewarding to properly apply evidence-based surgical practices to our patients and the author has taken a leading role in this endeavor. However, in severe destructive colonic injuries, often with surrounding devitalized tissue and major intra-abdominal vascular injuries, prompt damage control is necessary and an open abdomen results. I disagree with the author regarding primary colonic repair in such a clinical scenario, no matter how quickly one can suture the bowel. Definitive surgical procedures have no place in damage control. Colonic anastomoses are more vulnerable when they are exposed, as we have learned from exteriorized colonic repairs. In my view, the best possibility for a successful primary colonic anastomosis occurs when the surviving patient is returned to the operating room on a new day.

The author recommends routine placement of a closed-suction drain within the peritoneal cavity after performing a colonic anastomosis in trauma. I was surprised to read this comment, especially from an author whose innovative clinical studies have often challenged "routine" surgical practices. Closed-suction drains placed within the peritoneal cavity should be reserved for draining collections from hepatic, urinary tract, and pancreatic injuries.

Another major issue presented by the author is the revised treatment of rectal injuries. The traditional operative management has been debridement, diversion, drainage, and direct rectal lavage. Once again, the author clearly presents data pertaining to certain traditional practices which now, after proper study design and analysis, provide no benefit and may be potentially harmful to patients. However, the author considers proctosigmoidoscopy optional in patients with potential rectal injuries. My own bias is that even a negative digital rectal examination should always be followed by a rigid proctosigmoidoscopy to ensure the absence of rectal injury.

Expanded information regarding the management of impacted rectal foreign bodies would be useful in this chapter. Many of these patients experience domestic or drug violence or autoerotic and consensual sexual mishaps (Fig. 1). Although inexperienced physicians may attempt foreign-body removal in the emergency department, this practice is potentially dangerous for both the patient and the physician who may be injured by glass shards or sharp edges. These patients should be taken to the operating room for an examination under anesthesia and foreign-body removal.

As implied by the author, it is the continued refinement of surgical skill, critical review of the literature, and utilization of prudent judgment that still matter most in the care of critically ill and injured patients.

# Abdominal Vascular Injury

*Christopher J. Dente* ■ *David V. Feliciano*

The major sites of hemorrhage in patients sustaining blunt or penetrating abdominal trauma are the viscera, the mesentery, or the major abdominal vessels. Although any vessel in the abdomen can bleed, the term *abdominal vascular injury* generally refers to injury to major intraperitoneal or retroperitoneal vessels and may be classified as follows (with accompanying vessels):

- Zone 1: Midline retroperitoneum
  *Supramesocolic region:* suprarenal abdominal aorta, celiac axis, proximal superior mesenteric artery, proximal renal artery, and superior mesenteric vein (either supramesocolic or retromesocolic)
  *Inframesocolic area:* Infrarenal abdominal aorta, infrahepatic inferior vena cava

- Zone 2: Upper lateral retroperitoneum
  Renal artery, renal vein

- Zone 3: Pelvic retroperitoneum
  Iliac artery, iliac vein

- Portal-retrohepatic area
  Portal vein, hepatic artery, retrohepatic vena cava

## EPIDEMIOLOGY

In reviews of vascular injuries sustained in military conflicts, abdominal vascular injuries have been extraordinarily rare. For example, DeBakey and Simeone's classic article on 2471 arterial injuries during World War II included only 49 that occurred in the abdomen, an incidence of 2%.[1] Reporting on 304 arterial injuries from the Korean conflict, Hughes noted that only 7, or 2.3%, occurred in the iliac arteries.[2] In the review by Rich and colleagues of 1000 arterial injuries in the Vietnam conflict, only 29, or 2.9%, involved abdominal vessels.[3]

The data from civilian trauma centers are quite different. In 1979, 15% of patients with abdominal trauma treated at the Ben Taub General Hospital in Houston had injuries to major vascular structures.[4] In addition, abdominal vascular injury accounted for 27.5% of all arterial injuries treated over that same time period. A similar review from the same hospital in 1982 revealed that 31.9% of all vascular injuries occurred in the abdomen, including 18.5% of all arterial injuries and 47.5% of all venous injuries.[5] Finally, a 30-year review (1958 to 1988) at the same hospital, published in 1989, documented that 33.8% of 5760 cardiovascular injuries occurred in the abdomen.[6] In the last five years of the period covered by the report (1984 to 1988), abdominal vascular injuries accounted for 27.3% of all cardiovascular injuries.

Even with the recent decrease in the volume of penetrating trauma in some centers, many patients with abdominal vascular injuries continue to be treated. For example, there were 302 patients with 238 abdominal arterial and 266 abdominal venous injuries who underwent operative repair at the Los Angeles County Hospital (University of Southern California) from 1992 to 1997.[7] Similarly, there were 300 patients with 205 abdominal arterial and 284 abdominal venous injuries who underwent operative repair at the Grady Memorial Hospital (Emory University) from 1989 to 1998.[8]

The significantly higher number of abdominal vascular injuries treated in civilian as opposed to military practice reflects the modest wounding capacity of many handguns when compared to military ordnance, as well as the shorter prehospital transit times in most urban areas of the United States.

At present, the incidence of injury to major abdominal vessels in patients sustaining blunt abdominal trauma is estimated to be about 5 to 10%.[9,10] This is compared to patients with penetrating stab wounds to the abdomen, who will sustain a major abdominal vascular injury approximately 10% of the time[11] and patients with gunshot wounds to the abdomen, who will have injury to a major vessel 20 to 25% of the time.[12]

## PATHOPHYSIOLOGY

### Blunt Trauma

Rapid deceleration in motor vehicle crashes may cause two different types of vascular injury in the abdomen. The first is avulsion of small branches from major vessels. A common example of this is the avulsion of intestinal branches from either the proximal or distal superior mesenteric artery at sites of fixation. A second type of vascular problem seen with deceleration injury is an intimal tear with secondary thrombosis of the lumen, such as is seen in patients with renal artery thrombosis, or a full-thickness tear with a secondary pseudoaneurysm of the renal artery.[13–15]

Crush injuries to the abdomen, such as by a lap seat belt or by a posterior blow to the spine may also cause two different types of vascular injury. The first is an intimal tear or flap with secondary thrombosis of a vessel such as the superior mesenteric artery,[16] infrarenal abdominal aorta,[17,18] or iliac artery.[19,20] The "seat belt aorta" is a classic example of an injury resulting from this mechanism.[17,21–23] Direct blows can also completely disrupt exposed vessels, such as the left renal vein over the aorta[24] or the superior mesenteric artery or vein at the base of the mesentery,[25] leading to massive intraperitoneal hemorrhage, or even partly disrupt the infrarenal abdominal aorta, leading to a false aneurysm.[26,27]

### Penetrating Trauma

Penetrating injuries, in contrast, create the same kinds of abdominal vascular injuries as are seen in the vessels of the extremities, producing blast effects with intimal flaps and secondary thrombosis, lateral-wall defects with free-bleeding or pulsatile hematomas (early false aneurysms), or complete transection with either free bleeding or thrombosis.[28] On rare occasions, a penetrating injury may produce an arteriovenous fistula involving the portal vein and hepatic artery, renal vessels, or iliac vessels.

Iatrogenic injuries to major abdominal vessels are an uncommon but persistent problem. Reported iatrogenic causes of abdominal vascular injury have included diagnostic procedures (angiography, cardiac catheterization, laparoscopy), abdominal operations (pelvic and retroperitoneal procedures), spinal operations (removal of a herniated disk), and adjuncts to cardiac surgery (cardiopulmonary bypass, intra-aortic balloon assist).[29–31]

## DIAGNOSIS

As an abdominal vascular injury may present with free intraperitoneal hemorrhage, with a contained intraperitoneal or retroperitoneal hematoma or with thrombosis of the involved vessel, presenting symptoms are variable. For example, free intraperitoneal hemorrhage may be seen with blunt avulsion of mesenteric vessels and lead to secondary hypovolemic shock. Conversely, when thrombosis of the renal artery is present, the patient will be hemodynamically stable but may complain of upper abdominal and flank pain and will have hematuria 70 to 80% of the time.[15] Thrombosis of the proximal superior mesenteric artery

will cause severe abdominal pain, while thrombosis of the infrarenal abdominal aorta will cause pulseless lower extremities.

Penetrating truncal wounds from the nipples to the upper thighs, however, are the most common cause of abdominal vascular injuries. The exact vessel injured is generally related to the track of the missile or stab wound. For example, gunshot wounds directly on the midline most commonly involve the inferior vena cava or abdominal aorta. Gunshot wounds traversing the pelvis will often injure branches of the iliac artery and vein, while gunshot wounds in the right upper quadrant may involve the renovascular structures, hepatic artery, portal vein, or retrohepatic vena cava.

On physical examination, the findings in patients with abdominal vascular injury will obviously depend on whether a contained hematoma or active hemorrhage is present. Patients with contained hematomas in the retroperitoneum, base of the mesentery, or hepatoduodenal ligament, particularly those with injuries to abdominal veins, may be hypotensive in transit but will respond rapidly to the infusion of fluids. They may remain remarkably stable, with modest or even no peritoneal signs on examination, until the hematoma is opened at the time of celiotomy. Conversely, with free intraperitoneal hemorrhage, patients will often have a rigid abdomen and unrelenting hypotension. In a review by Ingram and colleagues of 70 consecutive patients undergoing laparotomy for an abdominal vascular injury, patients could generally be divided into two groups based on an admission systolic blood pressure greater than or less than 100 mm Hg.[32] In the former group, the mean base deficit on admission was –7.2, blood replacement in the operating room was 8.6 U, an isolated venous injury was present in 73.1% of patients, and survival was 96.2%. This was compared to a 43% survival and an average of 15.1 U of blood replacement in patients presenting with hypotension (Table 37-1). Indeed, admission base deficit was the only independent indicator of mortality in a recent series of patients with abdominal vascular injuries from Lincoln Hospital in New York City.[33]

The other major physical finding that may be noted in patients with abdominal vascular injury is loss of the pulse in the femoral artery in one lower extremity when the ipsilateral common or external iliac artery has been transected or is thrombosed. In such patients, the presence of a transpelvic gunshot wound associated with a wavering or an absent pulse in the femoral artery is pathognomonic of injury to the ipsilateral iliac artery.

**TABLE 37-1**

**Blood Pressure in the Emergency Department in Patients with Abdominal Vascular Injuries: Effect on Management and Prognostic Value**

| | SYSTOLIC BLOOD PRESSURE (SBP) | | |
|---|---|---|---|
| | >100 mmHg | <100 mmHg | p Value |
| Patients | 26 | 44 | — |
| Lowest SBP in emergency center | 123 | 62 | <0.001 |
| Admission base deficit | –7.2 | –14.7 | <0.001 |
| Blood transfusion in operating room (U) | 8.6 | 15.1 | 0.003 |
| Venous injury only | 73.1% | 40.9% | 0.009 |
| Injury to one vessel only | 76.9% | 52.3% | 0.04 |
| Survival | 96.2% | 43.2% | <0.001 |

(Source: Ingram WL, Feliciano DV, Renz BL, et al: Presented at the 55th Annual Meeting, American Association for the Surgery of Trauma. Halifax, Nova Scotia, Canada. September 27–30, 1995.)

In both stable and unstable patients, a rapid surgeon-performed ultrasound (FAST—Focused Assessment for the Sonographic Evaluation of the Trauma Patient) is useful in ruling out an associated cardiac injury with secondary tamponade or an associated hemothorax mandating the insertion of a thoracostomy tube.[34–37] In a *stable* patient with an abdominal gunshot wound, a routine flat-plate x-ray of the abdomen is of diagnostic value, so that the track of the missile can be predicted from markers placed over the wounds or from the position of a retained missile.

In earlier times, all patients who had suffered penetrating abdominal wounds and who were not in shock would undergo a one-shot intravenous pyelogram (IVP) in the emergency department (ED). The major purposes of this study were as follows: to evaluate the function of both kidneys, with lack of flow to one kidney suggesting either absence of the kidney or thrombosis of the renal artery; the presence of active hemorrhage from the kidney itself; and the position and status of the ureters. This study is no longer performed routinely and is indicated only in stable patients with a flank wound and gross hematuria when the computed tomography (CT) scanner is not available.[38]

In patients with blunt abdominal trauma, hematuria, modest to moderate hypotension, and peritonitis in the ED, a preoperative one-shot IVP during resuscitation would still be useful for documenting the presence of an intact kidney. If the kidney is mostly intact without extravasation of the dye, the surgeon will not have to open a perirenal hematoma at the subsequent laparotomy. Nonvisualization of one kidney on the IVP, suggesting thrombosis of the renal artery, was evaluated by renal arteriography in stable patients in the past. Experience with CT scanning of the abdomen in multiple patients with blunt trauma has documented that the absence of renal enhancement and excretion and the presence of a cortical rim sign are diagnostic of thrombosis of the renal artery, and arteriography is no longer indicated for this diagnosis.[39] Similarly, any stable patient with blunt trauma who does not require an immediate laparotomy and who has significant hematuria should undergo an immediate abdominal CT scan without a preliminary one-shot IVP.

Preoperative abdominal aortography should not be performed to document intra-abdominal vascular injuries after penetrating wounds. This is because most patients with such wounds are not stable enough to undergo the manipulation required for appropriate studies of large vessels in an angiographic suite. In patients with blunt trauma, aortography is used to diagnose and treat deep pelvic arterial bleeding associated with fractures[40] and to diagnose unusual injuries such as the previously mentioned intimal tears with thrombosis in the infrarenal aorta, the iliac artery, or the renal artery.

# INITIAL MANAGEMENT AND RESUSCITATION

## Prehospital Resuscitation

Resuscitation in the field in patients with possible blunt or penetrating abdominal vascular injuries should be restricted to basic airway maneuvers such as intubation or cricothyroidotomy and decompression of a tension pneumothorax at the scene. Insertion of intravenous lines for infusing crystalloid solutions is best attempted during transport to the hospital. Restoration of blood pressure to normal levels is critical to neurologic recovery in the rare patients with associated blunt intracranial injuries and possible abdominal vascular injuries.[41] In contrast, there is no consistent evidence to support either the aggressive administration of crystalloid solutions during the short prehospital times in urban environments versus the withholding of similar solutions ("delayed resuscitation") in patients with penetrating abdominal vascular injuries.[42–44] The same is true for the application of the pneumatic antishock garment (PASG).[45]

## Emergency Department Resuscitation

In the ED, the extent of resuscitation clearly depends on the patient's condition at the time of arrival. In the agonal patient with a rigid abdomen after a gunshot wound, ED thoracotomy with cross-clamping of the descending thoracic aorta may be necessary to maintain cerebral and coronary arterial flow, especially if the trauma operating room is geographically distant from the ED.[46] Although all trauma surgeons agree that performing a thoracotomy in the ED will complicate the patient's intraoperative course, the thoracotomy and cross-clamping are sometimes the only way to prevent irreversible ischemic changes in the patient's brain and heart until a celiotomy with vascular control can be performed. It must be recognized, however, that the need for ED thoracotomy is essentially predictive of a <5% survival for the patient with blunt or penetrating abdominal trauma.[47] In the large series by Feliciano and colleagues,[45] only one of 59 patients with isolated penetrating wounds to the abdomen survived after undergoing a preliminary thoracotomy in the ED.

In the patient arriving with blunt abdominal trauma, hypotension, and a positive surgeon-performed FAST *or* penetrating abdominal trauma and hypotension or peritonitis, a *time limit of less than five minutes in the ED is mandatory*. An identification bracelet is applied, an airway and thoracostomy tube are inserted if necessary, especially if the operating room is geographically distant, and blood samples for typing and cross-matching are obtained with the insertion of the first intravenous catheter. Whether more intravenous lines should be inserted in the ED or after arrival in the operating room is much debated. The authors have always believed that patients needing an emergency laparotomy should be in the operating room, as soon as the identification bracelet has been applied and a blood specimen has been sent to the blood bank.

There are now multiple large-bore catheters, specialized administration sets and heating elements commercially available for use in the ED or operating room. With short, large-bore (10-gauge or number 8.5 French) catheters in peripheral veins, flow rates of 1400 to 1600 mL/min of crystalloid solutions can be obtained when an external pressure device is exerting 300 mm Hg pressure.[48] Blood replacement during resuscitation is usually with type-specific blood, although universal donor type O-negative blood may be used when there is no time for even a limited cross-match.

Measures in the ED that will diminish the hypothermia of resuscitation include the following: a heated resuscitation room, the use of prewarmed (37 to 40°C [98.6° to 104.0°F]) crystalloid solutions, passage of all crystalloids and blood through high-flow warmers, and covering the patient's trunk and extremities with prewarmed blankets or heating units.[49,50]

## OPERATIVE PREPARATIONS

### Draping and Incisions

In the operating room, the entire trunk from the chin to the knees is prepared and draped in the usual manner. Before making the incision for celiotomy, the trauma surgeon should confirm that the following items are available: blood for transfusion, autotransfusion apparatus, a thoracotomy tray, an aortic compressor, a complete tray of vascular instruments, spongesticks with gauze sponges in place for later venous compression, as well as appropriate vascular sutures.

### Maneuvers to Prevent or Decrease Hypothermia

In addition to the maneuvers previously described for preventing hypothermia in the ED, operative maneuvers with the same purpose include warming the operating room to >85°F (29.4°C); covering the patient's head; covering the upper and lower extremities with a heating unit (Bair Hugger, Augustine Medical, Inc., Eden Prairie, MN); the irrigation of nasogastric tubes, thoracostomy tubes, and open body cavities with warm saline; and the use of a heating cascade on the anesthesia machine.[50]

### General Principles

A preliminary operating room thoracotomy with cross-clamping of the descending thoracic aorta is used in some centers when the patient's blood pressure on arrival is less than 70 mm Hg.[51–53] As previously mentioned, this maneuver will maintain cerebral and coronary arterial flow if the heart is still beating and may prevent sudden cardiac arrest when abdominal tamponade is released. Unfortunately, it has little effect on intra-abdominal vascular injuries because of persistent bleeding from backflow. Patients with unrelenting shock after cross-clamping of the descending thoracic aorta essentially never survive.[53]

A midline abdominal incision is made, and all clots and free blood are manually evacuated or removed with suction. A rapid inspection is performed to visualize contained hematomas or areas of hemorrhage. One intra-abdominal physical finding that may be of benefit to the surgeon is "black bowel," which has been seen in patients with total transection or thrombosis of the proximal superior mesenteric artery. In a patient with a penetrating upper abdominal wound, a large hematoma in the supramesocolic area and black bowel, an injury to the superior mesenteric artery is likely to be present.[54]

Active hemorrhage is controlled as quickly as possible before any other intraoperative maneuvers are undertaken. Hemorrhage from solid organs is controlled by packing, while standard techniques of vascular control are used to control the active hemorrhage from major intra-abdominal vessels. Finger pressure, compression with laparotomy pads, grabbing the perforated artery with a hand (common or external iliac artery), or formal proximal and distal control is needed to control any actively hemorrhaging major artery. Similarly, options for control of bleeding from major veins such as the inferior vena cava, superior mesenteric vein, renal veins, or iliac veins include finger pressure, compression with laparotomy pads or spongesticks, grabbing the perforated vein with a hand, Judd-Allis clamps to the edges of the perforation,[55] or the

application of vascular clamps. Once hemorrhage from the vascular injuries is controlled in patients with penetrating wounds, it may be worthwhile to rapidly apply Babcock clamps, Allis clamps, noncrushing intestinal clamps, or to rapidly use a surgical stapler to control as many gastrointestinal perforations as possible to avoid further contamination of the abdomen during the period of vascular repair. The abdomen is irrigated with an antibiotic-saline solution, the vascular repair is then performed, a soft tissue cover is applied over the repair, and the remainder of the operation is directed toward repair of injuries to the bowel and solid organs.

Conversely, if the patient has a contained retroperitoneal hematoma at the time of celiotomy, the surgeon occasionally has time to first perform necessary gastrointestinal repairs in the free peritoneal cavity, change gloves, and irrigate with an antibiotic-saline solution. The surgeon can then open the retroperitoneum to expose the underlying abdominal vascular injury.

Hematomas or hemorrhage associated with abdominal vascular injuries generally occur in Zone 1, midline retroperitoneum; Zone 2, upper lateral retroperitoneum; Zone 3, pelvic retroperitoneum; or in the portal–retrohepatic area of the right upper quadrant, as previously described. The magnitude of injury is best described using the Organ Injury Scale of the American Association for the Surgery of Trauma (AAST) (Table 37-2).[56]

## MANAGEMENT OF INJURIES IN ZONE 1: SUPRAMESOCOLIC REGION

### Exposure and Vascular Control

The midline retroperitoneum of Zone I is divided by the transverse mesocolon into a *supramesocolic* region and an *inframesocolic* region. If a hematoma or hemorrhage is present in the midline supramesocolic area, injury to the *suprarenal aorta, celiac axis, proximal superior mesenteric artery,* or *proximal renal artery* should be suspected. In such cases, there are several techniques for obtaining proximal vascular control of the aorta at the hiatus of the diaphragm. When a contained *hematoma* is present, as it frequently is with wounds to the aorta in the aortic hiatus, the surgeon usually has time to reflect all left-sided intra-abdominal viscera, including the colon, kidney, spleen, tail of the pancreas, and fundus of the stomach to the midline (left-sided medial visceral rotation (Fig. 37-1).[57–60] The advantage of this technique is that it provides extensive exposure for visualization of the entire abdominal aorta from the aortic hiatus of the diaphragm to the aortic bifurcation. Disadvantages include the time required to complete the maneuver (four to five minutes), risk of damage to the spleen, left kidney, or posterior left renal artery during the maneuver, and anatomic distortion that results when the left kidney is rotated anteriorly. One alternative is to leave the left kidney in its fossa, thereby eliminating potential damage to or distortion resulting from rotation of this structure. In either case, this maneuver provided the best exposure and allowed for the greatest survival in a series of 46 patients with suprarenal aortic injuries studied at Ben Taub General Hospital in Houston, Texas, in the 1970s.[59]

Because of the dense nature of the celiac plexus of nerves connecting the right and left celiac ganglia as well as the lymphatics that surround the supraceliac aorta, it is frequently helpful to transect the left crus of the aortic hiatus of the diaphragm at the two o'clock

**TABLE 37-2**

**AAST Abdominal Vascular Organ Injury Score**

| | OIS GRADE | ICD-9 | AIS-85 | AIS-90 |
|---|---|---|---|---|
| Grade I[a] | | | | |
| Nonnamed superior mesenteric artery or superior mesenteric vein branches | | 902.20/902.39 | NS | NS |
| Nonnamed inferior mesenteric artery or inferior mesenteric vein branches | I | 902.27/902.32 | NS | NS |
| Phrenic artery/vein | I | 902.89 | NS | NS |
| Lumbar artery/vein | I | 902.89 | NS | NS |
| Gonadal artery/vein | I | 902.89 | NS | NS |
| Ovarian artery/vein | I | 902.81/902.82 | NS | NS |
| Other nonnamed small arterial or venous structures requiring ligation | I | 902.90 | NS | NS |
| Grade II[a] | | | | |
| Right, left, or common hepatic artery | II | 902.22 | 3 | 3 |
| Splenic artery/vein | II | 902.23/902.34 | 3 | 3 |
| Right or left gastric arteries | II | 902.21 | 3 | 3 |
| Gastroduodenal artery | II | 902.24 | 3 | 3 |
| Inferior mesenteric artery, trunk or inferior mesenteric vein, trunk | II | 902.27/902.32 | 3 | 3 |
| Primary named branches of mesenteric artery (e.g., ileocolic artery) or mesenteric vein | II | 902.26/902.31 | 3 | 3 |
| Other named abdominal vessels requiring ligation/repair | II | 902.89 | 3 | 3 |
| Grade III[a] | | | | |
| Superior mesenteric vein trunk | III | 902.31 | 3 | 3 |
| Renal artery/vein | III | 902.41/902.42 | 3 | 3 |
| Iliac artery/vein | III | 902.53/902.54 | 3 | 3 |
| Hypogastric artery/vein | III | 902.51/902.52 | 3 | 3 |
| Vena cava, infrarenal | III | 902.10 | | 3 |
| Grade IV[a] | | | | |
| Superior mesenteric artery, trunk | IV | 902.25 | 3 | 3 |
| Celiac axis proper | IV | 902.24 | 3 | 3 |
| Vena cava suprarenal and infrahepatic | IV | 902.10 | 3 | 3 |
| Aorta, infrarenal | IV | 902.00 | 4 | 4 |
| Grade V[a] | | | | |
| Portal vein | V | 902.33 | 3 | 3 |
| Extraparerctymal hepatic vein | V | 902.11 | 3 (hepatic vein) 5 (liver vein) | 3 (hepatic vein) 5 (liver + veins) |
| Vena cava, retrohepatic or suprahepatic | V | 902.19 | 5 | 5 |
| Aorta, suprarenal, subdiaphragmatic | V | 902.00 | 4 | 4 |

This classification system is applicable for extraparenchymal vascular injures. If the vessel injury is within 2 cm of the organ parenchyma, refer to specific organ injury scale.

[a]Increase one grade for multiple grade III or IV injuries involving >50% vessel circumference. Downgrade one grade if <25% vessel circumference laceration for grade IV or V.

AAST: American Association for the Surgery of Trauma; AIS-85, Abbreviated Injury Scale; AIS-90, Abbreviated Injury Scale; ICD-9, International Classification of Diseases; OIS, organ injury scale.

*(Reproduced with permission from Moore EE, Cogbill TH, Jurkovich GJ, et al.: Organ injury scaling III: Chest wall, abdominal vascular, ureter, bladder, and urethra. J Trauma 33:337, 1992.)*

position to allow for exposure of the distal descending thoracic aorta above the hiatus.[61] With the distal descending thoracic aorta or abdominal aorta in the hiatus exposed, a supraceliac aortic clamp can be applied without difficulty.

Conversely, if active *hemorrhage* is coming from this area, the surgeon may attempt to control it manually or with one of the aortic compression devices.[62,63] An alternate approach is to divide the lesser omentum manually, retract the stomach and esophagus to the left, and digitally separate the muscle fibers of the aortic hiatus of the diaphragm from the supraceliac aorta to obtain the same exposure as described for the left-sided medial visceral rotation, but more quickly.[64] After either approach to the suprarenal abdominal aorta, cross-clamp time should be minimized to avoid the primary fibrinolytic state that occurs, presumably due to hepatic hypoperfusion.[65]

Distal control of the aorta in this location is awkward because of the presence of the celiac axis and superior mesenteric artery (Fig. 37-2). In several patients with injury confined to the supraceliac aorta, the celiac axis has been divided and ligated to allow for more space for the distal aortic clamp and subsequent vascular repair. Necrosis of the gallbladder is a likely sequelae, and cholecystectomy is generally warranted, although this may be done at repeat exploration when "damage control" techniques are required.[66]

## Suprarenal Aorta

With small perforating wounds to the aorta at this level, lateral aortorrhaphy with 3-0 or 4-0 polypropylene suture is preferred. If two small perforations are adjacent to one another, they should be

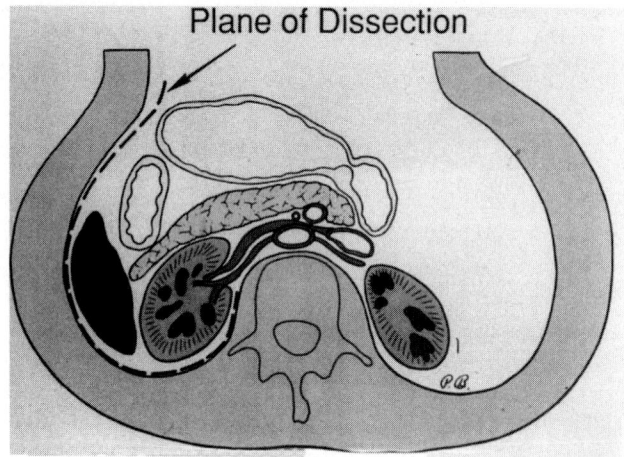

**FIGURE 37-1.** Left medial visceral mobilization is performed in the retroperitoneal plane behind all left-sided intra-abdominal viscera in a patient with a supramesocolic hematoma in the midline.
*(Reproduced with permission from Feliciano DV: Truncal vascular trauma. In Callow AD, Ernst CB, eds. Vascular Surgery. Theory and Practice. Stamford, CT: Appleton & Lange, 1995, p. 1059.)*

connected and the defect closed in a transverse fashion with the polypropylene suture. When closure of the perforations result in significant narrowing, or if a portion of the aortic wall is missing, patch aortoplasty with polytetrafluoroethylene (PTFE) is indicated. The other option is to resect a short segment of the injured aorta and perform an end-to-end anastomosis. Unfortunately, this is nearly impossible because of the limited mobility of both ends of the aorta at this level.

On rare occasions, patients with extensive injuries to the diaphragmatic or supraceliac aorta will require insertion of a synthetic vascular conduit or spiral graft after resection of the area of injury.[67–69] Many of these patients have associated gastric, enteric, or colonic injuries, and much concern has been expressed about placing a synthetic conduit, such as a 12-mm, 14-mm, or 16-mm woven Dacron, albumin-coated Dacron, or PTFE prosthesis, in the abdominal aorta

(Fig. 37-3). The data in the American literature describing young patients with injuries to nondiseased abdominal aortas do not support the concern about Dacron interposition grafts, and there are few reports describing the use of PTFE grafts in penetrating trauma to the abdominal aorta. Despite the available data, some clinicians continue to recommend an extra-anatomic bypass when injury to the abdominal aorta would require replacement with a conduit in the presence of gastrointestinal contamination.[21]

As previously noted, repairs of the intestine and the aorta should not be performed simultaneously. Once the perforated bowel has been packed away and the surgeon has changed gloves, the aortic prosthesis is sewn in place with 3-0 or 4-0 polypropylene suture. After appropriate flushing of both ends of the aorta and removal of the distal aortic clamp, the proximal aortic clamp should be removed very slowly as the anesthesiologist rapidly infuses fluids. If a long aortic clamp time has been necessary, the prophylactic administration of intravenous bicarbonate is indicated to reverse the "washout" acidosis from the previously ischemic lower extremities.[70] The retroperitoneum is then copiously irrigated and closed in a watertight fashion with an absorbable suture.

The survival rate of patients with penetrating injuries to the suprarenal abdominal aorta in eight series published from 1974 to 1992 was 34.8% (54/155)[59,69,71–76] (Table 37-3). Four more recent reviews have documented a significant decline in survival for injuries to the abdominal aorta (suprarenal and infrarenal), ranging from 21.1% to 50% (mean 30.2%, 62/205 patients) even when patients with exsanguination before repair or those treated with ligation only were excluded.[7,8,77,78] In one series in which injuries to the suprarenal and infrarenal abdominal aorta were separated, the survival rate in the suprarenal group was only 8.3% (3/36).[77] The reasons for this decrease in survival figures are not defined in the reviews described. A likely cause, however, is the shorter prehospital times for exsanguinated patients that have been realized with improvements in emergency medical services.

Blunt injury to the suprarenal aorta is extraordinarily rare. While blunt injury to the descending thoracic aorta is well-described throughout the trauma literature, only 62 cases of blunt trauma to

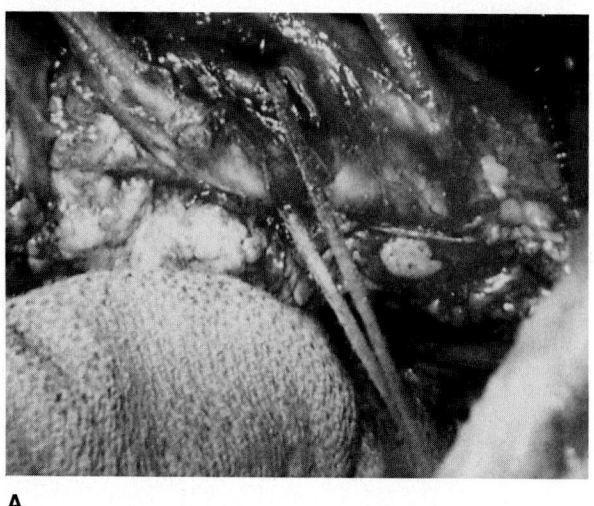

A

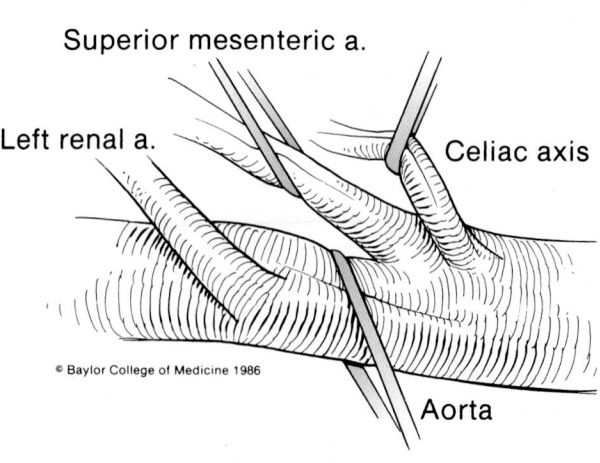

B

**FIGURE 37-2.** **(A)** View of suprarenal aorta and major branches after left-sided medial mobilization maneuver. **(B)** Diagrammatic representation of structures with labels.
*(Reproduced with permission from Baylor College of Medicine.)*

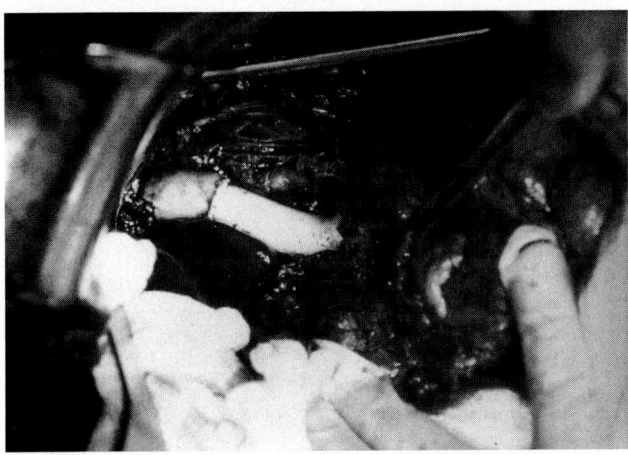

**FIGURE 37-3.** A 22-year-old man with a gunshot wound to the right upper quadrant had injuries to the prepyloric area of the stomach and to the supraceliac abdominal aorta. The aortic injury was managed by segmental resection and replacement with a 16-mm polytetrafluoroethylene (PTFE) graft. The patient was discharged 46 days after injury.
*(Reproduced with permission from Feliciano DV: Injuries to the great vessels of the abdomen. In Souba WW, Fink, MP, Jurkovich GJ, et al., eds. ACS Surgery Principles and Practice. New York, NY: Web MD, 2006, p. 1250.)*

the abdominal aorta were found by Roth et al. in a literature review in 1997.[79] Of these, only one case was noted to be in the suprarenal aorta. The most common location is between the origin of the inferior mesenteric artery and the aortic bifurcation (see below). These injuries generally present with signs and symptoms of aortic thrombosis, rather than hemorrhage, with the most common signs being a lack of femoral pulses (81%), abdominal tenderness (55%), lower extremity weakness or paralysis (47%), and paresthesias (20%).[79] Management of these injuries is discussed more extensively in the section on infrarenal aortic injuries.

## Celiac Axis

Injury to the trunk of the celiac axis is rare. One of the largest series in the literature, reported by Asensio et al., documented the treatment of 13 patients with this uncommon injury.[80] Penetrating injuries were the cause in 12 patients, and overall mortality was 62%. Eleven patients were treated with ligation and one with primary repair, with the final patient exsanguinating prior to therapy. Of the five survivors, four had undergone ligation. All deaths occurred in the operating room. This group also performed an extensive literature review and could only document 33 previously

reported cases, all the result of penetrating trauma. Furthermore, they could find no survivor treated with any sort of complex repair.[80] One case of injury to the celiac artery after blunt trauma was reported by Schreiber et al. and occurred in a patient with pre-existing median arcuate ligament syndrome.[81] Patients with injuries to the trunk of the celiac axis that are not amenable to simple arteriorrhaphy should undergo ligation, which should not cause any short-term morbidity other than the aforementioned risk of gallbladder necrosis.

When branches of the celiac axis are injured, they are often difficult to repair because of the dense neural and lymphatic tissue in this area and the small size of the vessels in a patient in shock with secondary vasoconstriction. There is clearly no good reason to fix major injuries to either the left gastric or proximal splenic artery in the patient with trauma to this area. In both instances, these vessels should be ligated. The common hepatic artery may have a larger diameter than the other two vessels, and an injury to this vessel may occasionally be amenable to lateral arteriorrhaphy, end-to-end anastomosis, or the insertion of a saphenous vein or prosthetic graft. In general, one should not worry about ligating the common hepatic artery proximal to the origin of the gastroduodenal artery, since the extensive collateral flow from the midgut through this vessel will maintain the viability of the liver.

## Superior Mesenteric Artery

Injuries to the superior mesenteric artery are managed based on the level of injury. In 1972, Fullen and coworkers[82] described an anatomic classification of injuries to the superior mesenteric artery that has been used intermittently by subsequent authors in the trauma literature.[54,83] If the injury to the superior mesenteric artery is beneath the pancreas (Fullen zone I), the pancreas may have to be transected between Glassman or Dennis intestinal clamps to control the bleeding point. Because the superior mesenteric artery has few branches at this level, proximal and distal vascular control is relatively easy to obtain once the overlying pancreas has been divided. Another option is to perform medial rotation of the left-sided intra-abdominal viscera, as previously described, and apply a clamp directly to the proximal superior mesenteric artery at its origin from the left side of the aorta. In this instance, the left kidney may be left in the retroperitoneum as the medial rotation is performed.

Injuries to the superior mesenteric artery also occur beyond the pancreas at the base of the transverse mesocolon (Fullen zone II, between the pancreaticoduodenal and middle colic branches of the artery). Although there is certainly more space in which to work in this area, the proximity of the pancreas and the potential

**TABLE 37-3**

| Survival with Injuries to the Abdominal Aorta | | | | | |
|---|---|---|---|---|---|
| | **ASENSIO ET AL. 2000**[7] | | **DAVIS ET AL. 2001**[8a] | **TYBURSKI ET AL. 2001**[77] | **COIMBRA ET AL. 1996**[78] |
| Abdominal aorta overall | Isolated Injury 21.7% (10/46) | With Other Arterial Injury 17.6% (3/17) | 39.1% (25/64) | 21.1% (15/71) | 50% (12/24) |
| Suprarenal aorta | 8 Series, 1974–1992[59,69,71–76] 34.8% (54/155) | | Tyburski et al. 2001 8.3% (3/36) | | – |
| Infrarenal aorta | 6 Series, 1974–1992[71,73–76,102] 46.2% (43/93) | | Tyburski et al. 2001 34.2% (12/35) | | – |

[a]Excludes patients with exsanguination before repair or ligation.

for pancreatic leaks near the arterial repair make injuries in this location almost as difficult to handle as the more proximal injuries.[54,82,83] If the superior mesenteric artery has to be ligated at its origin from the aorta or beyond the pancreas (Fullen zone I or II), collateral flow from both the foregut and hindgut should maintain theoretically the viability of the midgut in the distribution of this vessel.[84] In truth, exsanguinating hemorrhage from injuries in this area often leads to intense vasoconstriction of the more distal superior mesenteric artery. For this reason, collateral flow is often inadequate to maintain viability of the distal midgut, especially the cecum and ascending colon. In the hemodynamically unstable patient with hypothermia, acidosis, and a coagulopathy, the insertion of a temporary intraluminal shunt into the debrided ends of the superior mesenteric artery is most appropriate and fits the definition of *damage control*.[85] If replacement of the proximal superior mesenteric artery is necessary in a more stable patient, it is safest to place the origin of the saphenous vein or prosthetic graft on the distal infrarenal aorta, away from the pancreas and other upper abdominal injuries (Fig. 37-4).[54] A graft in this location should be tailored so that it will pass through the posterior aspect of the mesentery of the small bowel and then be sutured to the superior mesenteric artery in an end-to-side fashion without significant tension. It is mandatory to cover the aortic suture line with retroperitoneal fat or a viable omental pedicle to avoid an aortoduodenal or aortoenteric fistula at a later time. This is much easier to perform if the proximal origin of the graft is located on the distal aorta. Injuries to the more distal superior mesenteric artery (Fullen zone III, beyond the middle colic branch, and zone IV, at the level of the enteric branches) should be repaired, since ligation in this area is distal to the connection to collateral vessels from the foregut and the hindgut.[86] This may require microsurgical techniques.[87] If this cannot be accomplished because of the small size of the vessel, ligation may mandate extensive resection of the ileum and right colon.

The survival rate of patients with penetrating injuries to the superior mesenteric artery in six series published from 1972 to 1986 was 57.7% (67/116) (Table 37-4).[54,74,80,88–90] Four more recent reviews, including a large multi-institutional study,[83] had a mean survival of 58.7% (182/310).[7,8,77,83] In one of the older series, survival decreased to 22% when any form of repair more complex than lateral arteriorrhaphy was performed.[53] Independent risk factors for mortality in the multi-institutional study included injury to Fullen zone I or II, transfusion of >10 U of packed red blood cells, intraoperative acidosis or dysrhythmias, and multisystem organ failure.[83]

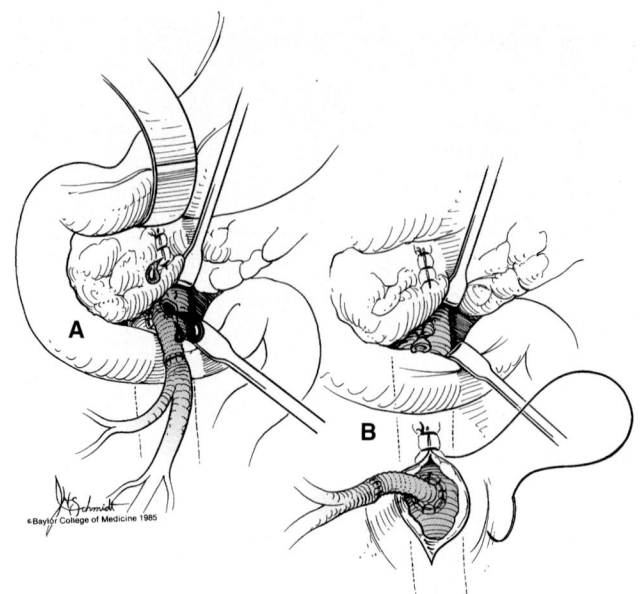

**FIGURE 37-4.** **(A)** When complex grafting procedures to the superior mesenteric artery are necessary, it may be dangerous to place the proximal suture line near an associated pancreatic injury. **(B)** The proximal suture line should be on the lower aorta, away from the upper abdominal injuries, and should be covered with retroperitoneal tissue. *(Reproduced with permission from Accola KD, Feliciano DV, Mattox KL, et al.: Management of injuries to the superior mesenteric artery. J Trauma 26:313, 1986.)*

## Proximal Renal Arteries

Injuries to the proximal renal arteries may also present with a Zone I, supramesocolic hematoma, or with hemorrhage in this area. The left medial visceral rotation maneuver described earlier allows visualization of much of the posterior left renal artery from the aorta to the kidney. This maneuver does not, however, allow for visualization of the proximal right renal artery. The proximal vessel is best approached through the base of the mesocolon beneath the left renal vein and between the infrarenal abdominal aorta and inferior vena cava. Options for repair of either the proximal or distal renal arteries are described later in this chapter (Zone 2).

## Superior Mesenteric Vein

One other major abdominal vessel, the proximal superior mesenteric vein, lying to the right of the superior mesenteric artery, may be injured at the base of the mesocolon. Injury to the most proximal

**TABLE 37-4**

| Survival with Injuries to the Superior Mesentery Artery | | | | |
| --- | --- | --- | --- | --- |
| **REFERENCE** | **YEAR** | **NO. PATIENTS** | **NO. SURVIVORS** | **SURVIVAL (%)** |
| 6 series[54,74,82,88–90] | 1972–1986 | 116 | 67 | 57.7 |
| Asensio et al.[7] (L.A. County) | 2000 | 27 (isolated injury) | 11 | 40.7 |
| | | 7 (with other artery) | 2 | 28.6 |
| Asensio et al.[83] (Multi-institutional) | 2001 | 233 | 143 | 61 |
| Davis et al.[8] | 2001 | 15 | 8 | 53.3 |
| Tyburski et al.[77] | 2001 | 41 | 20 | 48.8 |

aspect of this vessel near its junction with the splenic vein is difficult to manage. The overlying pancreas, proximity of the uncinate process, and close association with the superior mesenteric artery often preclude easy access to proximal and distal control of the vein. Therefore, as with injuries to the proximal superior mesenteric artery, the neck of the pancreas may have to be transected between noncrushing vascular or intestinal clamps to gain access to a perforation. More commonly, the surgeon will find a perforation inferior to the lower border of the pancreas. Often, the vein can be compressed manually or squeezed between the surgeon's fingers as an assistant places a continuous row of 5-0 polypropylene sutures into the edges of the perforation. If a posterior perforation is present, multiple collaterals entering the vein at this point will have to be ligated to roll the perforation into view. Occasionally, the vein will be nearly transected and both ends will have to be controlled with vascular clamps. With an assistant pushing the small bowel and its mesentery back toward the pancreas, the surgeon can reapproximate the ends of the vein without tension.

When multiple vascular and visceral injuries are present in the upper abdomen and the superior mesenteric vein has been severely injured, ligation can be performed in the young trauma patient. In three older reviews of injuries to the portal venous system, ligation of the superior mesenteric vein was performed in 27 patients, and 22 survived.[74,91,92] In one review of injuries to the superior mesenteric vein, survival was 85% among 33 patients treated with ligation, versus 64% in 77 patients who underwent repair.[93] Stone and associates have emphasized the need for vigorous postoperative fluid resuscitation in these patients as splanchnic hypervolemia leads to peripheral hypovolemia for at least three days after ligation of the superior mesenteric vein.[92] The survival rate of patients with injuries to the superior mesenteric vein in four series published from 1978 to 1983 was 72.1% (75/104) (Table 37-5).[74,90–92] Three more recent reviews had a mean survival of 58.3% (42/72).[7,8,77]

## MANAGEMENT OF INJURIES IN ZONE 1: INFRAMESOCOLIC REGION

### Exposure and Vascular Control

The second major area of hematoma or hemorrhage in the midline is the inframesocolic area. In this location, abdominal vascular injuries include those to the *infrarenal abdominal aorta* or *inferior vena cava*. Exposure of an inframesocolic injury to the aorta is obtained by duplicating the maneuvers used to gain proximal aortic control during the elective resection of an abdominal aortic aneurysm. The transverse mesocolon is pulled up toward the

patient's head, the small bowel is eviscerated toward the right (surgeon's) side of the table, and the midline retroperitoneum is opened until the left renal vein is exposed. A proximal aortic clamp should then be placed immediately inferior to the left renal vein. When a large retroperitoneal hematoma is present and proximal inframesocolic control is difficult to obtain, it should always be remembered that the hole in the aorta is under the highest point of the hematoma ("Mount Everest phenomenon"). Therefore, rapid finger splitting of the hematoma will generally bring the surgeon directly to the area of injury. Exposure to allow for application of the distal vascular clamp is obtained by dividing the midline retroperitoneum down to the aortic bifurcation, carefully avoiding the left-sided origin of the inferior mesenteric artery. This vessel, however, may be sacrificed whenever necessary for exposure.

If the aorta is intact and an inframesocolic hematoma appears to be more extensive on the right side of the abdomen than on the left, or, if there is active hemorrhage coming through the base of the mesentery of the ascending colon or hepatic flexure of the colon, injury to the inferior vena cava below the liver should be suspected. Although it is possible to visualize the vena cava through the midline retroperitoneal incision previously described, most trauma surgeons are more comfortable in visualizing the vena cava by mobilizing the right half of the colon and C-loop of the duodenum and leaving the right kidney in situ (right medial visceral rotation) (Fig. 37-5). This permits the entire vena caval system from the confluence of the iliac veins to the suprarenal vena cava below the liver to be visualized. It is often difficult to define precisely where a hole is in a large vein of the abdomen, such as the inferior vena cava, until much of the loose retroperitoneal fatty tissue is stripped away from the wall of the vessel. Once this is done, the site of hemorrhage can be localized.

If active hemorrhage appears to be coming from the anterior surface of the vena cava, a Satinsky-type vascular clamp should be applied directly to the perforation as it is elevated by a pair of vascular forceps or Allis clamps. When the vena cava has been extensively lacerated and partial occlusion cannot be performed, it is often helpful to compress the proximal and distal vena cava around the partial transection or extensive laceration using gauze sponges placed in straight spongesticks. Because of backbleeding from lumbar veins, it may be necessary to use large DeBakey aortic clamps and completely occlude the vena cava above and below some injuries. This maneuver carries a risk in the already hypotensive patient, since venous return to the right side of the heart is essentially interrupted. For this reason, the infrarenal abdominal aorta should be clamped simultaneously.

The two areas in which proximal and distal control of the inferior vena cava below the liver are especially difficult to obtain are at the confluence of the common iliac veins and at the caval junction

### TABLE 37-5

| Survival with Injuries to the Superior Mesenteric Vein | | | | |
| --- | --- | --- | --- | --- |
| REFERENCE | YEAR | NO. OF PATIENTS | NO. OF SURVIVORS | SURVIVAL (%) |
| 4 series[74,90-92] | 1978–1983 | 104 | 75 | 72.1 |
| Asensio et al.[7] | 2000 | 19 (isolated injury) | 9 | 47.4 |
| | | 14 (with other vein) | 5 | 35.7 |
| Davis et al.[8] | 2001 | 21 | 15 | 71.4 |
| Tyburski et al.[77] | 2001 | 32 | 18 | 56.3 |

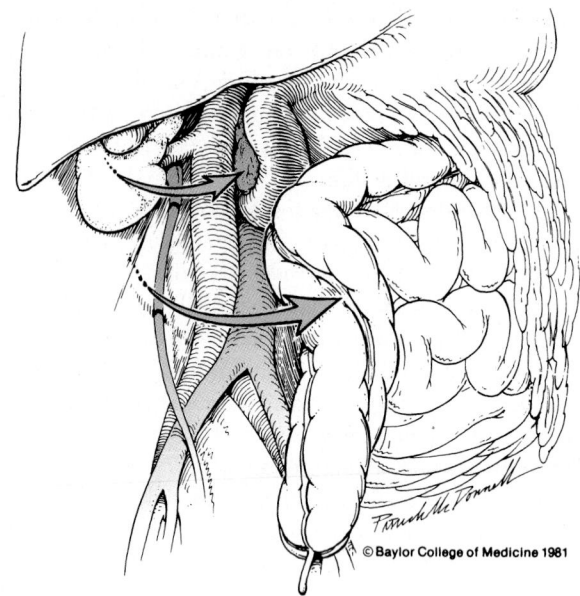

**FIGURE 37-5.** Medial mobilization of right-sided intra-abdominal viscera except the kidney allows for visualization of the entire infrahepatic inferior vena cava.
*(Reproduced with permission from Baylor College of Medicine.)*

with the renal veins. Although spongestick compression of the common iliac veins and the vena cava superiorly may control hemorrhage at the confluence, visualization of perforating wounds in this area is compromised by the overlying aortic bifurcation. In the case of difficult exposure, one technique is to divide and ligate the right internal iliac artery, which may allow for lateral and cephalad retraction of the right common iliac artery to expose the venous injury. An alternate and interesting approach is the temporary division of the overlying right common iliac artery itself, with mobilization of the aortic bifurcation to the left.[94] This technique provides wide exposure of the confluence of the common iliac veins and the distal vena cava. The venous injury can then be repaired in the usual fashion. The right common iliac artery is reconstituted by an end-to-end anastomosis. When the perforation occurs at the junction of the renal veins and the inferior vena cava, it should be directly compressed with either spongesticks or the fingers. An assistant then clamps or compresses the infrarenal vena cava and the suprarenal infrahepatic vena cava and loops both renal veins individually with vascular tapes to allow for the direct application of angled vascular clamps. When time does not allow for this dissection, medial mobilization of the right kidney may allow for the application of a partial occlusion clamp across the inferior vena cava at its junction with the right renal vein. This medial mobilization maneuver is also useful for exposing posterior perforations in the suprarenal infrahepatic vena cava.[95] Should this latter maneuver be performed, care must be taken to divide and ligate but not avulse the first lumbar vein on the right as it frequently enters the junction of the right renal vein and inferior vena cava. One other useful technique for controlling hemorrhage from the inferior vena cava in all locations is to use a Foley balloon catheter for tamponade.[96–98] Either a 5-mL or 30-mL balloon catheter can be inserted into a caval laceration, the balloon inflated in the lumen, and traction applied to the catheter. Once the bleeding is controlled, either a purse-string suture is inserted or a transverse

venorrhaphy is performed, taking care not to rupture the underlying balloon with the needle. The balloon catheter is then deflated and removed just before completion of the suture line.

## Infrarenal Aorta

As with injuries to the suprarenal aorta, penetrating or blunt injuries in the infrarenal abdominal aorta are repaired primarily with 3-0 or 4-0 polypropylene sutures or by patch aortoplasty, end-to-end anastomosis, or insertion of a woven Dacron graft, albumin-coated Dacron graft, or a PTFE graft—none of which require preclotting. Because of the small size of the aorta in young trauma patients, it is unusual to be able to place a tube graft larger than 12, 14, or 16 mm in diameter if one is required, as previously noted. The principles of completing the suture lines and flushing are exactly the same as for aortic repairs in the suprarenal area. Since the retroperitoneal tissue is often thin in young patients, it may be worthwhile to cover an extensive aortic repair or the suture line of a prosthesis with mobilized omentum before closure of the retroperitoneum.[99] The vascularized pedicle of omentum should prevent a postoperative aortoduodenal fistula.

While the vast majority of injuries to the infrarenal aorta are penetrating in nature, a small proportion occurs after blunt trauma. In the aforementioned review of 62 cases of blunt aortic trauma prior to 1997, reported by Roth et al., motor vehicle collisions accounted for 57% of the cases and 47% of the total were directly attributed to lap belts.[79] The patients generally present with symptoms of acute arterial insufficiency as stated above, though a small number present in a delayed fashion with claudication, impotence or, rarely, delayed rupture.[79,100,101]

The survival rate of patients with injuries to the infrarenal abdominal aorta in six series published from 1974 to 1992 was 46.2% (43/93) (Table 37-3).[71,73–76,102] As previously noted in the discussion of recent decreases in survival figures for injuries to the suprarenal abdominal aorta, the same has been true for injuries to the infrarenal abdominal aorta. In the one series, published in 2001, in which injuries to the suprarenal and infrarenal abdominal aorta were separated, the survival rate in the infrarenal group was only 34.2% (12/35).[77]

One peculiar and fortunately rare injury to the infrarenal abdominal aorta is rupture of a pre-existing aortic aneurysm or distal embolization from an aneurysm secondary to blunt abdominal trauma.[103,104]

## Infrahepatic Inferior Vena Cava

Anterior perforations of the inferior vena cava are best repaired in a transverse fashion using a continuous suture of 4-0 or 5-0 polypropylene. If vascular control is satisfactory and a posterior perforation can be visualized adequately by extending the anterior perforation, the posterior perforation can be repaired from inside the vena cava, with the first suture knot outside the lumen. When a significant longitudinal perforation is present, especially when adjacent perforations have been joined, the repaired vena cava will often take on the appearance of an hourglass. This narrowing may lead to slow postoperative occlusion of the vena cava. In the unstable patient who has developed a coagulopathy, no further attempt should be made to modify the repair. In the stable patient, there may be some justification for applying a large venous patch taken either from the resected inferior mesenteric vein or an ovarian vein or applying a PTFE patch.

In the case of a young patient who is exsanguinating and in whom extensive repair of the infrarenal inferior vena cava appears to be necessary, ligation of this vessel is usually well tolerated as long as certain precautions are taken. The first of these is to measure the pressures in the anterior compartments of the legs and to perform bilateral below-knee four-compartment fasciotomies at the first operation if the pressure is 30–35 mm Hg, depending on the patient's hemodynamic status. Bilateral thigh fasciotomies may be necessary, as well, within the first 48 hours after ligation. The second is to maintain circulating volume in the postoperative period through infusion of the appropriate fluids. The third is to apply elastic compression wraps to both lower extremities and keep them continuously elevated for approximately five to seven days after operation. Patients should wear the wraps when they start to ambulate, as well. If there is some residual edema even with the wraps in place at the time of hospital discharge, the patient should be fitted with full-length, custom-made support hose. While the majority of patients in the authors' experience will have no or minimal long-term edema, there have been occasional reports of severe edema in the postoperative period which has required later interposition grafting.[105] Again, this has not been necessary in patients treated by the authors.

Ligation of the suprarenal inferior vena cava is performed only when the patient has an extensive injury at this location and appears to have terminal shock at operation. Of interest, one report described a patient treated with suprarenal ligation who did not develop acute renal failure and who continued to do well two years after injury.[106] In order to avoid the risk of acute renal failure and massive edema of the lower half of the body that would ordinarily be associated with ligation at this level, several innovative approaches have been used. These include suprarenal insertion of a saphenous vein composite interposition graft, insertion of a Dacron or PTFE interposition graft, or insertion of a cavo-right atrial Dacron or PTFE bypass graft.[107,108] While long-term data are lacking for both Dacron and PTFE interposition or bypass grafts in the major veins of the abdomen, the use of an externally supported PTFE graft in combination with chronic anticoagulation would presumably offer the best long-term patency.

Survival rates for patients with injuries to the inferior vena cava obviously depend on the location of injury. If one eliminates suprahepatic and retrohepatic vena caval injuries from seven series

published from 1978 to 1994, the average survival for 515 patients with injuries to the infrahepatic vena cava was 72.2% (see Table 37-6).[74,76,95,110–113] Further eliminating juxtarenal injuries, the average survival for 318 patients with true infrarenal caval injuries was 76.1% (see Table 37-6).[74,76,95,110–112] It is difficult to compare more recent data, once again, because there is only one series[77] in which survival figures are correlated with the location of the caval injury. Overall, survival for injuries to the inferior vena cava appears to be decreased as compared to that of the past. This could only be confirmed if patients with exsanguination before repair or with injuries to the suprahepatic or retrohepatic vena cava were removed from all the recent reviews.

Short-term patency of repair of the inferior vena cava has been studied by Porter and colleagues.[114] In 28 patients with prior lateral venorrhaphy of the inferior vena cava, patency of the cava was documented by sonography, CT scan, or both in 24 (86%).

## MANAGEMENT OF INJURIES IN ZONE 2

### Exposure and Vascular Control

If a hematoma or hemorrhage is present in the lateral retroperitoneum, injury to the *renal artery, renal vein,* or *both,* as well as injury to the *kidney* should be suspected. Most patients with penetrating trauma to the abdomen are explored prior to extensive radiologic workup; however, in selected patients who are hemodynamically stable after sustaining penetrating wounds to the flank, CT scan has been used to document an isolated minor renal injury and operation has been avoided.[115] Conversely, patients found to have a perirenal hematoma at the time of exploration for a penetrating abdominal wound should have unroofing of the hematoma and exploration of the wound track. If the hematoma is not rapidly expanding and there is no free intra-abdominal bleeding, some surgeons will loop the ipsilateral renal artery with a vascular tape in the midline at the base of the mesocolon.[116] The left renal vein can be looped with a vascular tape in the same location; however, vascular control of the proximal right renal vein will have to wait for mobilization of the C-loop of the duodenum and unroofing of the vena cava at its junction with the renal veins (Fig. 37-6). It should be noted that obtaining proximal vascular control prior to exploration of a perirenal hematoma is controversial. Indeed, in one

**TABLE 37-6**

| Survival with Injuries to the Inferior Vena Cava | | | | | |
|---|---|---|---|---|---|
| | **ASENSIO ET AL. 2000[7a]** | | **DAVIS ET AL. 2001[8b]** | **TYBURSKI ET AL. 2001[77]** | **COIMBRA ET AL. 1996[78]** |
| Inferior vena cava overall | Isolated Injury 29.9% (12/41) | With other Venous Injury 22.3% (8/36) | 56.1% (47/84) | 42.9% (61/142) | 65.8% (27/41) |
| Pararenal to diaphragm | – | | – | 40.3% (31/77) | – |
| Infrahepatic inferior vena cava | 7 Series, 1978–1994 [74,76,107,110–113] 72.2% (372/515) | | – | – | – |
| Infrarenal inferior vena cava | 7 Series, 1978–1994 [74,76,107,109–113] 76.1% (242/318) | | – | 46.1% (30/65) | – |

[a]Excludes Retrohepatic vena cava.
[b]Excludes patients with exsanguination before repair or ligation.

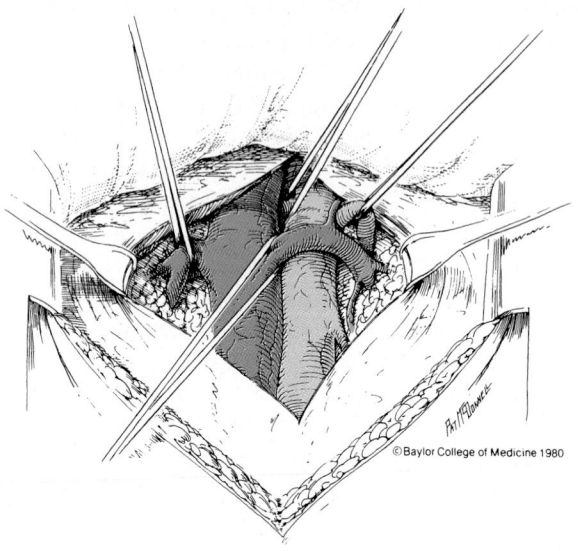

**FIGURE 37-6.** Midline looping of respective renal vessels is performed before entering any perirenal hematoma in some centers. *(Reproduced with permission from Baylor College of Medicine.)*

study, preliminary vascular control of the renal hilum had no impact on nephrectomy rate, transfusion requirements, or blood loss.[117]

Conversely, if there is active bleeding from the kidney through Gerota's fascia or from the retroperitoneum overlying the renal vessels, central renovascular control is not obtained. The surgeon should simply open the retroperitoneum lateral to the injured kidney and manually elevate the kidney directly into the wound. A large vascular clamp can be applied proximal to the hilum either at the midline on the left or just lateral to the inferior vena cava on the right to control any further bleeding.

Patients who present after blunt trauma may also have either a renovascular or renal parenchymal injury. Patients in the former group, however, generally present with renovascular occlusion, which will be discussed below. In patients who have suffered blunt abdominal trauma and have undergone a preoperative IVP, renal arteriogram, or CT of the kidneys which has demonstrated flow to the kidney and/or a low Organ Injury Scale grade of injury, there is no justification for exploring the perirenal hematoma should an emergency celiotomy be indicated for other reasons.

## Renovascular Injuries: Renal Artery

Renovascular injuries are difficult to manage, especially when the renal artery is involved. It is an extraordinarily small vessel that is deeply embedded in the retroperitoneum. Occasionally, small perforations of the artery from penetrating wounds can be repaired by lateral arteriorrhaphy or resection with an end-to-end anastomosis. Interposition grafting using either a saphenous vein or PTFE graft for extensive injuries is indicated only when there appears to be a reasonable hope for salvage of the kidney. Borrowed arteries, such as the splenic artery to replace the left renal artery and the hepatic artery to replace the right renal artery, have been used rarely, but are not often indicated in hypotensive trauma patients with significant renovascular injuries from penetrating wounds.[118] In these patients and those with multiple intra-abdominal injuries or a long preoperative period of ischemia, nephrectomy may be a better

choice, as long as intraoperative palpation has confirmed a normal contralateral kidney. The survival rate of patients with injuries to the renal arteries from penetrating trauma in two older studies was approximately 87%, with renal salvage in only 30 to 40%.[116,119] In three more recent series, the survival rate was 65.1% (28/43).[7,8,77]

Diagnosis of patients with blunt injury to the renal artery is more difficult. Intimal tears in the renal arteries may result from deceleration in motor vehicle crashes, automobile–pedestrian accidents, and falls from heights. These usually lead to secondary thrombosis of the vessel and complaints of upper abdominal and flank pain as previously noted. One older literature review noted that only 30% of patients with intimal tears in the renal arteries had gross hematuria, 43% had microscopic hematuria, and 27% had no blood in the urine.[120] Hence, the diagnosis may be missed, because a CT scan may not be performed expeditiously in stable patients with normal abdominal examinations.

If either an IVP or CT scan documents occlusion of a renal artery, the surgeon must decide on the need for operation. The time interval from the episode of trauma appears to be the most critical factor in saving the affected kidney.[116] In one study, there was an 80% chance of restoring some renal function at 12 hours, but this dropped to 57% at 18 hours after the onset of occlusion.[120] In a recent series, only two of five kidneys were salvaged after attempted revascularization, with one early salvage requiring a late nephrectomy at six months for severe hypertension, leading to a long-term salvage rate of only one kidney (20%). Of interest, only three of seven patients not undergoing revascularization required late nephrectomy.[15]

If surgery is performed, extensive mobilization of the injured renal artery will usually allow a limited resection of the area of the intimal tear 2–3 cm from the abdominal aorta, with an end-to-end anastomosis for reconstruction. An alternate approach is nephrectomy, perfusion of the kidney with Euro-Collins solution, and autotransplantation.[113] The latter approach is obviously only applicable to stable patients who, ideally, have isolated injuries. Documentation of a successful result is usually not possible until acute tubular necrosis resolves over several weeks.[121]

It is of interest that case reports in the literature have documented either spontaneous recovery or the late successful revascularization of one or both kidneys after presumed blunt thrombosis of the renal artery.[122] The authors of the report suggest that attempts at late revascularization may be occasionally rewarding and advise that early nephrectomy is unnecessary because of the low incidence of chronic hypertension in cases of renal artery thrombosis.[122]

One other blunt injury to the renal artery that is detected on selective renal arteriography is an intimal defect or dissection with intact flow to the ipsilateral kidney. Some of these lesions will heal, while others may lead to an early thrombosis. The insertion of an endovascular stent across such a lesion is one current approach, particularly when the magnitude of other injuries precludes the use of anticoagulation.[123]

In summary, because of the poor renal salvage rates after blunt occlusion of the renal artery discussed above, there is decreasing interest in renal revascularization especially after a delayed diagnosis or in a patient with a unilateral injury. Therefore, patients with injuries to only one renal artery should only be considered for revascularization if they are stable and have short warm ischemia times, ideally less than 5 hours. Other patients, assuming they have a normally functioning contralateral kidney should be observed.[15] Obviously, patients with bilateral renal artery injuries or those with injuries to a solitary kidney should be strongly considered for revascularization. In addition, prolonged follow-up should be arranged for all patients, as some of them will develop hypertension.[15]

## Renovascular Injuries: Renal Vein

Although blunt avulsion injuries of the renal vein may result in exsanguination, patients with penetrating wounds may be quite stable as a result of the previously described retroperitoneal tamponade. Either compression with a finger or the direct application of vascular clamps can be used to control bleeding from a perforation of the renal vein. Lateral venorrhaphy remains the preferred technique of repair. If ligation of the right renal vein is necessary to control hemorrhage, nephrectomy should be performed either at the initial operation or at the reoperation if damage control has been necessary. The medial left renal vein can be ligated as long as the left adrenal and gonadal veins are intact.[124] Repair is preferable if feasible, as a greater frequency of postoperative renal complications has been noted in older series when ligation was performed.[125] The survival rate for patients with penetrating injuries to the renal veins has ranged from 42 to 88% in the older literature, with the difference presumably due to the magnitude and number of associated visceral and vascular injuries.[112,115,116] In three recent reviews, survival ranged from 44.2 to 70% with a mean of 60.4% (58/96).[7,8,77]

Injuries to the renal parenchyma are covered in Chap. 39.

## MANAGEMENT OF INJURIES IN ZONE 3

### Exposure and Vascular Control

The fourth major area of hematoma or hemorrhage is the pelvic retroperitoneum. In this location, the *iliac artery, iliac vein,* or *both* may be injured. The majority of injuries reported in major series are the result of penetrating trauma. It is of interest, however, that major blunt abdominal trauma or pelvic fractures, particularly of the open type, have, in the past 25 years, become a more frequent cause of occlusion or laceration of the iliac arteries than previously noted.[19–21,126,127]

If a hematoma or hemorrhage is present after penetrating trauma, compression with a laparotomy pad or finger or simply grabbing the bleeding vessels with a hand should be maintained as proximal and distal vascular control is attained. The proximal common iliac arteries are exposed by eviscerating the small bowel to the right and dividing the midline retroperitoneum over the aortic bifurcation. In young trauma patients, there is usually no adherence between the common iliac artery and vein in this location, and vascular tapes can be passed rapidly around the proximal vessels. Distal vascular control is obtained at the point at which the external iliac artery comes out of the pelvis proximal to the inguinal ligament. The artery is readily palpable under the retroperitoneum and can be rapidly elevated into the field of view with a vascular tape. The major problem in this area is continued backbleeding from the internal iliac artery. This artery can be exposed by further opening the retroperitoneum on the side of the pelvis, elevating the vascular tapes on the proximal common iliac and distal external iliac arteries, and looking for the large branch of the iliac artery that descends into the pelvis.

When bilateral iliac vascular injuries are present, one of the former coauthors of this chapter (Jon M. Burch) has used the technique of total pelvic vascular isolation. This includes proximal cross-clamping of the abdominal aorta and inferior vena cava just above their bifurcations and distal cross-clamping of both the external iliac artery and vein with one clamp on each side of the pelvis. Backbleeding from the internal iliac vessels is minimal with this approach.

Injuries to the iliac veins are exposed through a technique similar to that described for injuries to the iliac arteries. It is not usually necessary to pass vascular tapes around these vessels, however, because they are readily compressible with either spongesticks or fingers. As previously noted, the somewhat inaccessible location of the right common iliac vein has led to the suggested temporary transection of the right common iliac artery in order to improve exposure at this location.[94] Similarly, transection and ligation of the internal iliac artery on the side of the pelvis will allow improved exposure of an injured ipsilateral internal iliac vein.[128]

### Common, External, and Internal Iliac Arteries

Injuries to the common or external iliac artery should be repaired or temporarily shunted if at all possible. Ligation of either vessel in the hypotensive patient will lead to progressive ischemia of the lower extremity and the need for a high above-knee amputation or a hip disarticulation in the later postoperative course. In fact, in World War II, ligation of these vessels led to amputation rates of approximately 50%. Furthermore, in a large review by Burch et al. in the 1980s, mortality associated with this technique was 90%.[129] In patients with severe shock, insertion of a temporary intraluminal shunt is a better choice for damage control. In contrast, an injured internal iliac artery can be ligated with impunity even with injuries that occur bilaterally.

Options in the management of more stable patients with injuries to the common or external iliac artery include the following: lateral arteriorrhaphy; completion of a partial transection and end-to-end anastomosis; resection of the injured area and insertion of a saphenous vein or PTFE graft (Fig. 37-7)[130,131]; mobilization of the ipsilateral internal iliac artery to serve as a replacement for the external iliac artery; or transposition of one iliac artery to the side of the contralateral iliac artery for wounds at the bifurcation.[132]

Extensive injuries to the common or external iliac artery in the presence of *significant* enteric or fecal contamination in the pelvis remain a serious problem for the trauma surgeon. Both end-to-end repairs and vascular conduits in this location have suffered postoperative pseudoaneurysm formation and even blowouts secondary to pelvic infection from the original intestinal contamination. Therefore, the authors have occasionally avoided an end-to-end anastomosis or the insertion of a saphenous vein or PTFE graft in either the common or external iliac artery in such a situation. Rather, the artery is divided just proximal to the injury, closed with a double-running row of 4-0 or 5-0 polypropylene sutures, and covered with noninjured retroperitoneum or a vascularized pedicle of omentum. If the patient's lower extremity on the side of the ligation appears to be in jeopardy at the completion of the abdominal operation, an extra-anatomic femorofemoral crossover graft

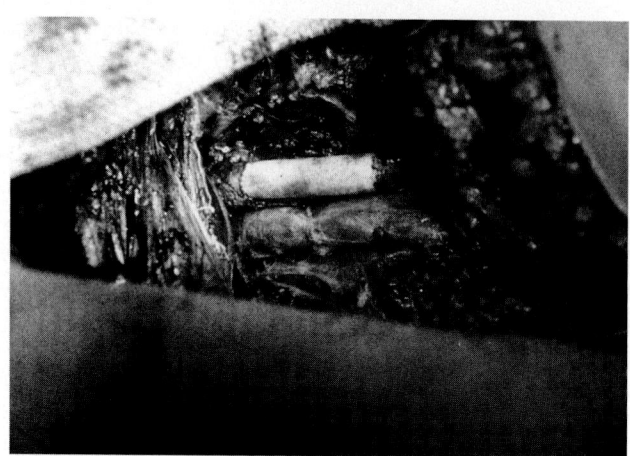

**FIGURE 37-7.** A 34-year-old man had a gunshot wound to the left external iliac artery and vein. The arterial injury was repaired with segmental resection and insertion of an 8-mm PTFE graft; the venous injury was repaired with segmental resection and an end-to-end anastomosis. *(Reproduced with permission from Feliciano DV: Injuries to the great vessels of the abdomen. In Souba WW, Fink, MP, Jurkovich GJ, et al., eds. ACS Surgery Principles and Practice. New York, NY: Web MD, 2006, p. 1250.)*

should be performed to return arterial inflow to the extremity.[24,67] If the surgeon chooses not to perform a femorofemoral crossover graft until the patient's condition has been stabilized in the surgical intensive care unit, an ipsilateral four-compartment below-knee fasciotomy should be performed, since ischemic edema below the knee will often lead to a compartment syndrome.

The survival rate among patients with injuries to the iliac arteries will vary with the number of associated injuries to the iliac vein, aorta, and vena cava, but was approximately 61% in 189 patients reviewed in four large series published from 1981 to 1990 (Table 37-7).[90,129,133,134] When patients with other vascular injuries, especially to the iliac vein, were eliminated, the survival rate among 57 patients in three series was 81% (see Table 37-7).[129,133,134] If the injury is large and free bleeding from the iliac artery into the peritoneal cavity has occurred during the preoperative period, the survival rate in one older series was only 45%.[133]

The survival rates in two recent series for patients with injuries to the common iliac artery (other vascular injuries not specified) ranged from 44.7% to 55.5% with a mean of 46.8%

(22/47; see Table 37-7).[8,77] In the same series the survival rate with injuries to the external iliac artery was a mean of 64.1% (50/78; see Table 37-7).[8,77] Finally, in another recent series, survival was correlated most heavily with preoperative base deficit, pH, and temperature. It was also noted that, even in busy trauma centers, significant delays to operative intervention occur, most notably prolonged ED time and anesthesia preparation times and these delays adversely affected patient outcome.[135] As such, every effort should be made to expedite operative intervention in a patient with a suspected abdominal vascular injury.

Blunt trauma to the iliac arteries is less common as they are protected by the bony pelvis and lie deep in the retroperitoneum. Partial transections, avulsions, or intimal injuries with secondary thrombosis have all been reported in association with pelvic fractures. Of the 10 patients with blunt thromboses reported in the literature, most have been treated with prosthetic interposition grafting, although several underwent primary repairs. Only one patient needed an amputation.[136]

## Common, External, and Internal Iliac Veins

Injuries to the common or external iliac vein are best treated either with lateral repair using 4-0 or 5-0 polypropylene suture or with ligation. Ligation in the young patient has been well-tolerated in the authors' experience and that of others if the same precautions used after ligation of the inferior vena cava are applied[137]; however, some centers strongly recommend repair rather than ligation for injuries of the common or external iliac veins.[138] When significant narrowing of the common or external iliac vein results from a lateral repair, postoperative anticoagulation is appropriate to lessen the risk of thrombosis and/or pulmonary embolism.

The survival rate of patients with injuries to the iliac veins is variable, but was approximately 70% in 404 patients reviewed in five large series published from 1981 to 1990 (see Table 37-7).[90,129,133,134,139] When patients with other vascular injuries, especially to the iliac artery, were eliminated, the survival rate among 137 patients in three series was 95% (see Table 37-7).[129,133,134] The survival rates in three recent series in patients with injuries to the iliac vein (not otherwise specified or common/external/internal combined) was a mean of 65.1% (121/186).[7,8,77]

---

**TABLE 37-7**

### Survival with Injuries to the Iliac Artery and Vein

| REFERENCE | YEAR | ILIAC ARTERY | | | ILIAC VEIN | | |
|---|---|---|---|---|---|---|---|
| | | No. Patients | No. Survivors | (%) Survival | No. Patients | No. Survivors | (%) Survival |
| Millikan et al.[133] | 1981 | 19 (6)[a] | 9 (5)[a] | 47.4 (83.3)[a] | 16 (8)[b] | 11 (8)[b] | 68.8 (100.0)[b] |
| Ryan et al.[134] | 1982 | 66 (17)[a] | 41 (15)[a] | 62.1 (88.2)[a] | 97 (48)[b] | 71 (45)[b] | 73.2 (93.8)[b] |
| Sirinek et al.[90] | 1983 | 21 | 15 | 71.4 | 28 | 23 | 82.1 |
| Burch et al.[129] | 1990 | 130 (34) | 80 (26)[a] | 61.5 (76.5)[a] | 214 (81)[b] | 153 (70)[b] | 71.5 (86.4)[b] |
| Wilson et al.[139] | 1990 | — | — | — | 49 | 24 | 48.9 |
| Davis et al.[8] | 2001 | 55 | 35 | 63.6 | 76 | 58 | 76.3 |
| Tybusrki et al.[77] | 2001 | 70 | 37 | 52.9 | 73 | 40 | 54.8 |
| Asensio et al.[7] | 2001 | — | — | — | 37 (22)[b] | 23 (18)[b] | 62.2 (81.8)[b] |
| Overall | | 361 (57)[a] | 217 (46)[a] | 60.1 (80.7)[a] | 590 (159)[b] | 403 (141)[b] | 68.3 (88.7)[b] |

[a]Isolated injury to iliac artery.
[b]Isolated injury to iliac vein.

## MANAGEMENT OF INJURIES IN THE PORTA HEPATIS

### Exposure and Vascular Control

If a hematoma or hemorrhage is present in the area of the portal triad in the right upper quadrant, there may be injury to the *portal vein*, *hepatic artery*, or *both*. Furthermore, this vascular injury may be in combination with an injury to the *common bile duct*. When a hematoma is present, the proximal hepatoduodenal ligament should be looped with a vascular tape, or a noncrushing vascular clamp should be applied (the Pringle maneuver) before the hematoma is entered. If hemorrhage is occurring, finger compression of the bleeding vessels will suffice until the vascular clamp is in place. The Pringle maneuver clamps the distal common bile duct as well as the bleeding vessels, but led to only one stricture of the common bile duct in one older series of hepatic injuries from the Ben Taub General Hospital in Houston, Texas.[140] Because of the short length of the porta in many patients, it may be difficult to place a distal vascular clamp right at the edge of the liver. In such patients, manual compression with forceps may allow distal vascular control until the area of injury can be isolated. Because of the proximity of the common bile duct, no sutures should be placed into the porta until the vascular injury is precisely defined.

Injuries to the portal vein in the hepatoduodenal ligament are isolated in much the same fashion as injuries to the hepatic artery. The posterior position of the vein, however, makes the exposure of these injuries more difficult. Mobilization of the common bile duct to the left and of the cystic duct superiorly, coupled with an extensive Kocher maneuver, will usually allow for excellent visualization of any suprapancreatic injury after proximal (and, if possible, distal) vascular control has been obtained. As with proximal wounds to the superior mesenteric artery or vein, division of the neck of the pancreas is necessary on rare occasions to visualize perforations in the retropancreatic portion of the portal vein. With the assistant compressing the superior mesenteric vein below and a vascular clamp applied to the hepatoduodenal ligament above, the surgeon should open both ends of the retropancreatic tunnel over the anterior wall of the portal vein by gently spreading a clamp or scissors. This maneuver may be prevented above by the position of the gastroduodenal artery, which should then be divided and ligated. When the tips of the surgeon's index fingers touch under the neck of the pancreas, two straight noncrushing intestinal (Glassman or Dennis) or slightly angled vascular (Glover) clamps are placed across the entire neck of the pancreas. The pancreas is divided between the clamps and retracted away until the perforations in the portal vein or proximal superior mesenteric or splenic veins are visualized.

### Hepatic Artery

Due to its small caliber, injury to any portion of the hepatic artery is rare. Indeed, because of its small size in this location, lateral repairs are often difficult and will frequently be followed by occlusion of the vessel in the postoperative period. Replacement of the injured artery with a substitute vascular conduit is rarely indicated, since most patients with a portal hematoma or hemorrhage also have significant injuries to the liver, right kidney, or inferior vena cava. As previously noted, ligation of the hepatic artery appears to be well-tolerated in the young trauma patient, even when performed beyond the origin of the gastroduodenal artery, owing to the extensive collateral arterial flow to the liver.[141–146]

Because of its rarity, few large studies have been performed on injuries to the hepatic artery. A relatively large multicenter experience was published in 1995 by Jurkovich et al., which documented the course of 99 patients with injury to the portal triad. Of this group, 28 patients had 29 injuries to a segment of the hepatic artery; 19 patients underwent ligation with eight survivors (mortality: 42%). Only one patient developed hepatic necrosis requiring debridement, and this patient had an associated extensive injury to that lobe. Seven patients had attempts at repair with only one survivor, and two other patients exsanguinated prior to therapy.[146] It should be noted, again, that selective ligation of the right hepatic artery warrants a cholecystectomy. Fortunately, injuries to the hepatic artery remain rare, and survival rates in cases of such injury are usually related to the number and magnitude of associated injuries.

### Portal Vein

As noted above, injuries to any portion of the portal vein are more difficult to manage than are injuries to the hepatic artery, owing to the posterior location of the vein, the friability of its wall, and the greater blood flow through it. Techniques for repair of the vein are varied, but lateral venorrhaphy with a 4-0 or 5-0 polypropylene suture is preferred. More extensive maneuvers that have occasionally been used with success include resection with an end-to-end anastomosis, interposition grafting, transposition of the splenic vein down to the superior mesenteric vein to replace the proximal portal vein, an end-to-side portacaval shunt, or a venovenous shunt from the superior mesenteric vein to the distal portal vein or inferior vena cava.[74,92,112,147–150] Such vigorous attempts at restoration of blood flow have resulted from the concern about viability of the midgut if the portal vein is ligated. Unfortunately, any type of portal–systemic shunt may have the undesirable effect of causing hepatic encephalopathy, since the direction of splanchnic venous flow with the shunt would mimic that in the patient with cirrhosis and hepatofugal flow in the obstructed portal vein. Ligation of the vein is compatible with survival, as both Pachter et al.[148] and Stone et al.[92] have emphasized. In the 1979 review of the literature on this subject by Pachter et al., one of six survivors of ligation of the portal vein developed portal hypertension.[148] The 1982 series by Stone et al. included nine survivors among 18 patients who underwent ligation of the portal vein.[92] In essence, ligation of the portal vein should be performed if an extensive injury is present and the patient is hypothermic and acidotic (damage control indicated). The surgeon must then be prepared to infuse tremendous amounts of fluids to reverse the transient peripheral hypovolemia secondary to splanchnic hypervolemia.[92]

To apply some perspective to the somewhat controversial area of injuries to the portal vein, a review of techniques for their management is helpful. The comprehensive older review by Graham et al. of 37 patients with injuries to the portal vein reported that 26 underwent lateral venorrhaphy, five had packing or clamping only, four (none of whom survived) had ligation, one had an end-to-end anastomosis, and one had a portacaval shunt.[91] In contrast, the aforementioned review by Stone et al. of 46 patients included 17 who had lateral venorrhaphy, 18 who had ligation (nine survived), seven in whom no repair was done, three who underwent an end-to-end anastomosis, and one who had a portacaval shunt.[92]

## TABLE 37-8

### Survival with Injuries to the Portal Vein

| REFERENCE | YEAR | NO. OF PATIENTS | NO. OF SURVIVORS | (%) SURVIVAL |
|---|---|---|---|---|
| Graham et al.[99] | 1978 | 37 | 18 | 48.6 |
| Petersen et al.[144] | 1979 | 28 | 17 | 60.7 |
| Stone et al.[102] | 1982 | 41 | 22 | 53.7 |
| Kashuk et al.[83] | 1982 | 9 | 3 | 33.3 |
| Sirinek et al.[93] | 1983 | 5 | 0 | 0.0 |
| Ivatury et al.[148] | 1987 | 14 | 7 | 50.0 |
| Overall | | 134 | 67 | 50.0 |

## TABLE 37-9

### Physiology Versus Outcome in 53 Patients with Iliac Vascular Injuries[135]

| PARAMETER | SURVIVORS[a] | DEATHS[a] | p VALUE |
|---|---|---|---|
| Initial | | | |
| OR temperature | 35.1 ± 1.47 | 33.8 ± 1.68 | 0.01 |
| OR pH | 7.27 ± 0.13 | 6.94 ± 0.20 | <0.0001 |
| OR base deficit | −7.8 ± 5.33 | −19.9 ± 7.23 | <0.0001 |
| Final | | | |
| OR temperature | 35.9 ± 1.41 | 33.6 ± 1.67 | <0.0001 |
| OR pH | 7.37 ± 0.06 | 7.22 ± 0.14 | <0.0001 |
| OR base deficit | −3.5 ± 3.51 | −9.1 ± 8.40 | <0.0005 |

[a]Values shown are number ± SD.

*(Reproduced, with permission, from Cushman JG, Feliciano DV, Renz BM, et al: Iliac vessel injury: Operative physiology related to outcome. J Trauma 42:1033, 1997.)*

## TABLE 37-10

### Physiology and Odds Ratio for Comparative Risk of Dying in 53 Patients with Iliac Vascular Injuries[135]

| PARAMETER | VALUE | ODDS RATIO | CONFIDENCE INTERVAL |
|---|---|---|---|
| Initial | | | |
| OR temperature | <34°C (93.2°F) | 3.7 | 1.0–13.9 |
| OR pH | <7.1 | 30.8 | 5.2–183.0 |
| OR base deficit | <−15.0 | 27.0 | 5.2–139.8 |
| Final | | | |
| OR temperature | <35°C (95°F) | 39.4 | 4.3–358.9 |
| OR pH | <7.3 | 14.4 | 2.8–73.0 |
| OR base deficit | <−6.0 | 11.0 | 2.2–53.8 |

*(Reproduced with permission from Cushman JG, Feliciano DV, Renz BM, et al: Iliac vessel injury: Operative physiology related to outcome. J Trauma 42:1033, 1997.)*

Ivatury has since reported on 14 patients with injuries to the portal vein, among whom exsanguination occurred in three, venorrhaphy was performed in ten (of whom six survived), and ligation was done in one (who survived).[151] Finally, Jurkovich reported on 56 injuries to the portal vein with 33 patients undergoing primary repair (42% mortality), one undergoing complex repair (died) and ten undergoing ligation (90% mortality). An additional 11 patients died before therapy. This led to an overall survival rate of 36% which is compared to the survival rate among 134 patients with injuries to the portal vein in six series from 1978 to 1987, which was approximately 50% (Table 37-8).[74,90–92,149,151]

Wounds of the retrohepatic and suprahepatic vena cava are discussed elsewhere in this text.

## ADJUNCTS TO OPERATIVE THERAPY

Essentially all patients who arrive in the operating room with active hemorrhage from a major abdominal vascular injury will require massive transfusion. It is clearly recognized that once 5 to 10 U of packed red blood cells from the blood bank are infused, many patients develop a significant coagulopathy. This problem appears to be related to the hypothermia and deficiency of coagulation factors associated with the use of stored blood, as well as to the dilution of coagulation factors associated with the massive infusion of crystalloids.[152] The major therapy for the resulting problem of non-mechanical hemorrhage is component replacement and early termination of the operative procedure. Most centers do not have fresh whole blood available and, therefore, infuse approximately 1 U of fresh frozen plasma for every 4 U of packed red blood cells infused. Conversely, in common practice, platelet packs have only been infused when nonmechanical hemorrhage is related to a platelet count of less than 50,000.[153] There is some evidence now, however, that more aggressive component therapy may be warranted, with a recent review on the topic of massive transfusion recommending 1 U of fresh frozen plasma and 1 U of platelets for each 1 U of packed red blood cells infused.[154] This same review noted that surprisingly few trauma centers have a massive transfusion protocol, so component therapy across the United States and the world continues to be somewhat variable.[154]

It is now clear that the metabolic state of the patient with an abdominal vascular injury on arrival at the trauma center is predictive of survival.[135] In the review of 53 patients with 92 iliac vascular injuries treated at Grady Memorial Hospital from 1989 to 1995, Cushman et al.

documented that an initial body temperature of less than 34°C (93.2°F), an initial arterial pH of less than 7.0, or an initial base deficit of less than −15 were all predictive of death in most patients (Table 37-9).[135] A failure to *significantly* improve any of these variables despite control of hemorrhage was ominous, as well (Table 37-10).

The combination of intraoperative hypothermia, metabolic acidosis, and coagulopathy is a lethal one and is responsible for up to 80% of all deaths in patients with abdominal vascular injuries. For this reason, surgery on individuals with such injuries should be of the damage control type (see Chap. 41). Once vascular injuries are repaired, techniques of visceral repair that decrease operating time include perihepatic packing, single-layer closure of the bowel, colonorrhaphy instead of colostomy, and packing of the pancreas rather than resection[12] Finally, the use of a temporary abdominal closure, which in its simplest form is a plastic silo sewn to the edges of the skin, will allow rapid wound closure and early transfer of the patient in shock at the completion of the operative procedure to the intensive care unit for continued resuscitation.[12,50,155]

There has also been recent interest in new methods of topical hemostasis. Hemostatics, such as fibrin glue, have long been used topically in cases of microvascular bleeding with good effect. Of interest, a recent report of ten patients, mostly with blunt hepatic trauma, showed good hemostasis of nonsurgical bleeding with a Modified Rapid Deployment Hemostatic Dressing. The Rapid Deployment Hemostat dressing (RDH, Marine

Polymer Technologies, Inc., Danvers, Ma) had been originally designed and has FDA approval for use on bleeding from an injured extremity after trauma. Nine of ten patients had complete cessation of bleeding and required no further transfusions after placement of this dressing in a damage control situation.[156]

Finally, the group at Los Angeles County/University of Southern California has begun to look at abdominal insufflation in animal models, as an adjunct to temporarily tamponade surgical bleeding. In a swine with a vena caval injury, they noted that blood loss could be reduced by 61% with insufflation of the abdomen to 20 mm Hg pressure for 15 minutes.[157] Whether this technique would be effective or safe in a hypotensive trauma patient in the field is not known.

## COMPLICATIONS

The complications of vascular repairs in the abdomen are much the same as those seen in the extremities. They include such problems as thrombosis, dehiscence of a suture line, and infection.[158] Occlusion is not uncommon when small, vasoconstricted vessels, such as the renal artery or superior mesenteric artery, undergo lateral arteriorrhaphy. In such patients, it may be valuable to perform a second-look operation

within 12 to 24 hours after the patient's temperature, coagulation abnormalities, and blood pressure have returned to normal. When this is done, correction of a vascular thrombosis may be successful.

Dehiscence of vascular suture lines in the abdomen has occurred in two locations in the authors' experience, and both have been previously discussed. First, a substitute vascular conduit inserted in the superior mesenteric artery near a pancreatic injury may be disrupted if a small pancreatic leak occurs in the postoperative period. For this reason, the proximal anastomosis of such a graft should be on the infrarenal abdominal aorta, far away from the pancreas, as previously noted. Second, the dehiscence of end-to-end anastomoses and conduit suture lines in the iliac arteries can be avoided by limiting the extent of repair if there is significant enteric or fecal contamination in the pelvis and considering early extra-anatomic bypass if the patient's limb is threatened.

Finally, a vascular complication unique to the abdomen is the postoperative development of vascular–enteric fistulas. This will occur most commonly in patients who have anterior aortic repairs, aortic grafts, or grafts to the superior mesenteric artery from the aorta. Again, this problem can be avoided by proper coverage of suture lines on the aorta with retroperitoneal tissue or a viable omental pedicle,[99] and on the recipient vessel with mesentery.

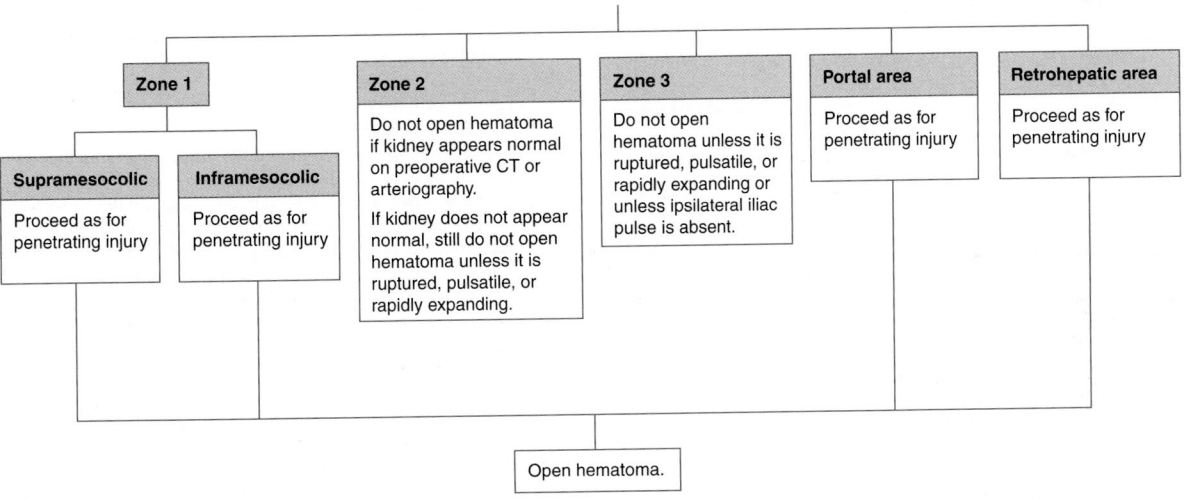

**FIGURE 37-8.** Patient with blunt abdominal trauma and intra-abdominal hematoma at laparotomy.

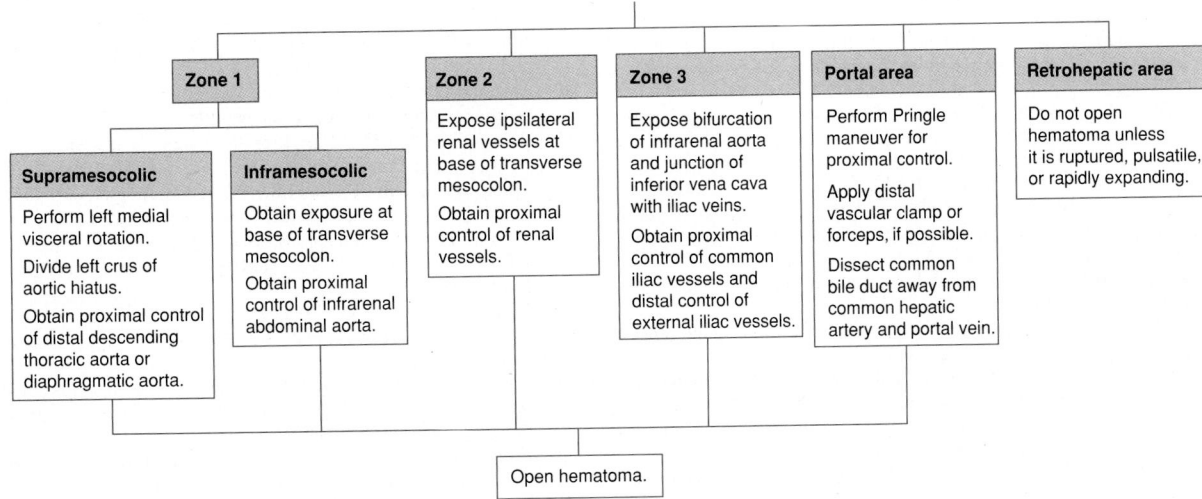

**FIGURE 37-9.** Patient with penetrating abdominal wound and intra-abdominal hematoma at laparotomy.

# SUMMARY

Abdominal vascular injuries are commonly seen in patients with penetrating wounds to the abdomen. They present with either a contained retroperitoneal, mesenteric, or portal hematoma or with active hemorrhage. When tamponade is present, proximal and distal vascular control should be obtained before opening the hematoma causing the tamponade. If active hemorrhage is present, direct compression of the bleeding vessels with a finger, hand, laparotomy pad, or spongestick at the site of injury is necessary until proximal and distal vascular control can be attained. Vascular repairs are generally performed with polypropylene sutures and can range from simple arteriorrhaphy or venorrhaphy to the insertion of substitute vascular conduits, much as in vascular injuries in the extremities. If hemorrhage can be rapidly controlled and there are no significant associated injuries, many patients with major abdominal vascular injuries can be salvaged with the techniques described in this chapter.[24,61,67,159]

# REFERENCES

1. DeBakey ME, Simeone FA: Battle injuries of the arteries in World War II: An analysis of 2,471 cases. *Ann Surg* 123:534, 1946.
2. Hughes CW: Arterial repair during the Korean War. *Ann Surg* 147:555, 1958.
3. Rich NM, Baugh JH, Hughes CW: Acute arterial injuries in Vietnam: 1,000 cases. *J Trauma* 10:359, 1970.
4. Rapaport A, Feliciano DV, Mattox KL: An epidemiologic profile of urban trauma in America—Houston style. *Tex Med* 78:44, 1982.
5. Feliciano DV, Bitondo CG, Mattox KL, et al.: Civilian trauma in the 1980's. A 1-year experience with 456 vascular and cardiac injuries. *Ann Surg* 199:717, 1984.
6. Mattox KL, Feliciano DV, Burch J, et al.: Five thousand seven hundred sixty cardiovascular injuries in 4459 patients. Epidemiologic evolution 1958 to 1987. *Ann Surg* 209:698, 1989.
7. Asensio JA, Chahwan S, Hanpeter D, et al.: Operative management and outcome of 302 abdominal vascular injuries. *Am J Surg* 180:528, 2001.
8. Davis TP, Feliciano DV, Rozycki GS, et al.: Results with abdominal vascular trauma in the modern era. *Am Surg* 67:565, 2001.
9. Fischer RP, Miller-Crotchett P, Reed RL II: Gastrointestinal disruption: The hazard of nonoperative management in adults with blunt abdominal injury. *J Trauma* 28:1445, 1988.
10. Cox CF: Blunt abdominal trauma. A 5-year analysis of 870 patients requiring celiotomy. *Ann Surg* 199:467, 1984.
11. Spjut-Patrinely V, Feliciano DV: Data from Ben Taub General Hospital, Houston, Texas, July 1985 to June 1988, unpublished.
12. Feliciano DV, Burch JM, Spjut-Patrinely V, et al.: Abdominal gunshot wounds: An urban trauma center's experience with 300 consecutive patients. *Ann Surg* 208:362, 1988.
13. Swana HS, Cohn SM, Burns GA, et al.: Renal artery pseudoaneurysm after blunt abdominal trauma: Case report and literature review. *J Trauma* 40:459, 1996.
14. Jebara VA, El Rassi I, Achouh PE, et al.: Renal artery pseudoaneurysm after blunt abdominal trauma. *J Vasc Surg* 27:362, 1998.
15. Haas CA, Dinchman KH, Nasrallah PF, et al.: Traumatic renal artery occlusion: A 15-year review. *J Trauma* 45:557, 1998.
16. Pezzella AT, Griffen WO Jr, Ernst CB: Superior mesenteric artery injury following blunt abdominal trauma: Case report with successful primary repair. *J Trauma* 18:472, 1978.
17. Michaels AJ, Gerndt SJ, Taheri PA, et al.: Blunt force injury of the abdominal aorta. *J Trauma* 41:105, 1996.
18. Siavelis HA, Mansour MA: Aortoiliac dissection after blunt abdominal trauma: Case report. *J Trauma* 43:862, 1997.
19. Nitecki S, Karmeli R, Ben-Arien Y, et al.: Seatbelt injury to the common iliac artery: Report of two cases and review of the literature. *J Trauma* 33:935, 1992.
20. Buscaglia LC, Matolo N, Macbeth A: Common iliac artery injury from blunt trauma: Case reports. *J Trauma* 29:697, 1989.
21. Roth SM, Wheeler JR, Gregory RT, et al.: Blunt injury of the abdominal aorta: A review. *J Trauma* 42:748, 1997.
22. Dajee H, Richardson IW, Iype MO: Seatbelt aorta: Acute dissection and thrombosis of the abdominal aorta. *Surgery* 85:263, 1979.
23. Warrian RK, Shoenut JP, Iannicello CM, et al.: Seatbelt injury to the abdominal aorta. *J Trauma* 28:1505, 1988.
24. Feliciano DV: Abdominal vascular injuries. *Surg Clin North Am* 68:741, 1988.
25. Courcy PA, Brotman S, Oster-Granite ML, et al.: Superior mesenteric artery and vein injuries from blunt abdominal trauma. *J Trauma* 24:843, 1984.
26. Matsubara J, Seko T, Ohta T, et al.: Traumatic aneurysm of the abdominal aorta with acute thrombosis of bilateral iliac arteries. *Arch Surg* 118:1337, 1983.
27. Bass A, Papa M, Morag B, et al.: Aortic false aneurysm following blunt trauma of the abdomen. *J Trauma* 23:1072, 1983.
28. Feliciano DV: Pitfalls in the management of peripheral vascular injuries. *Probl Gen Surg* 3:101, 1986.
29. Rich NM, Hobson RW II, Fedde CW: Vascular trauma secondary to diagnostic and therapeutic procedures. *Am J Surg* 128:715, 1974.
30. McDonald PT, Rich NM, Collins GJ Jr, et al.: Vascular trauma secondary to diagnostic and therapeutic procedures: Laparoscopy. *Am J Surg* 135:651, 1978.
31. Kozloff L, Rich NM, Brott WH, et al.: Vascular trauma secondary to diagnostic and therapeutic procedures: Cardiopulmonary bypass and intraaortic balloon assist. *Am J Surg* 140:302, 1980.
32. Ingram WL, Feliciano DV, Renz BM, et al.: Blood pressure in the emergency department in patients with abdominal vascular injuries: Effect on management and prognostic valve. Presented at the 55th Annual Meeting, American Association for the Surgery of Trauma, Halifax, Nova Scotia, Canada, September 27–30, 1995.
33. Eachempati SR, Robb T, Ivatury RR, et al.: Factors associated with mortality in patients with penetrating abdominal vascular trauma. *J Surg Res* 108:222, 2002.
34. Rozycki GS, Feliciano DV, Schmidt, JA, et al.: The role of surgeon-performed ultrasound in patients with possible cardiac wounds. *Ann Surg* 223:737, 1996.
35. Sisley AC, Rozycki GS, Ballard RB, et al.: Rapid detection of traumatic effusion using surgeon-performed ultrasonography. *J Trauma* 44:291, 1998.
36. Rozycki GS, Ballard RB, Feliciano DV, et al.: Surgeon-performed ultrasound for the assessment of truncal injuries. Lessons learned from 1540 patients. *Ann Surg* 228:557, 1998.
37. Rozycki GS, Cava RA, Tchorz KM: Surgeon-performed ultrasound imaging in acute surgical disorders. *Curr Prob Surg* 38:141, 2001.
38. Nagy KK, Brenneman FD, Krosner SM, et al.: Routine preoperative "one-shot" intravenous pyelography is not indicated in all patients with penetrating abdominal trauma. *J Am Coll Surg* 185:530, 1997.
39. Sclafani SJA: The diagnosis of bilateral renal artery injury by computed tomography. *J Trauma* 26:295, 1986.
40. Panetta T, Sclafani SJA, Goldstein AS, et al.: Percutaneous transcatheter embolization for massive bleeding from pelvic fractures. *J Trauma* 25:1021, 1985.
41. Chesnut RM: Avoidance of hypotension: Conditio sine qua non of successful severe head-injury management. *J Trauma* 42:S4, 1997.
42. Kaweski SM, Sise MJ, Virgilio RW: The effect of prehospital fluids on survival in trauma. *J Trauma* 30:1215, 1990.
43. Bickell WH, Wall MJ Jr, Pepe PE, et al.: Immediate versus delayed fluid resuscitation for hypotensive patients with penetrating torso injuries. *N Engl J Med* 331:1105, 1994.
44. Wall MJ Jr, Granchi T, Lisum K, et al.: Delayed versus immediate fluid resuscitation in patients with penetrating trauma: Subgroup analysis. Presented at the 55th Annual Meeting, American Association for the Surgery of Trauma, Halifax, Nova Scotia, Canada, September 27–30, 1995.
45. Mattox KL, Bickell W, Pepe PE, et al.: Prospective MAST study in 911 patients. *J Trauma* 29:1104, 1989.
46. Feliciano DV, Bitondo CG, Cruse PA, et al.: Liberal use of emergency center thoracotomy. *Am J Surg* 152:654, 1986.
47. Asensio JA, Wall M, Minei J, et al.: Practice management guidelines for emergency department thoracotomy. *J Am Coll Surg* 193:303, 2001.
48. Dutky PA, Stevens SL, Maull KI: Factors affecting rapid fluid resuscitation with large-bore introducer catheters. *J Trauma* 29:856, 1989.
49. Gentilello LM: Practical approaches to hypothermia. In Maull KI, Cleveland HC, Feliciano DV, et al. eds. *Advances in Trauma Critical Care*. St. Louis: Mosby, 1994, vol. 9, p. 39.
50. Feliciano DV, Rozycki GS: The management of penetrating abdominal trauma. In Cameron JL, et al. eds. *Advances in Surgery*. St. Louis: Mosby, 1995, vol. 28, p 1.
51. Samkaran S, Lucas C, Walt AJ: Thoracic aortic clamping for prophylaxis against sudden cardiac arrest during laparotomy for acute massive hemoperitoneum. *J Trauma* 15:290, 1975.
52. Ledgerwood AM, Kazmers M, Lucas CE: The role of thoracic aortic occlusion for massive hemoperitoneum. *J Trauma* 16:610, 1976.
53. Wiencek RG Jr, Wilson RF: Injuries to the abdominal vascular system: How much does aggressive resuscitation and prelaparotomy thoracotomy really help? *Surgery* 102:731, 1987.

54. Accola KD, Feliciano DV, Mattox KL, et al.: Management of injuries to the superior mesenteric artery. *J Trauma* 26:313, 1986.

55. Henry SM, Duncan AO, Scalea TM: Intestinal Allis clamps as temporary vascular control for major retroperitoneal venous injury. *J Trauma* 51:170, 2001.

56. Moore EE, Cogbill TH, Jurkovich GJ, et al.: Organ injury scaling III: Chest wall, abdominal vascular, ureter, bladder, and urethra. *J Trauma* 33:337, 1992.

57. DeBakey ME, Creech O Jr., Morris GC Jr: Aneurysm of thoracoabdominal aorta involving the celiac superior mesenteric and renal arteries. Report of four cases treated by resection and homograft replacement. *Ann Surg* 144:549, 1956.

58. Elkins RC, DeMeester TR, Brawley RK: Surgical exposure of the upper abdominal aorta and its branches. *Surgery* 70:622, 1971.

59. Mattox KL, McCollum WB, Jordan GL Jr, et al.: Management of upper abdominal vascular trauma. *Am J Surg* 128:823, 1974.

60. Fry WR, Fry RE, Fry WJ: Operative exposure of the abdominal arteries for trauma. *Arch Surg* 126:289, 1991.

61. Feliciano DV: Injuries to great vessels of the abdomen. In Holcroft JW, ed. *Scientific American Surgery.* Trauma Section. New York: Scientific American, 1998, p. 1.

62. Conn J Jr, Trippel OH, Bergan JJ: A new atraumatic aortic occluder. *Surgery* 64:1158, 1968.

63. Mahoney BD, Gerdes D, Roller B, et al.: Aortic compressor for aortic occlusion in hemorrhagic shock. *Ann Emerg Med* 13:29, 1984.

64. Veith FJ, Gupta S, Daly V: Technique for occluding the supraceliac aorta through the abdomen. *Surg Gynecol Obstet* 151:426, 1980.

65. Illig KA, Green RM, Ouriel K, et al.: Primary fibrinolysis during supraceliac aortic clamping. *J Vasc Surg* 25:244, 1997.

66. Kavic SM, Atweb N, Ivy ME, et al.: Celiac axis ligation after gunshot wound to the abdomen: Case report and literature review. *J Trauma* 50:738, 2001.

67. Feliciano DV: Approach to major abdominal vascular injury. *J Vasc Surg* 7:730, 1988.

68. Farret A, da Ros CT, Fischer CAC, et al.: Suprarenal aorta reconstruction using saphenous spiral graft: Case report. *J Trauma* 37:144, 1994.

69. Accola KD, Feliciano DV, Mattox KL, et al.: Management of injuries to the suprarenal aorta. *Am J Surg* 154:613, 1987.

70. Oyama M, McNamara JJ, Suehiro GT, et al.: The effects of thoracic aortic cross-clamping and declamping on visceral organ blood flow. *Ann Surg* 197:459, 1983.

71. Lim RC Jr, Trunkey DD, Blaisdell FW: Acute abdominal aortic injury. An analysis of operative and postoperative management. *Arch Surg* 109: 706, 1974.

72. Buchness MP, LoGerfo FW, Mason GR: Gunshot wounds of the suprarenal abdominal aorta. *Ann Surg* 42:1, 1976.

73. Brinton M, Miller SE, Lim RC Jr, et al.: Acute abdominal aortic injuries. *J Trauma* 22:481, 1982.

74. Kashuk JL, Moore EE, Millikan JS, et al.: Major abdominal vascular trauma—a unified approach. *J Trauma* 22:672, 1982.

75. Millikan JS, Moore EE: Critical factors in determining mortality from abdominal aortic trauma. *Surg Gynecol Obstet* 160:313, 1985.

76. Jackson MR, Olson DW, Beckett WC, et al.: Abdominal vascular trauma. *Am Surg* 58:622, 1992.

77. Tyburski JG, Wilson RF, Dente C, et al.: Factors affecting mortality rates in patients with abdominal vascular injuries. *J Trauma* 50:1020, 2001.

78. Coimbra R, Hoyt D, Winchell R, et al.: The ongoing challenge of retroperitoneal vascular injuries. *Am J Surg* 172:541, 1996.

79. Roth SM, Wheeler JR, Gregory RT, et al.: Blunt injury of the abdominal aorta: A review. *J Trauma* 42:748, 1997.

80. Asensio JA, Petrone P, Kimbrell B, et al.: Lessons learned in the management of thirteen celiac axis injuries. *South Med J* 98:462, 2005.

81. Schreiber JP, Fritz Angle J, Matsumoto AH, et al.: Acute visceral ischemia occurring subsequent to blunt abdominal trauma: Potential culpability of median arcuate ligament compression. *J Trauma* 45:404, 1998.

82. Fullen WD, Hunt J, Altemeier WA: The clinical spectrum of penetrating injury to the superior mesenteric arterial circulation. *J Trauma* 12:656, 1972.

83. Asensio JA, Britt LD, Borzotta A, et al.: Multi-institutional experience with the management of superior mesenteric artery injuries. *J Am Coll Surg* 193:354, 2001.

84. Ledgerwood A, Lucas CE: Survival following proximal superior mesenteric artery occlusion from trauma. *J Trauma* 14:622, 1974.

85. Reilly PM, Rotondo MF, Carpenter JP, et al.: Temporary vascular continuity during damage control: Intraluminal shunting for proximal superior mesenteric artery injury. *J Trauma* 39:757, 1995.

86. Nolan BW, Gabram SG, Schwartz RJ, et al.: Mesenteric injury from blunt abdominal trauma. *Am Surg* 61:501, 1995.

87. Pennington CJ, Gwaltney N, Sweitzer D: Microvascular repair of jejunal and ileal vessels for near complete mesenteric avulsion after seat-belt injury. *J Trauma* 48:327, 2000.

88. Graham JM, Mattox KL, Beall AC Jr, et al.: Injuries to the visceral arteries. *Surgery* 84:835, 1978.

89. Lucas AE, Richardson JD, Flint LM, et al.: Traumatic injury of the proximal superior mesenteric artery. *Ann Surg* 193:30, 1981.

90. Sirinek KR, Gaskill HV III, Root HD, et al.: Truncal vascular injury-factors influencing survival. *J Trauma* 23:372, 1983.

91. Graham JM, Mattox KL, Beall AC Jr: Portal venous system injuries. *J Trauma* 18:419, 1978.

92. Stone HH, Fabian TC, Turkleson ML: Wounds of the portal venous system. *World J Surg* 6:335, 1982.

93. Donahue TK, Strauch GO: Ligation as definitive management of injury to the superior mesenteric vein. *J Trauma* 28:541, 1988.

94. Salam AA, Stewart MT: New approach to wounds of the aortic bifurcation and inferior vena cava. *Surgery* 98:105, 1985.

95. Burch JM, Feliciano DV, Mattox KL, et al.: Injuries of the inferior vena cava. *Am J Surg* 156:548, 1988.

96. Ravikumar S, Stahl WM: Intraluminal balloon catheter occlusion for major vena cava injuries. *J Trauma* 25:458, 1985.

97. Linker RW, Crawford FA Jr, Rittenbury MS, et al.: Traumatic aortocaval fistula: Case report. *J Trauma* 29:255, 1989.

98. Feliciano DV, Burch JM, Mattox KL, et al.: Balloon catheter tamponade in cardiovascular wounds. *Am J Surg* 160:583, 1990.

99. Bunt TJ, Doerhoff CR, Haynes JL: Retrocolic omental pedicle flap for routine plication of abdominal aortic grafts. *Surg Gynecol Obstet* 158:591, 1984.

100. Munez AE, Haynes JH: Delayed abdominal aortic rupture in a child with a seat-belt sign and review of the literature. *J Trauma* 56:194, 2004.

101. Siavelis HA, Mansour MA: Aortoiliac dissection after blunt abdominal trauma: Case Report. *J Trauma* 43:862, 1997.

102. Cheek RC, Pope JC, Smith HF, et al.: Diagnosis and management of major vascular injuries: A review of 200 operative cases. *Am Surg* 41:755, 1975.

103. Carrillo EH, Ginzburg E, Namias N, et al.: Spontaneous rupture of abdominal aortic aneurysms in patients with non-related blunt traumatic injuries. *Kentucky Med* 15:64, 1997.

104. Ali MR Jr, Norcross ED, Brothers TE: Iliac and femoral artery occlusion by thromboemboli from an abdominal aortic aneurysm in the setting of blunt abdominal trauma. *J Vasc Surg* 27:545, 1998.

105. Nigro J, Velmahos GC: Delayed reconstruction of the inferior vena cava with prosthetic graft due to postligation edema. *Contemp Surg* 54:25, 1999.

106. Ivy ME, Possenti P, Atweh N, et al.: Ligation of the suprarenal vena cava after a gunshot wound. *J Trauma* 45:630, 1998.

107. Oldhafer KJ, Frerker M, Winkler M, et al.: Complex inferior vena cava and renal vein reconstruction after abdominal gunshot injury. *J Trauma* 46: 721, 1999.

108. Nigro J, Velmahos GC: Delayed reconstruction of the inferior vena cava with prosthetic graft due to postligation edema. *Contemp Surg* 54:25, 1999.

109. Frezza EE, Valenziano CP: Blunt traumatic avulsion of the inferior vena cava. *J Trauma* 42:141, 1997.

110. Graham JM, Mattox KL, Beall AC Jr: Traumatic injuries of the inferior vena cava. *Arch Surg* 113:413, 1978.

111. Kudsk KA, Bongard F, Lim RC Jr: Determinants of survival after vena caval injury: Analysis of a 14-year experience. *Arch Surg* 119:1009, 1984.

112. Wiencek RG, Wilson RF: Abdominal venous injuries. *J Trauma* 26: 771, 1986.

113. Klein SR, Baumgartner FJ, Bongard FS: Contemporary management strategy for major inferior vena caval injuries. *J Trauma* 37:35, 1994.

114. Porter JM, Ivatury RR, Islam SZ, et al.: Inferior vena cava injuries: Noninvasive follow-up of venorrhaphy. *J Trauma* 42:913, 1997.

115. McAninch JW, Carroll PR: Renal trauma: Kidney preservation through improved vascular control. *J Trauma* 22:285, 1985.

116. Carroll PR, McAninch JW, Klosterman P, et al.: Renovascular trauma: Risk assessment, surgical management, and outcome. *J Trauma* 30:547, 1990.

117. Gonzalez RP, Falimirski M, Holevar MR, et al.: Surgical management of renal trauma: Is vascular control necessary? *J Trauma* 47:1039, 1999.

118. Barone GW, Kahn MB, Cook JM, et al.: Traumatic left renal artery stenosis managed with splenorenal bypass: Case report. *J Trauma* 30:1594, 1990.

119. Brown MF, Graham JM, Mattox KL, et al.: Renovascular trauma. *Am J Surg* 140:802, 1980.

120. Maggio AJ Jr, Brosman S: Renal artery trauma. *Urology* 11:125, 1978.

121. Frassinelli P, Pasquale MD, Reckard C, et al.: Bilateral renal artery thrombosis secondary to blunt trauma: Case report and review of the literature. *J Trauma* 42:330, 1997.

122. Greenholz SK, Moore EE, Peterson NE, et al.: Traumatic bilateral renal artery occlusion: Successful outcome without surgical intervention. *J Trauma* 26:941, 1986.

123. Villas PA, Cohen G, Putnam SG III, et al.: Wallstent placement in a renal artery after blunt abdominal trauma. *J Trauma* 46:1137, 1999.

124. James EC, Fedde CW, Khuri NT, et al.: Division of the left renal vein: A safe surgical adjunct. *Surgery* 83:151, 1978.

125. Rastad J, Almgren B, Bowald S, et al.: Renal complications to left renal vein ligation in abdominal aortic surgery. *J Cardiovasc Surg* 25:432, 1984.
126. Rothenberger DA, Fischer RP, Perry JF Jr: Major vascular injuries secondary to pelvic fractures: An unsolved clinical problem. *Am J Surg* 136:660, 1978.
127. Tsai FC, Wang CC, Fang JF, et al.: Isolated common iliac artery occlusion secondary to atherosclerotic plaque rupture from blunt abdominal trauma: Case report and review of the literature. *J Trauma* 42:133, 1997.
128. Vitelli CE, Scalea TM, Phillips TF, et al.: A technique for controlling injuries of the iliac vein in the patient with trauma. *Surg Gynecol Obstet* 166:551, 1988.
129. Burch JM, Richardson RJ, Martin RR, et al.: Penetrating iliac vascular injuries: Experience with 233 consecutive patients. *J Trauma* 30:1450, 1990.
130. Feliciano DV, Mattox KL, Graham JM, et al.: Five-year experience with PTFE grafts in vascular wounds. *J Trauma* 25:71 1985.
131. Landercasper RJ, Lewis DM, Snyder WH: Complex iliac arterial trauma: Autologous or prosthetic vascular repair. *Surgery* 114:9, 1993.
132. Landreneau RJ, Mitchum P, Fry WJ: Iliac artery transposition. *Arch Surg* 124:978, 1989.
133. Millikan JS, Moore EE, Van Way CW III, et al.: Vascular trauma in the groin: Contrast between iliac and femoral injuries. *Am J Surg* 142:695, 1981.
134. Ryan W, Snyder W III, Bell T, et al.: Penetrating injuries of the iliac vessels. *Am J Surg* 144:642, 1982.
135. Cushman JG, Feliciano DV, Renz BM, et al.: Iliac vessel injury: Operative physiology related to outcome. *J Trauma* 42:1033, 1997.
136. Tsai FC, Wang CC, Fang JF, et al.: Isolated common iliac artery occlusion secondary to atherosclerotic plaque rupture from blunt abdominal trauma: Case report and review of the literature. *J Trauma* 42:133, 1997.
137. Mullins RJ, Lucas CE, Ledgerwood AM: The natural history following venous ligation for civilian injuries. *J Trauma* 20:737, 1980.
138. Agarwal N, Shah PM, Clauss RH, et al.: Experience with 115 civilian venous injuries. *J Trauma* 22:827, 1982.
139. Wilson RF, Wiencek RG, Balog M: Factors affecting mortality rate with iliac vein injuries. *J Trauma* 30:320, 1990.
140. Feliciano DV, Mattox KL, Jordan GL Jr, et al.: Management of 1000 consecutive cases of hepatic trauma (1979–1984). *Ann Surg* 204:438, 1986.
141. Mays ET, Wheeler CS: Demonstration of collateral arterial flow after interruption of hepatic arteries in man. *N Engl J Med* 290:993, 1974.
142. Mays ET, Conti S, Fallahzadeh H, et al.: Hepatic artery ligation. *Surgery* 86:536, 1979.
143. Flint LM Jr, Polk HC Jr: Selective hepatic artery ligation: Limitations and failures. *J Trauma* 19:319, 1979.
144. Bryant DP, Cooney RN, Smith JS, et al.: Traumatic proper hepatic artery occlusion: Case report. *J Trauma* 50:735, 2001.
145. Graham DD, May AK, Moore M, et al.: Management of hepatic artery injury: Case report. *Am Surg* 63:327, 1997.
146. Jurkovich GJ, Hoyt DB, Moore FA, et al.: Portal Triad Injuries. *J Trauma* 39:426, 1995.
147. Busuttil RW, Storm FK, Wilbur BG: Use of the splenic vein in the reconstruction of portal and superior mesenteric veins after traumatic injury. *Surg Gynecol Obstet* 145:591, 1977.
148. Pachter HL, Drager S, Godfrey N, et al.: Traumatic injuries of the portal vein. *Ann Surg* 189:383, 1979.
149. Petersen SR, Sheldon GF, Lim RC Jr: Management of portal vein injuries. *J Trauma* 19:616, 1979.
150. Busuttil RW, Kitahama A, Cerise E, et al.: Management of blunt and penetrating injuries to the porta hepatis. *Ann Surg* 191:641, 1980.
151. Ivatury RR, Nallathambi M, Lankin DH, et al.: Portal vein injuries. Noninvasive follow-up of venorrhaphy. *Ann Surg* 206:733, 1987.
152. Ferrara A, MacArthur JD, Wright HK, et al.: Hypothermia and acidosis worsen coagulopathy in the patient requiring massive transfusion. *Am J Surg* 160:515, 1990.
153. Reed RL II, Ciavarella D, Heimbach DM, et al.: Prophylactic platelet administration during massive transfusion. *Ann Surg* 203:40, 1986.
154. Malone DL, Hess JR, Fingerhut A: Massive transfusion practices around the globe and a suggestion for a common massive transfusion protocol. *J Trauma* 60:S91, 2006.
155. Feliciano DV, Burch JM: Towel clips, silos, and heroic forms of wound closure. In Maull KI, Cleveland, HC, Feliciano DV, et al. eds. *Advances in Trauma and Critical Care.* Chicago: Year Book Medical Publishers, 1991, p. 231.
156. King DR, Cohn SR, Proctor KG, et al.: Modified rapid deployment hemostat bandage terminates bleeding in coagulopathic patients with sever visceral injuries. *J Trauma* 57:756, 2004.
157. Sava J, Velmahos GC, Karaiskakis M, et al.: Abdominal insufflation for prevention of exsanguination. *J Trauma* 54:590, 2003.
158. Feliciano DV: Management of infected grafts and graft blowout in vascular trauma patients. In Flanigan DP, et al. eds. *Civilian Vascular Trauma.* Philadelphia: Lea & Febiger, 1992, p. 447.
159. Feliciano DV: Truncal vascular trauma. In Callow AD, Ernst CB, eds. *Vascular Surgery: Theory and Practice.* Stamford, CT: Appleton & Lange, 1995, p. 1059.

# Commentary ■ BRENT EASTMAN ■ SUNIL RAYAN

Abdominal vascular injuries are among the most challenging and potentially devastating problems facing the trauma surgeon today. Some of these injuries will result in ischemia to visceral organs which can create a cascade of deleterious physiological events. It is the combination of difficult exposures, and hemorrhage with hypovolemic shock, sometimes coupled with the insult of visceral ischemia, that makes abdominal vascular injuries so challenging.

This chapter by Drs. Dente and Feliciano provides a clear and logical approach to each vascular anatomical region and structure in the abdomen. The reader is clearly led through the anatomy, physiology, and operative interventions by surgeons who "have been there before…" In fact, much of the clinical expertise put forth in this chapter derives from the personal experience of Dr. Feliciano, about which he has published many sentinel articles which are appropriately referenced in this chapter. We fundamentally agree with the surgical approaches and procedures as outlined in this chapter, and will therefore limit our commentary to some issues not specifically discussed here which have served us well in our own trauma center.

The approach to major vascular injuries at our institution is that the initial resuscitation, assessment, and management be done by our small cadre of trauma surgeons whose practices focus exclusively on trauma, critical care, and acute care general surgery. Many vascular injuries are appropriately managed by these trauma surgeons; however, for more complex vascular injuries, we have two Board Certified vascular surgeons who are also an integral part of our trauma team, along with our interventional radiologists. This system has allowed us immediate access to experienced vascular surgeons who are doing major vascular surgical procedures virtually every day, and they are teamed with an experienced trauma surgeon. Their combined talents and expertise have resulted in excellent outcomes with complex abdominal vascular injuries.

In cases of multiorgan injury, complex vascular reconstruction may be required as detailed in this chapter. We often choose to perform extra-anatomic bypass, especially in the setting of a contaminated field, which is frequently the case. Patients, who have had severe intra-abdominal injury, as noted, will often require "damage control" procedures such as leaving the abdomen open with a "silo," or "second-look" re-operations to assess intestinal viability. We strongly endorse this approach. In extreme cases, we use activated Factor VII, and Factor specific intervention with thromboelstogram (TEG) to assist with control of hemorrhage in addition to vigorous resuscitation with crystalloid and blood products. We always prepare for blood salvage and auto transfusion with a high volume warming infusion machine.

The advances and availability of new imaging technology play an integral role in the management of complex trauma in our institution. After the initial evaluation by the trauma surgeon, patients with suspected intra-abdominal injury are immediately evaluated by a non-invasive imaging modality. If the patient is hemodynamically unstable, FAST ultrasound is performed in the trauma resuscitation room. The surgeon can then decide if the patient warrants immediate operative intervention, or a more detailed imaging study. Many of our patients undergo rapid CT in a high-resolution scanner with intravenous contrast. The image quality is so high that CT and CT angiogram scans have essentially obviated the use of invasive angiography as a diagnostic imaging tool unless a therapeutic vascular intervention is needed. High-resolution CT can reliably diagnose subtle and complex vascular injuries such as pseudo-aneurysms, dissections, thrombosis, and active hemorrhage. However, detailed imaging should *only* be utilized if the patient is hemodynamically stable enough to justify an interval in the CT scanner. This option is far more prevalent in patients presenting with blunt, as opposed to penetrating, trauma.

If the patient is hemodynamically stable, our vascular surgeons can employ either endovascular or open surgical solutions. Both our interventional radiologists and vascular surgeons use a flat-panel low-radiation angiographic suite to diagnose and manage vascular injuries. In the case of blunt organ trauma, pelvic vascular injury, or isolated visceral arterial injury, endovascular techniques are often employed. Splenic, hepatic, and pelvic embolizations are frequently performed to treat hemorrhage in hemodynamically stable patients. The established technology of using stents covered with polyester or polytetrafluoroethylene (PTFE) to treat abdominal aortic aneurysms has been successfully applied to traumatic vascular injuries in order to achieve a rapid and minimally invasive solution, especially in a patient with other injuries. Thoracic aortic, abdominal aortic, and visceral arterial stent grafting techniques have all been described in the literature and are employed at our institution to selectively treat vascular trauma. It is important to note that these minimally invasive methods should never preclude open repair should that become necessary. Immediate operation, rapid surgical exposure, control of hemorrhage, and direct vascular repair remain the "gold standard" of the management of abdominal vascular injuries.

Exposure for injuries of the retro hepatic cava may present the surgeon with major technical challenges. In some instances, we believe that the extension of a midline laparotomy incision to a median sternotomy incision provides optimal exposure of this anatomy to facilitate vascular isolation of the liver. We, therefore, ensure that our trauma surgeons are facile with performing a median sternotomy incision. It has proven helpful to have our trauma surgeons to occasionally scrub with our cardiac surgeons who perform median sternotomies several times a day for elective cardiac surgery. Another rare injury, but an operative approach of historical interest to me (ABE) is an injury to the renal artery of a solitary kidney. We, Drs. Lim; Eastman; Blaisdell, described "Renal autotransplantation. Adjunct to repair of renal vascular lesion," in *Arch Surg*. 1972; 105: 847–852. It behooves trauma surgeons dealing with abdominal vascular injuries to be familiar with this approach, which has obviously been refined since our initial description in 1972, as one possible surgical option in an attempt to salvage a solitary kidney.

The margin of error is narrow and the consequences of failure can be devastating when dealing with abdominal vascular injuries, hence the importance of this definitive chapter.

# Pelvic Fractures

*Thomas M. Scalea* ■ *Deborah M. Stein* ■ *Robert V. O'Toole*

Pelvic fractures represent a significant challenge for physicians caring for injured patients. The complex anatomic relations that exist within the bony pelvis put a myriad of structures at risk when the pelvis is fractured. The force required to fracture a pelvis is substantial. Thus, these injuries often occur in conjunction with serious injuries to other important structures. An increased recognition of pelvic fractures as a marker of injury severity, as well as improved algorithms for resuscitation, skeletal fixation, and critical care monitoring, have done much to advance the care of these severely injured patients. There is not, however, clear consensus as to the best management strategy for such patients. Decision-making can be problematic, and poor decision-making early on may seriously compromise a patient's chances for survival.

There are a large number of therapies within the clinician's armamentarium to care for these patients. These multiple options can create confusion in management, particularly at centers where the injury is less commonly seen. However, there are clearly defined principles, particularly in the acute management upon which most experienced clinicians would agree. The specifics of implementing some of these principles remain controversial and a subject of some discussion in the literature. Further, the optimal therapy for any patient is based both on the thorough knowledge of the magnitude of the physiologic insult and the potential resources available at that particular institution. Skilled judgment is therefore needed in order to select the most appropriate therapy in a timely fashion. The goal of this chapter is to provide the reader with a thoughtful discussion on the issue of pelvic fractures and present the rationales for the various diagnostic and treatment options that exist. We also present the specific algorithm for treatment of pelvic fractures at our institution.

## HISTORY

Surgeons caring for injury have recognized the importance of pelvic fractures as a cause for morbidity and mortality for over 100 years. Prior to 1900, the mortality rate for pelvic fractures was 80%, with the primary cause of death being blood loss. As blood loss in most pelvic fractures is self-limited, the advent of resuscitation fluids and the availability of banked blood radically reduced the mortality from pelvic fractures. Over the last 50 years, various modalities to treat hemorrhage from pelvic fractures that were not self-limited have continued to evolve. Utilization of pelvic binders and angiographic embolization of pelvic bleeders is now commonplace in most trauma centers. Although there is some disagreement about the order or timing of these interventions, it does seem that the combination of these therapies has continued to help reduce mortality from pelvic fracture bleeding. In fact, death from hemorrhage is now relatively rare and is usually associated with laceration of a large vessel. Thus, much of the management problems now have to do with associated life-threatening injuries and limiting the morbidity from the fracture.

The last of the major advances in the management of pelvic fractures has been the evolution of skeletal fixation. Most centers practice aggressive definitive fracture fixation as soon as possible in the patient's course. In some centers, definitive rigid fixation occurs within 24 to 72 hours. External fixation is sometimes used as a temporizing measure, allowing patients to receive the advantages of rigid skeletal fixation without the associated morbidity of a major operation soon after injury. This may then be used as a bridge to definitive therapy or may be used as definitive skeletal fixation in some cases.

Although management techniques for the pelvic fractures continue to evolve, the most important advancement in the treatment of patients has been the adoption of a multidisciplinary approach. General surgeons, orthopedic surgeons, emergency physicians, and interventional radiologists all have talents that are important in the care of acutely injured patients with pelvic fractures. It is only through cooperative efforts that the evolution can continue in a positive direction.

## PELVIC OSSEOUS ANATOMY

A ring of bone consisting of two innominate bones and the sacrum forms the pelvis. This pelvic ring is an excellent hard tissue marker that, when correctly assessed clinically and radiologically, can help identify the local blunt trauma pathology at the time of impact.

There is no inherent stability to the bones of the pelvis. The innominate bones and the sacrum are held in a structural unit primarily by the ligaments of the pelvis, which are among the strongest in the body. The sacroiliac (SI) joints gain their structural strength from the nearby anterior and posterior SI ligaments. The posterior ligaments are extremely strong across the entire posterior portion of the pelvis from iliac crest to iliac crest, as they incorporate the posterior surface of the sacrum. In addition, strong, shorter ligaments attach the medial portion of the posterior iliac wing directly to the sacrum, just posterior to the SI joints. There are also strong SI ligaments across the anterior portion of these joints as well as sturdy ligamentous complexes that connect both pubic bones across the cartilaginous pubic symphysis. These ligamentous complexes provide stability for the articulations of the pelvis.

There are two primary ligaments of the "pelvic floor," the sacrospinous and sacrotuberous ligaments (Fig. 38-1). These ligaments provide additional reinforcement to the pelvic floor by reinforcing the contents of the abdominal cavity with patients in the upright position and by providing additional stability and strength. The sacrospinous and sacrotuberous ligaments run from the lateral borders of the sacrum to the ischial spine and the ischial tuberosity, respectively. An understanding of this ligamentous and skeletal geometry provides the clinician with an appreciation of the pelvis in its normal state. This must be combined with an appreciation of both vascular and neuroanatomy (Figs. 38-2 and 38-3). More importantly, such anatomic knowledge combined with the history of the injury mechanism allows accurate diagnosis, help identify relevant therapeutic interventions, and predict indices with regard to associated injury patterns and resuscitative requirements.

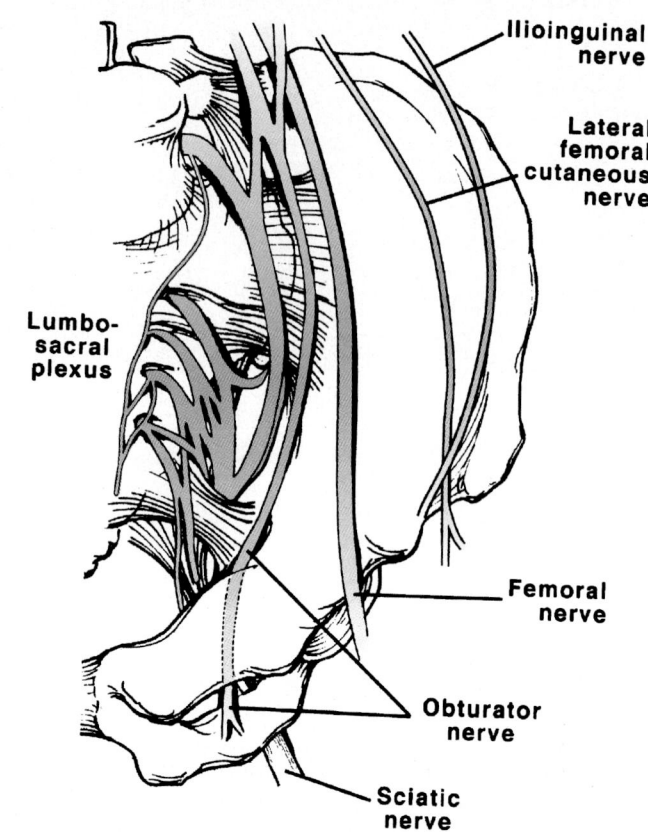

**FIGURE 38-2.** Neuroanatomy of the pelvis.

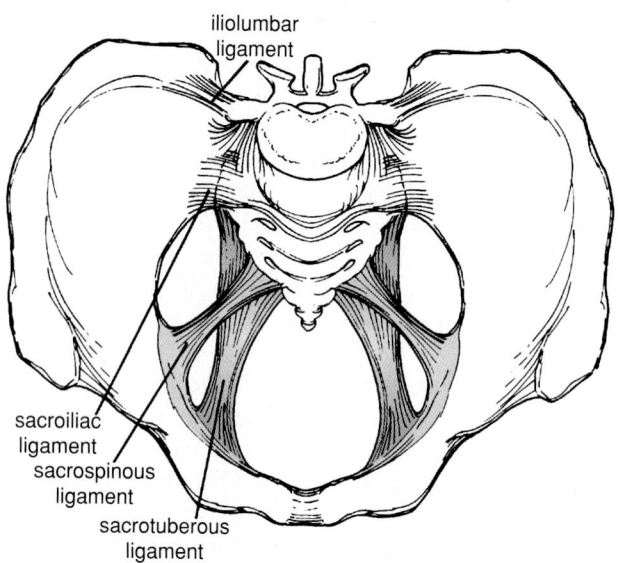

**FIGURE 38-1.** Ligamentous anatomy of the pelvis.

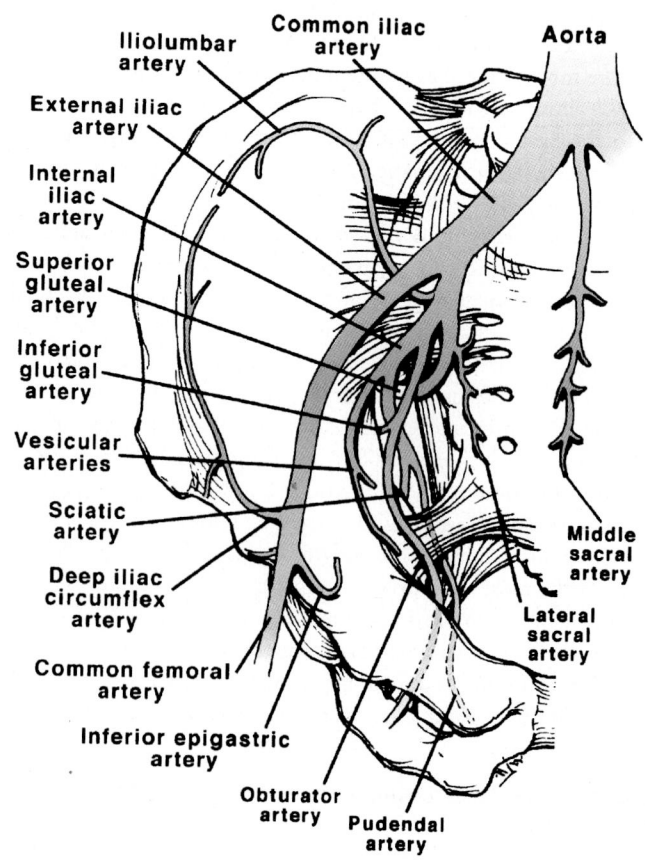

**FIGURE 38-3.** Vascular anatomy of the pelvis.

## BIOMECHANICS OF PELVIC FRACTURE

To understand pelvic injury, it is useful to consider three major vectors of force and the disruption they cause in the pelvic ring. First, and most common, are the lateral compression (LC) vectors, usually applied from the lateral side of the pelvic ring such as by a T-bone or intersectional motor vehicle crash (MVC), a pedestrian being struck from the side, or a fall from a height with the person landing on his or her side (Fig. 38-4).

Lateral compression produces an acute shortening of the diameter across the pelvis. Although LC fractures may be markers for severe injury to the human body, they typically do not destroy the ligamentous integrity of the pelvic ligaments and, hence, do not often "open the pelvis." Instead, they manifest as acute shortening of the arterial and venous vascular triplexes, primarily in the posterior pelvis. Although local vascular injuries with these types of pelvic fractures may occur from direct intrusion of bone fragments, this type of vector is generally forgiving to the vascular structures within the pelvic ring and typically do not produce large volume blood loss. Patients with this type of injury may, in fact, be critically injured, but it is usually from associated injuries to the solid visceral contents of the abdomen, to the thoracic contents (including lungs and aorta), and to the cervical spine.

The second most frequent force applied to the pelvic ring is one from an anterior or posterior (AP) direction, either via direct contact with the iliac spine or through secondary force transmitted from the femur, as in the person whose lower extremities are acutely spread apart in a motorcycle accident. This "AP" force causes the pelvic diameter to widen. In this situation, the pelvic injury may not be associated with a fracture and can involve ligament disruption only. The effect on the patient may be more severe than that of a major fracture. This pelvic injury usually manifests itself as a widened pubic symphysis and SI joints.

As the AP force increases, there is a progressive disruption of the ligaments of the pelvis. First, the symphyseal ligaments are disrupted (or there are fractures of the anterior pelvis). This is typically accompanied with disruption of the pelvic floor (sacrospinous and sacrotuberous ligaments) and the anterior SI ligaments creating an open book that is hinged only on the posterior SI ligaments (so called AP2 injury). These AP2 injuries are differentiated from AP3 injuries because the strong posterior ligaments remain intact (Fig. 38-5). Extremely high-energy subsets of this type of injury may also disrupt the posterior SI ligaments creating complete disassociation of the hemipelves from the axial skeleton (internal hemipelvectomy). This injury is often associated in its severe forms with substantial vascular damage secondary to the close anatomic relationships of the internal iliac artery and the accompanying veins with the posterior ligaments. Occasionally, the common or external iliac artery is injured as well. These injuries are frequently accompanied by a lumbosacral plexus injury. Other severe manifestations of this AP compression injury may include bilateral versions of either anterior or total SI disruption.

Vertical shear injuries are often seen in an individual who jumps from a height and lands on an extended lower extremity (Fig. 38-6). However, it may also occur as the result of structural collapses or in an individual who is subjected to this force while standing on an extended lower extremity, such as a motorcyclist at a stop. The vertical shear injury usually disrupts all the restraining

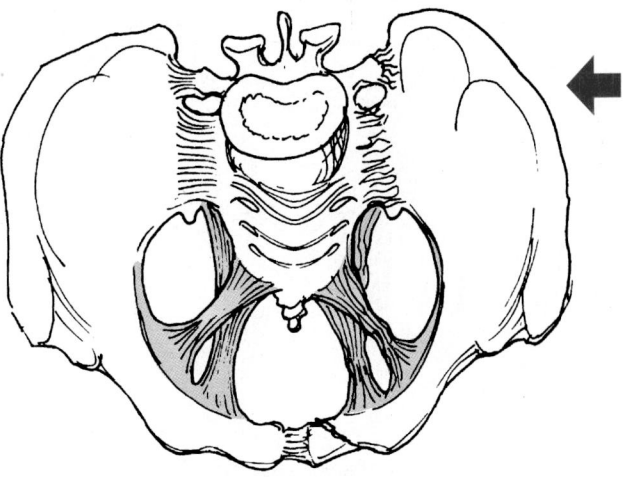

**lateral compression type I**

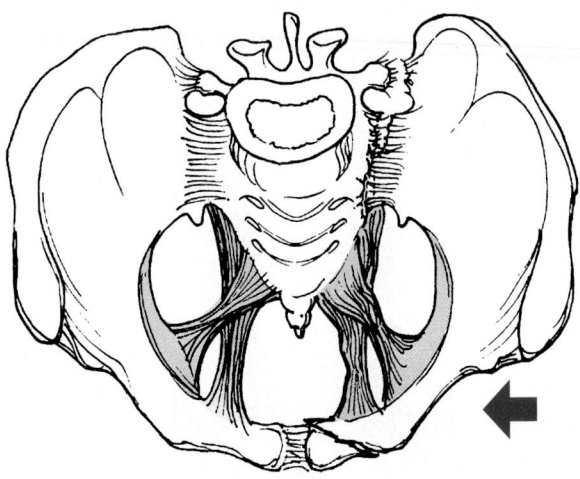

**lateral compression type II**

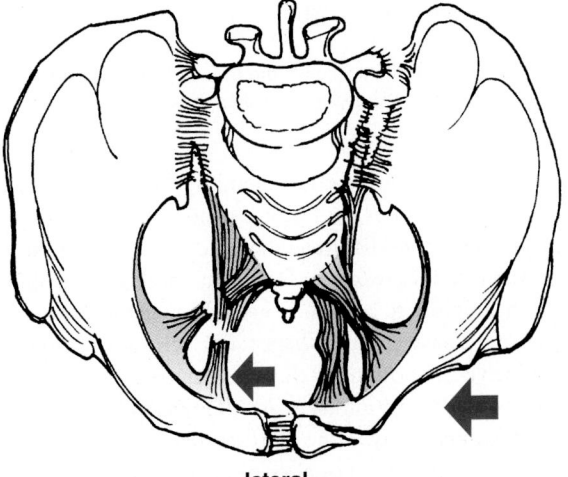

**lateral compression type III**

**FIGURE 38-4.** Lateral compression fractures are usually caused by T-bone motor vehicle crashes, pedestrians being struck from the side, or a fall from a height and produce acute shortening of the diameter across the pelvis.

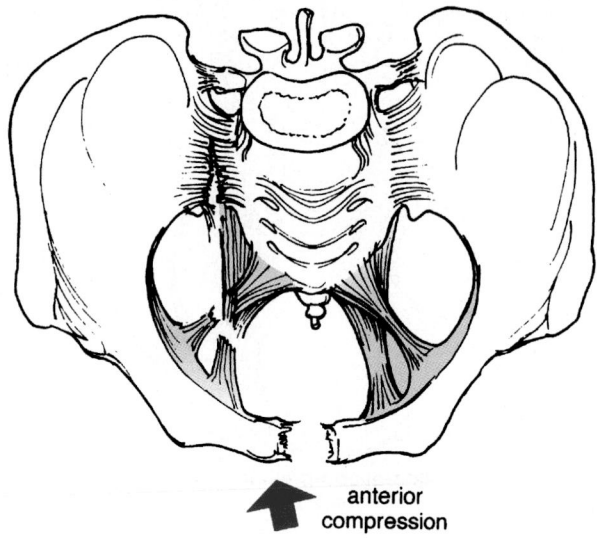

**FIGURE 38-5.** Anteroposterior compression injuries are usually caused by motor vehicle crashes from the front such as a crash in which force is transmitted through the femurs into the pelvis, or a straddle injury such as a motorcycle crash.

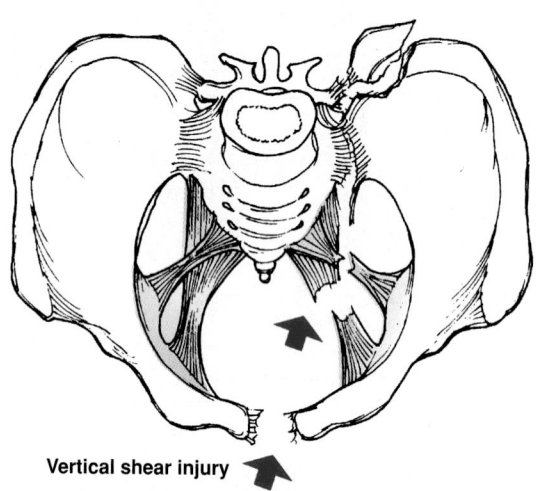

**FIGURE 38-6.** Vertical shear injuries are usually caused by a fall from a height and landing on extended lower extremities.

ligaments of the hemipelvis, including the symphyseal, sacrospinous, sacrotuberous, and SI ligaments. Although this may render the hemipelvis mechanically unstable as in the more severe AP compression injuries, work by Dalal and colleagues has shown the vertical shear injury to be slightly more forgiving with regard to the amount of associated hemorrhage.[1] The vertical displacement of the hemipelvis is shortening the vascular tree making it less likely to be disrupted, in contrast to an AP injury which places the vessels under tension. Only in the most severe cases does it involve major arterial injuries of the posterior pelvic vascular complexes.

It should be noted that most patients do not fall strictly into any of these three categories. Patients do not typically have a pure vector of injury that is 90º to the pelvis in an LC injury. As such the injury patterns can be a combination of LC and AP characteristics. In addition, radiographs are static images and may underestimate the degree of bony description at the time of impact. Serious LC fractures can damage the SI joints, sacrum, and symphysis. The pelvis will then open and may be incorrectly diagnosed as an open-book fracture. These injuries often behave clinically like an AP fracture so the distinction may be unimportant.

## PELVIC FRACTURE CLASSIFICATION

There are several pelvic fractures classifications. Early attempts concentrated on the anatomy and the location of the fracture with regard to the named structure that was injured. Later work by Tile concentrated on the exact rotational component of injury to address long-term reconstructive plans.[2,3] This system is based on pelvic stability: type A, stable both rotationally and vertically; type B, stable vertically but unstable rotationally; and type C, unstable both vertically and rotationally and is used at many centers.

Our center tends to use the classification of Young and Burgess[4–7] in assessing patients. This classification was described at our center and is based on early work of Tile and Pennal,[8,9] as later modified by Young and Burgess.[4–7] Understanding what happened to the pelvic ring at the moment of impact is quite valuable in the assessment of the relative risk of pelvic hemorrhage and associated injuries. Tile and Pennal regarded pelvic injury in terms of shortening of the pelvic diameter, implosion of the pelvic ring, and opening of the pelvic diameter from AP compression or vertical injury to the pelvis.[8,9] Young and Burgess describe these classifications, subdividing LC and AP compression injuries, according to increasing levels of energy and resultant associated risk.[4–7]

Using this system, pelvic fractures are subdivided according to the degree of displacement and/or degree of ligamentous instability (Table 38–1).[7] Dalal and colleagues showed this classification to be valuable in predicting pelvic fracture-related hemorrhage and other injuries,[1] although subsequent studies have not been as successful at confirming the ability of this classification to predict mortality and injury pattern.[10,11] The authors of this chapter have found it beneficial in assessing the risk of substantial local vascular injury.

**TABLE 38-1**

| Classification of Pelvic Fractures | |
|---|---|
| **Anteroposterior Compression** | |
| Type I | Disruption of the public symphysis of <2.5 cm of distansis; no significant posterior pelvic injury |
| Type II | Disruption of the pubic symphysis of >2.5 cm, with tearing of the anterior sacroiliac and sacrospinous and sacrotuberous ligaments |
| Type III | Complete disruption of the pubic symphysis and posterior ligament complexes, with hemipelvic displacement |
| **Lateral Compression** | |
| Type I | Posterior compression of the sacroiliac joint without ligament disruption; oblique pubic ramus fracture |
| Type II | Rupture of the posterior sacroiliac ligament; pivotal internal rotation of hemipelvis on the anterior SI joint with a crush injury of the sacrum and an oblique pubic ramus fracture |
| Type III | Finding in type II injury with evidence of an anteroposterior compression injury to the contralateral hemipelvis |

*Source: Young MR, Burgess AR, Brumback RJ, Poka A. Palvic fractures: Value of plan radiography in early assessment and management. Radiology 160:445, 1988.*

## DIAGNOSIS OF PELVIC FRACTURE

The presence of a pelvic fracture should be strongly suspected based on mechanism of injury and physical findings. All patients sustaining high-energy blunt trauma should be assumed to have a pelvic fracture until proven otherwise. Often, if awake and alert, patients will complain of pelvic pain. However, complaints may not be specific and may include reports of hip or lower abdominal pain. Some mechanisms are much more likely to produce pelvic fractures than are others. Vehicular crashes are the most common cause of pelvic injury in most environments.[12–16] These are followed in order of frequency by automobile–pedestrian collisions, falls from a height, motorcycle crashes, and crush injuries (Table 38–2).[13,17]

Physical findings seen commonly in patients with pelvic fractures include abrasions, contusions, or hematomas over the bony prominences of the pelvis. An examination of the perineum is important to identify scrotal or vulvar hematoma. A rectal exam should be performed, as well as a vaginal exam in women. These are particularly important in patients with perineal lacerations, as rectal or vaginal lacerations often accompany open pelvic fractures. A more careful and detailed examination such as a complete pelvic exam or a sigmoidoscopy may be necessary in some patients. This requires positioning that may be extremely painful in the awake patient. A complete evaluation may require general anesthesia.

A clinical examination should be performed to assess pelvic ring stability, prior to films being taken. This involves pushing both sides of the pelvis gently toward the midline with the examiner's hand on the interior superior iliac spine and then externally rotating the pelvis (again, with the examiner's hands on the anterior iliac spine). This simple exam combined with a single x-ray usually identifies those pelvic injuries that are most often associated

with substantial morbidity or mortality. It is important to emphasize that this maneuver must be done gently and not repeatedly by every person who is involved in the patients' care. Techniques for detecting pelvic instability that cause motion of fracture fragments such as rocking the pelvis are mentioned only to be condemned. They offer little additional information and risk destabilizing a stable hematoma and renewing active bleeding in a patient that otherwise had stopped. In a patient with a known pelvic injury by radiograph, the exam rarely provides any useful clinical information.

A single AP pelvic film is generally performed as one of the screening radiographs in most patients with blunt trauma. This is often done routinely when patients have significant blunt injury. However, data suggest that routine pelvic x-rays may not be necessary in a patient with a normal level of consciousness. Salvino and associates reviewed 779 patients who presented to their institution with blunt trauma.[18] All were awake and alert. Of the 779, 743 had no complaints of pain and a negative physical exam for pelvic tenderness. Only three of these patients were found to have pelvic fractures. These were all simple anterior rami fractures that required no treatment (a 0.4% incidence of missed pelvic fractures). All of the 36 patients who had more severe pelvic fractures had either pain or tenderness or both. It is important to emphasize that all of these patients were awake and alert and able to verbalize complaints. The authors concluded that routine radiographic examination of the pelvis is not necessary. Other authors have reached similar conclusions with reported sensitivity and specificity of 98 and 94%, respectively, for detection of posterior fractures with physical examination alone.[19] While this may be a reasonable policy for that subset of patients, it should not be applied universally. Patients who are unable to provide a good history (e.g., those who are impaired or have brain injuries), patients who are hemodynamically unstable, or patients who have injuries such as lower extremity fractures that may distract them from pelvic symptoms should undergo a single AP x-ray of the pelvis as part of their initial trauma evaluation.

Once a pelvic fracture has been identified, and the patient is hemodynamically stable, the next series of films generally obtained are inlet–outlet films. These radiographs are shot at 45° to the patient. The inlet film provides information about the AP displacement of the injury, such as posterior migration of the hemipelvis (Fig. 38-7). The outlet film provides information about vertical displacement and is particularly useful for diagnosing vertical shear injuries (Fig. 38-8). It should be noted that due to the orientation of the pelvis in the body, it is common to see some superior displacement of the hemipelvis with AP injuries, and the initial AP x-ray, but a vertical shear injury should have significant superior displacement on the outlet view.

Fracture orientation provides an important clue to the vector of the force causing injury. LC injuries tend to have a pelvic fracture demonstrating a transverse pattern (i.e., it crosses one of the anterior elements of the pelvis), while AP injuries tend to have vertical fractures or the ramus or symphysis disruptions. After the anterior pelvis is examined on x-ray, visual examination should include the integrity of the iliac wings bilaterally and, most importantly, the SI joints and the sacral foramina to identify subtle changes in sacral architecture that are best projected on the outlines of sacral foramen. The injury is defined by the side of the

### TABLE 38-2

| Mechanism of Injury of Pelvic Fracture | | |
|---|---|---|
| | **N** | **%** |
| Motor vehicle crash | 1532 | 44 |
| Automobile-pedestrian collision | 1007 | 29 |
| Falls from a height | 449 | 13 |
| Motorcycle crashes | 253 | 7 |
| Crush injuries | 89 | 3 |
| Other | 130 | 4 |
| Total | 3460 | 100 |

Source: Moreno C, Moore EE, Rosenberg A, et al.: Hemorrhage with major pelvic fracture: A multispecialty challenge. J Trauma 26:987, 1986. Dalal SA, Burgess AR, Siegel JH, et al: Pelvic fracture in multiple trauma: Classification by mechanism is key to pattern of organ injury, resuscitative requirements, and outcome. J Trauma 29:891, 1989. Evers BM, Cryer HM, Miller FB: Pelvic fracture hemorrhage: Priorities in management. Arch Surg 124:422, 1989. Burgess AR, Eastridge BJ, Young JWR: Pelvic ring disruptions: Effective classification system and treatment protocols. J Trauma 30:848, 1990. Klein SR, Sarovan RM, Raumgarten F, Bongard FS: Management strategy of vascular injuries associated with pelvic fractures. J Cardiovasc Surg 33:349, 1992. Gruen GS, Leit ME, Gruen RJ, Pietzman AB: The acute management of hemodynamically unstable multiple trauma patients with pelvic ring fractures. J Trauma 36:706, 1994. Demetriades D, Karaiskakis M, Toutouzas K, et al. Pelvic fractures: epidemiology and predictors of associated abdominal injuries and outcomes. J Am Coll Surg 195:1, 2002.

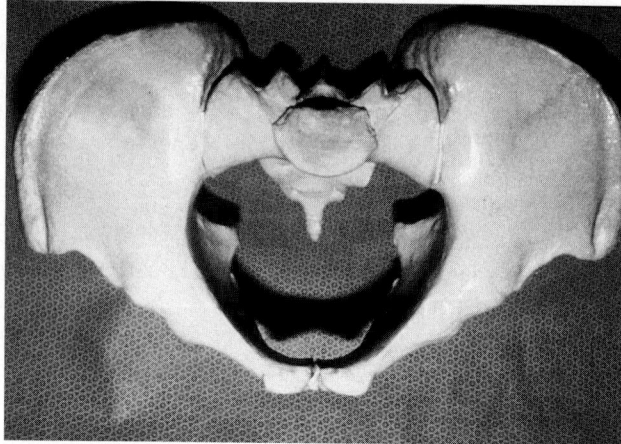

**FIGURE 38-7.**    Inlet view of the pelvis. Inlet views are taken at a 45° angle to the pelvis and give additional information about the sacrum and the anterior pubic bones.

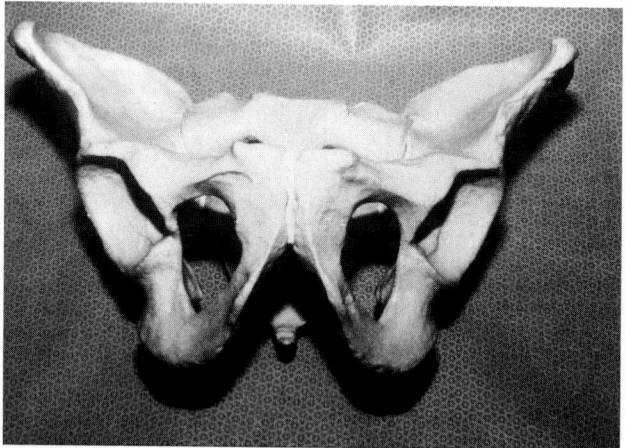

**FIGURE 38-8.**    Outlet view of the pelvis. Outlet views are taken at a 45° angle to the pelvis and provide additional information about the sacrum and SI joints.

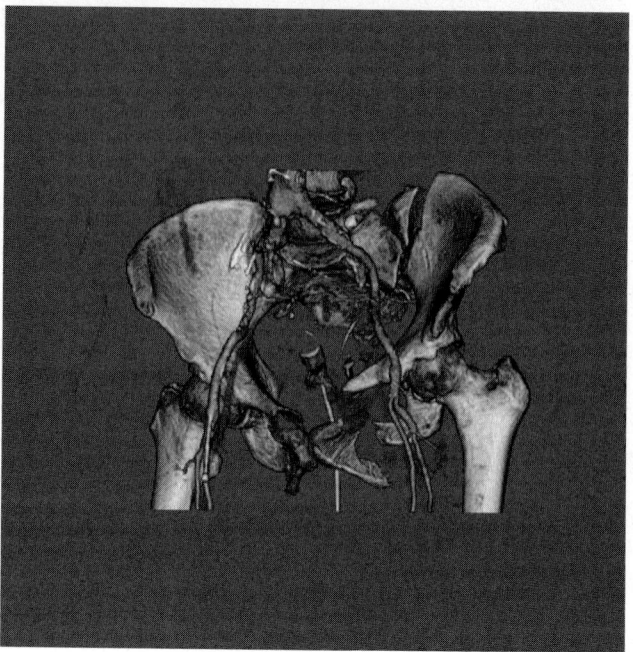

**FIGURE 38-9.**    The 3-D reconstruction of the patient with an LCII pelvic fracture allows for greater delineation of exact bony anatomy.

posterior injury, so the patient can have ipsilateral or contralateral ramus fractures. The acetabulae must also be carefully inspected as pelvic fractures can coexist with acetabular fractures. Judet views, which are AP views obtained with the patient's body rotated 45° to the long axis, are utilized in the evaluation of acetabular fractures and may not be needed unless there is an acetabular fracture.

Computed tomography (CT) scanning is now a routine part of the radiographic evaluation of patients with pelvic fractures. Its greatest utility may be in defining occult bony instability that is not apparent on clinical examination or the plain radiographs mentioned earlier.[17,20–23] In addition, it often adds significant information about the magnitude of the pelvic injury[23–25] and aids surgical planning. Plain radiographs, even when supplemented with inlet and outlet views, may not provide sufficient information about the posterior elements of the bony pelvis. CT scanning with 2 to 3mm cuts can provide this additional information. CT is particularly helpful in evaluating the integrity of the SI ligament complexes, the degree of posterior displacement and may demonstrate subtle sacral fractures. Finally, CT may be helpful in defining the degree

of bony pelvic instability. Pelvic instability is generally defined as the absence of an intact bony anatomy or the presence of posterior SI ligament insufficiency, enough to allow migration of the hemipelvis of more than 1 cm. There are a number of studies that suggest that in patients who are going to have a CT scan, plain radiographs in the stable patient with a suspected pelvic fracture may not be needed.[24,26] CT is a snapshot in time, just as any radiograph, and the displacement observed in the scanner, especially if the patient has a binder on, may be much less than was present at the time of injury.

Three-dimensional CT reconstruction is now available in many centers (Fig. 38-9). Although this does not replace the need for regular radiographs and standard CT scanning, it may be helpful in some cases, such as planning an operative approach, but this has been largely unstudied to date.

Not every patient with a pelvic fracture, however, requires CT scanning. This will depend on the patient's physiologic status, the pelvic pathology being evaluated, the need for other CT imaging, and the sophistication of the trauma center caring for the patient. In a high-volume center, simple AP films and physical examination may make the diagnosis of complete disruption of the hemipelvis. In this patient, CT scanning is not required before intervention. However, virtually all stable patients with a pelvic fracture will require abdominal CT scanning at some time because pelvic fractures are a marker for the magnitude of retroperitoneal injury and are often associated with intraperitoneal visceral injury. Even in the face of a negative abdominal ultrasound (US), abdominal CT scanning can be very helpful in patients with pelvic fractures, as a significant number of patients may have significant intra-abdominal injuries without hemoperitoneum.[27] CT of the pelvis can be accomplished at the time of abdominal CT, even if patients have already undergone intervention such as external fixation, application of the pelvic clamp, and/or pelvic angiography.

## MANAGEMENT

### Initial Management

The initial management of patients with pelvic fractures is not substantially different from any other injured patient; however, there are several issues that deserve some additional comment. As noted in Chaps. 10 and 11, airway management is the highest priority. Extra consideration should be given to definitive airway management for patients who have sustained serious pelvic injury. These patients are at high risk for developing hemodynamic instability and may do so with little warning. In addition, the evaluation process often requires transport to numerous parts of the hospital such as the x-ray suite, CT scanner, and angiography. Given the logistics of many hospitals, these may be located in areas that are remote from the resuscitation area. Definitive airway management early in the patient's course, while he or she is still located in the resuscitation suite, limits the possibility of the patient's requiring urgent airway management in a place where there may not be adequate personnel or equipment to handle this situation.

In addition, these patients may develop a unique type of respiratory failure.[28] As patients bleed into their retroperitoneum, intra-abdominal pressure rises, limiting thoracic excursion (see Chap. 40). Hypoxia may occur relatively late. These patients often present with tachypnea and relative hypercarbia because they can no longer move their diaphragms against the increased abdominal pressure. These findings are not specific and may be subtle. Hypoxia can then occur quickly, followed shortly by respiratory arrest. Thus, the clinician should have a low threshold for intubation in the patient with a significant pelvic fracture, particularly if accompanied by blood loss.

Once the airway is secure, a rapid assessment of the adequacy of oxygenation and ventilation becomes the highest priority. Approximately 20% of all patients with pelvic fractures have concomitant chest injuries.[29] Obviously, immediately life-threatening thoracic injuries must be managed expeditiously. In addition, a number of other potentially life-threatening injuries may be identified; evaluation for these injuries must be kept in mind and incorporated into the subsequent patient evaluation.

Circulation, or the adequacy of peripheral oxygen delivery, is the next highest priority. All patients with pelvic fractures are at risk for hemorrhage, which may be caused by the pelvic fracture or related to associated extrapelvic injuries. It is crucial to remember that the blood pressure and pulse rate are extremely crude methods of evaluating perfusion.[30] Though patients may be normotensive, the sophisticated clinician should recognize that all patients with pelvic fractures are at significant risk of shock even if blood loss is not obvious (see Chap. 9). All patients with pelvic fractures should have large-bore intravenous access established. If this is not reliably possible using peripheral veins, intravenous access should be obtained with large-bore central catheters. These lines should be located in upper-extremity peripheral veins or within the superior mediastinal venous structures. Because pelvic venous injury may accompany pelvic fractures, groin lines and lower extremity cutdowns should be avoided. Central venous oxygen saturation is an accurate method of estimating acute blood loss.[31] Thus, if a subclavian or internal jugular line is placed, obtaining a venous blood gas at the time of line placement may be very helpful in guiding therapy. In addition, arterial blood gases obtained in the emergency department (ED) are extremely valuable in assessing perfusion deficits as well as estimating the need for subsequent transfusion.[32] In general, a base deficit more negative than –6 is a cause for concern (see Chap. 12).

It is important to anticipate the need for blood administration. The mean 24-hour blood requirement in patients with pelvic fractures who are admitted with clear signs of shock is over 5 U, and approximately 20% of those patients will require more than 15 U.[29] Patients with pelvic fractures should always have blood available. In addition, it is important to anticipate the need for platelet and factor replacement (see Chap. 13). The blood bank should be alerted to have both platelets and fresh frozen plasma readily available. In addition to the consumptive coagulopathy that often occurs after 10 U of blood transfusion (see Chap. 57), the hypothermia and shock often seen in these patients can worsen any existing coagulopathy.[33] Thus, crystalloid and blood products should be delivered via a level 1 warmer or other similar device. Temperature must be monitored and hypothermia treated. If hypothermia becomes significant (35°C [95°F]) despite all efforts at therapy, consideration should be given to alternative means of treatment such as arteriovenous or veno-venous rewarming (see Chap. 49).

The remainder of the primary survey (a brief neurologic assessment and complete exposure of the patient) should be rapidly completed and the secondary survey begun. For patients with pelvic fractures, this should be directed toward identifying the source of hemorrhage. There are five cavities into which patients can lose large quantities of blood: the thorax, abdomen, muscle compartments, retroperitoneum, and "the street" (see Chaps. 10, 24, and 29).[34] Lower-extremity long-bone fractures commonly accompany pelvic fractures. While it may be difficult to assess the exact amount of blood loss into muscle compartments of the lower extremities in these patients, physical exam should identify patients with such blood loss. This noncavitary bleeding can be significant enough to cause hemodynamic instability.[35] Using the generally accepted rule of 2 U per long-bone fracture, it is easy to see that bilateral femoral fractures and a tibial fracture can cause class 4 hemorrhage, even in the absence of pelvic blood loss. Blood loss from intra-abdominal solid organs or mesenteric injuries can be considerable. Blood loss into the retroperitoneum from a pelvic fracture can likewise be impressive. While the fascial compartments in the lower extremities are able to stem some bleeding, no such planes exist in the retroperitoneum. Blood loss from a pelvic fracture can fill the pelvic retroperitoneum and extend superiorly behind the abdomen and the thorax to the level of the neck. Though uncommon, the authors have treated patients who have required in excess of 50 U of blood transfused for pelvic fracture bleeding.

Blood loss within the pelvis itself may originate from a variety of sources. One potential source of blood loss is from the fracture fragments themselves. Others are the veins and arteries that exist within the pelvis. While no data exists that accurately predict the relative distribution of vascular injuries, significant arterial injury occurs approximately 20% of the time.[17] These vascular injuries may be caused by lacerations from the fracture fragments at the time of the original injury or by subsequent displacement of these bones. Occasionally, blood loss from pelvic fractures occurs in major vessels, such as the external iliac arteries. More commonly, however, the bleeding occurs deeper within the pelvis in the hypogastric vascular distribution. This rich vascular network communicates via numerous collaterals with the contralateral hypogastric distribution. Thus, they are at particular risk for injury at the time of pelvic fracture. Rapid temporary control of hemorrhage secondary to pelvic fractures may be temporized with placement of a pelvic binder in patients with vascular injury secondary to opening of the pelvic ring.

## PRIORITIES IN POLYTRAUMA

Pelvic fractures commonly occur in association with other significant injuries, particularly in the abdomen. One of the most difficult dilemmas in the unstable polytrauma patient is the determination of intraperitoneal versus retroperitoneal blood loss (see Chap. 29). Some patients, however, are at particular risk for blood loss in one site as opposed to the other. For instance, patients with vertical deceleration injuries most often bleed from the combination of the retroperitoneum and long-bone fractures.[28] Although intra-abdominal injuries do occur in these patients, intra-abdominal blood is almost never the source of hemodynamic instability. This is in contrast to the constellation of injuries seen in motor vehicle collisions, in which significant solid organ injury is commonly seen in patients with severe pelvic fractures.[36,37]

There are various diagnostic tests available to help the clinician with this important decision. These are described in detail elsewhere (see Chaps. 10 and 29) but deserve some specific discussion as they relate to patients with pelvic fractures. Serial physical exam and serial laboratory evaluation may be appropriate for some patients, but they are not appropriate for patients with pelvic fractures. It is important to rapidly assess these polytraumatized patients for potential blood loss. Pelvic fractures and retroperitoneal blood loss may themselves cause abdominal tenderness, mimicking intra-abdominal injury. Evaluation based solely on physical exam risks faulty decision-making, which may have substantial consequences.

In the past, diagnostic peritoneal lavage (DPL) was the "gold standard" for the rapid evaluation of intra-abdominal bleeding. The role of DPL has largely been supplanted by the Focused Assessment with Sonography for Trauma (FAST) particularly in hemodynamically unstable patients. FAST is a noninvasive diagnostic test that provides rapid bedside determination of hemoperitoneum (see Chap. 16). The examination can be performed at the bedside while resuscitation is ongoing. The sensitivity and specificity of US in blunt trauma for detection of intra-abdominal fluid are over 80% and 98%, respectively, in the hemodynamically stable patient.[38–40] Since approximately 200 mL of intraperitoneal fluid are needed to detect on US, most hemoperitoneum causing significant hemodynamic instability will be detected with FAST.[41] In fact, one of the most compelling indications for US may be the unstable patient with pelvic trauma to locate the cavitary source of hemorrhage. Because US can be operator-dependent, some degree of training and expertise is necessary to make these sophisticated judgments.

In the setting of an equivocal FAST examination, repeat FAST or DPL can be of benefit in helping to determine the source of hemorrhage. For patients with pelvic fractures, DPL must be performed utilizing an open technique in a supraumbilical location (see Chap. 29). A negative DPL effectively rules out the intra-abdominal contents as a source of blood loss and allows the clinician to focus attention

elsewhere, particularly toward the issue of retroperitoneal bleeding. Unfortunately, there are some disadvantages to DPL. While still relatively rapid, open DPL takes considerably longer than does the closed percutaneous technique. In the authors' experience, it generally takes 15 to 20 minutes to perform open DPL, but times as long as 45 to 50 minutes have been reported.[42] In addition, DPL can be inaccurate. The false-positive rates have been reported to be as high as 30% when all patients with positive DPLs were explored.[43] The false positive resulted from entry into the retroperitoneal hematoma or diapedesis of red blood cells from tense retroperitoneal bleeding. Open DPL is an operative procedure requiring skilled surgeons, as well as good lighting and instruments. The catheter must be inserted into the abdomen carefully and gently to avoid entry into the retroperitoneal hematoma.

The hemodynamically unstable patient with a severe pelvic fracture presents a particularly difficult dilemma. Unstable patients with a positive FAST exam or positive DPL are best served by prompt laparotomy.[40,44,45] However, these judgments can have substantial impact on clinical decision-making. Clearly, not all intra-abdominal injuries require emergency laparotomy. The use of diagnostic angiography to identify ongoing blood loss and achieve hemostasis with embolization has become as widely utilized in the abdomen as it has in the treatment of pelvic injuries.[46] Thus, patients with splenic or hepatic injury accompanying pelvic fracture have the potential to have a definitive hemostasis achieved with a single technique. Judgments about the use and timing of therapy are critical (see Chap. 15).

There are several important reasons to limit the rate of nontherapeutic laparotomy. Renz and Feliciano have clearly documented the morbidity of a negative trauma laparotomy, with complication rates exceeding 40%.[47] Others have reported complication rates of 20%.[48] In addition, despite best efforts, the time involved in transport to the operating room, anesthetic induction, laparotomy, and abdominal closure is considerable. This is of particular concern in the patient with substantial retroperitoneal bleeding in whom time can be spent in far better ways. Finally, release of the tamponade afforded by an intact interior abdominal wall may allow bleeding to proceed more briskly. The surgeon is then faced with a patient in whom an abdominal closure is extremely problematic. Abdominal closure under tension may produce intra-abdominal hypertension with all of its physiologic consequences. Closure with mesh is more time-consuming and does not provide the same degree of tamponade until blood loss has continued for some time.

CT scanning can be extremely helpful in evaluating the abdomen of patients with pelvic fractures (see Chap. 15). It has become the diagnostic modality of choice in hemodynamically stable patients due to its simultaneous imaging of the retroperitoneum and intraperitoneal contents. There is more objectivity in the interpretation of CT scans than there is with US. However, CT scanning is relatively time-consuming and in many centers requires transportation out of the resuscitation suite. While it clearly has an important role in the assessment of patients with pelvic fractures, a more expeditious diagnostic test such as DPL or US should be performed to evaluate patients for intra-abdominal blood loss.

If patient stability permits, the additional information gained by abdominal CT scanning can be considerable (see Chap. 15). Patients found to have relatively minor abdominal injuries but significant retroperitoneal hematoma can have the issue of retroperitoneal bleeding dealt with first and vice versa. Even patients found to have abdominal injuries requiring surgery, such as a pancreatic transection or small bowel injury, may be best served by control of retroperitoneal bleeding preoperatively. Caution should be exercised in reviewing a CT scan after DPL because some lavage fluid and air will likely be present in the peritoneal cavity that may be misleading. However, CT is still useful for identifying solid-organ injury, and assessing the integrity of the mesentery, the presence or absence of contrast extravasation, as well as the status of the retroperitoneal organs.[49]

Although control of hemorrhage is the primary priority in the multiply injured patient after securing of the airway and establishment of adequate oxygenation and ventilation, recognition of other injuries, such as severe traumatic brain injuries is vital. Immediately life-threatening intracranial mass lesions should not wait to be addressed until after thorough diagnosis and treatment of pelvic fractures and other associated injuries has been completed. Clearly, secondary hypotension is associated with poorer outcomes in this setting and necessitates that hemorrhage must be evaluated and attenuated in the setting of TBI. Prompt recognition of these injuries, however, allows for concomitant intervention with a multi-disciplinary approach.

## CONTROLLING PELVIC HEMORRHAGE

Early identification of those patients with pelvic fractures who are at highest risk for pelvic hemorrhage is imperative. Information concerning the injury pattern and therefore the mechanism of injury may be helpful in localizing the source of hemorrhage. In general, patients with an injury that increases the bony volume of the pelvis (AP or "open book") are much more likely to have significant pelvic bleeding than those with injuries that reduce the volume of the pelvis (LC).

Clearly, one must first make the diagnosis of hemorrhage and ascertain its location. For patients who may have ongoing pelvic bleeding, resuscitation and treatment occur simultaneously. Reducing the pelvis is the first priority which can be accomplished using several techniques. Definitive hemostasis can be accomplished by angiographic embolization and/or operative techniques in patients who continue to bleed. Imaging studies in patients who are stabilized may also help. Patients with CT scans that demonstrate a contrast blush, strongly suggesting arterial injury, would almost certainly be at very high risk for bleeding.[50] This is particularly true if the fractures are skeletally unstable.[51,52]

Severe AP compression injuries are generally associated with the largest blood loss. The staging of fracture severity seems to have a direct relation to the amount of blood loss.[51,53] Fractures with complete disruption of the hemipelvis have the greatest hemorrhage and can easily produce hypotension.[54] This may be the sole source of hemorrhage or may be combined with extrapelvic blood loss, commonly from the abdomen. Blood loss from these fractures will most likely be from fracture surfaces and/or venous bleeding. Bleeding may also be arterial, such as from the pudendal or obturator arteries.[55] Although AP compression can produce dramatic images on x-ray, posterior element disruption can be missed even if the film is carefully scrutinized, particularly if the pelvis has already been reduced with a binder. In a series of 92 patients with pelvic fractures requiring over 6 U of blood

within 24 hours, Moreno and coworkers found that 28% of the patients had only unilateral anterior element fractures seen in the initial pelvic film.[56] They commented that this surprising rate of seemingly insignificant fractures may have been due to under diagnosis of the posterior injury, particularly the ligamentous injuries. The average transfusion requirement in these patients was 11.2 U.

Lateral compression pelvic injuries are frequently associated with lethal torso injuries but are generally thought to be injury least likely to cause pelvic blood loss.[57] The average transfusion requirement in LC fractures is generally between 2 and 4 U.[54] This pattern may change in the elderly because the vascular structures of the posterior pelvis have substantial atherosclerosis and may be more susceptible to shearing-type injuries.[37,58,59] LC fractures that produce fracture patterns exiting the superior border of the greater sciatic notch occasionally injure the superior gluteal artery or vein directly, causing these relatively rare vascular injuries. Direct intrusion of a fracture fragment into other arteries of the pelvis can also injure structures such as the obturator and pudendal arteries. Any patient with an LC fracture pattern and ongoing hemodynamic instability should be carefully reexamined to look for other injuries causing blood loss, such as intraabdominal injury.

## ROLE OF COMPRESSIVE DEVICES

In hemodynamically unstable patients with a pelvic disruption that increases the volume of the pelvis, application of a compressive device is an emergent treatment that should be given the highest priority after the initial assessment. The compression device is designed to reduce the volume of the pelvis and promote hemodynamic stability. Delaying this intervention would be akin to allowing an arterial injury from an extremity to exsanguinate without applying pressure to stop the bleeding. Application of the compressive device often has sudden dramatic improvement in blood pressure in these critically injured patients.

Attempts at stabilizing the bony pelvis with a compressive device after injury that has resulted from an LC force in an effort to control bleeding are seldom beneficial because LC injuries do not cause an increase in pelvic volume and the ligaments are often intact. However, data suggests that placement of devices such as pelvic binders is not harmful and when faced with a hemodynamically unstable patient poses little risk.[60,61] The type of fixation is not as important as is the ability to quickly reduce the pelvis in a hemodynamically unstable pelvis.

There are several efficacious methods of external stabilization available to the clinician to acutely control pelvic fracture bleeding. The first and most widely used is the pelvic binder. Trauma centers began to utilize commercially available pelvic girdles to reduce unstable pelvic fractures several years ago. There are several commercially available devices, such as the TPOD (Trauma Pelvic Orthotic Device, Cybertech). These devices can be rapidly and easily applied at the bedside and are effective in reducing the pubic diastasis in APC fractures.[61,62] Cadaveric studies of similarly applied devices (pelvic sling, pelvic circumferential compression device) have demonstrated comparable stabilization to C-clamps.[60,63,64] The pelvic binder consists of a wide belt and a velcro attached "buckle" pulley system. The garment is radiolucent, which allows radiographic imaging, CT scan, or angiography after they are applied (Fig. 38-10).

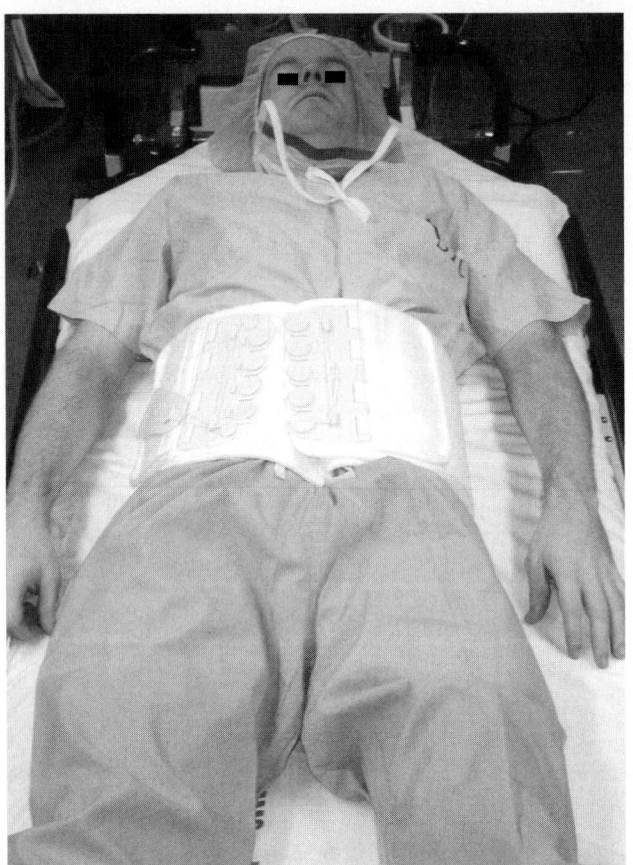

**FIGURE 38-10.** Pelvic binder placed on volunteer. This device is useful as external compression in patients with skeletal unstable pelvic fractures.

Virtually all the advantages of the pelvic binders can be achieved by using something as simple as a bedsheet (Fig. 38-11). Some high-volume centers routinely use a bedsheet to avoid the cost of the binders. There is some theoretic advantage of the binder in terms of spreading out the force over a larger area of skin to perhaps decrease risk of injury to the skin under the compressive device, but little data exists regarding this issue. Certainly a sheet

will do if a binder is not available, and this would be particularly appropriate before a patient is transferred from a community hospital to a higher level of trauma care.

The technique for applying any compressive device ideally involves three people. The device should be centered over the greater trochanters of the hip, not over the iliac wings. One person on each side of the patient applies pressure to the greater trochanters to reduce the pelvis and the third person tightens the binder or bedsheet. Holes can be cut in the binder to allow access for angiography. Laparotomy may be performed with the binder or bedsheet remaining in place. The binder may be left in place for some time, certainly up to 24 hours, but there is a risk of skin necrosis as the time in the binder increases. Nursing care to check the skin under the binder approximately every six hours or so is imperative.

After the binder is placed, the next step is to take a single AP pelvis to see if the binder has successfully reduced the volume of the pelvis. The patient's ankles and knees can be loosely bound together to aid in reduction, as abduction of the hips tends to open the pelvis. If the pelvis is not well reduced, a second attempt at tightening the binder is generally wise.

Diagnostics and therapeutics in patients with pelvic fractures often involve a number of modalities. Virtually all of these require transport from a stretcher to an imaging or operating room table, then back to a transport stretcher. If the fractured pelvic bones have not been stabilized, they are free to move as the patient is transported. Motion of these fracture fragments can aggravate old bleeding or may cause damage to the previously uninjured small vessels located adjacent to them. Use of the pelvic binder or other compressive devices may prevent such secondary vascular damage. The patient can be easily moved and transported with this device in place, allowing for good stability of the bony fragments. Our center's experience has been quite positive. Work is ongoing to examine the utility of these devices in the prehospital environment as well.[65]

Another option for compression of the pelvis to control hemorrhage is the MAST garment. The MAST garment is still the method of compression of choice in the prehospital environment in some emergency medical systems. Data suggest, however, that

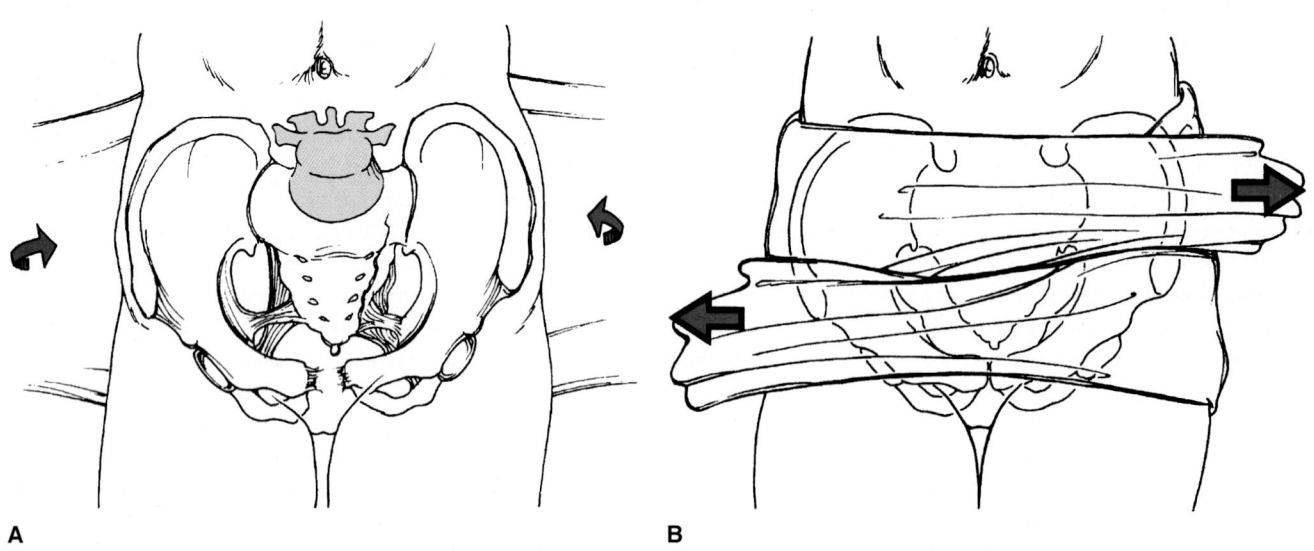

A                                                                 B

**FIGURE 38-11.** External compression with a bed sheet reduces pelvic volume.

the prehospital use of the MAST for patients with hypotension is of little value (see Chap. 7).[66] However, in the particular subset of patients with major pelvic trauma, military anti-shock trousers (MAST) may act as an effective splint.[67] It may help stop venous bleeding by raising intra-abdominal pressure above that of venous pressure. This is a double-edged sword since these increases in intra-abdominal pressure may also produce intra-abdominal hypertension (see Chap. 40) with associated ventilatory problems as well as cardiac and renal dysfunction.[68] In its role as a pelvic splint, the MAST may help limit bleeding from the pelvic fracture fragments themselves and prevent motion that can aggravate bleeding. Finally, MAST may decrease the effective volume of the pelvis by partially reducing displaced pelvic bones.

A number of pelvic clamps have been designed to reduce and compress the posterior fragments of a pelvic fracture.[69] This, theoretically, has the advantage of better reducing the posterior pelvis in some injury patterns, and thus may limit bone bleeding. While these clamps are placed in the resuscitation units in Europe, in most United States trauma centers, these clamps are placed in the operating room under general anesthesia using fluoroscopic guidance to avoid damage to neurovascular structures.

## ROLE OF EXTERNAL FIXATION

### External Fixation in the Emergency Room

Emergent external fixation of the pelvis is another technique that has been used to control blood loss in the acute management of hemodynamically unstable pelvic fractures, but has been almost completely replaced by binders and bedsheets. It can provide pelvic bony stability in a number of patients, though not all, with pelvic fractures.[70] External fixation can be applied quickly in the ED. In institutions in which this technique is commonly used, external fixation can be accomplished in less than 20 minutes although it should be noted that few institutions have these resources.[71] In a manner similar to pelvic binders, MAST, or pelvic clamps, external fixation almost certainly helps tamponade bleeding from bone edges as well as venous bleeding by reducing fracture fragments and decreasing the geometry of the pelvis. In addition, it seems to have the effect of "stabilizing the clot."[72] If bleeding is caused by damage to the superior gluteal artery or a large number of veins in the posterior venous plexus, controlling pelvic volume and bony elements stabilizes the clot that has already formed.

In fact, some series suggest that early application of pelvic external fixation decreases mortality.[73,74] Unfortunately, this degree of expertise is not available in all institutions. In addition, it is unlikely that external fixation can stop major arterial bleeding. The external fixator can serve to degrade the quality of CT images and may impede either the angiographer or the surgeon during the additional procedures necessary for the total care of the patient.

If external fixation is to be utilized in the emergency setting, the necessary infrastructure must be available at the institution to support such an effort. In the authors' institution, where the operating rooms are located adjacent to the resuscitation area, the patient can be rapidly transported to the operating room or the operating room personnel bring an operating room setup to the patient's bedside. When external fixation is done in the resuscitation unit, the

patient is anesthetized and the surgeon, scrub nurses, and circulating nurses all wear hats, masks, gowns, and gloves. The patient is prepped and draped, and the external fixator is applied with the same degree of sterility present in the operating room. These resources are not available in all institutions. However, at a minimum, it is important to have the instruments readily available in the form of a tray that includes the necessary drills to avoid the delay caused by searching for equipment in a situation when time is at a premium. Orthopedic surgeons must be immediately available to place the frame. Senior personnel from both general surgery and orthopedics, as well as any other consulting services necessary, must be available at the bedside to discuss the wisdom of external fixation within the context of resuscitation and the total patient care.

At our institution, external fixation is now rarely placed in the trauma resuscitation unit. Instead a binder is used as it is easier and quicker to place and has essentially all the advantages of the external fixator for acute management. Although there may be an indication for an external fixator initially in a patient who has a fracture pattern that is refractory to reduction by a pelvic binder, some would counter that a binder is actually better than an external fixator at reducing the pelvis. A binder provides circumferential compression, whereas an anterior external fixator tends to compress the anterior pelvis, and may in fact open up the posterior pelvis where it is most important to provide compression.

In the past, external fixation was the only real option for pelvic reduction. Thus, most trauma centers employed emergency external fixation early in the algorithm for hemodynamically unstable patients, particularly with AP compression fractures. This often involved mobilization of a significant number of resources and took time, perhaps the most precious resource. While there is no comparative data examining the efficacy of external fixation versus the binder, the immediate availability of the binder and ease of application make it extremely attractive.

## STAGED AND DEFINITIVE USE OF EXTERNAL FIXATORS

Although external fixation has fallen out of favor for the emergent resuscitation of the unstable patient in the trauma resuscitation unit, it still plays an important role in the staged and definitive management of many patients with pelvic fractures. The binder is clearly not a permanent solution. Placing an external fixator allows the patients' pelvis to be kept reduced without the skin issues associated with a binder. This is often performed in a more urgent manner when the patient is in the operating room already for a laparotomy. By placing a frame, the pelvis is kept stable while the surgical issues in the abdomen or elsewhere are addressed.

External fixation can also be used as definitive anterior fixation for open-book pelvic fractures and in injuries in which wound conditions or other parameters do not permit internal fixation. Comparable functional results have been reported by some, while others have found functional results following external fixation alone unacceptable compared with plate and screw fixation.[75–78]

External fixators can also be used as a bridge to internal fixation, as opening the pelvis acutely is not always advantageous, but getting the patient out of the binder is still desired. It is sometimes difficult to know early in the course of treatment whether a patient's overall status will tolerate the operative stress of open fixation of the pelvic fracture. Though it may not be ideal for long-term management of all pelvic fractures, external fixation provides some degree of bony stability, as well as limiting blood loss during application.[77,78] This "damage control" approach to pelvic fracture fixation has been found to be safe and effective.[79]

There are two main frames used at our institution: "resuscitation frames" and "Hannover frames." The resuscitation frames use three pins in each iliac wing and can be placed very rapidly without radiographic guidance. The disadvantage is that the bone is rather thin, the pins are often an issue in obese patients, and it is sometimes difficult to achieve good pin placement in a very displaced hemipelvis. In contrast, a Hannover frame uses one pin running from each anterior inferior iliac spine aimed posterior just above the sciatic notch. These pins pass through the strongest bone in the body and provide excellent purchase. We typically insert these under fluoroscopic guidance.

Regardless of frame type, it is advantageous to have two sets of bars (A frames) connecting the pins so that the location of the bars can be moved easily for access to the patient's abdomen without losing the reduction of the pelvis. Patients with high-energy injuries often swell substantially after surgery, so care must be taken to make sure the hardware is far from the skin. Rolls of kerlex gauze are used to keep the skin from contacting bar-pin clamps. The main downside to external fixation over plates and screws is infection at the pin sites and the need to have a cumbersome frame on the patient's pelvis. The rate of wound problems around the fixator pins is actually quite high. Further, a more anatomic reduction of the pelvis can usually be obtained with plates and screws than with external fixation, so orthopedists often try to use plate and screw fixation of the anterior ring injuries when possible.

## ROLE OF SELECTIVE EMBOLIZATION

Angiography has the potential to be both diagnostic and therapeutic in patients with serious blunt pelvic injury. Angiography precisely defines bleeding sites and allows for definitive therapy of pelvic bleeding via transcatheter embolization. Reported indications for angiography in patients with pelvic fractures include hemodynamic instability and large pelvic or retroperitoneal hematoma or presence of contrast blush on CT.[21,22,45,51,80–82] The absence of these CT findings does not exclude the need for angiography, however, if clinical suspicion of ongoing pelvic bleeding exists.[81] In patients in whom bleeding can be identified, transcatheter embolization definitively treats this bleeding 80 to 100% of the time.[53,83–88] One additional benefit of early angiography following major trauma is the ability to identify and treat abdominal solid organ injuries at the time of angioembolization of pelvic bleeding. Because trauma patients tend to be young, angiography is usually relatively risk free.

It is vitally important to identify a patient in need of angiography early in the patient's course. Even in trauma centers, where angiography is routinely used for hemostasis, time is required to mobilize the personnel and equipment needed to perform the study, particularly in off-hours. Arterial cannulation, diagnostic angiography, identification of the bleeding vessel, and subsequent embolization can all be time-consuming. Thus, the time from identification of need for angiography to definitive hemostasis can be prolonged.

In one series, the time required for angiography to control pelvic blood loss varied between 1 and 5 hours, averaging 2½ hours.[85]

If the decision is made to proceed with angiography, the patient should be transported as soon as possible to the angiography suite. It is important to recognize any limitations that may exist for ongoing resuscitation and evaluation while in the angiography suite. These limitations will vary from institution to institution. In complex, multiply injured patients such as these, critical care must be a concept and not a location. Ideally, the angiography suite should be equipped with critical-care-quality monitoring equipment and all the materials necessary for ongoing care of the patient. If this is not the case, it is necessary to transport these materials with the patient.

However, ongoing resuscitative efforts are bound to fail until the vascular injury has been controlled. The authors would contend that these patients are too sick not to go to angiography. They are no different than hypotensive patients with intra-abdominal bleeding. All would agree that patients with intraperitoneal hemorrhage are best served by rapid transport to the operating room and prompt hemostasis.

Once the arterial tree has been cannulated, diagnostic angiography is performed (see Chap. 15). In general, a flush aortogram should be performed first. Large vascular injuries within the pelvis may be identified and the angiographer can address these expeditiously. In addition, patients with pelvic fractures may have retroperitoneal bleeding in sites remote from the pelvis. The most common example is the patient who has lumbar vertebral fractures as well as a pelvic fracture. These patients may be bleeding from a lumbar arterial vascular injury, and this diagnosis can often be made at the time of aortography.[85,89]

If no pelvic vascular injury is identified at the time of aortography, the angiographer should proceed with selective pelvic angiography. The mechanism of injury and fracture pattern will dictate which hypogastric artery is at greatest risk for blood loss and should be imaged first. The entire pelvic vasculature must be completely imaged before the procedure is complete as patients will often bleed from multiple sites. In one series, 57% of the patients with definable vascular injuries had multiple bleeding sites.[55]

There are three basic principles that should guide the angiographer in performing embolization.[53] First, the purpose is to slow the bleeding to the extent that the body will control its own hemorrhage rather than creating large areas of ischemia or necrosis. Second, if ischemia or necrosis is unavoidable, it should be limited to the smallest area possible. Finally, the procedure must be done expeditiously. Keeping these three principles in mind, the angiographer can select the method of vascular occlusion based on the angiographic findings.

Ideally, embolization should be performed as selectively as possible. If the bleeding point can be reached selectively, Gelfoam is often the agent of choice for embolization. Each pledget of Gelfoam can be separately loaded into a syringe in a sterile manner and injected under fluoroscopic control. The Gelfoam usually lasts several weeks and is then absorbed. At this point, bleeding has ceased and the artery may recannulize. If the bleeding artery is too large to utilize Gelfoam, stainless steel coils are often used. Vascular occlusion produced by the coil is sometimes incomplete, but can be supplemented by Gelfoam, if necessary.[53,90,91]

Occasionally, the patient's blood loss may be substantial enough that selective embolization is simply not possible. In these cases, the patient is better served by blind embolization of the hypogastric circulation with small-particulate Gelfoam. Two millimeter pieces of Gelfoam are injected into the hypogastric artery. The Gelfoam will flow out and occlude the majority of the hypogastric circulation. Two-millimeter pledgets are large enough to prevent migration to the small vessels deep within the pelvis, thus preserving some degree of collateral flow. Usually, significant ischemic damage can be avoided with this technique,[53] although there are some case reports of significant ischemia following angiographic embolization of bilateral internal iliac or gluteal arteries.[92]

Coil blockade is a technique first described by Sclafani and colleagues to avoid the skin slough, lower extremity paresis, myonecrosis, and impotence that have been reported complications of distal embolization.[85] This technique spares the distal collateral circulation from Gelfoam occlusion by placing microcoils through coaxial catheters into the intact vessel located distal to injury. The proximal artery is then embolized with Gelfoam. The distal circulation is protected via the block afforded by the microcoils. Flow into the distal arteries via collaterals can be documented angiographically after embolization is completed. This technique allows isolation of the injured vessels and provides for occlusion of the injured portion of the vessel only.

Coils can also be used to control hemorrhage from proximal hypogastric arterial injuries.[93] In these cases, Gelfoam is placed distal to the injury. Care must be taken to cut the Gelfoam to the appropriate size to prevent migration of the Gelfoam too distally. The Gelfoam then blocks retrograde bleeding via collaterals. A coil is placed more proximally in the hypogastric artery occluding inflow.

The final technical point about embolization addresses vessels that are seemingly occluded at the time of angiography. Presumably, this represents a vascular injury that has stopped bleeding prior to angiography. While it may be tempting to ignore these injured arteries, the authors would caution against that treatment strategy. This is no different than a surgeon encountering a clotted artery at the time of operation. Virtually all surgeons would ligate that artery to prevent later hemorrhage. In addition, the intense spasm that accompanies some vascular injuries will make them appear occluded at the time of diagnostic study. As the spasm resolves, these vessels rebleed. Thus, transcatheter embolization of these vessels is advisable if technically possible.

The yield of angiography in patients with pelvic fractures varies widely. This is almost certainly due to the different indications for angiography used within each center. For instance, in institutions in which other methods of hemostasis are used primarily such as the MAST or external fixation, the yield of angiography has been reported to be as low as 3 to 5%.[56,67] However, in institutions in which angiography is used as a primary modality for hemostasis and is performed very early in the resuscitation, the yield has been as high as 20%.[29,85] When more selective criteria for angiography have been applied, including degree of hemodynamic stability, severity of pelvic fracture, and CT findings, the yield of angiography when utilized very early has been reported to be as high as 70–90%.[45,56,82,85,88]

The demographics of injury seen at various institutions may also affect the need for and yield of angiography. For instance, urban centers may see little in the way of high-speed vehicular injuries. Most often, in such centers, pelvic fractures are secondary to vertical shear mechanisms such as falls from a height. A compilation of data from several studies suggests that patients with high-risk pelvic fractures (i.e., posterior fractures, open-book fractures, and displaced fractures), who require more than 4 U of blood, have an incidence of pelvic arterial bleeding requiring embolization of approximately 20%.[17,29,67,94,95]

Often, the results of embolization are quite dramatic. Patients often immediately achieve hemodynamic stability and show very few signs of ongoing blood loss.[84,85] However, angiography will not stop all pelvic bleeding. Venous bleeding and bleeding from bony edges is not treated by angiographic embolization. Early reports suggested that a substantial number of patients required ongoing transfusions even after successful embolization. Matalon and Athanasoulis reported complete cessation of bleeding in only 40% of patients postembolization.[96] An additional 40% required between 3 and 10 U after embolization, and 20% required more than 10 U. There may be several reasons for this. First, vital signs or hematocrit often underestimates transfusion requirements. Additionally, ongoing transfusion requirements may have been due to the under recognition of initial blood loss, reequilibration of hematocrit, or blood loss from extrapelvic sources, in addition to ongoing pelvic bleeding.

The authors' indications for angiography are depicted in Table 38–3 (Figs. 38-12 and 38-13). Patients are generally divided

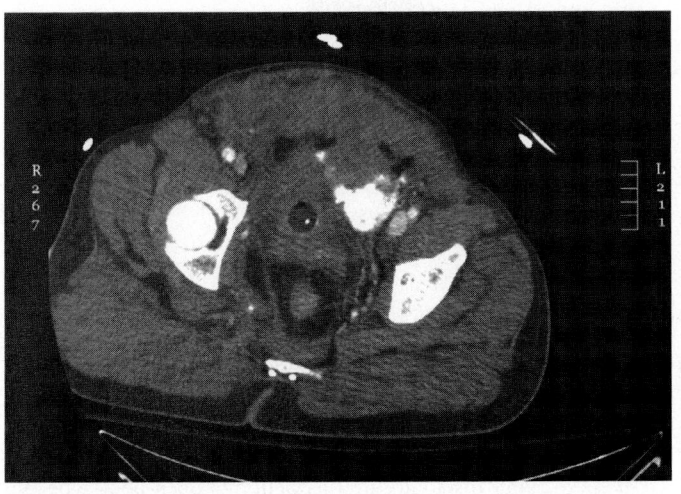
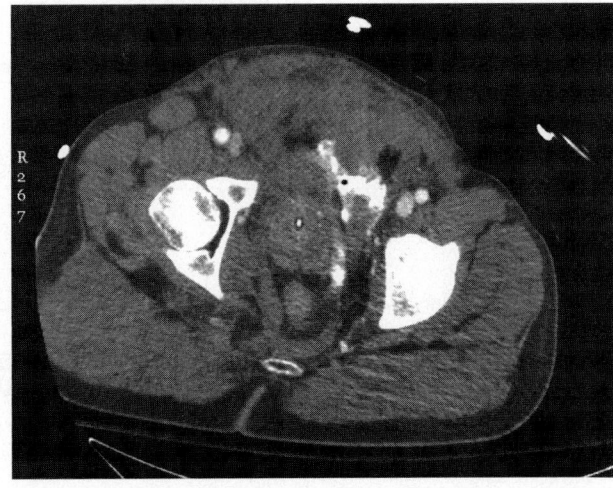

**A**          **B**

**FIGURE 38-12.** CT scan with active extravasation. This patient had undergone diagnostic angiography demonstrating a vascular lesion in the hypogastric arterial distribution.

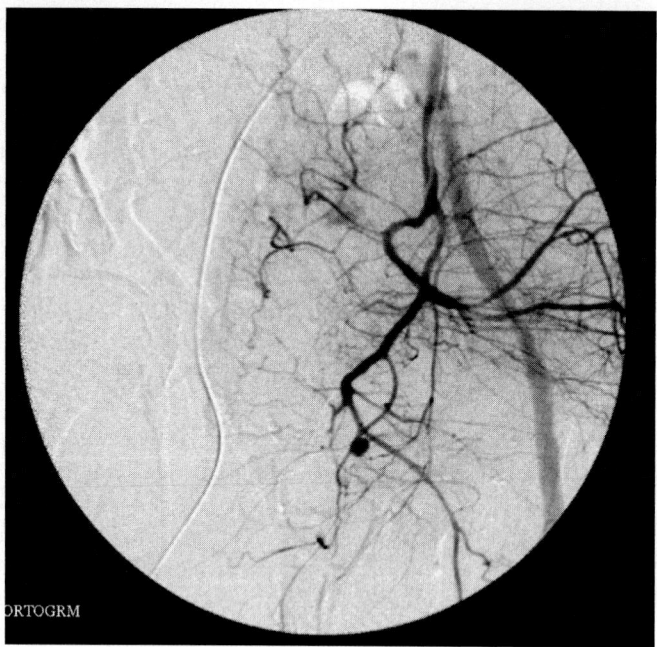
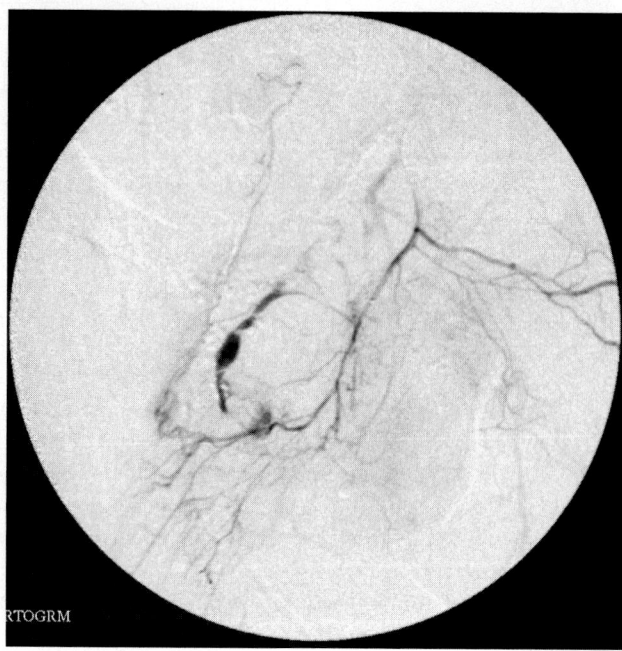
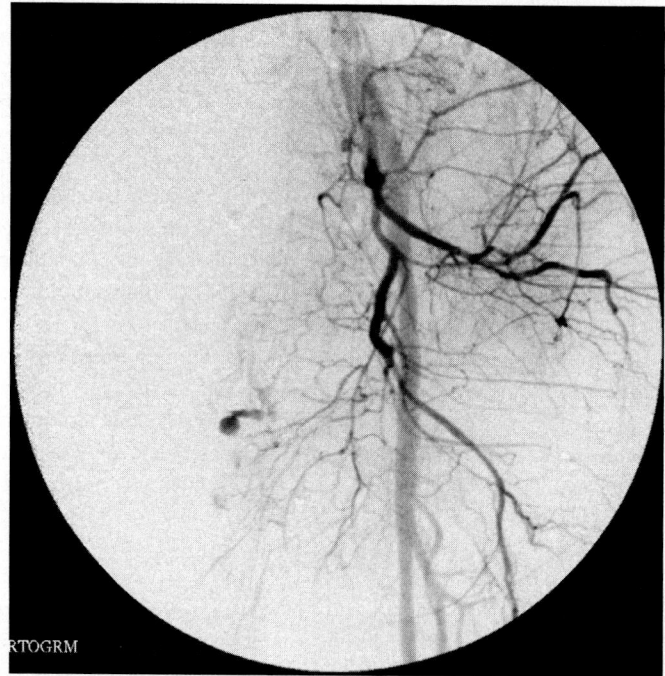

**FIGURES 38-13.** CT scan of patient from figure 38-12 demonstrating active contrast extravasation.

**TABLE 38-3**

**Indications for Angiography**

4 U transfused for pelvic bleeding in <24 h
>6 U transfused for pelvic bleeding in <48 h
Hemodynamic instability with a negative FAST or DPL
Large pelvic hematoma on CT
Pelvic pseudoaneurysm on helical CT
Large and/or expanded pelvic hematoma seen at the time of laparotomy

into two types. Patients with obvious blood loss often present hemodynamically unstable from pelvic fracture bleeding. They require immediate transfusion therapy and typically require 4 to 6 U of blood for initial stabilization. In those patients, we utilize angiography very early for hemostasis such as in patients who still have hemodynamic instability after reduction of open-book type injuries. The yield of diagnostic angiography should be reasonably high in these patients. The second group bled more slowly or intermittently. They often require 6 U of blood over the first several days or have a large retroperitoneal hematoma seen at the time of CT scanning. In these patients, it may be difficult to ascertain whether their decreasing hematocrit is secondary to ongoing pelvic blood loss, blood loss from another site, or re-equilibration and hemodilution. While the yield of angiography is much lower in such patients, it is not nil. The pelvis remains a potential source of blood loss in these types of patients and angiography can be helpful.

## ROLE OF OPERATIVE HEMOSTASIS

Many patients have concomitant intra-abdominal and pelvic bleeding at the time of laparotomy. Once intra-abdominal hemorrhage is controlled, rapid closure and immediate transport to the angiography suite is usually wise. It may be tempting for the surgeon to directly attack an expanding pelvic hematoma. While this may need to be employed as a last-ditch effort in institutions without the ability to provide rapid angiography, direct surgical control of hypogastric arterial bleeding is extremely difficult. In most people, the hypogastric artery branches many times soon after its origin making direct exposure of bleeding vessels almost impossible. While major hypogastric arterial bleeding may be controllable in this manner, deep pelvic arterial bleeding is not. In addition, once the peritoneum is widely opened and the hematoma explored, bone bleeding and venous bleeding may markedly increase as the tamponade effect of the intact peritoneum is lost.

There is, however, some enthusiasm in the literature for surgical exploration of blunt pelvic fracture bleeding. In 1979, Rothenberger and coworkers reported on 12 patients with pelvic fractures and major vascular injuries.[97] This represented a very small percentage of the patients with pelvic fractures seen over that period. The overall mortality in that series was 83%, primarily from blood loss. The authors pointed out that an unwillingness to directly explore these hematomas led to a significant delay and ongoing hemorrhage, which they believe, worsened the outcome. Since this manuscript was published in 1979, angiography has become far more readily available and is the mainstay for these types of patients.

Patients thought to have major vascular injuries such as common iliac or external iliac arterial injuries are probably best served by direct operative exploration. These patients almost always present in profound hemorrhagic shock and often have massive bony and soft tissue injury. The presence of a rapidly expanding abdomen and the absence of a unilateral palpable femoral pulse may be the only clues on physical exam that this patient has incurred this type of injury. These patients are probably appropriate candidates for laparotomy. In these patients, the hematoma is directly explored. Major arterial bleeding from the proximal hypogastric arteries should be controlled. Common or external iliac arterial injuries can be temporarily controlled using an intraluminal shunt (Figs. 38-14 and 38-15). If needed, decisions can be made regarding the advisability of direct bypass or extra-anatomic bypass to revascularize the lower extremities. Major venous injuries should be treated by ligation or temporary shunting. When major bleeding is controlled, the patient should then undergo standard angiography or intra-operative angiography to identify other potential sources of blood loss. These can be occluded using standard embolotherapy. Temporary packing may be helpful to control the smaller-caliber arterial bleeding while angiography is performed.

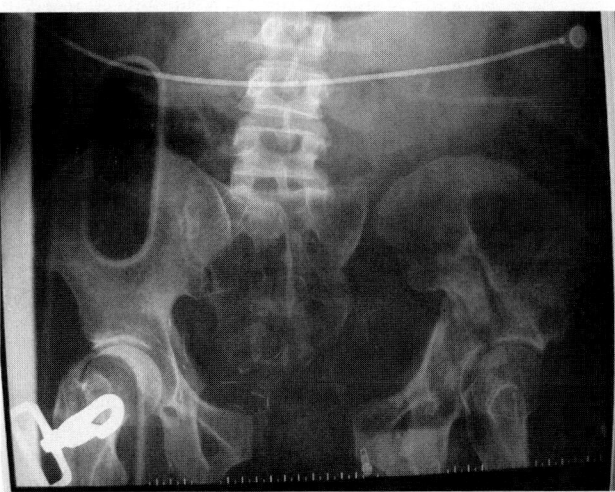

**FIGURE 38-14.** Internal hemi-pelvectomy in a patient who presented in profound hemorrhagic shock, unilaterally absent femoral pulse. This injury was treated with direct operative control and temporary shunting of the iliac artery and vein.

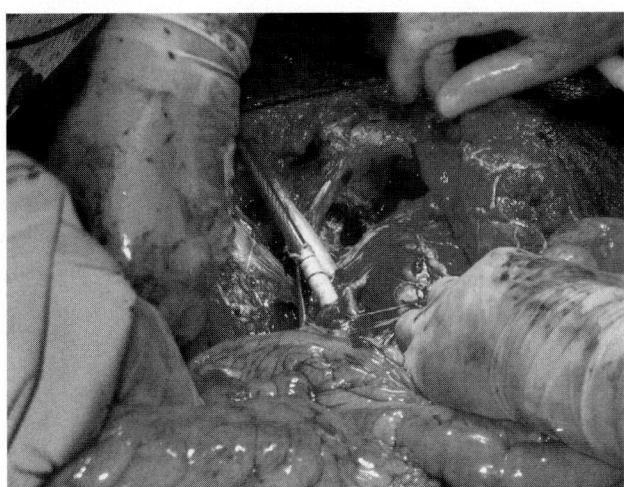

**FIGURE 38-15.** Operative intraluminal shunting of major pelvic vascular injury.

Occasionally, the surgeon will encounter a patient at the time of laparotomy who has pelvic bleeding to the extent that he or she does not believe that the patient will survive long enough to get to the angiography suite. The mortality for such a patient is extremely high. There are several techniques to help temporize under these circumstances. One attractive choice is to have the angiography team come to the operating room and perform intra-operative angiography and embolization with the patient on the table. Portable fluoroscopic equipment is available with sufficient resolution to identify major arterial bleeding. An institutional commitment is needed to have this equipment and personnel immediately available. Blind transcatheter Gelfoam embolization is often the most appropriate technique to use in these cases.

Proximal hypogastric arterial ligation may also be occasionally successful.[98] For several reasons, however, it is usually not the wisest choice if other methods of hemostasis are available. First, this maneuver is not often successful. Bilateral hypogastric ligation may be slightly more efficacious than unilateral ligation but is unwise most of the time. Since the collateral circulation in the pelvis is so rich, injuries may continue to bleed via the collaterals from the circumflex circulation. In addition, hypogastric ligation closes the angiographic window, making embolization later impossible. This may be true even if unilateral hypogastric ligation has been performed. Embolization via the contralateral hypogastric artery will be tremendously more time-consuming and rarely successful. If hypogastric ligation is used, packing the pelvis may be helpful. Another possibility is to perform blind hypogastric embolization in the operating room.[99] One or both hypogastric arteries are looped proximally, and a slurry of hemostatic agents are mixed and injected just distal to the vascular occlusion. One last option is the use of balloon catheters to help tamponade blood loss.[100] Both of these have been used anecdotally with some success.

Recently, the technique of direct retroperitoneal and pelvic packing as part of a damage control approach to major pelvic fractures with hemorrhage has been described. This technique has been described either through a midline incision or via a Pfannenstiel incision to avoid extension into the peritoneum

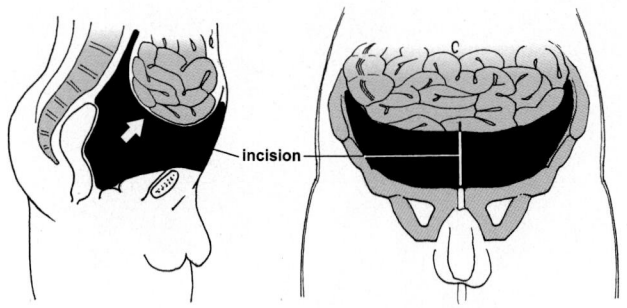

**FIGURE 38-16.** Preperitoneal packing is accomplished via a vertical or transverse incision. It is important not to enter the peritoneal cavity.

(Figs. 38-16 and 38-17). The fascia is incised and the space of retzius is opened taking care to avoid entry into the peritoneal cavity. The bladder is retracted laterally or posteriorly and the retroperitoneal space is bluntly dissected. Laparotomy pads are then packed into the retroperitoneum to tamponade hemorrhage. The retroperitoneum is closed with a running suture to maximize the tamponade effect. This may be efficacious if the patient requires concomitant laparotomy for intraabdominal injury. Successful use of this technique, in conjunction with bony stabilization, has been described in two case series.[101,102] At our institution and others, this technique has been used a number of times in conjunction with concomitant external fixation with notable results and rapid stabilization of the patient's hemodynamics.

## THE AUTHORS' APPROACH

The authors' general approach to the care of patients with pelvic fractures is based on the patient's hemodynamic stability and is detailed in Figs. 38-18 and 38-19. Certain aspects deserve some mention. As with almost every trauma algorithm, the first decision made involves hemodynamic stability. Patients who are stable are managed very differently from patients who are unstable. Clearly, this requires dynamic decision-making. Patients who are initially stable may rapidly become unstable. Thus, constant reassessment is necessary in order to avoid late recognition of a patient who is bleeding but it was not obvious at the time of initial presentation. If a stable patient becomes unstable, obviously the diagnostic and treatment algorithm must be rapidly adaptable.

The authors utilize surgeon-performed FAST as the screening exam for determining the presence of free intraperitoneal fluid. Patients who are hemodynamically unstable and have a positive FAST are urgently explored. The one exception to this may be the

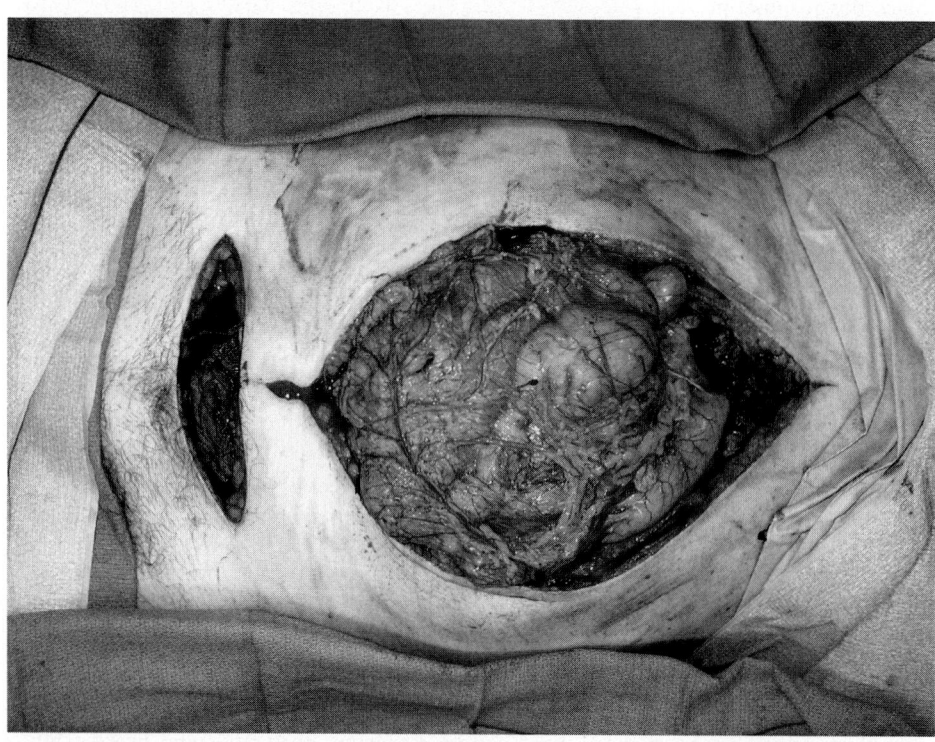

**FIGURE 38-17.** This patient had a damage control laparotomy and extraperitoneal pelvic packing. She was brought back to the operating room three days later when stable for unpacking.

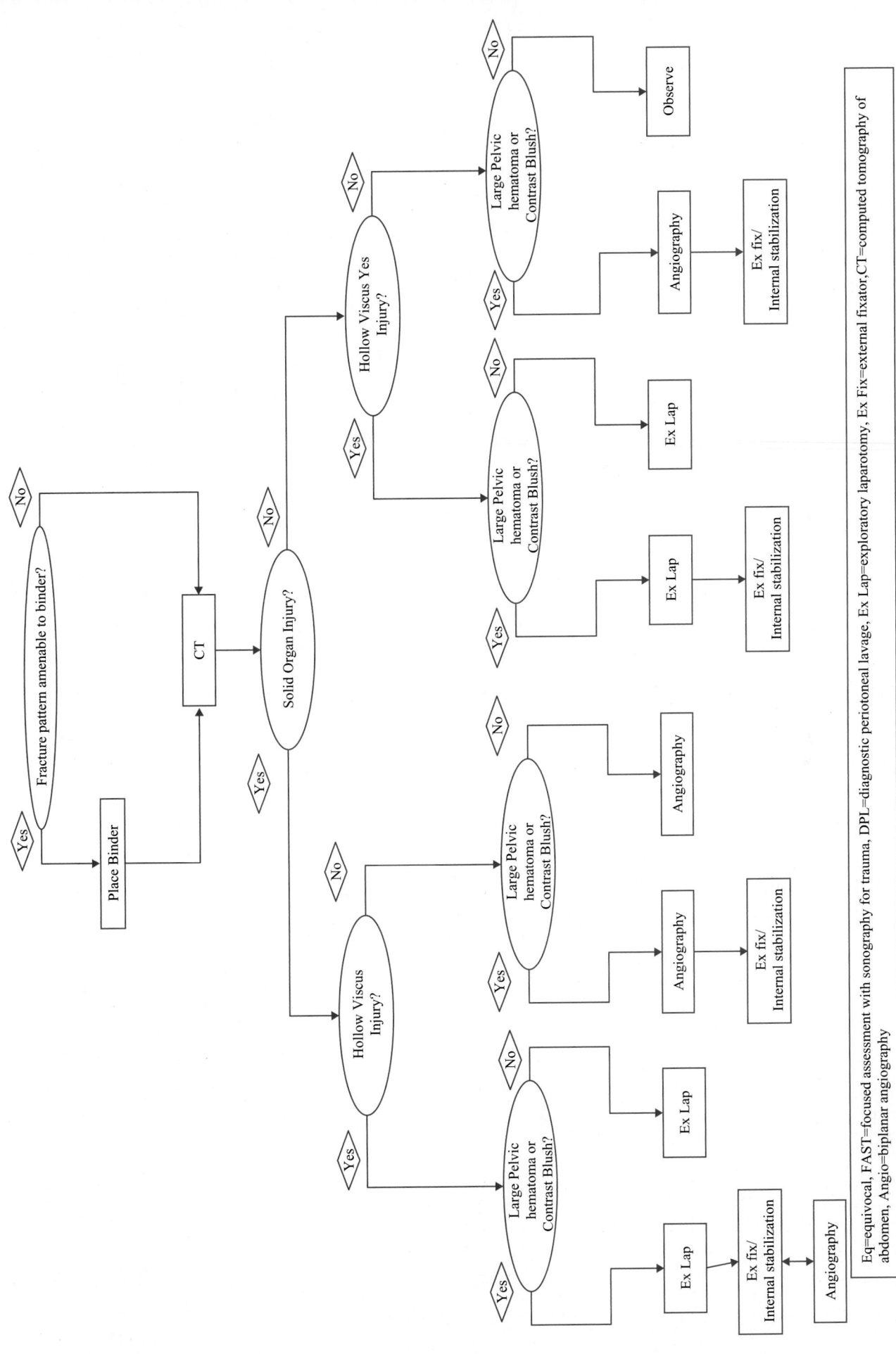

**FIGURES 38-18.** Shock Trauma Center algorithm for patients who are hemodynamically stable.

Eq=equivocal, FAST=focused assessment with sonography for trauma, DPL=diagnostic peritoneal lavage, Ex Lap=exploratory laparotomy, Ex Fix=external fixator, CT=computed tomography of abdomen, Angio=biplanar angiography

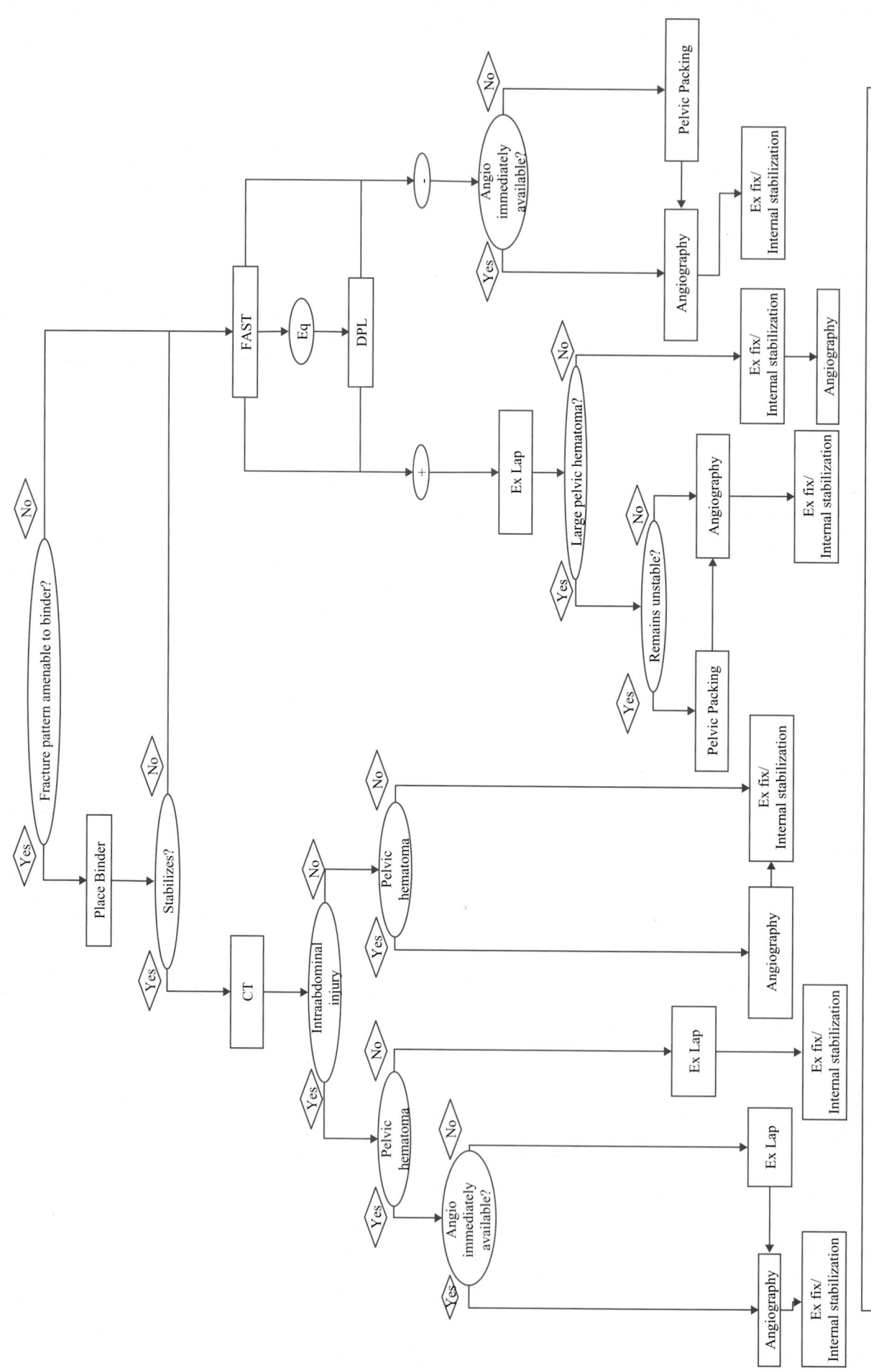

**FIGURES 38-19.**  Shock Trauma Center algorithm for patients who are hemodynamically unstable.

Eq=equivocal, FAST=focused assessment with sonography for trauma, DPL=diagnostic periotoneal lavage, Ex Lap=exploratory laparotomy, Ex Fix=external fixator, CT=computed tomography of abdomen, Angio=biplanar angiography patient with a severe pelvic fracture who rapidly stabilizes with placement of a pelvic binder. Because of the high associated rate of intra-abdominal injuries, even stable patients with pelvic fractures undergo abdominal screening with FAST. If this is positive and the patients remain stable, the authors may attempt to manage these patients nonoperatively. These patients undergo CT scanning and attempts at coil embolization to treat solid visceral injuries. Because FAST may fail to identify visceral injuries without hemoperitoneum in patients with pelvic fractures, even patients with a negative FAST undergo CT scan (see Chap. 29). FAST is important in these patients as it helps to determine relative priorities. Patients with a positive FAST are scanned at the earliest possible time. Patients with a negative FAST have their CT scan performed less urgently.

One particularly troubling subset of patients is those patients who have ongoing hypotension and a negative FAST. This is particularly problematic if they have a pelvic fracture pattern that is thought to be unlikely to produce significant blood loss. While all of the general surgery faculty at the authors' institution feel extremely comfortable with interpreting bedside ultrasounds, we also understood that there will be some false-negative examinations. If the patient is unlikely to have bled from pelvic fracture and has no other obvious blood loss injuries, generally an open supraumbilical diagnostic peritoneal lavage is performed to confirm the negative ultrasound exam. This technique is also utilized in the setting of a technically limited or equivocal FAST.

Frequently, the discussion about pelvic fracture bleeding centers around whether patients need fracture stabilization or angiography. With the increasing use of pelvic binders, the author's approach has changed dramatically over the past several years. Previously, patients with retroperitoneal blood loss underwent application of an external fixator if their fracture pattern (e.g., an AP compression or an open-book fracture) suggests that it would be helpful. This was often applied in the trauma resuscitation unit for patients who were unstable. If the fracture pattern was not favorable for external fixation, or if the patient showed signs of substantial blood loss following external fixation, angiography was performed as soon as possible.

The increasing use of pelvic binders for temporary fracture stabilization has virtually eliminated the need for emergent external fixators. Instead, at the authors' institution, the pelvic binder is placed and if hemodynamic stability is achieved, the patient may undergo additional diagnostic imaging, such as CT scan. Caution should be utilized, however, as the pelvic binder only provides temporary stabilization and the patient may rapidly clinically deteriorate should the binder shift or be moved. Removing the binder has the potential to cause hypotension and this should only be done in a very controlled setting. All patients who are to undergo additional imaging or angiography prior to definitive fracture stabilization must be closely monitored at all times.

The patient can undergo angiography with the binder in place and then more definitive fracture stabilization can be performed depending on the patient's other injuries and physiologic status. In patients who have achieved hemodynamic stability following angiography, we have started to perform definitive pelvic fixation with open reduction internal fixation (ORIF) in the acute setting, either alone or in conjunction with other procedures such as laparotomy. If the patient demonstrates evidence of ongoing shock secondary to continued hemorrhage or as a sequelae of their initial bleeding, external fixators are applied. The authors

have also left the pelvic binder in place and allowed the patient to be transported to the intensive care unit (ICU). Definitive fixation is then performed at 12–36 hours, after adequate resuscitation and warming.

Although these treatment algorithms describe the authors' standard practice, it is important to emphasize that care of any patient must be individualized. Associated injuries alter this scheme occasionally.

## MANAGEMENT OF OPEN PELVIC FRACTURES

Open pelvic fractures consist of open iliac wing fractures that do not destabilize the pelvic ring and open wounds associated with pelvic ring injuries. Whereas the iliac wing fractures tend not to cause damage to deep vasculature and organs, the open pelvic ring injuries can be devastating. While they can vary in severity, there are few situations more challenging than a patient with severe soft tissue, bony, and vascular injury located within or adjacent to the pelvis. Because of the severity of these injuries, many of these patients do not survive to reach medical attention. However, those surviving transport are potentially salvageable.

In a landmark study in 1982, Richardson and associates articulated four important treatment priorities for these devastating injuries: (a) control of hemorrhage, (b) debridement and management of the concomitant soft tissue injury, (c) recognition and treatment of associated injuries, and (d) treatment of the pelvic fracture itself.[103] The authors were able to achieve an impressive 94% survival in the 35 patients they treated using the aforementioned principles.[103] Ferrera and Hill reported similarly impressive results utilizing similar principles.[104] Morbidity and mortality rates associated with open pelvic fractures have varied considerably in the literature. Sinott and colleagues compiled data from eight studies that included 145 patients.[105] The overall mortality was 41% but exceeded 50% in some series. Despite advances in the treatment of pelvic fractures and the associated injuries, a mortality rate of 45% for patients with open pelvic fracture was published in a recent series.[106] Deaths from open pelvic fractures occur either early (<24 hours) secondary to exsanguination, or late (days to weeks following injury) secondary to sepsis and multiple organ dysfunction.

The major difference in the treatment priorities of patients with open pelvic fractures concerns the evaluation and treatment of the patient with hemorrhage. By definition, open pelvic fractures involve a communication between the fracture and the skin. This may include other perineal structures such as the vagina or the rectum. Arterial bleeding out of the wound can be massive. Presentation to the ED can be quite dramatic, especially if the patient has severe open soft tissue injury. Because of the direct communication to the environment, there is no longer any tamponade afforded by the peritoneum or any increase in intra-abdominal pressure. Thus, free blood loss will continue until the patient exsanguinates. Several management strategies exist to control this hemorrhage.

While the use of the MAST has been radically reduced, it may have real utility for patients with open pelvic fractures. It can be an effective means to tamponade blood loss, particularly if associated with significant soft tissue injury.[103,107] While this may be helpful in the prehospital phase of care as well as early in the ED, the authors would caution against its use for any prolonged period.

The MAST has been associated with significant injuries to lower extremities as well as local soft tissue.[108] Thus, use of the MAST should be limited and an alternative means of hemostasis used as soon as possible after the patient's arrival in the ED.

Direct compression is probably the best manner of achieving temporary vascular control. Depending on the size of the skin laceration, a variety of materials can be used to help tamponade blood loss. Simple gauze packing may suffice if the skin opening is relatively small. This can be supplemented with temporary skin closure to increase the tamponade effect. Patients with large perineal lacerations and soft tissue injuries may require larger packing such as laparotomy pads or towels. Skin closure may not be technically feasible for these patients, and direct hand pressure may be the only way to control blood loss.

Once bleeding is controlled temporarily, the patient should be resuscitated and plans made to provide more definitive hemostasis. One option is to take the patient directly to the operating room. Local wound exploration and hemorrhage control in the ED should never be employed. This maneuver requires good lighting, retractor systems, and deep instruments as well as skilled technicians. Blind manipulation in the ED may only compound an already desperate situation. In the operating room, the patient should be explored through the perineal wound and injured blood vessels individually identified and ligated. For all the aforementioned reasons, an approach via laparotomy will seldom result in adequate hemostasis. It is also important to remember that hemostasis may be incomplete even if it appears adequate after perineal exploration. Injured vessels may be difficult to expose via this approach. Once the patient is resuscitated, dramatic bleeding may again ensue.

The one time when a direct approach via laparotomy may be helpful is in the patient with near-total amputation at the level of the pelvis or hip. These patients generally present *in extremis* with obvious exsanguination. They often have major arterial injury at the level of the common iliac, proximal hypogastric, or external iliac artery. Vascular control via the perineal injury may be impossible. Laparotomy can be lifesaving in these patients. Concomitant bony, nervous, and soft tissue injuries may make these patients candidates for hemipelvectomy.[71] Most reports concerning pelvic fractures contain small numbers of these types of patients.[103,105] There are some case reports of patients who have undergone hemipelvectomy for this particular injury and survived.[109] The decision to perform hemipelvectomy cannot be made lightly. Frequently, the injury itself has already performed a good deal of the dissection, making the decision obvious. For other patients, damage control techniques may be useful. If hemorrhage can be arrested with surgical control or a combination of surgical control and angiographic embolization, the patient can be temporized and the decision about hemipelvectomy made as ongoing resuscitation occurs. In either case, because of the unstable nature of these patients, sophisticated imaging is usually not possible at the time of ED presentation. Decision must be made using limited data.

Angiographic embolization can be quite beneficial for patients with open pelvic fractures. The angiography service should be alerted at the time of patient presentation even if the patient is going to be transferred to the operating room in an effort to surgically control blood loss. Following attempts at hemostasis, the wound should be packed tightly with skin closure if possible. Patients can then be transferred to the angiography suite to evaluate for undiagnosed vascular injuries as a supplement to surgical hemostasis. One should avoid large dissections or prolonged attempts to control blood loss in the operating room. Obvious injuries should be treated and the patient packed and then taken to the angiography suite as quickly as possible.

Once hemostasis is secured, the soft tissue injury should be addressed. While this is a very high priority, pelvic sepsis is unlikely to be an issue for several days. Thus, if the patient has not been completely evaluated for potentially life-threatening associated injuries, this should take priority and be completed in order to allow proper sequencing of further diagnostics and therapeutics. All patients should have been evaluated with DPL or US, either in the operating room or ED, to rule out intra-abdominal blood loss. As they will be explored later for fecal diversion, further evaluation of the abdomen may not be necessary. The urinary system should be imaged completely. CT scanning should be considered at this point to examine the kidneys, bladder, and other retroperitoneal structures. Head, cervical spine, and thoracic imaging should be performed if there is concern about concomitant injury.

Once this survey is completed, a comprehensive treatment plan can be developed. If there are no other immediately life-threatening injuries identified, another assessment should be made as to the adequacy of resuscitation (see Chap. 10). It may be appropriate to take the patient to the ICU for invasive monitoring, further resuscitation, rewarming, and correction of coagulopathy. When the patient is fully resuscitated, they should be transferred to the operating room for management of the soft tissue injury. This should be accomplished within the first 48 hours of injury.[17,103] A complete evaluation of the perineum is then necessary. This includes a sigmoidoscopy in all patients and a pelvic exam in women. Associated injuries to the rectum and the genitourinary system are quite common, and must be fully evaluated. Rectal or vaginal lacerations should be repaired at this time. The abdomen should be explored and a diverting colostomy performed. This will help prevent subsequent pelvic sepsis. The wounds are packed open and the packing changed frequently. This obviates the need for other drainage such as presacral catheters. At the time of laparotomy, a decision can be made about the advisability of placing an intestinal feeding tube. The authors prefer a transgastric jejunal tube, though other options do exist. Some may be tempted to treat patients without fecal diversion, feeling that the wound is open and draining. The literature has substantiated the concerns originally raised by Richardson et al. concerning the importance of diversion as a part of the wound care management strategy.[95,105,110]

Devitalized and infected soft tissue must be thoroughly debrided and irrigated. The authors would also recommend a planned return to the operating room every day for further wound inspection and debridement as necessary. This can be supplemented with dressing changes in the ICU. These dressing changes are, in fact, surgical procedures that require expertise and equipment. Newer methods of conscious sedation allow patients to be comfortable during wound management in the ICU. The extent of debridement is an important decision. Prevention and/or treatment of pelvic wound sepsis will be a function of adequate debridement. In contrast, excessive debridement may limit the options for later reconstruction. These are not procedures that should be left to junior personnel. Kudsk and coworkers advocate copious pulsatile irrigation with 10 L of fluid daily to obtain good granulation.[111] Although this may be appropriate for many patients, it may not be so for patients with relatively small skin openings. Pelvic venous injury almost certainly complicates open pelvic fractures. Venous air embolus at the time of pulsatile irrigation for an open pelvic fracture has been reported.[112]

Despite best efforts, some patients will develop pelvic sepsis. Often, this is deep in the pelvis and may be hidden by a seemingly clean wound. These patients have the potential for infection in a multiplicity of sites. Pelvic CT scanning can be helpful but may reveal only retained clots within the pelvis. Direct exploration to drain these collections via laparotomy often fails. These are not pelvic abscesses.[103] The retroperitoneal clot itself can cause systemic inflammation, and the distinction between inflammation and true infection can be difficult. Serial CT scanning may be a useful way to follow these patients. Percutaneous sampling or drainage can also be helpful.

Once the patient has recovered and wounds are clean, options for closure must be addressed. This requires a multidisciplinary approach. These patients often have rectal sphincter and/or urethral injuries. It is often appropriate to provide temporary closure with split-thickness skin grafting and/or rotation flaps if there is sufficient tissue. Occasionally, free flap coverage may be necessary. Diagnostic evaluation of the integrity of the sphincters can be undertaken and sophisticated reconstruction efforts then staged over the ensuing months and years.

## DEFINITIVE TREATMENT OF PELVIC RING DISRUPTIONS

Definitive therapy of mechanically unstable pelvic fractures does not necessarily mean early rigid internal fixation. Definitive therapy may be, in fact, the continuation of external fixation. Conversely, external fixation may not be appropriate if early internal fixation is planned. Certain conditions such as open pelvic fractures make long-term external fixation the therapy of choice, particularly when there is substantial soiling from open bowel injuries. In addition, severe comminution of strategic portions of the pelvis, such as the pubic rami, may indicate that the patient would be better served by external rather than internal fixation. The choice of fixation in patients that need fixation is therefore based on the specifics of the pelvic disruption, the patient's soft tissue envelope, and other injuries, as well as the skillset of the orthopedic surgeons at a facility. The treatment is therefore not strictly algorithmic, but we attempt to present our typical treatment plans here.

Management of the AP injuries is relatively straightforward. An AP1 fracture is a very rare pattern that is mechanically stable and the patient typically can bear weight as tolerated with no intervention. AP2 fractures are an open-book injury that is hinged on the strong posterior SI ligaments. These injuries need surgery to restore a "tension band" in the front of the pelvis, and therefore can often be treated by addressing the anterior injury only. The options for this are plate and screw fixation or external fixation. Plate fixation is usually used when the disruption is at or near the symphysis, and external fixation is used more when the anterior displacement is through rami fractures or there are other reasons why external fixation is desirable. In the obese patient, or when fixation anteriorly is weak, the anterior fixation can be augmented with posterior fixation (percutaneous sacro-iliac screws). AP3 injuries typically need posterior fixation (SI screws or plate and screws) in addition to anterior fixation.

Management of LC injuries is less straightforward because even though the LC1 type is the most common (62% in a recent series of 1229 fractures at our institution) it is also the most heterogeneous. We divide the LC1 into "good" and "bad" LC1s. Good LC1s have a minor "sacral crunch" or incomplete sacral fractures. These are typically managed nonoperatively with no limitations to ambulation. Bad LC1s have complete sacral fractures and can have significant anterior injuries. The injury may even be so severe that the pelvis springs back and is actually opened up appearing like an AP2 or AP3 on plain films. These injuries are mechanically unstable and need at least posterior SI screws, protected weight bearing, and sometimes even anterior fixation. Injuries that fall between the good and bad LC1s are commonly encountered, making the treatment algorithm variable. LC2s often require treatment via "LC2" screws (a typical SI screws may miss the fracture) or iliac wing fixation. LC3 fractures are managed by the strategy for the individual AP and LC injuries on each side. Vertical shear injuries are treated like AP3 injuries.

Bladder rupture merits separate consideration as it may change management strategy and this injury is relatively common. If the patient has a pelvic injury that would typically be treated with a plate anteriorly, we often repair the bladder rupture to prevent bathing the plate in urine, even for extraperitoneal bladder ruptures that could heal without treatment. A bladder rupture is therefore a relative contraindication to plate fixation and may push the balance toward external fixation.

## TIMING OF OPERATIVE TREATMENT OF PELVIC RING DISRUPTIONS

The timing of surgery is often determined by associated injuries and their complications, such as pulmonary compromise and central nervous system injury. In some patients, very early internal fixation may be the best option. For instance, a patient with an open-book pelvic injury and a simple symphyseal disruption with intact posterior SI ligaments (APC II) who needs a laparotomy may be best served by laparotomy followed by symphyseal plating. Recent work at the authors' institution indicate that ORIF at the time of laparotomy for acute treatment of unstable pelvic fractures may be as safe as external fixator application and does not appear to be associated with any increased morbidity.[113]

In patients who do not need an emergent laparotomy, there is more flexibility regarding operative timing. The best management of pelvic ring injuries that require fixation may be staged surgery (see Chap. 40). If the patient is hemodynamically stable, the pelvic fracture that otherwise requires surgery does not necessarily require definitive fixation on the first day. For reasons of hemodynamic stability, coagulopathy, and hypothermia, surgery may be best delayed. However, most severe pelvic injuries require some type of surgical intervention early in the treatment regimen, whereas definitive and more rigid fixation may be more appropriately applied later (as previously discussed) when resuscitation is complete and management of other injuries have been addressed. This should be balanced against the advantages of earlier definitive fixation that allows for early patient mobilization which may benefit the patient in facilitating pulmonary toilet, terminating mechanical ventilation, and providing more aggressive early rehabilitation.

In general, open reduction of the anterior pelvis is typically attempted after some time (24 to 48 hours) has been allowed for clot to stabilize. Immediate plating is associated with increased blood loss and should not be entered into lightly in the patient who was previously hemodynamically unstable. However external fixation can be performed immediately with little blood loss. The advantage of immediate external fixation is that it allows for the removal of the binder in patients who needed a binder for hemodynamic compromise, particularly if the patient has ramus fractures that are not easily treated with plates and screws. Immediate percutaneous fixation of the SI joint or iliac wing fractures can also be performed immediately as there is only minimal blood loss with these injuries. Early posterior fixation is that percutaneous techniques require good fluoroscopic images and these may be difficult to obtain in the acute setting due to contrast from CT scans.

## TECHNIQUES OF FIXATION

In mechanically unstable pelvic ring disruptions, fixation options can be thought of addressing either the anterior ring or the posterior ring. The anterior ring is fixed with either an external fixator or with plate and screw fixation. Posterior ring injuries are either treated with percutaneous screw fixation or with open plating techniques, depending on the injury pattern and the soft tissue injuries.

There are two standard approaches for attaining access to the pubic symphysis for anterior plate and screw fixation. One is through the continuation of a midline laparotomy incision created for abdominal surgery. The second approach is through a Pfannenstiel incision two fingerbreadths cephalad to the superior pubic rami. Whichever skin approach is used, the plane of injury is then approached through the rectus abdominis muscle (one-half of which is almost always disconnected at its insertion to the symphysis). The nondisrupted portion of the rectus abdominis muscle is then elevated gently forward, and retractors are placed behind the remaining rectus to provide access to the superior portions of both pubic bones.

Reduction is then accomplished, often with simple surgical tenacula or pelvic reduction clamps. The surgeon must then make a decision about the cartilaginous disk between the pubic bones. It is often best addressed by resection, but if not, its position must be appreciated to permit symmetric application of the plate. The symphyseal plate is then held in place over the reduced symphysis, and large fragment screws fix it into position. Fluoroscopic guidance is useful to verify reduction. Anterior fixation of the pelvis has been achieved with various plate and screw constructs, as well as two plates placed at 90° to each other. At our institution we use at least two screws on each side of the pelvis for symphyseal disruptions. Longer plates are needed to span ramus fractures. Specially designed large fragment curved plates with either 6.5-mm or 4.5-mm screws are used for this application, as are 3.5-mm reconstruction plates. The screws running next to the symphysis are typically at least 50 mm long if directed in the correct plane (Fig. 38-20).

Definitive operative techniques for posterior pelvic ring injury are varied (Fig. 38-14). One approach is simply a surgical incision over the iliac crest with most of the reduction maneuvers occurring on the medial surface of the ilium after retraction of the iliacus. Exposure can be gained to address fractures of the iliac wing (LC2) as well as disruptions running all the way back to the SI joint (AP2, AP3). Open fixation of the SI joint can be done through this

approach and offers the advantage of direct visualization of the SI joint. Two perpendicular two-hole plates are traditionally used for fixation of the SI joint through this approach.

Another option to address posterior ring disruptions is a posterior approach to the ilium in a lateral or prone position with exposure made from the external surface of the ilium. This approach is needed to reduce certain "complete" sacral fractures. Large posterior approaches, and plating across the posterior pelvis (or "sacral bars") have been associated with high rates of wound complication[114] and should be avoided if possible.

Whenever possible, it is advantageous to perform percutaneous fixation of the posterior ring.[115–117] The advantage is the minimal blood loss and small surgical incisions. Open reduction techniques have the advantage of direct visualization, accuracy of reduction, and potentially more rigid fixation. However, in situations involving compromised skin and in patients whose other medical conditions do not permit certain surgical positioning, these techniques have considerable potential for complications. In addition, the wide exposure necessary for the benefit of direct visualization has the disadvantage of devascularization secondary to periosteal elevation, with all the attendant problems with wound infections.

The advantages of image-guided indirect reduction and percutaneous fixation of the posterior pelvic ring are best realized when the reduction can be accurately achieved. This relies on fluoroscopic visualization so the patient must not have contrast obscuring the radiographic views or be too obese to obtain good images. Disruptions of the SI joint, fractures of the sacrum, and certain iliac wing fractures are candidates for percutaneous fixation. Many reports have addressed this technique with regard to choice of approach, positioning of screws, and safety in these extremely high-risk areas.[115–117]

Although percutaneous posterior pelvic fixation of choice for most SI joint disruptions, fractures of the sacrum, and many LC2 iliac wing fractures, there is a very small margin of error. The obvious advantages of extremely minimal surgical fields and essentially no dissection may be outweighed by the inability to obtain direct reduction and, more importantly, by the unusually

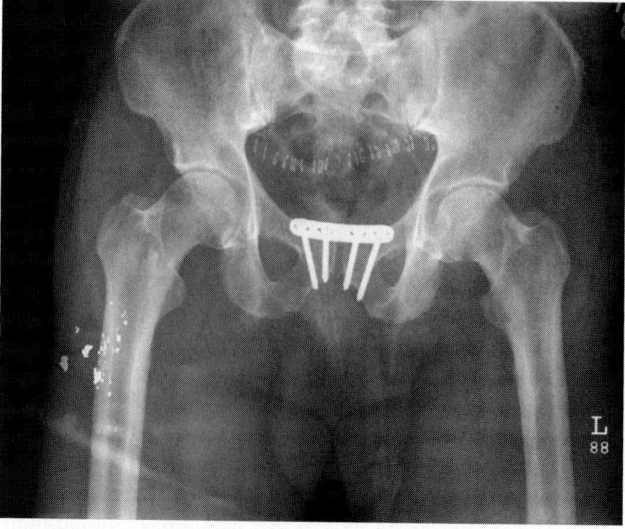

**FIGURE 38-20.** Patient with symphyseal disruption is treated operatively with an anterior pelvic plate.

small tolerances for error in screw placement. For example, iliosacral screws are placed through the ilium into the SI body via the first SI pedicle. The corridor of safety in this pedicle is extremely narrow because the great vessels of the posterior pelvis lie just anteriorly. Major nerve roots of L5 and S1 lie just cephalad and caudal to the path, and the spinal canal lies directly behind the path. With the corridor as narrow as perhaps $1.5 \times 1.5$ cm, accurate visualization and the hands of experienced surgeons are necessary for the benefits to outweigh the risks of this technique. This corridor is thought to shrink further with any malreduction of the sacro-iliac joint. These techniques should therefore only be attempted by experienced clinicians who are well trained in these techniques.

## ASSOCIATED INJURIES

Many patients do not have isolated pelvic fractures. As the understanding of pelvic fracture management continues to evolve, deaths from pelvic-fracture-related complications, particularly hemorrhage, have decreased. Thus, associated injuries have begun to play a more prominent role in morbidity and mortality. Table 38–4 depicts the most common injuries associated with pelvic fractures as compiled from the literature.[14,36,118] These specific injuries are dealt with in detail in other chapters. However, their management deserves some comment here, especially as it relates to relative priorities when a pelvic fracture is present.

In general, the management strategies should continue to follow basic principles of injury care. The bleeding from long-bone fractures must be quantified when one is assessing transfusion requirements and attempting to gauge the amount of blood loss that is referable to the pelvic fracture. External bleeding should be obvious on physical exam and must be promptly controlled by whatever means necessary. Intracavitary bleeding such as the thorax or abdomen is the next highest priority (see Chap. 29).

Traumatic brain injury is common in patients with pelvic fractures. CT scanning is the "gold standard" for the diagnosis and management of patients with closed-head injuries (see Chap. 19). Unfortunately, the hemodynamic status of patients may preclude safe transport to the CT scanner. Hypotension can substantially worsen long-term outcome from brain injury, even if transient.[119,120] Thus, the first priority must be resuscitation and treatment of hemorrhage. Patients who are most likely to have their treatment plan changed as a result of head CT scan (e.g., require craniotomy) are those who present with lateralizing neurologic signs on physical exam.[121]

One option for patients who are not able to have CT scanning is to have blind placement of intracranial pressure monitors. While this does give the clinician some measure of comfort about the patient's neurologic status, the information may not change the therapy.

Patients who have CT scans that demonstrate lesions requiring craniotomy can have that procedure performed concurrently with laparotomy or application of external pelvic fixation. Patients with retroperitoneal hemorrhage, hypotension, and brain injury requiring craniotomy represent a special subset. A decision must be made as to whether the patients can be stabilized with transfusions long enough to allow a full craniotomy or whether they are better served by angiography followed by craniotomy. Unfortunately, there is no cookbook way to approach this decision, but rather should be made at the level of best clinical judgment.

After hemorrhage and life-threatening brain injuries are addressed, the next priority is the repair of visceral injuries that are not accompanied by hemorrhage. Examples include intraperitoneal bladder rupture or a diaphragmatic injury. Occasionally, repair of these injuries must be staged in a manner similar to that of the patient treated with damage control techniques. For instance, patients with pelvic fractures and hypotension with positive FAST for free fluid should be taken to the operating room. Small bowel injuries can be stapled and bladder injuries temporized with sutures. If patients have ongoing pelvic hemorrhage, they should be rapidly taken to angiography and undergo embolization or have operative pelvic packing possibly followed by adjunctive angiography. Postembolization, patients can be returned to the operating room for a more complete exploration that allows for definitive management of important but non-life-threatening injuries.

The association between pelvic fractures and blunt aortic injury has been known for over ten years. Although the mechanism is unclear, it does seem that aortic injuries are most commonly seen in patients with AP and LC injuries.[122,123] As survival following aortic injury is directly related to the time to diagnosis, there must be a real premium on rapid evaluation of this potentially life-threatening injury. This is discussed in detail in Chap. 28. Richardson and associates have demonstrated that pelvic fractures occur approximately twice as often in patients with a widened mediastinum and aortic injury as in patients without aortic transection.[124] If the mediastinum is not normal, evaluation for the possibility of aortic injury should assume a high priority in the diagnostic evaluation. Fortunately, there are several tests that are commonly used in the care of patients with pelvic fractures that can be used to identify aortic injury.

**TABLE 38-4**

| Associated Injuries (%) | |
|---|---|
| Closed Head Injury | 50 |
| Long Bone Fracture | 48 |
| Peripheral Nerve Injury | 25 |
| Thoracic Injury | 21 |
| Bladder | 7 |
| Spleen | 7 |
| Liver | 7 |
| Gastrointestinal Tract | 5 |
| Kidney | 2 |
| Urethra | 3 |
| Mesentary | 1 |
| Diaphragm | 2 |
| N = 2.721 | |

Source: Evers BM, Cryer HM, Miller FB: Pelvic fracture hemorrhage: Priorities in management. Arch Surg 124:422, 1989. Burgess AR, Eastridge BJ, Young JWR: Pelvic ring disruptions: Effective classification system and treatment protocols. J Trauma 30:848, 1990. Klein SR, Sarovan RM, Raumgarten F, Bongard FS: Management strategy of vascular injuries associated with pelvic fractures. J Cardiovasc Surg 33:349, 1992. Parreira JG, Coimbra R, Rasslan S, et al: The role of associated injuries on outcome of blunt trauma patients sustaining pelvic fractures. Injury 31:677, 2000. Demetriades D, Karaiskakis M, Toutouzas K, et al.: Pelvic fractures: Epidemiology and predictors of associated abdominal injuries and outcomes. J Am Coll Surg 195:1, 2002. Inaba K, Sharkey PW, Stephen DJG, et al.: The increasing incidence of severe pelvic injury in motor vehicle collisions. Injury 35:159, 2004.

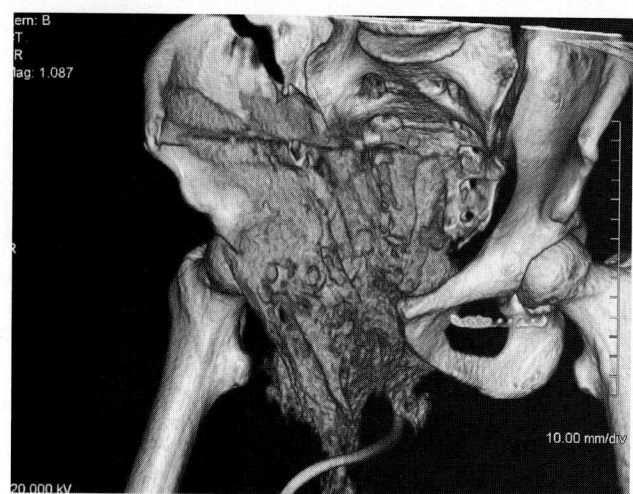

**FIGURE 38-21.** CT scan demonstrates obvious bladder disruption.

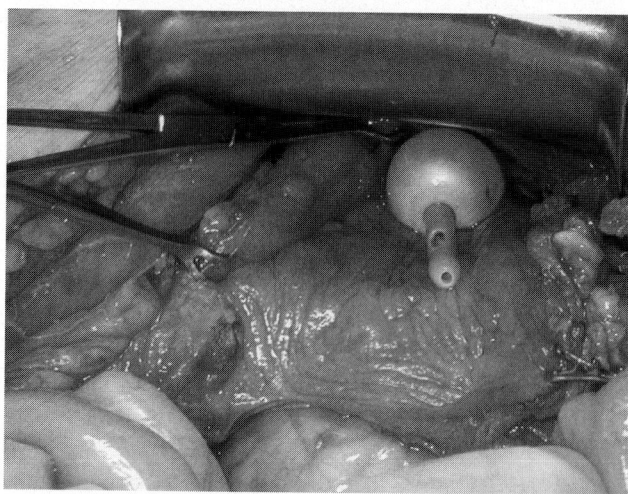

**FIGURE 38-22.** Intraoperative photo of intraperitoneal bladder rupture with the Foley catheter visible in the wound.

Helical CT has been shown to be an effective screening tool for blunt aortic injury.[125] Thus, patients who undergo CT scan as part of their workup for their pelvic fracture can undergo chest CT at the same time (see Chap. 15). Aortography can be utilized if other tests are equivocal.[126] Finally, transesophageal echocardiography (TEE) has been useful in the diagnosis of aortic injury.[127] This may be most appropriate for patients with a pelvic fracture and exsanguinating hemorrhage who are treated in the operating room, as TEE can readily be performed at the same time as laparotomy or pelvic fixation.

Genitourinary injuries commonly occur with pelvic fractures. Overall, they may be found in as many as 16% of the patients who present with pelvic fractures. Bladder injuries occur in as many as 7% of these patients (Figs. 38-21 and 38-22).[128,129] While the diagnosis of genitourinary injuries is discussed in Chap. 38, several additional comments are appropriate. All patients with pelvic fractures should have their lower urinary tract evaluated.

Urethral injuries occur in approximately 15% of males with pelvic fractures (Fig. 38-23).[129] If patients are stable, there is little reason not to perform a retrograde urethrogram prior to placement of a Foley catheter. The classic presentation of males with urethral injuries includes blood at the urinary meatus, a high-riding prostate, or scrotal hematoma. Unfortunately, these are nonspecific. While the presence of any of these signs is strongly suggestive of urethral injury, the absence does not necessarily rule out the injury. One series found that only 36% of patients with urethral injuries presented with blood at the meatus and another 21% had gross hematuria without meatal blood.[130] In a large retrospective review, Lowe and colleagues demonstrated that as many as 57% of male patients with urethral injuries present with none of the classic signs.[131] Although urethral injury is uncommon in females, it does exist. Some investigators quote an incidence as high as 6% associated with pelvic fractures.[132,133] Barach and coworkers have suggested that bilateral pubic rami fractures, significant vertical displacement of the pelvis, and symphyseal disruption are the fracture patterns most likely to be associated with urethral injuries in females.[133] These may be very difficult to diagnose. While lacerations of the vaginal mucosa have been reported with relative frequency, the finding of blood at the urinary meatus is virtually never present. Urethral injuries in the male are typically treated with suprapubic bladder drainage. They may require acute repair in the

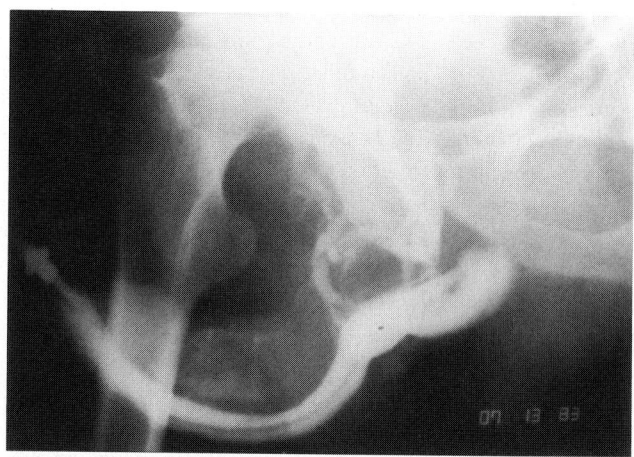

**FIGURE 38-23.** Retrograde urethrogram demonstrates extravasation of contrast. The patient was treated with suprapubic cystostomy.

setting of severe pelvic fractures for several reasons. Suprapubic tubes may interfere with bony fixation and early definitive repair may be associated with fewer long-term complications, such as stricture.[134,135] Urethral disruptions in females typically require operative repair.[136]

Bladder rupture also commonly accompanies pelvic fractures. It takes substantial energy to rupture an empty viscous bladder enclosed in a protective bony ring. A ruptured bladder is a good indicator of the severity of injury, particularly if the bladder was empty at the time of impact. Most patients present with gross hematuria, although in some instances hematuria may only be microscopic.[137–139]

The timing of diagnostics is crucial. While it is important not to delay the genitourinary evaluation, neither urethral injury nor bladder rupture is immediately life-threatening (see Chap. 38). Thus, their evaluation can be deferred until life-threatening injuries are addressed. Patients who require angiography for diagnosis and control of pelvic blood loss should not have a cystogram performed prior to the angiogram. Extravasation of contrast into the retroperitoneum may limit the angiographer's ability to identify vascular injury.

Extraperitoneal bladder rupture is the most common type of bladder rupture accompanying patients with pelvic fractures.[140] Treatment for this is simple decompression with a Foley catheter or suprapubic tube if a concomitant urethral injury is present (see Chap. 38). Extraperitoneal bladder ruptures may require operative repair if very extensive or if anterior plating of the pelvis is to be performed, to prevent contamination of implanted hardware. Conversely, an extraperitoneal bladder rupture may be a relative indication to use external fixation as a definitive strategy to avoid the potential for contamination of the hardware.

The genitourinary evaluation is not complete until the entire urinary tract has been examined and imaged. This includes an evaluation of the upper as well as the lower tract. Generally, CT scanning is the diagnostic test of choice to image the kidneys and ureters, while the urethra is evaluated with a retrograde urethrogram and the possibility of bladder injury by a cystogram (see Chap. 15). If a CT scan is being performed for other indications, a CT cystogram is an alternative to conventional cystography and may be as accurate.[141] Certainly, patients can have injuries at several levels. Thus, patients with gross hematuria and extraperitoneal bladder rupture should not be assumed to have hematuria as a result of the bladder rupture until the kidneys have been examined as well. Because the majority of renal injuries can be treated nonoperatively, it is acceptable to delay this evaluation for several hours until injuries of higher priority are addressed.

Nerve injury occurs relatively frequently with pelvic fractures, particularly if there is a significant posterior component.[142] Early documentation of this is important. The knowledge will not alter therapy over the short term; however, the information is significant when making long-term prognostic judgments. Unfortunately, a detailed neurologic evaluation may not be possible. The symptoms of pelvic nerve injury are often pain, which may be located in the back or may radiate to either lower extremity. Back pain is a common symptom of the pelvic fracture itself, and pain in the lower extremities may be easily explained by lower extremity fractures that may accompany the pelvic injury. Thus, the diagnosis may be difficult. When patient stability permits, a detailed neurologic assessment, with both sensory and motor examinations, directed at lumbar and sacral nerve root function should be performed. A neurologic consultation can be helpful to map out precise nerve root function. Occasionally, examinations such as electromyelograms can be used later in the patient's hospital course. Long-term functional results following pelvic fractures are markedly worse with concomitant neurologic injury.[143]

## DELAYED COMPLICATIONS

Pelvic fractures increase the risk of deep vein thrombosis (DVT).[144,145] Some combination of pneumatic sequential compression devices, lower extremity elastic stockings, and low-molecular weight or low-dose unfractionated heparin are generally employed as prophylaxis for DVT (see Chap. 57).[146,147] DVT may be difficult to assess on physical exam secondary to lower extremity swelling from fractures, operative fixation, or lymphedema. Duplex Doppler ultrasound screening may help to identify occult DVT. Unfortunately, thrombi may occur in the deep pelvic veins, making detection with US difficult. Patients with pelvic fractures

are at particular risk for thromboembolism, because they all have some degree of pelvic venous injury and are immobilized for some time. The best treatment strategy is an aggressive program of prevention. Pharmacologic manipulations combined with early fracture fixation and mobilization are probably the best way to prevent DVT. Unfortunately, this is not always possible. Despite aggressive therapy, some patients will develop deep thrombosis.

If DVT is diagnosed, consideration must be given to whether anticoagulation is safe. Certainly, anticoagulation is contraindicated for patients who have substantial blood loss, particularly from pelvic fractures. After several days, if patients have remained stable, they may be candidates for anticoagulation.

If there is any concern about the appropriateness of anticoagulation therapy, consideration should be given to placement of an inferior vena caval filter to prevent pulmonary embolism.[148] While the role of prophylactic caval filters has not been precise, the authors' practice is to give strong consideration to this procedure for patients with serious posterior pelvic fractures, especially if they are multiply injured. The development of retrievable filters makes this even more attractive. In particular, patients with pelvic fractures and significant traumatic brain injuries, spinal injury, or lower extremity fractures are often treated with prophylactic inferior vena caval filters.[148]

The diagnosis of pulmonary embolism must be suspected in any patient with a pelvic fracture. Unfortunately, these patients have a multiplicity of reasons to develop hypoxia other than that caused by pulmonary emboli, such as fat embolism from long-bone fractures, atelectasis from immobilization, or pneumonia. The diagnosis of pulmonary embolism must be aggressively pursued in order to make the diagnosis in a timely manner. A combination of chest x-ray, spiral chest CT, ventilation/perfusion lung scan, and pulmonary angiography should be utilized in order to make the diagnosis.

## OUTCOMES

The mortality for patients with pelvic fractures is approximately 6%.[17,29,49,56,67,150] In the past, most deaths were due to hemorrhage. More recently, this does not seem to be the case (Table 38-5). Presumably, a better understanding and earlier recognition of the pelvis as a potential source of blood loss has resulted in fewer people dying from pelvic bleeding. While approximately 40% of the people die secondary to hemorrhage, many of them have other sources of blood loss to explain this.[13,16,36,118,151,152] In one study, Poole and colleagues reviewed 236 patients with pelvic fractures treated over a one-year period.[152] Overall mortality was 7.6%. Of the 18 patients who died, approximately 39% died secondary to hemorrhage. However, only one of those deaths was caused by pelvic hemorrhage. All other deaths were due to hemorrhage from other sites. Another study from Los Angeles County of 1545 patients with pelvic fractures demonstrated a mortality rate of 13.5%, but less than 1% of deaths were attributed to hemorrhage from the pelvic fracture.[36] Other common causes of major morbidity and mortality include closed-head injuries, which accounts for approximately one-third of the deaths. Sepsis and multiple-organ failure account for the other 30% (see Table 38-5).

Unfortunately, patients surviving even major pelvic fractures often have long-term morbidity. Data from the 1980 and 1990s

## TABLE 38-5

### Mortality in Pelvic Fractures

|  | NUMBER | PERCENTAGE |
|---|---|---|
| Mortality | 83 | 6% of total |
| Bleeding | 32 | 39% of deaths |
| Head injury | 26 | 31% of deaths |
| Multiple-organ failure | 25 | 30% of deaths |
| N = 1399 |  |  |

Sources: Klein SR, Sarovan RM, Raumgarten F, et al.: Management strategy of vascular injuries associated with pelvic fractures. J Cardiovasc Surg 33:349, 1992. Evers BM, Cryer HM, Miller FB: Pelvic fracture hemorrhage: Priorities in management. Arch Surg 124:422, 1989. Flint L, Babikian G, Anderson M, et al.: Definitive control of mortality from severe pelvic fracture. Ann Surg 211:703, 1990. Gruen GS, Leit ME, Gruen RJ, et al.: The acute management of hemodynamically unstable multiple trauma patients with pelvic ring fractures. J Trauma 36:706, 1994 and Burgess AR, Eastridge BJ, Young JWR: Pelvic ring disruptions: Effective classification system and treatment protocols. J Trauma 30:848, 1990.

suggested that up to one-half of these patients may have serious pain and disability, especially if the fracture involves the sacrum or SI joints.[153-155] The nature of the fracture and the adequacy of reduction may play a significant role. McLaren performed a five-year follow-up on 43 patients with high-energy pelvic fractures.[154] Of patients who had a small amount of residual deformity (fracture displacement <1 cm), almost 90% had no pain and approximately 80% had normal function. However, patients who had residual deformity (displacement >1 cm posteriorly) had a 70% chance of having serious pain and a 70% chance of abnormal function. Other researchers have questioned this concept, however, claiming that degree of residual displacement may not have a significant effect on long-term functional outcome.[75,76,155,156] The functional results following a combination of operative approaches including internal reduction, percutaneous pinning, and external fixation of pelvic fractures are likely to be better than previously reported. Gruen conducted a one-year follow-up on 48 patients after ORIF for unstable pelvic ring fractures and found that the majority of patients were able to return to work and 77% reported only mild disability using the Sickness Impact Profile.[157] Other studies have similarly reported that over two-thirds of patients were able to return to their previous employment following severe pelvic ring fractures treated with internal fixation.[143,158] Fracture pattern may also have some bearing on long-term functional outcome. Patients with severe fractures seem to have a higher chance of long-term pain and disability, though even minor pelvic fractures can result in adverse outcomes. Open fractures are particularly associated with poor functional outcome.[159]

Other long-term complications exist. Though poorly documented in the literature, patients with pelvic fractures have been found to have significant problems with sexual function, impotence, and dyspareunia.[155,160-164] In addition, Copeland and associates noted surprisingly high numbers of females with pelvic fractures who had urinary tract symptoms (21%) and lower gastrointestinal symptoms (8%) more than 18 months after injury.[160] This was true despite a very low incidence of genitourinary and gastrointestinal trauma at the time of injury. Symptoms occurred more often in patients with residual pelvic fracture displacement (>5 mm) and in patients with residual lateral or vertical displacement. Cesarean sections were significantly more frequent in subjects with fractures initially displaced over 5 mm. Physicians caring for injured patients

must keep these symptoms in mind. Patients should be gently questioned because they are often reluctant to volunteer complaints of this nature to their physicians.

## REFERENCES

1. Dalal SA, Burgess AR, Siegel JH, et al.: Pelvic fracture in multiple trauma: Classification by mechanism is key to pattern of organ injury, resuscitative requirements, and outcome. J Trauma 29:891, 1989.
2. Pennal GF, Tile M, Waddell JP, et al.: Pelvic disruption: Assessment and classification. Clin Ortho 151:12, 1980.
3. Tile M: Acute pelvic fractures: I. Causation and classification. J Am Acad Orthop Surg 4:143, 1996.
4. Young JWR, Burgess AR: Radiologic Management of Pelvic Ring Fractures: Systematic Radiologic Diagnosis. Baltimore: Urban & Schwarzenberg, 1987.
5. Young JWR, Burgess AR: Fractures of the pelvis. In Mirvis SE, Young JWR, eds. Imaging in Trauma and Critical Care. Baltimore: Williams & Wilkins, 1992, p. 382.
6. Young JWR, Burgess AR, Brumback RJ, et al.: Lateral compression fractures of the pelvis: The importance of plain radiographs in the diagnosis and surgical management. Skeletal Radiol 15:103, 1986.
7. Young JWR, Burgess AR, Brumback RJ, et al.: Pelvic fractures: Value of plain radiography in early assessment and management. Radiology 160:445, 1986.
8. Tile M: Acute pelvic fractures: II. Principles of management. J Am Acad Orthop Surg 4:152, 1996.
9. Tile M, Pennal GF: Pelvic disruption: Principles of management. Clin Orthop 151:56, 1980.
10. Starr A, Griffin D, Reinert CM, et al.: Pelvic ring disruptions: Prediction of associated injuries, transfusion requirements, pelvic arteriography, complications, and mortality. J Ortho Trauma 16:553, 2002.
11. O'Sullivan RE, White TO, Keating JF: Major pelvic fractures identification of patients at high risk. J Bone Jt Surg Br 87B:530, 2005.
12. Poole GV, Ward EF, Muakkassa FF, et al.: Pelvic fracture from major blunt trauma. Ann Surg 213:532, 1991.
13. Poole GV, Ward EF: Causes of mortality in patients with pelvic fractures. Orthopedics 17:691, 1994.
14. Inaba K, Sharkey PW, Stephen DJG, et al.: The increasing incidence of severe pelvic injury in motor vehicle collisions. Injury 35:159, 2004.
15. Coppola PT, Coppola M: Emergency department evaluation and treatment of pelvic fractures. Emerg Med Clin North Am 18:1, 2000.
16. Gansslen A, Pohlemann T, Paul C, et al.: Pelvic fracture mechanism of injury in vehicular trauma patients. J Trauma 36:789, 1994.
17. Cryer HG, Johnson E: Pelvic fractures. In Feliciano D, Moore EE, Mattox K, eds. Trauma, 3rd ed. Stamford, CT: Appleton & Lange, 1996.
18. Salvino CK, Esposito TJ, Smith LD, et al.: Routine pelvic x-ray studies in awake blunt trauma patients: A sensible policy? J Trauma 33:413, 1992.
19. McCormick JP, Morgan SJ, Smith WR: Clinical effectiveness of the physical examination in diagnosis of posterior pelvic ring fractures. J Orthop Trauma 17:257, 2003.
20. Killeen KL, DeMeo JH: CT detection of serious internal and skeletal injuries in patients with pelvic fractures. Acad Radiol 6:224, 1999.
21. Cerva DS Jr, Mirvs SE, Shanmuganathan K, et al.: Detection of bleeding in patients with major pelvic fractures: Value of contrast-enhanced CT. AJR Am J Roentgenol 166:131, 1996.
22. Pereira SJ, O'Brien DP, Luchette FA, et al.: Dynamic helical computed tomography scan accurately detects hemorrhage in patients with pelvic fracture. Surgery 128:678, 2000.
23. Falchi M, Rollandi GA: CT of pelvic fractures. Eur J Radiol 50:96, 2004.
24. Guillamondegui OD, Pryor JP, Gracias VH, et al.: Pelvic radiography in blunt trauma resuscitation: A diminishing role. J Trauma 53:1043, 2002.
25. Herzog C, Ahle H, Mack MG, et al.: Traumatic injuries of the pelvis and thoracic and lumbar spine: Does thin-slice multidetector-row CT increase diagnostic accuracy? Eur Radiol 14:1751, 2004.
26. Stewart BG, Rhea JT, Sheridan RL, et al.: Is the screening portable pelvis film clinically useful in multiple trauma patients who will be examined by abdominopelvic CT? Experience with 397 patients. Emerg Radiol 9:266, 2002.
27. Chiu WC, Cushing BM, Rodriguez A, et al.: Abdominal injuries without hemiperitoneum: A potential limitation of focused abdominal sonography for trauma. J Trauma 42:617, 1997.
28. Scalea TM, Goldstein AS, Phillips TF, et al.: An analysis of 161 falls from a height, the "jumper syndrome." J Trauma 26:593, 1986.
29. Klein SR, Sarovan RM, Raumgarten F, et al.: Management strategy of vascular injuries associated with pelvic fractures. J Cardiovasc Surg 33:349, 1992.
30. Scalea TM, Henry SM: Inotropes in the intensive care unit. In Maull K, ed. Advances in Trauma and Critical Care. St. Louis: Mosby, 1992, p. 33.

31. Scalea TM, Holman M, Fuortes M, et al.: Central venous blood oxygen saturation: An early accurate measurement of volume during hemorrhage. *J Trauma* 28:725, 1988.

32. Rutherford EJ, Morris JA, Reed GW, et al.: Base deficit stratifies mortality and determines therapy. *J Trauma* 38:417, 1992.

33. Ferrara A, MacArthur JD, Wright HK, et al.: Hypothermia and acidosis worsen coagulopathy in patients requiring massive transfusion. *Am J Surg* 160:515, 1990.

34. Scalea TM, Duncan AO: Initial management of the critically ill trauma patient in extremis. *Trauma Q* 10:3, 1993.

35. Pedowitz RA, Shackford SR: Non-cavitary hemorrhage producing shock in trauma patients: Incidence and severity. *J Trauma* 29:219, 1989.

36. Demetriades D, Karaiskakis M, Toutouzas K, et al.: Pelvic fractures: Epidemiology and predictors of associated abdominal injuries and outcomes. *J Am Coll Surg* 195:1, 2002.

37. O'Brien DP, Luchette FA, Pereira SJ, et al.: Pelvic fracture in the elderly is associated with increased mortality. *Surgery* 132:710, 2002.

38. Healey MA, Simons RK, Winchell RJ, et al.: A prospective evaluation of abdominal ultrasound in blunt trauma: Is it useful? *J Trauma* 40:875, 1996.

39. Rozycki GS, Ochsner MG, Schmidt JA, et al.: P prospective study of surgeon-performed ultrasound as the primary adjuvant modality for injured patient assessment. *J Trauma* 39:492, 1995.

40. Rozycki GS, Ballard RB, Feliciano DV, et al.: Surgeon-performed ultrasound for the assessment of truncal injuries: Lessons learned from 1540 patients. *Ann Surg* 228:557, 1998.

41. Branney SW, Wolfe RE, Moore EE, et al.: Quantitative sensitivity of ultrasound in detecting free intraperitoneal fluid. *J Trauma* 39:375, 1995.

42. Mele TS, Stewart K, Marokus B, et al.: Evaluation of a diagnostic protocol using screening diagnostic peritoneal lavage with selective use of abdominal computed tomography in blunt abdominal trauma. *J Trauma* 46:847, 1999.

43. Hubbard SG, Bivins BA, Sachatello CR, et al.: Diagnostic errors with peritoneal lavage in patients with pelvic fractures. *Arch Surg* 114:844, 1979.

44. Ruchholtz S, Waydhas C, Lewan U, et al.: Free abdominal fluid on ultrasound in pelvic ring fracture: Is laparotomy always necessary? *J Trauma* 57:278, 2004.

45. Biffl WL, Smith WR, Moore EE, et al.: Evolution of a multidisciplinary clinical pathway for the management of unstable patients with pelvic fractures. *Ann Surg* 233:843, 2001.

46. Sclafani SJA, Weisberg A, Scalea TM, et al.: Blunt splenic injuries: Nonsurgical treatment with CT, arteriograph and transcatheter embolization of the splenic artery. *Radiology* 18:1, 1991.

47. Renz BM, Feliciano DV: Unnecessary laparotomies for trauma: A prospective study of morbidity. *J Trauma* 38:350, 1995.

48. Haan J, Kole K, Brunetti A, et al.: Related articles, links nontherapeutic laparotomies revisited. *Am Surg* 69:562, 2003. PMID: 12889616 [PubMed - indexed for MEDLINE

49. Baron BJ, Scalea TM, Sclafani SJ: A non-operative management of blunt abdominal trauma: The role of sequential diagnostic peritoneal lavage, CT and angiography. *Ann Emerg Med* 22:1557, 1993.

50. Schnurr MJ, Fabian TC, Gavarn M, et al.: Management of blunt splenic trauma: Computed tomography contrast blush predicts failure of non-operative management. *J Trauma* 35:907, 1995.

51. Eastridge BJ, Starr A, Minei J, et al.: The importance of fracture pattern in guiding therapeutic decision-making in patients with hemorrhagic shock and pelvic ring disruptions. *J Trauma* 53:446, 2002.

52. Metz CM, Hak DJ, Goulet JA, et al.: Pelvic fracture patterns and their corresponding angiographic sources of hemorrhage. *Orthop Clin N Am* 35:431, 2004.

53. Ben-Menachem Y, Coldwell DM, Young JWR, et al.: Hemorrhage associated with pelvic fractures: Causes, diagnoses and emergent management. *AJR Am J Roentgenol* 157:1005, 1991.

54. Burgess AR, Eastridge BJ, Young JWR: Pelvic ring disruptions: Effective classification system and treatment protocols. *J Trauma* 30:848, 1990.

55. O'Neill PA, Riina J, Sclafani S, et al.: Angiographic findings in pelvic fractures. *Clin Ortho Rel Res* 329:60, 1996.

56. Moreno C, Moore EE, Rosenberg A, et al.: Hemorrhage with major pelvic fracture: A multispecialty challenge. *J Trauma* 26:987, 1986.

57. Siegel JH, Dalal SA, Burgess AR, et al.: Pattern of organ injuries in pelvic fracture: Impact of force implications for survival and death in motor vehicle injuries. *Accid Anal Prev* 22:457, 1990.

58. Scalea TM, Kohn L: Geriatric trauma. In Feliciano DV, Moore EE, Mattox KL, eds. *Trauma*, 3rd ed. Stamford, CT: Appleton & Lange, 1996.

59. Henry SM, Pollak AN, Jones AL, et al.: Pelvic fractures in geriatric patients: A distinct clinical entity. *J Trauma* 53:15, 2002.

60. Bottlang M, Krieg JC, Mohr M, et al.: Emergent management of pelvic ring fractures with use of circumferential compression. *J Bone Joint Surg Am* 84-A:43, 2002.

61. Krieg JC, Mohr M, Ellis TJ, et al.: Emergent stabilization of pelvic ring injuries by controlled circumferential compression: A clinical trial. *J Trauma* 59:659, 2005.

62. Born CT, Fitzpatrick MK, Reilly P, et al.: Temporary stabilization of pelvic fractures with the Tpod device in the polytrauma patient. Poster #P247 presented at the *American Academy of Orthopedic Surgeons Annual Meeting*, San Francisco, CA, 2004.

63. DeAngelis NA, Wixted JJ, French BG: Use of the Trauma Pelvic Orthotic Device (T-POD) for provisional stabilization of anterior-posterior compression type pelvic injuries: A cadaveric study. Poster #97 presented at the *Orthopedic Trauma Association Annual Meeting*, Salt Lake City, Utah, 2003.

64. Ghanayem AJ, Stover MD, Goldstein JA, et al.: Emergent treatment of pelvic fractures comparison of methods for stabilization. *Clin Orthop Rel Res* 318:75, 1995.

65. Friese G, LaMay G: Emergency stabilization of unstable pelvic fractures. *Emerg Med Serv* 34:65, 2005.

66. Frank LR: Is MAST in the past? The pros and cons of MAST usage in the field. *J Emerg Med Services* 25:38, 2000.

67. Flint L, Babikian G, Anderson M, et al.: Definitive control of mortality from severe pelvic fracture. *Ann Surg* 211:703, 1990.

68. Cullen DJ, Cayle JP, Teplick R: Cardiovascular, pulmonary and renal effects of massively increased intra-abdominal pressure in critically ill patients. *Crit Care Med* 17:118, 1989.

69. Ganz R, Kroshell RJ, Jakob RP, et al.: The anti-shock pelvic clamp. *Clin Orthop* 126:71, 1991.

70. Burgess A: External fixation. In Tile M, ed. *Fractures of the Pelvis and Acetabulum,* 2nd ed. Baltimore: Williams & Wilkins, 1995.

71. Henry SM, Scalea TM, Tornetta P: Damage control for devastating pelvic and extremity injuries. *Surg Clin North Am* 77:879, 1997.

72. Burgess AR: The management of hemorrhage associated with pelvic fractures. *Int J Orthop Trauma* 2:101, 1992.

73. Gylling SF, Ward RE, Holcroft JW: Immediate external fixation of unstable pelvic fracture. *Am J Surg* 150:721, 1985.

74. Riemer B: Acute mortality associated with injuries to the pelvic ring: The role of early patient mobilization and external fixation. *J Trauma* 35:671, 1993.

75. Miranda MA, Riemer BL, Butterfield SL, et al.: Pelvic ring injuries: A long term functional outcome study. *Clin Orthop* 1:152, 1996.

76. Majeed SA: External fixation of the injured pelvis. The functional outcome. *J Bone Joint Surg Br* 72:612, 1990.

77. Lindahl J, Hirvensalo E, Bostman O, et al.: Failure of reduction with an external fixator in the management of injuries of the pelvic ring: Long-term evaluation of 110 patients. *J Bone Joint Surg Br* 81:955, 1999.

78. Mason WTM, Khan SN, James CL, et al.: Complications of temporary and definitive external fixation of pelvic ring injuries. *Injury* 36:599, 2005.

79. Taeger G, Ruchholtz S, Waydhas C, et al.: Damage control orthopedics in patients with multiple injuries is effective, time saving, and safe. *J Trauma* 59:409, 2005.

80. Miller PR, Moore PS, Mansell E, et al.: External fixation or arteriogram in bleeding pelvic fracture: Initial therapy guided by markers of arterial hemorrhage. *J Trauma* 54:437, 2003.

81. Brown CVR, Kasotakis G, Wilcox A: Does pelvic hematoma on admission computed tomography predict active bleeding at angiography for pelvic fracture? *Am Surg* 71:759, 2005.

82. Blackmore CC, Jurkovich JJ, Linnau KF, et al.: Assessment of volume of hemorrhage and outcome from pelvic fracture. *Arch Surg* 138:504, 2003.

83. Mucha P Jr, Welch TJ: Hemorrhage in major pelvic fractures. *Surg Clin North Am* 68:757, 1988.

84. Agolini SF, Shah K. Jaffe J, et al.: Arterial embolization is a rapid and effective technique for controlling pelvic fracture hemorrhage. *J Trauma* 43:395, 1997.

85. Panetta T, Sclafani SJA, Goldstein AJ, et al.: Percutaneous transcatheter embolization for massive bleeding from pelvic fractures. *J Trauma* 25:1021, 1985.

86. Agolini SF, Shah K, Jaffe J, et al.: Arterial embolization is a rapid and effective technique for controlling pelvic fracture hemorrhage. *J Trauma* 43:395, 1997.

87. Velmahos GC, Toutouzas KG, Vassiliu P, et al.: A prospective study on the safety and efficacy of angiographic embolization for pelvic and visceral injuries. *J Trauma* 53:303, 2002.

88. Fangio P, Asehnoune K, Edouard A, et al.: Early embolization and vasopressor administration for management of life-threatening hemorrhage from pelvic fracture. *J Trauma* 58:978, 2005.

89. Sclafani SJA, Florence L, Phillips TF, et al.: The radiologic diagnosis and management of lumbar arterial injuries. *Radiology* 165:709, 1982.

90. Ben-Menachem Y, Handel SF, Ray RD, et al.: Embolization procedures in trauma. *Semin Int Radiol* 2:125, 1985.

91. Sclafani SJA: Angiographic treatment of chronic post traumatic arteriovenous fistula of the extremities. *Sem Inter Radiol* 2:125, 1985.

92. Yasumura K, Ikegami K, Kamohara T, et al.: High incidence of ischemic necrosis of the gluteal muscle after transcatheter angiographic embolization for severe pelvic fracture. *J Trauma* 58:985, 2005.

93. Ben-Menachem Y: Embolotherapy in pelvic trauma. In Neal MP, Tisnado J, Chu SR, eds. *Emergency Interventional Radiology.* Boston: Little & Brown, 1989.

94. Cryer HM, Miller FB, Evers BM, et al.: Pelvic fracture classification: Correlation with hemorrhage. *J Trauma* 28:973, 1988.

95. Naam WH, Brown W, Hurd R, et al.: Major pelvic fractures. *Arch Surg* 118:610, 1983.

96. Matalon TS, Athanasoulis CA: Hemorrhage with pelvic fractures: Efficacy of transcatheter embolization. *Am J Med* 133:859, 1979.

97. Rothenberger DA, Fischer RP, Perry JF: Major vascular injuries secondary to pelvic fractures: An unsolved clinical problem. *Am J Surg* 136:660, 1970.

98. Seavers RM, Lynch J, Ballard R: Hypogastric ligation for uncontrollable hemorrhage in acute pelvic trauma. *Surgery* 55:516, 1963.

99. Saueracker AK, McCroskey RJ, Moore EE, et al.: Intra-operative hypogastric artery embolization for life threatening pelvic hemorrhage: A preliminary report. *J Trauma* 27:1127, 1987.

100. Sheldon GF, Winestuck DP: Hemorrhage from open pelvic fracture controlled intra-operatively with balloon catheter. *J Trauma* 18:68, 1978.

101. Ertel W, Keel M, Eid K, et al.: Control of severe hemorrhage using C-clamp and pelvic packing in multiply injured patients with pelvic ring disruption. *J Orthop Trauma* 16:362, 2002.

102. Smith WR, Moore EE, Osborn P, et al.: Retroperitoneal packing as a resuscitation technique for hemodynamically unstable patients with pelvic fractures: Report of two representative cases and a description of technique. *J Trauma* 59:1510, 2005.

103. Richardson JD, Harty J, Amin M, et al.: Open pelvic fractures. *J Trauma* 22:533, 1982.

104. Ferrera PC, Hill DA: Good outcomes of open pelvic fractures. *Injury* 30:187, 1999.

105. Sinott R, Rhodes M, Brader A: Open pelvic fractures: An injury for trauma centers. *Am J Surg* 163:283, 1992.

106. Dente CJ, Feliciano DV, Rozycki GS, et al.: The outcome of open book pelvic fractures in the modern era. *Am J Surg* 190:830, 2005.

107. Batalden DJ, Wickstrom PH, Rob E, et al.: Value of the G-Suit in patients with severe pelvic fractures. *Arch Surg* 109:326, 1974.

108. Brutman S, Browner BP, Cox EF: MAS Trousers improperly applied causing a compartment syndrome in lower extremity trauma. *J Trauma* 22:598, 1982.

109. Rodriguez-Morales A, Phillips T, Conn AK, et al.: Traumatic hemipelvectomy: Report of two survivors and review. *J Trauma* 23:615, 1983.

110. Maull KI, Sachatello CR, Ernst CB: The deep perineal laceration and injury frequently associated with open pelvic fractures: A need for aggressive surgical management. *J Trauma* 17:685, 1977.

111. Kudsk KA, McQueen MA, Voeller GR, et al.: Management of complex perineal soft tissue injuries. *J Trauma* 30:1155, 1990.

112. Brunicardi FC, Scalea TM, Bernstein MO, et al.: Air embolism during pulsed saline irrigation of an open pelvic fracture. *J Trauma* 24:700, 1989.

113. Crichlow RJ, Nascone J, Graf K, et al.: Immediate open reduction internal fixation (ORIF) vs. external fixation (ex-fix) in patients with unstable pelvic ring injuries undergoing trauma laparotomy. Poster #15 presented at the *Eastern Association for the Surgery of Trauma 19th Annual Scientific Assembly*, Orlando, Florida, 2006.

114. Kellam J, McMurtry R, Paley D, et al.: The unstable pelvic fracture: Operative treatment. *Orthop Clin North Am* 18:25, 1987.

115. Routt ML, Nork SE, Mills WJ: Percutaneous fixation of pelvic ring disruptions. *Clin Orthop Rel Res* 375:15, 2000.

116. Nork SE, Jones CB, Harding SP, et al.: Percutaneous stabilization of u-shaped sacral fractures using iliosacral screws: Technique and early results. *J Orthop Trauma* 15:238, 2001.

117. Griffin DR, Starr AJ, Reinert CM, et al.: Vertically unstable pelvic fractures fixwed with percutaneous iliosacral screws: Does posterior injury pattern predict fixation failure? *J Orthop Trauma* 17:399, 2003.

118. Parreira JG, Coimbra R, Rasslan S, et al.: The role of associated injuries on outcome of blunt trauma patients sustaining pelvic fractures. *Injury* 31:677, 2000.

119. Manley G, Knudson MM, Morabito D, et al.: Hypotension, hypoxia, and head injury: Frequency duration, and consequences. *Arch Surg* 136:1118, 2001.

120. Pietropoli JA, Rogers FB, Shackford SR: The deleterious effects of intraoperative hypotension on outcomes in patients with severe head injury. *J Trauma* 33:403, 1992.

121. Wisner DH, Victor NS, Holcroft JW: Priorities in the management of multiple trauma: Intracranial versus intra-abdominal injury. *J Trauma* 35:271, 1993.

122. Ochsner MG, Hoffman AP, DiPasquale D, et al.: Associated aortic rupture–pelvic fracture: An alert for orthopedic and general surgery. *J Trauma* 33:429, 1992.

123. Fabian TC, Richardson JD, Croce MA, et al.: Prospective study of blunt aortic injury: Multicenter trial of the American Association for the Surgery of Trauma. *J Trauma* 42:374, 1997.

124. Richardson JD, Wilson ME, Miller FB: The widened mediastinum: Diagnostic and therapeutic priorities. *Ann Surg* 211:731, 1990.

125. Gavant ML, Flick P, Menke P, et al.: CT aortography of thoracic aortic rupture. *AJR Am J Roentgenol* 166:955, 1996.

126. Weiss JP, Field M, Sclafani SJA, et al.: Traumatic rupture of the aorta. *Emerg Med Clin North Am* 9:789, 1991.

127. Vigon P, Boncoeur M, Francois B, et al.: Comparison of multiplane transesophageal echocardiography and contrast-enhanced helical CT in the diagnosis of blunt traumatic cardiovascular injuries. *Anesthesiology* 94:615, 2001.

128. Burgess AR, Jones AL: Fractures of the pelvic ring. In Rockwood CA, Green DP, eds. *Fractures in Adults*, 5th ed. Philadelphia: Lippincott, 2001.

129. Cass AS, Godec CJ: Urethral injury due to external trauma. *Urology* 11:607, 1978.

130. Malangoni MA, Buttner BK, Amin EA, et al.: Blunt urethral injury: Results and initial management. *Am Surg* 54:181, 1988.

131. Lowe MA, Mason JT, Luna GK, et al.: Risk factors for urethral injuries in men with traumatic pelvic fractures. *J Urology* 140:506, 1988.

132. Casselman RC, Schillinger JF: Fractured pelvis with avulsion of the female urethra. *J Urology* 117:385, 1977.

133. Barach E, Master G, Tomlanovich M: Blunt pelvic trauma with urethral injury in the female: Case report and review of the literature. *J Emerg Med* 2:101, 1984.

134. Mayher BE, Guyton JL, Gingrich JR: Impact of urethral injury management on the treatment and outcome of concurrent pelvic fractures. *Urology* 57:439, 2001.

135. Brandes S, Borrelli J: Pelvic fracture and associated urologic injuries. *World J Surg* 25:1578, 2001.

136. Perry MO, Husmann DA: Urethral injuries in female subjects following pelvic fractures. *J Urol* 147:139, 1992.

137. Carroll PR, McAnniach JW: Major bladder trauma: Mechanism of injury and a unified method of diagnosis and repair. *J Urology* 132:254, 1984.

138. Flancbaum L, Morgan AJ, Fleisher M, et al.: Blunt bladder trauma: Manifestations of severe injury. *Urology* 31:220, 1988.

139. Morey AF, Iverson AJ, Swan A, et al.: Bladder rupture after blunt trauma: Guidelines for diagnostic imaging. *J Trauma* 51:683, 2001.

140. Routt ML, Simonian PT, Defalco AJ, et al.: Internal fixation in pelvic fractures and primary repairs of associated genitourinary disruptions: A team approach. *J Trauma* 40:784, 1996.

141. Peng MY, Parisky YR, Cornwell EE, et al.: CT cystography versus conventional cystography in evaluation of bladder injury. *AJR* 173:1269, 1999.

142. Patterson FP, Morton KS: Neurological complications of fractures and dislocations of the pelvis. *J Trauma* 12:1013, 1973.

143. Tornetta P, Matta JM: Outcome of operatively treated unstable posterior pelvic ring disruptions. *Clin Orthop* 1:186, 1996.

144. Britt LD, Zolfaghari D, Kennedy E, et al.: Incidence and prophylaxis of deep vein thrombosis in a high risk trauma population. *Am J Surg* 172:13, 1996.

145. Rogers FB, Shackford SR, Wilson J, et al.: Prophylactic vena cava filter insertion in severely injured trauma patients: Indications and preliminary results. *J Trauma* 35:637, 1993.

146. White RH, Gouley JA, Brair TJ, et al.: Deep vein thrombosis after fracture of the pelvis: Assessment with serial duplex ultrasound screening. *J Bone Joint Surg* 72A:495, 1990.

147. Knudson MM, Ikossi DG, Khaw L, et al.: Thromboembolism after trauma: an analysis of 1602 episodes from the American College of Surgeons National Trauma Data Bank. *Ann Surg* 240:490, 2004.

148. Rogers FB, Shackford SR, Ricci M: Ruptured prophylactic vena cava filter: Insertion in severely injured trauma patients decreases the incidence of pulmonary emboli. *J Am Coll Surg* 180:641, 1995.

149. Evers BM, Cryer HM, Miller FB: Pelvic fracture hemorrhage: Priorities in management. *Arch Surg* 124:422, 1989.

150. Gruen GS, Leit ME, Gruen RJ, et al.: The acute management of hemodynamically unstable multiple trauma patients with pelvic ring fractures. *J Trauma* 36:706, 1994.

151. Wong Y, Wang L, Ng C, et al.: Mortality after successful transcatheter arterial embolization in patients with unstable pelvic fractures: Rate of blood transfusion as a predictive factor. *J Trauma* 49:71, 2000.

152. Poole GV, Ward EF, Muakkassa FF, et al.: Pelvic fracture from major blunt trauma. *Ann Surg* 213:532, 1991.

153. Goldstein AS, Phillips T, Sclafani SJA: Early open reduction and internal fixation of the disrupted pelvic ring. *J Trauma* 26:325, 1986.

154. McLaren A, Roraback CA, Halpenny J: Long-term pain and disability in relation to residual deformity after displaced pelvic ring fractures. *Can J Surg* 33:492, 1990.

155. Pohlemann T, Gansslen A, Schellwald O, et al.: Outcome after pelvic ring injuries. *Injury* 27:S31, 1996.

156. Nepola JV, Trenhaile SW, Miranda MA, et al.: Vertical shear injuries: Is there a relationship between residual displacement and functional outcome? *J Trauma* 46:1024, 1999.

157. Gruen GS, Leit ME, Gruen RJ, et al.: Functional outcomes of patients with unstable pelvic ring fractures stabilized with open reduction and internal fixation. *J Trauma* 39:838, 1995.

158. Van den Bosch EW, Van der Kleyn R, Hogervorst M, et al.: Functional outcome of internal fixation for pelvic ring fractures. *J Trauma* 47:365, 1999.

159. Brenneman FD, Katyal D, Boulanger BR, et al.: Long-term outcomes in open pelvic fractures. *J Trauma* 42:773, 1997.

160. Copeland CE, Bosse M, McCarthy ML, et al.: Effect of trauma and pelvic fracture in female femoral genitourinary sexual and reproductive fixation. *J Orthop Trauma* 11:73, 1997.

161. McCarthy ML, MacKenzie EJ, Bosse M, et al.: Functional status following orthopedic trauma in young women. *J Trauma* 39:828, 1995.

162. King J: Impotence after fractures of the pelvis. *J Bone Joint Surg* 57:1107, 1975.

163. Ellison M, Timberlake GA, Kerstein MD: Impotence following pelvic fracture. *J Trauma* 28:695, 1988.

164. Ramirez JI, Velmahos GC, Best CR, et al.: Male sexual function after bilateral internal iliac artery embolization for pelvic fracture. *J Trauma* 56:734, 2004.

# Commentary ■ LEWIS FLINT

The chapter by Scalea and associates is comprehensive and thorough. I agree with their emphasis upon the minority of pelvic fracture patients who continue to challenge trauma surgeons and continue to suffer significant mortality and morbidity because of simultaneous severe injuries outside the pelvis, pelvic fracture bleeding, and injury to visceral and neural structures within the pelvis. The frequency of severe pelvic fracture is likely to increase with time as lateral impact motor vehicle crashes and auto–pedestrian collisions increase particularly as motorists, unwilling to be delayed by a traffic signal, violate intersection rules. Motor vehicle size and weight differences (large, heavy vehicle impacting smaller vehicle) contribute to the occurrence of pelvic fractures in side-impact collisions not only because of the size and weight differences but because available side-impact air bags do not adequately protect the pelvis. Also, the perception of lower costs associated with motorcycles as a principle mode of transportation has resulted in increased numbers of riders and a concomitant increase in severe pelvic fracture. As the proportion of elderly patients increase in the population, pelvic fracture becomes an important marker for increased morbidity and resource utilization. In Florida trauma centers, any pelvic ring disruption and any thoracic injury visible on chest radiograph were markers strongly associated with underestimation of injury severity in patients more than 70 years of age. These findings have prompted re-evaluation of triage and transfer protocols for these patients. Patients older than 65 years comprise 24% of the population of Florida and are a group increasingly drawn to motorcycles as transportation. It is likely, therefore, that the lessons presented by Scalea will be valuable for surgeons caring for injured patients for the foreseeable future.

One form of pelvic disruption, complex acetabular fracture, is a challenging injury occasionally associated with lacerations of major arteries (common, internal, and external iliac). Endovascular approaches to these vessels may prove useful. More data is required to clearly identify the role of endovascular therapy as a means of hemorrhage control and maintenance of distal flow when major vessels are lacerated due to acetabular fractures. The definitive repair of acetabular fracture has become an area of specialty interest in orthopedic surgery. Trauma centers where expertise in acetabular repair exists will become regional resources for this service. Trauma surgeons will be involved in the care of these patients because of frequent associated injuries and comorbidities. It is useful to establish an agreed upon process for transfer and transport of such patients to the trauma center.

Life-threatening hemorrhage continues to be the principal challenge in the acute management of pelvic fracture. In no injury is the importance of a cohesive, rapidly responsive, multidisciplinary team more important. Trauma surgeons, orthopedic surgeons, emergency physicians, and anesthesiologists all have vital roles in the early care of patients with pelvic fracture bleeding. Prior agreement as to the roles each of these specialists will have is critical. Once the risk of pelvic fracture hemorrhage has been identified, all of the aforementioned specialists should be present in the resuscitation bay to participate in the decision process. Team consensus will determine the approach with the only minor disagreements concerning the management of pelvic fracture hemorrhage focusing upon sequencing of interventions.

Active simultaneous bleeding from the pelvis and intra-abdominal sites will dictate the use of open operation and pelvic packing. In our experience, this group of patients sustains lethal injuries in the majority of instances. Local biases and resource availability will determine the use of temporary pelvic fixation using external fixator devices; pelvic orthotic devices; and/or the employment of angiography with embolization. The pneumatic antishock garment is useful for temporary stabilization of the pelvis but is frequently not available. More recently, pelvic orthotic devices have been developed which can be easily applied in the resuscitation area. The downsides of these devices are occasional skin damage, which may delay definitive fixation, and over-correction of the pelvic deformity which may result in nerve injury. We employ a skin inspection protocol at eight-hour intervals after the orthotic device is applied as a precaution against this complication. Where possible, a careful neurologic examination prior to application of the device is useful. We attempt to correct the "open book" component of the pelvic ring deformity by 50% initially as determined by a postapplication pelvis radiograph. Patients who are hemodynamically unstable or who require six or more units of blood after application of the orthotic device are candidates for angiography and embolization. Occasionally, it will be necessary to transport a hemodynamically unstable patient to the angiography suite for embolization. As interventional radiology suites especially equipped for endovascular interventions have become more available, it has become possible to care for the patient in an environment that is essentially identical to the operating room in terms of monitoring and organ support capability. Our protocol requires that the unstable patient have continuous attendance by anesthesiologists and the trauma surgeon during the angiographic intervention.

Once bleeding has been controlled, efforts are directed toward expeditious definitive repair of the fracture. This will require continued participation by orthopedic specialists and careful imaging to facilitate planning of the repair. Our bias is that early definitive repair is associated with earlier ambulation and return to work. Overall, about half of pelvic fracture patients who require definitive operative repair of their fractures will return to work and this proportion is consistent with severely injured patients of all types. Sexual dysfunction remains a frustrating complication in men and women following pelvic fracture.

Deep vein thrombosis (DVT) and pulmonary embolus (PE) are troubling occurrences in this patient group. Our impression is that the risk of these events is largely independent of efforts at prophylaxis with anticoagulant drugs; that sequential calf compression devices are probably the most effective prophylactic intervention (but use of these is frequently prevented by the injury pattern); and that significant pulmonary embolus may occur during the first 24–48 hours after injury. We are liberal with the use of vena caval filters in patients with severe pelvic fracture and most often combine these with systemic anticoagulation when bleeding risk decreases.

Open pelvic fracture is an injury which continues to stimulate debate among trauma specialists. Suffice it to say that a high degree of suspicion is warranted to detect these injuries. The need for interventions such as diverting colostomy is determined on the basis of findings in the individual patient. The location of the surface laceration which communicates with the fracture site is the most useful physical finding which can facilitate the decision for or against colostomy. Perineal and vaginal wounds need diversion. Groin wounds do not usually need diversion and buttock wounds will require diversion based on proximity to the anus and the risk of fecal soilage of the wound. Colostomy placement as well as the decision to perform suprapubic bladder drainage for patients with bladder and/or urethral injuries require consultation with the orthopedic surgeon who will perform definitive repair so that optimum incision placement to perform the repair will be assured. Over the past several years, we have increasingly relied upon endoscopic-assisted placement of transurethral catheters in patients with urethral injuries. This has reduced the number of suprapubic tubes and facilitated anterior approaches to definitive fracture repair.

# Genitourinary Trauma

*Michael Coburn*

Genitourinary injury occurs in 2–5% of all trauma patients and in at least 10% of patients with abdominal trauma, emphasizing the need for a close collaboration between the general and urologic trauma surgeon. This unique relationship that the urologist and general trauma surgeon share in the management of urologic injuries requires that common philosophies of management be applied.

Controversies exist in the approach to urologic trauma, and recent efforts to achieve a broad consensus in the management of diverse urologic injuries have resulted in numerous publications. One such effort, sponsored by the World Health Organization and the Societe Internationale d'Urologie, involved a 25-year review of world literature focusing on levels of evidence and development of evidence-based management recommendations.[1-5] Another similar effort through the European Association of Urology (EAU) had a similar focus.[6] Both produced useful syntheses of a large body of literature. The current discussion will offer a broadly applicable approach to the management of urologic trauma based on current literature and local experience and perspective.

## ANATOMY

Beginning with surgical exposure for upper tract injuries, the contemporary approach to the injured kidney is through an anterior midline incision. Access to the kidneys and ureters is generally obtained by reflecting the colon on either side medially and exposing Gerota's fascial envelope. While modern descriptions of exposing the injured kidney often involve a discussion of first obtaining vascular control of the renal vessels prior to entering the perirenal hematoma, the important element in this practice is achieving access to the pedicle such that atraumatic vascular clamping can be achieved if significant bleeding is encountered. This can be accomplished through individually dissecting and "looping" the renal vessels through an incision in the posterior retroperitoneum over the aorta (which can allow access to either the left or right-sided artery and the left-sided vein) or by first

reflecting the colon on the side of injury and then obtaining vascular control or access to the pedicle. Obviously, the renal vessels should be approached first and dissected directly when there is suspicion of a renovascular injury (medial or perihilar hematoma, pulsatile hematoma). When suspicion of a renovascular injury is low, many urologic trauma surgeons successfully approach the kidney by first reflecting the colon and then achieving vascular control. This is achieved by individually dissecting the vessels, by using a vascular pedicle clamp, or through digital compression.

The kidney is located high and posteriorly in the retroperitoneum. The midline incision may need to be extended to the xiphoid process and additional upper abdominal retraction inserted for proper exposure. The kidney overlies the diaphragm, tranversus abdominis aponeurosis, and quadratus lumborum muscle laterally and psoas major muscle medially. Significant bleeding from these muscles and the deep muscles of the back can occur following penetrating trauma and may confuse the picture in which brisk bleeding is occurring in the renal fossa. The kidney is enclosed in a thin but strong fibrous capsule, which should be left intact during renal dissection and mobilization. As the capsule is usually lifted off the parenchyma by an underlying hematoma, the entire capsule may inadvertently be stripped off the kidney by the sweeping finger used to quickly elevate the kidney into the wound. Ideally, the kidney should be mobilized through sharp and blunt dissection working from a normal area toward the area of parenchymal injury to keep the capsule on the kidney. Stripping the capsule complicates the repair of the kidney and should be avoided.

Recognizing patterns of injury is important, and the trauma surgeon should anticipate injuries to adjacent organs based on the relational anatomy of the kidney and ureter and the trajectory of a penetrating injury (Fig. 39-1). The left kidney is crossed anteriorly in its upper portion by the tail of the pancreas and lies behind the lower portion of the spleen. On the right, the duodenum is immediately anterior to the hilar region. In the setting of a renal injury on the right side, the right colon, liver, and duodenum are

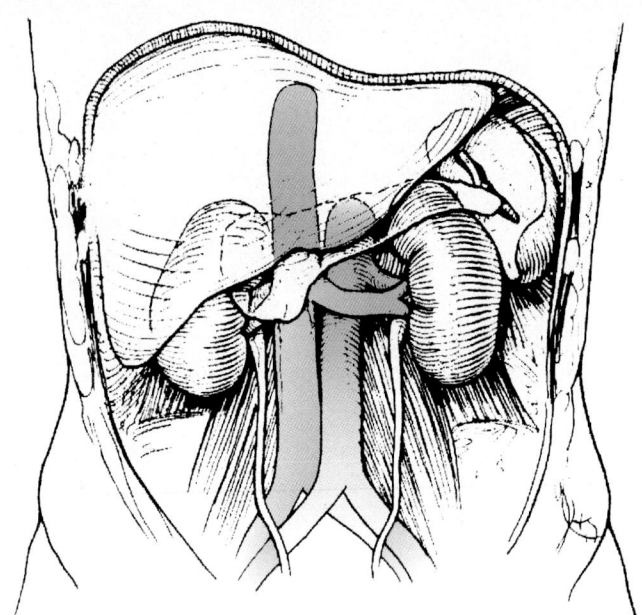

**FIGURE 39-1.** Renal anatomy: Relational anatomy of the kidney. Note proximity of great vessels, duodenum, liver, spleen, pancreas, and colon, relevant to predicting patterns of injury and likely sites of concomitant organ injury in renal trauma.

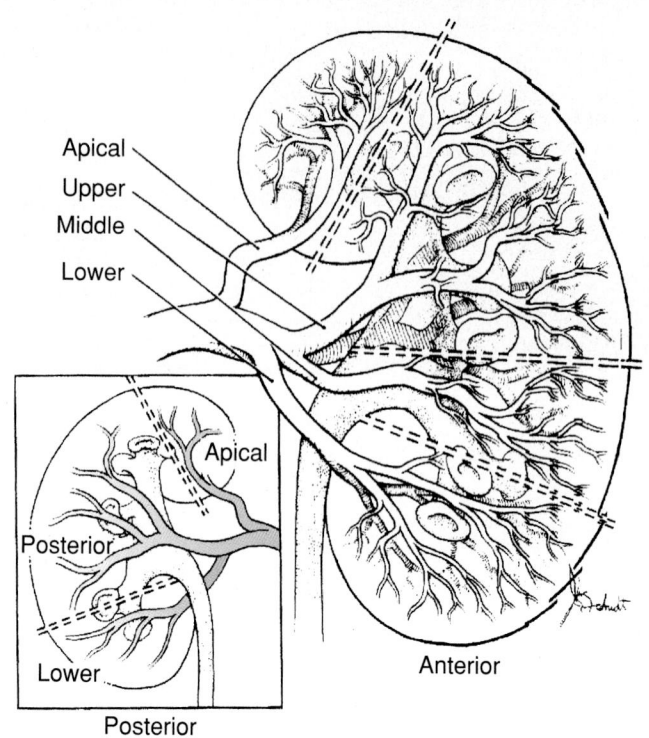

**FIGURE 39-2.** Intrarenal vascular anatomy: Vascular branches supplying various arterial segments of the renal parenchyma. Knowledge of intrarenal anatomy is critical to successful reconstructive efforts.

commonly injured in penetrating trauma. With blunt trauma, an associated hepatic laceration is most common. On the left-hand side, injuries to the left colon, stomach, spleen, and pancreas are common in penetrating trauma. And, lacerations of the spleen are particularly common with blunt trauma to the left upper quadrant. Injuries to the diaphragm are also common with penetrating renal injury and less common with blunt injury. The left adrenal gland is located medial to the upper pole of the left kidney, while the right adrenal gland is located in a more cephalad position relative to the right upper renal pole and may be in a retrocaval position.

At the level of the renal pedicle, there are most commonly single renal arteries and veins present bilaterally. The renal vein, artery, and renal pelvis are organized in an anterior-to-posterior orientation. On the right side, the gonadal vein arises from the vena cava at or slightly below the level of the renal pedicle. A lumbar vein, which may be quite large, often arises from the posterior aspect of the right renal vein, near the insertion with the inferior vena cava. The right adrenal vein enters directly into the vena cava, often on its posterolateral aspect. On the left, the main branches of the renal vein include the left gonadal, the adrenal, and one or more lumbar veins. This asymmetry of the collateral branches of the renal veins explains why the left renal vein can be safely ligated near the vena cava, with an 85% chance of renal preservation. In contrast, the right kidney will most likely develop venous thrombosis and become nonviable if the right renal vein is ligated.

For the urologic trauma surgeon who engages in intrarenal surgery and renal reconstruction, knowledge of the intrarenal anatomy is important (Fig. 39-2). The renal arterial supply consists of the following five segments: apical, superior (anterosuperior), middle (anteroinferior), lower (inferior), and posterior. The posterior branch crosses cephalad to the renal pelvis to reach its segment. About 25% of kidneys receive accessory arterial branches directly

from the aorta. These may enter through the renal sinus or at the upper or lower poles. Certain anomalies of the upper urinary tract, such as horseshoe kidney and congenital obstructive and duplication types, must be familiar to the trauma surgeon, as they may impact management.

The blood supply to the ureter is particularly important in surgery for urologic trauma (Figs. 39-3 and 39-4). The main sources are the renal artery from above, the aorta or common iliac arteries, and the vesical arteries from below. Branches approach the ureter primarily from the medial side; in the perirenal region, branches may approach the renal pelvis and ureter from a lateral direction. These branches form a long, predictable anastomotic chain usually with a single longitudinal vessel that runs the length of the ureter.

Anatomy of the urethra, perineum, and external genitalia may be less familiar to the general trauma surgeon. The gross anatomy and fascial layers of the genitalia and perineum are important in trauma, as they largely determine the manner in which blood and urine extravasate following urethral or genital trauma (Fig. 39-5).

## INJURY GRADING AND SCORING SYSTEMS FOR GENITOURINARY INJURIES

The American Association for the Surgery of Trauma (AAST) Injury Scaling Committee has devised a staging system for urologic injuries. The system, originally published in 1989 and since amended addresses injuries to the kidney, ureter, bladder, urethra, testis, scrotum, and penis (Table 39-1).[7] For some organs such as the kidney, the system has proven highly applicable and has come into common use. For other organs, such as bladder and ureter,

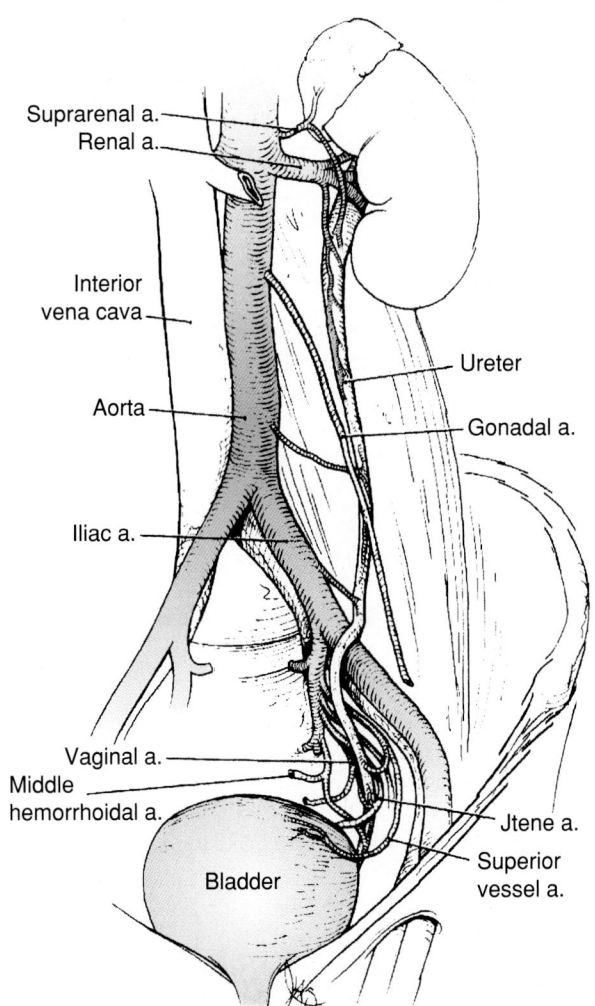

**FIGURE 39-3.** The ureteral blood supply originates from branches of the adrenal and renal arteries in the upper third, branches of the aorta and gonadal arteries in the middle third, and in the pelvic vessels as shown in the lower third. Knowledge of the ureteral blood supply and derangements due to preexisting pathology or prior surgery is important in maintaining ureteral viability during surgical mobilization and reconstruction.

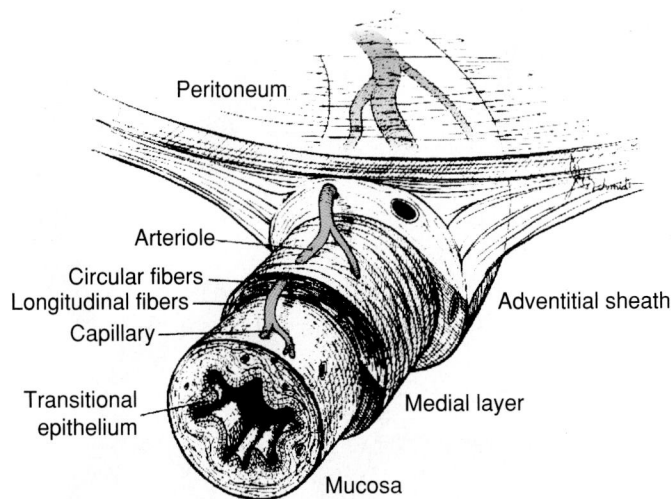

**FIGURE 39-4.** Ureteral anatomy: The longitudinal blood vessels run deep to the adventitial sheath; it is important to achieve a dissection plane superficial to this layer to avoid devascularization of the ureter during surgical mobilization.

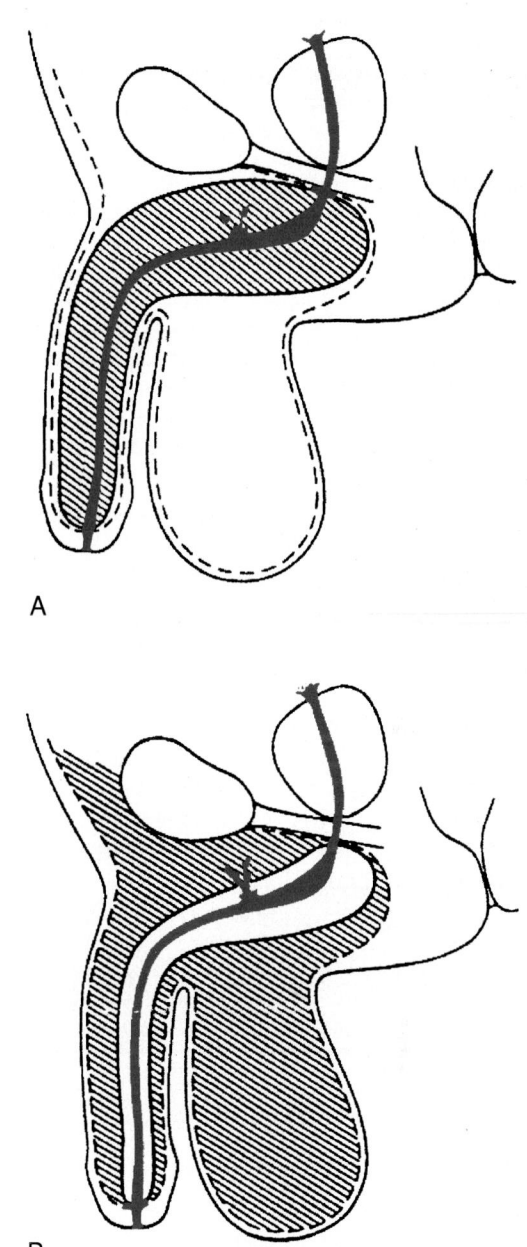

**FIGURE 39-5.** Diagram of sites of extravasation, associated with urethral disruption. **(A)** With an intact Buck's fascia, extravasation of blood and/or urine is isolated to the penile shaft. **(B)** With Buck's facial defect, extravasation extends into the scrotal tissues and compartments.

the AAST system has been less commonly utilized for a variety of reasons, largely relating to lack of specificity of available imaging approaches to provide the necessary data for assignment of a grade. The grading systems for urethra and external genitalia are coming into more common use and are of value in addressing outcomes following such injuries. Several aspects of the staging system have received attention regarding their clinical significance and impact on decision-making, complication rates, and patient outcomes.[8,9]

As noted, the renal Organ Injury Scale utilizes five grades of injury, ranging from contusion or subcapsular hematoma (I) to shattered kidney or avulsion of the hilum (V) (Fig. 39-6). It is

**TABLE 39-1**

## Urologic Injury Scale of the American Association for the Surgery of Trauma

| GRADE[a] | | INJURY DESCRIPTION[b] |
|---|---|---|
| **RENAL INJURY SCALE** | | |
| I | Contusion | Microscopic or gross hematuria; urologic studies normal |
| | Hematoma | Subcapsular, nonexpanding without parenchymal laceration |
| II | Hematoma | Nonexpanding perirenal hematoma confined to the renal retroperitoneum |
| | Laceration | <1 cm parenchymal depth of renal cortex without urinary extravasation |
| III | Laceration | >1 cm parenchymal depth of renal cortex without collecting-system rupture or urinary extravasation |
| IV | Laceration | Parenchymal laceration extending through the renal cortex, medulla, and collecting system |
| | Vascular | Main renal artery or vein injury with contained hemorrhage |
| V | Laceration | Completely shattered kidney |
| | Vascular | Avulsion of renal hilum that devascularizes kidney |
| **URETER INJURY SCALE** | | |
| I | Hematoma | Contusion of hematoma without devascularization |
| II | Laceration | ≤50% transection |
| III | Laceration | >50% transection |
| IV | Laceration | Complete transection with 2 cm devascularization |
| V | Laceration | Avulsion of renal hilum that devascularizes kidney |
| **BLADDER INJURY SCALE** | | |
| I | Hematoma | Contusion, intramural hematoma |
| | Laceration | Partial thickness |
| II | Laceration | Extraperitoneal bladder wall laceration ≤2 cm |
| III | Laceration | Extraperitoneal (>2 cm) or intraperitoneal (≤2 cm) bladder wall lacerations |
| IV | Laceration | Intraperitoneal bladder wall laceration >2 cm |
| V | Laceration | Intra- or extraperitoneal bladder wall laceration extending into the bladder neck or ureteral orifice (trigone) |
| **URETHRAL INJURY SCALE** | | |
| I | Contusion | Blood at urethral meatus; urethrography normal |
| II | Stretch injury | Elongation of urethra without extravasation on urethrography |
| III | Partial disruption | Extravasation of urethrographic contrast medium at injury site, with contrast visualized in the bladder |
| IV | Complete disruption | Extravasation of urethrographic contrast medium at injury site without visualization in the bladder; <2 cm of urethral separation |
| V | Complete disruption | Complete transection with >2 cm urethral separation, or extension into the prostate or vagina |

[a]Advance one grade for multiple injuries to the same organ.

[b]Based on most accurate assessment at autopsy, laparotomy, or radiologic study.

*Reproduced with permission from Moore EE, Shackford SR, Pachter HL, et al: Organ injury scaling: Spleen, liver, and kidney. J Trauma 29:1664, 1989.*

valuable to specifically distinguish the parenchymal lacerations from renovascular trauma in the group IV and V injuries when reporting experience, as management and outcomes differ between these entities. The varying degrees of renal injury as described in the scaling system are depicted diagramatically in Fig. 39-6. Recent data have shown support for the clinical utility and validity of the renal injury scale, indicating that this system is predictive of morbidity in blunt and penetrating renal injury, of mortality in blunt injury,[9] and of the risk of nephrectomy with exploration for renal trauma.[12]

As the percentage of the circumference of the ureter that has been disrupted is difficult to determine from imaging studies, the ureteral scaling system is mainly amenable to the operative setting. For the bladder, the distinction of intraperitoneal from extraperitoneal rupture is important and is addressed in the scaling system, but whether the length of the laceration in the bladder wall truly has clinical significance has not been demonstrated. For urethral injuries, the scaling system addresses anatomic factors that can often be determined from retrograde urethrography and provide advantages over the earlier system described by Calopinto and McCallum.[4] The current AAST system addresses urethral disruption based on whether the injury is complete or incomplete (i.e., whether

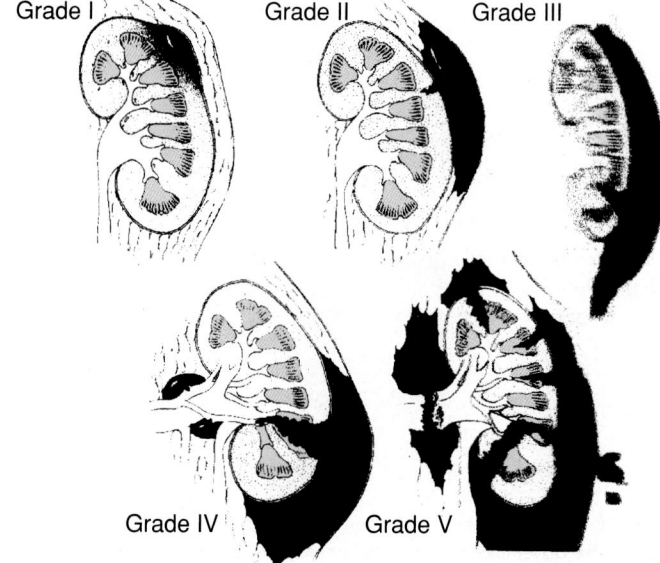

**FIGURE 39-6.** Organ injury scaling system for renal trauma.

contrast enters the bladder) and on the length of the urethral defect and presence of extension into prostate or vagina. Endoscopic assessment indicates that in some cases where the retrograde urethrogram would suggest a complete disruption, partial circumference continuity does exist, at times allowing for insertion of a catheter into the bladder. Nevertheless, despite some lack of specificity, the AAST organ injury scaling system has substantial usefulness.

The scaling system for organ specific injuries as applied to genitourinary trauma (Tables 19-22, 29-31 from AAST Website) has introduced a needed advance in the field.[7] The designations of the AAST system should be utilized whenever possible in clinical descriptions and published work on urologic trauma.

## CLINICAL PRESENTATION AND DIAGNOSIS OF RENAL TRAUMA

### Incidence and Patterns of Injury

Renal injuries occur in approximately 1–3% of all trauma patients and up to 10% of patients with abdominal trauma. The percentage of blunt and penetrating trauma varies dramatically depending on the healthcare institution and the population served. In some urban trauma centers, penetrating injuries predominate,[10] though overall, approximately 90% of significant renal injuries are due to blunt trauma in the United States.

For penetrating trauma, nearly all renal gunshot wounds are associated with injuries to other intra-abdominal organs; for renal stab wounds, approximately 60% of cases occur in combination with another intra-abdominal injury.

Kidneys with preexisting anatomic abnormalities appear to be more vulnerable to significant injury from seemingly minor blunt trauma.[11] Such entities would include obstruction of the ureteropelvic junction, large cystic lesions, and renal neoplasms. Injuries to nonurologic structures in the abdomen are found in approximately 20–33% of patients with blunt renal injuries.

### Clinical Presentation and Evaluation

A history of a blow to the flank, deceleration trauma, fall from a height, or penetrating abdominal, pelvic, and lower chest injury should raise the possibility of a renal injury. Hematuria is the most common sign of renal trauma, although the magnitude of the hematuria correlates poorly with the magnitude of injury.

Physical examination in patients at risk for renal injury should include careful assessment of the abdomen, back, flank, and chest, along with a complete genitourinary examination. Findings suggestive of a renal injury include tenderness in the flank, costovertebral angle or abdomen, a palpable flank mass, or ecchymosis in the flank, back, or abdomen. Complete inspection of the trunk for a penetrating injury is critical. Stab wounds posterior to the anterior axillary line carry a risk of renal injury, with only about 12% of such injuries being associated with injury to another organ.

Laboratory assessment should include urinalysis by dipstick, as well as microscopic examination for blood or infection. The first specimen in the emergency center should be analyzed for hematuria to optimize diagnostic accuracy. Determination of serum electrolytes, blood urea nitrogen (BUN) and serum creatinine, and hemoglobin are important. A blood sample for type and screen or cross-match should be obtained when clinically appropriate.

### Radiographic Imaging for Renal Trauma

Traditionally, all patients with abdominal trauma and any degree of hematuria were imaged in the emergency center upon presentation. Using this approach, some series of renal trauma have shown that greater than 90% of imaged patients will have only minor injuries, primarily contusions or other minor injuries not requiring intensive monitoring or intervention. With an eye toward cost-effectiveness and minimizing the time and potential morbidity of unnecessary imaging, several groups have assessed the safety and feasibility of establishing more selective approaches toward renal imaging in the trauma setting.[13] The disadvantages of imaging include expense, radiation exposure, possible allergic or nephrotoxic reactions to contrast, time expenditure, and the risk of moving the patient. These factors need to be balanced against the risk of missed injuries with a resultant delay in diagnosis. In 1985, the group from San Francisco General Hospital analyzed their renal trauma experience and found that the only findings that were predictive of significant renal injury were the presence of penetrating trauma, or blunt trauma with gross hematuria or with microhematuria and shock. Shock was defined as a systolic blood pressure <90 mm Hg at any time postinjury, including during transport by EMS. In a review of 812 patients with microhematuria but without shock, no significant renal injuries were detected. All 44 injuries in this original series were found among the 195 patients with gross hematuria or microhematuria and shock. This series has been extended over the years such that in the expanded patient group of 2254 patients with renal trauma approximately one-third were imaged and two-thirds were not. Within this group, no major renal injuries were missed using the established criteria.[5–7]

Other investigators have modified these imaging criteria according to their own experience and judgment. Some have suggested including standard imaging for those patients with injury to the brain, loss of consciousness, or altered mental status, with the belief that the loss of information on a physical examination and the magnitude of trauma in such patients may create a higher risk of a missed injury. Some have suggested extending imaging indications to those patients with mechanisms of injury consistent with deceleration trauma. This approach avoids missing injuries to the renal pedicle (e.g., intimal disruption in the renal artery and renal devascularization), which may present with no hematuria in 20 to 33% of patients. The presence of fractures of long bones, fractures of the lower ribs, or fractures of transverse spinous processes have also been suggested as indications to modify the previous imaging restrictions, possibly predicting a higher risk of occult renal injury. In the pediatric population (addressed in Pediatric Renal Trauma section later), imaging for patients with only microhematuria has been more liberally utilized.

As noted, the criteria involving limiting imaging to patients with gross hematuria or microhematuria with shock have not been extended to those with penetrating trauma. Patients with penetrating trauma with any degree of hematuria, injury proximity, or suspicion are appropriate candidates for imaging of the urinary tract, regardless of the presence or magnitude of hematuria. Significant penetrating injuries can present without hematuria, particularly if trauma to the major collecting system causes all urine from the injured kidney to exit into the retroperitoneum, preventing ureteral peristalsis.

In penetrating trauma, imaging would generally be obtained in assessing a patient's candidacy for nonoperative management in the appropriate clinical setting. The concept of obtaining preoperative renal imaging simply to demonstrate the presence of two functioning renal units prior to surgical intervention has become less popular in recent years. Instead, intraoperative examination and, when necessary, intraoperative intravenous pyelogram (IVP) may be used selectively during a trauma laparotomy to demonstrate renal function.[8] The selection of imaging modalities has evolved greatly since the advent and availability of computed tomography (CT) scanning to emergency center evaluation.[13] While the bolus intravenous pyelogram with nephrotomography had in the past been the standard imaging approach, the CT scan has, over the years, become the gold standard for precise staging of renal injuries (Fig. 39-7).

Although the IVP has in the past been described as being accurate for clinical staging purposes in 60–85% of patients, CT scanning offers a number of important advantages.[8,9] Nevertheless, trauma surgeons and urologists should remain familiar with the findings suggestive of renal injury on IVP, as routine use of CT for trauma assessment is not consistently available, especially when considering variations in international practice and infrastructure, and intraoperative IVPs may still be necessary at times. These IVP findings include the presence of a fracture of a transverse process on the scout film, presence of a mass effect in soft tissue, loss of the psoas margin on the involved side, and vertical displacement of the kidney. Loss of a clear renal cortical outline, gross extravasation of contrast, ipsilateral decrease in renal excretory function, and loss of opacification of portions of the collecting system should all be noted. The IVP allows confirmation of the presence of two renal units, gives general information of the extent of injury, and may show significant extravasation.

Estimates of the accuracy of IVP in detection of renal injury vary. In general, the IVP should be viewed as a crude means of detection, rather than as a means to obtain precise staging. Some studies indicate that as many as 20% of patients with significant renal injuries may have a normal IVP. In addition, up to half of patients with nonfunction of a kidney on IVP will have a reason for it other than arterial occlusion, including contusion, overhydration, and hypotension or hypoperfusion.

Advantages of CT over IVP include identification of contusion and subcapsular hematoma, definition of the location and depth of parenchymal lacerations, more reliable demonstration of extravasation of contrast, and identification of injuries to the pedicle and artery ("rim sign," "cut-off sign," etc.). There is also enhanced imaging of the perinephric space, other solid viscera (liver, spleen, pancreas), as well as delineation of many cases of perforation of a hollow viscus and identification of free intraperitoneal fluid. With the current spiral CT scanners, sequences are so rapid that it is important to be sure that delayed images are obtained to avoid missing extravasation from the collecting system or ureter, which may not be apparent from early images alone.[14]

Arteriography has had less of a role in the staging of a renal injury since CT has become popular, especially considering its cost, invasiveness, and the special expertise required. As the use of CT for diagnosis of a pedicle injury has become standard, far

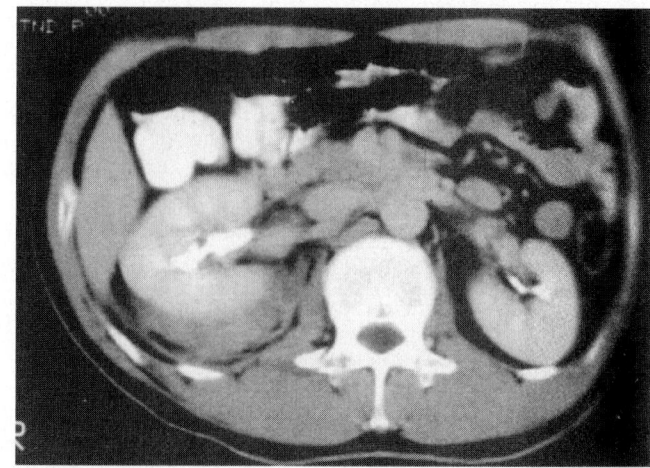

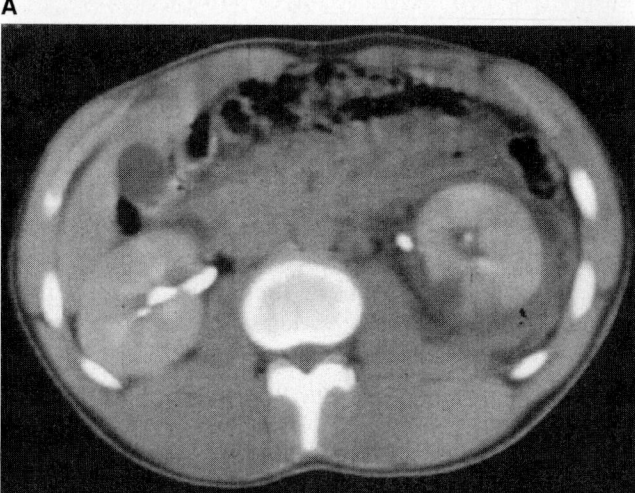

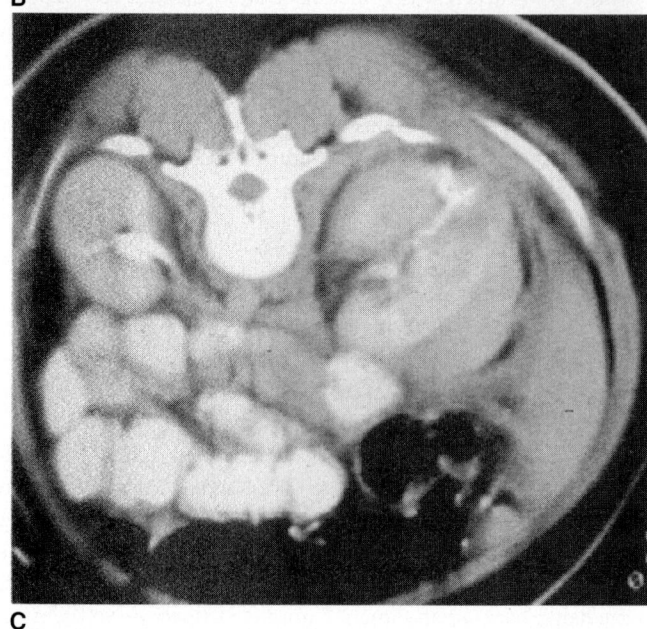

**FIGURE 39-7.** Staging computed tomography scans for blunt renal injury. **(A)** Grade II injury: Blunt trauma, small right posterior subcapsular and perirenal hematoma without obvious parenchymal laceration. **(B)** Grade II and III injury: Blunt trauma, laceration posteromedially in left kidney without collecting system injury. **(C)** Grade IV parenchymal injury: Blunt trauma, deeper laceration to right kidney, full-thickness parenchymal laceration with collecting system injury as indicated by contrast extravasation. Moderate-sized perinephric hematoma. No significant devitalized parenchyma noted.

fewer arteriograms are being obtained. Still, precise delineation of arterial anatomy and interventions for control of hemorrhage mandate the continued use of renal arteriography on a selective basis (Fig. 39-8). In Europe and other parts of the world, abdominal ultrasound has been extensively utilized in diagnosing and assessing blunt renal injury. In the United States and elsewhere the Focused Assessment for the Sonographic Evaluation of the Trauma Patient (FAST) study is performed to assess for free intra-abdominal fluid rather than the presence of an injury to parenchyma of solid organs. The ability to apply high-resolution Doppler

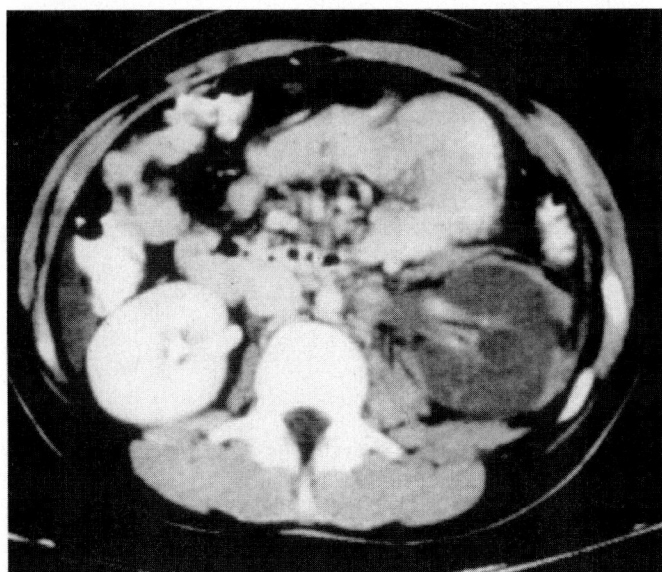

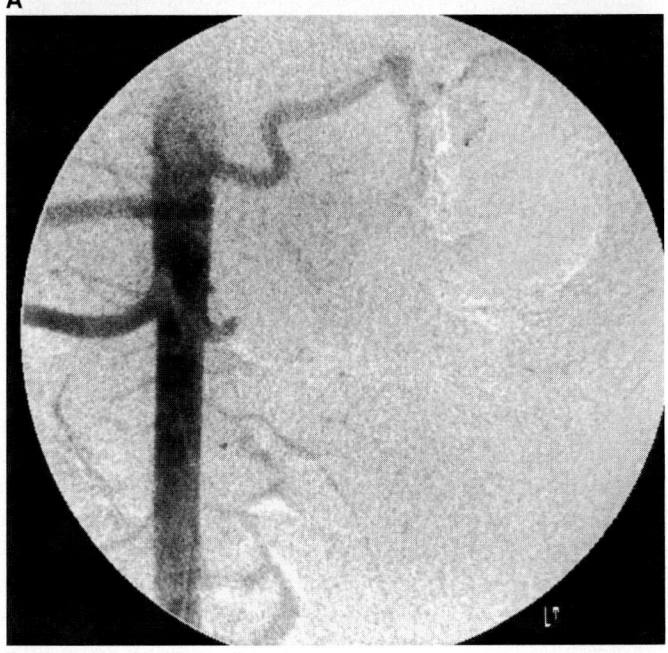

**FIGURE 39-8.** Renal artery occlusion due to intimal disruption following deceleration injury. Restrained driver in head-on motor vehicle collision. The left kidney is nonperfused and demonstrates minimal renal sinus vascular enhancement and cortical rim enhancement from capsular vessels. This finding is considered pathognomonic for this injury and does not require arteriographic confirmation unless the vascular surgeon believes further vascular imaging is necessary to plan therapy.

techniques to assess renal perfusion and vascular anatomy may extend the use of ultrasound for renal imaging in the future.

Retrograde pyelography plays a limited role in clearly defining anatomy of the ureter and collecting system when a pattern of medial extravasation or failure of ureteral opacification on CT or IVP is present.

## PEDIATRIC RENAL TRAUMA

Some studies suggest that the pediatric kidney is more vulnerable to trauma than is the adult kidney.[10] Reasons for this include the relatively larger size of the kidneys compared to the adult, the relative deficiency of perinephric fat in the child, and, probably, the higher incidence of preexisting renal abnormalities One recent review found that 8.3% of pediatric renal injuries occurred in the setting of preexisting renal abnormality,[11] with other estimates of preexisting renal abnormality described in as many as 23% of major pediatric renal injuries due to blunt trauma. Some data suggest that the kidney is the most commonly injured intra-abdominal organ in children.

It is nearly universally agreed that the presence of gross hematuria after trauma in the pediatric patient deserves further investigation with imaging of the urinary tract. As in the adult, the CT scan has the major role in staging such injuries for the same reasons as described earlier. Several studies suggest that only about 5% of pediatric patients with major renal injuries will develop signs of shock, further emphasizing the importance of an aggressive diagnostic approach. Pediatric patients can maintain a normal blood pressure despite significant blood loss, and persistent tachycardia is a particularly important parameter to note in the pediatric patient as a potential sign of significant blood loss.

The currently accepted approach in the adult is not applied liberally in the pediatric setting. Many authors suggest that all pediatric patients with any degree of hematuria after significant trauma should undergo renal imaging, while some have suggested modified criteria. One study has suggested that microscopic hematuria with greater than 50 red blood cells per high power field in the pediatric setting should be considered an imaging criterion, regardless of hemodynamic parameters.[11]

Certain types of renal injuries are clearly more common in the pediatric patient. These include laceration of the renal pelvis, avulsion of the ureteropelvic junction, and forniceal avulsion. When extensive medial extravasation is noted and/or the ureter does not opacify with contrast despite adequate excretion into the renal collecting system, a disruption of the major collecting system should be considered. In such cases, retrograde pyelography may be necessary to clarify the anatomy and achieve a diagnosis.

As in the adult, the use of the rapid spiral CT scanner can lead to a pitfall in diagnosis if a delayed sequence is not requested. Limiting the study to a nephrographic or early excretory phase may fail to demonstrate extravasation or asymmetrical opacification of the ureters, which would be readily visible on later images.

Overall, approximately 85% of pediatric renal injuries from blunt trauma are minor (contusions, superficial parenchymal lacerations) and are managed with bed rest and observation. Pedicle injuries comprise about 5% while major parenchymal injuries occur in 10–15% of patients. As in the adult, it is these latter groups for which management is somewhat controversial; however, it is largely agreed among pediatric urologists that operative decisions are based mainly on hemodynamic status rather than imaging criteria. The potential for successful management of kidneys that look very severely injured on imaging studies is remarkable in the pediatric population, and a nonoperative approach is the norm. Surgical treatment is generally reserved for patients with ongoing bleeding or hemodynamic instability, for those who have clearly failed an attempt at nonoperative management, and for penetrating injuries.

## CLINICAL PRESENTATION AND DIAGNOSIS OF TRAUMA TO THE URETER, BLADDER, URETHRA, AND EXTERNAL GENITALIA

### Ureter

Ureteral injuries are relatively uncommon, occurring in approximately 4% of patients with penetrating abdominal injuries and in less than 1% of those with blunt abdominal trauma. Concomitant visceral injury occurs in the majority of patients with ureteral injuries. While hematuria is an important sign of ureteral injury, it may be absent 15–45% of the time. As such, a high index of suspicion for ureteral injury is critical.[12–15] In fact, ureteral injury is one of the most common sites of missed injury at laparotomy, with one recent report noting a missed injury rate of 11% (15). While direct visualization of the ureter is the mainstay of detection of ureteral injury at the time of laparotomy, imaging modalities useful for detection of ureteral trauma include an IVP and contrast-enhanced CT scanning.[16] Modern spiral scanners move rapidly through the abdomen following administration of contrast, and, unless a delayed excretory phase is specifically requested, extravasation may be missed as previously described. Failure of the distal ureter to opacify on a CT scan should raise concern of an injury.[16] When noninvasive imaging fails to provide sufficient detail regarding ureteral anatomy or the specific nature of an injury, cystoscopy with retrograde pyelography may be indicated.

### Bladder

Sudden compression of the full bladder, shear forces, or a pelvic fracture may result in a blunt rupture. Rupture may be accompanied by lower abdominal pain, by an inability to void, and by perineal ecchymoses. The cardinal sign of injury to the bladder is gross hematuria, present in greater than 95% of cases, while only about 5% of patients will have microscopic hematuria alone.[17] Over 80% of patients with a bladder rupture have an associated pelvic fracture in centers with a high percentage of blunt trauma. An association of bladder rupture with disruption of the posterior urethra, also in the setting of pelvic fracture, may occur in 10–20% of patients.[18,19] Overall, recent data indicate that genitourinary injury occurs in approximately 15% of pelvic fractures in the pediatric setting[17] and that the incidence of injury to a pelvic organ is fairly comparable between adult and pediatric patients.[18]

Stress cystography is the standard study for diagnosis of injury to the bladder (Fig. 39-9).[20] It is important that the bladder be

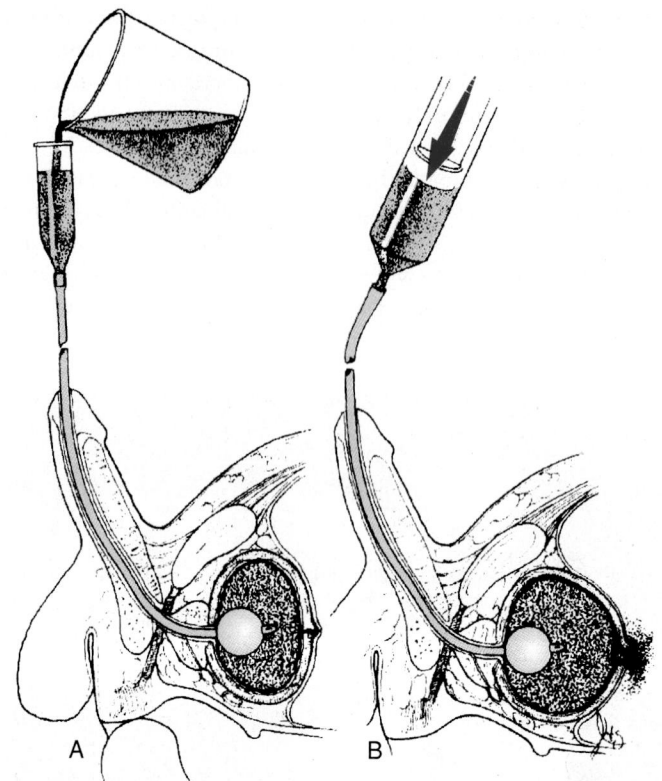

**FIGURE 39-9.** Stress cystogram: Through Foley catheter, the bladder is filled by gravity to a standard volume (300 to 400 mL typically in adult), or to the point of perceived fullness by patient. Plain radiograph obtained to allow visualization of upper and lower abdomen, followed by washout film.

adequately filled to avoid false-negative studies. For the adult bladder, the standard volume of filling is 300 to 400 mL of iodinated contrast (30% iodine commonly utilized), which is infused through the indwelling Foley catheter by gravity. Alternatively, the bladder can be filled by gravity to a point at which the patient describes a sense of bladder fullness. If the patient is obtunded or unable to indicate that there is a sense of fullness, using a standard filling volume is a useful methodology. A filling film is obtained that should be a vertically oriented abdominal image designed to show the entire abdomen. Patterns of contrast extravasation have been described for intraperitoneal, extraperitoneal, or combined ruptures (Fig. 39-10). Hematuria of bladder origin without contrast extravasation on a properly performed stress cystogram is consistent with a contusion or minimal mucosal injury, which is uniformly managed nonoperatively. Postdrainage washout films are generally recommended to avoid false-negative cystograms in which extravasated contrast may be missed if located only anterior or posterior to the distended bladder on an anteroposterior film.

Currently, stress cystography is commonly obtained using a CT technique (Fig. 39-11).[21] The same general principles apply as for static cystograms (i.e., adequate bladder filling is essential to avoid missed injuries) (Fig. 39-11b,c). Studies comparing the accuracy of standard radiographic stress cystography with CT cystography suggest equivalent capability in defining and staging bladder injuries, while the CT cystogram provides enhanced information regarding the perivesical space and adjacent structures. Simply clamping a bladder catheter following intravenous contrast administration is not adequate and will result in an

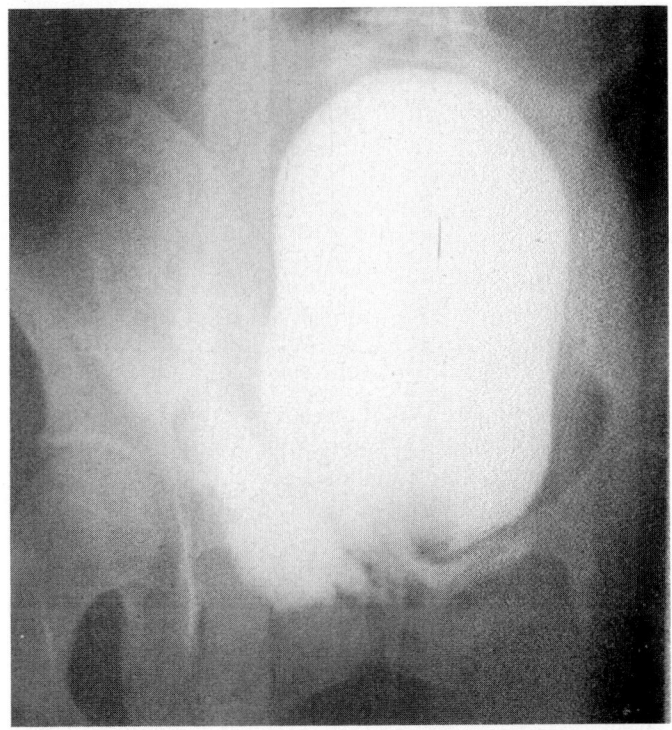

A

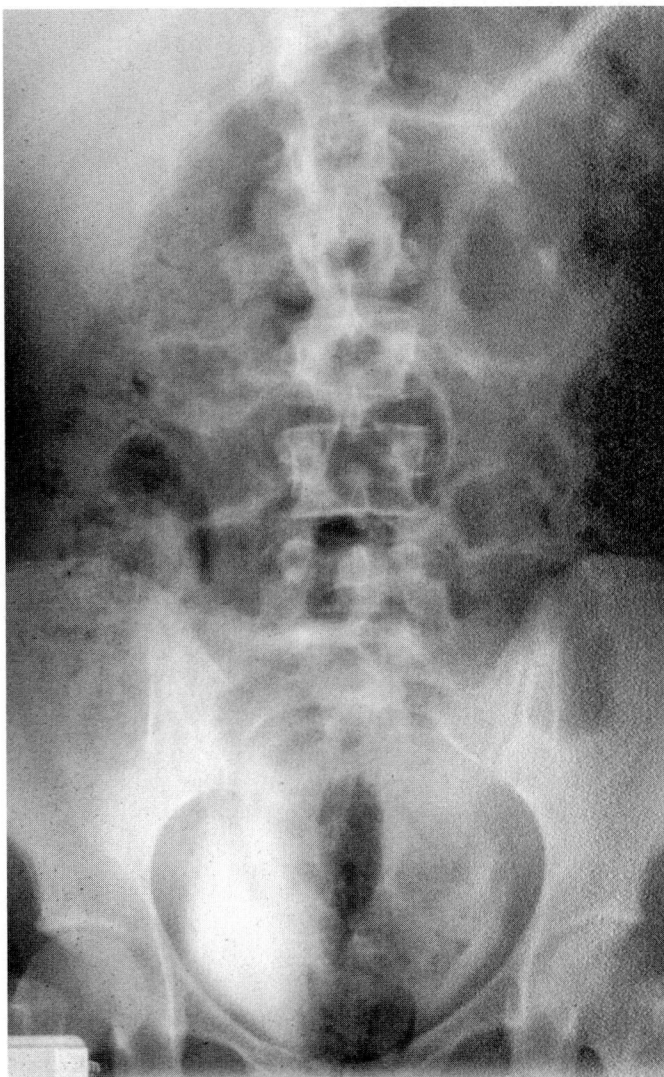

B

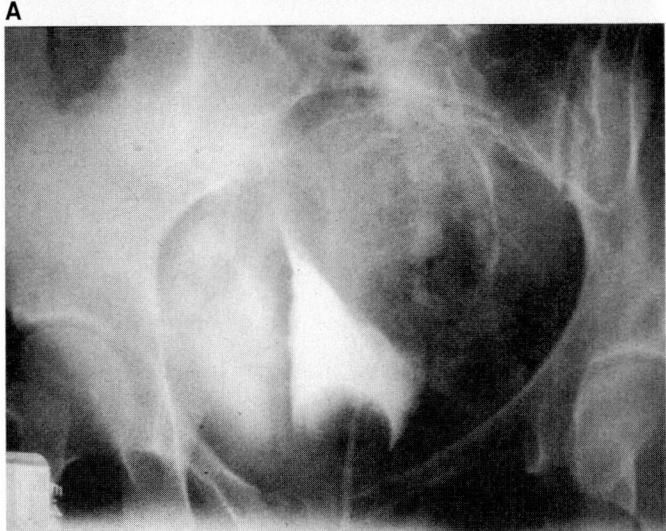

C

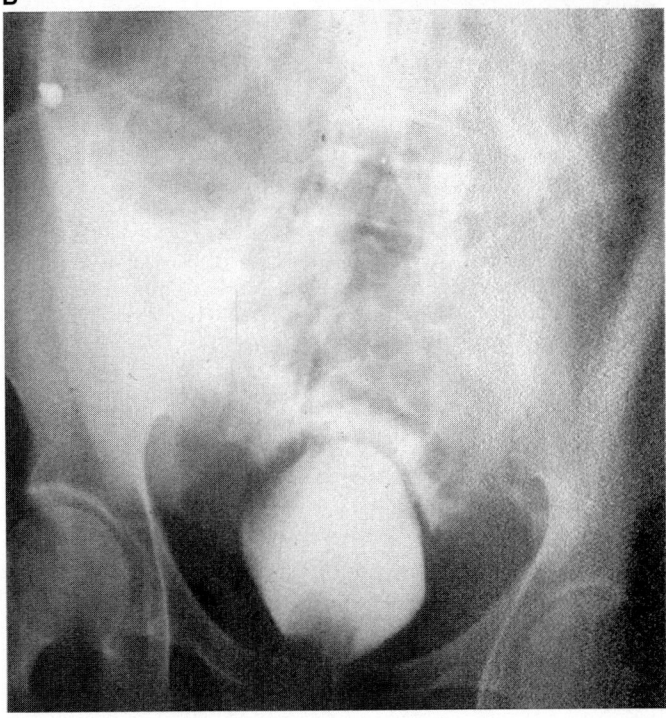

D

**FIGURE 39-10.** Bladder: Stress cystograms for assessment of suspected bladder injury following blunt trauma to pelvis. **(A)** Stress cystogram in patient with gross hematuria and pelvic fracture, demonstrating adequate bladder filling and typical pattern of extraperitoneal extravasation—flame-shaped contrast density lateral to right lower bladder segment. Injury managed successfully with 10 days of catheter drainage. **(B)** Washout phase following stress cystogram. Extraperitoneal extravasation pattern noted in right hemipelvis. Washout films may reveal extravasated contrast anterior or posterior to the contrast-filled bladder, which can be missed on films obtained when the bladder is filled with contrast. **(C)** Lateral compression of bladder from pelvic hematoma, along with extraperitoneal extravasation pattern in right pelvis, on an incomplete washout film. **(D)** Intraperitoneal bladder rupture. Note extravasated contrast outlining colic gutters, surrounding loops of small bowel, and occupying cul-de-sac in pelvis, indicative of intraperitoneal contrast.

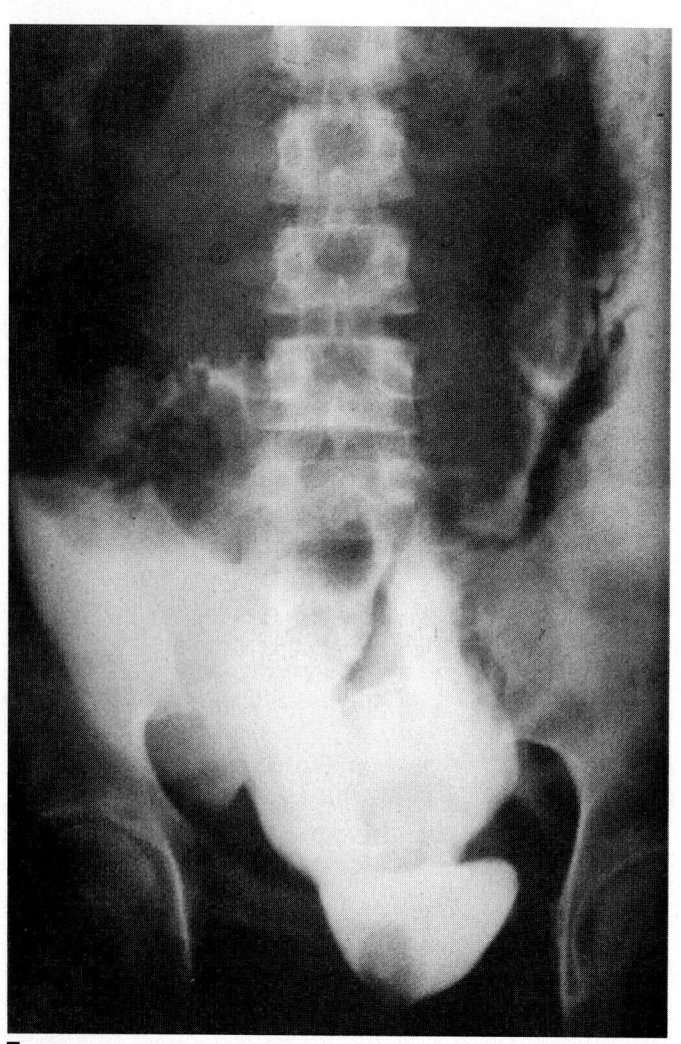

E

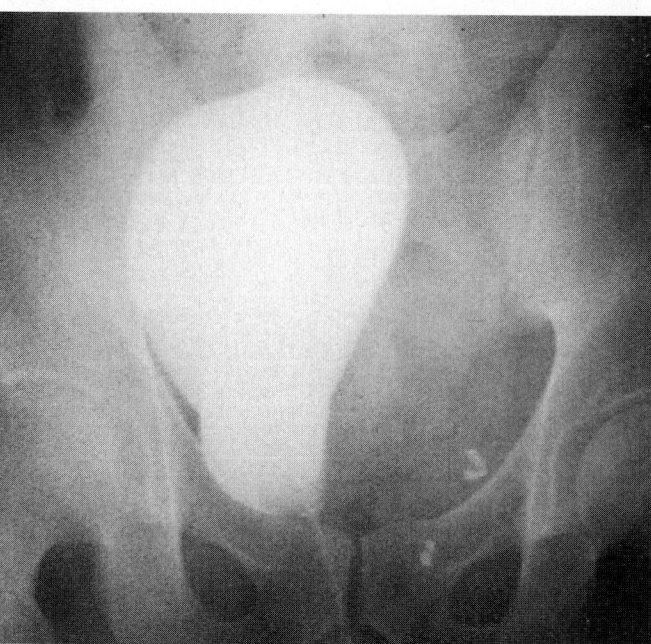

F

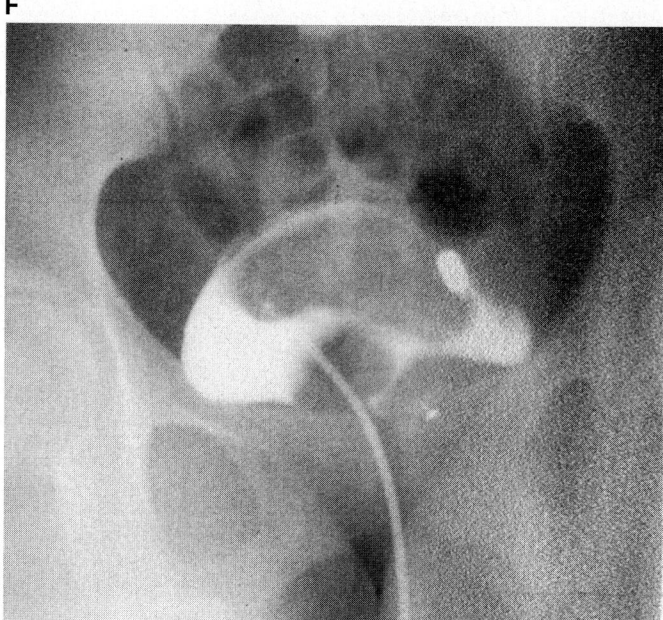

G

**FIGURE 39-10.** **(E)** Intraperitoneal bladder rupture. Again, note contrast in pelvis and outlining of right colon and small bowel in pelvis. Cystograms following penetrating pelvic trauma with hematuria. **(F)** Gunshot wound to pelvis in patient with microscopic hematuria. Bladder is intact, but is displaced to right due to large, left-sided pelvic hematoma. Obturator vessel injury noted, vessels ligated following evacuation of hematoma at laparotomy and pelvic exploration. **(G)** Gunshot wound to bladder with intravesical clot creating filling defect in bladder. Bladder incompletely filled; extravasation noted on subsequent film, following optimal filling of bladder.

unacceptably high percentage of false-negative examinations, with either the standard radiographic or the CT technique.[21]

## Urethra

Trauma to the anterior urethra may result from straddle injuries with sudden compression at the level of the mid- to deep-bulbous urethra against the inferior pubic arch. Urethral distraction injuries, or posterior urethral disruption, may accompany pelvic fracture in 4 to >10% of patients. Bilateral fractures of the pubic rami, especially when accompanied by an open pelvic ring (abnormally

distracted sacroiliac joint), may be present in patients who have suffered posterior urethral disruption as well. The classification system used to further describe urethral trauma is discussed in the section "Injury Grading and Scoring Systems for Genitourinary Injuries." It is important to determine from the urethrogram if an injury is partial (contrast passes proximal to the point of extravasation filling the more proximal urethra or bladder) or complete (all contrast extravasates, none enters the urethra proximal to injury or bladder), as this factor has an impact on selection of management.

Blood appearing at the urethral meatus, inability to void, presence of a perineal hematoma, and inability to clearly palpate the

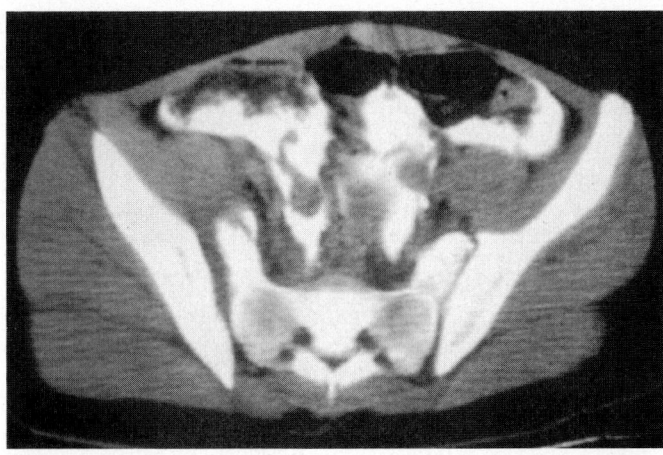

A

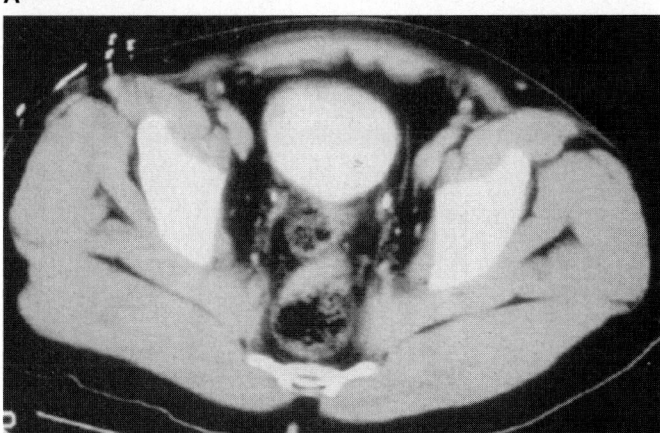

B

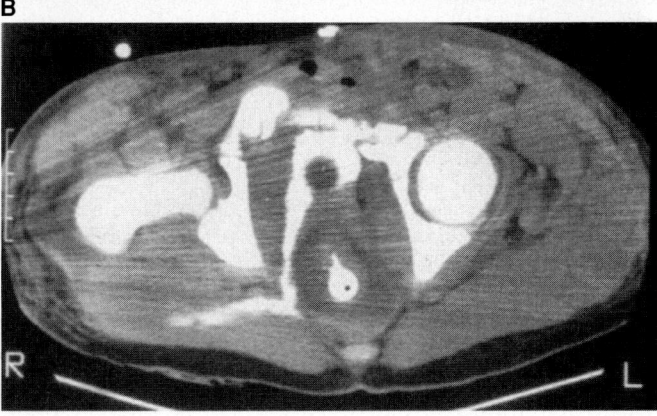

C

**FIGURE 39-11.** **(A)** Computed tomography (CT) cystogram demonstrating intraperitoneal bladder rupture. A standard stress cystographic technique has been employed, with instillation of 350 mL of contrast followed by scanning of upper, mid, and lower abdomen. Contrast is seen filling colic gutters and filling the true pelvis, in this case clearly outlining the ovaries. **(B)** False-negative CT cystogram. This image was obtained by clamping the indwelling Foley catheter and obtaining CT images of the pelvis with passive filling of the bladder following intravenous contrast administration. No extravasation is noted, but the bladder is not adequately filled to reliably exclude injury. A properly performed static cystogram following the CT revealed extensive intraperitoneal extravasation. Inadequate bladder filling is the most common reason for a false-negative cystogram. **(C)** Attempted CT cystogram following pelvic fracture in a 13-year-old male. Extravasation extends through the pelvic floor into the buttock, and no filling of the bladder is seen. The Foley balloon is actually positioned in the pelvic hematoma. The patient was found to have a bladder neck avulsion injury, which was initially managed with an open surgical cystostomy, then surgically reconstructed 72 h following injury.

prostate on rectal examination should make one suspicious of urethral injury (Fig. 39-12). When urethral injury is suspected, a retrograde urethrogram should be performed (Fig. 39-13). A Foley catheter is inserted into the fossa navicularis of the distal urethra and minimally inflated. This is followed by instillation of approximately 30 mL of iodinated contrast at which point a plain radiograph is obtained. A normal retrograde urethrogram should demonstrate contrast filling an intact urethra and entering the bladder without extravasation. No attempt at insertion of a bladder catheter should be pursued until a negative retrograde urethrogram is obtained to avoid further complicating a urethral rupture (Fig. 39-14).

Following placement of either a urethral catheter (if the urethra proved normal or by a urologist using direct vision techniques in selected incomplete injuries) or a suprapubic catheter (if urethral disruption was revealed), a stress cystogram should still be performed if hematuria is present. This is because 10–15% of patients with urethral disruptions from a pelvic fracture will have a concomitant injury to the bladder.

## External Genitalia

Genital injuries represent a diverse group of traumatic events.[22] These include the classic penile fracture, which occurs from forceful bending of the erect penis, often during intercourse, crush injuries with rupture of the testis, penetrating injuries, and industrial accidents. Amputation injuries of the penis or testicle can occur due to assaults, self-mutilation, or industrial trauma. After major blunt trauma to the scrotum, the risk of testicular rupture is approximately 50%. An ultrasound examination of the scrotum may be valuable to distinguish testicular rupture from a hematoma of the scrotal wall or hematocele (blood within the tunica vaginalis compartment). Nuclear scanning may have limited usefulness in the trauma setting to assess testicular viability, but generally does not provide sufficient anatomic detail to formulate decisions on management.

## NONOPERATIVE MANAGEMENT OF GENITOURINARY INJURIES

While nonoperative management for many urological injuries has become well-established, the selection of operative versus nonoperative management for certain genitourinary injuries remains controversial. Recent reviews of urologic management based on careful assessment of levels of evidence reveal a notable paucity of level 1, prospective management studies.[1-5] The relatively recent efforts to accurately and uniformly describe and stage the nature of injuries and the lack of long-term follow-up leave many questions as to the best way to manage many forms of genitourinary trauma.

### Kidney

It has long been accepted that low-grade renal injuries can be managed nonoperatively with a high success rate. Renal contusion and subcapsular hematomas are routinely managed expectantly and only rarely would surgical or other interventions be required in such cases. These

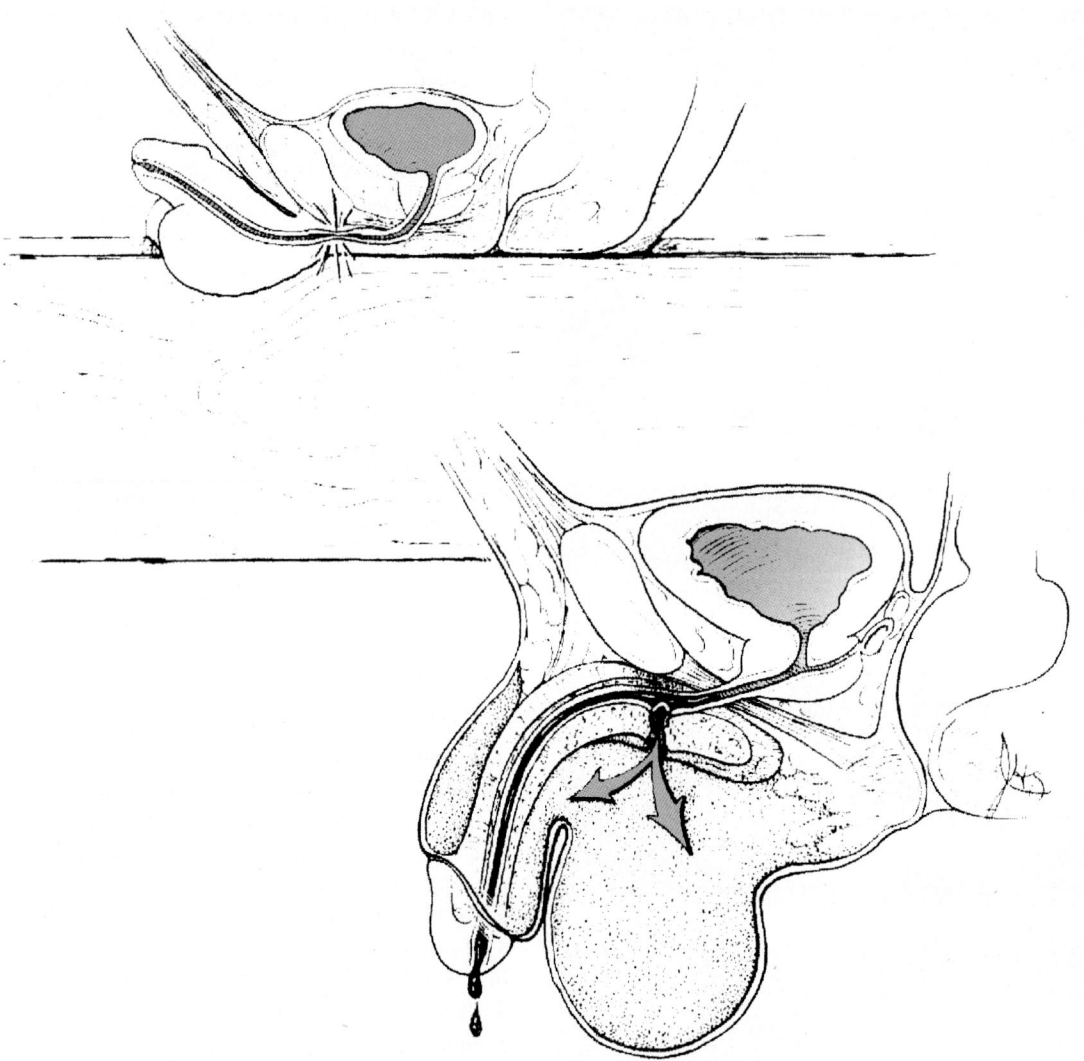

**FIGURE 39-12.** Mechanism of anterior urethral disruption due to straddle injury; extravasation pattern and hematoma limited in this case by Colles' fascia, due to rupture of Buck's fascia along with full thickness of urethral wall. Hematoma and urinoma may extend along shaft of penis and into scrotum and perineum.

injuries heal spontaneously with few exceptions as do low-grade parenchymal lacerations. Depending on the institutional bias and experience, some urologic trauma surgeons may limit operative management of renal injuries to those in which the patient is hemodynamically unstable, almost regardless of imaging findings. Alternatively, others would include those injuries in which the grade of injury is high, presumably translating into a higher incidence of postinjury complications with nonoperative management. A number of indications for renal exploration following injury have been suggested by McAninch and Carroll.[23] These include hemodynamic instability, ongoing hemorrhage requiring significant transfusion, pulsatile or expanding hematoma on exploration, or avulsion of the pedicle. Relative indications for surgical intervention have included high-grade injuries, large perirenal hematoma, presence of urinary extravasation on contrast studies, significant devitalized fragments of parenchyma, and findings in the operating room during laparotomy with an incompletely staged injury.

Proponents of the nonoperative management approach suggest that many high-grade injuries will heal without surgery, complications can frequently be managed with nonsurgical

techniques (percutaneous drainage, stenting, angiographic embolization), and renal salvage rates are better overall when renal exploration is avoided. This school of thought would maintain that, with few exceptions, it is only hemodynamic instability that should prompt surgical intervention for the injured kidney, not injury stage or other predetermined imaging criteria.

In contrast, proponents of a more aggressive surgical approach would suggest that higher grades of renal injury carry an unacceptably high complication rate and that such complications, when they occur, have a high likelihood of resulting in otherwise avoidable morbidity or nephrectomy (Fig. 39-15). Proponents would suggest that early exploration and repair offer the advantage of early debridement of devitalized tissue, definitive hemostasis, repair of injuries to the collecting system, and early institution of appropriate drainage. As such, postinjury infection, urinoma, and hemorrhage risk are minimized. Descriptions of "absolute" and "relative" indications for renal exploration for trauma have been suggested to attempt to provide assistance in this decision-making process.[23,24]

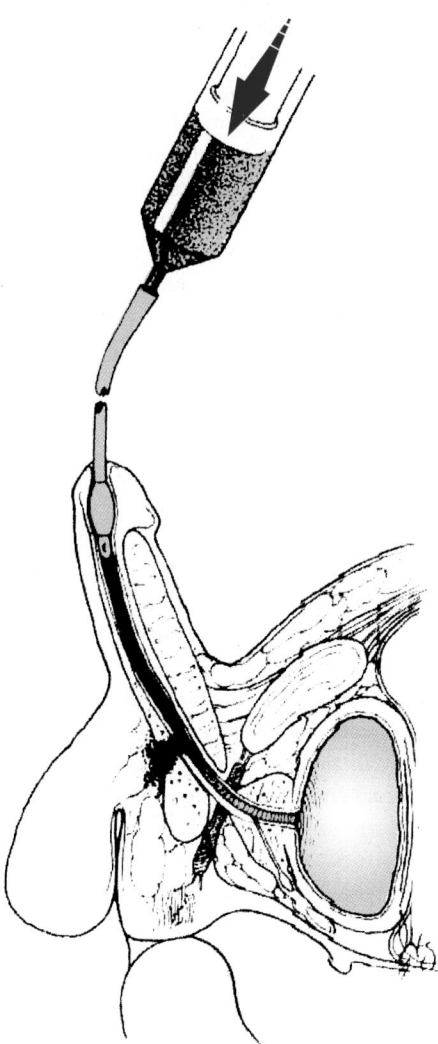

**FIGURE 39-13.** Technique of retrograde urethrogram. Retrograde urethrogram: Catheter is inserted into urethral meatus, with miminal balloon inflation to maintain position and allow hands to be out of x-ray field. Contrast is instilled to distend urethra.

For certain injuries, operative management is nearly universally accepted. These include blunt avulsion or penetrating lesions of the renovascular pedicle, AAST grade V parenchymal injuries, and ureteropelvic avulsion or complete avulsion of the fornices. While occasional case reports have suggested that grade V renal injuries can be managed nonoperatively, most studies demonstrate that 90–100% of such injuries require urgent nephrectomy.[19] In general, attempts at nonoperative management of true grade V renal injuries are not advised and may expose the patient to substantial risk.

Patients with significant ongoing bleeding from the injured kidney where angiographic control is not likely to correct the problem, is not available, or has failed also require prompt operative attention. For penetrating renal injuries in cases where laparotomy will occur regardless, especially when preoperative staging has not been performed or is incomplete, operative management is widely recommended.

When high-grade renal injuries are selected for nonoperative management, certain general principles apply. Such patients are at risk for continued bleeding or significant delayed bleeding, and it

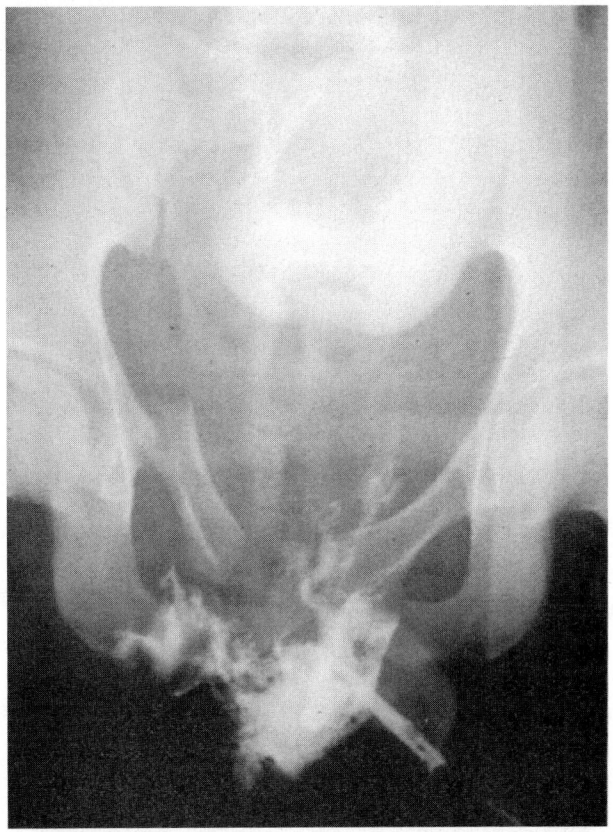

A

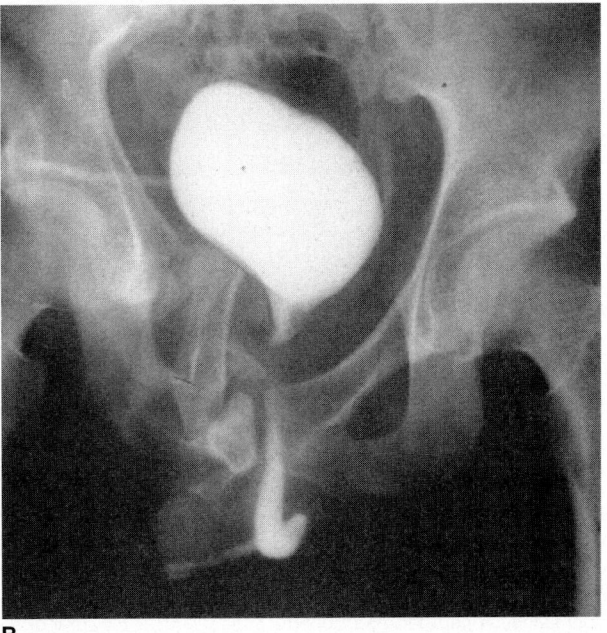

B

**FIGURE 39-14.** Urethra: Posterior urethral disruption with pelvic fracture. **(A)** Retrograde urethrogram demonstrates extravasation of contrast both above and below urogenital diaphragm and no filling of prostatic urethra or bladder neck, consistent with complete disruption. Note pubic ramus fracture and marked cephalad elevation of bladder (bladder filling with contrast excreted following intravenous administration for computed tomography scan). Hemodynamically unstable patient required angiographic embolization for pelvic hemorrhage. Urethral disruption managed with open suprapubic cystostomy. **(B)** Combined antegrade and retrograde contrast studies 6 months postinjury, demonstrating obliterated posterior urethral distraction defect, in preparation for reconstructive surgery.

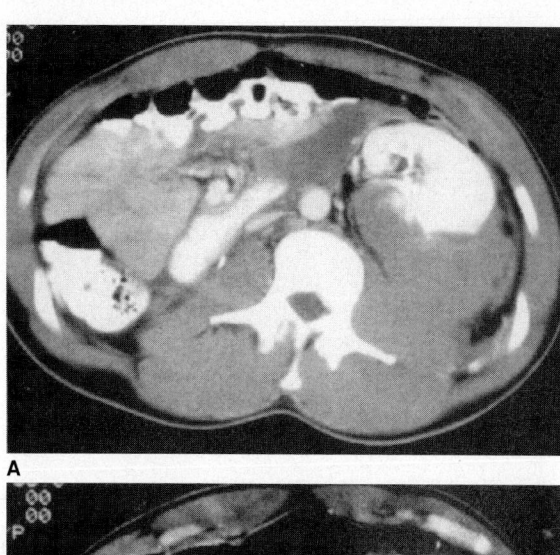

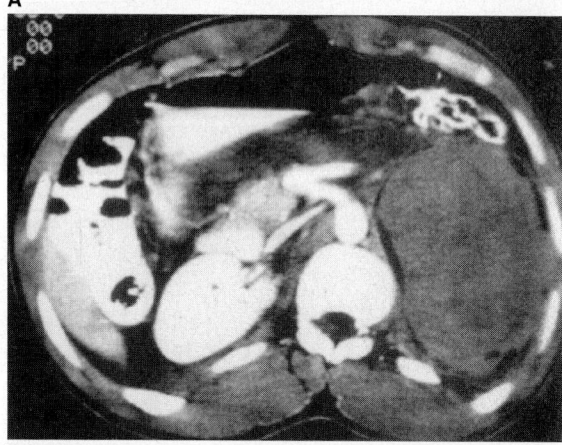

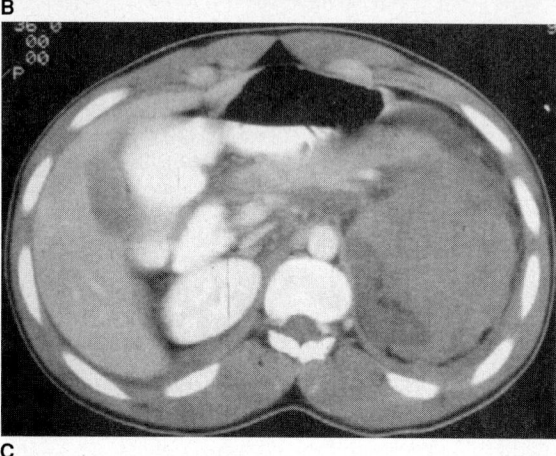

**FIGURE 39-15.** Grade V parenchymal injury. **(A)** This image through the upper abdomen demonstrates the upper pole of the left kidney to be elevated by a perinephric hematoma. The upper pole is well perfused and intact. **(B)** A lower section reveals a large, left retroperitoneal hematoma; the right kidney is perfused and appears normal. This is an early arterial and parenchymal phase, as indicated by the degree of enhancement of the aorta and right renal cortex. **(C)** A more caudal image demonstrates a large, devascularized fragment of the left kidney; this represents the lower third of the kidney that has been avulsed from the perfused portion of the kidney. This injury required operative repair, which involved removal of the avulsed parenchymal fragment, suturing of the large intrarenal vascular branches that were avulsed, and reconstruction of the collecting system and the level of the junction of the lower infundibulum with the renal pelvis. While some reports suggest that some grade V injuries may be manageable nonoperatively, most clinicians consider this anatomy of injury a surgical indication. Difficulties in classifying some parenchymal injuries as grade IV versus V may contribute to this apparent reported variability of opinion and outcome.

is important that they be observed in the surgical intensive care unit. Serial abdominal examinations are essential, as are serial laboratory studies including hemoglobin level and electrolyte status. Typed and cross-matched blood should be available for the first 24 to 48 hours. The patient's hemoglobin should be maintained in such a range that a sudden drop from renewed bleeding would not be catastrophic. Particular attention should be paid to the size of the perirenal hematoma on initial imaging. Large hematomas suggest bleeding from larger intrarenal vessels and, presumably, indicate cases in which the risk of continued bleeding is greater. Elderly patients or patients with cardiovascular disease should be transfused more liberally, with a low threshold for intervention, as any sudden substantial blood loss may not be tolerated. When managing high-risk renal injuries nonoperatively, it is advisable to reimage such injuries at 48 to 96 hours to allow early diagnosis of complications such as enlargement of the perirenal hematoma, formation of a urinoma, or evolution of ischemic parenchyma. Early knowledge of such untoward events allows for treatment before the patient demonstrates complications such as sepsis, azotemia, or severe anemia.

It is routine to impose a period of strict bed rest with nonoperative management of a major renal injury, though specific data to support this policy are lacking. Nevertheless, it seems reasonable to have the patient remain at bed rest for the first 24 to 72 hours or until significant gross hematuria resolves, then reinstitute ambulation cautiously and in a monitored environment. If nonoperative management has been successful, patients should be instructed to avoid significant physical exertion until follow-up imaging reveals adequate healing.

Selecting between renal exploration and observation when the incompletely staged renal injury is encountered intraoperatively is difficult. Some authors recommend that the unstaged kidney be routinely explored, while others suggest a more selective approach. If no radiographic information is available, an intraoperative intravenous pyelogram may be selectively obtained to assist in this decision. A standard technique would involve the bolus injection of iodinated contrast (2 mL/kg body weight), then obtaining a 10-minute excretion film. If significant anatomic distortion is observed, this is considered suggestive of major parenchymal disruption and/or injury to the collecting system, for which exploration may be of benefit. If the kidney appears grossly intact, observation would be selected, often with postoperative CT scanning for more precise imaging. Others would consider the size of the perirenal hematoma as an important parameter as well.

Injuries to branch renal arteries from blunt trauma, resulting in segmental devascularization without laceration, can be managed nonoperatively with a low complication rate.

Penetrating injuries to the kidney are accompanied by injury to nonurologic organs in a large proportion of cases, and the majority of these patients will undergo laparotomy. These patients may or may not be imaged preoperatively. The issue of whether to explore the (suspected) renal injury in such cases is addressed later in "Operative Management of Specific Genitourinary Injuries." When the general trauma surgeon sees no clear operative indication and penetrating renal injury is possibly present, the urologist will have to decide on operative versus nonoperative management based on the clinical status of the patient and, preferably, on the findings of a contrast-enhanced spiral CT scan. In general, patients with penetrating injuries to the kidney that involve the lateral and peripheral parenchyma, with small perirenal hematomas, minimal if any extravasation of contrast, and in which the pedicle and renal sinus structures are not at risk, may be safely managed nonoperatively (Fig. 39-16). Conversely, penetrating renal lesions that result in large perirenal hematomas, traverse the deep, medial renal parenchyma, renal sinus, or hilar region, or cause major urinary or vascular extravasation carry higher risks for nonoperative management (Fig. 39-17). The risk of delayed bleeding from such injuries is significant, and some authors have suggested prophylactic arteriography with embolization of violated arterial branches prior to nonoperative management. In addition, the risk of a missed associated visceral injury must be considered with nonoperative management of penetrating renal trauma. In one retrospective review of the nonoperative management of penetrating renal trauma, 55% of renal stab wounds and 24% of renal gunshot wounds were managed nonoperatively with a low complication rate.[25]

While an uncommon injury, blunt or penetrating trauma to the adrenal gland deserves brief mention. If an adrenal hematoma is not expansile, it is managed nonoperatively as with parenchymal injuries to other solid organs. If the adrenal is explored due to the path of a stab or bullet wound, suturing to achieve hemostasis is the standard approach, while extensive destruction of the gland is treated with adrenalectomy. As the adrenal glands each have several sources of arterial blood supply, devascularization from trauma is rare.

## Ureter

Nonoperative management of ureteral trauma has limited applications. When a ureteral injury is recognized intraoperatively, surgical repair is favored (see later).[15, 26] Reviews of outcomes of ureteral injuries indicate that most types of ureteral trauma fare better with early operative repair, as compared with delayed repair or attempts at nonoperative management, with the exception of limited iatrogenic injuries from endoscopy. This is the case for stab and gunshot wounds, as well as avulsion injuries from blunt trauma (Fig. 39-18). Nonoperative management is performed in selected patients with missed ureteral injuries or other settings of delayed diagnosis or in patients in whom damage control strategies are being adopted. Traditional urological teaching dictates that if ureteral trauma is recognized in the early days after injury, operative repair is performed. More significantly delayed recognition is managed with utilization of endoscopic or interventional radiologic techniques (stenting or percutaneous nephrostomy diversion) followed by delayed operative reconstruction as indicated. This approach has developed due to the long-standing recognition of problems such as inflammation, edema, friability, presence of a urinoma, and increased risks and complications of reconstructive efforts encountered when operative intervention is pursued greater than 3 to 5 days postinjury. Ureteral contusions recognized intraoperatively, due to either penetrating or blunt trauma, may be managed nonoperatively and simply observed; however, some reports suggest that the risk of late perforation and urinary extravasation may be reduced by intraoperative insertion of a ureteral stent.[27]

When nonoperative management is selected, retrograde ureteropyelography with attempted retrograde stent placement is often performed. Alternatively, percutaneous renal drainage may be the treatment of choice. The selection between these two approaches depends on the hemodynamic and metabolic stability of the patient, as well as specific anatomic and logistical factors. These include the appropriateness of performing a procedure under general anesthesia, the ability of the patient to undergo a procedure in a prone position (generally necessary for obtaining percutaneous renal access), the skill and availability of interventional radiology, and the expected ease of percutaneous access. The latter depends largely on the anatomy of and degree of distension of the collecting system and the presence of a perirenal hematoma. The finding of coagulopathy is often considered a relative contraindication to percutaneous renal drainage, as renal bleeding is always a risk of such procedures. Achievement of percutaneous access can be followed by antegrade ureteral stenting, if there is ureteral continuity and a guidewire can be placed across the injury into the bladder. Conversion of a nephrostomy tube to a percutaneous antegrade universal

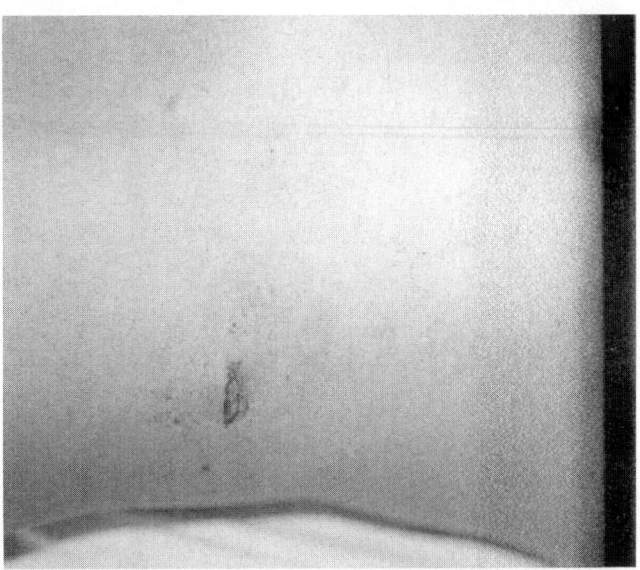

**A**

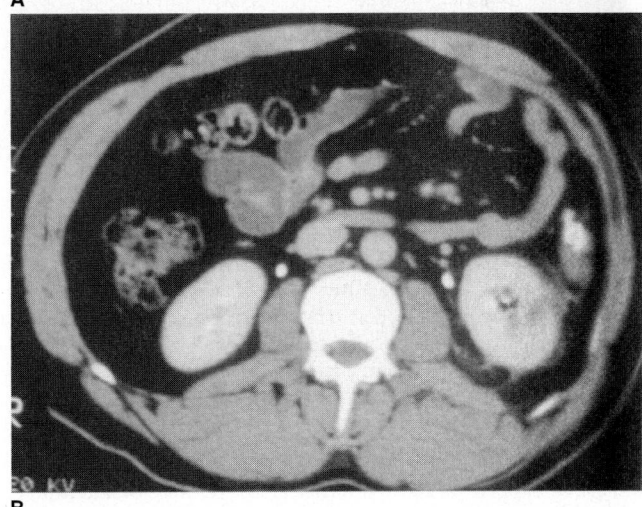

**B**

**FIGURE 39-16.** Penetrating renal injury, successful nonoperative management. **(A)** Stab wound to left flank, just posterior to midaxillary line; patient is hemodynamically stable, with gross hematuria that rapidly clears. **(B)** Staging computed tomography scan demonstrating laceration to lateral left kidney. There is minimal perinephric hematoma, no urinary extravasation, and no devitalized parenchyma. Injury is lateral and laceration does not extend into hilar region or renal sinus structures. Posterior descending colon is in proximity to injury, but general surgeons are prepared to manage nonoperatively. Ideal candidate for nonoperative management of a penetrating renal injury.

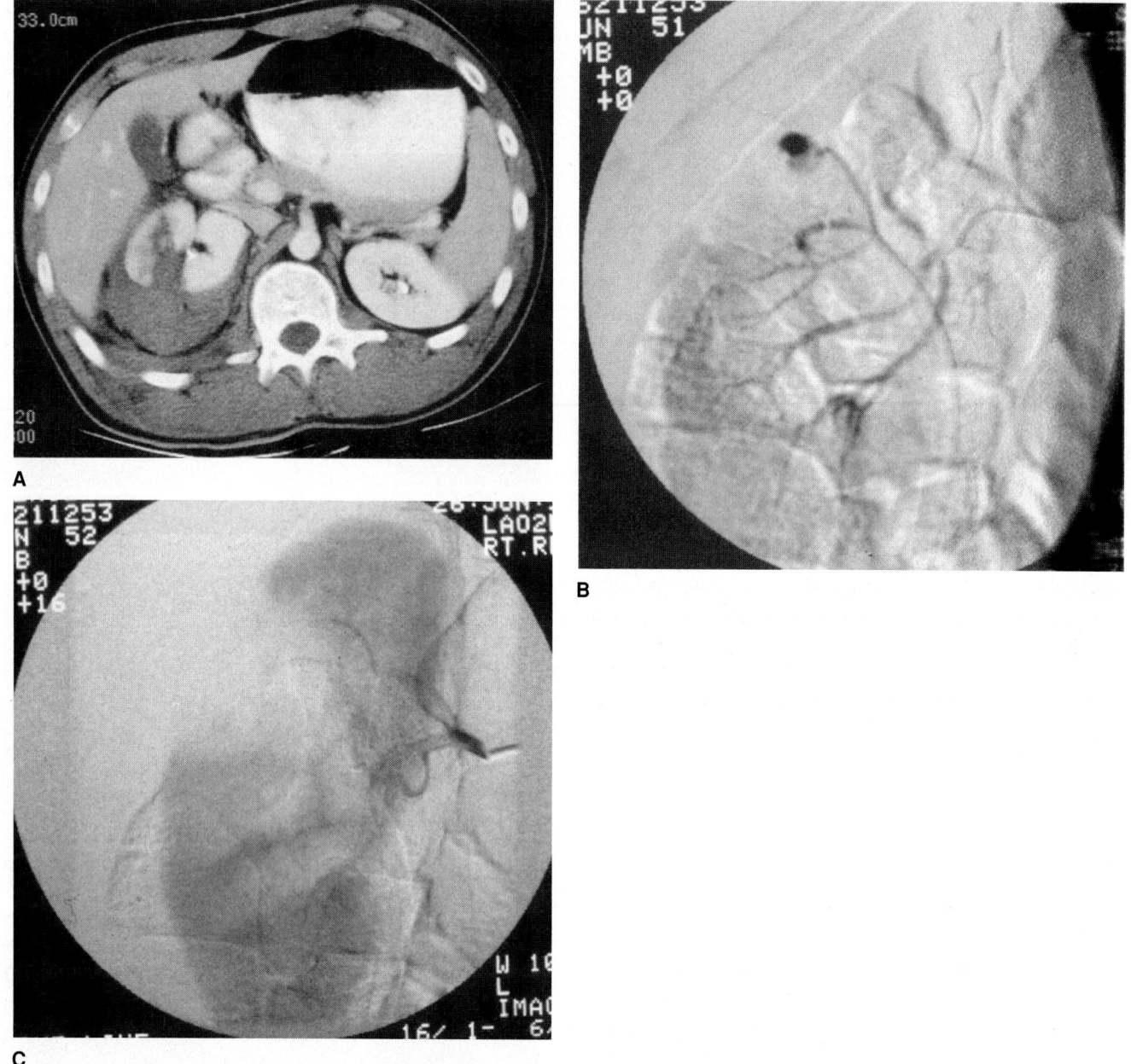

**FIGURE 39-17.**   Penetrating renal injury, complicated. **(A)** Staging CT scan of abdomen following single stab wound to right posterior flank, in patient presenting with gross hematuria. Deep laceration of right kidney with moderate-sized perinephric hematoma. Injury extends into renal sinus region, though no contrast extravasation is noted. After initial attempt at nonoperative management, patient develops major secondary hemorrhage manifested by profuse gross hematuria, resulting in hypotension, and requiring transfusion of 4 units packed red blood cells. **(B)** Arteriogram reveals two areas of arteriocalyceal fistula, successfully managed with subselective embolization. **(C)** Delayed arteriogram image demonstrates wedge-shaped infarct defect due to embolization. Remainder of hospital course uneventful. Embolization is ideal means of managing this problem, as the only indication for intervention is hemorrhage.

stent, which can be changed or manipulated and opened to external drainage or capped to allow internal drainage, may be attempted. Following an appropriate period, a pullback antegrade nephrostogram may be performed to determine if stent removal with clamping of the nephrostomy tube is appropriate.

When this type of management is utilized, a rate of ureteral strictures of up to 50% may be expected. A stricture may undergo an attempt at endourologic management, although delayed surgical reconstruction of the ureter is often necessary.

With blunt trauma, limited ureteral injuries with minimal extravasation may be treated nonoperatively with a retrograde stent. Retrograde pyelography is often necessary to document anatomy

amenable to such management. For penetrating injuries, small-gauge shotgun pellet wounds may create minute ureteral perforations that can be managed nonoperatively as well. Such injuries may be noted at laparotomy or may be seen on a contrast-enhanced CT or intravenous or retrograde pyelography. Again, such cases represent the rare exception to the general principles favoring early operative exploration and repair when technically and medically feasible.

## Bladder

Nonoperative management of extraperitoneal injury to the bladder has been the standard approach for over 10 years, largely as a

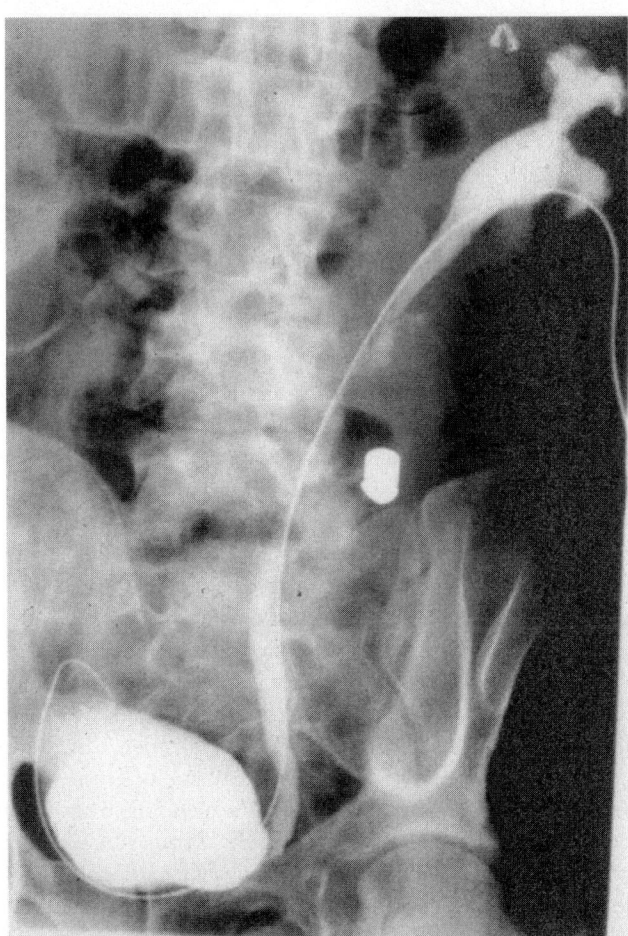

**FIGURE 39-18.** Ureter: Gunshot wound to ureter with missed injury, in a patient who had no hematuria on initial presentation. Patient developed abdominal fluid collection postlaparotomy; intravenous pyelogram demonstrated missed ureteral injury 5 days postoperatively. Injury initially managed with percutaneous nephrostomy and antegrade placement of universal stent. Long, densely fibrotic stricture of midureter developed, as shown here, ultimately requiring nephrectomy. A high index of suspicion is necessary to detect penetrating ureteral injuries at the time of initial laparotomy; outcomes are significantly improved with early recognition and prompt operative repair in such cases.

result of the studies of Corriere and associates and others in which catheter drainage alone was usually successful.[28,29] An 18 to 20 French or larger bladder catheter should be utilized to allow free drainage in the adult. The catheter is left indwelling for 10 to 14 days followed by a cystogram to confirm cessation of extravasation prior to removal. After this period, >85% of bladder injuries will show absence of extravasation. If extravasation persists, another 7 to 10 days of catheter drainage followed by repeat cystography is appropriate. Rarely, persistent extravasation will occur after a prolonged period of catheter drainage. In such cases, CT scanning and/or cystoscopy is indicated to be sure a foreign body such as a bony spicule from a pelvic fracture or some other anatomic cause is not resulting in failure of the laceration to heal properly. Indications for initial selection of operative management instead of catheter drainage alone include concomitant injury to the vagina or rectum, injury to the bladder neck in the female, avulsion of the bladder neck in any patient,[30] and the need for pelvic exploration for other surgical indications. If retropubic access is required for internal fixation of a pelvic fracture, surgical repair of the bladder is desirable to prevent

continued extravasation adjacent to orthopaedic hardware. Open pelvic fractures may also require operative repair of the bladder. The presence of combined extraperitoneal and intraperitoneal rupture or combined extraperitoneal bladder rupture and posterior urethral injury, for which catheter realignment is planned, would be considered appropriate settings to proceed with operative repair of the bladder as well. Finally, clot formation with troublesome occlusion of the drainage catheter may mandate operative repair.[31]

Intraperitoneal ruptures of the bladder are uniformly managed with operative repair. Most such injuries result in large, stellate tears in the dome of the bladder due to the sudden rise in pressure within a full bladder as from a blow to the lower abdomen or compression by a seatbelt. Rare exceptions to the routine application of operative repair for intraperitoneal bladder rupture include minimal intraperitoneal perforations. These usually occur during cystoscopic procedures, mainly when a resectoscope is being utilized for resection of a bladder tumor or during biopsies of lesions of the dome and anterior wall, or other minimal iatrogenic injuries. Several reports have appeared in recent years describing laparoscopic techniques of repair for iatrogenic injuries,[32] particularly when occurring during a primary laparoscopic procedure and when the urologist is capable of endosuturing. The application of techniques of laparoscopic repair to the management of intraperitoneal rupture of the bladder from blunt trauma is being explored at several centers.

For penetrating injury to the bladder, nonoperative management is occasionally applicable in carefully selected and fully evaluated patients with limited defects that are extraperitoneal.[33] Such patients often require proctoscopy and/or sometimes arteriography. Selectively, peritoneal lavage or laparoscopy may play a role in such cases to ensure that the peritoneal surface of the pelvis is intact. In our experience, cystoscopy and upper tract imaging (IVP or retrograde pyelography) has been helpful in assuring that the magnitude of the defect in the bladder is minimal and is likely to heal with catheter drainage alone. The considerations for conversion to operative management and postinjury monitoring and imaging and catheter management are comparable to those utilized with blunt extraperitoneal injuries.

## Urethra

The nature (blunt or penetrating), location of the injury (anterior vs. posterior urethra), completeness (partial vs. complete circumferential laceration), presence and seriousness of associated injuries, and the stability of the patient all impact the selection of management for urethral trauma.[34] When urethral trauma is suspected, retrograde urethrography (RUG) should be performed. If the RUG reveals minimal extravasation and flow of contrast past an anterior injury from blunt trauma into the proximal urethra and bladder, some authors have suggested that a single attempt at gentle passage of a bladder catheter should be performed. Other urologists believe that even minimal blind instrumentation of the injured urethra is ill-advised, preferring an endoscopically guided approach. In this author's opinion, endoscopically guided urethral instrumentation of the injured urethra is preferable to blind insertion of a catheter. The most conservative recommendation is to avoid any blind instrumentation of the injured urethra by the nonurologist. For incomplete anterior urethral injuries, urethral catheterization is reasonable therapy. Catheter-realignment techniques for posterior urethral trauma fall within the realm of the experienced urologist and constitute operative therapy and will be discussed later. Penetrating injuries to the anterior urethra are generally managed with operative exploration and repair.[35] Penetrating injuries to the posterior urethra may present complex challenges in management, may be complicated by adjacent rectal injury or other intrapelvic or visceral injury, and are also considered later.

## Genital Injuries

While penile fractures and testicular ruptures are best managed with early recognition and operative exploration and repair, certain genital injuries due to blunt trauma may be managed nonoperatively.[20] This would be the case when the injury is limited to the subcutaneous tissues, the tunica albuginea and urethra of the penis are intact, and the tunica albuginea of the testes is intact as well. For penile injuries, nonoperative management is appropriate for rupture of subcutaneous vessels resulting in limited ecchymoses or a hematoma. Scrotal trauma may be managed nonoperatively when the testis is intact and there is a limited hematocele that is not particularly uncomfortable for the patient. In most situations, however, significant genital trauma is best managed by operative exploration and repair. If physical findings are suspicious for significant injury to deep tissue or such injury cannot be ruled out by imaging studies, operative exploration is prudent. This is because the outcomes of nonoperative management of such injuries as penile fracture or testicular rupture are poor, as compared to the very high success rates of early operative repair of such injuries.[36] As the relative morbidity of surgical exploration of the external genitalia is minimal and the morbidity of missed injuries or delayed recognition is significant, one should err in the direction of operative management for such injuries.[22]

A scrotal ultrasound with a heterogeneous quality of the testicular parenchyma is predictive of testicular rupture, even if clear loss of continuity of the investing tunica albuginea cannot specifically be identified.[37] Certainly, if a clear defect in the continuity of the testicular tunic is noted on ultrasound, the diagnosis of testicular rupture should be suspected and operative repair undertaken. Patients with a significant hematocele (blood and/or clot within the tunica vaginalis compartment) with an intact testis may be observed, though they may often have a quicker recovery of activity and more rapid resolution of scrotal pain and swelling if this lesion is evacuated surgically. An intratesticular hematoma without testicular rupture is generally managed nonoperatively. At times, testicular ultrasound may demonstrate an abnormality in which a preexisting testicular lesion such as a germ cell neoplasm is suspected. Such may be the case when relatively minor trauma causes a significant intratesticular bleed or testicular rupture. When preexisting testicular pathology is suspected and nonoperative management is selected for the traumatic lesion, it is critical that the testis be reevaluated until the suspicious abnormality resolves or its continuing presence mandates further imaging and intervention.

For genital injuries involving significant loss of soft tissue or skin, nonoperative management may be appropriate as an initial approach, especially when more immediately life-threatening injuries demand priority. Wounds should be cleansed and a conservative approach should be adopted when determining whether to perform debridement of genital skin or soft tissues of marginal or questionable viability. Secondary operative management and delayed reconstruction with skin grafting or other tissue transfer techniques is often necessary when wounds are initially managed in this manner.[38]

## OPERATIVE MANAGEMENT OF SPECIFIC GENITOURINARY INJURIES

### Kidney

Renal exploration for trauma begins with prioritization of the injuries and determining that the initial operation is in fact the appropriate time to embark on the renal exploration (see "Damage Control Surgery," later). When contemplating exploration of an injured kidney in the absence of preoperative imaging, some assessment of the presence and normalcy of the contralateral kidney should be undertaken. While palpating the contralateral renal fossa for a grossly normal kidney is certainly appropriate and may be the only assessment feasible under many circumstances, an intraoperative IVP provides more precise information and may be indicated in selected cases. This can be performed by administering 1 to 2 mL/kg of iodinated contrast intravenously and then obtaining a 10-minute excretion film. This can occur while other general surgical tasks are being accomplished to avoid wasting time. While an intraoperative IVP provides some additional reassurance that a functional contralateral kidney is present when exploring an injured kidney, in our center we frequently proceed with exploration of the injured kidney based on contralateral renal palpation alone.

If it is jointly determined by the urologist and the general surgeon that renal exploration should occur, exploration is carried out through an anterior vertical incision in Gerota's fascia. There has been some controversy regarding the importance of first obtaining vascular control of the renal pedicle prior to renal exploration as previously described.[39,40] Some proponents claim a markedly reduced nephrectomy rate if the renal vessels are first dissected and controlled with vessel loops. Others claim that this maneuver is unnecessary to successful renal exploration and repair. This controversy is probably overstated, as even those who do not believe that individual dissection of the renal vessels is essential prior to renal mobilization generally use some other approach to control the pedicle or limit renal bleeding during examination and repair of the kidney. The bulk of the literature would suggest that the rate of otherwise unnecessary nephrectomies is minimized by having exposure and control of the renal pedicle prior to renal exploration. This can be achieved by the traditional maneuver of incising the posterior peritoneum lateral to the aorta and individually dissecting and looping the renal vessels on the side of injury (Fig. 39-19). This can also be achieved by reflecting the colon medially first, then clamping the pedicle if significant bleeding is encountered upon opening the Gerota's fascial envelope (Fig. 39-20). Alternatively, the pedicle or the renal parenchyma can be compressed digitally (most applicable to polar injuries) without having individual control over the renal vessels. Certainly if there is an injury to the pedicle, suggested by a large or expending medial hematoma in the vicinity of the great vessels, there is broad agreement that central vascular control should be the initial maneuver.

Following pedicle control or access, the colon and mesocolon on the side of injury is dissected medially following incision of the peritoneal reflection. When the anterior surface of Gerota's fascia is fully exposed, a generous, vertical, anterior incision is made through the fascia, and the kidney is fully mobilized. As indicated earlier in the section on surgical anatomy, it is important to dissect in an extracapsular plane and avoid inadvertently dissecting the renal capsule away from the underlying cortex. Accomplishing this is facilitated by beginning the dissection in an area of intact parenchyma rather than directly within the laceration. Completely

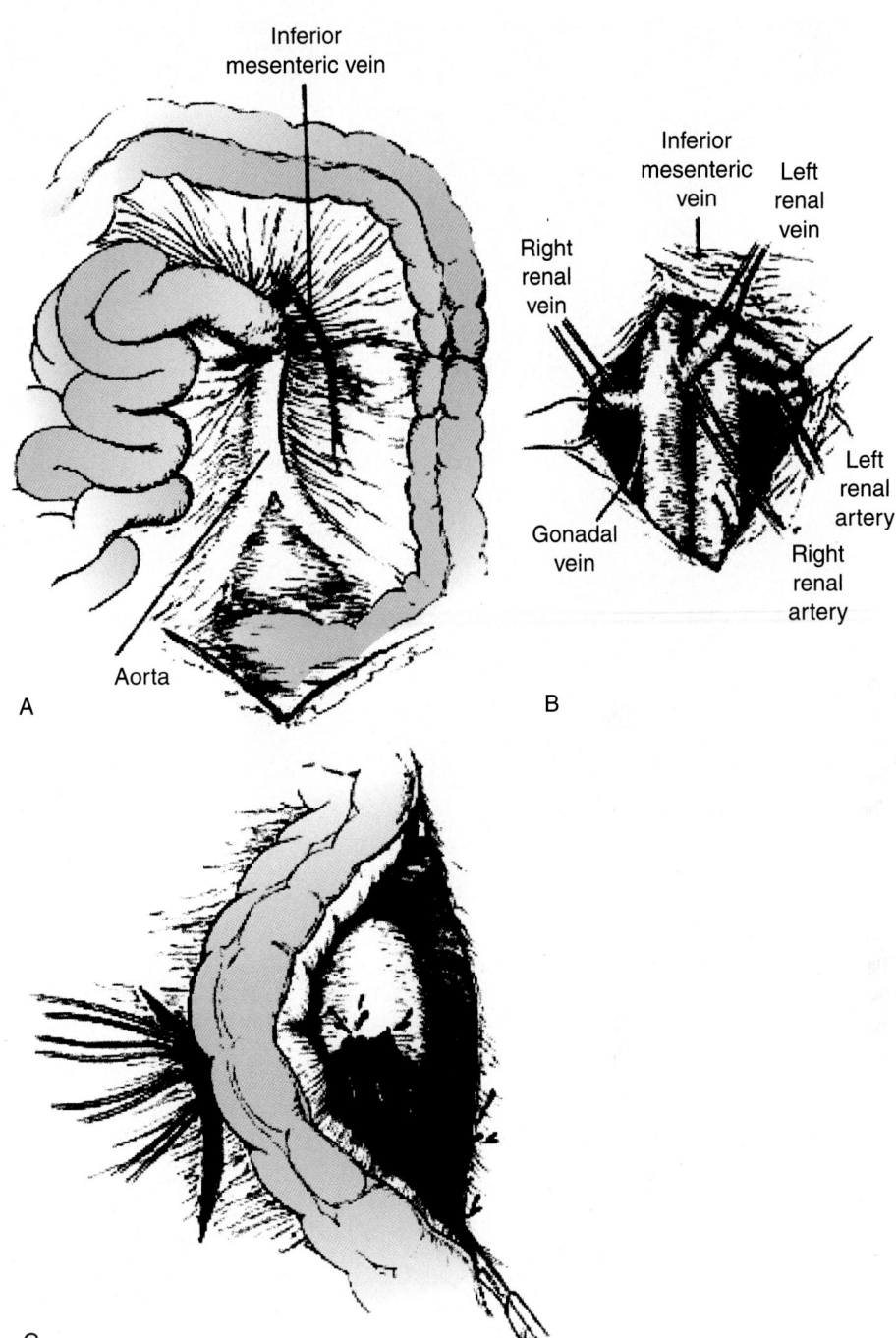

Inferior
mesenteric vein

Aorta

A

Inferior
mesenteric
vein

Left
renal
vein

Right
renal
vein

Gonadal
vein

Left
renal
artery

Right
renal
artery

B

C

**FIGURE 39-19.** Surgical management of renal trauma: vascular control. Diagram demonstrating early vascular control prior to renal exploration. **(A)** The posterior peritoneum is opened over the aorta medial to the inferior mesenteric vein. **(B)** The renal vessels are individually dissected and surrounded with vessel loops. **(C)** The colon is reflected medially exposing the perinephric hematoma. Some clinicians believe preliminary control of the renal vessels is not necessary when performing renal exploration for trauma, though best renal salvage rates are reported when vascular access or control is obtained.

mobilizing the kidney is very helpful, as it allows the kidney to be lifted anteriorly into the wound for complete inspection. If significant bleeding results during this maneuver, a noncrushing vascular clamp is applied to the renal artery, renal vein, or entire renal pedicle. An initial decision must be made regarding renal salvageability and the magnitude of the reconstructive effort that would be required to repair the injury. This is based largely on the amount of devitalized parenchyma, the degree of injury to the central vasculature and central collecting system, and the condition of the patient. If the kidney is felt to be reconstructible in an unstable patient, any significant intrarenal vascular injury can be rapidly sutured and the kidney can be packed off with laparotomy pads as other surgical injuries are treated (see Chap. 41). After repair of other injuries, or at the time of a secondary surgical procedure, formal exploration and reconstruction of the kidney is performed.

If, based on the anatomy of the injury, the kidney is not considered reconstructible, a nephrectomy is performed. It is preferable to separately ligate the renal artery and vein to avoid the potential for arteriovenous fistula. A rapid search is made for accessory or polar vessels, which must be ligated also. While urologists frequently suture or simply ligate the renal artery and a long stump of vein, vascular surgeons and some urologists prefer to oversew the short right renal vein with a continuous 3-0 Prolene suture. For trauma nephrectomies, the ureter and adjoining vessels are ligated near the kidney, while the gonadal vein is ligated and divided when necessary, with no need for concern for adverse impact on the gonadal structures.

If renal reconstruction is planned, several steps are generally followed (Fig. 39-21). Following evacuation of the hematoma, the kidney is carefully examined to identify lacerated vessels, the open collecting system, and devitalized parencyhyma. Large areas of lacerated,

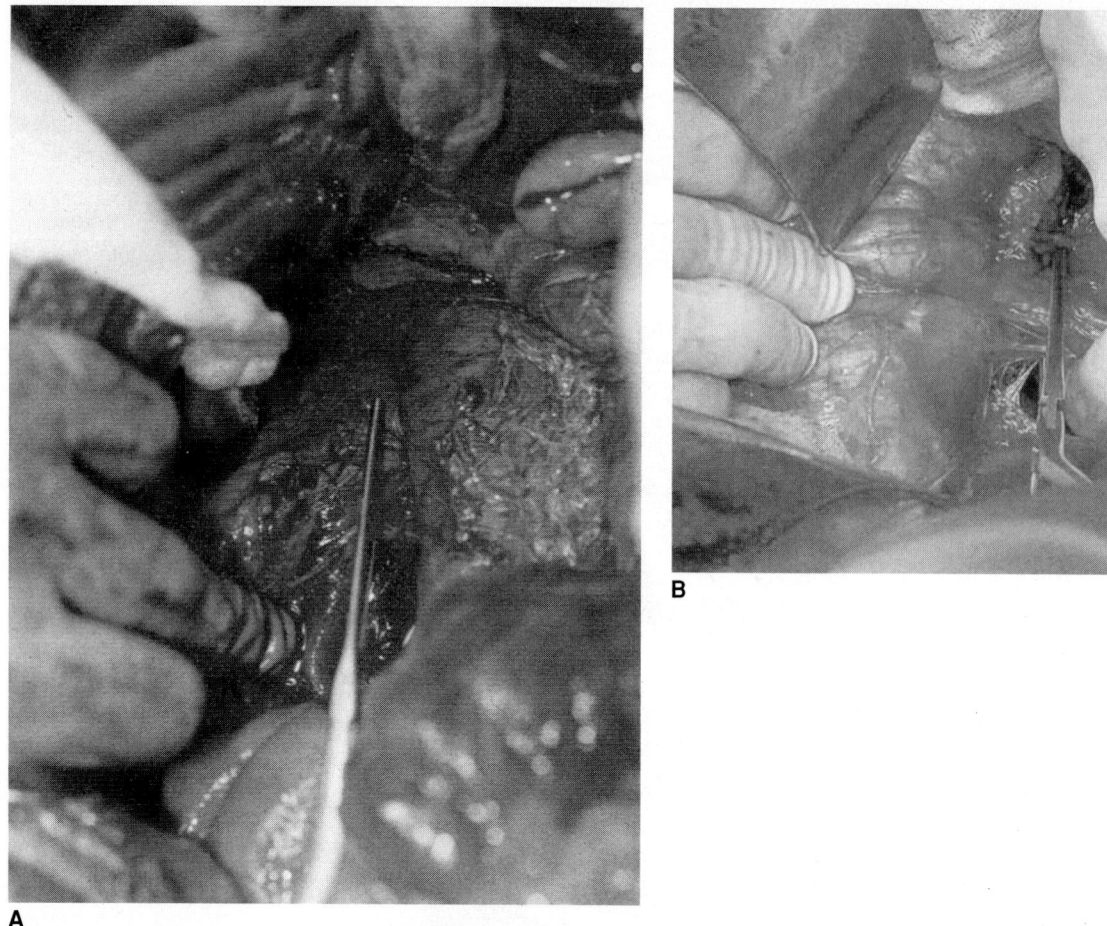

**FIGURE 39-20.** **(A)** Alternate means of obtaining vascular pedicle access prior to renal exploration. Colon is reflected medially initially. Blunt dissection lateral to vena cava allows creation of space anterior to psoas muscle for placement of pedicle clamp if necessary upon renal exposure. **(B)** Comparable technique on the left side, creating space for pedicle clamp lateral to aorta. This approach has been used successfully in the author's center.

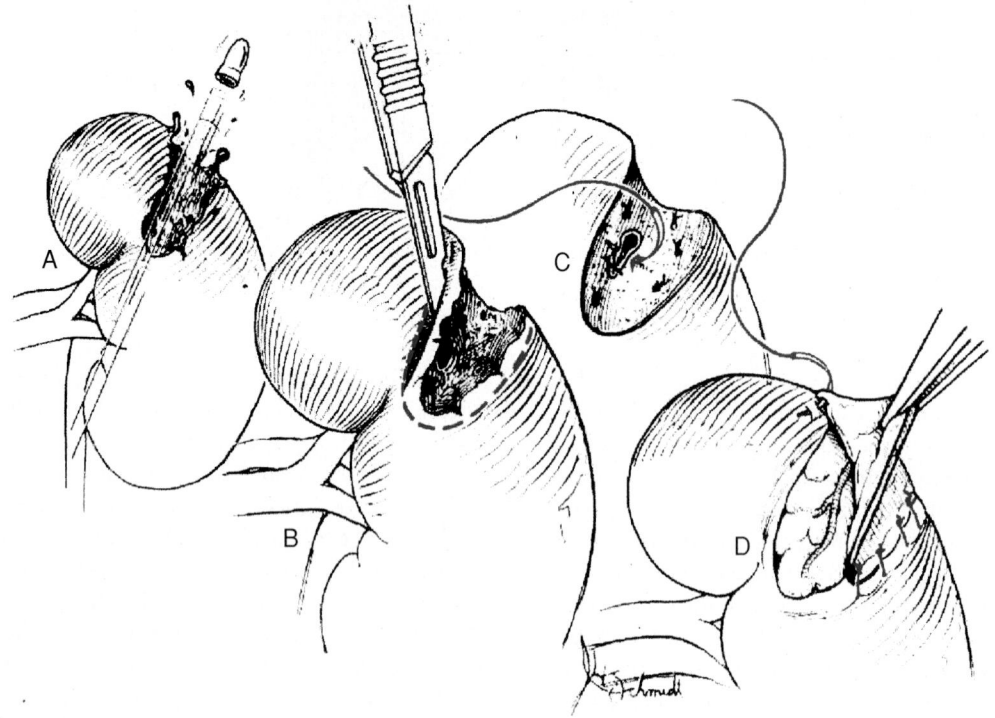

**FIGURE 39-21.** **(A,B)** Wedge resection of injured parenchyma. **(C)** Suturing of open collecting system and significant vessels with absorbable suture. **(D)** Capsule, if present, may be closed, or reconstructed using peritoneal patch, with absorbable gelatin sponge or local fat pedicle to aid in hemostasis

devitalized parenchyma are excised sharply, with smaller vessels controlled with an absorbable 3-0 or 4-0 suture. In general, an absorbable suture is utilized for intrarenal suturing, as a permanent suture may create a nidus for stone formation if in contact with the collecting system. If adequate closure of the collecting system is achieved, there is no need for stenting or a nephrostomy. If repair of the collecting system is tenuous or incomplete, placement of an internal stent (complemented by a bladder catheter) or a nephrostomy tube may decrease the risk of postoperative urinary extravasation and the formation of a urinoma.

Partial nephrectomy for polar lesions is performed by a "guillotine" technique, with the transected vessels and collecting system closed as noted earlier (Figs. 39-22 and 39-23). Topical hemostatic agents may be placed within a parenchymal defect to aid in hemostasis, with the capsule closed over the defect and the hemostatic material. If the capsule can be closed with mattress sutures or absorbable bolsters following debridement or partial nephrectomy, parenchymal hemostasis is aided considerably. If capsular closure is not feasible either due to the shape and location of the parenchymal defect or loss of the capsule from the injury or dissection, utilizing absorbable materials or native tissue as a patch may be helpful if hemostasis is still problematic. The argon beam coagulator has also been utilized successfully in the kidney to achieve hemostasis in the parenchyma, after suturing larger vessels and closing the collecting system. Topical hemostatic agents and tissue adhesives may be used on the kidney, collecting system, ureter, and other urologic repairs to aid in hemostasis and minimize the risk of postoperative urinary extravasation.[21] Some data exist to suggest that the application of fibrin sealant over a urinary tract suture line may decrease the likelihood of postoperative urinary leakage.[21] At times, wrapping the decapsulated kidney in absorbable mesh material has been utilized to provide mild temporary parenchymal compression for continued venous bleeding from lacerated parenchyma (Fig. 39-24).

Injuries to adjacent organs such as the liver, pancreas, duodenum, and colon generally do not change the indications for renal salvage versus nephrectomy,[41,42] as good results have been described

for renal repairs in the setting of injuries to these adjacent organs. It is desirable, however, to separate the renal injury from the adjacent visceral injury using available viable tissue. This can be accomplished by replacing the kidney within Gerota's fascia and closing the fascial layer over the kidney or by utilizing omentum in the form of a pedicle flap. Drains for renal injury are utilized when injury to the collecting system is present or there is concern for the need to evacuate blood postoperatively. Closed-suction drains are used as there is a lower risk of contributing to postoperative infection than open Penrose drains, though both types are used commonly by urologists. In the setting of injury to an adjacent organ, the organ sites should be drained separately.

Certain injuries are more common in the pediatric population and deserve specific mention. Avulsion of the fornices, ureteropelvic junction, and renal pedicle are more commonly seen in the pediatric population than they are in the adult.[10] Complete forniceal avulsion injuries are managed with nephrectomy as repair is nearly impossible. Avulsions of the ureteropelvic junction are amenable to repair through a direct anastomosis. Lacerations of the renal pelvis should also alert the trauma surgeon to the possibility of a preexisting obstruction of the ureteropelvic junction. Repair of the obstructing lesion may need to be performed with closure of the pelvis, or nephrectomy may be preferable if the kidney appears to have minimal parenchyma due to long-standing obstruction.

Renovascular injury from blunt or penetrating trauma presents certain challenges (see Chap. 37). As noted earlier, selected patients are taken to laparotomy for revascularization surgery based solely on a CT scan demonstrating the classic findings of renal nonperfusion following deceleration trauma. If exploration is undertaken based on the CT findings or if arteriographic imaging has been performed, the approach is similar. The artery is dissected from its origin at the aorta toward the kidney and the arterial pulse is palpated or assessed with a Doppler instrument. The artery is clamped near the aorta and opened at the circular ring of hematoma, resected to

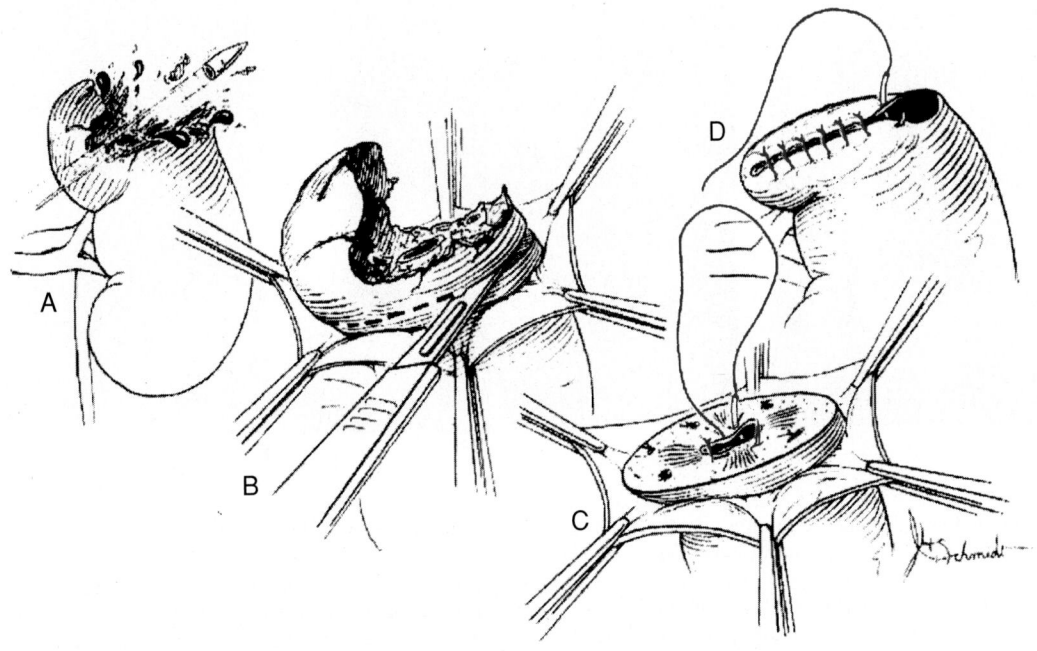

**FIGURE 39-22.    (A,B)** Partial nephrectomy for major injury to upper pole. **(C)** Repair of collecting system and suturing of bleeding vascular branches. **(D)** Mattress sutures of 2-0 chromic gut to reconstruct parenchyma and aid in hemostasis.

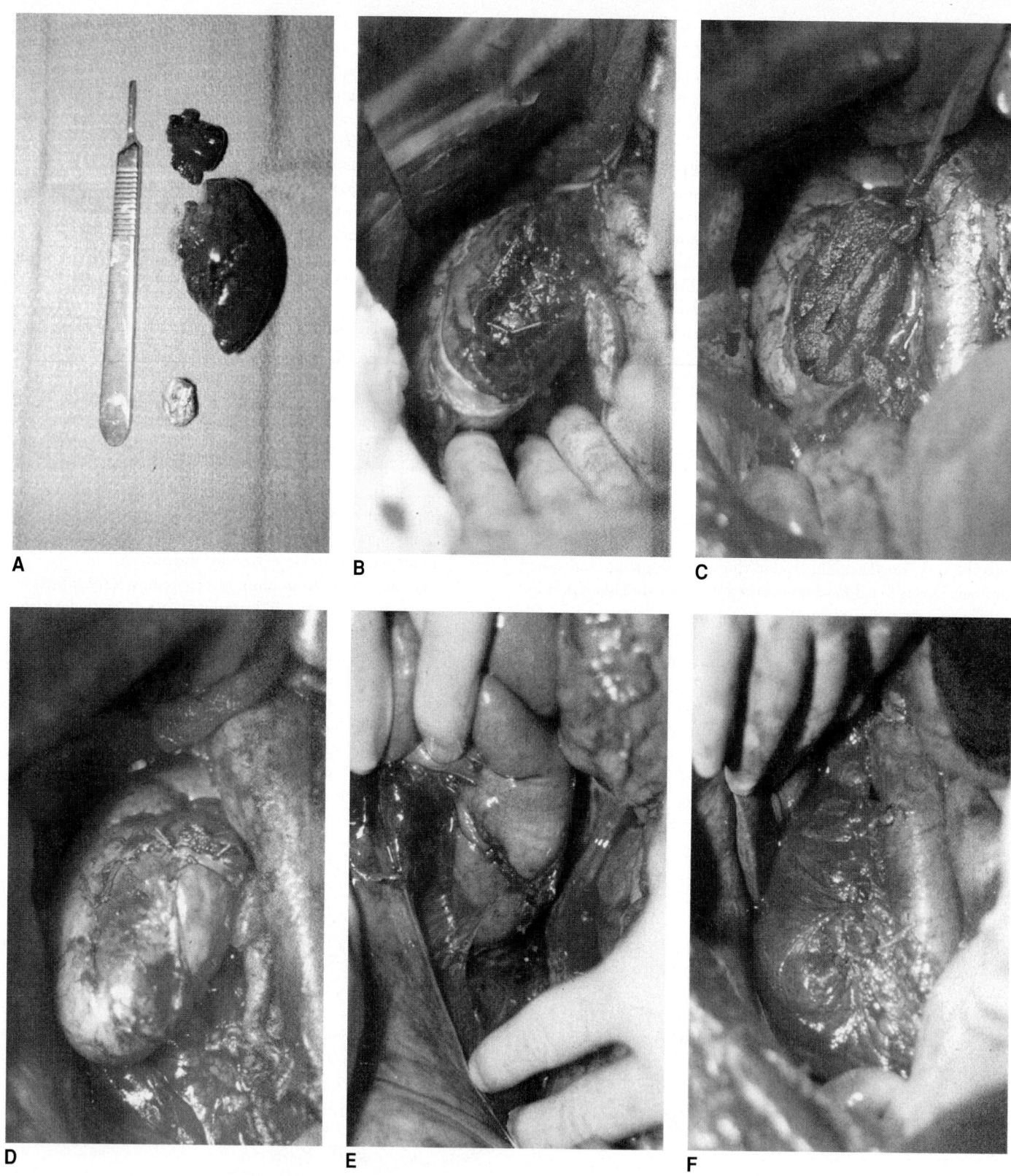

**FIGURE 39-23.** Surgical management of renal trauma. **(A)** Partial nephrectomy for lower pole laceration due to gunshot wound. Excised fragment of devascularized, lower pole parenchyma, debrided. Bullet removed, found immediately posterior to kidney. **(B)** Appearance of lower pole following suture repair of vessels and repair of collecting system. Capsule has been reflected back for completion of partial nephrectomy and will be used for coverage of defect. **(C)** Defect covered with absorbable gelatin sponge soaked in thrombin. Note vessel loops surrounding renal vessels. **(D)** Defect covered with adjacent capsule and peritoneal patch, to aid in hemostasis. **(E)** Duodenal injury, repaired, immediately anterior to the renal injury. It is desirable to separate such injuries with viable tissue interposition, when possible, to minimize the risk of postoperative leak from either source affecting the other repair. **(F)** Gerota's fascia closed over the kidney to separate the duodenal and renal injuries. Omental pedicle flaps are also very useful for this purpose. The renal repair was drained with an extraperitonealized closed-suction drain.

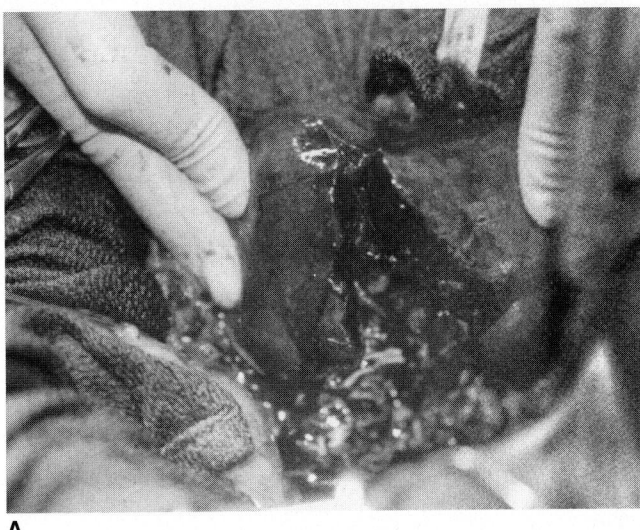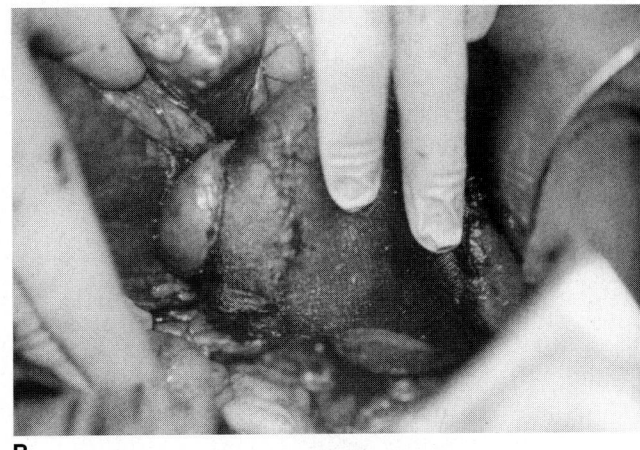

A

B

**FIGURE 39-24.** Surgical management of renal trauma: Renal parenchymal injury due to blunt trauma. **(A)** Large, deep laceration through posterior parenchyma, left kidney. Bleeding sites are sutured, collecting system closed with absorbable suture. Venous bleeding continues from lacerated cortex. **(B)** Due to absence of renal capsule (dissected away from parenchyma by hematoma), absorbable surgical mesh is used to wrap renal parenchyma providing gentle compression to assist in achieving hemostasis.

the point of normal anatomy, and a direct end-to-end anastomosis performed. When necessary, an autogenous vein graft or prosthetic graft is inserted. As in the pediatric population (in which the injury is more common), avulsion injuries involving the renovascular pedicle require urgent surgical intervention. Most such patients are managed with nephrectomy, although isolated vascular repairs have been described depending on the level of the avulsion. Avulsion of multiple branches from within the renal sinus is virtually impossible to repair in the trauma setting and generally requires nephrectomy as well. While current data suggest that the likelihood of achieving a favorable outcome with renal revascularization following renal injury is low,[22] patient selection is critical. In the appropriate clinical setting (brief warm ischemia time and a patient in suitable condition for surgery), the effort may be worthwhile in carefully selected patients. A collaborative approach involving the vascular surgeon and the urologist is highly applicable to cases in which renovascular reconstruction is planned. In selected cases in which an intimal disruption of the renal artery is documented arteriographically but perfusion is maintained, radiologic placement of a vascular stent may be applicable. Many limited penetrating injuries to the renal vein can be repaired, while arterial injuries have a high rate of nephrectomy. Injuries to branch vessels in a parenchymal laceration are ligated. When diagnosed on imaging studies in stable patients with intact parenchyma, nonoperative management is appropriate.

Bilateral renal injuries are rare and present special problems.[43] Assuming neither kidney is bleeding briskly, the kidney that seems to be less seriously injured (based on hematoma size and location, apparent orientation and location of entrance and exit wounds, etc.) is assessed to be sure that renal salvage is feasible. One kidney can also be packed off temporarily after obtaining gross hemostasis while the opposite kidney is assessed in an effort to avoid nephrectomy in these cases whenever possible.

Although rarely indicated, ex-vivo renal reconstructive surgery may be utilized in the trauma setting. This would be the case when

a solitary (functionally or anatomically) kidney is injured, and a complex reconstruction is needed for salvage.

## Ureter

The approach to ureteral repair depends largely on the level of the injury, the amount of ureteral loss, if any, and the condition of the local tissues. A ureteral laceration along with extensive destruction of the kidney from blunt or penetrating trauma is generally managed with nephrectomy. If the kidney is uninjured or the renal injury is limited and can be observed or repaired, ureteral repair is best performed at the time of recognition.[23]

Injuries to the ureter from blunt trauma require a high index of suspicion for diagnosis. Hematuria may be absent in such cases, and a delayed presentation is not uncommon. As noted earlier, the spiral CT scanners complete the initial renal imaging survey so rapidly that, unless a delayed excretory phase is requested, the study may be completed before the contrast has opacified the collecting system or injured ureter.

Blunt avulsion of the proximal ureter or ureteropelvic junction is best managed with limited debridement to viable tissue and a spatulated end-to-end anastomosis using fine absorbable suture (3-0, 4-0, or 5-0). In general, ureteral repairs performed after trauma are most often stented. This can be performed with an internal double-J-type stent or an externalized single-J stent. The single-J stent is usually exteriorized through a small stab incision in the anterior bladder wall and secured with a purse-string suture. Some surgeons also secure the stent to the bladder mucosa just outside the ureteral orifice with a fine absorbable suture (4-0 or 5-0). For tenuous repairs of the proximal ureter, diversion using a nephrostomy tube may be considered, but it is generally unnecessary.[44]

A blunt injury to the mid-ureter is uncommon, but when it is diagnosed, it is managed with a primary anastomosis. In the distal ureter (below the internal iliac artery), ureteral reimplantation into the bladder is preferred.

Injuries to the ureter from penetrating trauma also require a high index of suspicion for diagnosis. The presence of urine in the operative field may be difficult to appreciate, and the ureters, when at risk, must be thoroughly assessed by intraoperative inspection. The proximal and mid-ureters down to the internal iliac arteries are easy to visualize and examine. For very distal injuries, a vertical cystotomy with observation of efflux from the ureteral orifices and intraoperative retrograde pyelography may be a less morbid means of assessing the area of concern, rather than embarking on a difficult dissection of the ureter all the way to the bladder in the setting of a pelvic hematoma. Alternatively, intraoperative flexible cystoscopy with retrograde pyelography may be performed, avoiding the cystotomy. For proximal and mid-ureteral injuries, limited debridement of lacerated tissue and a spatulated end-to-end anastomosis is the procedure of choice (Fig. 39-25). For very distal injuries (generally below the

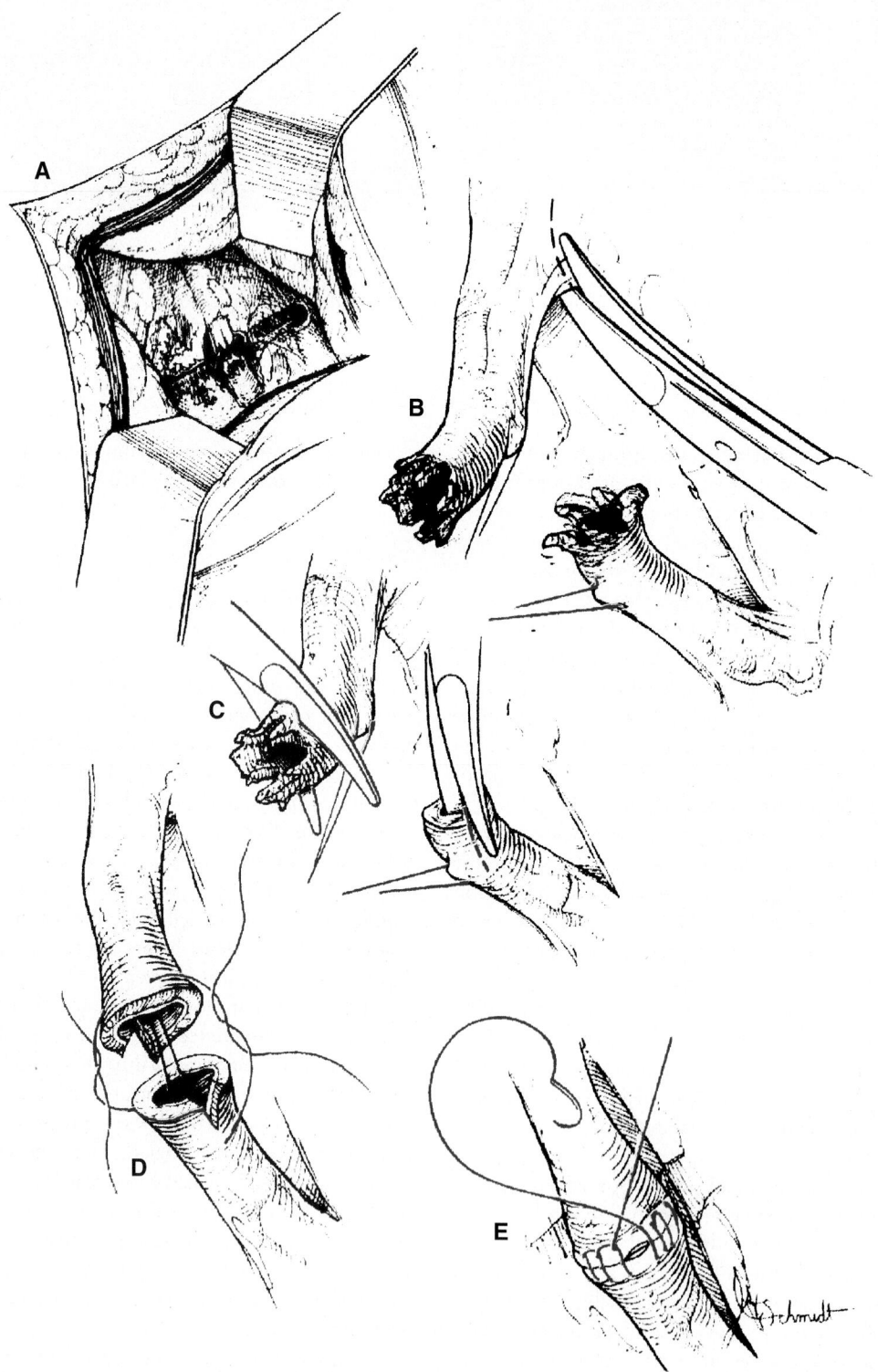

**FIGURE 39-25.** Techniques of ureteral reconstruction. Debridement and primary anastomosis for ureteral transection from gunshot wound. **(A,B)** Mobilization of ureter superficial to adventitial plane. **(C)** Limited debridement of lacerated ureter to viable tissue with spatulation for repair. **(D,E)** End-to-end anastomosis with fine absorbable suture, over stent (not shown).

internal iliac artery), reimplantation into the bladder is preferred as noted earlier as the blood supply to the distal ureteral stump may be compromised. A direct anastomosis to the bladder avoids the potential ischemic complications of a very distal ureter-to-ureter anastomosis. Stenting of such repairs is routine as described previously.

For injuries to the lower third of the ureter, it is not always possible to perform a direct anastomosis to the bladder without tension. In such cases, the bladder can be brought cephalad and lateral toward the injured side to achieve a tension-free anastomosis with the ureter by several techniques. The most commonly employed is the "psoas hitch" (Fig. 39-26). The bladder is opened anteriorly, lateral peritoneal attachments are divided as needed, and then the bladder body is displaced toward the side of the injury and sutured to the psoas muscle with 2-0 absorbable suture, taking care not to injure or entrap any major nerves. The ureter can then be reimplanted into the bladder either using a tunneled antirefluxing anastomosis, or the tunnel can be omitted if length is still a problem. It is important to ensure that no obstruction or acute angulation exists at the vesical hiatus where the ureter enters. If a psoas hitch cannot achieve a tension-free connection to the ureter, a bladder flap (Boari flap) can be created. This procedure has a higher complication rate than a psoas hitch and is performed only if the psoas hitch does not accomplish the required objective. The bladder flap may be performed in conjunction with the psoas hitch to maintain the cephalad extension of the bladder wall posterior to the flap. Again, a nonrefluxing tunneled or a refluxing repair can then be performed.

More complex techniques of ureteral reconstruction include transureteroureterostomy (TUU), ileal-ureteral replacement, and renal autotransplantation (Figs. 39-27 and 39-28). TUU is relevant when anastomosis to the bladder is not feasible due to inadequate length of the ureter or condition of the bladder, or when it is desirable to move the repair away from the ipsilateral hemipelvis due to local conditions of infection, prior pelvic radiation, etc. Ureteral replacement with the ileum is seldom performed in the acute trauma setting as it is preferable to have a fully prepped bowel when performing this procedure. Renal autotransplantation may be appropriate in the acute trauma setting if appropriate vascular surgical expertise is available and less complex options for ureteral replacement are not feasible. The proximal ureter can be anastomosed directly into the bladder, in the case of loss of the majority of the lower ureter, or an anastomosis can be performed to the lower ureter if it is clearly viable and not excessively distal.

When ureteral repairs are performed in direct apposition to adjacent vascular or visceral repairs, separation of the repairs by

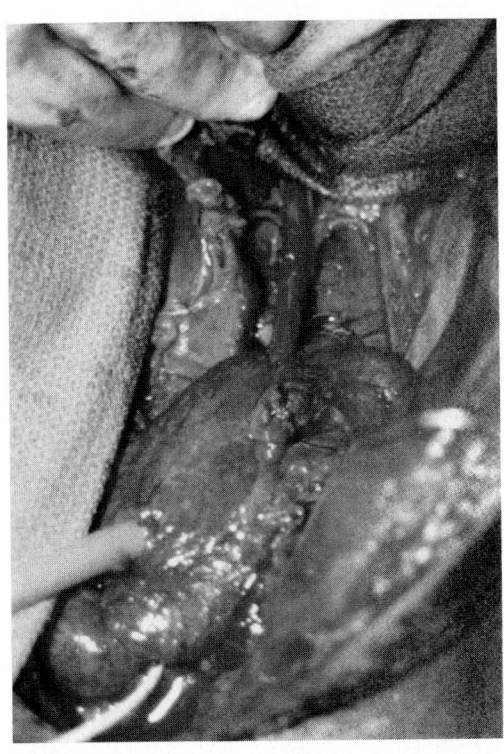
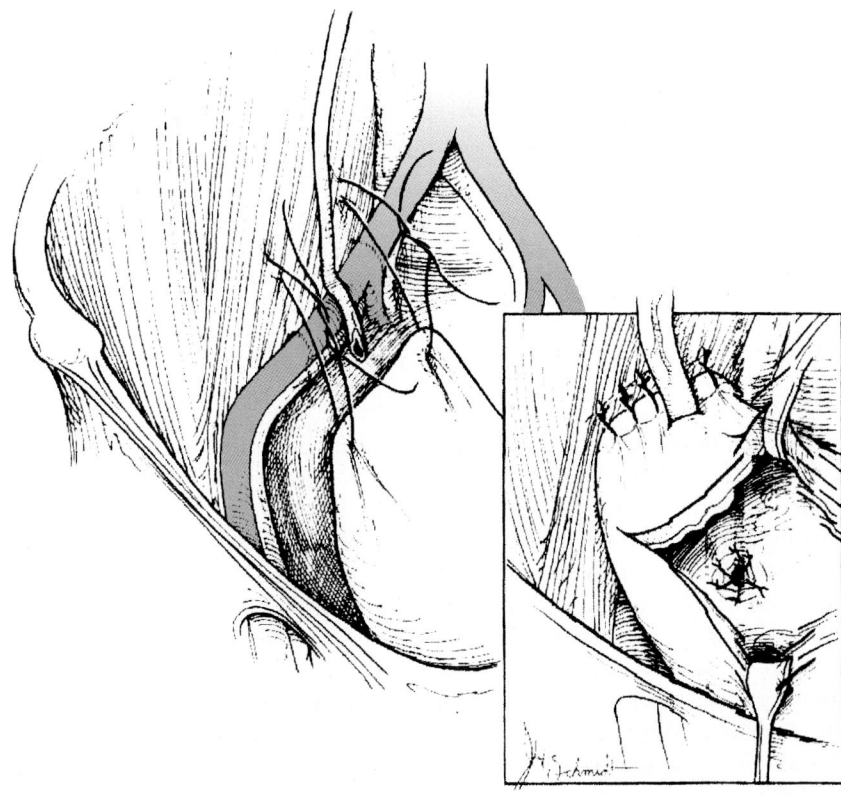

**A**    **B**

**FIGURE 39-26.** **(A)** Ureteral reimplantation with psoas hitch for lower ureteral injury: The bladder is opened either transversely or vertically and obliquely toward the side of injury, then hitched to the ipsilateral psoas muscle with 2-0 or 3-0 Vicryl suture. A tunneled, antirefluxing anastomosis of the ureter to the posterior wall of the bladder is performed, being certain that an adequate-width tunnel is created to prevent obstruction. If the available ureteral length is short, antirefluxing tunneling can be eliminated. Either an internal double-J-type stent or an externalized single-J stent can be used (not shown). **(B)** Psoas hitch ureteral reimplantation for penetrating injury to lower ureter, performed acutely during initial laparotomy in a hemodynamically stable patient. The bladder body can be seen sutured to the left psoas muscle, with the ureter entering cephalad. A single-J ureteral stent and suprapubic cystostomy exit from the bladder in the lower part of the photograph.

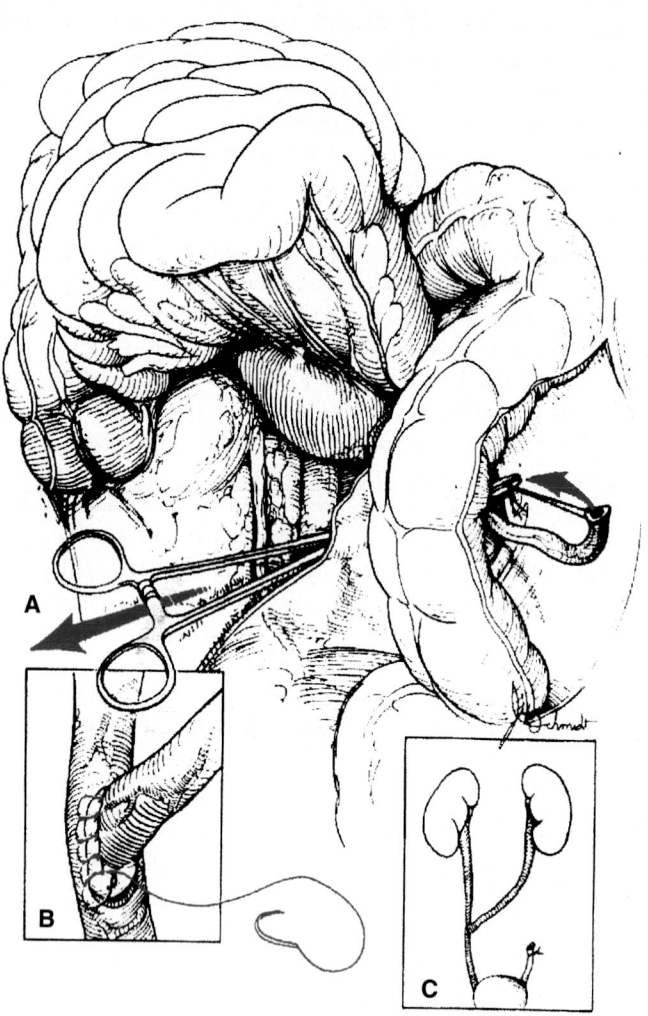

**FIGURE 39-27.** Transureteroureterostomy for reconstruction following extensive midlower ureteral injury. Prior bladder surgery or pelvic inflammatory or neoplastic disease, among other factors, may make psoas hitch or bladder flap repair undesirable. The injured ureter is mobilized and transposed to the contralateral side underneath the mesentery, then anastomosed with an end-to-side technique to the recipient ureter.

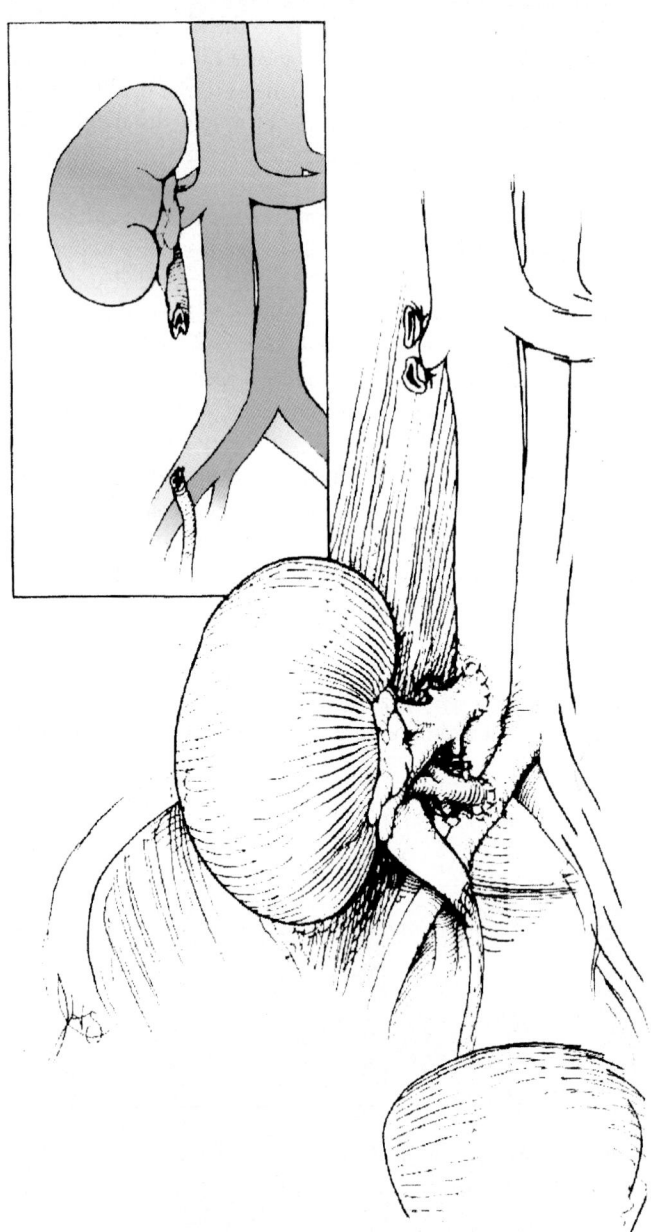

**FIGURE 39-28.** Renal autotransplantation for reconstruction following extensive loss of midureter, making direct union of upper ureter to bladder impossible. Alternative to ileal-ureteral replacement of most of the ureter. Nephrectomy must be tailored to include as much of the renal vessels as possible to aid in anastomosis to iliac vessels (in general, vein generally transected flush with vena cava on right, with artery transected more proximally, behind vena cava, than shown here). Anastomosis of proximal ureter to viable lower ureter.

an omental pedicle or other viable tissue is desirable to prevent a fistula or contact with urine at the site of the adjacent organ injury. External drainage of ureteral injuries, in addition to stenting or diversion, may be desirable, particularly if the repair is tenuous or the vascularity of the repaired tissues is questionable. Some urologists prefer Penrose drains for this purpose, to avoid having a closed-suction drain aspirating directly on a ureteral suture line. The author uses closed-suction drains, suturing them (with 4-0 chromic gut) to the psoas muscle or other adjacent soft tissue to prevent the drain from migrating directly onto the ureteral repair. In the postoperative period, antibiotic administration may be desirable, especially if urinary extravasation persists.

As noted later, ureteral injuries are also highly amenable to damage control strategies when the patient is not in suitable condition for repair at the time of the initial laparotomy. An external stent placed through the transected proximal ureteral stump allows maintenance of control of the urinary output while the patient is undergoing resuscitation in preparation for definitive delayed reconstruction.

## Bladder

Surgical repair of the bladder is performed for many iatrogenic injuries, for nearly all blunt intraperitoneal injuries, and for selected cases of blunt extraperitoneal rupture. Penetrating injuries to the bladder are also usually managed with operative repair.

Intraperitoneal ruptures of the bladder are approached through a midline abdominal incision. The large laceration is nearly always in the dome of the bladder as previously described (Fig. 39-29). The interior of the bladder is palpated and inspected through the laceration to verify that no other injuries are present and that there is clear efflux from both ureteral orifices. The laceration may be

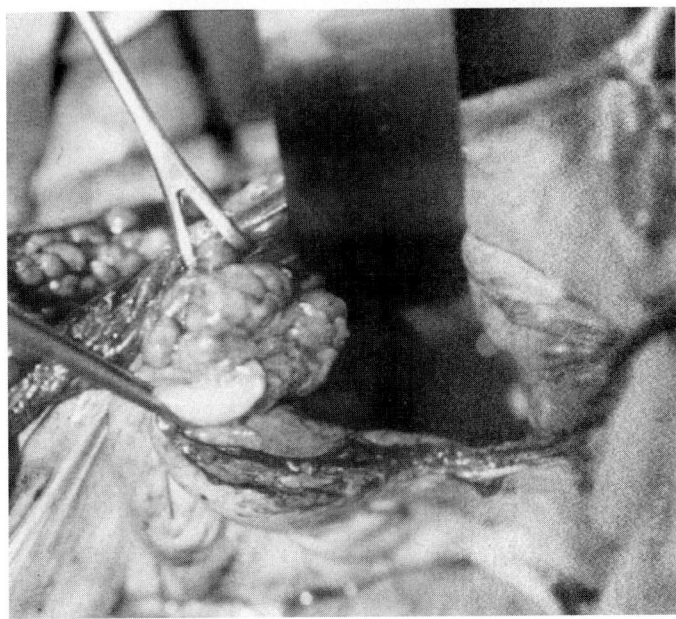
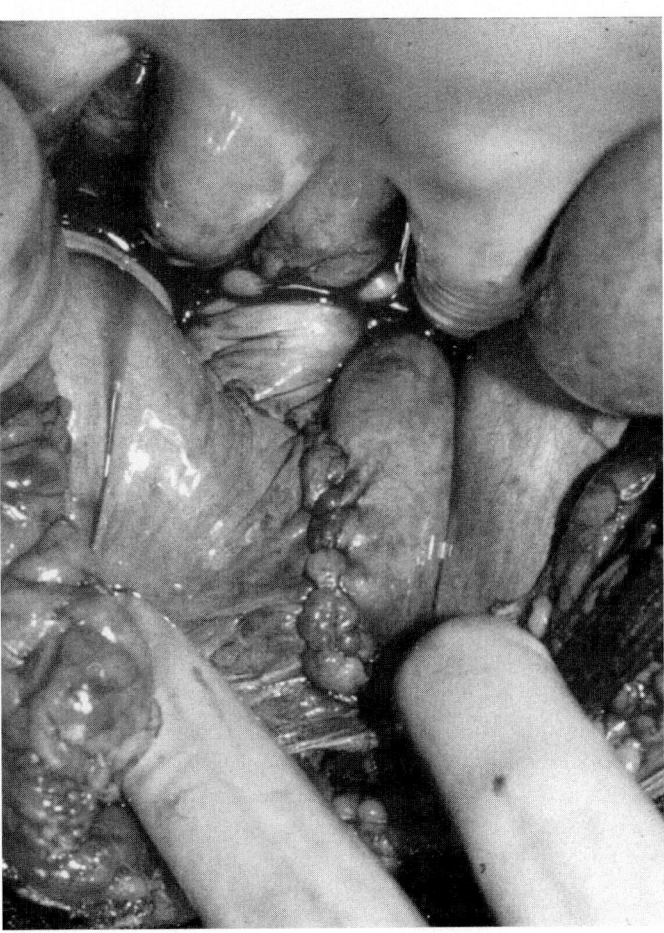

**A**

**B**

**FIGURE 39-29.** Operative appearance of intraperitoneal bladder injury from blunt trauma. **(A)** The anterior bladder wall is retracted at the top of the photograph, with the typical large, stellate defect noted in the bladder dome. **(B)** Appearance of the bladder dome after closure in two layers of 2-0 chromic gut.

extended into an anterior midline cystotomy if necessary for further assessment, but this is not usually necessary. The edges of the bladder laceration may require minimal debridement to remove devascularized tags of detrusor muscle or mucosa. The laceration is then closed using two layers of heavy absorbable suture. An adequate bore bladder catheter is used to allow free drainage of initially bloody efflux that clears in the first few days. The length of time of catheterization should consider the period needed for urinary efflux to clear and the ability of the patient to be ambulatory and void comfortably, but is usually 5 to 10 days. It is reasonable to perform a cystogram prior to removal of the catheter following any operative repair, and it is mandatory with nonoperative management. As a well-sutured repair carries an extremely low postoperative risk of extravasation, some practitioners do remove the catheter without prior contrast imaging with excellent success. Suprapubic cystostomy catheters are not generally needed after repairs of intraperitoneal ruptures. They should be inserted only when there will be the need for long-term bladder drainage, as in the patient with a significant injury to the brain, trauma to the pelvis or a lower extremity, or other factors that would be expected to substantially delay a return to ambulation.

For the selected cases in which extraperitoneal rupture of the bladder is managed with operative repair, there are several important differences when compared to intraperitoneal repairs. When

operating on the injured bladder during a laparotomy following a pelvic fracture, an effort should be made to avoid entering the retropubic hematoma. This avoids potentially serious hemorrhage from a site that is often tamponaded. If repair of the bladder is necessary in this setting (see "Nonoperative Management of Genitourinary Injuries" earlier), one should enter the bladder through an anterior cystotomy incision cephalad to the pelvic hematoma. The laceration, which is usually located in the lower anterior or anterolateral bladder, can be sutured transvesically by introducing Deaver or malleable retractors into the bladder and retracting them laterally. Often, only a single-layer, full-thickness closure is possible in this setting. It is useful to communicate with the orthopedic surgeons when operating on extraperitoneal bladder ruptures in the setting of a pelvic fracture to allow for coordinated care.

A penetrating injury to the bladder is most often managed operatively, though occasional patients as previously described may be candidates for nonoperative management.[33] If a patient is undergoing laparotomy and has gross hematuria following penetrating pelvic trauma, the peritoneal surface of the bladder is examined first. The retropubic space is then entered and an anterior, midline cystotomy is created. This may be easier to accomplish if the bladder is partly filled with irrigant. For laparotomies during which bladder surgery is likely, including the genitalia in the sterile field facilitates whatever manipulation may be necessary without abdominal contamination.

Following cystotomy, the interior of the bladder is thoroughly examined, as are the ureteral orifices and the bladder neck. The urinary efflux from both orifices should be observed; if it is bloody or absent, further investigation for trauma to the ureters or upper tract is indicated. Penetrating injuries to the bladder are closed with two layers of absorbable suture as described earlier.

In some patients, an iatrogenic or penetrating injury to the bladder may result in loss of a large portion of the detrusor of the bladder body. Closure over a bladder catheter is still recommended, as the bladder may expand to an acceptable volume with time. If minimal bladder capacity persists following a reasonable period of healing, augmentation cystoplasty can be performed electively.

As for renal and ureteral injuries, injuries to the bladder in the unstable trauma patient are amenable to damage control strategies. These include externalized stenting of the ureters with pelvic packing and delayed repair of complex lacerations.

Certain associated injuries impact on the management of bladder trauma. Contiguous injury to the vagina or rectum is such an example, requiring close collaboration between the clinical services involved in caring for these injuries. When such injuries are suspected, it is helpful to have the patient in a modified dorsal lithotomy position so simultaneous access to the perineum and abdomen can be obtained. During surgical repair, the bladder should be separated from the rectum or vagina by placing an interposition flap of viable tissue if the loss of tissue is significant and the injuries directly overlie each other. This effort at separation of the pelvic organs can be difficult in the trauma setting and, if the injuries do not directly overlie each other and tissue loss is minimal, simple transvesical closure is generally adequate. In this setting, longer indwelling catheter times, perioperative antibiotics, and radiographic imaging prior to removal of the catheter are recommended. Open pelvic fractures are among the most devastating injuries in orthopedic trauma, and injury to the lower urinary tract may complicate such injuries. A close interaction between the urologist, orthopedist, trauma surgeon, and interventional radiologist is necessary for management of such patients. Chronic disability is common following such injuries.[24]

Avulsion injuries of the bladder neck, more common in the pediatric population, require operative repair (Fig. 39-30).[30] Repair for these complex injuries may be best delayed until 24 to 72 hours postinjury to support a damage control strategy and to minimize the risk of excessive hemorrhage from an associated pelvic fracture.

## Urethra

Operative management for urethral trauma includes the broad topic of elective urethral reconstruction following traumatic injuries and surgical repair of urethral strictures. There are excellent reviews available on this latter topic.[45] This discussion will focus on immediate and subacute surgical intervention for urethral trauma.

Anterior urethral injuries that are incomplete may be managed with placement of a transurethral catheter or with suprapubic diversion. As noted above, the author favors using endoscopic guidance for any attempt to catheterize the traumatized urethra. If a blind attempt at catheterization is performed and any resistance is encountered, an endoscopically guided procedure should follow. Complete ruptures of the anterior urethra from blunt trauma are best managed with suprapubic diversion for three or more months, followed by elective end-to-end urethroplasty when the perineal

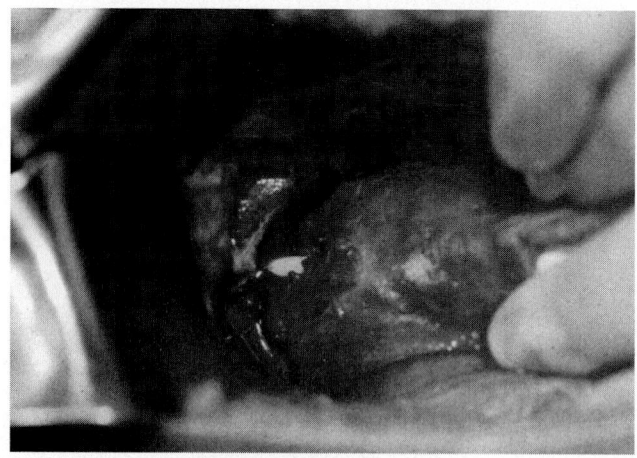

**FIGURE 39-30.** Bladder neck avulsion injury in an adult female with pelvic fracture. Operative appearance during surgical repair. An anterior midline cystotomy had been performed (to right in photo), with the tip of a Foley catheter protruding from the avulsed bladder neck for demonstration purposes. Anastomosis to urethral stump at level of pelvic floor performed over Foley catheter. The patient was initially managed with a percutaneous suprapubic cystostomy. This repair was performed 36 hours following injury, when the patient was hemodynamically stable and risk of excessive bleeding from the pelvic fracture would be lower.

hematoma and induration have fully resolved. Acute attempts at excision and repair are not recommended as it is unclear how much urethra to resect due to the crush injury and difficult to be sure that one is approximating viable, healthy tissue at the anastomosis.

Penetrating injuries to the anterior urethra may be managed with local exploration and repair or with suprapubic diversion. With stab wounds or gunshot wounds from low-velocity missiles, it is usually a simple matter to perform limited debridement and repair with a spatulated anastomotic technique. If the patient is not an appropriate candidate for immediate repair due to more pressing serious injuries, etc., suprapubic diversion or endoscopically guided insertion of a transurethral catheter placement is performed. Extensive loss of the urethra from penetrating trauma or industrial trauma may require a staged repair.

The management of disruption injuries of the posterior urethra is controversial. In the last decade, there has been increasing interest in early catheter realignment for such injuries. Techniques utilized have included endoscopic guidance, open surgical approaches, and the use of interlocking magnetic sounds (Fig. 39-31).[46-49] A potential advantage of endoscopic realignment is the possibility that the injury will heal free of intractable stricture. This would obviate the need for late urethroplasty, shorten the period of urinary intubation, and may improve the anatomic result as compared to the nonintubated state by reducing malalignment. The potential disadvantages of this approach are the risk of infecting the retropubic hematoma by the presence of the indwelling catheter with an adverse impact on late continence and sexual function and the high likelihood that a stricture will form anyway. When selected, catheter realignment should be performed by an experienced team in the operating room with endoscopic and fluoroscopic capability. Results are better for incomplete disruptions than they are for complete disruptions. Most patients managed in this manner do develop a stricture requiring endoscopic intervention, often involving

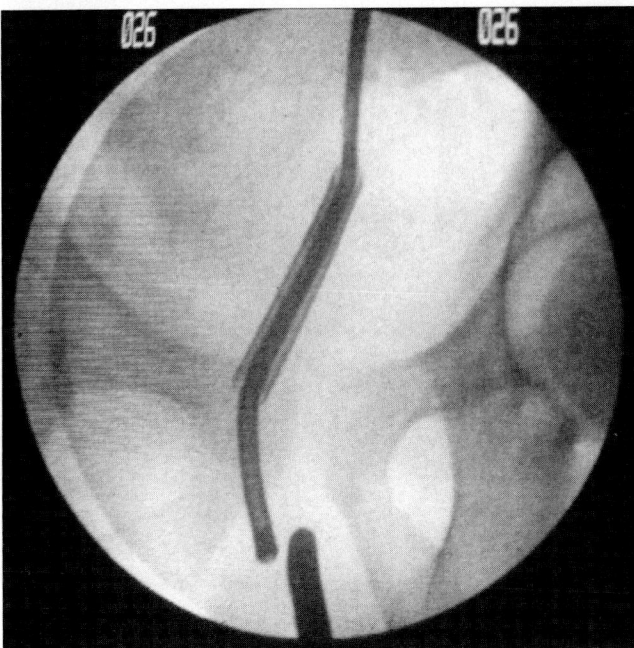

A

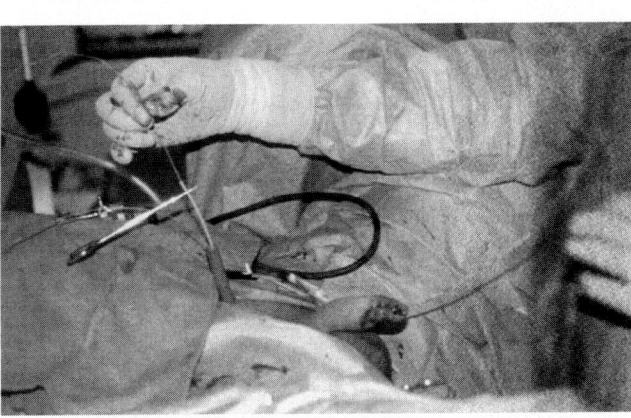

B

**FIGURE 39-31.** **(A)** Manipulating flexible cystoscope from above and rigid cystoscope sheath from below (beak placed at point of disruption at bulbomembranous junction), a guidewire is advanced across defect and continuity is achieved. A Foley catheter with end-hole punched is passed over the guidewire and positioned with balloon in bladder. Working sheath is removed after replacement of large-bore suprapubic catheter. This is one of a variety of techniques described for achieving catheter realignment using minimally invasive approaches. Primary urethral realignment for posterior urethral disruption. **(A,B)** Access to bladder, previously obtained via percutaneous cystostomy, is utilized for realignment. Retrograde flexible cystoscopy failed to demonstrate continuity; therefore, suprapubic tract was dilated and working sheath was placed into bladder using both direct vision and fluoroscopic guidance.

multiple procedures. Overall, patients managed with catheter realignment may avoid a subsequent urethroplasty about 50% of the time.

The traditional approach to disruption of the posterior urethra is diversion with a suprapubic cystostomy, followed by a period of observation of 3 to 6 months while the pelvic hematoma resolves and the anatomy stabilizes. Repeat antegrade and retrograde urethrograms are then performed, and definitive reconstructive surgery is planned. The ultimate success rate of this approach is over 90%; however, the

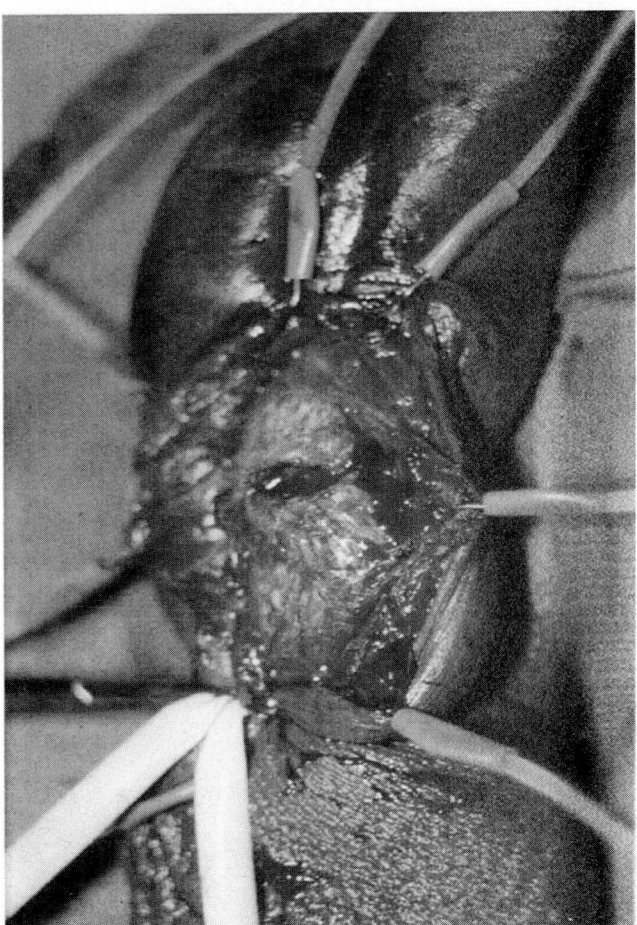

**FIGURE 39-32.** Penile fracture. Appearance of penis during surgical exploration for penile fracture sustained during sexual intercourse. Patient reported classic findings of pain, swelling, and detumescence following sudden marked bending of erect penis. Note marked swelling of distal phallus with subcutaneous hematoma. Penis is explored through a ventral, midline, penoscrotal incision. Dissection to area of palpable irregularity along penile shaft reveals transverse laceration of tunical albuginea of corpus cavernosum. A penile tourniquet, utilizing a Penrose drain, is in place to reduce bleeding during repair. The hooks are part of a ring-retractor system commonly used in genital surgery. The tunica albuginea defect is closed with running 3-0 Vicryl suture. Early exploration and repair for penile fracture injuries produces the best results. Circumcising, subglanular incision is preferred by some surgeons for this type of exploration and repair.

need for a long-term indwelling suprapubic tube while awaiting surgery may be frustrating for the patient. Nevertheless, newer techniques such as catheter realignment must be compared to the excellent outcomes of patients managed in this traditional manner.[50,51]

## Penis, Testis, and Scrotum

Penile trauma is nearly always managed through operative exploration and repair. For blunt penile fractures, the penis is explored either through a ventral midline penoscrotal incision or a circumcising subcoronal incision. The defect in the tunica albuginea is exposed and closed with absorbable suture (Fig. 39-32). The outcomes following early operative repair of penile fractures are far superior to those resulting from nonoperative management. Deformity, painful erection, pseudoaneurysm, and loss of erectile function are common in nonoperative management of such injuries (Fig. 39-33).[36]

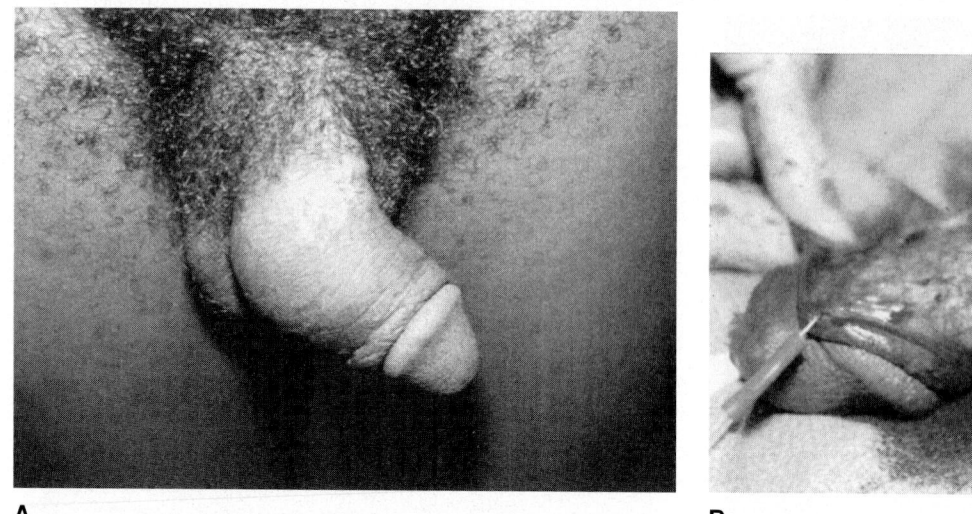
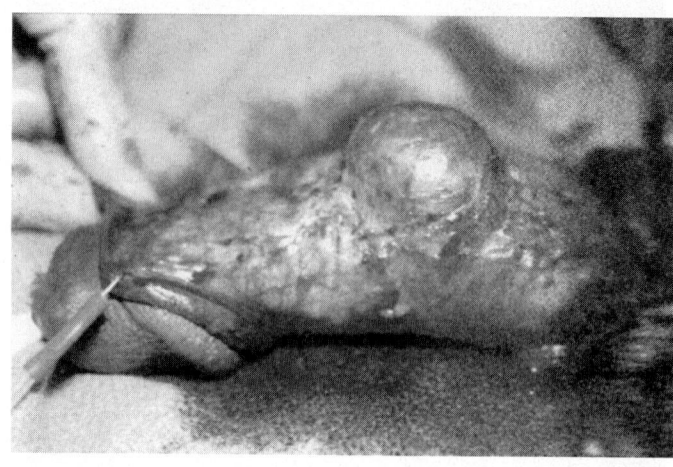

**A**                                                                    **B**

**FIGURE 39-33.** Delayed presentation following penile fracture. **(A)** Note marked angulation to left with mass effect on right lateral side of penile shaft following untreated rupture. Patient presents 6 weeks postinjury; the subcutaneous hematoma has resolved, while the defect in the corpus cavernosum remains, resulting in angulation and pain with erection. **(B)** Appearance of penis at surgical exploration through circumcising incision. Note large encapsulated hematoma under Buck's fascia, which, upon incision, still communicates with cavernosal space. Defect repaired with correction of deformity.

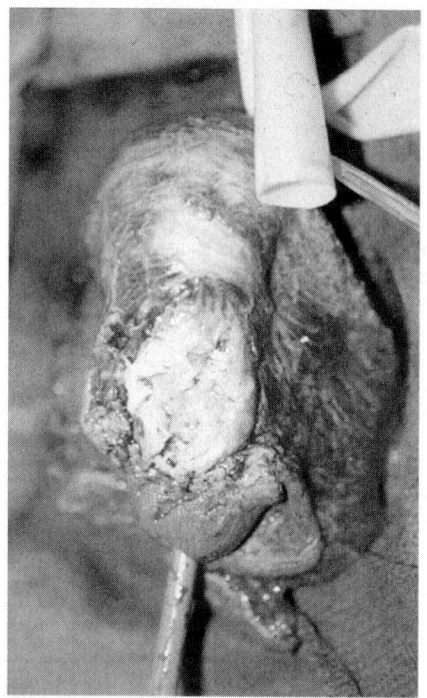
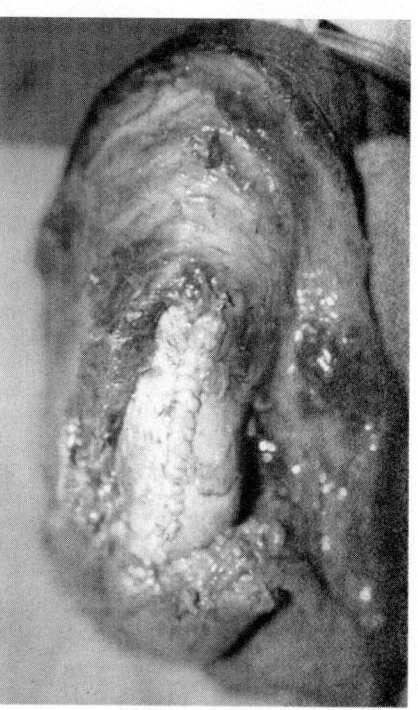
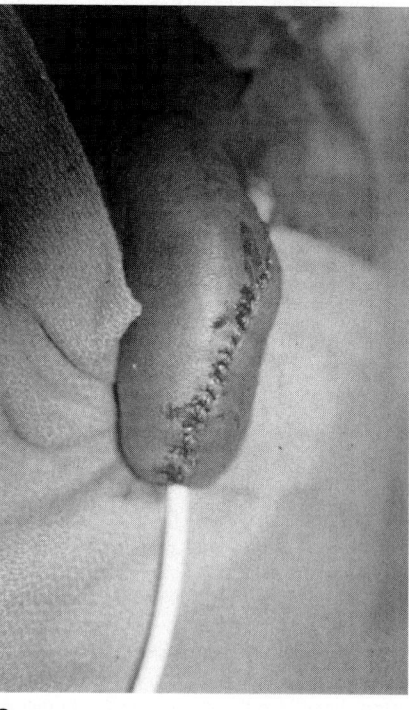

**A**                                    **B**                                    **C**

**FIGURE 39-34.** Gunshot wound to penis with entrance at dorsal penile base. **(A)** Extensive injury to skin and subcutaneous tissues and laceration of tunica albuginea of corpus cavernosum. Penile tourniquet in place to allow injury assessment while minimizing bleeding. **(B)** Tunica albuginea has been conservatively debrided and closed with running Vicryl suture. **(C)** Appearance of penis following reconstruction of glans and skin tube. Subsequent scar revision was necessary for necrosis of skin edges (not shown). Preservation of soft tissues and conservative debridement demonstrated.

Penetrating penile injuries, similarly, should be managed with operative exploration and repair (Figs. 39-34 and 39-35). As combined cavernosal and urethral injury occurs in roughly 10% of penile fractures, a preoperative urethrogram or flexible cystoscopy is useful in planning the repair.

In cases of penetrating penile injury, a similar surgical approach is utilized, with conservative debridement, repair of cavernosal and urethral injury, and microsurgical repair of dorsal neurovascular structures when possible. For limited injuries, direct wound exploration may be preferable approach. The possibility of adjacent

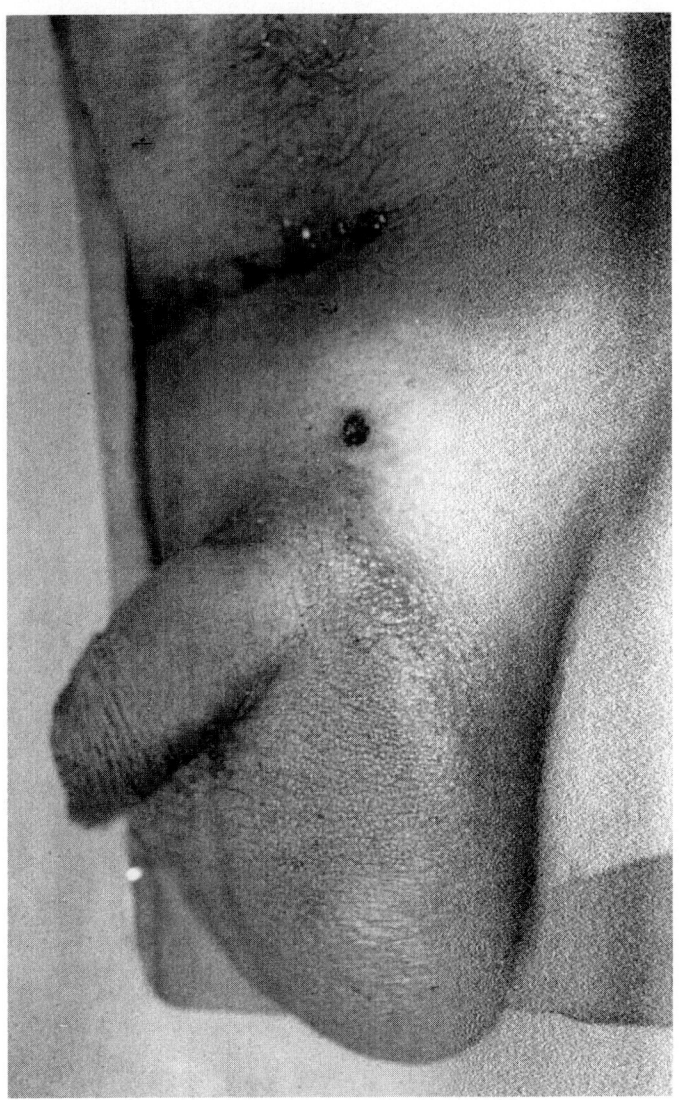
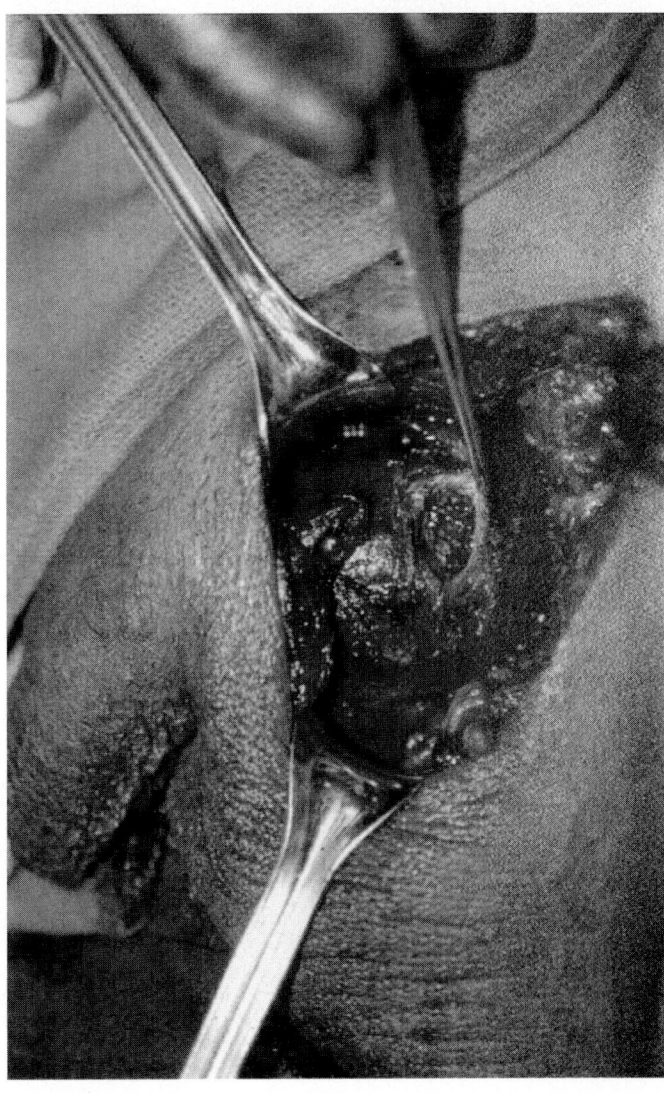

**A**

**B**

**FIGURE 39-35.** Gunshot wound to mons pubis region, cephalad and to left of penile base. **(A)** No palpable abnormality of penis is recognized. Small left scrotal hematoma present. **(B)** Surgical exploration of wound via oblique scrotal neck incision extends toward groin. Bleeding sites in left spermatic cord were controlled (not shown), followed by evacuation of hematoma resulting in significant bleeding. Dissection revealed complete transection of left corpus cavernosum at penile base, which was repaired. Case demonstrates importance of surgical exploration of penetrating injuries in proximity to male genitalia.

nonurologic injury (thigh, femoral vessels, pelvic organs) must always be considered in cases of penetrating genital injury.

Penile strangulation injuries due to constricting bands or other devices are managed with removal of the constricting object in as atraumatic a manner as possible. Distal penile skin, glans, cavernosal, or urethral necrosis can occasionally occur in such cases. A conservative approach to debridement of tissues of questionable viability and diversion with a suprapubic cystostomy tube if the urethra is compromised are principles of management.

Patients with traumatic amputation of the penis require specialized management (Fig. 39-36). Often, patients who suffer traumatic amputation through self-mutilation are psychotic and/or involved in substance abuse and require psychiatric as well as urologic intervention.[52] The severed organ should be cleansed and kept in cold saline-soaked gauze in a sealed bag, which is then placed in ice. Replantation surgery is well described.[53] In sequence, anastomosis of the corpora cavernosa,

urethra, dorsal blood vessels, and nerves should be performed with appropriate microsurgical expertise. Functional outcomes are variable with such replantation efforts, largely reflecting the condition of the severed organ and the time that elapses prior to replantation.

Scrotal trauma should be explored if there is a concern about testicular rupture. In blunt trauma, testicular ultrasound may be helpful in deciding if operation is indicated. In penetrating trauma, we often utilize an oblique upper scrotal incision that provides access to the groin, spermatic cord, penile base, and scrotal contents. Most scrotal injuries should be explored with the goal of evacuation of the hematoma, debridement of devitalized tissue, and repair and salvage of the testicle (Figs. 39-37 and 39-38). Reproductive outcomes are favorable following such management.[54]

Cases of scrotal and other soft tissue loss in the genital region should be managed with a conservative approach to debridement of marginally vascularized skin and soft tissues as previously

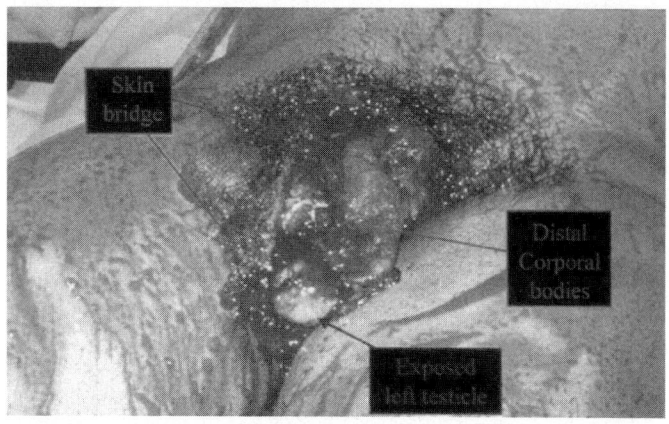

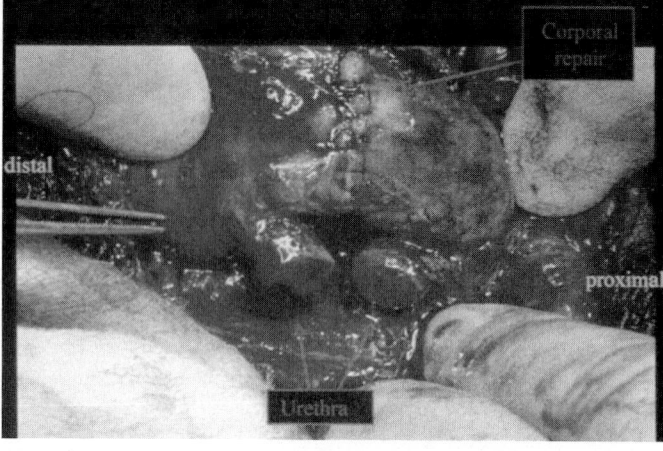

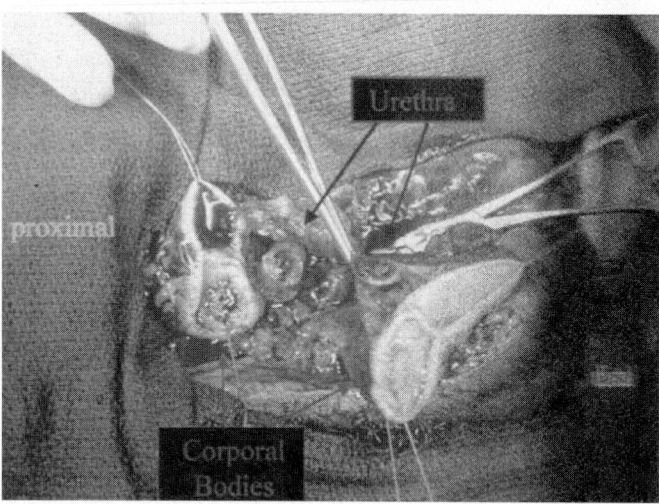

**FIGURE 39-36.** Subtotal penile amputation injury due to assault with knife. **(A)** Photograph demonstrates complete transection of body of penis with right-sided skin bridge attaching distal phallus to body. Left testis is exposed as well. **(B)** Preparing for surgical reconstruction-minimal debridement of corpora cavernosa and urethra, following extensive irrigation. **(C)** Corpora cavernosal anastomosis has been completed; urethral anastomosis about to be completed after spatulation and mobilization of distal ends to avoid tension on repair. Following completion of urethral repair over Foley catheter, microsurgical anastomosis of deep dorsal arteries, deep dorsal vein, and adjacent nerves was performed (not shown).

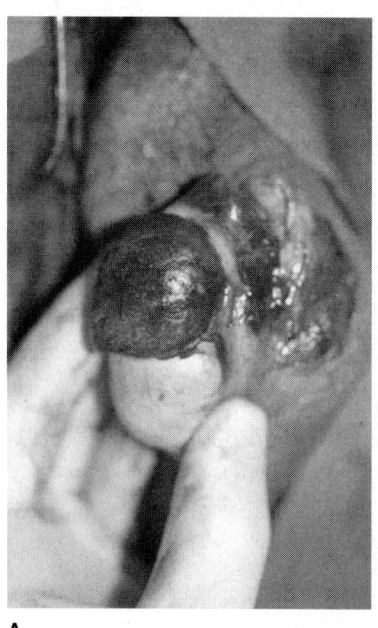

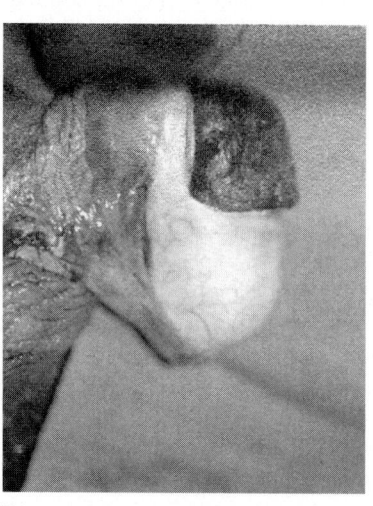

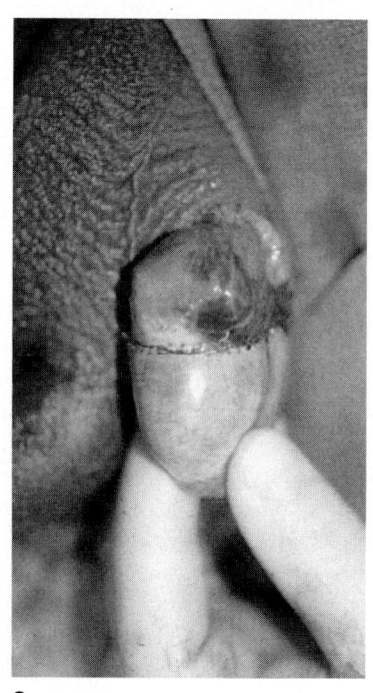

**FIGURE 39-37.** Testis: Testicular rupture due to blunt trauma. **(A,B)** Appearance of ruptured testis at surgical exploration following blunt trauma to scrotum. Note laceration of tunica albuginea with extruded seminiferous tubules. **(C)** Appearance of testis following minimal debridement of testicular parenchyma and repair of tunica albuginea with running 3-0 Vicryl suture.

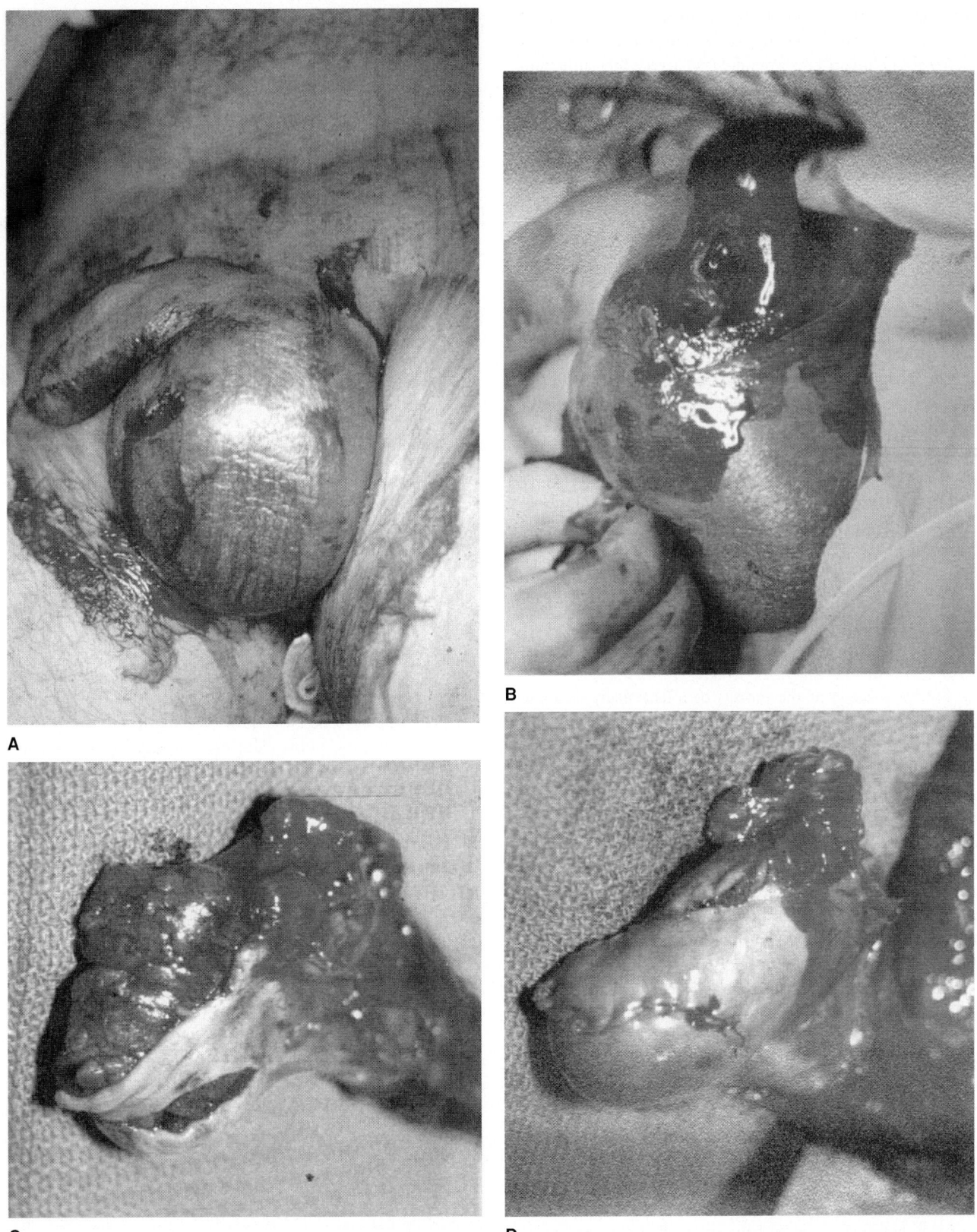

**FIGURE 39-38.** Scrotal exploration and testicular repair following gunshot wound to scrotum. **(A)** Entrance wound visible lateral to base of penis on left, exit just to the right of the median raphe; note marked left hemiscrotal swelling from hematoma. Surgical exploration is mandatory and preoperative scrotal imaging is unnecessary. **(B)** Scrotal exploration performed through high oblique scrotal incision for optimal exposure of scrotal contents and possible extension to groin if further spermatic cord exposure proves necessary. Entrance into tunica vaginalis visible. Testis introduced out of scrotum on spermatic cord pedicle. **(C)** Appearance of left testis demonstrating complex laceration of tunical albuginea with extruded testicular parenchyma. **(D)** Appearance of testis following limited parenchymal debridement and reconstruction of tunica albuginea. Testis is then returned to scrotum following evacuation of hematoma and extensive irrigation; Penrose drain placed through inferior stab incision in left hemiscrotum (not shown).

described. Delayed primary closure or reconstruction of significant scrotal loss using meshed split thickness skin grafting produces favorable results. Human bite wounds have a very high infection rate and should be left open if presenting in a delayed fashion (see Chapter 49).

## COMPLICATIONS OF GENITOURINARY TRAUMA

The management of complications of urological injury is an important issue facing the trauma surgeon. Extensive reviews of this topic are available.[55] Complications may be categorized as early or late occurrences and can occur in the setting of an early diagnosis of injury or a delayed diagnosis of injury. Early complications of injury to the upper urinary tract include bleeding, postinjury infections, problems related to urinary extravasation, and ischemic processes. Renal and ureteral injuries may also result in late complications including hypertension, hydronephrosis, and renal insufficiency. Functional abnormalities following trauma to the urinary tract may include a neurogenic bladder, urethral stricture, and sexual or reproductive dysfunction. Appropriate follow-up studies for high-risk injuries are critical in the early detection of complications of urologic trauma.

## DAMAGE CONTROL PRINCIPLES IN GENITOURINARY TRAUMA

Damage control surgery, or the process of intentionally delaying surgical interventions for lesions that are not immediately life-threatening, is an evolving strategy that is applicable to all surgical specialties.[56] With the exception of major, active bleeding from the kidney or renal pedicle, virtually any urologic injury can be handled in a delayed fashion without exposing the patient to significant risk. If the patient becomes stable, interval imaging (generally with contrast-enhanced CT or with arteriography if performed for another purpose) of a renal injury may allow selection of definitive nonoperative management. This avoids the time and potential morbidity of an unnecessary renal exploration at the second operative procedure. If, at the initial operation, bleeding from the kidney is not a major concern or hemostasis for significant bleeding has been obtained, the kidney can be packed. Renal reconstruction is then performed at a secondary laparotomy.

Ureteral injuries for which delayed management is necessary can be managed with externalized stenting (Fig. 39-39). A single-J urinary diversion stent can be passed up into the kidney through the lacerated or transected ureter, tied or sutured to the end of the proximal segment of ureter, and then externalized and attached to a drainage device. At secondary exploration, formal ureteral reconstruction can be completed. Alternatively, the injured ureter can be ligated or simply left to drain in situ, although these approaches have the disadvantages of either creating an obstruction or allowing urine to pool in the abdomen and increasing the risk of a postoperative infection.

Certain bladder injuries may be difficult to repair at the initial operation as well. Visibility may be compromised by pelvic bleeding requiring packing, the complexity of the repair may require more time and blood loss than the patient can tolerate, or the degree of debridement needed may be unclear, as may be the case

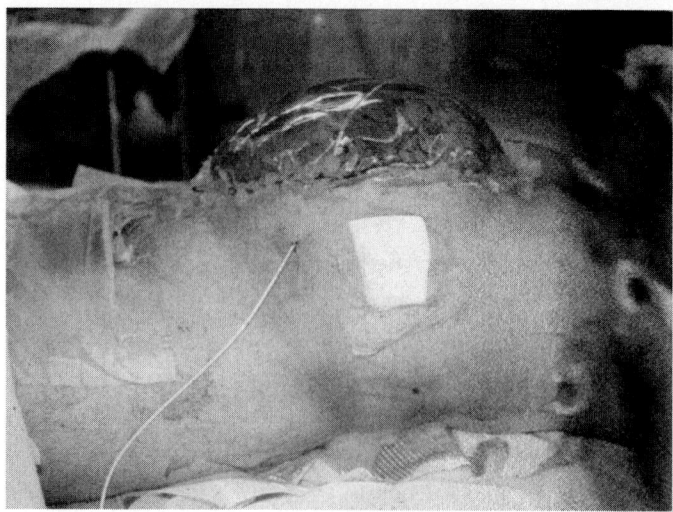

**FIGURE 39-39.** Patient managed with damage control laparotomy: Gunshot wound to abdomen with injuries to small bowel, left iliac artery and vein, and left ureter. Patient was hemodynamically unstable following vascular repair, so ureteral injury was managed with damage control approach. Single-J stent was passed up proximal ureter at injury site and secured to end of ureter with silk tie; stent was externalized, exiting from left lower quadrant, as shown. Abdomen was closed with "Bogota bag" silo due to bowel and mesenteric edema. On return to operating room at 36 hours postinjury, formal ureteral repair with psoas hitch and ureteroneocystostomy was performed.

with a high-velocity gunshot wound. Delaying definitive repair may be accomplished by inserting bilateral externalized ureteral stents. The pelvis can then be packed for bleeding, compressing the open bladder against the pubis. Alternatively, placing an externalized suprapubic catheter (Malecot or Foley) within the injured bladder is also an option. If the catheter prevents tamponade of pelvic bleeding, it can be clamped temporarily and then reopened to drainage when the patient's coagulopathy is corrected. The use of damage control principles for complex penetrating pelvic trauma in the battlefield setting has been recently reported. In this series, 43% of patients had urologic injury while 50% had major vascular injury. A 21% mortality rate in the first week postinjury was reported, while 36% of patients with combined vascular and rectal injuries died.[25] A staged, multidisciplinary approach to management and reconstruction was shown to be valuable in this experience.

Injuries to the urethra and external genitalia can be temporarily managed with suprapubic catheterization or dressing applications pending the patient's return to surgery for definitive management.

The results of damage control management for urologic injuries in appropriately selected patients appear to be acceptable in terms of patient survival, renal salvage, and functional outcome.[57]

## CONSULTATION AND INTERSERVICE INTERACTION

A specialty service such as urology offers skills that are different from those of the general surgeon. These include endoscopic capability and familiarity with reconstruction of the urinary tract in the elective setting. The urology service should be informed of signs of urologic injury as early as possible, preferably from the emergency department. This allows the urologist to be involved in preoperative imaging and interpretation, later operative sequencing, and use of damage control strategies. The experience of large trauma centers in which an interested and capable urologic trauma team is involved often results in reduced rates of nephrectomy and improvements in other outcome measures.

## MEDICOLEGAL CONSIDERATIONS

Urologists frequently become involved in the management of injuries that were not diagnosed at the initial operation. These are often recognized later in a patient's clinical course, often after a complication (urinary extravasation, bleeding, azotemia, sepsis) initiates further testing and imaging studies. In this setting, it is important to communicate to the patient and family what is occurring and to document the events that have occurred in the medical record. It is important to educate patients and their families that traumatic injuries are complex and that certain complications are common and to be expected. Also, functional outcomes may be disappointing to patients.

In urologic reconstruction, internal stents may be utilized, and patients may be discharged with indwelling catheters that may be invisible and/or require regular attention to avoid complications. As patients with internal stents placed in the trauma setting may be lost to follow-up, it is important that specific instructions be given

to a patient regarding outpatient care and for a date of return to the clinic. If a nephrostomy tube must be changed after being in place for a month, it is best to arrange for this intervention prior to discharge. Also, it is important to explain and document the potential consequences of neglecting internal tubes, including calcification and obstruction. As it is important to monitor a patient for hypertension for 2 years following certain major renal injuries, this should be explained and documented as well.

## CONCLUSIONS

Much of the current consensus on approaches to genitourinary injury is based on retrospective studies. In fact, there are very few prospective studies in the urologic literature, leaving levels of evidence at a suboptimal state for evidence-based medical practice. Nevertheless, attempts at achieving a broad international consensus regarding the management of urologic injuries are ongoing.[1-6] Important developments in body imaging, endoscopic approaches, endovascular stenting, and other radiologic and minimally invasive techniques have changed approaches to urologic trauma and selection of patients for operative versus nonoperative management. Further research will continue to impact the urologist's role and approach in dealing with genitourinary injury (Fig. 39-40).

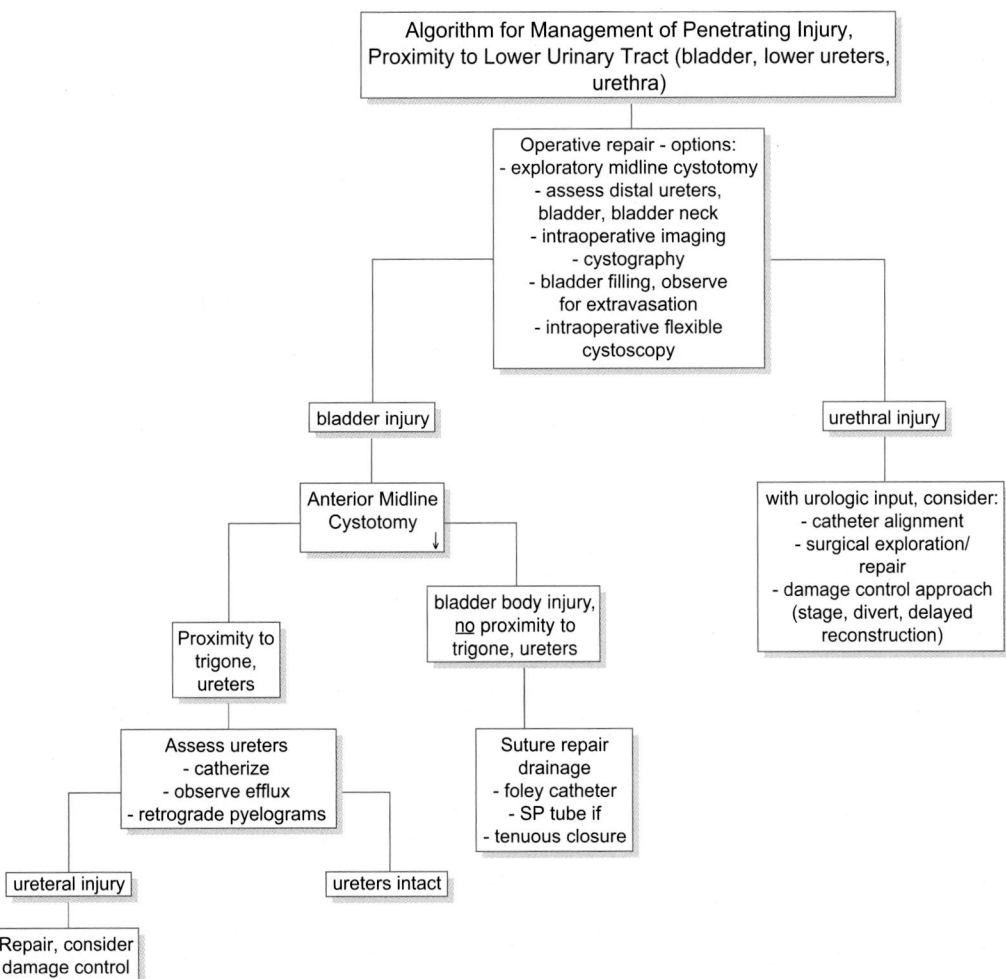

**FIGURE 39-40.** Algorithm for Management of Penetrating Injury, Proximity to Lower Urinary Tract (bladder, lower ureters, urethra).

## REFERENCES

1. Peterson NE: Genitourinary trauma. In Mattox KL, Feliciano DF, Moore EE (eds): *Trauma*, 4th ed. New York: McGraw Hill, 2000, p. 839.
2. Moore EE, Shackford SR, Pachter HL, et al.: Organ injury scaling: Spleen, liver and kidney. *J Trauma* 29:1664, 1989.
3. Moore EE, Cogbill TH, Jurkovich GJ, et al.: Organ injury scaling III: Chest wall abdominal vascular, ureter, bladder and urethra. *J Trauma* 33:227, 1992.
4. Calopinto V, McCallum RW: Injury to the male posterior urethra in fractured pelvis: A new classification. *J Urol* 118:575, 1977.
5. Nicolaisen GS, McAninch JW, Marshall GA, et al.: Renal trauma: Reevaluation of the indications for radiographic assessment. *J Urol* 133:183, 1985.
6. Mee SL, McAninch JW, Robinson AL, et al.: Radiographic assessment of renal trauma: A 10-year prospective study of patient selection. *J Urol* 141:1095, 1989.
7. Miller KS, McAninch JW: Radiographic assessment of renal trauma: Our 15-year experience. *J Urol* 154:352, 1995.
8. Morey AL, McAninch JW, Tiller BK, et al.: Single shot intraoperative excretory urography for the immediate evaluation of renal trauma. *J Urol* 161:1088, 1999.
9. Brown SL, Hoffman DM, Spirnack JP: Limitations of routine spiral computerized tomography in the evaluation of blunt renal trauma. *J Urol* 160:138, 1998.
10. McAleer IM, Kaplan GW: Pediatric genitourinary trauma. *Urol Clin North Am* 22:177, 1995.
11. Morey AF, Bruce JE, McAninch JW: Efficacy of radiographic imaging in pediatric blunt renal trauma. *J Urol* 156:2014, 1996.
12. Perez-Brayfield MR, Keane TE, Krisnan A, et al.: Gunshot wounds to the ureter: A 40-year experience at Grady Memorial Hospital. *J Urol* 166:119, 2001.
13. Azimuddin K, Milanesa D, Ivatory R, et al.: Penetrating ureteric injuries. *Injury* 29:363, 1998.
14. Palmer LS, Rosenbaum RR, Gershbaum MD, et al.: Penetrating ureteral trauma at an urban trauma center: 10-year experience. *Urol* 54:34, 1999.
15. Brandes SB, Chelsky MJ, Buckman RF, et al.: Ureteral injuries from penetrating trauma. *J Trauma* 36:766, 1994.
16. Townsend M, DeFalco AJ: Absence of ureteral opacification below ureteral disruption: A sentinel CT finding. *Am J Roentgen* 164:253, 1995.
17. Carroll PR, McAninch JW: Major bladder trauma: Mechanisms of injury and a unified method of diagnosis and repair. *J Urol* 132:254, 1984.
18. Cass AS: The multiple injured patient with bladder trauma. *J Trauma* 24:731, 1984.
19. Cass AS, Luxenberg M: Features of 164 bladder ruptures. *J Urol* 138:743, 1987.
20. Carroll PR, McAninch JW: Major bladder trauma: The accuracy of cystography. *J Urol* 130:887, 1983.
21. Peng MY, Parisky YR, Cornwell EE, et al.: CT cystography versus conventional cystography in evaluation of bladder injury. *Am J Roentgenol* 173:1269, 1999.
22. Cass AS, Luxenberg M: Testicular injuries. *Urol* 27:528, 1991.
23. McAninch JW, Carroll PR: Renal exploration after trauma: Indications and reconstructive techniques. *Urol Clin North Am* 16:203, 1989.
24. Husmann DA, Gilling PJ, Perry MO, et al.: Major renal lacerations with devitalized fragments following blunt abdominal trauma: A comparison between non-operative (expectant) versus surgical management. *J Urol* 150:1774, 1993.
25. McAninch JW, Carroll PR, Klosterman PW, et al.: Renal reconstruction after injury. *J Urol* 145:932, 1991.
26. Steers WD, Corriere JN, Benson GS, et al.: The use of indwelling ureteral stents in managing ureteral injuries due to external violence. *J Trauma* 25:1001, 1985.
27. Cass AS: Ureteral contusion with gunshot wounds. *J Urol* 24:59, 1984.
28. Hayes EE, Sandler CM, Corriere JN Jr: Management of the ruptured bladder secondary to blunt abdominal trauma. *J Urol* 129:946, 1983.
29. Corriere JN Jr, Sandler CM: Management of the ruptured bladder: 7 years experience with 111 cases. *J Trauma* 26:830, 1986.
30. Merchant WC, Gibbons MD, Gonzales ET: Trauma to the bladder neck, trigone and vagina in children. *J Urol* 131:747, 1984.
31. Kotkin L, Koch MO: Morbidity associated with nonoperative management of extraperitoneal bladder injuries. *J Trauma* 38:895, 1995.
32. Appeltans BMG, Schapmans S, et al.: Urinary bladder rupture: Laparoscopic repair. *Br J Urol* 81:764, 1998.
33. DeConcini DT, Coburn M: Penetrating bladder trauma: Indications for non-operative management. *South Central Section, American Urological Association 1997 Annual Meeting*, Bermuda.
34. Pierce JM Jr: Disruptions of the anterior urethra. *Urol Clin North Am* 16:329, 1989.
35. Husmann DA, Boone TB, Wilson WT: Management of low velocity gunshot wounds to the anterior urethra: The role of primary repair versus urinary diversion alone. *J Urol* 150:70, 1993.
36. Kalash SS, Young JD Jr: Fracture of the penis: Controversy of surgical versus conservative treatment. *Urol* 24:21, 1989.
37. Fournier GR, Laing FC, Jeffrey RB, et al.: High resolution scrotal ultrasonography: A highly sensitive but nonspecific diagnostic technique. *J Urol* 134:490, 1985.
38. Jordan GH: Scrotal trauma and reconstruction. In Graham DS, ed, *Glenn's Urologic Surgery*, 5th ed. Philadelphia, PA: Lippincott William & Wilkins, 1998, p. 539.
39. Scott RF Jr, Selzman HM: Complications of nephrectomy: Review of 450 patients and a description of a modification of the transperitoneal approach. *J Urol* 95:307, 1966.
40. Corriere JN, McAndrew JD, Benson GS: Intraoperative decision making in renal trauma surgery. *J Trauma* 31:1390, 1991.
41. Rosen MA, McAninch JW: Management of combined renal and pancreatic trauma. *J Urol* 152:22, 1994.
42. Wessels H, McAninch JW: Effect of colon injury on the management of simultaneous renal trauma. *J Urol* 155:1852, 1996.
43. Quesada ET, Coburn M: Bilateral penetrating renal injuries. *South Central Section, American Urological Association 1993 Annual Meeting*, Acapulco, Mexico.
44. Boone TB, Gilling PJ, Husmann DA: Ureteropelvic junction disruption following blunt abdominal trauma. *J Urol* 150:33, 1993.
45. Jordan GH, Schlossberg SM, Devine CJ: Surgery of the penis and urethra. In Walsh PC, Retik AB, Vaughan ED et al., eds. *Campbell's Urology*, 7th ed. Philadelphia, PA: Saunders, 1998, p. 3316.
46. Follis HW, Koch MO, McDougal WS: Immediate management of prostatomembranous urethral disruptions. *J Urol* 147: 1259, 1992.
47. Porter JR, Takayama TK, Defalco AJ: Traumatic posterior urethral injury and early realignment using magnetic urethral catheters. *J Urol* 158:425, 1997.
48. Jepson BR, Boullier JA, Moore RG, et al.: Traumatic posterior urethral injury and early primary endoscopic realignment: Evaluation of long-term follow-up. *Urol* 53:120-125, 1999.
49. Gheiler EL, Frontera JR: Immediate primary realignment of prostatomembranous urethral disruptions using endourologic techniques. *Urol* 49:596, 1997.
50. Corriere JN Jr, Rudy DC, Benson GS: Voiding and erectile function after delayed one-stage repair of posterior urethral disruptions in 50 men with a fractures pelvis. *J Trauma* 37:587, 1994.
51. Webster GD, Mathes GL, Selli C: Prostatomembranous urethral injuries: A review of the literature and a rational approach to their management. *J Urol* 130:898, 1983.
52. Romilly CS, Isaac MT: Male genital self-mutilation. *Br J Hosp Med* 55:427, 1996.
53. Jordan GH, Gilbert DA: Management of amputation injuries of the male genitalia. *Urol Clin North Am* 16:359, 1989.
54. Lin WW, Kim ED, Quesada ET, et al.: Unilateral testicular injury from external trauma: Evaluation of semen quality and endocrine parameters. *J Urol* 159:841, 1998.
55. Coburn M, Guerriero WG: Complications of genitourinary trauma. In Mattox KL, ed. *Complications of Trauma*, New York: Churchill Livingstone, 1994, p. 533.
56. Rotondo MF, Zonies DH: The damage control sequence and logic. *Surg Clin North Am* 77:761, 1997.
57. Coburn M: Damage control for urologic injuries. *Surg Clin North Am* 77:821, 1997.

## SUGGESTED READINGS

1. Santucci RA, Wessels H, Bartsch G, et al.: Consensus on genitourinary trauma. Evaluation and management of renal injuries: consensus statement of the renal trauma subcommittee. *Br J Urol* 93:937, 2004.
2. Chapple C, Barbagli G, Jordan G, et al.: Consensus on genitourinary trauma. Consensus statement on urethral trauma. *Br J Urol* 93:1195, 2004.
3. Gomez, RG, Ceballos, L, Coburn, M, et al.: Consensus on Genitourinary trauma. Consensus statement on bladder injuries. *Br J Urol* 94:27, 2004.
4. Brandes, S, Coburn, M, Armenakas, N, et al.: Consensus on genitourinary trauma. Diagnosis and management of ureteric injury: an evidence-based analysis. *Br J Urol* 94:277, 2004.
5. Morey, AF, Metro, MJ, Carney, KJ, et al.: Consensus on genitourinary trauma. Consensus on genitourinary trauma: external genitalia. *Br J Urol* 94:507, 2004.
6. Lynch, TH, Martinez-Pineiro L, Plas E, et al.: European Association of Urology. EAU guidelines on urologic trauma. *Eur Urol* 47:1, 2005.
7. Scaling system for organ specific injuries. From: AAST Website. http://www.aast.org, Trauma Resources, The AAST Injury Scale Tables (Tables 19-22, 29-31), 2007.

8. Mohr AM, Pham AM, Lavery RF, et al.: Management of trauma to the external genitalia: the usefulness of the American Association for the Surgery of Trauma organ injury scales. *J Urol* 170:2311, 2003.

9. Kuan JK, Wright JL, Nathens AB, et al.: American Association for the Surgery of Trauma Organ Injury Scale for kidney injuries predicts nephrectom, dialysis, and death in patients with blunt injury and nephrectomy for penetrating injuries. *J Trauma* 50:351, 2006.

10. Kansas BT, Eddy MJ, Mydio JH, et al.: Incidence and management of penetrating renal trauma in patients with multiorgan injury: extended experience at an inner city trauma center. *J Urol* 172:1355, 2004.

11. McAleer IM, Kaplan GW, LoSasso BE: Congenital urinary tract anomalies in pediatric renal trauma patients. *J Urol* 168:1808, 2002.

12. Davis KA, Reed RL, Santaniello J et al.: Predictors of the need for nephrectomy after renal trauma. *J Trauma* 60:164, 2006.

13. Jankowski JT, Spirnak JP: Current recommendations for imaging in the management of urologic traumas. *Urol Clin N Amer* 33:365, 2006.

14. Leslie CL, Zoha Z: Simultaneous upper and lower genitourinary injuries after blunt trauma highlight the need for delayed abdominal CT scans. *Am J Emerg Med* 22:509, 2004.

15. Kunkle, DA, Kansas BT, Pathak, A, et al.: Delayed diagnosis of traumatic ureteral injuries. *J Urol* 176:2503, 2006.

16. Medina d, Lavery R, Ross SE, et al.: Ureteral trauma: preoperative studies neither predict injury nor prevent missed injuries. *J Am Coll Surg* 186:641, 1998.

17. Spiguel L, Glynn L, Liu, D, et al.: Pediatric pelvic fractures: a marker for injury severity. *Am Surg* 72:481, 2006.

18. Demetriades D, Karaiskakis M, Velmahos GC, et al.: Pelvic fracture in pediatric adult trauma patients: are they different injuries? *J Trauma* 54:1146.

19. Baverstock R, Simons R, McLoughlin M: Severe blunt renal trauma: a 7-year retrospective review from a provincial trauma center. *Can J Urol* 8:1372, 2001.

20. Bandi, G, Santucci RA: Controversies in the management of male external genitourinary trauma. *J Trauma* 56:1362, 2004.

21. Evans LA, Ferguson KH, Foley JP, et al.: Fibrin sealant for the management of genitourinary injuries, fistulas and surgical complications. *J Urol* 169:1360, 2003.

22. Knudson MM, Harrison PB, Hoyt DB, et al.: Outcome after major renovascular injuries: a Western trauma association multicenter report. *J Trauma* 49:1116, 2000.

23. Elliott S, McAninch JW: Ureteral injuries from external violence: the 25-year experience from San Francisco General Hospital. *J Urol* 170:1213, 2003.

24. Brenneman FD, Katyal D, Boulander BR, et al.: Long-term outcomes in open pelvic fractures. *J Trauma* 42:773, 1997.

25. Arthurs Z, Kjorstad R, Mullenix P, et al.: The use of damage-control principles for penetrating pelvic battlefield trauma. *Am Surg* 191:604, 2006.

# Commentary  ■ FERNANDO J. KIM

Coburn's chapter on genitourinary (GU) trauma has provided a superior comprehensive and concise review of the current strategies for patients with urological trauma. This chapter discusses the controversies and the new trends in the management of GU trauma and provides an important and very enjoyable read for urological and trauma surgeons.

The author described the different evaluation and management schemes that cannot be overemphasized. Although the American Association for the Surgery of Trauma (AAST) injury scaling system (1989) has been widely utilized as a tool to assess the severity of injury in trauma patients providing a common language among surgeons to describe the injuries, overwhelmingly, the renal injuries grading system have successfully been adopted in urology, partly due to the lack of clinical relevance with other GU organs grading system. There is no doubt that a comprehensive update is sought-after.

The recent innovations in minimally invasive procedures allowed surgeons to adopt laparoscopic instrumentation and techniques to safely and rapidly perform emergent open procedures, such as hilar ligation with laparoscopic vascular staples during simple nephrectomies in unstable patients. Reports of Palmaz endovascular stents have shown increased organ salvage rate after renal vascular trauma.

Other minimally invasive complex reconstructive procedures post trauma have been demonstrated their feasibility with promising results, such as, laparoscopic repair of UPJ disruption with lower pole amputation and ureterocalicostomy, laparoscopic ureteral reimplantation and laparoscopic evaluation of pelvic fractures with concomitant bladder repair achieving great cosmetic results and faster recovery.[1,2]

The field of urological trauma is an exciting and dynamic surgical subspecialty. Advances in imaging technology, interventional and minimally invasive surgery has changed the way we evaluate and manage genitourinary trauma. Future research in the areas of hemostasis and bioengineering may have a great impact on the non-operative or minimally invasive surgical management of GU trauma and reconstructive surgery.

## References

1. Campagna A, Dall'Era J, Gewehr EV, et al.: Laparoscopic Ureteroneocystostomy (LUNC) in adults for distal ureteral injury. *J Endourol* 20:A46, 2006.

2. Brant W, Gewehr EV, Kim FJ: Laparoscopic Exploration and Repair of Intraperitoneal Bladder Ruptures. AUA South Central Section Annual Meeting. October 23–27, 2004. Dublin, Ireland.

# Reproductive System Trauma

*M. Margaret Knudson* ■ *Jennifer J. Wan*

Penetrating injuries to the gravid uterus date back to antiquity, when wounding instruments included spears, sticks, and animal horns. Ambroise Paré, famous for his skills as a military surgeon, was also an obstetrician and was among the first to describe the treatment of gunshot wounds to the uterus. Paré wrote, "When the womb is wounded, the blood cometh out at the privites, and all other accidents appeared..."[1] Maternal deaths resulting directly from pregnancy or the complications of labor and delivery have declined sharply in recent years. In contrast, *trauma* has emerged as the leading cause of death during pregnancy, accounting for nearly 50% of maternal deaths in one series.[2] An estimated 6 to 7% of pregnancies are complicated by trauma, and 0.4% of all pregnant patients require hospitalization for the treatment of injuries.[3] The true number of injured gravid women is grossly underestimated by these figures, however, as many injuries are unreported, especially those resulting from domestic violence. Thus, it is essential that all trauma care professionals recognize the anatomic and physiologic changes unique to pregnancy and appreciate how these changes impact the evaluation and treatment of the injured gravid patient. Complete evaluation of these patients includes an assessment of the fetus, and the treating physician must not only be cognizant of the signs of fetal distress, but must also be able to make rapid interventions in the interest of salvaging the pregnancy. Additionally, recognition and prompt treatment of pelvic trauma in the nongravid patient will optimize preservation of her sexual and reproductive function.

## EPIDEMIOLOGY OF TRAUMA IN PREGNANCY

Weiss and coworkers examined data from the Pennsylvania state trauma registry and found that among a total of 16,722 women of childbearing age who required hospitalization for injuries over a one-year period, 761 were pregnant (4.6%).[4] The leading causes of injury among pregnant women in this series were transportation-related (33.6%), falls, and assaults. Younger women (mean age 25) appeared to be at higher risk for injuries when compared to older gravid women. In a related study that included data from 16 states, 240 trauma-related fetal deaths were identified (3.7 fetal deaths per 100,000 live births).[5] Motor vehicle crashes were again the leading mechanism resulting in fetal death (82% of cases), followed by firearms (6%), and falls (3%). Placental injury was mentioned in 100 cases, and maternal death was the cause of fetal death in 11% of the cases. Again, pregnant mothers aged 15 to 19 years appeared to be at greatest risk for trauma-related fetal loss.

Young pregnant women are also at significant risk of sustaining injuries as the result of an assault. Battering can begin or escalate during pregnancy, and it is estimated that between 10 to 30% of women are abused during pregnancy, with fetal death resulting in 5%.[6] In a series of 41 injury-related deaths during pregnancy reported from North Carolina, half were known or suspected of having been abused.[7] Physical abuse is suggested by proximal and midline injuries rather than distal injuries, trauma to the neck, breast and face, and injuries to the upper arms and lateral thighs. Cigarette burns and bites should also raise the level of suspicion for the examiner.[8] A history of depression, substance abuse, or several emergency department (ED) visits are other factors that suggest domestic violence, which is not dependent on age, race, or marital status and cuts across all socioeconomic classes. Thus, it is imperative that all health care providers recognize the signs and symptoms of physical abuse and the opportunity to intervene and protect both the mother and her fetus (see Chap. 48).

Chang and others recently summarized data from the Pregnancy Mortality Surveillance System at the Center for Disease Control (CDC), focusing on risk factors for pregnancy-associated homicide.[9] According to this report, homicide was the third leading cause of injury-related death for all women of child-bearing age, pregnant or not. The pregnancy associated homicide ratio was 1.7 per 100,000 live births. Risk factors for homicide in this group included age younger than 20 years, Black race, and either late or no prenatal care. Firearms were the leading mechanism for homicide (56.5%). It is hoped that the new surveillance system developed by the CDC, the National Violent Death Reporting System, which captures information about pregnancy status, victim–perpetrator relationships, and the presence of intimate partner violence, will provide more comprehensive data on this important mechanism of injury among women.

Ikossi and coinvestigators utilized the American College of Surgeons' National Trauma Data Bank (NTDB) to develop a profile for mothers at risk for injury during pregnancy. Among the 77,321 women hospitalized after injury who were of childbearing age, 1195 (1.5%) were also pregnant.[10] The major mechanism of injury among the pregnant patients was motor vehicle crash (70%), followed by interpersonal violence (11.6%) and falls (9.3%). Young age, African-American or Hispanic ethnicity, and insurance status (none or underinsured) identified women at highest risk for injury during pregnancy and thus are the women most likely to benefit from primary trauma prevention efforts (see below).

## ANATOMIC AND PHYSIOLOGIC CHANGES UNIQUE TO PREGNANCY

Although the initial assessment and management priorities for resuscitation of the injured pregnant patient are the same as those for other traumatized patients (see Chap. 11), the specific anatomic and physiologic changes that occur during pregnancy may alter the response to injury and, hence, necessitate a modified approach to the resuscitation process. Most of these anatomic, physiologic, and biochemical adaptations occur in response to physiologic stimuli provided by the fetus. An understanding of these adaptations (summarized in Table 40-1) is necessary in order to provide appropriate and timely care to both mother and unborn child.

## Cardiovascular System

Plasma volume begins to expand at ten weeks' gestation and increases to 45% of pregravid levels by full-term. Other contributing factors to blood volume expansion include increases in estrogen, progesterone, renin, and aldosterone. Additionally, tubular resorption of sodium is increased. During a normal pregnancy, about 950 meq of sodium and an additional 6 to 8 L of total body water are retained.[11] This hypervolemic state is protective for the mother because fewer red blood cells are lost during hemorrhage and, hence, the oxygen-carrying capacity of her blood is less affected.[12] Furthermore, the hypervolemia prepares the patient for the blood loss that accompanies vaginal delivery (500 mL) or cesarean section (1000 mL). This pregnancy-induced hypervolemia, however, may create a false sense of security for the resuscitating physician because almost 35% of maternal blood volume may be lost before there are signs of maternal shock.

This 30 to 40% increase in plasma volume is accompanied by an erythroid hyperplasia in the bone marrow, resulting in a 15% increase in red blood cell mass and a "physiologic anemia." A hemoglobin level below 11 g/dL should be considered abnormal. This anemia of pregnancy is greatest at 30 to 32 weeks' gestation and will be most significant in patients who have not received iron supplements.[12] Although pregnancy is associated with a moderate leukocytosis, primarily comprising neutrophils, white blood cell counts as high as 25,000/mm³ are not uncommon during labor. Because there is a wide range of normal white blood cell values, more emphasis is put on the trend toward an increasing white blood cell count than it is on its absolute value. Factors VII, VIII, IX, X, and XII and fibrinogen are increased, fibrinolytic activity is reduced, and the net result is a hypercoagulable state, putting the patient at increased risk for thromboembolic events.

During the first trimester, maternal pulse rate increases by about 10 to 15 beats/minute and remains elevated until delivery. As the diaphragm becomes progressively more elevated secondary to the

**TABLE 40-1**

| **Alterations in Pregnancy** | | |
|---|---|---|
| **SYSTEM** | **CHANGE** | **POTENTIAL IMPLICATION** |
| Cardiovascular | ↓ Pheripheral vascular resistance, ↓ venous return, ↓ blood pressure (10–15 mmHg) | Supine hypotensive syndrom (10–15 mmHg) |
| Blood volume | ↑ Plasma volume, RBC volume, ↑ WBC (20,000 WBC/mm³) | Physiologic hypervolemia may mask hypotension secondary to blood loss |
| Coagulation | Hypercoagulable; ↑ fibrinogen; ↑ factors VII, VIII, IX, X, XII; ↓ fibrinolysis | ↑ Venous thromboembolism |
| Respiratory | ↑ Subcostal angle (68°–103°), ↑ chest circumference (5–7 cm), ↑ diaphragmatic excursion (1–2 cm), elevated diaphragm, ↑ tidal volume, ↑ minute ventilation, ↓ FRC, ↓ PCO₂, HCO₃ | Alteration in FRC and lung volume, chronic compensated respiratory alkalosis |
| Gastrointestinal | ↓ Motility, ↓ intestinal secretion, ↓ nutrient absorption, ↓ sphincter competency (progesterone) | Aspiration |
| Hepatobiliary | Organ displacement | Clinical examination unreliable |
|  | ↑ Gallbladder volume, ↓ gallbladder emptying, ↓ albumin, ↑ AP, ↓ bilirubin (free), ↓ GGT | Cholestasis, ↑ cholestasis saturation, ↑ chenodeoxycholic acid, ↑ gallstones |
| Renal | ↑ Glomerular filtration rate, ↑ renal plasma flow, ↑ creatinine clearance, ↓ serum creatinine, ↓ BUN | Hydronephrosis, hydroureter |
|  |  | Dilation of collecting system |
|  |  | Bladder/urethral muscle tone |
| Endocrine | ↑ Parathormone, ↑ calcitonin | ↑ Calcium absorption |
| Musculoskeletal | Pelvic ligaments soften (relaxin, progesterone) | Pelvic widening, lordosis, shift in center of gravity |

AP, alkaline phosphatase; BUN, blood urea nitrogen; FRC, functional residual capacity; GGT, γ-glutamyltransferase; RBC, red blood cell; WBC, white blood cell.

enlarging uterus, the heart is displaced to the left and upward, resulting in a lateral displacement of the cardiac apex. Moreover, each pregnant woman has some degree of benign pericardial effusion. Both of these changes result in an enlarged cardiac silhouette and increased pulmonary vasculature on the chest radiograph.[13]

Maternal blood pressure decreases during the first trimester, reaches its lowest level in the second trimester, and then rises toward prepregnancy levels during the final two months of gestation. The mean blood pressure values of 105/60 mm Hg for the first trimester, 102/55 mm Hg for the second trimester, and 108/67 mm Hg for the third trimester are important to note because significant elevations in these values may indicate pregnancy-induced hypertension.

By the end of the first trimester, cardiac output increases to 25% above normal. Although these values may vary with position of the patient, cardiac output continues to rise so that by term, measurements of about 6.2 ± 1 L (min are obtained.[14] In the healthy gravida, this increased workload on the heart is well tolerated.

When the patient is in the supine position and the inferior vena cava is partially obstructed by the gravid uterus, there is a decrease in blood return to the heart, resulting in a lower cardiac output, causing the supine hypotensive syndrome. This syndrome is marked by dizziness, pallor, tachycardia, sweating, nausea, and hypotension. Turning the mother onto her left side restores the circulation and increases cardiac output by about 30% after 20 weeks' gestation. A point worth emphasizing is that in the supine position, the enlarged uterus also compresses the aorta, reducing the pressure in the uterine arteries and decreasing some blood flow to the fetus.[15]

During labor and delivery, maternal hemodynamics are further altered. For example, with each uterine contraction, 300 to 500 mL blood is expelled from the uterus, increasing systemic blood volume and raising central venous pressure.[16] Immediately after delivery, there is a dramatic increase in cardiac output. The contracted uterus shunts blood from the uterine vessels into the systemic circulation, subsequently increasing venous return to the

heart. This results in approximately 1000 mL of autotransfusion at the time of delivery. This increase in postdelivery cardiac output persists for about one week. A summary of hemodynamic changes in pregnancy is included in Table 40-2.

## TABLE 40-2

### Cardiovascular Changes During Pregnancy and Postpartum

| TIME PERIOD IN WEEKS' GESTATION | | | | | POSTPARTUM |
|---|---|---|---|---|---|
| Indices | | | | | |
| | 10–18 | 18–26 | 26–34 | 34–42 | 6 Weeks |
| Cardiac output (L/min) | 7.3 | 7.6 | 7.4 | 6.4 | 6.5 |
| Stroke volume (mL) | 85 | 85 | 82 | 70 | 70 |
| Heart rate (beats/min) | 87 | 90 | 92 | 92 | 79 |
| SVR (dynes . s/cm$^5$) | 966 | 901 | 932 | 1118 | 1274 |
| Mean arterial pressure (mmHg) | 87 | 84 | 84 | 86 | 86 |

SVR systemic vascular resistance.

*Adapted from Van Oppen AC, van der Tweel I. Alsbach GP, et al: A longitudinal study of maternal hemodynamic during pregnancy. Obstet Gyhnecol 88:40, 1996 42, 1996, with permission from the American College of Obstetricians and Gynecologists*

## Respiratory System

Several changes in the maternal respiratory system occur during pregnancy to meet increased oxygen requirements. As the uterus enlarges, the diaphragm rises about 4 cm and the diameter of the chest enlarges by 2 cm, increasing the substernal angle by 50%.[17] These changes occur very early in pregnancy secondary to hormonal effects, and then later from mechanical pressure caused by the enlarged uterus. Care should be taken to consider these anatomic changes when thoracic procedures such as tube thoracostomies or thoracenteses are being performed. Figure 40-1 demonstrates the changes in pulmonary volumes and capacities that occur

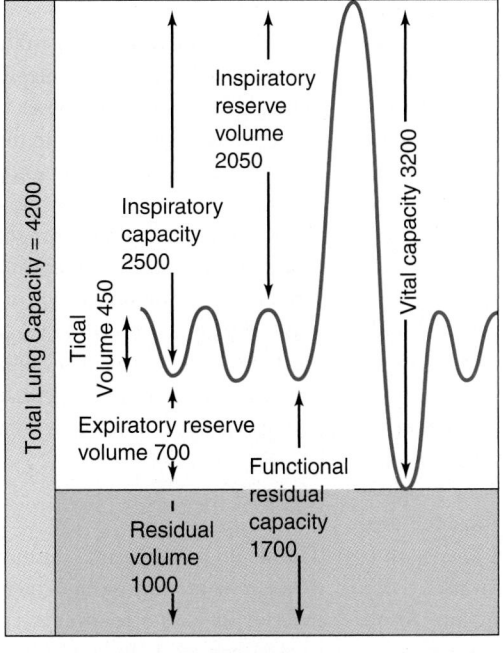

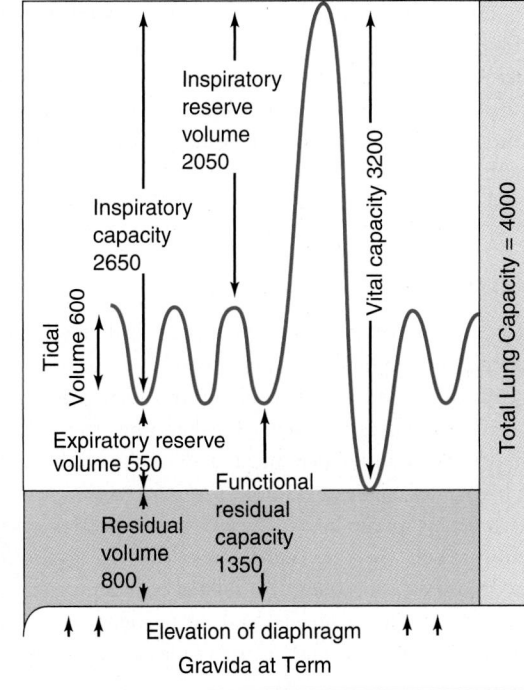

**FIGURE 40-1.** Pulmonary volumes and capacities during pregnancy, labor, and the postpartum period.

Nonpregnant

Gravida at Term

during pregnancy. The most notable changes are the progressive increases in tidal volume and minute ventilation. Functional residual capacity (FRC) decreases because of a decline in expiratory reserve and residual volumes. The net result is an unchanged arterial partial pressure of oxygen ($PaO_2$), a reduction in the partial pressure of carbon dioxide ($PCO_2$) to 30 mm Hg, and a slight compensatory decrease in plasma bicarbonate levels.[18] Therefore, pregnancy is a state of partially compensated respiratory alkalosis. Relative to these changes, the injured gravida tolerates apnea poorly because of the reduced FRC. Hence, supplemental oxygen is always indicated for these patients.

## Gastrointestinal System

Increased levels of progesterone and estrogen inhibit gastrointestinal motility, intestinal secretion, and nutrient absorption during pregnancy. Additionally, the angle of the gastroesophageal junction is altered such that the lower esophageal sphincter is displaced into the thorax. This alteration, along with hormonal changes, decreases the competency of the gastroesophageal sphincter, which increases the potential for aspiration as early as 8 to 12 weeks' gestation.[19] The hormone gastrin, produced by the placenta, raises the acid, chloride, and enzyme contents of the stomach during pregnancy. Studies have shown that parturients who have an elective cesarean section after an overnight fast have more than 25 mL of acidic (pH < 2.5) gastric contents at the time of surgery.[19] It is, therefore, prudent to insert a nasogastric tube to decompress the stomach and prevent aspiration. Furthermore, as the uterus enlarges, it displaces the intestines upward and laterally, stretching the peritoneum and making the physical examination unreliable.

Hepatomegaly does not occur during pregnancy, but hepatic physiology is altered. Although several hepatic enzymes have altered levels, the change in alkaline phosphatase is most notable. Alkaline phosphatase levels nearly double, a phenomenon largely attributed to the presence of placental isoenzymes of alkaline phosphatase.[20] Plasma albumin decreases to an average of 3.0 g/dL, as compared to 4.3 g/dL in nonpregnant patients.

High progesterone levels during the second and third trimesters result in impaired contraction of the gallbladder and a high residual volume of bile, resulting in an increased incidence of gallstone formation.[21] Progesterone inhibits cholecystokinin-mediated smooth-muscle stimulation, leading to bile stasis. This, coupled with the increased cholesterol saturation associated with pregnancy, explains the increased prevalence of cholesterol stones.

## Renal System

To accommodate both maternal and fetal metabolic and circulatory requirements, renal blood flow increases by 30% during gestation.[22] Consequently, blood urea nitrogen (BUN) and serum creatine levels are reduced. Furthermore, the kidneys enlarge by hypertrophy and hyperemia as early as the tenth week of gestation. This is caused by the smooth-muscle-relaxing effects of progesterone. As pregnancy progresses, the ureters and bladder are compressed by the uterus, resulting in hydronephrosis and hydroureter; consequently, a dilated collecting system visualized on imaging studies is normal and not evidence of obstruction. Also, the insertion of a urinary catheter may be necessary if urine output is to be monitored closely.

The growth hormone effect of placental lactogen, increase in blood volume, and increase in cardiac output during pregnancy accommodate the increase in glomerular filtration rate (GRF) and renal plasma flow (RPF). The increase in RPF is greater than that of GFR, reaching 80% over baseline by 26 weeks' gestation versus a 50% increase in GFR.[22] Therefore, more plasma is filtered, reducing the serum protein concentration and, hence, the plasma oncotic pressure.[22] There is some evidence that a decreased colloid oncotic pressure ($COP_p$) puts the pregnant patient at increased risk for pulmonary edema. This change also results in an increase in the renal clearance of many substances during pregnancy, and a review of the metabolism of pharmaceutical agents prior to their administration to pregnant patients is, therefore, recommended.[23]

## Endocrine System

The placenta produces human chorionic gonadotropin (hCG) and human placental lactogen (hPL), as well as progesterone, estrogen, thyroid-stimulating hormone (TSH), and adrenocorticotropic hormone (ACTH).[24] hPL, which is immunochemically similar to human growth hormone, affects the nutrient phase of maternal and fetal metabolism. Maternal utilization of glucose is decreased while maternal lipolysis is enhanced, making nutrients available to the fetus. hPL is the physiologic antagonist of insulin and contributes to the diabetogenic effect of pregnancy by causing increased peripheral resistance to insulin. The resulting increased level of maternal insulin promotes protein synthesis, thereby ensuring a source of amino acids for the fetus. Because estriol production depends on the adequate function of the fetal-placental unit, serial measurements of maternal estriol have been used as a clinical index of fetal and placental well-being.[16] The pituitary gland enlarges during pregnancy by approximately 135%,[24] and, consequently, has increased blood-flow demands. Shock may cause necrosis of the anterior pituitary gland, resulting in pituitary insufficiency or Sheehan's syndrome.

## Reproductive System

By the end of full-term gestation, the weight of the uterus has increased to 20 times its prepregnancy weight (i.e., from 60 g to about 1000 g). After the twelfth week of pregnancy, the uterus extends out of the pelvis, rotates slightly to the right, and ascends into the abdominal cavity to displace the intestines laterally and superiorly.

At 10 weeks' gestation, uterine blood flow is estimated to be about 50 mL/min. With progressive uterine enlargement, uterine blood flow increases dramatically, to approximately 500 mL/min at term, constituting up to 17% of the cardiac output.[25] Uterine veins may dilate up to 60 times their size in the prepregnant state, allowing for adequate venous drainage to accommodate the uteroplacental blood flow. This increased vascularity carries an attendant risk of massive blood loss with a pelvic injury.

## Central Nervous System

The hemodynamic and hormonal changes associated with pregnancy may predispose the gravid patient to cerebrovascular abnormalities such as arteriovenous malformations (AVMs). Hemodynamic changes include increases in blood volume, stroke volume, and cardiac output, while hormonal changes include increased estrogen levels, which may result in the dilation of already abnormal vessels.[26] Ensuing complications such as hydrocephalus, vasospasm, and rebleeding may mimic signs of injury to the brain, making computed tomography (CT) scanning or magnetic resonance imaging (MRI) necessary to determine the etiology of these effects. Intracerebral hemorrhage is the most common cause of death in patients with pregnancy-induced hypertension (PIH). Because PIH may be accompanied by tonic–clonic seizures, which also occur in patients with injuries to the brain, a complete neurologic examination is crucial in any patient who manifests signs of hypertension.

## Musculoskeletal System

The softening and relaxation of the interosseus ligaments during pregnancy cause increased mobility of the sacroiliac and sacrococcygeal joints and widening of the symphysis pubis. These changes, coupled with an enlarged uterus, disrupt the maternal center of gravity, for which the mother compensates by assuming a lordotic posture. This resultant change in stability of gait puts the gravida at increased risk for trauma, especially from falls.

# INITIAL ASSESSMENT AND MANAGEMENT

## Prehospital Care

Prehospital care is an extension of the trauma system (see Chap. 4) and must be appropriately adapted to the needs of the injured gravid patient. Prehospital personnel must be aware of the physiologic changes of pregnancy, as outlined previously. In particular, the importance of providing an adequate airway and supplemental oxygen to prevent fetal hypoxia must take priority during field transport. Additionally important is the recognition that the relative hypervolemia of pregnancy may mask the usual signs and symptoms of acute blood loss. Thus, intravenous fluids should be given liberally during transport in these patients. Patients who are in the second or third trimester of pregnancy should be transported on a backboard tilted to the left (while maintaining immobilization of the spine) in order to avoid the hypotension associated with uterine compression of the vena cava.[27] Any information on the length of the gestation and prenatal care and complications that can be obtained should be relayed to the receiving trauma center.

## Primary Survey

The priorities for treatment of an injured pregnant patient remain the same as those for the nonpregnant patient (see Chap. 11). As with any other injured patient, the primary survey of the injured pregnant patient addresses the airway, breathing, and circulation (volume replacement and hemorrhage control), with the mother receiving treatment priority. Ensuring an adequate maternal airway with supplemental oxygen is essential for preventing maternal and fetal hypoxia (see Chap. 12). Severe trauma stimulates the release of maternal catecholamines, which cause uteroplacental vasoconstriction and, hence, compromise of the fetal circulation. Because the oxyhemoglobin dissociation curve for fetal blood is different from that for maternal blood, small increments in maternal oxygen concentration improve the blood oxygen content and reserve for

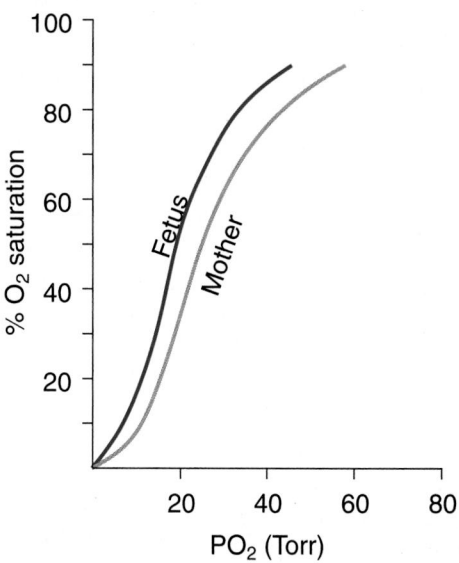

**FIGURE 40-2.** Maternal and fetal oxyhemoglobin dissociation curves demonstrating high affinity of fetal hemoglobin toward oxygen.

the fetus, even though the maternal arterial oxygen content does not change appreciably (Fig. 40-2).

As mentioned above, in the supine position the gravida may become hypotensive from the mechanical effects of her enlarged uterus causing aortocaval compression. Prevention of the supine hypotensive syndrome is accomplished by placing the patient in the left lateral decubitus position. Alternatively, the knee–chest (supine) or right lateral decubitus position can be used and, at 36 weeks' gestation, there is no marked difference in blood pressure when comparing these three positions.[27] Patients with suspected spinal injury can be secured on a backboard and then tilted to the left. As a final measure, the uterus can be manually displaced to the left side.

Hypovolemia should be suspected long before it becomes apparent (see Chap. 13). Because of the physiologic hypervolemia associated with pregnancy, signs of shock may be delayed; hence, vigorous crystalloid resuscitation is encouraged even for patients who appear normotensive.

## Secondary Survey and Maternal Assessment

Following the primary survey of the patient and performance of life-saving measures, the secondary survey is initiated (see Chap. 11). This consists of obtaining a thorough history, including an obstetric history, performing a physical examination in search of all injuries, and evaluating and monitoring the fetus. During the secondary survey, appropriate x-rays should be ordered as during any trauma evaluation (see later).

An accurate prenatal history is crucial because comorbid factors such as PIH, diabetes mellitus, and congenital heart disease may alter management decisions. Furthermore, a history of preterm labor, placental abruption, or placenta previa puts the patient at increased risk for the recurrence of these conditions. The obstetric history includes the date of the last menstrual period, expected date of delivery, and date of the first perception of fetal movement, and any problems or complications of the current and previous pregnancies.

Determination of the uterine size provides an approximation of gestational age and fetal maturity. Measurement of fundal height is

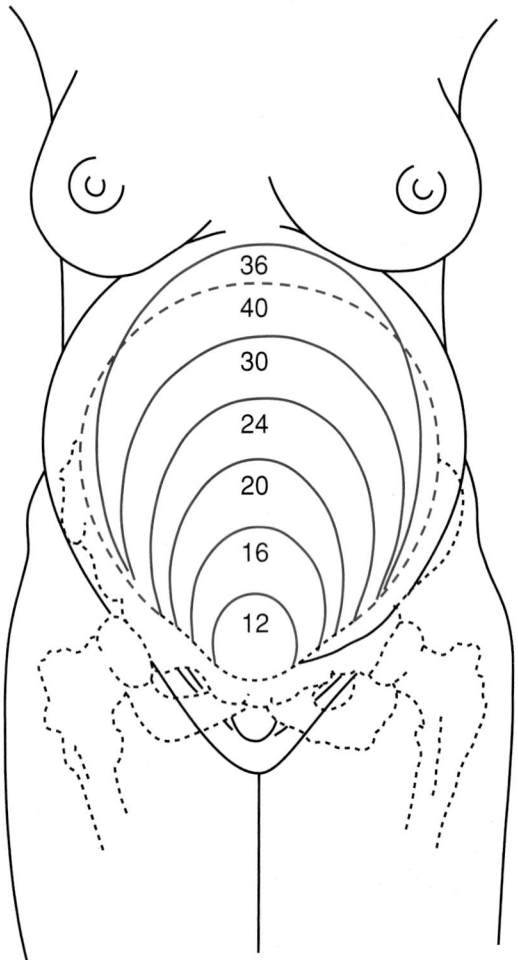

**FIGURE 40-3.**  Location and relative size of uterus at various weeks of gestation.
*(Reproduced with permission from Rozycki GS, Champion HR, Drass M J: Traumatic injuries in the pregnant patient. Hosp Physician 25:20, 1989.)*

a rapid method for estimating fetal age. If, for example, the most superior part of the fundus is palpated at the umbilicus, the fetal age is estimated to be 20 weeks (Fig. 40-3). A discrepancy between dates and uterine size may result from a ruptured uterus or intrauterine hemorrhage. Determination of fetal age and fetal maturity is an important factor in the decision matrix regarding early delivery. For example, a 26-week-old fetus is considered viable if given neonatal intensive care.

A sterile speculum examination should be performed before a bimanual examination and only in the absence of vaginal bleeding. The bimanual examination is generally performed by an obstetrician and in a setting where emergency cesarean delivery can be performed is necessary. The pelvic exam focuses on the following: (a) vaginal bleeding; (b) ruptured membranes (amniotic sac); (c) a bulging perineum; (d) the presence of contractions; and (e) an abnormal fetal heart rate and rhythm. These five conditions indicate the acute status of the pregnancy.

Vaginal bleeding prior to labor is abnormal and may indicate premature cervical dilation, early labor, placental abruption (separation of the placenta from the uterine wall), or placenta previa (location of the placenta over a portion of the cervical os).

If the amniotic sac has ruptured, prolapse of the umbilical cord can occur, resulting in compression of the umbilical vein and

arteries. This can be detected visually by observing cloudy white or green fluid coming from the cervical os or perineum. The presence of amniotic fluid can be confirmed by the change in color of nitrazine paper from blue-green to deep blue when the fluid is tested. Rupture of the amniotic sac is significant because of the potential for infection and prolapse of the umbilical cord, the latter being an obstetric emergency requiring immediate cesarean section.

Bloody amniotic fluid is an indication of premature separation of the placenta (placental abruption) or placenta previa. In the presence of known or continuous meconium staining (green amniotic fluid), continuous electronic fetal monitoring is necessary.

A bulging perineum is caused by pressure from a presenting part of the fetus. If this occurs during the first trimester, spontaneous abortion may be imminent.

Assessment of the pattern of uterine contraction is accomplished by resting the hand on the fundus and determining the frequency, duration, and intensity of contractions. Contractions are usually rated as mild, moderate, or strong. Strong contractions are associated with true labor and assessment for their presence is important so that appropriate preparation can be made for delivery and resuscitation of the neonate if necessary.

The Kleihauer–Betke (KB) test is used after maternal injury to identify fetal blood in the maternal circulation (i.e., fetomaternal transfusion). Adult hemoglobin (HbA) is eluted in the presence of an acidic buffer, whereas fetal hemoglobin (HbF) is resistant to elution. Fetal cells containing HbF are stained with erythrosin, while maternal cells containing HbA fail to stain and remain as "ghost cells" in the peripheral smear. Because the KB test can determine the risk of isosensitization in Rh-negative gravidas, it is recommended for detecting imminent fetal exsanguination in injured pregnant patients who are Rh-negative in the second or third trimester. If positive, the KB test should be repeated after 24 hours to identify ongoing fetomaternal hemorrhage. The initial dose of Rh-immune globulin is 300 µg, with an additional 300 µg given for every 30 mL of fetomaternal transfusion estimated by the KB test. While the KB test is a very sensitive marker for even a small amount of fetomaternal transfusion, its clinical utility in Rh-positive mothers is uncertain.[28] Indeed, the usefulness of the KB test after injury has been challenged recently by several authors. Authors from the R. Adams Cowley Shock Trauma Center in Baltimore reported that among 46 injured women who were KB-positive on admission, 44 had documented contractions.[29] Indeed, in that study, KB testing accurately predicted the risk of preterm labor after maternal trauma whereas clinical assessment was insensitive in identifying women at risk for this complication. On the other hand, a recent study from Cincinnati documented that 5% of low-risk women had a positive KB test, compared to only 2.6% of injured patients.[30] None of these positive results were associated with a clinical abruption or fetal distress. These authors concluded that the presence of a positive KB test alone does not necessarily indicate pathologic fetal–maternal hemorrhage in patients with trauma and that its routine use after injury should be abandoned.

## Fetal Assessment

Unfortunately, direct assessment of the fetus following trauma is somewhat limited. Currently, the most valuable information regarding fetal viability can be obtained by a combination of monitoring of the fetal heart rate and ultrasound imaging. Fetal heart tones can be detected with a Doppler device around the

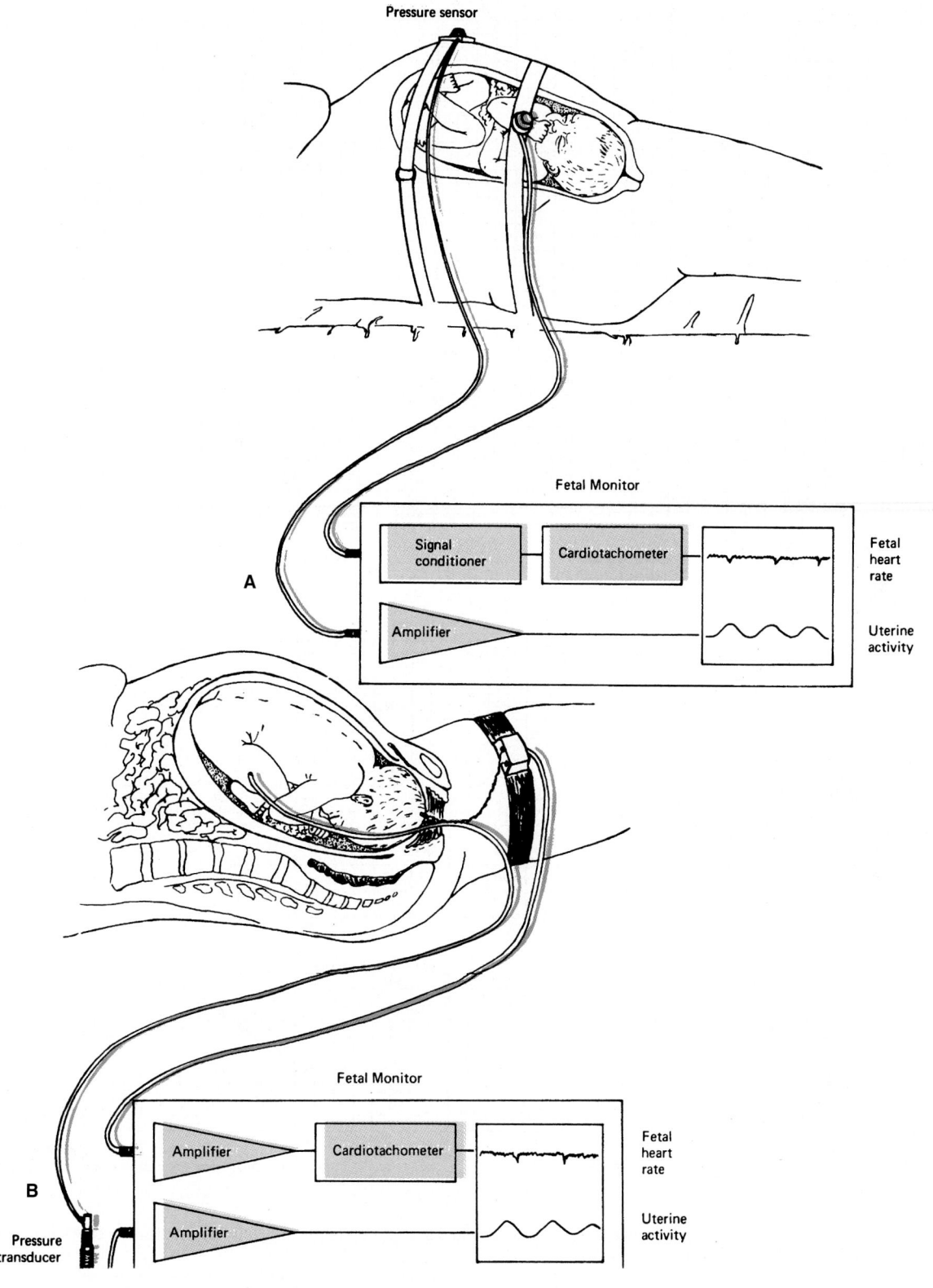

**FIGURE 40-4.** Indirect and direct monitoring of fetal heart rate and uterine contractions.

twelfth week of pregnancy. The normal fetal heart rate (FHR) is between 120 and 160 beats/minute. Because the fetal stroke volume is fixed, the initial response to the stress of hypoxia or hypotension is tachycardia. Severe hypoxia in the fetus, however, is associated with bradycardia (FHR < 120 beats/minute) and should be recognized as fetal distress, demanding immediate attention. Initial FHR monitoring of all pregnant patients with

potentially viable pregnancies (i.e., those that would survive if emergency delivery was required) is indicated, even following relatively minor abdominal trauma. This monitoring is best accomplished using cardiotocographic (CTM) devices, which record both uterine contractions and FHR (Fig. 40-4). A lack of variability in heart rate may also indicate fetal distress and if there is no response to conservative measures such as fluid administration,

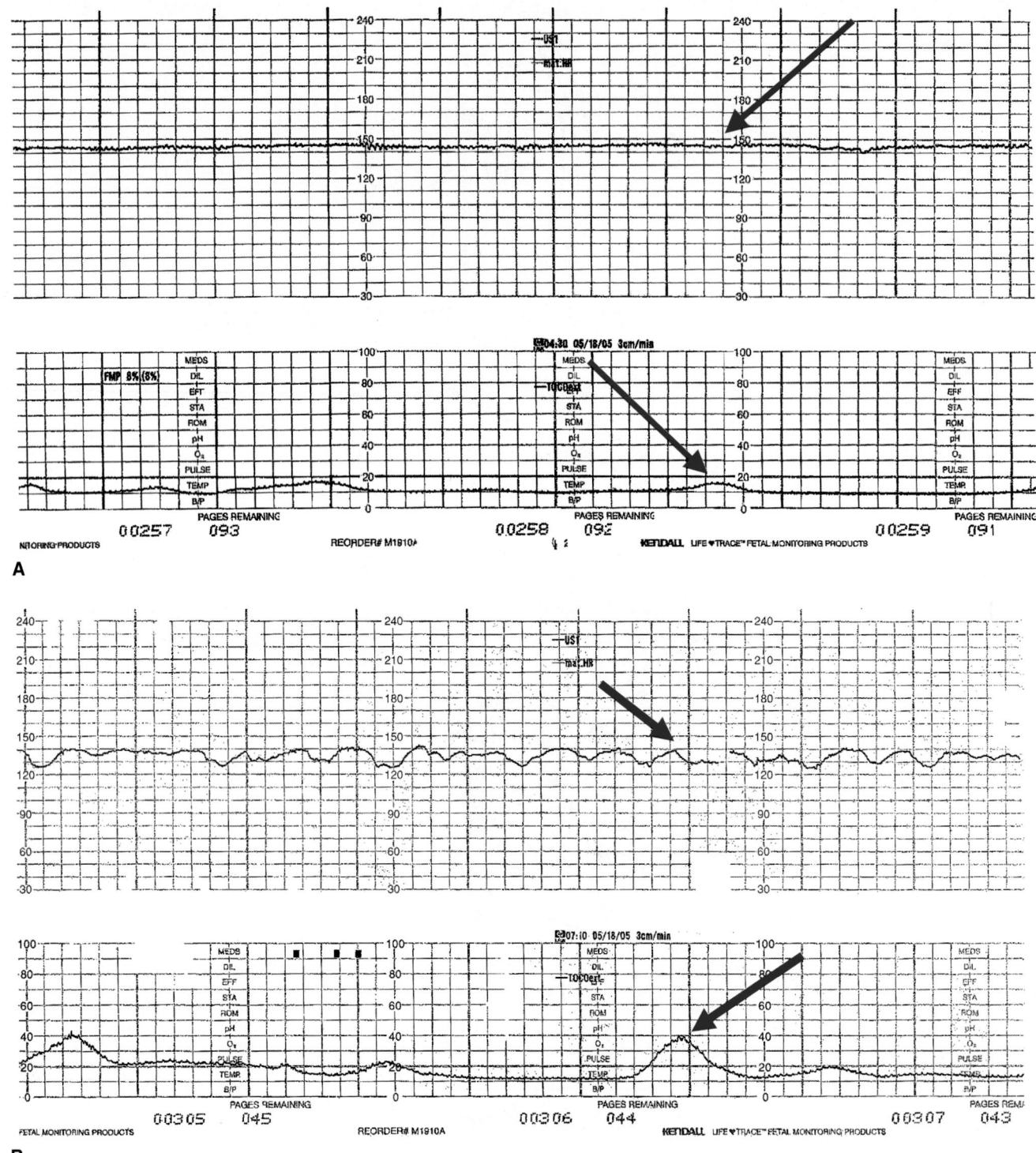

**FIGURE 40-5.**  **(A)** CTM Strip demonstrating poor beat to beat variability in the fetus. **(B)** Return of beat to beat variability after resuscitation; variable decelerations with uterine contractions are within normal limits.

increasing inspired oxygen, or change in maternal position, an emergency delivery should be considered (Fig. 40-5).

Blunt trauma to the abdomen can result in uterine rupture, but this event is uncommon, unlikely to be missed, and usually rapidly fatal for the fetus. A much more common event is placental separation from the uterus as the result of the shearing forces following blunt injury. This separation is termed *placental abruption.* Major cases of placental abruption (i.e., >50% separation) are uniformly

fatal for the fetus, but more minor cases may initially go undetected. In patients with placental abruption following trauma, CTM will detect early fetal distress, often manifested as a decelerated heart rate associated with uterine contractions. Most cases of placental abruption become evident within several hours of trauma.[31,32] A minimum of 24 hours of CTM is recommended for patients with frequent uterine activity (≥6 contractions per hour), abdominal or uterine tenderness, vaginal bleeding, or hypotension.[33] A study of 271 pregnant patients who had sustained blunt trauma identified the following risk factors for fetal loss: ejections, motorcycle and pedestrian collisions, maternal tachycardia, abnormal fetal heart rate, lack of restraints, Injury Severity Score (ISS) >9, gestational age >35 weeks, and a history of assaults.[34] Patients with any of these risk factors should be monitored for at least 24 hours. In the absence of these factors, asymptomatic patients should undergo at least six hours of CTM should be performed prior to considering discharge of a patient after trauma. These patients should be counseled to observe for decreased fetal movement, vaginal bleeding, abdominal pain, or frequent uterine contractions, as partial placental lacerations have been reported to progress over time.[35]

## Ultrasonography

High-resolution real-time ultrasonography (US) has proven valuable for the assessment of fetal age and well-being, recognition and categorization of fetal abnormalities, and treatment of disease processes in the unborn patient. In the trauma setting, US is used primarily to identify acute problems that may be due to maternal events such as placental abruption, placenta previa, or cord prolapse. Although placental abruption is difficult to detect, US can accurately locate the lower margin of the placenta and its relation to the cervical os, hence demonstrating placenta previa.[36] Additionally, it is routine to evaluate the fetus for gestational age, cardiac activity, and movement (Table 40-3). Biophysical profile scoring examines fetal breathing movements, gross body movements, body tone, reactive heart rate, and the volume of amniotic fluid. In a study of 216 patients with high-risk pregnancies, fetal biophysical profile scores corresponded well with perinatal outcome.[37] In another study by Towery and colleagues, the combination of CTM and US demonstrated all fetal or pregnancy-associated complications whereas the KB test was not useful in predicting posttraumatic complications.[38] US findings consistent with uteroplacental injury may include oligohydramnios secondary to uterine injury or ruptured membranes. Oligohydramnios should be suspected if less than a 1-cm layer of amniotic fluid surrounds the fetus.

## Radiographic Examination

Following the secondary survey and the initial assessment of the fetus, appropriate diagnostic studies should be utilized to fully evaluate the extent of maternal injuries. Although there is much concern about radiation exposure during pregnancy, a diagnostic modality

deemed necessary for maternal evaluation should not be withheld on the basis of its potential hazard to the fetus (see Chap. 16). There are three phases of radiation damage related to the gestational age of the fetus.[39] During preimplantation and early implantation (less than three weeks' gestational age), exposure to radiation can result in death of the embryo. During organogenesis (from 3 to 16 weeks' gestation), radiation can damage the developing fetal tube and result in the associated anomalies of exencephaly, dysraphism, single cerebral ventricle, hydrocephaly, and the hypoplastic brain syndrome. Skeletal and genital abnormalities, retinal pigmentation, and cataracts are associated with radiation received during the third and eleventh weeks of gestation. After 16 weeks, neurologic defects are the most common complication of radiation exposure, due to the sensitivity of neuroblasts, which persist in the human embryo from 16 days postconception until about two weeks after birth.[39] Prenatal x-ray exposure may also be associated with the later development of childhood cancers.[40]

Most of the human data on exposure to radiation is based on the large doses received in an atomic bomb blast (which includes neutrons and gamma ray), rather than on doses applied during normal diagnostic (x-ray) studies. The rad is the unit of measurement for absorbed radiation and corresponds to an energy transfer of 100 erg/g of tissue. Absorbed radiation is expressed in Gray (Gy) units, with 1 Gy equal to 100 rad. The dose to the uterus/fetus from x-ray procedures depends on several factors, including the x-ray tube potential, the current, the exposure time, the size of the patient, the type of procedure, the source-to-film distance, and the type of x-ray generator (see Table 40-4).

The American College of Obstetricians and Gynecologists (ACOG) has recently produced a consensus statement on the use of diagnostic imaging during pregnancy.[41] These authors emphasize the fact that *most diagnostic radiologic procedures are associated with little, if any, known significant fetal risk.* Specifically, exposure of the fetus to less than 5 rad has not been associated with an increase in fetal anomalies or pregnancy loss. A plain x-ray generally exposes the fetus to very little radiation, and the uterus is shielded for nonpelvic procedures during pregnancy. With the exception of barium enema or small bowel series, most fluoroscopic examinations result in fetal exposure of just millirads. Radiation exposure from CT varies depending on the number and spacing of adjacent image sections (see Table 40-4). CT pelvimetry can result in fetal exposures as high as 1.5 rad, but can be reduced by using a low-exposure technique as outlined by Moore and others.[42] Radiation exposure using helical CT is affected by slice thickness,

---

**TABLE 40-3**

| Ultrasonogrphic Examination of the Fetus by Trimester | | |
|---|---|---|
| **FIRST TRIMESTER** | **SECOND TRIMESTER** | **THIRD TRIMESTER** |
| Location | | |
| Intrauterine | Size for date | Size for growth |
| Extrauterine | | |
| Size | Anatomy | Anatomy |
| | Viability | Biophysical behavior |

*Adapted with permission from Reed K: Ultrasound in Obstetrics, in Scott JR, DiSaia PJ, Hammond CG, Spellacy WN (eds): Danforth's Obstetrics and Gynecology, 6th ed. Philadelphia: Lippincott, 1990 p 297.*

---

**TABLE 40-4**

| Estimated Fetal Exposure from Some Common Radiologic Procedures | |
|---|---|
| **PROCEDURE** | **FETAL EXPOSURE** |
| Chest x-ray (2 views) | 0.02–0.07 mrad |
| Abdominal film (single view) | 100 mrad |
| Hip film (single view) | >1 rad |
| CT scan of head or chest | <1 rad |
| CT scan or abdomen and lumbar spine | 3.5 rad |

*Modified from: Cunningham FG, Gant NF, Leveno KJ, et al.: General considerations and maternal evaluation: In Williams Obstetrics. 21st ed. New York, NY: McGraw-Hill 2001, p. 1143.*

the number of cuts obtained, and the pitch (a ratio defined as the distance the couch travels during one 360° rotation divided by the section thickness). In general, the exposure to the fetus from spiral CT is comparable to conventional CT.[43]

In summary, the ACOG Committee (41) recommends the following:

- Women should be counseled that x-ray exposure from a single diagnostic procedures does not result in harmful fetal effects. Exposure to less than 5 rads is not harmful to the fetus or the pregnancy

- Concern about possible effects of high-dose ionizing radiation should not prevent medically indicated diagnostic x-ray procedures from being performed during pregnancy

- Other imaging procedures not associated with ionizing radiation, such as ultrasonography or MRI, which are not associated with known adverse fetal effect, should be utilized when appropriate

- Consultation with an expert in dosimetry calculation may be helpful when multiple diagnostic x-rays are required.

For a more complete review of the effects of ionizing radiation in pregnancy, readers are referred to the recent publications by De Santis et al. and Mann and others.[44,45] For the injured patient, then, the following guidelines are suggested:

1. The minimum number of radiographs should be ordered to obtain the maximum information. Careful planning prevents duplication.

2. The patient's abdomen should be shielded with a lead apron. This reduces fetal exposure by a factor of 8.

3. When many radiographs are required over a long period, a thermoluminescent dosimeter or "radiation badge" may be attached to the patient to serve as a guide to the dosage of radiation delivered. This is particularly valuable for the critically ill patient, who may have a prolonged stay in the intensive care unit.

## Evaluation of Abdominal Trauma in Pregnancy

Evaluation of the abdomen following trauma is difficult and may be particularly challenging in the gravid patient. Because of the lack of sensitivity of physical findings, objective evaluation should be considered in patients with rib or pelvic fractures, unexplained hypotension, blood loss or abnormal base deficit, hematuria, and altered sensorium secondary to drugs, alcohol, or concomitant injury to the brain. Just as ultrasound has a major role in evaluating the fetus following trauma, focused abdominal sonography for trauma (FAST) can rapidly detect the presence of both intra-abdominal and intrapericardial fluid in the mother, thus making ultrasound the diagnostic modality of choice in the initial evaluation of the pregnant patient following blunt trauma (Fig. 40-6; see also Chap. 17). A study of 127 pregnant trauma patients undergoing FAST exams documented a sensitivity of 83% in the detection of peritoneal fluid.[46] In a related study, investigators from the Cowley Shock Trauma Center in Baltimore have discovered incidental pregnancies during the FAST exam and theorize that this early detection may be useful in decreasing exposure to radiation.[47] A recent report on the use of ultrasound by radiologists in pregnant patients with blunt abdominal trauma noted that ultrasound had a sensitivity of only 61% in detecting abdominal injuries (compared

to CT or laparotomy) but had a specificity of 94%.[48] The pattern of fluid accumulation was somewhat different when compared to the nonpregnant patients in that right and left upper quadrant locations were more common (compared to Morison's pouch being the most likely location in the nonpregnant population). This is an important finding that all surgeon or emergency physician sonographers should appreciate when using this modality to screen for free fluid in the pregnant patient (see Fig. 40-6). In our center, as in many other trauma centers, ultrasound has replaced DPL in the initial evaluation of the abdomen in pregnant patients (as well as in most other patients).

As mentioned earlier, abdominal CT scanning can also be safely performed in the pregnant patient and is capable of not only detecting blood loss and its source, but can also evaluate the fetus for injuries (Fig. 40-6). Patients undergoing abdominal CT scanning should receive both oral and intravenous noniodinated contrast agents, and hemodynamic stability must be ensured prior to transfer to the radiology suite.

## MANAGEMENT OF INJURIES DURING PREGNANCY

### Thoracic Trauma

The management of thoracic trauma during pregnancy differs little from the nonpregnant state; however, strict attention to oxygenation is essential in order to avoid fetal hypoxia (see above). Additionally, during placement of thoracostomy tubes in late pregnancy, the elevated location of the diaphragm must be considered. A few cases of traumatic aortic rupture during pregnancy have been reported, and there is evidence to suggest changes in the aortic wall during this period may make women particularly prone to these injuries.[49]

### Blunt Abdominal Trauma

Once diagnosed, the management of abdominal injuries during pregnancy differs little from the nonpregnant state. Nonoperative management of injuries to solid organs (liver, spleen, kidney) has been performed successfully in the gravid state and should be considered the treatment of choice in stable patients with these injuries. In contrast, *unstable* patients or those in whom an intestinal injury is likely benefit from early operative treatment, as both hypotension and intra-abdominal infection can be harmful and potentially lethal to the fetus. As with any other emergency laparotomy during pregnancy (i.e., for acute appendicitis, cholecystitis, etc.), the uterus should be left intact, unless it is directly injured or it presents a mechanical limitation for treatment of maternal injuries. The indications for cesarean section following trauma are discussed later.

Although the experience with abdominal operative procedures in injured pregnant patients is generally limited, the data about the safety and timing of other nonobstetrical abdominal surgeries in pregnancy is available. A review of 77 patients requiring laparotomy demonstrated that preterm labor occurred in 26% of the second-trimester patients and 82% of the third-trimester patients.[50] Preterm labor was most common in patients with appendicitis.

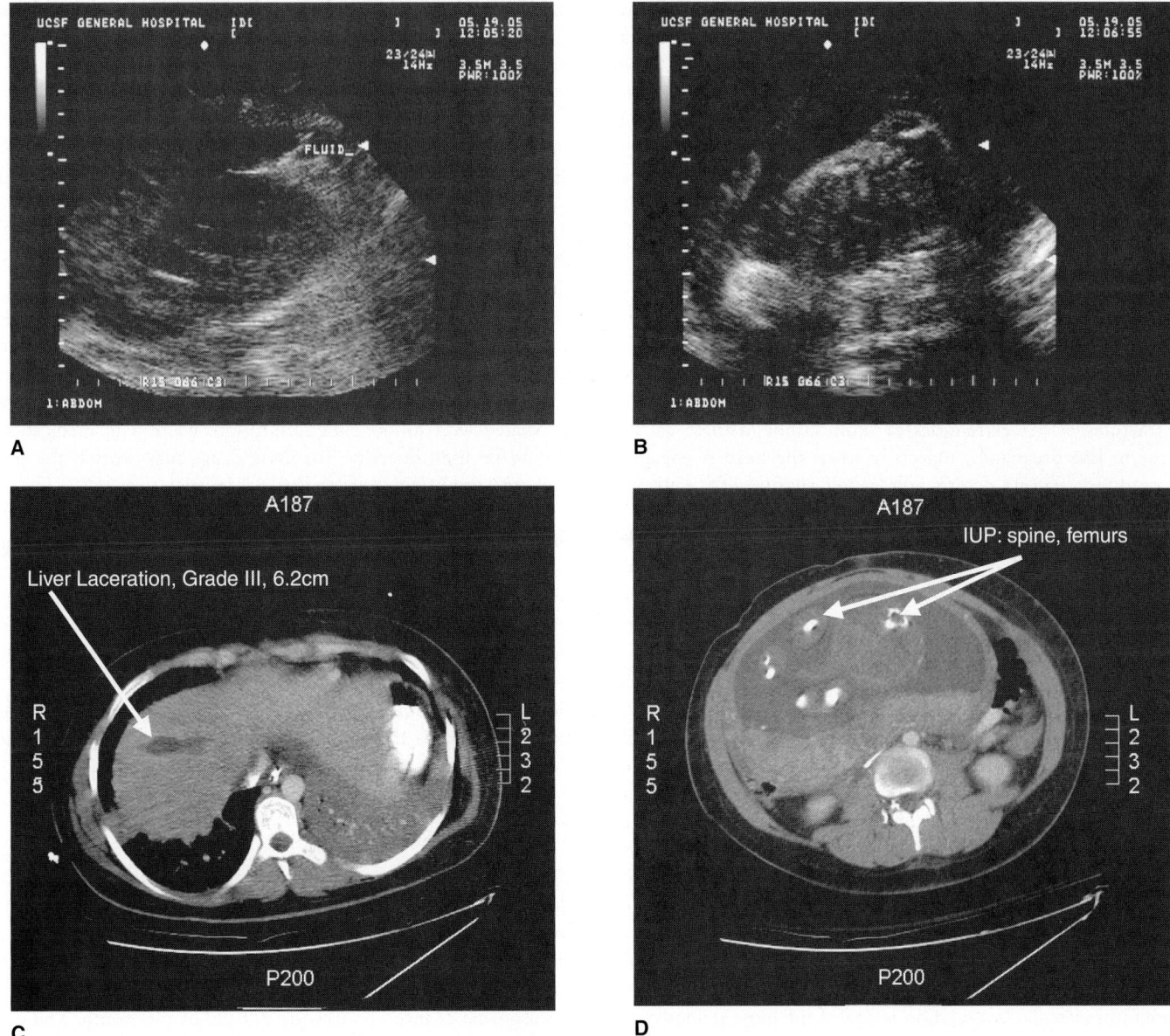

**FIGURE 40-6.** **(A)** Left upper quadrant ultrasound exam of an injured gravid patient demonstrating fluid above the spleen. **(B)** Ultrasound of the fetus in same patient showing ample amount of amniotic fluid and intact pregnancy. **(C)** CT of the mother showing liver laceration as cause of free fluid (blood) seen on ultrasound. **(D)** CT of fetus showing no injuries.

Although preterm labor was significantly higher in the last trimester, fetal loss was not. The authors concluded that the severity of the underlying disease, not the operation, was the most important factor in determining fetal and maternal outcome. There are also important anesthetic considerations when performing surgery during pregnancy. The basic objectives in the anesthetic management of these patients include the following: (a) maternal safety; (b) avoidance of teratogenic drugs; (c) avoidance of intrauterine fetal asphyxia; and (d) prevention of preterm labor.[51] While a complete review of this subject is beyond the scope of this chapter, most studies to date indicate that surgery and anesthesia during pregnancy are likely not to be associated with an increased incidence of congenital anomalies, but may produce a slightly increased risk of miscarriage. When emergency surgery is required, the optimal anesthetic for the mother should be chosen and modified by considerations for maternal physiologic changes and fetal

well-being.[51] An obstetrician and/or perinatologist should be consulted if there is time, and intraoperative fetal and uterine monitoring should be standard.

## Pelvic Fractures

The management of a pelvic fracture following blunt trauma may be particularly challenging during late pregnancy. Hemorrhage from massively dilated retroperitoneal vessels can obviously cause hemorrhagic shock.[52] Pelvic fracture is the most common injury to the mother that results in fetal death, with a fetal mortality rate as high as 35%.[53] Fetal death may result indirectly from maternal shock or placental laceration or may be caused by direct injury to the head. Although management of hemorrhage may include pelvic angiography and embolization of bleeding vessels, the dose of radiation associated with this approach usually exceeds the threshold considered safe during pregnancy, and these patients should be appropriately counseled. Operative fixation of unstable pelvic fractures, including acetabular fractures, has been reported during pregnancy, with good outcomes for both the mother and the fetus.[54,55] The dose of radiation can be minimized and procedures chosen that do not rely heavily on radiographic control. Some of these patients have gone on to have normal vaginal deliveries within weeks of their pelvic fracture surgery.

## Fetal Injuries Following Blunt Trauma

The fetus is generally well protected from blunt forces by the pelvic bones (until the third trimester) and by the cushion of amniotic fluid. Occasionally, blunt trauma to the fetus may result in fractures of the extremities or skull, although these usually occur in late pregnancy, especially when the head is engaged. Severe blunt trauma occasionally causes rupture of the uterus. Manifestations of uterine rupture include severe maternal shock, a uterus small for dates, and presence of fetal parts outside the uterus. While the diagnosis of this catastrophic event is usually not difficult, in less severe cases ultrasound is very sensitive in detecting uterine rupture and the presence of intraperitoneal hemorrhage.[56]

More commonly, blunt abdominal trauma causes separation of the placenta from the relatively inelastic uterine wall, a condition termed *placental abruption* (or *abruptio placenta*). While minor placenta abruptions may be tolerated by the fetus, major abruptions are the most common cause of fetal death if the mother survives. Separation of the placenta from the uterus reduces the area for feto-maternal exchange of respiratory gases and delivery of nutrients for the fetus. Perinatal death associated with placental abruption may be due to anoxia, prematurity, or exsanguination. The manifestations of placental abruption include vaginal bleeding (which may be relatively minor), abdominal pain, uterine tenderness, and contractions.[57] Disseminated intravascular coagulation is one of the most serious complications associated with abruption, as thromboplastins from the injured placenta enter into the maternal circulation. In the absence of clinical symptoms, pelvic ultrasound may be useful but will miss minor abruptions. As discussed earlier in the chapter, CTM is the most useful method of detecting clinically silent cases of placental separation that result in fetal distress.

## Penetrating Trauma

As the uterus expands out of the pelvis in the later stages of pregnancy, it frequently becomes the target for penetrating trauma. Low-velocity stab wounds rarely penetrate the thick uterine wall and usually present little risk to either the mother or her unborn child. Death of the mother after abdominal gunshot wounds is similarly uncommon, as only 20 to 30% have injuries outside of the uterus.[58] In contrast, gunshot wounds to the upper abdomen can result in severe maternal damage, as the abdominal organs and vasculature are compressed into this small space. Up to 70% of the fetuses will sustain injuries following abdominal gunshot wounds, and 40 to 65% will die, depending on the injury and the degree of prematurity.[59] If the bullet has penetrated the uterus and the fetus is both viable and alive, cesarean section should be performed and

the baby's injuries addressed surgically, if indicated. Successful outcome with this approach has been reported.

## Burns in Pregnancy

Burns occurring during pregnancy are not uncommon, particularly in major burn centers and in developing countries. While the treatment of the burned patient during pregnancy does not differ significantly from the patient in the nongravid state (see Chap. 50), there are certain caveats to be considered. First, fluid resuscitation should be particularly vigorous, given the expanded intravascular volume during normal pregnancy. Second, hypoxia must be avoided, and this may be particularly challenging in patients with inhalational injury associated with the burn. Silver sulfadiazine cream should be used sparingly because of the risk of kernicterus associated with sulfonamide absorption, while pain medications should be used liberally. Tocolytic drugs may worsen the pulmonary complications of inhalational injuries.

A review of reports on the outcomes of burn injuries during pregnancy shows relatively favorable results. Miscarriage is more common in the first trimester and is often related to septic complications.[60–62] Adequate treatment of shock and early excision with grafting result in improved maternal and fetal survival. In one prospective study of 50 pregnant burned patients, pregnancy did not alter maternal survival, and only the total body surface area was significant in predicting adverse outcome for the fetus and the mother.[63] Venous thrombosis may also complicate burn injuries during pregnancy.[64]

## Cesarean Section Following Injury

Guidelines for performing cesarean section following trauma as developed by the ACOG for the mother *in extremis* following a medical disaster (i.e., amniotic fluid embolism, major cardiac event) are summarized in Table 40-5. These guidelines apply to infants who are at least 25 weeks of gestation and thus would have a reasonable chance of surviving outside of the womb. The data suggest that if a fetus is delivered within five minutes of maternal death, the anticipated fetal survival rate is 70%.[65]

In a study representing nine major trauma centers, 441 pregnant trauma patients were reviewed, including 32 patients who required cesarean section for either maternal or fetal distress.[66] Fifteen (45%) of the fetuses and 23 (72%) of the 32 mothers survived. Thirteen of the fetuses delivered had no fetal heart tones and none survived, whereas 20 infants with both fetal heart tones and an estimated gestational age of 26 weeks or more had a 75% survival rate. Five of the infants who died were potentially salvageable (i.e., had both fetal heart tones and an estimated gestational age of ≥26 weeks), but there was delayed recognition of fetal distress among mothers with moderate injuries (ISS <16). The use of CTM was not universal among these patients even in these experienced trauma centers. The algorithm proposed from this study for emergency and perimortem cesarean section following maternal trauma is shown in Fig. 40-7.

In most trauma centers, an obstetrician should be readily available to perform a cesarean section for fetal or maternal distress. Should the trauma surgeon be in the position to perform this operation, the key to success is the use of large incisions. A long, vertical abdominal incision is used to access the uterus, followed by a midline vertical incision

## TABLE 40-5

### Postmortem Cesarean Section

**PREDICTORS OF SUCCESSFUL FETAL OUTCOME FOLLOWING POSTMORTEM CEASAREAN SECTION**

1. Duration of gestation
   Fetal viability generally is defined as = 26–28 weeks' gestation. This corresponds to a fundal height of approximately 26–28 cm above the pubis and/or uterus, halfway between the umbilicus and costal margin. At this age, the fetus, under optimal conditions, has a 40–70% estimated chance of survival without major handicap; therefore, cesarean section is indicated shortly after maternal death.
2. Time between maternal death and delivery
   <5 min, excellent
   5–10 min, good
   10–15 min, fair
   15–20 min, poor
   20–25 min, unlikely

**Procedure**

1. Establish viability
2. Complete the cardiopulmonary resuscitation (CPR) sequence
3. Make a vertical midline incision through the abdominal layers into the uterus
4. Remove the fetus from the uterine cavity, clamp the cord, and hand the neonate to appropriate personnel for resuscitation
5. Remove the placenta
6. Continue CPR and assess for maternal signs of life; maternal survival is still possible after the uterus has been emptied and the supine hypotension syndrome has been resolved.

Adapted with permission from Higgins SO: Perinatal protocol: Trauma in pregnancy. *J Perinatol.* 1988;8:288; and Seldin BS, Burke TJ: Complete maternal and fetal recovery after prolonged cardiac arrest. *Ann Emrg Med* 17:346, 1988.

through the upper uterine segment. The infant is removed immediately and suctioned, the cord is clamped and cut, and resuscitation initiated on the baby while the surgeon simultaneously tamponades bleeding from the placenta and uterine wall of the mother.

In the study using data from the **NTDB** cited above, Ikossi reported that among the 1195 pregnant women on whom data were available, 1178 survived, 17 died, and 66 pregnancies were lost.[10] Of those patients who delivered their infant during their trauma admission, 75% underwent cesarean section. This is a threefold greater rate than the national average of 13–22%. Also, 75% of these cesarean sections were performed within 24 hours of admission, implying urgent operation. The indications for delivery (fetal or maternal distress etc.) are not currently available in the NTDB, nor are the outcomes of the fetuses. Only 3% of records included fetal monitoring in the data submitted, but this is likely underreported as there is no separate coding field for CTM data in the NTDB. The data capture fields on both the infant and the mother contained in the NTDB will need to be expanded in order to get a more complete picture of the impact of trauma on fetal outcome.

## CRITICAL CARE OBSTETRICS

During pregnancy, the cardiorespiratory status of the patient is in a dynamic state. It is modified by gestational age, maternal position, labor, and peripartum blood loss. A basic understanding of these changes in maternal cardiorespiratory function is required for optimal care of the critically ill obstetric patient. As compared to the nongravid state, pregnancy is associated with significant increases in heart rate (17%), stroke volume (23%), and cardiac output (+43%) as previously noted. Table 40-2 illustrates the central hemodynamic changes associated with pregnancy.

Hyperventilation begins in early pregnancy, secondary to the effect of progesterone and continues as the uterus enlarges. The underlying chronic respiratory alkalosis is partially compensated by increased renal excretion of bicarbonate into the urine. Oxygen consumption and the basal metabolic rate increase by 21% and

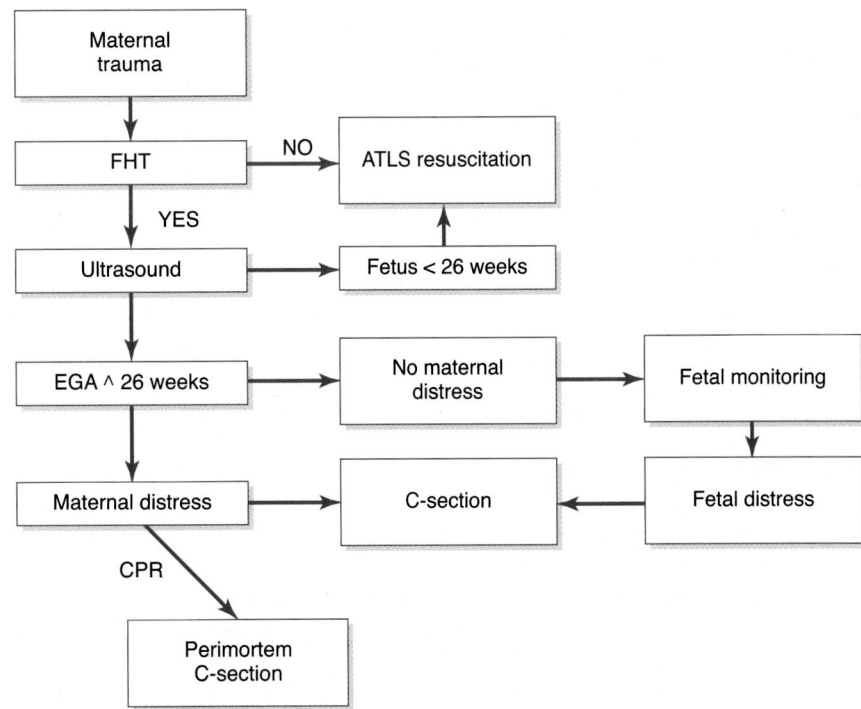

**FIGURE 40-7.** Algorithm for emergency cesarean section following trauma in pregnancy. CPR, cardiopulmonary resuscitation; EGA, estimated gestational age; FHT, fetal heart tones.
*(Reproduced with permission from Morris JA, Rosenbower TJ, Jurkovich GJ, et al.: Infant survival after cesarean section for trauma. Ann Surg 223:481, 1996.)*

14%, respectively.[16] Therefore, assessment of the critically ill mother and her fetus is based on an understanding of normal maternal-fetal physiology.

## Maternal-Fetal Physiology

The supply of oxygen from mother to fetus is affected by the oxygen saturation and oxygen-carrying capacity of maternal blood and by the magnitude of uterine blood flow. As oxygen is transported from the mother to the fetus through uterine and then umbilical vessels, there is a stepwise decrement in the $PaO_2$; however, the following mechanisms maximize fetal oxygenation:

1. Fetal oxygen uptake per unit body weight exceeds that of adults.
2. There is an increased affinity of fetal hemoglobin for oxygen because the fetus functions on a different oxyhemoglobin dissociation curve.

The advantage of this high oxygen affinity is that each fetal red blood cell that travels through the placenta returns to the fetus almost fully saturated with oxygen. Furthermore, the increase in maternal blood volume and uterine blood flow allow for adequate uterine perfusion and physiology, hence maximizing oxygen delivery to the placenta.

Whenever oxygen content of fetal blood is reduced by more than 50%, the fetus responds with brief episodes of bradycardia, which manifest themselves as late decelerations in heart rate. Major trauma with acute hemorrhage reduces the oxygen-carrying capacity of maternal blood and diminishes maternal cardiac output, hence restricting uterine blood flow. The release of catecholamines causes vasoconstriction and a redistribution of blood flow to other organs. As a protective mechanism, the fetus is able to reduce blood flow to viscera and, therefore, maximizes cerebral blood flow. All of these factors reduce fetal oxygenation, although maternal oxygen saturation may still be above 90%. Increasing the maternal $PaO_2$ by even small amounts results in favorable changes in the oxygen content of the fetus because the fetus is operating on the steep portion of the oxyhemoglobin dissociation curve (see Fig. 40-2). Similarly, a decrease in maternal $PaO_2$ to below 60 mm ;Hg results in an even greater decline in fetal oxygen content.[67] Because oxygenation depends on blood flow, uterine blood flow should be maximized in the critically ill gravida to ensure adequate fetal oxygenation. Avoidance of the supine position, with its potential to occlude the maternal vena cava, diminish preload, and reduce cardiac output, is essential in maintaining uterine blood flow.

Some diagnoses common to critically ill obstetric patients will be discussed in the light of these principles of maternal–fetal physiology.

## Pregnancy-Induced Hypertension

Although the diagnosis of PIH is based on the findings of hypertension, proteinuria, and edema, the most severe form is characterized by the following: (a) a systolic blood pressure of 160 mm Hg or more and a diastolic pressure of 110 mm Hg or more; (b) oliguria; (c) proteinuria of 5 g per 24 hour, or 3+ on urinalysis; (d) disturbances in cerebral function; and (e) pulmonary edema. Seizures may occur and persist for up to one week after delivery in patients with PIH. Although PIH occurs in approximately 5 to 10% of all pregnancies, the most severe form is recognized in only 0.1% of

pregnancies. Nulliparous patients with a family history of this condition are at greatest risk for its occurrence.

The most serious complications of severe preeclampsia are the eclamptic seizure itself (due to vasogenic cerebral edema), intracerebral hemorrhage, blindness, acute tubular/cortical necrosis, cardiac failure, pulmonary edema, and disseminated intravascular coagulation. From the standpoint of the fetus, intrauterine growth retardation (IUGR) is a common complication.

Although it resolves upon delivery, preeclampsia always worsens the longer the pregnancy continues. The first principle of treatment for preeclampsia at term is delivery. A dose of 4 to 6 g magnesium sulfate is given intravenously for the prevention of seizures. This dose is given over 20 minutes and then continued at 2 g/hour. Hydralazine hydrochloride (Apresoline) in a 5- to 10-mg intravenous bolus dose is the antihypertensive drug of choice, and it is given if the diastolic blood pressure is above 105 mm Hg. Neonatal thrombocytopenia and secondary bleeding have been associated with the use of hydralazine, which readily crosses the placenta. This potent antihypertensive agent should be administered cautiously to avoid a rapid, profound reduction in blood pressure, which would in turn decrease uteroplacental blood flow and reduce oxygen delivery to the fetus. Small incremental doses of 5 to 10 mg intravenously every 20 minutes are preferable. An intraarterial catheter is recommended for continuous measurement of the maternal blood pressure.

A low serum oncotic pressure and increased capillary permeability in pre-eclampsia result in significant fluid shifts. Considering the potential for multisystem organ dysfunction with this disease process, invasive hemodynamic monitoring with special attention to normovolemia is important, especially prior to antihypertensive therapy.

## Amniotic Fluid Embolism

Although uncommon, amniotic fluid embolism (AFE) is associated with a maternal mortality as high as 80%. This condition and pulmonary thromboembolism remain the leading causes of maternal mortality in the United States.[68] In addition to having hemodynamic instability and pulmonary compromise, 40% of patients surviving the initial injury may develop a coagulopathy ranging from minor disturbances in the platelet count to disseminated intravascular coagulation (see Chap. 61). Because the introduction of small amounts of amniotic fluid into the maternal circulation is considered relatively benign, it is thought that AFE is due to abnormal amniotic fluid containing abnormal substances entering the maternal pulmonary circulation. It is postulated that these abnormal substances may be leukotrienes or arachidonic acid metabolites.[69]

The classic presentation of AFE is that of sudden dyspnea and hypotension, often with subsequent cardiorespiratory arrest. The diagnosis is based on the clinical presentation and supportive laboratory studies. Treatment is directed toward oxygenation, maintenance of cardiac output and blood pressure, and correction of the coagulopathy.

## Deep Venous Thrombosis and Pulmonary Embolism

Thromboembolic disease remains the major cause of maternal morbidity and mortality during pregnancy and also during the

**TABLE 40-6**

### Changes in Hemostasis in Mid to Late Pregnancy

**Changes Promoting Thrombosis**
Increased levels of factors V, VII, VIII, IX, X and XII and fibrinogen
Placental inhibitors of fibrinolysis
Tissue thromboplastin released into the circulation at placental separation
Venous stasis of the lower extremities
Endothelial damage associated with parturition

**Changes discouraging thrombosis**
Decreased levels of factors XI and XIII
PAPP-A, a pregnancy-specific protein neutralizing AT III

*Adapted from Rutherford SE, Phelan P. Deep venous thrombosis and pulmonary embolism, in Clark SL. Cotton DB, Hankins GOV. Pheen JP (eds): Critical Care Obostetrics. 2nd ed. Boston: Blackwell, 1991, p 150. Adapted by permission of Blackwell Science, Inc.*

puerperium. Whether the clinician is dealing with major or minor trauma, the risks of thromboembolic disease should be minimized.

Pregnancy is a hypercoagulable state because of increased levels of factors XII, IX, VII, X, VIII, and V and fibrinogen in the maternal blood. In comparison, factors XI and XIII and plasma fibrinolytic activity decrease as a result of placental inhibitors. The increased tendency toward hypercoagulability is partly balanced by a pregnancy-specific protein called PAPP-A, which facilitates the neutralization of thrombin by antithrombin III.[70] The net effect on hemostasis is an increased potential for thrombosis that is most marked at term and in the immediate puerperium. Table 40-6 summarizes the changes in hemostasis in pregnancy.

In addition to these changes in hemostasis, other risk factors associated with deep venous thrombosis and pulmonary embolism (DVT/PE) during pregnancy include older maternal age, the presence of neurologic injuries, parity, prolonged immobilization, the presence of pelvic or lower extremity fractures, venous injuries, and inherited deficiencies in the natural inhibitors of coagulation. A history of a prior episode of DVT also greatly increases the risk of thromboembolism during both the postinjury period and pregnancy.[71,72] A large review that included 1602 episodes of venous thromboembolic (VTE) complications following trauma has helped to stratify the major risk factors after injury.[73] The odds ratios and 95% confidence intervals for the major risk factors for VTE following trauma are listed below:

| | |
|---|---|
| Age ≥ 40 years | OR = 2.01 (1.74–2.32) |
| Lower extremity fracture (AIS ≥ 3) | OR = 1.92 (1.64–2.26) |
| Head injury (AIS ≥ 3) | OR = 1.24 (1.05–1.46) |
| Ventilator days > 3 | OR = 8.08 (6.86–9.52) |
| Venous injury | OR = 3.56 (2.25–5.72) |
| Major operative procedure | OR = 1.53 (1.30–1.80) |

Unfortunately, no method of prophylaxis against thromboembolism has been shown to be both safe and 100% effective in the multisystem injured or gravid patient. To date, the most effective method appears to be the subcutaneous administration of the low molecular weight heparin (LMWH) enoxaparin twice daily in prophylactic doses (30 mg BID).[74] In pregnancy, enoxaparin is both safer and more effective than standard heparin. It does not cross the placenta and thus presents a low risk to the fetus. Should DVT or PE

develop despite prophylaxis, full dose (1 m/kg) enoxaparin can be safely administered to the gravid mother. The use of LMWH within two hours prior to cesarean section has been associated with an increased incidence of wound hematomas. Additional studies on the enoxaparin concentrations and dose adjustments during pregnancy where factor Xa is overexpressed (see Table 40-6) are indicated. Based on her extensive reviews, Knudson developed an algorithm for the use of prophylaxis based on the relative risks for VTE after trauma.[73] For patients with high-risk factors, LMWH is recommended if there is no contraindication. For patients with very high-risk factors (see odds ratios above) either a combination of LMWH and mechanical compression should be considered combined with surveillance scanning with color flow duplex. Experience with vena caval filters, either prophylactically in very high-risk patients or therapeutically for established thromboembolic complications, is very limited in both the trauma setting and during pregnancy.

## Premature Labor

Preterm labor may result from trauma, although the true incidence of this complication is unknown. Premature labor is defined as uterine contractions combined with cervical change (effacement or dilation). In one study of relatively minor trauma, less than 1% of patients demonstrated preterm labor, whereas following severe trauma, most patients will exhibit some degree of uterine contractile activity.[31,33] While most of these contractions will resolve spontaneously over time, some patients may benefit from the pharmacologic inhibition of labor by the administration of tocolytic drugs. Drugs currently available for tocolysis include sympathomimetics such as terbutaline, indomethacin, and calcium channel blockers (nifedipine).[3] All these drugs have side effects that may complicate their use in trauma patients. Magnesium sulfate may cause hypotension and mental status changes, whereas indomethacin has been associated with oligohydramnios and promotes closure of the ductus arteriosus in the fetus.[3] Additionally, indomethacin may produce bleeding in the trauma patient. Alpha-adrenergic drugs produce tachycardia, may mask blood loss, and may induce chest pain. The use of calcium channel blockers is associated with hypotension.[3] Tocolytic drugs should not be used in patients with active vaginal bleeding or suspected placental abruption, because blood may accumulate inside a relaxed uterus. Other contraindications to tocolysis include preeclampsia, eclampsia, uncontrolled diabetes mellitus, serious cardiac disease, and cervical dilatation greater than 4 cm. In patients in the last trimester of pregnancy who develop contractions or premature labor, dexamethasone is administered in order to hasten lung maturation in the premature baby should delivery be necessary.

## Infectious Complications in Pregnancy

In patients who survive their initial trauma, many will succumb to infections in the intensive care unit. Evidence suggests that abdominal infections may be particularly harmful to the fetus. Mays and others described three pregnancies complicated by acute appendicitis and refractory labor, resulting in the delivery of neonates with major intraventricular hemorrhage and periventricular leukomalacia.[75] These neonatal complications correlate with cerebral palsy, but the exact mechanism by which maternal infection causes injury to the fetal brain is unknown. In the pregnant trauma patient, missed intestinal injuries can produce such disastrous results, and these injuries must be diligently searched for and promptly treated. Similarly, established infections deserve aggressive antibiotic therapy and/or operative intervention when appropriate. Consultation from both obstetrical and infectious disease services in the use of antibiotics is recommended, as many drugs have adverse effects on the fetus. For a complete review of pharmacology in pregnancy, readers are referred to the excellent book by Briggs and colleagues and the ACOG bulletin on teratology.[23,76]

## Neurologic Injury During Pregnancy

The multi-institutional study by Kissinger and associates was the first to demonstrate the adverse effect of moderate and severe (Glasgow Coma Scale Score < 12) trauma to the brain on fetal outcome.[77] Severe injury to the brain also emerged as a significant risk factor for pregnancy loss in the investigation conducted by Ikossi and others.[10] Certainly, maternal hypothalamic and pituitary dysfunction may accompany catastrophic brain injuries, and replacement of cortisone, thyroid, and vasopressin hormones may be required.[78] Kelley and colleagues examined the function of both the anterior and posterior pituitary of 22 head-injured patients of both sexes and demonstrated some degree of hypopituitarism in 40% of patients with moderate to severe injuries to the brain.[79] Growth hormone and gonadotrophic deficiencies were the most commonly observed disorders. In addition, nutritional support, seizure control, and avoidance of infections and thrombotic complications are required to ensure normal growth and development.

The care of the pregnant patient with an acute injury to the spinal cord (see Chap. 24) is also challenging. For an extensive review of this subject, readers are referred to the excellent articles by Gilson and coworkers, and Popov and others.[80,81]

## PREDICTING OUTCOME FOLLOWING TRAUMA AND PREGNANCY

Although it is generally recognized that the most common cause of fetal death following trauma is maternal death, the actual ratio of fetal to maternal deaths ranges from 3:1 to 9:1.[77,82] Several attempts have been made to identify factors that would predict a poor fetal outcome following trauma during pregnancy.[10,77,82–90] While not all studies are in agreement, it appears that maternal physiologic variables are poor predictors of fetal outcome. Factors generally associated with risk to the fetus include the following:

- Maternal hypotension
- Traumatic brain injury
- High Injury Severity Score
- Pelvic fracture
- Ejection from a vehicle
- Severe abdominal injury

A recent population-based study by Schiff and others examined the outcomes of both mother and infant after injury during pregnancy in a ten-year review including 266 nonseverely injured gravid women (ISS of 1–8) and 28 severely injured women (ISS > 9) who delivered during their hospitalization

### TABLE 40-7

**Risk Factors for Loss of Pregnancy After Trauma**

| RISK FACTOR | ODDS RATIO |
| --- | --- |
| ISS > 15 | 9.17 |
| GCS < 8 | 5.24 |
| AIS > 3 | |
|     Head | 3.02 |
|     Thorax | 2.29 |
|     Abdomen | 5.63 |
|     Lower extremity | 3.98 |

(From: Ikossi DG, Lazar AA, MOrabito D, et al.: Profile of Mothers at Risk: An Analysis of Injury and Pregnancy Loss in 1,195 Trauma Patients. J Am Coll Surg 200:49, 2005.)

after injury.[88] Even the nonseverely injured pregnant women were at increased risk of placental abruption and their infants were at increased risk of suffering hypoxia and fetal death. Severely injured pregnant women were at a 17-fold increased risk of placental abruption and their infants were at increased risk of prematurity, low birth weight, and fetal distress, and had a 30-fold greater risk of fetal death. In a similar study from California, women who delivered at the trauma hospital (Group 1) were compared with women who had a history of trauma during their pregnancy but delivered during a second hospitalization (Group 2), and with nontrauma controls.[89] As would be anticipated, Group 1 women had the worst outcomes, with an odds ratio (OR) of 60 for maternal death, 4.7 for fetal death, 43 for uterine rupture, and 9.2 for placental abruption. Group 2 women sustained a 2.7-fold increase in premature labor and a four-fold increased risk of maternal death compared with uninjured women. Group 2 women also had higher rates of premature delivery and low birth weight at delivery compared to uninjured pregnant women, raising the suggestion that chronic abruptions secondary to trauma may lead to placental insufficiency and fetal compromise. In the large study compiled from data in the NTDB, the odds ratios for loss of a pregnancy after trauma were calculated based on the nature of the injury.[10] As can be seen in Table 40-7, injuries to the head and abdomen carried the highest risk, as did an overall ISS of >15.

## INJURY PREVENTION DURING PREGNANCY

These poor outcomes for both the mother and her fetus associated with even relatively minor trauma highlight the need for attention to injury prevention during pregnancy, and three areas of injury prevention deserve specific attention. The first involves the use of drugs and alcohol (see Chap. 45). An alarming number of women test positive for illegal drugs and/or alcohol when they are injured during their pregnancy. Ikossi reported that 13% of pregnant women tested positive for alcohol at the time of their trauma admission and 20% were using illicit drugs.[10] Not only are these substances known to be harmful to the unborn child, but the association between their use and both intentional and unintentional injuries has been well-documented.[76] Prenatal care must include education on the subject of substance abuse and provide opportunities for treatment for those women with a history of alcohol abuse.

The role of interpersonal violence as a cause of trauma in pregnancy has been largely ignored until recently.[6-8] McLeer and Anwar reported that after ED staff were trained to recognize signs of battery, the number of women seeking emergency care who were identified as being physically abused rose from 6 to 30%.[91] Similarly, McFarlane and coworkers, using a three-question Abuse Assessment Screen, detected a 17% prevalence of physical or sexual abuse during pregnancy, with 60% of women reporting two or more episodes of assault.[8] These investigators emphasize that pregnancy is the only time that healthy women come into frequent contact with health care providers, thus offering a unique opportunity to intervene in cases of abuse during pregnancy. In another study of 203 injured pregnant patients, 32% were victims of intentional injury.[91] In most cases, the husband or boyfriend was the offender. The incidence of fetal loss was surprisingly high in this group of battered women. In addition to fetal loss, abuse during pregnancy has been associated with low fetal birth weight, low maternal weight gain, maternal infections, anemia, and maternal alcohol and drug abuse.

Interpersonal violence is not dependent on race, age, marital status, or socioeconomic status (see Chap. 48), thus making all pregnant women potential victims of abuse.[92] A history of depression, substance abuse, or multiple visits to the ED should raise the level of suspicion for abuse, as should the presence of an overprotective partner.[92] Abused women may initially delay seeking medical attention or give an implausible explanation for injuries. A history of "spontaneous" abortion, miscarriages, and premature labor may also indicate violence occurring during pregnancy. Physical signs of abuse may include bruises on the breasts, abdomen, head, neck, or upper extremities, as well as the presence of injuries at multiple sites in various stages of healing. Recognition and intervention in cases of abuse can prevent subsequent serious injuries to both the mother and her fetus.

Despite the recognition that fetal deaths are far more common in women who are ejected from moving vehicles, Agran and her colleagues found that in nine cases of fetal deaths resulting from motor vehicular trauma in Orange County, California, none of the mothers were restrained.[93] In another study, unrestrained pregnant women were 1.9 times more likely to have a low-birth weight baby and 2.3 times more likely to give birth within 48 hours of a crash.[94] In New Mexico, where seat belt use was mandated in 1986, a 1992 study found that only 16% of women had received any information about the use of seat belts during pregnancy, one-third were uncertain about the safety of seat belts during pregnancy, and 26% did not know the correct way to position the seat belt during pregnancy[95] (see Fig. 40-8). Another study from California demonstrated that most women used restraints during pregnancy, but since only 21% were educated on their proper application during pregnancy, most were using them incorrectly.[96] A comprehensive biomechanical program aimed at improving the safety of pregnant women and their fetuses in motor vehicle crashes is currently under way in several states.[97,98] Although the experience with air bags is limited, Sims and associates concluded that the combination of air bags and lap/shoulder restraints had no untoward effect on pregnancy.[99] It seems intuitive that prenatal visits provide an excellent opportunity to educate women in these important areas of injury prevention.

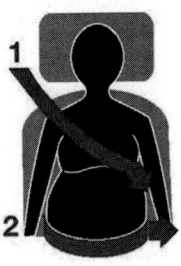

Source:
http://www.thinkroadsafety.gov.uk/campaigns/seatbelts/pregnant.htm

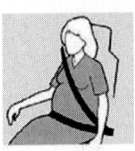

Source:
http://www.ghsp.ky.gov/seat_belt_ky_law.htm

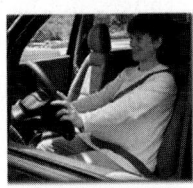

Source:
http://www.webmd.com/baby/tc/Pregnancy-Common-Concerns

**PREGNANT WOMEN**

- **Wear lap belt below abdomen.**
- **Wear shoulder belt across chest**
- **If your seat belt is too short, consult auto dealer for seat belt extender.**

**FIGURE 40-8.** Figure demonstrating proper use of restraint devices in pregnant patient.

## TRAUMA IN THE NONPREGNANT PATIENT

The female reproductive organs are usually well protected by their location deep within the pelvis, making injuries to these organs relatively uncommon except during pregnancy or states in which they are pathologically enlarged. Occasionally, severe blunt trauma may injure the female genital system. Such injuries should be suspected in the presence of pelvic fractures. In young girls, the three most common types of accidental injury to the external genitalia are straddle injuries, accidental penetration, and tearing due to sudden forced stretching of the perineum when the legs are abducted suddenly, such as in gymnastics or in falls.[100] Female athletes, in general, are also at risk for genital trauma. Sexual assault can result in genital injury, as well as other bodily injuries. Less commonly, a wandering missile from a firearm may injure the otherwise normal female reproductive organs. Missed or improperly treated female genital injuries can result in hemorrhage, sepsis, and the loss of endocrine and reproductive function.

### Etiology of Injury

**Penetrating Injury.** Although the true incidence of penetrating injuries to the female genital tract is largely unknown, isolated injuries to its organs are rare in the nongravid state.[101] These injuries are discovered during routine laparotomy following firearm-related trauma and in selected cases of abdominal stab wounds. The organ most commonly involved is the uterus, followed by the fallopian tubes, ovaries, and cervix. Often, these organs are either pathologically enlarged or the injuries occur in the early postpartum period. Impalement injuries represent another form of penetrating trauma that may involve the female genital tract. As with any perineal injury, associated intra-abdominal trauma must always be suspected in cases of female genital injury. Dowd and coworkers reviewed the charts of 100 patients with straddle injury, of which 72% were female.[102] Three of the 72 girls had injuries involving an unintentional penetrating mechanism including a fall onto the handle of a plunger, impalement on a sharp fencepost while climbing, and a fall on the steering column of a bicycle after the handlebars came off while riding. In one case, there was penetration into the peritoneum through the vagina. The resulting penetrating injuries were characteristically different from those caused by blunt mechanisms. In Onen's review of 80 girls suffering genital trauma, 14 girls or 18% sustained their injury after falling onto a penetrating object .[103] Isolated penetrating genital trauma was associated with sexual abuse over half the time (57%).

Blunt Trauma.    As stated earlier, the relative protection offered to the upper female genital tract guards these organs against injury in all but very severe forms of blunt trauma. The largest reported experience with such injuries was in the Maryland Institute for Emergency Medical Services Systems in 1984.[104] The authors of this report described 13 cases of hemorrhage into ovarian cysts, one case of ovarian laceration, and one case of uterine and vaginal lacerations that followed motor-vehicle-related trauma. The injuries were discovered at laparotomy, which was performed after a positive DPL. In 13 patients, the hemorrhage was produced by a follicular ovarian cyst. Seven of these 13 patients had an associated pelvic fracture, and nine had lacerations of the bladder or iliac veins.

In contrast to injuries of the upper genital organs, injuries to the perineum and lower tract occur relatively frequently. Children and athletes are particularly vulnerable to perineal trauma. Sports such as gymnastics, water-skiing, and bicycling are associated with straddle-type trauma. The injuries produced by straddle trauma are due to forced compression of the soft tissues between the object straddled and the underlying pubic symphysis and rami.[105] These injuries include hematomas or lacerations of the labia, clitoris, and vagina and urethral tears. Urinary retention may accompany this type of trauma. Both the urinary tract and the rectum must be carefully evaluated for associated injuries following sports-related genital trauma.[105] Several groups have investigated genital injuries in children. McAleer and associates examined a series of 117 pediatric patients (47 girls) with genitourinary trauma over a six-year period, with 98% sustaining injuries secondary to motor vehicle trauma.[106] Sadly, only 9% of these children were properly restrained. Eight of these children were found to have vaginal injuries. In another study examining 116 children seen for genital trauma, 39% of the 80 girls in the study sustained hymen or vaginal lacerations and 47% had associated anorectal injuries, while only 8% suffered intra-abdominal injury.[103] Once again, motor vehicle crash was the most common mechanism of injury (46%), followed by falls (32%).

Pokorny and coworkers summarized the acute genital injuries seen in 32 prepubertal girls.[107] Most of the injuries in these young patients resulted from falling on objects or bicycle bars. Although painful and sometimes hemorrhagic, most of these straddle injuries were not associated with injuries to intra-abdominal organs. In contrast, symmetrical injuries that transect the hymen indicate that the weakest point in the perineal floor has received the force of the causative agent and that internal pelvic and abdominal injuries are possible. Only two of the 32 injuries in the series reported by Pokorny and coworkers resulted from motor vehicle related trauma.

In a ten-year review of major perineal trauma in children seen at one Canadian trauma center, 22 children sustained perineal trauma sufficiently severe to injure the rectum, urethra, or vagina.[108] Traffic-related crashes were the main cause of urethral injuries, while impalement was the principal mechanism of injury in children with rectal tears. One-third of the children had more than one major perineal injury, emphasizing the need for a complete evaluation.

Sexual Assault.    Sexual assault must also be considered a potential cause of perineal injury when there is severe or extensive injury that does not correlate with the history or when there is a concomitant nongenital injury (e.g., facial or extremity bruising) and a large hymenal tear.[102] Other signs of intentional injuries include high vaginal lacerations or contusion, rectal mucosal trauma, the presence of abnormal secretions, and evidence of previous injuries.[109]

Many women who are victims of sexual assault do not suffer physical injury. Only 20 to 32% of sexual assault victims had evidence of genital trauma upon examination by a gynecologist within 72 hours.[110–112] Also, 46 to 68% of sexual assault victims suffered nongenital injuries, usually injuries to soft tissue.[110–112] Genital injury was almost exclusively found in women who also suffered other injuries.[110] In a specialized center reporting a series of 766 women presenting after sexual assault, healthcare providers specially trained to identify genital injuries utilizing colposcopy and nuclear stains determined the rate of genital injury to be as high as 69%.[113] Genital injuries from sexual assault can be severe. In a report of reproductive tract trauma presenting to a single Level I trauma center over 12 years, 19 coitus related injuries were reported, including 15 women with severe vaginal lacerations requiring repair and seven women who presented in shock.[114] The most common genital injuries involved the posterior fourchette (49%), the anus or perianal area (23%), the vestibulum (17%), and the hymen (18%).[111] Skeletal injuries, especially pelvic fractures, have also been identified in children who were sexually abused.[115]

Risk factors associated with injury after sexual assault include assault by a stranger, threat of violence by the assailant, women without prior sexual experience, and involvement of anal penetration.[103,110,112] Injury was also more common in adolescents, and in women over the age of 50.[112,116]

## EVALUATION AND TREATMENT

### Perineal Injuries

Perineal injuries are frequently associated with straddle injuries. The perineal body was the most commonly injured area among pediatric patients who sustained blunt urogenital trauma in one series.[109] Management of perineal injuries begins with a complete examination. This may be difficult in the patient who is in pain or in whom there is profuse bleeding in the area. In these cases, an examination under anesthesia is appropriate. Examination in the ED is especially difficult in the young girl who, in addition to pain, is likely feeling embarrassed or scared. Lynch and colleagues recommend that all prepubescent girls with blunt traumatic injuries in the urogenital region be evaluated under anesthesia.[109] In their series of 22 girls with blunt urogenital trauma seen over a 24-month period, all were first evaluated in the ED by an emergency physician and a pediatric surgeon. The initial findings were then compared to those found at the time of examination under anesthesia. Of these 22 patients, 16 had more severe injuries than were initially appreciated in the ED.

Regardless of the examination setting, a complete inspection of the genital area must be made. The vulvar area is carefully inspected for external laceration, and the urethral meatus should be examined as well. A full vaginal examination is then conducted, followed by anoscopy. Finally, cystourethrograms are obtained.[106] When sexual assault is suspected, an appropriate medical-legal exam should be performed by trained personnel if the patient's

clinical situation allows it. (See Chap. 48 for more information on diagnosis and management after sexual assault.)

Because the perineum is highly vascularized, hematomas are a frequent finding in cases of trauma to this area. Simple contusions may require only ice-pack therapy and analgesics. When a hematoma is expanding or is more than 5 cm in diameter, however, incision and drainage should be considered. If the source of bleeding is readily apparent after incision of the area, the causative vessel should be cauterized or ligated. Commonly, small venous vessels are responsible for the hematoma and are difficult to find. In these cases, simple packing may be the best therapy. Alternatively, the incision site can be closed over a drain. Antibiotics are generally not indicated in cases of perineal hematoma. In a study of conservative versus operative management of vulvar and vaginal hematomas, the conservative management of large hematomas (i.e., cross-sectional diameter $\geq$ 15 cm) was associated with more complications requiring antibiotics and transfusion.[117]

Lacerations of the vulvar area should be debrided of necrotic tissue and carefully closed. Deep lacerations may require multiple layers of suture (Table 40-8). The wounds are irrigated prior

**TABLE 40-8**

| Aast Organ Injury Scaling: Vulva, Vagina, Uterus, and Ovaries | | |
|---|---|---|
| **GRADE** | **INJURY DESCRIPTION** | **RATIONATE** |
| **Vulva Injury Scale** | | |
| I | Contusion/hematoma | No therapy |
| II | Superficial laceration (skin only) | Suture simple |
| III | Deep laceration (into fat/muscle) | Suture multiple layers, drain, and/or exploration |
| IV | Avulsion (skin/fat/muscle) | Grafts |
| V | Injury into adjacent organs (anus, rectum, urethra, bladder) | Extensive therapy |
| **Vagina Injury Scale** | | |
| I | Contusion/hematoma | No therapy |
| II | Superficial laceration (skin only) | Suture, simple |
| III | Deep laceration (into adjacent fat/muscle) | Suture, multiple layers, and/or drain |
| IV | Laceration—complex into cervix | Grafts |
| V | Injury into adjacent organs (anus, rectum, urethra, bladder) | Extensive therapy |
| **Uterus (nonpregnant) Injury Scale** | | |
| I | Contusion/hematoma | No therapy |
| II | Superficial laceration (= 1 cm) | Suture, single layer |
| III | Deep laceration (> 1 cm) | Layered suture, exploration |
| IV | Laceration involving uterine artery | Suture and control of vascular supply |
| V | Avulsion/devascularization | Hysterectomy or repair |
| **Uterus (pregnant) Injury Scale** | | |
| I | Contusion/hematoma (without placental abruption) | No therapy |
| II | Superficial laceration (= 1 cm) of partial placental abruption (<25%) | Fetal monitoring, evaluation for DIC |
| III | Deep laceration (> 1 cm) or placental abruption (>25% but <50%) | Monitoring and/or delivery, evaluation for DIC |
| IV | Laceration involving uterine artery, deep laceration (> 1 cm) with 50% placental abruption | Delivery, evaluation for DIC |
| V | Uterine rupture | Emergent exploration and repair of hysterectomy |
| | Complete placental abruption | |
| **Ovary Injury Scale** | | |
| I | Contusion hematoma | No theray |
| II | Superficial laceration (= 0.5 cm) | Suture |
| III | Deep laceration (> 0.5 cm) | Multiple suture |
| IV | Partial disruption of blood supply | Repair, determine viability |
| V | Avulsion or complete parenchymal destruction | Oophorectomy |

*Adapted with permission from Moore EE. Jurkovich GK. Knudson MM, et al. Organ Injury Scaling V. Exratepatic biliary, esophagus, stomach, vulva, uterus (nonpregnant uterus) pregnant, fallopian tube, may, J Trauma 39:1069, 1995.*

to closure, and the status of the patient with regard to tetanus should be addressed. For deep lacerations, perioperative antibiotics directed both at aerobic and anaerobic organisms are recommended. Avulsion-type injuries may require grafts for complete closure. If the urogenital diaphragm is involved, injuries to pelvic and(or intra-abdominal organs must be suspected. While relatively uncommon, associated colorectal injuries must be considered in all cases of urogenital trauma, especially when there is an impalement injury or a pelvic fracture. These can include a tear of the posterior vaginal wall through the sigmoid colon, or a laceration of the posterior fourchette and vaginal wall with a transected perineal body, which includes the internal rectal sphincter.[102,109] Rectal mucosal injuries must be ruled out in all cases of sexual abuse.

## Vaginal Injuries

The hallmark of vaginal injury is bleeding, which may be severe enough to cause shock.[101] A careful speculum examination of the vagina includes visualization of the anterior and posterior walls as well as both fornices. A bimanual examination is necessary to detect a retroperitoneal hematoma. Patients with retroperitoneal bleeding may be hemodynamically unstable but display no external signs of hemorrhage. These patients often complain of severe perineal pain that radiates to the vulva or rectum.

Vaginal lacerations are repaired with absorbable suture in simple or multiple layers (see Table 40-8). Superficial lacerations may be repaired under local anesthesia, but deeper injuries require regional or general anesthesia. Although temporary packing may be attempted, it usually proves ineffective in controlling hemorrhage because of the great vascularity of the vaginal mucosa.[101] The vascular supply to the vagina is such that bleeding sites are usually located along the cut edges of the mucosa, and a continuous suture that reapproximates the edges results in hemostasis. Penetrating injuries to the inferior lateral vaginal wall may involve the pudendal artery or vein, which require direct suture ligation. If the cul de sac has been penetrated with entrance into the peritoneum, a laparotomy and inspection of adjacent pelvic organs is indicated. Simple vaginal lacerations generally heal without complications. Patients with deeper injuries (i.e., AAST grades III to V) and those with large hematomas should receive perioperative broad-spectrum antibiotics.

## Injuries to the Uterus, Cervix, and Ovaries

As mentioned earlier, injuries to the intra-abdominal reproductive organs occur rarely in the nongravid patient and are usually discovered during laparotomy for associated injuries. After these other injuries have been managed and the patient has been stabilized, repair of the reproductive organs is accomplished, with all attempts made to preserve reproductive function. The uterus and cervix can be repaired with single or multiple layers of absorbable sutures (see Table 40-8). Hysterectomy is reserved for severe grade V injuries with avulsion and cases of uncontrollable hemorrhage. Similarly, ovarian or tubal lacerations can usually be repaired with simple suturing. If the blood supply is compromised and the ovary appears nonviable, a unilateral oophorectomy may be required.

## Open Pelvic Fractures

Open pelvic fractures are associated with a high mortality and an aggressive approach is warranted.[118,119] These fractures may be associated with lacerations to the vagina, rectum, or perineum. Lacerations of the vagina may be caused by direct penetration of a bone fragment through the vaginal wall or from a tearing force on the perineum. Foreign bodies present in the vagina at the time of impact, such as tampons or contraceptive devices, are associated with an increased risk of vaginal tears.

Although the hallmark of vaginal injury is bleeding, the diagnosis may be missed in patients who are menstruating. In some cases the vaginal injury produces spasm of the walls of the vagina, trapping blood in the vault. Any female patient with a pelvic fracture should undergo at least a limited vaginal and anoscopic examination. If vaginal or rectal bleeding is encountered, a full-speculum examination of the vagina and a sigmoidoscopic examination are performed under general anesthesia with the patient in the lithotomy position. Although injuries to the lower urinary tract (see Chap. 39) associated with pelvic fractures are much less common in women than in men, the diagnosis should be considered in female patients, particularly in the presence of deep vaginal lacerations, inability to void, and unsuccessful catheterization.[120] Because the most common urethral injury in females consists of a partial tear of the proximal anterior wall, it should be noted that voiding symptoms may be minimal and urinary catheters may pass easily.[121]

In a long-term follow-up of a large series of women with pelvic fractures, a small but statistically significant association was found between pelvic fractures and dyspareunia.[122] This was especially true when the pelvic fracture included a displacement of bone of 5 mm or more. Displaced pelvic fractures may also result in an increased risk of cesarean section, but these fractures are not associated with later miscarriage or infertility.

Management of open pelvic fractures begins with aggressive fluid and blood replacement while associated life-threatening injuries to the head, chest, and abdomen are assessed. Emergency laparotomy may be required for hemorrhage from solid organs or intra-abdominal vessels. In these cases, pelvic stabilization with an external fixation device should be considered. If intra-abdominal hemorrhage can be ruled out by US or DPL, control of hemorrhage may be best accomplished with pelvic angiography and the embolization of major disrupted pelvic vessels.

After hemorrhage is under control, the patient should undergo a thorough perineal, vaginal, and rectal inspection in the operating room under anesthesia. Vaginal lacerations are then irrigated, debrided, and closed. If there is extensive perineal trauma or an associated rectal laceration, a diverting colostomy and distal rectal washout are indicated. Perineal injuries can then be debrided and carefully reapproximated with anatomic precision. Broad-spectrum antibiotics are given, and regular dressing changes and debridements anticipated, often requiring multiple trips to the operating room. Complex perineal injuries require aggressive wound management targeted at preventing morbidity and mortality from pelvic sepsis. This includes diversion of the fecal stream, sufficient nutrition, adequate and regular debridement and irrigation, and early coverage when the wound is clean.[123] A coordinated team approach by trauma, orthopedic, urologic and gynecologic surgeons, as well as by the interventional radiologist and physical therapist, is required to optimize the outcome following these life-threatening injuries.

## Burns

The perineum is generally protected from burns by the thighs, but burns of the genital region can be debilitating.[124] In one large series, 50% of patients with genital burns and 20% with perineal or buttock burns required acute skin grafting. Aggressive physical therapy was required to prevent contractures, the most common delayed complication of these injuries. A series of 78 children with perineal and genital burns demonstrated that while 61% improved with conservative therapy including debridement and topical and parenteral antibiotics, others required more aggressive treatment.[125] They also noted that 47% of the cases were associated with child abuse.

## INJURY PREVENTION

Because most perineal and pelvic injuries result from motor vehicular trauma, injury prevention programs must continue to emphasize the importance of using restraint devices. Proper use of infant and child seats must be taught to all parents by both neonatologists and pediatricians. Pedestrian crashes are also common causes of perineal injuries, and both children and elderly women are at particular risk. Pedestrian safety programs require input from multiple parties, including police and highway safety officials. The dangers associated with water sports must be emphasized to all participants. Sporting equipment can also be redesigned with safety in mind. Burn injuries decrease dramatically with the use of smoke detectors and fire-retardant clothing and by lowering the temperature of the water heater. Public health and public policy measures targeted at the prevention of domestic violence, sexual assault, and child abuse certainly contribute to the prevention of these injuries. Prevention of secondary complications following the initial injury must include an organized team of trauma professionals, including trauma surgeons, orthopedic surgeons, urologists, gynecologists, and pediatricians.

## REFERENCES

1. Keynes G: *The Apology and Treatise of Ambroise Paré.* London: Falcon Educational Books, 1951.
2. Fields J, Reed L, Jones N, et al.: Trauma: The leading cause of maternal death. *J Trauma* 32:643, 1992.
3. Lavery JP, Staten-McCormick M: Management of moderate to severe trauma in pregnancy. *Obstet Gynecol Clin North Am* 22:69, 1995.
4. Weiss HB: Pregnancy-associated injury hospitalizations in Pennsylvania, 1995. *Ann Emerg Med* 34:626, 1999.
5. Weiss HB, Songer TJ, Fabio A: Fetal deaths related to maternal injury. *JAMA* 286:1863, 2001.
6. Guth AA, Pachter HL: Domestic violence and the trauma surgeon. *Am J Surg* 179:134, 2000.
7. Parsons LH, Harper MA: Violent maternal deaths in North Carolina. *Obstet Gynecol* 94:990, 1999.
8. McFarlane J, Parker B, Soeken K, et al.: Assessing for abuse during pregnancy: Severity and frequency of injuries and associated entry into prenatal care. *JAMA* 267:3176, 1992.
9. Chang I, Berg CJ, Saltaman LE, et al.: Homicide: a leading cause of injury deaths among pregnant and postpartum women in the United States, 1991–1999. *Am J Public Health* 95:471, 2005.
10. Ikossi DG, Lazar AA, Morabito D, et al.: Profile of mothers at risk: an analysis of injury and pregnancy loss in 1,195 trauma patients. *J Am Coll Surg* 200:49, 2005
11. Harvey MG: Physiologic changes of pregnancy. In Harvey CJ, ed. *Critical Care Obstetrical Nursing.* Gaithersburg, MD: Aspen, 1991, p. 1.
12. Smith CV, Phalen JP: Trauma in pregnancy. In Clark SL, Cotton DB, Hankins GDV, et al., eds. *Critical Care Obstetrics,* 2nd ed. Boston: Blackwell, 1991, p. 498.
13. Lee W, Cotton DB: Cardiorespiratory changes during pregnancy. In Clark SL, Cotton DB, Hankins GDV, et al., eds. *Critical Care Obstetrics,* 2nd ed. Boston: Blackwell, 1991, p. 2.
14. Metcalfe J, McAnulty JH, Ueland K: Cardiovascular physiology. *Clin Obstet Gynecol* 24:693, 1981.
15. Pirhone JP, Erkola RU: Uterine and umbilical flow velocity wave forms in the supine hypotensive syndrome. *Obstet Gynecol* 76:176, 1990.
16. Cunningham FG, MacDonald PC, Gant NF: Maternal adaptations to pregnancy. In *Williams Obstetrics,* 19th ed. Norwalk, CT: Appleton & Lange, 1993, p. 209.
17. Elkus R, Popovich J: Respiratory physiology in pregnancy. *Clin Obstet Gynecol* 24:693, 1981.
18. Awe R, Nicotta M, Newson T, et al.: Arterial oxygenation and alveolar-arterial gradients in term pregnancy. *Obstet Gynecol* 53:182, 1979.
19. Bynum TE: Hepatic and gastrointestinal disorders in pregnancy. *Med Clin North Am* 61:129, 1977.
20. Bacq Y, Zarka O, Brechot JF, et al.: Liver function tests in normal pregnancy: A prospective study of 103 pregnant and 103 matched controls. *Hepatology* 23:1030, 1996.
21. Braverman DZ, Johnson ML, Kern F Jr: Effects of pregnancy and contraceptive steroids on gallbladder function. *N Engl J Med* 302:362, 1980.
22. Dunlop W: Serial changes in renal hemodynamics during normal human pregnancy. *Br J Obstet Gynaecol* 88:1, 1981.
23. Briggs GC, Freeman RK, Yaffe SJ: *A Reference Guide to Fetal and Neonatal Risk: Drugs in Pregnancy and Lactation,* 3rd ed. Baltimore: Williams & Wilkins, 1990.
24. Gonzalez JG, Elizondo G, Saldiver D, et al.: Pituitary gland growth during normal pregnancy: An in vivo study using magnetic resonance imaging. *Am J Med* 85:217, 1988.
25. Grant NF, Worley RJ: Measures of uterine-placental blood flows in the human. In Rosenfeld CR, ed. *The Uterine Circulation.* Ithaca, NY: Perinatology Press, 1989, p. 5.
26. Cunningham FG, MacDonald P, Gant NF: Hypertensive disorders in pregnancy. In *Williams Obstetrics,* 19th ed. Norwalk, CT: Appleton & Lange, 1993, p. 763.
27. Clark SL, Cotton DB, Pivarnik JM, et al.: Positional change and central hemodynamic profile during normal third trimester pregnancy and post partum. *Am J Obstet Gynecol* 164:883, 1991.
28. Mattox KL, Goetzl L: Trauma in pregnancy. *Crit Care Med* 2005;33:S385.
29. Muench MV, Baschat A, Reddy UM et al.: Kleihauer-Betke testing is important in all cases of maternal trauma. *J Trauma* 57:1094, 2004.
30. Dhanraj D, Lambers D: The incidences of positive Kleihauer-Betke test in low-risk pregnancies and maternal trauma patients. *Am J Obstet Gynecology* 190:1461, 2004.
31. Pearlman MD, Tintinalli JE, Lorenz RP: A prospective controlled study of outcome after trauma during pregnancy. *Am J Obstet Gynecol* 162:1502, 1990.
32. Kaiser G: Do electronic fetal heart rate monitors improve delivery outcomes? *J Florida Med Assoc* 78:303, 1991.
33. Dahmus MA, Sibai BM: Blunt abdominal trauma: Are there any predictive factors for abruptio placentae or maternal-fetal distress? *Am J Obstet Gynecol* 169:1054, 1993.
34. Curet MJ, Schermer CR, Demarest GB, et al.: Predictors of outcome in trauma during pregnancy: Identification of patients who can be monitored for less than 6 hours. *J Trauma* 40:18, 2000.
35. Fries MH, Hankins G: Motor vehicle accident associated with minimal maternal trauma but subsequent fetal demise. *Ann Emerg Med* 18:301, 1989.
36. Deutchman M: Primary application of ultrasound. In Heller M, Jehle D, eds. *Pelvic Applications in Ultrasound in Emergency Medicine.* Philadelphia: Saunders, 1995, p. 106.
37. Manning FA, Platt LD, Sipos L: Antepartum fetal evaluation: Development of a fetal biophysical profile score. *Am J Obstet Gynecol* 136:787, 1980.
38. Towery R, English TP, Wisner D: Evaluation of pregnant women after blunt injury. *J Trauma* 35:731, 1993.
39. Eliot G, Rao D: Pregnancy and radiographic examination. In Haycock CE, ed. *Trauma and Pregnancy.* Littleton, MA: PSG Publishing, 1985, p. 69.
40. Harvey EB, Boice JD, Honeyman M, et al.: Prenatal exposure and childhood cancer in twins. *N Engl J Med* 312:541, 1985.
41. ACOG Committee Opinion No. 299: Guidelines for diagnostic imaging during pregnancy. *Obstet Gynecol* 104:647, 2004.
42. Moore MM, Shearer DR: Fetal dose estimates for CT pelvimetry. *Radiology* 171:265, 1989.
43. Parry RA, Glaze SA, Archer BR: The AAPM(RSNA physics tutorial for residents. *Radiographics* 19:1289, 1999.

44. DeSantis M, Di Gianantonio E, Straface G, et al.: Ionizing radiations in pregnancy and teratogenesis; a review of literature. *Reproductive Toxicology* 20:323, 2005.

45. Mann FA, Nathans A, Langer SG, et al.: Communicating with family: The risk of medical radiation to conceptuses in victims of major blunt force torso trauma. *J Trauma* 48:354, 2000.

46. Goodwin H, Holmes JF, Wisner DH: Abdominal ultrasound examination in pregnant trauma patients. *J Trauma* 50:689, 2001.

47. Bochicchio GV, Napolitano LM, Haan J, et al.: Incidental pregnancy in trauma patients. *J Am Coll Surg* 192:566, 2001.

48. Richards JR, Ormsby EL, Romo MV, et al.: Blunt abdominal injury in the pregnant patient: detection with US. *Radiology* 233:463, 2004.

49. Badmanaban B, Diver A, Ali N, et al.: Traumatic aortic rupture during pregnancy. *J Card Surg* 18:557, 2003.

50. Visser BC, Glasgow RD, Mulvihill KK, et al.: Safety and timing of nonobstetric abdominal surgery in pregnancy. *Dig Surg* 18:409, 2001.

51. Levinson G: Anesthesia for surgery during pregnancy. In Hughes SC, Levinson G, Rosen MA, eds. *Anesthesia for Obstetrics*. Philadelphia: Lippincott Williams and Wilkins, 2001, p. 249.

52. Lavin JP, Polsky SS: Abdominal trauma during pregnancy. *Clin Perinatol* 10:423, 1983.

53. Leggon RE, Wood GC, Indeck MC: Pelvic fractures in pregnancy: factors influencing maternal and fetal outcomes. *J Trauma* 53:796, 2002.

54. Loegters T, Briem D, Gatzka C et al.: Treatment of unstable fractures of the pelvic ring in pregnancy. *Arch Orthop Trauma Surg* 125:204, 2005.

55. Kloen P, Flik K, Helfet DL: Operative treatment of acetabular fracture during pregnancy: a case report. *Arch Orthop Trauma Surg* 125:209, 2005.

56. Harrison SD, Nghieum HV, Shy K: Uterine rupture with fetal death following blunt trauma. *Am J Roentgenol* 165:1452, 1995.

57. Green JR: Placenta previa and abruptio placentae. In Creasey RK, Resnik R, eds. *Maternal-Fetal Medicine: Principles and Practice*, 3rd ed. Philadelphia: Saunders, 1994, p. 602.

58. Patterson RM: Trauma in pregnancy. *Clin Obstet Gynecol* 27:32, 1984.

59. Sandy EA, Koerner M: Self inflicted gunshot wound to the pregnant abdomen: Report of a case and review of the literature. *Am J Perinatol* 6:30, 1989.

60. Jain ML, Garg AK: Burns with pregnancy: A review of 25 cases. *Burns* 19:166, 1993.

61. Chang CJ, Yang JY: Major burns in pregnancy. *Chang Keng I Hsueh Chang Gung Med J* 19:154, 1996.

62. Prassana M, Singh K: Early burn wound excision in "major" burns with "pregnancy": A preliminary report. *Burns* 22:234, 1996.

63. Akhtar MA, Mulawkar PM, Kulkarni HR: Burns in pregnancy: Effect on maternal and fetal outcomes. *Burns* 20:351, 1994.

64. Guo SS, Greenspoon JS, Kahn AM: Management of burn injuries during pregnancy. *Burns* 27:394, 2001.

65. Katz VL, Dottero OJ, Droegemueller W: Perimortem cesarean delivery. *Obstet Gynecol* 68:571, 1986.

66. Morris JA, Rosenbower TJ, Jurkovich GJ, et al.: Infant survival after cesarean section for trauma. *Ann Surg* 223:281, 1996.

67. Meschua G: Safety margin of fetal oxygenation. *J Reprod Med* 30:308, 1985.

68. Kauntiz AM, Hughes JM, Grimes DA: Causes of maternal mortality in the United States. *Obstet Gynecol* 65:605, 1985.

69. Azegami M, Mori N: Amniotic fluid embolism and leukotrienes. *Am J Obstet Gynecol* 155:1119, 1986

70. Brandt JT: Current concepts of coagulation. *Clin Obstet Gynecol* 28:3, 1985.

71. Morrison RB: Obstetrics. In Goldhaber SZ, ed. *Prevention of Venous Thromboembolism*. New York: Marcel Dekker, 1993, p. 445.

72. Tolia MR, Weg JG: Venous thromboembolism during pregnancy. *N Engl J Med* 335:108, 1996.

73. Knudson MM, Ikossi DG, Khaw L et al.: Thromboembolism after trauma; an analysis of 1602 episodes from the American College of Surgeons National Trauma Data Bank. *Ann Surg* 240:490, 2004.

74. Knudson MM, Morabito D, Paiement GD, et al.: The use of low molecular weight heparin in preventing thromboembolism in trauma patients. *J Trauma* 41:446, 1996.

75. Mays J, Verma U, Klein S, et al.: Acute appendicitis in pregnancy and the occurrence of major intraventricular hemorrhage and periventricular leukomalacia. *Obstet Gynecol* 86:650, 1995.

76. ACGO Educational Bulletin: *Teratology* 236: 1997.

77. Kissinger DP, Rozycki GS, Morris JA Jr, et al.: Trauma in pregnancy: Predicting pregnancy outcome. *Arch Surg* 126:1079, 1991.

78. Countee RW, Thompson JP, Staggers BA: Neurological injuries during pregnancy. In Haycock CE, ed. *Trauma and Pregnancy*. Littleton, MA: PSG Publishing, 1985, p. 154.

79. Kelly DG, Gonzalo IT, Cohan P et al.: Hypopituitarism following traumatic brain injury and aneuysmal subarachnoid hemorrhage: a preliminary report. *J Neurosurg* 93:743, 2000.

80. Popov I, Ngambu F, Mantel G, et al.: Acute spinal cord injury in pregnancy: an illustrative case and literature review. *J Obstet and Gyne* 23:596, 2003.

81. Gilson GJ, Miller AC, Clevenger FW, et al.: Acute spinal cord injury and neurogenic Shock in pregnancy. *Obstet Gynecol Surg* 50:556, 1995.

82. Hoft WS, D'Amerlio LF, Tinkoff GH, et al.: Maternal predictors of fetal demise in trauma during pregnancy. *Surg Gynecol Obstet* 172:175, 1991.

83. Esposito TJ, Gens DR, Smith LG, et al.: Trauma during pregnancy: A review of 79 cases. *Arch Surg* 126:1073, 1991.

84. Scorpio RJ, Esposito TJ, Smith LG, et al.: Blunt trauma during pregnancy: Factors affecting fetal outcome. *J Trauma* 32:213, 1992.

85. Ali J, Yeo A, Gana TJ, et al.: Predictors of fetal mortality in pregnant patients. *J Trauma* 42:782, 1997.

86. Shah KH, Simons RK, Holbrook T, et al.: Trauma in pregnancy; maternal and fetal outcomes. *J Trauma* 42:83, 1998.

87. Rogers FB, Rozycki GS, Osler TM, et al.: A multi-institutional study of factors associated with fetal deaths in injured pregnant patients. *Arch Surg* 134:1274, 1999.

88. Schiff MA, Holt VL, Daling JR: Maternal and infant outcomes after injury during pregnancy in Washignton State from 1989 to 1997. *J Trauma* 53:939, 2002.

89. Kady DL, Gilbert WM, Anderson J, et al.: Trauma during pregnancy: an analysis of maternal and fetal outcomes in a large population. *Am J Obstetric Gynecology* 190:1661, 2004.

90. Baerga-Varela Y, Zietlow SP, Bannon MT, et al.: Trauma in pregnancy. *Mayo Clin Proc* 75:1243, 2000.

91. McLeer S, Anwar R: A study of battered women presenting in an emergency department. *Am J Pub Health* 79:65, 1989.

92. Poole GA, Martin JN, Perry KG, et al.: Trauma in pregnancy: The role of interpersonal violence. *Am J Obstet Gynecol* 174:1873, 1996.

93. Agran PF, Dunkle DE, Winn DG, et al.: Fetal death in motor vehicle accidents. *Ann Emerg Med* 16:1355, 1987.

94. Schiff M, Kasnic T, Reiff K, et al.: Seat belt use during pregnancy. *West J Med* 156:655, 1992.

95. Wolf ME, Alexander MD, Rivara FP, et al.: A retrospective cohort study of seatbelt use and pregnancy outcome after a motor vehicle crash. *J Trauma* 34:116, 1993.

96. Tyroch AH, Kaups KL, Rohan J, et al.: Pregnant women and car restraints: Beliefs and practices. *J Trauma* 46:241, 1999.

97. Pearlman MD, Klinich KD, Schneider LW, et al.: A comprehensive program to improve safety for pregnant women and fetuses in motor vehicle crashes: A preliminary report. *Am J Obstet Gynecol* 182:1554, 2000.

98. Moorcroft DM, Stitzel JD, Duma GD, et al.: Computerized model of the pregnant occupant: predicting the risk of injury in automobile crashes. *Am J Obstet Gynecol* 189:540, 2003.

99. Sims CJ, Boardman GH, Fuller SJ: Air bag deployment following a motor vehicle accident in pregnancy. *Obstet Gynecol* 88:726, 1996.

100. Baldwin DD, Landa HM: Common problems in pediatric gynecology. *Urol Clin North Am* 22:171, 1995.

101. Gould SF, Delaney JJ: Obstetrical and gynecological injuries. In Zuidema GA, Rutherford RB, Ballinger WF, eds. *Management of Trauma*, 4th ed. Philadelphia: Saunders, 1985, p. 505.

102. Dowd MD, Fitzmaurice L, Knapp JF, et al.: The interpretation of urogenital findings in children with straddle injuries. *J Pediatric Surg* 29:7, 1994.

103. Onen A, Ozturk H, Yayla M, et al.: Genital trauma in children: classification and management. *Urology* 65:986, 2005.

104. Stone NN, Ances IG, Brotman S: Gynecologic injury in the nongravid female during blunt abdominal trauma. *J Trauma* 24:626, 1984.

105. Madell J, Cromie WJ, Caldamone AA, et al.: Sports-related genitourinary injuries in children. *Clin Sports Med* 1:483, 1982.

106. McAleer IM, Kaplan GW, Scherz HC, et al.: Genitourinary trauma in the pediatric patient. *Urology* 42:563, 1993.

107. Pokorny SF, Pokorny W, Kramer W: Acute genital injury in the prepubertal girls. *Am J Obstet Gynecol* 166:1461, 1992.

108. Reinberg O, Yazbeck S: Major perineal trauma in children. *J Pediatr Surg* 24:982, 1989.

109. Lynch JM, Gardner MJ, Albasense CT: Blunt urogenital trauma in prepubescent female patients: More than meets the eye! *Pediatr Emerg Care* 11:372, 1995.

110. Palmer CM, McNulty AM, D'Este C, et al.: Genital injuries in women reporting sexual assault. *Sex Health* 1:55, 2004.

111. Hilden M, Schei B, Sidenius K: Genitoanal injury in adult female victims of sexual assault. *Forensic Sci Int* 154:200, 2005.

112. Sugar NF, Fine DN, Eckert LO: Physical injury after sexual assault: findings of a large case series. *Am J Obstet Gynecol* 190:71, 2004.

113. Jones JS, Rossman L, Wynn BN, et al.: Comparative analysis of adult versus adolescent sexual assault: epidemiology and patterns of anogenital injury. *Acad Emerg Med* 10:872, 2003.

114. Fallat ME, Weaver JM, Hertweck SP, et al.: Late follow-up and functional outcome after traumatic reproductive tract injuries in women. *Am Surg* 64:858, 1998.
115. Johnson K, Chapman S, Hall CM: Skeletal injuries associated with sexual abuse. *Pediatr Radiol* 34:620, 2004.
116. Danielson CK, Holmes MM: Adolescent sexual assault: an update of the literature. *Curr Opin Obstet Gynecol* 16:383, 2004.
117. Benrubi G, Neuman C, Nuss RC, et al.: Vulvar and vaginal hematomas: A restrospective study of conservative versus operative management. *South Med J* 80:991, 1987.
118. Sinnott R, Rhodes M, Brader A: Open pelvic fractures: An injury for trauma centers. *Am J Surg* 163:283, 1992.
119. Davidson BS, Simmons GT, Williamson PR, et al.: Pelvic fractures associated with open perineal wounds: A survivable injury. *J Trauma* 35:36, 1993.
120. Patil U, Nesbitt R, Meyer R: Genitourinary tract injuries due to fracture of the pelvis in females: Sequelae and their management. *Br J Surg* 54:32, 1982.
121. Koraitim MM: Pelvic fracture urethral injuries: the unresolved controversy. *J Urol* 161:1433, 1999.
122. Copeland CE, Bosse MJ, McCarthy ML, et al.: Effect of trauma and pelvic fracture on female genitourinary, sexual, and reproductive function. *J Ortho Trauma* 11:73, 1997.
123. Kudsk KA, Hanna MK: Management of complex perineal injuries. *World J Surg* 27:895, 2003.
124. Alghanem AA, McCauley RL, Robson MC, et al.: Management of pediatric perineal and genital burns: Twenty-year review. *J Burn Rehabil* 11:308, 1990.
125. Angel C, Shu T, French D, et al.: Genital and perineal burns in children: 10 years of experience at a major burn center. *J Pediatr Surg* 37:99, 2002.

## Commentary ■ MARY C. McCARTHY ■ A. PETER EKEH

The authors of this chapter, Margaret M. Knudson and Jennifer J. Wan, provide an excellent and thorough review of the physiologic changes of pregnancy and the management of trauma to the female reproductive system. In this commentary, I would like to highlight a few areas of interest and of controversy.

A thorough history is important when assessing trauma to women, especially penetrating trauma or assault. All women presenting to the emergency department with injuries should undergo domestic violence screening. Pregnant women are at particular risk; with one in six being a victim.[1] The following questions should be asked:

1. Have you ever been emotionally or physically abused by your partner or someone important to you?

2. Within the last year, have you been hit, slapped, kicked, or otherwise physically hurt by someone?

3. Within the last year, has anyone forced you to have sexual activity?

Delay in the recognition and control of domestic violence may result in additional injury to the women and children in the home. The next episode of violence may cause permanent damage or even death. The patient should also be examined for the physical hallmarks of domestic violence listed in the chapter.

Evaluation of fetal risk in the presence of maternal trauma is challenging. The Kleihauer-Betke Test, an indicator of fetal blood in the maternal circulation, is no longer routinely ordered in our injured pregnant patients as it does not contribute to decision making. Heart rate and ultrasound imaging provide the best evidence of fetal compromise.

The authors of this chapter appropriately encourage the performance of necessary radiologic studies in trauma. One particular finding of note is the presence of physiologic pericardial fluid in pregnant women. With the increasing use of FAST, the presence of this fluid may raise concern for cardiac injury. Abdominal CT is also valuable in delineating abdominal injuries. The major cause of fetal demise in the mother who survives is abruptio placenta. However, since CT images of the pregnant woman are uncommon, radiologists may not be familiar with the radiographic appearance of placental abruption (Fig. 1). This image of the gravid uterus and placenta in a patient who was involved in a motor vehicle crash shows enhancing areas representing normal placental perfusion with interposed areas of hypoperfusion and hemorrhage.[2] The trauma surgeon should recognize these findings.

Treatment of injuries to the female reproductive system is also well covered in this chapter. Signs of maternal hypovolemia are delayed due to the physiologic changes of pregnancy; however, caution should be exercised with the proposal for "vigorous crystalloid resuscitation" in the pregnant patient. While adequate blood volume for uterine perfusion is critical in fetal outcome, pregnant patients have decreased plasma proteins, and therefore plasma oncotic pressure. Thus, they may be more prone to pulmonary edema. Central monitoring may be required to optimize perfusion in seriously injured patients.

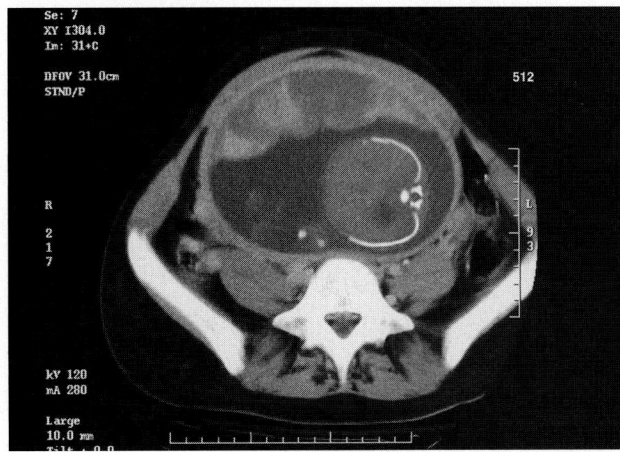

**FIGURE 1.** Abdominal CT scan demonstrating placental abruption after motor vehicle crash in 21-year-old woman who is 27 weeks pregnant. Enhancing areas represent normal placental perfusion with interposed areas of hypoperfusion and hemorrhage.
*(Reproduced with permission from Lippincott Williams & Wilkins, Ekeh AP, Anderson GA, Patterson L, et al.: Image of trauma: placental abruption. J Trauma 53:168, 2002)*

Thromboembolic disease is a major cause of maternal morbidity and mortality and patients are at even higher risk in the presence of injury. A special consideration in pregnant women is the recommendation that inferior vena cava filters be placed above the renal veins because of the possibility of caval perforation due to pressure from the gravid uterus. Intravascular ultrasound may be valuable in delineating the patency of the delivery route, the presence of thrombus, the presence of anatomical variants, the vena caval diameter, and the location of the renal veins reducing the use of fluoroscopy which exposes the fetus to higher doses of radiation.[3]

Increasingly, technological interventions can sustain life. The age of viability of the fetus is considered to be 24 weeks, 0 days. However, if a mother sustains a severe head injury in a motor vehicle crash, and the fetus is not yet viable, how long can (and should) a mother with death by neurologic criteria be maintained on life support to incubate a live but not yet viable fetus? Performing a caesarean section on a mother *in extremis* to deliver a potentially viable infant is another medical and ethical dilemma. The added insult of the surgical procedure will compromise the mother further, so it should only be performed in the case of recent or impending maternal death or in the case of maternal stability with fetal compromise.

## References

1. McFarlane J, Parker B, Soeken K, et al.: Assessing for abuse during pregnancy. *JAMA* 267:3176, 1992.
2. Ekeh AP, Anderson GA, Patterson L, et al.: Image of trauma: placental abruption. *J Trauma* 53:168, 2002.
3. Bonn J, Liu JB, Eschelman DJ, et al.: Intravascular ultrasound as an alternative to positive-contrast vena cavography prior to filter placement. *J Vasc Interv Rad* 10:843, 1999.

# Trauma Damage Control

*Amy D. Wyrzykowski* ■ *David V. Feliciano*

A number of new approaches to the management of patients with major truncal or extremity trauma have evolved over the past 20 years. These include the following: minimizing time at the scene of trauma and in the emergency department (ED); the presence of in-house attending surgeons, particularly in centers with a significant percentage of penetrating trauma; minimizing admission laboratory testing; initiating resuscitation in the operating room for patients with severe hypotension, cardiac arrest, or external hemorrhage; and early operative control of hemorrhage. All of these are now accepted as major factors in decreasing morbidity and mortality.[1–6] Another major change has been the recognition that conservative operative techniques and shortened operative times, even when all organ repairs have not been completed, will increase survival in civilian and military patients with cervical, truncal, or extremity injuries and intraoperative "metabolic failure."[5–22] Finally, it has been recognized that standard closure of a thoracotomy or the midline abdominal incision is impossible to achieve in many severely injured patients, is too time-consuming in others, and may cause an abdominal compartment syndrome in the postoperative period after a laparotomy.[23–33]

This chapter will describe the techniques used during "damage control" operations (as named by Rotondo and colleagues)[7]; prevention and sequelae of primary or secondary abdominal compartment syndrome; the alternate techniques for closure of a thoracic, abdominal, or extremity incision in patients with major trauma[34–43]; care of the patient in the surgical intensive care unit (SICU) after a damage control operation; the approach to reoperation; and late repair of incisional hernias when the abdomen has been left open at a reoperation.[41,44–47]

## DAMAGE CONTROL OPERATIONS

### Definition

Damage control operations are performed in injured patients with profound hemorrhagic shock and preoperative or intraoperative metabolic sequelae that are known to adversely affect survival. The widely accepted three stages of damage control are described as follows:

1. *Limited operation for control of hemorrhage and contamination.* Includes control of hemorrhage from the heart or lung; conservative management of injuries to solid organs; resection of major injuries to the gastrointestinal tract without reanastomosis; control of hemorrhage from major arteries and veins in the neck, trunk, or extremities; packing of organs or spaces to control the inevitable coagulopathy; and use of an alternate closure of a cervical incision, thoracotomy, laparotomy, or site of exploration of an extremity.

2. *Resuscitation in the SICU.* Includes vigorous rewarming of the hypothermic patient; restoration of a normal cardiovascular state by the infusion of fluids and blood and the use of inotropic and related drugs; correction of residual coagulopathy after hypothermia is reversed; and supportive care for stunned lungs and kidneys.

3. *Reoperation.* Completion of definitive repairs, search for missed injuries, and formal closure of the incision, if possible.

## Clinical Recognition of Patients Likely to Need Damage Control Operations

Reports to the hospital from prehospital providers or a rapid evaluation in the ED by experienced members of the trauma team are the mechanisms used to select patients for abbreviated resuscitation and immediate operation with damage control techniques in the operating room.

Patients in this small subset (Table 41-1) should stop in the ED only long enough to obtain control of the airway, decompression of an obvious pneumothorax, have blood drawn for type and cross-match, and for the application of an identification bracelet, unless a resuscitative thoracotomy is needed. These patients should then be transported immediately to the operating room. Patients arriving by air with hypotension or mangled extremities should bypass the emergency room entirely and be taken directly to the operating from the helipad.

## Intraoperative Indications to Perform Damage Control Operations

The primary indication to modify the conduct of an operation for major trauma to the neck, chest, abdomen, or an extremity is unresolved metabolic failure despite control of hemorrhage by suture, resection, or packing. Metabolic failure is characterized by severe hypothermia despite warming maneuvers initiated in the ED and continuing in the operating room, persistent acidemia despite vigorous resuscitation and control of hemorrhage, and a coagulopathy (nonmechanical bleeding) not amenable to operative control.[48–58] *Patients are more likely to die from their intraoperative metabolic failure than they are from the failure to complete organ repairs.*[5–9,12–14,51–58] Most have received transfusion of 1 to 2 blood volumes and are expected to have a survival of only 50 to 60% when severe injuries are present.[7,12–14,52,59–62]

**Hypothermia.**    Hypothermia continues to be a common problem in victims of major trauma. In one older series, 66% of severely injured patients admitted to a Level I trauma center were hypothermic (<36°C [96.8°F] on esophageal temperature probe), including 23% who were severely hypothermic (<34°C [93.2°F]).[63] Another older review documented that 57% of 74 trauma patients admitted directly to the operating room from the ED developed hypothermia (<36°C [96.8°F]) between the time of injury and the time they were moved out of the operating room.[64]

There are many causes of hypothermia in victims of major trauma. Hypovolemic shock in the preoperative period adversely affects oxygen delivery and leads to decreases in oxygen consumption and, therefore, production of heat.[65–67] Should the patient be intoxicated at the time of injury, vasodilatation will further compromise the ability to produce heat. The trauma team itself may be responsible for accelerating the loss of heat from a victim in shock. Undressing the patient in a cool resuscitation room, failing to cover the patient's head with a turban and the trunk and extremities with warm blankets or the Bair Hugger Patient Warming System (Augustine Medical, Inc., Eden Prairie, MN) during resuscitation, and infusion of unheated crystalloids and packed red blood cells are all sources of heat loss in the ED. Paralyzing the patient, which prevents shivering, and administering anesthetic agents, which prevents vasoconstriction; failing to cover areas of the body not undergoing operation; opening one or more body cavities in a cold operating room; and irrigating body cavities with unheated crystalloid solutions are further sources of heat loss during a thoracotomy or laparotomy. These multiple sources of heat loss cannot be fully compensated for by increasing heat production in the patient in shock, and the resuscitation and surgical teams are responsible for preventing or reversing hypothermia using the techniques listed in Table 41-2.[48]

The effect of hypothermia on mortality in severely injured patients is no longer controversial except for one study. In one large retrospective review, mortality among euthermic and hypothermic trauma patients was not significantly different when patients in both groups were stratified by physiologic and anatomic indicators of injury severity.[68] This is in marked contrast to the review of iliac vascular injuries by Cushman and colleagues which noted that the risk of dying was nearly four times greater when the patient's initial body temperature in the operating room was less than 34°C [93.2°F]. If the patient's last body temperature in the operating

---

**TABLE 41-1**

### Patients Likely To Need Damage Control Operations

Thoracic Trauma
- Penetrating thoracic wound and systolic blood pressure <90 mmHg
- Pericardial fluid on surgeon-performed ultrasound after blunt or penetrating thoracic trauma
- S/p emergency department thoracotomy for penetrating thoracic wound

Abdominal or Pelvic Trauma
- Penetrating abdominal wound and systolic blood pressure <90 mmHg
- Blunt abdominal trauma, systolic blood pressure <90 mmHg, and peritoneal fluid on surgeon-performed ultrasound or gross blood on diagnostic peritoneal tap
- Closed pelvic fracture, systolic blood pressure <90 mmHg, and peritoneal fluid on surgeon-performed ultrasound or gross blood on diagnostic peritoneal tap
- Open pelvic fracture

Trauma to an Extremity
- Shotgun wound to femoral triangle of thigh
- Mangled extremity from blunt trauma

General
- Emergency laparotomy to be followed by emergent craniotomy for compressive lesion, emergent thoracotomy for repair of ruptured descending thoracic aorta, or therapeutic embolization of pelvic bleeder related to fracture

---

**TABLE 41-2**

### Maneuvers to Prevent or Reverse Hypothermia During Damage Control Operations

Increase operating room temperature >85°F [29.4°C].

Infuse crystalloid solution and blood through a warming device such as the level I Fluid Warmer.[a]

Cover patient's head with a turban or warming device.

Cover body parts out of the operative field with a warming device such as the Bair Hugger[b] or Life-Air[c] system.

Irrigate nasogastric and thoracostomy tubes with warm saline during laparotomy.

Irrigate open pericardial cavity, pleural cavities, and peritoneal cavity during simultaneous sternotomy or thoracotomy and laparotomy.

[a]Level I Technologies, Inc., Rockland. MA.
[b]Augustine Medical, Inc., Eden Prarie, MN.
[c]Medical Products Group, Marshal, MN.

room was less than 35°C [95.0°F], the risk of death was nearly 41 times greater than it was for patients with a body temperature greater than 35°C.[69]

While hypothermia is helpful in certain elective operative procedures and has been used for cerebral protection in patients with injury to the brain, it has well-known adverse effects on the cardiovascular, respiratory, renal, gastrointestinal, endocrine, central nervous, and coagulation systems (see Chap. 51).[48,70,71] Both terminal cardiac dysfunction and irreversible nonmechanical bleeding have been noted in many injured hypothermic patients dying in the postoperative period after a trauma operative procedure. It would appear logical, therefore, to practice damage control and rapidly complete any trauma operation in which the patient's initial body temperature is less than 34° to 35°C (93.2° to 95.0°F) or the temperature decreases below this level at any time during the operation.[27,30,72] This is particularly true in patients undergoing thoracotomy or laparotomy because hypothermia will not be correctable until the chest or abdomen is closed.

Acidemia. Prolonged hypovolemic shock produces a state of persistent metabolic acidosis in the patient with major trauma. This leads to a "circle" phenomenon in which secondary decreases in cardiac output, hypotension, and an increased susceptibility to ventricular arrhythmias may be irreversible, despite adequate volume replacement.[8,49,50,55,58,73–75] Also, acidosis may cause the uncoupling of β-adrenergic receptors, with a secondary decrease in the patient's response to endogenous and exogenous catecholamines.[76] While acidosis by itself is an unusual reason to terminate a laparotomy being performed for trauma, it often accompanies hypothermia and a coagulopathy.[49,50,51,53,55] A persistent metabolic acidosis is a manifestation of anaerobic metabolism occurring during hypoperfusion. Markers of this phenomenon in the injured patient that should initiate damage control operations are listed in Table 41-3.[49,69,74,75,77]

Coagulopathy. Nonmechanical bleeding is common during emergency trauma thoracotomies, laparotomies, or operative procedures in patients with exsanguination from an injury to an extremity. Coagulopathy resulting in irreversible bleeding is a significant cause of mortality in the immediate postoperative period and, therefore, mandates aggressive therapy.[78] The historic replacement of volume losses with large amounts of crystalloid solutions

and cold-packed red blood cells (PRBCs) leads to clotting abnormalities secondary to dilution, deficiency of clotting factors, and hypothermia.[8,50,58,59,79–81] In particular, hypothermia has an adverse effect on enzymes associated with the coagulation cascade and on the function of platelets.[7,12,13,59,79–81] Traditionally, one unit of fresh frozen plasma was administered for each four units of packed red blood cells. Current expert opinion suggests that ratios of 2:3 or even 1:1 are advisable in the most severely injured patients. Such a vigorous replacement protocol may minimize the dilution of clotting factors in plasma and the exacerbation of the multifactorial coagulopthy.[82] The administration of recombinant activated factor VII (Novoseven, Novo Nordisk A/S, Bagsvaerd, Denmark) may also play a role in the management of a life-threatening coagulopathy. Originally approved for the treatment of hemophilia in patients with inhibitors, Factor VIIa has had promising results in several studies in trauma patients.[83–85] In two parallel randomized, placebo-controlled, double-blind clinical trials, administration of rFVIIa after transfusion of the eighth unit of PRBCs was an efficacious adjunct in the management of hemorrhage. It significantly reduced the transfusion requirements in patients with blunt trauma and produced a trend toward decreased transfusion in patients with penetrating trauma.[85] The administration of rfVIIa appears to be safe in the trauma population.[83–85]

When a coagulopathy does result, surgical attempts to control such nonmechanical bleeding, especially from the liver and retroperitoneum, are usually unsuccessful. In the major trauma patient who develops a coagulopathy characterized by an International Normalized Ratio (INR) or partial thromboplastin time 50% greater than normal during any major operative procedure after major sources of hemorrhage have been controlled, damage control would include the techniques to be described (see Table 41-3).

## Operative Techniques in Thoracic Trauma

Lung (see Chap. 26.). Exsanguinating hemorrhage from the lung is most rapidly controlled by the application of a DeBakey aortic clamp to the hilum or by twisting the hilum to kink the major vessels in the ED or operating room.[86] When the site of blood loss has been a stab wound deep into the pulmonary parenchyma or a gunshot wound completely through a lobe, the technique of *pulmonotomy* (sometimes called *nonneurosurgical "tractotomy"*) is used.[87–89] Pulmonotomy refers to the division of pulmonary parenchyma between noncrushing vascular clamps or by using a linear stapling and cutting device to expose injured parenchymal vessels. After selective ligation of these, the pulmonary parenchyma is closed in the usual fashion using a continuous 2–0 absorbable suture, with reinforcement material added to the staple line, as needed.

Heart (see Chap. 28.). Other than compression with a finger, the quickest way to control hemorrhage from a small wound or rupture of a ventricle in the ED or operating room is to apply 6-mm-wide skin staples (Auto Suture 35 W, United States Surgical Corporation, Norwalk, CT).[90,91] Formal cardiac repair with Teflon pledgets may then be accomplished over the staples or as they are sequentially removed in the operating room.

Larger wounds or ruptures of a ventricle in patients surviving by virtue of tamponade may be controlled by the insertion of a Foley

**TABLE 41-3**

| Intraoperative Indications to Perform Damage Control Operations[49,69,74,75,77] | |
|---|---|
| FACTOR | LEVEL |
| 1. Initial body temperature | <35°C [95.0°F][69] |
| 2. Initial acid-base status | |
| • Arterial pH | <7.2[69] |
| • Base deficit | <–15 mmol/L in patient <55 years of age[74,75] or <–6 mmol/L in patient >55 years of age[75,77] |
| • Serum lactate | >5 mmol/L[77] |
| 3. Onset of coagulopathy | prothrombin time and/or partial thromboplastin time >50% of normal[8,55] |

*Modified from Brasel KJ, KUJ, Baker CC: Damage Control in the critically ill and injured patient. New Horizons 7:73,1999.*

balloon catheter into the hole.[92] With the balloon inflated and traction applied to the catheter, Teflon-pledgeted sutures can then be passed through the ventricle from side to side over the balloon. The thin wall of the right ventricle puts the inflated balloon at significant risk of puncture as each suture is placed. Pushing the catheter and balloon into the ventricle with each bite of the suture will avoid this complication, although blood loss may be significant.

With a longitudinal perforation or significant rupture of a ventricle, the time-honored technique of inflow occlusion is useful in avoiding cardiopulmonary bypass.[93] Curved aortic or angled vascular clamps are first applied to the superior and inferior vena cavae. As the heartbeat slows, horizontal mattress sutures are inserted rapidly on either side of the defect and then crossed to control hemorrhage. A continuous suture is placed to close the defect, and before it is tied down, air is vented out of the elevated ventricle by releasing the clamps on the cavae.

## Operative Techniques in Abdominal Trauma

Liver (see Chap. 32.). The liver has a blood supply of 1500 mL/min and is the major site of synthesis of all the coagulation factors except factor VIII. Therefore, appropriate operative management of a major hepatic injury is a key component of a successful damage control laparotomy.

There is ample historical evidence that an emergency hepatic resection performed by a general or trauma surgeon with little experience in a similar elective procedure will result in a mortality rate of 20 to 44%.[94–99] This excessive mortality is certainly related to the magnitude of the hepatic injury, but also to the belated decision to resect at the same time that the aforementioned metabolic failure occurs in many patients. For this reason, more limited techniques of hemostasis should be applied when a hepatic injury is present and damage control is to be performed.[100,101]

Indirect control of hepatic hemorrhage may be accomplished by *extensive hepatorrhaphy,* using a continuous suture or interrupted vertical mattress sutures of absorbable material. While this technique is used much less frequently than it was in the past, it is appropriate for a damage control operation.

Damage control techniques in which the sources of hepatic hemorrhage are approached directly include hepatotomy with selective vascular ligation, resectional debridement with selective vascular ligation, or rapid resectional debridement.[100] Both former techniques are performed with a vascular clamp in place (Pringle maneuver), and experience with the finger fracture technique should allow for early control of hemorrhage.[100–102] When a coagulopathy is already present, hepatotomy or resectional debridement is not appropriate if the surgeon has only modest experience with hepatic trauma. After the Pringle maneuver is performed, rapid resectional debridement is initiated by applying a large Kelly clamp or vascular clamp just outside of a lateral area of partial avulsion or by applying two clamps around the contused sides of a central laceration. The tissue within the clamps is then rapidly debrided, and an O-chromic tie can then be placed around the clamp and all the enclosed tissue ligated en bloc. An alternate technique is to use deep horizontal mattress sutures on either side of the debrided laceration and fill the space between with a viable omental pack (Fig. 41-1).

Damage control techniques in which compression or tamponade rather than a suture or metal clip is used to control hepatic

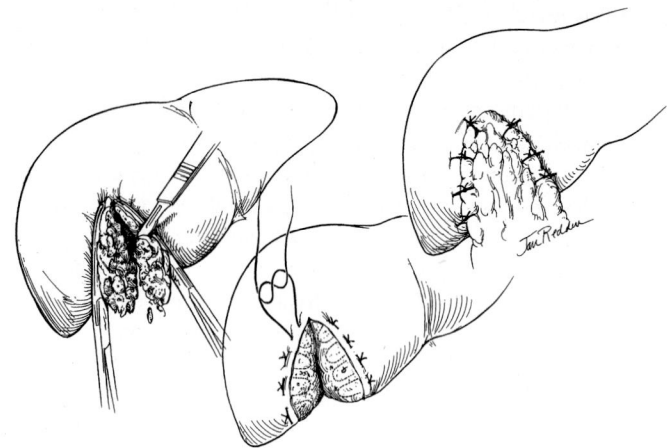

**FIGURE 41-1.** Technique of rapid resectional debridement using large vascular clamps, horizontal mattress sutures, and omental pack. *(Reproduced with permission from Feliciano DV, Pachter HL. Curr Prob Surg 26:453, 1989.)*

hemorrhage include *balloon catheter tamponade, absorbable mesh tamponade,* and *perihepatic packing.* Balloon catheter tamponade using a Foley or Fogarty balloon catheter or an inflated Penrose drain over a red rubber catheter is most useful to control hemorrhage from a deep lobar stab or missile track.[103,104] Inflation of the balloon is performed at different levels of the track until hemorrhage is controlled. Removal of the balloon catheter is performed at a reoperation when the patient's metabolic failure has been corrected. Absorbable mesh tamponade is used to reapproximate a disrupted lobe with viable fragments that are still attached to the hilum or to replace a disrupted Glisson's capsule after rupture of a subcapsular hematoma and may be an excellent alternative to major hepatic resection.[105,106] For the former, the technique involves mobilization of the injured lobe and circumferential wrapping with a mesh sewn to itself at various locations. Although it may be time-consuming in the patient with a severe coagulopathy, it does avoid the need for reoperation. The insertion of dry laparotomy pads as perihepatic packs continues to be necessary in less than 10% of patients undergoing operative repair of hepatic injuries. Primary indications, in addition to the onset of metabolic failure, include the need to transfer the patient to a center with more experienced hepatic surgeons, a desire to avoid opening a large subcapsular hematoma, and the presence of bilobar injuries.[57,107–109] The insertion of perihepatic packs mandates a reoperation and remains one of the classical indications for use of the alternate closures of the midline incision to be described. When placing perihepatic packs, one should be mindful of the possible need for hepatic angiography as an adjunct to laparotomy. If the radioopaque markers of the laparotomy pads are not strategically placed away from the hilum, they may obscure the visualization required for successful angiography.

Operative venovenous bypass of the liver, postoperative venous stenting, and postoperative arterial embolization are all adjuncts to the standard damage control techniques described earlier. All have been applied successfully in selected patients in recent years.[110–115]

Spleen (see Chap. 33.). With American Association for the Surgery of Trauma (AAST) Organ Injury Scale (OIS) grade III, IV, or V injuries, splenectomy remains the safest choice when damage

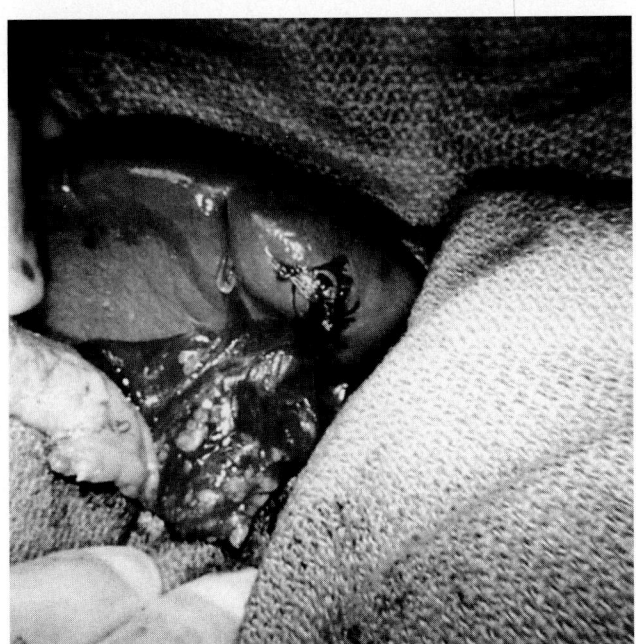

**FIGURE 41-2.** Rapid two-suture splenorrhaphy is faster than splenectomy for patients with AAST grade I or II injuries.
*(Reproduced with permission from Feliciano DV, Spjut-Patrinely V, Burch JM, et al. Splenorrhaphy: The alternative. Ann Surg 211:569, 1990.)*

control is necessary.[116,117] Should an AAST OIS grade I or II injury be present, rapid mobilization and direct suture may be faster than splenectomy and will avoid the creation of a denuded retroperitoneal area in the patient with a coagulopathy (Fig. 41-2). With rupture of the capsule, a topical agent such as microfibrillar collagen (Avitene, Bard, Murray Hill, NJ) or fibrin glue is applied to the parenchyma under an absorbable mesh. If the condition of the patient does not permit the time needed to suture absorbable mesh as a replacement capsule, a mesh sheet is compressed against the parenchyma with a laparotomy pad pack.

**Gastrointestinal tract (see Chaps. 34–36.).** Near transections of the duodenum are stapled shut, while an associated injury to the head of the pancreas is packed. At the reoperation after metabolic failure has been corrected, duodenal continuity can be restored with an end-to-end anastomosis. A pyloric exclusion with polypropylene suture (Fig. 41-3) and an antecolic gastrojejunostomy (Fig. 41-4) are added in selected patients with severe duodenal contusion, narrowing after a suture repair, or a combined pancreatoduodenal injury.[118,119]

In the patient with a limited number of enterotomies or colotomies from a penetrating wound, a rapid one-layer, full-thickness closure using a continuous suture of 3–0 or 4–0 polypropylene material is appropriate. Multiple large perforations within a short segment of the small bowel or colon are treated with segmental resection, using metallic clips for mesenteric hemostasis and staples to transect the bowel. In the unstable patient, neither an end-to-end anastomosis nor the maturation of a colostomy is performed until the reoperation in 12 to 72 hours.[120] Burch and colleagues have also described the use of umbilical tapes around the resected ends of the bowel or around segments containing perforations that have not been repaired.[56] With shotgun wounds and multiple partial and full-thickness perforations of the jejunum, a jejunectomy is appropriate as all of its absorptive capabilities are duplicated by the ileum.

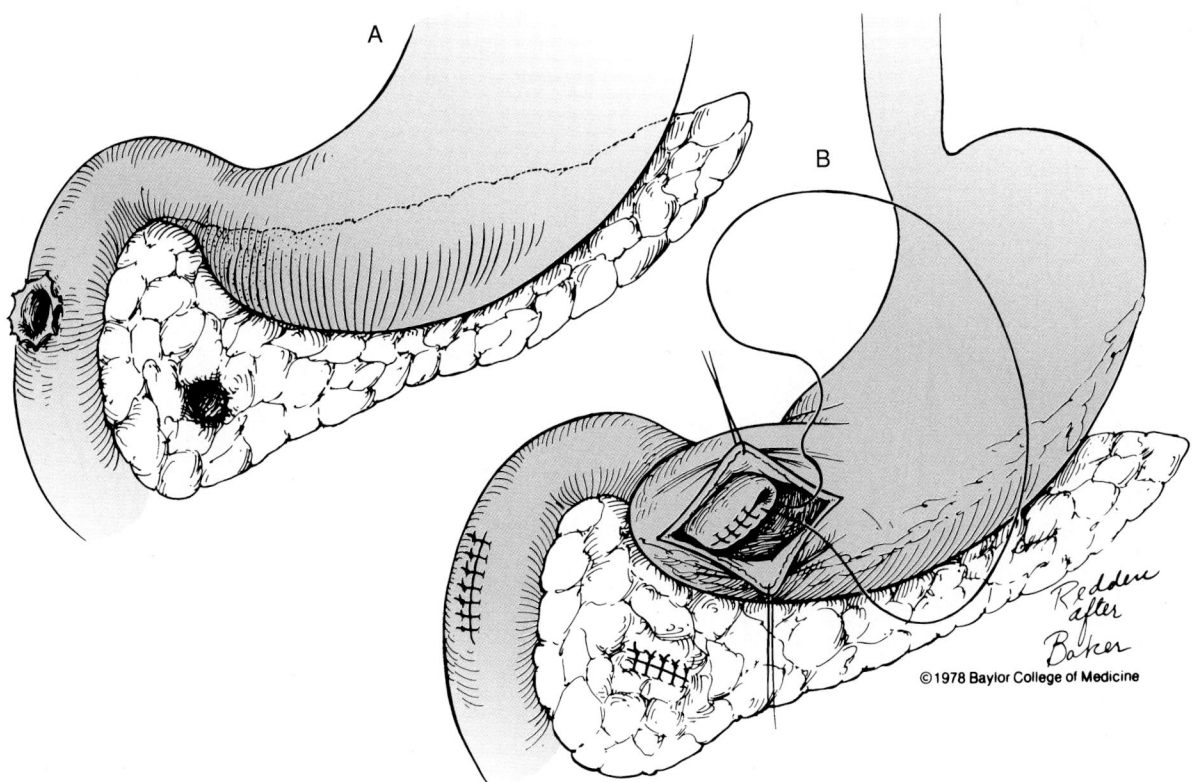

©1978 Baylor College of Medicine

**FIGURE 41-3.** Pyloric exclusion is performed through a dependent gastrotomy and completed with no. 1 polypropylene suture.
*(Reproduced with permission from Baylor College of Medicine.)*

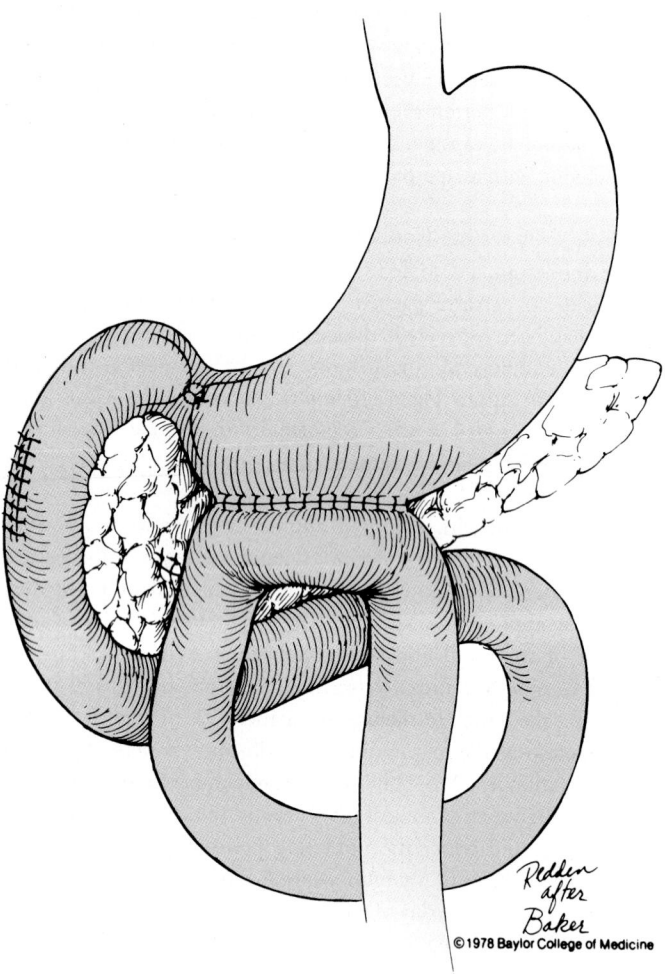

**FIGURE 41-4.** An antecolic gastrojejunostomy is added to the pyloric exclusion to allow for oral intake before the pyloric exclusion opens. *(Reproduced with permission from Baylor College of Medicine.)*

**Pancreas (see Chap. 35.).**    Parenchymal defects not involving the duct are either ignored at the damage control procedure or filled with omentum held in place by a tacking suture. The insertion of a closed-suction drain is delayed until the reoperation. Ductal transections to the left of the mesenteric vessels that do not involve the splenic vessels are packed or drained, with the distal pancreatectomy and splenectomy once again delayed until the reoperation (Fig. 41-5). Major parenchymal or ductal injuries in the head or neck of the pancreas are also packed or drained, once hemorrhage from the gland or underlying mesenteric–portal vessels is controlled. A needed pancreatoduodenectomy or reconstruction after a pancreatoduodenectomy caused by the original injury is obviously delayed until the reoperation as well.[120]

**Abdominal Arteries (see Chap. 37.).**    In any patient with multiple upper abdominal visceral and vascular injuries, a significant injury to the celiac axis is treated with ligation. An injury to the renal artery is also best treated with ligation and nephrectomy in the presence of a palpably normal contralateral kidney and multiple associated injuries. The use of a large intraluminal shunt (thoracostomy tube) is a theoretical consideration when there has been segmental loss of either the suprarenal or infrarenal aorta in a patient with profound shock; most experienced trauma surgeons, however, would choose to rapidly insert a 12-mm, 14-mm, or 16-mm woven Dacron, albumin-coated Dacron, or polytetrafluoroethylene (PTFE) interposition graft and accept a 20- to 25-minute longer operative procedure. The superior mesenteric artery or common or external iliac artery is smaller in young trauma patients, and an intraluminal Argyle, Javid, or Pruitt–Inahara shunt may be rapidly inserted under proximal and distal ties to avoid the need for ligation or interposition grafting.[121] Should arterial ligation be chosen rather than repair or shunting for a significant injury to the common or external iliac artery, a rapid ipsilateral two-skin incision, four-compartment

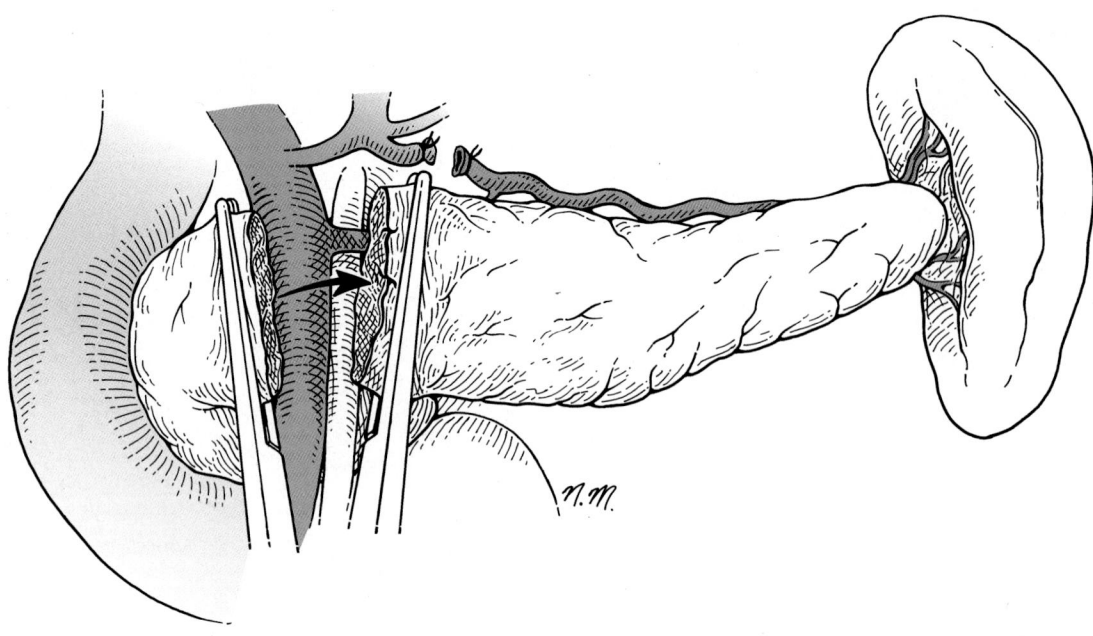

**FIGURE 41-5.**    Distal pancreatectomy with splenectomy may be completed at the reoperation rather than at the damage control laparotomy. *(Reprinted with permission from Cushman JG, Feliciano DV: Contemporary management of pancreatic trauma, in Maull KI, Cleveland HC, Feliciano DV, et al. eds. Advances in Trauma and Critical Care. St. Louis: Mosby, 1995, vol 10, pp 309-336.)*

below-knee fasciotomy may prevent myonecrosis with its associated renal and septic problems should the patient survive to undergo an early (within six hours) extra-anatomic revascularization procedure.[117]

When life-threatening *arterial* hemorrhage from either a blunt pelvic fracture or a penetrating wound occurs in the deep pelvis and cannot be controlled by packing, several innovative approaches are available. The first is to insert a Fogarty balloon catheter into the internal iliac artery beyond a proximal tie on the side of the hemorrhage. Once again, advancement of the balloon and sequential inflation is performed until the hemorrhage ceases.[123] The catheter may then be folded on itself, the excess cut off, and a ligature applied to maintain inflation of the balloon but avoid the need for reoperation.[92,123] The other option is for the surgical team to inject a slurry of autologous clot, two cans of microfibrillar collagen (Avitene, MedChem Products, Inc., Woburn, MA), one packet of bovine topical thrombin (Armour Pharmaceutical Co., Kankakee, IL), and 1 g calcium chloride into the distal internal iliac artery beyond a proximal ligature.[124]

### Abdominal Veins (see Chap. 37).

Ligation is the treatment of choice whenever there is a significant injury to the common or external iliac vein, infrarenal inferior vena cava, superior mesenteric vein, or portal vein in a patient with profound shock.[125–128] After ligation of the infrarenal inferior vena cava, bilateral four-compartment below-knee fasciotomies should be performed immediately if the anterior compartment pressure is greater than 25 to 35 mmHg, depending on the patient's hemodynamic status. Bilateral thigh fasciotomies will likely be necessary, as well, within the first 48 hours after ligation. When there are large defects in the sacrum or pelvic sidewall involving numerous pelvic veins or in the paravertebral area, a number of innovative approaches are available to rapidly control hemorrhage. Included among these are packing the missile track with several vaginal packs (to allow for postoperative pelvic or paravertebral arteriography), inserting fibrin glue, or placing a Foley catheter with a 30-mL balloon inflated at the site of hemorrhage as previously described. Placing packs outside the blast cavity in the deep pelvis or paravertebral area often fails to control hemorrhage in the patient who develops a coagulopathy. Bleeding from presacral veins can be controlled by inserting sterile tacks directly into the visible defect or by suturing a free piece of omentum into an obvious area of perforation.

### Intra-abdominal Packing.

When severe shock, hypothermia, acidosis, and massive transfusion have led to a coagulopathy and diffuse nonmechanical bleeding, the insertion of intra-abdominal packing for tamponade is appropriate.[57,107–109,129–131] Diffuse intra-abdominal packing has been found to be particularly useful when a coagulopathy occurs and extensive retroperitoneal or pelvic dissection has been necessary during a laparotomy for a trauma. Dry, folded laparotomy pads much as described for perihepatic packing are preferred followed by an alternate form of incisional closure. In general, a relaparotomy is performed to remove the packs, irrigate out old blood and clot, and rule out injuries missed at the original damage control laparotomy.

In the original series from Grady Memorial Hospital reported by Stone and associates, 17 trauma patients with intraoperative coagulopathies underwent damage control laparotomy including the insertion of diffuse packing with laparotomy pads. Reexploration was performed at 15 to 69 hours in 12 surviving patients, and 11 survived removal of the packs and definitive laparotomy.[129]

## Operative Techniques with Vascular Trauma in an Extremity (see Chap. 44)

Damage control operations on an extremity are appropriate when exsanguination has caused intraoperative metabolic failure (shotgun wound of femoral triangle); when multisystem injuries have occurred and an emergent craniotomy, thoracotomy, or laparotomy needs to be performed in addition to the vascular repair of the extremity (occlusion of superficial femoral artery from a femur fracture); or when the instability of an open fracture precludes formal repair of the associated vascular injury (mangled extremity).[132]

After rapid control of hemorrhage, an intraluminal Argyle or Javid shunt is inserted into the debrided ends of the injured femoral or popliteal artery and tied in place to preserve distal flow as the patient is resuscitated in the intensive care unit.[17,133] The Pruitt–Inahara shunt may be used also and has inflatable balloons on either end so that tying the shunt in place is not necessary. This shunt has a T-port, which allows for the infusion of heparin, a vasodilator such as tolazoline, or for arteriography in the postoperative period. In a review of eight patients who had extremity (5) or truncal (3) intraluminal arterial shunts placed as part of a damage control operation, thrombosis of the shunt occurred after operation in only one patient with a shunt in the superficial femoral artery despite the lack of heparinization.[133]

While ligation of major venous injuries in the extremities has been well tolerated in many stable patients,[134,135] patients undergoing damage control operations often have severe sequelae.[132] Among these are a compartment syndrome below the level of ligation in the lower extremity and excessive hemorrhage from soft tissue injuries and fasciotomy sites. Even if a compartment syndrome does not occur immediately, reperfusion injury as the patient undergoes resuscitation in the intensive care unit will usually cause the syndrome to develop. For these reasons, venous outflow after segmental resection of an injured femoral or popliteal vein should be restored with a temporary intraluminal shunt as part of a damage control operation. Short segments of thoracostomy tubes (size 24 to 28 French) are used as shunts for the popliteal, superficial femoral, or common femoral veins. After removal of the shunt at a reoperation, an externally supported PTFE graft is used for segmental replacement.[136]

When vascular control has been difficult to obtain with combined femoral or popliteal arterial and venous injuries, there may be some delay before the intraluminal shunts are inserted. In such a situation or when ligation of the femoral or popliteal vein has been necessary to prevent exsanguination, additional time should be spent to complete an ipsilateral four-compartment below-knee fasciotomy as part of the damage control operation. With two attending surgeons or senior residents performing these procedures, they can be completed within 20 minutes. The additional time involved prevents myonecrosis in the early postoperative period and allows the critical care team to focus on respiratory, cardiac, and renal resuscitation.

## INDICATIONS FOR ALTERNATE CLOSURES OF INCISIONS

### Intraoperative Metabolic Failure

In the previously described patients with hypothermia (temperature <35°C [95.0°F]), persistent acidemia (pH < 7.2), and/or the onset of an intraoperative coagulopathy, a damage control operation should be terminated with an alternate closure of the incision. A rapid closure of only the skin of the incision, if possible, will eliminate one source of heat loss and allow for immediate transfer of the unstable patient to the ICU. This technique has been used much less frequently in recent years as continued resuscitation in the intensive care unit has often led to a delayed abdominal compartment syndrome.

### Planned Reoperation

One of the fundamental principles of the damage control operation is that a reoperation will be necessary to complete repairs and resections, perform anastomoses, look for missed injuries, change thoracostomy tubes, insert drains, and attempt closure of the incision. There are also techniques utilized at first operations for trauma, whether damage control was necessary or not, that mandate an early reoperation. Patients in whom these techniques are used will also benefit from alternate forms of closure of the thoracic or abdominal incision and include the following:

- Insertion of perihepatic packing
- Insertion of intra-abdominal packing
- Planned second-look operation

Examples of patients who may require an early second-look procedure after laparotomy for abdominal trauma include those with primary repair of the renal or superior mesenteric artery and those with ligation of the superior mesenteric or portal vein. In the former group, repair of a small vasoconstricted artery in a hypotensive patient often leaves the surgeon with concern about an early postoperative thrombosis.[122,137] Early reoperation allows for visual inspection of the end organ after the patient has become hemodynamically stable. With major venous injuries, the dusky and congested appearance of the bowel after major splanchnic venous ligation during the initial operation often prompts concerns about secondary infarction of the involved intestine.[126–128] Planned reoperation is worthwhile in such patients, particularly if the base deficit does not correct in the first 8 to 12 hours after the ligation was performed.

### Closure of the Incision Cannot Be Performed or Will Cause an Abdominal Compartment Syndrome

Edema and distention of the midgut are commonly noted during prolonged laparotomies for trauma in which patients in shock have been treated with massive crystalloid resuscitation in addition to blood. Presumably, these changes are related to cellular edema from metabolic failure of the sodium pump in the cell membrane, a "capillary leak" phenomenon with secondary interstitial edema related to the release of vasoactive substances, reperfusion injury, the development of an ileus, or some combination of these.[23,24,138–141]

The volume of the midgut may increase significantly and, if perihepatic or intra-abdominal packs have been inserted as well, make formal fascial closure of the midline abdominal incision time-consuming and extraordinarily difficult. Should fascial closure be completed successfully, the increased volume and secondary increase in pressure (normal: 0 to subatmospheric) in the abdominal cavity may have severe adverse systemic effects, the so-called abdominal compartment syndrome.[23–33]

## ABDOMINAL COMPARTMENT SYNDROME

### Definition

The abdominal compartment syndrome refers to the decreased blood flow to the body wall and abdominal organs and secondary pressure effects on the respiratory, cardiovascular, and central nervous systems when the intra-abdominal pressure rises above a critical level.[23,24] While occasionally discussed in the literature since the 1800s, it is only in the past 20 years that the diagnosis has been made on a regular basis in patients on a variety of surgical and medical services.[25–33,142,143]

### Measurement of Intra-abdominal Pressure

Direct measurement of intra-abdominal pressure is accomplished by inserting an intraperitoneal catheter attached to a manometer or transducer.[144] In the clinical setting, indirect measurement is possible through a catheter inserted into the urinary bladder,[145,146] stomach,[147] or inferior vena cava.[148] The ease and accuracy of measuring intra-abdominal pressure at the level of the symphysis pubis through a saline column (50 to 100 mL) previously injected into an empty bladder and connected to a pressure transducer or manometer is well known and remains the technique of choice.[145,146] The validity of the bladder pressure as a measure of intra-abdominal pressure has been well documented.[149] A technique for the continuous measurement of intra-abdominal pressure via the urinary bladder has also been described utilizing the irrigation port of a three-way Foley catheter; this technique may theoretically allow for a more timely identification of elevated intra-abdominal pressures.[150]

### Clinical Manifestations of Intra-abdominal Hypertension

A comprehensive discussion of all the effects of intra-abdominal hypertension causing an abdominal compartment syndrome is beyond the scope of this chapter, and the reader is referred to published clinical and laboratory reviews and studies (Table 41-4).[24–33,142,143,151–178]

### Proposed Classification

The group at Denver Health Medical Center first proposed a grading system for the abdominal compartment syndrome in 1996.[24] This grading system was slightly modified in a subsequent publication and is presented along with recommendations for management based on an indirect measurement of intra-abdominal pressure in Table 41-5.[179] These recommendations were based on a

## TABLE 41-4

### Clinical and Laboratory Manifestations of Increased Intra-abdominal Pressure[24,25,137,138,145–172]

**Abdominal**

Body wall[145,146]

  Decreased blood flow

Gastrointestinal tract[147–151]

  Decreased mucosal blood flow and intramucosal pH

  Possible bacterial translocation

Hepatic[152,153]

  Decreased portal blood flow and hepatocyte mitochondrial funtion

Renal[154–160]

  Increased renal vein pressure

  Increased plasma renin and aldosterone

  Decreased renal blood flow, glomerular filtration rate, and urine output

**Thoracic**

Lung[157,161–163]

  Increased intrathoracic pressure, peak airway pressure, peak inspiratory pressure, and intrapulmonary shunt

  Decreased dynamic compliance

Heart/cardiovascular[157,161,164–168]

  Decreased venous return and cardiac output

  "False" increase of central venous pressure and pulmanary artery wedge pressure

  Increased systemic and pulmonary vascular resistance

**Central nervous system[169–172]**

  Increased intracranial pressure secondary to decreased venous return

  Decreased cerebral perfusion pressure

## TABLE 41-5

### Grading of the Abdominal Compartment Syndrome

| BLADDER PRESSURE | GRADE (mmHg) | RECOMMENDATION |
|---|---|---|
| I | 10–15 | Maintain normovolemia |
| II | 16–25 | Hypervolemic resuscitation |
| III | 26–35 | Decompression |
| IV | >35 | Decompression and reexploration |

Reproduced with permission from Meldrum DR, Moore FA, Moore EE et al.: Prospective characterization and selective management of the abdominal compartment syndrome. Am J Surg 174:667, 1997.

study of 145 acutely injured patients (ISS > 15) undergoing laparotomy, 21 of whom developed an abdominal compartment syndrome (Table 41-6). Of interest, this study validates an intra-abdominal pressure of 25 mm Hg as an indicator to decompress the abdominal compartment syndrome.

## Abdominal Perfusion Pressure

In one report, abdominal perfusion pressure defined as mean arterial pressure minus intra-abdominal pressure was compared to intra-abdominal pressure, arterial pH, base deficit, arterial lactate, and urinary output as an endpoint of resuscitation and as a predictor of survival.[180] The authors found that an abdominal perfusion pressure of 50 mm Hg was a potential endpoint for resuscitation in the patient with an elevated intra-abdominal pressure. Also, the abdominal perfusion pressure was statistically superior to

## TABLE 41-6

### Percentage of Patients with Respective Organ Dysfunction Per Grade of Abdominal Compartment Syndrome

| GRADE | UO <0.5 mL/kg/h | PAP > 45 | SVR >1000 | DO₂I <60 |
|---|---|---|---|---|
| I | 0% | 0% | 0% | 0% |
| II | 0% | 40% | 20% | 20% |
| III | 65% | 78% | 65% | 57% |
| IV | 100% | 100% | 100% | 100% |

$DO_2I$, oxygen delivery index (mL $O_2$/min/m²); PAP, peak airway pressure (cm $H_2O$); SVR, systemic vascular resistance (dyne/s/cm⁻⁵); UO, urine output (mL/min).

*Reproduced with permission from Meldrum DR, Moore FA, Moore EE, et al: Prospective characterization and selective management of the abdominal compartment syndrome. Am J Surg 174:667,1997.*

the other endpoints listed in predicting survival for patients with intra-abdominal hypertension and the abdominal compartment syndrome.

## Secondary Abdominal and Extremity Compartment Syndromes

There is now widespread recognition that the abdominal compartment syndrome can occur in the absence of intra-abdominal injuries.[28,30,31,33] This "secondary" abdominal compartment syndrome is thought to be due to an ischemia and reperfusion injury in the gastrointestinal tract as well as a capillary leak syndrome from abdominal viscera.[28,30] All patients who have developed this syndrome present with severe injuries, sepsis, or burns >41% and usually >70% total body surface area. Massive resuscitation has been necessary in all patients reported to date (mean of 19±5 L of crystalloid and 29±10 U of packed red blood cells in one report).[30] Of interest, the diagnosis of a secondary abdominal compartment syndrome was made from 3 hours to 9 days after injury in reports.[28,30,31] The mortality in four reports was 65.5% (19/29).[28,30,31]

Another related concern in the patient undergoing a massive resuscitation is the development of a secondary extremity compartment syndrome (SECS). Similar to secondary ACS, SECS is associated with extremely high morbidity and mortality (70%).[181] Serial measurement of creatine phosphokinase (CPK) and urine myoglobins may be appropriate in high-risk patients as a screening tool. Any individual with persistently rising CPKs or the unexplained development of myoglobinuria may benefit from measurement of extremity compartment pressures and fascial releases as appropriate.

## Prevention and Management of the Abdominal Compartment Syndrome

The abdominal compartment syndrome is prevented by leaving the midline celiotomy incision open in high-risk patients. Because the syndrome can have a delayed presentation after trauma and resuscitation or develop even though there are no abdominal injuries (secondary abdominal compartment syndrome), there are still critically injured or ill patients who will require treatment. Innovative approaches to avoiding a return to the operating room for abdominal decompression have included laparoscopic decompression or the insertion of an angiocatheter or peritoneal dialysis catheter to remove intraperitoneal fluid.[182,183] Another interesting approach used successfully in a laboratory model has been the application of a continuous negative abdominal pressure (CNAP) device.[178,184]

## OPERATIVE TECHNIQUES FOR THE OPEN ABDOMEN

Management of the open abdomen can be divided into two phases. In the acute phase, the goal is to provide some variant of temporary coverage to allow the patient to be taken from the operating room to the ICU for additional resuscitation and stabilization with the intent on returning to the operating room when normal physiology has been restored. In the second phase, which follows reoperation, the issue is the management of the abdominal wound and techniques range from delayed fascial closure to planned ventral hernia.

### Towel Clip or Suture Closure of the Skin

The simplest and most rapidly performed technique for temporary closure of a thoracic, abdominal, or groin incision in the unstable trauma or septic patient is towel clip or suture closure of only the skin.[23] Depending on the length of the incision, up to 25 to 30 standard towel clips may be necessary to complete closure of the wound during a two-minute period. In order to prevent manipulation of the towel clips and minimize secondary contamination of the chest, abdomen, or groin through the spaces between the towel clips, a large plastic adherent drape is placed over the towel clips and Jackson–Pratt drains lying lateral to the incision in the operating room prior to transfer to the SICU. When suture closure of only the skin is chosen, 2–0 nylon or thicker suture material is used, depending on the tension of the closure. These skin-closure-only techniques are used much less frequently than they were in the

past as increases in postoperative intra-abdominal pressure have led to the abdominal compartment syndrome in a significant number of patients.

### Temporary Silos

When the extent of edema and distention of the midgut or the presence of multiple intra-abdominal packs prevents towel clip or suture closure of the skin of the abdominal incision, the insertion of an abdominal silo to cover the exposed viscera is performed (Fig. 41-6). Complete coverage of the open abdomen using a polyvinyl plastic silo was first performed by Oswaldo Borraez G. at the San Juan de Dios Hospital in Bogota, Colombia, in March 1984. As the technique of complete silo coverage has become more acceptable since that time, a variety of materials and techniques have been used. When only a small- or moderate-sized silo is needed, a plastic wound drape (Steri-Drape, 3M, St. Paul, MN) applied to the skin edges with adhesive material or sewn to the skin edges with a continuous 2-0 nylon or polypropylene suture is appropriate. In patients with significant distention of the midgut or peritoneal contents secondary to packs, the soft plastic drape will not be adequate to maintain the midgut within the confines of the abdominal incision. A readily available stronger silo is a 3-L plastic bag of irrigating solution used by the urology service (Fig. 41-7).[185] A large silo of this material is constructed by cutting three seams of the bag open, and then gas-autoclaving the large rectangular piece that results. In an emergency, an unsterile silo is constructed in the same fashion. This silo is once again sewn to the skin edges of the abdominal wound. Another strong silo is Silastic sheeting (Dow Corning Corp, Midland, MI), but this is considerably more expensive than the bag of irrigating solution.[186] Even the "fish" available in every operating room has been used as a temporary silo.[187] Some groups have used gradual reduction in the size of the silo, much as has been described in the pediatric surgical literature for neonates with an omphalocele or gastroschisis.[188] In patients with significant distension of the

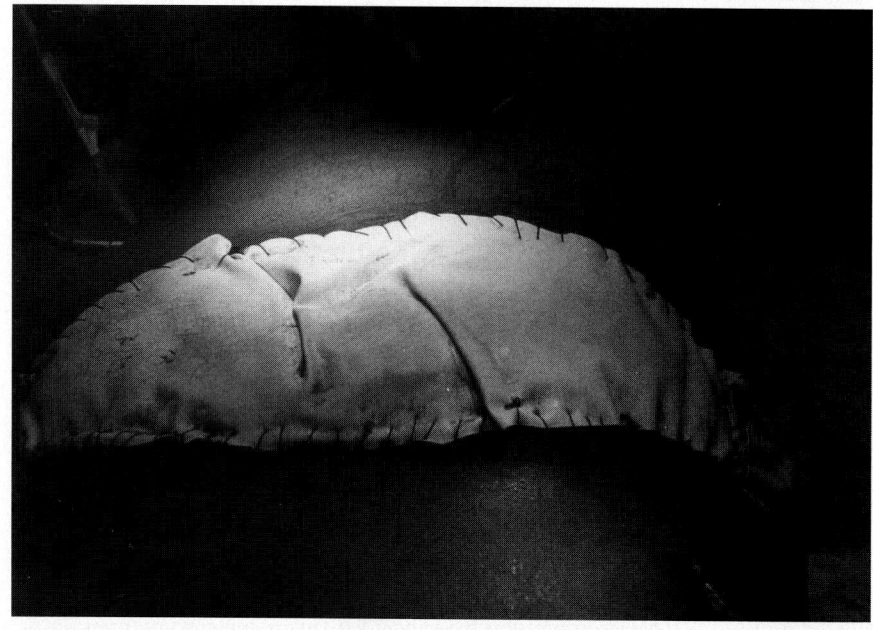

**FIGURE 41-6.** Esmarch bandage silo closure of bilateral anterolateral thoracotomy in patient with six missile perforations in the heart and inferior vena cava.

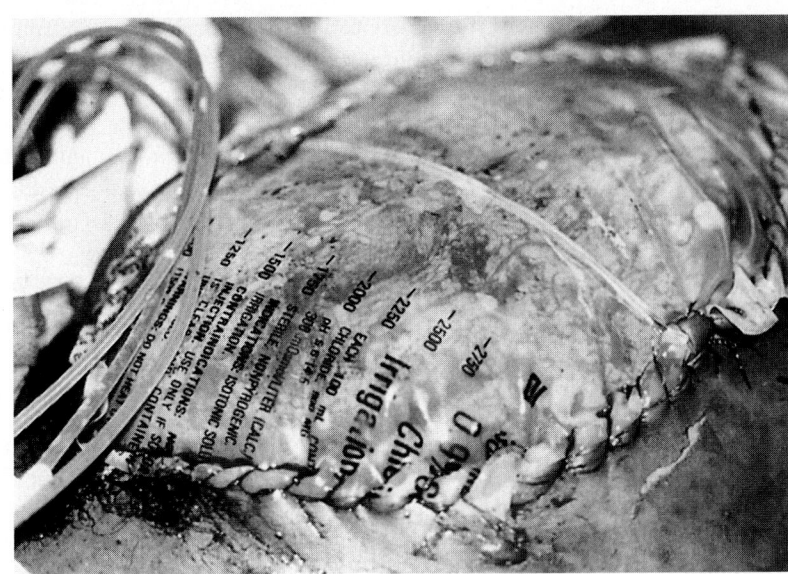

**FIGURE 41-7.** Plastic irrigating bag sewn to the skin edges of the abdominal wound makes an excellent silo.

midgut after removal of the temporary silo at a first reoperation, application of a vacuum assisted closure (VAC) device (Kinetic Concepts, Inc., San Antonio, TX) is now commonly performed (see below).

## Combination Closure

In patients with significant liver injuries requiring perihepatic packs, a combination of closures may be appropriate. In such a patient, it is sometimes desirable to have a "tight" closure of the upper abdomen to maintain tamponade of the injured liver. Partial fascial closure limited to the upper abdomen or partial towel clip closure of the same area may be used in conjunction with a silo placed over the lower abdomen. This arrangement maintains a tamponade effect on the injured liver while allowing ample room for expansion of the midgut to avert the development of an abdominal compartment syndrome.

## Vacuum-Assisted Wound Closure

A number of early reports described excellent results with "home-grown" vacuum pack coverage of the open abdomen.[189,190] The fundamental principle of applying suction to the open wound over the midgut is that it allows for the rapid removal of peritoneal fluid and collapses spaces between the viscera. As both these results will make the contents of the abdominal cavity smaller, there is a greater chance of formal aponeurotic closure of the midline incision. In the report by Barker et al.,[38] 216 vacuum packs were placed in 112 patients. While 22 patients (19.6%) died before abdominal closure was attempted, 62 (55.4%) went on to formal closure of the incision. The overall mortality rate in this large series was 25.9%.

As previously mentioned, The Kinetic Concepts, Inc., VAC system has been utilized in many centers.[39] A nonadherent occlusive plastic barrier (Steri-Drape; 3M Healthcare, St. Paul, MN) with small perforations placed in it is covered by an appropriately sized polyurethane foam sponge that is part of the VAC system. The suction tubing that is part of the system is attached, and the entire system is covered with an airtight occlusive drape. In the report by

Garner et al.,[39] 13 of the 14 injured patients in whom the system was used underwent formal closure of the midline incision before discharge.

## Open Packing

This older technique using nylon cloth material over the midgut has been used at Detroit Receiving Hospital for over 30 years.[36,191] The cloth is covered with "generous" gauze packs, while several widely spaced retention sutures are placed through the abdominal wall above the packs. Every effort is made to keep the midgut below the aponeurotic edges.

As midgut edema resolves, the patient is returned to the operating room for removal of the gauze and gradual tightening of the retention sutures until the linea alba can be closed. In the report by Bender et al.,[15,17] patients surviving longer than 24 hours had successful closure of the midline incision using the technique described.[191] There were no enterocutaneous fistulae or incisional hernias in the 14 long-term survivors. A number of related approaches have been described in the literature as well.[41,42]

## INTENSIVE CARE BEFORE REOPERATION

Following the control of surgical bleeding, patients are brought to the intensive care unit for ongoing resuscitation. The immediate goals are to provide both adequate oxygenation and reverse the effects of inadequate tissue perfusion and resultant metabolic failure. The lethal triad of hypothermia, coagulopthy, and acidosis must be aggressively rectified if the patient is to survive.

All the previously described warming maneuvers used in the emergency department and operating room—increased ambient temperature, external rewarming using a Bair Hugger or similar device, warming lights, warmed fluid and blood products—are also implemented in the intensive care unit. For refractory cases of hypothermia, Gentilello and associates have also described the use of a continuous arteriovenous rewarming (CAVR) device.[192] In the patient with a systolic blood pressure greater than 80 mm Hg, femoral arterial and venous catheters are connected through the heating mechanism of a standard countercurrent fluid warmer. The patient's own blood pressure drives the blood through heparin-bonded tubing; therefore, use of this system is limited in hypotensive patients. In a mixed group of 34 hypothermic patients (<35°C [95.0°F]) with trauma, major operations, or near-drowning, 16 patients treated with CAVR had resolution of their hypothermia in 39 minutes versus 3.23 hours in the group of 18 treated with the conventional methods described above. Inability to correct a patient's hypothermia after a damage control operation is a marker of inadequate resuscitation or irreversible shock.[69]

The multifactorial coagulopathy of the trauma patient must also be aggressively managed. Postoperatively, patients undergoing damage control procedures should have serial coagulation parameters monitored including routine measurement of fibrinogen levels to assess the need for cryoprecipitate in addition to fresh frozen plasma and PRBCs. As previously discussed, the administration of recombinant factor VIIa may also be appropriate.

Several parameters may be utilized to assess the adequacy of a resuscitation, with acidosis being one of the most common. It is generally accepted that resuscitation is not complete until the patient's oxygen debt is repaid; simple restoration of normal vital signs is not adequate as a patient may simply be in "compensated" shock while continuing to have occult hypoperfusion and ongoing tissue damage.[193] Extensive studies have been performed to determine the parameters that best define the endpoint of resuscitation. These endpoints can be divided into two broad categories, global and regional. In addition to acid-base status, parameters for monitoring global resuscitation include oxygen delivery, mixed venous saturation, right ventricular end diastolic volume, left ventricular stroke work index, and others.[193] From a regional perspective, gastric tonometry and intramucosal pH have been used to assess gastric perfusion. Additionally, both spectroscopy and electrodes have been applied to measure tissue $pO_2$, $pCO_2$, and pH in muscle and subcutaneous tissue to assess peripheral perfusion.[193,194] While all these techniques may provide data that can be used to predict outcome, none has been proven to be a superior marker of the endpoint of resuscitation.[193] Still, it is recommended that one of these endpoints be monitored in addition to the standard clinical parameters to assess that adequacy of resuscitation.[193]

Historically, there has been interest in "supranormal" resuscitation in previously shocky patients with a significant oxygen debt. In one often-quoted study by Moore and colleagues, 39 injured patients in the ICU were treated with a goal of attaining an oxygen delivery greater than 600 L/min/m² and an oxygen consumption of greater than 150 mL/min/m². In the group of 21 patients with a baseline oxygen consumption less than 150 mL/min/m², organ failure developed in 82% of those whose oxygen consumption remained less than 150 mL/min/m² 12 hours later. In contrast, organ failure developed in only 30% of those whose oxygen consumption was greater than 150 mL/min/m² 12 hours later.[195] Durham and coworkers[196] later compared 27 critically ill patients who were resuscitated to maintain similar endpoints as in the series by Moore and colleagues[195] to 31 patients resuscitated based on pulmonary artery wedge pressure, RVEDVI, mean arterial pressure, and cardiac index. No difference was found in the incidence of subsequent organ failure, and the authors concluded that "oxygen-based parameters are more useful as predictors of outcome than as endpoints for resuscitation."[196] Current expert opinion

recommends the observation of oxygen delivery parameters because "the ability of a patient to attain supranormal values correlates with an improved chance for survival."[193] There is not, however, adequate evidence to support the use of any specific interventions to drive a patient to supraphysiologic values at the present time.[193]

# REOPERATION

## Emergency Reoperation

Failure to attain the desired endpoints of resuscitation during the ICU phase of damage control may reflect continuing hemorrhage.[57,197] An early return to the operating room is a difficult decision because the hypothermia-related coagulopathy is often not resolved. Therefore, the surgeon must decide whether mechanical or surgical hemorrhage is occurring versus diffuse oozing from a coagulopathy in which an early reoperation may not be indicated. Morris and associates have suggested several indicators for an emergent return to the operating room based on continuing hemorrhage after a damage control laparotomy (Table 41-7).[198]

Another obvious indication for an early reoperation is the development of the previously described abdominal compartment syndrome. A progressive increase in inspiratory pressures on the ventilator coupled with oliguria and a "tight" abdomen mandate a rapid measurement of intra-abdominal pressure through the bladder catheter.[145,146] Reoperation is necessary when the clinical signs are accompanied by an intra-abdominal pressure greater than 25 mm Hg, as previously described.[24,179] Morris and colleagues[57,198] and many others have noted that sudden release of the abdominal compartment syndrome at the time of reoperation may lead to a reperfusion phenomenon and a cardiac arrest. For this reason, Morris has recommended that volume loading with 2 L of a solution composed of 0.45% normal saline, 50 g mannitol per liter, and 100 meq sodium bicarbonate per liter be performed before release of the abdominal wall.

## Routine Reoperation

When postoperative bleeding is not a concern, a return to the operating room is based on reversal of metabolic failure and normalizing of cardiovascular and pulmonary parameters as suggested by

---

**TABLE 41-7**

**Indications for Emergent Return to the Operating Room after A Damage Control Laparotomy**

| BLUNT TRAUMA | PENETRATING TRAUMA |
|---|---|
| Normothermic but bleeding >2 U/h | Bleeding >15 µ and hypothermia |
| Abdominal compartment syndrome with ongoing blood loss | Normothermic but bleeding >2 U/h |
| Abdominal compartment syndrome with ongoing blood loss | |

Reproduced with permission from Morris JA Jr, Eddy VA, Rutherford EJ: The trauma celiotomy: The evolving concepts of damage control. Curr Prob Surg 33:611, 1996.

**TABLE 41-8**

**Guidelines for Elective Return to the Operating Room After A Damage Control Laparotomy**

Temperature >30°C [96.8°F]
Acid-base balance
  Base deficit corrected to >–5 mmol/L if originally <–15 mmol/L
  Serum lactate normal or correcting gradually
Coagulation
  Prothrombin time <15 s
  Partial thromboplastin time <35 s
  Platelets >50,000/μL
Cardiovascular
  Cardiac index >3 L/min/m², with or without low-dose inotrope
Pulmonary
  Fraction of inspired oxygen <0.50
  O₂ saturation >95%

*Modified with permission from Morris JA Jr, Eddy VA, Rutherford EJ: The trauma celiotomy: The evolving concepts of damage control. Curr Prob Surg 33:611, 1996.*

Morris and coworkers (Table 41-8).[198] In a review of patients with perihepatic packs inserted to control hemorrhage, relaparotomy was performed at a mean time of 3.7 days from the original damage control operation.[107] The timing of reoperation, however, may be more critical than has previously been thought, as it may act as a "trigger" for sensitized leukocytes circulating during posttraumatic inflammation ("second hit phenomenom"). As multiple-organ failure may result, the timing of reoperation may turn out to be one of the more critical factors in determining survival after a damage control operation.[199–202] Another factor to consider is that the presence of intra-abdominal packs alone results in peritoneal endotoxin and accumulation of inflammatory mediators even when cultures are sterile.[203]

A patient who is normotensive, without a coagulopathy, and is in the diuretic phase of recovery after resuscitation from shock is an ideal candidate for reoperation. While this usually takes place within 48 to 72 hours of the damage control laparotomy, it may be delayed in patients with massive distention of the midgut so that a further diuresis may occur.

If towel clips were used to close the abdominal wall at the damage control laparotomy, five of every six are removed as the first stage of reoperation. The remainder are then elevated off the abdominal wall by placing them on a spongestick as scrubbing and painting of the abdominal wall are performed. After the surgical team has placed sterile towels around the wound, the final towel clips are removed. This technique prevents evisceration during the period of skin preparation.

Once the towel clips, skin sutures, or silos have been removed, clots and packs are evacuated manually and with the suction device. A complete examination of all abdominal contents is performed to detect any injuries missed at the damage control laparotomy.[23] Resections, anastomoses of the bowel, and maturation of colostomies are rapidly performed in the hemodynamically stable patient. Prior to closure, the abdominal cavity is vigorously irrigated with saline solution containing antibiotics. This solution is left in the abdominal cavity during the 3 to 5 minutes that it takes for the surgical team to change gloves and place towels around the wound. The irrigating solution is then aspirated from the abdominal cavity, and drains are inserted as indicated.

The linea alba is closed with permanent suture, while the subcutaneous tissue and skin are packed open with antibiotic-soaked mesh gauze.

## Techniques for the Management of the Open Abdomen at Reoperation

**Repeat Application of a Silo.** When a vacuum-assisted closure device is not available, a Steri-Drape or plastic silo may be reapplied at the reoperation in the distended patient as it protects the midgut, prevents evaporation, and allows for visual confirmation that the midgut is decreasing in size during the diuretic phase of recovery.[43]

**Vacuum-Assisted Fascial Closure.** Any of the vacuum dressing techniques discussed in the "acute" setting for management of the open abdomen can also be initiated following resuscitation at the reoperation. Cothren et al. reported a 100% fascial closure rate using vacuum assisted sequential fascial reapproximation. At the time of initial operation, a silo was applied. Following stabilization of the patient, they used a variant of the technique described by Miller et al. placing a nonadherent dressing over the viscera and under the fascia, using fascial sutures to provide moderate tension, placing a superficial sponge layer, and then placing the wound to suction. They returned patients to the operating room every two days for replacement of the sponges and gradual fascial closure. Using this technique, they achieved fascial closure in 100% of their patients.[204] Other authors have also reported excellent results with vacuum devices reporting closure rates ranging from 71.9% to 92% and few complications.[205–207] At the present time, this appears to be the preferred technique for management of the open abdomen.

**Zippers, Slide Fasteners, Velcro Analogue.** Originally described by Leguit in 1982,[190] the zipper closure of the abdominal wall was popularized by Stone and colleagues in the United States in their open treatment of patients with pancreatic abscesses.[208] Either a conventional zipper is sutured to the skin or fascia with a continuous suture of 0 or 2-0 nylon or polypropylene or a commercial zipper with adhesive side pieces is applied to the skin edges. The major advantage of using the skin is that it preserves the fascia for formal wound closure at an appropriate time.

Another option for septic or trauma patients reported by Teichmann and associates,[209] Wittmann and colleagues,[210] and Aprahamian and coworkers[211] is the Wittmann Patch (STARSURGICAL, Burlington, WI). In this system two sheets of Velcro-like biocompatible material are sewn to the aponeurotic edges of the midline incision. Closure is accomplished by the adherence between the overlapping Velcro-like sheets. As edema of the midgut resolves, excess patch material is trimmed, and the fascial edges can be pulled closer together. The major advantages of this system are in the ease of access for reoperations and the tension on the aponeurotic edges that prevents the usual lateral retraction. In one series, the Wittmann Patch was utilized in conjunction with a nonadherent dressing over the abdominal viscera and under the fascia to prevent the development of adhesions that sometimes prevent medial advancement of the fascia. The authors postulate that this revised technique may lead to a higher rate of closure of the open abdomen.[212]

**Permanent Meshes.**    For the trauma patient with marked distention of the midgut, a PTFE body wall patch is strong and water-tight and creates a smooth layer of granulation tissue that can be covered with a split-thickness skin graft when the prosthesis is removed. Unfortunately, this prosthesis is quite expensive, and similar results have been obtained with less expensive absorbable meshes as previously described.

Numerous clinicians have described short-term success with closure of the abdominal wall with Marlex mesh in the presence of extensive fasciitis or intra-abdominal sepsis.[213–216] Healing of the wound over the mesh has been reported in many patients, even in those in whom grossly purulent material surrounds the mesh.[217] Numerous long-term complications, however, may occur. In the report by Voyles and associates describing the use of Marlex (Bard, Murray Hill, NJ) mesh in 31 acute abdominal wall defects, nine wounds were closed by split-thickness grafts over granulated mesh.[215] In each instance, extrusion of the mesh and/or enteric fistulae developed. Nine other wounds healed by secondary intention, and six of these developed extrusion of the mesh or enteric fistulae. Stone and colleagues reported on the use of Marlex mesh in 23 patients with acute full-thickness loss of the abdominal wall from trauma or sepsis and noted that the mesh eventually had to be removed in all but two patients.[214] They also commented that "Marlex has twice the incidence of postoperative wound sepsis, almost six times as many associated bowel fistulas, and less than one-third as many successful skin graft takes for cover" compared to prolene mesh.

These data strongly suggest that a *permanent* rigid prosthesis such as Marlex or prolene mesh should not be inserted in abdominal wall defects in the presence of extensive contamination from a perforated gastrointestinal tract secondary to trauma, acute intra-abdominal sepsis, or necrotizing infection in the abdominal wall.[218] The risk of secondary infection and damage to the underlying bowel as the prosthesis develops "wrinkles" from contraction of the wound has now been documented on numerous occasions.

**Absorbable Meshes.**    Synthetic meshes such as polyglactin (Vicryl) and polyglycolic acid (Dexon) have been available to the surgeon for the past 30 years. They have been used primarily for renorrhaphy, splenorrhaphy, and hepatorrhaphy in abdominal trauma and for closure of the pelvic floor after abdominoperineal resection of the rectum. In laboratory studies using absorbable meshes to repair defects in the abdominal wall, bursting strength has been comparable to that of permanent meshes for the first eight weeks after insertion.[219–221] Unfortunately, as the mesh is absorbed, hernias or decreased bursting strength at the site of the mesh develop by 10 to 12 weeks after insertion.[219,221]

The primary clinical use of absorbable meshes as an alternate form of closure of the abdominal incision on the trauma service has been in patients with marked distention of the midgut at the time of removal of a plastic silo or vacuum assisted closure device.[213–215,222] It has also been used in patients with open abdomens from septic processes in the abdominal wall or in the abdominal cavity.[213,214] Fabian and associates have described four stages in the use of absorbable mesh to cover an open abdomen.[45] These include the following: (a) coverage of the midgut, preferably with an absorbable mesh; (b) removal of the mesh after granulation tissue has formed at two to three weeks (Fig. 41-8); (c) split-thickness skin grafting of granulation tissue or abdominal skin and subcutaneous flap closure over the granulation tissue several days later (Fig. 41-9); and (d) definitive reconstruction in 6 to 12 months.

One practical point in using absorbable mesh is that the Dexon variant has wider interstices that allow for drainage of intra-abdominal fluid.[74] Another is to use fine mesh gauze packing above the absorbable mesh. The gauze packing will aid in keeping the small bowel below the level of the fascia of the abdominal wall, much as has been described by Bender and colleagues with their technique.[191] This prevents the gradual dilation of the bowel and thinning of its wall as is commonly seen in patients in whom the abdomen has been left open and should significantly lower the incidence of enterocutaneous fistulae in such patients.

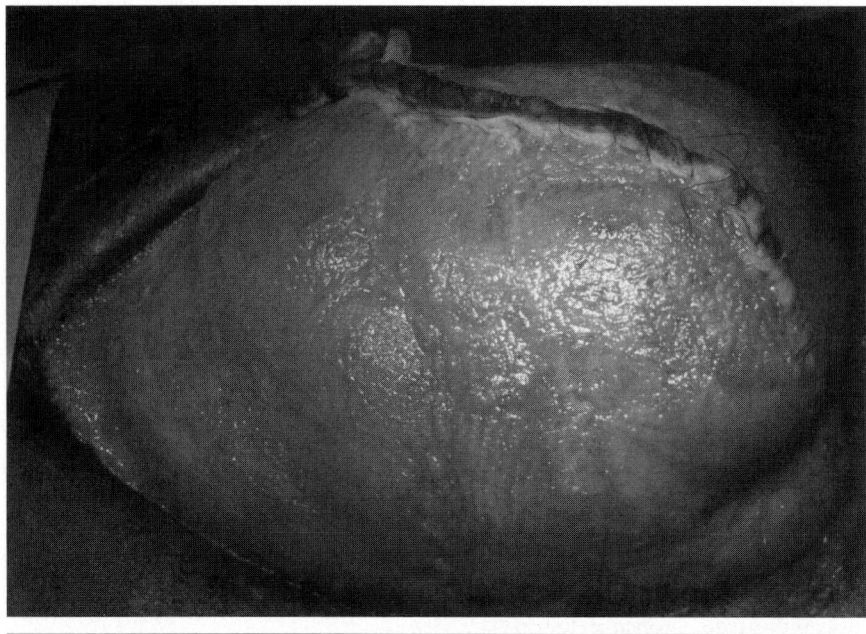

**FIGURE 41-8.**   Remains of double-layer absorbable mesh coverage of open abdomen on the day a split–thickness skin graft is to be applied. Patient sustained quadriplegia, rupture of the descending thoracic aorta, and a secondary abdominal compartment syndrome after being struck by a motor vehicle.

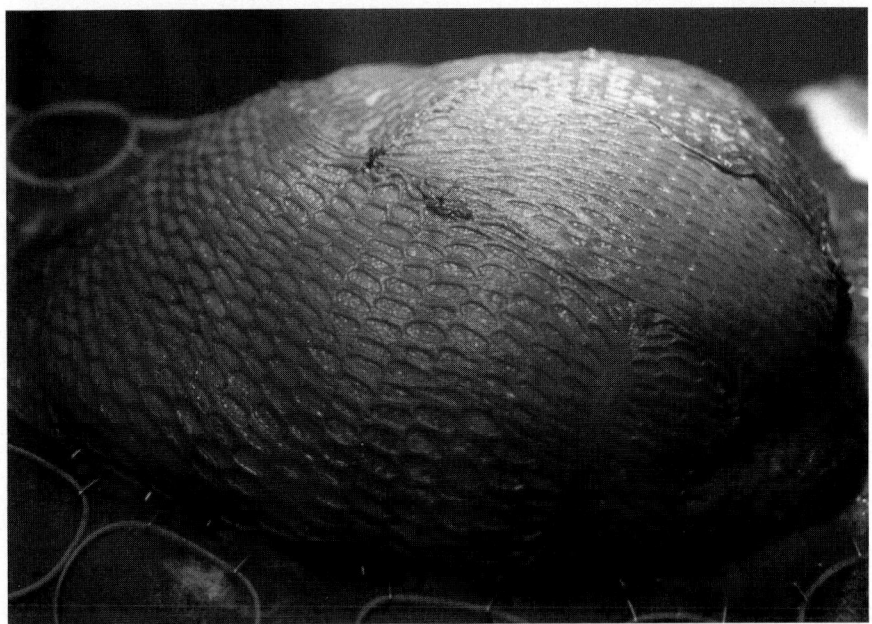

**FIGURE 41-9.**  A meshed split-thickness skin graft has been applied to the granulated abdomen of the same patient as in Fig. 41-8.

In patients with extensive manipulation of the heart during repair of a perforation or rupture or with internal cardiac massage, closure of the median sternotomy or bilateral anterolateral thoracotomy may compress the edematous heart and cause cardiac failure. An Esmarch bandage borrowed from the orthopedic surgery service should then be sewn to the skin edges as a temporary silo (Fig. 41-6). When cardiac edema has resolved, the patient is returned to the operating room, the congealed serum irrigated away, and a formal closure completed.

Should this occur, the silo is removed in the ICU and a double layer of absorbable mesh is applied over the midgut as previously described. Fine mesh gauze and a bulky pressure dressing are then used over the absorbable mesh to maintain the midgut below the level of the fascia. Split-thickness skin grafts are applied when granulation tissue completely covers the abdominal wound.

In summary, absorbable meshes avoid the major problems associated with permanent meshes (see above). When placed loosely over the midgut, they allow for distention and prevent abdominal compartment syndrome. Also, erosion into the bowel or infection of the mesh secondary to contamination from trauma or a septic process in the abdomen or abdominal wall is less likely. They help prevent evisceration when gauze packing is placed above the mesh, are soft and pliable, allow for drainage of contaminated abdominal fluid through the mesh, and permit the ingrowth of granulation tissue.[34,35,45,222] An incisional hernia occurs in all patients in whom the mesh is allowed to granulate, and repair is deferred until the patient has fully recovered from the original traumatic or septic event.

## WHAT HAPPENS TO PATIENTS WHEN A VACUUM-ASSISTED CLOSURE IS NOT USED ?

Tremblay et al. reported on 181 patients with an open abdomen over a four-year period managed with techniques other than vacuum assisted closure—silos, skin only or towel clip closure, open packing, and modified visceral packing. The morbidity in the series was high: 14% developed enterocutaneous fistulas, 5% suffered wound dehiscence, and almost half of the patients in the series were left with large incisional hernias at the time of discharge.[40] The results in this series do not compare favorably with the closure rates and complications associated with the use of the vacuum assisted closures (see above). It appears, then, that some method of vacuum assisted technique should be applied in the majority of patients.

## LATE CLOSURE OF THE INCISIONAL HERNIA

Only 10–20% of patients undergoing use of a vacuum assisted closure device are left with an incisional hernia after damage control procedures. When a hernia does result, either following an attempted closure or as the planned result following the use of vicryl mesh, it is appropriate to delay closure for 6 to 12 months. Any stomas should also be taken down in the same delayed fashion. This interval allows the patient to improve his nutritional status, fully recover from the original injuries, and complete the formation of adhesions and scars in the abdominal cavity and body wall. When assessing the patient with a massive ventral hernia preoperatively, one must carefully examine the abdominal skin graft. If the physician can pull the graft up and off of the underlying small bowel, i.e., if the patient passes the "pinch test," the timing is right for repair.[45] Additionally, one must determine if adequate skin will be available to cover the viscera and prosthetic, if used, once the skin graft to the abdomen has been excised. If it appears that skin will be lacking, tissue expanders should be placed two to three months prior to undertaking abdominal wall reconstruction.

In selected patients, the narrow midline defect that remains after excision of the skin graft over the midgut can be readily closed with a continuous or interrupted suture technique using no. 1 polypropylene material.[46] When it is not possible to close secondary to excessive tension on linea alba, lateral relaxing incisions should be made either unilaterally or bilaterally. The skin and fat is elevated off the underlying fascia through the midline incision until the flaps extend to several centimeters lateral to the rectus sheath. The external oblique aponeurosis is then divided parallel to the rectus sheath from the lower thoracic wall to just above the inguinal ligament. Each relaxing incision usually creates an additional 2 to 3 cm of width to the abdominal wall and often allows for closure of the midline. This is the second step of the components separation technique first described by Ramirez et al.[44] If this does not allow the midline to be reapproximated, the posterior rectus sheath is divided to complete the standard components separation. When a greater release is needed, the modified technique described by Fabian et al. can be used. After the rectus abdominis muscle is separated from the posterior rectus sheath, the internal oblique component of the anterior rectus sheath is divided from the epigastrium to the arcuate line. The final stage involves suturing the anterior rectus sheaths in the midline, as well as approximating the medial border of the posterior rectus sheath to the lateral border of the previously divided anterior rectus sheath. Using the technique described in nine patients, one patient developed a wound infection and a recurrent incisional hernia.[45]

If the midline can still not be reapproximated, a prosthetic patch should be used. In the presence of complete omental coverage over the midgut, a polypropylene or Marlex mesh can be utilized. In the absence of omentum, a PTFE body wall patch is appropriate.[23] If a colostomy is being taken down or there is other contamination during the procedure, a bioactive mesh may be preferable. Two options, Surgisis Gold 8-ply mesh (Cook Surgical, Bloomington, IN) and Alloderm (Life Cell Corporation, Branchburg, NJ) are widely available. The former is derived from porcine intestine, while the latter is processed cadaveric human acellular dermis. Both can be utilized in contaminated or infected fields. A recent study by Gupta et al. compared the use of these two biosynthetics for ventral hernia repair in a total of 74 patients. The initial 41 procedures used Surgisis, and the remaining 33 used Alloderm. The first 11 patients received unperforated Surgisis and 10 developed a significant seroma. The construction of fenestrations in the bioprosthetic dramatically reduced this complication (3/30). The Surgisis was placed in grossly contaminated fields in three patients with no adverse sequelae, and no patient developed a recurrent hernia (mean followup 29 months). Alloderm was placed in 33 patients. While seromas were uncommon in patients with alloderm, eight patients developed a recurrent hernia (mean follow-up 18 months). The authors concluded that while the biosynthetics may reduce infectious complications, they do have significant risks that should be considered before implantation.[223] Others have also reported problems with recurrent hernias with alloderm and have altered their operative techniques to improve outcome, using a two-layer Alloderm repair.[224,225] Similar problems have also been seen with Surgisis.[226]

## REFERENCES

1. Krausz MM, Bar-Ziv M, Rabinovici R, et al.: "Scoop and run" or stabilize hemorrhagic shock with normal saline or small-volume hypertonic saline? J Trauma 33:6, 1992.
2. Hoyt DB, Shackford SR, McGill T, et al.: The impact of in-house surgeons and operating room resuscitation on outcome of traumatic injuries. Arch Surg 124:906, 1989.
3. Frankel HL, Rozycki GS, Ochsner MG, et al.: Minimizing admission laboratory testing in trauma patients: Use of a microanalyzer. J Trauma 37:728, 1994.
4. Rhodes M, Brader A, Lucke J, et al.: Direct transport to the operating room for resuscitation of trauma patients. J Trauma 29:907, 1989.
5. Feliciano DV, Burch JM, Spjut-Patrinely V, et al.: Abdominal gunshot wounds. An urban trauma center's experience with 300 consecutive patients. Ann Surg 208:362, 1988.
6. Nicholas JM, Rix EP, Easley KA, et al.: Changing patterns in the management of penetrating abdominal trauma: The more things change, the more they stay the same. J Trauma 55:1095, 2003.
7. Rotondo MF, Schwab CW, McGonigal MD, et al.: "Damage control": An approach for improved survival in exsanguinating penetrating abdominal injury. J Trauma 35:375, 1993.
8. Moore EE, Burch JM, Franciose RJ, et al.: Staged physiologic restoration and damage control surgery. World J Surg 22:1184, 1998.
9. Ferrada R, Birolini D: New concepts in the management of patients with penetrating abdominal wounds. Surg Clin North Am 79:1331, 1999.
10. Eiseman B, Moore EE, Meldrum DR, et al.: Feasibility of damage control surgery in the management of military combat casualties. Arch Surg 135:1323, 2000.
11. Holcomb JB, Helling TS, Hirshberg A: Military, civilian, and rural application of the damage control philosophy. Military Med 166:490, 2001.
12. Shapiro MB, Jenkins DH, Schwab CW, et al.: Damage control: Collective review. J Trauma 49:969, 2000.
13. Johnson JW, Gracias VH, Schwab CW, et al.: Evolution in damage control for exsanguinating penetrating abdominal injury. J Trauma 51:261, 2001.
14. Hoey BA, Schwab CW: Damage control surgery. Scand J Surg 91:92, 2002.
15. Firoozmand E, Velmahos GC: Extending damage-control principles to the neck. J Trauma 48:541, 2000.
16. Vargo DJ, Battistella FD: Abbreviated thoracotomy and temporary chest closure: An application of damage control after thoracic trauma. Arch Surg 136:21, 2001.
17. Feliciano DV, Rozycki GS, Thourani VH, et al.: Changing indications for temporary intravascular shunts in peripheral vascular trauma. Am Surg (in press).
18. Granchi T, Schmittling Z, Vasquez J, et al.: Prolonged use of intraluminal arterial shunts without systemic anticoagulation. Am J Surg 180:493, 2000.
19. Scalea TM, Boswell SA, Scott JD, et al.: External fixation as a bridge to intramedullary nailing for patients with multiple injuries and with femur fractures: Damage control orthopaedics. J Trauma 48:613, 2000.
20. Pape HC, Hildebrand F, Pertschy S, et al.: Changes in the management of femoral shaft fractures in polytrauma patients: From early total care to damage control orthopedic surgery. J Trauma 53:452, 2002.
21. Pape HC, Giannoudis P, Krettek C: The timing of fracture treatment in polytrauma patients: Relevance of damage control orthopedic surgery. Am J Surg 183:622, 2002.
22. Kos X, Fanchamps JM, Trotteur G, et al.: Radiologic damage control: Evaluation of a combined CT and angiography suite with a pivoting table. Cardiovasc Intervent Radiol 22:124, 1999.
23. Feliciano DV, Burch JM: Towel clips, silos, and heroic forms of wound closure. In Maull KI, Cleveland HC, Feliciano DV, et al., eds. Advances in Trauma and Critical Care. Chicago: Year Book, 1991, p. 231.
24. Burch JM, Moore EE, Moore FA, et al.: The abdominal compartment syndrome. Surg Clin North Am 76:88, 1996.
25. Saggi BH, Sugerman HJ, Ivatury RR, et al.: Abdominal compartment syndrome. J Trauma 45:597, 1998.
26. Ertel W, Oberholzer A, Platz A, et al.: Incidence and clinical pattern of the abdominal compartment syndrome after "damage-control" laparotomy in 311 patients with severe abdominal and/or pelvic trauma. Crit Care Med 28:1747, 2000.
27. Offner PJ, de Souza AL, Moore EE, et al.: Avoidance of abdominal compartment syndrome in damage-control laparotomy after trauma. Arch Surg 136:676, 2001.
28. Biffl WL, Moore EE, Burch JM, et al.: Secondary abdominal compartment syndrome is a highly lethal event. Am J Surg 182:645, 2001.
29. Raeburn CD, Moore EE, Biffl WL, et al.: The abdominal compartment syndrome is a morbid complication of postinjury damage control surgery. Am J Surg 182:542, 2001.
30. Maxwell RA, Fabian TC, Croce MA, et al.: Secondary abdominal compartment syndrome: An underappreciated manifestation of severe hemorrhagic shock. J Trauma 47:995, 1999.
31. Kopelman T, Harris C, Miller R, et al.: Abdominal compartment syndrome in patients with isolated extraperitoneal injuries. J Trauma 49:744, 2000.
32. Mayberry JC, Goldman RK, Mullins RJ, et al.: Surveyed opinion of American trauma surgeons on the prevention of the abdominal compartment syndrome. J Trauma 47:509, 1999.
33. Ivy ME, Atweh NA, Palmer J, et al.: Intra-abdominal hypertension and abdominal compartment syndrome in burn patients. J Trauma 49:387, 2000.
34. Dayton MT, Buchele BA, Shirazi SS, et al.: Use of an absorbable mesh to repair contaminated abdominal wall defects. Arch Surg 121:954, 1986.
35. Mayberry JC, Mullins RJ, Crass RA, et al.: Prevention of abdominal compartment syndrome by absorbable mesh prosthesis closure. Arch Surg 132:957, 1997.
36. Saxe JM, Ledgerwood AM, Lucas CE: Management of the difficult abdominal closure. Surg Clin North Am 73:243, 1993.
37. Lyle WG, Gibbs M, Howdieshell TR: The tensor fascia lata free flap in staged abdominal wall reconstruction after traumatic evisceration. J Trauma 46:519, 1999.
38. Barker DE, Kaufman HJ, Smith LA, et al.: Vacuum pack technique of temporary abdominal closure: A 7-year experience with 112 patients. J Trauma 48:201, 2000.
39. Garner GB, Ware DN, Cocanour CS, et al.: Vacuum-assisted wound closure provides early fascial reapproximation in trauma patients with open abdomens. Am J Surg 182:630, 2001.
40. Tremblay LN, Feliciano DV, Schmidt J, et al.: Skin only or silo closure in the critically ill patient with an open abdomen. Am J Surg 182:670, 2001.
41. Paran H, Mayo A, Afanasiev A, et al.: Staged primary closure of the abdominal wall in patients with abdominal compartment syndrome. J Trauma 51:1204, 2001.
42. Koniaris LG, Hendrickson RJ, Drugas G, et al.: Dynamic retention. A technique for closure of the complex abdomen in critically ill patients. Arch Surg 136:1359, 2001.

43. Howdieshell TR, Yeh KA, Hawkins ML, et al.: Temporary abdominal wall closure in trauma patients: Indications, technique, and results. *World J Surg* 19:154, 1995.

44. Ramirez OM, Ruas E, Dellon AL: "Components separation" method for closure of abdominal-wall defects: An anatomic and clinical study. *Plast Reconstr Surg* 86:519, 1990.

45. Fabian TC, Croce MA, Pritchard E, et al.: Planned ventral hernia. Staged management for acute abdominal wall defects. *Ann Surg* 219:643, 1994.

46. Sleeman D, Sosa JL, Gonzalez A, et al.: Reclosure of the open abdomen. *J Am Coll Surg* 180:200, 1995.

47. Livingston DH, Sharma PK, Glantz AI: Tissue expanders for abdominal wall reconstruction following severe trauma: Technical note and case reports. *J Trauma* 32:82, 1992.

48. Gentilello LM: Temperature-associated injuries and syndromes. In Mattox KL, Feliciano DV, Moore EE, eds. *Trauma*, 4th ed. New York: McGraw-Hill, p. 1153.

49. Tremblay LN, Feliciano DV, Rozycki GS: Assessment of initial base deficit as a predictor of outcome: Mechanism of injury does make a difference. *Am Surg* 68:689, 2002.

50. Ferrara A, MacArthur JD, Wright HK, et al.: Hypothermia and acidosis worsen coagulopathy in the patient requiring massive transfusion. *Am J Surg* 160:515, 1990.

51. Krishna G, Sleigh JW, Rahman H: Physiological predictors of death in exsanguinating trauma patients undergoing conventional trauma surgery. *Aust N Z J Surg* 68:826, 1998.

52. Cinat ME, Wallace WC, Nastanski F, et al.: Improved survival following massive transfusion in patients who have undergone trauma. *Arch Surg* 134:964, 1999.

53. Eddy VA, Morris JA Jr, Cullinane DC: Hypothermia, coagulopathy, and acidosis. *Surg Clin North Am* 80:845, 2000.

54. Asensio JA, McDuffie L, Petrone P, et al.: Reliable variables in the exsanguinated patient which indicate damage control and predict outcome. *Am J Surg* 182:743, 2001.

55. Ku J, Brasel KJ, Baker CC, et al.: Triangle of death: Hypothermia, acidosis, and coagulopathy. *New Horizons* 7:61, 1999.

56. Burch JM, Ortiz V, Richardson RJ, et al.: Abbreviated laparotomy and planned reoperation for critically injured patients. *Ann Surg* 215:476, 1992.

57. Morris JA Jr, Eddy VA, Binman TA, et al.: The staged celiotomy for trauma. Issues in unpacking and reconstruction. *Ann Surg* 217:576, 1993.

58. Moore EE: Staged laparotomy for the hypothermia, acidosis, and coagulopathy syndrome. *Am J Surg* 172:415, 1996.

59. Phillips TF, Soulier G, Wilson RF: Outcome of massive transfusion exceeding two blood volumes in trauma and emergency surgery. *J Trauma* 27:903, 1987.

60. Wudel JH, Morris JA Jr, Yates K, et al.: Massive transfusion: Outcome in blunt trauma patients. *J Trauma* 31:1, 1991.

61. Kivioja A, Myllynen P, Rokkanen P: Survival after massive transfusions exceeding four blood volumes in patients with blunt injuries. *Am Surg* 57:398, 1991.

62. Hakala P, Lindahl J, Alberty A, et al.: Massive transfusion exceeding 150 U of packed red cells during the first 15 hours after injury. *J Trauma* 44:410, 1998.

63. Jurkovich GJ, Greiser WB, Luterman A, et al.: Hypothermia in trauma victims: An ominous predictor of survival. *J Trauma* 27:1019, 1987.

64. Gregory JS, Francbaum L, Townsend MC, et al.: Incidence and timing of hypothermia in trauma patients undergoing operations. *J Trauma* 31:795, 1991.

65. Chaudry CH: Cellular mechanisms in shock and ischemia and their correction. *Am J Physiol* 245:R117, 1983.

66. Weg JG: Oxygen transport in adult respiratory distress syndrome and other acute circulatory problems: Relationship of oxygen delivery and oxygen consumption. *Crit Care Med* 19:650, 1991.

67. Durham CM, Siegel JH, Weireter LJ, et al.: Oxygen debt and metabolic academia as quantitative predictors of mortality and the severity of the ischemic insult in hemorrhagic shock. *Crit Care Med* 19:231, 1999.

68. Steinemann S, Shackford SR, Davis JW: Implications of admission hypothermia in trauma patients. *J Trauma* 30:200, 1990.

69. Cushman JG, Feliciano DV, Renz BM, et al.: Iliac vascular injury: Operative physiology related to outcome. *J Trauma* 42:1033, 1997.

70. King RC, Kron IL, Kanithanon RC, et al.: Hypothermic circulatory arrest does not increase the risk of ascending thoracic aortic aneurysm resection. *Ann Surg* 227:702, 1998.

71. Clifton GL, Allen S, Barrodale P, et al.: A phase II study of moderate hypothermia in severe brain injury. *J Neurotrauma* 10:263, 1993.

72. Rutherford EJ, Fusco MA, Nunn CR, et al.: Hypothermia in critically ill trauma patients. *Injury* 29:605, 1998.

73. Yudkin J, Cohen RD, Slack B: The haemodynamic effects of metabolic acidosis in the rat. *Clin Sci* 50:177, 1976.

74. Brasel KJ, Ku J, Baker CC, et al.: Damage control in the critically ill and injured patient. *New Horizons* 7:73, 1999.

75. Davis JW, Kaups KL: Base deficit in the elderly: A marker of severe injury and death. *J Trauma* 45:873, 1998.

76. Davies AO: Rapid desensitization and uncoupling of human beta-adrenergic receptors in an *in vitro* model of lactic acidosis. *J Clin Endocrinol Metab* 59:398, 1984.

77. Abramson D, Scalea TM, Hitchcock R, et al.: Lactate clearance and survival following injury. *J Trauma* 35:584, 1993.

78. Kauvar DS, Lefering R, Wade CE: Impact of hemorrhage on trauma outcome: An overview of epidemiology, clinical presentations, and therapeutic considerations. *J Trauma* 60:S3-S11, 2006.

79. Reed RL, Johnston TD, Hudson JD, et al.: The disparity between hypothermic coagulopathy and clotting studies. *J Trauma* 33:465, 1992.

80. Watts DD, Trask A, Soeken K, et al.: Hypothermic coagulopathy in trauma: Effect of varying levels of hypothermia on enzyme speed, platelet function, and fibrinolytic activity. *J Trauma* 44:846, 1998.

81. Cosgriff N, Moore EE, Sauaia A, et al.: Predicting life-threatening coagulopathy in the massively transfused trauma patient: Hypothermia and acidoses revisited. *J Trauma* 42:857, 1997.

82. Ketchum L, Hess JR, Hiippala S: Indications for early fresh frozen plasma, cryoprecipitate, and platelet transfusion in trauma. *J Trauma* 60:S51, 2006.

83. Harrison TD, Laskosky D, Jazaeri O, et al.: "Low-dose" recombinant activated factor VII results in less blood and blood product use in traumatic hemorrhage. *J Trauma* 59:150, 2005.

84. Martinowitz U, Kenet G, Segal E, et al.: Recombinant activated factor VII for adjunctive hemorrhage control in trauma. *J Trauma* 51:431, 2001.

85. Boffard KD, Riou B, Warren B, et al.: Recombinant factor VIIa as adjunctive therapy for bleeding control in severely injured trauma patients: Two parallel, randomized, placebo-controlled, double-blind clincial trials. *J Trauma* 59:8, 2005.

86. Feliciano DV, Mattox KL: Indications, technique, and pitfalls of emergency center thoracotomy. *Surg Rounds* 4:32, 1981.

87. Wall MJ Jr, Hirshberg A, Mattox KL: Pulmonary tractotomy with selective vascular ligation for penetrating injuries to the lung. *Am J Surg* 168:655, 1994.

88. Asensio JA, Demetriades D, Berne JD, et al.: Stapled pulmonary tractotomy: A rapid way to control hemorrhage in penetrating pulmonary injuries. *J Am Coll Surg* 185:486, 1997.

89. Wall MJ Jr, Villavicencio RT, Miller CC, et al.: Pulmonary tractotomy as an abbreviated thoracotomy technique. *J Trauma* 45:1015, 1998.

90. Macho JR, Markison RE, Schecter WP: Cardiac stapling in the management of penetrating injuries of the heart: Rapid control of hemorrhage and decreased risk of personal contamination. *J Trauma* 34:711, 1993.

91. Bowman MR, King RM: Comparison of staples and sutures for cardiorrhaphy in traumatic puncture wounds of the heart. *J Emerg Med* 14:615, 1996.

92. Feliciano DV, Burch JM, Mattox KL, et al.: Balloon catheter tamponade in cardiovascular wounds. *Am J Surg* 160:583, 1990.

93. Trinkle JK, Toon RS, Franz JL, et al.: Affairs of the wounded heart: Penetrating cardiac wounds. *J Trauma* 19:467, 1979.

94. McClelland R, Shires T, Poulos E: Hepatic resection for massive trauma. *J Trauma* 4:282, 1964.

95. Aronsen KF, Bengmark S, Dahlgren S, et al.: Liver resection in the treatment of blunt injuries to the liver. *Surgery* 63:236, 1968.

96. Foster JH, Lawler MR Jr, Welborn MB Jr, et al.: Recent experience with major hepatic resection. *Ann Surg* 167:651, 1968.

97. Payne WD, Terz JJ, Lawrence W Jr: Major hepatic resection for trauma. *Ann Surg* 170:929, 1969.

98. Donovan AJ, Michaelian MJ, Yellin AE: Anatomical hepatic lobectomy in trauma to the liver. *Surgery* 73:833, 1973.

99. Lim RD Jr, Giuliano AE, Trunkey DD: Postoperative treatment of patients after liver resection for trauma. *Arch Surg* 112:429, 1977.

100. Feliciano DV, Pachter HL: Hepatic trauma revisited. *Curr Prob Surg* 26:453, 1989.

101. Pachter HL, Spencer FC, Hofstetter SR, et al.: Significant trends in the treatment of hepatic trauma. Experience with 411 injuries. *Ann Surg* 215:492, 1992.

102. Pachter HL, Feliciano DV: Complex hepatic injuries. *Surg Clin North Am* 76:763, 1996.

103. Poggetti RS, Moore EE, Moore FA, et al.: Balloon tamponade for bilobar transfixing hepatic gunshot wounds. *J Trauma* 33:694, 1992.

104. Thomas SV, Dulchavsky SA, Diebel LN: Balloon tamponade for liver injuries: Case report. *J Trauma* 34:448, 1993.

105. Stevens SL, Maull KI, Enderson BL, et al.: Total mesh wrapping for parenchymal liver injuries—A combined experimental and clinical study. *J Trauma* 31:1103, 1991.

106. Jacobson LE, Kirton OC, Gomez GA: The use of an absorbable mesh wrap in the management of major liver injuries. *Surgery* 111:455, 1992.

107. Feliciano DV, Mattox KL, Burch JM, et al.: Packing for control of hepatic hemorrhage. *J Trauma* 26:738, 1986.

108. Saifi J, Fortune JB, Graca L, et al.: Benefits of intra-abdominal pack placement for the management of nonmechanical hemorrhage. *Arch Surg* 125:119, 1990.

109. Sharp KW, Locicero RJ: Abdominal packing for surgically uncontrollable hemorrhage. *Ann Surg* 215:467, 1992.

110. Horwitz JR, Black T, Lally KP, et al.: Venovenous bypass as an adjunct for the management of a retrohepatic venous injury in a child. *J Trauma* 39:584, 1995.

111. Baumgartner F, Scudamore C, Nair C, et al.: Venovenous bypass for major hepatic and caval trauma. *J Trauma* 39:671, 1995.

112. Rogers FB, Reese J, Shackford SR, et al.: The use of venovenous bypass and total vascular isolation of the liver in the surgical management of juxtahepatic venous injuries in blunt hepatic trauma. *J Trauma* 43:530, 1997.

113. Denton JR, Moore EE, Coldwell DM: Multimodality treatment for grade V hepatic injuries: Perihepatic packing, arterial embolization, and venous stenting. *J Trauma* 42:964, 1997.

114. Biffl WL, Moore EE, Franciose RJ: Venovenous bypass and hepatic vascular isolation as adjuncts in the repair of destructive wounds to the retrohepatic inferior vena cava. *J Trauma* 45:410, 1998.

115. Asensio JA, Roldan G, Petrone P, et al.: Operative management and outcomes in 103 complex hepatic injuries AAST-OIS grades IV and V trauma. Surgeons still need to operate, but angioembolization helps. *J Trauma* 54:647, 2003.

116. Moore EE, Cogbill TH, Jurkovich GJ, et al.: Organ injury scaling: Spleen and liver (1994 revision). *J Trauma* 38:323, 1995.

117. Feliciano DV, Spjut-Patrinely V, Burch JM, et al.: Splenorrhaphy. The alternative. *Ann Surg* 211:569, 1990.

118. Martin TD, Feliciano DV, Mattox KL, et al.: Severe duodenal injuries. Treatment with pyloric exclusion and gastrojejunostomy. *Arch Surg* 118:631, 1983.

119. Feliciano DV, Martin TD, Cruse PA, et al.: Management of combined pancreatoduodenal injuries. *Ann Surg* 205:673, 1987.

120. Carrillo C, Folger RJ, Shaftan GW: Delayed gastrointestinal reconstruction following massive abdominal trauma. *J Trauma* 34:233, 1993.

121. Reilly PM, Rotondo MF, Carpenter JP, et al.: Temporary vascular continuity during damage control: Intraluminal shunting for proximal superior mesenteric artery injury. *J Trauma* 39:757, 1995.

122. Feliciano DV, Burch JM, Graham JM: Abdominal vascular injury. In Feliciano DV, Moore EE, Mattox KL, eds. *Trauma*. Stamford, CT: Appleton & Lange, 1996, p. 615.

123. Sheldon GF, Winestock DP: Hemorrhage from open pelvic fracture controlled intraoperatively with balloon catheter. *J Trauma* 18:68, 1978.

124. Saueracker AJ, McCroskey BL, Moore EE, et al.: Intraoperative hypogastric artery embolization for life-threatening pelvic hemorrhage: A preliminary report. *J Trauma* 27:1127, 1987.

125. Burch JM, Feliciano DV, Mattox KL, et al.: Injuries of the inferior vena cava. *Am J Surg* 156:548, 1988.

126. Pachter HL, Drager S, Godfrey N, et al.: Traumatic injuries of the portal vein. The role of acute ligation. *Ann Surg* 189:383, 1979.

127. Stone HH, Fabian TC, Turkleson ML: Wounds of the portal venous system. *World J Surg* 6:335, 1982.

128. Donahue TK, Strauch GO: Ligation as definitive management of injury to the superior mesenteric vein. *J Trauma* 28:541, 1988.

129. Stone HH, Strom PR, Mullins RJ: Management of the major coagulopathy with onset during laparotomy. *Ann Surg* 197:532, 1983.

130. Rumley TO: Improved packing technique in the control of diffuse hemorrhage of the abdomen. *Surg Gynecol Obstet* 156:82, 1983.

131. Talbert S, Trooskin SZ, Scalea T, et al.: Packing and re-exploration for patients with nonhepatic injuries. *J Trauma* 33:121, 1992.

132. Feliciano DV: Evaluation and treatment of vascular injuries. In Browner BD, Jupiter JB, Levine AM, Trafton PG, eds. *Skeletal Trauma*. Philadelphia: Saunders, 1998, p. 349.

133. Ballard RB, Salomone JP, Rozycki GS, et al.: "Damage control" in vascular trauma: A new use for intravascular shunts. Presented at the 28th Annual Meeting, Western Trauma Association, Lake Louise, Canada, Feb 22–28, 1998.

134. Mullins RJ, Lucas CE, Ledgerwood AM: The natural history following venous ligation for civilian injuries. *J Trauma* 20:737, 1980.

135. Timberlake GA, O'Connell RC, Kerstein MD: Venous injury: To repair or ligate, the dilemma. *J Vasc Surg* 4:553, 1986.

136. Feliciano DV, Herskowitz K, O'Gorman RB, et al.: Management of vascular injuries in the lower extremities. *J Trauma* 28:319, 1988.

137. Accola KD, Feliciano DV, Mattox KL, et al.: Management of injuries to the superior mesenteric artery. *J Trauma* 26:313, 1986.

138. Trunkey DD, Illner H, Wagner IY, et al.: The effect of hemorrhagic shock on intracellular muscle action potentials in the primate. *Surgery* 74:241, 1973.

139. Bock JC, Barker BC, Clinton AG, et al.: Post-traumatic changes in, and effect of colloid osmotic pressure on the distribution of body water. *Ann Surg* 210:395, 1989.

140. Doty DB, Hufnagel HV, Moseley RV: The distribution of body fluids following hemorrhage and resuscitation in combat casualties. *Surg Gynecol Obstet* 130:453, 1970.

141. McCord JM: Oxygen-derived free radicals in postischemic tissue injury. *N Engl J Med* 321:159, 1985.

142. Schein M, Wittmann DH, Aprahamian CC, et al.: The abdominal compartment syndrome: The physiological and clinical consequences of elevated intra-abdominal pressure. *J Am Coll Surg* 180:745, 1995.

143. Cheatham ML: Intra-abdominal hypertension and abdominal compartment syndrome. *New Horizons* 7:96, 1999.

144. Emerson H: Intra-abdominal pressures. *Arch Intern Med* 7:754, 1911.

145. Kron IL, Harman PK, Nolan SP: The measurement of intra-abdominal pressure as a criterion for abdominal re-exploration. *Ann Surg* 199:28, 1984.

146. Iberti TJ, Kelly KM, Gentili DR, et al.: A simple technique to accurately determine intra-abdominal pressure. *Crit Care Med* 15:1141, 1987.

147. Sugrue M, Buist MD, Lee A, et al.: Intra-abdominal pressure measurement using a modified nasogastric tube: Description and validation of a new technique. *Intensive Care Med* 20:588, 1994.

148. Lacey SR, Bruce J, Brooks SP, et al.: The relative merits of various methods of indirect measurement of intra-abdominal pressure as a guide to closure of abdominal wall defects. *J Pediatr Surg* 22:1207, 1987.

149. Fusco MA, Martin RS, Chang MC: Estimation of intra-abdominal pressure by bladder pressure measurement: Validity and methodology. *J Trauma* 50:297, 2001.

150. Balogh Z, Jones F, D'Amours S, et al.: Continuous intra-abdominal pressure measurement techniques. *Am J Surg* 188:679, 2004.

151. Mutoh T, Lamm WJ, Embree LJ: Volume infusion produces abdominal distension, lung compression, and chest wall stiffening in pigs. *J Appl Physiol* 72:575, 1992.

152. Diebel L, Saxe J, Dulchavsky S: Effect of intra-abdominal pressure on abdominal wall blood flow. *Am Surg* 58:573, 1992.

153. Diebel LN, Dulchavsky SA, Wilson RF: Effect of increased intra-abdominal pressure on mesenteric arterial and intestinal mucosal blood flow. *J Trauma* 33:45, 1992.

154. Diebel LN, Dulchavsky SA, Brown WJ: Splanchnic ischemia and bacterial translocation in the abdominal compartment syndrome. *J Trauma* 43:852, 1997.

155. Chang MC, Miller PR, D'Agostino R, et al.: Effects of abdominal decompression on cardiopulmonary function and visceral perfusion in patients with intra-abdominal hypertension. *J Trauma* 44:441, 1998.

156. Ivatury RR, Porter JM, Simon RJ, et al.: Intra-abdominal hypertension after life-threatening penetrating abdominal trauma: Prophylaxis, incidence, and clinical relevance to gastric mucosal pH and abdominal compartment syndrome. *J Trauma* 44:1016, 1998.

157. Friedlander MH, Simon RJ, Ivatury R, et al.: Effect of hemorrhage on superior mesenteric artery flow during increased intra-abdominal pressures. *J Trauma* 45:433, 1998.

158. Diebel LN, Wilson RF, Dulchavsky SA, et al.: Effect of increased intra-abdominal pressure on hepatic arterial, portal venous, and hepatic microcirculatory blood flow. *J Trauma* 33:279, 1992.

159. Nakatani T, Sakamoto Y, Kaneko I, et al.: Effects of intra-abdominal hypertension on hepatic energy metabolism in a rabbit model. *J Trauma* 44:446, 1998.

160. Shenasky JG, Gillenwater JY: The renal hemodynamic and functional effects of external counterpressure. *Surg Gynecol Obstet* 134:253, 1972.

161. Harman PK, Kron IL, McLachlan HD, et al.: Elevated intra-abdominal pressure and renal function. *Ann Surg* 196:594, 1982.

162. Richards WO, Scovill W, Shin B, et al.: Acute renal failure associated with increased intra-abdominal pressure. *Ann Surg* 197:183, 1983.

163. Cullen DJ, Coyle JP, Teplich R, et al.: Cardiovascular, pulmonary, and renal effects of massively increased intra-abdominal pressure in critically ill patients. *Crit Care Med* 17:118, 1989.

164. Sugrue M, Jones F, Janjua KJ, et al.: Temporary abdominal closure: A prospective evaluation of its effects on renal and respiratory physiology. *J Trauma* 45:914, 1998.

165. Bloomfield GL, Blocher CR, Fakhry IF, et al.: Elevated intra-abdominal pressure increases plasma renin activity and aldosterone levels. *J Trauma* 42:997, 1997.

166. Doty JM, Saggi BH, Blocher CR, et al.: Effects of increased renal parenchymal pressure on renal function. *J Trauma* 48:874, 2000.

167. Ridings PC, Bloomfield GL, Blocher CR, et al.: Cardiopulmonary effects of raised intra-abdominal pressure before and after intravascular volume expansion. *J Trauma* 39:1071, 1995.

168. Obeid F, Saba A, Fath J, et al.: Increases in intra-abdominal pressure affect pulmonary compliance. *Arch Surg* 130:544, 1995.

169. Simon RJ, Friedlander MH, Ivatury RR, et al.: Hemorrhage lowers the threshold for intra-abdominal hypertension-induced pulmonary dysfunction. *J Trauma* 42:398, 1997.

170. Richardson JD, Trinkle JK: Hemodynamic and respiratory alterations with increased intra-abdominal pressure. *J Surg Res* 20:411, 1976.

171. Diamant M, Benumof JL, Saidman LJ: Hemodynamics of increased intra-abdominal pressure: Interaction with hypovolemia and halothane anesthesia. *Anesthesiology* 48:23, 1978.

172. Kashtan J, Green JF, Parsons EQ, et al.: Hemodynamic effect of increased abdominal pressure. *J Surg Res* 30:249, 1981.

173. Barnes GE, Laine GA, Giam PY, et al.: Cardiovascular responses to elevation of intra-abdominal hydrostatic pressure. *Am J Physiol* 248:208, 1985.

174. Robotham JL, Wise RA, Bromberger-Barnea B: Effects of changes in abdominal pressure on left ventricular performance and regional blood flow. *Crit Care Med* 13:803, 1985.

175. Bloomfield GL, Dalton JM, Sugerman HJ, et al.: Treatment of increasing intracranial pressure secondary to the acute abdominal compartment syndrome in a patient with combined abdominal and head trauma. *J Trauma* 39:1168, 1995.

176. Bloomfield GL, Ridings PC, Blocher CR, et al.: Effects of increased intra-abdominal pressure upon intracranial and cerebral perfusion pressure before and after volume expansion. *J Trauma* 41:936, 1996.

177. Bloomfield GL, Ridings PC, Blocher CR, et al.: A proposed relationship between increased intra-abdominal, intrathoracic, and intracranial pressure. *Crit Care Med* 25:496, 1997.

178. Saggi BH, Sugerman HJ, Bloomfield GL, et al.: Nonsurgical abdominal decompression reverses intracranial hypertension in a model of acute abdominal compartment syndrome. *Surg Forum* 48:544, 1997.

179. Meldrum DR, Moore FA, Moore EE, et al.: Prospective characterization and selective management of the abdominal compartment syndrome. *Am J Surg* 174:667, 1997.

180. Cheatham ML, White MW, Sagraves SG, et al.: Abdominal perfusion pressure: A superior parameter in the assessment of intra-abdominal hypertension. *J Trauma* 49:621, 2000.

181. Tremblay LN, Feliciano DV, Rozycki GS: Secondary extremity compartment syndrome. *J Trauma* 53:833, 2001.

182. Corcos AC, Sherman HF: Percutaneous treatment of secondary abdominal compartment syndrome. *J Trauma* 51:1062, 2001.

183. Chen RJ, Fang JF, Lin BC, et al.: Laparoscopic decompression of abdominal compartment syndrome after blunt hepatic trauma. *Surg Endosc* 14:966, 2000.

184. Bloomfield G, Saggi B, Blocher C, et al.: Physiologic effects of externally applied continuous negative abdominal pressure for intra-abdominal hypertension. *J Trauma* 46:1009, 1999.

185. Fernandez L, Norwood S, Roettger R, et al.: Temporary intravenous bag silo closure in severe abdominal trauma. *J Trauma* 41:258, 1996.

186. DiGiacomo JC, Kustrup JF Jr: Alternatives in temporary abdominal closures. *Arch Surg* 129:884, 1994.

187. Rowlands BJ, Flynn TC, Fischer RP: Temporary abdominal wound closure with a silastic "chimney." *Contemp Surg* 24:17, 1984.

188. Schuster SR: A new method for the staged repair of large omphaloceles. *Surg Gynecol Obstet* 125:837, 1967.

189. Sherck J, Seiver A, Shatney C, et al.: Covering the "open abdomen": A better technique. *Am Surg* 64:854, 1998.

190. Leguit P Jr: Zip-closure of the abdomen. *Neth J Surg* 34:41, 1982.

191. Bender JS, Bailey CE, Saxe JM, et al.: The technique of visceral packing: Recommended management of difficult fascial closure in trauma patients. *J Trauma* 36:182, 1994.

192. Gentilello LM, Cobean RA, Offner PJ, et al.: Continuous arteriovenous rewarming: Rapid reversal of hypothermia in critically ill patients. *J Trauma* 32:316, 1992.

193. Tisherman SA, Barie P, Bokhari F, et al.: Clinical practice guideline: Endpoints of resuscitation. *J Trauma* 57:898, 2004.

194. Crookes BA, Cohn SM, Bloch S, et al.: Can near-infrared spectroscopy identify the severity of shock in trauma patients? *J Trauma* 58:806, 2005.

195. Moore FA, Haenel JB, Moore EE, et al.: Incommensurate oxygen consumption in response to maximal oxygen availability predicts post-injury multiple organ failure. *J Trauma* 33:58, 1992.

196. Durham RM, Neunaber K, Mazuski JE, et al.: The use of oxygen consumption and delivery as endpoints for resuscitation in critically ill patients. *J Trauma* 41:32, 1996.

197. Hirshberg A, Wall MJ Jr, Mattox KL: Planned reoperation for trauma: A two year experience with 124 consecutive patients. *J Trauma* 37:365, 1994.

198. Morris JA Jr, Eddy VA, Rutherford EJ: The trauma celiotomy: The evolving concepts of damage control. *Curr Prob Surg* 33:611, 1996.

199. Botha AJ, Moore FA, Moore EE, et al.: Postinjury neutrophil priming and activation: A vulnerable window. *Surgery* 118:358, 1995.

200. Botha AJ, Moore FA, Moore EE, et al.: Early neutrophil sequestration after injury: A pathogenic mechanism for multiple organ failure. *J Trauma* 39:411, 1995.

201. Partrick DA, Moore FA, Moore EE: Neutrophil priming and activation in the pathogenesis of postinjury multiple organ failure. *New Horizons* 4:194, 1996.

202. Waydhas C, Nast-Kolb D, Trupka A, et al.: Posttraumatic inflammatory response, secondary operations, and late multiple organ failure. *J Trauma* 41:624, 1996.

203. Adams JM, Hauser CJ, Livingston DH, et al.: The immunomodulatory effects of damage control abdominal packing on local and systemic neutrophil activity. *J Trauma* 41:792, 2001.

204. Cothren CC, Moore EE, Johnson JL, et al.: One hundred percent fascial approximation with sequential abdominal closure of the abdomen. *Am J Surg* 192:238, 2006.

205. Garner GB, Ware DN, Cocanour, et al.: Vacuum-assisted wound closure provides early fascial reapproximation in trauma patients with open abdomens. *Am J Surg* 182:630, 2001.

206. Stone PA, Hass SM, Flaherty SK, DeLuca JA, et al.: Vacuum-assisted fascial closure for patients with abdominal trauma. *J Trauma* 57:182, 2004.

207. Miller PR, Meredith JW, Johnson JC, et al.: Prospective evaluation of vacuum-assisted fascial closure after open abdomen. *Annals of Surgery* 239:608, 2004.

208. Stone HH, Strom PR, Mullins RJ: Pancreatic abscess management by subtotal resection and packing. *World J Surg* 8:341, 1984.

209. Teichmann W, Wittmann DH, Andreone PA: Scheduled reoperations (etappenlavage) for diffuse peritonitis. *Arch Surg* 121:147, 1986.

210. Wittmann DH, Aprahamian C, Bergstein JM: Etappenlavage: Advanced diffuse peritonitis managed by planned multiple laparotomies utilizing zippers, slide fastener, and Velcro analogue for temporary abdominal closure. *World J Surg* 14:218, 1990.

211. Aprahamian C, Wittmann DH, Bergstein JM, et al.: Temporary abdominal closure (TAC) for planned relaparotomy (etappenlavage) in trauma. *J Trauma* 30:719, 1990.

212. Fantus RJ, Mellett MM, Kirby JP: Use of controlled fascial tension and an adhesion preventing barrier to achieve delayed primary fascial closure in patients managed with an open abdomen. *Am J Surg* 192:243, 2006.

213. Gilsdorf RB, Shea MM: Repair of massive septic abdominal wall defects with Marlex mesh. *Am J Surg* 130:634, 1975.

214. Stone HH, Fabian TC, Turkleson ML, et al.: Management of acute full thickness losses of the abdominal wall. *Ann Surg* 193:612, 981.

215. Voyles CR, Richardson JD, Bland KI, et al.: Emergency abdominal wall reconstruction with polypropylene mesh: Short-term benefits versus long-term complications. *Ann Surg* 194:219, 1981.

216. Wouters DB, Krom RA, Slooff MJ, et al.: The use of Marlex mesh in patients with generalized peritonitis and multiple organ system failure. *Surg Gynecol Obstet* 156:609, 1983.

217. Usher FC, Ochsner J, Tuttle LLD: Use of Marlex mesh in the repair of incisional hernias. *Am J Surg* 24:969, 1958.

218. Jones JW, Jurkovich GJ: Polypropylene mesh closure of infected abdominal wounds. *Am J Surg* 55:73, 1989.

219. Lamb JP, Vitale T, Kaminski DL: Comparative evaluation of synthetic meshes used for abdominal wall replacement. *Surgery* 93:643, 1983.

220. Jenkins SD, Klamer TW, Parteka JJ: A comparison of prosthetic materials used to repair abdominal wall defects. *Surgery* 94:392, 1983.

221. Tyrell J, Silberman H, Chandrasoma P, et al.: Absorbable versus permanent mesh in abdominal operations. *Surg Gynecol Obstet* 168:227, 1989.

222. Smith PC, Tweddell JS, Bessey PQ: Alternative approaches to abdominal wound closure in severely injured patients with massive visceral edema. *J Trauma* 32:16, 1992.

223. Gupta A, Zahriya K, Mullens PL, et al.: Ventral herniorrhaphy: Experience with two different biosynthetic mesh materials, Surgisis and Alloderm. *Hernia* 10:419, 2006.

224. Kolker AR, Brown DJ, Redstone JS, et al.: Multilayer reconstruction of abdominal wall defects with acellular dermal allograft (Alloderm) and component separation. *Ann Plast Surg* 55:36, 2005.

225. Buinewicz B, Rosen B: Acellular cadaveric dermis (Alloderm): A new alternative for abdominal hernia repair: *Ann Plast Surg* 52:188, 2004.

226. Helton WS, Fisichella PM, Berger R, et al.: Short-term outcomes with small intestinal submucosa for ventral abdominal hernia. *Arch Surg* 140:549, 2005.

# Commentary ■ MICHAEL B. SHAPIRO

Damage control is now mainstream in trauma care, in both principle and practice. Twenty-four years after Stone and colleagues described the technique of truncated laparotomy, and fourteen years after Rotondo and colleagues applied the label and further expanded the concept, dozens of reports and thousands of patients whose mortality was imminent have been treated with this approach. Even the most junior of trauma trainees is familiar with the "lethal triad" represented by the deranged physiology of coagulopathy, hypothermia, and acidosis.

Adoption of damage control has happened even though it has never been evaluated in a randomized clinical trial. Nor should it be; the observation of Smith and Pell that "a survival benefit to skydivers of parachute use had never been validated in a randomized controlled trial," made clear that some questions should not be studied in this fashion. The use of staged surgical management, with intervening physiologic resuscitation, has spilled over into other specialties of surgery, including orthopedics, vascular surgery, urology, and thoracic surgery. Temporary vascular shunts and external skeletal fixation are but two examples of such applications. This practice has also taken root to some extent in general surgical emergencies, most commonly in patients with acute visceral perforation or hemorrhage, presenting in extremis, in whom survival of anesthesia and operation is a significant challenge. The practice has certainly not been accepted without reservation, and some skepticism with truncated laparotomy persists in many tertiary academic institutions. Nevertheless, the recently documented 75% survival in trauma patients undergoing damage-control laparotomy is an outcome that speaks for itself, and damage control as an operative and resuscitative strategy continues to take root because it makes sense.

In the present chapter, the authors have provided a comprehensive review of damage control for trauma. They review the indications to perform a damage-control operation. Patterns of injury, clinical conditions, and other factors that help to identify those patients likely to benefit from the damage-control approach are considered. The review describes operative techniques on an organ-specific basis, including detailed consideration of thoracic and abdominal viscera and extremity vascular injury. The discussion of abdominal compartment syndrome is concise but of seminal importance. It leads, in turn, to a thorough review of open abdominal wound management strategies. The chapter concludes with a review of reoperation, and strategies for definitive wound closure or management. The authors' extensive experience in developing our understanding of the physiology of exsanguination, abdominal hypertension, and the evolution of damage-control techniques provides valuable perspective.

Damage control is a dynamic topic, and there has been a continual evolution of this approach. Considerable attention has been given to the principle of immediate exploration for control of hemorrhage and contamination, with truncation of the initial procedure so as to restore normal physiology. "Damage-control resuscitation" is a newer concept that is taking on central importance in the management of the severely injured patient. Adoption of damage-control resuscitation has been driven to some extent by military practice. Massive transfusion protocols, emphasizing the use of a 1:1 ratio of packed red blood cells to fresh frozen plasma, along with increased utilization of platelets and other coagulation products have become a central focus. The role of recombinant factor VIIa in this context continues to be assessed. It has been suggested that this approach not only influences coagulation profiles, but also modulates the systemic inflammatory response to the stress of hemorrhage shock. The roles of decreased use of lactated Ringer's solution and use of hemoglobin substitutes as part of the resuscitation process remain of great interest, although considerable additional work is needed to validate these strategies.

The current military experience has also given rise to another new concept, "tactical damage control." In this instance, the driving force is less the presence of the lethal triad of exsanguinating injury but rather the expected continued influx of additional wounded personnel. In essence, tactical damage control is a triage decision, wherein the strained resources of the responding center may become the limiting factor in initial operative care rather than patient physiology.

Finally, there is clearly a need for development and ongoing assessment of better techniques for management of the open abdominal wound at reoperation. The authors describe their excellent experience with vacuum-assisted fascial closure. Several centers have reported experience with variations of progressive fascial tightening. Collectively ultimate fascial closure has been achieved in 70–100% of patients. Our own experience suggests that this reported success rate may be vastly overstated. Persistent visceral edema, lasting days or even weeks, has proved to be a significant impediment to restoring abdominal domain and primary fascial closure. Early lateral retraction of the fascial edges, compromised fascial integrity, and impaired perfusion can thwart efforts to achieve fascial closure. Although many patients do well with delayed abdominal-wall reconstruction, there are numerous reports of very morbid complications.

As our understanding of the damage-control approach continues to evolve, there is a need for refinement of current practice and for a better understanding of related aspects of physiology and resuscitation. The present chapter provides a superb grounding in the principles of damage control, and sets the stage for further inquiry in this field.

# Upper Extremity Injury

*Steven L. Peterson* ■ *Thomas P. Lehman*

## INTRODUCTION

Hand surgery has been considered a distinct surgical specialty in the United States since World War II. And while the treatment of congenital hand malformation was a significant part of this development, the major driving force in the evolution of the specialty was the treatment of the injured upper extremity, and the appreciation of the severe disability that could result from poor management.[1]

A primary theme throughout the development of hand surgery was the recognition that many injuries to the upper extremity are combined injuries, and that appropriate treatment could best be delivered by someone trained in management of both bone and soft tissue injury. Today, the successful approach to the treatment of many upper extremity injuries requires microsurgical skills to deal with soft tissue coverage, nerve repair and revascularization, in addition to fracture care. The same skills required for successful replantation apply to successful limb salvage.

## INITIAL EVALUATION

Upper extremity injury may occur as an isolated injury or in association with the multiple injuries that define the polytrauma patient. Prioritization in such a patient is required and even treatment of complex injuries, with the exception of vascular compromise, may require a delay before definitive care is rendered.

Whenever possible, however, a definitive history should be obtained. In addition to the patient's age, past medical history, tetanus prophylaxis status and medications; knowledge of occupation, hand dominance, and important activities are helpful in determining the demands the patient places on his upper extremity. Specifics about the mechanism of trauma are also important. This should include time of injury, whether the environment was clean or contaminated, whether the insult was a sharp cut or a crush and, very importantly, was the injury work related. Previous history of upper extremity injury should be solicited and establishment of any prior functional limitations should be explored.

The physical examination should focus on not only bony and ligamentous injury which can be evaluated by inspection, palpation, and passive range of motion, but also on the key soft tissue components of tendon, nerve, and artery. Distal vascular integrity should always be one of the first things established.

Circulation can initially be evaluated by observation of the color of the skin and nail bed, skin temperature, and rate of capillary refill after blanching the skin with light pressure. Findings are interpreted by comparison with an uninjured extremity (see Chap. 14). Arterial insufficiency produces a pale, cool limb with prolonged (>2 s) or absent capillary refill, and loss of turgor. Venous insufficiency will result in a purple, congested extremity with faster than normal capillary refill.

Arterial pulse evaluation begins proximally with palpation of the brachial artery followed by the radial and ulnar arteries. A manual Allen's test should be performed when the injury allows. The patient's arm should be elevated and while the examiner compresses the radial and ulnar arteries the patient should make a clenched fist three times followed by relaxation of the hand as the examiner releases pressure on the radial artery. Redness from arterial flow into the hand from the radial side should be observed. The test is then repeated, but this time releasing the ulnar artery. A positive test exists when perfusion is delayed with solo release of either the ulnar or radial artery indicating total or partial occlusion of the released vessel. This may be a result of the trauma or this tested individual may be one of the 10 to 15% of the normal population with an incomplete palmar arch. Whether ulnar or radial artery dominance is acquired or a baseline condition may have important implications in later treatment and should be appropriately interpreted and documented. Confirmation of a positive manual Allen's test can be further explored, when clinically indicated, by Doppler ultrasound, pulse oximetry, or angiography.[2,3]

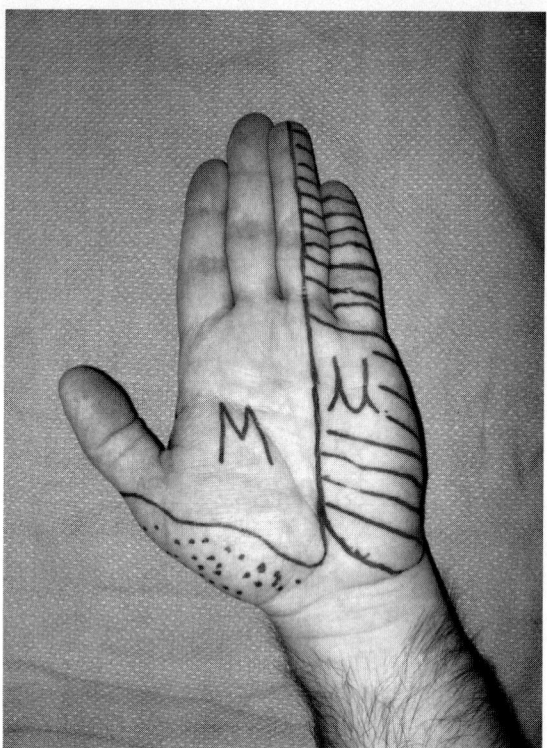 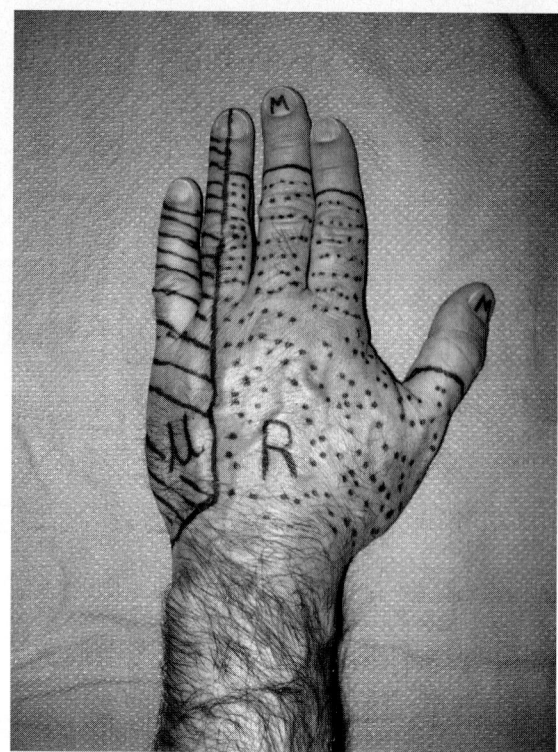

**FIGURE 42-1.** Autonomous zones of hand: M-clear areas correspond to median nerve; U-lined areas correspond to ulnar nerve; R-speckled areas correspond to redial nerve.

Sensation and motor function are essential to hand and upper extremity function and should be tested if there is any question of nerve injury. Although anatomical variations exist, in general, there are three autonomous zones in the hand (Fig. 42-1). The median nerve zone is the index fingertip, the ulnar nerve zone is the small finger tip, and the radial nerve zone is the dorsal side of the first web space over the first dorsal interosseous muscle. More proximally, standard dermatome maps can be utilized. For sensibility the most useful screening test is light touch perception which can be elicited by gently scratching or tapping the area of interest with a broken applicator stick. A more precise evaluation of distal innervation density can be accomplished by determining static and moving two-point discrimination at the finger tip. At the pulp, normal static two-point should be <6 mm and moving two point <3 mm. Occasionally threshold testing with a Semmes-Weinstein monofilament or vibration sensibility evaluation may be indicated.

Motor testing should begin distal to the level of suspected injury. Thus, when a possible traction injury to the brachial plexus has occurred, the evaluation must include all structures distal to the vertebral foramen. A systematic evaluation of each muscle based on innervation is the ideal (Tables 42-1 and 42-2). However, in the trauma setting this can be difficult and a reasonable option is to evaluate some simple motions that can then guide a more focused examination. Recreating the maneuvers of rock, paper, and scissors from the childhood game of "Ro-Sham-Bo" demonstrates median, radial, and ulnar nerve function, respectively (Fig. 42-2). Musculocutaneous, axillary, and suprascapular nerve integrity can be grossly evaluated by asking the patient to grasp a cup and simulate drinking. Whether a detailed examination is performed, or a more simple evaluation by basic maneuvers is done, both must be interpreted in light of any other soft tissue or bony injuries that might bias the examination.

The minimal radiographic examination includes the anterior–posterior (AP) or posterior–anterior (PA) and lateral view. However, complete evaluation at any articular level, or within the hand itself, usually requires additional views designed to better visualize specific injuries. These may include fluoroscopic motion views and stress views to help diagnose ligamentous instability. In addition, when dealing with a long-bone fracture, the joint above and below the injury must be visualized. More sophisticated radiographic studies such as arthrography, ultrasound, computed tomography (CT), and magnetic resonance imaging (MRI) may be important in future surgical planning, but are rarely indicated in the initial management of upper extremity trauma. Communication with consulting services regarding radiographic interpretation is greatly facilitated by a familiarity with common terms used in radiographic analysis (Table 42-3).

## SPECIFIC INJURIES

### Fractures and Dislocations

**Sternoclavicular Dislocation.** Sternoclavicular dislocation is a rare, high-energy injury. The clavicle typically dislocates in an anterior direction, but posterior dislocations do occur and are more commonly associated with damage to surrounding structures in the neck and chest.[4,5] Careful assessment of the patient is warranted, with particular attention paid to these structures. Plain radiographs are often difficult to interpret, but the injury and direction of displacement are generally identifiable on CT. Ultrasound has been advocated as a valuable imaging modality to assess the injury and adequacy of reduction.[6] If performed early and with general anesthesia,

**TABLE 42-1**

## Nerves and Muscles of the Upper Extremity

| NERVE | MUSCLES INNERVATED | TEST FOR FUNCTION | SENSORY DISTRIBUTION |
|---|---|---|---|
| Spinal accessory | Stemocleidomastoid | Ipsilateral head tilt contralateral head rotation | |
| | Trapezius | Scapular elevation rotation, adduction: head extension, rotation | |
| Dorsal scapular | Rhomboid | Seapular retraction; scapular stabilization | |
| Suprascapular | Supraspinatus | Arm abduction | |
| | Infraspinatus | Arm external rotation | |
| Long thoracic | Serratus anterior | Scapular protraction: scapular stabilization | |
| Subscapular | Subscapulans | Arm internal rotation adduction | |
| Thoracodorsal | Latissimus dorsi | Arm extension, internal rotation | |
| Pectoral (medical and lateral) | Pectoralis major and minor | Arm internal rotation, flexion, adduction | |
| Musculocutaneous | Biceps | Arm and forearm flexion; forearm supination | Lateral forearm (lateral antebrachial cutaneous) |
| | Coracobrachialis | Arm flexion, adduction | |
| | Brachialis | Forearm flexion | |
| Axillary | Deltoid | Arm abduction; internal, external rotation | Lateral aspect of shoulder |
| | Teres minor | Arm external rotation, adduction | |
| Radial | Triceps | Arm and forearm extension | Dorsoradial hand, thumb (superficial radial) |
| | Anconeus | Forearm extension | |
| | Brachioradialis | Forearm flexion | |
| | Extensor carpi radialis longus and brevis | Wrist extension | |
| | Extensor carpi ulnaris | | |
| | Supinator | Forearm supination | |
| | Extensor digitorum communis | Finger, thumb extension | |
| | Extensor indicis proprius | | |
| | Extensor digiti minimi | | |
| | Extensor pollicis brevis and longus | | |
| | Abductor pollicis longus | | |
| Median | Flexor carpi radialis | Wrist flexion | Volar thumb, index, long, radial half of ring finger; dorsum index, long, radial half of ring finger |
| | Pronator teres and quadratus | Forearm pronation | |
| | Flexor digitorum sublimis | Finger proximal interphalangeal joint flexion | |
| | Flexor digitorum profundus (index, long) | Finger distal interphalangeal joint flexion | |
| | Abductor pollicis brevis | Thumb abduction | |
| | Opponens pollicis | Thumb opposition | |
| | Flexor pollicis brevis (superficial head) | Thumb metacarpophalangeal joint flexion | |
| | Lumbricals (index, long) | Metacarpophalangeal joint flexion | |
| | | Interphalangeal joint extension | |
| Ulnar | Flexor carpi ulnaris | Wrist flexion | Volar and dorsum little. Ulnar half of ring finger; dorsal ulnar aspect of hand |
| | Flexor digitorum profundus (ring, little) | Finger distal interphalangeal joint flexion | |
| | Abductor digiti minimi | Little finger abduction | |
| | Flexor digiti minimi | Little finger metacarpophalangeal joint flexion | |
| | Abductor pollicis | Thumb adduction | |
| | Flexor pollicis brevis (deep head) | Thumb metacarpophalangeal joint flexion | |
| | Interossei (volar, dorsal) | Metacarpophalangeal joint flexion, interphalangeal extension | |
| | Lumbricals (ring, little) | Metacarpophalangeal joint flexion, interphalangeal extension | |

closed reduction is usually successful, but residual subluxation may persist, especially with anterior displacement. Correction of posteriorly displaced injuries may require a towel clamp or similar instrument to obtain reduction. It is important that a surgeon comfortable with vascular repair is available at the time of reduction to assess and address any injury to the associated structures. Later referral to a peripheral nerve surgeon may also be required.

Clavicle Fracture.    Clavicle fractures are among the most common upper extremity injures. While they generally heal without major

**TABLE 42-2**

## Cervical and Thoracic Nerve Roots and Function

| NERVE ROOT | TEST FOR FUNCTION (Muscle/Nerve) | SENSORY DISTRIBUTION | REFLEX |
|---|---|---|---|
| C5 | Shoulder abduction (deltoid/axillary) | Lateral upper arm | Biceps |
| C6 | Elbow flexion (biceps/musculocutaneous) | Lateral forearm, thumb, index finger | Brachioradialis |
| | Wrist extension (extensor carpi radialis longus and brevis/radial) | | |
| C7 | Elbow extension (triceps/radial) | Long finger | Triceps |
| | Wrist flexion (flexor carpi radialis/median: flexor carpi ulnaris/ulnar) | | |
| | Finger extension (extensor digitorum communis, extensor indicis proprius, extensor digiti minimi/radial) | | |
| C8 | Finger flexion (flexor digitorum superficialis, flexor digitorum profundus/median and ulnar) | Medial forearm, ring, little fingers | None |
| T1 | Finger abduction and adduction (dorsal and volar interossei/ulnar) | Medial forearm | None |

functional limitation, they can be associated with serious neurovascular injury, and afflicted patients should be evaluated with appropriate concern. Patients generally present following injury involving a fall or motor vehicle crash, with pain and reluctance to move the shoulder. Visual inspection and palpation often identify the location of injury. Most fractures can be identified on standard AP radiographs of the shoulder, but additional apical oblique views may assist in characterizing the injury.[7] CT or MRI studies are rarely required.

Clavicle fractures are classified by the location of the fracture in the proximal, central, or distal third of the bone. Eighty percent of clavicle fractures occur in the middle third, and most of these are amenable to closed management. Fractures of the proximal third are rare, but can usually be treated symptomatically if they are not associated with other injuries. Fractures of the distal third have a high incidence of nonunion and require careful attention.

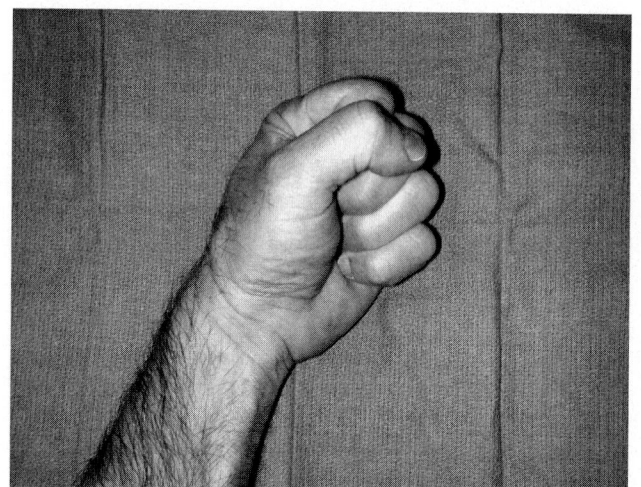
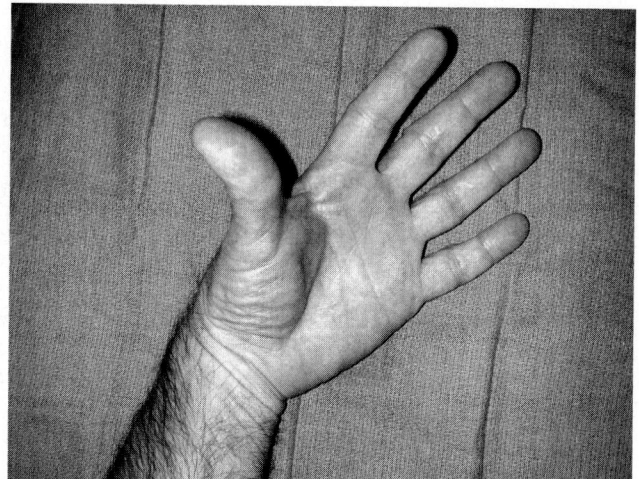
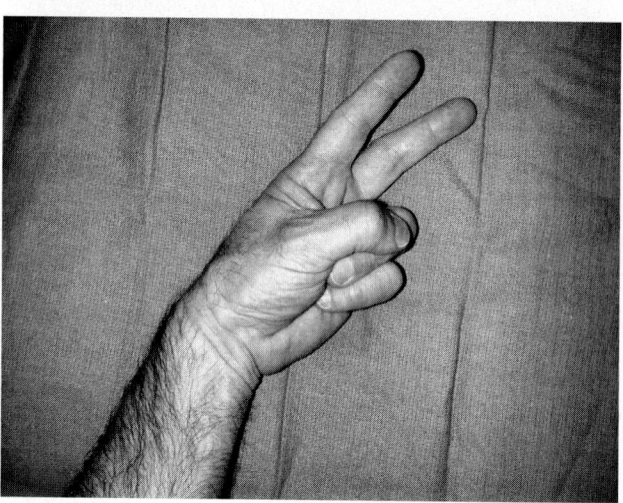

**FIGURE 42-2.** The simple childhood game maneuvers of rock, paper, scissors demonstrate (with some overlap), respectively, median, radial, and ulnar nerve integrity.

## TABLE 42-3

### Terms in Radiographic Analysis

| | |
|---|---|
| Location | Epiphysis, metaphysis, diaphysis |
| Pattern | Transverse, spiral, oblique |
| Comminution | Simple vs three or more pieces |
| Joint involvement | Extra-articular vs intra-articular |
| Alignment | Displacement, rotation, angulation |

Sling immobilization is adequate nonoperative treatment for most isolated clavicle fractures. Two to three weeks are sufficient for patient's symptoms to diminish so that they can tolerate pendulum exercises. As pain decreases the sling can be gradually discontinued and gentle activities resumed. Heavy activities are avoided for eight weeks or until union is achieved. Because of the clavicle's subcutaneous location, fracture callus is often palpable and may even be visible. Malunion of the clavicle can result in functional deficit, particularly if there is angulation or shortening due to comminution.[8] Malunited fragments or hypertrophic callus may also occasionally compress neurovascular structures requiring surgical treatment. In most patients, however, the concern is only cosmetic and slight misalignment does not interfere with daily activities.

Surgical treatment of clavicle fractures is generally reserved for fractures of the lateral clavicle, middle third fractures with >2 cm of shortening, open fractures, symptomatic nonunions, or fractures with associated neurovascular injury. Surgical stabilization of the clavicle may also be indicated in patients with a floating shoulder or other complex injuries to the shoulder girdle where addressing the clavicle may improve overall stability of the upper extremity. Because fractures of the distal third of the clavicle may be accompanied by injury to the coracoclavicular ligament complex and are at particular risk for nonunion, some recommend consideration of surgical stabilization if there is significant displacement. Surgical treatment of the clavicle is generally performed with plate and screw fixation, but intramedullary implants are an acceptable alternative.

Acromioclavicular Dislocation. Typically referred to as a "shoulder separation" is a common diagnosis, especially among athletes. Acromioclavicular (AC) joint injury typically occurs due to a fall onto the acromion. Stability of the AC joint is dependent upon both the AC and coracoclavicular (CC) ligaments. The severity and classification of the injury is based upon which of these structures are injured and to what degree (Table 42-4). Diagnosis

may be obvious clinically or with plain radiographs. Radiographs are often normal in mild injuries and, though they may confirm the diagnosis, stress radiographs are rarely indicated.

Some still consider Type III injuries a relative indication for surgical treatment, but most recommend initial nonoperative treatment for all injuries type I–III.[9,10] This typically consists of symptom reduction with activity modification, analgesics, and sling support for a few days to a few weeks. Successful early rehabilitation is possible, especially in injuries of lesser severity.

Types IV–VI are much less common, but generally require surgical reduction and ligament repair or reconstruction. Multiple surgical techniques have been described. AC joint injuries may also contribute to the late development of arthrosis and impingement necessitating distal clavicle excision.

Scapula Fractures. Scapular fractures comprise no more than 5% of shoulder fractures, but usually are the result of high-energy trauma. Because of this, patients with scapula fractures should be closely evaluated with a high index of suspicion for other serious, and possibly life threatening problems, including injury to the chest, cervical spine, or neurovascular structures. Initial evaluation of the patient should include a careful assessment of the neurologic and vascular status of the upper extremity. Scapular fractures can occur in the absence of obvious shoulder deformity, and may first be recognized on a routine chest radiograph. True AP, scapular Y, and axillary lateral views of the shoulder should always be obtained. CT scans are often required to fully evaluate the injury. Scapular fracture classification is anatomic (Table 42-5).

Treatment of scapular fractures has traditionally been nonoperative and many fractures of all types are amenable to initial treatment in a sling. Pendulum exercises may be initiated at three weeks, but strengthening should be delayed until six weeks when fracture healing may be expected.

Surgical reduction and fixation should be considered when a scapula fracture is part of a complex constellation of injuries to the shoulder girdle and fixation of the scapular component might be expected to result in functional improvement. With the exception of acromion and coracoid procedures, most scapular surgery is performed through a posterior approach, requiring the patient to be positioned prone or side lying. Because these patients often have complex associated chest and spine injuries, this may dictate that definitive surgical treatment be delayed until the patient is adequately stabilized.

Type I fractures are often avulsion injuries and Type IA fractures should be distinguished from a nonunited os acromiale. Operative

## TABLE 42-4

### Classification of AC Joint Injuries

| TYPE | LIGAMENT INJURY | FINDINGS |
|---|---|---|
| I | Incomplete AC ligament injury | No displacement or instability |
| II | Complete AC, Incomplete CC | No displacement, +Ant–Post instability |
| III | Complete AC, Complete CC | Inferior displacement of scapula, instability all planes |
| IV | Complete AC, Complete CC | Clavicle posteriorly dislocated through trapezius m |
| V | Complete AC, Complete CC | Deltoid & Trapesius tear allow +++ instability and displacement |
| VI | Complete AC, Complete CC | Clavicle locked inferior to coracoid process |

## TABLE 42-5

### Classification of Scapula Fractures

| | |
|---|---|
| **Type I** | **Apophyseal fractures** |
| IA | Acromion process |
| IB | Scapular spine |
| IC | Coracoid process |
| **Type II** | **Glenoid neck fractures** |
| IIA | Vertical, lateral to base of spine |
| IIB | Vertical, involving base of spine |
| IIC | Transverse fracture |
| **Type III** | **Fracture of glenoid articular surface** |
| **Type IV** | **Fracture of the scapular body** |

treatment may be indicated if the fracture represents an avulsion of a significant portion of the deltoid muscle, or when displacement of the avulsed fragment results in impingement of the subacromial space. Surgical treatment of scapular spine fractures (Type IB) is rarely indicated. Fractures of the coracoid process (Type IC) may require surgical fixation if the fracture extends into the glenoid fossa or is associated with an AC joint injury. Type II fractures with displacement may result in significant disruption of shoulder biomechanics. Surgical treatment has been recommended for fractures with >1 cm of medial displacement or >40 of angulation.[11] Type III fractures may require surgical treatment if there is significant articular displacement, particularly if this is accompanied by any glenohumeral instability. Suprascapular nerve injury has been reported in association with glenoid fractures and is a relative indication for surgical treatement.[12,13] Glenoid fractures with multiple small fragments are best managed with early mobilization.[14] Type IV fractures can also be treated nonoperatively. If the fracture displaces, however, painful scapulo-thoracic motion may result, and late debridement of the infrascapular prominence may be indicated.

### Floating Shoulder.
The term "floating shoulder" is used to describe a glenoid neck fracture with an associated clavicle fracture. This combination of injuries leaves the glenohumeral joint with no intact bony contact to the rest of the skeleton. Surgery is often considered in these injuries, even if the fractures individually might not otherwise meet the criteria for surgical treatment, particularly if the shoulder is displaced inferiorly.[15,16] Often stabilization of only one part of the injury, typically the clavicle, is necessary to impart some stability to the shoulder girdle.

### Scapulothoracic Dissociation.
Scapulothoracic dissociation is a rare but functionally devastating and potentially life-threatening injury which represents a closed amputation of the upper extremity. This should be suspected when the scapula appears laterally displaced on a nonrotated AP chest radiograph (Fig. 42-3). CT or MRI findings may confirm the diagnosis and identify damage to the surrounding soft tissues as well. An unusual intra-thoracic variant can occur, in which the inferior angle of the scapula penetrates an intercostal space and becomes lodged within the chest. This musculoskeletal injury is often accompanied by injury to the subclavian artery and brachial plexus. Emergent surgical treatment may be required to revascularize the upper extremity, simultaneous exploration of the plexus during this repair is strongly recommended to accurately access the degree of neurologic injury. If a global brachial plexus injury is detected at this initial exploration, consideration should be given to primary amputation, as the chance of meaningful neurologic recovery is minimal.[17,18]

### Glenohumeral Dislocation.
The glenohumeral joint is among the most commonly dislocated joints with a reported incidence of 2% in the general population and as high as 7% in athletes. Dislocation can occur with high-energy or low-energy injuries and may be anterior, posterior, or inferior in direction. Anterior dislocations account for 95% of glenohumeral dislocations with posterior dislocations comprising 4% and inferior dislocations only 0.5%. In approximately 1% of these cases, they may be associated with fractures.

In anterior dislocations the extremity is typically adducted and there is often a visible or palpable deformity of the anterior chest. Posterior dislocations present with less obvious gross deformity and

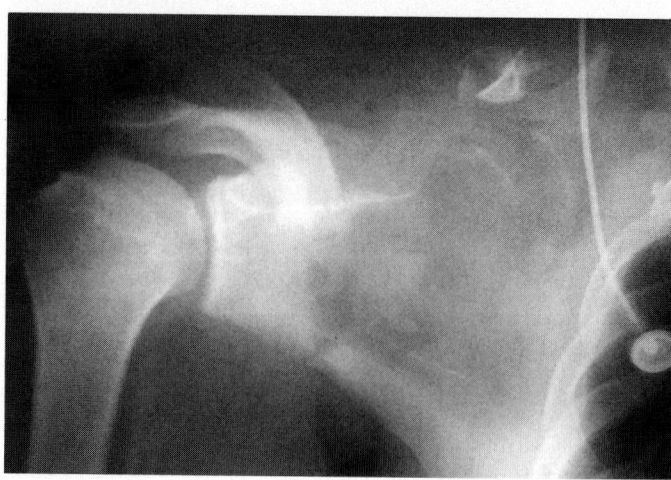

**FIGURE 42-3.** An example of scapulothoracic dislocation. Note the lateral translation of the scapula relative to the chest wall. A fracture of the clavicle and a nondisplaced fracture of the glenoid neck are also present. The patient was noted to have a complete brachial plexus palsy.

are often overlooked. Careful examination will show an inability to externally rotate the humerus and prominence of the humeral head posteriorly. Rarely, patients may present with an inferiorly dislocated shoulder locked in abduction with the forearm resting on the head *luxatio erecta.*[19] Inferior dislocations such as this are often associated with rotator cuff injury, labrial tears, and/or greater tuberosity fractures.

Radiographic evaluation of a suspected shoulder dislocation should include AP and axillary lateral views. The axillary lateral view, which includes the glenoid fossa and the humeral head, is of particular importance in evaluating the traumatized shoulder. AP radiographs of the shoulder may appear grossly normal despite dislocation of the glenohumeral joint, especially if the direction of the dislocation is posterior. Anterior or posterior displacement of the humeral head relative to the glenoid is readily apparent in the axillary lateral view (Fig. 42-4). Acutely injured patients are often reluctant to allow positioning of the shoulder in sufficient abduction to obtain an adequate radiograph. With gentle distraction and support of the extremity, this view can almost always be safely obtained with acceptable patient comfort. CT or MRI is only indicated if a more complicated injury is suspected.

Urgent reduction of a glenohumeral dislocation is the preferred treatment. Many closed reduction techniques have been described, but most dislocations can be successfully reduced in the emergency department (ED) by manipulation with or without sedation. In general, maneuvers involve either traction on the humerus or manipulation of the scapula.[20,21] Of the many named methods described for reduction, all have similar reported success rates of 70–90%. Failure to achieve reduction in the ED is an indication for general anesthesia and possible open reduction in the operating room.

After successful closed reduction, most shoulder dislocations can be successfully managed by a period of immobilization and early rehabilitation. The ideal duration and position of immobilization continue to be debated but adequate results are typically achieved with a simple sling and early, gentle pendulum exercises. Surgical indications include missed or recurrent dislocations, dislocations with associated injuries, and young, high-demand patients. Younger patients are at higher risk for recurrent dislocations and chronic instability leading some to advocate early repair

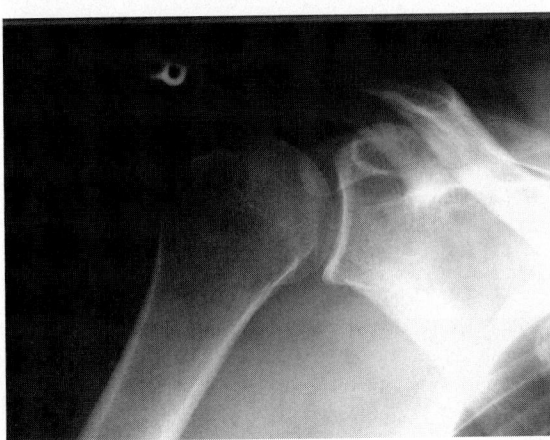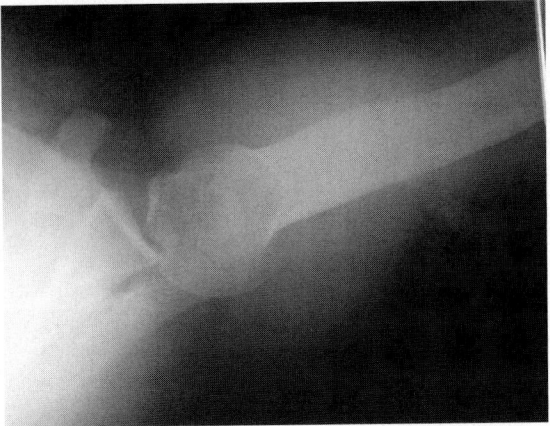

**FIGURE 42-4.** A posterior shoulder dislocation not readily apparent on a PA x-ray (left) becomes more obvious on a axillary lateral view (right).

of the capsule and labral detachment to reduce this risk.[22,23] Associated injuries are relatively common, dictating a carefully preformed and documented neurovascular examination on initial presentation, and again following reduction. Compression fractures, termed Hill-Sachs lesions, may occur in which the anterior glenoid impacts the posterior humeral head and can contribute to recurrent instability,[24] as can displaced fractures of the glenoid rim. Patients aged 40 years and over are at increased risk for rotator cuff tear,[25] which may also require repair. A common pattern of injury is shoulder dislocation that occurs with an associated fracture of the greater tuberosity of the humerus. This should be re-evaluated after closed reduction, and if there is persistent displacement of the fracture fragment, surgical treatment may be indicated. Vascular injuries should be explored and reconstructed. The most common neurologic injury is a traction neurapraxia of the axillary nerve and these typically recover fully without surgical treatment if early reduction is performed. More serious neurologic injuries may occur, including complete disruption of the brachial plexus.

Missed or unreduced shoulder dislocation can be functionally devastating. Late treatment often requires open reduction and additional bony and soft tissue procedures to attain stability. If the duration of dislocation exceeds six months or if there is extensive damage to the joint, glenohumeral arthroplasty may be indicated. Delayed treatment seldom results in the return of full function, highlighting the importance of accurate early diagnosis and treatment.

Patients who are able to voluntarily dislocate their shoulders deserve special consideration. Although voluntary relocation is often possible, they may occasionally present acutely for treatment. Dislocation can become a means to obtain frequent prescriptions for pain medication. These patients often have significant multidirectional instability of the gleno-humeral joint, which is difficult to alleviate. After reduction is obtained, nonsurgical treatment with strengthening exercises is recommended.

Proximal Humerus Fracture.    Proximal humeral fractures are relatively common and occur most often as the result of falls or motor vehicle trauma. The incidence increases with age and in the elderly the cause is typically a low-energy injury. Peripheral nerve injuries are common, especially involving the axillary nerve. Vascular injuries are also a concern, especially in the elderly who are at increased risk due to calcification in vessel walls. It is important to note that a vascular injury may be present even if a radial pulse is palpable, due to the presence of multiple collateral vessels around the shoulder. Shoulder dislocations and rotator cuff tears also commonly occur in association with proximal humeral fractures.

AP, trans-scapular lateral, and axillary lateral views should be obtained and carefully evaluated to assess possible displacement of the humeral head and tuberosities, and to rule out concomitant dislocation of the humeral head from the glenoid. CT may be useful for preoperative planning and angiography may be indicated if vascular injury is suspected (Fig. 42-5).

Displaced injuries are best classified by the system developed by Neer and are labeled two, three, or four part fractures.[26] The four potential parts are the humeral head, the greater tuberosity, the lesser tuberosity, and the shaft. A fragment must be displaced at least one centimeter or angulated at least 45° in order to be appropriately labeled a displaced part. Two-part fractures are most commonly displaced injuries of the humeral head or greater tuberosity, and three-part injuries are typically a combination of these two patterns.

When considering treatment options it is important to consider the age and functional expectations of the patient. Most nondisplaced fractures can be treated with a short period of sling immobilization. Early range of motion has been shown to improve functional outcomes.[27] For fractures of the humerus with valgus impaction of the head fragment, nonoperative treatment is often satisfactory, especially in the elderly. Other two-part fractures with a displaced head fragment may be amenable to closed reduction and percutaneous fixation. Two-part fractures of the greater tuberosity are best treated with open reduction and internal fixation if displaced more than 3–5 mm because there is increased risk of disability in patients who require overhead function.[28,29] Open reduction and internal fixation, typically through a deltopectoral approach, is indicated for most three-part fractures of the proximal humerus. Eventual osteonecrosis of the humeral head occurs in up to 27% of these injuries, but because it does not involve the entire head adequate shoulder function may be preserved.[30] Four-part fractures are at very high risk for development of complete osteonecrosis of the humeral head, resulting in functional limitation. For this reason, hemiarthroplasty of the shoulder is usually considered. One notable exception to this rule is four-part injuries in which the head fragment is impacted into the shaft, between the tuberosity fragments. In these injuries, the medial periosteal vessels maintain blood supply to the head, decreasing the risk of severe osteonecrosis.[31]

Humeral Shaft Fracture.    Fractures of the humeral shaft are common injuries. The incidence and mechanism of injury parallel

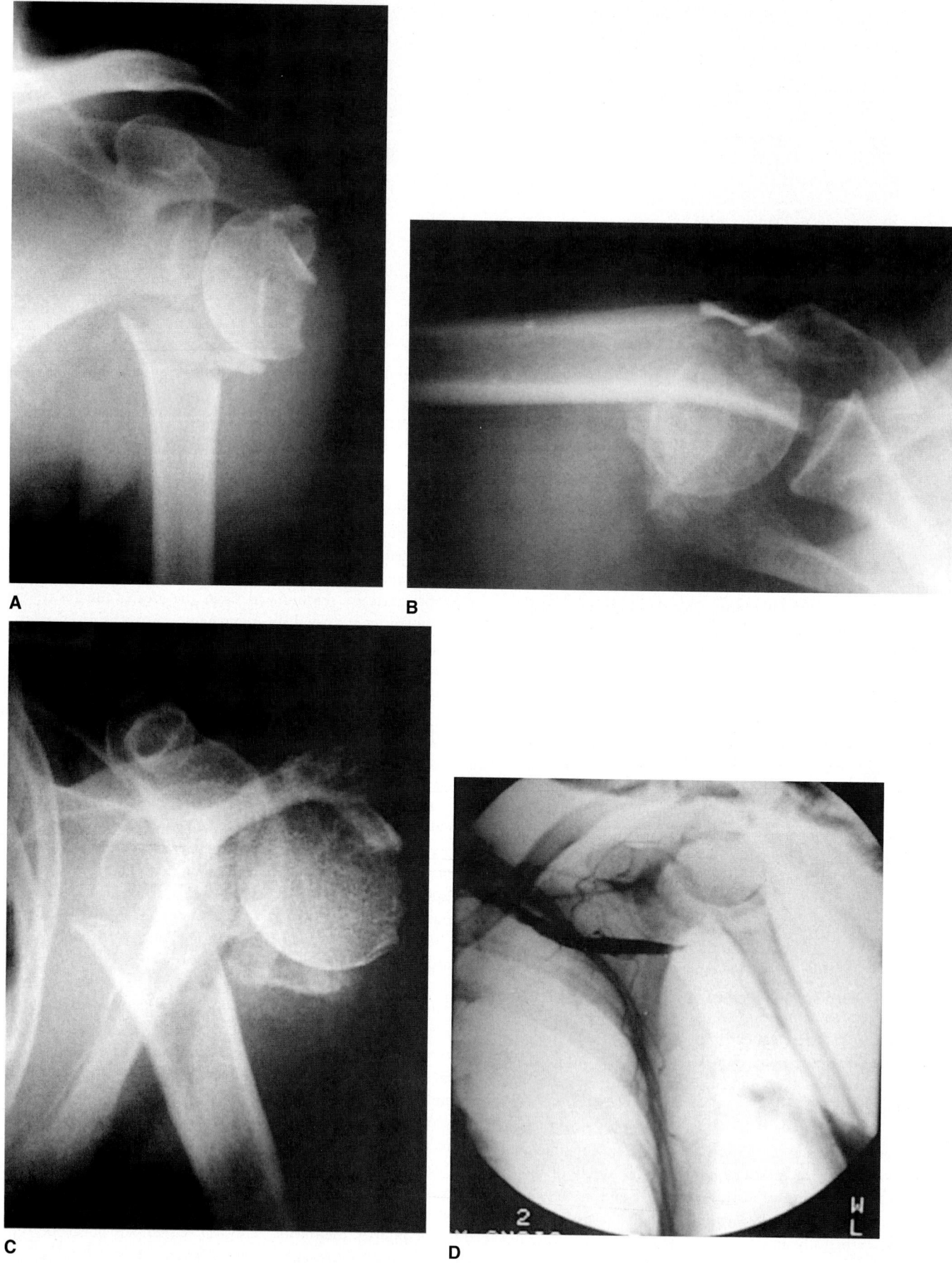

**FIGURE 42-5.** A displaced fracture of the proximal humerus is noted on the anteroposterior **(A)**, axillary lateral **(B)**, and transscapular lateral views **(C)**. An arteriogram displays an injury to the axillary artery at the level of the humeral neck **(D)**.

those of proximal humeral fractures. The unstable brachium is of significant discomfort to the patient who typically presents supporting the injured arm with the uninjured extremity. Standard AP and lateral views of the humerus are diagnostic, but the instability and crepitus at the fracture site are often readily apparent clinically. Because of the risk of neurovascular injury, a carefully performed and documented assessment of the patient's status should be completed immediately upon presentation and repeated after any treatment. Nerve injuries are commonly seen in association with fractures of the humeral shaft. The radial nerve is at highest risk, particularly in the distal third of the shaft where it is closely associated with the bone in the spiral groove (Fig. 42-6).

Nonoperative treatment is effective for most uncomplicated humeral shaft fractures. True cast immobilization of the brachium is impractical due to the inherent difficulty of immobilizing the shoulder. A coaptation splint can provide a more practical alternative. Gentle traction usually results in adequate reduction of even significantly displaced injuries. For this reason, some have advocated the use of a hanging arm cast for a brief period, especially early in the course of treatment. This consists of a long arm cast, which hangs from a loop around the patient's neck. The weight of the cast maintains longitudinal traction on the fracture fragments and helps to assure adequate alignment. This does improve patient comfort, but requires an upright posture to be effective. The use of a fracture brace, either initially or after a short period of long arm casting, has many benefits. It is usually effective in maintaining an adequate reduction and allows active elbow motion. Many patients prefer to sleep in a reclining chair for the first few weeks because this allows the longitudinal traction provided by gravity to be effective in controlling the fracture even when they are somewhat recumbent.

Surgical treatment for humeral shaft fractures is indicated for open injuries, failure to maintain acceptable alignment, and with polytrauma. In patients with multiple injuries, fixation of the humerus simplifies their care, improves pain control, and allows early mobilization. Surgical treatment is also considered in patients who are intolerant of the extreme activity modifications closed treatment requires, and in obese patients in whom it is a particular challenge to maintain an acceptable reduction because the fracture tends to assume a position of varus angulation when the arm rests on the abdomen. Operative fixation of the humerus classically involves plate and screw fixation, but intramedullary nailing is becoming more common and results are comparable.[32] When intramedullary nailing is performed, a limited approach to the fracture site will assure that the radial nerve is not interposed between the fracture fragments and at risk for iatrogenic injury.

Radial nerve injuries occur in 12% of humerus fractures and deserve special attention.[33] Most radial nerve injuries associated with closed humerus fractures are neurapraxias, and at least 70% will resolve with expectant management. During recovery, patients benefit from splinting of the wrist and digits to improve function. Failure to improve over three to four months is an indication for surgical nerve exploration. There has traditionally been a distinction between patients whose radial neuropathy is evident on initial presentation and those who develop neuropathy after fracture reduction. Early exploration has been advocated for the latter group, although secondary injuries often recover without surgical treatment. Early surgical exploration is also recommended in patients with open injuries where the risk of nerve transection is increased.

**Elbow Trauma.** The traumatized elbow should be approached systematically. It is important to remember that the elbow is not a single joint, but actually a complex set of articulations including the ulnohumeral, radio-capitellar, and proximal radio-ulnar joints. The result of these complex anatomic relationships is a very stable connection between the brachium and antebrachium that allows a large range of motion in flexion and extension as well as pronation and supination. Preservation of this motion is vital to normal functioning of the upper extremity and is secondary only to maintaining stability.

Elbow injuries present particular challenges to the surgeon charged with their repair and reconstruction. Small articular or peri-articular fractures can contribute to subtle but significant subluxation. If this is not recognized and corrected early, the resulting chronic instability may be functionally devastating. Further complicating treatment of elbow injuries is the tendency of this joint to become stiff and develop posttraumatic contracture, especially if it is immobilized for any length of time. For these reasons, the goal of treatment in most cases is to achieve enough stability to allow early range of motion and prevent stiffness. The challenges of reaching this goal have led to an ongoing expansion of techniques and implants designed to address particular injuries. Despite this,

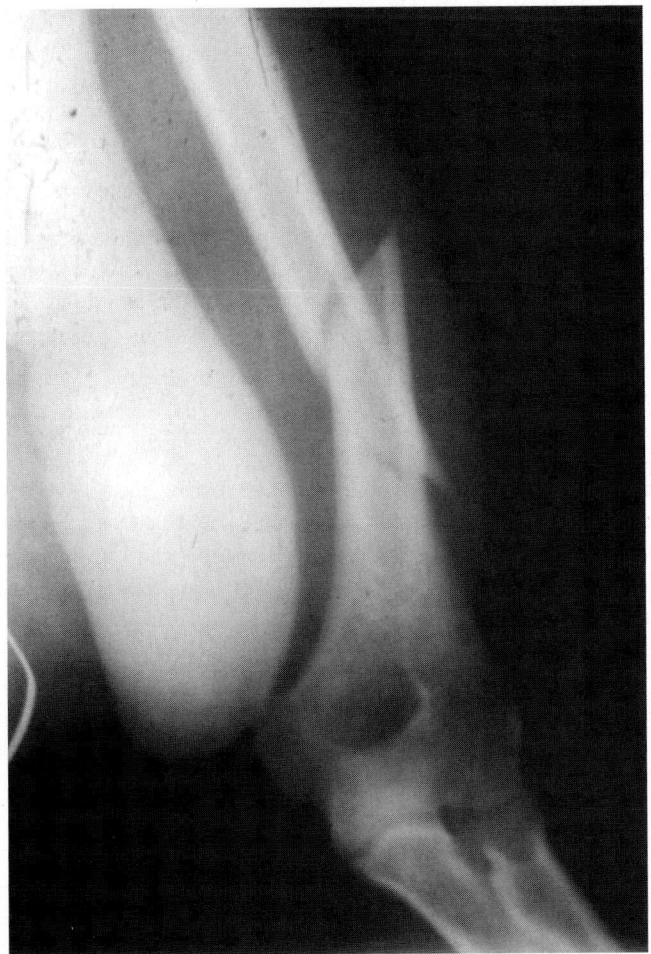

**FIGURE 42-6.** An AP x-ray of a spiral fracture of the distal third of the humerus. This fracture is called a Holstein-Lewis fracture. It is frequently associated with radial nerve palsy.

most patients who sustain severe elbow trauma continue to have some permanent limitation of motion. Preservation of an arc of motion from 30° short of terminal extension to 130° of flexion and at least 50° of pronation and 50° of supination is sufficient to allow patients to perform most routine tasks. In patients with more severe posttraumatic contracture, which does not respond to non-operative treatment, eventual closed manipulation or even open capsulectomy of the elbow may restore functional motion.

The elbow is frequently injured by falls from a standing height. This is particularly true in the elderly population. High-energy injuries are more common in younger patients and are typically sustained in falls from a distance or vehicular trauma. Patients with displaced fractures or dislocations often present with obvious deformity and instability of the elbow. However, potentially serious injuries may exist even if the only findings are pain, edema, and stiffness. The traumatized elbow should be carefully examined for crepitus, instability in any plane, and mechanical blocks to motion. Because of the relatively thin soft tissue envelope about the elbow, open fractures are common, and any open wound should be scrutinized with this in mind. Care should be taken to identify associated injuries, which may include trauma to the median, ulnar, and radial nerves, as well as the brachial artery.

Subjective complaints of pain or physical findings of bony injury should always be assessed radiographically. AP and lateral radiographs are sufficient to characterize most elbow trauma. It is especially important that the lateral radiograph be of good quality. A small amount of obliquity is sufficient to make subluxation or displaced, but functionally significant fractures, difficult to detect. Radiographs of the severely traumatized elbow with displaced fragments or segments may be difficult to interpret due to nonanatomic overlap of the injured parts. Gentle traction on the extremity may allow more anatomic positioning, facilitating interpretation. CT can be helpful in determining the size and location of small articular fragments and is sometimes valuable for preoperative planning.

Once the extent of the injury is established, efforts should be made to provisionally reduce any dislocation or displacement as anatomically as possible. Repeat radiographs should be carefully evaluated to assure that reduction is concentric and there are no fractures that were not identified in the original films. Definitive treatment should progress based on the pattern of injury.

### Distal Humeral Fractures.

The Orthopedic Trauma Association system for classification of supracondylar and intracondylar humeral fractures includes Type A, which are extra-articular, Type B, which are partial articular injuries of either the medial or lateral column, and Type C, complete articular injuries in which both columns of the distal humerus are fractured from the shaft and from each other. The elbow is usually grossly unstable but radiographs may be required to distinguish this from other types of elbow trauma. Isolated fractures of the medial or lateral epicondyle also occur and, although they are typically of lesser severity, they may require surgical treatment if significantly displaced.

Rarely is nonoperative treatment indicated for supracondylar humerus fractures. Occasionally a brief period of immobilization followed by early rehabilitation may be sufficient for a patient with very limited functional expectations due to preexisting diminished health. A preferred alternative to this technique in some elderly patients, particularly those with degenerative or rheumatoid

arthrosis, is total elbow arthroplasty.[34] In the vast majority of these cases, open reduction and internal fixation is indicated. Surgical treatment in these injuries is technically demanding especially if there is significant fragmentation of the joint surface.[35] The surgical approach to intra-articular injuries often requires an osteotomy of the olecranon. The ideal biomechanical construct continues to be debated, but most agree that plating of both the medial and lateral columns is usually indicated. The goal of surgical treatment is to obtain sufficient stability to allow early motion of the elbow while the fracture proceeds to union. Even when this goal is achieved, a permanent loss of some elbow motion is common.

Supracondylar humeral fractures in children are common injuries, especially in children aged 5–7 years. Almost all supracondylar humeral fractures in this age group are extra-articular with posterior displacement of the distal fragment. Type 1 injuires are non- or minimally-displaced, Type 2 injuries are displaced with an intact posterior cortex, and Type 3 injuries are completely displaced with disruption of the posterior cortex. Children may demonstrate only edema and pain in mild injuries or obvious hyperextension deformity in more severe cases. Most non- or minimally-displaced injuries may be managed with casting for approximately four weeks. Surgical treatment is indicated in displaced injuries. Because late stiffness is much less common in children, this typically consists of closed reduction and pinning followed by a period of immobilization. If satisfactory reduction cannot be obtained closed, it may be due to interposed tissues such as the brachialis muscle or neurovascular structures. Open exploration and reduction are indicated in these cases.[36] Associated nerve injuries most commonly involve the median nerve or its anterior interosseous branch and often recover with expectant management. Brachial artery injuries are also reported with some frequency. Because there is generally adequate collateral circulation vascular reconstruction may not be required if the extremity remains well perfused. The flexion of the elbow often required to maintain reduction of the fracture may further compromise blood flow and patients should be carefully monitored for any signs of worsening vascular status or compartment syndrome.[37]

### Capitellum Fractures.

Isolated fractures of the capitellum are relatively rare injuries, typically occurring due to relatively low-energy trauma, and are more common in women. Unless there is displacement, this injury may be easily missed on AP and lateral radiographs of the elbow. CT may be helpful if plain radiographs do not fully demonstrate the injury. Type I fractures are a complete fracture of the entire capitellum from the remainder of the articular surface; Type II injuries involve only a thin wafer of cartilage and subchondral bone; Type III injuries are comminuted fractures of the capitellum; Type IV fractures are coronal shear injuries in which the capitellum as well as a significant portion of the anterior trochlea are fractured. Unless fragments are nondisplaced, open reduction and internal fixation is recommended when possible.[38] In Types II and III, the fragments are often so small that stable internal fixation is not possible. In these cases, excision of the fragments may be a reasonable alternative.

### Elbow Dislocations and Fracture Dislocations.

Of all dislocated joints, the elbow is second in frequency only to the shoulder. Dislocation of the elbow typically refers to dislocation of the humerus from both the radius and ulna. Dislocations of the elbow are classified by the direction of displacement of the forearm segment. Posterior and lateral or posterior–lateral dislocations occur most frequently. Much less common are anterior, medial, and especially high-energy divergent dislocations in which the proximal radio-ulnar joint is also dislocated and the radius and ulna displace laterally and medially, respectively. Simple dislocations of the elbow result in injuries of the medial and lateral collateral ligament complexes without bony injury. Complex dislocations are those associated with fractures about the elbow. Isolated dislocations of the radial head also occur, especially in children. If this injury is suspected in an adult, care should be taken to assure that it is not a part of a Monteggia fracture-dislocation. Evaluation of the patient with an elbow dislocation reveals obvious deformity, and AP and lateral radiographs should confirm the diagnosis. Associated soft tissue injuries may involve the brachial artery, median, radial, and (most commonly) ulnar nerve.

Urgent closed reduction is recommended. Unless the joint has remained dislocated for some time, gentle traction on the distal segment and counter-traction on the humerus under heavy sedation is usually successful. In thin individuals, it may be possible to pull distally on the subcutaneous olecranon that is palpable posteriorly. Any medial or lateral malalignment is corrected before flexion completes the reduction. Forced maneuvers against resistance and extreme hyperextension should be avoided. General anesthesia and/or open reduction may be required. Difficulty obtaining stable closed reduction should increase suspicion of complex dislocation or other associated injuries. Once closed reduction is completed, the elbow should be passively flexed and extended to determine if there is a tendency to redislocate and the position at which this occurs should be noted. Simple dislocations are usually relatively stable following reduction and after immobilization in 90° of flexion for 7–10 days early range of motion activities may be safely initiated to minimize long-term stiffness.[39] Radiographs should be repeated after reduction and carefully scrutinized to confirm concentric reduction and identify any associated fractures that may not have been visible with the joint displaced. Simple dislocations rarely require surgical treatment.

Any complex dislocation of the elbow should be definitively addressed within a few days or as soon as the patient's overall condition allows. The longer the elbow remains in a dislocated or subluxated position, the more difficult it may be to achieve eventual stability. Complex dislocations are prone to redislocate if definitive treatment is delayed. In most cases, immobilization of the elbow in flexion and pronation imparts some stability. Patients immobilized in this way should be carefully monitored as this position may contribute to vascular compromise of the upper extremity as edema increases.

A notoriously unstable injury is the elbow dislocation with associated fractures of the radial head and coronoid process of the ulna. This pattern has been termed the "terrible triad of the elbow." Surgical treatment is required to restore stability to the elbow. Whenever possible this should include repair or reconstruction of the radial head, coronoid and, if necessary, the collateral ligaments. In severe injuries dynamic external fixation or even transarticular pin fixation may be required.[40] Restoration of full elbow function is rarely possible after severe injuries of this type.

### Fractures of the Proximal Ulna.

Injuries through the articular surface of the proximal ulna are frequent. Fractures with less than 1–2 mm of articular displacement may be treated nonoperatively with a 1–2-week period of splinting, followed by gentle early range

of motion activities. Frequent radiographic follow-up is important to assure that there is no increase in displacement. Most olecranon fractures have sufficient displacement to warrant operative treatment. The most common methods are tension band wiring and plate and screw fixation. Both may be effective in transverse or oblique injuries, but comminuted injuries require plate and screw constructs to prevent compression of the trochlear notch. Typically, sufficient stability can be obtained to allow early motion and satisfactory outcome is achieved. In extensively comminuted injuries, excision of up to half of the olecranon with advancement of the triceps may be considered.

Fractures of the coronoid process of the ulna represent the loss of the major anterior skeletal buttress preventing posterior subluxation of the elbow. Type I fractures are avulsions of the tip of the coronoid, Type II fractures involve <50% of the coronoid process, and Type III fractures involve >50% of the coronoid. These injuries are typically seen in association with a posterior elbow dislocation and the elbow should be carefully assessed and monitored for stability even if it appears well reduced. If not associated with significant instability, an avulsion fracture of the tip can be treated nonoperatively, similar to a simple elbow dislocation. Consideration should be given to fixation of some Type II and all Type III injuries and is required if there is instability of the elbow.[41] Posteriorly placed screw, suture, or wire fixation into or around the coronoid is often sufficient, but a more medial approach with an anterior buttress plate may be required to prevent redisplacement. If small coronoid fragments are not amenable to rigid fixation, they may be excised with repair of the anterior capsule.

Comminuted fractures of the olecranon that are accompanied by displacement of the coronoid process should be managed carefully. Even with anatomic fixation and union of the olecranon, the elbow may become unstable if the coronoid remains displaced. Stabilization of the coronoid process can be technically difficult. After olecranon fixation, access to the coronoid is extremely limited. Through a posterior approach, the proximal, fractured portion of the olecranon is retracted with the triceps and the remainder of the ulna is subluxated dorsally, allowing access to the anterior portion of the joint. The coronoid is reduced under direct visualization and stabilized as described above. Transolecranon fracture–dislocation of the elbow occurs when the distal humerus is driven distally through the proximal ulna. Displaced coronoid fragments are common in this injury pattern.[42]

### Radial Head Fractures.

Radial head fractures are common injuries and may occur in association with dislocation of the elbow. The fractures are classified by the system proposed by Mason. Type I fractures are nondisplaced, Type II fractures are single displaced fragments, Type III fractures are comminuted injuries, and Type IV are radial head fractures associated with an elbow dislocation. Patients may report relatively mild trauma and physical findings may be subtle. Injuries to neurovascular structures are uncommon with isolated radial head fractures. Standard radiographs are usually sufficient to make the diagnosis. Once a radial head fracture is identified, the elbow should be carefully evaluated for stability and range of motion. It is important to examine the wrist and forearm to identify any associated injuries to the distal radio-ulnar joint or interosseous membrane. If pain prevents motion, the intra-articular hematoma should be evacuated and lidocaine injected into the joint. A mechanical block to motion in the anesthetized joint is an indication for surgical treatment.

Type I and II injuries with <2 mm of displacement may be managed nonoperatively with early motion and follow-up to ensure there is no interval displacement. Displaced Type II injuries of the head and neck are typically treated with open reduction and internal fixation. It is important that implants do not interfere with the proximal radio-ulnar joint. The safe zone for implants in the radial head is the area between lines extended proximally from the radial styloid and Lister's tubercle, both of which are palpable at the wrist.[43] Headless screws may also be of value when fixation is necessary outside this safe zone.

Type III injuries are usually not amenable to open reduction and internal fixation. Excision of the radial head may be considered in some cases. This should not be performed if there is associated elbow dislocation, coronoid fracture, valgus instability of the elbow, or longitudinal instability of the forearm, which would indicate an interosseous ligament injury. A radial head fracture with an associated injury to the interosseous membrane is a pattern termed an *Essex-Lopresti* fracture–dislocation.[44] Clues to its presence include wrist pain, displacement at the distal radio-ulnar joint, and/or proximal migration of the radius evident on x-ray. If signs of instability in any plane are present, every attempt should be made to preserve the radial head or perform arthroplasty with a metallic radial head implant.

### The Floating Elbow.

The floating elbow occurs when there are ipsilateral fractures of the humerus and forearm. The elbow segment is unsupported proximally and distally, requiring stabilization of both injuries. These are the result of high-energy trauma, and are often associated with injuries to neuro-vascular structures. The prognosis for return of full function in these injuries is guarded, especially if the fractures are periarticular.[45]

### Monteggia Fracture Dislocations.

Monteggia injuries are fractures of the ulna with associated radial head dislocations.[46]

Isolated fractures of the ulna are rare in adults and should raise suspicion of this injury, as failure to recognize and treat the radial head dislocation will lead to significant disability. Radiographs of the forearm in the AP and lateral planes should characterize the ulnar shaft fracture, but may not clearly demonstrate the more proximal injury. AP and lateral elbow films should be obtained in any patient suspected of having a Monteggia fracture dislocation (Fig. 42-7).

Classification of these injuries is most simply based on the direction of displacement of the radial head. Anterior and anterior-lateral displacements are most common. Open reduction and internal fixation of the ulna with closed reduction of the radial head are indicated. Care must be taken to assure anatomic alignment of the ulna because persistent angulation may result in chronic instability of the radial head. This is particularly challenging in comminuted injuries. Failure to achieve closed reduction of the radial head despite satisfactory alignment of the ulna is an indication for open exploration and reduction of the radio-capitellar joint. Small osteochondral fragments of the radial head or interposed capsular tissue may prevent closed reduction.

### Ulnar Shaft Fracture.

Isolated ulnar shaft fractures, commonly referred to as "night-stick fracture," are usually amenable to a short period of long arm casting, followed by functional bracing, when there is less than 10–15% angulation and at least 50% contact area between fragments. Displaced fractures are usually treated with compression plating or, in the distal third, fixed angle, or locking plates. Intramedullary nailing in adults has limited application but may be indicated with some segmental fractures, those associated with severe soft tissue loss or in polytrauma. External fixation is really only indicated as a bridge to more definitive fixation.

Special circumstances in the management of ulnar fractures involve those associated with distal radial fractures, isolated ulnar head fractures, and Monteggia fractures.

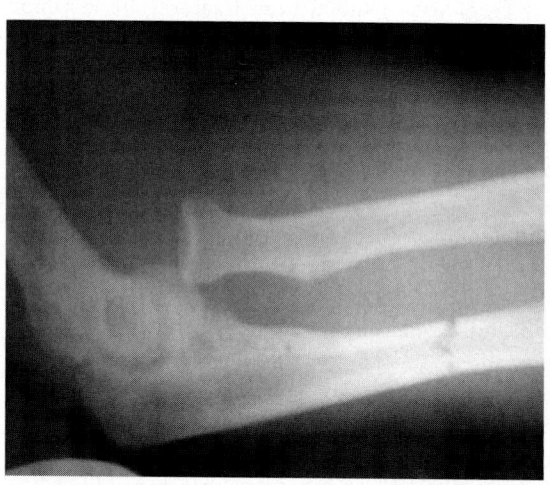
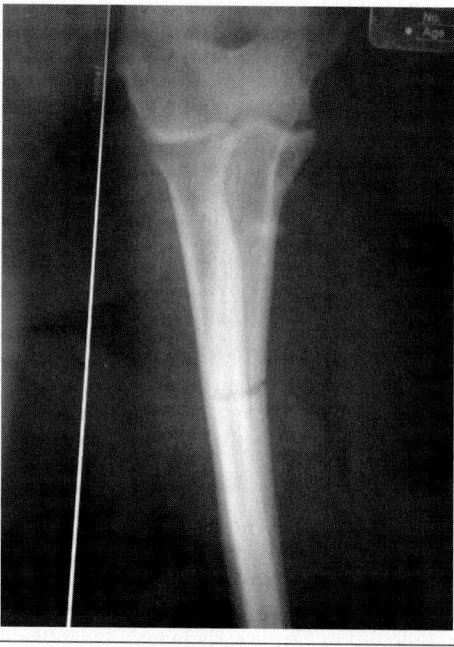

**FIGURE 42-7.** The lateral view of the elbow (left) much more dramatically demonstrates the dislocation of the radial head associated with a Monteggia fracture than the AP view (right).

Fracture of the distal ulna associated with distal radial fracture may or may not require fixation. However, when the integrity of the distal radial ulnar joint is compromised then consideration should be given to fixation.[47] Restoration can be by fixation of an ulnar styloid base or plating of the ulnar head; usually with a small condylar blade plate or a small locking plate. Addressing the ulnar component of these fractures in this manner can often greatly facilitate initiation of early motion.

Radial Shaft.   Galeazzi fracture–dislocation is a complex traumatic disruption of the distal radioulnar joint (DRUJ) that is associated with an unstable radial fracture.[48] In these fractures, the injury to the DRUJ can be a pure ligamentous disruption or can be associated with a fracture of the ulnar styloid. Most commonly, the site of fracture is the junction of the middle and distal thirds of the radius. This injury can be associated with a low-energy fall from a standing height or associated with a high-energy mechanism, such as a fall from a height or a motor vehicle accident. This fracture has also been referred to as a "reverse Monteggia fracture" or "the fracture of necessity" since, in adults, operative intervention is almost always required for a good outcome.

Radiographic evaluation of these fractures demonstrates a short appearing radius relative to the ulna, because of the pull of the pronator quadratus muscle (Fig. 42-8). On the PA view there will often appear to be an increase in space between the distal radius and ulna where they articulate.

Definitive treatment is by operative fixation of the radial shaft fracture, usually through a volar approach, followed by intraoperative examination of the DRUJ for instability, predominantly in supination. The intraoperative examination is the definitive test that determines a need to address the DRUJ, not the radiographs.[49] Treatment of the DRUJ instability is Kirschner wire fixation of the radius to the ulna in supination, with or without direct repair of the ligamentous component or styloid fracture. This is followed by six weeks of above elbow casting.

Distal Radius.   Distal radial fractures are the most common longbone fracture of the upper extremity accounting for 14% of all extremity injury and 17% of fractures treated in the ED.[50] Two primary age groups are involved with varying mechanisms. Highenergy comminuted intra-articular fractures occur primarily in young patients, while low-energy extra-articular fractures occur predominantly in the elderly. Despite the high prevalence of these fractures, and voluminous thought that has gone into development of a myriad of classification systems, no clear algorithm exists for their treatment. What is accepted, however, are the goals for anatomical restoration of radial length, radial inclination, and volar tilt and, ultimately, restoration of hand function.

The three anatomical goals are specific and are based on the normal distal radial anatomy, which demonstrates 21° of inclination, 12° of volar tilt and length defined by baseline relationship to the ulna, which can be determined in most instances from the uninjured wrist. The ability to restore and maintain these relationships, as well as restore articular congruity, is the prime determinant of the need for operative intervention. Because of the dorsal comminution that usually exists with the apex volar malformation, which usually accompanies these fractures, maintenance of what appears to be a good reduction in the ED requires continued vigilance and early operative intervention if loss of reduction occurs.

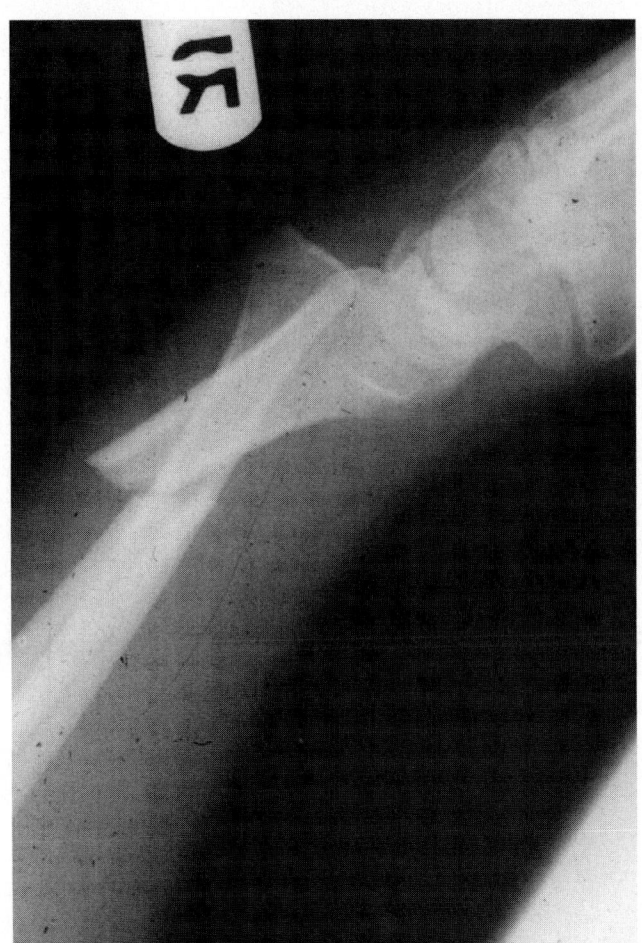

**FIGURE 42-8.**   A true lateral radiograph of the forearm showing a fracture of the distal third of the radius. The ulnar head is dorsal to the radius indicating a dislocation of the radial head. Anatomic reduction of the radius and internal fixation should reduce the distal radioulnar joint.

As previously pointed out, while no consensus algorithm exists for treatment of distal radial fractures, the recent addition of fixed angle locking plates and fragment specific fixation have led to more aggressive early treatment of both intra- and extra-articular fractures.[51,52] While there is still a role for closed reduction, and percutaneous pinning, and/or external fixation in the operative armamentarium stable plate fixation is being applied on an increased basis to even very comminuted fractures with encouraging early results (Fig. 42-9).[53]

Radius and Ulna.   Simultaneous fracture of both the radius and ulna are relatively common injuries. Patients present following trauma with forearm pain, swelling and, not uncommonly, grossly visible deformity. Associated neurovascular injury may occur and compartment syndrome may develop. AP and lateral x-rays should be obtained which include both the elbow and wrist. Fractures are classified based on their location as proximal, middle, or distal third fractures, with our without comminution. Careful inspection is necessary to rule out an open component.

While closed management is usually acceptable in children, in the adult this has historically led to reliable bony healing but usually in the pattern of a malunion with decreased rotation of the forearm. Because of this significant complication rate with closed reduction

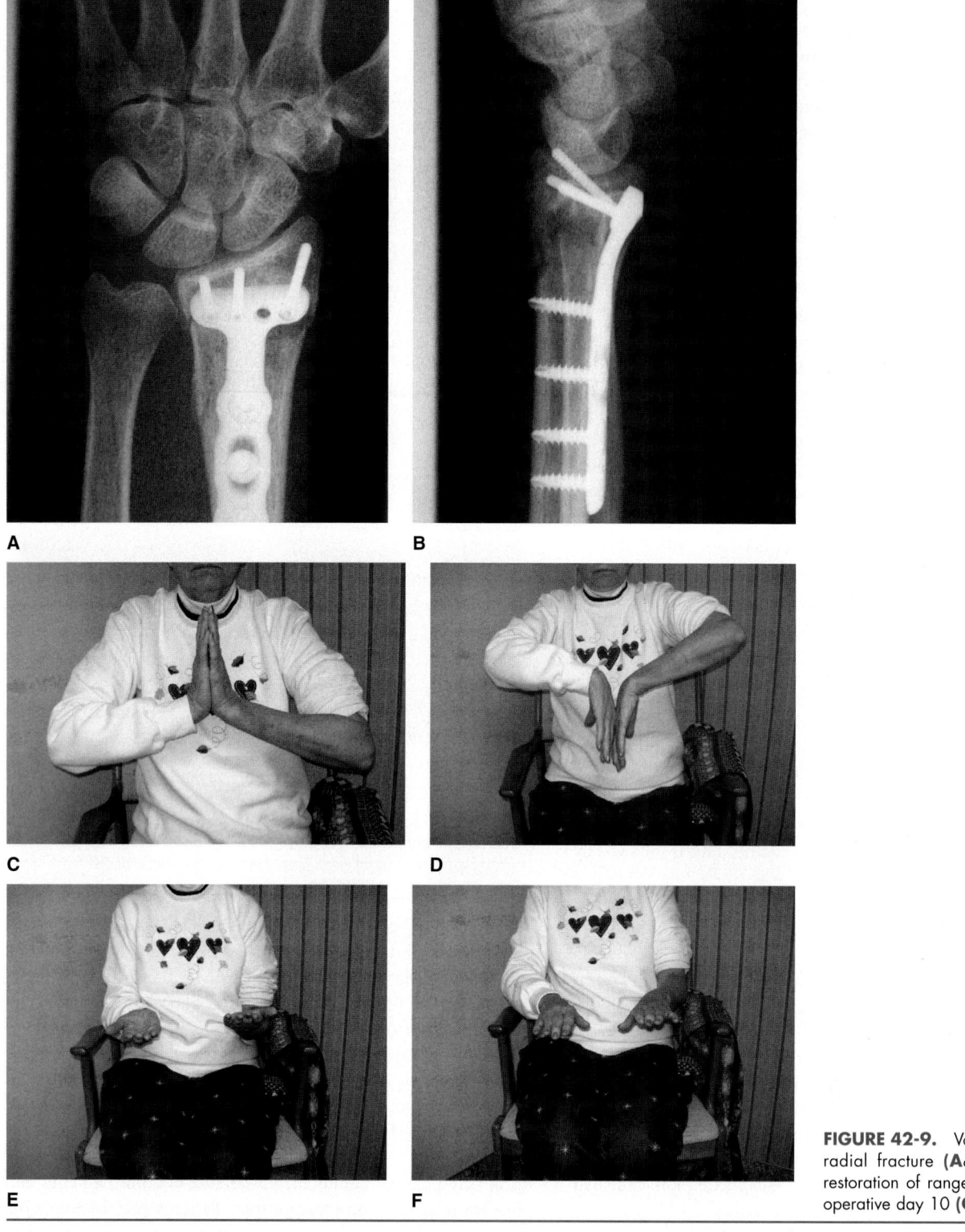

A

B

C

D

E

F

**FIGURE 42-9.** Volar plating of distal radial fracture (**A&B**) with excellent restoration of range of motion at postoperative day 10 (**C–F**).

and casting, open reduction with compression plate fixation has become the accepted standard of care for these fractures in adults.[54]

Scaphoid.    Fractures of the scaphoid account for over half of all detected isolated carpal bone fractures. The true incidence of injury to this bone, however, may be higher since many fractures are not appreciated until late when they convert to a symptomatic nonunion, and many may remain asymptomatic throughout life.[55]

Scaphoid fractures usually result from a fall onto an outstretched hand with the wrist extended and the forearm pronated. Fractures most commonly occur at the waist (75%), followed by the proximal pole (20%), and, least often, at the distal pole or tuberosity (5%). Location of the fracture is an important factor in prognosis for healing because of the blood supply of the scaphoid. As an intraarticular bone, the scaphoid receives its blood supply through ligamentous attachments, with the primary entry at the distal pole. This leaves the proximal pole with a consistently poor blood supply, which makes these fractures susceptible to nonunion or avascular necrosis.

Other factors playing a role in development of nonunion and malunion are stability of the fracture pattern and displacement.

Diagnosis of scaphoid fracture is first suggested by mechanism of injury, associated with onset of wrist pain and/or swelling. Examination may show tenderness on palpation within the anatomical snuff box and over the scaphoid tubercle. Pain may also be elicited by pronation and ulnar deviation or by applying axial load to the first metacarpal. However, no maneuver is specific for injury to the scaphoid and appropriate radiographs are critical.

Routine radiographs should include a posteroanterior, lateral, oblique in 45° of pronation and a posteroanterior view in slight ulnar deviation ("scaphoid view"). However, even with a thorough examination and appropriate radiographs, a nondisplaced fracture may be missed. An appropriate course of action in the presence of negative radiographs but positive clinical signs would be immediate MRI or application of a splint or short arm cast with more definitive test scheduled in 72 hours.[56]

The concept of immediate MRI is based on its sensitivity to detection of early fracture associated marrow edema. In addition, numerous studies have now demonstrated a cost benefit to this approach[57,58] versus the classic approach of repeat radiographs, followed by more definitive studies if these remain negative. Many centers, however, are not equipped to offer this treatment algorithm, and in this setting bone scan or a scheduled MRI in 72 hours are more efficacious than repeat films over the course of several weeks.

Surgical treatment is indicated for all displaced scaphoid fractures. An aggressive approach is supported by data reporting a 50–92% nonunion rate with displaced scaphoid fractures and development of degenerative joint disease with as little as 1mm of displacement. An open approach through a dorsal or volar incision, followed by screw placement, is the most common means of treating these fractures. However, percutaneous screw placement, with/or without arthroscopic guided reduction, is becoming increasing popular as a minimally invasive option (Fig. 42-10).[59–61]

This development of fluoroscopic or arthroscopic guided percutaneous screw fixation has brought into question the accepted protocol of prolonged casting for nondisplaced fractures. Advocates of this approach point to the advantage of earlier return to full function, as well as the potential elimination of the small percent of these fractures that go on to nonunion. Future prospective studies will determine whether surgical intervention is always indicated in scaphoid fracture.

Other Carpal Fractures. Fractures of carpal bones, other than the scaphoid, account for less than 45% of carpal fractures. Of the remaining seven bones in the carpus, the triquetrum is the next most frequently injured bone.[62] Dorsal avulsion fractures are the most common form of fracture and, while painful, surgical intervention is rarely indicated except to excise a persistently painful fragment. Body fractures and volar avulsion fractures may also occur and may be difficult to detect by plain radiographs. Both CT and MRI have been used to diagnose or more clearly delineate these fractures and, occasionally, body fractures will require fixation. However, in most instances, six weeks of immobilization in a short arm cast will resolve the pain associated with these fractures even though radiographic union may not occur.

The pisiform is rarely fractured and when this occurs it is usually the result of a direct blow to the hypothenar eminence. Palpation of the pisiform elicits pain and a carpal tunnel view and/or supinated oblique view are required to adequately image this bone with plain radiographs. CT may be indicated in the presence of persistent pain and negative plain films. A thorough evaluation of the integrity of the ulnar nerve is required when dealing with injuries to the pisiform because of its close proximity.[63] This is particularly important if surgical intervention is being considered.

Initial treatment with immobilization is recommended to decrease pain associated with wrist motion; however, there is no evidence this increases union rate. A persistently painful fractured pisiform can be excised as definitive treatment, with no significant sequelae.

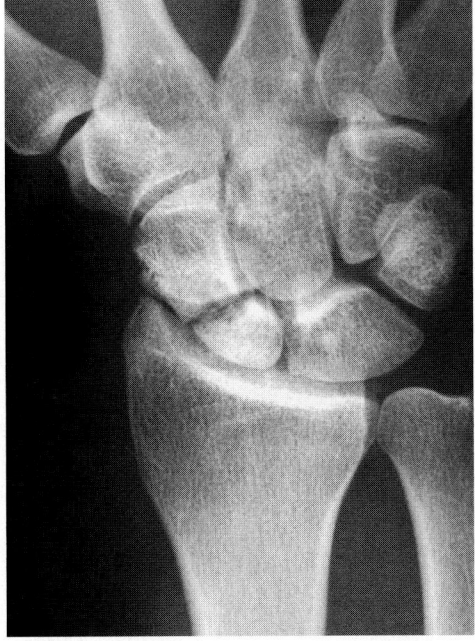
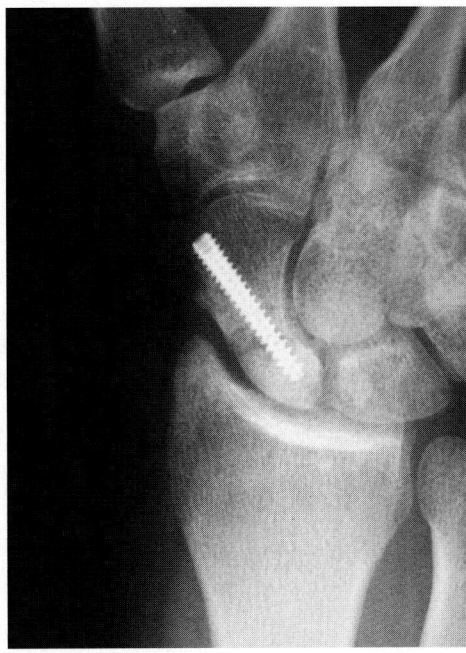

**FIGURE 42-10.** Right scaphoid fracture repaired by volar approach and cannulated screw placement.

Fractures of the trapezium, at the base of the thumb, are usually associated with fracture of the first metacarpal or distal radius. These fractures may involve the body, margin of the metacarpal articular surface, or volar ridge. Volar ridge fractures may be associated with median nerve injury and thorough examination of both motor and sensory components of this nerve should be documented. Cyclists appear to be prone to trapezial body fractures.

Radiographic diagnosis of any of these injuries requires a variety of special views including a hyperpronated "Roberts" view, a Bett's view, and a carpal tunnel view. CT may be required to further delineate a ridge fracture.

Except for displaced body fractures, the initial treatment of trapezial fractures should consist of a six-week period of immobilization. If, at the end of this time, persistent palmar pain is associated with a volar ridge fracture, then the fracture fragment should be excised. Displaced body fractures can usually be stabilized by lag screw fixation.[64]

Fractures of the trapezoid are exceedingly rare because of its protected position deep within the hand.[65] Injury to this protected bone is often associated with a high-energy fracture dislocation involving the index metacarpal. Radiographic diagnosis of this injury may be relatively straight forward; however, isolated injury or injury associated with a spontaneous reduction may require CT scan to define, since this bone is often poorly visualized even with a hyperpronated "Roberts" view targeting the scapho-trapezial-trapezoid articulation.

Treatment of nondisplaced isolated fractures is by six weeks of immobilization. Displaced fractures or those associated with carpometacarpal (CMC) dislocations require internal fixation or occasionally formal CMC arthrodesis with bone grafting to achieve stability and pain relief.

Capitate fractures may be isolated, associated with a scaphoid fracture ("scapho-capitate syndrome"), or associated with other carpal injury. Isolated fractures are often nondisplaced and occur at the waist. However, similar to proximal pole fractures of the scaphoid, the proximal pole of the capitate is dependent on a distal blood supply and prone to avascular necrosis.[66] Without treatment symptomatic nonunion is a common occurrence and can lead to the need for midcarpal fusion if ignored. Both open reduction and percutaneous methods of primary fixation have been described.

Scaphocapitate syndrome results in malrotation of the proximal capitate fragment and is the result of a direct blow to the dorsum of the hand while flexed or a fall onto an extended wrist.[67] Following closed reduction of the associated wrist dislocation, careful evaluation of the capitate is necessary to detect the persistent capitate malrotation. Open reduction with fixation of both the capitate and scaphoid is required to restore the normal relationships within the wrist and, hopefully, prevent avascular necrosis of the capitate.

Fractures of the hamate may involve the body, articular surfaces, and/or the hook/hamulus.[68] Clinically, pain and tenderness on the ulnar aspect of the hand is present often with associated swelling. Both ulnar and median nerve injury may be associated with hook fractures and a thorough examination of motor and sensory function should be documented. As with all carpal bone fractures, standard radiographs may be inadequate to image the injury. Additional views should include a carpal tunnel view and an oblique view with the hand in 45° of supination and the wrist in radial deviation. CT may be required if symptoms persist in the presence of negative plain radiographs.[69,70]

Isolated body fractures rarely displace and are usually amenable to a period of immobilization. Those associated with high-energy injuries, such as CMC fracture dislocations, require internal fixation as a fundamental component of the treatment of this complex injury pattern.

Hook fractures may be difficult to diagnose without CT, and this should be performed early when this fracture is clinically suspected. Delay in treatment of this fracture can result in flexor tendon rupture from attritional wear over the fracture site.[71] Untreated, this fracture can also be a nagging injury which causes pain with many of the activities of daily living. Treatment is by excision of the hook, or open reduction and screw fixation. Neither method has been shown to have an advantage over the other.[72]

Lunate fractures are rare when one excludes those associated with idiopathic avascular necrosis, or Kienbock's disease. Accurate imaging to rule out predisposing avascular necrosis usually requires CT and or MRI in addition to plain radiographs. Acute fractures may involve the volar or dorsal lips, or occur as transverse or sagittal fractures.[73] Sagittal fractures and dorsal lip fractures are usually stable because of ligamentous support and require only a 6–8 week period of immobilization. Volar lip fractures and transverse fractures have a tendency to displace and require open reduction and internal fixation.

Carpal Dislocations.    Compared with other types of injury to the wrist carpal dislocations are relatively infrequent in occurrence.[74] However, because these injuries are usually associated with high-energy trauma they have the potential to have devastating effects on future wrist function. Early diagnosis and aggressive treatment is indicated. Simple closed reduction rarely results in long-term wrist stability.

Based on anatomic patterns of injury these may be classified as perilunar, radiocarpal, midcarpal, axial, and isolated carpal dislocations. By far the most frequent traumatic carpal dislocations are perilunar dislocations and fracture dislocations. Radiocarpal and axial pattern dislocations are much less common but still more frequent than isolated carpal bone dislocations. Pure midcarpal dislocation without associated fracture is an extremely rare event.

Perilunar dislocations represent part of a staged pattern of injury centered around the lunate.[75] These can be purely ligamentous injuries, often referred to as lesser arc injuries, or can be associated with carpal bone fracture, greater arc injuries. These injuries are usually associated with motor vehicle trauma, a fall from height, or sports injury.

These injuries often appear as a dramatic deformity of the wrist that should not distract the examiner from performing a complete system examination to rule out other more life-threatening injuries. Once this is accomplished a focused examination of the upper extremity should include a documented neurologic examination because of the frequency of median nerve compromise with these dislocations. Posteroanterior, and lateral x-ray views of the wrist should be obtained (Fig. 42-11). The lateral projection is particularly helpful to evaluate the relationship of the lunate, capitate, and distal radius. With perilunate dislocation the lunate will retain its relationship with the radius, but the capitate will be displaced either palmarly or dorsally from the lunate. On a PA view the carpus will appear crowded due to overlap of the proximal and distal carpal rows.

Greater arc injuries will appear radiographically similar to lesser arc injuries but will include one or more carpal bone fractures

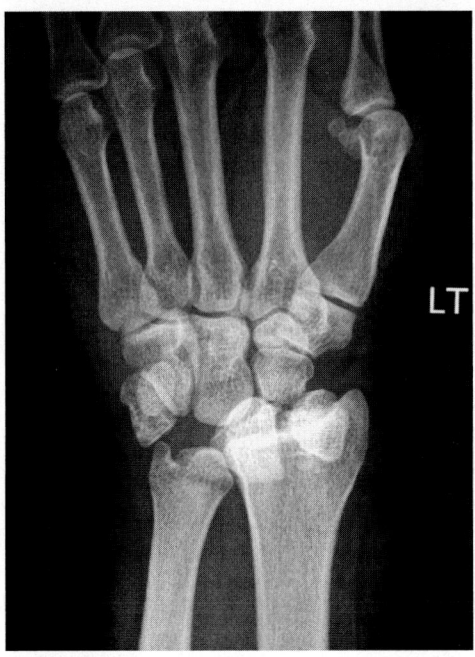 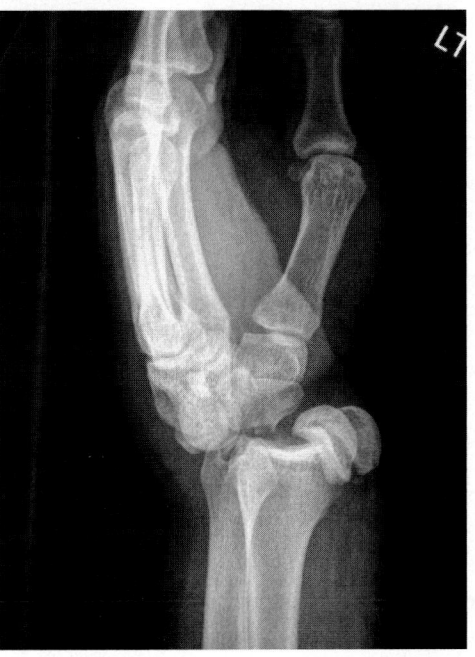

**FIGURE 42-11.** PA and lateral radiographs of a trans-scaphoid perilunate dislocation with translocation of both the lunate and proximal pole of the scaphoid into the carpal tunnel.

and/or radio-ulnar styloid fractures. Of these potential injures the most common is the trans-scaphoid perilunate fracture dislocation. Careful evaluation of these injuries is important not to miss the much less frequent trans-scaphoid/trans-capitate fracture dislocation often referred to as scaphocapitate fracture syndrome.

Treatment should be initiated as soon as the patient is able to be safely sedated or anesthetized. Closed reduction in the ED with splinting or application of a bivalved cast may be an appropriate short-term solution to decompress the median nerve and restore a semblance of normal anatomical alignment. However, this cannot be considered definitive long-term treatment since residual instability and misalignment should always be considered to present after this maneuver.

Operative treatment consisting of open reduction through a palmar and dorsal approach for ligamentous repair and anatomical alignment followed by pin stabilization should be considered emergently or relatively urgently.[76] When associated fractures are present these should also be stabilized, usually with screw fixation. Even with ideal treatment some loss of wrist motion should be anticipated.

### Metacarpal and Phalangeal.

Metacarpal and phalangeal fractures are the most common fractures of the upper extremity. The incidence peaks in males between the ages of 10 and 40. Unfortunately, metacarpal and phalangeal fractures are often trivialized, but in truth they account for a significant percentage of the >90 million days of restricted and >16 million days off work attributed to upper extremity injury.

Metacarpal fractures may involve the base, shaft, neck, or head, and may be articular or non-articular.[77] In addition, when the fracture is at the base, it may be associated with a dislocation.

The second and third carpometacarpal joints are relatively immobile and are injured less frequently than the more mobile fourth and fifth CMC joins. Thus, the most common metacarpal base fracture involves the small finger metacarpal and is almost always associated with dislocation. This injury is inherently unstable because of the pull of the extensor carpi ulnaris, and closed reduction and cast immobilization as definitive treatment is usually

doomed to failure. Therefore, initial splinting should be followed by scheduled outpatient closed reduction and pinning. At the time of ORIF, care must be taken during the approach to avoid injuring the dorsal sensory branch of the ulnar nerve or entrapping it in the fixation.

More complex injuries can result in the fourth metacarpal being dislocated with the fifth metacarpal, or disruption of the entire finger ray. Both these injuries represent high-energy disruptions of the ligamentous support of these joints and usually open reduction and internal fixation is necessary. In addition, concomitant ulnar nerve injury in these severe disruptions can lead to significant long-term morbidity.

Many metacarpal shaft fractures present as stable, nondisplaced fractures. These can be managed by placement into a clam-digger cast or thermoplast splint until the fracture is clinically nontender. At this point, despite a continued radiographically evident fracture line, the hand can be mobilized.

Isolated third and fourth metacarpal fractures, in particular, are amendable to this type of management because of continued support by the stout transverse metacarpal ligament. The border digits, index, and small, will more often develop some degree of malformation often expressed by crossing over of the fingers with flexion "scissoring." Therefore, these fractures should be treated by operative intervention. Modalities available include ORIF, closed reduction and percutaneous pinning with Kirschner wires, or closed reduction and intramedullary nailing.[78]

Multiple metacarpal fractures lead to an inherently unstable hand and operative intervention is always indicated. Often these injuries are combined injuries and will require not only fracture fixation but also soft-tissue and tendon reconstruction or repair. Principles of treatment of this type of injury are covered under the combined injury portion of this chapter.

Metacarpal neck fractures represent the most common metacarpal fracture and usually involve the fourth or fifth metacarpal. Acceptable closed reduction of these fractures depends on the digit involved, with fracture angulation of 50–70° tolerable in the fifth digit and only 10–20° in the index.[79,80] Fifth metacarpal neck fractures are commonly referred to as "Boxer's fractures" and are almost always associated with a clenched fist striking a solid object. This object is usually inanimate, not another individual. The result is an apex dorsal angulated fracture with volar comminution. This comminution is the reason that most acute reductions fail, with rapid relapse in a splint or cast to the postinjury state. Because of this high incidence of postreduction relapse, it has been recommended that the patient should initially be splinted in the intrinsic plus position, and then perform the reduction at 7–10 days when the fracture has begun to consolidate. Whether the hand is then splinted in extension to presumably enhance a "ligamentotaxis" effect and counteract the tendency to relapse into an apex dorsal deformity, or splinted or casted in the classic "cobra" cast position makes little or no difference to long-term outcome. Fours weeks should be the maximum period of immobilization after treatment of such a fracture.

Metacarpal head fractures are usually intra-articular fractures and are often associated with a clenched fist or "fight-bite" injury. Closed fractures with significant intra-articular displacement should undergo open reduction and screw fixation. When significant comminution is present, fixation is probably not possible. Either acute joint replacement should be performed or the fracture should be allowed to heal and, if significant morbidity develops, then joint replacement should occur at a later time.

Clenched fist or "fight bite" injuries occur when the patient strikes the mouth of another person.[81] This most commonly involves the metacarpal head of the long finger because of its prominence in the clenched position. The initial injury may appear quite innocuous; however, all injuries should be assumed to have penetrated deeper structures and to have entered the underlying joint. X-rays are mandatory for these injuries, not only to look for a head fracture, but also to rule out the presence of a retained tooth fragment. Even when seen acutely, these injuries should be explored by a formal arthrotomy in the operating room where cultures are obtained and the joint irrigated.

It is preferable to enter the joint by taking down the ulnar sagittal band to decrease the possibility of ulnar luxation or subluxation of the extensor hood. Operative intervention should be followed by intravenous antibiotics targeting *Staphylococcus sp.* for 24 to 48 hours (see Chap. 19).

Thumb metacarpal shaft fractures require less accurate reduction because of the mobility of the carpometacarpal joint. However, articular fractures of the base in the form of Bennett's and Rolando fractures (Fig. 42-12) do not have this latitude. Bennett's fracture is essentially a fracture-dislocation of the carpometacarpal joint. Axial loading results in the strong palmar oblique ligament retaining a fragment of bone while the metacarpal is dislocated radially and proximally by the pull of the abductor pollicis longus muscle. Posttraumatic arthritis is frequently a sequelae to a Bennett's type fracture and operative intervention is recommended. Either closed reduction percutaneous pinning, or open reduction internal fixation is acceptable and yield similar outcomes.[82]

The Rolando fracture is T- or Y-shaped fracture of the thumb metacarpal base, which has both the volar lip fracture seen in Bennett's fracture as well as a large dorsal fragment (Fig. 42-12). These fractures are extremely difficult to manage and frequently lead to posttraumatic arthritis regardless of what technique is used for management. Surgical options include multiple k-wires, tension band wires, plates and screws, and external fixation.

Phalangeal fractures are common in all age groups, with a reported incidence of 105 per 100,000 for women and 149 per 100,000 for men.[50] The signs of injury are obvious: swelling, tenderness, ecchymosis, deformity, and/or skin abrasions. The examination needs to differentiate between fracture, collateral ligament rupture, volar plate rupture, and tendon avulsion, all of which may have similar signs on cursory inspection. At a minimum, a PA, oblique, and lateral x-rays should be obtained.

Nondisplaced, stable proximal, and middle phalangeal fractures can be effectively managed by either buddy taping or splint

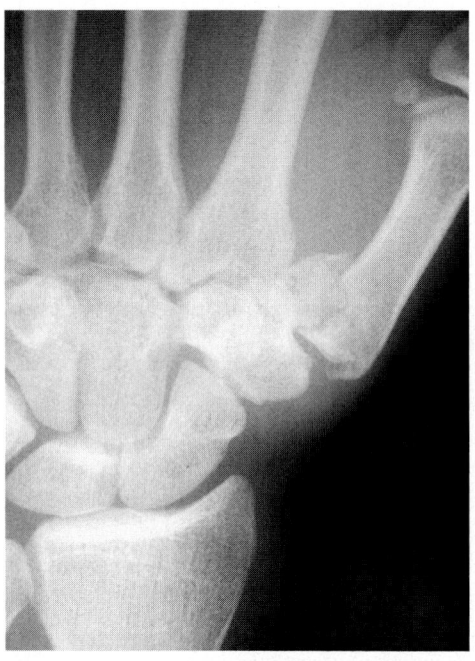
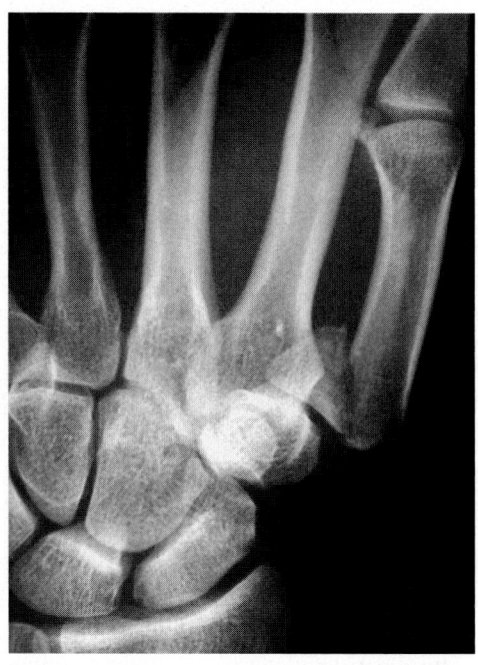

A                              B

**FIGURE 42-12.** Bennett's fracture **(A)** with a single fragment retained by the palmar oblique ligament and the metacarpal displaced proximally and radially by the pull of the abductor pollicis longus. Rolando fracture **(B)** demonstrating comminution of the first metacarpal base.

immobilization. However, many proximal and middle phalangeal fractures have articular involvement or have significant malformation because of the effect of the flexor tendons and/or extensor apparatus. Closed reduction to align displaced fractures can be performed by a combination of axial traction and reversal of the deformity. Even what initially appear to be nondisplaced articular fractures have the potential to displace. Therefore, if nonoperative management is selected as the primary treatment, then close follow-up and frequent radiographs are necessary to avoid missing displacement.

Operative treatment of articular fractures entails closed reduction with percutaneous screw or Kirschner wire placement. More ridged fixation allows early initiation of range of motion. Pilon-type injuries require some type of traction fixation to allow motion with maintenance of articular congruity.[83,84] Even with this type of approach, secondary arthroplasty procedures may be required.

Transverse, spiral, oblique, and comminuted phalangeal shaft fractures may occur. Proximal phalangeal fractures angulate apex volar, due to the strong pull of the interosseous muscles. Deformation of middle phalangeal fractures depends on the location of the shaft fracture with relation to the superficialis tendon insertion. Apex volar deformation result when the fracture is distal to the insertion of the superficialis tendon, while apex dorsal deformation results from fractures proximal to the superficialis insertion. A variety of methods have been employed to overcome these distracting forces. These include static casting in the intrinsic plus position for proximal phalangeal fracture, with early mobilization at four weeks with buddy tape support to the adjacent finger. Traction has also been utilized, with force exerted through the skin, pulp, nail plate, or skeleton. Difficulties with this technique include the awkwardness of the device, joint stiffness, and skin problems. Operative techniques include external fixation, percutaneous pinning and ORIF with plates, screw, or interosseous wires.

Of these techniques, percutaneous pin fixation seems to have the least long-term morbidity.

Metacarpophalangeal Dislocations. Dislocations of the finger metacarpophalangeal joints are relatively rare because of the stout ligamentous support and the associated flexor and extensor tendons. As would be expected, the border digits consisting of the index and small are much more vulnerable to this type of injury than the central two fingers. Most dislocations occur dorsally, and are associated with a hyperextension injury.[85] These injuries may be classified as simple or complex.

Simple metacarpophalangeal (MCP) joint dislocations are, in reality, subluxations and differ anatomically from complex or complete dislocations, in that the volar plate is draped over the metacarpal head and not entrapped above the metacarpal head. In a simple dislocation the proximal phalanx is locked in 60–80° of hyperextension. A key point in treatment of these injuries is to avoid hyperextension or traction during reduction attempts, which could result in conversion of this injury to a complex dislocation. The correct reduction maneuver for incomplete dislocations is flexion of the wrist to relax the flexor tendons and application of simple distal- and volar-directed pressure to the dorsal base of the proximal phalanx. This maneuver slides the proximal phalanx and its attached volar plate over the metacarpal head into the reduced position.

Patients with complex dislocations present, in contrast, with the finger held in only slight extension and inability to flex (Fig. 42-13).[86] Palpation of the palm will demonstrate a bony prominence corresponding to the metacarpal head. Radiographs will show a widened joint space and often a sesamoid will be present within the joint confirming entrapment of the volar plate.

Surgical reduction of a complex dislocation has been described by both a volar and dorsal approach. Limitations of the dorsal approach are the assumption that the volar plate is the only blocking structure;

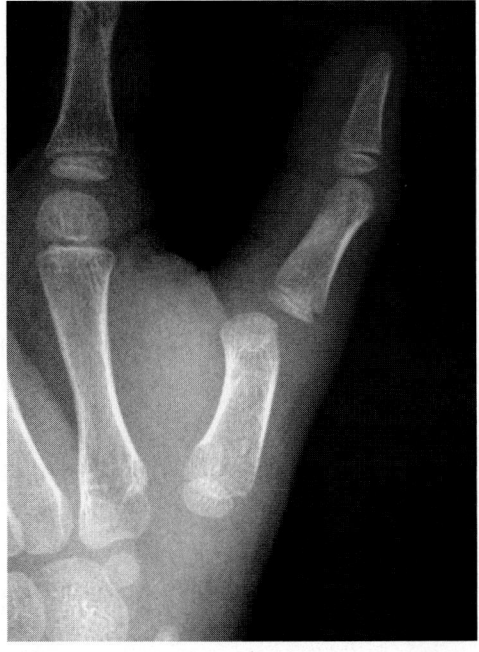

**A**

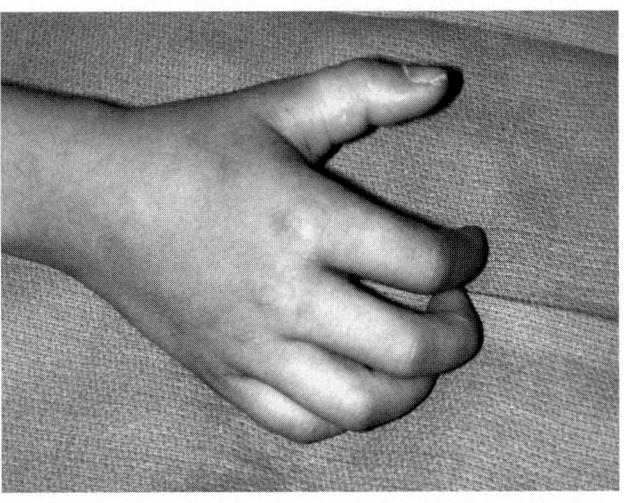

**B**

**FIGURE 42-13.** Radiograph of a complex dislocation of the thumb metacarpal phalangeal joint **(A)**, and view of the hand demonstrating only slight hyperextension of the involved joint **(B)**.

however, this approach allows access for any associated fracture fixation and is applicable in most instances. In the event that reduction cannot be obtained by longitudinally splitting the volar plate through a dorsal approach, a volar incision should be added.

Most dislocations of the thumb metacarpophalangeal joint are dorsal and may be simple or complex. Like finger MCP dislocations, the mechanism is hyperextension with rupture of the volar plate either proximal, distal, or through the sesamoids. Most dorsal dislocations are reducible, but entrapment of the flexor pollicis longus tendon, usually over the ulnar side of the metacarpal head, may create a noose in conjunction with the radially located intrinsics. Radiographs demonstrating entrapment of the sesamoid within the joint usually are consistent with a complex irreducible dislocation, whereas fracture of the sesamoids usually predicts successful closed reduction.

Again, closed management of these injuries should avoid longitudinal traction or hyperextension, which could convert a simple dislocation to a complex, irreducible dislocation. Instead, gentle pressure should be applied to the base of the proximal phalanx to push it over the head of the metacarpal. Failed attempts at reduction should be followed by operative intervention through a dorsal approach to split the volar plate longitudinally and remove other interposed tissue, thereby allowing reduction.

Once any MCP dislocation is reduced, collateral ligament integrity should be tested. If there is no injury to the collateral ligaments then the finger or thumb should be immobilized in flexion no longer than 14 days, at which point an active range of motion protocol should be initiated with a dorsal blocking splint.

Interphalangeal Joint Dislocations.    Dislocation of the proximal interphalangeal joint (PIP) joint may occur in any of three directions: dorsal, volar, or lateral with reference to the position of the middle phalanx, relative to the proximal phalanx. Of these possibilities, dorsal dislocation is the most common and is usually associated with hyperextension of the PIP joint, often during ball sports.[87]

Dorsal dislocation may be a purely soft tissue injury or a fracture dislocation. Greater axial force increases the likelihood that the volar lip of the middle phalanx will be sheared off. Reduction of dorsal dislocations is by longitudinal traction with local digital block. After reduction, radiographs should be obtained to assure a concentric reduction, and the integrity of the collateral ligaments confirmed by a passive lateral stress test in both full extension and 30° of flexion. If the joint is stable early motion should be encouraged by simple buddy taping. When instability exists, the point of dislocation is determined and the finger is flexed 10° further and an extension block splint is applied. Each week the block is decreased by 10° until full extension is achieved.

Volar PIP dislocations exist in two forms and are much less common than dorsal dislocations. In the first type the central slip is disrupted by a straight volar dislocation of the PIP joint. These injuries can be treated by closed reduction with longitudinal traction, and splinting of the PIP joint in extension for six weeks with the DIP joint free to flex and extend. The second type of dislocation is a volar rotary subluxation as a result of forces applied in a semi-flexed position. This results in a split between the central tendon and the lateral band with buttonholing of the condyle through this split. Closed reduction of this type of dislocation can be difficult but can be attempted by flexion of the MCP and PIP joints with gentle manipulation of the middle phalanx. Failure to

promptly achieve reduction should be followed by operative open reduction rather than repeated attempts at closed reduction. Following reduction if the central slip is intact early motion with buddy tape support should be utilized; however, if the central slip is disrupted then six weeks of PIP extension splinting is required as in any central slip rupture.

Lateral dislocations result from rupture of the volar plate and one collateral ligament. This results in asymmetric joint swelling with tenderness on the side of the collateral ligament rupture. Closed reduction is usually relatively easily accomplished by traction and manipulation. This is followed by two weeks of static splinting in extension followed by buddy tape protected motion.

DIP dislocations are most often dorsal or lateral and in many cases are open injuries because of the tightness of the soft tissue envelope at this level of the finger. Closed injuries can be reduced by longitudinal traction, open dislocations require appropriate antibiotics and irrigation of the joint followed by reduction. Occasionally irreducible dislocations may result from interposition of the proximal volar plate or the flexor tendon. Splinting should be in slight flexion for one week continuously followed by intermittent protected motion for an additional 1–2 weeks.

Fingertip and Nail Bed Injury.    The finger tip is the terminal end organ of the upper extremity. As such, it enables us to relate to the environment by touch so fine that Braille can be interpreted and sand can be sorted based on texture. Loss of this function can change one's career by making some previously performed tasks impossible after injury. In its position as the terminal end organ, the finger tip is extremely vulnerable to injury and, in fact, is frequently assaulted by slammed doors, hammers, saws, and a multitude of other sharp objects.

Fingernails serve to help protect the important tip and aid in the performance of certain fine tasks. Their loss can also be difficult to compensate for and, therefore, injury to these structures should not be trivialized.

Important points in the initial evaluation of the patient with a finger tip injury are overall medical condition, hand dominance, occupation, and finger involved. The injury should then be inspected and, in the case of amputation, both level and orientation should be noted. Oblique amputation can be categorized as dorsal, volar, or lateral oblique. Transverse amputations are primarily categorized by level in relation to the nail anatomy.

Distal amputations, without bone or tendon exposure and with skin loss less than 1 cm$^2$ are best managed conservatively with irrigation and frequent dressing changes. Healing of these injuries, however, can be protracted with up to nine weeks for complete epithelialization and even longer for complete sensory reeducation and resolution of hyperpathia and cold intolerance.[88]

Treatment of more complex lesions with exposed bone or tendon can be as simple as rongeuring back exposed bone, or can involve more complex techniques, such as full thickness skin grafting, local flaps, or regional flaps. Treatment of these injuries with full thickness skin grafts can be adequate and has been shown to result in a two-point discrimination of 10 mm or less occurred 86% of the time, and 50% of patients had 6 mm or less two-point discrimination. Donor site morbidity was minimal with this simple technique, and no cold intolerance or ulceration was reported.[89]

Kutler, in 1947, described radial and ulnar V–Y advancement flaps for treatment of finger tip injuries that are still utilized today.[90] In this technique, V-shaped flaps, with the apex at the distal crease, are designed and cut through the skin and subcutaneous tissues without disrupting the blood supply. Mobilization is by separation of the fibrous septa from the underlying bone. The flaps are sutured together across the tip of the finger.

This concept of a V–Y advancement flap was then modified by Atasoy and coworkers in 1970 to encompass the volar surface.[91] This modification presented a much simpler dissection and placed the scar at the skin nail bed junction, not over the tip, resulting in less problems with hyperpathia. Sensation in this flap has also been evaluated and, while protective, it is only approximately 73% of the contralateral digit.[92]

When either of the above flaps is inadequate, a common alternative is the cross-finger flap (Fig. 42-14). In this procedure, the dorsal skin overlying the middle phalanx of an adjacent digit is elevated and sewn to the injured tip. The donor site is then covered with a full thickness skin graft, usually harvested from the hypothenar area or wrist crease. This is a delayed flap and the sutured together fingers need to be protected for 10–14 days prior to separation and inset. Sensory recovery with this flap can be expected to be protective, with results comparable to a full thickness skin graft. Improvement in this sensitivity can be increased by transferring this flap as a sensate flap with microneural reconstruction.[93]

A multitude of other flaps have also been described for finger tip reconstruction, including the sensate heterodigital island flap, homodigital island flap, and dorsometacarpal island flaps, as well as free flaps from the toes or adjacent fingers. Successful replantation of pulp and Zone I injuries is also possible and should not be overlooked.

Nail bed injuries include subungual hematomas, laceration, crush injuries, and avulsion injuries.[94] When delaying care of these injuries, one should keep in mind that late reconstruction of the nail bed is much more technically demanding and fraught with complication than primary repair or reconstruction.

Subungual hematomas comprising 50% or less of the nail bed, and without an associated distal phalanx fracture, can be treated with drainage if symptomatic. There is no absolute requirement for drainage in this situation. For hematomas comprising greater than 50%, or those associated with a displaced fracture of the distal phalanx, removal of the nail plate and repair of the nail bed is advised.

For simple nail bed lacerations, repair can be accomplished with digital block and tourniquet. The nail is removed with a

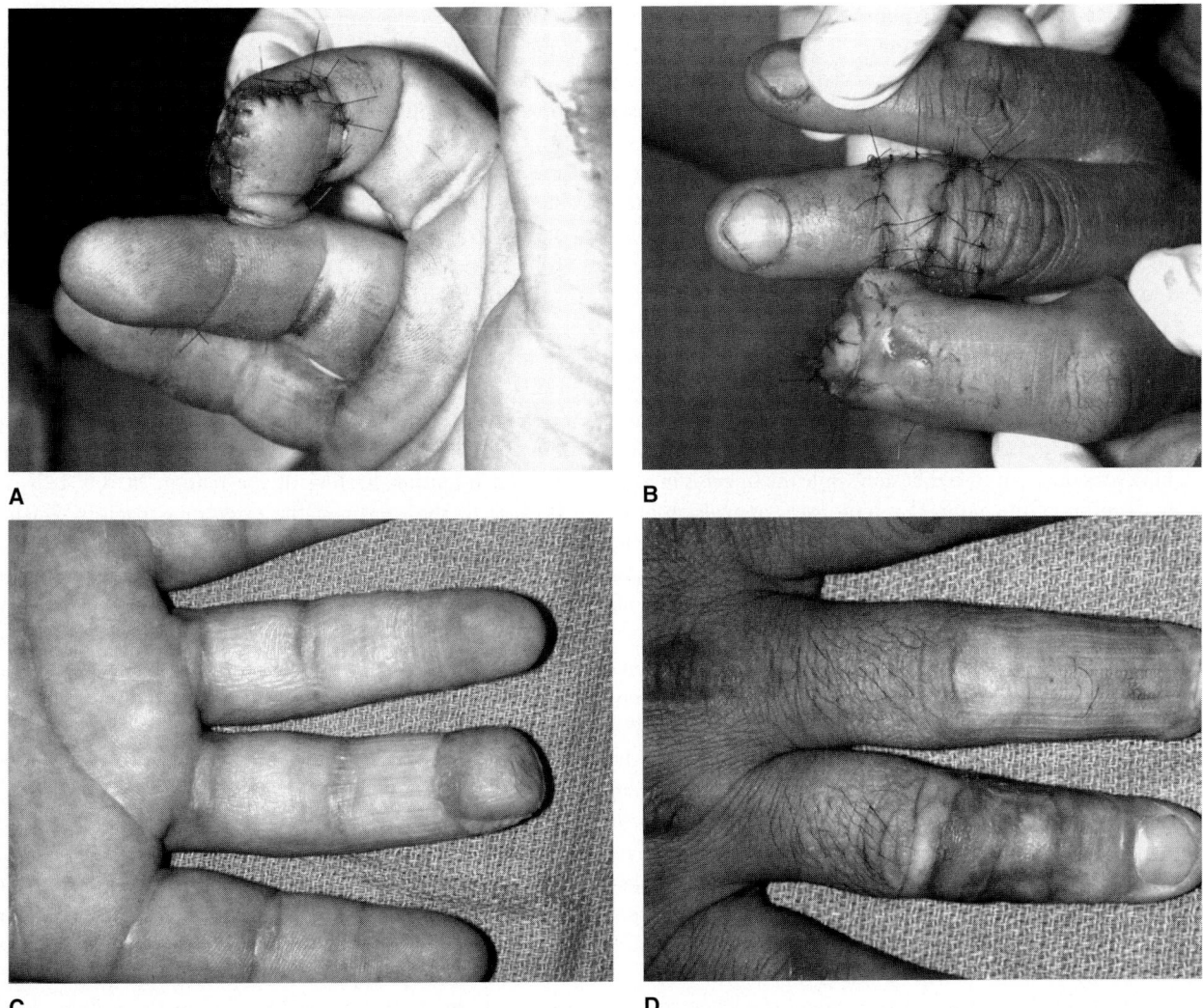

A

B

C

D

**FIGURE 42-14.** Long finger tip injury treated with cross-finger flap from ring finger (**A**) and full thickness skin graft to donor site (**B**). Follow-up demonstrating good restoration of tip (**C**) and healing of donor site (**D**).

Freer elevator, hemostat, or fine iris scissors. The matrix is then repaired with fine 6-0 or 7-0 chromic or plain gut, absorbable suture under loupe magnification. Following repair, the nail or a piece of x-ray film trimmed to mimic the nail can be slipped under the nail fold to prevent formation of a synechium. When properly placed this stent does not need to be sutured in place.

Severe crush injuries often result in avulsion of the nail plate with a portion of the nail matrix, or loss of portions of the nail matrix requiring replacement to affect repair. When the nail is present with attached matrix, this can be removed gently from the nail and sutured into the corresponding defect as a graft. If nail matrix is missing but length can be preserved, then an acute nail matrix graft may be harvested from the great toe or, in the instance of multiple digit injury, from adjacent parts that cannot be salvaged. Taking the time to restore nail integrity can be a worthwhile and rewarding experience for both the surgeon and patient.

Late presentation of nail loss or injury often requires complex reconstruction or nail ablation to result in a pain free, cosmetically acceptable situation.

## Tendon Injury

Extensor Tendons.    Extensor tendon injury is frequently not taken as seriously as flexor tendon injury. This was because it previously believed that recovery from these injuries is relatively benign with few long-term complications. However, the extensor tendon is the end organ of a complex mechanism, which involves input from both the extrinsic and intrinsic muscles of the hand to maintain the balanced finger function that is expected by most individuals. Disruption of any component of this balance, bone, skin, the musculotendinous system, or neurovascular structures, can lead to stiffness and poor functional outcome.

In the evaluation of extensor tendon injury the hand and distal forearm are divided into eight zones that aid in communication and, to a degree, guide treatment. Zone I injuries (mallet finger) involve disruption of the extensor mechanism over the distal interphalangeal joint resulting in the classic mallet finger deformity. Closed injury results from forced flexion while the finger is in rigid extension. Rupture of the terminal tendon itself, or avulsion of its insertion with a variable sized bony fragment, is the end result. The result is an inability to extend the distal phalanx. Lacerations or other open injuries, with combined skin and tendon loss, can result in a similar deformity.

Closed acute mallet fingers should be treated initially by continuous splinting in extension for six weeks.[95] The splint should not incorporate the other joints of the finger or hand, and active PIP motion should be encouraged. If resisted extension is present at the end of six weeks, the splint can be limited to nighttime use for an additional six weeks with close follow-up. Any relapse should be treated with three weeks of additional continuous splinting. Care must be taken during this prolonged period of splint use that skin maceration and necrosis do not occur. Occasionally, operative fixation by a variety of pinning methods is required for compliance or to more appropriately manage DIP joint subluxation.

Open mallet fingers can present a treatment challenge. Simple transverse lacerations are best treated by mass suturing with incorporation of the terminal tendon and skin with a series of interrupted, nonabsorbable sutures. Fingers with skin and tendon loss require soft tissue coverage and primary tendon grafting or late reconstruction. Emergency treatment consists of irrigation of the open wound/joint, dressing of the wound, antibiotic coverage, splinting in extension, and arranging urgent follow-up in the next 24 hours for surgical evaluation and treatment.

Zone II injuries occur over the shaft of the middle phalanx and are usually associated with laceration or open fractures. Lacerations involving less than 50% of the tendon width, and with no extensor lag, can be treated by wound care and splinting in extension for 7–10 days, followed by active range of motion. If more than 50% of the tendon is lacerated, or an extensor lag at the DIP joint exists, then the tendon should be repaired followed by splinting or pinning the DIP in extension for 6–8 weeks in a mallet finger protocol. Open fractures with tendon involvement require fracture and tendon repair and extensive therapy to regain range of motion.

Zone III injuries involve the central slip of the extensor tendon over the PIP joint and initially result in loss of extensor power at the PIP joint. Untreated, this injury results in palmar subluxation of the lateral bands and, within one to two weeks, development of the classic Boutonniere deformity. With this deformity, the finger rests in a position of flexion at the PIP joint and hyperextension at the DIP joint.

Physical examination will show weak or absent extension of the PIP joint with this injury. However, in closed rupture of the central slip, initial evaluation may be difficult due to pain and swelling at the PIP joint. Extension splinting of the PIP joint with follow-up and re-examination at seven days is a reasonable course of action in this situation. Splinting must not incorporate either the metacarpophalangeal joint or DIP joint. If, at one week, findings support the diagnosis of closed central slip rupture then splinting should continue for four to six additional weeks with weekly follow-up. Formal therapy is usually required at the completion of splinting to successfully regain full range of motion.

Open injury in Zone III requires wound management in the form of irrigation and debridement, formal arthrotomy if indicated, and soft tissue coverage if local tissue has been lost. Tendon repair may be primary or may be managed by transarticular pinning for four to six weeks to allow the tendon to heal on its own. Second intention healing of the tendon in this area is possible because of the design of the extensor apparatus which prevents retraction if the PIP joint is held in extension.

Zone IV lies over the proximal phalanx and injury at this level is often associated with proximal phalangeal fracture. Many tendon injuries at this level are incomplete, due to the broad nature of the extensor hood at this level. Like Zone III injuries, even complete laceration will not result in proximal migration of the tendon due to the constraints of the sagittal bands which tether the severed end.

Because of the broad tendon expanse at this level, most lacerations in Zone IV will need to be extended to allow complete exploration and repair. Repair in some individuals will be possible with a core stitch; however, often the tendon remains too thin at this level to support this type of repair and simple interrupted sutures or near-far/far-near sutures will suffice. Early motion in this zone by an active flexion passive extension protocol is recommended.

When Zone IV injuries are associated with proximal phalangeal fractures, stable fracture repair will greatly facilitate initiation of early tendon motion.

Open Zone V injuries are commonly associated with the "fight bite" wound and treatment is addressed in the *Infection* section of this chapter. Closed tendon injuries in this zone are less common and usually involve the radial sagittal band, which results in subluxation or luxation of the extensor digitorum communis tendon into the ulnar gutter. This injury should not be overlooked in the older patient with attritional rupture.

Conservative treatment of sagittal band injuries or attritional rupture is possible if diagnosed within the first two to three weeks. Splinting may be with the wrist neutral, the MP joints in extension and the PIP and DIP joints free,[96] or with a recently described finger based sagittal band bridge splint.[97] If splinting for six to eight weeks fails, or the injury is seen late, then operative re-centralization should be performed.

Zone VI injuries can occur distal or proximal to the juncturae tendini, the tendinous connections between the extensor digitorum communis (EDC) tendons. Injury to a single EDC tendon proximal to the juncturae may make diagnosis difficult, since the finger will still extend at the MP joints through the transmission of the adjacent tendon action through the juncturae. In this situation, exploration may be the only means of diagnosis, short of imaging techniques such as ultrasound or MRI. Diagnosis of Zone VI laceration of the extensor indicis pollicis (EIP) or extensor digitorum quinti (EDQ) can also be difficult because the EDC may still provide extension to the index and small fingers. In both the situation of laceration of the EDC proximal to the juncturae, and isolated EIP or EDQ tendon laceration, proximal retraction of the lacerated tendon will occur. With the EIP and EDQ tendons this retraction is often to the level of the wrist retinaculum. In these instances, exploration in the operating room is probably preferable to exploration in the ED. Core suture with an epitendinous suture is usually possible at this level.

Open injuries in Zone VI can have extensive soft tissue loss associated with them. Repair of such injuries often requires complex soft tissue coverage with immediate or delayed tendon reconstruction or transfer.

Zone VII injuries to the extensor tendons occur at the level of the wrist retinaculum where the tendons are divided into six compartments. In this zone retraction of the tendon ends always occurs, making formal operative exploration imperative. Repair needs to be meticulous to avoid adhesions to the overlying retinaculum which often needs to be expanded by z-plasty during closure. Failure to appropriately repair the retinaculum will result in bowstringing of the extensor tendons at the level of the wrist. Associated injury to the dorsal sensory branches of the radial and ulnar nerves can occur with these injuries and requires a high level of suspicion to prompt exploration and microneural repair. Ignoring these associated nerve injuries can not only lead to only loss of sensation over a portion of the dorsum of the hand, but also chronic neuropathic pain.

Zone VIII represents the musculotendinous junctions of the extensors. Injury at this level is always associated with penetrating trauma or massive soft tissue injury, often with associated open forearm fractures. Initial evaluation of penetrating trauma, usually by glass or knives, may show a relatively small wound that belies the damage that has been done internally. Even with what appears to be normal extension on examination, significant damage can be found with surgical exploration.[98] Repair of the musculotendinous junction itself is difficult because of the poor suture holding properties of the muscle. Large figure of eight sutures are required to restore continuity and repair should be followed by four to six weeks of splinting with the wrist in 20° of extension and the MCP

joints in 20° of flexion. If the injury is distal to the posterior interosseous nerve, good restoration of function is possible. Injury to this nerve requires thorough exploration and repair by an experienced microneural surgeon familiar with this complex anatomy to maximize functional recovery. Even with meticulous nerve repair, tendon transfer may be required at a later date.

In order to salvage a functionally threatened extremity, massive combined injury in Zone VIII requires application of the principles discussed in combined injury portion of this chapter.

Thumb Extensor Injury.    The thumb represents a unique structure in many contexts including its extensor anatomy. Because the thumb has only two phalanges, the Zones are slightly different and often referred to as T I–V. T I and T II are over the only interphalangeal joint of the thumb and the proximal phalanx, respectively. Injuries in these areas can result in Mallet deformity similar to Zone I injuries in the fingers. Treatment principles in these thumb zones remain the same as previously described for Zone I of the fingers.

T III is over the metacarpophalangeal joint of the thumb and, unlike the fingers, two tendons are vulnerable to injury at this level. The extensor pollicis brevis inserts here in the radial aspect of the base of the proximal phalanx, while the extensor pollicis longus passes ulnarly and inserts on the distal phalanx. Injury to the EPB at this level can be isolated or associated with injury to the dorsal capsule and radial collateral ligament. Examination of patients with injury at this level should include a thorough evaluation of the stability of the MCP joint and, at surgical exploration; all potentially injured structures should be evaluated and repaired. After surgical repair, both the thumb and wrist should be immobilized.

In T IV, the EPL and EPB tend to become more oval, making them amendable to core stitches as well as epitendinous suture. These two tendons remain closely associated at this level, and with isolated injury of one tendon, retraction may be prevented by the remaining intact tendon. However, one should be prepared for more proximal exploration, particularly with injury to the EPL.

T V injuries may involve the EPL, EPB, and/or abductor pollicis longus. In addition, injury to branches of the superficial radial nerve is often a component at this level. All three tendons have a tendency to retract at this level and more proximal exploration is often required. Failure to repair the superficial radial nerve branches can result in not only sensory loss in its distribution, but also a syndrome of chronic neuropathic pain.

Following repair at the T IV–V level, a short period of immobilization of the wrist and thumb should be followed by a therapist-directed early active range of motion program.

Flexor Tendon.    Because of its complexity, the treatment of flexor tendon injury is a major component of the history of the development of hand surgery.[99] Today, despite many advances in the surgical treatment of flexor tendon injury and rehabilitation, the care of these injuries remains a significant challenge.

Flexor tendon injury can be by laceration, avulsion, or crush; or associated with massive upper extremity trauma. Because of the proximity of neurovascular structures at all levels along the course of the flexors in the forearm, wrist, and hand, combined injury of these soft tissue structures is common and adds to complexity of care.

Examination of the flexor tendons of the fingers and thumb is based on the anatomical relationship of the flexors to specific joint function. In the fingers, both the DIP and PIP joints can be flexed by the flexor digitorum profundus (FDP), a muscle that has its radial component (index and long fingers) innervated by the anterior interosseous (median) nerve, and its ulnar component (ring and small fingers) innervated by the ulnar nerve. While the flexor digitorum superficialis (FDS) flexes, which PIP joint alone, is innervated only by the anterior interosseous (median) nerve. Specific simple maneuvers, however, can be done to separate FDP and FDS function during the hand examination (Fig. 42-15). The thumb is flexed predominantly by the flexor pollicis longus, which is innervated by the anterior interosseous nerve and is solely responsible for flexion of the IP joint.

Flexor tendon repair, in general, consists of both a core and epitendinous suture. A number of core stitches have been described and while all have been shown to be effective when applied correctly, the recent addition of preformed loop sutures offers several advantages in repair and should be considered for use.[100] These sutures allow easier placement of an increased number of strands, which proportionally increases the strength of the repair allowing earlier and more aggressive therapy.[101]

As with extensor tendon injury, various zones (I–V) have been defined for flexor tendon injury. This classification helps in communication when describing an injury and in determining appropriate rehabilitation program.

Zone I injuries involve the insertion of the FDP or FPL into the distal phalanx of the finger or thumb. These may be associated with a laceration or avulsion. Definitive laceration treatment in this zone depends on the length of the distal stump. If the stump is less than 1 cm, then suture repair will not be sufficient and the FDP should be advanced and reinserted into the bone. FDP avulsions at this level, often called "jersey fingers," occur as three patterns of decreasing severity.[102] Type I avulsions are the most severe and the most easily missed because of lack of radiographic evidence of injury. In this instance, the tendon pulls off the bone and ruptures the vincula within the finger; this allows complete retraction of the proximal tendon into the palm. Early recognition and treatment of this injury is necessary to avoid the need for two-stage tendon reconstruction. Repair can be accomplished early by pullout button or suture anchor with equal outcome.[103]

In Type II avulsions, the tendon is held at the level of the vincula, which does not rupture. This prevents flexor canal collapse proximal to the A-4 pulley and makes advancement and reinsertion

possible for up to six weeks. Clinical differentiation from Type I rupture is difficult in the absence of visualization of a bony fragment on x-rays.

In Type III avulsions, a large bony fragment is associated with the distal FDP, which causes the tendon to be retained at the level of the distal A-4 pulley. Repair in this instance is often possible by pull out stitch reinsertion or fixation of the bony fragment with a Kirschner wire or screw.

Zone II has historically been referred to as "no-man's land" because of the difficulty of rehabilitation with this level of injury.[99] This zone is defined by the presence of the adjacent FDS and FDP within the flexor sheath. Repair in this area requires skillful repair and early active or passive motion protocols for functional restoration. Preservation of the pulley system during this repair may require passage of the proximally retrieved with a small catheter that has been passed from the distal site of the injury. Even when all principles are adhered to, secondary tenolysis may be required due to the development of peritendinous adhesions.

Zone III injuries are in the palm between the distal extent of the carpal tunnel and the proximal border of the A-1 pulley. Because this zone is not constrained by the fibro-osseous canal the prognosis for recovery is markedly improved over Zone II injury. An important part of preoperative counseling is to prepare the patient for the possibility of a laceration in the palm really being a Zone II injury. This occurs because with a clenched fist the tendons will be maximally drawn into the palm at the time of injury, but will excurse into Zone II with relaxation. This means wounds may need to be operatively extended into the fingers and the rehabilitation may be protracted.

Zone IV (within the carpal tunnel) and Zone V injuries (distal to the musculotendinous junction) have a high probability of associated major vessel and/or nerve injury. Preoperative examination should include a thorough evaluation of the motor and sensory status of the patient with appropriate documentation. Hemorrhage in these situations can be quite dramatic, but can usually be controlled by direct pressure. Blind clamping or use of a tourniquet is discouraged in this situation and usually unnecessary. Only rarely, with laceration of both the ulnar and radial artery is the hand truly threatened by ischemia. Collateral circulation through the interosseous arteries will maintain adequate distal perfusion if not obstructed by application of a proximal tourniquet. Tendon repair in this zone can be by core suture alone; however, epitendinous

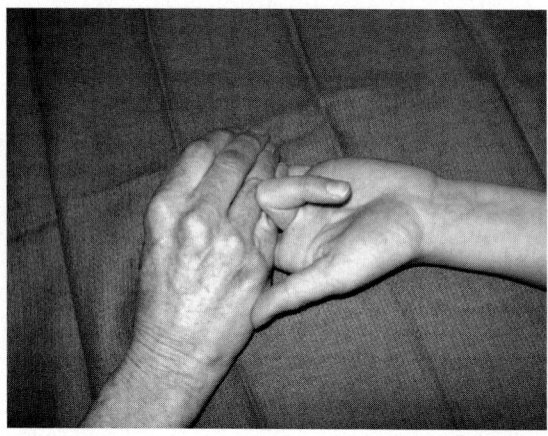 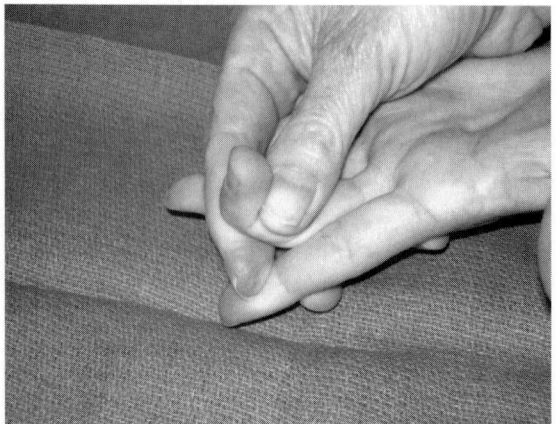

**A** **B**

**FIGURE 42-15.** Blocking maneuvers that allow isolation of the FDS **(A)** and FDP **(B)** to help elucidate individual involvement with injury.

suture use is encouraged to increase repair strength and preserve independent tendon excursion. Ultimately, the outcome of these injuries will be largely determined by precise nerve repair and successful re-innervation.

With laceration of the FPL to the thumb, proximal retraction to the level wrist is the rule, because of lack of vincular restraints. Retrieval requires location of the tendon at its proximal location and passage of a catheter from the distal laceration to the counter incision in the same manner depicted for passage under the pulley system in the fingers. The retrieved tendon can then be sutured to the catheter and retracted with the catheter to the distal site of injury. Early motion protocols are required to prevent adhesion within this well-defined sheath.

## Vascular Injury

Vascular injury can occur with either closed or open upper extremity trauma (see Chap. 44). Closed injury associated with arterial disruption includes scapulothoracic dissociation, shoulder dislocation, and elbow fractures and dislocations. Scapulothoracic dissociation represents a complex injury with a high incidence of both vascular disruption and concurrent brachial plexus rupture or avulsion. Successful treatment requires prompt diagnosis, preoperative angiography, and reconstruction by interpositional vein grafting.

Despite the frequency of shoulder dislocation or fracture, arterial injury remains a relatively rare complication. Anterior dislocation in the elderly is the most common scenario where vascular injury occurs with blunt shoulder trauma. Predisposing atherosclerotic disease with a more tortuous and noncompliant artery may play a role in this occurrence, and the injury is just as likely to occur during relocation, for the same reasons. Because of this, the distal vascular status should be assessed prior to reduction of any anterior dislocation. When this injury is encountered, only rarely is there adequate collateral flow to negate the need for reconstruction of the injured segment.

Supracondylar fractures in children infrequently involve the brachial artery; however, the extension type fracture with posterolateral displacement of the distal fragment and wide separation can result in vascular injury.[104] The ischemia present in this injury can be by direct impingement from the medial spike, or be secondary to vascular spasm and progressive soft tissue swelling. When vascular trauma is suspected, a gentle closed manipulation of the fracture and percutaneous pin fixation should be followed by repeat clinical examination. If distal pulses do not return with reduction, then angiography should be obtained. Surgery may only require release of the artery from entrapment in the fracture or formal repair to include interpositional vein grafting.

Open injury with pulsatile hemorrhage in the upper extremity should be managed initially with pressure alone, whenever feasible. Blind clamping and ligation can lead to devastating injury of closely associated nerves that can result in a successfully revascularized but worthless limb, requiring multiple procedures to restore less than satisfactory function. Similarly, use of the tourniquet should be limited to avoid contributing further to ischemic damage from occlusion of collateral flow. Once hemorrhage is controlled, few would argue that prompt surgical repair of subclavian, axillary, or brachial artery injuries is indicated. Less obvious is the treatment of single vessel injury in the forearm. Many have argued that, with documentation of adequate collateral flow from the remaining artery, it is more expeditious to ligate the injured vessel. However, with improvements in microvascular surgery, repair of arteries this size has become quite straightforward and the procedure itself adds little time to a wrist or forearm exploration where other associated injuries are being addressed.

## Peripheral Nerve Injury

Treatment of peripheral nerve injury represents a major component of upper extremity surgery and the end result of the care of this injury is often the major determinant of the degree of functional recovery in the injured upper extremity. Nerves do have the ability to regenerate but optimal regeneration will only occur with proper care.

The first step is recognition of the injury, which at times can be difficult in the polytrauma patient who is unable to cooperate in a neurosensory or motor examination (see *Examination* section of this chapter). In this instance a high level of suspicion based on anatomical location of injury, should trigger the response of serial examinations over the course of the patients' recovery. Also, if surgery is planned to deal with other injuries the opportunity for direct exploration of known at-risk nerves in the zone of injury being addressed should not be missed, this is particularly indicated in the presence of sharp penetrating trauma.

Injury to nerve has been clinically described as a continuum with variable potential for spontaneous recovery based on the degree of injury. The terms neurapraxia, axonotmesis, and neurotmesis commonly used to describe these degrees of the continuum and each term, in turn, correlates with potential for recovery. One or all degrees of injury may be present in a single injured upper extremity which further complicates the picture. More expanded classifications have also been described but are beyond the scope of this review.

Neurapraxia, the most minor form of injury, represents a conduction block with preservation of anatomical continuity. The neuropraxic injury may be complete or partial and although recovery will be complete it may take up to three months. Importantly, there is no nerve regeneration involved in this recovery and there is no advancing Tinel's sign because there is no axonal involvement. Neuropraxic injury can be associated with a concussive blow or a compressive injury such as a promptly released compartment syndrome, or a tourniquet-type injury.

In axonotmesis there is structural damage to the axon while the endoneurium and perineurium remain intact. A Tinel's sign is present in this form of injury, and can be followed during recovery as it progresses distally with axonal regrowth. In this injury, there is classic histological Wallerian degeneration distal to site of axon disruption. Because the axon sheaths remain essentially undisturbed, complete restoration of the original pattern of innervation is possible.

Neurotmesis represents complete severance of the nerve. Recovery in this situation is not possible without microsurgical repair. These injuries can result from traction and rupture, but are more commonly associated with penetrating trauma.

In large nerves it is possible to have all forms of injury present within the same nerve. This situation can complicate both initial diagnosis and interpretation of recovery as well as delay and complicate surgical intervention.

Surgical interventions in nerve injury include decompression, neurolysis, direct repair, and nerve grafting.[105] In complex injuries involving multiple nerve or nerve segments, all these techniques may be required. Direct nerve repair may be by epineural (Fig. 42-16) or fascicular suturing. While fascicular repair intuitively seems like it would give more precise anatomical alignment this has never been substantiated and the principle of less is more seems to apply. This means minimal foreign material in the form of suture, minimal or no tension, and minimal trauma are required for successful repair. When a tension-free repair is not possible, nerve conduit in the form autogenous nerve graft, or for short segment replacement vein or artificial conduit, must be utilized to fill the defect and serve as a guide for new axonal growth. A number of sensory nerves can be sacrificed with minimal deficit but the most common is the sural nerves from the lower legs.

Timing of nerve repairs can be defined as primary when repaired within one week of injury; nerve repairs after this time are considered secondary repairs. Direct end-to-end tensionless suture neuroraphy may not always be possible in the case of secondary repair and one should be prepared for interposition grafting or employment of other techniques to achieve successful reinnervation.

In general, nerve injuries associated with sharp penetrating open injuries should be explored early. If the injury is a sharp laceration immediate direct repair is usually the best option for optimal recovery. However, when the precise zone of injury to the nerve cannot be determined, as is often the case in crush injuries associated with significant soft tissue destruction, then a delayed repair is indicated so that the zone of injury is more clearly defined. Simple tagging of injured nerves at the time of exploration in itself probably serves no useful purpose since the experienced peripheral nerve surgeon will readily locate the injured nerve proximal and distal to the injury at the time of re-exploration. However, suture tagging the nerve to a stable adjacent structure may serve to prevent the inevitable retraction and minimize the distance that requires grafting at the time of definitive repair.

An exception to early exploration of penetrating open injuries is the gunshot wound. In these injuries the mechanism of injury is predominantly heat and shock wave effects and expectant management is usually appropriate. Vascular injury where the vessel is enclosed with the nerve in a common sheath, however, may lead to similar injury to both the nerve and vessel. In these situations it is imperative that during vessel repair the continuity of the nerve is verified.

Nerve transfer represents another option for dealing with both motor and sensory loss in what potentially would be a non-reconstructable injury.[105,106] The theory behind nerve transfer is to convert a high-level nerve injury into a low-level injury. This is accomplished by utilizing redundant or unimportant nerves or fascicles of the donor nerve to innervate critical motor or sensory targets. Initial experience with this concept was in brachial plexus surgery with the now classic intercostal to Musculocutaneous nerve transfer to restore elbow flexion. This technique has now been expanded in brachial plexus neurotization to a number of nerve transfers with specific functional targets and more recently to reconstruct a number of other nerve injuries.

An important example of a nerve transfer outside of the brachial plexus is the transfer of the distal anterior interosseous to the motor branch of the ulnar nerve to restore intrinsic function. This gives a very simple functional alternative to complex tendon transfer and preserves muscle mass within the hand resulting in a more cosmetic outcome.

Spaghetti Wrist.    On the volar side of the wrist there are 16 structures, including 12 tendons, two nerves, and two arteries in close proximity to the skin. This leaves these structures vulnerable to trauma when the integument is violated. Because of the appearance when the wrist at this level is lacerated resulting in exposure of numerous white string appearing structures the term "spaghetti wrist" has frequently been applied. Other colloquialisms include "full house wrist" and "suicide wrist."

Even when this injury is complete, with involvement of both the radial and ulnar arteries, only rarely is circulation to the hand compromised because of the abundant collateral circulation via the anterior and posterior interosseous arteries and dorsal branches from the ulnar and arteries. While blood loss may be dramatic, initial hemostasis can often be achieved by direct pressure, or brief tourniquet use and closure of the skin. These maneuvers should be followed by application of a splint and compressive dressing. Once this is accomplished, if this was a self-inflicted injury, the patient's inciting cause can be addressed and at least initial postoperative cooperation assured.

Repair of the "spaghetti wrist" is performed in a sequential manner from deep to superficial. This is undertaken in the operating room with tourniquet control. Initial steps include a thorough exploration and cataloging of injured structures. Imperative in this

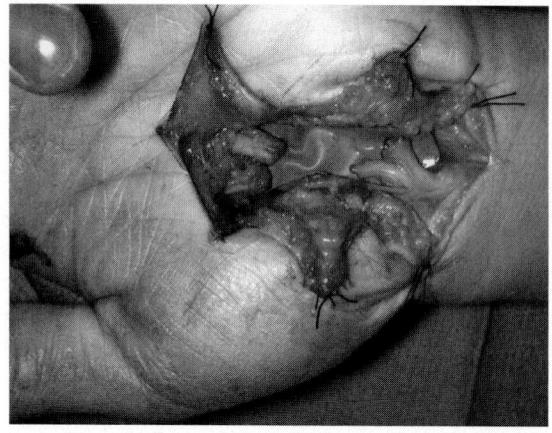

A

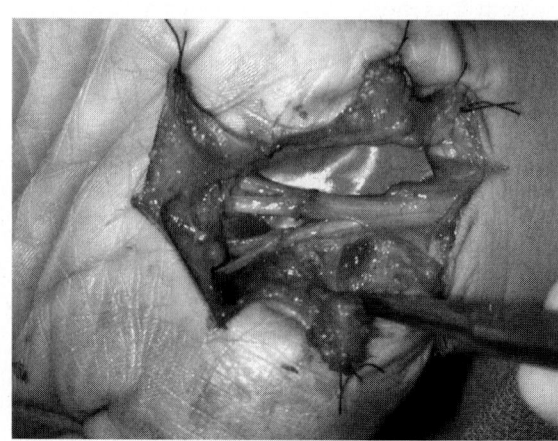

B

**FIGURE 42-16.**    Stab wound to median nerve in the hand (**A**) repaired by direct suturing of the epineureum (**B**).

exploration is assuring that multiple-level injury has not occurred due to repeated lacerations. Once this is assured the tendons are identified proximally and distally by anatomic arrangement and pulling on the distal stumps and observing joint and finger motion. Tendon repair is usually followed by microscopic nerve repair and finally repair of the ulnar and radial arteries. At this point the tourniquet is decompressed and final hemostasis is assured prior to skin closure. An initial dorsal blocking splint with the wrist neutral and the fingers in the intrinsic plus position is applied. A controlled tendon rehabilitation program is initiated as soon as patient cooperation can be assured.

As with most injuries of the upper extremity with nerve involvement, the final determining factor in degree of disability in this injury is successful nerve recovery.[107,108] Both sensory and motor recoveries are required for optimal result. Factors that affect outcome even with application of modern microsurgical nerve repair are age (<16 years with a better prognosis than >40 years), nerve repair before three months, and whether the ulnar nerve is involved. Sensory recovery is usually equal for both the ulnar and median nerve injury and repair; however, the failure to recover critical ulnar innervated intrinsic muscle function invariably leads to an unbalanced weak hand with significant long-term disability.

Brachial Plexus Injury.    Adult closed brachial plexus injury most often occur in young active males participating in extreme sporting activities or involved in high-speed motor vehicle accidents. This is a devastating injury that frequently leads not only to physical disability but also psychological distress and socioeconomic hardship. Often this injury is initially overlooked when faced with the polytrauma patient with more obvious life-threatening injuries. Even when detected, treatment historically has been delayed in hopes of some type of spontaneous functional recovery. This delay is largely unjustified today and is now known to potentially seriously compromise future reconstructive options.

A detailed knowledge of the anatomy of the brachial plexus is required of any surgeon operating in this anatomical region. Failure to appreciate the anatomy of this region of the neck, anterior chest, and axilla can further aggravate the initial injury, or result in additional devastating injury.

The brachial plexus is formed, in most instances, from the anterior branches of the four lowest cervical spinal nerves, C5–C8, and the first thoracic nerve, T1. The spinal nerves derive from the dorsal and ventral roots which arise from the spinal cord. The dorsal roots carry sensory fibers that originate in the dorsal root ganglion the lies within or just beyond the intervertebral foramen. The ventral roots contain motor fibers. Beyond the dorsal root ganglion the spinal nerve is formed as the dorsal and ventral roots coalesce.

Dural and arachnoid extensions are carried with the ventral and dorsal roots as they leave the spinal cord to form a root sleeve. In addition, there is a fibrous attachment of the spinal nerves to the transverse process in the fourth through seventh cervical roots. This firm fibrous attachment is not present on C8 and T1, explaining the increased incidence of root avulsion in the lower two roots of the plexus.

The spinal nerves unite to form three trunks, upper (C5 and C6), middle (C7), and lower (C8 and T1). Each trunk, in turn, divides into anterior and posterior divisions. Just distal to the clavicle the anterior divisions of the upper and middle trunks form the lateral cord and anterior division of the lower trunk is continued as the medial cord. The posterior divisions of all three trunks coalesce to form the posterior cord which lies posterior to the axillary artery.

Common terminology used to describe injury to the brachial plexus are root rupture, root avulsion, pre-ganglionic, post-ganglionic, supraclavicular, and infraclavicular.[109] Supraclavicular injury refers to injury of the spinal nerves, trunks, or divisions. Infraclavicular injury refers to injury of the cord and their terminal branches. When an injury causes tearing of the rootlets from the spinal cord proximal to the dorsal root ganglion, the injury is classified as pre-ganglionic or a root avulsion. When an injury is distal to the dorsal root ganglion it is called a postganglionic injury. This type of injury is often associated with rupture of the root.

There are practical implications to determining a lesion to be pre- or post-ganglionic. At this time a pre-ganglionic injury is not amenable to direct surgical repair and therefore alternative means of functional restoration must be explored. In contrast postganglionic injuries can potentially be restored by interpositional nerve grafting.

Importantly, there are features in the history and clinical examination that can indicate a pre-ganglionic versus a post-ganglionic injury. Horner's syndrome is characterized by ptosis, meiosis, anhydrosis of the cheek, and enophthalmos, and suggests a preganglionic avulsion of C8 and T1. Winging of the scapula suggests a pre-ganglionic avulsion of C6, as the serratus anterior is supplied by the long thoracic nerve that arises predominantly from the anterior division of C6 close to the intervertebral foramen. Inability to move the scapula medially indicates rhomboid dysfunction and is indicative of a C5 avulsion with compromise of the dorsal scapular nerve. This motion can be evaluated by asking the patient to attempt to bring the elbows together behind the back with the hands resting on the hips.

Post-ganglionic injury occurs at points of tethering of the plexus to surrounding structures. Erb's point where the suprascapular nerve comes off the upper trunk is a common, and historic, site of post-ganglionic injury. Rupture of C5 commonly occurs from the previously described fascial attachments from the transverse process. This is particularly strong at this segment and this anatomical feature may help preserve C5 for grafting when other roots have been injured by avulsion. The suprascapular nerve is also confined at the suprascapular notch and can be injured with upward displacement of the scapula during trauma. Injury to clavicle can result in injury to the brachial plexus at the level of the divisions where again they are relatively immobile. The axillary nerve is tethered both at its point of take-off from the posterior cord and as it passes through the quadrangular space and is vulnerable to injury at both these points.

Advances in ancillary diagnostic tests have paved the way for early surgical intervention. When used appropriately the combination of electrodiagnostic studies, CT myelography, and occasionally MRI can, when coupled with clinical finding, determine that significant recovery is not possible without surgical intervention.

Nerve conduction studies (NCS) and electromyography (EMG) are the primary electrodiagnostic studies that can aid in the evaluation of a patient with a brachial plexus injury.[110] With nerve injury other than neuropraxia, at 48–72 hours following injury, the axons distal to the lesion begin to undergo Wallerian degeneration and loose the ability to conduct. Unfortunately, it may take as long as four to six weeks after injury before fibrillation potentials are detected by EMG indicated muscle denervation. Nerve conduction studies can be utilized to help differentiate between pre- and post-ganglionic injury by evaluating the sensory nerve action potential (SNAP). This is possible because of the previously described location of the dorsal root ganglion outside the spinal cord proper. With a root avulsion the electrical circuit involved in SNAP recordings remains intact whereas with rupture distal to the dorsal root ganglion circuit is disrupted. This information can be extremely valuable both preoperatively and intraoperatively when trying to determine whether a root remains accessible for grafting. In practice, electrodiagnositic studies should be initially performed at four to six weeks post injury.

Both CT and MRI have a place in evaluation of brachial plexus pathology.[109,111] However, in the setting of traumatic brachial plexus injury CT myelography remains the "gold standard" for demonstration of root avulsion. MRI, while the preferred modality for compressive lesions or other nontraumatic brachial plexopathies, still suffers from too much motion artifact generated by pulsations of the cerebral spinal fluid to consistently demonstrate root avulsion and, thereby, aid in surgical planning. Early CT myelography timed to coincide with the initial electrodiagnostic studies can allow for surgery within two to three months of injury if not sooner. If these initial studies at four to six weeks are consistent with an in-continuity injury then follow-up electrodiagnositic may be performed six weeks later to evaluate for evidence of reinnervation. This second study is still within the three-month timeframe for early aggressive intervention if indicated.

While still a devastating injury, advances in the last 20 years have significantly improved the prognosis of some degree of functional recovery with traumatic brachial plexus injury. Surgical options include neurolysis, nerve grafting, and neurotization.

The first of these techniques, neurolysis is the surgical technique of freeing intact nerves from scar tissue. In traumatic brachial plexus injury this rarely is a definitive treatment when utilized on its own. More often neurolysis is an incidental technique that occurs during reconstruction of the plexus by nerve grafting or neurotization.

Prior to undertaking nerve grafting or brachial plexus neurotization, prioritization is essential. It is generally agreed that elbow flexion is the most important function to restore followed by active shoulder control and scapular stabilization. Triceps control through restoration of radial nerve function may also be achievable. However, restoration of useful median and ulnar nerve function by nerve surgery alone is probably not a realistic goal.

Nerve grafting requires a suitable lead-in nerve source. C5 and C6 may serve this purpose even in global brachial plexus injury. Grafting from these sources is targeted toward the above listed priorities via the suprascapular nerve and posterior division of the upper trunk to allow shoulder control. In the face of minimal suitable lead-in nerves further supplementation via nerve transfer will be required for elbow flexion. The classic transfer for this additional function is intercostals nerve transfer directly to the musculocutaneous nerve.

While the above approach has led to significant successful functional recovery, such a classic approach now needs to be weighed against more modern options that utilize nerve grafting in conjunction with more aggressive nerve transfers utilizing the terminal branch of the spinal accessory nerve and phrenic nerve, in conjunction with functional free muscle transfer with one or two gracilis

muscles revascularized and re-innervated via microsurgical techniques.[112] These aggressive techniques have led to successful restoration of simple grasp, a previously unheard of functional restoration.

While the focus of this review has been closed brachial plexus injury, penetrating trauma also accounts for 10–20% of brachial plexus injury. These injuries are often infraclavicular and represent more selective loss of function. Sharp, penetrating injuries are often associated with vascular injury and ideally someone comfortable in both vascular and nerve repair should be responsible for the initial exploration and repair. Alternatively, the vascular injury should be addressed with extreme care to avoid injury to closely associated nerves. The plexus should then be re-explored by a peripheral nerve surgeon as soon as possible.

Gunshot wounds present a more difficult dilemma.[113] Gunshots without vascular injury may be managed expectantly with serial examinations and sequential electrodiagnostic examinations at six and 12 weeks post-injury. If at 12 weeks no recovery is detected then exploration is probably indicated. In the instance of a vascular injury requiring surgical exploration the plexus must also be explored and any injuries defined. Acute repair is probably not indicated since the zone of injury to the nerve will be poorly defined and could result in inadequate resection and failed grafting. In these instances exploration at six weeks post-injury is recommended since nerve transaction has been confirmed and there is no hope of spontaneous recovery.

## Combined Injury

### The Mangled Upper Extremity.

Treatment of mangling injury of the upper extremity requires the ability to address all components of the injury both to preserve as much function as possible, and to set up the proper scenario for optimal future reconstructive options.[114] Inappropriate debridement or disposal of amputated parts can have long-term negative effects on any effort to restore upper limb function. Ideally, initial treatment should be by the individual who will ultimately be responsible for future reconstruction. Given that emergency settings may prevent this, the treating physician must make a maximum effort to preserve tissue and thereby preserve function. This should be followed promptly by evaluation by the reconstructive surgeon.

Because of the degree of force associated with these injuries, a complete trauma evaluation is required and other life-threatening injuries should take priority. When these injuries are such that timely care cannot be provided to the injured extremity, amputation may be necessary. Given the potentially morbid state of the patient and the limb, a thorough history and examination in the ED may not be possible. Instead, a focused history should be obtained from emergency personnel. This should target the time and mechanism of injury, and the environment in which it occurred. Similarly, the ED examination may need to focus on the vascular status to help determine the urgency of operative treatment. More thorough evaluation and tabulation of injured structures should then be deferred to the time of operative debridement.

Even at the time of initial operative intervention, the seven basic functions of the hand should be kept in mind; precision pinch, opposition pinch, key pinch, chuck grip, hook grip, span grasp, and power grasp. In addition, consideration should be given to the basic components necessary for hand function: an opposable thumb, the index and long fingers serving as the stable fixed unit of the hand for fine manipulation and power pinch, the ring and small fingers serving as the mobile unit of the hand for grasp, and the wrist. Complete restoration of these is the ultimate goal with the bare minimum goal being restoration of an opposition digit and a stable opposition post.

While classic teaching recommends debridement and skeletal fixation as the first steps, this may need to be amended to include re-establishment of blood flow if injury involves the brachial artery, or both the radial and ulnar arteries. This revascularization can be temporary by means of shunt, or definitive. Once adequate perfusion is assured, the initial debridement should be performed, while keeping in mind that this may be the single most important determinant of ultimate upper extremity function. This should not be a task relegated to junior staff or resident, experience and judgment are vital for both adequate debridement and appropriate preservation of questionable tissue. Whenever possible, debridement should be performed under tourniquet control so that identification of important structures is not obscured by active bleeding. Once the debridement is complete the tourniquet is then released to reassess distal flow and obtain hemostasis.

Skeletal fixation is the next step with the goals of restoration and preservation of maximal restorable length and stability. While the principles of damage control orthopedics may be applied to supply temporary fixation, it should be remembered that early stable fixation may allow earlier motion, thereby setting up a better situation for future reconstruction.

Once skeletal stabilization is complete, tendon, nerve and, if not already done, vessel repair should be performed. While revascularization must always occur, the availability of soft tissue coverage may determine whether successful tendon and nerve repair can be done at the time of initial treatment. The need for delay in definitive repairs is absolute if interpositional tendon or nerve grafting is necessary to re-establish continuity of the injured structure. Premature grafting for either injury may result in loss of valuable graft if coverage is not promptly performed. When the zone of injury for nerve is not clear, a delay in grafting for six to eight weeks is indicated and the appropriate level of resection is more clearly demarcated.

Soft tissue coverage may require use of local, regional, or free tissue flaps. Free flaps are often preferable to achieve the goal of early range of motion.

Replantation.    The replantation of a severed upper extremity or portion of the upper extremity represents a unique treatment subcategory of the combined injury. Replantation is distinct from revascularization and describes the reattachment of a completely amputated part by restoration of arterial inflow and venous outflow. Revascularization, in contrast, describes re-establishment of arterial inflow and/or venous outflow to a part that has not been completely amputated.

Malt and McKann described the first successful upper extremity replant, at the level of the upper arm, in 1962.[115] This was followed, in 1968, by the successful replantation of a thumb in Japan.[116] Since that time, replantation has been successfully performed at multiple levels in the upper extremity and has been extended to the lower extremity, genitals, and facial parts. Furthermore, the principles of microsurgery developed for these endeavors have aided in the development of free tissue transfer used from reconstruction from head to toe.

Experience gained from over 40 years of replantation has led to practical guidelines that have improved functional outcome. Merely putting on a part that is destined to be stiff, cold intolerant, and a potential impediment to limb function is no longer considered a surgical success. These published guidelines help avoid unnecessary transport of patients who are not candidates for replantation, thereby preserving healthcare resources.[117]

Absolute contraindications to replantation are significant associated injuries, multiple-level injuries to the amputated part, and systemic illness. Relative contraindications include patient's age, avulsion injuries, prolonged warm ischemia time (>6 hours for major limb amputations), massive contamination, underlying psychiatric illness, and single digit amputation. All these relative contraindications need to be interpreted in light of the actual injury and the patient assessment. Physiologic age and activities are more important than chronologic age and need to be assessed along with any underlying health problems. Massive contamination may preclude acute replantation but ectopic implantation with repeated debridement may be a viable option, which allows formal replantation at a later date when both stumps are clean. Self-inflicted injury may precede a later successful suicide attempt and some commitment to psychiatric care should be obtained prior to surgery whenever feasible. Single digit amputations should always be attempted in children; however, in the adult this is more controversial. Level of amputation plays a role in this decision-making process and more distal amputations that do not involve the flexor digitorum sublimis may be more practical than Zone II amputations. Single digit replantation may also be indicated in young females who may be more willing to accept a stiff, marginally functional digit than a manual laborer. Also, certain professionals (musicians) may require every attempt to preserve length and digit number.

Amputation situations where there is more uniform agreement to nearly always recommend attempted replantation are those involving the thumb, multiple digits, transmetacarpal, wrist level, distal two thirds of the forearm, and any amputation in children. Forearm amputations, like digit amputations, are dependent on level and mechanism. When a clean amputation occurs at or distal to the musculotendinous junctions, then replantation is absolutely indicated. However, when an amputation occurs in the proximal third of the forearm with considerable destruction of the forearm musculature, the outcome may be suboptimal and may require further functional muscle transfer to obtain adequate distal motion.

When faced with an amputated part in the field, appropriate treatment of that part should begin immediately, if possible, to minimize warm ischemia time and thereby increase the chance for successful replantation. Two methods have been advocated for preserving the amputated part: (1) wrapping the part in a saline or lactated Ringer's soaked gauze and placing the package into a specimen bag or cup that is then placed on ice or (2) placing the specimen directly into a container of saline or lactated Ringer's and again placing the container on ice. The amputated part should never be placed directly on ice, buried in ice, or transported with dry ice. Similar handling of the part should be done when the patient is initially seen at a facility that does not engage in replants. At such a facility, however, guidelines for replantable parts should be applied and, if the part or patient is not a candidate, then further transport is unnecessary and completion of the amputation can be performed then or often in a nonemergent fashion, after cleansing and dressing the wound.

In general, an ordered approach is recommended for successful replantation. With tourniquet control and prior to debridement, vessels and nerves should be tagged to protect these vital structures for later repair. Following debridement, bone shortening and fixation is accomplished. The degree of shortening should be limited to a functional length but be sufficient to avoid the need for interposition vein and nerve grafts, if possible. Next, the extensor tendons are repaired. While working on the dorsum of the hand repair of the veins may also be performed, or this may be put off as the final step prior to skin approximation. Many times with a major limb replantation, vein repair prior to arterial repair can decrease blood loss. Next, the flexor tendons, arteries, and nerves are repaired in this order. Finally, when reperfusion is established, loose approximation of the skin is indicated.

Deviation from this order may be required in major limb replantation where it may be necessary to temporarily establish an arterial shunt to reperfuse or give the amputated part "a drink" when one is approaching the limits for warm ischemia time. This allows more time for bony fixation and debridement but will lead to use of additional blood products. Compartment release is nearly always indicated and delayed wound closure with skin grafts is often the means of definitive wound closure.

## Compartment Syndrome

Compartment syndrome represents a unique vascular condition that can be the end result of a number of pathologic conditions; however, none is more common than trauma. While compartment syndrome has been described in the arm, it is much more common in the forearm and hand.[118] The forearm is composed of three distinct compartments: volar, dorsal, and the mobile wad. The hand has four dorsal and three volar interosseous compartments. After trauma, if acute swelling of the forearm or hand occurs, then one should be suspicious of potential compartment syndrome. Clinically, pain, pallor, pulselessness, and paresthesias or paralysis have been considered the classic signs of compartment syndrome. Of these, pain out of proportion to the clinical findings is probably the most reliable indication to pursue further diagnostics or take direct action. If compartment syndrome is suspected after application of a cast or splint, these should be immediately split to the underlying skin. Measurement of compartment pressures is a particularly valuable aid in diagnosis and may be the most useful tool in the unconscious or noncommunicative patient.

Controversy still exists over the compartment pressure at which fasciotomy is deemed necessary. Whitesides recommended fasciotomy when the pressure was measured at 10–30 mm Hg below the diastolic blood pressure.[119] Others have recommended that the compartment pressure alone be used as a guide for fasciotomy, but this recommendation has varied from 30–50 mm Hg in normotensive individuals. A safe guideline may be when the intracompartmental pressure of the affected limb is higher than the contralateral normal limb, and progressively rises above 30 mm Hg, and then prompt fasciotomy is indicated. Error should be on the side of early release to avoid devastating sequelae. Muscle damage begins within four hours of ischemic and is irreversible by six hours. In addition, nerve damage can put distal intrinsic function at risk and further limit reconstructive options.

## Burns

General Principles.    Key to management of any type of thermal or chemical burn to the hand is an understanding of the functional anatomy of the hand coupled with a standardized approach to treatment.[120] Total body surface area of the hands, including volar and dorsal surfaces, is approximately 5%. These two surfaces are, however, quite different in their ability to tolerate thermal exposure in particular. The dorsal surface presents thin, mobile, and flexible skin overlying a thin layer of subcutaneous tissue. Just below this layer is the extensor mechanism, initially as the extrinsic tendons and then, distal to the metacarpophalangeal joints, both the extrinsic and intrinsic components as a single fascial–tendon expansion with four firm attachments to the base of each phalanx and the volar plate of the MP joint. The volar surface is much thicker, hairless, nonpigmented, and relatively nonmobile due to numerous fibrous septae connecting it to the underlying palmar fascia. In the fingers themselves extensions of the palmar fascia are represented by Cleland's and Grayson's ligaments which encompass the neurovascular structures of the digit. Because of these differences in structure, management can vary with dorsal versus volar burns. In dorsal burns, coverage and restoration of movement needs to occur by 14 days post injury. With volar burns this time can sometimes be extended to 21 days with acceptable outcome.

Thermal Burns.    Accurate determination of the depth of injury is necessary to appropriately manage thermal burns of the hand (see Chap. 50). This is not an easy determination with one examination, as even in experienced hands, the first assessment will be wrong 50% of the time. Biopsy,[121] ultrasound,[122] laser Doppler,[123] static thermography,[124] and vital dyes[125] have all been used to try to increase the accuracy of the initial assessment but, despite some improvement with these techniques, the "gold standard" remains the serial examination. This may mean initial, labor intense, daily assessments to determine the potential for successful re-epithelialization.

Management of the thermally injured patient requires complete evaluation to rule out airway injury, or other secondary injury, followed by appropriate resuscitation. All burned upper extremities should be elevated to minimize edema and splinted in the intrinsic plus position with the interphalangeal joints in extension and metacarpo–phalangeal joints in 70% of flexion to maximize collateral ligament length. Careful initial evaluation of distal perfusion should be followed by hourly assessment. If circumferential full thickness burns are compromising distal circulation, then escharotomy is indicated. A radial full thickness incision, with either a scalpel or unipolar electrocautery, provides the safest pattern of initial decompression with only the superficial branch of the radial nerve being put at risk. Rarely axial escharotomies of the fingers are also indicated. More commonly, escharotomy of the hand should be performed to decompress the intrinsic compartments and hopefully preserve this vital function.

Superficial burns that will heal without surgical intervention within 14 days often only require polysporin or water-soluble bacitracin ointment. Slightly deeper burns are probably best treated with silver sulfadiazine cream. With either choice of ointment, daily cleansing with 4% chlorhexidine gluconate and application of nonadherent dressing is also necessary. Early referral to a hand therapist to assist in range of motion, edema control, and ultimately scar management is a major component of modern burn care.

**Tar and Chemical Burns.** Tar burns require specialized treatment to effectively remove the material by the process of emulsification. A number of agents have been described for this purpose, including Tween 80,[126] which can be found in the readily available ointments Polysporin and Neosporin. Following application of these ointments the tar can often be gently wiped off or cleansed off with a mild soap and water. The underlying burn is then evaluated and treated in the usual manner based on depth.

Hydrofluoric acid is another chemical that presents a unique situation.[127] This is commonly used in glass etching and in petrochemical refining. Rapid penetration through the epidermal barrier and into the subcutaneous tissues occurs with this agent. Once in the subcutaneous layer, the fluoride ion binds to calcium leading to intense pain and, with exposure greater than 2.5% total body surface area, systemic hypocalcemia occurs. Hydrofluoric acid exposure has a specific antidote in the form of 10% calcium gluconate applied topically or injected subcutaneously until pain relief occurs. Subcutaneous injection into the fingers and palm is not a possibility because of the constraints of the palmar fascial system. In these instances, 10 mL of 10% calcium gluconate in 40 mL of 0.9% saline can be delivered intravenously by Bier Block over 20 to 25 minutes. The same dose may also be administered intra-arterially using a low pressure infusion system over four hours until pain is eliminated.

**Electrical Injury.** Although electric injuries constitute only small percentage of admissions to United States burn centers, the upper extremity is the most frequently involved body part.[128] The severity of injury correlates with voltage, amperage, resistance, type of current, duration of contact, and pathway of the current through the body. For practical purposes, exposure is divided into low-voltage (<1000 volts) and high voltage (>1000 volts) injuries (see Chap. 50).

Low-voltage burns are generally localized cutaneous burns that can be managed expectantly by the previously described techniques for flame burns. High-voltage burns, in contrast, are devastating and often life-threatening injuries. Early management requires application of the general principles of resuscitation described elsewhere in this text. Usually there is both an entrance and exit wound with not only damage at these sites but to the intervening tissues as well. The main source of damage is the conversion of the electrical energy into heat, which affects all components of the exposed extremity. Compartment syndrome usually accompanies such exposure and should be addressed by early and complete release through both escharotomy and fasciotomy. These incisions should release not only muscle compartments but also the carpal tunnel, Guyon's canal, and the cubital tunnel. Despite this decompression, it should be anticipated that massive progressive muscle necrosis will ensue, requiring frequent and aggressive serial debridement. Because of intravascular thrombosis and damage to major vessels, vascular reconstruction may be required to salvage the limb. Once the progressive necrosis has stabilized and adequate debridement has been completed, reconstruction will require all the modalities at the reconstructive surgeons' disposal, including skin grafts, local flap, and microvascular free tissue transfer.[129,130] Despite these best efforts, amputation will frequently be necessary.[131,132]

## High-Pressure Injection Injury

High-pressure injection injury is an emergency requiring prompt surgical intervention. The velocity of the fluid is high enough in these exposures that direct contact with the source is not required for skin penetration, and penetration through gloves and other protective garments has been reported. Often the wound looks rather innocuous and the initial pain may be so minor that the patient will continue to work, thereby delaying care. While any digit may be involved, the non-dominant index finger is the most frequent. The degree of injury corresponds to the force of injection, type of material involved, and amount of material injected. Oil-based paints and industrial solvents cause the most direct damage and these injuries may be associated with an amputation rate of up to 50%. Radiographs may be helpful in the initial evaluation to determine the extent of proximal invasion of radio-opaque substance. Initial treatment should include tetanus prophylaxis, administration of antibiotics, analgesia, and elevation while arranging emergent surgical exploration. Surgery should be done under general anesthesia or regional blocks, Bier blocks should be avoided. Surgical decompression and meticulous debridement is necessary to salvage the digit. Re-operation within 24 hours for a second look and further debridement is almost always indicated. Delay in definitive treatment more than 10 hours increases the rate of amputation. Even with prompt treatment, cold intolerance, hypersensitivity, paresthesias, constant pain, and decreased range of motion and grip strength can be expected.[133]

## Infection

Infection is a common occurrence in the hand with most organisms introduced by direct inoculation via puncture, laceration, open fractures, or bites (see Chap. 19). The apparent vulnerability of the hand to infection is probably related to the multiple anatomical closed spaces present. Untreated infection in these spaces can lead to severe damage and ultimately diminished or lost function. History is important to determine not only possible accidental trauma, but also other predisposing factors such as immunocompromise or injectable drug abuse.

Despite a variety of initiating causes the infection itself is usually caused by common flora to the skin and mouth such as *Staphylococcus sp* and *Streptococcus sp*. And exception to this gram-positive preponderance is in diabetics and intravenous drug users where Gram-negative organisms are frequently encountered.[134]

Physical examination will often reveal erythema, warmth, tenderness, and swelling, as well as restricted function. Lymphangitic spread may be observed proximal to the site of infection. Careful palpation should seek areas of fluctuance that would require surgical drainage as opposed to monitored antibiotic treatment alone.

The most common infections of the hand are paronychias and felons. Paronychias, or nail fold infections, occur when bacteria gain entrance through a break in the seal between the nail and fold. Nail biting and excessive manicuring may predispose to this occurrence. During the cellulitic phase, soaks and antibiotic therapy targeting *Staphylococcus* species may lead to resolution. However, once fluctuance is noted under the nail fold, surgical drainage is indicated. A simple approach to drainage is to sharply elevate the nail fold from the nail plate in the region of the fluctuance. If any dissection of purulence is noted under the nail at this time, then the involved portion of the nail plate or the entire nail plate should be avulsed to allow complete drainage.

A felon is an abscess of the fingertip pulp which is confined by the many fibrous vertical septa that secure the relationship between the bony tuft and overlying skin. When undrained, this infection will ultimately liquefy the pulp fat and lead to tip malformation.

Surgical drainage is always indicated once an abscess has developed, and a number of incisions have been advocated. A straight mid-axial incision on the non-opposition side of the finger is preferred unless the abscess points volarly. In this instance, a straight longitudinal midline volar incision is acceptable.

Suppurative flexor tenosynovitis represents an infection of the flexor tendon sheath, another confined space of the hand. This condition is usually diagnosed clinically and has the characteristic signs of partially flexed resting posture of the finger, pain with passive extension, fusiform swelling of the entire finger, and volar tenderness along the course of the flexor sheath. Delayed treatment of this condition can lead to tendon scarring or necrosis and, in the small finger and thumb, because of anatomical communication through the radial and ulnar bursa, development of a horseshoe abscess.

Treatment with antibiotics alone is rarely successful for these infections unless initiated early after onset of symptoms. Furthermore, because of the severe sequelae associated with delay in definitive care, it is difficult to advocate medical management. Early surgical intervention with open or closed sheath irrigation remains the "gold standard."

Interdigital web space infections (Collar Button Abscess) and palmar space infections represent two additional closed space infections requiring prompt surgical intervention.

The term "collar button abscess" refers to the hourglass shape of the abscess that occurs in a web space infection and its resemblance to the collar button used in dress shirts in the 1900s. Inspection of the hand in this instance will usually show an associated fissured callus at the involved web space and the two adjacent fingers in repose of abduction. Physical examination will reveal tenderness and palpable swelling both dorsally and volarly. Because of this volar and dorsal component drainage is required, and should be designed as separate incisions that do not carry across the webspace.

The palm has three distinct anatomical spaces, all of which may trap infection. These are the thenar space, midpalmar space, and hypthenar space. Of these, the thenar and midpalmar spaces are most frequently affected by a suppurative process. Patients with these infections almost always have a history of penetrating trauma with/or without foreign body retention. The hand on inspection with be swollen and erythematous volarly and will be exquisitely tender to palpation. If doubt exists as to the presence of an abscess versus cellulitis, aspiration or ultrasound may be performed. However, as with suppurative flexor tenosynovitis, the severe sequela of a delay in treatment means that a negative aspirate should not negate surgical exploration. As in all infections, routine radiographs should be obtained to rule out the presence of radio-opaque material prior to exploration.

Dog and cat bite wounds to the hand are common as are human bites, and often serve as the means of introduction of the infectious material responsible for the above described closed space infection.[135] Whether prophylactic antibiotics can prevent this end result when initiated early has been the subject of a great deal of research. From this it would appear that there are good prospective data to support routine prophylactic antibiotic use in human bite wounds, while retrospective data supports antibiotic use in dog and cat bites, no similar prospective data exist.[136]

## REFERENCES

1. Littler JW: Plastic surgeons and development of reparative surgery of the hand. In Aston SJ, Beasley RW, Thorne CHM, eds. *Grabb and Smith's Plastic Surgery*, 5th ed. Philadelphia: Lippincott Raven, 1997, p. 791.

2. Greenwood MJ, Della-Siega AJ, Fretz EB, et al.: Vascular communications of the hand in patients being considered for transradial coronary angiography. Is the Allen's Test accurate? *J Am Coll Cardiol* 46:2013, 2005.

3. Jarvis MA, Jarvis CL, Jones PRM, et al.: Reliability of Allen's Test in selection of patients for radial artery harvest. *Ann Thorac Surg* 70:1362, 2000.

4. Wirth MA, Rockwood CA: Acute and chronic traumatic injuries of the sternoclavicular joint. *J Am Acad Orthop Surg* 4:268, 1996.

5. Ono K, Inagawa H, Kiyota K, et al.: Posterior dislocation of the sternoclavicular joint with obstruction of the innominate vein: Case report. *J Trauma* 44:381, 1998.

6. Siddiqui AA, Turner SM: Posterior sternoclavicular joint dislocation; the value of intra-operative ultrasound. *Injury* 34:448, 2003.

7. Weinberg B, Seife B, Alonso P: The apical oblique view of the clavicle: Its usefulness in neonatal and childhood trauma. *Skeletal Radiol* 20:201, 1991.

8. Kitsis CK, Marino AJ, Krikler, et al.: Late complications following clavicular fractures and their operative management. *Injury* 34:69, 2003.

9. Schlegel TF, Burks RT, Marcus RL, et al.: A prospective evaluation of untreated acute grade III acromioclavicular separations. *Am J Sports Med* 29:699, 2001.

10. Phillips AM, Smart C, Groom AF: Acromioclavicular dislocation: Conservative or surgical therapy. *Clin Orthop Relat Res* 353:10, 1998.

11. Ada JR, Miller ME: Scapular Fractures: Analysis of 113 cases. *Clin Orthop Relat Res* 269:174, 1991.

12. Edeland HG, Zachrisson HE: Fracture of the scapular notch associated with lesion of the suprascapular nerve. *Acta Orthop Scand* 46:758, 1975.

13. Solheim LF, Roaas A: Compression of the suprascapular nerve after fracture of the scapular notch. *Acta Orthop Scand* 49:338, 1978.

14. Goss TP: Fractures of the scapula: Diagnosis and treatment. In Iannotti JP, Williams GR, eds. *Disorders of the Shoulder: Diagnosis and Management.* Philadelphia: Lippincott Williams & Wilkins, 1999, p. 597

15. Egol KA, Connor PM, Karunakar MA, et al.: The floating shoulder: clinical and functional results. *J Bone Joint Surg Am* 83-A:1188, 2001.

16. van Noort A, te Slaa RL, Marti RK, et al.: The floating shoulder: A multicenter study. *J Bone Joint Surg Br* 83:795, 2001.

17. Clements RH, Reisser JR: Scapulothoracic dissociation: A devastating injury. *J Trauma* 40:146, 1996.

18. Damschen DD, Cogbill TH, Siegel MJ: Scapulothoracic dissociation caused by blunt trauma. *J Trauma* 42:537, 1997.

19. Matsumoto K, Ohara A, Yamanaka K, et al.: *Luxatio erecta* (inferior dislocation of the shoulder): A report of two cases and review of the literature. *Injury Extra* 36:450, 2005.

20. Ufberg JW, Vilke GM, Chan TC, et al.: Anterior shoulder dislocation: beyond traction-counter traction. *J Emerg Med* 27:301, 2004.

21. Sagarin MJ: Best of both (BOB) maneuver for rapid reduction of anterior shoulder dislocation. *J Emerg Med* 29:313, 2005.

22. Hovelius L, Augustini BG, Fredin H, et al.: Primary anterior dislocation of the shoulder in young patients: A ten-year prospective study. *J Bone Joint Surg Am* 78:1677, 1996.

23. Bottoni CR, Wilckens JH, De Berardino TM, et al.: A prospective, randomized evaluation of arthroscopic stabilization versus nonoperative treatment in patients with acute, traumatic, first-time shoulder dislocations. *Am J Sports Med* 30:576, 2002.

24. Hill HA, Sachs MD: The grooved defect of the humeral head: A frequently unrecognized complication of dislocations of the shoulder joint. *Radiology* 35:690, 1940.

25. Pevny T, Hunter RE, Freeman JR: Primary traumatic anterior shoulder dislocation in patients 40 years of age and older. *Arthroscopy* 14:289, 1998.

26. Neer CS II: Displaced proximal humeral fractures: I. Classification and evaluation. *J Bone Joint Surg Am* 52:1077, 1970.

27. Koval KJ, Gallagher MA, Marsicano JG, et al.: Functional outcome after minimally displaced fractures of the proximal part of the humerus. *J Bone Joint Surg Am* 79:203, 1997.

28. Park TS, Choi IY, Kim YH, et al.: A new suggestion for the treatment of minimally displaced fractures of the greater tuberosity of the proximal humerus. *Bull Hosp Jt Dis* 56:171, 1997.

29. Bono CM, Renard R, Levine RG, et al.: Effect of displacement of fractures of the greater tuberosity on the mechanics of the shoulder. *J Bone Joint Surg Br* 83:1056, 2001.

30. Schai P, Imhoff A, Preiss S: Comminuted humeral head fractures: a multicenter analysis. *J Shoulder Elbow Surg* 4:319, 1995.

31. Resch H, Povacz P, Frohlich R, et al.: Percutaneous fixation of three- and four-part fractures of the proximal humerus. *J Bone Joint Surg Br* 79:295, 1997.

32. Chapman JR, Henley MB, Agel J, et al.: Randomized prospective study of humeral shaft fracture fixation: intramedullary nails versus plates. *J Orthop Trauma* 14:162, 2000.

33. Shao YC, Harwood P, Grotz MR, et al.: Radial nerve palsy associated with fractures of the shaft of the humerus: a systematic review. *J Bone Joint Surg Br* 87:1647, 2005.

34. Gambirasio R, Riand N, Stern R, et al.: Total elbow replacement for complex fractures of the distal humerus. An option for the elderly patient. *J Bone Joint Surg Br* 83:974, 2001.

35. Ring D, Jupiter JB, Gulotta L: Articular fractures of the distal part of the humerus. *J Bone Joint Surg Am* 85:232, 2003.

36. Fleuriau-Chateau P, McIntyre W, Letts M: An analysis of open reduction of irreducible supracondylar fractures of the humerus in children. *Can J Surg* 41:112, 1998.

37. Copley LA, Dormans JP, Davidson RS: Vascular injuries and their sequelae in pediatric supracondylar humeral fractures: Toward a goal of prevention. *J Pediatr Orthop* 16:99,1996.

38. Sano S, Rokkaku T, Saito S, et al.: Herbert screw fixation of capitellar fractures. *J Shoulder Elbow Surg* 14:307, 2005.

39. Mehlhoff TL, Noble PC, Bennett JB, et al.: Simple dislocation of the elbow in the adult: Results after closed treatment. *J Bone Joint Surg Am* 70:244, 1988.

40. Ring D, Jupiter JB, Zilberfarb J: Posterior dislocation of the elbow with fractures of the radial head and coronoid. *J Bone Joint Surg Am* 84:547, 2002.

41. Regan W, Morrey B: Fractures of the coronoid process of the ulna. *J Bone Joint Surg Am* 71:1348, 1989.

42. Ring D, Jupiter JB, Sanders RW, et al.: Transolecranon fracture-dislocation of the elbow. *J Orthop Trauma* 11:545, 1997.

43. Caputo AE, Mazzocca AD, Santoro VM: The nonarticulating portion of the radial head: Anatomic and clinical correlations for internal fixation. *J Hand Surg [Am]* 23:1082, 1998.

44. van Riet RP, Morrey BF, O'Driscoll SW, et al.: Associated injuries complicating radial head fractures: A demographic study. *Clin Ortho* 441:351, 2005.

45. Yokoyama K, Itoman M, Kobayashi A, et al.: Functional outcomes of "floating elbow" injuries in adult patients. *J Orthop Trauma* 12:284, 1998.

46. Ring D, Jupiter JB, Simpson NS: Monteggia fractures in adults. *J Bone Joint Surg Am* 80:1733, 1998.

47. May MM, Lawton JN, Blazar PE: Ulnar styloid fractures associated with distal radius fractures: Incidence and implications for distal radioulnar joint instability. *J Hand Surg [Am]* 27:965, 2002.

48. Rettig ME, Raskin KB: Galeazzi fracture-dislocation: A new treatment-oriented classification. *J Hand Surg [Am]* 26:228, 2001.

49. Ring D, Rhim R, Carpenter C, et al.: Isolated radial shaft fractures are more common than Galeazzi fractures. *J Hand Surg [Am]* 31:17, 2006.

50. Chung KC, Spilson SV: The frequency and epidemiology of hand and forearm fractures in the United States. *J Hand Surg [Am]* 26:908, 2001.

51. Orbay JL, Fernandez DL: Volar fixation for dorsally displaced fractures of the distal radius: A preliminary report. *J Hand Surg [Am]* 27:205, 2002.

52. Orbay JL, Fernandez DL: Volar fixed-angle plate fixation for unstable distal radius fractures in the elderly patient. *J Hand Surg [Am]* 29:96, 2004.

53. Margaliot Z, Haase SC, Kotsis SV, et al.: A meta-analysis of outcomes of external fixation versus plate osteosynthesis for unstable distal radius fractures. *J Hand Surg [Am]* 30:1185, 2005.

54. Goldfarb CA, Ricci WM, Tull F, et al.: Functional outcome after fracture of both bones of the forearm. *J Bone Joint Surg Br* 87:374, 2005.

55. Kozin SH: Incidence, mechanism, and natural history of scaphoid fractures. *Hand Clin* 17:515, 2001.

56. Low G, Raby N: Can follow-up radiography for acute scaphoid fracture still be considered a valid investigation? *Clin Radiol* 60:1106, 2005.

57. Brooks S, Cicuttini FM, Lim S, et al.: Cost effectiveness of adding magnetic resonance imaging to the usual management of suspected scaphoid fractures. *Br J Sports Med* 39:75, 2005.

58. Saxena P, McDonald R, Gull S, et al.: Diagnostic scanning for suspected scaphoid fractures: An economic evaluation based on cost minimisation models. *Injury* 34:503, 2003.

59. Slade JF III, Jaswhich D: Percutaneous fixation of scaphoid fractures. *Hand Clin* 17:553, 2001.

60. Slade JF III, Geissler WB, Gutow AP, et al.: Percutaneous internal fixation of selected scaphoid nonunions with an arthroscopically assisted dorsal approach. *J Bone Joint Surg Am* 85-A: 20, 2003.

61. Shih JT, Lee HM, Hou YT, et al.: Results of arthroscopic reduction and percutaneous fixation for acute displaced scaphoid fractures. *Arthroscopy* 21:620, 2005.

62. Hocker K, Menschik A: Chip fractures of the triquetrium. Mechanism, classifications and results. *J Hand Surg [Br]* 19:584, 1994.

63. Matsunaga D, Uchiyama S, Nakagawa H, et al.: Lower ulnar nerve palsy related to fracture of the pisiform bone in patients with multiple injuries. *J Trauma* 53:364, 2002.

64. McGuigan FX, Culp RW: Surgical treatment of intraarticular fractures of the trapezium. *J Hand Surgery [Am]* 27:697, 2002.

65. Miyawaki T, Kobayashi M, Matsuura S, et al.: Trapezoid bone fracture. *Ann Plast Surg* 44:444, 2000.

66. Vander Grend R, Dell PC, Glowczewskie F, et al.: Intraosseus blood supply of the capitate and its correlation with aseptic necrosis. *J Hand Surg [Am]* 9:677, 1984.

67. Aspergis E, Darmanis S, Kastanis G, et al.: Does the term scaphocapitate syndrome need to be revised? A report of 6 cases. *J Hand Surg [Br]* 26:441, 2001.

68. Kapickis M, Looi KP, Khin-Sze Chong A: Combined fractures of the body and hook of hamate: A form of ulnar axial injury of the wrist. *Scand J Plast Reconstr Surg Hand Surg* 39:116, 2005.

69. Andresen R, Radmer S, Sparmann M, et al.: Imaging of hamate bone fractures in conventional x-rays and high-resolution computed tomography: An in vitro study. *Invest Radiol* 34:46, 1999.

70. Kato H, Nakamura R, Horii E, et al.: Diagnostic imaging for fracture of the hook of the hamate. *Hand Surg* 5:19, 2000.

71. Grant I, Berger AC, Ireland DC: Rupture of the flexor digitorum profundus tendon to the small finger within the carpal tunnel. *Hand Surg* 10:109, 2005.

72. Scheufler O, Andresen R, Radmer S, et al.: Hook of hamate fractures: Critical evaluation of different therapeutic procedures. *Plast Reconstr Surg* 115:488, 2005.

73. Teisen H, Hjarbaek J: Classification of fresh fractures of the lunate. *J Hand Surg [Br]* 13:458, 1988.

74. Murray PM: Dislocations of the wrist: Carpal instability complex. *J Am Soc Surg Hand* 3:88, 2003.

75. Mayfield JK, Johnson RP, Kilcoyne RK: Carpal dislocations: Pathomechanics and progressive perilunar instability. *J Hand Surg [Am]* 5:226, 1980.

76. Melone CP Jr., Murphy MS, Raskin KB: Perilunate injuries. Repair by dual dorsal and volar approaches. *Hand Clin* 16:439, 2000.

77. Weinstein LP, Hanel DP: Metacarpal fractures. *J Am Soc Surg Hand* 2:168, 2002.

78. Orbay J: Intramedullary nailing of metacarpal shaft fractures. *Tech Hand Up Extrem Surg* 9:69, 2005.

79. Ali A, Hamman J, Mass DP: The biomechanical effects of angulated boxer's fractures. *J Hand Surg [Am]* 24:835, 1999.

80. Leung YL, Beredjiklian PK, Monaghan BA, et al.: Radiographic assessment of small finger metacarpal neck fractures. *J Hand Surg [Am]* 27:443, 2002.

81. Perron AD, Miller MD, Brady WJ: Orthopedic pitfalls in the ED: fight bite. *Am J Emerg Med* 20:114, 2002.

82. Lutz M, Sailer R, Zimmermann R, et al.: Closed reduction transarticular wire fixation versus open reduction internal fixation in the treatment of Bennett's fracture dislocation. *J Hand Surg [Br]* 28:142, 2003.

83. Slade JF, Baxamuca TH, Wolfe SW: External fixation of proximal interphalangeal joint fracture dislocations. *Atlas of the Hand Clinics* 5:1, 2000.

84. Badia A, Riano F, Ravikoff J, et al.: Dynamic intradigital external fixation for proximal interphangeal joint fracture dislocations. *J Hand Surg [Am]* 30:154, 2005.

85. Green DP, Terry GC: Complex dislocation of the metacarpophalangeal joint. Correlative pathological anatomy. *J Bone Joint Surg [Am]* 55:1480, 1973.

86. Sodha S, Breslow GD, Chang B: Percutaneous technique for reduction of complex metacarpophalangeal dislocations. *Ann Plast Surg* 52:562, 2004.

87. Leggit JC, Meko CJ: Acute finger injuries: Part II. Fractures, dislocations and thumb injuries. *Am Fam Physician* 73:827, 2006.

88. Allen MJ: Conservative management of fingertip injuries in adults. *Hand* 12:257, 1980.

89. Schenck RR, Cheema TA: Hypothenar skin grafts for fingertip reconstruction. *J Hand Surg [Am]* 9:750, 1984.

90. Kutler W: A new method for fingertip amputation. *JAMA* 133:29, 1947.

91. Atasoy E, Ioakimidis E, Kasdan ML, et al.: Reconstruction of the amputated fingertip with a triangular volar flap. *J Bone Joint Surg Am* 52:921, 1970.

92. Tupper J, Miller G: Sensitivity following volar V-Y plasty for fingertip amputations. *J Hand Surg [Br]* 10:183, 1985.

93. Cohen BE, Cronin ED: An innervated crossfinger flap for fingertip reconstruction. *Plast Reconstr Surg* 72:688, 1983.

94. Zook EG, Guy RJ, Russell RC: A study of nail bed injuries: Cause, treatment and prognosis. *J Hand Surg [Am]* 9:247, 1984.

95. Bendre AA, Hartigan BJ, Kalainov DM: Mallet finger. *J Am Acad Orthop Surg* 13:336, 2005.

96. Rayan GM, Murray D: Classification and treatment of closed sagittal band injuries. *J Hand Surg [Am]* 19:590, 1994.

97. Catalano LW III, Gupta S, Ragland R III, et al.: Closed treatment of nonrheumatoid extensor tendon dislocations at the metacarpophalangeal joint. *J Hand Surg [Am]* 31:242, 2006.

98. Tuncali D, Yavuz N, Terzioglu A, et al.: The rate of upper extremity deep-structure injuries through small penetrating lacerations. *Ann Plast Surg* 55:146, 2005.

99. Newmeyer WL III, Manske PR. No mans's land revisited: The primary flexor tendon repair controversy. *J Hand Surg [Am]* 29:1, 2004.

100. Gill RS, Lim BH, Shatford RA, et al.: A comparative analysis of the six-strand double loop flexor tendon repair and three other techniques: A human cadaveric study. *J Hand Surg [Am]* 24:1315, 1999.

101. Viinikainen A, Goransson H, Huovinen K, et al.: A comparative analysis of the biomechanical behaviour of five flexor tendon core sutures. *J Hand Surg [Br]* 29:536, 2004.

102. Leddy JP, Packer JW: Avulsion of the profundus tendon insertion in athletes. *J Hand Surg [Am]* 2:66, 1977.

103. McCallister WV, Ambrose HC, Katolik LI, et al.: Comparison of pullout button versus suture anchor for zone I flexor tendon repair. *J Hand Surg [Am]* 31:246, 2006.

104. Gosens T, Bongers KJ: Neurovascular complications and functional outcome in displaced supracondylar fractures of the humerus in children. *Injury* 34:267, 2003.

105. Dvali L, McKinnon S: Nerve repair, grafting, and nerve transfers. *Clin Plast Surg* 30:203, 2003.

106. Chuang DC: Nerve transfers in adult brachial plexus injuries: My methods. *Hand Clin* 21:71, 2005.

107. Jaquet JB, vander Jagt I, Kuypers PDL, et al.: Spaghetti wrist trauma: Functional recovery, return to work, and psychological effects. *Plast Reconstr Surg* 115:1609, 2005.

108. Ruijs ACJ, Jaquet JB, Kalmijn S, et al.: Median and ulnar nerve injuries: A meta-analysis of predictors of motor and sensory recovery after modern microsurgical nerve repair. *Plast Reconstr Surg* 116:484, 2005.

109. Rankine JJ: Adult traumatic brachial plexus injury. *Clin Rad* 59:767, 2004.

110. Harper CM: Preoperative and intraoperative extrophysiologic assessment of brachial plexus injury. *Hand Clin* 21:39, 2005.

111. Amrani KK, Port JD: Imaging the brachial plexus. *Hand Clin* 21:25, 2005.

112. Doi K, Muramatsu K, Hattori Y, et al.: Restoration of prehension with the double free muscle technique following complete avulsion of the brachial plexus. Indications and long-term results. *J Bone Joint Surg [Am]* 82:652, 2000.

113. Kim DH, Murovic JA, Tiel RL, et al.: Penetrating injuries due to gunshot wounds involving the brachial plexus. *Neurosurgical Focus* 16:E3, 2004.

114. Gupta A, Shatford RA, Wolff TW, et al.: Treatment of the severely injured upper extremity. *Instr Course Lect* 49:377, 2000.

115. Malt RA, McKhann CF: Replantation of severed arms. *JAMA* 189:716, 1964.

116. Komatsu S, Tamai S: Successful replantation of a completely cut-off thumb. *Plast Reconstr Surg* 43:374, 1964.

117. Chang J, Jones NF: Twelve simple maneuvers to optimize digital replantation and revascularization. *Tech Hand Upper Ext Surg* 8:161, 2004.

118. Seiler JG, Olvey SP: Compartment syndromes of the hand and forearm. *J Am Soc Surg Hand* 3:184, 2003.

119. Whitesides TE Jr, Haney TC, Morimoto K, et al.: Tissues pressure measurements as a determinant of the need for fasciotomy. *Clin Orthop Relat Res* 113:43, 1975.

120. Cartotto R: The burned hand: Optimizing long-term outcomes with a standardized approach to acute and subacute care. *Clin Plast Surg* 32:515, 2005.

121. Watts AM, Tyler MP, Perry ME, et al.: Burn depth and its histological measurements. *Burns* 27:154, 2001.

122. Adams TS, Murphy JV, Gillespie PH, et al.: The use of high frequency ultrasonography in the prediction of burn depth. *J Burn Care Rehabil* 22:261, 2001.

123. Riordan CL, McDonough M, Davidson JM, et al.: Noncontact laser Doppler imaging in burn depth analysis of extremities. *J Burn Care Rehabil* 24:177, 2003.

124. Renkielska A, Nowakowski A, Kaczmarek M, et al.: Static thermography revisited – an adjunct method for determining the depth of the burn injury. *Burns* 31:768, 2005.

125. Still JM, Law EJ, Klavuhn KG, et al.: Diagnosis of burn depth using laser-induced indocyanine green fluorescence: A preliminary clinical trial. *Burns* 27:364, 2001.

126. Demling RH, Buerstatte WR, Perea A: Management of hot tar burns. *J Trauma* 20:242, 1980.

127. Hatzifotis M, Williams A, Muller M, et al.: Hydrofluric acid burns. *Burns* 30:156, 2004.

128. Arnoldo BD, Purdue GF, Kowalske K, et al.: Electrical injuries: A 20 year review. *J Burn Care Rehabil* 25:479, 2004.

129. Hallock GG: A history of the development of muscle perforator flaps and their specific use in burn reconstruction. *J Burn Care Rehabil* 25:366, 2004.

130. Baumeister S, Koller M, Dragu A, et al.: Principles of microvascular reconstruction in burn and electrical burn injuries. *Burns* 31:92, 2005.

131. Kennedy PJ, Young WM, Deva AK: Burns and amputations: A 24 year experience. *J Burn Care Res* 27:183, 2006.

132. Cancio LC, Jimenez-Reyna JF, Barillo DJ, et al.: One hundred ninety-five cases of high-voltage electric injury. *J Burn Care Rehabil* 26:331, 2005.

133. Wieder A, Lapid O, Plakht Y, et al.: Long-term follow-up of high pressure injection injuries to the hand. *Plast Reconstr Surg* 117:186, 2006.

134. Houshian S, Seyedipour S, Wedderkopp N: Epidemiology of bacterial hand infections. *Int J Inf Diseases*, 2006 (In Press).

135. Benson LS, Edwards SL, Schiff AP, et al.: Dog and cat bites to the hand: treatment and cost assessment. *J Hand Surg [Am]* 31:468, 2006.

136. Medeiros I, Saconato H: Antibiotic prophylaxis for mammalian bites. *Cochrane Database Syst Rev* (2):CD001738, 2001.

## Commentary ■ MARK WILCZYNSKI ■ GARY MCGILLIVARY

The authors of this chapter have orchestrated a comprehensive update of hand and upper extremity injuries. They provide a thorough and concise review of traumatic injury to the hand and upper extremity in which important information is provided for students, residents, and seasoned clinicians. The format of the chapter is logical and the text is easily readable. The content is augmented with plentiful graphics.

After a brief introduction, the authors discuss initial management of hand and upper extremity injuries. In this section, a basic neurologic and vascular examination of the upper extremity is described. However, the physical examination for tendon and other soft tissue injuries is described elsewhere in the chapter. Anatomy in the hand is highly concentrated and injuries to nerves and vessels are frequently accompanied by additional soft tissue injuries that should be identified at initial evaluation if possible.

In the following section, specific injuries are described. The authors methodically present fundamental information regarding osseous and soft-tissue injury, assessment techniques, and recommended intervention. Fractures and dislocations are addressed systematically from proximal to distal. This is followed by equally systematic and thorough reviews of tendon, vascular, and peripheral nerve injuries.

The chapter continues with combined injuries. Again, hand and upper extremity anatomy is dense and anatomical structures are intimately related. For this reason, injuries are frequently associated. This is perhaps most apparent in the mangled or amputated extremity that may require revascularization, multiple nerve and tendon repairs, as well as fixation of osseous injuries. These concepts are further developed in this section and management of complex injuries is suggested.

The final sections of the chapter address compartment syndromes, burns of the upper extremity, high-pressure injection injuries, and infection. The authors correctly emphasize pain out of proportion to the injury as the most reliable indicator of elevated intracompartmental pressure. However, in the obtunded patient intracompartmental pressures should be monitored if clinical suspicion of compartment syndrome exists. Compartment pressure at which fasciotomy is deemed necessary is a controversial issue. The authors advocate an absolute pressure of 30 mm Hg at which fasciotomy should be performed. At our institution, we adhere to the principle of perfusion pressure gradient and perform fasciotomy when the intracompartmental pressure is within 30 mm Hg of diastolic blood pressure.[1] Although the sequelae of missed compartment syndrome are devastating, fasciotomy is not without morbidity and should be avoided in those it is not required.

The authors are commended for condensing the broad topic of hand and upper extremity trauma into a single chapter. The important concepts have been identified and emphasized without focusing on minutiae. This chapter is an excellent first resource for the generalist seeking a concise reference for trauma to the hand and upper extremity.

## Reference

1. Whitesides TE Jr, Haney TC, Morimoto K, et al.: Tissues pressure measurements as a determinant of the need for fasciotomy. *Clin Orthop Relat Res* 113:43, 1975.

# Lower Extremity

*Wade R. Smith* ■ *Philip F. Stahel* ■ *Steven J. Morgan* ■ *Peter G. Trafton*

## INTRODUCTION

Acute lower extremity trauma is most commonly a result of road accidents, sports, recreational, or work-related activities. In children, the major cause is sports such as football, trampolining, biking and skiing, and accidental falls. In older patients, who have reduced muscle mass and bone strength, other premorbid conditions make them more vulnerable to falls and consequent fractures. The type of injury is a result of the mechanism (penetrating, twisting, jerking, bending, and crush). Significant injuries compromise function and can lead to pain, abnormal gait, and secondary degenerative joint disease. Their frequency, severity, and costs emphasize the impact of lower extremity fractures on society.[1,2] Fractures are typically the primary cause of more than half of all hospitalizations for trauma, and a significant majority of these involve the lower extremities. According to the Healthcare Cost and Utilization Project (HCUP), in 2003 more than 746,000 people were seen in hospital for lower limb fractures. In 2000 alone, 50 million injuries required medical treatment and cost $80 billion in medical care costs and $326 billion in productivity losses. The total productivity loss from upper and lower extremity injuries amounted to over $95 billion. In many of these cases, the ability to return to work after injury is dependent upon appropriate management and the final functional outcome.[3,4]

Lower extremity fractures may be caused by either low- or high-energy forces and occur both in isolation and as multiple injuries. With the increasing use of safety belts and airbags in vehicles, there are more survivors of high-energy crashes dealing with increasingly severe lower extremity injuries. In one series, lower extremity injuries accounted for 40% of the motor vehicle trauma treatment charges of hospitalized patients in Maryland during that year. In another study, a third of patients injured in motorcycle crashes sustained at least one open lower extremity fracture.[3,4] It is important to remember that potentially life-threatening injuries to the head and torso may be present with those of the extremities. It is thus essential to evaluate the whole patient and not focus exclusively on his or her injured limb.[5,6]

## HISTORICAL PERSPECTIVE

Orthopedic surgery has developed through the need to alleviate pain, correct deformity, and restore function following fracture. Evidence of splinted fractures and the first successful amputations has been found as far back as the fifth Egyptian dynasty, about 4500 years ago. The "Corpus Hippocrates" described the principles of traction, countertraction, and external fixation. Surgeons have built on these past foundations with the advancement of technology.[7] In England, Thomas described the traction splint that still bears his name. In France, Malgaigne described the external fixator, and Delbet reported use of a weight-bearing cast for tibial fractures. In the United States, Buck described skin traction, while Steinmann in Switzerland and Kirschner in Germany introduced skeletal traction. Küntscher, a German, made many contributions to modern intramedullary nailing. In Austria, Böhler established hospitals devoted to the care of injuries and published a comprehensive text on fracture surgery. Lambotte, a Belgian, is the father of modern internal fixation, which was advanced further by his countryman, Danis, who demonstrated that rigid fixation could result in direct bone healing without callus formation. The Swiss-based Arbeitsgemeinschaft für Osteosynthesefragen, or Association for the Study of Internal Fixation (AO/ASIF) was founded in 1958 by a group of Swiss surgeons to produce and disseminate a system of fracture care based on stable fixation with preservation of soft tissue, active motion, and functional rehabilitation.[8,9] This association has earned itself a worldwide reputation as an international authority in the treatment of trauma through its continuing research and development of instrumentation. Further advances continue, with emphasis on indirect reduction techniques, closed or minimally invasive fracture fixation, and stable but less rigid fixation that promotes rather than suppresses indirect, callus-dependent healing of bone.[7]

At about the same time in the Soviet Union, Professor Ilizarov, working in the Siberian town of Kurgan, developed and refined the concept of distraction osteogenesis, permitting healthy de novo bone to be created in vivo through distraction with a ring external fixator system with Kirschner-type wires. His work led to significant advances in the use of external fixators as definitive treatment for a variety of traumatic injuries and posttraumatic complications.

The increasing ability of orthopedic surgeons to obtain early fracture stability with relatively low complication rates has led to improvements in postinjury rehabilitation. Rehabilitation concepts have changed from the prolonged rest suggested by Thomas to the present emphasis on rapid restoration of skeletal stability that allows for prompt mobilization of injured extremities and patients. Early weight bearing is encouraged, whenever possible to promote bone healing and overall physiologic restoration. Detailed knowledge of a patient's musculoskeletal injuries, their treatment, and their response is crucial for appropriate decision making in both the acute and late phases of care. Therefore, the orthopedic surgeon should ideally be directly involved from the trauma bay through the entire recovery process.

## CURRENT CONCEPTS

The large volume of musculoskeletal tissue in the lower extremities, including the pelvis, increases the potential systemic effects of lower extremity injuries. Bleeding and accumulation of extracellular fluid may cause hypovolemia and contribute to systemic hypotension.[10] Several units of blood can be lost into severely injured thighs, and preoperative blood loss associated with a single femur fracture is up to 1500 to 2000 mL. A crushing wound of the lower extremity releases intravasated debris (e.g., bone marrow), myoglobin, related muscle breakdown products, and various inflammatory mediators. The release of these substances may cause fat embolism and adult respiratory distress syndrome (ARDS), acute renal failure, and multiple organ failure (MOF).[11,12] Life-threatening infections such as clostridial myonecrosis or necrotizing fasciitis can rapidly develop in the tissues of the lower extremities. While proper early operation may prevent these, immediate recognition and treatment are vital to the salvage of any patient who develops such an infection.[13]

As demonstrated by Tscherne, Bone, Trentz, and others, prompt surgical treatment for severe extremity injuries benefits the whole patient.[5,14–16] Early fracture stabilization reduces the systemic effects of fractures, including systemic inflammatory response syndrome (SIRS), sepsis, MOF, and ARDS. Early stabilization reduces pain and the need for analgesic medication, promotes mobilization of the patient with attendent benefits to the respiratory and gastrointestinal systems. While fracture fixation is particularly beneficial for the patient with injuries to the lower extremity and pelvis, "damage control" procedures should be undertaken if the patient is in shock, coagulopathic, hypothermic, or has an actively developing traumatic brain injury.[10,17–20] The concept of damage control orthopedics (DCO) emphasizes rapid provisional skeletal stabilization with simple external fixators, followed by delayed definitive fixation when the patient is stable and the inflammatory system is less primed, usually at 5–10 days post injury[5,14–16,19,21] (Fig. 43-1). While controversy exists concerning the utility of orthopedic damage control, the concept of rapid, minimally invasive fracture fixation, has been found safe and cost effective.

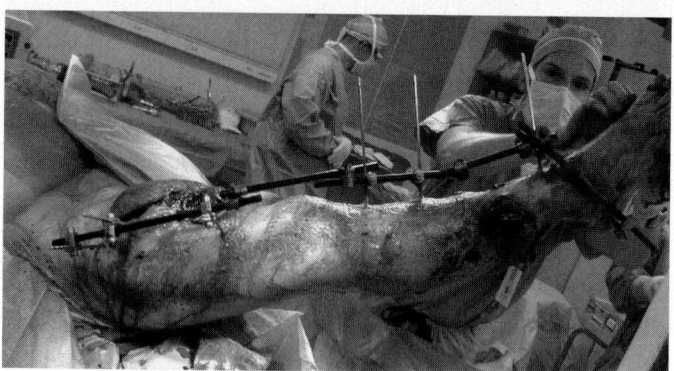

**FIGURE 43-1.** Concept of "damage control" orthopedic surgery for severely injured patients with associated long bone fractures of the lower extremity. Early external fixation of these fractures is time saving and helps to attenuate the systemic "trauma load" to the patient by attenuating stress and pain and reducing the extent of secondary injuries to the brain and the pulmonary endothelium. This concept allows an unrestricted positioning of the patient in the intensive care unit for adequate treatment of chest and brain injuries and to avoid pressure sores which may lead to severe soft tissue complications. Definitive fracture fixation by conversion to intramedullary implants or plate osteosynthesis is physiologically safe in the majority of cases during the "time window of opportunity" between days 5 to 10 after trauma.

A significant body of research has shown that the timing and type of fracture fixation may be critical in specific patient subsets. Intramedullary instrumentation of the femoral shaft can effect circulating neutrophil cell membranes causing surface receptor changes know as "priming" or "activation." The "primed" neutrophil when releases cytokines and other mediators which alter endothelial membrane permeability throughout the body, resulting in systemic inflammatory syndrome and fluid entering the alveoli.[22] A number of other physiologic changes may occur, including activation of the alternative complement pathway in the brain, alterations in the coagulation and immune systems.[15,23] All of these changes are part of the "second hit" phenomena in which the damage of the initial trauma (first hit) is augmented by further damage from a "second hit". The "second hit" may be caused by secondary procedures such as prolonged surgery with blood loss or instrumentation of the femoral canal.[16,19,20] The initial approach to fracture care in the polytraumatized patient must take into account these physiologic realities. However, the clinical implications of neutrophil changes and mediator release have not been directly correlated with clinical outcome, in part because of the large cohort numbers required to achieve statistical significance for such a study.

Fractures, whether isolated or in polytrauma, have far-reaching implications for the patient. The results of a "fracture" often depend more on damage to the soft tissues of the limb than on the isolated bony injury. Thus, accurate evaluation of an extremity injury requires assessment of the following: (a) skin and subcutaneous tissue; (b) muscles and tendons; (c) bones; (d) joints, including ligaments and articular cartilage; (e) arteries and veins; and (f) peripheral nerves. Acute as well as final functional outcome will depend on treatment of the entire spectrum of injury.

Quantification of injury severity has been attempted by many investigators. Tscherne emphasized that the severity of injury depends largely on the extent of damage to soft tissue in both closed and open fractures.[24,25] The Tscherne classification focuses on categorization of the soft tissue injury (Table 43-1). Open fractures require urgent

**TABLE 43-1**

| | Hannover Classification System for Soft Tissue Injuries According to Tscherne and Oestern | |
|---|---|---|
| SCORE | DESCRIPTION | EXAMPLE |
| 0 | No soft tissue injury, indirect trauma mechanism, simple fracture pattern | *Indirect torsion fracture of the tibia* |
| I | Superficial skin abrasion, skin contusion by internal pressure of fracture fragments | *Unreduced fracture-dislocation of the ankle* |
| II | Deep soft tissue contamination, skin contusion by direct force, impending compartment syndrome, complex fracture pattern | *Bumper injury to the lower leg* |
| III | Severe soft tissue contusion with skin necrosis, myonecrosis, degloving injury, acute compartment syndrome, comminuted fracture pattern | *High energy roll over trauma* |

surgical treatment for debridement and fracture stabilization. Closed fractures with high-energy soft tissue damage also require urgent stabilization as well as close monitoring for compartment syndrome.

Grading systems for open fractures have been proposed by Gustilo and colleagues, among others (Table 43-2). The Gustilo classification has significant interobserver variability but is well accepted amongst orthopedic surgeons.[26,27]

A relatively recent concept in lower extremity fracture care is that the majority of fractures can be treated entirely or in part with minimally invasive fixation. The evolution of techniques for percutaneous reduction and fixation of fractures, coupled with technological adaptation of fracture implants, has completely revolutionized fracture fixation. While intraarticular fractures usually require some form of open reduction to restore articular congruity, most diaphyseal and meataphyseal lower extremity fractures and many pelvis fractures can be treated with minimally invasive surgery.[28–30] The decreased blood loss, lowered risk of infection, and increased rate of healing have positive implications for the injured patient.

## LIMB SALVAGE VERSUS AMPUTATION

One of the most challenging decisions involved in the care of an injured patient is whether or not to attempt salvage of a severely injured limb.[31–39] Although every appropriate effort should be made to preserve functional and anatomic integrity, for some severe lower extremity injuries, an amputation and prosthesis may be more effective for the patient than a limb that is still attached but is of limited use (Fig. 43-2). In the acute phase, the decision to amputate will depend primarily on the immediate condition of the patient and the feasibility of stabilizing/revascularizing the injured limb. If the limb is initially salvaged then further decisions must be made regarding the desirability of maintaining the salvage effort, which usually involves further multiple operations. Key factors in this decision process include the patient status, the level of potential amputation as well as the wishes of the patient in those cases in which they are cognizant. In all situations involving a decision between limb salvage and amputation, the two primary concerns are (a) the systemic consequences of either alternative for the patient and (b) the likelihood of achieving a functional limb versus the problems associated with limb salvage (time involved, duration of disability, medical risks, socioeconomic costs, number of operations, and hospitalizations, etc.).[35] If a limb is severely injured, it is rare that either amputation or salvage will completely restore function.

In those cases in which the patient is hemodynamically unstable and revascularization cannot be accomplished without increasing the chance of death, amputation is the only choice. In these cases a guillotine-type amputation is appropriate, but every effort should be made to preserve length and coverage options. In particular, efforts to preserve the potential for a below-knee amputation (BKA) by preserving any viable distal muscle and /or skin, will improve the patient's outcome[40] (Fig. 43-2). Free tissue transfers, rotational flaps, and skin grafts can all be used effectively to improve length and provide a durable, useful stump. Many surgeons are unaware that skin grafting of well-padded stumps is feasible and highly successful. Similarly, latissimus dorsi free flaps, combined with skin grafts, preservation of vascularized heel pads, and turn down procedures, using vascularized portions of bone from the zone of injury, can effectively preserve a BKA despite severe soft tissue loss. Unfortunately, in many cases, the decision to amputate is made in the middle of the night, without opportunity for consultation with experienced salvage surgeons. Multidisciplinary decision making in these severe cases may provide increased reconstructive options whether the limb is salvaged in entirety or amputated.

The level of amputation greatly impacts future function. Proximal amputations have greater functional impairment and are often less satisfactory than prosthetic alternatives. Prosthetic replacement of the foot and ankle is highly functional. A through-knee or above-knee amputation, however, requires a prosthesis that requires more energy for ambulation and is less functional than one used after a BKA. Thus, every reasonable effort is appropriate to preserve the patient's own knee joint and enough proximal tibia (at least 10 cm below the joint) to provide for good prosthetic fitting. Prostheses for very proximal femoral amputation levels, hip disarticulation, or hemipelvectomies are rarely functional for ambulation; therefore, efforts are also appropriate to preserve an adequate above-knee amputation level.

**TABLE 43-2**

| | Classification of Open Fractures According to Gustilo and Anderson |
|---|---|
| SCORE | DESCRIPTION |
| I | Clean wound < 1 cm, inside-out perforation, little or no contamination, simple fracture pattern. |
| II | Skin laceration > 1 cm, surrounding soft tissue without signs of contusion, vital musculature, moderate to severe fracture instability. |
| III | Extensive soft tissue damage, wound contamination, exposed bone, marked fracture instability due to comminution or segmental defects. |
| IIIA | *Adequate soft-tissue coverage of the fractured bone.* |
| IIIB | *Exposed bone with periosteal stripping.* |
| IIIC | *Any open fracture with associated arterial injury requiring vascular repair.* |

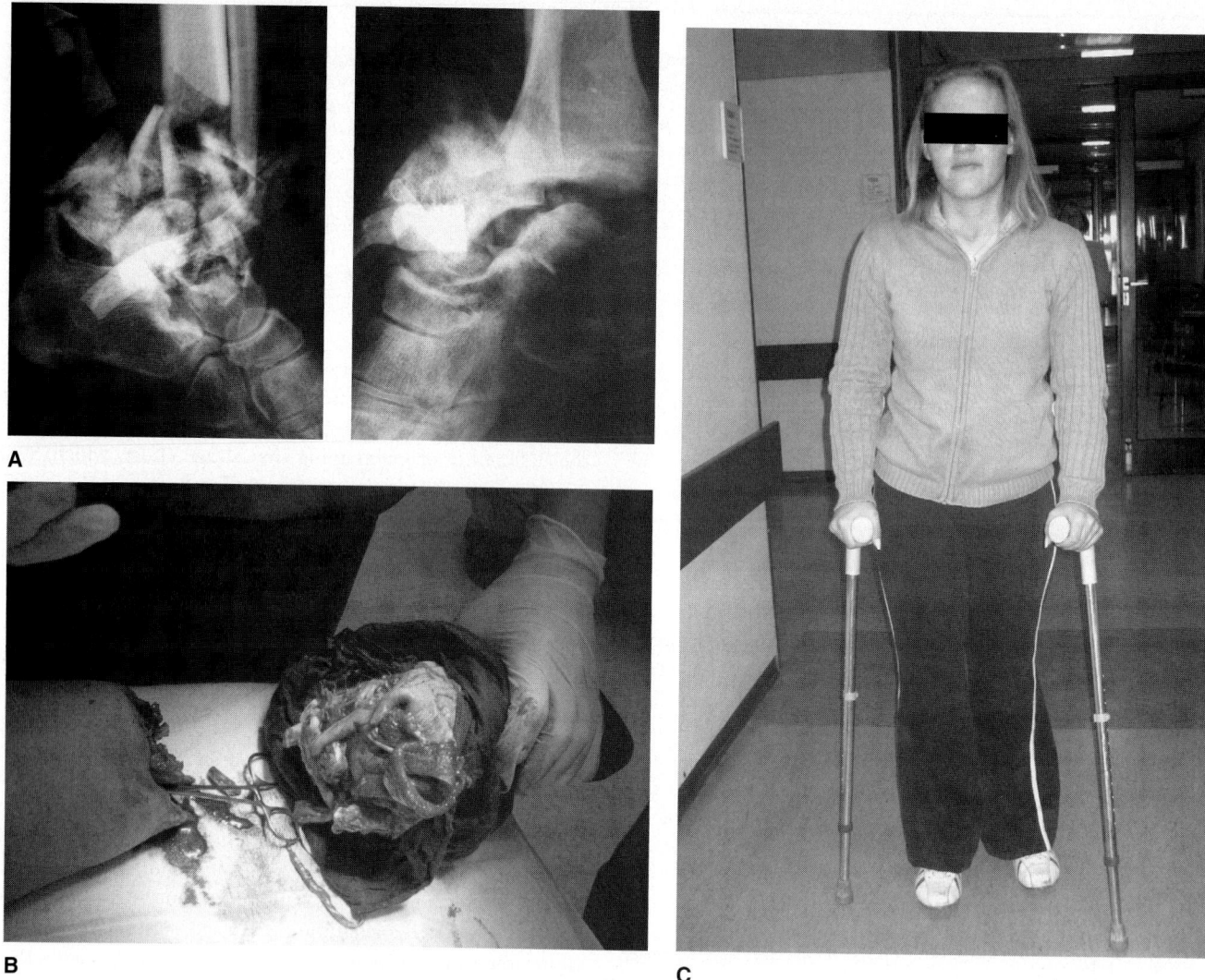

**FIGURE 43-2.** Severe crush injury with subtotal traumatic amputation of bilateral lower extremities in a 21-year-old girl who was rolled over by a train **(A,B)**. The injuries were associated with a severe soft tissue deglovement and gross contamination, bilateral tibial nerve crush injuries, and complete transection of the arterial blood supply to both feet (bilateral Gustilo-Andersen IIIC open fractures and "mangled extremity severity score" of 8 points). Under these circumstances, both lower extremities were assessed as nonsalvageable, and bilateral below-knee amputation was performed according to the Brückner technique. Panel **C** shows the rehabilitated patient walking on bilateral prostheses at two months after injury.

The classic injury requiring a decision of amputation versus salvage is an open tibial fracture, with arterial injury (Gustilo grade IIIC). Gregory et al. have defined a mangled extremity as one with significant injuries to three of the following four components: integument, bone, nerve, and vessel.[41] Some element of subjective assessment of severity is inevitably involved in the evaluation of severe limb injuries. Several predictive scoring systems have been proposed to aid decisions about limb salvage.[27,34,35,38,39,42,43] These necessarily require consideration of multiple factors. Unfortunately, none of these scoring systems reliably predict the need for amputation and, while they suggest which limbs may be salvaged, they do not correlate with functional outcome.

Variables that must be considered in the decision for limb salvage are both systemic and local. The severity and duration of shock, the severity of other injuries (Injury Severity Score [ISS]), the patient's age, and pre-existing medical conditions are crucial. Important features of the extremity injury include duration of ischemia, causative mechanism, fracture pattern, location of vascular injury, neurologic status, condition of the foot, and muscle

viability following revascularization. The patient's occupation and subjective desires merit consideration. One limb injury scoring scale is the mangled extremity severity score (MESS) developed by Johansen and colleagues[42] (Table 43-3). Such scales were originally described for open grade IIIC injuries, but their use has been extended by other investigators to complex lower extremity trauma.

A total MESS of 7 or more suggests the need for primary amputation, since limbs with such scores rarely are salvaged successfully (Fig. 43-2). The sensitivity and specificity of the MESS, however, have not gone unquestioned. Bonanni and coworkers have critically reviewed the MESS score, comparing it with three similar indices.[44] Applying these scores to 58 lower extremities with salvage attempts, they found that none of the scores had a predictive value significantly better chance than in determining which limbs would be successfully salvaged. Bosse and colleagues, in a large prospective multicenter study of patients with severe injuries to the lower extremity, demonstrated that current severity scores of limb injury cannot be used to effectively predict the need for amputation and functional outcome of the patient.[34,35] They also found

**TABLE 43-3**

**Mangled Extremity Severity Score (MESS), According to Johansen and Colleagues. The MESS is Calculated as the Sum of the Four Parameters (A+B+C+D). An Ischemic Time of >6 h After Injury Doubles the Ischemia Score (*). The Cut-off for a Mangled Extremity to be at Risk for Amputation has been Determined at a MESS of 7 Points**

| CRITERIA | POINTS | DESCRIPTION |
|---|---|---|
| (A) Skeletal /soft tissue injury | | |
| | 1 | Low energy (stab wound, low-velocity gun shot, simple fracture) |
| | 2 | Medium energy (open fractures, multiple fractures, fracture-dislocations) |
| | 3 | High energy (high-speed deceleration, high-velocity gun shot) |
| | 4 | Very high energy (high-speed trauma with gross contamination) |
| (B) Ischemia* | | |
| | 1 | Pulse reduced or absent, normal perfusion/capillary refill |
| | 2 | Pulseless, paresthesias, diminished capillary refill |
| | 3 | Cool, paralyzed, insensate, numb |
| (C) Shock | | |
| | 0 | Normotension |
| | 1 | Transient hypotension (<90 mm Hg) |
| | 2 | Persistent hypotension (<90 mm Hg) |
| (D) Age | | |
| | 0 | <30 years |
| | 1 | 30–50 years |
| | 2 | >50 years |

that patients with tibial nerve injury did not necessarily have a dismal outcome with salvage and that the two-year outcome differences between amputation and salvage patients, was minimal.[33]

## REPLANTATION

Technically, replantation is possible for complete and subtotal lower extremity amputations.[45] However, given the current near-impossibility of lower extremity nerve regeneration in adults, the functional outcome is questionable. In general, only cleanly separated traumatic amputations in young individuals without significant systemic risk factors, including smoking, deserve consideration for replantation. Revascularization in the face of severe neuromuscular injury may result in a viable but painful, dysfunctional limb. Consultation with an experienced replantation team is essential. Preservation of the amputated part is according to the same principles for upper extremity replantation. Care must be taken to not jeopardize the patients' life in lower extremity replantation and revascularization. Re-establishment of blood flow after a period of prolonged hypoxia can have a toxic effect, causing systemic inflammation and MOF. Consideration should be given to rapid external fixation and arterial shunt placement to "buy time" and permit an overall reassessment of the patient and of the desirability of reattachment of the limb.

## OPEN FRACTURES

All open fractures require urgent surgical treatment to reduce the risks of infection, soft tissue damage, and ongoing bleeding. In the emergency department (ED), the wound is kept covered with a sterile dressing, pressure is applied as necessary to control bleeding, and the limb is splinted. Tetanus prophylaxis and systemic antibiotics are given. Generally, a first-generation cephalosporin is used

for 24 to 48 hours following wound closure. For more severe wounds or contamination, additional coverage is added (e.g., an aminoglycoside or third-generation cephalosporin for grade III open fractures, or high-dose penicillin for "barnyard" injuries with risk of clostridial contamination).

As soon as the patient's condition permits, radiographs of the injured limb are obtained. Operative care of the open fracture must fit appropriately into the care of the patient's other problems. This should be done in an operating room with general or regional anesthesia. Debridement should preferably be performed within six hours of injury, unless more time is required for resuscitation of the patient or for treatment of injuries that pose a greater threat to life or limb. Longer delays probably increase the risk of infection. After thorough debridement of devascularized muscle, fascia, subcutaneous tissue, skin, and bone; removal of all foreign material; and copious irrigation, wound care is enhanced by appropriately chosen fracture fixation. Generally, this involves screw and/or plate fixation for joint fractures, intramedullary nails or external fixators for diaphyseal fracture. Intramedullary nails in the tibia and femur can safely be placed in reamed fashion, even in open fractures. However, in multiply injured, concern for marrow extravasation and subsequent development of SIRS has led to the use of unreamed, small diameter nails, temporary external fixators, or reamer-irrigator-aspirator (RIA) systems to decrease marrow embolization.[46,47]

After fracture fixation, the open fracture wound, extended as required for debridement and fixation, is left open initially, under a sterile moisture-retaining dressing. Recent randomized studies indicate that there may be a role for primary closure in well-debrided open injuries. Antibiotic-impregnated methyl-methacrylate beads placed in large or contaminated wounds may significantly reduce the risk of infection. Severe open fracture wounds mandate a return to the operating room within 24–48 hours to assess the adequacy of debridement and to further debulk potential bacterial contamination. Delayed primary closure, generally after three or four days, reduces the risk of wound infection. Unless the local tissues are

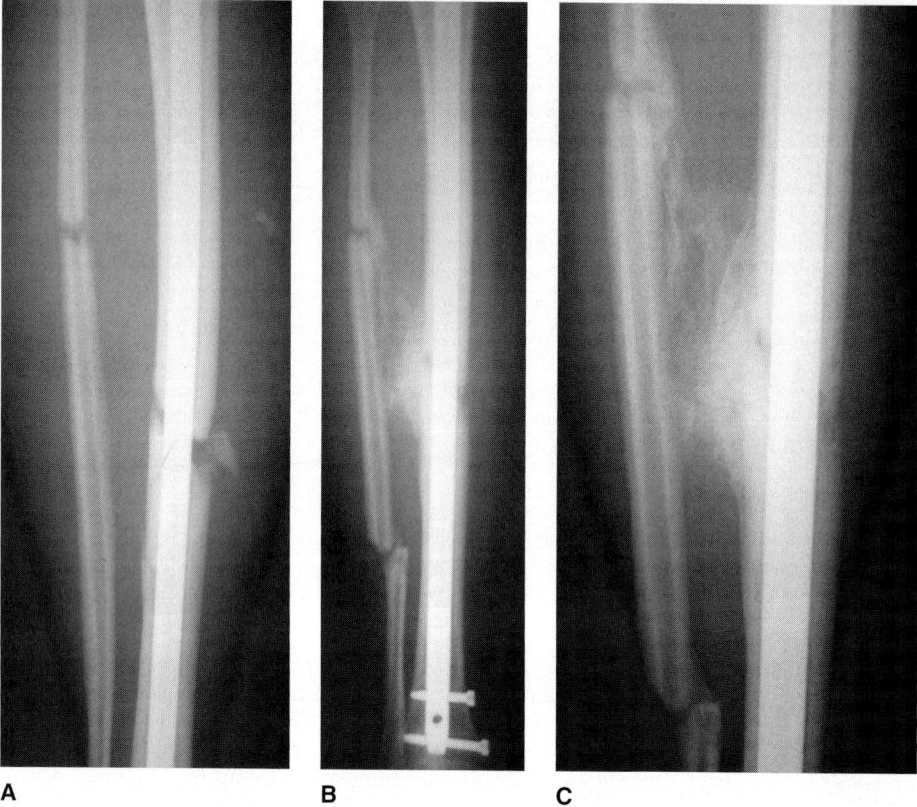

**FIGURE 43-3.**  Postero-lateral bone grafting for a midshaft tibia fracture with a bone defect and distraction after intramedullary nailing **(A)**. The progressive healing of the postero-lateral bone graft leads to a stable synostosis between tibia and fibula **(B,C)**.

intact enough to permit delayed suture closure, or split-thickness skin grafting, open wounds often require muscle flaps, either swung locally or brought in from a distance with microvascular anastomoses.[48,49] Severe open fractures often require bone grafting to gain union. While bone grafting may be essential, it should be postponed until the wound is securely healed, as the risk of infection is increased if bone grafting is performed at the time of initial open fracture surgery or at delayed closure of the wound (Fig. 43-3).

## IMPORTANCE OF EARLY RECOGNITION AND TREATMENT OF EXTREMITY INJURIES

Dislocations of the hip, knee, or more distal joints, as well as displaced fractures, may cause pressure on nerves, vessels, or skin, resulting in permanent deficits. Delay of more than a few hours in reducing a dislocated hip significantly increases the risk of avascular necrosis of the femoral head. Displaced intracapsular femoral neck fractures also have a high risk of avascular necrosis, which can be lowered by urgent reduction and fixation. In young patients, this injury may appropriately be considered as an ischemic surgical emergency. Failure to recognize an undisplaced fracture of the femoral neck may result in its displacement, with a much greater likelihood of poor outcome. Open fractures, particularly those of the lower extremities, are true emergencies, requiring surgical treatment within six to eight hours to minimize the risk of infection. Early stabilization (within 24 hours) of lower extremity fractures, especially the femur and pelvis, facilitates resuscitation, minimizes pulmonary complications, and shortens hospital stay (Fig. 43-1). Most importantly, prompt treatment of fractures and dislocations offers systemic benefits as well as relieving pain and facilitating rehabilitation.

## INJURY COMBINATIONS

Awareness of typical combinations of lower extremity injuries aids diagnosis and may decrease the risk of missing important injuries. One mechanism can produce several injuries. An unrestrained passenger in a head-on motor vehicle collision may strike his or her knee against the dashboard, sustaining a patellar fracture or injury to knee ligaments, depending on the point of impact. The force indirectly applied along the femur then dislocates the flexed hip, concurrently producing a posterior wall acetabular fracture and/or fracture of the femoral head. The association between femur fractures and pelvic or acetabular fractures is so strong that careful review of a pelvic x-ray is mandatory for all patients with femoral shaft fractures. Patients who fall from a height and land on their feet may have both calcaneal fractures and injuries to the thoracolumbar spine—another "classic" combination. Patients with fractures of the femoral shaft may have associated fractures of the femoral neck, either obvious or undisplaced and occult. The trauma surgeon should be aware of the association of ruptures of the thoracic aorta with pelvic fractures and of the frequently observed multiple injuries seen with "floating knees" (simultaneous ipsilateral femoral and tibial fractures), which also have a high incidence of associated injuries to soft tissue at the knee joint. Isolated fibular fractures may be associated with traction injuries of the peroneal nerve or with ligamentous disruptions of the knee or ankle. While fractures are often distractingly obvious on x-rays, injuries to joints such as subluxations and even dislocations may easily be overlooked unless one is suspicious.

## PATHOPHYSIOLOGY AND BIOMECHANICS

Fractures occur when the applied loads to the bone exceed its load-bearing capacity. Fracture patterns relate to bone strength and the forces that cause the injury. Young, active individuals have strong bone. Children's bones can undergo plastic deformation and may bend without breaking. Elderly, osteoporotic individuals have diffusely weak bone. Focal bone defects may weaken a bone so significantly that it fails under a load that normally would pose no problem, resulting in a pathologic fracture. Such pathologic fractures may be due to tumor, infection, or dysplasia, as well as more generalized conditions that severely weaken bone, such as osteoporosis (Fig. 43-4).

The amount of energy that produced a given fracture is suggested by the patient's history and the fracture pattern. Comminution (the presence of more than two fracture fragments) implies a higher-energy injury that will produce multiple fracture lines. Displacement and the extent of local damage to soft tissue also reflect the amount of absorbed energy. Spiral fractures are produced by indirect, torsional forces. Less local soft tissue damage is generally present, but a very comminuted spiral fracture may have required such force that each fracture fragment acted as a high-velocity "internal missile," producing significant damage in the surrounding tissues. Transverse fractures are caused by directly applied forces. A wedge or "butterfly" fragment is often seen on the side of the bone where the fracturing force was applied as a result of local compression, while the opposite cortex fails transversely in tension.

## DIAGNOSIS

### History

Obtaining a thorough patient history provides the physician with useful information to begin forming a list of differential diagnoses in his/her mind prior to radiographic examination of the patient. The history should specify the mechanism of injury, provide information

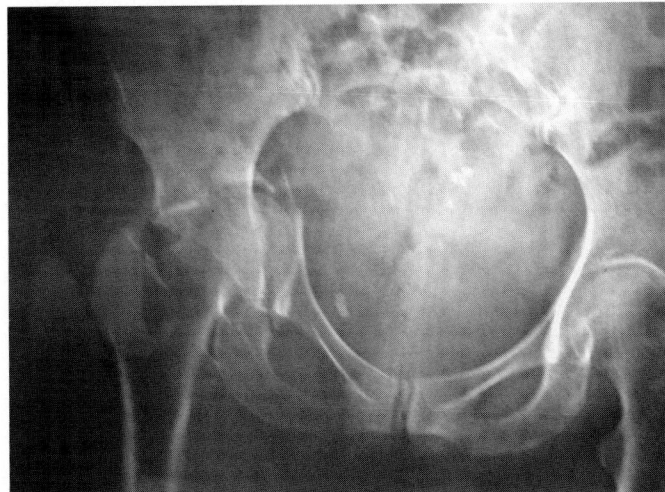

**A**

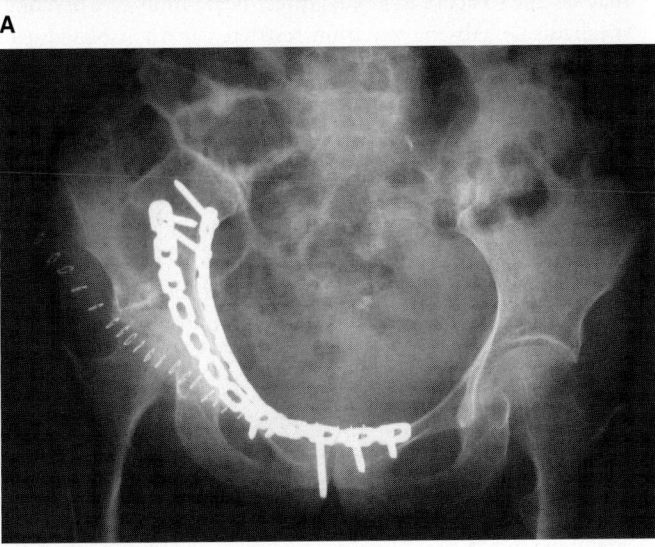

**B**

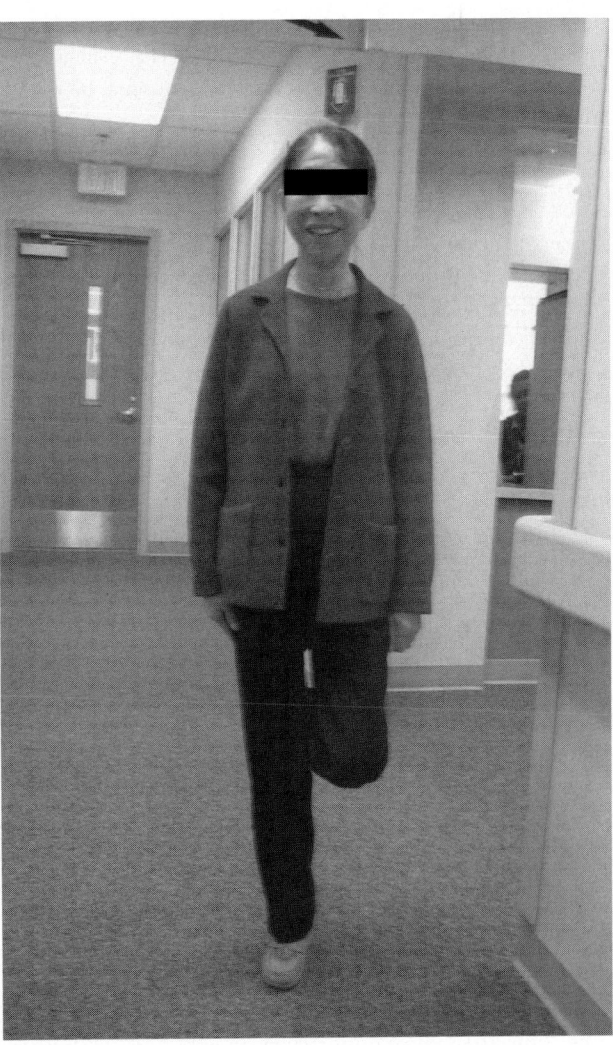

**C**

**FIGURE 43-4.** 74-year-old lady with severe osteoporosis who sustained a displaced right acetabular fracture after a fall **(A)**. The fracture was treated by angular stable bridge plating with two anterior locking plates **(B)**. Conventional, nonlocking screws and plates have a high risk of failure in osteoporotic cancellous bone. The patient is fully weight bearing on the right side, three months after surgery **(C)**.

regarding the severity of the applied forces, and alert the physician to associated injuries, illness, or medically relevant problems. While an accurate history may be difficult or impossible to obtain initially in a seriously injured patient, more details should always be sought and reconfirmed as the patient improves or more information becomes available. The history may be particularly helpful in managing open fractures by providing information on the following: the identification of the source and extent of contamination; the time elapsed from the moment of injury and, whether bone was initially protruding from an extremity wound.

A history inconsistent with the extent of injury suggests either a pathologic fracture or the possibility of abuse. A normal child, particularly under two years, should not fracture his or her femur while playing, even roughly, with a friend or parent. An elderly patient will not normally sustain a hip fracture from turning over in bed. Although pathologic fractures should be suspected in a patient with known malignant or metabolic disease and can be preceded by local pain, fractures may occur in completely asymptomatic patients as the initial presentation of an underlying disorder. In a young child, multiple fractures at various stages of healing are pathognomonic of child abuse, the diagnosis and appropriate management of which may be lifesaving. The report of pain or impaired function of an extremity requires careful evaluation to exclude a fracture or injury to a joint, nerves, muscles, or vascular structures.

## Physical Examination

Examination according to the advanced trauma life support (ATLS) protocol provides a systematic method of thoroughly examining the trauma patient and minimizing missed injuries.[6,50] In addition, the importance of continuous detailed documentation of the physical findings cannot be overemphasized. Assessment of patient progress may suffer due to a lack of re-examination and thorough documentation. Local tenderness at a fracture site may be masked or completely absent in a severely injured patient. Deformity, swelling, or both almost inevitably occur with fractures or dislocations of the lower extremity, though swelling may be delayed, especially if the patient arrives in a hypovolemic state. Truly occult fractures are rare indeed. Displaced long-bone fractures result in shortening, malrotation, or angulation. Immediate reduction and splint placement reduces pain and blood loss, and often restores circulation to a pulseless extremity. Dislocations typically assume characteristic positions, and may be masked by associated fractures. Intra-articular injuries usually cause a hemarthrosis unless the joint capsule is disrupted, in which case more diffuse soft tissue swelling occurs about the joint. Instability or abnormal motion when stressing the joint may be difficult to elicit if the region is tender, but is particularly important and useful in the anesthetized patient. Immediate relocation of a dislocated joint is warranted especially when circulatory compromise is apparent.

Swelling and pain is typical of compartment syndrome, which must be suspected in every injured lower extremity.[51,52] Impaired sensory or motor function in the setting of compartment syndrome is a late presentation and correlates with compartment necrosis. Compartment syndromes typically develop several hours or more after injury, before or after treatment has begun, and may be related to a cast or dressing that has become tight as the enclosed limb swells. Immediate release of such a constricting dressing aids diagnosis and may be therapeutic. Compartment syndrome is most effectively diagnosed by an experienced examiner and remains primarily a clinical diagnosis. Intra-compartmental monitoring with arterial lines or specialized "compartment monitors" can be helpful in the obtunded patient. In the awake patient, unremitting pain and a tense or swollen limb should be assumed to be compartment syndrome. Patients with suspected compartment syndrome should be taken to the operating room immediately and undergo fasciotomy of all compartments (3 in the thigh, 4 in the tibia, 9 in the foot). Partial fasciotomies, or the use of limited incisions, in general are not appropriate in the trauma patient.

The neurovascular status may be difficult to assess clinically in a severely injured patient or extremity. Therefore, a high level of suspicion is required for identifying and treating potentially catastrophic vascular injuries. Capillary filling is not, by itself, adequate clinical evidence of an intact proximal vascular tree. Distal pulses may be present after a significant arterial injury. Perhaps the most familiar arterial injury in the lower extremity involves the popliteal artery in association with knee dislocations or periarticular fractures. Late thrombosis of an initially non-occlusive injury may result in limb loss. Frequent assessment of pedal pulses is required for such patients. Any alteration of pedal pulses requires assessment, at least with Doppler pressure measurement. Measurement of ankle systolic blood pressure is an important adjunct to the physical exam. Pressure below 90% of that in the arms or the opposite leg requires prompt evaluation by a vascular surgeon. Color Doppler or contrast arteriography may be considered if pulses decrease, but should not delay consultation with a trauma surgeon. Risks factors for limb loss include delayed surgery, arterial contusion with consecutive thrombosis, and most importantly failed revascularization.

The neurological status of the extremity should be documented before any definitive treatment, whenever possible. The neurological examination, like the vascular examination, may be unreliable in the severely injured patient. Stocking hypoesthesia may be due to acute ischemia, direct nerve injury, or psychogenic mechanisms. Absent sensation restricted to the isolated sensory area of a peripheral nerve suggests injury to that nerve. Impaired motor function may be caused by pain and instability, a peripheral nerve injury, or a spinal cord injury. Peripheral nerve damage is associated with certain lower extremity injuries. Posterior dislocations of the hip may injure the sciatic nerve, most often its peroneal component. Knee dislocations or equivalent injuries may injure the common peroneal and/or tibial nerves in the popliteal fossa, a possible clue to an associated arterial injury. Pressure from a splint or cast may also injure the peroneal nerve as it encircles the neck of the fibula at the knee.

Open fractures should be quickly assessed upon arrival of the patient in the emergency room. The wound should be covered with a Betadine or saline dressing and only examined in the operating room in order to avoid further contamination and soft tissue damage. Extensive exploration or manipulation of exposed bone should not be attempted in the ED. Bleeding, even from amputation wounds, can almost always be managed with a pressure dressing. A tourniquet should be reserved for otherwise uncontrollable hemorrhage.

Because a significant percentage of injuries, particularly those involving the distal extremity and the major joints, are missed during the initial trauma evaluation, repeated exams are essential, especially as the patient's recovery permits more cooperation. At least one "tertiary" survey is an important part of each significantly injured patient's diagnostic evaluation.

## Radiography of Extremity Injuries

As per ATLS protocol, an antero-posterior (AP) chest and pelvis, and an adequate lateral cervical spine radiographs are indicated early in the evaluation and resuscitation of the injured patient during the primary survey.[6,50] Kaneriya et al. have demonstrated routine pelvic x-rays to be cost-effective in patients with blunt trauma.[53] X-rays of injured extremities are of much lower priority and fall into the secondary survey. The obviously injured extremity should be dressed and stabilized with a splint. Resuscitation of the patient should never be delayed or interrupted for x-rays of the extremities. X-rays can be taken after urgent surgical treatment for other life-threatening problems. In the unstable patient, care should be concurrent and not contiguous, implying that x-rays and fracture stabilization can occur concomitantly in the operating theater or resuscitation bay with life-saving maneuvers such as laparotomy or thoracotomy. If adequate extremity radiographs can be obtained without delaying other essential aspects of the evaluation and treatment of the trauma patient, they can be valuable in making the initial care plan.

Extremity x-rays should show both AP and lateral views of the entire bone in question. If the need for surgical treatment has been determined, further views may be better obtained in the operating room under anesthesia or after traction has realigned and separated the fracture fragments sufficiently to improve visualization. Certain complex articular fractures are best visualized with computerized tomography (CT) scans. If a patient is hemodynamically stable and requires other CT studies, extremity CTs may be obtained at the same time. Early involvement of the orthopedic surgeon ensures proper x-rays and avoidance of unnecessary studies. Pelvic CT scans are NOT part of the initial workup of the pelvic fracture patient with hemodynamic instability.[6,10]

## MANAGEMENT OF COMMON FRACTURES AND DISLOCATIONS

### Pelvic and Acetabular Fractures

Pelvic fractures are life-threatening injuries that require rapid and effective management by a multidisciplinary team. Patients at risk for pelvic fractures are any who have been exposed to high-energy forces (vehicular crashes, falls from heights, crushing forces, etc.), though these injuries may occur from simple falls as well. Pain in the pelvic region, as well as instability, deformity, open wound, and/or trouble moving the hip or thigh are all clues to a pelvic injury. Any injured patient with such complaints or findings requires at least a screening AP pelvis radiograph for evaluation. The same is true for any potentially injured patient with altered mental status. A careful review of this radiograph is required, because significant, unstable pelvic injuries can be easily overlooked. The value of the AP pelvic radiograph in the acutely unstable patient is solely to identify whether the pelvis could be a source of shock. A patient can be hemodynamically unstable from an isolated pelvic fracture that is minimally displaced. Once the patient

is stable, additional x-rays will be required to characterize the injury and make surgical decisions. This usually involves additional plain x-ray views, including inlet and outlet views for injuries to the pelvic ring and oblique (Judet) views for acetabular fractures. CT scans are helpful for both categories of pelvic injuries, but "bone windows" are necessary. While it is conventional to divide pelvic injuries into disruptions of the pelvic ring and acetabular fractures, both components of the pelvis may be involved.

### Pelvic Ring Injuries

The sacrum and the two innominate bones comprise the pelvic ring, which is both the base of the spine and the connection of the lower extremities to the trunk. The symphysis pubis and the two sacroiliac joints unite the three bony components of the ring, and their stability depends upon ligamentous integrity. Injuries that deform the pelvic ring or render it unstable must involve at least two different foci of damage, including bone, joint, or both components. The main ligaments that stabilize the pelvis are the posterior sacroiliac ligaments and the fibrocartilaginous pubic symphysis. Significant secondary stabilizers are the sacrotuberous and sacrospinous ligaments, which are major parts of the pelvic floor. They can be disrupted with severe pelvic displacement, particularly if widening or vertical shift occurs. The radiographic appearance of anterior pelvic injuries, generally fractures of the pubic rami and separations of the pubic symphysis, are easily noted on the AP pelvic radiograph. Anterior injuries are less significant, however, than the disruption of the posterior pelvic ring. The posterior injury determines the degree of pelvic instability, the likelihood of associated injuries, and the prognosis for late functional outcome. The posterior pelvis is intimately adherent to the presacral venous plexus, branches of the iliac arteries, and the lumbosacral nerve plexus. Bone displacement in this area usually causes significant injury to all of these structures and is a major cause of life-threatening bleeding. Because the pelvis rarely breaks at a single point, any anterior pelvic ring injury requires a careful search for posterior disruption.

Pennal and Tile grouped disruptions of the pelvic ring according to mechanism of injury, as revealed by the displacement pattern seen on inlet and outlet radiographs.[54] Lateral compression (LC), AP compression (APC), and vertical shear (VS) are the three basic types they described. While vertical shear displacement is necessarily unstable, the extent of pelvic instability associated with LC and APC injuries varies from stable to profoundly unstable. Several authors have correlated the degree and type of pelvic ring injury with specific patterns of associated injuries to the head, thorax, and abdomen.

Injuries of the pelvic ring, especially those that are mechanically unstable, may have associated life-threatening hemorrhage, the source of which is usually low-pressure bleeding from pelvic veins or intraosseous blood vessels.[55] Large clinical studies found that in less than 10% of patients with significant pelvic hemorrhage was the source an arterial bleeding, and only about 2% of the patients could be successfully be embolized.[56,57] This strongly suggests that most bleeding caused by pelvic fractures should first be addressed by promoting tamponade of the retroperitoneal hemorrhage, by splinting significant pelvic instability, and by reducing any pathologically increased pelvic volume. A pelvic wrap or binder, pelvic external fixation, and pelvic internal fixation can be used for the mechanical stabilization component of resuscitation. Acute retroperitoneal packing can be used in conjunction with acute mechanical stabilization to

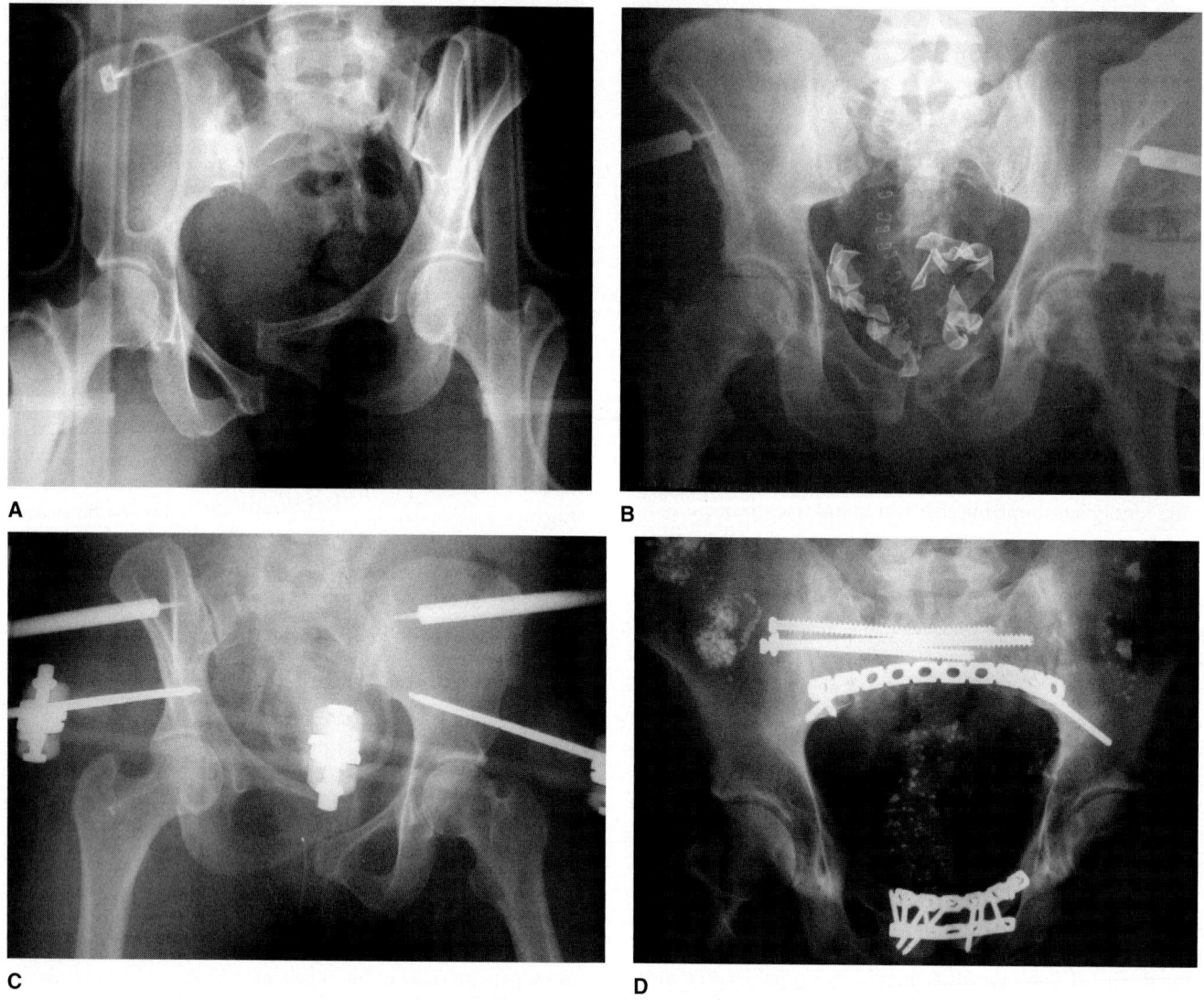

**FIGURE 43-5.** Complete disruption of the anterior and posterior pelvic ring in a 27-year-old patient who sustained a lateral compression type III (LC III) injury after a motor vehicle crash **(A)**. Due to massive retroperitoneal bleeding with hemorrhagic shock the patient was treated by a "damage control" including initial stabilization with a pelvic C-clamp and retroperitoneal packing **(B)**. The instability of the anterior pelvic ring was augmented by an anterior supraacetabular external fixator after depacking **(C)**, and the patient was converted to internal fixation at two weeks, after hemodynamic stabilization. The definitive osteosynthesis consisted of three sacro-iliac screws, a posterior tension banding plate, and double-plating of the anterior pelvic ring **(D)**.

reduce blood loss and decrease mortality[58–61] (Fig. 43-5). The need for angiography cannot be accurately determined by examining the type of fracture pattern. Considering the low percentage of patients who have embolizable pelvic bleeding (<10%), angiography should probably be reserved only for those patients who continue to bleed despite aggressive venous control measures such as graded resuscitation, retroperitoneal packing, surgical treatment of associated injuries, and mechanical stabilization[56,57,62,63] (Fig. 43-6).

Late disability associated with pelvic ring injuries is typically due to pain, which may be caused by residual instability from a posterior ligamentous injury (e.g., of the sacroiliac joint), an ununited fracture, or by deformity that affects sitting posture or gait. Neurologic and genitourinary dysfunctions are other important and frequent causes of disability after injury to the pelvic ring. If the pelvic outlet heals with deformity, vaginal delivery may be affected. Male and female patients suffer a relatively high rate of chronic sexual dysfunction. Pediatric pelvic fracture patients also have significant disability from their injuries. Long-term outcome

studies show that pediatric patients with significant pelvic asymmetry have functional outcome problems as adults, compared to those patients with minimal asymmetry. Pediatric pelvic fractures can be equally life threatening and disabling and thus deserve a similarly aggressive approach as in adult fracture management.

Isolated disruptions of the sacroiliac joint heal slowly and may result in chronic pain. Posterior fractures, however, usually heal within a few weeks. If deformity is not corrected promptly, it is exceedingly difficult to correct once healing progresses. Revision surgery for pelvic malunion has a high rate of neurovascular complications. Thus, early recognition and treatment of displaced pelvic ring injuries is important. Generally, significant posterior instability or deformity requires early posterior surgical stabilization, as anterior fixation alone is frequently unable to maintain alignment of the pelvis.

Stabilization surgery of the posterior pelvis is indicated for displacement or significant posterior instability. Definitive posterior fixation may often be deferred until 5–10 days after injury, as

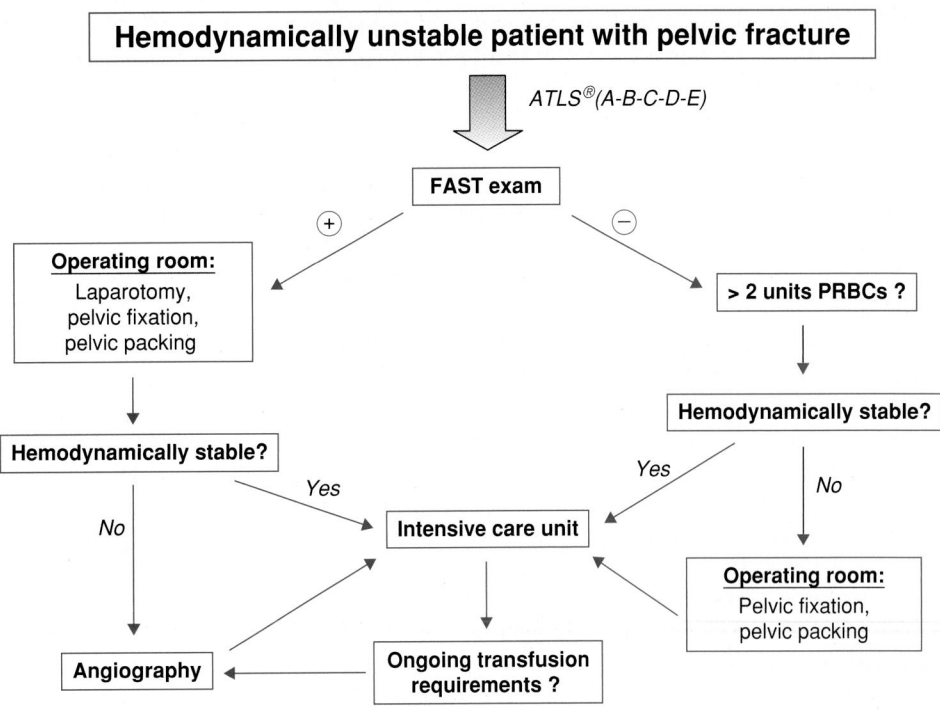

**Hemodynamically unstable patient with pelvic fracture**

ATLS®(A-B-C-D-E)

FAST exam

(+) (−)

Operating room:
Laparotomy,
pelvic fixation,
pelvic packing

> 2 units PRBCs ?

Hemodynamically stable?

Hemodynamically stable?

No | Yes | Yes | No

Intensive care unit

Operating room:
Pelvic fixation,
pelvic packing

Angiography ← Ongoing transfusion
requirements ?

**FIGURE 43-6.** Denver Health Medical Center institutional algorithm for the management of hemodynamically unstable patients with pelvic fractures. ATLS, advanced trauma life support; FAST, focussed assessment sonography in trauma; PRBC, packed red blood cell concentrate.

anterior fixation alone typically provides enough initial stability to aid control of hemorrhage (Fig. 43-5). Conversely, if posterior stabilization will be necessary later, and a patient is not actively bleeding, it may be better to delay any pelvic fixation until the entire task can be accomplished in one anesthetic. Vertical displacement should be corrected by applying skeletal traction through the distal femur or by placement in the operating room of a C clamp in the posterior position following traction–reduction of the pelvis. The type of definitive posterior fixation required, and the surgical approach, will be dictated by the anatomic location of the injury. Sacral fractures may be reduced with a closed technique or through an open posterior approach. Posterior exposures may lead to complications with wound healing if the local tissues have been injured. Generally performed with the patient supine, these approaches permit stabilization with a posterior plate or with iliosacral screws. Overcompression or malreduction of a sacral alar fracture may injure nerve roots exiting this lowest level of the spine. In some cases, transforaminal fractures with sacral displacement should be decompressed at the time of open reduction to lessen the chance of permanent sacral nerve root injury. Disruptions of the sacroiliac joints can be reduced and stabilized with cannulated screws inserted using fluoroscopic or CT control or via the first window of the ilioinguinal approach, anteriorly between the iliacus muscle and iliac wing. In some cases, using the same approach, plates can be applied across the anterior sacroiliac joint. Fractures of the iliac wing can be reduced and fixed with plates and screws via either anterior or posterior (lateral) approaches.

Disruptions of the anterior pelvic ring generally involve either fractures of the rami or separation of the symphysis pubis. The latter can be stabilized with plate fixation through either a lower midline or Pfannenstiel incision. Pubic rami fractures can be fixed with a plate generally via the ilioinguinal or Stoppa approaches with minimal insult to the patient. More recently, percutaneous fixation techniques have allowed surgeons to place long cannulated screws about the pelvis and anterior rami. Percutaneous

pelvic and acetabular surgery radically reduces blood loss without sacrificing stability (Fig. 43-7). However, numerous anatomic structures are at high risk, the learning curve is steep and obtaining an adequate reduction without incision remains challenging. Many rami fractures can be managed with closed reduction and simple anterior external fixation for five or six weeks.

Clearly, it is essential for all involved in the care of pelvic fracture patients—general/trauma surgeons, urologists, gynecologists, and orthopedists—to develop an overall plan for management before any one team member chooses a treatment element that

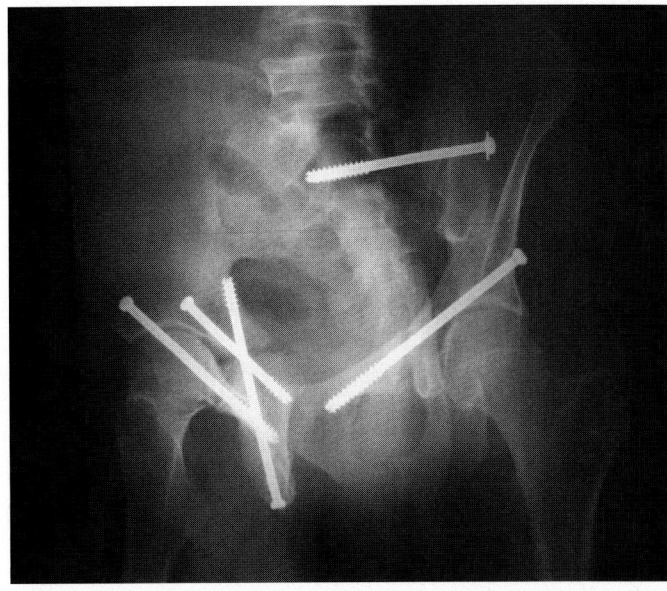

**FIGURE 43-7.** Polytrauma patient with combined pelvic ring and acetabular fractures. Due to the high risk constellation in this patient, all fractures were treated by closed reduction and percutaneous cannulated screw fixation.

precludes overall optimal care (e.g., placement of a diverting colostomy in the location of a planned anterior surgical approach to the pelvis).

## Acetabular Fractures

Fractures of the acetabulum are articular injuries with profound implications for the long-term function of the hip joint. Successful open reduction and internal fixation (ORIF) of displaced acetabular fractures significantly improves the prognosis of these potentially devastating injuries and permits early mobilization of a patient who might previously have been managed with many weeks of skeletal traction and bed rest (Fig. 43-4). Judet and Letournel's seminal work has led to our current classification, understanding, and management of acetabular fractures.[64,65] Oblique x-rays and CT scans are used to classify the acetabular fracture, to assess displacement, need for surgical treatment, and to determine the best surgical approach.[66] There are multiple surgical approaches to the acetabulum including the Kocher-Langenbeck, the ilioinguinal, the externded iliofemoral, the modified iliofemoral, the Stoppa, the Triradiate, combined anterior/posterior and percutaneous. The surgical approach is dictated by the fracture pattern and the overall condition of the patient. A complete three-dimensional understanding of the fracture is essential for formulating a preoperative surgical plan. Preservation of soft tissue attachments is needed to promote healing and avoid osteonecrosis. Vital neurovascular structures must be protected. A precise anatomic reduction must be achieved and fixed stably, generally with screws and plates, which must not encroach upon the articular surface. Intraoperative fluoroscopy has become a valuable tool for ensuring appropriate placement of orthopedic hardware around the acetabulum. Complications and poor results become less frequent with increasing experience of the acetabular surgeon. Acetabular fracture surgery remains among the most challenging procedures in orthopedics. These difficult and dangerous reconstructive surgeries should generally be done in specialized centers to ensure that each patient receives optimal treatment.

Acetabular fractures in osteoporotic individuals pose special problems. Comminution is often so severe and bone quality so poor that conventional fixation techniques are doomed to failure. In these instances, total hip arthroplasty with specialized acetabular reconstruction devices allows improved fixation and early weight bearing of the elderly patient. Because the femoral head is removed in total hip arthroplasty, extensile or combined exposures may not be required, and operative morbidity may be reduced.

Acetabular fractures are usually closed injuries, without need for immediate operation. If surgery is delayed for three to five days, operative bleeding is reduced, and preoperative planning may be improved. Patients with pelvic and acetabular fractures have a significant risk of thromboembolic disorders. Intermittent venous compression devices, anticoagulation with fractionated or low molecular heparin, and insertion of removable inferior vena cava filters for high-risk patients are all appropriate strategies for these injuries.

## Dislocations of the Hip

Posterior dislocations of the hip result from direct blows to the front of the knee or upper tibia of a sitting patient, most typically an unrestrained passenger in a motor vehicle (Fig. 43-8). A fracture of the posterior wall of the acetabulum occurs if the leg is more abducted and pure dislocations occur if the leg is adducted at the time of impact. The typical appearance of a patient with a posterior hip dislocation is with a hip that is flexed, adducted, internally rotated, and resistant to motion. This appearance may be lacking if a significant fracture of the posterior wall exists. An associated sciatic (often peroneal component alone) nerve palsy must be checked for. Anterior dislocations are rarer (5%) and are due to forced abduction and external rotation, which are also the characteristic deformity. An AP pelvis x-ray usually shows obvious signs of a hip dislocation or fracture dislocation. Additional views may be needed, however, to assess adequately the proximal femur where an associated fracture of the head or neck may be present (Fig. 43-8). A CT scan is required after reduction of a dislocated hip to assess its adequacy and the integrity of the acetabulum, as well as to exclude intra-articular bone fragments. Fractures of the femoral head occasionally occur with hip dislocations. They must be recognized and treated appropriately.

Dislocations of the hip are painful dramatic injuries that demand immediate reduction. Improvised splinting in situ with pillows or folded linen is unsatisfactory when compared to prompt reduction for pain relief. After initial x-rays, reduction can be done with intravenous analgesia, but may be gentler and easier for both patient and surgeon with general anesthesia and muscle relaxation. A rapid reduction (under six to eight hours, if at all possible) is crucial to minimize the risk of avascular necrosis of the femoral head. This disastrous complication results in destruction of the hip joint, with arthroplasty or arthrodesis almost always needed. Stability of the hip joint is usually restored by adequate reduction of pure dislocations, but the reduced joint must be checked for stability. Acetabular wall fractures of any significant size can result in instability, which, if present, is an indication for surgical repair within a few days after injury.

A stable, concentrically reduced dislocation of the hip usually becomes comfortable within a very few days. While applying weight to the hip in an unstable position (e.g., getting up from a low chair or toilet or getting into or out of a car) must be avoided until soft tissue healing has occurred, most patients can get out of bed and ambulate as soon as they can move and control their leg. Skeletal traction is required only for unstable hips, which will usually require surgery. Long-term outcome of hip dislocations includes an acknowledged significant risk of osteoarthritis, as well as some stiffness and limping that may never resolve. Avascular necrosis (AVN), the risk of which increases dramatically (from about 2% to 15%) if initial reduction is delayed more than a very few hours, usually appears during the first year, with essentially all cases evident three years after injury.

## Fractures of the Proximal Femur (Hip Fractures)

Proximal femur fractures mainly occur in elderly patients with osteoporosis due to low-energy trauma mechanisms, such as simple falls. These injuries represent an important socioeconomic factor due to the increasing life expectancy.[67,68] In industrialized countries, more than two million proximal femur fractures have been estimated to occur annually with more than 50% of the patients being over 85 years of age. Postoperative geriatric care is required in about 75% of all cases and six-month mortality in this cohort has been shown to be around 20%.

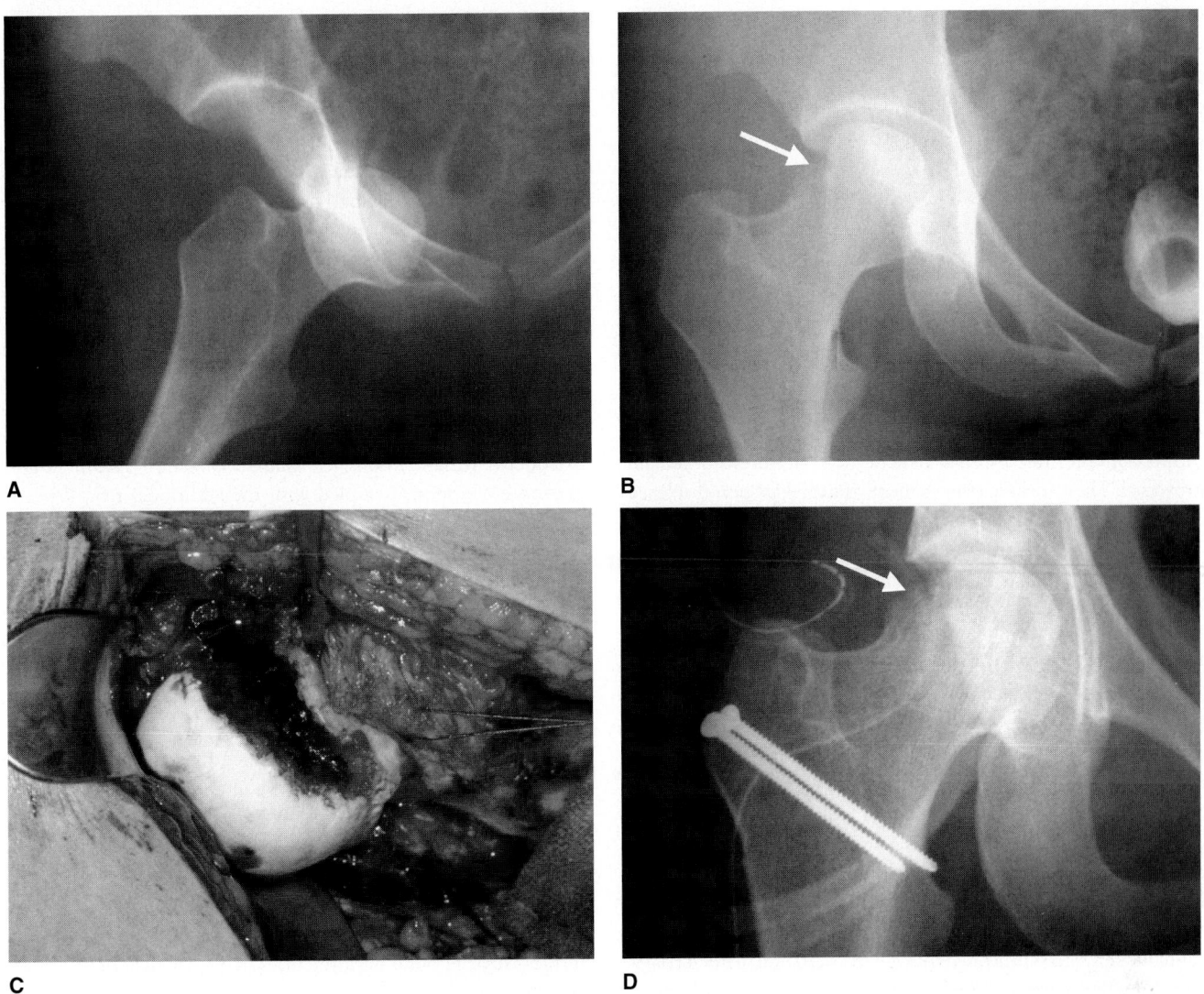

**FIGURE 43-8.** Traumatic posterior hip dislocation in a 25-year-old woman who sustained a high-velocity motorcycle accident (**A**). After closed reduction, a traumatic defect of the femoral head is seen on the a.p. X-ray, classified as a Pipkin type II fracture (**B**; arrow). A trochanteric Ganz osteotomy was performed with a surgical hip dislocation to assess and repair the defect (**C**). Postoperative x-ray shows the partially filled defect by an osteochondral autologous graft (**D**; arrow).

Measures to prevent falls, to reduce their consequences, and to prevent and treat osteoporosis are essential if we are to reduce the tremendous socioeconomic consequences of these injuries in the older population. In contrast, proximal femur fractures represent a rare entity in young patients and are usually the consequence of high-energy trauma. These patients are often severely injured and associated injuries to pelvis, abdomen, and chest are common. Early surgical fixation of proximal femur fractures is important in order to reduce the incidence of posttraumatic complications.[69] Patients with displaced proximal femur fractures usually have significant pain and obvious physical abnormalities, typically shortening and external rotation of the injured limb, with an inability to move the leg significantly because of hip pain, usually felt in the groin. Occasionally, hip fractures are undisplaced. These may be occult with pain and tenderness but no radiographic findings. The distinct anatomical regions of hip fractures which are typically distinguished radiographically include femoral neck fractures (intra-/extracapsular), trochanteric (per-/intertrochanteric), and subtrochanteric fractures.

The location of a hip fracture has important implications for treatment and outcome. In all cases, the goal of surgical treatment is to stabilize the bone sufficiently to allow mobilization of the patient, to minimize the risk of destruction of the hip joint, and also to restore normal anatomic shape of the proximal femur. This is important for normal hip function, which is crucial for most activities of work and daily living. Preoperatively, light skin traction, as with a padded Buck's traction boot, or skeletal traction for more unstable injuries, are appropriate for immobilizing hip fractures until surgery. Traction is not essential for elderly patients with low-energy hip fractures. Nonambulatory patients with osteoporotic bone quality are occasionally best treated nonoperatively.

## Femoral Neck Fractures

Fractures of the femoral neck are generally distinguished as intra- or extracapsular. In the German literature, the corresponding designations are medial and lateral femoral neck fractures. Intracapsular fractures involve the narrow part of the femoral neck just below the femoral head. These fractures are defined as 31-B type by the Arbeitsgemeinschaft für Osteosynthesefragen/Orthopaedic Trauma Association (AO/OTA) classification. They have a high risk of nonunion and of AVN of the femoral head, where the blood supply runs along the neck in extraosseous retinacular vessels that are torn or kinked by displaced fractures.[70-73] Furthermore, the expanding intracapsular hematoma may contribute to further hypoperfusion through compression of the nutrient vessels. These complications are so serious for younger patients that most orthopedic traumatologists consider fractures of the femoral neck in a young person to be a surgical emergency. Urgent anatomic reduction, decompressive capsulotomy, and secure fixation of a displaced femoral neck fracture provide the best opportunity for salvage of the patient's own hip joint.

Despite countless published data from clinical, experimental, and biomechanical studies in the past decades, several aspects on the treatment modalities for intracapsular femoral neck fractures still remain controversial. These include management strategies for non-displaced fractures (nonoperative vs. operative), for displaced femoral neck fractures (osteosynthesis vs. arthroplasty/hemiarthroplasty), timing of surgery, open vs. closed reduction, anatomic vs. valgus reduction, choice of implant, etc., as well as the differing strategies for postoperative rehabilitation and early weight bearing status.

Undisplaced fractures of the femoral neck (Garden types I and II) are generally at risk of secondary displacement and are best treated with internal fixation by minimally invasive procedures, e.g., by percutaneous screw fixation with three 6.5-mm short-threaded cancellous bone lag screws. In such cases where no decompressive capsulotomy is performed, tapping of the intracapsular hematoma for release of intracapsular pressure is advised. Regarding the issue of anatomic versus valgus reduction, recent clinical studies have suggested that in younger patients (age < 60 years) an anatomic reduction leads to better long-term results in Pauwels type I and Garden type II fractures, whereas a valgus reduction is recommended for Pauwels II/III and Garden III/IV type fractures due to the increased risk of a secondary loss of reduction.

A long-term complication of intracapsular femoral neck fractures is represented by the anterior femoro–acetabular impingement syndrome.[74] This syndrome is characterized by a persistent painful loss of motion and progressive joint-destruction due to a flat contour of the anterior head-neck-junction which may cause a cam-type impingement with subsequent damage of the anterior-superior acetabular cartilage adjacent to the rim. Thus, in patients with a healed femoral neck fracture and persisting chronic pain without signs of AVN, the possibility of an anterior femoro-actebaular impingement syndrome caused by retrotorsion of the proximal fragment should be taken into consideration. These symptoms can be relieved by surgical correction of the femoral head-neck-offset through a surgical hip dislocation, as first described by Reinhold Ganz in Switzerland.[75]

Internal fixation of femoral neck fractures usually results in union for young patients with adequate bone density. In elderly osteopenic patients, however, failure of fixation and/or nonunion are more common. Coupled with the additional risk of posttraumatic AVN of the femoral head, these problems render internal fixation less attractive for elderly patients. For these individuals, who are typically less active, a primary hip arthroplasty may be a better alternative. This involves the replacement of the femoral head only (hemiarthroplasty with a bipolar prosthesis) or a total hip replacement in patients with preexisting degenerative joint disease. Recent studies from Europe have suggested that intracapsular femoral neck fractures (Garden types I–III) in elderly patients over 70 years of age may also be treated by closed reduction and percutaneous screw fixation, with about 90% of the patients regaining their preoperative stage of mobility. While this concept may appear promising particularly in elder patients with significant comorbidity as well as from an economic point of view, this concept remains controversial. The current state-of-the-art based on published large meta-analyses recommends a primary joint replacement for displaced intracapsular femoral neck fractures in elderly patients, with an age cut-off somewhere between 65 and 70 years[76-79] (Fig. 43-9).

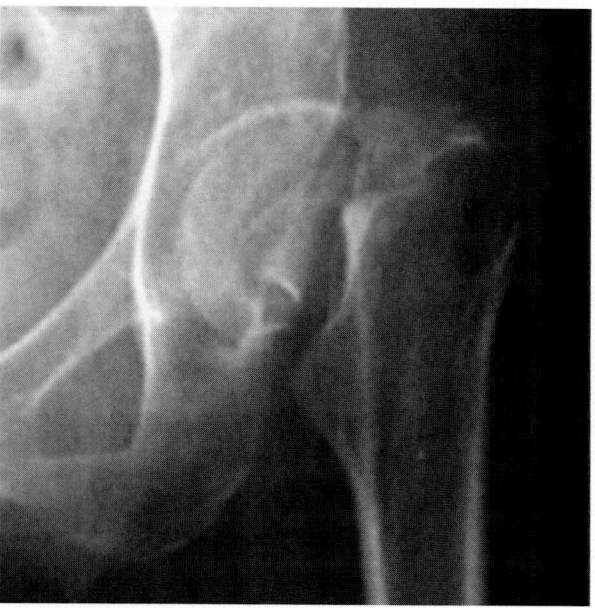

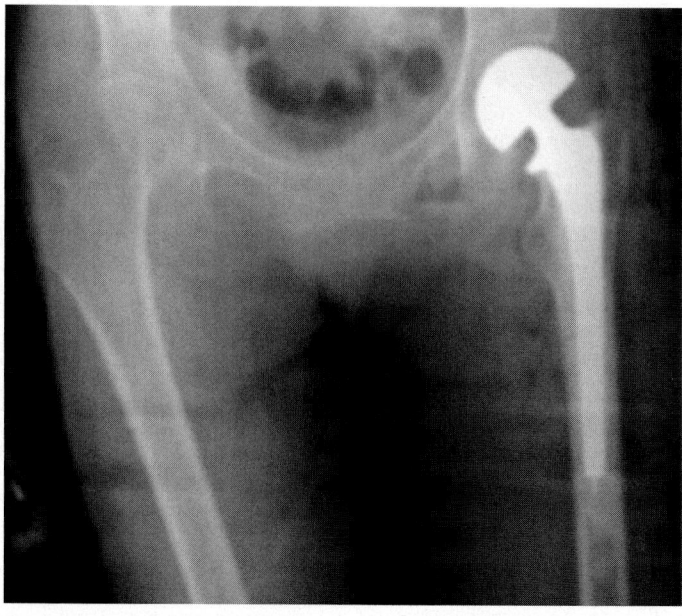

**A**                                    **B**

**FIGURE 43-9.**  Displaced intracapsular fracture of the femoral neck (Garden type IV) in a 75-year-old lady who fell down the stairs in a nursing home **(A)**. The fracture was treated by hemiarthroplasty with a bipolar cemented prosthesis which allows early mobilization with full-weight bearing **(B)**.

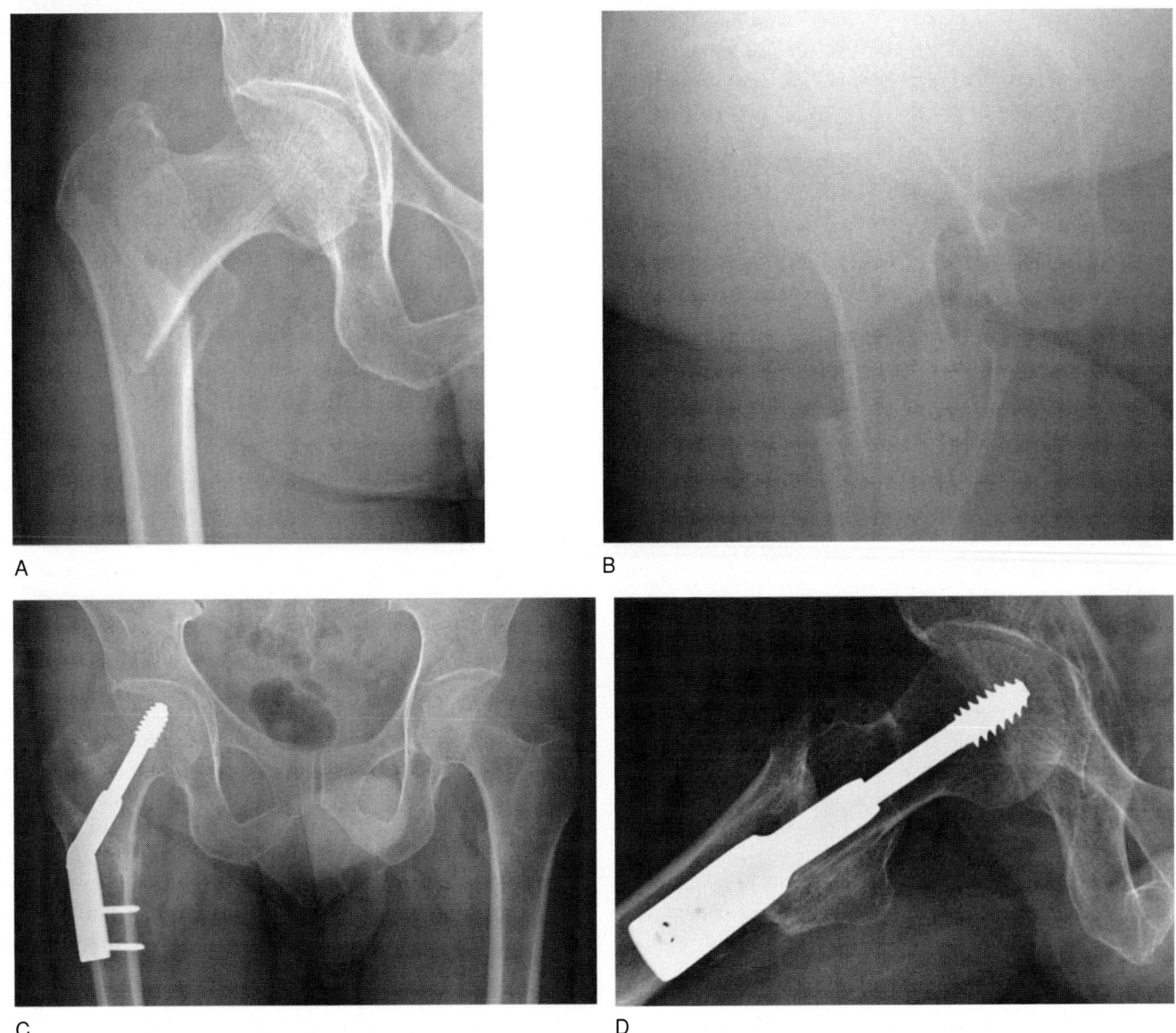

**FIGURE 43-10.** Displaced trochanteric femur fracture (AO/OTA type 31-A2.1) in a 51-year-old construction worker who sustained a fall from a ladder (**A, B**). The fracture was treated by closed reduction and fixation with a dynamic hip screw (DHS). X-rays taken at follow-up after four months show a healed fracture in anatomic position (**C, D**).

Extraarticular femoral neck fractures are less cumbersome to treat than intracapsular fractures and are not generally associated with the above-mentioned complications, such as posttraumatic AVN. The method of choice for stabilization of these fractures is a dynamic hip screw (DHS) and early functional rehabilitation with full weight bearing (Fig. 43-10).

## Trochanteric Fractures

Trochanteric fractures are located distal to the femoral neck and are classified by AO/OTA as the 31-A type. Hereby, a more stable fracture pattern with intact medial cortex/lesser trochanter is defined as 31-A1, whereas increased instability is associated with an avulsion fracture of the lesser trochanter (31-A2), an intertrochanteric—more transverse—fracture pattern (31-A3.2 and A3.3), and a so-called "reversed-type" fracture (31-A3.1) where the fracture line runs 180° converse to the fracture line between the major and lesser trochanters

of the "classical" A2-type fractures. All these fractures require operative stabilization in order to allow early postoperative weight bearing and functional rehabilitation and to avoid the risk of a varus malposition of the hip, which may contribute to the development of early posttraumatic arthritis.

With modern internal fixation devices properly applied, union is typically achieved within three months, with acceptable alignment and a low incidence of fixation failure, for all categories of trochanteric fractures (Fig. 43-10). Fixation is, naturally, more tenuous when osteoporosis is present. The fracture is initially reduced with the aid of a fracture table and image intensifier fluoroscope. Occasionally, actual open reduction is required in order to correct a varus malreduction. While the 31-A1 type represents a typical indication for an extramedullary two-part sliding hip screw, such as a DHS, the more unstable 31-A2 type fractures are generally stabilized either by a DHS or by an intramedullary nail with a sliding femoral neck component, such as the Gammanail or the proximal femoral nail (PFN). Large clinical trials have revealed no difference in outcome and in intra- and postoperative complications when comparing the DHS with intramedullary devices for these types of fractures.[80–83] Overall, the "cut out" rate of the femoral neck screw with requirement for revision surgery lies below a 10% margin in the literature. In contrast, the highly unstable A3-type fractures should generally be stabilized with long intramedullary force carriers to provide optimal stability and reduce the risk of a secondary loss of reduction.

Newer generation implants aimed at reducing the incidence of failure due to "cut-out" of the femoral neck screw by replacing the screw with a twisted blade. Biomechanical testing has suggested an improved "cut-out" resistance of these new implants, such as the trochanteric femoral nail. However, prospective clinical trials which provide a scientific evidence for the superiority of this new generation of intramedullary nails compared to conventional implants are still lacking.

Given the "key" importance of a correct screw position in the femoral head as the most predictive factor for mechanical failure in osteosynthesis for trochanteric fractures, a promising future avenue may consist in the concept of computer-assisted surgery (CAS) for proximal femur fractures. In this regard, preliminary studies have revealed a highly accurate positioning of the screw by CAS in conjunction with about 90% reduced intraoperative radiation time when compared to conventional fluoroscopic guidance.[84,85]

The optimal timing of surgery for trochanteric femur fractures is still an issue of debate. Particularly, the question of whether surgery should be performed at night for these types of fractures remains controversial. While the advocates of urgent circadian surgery postulate an increased incidence in pulmonary and cardiovascular complications due to immobility, stress and pain due to non-fixed fractures, opponents implied an increased risk for iatrogenic complications for nocturnal surgery under suboptimal conditions. Studies which prospectively assessed the outcome depending on the timing of the surgery for proximal femur fractures revealed that—given a medical team with equal qualifications—patients operated at night did not have a significantly higher mortality rate than patients undergoing surgery under more elective conditions during the day. Thus, patients with proximal femur fractures requiring surgical fixation should be operated on as soon as possible, depending on the local circumstances, infrastructural conditions, and the individual patients' comorbidity.

## Subtrochanteric Fractures

Subtrochanteric fractures are classified as a 32-X.1 region by the AO/OTA classification, as opposed to the 31-X type of classification for the trochanteric and femoral neck fractures. In young patients, subtrochanteric fractures result from high-energy forces, typically motor vehicle crashes and falls from heights, and usually extend into the femoral shaft. In accordance to the high-energy trauma mechanism, these young patients are usually severely injured and the traumatic impact is associated with severe soft tissue injuries and bleeding. In contrast, the subtrochanteric fracture pattern in older patients is different due to the usual low-energy mechanism of injury, similar to osteoporotic trochanteric fractures. A less frequent variety of hip fracture, subtrochanteric fractures still represent challenging injuries because of frequent failures of surgical fixation. Significant advances in understanding of

fracture healing and of fixation techniques have improved the management of these fractures. Each of the typical modalities for osteosynthesis of subtrochanteric fractures has its pitfall. When treated by closed reduction and intramedullary nailing, the proximal fragment is difficult to reduce adequately and tends to malreduce in varus position and anteflexion. Often, this problem is overcome intraoperatively by additional cerclage wires, which, however, may contribute to impaired periosteal blood supply to the fracture. The other option is the exact anatomic reduction by ORIF technique using a 95° angular blade plate. Such operative techniques which fully expose the fracture and devascularize bone fragments may produce a "nicer x-ray," but interfere significantly with fracture healing and thus lead to delayed union with loosening or fatigue failure of fixation. The location of a subtrochanteric fracture is important for choosing fixation. If there is a large enough proximal femoral segment to insert a long intramedullary nail, this type of fixation is preferred. If the lesser trochanter is intact, a standard proximal interlocking configuration can be used. If the lesser trochanter is involved, the usual proximal locking screw has insufficient anchorage, and a cephalomedullary ("reconstruction-type") nail is used instead, with locking screws inserted proximally into the femoral head. If the fracture involves the nail entry site, special care is required for intramedullary fixation. A blade-plate or screw-plate device, with indirect reduction technique, may be easier and more reliable.

Although technically demanding, indirect reduction techniques with blade-plate or screw-plate devices can leave the fracture site undisturbed and yield predictable healing without bone grafting or high risk of fixation failure. The key to such procedures is that they maintain the soft tissue envelope around the fracture site, thus providing an improved biologic environment for healing. This concept was recently advanced by the introduction of angular-stable locking plates for the proximal femur, which can be applied in a less-invasive technique and do not compress the bone, thus leaving periosteal vascularization intact.

## Rehabilitation of Patients with Proximal Femur Fractures

For all patients with hip fractures, the goals of surgery include maximal restoration of function, maintaining low morbidity and mortality, while rapidly mobilizing the patient out bed. Modern surgical techniques usually achieve these ends. Elderly patients may not be able to limit their weight bearing. Therefore, hemiarthroplasty, which offers greater mechanical stability than fracture fixation of osteopenic femoral neck fracture, may be the more appropriate treatment for these intracapsular fractures. Although today's hip screw devices generally permit weight bearing for patients with intertrochanteric fractures, significant osteoporosis or comminution may require protection until fracture consolidation has occurred. In young patients, limited weight bearing is generally easy with crutches and is routinely advocated initially. Early rehabilitation thus typically involves teaching the patient to do transfers and gait to the point of documenting safe ambulation with crutches or walker. Range-of-motion and strengthening exercises are routine. Depending on the injury and operative treatment, the patient may need to avoid certain activities such as loading the significantly flexed hip or crossing the legs in a way that might lead to prosthetic dislocation. Nutritional supplementation, prophylaxis against deep vein thrombosis, monitoring and managing intercurrent medical and psychiatric problems, and, in some cases, formal geriatric rehabilitation programs are also beneficial for patients with hip fractures.

Early stability of a repaired fracture depends on the quality of reduction, and of fixation, as well as bone density. These factors cannot be assessed by radiographic appearance alone and are not constant from patient to patient. No one is in a better position to judge them than is the surgeon who did the original fixation. Unless union occurs within a reasonable period, any fracture fixation implant will inevitably fail. For subtrochanteric fractures, this may take six to nine months or more. For these reasons, the operating surgeon remains an essential part of the patient's rehabilitation team and should direct graded progression of weight bearing and resumption of activities while maintaining personal follow-up.

## Fractures of the Femur Shaft

Femoral shaft fractures invariably represent severe injuries due to high-energy trauma and are associated with a significant blood loss of up to 1500 to 2000 mL. An isolated femur shaft fracture alone can be the cause of a traumatic-hemorrhagic shock. Most patients, however, suffer severe associated injuries to the torso, pelvis, and to soft tissues. Thus, every femoral shaft fracture must be appraised as a highly critical, potentially lethal injury pattern. Early fixation of femur fractures is essential, in order to avoid or reduce the incidence of complications such as fat embolism syndrome, acute lung injury (ALI), and the more severe and potentially lethal ARDS. Furthermore, early fracture fixation pays tribute to the intrinsic load to the patient by reducing stress and pain, which represents an important cardiovascular risk factors and may contribute to secondary deterioration of traumatic brain injuries due to increases in intracranial pressure.[15,19,86–88]

Intramedullary nailing of a femoral shaft fracture was performed for the first time by the German surgeon Gerhard Küntscher in November 1939. Despite the revolutionary innovation introduced by this new "biological" osteosynthesis, intramedullary nailing of long-bone fractures has fallen into oblivion for several decades and had its "renaissance" only in the late 1980s by the introduction of solid and cannulated nails. Currently, the concept of closed reduction and fixation with a reamed interlocked intramedullary nail represents the "gold standard" for the treatment of femoral shaft fractures (Fig. 43-11). This procedure is associated with about 99% union rates in the literature, a low complication rate, and the possibility of early functional aftercare with weightbearing. Intramedullary nailing provides generally reliable fixation for any femoral fracture with sufficient intact bone proximally and distally. Interlocking screws were adopted to improve control of comminuted fractures. Intramedullary reaming permits use of a larger-diameter nail with larger diameter locking bolts. Small femoral medullary canals may not permit insertion of an implant with sufficient strength and durability to avoid the risk of fixation failure. As a result, reaming has generally been routine. Awareness of intravasation of reaming debris (fat, bone marrow fragments, inflammatory mediators, etc.) has led to concerns that their embolization to the lung might increase the risk of pulmonary complications and induce ALI and ARDS. Clinical trials and experimental animal studies in recent years have ended the year-long debate on the clinical relevance of reaming the

intramedullary canal as opposed to using unreamed femoral nails. The current consensus implies that the reaming procedure does not increase the risk of intra- and postoperative pulmonary complications.[46,47,89] Thus, the reamed interlocking nail represents the current standard of care for femoral shaft fractures.

Further controversy exists on the optimal entry point of intramedullary nails (piriformis vs. trochanter). While the piriformis nails bear a theoretical risk of AVN due to iatrogenic injury to the nutrient artery,[90] and for an intraoperative femoral neck fracture due to an incorrect entry-point (too anterior and too medial), clinical trials have failed to prove a benefit in outcome for the femoral nails with a trochanteric entry point. A newer generation of trochanteric femoral nails has improved the design with regard to a more anatomic bending radius of 150 cm (as opposed to 120 cm in conventional nails) and a 6° angle of the proximal nail segment which allows insertion through the major trochanter. Future clinical studies will have to determine the potential benefits of these new implants, compared to the conventional piriformis nails, with regard to outcome.

Severely injured polytrauma patients (ISS > 17) as well as patients with a concomitant chest trauma (AIS for chest wall or lung injury > 2 pt) or significant head injury (GCS ≤ 13) should be treated by the damage control orthopedics (DCO) procedure, as described above. This implies an early fracture fixation by closed reduction and external fixation, followed by conversion to an intramedullary nail during the "time window of opportunity" between day 5 and 10 after trauma. A few highly critical patients with head or chest injuries and persisting morbidity due to increased intracranial pressure or ventilatory problems (ALI/ARDS) may be candidates for a minimal-invasive "biological" plating of femur shaft fractures, preferably by the use of modern angular-stable locking plates. This modality strictly avoids any potential "second hits" to the injured brain or the pulmonary endothelium caused by the intramedullary insertion of femoral nails.

Intramedullary nailing has been demonstrated to be a safe treatment modality also for open femur fractures (grade I, II, and Gustilo IIIA). Patients with severe open femoral shaft fractures (Gustilo grades IIIB and IIIC) need individualized decisions about fixation techniques. Preferably, external fixation represents a safe modality for early stabilization of these severe open injuries, followed by conversion to an internal fixation (nail or plate) at the time of definitive soft tissue coverage.

## Fractures of the Distal Femur

The osteosynthesis of supracondylar (AO/OTA type 33-A) and transcondylar distal femur fractures (type 33-C) has represented a significant challenge for a long time, due to high complication rates. A problem unique to these fractures is the loss of fixation of the distal femoral fragment, particularly in osteoporotic bone, by the use of conventional implants, such as the condylar buttress plate. Both the conventional plate osteosynthesis as well as intramedullary nailing procedures were associated with high rates of primary or secondary loss of reduction, malunions, nonunions, and infections. The recent emphasis on more "biological" approaches with minimally invasive techniques in conjunction with the development of angular-stable implants which allow the percutaneous placement of locking head screws has resulted in improved outcomes.[91–93] These include increased union rates without the need for additional bone grafting and decreased rates of infection and loss of reduction by the

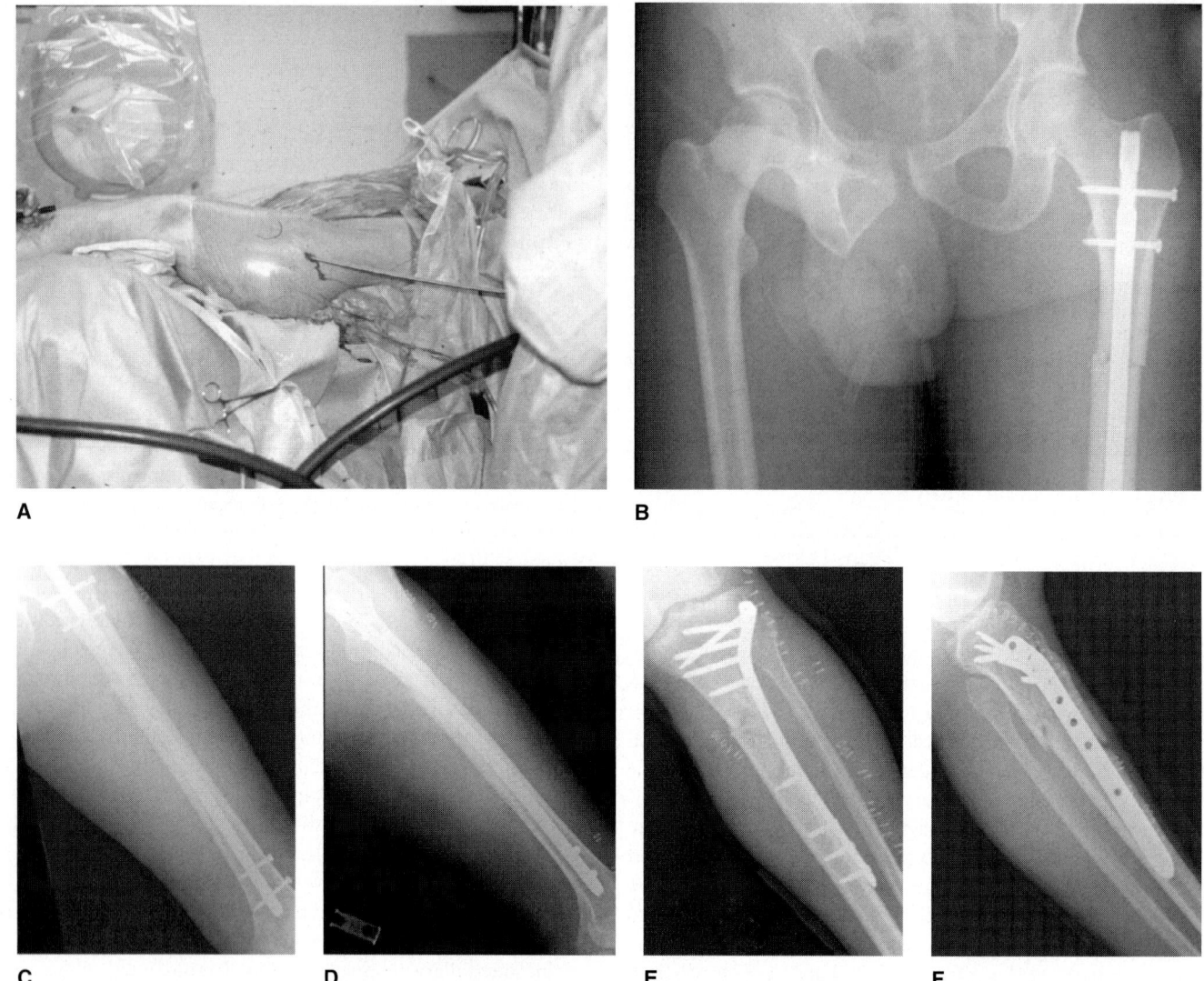

**A**

**B**

**C**        **D**        **E**        **F**

**FIGURE 43-11.** "True" percutaneous femoral nailing technique by the use of a cannulated femoral nail, which is reamed through a small 1-cm proximal skin incision **(A)**. This 51-year-old polytraumatized patient sustained a transverse femur shaft fracture (AO/OTA 32-A3), which was treated by closed reduction and stabilization with an interlocked cannulated femur nail **(B, C, D)**, and an ipsilateral, comminuted meta-diaphyseal proximal tibia fracture (AO/OTA 41-A3.3), which was stabilized by a minimally invasive locking plate **(E, F)**. Both measures are considered "biological" techniques since they spare the soft tissue envelope by the use of minimal invasive skin incisions.

use of minimal-invasive or less-invasive locked plating techniques or retrograde intramedullary nails (Fig. 43-12).

Generally accepted principles of management for articular fractures include anatomic reduction and fixation of the articular surface, with sufficiently stable fixation to permit immediate active and/or passive motion of the joint, and delayed weight bearing until the articular surface has recovered and the fracture has healed sufficiently. A classical implant developed in the 1960s by Maurice Müller in Switzerland is the 95° condylar blade plate which provides sufficient stability for treatment of distal femur fractures.[94,95] However, the technique of blade plating requires a high level of skill and experience and may result in failure if not applied properly (Fig. 43-13).

Partial intraarticular fractures of the femoral condyles (AO/OTA types 33-B) are usually treated by open reduction and internal screw fixation, in order to ensure anatomic reduction of fractures of the articular surface. A typical example is the "Hoffa fracture" which corresponds to a coronal split of the femur condyle (B3 type). Extra-articular components in C-type fractures can

often be managed by indirect reduction techniques to restore proper alignment of the articular segment to the limb, relying on proper use of specialized, minimal- or less-invasive implants, such as the new generation locking plates.

Much interest has developed in retrograde intramedullary nail fixation for distal femoral fractures. These nails are inserted in a minimal-invasive fashion via the knee joint, into the intercondylar notch of the distal femur, and across the fracture site (Fig. 43-12). Fractures of the articular surface must be reduced and fixed first, with precautions to avoid displacement or interference with hardware as the nail is inserted and its distal and proximal locking screws are placed. Retrograde femoral nail techniques and implants are still evolving. Operations to fix distal femoral fractures can pose formidable technical challenges, especially for the surgeon who does not frequently treat such injuries, with one of the major pitfalls being a malreduction of the distal fragment in varus/valgus or retrocurvatum. However, with appropriate application, this technique is suitable for all fractures of the distal third of the

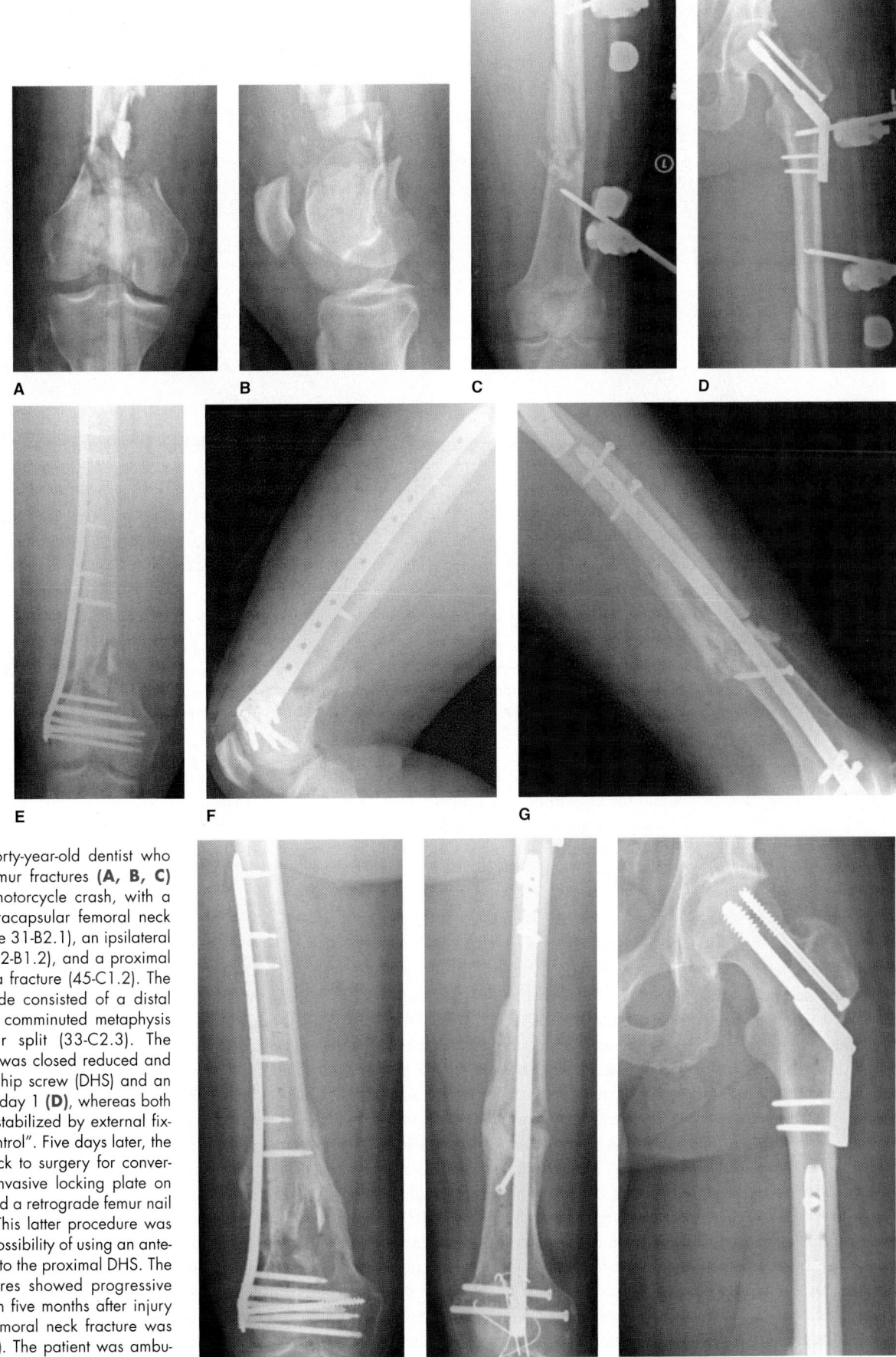

**FIGURE 43-12.** Forty-year-old dentist who sustained bilateral femur fractures (**A, B, C**) after a high-energy motorcycle crash, with a nondisplaced left extracapsular femoral neck fracture (AO/OTA type 31-B2.1), an ipsilateral femur shaft fracture (32-B1.2), and a proximal pole transverse patella fracture (45-C1.2). The injury on the right side consisted of a distal femur fracture with a comminuted metaphysis and an intraarticular split (33-C2.3). The femoral neck fracture was closed reduced and fixed with a dynamic hip screw (DHS) and an anti-rotation screw on day 1 (**D**), whereas both femur fractures were stabilized by external fixation for "damage control". Five days later, the patient was taken back to surgery for conversion to a minimally invasive locking plate on the right side (**E, F**) and a retrograde femur nail on the left side (**G**). This latter procedure was chosen due to the impossibility of using an antegrade nail secondary to the proximal DHS. The bilateral femur fractures showed progressive callus formation within five months after injury (**H, I**) and the left femoral neck fracture was healed at this time (**J**). The patient was ambulating with full-weight bearing bilaterally and a free range of motion of both knee joints.

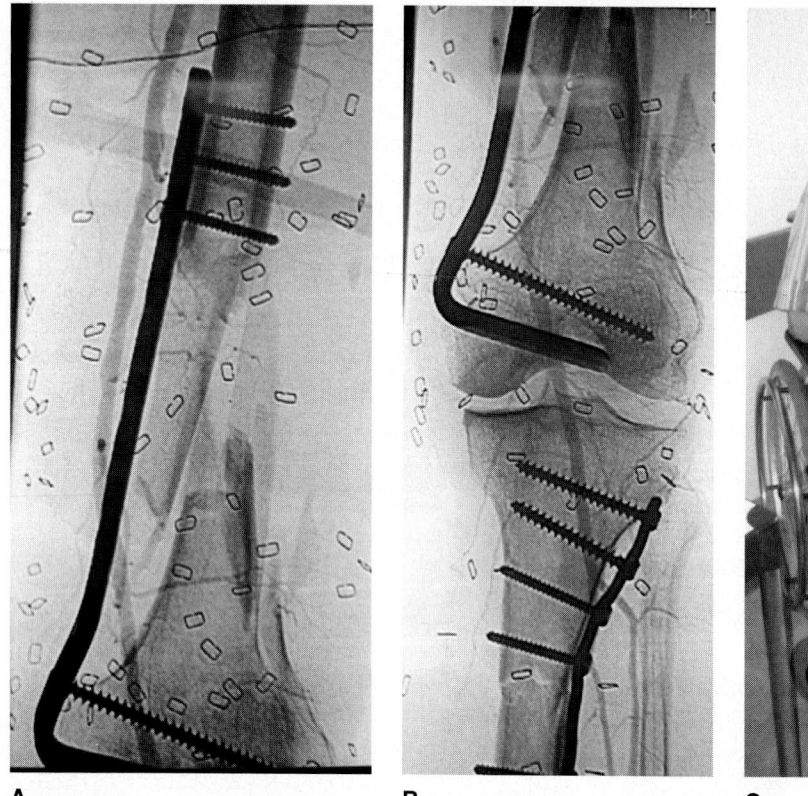
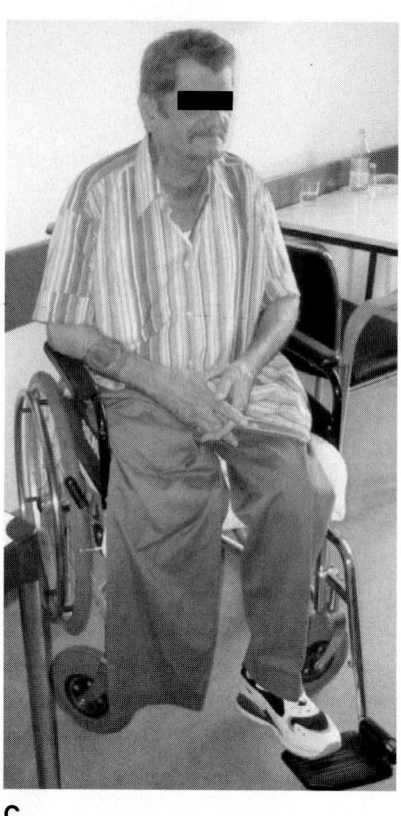

**A**          **B**          **C**

**FIGURE 43-13.** Wrong technique of plating for an open (Gustilo-Anderson grade IIIB) distal femur shaft fracture in a 55-year-old patient with an ipsilateral proximal tibia fracture and a "floating knee." The 95° condylar blade plate—which is designed for lateral insertion for fixation of distal femur fractures—was applied medially through the open wound, leading to a nonreduced fracture and an acute vascular compromise of the femoral artery, as revealed by the postoperative angiography **(A, B)**. Inadequate intraoperative decision making in conjunction with an inappropriate surgical technique led to chain of complicating events which ultimately resulted in an above-knee amputation of the injured extremity **(C)**.

femoral shaft including highly unstable bicondylar fractures without damage to the soft tissues and the knee joint. The primary aim of all surgical techniques applied for fixation of distal femur fracture consists in an early functional rehabilitation, preservation of knee joint range of motion, and an uneventful fracture healing.

## Fractures of the Patella

Patellar fractures are classified according to the classification system published by Speck and Regazzoni from Switzerland.[96] These injuries usually result from a direct blow to the flexed knee. Displaced transverse fractures lead to a loss of continuity of the extensor mechanism, which produces extension of the knee both by pulling through the patella (via quadriceps tendon proximally and patellar ligament distally) and through the medial and lateral patellar retinacula. Nonoperative treatment is recommended for undisplaced fractures with a clinically intact extensor mechanism, i.e., in those cases where the patient can raise the fully extended leg against gravity. In contrast, a surgical treatment by ORIF is indicated in all cases with a compromised extensor mechanism as well as in displaced fractures with an incongruity of the articular surface. Depending on the exact fracture type, location, and the amount of comminution, repair may involve ORIF by lag screws, tension banding, and rarely by primary partial or total patellectomy. In all cases, the patellar retinacula must be repaired. Treatment of a patellar fracture should allow early range of motion of the knee, but weight bearing on the flexed knee must be prevented

until healing is sufficient to tolerate the powerful tensile stresses produced by the quadriceps muscle. The usual postoperative concept consists of mobilization with touch-down bearing for four to six weeks and early limitation of knee flexion to about 60°, with progressive increase in the range of motion to about 90° until the fracture is consolidated.

## Knee Dislocations and Ligamentous Injuries

Knee dislocations may involve either the patello–femoral or the tibio–femoral joints. Lateral patellar dislocations typically occur in adolescent females with a genu valgus alignment. True tibiofemoral dislocations are much less common and generally require significant injury forces, although occasionally they are caused by a simple slip and fall. They are important to recognize because of extensive ligamentous disruption and risk of associated neurovascular injuries. A high level of suspicion for these associated injuries is mandatory when evaluating a patient with a tibiofemoral dislocation and the potential for limb loss due to a missed blunt injury to the popliteal artery must be kept in mind.

Patellar dislocations are usually lateral and involve indirect stresses applied by the patient pivoting on or forcefully extending a flexed knee in valgus. A hemarthrosis or effusion soon develops. Recurrent patellar dislocations are not infrequent, because anatomic abnormalities are often predisposing factors. The dislocated patella is palpable laterally, though it may have been reduced by straightening the knee for immobilization or x-ray. Closed reduction, if necessary, is obtained by passively extending the knee, flexing the hip to relax the rectus femoris, and applying medially directed pressure to the patella. Immobilization for four to six weeks allows healing of the medial retinacular tear that typically accompanies an initial dislocation, although acute repair of the medial patellofemoral ligament may be considered. Recurrent dislocations should be evaluated for elective surgical reconstruction.

Complete knee dislocations usually produce obvious deformity and difficulty moving the involved joint, as well as a radiographically evident dislocation, usually anteriorly or posteriorly, but sometimes medially or with rotation to any quadrant. Multiligamentous injuries in the knee with similar neurovascular concerns may be present without obvious deformity on exam or x-rays. It is often stated that these injuries are dislocations that have spontaneously reduced. Knee instability may be due to a purely ligamentous injury or may involve both ligament disruption and a fracture of the proximal tibia, typically a marginal avulsion (so-called "Segond fracture" or Moore type III fracture dislocation) or a fracture of the medial tibial condyle (Moore type I fracture dislocation).[97] Gross instability of the knee in more than one direction is the key diagnostic finding. With a torn articular capsule, hemarthrosis may be absent. With time, however, periarticular swelling is usually evident. Instability of the knee should always be considered when a patient presents with evidence of acute distal neurovascular compromise. A knee dislocation should be reduced as soon as possible after recognition. This can usually be done by traction and gentle manipulation in the ED.

The early recognition of an associated popliteal artery injury is crucial, which has been described in the literature in 14% to 34% of all cases with traumatic knee dislocations. While a complete arterial disruption may be obvious early after trauma due to clinical signs of peripheral ischemia, an incomplete dissection or intimal injury by stretching forces may be missed. Intimal tears can lead to delayed thrombosis and secondary limb ischemia in spite of the absence of apparent early clinical evidence for a vascular injury. Due to the often asymptomatic nature of blunt popliteal injuries, the amputation rate for blunt vascular trauma is about three times higher than after penetrating injuries and lies in the range of 15% to 20%. Thus, a high index of suspicion is required for blunt popliteal injuries in all cases of knee dislocation and defined algorithms should help establish early and an accurate diagnosis early on. Any pulse deficit or measurable reduction in ankle–brachial Doppler-assisted arterial pressure index, before or after manipulation, should be considered evidence of a vascular injury. This includes the reported absence of pulses at the accident site even when pulses return to normal after reduction of the knee dislocation. Based on large meta-analyses in the literature, the accuracy of pulse examination alone is very low, yielding a sensitivity of only about 79% for the detection of an arterial injury.[98] The five clinical "hard signs" for an arterial injury, which are present in about two-thirds of all cases, include:

Active or pulsatile hemorrhage

Presence of a pulsatile or expanding hematoma

Diminished or absent peripheral pulses

Bruit or thrill over the popliteal fossa, implying an AV-fistula

Clinical signs of limb ischemia

In cases of a suspected arterial injury, either an (on table) arteriography or a surgical exploration are mandatory, since observation alone will have detrimental consequences for the patient. Injuries to the peroneal or tibial nerve, with motor and/or sensory impairment, may be associated with an arterial occlusion. Such neurologic lesions also interfere with recognition of ischemic pain due to arterial occlusion or an acute compartment syndrome.

A popliteal artery injury associated with dislocation of the knee is repaired in the operating room with both vascular and orthopedic surgeons present. Adequate reduction and stabilization of the knee dislocation is required, and external fixation is well suited for provisional stabilization. A simple external fixator, connecting two self-drilling pins in the femur to two similar pins in the tibia with a bridging bar anterior to the knee, can be applied so rapidly that it will not delay arterial repair. It can readily be adjusted to allow intraoperative motion of the knee, should that help with vascular repair, and furthermore provides a nonconstricting splint for postoperative immobilization and protection of the vascular graft. With regard to ligamentous injuries, the currently favored concept of treatment consists of an early, but not immediate, surgical repair. While the incision for arterial repair must be chosen by the vascular surgeon, consideration should be given to the exposure required for secondary ligamentous repair and whether or not this might safely and appropriately be combined with the emergency vascular repair. Trauma teams that treat these relatively rare injuries may manage them more effectively by developing collaborative protocols for knee dislocations with concomitant injuries to the popliteal artery. Below-knee four-compartment fasciotomy is routinely advisable after popliteal artery repair in order to avoid a secondary compartment syndrome due to ischemia-reperfusion injuries.

Ligamentous and meniscal injuries without dislocation of the knee may occur in multiple trauma patients or as isolated injuries. Hemarthrosis, swelling, pain, tenderness, and impaired motion of the joint are typical findings. If a knee cannot be examined initially because of adjacent fractures, ligamentous stability must be assessed as soon as those fractures are stabilized. Associated knee injuries are not uncommon with femoral or tibial fractures and particularly when both are present in a so-called "floating knee." Inability to passively extend the knee suggests a mechanical block, usually a meniscal tear, whereas instability indicates a ligamentous injury. Both knees should be examined for comparison, because individuals have different amounts of intrinsic laxity. Initial examination of the knee requires x-rays to rule out associated fractures. Aspiration of a tense hemarthrosis under sterile conditions can relieve pain. Complete evaluation may also require arthroscopy or magnetic resonance imaging (MRI) to identify ligamentous or meniscal injuries, but such studies are rarely needed emergently. Although many acute ligamentous injuries of the knee can be treated nonoperatively, major reconstructions may be required to restore function. Accurate diagnosis of ligamentous injuries is crucial for planning appropriate treatment. Relatively infrequent disruptions of the posterolateral ligamentous complex should be repaired within the first two weeks. Isolated ruptures of the medial collateral ligament do well with nonoperative management in a hinged knee brace. Delayed reconstruction is often advisable for disruptions of the cruciate ligaments, unless avulsed with a bone fragment, e.g., in combination with Moore-type fracture dislocations of the tibial head.

## Fractures of the Tibia

Proximal Tibia. Proximal tibia fractures are differentiated as extra-articular metaphyseal fractures (AO/OTA 41-A type), intraarticular tibial plateau fractures (41-B/-C types and Schatzker classification), and fracture dislocations (Moore classification). While the typical split-depression type fractures (Schatzker type I-III) of the lateral condyle are usually due to low-energy, indirect valgus-stress mechanisms of injury, the more severe bicondylar fractures (Schatzker type V and VI) and fracture dislocations (Moore type I-V) are mainly due to direct high-energy forces with significant soft tissue compromise and a risk for acute compartment syndrome.[97] Those fractures are inherently unstable, difficult to reduce and stabilize, and associated with a high rate of complications, such as malreduction, secondary loss of reduction, infections, and nonunions. Isolated fractures of the medial condyle (Schatzker type IV and Moore type I) are more rare and often require special approaches for adequate reduction and stabilization, e.g., by a direct posterior approach[99] (Fig. 43-14).

For the accurate diagnosis of a tibial plateau fractures, routine x-rays of the knee should be complemented by a CT scan with two-dimensional reconstruction, in order to allow an adequate planning of surgical approaches and fixation strategies. Undisplaced proximal tibial fractures can usually be treated with early motion and touch-down weight bearing in a hinged knee brace for six to twelve weeks. The need to stabilize a severely injured limb, especially in a multiply injured patient, can be met initially with a spanning external fixator. Significant deformity of the articular surface, instability, and/or displacement are frequent indications for surgical treatment. To be successful, this must achieve stable fixation and early motion of an anatomically reduced articular surface. Unless these goals can be met, the results of surgery are typically worse than those of nonoperative care. The recent availability of angular-stable locking plates has enabled less-invasive approaches and diminished

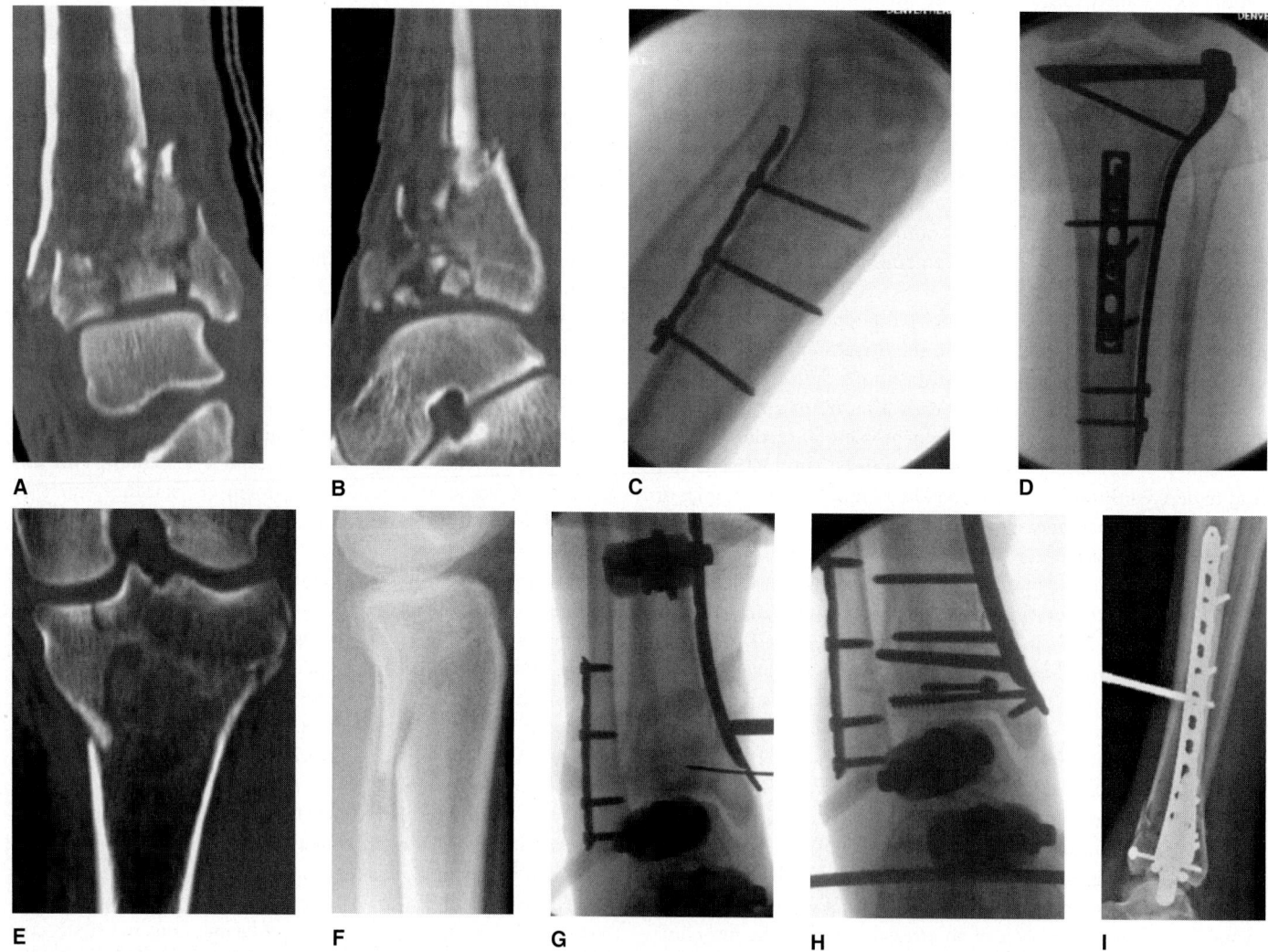

**FIGURE 43-14.** Bilateral complex tibia fractures in a 52-year-old lady who sustained a collision as a car driver against a truck. She sustained a severely comminuted tibial pilon fracture on the right side (AO/OTA 43-C3; panels **A, B**) as well as a contralateral, unstable bycondylar tibial head fracture (Schatzker type V; panels **E,F**). Both injuries were initially immobilized in an external fixator due to the critical soft tissue conditions. Once the soft tissue swelling subsided within 10 days, the fractures were converted to internal fixation. The bycondylar tibial head fracture was stabilized through a direct posterior approach with a posterior anti-glide plate and completed by a lateral buttress plating with a locking plate (**C, D**). The pilon fracture was stabilized by initially fixing the fibula for correct length and rotation and by open reduction of the articular part of the pilon fracture with two lag screws and minimal-invasive osteosynthesis with a locking plate (**G, H, I**). The patient recovered well without postoperative complications and was non-weight bearing bilateral for 10 weeks.

the requirement for primary bone grafting of metaphyseal defects. For example, intra-articular fractures of the lateral plateau (Schatzker type I-III) are nowadays frequently treated by less-invasive procedures, whereby the adequacy of articular reduction is intraoperatively assessed by arthroscopic or fluoroscopic control.

Tibial Shaft.    Fractures of the tibial shaft range from low-energy, indirect torsional injuries that do well with nonoperative treatment, to severe high-energy fractures with severe soft tissue damage and a high incidence of acute compartment syndrome. The amount of energy absorbed by the leg is suggested by the radiographic appearance of a fractured tibia. The severity of the soft tissue injury, whether open or closed, is most important for the overall outcome of tibial shaft fractures. For example, the presence of severely crushed soleus and gastrocnemius muscles make a plastic coverage of an open tibia fracture by a local rotational flap impossible. The soft tissue envelope on the medial border of the tibia is very thin; thus, minor open fractures may have major therapeutic implications for covering the exposed bone, ranging from skin grafts, to local or free microvascular flaps, to a lower limb amputation.

Compartment syndromes develop frequently in tibial shaft fractures due to direct compression forces. They are especially common if the soft tissues have been crushed or if a period of ischemia has occurred. The initial symptom is out of proportion leg or ankle pain to the physical signs and exacerbated by passive motion of the ankle and toes. Indurated swelling of the calf and, occasionally, the foot is noted. Hypesthesia of the foot and reduced motor strength are due to ischemia of the muscles and nerves within the calf compartments and represent late signs of a (missed) compartment syndrome. Skin perfusion and distal pulses remain intact until late in the evolution of compartmental syndromes, since the obstruction, within the involved spaces, is to capillary rather than arterial flow. The diagnosis is made clinically. Measurements of intracompartemental pressures are required in obtunded or comatose patients and to rule out compartment syndrome in unclear or borderline cases. The treatment for an acute calf compartment syndrome is immediate decompression by a four-compartment fasciotomy, which is performed with medial and lateral incisions.

Timing and treatment modalities for tibial shaft fractures are dependent on the severity of injury and associated problems. Limb-threatening complications such as open fractures, vascular injuries, and a compartment syndrome require immediate surgery. In absence of such complications, a provisional closed reduction and application of a long leg cast provide initial immobilization. In tibial shaft fractures of minor severity and dislocation, closed treatment is the method of choice.[100] Weight bearing begins as tolerated in the long leg cast, proceeding to a patella-tendon bearing short leg cast or brace, as soon as patient comfort and stability of the fracture permit. Although this approach can succeed, with more severe tibial shaft fractures, it is often associated with delayed union, deformity, and prolonged disability. Surgical fixation, which provides better control of alignment and allows motion of the foot and ankle, as well as the possibility of earlier weight bearing, is more appropriate for these injuries. Intramedullary nailing is the fixation of choice.[101] The indications for intramedullary nailing (Fig. 43-15) is increasingly expanding to more proximal and distal metaphyseal fractures due to the availability of new generation interlocking nails which allow three-dimensional interlocking in very proximal and distal areas of the tibia. One of the important risks of extending the indication for tibia nails to the proximal and distal metaphysis is a malalignment in valgus or varus, unless fractures are reduced adequately, e.g., by the use of blocking screws.

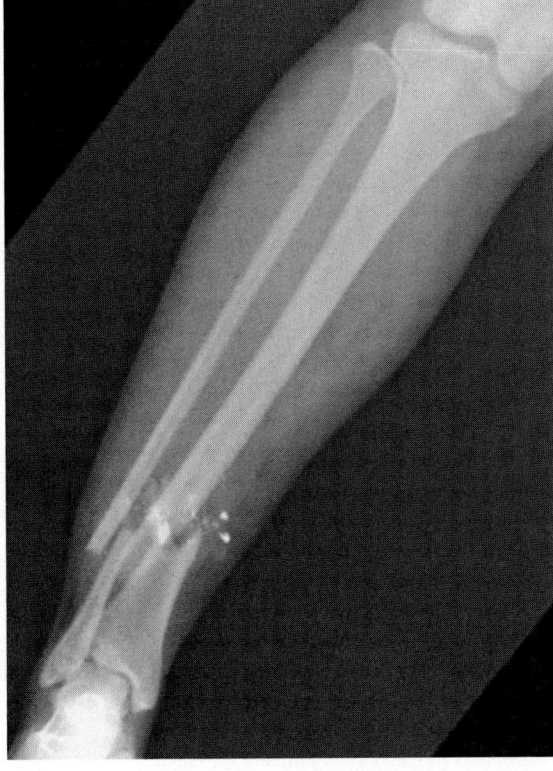
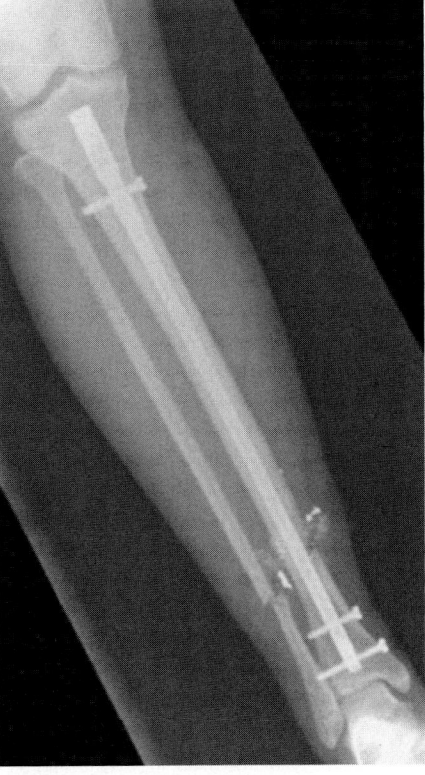

**FIGURE 43-15.** Nineteen-year-old girl who was accidentally shot in the right leg as a victim of a drive-by shooting. She was immediately taken to the OR and treated by local wound debridement and intramedullary fixation of her tibial shaft fracture. She did not have any neurovascular injuries. Her postoperative course was uneventful and she was allowed to ambulate with weightbearing as tolerated. No postoperative infection occurred.

A

B

Reaming of the tibial medullary canal permits use of nails with large enough diameters to provide adequate fixation for most tibial shaft fractures. Such nails have large enough diameters to permit the use of locking screws of adequate strength to ensure definitive control of alignment. The strength and fatigue life of smaller-diameter unreamed nails, and especially of their small-diameter locking screws, is not sufficient for keeping the reduction of tibial fractures throughout their healing period.[101–103] Thus, the unreamed tibia nail has been associated with a high risk of complications, such as breaking locking bolts, malunion, and nonunion. Multiple large clinical trials have demonstrated, that both the non-operative treatment and unreamed nailing strategies have the highest incidence of nonunion and malunion, as opposed to fracture fixation by reamed cannulated nails. Intramedullary nailing was furthermore shown to be an adequate treatment option also for open fractures, from grade I up to Gustilo grade IIIB.[104]

External fixation is still a valuable technique for selected tibial fractures. These include high-energy trauma with significant soft tissue injury, vascular injuries requiring repair, and in the setting of polytrauma patients, as a "damage control" procedure. External ring fixators may furthermore be applied for segment transport in situations with significant bone loss, and for correction of malunions and nonunions. Long-term use of an external fixator (>14 days) is associated with bacterial colonization of the pin tracts and a risk of infection from subsequent intramedullary nailing. Use of an external fixator for only a few days, however, can safely precede intramedullary nailing for definitive management of tibial shaft fractures.

A variety of fixator designs are available, with no clearly established proof that one is better than another. Generally, transfixion pins or wires are used only in the very proximal or distal zones of the tibia, and "half-pins," screws with long shafts inserted through the subcutaneous anteromedial surface of the tibia are used to anchor the external fixator frame (Fig. 43-16). Leaving the external fixator in place until the fracture is healed helps prevent the typical complication of late loss of alignment, commonly seen with premature removal of the fixator. Early posterolateral bone grafting may be advisable to accelerate union of tibial shaft fractures with primary bone loss (Fig. 43-3).

Plate fixation of acute fractures of the tibial shaft is generally reserved for periarticular injuries too proximal or distal for intramedullary nailing. If severe injuries to soft tissue are present, such plating involves a significant risk of sloughing of the incision and/or infection. Techniques of plating that emphasize gentle handling of soft tissues, the avoidance of devascularizing flaps, and use of indirect reduction methods can further reduce the risk of surgical complications of plate fixation. Locking plates that allow less-invasive or minimal-invasive plating techniques are ideal for bridging comminuted metaphyseal fractures which may be too proximal or too distal for intramedullary nailing techniques (Fig. 43-17).

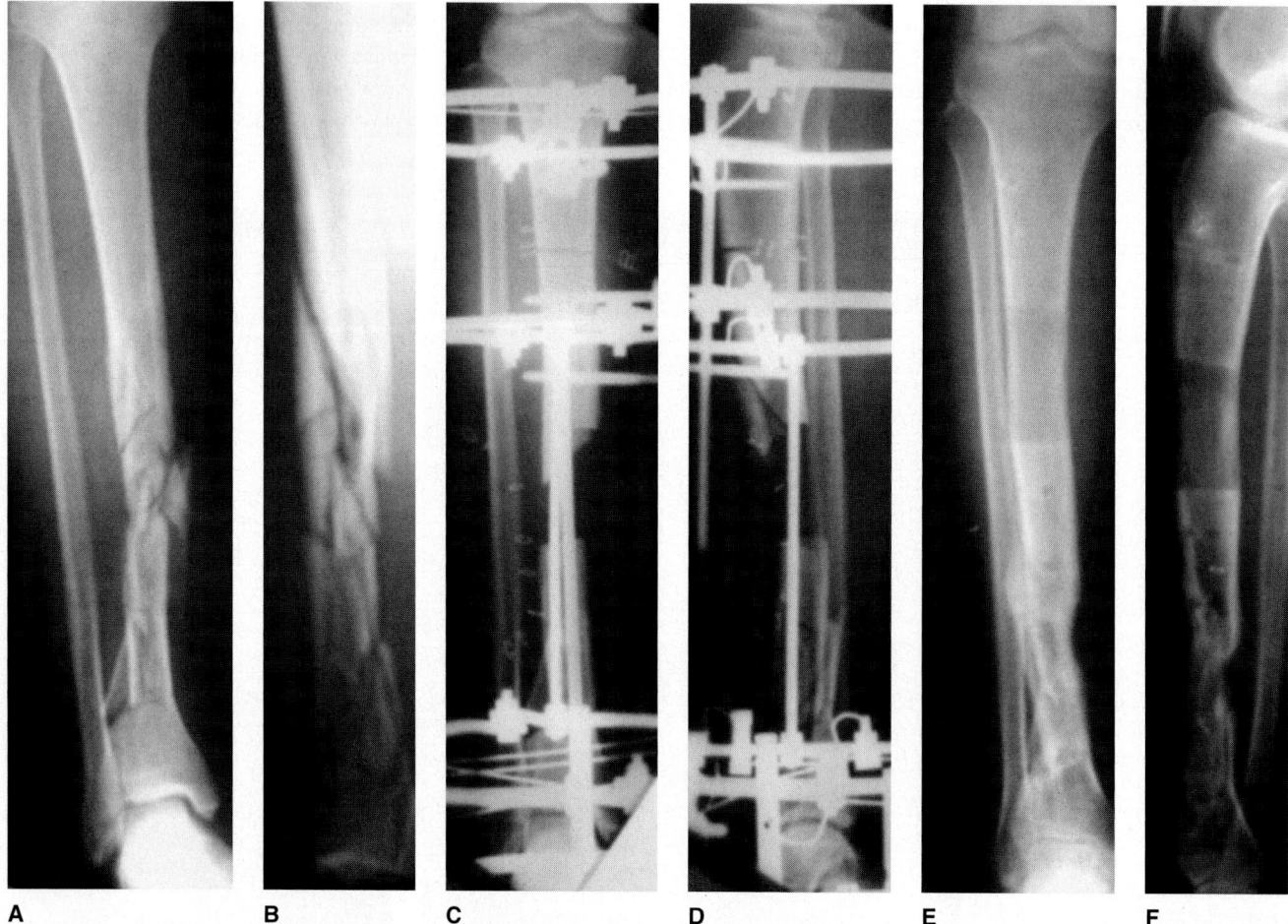

A          B          C          D          E          F

**FIGURE 43-16.**   Segment transport using an external Ilizarov frame in case of a severely comminuted and contaminated tibial shaft fracture **(A, B)**. After a proximal corticotomy **(C, D)**, the bone loss was replaced by means of a distraction osteogenesis, and the distal docking site healed uneventfully **(E, F)**.

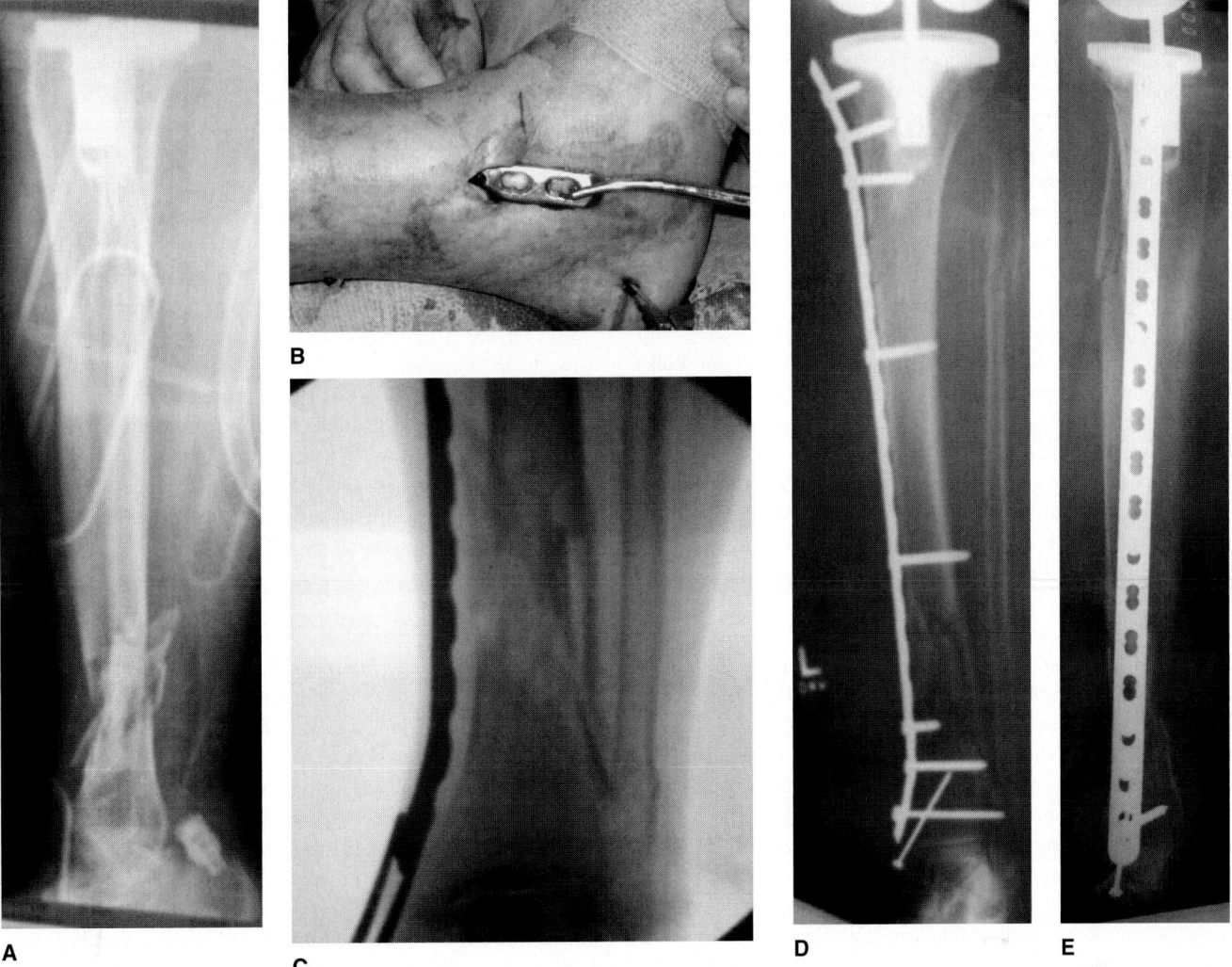

**FIGURE 43-17.** Combination of a comminuted distal tibia shaft fracture with an ipsilateral periprosthetic proximal tibia fracture **(A)**. The fractures were treated by minimal-invasive angular-stable osteosynthesis with an internal plate fixator by fluoroscopic control of the reduction **(B, C)**. This locking plate allows the placement of unicortical screws in the area of the periprosthetic fracture **(D)** and bridging of the zone of comminution **(D, E)**.

Pilon Fractures.    Tibial pilon fractures are highly challenging intra-articular injuries of the distal tibia which are typically caused by axial loading forces with concurrent distortion and of the ankle, leading to a disruption of the tibial articular surface by the twisted and rotated body of the talus. Pilon fractures are classified as AO/OTA types 43-B (partial intraarticular) and 43-C (complete intraarticular) (Fig. 43-14). These fractures typically involve a significant damage to soft tissue, whether or not an open wound is present. Traditional ORIF techniques have a high risk of wound dehiscence and infection, particularly if surgery is performed during the phase of posttraumatic inflammation and soft tissue swelling within the first days after trauma. Clinical studies have revealed an improved outcome of tibial pilon fractures when staged procedures were applied, such as early external fixation and later conversion to ORIF once the soft tissue swelling has subsided.[105–109] The concept of definitive surgery for pilon fractures involves a standard technique in four "classical" steps, according to Sommer and Rüedi: (1) plating of the fibula for anatomic length of the lower leg; (2) anatomic reconstruction of the tibial articular surface; (3) bone grafting of the metaphyseal gap; and (4) buttress plating of the distal tibia. Depending on the degree of comminution,

the individual bone quality and on the extent of soft tissue compromise, the postoperative rehabilitation of pilon fractures is either by early functional aftertreatment or by immobilization in a lower leg cast for about six weeks. As for all metaphyseal fractures, weight bearing status must be restricted to touch down weight bearing until the fracture is healed, usually for 10 to 12 weeks.

## Ankle Injuries

Overall, ankle injuries represent the most frequent musculoskeletal injuries.110 The ankle is a hinge joint, in which the body of the talus dorsiflexes and plantarflexes within a mortise-like socket formed by the distal tibia (medial malleolus and plafond) and distal fibula (lateral malleolus). Integrity of the mortise is maintained by the ligamentous connections between tibia and fibula, just above the ankle joint (anterior and posterior syndesmosis). Widening of this mortise results in talar instability, which predisposes to posttraumatic arthritis. The lateral malleolus is the prime determinant of talar alignment. Restoration of its proper relation with the distal tibia is "key" to treating malleolar injuries. This may require anatomic ORIF of a displaced lateral malleolar fracture and/or restoration of the disrupted syndesmosis by returning the fibula precisely to its location adjacent to the tibia. Stable, minimally displaced lateral malleolar fractures can be managed nonoperatively with closed treatment, typically with about six weeks of immobilization, followed by rehabilitative exercises to restore the range of motion. If the syndesmosis is unstable, it will need to be temporarily fixed with a syndesmotic screw until ligamentous healing is secure, usually for six weeks.[111] Medial ankle disruptions may involve the medial malleolus, which should be reduced and fixed, or the deltoid ligament, which need not be repaired if the remainder of the joint is reduced and repaired properly. The posterior lip of the tibial plafond, the so-called "posterior malleolus" or Volkmann's triangle, is frequently fractured in malleolar injuries. The designation of a "trimalleolar" fracture implies those injuries which involve the posterior tibial plafond in addition to the medial and lateral malleoli. Large posterior tibial plafond fractures of more than one-fifth of the articular surface should be reduced and fixed to avoid posterior subluxation of the talus and/or incongruency of the joint. Malleolar fractures are produced by indirect forces, generally caused by the body's momentum when the foot is planted on the ground in one of several typical positions. Depending on the position of the foot and direction of motion, typical combinations of fractures and ligamentous injuries result, with progressively greater damage and displacement, up to and including talar dislocation. Knowledge of these patterns improves the surgeon's understanding and treatment of such injuries. The basic principle of treatment remains open reduction of displaced injuries, with anatomic reduction and rigid fixation. If significant displacement is present, prompt closed reduction is urgent, while definitive fixation can be delayed, depending on the quality of the individual soft tissue situation. As with pilon fractures, significant swelling is an indication for a delay in surgery to decrease complications with wound healing. Some authors have suggested a staged protocol for complex ankle fractures with significant soft tissue compromise, with initial closed reduction and transarticular pin-fixation, followed by delayed ORIF once the soft tissue swelling has subsided.[112] The soft tissue envelope about the ankle and foot is thin, with little muscle coverage. This renders simple lateral malleolar fractures susceptible to significant soft tissue complications, including skin necrosis, wound dehiscence, and infections. Open fractures of the malleoli may require a microvascular free-flap transfer due to the bad quality soft tissue coverage and the impossibility of local rotational flap in this distal area of the leg. Recognition and appropriate management of open ankle injuries is essential to minimize complications and avoid adverse outcome, which may require a below-knee amputation. This notion emphasizes again, as mentioned above for the pilon and tibial shaft fractures, the "key" aspect of the soft tissues for uneventful fracture healing.[106]

Ligamentous injuries of the ankle most commonly involve the lateral collateral ligament complex, which provides inversion stability of the talus within the mortise. Inversion of the foot normally occurs at the subtalar joint, between the talus and calcaneus. If forced to the limit, however, the lateral collateral ligament stretches or ruptures, producing the typical "sprained ankle" with lateral pain, swelling, and ecchymosis and tenderness over the injured ligament distal and anterior to the lateral malleolus. Minor ankle sprains can be treated symptomatically, with restricted activities, elevation, ice, and support as needed for comfort. More severe sprains require immobilization and/or crutches for comfort and to decrease the risk of late instability, which is manifested by recurring episodes of "giving way" of the ankle. After a brief period of rest, most injuries to the lateral collateral ligament of the ankle are effectively treated with a functional brace.

Since it is difficult to differentiate a simple sprain from a fracture in the acute phase, due to nonspecific symptoms such as pain, tenderness, and swelling, a precise diagnosis usually requires adequate radiographs. A "true" anteroposterior view of the ankle (so-called "mortise" view) requires internal rotation of about 15–20° to position the joint axis, which runs between the tips of the two malleoli, in a plane parallel to the x-ray film. The mortise view and a lateral view are usually sufficient to adequately diagnose most ankle fractures. Oblique views and foot x-rays may be required to identify more occult or associated injuries, such as a base of the fifth metatarsal avulsion fracture, lateral process of talus ("snowboarder's injury"), or anterior process of calcaneus fractures.

## Fractures and Dislocations of the Foot

Injuries of the foot typically result from a direct blow or crushing force. Extreme dorsiflexion or plantarflexion and rotation outward (pronation) or inward (supination) can also produce significant bony and joint injuries of the foot. These injuries may be unrecognized or underestimated, especially in a multiply injured patient, and a delay in definitive treatment may compromise outcome (Fig. 43-18). Disability due to a significant foot injury is often far greater than that resulting from more dramatic injuries to long bones. Open fractures may result from crushing injuries, which can severely damage the surrounding skin envelope, as well as from lacerations and gunshot wounds. Neurovascular structures and tendons may be involved, and their function must be carefully assessed with any injury. Compartment syndromes occasionally develop due to severe crush mechanisms; however, they are much rarer in the foot than in the lower leg.

A swollen, tender, or painful foot following trauma should be assumed to be a fracture or dislocation until proven otherwise. Radiographs must be obtained to demonstrate suspected or obvious fractures and to locate possible foreign bodies. Major injuries such as tarso-metatarsal dislocations often have subtle x-ray findings, while less severe fractures may be quite obvious. Fractures of the talus and calcaneus result from a direct blow to the plantar surface, usually transmitted through the heel. Undisplaced and extra-articular fractures of the calcaneus can be managed nonoperatively. Improved surgical approaches and fixation techniques, coupled with detailed demonstration of the pathologic anatomy of calcaneal fractures provided by CT scanning, have focused surgical treatment on restoration of the typical posttraumatic varus deformity as well as reconstruction of the frequently involved subtalar articular surface (so-called "posterior facette") and the calcaneo-cuboideal joint.[113] Interestingly, large prospective trials have impressively shown that the nonoperative treatment of displaced intra-articular calcaneus fractures yields similar long-term results as in operative cases where the articular surfaces have been anatomically restored. Furthermore, operative interventions bear a high risk for severe soft tissue complications, since the surgical approach typically dissects through the thin skin envelope over the lateral calcaneus. For this reason, ORIF

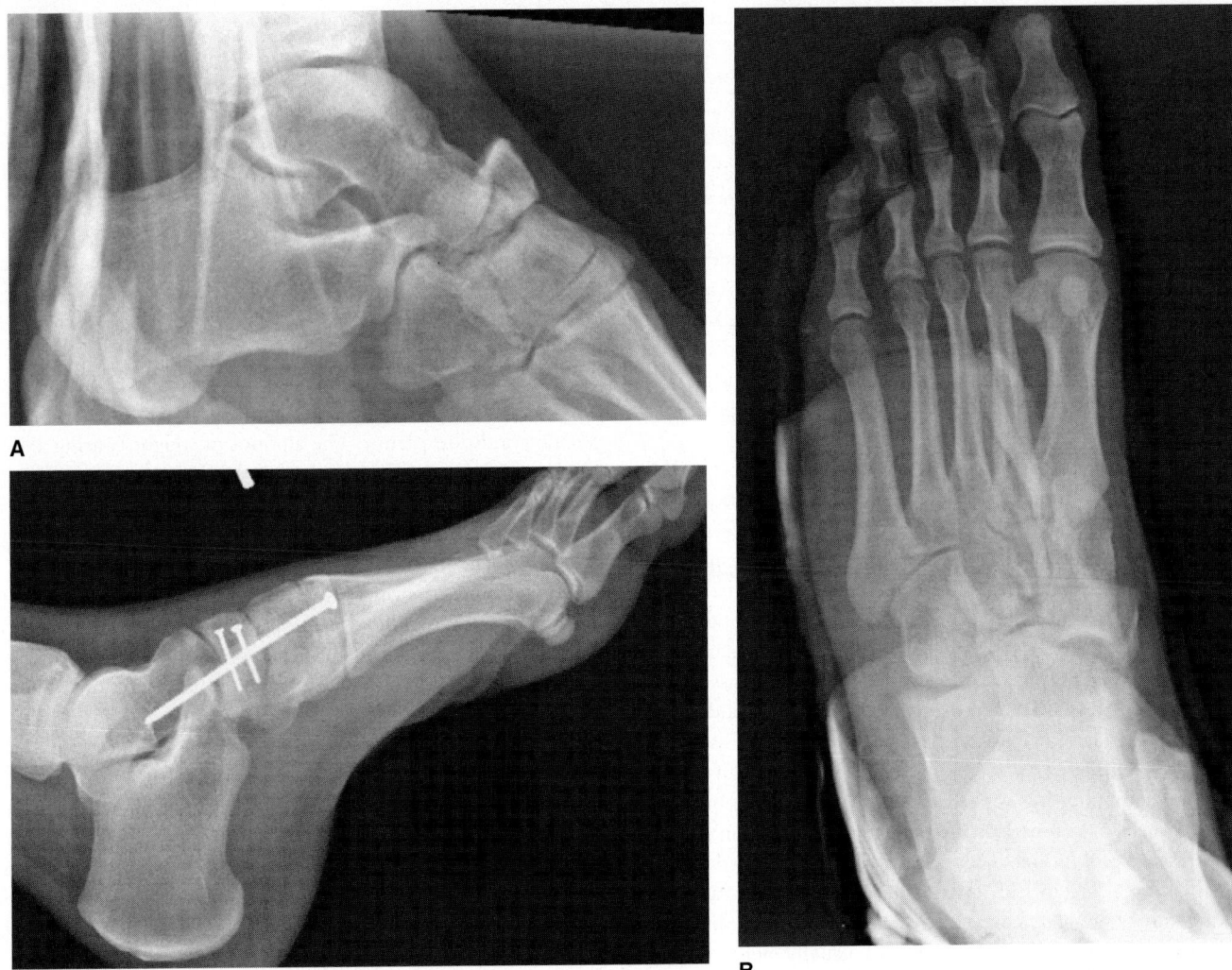

**FIGURE 43-18.**   Combined navicular fracture-dislocation and metatarsal I Lisfranc dislocation of the left foot **(A, B)** in a severely injured polytrauma patient. The foot injury was treated by open reduction and internal fixation of the navicular fracture with two 2.0-mm Mini-AO screws and a 3.5-mm joint-transfixing screw as temporary arthrodesis **(C)**. This screw was removed after three months and the patient could walk with full-weight bearing without pain.

should be delayed until soft tissue swelling is completely resolved. This may take up to two to three weeks for severely displaced and comminuted calcaneus fractures.[114–116]

Displaced fractures and fracture dislocations of the talus require precise reduction and rigid fixation with an interfragmentary screw. Displaced talar neck fractures represent a surgical emergency due to the high risk of posttraumatic AVN. This risk gradually increases with the severity of injury, as graded by the Hawkins classification (I–IV). Posttraumatic arthritis and AVN may require an ankle fusion in the end-stage.[117]

Isolated, minimally displaced, or undisplaced metatarsal fractures are treated nonoperatively. Treatment options include a hard-soled stiff shoe, a brace or cast for comfort, with weight bearing allowed as tolerated. Displaced midfoot fractures and dislocations require anatomic reduction, which is best done by an open technique. Typical fracture dislocations at the Lisfranc or Chopart joints require open reduction and internal fixation by temporary arthrodesis, usually with small-fragment or mini-fragment screws for about three months. While dislocations of a toe should be reduced promptly, phalangeal fractures generally require little specific treatment. Open fractures of the foot are treated with debridement,

repair of critical structures, and fixation of fractures as needed to preserve stability and alignment. Loss of skin at the foot represents a serious problem, which can be addressed in part with skin grafting but may require free-tissue transfer or even amputation. Mangling injuries of the toes are usually treated with primary amputation.

## REHABILITATION

Rehabilitation after injury to a lower extremity begins as soon as possible and must have a multidisciplinary approach to provide the physical, emotional, and other needs of the patient. Physicians, therapists, psychologists, and other orthopedic health care workers such as orthotists and social workers are normally involved. The patient's pre-existing medical status; other injuries; physiologic and psychological condition; status of family, friends, home environment, vocational, and recreational opportunities; and available supporting resources must all be considered in addition to the magnitude of the injury to the lower extremity. The general goals are to maximize the functional potential remaining after injury through correcting limb deformities, maximizing muscle strength and motor control, while minimizing the risk and severity of any complications. However, specific realistic goals must be outlined for each patient's rehabilitation including appropriate functional endpoints and a timeline for their achievement. Depending on the injury, many months may be required for complete recovery. Stiffness and contractures should be avoided after a significant injury to a lower extremity. A contracture occurs when a body part is stiff in a nonfunctional position (e.g., an equinus position plantarflexion of the ankle), which interferes with standing and walking. Effective splinting and range-of-motion exercises can prevent or minimize such problems, unless severe neuromuscular problems such as spasticity from injury to the brain or spinal cord are present. In such cases, surgical release of contractures and/or surgery to eliminate or redirect deforming forces (tendon releases, lengthening, or transfer) may be required.

Immobilization may be required to maintain reduction of the fracture, to facilitate wound management, or to avoid contractures. For more severe injuries, internal or external fixation is generally preferred over traction, casts, or splints, although these may be required as supplements. Whenever possible, joints outside the injured zone should not be immobilized. Great care must be taken to avoid focal pressure over bony prominences, particularly the heel, the malleoli, the patella, and the proximal fibula with its closely related peroneal nerve. Extra noncompressible padding of casts or splints is required in these locations. Room for swelling must always be provided for acute injuries. The patient with a rigid or circumferential dressing applied to a fresh injury must be carefully monitored for compartmental ischemia, often first indicated by progressive discomfort. Casts and splints may need to be changed, and reinforcement is often required for walking casts.

Wounds may be safely covered with casts. Blood staining of a fresh postoperative cast is common and usually benign after extremity surgery. Increasing pain, a foul odor, or a patient with impaired pain sensation, however, requires inspection of the incision or wound. Immobilization may need to be continued until an unstable wound has healed.

Injured extremities can often be immobilized with removable, bi-valved casts or splints, thus permitting supervised or assisted motion of joints that might otherwise become stiff from disuse. Such motion should begin as soon as possible and can rapidly progress, limited only by the protection necessary for unstable injured tissues. If active motion is not possible, passive movement can be provided by the patient, the therapist, or by a continuous passive motion (CPM) machine. Additionally, exercises for strengthening weakened muscles are important, particularly in patients whose injuries are severe and whose recovery will be slow. These can initially involve isometric muscle contractions, with progressive resistance exercises as recovery permits. The assistance of physical therapists, under direction of the orthopedist, is invaluable especially when patients are unable to undertake their own rehabilitation. Rehabilitative exercises, especially passive motion and positioning to avoid contractures, must begin as soon as possible in the acute care setting and should never be deferred "until transfer to rehabilitation."

Mobilization of the patient is as essential as is that of the injured limbs. As soon as the medical condition and skeletal stability permit, upright posture should be encouraged. At first, this may require elevation of the head of the bed or use of a "mobilizer" chair. Significant passive and/or active exercises are not only helpful but are required for bed-bound patients unless prohibited by an elevated intracranial pressure or other injury. An overhead frame and trapeze should always be provided for a patient with an injury to a lower extremity unless unstable injuries of the spine or upper extremities make use of a trapeze unsafe. As soon as the patient's condition permits, transfers from bed to chair are encouraged. The level of assistance for transfers must be specified, based on the patient's abilities and skeletal stability. Transfers may be accomplished with total assistance, with a sliding board that eliminates the need for lower extremity weight bearing, by standing and pivoting on a sufficiently stable leg, or by nearly normal ambulation, depending on safety.

Ambulation is the eventual goal of treating a fracture of a lower extremity and should begin as soon as the patient's injuries and general condition permit. The amount of weight bearing allowed for an injured limb must be specified. For articular injuries, weight bearing may need to be minimal for three months or more. For practical purposes, it is impossible to walk without allowing full weight bearing on at least one leg. Similarly, the status of the spine and upper extremities must be considered. A patient who cannot or must not bear significant weight on his or her arms cannot use them for transfers, for arising from a chair, or for crutches or a walker to assist with ambulation. Rather than complete avoidance of weight bearing, limited loading of an injured leg can facilitate rehabilitation and may actually decrease the stress on the injured limb compared with strict non-weight-bearing. Instructions for partial weight bearing should specify how much weight is allowed.

Prosthetic rehabilitation of the individual who has undergone an amputation of a lower extremity begins before the amputation, when possible, with exercises and discussions about the forthcoming prosthesis. Ambulation begins as soon as possible after amputation as the immediate postoperative use of a prosthesis has proved effective in reducing the time to definitive prosthetic fitting and limb maturation. A cast is advisable for below-knee or more distal amputations, and sometimes this can be adapted for weight bearing if stability of the wound permits. Control of edema is provided by elastic supports and the leg is elevated when the patient is not walking. Definitive fitting of a prosthesis should be accomplished in a matter of weeks rather than months.

Common problems obstructing rehabilitation include poor nutritional status, urinary tract infections, impaired bladder control, and pressure sores. Patient assessment to provide adequate nutrition, prophylaxis for pressure sores such as regular turning and padding of pressure points, and avoiding prolonged urinary catheterization and basic hygiene can help to prevent the above problems from occurring.

## LATE COMPLICATIONS

### Nonunion

A diagnosis of nonunion is made when there is failure of complete healing within a six to nine month time period following definitive fracture care. Fractures have different expected time periods of healing depending on the type of fracture and the location. Tibia fractures are relatively slow healing, particularly open fractures. Femur fractures heal more rapidly. Nonunions complicated by bone loss, significant malalignment, or infection are extremely difficult challenges for the patient and surgeon (Fig. 43-19). Treatment to gain union may require two to five years and numerous operations.

Nonunions are categorized as hypertrophic, normotrophic, and atrophic. These distinctions are critical in that they describe the underlying cause of the nonunion and therefore point toward correct treatment options. Hypertrophic nonunions are fractures that have failed to heal in spite of a good local blood supply and obvious formation of callus. Mechanical stabilization alone usually produces union in this situation. Normotrophic nonunions show minimal callous formation but no bony resorption. These need mechanical stabilization and some improvement of the local biology, usually by local autogenous bone grafting. Atrophic nonunions show little or no callus formation and have local bone resorption. The atrophic nonunion has poor local blood supply and will require rigid mechanical stabilization, local bone grafting, and in many cases resection of dead bone and flap coverage. If the bone resection is significant, distraction osteogenesis with a ring or monolateral transport external fixator will be necessary. If deformity coexists with a nonunited fracture, both problems should be addressed simultaneously, if possible.[118]

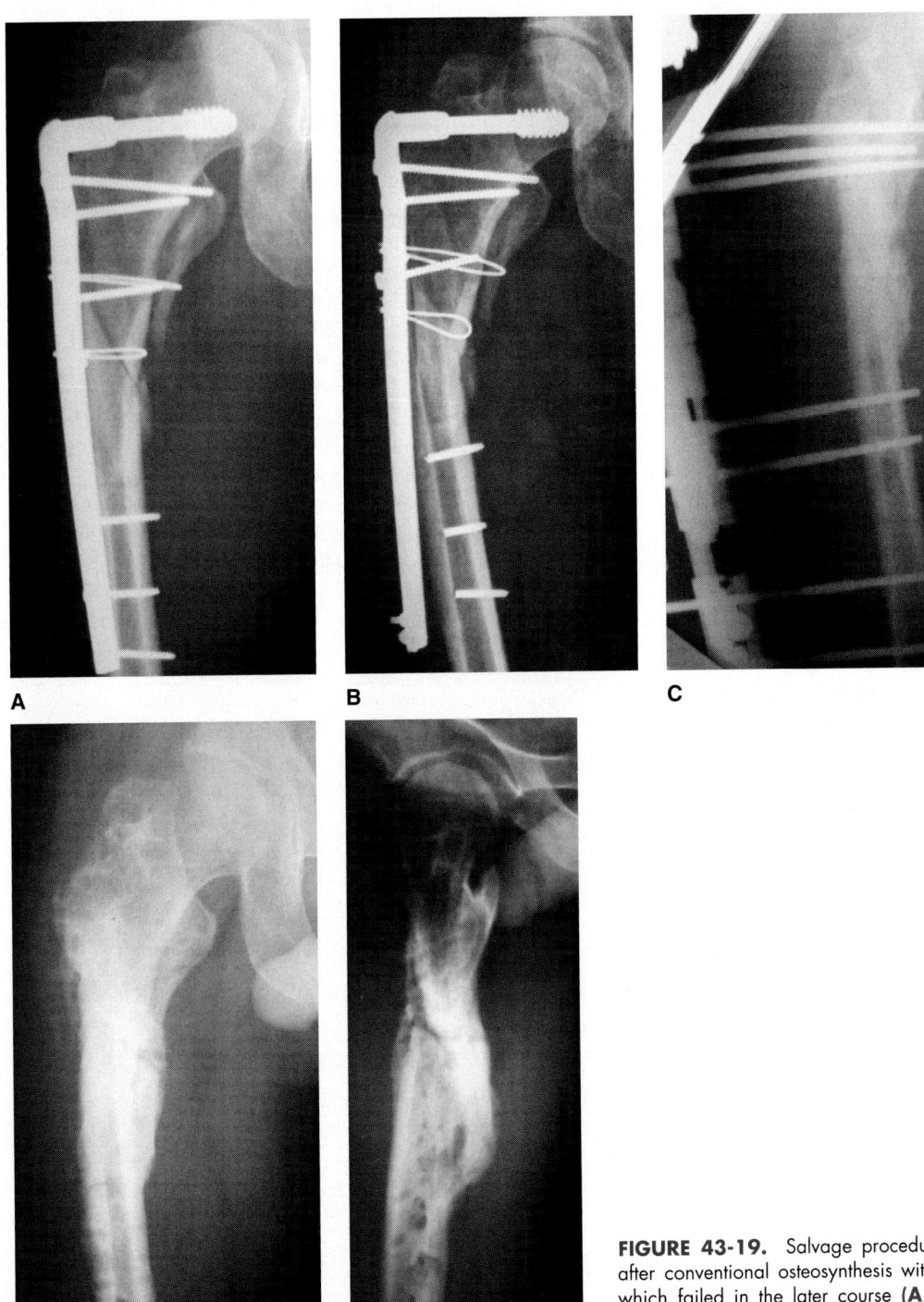

**A** **B** **C** **D** **E**

**FIGURE 43-19.** Salvage procedure of a subtrochanteric femoral nonunion after conventional osteosynthesis with a dynamic condylar screw (DCS) plate, which failed in the later course **(A, B)**. During revision surgery, an infected nonunion was apparent. The patient was therefore treated by antibiotics and the nonunion was fixed in a unilateral fixator under compression **(C)**. A healed fracture with strong callus formation was evident on x-ray six months after revision surgery **(D, E)**.

## Malunion

Malunion involves shortening, angulation, and/or malrotation following fracture. While some amount of shortening is well-tolerated, shortening greater than 2 cm in the lower extremity requires a built-up shoe to equalize leg length for stance and gait. Elective limb lengthening, contralateral extremity shortening and even amputation are surgical alternatives to a significant leg length discrepancy. A variety of techniques are available using external fixators or specialized lengthening intramedullary nails to regain limb length.

Rotational and angular deformities may be better tolerated in the femur than in the tibia. Varus or valgus deformity may be cosmetically unacceptable and can produce knee and ankle symptoms that warrant corrective osteotomy. Significant deformity may also predispose to progressive osteoarthritis from asymmetric loading of joints. Malunion of hindfoot or metatarsal fractures may result in painful weight bearing, requiring osteotomy for realignment, with or without arthrodesis of adjacent joints.

## Sequelae of Joint Trauma

Stiffness, ankylosis, and contracture may follow an injury to a joint or to the proximal muscles that control it. Direct injury to articular cartilage, joint malalignment, or incongruity increases the risk of post traumatic arthritis. Significant arthritis leads to pain with weight bearing and eventually loss of normal functional activities, necessitating joint replacement or fusion.

Anatomic reduction and early motion of injured joints provides the best chance of preventing posttraumatic arthrosis. Unfortunately, perfect postoperative reductions do not guarantee perfect functional outcomes. Factors out of the control of the surgeon such as cartilage damage occurring at the time of injury, soft tissue injuries and post injury psychological distress have significant impact on the overall outcome.

Flexion contractures of the hip, knee, and ankle may occur in patients who do not perform frequent prophylactic extension stretching exercises of these joints. This is particularly true for intensive care patients who remain intubated for extended periods of time. Equinus ankle contractures predictably develop if appropriate splinting and stretching exercises are not provided for the posterior calf muscles. Flexion contractures of the toes may follow injuries to the leg and foot. Passive toe stretching is required to ensure adequate dorsiflexion for normal gait. Toe clawing is the result of contractures of the leg and/or foot muscles following injury, scarring, traumatic neuropathy, or ischemic contractures from a compartment syndrome. Surgical correction may be required. Prevention of contracture with appropriate splinting and early exercises is more effective than late correction.

Traumatic arthritis may develop in any injured joint. While ankle and subtalar joint arthrosis is usually evident within a year, the hip and knee may require several years before symptoms are significant. Rapid deterioration of the hip joint may be caused by avascular necrosis, typically after delayed reduction of a hip dislocation or a displaced femoral neck fracture. Avascular necrosis eventually results in segmental joint collapse, typically seen in the first year or two after injury. Pain and disability do not always correlate with x-ray findings. Pain with activity is the typical major symptom of posttraumatic arthritis. If symptoms are not too disabling, then conservative measures such as a cane or brace or intermittent use of anti-inflammatory drugs are indicated. Although arthroplasty of the hip or knee is a satisfactory reconstructive procedure for elderly adults with severe symptoms of traumatic arthritis, there is still no uniformly satisfactory procedure for alleviating the condition in the young, vigorous patient.

## CONCLUSION

Lower extremity injuries have a huge impact on the acute and long-term functional outcome of the traumatically injured patients. Advances in orthopedic trauma care center upon multidisciplinary cooperation and management, with an emphasis on prudently aggressive stabilization of the polytraumatized patient. The plethora of effective techniques and approaches to early stabilization mandate an ongoing conversation between the orthopedic surgeon, general/trauma surgeon, and neurosurgeon regarding the management of individual patients. Clearly, in this day and age, the placement of multisystem trauma patients in splints and traction is suboptimal for most major lower extremity and pelvic injuries. Whether "damage control" external fixation or definitive minimally invasive fixation is chosen, early aggressive care is part of an optimal management paradigm.

Isolated lower extremity injuries can be devastating with potential loss of life and limb or appear to be relatively benign. Unfortunately, nondramatic injuries such as foot fractures can have lifetime consequences and prevent a patient from returning to their work and life activities. Therefore, each injury should be carefully evaluated, thoughtfully treated and followed long term to insure the best possible physical and psychological result.

## REFERENCES

1. MacKenzie EJ, Bosse MJ, Kellam JF, et al.: Early predictors of long-term work disability after major limb trauma. *J Trauma* 61:688, 2006.
2. Butcher JL, MacKenzie EJ, Cushing B, et al.:Long-term outcomes after lower extremity trauma. *J Trauma* 41:4, 1996.
3. Coben JH, Steiner CA, Barrett M, et al.: Completeness of cause of injury coding in healthcare administrative databases in the United States, 2001. *Inj Prev* 12:199, 2006.
4. Dischinger, Read K, Kufera JA, et al.: Consequences and costs of lower extremity injuries. *CIREN Report* DOT HS 809 871:1, 2005.
5. Pape HC, Giannoudis PV, Krettek C, et al.: Timing of fixation of major fractures in blunt polytrauma: Role of conventional indicators in clinical decision making. *J Orthop Trauma* 19:551, 2005.
6. Stahel PF, Heyde CE, Ertel W: Current concepts of polytrauma management. *Eur J Trauma* 31:200, 2005.
7. Colton CL: The history of fracture treatment. In Browner BD, Jupiter JB, Levine AM, et al. eds. *Skeletal Trauma.* Philadelphia, PA: Saunders, 1998.
8. Helfet DL, Haas NP, Schatzker J, et al.: AO philosophy and principles of fracture management-its evolution and evaluation. *J Bone Joint Surg Am* 85-A:1156, 2003.
9. Perren SM, Matter P: Evolution of AO philosophy. *Acta Chir Orthop Traumatol Cech* 70:205, 2003.
10. Rossaint R, Cerny V, Coats TJ, et al.: Key issues in advanced bleeding care in trauma. *Shock* 26:322, 2006.
11. Gattinoni L, Carlesso E, Valenza F, et al.: Acute respiratory distress syndrome, the critical care paradigm: what we learned and what we forgot. *Curr Opin Crit Care* 10:272, 2004.
12. Ciesla DJ, Moore EE, Johnson JL, et al.: Decreased progression of postinjury lung dysfunction to the acute respiratory distress syndrome and multiple organ failure. *Surgery* 140:640, 2006.
13. Varma R, Stashower ME: Necrotizing fasciitis: Delay in diagnosis results in loss of limb. *Int J Dermatol* 45:1222, 2006.
14. Tscherne H: John Border Memorial Lecture. Trauma Care in Europe before and after John Border: The evolution in trauma management at the University of Hanover. *J Orthop Trauma* 12:301, 1998.

15. Keel M, Trentz O: Pathophysiology of polytrauma. *Injury* 36:691, 2005.
16. Bone LB, Johnson KD, Weigelt J, et al.: Early versus delayed stabilization of femoral fractures: A prospective randomized study. 1989. *Clin Orthop Relat Res*:11, 2004.
17. Poole GV, Miller JD, Agnew SG, et al.: Lower extremity fracture fixation in head-injured patients. *J Trauma* 32:654, 1992.
18. Grotz MR, Giannoudis PV, Pape HC, et al.: Traumatic brain injury and stabilisation of long bone fractures: An update. *Injury* 35:1077, 2004.
19. Giannoudis PV, Veysi VT, Pape HC, et al.: When should we operate on major fractures in patients with severe head injuries? *Am J Surg* 183:261, 2002.
20. Stahel PF, Ertel W, Heyde CE: Traumatic brain injury: Impact on timing and modality of fracture care. *Orthopade* 34:852, 2005.
21. Scalea TM, Boswell SA, Scott JD, et al.: External fixation as a bridge to intramedullary nailing for patients with multiple injuries and with femur fractures: Damage control orthopedics. *J Trauma* 48:613, 2000.
22. Ciesla DJ, Moore EE, Zallen G, et al.: Hypertonic saline attenuation of polymorphonuclear neutrophil cytotoxicity: Timing is everything. *J Trauma* 48:388, 2000.
23. Schmidt OI, Heyde CE, Ertel W, et al.: Closed head injury - an inflammatory disease? *Brain Res Rev* 48:388, 2005.
24. Tscherne H: Principles of primary treatment of fractures with soft tissue injury. *Orthopade* 12:9, 1983.
25. Oestern HJ, Tscherne H: Pathophysiology and classification of soft tissue damage in fractures. *Orthopade* 12:2, 1983.
26. Gustilo RB, Mendoza RM, Williams DN: Problems in the management of type III (severe) open fractures: A new classification of type III open fractures. *J Trauma* 24:742, 1984.
27. Gustilo RB, Gruninger RP, Davis T: Classification of type III (severe) open fractures relative to treatment and results. *Orthopedics* 10:1781, 1987.
28. Sommer C, Bereiter H: Actual relevance of minimal invasive surgery in fracture treatment. *Ther Umsch* 62:145, 2005.
29. Perren SM: Evolution of the internal fixation of long bone fractures. The scientific basis of biological internal fixation: Choosing a new balance between stability and biology. *J Bone Joint Surg Br* 84:1093, 2002.
30. Zobrist R, Messmer P, Levin LS, et al.: Endoscopic-assisted, minimally invasive anterior pelvic ring stabilization: a new technique and case report. *J Orthop Trauma* 16:515, 2002.
31. Archer KR, Castillo RC, Mackenzie EJ, et al.: Physical disability after severe lower-extremity injury. *Arch Phys Med Rehabil* 87:1153, 2006.
32. Smith JJ, Agel J, Swiontkowski MF, et al.: Functional outcome of bilateral limb threatening: Lower extremity injuries at two years postinjury. *J Orthop Trauma* 19:249, 2005.
33. Bosse MJ, McCarthy ML, Jones AL, et al.: The insensate foot following severe lower extremity trauma: An indication for amputation? *J Bone Joint Surg Am* 87:2601, 2005.
34. Bosse MJ, MacKenzie EJ, Kellam JF, et al.: A prospective evaluation of the clinical utility of the lower-extremity injury-severity scores. *J Bone Joint Surg Am* 83-A:3, 2001.
35. Bosse MJ, MacKenzie EJ, Kellam JF, et al.: An analysis of outcomes of reconstruction or amputation after leg-threatening injuries. *N Engl J Med* 347:1924, 2002.
36. MacKenzie EJ, Bosse MJ, Pollak AN, et al.: Long-term persistence of disability following severe lower-limb trauma. Results of a seven-year follow-up. *J Bone Joint Surg Am* 87:1801, 2005.
37. Mackenzie EJ, Bosse MJ: Factors Influencing Outcome Following Limb-Threatening Lower Limb Trauma: Lessons Learned From the Lower Extremity Assessment Project (LEAP). *J Am Acad Orthop Surg* 14:S205, 2006.
38. Rajasekaran S, Sabapathy SR: A philosophy of care of open injuries based on the Ganga hospital score. *Injury*, 2006.
39. Rajasekaran S, Babu JN, Dheenadhayalan J, et al.: A score for predicting salvage and outcome in Gustilo type-IIIA and type-IIIB open tibial fractures. *J Bone Joint Surg Br* 88:1351, 2006.
40. Stahel PF, Oberholzer A, Morgan SJ, et al.: Surgical concepts of transtibial amputation: Burgess technique vs. modified Brückner procedure. *ANZ J Surg* 76:942, 2006.
41. Gregory RT, Gould RJ, Peclet M, et al.: The mangled extremity syndrome (M.E.S.): A severity grading system for multisystem injury of the extremity. *J Trauma* 25:1147, 1985.
42. Johansen K, Daines M, Howey T, et al.: Objective criteria accurately predict amputation following lower extremity trauma. *J Trauma* 30:568, 1990.
43. Helfet DL, Howey T, Sanders R, et al.: Limb salvage versus amputation. Preliminary results of the Mangled Extremity Severity Score. *Clin Orthop Relat Res* 80, 1990.
44. Bonanni F, Rhodes M, Lucke JF: The futility of predictive scoring of mangled lower extremities. *J Trauma* 34:99, 1993.
45. Pelissier P, Boireau P, Martin D, et al.: Bone reconstruction of the lower extremity: Complications and outcomes. *Plast Reconstr Surg* 111:2223, 2003.
46. Pape HC, Zelle BA, Hildebrand F, et al.: Reamed femoral nailing in sheep: Does irrigation and aspiration of intramedullary contents alter the systemic response? *J Bone Joint Surg Am* 87:2515, 2005.
47. Giannoudis PV, Tzioupis C, Pape HC: Fat embolism: the reaming controversy. *Injury* 37 Suppl 4:S50, 2006.
48. Parrett BM, Matros E, Pribaz JJ, et al.: Lower extremity trauma: Trends in the management of soft-tissue reconstruction of open tibia-fibula fractures. *Plast Reconstr Surg* 117:1315, 2006.
49. Dornseifer U, Ninkovic M: Timing of management of severe injuries of the lower extremity by free flap transfer. *Bosn J Basic Med Sci* 5:7, 2005.
50. Gwinnutt C: ATLS approach to trauma management. *Acta Anaesthesiol Belg* 56:403, 2005.
51. Blaisdell FW: The pathophysiology of skeletal muscle ischemia and the reperfusion syndrome: a review. *Cardiovasc Surg* 10:620, 2002.
52. Finkelstein JA, Hunter GA, Hu RW: Lower limb compartment syndrome: Course after delayed fasciotomy. *J Trauma* 40:342, 1996.
53. Kaneriya PP, Schweitzer ME, Spettell C, et al.: The cost-effectiveness of routine pelvic radiography in the evaluation of blunt trauma patients. *Skeletal Radiol* 28:271, 1999.
54. Pennal GF, Tile M, Waddell JP, Garside H: Pelvic disruption: assessment and classification. *Clin Orthop Relat Res*:12, 1980.
55. Giannoudis PV, Pape HC: Damage control orthopaedics in unstable pelvic ring injuries. *Injury* 35:671, 2004.
56. Miller PR, Moore PS, Mansell E, et al.: External fixation or arteriogram in bleeding pelvic fracture: Initial therapy guided by markers of arterial hemorrhage. *J Trauma* 54:437, 2003.
57. Eastridge BJ, Starr A, Minei JP, et al.: The importance of fracture pattern in guiding therapeutic decision-making in patients with hemorrhagic shock and pelvic ring disruptions. *J Trauma* 53:446, 2002.
58. Tscherne H, Pohlemann T, Gansslen A, et al.: Crush injuries of the pelvis. *Eur J Surg* 166:276, 2000.
59. Ertel W, Keel M, Eid K, et al.: Control of severe hemorrhage using C-clamp and pelvic packing in multiply injured patients with pelvic ring disruption. *J Orthop Trauma* 15:468, 2001.
60. Cothren CC, Moore EE, Smith WR, et al.: Preperitoneal pelvic packing in the child with an unstable pelvis: A novel approach. *J Pediatr Surg* 41:e17, 2006.
61. Smith WR, Moore EE, Osborn P, et al.: Retroperitoneal packing as a resuscitation technique for hemodynamically unstable patients with pelvic fractures: Report of two representative cases and a description of technique. *J Trauma* 59:1510, 2005.
62. Sarin EL, Moore JB, Moore EE, et al.: Pelvic fracture pattern does not always predict the need for urgent embolization. *J Trauma* 58:973, 2005.
63. Gansslen A, Giannoudis P, Pape HC: Hemorrhage in pelvic fracture: Who needs angiography? *Curr Opin Crit Care* 9:515, 2003.
64. Judet R, Judet J, Letournel E: Fractures of the acetabulum: Classification and surgical approaches for open reduction. Preliminary Report. *J Bone Joint Surg Am* 46:1615, 1964.
65. Beaule PE, Dorey FJ, Matta JM: Letournel classification for acetabular fractures. Assessment of interobserver and intraobserver reliability. *J Bone Joint Surg Am* 85-A:1704, 2003.
66. Ohashi K, El-Khoury GY, Abu-Zahra KW, et al.: Interobserver agreement for Letournel acetabular fracture classification with multidetector CT: Are standard Judet radiographs necessary? *Radiology* 241:386, 2006.
67. Fierens J, Broos PL: Quality of life after hip fracture surgery in the elderly. *Acta Chir Belg* 106:393, 2006.
68. Beringer TR, Clarke J, Elliott JR, et al.: Outcome following proximal femoral fracture in Northern Ireland. *Ulster Med J* 75:200, 2006.
69. Gurman GM: Surgery for hip fracture: How urgent? *Isr Med Assoc J* 8:663, 2006.
70. Lafforgue P: Osteonecrosis of the femoral head. *Rev Prat* 56:817, 2006.
71. Damany DS, Parker MJ, Chojnowski A: Complications after intracapsular hip fractures in young adults. A meta-analysis of 18 published studies involving 564 fractures. *Injury* 36:131, 2005.
72. Lavigne M, Kalhor M, Beck M, et al.: Distribution of vascular foramina around the femoral head and neck junction: Relevance for conservative intracapsular procedures of the hip. *Orthop Clin North Am* 36:171, 2005.
73. Gautier E, Ganz K, Krugel N, et al.: Anatomy of the medial femoral circumflex artery and its surgical implications. *J Bone Joint Surg Br* 82:679, 2000.
74. Leunig M, Beck M, Dora C, et al.: Femoroacetabular impingement: trigger for the development of coxarthrosis. *Orthopade* 35:77, 2006.
75. Ganz R, Gill TJ, Gautier E, et al.: Surgical dislocation of the adult hip a technique with full access to the femoral head and acetabulum without the risk of avascular necrosis. *J Bone Joint Surg Br* 83:1119, 2001.
76. Bjorgul K, Reikeras O: Hemiarthroplasty in worst cases is better than internal fixation in best cases of displaced femoral neck fractures: A prospective study of 683 patients treated with hemiarthroplasty or internal fixation. *Acta Orthop* 77:368, 2006.
77. Macaulay W, Pagnotto MR, Iorio R, et al.: Displaced femoral neck fractures in the elderly: Hemiarthroplasty versus total hip arthroplasty. *J Am Acad Orthop Surg* 14:287, 2006.

78. Raaymakers EL: Fractures of the femoral neck: A review and personal statement. *Acta Chir Orthop Traumatol Cech* 73:45, 2006.

79. Sierra RJ, Schleck CD, Cabanela ME: Dislocation of bipolar hemiarthroplasty: Rate, contributing factors, and outcome. *Clin Orthop Relat Res* 442:230, 2006.

80. Hoffmann R, Schmidmaier G, Schulz R, et al.: Classic nail versus DHS. A prospective randomised study of fixation of trochanteric femur fractures. *Unfallchirurg* 102:182, 1999.

81. Klinger HM, Baums MH, Eckert M, et al.: A comparative study of unstable per- and intertrochanteric femoral fractures treated with dynamic hip screw (DHS) and trochanteric butt-press plate vs. proximal femoral nail (PFN). *Zentralbl Chir* 130:301, 2005.

82. Nuber S, Schonweiss T, Ruter A: Stabilisation of unstable trochanteric femoral fractures. Dynamic hip screw (DHS) with trochanteric stabilisation plate vs. proximal femur nail (PFN). *Unfallchirurg* 106:39, 2003.

83. Parker MJ, Pryor GA: Gamma versus DHS nailing for extracapsular femoral fractures. Meta-analysis of ten randomised trials. *Int Orthop* 20:163, 1996.

84. Gebhard F, Kinzl L, Arand M: Computer-assisted surgery. *Unfallchirurg* 103:612, 2000.

85. Hufner T, Kfuri M, Jr., Kendoff D, et al.: [Navigated osteosynthesis of the proximal femur. An experimental study]. *Unfallchirurg* 106:975, 2003.

86. Pape HC, Auf'm'Kolk M, Paffrath T, et al.: Primary intramedullary femur fixation in multiple trauma patients with associated lung contusion—a cause of posttraumatic ARDS? *J Trauma* 34:540, 1993.

87. Pape HC, Grimme K, Van Griensven M, et al.: Impact of intramedullary instrumentation versus damage control for femoral fractures on immunoinflammatory parameters: Prospective randomized analysis by the EPOFF Study Group. *J Trauma* 55:7, 2003.

88. Harwood PJ, Giannoudis PV, van Griensven M, et al.: Alterations in the systemic inflammatory response after early total care and damage control procedures for femoral shaft fracture in severely injured patients. *J Trauma* 58:446, 2005.

89. Bosse MJ, MacKenzie EJ, Riemer BL, et al.: Adult respiratory distress syndrome, pneumonia, and mortality following thoracic injury and a femoral fracture treated either with intramedullary nailing with reaming or with a plate. A comparative study. *J Bone Joint Surg Am* 79:799, 1997.

90. Dora C, Leunig M, Beck M, et al.: Entry point soft tissue damage in antegrade femoral nailing: A cadaver study. *J Orthop Trauma* 15:488, 2001.

91. Marti A, Fankhauser C, Frenk A, et al.: Biomechanical evaluation of the less invasive stabilization system for the internal fixation of distal femur fractures. *J Orthop Trauma* 15:482, 2001.

92. Wong MK, Leung F, Chow SP: Treatment of distal femoral fractures in the elderly using a less-invasive plating technique. *Int Orthop* 29:117, 2005.

93. Ricci AR, Yue JJ, Taffet R, et al.: Less Invasive Stabilization System for treatment of distal femur fractures. *Am J Orthop* 33:250, 2004.

94. Jaakkola JI, Lundy DW, Moore T, et al.: Supracondylar femur fracture fixation: Mechanical comparison of the 95 degrees condylar side plate and screw versus 95 degrees angled blade plate. *Acta Orthop Scand* 73:72, 2002.

95. Albert MJ: Supracondylar Fractures of the Femur. *J Am Acad Orthop Surg* 5:163, 1997.

96. Speck M, Regazzoni P: Classification of patellar fractures. *Z Unfallchir Versicherungsmed* 87:27, 1994.

97. Moore TM: Fracture-dislocation of the knee. *Clin Orthop Relat Res* 128, 1981.

98. Barnes CJ, Pietrobon R, Higgins LD: Does the pulse examination in patients with traumatic knee dislocation predict a surgical arterial injury? A meta-analysis. *J Trauma* 53:1109, 2002.

99. Galla M, Lobenhoffer P: The direct, dorsal approach to the treatment of unstable tibial posteromedial fracture-dislocations. *Unfallchirurg* 106:241, 2003.

100. Sarmiento A, Latta LL: Functional fracture bracing. *J Am Acad Orthop Surg* 7:66, 1999.

101. Finkemeier CG, Schmidt AH, Kyle RF, et al.: A prospective, randomized study of intramedullary nails inserted with and without reaming for the treatment of open and closed fractures of the tibial shaft. *J Orthop Trauma* 14:187, 2000.

102. Mertens P, Broos P, Reynders P, et al.: The unreamed locked intramedullary tibial nail: A follow-up study in 51 patients. *Acta Orthop Belg* 64:277, 1998.

103. Markmiller M, Tjarksen M, Mayr E, et al.: The unreamed tibia nail. Multicenter study of the AO/ASIF. Osteosynthesefragen/Association for the Study of Internal Fixation. *Langenbecks Arch Surg* 385:276, 2000.

104. Joshi D, Ahmed A, Krishna L, et al.: Unreamed interlocking nailing in open fractures of tibia. *J Orthop Surg (Hong Kong)* 12:216, 2004.

105. Chen SH, Wu PH, Lee YS: Long-term results of pilon fractures. *Arch Orthop Trauma Surg*, 2006.

106. Strauss EJ, Petrucelli G, Bong M, et al.: Blisters Associated With Lower-Extremity Fracture: Results of a Prospective Treatment Protocol. *J Orthop Trauma* 20:618, 2006.

107. Marin LE, Wukich DK, Zgonis T: The surgical management of high- and low-energy tibial plafond fractures: A combination of internal and external fixation devices. *Clin Podiatr Med Surg* 23:423, 2006.

108. Kapukaya A, Subasi M, Arslan H: Management of comminuted closed tibial plafond fractures using circular external fixators. *Acta Orthop Belg* 71:582, 2005.

109. Khoury A, Liebergall M, London E, et al.: Percutaneous plating of distal tibial fractures. *Foot Ankle Int* 23:818, 2002.

110. Frey C: Ankle sprains. *Instruct Course Lect* 50:515, 2001.

111. Moore JA Jr, Shank JR, Morgan SJ, et al.: Syndesmosis fixation: A comparison of three and four cortices of screw fixation without hardware removal. *Foot Ankle Int* 27:567, 2006.

112. Przkora R, Kayser R, Ertel W, et al.: Temporary vertical transarticular pin fixation of unstable ankle fractures with critical soft tissue conditions. *Injury* 37:905, 2006.

113. Lauder AJ, Inda DJ, Bott AM, et al.: Interobserver and intraobserver reliability of two classification systems for intra-articular calcaneal fractures. *Foot Ankle Int* 27:251, 2006.

114. McGarvey WC, Burris MW, Clanton TO, et al.: Calcaneal fractures: Indirect reduction and external fixation. *Foot Ankle Int* 27:494, 2006.

115. Zgonis T, Roukis TS, Polyzois VD: The use of Ilizarov technique and other types of external fixation for the treatment of intra-articular calcaneal fractures. *Clin Podiatr Med Surg* 23:343, 2006.

116. Pisani PC, Parino E, Acquaro P: Treatment of late complications of intra-articular calcaneal fractures. *Clin Podiatr Med Surg* 23:355, 2006.

117. Higgins T, Baumgaertner M: Diagnosis and treatment of fractures of the talus: A comprehensive review of the literature. *Foot Ankle Intern* 20:595, 1999.

118. Cierny GI, Zorn KE: Segmental tibial defects: Comparing conventional and Ilizarov methodologies. *Clin Orthop Relat Res* 301:118, 1994.

# Commentary ■ BRUCE H. ZIRAN

This chapter is an excellent description of the current state of the art. Because of the ongoing fragmentation of surgical specialties into subspecialty care, there is growing need for the general trauma surgeon to understand all aspects of patient injury. With declining call panels for orthopedic surgery and neurosurgery in developed countries, and lack of availability in underdeveloped countries, the trauma surgeon cannot solely rely on consultation for the treatment of polytrauma. A clear understanding of the impact of musculoskeletal injury on the acute and long-term care of the injured patient will facilitate better interdisciplinary conversation and decision making. Understanding the implications of open fractures, and more importantly the soft tissue envelope is a fundamental aspect of orthopedic trauma. Furthermore, modern concepts of damage control and interaction with the general surgical team has altered the traditional approach to such extremity injuries.

The authors have emphasized that lower extremity trauma can be lethal and have an additive effect on the inflammatory burden of the patient, and that often relatively simple maneuvers can be used to mitigate such effects. I recommend in particular that trauma surgeons follow the authors' direction and review and thoroughly understand the current literature regarding the systemic effects of lower extremity trauma and treatment. The concept of *orthopaedic* damage control has now been well described and, as advocated by the authors, will hopefully end the archaic practices of femoral and pelvic traction, delayed treatment of spine fractures and arguments about patients being "too sick" to undergo timely and basic stabilization procedures. Conversely, the authors correctly make the point that orthopaedic surgeons need to understand the physiologic challenges of shock, systemic inflammation and brain trauma and become full fledged, informed participants on the trauma team, as opposed to technicians making brief cameo appearances or insisting on a "fix it all and fix it now" approach. In fact, just like the authors of this chapter, we have worked closely with the trauma surgeon to understand and learn their perspective, and we have tried to emulate the authors' approach. Thus, we strive to be versatile enough that we tailor our treatment based on the state of the patient. Instead of negotiating for our own convenience, we ask the traumatologist "How much time and how much blood loss can the patient tolerate?" and then tailor

our treatment appropriately. Toward this end, surgeons learning more about each other's specialty and working together collegially are the vital keys toward progressive trauma care. Unfortunately, the world of orthopedics is becoming more specialized and fragmented, which has resulted in a major attrition of orthopedic surgeons who participate in trauma care. As a result, there has been the advent of the Acute Care Surgery concept, which aims to fill in significant gaps in acute orthopedic trauma care. No matter what side of the debate one sits, patient care cannot be the currency of such controversy, and acute care surgery may be a necessity in some areas. While it has the potential to enhance trauma care by providing acute care of limb and life-threatening extremity trauma, we must also note that if done without proper sensitivity and knowledge, it may also cause further divisions and a big step backwards.

The authors of this chapter should be commended in their fine work and efforts to bridge the gap and provide a valuable resource to anyone involved in the care of skeletal trauma.

# Peripheral Vascular Injury

*Eric R. Frykberg* ■ *Miren A. Schinco*

## HISTORICAL PERSPECTIVE

> "One of the chief fascinations in surgery is the management of wounded vessels"
>
> —William S. Halsted, 1912

The same year that Halsted made this statement, Alexis Carrel received the Nobel Prize for his body of work, which included a demonstration of the feasibility and technical principles of vascular anastomosis. By the beginning of the 20th century, several others also had shown in animals and humans that direct repair of vascular injuries can be successfully accomplished.[1–3] In 1910, Stich published 146 cases of direct vascular repair by lateral suture and end to end anastomosis.[2] Soubbotitch, a Serbian military surgeon, was the first to document the feasibility of large scale repair of combat vascular injuries, with 32 successful repairs by lateral suture and anastomosis in 1913.[4] All these cases, however, involved the repair of chronic complications of vascular trauma, after long periods of delay, including false aneurysms and arteriovenous fistulae (AVF). Acute repair was not feasible at that time. The standard of care for management of vascular injury remained arterial and venous ligation until the 1950s, a technique that dated back to the 16th century. This was because of the complexity of the wounds, exigencies of managing multiple casualties with slow evacuation methods, lack of antibiotics, lack of effective asanguinous resuscitation fluids and blood, lack of anticoagulation and blood banking, the often moribund state of the patient, and the high rate of infection and secondary hemorrhage following vascular repair. These considerations dictated ligation to prevent death from exsanguination and sepsis, rather than repair to salvage a limb. As a result, amputation was common after peripheral vascular injury.

DeBakey and Simeone, in their now-classic work describing 2471 vascular injuries sustained by American forces in World War II, stated that ligation was "not a procedure of choice. It is a procedure of stern necessity, for the purpose of controlling hemorrhage."[5] In extremities that survived vascular ligation, the thrombosis, false aneurysms, and AVFs that later developed then could be repaired electively; however, even salvaged limbs following arterial ligation had severe functional disability.[6] Nonetheless, such delayed repair of vascular trauma was believed superior to immediate repair, because it was thought to provide the opportunity for collateral circulation to develop to improve the chances of ultimate viability of the limb. This philosophy and practice persisted into the early part of the Korean War.[7] DeBakey and Simeone[5] advocated this approach by noting (p 563), "The almost negligible incidence of loss of limb after excision of false aneurysms prompts the rather paradoxical statement that the best safeguard for the survival of a limb is to permit an acute arterial wound to develop into an aneurysm."

Makins[8] documented an amputation rate of 16.4% in the British casualties of World War I, while DeBakey and Simeone reported an amputation rate of 49%.[5] The lower amputation rate in World War I is reflective of a selection bias from the prolonged evacuation and delay to treatment, averaging over 24 hours, during which time patients died from exsanguination from peripheral vascular injuries, and ligation and amputation were not necessary. Suture repair of acute vascular trauma was attempted in only 81 cases (3.3%) in American casualties in World War II, in three cases by end-to-end anastomosis. In this group the "significantly better" amputation rate of 35% was the first indication in a large scale clinical setting that acute repair may be superior to ligation.[5]

With the advent of antibiotics, advanced vascular surgical techniques, and an average evacuation time to definitive care that had improved from 10 hours in World War II to 2–4 hours with the introduction of helicopter transport during the Korean War, the repair of injured arteries became more common. Consequently the amputation rate in the Korean War decreased to 13% among 227 cases of acute suture repair.[7,9] This confirmed the benefit of routine repair of acute vascular injuries in a combat setting and finally resolved the concerns that vascular repair may result in a high incidence of thrombophlebitis and embolism.

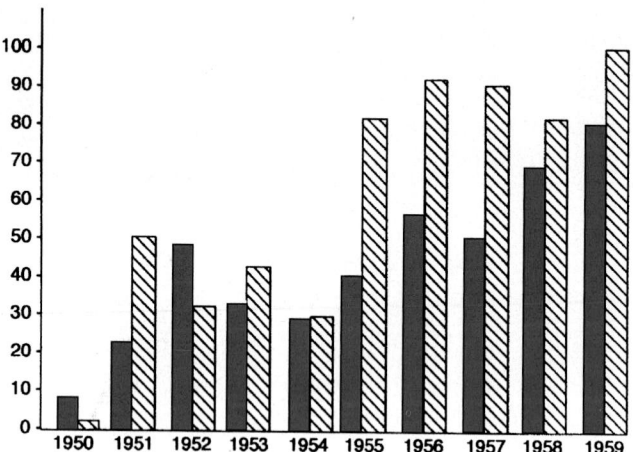

**FIGURE 44-1.** Ten-year trend in the early treatment of civilian arterial injuries by repair rather than ligation.
*(Reproduced with permission from Ferguson IA, Byrd WM, McAfee DK: Experiences in the management of arterial injuries. Ann Surg 153:980,1961.)*

The principles derived from this Korean War experience rapidly became established in the civilian sector. Ferguson and coworkers[10] documented a 10-fold increase in the percentage of peripheral vascular injuries undergoing repair rather than ligation, and a doubling of the number of successful repairs, among 200 cases treated in Atlanta, Georgia, during the 1950s (Fig. 44-1). Their 13.6% amputation rate, identical to that achieved in Korea, confirmed their emphasis on the importance of early diagnosis and treatment, the technique of intimal approximation, the need to achieve and maintain palpable distal pulses, and resection of grossly damaged arterial segments. These principles echoed the assertions of J.B. Murphy 65 years earlier.[1]

The Vietnam War provided further opportunity for advances in the management of vascular trauma with the establishment of the Vietnam Vascular Registry at Walter Reed Army Medical Center. In 1970, Rich and coworkers reported a 13.5% amputation rate among 1000 acute combat arterial injuries, 98.5% of which underwent repair. This was identical to the results from Korea, despite the more frequent use of high-velocity weapons and antipersonnel devices.[11] A major contributor to these results was the most rapid access to definitive care ever achieved in war. Over 95% of all casualties were evacuated by helicopter, within an average of 65 minutes.[3,12]

Over the ensuing 30 years, the civilian sector has provided the predominant experience in vascular trauma in the United States, with some extrapolation to recent combat experiences in the Middle East. Building on the principles developed from military experience, amputation rates following most civilian extremity vascular injury currently are less than 5%.[13–15] The following chapter reviews our current knowledge of the epidemiology, pathology, prognosis, diagnosis, and treatment of extremity vascular trauma that has evolved from these experiences of past years.

## EPIDEMIOLOGY

Peripheral vascular trauma typically occurs in males (72% to 90%) between the ages of 20 and 40 years.[14] Like most trauma, injuries typically present outside normal working hours, most commonly around midnight.[15] The incidence of vascular injury among all forms of trauma is very low, ranging from 0.2% to 2% in military series, and up to 3.7% in civilian series[16–18] (Table 44-1).

Vascular injuries occur most commonly in the extremities. This is due partly to selection bias, in that great vessel injuries of the torso, head, and neck are highly lethal, as well as to the greater exposure of the extremities to injury. Dennis and coworkers[19] showed that most extremity arteries are injured in less than 10% of all penetrating wounds placing them at risk, with the brachial artery having the greatest vulnerability to injury (15.7% of all penetrating wounds to the arm). Combat injuries emphasize these points. The extremities represent 61% of the total body area exposed in combat.[20] Although 66% of all wounds among American casualties in WWII occurred in the extremities, 97.5% of all vascular injuries occurred there; however, only 1.4% of all extremity wounds resulted in vascular injury.[5] In 4977 published cases of vascular trauma in surviving troops from WWI, WWII, Korea and Vietnam,[5,8,9,11] 4665 (93.7%) were in the extremities. Most of these (62%) were in the lower extremities, reflecting the wartime use of antipersonnel devices such as land mines and bungi sticks. The published civilian experience with vascular trauma since 1960 documents a lower incidence of the extremity as a site of vascular injuries, and a greater predominance of the upper extremity (Table 44-2). This is most likely due to the lesser wounding power and lethality of civilian weaponry, as well as the rapid prehospital transport and prompt aggressive treatment of shock and injury that has characterized the civilian sector in recent years. These result in greater survival of patients with truncal or head and neck wounds.[14,37]

The great majority of vascular injuries are due to penetrating trauma. In the military setting, only 1.1% of such injuries were due to blunt trauma,[11] with the most common penetrating mechanisms being shrapnel wounds from bombs, land mines, and grenades (60%), followed by high-velocity gunshots (34%). Blunt mechanisms are responsible for a greater proportion of civilian vascular injuries (10–15%), especially in the rural population,[17,18,34,36] although penetrating wounds remain the predominant etiology (see Table 44-2). In the civilian sector, approximately 6% of all

### TABLE 44-1

| Incidence of Military and Civilian Vascular Trauma | | |
|---|---|---|
| **REFERENCE** | **SETTING** | **INCIDENCE VASCULAR TRAUMA**[a] |
| Soubbotitch[4] | Balkan Wars | 0.4 |
| DeBakey and Simeone[5] | World War II | 0.96 |
| Beebe and DeBakey[16] | World War I | 0.25 |
| Vollmar[17b] | Germany | 0.2 |
| Rich et al.[3] | Vietnam War | 2.0 |
| Frykberg et al.[15b] | Florida | 0.8 |
| Oller et al.[18b] | North Carolina | 3.7 |

[a]Percentage among all cases of trauma.
[b]Civilian series.

**TABLE 44-2**

### Civilian Vascular Injuries of the Extremities: Incidence and Mechanism

| REFERENCE | TOTAL NO. VASCULAR INJURIES | NO. PENETRATING | NO. IN EXTREMITIES Upper | Lower | Total |
|---|---|---|---|---|---|
| Morris et al.[21] | 220 | 0 | 107 | 55 | 162 |
| Ferguson et al.[10] | 200 | 191 | 93 | 59 | 152 |
| Smith et al.[22] | 61 | 42 | 25 | 21 | 46 |
| Patman et al.[23] | 271 | 0 | 132 | 66 | 198 |
| Treiman et al.[24a] | 251 | 152 | 79 | 74 | 153 |
| Dillard et al.[25] | 85 | 66 | 36 | 31 | 67 |
| Drapanas et al.[26] | 226 | 204 | 97 | 59 | 156 |
| Perry et al.[27] | 508 | 235 | 236 | 141 | 377 |
| Cheek et al.[28a] | 250 | 237 | 54 | 72 | 126 |
| Hardy et al.[29] | 360 | 312 | 98 | 116 | 214 |
| Kelly and Eiseman[30] | 175 | 127 | 55 | 47 | 102 |
| Burnett et al.[31] | 94 | 78 | 25 | 42 | 67 |
| Robbs and Baker[32] | 267 | 191 | 112 | 114 | 226 |
| Reynolds et al.[33] | 191 | 145 | 69 | 73 | 142 |
| Saide et al.[34a] | 167 | 112 | 50 | 55 | 105 |
| Sharma et al.[35] | 211 | 169 | 64 | 111 | 175 |
| Mattox et al.[14a] | 5760 | 5375 | 1027 | 1104 | 2131 |
| Oller et al.[18a] | 978 | 615 | 361 | 271 | 632 |
| Humphrey et al.[36a] | 248 | 146 | 117 | 65 | 182 |
| Diamond et al.[13] | 56 | 28 | 28 | 28 | 56 |
| Total | 10,579 | 8,425 (80%) | 2865 | 2604 | 5469 (51.7%) |

[a]Includes both arterial and venous injuries.

*Source: Modified with permission from Frykberg ER: Vascular trauma. In Callow AD, Ernst CB, eds. Vascular Surgery-Theory and Practice, New York, McGraw-Hill, 1995, p.989.*

penetrating extremity wounds result in vascular injury,[15] while less than 1% of all blunt extremity trauma results in vascular injury.[38] Gunshots, mostly low velocity, are the most common penetrating agents causing civilian extremity vascular injury, accounting for approximately 50% of all cases, followed by stabs and lacerations (34%) and shotgun wounds (5%).[14,24,26,27,30,33,39]

Among 6808 published cases of both military and civilian extremity vascular injuries, the femoral artery was the most commonly injured (35%) (Table 44-3).

A total of 2569 injured body structures associated with arterial injuries in seven published series[10,11,23,27,29,36,42] shows that adjacent major veins are the most common site of associated injury, making up 31% of all cases, followed by nerve (27%), skeletal (26%), and miscellaneous injuries to the head, soft tissue, and torso (16%).

Mattox and coworkers documented a 400% increase in civilian cardiovascular injuries in Houston between 1958 and 1988, with 50% of all vascular injuries over this 30-year period occurring in the last 10 years of this study.[14] This pattern may be changing with the decline in urban violence and penetrating trauma that has occurred in the United States over the past decade.

Some of this increase was attributed to iatrogenic injuries, which increased from 0.6% of all vascular injuries between 1958 and 1963 to 2.3% of those between 1984 and 1988[44,45] with 85% of these cases occurring in the last five years of the study.[14] Youkey and coworkers also documented a 44% increase in iatrogenic vascular trauma between the periods of 1966–1973 and 1974–1982, with cardiac catheterization, angiography, and surgical procedures each responsible for approximately one-third of all cases. The

femoral and brachial arteries are the most commonly involved in iatrogenic vascular injuries.[46]

## PATHOPHYSIOLOGY

Arteries and veins are composed of three tissue layers including the outer adventitia of connective tissue, the central media of smooth muscle and elastic fibers, and the inner intima or endothelial cell layer. The specific response of blood vessels to injury depends on the magnitude of dissipated energy and its duration. Gunshot wounds produce greater injury than stabs, and high-velocity (>2500 ft/sec) gunshots result in massive injuries to vessels, soft tissue, nerve and bone, due to their greater kinetic energy. Blunt injury causes a similar level of destructive energy to surrounding tissues, which may disrupt collateral circulation and contribute to loss of perfusion and limb loss in any instance of direct vascular injury. Major blood vessels may be injured by the indirect force of the dissipating energy or shock wave, even though not directly impacted, an effect not seen in simple stabs or low-velocity gunshot wounds. The remarkably low incidence of extremity vascular injury following both blunt and penetrating trauma is due in part to the elasticity of major arteries, which allows them to stretch out of the path of injurious agents. This protective action may itself cause some forms of vascular injury through vessel wall contusion and intimal disruption.[43]

There are several types of vessel injuries (Fig. 44-2). The most common forms of injury to both arteries and veins documented in

**TABLE 44-3**

### Incidence of Major Extremity Artery Injury[a]

| REFERENCE | SUBCLAVIAN | AXILLARY | BRACHIAL | FEMORAL | POPLITEAL | TOTAL |
|---|---|---|---|---|---|---|
| Makins[8b] | 45 | 108 | 200 | 366 | 144 | 863 |
| DeBakey and Simeone[5b] | 21 | 74 | 601 | 517 | 502 | 1715 |
| Hughes[9b] | 3 | 20 | 89 | 95 | 79 | 286 |
| Morris et al.[21] | 7 | 12 | 55 | 36 | 14 | 124 |
| Ferguson et al.[10] | 8 | 10 | 29 | 42 | 14 | 103 |
| Patman et al.[23] | 11 | 24 | 46 | 49 | 7 | 137 |
| Dillard et al.[25] | 4 | 6 | 26 | 21 | 10 | 67 |
| Drapanas et al.[26] | 16 | 12 | 39 | 38 | 14 | 119 |
| Rich et al.[11b] | 8 | 59 | 283 | 351 | 217 | 918 |
| Perry et al.[27] | 23 | 38 | 78 | 112 | 17 | 268 |
| Smith et al.[40] | 3 | 10 | 28 | 35 | 7 | 83 |
| Cheek et al.[28] | 16 | 7 | 21 | 34 | 15 | 93 |
| Kelly and Eiseman[30] | 0 | 2 | 37 | 27 | 6 | 72 |
| Burnett et al.[31] | 0 | 7 | 12 | 29 | 8 | 56 |
| Robbs and Baker[32] | 24 | 33 | 55 | 51 | 47 | 210 |
| Reynolds et al.[33] | 15 | 14 | 40 | 37 | 36 | 142 |
| Menzoian et al.[41] | 2 | 5 | 18 | 27 | 15 | 67 |
| Mattox et al.[14] | 168 | 143 | 446 | 500 | 156 | 1413 |
| Humphrey et al.[36] | 3 | 9 | 30 | 15 | 15 | 72 |
| Total | 377 (5.5%) | 593 (9%) | 2133 (31%) | 2382 (35%) | 1323 (19.5%) | 6808 |

[a]Number of cases reported.

[b]Military series.

*Source: Modified with permission from Frykberg ER: Vascular trauma. In Callow AD, Ernst CB, eds. Vascular Surgery: Theory and Practice, New York, McGraw-Hill, 1995, p. 991.*

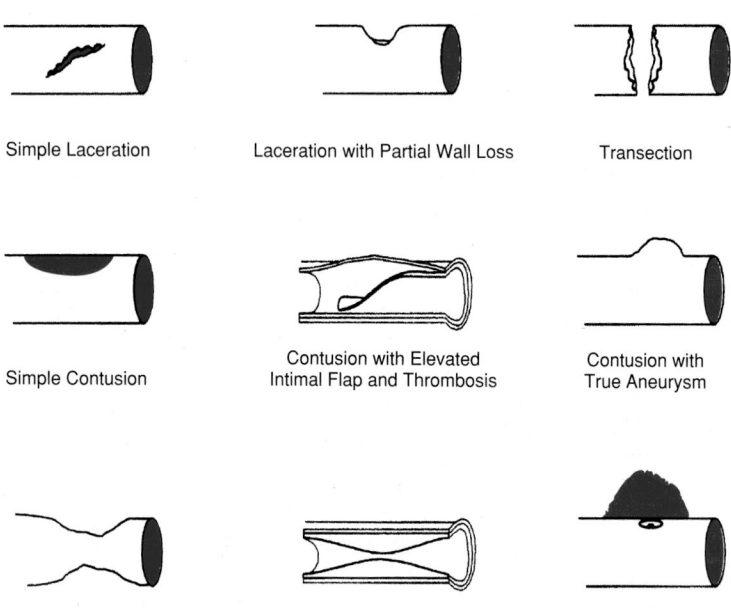

Simple Laceration    Laceration with Partial Wall Loss    Transection

Simple Contusion    Contusion with Elevated Intimal Flap and Thrombosis    Contusion with True Aneurysm

Contusion with Spasm    Contusion with Subintimal Hematoma    False Aneurysm

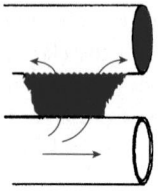
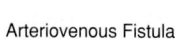

Arteriovenous Fistula

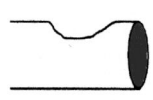

Extrinsic Compression

**FIGURE 44-2.** Morphology of vascular injuries.
*(Reproduced with permission from Frykberg ER: Vascular trauma. In Callow AD, Ernst CB, eds. Vascular Surgery: Theory and Practice, McGraw-Hill, 1995, p. 992.)*

**TABLE 44-4**

**Clinical Pathology of Arterial Injuries[a]**

| REFERENCE | TRANSECTIONS | LACERATIONS | CONTUSIONS | SPASM | FALSE ANEURYSMS | AVFS | TOTAL |
|---|---|---|---|---|---|---|---|
| Morris et al.[21] | 107 | 98 | 11 | 4 | 0 | 0 | 220 |
| Patman et al.[23] | 113 | 139 | 14 | 5 | 0 | 0 | 271 |
| Rich et al.[43] | 73 | 23 | 4 | 0 | 0 | 0 | 100 |
| Drapanas et al.[26] | 59 | 133 | 24 | 0 | 2 | 8 | 226 |
| Perry et al.[27] | 99 | 151 | 7 | 2 | 0 | 0 | 259 |
| Hardy et al.[29] | 140 | 111 | 21 | 2 | 39 | 38 | 351 |
| Gill et al.[42] | 26 | 6 | 14 | 3 | 4 | 1 | 54 |
| Humphrey et al.[36] | 117 | 91 | 29 | 0 | 7 | 4 | 248 |
| Total | 734 (42.5%) | 752 (43.5%) | 124 (7%) | 16 (1%) | 52 (3%) | 51 (3%) | 1729 |

[a]Number of cases reported.

AVF = arteriovenous fistula.

*Source: Modified with permission from Frykberg ER: Vascular Trauma. In Callow AD, Ernst CB, eds. Vascular Surgery-Theory and Practice. New York, McGraw-Hill, 1995, p. 993.*

clinical series are lacerations and transections (Table 44-4). Lacerations are full-thickness tears of the vessel in which part of the wall remains intact and vessel continuity is maintained. They are classified as mild when less than 25% of the vessel wall is involved, moderate when 25–50% is involved, and severe when more than 50% is involved (Fig. 44-3). Transection involves a complete division of the vessel with loss of continuity, in which case the severed ends tend to retract and constrict, with cessation of hemorrhage and some degree of proximal and distal thrombosis (Fig. 44-4). This results in loss of distal pulses and clinical signs and symptoms of tissue ischemia (the 6 Ps: pulseless, pain, pallor, paralysis, paresthesias, and poikilothermy or coolness). Both are most commonly caused by penetrating trauma. Hemorrhage can follow either transection or laceration, but is generally more severe with lacerations, because reflex smooth muscle contraction tends to open the tear further. Severe hemorrhage may result in shock and death if not treated promptly. Lacerations may lead to some difficulty in diagnosis,

because distal pulses and perfusion usually persist.[47] Bleeding from injured vessels can be contained within muscle and fascial compartments to create an acute pulsatile hematoma or false aneurysm. An AVF may result from contiguous wounds to both an artery and vein. Both these lesions may lead to major complications such as impingement on surrounding nerves, rupture, thrombosis, embolization, infection, or high-output cardiac failure.[48,49]

A contusion is a bruise of the arterial wall and comprises less than 10% of all vascular injuries. It may involve as little as an isolated adventitial hematoma with no adverse sequelae. Extension to a subintimal hematoma can constrict or occlude the vessel lumen, or may rupture the intima with elevation and prolapse of an intimal flap, both potentially resulting in thrombosis. One more consequence of contusion is full-thickness weakening of the arterial wall that results in a true aneurysm.[3,22,29,43,50] Histologic studies of contused arteries have shown that intimal damage tends to be more extensive than is evident by gross inspection, which led in past

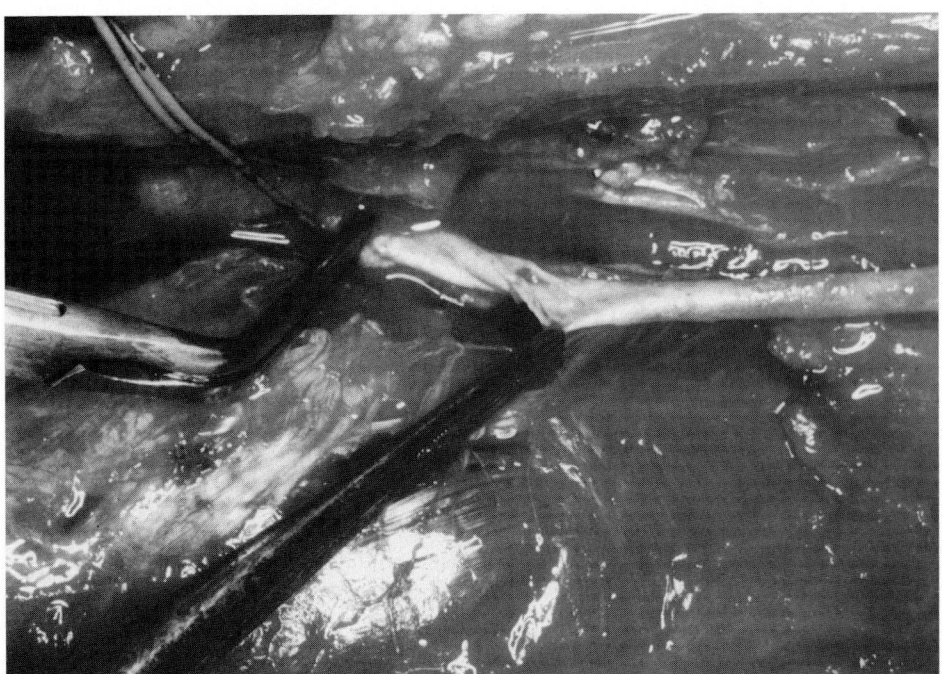

**FIGURE 44-3.** Severe laceration of superficial femoral artery following gunshot wound of thigh, requiring resection and end-to-end anastomosis.

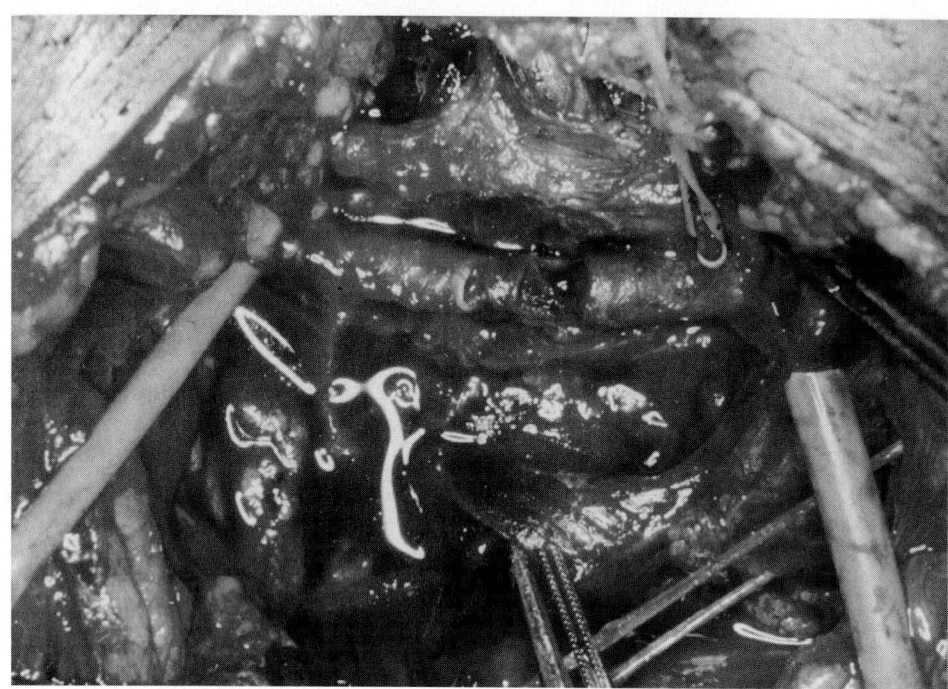

**FIGURE 44-4.** Transected popliteal artery with proximal and distal control obtained. Note thrombus in distal segment.

years to resection of damaged arteries for a distance of 1–2 cm beyond the grossly visualized injury before repair.[3,29,51] This debridement of any more than the grossly damaged arterial wall was demonstrated to be unnecessary in the Vietnam War.[3,43]

Spasm is a reflex myogenic response of arteries to injury and can be experimentally demonstrated by repetitive stretching of an artery. It manifests as a segmental constriction or a focal area of smooth narrowing on arteriography or by direct visualization. This may be indistinguishable from other more dangerous lesions such as subintimal hematoma or intimal dissection and has long been perceived to carry a high risk of thrombosis and require urgent surgery and resection if found. This was largely a misperception, arising from the tendency of some surgeons to inordinately delay repair of an already thrombosed vessel by attributing the signs of acute vascular insufficiency to spasm, rather than from any data of a patent vessel with spasm having any risk of subsequent thrombosis.[3,27,52]

Both contusion and spasm usually result from blunt mechanisms that acutely crush or stretch an artery. Some forms of penetrating trauma may also result in these lesions, especially high-velocity missile injuries in which an artery can be injured indirectly by the temporary tissue cavitation of a blast wave, without being directly hit.[3]

Acute interruption of blood flow to an extremity results in a number of pathophysiologic disturbances that may threaten life as well as the affected limb. Ischemia results from a failure of oxygen delivery to meet tissue metabolic needs. The vulnerability of a tissue to ischemia depends on its basal energy requirement, substrate stores and length and severity of the ischemic insult. Peripheral nerves are extremely vulnerable to ischemic damage in a short period of time, because they have a high basal energy requirement and virtually no glycogen stores. Therefore, motor and sensory deficits are often the first manifestations of arterial injury, which may lead to permanent neurologic disability after just a few hours delay in reperfusion.

Skeletal muscle is more tolerant of decreased blood flow, with no histologic changes evident after four hours of ischemia, and reversible changes with reperfusion after more than six hours of ischemia.[53] The more complete the interruption of arterial inflow, and the more severe the ischemia, the greater is the degree of ischemic damage that can occur in as little as three hours, and such damage may be extended rather than reversed by reperfusion.

This "reperfusion injury" is initiated by the generation of large amounts of superoxide anion as hypoxanthine, a metabolic product of anaerobic metabolism in ischemic tissue, is converted to xanthine with the reintroduction of oxygen. Leukocytes are thought to be the major source of free radicals in muscle.[54] Superoxide anion exerts a number of adverse effects on endothelial integrity, vasoconstriction, and activation of an inflammatory cascade, resulting in microvascular obstruction and elevated interstitial fluid pressure. This leads to a "no-reflow" phenomenon, and, ultimately, a compartment syndrome or irreversible ischemia and necrosis of both nerve and muscle.[55] The dissemination of toxic metabolites into the circulation leads to damage to distant organs.[56] With muscle necrosis or rhabdomyolysis, myoglobin and potassium are released into the circulation, which may lead to fatal arrhythmias and renal failure. Thus, in addition to potential local and regional effects on limb dysfunction and limb loss, acute interruption of extremity blood flow can have systemic consequences of organ failure and death if not recognized promptly and treated aggressively.

## PROGNOSTIC FACTORS

Over the past five decades of experience in the management of extremity vascular trauma, a number of factors have been identified which directly influence outcome. These include the time interval between injury and treatment, mechanism, anatomic location, associated injuries, age and comorbidity, and clinical presentation.

Knowledge of these prognostic factors is essential for the appropriate evaluation and treatment of afflicted patients.

The time interval from injury to treatment is perhaps the most critical determinant of salvage of both life and limb following extremity vascular injury, as it is for all forms of trauma. This is explained by the time-dependent nature of the two major consequences of vascular injury, hemorrhage and ischemia. A linear correlation between delay in treatment of arterial injuries and limb loss was shown in WWII.[5] This association has become even stronger in both experimental and clinical studies since then which involve prompt repair and restoration of blood flow following acute arterial injury. In 1949, Miller and Welch[57] showed increasing rates of limb loss with increasing time delay of reperfusion of canine hind limbs after femoral artery ligation. This relation was also demonstrated in wounded soldiers in subsequent military conflicts in Afghanistan[58] and Lebanon,[59] where amputation rates rose from 22% and 3%, respectively, among injuries revascularized within 6–12 hours, to as high as 93% when revascularization was delayed more than 12 hours. Several civilian clinical series have since confirmed this close correlation of limb loss with delay in revascularization, especially when extremity arterial injury is complicated by associated injuries to vein, soft tissue, and bone.[24,26,29,33,36,38,60,61] Even salvaged limbs following treatment delay are subject to functional disability from nerve and muscle damage, as well as the development of potentially dangerous vascular complications such as false aneurysms and AVFs (Fig. 44-5). These latter lesions are more difficult to repair than acute vascular injuries and have a greater perioperative morbidity and mortality in some series.[31,48,49] These results have established the critical time interval for restoration of limb perfusion and optimal limb salvage to be at most 6–8 hours following extremity vascular trauma. The degree of ischemia and extent of collateral circulation affect tissue tolerance of delay. Therefore, prompt diagnosis and treatment of vascular injuries must be a major goal of management of all extremity trauma.[62,63] The low incidence of false aneurysms and AVFs in large series of vascular injuries (see Table 44-4) demonstrates how well this principle has been learned.

Blunt mechanisms of injury involve a wider application of force, with greater damage to extremity vessels and surrounding structures than is imparted by penetrating trauma. Blunt vascular injuries are associated with a more difficult diagnosis, and higher rates of amputation and severe dysfunction, than simple penetrating vascular injuries, which are typically clean, isolated, and more easily diagnosed and repaired.[17,21,23,25,29,31,37,64,65] Among penetrating injuries, stabs impart the least destructive force and are associated with a small and discrete area of injury.[66] As discussed earlier, high-velocity gunshot and shotgun wounds create a level of damage similar to blunt trauma, in terms of the complexity and extent of the damage, the difficulty of diagnosis and treatment, and the higher rate of limb loss.[67] This increased wounding power of high-velocity firearms largely accounts for the differences between military and civilian reports of extremity vascular trauma.[3,11,14]

There is a differential susceptibility of extremity arteries to amputation following injury, most related to the extent of collateral flow that may still perfuse a limb with its artery occluded. This was demonstrated in WWII,[5] in which the incidence of upper extremity amputation following brachial artery ligation was only 24%, compared with a 50% loss of lower extremities following femoral artery ligation, due to the more tenuous collaterals of the

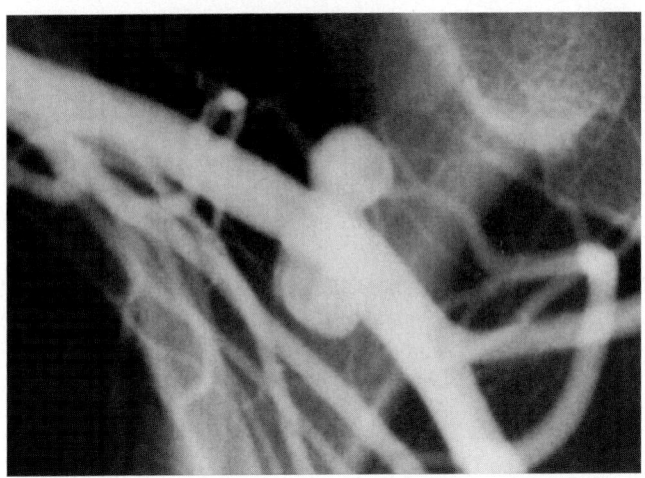

**FIGURE 44-5.** False aneurysm of axillary artery detected four months after gunshot wound to thoracic outlet that manifested no hard signs initially. Surgically repaired by resection and end-to-end anastomosis without complication.

latter. In either location, ligation above the profunda branches resulted in higher rates of limb loss than ligation below these branches. Acute occlusion of the popliteal artery results in the highest rate of limb loss (72.5%) of any peripheral vessel because it is a true end artery with tenuous collateral flow. This information allows the surgeon to assess the urgency required in detecting and treating various arterial injuries, and allows accurate prioritization of management in multiply injured patients.

Associated injuries to other tissues and body systems in patients with extremity vascular injury clearly worsen the prognosis for morbidity, mortality, and limb salvage. Most deaths and morbidity in these patients are due to associated injuries to the head and torso.[3,5,11,24,26,37] Such life-threatening problems are among the few remaining indications to ligate injured extremity arteries. Associated vein and skeletal injuries substantially increase the rate of limb loss over isolated vascular injuries.[26,31,38,39,47,63,64,68–70] Nerve injuries occur in up to 50% of patients with extremity vascular trauma and are the most important determinant of long-term limb disability in this setting.[34,38,71] Extensive soft tissue damage disrupts collateral flow and makes coverage of vascular repairs difficult, which increase the risk of limb loss.[3,67]

Age and comorbidity impart a poor prognosis on most forms of trauma, and must influence the judgment as to the proper management of any extremity vascular injury. Medical comorbidity affects the response to shock, ischemia, and general anesthesia and may require a truncated, damage control approach to extremity injuries that is not often necessary in young healthy patients. Older victims tend to have more diseased, brittle, and chronically occluded vessels which are more prone to injury, less tolerant of acute ischemia, and which render the physical findings of pulse deficit and ischemic changes unreliable determinants of acute vascular injury.[3,22,28,30,62]

The clinical presentation of extremity vascular trauma reflects the severity of the insult and the urgency of the threat to both life and limb. Active hemorrhage, manifested by external bleeding or large and expanding hematomas, is typically accompanied by shock. This is associated with a worse prognosis and requires more immediate attention than a stable patient without active blood loss.

The clinical findings of ischemia in an acutely injured extremity are also ominous and reflect the onset of tissue damage as well as the potential for reperfusion injury, limb disability, and compartment syndrome. This presentation indicates an urgent need for immediate revascularization in contrast to cases of incomplete occlusion in which distal perfusion is preserved.

## DIAGNOSIS

> "Perfection of tools and confusion of goals are the characteristics of our time"
>
> —Albert Einstein

All injured extremities must be evaluated for the presence of vascular trauma, and a prompt and accurate diagnosis is necessary to maximize limb salvage and function. The approach to diagnosis of extremity vascular trauma has been the subject of much debate, and has evolved rapidly in recent years. Most basically it requires a thorough understanding of the clinical manifestations of vascular injury and the appropriate roles and most efficient use of available diagnostic modalities in order to minimize the time to treatment.

### Clinical Manifestations

A history of active bleeding, or of pain out of proportion to physical findings typical of ischemia, may be the first indication of a vascular injury. Most extremity vascular injuries manifest one or more of the obvious physical findings or "hard signs" of hemorrhage: large, expanding or pulsatile hematoma, absent distal pulses, a palpable thrill or audible bruit over the wound, and distal ischemia (the 6 Ps mentioned earlier). These hard signs reflect a high probability of major vascular injury requiring surgical repair in the setting of injured extremities[15,24,63,72,73] and mandate that vascular injury be suspected and excluded. Overlooking hard signs of vascular trauma on the initial evaluation of injured extremities is the most common reason for the development of limb-threatening complications such as gangrene, false aneurysm and AVF.[22,26,31,48,49,74–78]

"Soft" signs are described in older literature as a set of more equivocal physical findings in injured extremities that are associated with a lower probability of major vascular trauma. These include small, stable hematomas, injury to an adjacent nerve, unexplained hypotension, history of hemorrhage at the scene no longer present in the hospital, and proximity of penetrating wounds to a major vessel.[15,63,65,78] Richardson and coworkers[79] found only a 58% incidence of arterial injuries in extremities with a combination of hard and soft signs. Other studies have shown that soft signs have no more correlation with the presence of extremity vascular injury than no signs at all and should not influence the treatment decision.[15,19,80,81] These signs are most likely caused by associated injury to adjacent muscle, nerves, bone and soft tissue, and any significant vascular injury present appears to be coincidental, and reflected by concomitant hard signs. Although soft signs are still described in some recent studies, it has become less relevant due to a demonstrated absence of clinical significance or utility in the diagnosis of vascular injury. The key clinical decisions in the evaluation of injured extremities for vascular trauma need only be based on the presence or absence of hard signs.[15,19,81,82]

Penetrating extremity wounds and wound tracks which are near enough to major blood vessels to have potentially injured them have posed a special diagnostic dilemma for surgeons, especially when the patient is asymptomatic (i.e., the absence of hard signs). These clinically occult "proximity" injuries illustrate an apparent weakness of the physical examination, because vascular injury has been documented in 5% to 24% of cases.[15,19,26,27,80,83–88] This led to aggressive diagnostic evaluation of all injured extremities in past years, regardless of clinical manifestations, so as to avoid the limb-threatening consequences of missed vascular injuries.[27]

### Contrast Arteriography

Although imaging of arteries through the intraluminal injection of radiopaque contrast is now a common tool for the evaluation of extremity trauma for vascular injury, it took several decades for this role to develop. As repair of vascular injuries became established in the military and civilian sectors in the 1950s, and the dangers of missed or delayed diagnosis became evident, immediate surgical exploration was the standard diagnostic modality applied to all limbs at risk for vascular injury through the 1970s.[10,22,23,25,27,30,31] This was questioned by many in view of its costs, complication rate, and a rate of negative explorations as high as 80%.

Arteriography was arbitrarily applied to the diagnosis of extremity vascular trauma during the 1960s and 1970s.[47,72,89,90] It was very accurate at confirming most vascular injuries in symptomatic limbs, but this was superfluous, unnecessarily costly and time-consuming, in view of how reliably hard signs on physical examination already do this.[15] Also, several clinical and experimental studies had indicated a poor accuracy at excluding vascular trauma in asymptomatic injured limbs.[10,31,91] By the mid- to late 1980s, as arteriography became more technically sophisticated, several studies, including one long-term follow-up,[79] established this modality to be as accurate as surgical exploration at excluding extremity vascular injury, even in the most problematic setting of asymptomatic penetrating proximity trauma.[85,86,92–95] Such "exclusion" arteriography led to large cost reductions in the evaluation of injured limbs for vascular injury, reducing negative limb explorations to as low as 20%, and with low false-negative rates, and sensitivities of 95–99%, entirely comparable to surgery (Table 44-5). It is a safer modality than surgery, with major complication rates of considerably less than 1%.[99–102]

## TABLE 44-5

### False-Negative (Missed Injury) Rates of Contrast Arteriography

| REFERENCE | NO. NEGATIVE ARTERIOGRAMS | NO. FALSE NEGATIVES (%) |
|---|---|---|
| Drapanas et al[26] | 56 | 2 (3.6) |
| Snyder et al.[92] | 133 | 1 (0.75) |
| O'Gorman et al.[96] | 385 | 1 (0.3) |
| Sclafani et al.[94] | 956 | 5 (0.5) |
| Lipchik et al.[97] | 63 | 1 (1.6) |
| Richardson et al.[79] | 455 | 9 (2) |
| Rose and Moore[95] | 17 | 1 (5.9) |
| Tohmeh and Perler[98] | 40 | 0 |
| Total | 2105 | 20 (0.95) |

*Source: Used with permission, from Frykberg ER: Angiography in extremity injury. In Ivatury RR, Cayten CG, eds. The Textbook of Penetrating Trauma. Baltimore, Lippincott, Williams and Wilkins, 1996, p. 409.*

It does have some drawbacks, however, including a still considerable charge to the patient that ranges between $1000 and $2000, and, like surgery, a high rate of negative studies. It typically involves delays of up to three hours even in the most experienced trauma centers,[80,83] a critical factor in limb salvage. Cargile and coworkers documented a significantly longer average delay to surgery among patients undergoing preoperative arteriography (6.8 hours) than among those without this study (2.5 hours).[103] Further, as many as 16% of studies may be technically suboptimal.[95]

The overriding advantages led arteriography to supplant routine surgical exploration as the diagnostic modality of choice for the evaluation of injured extremities by the mid-1980s, especially for the exclusion of occult vascular injuries in proximity wounds. The major indication for its application is any setting in which the clinical picture does *not* answer the two crucial questions on which treatment depends: Is there a vascular injury, and where is it located? Blunt or complex injuries, chronic vascular disease, multiple potential sites of injury, and thoracic outlet and shotgun wounds are examples of such indications. It may also be used to characterize the nature and extent of vascular injury when this will affect the management, as in intraoperative or postoperative assessment of a repaired vessel,[88] in cases of delayed presentation when the time element is no longer important, and to confirm abnormal findings from noninvasive tests. Arteriography should be performed only in hemodynamically stable patients, as life-threatening conditions require immediate surgery and must take precedence over injuries that threaten limbs (Table 44-6). The surgeon should always review the arteriogram with the radiologist, in order to judge the clinical significance of any abnormal finding and its appropriate management.

The prolonged time interval required for formal arteriography by a radiologist can be avoided in very urgent settings by a percutaneous one- or two-shot hand injected arteriogram performed by the surgeon in the emergency center or on the operating table (ECA). This technique is easy to perform, can be accomplished within 15 minutes, is cost-effective, and has an accuracy in confirming or excluding arterial injury that is entirely comparable to formal arteriography.[63,89,90,92,96,101] The artery to be studied is cannulated with an 18-gauge catheter (prograde in the femoral artery at the groin, retrograde into the brachial artery above an inflated blood pressure cuff at the elbow). With a portable x-ray unit and a plate placed under the extremity, 20–50 mL of radio-opaque contrast is injected, and an exposure is made while injecting the last 5 mL. For

**TABLE 44-6**

| Indications for Arteriography Following Extremity Injury |
| --- |
| Hemodynamic stability |
| Follow-up of nonoperatively managed arterial injuries |
| Intraoperative evaluation[a] |
| Postoperative evaluation[a] |
| Thoracic outlet or shotgun wounds |
| Confirmation of abnormal noninvasive tests |
| Any of the following that manifest hard signs: |
|   Blunt or complex injuries[a] |
|   Missile that parallels the course of an artery |
|   Multiple potential sites of injury (i.e., blast shrapnel) |
|   Chronic vascular insufficiency |

[a]Consider percutaneous hand-injected study in E.R. or O.R.

visualization of distal vessels in the leg, 50 mL should be injected and the x-ray taken 5 seconds after injection has been completed. The use of fluoroscopy simplifies the process by coordinating exposure with the visualization of the area of concern. Two exposures improve the success of this method; approximately 70% of diagnostic errors occurred in cases in which only one film was obtained. This technique is most useful for rapidly confirming or excluding vascular trauma in patients with equivocal clinical manifestations and multiple injuries, to help prioritize management (Fig. 44-6).

## Other Contrast Imaging Techniques

Intra-arterial digital subtraction arteriography (IADSA) has also been used to study arterial injury.[104] It has a sensitivity and specificity similar to arteriography and has several advantages, including a shorter time to complete the examination, less exposure to radiation, reduced cost, reduced dye load, less discomfort, and better contrast resolution. Because a smaller catheter is used, IADSA may lessen the chances of an iatrogenic injury. Its usefulness is limited, however, in shotgun injuries, in which metallic fragments may distort the images, and in detection of subtle intraluminal defects.

Digital venous arteriography and magnetic resonance angiography lack sufficient resolution to detect significant intimal injuries. In addition, these studies require intense cooperation of the patient to remain motionless. Magnetic resonance angiography is performed in an environment that is not user friendly to the critically ill patient and would be contraindicated in those patients with penetrating injuries and retained metallic fragments. Thus, these two modalities are not practical in the patient with peripheral vascular trauma.

Helical computed tomographic arteriography (CTA) has shown increasing feasibility and usage for imaging injured extremities for vascular trauma in recent years. This modality has demonstrated levels of accuracy, resolution, and cost that are comparable to conventional arteriography. Additionally, rapid data acquisition facilitates rapid multiorgan CT examinations in critically injured patients who will require such imaging anyway, avoiding the need for calling in an angiographic team with its inevitable delay. The three-dimensional reconstructions made possible by CTA are also superior to conventional arteriography, all of which may result in this modality becoming the standard form of arterial imaging in trauma.[105]

Venography has been used to evaluate patients for extremity venous injury.[103,106] Most venous injuries requiring surgical repair are found on exploration of concomitant arterial injuries or manifest hard signs that mandate surgery.[72,83] The only benefit of preoperative venography would be to detect asymptomatic venous injuries, but the absence of any evidence of adverse sequelae of missed venous injury, or of benefit of screening venography, makes such extensive diagnostic effort unnecessary.[84,92,99,107] Gagne and coworkers[108] found venography to be a poor screening tool for extremity venous injury, with 50% of studies technically unsuccessful, and only 43% of all venous injuries detected.

## Physical Examination

Before vascular imaging was feasible or widely accepted, physical findings were the sole means of diagnosing extremity vascular

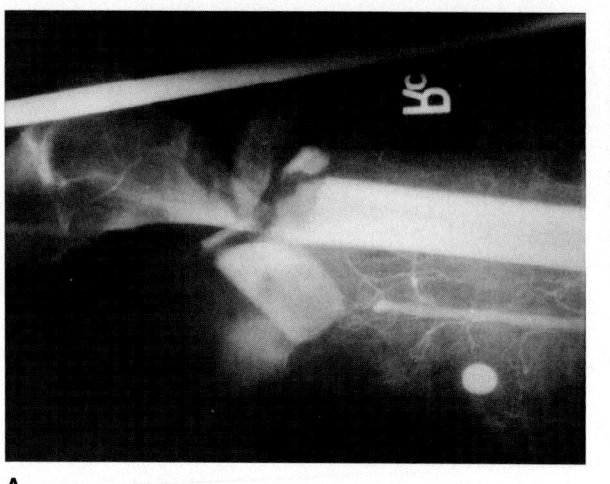
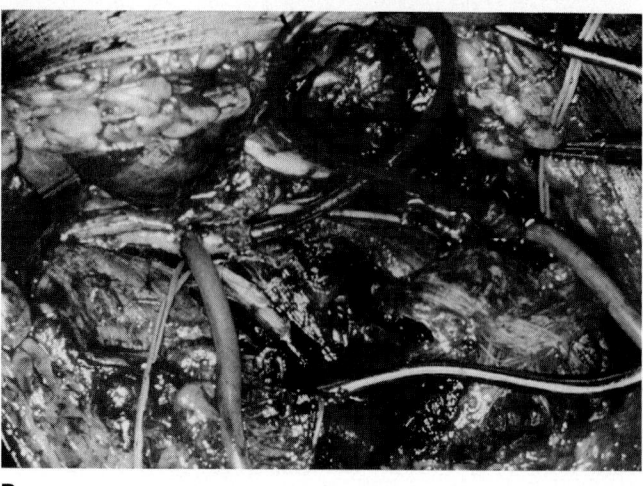

**A**                                    **B**

**FIGURE 44-6.** **(A)** Comminuted open supracondylar femur fracture with no distal pulses, on-table hand-injected arteriogram in operating room confirms popliteal artery injury. **(B)** Immediate shunting of transected popliteal artery allows external fixation across knee joint and soft tissue debridement, then definitive end to end anastomosis of artery with minimal warm ischemia.

trauma and the only basis for the decision to operate.[3,5,7–11,22,72] The close correlation of hard signs with the presence of a significant vascular injury became evident from this experience. It has been shown that hard signs are best considered as a unit, and that a positive physical examination following simple penetrating extremity trauma, defined as the presence of any one or more hard signs, predicts a major vascular injury requiring surgical repair with an accuracy that approaches 100%.[15,73] In this setting, further diagnostic work-up is superfluous, costly, and potentially dangerous in terms of the delay required for such modalities as arteriography.

There are exceptional circumstances in which a positive physical examination (i.e., hard sign present) does *not* accurately reflect either the presence or location of a vascular injury, and adjunctive diagnostic imaging still may be necessary (see Table 44-6). Thoracic outlet wounds (medial to the deltopectoral groove) are especially challenging and generally require arteriographic evaluation as the surrounding shoulder girdle may mask hard signs and, even if they are manifest, the surgical approach will be dependent on the exact location of the vascular injury[15,19,83,109,110] (see Fig. 44-5). Only 67% of all vascular injuries in the thoracic outlet are clinically evident, compared with 90% of all other upper extremity vascular injuries.[111] Blunt extremity trauma and complex injuries to bone and soft tissue from penetrating trauma have a high false-positive rate of physical examination, because hard signs may be manifested only by the associated tissue damage even in the absence of a major vascular injury.[65,83] Applebaum and coworkers[112] prospectively documented major vascular injury in only 13% of all patients with hard signs following blunt extremity trauma. Thus, unlike uncomplicated penetrating trauma, in which hard signs mandate immediate surgery, complex extremity wounds with hard signs mandate exclusion arteriography. This will minimize unnecessary surgical explorations in a large majority of these already compromised limbs.[38,65]

Soft signs of vascular injury generally have been an indication for further diagnostic work-up, having some correlation with vascular injury, but less than hard signs.[63,86,95] A series of studies at the University of Florida, however, has shown that soft signs have no

more statistical correlation with vascular injury than no signs at all.[15,19,80,81] Therefore, they should be placed in the category of a negative physical examination. Others have corroborated this observation.[112] Thus, in evaluating extremity trauma for vascular injury, a positive or negative physical examination should depend only on the presence or absence of hard signs.

A long-standing dilemma has involved the clinical implications of injured extremities with wounds placing major arteries at risk (i.e., penetrating proximity wounds or high risk blunt injuries such as supracondylar long bone fractures and knee or elbow dislocations), yet which do not manifest hard signs. The diagnostic approach here has substantial economic and logistical implications, because this is how most extremity trauma presents. Asymptomatic penetrating proximity injuries are known to be associated with vascular injury in 5–24% of cases (see previous section on Contrast Arteriography), suggesting that an absence of physical findings could not by itself reliably exclude extremity vascular injury. This prompted routine surgical exploration and, by the mid-1980s, routine arteriography, of all proximity injuries of the extremities to avoid the hazards of missing vascular injuries. The high incidence (up to 95%) of negative explorations and then negative exclusion arteriograms in this setting led to a question as to the validity and necessity of this costly approach.[87]

Several studies confirmed that occult vascular injury is found in approximately 10% of all asymptomatic proximity injuries, but analysis of the vascular injuries found in this unique setting showed that most had a benign and self-limiting natural history and seldom required surgical intervention. One study showed that routine arteriography of proximity injuries required over $66,000 in charges in order to detect a single vascular injury requiring surgical repair, clearly not a cost-effective screening tool.[80] All occult vascular injuries were found to be nonocclusive lesions, including intimal flaps, focal narrowing, and small false aneurysms and AVFs, explaining why they do not manifest physical findings.[19,81,113] Every study of this issue to date has corroborated these findings. A compilation of 3976 published cases of asymptomatic penetrating injuries in proximity to extremity arteries in which all were evaluated with arteriography (Table 44-7) confirms that, although occult vascular

**TABLE 44-7**

### Profile of Asymptomatic Penetrating Wounds in Proximity To Extremity Arteries[a]

| REFERENCE | NO. OF PROXIMITY WOUNDS | NO. OF OCCULT VASCULAR INJURIES (%) | NO. OF OCCULT VASCULAR INJURIES REQUIRING SURGERY (%)[b] |
|---|---|---|---|
| McDonald et al.[114] | 85 | 5 (6) | 0 |
| McCorkell et al.[115] | 57 | 7 (12) | 0 |
| Gomez et al.[87] | 72 | 17 (24) | 1 (1.4) |
| Hartling et al.[66] | 36 | 5 (14) | 0 |
| Lipchik et al.[97] | 59 | 3 (5) | 1 (1.7) |
| Rose and Moore[95] | 97 | 0 | 0 |
| Dennis et al.[19c] | 254 | 25 (10) | 2 (0.8) |
| Tohmeh and Perler[98] | 58 | 1 (1.7) | 0 |
| Weaver et al.[120c] | 157 | 17 (11) | 1 (0.6) |
| Francis et al.[116c] | 160 | 17 (11) | 7 (4.4) |
| Smyth et al.[117] | 65 | 2 (3) | 1 (1.5) |
| Itani et al.[101] | 1712 | 216 (14) | 28 (1.6) |
| Kaufman et al.[118c] | 92 | 22 (24) | 0 |
| Trooskin et al.[102c] | 153 | 7 (4.6) | 2 (1.3) |
| Gahtan et al.[119] | 394 | 37 (9.4) | 7 (1.8) |
| Gagne et al.[108c] | 43 | 4 (10) | 0 |
| Norman et al.[121c] | 61 | 17 (28) | 1 (1.6) |
| Gonzalez et al.[73] | 421 | 4 (0.95) | 20 (0.5) |
| Total | 3976 | 406 (10.2) | 53 (1.3) |

[a]Includes only wounds in extremity proper, excluding shotgun and thoracic outlet wounds.

[b]Percentage of all proximity wounds, excluding negative explorations.

[c]Prospective study.

Source: Modified with permission from Dennis JW, Frykberg ER, Veldenz HC, et al.: Validation of nonoperative management of occult vascular injuries and accuracy of physical examination alone in penetrating extremity trauma: 5- to 10-year followup. J Trauma 44:249, 1998.

injury was found in 10%, surgical intervention was performed in only 1.3% of all proximity injuries. In 468 of these proximity wounds from seven series, among which 44 occult vascular injuries were detected (9.4%), no surgery was required at all.[66,95,98,108,114,115,118] All vascular injuries requiring surgery in these studies were detected within two weeks by the subsequent appearance of hard signs and repaired at that time with no complications related to the delay. This further confirms the accuracy, safety, and reliability of physical examination at excluding *surgically significant* vascular injuries.

These data suggest that without arteriography, the absence of hard signs (i.e., a negative physical examination) alone following penetrating extremity trauma reliably excludes surgically significant vascular injuries with 98.7% accuracy. The only vascular injuries not excluded are those that rarely need intervention, and thus do not require detection. This false negative rate of 1.3% for physical examination (range 0–4.4%) should be acceptable, as it is entirely comparable to that of both arteriography and surgery (range 0.5–6%) (see Table 44-5),[76] but at less expense, risk, use of resources, and time delay.

These considerations support replacing arteriography with physical examination alone as the standard for evaluation of most penetrating extremity injuries for vascular trauma. Several studies have confirmed the safety of this approach. Frykberg and coworkers[15] documented a false-negative (i.e., missed injury) rate of 0.8% for physical examination of 366 penetrating extremity wounds with 99.5% diagnostic accuracy (100% when positive, 99.2% when negative), and a savings of over $255,000

in arteriography charges alone. Gonzalez and coworkers[73] reported 98.7% diagnostic accuracy for physical examination of 460 penetrating extremity wounds (95% when positive, 99% when negative), and a savings in radiology services of over $800,000. No instance of limb loss or limb morbidity has ever yet been reported to result from this approach. Concerns as to the long-term sequelae and safety of undetected and untreated occult vascular injuries were addressed with a follow-up of 309 asymptomatic penetrating proximity extremity wounds which had never undergone surgery or arteriography, over a mean interval of 5.4 years.[82] Among 90 (29%) injuries available for follow-up, four (1.3%) required surgery for delayed presentation of vascular injuries, all within two weeks of injury, and without any complications resulting from the delay. These results confirm those predicted by all published short-term studies (see Table 44-7).

Evidence also indicates that the absence of hard signs following blunt or complex penetrating extremity trauma excludes surgically significant vascular injury as reliably as it does in simple penetrating trauma, even in the setting of high-risk skeletal injuries. Applebaum and coworkers[112] found three arterial injuries in 22 cases of asymptomatic blunt extremity trauma (13.6%), none of which ever required surgery. Gillespie and coworkers[122] found 16 asymptomatic injuries to major arteries among 93 patients (17%) with both blunt and penetrating extremity trauma, none of which ever required surgery. Miranda and coworkers[123] reported no vascular injuries requiring surgical intervention among 27 patients with posterior knee dislocations and no hard signs, and confirmed this with a 13-month mean follow-up of 44% of these patients. As in simple penetrating trauma, the asymptomatic arterial injuries that occur in these complex cases have a largely benign natural history that does not require surgery, and thus does not require detection (Fig. 44-7).[121]

Physical examination thus appears to be as accurate in the confirmation and exclusion of most cases of extremity vascular injury *that require surgical intervention* as any other diagnostic modality applied in this setting. It is reliable only for those portions of the extremity properly amenable to examination (distal to the inguinal ligament and deltopectoral groove). These patients must be counseled as to the risks of this approach and the need for follow-up if any hard signs develop. The avoidance of screening arteriography in most extremity trauma not only reduces costs, but may impact on limb salvage by eliminating treatment delays.[103] The success of physical examination in this role, using only the presence or absence of hard signs for the treatment decision, validates the benign natural history of most asymptomatic vascular injuries, as well as the clinical irrelevance of the old category of soft signs. The fact that the great majority (50–90%) of all cases of extremity trauma present as blunt or penetrating proximity wounds without hard signs[15,66,86,92,95,97,99,102,114,115,120] emphasizes the considerable economic and logistical implications of avoiding routine arteriography and surgery in this setting, in view of the limited resources of most trauma centers.

## Noninvasive Studies

Noninvasive testing has been applied to the diagnosis of extremity vascular trauma, using ultrasonic flow detection (Doppler principle) to quantify blood flow and duplex ultrasonography to image vessels at risk.[124–126] This is a natural extrapolation from the demonstrated benefits of these tests since the early 1970s in the setting of chronic vascular insufficiency.

Hand-held Doppler flow detectors screen for arterial injury by measuring the arterial pressure index (API), determined by dividing the systolic pressure in the injured limb by the systolic pressure in an uninjured arm. The determination of phasic Doppler signals by an experienced examiner provides further qualitative evidence regarding collateral flow.[62] The absence of flow signals objectively establishes the hard sign of pulselessness, which may be helpful for the inexperienced physician, nurse, or paramedic. A dangerous pitfall, however, is the erroneous assumption that Doppler signals in the absence of a palpable

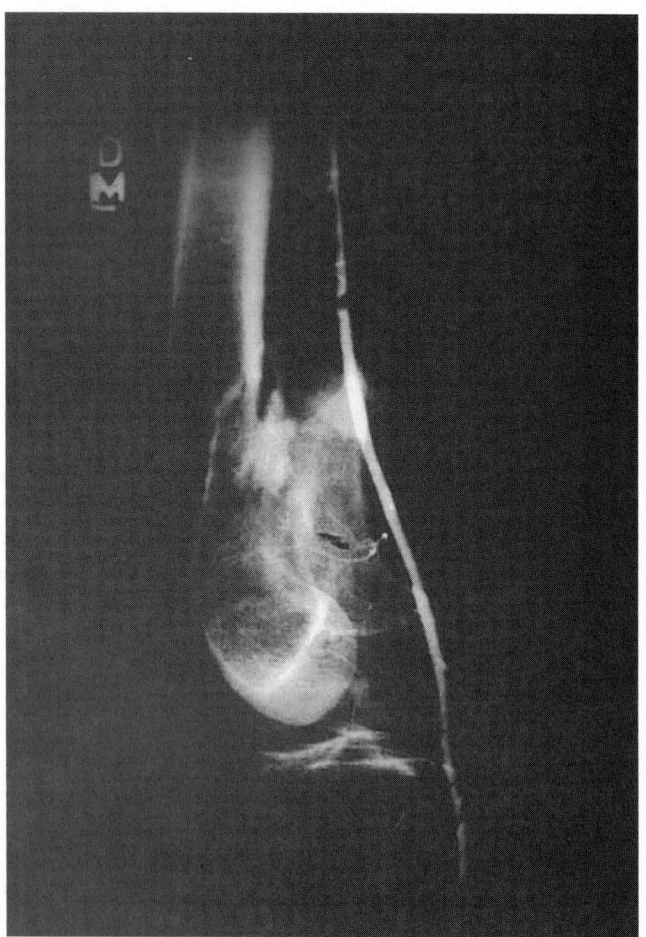

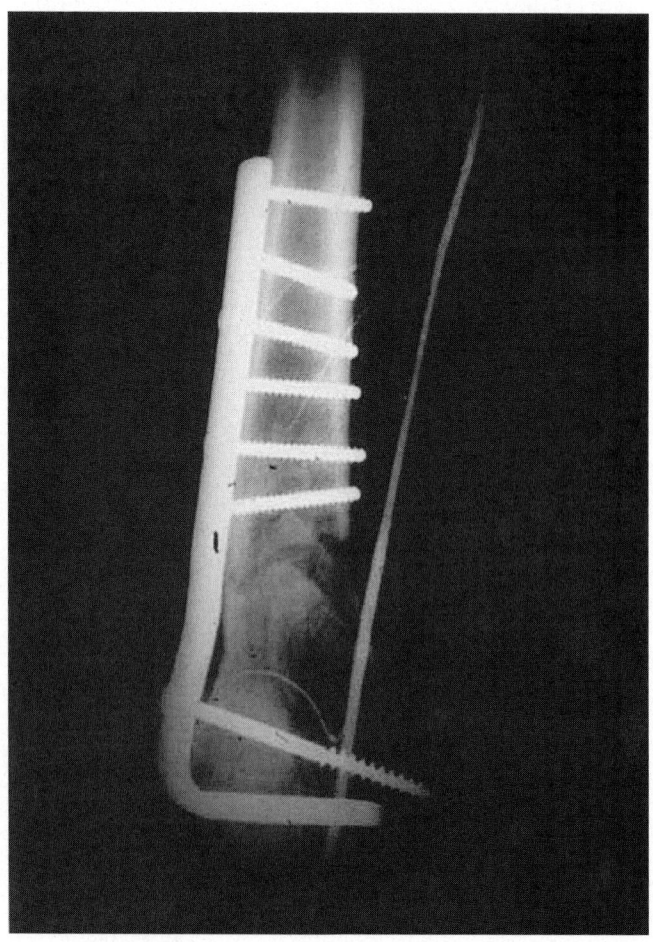

A                                                              B

**FIGURE 44-7.** **(A)** Asymptomatic nonocclusive intimal flap of popliteal artery following blunt supracondylar femur fracture, nonoperatively observed. **(B)** Complete resolution of intimal flap six weeks later following internal fixation of femur.
*(Reproduced with permission from Frykberg ER, Vines FS, Alexander RH, et al.: The natural history of clinically occult arterial injuries. J Trauma 29:77, 1989.)*

pulse exclude a vascular injury. Flow signals can occur from collateral flow around a transected or thrombosed vessel, while a pulse can only be conducted through an intact vessel. Therefore, clinical management of injured extremities must be governed primarily by the presence or absence of a pulse, in addition to the other hard signs.

Johansen and coworkers have found the Doppler-derived API to be highly reliable in excluding arterial injury in both blunt and penetrating extremity trauma.[127,128] An API <0.9 had a diagnostic accuracy of 95% for the prediction of a clinically significant arterial trauma, and they recommend confirming this finding with arteriography. Mills and coworkers reported this same finding in a prospective study of 38 patients with knee dislocation.[129] Others recommend arteriography when the systolic pressure in the injured limb is 10–20 mm Hg lower than the uninjured contralateral limb.[62,125] Weaver and coworkers[120] required the threshold API to be 0.99 or less to predict only 80% of arterial injuries, but at the expense of a very low specificity. They found an API of 0.90 to markedly reduce its sensitivity (i.e., miss injuries). Johansen and coworkers demonstrated a savings of over $65,000 in technical charges and over 180 hours of management time in 100 patients due to reduced utilization of arteriography. Nonocclusive arterial injuries that do not alter or obstruct blood flow, such as false aneurysms, AVFs, and intimal flaps, are not reliably detected by this modality.

As noted above, duplex ultrasonography combines real-time B-mode (brightness modulation) ultrasound imaging with a steerable pulsed-Doppler flow detection. The direction of flow can be represented by the addition of colorized imaging, which has been termed "triplex," or color-flow Doppler. Duplex scanning has been demonstrated to screen for extremity vascular injury at least as reliably as arteriography with nearly as much imaging resolution, but more safely and at less expense.[130–132] It can detect some of those minimal arterial injuries that are missed by physical examination and Doppler examination and has shown promise in diagnosing venous injuries as well.[108,131] It is an efficient and reliable method for intraoperative and postoperative monitoring of vascular repairs and extremity perfusion, as well as nonoperatively managed injuries.

On the other hand, poor sensitivity has been reported. Gagne and coworkers[108] reported that 67% of arterial injuries were missed by color-flow scanning, and Bergstein and coworkers[133] reported a sensitivity of only 50%, although the low number of true-positives in these studies may not reflect the true accuracy. Furthermore, the instrumentation is expensive, with duplex scanners selling for approximately $35,000, and color-flow devices for as much as six times this cost. This has led to the suggestion that these modalities be used selectively only in the cohort of patients with an abnormal API.[134]

The reliability of noninvasive modalities for the screening of injured extremities is not yet sufficiently established to either understand its proper role, or to allow management decisions based solely on its results.[62,82,108,112,135] Many studies have not confirmed the reported true-negative results by arteriography or surgery, nor by any documentation of the length of follow-up, thereby invalidating any clear expression of accuracy.[126–128,131,132] The diagnostic criteria that apply to chronic occlusive vascular disease cannot necessarily be extrapolated to acute arterial trauma. The accuracy of noninvasive tests is suspect in the setting of blunt trauma, patient discomfort, open wounds, large hematomas, bulky dressings, and traction devices, when it can be expected that Doppler signals and ultrasound images may be impaired and may limit appropriate interrogation of the vessel. Of interest, one recent prospective study of API in 38 patients with blunt knee dislocation concluded that it has a high diagnostic accuracy.[129] The training, experience and skill required for the necessary level of interpretation of this sophisticated technology is not available in most trauma centers around the clock to evaluate patients when they commonly present. Finally, noninvasive tests have yet to be compared directly with, or to demonstrate any advantage over, physical examination alone of injured extremities, which has an entirely comparable accuracy, and is simpler and less expensive than any other screening method currently applied to traumatized limbs.[82,108] For these reasons, further evaluation of this role for noninvasive tests has been recommended, and they should be used for this purpose only in the context of a controlled study.[135]

## Summary of the Diagnostic Approach

The first priority in the evaluation of extremity trauma must be the exclusion of major vascular injury. The proliferation of diagnostic technology in recent years can make this confusing. In most cases, the physical examination is sufficient for clinical decision-making. Uncomplicated penetrating extremity trauma that manifests one or more hard signs mandates immediate surgery for repair of the vascular injury that is reflected with almost 100% reliability by this presentation. The wound reveals the location of the vascular injury. No further imaging or testing is necessary or justified in this setting.

More complex extremity injuries manifesting hard signs, which do not as reliably reflect the presence or location of a vascular injury, or in which further characterization of the injury is needed for operative planning (i.e., complications of delayed presentation, thoracic outlet wounds, shotgun wounds, chronic vascular disease, associated skeletal and soft tissue injuries, multiple possible sites of injury), should undergo imaging with contrast arteriography in order to minimize unnecessary limb explorations and unexpected findings at surgery. CTA may prove to be a more rapid and feasible alternative for imaging in this setting, especially if the patient requires CT imaging of other body systems.[105] Consideration should be given in urgent circumstances to ECA. A positive arteriogram, showing occlusion or gross contrast extravasation from a major vessel, mandates surgical repair. A negative arteriogram, or the finding of a nonocclusive arterial lesion, rules out surgical intervention and may be followed nonoperatively by physical examination, repeat arteriography, or noninvasive testing.

Any injured extremity that manifests no hard signs of vascular trauma does *not* require any further vascular imaging or surgery for vascular exploration, regardless of the mechanism or complexity. Certainly if there is any doubt about physical findings, such as a borderline hematoma, or a question as to whether a pulse is present, arteriography is warranted. Any subsequent development of hard signs also mandates arteriography. Some trauma centers use noninvasive tests to aid in initial evaluation, but their reliability and role for this purpose remain uncertain, especially in blunt and complex extremity trauma, and require further study to clarify.

**TABLE 44-8**

**Comparison of Accuracy, Cost and Scientific Validity of Available Modalities for Evaluation of Penetrating Extremity Trauma for Vascular Injury**

|  | SURGERY | ARTERIO-GRAPHY | NON-INVASIVE | PHYSICAL EXAMINATION |
|---|---|---|---|---|
| Prospectively studied | 0 | ++ | + | ++ |
| Long-term follow-up available | ++ | ++ | +[a] | +++ |
| Cost | ++++ | ++ | + | 0 |
| Morbidity | ++ | + | 0 | 0 |
| Diagnostic accuracy | ++ | ++ | +[b] | ++ |

[a]One report of median one-year follow-up of 76% of patients (reference 108).

[b]Two reports of low sensitivity for arterial injuries (references 108, 133), and confirmatory arteriography required for all abnormal results.

*Source: Modified with permission from Dennis JW, Frykberg ER, Veldenz HC, et al.: Validation of nonoperative management of clinically occult vascular injuries and accuracy of physical examination alone in penetrating extremity trauma: 5- to 10-year follow-up. J Trauma 44:249, 1998.*

Abnormal results of flow detection and duplex scanning require confirmatory arteriography.

A comparison of all the major modalities currently used to evaluate extremity trauma for surgically significant vascular injury demonstrates essentially equivalent diagnostic accuracy and scientific validity, but large differences in cost and morbidity (Table 44-8). Physical examination alone should be the modality of choice in most settings. Arteriography (conventional, CTA or ECA) remains the modality of choice in that minority of circumstances when imaging is necessary (Fig. 44-8).

## MANAGEMENT

### General Principles

All patients with extremity vascular injury must be assessed for other life-threatening injuries, and overall supportive care must be assured. This includes establishing a patent airway, confirming adequate ventilation, supporting circulation and organ perfusion, and diagnosing and treating visceral injuries of the head and torso. Extremity trauma should not lead to mortality. The only immediately life-threatening problem that extremity trauma may present is hemorrhage, which must be controlled immediately with digital pressure or careful packing and application of pressure dressings. Blind probing and application of clamps in open wounds must be avoided, since it may cause more damage than benefit. Tourniquets should be only a last resort to control exsanguinating hemorrhage. When effective, tourniquets occlude collateral circulation and can lead to irreversible ischemia. When ineffective, they increase hemorrhage by failing to occlude arterial inflow while impeding venous return and increasing blood loss through injured veins.[3] Hemorrhagic shock is a common consequence of extremity vascular trauma,[10,26] which must be corrected promptly with repletion of intravenous volume in order to minimize morbidity and mortality.

Broad spectrum antibiotics should be administered as soon as possible after injury, especially if open fractures, severe soft tissue injury or contamination are present, or if prosthetic grafts are anticipated. Tetanus prophylaxis is indicated for any open wounds. When obvious ischemia is manifest in an injured extremity, systemic anticoagulation with heparin should be instituted immediately if there are no other sites of hemorrhage or intracranial trauma. This may prevent thrombosis or propagation of thrombus distal to an arterial injury during the preoperative preparation for surgical repair, and enhance limb salvage. Open wounds should be

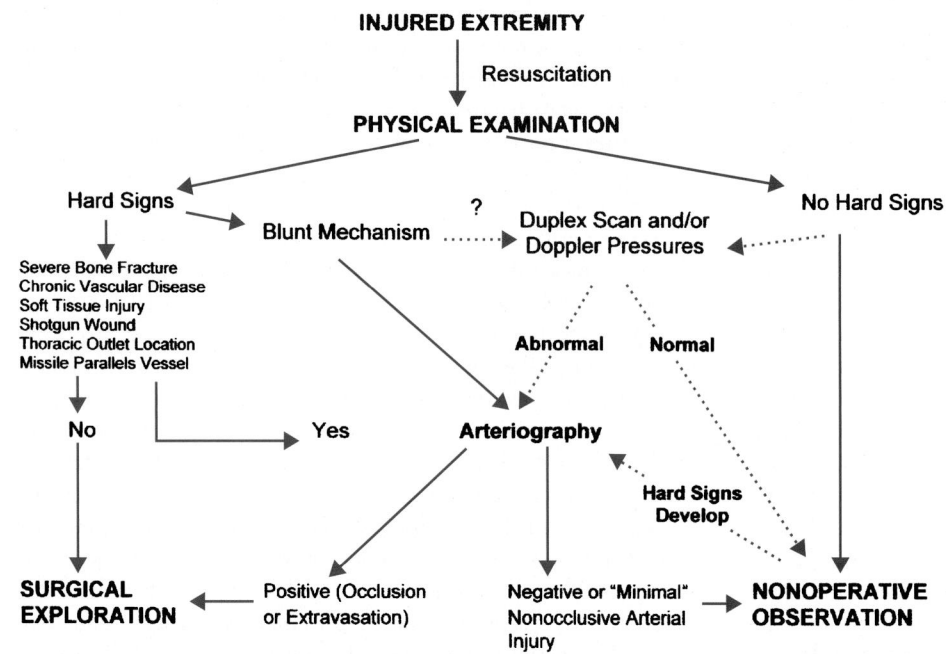

**FIGURE 44-8.** Algorithm for evaluation of injured extremities for vascular trauma. Dotted lines indicate possible alternative modalities that require further study.
*(Reproduced with permission from Frykberg ER: Advances in the diagnosis and treatment of extremity vascular trauma. Surg Clin North Am 75:207, 1995.)*

explored only in the operating room under controlled conditions, as dislodgement of a clot may lead to uncontrolled hemorrhage.

All resuscitative and diagnostic efforts must be directed at minimizing the time lag to definitive treatment. This is best accomplished within six hours, in which case a successful result can be expected in over 95% of cases.[3,13,63,88,103]

## Surgical Exposure and Preparation

Exploration of an injured extremity for direct repair of a vascular injury is best achieved under general anesthesia in the operating room, using loupe magnification and coaxial lighting (headlamp). The entire injured extremity should be prepared and draped into the operative field, allowing the foot or hand to be examined for return of distal pulses, color, warmth, and capillary refill. One uninjured extremity should also be prepped and draped to allow harvesting of the cephalic or saphenous vein. The first priority is to obtain proximal and distal control of the injured vessel through incisions placed directly over the area of injury and extended parallel to the course of the vessel. An S-shaped curvature should be made if the incision must cross a joint. Sharp debridement and copious irrigation of devitalized and contaminated tissue is necessary to reduce the chance of infection and optimize the success of vascular repair.

Exposure of the injured vessel is best done through uninjured tissue adjacent to the injury site, although active bleeding may require an approach directly through the traumatic wound. Digital pressure can be used to control hemorrhage until enough normal vessel can be sharply dissected free to allow clamping or vessel loop occlusion proximal and distal to the injury. Another method to control bleeding during exposure is by inserting a balloon-tipped catheter into the open proximal end of the vessel and inflating the balloon. Obtaining proximal control at some distance from the injury (i.e., at the groin for a mid-superficial femoral artery injury) generally is not effective, especially in the upper extremity, due to backbleeding from intervening branches.

Once control of the injured artery or vein is obtained, thrombus should be removed by the careful and gentle passage of balloon-tipped embolectomy catheters down the proximal and distal vessel segments, continuing these efforts until no further clot is obtained and vigorous backbleeding and forward bleeding occurs. Heparinized saline (15–30 mL of a solution of 50–100 U/mL) should be instilled into the proximal and distal vessel segments for regional anticoagulation during vascular repair. Systemic heparinization may be considered in the absence of contraindications from associated injuries.

The obviously damaged vessel ends should be sharply debrided only back to grossly normal vessel wall. Even though microscopic intimal damage may be more extensive, studies have shown that injured arteries heal without problem with conservative debridement.[3,43]

## Techniques of Arterial and Venous Repair

Repair of injured extremity arteries and veins generally is performed with synthetic nonabsorbable monofilament suture on atraumatic needles (5-0 polypropylene for larger arteries such as the subclavian, axillary, and femoral, and 6-0 or 7-0 for veins and smaller arteries such as the brachial, radial, ulnar, popliteal and tibials).

Interrupted suture is most effective in smaller vessels to prevent a purse-string constriction, while a continuous suture technique is best for circumferential repairs using an end-to-end anastomosis or insertion of an interposition graft in larger vessels. One or two sutures are used in circumferential running repairs, with perpendicular bites carefully taken 1mm back from the edge and 1mm apart. The distal clamp is released as the last suture is placed to allow backbleeding to wash out air and debris, then reclamped. The proximal clamp is then released for a final washout as the last suture is tied down, after which the distal clamp is again released, so as to prevent any remaining clot, air, or debris from flowing distally. A pulse should be palpated in the distal vessel and in the hand or foot to assure distal patency.

Only 10–15% of arterial injuries are amenable to lateral arteriorrhaphy. This technique is appropriate only for small punctures or clean lacerations, as any wound with a length greater than the vessel diameter will constrict the vascular lumen when sutured longitudinally. Patch angioplasty with autogenous vein or prosthetic patch may be considered to avoid vessel constriction with larger lacerations of intact vessels, but this is used in only 1% of all vascular repairs.[9,11,27,32,65,88,103,111]

Most vascular injuries have been managed by resection and either end-to-end anastomosis or insertion of autogenous vein or prosthetic interposition grafts.[9,11,63,88,103] Primary end-to-end anastomosis is preferred when possible, but should be performed only when the severed ends of the injured vessel can be approximated easily without undue tension (see Fig. 44-4). Substantial mobilization of vessels by sharply dissecting them free of surrounding tissue can achieve added length, but division of collateral branches for this purpose should be avoided, especially at the level of the popliteal artery. A direct repair should not be performed with a flexed joint, to be certain that there is adequate length and no tension or kinking of the repair. If an interposition graft is necessary, autogenous saphenous vein harvested from an uninjured extremity remains the conduit of choice, even in combat casualties with contaminated wounds.[11,136] The lesser saphenous and cephalic veins are acceptable alternatives. If autogenous vein is not available, is of inadequate quality, or if the patient's condition mandates a more rapid approach, prosthetic grafts of both Dacron and polytetrafluoroethylene (PTFE) have been used successfully as alternative conduits for the repair of both arterial and venous injuries. Although the long-term patency of synthetic grafts appears to be lower than autogenous vein, especially in the popliteal and tibial locations, previous concerns about their vulnerability to infection have not borne out and should not be a barrier to their consideration.[88,137–140]

Although surgical repair remains the approach of choice for all extremity artery injuries, there are circumstances in which arterial ligation may be necessary.[11,27,32,63,88,103,111] In hemodynamically unstable, acidotic, and hypothermic patients ligation should be considered as a damage control measure to cut short the operation and avoid mortality from an extremity injury. After the patient has been resuscitated, warmed, and stabilized, the limb then can be revascularized under more controlled conditions. Noncritical branch vessels, as from the profunda femoris or musculocutaneous arteries, can be ligated routinely. Injuries of the radial, ulnar, or tibial arteries can be ligated as long as one artery to the hand or foot remains intact and adequate perfusion is documented.[3,141] In the uncommon event that claudication or other ischemic symptoms develop, elective reconstruction can be done at a later date. Ligation of upper extremity arteries is tolerated better than in the lower extremity.[71,111]

## Postoperative Considerations

Postoperatively, limb perfusion must be monitored continuously by examination of skin temperature, color, and capillary refill, as well as palpation of the pulses. Frequently, peripheral pulses are not immediately palpable following vascular repair, even with a patent anastomosis and open runoff, due to reflex spasm. As long as an open repair has been documented at surgery, Doppler signals and pressures may be used to follow limb perfusion along with skin warmth and brisk capillary refill. Any evidence of loss of perfusion, and certainly any loss of pulses after they have been present, mandates either immediate investigation by arteriography or immediate return to the operating room.

Heparinization is not indicated routinely following vascular repair, since it offers no benefit at optimizing the success of repair, risks bleeding complications that may jeopardize a repair, and cannot substitute for technical perfection. The use of low molecular weight Dextran, however, has been helpful in maintaining the patency of venous repairs. Aspirin and other antiplatelet agents may also be given by suppository in the early postoperative period.

Suture line or soft tissue bleeding must be controlled to avoid hematomas that may become infected. There should be very little if any role for drains in these wounds. Drains should never be placed adjacent to vascular repairs, because they may erode or infect the suture line. Wound infections must be treated aggressively and promptly with open drainage, debridement, and antibiotics to avoid anastomotic disruption.

An associated injury to a peripheral nerve has been shown to be the most significant factor to affect long-term limb function adversely following vascular injury. This may require physical therapy and rehabilitation.

Elevation of the injured extremity will reduce the edema that may accompany resuscitation and reperfusion. Splinting of the extremities can be useful in preventing sudden movements that will stress vascular repairs.

Any complication or reoperation following repair of a vascular injury increases the risk of limb loss, especially if it involves repeated ischemic insults. This emphasizes the importance of prompt and appropriate initial management.

## Surgical Adjuncts

### Completion Arteriography.

Intraoperative "completion" arteriography should be a standard practice following arterial repair to document patency of the anastomosis and distal runoff and to ensure the absence of additional vascular injuries, especially if the success of repair is in any doubt. This can be performed on the operating table by simple needle puncture of the artery proximal to the repair, injection of 30 mL of water-soluble contrast with or without inflow occlusion, and a one-shot radiograph that includes the area of repair and the distal circulation. Repair should be considered complete only with the return of a palpable distal pulse, or a patent vessel on the completion arteriogram. As much as a 10% rate of clinically unsuspected problems with the

arterial repair has been reported with the routine use of completion arteriography.[3,88]

### Tissue Coverage.

Vascular repairs should be covered by full thickness vascularized tissue at the initial operation, to prevent the inevitable desiccation, infection, and disruption of exposed vessels, grafts, and suture lines. In most cases, coverage can be achieved by primary closure of muscle, subcutaneous and skin incisions, or by simple mobilization of adjacent soft tissue. Complex and contaminated wounds, however, are seen increasingly following crush injuries and shotgun blasts, in which primary closure may not be possible due to extensive tissue loss and debridement of devitalized areas. Primary closure may also be undesirable in the face of extensive contamination. These wounds should be closed with full thickness tissue, using pedicled transposed muscle flaps, free tissue muscle or myocutaneous flaps, or fasciocutaneous flaps.[142] Rarely, the soft tissue defect is so large that flap coverage is inadequate, or the level of contamination poses a prohibitive risk of infection. In these cases, porcine xenografts or cadaveric homografts of partial thickness skin have been used successfully to provide temporary coverage until the wound is clean enough to allow definitive full-thickness closure.[143]

A valuable option to consider is extra-anatomic bypass, in which an interposition graft is tunneled through clean uninjured tissue planes. This provides immediate coverage of the graft and suture lines, and allows appropriate and deliberate debridement and secondary closure of open complex wounds without the concern of an involved vessel. The posterior and lateral thigh, arm, and lower legs are common sites for these bypasses. When performing extra-anatomic bypass, it is essential that the proximal and distal artery be dissected well away from the site of injury and contamination, which is draped out of the surgical field. Autologous vein is the preferred graft conduit, although externally supported PTFE may be used as well. This method may be used as a definitive reconstruction, or it may be a temporary expedient, with arterial reconstruction through the native bed undertaken after healing has occurred.[144]

### Intraluminal Shunting.

There are circumstances in which extremity arterial repairs must be deferred for other priorities, such as life-threatening injuries elsewhere associated with systemic problems (shock, hypothermia, acidosis, and coagulopathy) or skeletal instability, which would jeopardize a vascular suture line. Such delay is a major risk to limb viability if it prolongs revascularization for more than six hours. This risk can be avoided by the use of plastic tubing that is inserted temporarily into the severed ends of injured vessels to immediately restore limb perfusion. In combined arterial and venous injuries, arterial flow can be restored while the vein is repaired. Parry and coworkers reported the successful use of temporary shunts in injured veins as an alternative to ligation and to maintain outflow until the patient can undergo definitive repair.[145] Intraluminal shunts also can be used while an amputated limb is evaluated and prepared for replantation, removing any concern about ongoing ischemia and tissue damage while other more urgent considerations are addressed.

Shunts can be constructed from sterile intravenous tubing or can be obtained commercially in a variety of forms and sizes. They can be placed in a matter of minutes. Following proximal and distal vascular control, balloon catheter thrombectomy, and regional heparinization, the shunt tubing is inserted proximally, blood is flushed through, then inserted into the distal vessel segment and secured with a ligature or vessel loop. If an interposition graft is required, it can be slipped over the shunt, the first anastomosis performed with the shunt in place, and the shunt then can be removed through the second anastomosis before the last few sutures are placed.

Intraluminal shunts minimize ischemia time in the setting of complex peripheral vascular injuries in multiply injured patients, when management priorities may not allow definitive vascular repair to proceed immediately (see Fig. 44-6). Rapid restoration of both perfusion and venous outflow by this method has been shown to improve limb salvage from combined skeletal, venous, and arterial injuries in an extremity.[38,125,146–149] Shunts are also an excellent damage control measure in unstable patients when definitive arterial or venous repair is not possible, providing a welcome alternative to ligation and limb loss.[148] Strict attention must be focused on indwelling shunts to assure patency by direct visualization in the wound, palpation of distal pulses, and the use of Doppler flow detection over the intact distal artery. Patency has been documented for up to 52 hours without systemic anticoagulation.[149] Thrombosis of the shunt should be corrected immediately by balloon catheter thrombectomy and reinsertion, maneuvers that can be performed easily in the operating room or at the bedside.

Fasciotomy.    Compartmental hypertension is a potentially devastating complication of extremity injury that can lead to limb loss even after successful revascularization. This results from a compromise in capillary perfusion of tissues within a limited space from increased pressure within that space, usually a fascial compartment of the lower leg. Venous hypertension usually begins this process. If allowed to progress, a vicious cycle develops that leads to necrosis of nerve and muscle. This may be followed by limb dysfunction and limb loss and by the life-threatening systemic manifestations of rhabdomyolysis, myoglobinuria, renal failure, hyperkalemia, and sepsis. Reperfusion of ischemic tissue following arterial injury is among the most common causes of this condition as a result of the capillary permeability and intracompartmental edema that follows the inflammatory response of reperfusion injury (see previous section on Pathophysiology). Ligation of a major vein can also lead to this problem. The upper extremity is less prone to develop compartment syndrome than the lower extremity due to its more extensive venous drainage, explaining why less than 10% of all brachial artery injuries are complicated by this problem.[150,151]

Compartment syndrome can develop insidiously, and tissue damage can occur in the absence of overt signs and symptoms. The classic clinical manifestations of pain out of proportion to apparent injury, especially when worsened by passive stretch, sensorimotor deficits, and palpable tenseness and swelling of the limb, are relatively insensitive, and may indicate irreversible necrosis by the time they first appear. Palpable distal pulses do not at all exclude this condition, as muscle and nerve necrosis can occur well before major arterial inflow is occluded, which is why pulses should never be used to monitor the development of a compartment syndrome. Absent pulses are virtually always due to arterial injury and not compartment syndrome.

A major goal of management of this complication must be prompt detection before tissue damage is established. Physical examination is clearly unreliable at permitting an early diagnosis,

especially in patients with altered mental status from a traumatic brain injury, drugs or alcohol ingestion, or who are undergoing general anesthesia for vascular repair or associated injuries, or patients with injury to the spinal cord. Therefore, the most effective early detection must involve a high index of suspicion, which requires a knowledge of the following clinical scenarios that pose a high risk for the development of compartment syndrome: any popliteal artery injury; any combined arterial and venous injury of the extremity; prolonged extremity ischemia of greater than four to six hours; any extremity vascular injury associated with shock; crush injuries; combined skeletal and vascular extremity trauma, and the ligation of a major extremity vein or artery, especially the popliteal vessels. It is also possible to measure compartment pressures directly in high-risk patients by needle puncture with a hand-held solid state transducer device (Stryker Surgical, Kalamazoo, Mi). Normal tissue pressures are 5 mm Hg. Any pressure above 25 mm Hg mandates immediate intervention.[152,153]

The definitive treatment of compartment hypertension is decompression of the afflicted compartments by incision of their investing fascia, which is called fasciotomy. This also allows direct visualization of the underlying tissue to assess the degree of damage and the need for debridement of devitalized areas. Most authors recommend a complete division of overlying epimysium and skin as well, to prevent them from also serving as limiting envelopes and visual barriers to evaluate viability.[32,154]

Proper treatment mandates knowledge of the anatomy of extremity compartments and their contents, especially of the most commonly afflicted four compartments of the lower leg. Although a single lateral incision can successfully expose all four lower leg compartments, either with or without fibulectomy, the most commonly used technique, and probably the quickest and safest, is the double-incision four compartment fasciotomy.[154] This involves a lateral longitudinal incision extending the length of the lower leg 2 cm anterior to the fibula, then longitudinally incising the fascia overlying the anterior and lateral compartments separately, taking care to avoid the superficial peroneal nerve. The superficial and deep posterior compartments are released through a similar skin and fascial incision medially, 2 cm posterior to the tibia, taking care to avoid the greater saphenous vein (Fig. 44-9). Whenever fasciotomy is indicated, all compartments should be released. The deep posterior compartment is the most hidden, but the most important to release as it contains the tibial nerve and two of the three arteries to the foot (peroneal and posterior tibial).

In recent years there has been increased emphasis on performing fasciotomy as early as possible, and even prophylactically, before any morbid sequelae or symptoms of compartmental hypertension develop.[151] This aggressive approach generally involves performing the fasciotomy before the vascular repair or reperfusion, to assure adequate outflow and prevent compartment syndrome from ever developing, and thus maximize limb salvage and function. Prophylactic fasciotomy is indicated in any of the high-risk settings for compartment syndrome mentioned above in this section, preferably before any physical findings are present. Several studies have attributed significant improvement in limb salvage following high-risk extremity trauma to this liberal application of early and prophylactic fasciotomy.[37,38,125,155,156] Another advantage of early fasciotomy is that the incisions can be closed primarily with good cosmetic results.[154] The use of a shoe-lacing technique with elastic

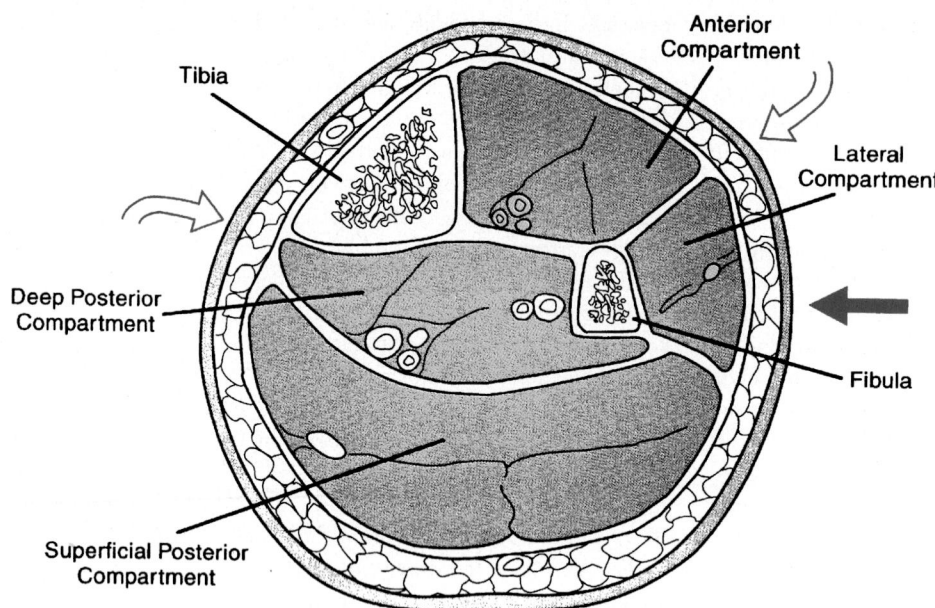

**FIGURE 44-9.** Cross-section of mid-calf showing the four fascial compartments and their contents. Open arrows show sites of double-incision fasciotomy, closed arrow shows site of single-incision fasciotomy. *(Reproduced with permission from Frykberg ER: Compartment Syndrome. In Cameron JL, ed. Current Surgical Therapy, 5th ed. 1995, p. 850.)*

vessel loops stapled to the skin edges allows gradual closure of the wound at the bedside without requiring an additional operative procedure (Fig. 44-10). Late fasciotomy done for established compartment syndrome is associated with significant muscle bulging that requires skin grafting to close.

Fasciotomy is a safe technique with low complication rates, most of which are related to technical pitfalls such as excessive bleeding and iatrogenic damage to nerves and vessels. The most common reported complication is infection, although this is due more to underlying tissue necrosis in cases of delay than to the fasciotomy itself. Some have advocated that when compartment syndrome has been established for more than 12 hours, fasciotomy should not be done, as the exposure of dead muscle will lead to infection and sepsis that may not occur if the skin is left intact.[157] The consensus of most experts is that an aggressive and early approach to diagnosis and treatment of compartment hypertension is best. Although there remains a role for nonoperative monitoring of injured extremities for the development of compartment syndrome, this approach must include frequent direct measurement of compartment pressure, and a liberal application of fasciotomy for any evidence of compartment syndrome.

## Nonoperative Approaches

*Observation.* The widespread use of arteriography in past decades has led to the detection of a variety of subtle arterial lesions of questionable significance, which obviously had been left untreated in the past. All arteriographic abnormalities were believed to require aggressive intervention, no matter how small or clinically insignificant, as all were assumed, in the absence of any data, to lead to a high rate of occlusion and limb loss unless surgically "repaired."[10,27,31,36,47,50,52,78,85,86,88,90,92] It is widely agreed that all *symptomatic* lesions presenting with arterial occlusion or gross extravasation must be repaired, as these will progress to limb-threatening complications if not treated; however, intervention for asymptomatic nonocclusive arterial injuries has been increasingly

questioned. This latter distinct category of vascular trauma includes segmental arterial narrowing, intimal flaps and irregularities, and small false aneurysms and AVFs, as described earlier.

A substantial body of clinical and laboratory evidence has demonstrated that a large majority of nonocclusive arterial injuries have a benign and self-limiting natural history which does not require intervention, and that nonoperative observation may be applied safely to these injuries.[95,112-114,158-160] A series of prospective studies from the University of Florida documented that approximately 90% of nonocclusive arterial injuries which did not manifest hard signs were successfully managed by nonoperative observation, with most of them resolving spontaneously over a mean follow-up of three months (Fig. 44-11). The minority that deteriorated all evolved into false aneurysms within a few weeks of injury, all of which were surgically repaired at that time without any morbidity related to the treatment delay.[19,80,81,161] Not a single instance of arterial occlusion, ischemic damage, limb morbidity, or limb loss has yet been reported in any published clinical study of this approach, regardless of injury mechanism or anatomic location of the injured artery (see Fig. 44-7). Dennis and coworkers[82] have confirmed these short-term results with a long-term follow-up of 44 untreated asymptomatic nonocclusive arterial injuries over a mean interval of 9.1 years, in which only 9% ultimately required surgery without adverse sequelae, among 58% of the study group available for follow-up. Arterial narrowing has been shown to be the safest form of nonocclusive injury to observe, with no deterioration ever documented, while 14% of intimal flaps and 40% of small AVFs and false aneurysms may ultimately require surgical intervention.[81]

Hoffer and coworkers[160] documented a 24% incidence of deterioration among 105 nonoperatively observed arterial injuries; however, they included symptomatic patients manifesting hard signs, as well as arterial occlusions, in their study population. Nonetheless, they still noted no significant limb morbidity or limb loss to result from treatment delay of these cases, and concluded, as have all other clinical series, that nonocclusive and asymptomatic arterial injuries may be observed with minimal risks.

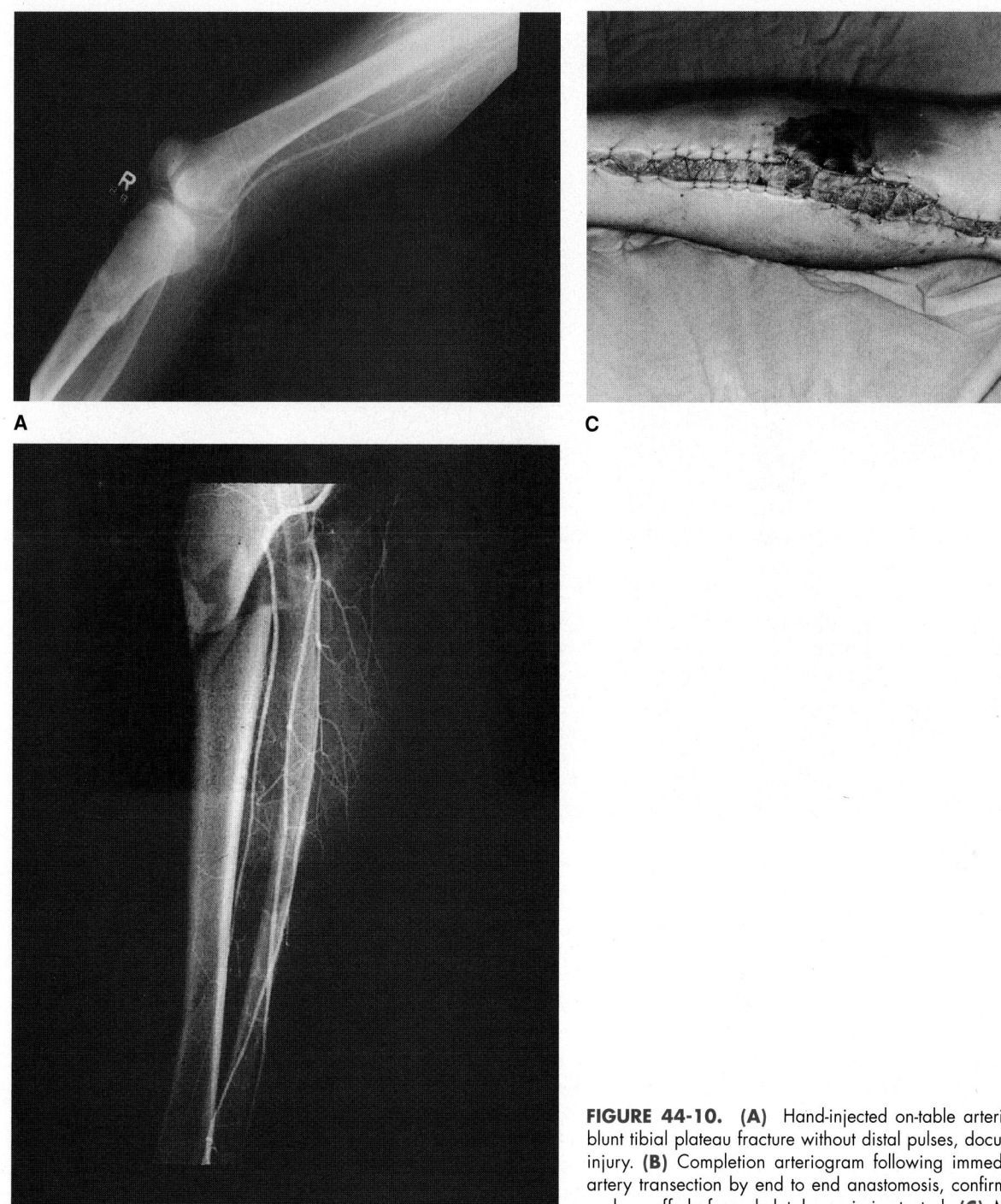

**FIGURE 44-10. (A)** Hand-injected on-table arteriogram of nondisplaced blunt tibial plateau fracture without distal pulses, documenting popliteal artery injury. **(B)** Completion arteriogram following immediate repair of popliteal artery transection by end to end anastomosis, confirming patent anastomosis and runoff, before skeletal repair is started. **(C)** Medial incision of four-compartment fasciotomy, extended superiorly for popliteal artery repair. Note shoelace wound closure technique.

Experimental studies of surgically created intimal flaps in canine femoral arteries have demonstrated a 40% rate of thrombosis over follow-up intervals ranging from five days to three weeks.[162,163] These models involved longitudinal arteriotomies with sharp intimal incision, which were highly and artificially thrombogenic due to post-surgical stricturing, and did not at all represent the actual mechanism of nonocclusive arterial injury following real trauma in humans. Nonetheless, 83% of these experimental injuries remained patent over follow-ups up to five months.[163] These and other authors[113] concluded that intimal flaps or narrowing that reduce the arterial lumen by at least 75%, and those directed "upstream," pose a high risk of thrombosis and should be surgically "repaired"; however, a number of large and upstream-directed flaps from clinical cases have been shown to completely resolve and cause no problems[82] (see Figs. 44-7 and 44-11), emphasizing the caution necessary in interpreting laboratory results. In fact there has been no relation shown between the radiographic appearance of nonocclusive arterial injuries and their outcome. Glover and Urbaniak[159] created histologically confirmed intimal tears in 50 rat femoral arteries by manual stretching, and found no thrombosis after 48 weeks of observation.

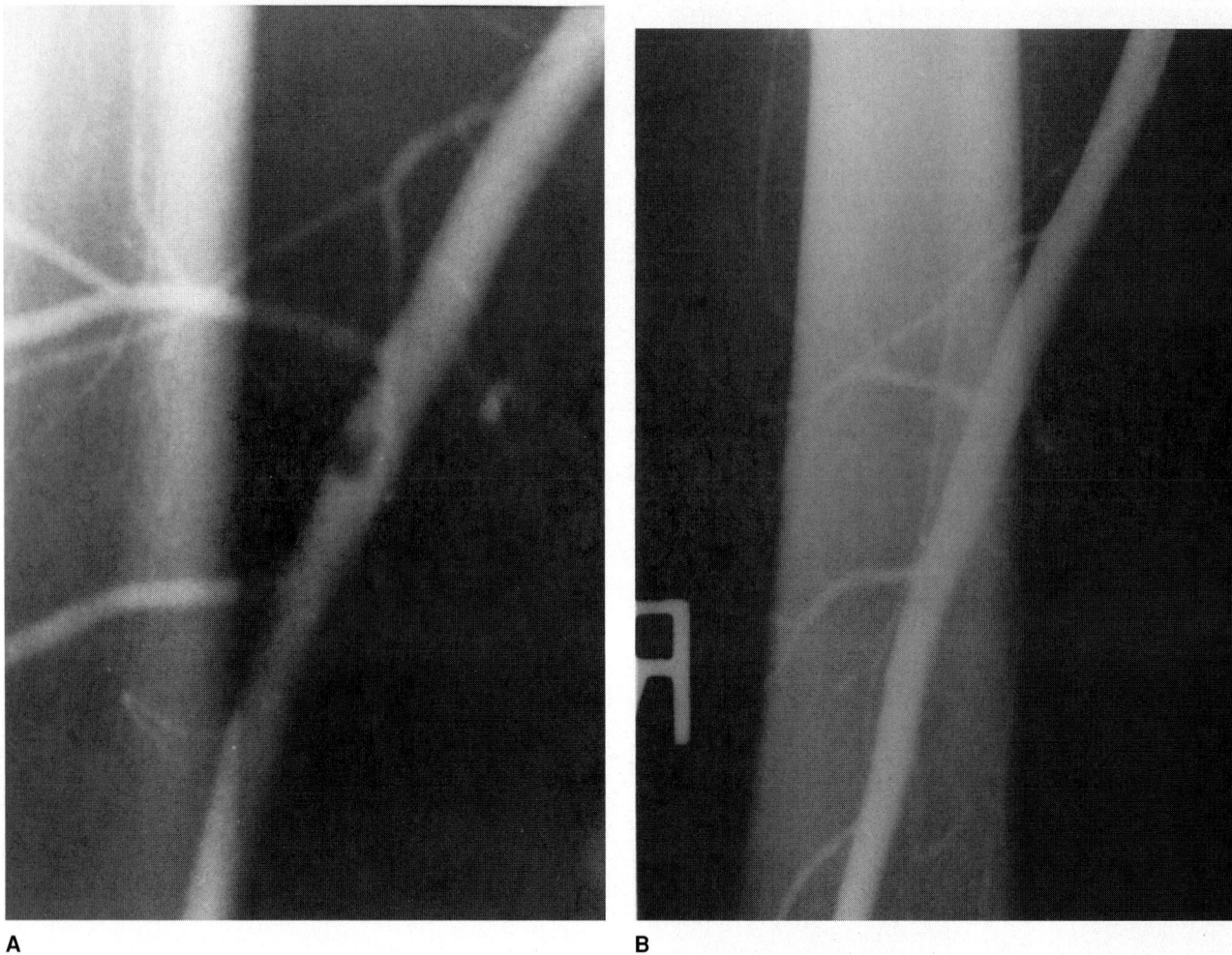

A                                              B

**FIGURE 44-11.** **(A)** Asymptomatic nonocclusive intimal flap of superficial femoral artery following proximity gunshot wound of thigh, nonoperatively observed. **(B)** Complete resolution after one week.
*(Reproduced with permission from Dennis JW, Frykberg ER, Crump JM, et al.: New perspectives on the management of penetrating trauma in proximity to major limb arteries. J Vasc Surg 11:84, 1990. Copyright 1990.)*

Successful nonoperative observation of vascular trauma dates back to at least WWI, and should not surprise contemporary surgeons. Soubbotitch[3,4] advocated observation of acute arterial trauma in 1913, believing the chronic sequelae of false aneurysms and AVFs would be easier to manage than acute injuries. As mentioned earlier, deliberate observation of arterial injuries was recommended and practiced in WWII and Korea, to encourage the development of chronic false aneurysms and collateral blood supply so as to optimize limb salvage following arterial ligation.[5,7] Rich and coworkers showed that asymptomatic arterial injuries that were initially overlooked from the Vietnam War, and developed into chronic AVFs and false aneurysms, had surprisingly few adverse sequelae.[164] The lesson derived from these historical experiences, that a number of arterial injuries have a benign natural history and never require surgery, was largely forgotten in subsequent decades as surgical repair became the standard therapeutic approach.

Reports of anecdotal cases of limb-threatening complications from missed vascular injuries have been advanced to criticize the concept of nonoperative observation.[165,166] These reports fail to specify the initial physical findings of these patients, the arteriographic appearance of the initial injuries, and how they were initially managed. Most limb-threatening complications of delayed treatment of arterial injuries occur when hard signs are initially overlooked, rather than no signs. These contentions are refuted by the abundant evidence cited above which supports nonoperative observation under strictly defined criteria, namely, no hard signs and an intact and open vessel on arteriography without gross extravasation.

Certainly false aneurysms and AVFs that complicate the delayed diagnosis of some arterial injuries have potential dangers, and their risks should be taken seriously. The available published evidence shows that these risks following asymptomatic arterial trauma appear to be much lower than the dogma of past years suggests. The morphologic characteristics and outcome following treatment of 783 published cases of delayed diagnosis of initially asymptomatic arterial injuries, most of which presented as AVFs and false aneurysms, from both civilian and military series, documents only a 1.4% incidence of limb loss (Table 44-9). No limbs were lost in any civilian series, even with treatment delays of almost four years. All cases of limb loss occurred in two military series from Vietnam,[76,164] in which there was only a

**TABLE 44-9**

**Morphology and Outcome of Complications of Delayed Diagnosis of Extremity Arterial Injurie**

| REFERENCE | NO. MISSED INJURIES | NO. AVF/FALSE ANEURYSM | MEAN DELAY (MONTHS) | NO. AMPUTATIONS |
|---|---|---|---|---|
| Fomon and Warren[74] | 16 | 10/6 | 46 (40% within 1 year) | 0 |
| Winegarner et al.[76a] | 40 | 12/20 | 1 | 3 (7.5%) |
| Moore et al.[167] | 26 | 8/18 | Not reported | 0 |
| Rich et al.[164a] | 558 | 262/296 | 1[b] (94% within 6 months) | 8 (1.4%) |
| Escobar et al.[77] | 58 | 35/23 | 37 | 0 |
| Feliciano et al.[78] | 28 | 10/12 | 0.35 (93% within 10 weeks) | 0 |
| Richardson et al.[79] | 17 | 4/8 | Not reported | 0 |
| Yilmaz et al.[168a] | 40 | 35/21 | 2[b] (80% within 3 months) | 0 |
| Total | 783 | 376/404 | | 11 (1.4%) |

[a]Military series.

[b]Median time interval.

Source: Modified with permission from Dennis JW, Frykberg ER, Veldenz HC, et al.: Validation of nonoperative management of occult vascular injuries and accuracy of physical examination alone in penetrating extremity trauma: 5- to 10-year followup. J Trauma 44:250, 1998.

1.8% amputation rate among all 598 extremity false aneurysms and AVFs, despite the fact that 50% of patients underwent arterial ligation.[164] Even one military series reporting 40 false aneurysms and AVFs complicating treatment delay reported no limb loss.[168] These results echo DeBakey's observation of the relatively benign course of these lesions in WWII as quoted earlier.[5] A number of other studies have documented spontaneous resolution of small false aneurysms and AVFs, confirming the safety of nonoperative observation of these lesions.[81,95,158,160] Any such lesion that is initially symptomatic, larger than 2 cm, or that becomes larger or symptomatic during observation, should undergo operative repair (see Fig. 44-5).

The benefits of nonoperative observation of asymptomatic nonocclusive arterial injuries are most apparent in multiply injured and unstable patients, and for arterial injuries in locations difficult to surgically access and which pose substantial surgical risks (such as Zone 3 of the neck and the thoracic inlet). These injuries should be documented carefully and closely followed when detected on arteriography, and the patients must be counseled as to potential risks, and to return for the development of any hard signs. Antiplatelet agents and anticoagulation are not necessary in managing these lesions.[82] The benign behavior of occult arterial injuries is what justifies the avoidance of routine imaging of asymptomatic blunt or penetrating extremity trauma, as it is only this category of nonocclusive arterial injuries that occurs in this setting.

Endovascular Management.    Endovascular techniques using arteriographic interventional modalities have been applied historically to the treatment of a select group of arterial injuries in which surgery poses a prohibitive risk, such as in anatomic locations difficult to expose and control, and in patients with medical comorbidity. Therapeutic embolization has been used successfully to treat hemorrhage from transected noncritical vessels, and to ablate false aneurysms and AVFs, using such materials as autogenous clot, gelatin sponge fragments (GelFoam, Upjohn, Kalamazoo, Mi), 95% alcohol, thrombin, steel coils, and detachable silicon balloons.[94,102,113,169] Intra-arterial pharmacotherapy has been used to treat severe vasospasm in small digital vessels by injection of a vasodilator. Embolized missiles within the vascular system have

been removed by endovascular catheters. Scalea and Sclafani have demonstrated the advantages of endovascular balloon placement for proximal and distal vascular control prior to surgical repair of arterial injuries in difficult locations, such as at the thoracic inlet or base of the skull.[170]

Endovascular grafting has been applied to the treatment of traumatic false aneurysms and AVFs, using synthetic grafts sutured to balloon-expandable stents which are introduced by the Seldinger technique from a remote site and fluoroscopically guided across the site of injury.[171] Marin and coworkers have used this technique in seven patients with penetrating arterial trauma, with no graft occlusion or infection over a 14-month follow-up.[172] Endovascular grafting is likely to have its most frequent application in stable patients with acute arterial injuries in difficult locations requiring repair, or in delayed presentation of traumatic false aneurysms and AVFs.[113] Surgeons should be cautious not to apply this treatment to lesions that typically resolve spontaneously, as discussed in the previous section.

## SPECIAL PROBLEMS

### Combined Arterial and Skeletal Extremity Trauma

History and Epidemiology.    Complex extremity trauma involving both arterial and skeletal injuries remains challenging. This combination of injuries is rare, comprising only 0.2% of all military and civilian trauma, and only 0.5–1.7% of all extremity fractures and dislocations.[38] Vascular and trauma surgeons are more likely than orthopedic surgeons to encounter these injuries, as 10–70% of all extremity arterial injuries are associated with skeletal trauma.[173] In past years, the great majority of complex extremity injuries in the civilian sector have been caused by blunt trauma,[38,63,65,174,175] although in some recent series penetrating trauma has caused a majority of these injuries.[156,173] Combat injuries of this type from military series usually are due to high velocity penetrating trauma.[5,68]

Combined arterial and skeletal extremity trauma imparts a substantially higher risk of limb loss and limb morbidity than does isolated skeletal and arterial injuries. Debakey and Simeone[5] documented this in WWII battle casualties, in which all injured arteries were ligated, reporting amputation in 60% of all combined injuries and 42% in isolated arterial injuries. Although McNamara and coworkers[68] reported a substantial improvement in limb salvage from isolated arterial injuries in the Vietnam War, combined injuries still had a ten-fold greater rate of limb loss (23% vs. 2.5%). These authors also documented a higher incidence of failed vascular repair among combined extremity injuries (33%) than among isolated extremity arterial injuries (5%). Romanoff and coworkers[176] reported more than a three-fold increase in limb loss in combined combat extremity trauma compared to isolated arterial injuries (36% vs. 11%) in the hostilities in Israel. This trend has continued into recent years in the civilian sector, even in the most experienced trauma centers, where amputation rates approaching 70% still are reported from combined arterial and skeletal extremity trauma,[38,64,174] while less than 5% of limbs currently are lost following isolated arterial or skeletal trauma.[63,103] Limb loss most commonly is attributed to delay in diagnosis and revascularization in most published series of this unique trauma. Major nerve damage, extensive soft tissue injury which disrupts collaterals and prevents adequate vessel coverage, infection, and compartment syndrome are other reasons for such a high rate of loss of these severely compromised limbs. Furthermore, patients with such complex extremity trauma have been shown to have a significantly greater hospital length of stay, consumption of hospital resources, and long-term disability than other trauma patients with similar Injury Severity Scores.[177]

Diagnosis.  Prompt diagnosis is essential if rapid treatment and optimal limb salvage is to be achieved in these complex extremity injuries. This requires that a high index of suspicion of arterial trauma be applied to every injured extremity by noting whether any hard signs are present. As discussed earlier (see section on Diagnosis), the presence of hard signs in any blunt or complex extremity trauma requires immediate arteriography due to the relatively low incidence of surgically significant arterial injury in this setting.[65,112] This is best done by the surgeon as a percutaneous hand-injected ECA in the trauma center, or on the operating table (see Fig. 44-6), to minimize time delay while achieving excellent accuracy.[64,96,101] The absence of hard signs excludes major arterial injury with sufficient accuracy to allow further diagnostic workup to be avoided.[112,121] Since most complex extremity trauma does not manifest hard signs,[112] avoiding the considerable expense of arteriography in this population has substantial economic advantages.

This principle holds true even for the especially high-risk injury of a posterior knee dislocation, in which setting routine arteriography has been advocated in all cases, due to a substantial risk of popliteal artery disruption and its associated high rate of limb loss.[176] Those published studies, however, that have compared the clinical manifestations of a total of 494 patients having posterior knee dislocation with outcome have shown no surgically significant arterial injuries in that majority of patients (78.5%) who have no hard signs (Table 44-10). This has been confirmed by follow-ups of up to two years.[171–173,175,185] Again, the fact that most cases present without hard signs emphasizes the major resource savings, at no harm to the patient, by using only physical findings to exclude arterial injury. Arteriography is indicated only in that minority of patients with knee dislocation presenting with hard signs (21.5%), to exclude the need for surgery in those patients who do not have an arterial injury (44% of all with hard signs). Immediate surgery without imaging may be undertaken if the manifest hard signs clearly indicate vascular injury (i.e., absent pulse, cold ischemic foot, pulsatile bleeding). One published meta-analysis concluded that the pulse examination did not reliably predict vascular injury following knee dislocation, although it did not include all hard signs as a unit in this analysis.[186]

There has been no clear role for noninvasive testing in complex extremity injuries, due to a paucity of studies of this category of trauma, and uncertainty over its accuracy in the presence of severe tissue disruption; however, the use of noninvasive testing in this population is evolving. Mills and coworkers reported a 100% diagnostic accuracy of the ankle–brachial index for confirming or excluding vascular injury following knee dislocation, though they did not correlate their results with the presence of all hard signs to document any advantage over clinical findings.[129] Further study is necessary to clarify this.

## TABLE 44-10

### Relation of Physical Findings of Vascular Injury to Outcome Following Knee Dislocation

| REFERENCE | NO. KD | HARD SIGNS PRESENT | | HARD SIGNS ABSENT | |
|---|---|---|---|---|---|
| | | No. (%)[a] | No. Surgery (%)[b] | No. (%)[a] | No. Surgery (%) |
| Kaufman et al.[177] | 19 | 4 (21) | 4 (100) | 15 (79) | 0 |
| Treiman et al.[178] | 115 | 29 (25) | 22 (75) | 86 (75) | 0 |
| Dennis et al.[179] | 38 | 2 (13) | 2 (100) | 36 (87) | 0 |
| Kendall et al.[180] | 37 | 6 (16) | 6 (100) | 31 (84) | 0 |
| Miranda et al.[123] | 32 | 8 (25) | 6 (75) | 24 (75) | 0 |
| Martinez et al.[181] | 23 | 11 (48) | 2 (18) | 12 (52) | 0 |
| Hollis et al.[182] | 39 | 11 (28) | 7 (64) | 28 (72) | 0 |
| Stannard et al.[184] | 134 | 10 (7.5) | 9 (90) | 124 (92.5) | 0 |
| Klineberg et al.[183] | 57 | 25 (44) | 7 (58) | 32 (56) | 0 |
| Total | 494 | 106 (21.5) | 65 (56) | 388 (78.5) | 0 |

[a]Percentage of all knee dislocations.

[b]Percentage of all patients with hard signs who required surgical repair of a vascular injury.

KD = Knee dislocation.

Management Priorities and Techniques. Appropriate prioritization of the management of the vascular and skeletal injuries is a major determinant of limb salvage. Initial stabilization and fixation of fractures has been advocated in past years in the absence of overt ischemia,[3,173] due to concerns that an established vascular repair will be disrupted by subsequent orthopedic manipulation. Published evidence has refuted such concerns, showing minimal disruption of initial vascular repairs in this setting, and no adverse impact of prompt revascularization on outcome.[7,38] Also, substantial tissue damage can still occur in the absence of clinical signs of ischemia, as our understanding of compartment syndrome has made clear. Further, clinical studies have shown a substantially higher rate of limb salvage among combined vascular and skeletal extremity injuries in which revascularization is performed first, compared with those in which it is delayed until the skeleton is addressed.[176]

In fact, definitive vascular repair *should* be delayed in cases of unstable or severely comminuted fractures or dislocations, segmental bone loss, or severe soft tissue destruction and contamination. These may impart risks of undue tension or slack on the repaired vessel, of infection and anastomotic disruption, and of the possibility of disruption from skeletal manipulation. But, these circumstances should not ever delay immediate restoration of perfusion to the extremity, which can be accomplished rapidly by temporary intraluminal shunting until skeletal stabilization and soft tissue debridement has been completed[36,38,125,146–149] (see Fig. 43-6). Alternatively, definitive vascular repair should be the means of initial revascularization in the setting of uncomplicated and stable skeletal injuries, or any setting in which minimal subsequent manipulation and length discrepancy is anticipated, and little jeopardy to the vascular repair is judged (see Fig. 44-10).

External fixation is preferred when rapid skeletal stabilization is necessary in open, comminuted and unstable fractures or in the presence of severe soft tissue disruption and contamination.[3,68] Internal fixation has been used successfully in this setting and is preferred if the patient's condition permits.[156,173,175]

The consensus of authorities now favors limb revascularization as the first priority in all combined vascular and skeletal extremity trauma.[38,155,156,175,176] How the revascularization is accomplished (i.e., definitive repair or temporary shunting) is a matter of judgment based on the nature of the skeletal and soft tissue injuries and the condition of the patient. Only with a cooperative multidisciplinary effort between the trauma, vascular, orthopedic, and plastic surgeons can the outcome of these injuries be optimized.

Surgical Adjuncts. In addition to prompt diagnosis with on-table arteriography, liberal use of a number of surgical adjuncts has improved limb salvage following combined arterial and skeletal extremity trauma. Some of these have been discussed above in the context of the overall management of vascular trauma (see the section on Management). Intraoperative completion arteriography is important to document patency of the repair, as any technical errors could easily result in limb loss in these severely compromised limbs (see Fig. 44-10). Four-compartment fasciotomy should be applied liberally and prophylactically in this setting due to the high risk of compartment syndrome following reperfusion.[38,156,173,175] Extra-anatomic bypass and pedicled or free-tissue flap coverage should be considered in the setting of severe contamination and soft tissue injury or loss to protect the vascular repair.[142,144] Careful

attention to all of these considerations, as well as to avoiding unnecessary surgery for nonocclusive arterial lesions (see Fig. 44-7), and meticulous postoperative surveillance, has led to dramatic improvements in limb salvage. Recent amputation rates, even in these complex injuries, have fallen below 10%[156,173,175] (Fig. 44-12).

The Decision for Amputation. Among the most difficult challenges in the management of complex extremity trauma is the decision as to whether and when amputation is indicated. Recent advances in the ability to salvage limbs have led to prolonged and aggressive reconstruction efforts following injuries which would have undergone amputation in the past. Such heroic efforts actually may harm patients in terms of prolonging hospitalization and time lost from work, as well as increasing sepsis, operative procedures, and even mortality.[174,187] These outcomes are especially undesirable if amputation or severe limb dysfunction ultimately occur anyway.

Although it is often difficult to predict soon after injury which extremities will require amputation, there are injuries of such destruction and severity that a decision for immediate amputation can be made easily. These are injuries in which it is obvious that attempts at revascularization are futile due to the extent of trauma to soft tissue, bone, and nerve or due to the presence of other life-threatening injuries. Gustilo III-C injuries (comminuted open tibial-fibular fractures with arterial injury) are an example of limb trauma in which immediate amputation is often considered.

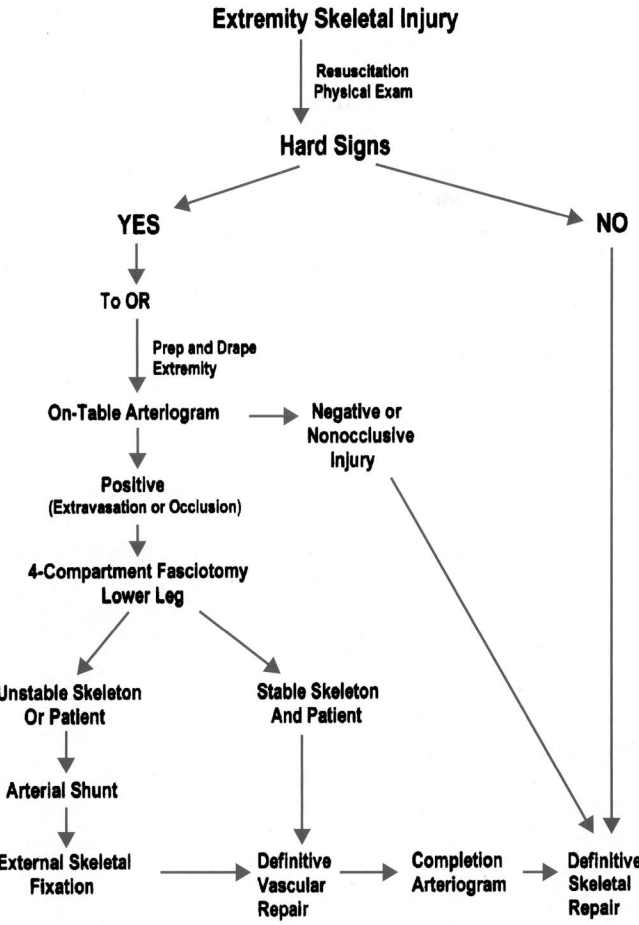

**FIGURE 44-12.** Algorithm for evaluation and treatment of combined arterial and skeletal extremity trauma.

Most complex extremity injuries are not that clear-cut. In these cases, in which the major nerves are intact, immediate revascularization should be performed, along with important surgical adjuncts such as shunts, fasciotomy, or extra-anatomic bypass, the skeleton should be stabilized promptly by either traction or external fixation, and then the extremity should be observed over the next 24–48 hours to determine what level of function and tissue viability returns. Nerve transaction should be determined by direct visualization, as vascular insufficiency or muscle damage alone may cause profound deficits that can be confused with nerve damage. If revascularization fails, tissue loss is severe or worsens, systemic sepsis or crush syndrome develops, or profound neurologic or functional deficits persist, amputation then should be performed. If improvement occurs, limb salvage may proceed, but should be assessed just as critically at each successive stage to minimize unnecessarily prolonged, costly, and futile efforts.

A number of scoring systems have been developed to objectify this difficult decision that is so often clouded by subjective and wishful thinking, often at the patient's expense.[38,174] Although none have been found to be prospectively useful in predicting amputation or the degree of functional impairment,[187] they do focus attention on those factors which most closely correlate with outcome and which must be a part of the treatment decision (Table 44-11). A major consideration in this decision is whether the injury is in the upper or lower extremity, as the former is less likely to require amputation, being more tolerant of deficits in protective sensation, motor function, weight-bearing concerns, and length discrepancy, and prostheses tend to be less satisfactory.[174,187]

Recent studies that analyze data from the prospective Lower Extremity Assessment Protocol (LEAP) have suggested that there is greater capacity for anatomic and functional salvage of limbs with complex injuries than indicated by the above criteria. A multivariate analysis showed that muscle and soft tissue injury, absence of plantar sensation, and vascular injury have the greatest influence on the clinical decision to amputate a limb.[188] Bosse et al. have shown that in injured limbs at high risk for amputation according to the above factors, two-year outcomes following either amputation or reconstruction are similar, although those in the reconstructed group still had higher risk of complications and more operations and hospital admissions.[189]

---

**TABLE 44-11**

**High-Risk Factors for Ultimate Limb Loss or Severe Dysfunction Following Combined Vascular and Skeletal Extremity Trauma**

Gustilo III — C skeletal injuries
Transected tibial or sciatic nerve
Transection of 2 of 3 upper extremity nerves
Prolonged ischemia (>6–12 hours)
Shock and life-threatening associated injuries
Below-knee arterial injury
Extensive soft tissue loss
Crush injury
Multiple fractures
Elderly with medical comorbidity
Severe contamination
Patient preference

---

This decision must be a matter of clinical judgment for the individual patient, and it must always involve a consensus of the trauma, orthopedic, vascular and plastic surgeons, rehabilitation specialist, psychologist, nursing, and, most importantly, the patient and family. The sophistication of limb prostheses, prompt return to work, short hospitalizations and lower costs, and morbidity following early amputation are often preferable to salvage efforts which may take months or years and still fail. The ultimate goal is to return the patient to a comfortable, self-sufficient, and productive life as quickly as possible.

## Management of Venous Injuries

**History and Epidemiology.**    The recorded history of venous trauma dates back to the 19th century. Schede, a German surgeon, is credited with the first lateral suture repair of the femoral vein in 1882. Multiple similar reports followed in the late 1800s.[190] During that time, it was felt that combined arterial and venous injury carried a significantly worse prognosis than did arterial injury alone. During WWI, ligation of both injured and uninjured veins at the time of arterial repair was advocated because of the theoretical advantage of increasing the blood pressure and blood "dwell time" within the limb.[8] Comparative review of these results and those of the American experience in WWII, when routine venous ligation was not practiced, failed to demonstrate any difference in amputation rates.[5] More information was obtained in the Korean War, when 71 of the 180 vascular injuries treated were major venous injuries and 82% of these were ligated.[9] Through this experience came the idea that repair of these injuries might decrease the postoperative complications associated with venous hypertension. During the Vietnam War, 33% of venous injuries were repaired, and reports from this setting suggest that patients who had venous repair had significantly better outcomes than those with ligation.[69] Prior concerns for increased thrombophlebitis and pulmonary embolism with venous repair were unsubstantiated. Stimulated by this experience, an aggressive approach to the treatment of venous injuries emerged. Gaspar and Treiman were among the first civilian surgeons to examine this question and to show venous repair to be safe.[191] Despite several studies of this issue in the last 40 years, the appropriate treatment of venous injuries remains unresolved.

Many peripheral venous injuries are not clinically significant and, therefore, are not identified. As such, the true incidence of this entity is unknown. They comprised 39% of vascular injuries in the Korean War and 27% in the Vietnam War. In military as well as civilian reports, the incidence of associated arterial and venous injury is noted to be 80–90%.[9,107,192] In the civilian experience, venous injury comprises 13–51% of vascular injuries and 35–63% of extremity vascular trauma.[63,70,107,192–196] Venous injuries are most commonly due to stab and gunshot wounds. Blunt venous injury is much more unusual and comprises only 5–15% of civilian vascular trauma.[193] Significant iatrogenic injury from catheterization and orthopedic surgery has been reported.

**Diagnosis.**    The diagnosis of venous injuries is usually straightforward. When isolated, venous injury is frequently tamponaded by surrounding structures due to the low-pressure nature of the system, and it is never detected. As most venous injuries accompany an arterial injury, the majority of them are found on exploration

**TABLE 44-12**

**Extremity Venous Injuries: Mechanism Presentation and Management**

| REFERENCE | TOTAL NO. | NO. PENETRATING | NO. ISOLATED | NO. REPAIRED |
|---|---|---|---|---|
| Rich[69a] | 377 | 377 | 53 | 124 |
| Sullivan[197a] | 26 | 26 | 8 | 21 |
| Agarwal[198] | 57 | 53 | 18 | 34 |
| Phifer[199] | 25 | 25 | 0 | 19 |
| Ross[193] | 22 | 0 | 1 | 12 |
| Pasch[70] | 82 | 0 | 4 | 53 |
| Borman[107] | 82 | 71 | 20 | 74 |
| Meyer[192] | 36 | 34 | 2 | 36 |
| Yelon[194] | 79 | 78 | 31 | 31 |
| Timberlake[195] | 322 | 292 | 83 | 98 |
| Parry[145] | 86 | 75 | 15 | 64 |
| Total | 1194 | 1031 (95.5%)[b] | 235 (20%) | 566 (47%) |

[a]Military Series.
[b]Based on 1079 evaluable injuries.

*Source: Modified from Frykberg ER: Vascular Trauma. In Callow AD, Ernst CB, eds. Vascular Surgery: Theory and Practice, McGraw-Hill, 1995, p. 1017. (with permission)*

for the latter (Table 44-12). They exhibit hard signs of vascular injury, which are not specific for venous injury.[83] Surgery for the presence of any hard signs will detect most venous injuries requiring repair.

The two diagnostic modalities that image the venous system are contrast venography and duplex scanning. In the past, routine venography of injured limbs was advocated to identify venous injuries regardless of clinical presentation. In 1976, Gerlock was able to identify venous injury in five of 30 consecutive patients with penetrating extremity trauma undergoing venography.[106] Most of the demonstrated injuries (four of five) had associated arterial injuries and, therefore, would have been found anyway. Additionally, the accuracy of this testing was noted to be suboptimal and it was difficult to perform. Gagne et al. reported similar results in 1995, with over 50% of attempts at venography unsuccessful, and only 43% of venous injuries detected (see previous section on Diagnosis).[108] This group also looked at the advisability of performing duplex ultrasonography in this scenario. They screened 37 patients with penetrating proximity extremity trauma and found eight (22%) occult venous injuries.

Currently, most centers do not perform routine venous imaging. In cases presenting with hard signs, imaging is contraindicated as immediate surgery is necessary. In the absence of such signs, there is no evidence of adverse sequelae or of a need to intervene for occult venous trauma. If delayed symptoms occur, then venous imaging may be warranted.

Management—Repair. Initial management includes standard resuscitation and stabilization. The general principles applicable to the management of arterial injury are appropriate for venous injury. Prompt manual compression is applied to control active bleeding. Fluid resuscitation is accomplished through large bore peripheral intravenous catheters placed away from the site of injury. A longitudinal incision is made over the injured vessel. As dissection is carried out in order to obtain proximal and distal control of the injured vessels, control of bleeding is accomplished

through use of a tourniquet, digital or spongestick compression, occluding clamps, or intraluminal balloons. Thrombectomy is performed manually by gentle milking of the injured vein and with limited use of balloon catheters being careful not to cause damage to venous valves.

There is significant histopathologic difference between arterial and venous injury. Arterial injuries are characterized by intimal damage that often extends well beyond the gross area of injury and may require debridement of the vessel to reach normal tissue. This is not necessary in venous repair because they tend to have little injury beyond the cut margin.

Due to high thrombosis rates after suture repair, it is clear that meticulous surgical technique must be employed for repair of venous injuries. This includes gentle handling of the endothelium to prevent further damage and precise suturing techniques. Simple lateral venorrhaphy of small lacerations should be attempted if possible. Significant narrowing of the lumen is to be avoided so as to reduce the risk of thrombosis. Patch angioplasty of lacerations that may narrow the lumen when sutured can be accomplished, preferably using autogenous vein. An end-to-end anastomosis is preferred for transection with little loss of vessel length. Interposition grafting has been reported with autogenous as well as prosthetic material. While autogenous material is felt to be far superior,[192] availability of an adequate conduit is a significant problem, as the greater saphenous vein is frequently too small. Complex repairs involving interposition grafts, or the construction of panel or spiral grafts have had poorer results than simple repairs,[196] although the use of externally supported grafts and aggressive use of adjuncts such as anticoagulation, limb elevation, and compression wrapping have led to patency rates as high as 74% in this setting.[145] Feliciano and coworkers have found that severe bleeding from complex extremity injuries following soft tissue destruction and venous ligation can be relieved by the temporary provision of venous drainage with PTFE grafts, even with their decreased patency rates. Formal venous repair with autogenous tissue can then be performed electively at a later time.[139]

In combined arterial and venous injury, there is debate over which vessel to repair first. Initial repair of the venous injury allows optimal outflow for the subsequently repaired artery. An intraluminal arterial shunt should be used here to minimize warm ischemia time.[146] Another technique involves initial arterial repair while shunting the venous side in order to maximize the time for definitive venous repair without concern for distal perfusion.[145]

The enthusiasm for venous repair was initiated in the Korean War following the observation that there was a significantly lower incidence of extremity edema and other signs of venous insufficiency with the restoration of venous outflow as compared to ligation. These observations were corroborated in the Vietnam War where an aggressive approach to venous repair led to dramatic improvement in limb salvage and function without the risk of thromboembolism.[200] The natural history of surgically repaired venous injury shows a significantly higher rate of thrombosis than that following arterial repair. Despite this, many studies report a lower incidence of adverse sequelae following repair rather than ligation.[70,107,192,197,198] This is thought to be due to the formation of venous collaterals that the slow thrombosis of venous repairs allows. Additionally, there is a high rate of later recanalization of thrombosed venous repairs that cannot happen with ligation.[199,201,202]

A number of adjuncts to venous injury repair have improved postoperative results. Temporary distal arteriovenous shunts and fistulae have improved patency rates.[203] They tend to increase extremity edema due to the higher than normal venous flow, and require reoperation to reverse, for which reasons they are no longer used. Systemic anticoagulation and antiplatelet therapy have not been shown to improve results; however, low molecular weight dextran has shown some evidence of improvement of venous patency rates.[204] Pneumatic compression devices, though they possess some theoretical advantage, have not been evaluated in this setting.

### Management—Ligation.

Since the Vietnam War, enthusiasm for venous repair has been tempered by civilian studies showing surprisingly uncomplicated courses following ligation of major veins in injured extremities.[194,195,205] Varying levels of edema have been reported in about half of the cases.[9,199,205] A compilation of 1194 published cases of venous injuries shows that most have been ligated in recent years in the civilian sector (see Table 44-12). There has been no limb loss attributed to venous ligation in this experience. Ligation of upper extremity veins has been better tolerated due to the more extensive collateral drainage that exists in the arm. Successful outcome following this management strategy mandates the use of adjunctive measures to promote venous drainage, including elastic bandages and bedrest with elevation of the extremity, especially with ligation of the popliteal vein. Prophylactic fasciotomy should be considered following ligation of major veins, as there is a high incidence of compartment syndrome.[198]

Although the literature appears divided as to whether repair or ligation is indicated, it is clear that each is successful under certain conditions. Venous ligation in the military setting may result in worse outcome because of the greater damage to soft tissue, collaterals, and bone from the more destructive weaponry. Injury in the civilian setting results in less destructive wounds, and venous ligation is better tolerated.

### Indications for Repair and Ligation.

Although most authorities agree that injury to major veins, particularly in the lower extremity, should undergo repair, some circumstances may prevent this management strategy. Hemodynamic instability, ongoing hemorrhage, and life-threatening associated injuries may mandate venous ligation as repair takes more time. Potentially preventable deaths have been attributed to the added time required for venous repair, as well as for the use of complex repairs in unstable patients. If a repair cannot be accomplished by lateral suture or end-to-end anastamosis, ligation is preferable to the time required for more complex repairs, which also have a higher rate of thrombosis than simple repairs. Parry and coworkers have shown, however, that in stable patients, complex repairs can in fact be accomplished successfully.[145] Patients generally tolerate ligation of any peripheral vein if adjunctive measures are applied. Furthermore, elective repair can be considered in that minority of cases in which complications develop.

There are circumstances under which venous repair should be attempted even under suboptimal conditions of instability or multisystem trauma. These include the following: massive tissue destruction where the venous outflow may be critical[139]; in combined arteriovenous injury where the venous outflow may be required for arterial patency[70,194]; popliteal vein injury in which ligation results in limb-threatening morbidity[63,125,197]; and in the

case of bilateral internal jugular vein injury, to allow adequate cranial venous outflow. Temporary intraluminal shunts may be used as a damage control measure to delay definitive repair while maintaining venous outflow of the injured extremity until after stabilization.[145]

Although early routine follow-up imaging of venous repairs may hold some interest, the natural history of a high rate of thrombosis typically followed by recanalization makes this unnecessary, especially in the absence of symptoms. Most thrombosed repairs do well. Imaging should be reserved for those patients who are symptomatic with deep vein thrombosis, edema, or chronic venous insufficiency. In these cases, anticoagulation or surgical revision may be indicated.

## Missile Embolism

Migration of bullets, shotgun pellets, or other wounding foreign bodies through the bloodstream is rare, occurring in less than 1% of all vascular trauma. Rich and coworkers reported only 22 cases (0.3%) from the Vietnam War.[206] Extremity blood vessels are frequently involved, either as the entrance point from which a missile migrates centrally, or as the final distal lodging point from central vascular injuries.

A high index of suspicion for missile embolism is a necessary first step in its detection. All patients with bullet or shotgun wounds must be evaluated for the location of the missiles. Embolism should be suspected in the absence of radiographic evidence of a bullet, especially if there is no exit wound or an odd number of wounds, and a radiographic search of the body should be undertaken in these instances. Arterial emboli typically travel in the direction of blood flow and become caught in distal arteries, where they cause acute occlusion and ischemia. These emboli must be removed, either from a distant site by balloon catheter embolectomy or through an arteriotomy directly over the missile.[207] Careful attention should be directed at obtaining proximal and distal control in these areas to prevent further migration during retrieval. In addition to retrieval, the entry site of the missile into the arterial circulation must be repaired, although there are reports of asymptomatic patients in which the site could not be found or repaired and no problems developed.

Missiles in the venous circulation typically embolize into the heart or pulmonary artery, although they may travel retrograde to more distal sites from the force of gravity. Cardiac or pulmonary emboli of bullets may cause complications of thrombus, endocarditis, myocardial damage, or pulmonary infection and infarction, in which case they should be removed. Percutaneous interventional methods for retrieval may allow thoracotomy to be avoided; however, evidence suggests that asymptomatic missiles may be left safely in both the heart and lungs, clearly a cost-effective option.[207–209]

## COMPLICATIONS AND OUTCOME

The most immediate and potentially dangerous complication of an extremity vascular repair is thrombosis, which is indicated by disappearance of the distal pulses and signs of distal ischemia following arterial repair and by limb swelling and edema following a venous repair. Regular postoperative surveillance following vascular repair allows these signs to be detected early, at which time a prompt return to surgery to revise the repair and restore perfusion or venous drainage still may allow full limb salvage and function. In the absence of signs of ischemia, indicating sufficient collateral blood flow to maintain limb viability, revascularization may be delayed as other problems require, or for further evaluation by arteriography.

Delay in the initial diagnosis and treatment of a vascular injury could lead to a failed arterial repair from the development of irreversible tissue damage. Even if the limb remains viable after revascularization following an ischemic interval, disability may result from damage to nerves and muscles.[6] This emphasizes the importance of rapid assessment for hard signs, selective use of on-table arteriography, and prompt operation.

Technical errors are another cause of failure of arterial repair, and, therefore, must be avoided. These failures typically occur early. Avoiding this problem requires strict attention to the following: gentle dissection; thorough debridement of vessels and soft tissue; appropriate prioritization of multiple injuries; meticulous technique in suturing arteries and veins; distal thrombectomy and regional heparinization; avoiding a stenotic anastomosis; proper choice of repair technique to avoid undue tension or damage to collaterals; full-thickness coverage of the repair; and confirmation of revascularization by restoration of pulses, clinical signs of perfusion, and completion arteriography. There is generally no role for postoperative anticoagulation following surgical repair of vascular injuries except in the rare instance of a true hypercoagulable state in the patient or some other unrelated indication (i.e., prosthetic heart valve). As mentioned above in the section on Venous Injuries, postoperative anticoagulation may sometimes be beneficial after repair of injured veins.[145] Anticoagulation generally cannot substitute for a technically perfect suture repair and should not be instituted to "make up" for a poor anastomosis, poor clinical judgment, or other suboptimal conditions such as poor sterile technique or inadequate tissue debridement and cleansing. Each instance of failure of an arterial repair substantially reduces the chance of ultimate limb salvage, which indicates how important it is that the initial diagnosis and management be done correctly.

Infection at the site of vascular repair is a dreaded complication that may lead to thrombosis, false aneurysm, or disruption with hemorrhage. This has to be acted upon immediately by ligation and resection of the involved area of vessel, followed by extra-anatomic bypass through a clean field. Failure to recognize infection as the cause of a failed repair will lead to futile attempts at continued repairs in the same contaminated tissue bed.

A minority of nonoperatively treated arterial injuries, or injuries that were frankly missed initially, may develop into false aneurysms and AVFs. If treated early by resection and repair, morbidity is minimal (see Table 44-9). Endovascular management of these problems may allow surgery to be avoided altogether.

Compartment hypertension is an insidious complication that can lead to limb loss even after successful revascularization and in the presence of normal pulses. It is best managed by prevention, through early or prophylactic fasciotomy in high-risk settings as discussed earlier.

The two measures of successful outcome of extremity arterial injury management are limb salvage and limb function. Mortality has been reported from these injuries, but it is rare and usually due to complications of shock, sepsis, pulmonary embolus, and multiple organ failure, most commonly from other associated injuries.[63] The salvage of a viable limb does not necessarily mean that function has been restored to normal. The neurologic, muscular, and skeletal function of the salvaged extremity, as well as its cosmetic appearance, can impact substantially on the patient, and may be detrimental enough that amputation would be preferred. The rate of amputation reported in most large series of extremity vascular trauma falls below 5%, even following such high-risk circumstances as popliteal artery trauma and combined extremity trauma.[63,88,103,125,155,156,173] This confirms the current understanding of prognostic factors in diagnosis and management that affect outcome, and the success of an aggressive application of surgical adjuncts and prioritization to maintain life and limb.

Increasing amounts of data are available on the level of functional recovery, late amputation, and long-term complications, despite the difficulties of following the young and transient trauma population.[82,177,188,189,210] These late results indicate that major extremity vascular trauma has many adverse long-term consequences, but also that recent advances in diagnosis and management have greatly improved many aspects of long-term survival. Further study of outcomes is warranted to help us improve the management of these patients.

# REFERENCES

1. Murphy JB: Resection of arteries and veins injured in continuity-end-to-end to suture-experimental and clinical research. *Med Record* 51:73, 1897.
2. Nolan B: Vascular Injuries. *JR Coll Surg* 13:72, 1968.
3. Rich NM, Spencer FC: *Vascular Trauma*. Philadelphia: WB Saunders, 1978.
4. Soubbotitch V: Military experiences of traumatic aneurysms. *Lancet* 2:720, 1913.
5. De Bakey ME, Simeone FA: Battle injuries of the arteries in World War II: An analysis of 2,471 cases. *Ann Surg* 123:534, 1946.
6. Bigger IA: Treatment of traumatic aneurysms and arteriovenous fistulas. *Arch Surg* 49:170, 1944.
7. Jahnke EJ, Seeley SF: Acute vascular injuries in the Korean War: An analysis of 77 consecutive cases. *Ann Surg* 138:158, 1953.
8. Makins GH: *Injuries to the blood vessels, in Official History of the Great War Medical Services: Surgery of the War*. London, England: His Majesty's Stationery Office, 1922, p. 170.
9. Hughes CW: Arterial repair during the Korean War. *Ann Surg* 147:555, 1958.
10. Ferguson IA, Byrd WM, McAfee DK: Experiences in the management of arterial injuries. *Ann Surg* 153:980, 1961.
11. Rich NM, Baugh JH, Hughes CW: Acute arterial injuries in Vietnam: 1,000 cases. *J Trauma* 10:359, 1970.
12. Rich NM: Vietnam missile wounds evaluated in 750 patients. *Mil Med* 133:9, 1968.
13. Diamond S, Gaspard D, Katz S: Vascular injuries to the extremities in a suburban trauma center. *Am Surg* 69:848, 2003.
14. Mattox KL, Feliciano DV, Burch J, et al.: Five thousand seven hundred sixty cardiovascular injuries in 4,459 patients: Epidemiological evolution 1958 to 1987. *Ann Surg* 209:698, 1989.
15. Frykberg ER, Dennis JW, Bishop K, et al.: The reliability of physical examination in the evaluation of penetrating extremity trauma for vascular injury: Results at one year. *J Trauma* 31:502, 1991.
16. Beebe GW, De Bakey ME: *Battle Casualties: Incidence, Mortality and Logistic Considerations*. Springfield, IL: Charles C. Thomas, 1952.
17. Vollmar J: Surgical experience with 197 traumatic arterial lesions (1953–1966). In Hiertonn T, Rybeck B, eds. *Traumatic Arterial Lesions*. Stockholm, Sweden: Forsvaretsforskningsanstalt, 1968.
18. Oller DW, Rutledge R. Clancy T, et al.: Vascular injuries in a rural state: A review of 978 patients from a state trauma registry. *J Trauma* 32:740, 1992.
19. Dennis JW, Frykberg ER, Crump JM, et al.: New perspectives on the management of penetrating trauma in proximity to major limb arteries. *J Vasc Surgery* 11:84, 1990.
20. Carey ME: An analysis of U.S. Army combat mortality and morbidity data. *J Trauma* 28:S183, 1988.
21. Morris GC, Beall AC, Roof WR, et al.: Surgical experience with 220 acute arterial injuries in civilian practice. *Am J Surg* 99:775, 1960.
22. Smith RF, Szilagyi DE, Pfeifer JR: Arterial trauma. *Arch Surg* 86:825, 1963.

23. Patman RD, Poulos E, Shires GT: The management of civilian arterial injuries. *Surg Gynecol Obstet* 118:725, 1964.

24. Treiman RL, Doty D, Gaspar MR: Acute vascular trauma: A fifteen year study. *Am J Surg* 111:469, 1966.

25. Dillard BM, Nelson DL, Norman HG: Review of 85 major traumatic arterial injuries. *Surgery* 63:391, 1968.

26. Drapanas T, Hewitt RL, Weichert RF, et al.: Civilian vascular injuries: A critical appraisal of three decades of management. *Ann Surg* 172:351, 1970.

27. Perry MO, Thal ER, Shires GT: Management of arterial injuries. *Ann Surg* 173:403, 1971.

28. Cheek RC, Pope JC, Smith HF, et al.: Diagnosis and management of major vascular injuries: A review of 200 operative cases. *Am Surg* 41:755, 1975.

29. Hardy JD, Raju S, Neely WA, et al.: Aortic and other arterial injuries. *Ann Surg* 181:640, 1975.

30. Kelly GL, Eiseman B: Civilian vascular injuries. *J Trauma* 15:507, 1975.

31. Burnett HF, Parnell CL, Williams GD, et al.: Peripheral arterial injuries: A reassessment. *Ann Surg* 183:701, 1976.

32. Robbs JV, Baker LW: Major arterial trauma: Review of experience with 267 injuries. *Br J Surg* 65:532, 1978.

33. Reynolds RR, McDowell HA, Diethelm AG: The surgical treatment of arterial injuries in the civilian population. *Ann Surg* 189:700, 1979.

34. Saide R, Jacobsen DC, Bloch JH, et al.: Management of peripheral vascular trauma. *Am Surg* 47:429, 1981.

35. Sharma PVP, Babu SC, Shah PM, et al.: Changing patterns in civilian arterial injuries. *J Cardiovas Surg* 26:7, 1985.

36. Humphrey PW, Nichols W, Silver D: Rural vascular trauma: A twenty-year review. *Ann Vasc Surg* 8:179, 1994.

37. Feliciano DV, Bitondo CG, Mattox KL, et al.: Civilian trauma in the 1980's: A 1-year experience with 456 vascular and cardiac injuries. *Ann Surg* 199:717, 1984.

38. Howe HR, Poole GV, Hansen KJ, et al.: Salvage of lower extremities following combined orthopaedic and vascular trauma: A predictive salvage index. *Am Surg* 53:205, 1987.

39. Hafez HM, Woolgar J, Robbs JV: Lower extremity arterial injury: Results of 550 cases and review of risk factors associated with limb loss. *J Vasc Surg* 33:1212, 2001.

40. Smith RF, Elliott JP, Hageman JH, et al.: Acute penetrating arterial injuries of the neck and limbs. *Arch Surg* 109:198, 1974.

41. Menzoian JO, Doyle JE, Cantelmo NL, et al.: A comprehensive approach to extremity vascular trauma. *Arch Surg* 120:801, 1985.

42. Gill SS, Eggleston FC, Singh CM, et al.: Arterial injuries of the extremities. *J Trauma* 16:766, 1976.

43. Rich NM, Manion WC, Hughes CW: Surgical and pathological evaluation of vascular injuries in Vietnam. *J Trauma* 9:279, 1969.

44. Rich NM, Hobson RW, Fedde CW: Vascular trauma secondary to diagnostic and therapeutic procedures. *Am J Surg* 128:715, 1974.

45. Mills JL, Wiedeman JE, Robison JG, et al.: Minimizing mortality and morbidity from iatrogenic arterial injuries: The need for early recognition and prompt repair. *J Vasc Surg* 4:22, 1986.

46. Youkey JR, Clagett GP, Rich NM, et al.: Vascular trauma secondary to diagnostic and therapeutic procedures: 1974 through 1982 *Am J Surg* 146:788, 1983.

47. Saletta JD, Freeark RJ: The partially severed artery. *Arch Surg* 97:198, 1968.

48. Robbs JV, Naidoo KS: Nerve compression injuries due to traumatic false aneurysm. *Ann Surg* 200:80, 1984.

49. Kollmeyer KR, Hunt JL, Ellman BA, et al.: Acute and chronic traumatic arteriovenous fistulae in civilians. *Arch Surg* 116:697, 1981.

50. Hare RR, Gaspar MR: The intimal flap. *Arch Surg* 102:552, 1971.

51. Jahnke EJ: Late structural and functional results of arterial injuries primarily repaired: A study of one hundred fifteen cases. *Surgery* 43:175, 1958.

52. Samson R, Pasternak BM: Traumatic arterial spasm — rarity or nonentity. *J Trauma* 20:607, 1980.

53. Malan E, Tattoni G: Physio- and anatamopathology of acute ischemia of the extremities. *J Cardiovasc Surg* 4:212, 1963.

54. Cambria RA, Anderson RJ, Dikdan G, et al.: Leukocyte activation in ischemia - reperfusion injury of skeletal muscle. *J Surg Res* 51:13, 1991.

55. Menger MD, Pelikan S, Steiner D, et al.: Microvascular ischemia-reperfusion injury in striated muscle: Significance of "reflow paradox." *Am J Physiol* 263 (*Heart Circ Physiol* 32): H-1901, 1992.

56. Klausner JM, Paterson IS, Kobzik L, et al.: Leukotrienes but not complement mediate limb ischemia-induced lung injury. *Ann Surg* 209:462, 1989.

57. Miller HH, Welch CS: Quantitative studies on the time factor in arterial injuries. *Ann Surg* 130:428, 1949.

58. Gosselin RA, Siegberg CJY, Coupland R, et al.: Outcome of arterial repairs in 23 consecutive patients at the ICRC-Peshawar Hospital for war wounded. *J Trauma* 34:373, 1993.

59. Dajani OM, Haddad FF, Hajj HA, et al.: Injury to femoral vessels: The Lebanese War experience. *Eur J Vasc Surg* 2:293, 1988.

60. Pretre R, Bruschweiler I, Rossier J, et al.: Lower limb trauma with injury to the popliteal vessels. *J Trauma* 40:595, 1996.

61. Razuk AF, Nunes H, Coimbra R, et al.: Popliteal artery injuries: Risk factors for limb loss. *Panam J Trauma* 7:93, 1998.

62. Rutherford RB: Diagnostic evaluation of extremity vascular injuries. *Surg Clinic North Am* 68:683, 1988.

63. Feliciano DV, Herskowitz K, O'Gorman RB, et al.: Management of vascular injuries in the lower extremities. *J Trauma* 28:319, 1988.

64. Rozycki GS, Tremblay LN, Feliciano DV, et al.: Blunt vascular trauma in the extremity: Diagnosis, management, and outcome. *J Trauma* 55:814, 2003.

65. Ransom KJ, Shatney CH, Soderstrom CA, et al.: Management of arterial injuries in blunt trauma of the lower extremity. *Surg Gynecol Obstet* 153:241, 1981.

66. Hartling RP, McGahan JP, Blaisdell FW, et al.: Stab wounds to the extremities: Indications for angiography. *Radiology* 162:465, 1987.

67. Meyer JP, Lim LT, Schuler JJ, et al.: Peripheral vascular trauma from close range shotgun injuries. *Arch Surg* 120:1126, 1985.

68. McNamara JJ, Brief DK, Stremple JF, et al.: Management of fractures with associated arterial injury in combat casualties. *J Trauma* 13:17, 1973.

69. Rich NM, Hughes CW, Baugh JH: Management of venous injuries. *Ann Surg* 171:724, 1970.

70. Pasch AR, Bishara RA, Schuler JJ, et al.: Results of venous reconstruction after civilian vascular trauma. *Arch Surg* 121:607, 1986.

71. Hardin WD, O'Connell RC, Adinolfi MF, et al.: Traumatic arterial injuries of the upper extremity: Determinants of disability. *Am J Surg* 150:266, 1985.

72. Spencer AD: The reliability of signs of peripheral vascular injury. *Surg Gynecol Obstet* 114:490, 1962.

73. Gonzalez RP, Falimirski ME: The utility of physical examination in proximity penetrating extremity trauma. *Am Surg* 65:784, 1999.

74. Fomon FJ, Warren D: Late complications of peripheral arterial injuries. *Arch Surg* 91:610, 1965.

75. Goldman BS, Firor WB, Key JA: The recognition and management of peripheral arterial injuries. *Can Med Assoc J* 92:1154, 1965.

76. Winegarner FG, Baker AG, Bascom JF, et al.: Delayed vascular complications in Vietnam casualties. *J Trauma* 10:867, 1970.

77. Escobar GA, Escobar SC, Marquez L, et al.: Vascular Trauma: Late sequelae and treatment. *J Cardiovasc Surg* 21:35, 1980.

78. Feliciano DV, Cruse PA, Burch JM, et al.: Delayed diagnosis of arterial injuries. *Am J Surg* 154:579, 1987.

79. Richardson JD, Vitale GC, Flint LM: Penetrating arterial trauma: Analysis of missed vascular injuries. *Arch Surg* 122:678, 1987.

80. Frykberg ER, Crump JM, Vines FS, et al.: A reassessment of the role of arteriography in penetrating proximity extremity trauma: A prospective study. *J Trauma* 29:1041, 1989.

81. Frykberg ER, Crump JM, Dennis JW, et al.: Nonoperative observation of clinically occult arterial injuries: A prospective evaluation. *Surgery* 109:85, 1991.

82. Dennis JW, Frykberg ER, Veldenz HC, et al.: Validation of nonoperative management of occult vascular injuries and accuracy of physical examination alone in penetrating extremity trauma: 5 to 10-year follow-up. *J Trauma* 44:243, 1998.

83. Turcotte JK, Towne JB, Bernhard VM: Is arteriography necessary in the management of vascular trauma of the extremities? *Surgery* 84:557, 1978.

84. McCormick TM, Burch BH: Routine angiographic evaluation of neck and extremity injuries. *J Trauma* 19:384, 1979.

85. Menzoian JO, Doyle JE, LoGerfo FW, et al.: Evaluation and management of vascular injuries of the extremities. *Arch Surg* 118:93, 1983.

86. Geuder JW, Hobson RW, Padberg FT, et al.: The role of contrast arteriography in suspected arterial injuries of the extremities. *Am Surg* 51:89, 1985.

87. Gomez GA, Kreis DJ, Ratner L, et al.: Suspected vascular trauma of the extremities: The role of arteriography in proximity injuries. *J Trauma* 26:1005, 1986.

88. Pasch AR, Bishara RA, Lim LT, et al.: Optimal limb salvage in penetrating civilian vascular trauma. *J Vasc Surg* 3:189, 1986.

89. Lumpkin MB, Logan WD, Couves CM, et al.: Arteriography as an aid in the diagnosis and localization of acute arterial injuries. *Ann Surg* 147:353, 1958.

90. Freeark RJ: Role of angiography in the management of multiple injuries. *Surg Gynecol Obstet* 128:761, 1969.

91. Lain KC, Williams GR: Arteriography in acute peripheral arterial injuries: An experimental study. *Surg Forum* 21:179, 1970.

92. Snyder WH, Thal ER, Bridges RA, et al.: The validity of normal arteriography in penetrating trauma. *Arch Surg* 113:424, 1978.

93. Sirinek KR, Gaskill HV, Dittman WI, et al.: Exclusion angiography for patients with possible vascular injuries of the extremities — a better use of trauma center resources. *Surgery* 94:598, 1983.

94. Sclafani SJA, Cooper R, Shaftan GW, et al.: Arterial trauma: Diagnostic and therapeutic angiography. *Radiology* 161:165, 1986.

95. Rose SC, Moore EE: Trauma Angiography: The use of clinical findings to improve patient selection and case preparation. *J Trauma* 28:240, 1988.

96. O'Gorman RB, Feliciano DV, Bitondo CG, et al.: Emergency center arteriography in the evaluation of suspected peripheral vascular injuries. *Arch Surg* 119:568, 1984.

97. Lipchik EO, Kaebnick HW, Beres JJ, et al.: The role of arteriography in acute penetrating trauma to the extremities. *Cardiovasc Intervent Radiol* 10:202, 1987.

98. Tohmeh AG, Perler BA: Angiography in the evaluation of proximal arterial injury. *Surg Gynecol Obstet* 170:117, 1990.

99. Rees R, Bonneval M, Batson R, et al.: Angiography in extremity trauma: A prospective study. *Am Surg* 44:661, 1978.

100. Reid JDS, Weigelt JA, Thal ER, et al.: Assessment of proximity of a wound to major vascular structures as an indication for arteriography. *Arch Surg* 123:942, 1988.

101. Itani KMF, Burch JM, Spjut-Patrinely V, et al.: Emergency center arteriography. *J Trauma* 32:302, 1992.

102. Trooskin SZ, Sclafani SJA, Winfield J, et al.: The management of vascular injuries of the extremity associated with civilian firearms. *Surg Gynecol Obstet* 176:350, 1993.

103. Cargile JS, Hunt JL, Purdue GF, et al.: Acute trauma of the femoral artery and vein. *J Trauma* 32:364, 1992.

104. Howard CA, Thal ER, Redman HC, et al.: Intra-arterial digital subtraction angiography in the evaluation of peripheral vascular trauma. *Ann Surg* 210:108, 1989.

105. Busquets AR, Acosta JA, Colon E, et al.: Helical computed tomographic angiography for the diagnosis of traumatic arterial injuries of the extremities. *J Trauma* 56:625, 2004.

106. Gerlock AJ, Thal ER, Snyder WH: Venography in penetrating injuries of the extremities. *AJR* 126:1023, 1976.

107. Borman KR, Jones GH, Snyder WH: A decade of lower extremity venous trauma: Patency and outcome. *Am J Surg* 154:608, 1987.

108. Gagne PJ, Cone JB, McFarland D, et al.: Proximity penetrating extremity trauma: The role of duplex ultrasound in the detection of occult venous injuries. *J Trauma* 39:1157, 1995.

109. Hewitt RL, Smith AD, Becker ML, et al.: Penetrating vascular injuries of the thoracic outlet. *Surgery* 76:715, 1974.

110. Aboujoud MS, Obeid FN, Horst HM, et al.: Arterial injuries of the thoracic outlet. A ten-year experience. *Am Surg* 59:590, 1993.

111. Borman RR, Snyder WA, Weigelt JA: Civilian arterial trauma of the upper extremity: An 11-year experience in 267 patients. *Am J Surg* 148:796, 1984.

112. Applebaum R, Yellin AE, Weaver FA, et al.: Role of routine arteriography in blunt lower extremity trauma. *Am J Surg* 160:221, 1990.

113. Stain SC, Yellin AE, Weaver FA, et al.: Selective management of nonocclusive arterial injuries. *Arch Surg* 124:1136, 1989.

114. McDonald EJ, Goodman PC, Winestock DP: The clinical indications for arteriography in trauma to the extremity: A review of 114 cases. *Radiology* 116:45, 1975.

115. McCorkell SJ, Harley JD, Morishima MS, et al.: Indications for angiography in extremity trauma. *AJR* 145:1245, 1985.

116. Francis H, Thal ER, Weigelt JA, et al.: Vascular proximity; is it a valid indication for arteriography in asymptomatic patients? *J Trauma* 31:512, 1991.

117. Smyth SH, Pond GD, Johnson PL, et al.: Proximity injuries: Correlation with results of extremity arteriography. *J Vasc Intervent Radiol* 2:451, 1991.

118. Kaufman JA, Parker JE, Gillespie DL, et al.: Arteriography for proximity of injury in penetrating extremity trauma. *J Vasc Intervent Radiol* 3:719, 1993.

119. Gahtan V, Bramson RT, Norman J: The role of emergent arteriography in penetrating limb trauma. *Am Surg* 60:123, 1994.

120. Weaver FA, Yellin AE, Bauer M, et al.: Is arterial proximity a valid indication for arteriography in penetrating extremity trauma? A prospective analysis. *Arch Surg* 125:1256, 1990.

121. Norman J, Gahtan V, Franz M, et al.: Occult vascular injuries following gunshot wounds resulting in long bone fractures of the extremities. *Am Surg* 61:146, 1995.

122. Gillespie DL, Woodson J, Kaufman J, et al.: Role of arteriography for blunt or penetrating injuries in penetrating injuries in proximity to major vascular structures: An evolution in management. *Ann Vasc Surg* 7:145, 1993.

123. Miranda FE, Dennis JW, Veldenz HC, et al.: Confirmation of the safety and accuracy of physical examination in the evaluation of knee dislocation for popliteal artery injury: A prospective study. *J Trauma* 49:375, 2000.

124. Lavenson GS, Rich NM, Strandness DE: Ultrasonic flow detector: Value in the management of combat incurred vascular injuries. *Arch Surg* 103:644, 1971.

125. Shah D, Naraynsingh V, Leather RP, et al.: Advances in the management of acute popliteal vascular blunt injuries. *J Trauma* 25:793, 1985.

126. Bynoe RP, Miles WS, Bell RM, et al.: Noninvasive diagnosis of vascular trauma by duplex ultrasonography. *J Vasc Surg* 14:346, 1991.

127. Johansen K, Lynch K, Paun M, et al.: Non-invasive vascular tests reliably exclude occult arterial trauma in injured extremities. *J Trauma* 31:515, 1991.

128. Lynch K, Johansen K: Can Doppler pressure measurement replace "exclusion" arteriography in the diagnosis of occult extremity arterial trauma? *Ann Surg* 214:737, 1991.

129. Mills WJ, Barei DP, McNair P: The value of the ankle-brachial index for diagnosing arterial injury after knee dislocation: A prospective study. *J Trauma* 56:1261, 2004.

130. Panetta TF, Hunt JP, Buechter KJ, et al.: Duplex ultrasonography versus arteriography in the diagnosis of arterial injury: An experimental study. *J Trauma* 33:627, 1992.

131. Fry WR, Smith RS, Sayers DV, et al.: The success of duplex ultrasonographic scanning in diagnosis of extremity vascular proximity trauma. *Arch Surg* 128:1368, 1993.

132. Knudson MM, Lewis FR, Atkinson K, et al.: The role of duplex ultrasound arterial imaging in patients with penetrating extremity trauma. *Arch Surg* 128:1033, 1993.

133. Bergstein JM, Blair JF, Edwards J, et al.: Pitfalls in the use of color-flow duplex ultrasound for screening of suspected arterial injuries in penetrated extremities. *J Trauma* 33:395, 1992.

134. Meissner M, Paun M, Johansen K: Duplex scanning for arterial trauma. *Am J Surg* 161:552, 1991.

135. DeGiannis E, Levy RD, Sofianos C, et al.: Arterial gunshot injuries of the extremities: A South African experience. *J Trauma* 39:570, 1995.

136. Mitchell FL, Thal ER: Results of venous interposition grafts in arterial injuries. *J Trauma* 30:336, 1990.

137. Shah DM, Leather RP, Corson JD, et al.: Polytetrafluoroethylene grafts in the rapid reconstruction of acute contaminated peripheral vascular injuries. *Am J Surg* 148:229, 1984.

138. Stone KS, Walshaw R, Sugiyama GT, et al.: Polytetrafluoroethylene versus autogenous vein grafts for vascular reconstruction in contaminated wounds. *Am J Surg* 147:692, 1984.

139. Feliciano DV, Mattox KL, Graham JM, et al.: Five-year experience with PTFE grafts in vascular wounds. *J Trauma* 25:71, 1985.

140. Martin LC, McKenney MG, Sosa JL, et al.: Management of lower extremity arterial trauma. *J Trauma* 37:591, 1994.

141. Johnson M, Ford M, Johansen K: Radial or ulnar laceration. *Arch Surg* 128:971, 1993.

142. Mellisinos EG, Parks DH: Post-trauma reconstruction with free tissue-transfer-analysis of 442 consecutive cases. *J Trauma* 29:1095, 1989.

143. Ledgerwood AM, Lucas CE: Biologic dressings for exposed vascular grafts: A reasonable alternative. *J Trauma* 15:567, 1975.

144. Feliciano DV, Accola KD, Burch JM, et al.: Extraanatomic bypass for peripheral arterial injuries. *Am J Surg* 158:506, 1989.

145. Parry NG, Feliciano DV, Burke RM, et al.: Management and short-term patency of lower extremity venous injuries with various repairs. *Am J Surg* 186:631, 2003.

146. Khalil IM, Livingston DH: Intravascular shunts in complex lower limb trauma. *J Vasc Surg* 4:582, 1986.

147. Reber PU, Patel AG, Sapio NLD, et al.: Selective use of temporary intravascular shunts in coincident vascular and orthopaedic upper and lower limb trauma. *J Trauma* 47:72, 1999.

148. Porter JM, Ivatury RR, Nassoura ZE: Extending the horizons of damage control in unstable trauma patients beyond the abdomen and gastrointestinal tract. *J Trauma* 42:559, 1997.

149. Granchi T, Schmittling Z, Vasquez J, et al.: Prolonged use of intraluminal arterial shunts without systemic anticoagulation. *Am J Surg* 180:493, 2000.

150. Mubarak SJ, Hargens AR: Acute compartment syndromes. *Surg Clinic North Am* 63:539, 1983.

151. Williams AB, Luchette FA, Papconstantinou HT, et al.: The effect of early versus late fasciotomy in the management of extremity trauma. *Surgery* 122:861, 1997.

152. McDermott AGP, Marble AE, Yabsley RH, et al.: Monitoring acute compartment pressures with the STIC catheter. *Clinic Orthoped* 190:192, 1984.

153. Feliciano DV, Cruse PA, Spjut-Patrinely V, et al.: Fasciotomy after trauma to the extremities. *Am J Surg* 156:533, 1988.

154. Mubarak SJ, Owens CA: Double incision fasciotomy of the leg for decompression in compartment syndromes. *J Bone Jt Surg* 59:184, 1977.

155. Lim LT, Michuda MS, Flanigan DP, et al.: Popliteal artery trauma: 31 consecutive cases without amputation. *Arch Surg* 115:1307, 1980.

156. Attebery LR, Dennis JW, Russo-Alesi F, et al.: Changing patterns of arterial injuries associated with fractures and dislocations. *J Am Coll Surg* 183:377, 1996.

157. Finkelstein JA, Hunter GA, Hu RW: Lower limb compartment syndrome: Course after delayed fasciotomy. *J Trauma* 40:342, 1996.

158. Schumacker HB, Wayson EE: Spontaneous cure of aneurysms and arteriovenous fistulas, with some notes on intrasaccular thrombosis. *Am J Surg* 79:532, 1950.

159. Glover MG, Urbaniak JR: Intimal tears and their relationship to long-term patency in the rat femoral artery. *MicroSurgery* 7:124, 1986.

160. Hoffer EK, Sclafani SJA, Herskowitz MM, et al.: Natural history of arterial injuries diagnosed with arteriography. *J Vasc Intervent Radiol* 8:43, 1997.

161. Frykberg ER, Vines FS, Alexander RH: The natural history of clinically occult arterial injuries: A prospective evaluation. *J Trauma* 29:577, 1989.

162. Sawchuck AP, Eldrup-Jorgensen J, Tober C, et al.: The natural history of intimal flaps in a canine model. *Arch Surg* 125:1614, 1990.

163. Neville RF, Hobson RW, Watanabe B, et al.: A prospective evaluation of arterial intimal injuries in an experimental model. *J Trauma* 31:669, 1991.

164. Rich NM, Hobson RW, Collins GJ: Traumatic arteriovenous fistulas and false aneurysms: A review of 558 lesions. *Surgery* 78:817, 1975.

165. Perry MO: Complications of missed arterial injuries. *J Vasc Surg* 17:399, 1993.

166. Tufaro A, Arnold T, Rummel M, et al.: Adverse outcome of nonoperative management of initial injuries caused by penetrating trauma. *J Vasc Surg* 20:656, 1994.

167. Moore CH, Wolma FJ, Brown RW, et al.: Vascular trauma: A review of 250 cases. *Am J Surg* 122:576, 1971.

168. Yilmaz AT, Arslan M, Demirkiyc V, et al.: Missed arterial injuries in military patients. *Am J Surg* 173:110, 1997.

169. Kang SS, Labropoulos N, Mansour MA, et al.: Percutaneous ultrasound guided thrombin injections: A new method for treating post catheterization femoral pseudoaneurysms. *J Vasc Surg* 27:1032, 1998.

170. Scalea TM, Sclafani SJA: Angiographically placed balloons for arterial control: A description of a technique. *J Trauma* 31:1671, 1991.

171. Stecco K, Meier A, Seiver A, et al.: Endovascular stent-graft placement for treatment of traumatic penetrating subclavian artery injury. *J Trauma* 48:948, 2000.

172. Marin ML, Veith FJ, Panetta TF, et al.: Transluminally placed endovascular stented graft repair for arterial trauma. *J Vasc Surg* 20:466, 1994.

173. Bishara RA, Pasch AR, Lim LT, et al.: Improved results in the treatment of civilian vascular injuries associated with fractures and dislocations. *J Vasc Surg* 3:707, 1986.

174. Johansen K, Daines M, Howey T, et al.: Objective criteria accurately predict amputation following lower extremity trauma. *J Trauma* 30:568, 1990.

175. Palazzo JC, Ristow AB, Cury JM, et al.: Traumatic vascular lesions associated with fractures and dislocations. *J Cardiovasc Surg* 27:688, 1986.

176. Romanoff H, Goldberger S: Combined severe vascular and skeletal trauma: Management and results. *J Cardiovasc Surg* 20:493, 1979.

177. Fern KT, Smith JT, Zee B, et al.: Trauma patients with multiple extremity injuries: Resource utilization and long-term outcome in relation to injury severity scores. *J Trauma* 45:489, 1998.

178. Kaufman SL, Martin LG: Arterial injuries associated with complete dislocation of the knee. *Radiology* 184:153, 1992.

179. Treiman GS, Yellin AE, Weaver FA, et al.: Examination of the patient with a knee dislocation: The case for selective arteriography. *Arch Surg* 127:1056, 1992.

180. Dennis JW, Jagger C, Butcher JL, et al.: Reassessing the role of arteriograms in the management of posterior knee dislocations. *J Trauma* 35:692, 1993.

181. Kendall RW, Taylor DC, Salvian AJ, et al.: The role of arteriography in assessing vascular injuries associated with dislocations of the knee. *J Trauma* 35:875, 1993.

182. Martinez D, Sweatman K, Thompson EC: Popliteal artery injury associated with knee dislocations. *Am Surg* 67:165, 2001.

183. Hollis JD, Daley BJ: 10-year review of knee dislocations – is arteriography always necessary? *J Trauma* 59:672, 2005.

184. Klineberg EO, Crites BM, Flinn WR, et al.: The role of arteriography in assessing popliteal artery injury in knee dislocations. *J Trauma* 56:786, 2004.

185. Stannard JP, Sheils TM, Lopez-Ben RR, et al.: Vascular injuries in knee dislocations: The role of physical examination in determining the need for arteriography. *J Bone Joint Surg* 86-A:910, 2004.

186. Barnes CJ, Pietrobon R, Higgins LD: Does the pulse examination in patients with traumatic knee dislocation predict a surgical arterial injury? A meta-analysis. *J Trauma* 53:1109, 2002.

187. Durham RM, Mistry BM, Mazuski JE, et al.: Outcome and utility of scoring systems in the management of the mangled extremity. *Am J Surg* 172:569, 1996.

188. Swiontkowski MF, MacKenzie EJ, Bosse MJ, et al.: Factors influencing the decision to amputate or reconstruct after high-energy lower extremity trauma. *J Trauma* 52:641, 2002.

189. Bosse MJ, MacKenzie EJ, Kellam JF, et al.: An analysis of outcomes of reconstruction or amputation of leg-threatening injuries. *New Engl J Med* 347:1924, 2002.

190. Rich NM, Hobson RW II: Historical background of repair of venous injuries. In Witkin E, et al., eds. *Venous Diseases, Medical and Surgical Management.* Presented at the American European Symposium on Venous Diseases. The Hague, Netherlands, New York: Mouton, 1974.

191. Gaspar MR, Treiman RL: The management of injuries to major veins. *Am J Surg* 100:171, 1960.

192. Meyer J, Walsh J, Shuler J, et al.: The early fate of venous repair after civilian vascular trauma. *Ann Surg* 206:458, 1987.

193. Ross SE, Ransom KJ, Shatney CH: The management of venous injury in blunt extremity trauma. *J Trauma* 25:150, 1985.

194. Yelon JA, Scalea TM: Venous injuries of the lower extremities and pelvis: Repair versus ligation. *J Trauma* 33:532, 1992.

195. Timberlake GA, Kerstein MD: Venous injury: To repair or ligate, the dilemma revisited. *Am Surg* 61:139, 1995.

196. Bermudez KM, Knudson MM, Nelken NA, et al.: Long-term results of lower extremity venous injuries. *Arch Surg* 132:963, 1997.

197. Sullivan WG, Thornton FH, Baker LH, et al.: Early influence of popliteal vein repair in the treatment of popliteal vessel injuries. *Am J Surg* 122:528, 1971.

198. Agarwal N, Shah PM, Clauss RH, et al.: Experience with 115 civilian venous injuries. *J Trauma* 22:827, 1982.

199. Phifer TJ, Gerlock AJ, Rich NM, et al.: Long-term patency of venous repairs demonstrated by venography. *J Trauma* 25:342, 1985.

200. Rich NM: Principles and indications for primary venous repair. *Surgery* 91:492, 1982.

201. Nypaver TJ, Schuler JJ, McDonnel P, et al.: Long-term results of venous reconstruction after vascular trauma. *J Vasc Surg* 16:762, 1992.

202. Smith LM, Block EF, Buechter KJ, et al.: The natural history of extremity venous repair performed for trauma. *Am Surg* 65:116, 1999.

203. Hobson RW, Croom RD, Swan KG: Hemodynamics of the distal arteriovenous fistula in venous reconstruction. *J Surg Res* 14:483, 1973.

204. Hobson RW, Croom RD, Rich NM: Influence of heparin and low molecular weight dextran on the patency of autogenous vein grafts in the venous system. *Ann Surg* 178:773, 1973.

205. Mullins RJ, Lucas CE, Ledgerwood AM: The natural history following venous ligation for civilian injuries. *J Trauma* 20:737, 1980.

206. Rich NM, Collins GJ, Anderson CA, et al.: Missile emboli. *J Trauma* 18:236, 1978.

207. Bongard F, Johs SM, Leighton TA, et al.: Peripheral arterial shotgun missile emboli: Diagnostic and therapeutic management-case reports. *J Trauma* 31:1426, 1991.

208. Bland EF, Beebe GW: Missiles in the heart. *N Engl J Med* 274:1039, 1966.

209. Kortbeek JB, Clark JA, Carraway RC: Conservative management of a pulmonary artery bullet embolism: case report and review of the literature. *J Trauma* 33:906, 1992.

210. Lin C-H, Weif-C, Levin LS, et al.: The functional outcome of lower extremity fractures with vascular injury. *J Trauma* 43:480, 1997.

# Commentary ■ IAN CIVIL

Peripheral vascular injuries are relatively uncommon and as such present a challenge to both busy and occasional trauma surgeons alike. As is true with other organ system injuries, whether the mechanism is penetrating or blunt is of crucial importance in regard to making a diagnosis of peripheral vascular injury and determining the best management strategy.

While penetrating trauma with major vascular injury can be associated with massive local trauma, it is more usually associated with limited soft tissue and musculo-skeletal injury. In this context

it is usually straightforward to diagnose the injury and treatment requires operative intervention at the point of injury. On the other hand, penetrating trauma without obvious vascular injury can be problematic in that the possibility of injury exists but physical signs are often minimal. Historically, this has generated a wide range of algorithms designed to comprehensively evaluate the vasculature and avoid missing what is almost inevitably a minor injury. While the principle of ensuring that all injuries are diagnosed in any trauma patient is laudable, when the injuries are both infrequent and associated with minimal morbidity if not diagnosed immediately, the merits of such an approach have to be questioned. The overall financial costs of healthcare are an increasing issue for both developed and developing countries and any investigation, particularly an invasive one, such as angiography, has a morbidity cost for the patient as well. Recent studies have made it clear that the consequences of not diagnosing trivial vascular injuries are minimal. Concentrating on hard signs and relying on clinical examination where at all possible are important messages both for the trauma patient with peripheral vascular injury and for the healthcare system as a whole.

Outside military conflict and certain geographic areas of the world, the predominant mechanism of injury is blunt. In that context, peripheral vascular injuries usually occur in conjunction with musculo-skeletal and soft tissue injuries and commonly present a much more difficult problem in terms of diagnosis and management. Where there is gross musculo-skeletal derangement there is usually evidence of vascular impairment. Whether the musculo-skeletal derangement is the only reason for the poor vascularity is one of the first questions that must be answered in the blunt trauma patient. Realignment of fractures and relocation of dislocations is often the first step in assessment of potential peripheral vascular injury. Where vascular impairment remains, the possibility of spasm, minor injury, or major vascular trauma all exist. Not only does the presence or otherwise of vascular injury need to be resolved, the location of vascular injury in blunt trauma is often not as self-evident as in penetrating trauma. A range of investigative approaches have been proposed and new imaging technologies, such as CT angiography, can be very helpful particularly if the patient is already having a CT scan for the diagnosis of other injuries. On the other hand, in an isolated extremity injury CT may not add anything to a well-performed angiogram and compared to an angiogram done in the operating room they may occasion significant delay. Quite apart from the presence or otherwise of a vascular injury, if there is a period of ischemia and soft tissue injury is present, a compartment syndrome may develop. The trauma surgeon dealing with a peripheral vascular injury needs to remain cognizant of this fact and treat it either as part of the repair of a vascular injury, or subsequent to it. Treating potential compartment syndrome should be part of the trauma surgeon's overall responsibility to damage control. To a lesser degree than in penetrating trauma, a range of injuries with a possibility of vascular trauma, e.g., knee dislocation, have generated algorithms designed to ensure that potential injuries are not missed. The likelihood of these studies being positive in the absence of physical findings and/or bedside investigations is relatively low and the question again needs to be asked as to whether the overall financial and morbidity costs of these investigations are warranted.

Interventional radiology has made huge strides in the last decade under the guidance of both vascular surgeons and interventional radiologists. While the relative dominance and/or cooperation of these two groups varies greatly around the world, their separate or combined skills represent a great resource for the trauma patient with peripheral vascular injury. The use of interventional radiological techniques can be crucial for both stemming bleeding by way of balloon exclusion or embolization and occasionally for maintaining patency by way of stenting. Some of the more difficult injuries can either have temporary or definitive management undertaken by the radiologic interventionalist allowing the trauma surgeon valuable time to stabilize the patient before embarking on treatment. Given recent progress in the use of such techniques, the appropriate management of peripheral vascular injuries needs to be under constant review to ensure that the options available in acute and elective peripheral vascular surgery are similarly available to the trauma patient with peripheral vascular injury.

Looking to the future, patient care algorithms are being developed that incorporate body imaging such as CT after the ABCs in the trauma bay prior to the clinical secondary survey. This will not only allow identification of bleeding and occlusive peripheral vascular injuries within minutes of arrival, it will demand appropriate treatment decisions be made in the same timeframe. The presence of both the surgeon with decision making and operative skills in the trauma bay and either the surgeon or interventional radiologist with vascular radiological skills will be crucial for optimal care of the patient with peripheral vascular injury. Decisions about further investigations, if any, and the range of options available to treat the injuries need to be available immediately. Generating this sort of input for injuries which are uncommon will be a significant challenge for trauma systems in many parts of the world. However, the stakes are high. Exsanguinating hemorrhage and/or limb loss are not minor outcomes and the trauma patient with peripheral vascular injury has a lot to lose if the system is not up to his/her demands.

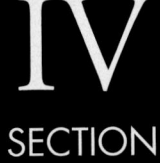

# SECTION IV

# SPECIAL PROBLEMS

# Alcohol and Drugs

*Larry M. Gentilello* ■ *Chris Dunn*

## INTRODUCTION

Excessive use of alcohol and other drugs is the leading risk factor for injury, making this behavior the most promising target for injury prevention programs. The American College of Surgeons-Committee on Trauma (ACSCOT) recently added the following two new criteria that hospitals must meet in order to be verified as a trauma center: Level I and II centers must have a mechanism in place to identify trauma patients who have an alcohol problem, and Level I centers must have a mechanism in place to offer an intervention to patients who screen positive.[1]

These criteria are based on a number of factors. Nearly 50% of patients admitted to a trauma center have a drinking problem. It is more common for a patient with a drinking problem to receive treatment for an injury than it is for them to seek treatment for the drinking problem itself, and injuries are the most common medical condition for which patients with an alcohol use disorder seek medical attention.[2] Nearly 50% of alcohol-related deaths are due to an injury, which makes trauma, not cirrhosis, hepatitis, pancreatitis, or other medical conditions, the leading cause of death in problem drinkers.[3] Patients with an alcohol problem are three and one-half times more likely to be reinjured and require readmission to a trauma center within two years than patients without a problem.[4] Finally, two recent nationwide surveys of trauma surgeons reported that nearly 85% support implementing screening and intervention services in trauma centers.[5,6]

The purposes of this chapter are to review the pathophysiologic effects of alcohol and other drug use as they relate to acute management and trauma outcome, to review current recommendations for managing withdrawal syndromes, and to provide guidelines for screening and counseling patients with such problems on a trauma service.

## MAGNITUDE OF THE PROBLEM

Pooled data from six regional trauma centers involving 4063 patients indicate that 40% of patients have a positive blood alcohol concentration (BAC) on admission.[7,8] If drug use is included, up to 70% of patients test positive for one or more intoxicants.[9] Most trauma patients with a positive BAC meet criteria for having an alcohol problem. In one study the Michigan Alcohol Screening Test (MAST), a questionnaire to identify patients with a potential alcohol problem, was administered to 2657 intoxicated trauma patients, and 75% screened positive.[10] Alcohol problems were so common that 26% of nonintoxicated patients also had a positive MAST.

In comparison to alcohol use, epidemiologic studies that document the prevalence of drug use in trauma patients are much less common. The frequency and type of use may reflect local, rather than national patterns; however, it is clear that the prevalence of drug use in trauma patients far exceeds the national norm.

One group performed urine tests and drug screening interviews on all patients admitted to an urban trauma center.[9] The prevalence of a drug problem was 20% for men, 11% for women, 10% for patients with an unintentional injury mechanism, and 36% for victims of violence. The most commonly used drugs were cocaine (11%), marijuana (7%), and opiates (10%). Overall, 70% of patients tested positive for either alcohol or drugs. The most comprehensive study to date performed routine toxicology screens over a 16-year period, generating a database of over 53,000 toxicology screens in trauma patients.[11] Cocaine positive and opiate positive results in patients with unintentional injuries were 9% and 18%, respectively.

## EFFECTS OF ALCOHOL OR DRUG USE ON TRAUMA MANAGEMENT AND OUTCOME

### Alcohol

Alcohol use affects the management of trauma patients in a variety of ways. Intoxicated patients are more than twice as likely to require intubation for airway control.[12] Tests such as diagnostic peritoneal lavage and computed tomography (CT) scans of the abdomen and brain are more frequently needed because the reliability of physical examination is reduced. Intoxication also results in an overestimation of the severity of injury to the brain. In one study, intoxicated patients were 50% more likely to receive an intracranial pressure monitoring device than nonintoxicated patients with similar injuries.[13]

Alcohol also appears to increase the risk of death from serious injury. The most detailed study used a statewide registry to obtain data from more than a million drivers involved in a crash.[14] When the effects of injury-related variables such as safety belt use, vehicle deformation, speed, driver age, weather conditions, and vehicle weight were taken into account, the drinking driver was more than twice as likely to suffer serious injury or death, compared with the nondrinking driver in a crash involving similar forces.

There are a number of mechanisms by which alcohol may adversely affect outcome. Patients with chronic excessive use are more likely to have serious complicating medical conditions. Nearly half of all cases of cardiomyopathy result from chronic use of alcohol. Most heavy drinkers have some degree of chamber dilatation and decreased cardiac output, and many of these cases are subclinical. Alcohol also reduces the threshold for fibrillation, and even an isolated episode of heavy drinking increases the risk of dysrhythmia (holiday heart). In a study involving severe blunt trauma to the chest in a dog model, 92% of those pretreated with alcohol died, compared to 11% of controls, and mortality was primarily due to cardiac dysfunction.[15]

Alcohol is also a peripheral vasodilator, which limits the ability to compensate for blood loss. One study measured the amount of hemorrhage required to induce hypotension in dogs and found that pretreatment with alcohol decreased the required volume by one-third.[16] This may be a particularly devastating consequence in patients with traumatic brain injury. In an animal study, pretreatment with ethanol prior to percussion injury resulted in increased cerebral oxygen extraction and cerebral venous lactate and reduced survival time due to impaired hemodynamic compensation.[17]

An elevated alcohol level also causes respiratory depression and compromise of the airway, especially in obtunded patients with traumatic brain injuries, resulting in the loss of a vital mechanism needed to compensate for hypoxia and metabolic acidosis. Beverages with high alcohol content decrease gastric motility, resulting in an increased risk of vomiting and aspiration.

The effects of alcohol-induced hepatic disease on production of clotting factors are well known. Of interest, a single episode of even moderate drinking also impairs the formation of clot. The reduction in adverse coronary events associated with moderate alcohol intake has been partially attributed to this effect. The mechanism is similar to the clotting dysfunction induced by aspirin, and is due to reduced production of thromboxane $A_2$ and degranulation of platelets. Alcohol also causes release of tissue plasminogen activator, which accelerates the lysis of clot. These effects may be responsible

for the observation that intoxicated but otherwise healthy patients with isolated splenic injuries have more blood loss and a higher incidence of splenectomy than nonintoxicated patients.[18]

Patients with chronic dependence on alcohol have an increased incidence of infections because malnutrition and hepatic disease affect the immune response; however, acute alcohol intoxication is also immunosuppressive. Documented effects include impaired response of monocytes and macrophages, reduced activity of natural killer cells, and altered humoral immunity. Neutrophil function is reduced due to impaired production of oxidants, reduced degranulation, and downregulation of the expression of adhesion molecules.

Acutely intoxicated animals have decreased pulmonary clearance of aerosolized bacteria and develop pneumonia and bacteremia more frequently than nonintoxicated controls. An elevated level of blood alcohol also decreases the clearance of peritoneal bacteria by macrophages. These effects of alcohol on host resistance are consistent with clinical data. One investigation analyzed infectious complications in patients with penetrating abdominal trauma and injury to a hollow viscus.[19] After controlling for chronic use, a blood alcohol concentration of 200 mg/dL or more at the time of arrival to the emergency department was associated with a 2.6-fold increase in infectious complications in the abdomen.

Alcohol causes calcium loss through the urinary and gastrointestinal systems, and patients with heavy chronic use typically have an elevated parathormone level, which results in a reduction in bone mass, a propensity for fractures, and impaired bone healing. A reduction in bone mass has been reported in over 50% of alcohol dependent patients, and the high incidence of fractures in alcohol impaired patients is attributable not only to an increased risk of falls, but also to the prevalence of osteopenia.

### Other Drugs

In the year 2004, 10.6 million people reported driving while under the influence of an illicit drug.[20] It is estimated that drugs are involved in up to 18% of fatalities in motor vehicle crashes.[21] Unlike alcohol, most states do not have standards that define a drug level at which one would be considered too impaired to drive because any illicit drug use is illegal. Prosecution for impaired driving is rare, as there are no devices analogous to a Breathalyzer test to detect alcohol, and, with no legal standard for impairment, it is difficult to prove intoxication.

The effect of drug use on trauma management and outcome has not been subject to intensive investigation. The performance of such studies would be difficult because patients who use drugs often use more than one, and drug intoxication is frequently combined with alcohol consumption; however, a number of adverse effects could be anticipated.

Heroin causes histamine release, which decreases systemic vascular resistance, and may decrease blood pressure after major hemorrhage. Injection continues to be the most common route for addicted users, but tracks and needle scars may be absent, as sniffing or snorting is currently the most widely used means of ingestion among users admitted for treatment. Many addicts do not fit the stereotypical profile of the street addict, as the availability of high purity heroin that can be sniffed or smoked has resulted in its appearance in many affluent communities.

Cocaine and its free-base form "crack" have acute effects that include peripheral vasoconstriction, dilated pupils, tachycardia, and hypertension. Its neuropsychological effects are mediated by blockage of dopamine reuptake in the central nervous system. Prolonged use causes downregulation of serotonin and dopamine receptors and clinical depression, which are often responsible for severe craving and continued use. In 2001, more than 1.1 million new users tried cocaine, a level of first use not seen since 1988.[21]

Methamphetamine (speed, ice) taken orally, nasally, by injection or smoking is a strong stimulant drug that causes release of high levels of dopamine. Users become addicted very quickly, and prolonged use causes irreversible damage to neuronal receptors. As with other potent stimulant drugs, tachycardia, and vasoconstriction can cause severe hypertension, cardiac stress, myocardial infarction, and stroke. Methamphetamine use is epidemic in some cities and rural communities, as it can be made using ingredients that can be purchased over the counter. The number of people seeking treatment for methamphetamine addiction has quadrupled in past ten years, from 28,000 in 1993 to 136,000 in 2003.[22]

One characteristic sign of use that should raise suspicion is "meth mouth." Methamphetamine is made with anhydrous ammonia, lithium from batteries, muriatic acid, and red phosphorous. When the route of ingestion is smoking or snorting, the teeth of chronic users are generally eroded down to the gumline as these are all highly caustic and corrosive.

## WITHDRAWAL SYNDROMES

The goals of prophylaxis and treatment of withdrawal syndromes are to minimize the risk of serious complications such as seizures, delirium tremens, and the cardiovascular morbidity that occurs as a result of sympathetic overload. Clinicians should also consider treating withdrawal as the first step in a plan aimed at facilitating abstinence.

Withdrawal syndromes are characterized by signs and symptoms that are the opposite of the pharmacologic effects of the discontinued drug. The four primary categories are alcohol, sedative–hypnotics (benzodiazepines, barbiturates), opiates, and stimulants. All drugs in each category are associated with similar withdrawal syndromes, but they differ in their intensity, timing of onset, and duration. Symptoms from cessation of short acting drugs like alcohol may emerge within 6–24 hours, while withdrawal from long acting drugs like chlordiazapoxide or methadone may not emerge for several days.

Alcohol and sedative–hypnotic drugs have similar pharmacologic effects, and withdrawal may cause life-threatening physiologic disturbances. Withdrawal from opiates is highly stressful, but is not dangerous except in patients with severe underlying comorbid conditions. Cessation of stimulant use is characterized by depression and a substantial risk of suicidal behavior.

### Alcohol

Scoring systems such as the Clinical Institute Withdrawal Assessment-Alcohol (CIWA-A) are useful for predicting and assessing the severity of withdrawal. A revised short form (CIWA-Ar) that rates 10 signs and symptoms on a 0–7 scale (nausea, tremor, autonomic hyperactivity, anxiety, agitation, tactile, visual, and auditory disturbances, headache, disorientation) is available, as well.[23]

Two main types of prophylactic regimens exist. The first is symptom-triggered therapy using results from a scoring instrument, and the second is fixed scheduled dosing with a taper. In randomized prospective trials symptom-triggered therapy reduced the amount of medication administered, reduced the duration of treatment, and many patients developed only mild symptoms that did not require therapy.[24] These studies used frequent assessments with the CIWA-Ar administered by nurses with special training and experience in managing alcohol problems and were conducted in alcohol treatment centers.

Use of the CIWA-Ar has also been reported in general medical and surgical wards; however, given the subjective nature of the assessment, the training required, and the need for frequent repeat administration, it is probably not feasible in most trauma centers and cannot be administered to patients who are intubated.

For these reasons, scheduled dosing with a taper is a reasonable alternative in high-risk patients. Patients at highest risk are those who have had prior episodes of delirium tremens characterized by tremor and restlessness. Any trauma patient who develops evidence of hand tremor without another medical cause should be considered as potentially having a withdrawal syndrome, while the absence of tremor makes the condition very unlikely. Tachycardia, fever, and hypertension are also usually present, but are nonspecific.

The efficacy of benzodiazepines for both prophylaxis and treatment has been established in numerous clinical trials. They have an excellent safety profile and are first line agents for the treatment of seizures. All currently existing evidence-based guidelines recommend the use of benzodiazepines as primary therapy.[25]

Benzodiazepines with a long half-life, such as diazepam, are preferred because they result in a gradual decline in blood levels. In a typical scheduled dose prophylactic regimen, 10 mgs is given PO or IV every 6 hours for 4 doses, then 5 mg is provided every 6 hours for 8 doses. If the patient already has symptoms, 10–20 mg PO every hour, or 5 mg IV every 10–15 minutes, should be administered until the patient is drowsy or has slurred speech. Induction of hepatic enzymes may result in the need for much larger doses. Because of the long half-life of diazepam additional dosing is generally not required after an adequate loading regimen. In an occasional patient tapering using the above regimen is needed after gaining control.

Chlordiazapoxide (Librium) is the preferred agent for patients who are able to take oral medication. Its very long half-life results in a gradual taper after adequate loading. Lorazepam or oxazapam, which do not have active metabolites, are preferred agents for elderly patients or those with significant hepatic disease. Occasionally, patients are resistant to benzodiazepines but are responsive to propofol, which can be used in the intensive care unit if the airway is controlled.

The administration of alcohol for prophylaxis is no longer considered acceptable. Alcohol blocks some of the autonomic effects of withdrawal, but it lowers the seizure threshold. Convulsions occur in alcohol dependent patients even when they have alcohol in their bloodstream. Intravenous alcohol is toxic to tissues in the event of extravasation, it increases the risk of gastric mucosal bleeding, may increase hepatic enzymes, and may precipitate acute hepatic failure in critically ill patients with reduced hepatic reserve.

There are several useful adjunctive agents such as beta-blockers, clonidine, and neuroleptics, but they should not be used as primary therapy. None have anticonvulsant properties, and all may increase the incidence of delirium by selectively reducing autonomic manifestations, or masking the emergence of other withdrawal symptoms such as hallucinations and confusion that would otherwise be recognized and treated.

## Other Drugs

The principles of preventing and treating sedative–hypnotic withdrawal are similar to those used for alcohol. Management consists of switching short acting agents for longer acting ones, then tapering the dose by 20% per day over five days. Patients with opiate dependence may experience flu-like symptoms as the drug is tapered. Clonidine can reduce autonomic signs and symptoms, diphenoxylate may be needed to control diarrhea, and many patients also require an anti-emetic.

Patients who are on methadone maintenance should be continued on their regular dose, with supplemental morphine provided to control pain as needed. If the patient desires, a referral to an abstinence oriented program can be made upon discharge. Four randomized trials, two comparing methadone with no treatment and two using placebo controls, have established methadone maintenance as an accepted medical treatment for opiate addiction.[26,27,28,29] One of these trials, using intention to treat analysis, found that control patients were 92 times more likely to be using heroin daily, and were 53 times more likely to be reincarcerated. Other studies have documented reduced transmission rates of HIV and hepatitis, higher employment rates, and a number of other social benefits.

## ALCOHOL SCREENING AND INTERVENTIONS IN TRAUMA CENTERS

The rationale behind a brief intervention is that not all patients with a drinking problem are "alcoholics." Alcohol dependence (alcoholism) is a distinct alcohol use disorder defined by tolerance, withdrawal symptoms, inability to control drinking, craving, and significant social, legal, and medical consequences. There are many patients who drink at levels that result in adverse consequences, but who do not have an addiction to alcohol.

For example, more injuries occur as a result of binge drinking, defined as more than four drinks per drinking occasion for males, or more than three drinks for females, than as a result of alcohol dependence. Heavy drinking, defined as more than 14 drinks per week for a male, or more than seven for a female, is also associated with harmful health effects, even though dependence may not be present.[30]

It is estimated that nearly one out of three people who use alcohol exceed recommended daily or weekly limits, but only 3–4% of the US population is alcohol dependent. Thus, the majority of patients with an alcohol use disorder are candidates for brief interventions and do not need access to more expensive, difficult to access, in- or out-patient treatment programs for alcoholism. The rationale for interventions in the trauma center is based on a public health approach that addresses harmful or at-risk drinking in a broad population, as opposed to being focused on getting more patients into centers for the treatment of alcoholism (Fig. 45-1).

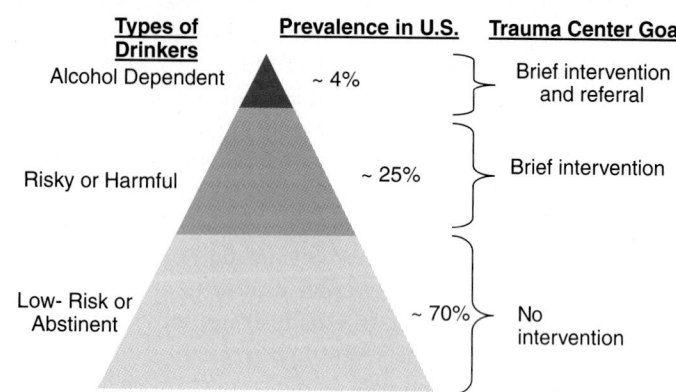

**FIGURE 45-1.** Matching interventions to problem severity for trauma patients who use alcohol or drugs.
*(Reproduced with permission from Daniel Hungerford, PhD, Centers for Disease Control).*

## Classification of Drinking Problems

Terms that have been used to classify alcohol problems along a continuum from mild to severe are hazardous or risky drinking (at risk but not yet incurring harm), harmful drinking or alcohol abuse (has already incurred injury or other consequences, but is not addicted), and alcohol dependence. The term "substance abuse" is likely to be deleted from future editions of the Diagnostic and Statistical Manual (DSM) as it is pejorative and stigmatizing and is confusing because it is often inappropriately applied to patients with alcohol dependence.

Physicians tend to place their focus on "alcoholics," the patients that are most difficult to treat, and generally do not recognize those with other types of drinking problems, such as binge drinking.

For trauma center purposes, one needs to recognize patients with unsafe levels of alcohol use who are candidates for brief interventions. In contrast, patients with signs of dependence should receive an intervention designed to motivate them to accept and follow through on a referral to an alcohol treatment specialist or treatment center, or to a self-help group such as Alcoholics Anonymous.

Since most brief intervention protocols last from three to 20 minutes they are consistent with the scope, mission, financial resources, and responsibilities of trauma centers. A recent multicenter feasibility study documented that even the busiest trauma centers in the country can meet their screening and intervention needs with one half-time employee.[31] Trauma center funding and staffing patterns should reflect the fact that interventions can be provided at a small cost in comparison to the enormous costs of alcohol and drug use on trauma centers.

## Studies on the Outcome of Brief Intervention

In recent years there have been over 50 reports on brief interventions (BI) involving over 9000 patients, including over 15 randomized trials conducted in outpatient family practice and medicine clinics, orthopedic units, emergency departments, and trauma centers.[32] In the studies conducted on injured patients, brief interventions have been associated with the following: a significant reduction in alcohol intake, a nearly 50% decrease in injuries requiring trauma center readmission, a similar reduction in injuries requiring treatment in the emergency department, reduced injuries and drinking in adolescent trauma patients, decreased binge-drinking in teenagers, reduced arrests for driving while under the influence (DUI), and a significant reduction in healthcare costs.

One study analyzed the efficacy of brief interventions on injury recurrence in patients in the emergency room by randomly assigning 94 patients aged 18 or 19 years to receive either a 30-minute brief intervention, or standard care.[33] At six months follow-up the intervention group had a significant reduction in drinking and driving, moving violations, alcohol-related problems, and less than half as many alcohol-related injuries as the patients randomized to no intervention. In another randomized study of injured adolescents, those who screened positive for problem drinking and were randomized to receive an intervention reduced their binge drinking significantly more than those assigned to the control group.[34]

Another randomized prospective trial was performed on 762 patients admitted to a Level 1 trauma center.[35] Patients who screened positive for an alcohol problem were randomized to a single 30-minute brief intervention or to conventional trauma care. At one year follow-up the intervention group decreased their alcohol intake by 22 drinks per week compared to a two drink reduction in the conventional care group. A statewide registry was used to detect readmission to any hospital for treatment of an injury over a three-year follow-up period. There was a 47% reduction in trauma readmission in the intervention group, compared to controls. There was also a 48% reduction in returns to the emergency department for treatment of another injury (Fig. 45-2).

A study on cost-benefits demonstrated that the reduction in repeated injuries that occurs after a brief intervention saves $3.81 for every dollar spent and generates savings of $380 in direct medical costs for every intervention performed.[36] Another randomized prospective trial demonstrated that the provision of a brief intervention during trauma center admission, even with dependent drinkers, decreased DUI arrest rates by 66% at three-year follow-up.[37]

Although there are fewer data on brief interventions for drug use disorders, one randomized clinical trial conducted in an inner-city teaching hospital assessed patients for continued drug use by analyzing hair samples with a radioimmunoassay. The intervention group was more likely to be abstinent for cocaine alone (22.3% vs. 16.9%), heroin alone (40.2% vs. 30.6%), and for both drugs (17.4% vs. 12.8%). Cocaine levels in hair were reduced by 29% in patients in the intervention group and by only 4% in controls.[38]

## Screening Trauma Patients for an Alcohol Problem

Screening can be conducted by performing blood alcohol testing, with additional testing for urine toxicology, or by use of screening questionnaires. In either case, screening should be routine and not depend upon clinical suspicion. Clinicians are unable to identify over one-third of patients with a BAC greater than 0.8 mg/dL, especially when patients are severely injured, in shock, have injuries to the brain, or are intubated.[39] Clinical suspicion fails to identify over one-half of patients who meet criteria for dependence. Also, patients are frequently misclassified as being intoxicated or alcohol dependent when they are not, and these distinctions are often based on gender, insurance status, and socioeconomic considerations. Finally, ethnic patients and racial minorities admitted to trauma centers are more frequently tested for alcohol and drugs than nonminority patients.[40]

The ACSCOT criterion for screening trauma patients provides several options, ranging from the least intensive practices to a "best practices" model. The best practices model combines a standardized questionnaire with laboratory tests such as a BAC and urine toxicology. Each trauma center should select the screening method that establishes an optimal balance between quality and cost for their institution.

The screening method should be sensitive enough to detect the full spectrum of alcohol problems. In resolving the trade-off between sensitivity and specificity it is better to use a more sensitive test because the harm of a false positive is very low. Also, a more sensitive screen will identify more patients with less severe drinking problems, as compared to a more specific screen that will primarily be sensitive to alcohol dependence.

A BAC can be obtained with minimal expense and disruption when admission labs are drawn for other purposes. In the case of drugs other than alcohol, any urinalysis found to be positive for a stimulant (cocaine, methamphetamine) or marijuana is considered a positive screen, whereas the presence of an opiate or benzodiazepine may reflect administration of these drugs as part of emergency care.

An alternative to BAC testing is to use a questionnaire such as the CAGE or AUDIT.[41,42] A questionnaire may detect patients with an alcohol problem who were not drinking at the time of the injury. Many physicians are mistrustful of patient self-report, but when asked in a respectful, concerned, and confidential manner, patients with an alcohol problem do not typically underreport their drinking.[43]

There are, however, circumstances where patients may be less inclined to admit alcohol use, such as after a crash where others have been seriously injured or if the alcohol or drug use would constitute a parole violation. Also, screening questionnaires are primarily aimed at detecting patients who are likely to have a DSM-IV diagnosis of a substance use disorder. For trauma center purposes, patients who injure themselves while intoxicated are appropriate candidates for preventive counseling, regardless of whether or not they meet formal criteria for a substance use disorder.

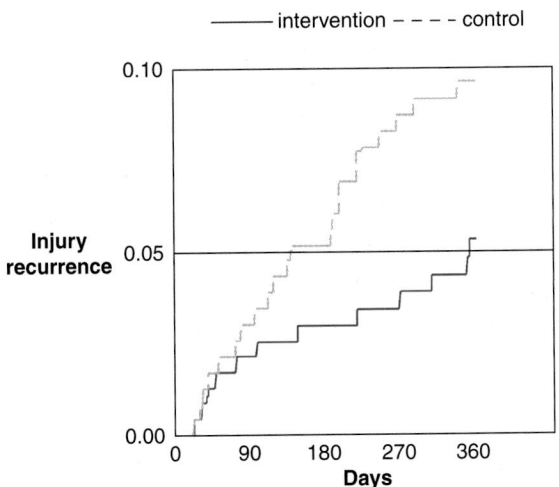

**FIGURE 45-2.** Rate of reinjury requiring emergency department treatment or trauma center admission in trauma patients. There was a 48% reduction in the intervention group compared to standard care.

Overall, a combination of a screening questionnaire and a BAC is most likely the best means of enhancing both sensitivity and specificity. The CAGE test is a simple screening tool with its name derived from the key words in four questions that can easily be incorporated into an admission history or during subsequent rounds. "Have you ever Cut down on your drinking?" "Have you ever been Annoyed by people complaining about your drinking?" "Have you ever felt Guilty about your drinking?" and "Have you ever had a drink in the morning to feel better ("Eye-opener?"). The CAGE has a high rate of agreement with more time-consuming questionnaires, demonstrates strong concordance with an admission BAC, has been validated in trauma patients, and is easy for clinicians to remember.

Traditionally, two or more positive responses constitute a positive screen; however, the CAGE was designed to detect alcohol dependence, and is less sensitive to less severe problems. Therefore, some have recommended using a cutoff score of 1 as a positive CAGE. A modification of the CAGE, where the same questions are used but the phrase "or drugs" is added to each, has been shown to be a reasonably sensitive and specific method of screening for drug problems.

The Alcohol Use Disorders Identification Test (AUDIT) is a 10-question, self-report screening tool developed by the World Health Organization, and it has been validated in trauma patients. It was designed to be sensitive to a broad spectrum of harmful drinking levels. It assesses drinking quantity and frequency (three questions), problems caused by alcohol (four questions), and symptoms of dependence (three questions). It takes less than five minutes to ask these 10 questions and to score them. A score of 8 or more is considered a positive screen. Because the safe recommended level of alcohol intake differs between males and females, the three quantity and frequency questions decrease the sensitivity of the AUDIT in females, and a lower cut-off score of five points has been recommended (Table 45-1).[44]

Another screening strategy is to use a combination of the three quantity and frequency questions of the AUDIT, combined with a BAC. These three questions allow the screener to calculate typical weekly alcohol consumption and to compare it to established guidelines for low-risk drinking (no more than four or three drinks per occasion for males and females, or 14 or 7 drinks per week for each). During the intervention the patient can be informed that his/her drinking exceeds these guidelines. The BAC facilitates the intervention because it underlines the fact that the patient was intoxicated when injured.

At a minimum, reasonably effective screening for drinking above safe guidelines can be performed by asking only one question. In a study of 1537 patients who presented to the emergency department with an injury, researchers asked the question, "When was the last time you had more than five drinks in a day (four drinks for women)?" Formal interviews by trained staff were then conducted to determine if an alcohol problem was present. The question about consumption in a day, when answered, "in the past 3 months," had sensitivities and specificities of 85% and 70% in males, and 82% and 77% in females. This indicates that asking only one straightforward question can be used as a brief screening method.[45]

## HOW TO PERFORM A BRIEF INTERVENTION

A brief intervention is an empathic, nonconfrontational style of counseling derived from Motivational Interviewing. It is based on the theory that people often change toward a more positive lifestyle when they become too uncomfortable with the discrepancy between their current situation and how they would prefer things to be. Although formal treatment or counseling is useful and may

---

**TABLE 45-1**

**The Alcohol Use Disorders Identification Test (AUDIT) was Designed to Detect Alcohol Problems Across a Range of Severity, Including Harmful or Nondependent Drinking**

**AUDIT QUESTIONNAIRE**

**Hazardous Use**

1. How often do you have a drink containing alcohol?

| Never | Monthly or less | 2–4 times/month | 2–3 times/week | ≥ 4 times/week |
|---|---|---|---|---|

2. How many drinks of alcohol do you have on a typical day when you are drinking?

| 1–2 | 3–4 | 5–6 | 7–9 | 10 or more |
|---|---|---|---|---|

3. How often do you have six or more drinks on one occasion?

**Symptoms of Dependence**

4. How often during the last year have you found that you were not able to stop drinking once you had started?
5. How often during the last year have you failed to do what was normally expected from you because of drinking?
6. How often during the last year have you needed a first drink in the morning to get yourself going after a heavy drinking session?
7. How often during the last year have you had a feeling of guilt or remorse after drinking?
8. How often during the last year have you been unable to remember what happened the night before because you had been drinking?

**Responses to Questions 3–8.**

| Never | Less than monthly | Monthly | Weekly | Daily or almost daily |
|---|---|---|---|---|

**Consequences of Drinking**

9. Have you or has someone else been injured as a result of your drinking?
10. Has a relative or friend, or a doctor or other health worker been concerned about your drinking or suggested you cut down?

**Responses to Questions 9–10.**

| No | Yes, but not in the last year | Yes, during the last year |
|---|---|---|

Questions 1-8 are scored 0, 1, 2, 3, or 4 points. Questions 9 and 10 are scored 0, 2, or 4 points only. A total score of 8 or more points indicates a strong likelihood of hazardous or harmful alcohol consumption.

enable change to occur at a sooner point in a patient's life, most patients who have successfully quit or reduced their drinking to safe limits have done so without formal help.

Aggressive, authoritarian counseling is unlikely to be successful in a trauma center. Research has failed to support the concept that patients with alcohol problems have consistent personality traits such as poor motivation and rigid defense mechanisms such as denial.[46] Rather, these factors are an outcome of the style of interaction between the clinician and patient. When patients "in denial" are heard to argue in favor of the status quo, it is usually because they are trying to defend themselves against a confrontational counselor. These tactics are particularly counterproductive in a trauma center because the denial they provoke requires too much time and skill to overcome.

## A Model for Stages of Change

Currently, the most useful organizing concept for understanding how people move away from harmful behaviors and towards a healthier lifestyle is called the Trans-theoretical Stages of Change Model.[47] The model emerged from the discovery of a common sequence of psychological benchmarks that patients experience as they prepare to change. Although there are five stages in the Model, only the first three need to be considered in trauma patients: *pre-contemplation*, *contemplation*, and *preparation*. These stages can be summarized as not-ready, unsure, or ready-to-change. The two later stages are *action* and *maintenance*, and will hopefully occur after discharge from the trauma center (Fig. 45-3).

Standardized questionnaires for determining the patient's readiness to change exis however, a simple means of doing so is to ask the patient to rate on a scale of 1–10, "How important is it for you to change your drinking?"[48] Those who score in the middle range (4–6) are contemplators (unsure), and those scoring higher should be considered as more ready to change.

Patients who are in the precontemplation stage have little awareness of the negative impact of their drinking or drug use and have no intention of changing. Patients at this stage perceive a benefit to using substances, are not aware of any disadvantages, and say phrases such as, "Alcohol isn't a problem for me; if anything, it is a fun way to deal with my boredom."

Contemplation (unsure) is the second stage, where patients have become aware of the negative consequences of drinking and are considering the need for change, but are not yet committed to doing so. They are ambivalent about their drinking, and this is sometimes characterized by, "yes, but" statements: "I suppose my drinking had something to do with my injury, but I'm really not an alcoholic."

The third stage is preparation, in which the patient is determined to quit or cut down, and develops a change plan: "I'm going to quit drinking, and I'm going to go back to AA to do it." The final two stages in the Model are characterized by the length of time new behaviors are sustained. In the action stage the new behavior is sustained for less than six months and, in the maintenance stage, it is sustained for more than six months.

Individuals do not necessarily move through the stages of change in sequential or linear fashion. They often move backward as well. Relapse commonly occurs among patients with chronic diseases such as diabetes, asthma, or hypertension. As with treatment of these conditions, an alcohol intervention should not be considered a failure if symptoms recur, especially after a significant period of reduced drinking or abstinence. Brief interventions have treatment efficacy that is actually better than treatment for these other chronic medical disorders with respect to patient compliance, relapse rates, and need for additional treatment. Also, a small but significant number of patients successfully quit drinking permanently, often after years of repeated relapses.

The goal of staff within a trauma center should be to capitalize on the effects of the injury and attempt to move the individual from the precontemplation or contemplation phase and closer to the preparation/action phase of the change process. One of the appealing features of the model is that an intervention can be considered successful even if the patient does not agree to quit drinking. For example, an intervention in a precontemplator may be considered successful if it generates doubt in the patient that his or her drinking is okay, or if it increases a contemplator's ambivalence about his or her drinking by making them more aware that the "pros" of continuing to drink are beginning to be outweighed by the "cons."

## The Three Components of an Intervention

The three basic elements of a brief intervention can be summarized by the acronym, **SUM**: Screening feedback, Understanding the patient's views, and providing a Menu of change options. The relative emphasis placed on each component is determined by how ready the patient is to change (not ready, unsure, ready). All three **SUM** components can be delivered in as few as 5 minutes, or alternatively, a single component might take as much as 15 minutes.

Screening Feedback is different from education and refers to providing the patient with the results of his or her screening tests. Unlike general education, information that patients can distance themselves from, screening results are uniquely relevant to a particular patient. For example, instead of telling the patient, "Excessive drinking can cause liver damage," the interventionist would tell the patient, "When you were injured your blood alcohol level was 0.16 mg/dL, which is two times the legal limit for driving." The screening feedback process should be interactive, with the clinician encouraging a reaction from the patient, and then listening in an empathic manner. This provides the clinician with information about the patient's readiness to change, and provides the

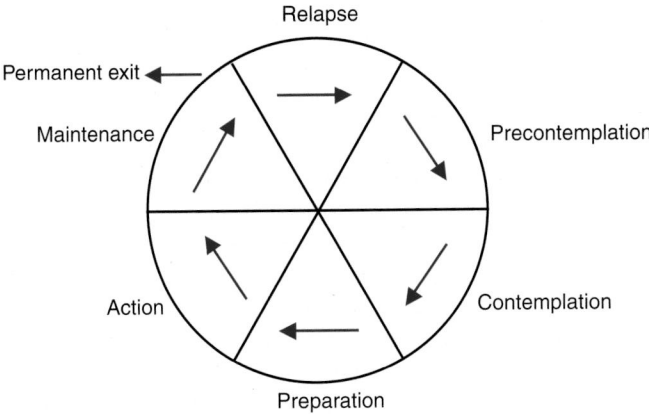

**FIGURE 45-3.** Trans-Theoretical Model of Change.

patient with an opportunity to express concerns about their drinking that can be used to increase their motivation to change.

The two main sources of feedback for trauma patients are their admission BAC and how their score on a screening questionnaire compares to normative standards. This might include telling the patient the score that represents normal or low-risk drinking, and then providing the patient with his or her own score. A simple five-step acronym ("RANGE") can be used to provide feedback about the patient's BAC. Tell the patient the Range of possible BAC results, from 0 (sober) to 500 mg/dL (fatal). Mention that all drivers know that .08 mg/dL is the definition of drunk driving, and that Normal drinkers usually stay under .08 mg/dL, even when not driving. Give the patient his or her BAC result and interpret it in relation to .08 mg/dL: "Your BAC was twice the legal limit for drunk driving." Then, elicit the patient's reaction.

If the patient was injured in a crash, feedback about the risk of driving while intoxicated should be provided. This can be done by showing a graph that indicates the risk of crashing at a given level of blood alcohol. For example, the physician might state, "The best way to explain this is to show you an illustration that indicates that at your blood alcohol concentration of 0.14 mg/dL you were 48 times more likely to have a serious crash than if you had not been drinking." When providing feedback it is important to inform the patient that you are not concerned with labels ("alcoholism"), but instead express, "I am concerned that alcohol is hurting you."

The next part, Understanding the patient's views, can be done by asking the patient about the "pros and cons" of their drinking. After the clinician has asked the patient what they like about their drinking, he or she listens to what the patient believes are benefits, such as, "It helps me to relax," "It makes it easier to interact with others," or, "It helps me to have a good time." The clinician then asks the patient to explore the "cons" by asking, "What are some of the things you don't like about drinking?" For example, if the patient indicates that one of the negative aspects of drinking has been frequent arguments with family members, the clinician might ask, "How does your alcohol use affect your ability to have a stable family life?" The goal is not to demand change, but to raise doubt by having the patient, rather than the clinician, articulate how alcohol use is having an adverse effect on their family, health, work, finances, driving record, or legal status.

If the patient is unable to provide any negative statements about their drinking the clinician might supply such information, and ask if it is true for him or her. Asking for, then summarizing the pros and cons of drinking, is a key technique in brief intervention. It conveys that the clinician is interested in the patient's point of view. Also, it is a key step in establishing rapport and allows the patient to state the ways that their use of alcohol is adversely affecting them so that recommendations for change are based upon the patient's own goals and values. Clinicians should emphasize the risk of injury because most patients are not aware of its extent and they value avoiding readmission to the trauma center.

The menu of options is simply a list of choices available to the patient that is presented in the following ascending order of commitment: no change whatsoever, merely think about it and notice more about your drinking in the future, cut down, or quit. If the patient selects one of the latter three options, a plan for achieving this goal can be discussed.

By offering a menu of options for change the patient is more likely to find an approach that is acceptable to his or her own particular situation. For example, a patient may refuse a referral to formal treatment or to a self-help group, but may be willing to accept an incremental change such as setting specific limits on their alcohol intake and agree to seek further help if they are unable to stay within the limit. Or, the patient may be willing to agree to avoid drinking and driving and agree to become involved with a self-help group if they are unable to do so.

The interventionist should remind the patient that it is his or her responsibility to decide whether or not to change. By emphasizing personal responsibility instead of making demands, interventionists are less likely to encounter resistance or denial. A sense of personal control is a widely recognized element of motivation for behavioral change.

Self-efficacy theory holds that behavioral change requires a belief that change will be rewarding and that the patient believes that he or she is capable of changing. This is accomplished by interacting with the patient in a manner that is meant to increase their sense of personal efficacy and optimism by noting their strengths and attempting to highlight them. This might include pointing out that he or she was able to successfully quit their drinking in the past or has shown perseverance or skill in other areas of their life.

Giving advice is also an important part of the intervention. It is best to first elicit the patient's own viewpoint, but it is then appropriate for the clinician to provide an opinion. After discussing the negative aspects of the patient's drinking the clinician might provide advice by stating, "The best way to eliminate these problems is to cut down on the amount that you drink, or to drink less frequently, or to abstain entirely from alcohol." The degree of emphasis on the options presented, and the advice provided, should vary as a function of the patient's readiness to receive it and on the severity of the alcohol problem.

For patients considered to have a mild problem, the interventionist might focus on general strategies to cut down or eliminate alcohol intake. This might include a discussion of guidelines for low-risk drinking, setting specific limits on alcohol consumption, pacing one's drinking, and coping with problems that may lead to drinking.

Statements that patients make during the intervention in favor of change ("change talk") strongly predict healthy change, and statements they make against change (resistance) strongly predict more drinking. Therefore, the amount of change talk or resistance the counselor hears during the interview is a real-time indicator of how well the intervention is proceeding. The clinician's behavior during the intervention strongly influences how the patient talks about his or her drinking. Genuine concern facilitates change talk, whereas a style that the patient experiences as attacking or confrontational provokes resistance and slows the process of change.

## Application of Stages of Change Model

The stage of change informs the clinician about which of the three intervention components to emphasize during the intervention. The clinician should recognize that patients at different stages of change have different needs at the time of intervention. This avoids the ineffective dynamic where the clinician recommends quitting drinking to a precontemplator (not-ready) who is not aware of having a drinking problem and who does not perceive any discrepancy between their continued drinking and how they want their life to be.

Rather than advising such a patient to quit drinking, a patient characterized as "not-ready" may benefit from Screening Feedback that raises doubt or ambivalence about their drinking, such as information that their liver function tests were abnormal.

A patient characterized as "unsure" is aware of the adverse effects of their drinking, but is still unwilling to part with the perceived benefits. The emphasis of the intervention in an "unsure" patient is to raise awareness of their ambivalence. After asking for statements about the pros and cons of drinking, the interventionist should attempt to elicit statements that emphasize the seriousness of the cons.

This might be accomplished by asking the patient a question such as "You have told me that you have several concerns about your drinking, and I was wondering if you could tell me which of these concerns you the most?" The clinician should provide information about the seriousness of the adverse effects in order to make them more salient than the perceived benefits, thus altering the decisional balance between drinking and not drinking. The clinician should attempt to heighten the sense of ambivalence by asking the patient to discuss how their situation might improve if their drinking was under control. The objective is to elicit statements about why change might be beneficial, so that the patient is the one making the argument for change (Fig. 45-4).

Patients assessed as being in the preparation (ready) stage are already aware that the negative aspects of drinking outweigh the benefits. The goals are the following: to strengthen the commitment to change; to elicit and reflect patient statements about the benefits of changing; to assist the patient in exploring various strategies for change (e.g., self-change, brief treatment, intensive treatment, self-help group attendance); to encourage them to think out loud about possible solutions; to help them identify and avoid drinking triggers; and to support their commitment to change.

## Who Should Do the Brief Intervention

Most intervention studies with positive outcomes used nonspecialists in substance abuse to perform the procedure, including college students, psychologists, nurses, chaplains, volunteers, social workers, or substance abuse counselors. In other words, anyone who is willing to learn the techniques and is capable of showing respect and concern for injured patients who sometimes drink too much and take dangerous risks.

## Confidentiality

It is important for trauma surgeons to be familiar with the applicability of federal laws and regulations governing the confidentiality of records regarding substance use. Fewer people now regard problems with substance use as a moral failure, and there is greater recognition of medical, genetic, environmental, and social factors, and increasing emphasis on identification and treatment. Even so, patients with these disorders are at risk of problems with insurance, employment, family, and the law.

In the early 1970s the federal government passed laws intended to increase the willingness of patients to accept treatment by passing legislation to provide confidentiality of medical records related to disorders of alcohol and drug use. The rules were designed to ensure that a person who admits his or her problem to a healthcare provider is not made more vulnerable to adverse consequences than a person who avoids treatment or refuses to discuss his or her problem.[49]

The motivating reason for alcohol or drug screening determines the level of confidentiality of the resulting information. A trauma surgeon who obtains a BAC or toxicology screen because the information is needed to manage the patient's injuries is not required to protect that information beyond HIPAA rules. In contrast, trauma center staff whose primary purpose is to screen patients for a disorder of substance use and to provide interventions, counseling, or referrals for counseling must protect all information obtained for such purposes. Therefore, this information is segregated from the general medical record and is released only if the patient signs a special release form. Without consent this information can only be released by a court order, and a subpoena is insufficient.[50]

## Myths about Brief Interventions

1. *To do an effective intervention, one must know a great deal about the subject of how to provide alcohol counseling and psychological help to patients.* A brief intervention focuses less on the "how" of change, and more on the "why" of change, because lack of change is usually due more to lack of patient motivation than to lack of skills.

2. *I can't do a brief intervention unless I know of readily available treatment resources in the community to refer the patient to.* With the exception of patients with significant dependence, most trauma patients do not have access to formal treatment, nor do most of them need it. Many patients with less severe problems are able to change and reduce their injury risk on their own with minimal intervention.

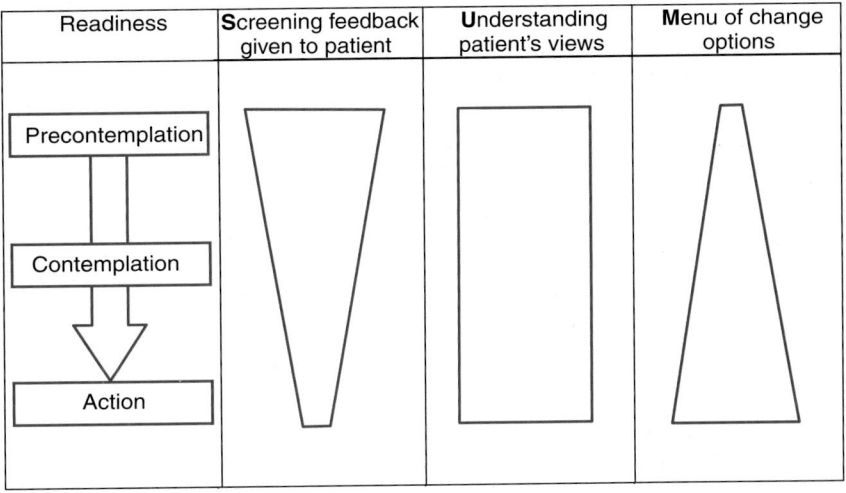

**FIGURE 45-4.** Degree of emphasis placed on **SUM** intervention components according to patient's readiness to change (not ready, unsure, ready).
**S** = Screening feedback (give BAC results, give score on screening questionnaire)
**U** = Understanding patients views (listening and summarizing their views on drinking and change)
**M** = Menu of options (giving patients choices for action such as cut down or quit)

## CONCLUSION

The use of alcohol and other drugs and the high-risk behavior that goes along with their use is the most common comorbid condition found in trauma patients and the most common cause of preventable injury. The procedures for brief intervention discussed in this chapter have been tested and applied in a variety of healthcare settings, and a large number of research studies have established them as evidence-based. When receiving medical care, all patients have the right to expect that the underlying causes of their disease will be sought and addressed. Trauma surgeons are responsible for making sure that this occurs when caring for a patient with an alcohol related injury.

## REFERENCES

1. Resources for Optimal Care of the Injured Patient. Chicago, IL: American College of Surgeons, 2006.
2. Blose JO, Holder HD: Injury-related medical care utilization in a problem drinking population. *Am J Pub Health* 81:1571, 1991.
3. National Institute on Alcohol abuse and Alcoholism. Fourth Special Report to the US Congress on Alcohol and Health. Washington DC: US Government Printing Office, 1981, p. 83.
4. Rivara FP, Koepsell TD, Jurkovich GJ, et al.: The effects of alcohol abuse on readmission for trauma. *JAMA* 270:1962–1963.
5. Gentilello LM, Donato A, Nolan S, et al.: Effect of the uniform accident and sickness policy provision law on alcohol screening and intervention in trauma centers. *J Trauma* 59:624, 2005.
6. Schermer CR, Gentilello LM, Hoyt DB, et al.: National survey of trauma surgeons' use of alcohol screening and brief intervention. *J Trauma* 55:849, 2003.
7. Walsh JM, Flegel R, Cangianelli LA, et al.: Epidemiology of alcohol and other drug use among motor vehicle crash victims admitted to a trauma center. *Traffic Inj Prev* 5:254, 2004.
8. Soderstrom CA, Dischinger PC, Smith GS, et al.: Psychoactive substance dependence among trauma center patients. *JAMA* 267:2756, 1992.
9. Madan AK, Yu K, Beech DJ: Alcohol and drug use in victims of life-threatening trauma. *J Trauma* 47:568, 1999.
10. Rivara FP, Jurkovich GJ, Gurney JG, et al.: The magnitude of acute and chronic alcohol abuse in trauma patients. *Arch Surg* 128: 907, 1993.
11. Dischinger PC, Mitchell KA, Kufera JA, et al.: A longitudinal study of former trauma center patients: The association between toxicology status and subsequent injury mortality. *J Trauma* 51:877, 2001.
12. Gurney JG, Rivara FP, Mueller BA, et al.: The effects of alcohol intoxication on the initial treatment and hospital course of patients with acute brain injury. *J Trauma* 33:709, 1992.
13. Jurkovich GJ, Rivara FP, Gurney JG, et al.: Effects of alcohol intoxication on the initial assessment of trauma patients. *Ann Emerg Med* 21:704, 1992.
14. Waller PF, Stewart JR, Hansen AR: The potentiating effects of alcohol on driver injury. *JAMA* 19;256:1461, 1986.
15. Liedtke AJ, DeMuth WE: Effects of alcohol on cardiovascular performance after experimental nonpenetrating chest trauma. *Am J Cardiol* 35:243, 1975.
16. Moss LK, Chenault OW, Gaston EA: The effects of alcohol ingestion on experimental hemorrhagic shock. *Surg Forum* 10:390, 1959.
17. Zink BJ, Stern SA, Wang X, et al.: Effects of ethanol in an experimental model of combined traumatic brain injury and hemorrhagic shock. *Acad Emerg Med* 5:9, 1998.
18. Rappaport WD, McIntyre KE, Stanton C, et al.: The effect of alcohol in isolated blunt splenic trauma. *J Trauma* 30:1518, 1990.
19. Gentilello LM, Cobean R, Wertz M, et al.: Acute ethanol intoxication increases the risk of infection after penetrating abdominal trauma. *J Trauma* 34:669, 1993.
20. Jones RK, Shinar D, Walsh JM: State of knowledge of drug-impaired driving. Dept of Transportation (US), National Highway Traffic Safety Administration (NHTSA); 2003.
21. 2002 National Survey on Drug Use and Health. Substance Abuse and Mental Health Services Administration, 2003, Washington, DC. Available at: http://www.oas.samhsa.gov/nhsda.htm
22. Admissions to Treatment for Methamphetamine Abuse Rise Sharply. Substance Abuse and Mental Health Services, Press Release # 240-276-2130, Washington, DC, 2006.
23. Sullivan JT, Sykora K, Schneiderman J, et al.: Assessment of alcohol withdrawal: The revised clinical institute withdrawal assessment for alcohol scale (CIWA-Ar). *Br J Addiction* 84:1353, 1989.
24. Saitz R, Mayo-Smith MF, Roberts MS, et al.: Individualized treatment for alcohol withdrawal: A randomized double-blind controlled trial. *JAMA* 272:519, 1994.
25. Mayo-Smith MF. Pharmacologic management of alcohol withdrawal: A meta-analysis and evidence-based practice guideline. American society of addiction medicine working group on pharmacological management of alcohol withdrawal. *JAMA* 278:144, 1997.
26. Strain EC, Stitzer ML, Liebson IA, et al.: Dose-response effects of methadone in the treatment of opioid dependence. *Ann Intern Med* 119:23, 1993.
27. Newman RG, Whitehill WB: Double-blind comparison of methadone and placebo maintenance treatments of narcotic addicts in Hong Kong. *Lancet* 2:485, 1979.
28. Dole VP, Robinson JW, Orraca J, et al.: Methadone treatment of randomly selected criminal addicts. *N Engl J Med* 280:1372, 1969.
29. Gunne L-M, Gronbladh L. The Swedish methadone maintenance program: A controlled study. *Drug Alcohol Depend* 7:249, 1981.
30. Understanding Alcohol. National Institutes of Health. Accessed 3/7/06 at: http://science.education.nih.gov/supplements/nih3/alcohol/default.htm.
31. Schermer CR: Feasibility of alcohol screening and brief intervention. *J Trauma* 59:S119, 2005.
32. Bien TH, Miller WR, Tonigan JS: Brief interventions for alcohol problems: A review. *Addiction* 88:315, 1993.
33. Monti PM, Colby SM, Barnett NP, et al.: Brief intervention for harm reduction with alcohol-positive older adolescents in a hospital emergency department. *J Consult Clin Psychol* 67:989, 1999.
34. Spirito A, Monti PM, Barnett NP, et al.: A randomized clinical trial of a brief motivational intervention for alcohol-positive adolescents treated in an emergency department. *J Pediatr* 145:396, 2004.
35. Gentilello LM, Rivara FP, Donovan, DM, et al.: Alcohol interventions in a trauma center as a means of reducing the risk of injury recurrence. *Ann Surg* 230:473, 1999.
36. Gentilello LM, Ebel BE, Wickizer TM, et al.: Alcohol interventions for trauma patients treated in emergency departments and hospitals: A cost benefit analysis. *Ann Surg* 241:541, 2005.
37. Schermer CR, Moyers TB, Miller WR.: Trauma center brief interventions for alcohol disorders decrease subsequent driving under the influence arrests. *J Trauma* 60:29, 2006.
38. Bernstein J, Bernstein E, Tassiopoulos K, et al.: Brief motivational intervention at a clinic visit reduces cocaine and heroin use. *Drug Alcohol Depend* 7:77;49, 2005.
39. Gentilello LM, Villaveces A, Ries RR, et al.: Detection of acute alcohol intoxication and chronic alcohol dependence by trauma center staff. *J Trauma* 47:1131, 1999.
40. Kon AA, Pretzlaff RK, Marcin JP: The association of race and ethnicity with rates of drug and alcohol testing among US trauma patients. *Health Policy* 69:159, 2004.
41. Mayfield D, McLeod G, Hall P: The CAGE questionnaire: Validation of a new alcoholism screening instrument. *Am J Psychiatry* 131:1121, 1974.
42. Saunders JB, Aasland OF, Babor TF, et al.: Development of the Alcohol Use Disorders Identification Test (AUDIT): WHO collaborative project on early detection of persons with harmful alcohol consumption-II. *Addiction* 88:791, 1993.
43. Donovan DM, Dunn CW, Rivara FP, et al.: Comparison of trauma center patient self-reports and proxy reports on the Alcohol Use Identification Test (AUDIT). *J Trauma* 56:873, 2004.
44. Neumann T, Neuner B, Gentilello LM, et al.: Gender differences in the performance of a computerized version of the alcohol use disorders identification test in subcritically injured patients who are admitted to the emergency department. *Alcohol Clin Exp Res* 28:1693, 2004.
45. Canagasaby A, Vinson DC: Screening for hazardous or harmful drinking using one or two quantity-frequency questions. *Alcohol* 40:208, 2005.
46. Miller WR: Motivation for treatment A review with special emphasis on alcoholism. *Psychol Bull* 98:84, 1985.
47. Prochaska JO, DiClemente: Transtheoretical therapy: Toward a more integrative model of change. *Psychother Theor Pract* 19:276, 1982.
48. Miller WR: *Enhancing motivation for change in substance abuse treatment.* Rockville, MD: U.S. Department of Health and Human Services, SAMHSA/CSAT, 1999.
49. Code of Federal Regulations. 42 C.F.R. Part 2. Confidentiality of Alcohol and Drug Abuse Patient Records. National Archives and Record Administration. Available at: http://www.access.gpo.gov/nara/cfr/waisidx_02/42cfr2_02.html.
50. Gentilello LM, Samuels P, Henningfield J, et al.: Alcohol interventions in trauma centers: confidentiality and legal concerns. *J Trauma* 59:1250, 2005.

# Commentary ■ CAROL R. SCHERMER

Gentilello and Dunn provide a comprehensive chapter on the problem of alcohol and injury. They discuss the impact of acute and chronic alcohol use on injury resuscitation and outcomes; they discuss therapy for alcohol withdrawal and discuss how to prevent subsequent injury by performing brief interventions.

Alcohol affects all phases of injury, but the most important phase is that of the epidemiology of injury, specifically the one that can be decreased through injury prevention and control measures. If alcohol related injury is decreased, not only will the overall number of injuries be decreased, it follows that the adverse sequelae such as immunosuppression, infection, poor bone healing, and increased costs will also be decreased.

Recognition that a trauma patient is intoxicated may help explain a myriad of problems in diagnosis and management that are not explained by injury alone. As the authors state, alcohol affects the surgeon's ability to evaluate a patient and hence leads to increased use of tests including abdominal and head CT scanning to elucidate injuries. In addition, the physiologic responses to injury can be exaggerated in the intoxicated patient resulting in large volume fluid resuscitation and increased resource utilization.

The alcohol withdrawal syndrome (AWS) is perceived as a large problem in trauma centers but its incidence has not been well studied. The prevalence of alcohol dependence will vary greatly by trauma center. Overall, from an epidemiologic standpoint most injuries occur as a result of binge drinking. Hence, the majority of patients who drink alcohol and end up in trauma centers are not dependent drinkers, and therefore are unlikely to suffer from AWS.

The AWS is due to the rapid removal of the depressant effects of alcohol in the central nervous system. AWS occurs when a patient who is physiologically dependent on alcohol ceases or severely reduces alcohol consumption. The majority of these patients experience 24–48 hours of mild to moderate symptoms due to central nervous system and sympathetic hyperactivity including insomnia, tremulousness, mild anxiety, gastrointestinal upset, headache, diaphoresis, palpitations, or anorexia. Other more serious aspects of AWS include withdrawal seizures of the generalized tonic-clonic variety, alcoholic hallucinosis, and delirium tremens. Benzodiazepines are suitable and recommended agents for alcohol withdrawal. The choice among different agents should be guided by duration of action, rapidity of onset, and cost. Dosage should be individualized, based on withdrawal severity measured by withdrawal scales, but adjusted for comorbid illness, and history of withdrawal seizures. Beta-blockers, clonidine, carbamazepine, and neuroleptics may be used as adjunctive therapy but are not recommended as monotherapy.[1]

As the authors note, AWS can be a life-threatening withdrawal syndrome due to its effect on the autonomic nervous system. Clinicians should know how to evaluate and treat a person for AWS. In general, as the authors state, withdrawal syndromes manifest themselves as the opposite effects of the ingested drug, so sedatives such as alcohol and heroin have agitated withdrawal states, and stimulants such as methamphetamine and cocaine have sedating withdrawal

states. Early signs and symptoms include tremulousness and mild anxiety. Waiting for the patient to develop signs and symptoms such as tachycardia and agitation, which occur later in the withdrawal stages should not occur in a healthcare environment where patients are being adequately observed.

Many trauma centers automatically "prophylax" patients with a high BAC for the alcohol withdrawal syndrome. Gentilello and Dunn recommend a prophylaxis regimen for withdrawal because they argue that it may be difficult and time consuming to make the diagnosis of AWS and provide symptom triggered therapy. Because studies in intensive care units and outpatient settings[2] have shown that prophylaxis leads to a greater use of drug and to more diagnostic tests than does symptom triggered therapy, I do not endorse prophylaxis for AWS. In an ICU patient population, Spies and colleagues have shown that symptom-oriented bolus-titrated therapy decreased the severity and duration of AWS and of medication requirements, with clinically relevant benefits such as fewer days of ventilation, lower incidence of pneumonia, and shorter ICU stay.[3] In another ICU study, DeCarolis and colleagues showed that the use of a symptom-driven protocol was associated with significantly decreased time to symptom control, amount of sedative required, and time spent receiving benzodiazepine infusion compared with historical controls.[4]

In patients presenting with a positive BAC, agitation is often assumed to be due to AWS and treatment is initiated. Trauma patients may have a number of serious reasons other than AWS to be agitated such as hypoxia, electrolyte disturbances, shock, and progression of a traumatic brain injury. However, it is frequently assumed that agitation is due to AWS and then the incorrect treatment may be provided and delay the evaluation of other serious sources of agitation. As the authors mention, the best predictor of withdrawal is a prior history of withdrawal symptoms. We need to move away from a culture of responding automatically to a laboratory result to one in which we talk to patients about their alcohol use. Obtaining a good drinking history can both prevent overuse of therapy for "prophylaxis" for AWS and can further set the stage for screening and brief intervention.

Alcohol screening and brief interventions (BI) are one important mechanism for decreasing the impact of alcohol on injury. Trauma is a disease primarily of young people and as such is the largest contributor to years of productive life lost. Trauma centers can also be involved in local and state legislation. Underage drinking, and in particular binge drinking are issues that respond to legislation and enforcement. Trauma centers can work jointly with local high schools, colleges and state legislatures to combat this devastating problem. Some effective legislative interventions include increased alcohol excise taxes which have their greatest impact on underage drinkers, DUI checkpoints, alcohol per se laws, and open container laws.

I agree with the authors that all trauma patients should be screened for alcohol use disorders in a nonbiased manner, and all exceeding the screening cut-off scores should be referred for BI. BI essentially serves as "treatment" for people who are hazardous and harmful drinkers, and facilitates treatment entry for those who are dependent drinkers. A large meta-analysis of BI in many different types of settings showed that BI performed in "opportunistic" settings has a larger effect size than BI performed in people seeking treatment for alcohol use disorders. This means that when trauma centers seize the opportunity to intervene while people are hospitalized for injury, they can expect better results than if they wait for these individuals to present to treatment on their own. This success probably represents a window of opportunity that makes the most of the motivating effects of the injury.

The authors present a particular model for performing BI. Rather than endorsing a particular model such as the SUM here, I think it is more important for trauma surgeons to understand the general concepts of BI. One important concept for providers to understand is that most people change behaviors on their own without formal treatment. BI is designed to facilitate this natural change process. There are many ways to perform BI but most successful BIs are based on the principles of Motivational Interviewing (MI) described by Miller and Rollnick. Motivational interviewing is a "client centered, directive method for enhancing intrinsic motivation to change by exploring and resolving ambivalence."[5] It is centered on notion that most people are ambivalent about change. The spirit of MI is to minimize resistance to change through skillful listening.

Although BI performed in trauma centers is not motivational interviewing, its overall spirit and goals are the same. The important pieces are that its purpose to enhance a person's intrinsic motivation to change. The exploration and resolution of ambivalence are done through careful reflective listening. This is done by reflecting what the person says in order to evoke their ideas and reasons for change, to direct the conversation and to convey provider understanding of what the patient is saying. Motivational interviewing is a collaborative rather than authoritarian approach to counseling that supports a person's autonomy to decide if they should change and how to change. Motivational interviewing is a difficult style to master but its principles and spirit are not. The principles and spirit of motivational interviewing are conveyed in BI through respect for the patient and recognition that the decision and method for change is up to them. BI does require a specific set of skills based on these principles but most clinicians can learn them provided they believe that people can and will change behaviors.

## References

1. Mayo-Smith MF: Pharmacological management of alcohol withdrawal. A meta-analysis and evidence-based practice guideline. american society of addition medicine working group on pharmacologic management of alcohol withdrawal. *JAMA* 278:144, 1997.
2. Daeppen JB, Gache P, Landry U, et al.: Symptom-triggered vs. fixed-schedule doses of benzodiazepine for alcohol withdrawal. *Ach Intern Med* 162:1117, 1992.
3. Spies CD, Otter HE, Husker B, et al.: Alcohol withdrawal severity is decreased by symptom oriented adjusted bolus therapy in the ICU. *Intensive Care Med* 12:2230, 2003
4. Decarolis DD, Rice KL, Ho L, et al. Symptom-driven lorazepam protocol for treatment of severe alcohol withdrawal delirium in the intensive care unit. *Pharmacotherapy* 27:510, 2007.
5. Miller WR, Rollnick S. *Motivational Interviewing: Preparing People for Change.* 2nd ed., New Yark: Guilford Press, 2002, p. 25.

# Pediatric Trauma

*David W. Tuggle* ■ *Jennifer Garza*

Pediatric trauma is the number one cause of death of children, as well as the number one cause of permanent disability in this population. It has often been said that children are not merely small adults, and this is never more accurate than in pediatric trauma.[1] Although the principles of trauma care are the same for children as with adults, the differences in care required to optimally treat the injured child do require special knowledge, careful management, and attention to the unique physiology and psychology of the growing child or adolescent. With this in mind, it is important to view pediatric trauma as a similar but separate entity from adult trauma. Those who take care of children are deeply indebted to pioneers in pediatric trauma care such as J. Alex Haller, Ide Smith, and Judson Randolph. It was Haller of the Johns Hopkins University who stressed the importance of regional trauma systems for pediatric patients. His system for safe care included two-way communication, dependable transportation, emergency medical technicians trained in the care of newborns, infants, and children, a designated pediatric ICU, and rehabilitation.[2] His work has helped shape and improve our pediatric trauma care significantly.

## EPIDEMIOLOGY OF THE INJURED CHILD

Although medical science has made vast strides in the surgical care of the neonate and child, injury remains the leading cause of childhood death in patients under 14 years of age.[3] As less well developed countries become more sophisticated, injury becomes the leading cause of death in children.[4] Of interest, there was a 45.3% reduction in the mortality rates from unintentional injury in children in the United States from 1979 to 1996.[5] This reduction is crucial if one accepts the 347 billion dollar annual cost of unintentional childhood injury—17 billion dollars in medical costs, 72 billion dollars in future work lost, and 257 billion dollars in lost quality of life. This is based upon the estimate that 1 in 4 children sustain an unintentional injury requiring medical care each year.[6] Using the Centers for Disease Control Web-based Injury Statistics Query and Reporting System (WISQARS), anyone can run a death and injury report for any age group and any type of injury. Both crude and adjusted mortality rates are provided.

Children have different patterns and causes of injury depending on age, further strengthening the idea of regional pediatric trauma centers. The defined age range constituting a pediatric age group, however, varies between institutions. The Centers for Disease Control and Prevention (CDC) define a pediatric (children and adolescent) patient as under the age of 19 years in many instances.

The mechanism of injury and mortality in children has remained remarkably consistent. In children over one year and under 14 years of age, motor vehicle crashes cause 46.5% of all pediatric trauma deaths (2002). Drowning is the second cause followed by burns. A detailed view of mortality statistics reveals the home as an area of continuing concern.[3] Other areas of concern include falls, bicycle-related injuries, and injuries associated with all terrain vehicle crashes.[7]

Childhood injuries most commonly occur as energy is transferred abruptly by rapid acceleration, deceleration, or a combination of both. The body of a child is very elastic, and energy can be transferred creating internal injuries without significant external signs. Due to the closer proximity of vital organs, children can have multiple injuries from a single exchange of energy, more so than in older patients. Penetrating trauma is a much less common form of injury in small children, accounting for 1–10% of admissions to pediatric trauma centers. No matter the type of injury, the healthcare professional evaluating the injured child should keep in mind these significant differences during evaluation and management.

## INITIAL ASSESSMENT AND RESUSCITATION OF THE INJURED CHILD

Primary survey with simultaneous resuscitation and secondary survey with definitive care, as promoted by the Advanced Trauma Life

Support (ATLS) course of the American College of Surgeons Committee on Trauma (ACSCOT), applies to a child as well as an adult. Multiple organ system injury is much more common in the child than the adult and, as a result, it is best to manage children as if every organ is injured until proven otherwise.

The care of the injured child often starts with a brief evaluation in the prehospital setting. The ASCOT has published a minimum set of criteria for the definition of a "major resuscitation" once the patient arrives at the hospital.[8] A patient who needs major resuscitation is typically a child who would benefit from the trauma surgeon being present at the bedside at this point. This condition is ideally determined in the field as noted above or from a referring hospital. Although these criteria are the same for injured patients of all ages, hypotension is age specific (see Chap. 4).

## Airway Management

Assessment of the child's airway is the first step. Most children do not have preexisting pulmonary disease so a room air saturation of greater than 90% indicates effective gas exchange. Children also tolerate lower oxygen saturations than adults, up to a point. If oxygenation is difficult, then an injury to the lung, a pneumothorax, or aspiration should be considered. In children, hypoventilation is common in the presence of a traumatic brain injury or shock. If any of these conditions exist, intubation is appropriate. Respiratory compromise requiring intubation commonly indicates a very severe injury. Although none of the previously mentioned criteria to determine a major resuscitation has been validated in children, compromise of the airway and intubation suggest a population that has a higher mortality when compared to those injured children who do not have airway issues.[9] A child who is comatose or unresponsive is fairly easy to intubate with an appropriately sized orotracheal tube. Typically, this tube is not cuffed in children less than 8 years of age since the narrowest part of the airway, the cricoid ring, will stabilize the tube without the need for a cuff.

Children who are combative from hypoxia or from emotional distress may also need to be intubated to facilitate the work-up, including computed tomography (CT) scanning. For intubation, the injured child is best managed with a protocol for rapid sequence intubation (RSI). Table 46-1 describes a rapid sequence intubation protocol that is both safe and effective. If there is time, preoxygenating the child is useful. The tube size can be roughly approximated by either the width of the nail or the size of the child's fifth finger. These rough calculations may not be accurate in children of Chinese descent.[10] The use of the Broselow Pediatric Resuscitation Measuring Tape has become the standard for determining height, weight, and the appropriate size for resuscitative equipment in a child. The use of the Broselow cart has been found to be more useful than older "standard" carts for children.[11] In addition, this tape has been useful in determining drug doses and drip concentrations throughout the hospitalization.[12]

Intubating the injured child can be a very stressful event for those who are less familiar with the technique. The head should be held in line with cervical traction. After selecting the appropriate sized noncuffed tube and employing pharmacological adjuncts as needed for RSI, the airway is approached with a properly sized laryngoscope. The smaller the child the more likely successful intubation can be achieved with a straight blade. Gentle cricoid pressure is useful to guide the larynx into view and to help close the esophagus during

### TABLE 46-1

**Pediatric Rapid Sequence Intubation (RSI)**

Pre-oxygenate
↓
Atropine Sulfate IV
0.1–0.5 mg
↓
Sedation
↓

| Hypotensive | Normotensive |
|---|---|
| Etomidate 0.3 mg/kg Or Midazolam 0.1 mg/kg (max 5mg) | Etomidate 0.3 mg/kg Or Midazolam 0.1 mg/kg (max 5mg) |

↓
Cricoid Pressure
↓
Paralysis
Succinylcholine[a]
<10 kg give 2mg/kg
>10 kg give 1 mg/kg
↓
Intubate
Check tube position
Release Cricoid pressure

[a]Vecuronium 0.2 mg/kg is another option.

manipulation of the oropharynx. The endotracheal tube should be advanced about 3 cm beyond the vocal cords. Bilateral breath sounds along with symmetric chest excursion are assessed, followed by confirmation with a device that measures exhaled carbon dioxide. Due to the thin tissues of the chest wall, gastric insufflation may be confused with normal breath sounds. A chest x-ray should be obtained to confirm the correct position of the tube since a right mainstem intubation is the most common complication of pediatric intubation after missed intubation. Nasotracheal intubation is generally not used in small children in the emergency setting.

The need for invasive emergency airway access for acute pediatric airway obstruction is a very uncommon event. If needed, a 14 or 16 gauge angiocatheter may be placed through the cricothyroid membrane or even the tracheal wall. Care should be taken to not penetrate the posterior tracheal membrane. Oxygen can then be administered through the catheter, allowing time for attempts at orotracheal intubation. The needle cricothyroidotomy is preferred in patients under 10 years of age as the cricoid cartilage is very delicate and could be injured easily with a surgical incision. The needle cricothyroidotomy may then be followed by tracheostomy in a more organized fashion.

Post-intubation issues include gastric decompression and surveillance for a pneumothorax. Gastric decompression with a nasogastric or orogastric tube should be employed in every patient since gastric distention will impair diaphragmatic excursion and cause respiratory compromise in the small child. A pneumothorax is especially treacherous in the child due to mediastinal mobility. A tension pneumothorax in a patient with a mobile mediastinum causes compression of the contralateral and ipsilateral lungs, as well as vascular compromise. If a pneumothorax is present, needle decompression can be employed, but this should be followed by immediate tube thoracostomy.

## Vascular Access

As in injured adult patients it is important, to obtain reliable, quick, and safe intravenous access. Simpler measures should be attempted first and, if not successful, proceeding to more invasive measures may be necessary (Table 46-2). The ideal initial sites for vascular access for children are the peripheral veins in the upper extremities, especially the antecubital fossa. A percutaneous femoral venous catheter is the next best choice and the most commonly used route for emergency venous access in the child.[13] This should be done without attempting a cutdown, preferably using the Seldinger technique. If the trauma team is unable to establish intravenous access using these techniques, a cutdown on the saphenofemoral junction will also work in the emergency setting.[14] Surgeons who are familiar with subclavian catheterization in the child may utilize this route as the next choice as there are very few complications. This is especially true if a chest tube is already in place on the selected side of the subclavian venipuncture.

If the conditions for intraosseous access are satisfied, this is a very useful technique for problematic trauma victims without intravenous access. Contraindications include proximal fractures and sites of infection. The anteromedial surface of the proximal tibia is used, 2 to 4 cm distal to the tibial tuberosity. For insertion in the proximal tibia, the needle is directed inferiorly at a 45° angle from the perpendicular. If the insertion site is the distal tibia, the needle should be angled 45° superiorly. In both instances the goal is to angle away from the region of the growth plate and/or joint.

There are specialized needles readily available to use with this technique, but, if these are not available, a spinal needle with a trochar may be employed. Multiple entries into the medullary cavity should be avoided as the leakage that occurs with multiple attempts may cause an iatrogenic compartment syndrome. For surgeons who are not familiar with peripheral, central, or intraosseous access in children, a cutdown of the saphenous vein at the ankle may be employed.

## Restoration of Circulation

Age specific hypotension is an indication for major resuscitation of an injured child. In an analysis of the National Pediatric Trauma Registry, 38% of recorded deaths occurred in children whose systolic blood pressure was less than 90 mm Hg.[15] This group represented 2.4% of the study population. To determine which child has "age specific hypotension" requires knowledge of normal blood pressures in children. New national guidelines for the ranges of normal childhood blood pressures based on age were published in 2004.[16] The healthcare professional caring for injured children should be familiar with these new numbers for normal blood pressure depending on age (Table 46-3).

A child with an injury that produces significant blood loss may present with a normal blood pressure. The otherwise healthy child can readily compensate for blood loss by mounting a significant tachycardia coupled with peripheral vasoconstriction. Therefore, a normal blood pressure in a child does not mean that circulating blood volume is at normal levels. A more accurate determination includes a blood pressure evaluation along with monitoring heart rate and assessing peripheral perfusion. Clinical signs of poor perfusion in conjunction with altered mentation are the classic findings in pediatric hypovolemic shock. If these are present, then an immediate bolus of 20 mL/kg of an isotonic crystalloid solution is in order. If a second bolus of this amount is needed, and there is little improvement, type-specific packed red blood cells or O-negative blood should be administered immediately followed by the standard infusions of fresh frozen plasma and platelets. As noted above, this scenario occurs in less than 3% of injured children. Caution must be employed as overresuscitation may be as problematic as underresuscitation, especially in the presence of a traumatic brain injury. Overtreatment with crystalloid solutions may exacerbate

### TABLE 46-2

**Sequencing of Venous Access in Children**

**Peripheral Veins x 2**
Preferably antecubital fossa
↓ If unable

**Intraosseous access**
↓ If unable

**Percutaneous Central Venous Access Femoral vein**
↓ If unable

**Venous cutdown**
(Distal saphenous preferred)
↓ If unable

**Percutaneous External Jugular/Subclavian/Internal Jugular**

### TABLE 46-3

**Vital Functions for Children**

| AGE GROUP (in years) | WEIGHT RANGE (in kg) | HEART RATE (beats/min) | BLOOD PRESSURE (mmHg) | RESPIRATORY RATE (breaths/min) |
|---|---|---|---|---|
| Infant 0–1 | 0–10 | <160 | >60 | <60 |
| Toddler 1–3 | 10–14 | <150 | >70 | <40 |
| Preschool 3–5 | 14–18 | <140 | >75 | <35 |
| School age 6–12 | 18–36 | <120 | >80 | <30 |
| Adolescent >12 | 36–70 | <100 | >90 | <30 |

Source: ATLS, 8th Edition, In Press.

cerebral edema in certain circumstances. In adults, excess infusion of crystalloid infusions may result in poor formation of clot, worsening of the compromised hemorrhagic state, and may have no impact on survival.[17] One study in injured adults showed that supranormal trauma resuscitation increased the likelihood of the abdominal compartment syndrome, and there are anecdotal reports of the same problem in children.[18]

Hypothermia is an extremely common occurrence in injured children and may occur at any time of the year, even in the heat of summer. The response to hypothermia includes catecholamine release and shivering, with an increase in oxygen consumption and metabolic acidosis. Hypothermia as well as acidosis then contributes to a post-traumatic coagulopathy.[19] A warm room, warmed fluids, heated air-warming blankets, or externally warmed blankets should be utilized during the initial resuscitation of an injured child. This aggressive approach to rewarming should be extended to the radiology suite during evaluation. If at all possible the room should be warmed to 37°C or warmer, even if the trauma team feels some discomfort. Fluids and blood should be warmed to 39°C if the child is cool (<36°C). Conversely, care should be taken to avoid hyperthermia in the child with a traumatic brain injury[20]; therefore, maintenance of a normal core temperature is the goal for management. There is some evidence, however, to suggest that early, carefully controlled hypothermia in the child with a severe injury to the brain and no other injuries may be beneficial, but this treatment option is still experimental.[21]

## DIAGNOSTIC ASSESSMENT

The physical examination is a crucial first step in diagnosis as it will direct all other forms of assessment. It also becomes the baseline for serial physical examinations by the trauma team performed later in the hospitalization. After the physical examination, other diagnostic adjuncts may be employed.

Although the patient is undergoing examination and resuscitation in the emergency department (ED), diagnostic testing with standard radiographs is performed with a portable x-ray machine or one dedicated to the trauma room, thus avoiding movement of the patient. The initial most frequently ordered imaging studies in the ED include plain radiographs of the chest, abdomen, pelvis, cervical spine, and extremities. Thoracic and lumbar spinal x-rays are commonly ordered when neurological injuries are suspected or when the physical examination reveals point tenderness over the spine. The role of cervical, thoracic, or abdominal CTs with reconstruction to evaluate the vertebral column in children is still being evaluated at this time. Detecting a pneumothorax, pneumoperitoneum, pelvic fracture, or fracture of a long bone is an important component of the initial care of an injured child. Some previously common studies have been shown to be of limited use. Plain x-rays of the skull may document fractures, but they have little value in directing management of the child with an injury to the brain, except for a penetrating injury or suspected child abuse.[22,23] The inability of plain radiographs in predicting intracranial bleeding in the injured child has also been documented.[24]

In the past decade, surgeon-directed ultrasonography has been popularized in the United States. Several recent studies by adult and pediatric trauma surgeons have attempted to determine the role of the focused assessment for the sonographic examination of the trauma patient (FAST) in the evaluation of the injured child (see Chap.17). The most common FAST evaluation examines the pericardium, right and left upper quadrants, and the pelvis for fluid. Some surgeons include a thoracic evaluation to detect a hemothorax or pneumothorax.

The technique of B-mode ultrasound in the hands of an experienced ultrasonographer should be as accurate in detecting blood in the abdomen as CT scanning or diagnostic peritoneal lavage (DPL).[25–27] In a collected series of over 4900 patients, surgeons who performed ultrasound to detect hemoperitoneum and visceral injury demonstrated a sensitivity of 93.4%, a specificity of 98.7%, and an accuracy of 97.5%.[25–28] This can be compared to a group of 1043 patients in whom the ultrasonographic study was performed by radiologists. This collected series showed a sensitivity of 90.8%, a specificity of 99.2%, and an accuracy of 97.8%.[29–33] Both of these series include adults as well as children.

Currently, surgeon-performed ultrasound evaluation in children should be coupled with the physical examination[34] and not be considered a conclusive diagnostic study except in patients with fluid in the pericardium or in hypotensive patients with fluid in the peritoneal cavity. Because its sensitivity, specificity, and accuracy are high, however, it is used in both hypotensive and normotensive patients as a screening tool to determine the need for more indepth imaging studies or invasive evaluation. The typical FAST examination takes three to five minutes when performed by a physician experienced in its use. A 3.5 MHz (megahertz) probe is used for children over 10 kg, while either a 3.5 or a 5 MHz probe can be used for children under 10 kg. The relative lack of subcutaneous tissue in most children makes this an easy study to perform as compared to adolescents and adults. Obvious benefits of the FAST evaluation include its portability, eliminating the need to transport the child to the radiology suite, and the decreased radiation exposure to the child.

Computerized tomography scans of the head, chest, and abdomen are the accepted diagnostic radiologic studies of choice in the vast majority of hemodynamically stable injured children suspected of having a potentially life-threatening injury. Despite the liberal use of CT scans of the head, it is possible for the child with a severe neurological injury to have a normal initial scan or for a child to develop late manifestations of a neurologic injury or cerebral edema despite an initial study that was normal.[36] The majority of children with suspected intra-abdominal injuries, providing they are stable, should have a CT scan performed prior to instituting operative or nonoperative management unless an absolute indication for surgery is present. Although CT scanning is the imaging modality of choice in the evaluation of a stable injured child, it is generally accepted that a high percentage of those scans will reveal no injuries. The CT scans of 1500 consecutive children were evaluated for blunt abdominal trauma, and abnormal CT scans were seen in only 26% of patients.[36] A normal study was found to strongly predict a lack of deterioration as only one delayed laparotomy was required in the 1112 children in this group. In addition, a CT scan affected the decision to operate on children with a solid organ injury in a very small subset of patients (5 of 1500 CT scans).

The optimal technique for performing an emergency CT scan on an injured child, with regard to the use of contrast material, remains unclear. Most institutions will perform an initial CT of the head without using intravenous contrast. The use of intravenous contrast during a CT scan to evaluate intrathoracic or intra-abdominal trauma improves its diagnostic accuracy, but is not required and can be omitted during the initial scan depending upon the experience and protocols of the particular trauma center. The benefit of using oral contrast for an abdominal CT in injured children is also a matter of debate. In a randomized prospective clinical trial in adults, the addition of oral contrast to an acute abdominal CT scan for trauma was found to be unnecessary and caused a delay in the time to CT scanning.[37] In a review of 2162 patients with blunt trauma and an abdominal CT, Tsang and colleagues found that all 7 patients with an intestinal perforation had studies that showed neither extraluminal air nor extraluminal oral contrast.[38] In some centers, due to the length of time needed to fill the bowel with contrast and the resultant full stomach that increases the risk of vomiting with aspiration, gastrointestinal (GI) contrast is avoided in the initial CT scan of the abdomen in the injured child. Other centers suggest that it improves the accuracy of abdominal CT scans when intestinal or retroperitoneal injury is suspected and that oral contrast in adults and children is safe and has a minimal incidence of aspiration.[39,40] In summary, the use of GI contrast in emergency CT scans of the abdomen for trauma is a matter of institutional preference at the present time.

Evidence of intra-abdominal injuries requiring operative correction on the CT scan may be subtle. Findings of free intraperitoneal or retroperitoneal air, extravasation of GI contrast, defects in the bowel wall, and active hemorrhage are often obvious and have a high correlation with an injury to the intestine that will require operative intervention.[41] There are, however, potentially life-threatening intestinal injuries that may be manifest only by focal thickening of the bowel wall or the presence of peritoneal fluid without injury to a solid organ.[42] Other less specific findings associated with intestinal injuries include mesenteric stranding, fluid at the mesenteric root, focal hematomas, mesenteric pseudoaneurysm, and the hypoperfusion complex.

Other diagnostic adjuncts to the management of the injured child may include interventional radiologic techniques, magnetic resonance imaging (MRI), and invasive and noninvasive vascular studies.

## Laboratory Studies

The routine use of laboratory studies in the ED, in general, has not been shown to be of significant value in the pediatric trauma population.[43–45] Some specific clinical laboratory testing such as urinalysis and arterial blood gases with base deficit may be of limited benefit in selected circumstances.[46] More often, laboratory testing delays the clinical decision-making process occurring in the ED during evaluation and resuscitation, and point of care testing has not altered this concept.[47] In the presence of a possible injury to the brain, testing for a coagulopathy, thrombocytopenia, or hyperglycemia may be of benefit to establish a baseline for later determinations or to assist in assessing morbidity or mortality risks.[48–50] During hospitalization, routine laboratory testing is appropriate as long as specific indications exist for monitoring, such as nonoperative management of an injury to the spleen or pancreas.

## MANAGEMENT OF SPECIFIC INJURIES

### Injury to the Head and Central Nervous System

Acute traumatic brain injury is the most common cause of death and disability in the pediatric population.[51] In those who survive, minor injuries can be associated with reversible defects while major injuries can result in severe disabilities. The mechanisms of injury to the brain in children are related to age. Infants typically suffer more from falls such as from a table or the arms of a caregiver. Intentional injury is a common cause of death in children under 2 years of age. Injury with intention, independent of severity, raises the mortality in children with traumatic brain injuries.[52] In older children the usual cause of injuries to the brain is from vehicle-related accidents or recreational activities. Although children have a better survival rate with injury to the brain than adults do, this does not mean they have a lesser morbidity with similar injuries. Children have a plasticity of the neuron related to myelination and the establishment of neuronal interconnections. This allows a given focal injury to produce a less severe deficit when compared to a mature brain. This same lack of maturity may also make the child more susceptible to a diffuse injury with greater cognitive impairment.[53]

The head of an infant constitutes 15% of the total body mass, while the head of an adult makes up only 3%. Acceleration and deceleration injury in pediatric trauma, therefore, yields a greater amount of force applied to the brain. The neck muscles do not support this relatively larger head as well as they do in teenagers and adults. Also, the skull of the infant is thin and soft, and the closure of fontanelles and sutures is not completed until age 3. In addition, the volume of cerebrospinal fluid is smaller than those of the adult and the child's brain has greater water content. Finally, myelination occurs between 6 and 24 months, making the brain very soft and prone to disruption prior to completion of this process.

Injuries to the brain are classified as primary or secondary. Primary injuries are those inflicted immediately by the trauma, while secondary injuries are those resulting from ischemia, hypoxia, hypotension, infection, hydrocephalus, seizures, or increased intracranial pressure (ICP) in addition to the primary injury. Children are more likely to have low pressure venous bleeding from an overlying skull fracture than they are arterial injuries resulting in an epidural hematoma. The very young infant can actually have a critical reduction in blood volume from intracranial bleeding due to the relatively large size of the brain compared to the body mass. Much as in adults diffuse axonal injury or a shear stress to the brain caused by acceleration/deceleration mechanisms and often with angular or rotational motion occurs in children. Even minor shearing can cause severe neurologic deficits.

Secondary injury is most often the result of an elevated ICP. An elevated ICP may be caused by increased cerebral blood volume, increased brain volume, or hematomas. An elevated ICP can cause direct injury due to compression resulting in herniation under the falx cerebri or through the tentorium cerebelli. Increased ICP can also cause a reduction in cerebral perfusion pressure (CPP). The CPP should be 60–80 mm Hg in older children and at least 50 mm Hg in children under the age of 8. As injury to the brain can impair autoregulation so that inappropriate vasodilation occurs, there can be a significant rise in tissue volume and ICP.

**TABLE 46-4**

| SCORE | EYES OPEN | VERBAL | MOTOR |
|-------|-----------|--------|-------|
| 6 | — | — | spontaneous |
| 5 | — | age appropriate | localizes |
| 4 | spontaneous | cries/consolable | withdraws |
| 3 | to voice | irritable | flexion posture |
| 2 | to pain | restless | extension posture |
| 1 | none | none | none |

**Glasgow Coma Scale**

With this deranged physiology, even minor injuries to the brain in children can lead to global hyperemia and death.[54]

The Brain Trauma Foundation has recently published guidelines for the management of trauma to the brain in children.[55] These recommendations are based upon the available literature, at times drawing from adult data. There are no standards of care and very few guidelines, and the majority of the recommendations are options that are commonly used in the clinical setting. The Glasgow Coma Scale (GCS) can be used for children over the age of 5, while some modification is often used for children under 5 (Table 46-4). If a score of less than 9 is determined, that patient typically requires airway management and measurement of the ICP.

During the initial evaluation and resuscitation of the child with an injury to the brain, care should be taken to avoid a secondary injury due to the causes noted above. Also, clinical and radiologic evaluation of the cervical spine is important to rule out injury. The presence of cervical tenderness mandates the application of a rigid collar and x-rays aimed at identifying the possible injury. Three view radiographs of the cervical spine are a necessary start followed by a CT scan or MRI as needed.

Once the patient has undergone an initial evaluation, causes of secondary brain injury have been managed and the cervical spine has been stabilized, a CT of the head and brain should be obtained, ideally 30–60 minutes after arrival depending on the hemodynamic stability of the patient. If there is evidence of swelling of the brain, monitoring of ICP is indicated. This is best done with a ventriculostomy that allows for drainage of cerebrospinal fluid. The ICP should be maintained under 20 mm Hg, while cerebral perfusion pressure (CPP = MAP-ICP) should ideally be in the range of 40–65 mm Hg as noted previously.

Avoiding hyperthermia is important as this may cause a secondary injury to the brain. Another management technique is hyperosmolar therapy with hypertonic saline or mannitol. Hypertonic saline is delivered in a continuous 3% solution at 0.1 to 1.0 mL/kg/hour on a sliding scale to keep ICP <20 mm Hg, while mannitol is used as a bolus at 0.25 gm/kg to 1 gm/kg of body weight. Euvolemia should be maintained with appropriate administration of intravenous fluids. The serum osmolarity should be maintained at 320 mOsm for mannitol, and below 360 mOsm with hypertonic saline. Other methods to decrease ICP and protect the injured brain include sedation, the rare use of hyperventilation, the administration of barbiturates and decompressive craniectomy. The latter approach should only be considered in children with cerebral edema and medically uncontrolled intracranial hypertension. It is not likely to be useful in children who have suffered an extensive secondary injury to the brain or in those who have an admission GCS of 3 and

no improvement with therapy. Nutritional support, avoiding the use of steroids, and treating post-injury seizures are also important aspects of the care of the child with an injury to the brain.

## Injury to the Cervical Spine

Injuries to the cervical spine represent less than 1% of all pediatric fractures.[56] Trauma to the upper cervical spine tends to occur in younger children (less than 8 years), while mid-cervical injuries occur in older children. Motor vehicle crashes are the primary cause of associated injuries to the spinal cord in younger children while sporting activities are more common in older children.[57]

Currently there are no procedural nor diagnostic standards for clearance of the cervical spine in children, but protocols have been suggested based on the distinct anatomic differences between children and adults. For example, children have more flexible interspinous ligaments and joint capsules, their vertebral bodies are wedged anteriorly and tend to slide forward with flexion, and their facet joints are flat. Their head to neck ratio is also different placing them at risk for different injuries than in adults.

The diagnosis of injuries may be challenging as radiologic differences exist, as well. There may be anterior displacement of C2 on C3 appearing as a subluxation. This is a normal pediatric variant described as a pseudosubluxation (Figs. 46-1A–C). In addition, skeletal growth centers may be easily confused for fractures. A careful physical exam is always warranted, as spinal cord injury without radiographic abnormalities (SCIWORA) has been shown to occur in as many as 66% of children.[59] When plain films do not demonstrate an injury, but the physical examination is positive, a CT scan or MRI may be helpful. In the interim the child's head and neck should remain immobilized at all times.

## Injury to the Thorax

Thoracic trauma is an important cause of morbidity and mortality in children. It accounts for 4–25% of pediatric injuries and is associated with a greater mortality rate when compared to injuries in other systems.[60,61] Isolated thoracic trauma in a child is associated with a mortality rate of approximately 5%[60] and is largely due to penetrating trauma. About 80% of thoracic injuries in children are from a blunt mechanism, and children with associated neurosurgical trauma, thoracic trauma, and abdominal trauma may have a mortality rate that approaches 40%. Thoracic trauma is likely to be present in children who present with a low systolic blood pressure, an elevated respiratory rate, abnormalities on physical examination of the thorax, and the presence of a fracture of the femur.[62]

The child's thorax has unique anatomic and physiological properties that are important to the diagnosis and treatment of thoracic trauma. The trachea is shorter relative to body size and is more anterior, narrower, and more easily compressed as compared to the adult. Also, the subglottic region is the narrowest part of the airway in children because of its small cross sectional diameter. Therefore, the pediatric airway is more susceptible to mucus plugging and edema. The chest wall is more compliant in children with less muscle mass, and this allows a greater transmission of energy to underlying organs when injury occurs. Finally, the mediastinum is more mobile than in older patients, especially in young children. Unilateral changes in thoracic pressure such as with a tension pneumothorax can

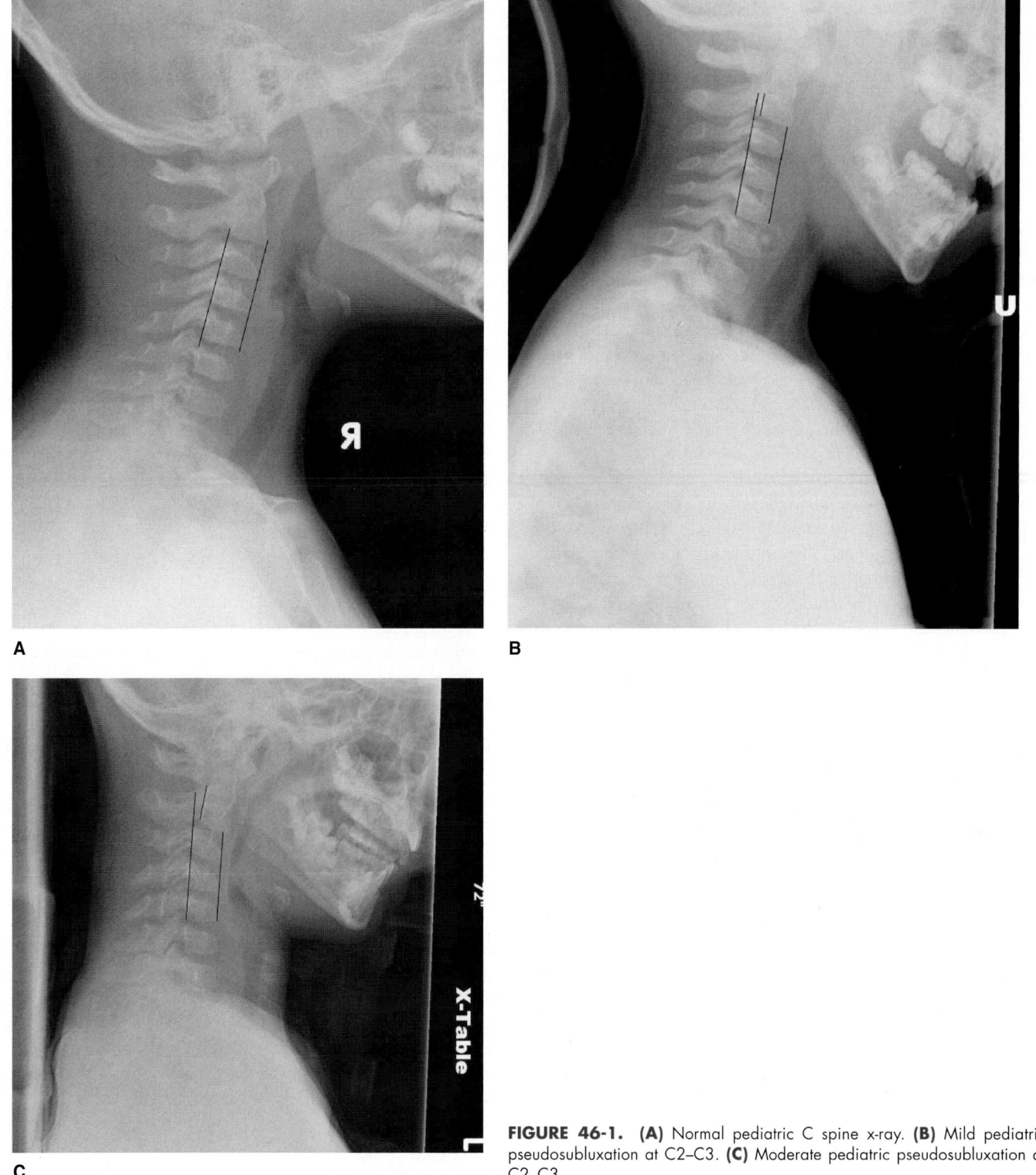

A

B

C

**FIGURE 46-1.** **(A)** Normal pediatric C spine x-ray. **(B)** Mild pediatric pseudosubluxation at C2–C3. **(C)** Moderate pediatric pseudosubluxation at C2–C3.

lead to a shift of the mediastinum to the extent that venous return is markedly reduced much as in hypovolemic shock. This response is more pronounced than typically seen in an adult.

Young children have a compliant thorax that becomes more adult-like at 8 to 10 years of age. As a consequence, rib fractures are relatively uncommon in young children and occur more frequently in adolescents. Even though rib fractures are uncommon, injuries to the lung, liver, and spleen lying underneath the ribs are quite common. One of the most common thoracic injuries in children is

a pulmonary contusion, which can occur with blunt or penetrating trauma. The presence of a pulmonary contusion contributes to decreased pulmonary compliance, hypoxia, hypoventilation, and a ventilation perfusion mismatch. A chest x-ray taken during the initial assessment may demonstrate a pulmonary contusion, while a thoracic CT scan may show areas of pulmonary contusion not appreciated on the x-ray. Treatment of a pulmonary contusion includes appropriate fluid resuscitation, supplemental oxygen, pain management, and strategies to prevent atelectasis and pneumonia.

Unfortunately, some patients may develop pneumonia or the respiratory distress syndrome (RDS) after sustaining a pulmonary contusion.[63] In an occasional patient, a large pulmonary contusion may cause life-threatening hypoxia that cannot be supported with conventional or advanced techniques of ventilation including high frequency oscillation. Extracorporeal life support has been used in extreme circumstances to support patients with severe pulmonary contusions and secondary RDS.

A pneumothorax is typically treated with a tube thoracostomy appropriately sized for the patient, while a hemothorax is treated with the largest tube that can be inserted. Intrathoracic blood loss of 15 mL/kg immediately or ongoing losses of 2 to 3 mL/kg/hour for three or more hours mandate thoracic exploration to control bleeding in children.[64,65] Cardiac injuries are extremely rare, as are tracheobronchial or esophageal injuries. They do occur however, and should be ruled out in any child with cervicothoracic injuries. Similarly, injuries to the great vessels occur in children with rapid deceleration injuries, and these types of injuries should be considered in any child with the appropriate mechanism.[66]

Injuries to the thoracic aorta are rare in the pediatric population, but they are lethal. Aortic injury is the second leading cause of death in the pediatric population next to injuries to the brain and account for 14% of trauma deaths.[67] The age range of victims of aortic injury has been shown to be anywhere from 6 to 17 years old, and most are victims of motor vehicle crashes. It has been demonstrated that there are identifiable risk factors that have been associated with blunt injury to the thoracic aorta. A correlation has been seen in older children in motor vehicle crashes that cause severe injuries to the brain, torso, and lower extremities.[68] Clinical predictors that have been noted include a low systolic blood pressure on admission, increased respiratory rate, abnormal thoracic exam and auscultation, an associated fracture of the femur, and a GCS of less than 15.[69] If there is an index of suspicion based on history, physical examination or an x-ray of the chest, then further testing is required. Helical chest CT and transesophageal ECHO (TEE) have been found to be equally as sensitive as aortography in the detection of an aortic injury. Once the injury is found, the treatment of thoracic aortic injuries is similar to that in adults. Beta-blockers should be started early, while treatment options include nonoperative management, operative management and the use of an endovascular stent graft if a correctly sized graft is available. The long-term outcome of endovascular stenting in children is unknown.[70]

## Injury to the Abdomen

Due to the relatively thin nature of the pediatric abdominal wall, a modest amount of force may cause a significant injury to one or more organs in the abdomen. Also, multiple organs may be injured from a single blow due to proximity. The assessment for abdominal injury begins with the physical examination. Inspection may reveal bruising, a mark from a lap seatbelt, or abdominal distention. Tenderness on physical examination should prompt a higher level of evaluation with CT scanning. A nasogastric or orogastric tube should be placed to decompress the stomach.

With the emphasis on nonoperative management of abdominal injuries in children, injuries requiring operative management have been missed for hours to days. It has been noted that a delay in diagnosis, however, is not usually associated with an increased mortality, through an increase in septic complications has been seen when

operative intervention is delayed more than 24 hours post injury. This phenomenon is peculiar to children and, as a result, in-hospital observation with serial examinations should be employed in all children with abdominal examinations that are not perfectly normal. The use of repeat ultrasound is particularly useful in this subset of patients. When abdominal injuries occur under suspicious circumstances, the diagnosis of child abuse should be entertained.

Blunt diaphragmatic rupture is an uncommon occurrence in a child. The left diaphragm is involved more often, but bilateral ruptures have occurred. The frequency of associated injuries, especially to the liver and spleen, is very high.[71] An abnormal contour of the diaphragm, a high riding diaphragm, or a questionable overlap of abdominal visceral shadows may indicate injury on a chest x-ray. Visceral herniation, the abnormal position of a nasogastric tube overlaying the hemithorax, or early intestinal obstruction after trauma make the diagnosis likely. Computerized tomography has been used to establish this diagnosis, but may appear normal in some patients. Therefore, thin cuts of the CT scan through the diaphragm are mandatory. Many diaphragmatic ruptures are not identified in the first few days after injury and may not be detected for a considerable period of time.[72] Repair of an acute diaphragmatic rupture is best accomplished with an abdominal approach. If a late diagnosis of a diaphragmatic injury is made, a thoracic approach to repair is often considered secondary to the scarring and adhesions that might have formed much as in adults.

Blunt injuries to the stomach are the third most common perforation of the gastrointestinal tract in the injured child and occur relatively more frequently in children than in adults.[73] The site of perforation is most often the greater curve of the stomach. The diagnosis is usually made quickly, due to the common occurrence of peritonitis and free air seen on initial x-rays in the ED or a bloody nasogastric aspirate. At operation, the stomach is closed in two layers when possible, with the use of a decompressive gastrostomy considered when a massive injury is present. Every effort should be made to salvage the spleen during repair of the gastric injury.

Duodenal injuries are uncommon in children. The child with a duodenal injury that requires surgery most often presents with abdominal distention, bilious vomiting, peritonitis, and a pneumoperitoneum on an abdominal x-ray. In a recent review from two busy pediatric trauma centers, 42 patients with a duodenal injury were identified in 10 years.[74] There were 33 blunt and 9 penetrating injuries. Operative management was necessary in 24 patients and included primary repair, duodenal resection, and gastrojejunostomy with pyloric exclusion. In contrast, a duodenal hematoma is usually treated nonoperatively with nasogastric decompression and total parenteral nutrition. This management has a high rate of success, but it may take as long as 3 weeks for the obstruction to resolve. A late diagnosis of duodenal perforation can occur with this injury and is usually associated with an increase in complications, but not mortality.

The jejunum and ileum are the most common parts of the gastrointestinal tract to sustain injury in the child. The mechanism of injury to the small bowel is a crush injury between the delivered force and the vertebral column. Adult-sized seatbelts are often employed by conscientious parents and, as a result, the risk of injury to the small bowel increases, especially for children under 100 pounds in weight. The use of a seatbelt should always be asked about when an injured child from a motor vehicle crash is evaluated.

If a hematoma from a seat belt is present on the abdominal wall, the risk of an intra-abdominal injury is 232 times more likely. Therefore, a higher index of suspicion should be employed.[75] Children with rupture of the small bowel due to blunt trauma invariably have an abnormal physical examination. Free fluid seen on ultrasound (FAST) or CT scan, coupled with a tender abdomen and no injury to a solid organ on the CT mandates an abdominal exploration for a suspected injury to the small bowel. Even if no perforation is identified at surgery, care should be taken to repair mesenteric rents, evacuate large hematomas, and rule out retroperitoneal injuries. In this same setting, an associated compression injury of the lumbar vertebrae (Chance fracture) is often present.

Injuries to the colon and rectum are not common in children. Accidental causes of colon and rectal injuries include motor vehicle crashes with pelvic fractures and penetration of the rectum by bone shards, occasional deserosalization injuries from seat belts, and straddle injuries. Nonaccidental injuries are invariably related to abuse, typically from instrumentation. If the mucosa is injured or the injury is superficial, observation is appropriate. Full-thickness injuries of the distal rectum can be managed with primary repair in many cases. Devastating colon injuries above the peritoneal reflection occasionally need temporary fecal diversion, much as in adults.[76]

The injured spleen in a child will almost always stop bleeding without any intervention, so nonoperative management is widely accepted.[77] Occasionally, a child with a severely injured spleen may develop a pleural effusion in the left hemithorax (Figs. 46-2A and 2B). If a study for occult diaphragmatic injury is negative, this can typically

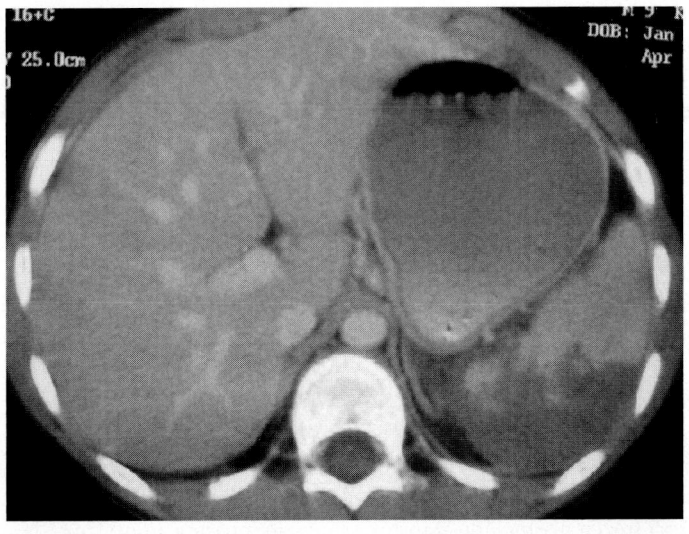

A

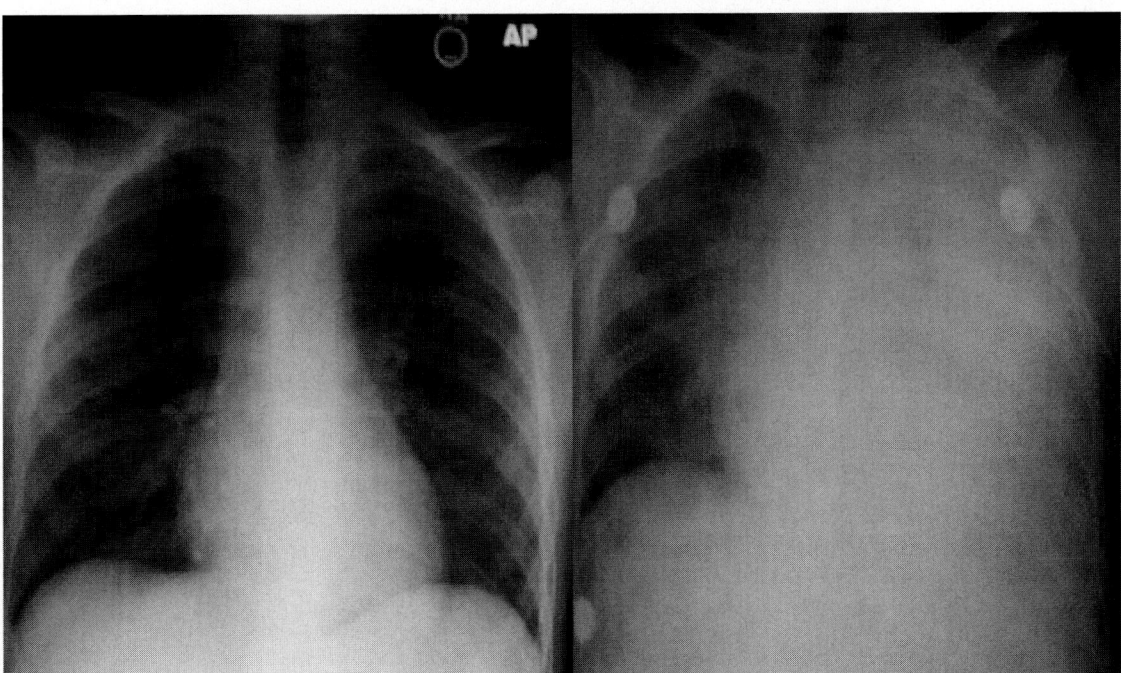

B

**FIGURE 46-2.** **(A)** Note the grade 4 spleen injury. **(B)** The admission chest x-ray of the injured child shown in Figure 46-1A, and the chest x-ray 4 days later showing a pleural effusion.

be treated with a tube thoracostomy. Children who require surgery are those who have uncorrectable physiologic instability, those who have received or are likely to receive half their blood volume in transfusions within 24 hours of injury (40 mL/kg), or those who have progression of the rupture during nonoperative management. The physiologic response to splenic injury correlates with the grade of splenic injury, and children who need operative intervention often need splenectomy.[78] If splenectomy must be performed, postsplenectomy immunization and antibiotic therapy is appropriate and necessary based on available guidelines.[79] The administration of pneumococcal vaccine, hemophilus influenza vaccine, and meningococcal vaccine should be considered at 14 days after splenectomy. In addition, many children are given penicillin on a daily basis if the splenectomy is performed before the age of 5 years. If immunosuppression is suspected, hepatitis B vaccine should also be administered.

When only the parenchyma of the liver is injured, without involvement of a major intrahepatic vessel or bile duct, then observation will almost always succeed. This is especially true in patients with isolated hepatic injuries; however, hepatic injuries are associated with a slightly higher mortality rate than with splenic injuries. The combination of hepatic and splenic injuries is clearly associated with a higher mortality rate, which goes up as the severity of injury rises.[80] The concept of operation when half of the blood volume has been transfused as noted for splenic injury is valid for injury to the liver. If a blush is seen on CT, however, angioembolization may replace operation in the stable patient. Others have advocated early operative packing in more unstable patients, coupled with embolization and early reoperation as a means to improve survival.[81] The physiologic and hematologic effects of massive transfusion in the child often make the operative management of a major hepatic injury very difficult unless the new paradigm of a 1:1 red blood cell unit: fresh frozen plasma unit transfusion is followed. When perihepatic packing has been necessary or the midgut is edematous after a major hepatic repair, a commercially available vacuum system or off-the-shelf supplies such as soft bowel bags, laparotomy packs, adhesive dressings, and silastic

drains placed on suction can provide a very effective damage control dressing. With attention to detail, fascial closure should be able to be accomplished with most survivors.[82]

Pediatric pancreatic injuries, especially following trauma involving bike riding, are uncommon and are most often due to blunt trauma.[83] The majority of pancreatic injuries in children may be treated successfully with nonoperative management including gut rest, intravenous nutrition, and occasionally pancreatic antisecretory medication. Conservative management of children with a pancreatic transection is much more controversial. A small group of patients with a prolonged median hospitalization and incomplete follow-up has been reported, and nonoperative management was advocated.[84] Late pancreatic pseudocysts were common and required intervention. Others have reported the beneficial effects of a spleen-sparing distal pancreatectomy even in the face of a delayed diagnosis.[85] Operative intervention allowed an earlier return to normal activities and avoided the stress of prolonged hospitalization. When the capabilities for pediatric ERCP are available, ductal stenting may be of significant benefit.[86] Some surgeons have been able to employ laparoscopic distal pancreatectomy with splenic salvage for pancreatic transection when stenting could not be accomplished.[87]

Blunt trauma is the most common mechanism of renal injury in children (Fig. 46-3), contusion is the most common injury seen, and renal injury can occur in the absence of hematuria. Nonoperative management of most pediatric renal injuries (grades I–IV) can be accomplished safely, but operative renal salvage for grade V injuries appears to be uncommon.[88,89] Some investigators have noted a good salvage rate with nonoperative management of grade V injuries, but scarring and loss of parenchymal volume loss did occur.[90] Ureteral stenting for urine leaks may be needed in patients with injuries of the collecting system. Rarely, nephrectomy for exsanguinating injury may be needed, and it would typically be when 40 mL/kg of blood transfusion had been administered. Angioembolism may be considered in selected cases of intraparenchymal bleeding, but the majority of patients will not require an emergency intervention. Since most injured children now

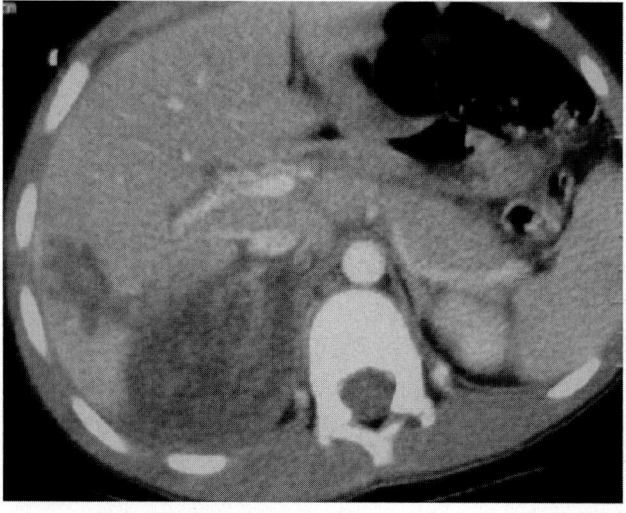
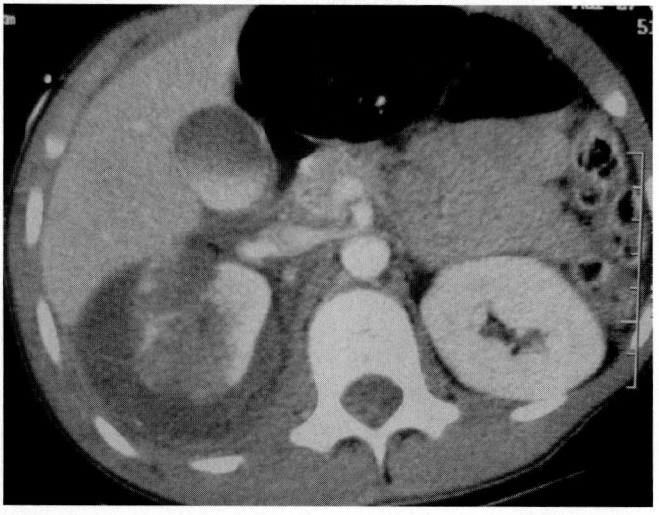

A                                                                 B

**FIGURE 46-3.** **(A)** CT scan of a child with a hepatic injury, adrenal injury, and renal injury. **(B)** CT scan of the same patient with a renal injury. This child did not have surgery and retained bilateral renal function without complications.

undergo abdominal CT scanning, CT cystography should be considered on every child to evaluate for the presence of an injury to the bladder.[91] The majority of bladder ruptures can be treated successfully with urethral catheters, without the need for additional suprapubic drainage.[92]

## Injury to Blood Vessels

Injuries to vessels in the extremities are equally divided between blunt and penetrating mechanisms.[93] Such injuries in children are uncommon, and children can tolerate complete vascular occlusion to the extremities to a greater extent than adults. Due to the elastic nature of the child's body, injuries to large vessels do not occur as often as adults. Limb salvage is typically greater than 95% using a team approach to care for associated orthopedic and soft tissue injuries. Pediatric peripheral vascular injuries requiring resection are repaired with autologous tissue whenever possible.[94] Injuries to the abdominal aorta have been caused by seat belts, bicycle crashes, and ATV crashes.[95] These are repaired immediately, and missed abdominal aortic injuries have resulted in late deaths.[96] The rare injuries to the thoracic aorta in children have been treated like those in adults with good results.[97] The use of endovascular stents in children, while successful in the short-term, has not been evaluated for long-term use, and especially in the growing child as noted above.

## Injury to the Skeletal System

Orthopedic injuries are the greatest cause of operative intervention required in the injured child. These injuries often are painful enough that they distract the child from complaining of other more serious injuries. Orthopedic injuries are also a source of missed injury in the injured child, and these missed injuries are the most important reason that a tertiary examination should be considered for all children admitted to the hospital.[98] As previously discussed, injuries to the cervical spine are often misdiagnosed, and most of the missed injuries are due to normal variants.[99]

Orthopedic injuries in children differ from adults in that they may involve the growth plate. The physis, also known as the growth plate, exists in the immature skeleton and can cause potential confusion on diagnostic studies and with treatment. New bone is laid down by the physis near the articular surfaces causing lengthening of the bone. When an injury occurs before the physis has closed, this may cause retardation of normal growth or development of the bone.

As children grow and bones mature, there is a change in porosity, composition of collagen fibers, and mineral content causing a certain laxity. Due to the immature, elastic nature of the bones there are fractures that are specific to children. Greenstick fractures are incomplete with angulation supported by cortical splinters on the concave surface. Buckle fractures are also a result of the growing bone of children and involve angulation due to cortical impaction. Other fractures that may cause injury to the growth plate include supracondylar fractures of the humerus or femur, and these are associated with vascular injuries, as well.

A good history including mechanism, force, and time of injury in addition to the physical examination and x-rays allows for easier and more accurate diagnosis. Fractures from different time periods as well as long bone fractures in children under 3 years of age should alert the clinician to the possibility of child abuse.

Blood loss is associated with fractures of long bones and the pelvis, but it is proportionately less than in adults and usually not enough to cause shock. If hemodynamic instability exists with an isolated fracture of the femur or pelvis, an evaluation for other sources of blood loss should be undertaken starting with the abdomen.

The key principle of the treatment of fractures is immobilization, and splinting of fractured extremities is necessary until more definitive treatment is undertaken. Also, it is important to obtain a good vascular exam in every patient with fracture of a long bone. Compromise of arterial inflow requires an early diagnosis, realignment of the fracture, and an occasional revascularization procedure to prevent permanent dysfunction or loss of tissue. Finally, it is important to be aware that a compartment syndrome secondary to hemorrhage from the fracture may occur and should be addressed within 6 hours of injury to prevent permanent damage.

## PEDIATRIC CRITICAL CARE

Trauma is a leading cause of morbidity and mortality in the pediatric population, often necessitating management in an intensive care unit (ICU). In general, hemodynamic instability, traumatic brain injury, altered mental status, significant injuries of the spleen, liver, or pancreas, multiple orthopedic injuries, severe pulmonary contusion, and polytrauma require more care than can be provided in a general hospital setting. Patient management in the ICU allows for hourly checks of vital signs, oxygen saturation levels, urine output, and neurological exams, which are essential to care. There are data that suggest that the care of injured children in a pediatric ICU improves survival.[100]

Monitoring in the ICU may be noninvasive or invasive. Arterial lines, which allow for closer observation of blood pressure and for drawing of blood gases, should be placed in the ICU. Central venous pressures may also easily be obtained and used for monitoring. For some injured children, especially those on ventilators, multiple drips may be necessary. Table 46-5 demonstrates the most common medications used in the intensive care setting.

Acute respiratory distress syndrome (ARDS) may occur within 3 to 4 days after major trauma, and ventilation modes are somewhat similar to adults in concept. The two common modes of ventilation are based on pressure and volume. Pressure control is rapid variable flow that provides a peak inspiratory pressure throughout inspiration. Volume control provides a constant tidal volume and minute ventilation regardless of pulmonary compliance. Pressure-regulated volume control is a combination that has a set tidal volume and inspiratory time, but allows the ventilator to adjust the flow rate. If the patient's respiratory status is refractory to conventional modes of ventilation, then the oscillator or high-frequency ventilation may be necessary. This allows for continuous high airway pressures, low tidal volumes, and a very fast rate. If all modes of ventilation have failed and the patient is a candidate, then extracorporeal membrane oxygenation (ECMO) may be necessary as previously mentioned. It is important to note that ECMO does not reverse any disease process, but it allows the heart and lungs to rest in order to heal the primary process.

## TABLE 46-5

### Dosages of Commonly Used Drugs in Injured Children

| Paralytic drugs | | |
|---|---|---|
| Succinylcholine | | 1.0–3.5 mg/kg |
| Vecuronium | | 0.2 mg/kg |
| Etomidate | | |
| Cistraconium | | 1–2 mcg/kg/min |
| **Sedation** | | |
| Ativan | | 0.05–0.2 mg/kg/hr |
| Versed | | 0.05–0.2 mg/kg/hr |
| Ketamine | | 0.5–2 mg/kg |
| **Analgesics** | | |
| Fentanyl | | 1–5 mcg/kg/hr |
| Morphine | | 0.05–0.2 mg/kg/hr |
| **Cardiovascular** | | |
| Dopamine | Low | 2–5 mcg/kg/min |
| | Intermediate | 5–15 mcg/kg/min |
| | High | 15–20 mcg/kg/min |
| Dobutamine | | 2–15 mcg/kg/min |
| Epinephrine | Bolus | 1.0–10 mg/kg/min |
| | Maintenance | 0.1–2.0 mcg/kg/min |
| Atropine | | 0.02 mg/kg (min 0.1 mg, max 0.5 mg) |
| **Bronchodilators** | | |
| Albuterol | | 0.05–15 mg/kg nebulized |
| Racemic epinephrine | | 0.05 cc/kg/dose nebulized (dilated to 3 cc NS) |

## PEDIATRIC REHABILITATION (See Chap. 54)

Rehabilitation is an important part of the recovery from injury for both children and adults. A rehabilitation facility is where an injured individual with new onset disabilities and impairments due to trauma may go to regain function and autonomy. The rehabilitation team focuses on medical issues as well as teaching compensatory techniques, lifestyle modifications, use of adaptive equipment depending on injury, how to deal with post-traumatic psychological impairment, and prevention of deterioration. The major difference between adult and pediatric rehabilitation is that growth and development must be taken into account with children. The age of the child must be considered at every stage of the process to ensure that appropriate goals are set and being met if possible.

Rehabilitation begins by carefully outlining all the injuries, disabilities, and impairments. Based on age, a multidisciplinary team formulates a plan with the family and patient (if possible). It is important to acknowledge and treat any grief, sadness, anger, or depression that is present and may impede the process of rehabilitation. Prior to discharge a plan with the family and patient should be in place. Follow-up with the surgical team should continue throughout rehabilitation and after as needed.

## CHILD ABUSE

Child abuse is a serious problem and represents 3% to 4% of all traumatic injuries seen in pediatric trauma centers.[101] It is important for clinicians to know the signs of potential child abuse in order to protect and care for those who cannot protect themselves. A thorough history and physical examination are paramount. Suspicion should be raised if there is a discrepancy between the history and the extent of injury, there are explanations that do not fit, and a long period of time has passed from the incident to when medical advice was sought. Unexplained events such as loss of consciousness should be questioned. A history of repeated trauma treated at different emergency rooms with "doctor shopping" is also ominous. In addition, if the history changes between caregivers and there is inappropriate behavior displayed from parents or caregivers in regard to the medical advice given, a suspicion should be raised. It is important to observe the relationship between the child and the parents and decipher whether the relationship appears strained or abnormal.

On examination, it is very important to observe multicolored bruises signifying different stages of healing and evidence of frequent injuries demonstrated by old scars or healed fractures on x-ray. Long bone fractures in children younger than 3 years old, multiple subdural hematomas, especially without a new skull fracture, and retinal hemorrhage are suspect injuries. Other injuries that should "raise a red flag" are those in odd places such as the perioral, genital, or perianal areas. Ruptured internal viscera without a history of major blunt trauma has also been associated with abuse. Finally, it is important to recognize and thoroughly investigate abnormal injuries such as bites, cigarette burns, or rope marks as well as sharply demarcated second- and third-degree burns in odd locations.

The work up should include a skeletal survey to look for other or old fractures. CT scans and MRIs should be obtained accordingly. It is important to emphasize that it is a requirement for the examining physician in all 50 states to report any questionable circumstance to Child Protective Services (CPS). Once reported, it is up to CPS to investigate and proceed with the appropriate measures.

## EMERGENCY DEPARTMENT MANAGEMENT AND FAMILY RELATIONS

The ED of a hospital that is not pediatric trauma center should still have the equipment, supplies, and the mindset to care for an injured child, since the majority of injured children are not cared for at pediatric trauma centers.[102] Because of this fact, many nontrauma centers see children with injuries that are beyond their capabilities. With this in mind, establishing good communication and plans for transfer to referral centers that do care for large volumes of children is mandatory. Also, many pediatric trauma centers are allowing families at the bedside of children with severe injuries,[103] after or during the initial resuscitation. Some centers even have the family at the bedside while cardiopulmonary resuscitation is in progress. This takes a serious commitment to professionalism and sensitivity during a time when stress in the emergency room is at its highest.

## Acknowledgment

This work is supported in part by the Paula Milburn Miller/CMRI Chair in Pediatric Surgery.

# REFERENCES

1. Kissoon N, Dreyer J, Walia M: Pediatric trauma. Differences in pathophysiology, injury patterns and treatment compared with adult trauma. *Can Med Assoc J* 142:27, 1990.

2. Haller A: Toward a comprehensive emergency medical system for children. *Pediatrics* 86:120, 2002.

3. Vyrostek SB, Annest JL, Ryan GW: Surveillance for fatal and nonfatal injuries–United States, 2001. *MMWR Surveill Summ* 3:1, 2004.

4. Inon AE, Haller JA: Caring for the injured children of our world: A global perspective. *Surg Clin North Am* 82:435, 2002.

5. Rivara FP: Pediatric injury control in 1999: Where do we go from Here? *Pediatrics* 103:883, 1999.

6. Danesco ER, Miller TR, Spicer RS: Incidence and costs of 1987–1994 childhood injuries: demographic breakdowns. *Pediatrics* 105:e27, 2000

7. Killingsworth JB, Tilford JM, Parker JG, et al.: National hospitalization impact of pediatric all-terrain vehicle injuries. *Pediatrics* 115:e316, 2005.

8. Resources for Optimal Care of the Injured Patient 2006. American College of Surgeons Committee on Trauma. Chapter 10, p. 59.

9. Edil BH, Tuggle DW, Jones S: Pediatric major resuscitation–respiratory compromise as a criterion for mandatory surgeon presence. *J Pediatr Surg* 40:926, 2005.

10. Wang TK, Wu RS, Chen C, et al.: Endotracheal tube size selection guidelines for Chinese children: prospective study of 533 cases. *J Formos Med Assoc* 96:325, 1997.

11. Agarwal S, Swanson S, Murphy A, et al.: Comparing the utility of a standard pediatric resuscitation cart with a pediatric resuscitation cart based on the Broselow tape: A randomized, controlled, crossover trial involving simulated resuscitation scenarios. *Pediatrics* 116:e326, 2005.

12. Luten R: Error and time delay in pediatric trauma resuscitation: Addressing the problem with color-coded resuscitation aids. *Surg Clin North Am* 82:303, 2002.

13. Chiang VW, Baskin MN: Uses and complications of central venous catheters inserted in a pediatric emergency department. *Pediatr Emerg Care* 16:230, 2002.

14. Rogers FB: Technical note: a quick and simple method of obtaining venous access in traumatic exsanguination. *J Trauma* 34:142, 1993.

15. Tepas JJ, Schinco MA: Pediatric Trauma. In: Moore EE, Feliciano DV, Mattox KL, eds. *Trauma*. Fifth Edition. New York, NY: p. 1025, 2004.

16. National High Blood Pressure Education Program Working Group on High Blood Pressure in Children and Adolescents. The fourth report on the diagnosis, evaluation, and treatment of high blood pressure in children and adolescents. *Pediatrics* 114:555, 2004.

17. Dula DJ, Wood GC, Rejmer AR, et al.: Use of prehospital fluids in hypotensive blunt trauma patients. *Prehosp Emerg Care* 6:417, 2002.

18. Balogh Z, McKinley BA, Cocanour CS, et al.: Supranormal trauma resuscitation causes more cases of abdominal compartment syndrome. *Arch Surg* 138:637, 2003.

19. Martini WZ, Pusateri AE, Uscilowicz JM, et al.: Independent contributions of hypothermia and acidosis to coagulopathy in swine. *J Trauma* 58:1002, 2005.

20. Selden PD, Bratton SL, Carney NA, et al.: Guidelines for the acute medical management of severe traumatic brain injury in infants, children, and adolescents following severe pediatric traumatic brain injury. The role of temperature control. *Pediatr Crit Care Med* 4:S53, 2003.

21. Adelson PD, Ragheb J, Kanev P: Phase II clinical trial of moderate hypothermia after severe traumatic brain injury in children. *Neurosurgery* 56:740, 2005.

22. Merten DF, Carpenter BLM: Radiologic imaging of inflicted injury in the child abuse syndrome. *Pediatr Clin North Am* 37:815, 1990.

23. Lloyd DA, Carty H, Patterson M, et al.: Predictive value of skull radiography for intracranial injury in children with blunt head injury. *Lancet* 349:821, 1997.

24. Wang MY, Griffith P, Sterling J, et al.:A prospective population based study of pediatric trauma patients with mild alterations in consciousness (GCS 13-14). *Neurosurgery* 46:1093, 2000.

25. Kimura A, Otsuka T. Emergency Center ultrasonography in the evaluation of hemoperitoneum: A prospective study. *J Trauma* 31:20, 1991.

26. Tso P, Rodriguez A, Cooper C, et al.: Sonography in blunt abdominal trauma: a preliminary progress report. *J Trauma* 33:39, 1992.

27. Hoffman R, Nerlich M, Muggia-Sullam M, et al.: Blunt abdominal trauma in cases of multiple trauma evaluated by ultrasonography: a prospective analysis of 291 patients. *J Trauma* 32:452, 1992.

28. Rozycki GS, Ochsner MG, Jaffin JH, et al.: Prospective evaluation of surgeons' use of ultrasound in trauma patients. *J Trauma* 34:516, 1993.

29. Mutabagani KH, Coley BD, Zumberge N, et al.: Preliminary experience with focused abdominal sonography for trauma (FAST) in children: is it useful? *J Pediatr Surg* 34:48, 1999.

30. Luks FI, Lemire A, St. Vil D, et al.: Blunt abdominal trauma in children: the practical value of ultrasonography. *J Trauma* 34:607, 1993.

31. Sarkisian AE, Khondkarian A, Amirbekian NM, et al.: Sonographic screening of mass casualties for abdominal and renal injuries following the 1988 Armenian earthquake. *J Trauma* 31:247, 1991.

32. Bode PJ, Niezen RA, Van Vugt AB, et al.: Abdominal ultrasound as a reliable indicator for conclusive laparotomy in blunt abdominal trauma. *J Trauma.* 34:27, 1993.

33. Shackford SR: Credentialing, Liability, and Turf Wars. American College of Surgeons- Ultrasound Instructors Course, April 2001; p. 45.

34. Suthers SE, Albrecht R, Foley D, et al.: Surgeon-directed ultrasound for trauma is a predictor of intra-abdominal injury in children. *Am Surg* 70:164, 2004.

35. Ruess L, Sivit CJ, Eichelberger MR, et al.: Blunt abdominal trauma in children: Impact of CT on operative and nonoperative management. *AJR* 169:1011, 1997.

36. O' Sullivan MG, Statham PF, Jones PA, et al.: Role of intracranial pressure monitoring in severely head injured patients without signs of intracranial hypertension on initial computerized tomography. *J Neurosurg* 80:46, 1994.

37. Stafford RE, McGonigal MD, Weigelt JA, et al.: Oral contrast solution and computed tomography for blunt abdominal trauma: a randomized study. *Arch Surg* 134:622, 1999.

38. Tsang BD, Panacek EA, Brant WE, et al.: Effect of oral contrast administration for abdominal computed tomography in the evaluation of acute blunt trauma. *Ann Emerg Med* 30:7, 1997.

39. Federle MP, Yagan N, Peitzman AB, et al.: Abdominal Trauma: Use of oral contrast material for CT is safe. *Radiology* 205:91, 1997.

40. Lim-Dunham JE, Narra J, Benya EC, et al.: Aspiration after administration of oral contrast material in children undergoing abdominal CT for trauma. *AJR* 169:1015, 1997.

41. Strouse PJ, Close BJ, Marshall KW, et al.: CT of bowel and mesenteric trauma in children. *Radiographics* 19:1237, 1999.

42. Cox TD, Kuhn JP: CT scan of bowel trauma in the pediatric patient. *Radiol Clin North Am* 34:807, 1996.

43. Keller MS, Coln CE, Trimble JA, et al.: The utility of routine trauma laboratories in pediatric trauma resuscitations. *Am J Surg* 188:671, 2004.

44. Ford EG, Karamanoukian HL, McGrath N, et al.: Emergency center laboratory evaluation of pediatric trauma victims. *Am Surg* 56:752, 1990.

45. Bryant MS, Tepas JJ III, Talbert JL, et al.: Impact of emergency room laboratory studies on the ultimate triage and disposition of the injured child. *Am Surg* 54:209, 1988.

46. Peterson DL, Schinco MA, Kerwin AJ, et al.: Evaluation of initial base deficit as a prognosticator of outcome in the pediatric trauma population. *Am Surg* 70:326, 2004.

47. Asimos AW, Gibbs MA, Marx JA, et al.: Value of point-of-care blood testing in emergent trauma management. *J Trauma* 48:1101, 2000.

48. Carrick MM, Tyroch AH, Youens CA, et al.: Subsequent development of thrombocytopenia and coagulopathy in moderate and severe head injury: Support for serial laboratory examination. *J Trauma* 58:725, 2005.

49. Cochran A, Scaife ER, Hansen KW, et al.: Hyperglycemia and outcomes from pediatric traumatic brain injury. *J Trauma* 55:1035, 2003.

50. Tepas JJ, DiScala C, Ramenofsky ML, et al.: Mortality and head injury: the pediatric perspective. *J Pediatr Surg* 25:92, 1990.

51. Sills MR, Libby AM, Orton HD: Prehospital and in-hospital mortality: A comparison of intentional and unintentional traumatic brain injuries in Colorado children. *Arch Pediatr Adolesc Med* 159:665, 2005.

52. Kriel RL, Krach LE, Panser LA: Closed head injury: comparison of children younger and older than 6 years of age. *Pediatr Neurol* 5:296, 1989.

53. Bauer R, Fritz H: Pathophysiology of traumatic injury in the developing brain: an introduction and short update. *Exp Toxicol Pathol* 56:65, 2004.

54. American Association for the Surgery of Trauma; Child Neurology Society;International Society for Pediatric Neurosurgery; International Trauma Anesthesia and Critical Care Society; Society of Critical Care Medicine, et al. Guidelines for the acute medical management of severe traumatic brain injury in infants, children, and adolescents. *J Trauma* 54:S235, 2003.

55. Peclet MH, Newman KD, Eichelberger MR, et al.: Thoracic trauma in children: An indicator of increased mortality. *J Pediatr Surg* 25:961, 1990.

56. Gray A: Pediatric Orthopedia Trauma. In: Wesson DE, Cooper A, Scherer LRT, et al., eds. *Pediatric Trauma*. New York: Taylor and Francis, p.325, 2006

57. Platzer P, Jaindl M, Thalhammer G, et al.: Cervical spine injuries in pediatric patients. *J Trauma* 62:389, 2007.

58. Anderson RCE, Scaife ER, Fenton SJ, et al.: Cervical spine clearance after trauma in children. *J Neurosurg* 105:361, 2006.

59. Duckman CA, Zambranski ZM, Hadley MN, et al.: Pediatric spinal cord injury without radiographic abnormalities: Report of 26 cases and review of the literature. *J Spinal Discord* 4:296, 1991.

60. Peterson RJ, Tepas III JJ, Edwards FH, et al.: Pediatric and adult thoracic trauma: Age related impact on prsentation and outcome. *Ann Thorac Surg* 58:14, 1994.

61. Holmes JF, Sokolove PE, Brant WE, et al.: A clinical decision rule for identifying children with thoracic injuries after blunt torso trauma. *Ann Emerg Med* 39:492, 2002.
62. Allen GS, Cox CS: Pulmonary Contusion in children: Diagnosis and management. *So Med J* 91:1099, 1998.
63. Rielly JP, Brandt ML, Mattox KL, et al.: Thoracic trauma in children. *J Trauma.* 34:329, 1993.
64. Peterson RJ, Tiwary AD, Kissoon N, et al.: Pediatric penetrating thoracic trauma: A five-year experience. *Pediatr Emerg Care* 10:129, 1994.
65. Tiao GM, Griffith PM, Szmuszkovicz JR, et al.: Cardiac and great vessel injuries in children after blunt trauma. An institutional review. *J Pediatr Surg* 35:1656, 2000.
66. Canty TG Sr, Canty TG Jr, Brown C: Injuries of the gastrointestinal tract from blunt trauma in children: A 12-year experience at a designated pediatric trauma center. *J Trauma* 46:234, 1999.
67. Cooper A: Thoracic injuries. *Semin Pediatr Surg* 4:109, 1995.
68. Heckman SR, Trooskin SZ, Burd RS: Risk factors for blunt thoracic aortic injury in children. *J Ped Surg* 40:98, 2005.
69. Holmes JF, Sokolove PE, Brant WE, et al.: A clinical decision role for identifying children with thoracic injuries after blunt torso trauma. *Ann Emer Med* 39:492, 2002.
70. Karmy-Jones R, Hoffer E, Meissner M, et al. Management of traumatic rupture of the thoracic aorta in pediatric patients. *Ann Thor Surg* 75:1513, 2003.
71. Kisson N, Dreyer J, Walia M. Pediatric trauma: Differences in pathophysiology, injury patterns and treatment compared with adult trauma. *Can Med Asso J* 142: 27, 1990.
72. Guth AA, Pachter HL, Kim U: Pitfalls in the diagnosis of blunt diaphragmatic injury. *Am J Surg* 170:5, 1995.
73. Ciftci AO, Tanyel FC, Salman AB, et al.: Gastrointestinal tract perforation due to blunt abdominal trauma. *Pediatr Surg Int* 13:259, 1998.
74. Clendenon JN, Meyers RL, Nance ML, et al.: Management of duodenal injuries in children. *J Pediatr Surg* 39:964, 2004.
75. Lutz N, Nance ML, Kallan MJ, et al.: Incidence and clinical significance of abdominal wall bruising in restrained children involved in motor vehicle crashes. *J Pediatr Surg* 39:972, 2004.
76. Haut ER, Nance ML, Keller MS, et al.: Management of penetrating colon and rectal injuries in the pediatric patient. *Dis Colon Rectum* 47:1526, 2004.
77. Stylianos S: Compliance with evidence-based guidelines in children with isolated spleen or liver injury: A prospective study. *J Pediatr Surg* 37:453, 2002.
78. Mooney DP, Downard C, Johnson S, et al.: Physiology after pediatric splenic injury. *J Trauma* 58:108, 2005.
79. Howdieshell TR, Heffernan D, Dipiro JT; Therapeutic Agents Committee of the Surgical Infection Society. Surgical infection society guidelines for vaccination after traumatic injury. *Surg Infect (Larchmt)* 7:275, 2006.
80. Paddock HN, Tepas JJ III, Ramenofsky ML, et al.: Management of blunt pediatric hepatic and splenic injury: Similar process, different outcome. *Am Surg* 70:1068, 2004.
81. MacKenzie S, Kortbeek JB, Mulloy R, et al.: Recent experiences with a multidisciplinary approach to complex hepatic trauma. *Injury* 35:869, 2004.
82. Markley MA, Mantor PC, Letton RW, et al.: Pediatric vacuum packing wound closure for damage-control laparotomy. *J Pediatr Surg* 37:512, 2002.
83. Gross JA, Vaughan MM, Johnston BD, et al.: Handlebar injury causing pancreatic contusion in a pediatric patient. *AJR Am J Roentgenol* 179:222, 2002.
84. Wales PW, Shuckett B, Kim PC: Long-term outcome after nonoperative management of complete traumatic pancreatic transection in children. *J Pediatr Surg* 36:823, 2001.
85. Meier DE, Coln CD, Hicks BA, et al.: Early operation in children with pancreas transection. *J Pediatr Surg* 36:341, 2001.
86. Canty TG Sr, Weinman D: Management of major *pancreatic* duct injuries in children. *J Trauma* 50:1001, 2001.
87. Sayad P, Cacchione R, Ferzli G: Laparoscopic distal pancreatectomy for blunt injury to the pancreas. A case report. *Surg Endosc* 15:759, 2001.
88. Nance ML, Lutz N, Carr MC, et al.: Blunt renal injuries in children can be managed nonoperatively: Outcome in a consecutive series of patients. *J Trauma* 57:474, 2004.
89. Rogers CG, Knight V, MacUra KJ, et al.: High-grade renal injuries in children–is conservative management possible? *Urology* 64:574, 2004.
90. Keller MS, Coln EC, Garza JJ, et al.: Functional outcome of nonoperatively managed renal injuries in children. *J Trauma* 57:108, 2004.
91. Deck AJ, Shaves S, Talner L, et al.: Computerized tomography cystography for the diagnosis of traumatic bladder rupture. *J Urol* 164:43, 2000.
92. Parry NG, Rozycki GS, Feliciano DV, et al.: Traumatic rupture of the urinary bladder: is the suprapubic tube necessary? *J Trauma* 54:431, 2003.
93. Harris LM, Hordines J: Major vascular injuries in the pediatric population. *Ann Vasc Surg* 17:266, 2003.
94. Milas ZL, Dodson TF, Ricketts RR: Pediatric blunt trauma resulting in major arterial injuries. *Am Surg* 70:443, 2004.
95. Lin PH, Barr V, Bush RL, et al: Isolated abdominal aortic rupture in a child due to all-terrain vehicle accident–a case report. *Vasc Endovascular Surg* 37:289, 2003.
96. Tracy TF Jr, Silen ML, Graham MA: Delayed rupture of the abdominal aorta in a child after a suspected handlebar injury. *J Trauma* 40:119, 1996.
97. Karmy-Jones R, Hoffer E, Meissner M, Bloch RD. Management of traumatic rupture of the thoracic aorta in pediatric patients. *Ann Thorac Surg* 75:1513, 2003.
98. Soundappan SV, Holland AJ, Cass DT: Role of an extended tertiary survey in detecting missed injuries in children. *J Trauma* 57:114, 2004.
99. Avellino AM, Mann FA, Grady MS, et al.: The misdiagnosis of acute cervical spine injuries and fractures in infants and children: The 12-year experience of a level I pediatric and adult trauma center. *Childs Nerv Syst* 21:122, 2005.
100. Odetola FO, Miller WC, Davis MM, et al.: The relationship between the location of pediatric intensive care unit facilities and child death from trauma: A county-level ecologic study. *J Pediatr* 147:74, 2005.
101. Cox C: Trauma from Child Abuse. In: Wesson DE, Cooper A, Scherer LRT, et al., eds. *Pediatric Trauma: Pathophysiology, Diagnosis, and Treatment.* New York: Taylor & Francis p. 73, 2006.
102. Segui-Gomez M, Chang DC, Paidas CN, et al.: Pediatric trauma care: An overview of pediatric trauma systems and their practices in 18 US states. *J Pediatr Surg* 38:1162, 2003.
103. Morse JM, Pooler C: Patient-family-nurse interactions in the trauma-resuscitation room. *Am J Crit Care* 11:240, 2002.

# Commentary ■ STEVEN STYLIANOS

Doctors Tuggle and Garza have provided a focused summary of key concepts in the epidemiology, initial assessment and specific treatment of injured children. Although morbidity and mortality figures have decreased in designated pediatric trauma centers it is crucial to note that the vast majority of injured children are treated at centers with variable knowledge of trauma care and even less knowledge in the care of critically injured children. The impact of state trauma systems in the triage of injured children to designated trauma centers is increasing, however, all treating facilities could benefit by preparing for future injured children utilizing the points outlined in the chapter above.

I'd like to emphasize several of the key points:

1. Benefits of the Broselow Pediatric Resuscitation Measuring Tape for rapid determination of appropriate tube size and medication dosages.

2. Children can maintain "normal," age-specific blood pressure despite significant blood loss.

3. Hypothermia can occur quickly in injured children and exacerbate the physiologic and metabolic consequences of injury.

4. Children with significant CNS injury can have a "normal" initial head CT.

5. Unique anatomic features in infants that increase the risk of CNS injury.

6. Mobile mediastinum that creates physiologic havoc is acutely shifted.

7. Marked increase in significant intraabdominal injury when a child presents with a seat-belt bruise across the lower abdomen.

8. The importance of physician interactions with family members and parent participation during the critical care of injured children.

The nonoperative treatment of abdominal solid organ injuries in hemodynamically stabile children is well accepted and practiced in most pediatric trauma centers. It is alarming that rates of operative intervention are significantly increased when physician or instituitional expertise in pediatric trauma care is lacking. The use of operative rates for children with blunt spleen injury may be useful audit filters in assessing performance in a trauma system.

## Recommended Reading

Stylianos S, Egorova N, Guice KS, et al.: Variation in treatment of pediatric spleen injury at trauma centers versus non-trauma centers: A call for dissemination of APSA benchmarks and guidelines. *JACS* 202:247-251, 2006.

Jurkovich GJ, Pierce B, Pananen L, et al.: Giving bad news: The family perspective. *J Trauma* 48:865-873, 2000.

Montgomery V, Oliver R, Reisner A, et al.: The effect of severe traumatic brain injury on the family. *J Trauma* 52:1121-1124, 2002.

# Geriatric Trauma

Carl I. Schulman  ■  Reginald Alouidor  ■  Mark G. McKenney

## DEMOGRAPHICS

As one of the fastest growing age groups of the population, the elderly will comprise an increasingly important proportion of trauma victims. As of 2002, trauma is the fifth leading cause of death in all age groups and the ninth leading cause for those 65 years and older.[1] The rate per 100,000, however, is 56.0 for all groups and 113.2 for those older than 65.[2] In 2000, the 65 and older group comprised 35 million people. This represents a 12% increase since 1990, when 31.2 million older people were counted, but is the first time in census history that the 65 years and over population did not grow faster than the total population. This is due to a decrease in the birth cohort that is expected to reverse as baby boomers (born from 1946 to 1964) reach age 65, starting in 2011. Within this group, 18.5 million people or 53% were aged 65 to 74, 12.3 million or 35% were aged 75 to 84, and 4.2 million or 12% were aged 85 and over. In the population 65 and over, 42% reported some type of long-lasting condition or a disability. In those aged 65 to 74, 32% reported at least one disability, in contrast with 72% of people 85 and over.[3,4]

Perhaps the most important issue is what exactly defines a geriatric trauma patient. Is it chronological age, physiological age, the presence of preexisting conditions, or a combination of these factors? This is extremely important not only in being able to identify a geriatric patient who may be at increased risk, but also in understanding that the data we use to make such decisions are based on studies with a myriad of age ranges and definitions of the geriatric trauma patient.

By strict census criteria the most common age cutoff for the group of elderly or geriatric trauma patients is 65 years old. There are, however, some data to suggest that those even as young as 45 years old may have poorer outcomes than their younger counterparts, and that those greater than 75 years old may be at especially high risk.[5,6]

## ALTERED PHYSIOLOGY AND COMORBIDITY

Multiple studies have consistently shown elderly trauma patients have a higher level of injury related mortality than younger trauma patients. Much of this increased risk of death is due to preexisting medical conditions (PEC) in the elderly population and is greatest in patients with the least severe injuries, with a lesser effect on those with moderate injuries.[7,8] This risk of death will vary according to the type and number of medical conditions.

There are significant differences in the reported rates of comorbid diseases in the elderly population. These differences are due to the heterogeneity in the definitions of comorbid conditions, to subjective bias in the identification and reporting of these conditions, and, finally, because individuals significantly impaired by disease lead a less active lifestyle and are frequently underrepresented.

Milzman documented the prevalence of preexisting conditions in the trauma population by increasing age. By the fourth decade the prevalence is estimated to be 17%, by the sixth decade 40%, and by age 75, 69% of the population has one or more chronic medical conditions.[9] Bergeron, in a study on Trauma Score-Injury Severity Score (TRISS) methodology by age categories, noted the prevalence of comorbidities among the overall study population to be 26.8%. It was 4.6% in the population younger than 55 years old and 57.2% in those over 55. For those over 65 the prevalence increased to 66.5%, and, over 95, to 81.5%.[10] A review of the New York State Trauma Registry (1994–1998) looking at elderly trauma inpatients documented the incidence of preexisting conditions to be only 3.5% in patients younger than 40. This incidence jumped to 34.7% in patients 75–84 years old and to 37.3% in patients 85 years old and older.[11] Clearly the prevalence of preexisting conditions increases with age and can be as high as 80% in those over 95.

Preexisting conditions make it difficult for older patients to tolerate perturbations of their normal physiologic parameters when confronted with the acute stress of trauma or major surgery. In most elderly trauma patients, "resting organ function often is preserved but the ability to augment performance in response to stress is greatly compromised."[12] A summary of the age-related and physiologic changes is presented in Tables 47-1 and 47-2, with a discussion below.

## Cardiovascular System

The most frequent comorbidities in the geriatric population involve the cardiovascular system. It is often difficult to differentiate the changes that derive from aging versus those that are due to the interaction of the natural aging process with lifestyle and chronic disease.[13] As the heart ages there are changes in the tissue concentrations and the level of activity of growth factors such as angiotensin II, endothelin, TGF-B, FGF, and IGF. These growth factors influence the function of myocardial and vascular cells and their extracellular matrices. The myocytes and conductive pathways are slowly replaced with fat and fibrous tissue, which predisposes to arrhythmias and creates a stiffer heart. There are changes in the concentrations of elastin, collagen, and calcium, which lead

to thickening of the valves and blood vessels with loss of elasticity. As a result the walls of large arteries dilate and the intima in particular becomes thickened. Older patients experience a decrease in the response to catecholamines with reduced activity of B-adrenergic modulation of the vasculature and the heart, thus limiting maximal heart rate.[14]

The consequences of these combined effects are an age-associated increase in afterload on the heart, which is reflected in a modest increase in systolic blood pressure at rest. In healthy individuals these vascular changes are compensated for in large part by age-associated changes in the architecture and contractile properties of the heart, which, despite reductions in aortic distensibility, allow the older heart to pump a normal quantity of blood at rest.[14]

Coronary artery disease is ubiquitous in the elderly population and reduces the ability to autoregulate blood in the coronary circulation. Patients with coronary artery disease frequently present with fixed coronary lesions, which, in the presence of increased myocardial activity, can precipitate failure of the cardiac pump. The elderly cardiovascular system has limited capacity to adjust. In times of increased demand, the elderly heart can experience occult or overt ischemia.[14]

While most of the effects of aging on the heart are functionally minor, the effects of aging on the vascular system are more significant. The increased impedance of the central elastic vessels with aging impairs ventricular performance, reduces ventricular ejection fraction,

### TABLE 47-1

#### Age-Related Anatomic Changes

**ANATOMIC CHANGES**

**Central Nervous System**
- Cortical brain atrophy
- Increased volume CSF
- Decreased epidural space
- Increased subdural space

**Cardio-Vascular System**
- Thickening of the heart valves and great vessels
- Loss of elasticity of the large vessels
- Development of fixed coronary lesions
- Decreased vital capacity
- Increased alveolar surface area
- Increased stiffness chest wall
- Decreased elastic lung recoil/increased closing volume

**Renal System**
- Decreased renal cell mass (cortical cell mass)
- Thickening of the basement membrane
- Decrease in total body water
- Glomerular sclerosis/Interstitial fibrosis
- Decreased number functional nephrons

**Musculo-Skeletal System**
- Decreased lean body mass
- Decreased muscle mass
- Increased proportion of adipose tissue
- Bone loss/decreased bone density
- Thickened intervertebral discs/shortening vertebral bodies
- Increased density subchondral cartilage
- Atrophy skin (all layers)

**Gastrointestinal/Hepatobiliary System**
- Decreased gastrointestinal blood flow
- Decreased hepatic volume (decreased cell mass)
- Atrophy gastric mucosa
- Decreased volume of thymus
- Fibrosis thyroid gland

### TABLE 47-2

#### Age-Related Physiologic Changes

**PHYSIOLOGIC CHANGES**

**Central nervous system**
- Decreased efficiency of the BBB
- Alteration in autonomic system functions
- Alterations in neurotransmitters
- Decreased cerebral oxygen consumption

**Cardio-vascular system**
- Decreased inotropic and chronotropic response to beta adrenergic stimuli
- Increased peripheral vascular resistance
- Slowed ventricular filling/increased reliance on atrial contribution

**Respiratory system**
- Decreased chemoreceptor response to hypoxia/hypoxemia
- Decreased strength and endurance of respiratory muscles
- Decreased diffusion capacity
- Decreased cough reflex

**Renal system**
- Decreased response to vasopressin/ADH and aldosterone
- Decreased drug elimination
- Decreased thirst response
- Decreased hydroxylation of vitamin D

**Musculo-skeletal system**
- Decreased epithelial cell regeneration

**Gastrointestinal/hepatobiliary system**
- Decreased bicarbonate secretion

**Immune system/metabolism**
- Decreased cell mediated immunity
- Decreased antibody titers
- Loss effective mechanisms heat production/conservation/dissipation
- Blunting febrile response

and decelerates aortic flow even in the absence of heart failure in the elderly. The result is that maximal heart rate, stroke volume, cardiac output, ejection fraction, and oxygen uptake all decrease, whereas both end-systolic and end-diastolic volumes increase.[15]

Older trauma patients do not respond to hypovolemia as do their younger counterparts. Instead of increased heart rate and cardiac output, they respond with increased systemic vascular resistance which can result in a deceptively reassuring blood pressure. Reduction of blood pressure from baseline hypertension in these patients can also mask the effects of volume loss to the limits of compensatory mechanisms. Apparently normal blood pressures in elderly trauma patients may actually correspond to profound shock as evidenced by laboratory endpoints of perfusion (rising lactic acid level and base deficit) and early aggressive invasive monitoring. In some series over 50% of the patients had evidence of occult cardiogenic shock and, subsequently, had an adverse outcome.[12,16] Finally, patients with preexisting cardiovascular disease experience a higher incidence of posttraumatic cardiac events. Gallagher, in a retrospective study using a modified cardiac risk score, demonstrated a positive predictive value (PPV) of 76% for occurrence of a posttraumatic cardiac event in patients with a high risk score.[17]

## Respiratory System

The respiratory system undergoes well-documented age related changes. There is a decrease in the alveolar surface area by 4% per decade after age 30. The decrease in alveolar surface area reduces alveolar surface tension, with a negative effect on alveolar gas exchange and forced expiratory flow.[18] The alveoli flatten and shallow out, thereby reducing the area for gas exchange. It has been demonstrated that the gas exchange rate decreases by 0.5% per year.[19] In addition, the alveolar ducts enlarge and the alveolar walls thin and contain fewer capillaries. Diffusion capacity decreases as well because of a decrease in the total functional surface area and an increase in alveolar–capillary membrane thickness.[20]

Gross anatomic changes in the elderly include the development of thoracic kyphosis with rib calcification and decalcification, reducing the transverse thoracic diameter. This results in loss of bone density and increasing rigidity of the chest wall. There is thinning of the intervertebral discs and shortening of the vertebral bodies. The chest takes on a barrel shape, which is not believed to have a significant functional importance.[18] Compliance of the chest wall is decreased so that the 70-year-old utilizes 70% of the total elastic work of breathing on the chest wall compared to 40% in the 20-year-old.[21] Muscle mass is reduced causing the respiratory muscles to weaken in strength and endurance, and more dependence is placed on the accessory muscles of the abdominal wall. The elastic recoil of lung tissue decreases with age resulting in decreased compliance and increased closing volume. Compliance is further compromised as the chest wall stiffens, leading to increased air trapping, increased closing capacity, and frequency-dependent problems with compliance and gas exchange.[22] The elderly also experience decreased cough reflex and strength, decreased mucociliary clearance (because of atrophy of the pseudo-ciliated bronchial mucosa), decreased response to foreign antigen, and increased oropharyngeal colonization with Gram-negative bacteria. These changes, coupled with a higher risk of aspiration because of decreased lower esophageal sphincter tone, lend themselves to an increased risk of nosocomial and ventilator-associated pneumonia.

In the presence of trauma one should be prepared for a more difficult airway in the elderly patient. Elderly patients can present with fixed flexion deformities of the cervical spine secondary to rheumatoid arthritis and ankylosing spondylitis, leading to increased difficulty of intubation. Degenerative changes of the temporomandibular joint may also restrict opening of the mouth.[23] The presence of preexisting pulmonary disease, either restrictive or obstructive, will result in decreased pulmonary reserve. These patients have decreased baseline $PaO_2$ and increased $PaCO_2$ and are at risk for rapid decompensation. The diminished vital capacity as well as changes in ventilation–perfusion mismatch will further decrease baseline arterial oxygen tension, which is less responsive to supplemental oxygen.

As noted previously the chest wall is fused and brittle, and this increased chest wall rigidity and osteoporosis places geriatric patients at higher risk for rib fractures and more severe underlying lung contusions. Multiple rib fractures in elderly patients, in particular when accompanied by a flail chest, are associated with significant morbidity (atelectasis, pneumonia, respiratory failure) and mortality.[24,25] In those with multiple rib fractures and flail chest, age has been shown to be the strongest predictor of outcome and is directly proportional to mortality.[26] The elderly with thoracic trauma have twice the morbidity and mortality than younger patients with similar injuries. For each rib fractured, the risk of pneumonia increases by 27% and the risk of mortality by 19%.[27] There is also a complex relationship between age and the development of adult respiratory distress syndrome (ARDS) in older trauma patients. Johnston et al. demonstrated an increasingly higher risk of development of ARDS up to the 60- to 69-year-old age group, independent of the severity of trauma.[28]

## Central Nervous System

Normal aging is accompanied by progressive cortical atrophy with a reduction in cortical brain volume of approximately 15–20% between the fifth and tenth decades.[29] The volume in the frontal region, the temporoparietal region, and the parieto-occipital region all decrease with age. This is accompanied by an increase in the volume of cerebrospinal fluid in the lateral ventricles and in the third ventricle.[30] The brain in the elderly patient occupies only 82% of the cranial vault, as opposed to 92% in younger individuals.[31] Despite this, neuronal loss in the absence of neurodegenerative processes may be minimal.[32] There is normally a loss of brain weight of 6–11% in subjects over 80 years old.[33] Cerebral blood flow also decreases, but autoregulation is preserved. Cerebral oxygen consumption decreases with age, particularly in areas with decreased gray and white matter.[34]

In the elderly, the dura adheres tightly to the skull and the brain pulls away because of atrophy, thereby increasing the subdural space. In addition, the parasaggital and branching veins in the subdural space are under tension and are more susceptible to rupture.[35] Subdural hematomas (SDH) are three times more common than in the younger population. On the contrary, the epidural space is potentially eliminated which translates into a decreased risk of epidural hematoma (EDH).

In the elderly patient, the initial Glasgow Coma Scale (GCS) may be less reliable and may reflect chronic disease of the central nervous system or systemic disease. Determination of normal mental status in the elderly is often confounded by dementia or severe impairment of hearing. To compound this problem, baseline neurological status in many older individuals fluctuates over time. After admission to the hospital many elderly patients, even in the absence of pathology, can experience episodes of confusion, depression, delirium, and agitation.

In the geriatric population, significant traumatic brain injury (TBI) can result from apparently minor trauma. Any change in mental status in the elderly should prompt a thorough evaluation for TBI. The enlarged subdural space can accommodate more blood volume before the pressure volume curve is exceeded; therefore, these patients may be asymptomatic at the time of initial assessment.[36] Any history of trauma, even trivial (i.e., fall from standing height), should be taken seriously. When it does occur, injury to the underlying brain tissue is usually more severe. Elderly patients with isolated trauma to the brain have worse outcomes than younger patients at one year after trauma, despite what appears to be a less severe TBI on admission.[37]

## Renal System

Progressive sclerosis of the glomeruli occurs with normal aging. After the age of 40, there is a decrease in the number of functioning nephrons by 10% per decade while the remaining functional units hypertrophy. Between the ages of 30 and 85 there is a 20–25% decrease in renal mass mostly secondary to renal cortical loss, whereas the renal medulla maintains most of its volume.[38] From age 50 to 80, the weight of the kidneys progressively decreases from a mean of 250 g to 180 g. There is decreased renal filtering ability as measured by the glomerular filtration rate (GFR) by about 45%, typically declining by 0.75 to 1 milliliter per minute per year. This is not detected by a baseline evaluation of renal function because of a concomitant decrease in total muscle mass and production of creatinine. This decrease in renal function can be estimated by the Cockroft-Gault formula.[39]

Structural changes include a decrease in the length of renal tubules, thickening of the basement membranes, development of interstitial fibrosis, and atherosclerosis of the surrounding capillary bed. This leads to loss of effective secretion of solutes (potassium and hydrogen) and loss of resorption capacity (sodium) but, in a healthy elderly patient, serum sodium and potassium levels do not change significantly because of decreased muscle mass.

Geriatric patients have a diminished ability to concentrate urine because of decreased glomerular filtration rate and the frequent use of diuretics. The normal response to ADH and aldosterone is blunted, further impeding concentrating ability. The maximum concentrating ability of the kidney in an octogenarian is only 70% of the ability of the 30-year-old kidney.[40] As a result, urine output is less reliable as a surrogate for renal perfusion in elderly patients. Even dehydrated, elderly patients can maintain a deceptively normal urine output.

The gradual loss of nephrons and the diminished clearance of drugs put older patients at increased risk for volume and electrolyte abnormalities. They are at increased risk for the development of acute renal failure (ARF) following trauma. They also have a higher risk of developing volume overload and hyperchloremic metabolic acidosis following aggressive resuscitation with normal saline. Additionally, precautions must be taken with drugs excreted through the kidneys to prevent accumulation of toxic doses.

## Musculo–Skeletal System and Skin

Some of the more visible changes that come with aging involve the musculo–skeletal system. Older individuals undergo a progressive decrease in lean body mass by about 4% every 10 years after the age of 25. This increases to 10% after age 50 and is accompanied by an increase in the proportion of adipose tissue. The loss of muscle mass is proportional to the decrease in strength that accompanies aging.

Osteoporosis is a common feature of aging with loss of up to 60% of trabecular bone mass and 35% of the cortical bone mass.[36] This leads to an increased risk of fractures involving the vertebrae (compression fractures), hip, and distal forearm. At the level of the cartilages and joints, there is increasing density of the subchondral bone and formation of osteophytes accompanied by atrophy of the fibrocartilaginous and the synovial tissues. The end result is osteoarthritis and degenerative disorders affecting hips, knees, feet, and hands. The elderly experience increasing instability of joints and pain with ensuing impaired balance and mobility.[20]

The degenerative osseous changes associated with aging influence the site of injuries to the cervical spine. In younger individuals the most mobile segments are between C4 and C7, and, as a consequence, most fractures occur at this level. In older individuals, degenerative changes make these segments less mobile and the C1–C2 segment becomes the most mobile portion of the cervical spine. Studies indicate a high frequency of injury to the upper cervical spine, particularly odontoid fractures and injuries involving the atlantoaxial complex in elderly patients.[41] In this population, even falls from standing place the patient at risk for fracture so it is important to always maintain a high index of suspicion for injuries to the cervical spine, even in the presence of relatively minor trauma.[42] In the lower spine, trabecular bone loss leads typically to fractures of the anterior vertebral body with intact posterior elements. In this type of vertebral injury neurologic deficits are not frequent.

The skin atrophies with aging causing a loss of water, subcutaneous fat, and tonicity. The cutaneous microcirculation is impaired, as well. The skin is, therefore, more fragile and prone to breakdown in patients who are immobile after trauma.[43] For example, spinal boards used for transport can cause pressure ulcers within two hours and should be removed as soon as possible.

## Gastrointestinal System

Age-related changes involving the gastrointestinal tract are usually divided into the following three groups: changes involving neuromuscular function, changes involving secretion and absorption, and changes involving the bowel wall.[44] In the liver, enzyme activity per gram of hepatic tissue is virtually identical in the young and old, but there is a loss of hepatic mass by about 40% at age 80 resulting in decreased hepatic function in the elderly.[45,46]

The role of preexisting conditions of the gastrointestinal tract on trauma is less well researched than in other organ systems. The liver is the organ most frequently studied. In a case controlled study on trauma mortality, Morris documented the presence of cirrhosis to be associated with an odds ratio for mortality of 4.6. This was ahead of chronic obstructive pulmonary disease, ischemic heart disease, and diabetes mellitus.[8] In a retrospective study from the National Trauma Data Base (NTDB), McGwin and colleagues also documented preexisting hepatic disease to be associated with increased mortality in elderly trauma patients with less severe injuries.[7] Similarly, a study using the Pennsylvania State Trauma Data Bank showed that the preexisting condition with the strongest impact on mortality was hepatic disease.[47]

In the presence of trauma, the elderly are more likely to sustain injuries to the bowel and mesenteric infarction. The diagnosis may be more difficult because the clinical evaluation of the abdomen is less reliable. The elderly do not always manifest peritoneal signs and tend to localize pain poorly. Overall, gastrointestinal tract injuries in the elderly are associated with a three- to four-fold increase in mortality when compared to younger adults with similar injuries.[48]

## Metabolism, Nutrition, and the Immune System

The changes in the immune and endocrine systems that accompany aging are subtle, but have profound effects on the homeostatic mechanisms of the body. The solid lymphoid organs (liver, spleen, thymus) decrease in volume. The thymus at age 50 is only 15% of its original weight, mostly replaced by fat, though some functional thymic tissue remains until at least the sixth decade.[49] Cell mediated immunity is diminished with a decrease in peripheral T-cell count and function. The antibody response to stimuli is depressed, and this places the elderly at increased risk for infection.[50,51] In the presence of severe trauma, they may be more prone to the development of the multiple organ failure syndrome.

The thyroid gland undergoes fibrosis, cellular infiltration, and nodularity. There is a decrease in T3 secretion and a lower basal metabolic rate. Normal thermoregulatory mechanisms become less responsive. The two primary responses to cold stimuli (cutaneous vasoconstriction and shivering) are less effective, making the elderly more susceptible to hypothermia in cold environments.[52,53] Efforts aimed at preventing hypothermia in trauma patients are even more important in the elderly and must be started immediately upon admission.

Cortisol production remains relatively constant with age. Levels of dehydroepiandrosterone (DHEA) and dehydroepiandrosterone sulphate (DHEAS) decrease gradually, reaching only 10–20% of their maximum by the eighth decade.[54] The elderly are thus in a relative state of glucocorticoid excess with a negative impact on immune function and glucose metabolism. In the presence of trauma, the production of cortisol is further increased.[55] In addition, the elderly develop age-related glucose intolerance due to a combination of decreased secretion of insulin and increased resistance to insulin.[56]

Nutritional deficiencies in elderly trauma patients are common.[57] These deficiencies are multifactorial, resulting from a combination of poor intake and inadequate absorption. Nutritional support is essential in this population and affects length of stay and outcome.[58]

## PATTERNS OF INJURY

Elderly trauma patients frequently present with injuries similar to their younger counterparts though the mechanisms of injury may be different. In younger patients, assaults and motor vehicle crashes (MVC) are frequent causes of trauma. In the elderly, most injuries are the result of falls (falls accounted for 62% of all nonfatal elderly visits to the emergency department [ED] in 2001), followed by MVCs, automobile versus pedestrian collisions, assaults, and burns.[59,60] Hospital inpatient data from the Florida Agency for Healthcare Administration documented a precipitous rise in falls at the age of 65, peaking at age 75–84, and then declining somewhat (Table 47-3). The less active elderly are more likely to be injured as a result of activities of daily living (ADL), while the more active elderly have increased exposure to mechanisms of higher energy (e.g., motor vehicle collisions as compared to falls).

## Falls and Household Injuries

The most common mechanism of injury in the geriatric population is falls. One-third of individuals 65 years old and older living in the community and half of those living in institutions fall every year, and about half of those who fall do so repeatedly.[61,62] It is estimated that 6% of all medical expenditures in those over 65 go to the management of falls and related injuries.[63] The healthier and more active elderly sustain falls with mechanisms similar to younger individuals. They are more likely to fall from a greater height and have a higher number and severity of injuries. They represent the majority of the trauma center admissions in this age category.[64]

Studies from Finland have shown an increase in the absolute as well as the relative number of fall-induced injuries in the older population between 1970 and 1995. This was accompanied by an increase in fall-induced deaths in this population, which was greatest in the over 80 year-old category. In the United States, similar findings for fall-related deaths were observed from 1987–1996.[65] It is believed that comparable trends exist in other industrialized western countries with a predominantly white population, though there are no solid data to confirm this.[66] This increasing rate of falls is due to a proportional increase in the population of the older elderly (those greater than 75). The aging of the population and the prolonged survival of the older elderly produce more frail and ill individuals. Older elderly patients have a higher incidence of coexisting medical problems, poorer mobility and neuromuscular function, and more frequent use of medications (drugs and related substances) that can induce falls.[66] Young elderly patients (those from 65 to 75), on the other hand, benefit from improved health

### TABLE 47-3

**Mechanism of Injury In Patients ≥55 Years of Age Hospitalized in Florida, 2002–2004**

| AGE | 55–64 | 65–74 | 75–84 | 85+ | TOTAL |
|---|---|---|---|---|---|
| Number of injury patients | 27,661 | 34,699 | 62,137 | 51,204 | 175,701 |
| Incidence of injury by mechanism (%) | | | | | |
| Fall | 38 | 52 | 65 | 73 | 60 |
| Motor vehicle traffic crash | 13 | 8 | 4 | 2 | 6 |
| PHBC | 2 | 1 | <1 | <1 | <1 |
| Assault/abuse | 2 | <1 | <1 | <1 | <1 |

Data Source: With Permission from the Hospital Inpatient Data File, Florida Agency for Health Care Administration.

and functional capacity and, in turn, engage in activities that place them at a higher risk for falls.[66] Elderly victims of falls have a high injury rate (up to 71% in some studies), high admission rates (up to 57%), and prolonged hospitalizations (10 days or more in over 33% of patients admitted). The most common injuries are fractures (femoral neck, upper extremities, and pelvis), soft tissue injuries, and lacerations.[67]

Elderly patients who fall must undergo appropriate assessment and management of acute injuries. Once stabilized, these patients should have a thorough medical evaluation to determine the cause of the fall. Ideally, this assessment would begin with a preinjury appraisal of fall risk. The etiologies of falls are too numerous to be reviewed here, but they are divided into extrinsic factors related to the environment and intrinsic factors related to the patient. The intrinsic factors include age-associated changes in components of the sensory-neuromuscular systems related to balance, as well as pathology affecting any of these systems. The use and abuse of prescription and over-the-counter drugs, especially sedatives, is often considered an intrinsic factor.[68]

## Motor Vehicle Crashes (MVC)

Motor vehicle crashes are the second most common mechanism of injury in persons aged 65 and older. MVCs account for 28% of all injuries in this age group and represent the most common type of fatal event in the elderly through age 80. Unfortunately, older drivers are overrepresented among motor vehicle fatalities. In 2004, 141,000 older individuals were involved in traffic crashes, accounting for 5% of all injuries and 12–14% of all traffic fatalities.[69]

In general, older individuals drive less miles and their travel patterns are different than the rest of the population. They travel less at night and more on familiar roads with lower speed limits, yet they have a higher rate of MVC per mile driven and they are at increased risk for hospitalization and fatality. Drivers over 85 have a fatality rate that is seven to nine times that of younger drivers.[70,71] For similar injuries, older adults in general are five to six times more likely to die than their younger counterparts.[36] The older elderly drivers are the most at risk, with two-thirds of MVC-related deaths involving drivers 75 and older.[72]

There are multiple risk factors that account for MVCs in the older population. Older drivers can have a large blind spot due to decreased peripheral vision and limited cervical mobility. They have slower reaction times, poorer merging behavior (entering into traffic), and, frequently, have cognitive impairments and decreased hearing. Chronic medical conditions such as diabetes mellitus and heart disease can cause a dysrhythmia, syncope, stroke, or myocardial infarct that can precipitate an accident. These conditions require investigation and management along with the traumatic injuries. Alcohol plays a lesser role in MVCs involving the elderly, and older drivers have the lowest levels of intoxication.[69,73]

The general opinion is that the elderly are high-risk drivers, yet, in reality, drivers in their teens and twenties represent the highest risk on the road to themselves, their passengers, and other road users for fatal and nonfatal injuries.[72] When a death occurs, the probability that it is a traffic fatality for someone in their 20s is over 20%, while, at 65, it is less than 1% and, at 80, it is less than half a percent.[74]

## Pedestrians Hit by Automobiles (PHBC)

In 2003, National Highway Traffic Safety Administration (NHTSA) reported 4749 pedestrian traffic-related deaths and 7000 nonfatal injuries.[75] In 1998, pedestrian fatalities were the second leading cause of motor vehicle deaths and 13% of all motor vehicle-related deaths.[76] In fact, one pedestrian is killed in a traffic crash every 111 minutes and one pedestrian is injured in a traffic crash every eight minutes.[77] Pedestrians greater than 65 years old comprise 10% of the population, yet account for 21% of pedestrian fatalities and their death rate of 2.95 per 100,000 is the highest for any age group.[75,77,78] More than half of crashes occur at night when less than optimal visual acuity may play a role.[76] Substance abuse is also a problem with either the driver or pedestrian having measurable blood alcohol levels in almost half of all crashes.[77]

Haddon and colleagues performed the landmark study of pedestrian injury in 1961. They noticed an increased risk of pedestrian crashes and fatalities with increasing age and that those killed were 17 years older than those similarly exposed, but not killed (mean age killed 58.8 years vs. controls 41.6 years).[79] Since Haddon's landmark study, numerous other researchers have corroborated and added to our knowledge of pedestrian injury. It has been demonstrated that mortality in the elderly pedestrian increases with age and that the incidence of fractures, the need for admission to an intensive care unit (ICU) and ventilator support, and hospital stay all increased with age, as well.[80] Elderly patients have been found to be overrepresented in fatal cases with 37% of pedestrian fatalities in those greater than 65 years old. This suggested the risk was greater for elderly pedestrians who move slower and spend a longer time on the street and in traffic.[81] Some might expect that elderly individuals would adjust their behavior to compensate for these disabilities, but they may not be doing so. Older pedestrians often fail to recognize dangerous situations while walking.[82] This may be due to mental confusion or sensory changes (hearing and vision) associated with aging.[78,83] In addition, pedestrians commonly overestimate their actual visibility.[84]

A prospective population based study demonstrated that injured pedestrians were older (mean age 56 years) than injured car occupants (mean age 26 years). The median Injury Severity Score (ISS) for pedestrians was an astonishing 34 (ISS >15 is considered a severe life-threatening injury). Even once they arrived to the trauma center, mortality for occupants of a car was only 13% compared to 30% for pedestrians.[85]

There is a large body of evidence to suggest that elderly trauma patients, including pedestrians, have worse clinical outcomes than similarly injured younger patients. The mortality rate is higher for those >60 years old versus <60 years old with elderly patients much more likely to die (44.6% vs. 10.4%). Elderly pedestrians have higher hospital mortality (52.5% vs. 21.5%), thereby consuming extensive resources at the end of their lives. Pedestrians >65 years old had a mortality rate 2.6 to 5.7 times higher than younger pedestrians. It has been suggested that improved in-hospital care would decrease elderly mortality rates and that the elderly were dying of complications that younger pedestrians survive.[86] Similar studies have documented that people greater than 60 years old have a significantly higher risk of traffic-accident death than younger people for both passenger and pedestrian groups and that, while those age 65 or greater comprised only 8% of pedestrian cases, they had a mortality of 27.8%.[87] In addition, 78% of elderly pedestrians injured had at least temporary disability on discharge. The death rate per 100,000 in various age groups is shown in Fig. 47-1.

Attempts have been made to identify specific risk factors for elderly patients with pedestrian-type injuries. Apache score, intracranial hemorrhage with mass effect, and cardiac complications were found to be independent predictors of mortality.[88] Adult pedestrian injuries are more common in lower socioeconomic groups, consistent with the finding that socioeconomic status is often associated with health outcomes.[89] A study of crossing speeds in elderly pedestrians demonstrated that 27% were unable to reach the opposite curb before the light changed to allow cross traffic to enter the intersection, and one-fourth of this group were stranded by at least a full traffic lane away from safety.[90] Attempts to understand and modify the elements of the injury-producing sequence are important because the pedestrians who are most likely to be killed are often those who are the hardest to influence.

## Assault and Domestic Abuse

Violence is frequently viewed as a problem of the young. It is perceived as less of a public health concern in the elderly, yet there are little data to support this. Actually, violence is an increasing cause of injury in the elderly. In 2001, an estimated 33,026 persons over 60 years old were treated in EDs in the United States for nonfatal assault-related injuries (rate 72 per 100,000 population). The Department of Justice estimated that there were 165,000 lethal violent crimes a year against individuals 65 and older between 1992 and 1997 in the United States.[91] The majority of the injuries were contusions or abrasions (31.9%), lacerations (21.1%), and fractures (12.7%). Most patients were treated in the ED and released (91.3%), while only 8.3% required hospitalization.[92] In 2000, close to 1000 of these assaults resulted in a fatality.[93] In the United States, 5% of all homicides are committed against people age 65 and older.[94]

Abuse is another serious health concern in the geriatric population. The shocking images of abused children are ever too present in the media, yet abuse of elderly patients is frequently overlooked in the broader context of domestic violence. In the United States, it is believed that two million older adults are abused or mistreated every year.[95] In 1996, there were 551,011 documented cases of persons over the age of 60 who were victims of abuse, neglect, or self-neglect.[96] It is estimated that for every case reported, five cases go unreported for different reasons including guilt, embarrassment, distrust of law enforcement, or fear of retribution.[93,97] The overall incidence of abuse in elderly patients is estimated to be between

2 and 10%. The abuse can take on many forms including physical, emotional, sexual, and financial. This is a complex social phenomenon that will not be reviewed here in detail, except to note that abuse should always be considered when evaluating the older trauma patient. Injuries (fractures, contusions, bruises, head injuries, lacerations) related to falls and other mechanisms are frequently the result of abuse or mistreatment. Findings such as unexplained bruising or fractures or injuries with inconsistent mechanisms should raise suspicion and prompt an evaluation for abuse of the elderly patient. This is highlighted by the finding that elderly victims of abuse were three times more likely to die during a three-year period than those who did not experience abuse.[98]

## Penetrating Trauma

There are few studies of penetrating trauma in elderly individuals. Penetrating injuries represent 8–14% of injuries in the elderly population with the majority of these injuries being suicide.[99,100] Roth and colleagues demonstrated a clinically significant trend to longer lengths of stay in the ICU and in the hospital for older patients with penetrating injury, yet mortality rates were similar to their younger counterparts.[100] A similar study by Kimberly and colleagues also demonstrated that these patients did not have a greater rate of complications than younger patients.[99] Outcomes were generally good, with 87% of patients ultimately discharged to home, most without assistance. The data suggest that elderly patients do nearly as well as their younger counterparts with penetrating trauma and justifies aggressive efforts in the management of penetrating injuries in older patients despite age and preexisting conditions.

## Self-Inflicted Injury and Suicide

Suicide is the third leading cause of death from injury between the ages of 65 and 74.[1] In the population over 85 years old, the suicide rates are five-fold higher than in the general population. In 2000, the incidence of suicide in the general population was 10.7 per 100,000 people compared to the population over 65 where it was 15.3 per 100,000 people.[101] Elderly individuals have the highest rate of completed suicide (one in four) compared to the general population (one in 25), which is attributed to the lethality of the techniques used.[101] The most common mechanism for suicide in elderly individuals in the United States is the use of firearms in 73%, though geographical variations do exist such as a preference for fall from a height in some major cities where access to tall buildings is easy.[102,103]

**FIGURE 47-1.** PHBC death rates by age.
*(Reproduced with permission from Demetriades D, Murray J, Sinz B, et al.: Epidemiology of major trauma and trauma deaths in Los Angeles County. J Am Coll Surg 187:373, 1998.)*

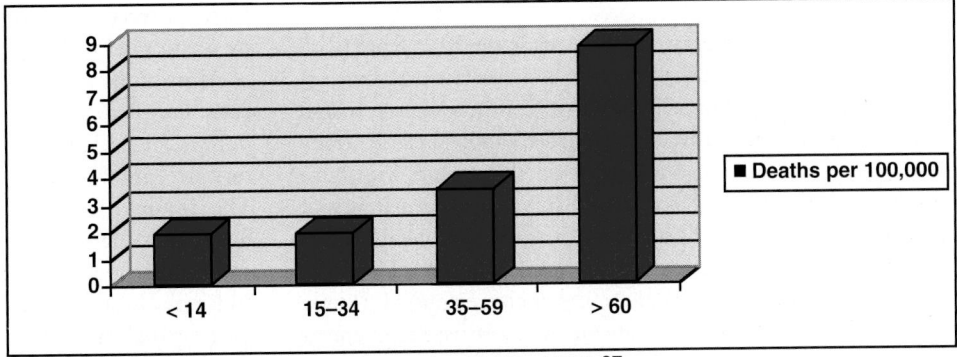

Data Adapted from Demetriades et al., JACS, 1998.[87]

The etiology of suicide in the elderly is multifactorial and not well understood.

Using the technique of "psychological autopsy," major depression and other mood disorders were documented in 60–90% of elderly suicide victims. Other important etiological factors are the role of physical illness and general poor health, the role of social isolation, loneliness and loss of a significant other, and the role of neurobiological factors such as lower concentrations of 5-hydroxyindoleacetic acid (HIAA) and homovanillic acid (HVA) in cerebrospinal fluid. Substance abuse plays a less important role than in younger populations.[104]

## Burns

Burn injuries comprise 8% of elderly trauma cases. Burns and fires represent the fifth leading cause of death from accidental injury in the population over 65 years old and accounted for a total of 500,000 ED visits in the United States in 2001.[105] The overwhelming majority of burns in the elderly population are due to domestic accidents (86–90%).[106,107] Flame burns are responsible for 50% of burn injuries, scalds account for 19%, and flammable liquids 10%. Chemical and electrical burns (about 1–2% each) are rare in this population.[106]

Many of these burns injuries are preventable, and 81% of burns in elderly individuals were a result of their own actions. These accidents are mostly due to neglected cigarettes or fires forgotten on the stove. Burn injuries involving occupational and recreational activities are much less common than in the younger population. Burn injuries in the elderly are frequently related to impaired judgment, limited mobility, or a combination of both. Impaired judgment may result from Alzheimer's disease or other forms of dementia. Occasionally, intoxication or mental illness may also play a role in the inaccurate evaluation of the threat of a situation. Limited mobility in an elderly individual can result in decreased reaction time and incapacity to quickly flee from danger. This causes prolonged exposure, deeper burn injuries, larger total body surface areas (TBSA) burned, and more severe injuries from smoke inhalation.[108] Thin, fragile skin and poor microcirculation in the elderly also contribute to deeper burn injuries. The more fragile skin has decreased ability to heal and leads to higher rates of wound infection when combined with the decreased ability to fight infection in the elderly.

Another important aspect of burn care is the fact that many elderly individuals live alone. Some cannot call for help while others, because of mental or physical incapacities, do not seek help in a timely fashion; therefore, the injury may progress significantly before treatment is started.[107]

Advances in modern burn care have made the Baux score (Risk of mortality = age in years + percent body surface area burned) less accurate, although burns in the elderly continue to carry a high risk of mortality.[109] Extensive burns in elderly individuals generally have a poor prognosis. In a review of elderly patients with burn injuries, no patient over 80 years old survived a burn injury of more than 40% total body surface area.[110] In fact, many studies show high mortality rate with lesser burns (10–39% TBSA).[108] This is important to consider in the management of elderly patients with burns. In some patients conservative management and comfort care are acceptable forms of treatment. In no way should the decision to withhold care or withdraw care be based solely on age. Age should be a consideration in the decision algorithm along with other factors such as preexisting medical conditions, the preinjury level of function, the presence of inhalation injury, and, if known, the patient's wishes. There is a need for research in this area to determine the role of early operative intervention and to help guide end-of-life decisions in this population.[111]

Discharge of elderly patients with burns must be well planned. For minor injuries, these individuals can frequently return to their previous level of function with assistance. For more extensive injuries, they might require rehabilitation and physical therapy or prolonged admission to skilled nursing facilities. A study of survivors of serious burns aged 59 or greater revealed that fewer than half were discharged to independent living, one-third to assisted living homes, and one-fifth to nursing facilities. For those who return home, an evaluation of home safety and environmental modifications are important to prevent repeat injuries.

Despite the limitations imposed by preexisting medical conditions, elderly burn victims are 58% less likely to die from their injuries as compared to the 1970s.[112] The main reasons for improved survival are the advances in burn care. As stated earlier, early excision of the burn wound and the standard of care in younger populations has had questionable success in the elderly.

## MANAGEMENT

### Triage Issues

Triage has been defined as the process of sorting patients based on their need for immediate medical treatment as compared to their chance of benefiting from such care (see Chap. 8). In short, triage attempts to maximize patient benefit based on available resources. This includes the initial triage from the field to the hospital, further triage within the hospital to a greater or lesser level of care, and, finally, the potential decision to withhold or withdraw care based on inability to achieve the desired outcome.

In *Resources for Optimal Care of the Injured Patient—2006* from the American College of Surgeons Committee on Trauma, it is suggested that patients greater than 55 years old should be considered for transport to a trauma center.[113] Unfortunately, exactly the opposite tends to occur. Several studies have documented that undertriage is much more common in patients over the ages of 55 and even worse for those over 65.[114–116] Clearly, better criteria and recognition of the importance of such criteria by prehospital and hospital providers is essential.

Most of the scoring systems (RTS, GCS, APACHE, etc.) have been shown to correlate with outcome in the geriatric population. More basic measures such as initial blood pressure, respiratory rate, and base deficit have also correlated well with outcome. The Trauma Score (TS) varies from 0 to 16 and contains the blood pressure, respiratory rate, respiratory effort, GCS score, and capillary refill and may be the most useful in the prehospital and early hospital setting as a triage tool. Several studies have documented the correlation between the TS (or Revised Trauma Score) on mortality in the geriatric population. A case-matched review of 100 elderly patients showed that no patient hospitalized

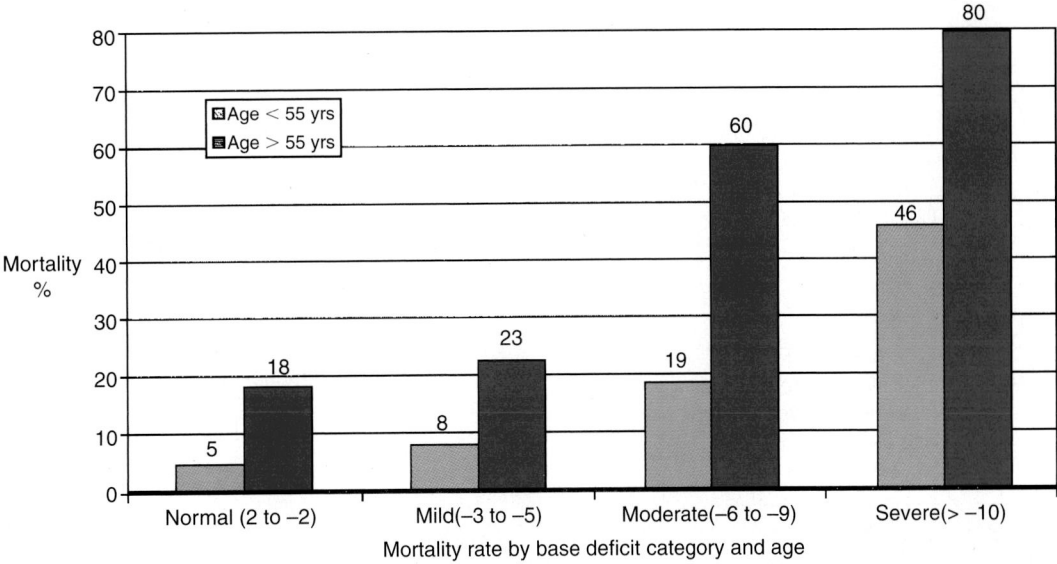

**FIGURE 47-2.** The mortality rate (y axis) in each base deficit category (x axis) by patient group, age <55 years and age ≥55 years. The difference in mortality between age groups at each base deficit category was significant ($p < 0.001$; ANOVA), and the increase in mortality with each successive base deficit category within age groups was significant as well ($p < 0.001$; ANOVA).
*(Reproduced with permission from Davis JW: J Trauma, 45: 873, 1998, with permission from Lippincott Williams & Wilkins.)*

with severe injuries survived with a TS <9 and no elderly patients with a TS <7 even survived to reach the hospital.[117] Another study of 852 elderly trauma patients also demonstrated a 100% mortality with a TS <7.[118] Similar correlations with the TS have been reported for elderly patients admitted to the ICU. While these population-based studies cannot be directly translated to individual patients, they may provide some guidance when counseling families about the expected outcomes and making end-of-life decisions.

As in the general trauma population, arterial base deficit has been correlated with mortality in the geriatric population, as well. In a study of elderly (>55) trauma patients those with a severe base deficit (–10 or worse) had an 80% mortality, those with a moderate (–6 to –9) base deficit had a 60% mortality, and those with a mild base deficit (–3 to –5) had a 23% mortality. Interestingly, even those with a normal base deficit (2 to –2) had a 18% mortality (Fig. 47-2).[119]

The ISS is a good predictor of survival in most trauma populations, and this most likely extends to the elderly population, as well. Unfortunately, it is not useful as a triage tool due to the delay in obtaining the data required to calculate the score. This leaves basic physiologic variables such as those contained in the TS and base deficit as the only possible predictors. Unfortunately, none of these markers is specific enough to make decisions on definitive care, although they may provide some guidance in the decision to start early aggressive care and monitoring as well as, once again, aid in the decisions at the end-of-life.

## Resuscitation and Invasive Monitoring

In addition to inaccurate triage, geriatric trauma patients are more likely to present in shock than younger patients matched for trauma and ISS.[120] For these patients the decision to start aggressive care and monitoring is less difficult. Otherwise, the decision to institute aggressive monitoring and resuscitation may be harder to determine.

Scalea and colleagues performed a study of 30 patients more than 65 years of age who presented with a pedestrian–motor vehicle mechanism, initial BP less than 150 mm Hg Hg, acidosis, multiple fractures, and head injuries. Patients meeting this criteria were treated with invasive hemodynamic monitoring including a pulmonary artery catheter and moved to the ICU as soon as possible. Hemodynamic parameters including cardiac index and oxygen consumption were optimized. There was a statistically significant difference in the ability to optimize cardiac output and systemic vascular resistance in survivors compared to nonsurvivors. All of the patients treated in this manner were hemodynamically stable upon initial presentation, yet 13 of 30 (43%) of patients were found to be in cardiogenic shock and 54% of these patients died.[16] This underscores the fact that geriatric trauma patients with significant underlying physiologic abnormalities may be difficult to identify early in the course of treatment and may be at greater risk for mortality.

McKinley and colleagues looked at the responses of old (≥65 years old) and young (<65 years old) trauma patients resuscitated using a standardized protocol to attain and maintain an oxygen delivery index of 600 mL/min/m$^2$ or greater (DO$_2$I ±600) for the first 24 hours in the ICU. Patients were selected if they were at high risk of postinjury multiple organ failure because one of the following was present: major organ or vascular injury and/or skeletal fractures, initial base deficit of 6 mEq/L or greater, need for six units or more of packed red blood cells in the first 12 hours, or age of 65 years or older with any two previous criteria. They used a pulmonary artery catheter, infusion of crystalloid solutions, transfusion of packed red blood cells, and moderate inotropic support as needed in that sequence, to attain a DO$_2$I ≥600. During the 19-month study period, 12 old patients and 54 young patients were resuscitated according to the protocol. For old patients, nine (75%) attained DO2I ≥600, and 11 (92%) survived seven or more days, and five (42%) 30 or more days. For young patients, 45 (83%) attained the DO$_2$I goal, and 48 (89%) survived 30 or more days. They concluded that although ultimate outcome is poorer than in the younger cohort, resuscitation is not futile.[121] This study is limited by the lack of a control group of elderly patients who were not resuscitated with the study protocol.

The only randomized trial of resuscitation in geriatric trauma patients studied 70 hip fracture patients. The control group received a central venous line and the treatment group received a

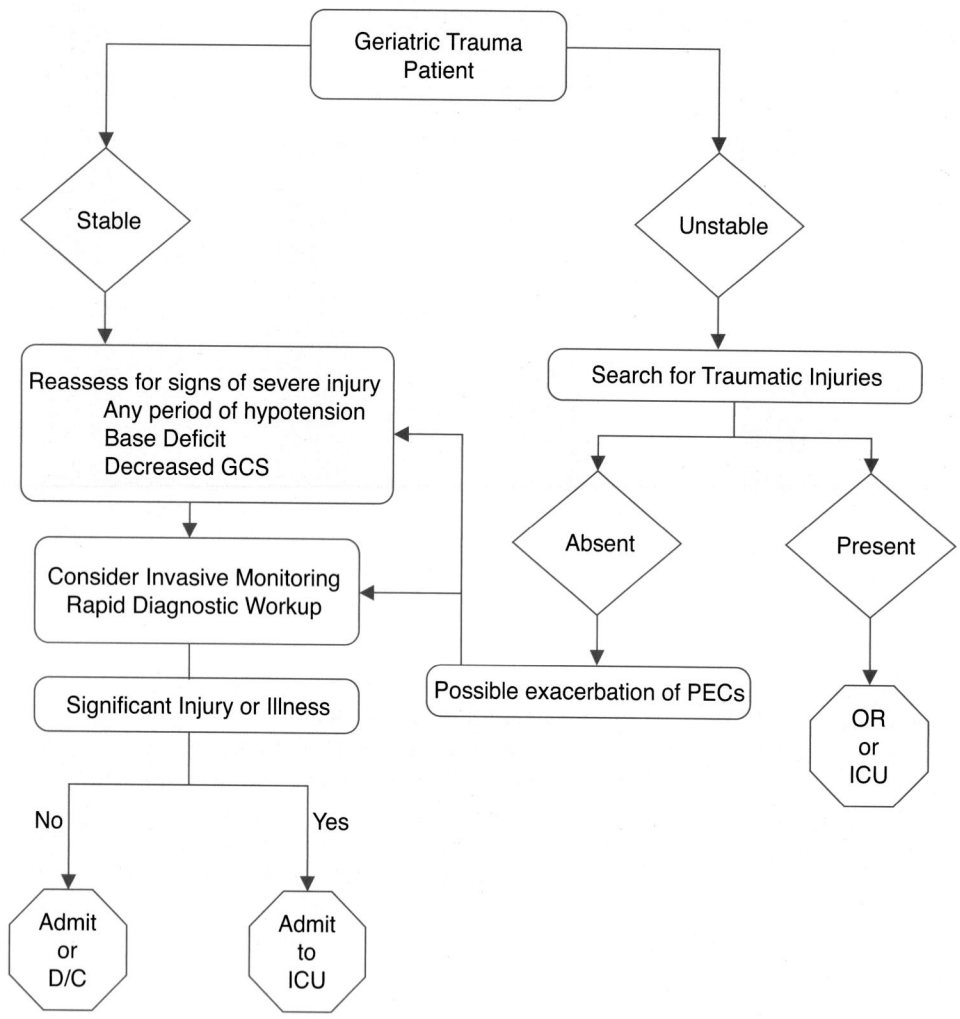

**FIGURE 47-3.**  Treatment algorithm.

pulmonary artery catheter. A significant increase in mortality was noted in the nonmonitored group (29% vs. 2.9%).[122] Unfortunately, the study did not include the multiply injured trauma patient, and the exact protocol by which patients were optimized with the use of the PA catheter is not clear.

The selection criteria for which elderly patients need aggressive resuscitation and monitoring have yet to be determined; however, the data using scoring systems for triage, the severity of the base deficit, and the presence of shock may provide some guidance. A trauma score <15, a base deficit of −6 or worse, or the presence of shock (SBP < 90) have all been associated with worse outcomes and may help identify patients who would benefit from aggressive resuscitation.[118,119,123,124] The important message is that a single criterion or an initial set of normal vital signs should not lull the practitioner into a false sense of security. Early, aggressive resuscitation and invasive monitoring may be warranted in a large number of elderly patients with injuries (Fig. 47-3).

## OUTCOMES

### At Present

The main question is whether age itself is a direct predictor of outcome in the seriously injured trauma patient. The literature is unclear on this question, mainly due to differences in age ranges studied, the heterogeneity of the populations studied, and the definition of a bad outcome. The latter includes poor functional outcome, in-hospital mortality, or anywhere from six-month to three-year long-term survival. Additionally, since age is a continuous variable, outcomes are likely to vary along a continuous spectrum and not vary drastically at specific age cut-offs.[125]

The largest study examined almost 200,000 trauma admissions in patients older than 15 years in California during 1986. Logistic regression showed ISS to be the best predictor of mortality (defined as in-hospital death), but also found that age, gender, and preexisting medical conditions were independent predictors of mortality. A more recent study of 448 patients suggested age was an independent predictor of both early (<24 hours) and late (>24 hours) mortality. For those greater than 65 years old, there was a 2.46-fold increased risk of early mortality and a 4.64-fold increased risk of late mortality.[126] There are, however, other studies which did not demonstrate a direct effect of age on mortality.[117,118] These studies may have been underpowered or utilized different criteria in performing their regression analysis. Likewise, it appears that once admitted to the ICU, elderly patients do not demonstrate a significantly worse in-hospital mortality compared to their younger counterparts, but there is a paucity of data on this particular subset of patients.

The long-term outcome of geriatric trauma patients has also been the subject of several studies with differing results. Most of the recent literature, however, suggests age may not be a good independent predictor of poor long-term outcome, defined generally as survival less than six months following hospital discharge.[127,128] Long-term outcome by itself may not be as important as long-term functional outcome. Again, multiple studies suggest that favorable long-term outcomes (defined as functioning independently at home) are achievable in the geriatric trauma population in up to 85% of cases.[127,129,130] The simple conclusion is that advanced age, by itself, may not be a good predictor of long-term outcome or function.

Perhaps, TBI in elderly patients deserves special mention. While the literature is far from conclusive, it is all supportive of the fact that outcomes for geriatric trauma patients with TBI are far worse than their younger counterparts. A TBI has been shown to increase mortality from 38% to 80% in one series and from 18% to 74% in another.[131,132] Similarly, low admission GCS has been correlated with poor outcome, although an exact cut-off has not been established. It appears, however, that elderly trauma patients have very poor outcomes when the admission GCS is ≤8.[125,133] In addition to worse mortality, elderly traumatic patients with a TBI have a worse functional outcome even though their injury to the brain and overall injuries are seemingly less severe than nonelderly patients.[134]

Based on existing evidence and the inability to definitively predict outcome for an individual geriatric trauma patient, it seems prudent to establish an aggressive approach to care for all. Subsequent clinical course and identification of other risk factors and poor prognostic characteristics may give some guidance for further care. If successful, it appears that outcome and long-term functional survival is reasonable and justifies the effort.

## Influence of Comorbidities

If age itself is not a good predictor of outcome, then perhaps the patients' functional status or "physiologic age" would be a better predictor. The presence of preexisting conditions is often used as a surrogate for this physiologic age. Morris and colleagues examined hospital discharge data for trauma patients in the state of California and found that preexisting conditions were important predictive factors of mortality independent of age.[6,8] A similar study of 8000 trauma patients demonstrated a threefold increase in mortality in patients with preexisting conditions, compared to those without preexisting conditions.[9] Both these authors did note, however, that the effect of preexisting conditions diminished with advancing age beyond 65 years, perhaps as chronological age begins to catch up with physiologic age.

In one review of 30,000 records in a state trauma database over a 13-year period, the overall mortality was 7.6% with an increase of 6.8% for each year over age 65. After controlling for initial vital signs, GCS score and ISS, preexisting conditions were still found to have an independent effect on mortality. The strongest effects were seen for hepatic disease (odds ratio 5.1), renal disease (odds ratio 3.1), and cancer (odds ratio 1.8) (Table 47-4). Interestingly, warfarin therapy was not an independent predictor of mortality.[47]

## Ability to Influence Outcome

Clearly, the ability to influence outcomes relies on the ability to identify those patients in need of a higher level of care. As discussed

**TABLE 47-4**

### Conditional Odds Ratios for Effect of Pre-existing Conditions (PECSs) On Mortality in Geriatric Trauma (N = 33,781)

| VARIABLE | ODDS RATIO | UCL | LCL |
|---|---|---|---|
| Dementia | 0.726 | 0.584 | 0.896 |
| Neurologic | 1.06 | 0.887 | 1.26 |
| Cardiac | 0.951 | 0.848 | 1.06 |
| CHF | 1.74 | 1.46 | 2.08 |
| Diabetes (IDDM) | 1.04 | 0.788 | 1.36 |
| Diabetes (NIDDM) | 1.05 | 0.861 | 1.28 |
| Gastrointestinal | 1.14 | 0.860 | 1.48 |
| Hematologic | 1.22 | 0.960 | 1.53 |
| Coumadin | 1.21 | 0.932 | 1.55 |
| Psychiatric | 0.848 | 0.654 | 1.09 |
| Immunocompromise | 2.05 | 0.940 | 4.13 |
| Steroids | 1.59 | 1.03 | 2.40 |
| Liver disease | 5.11 | 3.09 | 8.21 |
| Cancer | 1.84 | 1.37 | 2.45 |
| Arthritis | 0.868 | 0.524 | 1.37 |
| Obesity | 0.704 | 0.469 | 1.03 |
| Drug abuse | 0.318 | 0.017 | 1.66 |
| Alcohol abuse | 0.993 | 0.718 | 1.35 |
| Pulmonary | 1.06 | 0.770 | 1.43 |
| COPD | 1.49 | 1.22 | 1.80 |
| Renal | 3.12 | 2.25 | 4.28 |

UCL upper confidence limit; LCL, lower confidence limit; CHF, congestive heart failure; IDDM, insulin-dependent diabetes mellitus; NIDDM, non-insulin-dependent diabetes millitus; COPD, chronic obstructive pulmonary disease.

*(Reproduced with permission from Grossman MD: J Trauma, 52:242, 2002; with permission from Lippincott Williams & Wilkins.)*

previously, markers such as a low Trauma Score, base deficit, or initial blood pressure can be used to identify this subgroup of injured elderly patients. Some studies have documented the triage bias that exists leading to elderly patients being mistriaged to nontrauma center facilities. Recent evidence clearly suggests that outcomes are better for all age groups, including the elderly, when they are appropriately triaged and treated at trauma centers.[135,136]

After arrival at the hospital, Demetriades and colleagues have shown that a heightened level of alertness may lead to better outcomes for geriatric trauma patients. They changed their protocol for trauma team activation to include all patients ≥70 years old. In addition there was "liberal" use of noninvasive and invasive monitoring in these patients, although a specific protocol was not followed. A subsequent review of their trauma registry before and after the age criterion was implemented documented that mortality was reduced from 53.8% to 34.2% (p = 0.003) with a relative risk of 1.57 (95% CI 1.13 to 2.19). In those patients with an ISS greater than 20, the mortality decreased from 68.4% to 46.9% (p = 0.01) with a relative risk of 1.46 (95% CI 1.06 to 2.00).[137]

The ultimate ability to influence outcome lies in the reduction of injuries. Injury prevention has proven to be successful for a wide variety of traumatic injuries. Since the majority of elderly injuries result from falls, this has been the most studied area. Many methods and programs already exist and have been proven effective in elderly populations. Some examples include regular exercise, supplementation of vitamin D and calcium, withdrawal of psychotropic medication, cataract surgery, professional assessment and modification of environmental hazards, hip protectors, and multifactorial prevention programs.[138] It is worthwhile for the trauma surgeon to be aware of such programs and serve as a source of information, referral, and, perhaps, even program implementation in high-need, underserved areas.

## COSTS OF INJURY AND CARE

Unintentional injury is the leading cause of years of potential life lost before the age of 65 and remains the third leading cause for those under age 85.[139] The landmark report *Cost of Injury in the United States: A Report to Congress*, published in 1989, highlighted for the first time the tremendous financial burden of injury in the United States. For the 57 million persons injured in 1985, the cost amounted to $157.6 billion, or $2772 per injured person. Premature death due to injury is extremely costly to the nation, amounting to an estimated annual loss of 5.3 million life years, or 34 years per death. The loss to the economy amounted to $47.9 billion or $307,636 per death. For the direct costs of injury, the 25–44 age group ranked highest (28%), followed by those 65 years and over (24%). The high direct cost for injured elderly patients reflects the large number of falls leading to long stays in hospitals and nursing homes.[140]

Several studies have demonstrated the increased cost for a given injury severity in the elderly patient as compared to a younger patient. A 1988 study by DeMaria and colleagues of elderly patients with injuries documented that mean hospital costs dramatically exceeded mean projected reimbursement in patients over the age of 80 ($18,197 ± 3,682 vs. $7,069 ± 700; $p < 0.001$), in patients with severe overall injury ($18,992 ± 3,540 vs. $8,508 ± 643; $p < 0.001$), and in patients with more than one complication ($25,504 ± 3,959 vs. $7,247 ± 626; $p < 0.001$). Hospital costs were also increased in elderly patients discharged to a nursing home ($22,811 ± 3,664) primarily as a result of a prolonged hospital stay. The daily cost for trauma care in elderly patients who died was a staggering $1735 ± 366, reflecting the aggressive care given these patients.[141]

Another study in1988 noted that length of stay and gross financial charges were found to be significantly associated with age and TS. Daily charges were associated with length of stay and TS, while rates of reimbursement were inversely associated with age and length of stay.[142]

Ross and colleagues compared charges in a group of 60 elderly patients and a group of 60 younger patients admitted to the hospital. The older group had an average hospital charge of $15,769.55 more

than the younger group, partly due to a longer hospital length of stay.[143] On the contrary, Sartorelli and colleagues compared pediatric versus geriatric costs and reimbursements in a Level I trauma center. They found the Reimbursement Ratio (RR = reimbursement/cost; RR > 1 = profit, RR < 1 = loss) for geriatric patients (age > 64, RR = 0.99) was significantly lower than for pediatric patients (age < 17, RR = 1.15) and adult patients (age 17–64, RR = 1.16). Cost per patient and length of stay were less in pediatric versus adult and geriatric patients ($p < 0.05$), suggesting reimbursement for trauma care in elderly patients is inadequate, whereas pediatric trauma care costs less to deliver and is profitable to the trauma center.[144]

Young and colleagues examined the differences in outcome and cost between elderly and younger patients and the financial burden imposed by care for elderly patients after trauma. Medicare, the single-payer insurance plan for elderly individuals, reimburses at a lower rate than standard private insurance carriers. Only 2% of elderly patients were uninsured (76% were insured by Medicare), whereas 25% of younger patients were uninsured. Medicare reimbursement rates actually exceeded those of all other carriers (114% of costs). As injury severity increased, profit per case increased in the elderly and decreased in the younger group. The per capita cost of hospital care for the elderly patient was lower than for younger patients, whereas reimbursement was higher, primarily because 98% of elderly patients were insured.[145] Therefore, care of the elderly trauma patient may be financially sound in areas where there is a high rate of uninsured trauma patients.

A more recent study of hospital discharge records in ten European countries demonstrated that costs per capita increase exponentially in older age groups (age ≥ 65 years) due to the combined effect of high incidence and high costs per patient. Elderly patients aged 65 years and older, especially women, consume a disproportionate share of hospital resources for trauma care (Fig. 47-4), mainly caused by hip fractures and fractures of the knee/lower leg, which indicates the importance of prevention and investing in trauma care for this specific patient group.[146]

## WITHHOLDING CARE

The combination of age, injury severity, and underlying disease makes even the most advanced modern medical care futile for certain patients. This, however, is a very individualized decision. Some patients and families might consider a 1% chance of any type of

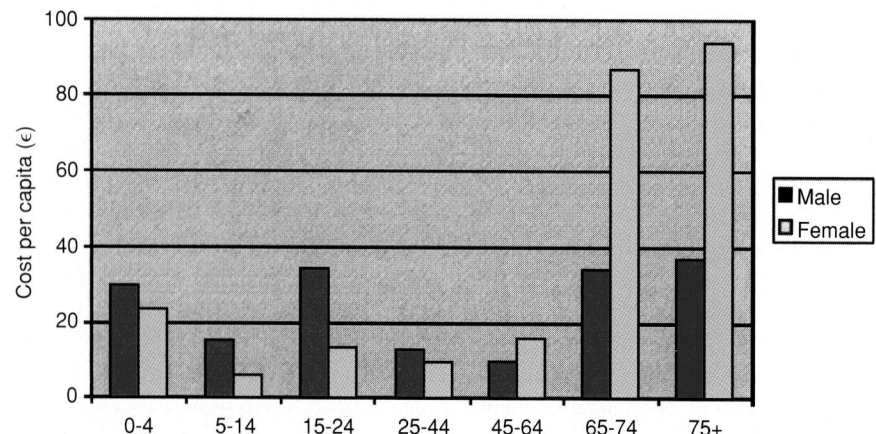

**FIGURE 47-4.** Hospital cost per capita ([Euro sign]) for admitted injury patients by age and sex for the EUROCOST countries.
*(Reproduced with permission from Polinder S: J Trauma 59:1283, 2005; with permission from Lippincott Williams & Wilkins.)*

survival (i.e., even a poor functional outcome) acceptable and desire all possible medical efforts. Patients who cannot reasonably be expected to maintain their quality of life as the result of severe injuries may not wish to continue with possible life-saving treatment. While no prospective trial will ever be done to definitively identify the criteria by which care should be withheld, there are several studies which attempt to provide some insight.

A review of the NTDB by Nirula and Gentilello is the largest and most recent attempt to provide criteria for the futility of resuscitation in elderly trauma patients. Moreover, they stratified the patients into "young" old (65–74 years) and "old" old (75–84 years). A multiple regression analysis of over 76,000 records was performed to identify predictors of a 95% probability of death. This was the authors' cutoff to determine a futile effort and is, of course, subject to controversy and individual interpretation. The strongest anatomic injury predictors of mortality were injuries to the brain, chest, and abdomen ($p < 0.001$ for all), while the strongest physiologic predictors of mortality were worsening base deficit and systolic blood pressure less

than 90. In the 65–74 year-old age group, only hypotensive patients admitted with a severe thoracic and/or abdominal injury who also had severe injuries to the brain (AIS $\geq$ 4) or profound shock (BD $\leq$ −12) had a less than 5% chance of survival. For those aged 75 to 84, even moderate injury to the brain (AIS $\leq$ 3) and moderate shock (BD $\leq$ −6) were associated with a less than 5% chance of survival (Fig. 47-5). Finally, for those age 85 or older, profound shock or the combination of moderate shock and moderate injury to the head was associated with a less than 5% chance of survival.[147]

## CONCLUSION

Trauma in geriatric patients remains a significant cause of morbidity and mortality. Practitioners need to be aware of the anatomic, physiologic, and mechanistic differences encountered in this population. The effects of preexisting medical conditions place the elderly patient at increased risk and make it difficult for them to compensate in the face of injury. In addition, geriatric trauma patients may have atypical presentations making diagnosis more difficult and challenging.

Falls and motor vehicle collisions remain the leading injury mechanisms in the geriatric population, yet pedestrian injuries lead to the greatest mortality. Suicide is also a common cause of mortality, and depression is the leading etiology. Elder abuse must also be suspected in patients with unexplained findings.

These differences place the geriatric trauma patient at increased risk for complications such as infection and mortality. A heightened level of suspicion, starting with appropriate triage to a trauma center and continuing throughout the spectrum of care is the only way to avoid poor outcomes. A TS <15, a base deficit of –6 or worse, or the presence of shock (SBP < 90) have all been associated with worse outcomes and may help identify patients who would benefit from aggressive resuscitation. It does appear, however, that those patients who do survive have an acceptable quality of life, justifying aggressive treatment in all but the most severely injured patients (Table 47-5).

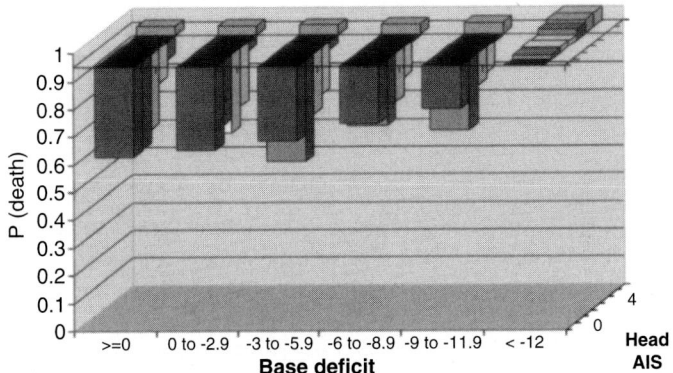

**A**

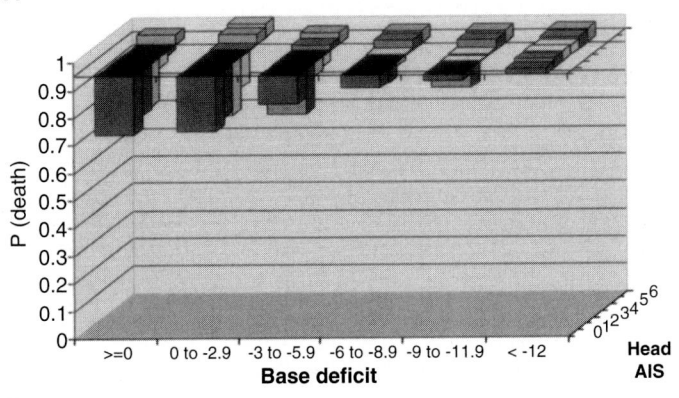

**B**

**FIGURE 47-5.** Probability of death among patients aged 65 to 74 years (**A**) and 75 to 84 years (**B**) with chest and/or abdominal AIS score >3 and admission SBP < 90 mmHg, stratified by base deficit and head AIS score. A 95% plane emphasizes those groups of patients whose probability of survival is low. Those categories where the bars are above the 95% plane have a probability of survival of less than 5%. For those aged 65 to 74 years, only patients with profound shock or severe head injury have a less than 5% probability of death. For those aged 75–84, patients with even mild shock and moderate to severe head injury have less than a 5% chance of survival. Blue head, AIS score of 0; purple head, AIS score of 1; cream head, AIS score of 2; yellow head, AIS score of 3; red head, AIS score of 4; green head, AIS score of 5; and orange head, AIS score of 6.
*(Reproduced with permission from Nirula R: J Trauma, 57:37–41, 2004; with permission from Lippincott Williams & Wilkins.)*

**TABLE 47-5**

| Highlights in Management |
|---|
| Patients greater than 55 years old should be considered for transport to a trauma center |
| Geriatric trauma patients are more likely to present in shock than younger patients |
| A trauma score < 15, a base deficit of –6 or worse, or the presence of shock (SBP< 90) have all been associated with worse outcomes and may help identify patients who would benefit from aggressive resuscitation |
| Significant underlying physiologic abnormalities may be difficult to identify |
| Older trauma patients do not respond to hypovolemia as do their younger counterparts |
| Findings such as unexplained bruising or fractures or injuries with inconsistent mechanisms should raise suspicion and prompt an evaluation for elder abuse |
| Appropriate recognition and treatment requires a high index of suspicion to maintained at all times |
| Early, aggressive resuscitation and invasive monitoring may be warranted in a large number of cases |
| Heightened level of alertness may lead to better outcomes for geriatric trauma patients |

# REFERENCES

1. CDC: *10 Leading Causes of Death*, United States. Vol. 2006: National Center for Injury Prevention and Control, 2002.
2. CDC: *All Injury Deaths and Rates per 100,000*. Vol. 2006: National Center for Injury Prevention and Control, 2002.
3. Gist Y, Hetzel L: *We the People: Aging in the United States*. US Census Bureau, 2004.
4. Hetzel L, Smith A: *The 65 Years and Over Population: 2000*. US Census Bureau, 2001.
5. Champion HR, Copes WS, Buyer D, et al.: Major trauma in geriatric patients. *Am J Public Health* 79:1278, 1989.
6. Morris JA Jr, MacKenzie EJ, Damiano AM, et al.: Mortality in trauma patients: The interaction between host factors and severity. *J Trauma* 30:1476, 1990.
7. McGwin G Jr, MacLennan PA, Fife JB, et al.: Preexisting conditions and mortality in older trauma patients. *J Trauma* 56:1291, 2004.
8. Morris JA Jr, MacKenzie EJ, Edelstein SL: The effect of preexisting conditions on mortality in trauma patients. *JAMA* 263:1942, 1990.
9. Milzman DP, Boulanger BR, Rodriguez A, et al.: Pre-existing disease in trauma patients: A predictor of fate independent of age and injury severity score. *J Trauma* 32:236, 1992; discussion 243.
10. Bergeron E, Rossignol M, Osler T, et al.: Improving the TRISS methodology by restructuring age categories and adding comorbidities. *J Trauma* 56:760, 2004.
11. Hannan EL, Waller CH, Farrell LS, et al.: Elderly trauma inpatients in New York state: 1994–1998. *J Trauma* 56:1297, 2004.
12. Scalea T: Invited Commentary (for MacMahon et al.: Co-morbidity and Trauma in the Elderly). *World J Surgery* 20:119, 1996.
13. Lakatta EG: Age-associated cardiovascular changes in health: Impact on cardiovascular disease in older persons. *Heart Fail Rev* 7:29, 2002.
14. Lakatta EG, Levy D: Arterial and cardiac aging: major shareholders in cardiovascular disease enterprises: Part II: The aging heart in health: links to heart disease. *Circulation* 107:346, 2003.
15. Westerhof N, O'Rourke MF: Haemodynamic basis for the development of left ventricular failure in systolic hypertension and for its logical therapy. *J Hypertens* 13:943, 1995.
16. Scalea TM, Simon HM, Duncan AO, et al.: Geriatric blunt multiple trauma: Improved survival with early invasive monitoring. *J Trauma* 30:129, 1990; discussion 134–136.
17. Gallagher SF, Williams B, Gomez C, et al.: The role of cardiac morbidity in short- and long-term mortality in injured older patients who survive initial resuscitation. *Am J Surg* 185:131, 2003.
18. Carpo RO CE: Aging of the respiratory system. In Fisherman, ed. *Pulmonary Diseases and Disorders*. New York, NY: McGraw-Hill, 1998, p. 251.
19. Oskvig RM: Special problems in the elderly. *Chest* 115:158S, 1999.
20. Russel R: *The Liverpool Hospital Trauma Manual, Ch. 8, Special Situations: The Elderly*. 6th ed. Sydney, Australia: Trauma Department Liverpool Hospital 2002, p. 269.
21. Chen HI, Kuo CS: Relationship between respiratory muscle function and age, sex, and other factors. *J Appl Physiol* 66:943, 1989.
22. Chan ED, Welsh CH: Geriatric respiratory medicine. *Chest* 114:1704, 1998.
23. Young L, Ahmad H: Trauma in the elderly: A new epidemic? *Aust N Z J Surg* 69:584, 1999.
24. Stawicki SP, Grossman MD, Hoey BA, et al.: Rib fractures in the elderly: A marker of injury severity. *J Am Geriatr Soc* 52:805, 2004.
25. Alexander JQ, Gutierrez CJ, Mariano MC, et al.: Blunt chest trauma in the elderly patient: How cardiopulmonary disease affects outcome. *Am Surg* 66:855, 2000.
26. Albaugh G, Kann B, Puc MM, et al.: Age-adjusted outcomes in traumatic flail chest injuries in the elderly. *Am Surg* 66:978, 2000.
27. Bulger EM, Arneson MA, Mock CN, et al.: Rib fractures in the elderly. *J Trauma* 48:1040, 2000; discussion 1046–1047.
28. Johnston CJ, Rubenfeld GD, Hudson LD: Effect of age on the development of ARDS in trauma patients. *Chest* 124:653, 2003.
29. Mouton PR, Martin LJ, Calhoun ME, et al.: Cognitive decline strongly correlates with cortical atrophy in Alzheimer's dementia. *Neurobiol Aging* 19:371, 1998.
30. Coffey CE, Saxton JA, Ratcliff G, et al.: Relation of education to brain size in normal aging: Implications for the reserve hypothesis. *Neurology* 53:189, 1999.
31. Feldman M: Aging changes in the morphology of cortical dendrites. In Terry RD, Gershon S, ed. *Neurobiology of Aging*. New York, NY: Raven Press, 1976.
32. Terry RD, DeTeresa R, Hansen LA: Neocortical cell counts in normal human adult aging. *Ann Neurol* 21:530, 1987.
33. DelaTorre J, Fay L: *Effects of Aging on the Human Nervous System*. New York, NY: Springer-Verlag, 2001.
34. Yam AT, Lang EW, Lagopoulos J, et al.: Cerebral autoregulation and ageing. *J Clin Neurosci* 12:643, 2005.
35. Cagetti B, Cossu M, Pau A, et al.: The outcome from acute subdural and epidural intracranial haematomas in very elderly patients. *Br J Neurosurg* 6:227, 1992.
36. Mandavia D, Newton K: Geriatric trauma. *Emerg Med Clin North Am* 16:257, 1998.
37. Livingston DH, Lavery RF, Mosenthal AC, et al.: Recovery at one year following isolated traumatic brain injury: A Western trauma association prospective multicenter trial. *J Trauma* 59:1298, (discussion 1304), 2005.
38. Beck LH: The aging kidney. Defending a delicate balance of fluid and electrolytes. *Geriatrics* 55:26, 2000.
39. Cockcroft DW, Gault MH: Prediction of creatinine clearance from serum creatinine. *Nephron* 16:31, 1976.
40. Bell R: Trauma in the Elderly: More than just age. *Sydney South West Area Health Service News Letter* 3: 1998. www.swahs.nsw.gov.au/livtrauma/educationnewsletters/mar98.asp.
41. Lowery DW, Wald MM, Browne BJ, et al.: Epidemiology of cervical spine injury victims. *Ann Emerg Med* 38:12, 2001.
42. Spivak JM, Weiss MA, Cotler JM, et al.: Cervical spine injuries in patients 65 and older. *Spine* 19:2302, 1994.
43. Goode P, Allman R: Pressure Ulcers. In Duthie EH, ed. *Practice of Geriatrics*. Philadelphia, PA: W B Saunders, 1998, p. 228.
44. Aalami OO, Fang TD, Song HM, et al.: Physiological features of aging persons. *Arch Surg* 138:1068, 2003.
45. Woodhouse KW, Mutch E, Williams FM, et al.: The effect of age on pathways of drug metabolism in human liver. *Age Ageing* 13:328, 1984.
46. Kampman KW SJ, Moller-Jorgensen I: Effect of Agind on liver function. *Geriatrics* 30:91, 1975.
47. Grossman MD, Miller D, Scaff DW, Arcona S: When is an elder old? Effect of preexisting conditions on mortality in geriatric trauma. *J Trauma* 52:242, 2002.
48. Schwab CW, Kauder DR: Trauma in the geriatric patient. *Arch Surg* 127:701, 1992.
49. Haynes BF, Markert ML, Sempowski GD, et al.: The role of the thymus in immune reconstitution in aging, bone marrow transplantation, and HIV-1 infection. *Annu Rev Immunol* 18:529, 2000.
50. Gavazzi G, Krause KH: Ageing and infection. *Lancet Infect Dis* 2:659, 2002.
51. High KP: Infection as a cause of age-related morbidity and mortality. *Ageing Res Rev* 3:1, 2004.
52. Wagner JA, Robinson S, Marino RP: Age and temperature regulation of humans in neutral and cold environments. *J Appl Physiol* 37:562, 1974.
53. Inoue Y, Nakao M, Araki T, et al.: Thermoregulatory responses of young and older men to cold exposure. *Eur J Appl Physiol Occup Physiol* 65:492, 1992.
54. Ferrari E, Cravello L, Muzzoni B, et al.: Age-related changes of the hypothalamic-pituitary-adrenal axis: pathophysiological correlates. *Eur J Endocrinol* 144:319, 2001.
55. Butcher SK, Lord JM: Stress responses and innate immunity: Aging as a contributory factor. *Aging Cell* 3:151, 2004.
56. Scheen A: Diabetes mellitus in the elderly: Insulin resistance and/or impaired insulin secretion? *Diabetes Metab* 31:27, 2005.
57. Demling RH: The incidence and impact of pre-existing protein energy malnutrition on outcome in the elderly burn patient population. *J Burn Care Rehabil* 26:94, 2005.
58. Avenell A, Handoll HH: Nutritional supplementation for hip fracture aftercare in the elderly. *Cochrane Database Syst Rev* 1:CD001880, 2004.
59. Kocher K, Dellinger A: Nonfatal injuries among older adults treated in hospital emergency departments-United States, 2001. *MMWR Morb Mortal Wkly Rep* 52:1019, 2003.
60. Spaite DW, Criss EA, Valenzuela TD, et al.: Geriatric injury: An analysis of prehospital demographics, mechanisms, and patterns. *Ann Emerg Med* 19:1418, 1990.
61. Rubenstein LZ, Josephson KR, Robbins AS: Falls in the nursing home. *Ann Intern Med* 121:442, 1994.
62. Tinetti ME, Speechley M: Prevention of falls among the elderly. *N Engl J Med* 320:1055, 1989.
63. Guideline for the prevention of falls in older persons. American Geriatrics Society, British Geriatrics Society, and American Academy of Orthopaedic Surgeons Panel on Falls Prevention. *J Am Geriatr Soc* 49:664, 2001.
64. Nevitt MC, Cummings SR, Kidd S, et al.: Risk factors for recurrent nonsyncopal falls. A prospective study. *Jama* 261:2663, 1989.
65. Stevens JA, Hasbrouck LM, Durant TM, et al.: Surveillance for injuries and violence among older adults. *MMWR Morb Mortal Wkly Rep CDC Surveill Summ* 48:27, 1999.
66. Kannus P, Parkkari J, Koskinen S, et al.: Fall-induced injuries and deaths among older adults. *Jama* 281:1895, 1999.
67. Bell AJ, Talbot-Stern JK, Hennessy A: Characteristics and outcomes of older patients presenting to the emergency department after a fall: A retrospective analysis. *Med J Aust* 173:179, 2000.
68. Hill K, Schwarz J: Assessment and management of falls in older people. *Intern Med J* 34:557, 2004.
69. NHTSA: *Traffic Safety Facts 2004. Pedestrians/Older Population*. National Highway Traffic Safety Administration, 2004.

70. NHTSA: *Traffic Safety Facts 2000. Older Population*. National Highway Traffic Safety Administration, 2001.

71. Cook LJ, Knight S, Olson LM, et al.: Motor vehicle crash characteristics and medical outcomes among older drivers in Utah, 1992–1995. *Ann Emerg Med* 35:585, 2000.

72. Braver ER, Trempel RE: Are older drivers actually at higher risk of involvement in collisions resulting in deaths or non-fatal injuries among their passengers and other road users? *Inj Prev* 10:27, 2004.

73. Rehm CG, Ross SE: Elderly drivers involved in road crashes: A profile. *Am Surg* 61:435, 1995.

74. Evans L: Risks older drivers face themselves and threats they pose to other road users. *Int J Epidemiol* 29:315, 2000.

75. Gower BA, Nagy TR, Goran MI, et al.: Leptin in postmenopausal women: Influence of hormone therapy, insulin, and fat distribution. *J Clin Endocrinol Metab* 85:1770, 2000.

76. Butler JC, Schuchat A: Epidemiology of pneumococcal infections in the elderly. *Drugs Aging* 15:11, 1999.

77. *NHTSA Traffic Safety Facts, 1998: Pedestrians.*, Vol. 2000. Washington, D.C.: National Highway Traffic Safety Administration, 1999. DOT HS 808 958., 1998.

78. Aronson SC, Nakabayashi K, Siegel M, et al.: Traffic fatalities in Rhode Island: Part IV. The pedestrian victim. *R I Med J* 67:485, 1984.

79. Haddon W, Valien P, McCarroll J, et al.: A controlled investigation of the characteristics of adult pedestrians fatally injured by motor vehicles in manhattan. *J Chron Dis* 14:655, 1961.

80. Brainard BJ, Slauterbeck J, Benjamin JB, et al.: Injury profiles in pedestrian motor vehicle trauma. *Ann Emerg Med* 18:881, 1989.

81. Lane PL, McClafferty KJ, Nowak ES: Pedestrians in real world collisions. *J Trauma* 36:231, 1994.

82. Jonah B, Engel G: Measuring the relative risk of pedestrian accidents. *Accid Anal Prev* 15:193, 1983.

83. Ferrera PC, Bartfield JM, D'Andrea CC: Outcomes of admitted geriatric trauma victims. *Am J Emerg Med* 18:575, 2000.

84. Allen M, Hazlett P, Tacker H: Actual pedestrian visibility and the pedestrian's estimate of his own visibility. Proceedings of the American Association for Automotive Medicine, Thirteenth Annual Conference 1969: p. 293.

85. Hill DA, Delaney LM, Duflou J: A population-based study of outcome after injury to car occupants and to pedestrians. *J Trauma* 40:351, 1996.

86. Sklar DP, Demarest GB, McFeeley P: Increased pedestrian mortality among the elderly. *Am J Emerg Med* 7:387, 1989.

87. Demetriades D, Murray J, Sinz B, et al.: Epidemiology of major trauma and trauma deaths in Los Angeles County. *J Am Coll Surg* 187:373, 1998.

88. Hui T, Avital I, Soukiasian H, et al.: Intensive care unit outcome of vehicle-related injury in elderly trauma patients. *Am Surg* 68:1111, 2002.

89. Lyons RA, Jones SJ, Deacon T, et al.: Socioeconomic variation in injury in children and older people: A population based study. *Inj Prev* 9:33, 2003.

90. Hoxie RE, Rubenstein LZ: Are older pedestrians allowed enough time to cross intersections safely? *J Am Geriatr Soc* 42:241, 1994.

91. Klaus P: Crimes against Persons Age 65 or Older, 1992–1997. Vol. 2006: US Department of Justice, 2000.

92. Mitchell R, Hasbrouk L, Ingram E, et al.: Public health and aging: Nonfatal physical assault-related injuries among persons aged ≥ 60 years treated in hospital emergency departments–United States, 2001. *MMWR Morb Mortal Wkly Rep* 54:812, 2003.

93. Chu L, Kraus J: Predicting Fatal Assault Among the Elderly Using the National Incident-Based Reporting System Crime Data. *Homicide Studies* 8:71, 2004.

94. *Homicide trends in the U.S.* U.S.: Department of Justice, 2004.

95. Tatata T: *Summaries of National Elder Abuse Data: An Exploratory Study of State Statistics*. National Aging Resource Center on Elder Abuse, 1990.

96. National elder abuse incident final report. Administration for Children and Families, Administration on Aging, US Department on Health and Human Services, 1998.

97. The National Elder Maltreatment Incidence Study–Final Report. Vol. 2005: US Department of Health and Human Services. Administration for Children and Administration on Aging, 1998.

98. Lachs MS, Williams CS, O'Brien S, et al.: The mortality of elder mistreatment. *JAMA* 280:428, 1998.

99. Nagy KK, Smith RF, Roberts RR, et al.: Prognosis of penetrating trauma in elderly patients: A comparison with younger patients. *J Trauma* 49:190, 2000; discussion 193.

100. Roth BJ, Velmahos GC, Oder DB, et al.: Penetrating trauma in patients older than 55 years: A case-control study. *Injury* 32:551, 2001.

101. Minino A, Arias E, Kchanek K, et al.: *Deaths: final data for 2000*. National Vital Statistics Report, 2002.

102. CDC: *Suicide: Fact Sheet*. Vol. 2004, 2004.

103. Abrams RC, Marzuk PM, Tardiff K, et al.: Preference for fall from height as a method of suicide by elderly residents of New York City. *Am J Public Health* 95:1000, 2005.

104. Cattel H: Suicide in the elderly. *Advances in Psychiatric Treatment* 6:102, 2000.

105. CDC: *Burn Statistics in the Elderly*. National Center for Health Statistics, 2003.

106. Cutillas M, Sesay M, Perro G, et al.: Epidemiology of elderly patients' burns in the South West of France. *Burns* 24:134, 1998.

107. Ho WS, Ying SY, Chan HH: A study of burn injuries in the elderly in a regional burn centre. *Burns* 27:382, 2001.

108. McGill V, Kowal-Vern A, Gamelli RL: Outcome for older burn patients. *Arch Surg* 135:320, 2000.

109. Baux S: *Contribution a l'Etude du traitement local des brulures thermigues etendues*. Paris, 1961.

110. Stassen NA, Lukan JK, Mizuguchi NN, et al.: Thermal injury in the elderly: When is comfort care the right choice? *Am Surg* 67:704, 2001.

111. Wibbenmeyer LA, Amelon MJ, Morgan LJ, et al.: Predicting survival in an elderly burn patient population. *Burns* 27:583, 2001.

112. Lionelli GT, Pickus EJ, Beckum OK, et al.: A three decade analysis of factors affecting burn mortality in the elderly. *Burns* 31:958, 2005.

113. Committee on Trauma ACoS: *Resources for the optimal care of the injured patient*. Vol. 14. Chicago: American College of Surgeons, 1999.

114. Ma MH, MacKenzie EJ, Alcorta R, et al.: Compliance with prehospital triage protocols for major trauma patients. *J Trauma* 46:168, 1999.

115. Phillips S, Rond PC III, Kelly SM, et al.: The failure of triage criteria to identify geriatric patients with trauma: Results from the Florida Trauma Triage Study. *J Trauma* 40:278, 1996.

116. Zimmer-Gembeck MJ, Southard PA, Hedges JR, et al.: Triage in an established trauma system. *J Trauma* 39:922, 1995.

117. Osler T, Hales K, Baack B, et al.: Trauma in the elderly. *Am J Surg* 156:537, 1988.

118. Knudson MM, Lieberman J, Morris JA Jr, et al.: Mortality factors in geriatric blunt trauma patients. *Arch Surg* 129:448, 1994.

119. Davis JW, Kaups KL: Base deficit in the elderly: A marker of severe injury and death. *J Trauma* 45:873, 1998.

120. Clancy TV, Ramshaw DG, Maxwell JG, et al.: Management outcomes in splenic injury: A statewide trauma center review. *Ann Surg* 226:17, 1997.

121. McKinley BA, Marvin RG, Cocanour CS, et al.: Blunt trauma resuscitation: The old can respond. *Arch Surg* 135:688, 2000; discussion 694.

122. Schultz RJ, Whitfield GF, LaMura JJ, et al.: The role of physiologic monitoring in patients with fractures of the hip. *J Trauma* 25:309, 1985.

123. Pellicane JV, Byrne K, DeMaria EJ: Preventable complications and death from multiple organ failure among geriatric trauma victims. *J Trauma* 33:440, 1992.

124. van Aalst JA, Morris JA Jr, Yates HK, et al.: Severely injured geriatric patients return to independent living: A study of factors influencing function and independence. *J Trauma* 31:1096, (discussion 1101), 1991.

125. Jacobs DG, Plaisier BR, Barie PS, et al.: Practice management guidelines for geriatric trauma: The EAST Practice Management Guidelines Work Group. *J Trauma* 54:391, 2003.

126. Perdue PW, Watts DD, Kaufmann CR, et al.: Differences in mortality between elderly and younger adult trauma patients: Geriatric status increases risk of delayed death. *J Trauma* 45:805, 1998.

127. Battistella FD, Din AM, Perez L: Trauma patients 75 years and older: Long-term follow-up results justify aggressive management. *J Trauma* 44:618, 1998; discussion 623.

128. Tornetta P III, Mostafavi H, Riina J, et al.: Morbidity and mortality in elderly trauma patients. *J Trauma* 46:702, 1999.

129. Zietlow SP, Capizzi PJ, Bannon MP, et al.: Multisystem geriatric trauma. *J Trauma* 37:985, 1994.

130. Day RJ, Vinen J, Hewitt-Falls E: Major trauma outcomes in the elderly. *Med J Aust* 160:675, 1994.

131. Vollmer DG, Dacey RG Jr. The management of mild and moderate head injuries. *Neurosurg Clin N Am* 2:437, 1991.

132. Howard MA III, Gross AS, Dacey RG Jr, et al.: Acute subdural hematomas: An age-dependent clinical entity. *J Neurosurg* 71:858, 1989.

133. Gan BK, Lim JH, Ng IH: Outcome of moderate and severe traumatic brain injury amongst the elderly in Singapore. *Ann Acad Med Singapore* 33:63, 2004.

134. Susman M, DiRusso SM, Sullivan T, et al.: Traumatic brain injury in the elderly: Increased mortality and worse functional outcome at discharge despite lower injury severity. *J Trauma* 53:219, 2002; discussion 223.

135. MacKenzie EJ, Rivara FP, Jurkovich GJ, et al.: A national evaluation of the effect of trauma-center care on mortality. *N Engl J Med* 354:366, 2006.

136. Meldon SW, Reilly M, Drew BL, et al.: Trauma in the very elderly: A community-based study of outcomes at trauma and nontrauma centers. *J Trauma* 52:79, 2002.

137. Demetriades D, Karaiskakis M, Velmahos G, et al.: Effect on outcome of early intensive management of geriatric trauma patients. *Br J Surg* 89:1319, 2002.

138. Kannus P, Sievanen H, Palvanen M, et al.: Prevention of falls and consequent injuries in elderly people. *Lancet* 366:1885, 2005.

139. CDC N: *WISQARS Years of Potential Life Lost (YPLL) Reports*, 1999–2002. Vol. 2006, 2002.

140. CDC: *Cost of Injury - United States: A Report to Congress*, 1989.

141. DeMaria EJ, Merriam MA, Casanova LA, et al.: Do DRG payments adequately reimburse the costs of trauma care in geriatric patients? *J Trauma* 28:1244, 1988.
142. Weingarten MS, Wainwright ST, Sacchetti AD: Trauma and aging effects on hospital costs and length of stay. *Ann Emerg Med* 17:10, 1988.
143. Ross N, Timberlake GA, Rubino LJ, et al.: High cost of trauma care in the elderly. *South Med J* 82:857, 1989.
144. Sartorelli KH, Rogers FB, Osler TM, et al.: Financial aspects of providing trauma care at the extremes of life. *J Trauma* 46:483, 1999.
145. Young JS, Cephas GA, Blow O: Outcome and cost of trauma among the elderly: A real-life model of a single-payer reimbursement system. *J Trauma* 45:800, 1998.
146. Polinder S, Meerding WJ, van Baar ME, et al.: Cost estimation of injury-related hospital admissions in 10 European countries. *J Trauma* 59:1283, (discussion 1290), 2005.
147. Nirula R, Gentilello LM: Futility of resuscitation criteria for the "young" old and the "old" old trauma patient: A national trauma data bank analysis. *J Trauma* 57:37, 2004.

# Commentary  ■ HEIDI L. FRANKEL  ■ MARK GUNST

Alas, the "baby boomers" are aging! The slow, steady population growth experienced by the aged population over the last several decades is shortly going to be replaced by more accelerated expansion. As Drs. Schulman and colleagues note, starting in 2011, when the first boomer reaches age 65, the trauma surgeon's practice will change dramatically. A mobile, adventurous, and physically active generation (not accustomed to being denied much of anything) will soon descend upon trauma centers and trauma ICUs. These patients will likely require comprehensive diagnostic evaluations and more aggressive invasive monitoring in the ICU. It is, therefore, essential for those involved in trauma care to be aware of this paradigm shift so that hospital resources aren't overwhelmed and are utilized appropriately.

Increasing age places an injured patient at higher risk. Elderly patients sustaining major trauma have higher complication and mortality rates than their younger counterparts. In fact, mortality rates start to increase in injured patients after the age of 40. Thus, as the authors point out, the very definition of a geriatric trauma patient is at question. What becomes apparent is that it is not simply chronological age. A combination of pre-existing medical conditions, changes in physiology and mechanics, and the use of certain medications contribute to the "altered" response of a geriatric patient to trauma stress. As people age, the number of comorbid conditions increases and this is, at least in part, influenced by lifestyle habits. Smoking, lack of exercise, and an unhealthy diet, in addition to the natural process of aging, all predispose patients to alterations in cardiovascular and pulmonary physiology and compromise their ability to adapt to even relatively minor stress.

As the population ages, the proportion of patients in this cohort will continue to rise and it is the responsibility of the trauma surgeon to be familiar with the physiologic changes that accompany the aging process to ensure optimal care of the injured patient. Just as pediatric patients are not little people, geriatric patients should not be considered an older version of healthy adults. As this chapter describes, there are many considerations that must be taken into account.

The authors comprehensively document the altered physiology and comorbidities inherent in the geriatric population and the consequences of their treatment. Several are worth noting, namely, the use of coumadin, beta blockers, and statins and the consequences of altered renal and musculoskeletal physiology. Medications, especially anticoagulants and cardiac medications such as B-blockers, often confound what appears to be a straightforward, manageable problem. Small intracerebral contusions may blossom in the anticoagulated patient and cause otherwise unexpected morbidity and

mortality. Rapid identification of the coumadinized patient at risk for intracerebral (or torso) hemorrhage is key to initiate prompt therapy. Judicious use of prothrombin complex, Vitamin K, and even factor VII may minimize volume required to correct pT and improve outcome. Because the prevalence of hypertension increases with age, along with the use of B-blockers and other antihypertensive medications, a seemingly stable patient may promote a false sense of security when, in fact, the patients is in profound shock. On the other hand, use of beta blockers in the injured patient population may prove cardioprotective. It certainly seems as if statin use is associated with a lower risk of sepsis. The authors note that renal dysfunction in the elderly may be protean. This is extremely important to consider with an increasing reliance on diagnostic modalities using intravenous contrast, particularly as effective prophylactic strategies exist. Finally, unique musculoskeletal challenges in the geriatric population, including the epidemic of obesity, will affect trauma care.

The chapter notes that patterns of injury are different for the elderly. The most common mechanism in this patient population is falls related to both intrinsic and extrinsic factors. Automobile-related injuries, burns, and assaults follow, and are becoming increasingly more common as are injuries related to violence. Because of the patient's inability to adapt physiologically, chest wall and other musculoskeletal fractures, blunt cardiac injury, and pulmonary contusions dramatically increase the risk of complications such as infection and multiple organ system dysfunction and death.

Despite the challenges of trauma in the elderly, trauma surgeons can positively impact outcome. Aggressive management consisting of early invasive monitoring, trauma team involvement, and use of geriatricians can lower mortality and morbidity. How the use of less invasive monitors instead impacts outcome remains to be determined. Finally, with an ever-increasing number of elderly patients, it becomes necessary to encourage a more proactive approach in the prevention of these injuries. Prevention may have as important a role as recognition of treatment in order to reduce the undue burden of complications and death. At the other end of the spectrum, trauma providers will need to more comfortably address the issues of withdrawing and withholding care.

The authors of this chapter provide a very thorough review of physiologic changes associated with aging, mechanisms of injury in the elderly, and the consequences of both. For trauma surgeons in the present and future, it will be imperative to be well informed and familiar with these patterns of injury. This will allow for prevention of many unnecessary injuries and an ability to optimally manage those that do occur.

# Family and Youth Violence

*Kathleen R. Liscum* ■ *Edward E. Cornwell, III* ■ *H. Scott Bjerke* ■ *David C. Chang*

Trauma care by its very nature is fast-paced, problem-focused, and outcomes-driven. We are accustomed to making decisions with incomplete information and are acutely aware that indecisiveness can be fatal. However, if we are not careful, this approach may become our only modus operandi and may hinder us in the complete care of the trauma patient. Excellence in trauma care should incorporate consideration of the psychosocial aspects of each patient's injuries as well as the needs of and impact on the larger health care system. While no patient exists in a vacuum, trauma patients in particular, often present unique challenges in this regard. This is especially true for those who are victims of intentional violence. Patients who are victims of family and youth violence may have relatively simple traumatic injuries but often have very complex psycho-social issues that affect their response to injury. This should affect our interventions. Likewise, we will never dramatically improve trauma care only by becoming more efficient and effective in treating the resultant injuries. Early detection and prevention of interpersonal violence must be our goals.

We tend to become desensitized to violence. In addition to the day-in and day-out exposure to patients who are victims of violent acts such as stabbings and gunshot wounds, we are bombarded with images of violence in the media and from the entertainment industry. We read about sensational violent incidents such as road rage, school shootings, and home invasions and are repeatedly exposed to glamorized versions of violence in movies and television programs. What should be, by any standard, deviant behavior has become the "norm". It may be somewhat self-protective to shield ourselves from some of the misery our patients suffer, however, we must recognize that our failure to address psycho-social issues such as domestic and youth violence may be seen as passively condoning these activities.

Violence, for the purposes of this chapter is "the intentional use of physical force against another person or against oneself, which results in or has a high likelihood of resulting in injury or death."[1] Its frequency is documented in the following facts. Homicides and suicides are the second and third leading causes of death among children and youth under the age of 21.[2] Domestic violence is the most common cause of injury to women in the United States.[3] One person dies every four minutes as a result of intentional injury.[4] The literature is replete with studies identifying the scientifically proven risk factors for interpersonal violence.[2,5-7] Despite this potential knowledge base, physicians are often hesitant to utilize this information.[8-10] Early recognition and intervention may prevent future incidents and decrease rates of complications such as posttraumatic stress disorder.[2,10-12]

The statistics on death and injury from intentional violence are only the tip of the iceberg. The cost to society of violent behavior is composed of the price of legal battles, incarceration, and the economic effects on the health care system as a whole, as well as the psychological stress to victims and the families of victims.[3,4]

Physicians care for the victims and the perpetrators of this violence. Despite its prevalence, many have historically taken a "don't ask, don't tell" approach to interpersonal violence. We have treated the physical injuries and disabilities of the victims without attending to the complex set of interactions that may have caused the injury and may affect their ultimate outcome.

More than 20 years have passed since the identification of interpersonal violence as a serious public health concern.[13] A few improvements have been noted. Since the mid-1990s a decrease in the rates of homicides and violent assaults has been documented. The causes of this decrease are likely multiple but may in some part be related to improvements in the health care system. However, much work remains to be done.

Studies document significant deficits in the health care system and our communities in dealing with interpersonal violence.[14] A large, national, multispecialty survey of physicians found that half of the respondents screen less than 10% of the patients they see.[10] Cohen and coworkers performed a qualitative evaluation of five communities to assess how each deals with issues of domestic violence. They found that the communities unanimously felt they were doing an inadequate job of responding to victims of this complicated problem.[15] Another study found that while the majority of both internists and surgeons (84% and 72%, respectively) felt they should be involved in firearm injury prevention, only 20% of the respondents actually engage in any form of prevention in their practices.[16] The literature documents that patients strongly desire physician involvement.[17-19]

The purpose of this chapter is to provide the practicing surgeon with some basic information on intentional violence with a focus on intimate partner and youth violence, so that he or she may be a better provider of care for these patients with special needs. Barriers to care, as well as possible interventions, will be reviewed, and methods to impact the larger public health problem will be addressed. The authors hope to stimulate the reader to peruse opportunities to affect a decrease in the epidemic level of violence in our society.

## DOMESTIC/FAMILY VIOLENCE

Domestic violence refers to those acts of interpersonal violence resulting in physical or psychological injury to members of the same family or household or to intimate acquaintances in heterosexual, homosexual, or lesbian relationships. Women are most often the victims of this type of violence, but they may also be the perpetrators. Children, the elderly, and men may all be casualties of this hidden war. In addition to emotional and psychological abuse, individuals may be the victims of neglect, abandonment, and exploitation. Additional factors such as alcohol or drug abuse, mental illness, and poverty often complicate this picture. Domestic violence is in direct contrast to violence as a result of criminal activity, which is usually male-dominated and among strangers.

Domestic violence is not just a product of 20th century progress; human society has been grappling with the issue for centuries. The Koran and the New Testament of the Bible codified acceptable behavior toward women, children, and the elderly in ancient times. English Common Law addressed such issues with the Rule of Thumb in 1895, stating that a husband could not beat his wife with a switch greater in diameter than the width of his thumb. Once considered improper for polite or public discussion, the issue of domestic and intimate violence has now become a significant societal and political issue. The modern era's interest in issues of intimate violence stems in great part from compilation of data from police organizations in the late 1970s and early 1980s reported by the Federal Bureau of Investigation (FBI) and the National Institute of Justice. The magnitude of the problem was so disturbing that after minimal debate; the U.S. Congress passed the Family Violence and Prevention Act of 1984. The initial impact of this legislation was to provide funds for police agencies to examine new ways to combat the growing problem and for social agencies to provide support for its victims. At the same time, the U.S. Surgeon General brought attention to what he termed the biggest public health problem for women between the ages of 15 and 44 in a national workshop on domestic violence in 1985. The Surgeon General's Office estimated that over six million women a year are beaten or physically abused by boyfriends or husbands in the United States, with an act of domestic violence occurring every 18 seconds. He also noted that battery and assault against women occurred more frequently than rape, mugging, and

**TABLE 48-1**

| Average Annual Rate of Violent Victimization per 1000 Persons (Female, Male) | | |
| --- | --- | --- |
| **Old Survey Methodology, 1987–1991** | | |
| Intimate | 5.4 | 0.5 |
| Other relative | 1.1 | 0.7 |
| Acquaintance/friend | 7.6 | 13 |
| Stranger | 5.4 | 12.2 |
| **New NCVS Methodology, 1992–1993** | | |
| Intimate | 9.4 | 1.4 |
| Other relative | 2.8 | 1.2 |
| Acquaintance/friend | 12.9 | 17.2 |
| Stranger | 7.4 | 19 |

Source: U.S. Department of Justice: Violence Against Women: Estimates from the Redesigned Survey. Special Report. Washington. DC: U.S. Department of Justice, August 1995, NCJ-154348.

motor vehicle accidents combined. Unfortunately, much of the original data derived from police and FBI sources was biased or skewed or incomplete, a fact that has fueled the emotional aspect of the debate over the realities of domestic violence and its importance in modern society. In an attempt to rectify the lack of good and unbiased data, the Violence Against Women Act of the Violent Crime Control and Law Enforcement Act of 1994 brought about fundamental changes in how the data on domestic violence are collected and analyzed. The authors of the National Institute of Justice Research Report, *Domestic and Sexual Violence Data Collection: A Report to Congress Under the Violence Against Women Act,* state in their foreword:

As we seize the opportunity to make a difference in the lives of women and children victimized by violence, we want to be sure to proceed on the basis of knowledge. We need sound data to guide our policy making. The Congress recognized this need by calling for a study to learn how the States could centralize data collection on the incidence of sexual and domestic violence offenses and to examine statistical record keeping at the Federal level for domestic violence-related criminal complaints.[20]

More precise data from the redesigned National Crime Victimization Survey (NCVS) was published in the Bureau of Justice Statistics Special Report in August 1995 and is presented in Table 48-1. The NCVS also documented the following:

Women age 12 or older annually sustained almost five million violent victimizations in 1992 and 1993. About 75% of all lone-offender violence against women and 45% of violence involving multiple offenders was perpetrated by offenders whom the victim knew. In 29% of all violence against women by a lone offender, the perpetrator was an intimate (husband, boyfriend, ex-boyfriend).

Women were about six times more likely than men to experience violence committed by an intimate.

Women of all races and Hispanic and non-Hispanic women were equally vulnerable to violence by an intimate.

Women aged 19 to 29 and women in families with an annual income below $10,000 were more likely than other women to be victims of violence by an intimate.

Among victims of violence committed by an intimate, the victimization rate of women separated from their husbands was about three times higher than that of divorced women and about 25 times higher than that of married women.

Female victims of violence by an intimate were more often injured by the violence than females victimized by a stranger.[21]

Between 1993 and 1999, Bureau of Justice Statistics have shown a small, but evident decrease in the incidence of intimate violence reported to police agencies. Women in the 16 to 24 age group remain the most vulnerable to intimate violence, but women aged 35 to 49 are the most vulnerable to intimate murder.[22] While the epidemiology remains essentially unchanged, the reasons for the decrease in domestic violence are not entirely clear. They have been attributed to requiring mandatory reporting of domestic violence, better physician and healthcare worker awareness, activity of community support groups, improved education of the population. While arrests for domestic violence have increased slightly over the last ten years and this has been shown to be a small deterrent,[23] most experts feel the combined societal reaction to the subject is responsible for the decrease, but that society still has a long way to go to eradicate the problem.

While many victims of domestic violence will not seek medical attention, it is estimated that over 20% of women who use hospital emergency surgical services, or nearly one million women per year do so as a result of domestic violence. Stark and Flitcraft estimated in 1982 that only 4% of these one million emergency department (ED) visits were properly attributed to domestic violence by physicians allowing for counseling and social service interventions.[24] The medical cost of domestic violence is estimated at $3 billion to $5 billion annually, with another $100 million in lost wages and absenteeism from work per year.[25] It is estimated that 4000 women will die as a result of domestic violence each year, many of whom will have been seen in the regional trauma center prior to this tragedy.

While society expects physicians and healthcare workers to recognize the signs of domestic violence, not all states require mandatory reporting by law even in 2001.[26] Surveys of female emergency room patients shows that only 55% of battered women while 70% of nonbattered women support mandatory reporting by law without the patients consent.[27] This puts the physician and nurse as patient advocate in a difficult position.

In response to these facts, organized medical groups are educating their members and attempting to be pre-emptive rather than reactive. The American Association of Family Practice, the American College of Obstetrics and Gynecology, the American College of Emergency Physicians, and the American Medical Association have all produced position papers on domestic violence and recommendations for physicians who encounter the victims of intimate violence. In 1992, the Joint Commission for Accreditation of Hospitals initiated the requirement that written guidelines be available in hospital EDs for staff regarding domestic violence and the services available for its victims. Unfortunately, hospital admissions data document that most abuse occurs outside of the 9:00 to 5:00 workday, when most special services are available. It therefore falls on the physician and nursing staff in many situations to know about and screen for domestic violence and to provide victims with information for access to social and psychiatric counseling, shelters, and legal and personal counseling services. Much of this information is easily available on the Internet. Some national groups dealing with domestic violence are listed in Table 48-2. A directed query on domestic violence and a city name will provide an enormous

## TABLE 48-2

### National Groups with Domestic Violence Focus

**Hotlines and Telephone Resources**
National Domestic Violence Hotline 800-799-SAFE, 800-787-3224 (TDD)
National Resource Center on Domestic Violence 800-537-2238
National Coalition Against Domestic Violence 202-638-6388, 303-839-1852

**World Wide Web Sites**
U.S. Department of Justice
  www.usdoj.gov/ovw
Justice Information Center
  http://www.ncjrs.org
Family Peace Project
  http://www.family.mcw.edu/ahec/ec/medviol.html
Domestic Violence http://www.sfms.org/domestic.html
Domestic Violence Shelters
  http://www.dvsheltertour.org/links.html
Domestic Violence Info Center
  http://www.feminist.org/other/dv/dvhome.html
Minnesota Center Against Violence & Abuse
  http://www.umn.edu/mincava
Electronic Journal of Intimate Violence
  http://gort.ucsd.edu/newjour/e/msg00129.html

## TABLE 48-3

### Warning Signs of Domestic Violence

Recurrent visits for minor injuries
Vague or incomplete history of injury
Delay between injury and seeking medical evaluation
Contusions or minor lacerations to face, breasts, or abdomen
Increasing severity of injuries with time

amount of information in a short time. Most cities also have telephone listings for domestic violence crisis and support lines available through the local phone company information service.

As professionals in a team caring for traumatized victims, our greatest opportunity to change the devastating effects of domestic violence exist in first recognizing abuse in a nonjudgmental manner, then providing access to information regarding services in a nonthreatening fashion.

While primary care and emergency nurses and physicians will first see the majority of domestic violence incidents, trauma team members are not exempt from their responsibility to recognize the signs of domestic violence and to intervene when possible. Studies have shown surgeons in general are poorly informed about injury prevention in general and domestic violence in particular.[8] An initial attempt to educate surgeons by incorporation of information into the 1997 ATLS course curricula has not been proven to be as effective as anticipated and further work needs to be done.[8] Educational activities regarding domestic violence for physicians, and surgeons in particular, are helpful and more prevalent, but need to be continued and monitored to determine the most effective methods to combat physician ignorance of this epidemic.[28–31]

Table 48-3 lists the common presenting signs of domestic abuse in women, similar to that seen in child and elder abuse. Surgeons, especially trauma surgeons will infrequently see the early signs of domestic violence, but can expect to commonly see its more terminal effects when the violence goes undiagnosed and unchecked

**TABLE 48-4**

**Medical Response to Domestic Violence**

Consider domestic violence as a cause of violent trauma in women, men, and the elderly.

If domestic violence is suspected, ask the patient, "Are you safe?"

Provide information on shelters and counseling.

Remain supportive and nonjudgmental.

for years. One such patient presented with abdominal pain. Direct questioning revealed a history of multiple assaults by a boyfriend, which had been escalating in severity for over a year, related to substance abuse in both parties. Though previous numerous visits to the ED were documented, no documentation or questioning had previously been directed toward domestic violence. The patient underwent splenectomy and postoperatively was offered counseling with police, legal, and drug rehabilitation support, which she accepted. After hospital discharge, the patient successfully completed a drug rehabilitation program and moved in with family members, ending her violent relationship. While not all such situations will end up on such a positive note, recognition and nonjudgmental support and education of domestic violence issues improves the chances for a "complete cure" (Table 48-4).

Not all cases have such a fairy-tale ending, however. The following case reflects some of the more common and real themes in the ongoing epidemic of domestic violence.

A middle-aged, middle-income Caucasian woman, in the process of divorcing her husband, became embroiled in an argument with him in their shared home in a rural community. The argument escalated. After being knocked to the floor, she was shot at close range eight times with a .22 caliber weapon in the thorax, abdomen, and head. The husband, suddenly remorseful, called 911 then put her in his car to drive to the hospital. He was stopped en route by police for driving erratically and speeding. The police informed the emergency medical system (EMS) which dispatched an ambulance to the arrest site to transfer the patient. The patient arrived in the community hospital as a known domestic violence incident reported by the EMS crew and the medical staff immediately requested the patient be transferred by helicopter to a Level 1 trauma center. The patient maintained reasonably stable vital signs and was taken emergently to the operating room at the Level 1 trauma center nearly four hours after the initial event. Multiple abdominal hollow viscus injuries were repaired, chest tubes placed, and an intraoperative cardiac echo revealed pericardial fluid prompting a median sternotomy. A single, tangential 1.2 cm tear of the intrapericardial inferior vena cava was discovered and repaired. The patient had an uneventful postoperative course with social work and justice system involvement related to her domestic violence incident. Mutual friends with her husband/assaulter were barred from visiting, discharge arrangements were made for follow-up in another state trauma center to allow her to recover with family members away from her home and separated husband, and she and her daughters received intensive counseling. Six weeks later she returned to her community and her house with her husband where she requested the Superior Court Judge drop the order barring her husband from having contact with her. She announced to the local newspaper that her recovery was a miracle but "I knew I was responsible for what happened. There was no one to blame but myself." She informed the Prosecutor's Office that she would refuse to testify against her husband in any situation and charges were not filed.

This case points out some of the more common issues in domestic violence. Domestic violence occurs in all age groups but intimate murder is more common in middle-aged women. Most documented injuries result from male-perpetrated violence. Much of the violence results from poor impulse control in the heat of the moment, usually aggravated by intoxication with alcohol or drugs, with the injurer becoming remorseful shortly after the event. The severity of the injuries tends to increase with time, with a higher risk of fatal injuries seen more commonly in middle-aged women. Many abused spouses will reconcile with their abusers and refuse to press charges, even with social services and community support, even in "miraculous" medical recoveries. We are making progress in this epidemic, but as physicians and surgeons, we still have, in the words of a famous poem, "miles to go before we sleep."

As in much of what we see in trauma care, the basic causes and effects of domestic violence and intrapersonal violence have not changed much since the last edition of this textbook. The basics are still the same but our understanding and the effect that trauma programs, EDs, police agencies, federal agencies, and social agencies are beginning to reveal themselves. Domestic violence is a multifactoral problem, and will not be solved by any one group. Through interactive participation and individual effort we are seeing an effect.

While not absolutely specific to domestic violence, Bureau of Justice Statistics data from the last 15 years shows a progressive decrease in nonfatal intimate partner violence, especially against women (Table 48-5). The decrease has been significant, 49.3% during the period 1993 to 2001. While many groups still debate the available evidence, it is clear that better education, better screening, better identification, and better and more social programs directed toward domestic violence are having a positive effect. We, as a society, are making headway in nonfatal injuries but have yet to significantly impact the reported fatality rate in intimate violence[32] (Table 48-6).

Trends in our ability to combat violence highlight some interesting facts. Where we used to debate whether screening was appropriate or not we are now evaluating how we screen possible victims.[33–35] Emerging data suggest battered women prefer non-face to face screening.[36] Physicians and surgeons, with enormous time constraints

**TABLE 48-5**

**Bureau of Justice Statistics Data Published in Intimate Partner Violence 1993–2001**

**RATES OF INTIMATE PARTNER VIOLENCE, BY THE GENDER OF VICTIMS, 1993–A1052001**

Number of nonfatal intimate victimizations per 1000 persons

| | 1993 | 1994 | 1995 | 1996 | 1997 | 1998 | 1999 | 2000 | 2001 | Percent change, 1993–2001 (indicates a significant difference[a]) |
|---|---|---|---|---|---|---|---|---|---|---|
| Total | 5.8 | 5.5 | 4.9 | 4.7 | 4.3 | 4.8 | 3.5 | 2.8 | 3 | −48.4[a] |
| Male | 1.6 | 1.7 | 1.1 | 1.4 | 1 | 1.5 | 1.1 | 0.8 | 0.9 | −41.8[a] |
| Female | 9.8 | 9.1 | 8.5 | 7.8 | 7.5 | 7.8 | 5.8 | 4.7 | 5 | −49.3[a] |

Note: These rates are based on the data-year only and do not include fatal violence. Nonfatal violence includes rape, sexual assault, robbery, aggravated assault, and simple assault.

These rates differ from rates published in Intimate Partner Violence (May 2000, NCJ 178247), which included fatal violence and some collection-year data. Percent changes are based on unrounded rates.

**TABLE 48-6**

| Murder Victims of an Intimate Partner | | | |
|---|---|---|---|
| | MALE NUMBER | PERCENT OF ALL MURDERS % | FEMALE NUMBER | PERCENT OF ALL MURDERS % |
| 1976 | 1,357 | 9.6 | 1,600 | 34.9 |
| 1980 | 1,221 | 6.9 | 1,549 | 29.6 |
| 1990 | 859 | 4.7 | 1,501 | 29.3 |
| 1993 | 708 | 3.7 | 1,581 | 28.5 |
| 2000 | 440 | 3.7 | 1,247 | 33.5 |

Note: Categories used for intimate in this table are spouses, former spouses, boyfriends, and girlfriends (including homosexual relationships).

Sources: FBI, Supplementary Homicide Reports, 1976–2000 and (www.ojp.usdoj.gov/bjs/homicide/intimates).

within the healthcare system, are not viewed by victims as being especially helpful in their individual situations, while police and social workers score high marks.[37–38] Computer and survey screening appear to be more acceptable, non-confrontational, methods to identify victims in the hospital and ED environment. These allow a victim to be approached by health care personnel and social service providers.[39] Screening works, both prospectively and retrospectively. Adult and pediatric trauma databases can be shown retrospectively to correlate with future nonfatal and fatal risk and may provide another method besides individual screening to identify those at risk.[40] Pooled database information is also allowing the healthcare system to identify injury patterns and types suggestive of domestic violence in an earlier fashion before it has progressed to fatal incidents.[41–42]

The literature also shows that trauma centers are becoming more active in the fight.[9,43–45] The number of papers in the medical literature, especially in the surgical literature has increased by a factor of 10 in the last 10 years. And we are now assessing our efforts and our progress in a true scientific fashion. Data on the effects of initial Advanced Trauma Life Support (ATLS) domestic violence education has been disappointing, but this program continues to evolve and improve and provides exposure that can only be positive in the fight against this problem. Continued education, both of health care providers and the public exposing the magnitude of the problem as well as providing direction to helpful resources continues to improve our effectiveness.

As physicians, data suggests the victims of interpersonal violence don't find us as helpful on an individual basis when compared with others but we are one of the most important first steps in the eradication of domestic violence. Initial recognition of risk, participating in screening, recognition of specific injury types, and patient direction to social resources as well as continued research and education are our most useful tools in fighting this epidemic.

## YOUTH VIOLENCE

### History of the Problem

The issue of interpersonal violence as a public health problem gained a significant national spotlight through a workshop in October 1985 convened by the Surgeon General of the United States to address the problem. A challenge went out to health care providers, administrators, and the public at large to consider violence as a public health problem, and to seek its causes and most effective treatment. In the ensuing two years, more Americans died from gunshot wounds than during the entire 8 $\frac{1}{2}$ years of war in Vietnam. By 1994, intentional injury was the tenth leading cause of death in America (20,000 per year) and the leading cause of premature mortality.[46]

An interesting phenomenon began to occur in the mid-1990s. Most major cities, and the United States overall, saw a gradual decrease in the rates of homicide and violent assault. Perhaps the most compelling of the many potential explanations of this phenomenon can be found in the population demographics of the United States. The youngest amongst the population spike of "Baby Boomers" (Americans born from 1946–1964) departed their "crime-prone" years (14–29) by the mid-1990s. By this time, record numbers of Americans had been killed or incarcerated because of interpersonal violence. The progression of the Baby Boomer generation into middle-age closely coincides with the decreasing patterns of violence in the United States.

If the aforementioned explanation is convincing, it carries with it the sobering reality that the post-Baby Boomer generation has record number of youths entering their potential crime-prone years. More so than any generation in American history, children of this generation: (a) are less likely to come from a home with a nonviolent male role model, (b) are more likely to have witnessed or experienced violence in their immediate environment, and (c) have easier access to guns. Indeed, the aforementioned observations regarding the Baby Boomers and their offspring may provide an explanation as to why the trend of decreasing violence overall was matched by a pattern of younger ages amongst victims of violent assaults and penetrating injuries.

This chapter discusses the potential role of a trauma center in violence prevention.

## Impact of Enhanced Trauma Commitment on Patient Outcomes

While a landmark study by MacKenzie and the investigators of the National Study on Costs and Outcomes of Trauma (NSCOT) suggested a significantly lower mortality amongst patients cared for at trauma centers, as compared to those who were treated at non-trauma center hospitals,[47] the result of several studies from the Division of Trauma at Johns Hopkins Hospital suggested that additional improvement in trauma patient outcome will need to come from violence prevention.

It began with a study showing that while the implementation of a multidisciplinary trauma program resulted in significant improvement in patient outcomes, no improvement was seen among patients with gunshot wounds, the majority of whom were youths (ages 15–24). This observation was explained by a disturbing pattern showing an increasing prevalence of gunshot wound patients arriving *in extremis* or dead on arrival (DOA) from multiple gunshot wounds to the head and/or chest. While 99% of patients leaving the emergency department alive ultimately survived their hospital visit, the ever-growing incidence of patients who are DOA suggests that the "glass ceiling" is being approached in terms of benefits in patient outcomes to be gained from in-hospital performance improvement endeavors. In the year 2005, 61 of the 88 trauma deaths (69%) seen at Johns Hopkins Hospital were declared dead in the emergency department in an average of six minutes after arrival. Of the remaining 27 patients, 14 were declared dead in the intensive care unit from devastating brain injuries. This suggests that in an entire calendar year, at an urban, university-affiliated Level I trauma center, only 13 of 88 patients who died (15%) were even theoretically salvageable.[48–49] This is perhaps the most compelling argument suggesting further incremental improvement in injury outcomes are likely to be realized from prevention activities in the prehospital arena.

A follow-up study involved a geographic analysis showing that the majority of trauma patients admitted to Johns Hopkins Hospital came from a five-mile radius, incorporating some of Maryland's most impoverished neighborhoods, and confirmed the previously described predominance of youths (ages 15–24) amongst gunshot wound patients.[50] These data led to the conclusion that the injury prevention program should take the form of violence prevention activities for at-risk youths.

## In-Hospital Prevention: Shortcomings

A third project sought to duplicate the experience with alcohol and drug abuse intervention described at other centers amongst predominantly blunt trauma populations. Given the recognized comorbid incidence of alcohol and substance abuse among perpetrators and victims of interpersonal violence, a project was undertaken that sought to analyze introspection and readiness to change among young patients (ages 15–24) surviving an injury and demonstrating a positive toxicology screen. In contrast to other reports in the literature, this project demonstrated a depressingly low incidence of "readiness to change", and an even lower incidence in accessing available counseling services.[51] This study suggests a major shortcoming of an in-hospital violence prevention program: the potential beneficiaries are random and are based on the trajectory of a bullet, rather than the presence of psychosocial risk factors.

## Effectiveness of a Violence Prevention Program

Baltimore is one of the most appropriate cities in America in which to pursue initiatives in youth violence prevention. It is the nation's 13th largest city, and the largest American city that did not enjoy the decrease in violence seen nationally in the mid-1990s. Baltimore ranks at or near the top of the nation in the following high risk indicators: (1) rate of births to unwed teenage mothers, (2) episodes of assault and suspension among students in Baltimore City Elementary Schools (K-5), (3) drop-out rate for Baltimore City Public High Schools (76% for black males), and (4) juvenile arrest rate for murder.

A project was undertaken to evaluate the effectiveness of a violence-prevention initiative geared toward changing attitudes about interpersonal conflict among at-risk youths from a previously described catchment area. Participants were given a package survey of six previously validated scales, both pre- and post-intervention, to assess their attitudes about interpersonal conflicts. This package included:

1. Beliefs supporting aggression
2. Attitude toward conflicts
3. Attitudes toward school
4. Achievement motivation
5. Likelihood of violence and delinquency
6. Violent intentions from teen conflict survey

After parental consent and youths' self-assent, the children would be administered the survey package as a preintervention test at their Police Athletic League (PAL) center. They would then be brought to the hospital in groups on a day convenient for the officer at the PAL center to accompany them. The tour included video and slide presentations that graphically depicted the results of gun violence, followed by open discussions. The children would be given T-shirts on completion of their tour and their postintervention tests.

Among the first 90 participants in the program, there was statistically significant reduction in the 'beliefs supporting aggression' scale and a trend toward reduce 'likelihood of violence'. This suggested a multidisciplinary violence-prevention program can produce short-term improvement in beliefs supporting aggression among at-risk youth.[52]

## Culture of Violence and Understanding the Problem

Recent visits by the authors to the executive offices of media production companies have emphasized the dominance of an American culture that glamorizes violence. Images that sensationalize violent acts reach millions of young people every day, while the previously described outreach program reached only 90 kids over one year. Although the American College of Surgeons require that a Level I trauma center be actively involved in injury control, the trauma surgeon dealing with resuscitation, operative intervention, and postoperative critical care requires guidance from a vast array of professionals in order to understand and prevent injuries due to interpersonal violence.[53] For this reason, a growing cadre of surgeons and other physicians and public health professionals are now committed to extend the sphere of their influence beyond the hospital and university walls, and interact with a larger audience beyond our typical professional societies and scientific publications. The process of changing a culture of violence will require a sustained generational effort from multiple disciplines.

## SURGEON'S ROLE

Physicians are poised in key positions from which to impact the lives of victims of interpersonal violence.[54] The timing and proximity of our contact with the patient are crucial components of the formula for successful intervention. The previous sections have elucidated the futility of treating only the symptoms of this complex public health problem and have demonstrated the need for change. Reluctance to address issues of interpersonal violence are due to multiple barriers[3,10,13,19,55–59] These barriers can be grouped into those directly related to the patient, those that are characteristics of the individual physician and those that are larger system issues.

Firstly, the patient may serve as a blockade to appropriate treatment. Gang allegiance or shame and humiliation for victims of youth and domestic violence, respectively, may result in reluctance to share the circumstances of his or her injuries, effectively preventing any potential intervention. In addition, many individual victims and perpetrators do not see themselves as being in abusive relationships.[60] Secondly, health care providers must be cognizant of the role their personal views, experiences, knowledge, and skills have on their effectiveness in exploring for possible interpersonal violence. Dealing with issues that strike a familiar chord may be difficult. A survey of 390 medical students at three New England medical schools revealed that 38% of the students had some personal history of abuse.[61] A similar study of medical students and faculty at the University of Rochester Medical Center reported a 34% lifetime exposure rate to physical and sexual violence among medical students and a 20% lifetime exposure rate among faculty.[62] Identifying with the patient may prove to be too uncomfortable and result in impairment of the physician's ability to intervene with patients who are victims of abuse. Cultural backgrounds and personal attitudes such as beliefs about individual versus societal responsibility, gender roles, and concepts of power and control may also affect the practitioner's ability to interact with patients effectively.[17,63,64] In a study sponsored by the Robert Wood Johnson Foundation, investigators studied barriers to identifying, referring, and treating victims of family violence in five diverse communities.[15] Interviews with 480 physicians and other health care workers documented considerable "cultural distance" between the health care workers and their patients. Nearly all of those interviewed felt that family violence was a disease of people in poverty. Some physicians see intimate partner abuse as a situation between two consenting adults who are individually responsible for their own experiences (in contrast to child or elder abuse in which the abused is dependent on the abuser).[63] The female physician may be less likely to correctly identify spousal abuse in her female patients in an unconscious effort to avoid the victimizing diagnosis.[65] The use of biased language and a lack of sensitivity to gender identity and orientation also serve as barriers to the identification of interpersonal violence in the gay patient population.[66]

Feeling inadequately trained and concerned about insufficient resources to deal with the problems identified, the so-called "Pandora's Box" phenomenon[67] helps explain some individual physician's detachment. Alternatively, a sense of control is gained through dealing with the physical maladies – familiar exercises in surgical techniques and clinical problem solving. The patient's physical needs are met, while the more emotionally laden issues of family and youth violence are avoided; thus, the familiar pattern develops. Additionally, concerns about time constraints, legal entanglements, and the physician's professional and/or personal relationship with the abuser and the abused also serve as barriers.

A genuine lack of knowledge and experience can be real barriers to providing appropriate care. Deficient knowledge can lead to missing clues that may identify patients as victims of abuse. Inadequate skills in communication can lead to the premature termination of conversations with the patient and prevent disclosure. A recent study has shown that identifying domestic abuse can be difficult even for those with a clear commitment to helping this group of patients.[68]

There are few training resources available to help physicians deal with youth violence, especially with regard to prevention.[69]

Despite these barriers, physicians can and should address the issue of intentional violence. Many professional organizations have published position statements and/or guidelines. For each of the barriers listed above there are specific opportunities to affect better outcomes for these patients. Most guidelines advocate for the routine incorporation of questions regarding safety and exposure to interpersonal violence into the history. Alpert and colleagues have made a list of age-specific screening questions that can be easily covered.[70] The value of this routine asking is only in part about identifying individual victims. Many see this as an opportunity to improve overall health care. Routine screening provides physicians with opportunities to express concern for the patient and to express the antiviolence message.[68] Indeed, when patients were given an opportunity to tell physicians how to intervene in family conflict, the overwhelming majority thought physicians should ask.[10] This move toward routine attention to the violence our patients experience also help move us to the more appropriate position of listener and empowerer instead of problem-solver.[71]

Surgeons in academic positions must work with the curriculum committees of medical school and residency programs to include adequate coverage of this material to help new physicians gain the knowledge, attitudes, and skills necessary to care for patients who are victims and perpetrators of intentional injury. In addition,[70,72,73] it is their charge to further the knowledge base in this area through research. Surgeons in trauma centers should become involved in prevention programs for youth violence as well as outreach programs.[69]

Detailed, thorough documentation is of particular importance for the victims of intentional injury. In addition to the usual information included in a thorough medical and social history, the chart should include specifics about the abusive or violent event using the patient's own words in quotes.[52–54] The patient's injuries should be described in detail. Notations on body charts or drawings may be helpful. If possible, Polaroid or digital pictures should be taken. (Polaroid images are immediate and more difficult to tamper with than prints from negatives.)[74] In addition to the detailed documentation, the physician should make an assessment about the adequacy of explanation of injuries. If abuse is suspected, then the chart should clearly reflect this.[75]

The role of facilitator rather than rescuer may be an unfamiliar one for the surgeon. Simply allowing the patient to ventilate and making the appropriate referrals are interventions that may seem inadequate at first. However, it is essential that the surgeon realize that helping the victims to feel in control and self-directed are of paramount importance.[75] Victims of violence are at risk for the development of posttraumatic stress disorder. Attending to the psychosocial aspects of the patient's injuries in a timely fashion allows the patient to begin to work on addressing fears and feelings of powerlessness, shame, and guilt and interrupts the development of maladaptive responses. A traumatic event can stimulate the fight-or-flight mechanism, resulting in release of cortisol. If cortisol release becomes unregulated, the patient can develop sleep and appetite disturbances and impairment of the immune system and wound healing.[76] Instead, if as a result of receiving information regarding counseling, shelters, or legal services the patient makes an early connection with the appropriate support systems, he or she may begin to deal with the traumatic event and learn helpful coping skills. With the help of these interventions, healing can begin.

Due to the prevalence of intentional injury in the trauma patient population, it is the obligation of every trauma surgeon to independently identify and address his or her inadequacies in violence-specific knowledge and skills. We should also reflect on how our perceptions and experiences may be affecting our attitude toward this patient group.

## SUMMARY

Violence in our society represents a complex, multifaceted problem. In many ways, violence is like a chronic disease and the bullet is a common pathogen. This "disease" is related to both lifestyle and environment.[77] Characteristics associated with trauma include substance abuse, unemployment, poverty, drug trafficking, and crime convictions.[77–79] Sims and coworkers at Henry Ford Hospital found that trauma is a recurrent disease. In their study of 501 consecutive victims of violent trauma (gunshots, stabbings, and assaults), 263 patients were seen again in a medical setting (the remainder were lost to follow-up). Forty-four percent of these patients had recurrent trauma.[77] A five-year mortality rate of 20% clearly demonstrates that this "disease" should not be ignored.

An explosion of street gangs and the increased availability of firearms are two additional examples of societal ills that are related to the mortality rate from interpersonal violence. More than 94% of cities with a population greater than 100,000 have street gangs, and 40–50% of American households have guns.[80] When conflicts result in assault, they are five times more likely to end in death if a gun is available than those involving a knife.

Many of the victims of interpersonal violence are "innocent bystanders." Disturbing evidence exists that indicates that early life events such as exposure to intentional violence may make children high-risk for becoming antisocial.[2,6] Sixty-five percent of children entering the adult criminal system come from foster care.[81] Individuals who do not abuse alcohol or illicit drugs but live in the same household as these individuals are also at increased risk of violent death.[79]

The enormity of this problem requires an ordered, disciplined approach such as that developed by the public health community to address infectious diseases.[1] This approach should include event surveillance, epidemiologic analysis, intervention design and evaluation, and a focus on prevention. Our educational efforts should be based on clear competencies[69] and interventions should be evidence-based. It is our duty as physicians to go beyond treating only the physical injuries our patients incur. We are optimally placed to help our patients achieve real healing—a restoration to soundness.

## REFERENCES

1. Rosenberg ML, O'Carroll PW, Powell KE: Let's be clear, violence is a public health problem. *JAMA* 267:3071, 1992.
2. Centers for Disease Control and Prevention: Web-based Injury Statistics Query and Reporting System (WISQARS) [Online]. (2006). National Center for Injury Prevention and Control, Centers for Disease Control and Prevention (producer). Available from: URL: http://www.cdc.gov/ncipc/wisqars/. [Accessed April 13, 2006].
3. Chambliss LR, Bay RC, Jones RF: Domestic violence: An educational imperative? *Am J Obstet Gynecol* 172:1035, 1995.
4. Fleming AW, Sterling-Scott RP, Carabello G, et al.: Injury and violence in Los Angeles: Impact on access to health care and surgical education. *Arch Surg* 127:671, 1992.
5. Burke LK, Follingstad DR. Violence in lesbian and gay relationships: Theory, prevalence, and correlational factors. *Clin Psychol Rev* 19:487, 1999.
6. Durant RH, Altman D, Wolfson M, et al.: Exposure to violence and victimization, depression, substance use, and the use of violence by young adolescents. *J Pediatr* 137:707, 2000.
7. Kyriacou DN, Hutson HR, Anglin D, et al.: The relationship between socioeconomic factors and gang violence in the City of Los Angeles. *J Trauma* 46:334, 1999.
8. Knudson MM, Vassar MJ, Straus EM, et al.: Surgeons and injury prevention: What you don't know can hurt you! *J Am Coll Surg* 193:119, 2001.
9. Guth AA, Pachter HL: Domestic violence and the trauma surgeon. *Am J Surg* 179:134, 2000.
10. Rusch MD, Gould LJ, Dzwierzynski WW, et al.: Psychological impact of traumatic injuries: What the surgeon can do. *Plast Reconstr Surg* 109:18, 2002.
11. Nelson BV, Patience TH, MacDonald DC: Adolescent risk behavior and the influence of parents and education. *J Am Board Fam Pract* 12:436, 1999.
12. Fein JA, Ginsburg KR, McGrath ME, et al.: Violence prevention in the emergency department: Clinician attitudes and limitations. *Arch Pediatr Adolesc Med* 154:495,2000.
13. Cohen S, De Vos E, Newberger E: Barriers to physician identification of treatment of family violence: Lessons from five communities. *Acad Med* 72:19, 1997.
14. Koop CE, Rosenberg ML, Mercy JA, et al.: Violence as a Public Health Problem. Background papers prepared for the Surgeon General's Workshop on Violence and Public Health, October 27–29, 1985, Leesburg, VA. Atlanta, GA, The Violence Epidemiology Branch, Center for Health Promotion and Education, Centers for Disease Control, U.S. Public Health Service, 1985.
15. Tellez ML, Mackersie RC: Violence prevention involvement among trauma surgeons: Description and preliminary evaluation. *J Trauma* 40:602, 1996.
16. Cassel CK, Nelson EA, Smith TW, et al.: Internists' and surgeons' attitudes toward guns and firearm injury prevention. *Annals of Int Med* 128:224, 1998.
17. Friedman LS, Samet JH, Roberts MS, et al.: Inquiry about victimization experiences. A survey of patient preferences and physician practices. *Arch Intern Med* 152:1186, 1992.
18. McCauley J, Yurk RA, Jenckes M, et al.: Inside "Pandora's box" Abused women's experiences with clinicians and health services. *J Gen Intern Med* 13:549, 1998.
19. Burge SK, Schneider FD, Ivy L, et al.: Patients' advice to physicians about intervening in family conflict. *Annals of Fam Med* 3:248, 2005.
20. Domestic and Sexual Violence Data Collection (National Institute of Justice Research Report), July 1996.
21. Violence Against Women: Estimates from the Redesigned Survey Bureau of Justice Statistics Special Report. U.S. Department of Justice, August 1995.
22. Intimate Partner Violence and Age of Victim 1993–1999, Bureau of Justice Statistics Special Report October 2001, NCJ187635.
23. Maxwell CD, Garner JH, Fagan JA: The Effects of Arrest on Intimate Partner Violence: New Evidence from the Spouse Assault Replication Program, NIJ Research in Brief publication, July 2001.
24. Stark, Flitcraft: *Medical Therapy as Repression: The Case of the Battered Woman*, 1982.
25. *Domestic Violence for Healthcare Providers*. 3rd ed. Colorado Domestic Violence Coalition, 1991.
26. Houry D, Sachs CJ, Feldhaus KM, at al.: Violence-inflicted injuries: Reporting laws in the fifty states. *Ann Emerg Med* 39:56, 2002.
27. Rodriguez MA, McLoughlin E, Nah G, et al.: Mandatory reporting of domestic violence injuries to the police: What do emergency department patients think? *JAMA* 286:580, 2001.
28. Guth AA, Pachter LL: Domestic violence and the trauma surgeon. *Am J Surg* 179:134, 2000.
29. Zillmer DA: Domestic violence: The role of the orthopaedic surgeon in identification and treatment. *J Am Acad Orthop Surg* 8:91, 2000.r
30. Le BT, Dierks EJ, Ueeck BA, et al.: Maxillofacial injuries associated with domestic violence. *J Oral Maxillofac Surg* 59:1277, 2001.
31. Gadomski AM, Wolff D, Tripp M, et al.: Changes in health care providers' knowledge, attitudes, beliefs, and behaviors regarding domestic violence, following a multifaceted intervention. *Acad Med* 76:1045, 2001..
32. Wadman MC, Muelleman RL: Domestic violence homicides: ED use before victimization. *Am J Emerg Med* 17:689, 1999.
33. Larkin GL, Rolniak S, Hyman KB, et al.: Effect of an administrative intervention on rates of screening for domestic violence in an urban emergency department. *Am J Public Health* 9:1444, 2000.
34. Krasnoff M, Moscati R: Domestic violence screening and referral can be effective. *Ann Emerg Med* 40:485, 2002.
35. Halpern LR, Perciaccante VJ, Hayes C, et al.: A protocol to diagnose intimate partner violence in the emergency department. *J Trauma* 60:1101, 2006.
36. MacMillan HL, Wathen CN, Jamieson E, et al.: Approaches to screening for intimate partner violence in health care settings: A randomized trial. *JAMA* 296:530, 2006.
37. Krugman SD, Witting MD, Furuno JP, et al.: Perceptions of help resources for victims of intimate partner violence. *J Interpers Violence* 19:766, 2004.
38. Bacchus L, Mezey G, Bewley S: Experiences of seeking help from health professionals in a sample of women who experienced domestic violence. *Health Soc Care Community* 11:10, 2003.
39. Rhodes KV, Lauderdale DS, He T, et al.: Between me and the computer: Increased detection of intimate partner violence using a computer questionnaire. *Ann Emerg Med* 40:476, 2002.
40. Chang DC, Knight V, Ziegfeld S, et al.: The tip of the iceberg for child abuse: The critical roles of the pediatric trauma service and its registry. *J Trauma* 57:1189 (discussion 1198), 2004.

41. Corrigan JD, Wolfe M, Mysiw WJ, et al.: Early identification of mild traumatic brain injury in female victims of domestic violence. *Am J Obstet Gynecol* 188:S71, 2003.

42. Wiebe DJ: Sex differences in the perpetrator-victim relationship among emergency department patients presenting with nonfatal firearm-related injuries. *Ann Emerg Med* 42:405, 2003.

43. Davis JW, Kaups KL, Campbell SD, et al.: Domestic violence and the trauma surgeon: results of a study on knowledge and education. *J Am Coll Surg* 191:347, 2000.

44. Davis JW, Parks SN, Kaups KL, et al.: Victims of domestic violence on the trauma service: Unrecognized and underreported. *J Trauma* 54:352, 2003.

45. Melnick DM, Maio RF, Blow FC, et al.: Prevalence of domestic violence and associated factors among women on a trauma service. *J Trauma* 53:33, 2002.

46. Koop CE, Lundberg GD: Violence in America: A public health emergency. *JAMA* 267:3075, 1996.

47. MacKenzie EJ, Rivara FP, Jurkovich GJ, et al.: A national evaluation of the effect of trauma-center care on mortality. *N Engl J Med* 354:366, 2006.

48. Cornwell EE, Chang DC, Phillips J, et al.: Enhanced trauma program commitment at a Level I trauma center: Impact on the process and outcome of care. *Arch Surg* 138:838, 2003.

49. Efron D, Haider A, Chang DC, et al.: The alarming surge in non-survivable urban trauma and the case for violence prevention. *Arch Surg* 141:800, 2006.

50. Chang DC, Cornwell EE, Phillips J, et al.: Community characteristics and demographic information as determinants for a hospital-based injury prevention outreach. *Arch Surg* 138:1344, 2003.

51. Yonas M, Baker D, Cornwell EE, et al.: Inpatient counseling for alcohol/substance abusing youths with major trauma... Ready or not? *J Trauma* 59:466, 2005.

52. Chang DC, Sutton ER, Cornwell EE, et al.: Evaluating the efficacy of a multidisciplinary youth violence prevention initiative: Changing attitudes regarding interpersonal conflict? *J Am Coll Surg* 201:721, 2005.

53. Cornwell EE III, Jacobs D, Walker M, et al.: National Medical Association Surgical Section position paper on violence prevention. A resolution of trauma surgeons caring for victims of violence. *JAMA* 273:1788, 1995.54.
McAfee RE: Physicians and domestic violence: Can we make a difference? *JAMA* 273:1790, 1995.

55. Council on Ethical and Judicial Affairs, American Medical Association: Physicians and domestic violence: Ethical considerations. *JAMA* 267:3190, 1992.

56. American Medical Association Council on Scientific Affairs: Violence against women: Relevance for medical practitioners. *JAMA* 267:3184, 1992.

57. Flitcraft AH, Hadley SM, Hendricks-Matthews MK, et al.: American Medical Association Diagnostic and Treatment Guidelines on Domestic Violence. *Arch Fam Med* 1:39, 1992.

58. Baker NJ: Strategic footholds for medical education about domestic violence. *Acad Med* 70:982, 1995.

59. Neufeld B: SAFE Questions: Overcoming barriers to the detection of domestic violence. *Am Fam Phys* 53:2575, 1996.

60. Ferris LE, Norton PG, Dunn EV, et al.: Guidelines for managing domestic abuse when male and female partners are patients of the same physician. *JAMA* 278:851, 1997.

61. Cullinane PM, Alpert EJ, Freund KM: First-year medical students' knowledge of, attitudes toward, and personal histories of family violence. *Acad Med* 72:48, 1997.

62. deLahunta EA, Tulsky AA: Personal exposure of faculty and medical students to family violence. *JAMA* 275:1903, 1996.

63. Gremillion DH, Kanof EP: Overcoming barriers to physician involvement in identifying and referring victims of domestic violence. *Ann Emerg Med* 27:769, 1996.

64. Sugg NK, Inui T: Primary care physicians' response to domestic violence: Opening Pandora's box. *JAMA* 267:3157, 1992.

65. Saunders DG, Kindy P Jr: Predictors of physicians' responses to woman abuse: The role of gender, background, and brief training. *J Gen Int Med* 8:606, 1993.

66. Nelson JA: Gay, lesbian, and bisexual adolescents: Providing esteem-enhancing care to a battered population. *Nurse Pract* 98, 1997.

67. Flitcraft A, Zuckerman D, Gray A, et al.: *Wife Abuse in the Medical Setting: An Introduction for Health Care Personnel.* Monograph 7. Washington, DC, Office of Domestic Violence, 1981.

68. Gerbert B, Caspers N, Bronstone A, et al.: A qualitative analysis of how physicians with expertise in domestic violence approach the identification of victims. *Ann Intern Med* 131:578, 1999.

69. Knox LM, Spivak H: What health professionals should know: Core competencies for effective practice in youth violence prevention. *Am J Prev Med* 29:191, 2005.

70. Alpert EJ, Sege RD, Bradshaw YS: Interpersonal violence and the education of physicians. *Acad Med* 72:41, 1997.

71. Director TD, Linden JA. Domestic violence: An approach to identification and intervention. *Emerg Med Clin North Am* 22:1117, 2004.

72. Alpert EJ: Making a place for teaching about family violence in medical school. *Acad Med* 70:974, 1995.

73. Alpert EJ, Tonkin AE, Seeherman AM, et al.: Family violence curricula in U.S. medical schools. *Am J Prev Med* 14:273, 1998.

74. Taliaferro E: Domestic violence: The need for good documentation. PVS Action Notes, 1997.

75. Steiner RP, Vansickle K, Lippman SB: Domestic violence: Do you know when and how to intervene? *Domestic Violence* 100:103, 1996.

76. Doiron RG, Tselikis P: Finding trauma behind diseases. *Strategic Med* 1:43, 1997.

77. Sims DW, Bivins BA, Obeid FN, et al.: Urban trauma: A chronic recurrent disease. *J Trauma* 29:940, 1989.

78. Stanton B, Galbraith J: Drug trafficking among African-American early adolescents: Prevalence, consequences, and associated behaviours and beliefs. *Pediatrics* 93:1039, 1994.

79. Rivara FP, Mueller BA, Somes G, et al.: Alcohol and illicit drug abuse and the risk of violent death in the home. *JAMA* 278:569, 1997.

80. Zuckerman DM: Media violence, gun control, and public policy. *Am J Orthopsych* 66:378, 1996.

81. Lamberg L: Kids who kill: Nature plus (lack of) nurture. *JAMA* 275:1712, 1996.

# Commentary ■ GERALD B. DEMAREST

The occurrence of interpersonal violence among humankind has been present since the beginning of our history. Unfortunately, it appears to be an integral part of our social fabric. As stated by the authors, "As a consequence of the day-in and day-out exposure to patients who are victims of violent acts, we tend to become desensitized to violence. The end result of the pervasiveness of violent acts in our society, the recognition that our failure to address psychosocial issues such as domestic and youth violence may be seen as passively condoning these activities."

As healthcare providers we have only recently begun to look at the psychological effects of violent acts. More than 20 years have passed since the identification of interpersonal violence as a serious public health concern in the United States. This recognition coupled with various interventions has resulted in a decrease in the rates of homicides and violent assaults during this 20-year period. Sadly, we as a society have only just begun to recognize and deal with the devastating effects of violent acts.

In this chapter the authors provide an extensive analysis of the violence perpetrated against women and children. It also documents medicine's attempts to deal with this social issue. The American Association of Family Practice, the American College of Obstetrics and Gynecology, the American College of Emergency Physicians, and the American Medical Association have all produced position papers on domestic violence and recommendations for physicians who encounter the victims of intimate violence. The Joint Commission for Accreditation of Hospitals initiated the requirement that written guidelines be available in hospital EDs for staff regarding domestic violence and the services available for its victims. This is just a beginning in our efforts to deal with this hidden issue.

The authors conclude that domestic violence is a multifactoral problem, and will not be solved by any one group, but by interactive participation and individual effort. Better education, better screening, better identification, and better and more social programs directed toward domestic violence are having a positive effect. Trauma centers are becoming more active in this issue. Recognition of specific injury types and patient direction to social resources as well as continued research and education are our most useful tools in fighting this epidemic.

# Wounds, Bites, and Stings

*Charles A. Adams, Jr.* ▪ *Walter L. Biffl* ▪ *William G. Cioffi*

## WOUNDS

### INTRODUCTION

This chapter will review the broad topic of wounds and wound healing and will focus on general principles and concepts rather than specific topics since the majority of these are dealt with in greater detail in other sections of this text. In the first section, the biology and pathophysiology of wound healing will be explored in depth. The next section will deal with bites and stings and will similarly cover general treatment concepts and offer treatment algorithms.

Traumatic wounds are a fact of life and affect millions of patients in the United States each year. The overwhelming majority of these wounds are simple and are treated by nonhealthcare trained individuals or the patients themselves. In practical terms, satisfactory wound healing would take place regardless of the treatments that they received. The focus of this chapter will be on more severe wounds or those wounds that would not have a satisfactory outcome without special attention. The main principles in treating these wounds are preventing infection, retaining maximal function, and achieving acceptable cosmesis. Such wounds are typically managed by a variety of healthcare personnel including emergency medicine physicians, advanced-practice nurses, family physicians, surgeons, and surgical sub-specialists, but the treatment philosophy is basically the same. The nature and mechanism of the wound, its anatomic location, pre-existing comorbidities, and the current clinical situation all dictate the approach to the wound. Figure 49-1 provides a treatment algorithm for acute wounds that is applicable to a wide array of clinical scenarios and wounds.

Since the time of the early Egyptians as evidenced by the Edwin S. Smith papyruses, individuals have been concerned with wound healing.[1] The ancients observed that dead tissue and foreign bodies had to be removed in order for normal wound healing to progress and that cleanliness prevented infection. They recognized that organized collections of pus required drainage and that honey (a hypertonic, hygroscopic, and bactericidal fluid) could prevent infections while dirt and dung promoted them; however, the biology of this effect was a mystery to them.[2] Later in the 1500s the scholarly treatise on wounds by French surgeon Ambroise Pare established a truism that is still applicable today; "Do not put anything in a wound that you would not put in your own eye." Despite the seminal contributions of Lister, Semmelweis, Ehrlich, Fleming, and Florey, it was not until the very end of the 20th century that our understanding of the biology of wound healing grew to the point that physicians are now able to manipulate wounds utilizing translational techniques taken from cellular and molecular biology.

Wounds are generally classified into one of the two categories; i.e., acute and chronic. Acute wounds follow a systematic, organized series of stages that ultimately result in restoration of skin integrity. In contrast, chronic wounds follow many of the same steps but do not result in re-establishment of skin integrity. As a rule of thumb a wound that fails to fully heal by three months is said to be a chronic wound, but this arbitrary definition fails to take into consideration the size or anatomic location of the wound or other impediments to healing. We will focus on the healing of acute, cutaneous wounds since they represent the majority of traumatic wounds.

### NORMAL WOUND HEALING

It is paradoxical that the "highest" forms of life on earth, mammals, heal their wounds through a more primitive mechanism than "lower" forms of life. Many lower life forms have the ability to regenerate after wounding. In humans only the liver retains the ability to heal by regeneration. With the exception of bone, all other mammalian tissues heal through scar formation. The steps of scar

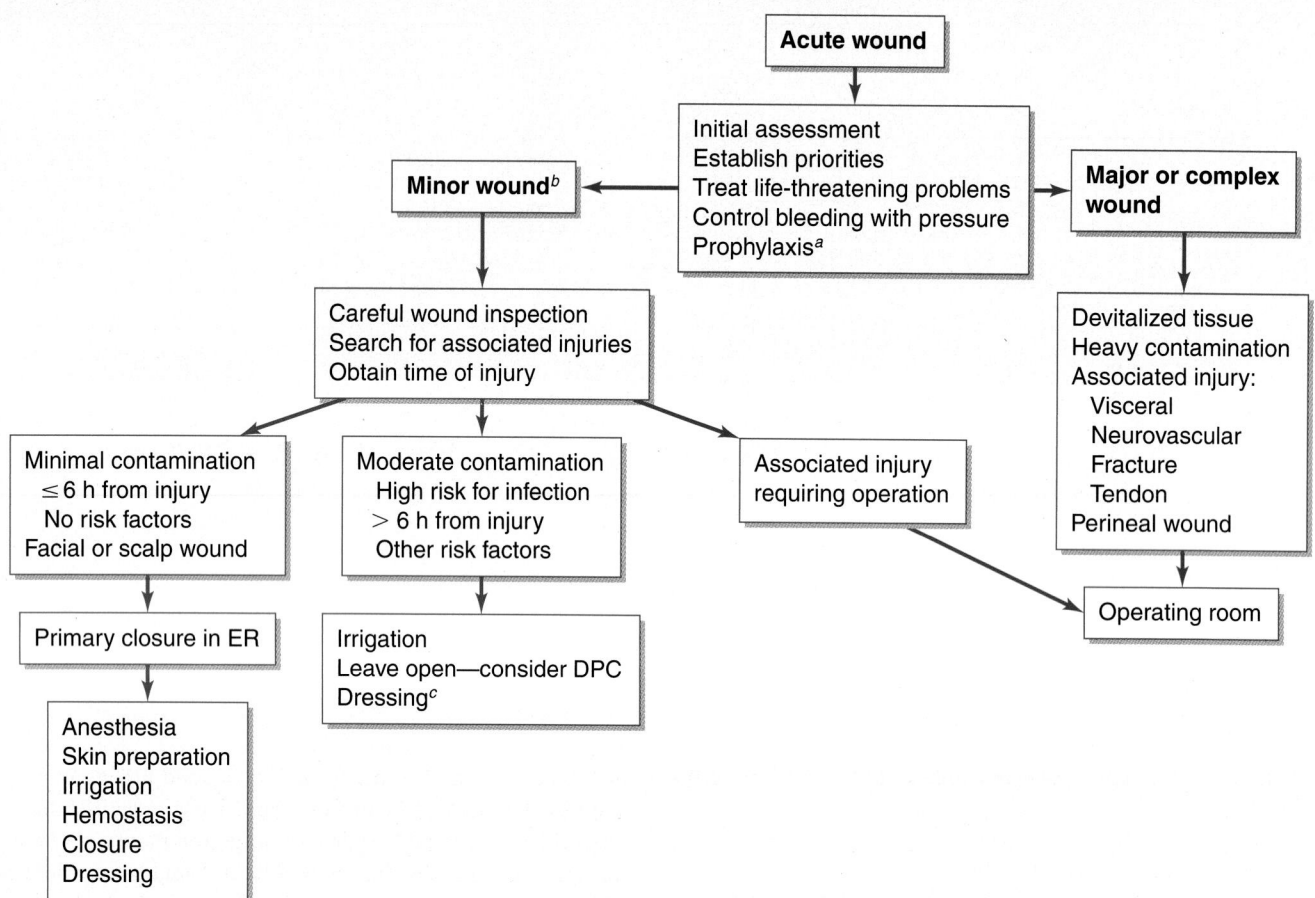

**FIGURE 49-1.** Algorithm for the treatment of an acute wound. <sup>a</sup>Appropriate tetanus, rabies, and antibiotic prophylaxis. <sup>b</sup>Intermediate-risk wounds require more judgment. <sup>c</sup>See Table 49-9.

formation or wound healing are classically divided into three distinct phases including inflammatory, proliferative, and remodeling (Table 49-1). These phases usually take place in a stepwise fashion although, as we will discuss later, there are varying degrees of overlap, and in certain wounds, all phases may coexist simultaneously.

## Inflammatory Phase

The first phase of wound healing is the inflammatory (also called reactive) phase and it commences the instant an injury occurs. The main therapeutic goals of this stage are to stop bleeding, prevent infection, and remove devitalized tissue. Wounding invariably leads to disruption of blood vessels with ensuing bleeding which ranges from a slow ooze from capillaries to an exsanguinating hemorrhage if large arteries or veins are involved. In order to stop the bleeding, coagulation of blood must occur in a tightly regulated fashion so that clotting is confined to the site of injury but not at remote vascular locations. Blood vessel injury leads to the exposure of subendothelial, procoagulant substances that bind and activate platelets. Platelet activation leads to a chain reaction culminating in

the formation of a platelet "plug." Simultaneously, activated platelets serve as the platform upon which clotting factors interact so that an insoluble fibrin meshwork is generated from soluble, circulating fibrinogen. This fibrin mesh is cross-linked and traps circulating erythrocytes and activates additional platelets resulting in a tight, hemostatic plug.[3] Shortly after coagulation is initiated, the complement cascade is set in motion and causes the release of potent neutrophil chemotactic factors such as C5a. Complement is also involved in the destruction of bacteria through formation of the membrane attack complex, as well as opsonizing bacteria which facilitates phagocytosis.

Effective hemostasis leads to a relative lack of blood flow to the wound micro-environment. This coupled with anaerobic metabolism by leukocytes leads to a locally hypoxic and acidotic wound environment. Such settings are known to be a stimulus for leukocyte activation so that coagulation is quickly followed by inflammation, but there is some overlap in these processes.[4] Activated platelets and endothelial cells release cytokines that attract neutrophils and macrophages to the area. If thrombin is present, endothelial cells exposed to leukotrienes $C_4$ and $D_4$ will release platelet activating factor (PAF) which enables neutrophil adhesion. Accordingly, by the end of the first hour and for the first two to three days after wounding, the dominant cell type is the neutrophil. The main purpose of the neutrophil is destruction of bacteria through phagocytosis and the generation of reactive oxygen species through a process called "respiratory burst." Respiratory

**TABLE 49-1**

| |
|---|
| INFLAMMATION |
| PROLIFENATIVE |
| REMODELING |

burst results in the formation of many reactive oxygen species such as superoxide anion ($SO_2^-$), hydrogen peroxide, hydroxyl radicals, and hypochlorous acid. They also debride the wound by elaborating activated proteases and elastases that breakdown devitalized tissues and cells. Unfortunately, the release of activated lysosomal enzymes along with reactive oxygen species leads to the indiscriminant damage of otherwise healthy host cells, as well.[5] Ultimately, the action of neutrophils leads to the generation of pus which is a simply a collection of dead neutrophils and bacteria and tissue breakdown products. Once neutrophils have completed their job they undergo apoptosis, or programmed cell death, and are eliminated by macrophages in a process that is remarkably free of inflammation.

Of all the cells involved in wound healing, none is as critical as the macrophage.[6] Activation of platelets and endothelial and other cells in the wound lead to the generation of inflammatory substances like histamine, serotonin, prostaglandins, kinins, platelet-derived growth factor (PGDF), transforming growth factor beta (TGF-β), insulin-like growth factor-1 (IGF-1), fibronectin, fibrinogen, von Willebrand factor, thrombospondin, and thromboxanes. These substances have many varied effects including increasing capillary permeability by disrupting the integrity of the endothelium, both vasoconstriction and vasodilatation, and the recruitment of several other inflammatory cell types. Monocytes respond to chemotatic signals such as fibrin and fibrinopeptides and leave the blood vessels via diapedesis. This migration is facilitated by capillary leak and interstitial edema that results from the action of inflammatory substances such that, by the end of one and a half days postinjury, the numbers of monocytes in the wound reaches its peak. The inflammatory milieu of the wound then stimulates the monocyte to become a macrophage, and it is these macrophages in conjunction with resident tissue macrophages that orchestrate wound healing.

Macrophages release over 20 different growth factors and cytokines and can perform a wide range of functions so that they are truly the central cell in wound healing.[7] Just like the neutrophil, macrophages contribute to clearing the wound of bacteria, although neutrophils remain the prime anti-bacterial cell in the wound. The phagocytic function of macrophages is not limited to bacteria alone since they also clear away apoptotic neutrophils and other cells via phagocytosis. Unlike the neutrophils, phagocytosis is not the main function of the macrophage and this activity is typically manifested only in the very early stages of wound healing. As the wound is cleared of bacteria, the macrophages release growth factors that reinforce endothelial cell activation and are chemotatic signals for various cells. Activated endothelial cells display adhesion molecules so that additional inflammatory cells can bind to the activated endothelium and be recruited into the wound. The combination of endothelial cell activation and the release of chemotatic and growth factors leads to the next stage of wound healing, the migratory phase.

## Migratory Phase

The next phase of wound healing is the migratory phase. The interaction of activated endothelial cells with circulating inflammatory cells leads to the margination of leukocytes. They traverse the blood vessel wall through diapedesis and migrate along chemotatic gradients to the site of injury. At this point of wound healing,

macrophages are progressing from bacterial phagocytosis to the coordination of the complex cell–cell interactions and are now the dominant cell type in the wound. The relatively hypoxic wound environment causes macrophages to release angiogenic growth factors, which along with PDGF released by activated platelets lead to the creation of new blood vessels or angiogenesis.[8-9] PDGF also stimulates fibroplasia by stimulating the normally present but quiescent fibroblasts to begin replicating by releasing them from their $G_0$ arrest. Cytokines like IGF-1 and epidermal growth factor (EGF) released from activated macrophages and platelets cause the fibroblasts to begin replicating. Additional fibroblasts from outside the wound environment arrive by traveling over the scaffold of the fibrin clot by binding to fibronectin within it. While angiogenesis and fibroblast proliferation occur simultaneously, it is obvious that like all cellular synthetic functions, fibroblast synthetic function is dependent on oxygen. Thus, in the healing wound, angiogenesis and fibroplasia are interconnected processes.[10]

Angiogenesis is dependent on the action of endothelial cells derived from the nearby uninjured portion of blood vessels.[11] These endothelial cells first generate plasminogen activator to degrade the clot at the site of vessel injury so that they can migrate out into the extracellular matrix.[10] This action is dependent on the activity of zinc-dependent metalloproteinases which are required to dissolve the basement membrane and collagenases.[11] The newly "liberated" endothelial cells then migrate through the surrounding extracellular matrix by extending pseudopodia, just like leukocytes do, in response to chemotatic signals released by platelets and macrophages. The relatively hypoxic local wound environment leads to the formation of lactic acid through anaerobic metabolism, which has been shown to be a potent stimulus for macrophages to release endothelial cell growth factors.[7] When tissue oxygen tension improves and the macrophages are no longer hypoxic, they stop elaborating endothelial cell growth factors in an elegant feedback loop controlling angiogenesis. Thus, wound re-vascularization removes the stimulus for endothelial cell growth and migration, and like the preceding neutrophils, the endothelial cells also undergo apoptosis. The typical beefy red color of granulation tissue is a result of dense collections of capillaries formed through the process of angiogenesis.

While angiogenesis is occurring within the wound, re-epithelialization is occurring at the margin of the wound. This process begins approximately 24 hours postinjury and is driven primarily by transforming growth factor alpha (TGF-α) which is released by platelets and macrophages. If a wound is sufficiently deep enough to destroy the stratum basale of the skin, keratinocytes from the wound edges or from deep skin appendages such as hair follicles, sweat glands, or sebaceous glands spared by the wounding insult serve as the source for re-epithelialization. Interestingly, re-epithelialization of the wound is almost entirely dependent on migration of keratinocytes, which occurs as sheets of cells move in from the wound periphery, rather than mitosis of keratinocytes within the wound. In order for keratinocytes to migrate they must detach themselves from their basement membrane by dissolving their anchoring desmosomes. Following this they display integrins and migrate across the early wound matrix using fibronectin cross-linked with fibrin as adhesion sites exactly like the fibroblasts before them. As the keratinocytes migrate they elaborate matrix metalloproteinases (MMPs), collagenases, plasminogen activator, and other proteases to dissolve debris as well as phagocytosing dead cells blocking their path.

As the sheet of migrating epithelial cells advances, new cells are formed at the wound margin by greatly upregulated mitosis to replenish the advancing cells. The rate of mitosis at the wound margin may be 17 times higher than that seen in normal tissue and remains the only focus of epithelial cell mitosis in the wound.[12] The migration continues until keratinocytes encounter other cells, which stops their advancement through contact inhibition, and down regulation of their fibronectin receptors that are necessary for their movement.[10] Re-epithelialization proceeds more rapidly if the basement membrane is intact, otherwise new basement membrane substances must be secreted.[13] Keratinocytes will then reanchor themselves to the basement membrane and each other using desmosomes and hemi-desmosomes, and normal skin stratification is established by cell division of the basal layer of cells.

Thus, by the conclusion of the migratory phase, new blood vessels are being formed and fibroblasts are appearing in the wound and begin replicating so that fibroplasia may take place, while, at the wound margin, an advancing sheet of epithelial cells moves inward. Table 49-2 reviews some of the more important cytokines and growth factors involved in the regulation of wound healing.

## Proliferative Phase

The migration of multiple cell types including monocytes, lymphocytes, and endothelial cells into the wound along with the emergence of active fibroblasts leads to the next phase of wound healing, the proliferative phase. This phase usually commences around day five and is characterized by the dramatic increase in the number of cells and the production of collagen. While the production of collagen may be detected as early as 10 hours after injury, it is not until day seven that its rate of production reaches its maximum velocity. Collagen synthesis continues at a vigorous pace until approximately day 21 when the wound approaches its peak of collagen content and collagen production plateaus. It is not coincidental that retention sutures used to reinforce tenuous laparotomy closures are left in place until day 21.

Eventually, granulation tissue is formed as the fibrin-fibronectin network that comprises the blood clot along with the makeshift wound matrix of proteoglycans, glycosaminoglycans, and hyaluronic acid is replaced by a combination of collagen, new capillaries, and numerous inflammatory cells and fibroblasts. This process is largely accomplished by fibroblasts that interact with several adhesive ligands in the wound matrix such as laminin, tenascin, and fibronectin while they release hyaluronidases that degrade the provisional wound medium. This early wound continues to evolve as collagen is haphazardly laid down upon the fibronectin and glycosaminoglycan scaffold. The amount of granulation tissue in the wound is dependent on the size and depth of wounds that are allowed to heal by secondary intention. Large wounds need to "fill in" with granulation tissue so that epithelial cells from the wound margin can migrate across and re-epithelialize the wound. Alternatively, the development of a healthy bed of granulation tissue is the sign that a wound is ready to accept an autologous skin graft. It is the rich network of capillaries along with the relatively aqueous environment that supports the transplanted epithelium by bathing it in a flow of nutrient containing fluid and oxygen. Full-thickness skin grafts are an important modality to mitigate the next step of wound healing, which is contraction.

Wounds that are allowed to heal by secondary intention and, to a much lesser degree, wounds closed primarily, all undergo the phenomenon of wound contraction which is a process whereby the wound edges and surrounding skin are pulled in toward the center of the wound. Contraction usually starts around one week after wounding, peaks in intensity around day 10 and may persist for weeks with a reported speed of nearly 0.75 mm per day. This process is a highly efficient way of reducing the surface size of the wound and decreases the amount of re-epithelialization that needs to occur. Unfortunately, this process can be particularly debilitating if the wound overlies a joint, flexible part of the body or crucial orifice such as the eye or mouth. Significant loss of function due to the presence of a contracting wound is clinically called a "contracture." Differences in the thickness of skin in various anatomic locations along with the laxity of the surrounding skin leads to variable degrees of contraction. Typically, the perineum and trunk experience the greatest degree while the extremities exhibit the least. The head and neck exhibit an in-between amount of wound contraction. The exact mechanism of wound contraction is not well elucidated but appears to be dependent on modified fibroblasts that contain microfilaments and alpha smooth muscle actin and phenotypically resemble smooth muscle cells.[14] These myofibroblasts are richly endowed with adhesion molecules in order to complex with a vast array of components making up the early wound environment. It is these attachments that allow them to bind and draw the wound edges together. As the wound contracts, other fibroblasts continue to synthesize collagen which effectively holds the wound together.

Nearly 20 different types of collagen have been identified and all share a common structural similarity known as the right-handed triple helix. Each type of collagen has unique structural properties which are attributed to specific breaks in the triple helix pattern. In general, collagen triple helices comprise three alpha peptide chains which undergo extensive modification both in and outside the fibroblast. Collagen is the major component of all human tissues and is distinctive in that it contains large quantities of the unique amino acids hydroxyproline and hydroxylysine. The hydroxylation of specific prolines in the early peptide chain is extremely important because error at this stage of collagen synthesis leads to the creation of an unstable collagen that is quickly degraded in the extracellular environment. The hydroxylation of proline and lysine requires ascorbic acid (vitamin C) which is the mechanism whereby vitamin C deficiency leads to impaired wound healing, and even opening of previous healed wounds, as seen in the disease scurvy.

Regulation of collagen synthesis occurs at many levels, beginning with the transcription. Collagen transcription takes place on several different chromosomes from discontinuous genes resulting in a large precursor molecule that must be modified within the nucleus, thus only limited amounts of messenger RNA is created. This highly modified mRNA then undergoes translation on ribosomes of the endoplasmic reticulum so that by the time the collagen molecule is ready to leave the golgi apparatus, it has undergone significant glycosylation with glucose and galactose. Also, it has had "extension" peptides placed on its amino and carbon terminals to facilitate its orientation and handling. These procollagen monomers leave the cell where additional modification takes place extracellularly, resulting in highly cross-linked collagen fibers. The extracellular modification process is fairly unique to collagen, and it is during this juncture that the extension peptides are cleaved

**TABLE 49-2**

## Cytokines and Growth Factors

| PEPTIDE | SITE OF SYNTHESIS | REGULATION | TARGET CELLS | EFFECTS |
|---|---|---|---|---|
| G-CSF | Fibroblasts, monocytes | Induced by IL-1, LPS, IFN-$aL | Committed neutrophil progenitors (CFU-G, Gran) | Supports the proliferation of neutrophil-forming colonies. Stimulates respiratory burst. |
| GM-CSF | (IL-3 has almost identical effects) | Endothelial cells, fibroblasts, macrophages, T lymphocytes, bone marrow | Induced by IL-1, TNF | Granulocyte-erythrocyte-monocyte-megakaryocyte progenitor cells (CFU-GEMM, CFU-MEG, CFU-Eo, CFU-GM) Supports the proliferation of macrophage-, eosinophil-, neutrophil-, and monocyte-containing colonies |
| IFN$aL, −$bT, −$gM | Epithelial cells, fibroblasts, lymphocytes, macrophages, neutrophils | Induced by viruses (foreign nucleic acids), microbes, microbial foreign antigens, cancer cells | Lymphocytes, macrophages, infected cells, cancer cells | Inhibits viral multiplication. Activates defective phagocytes, direct inhibition of cancer cell multiplication, activation of killer leukocytes, inhibition of collagen synthesis. |
| IL-1 | Endothelial cells, keratinocytes, lymphocytes, macrophages | Induced by TNF-$aL, IL-1, IL-2, C5a. Suppressed by I L-4, TGF-$bT | Monocytes, macrophages, T cells, B cells, NK cells, LAK cells | Stimulates T cells, B cells, NK cells, LAK cells. Induces tumoricidal activity and production to other cytokines, endogenous pyrogen (via PGE$_2$ release). Induces steroidogenesis, acute phase proteins, hypotension; chemotactic neutrophils. Stimulates respiratory burst. |
| IL-1ra | Monocytes | Induced by GM-CSF, LPS, IgG | Blocks type 1 IL-1 receptors on T cells, fibroblasts, chondrocytes, endothelial cells | Blocks type 1 IL-1 receptors on T cells, chondrocytes, endothelial cells. Ameliorates animal models of arthritis, septic shock, and inflammatory bowel disease. |
| IL-2 | Lymphocytes | induced by IL-1, IL-6 | T cells, NK cells, B cells, activated | Stimulates growth of T cells, NK cells, and B cells monocytes |
| IL-4 | T cells, NK cells, mast cells | Induced by cell activation, IL-1 | All hematopoietic cells and many others express receptors | Stimulates B cell and T cell growth. Induces HLA class II molecules. |
| IL-6 | Endothelial cells, fibroblasts, lymphocytes, some tumors | Induced by IL-1, TNF-$aL | T cells, B cells, plasma cells, keratinocytes, hepatocytes, stem cells | B cell differentiation. Induction of acute phase proteins, growth of keratinocytes. Stimulates growth of T cells and hematopoietic stem cells. |
| IL-8 | Endothelial cells, fibroblasts, lymphocytes, monocytes | Induced by TNF, IL-1, LPS, cell adherence (monocytes) | Basophils, neutrophils, T cells | Induces expression of endothelial cell LECAM-1 receptors, $bT_2$ integrins, and neutrophil transmigration. Stimulates respiratory burst. |
| M-CSF | Endothelial cells, fibroblasts, monocytes | Induced by IL-1, LPS, I | | |
| FN-$aL | Committed monocyte progenitors (CFU-M, Mono) | Supports the proliferation of monocyte-forming colonies. Activates macrophages. | | |
| MCP-1, MCAF | Monocytes. Some tumors secrete a similar peptide. | Induced by IL1, LPS, PHA | Unstimulated monocytes | Chemoattractant specific for monocytes |
| TNF-$aL (LT has almost identical effects) | Macrophages, NK cells, T cells, transformed cell lines, B cells (LT) | Suppressed by PGE$_2$, TGF-$bT, IL-4. Induced by LPS. | Endothelial cells, monocytes, neutrophils | Stimulates T cell growth. Direct cytotoxin to some tumor cells. Profound proinflammatory effect via induction of IL-1 and PGE$_2$. Systemic administration produces many symptoms of sepsis. Stimulates respiratory burst and phagocytosis. |

Key: CFU = Colony-forming unit; G-CSF = Granulocyte colony-stimulating factor; GM-CSF = Granulocyte-macrophage colony-stimulating factor; IFN = Interferon; IL = Interleukin; IL1ra = Interleukin-1 receptor antagonist; LPS = Lipopolysaccharide; LT = Lymphotoxin; MCAF = Monocyte chemotactic and activating factor; M-CSF = Macrophage colony-stimulating factor; MCPO-1 = Monocyte chemotactic peptide-1; NK = Natural killer (cell); PHA = Phytohemagglutinin; TGF-$bT = Transforming growth factor beta; TNF-$aL = Tumor necrosis factor alpha

from the end of procollagen, which are then taken back into the cell and down regulate collagen expression. At the end of this stage of wound healing, sufficient collagen fibers have been synthesized and the wound is more appropriately called a scar.

## Remodeling Phase

Although it seems contradictory, it is true that collagen must be degraded at the same time it is created in order for normal wound healing to occur. When the rate of collagen synthesis is balanced by an equal rate of collagen degradation, the wound is said to have reached the remodeling or maturational phase. This phase of wound healing may last for several months or even years for large wounds that heal by second intention. The tensile strength of the wound increases over time as the disorganized type III collagen that was laid down initially is degraded by MMPs and slowly replaced by type I collagen. The activity of the MMPs is itself regulated by tissue inhibitors of matrix metalloproteinases (TIMPs) so that a balance between synthesis, deposition, and degradation of extracellular matrix is maintained.[15]

As type I collagen is laid down and oriented parallel to lines of stress, the tensile strength of the wound increases. This increase is most rapid during the first six weeks, and then slows down but may persist for over a year. The tensile strength of the wound approaches 50% of normal skin by three months after injury and plateaus out about 80% by the end of remodeling, although this process continues on at an extremely slow rate for several more years. The increase in tensile strength is attributed to collagen cross-linking since the collagen content of the wound does not change beyond the third week. The scar which was originally red or purple in color due to the tremendous amount of capillaries it contains gradually turns white as these are re-adsorbed and replaced with type I collagen. The final result of the repair is an inelastic, avascular, brittle scar that is devoid of skin appendages such as hair follicles and sweat glands and never recovers more than 80% of the tensile strength of unwounded skin.

## CLINICAL MANAGEMENT OF WOUNDS

### Types of Wound Closure

Wound closure falls into one of four general categories: primary, secondary, delayed-primary closures, and tissue-transfer closures. In primary closure, the cutaneous defect is approximated through the use of sutures, staples, adhesive dressings, or topical sealants, and the previously described phases of wound healing occur albeit on a limited scale. These wounds are typically closed in layers along tissue planes and derive their strength from collagen-rich layers such as dermis or fascia. The duration of healing and the final cosmetic result are closely linked to the amount of devitalized tissue, bacteria, and blood left in the wound at the time of closure. Meticulous debridement of the wound along with scrupulous hemostasis minimizes the inflammatory phase of wound healing and allows the wound to progress rapidly to the migratory and proliferative phases of the healing process and promotes earlier wound closure with improved cosmesis, as well. The decision to close a wound primarily is based on the judgment by the clinician that the wound is at minimal risk for wound infection or that subsequent wound infection after primary closure is less detrimental than open management of the wound.

Wounds that are felt to be at excessive risk for infection are best left open to heal by secondary intention. Spontaneous or secondary intention closure occurs when the wound edges are not re-approximated and the wound must undergo contracture, granulation, and re-epithelialization in order to close. Open wounds are much less likely to become infected, but they are not immune to wound infection. The presence of increased bacteria and tissue debris leads to a longer, more intense inflammatory phase which results in more scaring and decreased cosmesis. Failure of healing by secondary intention leads to a chronic wound and in large part is due to a fundamental shift in the type and quality of wound inflammation. Chronic wounds, which are practically defined as a wound that has failed to close within three months, exhibit much higher levels of collagenases and matrix metalloproteinases, yet have reached a point of stasis and do not ultimately heal.

In delayed primary closure, a wound is left open for a few days and is treated much the same as a wound that is healing by second intention. The difference is that after a certain time the wound is then closed primarily. The main reason that a wound is handled in this fashion is that there is too much bacterial contamination, tissue trauma, or foreign bodies to allow a primary closure, and the wound is left open so that wound care and dressing changes can remove these impediments to infection-free healing.[16] There tends to be more inflammation in wounds that are managed by delayed primary closure than primary closure, but eventually these wounds exhibit the same tensile strength and cosmesis as wounds that were initially closed primarily and with lower infection rates.[16]

Open wounds and those with extensive soft-tissue loss that are technically difficult to close are best treated by application of a skin graft or tissue transfer. In general the simplest technique that will result in a closed wound should be employed so that a flap should not be used when a skin graft would suffice, and a free flap should be avoided if a rotational flap will be satisfactory. The timing of grafting or creating a flap is somewhat controversial and is best determined by the overall physiologic condition of the patient. Vascular anastomoses and exposed blood vessels are special cases and need to be covered as soon as possible to prevent catastrophic blowouts. In patients with an open abdomen it is highly desirable to get coverage of intestinal anastomoses with omentum, absorbable mesh or the abdominal wall since they have a tendency to break down leading to devastating "entero-atmospheric fistulas."[27] Split-thickness skin grafts are usually applied five days after injury but this is based more on tradition than physiology.

### Decision Making in Wound Management

The way a wound is treated is dependent on several decisions that can loosely be defined as clinical judgment. The first determination in whether to close a wound or treat it open is related to the time since injury. In general, wounds that have been open for more than six to eight hours should be left open, otherwise primary closure is advantageous. Obviously there are many exceptions to this "rule" since open wounds on the face or scalp tend to do well even when closed more than eight hours after wounding. This observation is due to the relatively low levels of commensal bacterial colonization coupled with an outstanding blood supply in these locations. On the other end of the spectrum, a four-hour old wound in an ischemic extremity in a patient with diabetes mellitus is best left open since neither bacterial flora nor blood supply favors infection-free healing.

The next consideration in establishing a treatment plan for the wound is based on the mechanism of wounding. High-velocity gunshot wounds, crush injuries, close-range shotgun wounds, and high-energy open fractures are all characterized by extensive destruction of soft tissue and are frequently complicated by a wound infection.[17] Heavily contaminated wounds such as human bites, farming-related accidents, and wounds with gross contamination, especially soil, are at exceedingly high risk for subsequent wound infection and are best managed open. These contaminated wounds are at risk for tetanus and the patient should receive tetanus prophylaxis, as well. Tetanus prophylaxis is detailed in Table 49-3, while Table 49-4 reviews the characteristics of a wound that is tetanus prone.

**TABLE 49-3**

| Tetanus Prophylaxis | | | | |
|---|---|---|---|---|
| **NOTETANUS-PRONE WOUNDS** | | | **TETANUS-PRONE WOUNDS** | |
| History of adsorbed tetanus toxoid (doses) | Td[a] | TIG | Td | TIG |
| Unknown or less than three doses | Yes | No | Yes | Yes |
| Three or more doses[b] | No[c] | No | No[d] | No |

[a]For children younger than 7 years old: diphtheria-telanus-pertussls (DPT) vaccination (DT, if pertussis vaccine is contraindicated) is preferred to tetanus toxoid alone. For persons 7 years old or more. Td is preferred to tetanus toxoid alone.
[b]If only three dosses of fluid toxoid have been given, a fourth dose of toxoid, perferably an adsorbed toxoid, should be given.
[c]Yes, if more than 10 years since last dose.
[d]Yes, if more than 5 years since last dose.
Td, tetanus and diphtheria boxoids adsorbed (for adult use): TIG, tetanus immune globulin (human).
Tetanus toxoid and TIG should be administered with different syringes at different sites.

**TABLE 49-4**

| Wound Characteristics Relating to Likelihood of Tetanus | | |
|---|---|---|
| **CLINICAL FEATURES** | **NONTETANUS-PRONE WOUNDS** | **TETANUS-PRONE WOUNDS** |
| Age of wound | ≤6 h | >6 h |
| Configuration | Linear | Stellate wound, avulsion, abrasion |
| Depth | ≤1 cm | >1cm |
| Mechanism of injury | Sharp surface | Crush, bum, missile wound, other |
| Signs of infection | Absent | Present |
| Devitalized tissue | Absent | Present |
| Contaminants (dirt, feces, soil, etc.) | Absent | Present |
| Ischemic or denervated tissue | Absent | Present |

**TABLE 49-5**

| Threats Infection-Free Wound Healing |
|---|
| Necrotic tissue |
| Inadequate hemostasis |
| Foreign body |
| Heavy contamination |
| Local ischemia |
| Local conditions |
| Shock |
| Systemic conditions |
| Malnutrition |
| Immunosuppression |
| Shock |
| Diabetes |
| Renal insufficiency |
| Steroids |
| Cytotoxic drugs |
| Vitamin and trace metal deficiency |
| Collagen vascular disease |

In addition to local wound factors, systemic conditions can also greatly increase the incidence of wound infection. Hemorrhagic shock has been identified as strong risk factor for wound infection.[18-19] This phenomenon is likely multifactorial since trauma and hemorrhage affects blood flow on both the global and tissue level and causes dysfunction of the immune,[20] hemtapoeitic,[21] and myelopoeitic[22] systems. Diabetes mellitus,[23] connective tissue disorders,[24] advanced cancers,[25] immunosuppressed states, atherosclerosis, hypothermia, malnutrition,[26] chronic obstructive pulmonary disease, corticosteroid therapy, and a multitude of other systemic disease processes all negatively impact wound healing and need to be considered in the plan for wound treatment. Thus, the decision to close a wound is based on a series of assessments of the mechanism of injury, anatomic location, degree of contamination, and physiologic and medical condition of the patient.

In addition to the factors predisposing to wound infection discussed above, additional variables leading to wound infections have been identified. These threats to infection-free healing are listed in Table 49-5. Devitalized tissue is a common finding in high-velocity gunshot and high-energy wounds and represents a major risk factor for wound infection. Such tissue is a culture medium for bacteria, poorly penetrated by immune cells and antibiotics, and incites an increased inflammatory response. Debridement is an effective way of removing this source of infection and inflammation and is an integral part of wound care.[28]

Meticulous hemostasis is often cited as a key component to normal wound healing, but the reason is mentioned infrequently. Iron is an essential component for bacterial replication,[29] so it is tightly regulated in vivo by sequestration in macrophages as well as by hepcidin, an iron-binding protein released by the liver in response to inflammation.[30] Wound hematomas lead to increased infections by overwhelming the body's ability to restrict iron and inhibit bacterial growth. Thus, they render a wound susceptible to infection by smaller bacterial numbers. In a similar fashion, contamination with a foreign body also leaves a wound more susceptible to smaller bacterial burdens by reducing phagocytosis by granulocytes. If adequate hemostasis cannot be obtained due to a coagulopathy or extensive injury or if debridement is inadequate, it is best to postpone primary closure until these conditions are corrected. Such wounds can be managed as open wounds and then treated by delayed primary closure at the bedside or taken to the operating room for further debridement and eventual closure.

## Operative versus Nonoperative Management of the Wound

Similar to the decision process regarding closure of a wound, the setting of wound care is equally important. In general, large complex contaminated wounds containing foreign bodies or devitalized tissue are best managed in the operating room. Anatomic location can be critical as well since perineal, facial, and severe hand injuries can have serious consequences if initially mismanaged. Noncompliant patients and those with hazardous communicable diseases are best treated in the operating room for safety reasons for the patient and clinician alike. Although a wound may be impressive, it is frequently the associated injury that is most threatening to the patient. A two centimeter neck wound is not impressive, but it may lead to a disastrous sequence of events if it overlies the carotid artery. In general, attempting to manage a major wound without adequate light, exposure, anesthesia, equipment, or patient cooperation leads to missed injuries, retained foreign bodies, inadequate debridement, wound hematomas, and soft tissue infections. Table 49-6 summarizes some conditions mandating operative management of a wound.

## Operative Issues

Once the decision is made to proceed to the operating room, the next step is to consider positioning of the patient and preparation of the skin. In general, the patient should be positioned in such a way so that access to other body cavities and surfaces is maintained. The lateral decubitus position offers excellent access to a hemithorax, but does so at the expense of access to the contralateral chest and abdomen. Extremities are best fully prepped and free draped to maximize exposure and operative options.

After positioning, the patient's skin is prepared with an antiseptic. As part of this preparation, body hair may need to be removed to facilitate wound exploration and exposure and to prevent hair from becoming trapped in the wound. Shaving hair should be avoided since it has been shown to lead to higher wound infection rates when compared to depilatories or clippers.[31] While depilatories may be useful in elective surgery, they have little role in the management of urgent traumatic wounds. Thus, surgical clippers with disposable heads are readily available in the emergency department (ED) and operating room. Hair should be removed in an atraumatic fashion so as not to cause additional injury. Loose foreign bodies and debris should be removed, as well. Eyebrows should not be removed since in a minority of patients their regrowth can be inadequate.[32]

The most common skin antiseptics are povidone-iodine solution (BD E-ZScrub; Becton, Dickinson and Co.,Franklin Lakes, NJ) and chlorhexidine gluconate solution (BD EZ-Scrub 107 with 4% chlorhexidine, Becton, Dickinson and Co., Franklin Lakes, NJ). Both agents are rapidly bactericidal, but emerging evidence shows that chlorhexidine is a superior prep agent since it has more residual activity and is associated with lower rates of infection.[33–36] Povidone-iodine and chlorhexidine are both toxic to normal tissue so they should only be used as prepatory agents rather than as topical wound treatments.[37] Ambroise Pare admonished against putting anything into a wound that would not be tolerated in one's eye, but this is especially true for chlorhexidine since it causes corneal injury.[38–39] Povidone-iodine or hexachlorophene solution

(PHisoHex®) should be used for prepping the face to avoid corneal damage and possible blindness.[40]

One of the hallmarks of operative management of heavily contaminated wounds centers on the use of high-pressure pulse lavage systems. In the past, it was felt irrigation had to be performed at high pressure in order to effectively remove microparticulate contaminants and bacteria.[41] Lavage of contaminated wounds with a bulb syringe or low-pressure systems was thought to be ineffective. While commercially available high-pressure irrigating systems are undoubtedly effective, their destructive effects on already injured tissues is frequently overlooked. In addition to the increased devitalization of the wound, high-pressure irrigation can also have detrimental effects on immune function and wound healing.[42] Emerging evidence suggests that in addition to local trauma, high-pressure irrigation may not be as effective in removing contamination as gentler methods and may in fact drive bacteria deeper into tissues.[43] Sharp debridement, curettage, suction, and irrigation of all non-variable and grossly infected tissue should be undertaken until the wound is left with only clean, healthy, and well-perfused tissues. Outside of the operating room, one of the simplest irrigation systems can be made by punching several holes in the top of a half-liter bottle of saline utilizing an 18-gauge needle. Alternatively, a syringe and angiocatheter can be fashioned into an effective irrigator as demonstrated in Fig. 49-2.

### TABLE 49-6

| Conditions Requiring Management in Operating Room |
|---|
| Large or complicated soft tissue injury |
| Extensive amount of necrotic or ischemic tissue |
| Heavy contamination |
| Associated injury |
| Visceral |
| Vascular |
| Fracture |
| Perineal wounds |
| Compartment syndrome |
| High-pressure injection injuries |

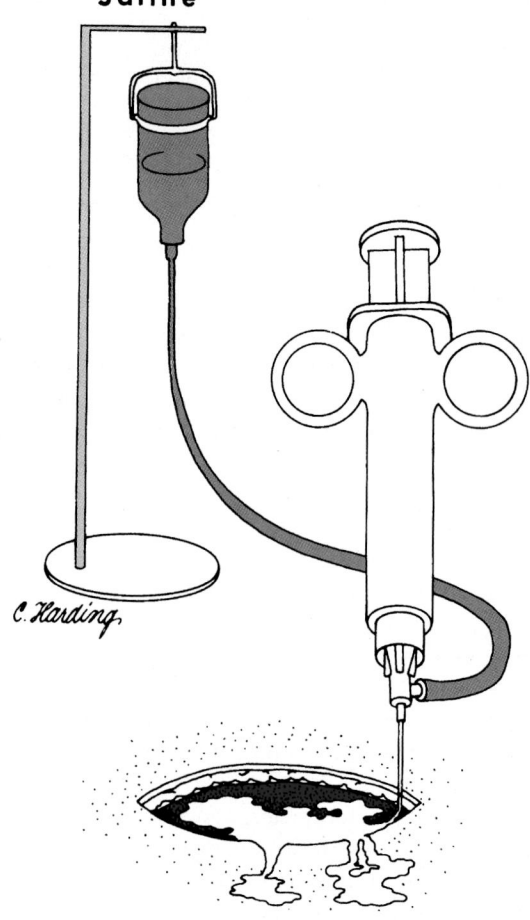

**Saline**

C. Harding

**FIGURE 49-2.** Technique for high-pressure syringe irrigation of a wound.

## Local Anesthetics

Operative treatment of a wound gains the added benefit of effective analgesia and anesthesia administered by an anesthesiologist. For wounds cared for in other venues, local anesthesia plays a crucial role and is personally administered by the clinician caring for the wound. Local anesthesia facilitates excision of devitalized tissue, removal of foreign bodies, and enhances patient comfort and cooperation during closure of the wound. Most local anesthetics work by binding neural cell membrane sodium channels to block depolarization and conduction of noxious stimuli. These drugs are weak polar bases that are structurally composed of an aromatic, hydrophobic ring, a hydrophilic tertiary amino group and an intermediary chain. It is the presence of an ester or amide linkage in the intermediary chain that is used to broadly classify the local anesthetics.[44] Ester local anesthetics are rapidly metabolized by plasma pseudocholinesterases, and the resultant hydrophilic metabolites are excreted through the kidney. In contrast, amide anesthetics are metabolized by the liver. Hence, their clearance is a much slower process and the potential for adverse effects is greater due to accumulation of the drug or impaired clearance secondary to hepatic dysfunction.[45]

The lipid solubility of a local anesthetic is proportional to the drug's potency while its protein binding helps regulate its duration of action. The duration of action of local anesthetics may be enhanced by the addition of dilute concentrations of epinephrine in order to cause vasoconstriction and impair the clearance of the drug from the tissues. The addition of epinephrine to the local anesthetic increases the maximum dose since vasoconstriction reduces systemic absorption. Obviously, local anesthetics containing epinephrine should not be injected into tissues perfused by end arterioles such as fingers, toes, nose, penis, or ear since vasoconstriction may result in tissue necrosis. Although some recent literature has challenged this dogma, it is still prudent to avoid this possible complication altogether.[46–47] Inadvertent intravascular injection is another potential pitfall that can be avoided by aspirating the syringe slightly to exclude this possibility prior to injecting the drug. Lastly, there is some concern that the injection of epinephrine into a contaminated wound may result in an increased incidence of wound infection.[48]

Injections of local anesthetics are inherently painful; however, several simple techniques can be utilized in order to minimize patient discomfort. Small gauge needles, as fine as 30-gauge, should be utilized and the drug administered by a technique of slow infiltration. Beginning the process through the existing break in the dermis rather than injecting into intact skin can also lessen pain. Intradermal injections should only be administered when needed and only after attempts of subdermal administration fail. Perhaps the most effective method for reducing the pain associated with local anesthetics can be achieved through the addition of sodium bicarbonate to buffer the pH of the anesthetic.[49–52] What remains puzzling is why this well described and efficacious technique is so underutilized in medicine today.[53]

In 1884, shortly after Carl Koller popularized the local anesthetic properties of cocaine, clinicians began noting serious unintended side effects.[54] While cardiac toxicity is most pronounced with cocaine, it is seen with all local anesthetics and is related to their effect on sodium channels in excitable membranes. Like the cardiovascular system, the central nervous system (CNS) also contains excitable cell membranes and is the other major site of toxicity

**TABLE 49-7**

### Symptoms of Local Anesthetic Overdose

**CENTRAL NERVOUS SYSTEM**
Excitability
Dizziness
Tinnitus
Nystagmus
Seizures

**CARDIOPULMONARY**
Hypotension
Myocardial collapse
Respiratory arrest

of local anesthesia. Increasing concentrations of local anesthetics lead to blockade of the inhibitory pathways in the amygdala and results in excess neural stimulation.[55] The CNS toxicity of a local anesthetic is initially manifested as muscle twitching, tinnitus, and agitation which can progress to seizures, coma, and death as levels continue to rise. The cardiovascular system is relatively more resistant than the CNS to the toxicity of local anesthetics, but arrhythmias and cardiovascular collapse are the most feared complications. Unfortunately, as the potency of a local anesthetic increases, so does its potential for cardiac depression and arrhythmias.[56] This observation is borne out by the fact that the potent anesthetic bupivacaine exerts a greater degree of cardiac toxicity than the weaker related amide anesthetic lidocaine. See Table 49-7 for a review of the symptoms of toxicity of local anesthetics.

Lidocaine and bupivacaine are the two most commonly used local anesthetics in the United States. Both are amide-type anesthetics and are available in combination with dilute concentrations of epinephrine (1:100,000 to 1:400,000), which lessens systemic absorption of the anesthetic due to vasoconstriction. As a result the maximum dosage for lidocaine for infiltrative anesthesia goes from 4.5 mg/kg for plain lidocaine to 7 mg/kg when it is combined with epinephrine. The best way to avoid toxicity from a local anesthetic is to be cognizant of the total dose being administered. Bupivacaine is far more potent, as well as toxic, than lidocaine due to its lipophilicity. It also has a much longer onset of action than lidocaine, thus lidocaine is the most commonly used local anesthetic in clinical medicine. Lidocaine is occasionally administered in combination with bupivacaine in order to capitalize on lidocaine's short onset of action coupled with the high potency and long half life of bupivacaine. Please refer to Table 49-8 for a summary of both agents.

For large areas where the dose of anesthetic required to achieve anesthesia would be prohibitive or areas that are technically difficult to infiltrate, a regional block may be an excellent way to achieve anesthesia.[57] Local blocks can be more efficacious than infiltrative anesthesia with less pain and a smaller volume of anesthetic used. Knowledge of the neural anatomy relevant to the sensory innervation of the region to be blocked is critical and allows for complete anesthesia. Two of the most commonly employed peripheral blocks are the median and ulnar nerve blocks, which are reviewed in Figs. 49-3 and 49-4, respectively. Figure 49-5 illustrates the ubiquitous digital block which is an extremely helpful technique utilized in the management of trauma to the fingers.

**TABLE 49-8**

| Local Anesthesia | | | | | |
| NAME | CLASS | ONSET | DURATION | MAXIMUM DOSE | METABOLISM |
| --- | --- | --- | --- | --- | --- |
| Lidocaine HCl (Xylocaine, Dilocaine, Nervocaine) | Amide | 1–5 min | 30–120 min | 4.5 mg/kg 7–8 mg/kg with epinephrine | Liver |
| Bupivacaine (Marcaine, Sensorcaine) | Amide | 2–10 min | 3–7 h | 175 mg 0.3 mg/kg (not for use in children) | Liver |

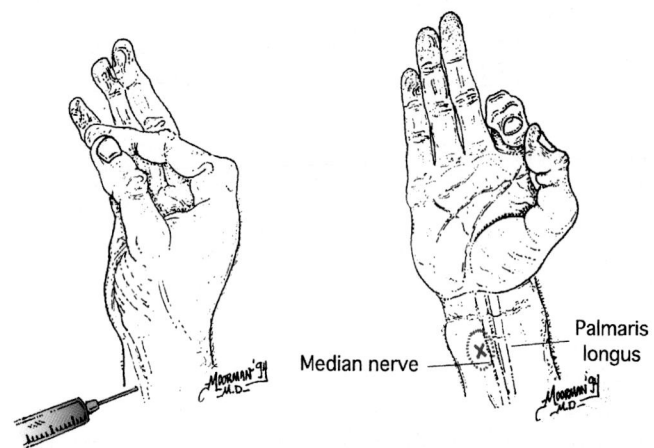

**FIGURE 49-3.** Technique of median nerve block anesthesia.

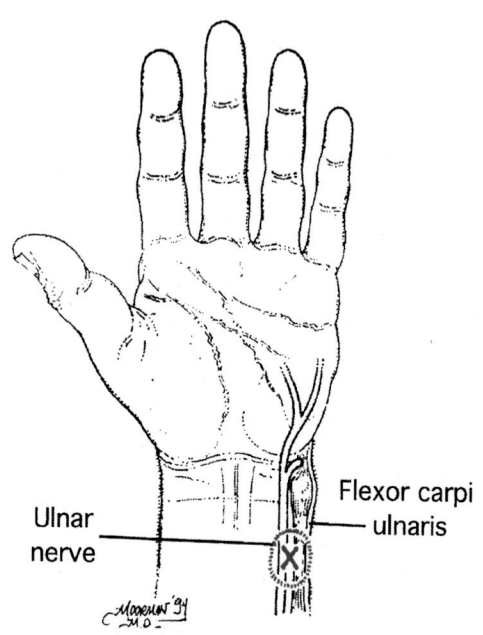

**FIGURE 49-4.** Technique of ulnar nerve block anesthesia.

## Use of Antibiotics for Acute Wounds

For over 50 years it has been known that administering an antibiotic well in advance of bacterial inoculation is a highly effective method of reducing wound infection; however, when dealing with traumatic wounds this is simply not possible. Since traumatic wounds are always contaminated with bacteria prior to their clinical presentation, the use of antibiotics for acute wounds is considered empiric rather than prophylactic. Accordingly, there is little role for empiric antibiotics in the management of open wounds except for a few special circumstances. Although controversial, most clinicians would agree to the use of antibiotics in the following situations:

1. *Open fractures or open joints.* An open fracture, defined as communication of a fracture site with the outside environment through an associated wound in the skin, can have devastating long-term consequences if nonunion or osteomyelitis sets in. Similarly, bacterial destruction of the articular surfaces of a joint can also lead to significant morbidity. Accordingly, these wounds are best treated with antibiotics; however, in this capacity, the antibiotics are an adjunct to basic wound and fracture care consisting of surgical debridement, irrigation of the joint, and fixation of the fracture.[58–60]

2. *Heavily contaminated extensive soft-tissue wounds.* Similar to traumatic orthopedic injuries, antibiotics serve an adjunctive role in the management of heavily contaminated soft tissue injuries; however, the mechanism of injury and degree of contamination remain far more predictive of subsequent wound infection than the choice of antibiotic.[61] Data are lacking about the duration of antibiotic usage in such wounds, but short courses are desirable if bacterial resistance is to be avoided.

3. *Delayed presentation.* Traumatic wounds that present in a significantly delayed fashion are well along on the continuum from contaminated to infected and likely benefit from antimicrobial therapy.

4. *Host factors.* Patients with profound immunosuppression, indwelling foreign bodies such as mechanical heart valves, and those unable to tolerate transient bacteremias are all likely to derive benefit from antibiotic therapy in the management of an acute wound. This decision is not based on evidence-based recommendations but rather on clinical judgment since trials of efficacy in these populations will never be undertaken for ethical reasons.

## Wound Dressings

For over 100 years the benefits of keeping a wound moist have been known[62,63]; however, it was not until the seminal article by Winter in 1962 showing that an occlusive dressing led to 40% faster healing than wounds left open to air did the concept of "wet" wound healing take hold.[64] Unfortunately, for many clinicians the choice of wound dressings is based on tradition and experience rather than data.[65] Therefore, one of the most painful, labor-intensive dressings remains the most commonly used; i.e., the wet to dry gauze dressing. This dressing comprises saline moistened gauze in

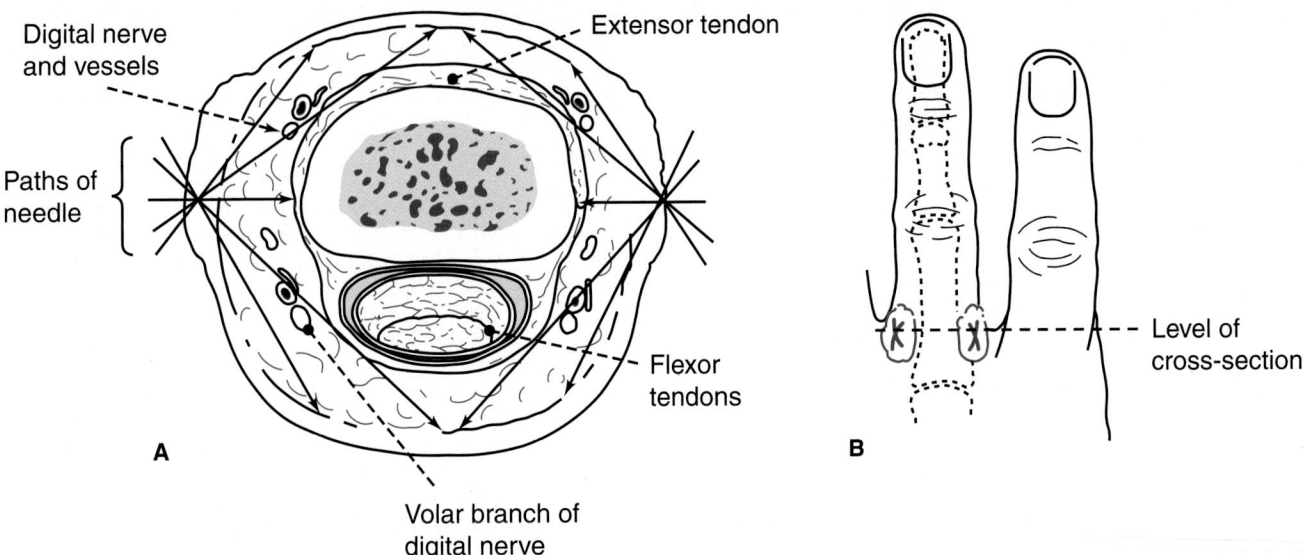

**FIGURE 49-5.   A.** Method of executing a digital block. **B.** Position of skin wheals and level of cross-section.

close contact with the wound covered by several layers of dry gauze. By the time this dressing is changed it typically dries out and sticks to the wound so its removal debrides the wound of necrotic tissue, secretions, and bacteria while causing significant pain and occasional bleeding.

One particularly useful type of dressing is a modification of the technique used on split-thickness skin graft donor sites to treat asphalt abrasions or "road rash." Road rash is a common finding after motorcycle or bicycle collisions, ejection from automobiles, or in pedestrians struck by automobiles. These wounds are typically contaminated with small stones, dirt, and other road substances and can present a serious challenge to the treating physician. For patients with small wounds, a combination of a topical viscous lidocaine solution with systemic analgesics can facilitate scrubbing and debridement in the operating room. For larger wounds treated under general anesthesia, the wound can be scrubbed clean of all foreign bodies using a pre-surgical scrub brush. Failure to fully debride the wound will lead to "tattooing" or retention of foreign bodies in the healing wound causing discoloration. Following debridement, the wound can be treated like a donor site. Hemostasis is achieved through the application of epinephrine-soaked lap sponges followed by a petrolatum-impregnated dressing which will adhere to the wound. This dressing can then be trimmed as re-epitheliazation takes place underneath it.

Wound dressings can be roughly broken down into several groups, including gauzes, semipermeable occlusive film dressings, foam dressings, alginates, and hydrocolloids all of which are reviewed in Table 49-9. The perfect dressing does not exist, but an excellent one would have the following properties:

1. *Encourage a moist but not macerated wound environment.* As discussed earlier, moist wound healing is far superior to dry wound healing; however, a major concern is maceration of the skin under moist dressings. Macerated skin can serve as a portal of entry for skin bacteria and may lead to infection.

2. *Avoid the presence of toxic substances.* Previously we have learned that povidone-iodine, chlorhexidine, acetic acid solutions, and dilute sodium hypochlorite solutions (Dakin's) all exhibit some degree of toxicity to fibroblasts or keratinocytes and should be avoided.

3. *Avoid leaving foreign bodies in the wound.* Foreign bodies are undesirable because they retard phagocytosis and delay wound healing.[66]

4. *Prevent bacterial contamination.* The dressing must not be penetrable to the outside environment and bacteria.

5. *Maintain optimal temperature and pH.* Wound healing proceeds faster at physiological temperature and pH.[67]

6. *Require less frequent dressing changes.* Many of the newer hydrocolloid, alginate and foam dressings are very expensive, but they may be cost-effective if the need for them to be changed is infrequent. Regrettably, studies confirming this advantage are still lacking.

7. *Cause less patient discomfort.*

8. *Serve as a vehicle to deliver adjuncts to wound care.* Topical silver,[68] anti-infectives,[69] and growth factors[70] have all been delivered by some of the newer surgical dressings.

## Sub-atmospheric Sponge Dressings

One of the biggest advances in wound management of the last decade has centered on the use of the "vac sponge." Vacuum-assisted closure of difficult wounds as initially described by Argenta[71] consists of an open-cell foam sponge, connected to a controlled vacuum device. The sponge is covered by a thin, adhesive occlusive dressing so that the wound environment remains sub-atmospheric. Kinetic Concepts, Inc. (San Antonio, TX) has patented Argenta's system (V.A.C.® System) and offers a vast array of vacuum dressing products and wound therapies such as ionic silver

**TABLE 49-9**

## Wound Dressing Materials

| CLASSIFICATION | MATERIAL | FUNCTIONS | USE | EXAMPLES | DISADVANTAGE | ADVANTAGES |
|---|---|---|---|---|---|---|
| Gauze | Cotton gauze | Absorbs fluid, removes exudate with changes | Open or infected wounds | Kertex Fluffs 4x4s | Frequent changes, foreign body in wound, desiccation if not kept moist | Readily available |
| Hydrocolloid | Hydrophilic colloidal particles with adhesive matrix (usually as a film or foam covered by a piece of release paper) | Maintains moist wound environment with optimum temperature and pH, adherence without adhesion, promotes granulation and epithelialization, seals and protects wound, wound debridement by autolysis | Full- or partial-thickness wounds, decubitus ulcers, primary dressing for closed wounds | Duoderm, Granuflex, Restore, Comfeel, Intrasite Ultec, J&J ulcer dressing, Tegasorb, Dermiflex Intrasite, Biofilm | Some seepage with heavily exudative wounds, difficult to seal wounds of complex shape, probably not indicated for infected wounds | Optimal wound environment, improved healing of some wounds, infrequently needs changing, decreased pain, no foreign body residual |
| Absorptive powders and pastes | Colloidal hydrophilic particles | See above (hydrocolloids) | Full-thickness wounds, deep angles, wound, with heavy exudate | Duoderm granules, Hydrogran, Hollister exudate absorber, Gelipe rm, Spand Gel | Probably not for use in infected wounds | High absorbancy, debridement with autolysis (see Hydrocolloid above) |
| Aiginates | Calcium alginate fibers (brown seaweed species) | Absorbs fluid and exudate, maintains moist wound environment | Open or infected wounds | Sorbsan, Kaltostat, Tegagal, Ultraplast, Stop Hemo | Not for use in wounds with little or no exudate as it does not form a gel | May be used in infected or contaminated wounds, infrequent dressing changes |
| Films | Semipermeable membranes (polyurethane or copolyester) | Occlusive dressing | IV site dressings, partial-thickness, minimally exuding wounds | Op-site, Opsite 3000, Tegaderm, Bioclusive, Blisterfilm, Visulin | Highly variable water vapor permeability among diferent products; not for use alone in heavily exuding wounds; skin maceration with bacterial overgrowth in products with low $H_2O$ permeability | Mimics skin performance, seals wound, may be used in combination with other dressings (i.e., alginates) |

impregnated sponges, irrigating vacuum systems, and polyvinyl alcohol sponges for use in tunnels and on top of skin grafts.

Sub-atmospheric dressings have simplified wound care, wound closures and reconstructions, and skin grafting, as well. These dressings have been shown to speed up the development of granulation tissue[72] and often allow a simple skin graft to be placed instead of a complex flap procedure. The reason why these dressings speed up the healing process is poorly understood and may be related to reducing wound edema, increasing blood flow,[72] increasing cellular proliferation,[73] or removing inhibitor substances from the milieu of the wound. Additional benefits of these types of dressings include keeping the wound environment moist and drawing the edges of the wound closer together. Combined with the natural process of wound contraction this leads to faster closure times and reduced wound size.

While negative pressure wound therapy represents a major advance in the care for both acute and chronic wounds, it is not a panacea for all wounds. Failure to fully debride a necrotic wound before placing the sponge can lead to ongoing necrosis, infection, and clinical deterioration. The currently recognized contraindications to negative pressure wound therapy include wounds with necrotic tissue, malignancy within the wound, exposed arteries, veins or vascular grafts, untreated osteomyelitis, and fistulas between epithelial surfaces. Wound ischemia and severe malnutrition are relative contraindications. Some physicians have reported success treating fistulas, but this is an off-label use.[74]

## BITES AND STINGS

### Human Bites

Human bites may be the most common bites seen in many urban emergency rooms. The main clinical problem in human bites relates to soft tissue infection since human saliva contains up to $10^{11}$ bacteria per milliliter and plaque on teeth has even greater numbers of bacteria. Common infecting organisms include *Streptococcus viridans, Staphylococcus spp., Eikenella corrodens, Bacteroides spp.*, and microaerophilic streptococci. The most common serious infections develop when there has been penetration of the joint capsule, which typically occurs when a clenched fist strikes the tooth of the person being assaulted ("fight bite"). These wounds usually involve the metacarpophalangeal (MCP) or the proximal interphalangeal joints (PIP). These are usually benign-appearing wounds and are frequently missed unless the examiner is aware of the potential problems of joint penetration. Such wounds may not be directly over the MCP joint unless the hand is examined with the fist clenched. These wounds should be seen in consultation with a hand surgeon and are usually best treated with intraoperative irrigation, intravenous antibiotics, and elevation of the hand and arm in an inpatient setting. In general, human bites should not be closed, with the exception of wounds on the face.

Antibiotic prophylaxis for human bites consists of ampicillin plus a β-lactamase inhibitor (intravenous ampicillin/sulbactam or amoxicillin/clavulanate). Alternative agents include cefoxitin or ampicillin alone or in combination with clindamycin. Although the incidence is unknown, hepatitis and infection with human immunodeficiency virus (HIV) are potentially transmissible by human bites. As with other exposures, the risk of infection depends on the size of the inoculum and the virulence of the viral agent. HIV exists in relatively low concentrations in human saliva and is relatively fastidious, presumably making its transmission difficult. Hepatitis B and C require a much smaller inoculum, and their transmission in a human bite is theoretically a greater risk. If the individual responsible for the bite is known or available for evaluation, serologic testing for HIV and hepatitis B and C is recommended. If the individual responsible for the bite is unavailable for testing, the administration of gamma globulin and hepatitis B vaccination should be considered in non-immunized patients. Tetanus immunization should be given if indicated (see Table 49-4).

## Cat Bites

Cat bites, like human bites, tend to be heavily contaminated. Cats tend to leave deep, small punctures that may penetrate all the way to the bone. Commonly isolated organisms include *Pasteurella multocida* and *Staphylococcus* spp. Ampicillin plus a β-lactamase inhibitor provides reasonable empiric coverage and tetanus and rabies prophylaxis should be given if indicated (Tables 49-3, 49-4, 49-10, and 49-12).

## Dog Bites

Dog bite wounds are another common clinical problem. Wound concerns center around injury to soft tissue since large dogs can generate tremendous force with their muscles of mastication. Soft tissue infections following dog bites are not as common as after cat and human bites, but they do occur. The bite wound should be copiously irrigated, and empiric preventive antibiotics are generally recommended. Facial dog bite wounds are usually closed, while wounds in other locations are managed with delayed primary closure or healing by secondary intention. Common infecting organisms include *Pasteurella multocida*, *Streptococcus viridans*, *Bacteroides*

**TABLE 49-10**

### Treatment Recommendations and Estimates of the Risk of Rabies, According to Type of Exposure and Geographic Area

| GEOGRAPHIC AREA | ANIMALS[a] | TREATMENT RECOMMENDATIONS[b,c] | | CASES OF RABIES/10,000 UNTREATED EXPOSURES[c] | |
|---|---|---|---|---|---|
| | | Bite | No Bite | Bite | No Bite |
| Group 1: Rabies endemic or suspected in species involved in the exposure | Bats anywhere in the United States; raccoons, skunks, foxes; mongooses in Puerto Rico; dogs in most developing countries and in the United States along Mexican border (3–80% rabid) | Treat | Treat | 150–5,000 | 0.3–160 |
| Group 2: Rabies not endemic in species involved in the exposure, but endemic in other terrestrial animals in area | Most wild carnivores (wolves, bobcats, bears) and groundhogs (2–20% rabid) | Treat | Treat or consult | 10–1200 | 0.2–40 |
| | Dogs and cats (0.1–2% rabid) | Observe or consult | Observe or consult | 0.5–120 | 0.01–4 |
| | Rodents and lagomorphs except groundhogs (about 0.01% rabid) | Consult or do not treat | Do not treat | 0.05–0.6 | 0.001–0.02 |
| Group 3: Rabies not endemic in species involved in the exposure or in other terrestrial animals in the area | Dogs, cats, many wild terrestrial animals in Washington, Idaho, Utah, Nevada, Colorado (0.1–0.01% rabid) | Consult or do not treat | Consult or do not treat | 0.05–6 | 0.001–0.2 |

[a]Percentages are the approximate proportions of indicated species found rabid when submitted and tested in state health department laboratories.

[b]"Consult" denotes consultation with a state or local health department. If the risk of rabies in the species involved in the exposure is low and the animal's brain is available, treatment is sometimes delayed up to 48 hours pending the results of laboratory testing. A healthy domestic dog or cat that bites a person should be confined and observed for 10 days. Any illness in the animals should be evaluated by a veterinarian and reported immediately to the local health department. If signs suggestive of rabies develop, treatment is begun immediately. If the animal is a stray or unwanted dog or cat, it should be killed immediately and the head removed and shipped, under refrigeration, for examination by a qualified laboratory.

[c]Rabies develops in 50 to 60% of untreated humans bitten by a rabid animal, and in 0.1 to 2% of those exposed to a rabid animal but not bitten (scratched or licked on an open wound or mucous membrane). The number of cases per 10,000 untreated patients was derived by multiplying the prevalence of rabies in a geographic area by the proportion of untreated humans in whom rabies would be expected to develop after exposure to a rabid animal.

spp., *Fusobacterium,* and *Capnocytophaga.* As in the case of human and cat bite wounds, ampicillin plus a β-lactamase inhibitor provides reasonable empiric coverage for dog bite wounds. Tetanus and rabies prophylaxis should be administered if indicated (see Tables 49-3, 49-4, 49-10, and 49-12).

## Rabies Prophylaxis

A number of different strains of highly neurotropic viruses cause clinical rabies infection. Most of these viruses belong to a single serotype in the genus *Lyssavirus,* family Rhabdoviridae. The virion contains a single-stranded, nonsegmented, negative-sense ribonucleic acid (RNA) genome, which encodes for five structural proteins.[75]

Susceptibility to rabies infection varies according to species, although most wild mammals can become infected with the virus. Foxes, coyotes, wolves, and jackals are most susceptible; skunks, raccoons, bats, bobcats, mongooses, and monkeys are intermediate; and opossums are surprisingly resistant.[75]

In the United States, rabies is found in terrestrial animals in ten distinct geographic areas. In each of these areas, one species is the predominant reservoir, with one of the distinct antigenic variants predominating. Bats account for an additional eight variants, accounting for sporadic outbreaks throughout the United States. The majority of the cases of rabies encephalitis acquired in the United States probably originate from exposure to bats. The epidemiology of human rabies reflects the geographic distribution of animals, emphasizing the fact that rabies is primarily a disease of nonhuman mammals. Vaccination programs for domestic animals in the United States have been responsible for a dramatic decline in rabies acquired from domestic dog and cat bites (Table 49-10 and 49-11). Internationally, the majority of human rabies is still acquired from dog bites, where canine rabies is still endemic.[75]

In humans, the established disease is almost always fatal. The diagnosis is relatively straightforward when a history of an animal bite is obtained; however, the history of a probable bite is inconsistently reported. Clinical symptoms of human rabies include pain at the bite site, dysphagia, pharyngeal spasms, paralysis, hydrophobia, and seizures. Distinguishing rabies from other causes of viral encephalitis or tetanus can be difficult. An effective vaccine is available for preventing the onset of clinical rabies. The dismal prognosis of rabies encephalitis emphasizes the importance of appropriate use of the vaccine and immunoglobulin preparations to prevent infection.

The risk of acquiring rabies depends on the probability of rabies infection in the animal and the amount of inoculum delivered into the wound, with the greatest risk from a bite. All animal wounds should be irrigated and cleansed with soap or a detergent. This has been shown to protect 90% of experimental animals from infection following inoculation of rabies virus into a wound.

Because public health officials monitor the incidence of rabies in populations of domestic and wild animals, a treating physician should be familiar with the local incidence of rabies in his or her region. Several historical clues may be of benefit in determining the likelihood that the animal was rabid. If the bite was unprovoked or the animal was behaving erratically prior to the bite, the chance of rabies inoculation is increased. Bites from most wild carnivores, skunks, raccoons, and bats should be considered as rabid, while bites from immunized animals should be considered low risk. Healthy dogs and cats in nonendemic areas are low risk. Tables 49-10 and 49-12 summarize recommendations regarding the risk of transmission of rabies and treatment. If there is any question concerning prophylaxis, public health officials should be promptly consulted.

---

**TABLE 49-12**

**Schedule of Prophylaxis Recommended in the United States After Possible Exposure to Rabies**

| VACCINATION STATUS | REGIMEN[a] |
|---|---|
| **NOT PREVIOUSLY VACCINATED** | |
| Local wound cleansing | Immediate cleansing with soap and water |
| Rabies Immune globulin | 20 IU/kg of body weight (If anatomically feasible, up to half the dose be infiltrated around the wound or wounds and the rest should be administered intramuscularly in the gluteal area. Never give more than the recommended dose. Do not use the syringe used for vaccine or inject into the same anatomic site.) |
| Vaccine | 1.0 mL of HDCV or RVA intramuscularly in the deltoid area[b] on days 0, 3, 7, 14, and 28 |
| **PREVIOUSLY VACCINATED[c]** | |
| Local wound cleansing | Immediate cleansing with soap and water |
| Rabies immune globulin | Should not be given |
| Vaccine | 1.0 mL of HDCV or RVA Intramuscularly in the deltoid area[b] on days 0 and 3 |

HDCV, human diploid cell vaccine; RVA, rabies vaccine adsorbed.
[a]The regimens are applicable to all age groups, including children.
[b]The deltoid area is the preferred site of vaccination for adults and older children. For younger children, the outer aspect of the thigh may be used. Vaccine should never be administered in the gluteal area.
[c]"Previously vaccinated" indicates previous vaccination with HDCV or RVA, or any other type of rabies vaccine and a documented history of antibody response.

---

**TABLE 49-11**

**Jman Rabies Cases in the United States by Exposure Category, 1946–1995[a]**

| | EXPOSURE SOURCE | | | | |
|---|---|---|---|---|---|
| YEARS | Domestic | Wildlife | Other | Unknown (%) | CASE TOTAL |
| 1946–1955 | 86 | 8 | 0 | 26(22) | 120 |
| 1956–1965 | 21 | 7 | 0 | 10(26) | 38 |
| 1966–1975 | 6 | 7 | 1 | 2(13) | 16 |
| 1976–1985 | 6 | 1 | 2 | 11(55) | 20 |
| 1986–1995[a] | 2 | 2 | 0 | 14(78) | 18 |

[a]Through October 1995.

**TABLE 49-13**

**Crotalidae of North America**

| GENUS | COMMON NAME | CHARACTERISTICS | RANGE |
|---|---|---|---|
| *Agkistrodon* | Moccasins, copperheads | No rattles, large plates on crown | North America, Southeastern Europe, Asia |
| *Crotalus* | Rattlesnakes | Rattles, small scales on crown | North, Central, and South America |
| *Sistrurus* | Massasaugas and pygmy rattlesnakes | Rattles, large plates on crown | North America |

## Snake Bites

Snakebite is a challenging but rare problem that is more common in the southern United States and Mexico than elsewhere in North America. Like most other traumatic illnesses, it is more common in men than it is in women. Approximately 50% of patients are bitten during recreational activity or while working out of doors, while the remaining half are bitten by pet snakes or snakes being handled for some other reason. Snakebites are responsible for an average of only 12 deaths per year in the United States with rattlesnakes causing the majority of severe envenomations. Venomous snakes indigenous to the continental United States are either crotalids, which include rattlesnakes, copperheads, and cottonmouths, or elapids, of which coral snakes are the only indigenous species. Table 49-13 reviews the common Crotalidae of North America.

Since no evidence-based recommendations can be made for the treatment of snakebite, treatment recommendations are based on clinical series, animal studies, and common sense. While the clinical data are conflicting, the experimental animal data are clear. In this chapter, a treatment regimen for snakebite is proposed, pertinent controversies are discussed, and a rationale for the treatment scheme is presented (Fig. 49-6).

**Identification of the Snake.** Because the majority of snakebites in the United States are nonvenomous, an attempt should be made to identify the snake. This is possible by history as well as direct observation; however, the patient must bring the snake to the ED for this to occur. If at all possible, the snake should be identified by someone knowledgeable in herpetology. No identification should be attempted by hospital personnel unless the snake is dead or completely contained. For patients who are snake handlers or those bitten by pet snakes, the patient themselves will be the best resource to identify the type of snake. Figure 49-7 summarizes the physical characteristics of crotalid snakes. The three important genera of Crotalidae in the United States are *Crotalus* and *Sistrurus* (rattlesnakes) and *Agkistrodon* (copperheads and water moccasins; Table 49-13). These snakes are characterized by a broad triangular head, relatively thick body, elliptical pupils, and facial pits. All but one species of rattlesnakes have rattles, which distinguishes them from copperheads and water moccasins. The only other snakes of clinical importance in the continental United States are the coral snakes. The two species that are common to the United States are *Micrurus fulvius fulvius* (Eastern coral snake) and the *Micrurus fulvius tenere* (the Texas coral snake). The Sonoran coral snake *(Micrurus euryxanthus)* is present

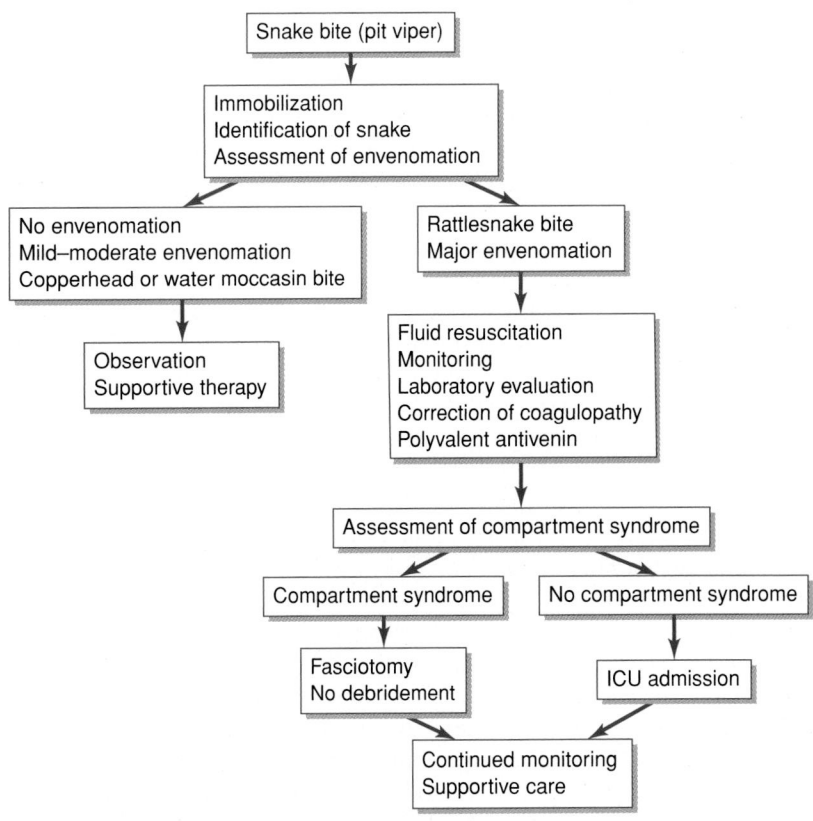

**FIGURE 49-6.** Algorithm for the treatment of snakebite, only in a setting in which anaphylaxis can be treated.

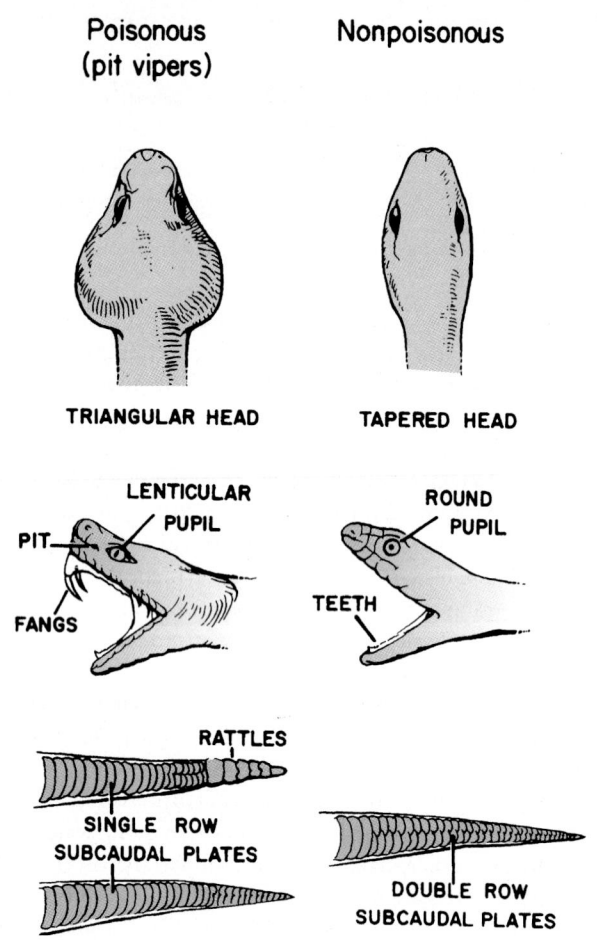

| Poisonous (pit vipers) | Nonpoisonous |
|---|---|
| TRIANGULAR HEAD | TAPERED HEAD |

PIT
LENTICULAR PUPIL
FANGS
ROUND PUPIL
TEETH

RATTLES
SINGLE ROW SUBCAUDAL PLATES
DOUBLE ROW SUBCAUDAL PLATES

**FIGURE 49-7.** Characteristics of poisonous and nonpoisonous snakes.

in a small area of southern Arizona, but is mostly indigenous to Mexico. These snakes are brightly colored, with red, yellow, white, and black rings. They are relatively small bodied and have small nontriangular heads without facial pits. Their rings encircle the body and the mouth area is black. Their characteristic coloring pattern of a red band adjacent to a yellow one distinguishes coral snakes from other snakes that are brightly colored but nonvenomous. This is the justification for the idiom, "Red on yellow, kill a fellow, red on black, venom lack." Coral snakes belong to the family Elapidae, or elapid, which includes cobras, kraits, mambas, and the poisonous snakes of Australia. Coral snakes tend to be secretive, burrowing, and nonaggressive, accounting for the low incidence of bites by these animals. They do not have large fangs and, when they do bite, they tend to chew on the offending animal or part.

Crotalid Envenomation.   An assessment for envenomation must be made in cases of bites by poisonous snakes. If there are no fang marks, envenomation is not possible and even with the presence of fang marks, approximately 20 to 25% of patients will not have been envenomated. It is estimated that another 50% have minimal to mild envenomation, which would not be a threat to life or limb. *Agkistrodon* (moccasin and copperhead) bites tend to be less severe than rattlesnake bites and rarely require antivenin or invasive treatment. With rattlesnake bites, it is usually easy to assess whether envenomation has occurred. Crotalid venoms are a mixture of

enzymes, polypeptides, and glycosylated peptides that have broad biologic actions; however, one of the common features of these venoms is local tissue destruction. This locally destructive action is an accurate marker of the degree of envenomation. A great deal of pain, edema, and discoloration or formation of bullae is associated with envenomation. Recent data appear to point to the presence of metalloproteinases in crotalid venom as a major source of local and systemic adverse effects.[76]

Since the signs and symptoms of envenomation have a rapid onset, it is probable that, if the patient arrives without edema or pain, a significant envenomation has not occurred. The other possibility is that the patient was bitten by a moccasin or copperhead. These points are emphasized because no treatment advocated for a rattlesnake bite is free of risk (most actually have a relatively high risk). Also, in the absence of envenomation or with mild exposure only, supportive care alone will suffice. This point is one that makes evaluation of the snakebite literature difficult. If the clinical series in question includes a large number of *Agkistrodon* bites or patients with mild envenomations, the outcome will almost always be favorable, regardless of the treatment applied. The real concern in the treatment of snakebite relates to the patient with a severe envenomation associated with extensive destruction of local tissue or systemic signs of toxicity. The outcome for this type of patient is harder to assess from clinical series involving humans.

First Aid.   First aid is defined as the care delivered to the patient prior to arrival in the hospital. "First do no harm" should be loudly emphasized for first aid in the treatment of snakebites. A large number of first aid measures have been proposed for the treatment of venomous snakebites, and many, if not most, have carried a high risk of harm to the patient. The atmosphere at the scene of a snakebite is usually characterized as chaotic at best, punctuated by poorly trained first aid providers. This combination sets the stage for a therapeutic disaster if overly aggressive therapy is initiated at the scene of the bite. The most common potentially harmful treatments include incision and suction, electrical shock therapy, use of a tourniquet, and immersion in ice.

Incision and suction have been shown experimentally to remove subcutaneously injected venom from animals; however, unless this is done very soon after envenomation, the yield of extracted venom is low.[77] The risk of incision and suction is significant when one considers that the person making the incision is probably doing it for the first time, the patient is in pain and unanesthetized, and there is probably no knowledge of anatomy by either person involved in the procedure. It should also be remembered that 25% of the victims of snakebite will have no envenomation or a trivial one. For these reasons, incision and suction has fallen into disfavor as a first aid measure.

In a series of letters to the editor of the *Lancet*, a group of physicians practicing medicine in Ecuador advocated the use of electrical shock therapy for snakebite. They presented a series of 34 patients who were treated with electrical current using a modification of a stun gun.[78] A stun gun is a personal protective device that delivers an extremely high voltage with very little current. When used on attackers, it temporarily disables them. The Ecuadorean investigators used this device on a group of patients with snakebite, probably from *Bothrops atrox*. All of the patients were said to have fared well, with immediate improvement. Follow-up in this series was not described, and there were no controls. This report led to the widespread use and indeed to the marketing of the stun gun for use in human snakebite. This treatment is typical of snakebite therapy throughout history. A theoretical treatment plan, usually with the potential for great pain or harm, is proposed, implemented, and adopted without any degree of scrutiny. Several controlled animal studies have now shown electrical shock therapy to be ineffective in the treatment of snakebite.

Ice therapy for snakebite has been advocated on the basis of decreasing the optimal temperature range for the enzyme component of the venom, and thus decreasing local tissue damage.[79] This topic has been hotly debated without any clear resolution; however, the weight of the evidence would suggest that ice therapy is not efficacious. It has the potential for harm in cases of snakebite, and its use is discouraged. While putting a topical ice pack on the wound carries no risk, it is immersion of the extremity containing a bite or adding salt to the ice that has been associated with problems.

The use of a tourniquet has also been a debated issue in first aid for snakebite. A loosely applied venous tourniquet may decrease systemic absorption of the venom and delay the onset of symptoms; however, it certainly does not help the affected extremity and, if applied too tightly or if excessively tightened by the formation of edema, it carries the potential for causing great harm. Data from Australia suggest a logical and safer treatment. This involves the application of a compression bandage and immobilization of the bitten extremity, without using tourniquet. With a compression bandage alone there is a great delay in the systemic absorption of venom.[80] A splint and elastic bandage wrap or an inflatable air splint could also be used for this purpose. These measures have much less associated risk than placing a tourniquet on the involved extremity.

In summary, immobilization, neutral positioning, and a compression dressing of some sort are recommended as first aid in cases of snakebite, followed by rapid transport of the patient to a hospital. If a *skilled surgeon* is present and there is obvious envenomation, immediate incision and suction or local excision of the bite wound is recommended.[81]

**Definitive Care.** The care of the patient in the hospital is no less controversial than is first aid for snakebite.[82] Current debates center around the use of antivenin therapy, aggressive debridement, and fasciotomy, and, more recently, observation with supportive care alone. For severe bites, antivenin use is favored along with the aggressive use of supportive care. Antivenin limits the amount of tissue damage and systemic action of the venom if administered early. The problem is not efficacy but safety. Antivenin therapy carries a definite risk of anaphylaxis and serum sickness; however, the risk of its use is outweighed by the potential benefits in victims with life- or limb-threatening bites. Fasciotomy is used only in the treatment of a compartment syndrome. Immediate surgical debridement for the purpose of removal of venom and nonviable muscle is also not recommended. Experimentally, this approach does not remove the venom, and it is impossible to determine if muscle tissue is viable on the basis of the usual clinical criteria.[83] Supportive care alone is not recommended for severe envenomations, although patients with all but the most massive envenomations could probably survive with aggressive modern intensive care and replacement of blood factors.[84]

**Antivenin Therapy.** A polyvalent equine antivenin (Wyeth-Ayerst Laboratories, Marietta, PA) and an ovine Crotalidae polyvalent immune Fab antivenin, consisting of cleaved Fab antibody fragments (CroFab; Protherics, Inc., Nashville, TN), are currently commercially available for the treatment of crotalid envenomations. These products are manufactured by immunizing animals to crotalid venoms and then pooling the globulin fraction containing the antibodies. The ovine Fab product, CroFab, undergoes further modification by cleavage of the Fab antibody fragments and purification with affinity chromatography. Experimentally, antivenin has been shown to be effective in preventing death following the injection of rattlesnake venom. In an animal model, it also preserves muscle function and minimizes the systemic side effects of the venom.

Like all antibody therapies, the equine antivenin is most effective if given immediately before envenomation; however, it is also effective when given after envenomation.[83] It has also been shown to be effective if given up to four hours after envenomation, although there is little evidence to support its use beyond four hours. There have been anecdotal reports of clinical responses when it is given later than this, however, and it is recommended for use in life-threatening envenomations for up to 24 hours following a crotalid bite. Nevertheless, it must be emphasized that if antivenin therapy is going to be used, it should be used as soon as possible after envenomation.

Although widely used clinically, there are significant problems with the unmodified polyvalent equine antivenin. It is a foreign, impure horse-serum protein fraction and has been associated with severe and even life-threatening anaphylactic reactions. The exact incidence of such reactions is unclear, ranging from 1% to as high as 39%. The antivenin infusion should be started at a very slow rate and stopped with any signs of an allergic reaction. The antivenin may also cause a dose-dependent, delayed-type serum sickness, which is much less severe than an anaphylactic response, although probably more common with massive infusions of antivenin. These side effects have fueled a debate over use of the antivenin. CroFab is an attempt to make the immunotherapy safer by purification of immunoglobulin and cleavage of the Fc fragment to produce Fab fragments.[85] An increasing body of evidence supports the safety and efficacy of the Fab product, although additional post-marketing clinical data will ultimately be required.[86] The Fab fragment has not been directly compared to other antivenin products. CroFab appears to be different than the older equine antivenin in that it probably requires repeat dosing in the immediate period after administration.[85-86]

In addition to being given as early as possible and in doses large enough to effect a difference, antivenin should not be administered in any setting in which anaphylaxis cannot be treated (i.e., in the field) and should initially be infused very slowly as noted above. The dose of antivenin to be given is empiric and based on the physician's assessment of the amount of venom injected. The dose is the same in children as in adults, again being based on the amount of venom to be neutralized rather than on the weight of the patient. A minimum of six to ten vials of CroFab is used for severe bites, although this amount is increased as needed. Various schemes have been devised for assessing the dose of antivenin based on the severity of envenomation. As the antivenin should not be used for mild or uncomplicated, moderate envenomations, these classification schemes are not clinically useful. Skin testing prior to antivenin

**TABLE 49-14**

**Treatment for Anaphylaxis**

1. Airway control
2. Epinephrine, 0.5 mg SQ (may be given IV with major anaphylactic reaction). May be repeated every 20 min
3. Volume expansion
4. H$_1$ antagonists (diphenhydramine, 25–50 mg IV or IM)
5. H$_2$ antagonists (ranitidine, 50 mg IV)
6. Glucocorticoids (hydrocortisone, 125 mg IV). No effect for several hours, but may prevent recurrence of symptoms
7. Inhaled β$_2$ agonist for recurrent bronchospasm (albuterol, 0.5 mg)
8. Removal of bee stinger IM, intramuscularly; IV, intravenously; SQ, subcutaneously.

administration should probably be eliminated and replaced by a very small, very slow intravenous injection of the antivenin, with constant monitoring for signs of anaphylaxis. The manufacturer recommends skin testing, but there have been anaphylactic reactions to the skin test, and the presence or absence of a wheal does not always predict anaphylaxis. The treatment of anaphylaxis is reviewed in Table 49-14.

*Fasciotomy.* An ongoing debate during the past several decades has concerned the role of surgery in treating a rattlesnake bite. The theoretical rationale for surgical intervention is based on several observations. Crotalid venoms have very powerful, locally destructive effects. Part of the venom can be removed by incision and suction when this follows immediately after injection of the venom. Intramuscular injection of the venom, however, produces extensive edema which can lead to a compartment syndrome. These three observations lead to the conclusion that a rattlesnake bite is a local problem that should be amenable to local therapy (i.e., excision of the venom, dead muscle, and relief of a compartment syndrome). Excellent results have been claimed in clinical series in which this approach has been used.[87] Unfortunately, no controlled trials have been conducted, and there are large series in which excellent results have been reported without operative intervention.[88]

An animal study performed in rabbits using an intracompartmental injection of venom from a Western diamondback rattlesnake (*Crotalus atrox*) has yielded interesting results.[83] In this study, animals were randomized to undergo fasciotomy with debridement alone, antivenin alone, fasciotomy with debridement plus antivenin, or to have no treatment. Antivenin therapy prevented loss of muscle and improved survival, while surgery alone did not. It was also clear that muscle that would have survived was removed in the group that had the combination of antivenin plus surgery, since late muscle function was significantly worse in this group than it was in that treated with antivenin alone. The authors concluded, therefore, that although the theory of local treatment of rattlesnake bite was attractive, it was not supported by the data. The issue of fasciotomy alone was not addressed in this study. Based on these unanswered questions, fasciotomy should be done infrequently and should be reserved for the usual indication of compartment syndrome caused by an intramuscular or intracompartmental envenomation.[84] Although rare, this does occur, being more common over the anterior leg, fingers, and the hand. If there is a tight compartment with evidence of compartment syndrome, a fasciotomy

should be performed.[84] No debridement should be done acutely, as injured muscle may be salvaged with immunotherapy.[89]

Supportive care should consist of fluid resuscitation, tetanus prophylaxis, appropriate monitoring, and the correction of coagulopathy. The bacteriology of rattlesnake mouths has been studied. Commonly present organisms include *Pseudomonas* spp., Enterobacteraciae, *Staphylococcus* spp., and *Clostridia*.[90–91] An extended-spectrum penicillin with a β-lactamase inhibitor would provide reasonable empiric coverage; however, the weight of evidence supports not using empiric antibiotics.[92–93] Coagulopathy due to fibrinolysis is a common sequela of envenomation and should be corrected with infusions of fresh frozen plasma and cryoprecipitate. The patient's prothrombin time/international normalized ratio, partial thromboplastin time, fibrinogen concentration, and platelet count should all be monitored, with replacement therapy based on these values and evidence of clinical bleeding.[94]

*Envenomation by the Coral Snake.* The symptoms of coral snake envenomation include local pain at the bite site, but the venom has primarily systemic effects consisting of respiratory depression and changes in CNS function.[95] Antivenin and supportive care are the mainstays of treatment for coral snake envenomations. A commercially available antivenin exists for subspecies of *Micrurus fulvius* (the Eastern and Texas coral snake). This product probably has little cross-reactivity with the venom of *Micrurus euryxanthus* (the Sonoran coral snake). Patients with fang marks or fang scratches should be admitted for observation. Any signs or symptoms should be treated with between three to five vials of antivenin. It is probably not wise to wait for full-blown systemic symptoms to develop before initiating treatment. If signs of respiratory distress develop, the patient should be treated supportively with intubation and mechanical ventilation as needed.

## BITES AND STINGS BY MARINE ANIMALS

### Marine Invertebrates

Marine invertebrates (Cnidaria) are a heterogeneous group of phylogenetically primitive animals that are responsible for a large number of sea-water envenomations.[96] The phylum is divided into four major groups including Schyphozoa (true jellyfish), Hydrozoa (Portuguese man o' war and hydras), Anthozoa (corals and anemones), and Cubozoa (box jellyfish and sea wasps). All these animals have specialized organelles known as nematocysts for poisoning and capturing prey. Most nematocysts cannot penetrate human skin and cause only a painful superficial skin reaction; however, full-thickness penetration can lead to serious illness and even death. Common manifestations of jellyfish stings include local pain and eruption, edema, urticaria, anaphylaxis, and, rarely, cardiorespiratory arrest. The principles in the management of such stings are to minimize the number of nematocysts being discharged and minimize the harmful effects of discharged nematocysts. Any adherent tentacles should be carefully removed. Unexploded nematocysts should be deactivated with either a sodium bicarbonate slurry, papain (meat tenderizer), or a vinegar soak. The management of systemic side effects is largely supportive. Hypotension is treated with fluids and inotropic agents if necessary, while pain should be controlled with systemic narcotics. Calcium gluconate may improve the muscle spasms sometimes seen in cases of stings by marine invertebrates.

## Venomous Fish

Most venomous fish are slow swimmers that are relatively nonmigratory and are not typically found in North American waters. Stingrays are the most clinically significant with regard to causing stings and envenomation. Typically this occurs when the stingray is stepped on by a swimmer. The wounds are a combination of laceration and puncture. Treatment consists of irrigation and soaking of the wound in warm water. Much of the venom may be removed by simple mechanical irrigation. Tetanus prophylaxis should be given; however, no antivenin exists for envenomation by a stingray.[97]

Travelers to tropical waters and aquarium workers may encounter other venomous creatures such as the Blue-ringed octopus (*Haplochlaena spp.*), Stonefish (*Synanceia spp.*), Lionfish (*Pterois volitans*), and Cone shells that posses potent venoms, some of which can be fatal to humans. Only an antivenin to Stonefish toxin has been created, which is helpful in ameliorating the excruciating, narcotic-resistant pain associated with this venom.[97] This antivenin may have some usefulness in the treatment of Lionfish stings, which may be of particular interest to aquarium workers.[98]

## Shark Bites

The chance of being bitten by a shark is exceedingly rare, but these wounds do occur in all coastal areas of the world.[99] The principles described in the preceding section on wounds should be employed for the management of complex shark bites. These wounds should be considered tetanus prone and preventive antibiotics are generally recommended, especially against *Vibrio spp. and Aeromonas spp.*[99]

## Insect and Bug Bites

Insect bites are usually more of a nuisance than a serious medical problem, and most are not seen by a physician. Allergic reactions are the most common serious problem following insect bites. Because of their widespread distribution and proximity to humans, bees and wasps kill more people per year through fatal anaphylactic reactions to their venoms than do all other venomous animals combined.

Fire ants were imported to Mobile, Alabama, in the early part of the 20th century. The black fire ant (*Solenopsis richteri*) was the first species to be imported from Uruguay and Argentina and has a limited range along the Mississippi–Alabama border. The red fire ant (*Solenopsis invicta*), which originates from Brazil and northern Argentina, has had tremendous success in colonization and now has a range extending over most of the southeastern United States.[100] Its adaptability and aggressiveness have been remarkable. *Solenopsis invicta* tends to give multiple bites which are usually limited, but near-fatal cases of multiple bites have been reported. The bites of the imported fire ant have a typical appearance consisting of an initial vesicle, followed by the development of a sterile pustule. The venom of the fire ant is unique among that of venomous

animals. It consists of 95% nonprotein alkaloid, in contrast to most other venoms, of which protein is a major component. Allergy to a fire ant bite is relatively common, with anaphylaxis being the most common major problem with bites from imported fire ants. Treatment consists of immediately scrubbing the wounds with soap and water, since much of the venom may be removed by mechanical action. Anaphylaxis should be treated as described in Table 49-14.

## Spider Bites

All spiders have a venom apparatus for killing other insects or spiders although most pose no danger to humans. Of the two common species dangerous to humans in the continental United States, bites by the brown recluse spider (*Loxosceles reclusa*) are the most clinically significant. This is a brown spider with three pairs of eyes (dyads), one anterior and two lateral, with a violin-shaped carapace on its body, although this may be absent or difficult to discern.[101] Usually, there is minimal pain following a brown recluse bite, which often makes exact identification of the location of the bite difficult. In serious bites, a hemorrhagic blister develops with progression to a dark black necrotic area that may extend over several centimeters. Systemic symptoms may be present, but these are usually mild and respond well to supportive care. Initial reports[102] that early treatment with dapsone prevented ulceration or hastened healing have been largely superseded by evidence showing that adverse effects of dapsone are common and its efficacy is doubtful.[101,103]

Bites by the black widow spider (*Lactrodectus macrotans*) are characterized by a systemic toxic reaction. Only the female black widow spider, identified by her large size and shiny black body with a red hourglass on the underside of her abdomen, contains sufficient venom to evenomate a human.[104] Symptoms of envenomation are usually rapid, beginning within one hour of biting, and include pain, muscle rigidity, altered mental status, and seizures. Death rates from severe bites have been reported to be as high as 5%. Treatment is supportive, although an equine antivenin is available for use in severe cases. Muscle rigidity has been effectively treated with dantrolene,[105] as well as calcium and methacarbamol.[106]

## Bee and Wasp Stings

Bee and wasp stings are very common throughout the world but most victims never seek medical attention and recover uneventfully. The most serious problem in cases of bee and wasp stings relates to the development of an immediate hypersensitivity reaction. Owing to the large number of bees in the United States and the frequent proximity to humans, anaphylactic reactions from bee stings are responsible for more deaths than all other venomous animal bites and stings, as previously noted. Honeybees were not indigenous to the Americas, but were imported to the continent in the 1600s (the European honeybee). While exceedingly popular in the media, the Africanized honeybee ("killer bees") is still a member of the same species as the European honeybee (*Apis mellifera*). Africanized honeybees are a population that has evolved under different environmental conditions and has significantly different behavior than the common honeybee.

African honeybees were imported to Brazil in 1956 with the hope of creating bees that would be more suited to a tropical environment. Unfortunately, they escaped and bred with the local European honeybees and have been slowly migrating northward ever since. The first Africanized honeybee colony in the United States was discovered in south Texas in 1990. Africanized honeybees tend to be aggressive, and persons stung by them are more likely to sustain multiple stings, although the stings themselves are no different than those of other honeybees. Bees sting with double-barbed lancets, which tend to anchor the bee to the victim's skin. When the bee dislodges itself, it usually leaves its stinging apparatus behind, thus killing the bee. The exuded venom sac of the bee should be scraped with a knife, instead of squeezing the skin to get the poison sac out, in order to avoid injecting the venom remaining in the sac. Application of an ice pack to the local area tends to alleviate the associated pain. The treatment of anaphylaxis from bee stings and other bites and stings is outlined in Table 49-14. Patients who have a known sensitivity to bee or wasp stings should carry an emergency kit for the injection of epinephrine (EpiPen®, Dey, Inc., Napa, CA) and should wear a medical identification bracelet identifying their hypersensitivity.

# REFERENCES

1. Atta HM: Edwin Smith surgical papyrus: The oldest known surgical treatise. *Am Surg* 65:1190, 1999.
2. Namias N: Honey in the management of infections. *Surg Infect* 4:219, 2003.
3. Santoro MM, Gaudino G: Cellular and molecular facets of keratinocytes reepithelization during wound healing. *Experimental Cell Research* 304:274, 2005.
4. Jensen JA, Hunt TK, Scheuenstuhl H, et al.: Effect of lactate, pyruvate, and pH on secretion of angiogenesis and mitogenesis factors by macrophages. *Lab Invest* 54:574, 1986.
5. Szpaderska AM, DiPietro LA: Inflammation in surgical wound healing: Friend or foe? *Surgery* 137:571, 2005.
6. Leibovich SJ, Ross R: The role of the macrophage in wound repair. A study with hydrocortisone and antimacrophage serum. *Am J Pathol* 78:71, 1975.
7. DiPietro LA: Wound healing: The role of the macrophage and other immune cells. *Shock* 4:233, 1995.
8. Trabold O, Wagner S, Wicke C, et al.: Lactate and oxygen constitute a fundamental regulatory mechanism in wound healing. *Wound Repair Regen* 11:504, 2003.
9. Thakral KK, Goodson WH, Hunt TK, et al.: Stimulation of wound blood vessel growth by wound macrophages. *J Surg Res* 26:430, 1979.
10. Stadelmann WK, Digenis AG, Tobin GR: Physiology and healing of chronic cutaneous wounds. *Am J Surg* 176:26S, 1998.
11. Bauer SM, Bauer RJ, Liu ZJ, et al.: Vascular endothelial growth factor-C promotes vasculogenesis, angiogenesis, and collagen constriction in three-dimensional collagen gels. *J Vasc Surg* 41:699, 2005.
12. Deodhar AK, Rana RE: Surgical physiology of wound healing: A review. *J Postgrad Med* 43:52, 1997.
13. Marinkovich MP, Ishii M, Chanoki M, et al.: Cellular origin of the dermal-epidermal basement membrane. *Dev Dyn* 197:255, 1993.
14. Gabbiani G: Evolution and clinical implications of the myofibroblast concept. *Cardiovasc Res* 38:545, 1998.
15. Bullard KM, Lund L, Mudgett J, et al.: Impaired wound contraction in Stromelysin-1-deficient mice. *Ann Surg* 230:260, 1999.
16. Lowry KF, Curtis GM: Delayed suture in the management of wounds: Analysis of 721 traumatic wounds illustrating the influence of time interval in wound repair. *Am J Surg* 80:280, 1950.
17. Grande CM: Mechanisms and patterns of injury: The key to anticipation in trauma management. *Crit Care Clin* 6:25, 1990.
18. Livingston DH, Malangoni MA: An experimental study of the susceptibility to infection after hemorrhagic shock. *Surg Gynecol Obstet* 168:182, 1989.
19. Angele MK, Knoferl MW, Schwacha MG, et al.: Hemorrhage decreases macrophage inflammatory protein 2 and interleukin-6 release: A possible mechanism for increased wound infection. *Ann Surg* 229:651, 1999.
20. Angele MK, Chaudry IH: Surgical trauma and immunosuppression: Pathophysiology and immunomodulatory approaches. *Langenbecks Arch Surg* 390:333, 2005.
21. Livingston DH, Gentile PS, Malangoni MA: Bone marrow failure after hemorrhagic shock. *Circ Shock* 30:255, 1990.
22. Livingston DH, Anjaria D, Wu J, et al.: Bone marrow failure following severe injury in humans. *Ann Surg* 238:748, 2003.
23. Falanga V: Wound healing and its impairment in the diabetic foot. *Lancet* 366:1736, 2005.
24. Busti AJ, Hooper JS, Amaya CJ, et al.: Effects of perioperative antiinflammatory and immunomodulating therapy on surgical wound healing. *Pharmacotherapy* 25:1566, 2005.
25. Buck M, Houglum K, Chojkier M: Tumor necrosis factor-alpha inhibits collagen alpha 1 gene expression and wound healing in a murine model of cachexia. *Am J Pathol* 149:195, 1996.
26. Harris CL, Fraser C: Malnutrition in the institutionalized elderly: The effects of wound healing. *Ostomy Wound Manage* 50:54, 2004.
27. Miller RS, Morris JA Jr, Diaz JJ Jr, et al.: Complications after 344 damage-control open celiotomies. *J Trauma* 59:1365, 2005.
28. Fowler E, van Rijswijk L: Using wound debridement to help achieve the goals of care. *Ostomy Wound Manage* 41:23S, 1995.
29. Schaible UE, Kaufmann SH: Iron and microbial infection. *Nat Rev Microbiol* 2:946, 2004.
30. Ganz T: Hepcidin, a key regulator of iron metabolism and mediator of anemia of inflammation. *Blood* 102:783, 2003.
31. Alexander JW, Fischer JE, Boyajian M, et al.: The influence of hair-removal methods on wound infections. *Arch Surg* 118:347, 1983.
32. Fezza JP, Klippenstein KA, Wesley RE: Cilia regrowth of shaven eyebrows. *Arch Facial Plastic Surg* 1:223, 1999.
33. Chaiyakunapruk N, Veenstra DL, Lipsky BA, et al.: Chlorhexidine compared with povidone-iodine solution for vascular catheter-site care: A meta-analysis. *Ann Intern Med* 136:792, 2002.
34. Bibbo C, Patel DV, Gehrmann RM, et al.: Chlorhexidine provides superior skin decontamination in foot and ankle surgery: A prospective randomized study. *Clin Orthop Relat Res* 438:204, 2005.
35. Kinirons B, Mimoz O, Lafendi L, et al.: Chlorhexidine versus povidone iodine in preventing colonization of continuous epidural catheters in children: A randomized, controlled trial. *Anesthesiology* 94:239, 2001.
36. Adams D, Quayum M, Worthington T, et al.: Evaluation of a 2% chlorhexidine gluconate in 70% isopropyl alcohol skin disinfectant. *J Hosp Infect* 61:287, 2005.
37. Wilson JR, Mills JG, Prather ID, et al.: A toxicity index of skin and wound cleansers used on in vitro fibroblasts and keratinocytes. *Adv Skin Wound Care* 18:373, 2005.
38. Varley GA, Meisler DM, Benes SC, et al.: Hibiclens keratopathy: A clinicopathologic case report. *Cornea* 9:341, 1990.
39. Murthy S, Hawksworth NR, Cree I: Progressive ulcerative keratitis related to the use of topical chlorhexidine gluconate (0.02%). *Cornea* 21:237, 2002.
40. Mac Rae SM, Brown B, Edelhauser HF: The corneal toxicity of presurgical skin antiseptics. *Am J Opthalmol* 97:221, 1984.
41. Gross A, Cutright DE, Bhaskar SN: Effectiveness of pulsating water lavage in the treatment of contaminated crushed wounds. *Am J Surg* 124:373, 1972.
42. Wheeler CB, Rhodeheaver GT, Thacker JB, et al.: Side effects of high pressure irrigation. *Surg Gynecol Obstet* 143:775, 1976.
43. Draeger RW, Dahners LE: Traumatic wound debridement: A comparison of irrigation methods. *J Orthop Trauma* 20:83, 2006.
44. Tetzlaff JE: The pharmacology of local anesthetics. *Anesthesiol Clin North America* 18:217, 2000.
45. McLure HA, Rubin AP: Review of local anesthetic agents. *Minerva Anestesiol* 71:59, 2005.
46. Krunic AL, Wang LC, Soltani K, et al.: Digital anesthesia with epinephrine: An old myth revisited. *J Am Acad Dermatol* 51:755, 2004.
47. Wilhelmi BJ, Blackwell SJ, Miller J, et al.: Epinephrine in digital blocks: Revisited. *Ann Plast Surg* 41:410, 1998.
48. Stratford AF, Zoutman DE, Davidson JS: Effect of lidocaine and epinephrine on Staphylococcus aureus in a guinea pig model of surgical wound infection. *Plast Reconstr Surg* 110:1275, 2002.
49. Bartfield JM, Crisafulli KM, Raccio-Robak N, et al.: The effects of warming and buffering on pain of infiltration of local. *Acad Emerg Med* 2:254, 1995.
50. Masters JE: Randomised control trial of pH buffered lignocaine with adrenalin in outpatient operations. *Br J Plast Surg* 51:385, 1998.
51. Colaric KB, Overton DT, Moore K: Pain reduction in lidocaine administration through buffering and warming. *Am J Emerg Med* 16:353, 1998.
52. Fitton AR, Ragbir M, Milling MA: The use of pH adjusted lignocaine in controlling operative pain in the day surgery unit: a prospective, randomized trial. *Br J Plast Surg* 49:404, 1996.
53. Mader TJ, Playe SJ: Reducing the pain of local anesthetic infiltration: Results of a national clinical practice survey. *Am J Emerg Med* 16:617, 1998.
54. Calatayud J, Gonzalez A: History of the development and evolution of local anesthesia since the coca leaf. *Anesthesiology* 98:1503, 2003.
55. Buckenmaier CC III, Bleckner LL: Anaesthetic agents for advanced regional anaesthesia: a North American perspective. *Drugs* 65:745, 2005.

56. Mather LE, Copeland SE, Ladd LA: Acute toxicity of local anesthetics: Underlying pharmacokinetic and pharmacodynamic concepts. *Reg Anesth Pain Med* 30:553, 2005.
57. Crystal CC, Blakenship RB: Local anesthetics nd peripheral nerve blocks in the emergency department. *Emerg Med Clin N Am* 23:477, 2005.
58. Patzakis MJ, Harvey JP, Ivler D: The role of antibiotics in the management of open fractures. *J Bone Joint Surg Am.* 56:532, 1974.
59. Bergman BR: Antibiotic prophylaxis in open and closed fractures. A controlled clinical trial. *Act Orthop Scand* 55:57, 1982.
60. Benson DR, Riggins RS, Lawrence RM, et al.: Treatment of open fractures: A prospective study. *J Trauma* 23:25, 1983.
61. Weigelt JA: Isk of wound infection in trauma patients. *J Trauma* 150:782, 1985.
62. Vermeulen H, Ubbink DT, Goossens A, et al.: Systematic review of dressings and topical agents for surgical wounds healing by secondary intention. *Br J Surg* 92:665, 2005.
63. Rose A: Continuous water baths for burns. *JAMA* 47:1042, 1906.
64. Winter GD: Formation of the scab and the rate of epithelialization of superficial wounds in the skin of the young domestic pig. *Nature* 193:293, 1962.
65. Lewis R, Whiting P, ter Riet G, et al.: A rapid and systematic review of the clinical effectiveness and cost-effectiveness of debriding agents in treating surgical wounds healing by secondary intention. *Health Technol Assess* 5:1, 2001.
66. Truscott W: Impact of microscopic foreign debris on post-surgical complications. *Surg Technol Int* 12:34, 2004.
67. McGuiness W, Vella E, Harrison D: Influence of dressing changes on wound temperature. *J Wound Care* 13:383, 2004.
68. Ip M, Lui SL, Poon VK, et al.: Antimicrobial activities of silver dressings: An in vitro comparison. *J Med Micobiol* 55:59, 2006.
69. Phaneuf MD, Bide MJ, Hannel SL, et al.: Development of an infection-resistant. Bioactive wound dressing surface. *J Biomed Mater Res A* 74:666, 2005.
70. Lee AR: Enhancing dermal matrix regeneration and biomechnical properties of 2nd degree-burn wounds by EGF-impregnated collagen sponge dressing. *Arch Pharm Res* 28:1311, 2005.
71. Argenta LC, Morykwas MJ: Vacuum-assisted closure: a new method for wound control and treatment: Clinical experience. *Ann Plast Surg* 38:563, 1997.
72. Morykwas MJ, Argenta LC, Shelton-Brown EI, et al.: Vacuum-assisted closure: A new method for wound control and treatment: animal studies and basic foundation. *Ann Plast Surg* 38:553, 1997.
73. Olenius M, Dalsgaard C, Wickman M: Mitotic activity in the expanded human skin. *Plast Reconstr Surg* 91:213, 1993.
74. Erdmann D, Drye C, Heller C, et al.: Abdominal wall defect and enterocutaneous fistula treatment with the Vacuum-Assisted Closure (V.A.C.) system. *Plast Reconstr Surg* 108:2066, 2001.
75. Fishbein D, Robinson L: Rabies. *N Engl J Med* 329:1632, 1993.
76. Teixeira Cde F, Fernandes CM, Zuliani JP, et al.: Inflammatory effects of snake venom metalloproteinases. *Mem Inst Oswaldo Cruz* 100:181, 2005.
77. Snyder C, Pickins J, Knowles R, et al.: A definitive study of snake bite. *J Fla Med Assoc* 55:330, 1968.
78. Gudarian R, MacKenzie C, Williams J: High voltage shock treatment for snakebite. *Lancet* 2:229, 1986.
79. Glass TG: *Management of Poisonous Snakebite.* San Antonio, TX: Crumrine, 1986.
80. Sutherland SK, Coulter AR, Harris RD: Rationalisation of first-aid measures for elepid snakebite. *Lancet* 1:183, 1979.
81. Gold BS, Barish RA, Dart RC: North American snake envenomation: Diagnosis, treatment, and management. *Emerg Med Clin North Am* 22:423, 2004.
82. Lindsey D: Controversy in snakebite—Time for a controlled appraisal. *J Trauma* 25:462, 1985.
83. Stewart RM, Page CP, Schwesinger WH, et al.: Antivenin and fasciotomy/debridement in the treatment of the severe rattlesnake bite. *Am J Surg* 158:543, 1989.
84. Hall EL: Role of surgical intervention in the management of crotaline snake envenomation. *Ann Emerg Med* 37:175, 2001.
85. Burch JM, Agarwal R, Mattox KL, et al.: The treatment of crotalid envenomation with antivenin. *J Trauma* 28:35, 1988.
86. Schmidt JM: Antivenom therapy for snakebites in children: Is there evidence? *Curr Opin Pediatr* 17:234, 2005.
87. Dart RC, Seifert SA, Boyer LV, et al.: A randomized multicenter trial of crotalinae polyvalent immune Fab (ovine) antivenom for the treatment for crotaline snakebite in the United States. *Arch Intern Med* 161:2030, 2001.
88. Glass TG: Early debridement in pit viper bites. *JAMA* 235:2513, 1976.
89. Russell FE, Carlson RW, Wainschel J, et al.: Snake venom poisoning in the United States: Experiences with 550 cases. *JAMA* 233:341, 1975.
90. Ledbetter EO, Kutscher AE: Aerobic and anaerobic flora of rattlesnake fangs and venom. *Arch Environ Health* 19:770, 1969.
91. Clark RF, Selden BS, Furbee B: The incidence of wound infection following crotalid envenomation. *J Emerg Med* 11:583, 1993.
92. Kerrigan KR, Mertz BL, Nelson SJ, et al.: Antibiotic prophylaxis for pit viper envenomation: Prospective, controlled trial. *World J Surg* 21:369, 1997.
93. Blaylock RS: Antibiotic use and infection in snakebite victims. *South African Med J* 89:874, 1999.
94. White J: Snake venoms and coagulopathy. *Toxicon* 45:951, 2005.
95. McCollough NC, Gennaro JR Jr: Coral snake bites in the United States. *J Fla Med Assoc* 49:968, 1963.
96. Nimorakiotakis B, Winkel KD: Marine envenomations. Part 1 – Jellyfish. *Aust Fam Physician* 32:969, 2003.
97. Nimorakiotakis B, Winkel KD: Marine envenomations. Part 2 – Other marine envenomations. *Aust Fam Physician* 32:975, 2003.
98. Church JE, Hodgson WC: Adrenergic and cholinergic activity contributes to the cardiovascular effects of lionfish (Pterois volitans) venom. *Toxicon* 40:787, 2002.
99. Caldicott DG, Mahajani R, Kuhn M: The anatomy of a shark attack: A case report and review of the literature. *Injury* 32:445, 2001.
100. Burke WA: The red imported fire ant (Solenopsis invicta). A problem in North Carolina. *N C Med J* 52:153, 1991.
101. Swanson DL, Vetter RS: Bites of brown recluse spiders and suspected necrotic arachnidism. *N Engl J Med* 352:700, 2005.
102. King LE Jr, Rees RS: Dapsone treatment of a brown recluse bite. *JAMA* 250:648, 1983.
103. Mold JW, Thompson DM: Management of brown recluse spider bites in primary care. *J Am Board Fam Pract* 17:347, 2004.
104. Saucier JR: Arachnid envenomation. *Emerg Med Clin North Am* 22:405, 2004.
105. Ryan PJ: Preliminary report: Experience with the use of dantrolene sodium in the treatment of bites by the black widow spider *Latrodectus hesperus. J Toxicol Clin Toxicol* 21:484, 1983.
106. Key GF: A comparison of calcium gluconate and methocarbamol (Robaxin) in the treatment of latrodectism (black widow spider envenomation). *Am J Trop Med Hyg* 30:273, 1981.

# Commentary ■ KIMBERLY A. DAVIS

"The optimist already sees the scar over the wound; the pessimist still sees the wound underneath the scar."
—ERNST SCHRODER

Millions of healthy individuals are traumatically injured each year. Their wounds range significantly in severity from minor, easily treated "cuts and scrapes," to massive soft tissue injuries and complex open wounds. The scars resulting from these wounds serve as daily reminders to our patients of the extent of their injuries, and can result in long-term body image issues. As

physicians involved in the care of the critically ill and injured, it is incumbent upon us to minimize external scarring and preserve function.

Drs. Adams, Biffl, and Cioffi have authored a well-written and extensive chapter outlining the critical points that require consideration when managing traumatic wounds. They have focused on the key charges of preventing infection, retaining maximal function, and achieving acceptable cosmesis, and have provided an excellent review of the acute phases of wound healing and of wound closure techniques.

As alluded to in the chapter, the key priorities in the management of traumatic wounds can be divided into three phases. The first phase involves an assessment of the patient as a whole, and treatment in this phase is directed toward the management of life-threatening injuries. The most apparent wound, regardless of its dramatic nature, may not be the most important. Wound management in this phase should be directed at the control of hemorrhage, which is usually obtained by the application of direct pressure.

The second phase of wound management addresses the specific wound in question, and the manner in which it should be most efficiently addressed. In this phase, threats to wound healing should be identified, including the presence of ischemia and/or necrosis, the level of bacterial contaminations, the presence of foreign body contamination, and the presence of associated injuries. Identification of the systemic factors that may negatively impact wound healing is important and includes patient co-morbidities (malnutrition, immunocompromise etc.) and the circumstances of the wounding (the mechanism of injury, the presence of hemorrhagic shock, and systemic inflammatory response syndrome etc.). The assessment of the above factors should guide the surgeon in the management of the wounds, including whether the wound should be managed operatively or whether it could be safely managed outside of the operating theatre. The third phase of wound management relates to the actual wound closure, be it primary or secondary, delayed primary, or whether tissue transfer techniques would be of benefit.

However, it is the first two phases of the decision-making regarding wound management that are the most critical. It is the physician's judgment and the soundness thereof that determines the outcome of a wound. While technical aspects remain important, there is no substitute for careful assessment and sound surgical judgment in the management of a traumatic wound. Most poor outcomes in wound management can be related to errors in judgment rather than to errors in technique.

The authors have nicely diagrammed in broad strokes the general techniques of wound management. However, two specific difficult wounds deserve special mention. The first of these are the perineal degloving injuries, a complex injury pattern associated with mortalities as high as 30%, generally due to hemorrhagic shock or pelvic sepsis. These wounds require early, aggressive debridement coupled with fecal diversion and distal rectal

washout, particularly if the wounds involve the rectal sphincters. Subsequent daily debridement is recommended with pulsatile lavage until the wound is declared clean, to minimize the development of late pelvic sepsis.[1] These wounds should be allowed to heal by secondary intention; although anecdotal experience with vacuum-assisted closure techniques has suggested more rapid wound closure may be obtained. Delayed split-thickness skin grafting or closure with myocutaneous flaps may be useful in very large wounds.

The second difficult wound requiring complex management techniques is the closed internal degloving injury or the so-called Morel-Lavallee lesion. Commonly associated with pelvic ring and acetabular fractures, this injury involves a shearing mechanism whereby the subcutaneous tissues tear away from underlying fascia, resulting in a cavity filled with hematoma and liquefied fat. While this lesion is most common over the greater trochanter, it can also occur in the flank and lumbodorsal regions. Classic management of these lesions includes aggressive, repeat debridement before or at the time of fracture fixation, followed by secondary closure with or without vacuum-assisted techniques.[2] Recently, a method of percutaneous management has been described with good results. The percutaneous technique involves two small incisions (one over the distal most aspect and one over the most superior and posterior aspect) to evacuate the cavity, followed by mechanical debridement of the liquefied fat using a brush and pulsatile lavage. The cavity is then drained by a suction drain.[3]

In summary, the variety of wounds after trauma is extensive, and Drs. Adams, Biffl, and Cioffi have provided a thoughtful and comprehensive overview of the approaches to the traumatic wound. A thorough understanding of the physiology, decision-making strategies, and techniques described herein, coupled with sound surgical judgment, should allow the surgeon to achieve the three goals of wound management: the prevention of infection, the preservation of maximal function, and acceptable cosmesis.

## References

1. Kudsk KA, Hanna MK: Management of comples perineal injuries. *World J Surg.* 27:895, 2003.
2. Hak DJ, Olson SA, Matta JM: Diagnosis and management of closed internal degloving injuries associated with pelvic and acetabular fractures: the Morel-Lavallee lesion. *J Trauma* 42:1, 1997.
3. Tseng S, Tornetta P III: Percutaneous management of Morel-Lavallee lesions. *J Bone Joint Surg Am* 88:92, 2006.

# Burns and Radiation Injuries

*Jong O. Lee* ■ *David N. Herndon*

## BURNS

Nearly 1.25 million people are burned in the United States every year; however, the number of burn injuries is decreasing.[1] About 60,000 to 80,000 burns per year require hospitalization, and roughly 5500 of these patients die.[1,2] Burns requiring hospitalization typically include burns of greater than 10% of the total body surface area (TBSA) or significant burns of the hands, face, perineum, or feet.

The highest incidence of burn injury occurs during the first few years of life and between 20 and 29 years of age. The major causes of severe burn injury are flame burns and liquid scalds; flame burns cause most of the burn deaths while liquid scald burns account for the second largest number of deaths.

Between 1971 and 1991, burn deaths decreased by 40%, with a concomitant 12% decrease in deaths associated with inhalation injury.[2] Since 1991, burn deaths per capita have decreased another 25% according to statistics from the Centers for Disease Control and Prevention (www.cdc.gov/ncipc/wisqars). These improvements were probably due to prevention strategies resulting in fewer burns of lesser severity, as well as significant progress in treatment techniques. Improved care of severely burned patients has undoubtedly improved survival, particularly in children. In 1949, Bull and Fisher first reported the expected 50% mortality rate for burn sizes in several age groups based upon data from their unit.[3] They reported that approximately one-half of children aged 0 to 14 with burns of 49% TBSA would die.[3] This dismal statistic has dramatically improved, with the latest reports indicating 50% mortality for 98% TBSA burns in children 14 and under.[4,5] A healthy young patient with any size burn might be expected to survive.[6] The same cannot be said, however, for those aged 45 years or more, where the improvements have been much more modest, especially in patients over 65 years of age where a 35% burn still kills half of the patients.[7] These dramatic improvements in mortality after massive burns are due to advances in understanding of resuscitation, improvements in wound coverage by early excision and grafting, better support of the hypermetabolic response to injury, early nutritional support, more appropriate control of infection, and improved treatment of inhalation injuries. Aggressive treatment of patients with severe burns has improved outcomes to the point that survival in massive injuries is common. Future breakthroughs in the field are likely to be in the area of faster and better return of function and improved cosmetic outcomes.

Some burn patients benefit from treatment in specialized burn centers. These centers have dedicated resources and the expertise of all the required disciplines to maximize outcomes from such devastating injuries.[8] The American Burn Association and the American College of Surgeons Committee on Trauma have established guidelines about which patients should be transferred to a specialized burn center. Patients meeting the following criteria should be treated at a designated burn center:

1. Second- and third-degree burns of greater than 10% TBSA

2. Full-thickness burns in any age group

3. Any burn involving the face, hands, feet, eyes, ears, or perineum that may result in cosmetic or functional disability

4. Electrical injury

5. Inhalation injury or associated trauma

6. Chemical burns

7. Burns in patients with significant comorbid conditions (e.g., diabetes mellitus, chronic obstructive pulmonary disease, cardiac disease)

Patients meeting the following criteria can be treated in a general hospital setting:

1. Second-degree burns of less than 10% TBSA

2. No burns to areas of special function or risk, and no significant associated or premorbid conditions

## Pathophysiology

Burns are classified into six causal categories, three zones of injury, and five depths of injury (Table 50-1). The causes include injury due to fire, scald, contact, chemical, electrical, and radiation. Fire burns are divided into flash and flame burns, scald burns into those caused by liquids, grease, or steam, and liquid scald burns can be further divided into spill and immersion scalds.

Flame, scald, and contact induce cellular damage primarily by the transfer of energy that induces coagulative necrosis, while direct injury to cellular membranes is the cause of injury in chemical and electrical burns.

The skin generally provides a robust barrier to further transfer of energy to deeper tissues. After the inciting focus is removed, however, the response of local tissues can lead to further injury. The necrotic area of a burn is termed the *zone of coagulation*. The area immediately surrounding the necrotic zone has a moderate degree of injury that initially causes a decrease in tissue perfusion. This is termed the *zone of stasis* and, depending on the environment of the wound, can progress to coagulative necrosis if local blood flow is not maintained. Thromboxane $A_2$, a potent vasoconstrictor, is present in high concentrations in burn wounds, and local application of thromboxane inhibitors has been shown to improve blood flow and may decrease this zone of stasis.[9] Antioxidants[10] and inhibition of neutrophil-mediated processes[11] may also improve blood flow and preserve this tissue and affect the depth of injury. Endogenous vasodilators such as calcitonin gene-related peptide and substance P, whose levels are increased in the plasma of burned patients,[12] may also play a role. Local cellular interactions such as neutrophil aggregation are also likely to be active in forming the zone of stasis. The last area is the *zone of hyperemia* related to vasodilation from inflammation surrounding the burn wound. This zone contains the clearly viable tissue from which the healing process begins (Fig. 50-1).

## Burn Depth

Burn depth determines outcome in terms of scarring and survival. Burn depth is most accurately assessed by the judgment of experienced physicians, though technologies such as the heatable laser Doppler flow meter with multiple sensors hold promise for quantitatively determining burn depth. These measurements may give objective evidence of loss of tissue and thus assist the physician in

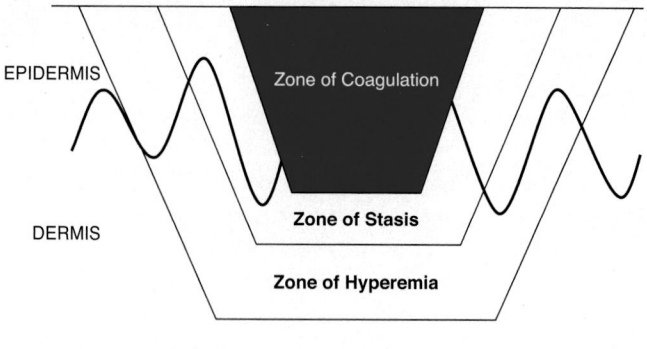

**FIGURE 50-1.** Illustration of the zones of injury after burn. Factors likely to affect the zone of stasis determine the extension of injury from the original zone of coagulation.

the proper choice of treatment.[13] Determination of depth is critical because as there are wounds that will heal with local treatment versus those that will require operative intervention for timely healing.

First-degree burns are confined to the epidermis. These burns are painful, erythematous, and blanch to the touch with an intact epidermal barrier without blister. Examples include sunburn or a minor scald. These burns will heal in three to six days. These burns will not result in scarring, and treatment is aimed at comfort with the use of topical soothing salves with or without aloe and nonsteroidal anti-inflammatory drugs or acetaminophen.

Second-degree (partial thickness) burns are divided into two types, superficial and deep. All second-degree injuries have some amount of dermal damage, and the division is based on the depth of injury into this structure. Superficial dermal burns are erythematous, painful, wet, blanch to touch, and often form blisters. Blistering may not occur for some hours following injury. Burns thought to be first degree may subsequently be diagnosed as second degree burns by the second day. These wounds will spontaneously reepithelialize from retained epidermal structures in the rete ridges, hair follicles, and sweat glands in 7 to 14 days. The injury may cause skin discoloration over the long term. Deep dermal burns into the reticular dermis will appear more pale than pink, or mottled, will not blanch to touch, but will remain painful to pinprick. In deeper second-degree burns the sensation becomes blunted (less sensitive to pinprick than surrounding normal skin). Capillaries may refill slowly after compression or not at all. These burns will heal in 21 to 28 days or longer by reepithelialization from hair follicles and keratinocytes in sweat glands, often with hypertrophic scarring. The longer the wound takes to heal, the worse the scarring will be.

Third-degree burns are full thickness burns through the dermis and are characterized by a firm leathery eschar that is painless and black, white, or cherry red in color. An eschar is insensitive to pinprick. No epidermal or dermal appendages remain, and these wounds must heal by re-epithelialization from the wound edges by contraction. Deep dermal and full-thickness burns require excision and grafting with autograft skin in order to heal the wounds in a timely fashion.

Fourth-degree burns involve other organs beneath the skin, such as muscle, tendon, and bone. They have a charred appearance that usually results from prolonged duration of contact with fire or an object such as a hot muffler or from high-voltage electrical injury.

### TABLE 50-1

| Definition of Burn Types, Zones, and Depth of Injury | | |
|---|---|---|
| **BURN CATEGORIES** | **ZONES OF INJURY** | **BURN DEPTH** |
| Fire — Flash, Flame | Zone of coagulation | First Degree (epidermal) |
| Scald — Liquid – Spill – Immersion | Zone of stasis | Superficial second degree (superficial dermal) |
| Grease | Zone of hyperemia | Deep second degree (deep thermal) |
| Steam | | Third degree (full thickness) |
| Contact | | Fourth degree (deep organ involvement) |
| Chemical | | |
| Electrical | | |
| Radiation | | |

## Inflammatory Response to a Burn

Massive release of inflammatory mediators is seen with a significant burn, both in the wound and in other tissues. These mediators produce vasoconstriction and vasodilation, increased capillary permeability, and edema locally and in distant organs. Many mediators have been proposed to explain the changes in permeability after burns, including prostaglandins, catecholamines, histamine, bradykinin, vasoactive amines, leukotrienes, and activated complement.[14] Mast cells in the burned skin release histamine in large quantities immediately after injury,[15] which will cause a characteristic response in venules by increasing the space in intercellular junctions.[16] The use of antihistamines in the treatment of burn edema, however, has had limited success with the possible exception of $H_2$-receptor antagonists.[17] In addition, aggregated platelets release serotonin, which plays a major role in the formation of edema. This agent acts directly to increase pulmonary vascular resistance and indirectly aggravates the vasoconstrictive effects of various vasoactive amines. Serotonin blockade has been shown to improve cardiac index, decrease pulmonary artery pressure, and decrease oxygen consumption after burns.[18]

Another mediator likely to play a major role in changes in vascular permeability and tone is thromboxane $A_2$. It has been shown that levels of thromboxane increase dramatically in the plasma and wounds of burned patients.[19,20] This potent vasoconstrictor leads to platelet aggregation in the wound contributing to expansion of the zone of stasis. It also causes prominent mesenteric vasoconstriction and decreased blood flow to the gut in animal models that compromise gut mucosal integrity and immune function.[21]

## Changes in Organ Function

Cardiopulmonary effects include marked loss of plasma volume, increased peripheral vascular resistance, and decreased cardiac output.[22] These changes are associated with mild direct cardiac damage[23] and a slight decrease in pulmonary static compliance.[24] Renal blood flow decreases with a fall in glomerular filtration rate, which may result in renal dysfunction. Metabolic changes are highlighted by an early depression followed by a marked, sustained increase in resting energy expenditure, increased lipolysis and proteolysis, and an increase in oxygen consumption. This is driven in part by an increase in production of catecholamines, cortisol, and glucagon.[25] There is a generalized impairment in host defenses with depressed production of immunoglobulin, decreased opsonic activity, depressed bactericidal activity, and increase in anergy to exposed antigens.[26] This causes the burned patient to become especially prone to infection.

## Initial Care and Resuscitation

A patient is removed from the source of burn, and clothing and jewelry are removed immediately. After the burning process is stopped, the patient should be kept warm by being wrapped in a clean sheet or blanket. The immediate treatment of a burn patient should proceed as with any trauma patient, and any potential life-threatening injuries should be identified and treated.

The airway should be assessed first. 100% oxygen is administered, and oxygen saturation is monitored using pulse oximetry. Wheezing, tachypnea, stridor, and hoarseness indicate impending airway obstruction due to an inhalation injury or edema, and immediate treatment is required. If the patient is not breathing or has labored respirations or signs of obstruction, immediate orotracheal intubation should be performed with in-line stabilization of the neck if an injury to the cervical spine is a consideration.

Measurements of arterial blood gases (ABG) and carboxyhemoglobin are obtained when appropriate. The presence of carbon monoxide (CO) in the blood, which has an affinity 280 times that of oxygen for hemoglobin, can falsely elevate oxygen saturation levels that are determined colorimetrically. The treatment for CO inhalation is 100% $O_2$ by endotracheal tube or face mask. This will decrease the half-life of CO from four hours at room air to 40 min with 100% $O_2$. It must be emphasized that as edema develops in the course of resuscitation, compromise of the airway may mandate intubation. Full-thickness circumferential burns of the chest can interfere with ventilation. Bilateral expansion of the chest should be observed to document equal air movement. If the patient is on a ventilator, airway pressure and $pCO_2$ should be monitored. If ventilation is compromised, an escharotomy should be performed to allow better movement of the chest and improve ventilation. Measurement of a cuff blood pressure may be difficult in patients with burned extremities, and these patients may need an arterial line to monitor their blood pressure during transfer or resuscitation. A radial arterial line may not be reliable in patients with extremity burns and is difficult to secure. Therefore, the insertion of a femoral arterial line may be appropriate.

## Fluid Resuscitation

In the hours after a serious burn, there is a systemic capillary leak that increases with burn size. Capillaries usually regain competence after 18–24 hours if resuscitation has been successful. Increased times to beginning resuscitation of burned patients result in poorer outcomes, and delays should be minimized.[27] The best venous access is with short peripheral catheters through unburned skin; however, veins beneath burned skin can be used to avoid a delay in obtaining intravenous access. Central venous lines or saphenous vein cutdowns are required when percutaneous access is difficult. In children under six years of age, intramedullary access can be utilized in the proximal tibia until intravenous access is accomplished. Lactated Ringer's solution without dextrose is the fluid of choice except in children under two, who should receive some 5% dextrose in lactated Ringer's solution. The initial rate can be rapidly estimated by multiplying the estimated TBSA burned by the weight in kilograms, which is divided by 4. Thus the rate of infusion for a 80-kg man with a 40% TBSA burn would be 80 kg × 40% TBSA/4 = 800 mL/hour for first eight hours.

Different formulas, all originating from experimental studies on the pathophysiology of burn shock, have been devised to assist the clinician in determining the proper amount of resuscitation fluid. Early work by Baxter and by Shires established the basis for modern protocols for fluid resuscitation.[28] They showed that edema fluid in burn wounds is isotonic and contains the same amount of protein as plasma and that the greatest loss of fluid is into the interstitial fluid compartment. They used various volumes of intravascular fluid to determine the optimal delivered amount in terms of cardiac output and extracellular volume in a canine burn model. These findings led to a successful clinical trial of the "Parkland formula" in resuscitating burned patients (Table 50-2). It was also

### TABLE 50-2

**Resuscitation Formulas**

| FORMULA | CRYSTALLOID VOLUME | COLLOID VOLUME | FREE WATER |
|---|---|---|---|
| Parkland | 4 mL/kg/% TBSA burn | None | None |
| Brooke | 1.5 mL/kg/% TBSA burn | 0.5 mL/kg/% TBSA burn | 2.0 L |
| Galveston (pediatric) | 5000 mL/m²burned + 1500 mL/m² total | None | None |

TBSA, total body surface area.

shown that changes in plasma volume were not related to the type of resuscitation fluid used in the first 24 hours, but, thereafter, colloid solutions could increase plasma volume. From these findings, it was concluded that colloid solutions should not be used in the first 24 hours until capillary permeability returned closer to normal. Others have argued that normal capillary permeability is restored somewhat earlier after a burn (six to eight hours) and, therefore, suggest that colloids can be used earlier.[29]

Moncrief and Pruitt also studied the hemodynamic effects of fluid resuscitation in burns, which resulted in the Brooke formula (Table 50-2). They showed that fluid loss in moderate burns resulted in an obligatory 20% decrease in both extracellular fluid and plasma volume during the first 24 hours after injury. In the second 24 hours, plasma volume returned to normal with the administration of colloid. Cardiac output was low the first day in spite of resuscitation, but subsequently increased to supernormal levels as the flow phase of hypermetabolism was established.[22] Since these studies, it has been found that much of the fluid needs are due to capillary leak that permits passage of large molecules and water into the interstitial space. Intravascular volume follows the gradient into the burn wound and non-burned tissues. Approximately 50% of fluid resuscitation needs are sequestered in nonburned tissues in 50% TBSA burns.[30]

Hypertonic saline solutions have theoretic advantages in the resuscitation of burned patients. These solutions have been shown to decrease net fluid intake,[31] decrease edema,[32] and increase lymph flow probably by the transfer of volume from the intracellular space to the interstitium. When using these solutions, care must be taken to avoid serum sodium concentrations greater than 160 mEq/dL.[14] Of note, it has been shown that patients with over 20% TBSA burns who were randomized to resuscitation with either hypertonic saline or lactated Ringer's solution did not have significant differences in total volume requirements or in changes in percent weight gain over days after the burn.[33] Other investigators have found an increase in renal failure with hypertonic solutions that has tempered further enthusiasm for their use in resuscitation.[34] Some burn units have successfully used a modified hypertonic solution by adding 1 ampule of sodium bicarbonate to each liter of lactated Ringer's solution.[35] Further research will need to be done to determine the optimal formula to reduce formation of edema as well as maintain adequate cellular function.

Of interest, it has been shown that resuscitation volumes required in the severely burned patient decreased when high-dose intravenous ascorbic acid was administered during resuscitation. This was associated with decreased weight gain and improved oxygenation.[36]

Most burn centers around the country use something similar to the Parkland or Brooke formula in which varying amounts of crystalloid and colloid solutions are administered for the first 24 hours postburn (Table 50-2). Intravenous fluids are generally changed in the second 24 hours to more hypotonic solutions. These formulas are guidelines to the amount of fluid necessary to maintain adequate perfusion. This is easily monitored in burned patients by following the volume of urine output, which should be maintained at 0.5 mL/kg/hour in adults and 1.0 mL/kg/hour in children. Other parameters such as heart rate, blood pressure, mental status, and peripheral perfusion are also monitored. Changes in the rates of intravenous fluid infusion should be made on an hourly basis as determined by the response of the patient to the particular fluid volume administered.

In children with burns, the commonly used formulas are modified to account for changes in surface area to mass ratios. Compared to adults, children have a larger body surface area relative to their weight than do adults and generally have somewhat greater fluid needs during resuscitation. The Galveston formula based on body surface area uses 5000 mL/m² TBSA burn in m² + 1500 mL/m² TBSA for maintenance in the first 24 hours (Table 50-2). This formula accounts for both maintenance needs and the resuscitation fluid requirements of a child with a burn. All of these formulas calculate the amount of volume given in the first 24 hours, one-half of which is given in the first eight hours and next one-half given over next 16 hours. Some dextrose is added to the resuscitation fluid in children under two to prevent hypoglycemia because they have limited glycogen stores. It is best to use two intravenous fluids in infants, lactated Ringer's solution for resuscitation, and 5% dextrose in lactated Ringer's solution for maintenance.

Administration of narcotic analgesia is not generally necessary in the prehospital setting. Once the patient has arrived at a hospital and is receiving resuscitation fluid it is reasonable to give small increments of morphine sulfate intravenously. Other routes of administration are not advisable because washout of either oral or intramuscular narcotics with re-establishment of adequate perfusion will induce significant respiratory depression. The overuse of narcotics for these painful injuries is a very common cause of respiratory arrest, especially in children, occasionally resulting in death even in patients with small burns. Caution with the use of analgesia must be maintained through a contemplated transfer to another facility to prevent unnecessary morbidity.

## Other Injuries

Other traumatic injuries such as fractures and abdominal injury may be present in patients who have been burned. Each patient should be fully evaluated for associated injuries that may be more life-threatening in the short term. The burn wounds can be addressed after standard evaluation and resuscitation. Burned patients should initially be placed on sterile or clean sheets. Cold water and ice may, in large burns, harm patients by inducing hypothermia and should be avoided. Placement of various ointments and antimicrobials at the receiving hospital may alter the appearance of the wound and could adversely affect treatment decisions at a burn center. The patient should be kept warm and the wounds clean until assessment by the physicians responsible for definitive care of the burns. Nasogastric tubes and bladder catheters are placed in patients requiring transfer to a burn center to decompress the stomach and to monitor the progress of resuscitation.

## Determination of Burn Size

The "rule of nines" is used for determination of burn size in adults (Fig. 50-2). Briefly, each upper extremity and the head and neck

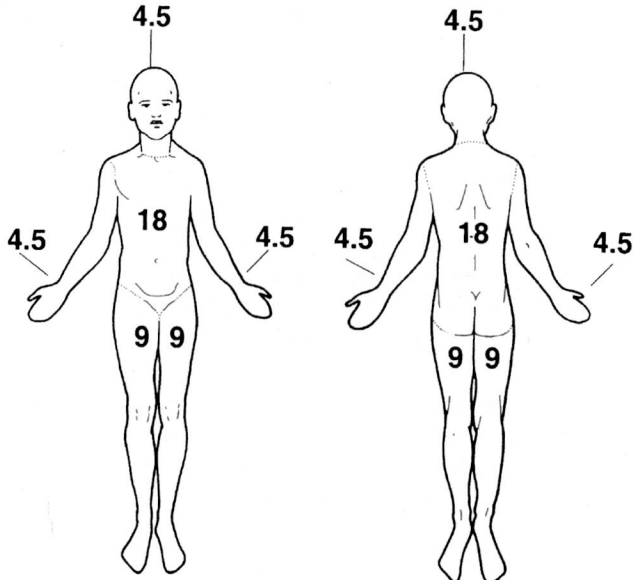

**FIGURE 50-2.** Determining burn size by the "rule of nines."

are 9% of the TBSA, the lower extremities, and the anterior and posterior trunk are 18% each, and the perineum and genitalia are assumed to be 1% of the TBSA. Another method of estimating smaller burns is the area of the patient's open hand; this is approximately 1% TBSA and can be transposed visually onto the wound for a determination of the burn size.

Children have a relatively larger portion of the body surface area in the head and neck and smaller surface area in the lower extremities. Infants have 21% of the TBSA in the head and neck and 13% in each leg, which incrementally approaches the adult proportions with increasing age. The Berkow formula can be helpful in determining burn size in children (Table 50-3).

## Escharotomies

With circumferential deep second- and third-degree burns to an extremity, peripheral circulation to the limb can be compromised. Development of generalized edema beneath a nonyielding eschar impedes venous outflow and will eventually affect arterial inflow to the distal beds. This can be recognized by numbness and tingling

### TABLE 50-3

**Berkow Chart for Estimation of Burn Size in Children**

| AREA | 1 YR | 1–4 YRS | 5–9 YRS | 10–14 YRS | 15 YRS |
|---|---|---|---|---|---|
| Head | 19 | 17 | 13 | 11 | 9 |
| Neck | 2 | 2 | 2 | 2 | 2 |
| Ant. trunk | 13 | 13 | 13 | 13 | 13 |
| Post. trunk | 13 | 13 | 13 | 13 | 13 |
| Buttock | 2.5 | 2.5 | 2.5 | 2.5 | 2.5 |
| Genitalia | 1 | 1 | 1 | 1 | 1 |
| Upper arm | 4 | 4 | 4 | 4 | 4 |
| Lower arm | 3 | 3 | 3 | 3 | 3 |
| Hand | 2.5 | 2.5 | 2.5 | 2.5 | 2.5 |
| Thigh | 5.5 | 6.5 | 8 | 8.5 | 9 |
| Leg | 5 | 5 | 5.5 | 6 | 6.5 |
| Foot | 3.5 | 3.5 | 3.5 | 3.5 | 3.5 |

in the limb and increased pain in the digits. Arterial flow can be assessed by pulse oximetry and determination of Doppler signals in the digital arteries and the palmar and plantar arches in affected extremities. Capillary refill is also assessed. Extremities at risk are identified on either clinical examination or measurement of tissue pressures greater than 40 mm Hg, which mandate an escharotomy performed at the bedside. The release of a burn eschar is performed by lateral and medial incisions on the extremity with an electrocautery unit. The entire constricting eschar must be incised to relieve the obstruction to blood flow. If the hand is involved, two dorsal incisions are made on the dorsal surface and along the lateral sides of the digits with care not to damage the neurovascular bundles. These bundles are located slightly to the palm side of the digit. If it is clear that the wound will require excision and grafting because of its depth, escharotomies are the safest route to restore perfusion to the underlying nonburned tissues. If vascular compromise has been prolonged, reperfusion after an escharotomy may cause a reactive hyperemia and further formation of edema in the muscle making continued surveillance of the distal extremities necessary. Increased pressures in the underlying musculofascial compartments are treated with standard fasciotomies.

As previously noted a circumferential burn of the chest with a constricting eschar can cause a similar phenomenon, except the effect is to decrease ventilation by limiting excursion of the chest wall. Any decrease in ventilation (increase in peak airway pressure and $pCO_2$) of a burned patient should be followed by inspection of the chest with appropriate escharotomies performed to relieve the constriction and allow adequate ventilation. This will become evident in a patient on a volume control ventilator where peak airway pressures will fall following the escharotomy.

## Chemical Burns

A chemical burn should be copiously irrigated with water or saline. Care must be taken to direct the drainage of the irrigating solution away from unburned areas to limit the area of skin exposed to noxious chemicals. Attempts at neutralization of either acidic or basic solutions will occasionally result in heat production and extend the injury. Generally, acids cause coagulative necrosis and are confined to the skin, while basic solutions cause liquefactive necrosis and extend further into the tissues until removal. Emergent operative debridement with pH testing of each tangential slice may be necessary to ensure no further injury after exposure to solutions with a high pH. After the chemical injury has been controlled, the remaining burn is treated in the same way as thermal injuries.

Hydrofluoric acid is used widely in industrial and domestic settings. When it is exposed to biological tissues, the fluoride ion precipitates calcium and may cause systemic hypocalcemia. This may occur even with a very small burn. Management of burns caused by this substance differs from burns caused by other acids. In addition to copious irrigation of the burned area, the exposed skin should be treated with 2.5% calcium gluconate gel to provide pain relief and limit the spread of the fluoride ion. For hand burns, even intra-arterial calcium gluconate has been advocated. Patients should be monitored closely for prolongation of the QT interval, torsade de pointes, or ventricular fibrillation. Changes in the QT interval should be treated with 20 mL of 10% calcium gluconate repeated as needed to maintain normal levels of serum calcium. Other serum electrolytes such as magnesium must also be closely monitored.

## Electrical Burns

Electrical burns are unique in that the location of the injury may be mostly internal. Electrical current proceeds down the path of least resistance, which is via nerves, blood vessels, bones and muscle, thus sparing the skin except at the entry and exit points of the electrical current. For these reasons, inspection of the entry and exit sites of the electrical burn will significantly underestimate the amount of internal damage. If the resistance of entry and exit sites of high-voltage current is high, the local injury may be extensive, with loss of digits or even entire extremities.

With any significant electrical injury, vigorous intravenous resuscitation should be given with attention to myoglobinuria from muscle damage. Urine output should be maintained at greater than 1 mL/kg/hour with fluid administration and mannitol diuresis to increase renal tubular flow if needed. The administration of intravenous bicarbonate to alkalinize the urine should be considered to decrease precipitation of hemochromogens in the renal tubules. Patients should be monitored for cardiac arrhythmias for 24 to 48 hours after admission.

Serial examinations of the extremities are necessary to detect any vascular compromise, and fasciotomies are often necessary. Debridement of nonviable tissue in decompressed sites is appropriate. If operative exploration is necessary, complete fasciotomies with inspection of deep tissues should be undertaken. Acute and chronic neuropathies are common and may be permanent. Development of cataracts is also common after severe electrical injury and may be delayed for months; therefore, close ophthalmologic follow-up is necessary.

## The Burn Wound

Improvements in the treatment of burn wounds and utilization of antimicrobial dressings have dramatically decreased the incidence of fatal sepsis in burned patients.[37] The previous technique of allowing separation of eschar with lysis by bacterial enzymes has given way to wound closure using early excision and grafting. In those wounds that will heal spontaneously without skin grafts, topical antimicrobial agents limit wound contamination and provide a moist environment for healing. Current therapy for burn wounds can be divided into the following three stages: assessment, management, and rehabilitation. Once the extent and depth of the wounds have been assessed and the wounds thoroughly cleaned and debrided, the management phase begins. Each wound should be dressed with an appropriate covering that serves three functions. First, it protects the damaged epithelium. Second, the dressing should be occlusive to reduce evaporative heat loss and minimize

cold stress. Third, the dressing should provide comfort over the painful wound.

The choice of dressing should be individualized based on the characteristics of the treated wound. First-degree wounds are minor with minimal loss of barrier function. These wounds require no dressing and are treated with topical salves to decrease pain and keep the skin moist. Second-degree wounds can be treated by daily dressing changes with an antibiotic ointment such as silver sulfadiazine covered with several layers of gauze under elastic wraps. Alternatively, the wounds can be covered with a temporary biologic or synthetic covering to close the wound. These coverings eventually slough as the wound re-epithelializes underneath. These types of dressings provide for stable coverage without painful dressing changes, provide a barrier to evaporative losses, and decrease pain. They may also have the added benefit of not inhibiting epithelialization that is a feature of most topical antimicrobial agents. As synthetic coverings have no antimicrobial property, therefore close observation is required. These coverings include allograft (cadaver skin), xenograft (pigskin), and Biobrane (Bertek, Morgantown, WV).[38,39] The advantages and disadvantages of the various coverings are listed in Table 50-4. These should generally be applied within 24 hours of the burn before high bacterial colonization of the wound occurs.

Deep second- and third-degree burns will not heal in a timely fashion without autografting. These burned tissues serve as a nidus for inflammation and infection that can lead to death of the patient. Early excision and grafting of these wounds is now practiced by most burn surgeons in response to reports showing benefit over serial debridement in terms of survival, blood loss, and length of hospitalization.[40–42]

These excisions can be performed with tourniquet control or with application of topical epinephrine and thrombin to minimize blood loss. After a burn wound has been excised, the wound must be covered with either autograft skin or some other covering. This covering is ideally the patient's own skin. Wounds less than 20 to 30% TBSA can usually be closed at one operation with autograft skin taken from the patient's available donor sites. In these operations, the skin grafts are either not meshed or meshed with a narrow ratio (2:1 or less) to improve cosmetic outcomes. In major burns, donor skin may be limited to the extent that the entire wound cannot be covered with autograft. The availability of cadaver allograft skin to cover these wounds has changed the course of modern treatment for massive burns. A typical method of treatment is to use widely expanded autografts (4:1 or greater) covered with allograft skin to completely close the wounds for which autograft is available. The 4:1 skin heals underneath the allograft skin in approximately 21 days, and the allograft skin will slough.

**TABLE 50-4**

| Advantages and Disadvantages of Alternative Wound Coverings | | | |
| --- | --- | --- | --- |
| **COVERING** | **MATERIAL** | **ADVANTAGES** | **DISADVANTAGES** |
| Homograft | Cadaver skin (fresh or frozen) | Reduces bacterial colonization, vascularizes | Expensive, limited availability, exposure to hepatitis and CMV |
| Xenograft | Pigskin | Vascularizes, readily available | Does not resist infection |
| Transcyte | Biobrane with impregnated killed fetal fibroblasts | Stable coverage, readily available, some anti-infective effects | Expensive |
| Biobrane | Synthetic nylon and silicon | Readily available | Must be placed early, infections are common |

CMV, cytomegalovirus.

Massively burned patients are profoundly immunosuppressed, and rejection of allograft skin is rarely a problem. Portions of the wound that cannot be covered with widely meshed autograft are covered with allograft skin in preparation for autografting when donor sites are healed and ready for reharvesting. Ideally, areas with less cosmetic importance are covered with the widely meshed skin to close most of the wound prior to using nonmeshed grafts for the cosmetically important areas, such as the hands and face.

Most surgeons excise the burn wound within the first week, sometimes in serial operations, removing 20% of the burn wound per operation on subsequent days. Others remove the whole of the burn wound in one operative procedure; however, this can be difficult in patients with large burns and complicated by the development of hypothermia or massive blood loss. It is the authors' practice to perform the excision immediately after stabilization of the patient, because blood loss diminishes if the operation can be performed the first day after injury. This may be due to the relative predominance of vasoconstrictive substances such as thromboxane and catecholamines in the circulation and the natural edema planes that develop immediately after the injury. When the wound becomes hyperemic after two days, blood loss during excision can be a considerable problem.

Early excision should be reserved for third-degree wounds typically caused by flame. This is highlighted because scald burns are very common. These injuries are often partial thickness or a mixture of partial and full thickness and should be covered with substances such as allograft, porcine xenograft, or Biobrane, allowing the wound, which will heal, to be protected. A deep second-degree burn can appear clinically to be a third-degree wound at 24 to 48 hours after injury, particularly if it has been treated with topical antimicrobials that combine with wound drainage to form a pseudoeschar. A randomized prospective study comparing early excision versus conservative therapy with late grafting with scald burn showed that those excised early had more wound excised, more blood loss, and more time in the operating room. No difference in hospital length of stay or rate of infection was seen.[43]

Loss of skin grafts is due to one or more of the following reasons: presence of infection; fluid collection under the graft; shearing forces that disrupt the adhered graft; or an inadequate excision of the wound bed leaving residual necrotic tissue. Infection is controlled by the appropriate use of perioperative antibiotics and covering the grafts with topical antimicrobial agents at the time of surgery. Meticulous hemostasis, appropriate meshing of grafts, or "rolling" of sheet grafts postoperatively and/or use of a bolster dressing over appropriate areas minimizes fluid collections. Shearing is decreased by immobilization of the grafted area. Inadequately excised wound beds are uncommon in the practice of experienced surgeons. Punctate bleeding or color of the dermis or fat in areas excised under a tourniquet denotes the proper level of excision.

## Control of Infection

Decreasing invasive infections in the burn wound is due to early excision and closure and the timely and effective use of antimicrobials. As stated previously, the infected burn wound filled with invasive organisms is uncommon in most burn units due to the effective use of antibiotics and techniques of wound care. The antimicrobials that are used can be divided into those given topically and those given systemically.

Available topical antibiotics can be divided into salves and soaks. Salves are generally applied directly to the wound with dressings placed over them, and soaks are generally poured into dressings on the wound. Each of these classes of antimicrobials has its advantages and disadvantages. Salves may be applied once or twice a day, but may lose their effectiveness in between dressing changes. More frequent dressing changes can result in shearing with loss of grafts or underlying healing cells. Soaks will remain effective because antimicrobial solution can be added without removing the dressing; however, the underlying skin can become macerated.

Topical antibiotic salves include 11% mafenide acetate (Sulfamylon), 1% silver sulfadiazine (Silvadene), polymyxin B, neomycin, bacitracin, and mupirocin. No single agent is completely effective, and each has advantages and disadvantages. Mafenide acetate has a broad spectrum of activity through its sulfa moiety, particularly for *Pseudomonas* and enterococcus species. It also has the advantage of penetration of eschar. Disadvantages include pain on application, an allergic skin rash, and inhibition of carbonic anhydrase activity that can result in a metabolic acidosis when applied over large surfaces. For these reasons, mafenide sulfate is typically reserved for small full-thickness injuries and ear burns to prevent chondritis. Silver sulfadiazine, the most frequently used topical agent, has a broad spectrum of activity from its silver and sulfa moieties that cover gram-positive organisms, most gram-negative organisms, and some fungi. Some *Pseudomonas* species, however, possess plasmid-mediated resistance. It is painless upon application, has a high patient acceptance, and is easy to use. Occasionally, patients will complain of some burning sensation after it is applied, and some patients will develop a transient leukopenia two to four days following its continued use. This leukopenia is generally harmless and resolves with cessation of treatment in two to three days. When the leukopenia resolves, silver sulfadiazine may be reapplied without recurrence of this problem. Petroleum-based antimicrobial ointments with polymyxin B, neomycin, and bacitracin are clear on application, painless, and allow for observation of the wound. These agents are commonly used for the treatment of facial burns, graft sites, healing donor sites, and small partial-thickness burns. Mupirocin is a relatively new ointment that has improved activity against gram-positive bacteria, particularly methicillin-resistant *Staphylococcus aureus,* and selected gram-negative bacteria. Nystatin in powder form can be applied to wounds to control fungal growth, and nystatin powder can be combined with topical agents such as polymyxin B to decrease colonization of both bacteria and fungi.

Available agents for application as a soak include 0.5% silver nitrate solution, 0.5% sodium hypochlorite, 5% acetic acid, and 5% mafenide acetate solution. Silver nitrate has the advantage of painless application and almost complete antimicrobial coverage. The disadvantages include its staining of surfaces to a dull gray or black when the solution is exposed to light. The solution is hypotonic and continuous use can cause leaching of electrolytes, with rare methemoglobinemia as another complication. Hypochlorite is a basic solution with effectiveness against most microbes, but it also has cytotoxic effects on wounds, thus inhibiting healing. Low concentrations of sodium hypochlorite (0.025%) have less cytotoxic effects while maintaining the antimicrobial effects. In addition, hypochlorite ion is inactivated by contact with protein, so the solution must be continually changed. The same is true for acetic acid solutions, though this solution may be more effective against

*Pseudomonas.* Mafenide acetate solution has the same characteristics as the mafenide acetate cream.

The use of perioperative systemic antimicrobials also has a role in decreasing sepsis in the burn wound until it is healed. Common organisms that must be considered when choosing a perioperative regimen include *Staphylococcus aureus* and *Pseudomonas* sp., which are prevalent in wounds. After massive excisions, gut flora are often found in the wounds mandating coverage of these species as well.

## Management of Organ Systems

Large burns result in a number of effects to organ systems in addition to injury to the skin. The immense inflammatory focus incited by the burn causes the release of numerous cytokines and inflammatory mediators that have many systemic effects and, ultimately, may result in multiorgan dysfunction and death. The systemic inflammatory response syndrome (SIRS) is present in every major burn, but with differing severity, and the kidneys, liver, heart, lungs, hematopoietic system, and coagulation system may be affected. Each of these systems must be supported through the course of the burn injury until function returns.

After resuscitation and stabilization, evaporative losses through open wounds including the area of burn and any donor sites remain high. Many of these patients are placed in air beds to prevent decubiti and decrease shearing of grafts, which also increases evaporative losses. Approximately 3750 mL/m$^2$ of free water is lost through open wounds, and an additional 1 L/m$^2$/day is lost through continuous airflow past open wounds if treated in an air bed. These insensible losses must be added to urine output, stool volume, and respiratory losses in determining fluid balances. Daily weights are useful in determining the response to fluid management. Sodium, potassium, calcium, magnesium, and phosphate are also lost into burn dressings and will require constant monitoring and replacement. Renal failure after a burn occurs in a bimodal fashion, with an early peak that is due to acute tubular necrosis from inadequate early resuscitation and a later peak at two to four weeks that is likely due to sepsis and nephrotoxic medications.[44,45] Treatment is as with any cause for renal failure. Indications for dialysis include life-threatening congestive heart failure, pulmonary edema, and hyperkalemia and metabolic acidosis refractory to medical management. Continuous venovenous hemodialysis (CVVHD) may have some advantages over routine hemodialysis because of slower fluid fluxes. Peritoneal dialysis is also an option in these patients, with the same advantages as CVVHD. Catheters can be placed through burned tissue, although intact skin is preferable.

Hepatic dysfunction can occur because of toxins associated with chemical injury or flame burns in which the patient was doused with chemicals, particularly gasoline. The direct hepatotoxicity that results is manifested by early increases in hepatocellular enzymes. Support through the recovery period is indicated. Later evidence of hepatic injury from sepsis is also common. A striking finding associated with the larger burns is the development of a fatty liver, which can increase hepatic size two- to threefold.[46] The primary determinant seems to be a relative decrease in efficiency of the very low density lipoprotein system to handle the massive increase in delivery of free fatty acids from peripheral lipolysis induced by sustained elevations in serum catecholamines. Fat that cannot be exported is thus deposited in the liver.

Coagulopathies from decreased hepatic synthetic function of coagulation factors, thrombocytopenia, or dilutional effects of massive blood transfusions can occur after a major burn. Treatment is directed toward prevention of massive blood loss through the use of tourniquets, epinephrine and thrombin topical sprays, and prevention of sepsis through timely operative treatment and use of antibiotics.

## Inhalation Injury

An associated inhalation injury is one of the factors that contributes to mortality in burns. Inhalation injury adds another inflammatory focus to the burn and impedes the normal gas exchange that is vital for critically injured patients. It has been shown that inhalation injury increases with burn size. In addition, the presence of such an injury can be used as a significant predictor of outcome in massive burns. In one study, the amount of time spent on a ventilator in the first 28 days was the strongest predictor of mortality in a group of children with over 80% TBSA burns; inhalation injury was present in the majority of these children.[27] Early diagnosis and prevention of complications are necessary to decrease morbidity and mortality related to inhalation injury.

Damage is caused primarily by inhaled toxins in most inhalation injuries. Heat is generally dispersed in the upper airways, whereas the cooled particles of smoke and toxins are carried distally into the bronchi and alveoli. Thus, the injury is principally chemical in nature. The response is an immediate dramatic increase in blood flow in the bronchial arteries to the bronchi with formation of edema and increases in lung lymph flow. The lung lymph in this situation is similar to serum, indicating that permeability at the capillary level is markedly increased. The edema that results is associated with an increase in lung neutrophils, and it is postulated that these cells may be the primary mediators of pulmonary damage with this injury. Neutrophils release proteases and oxygen-free radicals that can produce conjugated dienes by lipid peroxidation. High concentrations of these conjugated dienes are present in the lung lymph and pulmonary tissues after inhalation injury, suggesting that increased neutrophils are active in producing cytotoxic materials. When neutrophils are depleted prior to injury by nitrogen mustard, increases in lung lymph flow and conjugated diene levels are markedly reduced.[47]

Separation of the ciliated epithelial cells from the basement membrane followed by formation of exudate within the airways is another hallmark of inhalation injury. The exudate consists of proteins found in the lung lymph and eventually coalesces to form fibrin casts. Clinically, these fibrin casts can be difficult to clear with standard techniques of airway suction, and bronchoscopy is often required. These casts can also add barotrauma to localized areas of lung by forming a "ball-valve." During inspiration, the airway diameter increases, and air flows past the cast into the distal airways. During expiration, the airway diameter decreases, and the cast effectively occludes the airway, preventing the inhaled air from escaping. Increasing volume leads to localized increases in pressure that are associated with numerous complications, including pneumothorax and decreased lung compliance. Therapy aimed at clearing the airway and minimizing complications would likely improve outcomes after this injury.

Patients with smoke inhalation often present with a history of exposure to smoke in a closed space, hoarseness, wheezing, carbonaceous sputum, facial burns, and singed nasal vibrissae. Each of these findings has poor sensitivity and specificity; therefore, the diagnosis is often established by the use of bronchoscopy. Bronchoscopy can reveal early inflammatory changes such as erythema, edema, ulceration, sloughing of mucosa, and prominent vasculature in addition to infraglottic soot. Many of these patients will require mechanical ventilation to maintain gas exchange, and repeated bronchoscopies may reveal continued ulceration of the airways with the formation of granulation tissue and exudate, inspissation of secretions, and focal edema. Eventually, the airway heals by replacement of the sloughed cuboidal ciliated epithelium with squamous cells and scar.

Management of inhalation injury is directed at maintaining open airways and maximizing gas exchange while the lung heals. A coughing patient with a patent airway can clear secretions very effectively, and efforts should be made to treat patients without mechanical ventilation, if possible. If respiratory failure is imminent, intubation should be instituted early, with frequent chest physiotherapy and suctioning performed to maintain pulmonary hygiene. Frequent bronchoscopies may be needed to clear inspissated secretions. Mechanical ventilation should be used to provide gas exchange with as little barotrauma as possible. Inhalation treatments have been effective in improving the clearance of tracheobronchial secretions and decreasing bronchospasm. Intravenous heparin has been shown to reduce the formation of tracheobronchial casts, minute ventilation, and peak inspiratory pressures after smoke inhalation. When heparin was administered directly to the lungs in a nebulized form to reduce bleeding problems, it was shown to have similar effects on casts without causing a systemic coagulopathy. When N-acetylcysteine treatments are added to nebulized heparin in burned children with inhalation injury, reintubation rates and mortality are decreased.[48] In addition to the preceding measures, adequate humidification and treatment of bronchospasm with alpha-agonists is indicated. Steroids have not been shown to be of benefit in inhalation injury and should not be given unless the patient is steroid-dependent before injury or has bronchospasm resistant to standard therapy.[42]

In addition to conventional ventilator methods, novel ventilator therapies have been devised to minimize barotrauma, including high-frequency percussive ventilation. This method combines standard tidal volumes and respirations (ventilator rates 6 to 20 breaths/minute) with smaller high-frequency respirations (200 to 500 breaths/minute) and has been shown to permit adequate ventilation and oxygenation in patients who had failed conventional ventilation. An explanation for the greater utility of this method is the ability to recruit alveoli at lower airway pressures.[49] This ventilator method may also have a percussive effect to loosen inspissated secretions and improve pulmonary hygiene.

## Hypermetabolism in Burns

Burn patients have the highest metabolic rate of all critically ill or injured patients.[50,51] The metabolic response to a severe burn injury is characterized by a hyperdynamic cardiovascular response, increased energy expenditure, accelerated breakdown of glycogen and protein, lipolysis, loss of lean body mass and body weight, delayed wound healing, and immune depression.[52,53] This response is mediated by increases in circulating levels of the catabolic hormones including catecholamines, cortisol, and glucagon.[54]

Marked wasting of lean body mass occurs within a few weeks of injury. Modern techniques using immediate total burn excision, rapid wound closure, and adequate early enteral feeding have resulted in a significant reduction in mortality. Hypermetabolism and catabolism of muscle protein continue up to six to nine months after a severe burn.[55] Therefore, nutritional support of acute burn patients becomes an essential part of treatment during their hospitalization. Pharmacological agents have been used to attenuate catabolism and to stimulate growth after burn injury, as well. To further minimize erosion of lean body mass, administration of anabolic hormones such as growth hormone, insulin, insulin-like growth factor (IGF)/IGF-binding protein-3 (IGFBP-3), oxandrolone or testosterone, and catecholamine antagonists such as propranolol have been used. These agents contribute to maintenance of lean body mass as well as promoting wound healing.[56–61]

## Nutritional Management of Burn Patients

Nutritional support of the hypermetabolic response in severely burned patients is best accomplished by early enteral nutrition that can abate the hypermetabolic response to a burn.[62,63] Early enteral feeding preserves gut mucosal integrity and improves intestinal blood flow and motility, as well.[62] Therefore, duodenal or jejunal tube feeding should be commenced as early as within the first six hours postburn.

The caloric requirements needed to reach weight and nitrogen balance have been calculated from linear regression analysis of weight change versus predicted dietary intakes in adults at 25 kcal/kg plus 40 kcal/% TBSA burn for 24 hours (Table 50-5).[64] The pediatric formulas have been derived from retrospective analyses of dietary intake, which was associated with maintenance of body weight average over hospital stay (Table 50-6).[65–70]

## RADIATION INJURIES

Since the discovery of radiation by Becquerel over 100 years ago, our society has used radioactivity to its benefit as an energy source, defensive weapon, and diagnostic and therapeutic medical tool. With these benefits come hazards in the form of accidents in

### TABLE 50-5

**Curreri Formula for Estimating Caloric Requirements for Adults Burn Patients[37]**

| 16–60 years | 25 kcal/kg/day + 40 kcal/% burn/day |
| >60 years | 25 kcal/kg/day + 65 kcal/% burn/day |

### TABLE 50-6

**Formulas for Estimating Caloric Requirements for Pediatric Burn Patients[48–53] (Shriners Hospitals for Children at Galveston, Texas)**

| 0–1 year | 2100 kcal/m² TBSA/day + 1000 kcal/m² TBSA burn/day |
| 1–11 years | 1800 kcal/m² TBSA/day + 1300 kcal/m² TBSA burn/day |
| 12–18 years | 1500 kcal/m² TBSA/day + 1500 kcal/m² TBSA burn/day |

TBSA = Total Body Surface Area; TBSAB = Total Body Surface Area Burn nuclear power plants, threat of nuclear war, and potential for radiation injuries from improper use of radioactive isotopes and ionizing radiation. The threat of nuclear or radiation accidents resulting in mass casualties is real and has never been greater as radiation sources are ubiquitous and are available from medical, industrial, and military sources. Major industrial accidents at Three Mile Island, Chernobyl, and Goiania, Brazil, have highlighted the need for knowledge of radiation effects and treatment.

Exposure to radiation can be classified into the following three types[71]:

1. Small, contained events affecting one or more persons, either localized or affecting the whole body; e.g., laboratory accident or damage from x-ray machines.

2. Industrial accident affecting large numbers of people with varying degrees of severity; e.g., meltdown of a nuclear power plant.

3. Detonation of a nuclear device with injuries to hundreds or thousands with associated trauma.

Specific changes noted in association with radiation make these injuries unique and require consideration as a separate form of trauma.[72] In explosions, however, the release of kinetic energy can cause other more standard injuries commonly associated with blunt mechanisms. The patients may present with trauma and burns in addition to radiation exposure and explosions. The intent of this part of this chapter is to provide information regarding the terminology associated with radiation, pathophysiology of injury, and diagnosis and treatment of these injuries, including triage and decontamination.

## Measuring Exposure to Radiation

Radiation consists of both particles ($\alpha$, $\beta$, and neutrons) and photons ($\gamma$ and x-rays), which have specific energies and tissue penetrance (Table 50-7). Ionizing radiation can strip electrons from atoms to cause chemical change, resulting in biological damage. The potential for biologic injury for each of these depends on the amount of energy transmitted by the particle or photon when it interacts with the target. Each type of radiation has different qualities, and each will be absorbed in differing amounts in tissue.

Distance, time, and shielding can reduce exposure from a radiation source. The delivered dose of radiation diminishes over distance from its source by the inverse law.[73] If the distance between an object and the source of exposure is doubled, exposure is reduced to one-fourth its original value.

Dosimetry is the measurement of radiation exposure by detectors that indicate the type, quality, flux, and rate of exposure dependent on the distance of the detector from the source. Geiger-Mueller instruments detect $\beta$ and $\gamma$ radiation and are useful in the assessment of the effectiveness of decontamination procedures.[74] These instruments read counts per minute or milliroentgens per hour of $\beta$ and $\gamma$ irradiation. To determine individual exposure to radiation, radiation badges that contain a thermoluminescent dosimeter to record the cumulative dose of ionizing radiation on a photographic emulsion are useful. Pocket dosimeters, which give an immediate determination of radiation exposure as well as a running record of individual exposures, can be used as well. Such an online measure may be useful during an emergency response.

## Radiation Incidents

Radiation incidents within the United States must be reported to the Radiation Emergency Assistance Center/Training Site (REAC/TS) at the Oak Ridge Institute for Science and Education, Oak Ridge Associated Universities in Oak Ridge, Tennessee (http://www.orau.gov/reacts). This agency is funded by the U.S. Department of Energy and provides assistance in the response to all types of radiation accidents or incidents on a 24 hour/day basis. The agency has the capability of providing medical attention and should be contacted to both inform and receive advice about specific incidents. They can assist with calculations of absorbed dose. The telephone number for REAC/TS is (865) 576-1005.

The majority of incidents are associated with sealed highly radioactive sources often used in industrial radiography followed by those associated with x-ray machines or the use of unsealed radioisotopes in medicine and uranium products. When fissionable material, usually enriched uranium, has enough neutron flux to undergo a spontaneous nuclear reaction, the material has reached "critical mass," with the release of uncontrolled radiation. A total of 103 deaths associated with this circumstance have occurred to date. The majority of these deaths occurred after 1975, with most (>40) being associated with the Chernobyl incident in 1986.

The most devastating loss of life associated with radiation was with the detonation of atomic bombs in Nagasaki and Hiroshima in World War II. Fifty percent of the deaths were related to burn injuries, 30% of which were flash burns from the explosion. Physicians caring for the victims noticed that the burns began to heal, and then, at one to two weeks after the injury, began to deteriorate with infection and disordered formation of granulation tissue. A gray, greasy coating of the wounds was described. Associated thrombocytopenia caused bleeding into the wounds and gastrointestinal tract with ultimate demise of most of these patients. These observations have led to studies into the pathophysiology of these injuries.

## Pathophysiology

Radiation damage to cells is caused by the transfer of kinetic energy from particles or photons to existing molecules, causing ionization of mostly oxygen and formation of free radicals (such as the hydroxyl radical). These highly toxic compounds then react with normal biologic molecules to cause cellular damage, mostly to the phospholipid membranes and deoxyribonucleic acid.[75] Cell types have different sensitivities to radiation based on individual characteristics. Cells with high proliferation rates are the most sensitive, while those with very low proliferation rates are relatively resistant (Table 50-8). For organs made up of resistant cells, most of the effects are on the microvasculature.

**TABLE 50-7**

### Types of Radiation, Relative Energies, Penetrance, and Relative Hazard

| | RELATIVE ENERGY (MeV) | PENETRANCE INTO TISSUE (CM) | RELATIVE HAZARD |
|---|---|---|---|
| $\alpha$ | 1–5 | .0007–.004 | Low |
| $\beta$ | 0.2–1.0 | .017–.34 | Moderate |
| $\gamma$ | 0.1–10 | 20–150 | High |

**TABLE 50-8**

| Radiosensitivity of Human Cell Types | |
|---|---|
| RADIOSENSITIVITY | CELL TYPES |
| Very high | Lymphocytes |
| | Hematopoietic cells |
| | Intestinal epithelium |
| | Spermatogonia, ovarian follicular cells |
| High | Urinary bladder epithelium |
| | Esophageal epithelium |
| Intermediat | Endothelium |
| | Fibroblasts |
| | Pulmonary epithelium |
| | Renal epithelium |
| | Hepatocytes |
| Low | Hematopoietic STEM Cells |
| | Myocytes |
| | Chondrocytes |
| | Neural cells |

**TABLE 50-9**

| Four Phases of Acute Radiation Syndrome | |
|---|---|
| Prodromal Phase | Nausea, vomiting, fever |
| Latent Phase | Symptom free interval following acute nausea/vomiting |
| Manifest Phase | Symptoms of hematopoetic, gastrointestinal, and neurologic injury |
| Recovery Phase | Variable |

The overall effect depends on the extent of cellular mass exposed, the duration of exposure, and the homogeneity of the radiation field. Radiation injuries are either localized or whole body, depending on the circumstances of the exposure. The term *localized radiation injury* refers to an injury involving a relatively small portion of the body that does not lead to systemic effects.[73] This is mostly associated with local exposure to low-energy radiation, such as handling of sealed radiation sources of $^{60}$Cobalt or $^{192}$Iridium for industrial purposes or inadvertent exposure to x-ray beams from machines thought not to be operating.[74]

Injury severity is dependent on the dose of exposure. Erythema of the skin is often the first sign, and the sooner its appearance, the higher the dose of exposure. It often appears as a first-degree burn at the following intervals of time: (a) early, which will be transitory and short-lived; (b) secondarily, often two to three weeks after exposure and immediately preceding moist desquamation; and (c) late, 6 to 18 weeks after exposure, heralded by vasculitis, swelling, and pain. Depilation (loss of hair) is also used to determine the extent of localized injury and may occur as early as seven days after exposure. It is usually associated with doses of 7 to 10 Gy, and the hair loss is permanent. Alternatively, with lower doses of 3 to 5 Gy, depilation occurs at 18 to 30 days and the hair loss is temporary.

Moist desquamation is equivalent to a second-degree burn. This develops over a period of three weeks and occurs with doses of 12 to 20 Gy. The latency period is shorter with higher doses. Full-thickness ulceration and necrosis are caused by doses in excess of 25 Gy, and the onset varies from weeks to months after exposure. The microvasculature is changed in a characteristic pattern, with surviving superficial vessels becoming telangiectatic and deeper vessels developing obliterative endarteritis. Occlusion of deeper vessels results in full-thickness necrosis.

## Acute Radiation Syndrome

Detonation of a nuclear device can result in enough radiation exposure to cause immediate death for those exposed individuals within the lethal area of the blast. The symptoms and severity of injury from the acute radiation exposure are directly related to the effective dose of radiation to the whole body. Radiation exposure of less than 1 Gy is associated with minimal symptoms and no mortality, but exposure at greater than 8 Gy has 100% mortality.[76]

$LD_{50/60}$ is a lethal dose required to kill 50% of the population within 60 days. $LD_{50/60}$ for human beings is 250 to 450 rad. The hematopoietic and gastrointestinal systems are affected by radiation because they have rapidly dividing cell lines. Loss of stem cells and rapidly dividing cells from hematopoietic, and gastrointestinal tissues can lead to bleeding, infection, and diarrhea.

Acute radiation syndrome has four phases of severity of signs and symptoms (Table 50-9). In the prodromal phase, onset is related to total dose of radiation received. It can be minutes, if a lethal dose (>8 Gy) is received, to hours if <2 Gy is received. Nausea, vomiting, fever, and anorexia may last for two to four days or longer if a higher dose is received. Gastrointestinal symptoms appearing within two hours of radiation usually indicate a fatal outcome. When signs and symptoms regress, the latent phase starts. This may last few hours to two to three weeks or longer depending on the dose of radiation. As the dose of radiation increases, the latent phase becomes shorter. Symptoms of hematopoietic, gastrointestinal, and neurologic syndromes are expressed in a manifest phase following the latent phase. Nausea, vomiting, diarrhea, and bleeding characterize this phase. A recovery phase follows the manifest phase. This phase is variable and may last weeks to months and, if the dose is high enough, death ensues.

## Whole-Body Exposure

As with localized injury, effects of whole-body exposure depend on the dose of radiation absorbed by all tissues of the body. As opposed to local exposure to just the skin, whole body exposure will lead to much more absorption of energy. For instance, a 5 Gy exposure to the skin of a finger (10 g of tissue) will be a total amount of absorbed energy equaling 500,000 ergs. For an absorbed dose of 5 Gy over the whole body (100 kg = 100,000 g), the absorbed energy will total 5,000,000,000 ergs. Thus, a lower absorbed dose may actually mean a much higher amount of absorbed energy when considered over the whole body. The effects are primarily on the hematopoietic, gastrointestinal, cardiovascular, and central nervous systems. With relatively lower doses bleeding, infection, and loss of electrolytes can occur from damage to the intestinal mucosa and blood cell components. Higher doses will cause cardiovascular collapse and circulatory failure.

The dose absorbed will determine one of the three following courses:

1. Hematopoietic Syndrome—Exposure to 1 to 4 Gy causes pancytopenia with an onset of 48 hours and a nadir at 30 days.

Opportunistic infections can occur from granulocytopenia, and spontaneous bleeding can occur from thrombocytopenia.

2. Gastrointestinal Syndrome—Exposure to 8 to 12 Gy will cause gastrointestinal symptoms in addition to pancytopenia. Severe nausea, vomiting, cramping, and watery diarrhea occur within hours of the exposure. This resolves, then the epithelium of the bowel sloughs in four to seven days, which causes bloody diarrhea and loss of the intestinal barrier. Sepsis and massive fluid losses ensue and cause hypovolemia, acute renal failure, anemia, and death.

3. Neurovascular Syndrome—An exposure to >15 Gy causes immediate total collapse of vascular tone that is superimposed on the preceding syndromes. This may be caused by the massive release of vasodilatory mediators or destruction of the endothelium.[77] This progresses rapidly to shock and death.

Regardless of the dose, the first symptom encountered is usually nausea and vomiting that may resolve before the onset of the other symptoms.

## Assessment

Like other disaster situations, need for effective evacuation of casualties and field triage is important. In addition, one needs an effective decontamination plan.

During stabilization of the patient, information about the incident including the type of radiation, whether the source was sealed, the duration of the exposure, and the distance from and direct contact with the source should be obtained. This information will be necessary to calculate the dose. Other important information is the background radiation level of the involved area at the time of a radiation incident. Average radiation background in the United States is 360 mrem/year. Any radiation above background level is considered contamination. The history should also include any previous exposures to ionizing radiation.

The individual radiation dose is assessed by determining the time to onset and severity of nausea and vomiting, decline in absolute lymphocyte count over several hours or days after exposure, and appearance of chromosome aberrations (including dicentric and ring forms) in lymphocytes in peripheral blood. Documentation of clinical signs and symptoms affecting the hematopoietic, gastrointestinal, cerebrovascular, and cutaneous systems over time is essential for triage of victims, selection of therapy, and assignment of prognosis.

A complete blood count with differential should be performed as soon as possible and every four hours, with particular attention to the total lymphocyte count (TLC) as the most accurate indication of radiation injury. The rate of decrease in TLC varies inversely with the dose and, therefore, portends the prognosis. A decrease in the TLC by 50% or an absolute TLC of <1200/mm$^3$ within 48 hours of exposure indicates that at least a moderate dose of radiation has been encountered (Table 50-10).[78] Increases in serum amylase and diamine oxidase (specific to enterocytes) may be helpful to determine injury to the intestinal mucosa.[79] In patients who received a large dose of radiation, chromosome dicentric counting should be obtained. Chromosomal analysis of lymphocytes allows for accurate prediction of the received dose at 48 hours; however, this is impractical in determining the dose acutely.[80]

**TABLE 50-10**

| Significance of Absolute Lymphocyte Count on Prognosis | |
|---|---|
| **LYMPHOCYTE COUNT** | **SIGNIFICANCE AND PROGNOSIS** |
| 2000/mm$^3$ | Normal; no injury suspected; prognosis good |
| 1200–2000 mm$^3$ | Mild exposure; significant but probably not fethal |
| 500–1200 mm$^3$ | Moderate exposure; prognosis guarded |
| 100–500 mm$^3$ | Severe exposure; prognosis poor |
| <100 mm$^3$ | Lethal |

Doses under 1 Gy usually will cause no symptoms and do not require admission to the hospital. Those that are asymptomatic for 24 hours have no major injury.

## Treatment

Major radiation accidents and exposures can quickly overwhelm any response system. Treatment facilities may be destroyed, supply distribution may be hampered, and healthcare workers can be among the injured. For these reasons, triage with resources directed toward those likely to survive is paramount to limit casualties. Unfortunately, the extent of radiation injury may not be initially apparent.

Victims should be evacuated as quickly as possible to limit exposure with normal resuscitation procedures as the first priority. The patient's injuries including burn or traumatic injury should be treated, and then symptomatic treatment for the radiation illness should commence. Personnel involved in the treatment of the irradiated must recognize that there is rarely a hazard to healthcare workers from irradiated casualties. Only with extremely high radiation exposure will any of the tissues of irradiated patients actually become radioactive sources themselves. Individuals suffering from radiation injury are not radioactive, but the clothing they are wearing could be contaminated and radioactive.

Thermal burns are likely to occur in combination with radiation injury, which makes for a deadly combination. As previously noted, over 50% of the deaths in Hiroshima and Nagasaki were from thermal burns.[81] A thermal burn and radiation are synergistic, as animals that receive both injuries have a higher mortality beyond that expected for either alone or added together.[82,83] In case of a nuclear explosion, it has been proposed that patients with burns alone between 20 and 70% should receive the most attention, as they can be expected to survive with adequate treatment. With the addition of a significant radiation injury, only those with less than 30% could be expected to survive.[84] Therefore, available resources should be directed at this group if the system is overwhelmed.

Under most circumstances, the immediate resuscitation and treatment of life-threatening injuries supersedes treatment for radiation exposure, as the effects of radiation are relatively delayed.

## Decontamination

The first priority in treatment of radiation injury is the stabilization of the patient. Once the resuscitation has begun and the initial assessment is complete, decontamination should be started. Decontamination should occur before access to hospital or treating facility to reduce continued radiation exposure to the patient and eliminate radiation risk to others. Removal of clothing and jewelry and irrigation or washing of the body is an effective way of removing any radioactive contamination. Simply removing the clothes eliminates 90% of the contamination. Decontamination begins with the areas of highest levels of contamination. Contaminated wounds should be decontaminated prior to decontaminating intact skin. Nasal swabs from each nostril and a throat swab are performed to detect inhalation or radioactive contaminants. If patient has ingested or inhaled radioactive material, urine and stool samples are obtained to measure insoluble radioactive isotopes.

Open wounds should be covered with a clean dressing. These wounds are assumed to be contaminated with radioactive material and should be gently irrigated with copious quantities of water, saline, or 3% sodium hydroxide solution. The irrigant should be rinsed to a safe drain with the goal to dilute any radioactive particles without spread to adjacent uncontaminated areas. Irrigation is continued until the area indicates a steady state, absence of radiation with a Geiger counter, or reaches the background radiation level.

Attention should then be turned to the intact skin, where decontamination involves gentle scrubbing of the contaminated sites with a soft brush under a steady steam of water. A three- to four-minute scrub with a mild soap or detergent is also adequate. Following this, an application of povidone iodine or hexachlorophene solution and a two-minute scrub is recommended. This should be repeated until the skin has a steady state of radiation. After two rounds of the preceding treatment, a diluted mixture of one part commercial bleach to 10 parts water can be used to remove further radioactive particles.

## Management of Localized Injuries

Most radiation injuries are local injuries, frequently involving the hands. These local injuries seldom cause the classical signs and symptoms of the acute radiation syndrome. Local injuries to the skin evolve very slowly over time and symptoms may not occur for days to weeks after exposure.

After decontamination, efforts should be made to decrease any further irritation by decreasing exposure to the sun or further abrasive cleaning solutions. Mild erythema should be treated conservatively with light dressings, if needed. The lesion may progress to ulceration or chronic radiodermatitis. If no signs or symptoms develop in the first 48 hours, a less severe course can be expected. Any dry desquamation can be treated with lotions to moisturize the skin under loose fitting clothes. Moist desquamation should be treated as a second-degree wound with daily dressing changes and topical antimicrobials. Wounds with high radiation exposure may ultimately convert to full-thickness necrosis from obliterative endarteritis and may require skin grafting, flap coverage, or amputation. Early skin grafts may be successfully used on injuries from β radiation, as these particles do not penetrate as deeply. For other types of radiation, vascularized tissue is preferable to skin grafts laid on a bed with a questionable long-term blood supply. The decision regarding operative treatment of these wounds is difficult due to the slow progression of the injury. If intervention is performed too early, failure may occur due to progression of the injury; and, if performed too late, will result in undue suffering and may be associated with an increased risk of infection.

## Management of Whole-Body Injuries

The management of whole-body irradiation is aimed primarily at symptoms of cellular loss until these systems can regenerate themselves. Except for removal of internal radiation, no treatment can interrupt the process. Antiemetics to provide symptomatic relief from nausea and vomiting are indicated. Resuscitation needs may also be high to maintain euvolemia and urine output because of volume losses.

Patients with less than 1 Gy of exposure can be treated as outpatients if there are no other injuries. For those with more than 1 Gy, the patients should be admitted to the hospital until the symptoms have subsided. Gastrointestinal bleeding, diarrhea, infections, anemia, and diffuse bleeding from pancytopenia may occur with varying degrees of severity. If the exposure is more than 2 Gy, a bone marrow transplant as a salvage maneuver should be considered. This treatment is performed within five days of exposure (transplant will not function for 10 to 14 days) in a designated center with experience in the techniques and management of bone marrow transplantation. The blood analysis and cell typing should be completed promptly. A unique and important feature of radiation injury is that a severe exposure may so rapidly deplete the peripheral lymphocytes that none remain to serve as a basis for identification of a donor after the process has begun.[85]

Infections become problematic in these patients who are profoundly immunosuppressed. Opportunistic organisms are often the cause, and a thorough search for these should ensue when a clinical infection develops. The treatment by physicians experienced in the management of profoundly immunosuppressed patients, particularly those with transplants, is important for success in these situations. All blood products should be irradiated to prevent graft versus host disease. Transplants should be performed at the peak of immunosuppression, which is between three and five days after a high-dose exposure. The use of hemopoietic growth factors such as granulocyte colony stimulating factor (G-CSF) and granulocyte-macrophage colony stimulating factor (GM-CSF) has been shown to increase survival in animals and primates, but their success has not yet been proven in humans.[86]

## SUMMARY

The treatment of burns and radiation injuries is complex. Knowledgeable physicians can treat minor injuries in the community. Moderate and severe injuries, however, require treatment in dedicated facilities with resources to maximize the outcomes from these often devastating injuries. The care of patients has markedly improved over the last 30 years, and most patients with massive injuries now survive. Challenges for the future will be in modulation of the scar formation and in shortening the time to a functional and visually appealing outcome.

## REFERENCES

1. Brigham PA, McLoughlin E: Burn incidence and medical care in the United States: Estimates, trends, and data sources. *J Burn Care Rehab* 17:95, 1996.
2. Pruitt BA, Goodwin CW, Mason AD Jr: Epidemiologic, demographic, and outcome characteristics of burn injury. In Herndon DN, ed. *Total Burn Care.* London: Saunders, 2002, p. 16.

3. Bull JP, Fisher AJ: A study in mortality in a burn unit: Standards for the evaluation for alternative methods of treatment. *Ann Surg* 130:160, 1949.

4. Herndon DN, Gore DC, Cole M, et al.: Determinants of mortality in pediatric patients with greater than 70% full thickness total body surface area treated by early excision and grafting. *J Trauma* 27:208, 1987.

5. McDonald WS, Sharp CW, Deitch EA: Immediate enteral feeding is safe and effective. *Ann Surg* 213:177, 1991.

6. Sheridan RL, Remensnyder JP, Schnitzer JJ, et al.: Current expectations for survival in pediatric burns. *Arch Pediatr Adolesc Med* 154:245, 2000.

7. Stassen NA, Lukan JK, Mizuguchi NN, et al.: Thermal injury in the elderly: When is comfort care the right choice? *Am Surg* 67:704, 2001.

8. Committee on Trauma, American College of Surgeons: Resources for optimal care of the injured patient: 1999. Chicago, IL: *ACS*, 1998, p. 55.

9. DelBeccaro E, Robson M, Heggers J, et al.: The use of specific thromboxane inhibitors to preserve the dermal microcirculation after burning. *Surgery* 87:137, 1980.

10. Demling R, LaLonde C: Early post-burn lipid peroxidation: Effect of ibuprofen and allopurinol. *Surgery* 107:85, 1990.

11. Nwariaku F, Sikes PJ, Lightfoot E Jr, et al.: Inhibition of selectin- and integrin-mediated inflammatory response after burn injury. *J Surg Res* 63:355, 1996.

12. Onuoha GN, Alpar EK: Levels of vasodilators (SP, CGRP) and vasoconstrictor (NPY) peptides in early human burns. *Eur J Clin Invest* 31:253, 2001.

13. Yeong EK, Mann R, Goldberg M, et al.: Improved accuracy of burn wound assessment using laser Doppler. *J Trauma* 40:956, 1996.

14. Warden GD: Fluid resuscitation and early management. In Herndon DN, ed. *Total Burn Care*. Philadelphia: Saunders, 1996, p. 53.

15. Leape L: Initial changes in burns: Tissue changes in burned and unburned skin of rhesus monkeys. *J Trauma* 10:488, 1970.

16. Carvahal HF, Brouhard BH, Linares HA: Effect of anti-histamine, anti-serotonin, and ganglionic blocking agents upon increased capillary permeability following burn trauma. *J Trauma* 15:969, 1975.

17. Boykin JV, Crute SL, Haynes BW: Cimetidine therapy for burn shock: A quantitative assessment. *J Trauma* 25:864, 1985.

18. Holliman CJ, Meuleman TR, Larsen KR, et al.: The effect of ketanserin, a specific serotonin antagonist, on burn shock hemodynamic parameters in a porcine burn model. *J Trauma* 23:867, 1983.

19. Herndon DN, Abston S, Stein MD: Increased thromboxane A$_2$ levels in the plasma of burned and septic burned patients. *Surg Gyn Obstet* 159:210, 1984.

20. Heggers JP, Loy GL, Robson MC, et al.: Histological demonstration of prostaglandins and thromboxanes in burned tissues. *J Surg Res* 28:110, 1980.

21. Tokyay R, Loick HM, Traber DL, et al.: Effects of thromboxane synthetase inhibition on post-burn mesenteric vascular resistance and the rate of bacterial translocation in a chronic porcine model. *Surg Gyn Obstet* 174:125, 1992.

22. Pruitt BA, Mason AD, Moncrief JA: Hemodynamic changes in the early post-burn period: The influence of fluid administration and of a vasodilator (hydralazine). *J Trauma* 11:36, 1971.

23. Murphy JT, Horton JW, Purdue GF, et al.: Evaluation of troponin-I as an indicator of cardiac dysfunction after thermal injury. *J Trauma* 45:700, 1998.

24. Pruitt BA, Erickson DR, Morris A: Progressive pulmonary insufficiency and other pulmonary complications in thermal injury. *J Trauma* 15:369, 1975.

25. Wilmore DW, Long JM, Mason AD Jr, et al.: Catecholamines: Mediator of the hypermetabolic response to thermal injury. *Ann Surg* 180:653, 1974.

26. Takagi K, Suzuki F, Barrow RE, et al.: Growth hormone improves immune function and survival in burned mice infected with herpes simplex virus type 1. *J Surg Res* 69:166, 1997.

27. Wolf SE, Rose JK, Desai MH, et al.: Mortality determinants in massive pediatric burns: An analysis of 103 children with greater than 80% TBSA burns (70% full-thickness). *Ann Surg* 225:554, 1997.

28. Baxter CR: Fluid volume and electrolyte changes in the early post-burn period. *Clin Plast Surg* 1:693, 1974.

29. Carvajal HF, Parks DH: Optimal composition of burn resuscitation fluids. *Crit Care Med* 16:695, 1988.

30. Demling RH, Mazess RB, Witt RM, et al.: The study of burn wound edema using dichromatic absorptiometry. *J Trauma* 18:124, 1978.

31. Demling RH, Gunther RA, Haines B, et al.: Burn edema. Part II: Complications, prevention and treatment. *J Burn Care Rehab* 3:199, 1982.

32. Monafo WW: The treatment of burn shock by the intravenous and oral administration of hypertonic lactated saline solution. *J Trauma* 10:575, 1970.

33. Gunn ML, Hansbrough JF, Davis JW, et al.: Prospective randomized trial of hypertonic sodium lactate versus lactated Ringer's solution for burn shock resuscitation. *J Trauma* 29:1261, 1989.

34. Huang PP, Stucky FS, Dimick AR, et al.: Hypertonic sodium resuscitation is associated with renal failure and death. *Ann Surg* 221:543, 1995.

35. Du G, Slater H, Goldfarb IW: Influence of different resuscitation regimens on acute weight gain in extensively burned patients. *Burns* 17:147, 1991.

36. Tanaka H, Matsuda T, Miyangatani Y, et al.: Reduction of resuscitation fluid volumes in severely burned patients using ascorbic acid administration: A randomized prospective study. *Arch Surg* 135:326, 2000.

37. Merrell SW, Saffle JR, Larson CM, et al.: The declining incidence of fatal sepsis following thermal injury. *J Trauma* 29:1362, 1989.

38. Barret JP, Dziewulski P, Ramzy PI, et al.: Biobrane versus 1% silver sulfadiazine in second-degree pediatric burns. *Plast Reconstr Surg* 105:62, 2000.

39. Lal SO, Barrow RE, Wolf SE, et al.: Biobrane improves wound healing in burned children without increased risk of infection. *Shock* 14:314, 2000.

40. Cryer HG, Anigian GM, Miller FB, et al.: Effects of early tangential excision and grafting on survival after burn injury. *Surg Gyn Obstet* 173:449, 1991.

41. Herndon DN, Parks DH: Comparison of serial debridement and autografting and early massive excision with cadaver skin overlay in the treatment of large burns in children. *J Trauma* 26:149, 1986.

42. Thompson P, Herndon DN, Abston S, et al.: Effect of early excision on patients with major thermal injury. *J Trauma* 27:205, 1987.

43. Desai MH, Rutan RL, Herndon DN: Conservative treatment of scald burns is superior to early excision. *J Burn Care Rehab* 12:482, 1991.

44. Jeschke M, Wolf SE, Barrow RE, et al.: Mortality in burned children with acute renal failure. *Arch Surg* 134:752, 1998.

45. Holm C, Horbrand F, von Donnersmarck GH, et al.: Acute renal failure in severely burned patients. *Burns* 25:171, 1999.

46. Barret JP, Jeschke MG, Herndon DN: Fatty infiltration of the liver in severely burned pediatric patients: Findings and clinical implications. *J Trauma* 51:736, 2001.

47. Basadre JO, Sugi K, Traber DL, et al.: The effect of leukocyte depletion on smoke inhalation injury in sheep. *Surgery* 104:208, 1988.

48. Desai MH, Mlcak R, Richardson J, et al.: Reduction in mortality in pediatric patients with inhalation injury with aerosolized heparin/N-acetylcysteine. *J Burn Care Rehabil* 19:210, 1998.

49. Cioffi WG, Graves TA, McManus WF, et al.: High frequency percussive ventilation in patients with inhalation injury. *J Trauma* 29:350, 1989.

50. Yarborough MF, Herndon DN, Curreri PW: Nutritional management of the severely injured patient: (1) Thermal injury. *Contemp Surg* 13:15, 1978.

51. Wilmore DW: Nutrition and metabolism following thermal injury. *Clin Plas Surg* 1:603, 1974.

52. Lee JO, Herndon DN: Modulation of the post-burn hypermetabolic state. In Cynober L, Moore FA, eds. *Nutrition and Critical Care* (Vol. 8). Switzerland: Nestec Ltd, 2003, p. 39.

53. Herndon DN: Mediators of metabolism. *J Trauma* 21:701, 1981.

54. Fleming RYD, Rutan RL, Jahoor F, et al.: Effects of recombinant human growth hormone on catabolic hormones and free fatty acids following thermal injury. *J Trauma* 32:698, 1992.

55. Hart DW, Wolf SE, Mlcak RP, et al.: Persistence of muscle catabolism after severe burn. *Surgery* 128:312, 2000.

56. Pierre E, Barrow R, Hawkins H, et al.: Effects of insulin on wound healing. *J Trauma* 44:342, 1998.

57. Wolf SE, Barrow RE, Herndon DN: Growth hormone and IGF-I therapy in the hypercatabolic patient. *Baillieres Clin Endocrinol Metabol* 10:447, 1996.

58. Herndon DN, Ramzy PI, DebRoy MA, et al.: Muscle protein catabolism after severe burn: Effect of IGF-1/IGFBP-3 treatment. *Ann Surg* 229:713, 1999.

59. Hart DW, Wolf SE, Ramzy PI, et al.: Anabolic effects of oxandrolone after severe burn. *Ann Surg* 233:556, 2001.

60. Ferrando AA, Sheffield-Moore M, Wolf SE, et al.: Testosterone administration in severe burns ameliorates muscle catabolism. *Crit Care Med* 29:1936, 2001.

61. Herndon DN, Hart DW, Wolf SE, et al.: Reversal of catabolism by beta-blockade after severe burns. *N Engl J Med* 345:1223, 2001.

62. Mochizuki H, Trocki O, Dominioni L, et al.: Mechanism of prevention of postburn hypermetabolism and catabolism by early enteral feeding. *Ann Surg* 200:297, 1984.

63. Dominioini L, Trocki O, Fang CH, et al.: Enteral feeding in burn hypermetabolism: Nutritional and Metabolic effects at different levels of calorie and protein intake. *JPEN* 9:269, 1985.

64. Curreri PW, Richmond D, Marvin J, et al.: Dietary Requirements of Patients with Major Burns. *J Am Diet Assoc* 65:415, 1974.

65. Hildreth M, Carvajal HF: Calorie requirements in burned children: A simple formula to estimate daily caloric requirements. *J Burn Care Rehabil* 3:78, 1982.

66. Hildreth MA, Herndon DN, Parks D, et al.: Evaluation of a caloric requirement formula in burned children treated with early excision. *J Trauma* 27:188, 1987.

67. Hildreth MA, Herndon DN, Desai MH, et al.: Caloric needs of adolescent patients with burns. *J Burn Care Rehabil* 10:523, 1989.

68. Hildreth MA, Herndon DN, Desai MH, et al.: Reassessing caloric requirements in pediatric burn patients. *J Burn Care Rehabil* 9:616, 1988.

69. Hildreth MA, Herndon DN, Desai MH, et al.: Current treatment reduces calories required to maintain weight in pediatric patients with burns. *J Burn Care Rehabil* 11:405, 1990.

70. Hildreth MA, Herndon DN, Desai MH, et al.: Caloric requirement of burn patients under 1 year of age. *J Burn Care Rehabil* 14:108, 1993.

71. Eckerman KF: Annual limits on intakes of radionuclides. In Lide OR, ed. *CRC Handbook of Chemistry and Physics.* New York: CRC Press, 2002, p. 16.
72. Conklin JJ, Walker RI, Hirsch EF: Current concepts in the management of radiation injuries and associated trauma. *Surg Gyn Obstet* 156:809, 1983.
73. Nenot JC: Medical and surgical management for localized radiation injuries. *Intern J Rad Biol* 57:784, 1990.
74. Kelsey CA, Mettler FE: Instrumentation and physical dose assessment of radiation accidents. In Mettler FA, Kelsey CA, Ricks RC, eds. *Medical Management of Radiation Accidents.* Boca Raton: CRC Press, 1990, p. 294.
75. Neel JV: Update on the genetic effects of ionizing radiation. *JAMA* 32:698, 1991.
76. Guskova AK, Baranov AE, Gusev IA: Acute radiation sickness: Underlying principles and assessment. In Guskova AK, Mettler FA Jr, eds. *Medical Management of Radiation Accidents.* 2nd ed. Boca Raton, FL: CRC Press, 2001, p. 33.
77. Kelleher D: Acute effects of ionizing radiation, in United States Navy: *Royal Navy Workshop on Nuclear Warfare Combat Casualty Care* 1983, p. 71.
78. Browne D, Weiss JF, MacVittie TJ, et al. (eds): Consensus summary. *Treatment of Radiation Injuries.* New York: Plenum, 1990, p. 10.
79. Walden TL, Farzaneh MS: Biological assessment of radiation damage. In Walker RI, Cerveny TJ, eds. *Textbook of Military Medicine, Vol. 2.* Virginia: TMM Publications, 1989.
80. Hirsch EF, Bowers GJ: Irradiated trauma victims: The impact on ionizing radiation on surgical considerations following a nuclear mishap. *World J Surg* 16:918, 1992.
81. Glasstone S, Dolan PJ (eds): Biological effects. In Glasstones, ed. *The Effects of Nuclear Weapons.* Washington DC: US Atomic Energy Commission, 1977, p. 541.
82. Brooks JW, Evans EI, Han WT: The influence of external body radiation on mortality from thermal burns. *Ann Surg* 136:533, 1953.
83. Alpen EL, Sheline GE: Combined effects of thermal burns and whole body X irradiation on survival time and mortality. *Ann Surg* 140:113, 1954.
84. Becker WK, Buesher TM, Cioffi WG: Combined irradiation and thermal injury after nuclear attack. In Browne D, Weiss JF, MacVittie TJ, et al. (eds): *Treatment of Radiation Injuries.* New York: Plenum, 1990, p. 245.
85. Gale RP: The role of bone marrow transplantation following nuclear accidents. *Bone Marrow Transplantation* 2:1, 1987.
86. Dubos M, Neveux Y, Monpeyssin M, et al.: Impact of ionizing radiation on response to thermal and surgical trauma. In Walker RI, Gruber DF, MacVittie TJ, et al. (eds): *The Pathophysiology of Combined Injury and Trauma.* Baltimore: University Press, 1985.

# Commentary ■ RICHARD L. GAMELLI

Burn injuries remain a relatively frequent event albeit the overall incidence of major burn injuries has been reduced in the United States over the past several decades. On a worldwide basis, burn injuries remain a significant health problem with World Health Organization estimates of 322,000 fire-related deaths in 2002. The great majority of these deaths occurred in developing countries. More than half of these deaths occurred in South-East Asia with two-thirds of the deaths being in females with the age group of 15–45 years being responsible for 26% of all global fire deaths. Scald injury remains the major cause of injury in the pediatric population particularly in the United States in children less than two years of age. In many nations around the world burn injuries to children are related to the family ritual of cooking. The tragedy of these injuries in children is that these events are totally preventable events.

Lee and Herndon in their chapter, *Burns and Radiation Injury,* have well-outline the current thinking and approaches to the management of burn injured persons and those affected by radiation injury. Building upon the current understanding of the mechanisms of the body's response to injury the authors go through in careful detail the current management strategies for burn and radiation injuries. The advances in burn care can be related to scientific advances in the understanding of the body's response to injury, the importance of early burn wound closure, improvements in critical care, and the development of the burn team. Early closure of the burn wound is critical to reducing postburn mortality and morbidity. The care of patients with large body surface area burns where skin graft donor sites are the limiting factor in survival is facilitated by the alternatives to autografting such as a fabricated neodermis and cultured skin substitutes. The development of readily available and permanent alternatives to autografting represents the Holy Grail for burn surgeons. Understanding the metabolic response to a burn injury has not only led to improvements in nutritional support but also pharmacologic manipulation of the postburn metabolic response. This has proven to be particularly efficacious in children during the acute phase of burn care and during the months of recovery with enhancements in the restoration of functional protein mass, bone health, and growth recovery. There is now early evidence that similar approaches maybe of benefit in adults.[1]

Burn patients who also suffer from an inhalation injury continue to experience a level of mortality and morbidity beyond that of the burn alone. The diagnosis of an inhalation is best made with bronchoscopy. The primary advances in treating such patients have mostly come from employing the principles of gentle lung ventilation strategies. The goal in the care of the inhalation damaged lung is avoidance of barotrauma, volutrauma, shear stress, and use of permissive hypercapnia. While a burn center may use different modes of ventilation as their standard of care, failure to adhere to these principles can lead to an increase in pulmonary complications. The adjunctive use of aerosolized heparin and *N*-acetylcysteine to assist in the removal of retained carbonaceous material while seemingly logical as of yet lacks clear evidence that patient or pulmonary outcome is greatly improved with this form of therapy. Lungs damaged by an inhalation injury in a burn patient requiring intubation and mechanical ventilation are at significant risk for development of ventilator associated pneumonia (VAP). Episodes of VAP can occur early postinjury and maybe secondary to contamination of the damaged airway at the time of intubation and failure of local host defenses to clear the microbial inoculum.

The fluid formulas that exist today would seem to make the resuscitation of a burn patient a relatively straightforward matter; unfortunately this is not the case. While in the past under-resuscitation was a risk, the more concerning issues today is over-resuscitation. Burn patients receiving greater than expected volumes are at increased risk for extremity and abdominal compartment syndromes and fluid induced impairments in ventilation and gas exchange. The notion of "fluid creep" has become a real phenomenon in the care of burn patients.[2,3] Increasing doses of narcotic and benzodiazepine medications have been correlated with need for increased resuscitation volumes in a near proportionate manner. Also, fluid needs can be increased with delayed resuscitation, burns in combination with a severe inhalation injury, burn plus trauma, or a massive body surface area burn; as such patients likely represent resuscitation outliers and should not expected to follow the formulaic calculations. The resuscitation endpoints are the net result of the patient's response to the injury and subsequent treatments. Simply administering fluid volumes beyond 150% of calculated values is often an overly simplistic approach and may further exacerbate fluid needs. In patients failing to respond to fluid administration the clinician must understand that there may be the need for an alternative type of volume support such as the early use of colloid or fresh frozen plasma, recognize and promptly treat an impending abdominal or extremity compartment syndrome, institution of low dose vasopressin, reevaluate the patient for a missed injury, or directly assess the central hemodynamic response.

An importation consideration for the combined trauma and burn community is the ability to manage a large number of burn patients as the result of a natural disaster or terrorist event. While there are systems in place for the initial care and triage of victims at the state and federal level burn patients often require prolonged hospitalizations. A burn patient with a 50% TBSA burn will typically require 50 days of intensive care unit care and the unique resources provided by a burn center and its multidisciplinary burn team. Factors integral to capacity include the availability of burn beds, burn surgeons, burn nurses, other support staff, operating rooms, equipment, supplies, and related resources. Surge capacity is the capacity to handle up to 50% more than the normal maximum number of burn patients in the event of a mass burn casualty disaster. The Verification Program of the American Burn Association (ABA) in partnership with the American College of Surgeons has developed burn verification center criteria that at any point in time averages 45 or less verified centers. A significant proportion of the nation's nearly 1900 burn beds resided within these centers that often have an average daily census of 80% of capacity. A requirement of verified burn centers is participating in the national burn bed availability report coordinated though the Office of Public Health and Emergency Preparedness U.S. Department of Health and Human Services. This program that is a partnership between the ABA, verified and non-verified burn centers, and the Federal government is an important first step in improving our nation's ability to meet the challenges of a mass casualty burn or radiation exposure event.

## References

1. Wolf SE, Edelman LS, Kemalyan N, et al.: Effects of oxandrolone on outcome measures in the severely burned: A multi-center prospective randomized double-blind trial. *J Burn Care Rehabil* 27:131, 2006.
2. Cancio LC, Chavez S, Alvarado-Ortega M, et al.: Predicting increased fluid requirements during the resuscitation of thermally injured patients. *J Trauma* 56:404 (discussion 13), 2004.
3. Engrav LH, Colescott PL, Kemalyan N, et al.: A biopsy of the use of the Baxter formula to resuscitate burns or do we do it like Charlie did it? *J Burn Care Rehabil* 21:91, 2000.

# Temperature-Associated Injuries and Syndromes

*R. Lawrence Reed, II* ■ *Larry M. Gentilello*

Human physiology functions optimally within a relatively narrow core temperature range. This optimal temperature is maintained by a variety of physiologic responses designed to either preserve or lose heat, the failure of which is associated with pathophysiologic consequences. There are two major thermal overload syndromes; heat exhaustion and heat stroke. There are three major categories of cold injuries: systemic hypothermia and the two forms of local hypothermia; non-freezing tissue injuries (such as trench foot and chilblains), and freezing injuries (frostbite).

## SYSTEMIC HYPOTHERMIA

### Primary Accidental Hypothermia

Primary accidental hypothermia is defined as a core temperature reduction below 35°C due to excessive exposure to snow, wind, water, or altitude. It is considered primary because it occurs in patients who have a normal thermoregulatory mechanism, but who become hypothermic due to overwhelming cold stress. During its initial phases, it is associated with a marked increase in oxygen consumption, due to the body's attempt to maintain core temperature by a shivering-induced increase in heat production. When core temperature falls below 30–32°C, shivering ceases and core temperature may fall rapidly, leading to cardiac rhythm disturbances and circulatory arrest, the leading causes of mortality in such patients.

Due to reduced chest wall and myocardial compliance, cardiac output during cardiopulmonary resuscitation (CPR) for hypothermic cardiac arrest is only 50% of that achieved during normothermic CPR.[1] Palpation of a weak, bradycardic pulse in cold, stiff, hypothermic patients may be difficult, and the presence of an organized rhythm on electrocardiography makes CPR inadvisable. An organized rhythm may provide diminished, but

sufficient circulation in patients with severely reduced metabolism, and it is not worth the risk of precipitating ventricular fibrillation by performing vigorous chest compressions.

It is important to remember that almost every winter there are reports of patients with hypothermic cardiac arrest who have been successfully resuscitated after many hours of CPR. Therefore, CPR should be continued until the absence of cardiac activity is documented after raising the body temperature to a level that does not preclude successful defibrillation (>28°C). Endotracheal intubation is not a known risk factor for ventricular fibrillation, and should be undertaken according to standard indications.

Survival depends on the ability to rewarm the patient and restore circulation before irreversible neurologic and cardiac damage occurs. Patients who present with an organized rhythm have different treatment priorities, and initial management should focus on whether complications such as acidosis, electrolyte disturbances, dehydration, hypoxia, respiratory failure, or pulmonary edema are present. These complications may become progressively more severe during rewarming.

Treatment of these abnormalities may be more important determinants of outcome than the specific method of rewarming used. Correction of physiologic problems while maintaining an appropriate balance between oxygen supply and demand produces satisfactory survival rates when using rewarming methods ranging in intensity from heating blankets to full cardiopulmonary bypass. For example, in one series of 428 patients with a mean core temperature of 30.6°C, mortality was only 17%, with most of the deaths occurring in patients with serious underlying comorbidity.[2] Therefore, the emphasis should be placed on maintaining metabolic control to prevent the frustrating consequence of having the hypothermic patient die from physiologic aberrations despite a dramatic rescue and transport.

The rate of evolution of metabolic complications that occur during rewarming depends to some extent on the rewarming rate. Reports of successful resuscitation of patients treated in small hospitals or aid stations without access to sophisticated rewarming methods or advanced monitoring techniques may be attributable to the fact that the slower rewarming methods typically used in these settings provided sufficient time for the clinician to respond to the fluid shifts and metabolic changes that typically accompany rewarming. Methods such as cardiopulmonary bypass that rewarm very rapidly also require more frequent physiologic analyses of the patient's condition. The primary advantage of cardiopulmonary bypass would appear to be in patients with asystole or a nonconvertible fibrillating rhythm, who would otherwise require several hours of manual CPR if slow rewarming methods were used.

Although patients with primary hypothermia who are otherwise healthy will usually survive if physiologic control during rewarming is maintained, aggressive core rewarming may still be indicated in selected patients. Patients with core temperatures ≤30°C produce relatively little metabolic heat. The body temperature of a hypothermic patient may continue to decrease even after removal from the cold and may be refractory to simple rewarming methods. A continued decrease in core temperature to below 30°C may provoke a noncirculating cardiac rhythm in a previously stable patient. The duration of hypothermia, the rapidity of its onset, and the patient's underlying condition are additional points to be considered. A core temperature of 30°C in a patient who has been rescued from a mountain after several days may be complicated by exhaustion, with absence of the energy stores needed for spontaneous rewarming. In addition to the risks of a continued decrease in body temperature, prolonged hypothermia is also associated with fluid shifts and severe alterations in physiology which are likely to emerge during rewarming. These developments may lead to pulmonary or even cerebral edema in a patient who arrived to the hospital in a hypovolemic state.

Patients who are elderly or malnourished are also less likely to be able to rewarm spontaneously, and are probably candidates for more aggressive rewarming methods. Since the risk of ventricular fibrillation rises rapidly as core temperature reaches 28°C, below which treatments usually fail to correct such abnormal cardiac rhythms, rewarming should be considered urgent as core temperature drops below 30°C in patients who are unlikely to rewarm spontaneously.

The continued decrease in core temperature that sometimes occurs after removal from the cold has been referred to as the "afterdrop." There are many reports of patients who die during rewarming due to a dysrhythmia that is provoked during the afterdrop. Since an afterdrop is more common when external rewarming techniques are used, one suggested mechanism for this phenomenon is peripheral vasodilatation, resulting in central hypovolemia and cardiovascular collapse. Others have implicated the return of cold, acidotic blood sequestered in the periphery to the central circulation as a result of external heating, which causes a decrease in myocardial temperature and an increase in cardiac irritability.

There is little evidence to support either of these mechanisms for the afterdrop. Only a small amount of blood remains in the vasoconstricted periphery of a hypothermic patient, so the return of a bolus of sequestered blood to the heart is unlikely. Several studies have measured peripheral blood flow during external rewarming, and have noted minimal flow through skin and muscle while the afterdrop was occurring. The afterdrop has also been observed in fibrillating patients without any circulation, and has been

reproduced in isolated legs of beef and blocks of gelatin upon removal from cold water.[3–7]

The afterdrop most likely occurs as a simple function of the laws of thermodynamics. Heat flows from an area of higher temperature to one of lower temperature as a function of the second law. The temperature of the skin and outer layers of the body are usually 15–25°C cooler than the temperature of the core of a hypothermic patient. External rewarming techniques cannot transfer heat from the shell to the core against a temperature gradient until the temperature of the shell is raised to at least the temperature of the core. Until the abnormal core to periphery temperature gradient is abolished heat continues to flow from the core to the periphery, and central temperature may continue to decrease despite the application of external heat. The afterdrop should therefore not be considered a deterrent to external rewarming, but as an indication that insufficient heat is being transmitted to the patient. Intensive core rewarming to offset the dissipation of central heat, and even more aggressive external rewarming to abolish abnormal temperature gradients are the best methods of decreasing the duration of the afterdrop.

## Secondary Accidental Hypothermia

Secondary hypothermia occurs when a patient becomes cold despite an environmental temperature that does not result in hypothermia in otherwise healthy patients. It occurs in individuals who have abnormal heat production and heat conserving mechanisms. Considerable confusion has resulted from discussing all forms of systemic hypothermia as a single entity, as primary and secondary accidental hypothermia have significantly different mortality rates and clinical implications.

The mortality rate associated with secondary hypothermia is far higher than that of accidental hypothermia, primarily due to its association with severe underlying diseases that affect thermoregulation (i.e., trauma, stroke, endocrinopathy, etc.). This very high mortality is especially true for the trauma patient (Fig. 51-1). A prospective study of 44 patients with primary accidental

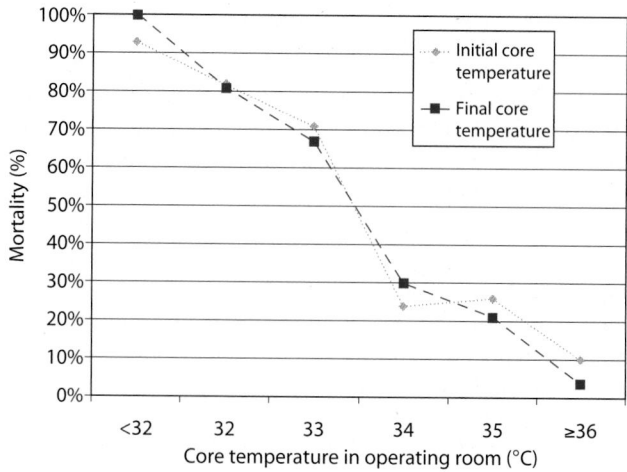

**FIGURE 51-1.** Stepwise mortality increases associated with progressive hypothermia identified by core temperatures obtained in the operating room on patients with abdominal vascular injuries.
*(Reproduced with permission from Tyburski JG, Wilson RF, Dente C, et al.: Factors affecting mortality rates in patients with abdominal vascular injuries. J Trauma 50:1020, 2001.)*

hypothermia (range of 20.0°C to 34.3°C) demonstrated a mortality rate of 27% with external rewarming only, and nearly all deaths occurred in elderly patients with underlying comorbidity.[8] In contrast, a study on outcome from hypothermia in trauma patients demonstrated a mortality rate of 40% when core temperature was less than 34°C, 69% when temperature dropped to less than 33°C, and 100% with hypothermia to 32°C or less.[9]

## Hypothermia in Trauma

Hypothermia and Coagulation.    In the trauma patient, a particularly detrimental effect of hypothermia is its effects on clotting. Hypothermia can affect blood coagulation in each of the major phases of the clotting process: vascular, platelet, and clotting factor activation. For example, systemic hypothermia has long been known to provoke cutaneous vasoconstriction. No doubt because of this observation, the topical application of cold has been used as a method to stop bleeding. Hippocrates, for example, listed hemorrhagic control as one of the primary uses of cold application.[10] Laypersons commonly use ice packs to control nosebleeds or to limit hematoma formation. For over two decades, iced saline lavage was used as a technique for controlling upper gastrointestinal hemorrhage due to acute peptic ulceration or ruptured esophageal varices.[11–13]

The underlying assumption was that because systemic hypothermia induced vasoconstriction, active bleeding could be reduced as a consequence of the vasoconstriction. Yet, topical exposure to cold appears to be different from systemic hypothermia. Local cooling actually elicits skin and skeletal muscle vascular dilation, as the primary risk of focal cold exposure is tissue damage due to frostbite, rather than systemic hypothermia. Cutaneous vasodilation may be a teleological mechanism designed to increase the flow of blood to threatened tissue. In contrast, core hypothermia represents a risk to the organism as a whole, and peripheral vasoconstriction is an available mechanism to reduce ongoing losses.[14]

Early studies of hypothermia suggested that a thrombocytopenia could develop at severe degrees of temperature reduction. However, this was reversible and is typically seen at temperatures below 25°C, which, in turn, is rarely associated with survival in trauma patients. A much more likely problem in trauma patients could be hypothermia's ability to alter platelet function. Valeri et al.[15] demonstrated evidence in baboons of a reversible platelet dysfunction that occurs during hypothermia and correlates with reduced local production of thromboxane B2 (the stable breakdown product of thromboxane A2, which is a potent vasoconstrictor and platelet aggregating agent).[16]

With respect to clotting factor function, the extent to which hypothermia intensifies coagulopathic bleeding is often underestimated clinically because standard functional coagulation assays (such as the partial thromboplastin time [PTT] and the prothrombin time [PT]) are performed by hospital laboratory after heating the blood to 37°C. Thus, these tests provide information about clotting factor depletion, but are corrected for any potential effect of hypothermia on clotting factor function.

Studies have demonstrated that when coagulation is measured at temperatures below 35°C, PT and PTT are significantly prolonged due to clotting enzyme inhibition.[17,18] A dilutional coagulopathy often coexists with hypothermia in the trauma patient.

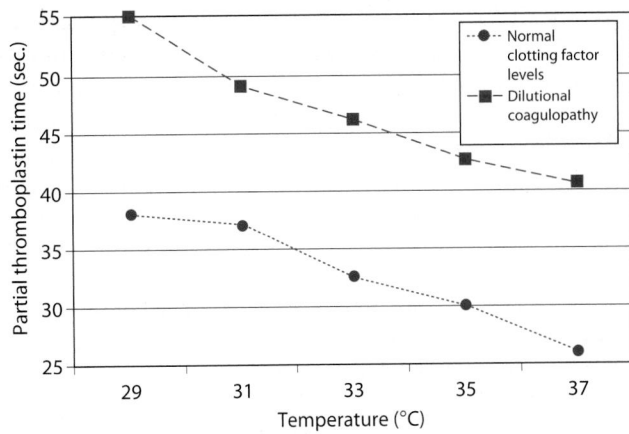

**FIGURE 51-2.** This graph depicts the prolongation of partial thromboplastin time (PTT) that results from cooling of the blood in samples with normal clotting factor levels, and in samples of blood with diluted clotting factor levels.
*(Reproduced with permission from Gubler KD, Gentilello LM, Hassantash SA, et al.: The impact of hypothermia on dilutional coagulopathy. J Trauma 36:847, 1994.)*

Reduced concentrations clotting factors, combined with severe inhibition of clotting enzyme kinetics due to cooling of the blood may make all attempts at achieving hemostasis futile, and may lead to persistent oozing and noncavitary hemorrhage in the pelvis or retroperitoneum (Fig. 51-2).

Effects of Hypothermia on Other Body Systems.    Hypothermia exerts several adverse effects on the circulation. Bradyarrhythmias and ventricular fibrillation have been observed as patients become hypothermic. Unless the hypothalamus is controlled by general anesthesia, or shivering is prevented with paralytic agents, hypothermia results in a three- to fivefold increase in oxygen consumption, which may be particularly detrimental in hypoxic patients with an already stressed circulatory system.

The immune response also appears to be impaired due to hypothermia, much of it poorly studied. Hypothermia reduces the enzymatic functions of white blood cells. For example, there is evidence that hypothermia reduces production of reactive oxygen intermediates by polymorphonuclear leukocytes and reversibly inhibits the transcription and expression of E-selectin.[19] Conceptually, hypothermia puts the immune system at a disadvantage in that it is pitted against bacteria, which are not homeothermic organisms. Clinical studies provide evidence that mild hypothermia is associated with increased risk for surgical site infection, pneumonia, and other infectious complications.[20,21]

Metabolically, hypothermia could be potentially beneficial in ischemic or shock states through its potential to reduce the metabolic rate at a time when oxygen delivery is compromised. On the other hand, hypothermia could be potentially harmful. For example, it often prolongs the duration of action of several drugs.

Neurologically, hypothermia can be detrimental and produces mental status changes (as in primary accidental hypothermia). Presumably, this results through a combination of its effect on neurotransmitter systems, reduction of the membrane resting potential, and reduction of the amplitude and duration of the action potential. Nerve conduction velocity is also decreased during hypothermia.

**Studies of Hypothermia in Trauma.** Although hypothermia is associated with a marked increase in mortality in trauma patients, there has been considerable controversy over whether the increased mortality occurs because hypothermia is more common and more profound in more seriously injured patients, or because hypothermia independently increases the risk of mortality. A recent large study analyzing the National Trauma Data Bank (NTDB) found that hypothermia was an independent predictor of mortality by using stepwise logistic regression (odds ratio 1.54, 95% CI 1.40–1.71).[22] On the other hand, some have proposed that hypothermia may serve a protective role in trauma patients by virtue of its potential to reduce oxygen consumption requirements during periods where oxygen availability is compromised.[23–26]

Retrospective studies have stratified patients by ISS and have demonstrated that patients who developed hypothermia had higher mortality rates than similarly injured patients who remained warm.[9,27,28] However, since oxygen consumption and heat production decrease during the process of dying, the development of hypothermia may simply have identified the patients in each ISS subgroup who were dying from their injuries; in such circumstances, hypothermia occurs as a normal consequence in the process of dying, but is not itself the cause of death. These factors have made it difficult to determine the effects of hypothermia on outcome from trauma using retrospective data.

However, prospective studies have continued to demonstrate an adverse effect of hypothermia on trauma patients. One study used an continuous arteriovenous heat exchanger (CAVR) to decrease the duration of hypothermia experienced by cold trauma patients. When their outcomes were compared with a matched group of patients treated the previous calendar year with less aggressive rewarming methods, the more aggressive treatment was associated with a significant decrease in blood loss and fluid resuscitation requirements.[29]

A subsequent study prospectively randomized hypothermic (<34.5°C) trauma patients to receive standard (slower) rewarming methods or rapid rewarming using CAVR. This study again produced two groups of patients with significantly different durations of hypothermia exposure. The aggressively rewarmed group required significantly less resuscitation fluid and blood products administered during the first 24 hours. Twelve of 28 patients (43%) randomized to receive the standard rewarming failed to rewarm, and all 12 died early because they could not be resuscitated from shock. In contrast, only two of 29 patients (7%) randomized to receive the more efficient heat transfer method could not be rewarmed, resulting in only two deaths during resuscitation ($p = 0.002$).[30] Overall, there was a significant improvement in the Kaplan–Meier survival curves in the group randomized to receive rapid rewarming methods, which more quickly replaced caloric losses (Fig. 51-3). Current evidence therefore suggests that every attempt should be made to prevent hypothermia in the trauma patient and to aggressively treat it once it has occurred (Fig. 51-4).

**Metabolic Protection.** There has been some interest in the use of hypothermia as a means of improving outcome from traumatic brain injury. Preliminary studies suggested that inducing mild hypothermia may improve outcome in patients with moderately severe brain injuries.[31–33] However, these studies typically exclude unstable patients with a history of hypoxia or hypotension, and they involved mainly patients with isolated brain injuries. However, a subsequent large well-conducted prospective randomized

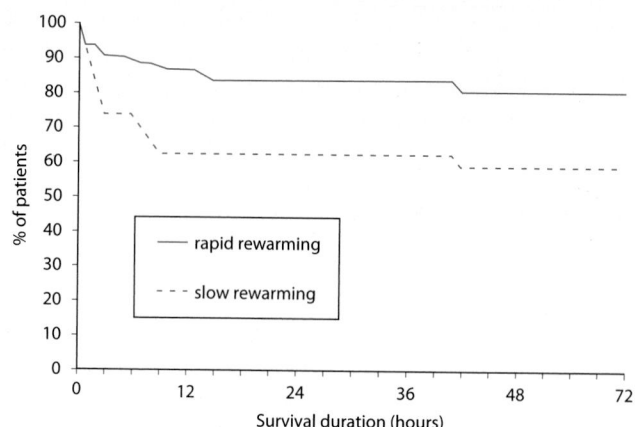

**FIGURE 51-3.** Adjusted cumulative survival (Kaplan-Meier) of patients randomized to rapid or slow rewarming, demonstrating an increase in mortality during resuscitation with slow rewarming ($p = 0.047$). (Reproduced with permission from Gentilello LM, Jurkovich GJ, Stark MS, et al.: Is hypothermia in the victim of major trauma protective or harmful? A randomized, prospective study. Ann Surg 226:439, 1997.)

trial demonstrated that mild hypothermia failed to provide benefit.[34] Given the detrimental effect of systemic hypothermia on patients during trauma resuscitation, therapeutic use of hypothermia may require methods to selectively cool the brain in patients with multiple injuries.

**Metabolic Exhaustion.** Trauma patients are at risk for developing hypothermia even in warm climates. This can be explained by understanding that hypothermia in trauma patients is a secondary phenomenon. Humans produce heat by combustion, or as a byproduct of their oxygen consumption. The definition of shock is a decrease in oxygen delivery that results in a pathologic decrease in oxygen consumption, with a consequent decrease in heat production. This mechanism explains why there is no seasonal variation in the incidence of hypothermia, and why the incidence of hypothermia is similar in trauma centers located in warm, temperate climates such as San Diego and Alabama, and in centers located in northern states such as Wisconsin and Ohio.[23,28,35,36]

This also appears to be the mechanism for the strong correlation between hypothermia and injury severity. It is consistent with early descriptions of the metabolic response to injury, which described the presence of an "ebb phase" during which a reduction in oxygen consumption and a fall in body temperature occurred.[37,38] The ebb phase and consequent fall in body temperature is characteristic of anaerobic metabolism, and a nonphysiologic reduction in heat production.

Some very intriguing data further support this concept. Seekamp and associates[39] performed a prospective study of ATP levels in plasma in three groups of patients: normothermic patients undergoing elective surgery, hypothermic coronary artery bypass surgery patients undergoing elective surgery, and hypothermic trauma patients. Plasma ATP levels were drawn preoperatively and at 2, 4, and 24 hours postoperatively in the elective surgery patients; levels were drawn on admission and 24 hours following admission in the trauma patients. Only transient decreases in plasma ATP levels were observed postoperatively in the elective surgery patients, with recovery to normal levels by 24 hours. However, trauma patients

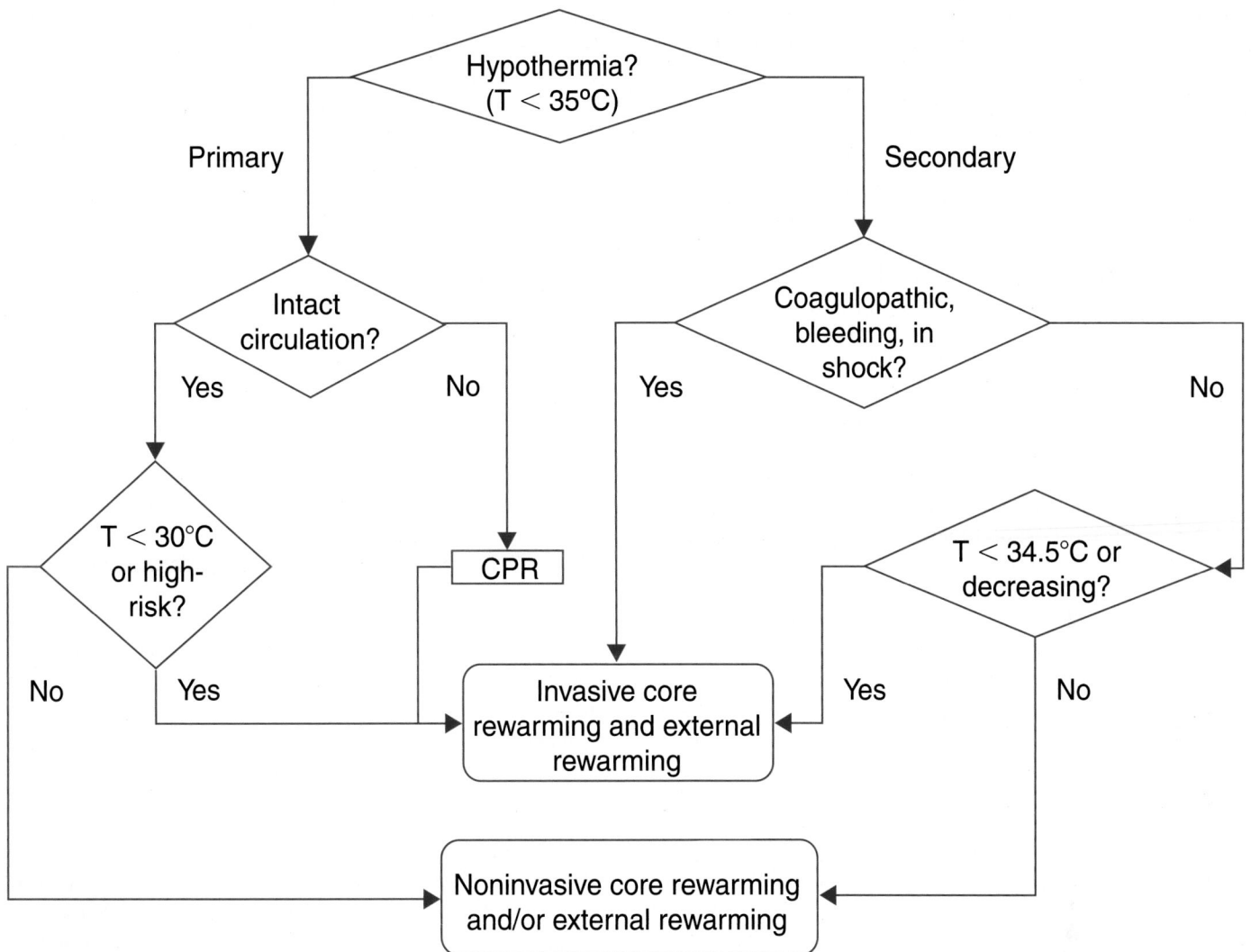

**FIGURE 51-4.** Management algorithm for treatment of hypothermia. All patients should also be closely monitored for physiologic complications associated with hypothermia.

exhibited a significant drop in ATP levels, especially in the most severely injured trauma patients (Injury Severity Score >30), which had not recovered by 24 hours postinjury.

Thus, credence can be given to the concept that the hypothermia observed in a trauma patient is reflective of metabolic exhaustion. This contrasts with the concept of hypothermia's ability to provide metabolic protection by conserving ATP stores in elective settings. Aggressive resuscitation is therefore the key management issue for prevention and treatment of secondary hypothermia in the trauma patient, and for restoring already depleted stores of ATP.

## LOCALIZED HYPOTHERMIA

### Frostbite

Frostbite is defined as local freezing of tissues resulting in ice crystal formation within the extracellular space. This initially causes osmotic transport of water out of the cell and severe cellular dehydration. If prolonged, the process leads to progressive mechanical tissue injury due to growing ice crystals that produce destruction as

they stretch membranes and other structures. Frostbite occurs almost exclusively in humans, who have a significant propensity for vasospasm, and is not suffered by other mammals such as deer, bear, or wolves, even when walking in the snow at −70°C. This is due to the unique human capacity for peripheral vasoactivity, which can increase cutaneous blood flow from approximately 400 mL/minute under normal conditions up to 8000 mL/minute for heat dissipation, and down to 20 mL/minute under cold conditions. The nose, ears, hands, and feet are the areas most richly supplied with arteriovenous anastomoses. Therefore, they are most at risk for shunting of blood flow with resultant tissue freezing due to inadequate circulation with warmed blood. Predisposing conditions include tight garments, nicotine, previous cold injury, and Raynaud's phenomena.

Pain and numbness are typical features of frostbite, and the discomfort usually becomes severe during thawing. The physical exam may reveal a waxy, white extremity, but findings may depend on whether or not the body part is still frozen at the time of hospital presentation. Following thawing, further injury takes place due to severe hyperemia, edema, and red cell and platelet clumping, which leads to profound circulatory stasis. This may result in severe ischemia, progression to gangrene, and autonomic dysfunction due to neuropathic changes. Edema may be prominent, along with blebs and vesicle formation. The absence of edema, as well as cyanosis that does not blanch with pressure, are poor prognostic signs.

Treatment protocols for frostbite have undergone significant improvements in recent years. Early protocols for treating this condition were based on sporadic, uncontrolled reviews of early military experiences. For example, rapid thawing of frozen body parts was considered contraindicated until relatively recently, leading to increased tissue loss in many patients. Others advocated treating the frostbitten body part as a burn, with early debridement and grafting and/or amputation, to prevent subsequent infection.

The Alaskan surgical experience has contributed substantially to the current approach to frostbite. Previously, patients in this region frequently experienced high-level amputations as a result of cold injuries sustained as a result of shipwrecks in fishing communities. An organized approach was developed with a goal of preserving tissue viability. As a result, the notion is now accepted that decreasing the duration of time during which the tissues are exposed to damaging temperatures decreases the extent of damage and reduces the progression of injury.

The currently accepted treatment of frostbite is immersion in a warm water bath (40–42°C) until rewarming is complete with the observation of flushing down to the tips of the fingers or toes and the return of sensation. A second important principle is absolute avoidance of surgical debridement, even in the face of obvious gangrene, unless sepsis occurs. Debridement should not take place and surgery should be postponed for as long as three to four months; letting the necrotic tissue spontaneously amputate maximizes tissue preservation.

In most cases sufficient healing takes place such that the amount of resection required is considerably less than anticipated. In a report summarizing 200 cases, Mills, using the Alaska protocol (consisting of rapid rewarming in a water bath and postponement of surgical debridement), noted that only one major amputation was required. Only 10.5% of patients lost tissue, consisting of only portions of phalanges. In contrast, in 70 cases where other treatments were used, 50% of patients lost tissue and there was an 18.6% major amputation rate.[40] The role of early surgical treatment for frostbite is primarily restricted to the treatment of compartmental syndrome, which may become manifest after thawing.

Local treatment while awaiting demarcation of irreversible tissue loss consists of elevating the affected area to minimize edema, gentle daily local nonabrasive cleaning (preferably with a whirlpool bath), air drying of tissues, placing cotton between digits to minimize maceration, using a tent or cradle to prevent tissue abrasion, and avoiding pressure spots. Anti-tetanus prophylaxis should be assured, but prophylactic antibiotics are not useful. Blisters should probably be left intact, as they provide sterile coverage of underlying tissues until re-epithelialization occurs. After resolution of edema, digits should be exercised during the whirlpool bath, and physical therapy should be initiated.

## Nonfreezing Cold Injuries (Trench Foot)

Trench foot, or nonfreezing cold injury, is due to repeated long-term exposure to cold water at near-frozen temperatures. There is no ice crystal formation, and the pathophysiology appears to be related to severe local cooling, resulting in intense arterial vasospasm as the body attempts to preserve core temperature. Peripheral myelin sheaths are particularly cold sensitive, and when combined with local ischemia, they undergo degeneration and chronic neuropathic changes.

The feet initially feel cold and painful, and they appear waxen and cold, but not frozen. After rewarming, a hyperemic phase ensues, with intense burning and blister formation, but there is no necrosis. This is associated with local warmth and intense pain that may last for several weeks. Afterwards, a chronic phase may occur, manifested by pain and cold sensitization, Raynaud's phenomena, loss of sensation, and motor nerve abnormalities. Treatment consists of rewarming, elevation, pain control, and range of motion exercises to minimize chronic disability.

## HEAT OVERLOAD SYNDROMES

Heat overload syndromes are not rare, and cause more annual deaths in the United States than primary accidental hypothermia. There are approximately 500 deaths per year due to excessively cold conditions, whereas in July 1995, there were over 700 deaths during a Midwestern heat wave in the city of Chicago alone, and thousands died during a recent heat wave in Europe.[41] Heat waves are defined by the National Weather Service as three or more consecutive days of temperatures of 32.2°C (90°F) or higher. Deaths are classified as due to heat stroke or hyperthermia if the patient's core temperature exceeds 40.6°C (105°F). However, these deaths comprise only a small portion of mortality attributable to heat excess, as most deaths are due to exacerbation of cardiac, respiratory, and other chronic diseases in elderly patients who are often indigent, immobile, and live in housing environments that offer minimal protection.

There are two main categories of heat-related illness: heat exhaustion and heat stroke. Heat exhaustion is characterized by progressive hypovolemia. Its symptoms include tachycardia, tachypnea, headache, dizziness, and profound fatigue. Sweating is usually profuse. Treatment consists of removing the patient from the heat and restoring circulatory volume. Cooling measures should consist of restoring circulating volume, removal of clothing, and increasing evaporative and convective losses by fanning to increase air turnover rates, or by placing the patient in a cooled environment or bath. Fans may actually increase heat stress, depending on the ambient temperature. When air temperature is greater than 37.8°C (100°F), fanning actively transfers heat to the patient. Also, fanning is ineffective in areas of high humidity. For example, when temperatures exceed 90°F, fanning does not result in cooling if humidity exceeds 35%.

Heatstroke is a severe illness and occurs when complete thermoregulatory dysfunction occurs, with absence of sweating and hyperpyrexia. Mortality rates are reported as ranging from 17% to 80%.[42] The universal sign that distinguishes heat stroke from heat exhaustion is the presence of neurologic signs and symptoms. Symptoms ranging from stupor, coma, and convulsions are present in virtually all patients with heat stroke.[43] Early treatment usually results in complete resolution, whereas significant delays in cooling result in permanent sequelae in most cases.

The body responds to the buildup of heat by carrying blood to the skin surface. Under most conditions, the most effective means of dissipating heat is through evaporation of sweat from the skin surface. When the air surrounding the patient is already saturated with humidity, sweat runs off the body without evaporation and heat dissipation becomes inefficient. Dehydration is the primary cause of most cases of heat overload. Individuals with adequate access to water rarely have a significant elevation in body temperature, and volume depletion is typically the key underlying risk factor.

Adverse effects of heat on the heart are also common, with many patients demonstrating ischemia or conducting defects.[44] In addition to acute neurologic effects, a hyperinflammatory state often occurs following heat stroke. High levels of endogenous pyrogens with pro-inflammatory effects, such as TNF, IL-1, and γ-interferon, have been detected in victims of heat stroke. They have been proposed as mediators of the multiple organ failure syndrome that frequently ensues when treatment is delayed.[45–47] Multiple organ failure with pulmonary injury, hepatic failure, disseminated intravascular coagulation, and renal failure are the most frequent causes of death that can occur despite cooling.

Since the duration of hyperpyrexia is the primary determinant of neurologic outcome, treatment priorities consist of establishing an airway, infusing intravenous fluids at 18–20°C, whole body cooling, controlling neurologic symptoms such as seizures, managing acid-base and electrolyte abnormalities, and assessing the degree of multisystem involvement. Fluid replacement may need guidance with central pressure monitoring due to the frequent effects of hyperpyrexia on cardiac function. Also, at the time of collapse, patients may be peripherally dilated, but vasoconstriction may occur during cooling vasoconstriction. This makes accurate determination of volume status difficult. In a study of 34 dehydrated patients with heat stroke during pilgrimage in the Saudi Arabian desert, central venous pressures ranged from 0–26 mm Hg during the course of therapy. As a result, an unmonitored brisk fluid challenge may predispose to either continued dehydration, or to pulmonary edema.[48]

## REFERENCES

1. Maningas PA, DeGuzman LR, Hollenbach SJ, et al.: Regional blood flow during hypothermic arrest. *Ann Emerg Med* 15:390, 1986.
2. Danzl DF, Pozos RS, Auerbach PS, et al.: Multicenter hypothermia survey. *Ann Emerg Med* 16:1042, 1987.
3. Savard GK, Cooper KE, Veale WL: Possible mechanisms for the afterdrop of core temperature upon rewarming from mild hypothermia. *Presentation at the Sixth International Symposium on Circumpolar Health, Anchorage, Alaska:* Abstract pg. 77.
4. Webb P: Afterdrop of body temperature during rewarming: An alternative explanation. *J Appl Physiol* 60:385, 1986.
5. Paton BC, Pozos RE, Wittmer LE: *Cardiac function during accidental hypothermia.* Minneapolis, MN: University of Minnesota Press, 1983, p. 133.
6. Golden FS, Hervey GR: The mechanism of the after-drop following immersion hypothermia in pigs [proceedings]. *J Physiol* 272:26P, 1977.
7. Cooper KE, Ferguson AV, Pozos RS, et al.: *Thermoregulation and hypothermia in the elderly.* Minneapolis, MN: University of Minnesota Press, 1983, p. 35.
8. Ledingham IM, Mone JG: Treatment of accidental hypothermia: A prospective clinical study. *Br Med J* 280:1102, 1980.
9. Jurkovich GJ, Greiser WB, Luterman A, et al.: Hypothermia in trauma victims: An ominous predictor of survival. *J Trauma* 27:1019, 1987.
10. Hippocrates: Aphorisms, Section V.23. In Hutchins RM, ed.; Adams F, trans. *Hippocratic Writings.* Chicago: Encyclopaedia Britannica, Inc., 1980, p. 138.
11. Law D, Gregory D: Gastrointestinal bleeding. In Sleisinger MFJ, ed. *Gastrointestinal diseases.* Philadelphia: WB Saunders Co., 1973, p. 199.
12. Bogoch H, Bockus HL: *Hematemesis and melena.* Philadelphia: WB Saunders Co., 1974, p. 814.
13. Lekagul S, Smyth NP, Brooks MH, et al.: The control of upper gastrointestinal hemorrhage in the dog by peritoneal cooling. An experimental study. *J Surg Res* 10:423, 1970.
14. Major TC, Schwinghamer JM, Winston S: Cutaneous and skeletal muscle vascular responses to hypothermia. *Am J Physiol* 240:H868, 1981.
15. Valeri C, Feingold H, Cassidy G, et al.: Hypothermia-induced reversible platelet dysfunction. *Ann Surg* 205:175, 1987.
16. Moncada S, Vane JR: Arachidonic acid metabolites and the interactions between platelets and blood-vessel walls. *N Engl J Med* 300:1142, 1979.
17. Reed R, Johnson T, Hudson J, et al.: The disparity between hypothermic coagulopathy and clotting studies. *J Trauma* 33:465, 1992.
18. Johnston T, Chen Y, Reed R: Functional equivalence of hypothermia to specific clotting factor deficiencies. *J Trauma* 37:413, 1994.
19. Haddix TL, Pohlman TH, Noel RF, et al.: Hypothermia inhibits human E-selectin transcription. *J Surg Res* Aug 64:176, 1996.
20. Kurz A, Sessler DI, Lenhardt R: Perioperative normothermia to reduce the incidence of surgical-wound infection and shorten hospitalization. Study of Wound Infection and Temperature Group. *N Engl J Med* 334:1209, 1996.
21. Flores-Maldonado A, Medina-Escobedo CE, Rios-Rodriguez HM, et al.: Mild perioperative hypothermia and the risk of wound infection. *Arch Med Res* 32:227, 2001.
22. Martin RS, Kilgo PD, Miller PR, et al.: Injury-associated hypothermia: An analysis of the 2004 National Trauma Data Bank. *Shock* 24:114, 2005.
23. Blalock A: A comparison of the effects of the local application of heat and of cold in the prevention and treatment of experimental traumatic shock. *Surgery* 11:356, 1942.
24. Jurkovich GJ, Pitt RM, Curreri PW, et al.: Hypothermia prevents increased capillary permeability following ischemia-reperfusion injury. *J Surg Res* 44:514, 1988.
25. Sori AJ, el-Assuooty A, Rush BF Jr., et al.: The effect of temperature on survival in hemorrhagic shock. *Am Surg* 53:706, 1987.
26. Kim SH, Stezoski SW, Safar P, et al.: Hypothermia and minimal fluid resuscitation increase survival after uncontrolled hemorrhagic shock in rats. *J Trauma* 42:213, 1997.
27. Luna GK, Maier RV, Pavlin EG, et al.: Incidence and effect of hypothermia in seriously injured patients. *J Trauma* 27:1014, 1987.
28. Steinemann S, Shackford SR, Davis JW: Implications of admission hypothermia in trauma patients. *J Trauma* 30:200, 1990.
29. Gentilello LM, Cobean RA, Offner PJ, et al.: Continuous arteriovenous rewarming: Rapid reversal of hypothermia in critically ill patients. *J Trauma* 32:316, (discussion 325), 1992.
30. Gentilello LM, Jurkovich GJ, Stark MS, et al.: Is hypothermia in the victim of major trauma protective or harmful? A randomized, prospective study. *Ann Surg* 226:439 (discussion 447), 1997.
31. Marion DW, Penrod LE, Kelsey SF, et al.: Treatment of traumatic brain injury with moderate hypothermia. *N Engl J Med* 336:540, 1997.
32. Chen L, Piao Y, Zeng F, Lu M, et al.: Moderate hypothermia therapy for patients with severe head injury. *Chin J Traumatol* 4:164, 2001.
33. Clifton GL, Allen S, Barrodale P, et al.: A phase II study of moderate hypothermia in severe brain injury. *J Neurotrauma* 10:263 (discussion 273), 1993.
34. Clifton GL, Miller ER, Choi SC, et al.: Lack of effect of induction of hypothermia after acute brain injury. *N Engl J Med* 344:556, 2001.
35. Gregory JS, Bergstein JM, Aprahamian C, et al.: Comparison of three methods of rewarming from hypothermia: Advantages of extracorporeal blood warming. *J Trauma* 31:1247, (discussion 1251), 1991.
36. Gregory JS, Flancbaum L, Townsend MC, et al.: Incidence and timing of hypothermia in trauma patients undergoing operations. *J Trauma* 31:795, (discussion 798), 1991.
37. Stoner HB: Responses to trauma: Fifty years of ebb and flow. *Circ Shock* 39:316, 1993.
38. Edwards JD, Redmond AD, Nightingale P, et al.: Oxygen consumption following trauma: A reappraisal in severely injured patients requiring mechanical ventilation. *Br J Surg* 75:690, 1988.
39. Seekamp A, van Griensven M, Hildebrandt F, et al.: Adenosine-triphosphate in trauma-related and elective hypothermia. *J Trauma* 47:673, 1999.
40. Mills WJ Jr.: Frostbite. A discussion of the problem and a review of the Alaskan experience. 1973. *Alaska Med* 35:29, 1993.
41. Semenza JC, Rubin CH, Falter KH, et al.: Heat-related deaths during the July 1995 heat wave in Chicago. *N Engl J Med* 335:84, 1996.
42. Seraj ME: Heat stroke during Hajj (Pilgrimage)–an update. *Middle East J Anesthesiol* 11:407, 1992.
43. Dixit SN, Bushara KO, Brooks BR: Epidemic heat stroke in a midwest community: Risk factors, neurological complications and sequelae. *Wis Med J* 96:39, 1997.
44. Akhtar MJ, al-Nozha M, al-Harthi S, et al.: Electrocardiographic abnormalities in patients with heat stroke. *Chest* 104:411, 1993.
45. Chang DM: The role of cytokines in heat stroke. *Immunol Invest* 22:553, 1993.
46. Bouchama A, Parhar RS, el-Yazigi A, et al.: Endotoxemia and release of tumor necrosis factor and interleukin 1 alpha in acute heatstroke. *J Appl Physiol* 70:2640, 1991.
47. Bouchama A, al-Sedairy S, Siddiqui S, et al.: Elevated pyrogenic cytokines in heatstroke. *Chest* 104:1498, 1993.
48. Seraj MA, Channa AB, al Harthi SS, et al.: Are heat stroke patients fluid depleted? Importance of monitoring central venous pressure as a simple guideline for fluid therapy. *Resuscitation* 21:33, 1991.
49. Tyburski JG, Wilson RF, Dente C, et al.: Factors affecting mortality rates in patients with abdominal vascular injuries. *J Trauma* 50:1020, 2001.

# Commentary ■ DAVID H. AHRENHOLZ

Drs. Reed and Gentilello have provided a comprehensive review of the physiology and treatment of cold and hyperthermia injuries. My comments are offered to emphasize some of the significant clinical points they have made, or emphasize some newer treatments for these conditions.

The optimal management of hypothermia includes real-time monitoring of the core temperature to detect after drop. This is most easily achieved with a thermister tipped Foley catheter. Patients with moderate to severe systemic hypothermia have an obligatory diuresis and present with a contracted circulating blood volume. This should be replaced with rapid infusion of warm parenteral fluids with concomitant CVP monitoring. Urine volume is an unreliable marker of adequate intravascular volume, until the temperature rises to a near normal level.

For life-threatening hypothermia, core rewarming is most rapidly achieved with cardiopulmonary bypass, or by an external heat exchanger system connected by heparinized tubing to large-bore femoral arterial and venous catheters. The latter system is available as a commercial kit (Smiths-Level 1 Inc., continuous arteriovenous rewarming device [CAVR]). Immersion of the patient in a whirlpool of 104 ° F (40 °C) water is also extremely effective, but is contraindicated in combative patients, those receiving CPR, or those with major trauma such as open wounds, unstable long-bone or spine fractures, or any trauma requiring an immediate surgical procedure. We do not rewarm frostbitten extremities until the core temperature has reached at least 32°C; then each extremity is sequentially immersed in 40°C water.

Exposure to ultra cold agents, such as liquefied oxygen, nitrogen, or propane (LP) gas, or contact with dry ice (solid $CO_2$) can produce a flash freeze injury. Huge ice crystals form both extracellularly and intracellularly, immediately rupturing the affected cells. The injury may have the appearance of a thermal burn and can affect any body part, since escaping gas can pass rapidly through layers of clothing. Soft tissue loss requiring a skin graft is extremely common.

In contrast, frostbite occurs under conditions of less rapid tissue cooling, and ice crystals form first in the extracellular fluid.[1] Proximal vasoconstriction preserves core body heat as the distal body parts cool, so the injury is most severe in the distal body parts, including tips of digits, ears, and nose. Rapid rewarming in 104°F (40°C) water restores blood flow to tissues as the metabolic rate increases, to minimize local ischemic injury.

Bullae may develop over a period of several hours after thawing a frostbite injury. The appearance of hemorrhagic blisters or proximal blisters with purplish digits is associated with subsequent extensive tissue necrosis. We have had experience performing angiography within 12 hours of such injury and using catheter-directed thrombolytic agents to restore blood flow in highly selected patients. This intervention is not indicated in patients with hemorrhagic strokes, major solid organ injury, recent surgical procedures, or other trauma, freeze-thaw-refreeze injuries, or delay of greater than 24 hours after thawing.[2] Severe arthritis and joint pain secondary to loss of articular cartilage are the most common sequelae of frostbite, associated with prolonged severe cold sensitivity or even Raynaud's phenomenon.

Systemic hyperthermia begins as heat stress and progresses to heat exhaustion as fluid losses mount and core temperature increases. The hallmarks are intense thirst, weakness, confusion, slurred speech, and incoordination, progressing to muscle cramps, nausea, and vomiting. Continued heat exposure leads to autonomic shutdown and the red, hot, sweaty skin surface suddenly becomes pale and cool to the touch. The accompanying profound neurologic deficits may be incorrectly attributed to hemorrhagic or ischemic stroke, unless the victim's core temperature is measured. Survival is unlikely unless immediate steps are taken to lower the elevated core temperature. An ice bath is the treatment of choice but any cooling efforts may be life saving.

Iatrogenic hyperthermia occurs as a complication of administered drugs such as psychotropic agents, which rarely cause neuroleptic malignant syndrome, or exposure to halogenated anesthetic agents in susceptible individuals. For the latter condition, immediate treatment includes immediate external cooling, hyperventilation using 100% inspired oxygen to remove the anesthetic agent, and intravenous administration of dantrolene.

## References

1. Ahrenholz DH: Frostbite injuries. *Probl Gen Surg* 20:129, 2003.
2. Ahrenholz DH, Rood J, Moudry B, et al.: Catheter directed TPA improves digital perfusion and digit survival following acute frostbite injury. Presented at American Burn Association 35th Annual Meeting, Miami Beach, FL April 1–4, 2003.

# Organ Procurement for Transplantation

*Aditya K. Kaza* ■ *Max B. Mitchell*

This chapter is relevant to all surgeons caring for victims of trauma because traumatic injury is a leading cause of brain death and subsequent organ donation. Because of the severe shortage of organ donors, it is critical that traumatologists recognize potential organ donors as early as possible and care for these patients assuming that organ donation may occur. It is important for physicians to understand the criteria for brain death and the local requirements for the pronunciation of brain death.

This chapter provides an overview of the procurement organization and how organs are allocated. The responsibilities of the local organ procurement organizations (OPOs) are underscored in this chapter (i.e., community education, evaluation and screening of potential donors, local hospital coordination, and family counseling). The trauma team's role is to resuscitate the patient and maintain perfusion of the organs. Once a potential donor is identified the trauma team must coordinate its efforts with the OPO. Once a patient is declared brain dead the trauma team's role does not end. Cooperation between the trauma team and representatives of the OPO will help to maximize donation of organs and is important for preserving the function of donated organs.

## INTRODUCTION

The combined developments of effective immunosuppressant therapy and sophisticated surgical techniques have made organ transplantation very successful in treating the end-stage failure of most solid organs. Transplantation is now the treatment of choice for end-stage heart, lung, liver, and renal disease for patients who have no contraindications to transplantation. Pancreas transplantation has also proven successful in the treatment of diabetes mellitus. In addition, there is increasing demand for bone, skin, and other tissues used in the treatment of other disease processes. Despite advances in living-related solid organ transplantation,[1] the majority of transplant recipients remain dependent on cadaveric organ donors.[2] Improved

supportive care for patients with advanced organ failure and expanded indications for transplantation have increased the numbers of patients waiting for organs. In contrast, efforts at increasing the pool of suitable organ donors have had comparatively little success in increasing the supply of organ donors; however, there is a slow increase in living donors as noted from 1988 to 2005 (Fig. 52-1). Consequently, the number of patients on the various transplant waiting lists continues to outpace the available donor pool. In the year 2000, an average of 114 patients were placed on waiting lists each day while an average of 63 patients per day received organ transplants.[3] During the same year an average of 16 patients per day died awaiting transplantation.[3]

Traumatic brain injury is the most common cause of death leading to cadaveric solid organ donation.[4] Clinicians caring for severely injured patients necessarily play a key role in the initiation and implementation of the transplantation process. Early recognition of potential organ donors is critical to maximizing the available pool of donor organs and the number of transplantable organs per donor. It is essential for those caring for potential organ donors to be knowledgeable about the criteria and process for declaring brain death and the physiologic effects of brain death. Familiarity with local organ procurement organizations is important because of the vital role they play in counseling the families of potential organ donors and coordinating the transplant process. Lastly, following the declaration of brain death, treatment priorities aimed at minimizing brain injury require adjustment. Physiologic support directed at maintaining perfusion of potentially transplantable organs assumes priority, and timely initiation of this support is crucial to increasing the probability of successful transplantation.

## ORGAN DONATION AND ALLOCATION

Under the National Organ Transplant Act (Pub.L. No.98-507, Title I, 1984), the United States Congress established The Organ Procurement and Transplantation Network (OPTN). The OPTN

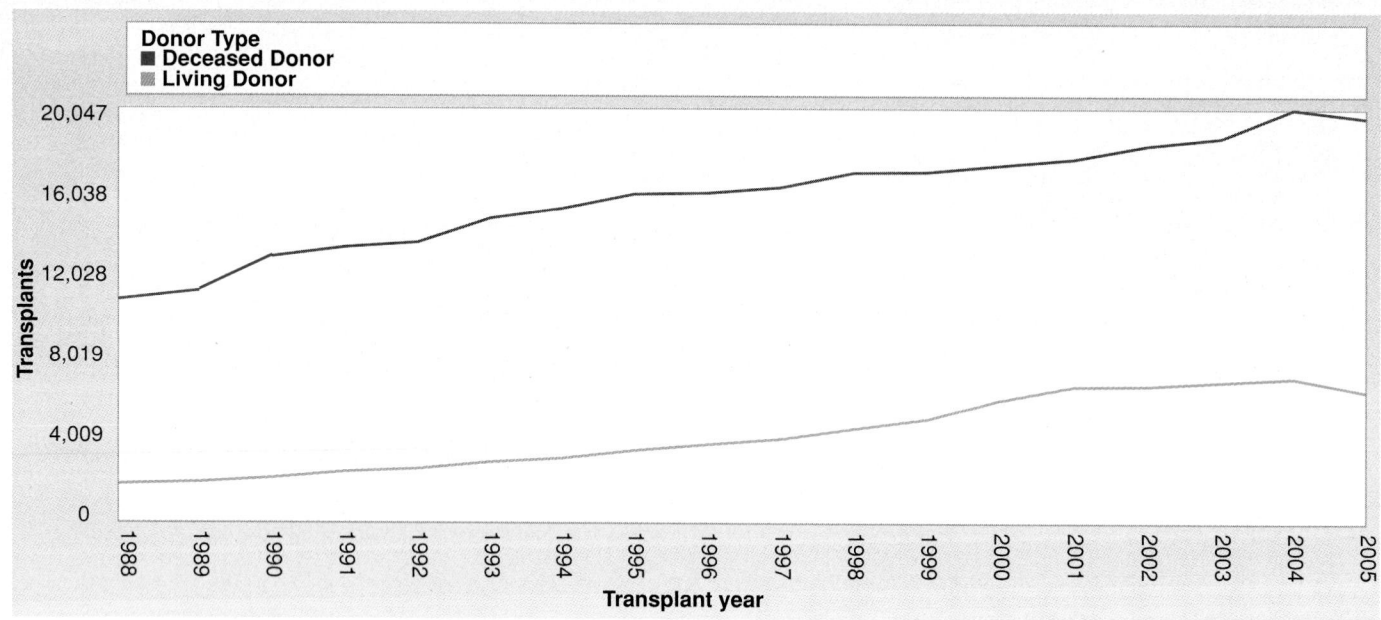

**FIGURE 52-1.** Total patients in the U.S. who underwent organ transplantation from deceased and living donors from 1988 to 2005. *(Reproduced with permission from United Network for Organ Sharing website, accessed Feb 2005: http://www.unos.org/Data).*

is a unique public–private partnership linking professionals involved in the organ donation and transplantation system. Subsequent federal legislation mandated that all U.S. transplant centers and organ procurement organizations must be members of the OPTN to receive any funds through Medicare or Medicaid (H.Rep.No. 100-383, 1987, and Pub.L. No. 100-607, Title IV, 1988). Other members of the OPTN include independent histocompatibility laboratories involved in organ transplantation; relevant medical, scientific and professional organizations; voluntary health and patient advocacy organizations; and members of the general public with a particular interest in organ transplantation.

The OPTN is administered by the United Network for Organ Sharing (UNOS). UNOS is a private nonprofit charitable organization contracted by the Health Resources and Services Administration of the U.S. Department of Health and Human Services (DHHSS) to develop organ transplantation policy.[5] Policy recommendations are then adopted and enforced by the DHHSS. UNOS facilitates organ transplantation by organizing the medical, scientific, public policy, and technological resources required to maintain an efficient national transplantation system. UNOS is responsible for developing recipient priority policies and for managing the national transplant waiting lists. UNOS also sets professional standards for efficiency and patient care for transplant centers. UNOS maintains the national transplant database, plays a very important role in raising public awareness of the importance of organ donation, and helps to keep patients informed about transplant issues and policy.[6]

Organ donation, allocation, and procurement require a closely coordinated and complex series of efforts. In the United States this process is coordinated by independent local OPOs. OPOs employ specially trained professionals who assist with the evaluation of potential organ donors, the declaration of brain death, counseling of donor family members, management of the donor, organ allocation, and the procurement process. When an organ donor is identified the local OPO serves to ensure that brain death has been established and assists in obtaining consent for organ donation. Thereafter, coordination of organ placement and the procurement of the organs are facilitated by

the OPO. There are currently 51 cooperating OPOs in the United States distributed among 11 geographic regions. The regional system plays a pivotal role in the current process of allocating organs for transplanation. It was established to help reduce organ preservation time and improve organ quality and survival outcomes. In addition it was intended to reduce the costs of organ transplantation and provide equal access to transplantation for patients regardless of where they live.

Donor organs are matched to individual patients according to waiting lists developed and coordinated by UNOS. Each organ waiting list incorporates specific criteria to establish individual patient ranking on the list. All lists incorporate patient waiting time and patient ABO blood grouping. For lung transplantation these are the primary factors. The kidney waiting list also incorporates the degree of human lymphocyte antigen matching so that top priority is given to patients with a perfect human leukocyte antigens (HLA) match. This is not done for other organs. The heart and liver waiting lists differ by including organ-specific criteria to establish severity of illness prioritizing the sickest patients. All lists are patient specific so that organs are offered to an individual patient on a center's list as opposed to the center. Organs are first offered locally within the boundaries of the involved OPO. If the organ is declined by all local centers, it is then offered regionally followed by national offers. There has been significant recent debate regarding the current allocation system with some parties advocating a nationally based system.[7] Such a system would be predicated primarily on the severity of illness followed by waiting time while eliminating consideration of the region from which the organ originates. At this time no changes in this system have been adopted.

## DONOR SCREENING

The screening process for organ donors begins when a potential organ donor is identified. All patients who have suffered severe brain injuries and are either brain dead or likely to progress to brain

**TABLE 52-1**

### Contraindications to Organ Donation[a]

| ABSOLUTE | RELATIVE |
|---|---|
| Uncontrolled sepsis | Bacteremia |
| Extracranial malignancy | Fungemia |
| Chronic transmissible infections: | High-risk social history |
|     Tuberculosis | |
|     HIV | |
| Coroner exclusion | |

[a]Organ-specific exclusions also exist.

**TABLE 52-2**

### Defining Brain Death: Guidelines of the President's Commission for the Study of Ethical Problems in Medicine (1981)

**Preconditions**
    Coma with known cause
    Documentation of irreversible structural brain injury
    Exclusions (preclude diagnosis of coma)
    Hypotension
    Hypothermia
    Hypoxemia
    Drug intoxication
    Metabolic derangements
**Tests**
    Absence of brain stem function Pupillary, corneal, oculovestibular, gag, cough reflexes absent
    Apnea (strict definition)
**EEG not Indicated**

death should be considered for organ donation regardless of their age, underlying cause of illness, and overall social history. Although perceived contraindications to donation may exist, they should be discussed with a representative of the local OPO before concluding that a given patient is not a candidate for organ donation (Table 52-1). The physician caring for the patient is responsible for notifying the local OPO of such patients. In many states physicians are legally required to notify the local OPO of each in-hospital death. All OPOs employ personnel who are responsible for advising health care providers on the suitability of an individual patient for organ donation. Communication with local forensic authorities is extremely important. The OPO will contact the medical examiner or coroner in order to obtain permission to proceed with organ donation. Once a donor is identified the OPO is responsible for obtaining family consent for organ donation. Organ procurement specialists are trained in counseling families about the importance and process of organ donation, and it is advisable to refer families to these specialists when potential organ donation is discussed. These individuals also perform a careful review of the potential donor's social and past medical history. The circumstances leading to brain death are very important, as is any history of the occurrence and duration of cardiopulmonary arrest. Screening also includes an extensive laboratory and serologic evaluation to exclude chronic disease and transmissible infections. A donor profile is then generated and includes current hemodynamics as well as an assessment of current organ function. The assessment of organ function is individualized to the donor based on the donor profile, the specific organs under consideration, and the level of medical support required to maintain the donor. The overall profile that is generated is crucial for transplant physicians who must evaluate the suitability of a given organ donor for the individual recipient.

## DECLARATION OF BRAIN DEATH

Ethical standards in the United States mandate that all organ donors must be declared dead before organ donation can proceed. Brain death must therefore constitute a sufficient basis on which to declare a person legally dead. Despite continued interest in non-heart beating donors, the vast majority of cadaveric organs are procured from donors whose deaths are declared on the basis of brain death. Consequently, cadaveric solid organ donation is dependent on the ability to reliably determine that a patient is brain dead.[8] Unfortunately, many clinicians remain poorly informed about brain death and how it is defined. The current concept of brain death used in the United States is based on guidelines published in

1981 by the President's Commission for the Study of Ethical Problems and adopted under the Uniform Determination of Death Act (Table 52-2).[9,10] This act states that death has occurred when there is irreversible cessation of all functions of the brain including the brain stem. Each state government has adopted these guidelines in legislating local criteria for the determination of brain death. The qualifications and number of physicians who must agree on the diagnosis of brain death in order to legally declare a patient brain dead vary considerably among the 50 states. Some states require two separate declaration procedures with a defined time interval between the two examinations. Some states require that the declaration be made by two separate physicians. In other states a single physician may declare a patient brain dead on the basis of one examination. In no case can the declaring physician take part in the recovery or transplantation of organs from the donor. Most hospitals have established policies within state guidelines for physician qualifications required to make the diagnosis of brain death. Physicians caring for these patients should be aware of local requirements and hospital guidelines in order to facilitate the declaration process and allow termination of care for brain dead patients who will not be organ donors.

Symptoms that support the diagnosis of brain death are the absence of brain stem reflexes, absence of cortical activity, and the demonstration of the irreversibility of this state.[8] Therefore, in order to declare brain death there must be proof of the cause of brain injury; otherwise, the irreversibility requirement cannot be met.[11] A patient found unresponsive with no clear cause of brain death generally cannot be an organ donor. Secondly, all reversible causes of coma must be excluded. Causes of reversible coma include hypothermia, hypoxia, hypoglycemia, hyperglycemia, uremia, hepatic failure, Reye's syndrome, hyponatremia, hypercalcemia, myxedema, adrenal failure, and CNS depressants. The presence of CNS depressing agents such as narcotics, sedatives, anticonvulsants, anesthetics, and alcohol must be assessed. If any of these agents are present, confirmatory testing is usually required to declare brain death.[12] In the brain dead patient, all cranial nerve function will be absent. The absence of brain stem reflexes must be confirmed by careful neurologic examination. Neuromuscular conduction must be intact in order to allow adequate examination; consequently, the presence of neuromuscular blocking agents must be excluded.

The most definitive finding supporting the diagnosis of brain death is the presence of apnea. The apnea test remains one of the most important parts of the neurological evaluation of potential organ donors.[13] To perform a reliable apnea test the $PaCO_2$ is normalized to 40 mm Hg. The patient is preoxygenated with 100% $O_2$ for at least five minutes. The patient is then disconnected from the ventilator and placed on 100% $O_2$ delivered passively to the endotracheal tube via a T-piece at 8–12 liters per minute. The $PaCO_2$ is allowed to rise to 60 mm Hg, confirmed by a blood gas drawn after approximately 10 minutes. If hemodynamic instability occurs, the patient should be immediately returned to mechanical ventilation and a blood gas should be drawn to assess the $PaCO_2$. If there is any evidence of respiratory activity the patient is not brain dead and should be immediately returned to the ventilator. If there is no evidence of spontaneous respiratory activity, the $PaCO_2$ has reached 60 mm Hg, and the pH is acidotic, apnea is established and is strongly supportive of brain death.

In many cases confirmatory testing must be performed in addition to a careful neurologic examination in order to firmly establish the diagnosis of brain death. Patients with cervical fractures above the level of C4 may not have intact diaphragmatic function precluding a reliable apnea test. Apnea testing is also unreliable in cases involving overdoses of substances that depress respiratory drive such as alcohol, anti-seizure medications, and sedatives. Hemodynamic instability during apnea testing will also preclude the establishment of the diagnosis of brain death on the basis of apnea. In other cases local requirements and or hospital policy may dictate the use of additional confirmatory testing. Confirmatory tests may also be useful in demonstrating a clear etiology for brain death or severe anatomic damage and can decrease the observation period required to establish the diagnosis of brain death.[12]

Confirmatory tests of brain death include electro encephalogram (EEG), testing of brainstem auditory evoked response (BAER), and methods of demonstrating the absence of cerebral blood flow. EEGs are not entirely reliable and are now rarely used for this purpose with the exception of brain death determination in young infants. BAER testing involves measuring electrical waveforms generated in the brainstem in response to an auditory stimulus transmitted by headphones. In the brain dead patient no waveform will be detectable. BAER testing is rarely used at this time. Demonstration of the absence of cerebral blood flow is the most common confirmatory test currently in use. Methods used to make this determination include cerebral angiography, cerebral blood flow Doppler ultrasound scanning, and radionucleide cerebral blood flow scanning. The latter two methods are noninvasive, low risk, relatively inexpensive, and are more readily available than cerebral angiography. These tests are highly accurate in verifying the absence of cerebral blood flow and are useful in reducing the time required to establish the diagnosis of brain death. Conversely, an exam that indicates continued cerebral blood flow does not necessarily exclude the diagnosis of brain death. Uncommonly, cerebral blood flow may persist despite brain death due to testing before increasing intracranial pressure completely shuts down flow, skull pliability in infancy or in the presence of decompressing fractures, ventricular shunts, ineffective deep brain flow, reperfusion, brain herniation, jugular reflux, the presence of emissary veins, and pressure injection artifacts.[14]

Appropriate documentation of brain death is very important in facilitating organ donation for a brain dead patient. The diagnosis of brain death must be documented in writing and it must be unequivocal. The circumstances leading to brain injury, the specific findings of the neurologic examination, and the results of any confirmatory tests should be clearly recorded. Lastly, the date and time of the declaration of brain death must be noted before OPO personnel may obtain the permission of local authorities and the consent of the potential donor's family. Despite the presence of evidence indicating a person's desire to be an organ donor, family consent for donation must be obtained. Family refusal is the most common reason that otherwise suitable donors do not become organ donors. If consent for donation is declined, appropriate testing and documentation of brain death is necessary in order to initiate the withdrawal of care.

## PHYSIOLOGIC CONSEQUENCES OF BRAIN DEATH

Brain death has profound effects on virtually all organ systems either directly or secondarily as a consequence of the accompanying effects on the cardiovascular and respiratory systems.[15] Disruption of normal autonomic innervation may lead to profound vasodilation and hypotension. In turn decreased organ perfusion is injurious to potentially transplantable organs. Direct myocardial depression may occur and is largely due to increased sympathetic outflow as a response to sudden increases in intra-cranial pressure.[15] This may lead to arrhythmias, myocardial ischemia, and in some cases myocardial infarction. Circulatory instability impairs distal organ perfusion leading to significant injury that may preclude organ donation. Respiratory dysfunction associated with brain death will have profound effects on all other organ systems. Impaired gas exchange is common in brain dead patients who have required mechanical ventilation for any length of time. Pulmonary infection and or aspiration injury frequently occur in potential organ donors either prior to or early after the time of endotracheal intubation. Neurogenic pulmonary edema is another cause of impaired gas exchange that may accompany brain death.[16] Myocardial dysfunction may also contribute to lung dysfunction due to increases in left atrial pressure thereby potentiating pulmonary edema. Similarly, hypoxemia will further impair myocardial function leading to a precarious hemodynamic state. Endocrine dysfunction is also common. The absence of hypothalamic function leads to the loss of thermoregulation and is manifested by the development of hypothermia. Impaired thyroid regulation contributes to hypothermia, and circulatory instability. Diabetes insipidus is common because antidiuretic hormone is no longer released from the posterior pituitary. If not managed appropriately diabetes insipidus will have a profound effect on fluid and electrolyte balance. The systemic release of substances from necrotic brain tissue may lead to disseminated intravascular coagulation producing a consumptive coagulopathy that is often exacerbated by hypothermia. Without appropriate intervention brain death is followed by severe injury to all other organs, and circulatory collapse will usually occur within 48 hours.

## DONOR MANAGEMENT

Prior to the declaration of brain death the treatment of patients with severe brain injury is directed at controlling intracranial pressure and preserving cerebral perfusion pressure in order to limit secondary brain injury. Once the diagnosis of brain death is established and a patient is recognized as a potential organ donor, treatment priorities must shift in favor of preserving the function of potentially transplantable organs. Preservation of organ function requires maintenance of adequate organ perfusion. Therefore, the goal of donor management should be to normalize hemodynamics and maintain biochemical parameters of organ function in as normal a condition as possible. Because of the profound effects on the cardiovascular system, invasive hemodynamic monitoring is essential to guide the appropriate resuscitation of brain dead patients. Central venous access should be obtained to allow measurement of volume status and to provide a reliable means of administering vasoactive drugs. Arterial access is required to facilitate continuous monitoring of blood pressure and frequent measurements of acid-base status, gas exchange, and serum biochemical parameters.

Hypovolemia is common in brain dead patients due to vasodilation and in some cases blood loss as a result of trauma or fluid loss due to diabetes insipidus. In general, patients should be resuscitated with crystalloid and appropriate blood products based on measurements of hematocrit and coagulation status. Resuscitation should be guided by frequent monitoring of central venous pressure or pulmonary capillary wedge pressure. Body temperature must be monitored and should be maintained above 36°C using passive warming as needed. Urine output should be maintained at 2 mL/kg/hour. Renal dose dopamine (3–5 μg/kg/minute) is recommended for nearly all donors unless higher doses are required to maintain perfusion. Vasopressin should be infused to treat diabetes insipidus when present, and fluids should be adjusted on the basis of electrolyte measurements.[17] This will usually require the administration of 5% dextrose solution. Serum sodium and osmolarity should be kept as normal as possible. Replacement fluids should be based on measurements of serum electrolytes and urine output. Frequent serum glucose measurements are required to facilitate treatment of hyperglycemia. Excess fluid administration may lead to pulmonary edema causing the lungs to become unsuitable for transplantation. Therefore, judicious fluid resuscitation is important in order to maximize the number of transplantable organs.

Inotropic support should be introduced to support blood pressure if initial volume resuscitation fails to restore adequate perfusion pressure.[18] Dopamine is usually the first agent of choice. Pure vasoconstrictors such as norepinephrine should be avoided whenever possible due to deleterious effects on myocardial, and splanchnic perfusion. Dobutamine is frequently added to increase cardiac output. If these agents are not effective at restoring hemodynamic stability, an epinephrine infusion should be initiated and titrated to the lowest dose required to achieve adequate support. Thyroxine (T4) or triiodothyronine (T3) infusions are commonly used due to their inotropic effects and potentiation of myocardial catecholamine sensitivity.[19] However, there is continuing controversy regarding whether or not the use of thyroid hormone infusions have a beneficial effect on organ function following transplantation. Consequently, thyroid infusions should be used primarily at the discretion of OPO representatives in consultation with their medical directors and the involved transplant physicians.

Ventilator management in potential organ donors is dependent on the respiratory function of the donor. Pulmonary injury is common in brain dead patients, and all attempts should be made to preserve the possibility of lung donation. As mentioned previously, fluids must be managed carefully and should be guided by measurements of central venous pressure. Chest radiographs should be obtained to assess pulmonary expansion, guide appropriate intervention to counteract atelectasis, and assess the suitability for transplantation. A nasogastric tube should be placed and kept on suction in order to minimize gastric distension and the risk of aspiration. An endotracheal tube with an internal diameter of 7.5 mm or larger should be inserted whenever possible in order to accommodate a therapeutic size fiberoptic bronchoscope. This will assist in the evaluation of potential lung donation and will facilitate clearing secretions to optimize lung expansion. Excessive mean airway pressures should be avoided. Tidal volumes and physiologic levels of positive end-expiratory pressures (PEEP) should be maintained to provide adequate lung expansion and minimize atelectasis. High concentrations of inspired oxygen are injurious to the lungs and should be avoided. The inspired oxygen concentration should be tritrated to maintain an oxygen saturation of 95%. In patients with significant pulmonary injury, lung donation is unlikely; therefore increased levels of PEEP and higher inspired oxygen concentrations may be required.

## ORGAN PROCUREMENT

The actual process of multiorgan procurement occurs in the operating room environment under the usual sterile conditions.[20] Representatives of the local OPO will coordinate the use of the operating room with the arrival of the various transplant procurement teams involved with a particular donor. Frequently this procedure may involve several teams whose members are operating together for the first time. In addition, the initial phases of the transplant operations for heart and lung recipients are commonly carried out simultaneously with the donor procurement procedure in order to minimize graft ischemia time.

An anesthesiologist is required to provide physiologic support of the donor during the procurement procedure. The donor patient is prepped and draped to allow an incision from the sternal notch to the pubis. In this manner the thoracic and abdominal organs can be evaluated and procured simultaneously. In all cases the final determination of organ suitability for transplantation is made after visual inspection and manual palpation of the organ. Biopsy of any suspicious lesions should be performed, and pathologic evaluation of frozen sections must be confirmed before the recipient transplant operation is initiated. Similarly, a liver biopsy may be required to evaluate the degree of fatty infiltration present in some donors. Following inspection the thoracic and abdominal organs are dissected to allow rapid removal after flushing with the appropriate preservation solution. There are numerous preservation solutions in use and vary according to the organ being procured and the preference of the procuring institution. All preservation solutions are kept at approximately 4°C because hypothermia is a key element of organ preservation. After all intended organs are dissected, the patient is systemically anticoagulated with heparin. Appropriate vascular cannulas are inserted in the abdominal and thoracic vessels to allow rapid flushing of the organs being procured. When all members of the procuring teams are prepared the superior vena cava, ascending aorta, and the supra-celiac aorta are clamped. The inferior vena cava is transected at the cavo-atrial junction and blood is suctioned from the open inferior vena cava exsanguinating the patient. The left atrium is vented in order to prevent left ventricular distension and back-pressure on the pulmonary vascular bed. Preservation fluids are infused through the previously placed cannulas flushing the procured organs of blood and rapidly lowering their temperature. Topical ice is applied augmenting rapid cooling. Thereafter, the heart and lungs are usually removed first. Donor hepatectomy is then carried out followed by removal of the kidneys. Variations in this sequence are required when the pancreas and or small bowel are also procured. The iliac vessels and occasionally segments of the descending thoracic aorta are then removed to provide additional vascular conduits that are sometimes necessary for complex vascular reconstructions at the time of organ implantation. All organs are inspected on the back table to ensure that no surgical damage has occurred. Finally, the organs are placed in sterile containers containing cold preservation solution or saline. The containers are then packed in ice in preparation for transport to the location where transplantation will occur. Once all solid organs are removed any additional tissues approved for donation are removed.

## CONCLUSION

Organ transplantation benefits thousands of people every year in the United States alone. However, donor organs remain a precious resource as evidenced by increasing recipient waiting times and the increasing number of patients who die waiting for donor organs. Efforts at expanding the available donor pool have not kept up with the need for organs. More recent efforts include the use of non-heart beating donation strategies,[21] the relaxation of donor organ criteria for recipients who would otherwise not be candidates for transplantation,[22] and other strategies. In general these measures have not been widely adopted and the donor to recipient disparity will undoubtedly continue. Advances in the development of artificial organs and xenotransplantation hold great promise in relieving this situation. Nevertheless, healthcare providers who care for traumatically injured patients will continue to play an important role in the identification and critical care management of potential organ donors for the foreseeable future.

## REFERENCES

1. Bak T, Wachs M, Trotter J, et al.: Adult-to-adult living donor liver transplantation using right-lobe grafts: Results and lessons learned from a single-center experience. *Liver Transpl* 7:680, 2001.
2. UNOS Website: 2000 Annual report of the U.S. Scientific Registry for transplant recipients and the Organ Procurement and Transplant Network transplant data: 1990–1999: http://www.unos.org/Data/anrpt00/ar00_data_fig_01.htm; accessed 1/6/2002.
3. UNOS Website: http://www.unos.org/Newsroon/archive_newsrelease_20011220_statquote.htm; accessed 1/12/2002.
4. UNOS Website: 2000 Annual report of the U.S. Scientific Registry for transplant recipients and the Organ Procurement and Transplant Network transplant data: 1990–1999: http://www.unos.org/Data/anrpt00/ar00_table12_05_alld.htm; accessed 1/6/2002.
5. UNOS Website: http://www.unos.org/About/who_main.htm; accessed 1/12/2002.
6. UNOS Website: http://www.unos.org/About/what_main.htm; accessed 1/12/2002.
7. Fung J: Survival of the sickest. Organ allocation should be based on patients' medical need, not location. *Mod Healthc* 28:29, 1998.
8. Beresford HR: Brain death. *Neurol Clin* 17:295, 1999.
9. President's Commission for the Study of Ethical Problems in Medicine and Biomedical Behavioral Research: Defining Death: *A Report on the Medical, Legal, and Ethical Issues in Determination of Death.* Washington, D.C.: U.S. Government Printing Office, 1981, p. 1.
10. Beecher HK, Adams RD, Banger AC: A definition of irreversible coma. Report of the Ad Hoc Committee of the Harvard Medical School to Examine the Definition of Brain Death. *JAMA* 205:337, 1968.
11. Lazar NM, Shemie S, Webster GC, et al.: Bioethics for clinicians: 24. Brain death. *CMAJ* 164:833, 2001.
12. Lopez-Navidad A, Caballero F, Domingo P, et al.: Early diagnosis of brain death in patients treated with central nervous system depressant drugs. *Transplantation* 70:131, 2000.
13. Lessard M, Mallais R, Turmel A: Apnea test in the diagnosis of brain death. *Can J Neurol Sci* 27:353, 2000.
14. Flowers WM Jr, Patel BR: Persistence of cerebral blood flow after brain death. *South Med J* 93:364, 2000.
15. Power BM, Van Heerden PV: The physiological changes associated with brain death–current concepts and implications for treatment of the brain dead organ donor. *Anaesth Intensive Care* 23:26, 1995.
16. Rogers FB, Shackford SR, Trevisani GT, et al.: Neurogenic pulmonary edema in fatal and nonfatal head injuries. *J Trauma* 39:860, 1995.
17. Powner DJ, Kellum JA, Darby JM: Abnormalities in fluids, electrolytes, and metabolism of organ donors. *Prog Transplant* 10:88, 2000.
18. Powner DJ, Darby JM: Management of variations in blood pressure during care of organ donors. *Prog Transplant* 10:25, 2000.
19. Roels L, Pirenne J, Delooz H, et al.: Effect of triiodothyronine replacement therapy on maintenance characteristics and organ availability in hemodynamically unstable donors. *Transplant Proc* 32:1564, 2000.
20. Van Buren CT, Barakat O: Organ donation and retrieval. *Surg Clin North Am* 74:1055, 1994.
21. Fung JJ: Use of non-heart-beating donors. *Transplant Proc* 32:1510, 2000.
22. Laks H, Marelli D: The alternate recipient list for heart transplantation: A model for expansion of the donor pool. *Adv Card Surg* 11:233, 1999.

# Commentary ■ DAVID A. GERBER

With the evolution of solid organ transplantation from an experimental procedure in the 1950s and 1960s to a standard of care for patients diagnosed with select end stage organ diseases there has been an associated increasing awareness related to the organ donor. This chapter by Kaza and Mitchell provides an overview of the issues that are pertinent to organ donation and organ procurement as they relate to the pre-transplant and peritransplant activities. The authors have laid out a structure that addresses the topics of brain death, donor screening and management followed by a description of organ procurement and allocation. These topics can be viewed as a foundation by which organ transplantation has increased its presence in the healthcare community.

Beginning with a summary of the role of the National Organ Transplant Act that established the OPTN the authors provide the groundwork for understanding the roles of the federal government and local jurisdictions with respect to processes and policies around organ donation. In the more than two decades since the publication of this act there has been a significant increase in donor activity along with an enhanced coordination of the complex activities surrounding organ donation and subsequent organ transplantation. The authors address the fact that federal policy is essentially implemented on a local level with independent local organ procurement organizations that are distributed throughout the United States and Puerto Rico. These OPOs are governed by rules that are laid out in the OPTN which is currently administered by the United Network of Organ Sharing (UNOS). UNOS can be viewed as the integrating organization for policies that are associated with organ donation and subsequent organ transplantation.

Deceased organ donation (formerly known as cadaveric organ donation) typically begins with the pronouncement of brain death. The authors have detailed the definition of brain death as occurring when there is irreversible cessation of all functions of the brain including the brain stem. Yet while there is a uniform definition for brain death the diagnosis and pronouncement of this condition is variable from state to state and even within a state there are potential variations in the procedural diagnosis at individual hospitals. The authors have taken the time to help educate the reader in understanding that across the spectrum from definition to implementation the traumatologist has to be aware of current practices at the medical center where they provide medical care.

The authors have appropriately emphasized the distinction of medical practice directed for the trauma patient and the subsequent consultation to the OPO when brain death is determined or imminent. This separation of responsibilities and the utilization of trained professionals to approach the family or next-of-kin is critical in the process of obtaining consent for organ donation and extremely important for all of the involved parties (i.e., traumatologists, OPO personnel, decedents, and family).

The phases of organ procurement are detailed as beginning from the declaration of brain death to the ensuing phase that requires resuscitation of the organs within the donor during the pre-donation phase. This often requires vastly different approaches in the management as the authors point out the necessity of achieving a euvolemic state; something that is critical with respect to the ensuing ischemia/reperfusion phase that the organs will go through at the time of procurement and subsequent transplantation. As pointed out by the authors the role of hypothermia and newer preservation solutions has allowed us to maximize the recovery and subsequent use of organs with fewer limitations than we had several decades ago. Nevertheless, all these organs will go through an ischemia/reperfusion period and this stage along with their status pre-procurement can impact subsequent organ function after transplantation.

Following the resuscitation period is the organ procurement procedure. This is one of the more complex activities that occurs in the operating room because it frequently involves multiple recovery teams from different medical centers who often have to travel several hours to get to the procurement. The coordination of these travel plans places an increased burden on most medical centers whether it is a rural hospital or a large academic medical center. The procurement requires anesthesia support at the start of the procedure along with an operating room team throughout the time that the solid organs are procured. This effort translates into hours of operating room time; something that can place an increased stress on an already busy operating room.

Another critical factor associated with the expansion of organ transplantation is the natural evolution in the type of organ donor. No longer do we only see the "young" trauma victim; not surprisingly our donor population resembles our general population as it goes through an "aging period." We are routinely spending more time evaluating donors in their sixth and seventh decades of life. As such we have to become more cognizant of the distinct stages that lead to a successful organ procurement and subsequent transplant. As with most surgical procedures involving our aging population there is less reserve for these organs if attention to detail is lost at any step in this process.

In summary, the impact of organ procurement for transplantation impacts multiple areas of the medical center and this chapter helps provide insight into this role as it relates to the trauma team.

# Reconstructive Surgery After Trauma

*Albert Losken* ■ *Timothy G. Schaefer*

## PRINCIPLES OF PLASTIC SURGERY

Plastic surgical emergencies (including hand-related trauma) account for a significant number of emergency room visits. The acute management of the injured patient should always begin with a succinct, goal-directed history, and accurate physical exam. As the injuries treated by plastic surgeons are often not life threatening, the patient first needs to be evaluated and stabilized by the trauma team. The plastic surgeon can then appropriately evaluate the patient's condition based on an understanding of the regional anatomy of the injured part and the pathophysiology of the injury.

### Initial Evaluation

The history should identify the time and mechanism of injury, patient comorbidities, patient symptoms, and status of tetanus immunization. Appropriate imaging studies and wound exploration augment the physical exam. One of the most important initial decisions is whether the particular injury needs to be managed in the operating room (either acutely or in a few days) or in the emergency room. This decision will often depend on the patient's age, ability to cooperate, and availability of facilities.

### Wound Healing

Management of wounds is integral to the care of the trauma patient. Therapy is guided by an understanding of the basic phases of wound healing (inflammatory phase, phase of fibroplasia, and maturation phase). Clinically, wound healing is separated into primary intention (acute closure), secondary intention (contraction granulation and re-epithelialization), and third intention (delayed primary closure).

## INJURIES TO SKIN AND SOFT TISSUE

### The Treatment of Wounds

The management of any wound must be individualized. Injuries to soft tissue with involvement of deeper structures such as bone, tendon, or nerve complicate the process, but the basic tenets remain the same. The key to managing traumatic wounds is adequate sharp debridement. This entails removal of all infected, nonbleeding tissue; however; skin is highly vascular and excessive removal is often unnecessary and further complicates reconstruction. Areas of questionable viability can be managed by allowing the area to demarcate with plans for repeat debridement 24 to 48 hours later. Another option is the administration of intravenous fluorescein 10–15 mg/kg and examination of the skin 15 minutes later with a Wood's lamp (mercury arc lamp to document fluorescence and confirm blood flow). This can offer accurate delineation of devitalized skin. Clinical impression should always take precedence, and it is safer to leave marginally viable tissue even if it does not flouresce, as it may go on to survive. Also, wounds should be explored for foreign bodies, and these must be removed prior to closure.

All open wounds should be considered contaminated, and irrigation to remove bacteria and particulate matter is essential for optimal healing. As irrigation with a bulb syringe is marginally effective and removes only surface bacteria, irrigation of wounds through a 35-mL syringe and 19 gauge needle (>8 PSI) is necessary to adequately cleanse a wound.[1] Pressure irrigation systems at 70 PSI are indicated in heavily contaminated wounds with the caveat that healthy tissue may sustain trauma. The appropriate volume for an uncomplicated wound is 50–100 mL/cm$^2$ of wound. Higher risk wounds or those grossly contaminated are better irrigated with 3–6 liters of fluid.

Tap water is an acceptable irrigant, but sterile solutions are most commonly used.[2] Frequently, sterile solutions containing

Neosporin, polymixin B, bacitracin, or other antibiotics are used as additives in the hopes of reducing bacterial loads despite the lack of evidence supporting their use or safety.[3–5] Antiseptic solutions containing additives such as hydrogen peroxide or betadine may be toxic to healthy tissues and are not recommended.[6] Recent studies have suggested that any improvement irrigation with Bacitracin is probably achieved due to detergent-like mechanisms rather than bactericidal properties. Compared with detergent solutions for irrigation, irrigation with Bacitracin offered no advantage in preventing infection and was associated with increased problems with soft tissue healing in one study.[7]

It has been shown that 80% of unselected wounds presenting to the emergency department fall into the clean category, and it is the other 20% that can lead to later infections.[8] Quantitative microbiology is available for wounds that are known to be contaminated (i.e., human bites); however, decisions are usually made on clinical suspicion. Heavily contaminated wounds are generally debrided, irrigated, packed with gauze soaked in saline, and left to heal by second or third intention.

The decision to close a wound primarily should depend on the degree of contamination, the time it has been open, and the underlying injury. If severe swelling or the need for a second debridement is anticipated, the wound should be packed open or temporarily closed. In the course of debriding wounds in the extremities, injured nerves or tendons are often encountered. If primary closure is not planned, these structures should be tagged with 5-0 nylon sutures to ensure identification in the future. Also, nerves should be gently approximated with 7-0 nylon or polypropylene suture to limit subsequent retraction.

Irrigation alone is not sufficient to obtain a clean environment for wounds with nonviable tissue. Nonselective debridement includes mechanical methods using wet-to-dry, dry-to-dry, or wet-to-wet dressings. As these dressings lose moisture through water vapor, necrotic tissue, wound exudates, and bacteria are removed from the wound with the gauze at the next dressing change. The wetting solution for these dressing changes can be saline, hydrogen peroxide, or Dakin's solution depending on the status of the wound. These types of dressing changes should be reserved for wounds containing necrotic tissue and exudate as they damage healthy granulation tissue.

Selective debridement also comes in numerous forms. Surgical debridement is a form of mechanical debridement that is effective, rapid, and complete. Enzymatic debridement is a form of chemical debridement using naturally occurring enzymes such as collagenase, papain-urea, or trypsin to selectively remove devitalized tissue.[9] Autolytic debridement encourages a patient's own enzymes to remove devitalized tissue by providing a moist environment with occlusive or semiocclusive dressings.[10] Biological debridement in the form of maggots was used in the early 1900s only to regain popularity in the 1990s. Sterile maggots are grown and placed in the wound for 1–3 days. Not only is this an effective method for debridement of necrotic tissue, but some secretions of maggots are bactericidal.[11]

## Primary Wound Closure

Most wounds associated with blunt trauma have a zone of surrounding damaged skin, which should be removed for optimal cosmetic results. Edges are generally trimmed perpendicular to the skin surface, except in hair-bearing regions where the edges should be beveled in the direction of the follicles. Wounds are closed to coincide with Langer's lines or lines of minimal skin tension, if possible, to ensure a better aesthetic result. A ladder of complexity exists when it comes to wound closure, and this depends on the extent of the injury, age of the patient, and the nature and location of the wound. Simple superficial lacerations may be managed with adhesive strips or adhesive glues assuming adequate alignment of wound edges can be obtained. It is also important that the lacerations are favorably located (i.e., eyelids, children) and not under tension at rest. For the deeper, more complex lacerations or ones that are widely separated at rest, a layered tension-free closure is required.

## Suture Technique

The width of a scar is directly proportional to the tension on the skin. Ways to minimize tension and subsequent scarring include undermining at the subdermal or fascial layer and layered closure. The strength layer is the dermis, which should be reapproximated with buried resorbable deep dermal sutures (3-0 or 4-0 Monocryl) (Ethicon Inc., Somerville, NJ). When done correctly, the skin edges should be well aligned and slightly everted. The skin suture is then used for precise approximation of the skin edges. Clean, debrided, or straight line lacerations can be approximated with a subcuticular monofilament suture, especially on the face to minimize visible scarring; however, deeper dermal sutures will allow early removal of interrupted sutures in the face if necessary. Simple interrupted or running sutures are used when edges need more assistance with skin alignment (i.e., in jagged, stellate lacerations). It is important that the skin edges are everted, and this can also be accomplished when necessary using horizontal or vertical mattress-type sutures.

Sutures in the face are generally removed at five days and earlier in children. Sutures in the remainder of the body are left in place for 7 to 10 days. Sutures in the hand, areas of motion such as across joints, lower extremity, and lacerations in patients with suspected poor wound healing (i.e., steroid medication, peripheral vascular disease, radiation damage) should be left in for 12 to 14 days. Leaving sutures in for an excessive period of time may result in permanent suture marks due to epithelial migration down the suture tract during the course of healing.

## Suture and Needle Selection

Most sutures used in the emergency room are the swaged type. The conventional cutting needle (3/8 circle) is most frequently used for skin closure. Both resorbable and permanent suture material which differ with respect to tensile strength, absorption rate, tissue reaction, and manageability are available. Resorbable suture material is generally used for deeper layers.

Sutures are primarily responsible for keeping the wound together in the early stages of wound healing. At one week, tensile strength is less than 5% of unwounded skin and increases to 10% at two weeks, 25% at four weeks, and 80% at 8–10 weeks. Monofilament absorbable suture such as poliglecaprone 25 (Monocryl) is frequently chosen for its handling ability and low reactivity. It maintains tensile strength for 2–4 weeks with absorption complete at 3–4 months. When closing deeper fascial layers or layers with a material that holds its tensile strength for a long time, a suture such as polydioxanone (PDS) (Ethicon Inc., Somerville, NJ), polyglycolic acid (Dexon) (U.S. Surgical, Norwalk, CT), polyglyconate (Maxon) (Sherwood Medical, St. Louis, MO), or polyglactin 910 (Vicryl) (Ethicon Inc., Somerville, NJ) is more desirable. Continuous subcuticular closures can be performed with absorbable sutures or permanent sutures. A permanent suture such as polypropylene (Prolene) (Ethicon Inc., Somerville, NJ) can be used, as it produces little inflammatory reaction, maintains tensile strength, and can be easily removed. For running or interrupted sutures in the skin, a permanent suture such as nylon or polypropylene is frequently the best choice. In situations where suture removal is felt to be difficult, as in children, rapidly absorbing 5-0 or 6-0 plain gut sutures are often used. Wounds that are bleeding, such as in the scalp, can be closed faster and more expeditiously with staples. Staples actually cause less inflammatory reactions than sutures.

## Dressings

The process of wound healing includes an initial inflammatory phase followed by a proliferative phase and ending in a remodeling phase. This process continues for 12 months from the time of injury. Optimal healing is a delicate balance between an underactive process that results in a chronic wound and an overactive process that results in hypertrophic scarring or formation of a keloid.

Once a clean wound is attained, numerous options exist for further management of the wound. It has been found that moist wounds heal faster than dry wounds.[12] Semiocclusive dressings provide such a moist environment while allowing the transfer of gases and the escape of moisture vapor to prevent excess accumulation of fluid that can result in maceration of tissues.[13] Care must be taken to ensure a clean wound under this type of dressing because an infection can occur if pathogens are introduced into this closed space. Alginates produce an occlusive, moist environment by transforming into a hydrophilic gel when in contact with heavy wound exudates. Once the gel weeps, the dressing must be changed.[14]

Topical agents for protected wound healing include creams and ointments that may contain antibiotics for preventing bacterial infection or growth factors for accelerating the healing process. Many of the commercially available preparations containing platelet derived growth factor (PDGF) or granulocyte/monocyte colony stimulating factor (GM-CSF) are indicated for chronic wounds in the lower extremities. Commonly used topical antibiotic creams include silvadene, bacitracin, and sulfamylon. Although silvadene is an excellent topical agent that can prevent sepsis in patients with large burns, it may not be the best choice for smaller wounds with a low risk of infection because it retards epithelialization.

Other adjuncts to wound healing including hyperbaric oxygen therapy, ultrasound, electrostimulation, and lasers have been used with some efficacy. Perhaps, the most commonly used and most effective adjunctive measure for wound management is negative pressure wound therapy approved by the Food and Drug Administration (FDA) in 1995. This modality has several mechanisms which theoretically improve rates of wound healing. Based on animal studies, negative pressure wound therapy increases local perfusion, accelerates the rate of formation of granulation tissue,

and decreases tissue levels of bacteria.[15,16] It is theorized that by removing interstitial fluid, growth inhibitors are removed, thereby accelerating rates of wound healing over wet to dry dressings.[17] Other mechanisms are also believed to stimulate growth factors through cellular and micromechanical deformational forces.[18]

## Flaps and Grafts

Some wounds are not amenable to primary closure or healing by secondary intention. These include wounds with a large surface area because of loss of tissue (i.e., burns or avulsions) and wounds where deeper structures (i.e., bones, vessels, and bowel) are exposed. In this situation, a skin graft or a flap is required. Skin grafts will only take over a vascularized wound and provide little protective covering if subjected to high shear stresses. These are usually split thickness skin grafts harvested at a thickness of 0.012–0.018 inches using a dermatome. Grafts are avascular and survive for 48 hours by plasmic imbibition or absorption from the wound bed. A hematoma, edema or shearing forces may disrupt this process and must be avoided by nonadherent dressings, tie-over bolsters, and meshing of the graft. Recently, use of a vacuum assisted closure device (VAC, KCI, and San Antonio, TX) has been placed on top of skin grafts in areas where contour irregularities exist to ensure contact with the graft and the bed. The bolster or VAC. is left on for four to five days, at which point the graft is examined.

Although a skin graft can survive when placed over bone with periosteal covering or over tendon as long as the paratenon is intact, this is often not the most durable coverage, and a flap is often chosen instead. A flap carries its own blood supply and is not dependent on the wound bed for revascularization. It is classified by blood supply or tissue type. Local cutaneous or fasciocutaneous flaps are either random flaps based on the subdermal plexus or axial based on a known blood supply through the skin or fascia. Muscle flaps with or without skin are based on known vascular pedicles. For the most part, local flaps are available to cover wounds. In situations where this does not provide sufficient tissue, or limited local options are available, distant flaps must be elevated along with their blood supply and transferred to the wound bed. The blood supply of the flap is then attached to recipient vessels in the vicinity of the wound using the microscope or loupe magnification. This technique of free tissue transfer has revolutionized the treatment of complex wounds, especially in the lower extremities where local options are limited and skin coverage is minimal. Postoperatively, these flaps must be monitored closely for three to five days to detect vascular compromise which occurs most frequently in the venous anastomosis.

## MAXILLOFACIAL TRAUMA (See Chap. 22)

Maxillofacial injuries are the second most common type of plastic surgery injury seen in the emergency room after injuries to the hand. These injuries are often complex and can involve skin, nerves, vessels, bone, and/or brain. Meticulous evaluation and work-up in a system-oriented, anatomically based manner is crucial to ensure a favorable aesthetic and functional outcome. The complexity of these injuries requires cooperation with multiple specialists including trauma surgeon, neurosurgeon, ophthalmologist, otolaryngologist, oral surgeon, and plastic surgeon.

## Injuries to Soft Tissue

Facial Nerve and Parotid Duct.    Deep lacerations across the cheek or temporal region may result in transection of the facial nerve. Physical exam should focus on forehead elevation (frontal branch), forced eyelid closure (zygomatic branch), upper lip elevation (buccal branch), lower lip depression (marginal branch), and platysma flare (cervical branch). The surgeon must be familiar with the branches and location of the facial nerves (Fig. 53-1). Facial nerve branches transected lateral to the lateral canthus should be explored and repaired by primary anastomosis. This requires microsurgical techniques and should not be attempted in the emergency room. The time course of this is critical as it becomes difficult to stimulate the distal nerve endings for identification after 4–5 days. Repair is performed using 9-0 and 10-0 nylon sutures in the epineurium under no tension. In late repairs, or when a segment of nerve is missing, a nerve graft using the greater auricular nerve is preferred.

The parotid duct travels within the parotid gland above the masseter muscles and pierces the buccinator muscle to enter the mouth. Function can be examined by gently massaging the gland and observing for clear saliva fluid within the mouth. The level of injury can be assessed by probing Stenson's duct within the mouth (upper second molar). Repair is possible over a stent with 7-0 Nylon or absorbable sutures. Ligation is an option if the duct cannot be repaired primarily; however, the gland will become swollen for a few days before it ceases to function and atrophies. Injury to the buccal branch of the facial nerve should be suspected with lacerations involving the parotid duct.

Eyelid.    Simple lacerations of the eyelids can be repaired primarily with minimal scarring. A full thickness laceration to the eyelid margin requires a complete ophthalmologic examination and precise alignment of the tissues to obtain a good outcome. Initial repair must ensure alignment of the gray line of the margin which corresponds with the attachment line of the tarsus. Even minor deformities

(<1–2 mm) are noticeable if not exactly aligned. This is reapproximated with a horizontal mattress suture to ensure skin eversion. The edge of the eyelid should be sutured with a soft multifilament nylon suture (6-0 Nurolon) to prevent corneal irritation. The remainder of the defect is closed in layers, beginning with a resorbable suture placed in the tarsal plate of the lid, located in the posterior lamella. The skin is closed primarily with resorbable or permanent sutures. Closure of the conjunctiva is possible with 6-0 buried plain gut sutures; however, corneal irritation is possible especially in the upper lid. The conjunctival layer can be left open in this situation. Canthal tightening and lower lid support is often necessary in complex avulsion type injuries of the lower lids to minimize the potential for developing ectropion, entropion, or lagophthalmos. An unrepaired tear or avulsion of the levator apparatus in the upper lid results in a ptosis deformity. Levator repairs are performed under local anesthesia to allow for voluntary excursion of the lid.

Medial lacerations risk damaging the canaliculus draining the lacrimal system. The canaliculus extends 1–2 mm perpendicular to the lid margin and then courses parallel to the lid margin under the medial canthal region. A lacrimal probe can be passed through the canaliculus and ductal system to determine patency. These ducts are very fragile and repair is often not feasible. In such a situation a Silastic lacrimal stent needs to be placed through the duct into the nasal cavity for six months.

Lip.    The lip is functional and aesthetically prominent. Full thickness lacerations of the lip should be closed in three layers including the mucosa, muscle, and skin. The two critical components to keep in mind when repairing lip lacerations are the vermillion border and the orbicularis muscle. Discrepancies in the red–white transition of the lip as little as 1mm can be noticed at conversational distance. Repair of the orbicularis muscle is performed with several buried absorbable sutures to complete the sphincter function of this muscle. Failure to do so will result in bunching of the muscle on either side with attempted lip animation and may cause scar contracture and shortening of the lip. Mucosal approximation is typically performed using absorbable sutures. Intraoral hygiene and antibiotic coverage against Staphylococcus aureus and anaerobes is important to prevent subsequent infection. Lip defects less than one-third of the lip length can be closed primarily.

Ear.    When attempting to identify and repair landmarks of the injured ear, comparisons are made to the opposite side. Also, physical examination must always rule out injury to the structures of the middle or inner ear. Copious irrigation is important to minimize infection, especially with exposed cartilage. A delayed presentation with secondary chondritis is a medical emergency and can result in a permanent deformity of the ear. Exact alignment of the skin edges is critical to prevent noticeable notching, and horizontal mattress sutures are placed to create eversion of the skin. Placing sutures in the cartilage is generally not necessary as the skin on the lateral aspect of the ear is intimately adherent to the cartilage. Hematomas beneath the skin must be drained or prevented using a compression dressing as they may become secondarily infected and lead to a disfiguring "cauliflower" ear deformity. Ear amputations or avulsion injuries can be salvaged by microsurgical replantation or therapy with leeches if the ear has venous congestion. Other options for ear reconstruction can be performed if microsurgical replantation is not an option, but a description of these techniques is beyond the scope of this chapter.

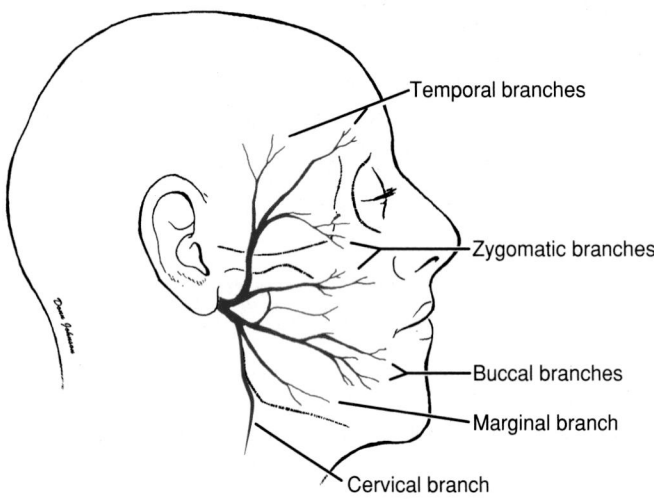

**FIGURE 53-1.** Facial nerve anatomy.

## Facial Fractures

Nasal Fractures. Nasal bones are the most commonly fractured facial bones, and these occur in frontal and lateral patterns. Treatment starts with a complete external and intranasal examination. Septal fractures, hematomas, and dislocations are common and may result in serious functional consequences. A septal hematoma should be treated urgently with drainage, light packing, and prophylactic antibiotics. Signs of nasal fractures include edema, lacerations, nasal displacement, angulation, epistaxis, crepitis, and rhinorrhea. As x-rays are of limited value, the diagnosis and decision to operate is typically made on clinical exam. Immediate treatment includes controlling the intranasal issues and closure of lacerations. Immediate closed reduction is possible in the emergency room if swelling is minimal. Delayed treatment is indicated in patients with extensive nasal edema, comminuted nasal fractures, or a septal fracture. This should be performed within seven days in children and 2–3 weeks in adults. Open reduction is required when the fractures are immobile. Late complications include obstruction of the nasal airway, saddle nose deformity, nasal deviation, epistaxis, headache, and synechiae causing obstruction of air flow.

Mandibular Fractures. The mandible is fractured in 50–67% of all facial fractures.[19] It plays a functional role (eating, breathing, talking) and contributes to facial profile. Occlusion is the most important aspect of the diagnosis and treatment of mandibular fractures, and discrepancies as little as 1mm are noticeable to most patients and may indicate an underlying injury. Fractures are classified based on location or on whether they are open or closed, displaced or nondisplaced, and favorable or unfavorable. Mandibular fractures are multiple 50% of the time, and 11% have associated injuries to the cervical spine. Diagnosis is based on clinical exam and radiographic imaging. Panorex and three-dimensional computed tomography (CT) scans provide valuable anatomic information regarding location and orientation of the fracture (Fig. 53-2). Treatment begins with an evaluation of the airway, cervical spine, and intraoral cavity. Teeth in the fracture line that are damaged, carious, or interfering with reduction should be removed. Most fractures are

open to the oral cavity and prophylactic antibiotics against Staphylococcus aureus and anaerobes and oral hygiene measures should be used. Treatment is aimed at re-establishing the patient's original occlusion by reducing and immobilizing the fracture line. Fixation includes mandibular-maxillary fixation (MMF), interosseous wiring, metal plates and screws, external fixation devices, or intraoral splints. Nonunion and malocclusion are the two most significant complications associated with the treatment of mandibular fractures.

Malar Fractures. A reproducible pattern of complex fractures of the zygoma frequently occurs. Patients typically present with periorbital swelling, ecchymosis, pain, unilateral epistaxis, V2 anesthesia, trismus, and flattening of the malar prominence or the zygomatic arch. A palpable stepoff is often felt at the zygomaticofrontal suture, infraorbital rim, and zygomaticomaxillary buttress. Fractures typically extend from zygomaticofrontal region and into the orbit at the zygomaticosphenoid suture. They then travel inferiorly to the maxilla through the zygomaticomaxillary buttress and zygomatic arch. Diagnosis is made on CT scan with attention paid to the axial and coronal cuts through the lateral orbital wall (Fig. 53-3). Definitive

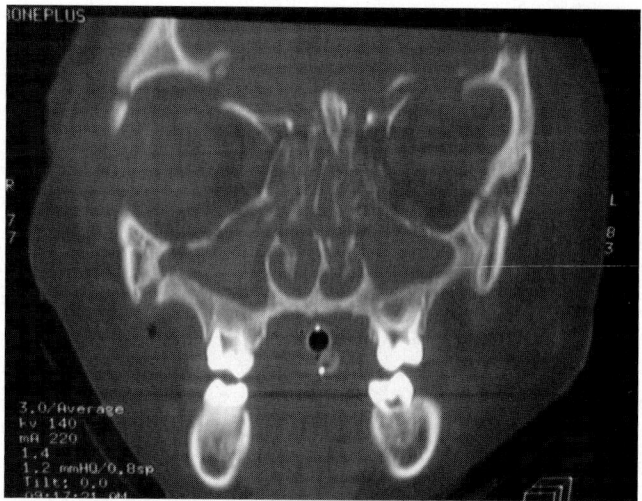

A

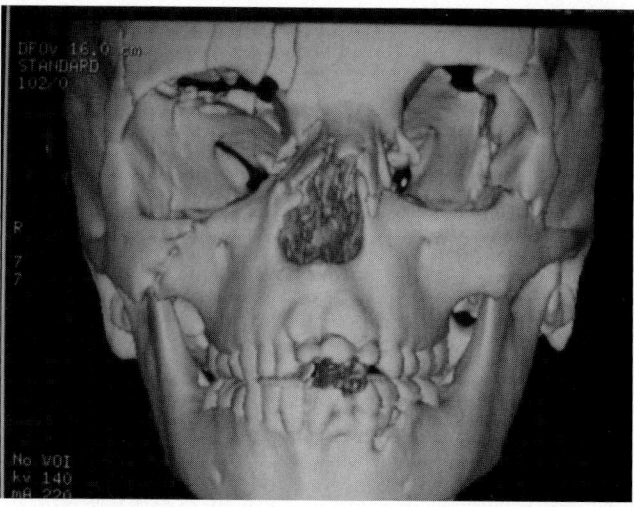

B

**FIGURE 53-2.** Three-dimensional CT scan showing anatomic location of left mandibular parasymphyseal fracture in relation to important landmarks, i.e., mental foramen. Note excellent visualization of midface.

**FIGURE 53-3.** (A,B) Coronal CT scan and three-dimensional CT scan demonstrating significant midface and naso-orbital ethmoidal fractures.

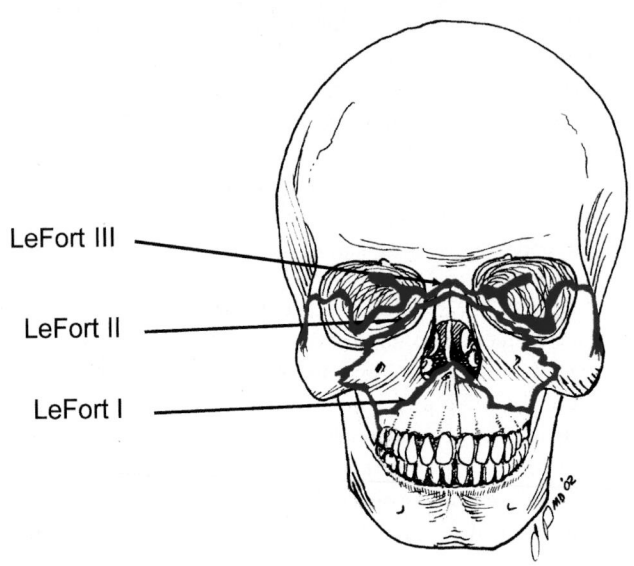

**FIGURE 53-4.** LeFort classification of maxillary fractures.

treatment can be postponed until edema has resolved. The goal in treating midface fractures is to correct the occlusion and restore facial width and height. Nondisplaced fractures should be observed conservatively with the patient on a soft diet and restricted activities. Any displacement may result in enophthalmos and malar recession requiring operative intervention, and displaced fractures often require open reduction and internal fixation through multiple approaches. Resorbable plates and screws can be used in nonweight bearing bones or in pediatric facial fractures.[20–22] New studies have demonstrated effective use of absorbable plates and screws in load bearing locations as much as with the mandible.[23]

Maxillary Fractures.    Maxillary fractures are caused by high-impact forces and classified according to the Le Fort Classification (Fig. 53-4). They all have fractures of the pterygoid, and there is potential for mobility, malocclusion, airway obstruction, epistaxis, and change in facial height. Mobility of the maxillary segment may be demonstrated on exam by stabilizing the patient's head and manipulating the maxilla. This is often misleading, and CT scans will provide a more definitive diagnosis. Le Fort II and III fractures involve the orbital walls and may produce periorbital edema and ecchymosis. Treatment is aimed at restoring facial profile and occlusion by re-establishing the three structural pillars of the midface (nasomaxillary buttress, zygomaticomaxillary buttress, and pterygomaxillary buttress). Reduction and fixation depend on the extent of displacement. Options range from closed reduction with MMF to open reduction and internal fixation.

Orbital Fractures.    Immediate ophthalmologic consultation is required for blurred vision, blindness, scotoma, eye pain, afferent papillary defect, hyphema, ruptured globe, and retrobulbar hematoma.[24] Post traumatic optic neuropathy may preclude early operative intervention and often requires steroids to diminish swelling and subsequent risk to the optic nerve and vision.[24,25]

The most common isolated orbital fracture involves the floor and lower portion of the medial orbit. Signs include periorbital edema, ecchymosis, subconjunctival hemorrhage, hypoaesthesia in the distribution of the infraorbital nerve (seen in 90–95%), and a palpable bony step-off (anterior fractures). Dysfunction of extraocular muscles is often due to trauma to the muscles or, less often, due to entrapment of the orbital contents within the fracture. Diagnosis is made based on clinical exam and CT scan, while entrapment is diagnosed in the comatose patient using the forced duction test. Diplopia is often transient and rarely an indication for surgery. Treatment is needed to reduce/release herniated or entrapped orbital contents and restore normal orbital architecture and volume. Increased orbital volume is seen in significant fractures or those fractures causing displacement of the globe (enophthalmos and globe dystopia). There are multiple approaches to the orbit, with bone grafts or alloplastic materials being used to reconstruct the floor. Enophthalmos and diplopia are the most frequent results of inadequately treated orbital fractures.

## TRAUMA TO THE HAND AND UPPER EXTREMITY (See Chap. 42)

"Next to the brain, the hand is the greatest asset to man, and to it is due to the development of Man's handiwork" (Sterling Bunnell, 1882–1957). This quotation summarizes the importance and complexity related to the management of hand injuries. Although injuries to the hand can be functionally devastating and disfiguring, they are rarely fatal. A thorough knowledge of the anatomy and functional intricacies within the hand and upper extremity is critical for appropriate management of these injuries.

The examination should begin with inspection of the hand for color or temperature changes. *Vascularity* should be tested by checking the capillary refill (should be two seconds or less), pulp turgor of each digit, and an Allen's test should be performed to assess patency of the radial and ulnar arteries. If perfusion is questionable, this can also be evaluated by Doppler examination of the named vessels, pulse oximetery, or pinprick. Nerve injuries are tested by evaluating *sensation* in the distribution of the radial, ulnar, and median nerves, and comparisons are made to the uninjured hand. Sensation is determined by light touch or two-point discrimination (normal value 2–3 mm at the pulp of the finger). The three major nerves can be tested by assessing sensation at the ulnar aspect of the small finger (ulnar nerve), dorsal aspect of the first web space (radial nerve), and the radial aspect of the index finger (median nerve). *Motor function* is determined by isolating movements and muscle groups innervated by particular nerves. The ulnar nerve is evaluated by having the patient extend the index finger and resist a force directed along the radial side. Inability to perform this action demonstrates weakness in the first dorsal interosseous muscle, the last muscle innervated by the ulnar nerve. Inability to elevate the thumb superiorly against resistance with the palm on the table demonstrates weakness in the thenar muscles, the last group of muscles innervated by the median nerve. Radial nerve function is best assessed by having the patient extend the wrist or fingers against resistance. *Flexor and extensor tendons* should be assessed in active motion and at rest. The deep and superficial flexor tendons to each finger should be examined separately. The function of the flexor digitorum profundus (deep) tendons is checked by blocking and allowing only flexion of the distal interphalangeal joint. To isolate function of the flexor digitorum superficialis tendon, the remaining fingers are held in extention which eliminates any contribution from the flexor profundus system and the involved finger is flexed. The flexor pollicis longus muscle tendon is examined by asking the patient to flex the interphalangeal joint of the thumb. Extensor tendons are similarly isolated and evaluated. Skeletal injuries are diagnosed based on extent of injury, exam, and x-ray findings (three views).

Injuries to the upper extremity can involve soft tissue, bone, vessels, or nerves. Injuries to extensor tendons, simple lacerations, and isolated skeletal injuries can be managed in the emergency room. Injuries to flexor tendons or nerves are managed in the operating room within 7–10 days. Vascular injuries obviously require emergent management in the operating room.

## COMPARTMENT SYNDROME (See Chap. 44)

Compartment syndromes of the fingers, hand, and forearm can occur following severe trauma to the upper extremity, crush injuries, or following a compromise of the arterial inflow into the arm. Swelling occurs within the fascial compartments, which lead to increased pressures, compromising the viability of neuromuscular structures. Pain with passive range of motion is an early finding. Paresthesias or ischemic compromise to the hand are late findings and suggest that irreversible damage has occurred.

A compartment syndrome should always be ruled out whenever concerns exist. Pressures can be measured directly with a large bore needle attached to a pressure transducer into either the flexor or extensor compartments (>30 mm Hg abnormal). The differential between compartment pressure and diastolic pressure may be more important, with neuromuscular deficits appearing when the difference is less than 35–40 mm Hg (11), especially in hypotensive patients.

Fascial release of the flexor muscle compartment, the extensor compartment, and the "mobile wad" muscles, including the brachioradialis and extensors of the forearm should be performed. A curvilinear incision is made on the volar aspect beginning at the medial epicondyle extending distally and radially to the wrist. The carpal tunnel should be released, and a skin flap raised to cover the median nerve and flexor tendons (Fig. 53-5). Dorsal release is performed by a straight line incision over the extensor surface of the forearm. If there is a compartment syndrome in the hand, release is performed by opening four dorsal and three volar interosseous compartments, the thenar and hypothenar compartments, and the compartment containing the adductor pollicis muscle. The skin can often be closed primarily once the swelling has diminished, frequently within one to two weeks. Vessel loops can be placed in the skin at the time of fasciotomy and sequentially tightened at the bedside with delayed primary closure. Occasionally, a skin graft is placed secondarily when swelling of the muscles persists.

## TRAUMA TO THE LOWER EXTREMITY

### Evaluation

As with any traumatic injury, advanced trauma life support (ATLS) protocol dictates management of patients. Skeletal integrity, vascular status, function of motor and sensory nerves, and the extent of soft tissue destruction in the lower extremity must be assessed in the

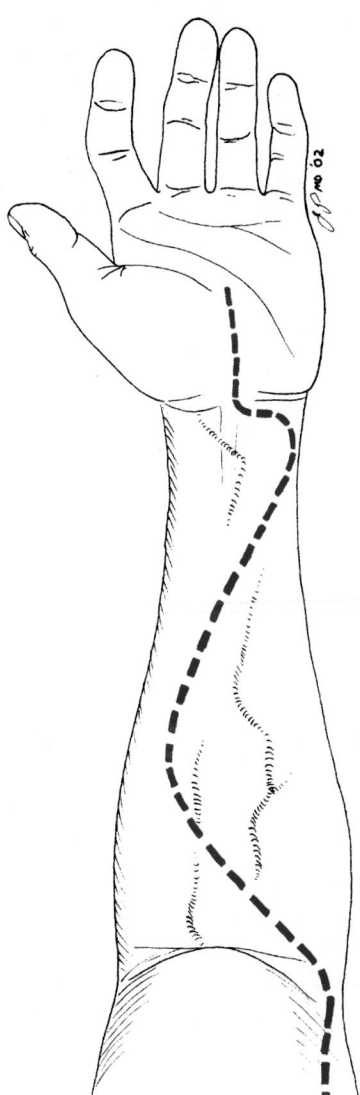

**FIGURE 53-5.** Volar incision used for upper extremity fasciotomy.

secondary survey. In patients with crush injuries or in those with ischemia and subsequent reperfusion, there should be a high index of suspicion that a compartment syndrome will develop.[27]

### Limb Salvage

Occasions arise where the technical capability may be present to salvage an extremity, but the functional outcome of the reconstructed limb would be poor.[29] Assessments of patients with severe trauma to the lower extremity who have undergone reconstruction have demonstrated that nearly two-thirds develop infectious complications, each patient requires nearly nine surgical procedures, and hospital stays range from 1.5 to 2 months.[30] These assessments have also demonstrated similar rates for return to work for patients who become ambulatory early after reconstruction compared with those patients who undergo primary amputations.[31] A number of studies and scoring systems have been developed to better define those injuries that should be amputated versus those where reconstructive attempts are warranted.[32]

The LEAP study documented that a patient is more likely to require amputation when injuries result in the loss of plantar sensation, severe damage to muscle compartments, and vascular disruption.[33,34] Other factors that have been predictive of poor outcomes include crush injuries, segmental tibial injuries, and ischemia lasting longer than six hours, and indications for primary amputation have been suggested.[35] Reconstruction, in general, has been advocated where there is a reasonable expectation for ambulation within one year after the injury with the main goal of achieving bony union and ambulation as soon as possible.[36,37]

## Debridement

Early debridement within the first three hours of injury is more effective at removing bacterial contamination than later debridement as previously noted.[38] For severely contaminated wounds and those with questionable viability, serial debridement every 24–48 hours are warranted. Vacuum-assisted wound closure has become commonplace between debridements for its relatively low nursing requirements, decreased level of bacterial colonization, and increased rate of formation of granulation tissue.

## Amputation Stump

Maintenance of the longest possible stump with the preservation of distal sensation will yield the most functional limb with the least amount of energy expenditure for prosthetic-assisted ambulation. A below-knee amputation will require an additional 25% energy expenditure for ambulation as compared to an above-knee amputation that requires an additional 65%. Traumatic amputation stumps may require reconstruction with local muscle, musculocutaneous or fasciocutaneous flaps, or free tissue transfer for complete coverage. Donor tissue for pedicled or free tissue transfer may well be the amputated or partially amputated part itself.[26]

## Bone Gaps (See Chap. 43)

Techniques available for reconstructing bone gaps include grafting of free cancellous bone, transfer of vascularized bone, and distraction osteogenesis (Ilizarov technique). Nonvascularized bone grafts are the reconstruction of choice for small defects (<6 cm in length). Injuries with soft tissue defects and bone gaps <3 cm are frequently filled with antibiotic beads and stabilized with an external fixator while providing soft tissue coverage with pedicled or free tissue transfer. Eight to 10 weeks later, the soft tissue coverage is elevated, the beads are removed, and the bone gap is filled with cancellous bone. The soft tissue coverage is reapproximated, and the bone is allowed to heal with external fixation in place. Defects measuring 6–12 cm are often managed by distraction osteogenesis. This requires that a corticotomy is made some distance from the bone gap with a dynamic type external fixator placed with pins proximal and distal to the corticotomy sites. Using the device, traction is placed across the corticotomy site, expanding approximately 1mm per day, until bone fills the gap. The device is then left in place for consolidation of the bone. Gradual weight bearing achieves bone hypertrophy and eventual structural stability.

For injuries ≥12 cm in length, vascularized bone grafts are needed to fill the bone gap. Donor sources of vascularized bone are the fibula, iliac crest, rib, and scapula. These may be harvested and transferred with skin for soft tissue coverage as well. For injuries with large soft tissue defects and bone gaps >6 cm, another good option is free flap coverage and distraction osteogenesis. Studies have shown that soft tissue can be expanded concomitantly with distraction osteogenesis to achieve coverage in some patients.[40,41]

## Timing

In patients with open fractures, complications increase from 18% if soft tissue reconstruction is completed within six days of injury to 40–50% for injuries treated with flaps after one week.[42] Other authors have achieved similar low complication rates with subacute wounds, approximately two weeks after injury, by implementing more aggressive debridement.[43,44] Godina et al. studied a large number of severe open tibial fractures and noted significant improvements in viability of flaps, infection rate, and time to union when soft tissue was covered within 72 hours of injury.[45]

## Healing by Secondary Intention

Defects in patients with severe concomitant injuries or comorbid conditions may be best served by wound care in the absence of exposed vital structures. Treatment with negative pressure wound therapy has been instrumental in accelerating wound closure rates for lower extremity wounds or reducing the size of the wound so a lesser reconstructive option may be used. Some studies have even shown the successful development of granulation tissue over exposed bone and hardware with negative pressure therapy.[46]

## Soft-Tissue Reconstruction

Soft-tissue injuries to the thigh are typically amenable to local tissue transfer because of the availability of large muscle masses. Commonly used muscle flaps are the rectus femoris, the vastus lateralis, the vastus medialis, and the gracilis. The sartorius muscle is used effectively for coverage of soft tissue defects in the femoral triangle with exposed neurovascular structures. Frequently, final closure can be attained with a skin graft. If large soft tissue defects require tissue from adjacent areas, the rectus abdominis muscle can be rotated based on the deep inferior epigastric artery. Skin islands oriented vertically (VRAM) or horizontally (TRAM) may be taken along with the muscle for coexisting defects in the skin.

Options for local tissue transfer become less abundant as the injury moves more distally on the lower extremity (Fig. 53-6). Defects about the knee may be covered with one of the quadriceps muscles or from the medial head of the gastrocnemius muscle. Dividing the leg into conceptual thirds, defects in the proximal third are most commonly covered by pedicled gastrocnemius flaps. The medial head is larger and capable of more wound coverage, but both heads can be used for reconstruction based proximally on the sural artery. The medial head of the gastrocnemius muscle can be rotated to cover defects within the proximal third of the leg to as high as 10 cm proximal to the knee.

Defects in the middle third of the leg can generally be covered by the soleus muscle when it is detached from the Achilles tendon and based proximally. The blood supply is provided from branches of the posterior tibial and peroneal arteries. Little functional deficit occurs from harvesting the soleus. Although it may reach to cover a wound in the distal third of the leg, the reliability of the distal aspect of the flap is poor. Other local muscles can be used in the middle third of the leg, but they are only suitable for small defects.

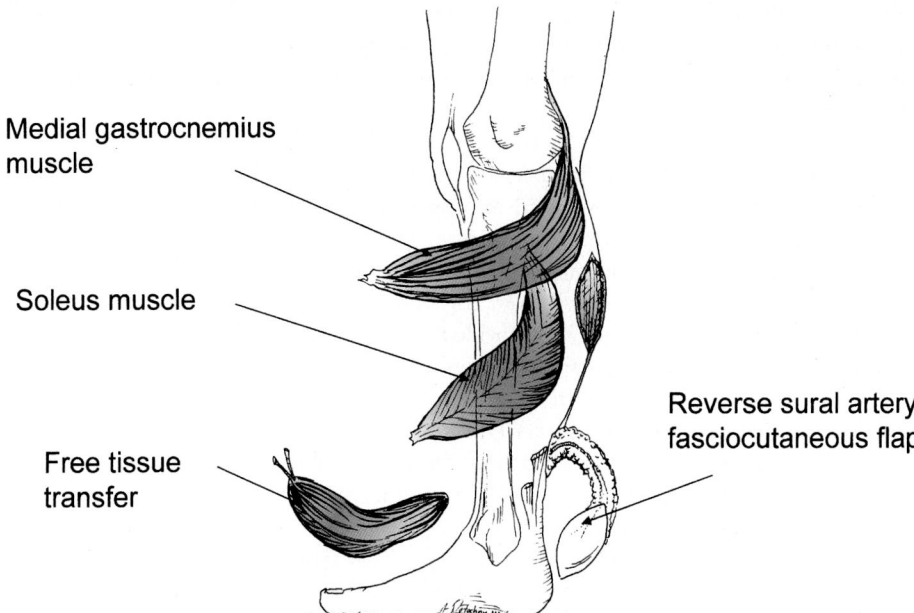

Medial gastrocnemius muscle

Soleus muscle

Free tissue transfer

Reverse sural artery fasciocutaneous flap

**FIGURE 53-6.** Flaps available for soft-tissue reconstruction of lower extremity wounds.

Defects of the distal third of the leg typically require a local fasciocutaneous flap or a free tissue transfer. Commonly used fasciocutaneous flaps, designed with either antegrade or retrograde arterial supply, are the sural artery flap and the lateral supramalleolar flap.[47,48] When used for distal third coverage, they are commonly based on retrograde blood flow. The workhorse donor sites for free muscle tissue transfer include the latissimus dorsi, the rectus abdominus, the serratus anterior, and the gracilis. The omentum has also been used successfully for the dual purpose of acting as a flow through flap for distal revascularization and soft tissue coverage.[49] Minimizing donor site morbidity has popularized the use of perforator flaps as donor sites for reconstruction of the lower extremity, as these flaps leave the functioning muscles. A well used perforator flap for reconstruction of the lower extremity is the anterolateral thigh flap based on the descending branch of the lateral circumflex femoral vessels. In some cases, it may be possible to achieve wound coverage with either a free muscle flap or a local flap. In severe open fractures of the tibia the LEAP study has demonstrated significantly lower six-month morbidity requiring operative intervention for free flaps than for local flaps.[50]

There are a number of general principles for free tissue transfer in the lower extremity. To minimize anastomotic complications, the vascular coupling should be located outside the zone of injury. It is acceptable to locate the anastomosis distal to the zone of injury via antegrade or retrograde flow, provided pulsatile flow is present.[51,52] End-to-side arterial anastomoses are recommended, when possible, to preserve distal blood flow. Donor tissue should be selected based on the location of the injury, local vascular availability, volume of soft tissue defect, and final cosmesis. In general, free flaps are successful approximately 95–97% of the time. They have been used successfully in both the elderly and in children. Failure rates do increase for free tissue transfer done for traumatic indications, those with concomitant vascular injuries, those with large bony defects, and those requiring vein grafts.

Numerous local tissue transfers for small defects of the foot exist, as well.[53] Larger, nonweight bearing defects of the foot can sometimes be covered with skin grafts. For large defects in weight bearing locations, skin grafts can be combined with free tissue transfer. Other options for weight bearing areas include local flaps based on the medial and lateral plantar arteries for transfer of specialized plantar tissue with thick, protective epidermis.

## Replantation

Infrequently, replantation of a lower extremity may be indicated. Long-term success is predicated on the return of protective sensation to the plantar aspect of the foot. Optimum results in most studies have been observed with amputation levels at or distal to the ankle.[54] Success of replantation should be compared to function with amputation and a proper prosthetic. Consideration of replantation is warranted in children with minimal bone loss and when the return of protective sensation is reasonably expected.[55]

## RECONSTRUCTION OF THE ABDOMINAL WALL (See Chap. 41)

The success of "damage control" surgery for abdominal trauma has led to a rise in complicated abdominal wounds requiring plastic surgery techniques for closure. The goal in reconstruction of the abdominal wall is to protect the intra-abdominal viscera, repair and prevent herniation, and achieve acceptable contour. When evaluating abdominal wounds it is important to consider the underlying disease process, stability of the wound, partial or full thickness defect, lower versus upper versus entire abdomen, and the presence of a gastrointestinal fistula. In the trauma setting, primary closure is often not possible due to massive fluid resuscitation and edema of the bowel, gross enteric or fecal contamination, secondary infection, or loss of soft tissue. It is important that abdominal wounds are not closed under too much tension because of the risk of the abdominal compartment syndrome.[56] This can result in cardiopulmonary and renal compromise, as well as a reduction in blood flow to the abdominal wall with associated problems with wound healing.[57]

If closure is deferred, the wounds can be treated by temporizing measures with coverage using a large irrigation bag, and, more recently, a VAC. The wound VAC is beneficial as it can prevent loss of domain while waiting for bowel edema and inflammation to decrease. Some complex abdominal wounds can often have primary closure of the midline aponeurosis within 24–72 hours without complications. Patients with more complex problems are managed by surgical debridement, dressing changes or use of the wound VAC, and eventual coverage of the open abdomen to eliminate fluid and protein losses. Options include coverage of the exposed bowel with a polytetrafluoroethylene patch for 7–10 days followed by removal and placement of a split thickness skin graft (STSG).[58] A STSG placed directly on exposed viscera has become less popular as it lacks the resilience to protect internal organs, promotes adhesions, and has a higher early fistula rate. Another option is to place an absorbable mesh and allow for wound granulation and then coverage with a delayed STSG. These options are somewhat limited when a gastrointestinal fistula is present. Patients who undergo decompressive laparotomy for abdominal compartment syndrome are best managed by staged closure of the abdominal wall (i.e., temporary coverage with absorbable mesh and then a STSG, followed by definitive abdominal wall closure with components separation in a delayed fashion.)[59]

The two issues that need to be addressed for definitive coverage are restoration of integrity of the abdominal wall to protect viscera and prevent hernia and soft tissue coverage.

If temporary coverage has been performed in the acute setting, definitive closure is usually undertaken 6–8 months later and is technically more feasible when the skin graft and underlying bowel demonstrate some degree of independent mobility on exam. The skin graft is usually excised, and the abdominal wall is reconstructed focusing on aponeurotic reconstruction and soft tissue coverage. The midline remnants of the linear alba are re-approximated primarily in smaller defects and through components separation in larger defects. Use of synthetic meshes for reconstruction is now less common, and these are only used when the defect is extremely large (>20 cm) with severe loss of domain or the abdominal wall is missing (infection or blast injury).[60,61]

Soft tissue coverage includes use of local musculofascial or musculocutaneous flaps, free flaps, tissue expansion, or omentum.

Some flaps contain a fascial component and can be used for both support and soft tissue coverage (i.e., tensor fascia lata flap). The most frequently used muscle flaps include the rectus femoris (suprapubic region) and tensor fascia lata, both with a reliable vascular pedicle from the lateral femoral circumflex artery. The rectus abdominis muscle and the omentum also play a major role in abdominal wall reconstruction with their dual blood supply and excellent arc of rotation. The omentum can also be used to reduce formation of adhesions by separating reconstructions with synthetic mesh from the underlying viscera. Local fasciocutaneous flaps can also provide thin pliable coverage and include the thoracoepigastric flap supplied by branches of the superior epigastric artery for the chest and proximal abdomen and the groin flap based on the superficial circumflex iliac vessels for infraumbilical defects. Gracilis and sartorius muscle flaps also play a role in covering major vessel repairs and salvage of infected peripheral vascular prostheses in the groin and thigh.[62]

Additional options for local tissue flaps also include components separation, fascial partition release, and tissue expansion. Components separation consists of releasing the external oblique fascia 1–2 cm lateral to the linea semilunaris and dissecting posteriorly[63] (Fig. 53-7). Preservation of paraumbilical perforators improves the viability of the skin flaps. Release of the posteromedial rectus fascia from beneath will provide further advancement. The rectus abdominis muscle is then advanced medially with the internal oblique and transversus abdominis muscles attached at the lateral margin of the rectus sheath, with the undermined external oblique muscle in its original position. Unilateral dissection will allow 3–5 cm advancement in the epigastrium, 7–10 cm at the umbilicus, and 1–3 cm in the suprapubic region. Fascial partition release is another method used to minimize tension on the closure. This involves parasagittal relaxing incisions in the external oblique and transversus abdominis muscles. Tissue expansion has also been used to expand local skin and fascial flaps for eventual closure.[64] For larger and more complex defects, separation techniques, insertion of mesh, rotation muscle flaps, and free flaps are often required.

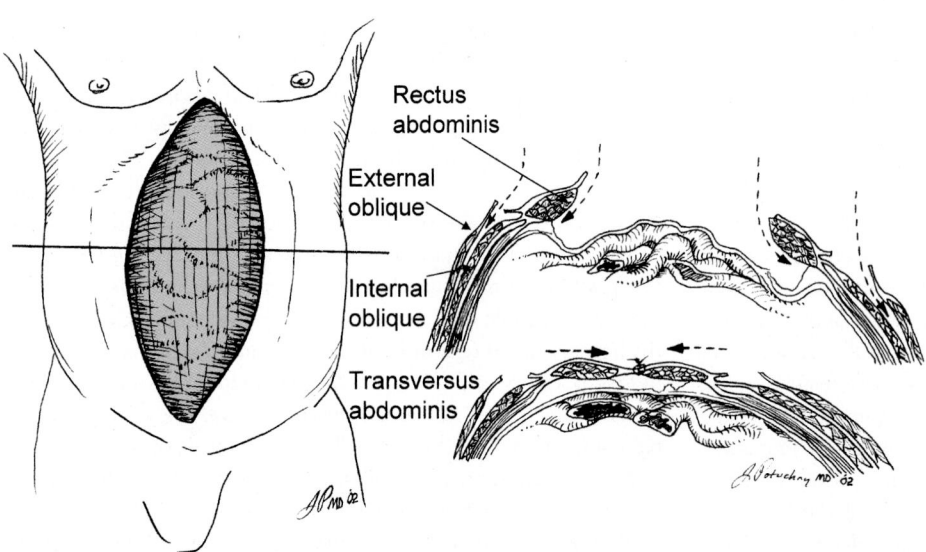

Rectus abdominis

External oblique

Internal oblique

Transversus abdominis

**FIGURE 53-7.** Component separation technique of abdominal wall closure.

## RECONSTRUCTION OF THE CHEST WALL

The management of thoracic trauma includes the reconstruction of complex defects in the chest wall, treatment of sternal wound infections, flap reinforcement of repaired tracheoesophageal or great vessel injuries, and assistance with empyema and bronchopleural fistulas. General principles include the following : (1) wide debridement of devitalized soft tissue, cartilage, and bone; (2) local wound care and culture specific antibiotics; (3) definitive coverage with well vascularized tissue (omentum or muscle); (4) obliteration of intrathoracic dead space; and (5) restoration of skeletal stability.

A thorough analysis of the defect in the chest wall is important and will essentially dictate the reconstructive goals. Restoration of skeletal stability is often required to ensure protection of the intrathoracic contents and preserve the mechanical forces that allow respiration. Integrity of the diaphragm and accessory muscles of inspiration should always be considered when assessing the skeletal defect and when deciding on appropriate local flap coverage, if necessary. In defects involving four or more ribs, the time on a respirator decreased from 8.6 to 1.1 days in one study when a permanent mesh was used, with a corresponding decrease in hospitalization.[65] The synthetic materials available today are diverse and provide adequate support and stability. The ideal characteristics of a prosthetic material for reconstruction of the chest wall include rigidity, malleability, inertness, and radiolucency. Prolene and Marlex meshes provide semirigid fixation and good skeletal support when sutured under tension. They can be used for the majority of patients as they have good in-growth and pliability. If rigidity is considered crucial, then methyl methylacrylate can be used alone or incorporated into the mesh in a sandwich fashion. This is often required following sternal resection when stability and protective coverage is essential over the exposed heart or great vessels. Deschamps showed no significant difference in the postoperative outcome or complications between Prolene mesh and polytetrafluoroethylene (PTFE) soft tissue patch for reconstruction of the chest wall.[66] Prolene mesh was often doubled or quadrupled on itself for additional support. This is similar to the double-knit prolene mesh technique proposed by Arnold et al.[67] Vicryl mesh can be used as a temporary cover in situations where there has been wound contamination or infection. Heavily contaminated wounds can also be treated with split rib grafts enshrouded with well vascularized muscle flaps such as the latissimus dorsi, which can also carry a vascularized rib segment.[68]

Numerous factors influence the decision process regarding which defects require reconstruction with mesh. It has generally been accepted that a two-rib segmental chest wall resection requires soft tissue coverage, alone. Location of the defect and a history of radiation therapy also influence the need for skeletal stability. Also, mesh reconstruction is required more often for lateral defects, likely due to the lack of sternal or spinal stability in that location.[69] Radiated defects in the chest wall often do not require mesh, regardless of the number of ribs removed, given the inherent stability and fixation of the previously irradiated tissue. Muscle flaps alone often provide enough stabilization for large radiated defects without causing flail segments. The smaller defects (less than 5 cm) and those located posteriorly beneath the scapula and above the fourth rib can usually be closed with soft tissue only, ignoring the skeletal component.

Numerous options exist for reconstruction of the chest wall depending on depth and location. While superficial defects of the chest wall are easily closed with skin grafts, full thickness defects are more challenging. Muscle flaps or omentum are frequently employed to cover deeper wounds because their robust vascularity promotes wound healing, eradicates residual bacterial colonization, promotes delivery of antibiotics, obliterates dead space, and provide coverage of synthetic material (Fig. 53-8). The greater omentum provides well-vascularized tissue to areas of extensive radiation damage or infection where other local flaps have failed

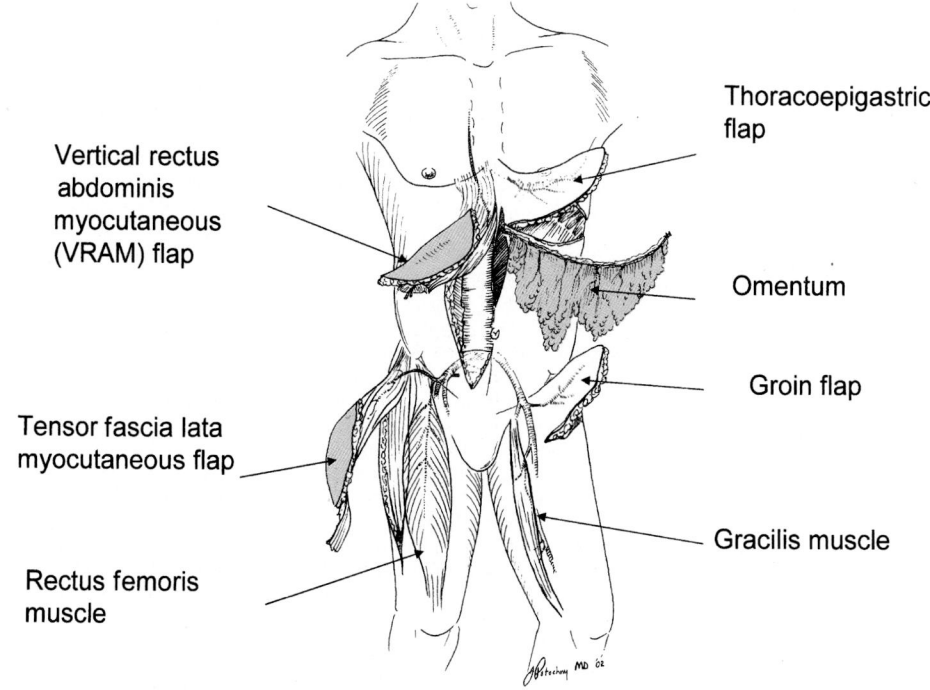

Vertical rectus abdominis myocutaneous (VRAM) flap

Tensor fascia lata myocutaneous flap

Rectus femoris muscle

Thoracoepigastric flap

Omentum

Groin flap

Gracilis muscle

**FIGURE 53-8.** Flaps available for abdominal and chest wall reconstruction.

or are insufficient; however, use of the omentum is not without the risk of possible intra-abdominal complications.[70] The principal muscle flaps used for reconstruction of the chest wall include the pectoralis major, latissimus dorsi, serratus anterior, rectus abdominis, and trapezius. The pectoralis muscle is useful for midline and anterior defects in the chest wall. It can be transposed on its thoracoacromial pedicle or utilized as a turnover flap perfused by perforators from the internal mammary artery. The pectoralis, latissimus, and serratus muscles can all be dropped into the thoracic cavity after segmental resection of the second rib for infection control or to buttress a bronchial stump or fistula. The latissimus dorsi can be raised on the thoracodorsal vessels and utilized for anterior and lateral defects or it can be advanced or turned over based on the medial paraspinous perforators for defects in the posterior midline. A thorough knowledge of the anatomy is essential as the latissimus dorsi pedicle can be damaged during a standard thoracotomy incision, as can the internal mammary vessels during a sternotomy incision. The serratus muscle is another alternative if the latissimus dorsi has been damaged. This muscle is elevated on branches of the thoracodorsal vessels and is primarily used for intrathoracic defects. The trapezius muscle, supplied by the transverse cervical artery, is well-suited for covering defects of the posterior neck and paraspinous region. The need for free tissue transfer is infrequent, and it is reserved for situations where regional flaps are unavailable, insufficient, or have previously failed.

The omental flap with its rich lymphatic plexus and extensive vascularity plays an important role in reconstruction of the chest wall because of its large surface area and ability to eradicate residual bacteria. The flap is based on either the left or right gastroepiploic artery and used for defects from the head and neck down to the perineum. It can be tunneled through the diaphragm or transposed above the costal margin for anterior defects in the chest wall or to obliterate intrathoracic defects.

Other infectious complications such as mediastinitis, empyemas, and bronchopleural fistulae are also managed by aggressive debridement of all nonviable tissue and coverage with well-vascularized tissue under suction drainage. Occasionally, definitive coverage is deferred until all infection is resolved. While *Staphylococcus aureus* is the most frequently isolated organism in such infections, broad-spectrum, empiric intravenous antibiotics should be utilized until definitive cultures of bone and soft tissue available.[71] The mortality from sternal wound infections has been reduced from 50% to less than 5% by employing the regimen of aggressive debridement, coverage with well-vascularized flaps, and 6–8 weeks of culture specific antibiotics.[72]

Intrathoracic transposition of muscle flaps and omentum is an effective means of reinforcing bronchial repairs while obliterating dead space. Bronchopleural fistulae have been successfully closed with a one-stage reconstruction following debridement, primary closure of the fistula, and complete obliteration of the thoracic cavity with omentum and a series of local muscle flaps.[73] Others advocate closure of the fistula, coverage of the repair with vascularized tissue, and packing the chest with gauze saturated with a (20:1) solution of povidone-iodine and saline. When healthy granulation tissue is present, the patient is returned to the operating room, where the chest is filled with antibiotic solution (0.5 g neomycin, 0.1 g polymyxin B sulfate, and 80 mg gentamicin per liter NS). A watertight closure of the chest is then performed (Clagett procedure).[74]

Thoracoplasty remains a salvage procedure for the treatment of recurrent or chronic empyema. Resection of multiple ribs promotes inward collapse of the chest wall. This volume reduction in conjunction with the natural shift of the mediastinum yields a space that can be obliterated with muscle flaps or omentum.

## CONCLUSION

Trauma patients are best managed through a multidisciplinary approach. In order to provide safe and effective reconstruction, the plastic surgeon needs to have a thorough knowledge of the wound defect as it relates to the traumatic event, understands the patient's anatomy and systemic conditions, and has close interactions with the trauma service.

## REFERENCES

1. Stevenson TR, Thacker JG, Rodeheaver GT, et al.: Cleansing the traumatic wound with high pressure syringe irrigation. *JACEP* 5:17, 1976.
2. Valente JH, Forti RJ, Frendlich LF, et al.: Wound irrigation in children: Saline solution or tap water? *Ann Emerg Med* 41:609, 2003.
3. Stevenson J, McNaughton G, Riley J: The use of prophylactic flucloxacillin in treatment of open fractures of the distal phalynx within an accident and emergency department: A double-blind randomized placebo-controlled trial. *J Hand Surg* 28:388, 2003.
4. Roth RM, Gleckman RA, Gantz NM, et al.: Antibiotic irrigations. A plea for controlled clinical trials. *Parmacotherapy* 5:222, 1985.
5. Golightly LK, Branigan T: Surgical antibiotic irrigations. *Hosp Pharm* 24:116, 1989.
6. Anglen JO: Wound irrigation in musculoskeletal injury. *J Am Acad Orthop Surg* 9:219, 2001.
7. Anglen, JO: Comparison of Soap and Antibiotic solutions for irrigation of lower-limb open frature wounds: A prospective, randomized study. *J Bone Joint Surg* 87A:1415, 2005.
8. Robson MD, Krizek TJ, Heggers JP: Biology of the surgical infection. In Ravitch MM, Austen WG, Scott HW, et al., eds. *Current Problems in Surgery*. Chicago: Year Book, 1973, p. 1.
9. Ayello EA, Cuddigan JE: Debridement: Controlling the necrotic/cellular burder. *Adv Skin Wound Care* 17:66, 2004.
10. Mertz PM: Dressing effects on wound healing. *Nurs RSA* 7:12, 1992.
11. Bonn D: Maggot therapy: An alternative for wound infection. *Lancet* 356:1174, 2000.
12. James JH, Watson ACH: The use of opsite, a vapour permeable dressing, on skin graft donor sites. *Br J Plast Surg* 28:107, 1975.
13. Carver N, Leigh IM: Synthetic dressings. *Int J Dermatol* 31:10, 1992.
14. Piacquadio D, Nelson DB: Alginates. A "new" dressing alternative. *J Dermatol Surg Oncol* 18:992, 1992.
15. Morykwas MJ, Argenta LC, Shelton-Brown El, et al.: Vacuum-assisted closure: A new method for wound control and treatment: Animal studies and basic foundation. *Ann Plast Surg* 38:553, 1997.
16. Argenta LC, Morykwas MJ: Vacuum-assisted closure: A new method for wound control and treatment: Clinical experience. *Ann Plast Surg* 38:563, 1997.
17. Bucalo B, Eaglstein WH, Falanga V: Inhibition of cell proliferation by chronic wound fluid. *Wound Rep Regen* 1:181, 1993.
18. Saxena V, Hwang CW, Huang S, et al.: Vacuum-assisted closure: Microdeformations of wounds and cell proliferation. *Plast Reconstr Surg* 114:1086, 2004.
19. Ellis E, Moosk F, El Attar A: Ten years of mandible fractures: Analysis of 2, 137 cases. *Oral Surg* 59:129, 1985.
20. Enislidis G, Pichorner S, Kainberger F, et al.: Lactosorb panel and screws for repair of large orbital floor defects. *J Craniomaxillofac Surg* 25:316, 1997.
21. Enislidis G, Pichorner S, Lambert F, et al.: Fixation of zygomatic fractures with a new biodegradable copolymer osteosynthesis system: Preliminary results. *Int J Oral Maxillofac Surg* 27:352, 1998.
22. Haers PE, Sailer HF: Biodegradable self-reinforced poly-L/DL-lactide plates and screws in bimaxillary orthognathic surgery: Short term skeletal stability and material related failures. *J Craniomaxillofac Surg* 28:363, 1998.
23. Yerit KC, Hainich S, Turhani D, et al.: Stability of biodegradable implants in treatment of mandibular fractures. *Plast Reconstr Surg* 115:1863, 2005.
24. Wang BH, Robertson BC, Girotto JA: Traumatic optic neuropathy: A review of 61 patients. *Plast Reconstr Surg* 107:1655, 2001.
25. Amrith S, Saw SM, Lim TC, et al.: Ophthalmic involvement in crainio-facial trauma. *J Craniomaxillofac Surg* 28:140, 2000.
26. Stiebel M, Lee C, Fontes R: Calcaneal fillet of sole flap: Durable coverage of the traumatic amputation stump. *J Trauma* 49:960, 2000.

27  Mubarak SJ, Owen CA, Hargens AR, et al: Acute compartment syndromes: Diagnosis and treatment with the aid of the wick catheter. *J Bone Joint Surg* 60- A:1091,1978

28  Moehring HD, Gravel C, Chapman MW, Olson SA: Comparison of antibiotic beads and intravenous antibiotics in open fractures. Clin *Orthop* 3 72:254, Mar 2000

29  Gustilo RB, Mendoza RM, Williams DN: Problems in the management of type III (severe) open fractures: a new classification of type III open fractures. J Trauma 24:742, 1984

30  Pelissier P, Boireau P, Martin 0, Baudet J: Bone reconstruction of the lower extremity: complications and outcomes. *Plast Reconstr Surg* 111:2223, 2003.

31  Bosse MJ, MacKenzie EJ, Kellam JF, et al: An analysis of outcomes of reconstruction or amputation after leg-threatening injuries. N Eng J Med 347:1924, 2002.

32  Russell WL, Sailors DM, Whittle TB, et al: Limb salvage versus traumatic amputation. A decision based on a seven-part predictive index. Ann Surg 213(5):473, 1991.

33  Bosse MJ, MacKenzie EJ, Kellam JF, et al: A prospective evaluation of the clinical utility of the lower-extremity injury-severity scores. *J Bone Joint Surg* 83A:3, 2001.

34  MacKenzie EJ, Bosse MJ, Kellam JF, et al: Factors influencing the decision to amputate or reconstruct after high-energy lower extremity trauma. *J Trauma* 52:641, 2002.

35  Lange RH: Limb reconstruction versus amputation decision-making in massive lower extremity trauma. *Clin Orthop 243:92, 1989*

36  Bosse MJ, MacKenzie EJ, Kellam iF, et al: An analysis of outcomes of reconstruction or amputation after leg-threatening injuries. N Engl Med 347:1924, 2002

37  Hertel R, Strebel N, Ganz R: Amputation versus reconstruction in traumatic defects of the leg: outcome and costs. J Orthop Trauma 10:223, 1996

38  Bhandari M, Schemitsch EH, Adili A, etal: High and low pressure pulsatile lavage of contaminated tibial fractures: an in vitro study of bacterial adherence and bone damage. J Orthop Trauma 13:526, 1999

39  Stiebel M, Lee C, Fontes R: Calcaneal fillet of sole flap: durable coverage of the traumatic amputation stump. J Trauma 49:960, 2000

40  Bundgaard KG, Christensen KS: Tibial bone loss and soft-tissue defect treated simultaneously with llizarov-technique–a case report. Acta Orthop *Scand* 71:534, 2000.

41  Lemer A, Ullman Y, Stein H, Peled U: Using the llizarov external fixation device for skin expansion. *Ann Plast Surg 45:535, 2000*

42  Byrd HS, Spicer TE, Cierny G III: Management of open tibial fractures. *Plast ReconstrSurg 76:719, 1985.*

43  YaremchukMj, Brumback Ri, Manson PN, et al: Acute and definitive management of traumatic osteocutaneous defects of the lower extremity. *Plast Reconstr Surg 80:1, 1987*

44  Francel Ti et al: Microvascular soft-tissue transplantation for reconstruction of acute open tibial fractures: Timing ofmcoverage and long-term functional results. *Plast Reconstr Surg 89:4 78, 1992*

45  Godina M: Early microsurgical reconstruction of complex trauma of the extremities. *Clin Plast Surg 13(4):619, 1986.*

46  DeFranzo AJ. Argenta LC. Marks MW. Molnar JA. David LR. Webb LX. Ward WG. Teasdall RG. The use of vacuum-assisted closure therapy for the treatment of lower-extremity wounds with exposed bone *Plastic & Reconstructive Surgery.* 108(5):1184-91, 2001 Oct

47  Singh 5, Naasan A: Use of distally based superficial sural island artery flaps in acute open fractures of the lower leg. *Ann Plast Surg 47:505, 2001*

48  Touam C, Rostoucher P, Bhatia A, Oberlin C: Comparative study of two series of distally based fasciocutaneous flaps for coverage of the lower one-fourth of the leg, the ankle, and the foot. *Plast Reconstr Surg 707:383, 2001*

49  Maloney CT Jr, Wages D, Upton J, Lee WP: Free omental tissue transfer for extremity coverage and revascularization. *Plast Reconstr Surg 117:1899, 2003*

50  Pollak AN, McCarthy ML, Burgess AR: Short-term wound complications after application of flaps for coverage of traumatic soft-tissue defects about the tibia. The Lower Extremity Assessment Project (LEAP) Study Group. *J Bone Joint Surg 82A:1681, 2000*

51  Minami A, Kato H, Suenaga N, Iwasaki N: Distally-based free vascularized tissue grafts in the lower leg. *J Reconstr Microsurg 7 5:495, 1999*

52  Park 5, Han SH, Lee Tj: Algorithm for recipient vessel selection in free tissue transfer to the lower extremity. *Plast Reconstr Surg 103:1937, 1999*

53  Attinger CE, Ducic I, Zelen C: The use of local muscle flaps in foot and ankle reconstruction. *Clin Podiatr Med Surg 17:681, 2000*

54  Cayle LB, Lineaweaver WC, Buncke GM, et al: Lower extremity replantation. *Clin Plast Surg 18(31:437, 1991*

55  Griffin JR, Thorton JF. Lower Extremity Reconstruction. *Selected Readings in Plastic Surgery Vol 10, No. 5, Part 1 2005*

56  Ledgerwood AM, Lucas CE: Postoperative complications of abdominal trauma. *Surg Clin North Am* 70:715, 1990.

57  Ivatury RR, Diebel L, Portes JM, et al: Intra-abdominal hypertension and the abdominal compartment syndrome. *Surg Clin North Am* 77:783, 1997.

58  Cohen M, Morales R Jr, Fildes J, et al: Staged reconstruction after gunshot wounds to the abdomen. *Plast Reconstr Surg* 108:83, 2001.

59  Hultman CS, Pratt B, Cairns, CA et al. Multidisciplinary Approach to Abdominal Wall Reconstruction after Decompressive Laparotomy for Abdominal Compartment Syndrome. *Ann Plast Surg.* 54(3), March 2005, pp 269-275.

60  Butler CE, Langstein HN, Kronowitz SJ. Pelvic, abdominal and chest wall reconstruction with Alloderm in patients at increased risk for mesh-related complications *Plast Reconstr Surg* 116(5): 1263-75, 2005.

61  Hamilton JE: The repair of large or difficult hernia with mattress onlay grafts of fascia lata: A 21 year experience. *Ann Surg* 167:87, 1968.

62  Meland BN, Arnold PG, Pairolero PC et al: Muscle-flap coverage for infected peripheral vascular prostheses. *Plast Reconstr Surg* 93:1005, 1994.

63  Ramirez OM, Ruas E, Dellon AL. "Components Separation" method for closure of abdominal wall defects: an anatomic and clinical study. *Plast Reconstr Surg* 86:519-526, 1990.

64  Carlson GW, Elwood E, Losken A, Galloway JR. The Role of Tissue Expansion in Abdominal Wall Reconstruction. *Ann. Plast. Surg.* 44(2): 147-153, 2000.

65  Kroll SS, Walsh G, Ryan B, et al: Risk and benefits of using marlex mesh in chest wall reconstruction. *Ann Plast Surg* 31:303, 1993.

66  Deshamps C, Tirnaksiz BM, Darbandi R et al. Early and long term results of prosthetic chest wall reconstruction. *J Thorac Cardiovasc Surg* 1999, 117:588- 92.

67  Arnold PG, Pairolero PC. Chest wall reconstructions: an account of 500 consecutive cases. *Plast Reconstr Surg* 1996, 98(5):804.

68  Hirase Y: Composite reconstruction for chest wall and scalp using multiple ribs-latissimus dorsi osteomyocutaneous flaps as pedicled and free flaps. *Plast Reconstr Surg* 87:555, 1991.

69  Losken A, Thourani VH, Carlson GW, Jones GE, Culbertson JH, Miller Jl, Mansour KA. A Reconstructive Algorithm for Plastic Surgery Following Extensive Chest Wall Resection. *British J. Plast .Surg.* 57(4): 295-302, 2004

70  Hultman CS, Culbertson JH, Jones GE, Losken A et al. Thoracic reconstruction with the omentum:indications, complications and results. *Ann Plast Surg* 2001, 46:242-9.

71  Francel TJ, Kouchoukos NT: A rational approach to wound difficulties after sternotomy: The problem. *Ann Thorac Surg* 72: 1411, 2001.

72  Nahai F, Rand RP, Hester TR, et al: Primary treatment of the infected sternotomy wound with muscle flap. A review of 211 consecutive cases. *Plast Reconstr Surg* 83:434, 1989.

73  Miller Jl: Single-stage complete muscle flap closure of the postpneumonectomy empyema space: A new method and possible solution to a disturbing complication. *Ann Thorac Surg* 38:227, 1984.

74  Johnson CH, Arnold PG: Chest and abdominal wall reconstruction (discussion), in. Goldwin R, Cohen M *(eds):The Unfavorable Result in Plastic Surgery.* Philadelphia: Lippincott Williams & Wilkins, 2001:687.

## Commentary ■ DAVID A. KAPPEL

The adherence to basic principles in the plastic surgical approach to managing traumatic wounds cannot be overemphasized. The key elements of a thorough physical examination, i.e., observation and palpation combined with the judicious use of adjunct technology will provide the foundation for successful wound closure. Reducing a complex wound problem to its basic elements will allow formation of a logical treatment algorithm and methodical approach. The complexity of treatment should mirror the complexity of the wound.

Management of injured soft tissue should err on the side of conservatism. Debridement should be adequate but not overenthusiastic. Marginal tissue can be re-evaluated at appropriate intervals. Doing "no further harm" in terms of solutions, irrigations, antibiotics, and surgical debridement remains a basic tenet.

Chronic or indolent wounds may require additional manipulation through topical treatment to obtain satisfactory granulation and/or epithelialization. The choice for this therapy should be based on previous successful experience and not necessarily the latest technology. On rare occasions, particularly refractory wounds may necessitate expensive and complex approaches. Most open wounds, however, can be managed by time-honored traditional techniques.

Secondary coverage is dictated by the need for function and cosmesis. Wounds of the extremities require functional coverage as a primary consideration with appearance secondary. With secondary coverage of the face and neck, however, appearance becomes of paramount importance. The choices between split thickness and full thickness grafts versus flap coverage will be determined based on these considerations. As the detailed anatomy of the soft tissues of the body has been defined, multiple reliable local flaps are now part of the plastic surgeon's armamentarium.

Microvascular free flap transfer is a very effective "hammer" but not every wound is a "nail."

Utilization of specialty resources in terms of manpower, operating room time and expense will increase as the complexity of the injury increases. Complex maxillofacial, trunk, and extremity injuries will of necessity require specialty involvement. The absence of local resources may require transfer to a regional center as the most complex injuries will require a team of experienced providers. The nutrition and rehabilitation needs of the patient should be considered early with involvement of the appropriate areas of expertise.

Extremity injuries will require the input of physical medicine and often the prosthetist in the consideration of amputation or reconstruction decisions. The patient's vocation and hobbies, age and lifestyle all become part of the decision algorithm.

The systematic management of complex wounds parallels the system management of the trauma patient. The patient's wounds should be treated with an appropriate level of care in an expeditious but thoughtful manner. The complexity and severity of the wound should be matched by the level of skill, knowledge, and resources applied to the problem.

# Rehabilitation

*Elliot B. Bodofsky* ■ *Steven E. Ross*

In the landmark 1966 paper "Accidental Death and Disability: The Neglected Disease of Modern Society," priorities were identified for the development of trauma care in America.[1] Rehabilitation of the injured was one of the significant problems identified in that document. Major strides have been made in both the techniques and organization of prehospital care, resuscitation, surgery, and intensive care. The development of rehabilitation services continues to lag behind that of acute care.

In 2003, there were over 164,000 deaths due to injury and over 29 million nonfatal injuries in the United States.[2] The total cost of unintentional trauma in 2003 including medical, wage losses, and property damage was over $600 billion.[3] Inpatient acute care hospital admissions for trauma totaled 2.7 million, with acute hospital costs of over $50 billion.[3] Brain injuries cause 100,000 deaths per year and result in serious permanent disability for another 100,000. Spinal cord injuries result in 10,000 cases per year of permanent quadriplegia or paraplegia. Trauma systems must strive to reduce impairment due to injury and return individuals to their highest possible functional role.

Brain injury and spinal cord injury, because of their tremendous impact on function, necessitate the greatest application of rehabilitative resources.[4] While orthopedic injuries also require special services and lead to significant disability, many life-threatening visceral injuries do not lead to long-term disability.[5]

## DEFINITIONS

*Impairment* is any loss or abnormality of psychological, physiologic, or anatomic structure or function. *Disability* is any restriction or lack resulting from an impairment of ability to perform an activity in the manner or within the range considered normal for a human being. *Handicap* is a disadvantage for a given individual resulting from an impairment or disability that limits or prevents the fulfillment of a role that is normal for that individual.[6]

## THE REHABILITATION TEAM

Rehabilitation is best provided by an interdisciplinary team, orchestrating different therapies in a coordinated manner. Good communication between the disciplines and physician supervision and interaction with the therapists are crucial.

Mobility, activities of daily living, communication, and sexual function are issues that must be addressed by the team. The psychological well-being of the injured individual must also be considered. The team must provide vocational training in order to assist the victim in returning to (or developing) a productive role in society. Finally, the patient's need for financial and social support must be assessed and a plan for access to ongoing services developed.

Overall leadership of the team should be held by the rehabilitation physician (physiatrist), but leadership of a specific phase may be held by any member of the team based on his or her expertise. It is best if the entire team hold team meetings during which each patient is discussed.

### Physiatrist

The physiatrist reviews the history, and examines the patient thoroughly to determine the patient's abilities and disabilities, and then prescribes appropriate therapies. Physiatrists also order adaptive equipment, prosthetics, and orthotics. This physician has a crucial role in communication with the patient, family, rehabilitation team, and other members of the hospital staff. Physiatrists prescribe medications to alleviate pain and spasticity; bowel and bladder programs to provide safe, hygienic elimination after nerve injury; electromyography/nerve conduction studies to diagnose nerve and muscle pathology; and edema management.

### Orthopedist

The orthopedist assesses and treats patients with musculoskeletal injury. Before and after surgical intervention, the rehabilitation team follows guidelines for weight bearing and range of motion set by the orthopedist. In patients with isolated orthopedic injuries, the orthopedist often directs the rehabilitation process.

## Physical Therapist

Physical therapy is the most commonly involved discipline. The therapist evaluates the patient's strength, range of motion, balance, and coordination, and leads the patient in exercises to improve function. The physical therapist instructs the patient in ambulation, use of ambulation aids, wheelchair usage, stairs, curbs, and ramps. Modalities for pain relief and wound management, such as heat, cold, electrical stimulation, hydrotherapy, massage, and traction, are an important part of physical therapy. Physical therapists also instruct the patient in the use of lower extremity prosthetics and orthotics.

## Occupational Therapist

Occupational therapists evaluate upper extremity range of motion, strength, coordination, and self-care skills. They instruct patients in these areas as well as in transfers needed for self-care. They can fabricate upper extremity splints as well as guide patients in the use of adaptive equipment, splints, and upper extremity prostheses. Occupational therapists conduct cognitive and perceptive evaluations and treat deficits in these areas. Physical and occupational therapists also conduct home evaluations to assess barriers and the patient's ability to manage activities of daily living, and they are involved with family training.

## Speech Therapist

Speech therapists are involved in the evaluation and treatment of communication disorders such as aphasias, dysarthrias, and apraxias. Aphasia is a cognitive impairment involved with speech, and can be receptive, expressive, or both. A dysarthria, by contrast, is abnormal speech because of muscle weakness or spasm. An apraxia is an impairment of sequencing, and can involve activities other than speech.

Diagnostic testing for and therapy of swallowing disorders is a crucial component of speech therapy. Speech therapists are involved with the evaluation and treatment of cognitive deficits and instruct patients in the use of augmentative communication devices.

## Rehabilitation Nurse

Rehabilitation nurses specialize in the personal care of physically impaired patients. This includes medication management, hygiene, bowel and bladder programs, and the use of adaptive equipment.

## Psychologist and Neuropsychologist

The rehabilitation psychologist and neuropsychologist are primarily involved in the testing of perception, memory, and reasoning. They also evaluate personality and psychological status as well as coping skills. Psychologists aid patients in the development of problem-solving skills and help patients and families adapt to disabilities. Neuropsychologists evaluate cognitive function and attendant skills (e.g., reading, mathematics) and implement training programs to overcome or circumvent deficits.

## Psychiatrist

The psychiatrist is primarily involved in the identification and treatment of psychopathology—either pre-existing or secondary to brain injury—or normal/abnormal psychological reactions to injury. Drug therapy for sleep deprivation, treatment for substance dependence, and management of alterations of behavior in brain injured patients are all the province of the psychiatrist.

## Recreational Therapist

The recreational therapist uses leisure activities to promote recovery. This starts with a thorough assessment of the patient's interests and capabilities. Recreational activities are then used to improve strength, endurance, and concentration. These activities also aid in the patient's reintegration to the community. Play therapy may be extremely important in the treatment of the injured child.

## Vocational Counselor

The vocational counselor evaluates vocational interests, aptitudes, and skills. he or she counsels patients who must change or adjust their jobs. Vocational counselors also provide information on job training and placement.

## Prosthetist/Orthotist

The prosthetist/orthotist is a key member of the rehabilitation team, responsible for the evaluation of patients requiring braces and artificial limbs as well as the design and fabrication of these devices. It is important that the team, particularly the physiatrist and orthopedist, work closely with the prosthetist/orthotist to explain the patient's restrictions and needs.

## Nursing Staff

The trauma nurse must function as a member of the rehabilitation team. As the bedside patient advocate, the nurse frequently identifies the physical, psychological, and behavioral needs of the patient (and his or her family) earlier than any other member of the team. Prevention of decubitus ulcers and contractures is part of the trauma nurse's primary role; however, impairments of bowel, bladder, speech, motor, and swallowing function are more readily apparent to the nurse than to any other member of the team.

## Respiratory Therapist

The respiratory therapist's involvement in rehabilitative care has increased as a result of the movement of ventilator-dependent patients into rehabilitation facilities. In addition to efforts for weaning of these patients from ventilatory support, these therapists help the spinal cord-injured patient learn techniques of cough and airway clearance.

## Social Worker

The social worker's role in the rehabilitation team varies on an institutional basis. In some hospitals, the social worker is primarily involved in financial and placement issues, identifying the appropriate rehabilitation facility for transfer from an acute care center, and arranging such transfer. In others, the social worker may participate in patient and family counseling and social support. This family/patient support service is important in helping the patient and his or her family to cope with the immediate changes that may occur after injury and to develop plans for ongoing coping.

## SPECIFIC ORGAN-SYSTEM INJURY

### Brain Injury

There are approximately 1 million cases of brain injury annually in the United States, and 260,000 hospital admissions for brain injury.[3] More than 100,000 individuals suffer long-term disability due to brain injury annually.[3] Although a small percentage of survivors of brain injury never recover independent function, the majority develop some level of independence or even return to work with appropriate rehabilitation.

Assessment of the rehabilitative needs of the brain-injured patient is an ongoing process. Initial prediction of neurologic outcome is problematic. Injury severity scales are useful in stratifying patient populations, assessing survival/recovery risk for such groups, and planning institutional resource requirements. Early assessment of needs is possible in patients with mild (Glasgow Coma Scale [GCS] >12) injury, but caution must be exercised for moderate (GCS 9 to 12) and severe (GCS <9) injury. Posttraumatic coma lasting for prolonged periods is associated with poor survival and functional outcome. Higher initial GCS are associated with better cognitive functioning at time of discharge from rehabilitation,[7] and six months post injury.[8]

Initial rehabilitative efforts for the moderate to severe brain-injured patient focus on physical needs. Many patients are immobile, either due to injury or therapeutic sedation or paralysis. Nearly all will require mechanical ventilation. Abnormal muscle tone due to posturing or spasticity may occur. Mild spasticity is best managed with range-of-motion exercises and positioning. More severe spasticity that prevents range-of-motion exercises from being carried out usually requires medications (Table 54-1). Early efforts must address prevention of decubitus ulcers through changes in position and specially designed beds. In addition to the usual sites of decubiti, extended use of cervical orthoses may lead to occipital or shoulder ulcers. Range-of-motion exercises and splinting of major extremity joints may prevent contractures.

In less severely injured patients and in those recovering from severe injury, evaluation for cognitive deficits, behavioral abnormalities, and personality changes can proceed. A few studies now show that cognitive rehabilitation improves cognitive function.[9] Various scales describing a patient's current cognitive state and progress over time have been used in attempts to assess potential for recovery.

Based on available data, an integrated brain injury program should be initiated once life-threatening physiologic disturbances have been corrected. Earlier initiation of cognitive rehabilitative cannot be supported. Shock and multiple extracranial injuries have been demonstrated to reduce cognitive outcome.[10]

Behavioral abnormalities are common among patients recovering from severe brain injury. They may require drug therapy to modify behaviors such as agitation, aggression, inattention, and depression (Fig. 54-1).[11–15] Antidepressants may also help to improve attention. Stimulants may decrease agitation in many brain-injured patients by improving the level of awareness, thereby decreasing confusion.[13] Many of these drugs have significant side effects, and careful monitoring of their use is important.

Minor head injury cannot be ignored in the development of brain injury rehabilitation programs. Patients with "postconcussive syndrome" frequently sustain significant disability. Persistent subjective complaints of neurologic symptoms—such as headache, vertigo, nausea, fatigue, irritability, memory or concentration difficulties, insomnia, emotional liability, or other nonspecific symptoms—should alert the clinician to the possibility of this disorder.[16]

### Spinal Cord Injury

There are approximately 11,000 new cases of spinal cord injury (SCI) in the United States each year[3,17]; there is a population of about 200,000 tetraplegics and paraplegics at any one time. Acute care, including surgical decompression, surgical stabilization and/or bracing, megadose steroid administration, and respiratory care, must be designed to limit extension of spinal cord damage as well as to prevent respiratory compromise and complications of infection. Rehabilitation begins immediately following resuscitation and evaluation, during acute medical care.

Passive range-of-motion exercise and splinting for joints below the level of paralysis should be started as soon as possible. Particularly in low tetraplegics and paraplegics, active range-of-motion therapy for the upper extremities should also be started. Contractures and decubiti are a risk, and steps to prevent them are important. In the supine patient, the occiput, scapulae, vertebrae, elbows, sacrum, coccyx, and heels are pressure points: other positions subject other points to pressure. The prevention of decubitus ulcers must be a lifelong activity for patients with spinal cord injury. Spasticity can be treated with the medications listed in Table 54-1.

As soon as bony spinal stability is established, active mobilization of the patient should be initiated. Expectations for the level of

**TABLE 54-1**

| Medications for Spasticity | | | |
| --- | --- | --- | --- |
| MEDICATION | STARTING DOSE | MAXIMUM DOSE | SIDE EFFECTS |
| Baclofen | 10 po tid | 30 po tid | Sedation, dizziness, nausea, seizures |
| Tizanidine | 2 po bid | 8 po tid | Dizziness, sedation, dry mouth |
| Dantrolene | 25 po/day | 400 po/day | Sedation, dizziness, nausea, liver dysfunction |
| Botulinum toxin A | 100–400 U IM[a] | 100–400 U IM[a] | Rash, fevers |

[a]Botox A should only be injected by physicians experienced in its usage under EMG guidance.

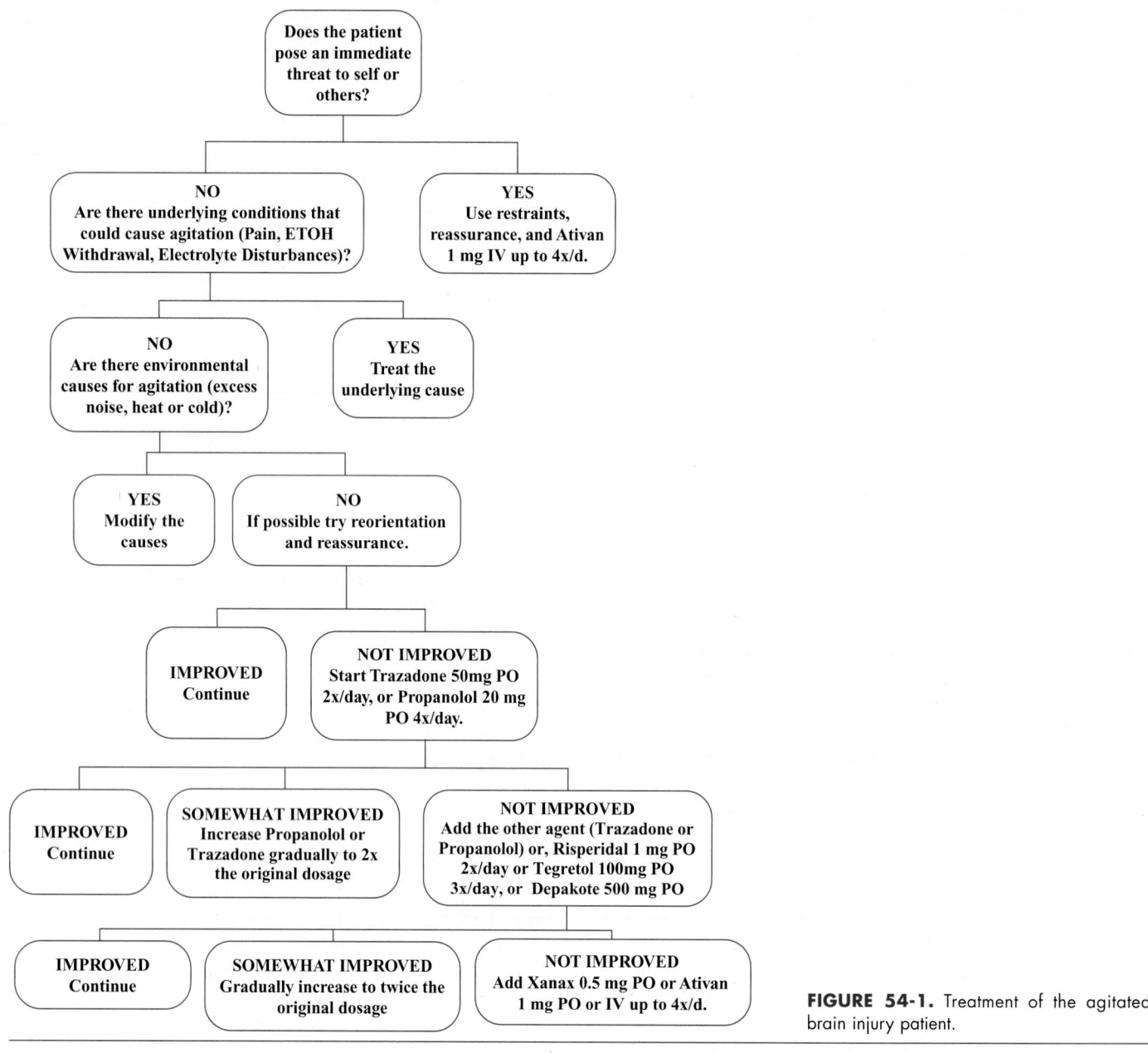

**FIGURE 54-1.** Treatment of the agitated brain injury patient.

independence (based on the level of the cord injury) should be established for the patient, and physical rehabilitation and long-term planning targeted to reach or exceed that goal. Mobility may require the use of motorized or manual wheelchairs or braces and crutches.

A bowel regimen with stool softeners and suppositories should be instituted. Bladder training should not begin until urine output is low enough to allow safe intermittent catheterization less frequently than six times daily of 400 mL or less each time. Whenever possible, the patient should be trained to do self-catheterization until reflex voiding patterns are established.

Planning modifications of the home environment to accommodate a wheelchair and transfer from it as well as the provision of special equipment must be undertaken. Planning with inpatient social services, insurance company rehabilitation nurses, and community support services must be started early.

## Orthopedic Injuries

Extremity fractures affect a large proportion of patients with injury. The early fixation of lower extremity fractures has become widespread. Although this is undertaken to reduce respiratory and infectious complications, it also affords the opportunity to institute early rehabilitative care. Transfer and gait training may be the all that is needed for patients with isolated injury; but in those requiring complex multifracture management, extensive physical rehabilitation may be necessary. Early use of continuous passive motion devices to maintain joint mobility, particularly in patients with other injuries to other systems, can be of benefit. When early placement in subacute care facilities occurs following isolated orthopedic injury, it is important that continuity of both medical and rehabilitative care be maintained.

Nearly three-quarters of all patients with lower extremity injury will return to work by one year, and more than 60% will have no residual disability at 30 months. Less than 10% will have severe disability.[18] Although severe pelvic fracture poses a greater risk to life than other fractures, with aggressive stabilization and rehabilitation, the functional outcome is similar to that of lower extremity injuries.[19]

Heterotopic ossification (myositisis ossificans traumatica) is a concern related to traumatic injury of soft tissue and fractures as well as brain and spinal cord injury. It is the deposition of mature lamellar bone into major muscle groups. Risk factors include spasticity, paralysis, loss of consciousness for longer than two weeks, and the proximity of muscle groups to long-bone fractures. Frequent sites for this complication are the quadriceps muscles, the abductors muscles of the hip, and the brachialis muscle.

In the early phase of heterotopic ossification, calcium deposition occurs and heterotopic bone forms. The process of inflammation sets in during the intermediate phase, followed by bone remodeling and maturation. Complete ossification of the soft tissue occurs between 6 to 18 months after the start of the process.

After heteropic ossification occurs, treatment options are limited. Injured patients with increasing pain over areas of soft tissue and/or a rapid decrease in range of motion should be evaluated for heterotopic ossification. Plain radiographs and a cold bone scan should be obtained. Biphosphonates, such as etidronate disodium, have been shown to slow down the deposition of lamellar bone in patients who have suffered spinal cord injuries. Patients at very high risk, such as those with fractures of the hip and pelvic girdle, may benefit from prophylactic use of indomethacin or local radiation therapy early after injury or surgery.[20] If range of motion is severely limited, manipulation under anesthesia should be performed. If surgical resection is necessary, it is best to wait until the process has completed.

## Multisystem Trauma

Victims of multisystem trauma pose challenges to the rehabilitation system just as they do to acute care. In 1988, Rhodes and associates found that 70% of survivors of severe injury returned to their prior work status and that few remained severely disabled or in a persistent vegetative state.[21] Holbrook and coworkers found that only 18% of victims of major trauma had normal levels of function one year following injury.[22] Severity of injury has consistently been a poor predictor of return to work; specific injuries—such as brain, spinal cord, and extremity injury—are more predictive of functional outcome.[5]

Return-to-work statistics may not accurately reflect the impact of multisystem injury. Although the majority of trauma patients surviving to discharge return to work, 80% have some impairment, 76% have some nonvocational disability, and 19% of the employed have vocational disability.[23] Nearly 40% of survivors of multisystem trauma and prolonged stay in an intensive care unit, returned to their former employment, and only 23% retired or were on prolonged sick leave.[24] Return to social function is likely after multisystem trauma.

## Pediatric Trauma

Systems for pediatric trauma care have developed more recently than those for adults; consequently, rehabilitation systems for injured children have lagged. Availability and integration of acute rehabilitation services for injured children is critical to postinjury function. Injuries to children result in impairment; without rehabilitative services, such children may not recover or adapt, resulting in accentuated disability or handicap. Some 55% of children are found to have functional limitations one year after severe injury, and even those with good outcome after brain injury frequently have major deficits of cognitive, motor, or neuropsychological function.[25]

Play therapy has an important role in pediatric rehabilitation. Psychosocial specialists with pediatric training and experience are critical to this effort. The child's family must be intimately involved in their child's physical, cognitive, and social rehabilitation. Psychosocial support should be available for the family, especially when the victim has brain or spinal cord injury. Eventual transfer from acute care to an institution (or outpatient program) that provides specialized pediatric rehabilitative care, rather than a general rehabilitation center, is important for children with severe injury.

## SPECIAL PROBLEMS IN TRAUMA REHABILITATION

### Amputee Rehabilitation

Trauma is the second leading cause of lower extremity amputations, the leading cause of upper extremity amputations, and in patients aged 11 to 40.[26] In many cases, the need for amputation after trauma is clear. While salvage of a damaged limb is usually desirable, it should be attempted only if it appears likely that the limb will be functional and relatively pain-free. For example, in the case of severe open foot and ankle injuries with tibial nerve disruption, it is usually better to amputate. Prolonged unsuccessful attempts to salvage a painful limb may increase the likelihood of developing phantom limb pain.[26]

In general, the goal is to preserve as much length as possible. There are some exceptions. Lisfranc and Chopart (Hindfoot) amputations usually lead to ankle deformities and skin breakdown and should not be performed. Below-knee amputees function better than above-knee amputees; however, below-knee amputees with a tibial length of less than 2 cm are very difficult to fit with a prosthesis, and a tibial length less than 6 cm requires a more complex knee joint mechanism. The knee disarticulation functions very well. In the upper extremity, wrist and elbow disarticulations have very poor cosmesis; these amputations should be at least 6 cm proximal to the joints.[27]

In children under 12 years of age, bony overgrowth at the amputated end can become a major problem.[28] These are painful and often require surgical revision. When possible, it is better to amputate through a joint than through bone in children.[29]

The surgeon can improve postamputation function and decrease the likelihood of subsequent pain by transecting nerves sharply, beveling the ends of bones, placing skin incisions to avoid adherence to bone, and using an appropriate myofascial closure.

Stump dressings affect functional outcome. When soft elastic bandages are used, the stump should be wrapped in a figure-eight configuration to create even pressure. Whirlpool therapy should not be used on uninfected wounds because it promotes edema. There is evidence that stumps heal more quickly with rigid dressings (casts) and may have a lower incidence of phantom pain. However, the rigid dressing does not allow for frequent viewing of wounds.

The physiatrist should be consulted preoperatively if possible, and if not, immediately postoperatively, in order to assess the patient and discuss the rehabilitation process as well as long-term goals. Immediate postoperative goals include maintaining range of motion, edema control, pain management, and strengthening of uninvolved extremities. As wounds heal, strengthening of the residual limb is helpful. In the traumatic lower extremity amputee, transfer training and ambulation with crutches or a walker should begin as soon as possible. Likewise, activities of daily living (ADL) training for the upper extremity amputee should begin quickly. Traumatic amputees have much better functional outcomes than amputees who have lost their limbs because of peripheral vascular vascular disease or tumor.[28,29]

Pain management may be problematic after traumatic amputation. Stump pain usually begins to resolve several days postoperatively but can continue up to several months. Pain that fails to resolve is often due to neuromas, adhesions, or limited muscle padding over bone ends. Phantom sensation occurs in 70–80% of amputees, is not a problem, but can worry the patient. Reassurance that phantom sensation is not delusional thinking is all that is needed. Phantom pain, by contrast, occurs in about 20% of cases and is difficult to treat.[28] Phantom pain is central in origin; local treatments to the stump have no effect. Modalities such as transcutaneous electrical nerve stimulation (TENS), massage, biofeedback, and acupuncture can be helpful. Analgesic medications, tricyclic antidepressants, anticonvulsants, and beta blockers can also alleviate the pain. Only the tricyclics, tramadol, and gabapentin have been conclusively proven to be beneficial in studies.[29,30] Such medications should be used systematically. The chronic use of long-acting narcotic medications may be indicated in some of these patients.

Replantation in upper extremity amputation has become more commonplace, and success in revascularization and limb survival is high. Return-to-function rates are in the range of 40–60%.[31] Recovery is significantly better for upper extremity replantation than for early amputation and prosthesis. Functional recovery depends on nerve recovery, but a large component depends on patient motivation, as the rehabilitative period may be quite long.[32] Early after replantation, attention to edema management as well as the avoidance of smoking, the use of caffeine, and cold environments is important, as is careful splinting. Early passive and controlled active range-of-motion exercises should be instituted under direct supervision. Later, active range-of-motion exercise, dynamic splinting, and early strengthening exercises may begin. The lack of protective sensation must be considered in any therapy so as to prevent pressure or thermal injury. Manual skill development and occupational therapy must be planned for patient reintegration into prior activities.

## Hand Injuries

Hand injuries—including fractures, dislocations, burns, and sprains—are quite common. Keys to treatment include edema control, maintenance of range of motion, splinting, scar suppression, pain reduction, and muscle reeducation.

Significant edema frequently occurs with hand injuries. It can also occur without direct hand trauma in patients with more proximal upper extremity injuries or those with decreased serum proteins as well as through lack of movement. Edema leads to fibrosis, with resulting loss of function, and predisposes to infection. Range-of-motion exercises, massage, elevation of the hands, splinting, elastic wraps, and compression pumps are useful for edema control.

Splinting is useful after many hand injuries. Static splints maintain positioning, prevent contractures, and reduce edema. Dynamic splints allow motion over a controlled range. Precise fitting of orthotics is crucial. Strengthening and coordination exercises are a key component of hand rehabilitation. At the same time, muscle reeducation is important.

Pain is a common problem after hand injuries and can be disabling. The hand has intense sensory innervation and can become extremely painful after injury. Desensitization is often successful. This involves gradual exposure of the hand to increasing cutaneous stimulation to build up tolerance. Massage and pain-relieving modalities such as fluidotherapy, hot packs, ultrasound, paraffin, and TENS can be helpful. Heating modalities should not be used in patients with infected hands, impaired sensation, or cognitive deficits. Medications—including nonsteroidal anti-inflammatory drugs, tricyclic antidepressants, anticonvulsants, alpha-adrenergic blockers, and narcotics—are also useful adjuncts to the pain management program. In more severe cases, nerve blocks may be necessary.

## Nerve Injuries

Peripheral nerve and plexus injuries are common. Some 65% of patients with amputation, 55% with fractures, 45% with spinal cord injuries, and 32% with traumatic brain injury suffered plexus or peripheral nerve injuries as part of their injury complex during the first Persian Gulf War.[33] Some 21% of upper extremity nerve entrapments are road crash-related.[34] Patterns of nerve injury vary with the cause. The majority of crash-related nerve injuries occur in the upper extremity.[24] Multiple injuries are common. In road crashes, 91% of such injuries are sustained by drivers. The driver of the vehicle often sustains median nerve injury at the wrist and ulnar nerve injury at the elbow.

Brachial plexus injury is frequently due to traction on an abducted arm.[35] Complete brachial plexus injuries are usually secondary to road crashes and cause complete upper extremity paralysis and sensory loss just below the shoulder. The most common injury is to the lower brachial plexus and results in a claw-hand deformity and decreased sensation in the ulnar zone. Brachial cord injuries are common with stab and gunshot wounds. The axillary nerve is frequently entrapped by shoulder dislocations and humeral neck fractures, while the musculocutaneous nerve is occasionally injured in humeral fractures. Radial nerve lesions are frequently in humeral fractures. They produce elbow, wrist, and finger extension paralysis and decreased sensation on the dorsal forearm and radial dorsal hand. Median nerve compression is seen in shoulder dislocation, wrist fractures, and gunshot wounds; it causes weakness of pronation and finger flexion. Ulnar nerve injuries are seen in wrist and elbow fractures as well as stab and gunshot wounds, producing decreased sensation in the ulnar distribution and claw-hand deformity.

Lumbosacral plexus injuries are usually associated with pelvic fracture and are usually incomplete. The sciatic nerve is injured by pelvic and femoral fractures as well as gunshot wounds to the buttock and thigh. These injuries produce knee flexion paralysis,

paralysis at the ankle, and decreased sensation over the posterior thigh, posterior and lateral leg, and sole of the foot. The common peroneal nerve is frequently injured in fibular head fractures. This produces dorsiflexion weakness and numbness on the dorsum of the foot. The tibial nerve is occasionally injured in tibial and ankle fractures, causing plantarflexor weakness and decreased sensation on the plantar surface of the foot.

The clinical examination is crucial in diagnosing plexus and peripheral nerve injuries. Plain x-rays will not show nerve injuries but can indicate the types of fractures likely to cause nerve entrapment. Magnetic resonance imaging (MRI) may be helpful in diagnosing plexus injuries. Electrodiagnosis may be useful in the diagnosis of both peripheral nerve and plexus injuries. In some situations, it may be 2–3 weeks postinjury before electrodiagnosis is conclusive.

Treatment varies with the type of injury, its severity, and the patient's clinical status. Surgery can be useful to relieve compression and for nerve grafting. Bracing to maintain range of motion and function in injuries of the median, ulnar, and peroneal nerves may be useful. Physical and occupational therapists work to maintain range of motion, strengthen alternative muscles, instruct in proper use of braces, ambulation, and ADLs. It is crucial to make clear to patients that nerve injuries may require many months to resolve, and that their deficits may be permanent.

## Pain Management

Pain management is of particular importance in the care of patients undergoing the rehabilitation process.[36] Acute pain must be reduced to allow patient cooperation with range of motion and strengthening, particularly for those with extremity injury. Chronic pain syndromes present challenges for those with amputation, extremity injury, brain injury, or SCI and frequently require a multidisciplinary approach. Traditional drug therapy must often be supplemented by novel approaches, and nontraditional therapists. Anesthesiologists, physiatrists, and/or psychiatrists may provide leadership for pain management.

## Complex Regional Pain Syndrome

Complex regional pain syndrome (CRPS) was originally recognized by Weir Mitchell in 1864.[37] Other names commonly used for this syndrome include *causalgia* and *reflex sympathetic dystrophy*. The diagnostic criteria for CRPS include the presence of an initiating noxious event or a cause of immobilization. In type I CRPS, no specific nerve injury or causalgia can be identified, while in type II CRPS, nerve injury is present. Continuing and/or spontaneous pain, allodynia (pain provoked by innocuous stimuli), and hyperalgesia disproportionate to any inciting event. These three correlate to abnormal pain processing. Autonomic nervous system dysfunction that manifests itself as edema, changes in skin blood flow, or sudomotor activity in the region of pain, and the exclusion of all other diagnoses.[38]

Patient assessment should include attempts to identify the initiating event. Most cases of CRPS I develop after trauma. The most common are fractures, surgery, or crush injury. Less common events include vascular trauma and immobilization from casting. CRPS II develops as a result of injury to peripheral nerves.

The evaluation should include a description of both the quality and severity of pain and the interval between the inciting event and the time when the pain became out of proportion to the perceived cause. The examiner must seek signs of autonomic nervous system dysfunction (vasomotor changes), sudomotor dysfunction (asymmetrical sweating), movement dysfunction, and the presence of edema. Other disorders must be excluded. Diagnostic studies such as plain radiographs, electromyography, MRI, autonomic nervous system testing, or quantitative sensory testing may be warranted.

Patients with CRPS may develop myofascial pain syndrome surrounding the joint supporting the affected limb. This syndrome develops as a result of abnormal posturing or bracing of the limb. Patients with CRPS often use protective positioning in order to avoid stimulation that increases pain. Patients with myofascial pain syndrome develop a deep aching pain associated with muscle spasm and detectable trigger points, unlike the symptoms of CPRS itself.

It is important to diagnose CRPS early so that therapy/treatment can be started before irreversible changes occur. Nonsteroidal anti-inflammatory drugs aid in reducing neurogenic inflammation as well as decreasing the symptoms of myofascial pain syndrome. Tricyclic antidepressants block peripheral sodium channels, which accumulate on injured axons, inhibit norepinepherine and serotonin reuptake, and block the *N*-methyl d-aspartate receptor found in the dorsal horn of the spinal cord. Antiepileptic agents block the GABA receptor. Sympathetic blocks may be performed for pain reduction. Often several different treatments must be tried before finding one that works.

Rehabilitative maneuvers should be performed with caution in patients with CRPS. Extremes of heat and cold must be avoided. More than 90% of these patients' disease is a result of either a trauma and/or a surgical procedure. Non-weight-bearing, low-resistance exercises should be prescribed. Range-of-motion exercises should be done to prevent contractures from forming. Attention should be focused on the release of trigger points and muscle spasm.

## Comorbidity and Age

There have been few studies regarding the impact of preinjury medical conditions or age on functional outcome in trauma. Oreskovich described a population of elderly trauma victims in which only 8% returned to their previous level of function.[39] Since that time, other investigators have found that approximately 70% of injured elderly return to independent function after surviving injury.[40,41] Injury-related factors that affect outcomes are central nervous system injury, shock, and sepsis.

Pre-existing medical conditions may necessitate modification of the rehabilitation plan. Neuropsychiatric problems and drug dependency must be addressed as part of rehabilitation, and care should be taken to reduce physical expectations of those with limits imposed by cardiac, pulmonary, peripheral vascular or other disease.

Age alone is not a contraindication to rehabilitative efforts, but age related poorer outcome occurs even among those over 45 years of age, especially those with brain injury.[42] Those at extreme old age have a high likelihood of poor outcome.

## OUTCOME SCALING AND PREDICTION

Injury scaling has been important in the assessment of both patient status and system performance. Although some of these scales, such as the GCS, are useful in the management of individual patients, most are useful primarily for studying populations, not single patients. Numerous scales have been devised to assess the functional outcome of illness and injury. These scales address brain injury, disabilities, communication function, cognitive function, and general outcomes of function and wellness; many have both objective and subjective components.[42] A complete discussion of individual scales is beyond the scope of this chapter. Most of these scales are research tools and not intended for clinical use. Simple scales such as the GCS or Rancho Los Amigos Scale for head injury are useful for clinical outcome scoring.

The use of common scales by both trauma and rehabilitation centers is important to both patient follow-up and research. It is important to collect functional outcome data in trauma center databases.[43]

Attempts to apply anatomic or physiologic injury severity scoring to the predictions of functional outcome have had limited success. Rehabilitation scores that can predict functional outcome are difficult to perform early in the course of severe injuries. At present, prediction of functional outcome for individual patients is often difficult, with predictions being based on injury patterns, a knowledge of the literature, and, to a large extent, the personal experience of the treating team. The importance of such prognostication has been emphasized by the increased use of patients' rights of self-determination, such as the use of advance directives, and decisions regarding the need to limit (or withdraw) therapy for patients who have little or no chance of independent function. In such cases, evaluation and prognostication by multiple members of the treating team may be necessary in order to assure that decisions to withhold or withdraw care are made in an ethical and informed manner.

## ACCESS TO REHABILITATION

Recent advances in rehabilitation services have allowed disabled individuals to lead more productive lives—at a price. Rehabilitation services are expensive. In 2004, the total cost of SCI in the United States was at least $8 billion. Lifetime costs per SCI case ranged from $453,000 for older paraplegics, to $2.8 million for young high tetraplegics.[44]

Rehabilitation services are often difficult (or impossible) to arrange for patients with limited financial resources, poor social support, or both. Medicare and Medicaid generally do not pay for inpatient or outpatient traumatic brain injury (TBI) programs. Undocumented aliens frequently have neither funding nor eligibility for government programs to fund acute care or rehabilitative services. In some states, funds for auto crash victims may be held up until court cases settle. Many patients have no insurance, while others exhaust their insurance funds while still in acute care. Shortly after admission, Social Services should investigate insurance coverage, financial resources, support systems, and patient preferences. Cultural issues must be considered in the assessment of these factors.

Not all seriously injured trauma patients are rehabilitation candidates. All insurance companies monitor patient progress, both to justify the need for rehabilitation hospitalization and continued rehabilitative treatment.

Case management programs are designed to optimized resource utilization for the individual patient. The role of the case manager is to assess, plan, implement, coordinate, and monitor an injured patient's health needs as a means of controlling health care costs. Case managers' goals in management may be dependent upon their relationship to the patient. Institutional case managers attempt to optimize institutional resource utilization, and work with the patient to monitor and expedite the injured patient's progress through the system. The external case manager manages the claim for an employer or insurance company in order to assure that the patients receive care in a manner which controls costs for the payer.

Rehabilitation services should not be continued for patients failing to progress. Patients who have not shown progress in therapy in the acute care setting may not be accepted for admission to rehabilitation facilities.

It is crucial to refer patients to the appropriate rehabilitation program. Most patients with moderate to severe brain injury should be referred to facilities specializing in TBI, preferably with a dedicated unit. Likewise, spinal cord-injured patients are better cared for at facilities with a large experience with such patients. Acute rehabilitation centers provide an average of five hours per day of coordinated therapies. Subacute rehabilitation centers offer a coordinated therapy program with less intensity. Patients typically receive 2.5 hours per day of therapy, at lower costs. These programs may be more appropriate for patients with complicated medical illness or decreased endurance. For patients with more limited rehabilitation potential, nursing homes with a limited therapy program may be more suitable.

As patients progress, day hospital programs may provide coordinated therapies in an outpatient environment. These programs are particularly successful with TBI patients, often after an acute rehabilitation stay. These programs cost much less than acute or subacute rehabilitation, but require that the patient be mobile, and stable medically. Many patients benefit from home rehabilitation services and home health services, either directly after discharge from the hospital or after a stay in a rehabilitation facility. Such arrangements are often viewed quite favorably by patients.

Ultimately the goal of rehabilitation is to return each patient to as much independent function as is possible. Activities of daily living, return to previous employment (work, school, domestic), retraining for new employment, return to driving, and return to recreational activities all need to be considered in planning care for the individual and evaluating both individual and system outcomes.

## REFERENCES

1. National Research Council: *Accidental Death and Disability: The Neglected Disease of Modern Society.* Washington, DC: U.S. Government Printing Office, 1966.
2. Web-based Injury Statistics Query and Reporting System [database on the Internet]: National Center for Injury Prevention and Control, 2005; available from: http://www.cdc.gov/ncipc/wisqars
3. Report on Injuries in America, 2003 in: National Safety Council *Injury Factbook* 2004. National Safety Council, Itasca, NY.
4. Frankowski RF, Annegers JF, Whitman S: Epidemiological and descriptive studies. Part I: Descriptive epidemiology of head trauma in the United States. In Becker DP, Povlishock JT, eds. *Central Nervous System Trauma Status Report.* Bethesda, MD: National Institute of Neurologic and Communicative Disorders and Stroke, National Institute of Health, 1985.
5. MacKenzie EJ, Shapiro S, Smith RT, et al.: Factors influencing return to work following hospitalization for traumatic injury. *Am J Public Health* 77:329, 1987.
6. World Health Organization: *International Classification of Impairments and Handicaps.* Geneva, WHO, 1980.
7. Niemeier JP, Kreutzer JS, Taylor LA: Acute cognitive and neurobehavioral intervention for individuals with acquired brain injury: Preliminary outcome data. *Neuropsychol Rehab* 15:129, 2005.

8. de Guise E, Leblanc J, et al.: Prediction of the level of cognitive functional independence in acute care following traumatic brain injury. *Brain Injury* 19:1087, 2005.

9. Tiersky LA, Anselmi V, et al.: A trial of neuropsychological rehabilitation in mild-spectrum traumatic brain injury. *Arch PM&R* 86:1565, 2005.

10. Groswassner Z, Cohen M, Blankstein E: Polytrauma associated with traumatic brain injury: Incidence, nature, and impact on rehabilitation outcome. *Brain Injury* 4:161, 1990.

11. Nickels JL, Schneider WN, Dombovy ML, et al.: Clinical use of amantadine in brain injury rehabilitation. *Brain Injury* 8:709, 1994.

12. Kraus MF, Maki P: The combined use of amantadine and I-dopa/carbidopa in the treatment of chronic brain injury. *Brain Injury* 11:455, 1997.

13. Whyte J, Hart T, Schuster K, et al.: Effects of methylphenidate on attentional function after traumatic brain injury. *Am J Phys Med Rehabil* 76:440, 1997.

14. Meythaler JM, Depalma L, Devivo MJ, et al.: Sertraline to improve arousal and alertness in severe traumatic brain injury secondary to motor vehicle crashes. *Brain Injury* 15:321, 2001.

15. Reinhard DL, Whyte J, Sandel ME: Improved arousal and initiation following tricyclic antidepressant use in severe brain injury. *Arch PM&R* 77:8, 1996.

16. Cattelani R, Gugliotta M, Maravita A, et al.: Post-concussive syndrome: Paraclinical signs, subjective symptoms, cognitive function and MMPI profiles. *Brain Injury* 10:187, 1996.

17. Burney RE, Maio RF, Maynard F, et al.: Incidence, characteristics and outcome of spinal cord injuries at trauma centers in North America. *Arch Surg* 128:596, 1993.

18. Butcher JL, MacKenzie EJ, Cushing B, et al.: Long term outcomes after lower extremity trauma. *J Trauma* 41:4, 1996.

19. Gruen GS, Leit ME, Gruen RJ, et al.: Functional outcome of patients with unstable pelvic ring fractures stabilized with open reduction and internal fixation. *J Trauma* 39:838, 1995.

20. Burd TA, Lowry KJ, Anglen JO: Indomethacin compared with localized irradiation for the prevention of heterotopic ossification following surgical treatment of acetabular fractures. *J Bone Joint Surg Am* 83:1783, 2001.

21. Rhodes M, Aronson J, Moerkirk G, et al.: Quality of life after the trauma center. *J Trauma* 28:931, 1988.

22. Holbrook TL, Anderson JP, Sieber WJ, et al.: Outcome after major trauma: 12-month and 18-month follow-up results from the Trauma Recovery Project. *J Trauma* 46:765, 1999.

23. Anke AGW, Stanglelle JK, Finset A, et al.: Long-term prevalence of impairments and disabilities after multiple trauma. *J Trauma* 42:54, 1997.

24. Grotz M, Hohensee A, Remmers D, et al.: Rehabilitation results of patients with multiple injuries and multiple organ failure and long-term intensive care. *J Trauma* 42:919, 1997.

25. Anderson V, Catroppa C: Recovery of executive skills following paediatric traumatic brain injury (TBI): a 2-year follow-up. *Brain Inj* 19:459, 2005.

26. Kay HW, Newman JD: Relative incidences of new amputations. *Orthot Prosthet* 29:3, 1975.

27. Esquenazi A, Meier RH: Rehabilitation in limb deficiency: 4. Limb amputation. *Arch Phys Med Rehabil* 77:S18, 1996.

28. Jain S: Rehabilitation in limb deficiency: 2. The pediatric amputee. *Arch Phys Med Rehabil* 77:S9, 1996.

29. Bone M, Critchley P, Buggy, DL: Gabapentin in postamputation phantom limb pain: a randomized, double-blind, placebo-controlled, cross-over study. *Reg . Anesth Pain Med* 27:481, 2002.

30. Wilder-Smith CH, Hill LT, Laurent S: Postamputation pain and sensory changes in treatment-naïve patients: characteristics and responses to treatment with tramadol, amitriptyline, and placebo. *Anesthesiology* 103:619, 2005.

31. Graham B, Adkins P, Tsai TM, et al.: Major replantation versus revision amputation and prosthetic fitting in the upper extremity: A late functional outcomes study. *J Hand Surg* 23A:783, 1998.

32. Papanastasiou S: Rehabilitation of the replanted upper extremity. *Plast Reconstr Surg* 109:978, 2002.

33. Dillingham TR, Spellman NT, Braverman SE, et al.: Analysis of casualties referred to army physical medicine during the Persian Gulf conflict. *Am J Phys Med Rehabil* 72:214, 1993.

34. Coert JH, Dellon AL: Peripheral nerve entrapment caused by motor vehicle crashes. *J Trauma* 37:191, 1994.

35. Adams RD, Victor M (eds): *Principles of Neurology*, 5th ed. New York: McGraw-Hill, 1993, p. 1156.

36. Cohen SP, Christo PJ, Moroz L: Pain Management in Trauma Patients. *Am J Phys Med Rehabil* 83:142, 2004.

37. Mitchell SW, Morehouse GR, Keen WW: *Gunshot Wounds and Other Injuries of Nerves*. Philadelphia: Lippincott, 1864.

38. Schwartzman RJ, Popescu A: Reflex sympathetic dystrophy. *Curr Rheumatol Rep* 4:165, 2002.

39. Oreskovich MR, Haward JD, Copass MK, et al.: Geriatric trauma: Injury patterns and outcome. *J Trauma* 24:565, 1984.

40. vanAalst JA, Morris JA, Yates HK, et al.: Severely injured geriatric patients return to independent living: A study of factors influencing function and independence. *J Trauma* 1096, 1991.

41. Carillo EH, Richardson JD, Malias MA: Long term outcome of blunt trauma care in the elderly. *SG&O* 176:559, 1993.

42. Livingston DH, Lavery RF, Mosenthal AC, et al.: Rovocovery at one year following isolated traumatic brain injury. *J Trauma* 59:1298, 2005.

43. Copes WS, Stark MM, Lawnick MM, et al.: Linking data from national trauma and rehabilitation registries. *J Trauma* 40:428, 1996.

44. Spinal Cord Injury facts and figures at a glance (June, 2005) Spinal Cord Injury Information Network. National Institute for Spinal Cord Injury Statistics, National Institute for Disability and Rehabilitation Research (NIDRR), 2005. Available from: http://www.spinalcord.uab.edu/Spinal Cord

# Commentary ■ R. STEPHEN SMITH

Rehabilitation of the multiply injured patient is a vital component in the spectrum of optimal trauma care. Despite its importance, rehabilitation is often not appropriately emphasized in the early treatment of the injured. The positive impact of early rehabilitation is poorly understood and underappreciated by many health care providers involved in initial treatment of the trauma patient, even those that practice in Level 1 trauma centers. This important aspect of care should begin during the first day of hospitalization, as the ultimate goal for injured patients is to restore as much function as possible, as quickly as possible. Every member of the trauma team should be acutely aware of the importance of early rehabilitation.

In this chapter, Bodofsky and Ross have provided a thorough overview of current principles of rehabilitation for injured patients. They have provided a sound review of rehabilitation practices that are essential to optimal outcome. Additionally, they have provided significant insight into the positive social and economic impact of optimal rehabilitation of the injured. As Bodofsky and Ross point out, inadequate efforts toward rehabilitation have been identified as problematic in trauma care for a number of decades. In many otherwise excellent trauma centers, the development of rehabilitation services continues to trail behind other aspects of care for the injured patient.

This chapter offers accurate and up to date information that may be used to organize or upgrade trauma rehabilitation services. Bodofsky and Ross have, in fact, written a primer in rehabilitation medicine for the trauma surgeon. One of the greatest assets of this chapter is an exhaustive description of functions of members of the rehabilitation team and the roles they play in facilitating optimal recovery. Upon completion of this chapter, the reader will clearly understand the essential interaction of the members of the multidisciplinary rehabilitation team.

The rehabilitation efforts for patients with specific injuries to the various anatomic regions and organ systems must be individualized.

While general principles of rehabilitation hold true for patients with medical and surgical illnesses, trauma patients have specific needs and requirements that differentiate them from the general rehabilitation population. Drs. Bodofsky and Ross provide an exceptional overview of rehabilitation requirements for patients with a variety of specific organ system injuries. Their discussion of traumatic brain injury and the special problems and needs associated with this group of patients includes many aspects of rehabilitation that are not readily apparent to those involved in the acute care of trauma, including trauma surgeons and neurosurgeons. This discussion includes topics as far ranging as prediction of neurologic outcome to prevention and treatment of decubitus ulcers. Their discussion of rehabilitation for the patient with minor and moderate brain injuries reminds us that the problems of these patients are frequently overlooked. Issues regarding the particular problems associated with SCI and paralysis, as well multiple orthopedic injuries and polytrauma are fully discussed. The special problems involved with rehabilitation of pediatric patients are emphasized.

Severe injury to an extremity requiring amputation is one of the most devastating scenarios for the injured patient and requires rehabilitation efforts on the psychological and social, as well as, physical fronts. These patients present a number of special problems. This chapter provides an in-depth discussion of the issues and problems associated with specific types of amputations. The discussion of pain management after amputation for trauma is informative and practical. Members of the trauma team understand that pain management is a vital component of the initial care of injured patients. Less well understood is the impact of chronic pain and its effect on outcome. Drs. Bodofsky and Ross provide an excellent overview of the principles of pain management for injured patients and their discussion of the complex regional pain syndrome is extensive. The authors describe one of the most significant obstacles to optimal return of function: limited access to rehabilitation services. Practitioners at busy trauma centers are frequently confronted with the almost impossible task of placing injured patients in appropriate rehabilitation facilities. This task is frequently insurmountable if patients are unfunded or underinsured. The authors provide an excellent discussion that will enable trauma surgeons to understand the problems of access to rehabilitation and streamline their efforts toward obtaining rehabilitation services for their patients.

In summary, this is an excellent overview of the issues regarding rehabilitation of trauma patients. A thorough reading is recommended to all who care for injured patients.

## References

1. American College of Surgeons Committee on Trauma: *Resources for Optimal Care of the Injured Patient*, 2006.
2. Holbrook TL, Hoyt DB, Anderson JP, et al.: Functional limitation after major trauma: A more sensitive assessment using the quality of well-being scale: The Trauma Recovery Project. *J Trauma* 36:74, 1994.
3. Mock C, MacKenzie E, Jurkovich G, et al.: Determinants of disability after lower extremity fracture. *J Trauma* 49:1002, 1993.

# Modern Combat Casualty Care

*Peter Rhee* ■ *John Holcomb* ■ *Donald Jenkins*

## PREFACE

In military medicine, there is no greater honor and privilege than the opportunity to serve the men and women of the armed forces during war time. Caring for combat casualties is the ultimate reward for all military medical personnel. Working in an austere environment with limited resources and saving lives is a humbling and intensely emotional experience. The opportunity to help the injured, regardless of the casualty's political background is gratifying and constitutes a selfless and charitable action.

Wars have always fostered advances in trauma care.[1] During the decades of relative peace since the Vietnam conflict, the military has benefited tremendously from the civilian trauma community. Practice patterns at the beginning of the current conflict (November 2001) were dictated by the teachings and the advancements made by the leaders in the civilian trauma sector. Like all previous wars we will eventually bring home many lessons learned that will benefit the civilian sector. Since much has been written on the evolution and historical aspects of military surgery, the intent of this chapter is to enlighten those who are not in the military and those who are relatively new to the military system on the current state of affairs. Although there are many aspects of this war that remain unchanged, the important advances will be discussed. The way we treat casualties are revolutionary compared to the Vietnam era in many ways, and the hope is that the information provided will aid in future conflicts by minimizing reinvention of the wheel and allow progress to occur.

Modern warfare in many ways is different in comparison to historic wars. Previously battles were won by attrition of forces and those with the larger army claimed victory. Recent changes in modern warfare can be attributed much to our country's relative prosperity and resulting advancements in technology. This translated into superior equipment, logistics, maneuverability, and training. This equates to the use of a relatively small force in the rapid and nonlinear battlefield, which means that instead of gaining territory the battles are fought with precision with specific objectives and thereby eliminating the need to control all territories with a large military force. Many of these capabilities are due to advancements in technology (Fig. 55-1). Our current US military is without question unrivaled in capability. It can quickly mount an offensive maneuver with relatively small size and conduct a rapid, lethal, nonlinear warfare to win battles against enemies that are up to ten times larger in number and with a kill ratio ranging from 10–100 to one. For example, the Gulf war in 1991 was over in 100 hours and the "invasion phase" of the Iraqi war (Operation Iraqi Freedom I) was over in three weeks. Just as we remember the dominant armies of the past such as the Roman and the British Empire, our current military force will be recorded in history as most dominant force of our current modern civilization. In no previous time in history has a military been able to fight forces many times larger in numerous places in the world so rapidly. This era could arguably be recorded in the future as the American Empire.

This has also lead to changes in the way we provide surgical care in the field. This advancement in technology has resulted in better efficient care in many aspects. However, as in all wars, resources are not equivalent to modern civilian trauma centers and the well-trained surgeons who can rely on their clinical skills are still the backbone of combat casualty care. In the war in Iraq and Afghanistan, the fighting force was relatively small compared to the past. As we were able to do more with less, this affected our management of casualties.

## COMBAT TRAUMA EPIDEMIOLOGY

The focused experience of thousands of severe casualties galvanizes the military medical community to improve care in revolutionary ways. Wars have always served to accelerate improvements in trauma care. However, due to the fortunes of relative peace time, recent advances have been from the civilian trauma sector to the military

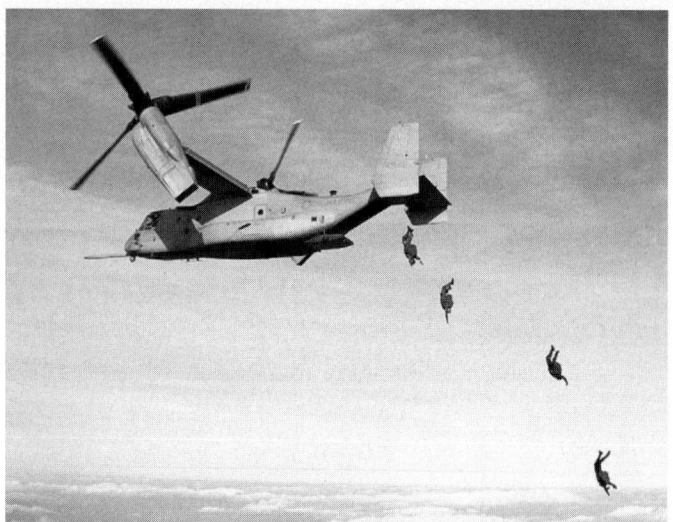

**FIGURE 55-1.** VR22 osprey allows for transport of troops and supplies over much longer distances. It can perform vertical landings and take off like a helicopter but can fly longitudinally like an airplane.

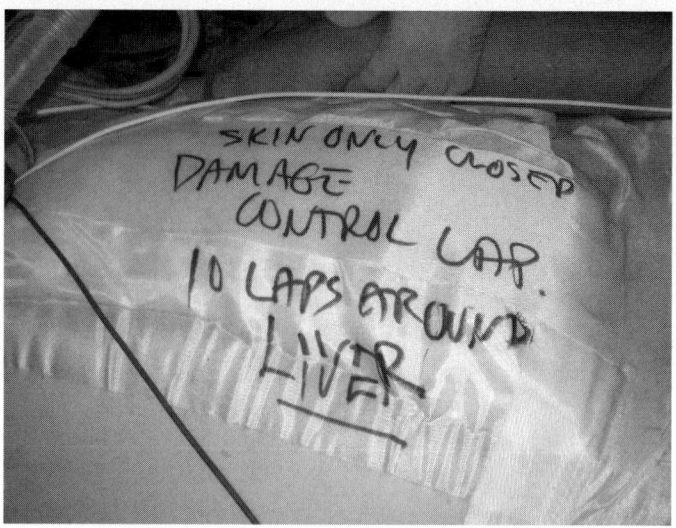

**FIGURE 55-2.** Abdominal dressing with information written on it after surgery. (Picture courtesy of H.R. Bockmon.)

sector. One such example is trauma registries. The backbone for advances has been, and will continue to be trauma registries. It is critical to know what is happening to our deployed troops in order to react and make continual improvements.

In response to the lack of a Department of Defense trauma registry, a joint theater trauma registry (JTTR) was recently developed taking into consideration the lessons learned from the civilian trauma sector. Through the efforts of the three Surgeons Generals and the Department of Health Affairs, a policy paper was published recently describing the minimum essential data elements needed to comprise uniform trauma data collection on the battlefield and to establish a JTTR.[2] The repository for this data is at the US Army Institute of Surgical Research at Ft Sam Houston, TX. This will allow feedback to commanders, researchers, soldiers, and physicians, allowing for data-driven changes to new tactics and interventions.

In addition to providing information to guide future changes, the intent of this databank is also to aid in the present treatment of combat casualty care as the fundamental electronic medical record. Access to this information worldwide by military providers would be tremendous leap in combat casualty care and would be an example for the civilian sector to follow. Advances in computer technology with portable thumb drives or other off-the-shelf memory devices may eventually function as an electronic dog tag and allow for electronic data to be transferred with the casualty throughout the multiple levels of care. At the beginning of the war, record transmission was difficult due to the rapid and urgent transport of severely injured and critically ill casualties across three continents in an unprecedented time (Fig. 55-2). The hope is that one day seamless transfer of information including trauma history and physicals, operative reports, digital pictures, digital videos, x-rays, and daily documentation may be deposited to a server in addition to traveling with the casualty.

While accurate understanding of the epidemiology and outcome of battle injury is essential to improving combat casualty care, data are acquired under notoriously difficult circumstances and involve variables unfamiliar to most who has not been in the field. How to account for injury time, wear of body armor, ground versus air evacuation, where and how to acquire injury data, the enormous impact of troop rotations and different services, etc. are significant obstacles for accurate data collection. The US Department of Defense (DoD) maintains two Internet websites providing information on combat casualties. The Defense link website (http://www.defenselink.mil/) has data on return to duty (RTD) casualties while the site maintained by the Directorate for Information Operations and Reports (http: //www.dior.whs.mil/mmid/casualty/castop.htm) provides information from the current and past conflicts in sufficient detail for calculation of proportional mortality (the fraction of an exposed group — those injured in combat — who die, expressed as a percent).

## Definitions

The term "casualty" must be approached with caution when reviewing military medical data. "Casualty" in customary military usage means active duty personnel lost to the theatre of operations for medical reasons.[3] The term therefore includes illness and noncombat injuries as well as combat injuries which are injuries sustained in combat during hostile engagement with a military enemy. However, using this definition, subgroups of casualties may be included or excluded from a given set of summary statistics, depending on the definitions in use at the time. The following definitions, taken from Bellamy, standardize the numbers to allow a reasonable retrospective comparison between conflicts:

*Wounded in Action (WIA)* is a key term used to define combat-injured casualties and is the sum of three subgroups as shown in Fig. 55-3. Conventionally, the subgroup of surviving WIAs who return to duty (RTD) within 72 hours is excluded from denominators when proportional statistics are presented. This is significant because this group traditionally represents about 50% of all wounded in action. The number and classification of wounded and deaths from combat is classically used to provide insights into the lethality of the battle, the effectiveness of the systems of care and evacuation, and focus attention on required areas of research.

*Case Fatality Rate (CFR)* refers to the fraction of an exposed group—all those wounded in action including all those who die (at any level), expressed as a percent. This summary statistic provides

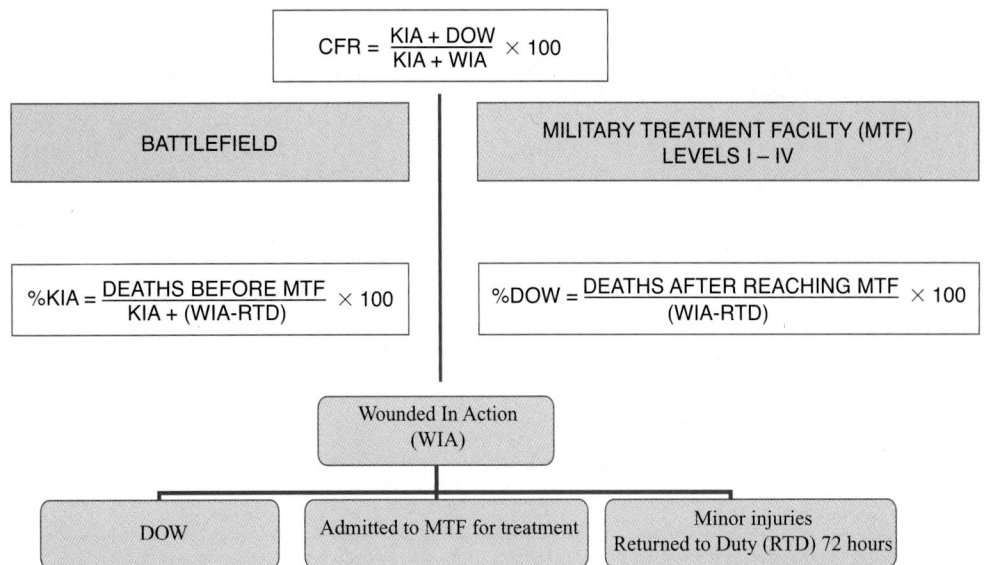

$$CFR = \frac{KIA + DOW}{KIA + WIA} \times 100$$

BATTLEFIELD

MILITARY TREATMENT FACILTY (MTF)
LEVELS I – IV

$$\%KIA = \frac{DEATHS\ BEFORE\ MTF}{KIA + (WIA\text{-}RTD)} \times 100$$

$$\%DOW = \frac{DEATHS\ AFTER\ REACHING\ MTF}{(WIA\text{-}RTD)} \times 100$$

Wounded In Action
(WIA)

DOW

Admitted to MTF for treatment

Minor injuries
Returned to Duty (RTD) 72 hours

**FIGURE 55-3.** CFR — case fatality rate, KIA — killed in action, DOW — died of wounds, WIA — wounded in action, MTF — military treatment facility, RTD — return to duty.

a measure of the overall lethality of the battlefield in those who receive combat wounds. It includes the RTDs that are excluded in the denominator of DOW and killed in action (KIA) rates defined below. However, this statistic has been used both with and without the RTD population, creating a major source of confusion when comparing data sets. Insufficient detail is provided by a CFR for detailed medical planning for reasons discussed below. The CFR is not a total mortality rate which would describe all deaths relative to the entire deployed population at risk.

*Killed in Action (KIA)* refers to the number of combat deaths that occur prior to reaching an MTF (battalion aid station, forward surgical, combat support, and higher levels of hospital care where a medical officer is present), expressed as a percent of the Wounded in Action minus the RTDs. This statistic provides a measure of (1) the lethality of the weapons (currently 82% of KIAs are near-instant deaths from nonsurvivable injuries that result from the massive destructive nature of military weapons); (2) the effectiveness of point-of-wounding and medic care; and (3) the availability of evacuation from the tactical setting. Factors that change KIA include body and vehicle armor, effectiveness of the trauma system in place, time from wounding to MTF, and care in the field either by the casualty, buddy, or medic/corpsman.

*Died of Wounds (DOW)* is the number of all deaths that occur after reaching an MTF, expressed as a percentage of total wounded minus the RTDs. This statistic provides a measure of the effectiveness of the MTF care and perhaps also of the appropriateness of field triage, initial care, optimal evacuation routes, and application of a coordinated trauma systems approach in mature combat settings. Deaths that occur at anytime after admission to an MTF are included in this category.

It is important to note that the above two statistics, %KIA and %DOW, have different denominators. The latter does not include deaths prior to reaching a medical treatment facility (or those who are dead on arrival at an MTF). This focuses %DOW as a measure of MTF care. However, both denominators use the same definition of a battle injury: the first two subgroups of WIA. The main difference is that the KIAs are excluded from the DOW calculations.

Over the past century, the %KIA has consistently remained between 20% and 25%. The %DOW dropped significantly towards the latter half of World War II when improved evacuation,

anesthesia, antibiotics, blood transfusion, and surgical techniques all coalesced to bring the %DOW to less than 5%, where it has stayed for the latter half of the 20th century. To put into perspective the previous and current wars the deaths incurred at the current time is shown on Table 55-1.

For Vietnam, the final compilations appear relatively complete and have been reviewed and revised officially.[4] Data sets of well-defined samples have been compiled and analyzed.[5,6] The Wound Data and Munitions Effectiveness Team (WDMET) database from the Vietnam War is arguably the most largest, complete, and detailed source of information to date on weapons and wounding but is on a sample of only 4% of the total Vietnam casualties between 1965 and 1969. This initiative provided a model for field data retrieval. However, early reporting on the medical consequences of both Vietnam and the current conflict have relied on reporting of data from individual medical units, with little or no outcome data available from the follow-on levels of care and are thus skewed.

The raw battle casualty data from the U.S. military engagement in Afghanistan and Iraq are available on the DIOR website. The Defense link website, which provides military casualty data for the conflict, distinguishes between the RTD and those more seriously wounded. By combining data from both websites, it is possible to adjust the Afghanistan/Iraq data to more accurately equate with the denominator provided by the DIOR site for Vietnam. Table 55-2 displays the summary data available from the two websites for the major categories of interest for Iraq and Afghanistan.

In the war in Iraq, Afghanistan case fatality rate for combat injury among U.S. military personnel was significantly lower than that seen during World War II and Vietnam. Some of this reduction may be due to widespread use of improved body armor as chest wounds are relatively decreased compared to previous conflicts.[7] However, there are many other factors including different tactics and technology, and use of armored vehicles. Additional contributing factors may include the successful transition of products from the 10-year DOD research program on improved hemorrhage control and increased focus on prehospital Tactical Combat Casualty Care training,[8] coupled with rapid evacuation. Some degree of reciprocity between KIA and DOW rates is expected[9,10] as many of the more severely injured casualties who in the past would have died before reaching MTF

**TABLE 55-1**

| US Military Deaths | | | | |
|---|---|---|---|---|
| | TOTAL DEATHS | DEATHS PER YEAR | US POPULATION DURING THE WAR | DEATHS/YEAR/ 100,000 |
| Revolution (1775–1783) | 4,435 | 493 | 3,929,884 | 12.6 |
| War Of 1812 (1812–1815) | 2,260 | 565 | 7,036,509 | 8.0 |
| Mexican War (1846–1848) | 13,283 | 4,428 | 17,019,678 | 26.0 |
| Civil War (1861–1865) | 623,026 | 124,605 | 30,383,684 | 410.1 |
| Spanish–American War (1898) | 2,446 | 2,446 | 61,116,815 | 4.0 |
| World War I (1917–1918) | 116,516 | 58,258 | 91,641,186 | 63.7 |
| World War II (1941–1945) | 405,399 | 81,080 | 130,962,661 | 62.6 |
| Korean War (1950–1953) | 36,574 | 9,144 | 149,895,183 | 6.2 |
| Vietnam War (1964–1975) | 58,200 | 5,291 | 178,554,916 | 3.0 |
| Persian Gulf War (1990–1991) | 382 | 382 | 248,709,873 | 0.05 |
| Afganistan War (Oct 7, 2001–2005) | 255 | 51 | 290,809,777 | 0.02 |
| Iraq War (March 19, 2003–2005) | 1,739 | 580 | 293,655,404 | 0.2 |

Afganistan and Iraq war was ongoing at the time of this table generation. The Iraq war excludes the 485 nonbattle injury deaths.

**TABLE 55-2**

| Comparison of Proportional Statistics for Battle Casualties, US Military Ground Troops, World War II, Vietnam, Afghanistan/Iraq | | | | | |
|---|---|---|---|---|---|
| | WW II[8,9] | VIETNAM[4] | TOTAL IRAQ/ AFGHANISTAN[1,2] | AFGHANISTAN[1,2] | IRAQ[1,2] |
| %KIA | 20.2[a] | 20.0[b] | 13.8[c] | 18.7 | 13.5[d] |
| %DOW | 3.5[a] | 3.2[b] | 4.8[c] | 6.7 | 4.7[d] |
| CFR | 19.1[a] | 15.8[b] | 9.4[c] | 16.4 | 9.1[d] |

Comparisons between WWII, Vietnam, and Total Iraq/Afghanistan, a,b,c, < 0.05.

Comparison between Iraq and Afghanistan, [d]p < 0.05.

care (KIA), now die after rapid evacuation to MTFs, changing their classification to DOW. The observed increase ($p < 0.01$) in DOW rates would likely be higher if not for the improvements in surgical management utilizing tactical damage control techniques, improved intensive care unit (ICU) care, liberal use of fresh whole blood, and recombinant factor VIIa (rFVIIa), among other new techniques.

Thoughtful review of KIA, DOW, and CFR rates for combat trauma are important for optimal medical planning, training, research, and resource allocation. The need to bring combat casualty epidemiology to a civilian standard requires utilization of both technology and organization that are routinely utilized in the U.S. civilian trauma community. Thanks to efforts by the Deputy Assistant Secretary of Defense for Health Affairs and the Surgeons General of each of the armed services, raw data appropriate for this effort are now being collected. Standard operational definitions are in use for the cataloging and analysis of this complex information. Injury severity data are recorded, scored, and analyzed by methods that both meet trauma-community standards and are appropriate to meet the unique aspects of battle injuries. If these efforts are successful, the current war will be the first in history from which detailed, concurrent analyses of the epidemiology, nature and severity of injuries, care provided, and patient outcomes can be used to guide research, training, and resource allocation for improved combat casualty care.

## Weapons of Mass Destruction (WMD)

This is an important topic that we must now learn to live with. WMD is a reality and the surgeon does need to be familiar with some of the potential agents that might be used. Biologic Warfare (BW) agents infect the body via the same portals of entry as infectious organisms that occur naturally. These include *inhalation* into the respiratory tract, *ingestion* into the GI tract, and absorption through mucous membranes, eyes, or wounds. Usually, the disease produced by a BW agent will mimic the naturally occurring disease but the clinical presentation can be different if delivery of an agent occurs through a portal that differs from the natural portal.

Detection of BW injury is suspected when there is a compressed epidemiology with record numbers of sick and dying in a short time, high attack rates (60–90%), high incidence of pulmonary involvement when usual form of infection is not (i.e., anthrax), incidence of a particular disease in an unlikely location, increased deaths of animals of all species, near simultaneous outbreaks of several different epidemics at the same site, or direct evidence of an attack such as contaminated or unexploded munitions.

The best defense against BW is prevention, to include immunizations (e.g., anthrax, smallpox, and plague), pre- or post-exposure chemoprophylaxis (e.g., anthrax, plague, Q fever, and tularemia) and use of protective clothing and mask. Infection control procedures should be reinforced for mass casualty situations involving BW agents. Universal precautions are appropriate for BW agents once they have been identified. For an undifferentiated febrile illness following a BW agent attack: place patients together in an isolated setting such as a designated tent or other structure; surgical masks may be placed on patients when isolation is not possible, and employ respiratory droplet precautions along with universal precautions until diseases transmissible by droplet (such as plague and smallpox) have been excluded.

Chemical agents fall into broad categories and treatment algorithms are readily available, based on presenting symptoms and suspected agents. These agents include: nerve agents (GA, GB, GD, GF, and VX); vesicants (HD, H, L, and CX); pulmonary (choking) agents (phosgene (CG), diphosgene (DP), and chlorine (CL)); the cyanides (Blood Agents AC and CK); and incapacitation agents (BZ and Agent 15).

Wound decontamination in chemical injury combined with traumatic injury presents the surgeon with a unique challenge. The initial management of a casualty contaminated by chemical agents will require removal of mission-oriented protective posture (MOPP) gear and initial skin and wound decontamination with 0.5% hypochlorite before treatment. This decontamination has several specific considerations: bandages are removed, wounds are flushed, and bandages replaced; tourniquets are replaced with clean tourniquets after decontamination; splints are thoroughly decontaminated; and bandages are removed in operating room (OR) and disposed of (submerged in 5% hypochlorite, or sealed in a plastic bag). Of note, only the vesicants and nerve agents present a hazard from wound contamination. Cyanide is so volatile that it is extremely unlikely it would remain in a wound.

During formal wound exploration and debridement in the ORs, surgeons and assistants should wear a pair of well-fitting, thin, butyl rubber gloves or double latex surgical gloves. Gloves should be changed often until certain that there are no foreign bodies or thickened agents remaining in the wound. Wound excision and debridement should be conducted using a no-touch technique. Removed fragments of tissue should be dumped into a container of 5–10% hypochlorite. Superficial wounds should be wiped thoroughly with a 0.5% hypochlorite solution and then irrigated with copious amounts of normal saline. Following the surgical procedure, instruments that come into contact with possible contamination should be placed in 5% hypochlorite for ten minutes prior to normal cleansing and sterilization. Reusable linen should be checked with the CAM, M8 paper, or M9 tape for contamination.

Radiological casualties on the battlefield may occur with conventional nuclear devices or radiological dispersal devices ("dirty bombs"). A nuclear detonation generally causes injuries with the following distribution: blast injury 50%; thermal injury 35%; and ionizing radiation injury 15%. If triage is occurring soon after a nuclear detonation, many victims may not yet manifest the symptoms of acute radiation injury. Therefore, conventional injuries (blast, burn, etc.) should be treated first and initial triage should be based on these injuries. Once there are clinical signs of acute radiation exposure (mainly GI symptoms of nausea, vomiting, and diarrhea), triage can be done again, likely placing many patients with combined radiation and other injuries in the expectant category. Hypotension should be always be assumed to be hypovolemia and not due to radiologic injury. Hyperthermia is common. Decontamination is paramount as early as possible after radiation exposure. Removal of the victim's clothing can remove as much as 80% of the radiologic contamination. The first priority of surface decontamination should be open wounds, then other areas. To prevent rapid incorporation of radioactive particles, wounds should be copiously irrigated with physiological saline for several minutes. The eyes, ears, nose, mouth, areas adjacent to uncontaminated wounds, and remaining skin surface should be decontaminated.

The usual methods of treatment for blast injuries must be modified in those casualties simultaneously exposed to ionizing radiation.

Traditionally, combat wounds are left open; however, wounds left open to heal by secondary intention in the irradiated patient will serve as a nidus of infection. Wounds exposed to ionizing radiation should be debrided and closed at a second look operation within 36–48 hours. Amputation should be seriously contemplated when the contamination burden is great and severe radionecrosis is likely. Radiological injuries increase the morbidity and mortality of injuries due to compromise of the normal hematopoietic and immune responses to injury. Surgical procedures may need to be delayed during bone marrow suppression if at all possible.

## CAUSES OF INJURIES

The causes of injuries during the Iraq/Afghanistan war are really no different than previous wars.[11,12] The vast majority are penetrating injuries with various velocities. They can be direct gunshot wounds but more common is the fragmentation injury after an explosion, whether they are caused by rockets, mortars, grenades, or improvised explosive devices[13] (Fig. 55-4). Accompanying blunt trauma injury can occur but is rather the exception than the rule. In the Iraqi war the distinct difference is that the fragmentation injuries are not from artillery or land mines but from "improvised explosive devices" or IEDs.[14] During the invasion phase of OIF I, injury from small arms was a higher source of injury but during the occupation phase, the fragmentation injury from IEDs is the main cause of wounding (Fig. 55-5). When referring to small arms fire, it has to be stressed that high-velocity rounds from hand-carried weapons which can cause tremendous tissue injury are included in this category.[15,16] IEDs are placed by insurgents and terrorists. Insurgents, which is a relatively new and popular term, is defined by Webster as a person who takes part in an armed rebellion against the constituted authority or a member or an irregular armed force that fights a stronger force by sabotage and harassments.

Whether they are from small arms fire or IED injuries, the common denominator is that the individual wounds are much worse than what is normally seen in urban civilian trauma,[17–19] and

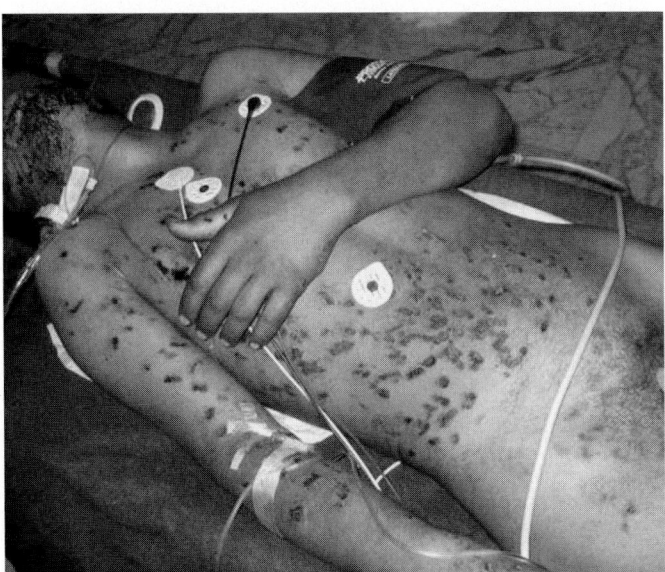

**FIGURE 55-4.** Fragmentation injuries causing ("peppered") multiple wounds.

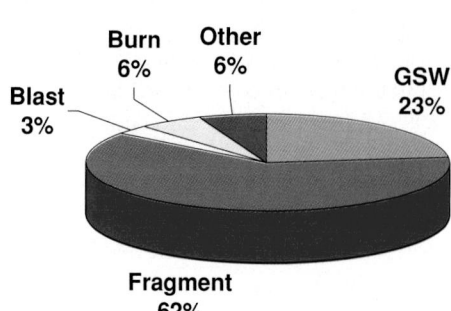

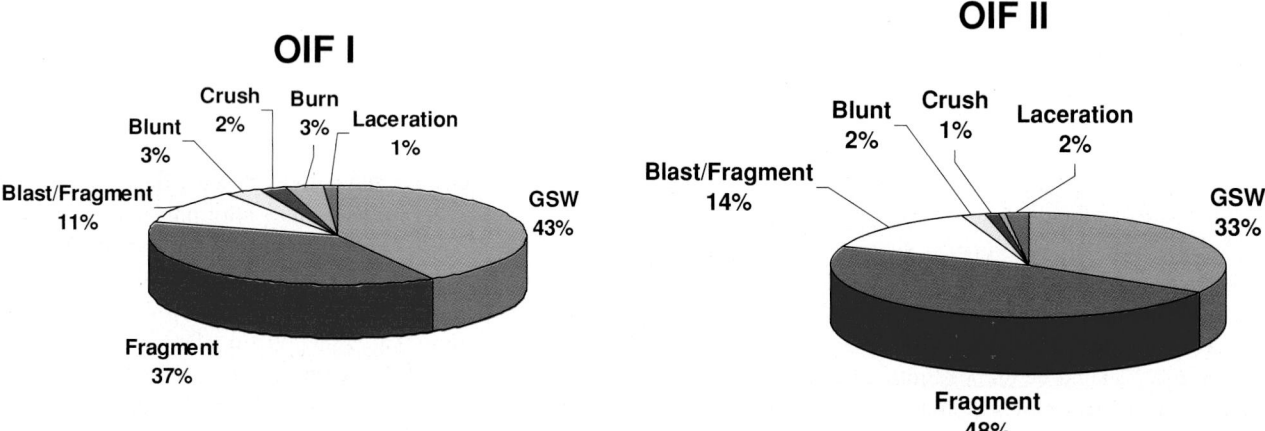

**FIGURE 55-5.** Mechanism of Injury. OIF I — Operation Iraqi Freedom I which was the invasion phase of the war beginning in March of 2002. OIF II — Operation Iraqi Freedom II was the occupation phase of the war which followed the invasion phase.

are frequently multiple. What is seemingly innocuous at the skin does not reflect the energy absorbed by the casualty. Sometimes a casualty may present with only one tiny small punctuate hole on the skin from a pellet dispersed from a suicide bomber.[20] This tiny pellet can traverse the entire thorax causing injury to both thoracies, transection of the spine, and penetration of the heart. The difference between civilian trauma and military wounds can be quite dramatic and this difference cannot be overemphasized.[21]

Due to the evolution of IEDs, the military vehicles had to be modified in theater to deal with the new weaponry of modern insurgents.[22,23] While in the past personal landmines were decreased in explosive power to cause a maiming injury to incapacitate and draw out more soldiers, the new IEDs are more similar to antitank mines and have been increased in explosive capability as they try to overcome the modern fortified equipment (Fig. 55-6). The result is that the energy transferred is much greater. Often there is no penetration into the compartments of the vehicles but occupants are sometimes killed from other bodies being projectiles within the vehicle (Fig. 55-7). Even if the vehicle is not penetrated, they can still cause severe injuries (Fig. 55-8).

The explosive devices are ingenious and they use any opportunity available with relatively small costs.[24] Military artillery rounds are commonly used as they are rigged with simple timing devices and triggering mechanisms. The fuses for the explosive devices are common household items including baker's time clocks to

garage door openers to cell phones. The trend now has been to incapacitate the vehicle with an IED that is buried, wait for the dismounting of the vehicles by the survivors, or the quick reaction team to come to the scene before a second or third IED is set off from the side or above from structures such as trees and poles. In addition, snipers are at the ready for the dismounted soldiers. The snipers have also learned the soft spots of the body armor which includes the sides of the torso and base of the neck in the front. Sniper rifles can penetrate the standard Kevlar helmet and while protection is offered and the projectile is slowed by the helmet, it is by no means foolproof[25–27] (Fig. 55-9). The protective effect of body armor is obvious during OIF, and this is best exemplified by comparing the distribution of injuries between the US forces and civilian casualties (Fig. 55-10). With the use of body armor the US versus Iraqi casualties in proportion are more likely to have extremity injuries. These injuries often are mangled extremities.

Explosive devices are also loaded into cars and these vehicle-borne improvised explosive devices (VBIED) can be highly lethal as the amount of explosive power that they carry leaves no wounded at times. Suicide improvised explosive devices (SIED) may not be new to some countries,[28–32] but the current US military is a novice in this arena. They cause tremendous explosions and hope for survival are slim if the soldier is in close proximity. In Ar Ramadi, Iraq, one suicide bomber caused 200 casualties as the bomber was mingling in the crowd during police recruitment.

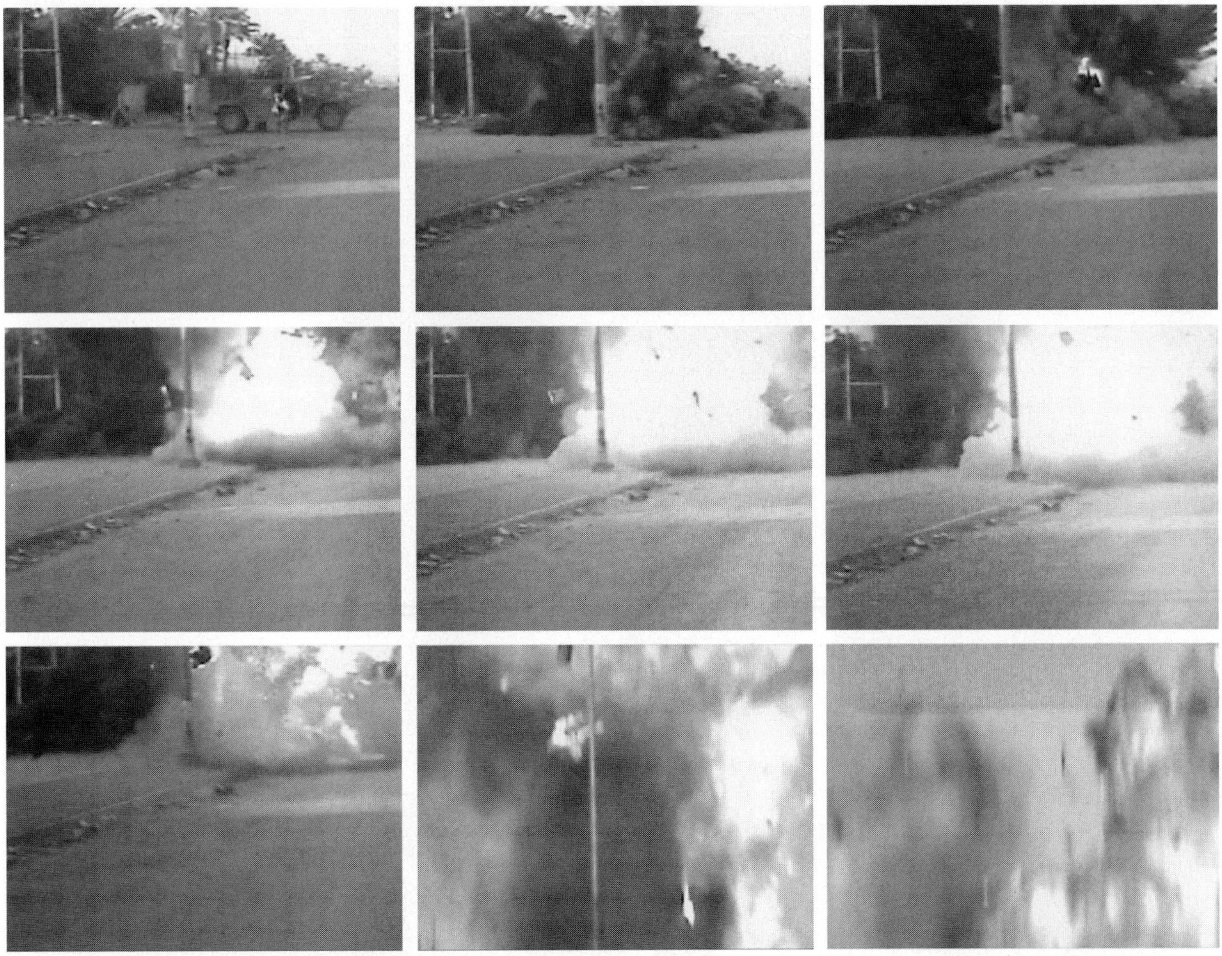

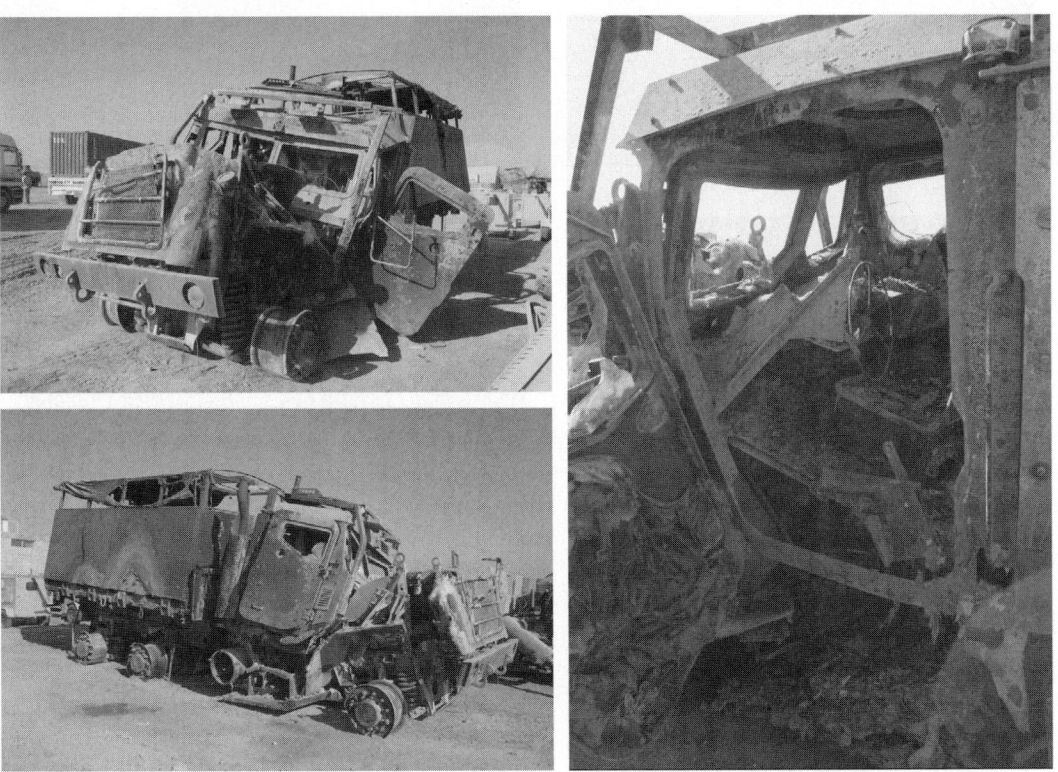

**FIGURE 55-6.** Example of the improvised explosive devices (IEDs) and their capability.

**FIGURE 55-7.** Vehicles destroyed by improvised explosive devices (IEDs).

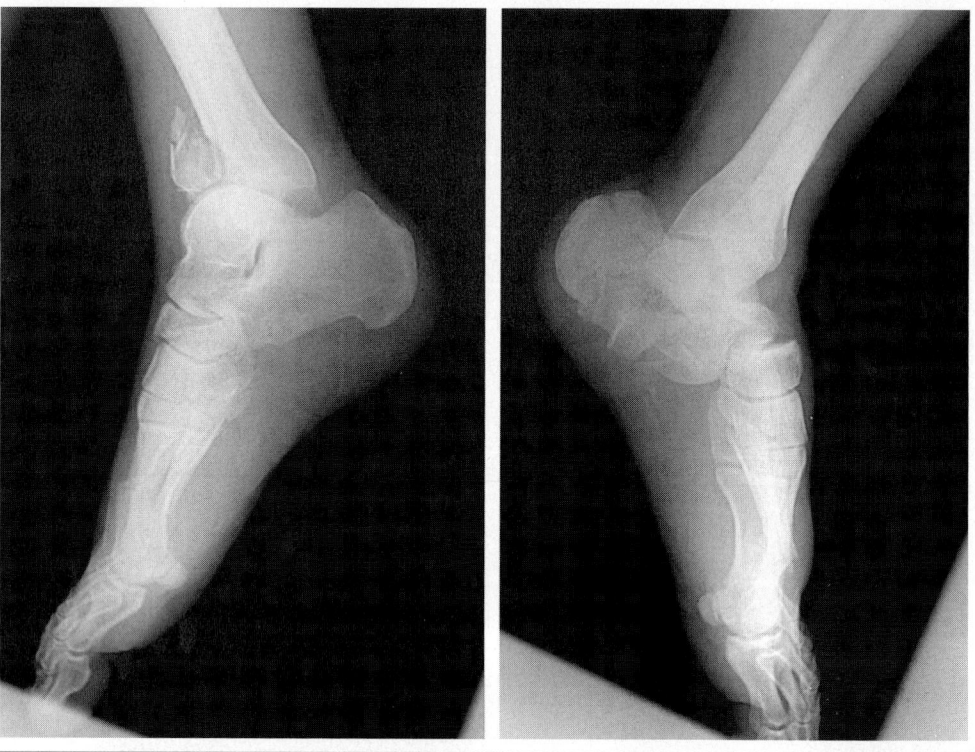

**FIGURE 55-8.** Bilateral ankle fractures from the fortified vehicle being hit by an IED underneath the vehicle. Even if the explosion is minor, the energy transmitted can cause serious injury.

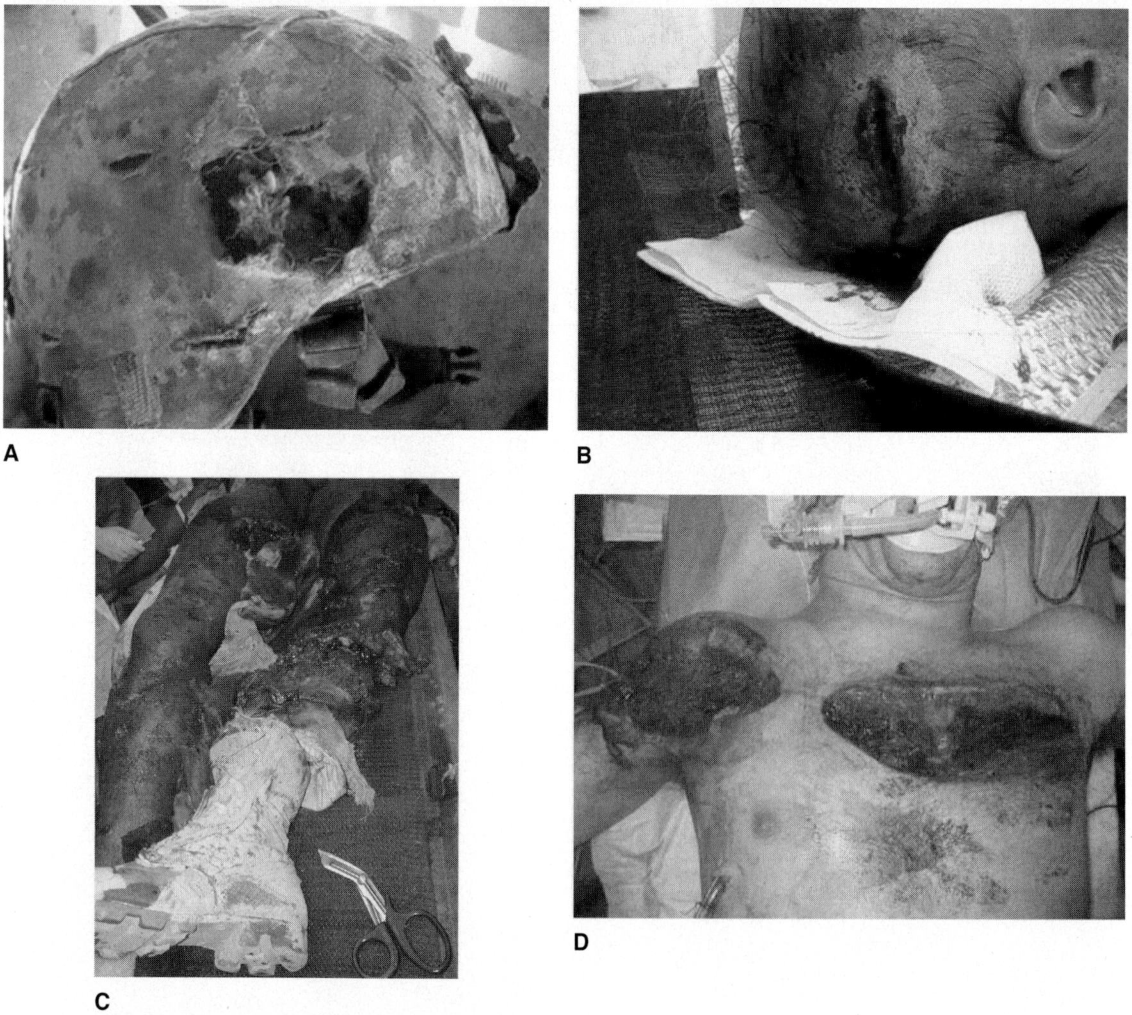

A

B

C

D

**FIGURE 55-9.** **(A,B)** Fortunate Marine who received sniper fire from AK74, and penetrated the Kevlar helmet but only grazed his scalp. **(C)** wounds to lower extremity which is not well protected by current body armor. **(D)** High-velocity round that went under the Kevlar.

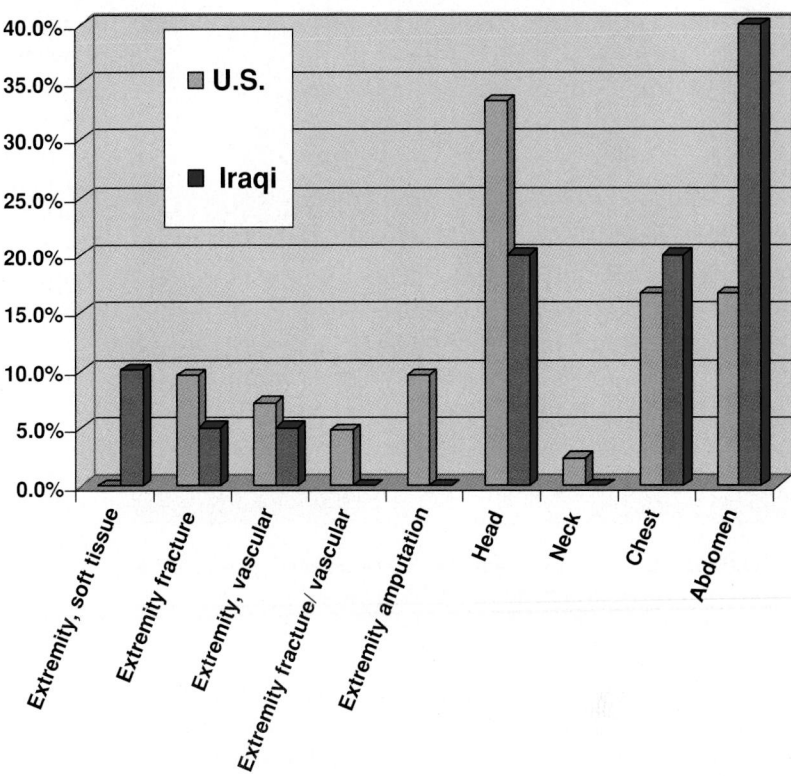

**FIGURE 55-10.** Difference in wounding between US forces and Iraqi who did not have robust body armor.

Survivors sustain injuries that are truly incomparable to civilian trauma (Fig. 55-11). One US casualty during this incident did have body armor on and had no discernible injuries on the exterior but was killed most likely instantaneously from the blast. In addition to the IEDs, mortars, shoulder-mounted rocket-propelled grenades are frequently used (Fig. 55-12). The number of injuries caused during the Iraq war has not been as high as it could potentially be as the accuracy of the rocket attacks on to the many military bases is extremely limited. Tubes are placed on rocks and aimed at military bases with minimal aiming capability or true knowledge of ballistics. Although on occasion they do cause damage to the base and personnel, most are harassing but not really effective.

Motor vehicle injuries cause a number of injuries and can be associated with IEDs as well. Although pure motor vehicle collisions (MVC) do occur, one must keep in mind that the velocity is lower and due to the weight of the military transport vehicles, the change in velocity which is one of the primary determinants in causes of injury is less than what is typically seen in civilian trauma centers. On the other hand, the military vehicles are not built for passenger safety like civilian vehicles and have rough and sharp edges within the compartments. Therefore, while severe solid organ injuries and fractures may be less likely, superficial lacerations are seemingly more common and severe.

*Wound Care:* The wounds are massive and aggressive debridement is the rule. This aspect is no different than previous historical wounds of the last century, where extremity injuries have always accounted for 60–70% of all injuries. The principles learned from the past still apply here. This includes aggressive cleansing of the wounds, with removal of foreign bodies and nonviable tissues. In addition, it is always best to leave wounds open in cases of massive tissue destruction. Some wounds are wide open and obvious as to

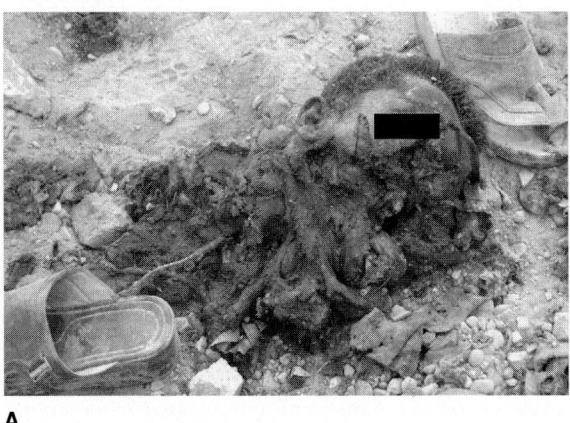

A

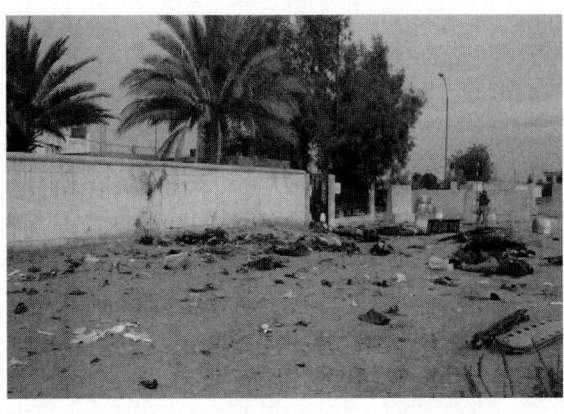

B

**FIGURE 55-11.** Panel **A** is the remains of the suicide bomber and Panel **B** is the surrounding area of the bombing after the surviving casualties have been removed.

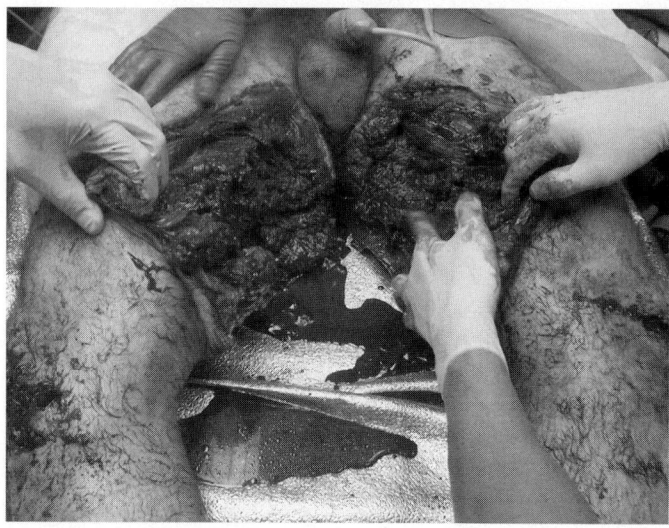

**FIGURE 55-12.** Wounds to legs after rocket propelled grenade (RPG) passed through the cabin of the vehicle killing the driver and injuring the posterior aspect of the legs of this passenger.

the extent of injury but many present with only small puncture wounds. These wounds vary highly in originating forces behind the projectile and thus the depth of penetration is also extremely variable. Some casualties are "peppered" with hundreds of small superficial fragmentations from surrounding material such as dirt or concrete buildings. While appearing worrisome they are sometimes very innocuous. One should try and avoid "swiss cheese" surgery in an attempt to excise all wounds and retrieve fragments. Simply cleanse the wounds with antiseptic and scrub brush. Superficial penetrating fragment injuries usually do not require surgical exploration but deciding whether a wound is superficial or not is the key as some other injuries are seemingly innocuous but highly lethal.

Primary surgical wound care for deep penetrating fragments involves long-standing combat surgery principles which include limited longitudinal incisions with excision of foreign material and devitalized tissue. They are then irrigated copiously and left open. The incisions should be parallel to the long axis of the extremity, to expose the entire deep zone of injury. At the flexion side of joints, the incisions are made obliquely to the long axis in order to prevent the development of flexion contractures. The use of longitudinal incisions, rather than transverse ones, allows for proximal and distal extension, as needed, for more thorough visualization and debridement. For skin, a conservative excision of 1–2 mm of damaged skin edges is all that is required. Excessive skin excision is avoided; questionable areas can be assessed at the next debridement. Damaged and contaminated fat should be generously excised. Damage to the fascia is often minimal, relative to the magnitude of destruction beneath it. Shredded, torn portions of fascia are excised, and the fascia is widely opened through longitudinally incision to expose the entire zone of injury beneath. Nerves and tendons do not require debridement, except for trimming frayed edges and grossly destroyed portions. Following surgical removal of debris and nonviable tissue, irrigation is performed until clean. While sterile physiologic fluid is preferred, do not deplete resuscitation fluid resources as potable water is a viable alternative. When local soft tissue coverage is inadequate, the development and rotation of formal flaps for this purpose should not be done during primary

surgical wound care. Local soft tissue coverage through the gentle mobilization of adjacent healthy tissue in order to prevent drying, necrosis and infection is recommended. Saline soaked gauze is an alternative.

Wound management after initial surgery is just as important as initial wound management in limiting infection and subsequent morbidity and mortality. The wound should undergo a planned second debridement and irrigation in 24–72 hours, and subsequent procedures until a clean wound is achieved. Between procedures there may be better demarcation of nonviable tissue or the development of local infection. Early soft tissue coverage is desirable within 3–5 days if the wound is clean. Delayed primary closure (3–5 days) requires a clean wound that can be closed without undue tension. This state may be difficult to achieve in war wounds. There is currently extensive experience with delayed wound closure and the use of negative pressure dressings. In some reports, wounds are able to successfully undergo delayed closure in as little as 4–5 days with very low infection rates. Soft tissue war wounds heal well without significant loss of function through secondary intention. Definitive closure with skin grafts and muscle flaps should not be done in theater.

*Open fractures* should be addressed as early as tactically feasible. The fragments of bone with soft tissue attachments and large, free, articular fragments are preserved. All devitalized, avascular pieces of bone smaller than thumbnail size that have no soft tissue attachment should be removed. The bone ends of any fracture should be cleaned independently, by cleaning out the ends of the medullary canal and the exposed surfaces of the bones irrigated with sterile fluids.

*Compartment syndrome* is common. The fascial defect caused by the injury itself is not often adequate to fully decompress the compartment. Mechanisms of injury frequently associated with compartment syndrome include: open and closed fractures; penetrating wounds; crush injuries; vascular injuries; and reperfusion following vascular repairs. The early clinical diagnosis of compartment syndrome is classically described to include the following findings: pain out of proportion; pain with passive stretch; and tense, swollen compartment. Once compartment syndrome has begun to cause irreversible cellular damage, several late clinical diagnostic findings develop: paresthesia, pulselessness, pallor, and paralysis. The diagnosis of a compartment syndrome is made on clinical grounds and the measurement of compartment pressures can be helpful, if available. However, it is always better to just perform the fasciotomy if it is considered as the follow-up through many levels of transport is not ideal. During the fasciotomy, the removal of dead muscle is important to prevent infection but accurate initial assessment of muscle viability is difficult. Tissue sparing debridement is acceptable if follow-on wound surgery will occur within 24 hours. More aggressive debridement is required if subsequent surgery will be delayed for more than 24 hours. To do this, sharply excise all nonviable, severely damaged, avascular muscle. The "4 Cs" (Contractility, Capacity to bleed, Color, Consistency) may be unreliable for initial assessment of muscle viability. Color is the least reliable sign of muscle injury. Surface muscle may be discolored due to blood under the myomesium, contusion, or local vasoconstriction. Contractility is assessed by observing the retraction of the muscle with the gentle pinch of a forceps or with the use of electorcautery. Consistency of the muscle may be the best predictor of viability. In general, viable muscle will rebound to its original shape when grasped by a forceps, while muscle that retains the mark has questionable viability.

*Infection in the field hospital setting:* All wounds incurred on the battlefield are heavily contaminated with all forms of foreign bodies including dirt, clothing, projectile fragments including tissue and bones from other casualties. Thus, the bacterial load is also heavy. Most will become infected unless appropriate treatment is instituted quickly. The battlefield environment is conducive to wound infection due to the associated devitalized tissue, contaminated hematomas, and delay in casualty evacuation. Surgery plays the most important role in the empiric treatment of war-wound infection. Surgical treatment of war wounds always includes the early and thorough excision of all dead tissue, removal of foreign bodies, and assurance that remaining tissue is healthy, viable, with a good blood supply. The current recommendation is antibiotics for all open wounds. If the debrided wound still has possibly ischemic tissue or retained foreign material, the patient is returned to the OR every one to two days for redebridement, until absolute assurance of healthy, clean tissue is achieved. Other infectious complications, particularly the nosocomial infections typically seen in an ICU, such as ventilator associated pneumonia or blood stream infections, are equally common in the field hospital. There is no difference in the diagnosis and treatment of such infections in the military environment.

## TRIAGE

Triage, is the art of sorting casualties to do the most good with what you have. The implications of doing the most good for the most people are obvious. Because triage is a broad topic, and occurs at many locations on the battlefield, we will concentrate on triage at facilities with surgical assets. The most important aspect of dealing with mass casualty situations is proper planning and practice.[33-35]

Mass casualty scenarios are more often the case than the trickle effect that is more common in civilian trauma centers. There can be long periods of inactivity quickly followed by large number of casualties. Mass casualties of 10–30 injured soldiers at one time a fairly common. The scenario of the surgeon sorting through bodies laid out side-by-side outside on the ground is largely unrealistic. While the total number of casualties for a specific event may be large for the triage officer, they do not all simultaneously appear. This is because the casualties arrive in vehicles. On the average, whether the transport is by ground or air, they come in batches of three to four. This is true whether the casualties are brought in by ambulance, Humvee, combat vehicles, civilian sedans, or pick-up truck. This is also true when they are brought in by rotary wing aircraft. Only on an extremely rare occasions will there be a vehicle carrying 20 casualties. On January 4, 2006, a mass casualty event occurred just outside a compound in Camp Ramadi, Iraq. Over a 30-minute period, approximately 25 vehicles brought in 83 casualties and each vehicle had on the average 2–4 casualties. This point is very important to develop an efficient triage system.

Military doctrine typically teaches that a designated area be set aside for triage. While this has worked historically, this system is not necessary or efficient. There is no true necessity to have a triage staging area where the casualties are all placed, examined, and

sorted. An alternate and effective method has been to quickly assess the casualties as they are brought out of the ambulance or by the triage officer climbing into a vehicle and getting a quick feel for who needs the urgent attention. The examination that is performed is a 2–3 second look to see if the patient is responsive, pulse character, and whether there is a lot of blood on the casualty. There is no place for a stethoscope or blood pressure cuff during this scenario. It cannot be overemphasized that the triage is a sorting process and not a treatment process. There is no equipment necessary for triage. In most circumstances, the person with the casualties or the casualties themselves will tell you who is in need of immediate attention. Then the triage officer verifies and directs flow of traffic. The dead are kept on the vehicle, and the talking patients, which will be the majority of the casualties, can be directed to either the treatment area or the minimal care area. In cases of overwhelming numbers, an option is to keep the casualties that have minor injuries and direct them to a Battalion Aid Station (BAS) or other level I treatment facility for treatment and temporary holding if one is available nearby. If the option of using a triage area is utilized to examine and sort casualties, it should also be stressed that obtaining as much help to run this area as possible is extremely helpful. The triage officer should be experienced enough to quickly determine the dead, sick, and not sick. He then directs flow of casualty traffic. The main role of the triage officer is to ensure that the right people go to the right place at the right time. The triage officer should not be thoroughly examining each casualty. Realistically, there is no time for this and if practiced the triage process will instantly become a bottleneck.

In the military, there is also an important aspect of triage that must be mentioned. Often the triage officer and treating medical personnel are very anxious to get to the patient to determine the injuries but have to wait for the ordinance or Sergeant-at-arms to inspect the casualty for arms, ammunition, or unexploded ordinance.[36] This is a required process that should take place quickly for all casualties if it has not already been done. One should also be aware that many of the casualties can be civilians or enemy. They and coalition forces do have to be searched for weapons and this cannot really be avoided and is best for all involved. However, this process can be quick and efficient and some places that have been less active sometimes have a very robust search process which can be extremely distressing for medical personnel if the casualty is in extremis.

*Triage categories:* The military doctrine typically uses the four-tier system. This again is a tested and useful option. However, during OIF, the three-tier system was typically used and found to be more effective and faster. This separates the casualties into the dead or dying, sick, and not sick. The sick are those who will need immediate treatment and not sick are those who can wait. Those who can lift and support their own head, look around, and can verbally respond are usually less urgent patients. The dead and dying patients can be sent to one area, the "sick" to another, and the "not sick" to the third. In the sick category, unresponsive patients with blood on them usually need to be in the OR and can be taken directly there without going to the resuscitation or treatment area. The resuscitation can be performed in the OR and stopping at a treatment area only delays the control of bleeding. This step of taking all patients to a resuscitation area is not mandatory neither a prerequiste. The casualties that need the highest level of attention and most urgent procedures such as airway control, chest tubes, and central lines can be better performed in the OR. Thus, the occasional urgent airway should also be considered to be taken directly to the OR. Compared to civilian trauma centers where many patients are nonoperative, combat casualties in extremis almost always belong on the OR table as surgical control of hemorrhage is almost always required. Even if they do not need a named operation, the OR is the most well equipped, lighted room with the most amount of trauma expertise. For example, in some locations, when treating an isolated penetrating injury to the head, it can be argued that taking these patients directly to the OR is preferred. Anesthesia providers are the most experienced with difficult airways and their gear is in the OR. This type of planning should be discussed ahead of time and evaluated for appropriateness of each individual facility. Also important is planning ahead of time on how to evacuate mass casualties from your facility. Each location will have specific peculiarities that must be addressed.

On extremely rare circumstances, "reverse triage" is necessary in the military. This is a circumstance when the facility is being overrun or the tactical scenario dictates that all wounded soldiers capable of returning to the battle is required to be treated first. Thus, someone with an extremity injury may need to be assessed quickly, appropriately treated, and returned to the battlefield before treating someone with torso injury that is not capable of fighting. The rationale for this is that this would result in the least number of injured and dead overall.

*Triage officer:*   Although military doctrine has classically taught that the dental officer is the triage officer is antiquated and should be eliminated. The triage officer should be the most senior trauma experienced person on shift. Most often the surgeons fulfill this requirement and should be the initial triage officer. If the triage officer is the senior surgeon and is needed to be in the OR, the next most experienced person should take over the role no matter the specialty. It does not make sense to have the most capable person waiting in the OR or resuscitation area when their expertise could be better utilized in the triage area. In a mass casualty scenario, the roles need to be clearly identified and markings or identifying clothing such as ball caps or vests that marks a person's role is crucial to making the process work as many people will have different roles as the process is dynamic. As such, to clearly mark the triage officer is vital to this process especially when the task is passed off to another person.

## Geneva Convention and Noncoalition Care

Fortunately, the care provider does not have to face the difficult daily decisions of the soldiers regarding friend or foe. They are fortunate that they can be blinded to what political side the casualty is on. Medical triage and not political triage is the policy and practice of US Military Medicine. This is also the policy of the Geneva Conventions. The Geneva Conventions define medical personnel as those individuals "exclusively engaged in the search for, or the collection, transport, or treatment of the wounded or sick, or in the prevention of disease, (and) staff exclusively engaged in the administration of medical units and establishments" (Geneva I, Article 24). The 1949 Geneva Convention refers to the protection of civilians in the time of war and Article 13 states: "that the whole of the populations of the countries in conflict, without any adverse distinction based, in particular, on race, nationality, religion or political openion, and are intended to alleviate the sufferings cause by war." Deployed medical providers must provide appropriate treatment to all who require it on the basis of medical need alone, within the constraints of triage and medical resources. The current practice policy is to care for the human that is in the most need of care. It is not uncommon for US soldiers to be brought in simultaneously with enemy casualties and universally the Geneva Conventions are followed.

## TACTICAL COMBAT CASUALTY CARE

The military surgeon should be aware that there has been an evolution in military medical tactics and performing civilian style trauma care is sometimes inappropriate in the field. In order to make recommendations on policy of prehospital combat casualty care, a committee was formed to examine the latest literature and science to make recommendations on care in the field. This standing Committee on Tactical Combat Casualty Care (COTCCC) consists of civilian and military medical providers. The military personnel are of various subspecialties and include medical officers and enlisted. This committee continually reviews the state-of-the-art in trauma and makes recommendations that are applicable to those who practice in the military. The first set of recommendations was published in the fourth edition of *Prehospital Trauma Life Support*, and since then a military edition has been published,[37] with the latest edition available in 2006. The unique product of this committee is that they have been able to separate the type of care rendered into three categories. This makes the permutations of field care manageable. The categories include "care under fire" which dictates what the care should be when under hostile fire. When the hostility has diminished the care giver switches to "tactical field care." Finally, the last category is CASEVAC care which is the care during movement of the casualty from the point of injury to a medical facility. The basic recommendations are shown in Table 55-3. The recommendations are similar to civilian trauma care, but they do have distinct differences that military surgeons need to be aware of. Although much of it may be intuitive, this set of recommendations allows the medic/corpsman the license to parallel civilian trauma care but with important distinctions. These differences includes for example in the care under fire phase, the ABCs (airway, breathing, circulation) of trauma care classically taught are not applicable and could cause further harm. Instead, when under fire, the emphasis is on preventing additional casualties and the only real emphasis is on hemorrhage control bypassing the rare airway compromise, and breathing problems which cannot be adequately addressed when under attack in austere environment. Other changes includes the widespread use of new and effective tourniquets, novel local hemostatics, permissive hypotension, low volume resuscitation, oral fluids, only using cervical collar on blunt symptomatic patients, prehospital antibiotics, improved pain control, and prevention of hypothermia, as outlined in Table 55-3.

## MILITARY MEDICAL CARE STRUCTURE

There are five basic levels of care (previously referred to as Echelons, and not to be confused with ACS designation of US trauma centers (Table 55-4)). Different levels denote differences in

**TABLE 55-3**

| Tactical Combat Casualty Care | | |
| --- | --- | --- |
| **CARE UNDER FIRE** | **TACTICAL FIELD CARE** | **CASEVAC CARE** |
| 1  Return fire take cover<br>2  Direct expect casualty to remain engaged as a combatant, if appropriate | Casualties with an altered mental status should be disarmed immediately<br>Airway management<br>  a. Unconscious casualty without airway obstruction:<br>    • Chin-lift or jaw-thrust maneuver<br>    • Nasopharyngeal airway<br>    • Place casualty in recovery position<br>  b. Casualty with airway obstruction or impending airway obstruction<br>    • Chin-lift or jaw-thrust maneuver<br>    • Nasopharyngeal airway<br>      – Allow conscious casualty to assume any position that best protects the airway, to include sitting up.<br>      – Place unconscious casualty in recovery position If measures above unsuccessful,<br>    • Surgical cricothyroidotomy (with lidocaine if conscious) | Airway management<br>  a. Unconscious casualty without airway obstruction:<br>    • Chin-lift or jaw-thrust maneuver<br>    • Nasopharyngeal airway<br>    • Place casualty in recovery position<br>  b. Casualty with airway obstruction or impending airway obstruction<br>    • Chin-lift or jaw-thrust maneuver<br>    • Nasopharyngeal airway<br>      – Allow conscious casualty to assume any position that best protects the airway, to include sitting up.<br>      – Place unconscious casualty in recovery position If measures above unsuccessful,<br>    • Surgical cricothyroidotomy (with lidocaine if conscious) or<br>    • Laryngeal mask airway/ILMA or<br>    • Combitube or<br>    • Endotracheal intubation or<br>    • Surgical cricothyroidotomy (with lidocaine if conscious)<br>  c. Spinal immobilization is not necessary for casualties with penetrating trauma |
| 3  Direct casualty to move to cover/apply self aid if able | Breathing<br>  a. Consider tension pneumothorax and decompress with needle thoracostomy if casualty has torso trauma and respiratory distress<br>  b. Sucking chest wounds should be treated by applying a Vaseline gauze during expiration, covering it with tape or a field dressing, and monitoring for development of a tension pneumothorax | Breathing<br>  a. Consider tension pneumothorax and decompress with needle thoracostomy if casualty has torso trauma and respiratory distress<br>  b. Consider chest tube insertion if no improvement and/or long transport anticipated<br>  c. Most combat casualties do not require oxygen, but administration of oxygen may be of benefit for the following types of casualties:<br>    • Low oxygen saturation by pulse oximetry<br>    • Injuries associated with impaired oxygenation<br>    • Unconscious patient<br>    • TBI patients (maintain oxygen saturation >90)<br>    • Casualties in shock<br>    • Casualties at altitude<br>  d. Sucking chest wounds should be treated by applying a Vaseline gauze during expiration, covering it with tape or a field dressing, and monitoring for development of a tension pneumothorax |
| 4  Try to keep the casualty from sustaining additional wounds | Bleeding<br>  a. Assess for unrecognized hemorrhage and control all sources of bleeding<br>  b. Assess for discontinuation of tourniquets once bleeding is controlled by other means. Before releasing any tourniquet on a patient who has been resuscitated for hemorrhagic shock, assure a positive response to resuscitation efforts (i.e. a peripheral pulse normal in character and normal mentation if there is no TBI). | Bleeding<br>  a. Assess for unrecognized hemorrhage and control all sources of bleeding<br>  b. Assess for discontinuation of tourniquets once bleeding is controlled by other means. Before releasing any tourniquet on a patient who has been resuscitated for hemorrhagic shock, assure a positive response to resuscitation efforts (i.e. a peripheral pulse normal in character and normal mentation if there is no TBI). |

*(Continued)*

**TABLE 55-3** *(Continued)*

**Tactical Combat Casualty Care**

| CARE UNDER FIRE | TACTICAL FIELD CARE | CASEVAC CARE |
|---|---|---|
| 5   Airway management is generally best deferred until the Tactical Field Care phase | IV<br>a. Start an 18-gauge IV or saline lock, if indicated<br>• If resuscitation is required and IV access is not obtainable, use the intraosseous route | IV<br>a. Reassess need for IV access<br>• If indicated, start an 18-gauge IV or saline lock<br>• If resuscitation is required and IV access is not obtainable, use intraosseous route |
| 6   Stop life-threatening external hemorrhage if tactically feasible:<br>• Direct casualty to control hemorrhage by self aid if able.<br>• Use a tourniquet for hemorrhage that is anatomically amenable to tourniquet application.<br>• For hemorrhage that cannot be controlled with a tourniquet, apply HemCon dressing with pressure | Fluid resuscitation<br>Assess for hemorrhagic shock; altered mental status in the absence of head injury and weak or absent peripheral pulses are the best field indicators of shock.<br>a. If not in shock:<br>• No IV fluids necessary<br>• PO fluids permissible if conscious<br>b. If in shock:<br>• Hextend® 500 mL IV bolus<br>• Repeat once after 30 min if still in shock<br>• No more than 1000 mL of Hextend®<br>c. Continued efforts to resuscitate must be weighed against logistical and tactical considerations and the risk of incurring further casualties<br>d. If a casualty with TBI is unconscious and has no peripheral pulse, resuscitate to restore the radial pulse | Fluid resuscitation<br>a. Re-assess for hemorrhagic shock; altered mental status (in the absence of brain injury) and/or abnormal vital signs<br>b. If not in shock:<br>• No IV fluids necessary<br>• PO fluids permissible if conscious<br>c. If in shock:<br>• Hextend 500 mL IV bolus<br>• Repeat once after 30 min if still in shock<br>• No more than 1000 mL of Hextend<br>d. Continue resuscitation with PRBC, Hextend, or LR as indicated<br>e. If a casualty with TBI is unconscious and has a weak or absent peripheral pulse, resuscitate as necessary to maintain a systolic blood pressure of 90 mm Hg or above |
| 7   Prevent hypothermia:<br>Wrap casualty in Blizzard Rescue Blanket Cover scalp with Thermolite cap | Prevention of Hypothermia<br>a. Minimize casualty's exposure to the elements. Keep protective gear on or with the casualty if feasible.<br>b. Replace wet clothing with dry if possible<br>c. Apply Ready-Heat™ blanket to torso<br>d. Wrap in Blizzard™ Rescue Blanket<br>e. Put Thermo-Lite® Hypothermia Prevention System Cap on the casualty's head, under his/her helmet<br>f. Apply additional interventions as needed/available<br>g. If mentioned gear is not available, use dry blankets, poncho liners, sleeping bags, body bags, or anything that will retain heat and keep the casualty dry | Prevention of Hypothermia<br>a. Minimize casualty's exposure to the elements. Keep protective gear on or with the casualty if feasible.<br>b. Continue Ready-Heat™ Blanket, Blizzard™ Rescue Blanket and Thermo-Lite® cap<br>c. Apply additional interventions as needed (see Table 3-1)<br>d. Utilize the Thermal Angel™ or other portable fluid warmer on all IV sites, if possible.<br>e. Protect the casualty from wind if doors must be kept open |
| 8   Communicate with the patient if possible:<br>a. Offer reassurance and encouragement.<br>b. Explain first aid actions | Monitoring – Pulse oximetry should be available as an adjunct to clinical monitoring. Readings may be misleading in the settings of shock or marked hypothermia. | Monitoring – Institute electronic monitoring of pulse oximetry and vital signs if indicated |
| 9 | Inspect and dress known wounds | Inspect and dress known wounds if not already done |
| 10 | Check for additional wounds | Check for additional wounds |
| 11 | Analgesia as necessary<br>a. Able to fight:<br>*These medications should be carried by the combatant, and self-administered as soon as possible after the wound is sustained.*<br>• Mobic® 15 mg PO qd<br>• Tylenol®, 650 mg bi-layer caplet, 2 PO q 8 h<br>b. Unable to fight:<br>NOTE: *Have naloxone readily available whenever administering opiates*<br>• Does not otherwise require IV/IO access:<br>  i. Oral Transmucosal Fentanyl Citrate 400 micrograms transbuccally | Analgesia as necessary<br>a. Able to fight:<br>*These medications should be carried by the combatant, and self-administered as soon as possible after the wound is sustained.*<br>• Mobic® 15 mg PO qd<br>• Tylenol®, 650 mg bi-layer caplet, 2 PO q 8 h<br>b. Unable to fight:<br>NOTE: *Have naloxone readily available whenever administering opiates*<br>• Does not otherwise require IV/IO access:<br>  i. Oral Transmucosal Fentanyl Citrate 400 micrograms transbuccally |

**TABLE 55-3** *(Continued)*

**Tactical Combat Casualty Care**

| CARE UNDER FIRE | TACTICAL FIELD CARE | CASEVAC CARE |
| --- | --- | --- |
| | – Recommend taping lozenge-on-a-stick to casualty's finger as an added safety measure | – Recommend taping lozenge-on-a-stick to casualty's finger as an added safety measure |
| | – Reassess in 15 min | – Reassess in 15 min |
| | – Add second lozenge, in other cheek, as necessary to control severe pain | – Add second lozenge, in other cheek, as necessary to control severe pain |
| | – Monitor for respiratory depression | – Monitor for respiratory depression |
| | • IV or IO access obtained: | • IV or IO access obtained: |
| |    i. Morphine Sulfate 5 mg IV/IO |    i. Morphine Sulfate 5 mg IV/IO |
| | – Reassess in 10 min | – Reassess in 10 min |
| | – Repeat dose q 10 min as necessary to control severe pain | – Repeat dose q 10 min as necessary to control severe pain |
| | – Monitor for respiratory depression | – Monitor for respiratory depression |
| |    ii. Promethazine 25 mg IV/IO/IM q 4 h, for synergistic analgesic effect, and as a counter to potential nausea |    ii. Promethazine 25 mg IV/IO/IM q 4 h, for synergistic analgesic effect, and as a counter to potential nausea |
| | Splint fractures and recheck pulse | Re-assess fractures and re-check pulses |
| | Antibiotics: recommended for all open combat wounds | Antibiotics: recommended for all open combat wounds |
| 12 | a. If able to take PO | a. If able to take PO |
| 13 | • Gatifloxacin 400 mg PO qd | • Gatifloxacin 400 mg PO qd |
| | b. If unable to take PO (shock, unconsciousness) | b. If unable to take PO (shock, unconsciousness) |
| | • Cefotetan 2 g IV (slow push over 3-5 minutes) or IM q12 h or | • Cefotetan 2 g IV (slow push over 3-5 min) or IM q 12 h or |
| | • Ertapenem 1 gm IV or IM q 24 h | • Ertapenem 1 gm IV or IM q 24 h |
| | Communicate with the patient if possible | Pneumatic antishock garment (PASG) may be useful for stabilizing pelvic fractures and controlling pelvic and abdominal bleeding. Their application and extended use must be carefully monitored. They are contraindicated for casualties with thoracic and brain injuries |
| 14 | a. Encourage, reassure | |
| | b. Explain care | |
| | | Document clinical assessments, treatments rendered, and changes in casualty's status. Forward this info with the casualty to the next level of care. |
| | Cardiopulmonary resuscitation | |
| 15 | Resuscitation on the battlefield for victims of blast or penetrating trauma who have no pulse, no ventilations, and no other signs of life will not be successful and should not be attempted. | |
| | Document clinical assessments, treatments rendered, and changes in casualty's status. Forward this info with the casualty to the next level of care | |
| 16 | | |

capability, not the quality of care. Each level has the capability of the level forward of it, and expands on that capability. Soldiers with injury or illness effectively treated at any level should be returned to duty at that level. All others are prepared for safe transport to a higher level.

*Level I:* First aid and immediate life-saving measures delivered at the scene. Care is administered by the injured soldier himself, "self aid and buddy aid," a combat lifesaver (squad member trained to assist in first aid) or the combat medic or corpsman (trained as an Emergency Medical Technician-Basic). The most forward medical facility is the Battalion Aid Station (BAS). They can be in a tent or any opportune hardened facility. They can perform treatment and triage. Typically, the highest level medical provider is a physician assistant (PA) or nonsurgical physician. "Flight surgeons" sometimes are located in BAS but again these are not surgeons who perform surgery. In the military the term "surgeon" is frequently synonymous with a "doctor" and can be misleading. The BAS will either treat and return the casualty to duty, or evacuate to the next higher level of care as they only have the holding capability of up to six hours.

*Level IIA:* Medical Company. Generally, these are facilities and have approximately 70 medical providers. They have limited inpatient bed space and can hold and treat casualties for up to 72 hours. The services that are typically available at this level include primary care (sick call), and dental. They have laboratory and x-ray capability. Sometimes they have optometry and psychiatry rotating through when possible. Each service has a slightly different unit at this level. For example, the Navy equivalent of a medical company is the Shock Trauma Platoon (STP).

*Level IIB:* The medical company or BAS can be augmented with surgical capability. The Army does this with the addition of a forward surgical team (FST—20-member team),[38–40] the Navy with a forward resuscitative and surgical system (FRSS—8-member team),[41] and the Air Force with the Mobile Field Surgical Team

**TABLE 55-4**

| **Eschelons of Care** | | |
|---|---|---|
| **MILITARY DESIGNATION ECHELON OF CARE** | **DESCRIPTION** | **US CIVILIAN DESIGNATION** |
| V (e.g., BAMC/ISR & WHMC) | Major Trauma Center with Teaching and Research | I |
| IV (NNMC, WRAMC) | Major Trauma Center | II |
| III (e.g., Landstuhl, Germany & Theater Hospitals in Iraq) | Regional Trauma Center, Limited Capability, 30-day ICU holding capability | III |
| IIB (e.g., Surgical Company, FRSS, FST, EMEDS) | Community Hospital with Limited Emergency Surgery Capability | IV |
| IIA | Outpatient Clinic | – |
| I | EMS/Corpsman/Medic | – |

BAMC/ISR – Books Army Medical Center/Institute of Surgical Research, WHMC – Wilford Hall Medical Center, both at San Antonio, TX; level V also provides rehabilitation centers. NNMC – National Naval Medical Center in Bethesda, MD, Walter Reed Medical Center in Washington DC. FRSS – Forward Resuscitative Surgical System, FST – Forward Surgical Team, EMEDS – Expeditionary Medical Support.

**TABLE 55-5**

| **Level II B Augmentation** | | |
|---|---|---|
| **ARMY** | **NAVY** | **AIR FORCE** |
| 24 member team | 8 member team | 5 member team |
| 40 operations | 18 operations | 10 operations |
| 3 general surgeons | 2 general surgeons | 1 general surgeon |
| 1 orthopedic surgeon | | 1 orthopedic surgeonII |
| 2 anesthetists | 1 anesthesiologist | 1 anesthetists |
| Critical care nursing and operative tech support. | Critical care nursing and operative tech support. | Critical care nursing and operative tech support. |

(MFST — 5-member team). Their basic capability is to provide life and limb salvage resuscitative surgery. Using these building blocks these highly mobile teams can typically provide one to two operating room tables within one hour. They can be set up in mobile environment controlled tents or in shelters of opportunity. [42] They carry enough equipment and supplies to perform 10–40 operations. While designed for 24–72 hours of continuous operations without resupply, they can be employed in a nondoctrinal configuration and provide ongoing support to small maneuver elements, given adequate resupply[43] (Table 55-5). These facilities do not usually have any significant holding capability, and do not have the ability to perform split operations.

The Navy serves two populations and they are either sailors or marine soldiers. While surgical capability is available on board aircraft carriers and surrounding support ships, this capability is for daily elective and semi-urgent surgery as there is only one surgeon on board. When the aircraft is deployed as a "Carrier Group" which consists of approximately 8–13 ships, this one surgeon, who is typically a recent residency graduate, provides surgical support for up to 13,000 sailors while at sea. Since there is no real surface threat for blue water battles, this has proven to suffice for surgeries such as appendectomies, cholecystectomies, hernia repairs, and other routine semi-urgent surgeries. The Navy in support of the Marines provides Level II surgical support in two other ways than what was described above and deserve mention.

One of these capabilities includes the Casualty Receiving and Treatment Ships (CRTS). These are aircraft carriers whose primary function is transport of the marine expeditionary unit (MEU). The secondary function is for the ship to function as a casualty receiving and treatment ship. They typically have on board a fleet surgical team which is an 18-member team consisting of one surgeon. Since the ships typically function as a member of a strike force with three to eight ships, when heavy casualties are anticipated, a mobile augmentation team of up to 81 members can be rapidly deployed. In this scenario, they will have up to four surgeons and the ships can make available four operating rooms with 15 intensive care bed. These ships have radiology and blood bank capabilities.

When surgical capability is required on land, a surgical company is available and these facilities can have ready three operating tables with a 60-bed holding capability for a mini-field hospital. This set up includes when maximally deployed, up to six surgeons. However, due to the limitation of general surgeons in the Navy, urologists and obstetricians can substitute a general surgeon.

*Level III:* Represents the highest level of medical care available within the theater, with the bulk of inpatient beds located here.[44] Most deployable hospitals are modular, allowing the commander to tailor his medical response to the expected or actual demand. These hospitals can be set up in a mobile fashion but will use buildings such as churches or abandoned hospitals when opportunities arise. The Army's nomenclature for these units is the Combat Support Hospital (CSH) which has replaced the historical Mobile Army Surgical Hospital (MASH). The Navy has the fleet hospital which is now termed Expeditionary Medical Units (EMU) and the Air Force the Expeditionary Medical Support (EMEDS). The difference in capability between the Level II an III is that they have can have subspecialty care available (neurosurgery, ENT, urology, OMFS, etc.), and other services to typically include computerized tomography (CT) and increased blood bank and laboratory capability. They have increased number of ICU and ward beds. While they can fully recover patients in theater as they did in Vietnam, the current policy is to send the casualty back to the United States and this can occur as early as 12–48 hours after injury. Basically, as soon as the casualty is stable enough for transport, they will be moved. During the Vietnam conflict, the doctrine was that patient transport was only performed on highly stable casualties but this change in mind frame has been due to the Air Force's capability of providing critical care during transport. Since the US military forces are sent home so rapidly, the majority of the long-term patients at these Level III facilities are host nation civilians and combatants. Their size range is large and now has been modularized to provide from 25 to 500 beds in theater. The downside with these facilities is lack of mobility and footprint on the ground as some may take up to 1000 personnel using 450 tents over 28 acres. The last Level III that needs mentioning is the two hospital ships the (TAH)- USNS Mercy and USNS Comfort which can be ramped up to function as a 1000 bed floating hospital. In the current war, these hospital ships have been used for humanitarian missions and have not had an active role in Iraq or Afghanistan.

*Level IV:* The Level IV represent the larger more capable military hospitals in Germany and the United States. Although the three services have many hospitals worldwide only a few select hospital receives casualties from the war. The Landstuhl Regional Medical Center is the hub for all casualties being transported out of theater. This facility has recently increased its acute care capability, as many of the casualties being transported are significantly injured and require intensive care.[45]

*Level V:* Represents the Zone of the Interior, continental United States (CONUS)-based hospitals outside the communication zone, including military medical centers, other federal hospitals, and civilian contracted hospitals. This represents the most definitive care possible and includes burn care, long-term convalescence, and specialized rehabilitation.

## TRAUMA SYSTEMS

Military doctrine previously had been fashioned for the linear battlefront. While this system has served us well, in the modern nonlinear battlefield, the casualty would not have to progress through all the various levels of care. In the current war in Iraq, there are many facilities of various levels in close proximity. The extensive civilian trauma system experience has taught us that integrating the various levels of trauma centers into a coherent trauma system, improves patient outcome. For the severely injured, transport to the most capable center in the shortest amount of time is the key to optimal outcome. Ideally, the severely injured are not taken to the nearest health care facility but to the highest designated trauma centers depending on their injury. However, the role of the Level II–III trauma centers are also important serving the local community and sharing the burden of the sometimes overwhelming workload of the Level I trauma centers. Triage is performed by the civilian EMS personnel, so as not to overload the Level 1 trauma center. Appropriate triage in the civilian results in a 50% overtriage rate, therefore avoiding the moving severely injured patients to an inadequate facility. This trauma systems approach should be transferred to the military sector as well.[46]

In the same regard, the BAS while serving a multitude of roles has no role in treating traumatic casualties and should be bypassed when possible. The BAS has many vital roles including running daily sick call[47] and promotion of readiness status but it is ill-equipped and manned for trauma and can delay transport to a higher level facility. It would be better to bypass the BAS and directly transport to a highest level of care that the casualty can tolerate. Other than the rare chest tube or airway, no other definitive care is really provided at the BAS level that cannot be provided by a medic or corpsman. It has to be also realized that placing a chest tube in the BAS type facility takes time and since it is a relatively rare life-saving procedure with inexperienced person performing the procedure with inexperienced assistance, the set up and packaging of the chest tube can take considerable time and this time spent at that level is precious. Hemorrhage control can be obtained with pressure or tourniquets and in the case of ongoing uncontrolled truncal hemorrhage, the casualty would benefit more from shorter transport time to a surgical facility, more than resuscitating at the BAS level. The BAS also does not typically have x-ray capability for minor injuries and for the more severe casualty they can delay surgical treatment. The casualty should only be taken to a BAS when it is in a remote location with no supporting Level IIb or III facility.

The same principle should also apply to Level IIb facilities.[48] The casualty would be better served if they were bypassed and transported directly to a Level III facility unless the casualty cannot tolerate the delay in treatment or if it is anticipated that the casualty will not need Level III care. In contrast, casualties that are anticipated to eventually return to duty should not be transported out of the local region. An example is an open fracture. It is rare that these casualties will remain in theater and definitive care at a Level IIb facility will not be justified. Thus, if this injury is isolated without vascular compromise, then directly transporting them to a Level III facility without going through the Level I and II facility would be in the casualties' best interest and aid the efficiency of the trauma care systems capability.

The Level IIb facility provides surgical capability to a region without the larger footprint and personnel. These facilities have a long history within the military and are an integral aspect of military medicine. While supposedly only a "life and limb sparing" facility, it can also function usefully in many other circumstances. It can often provide elective and semielective surgery without compromising the patient depending on the facility. Appendectomies, testicular torsions, abscess drainages, and symptomatic hernia repairs can be performed at Level IIb facilities benefiting the system and retaining the fighting force. These patients can be returned to duty within a relatively short period of time and thereby decreases transport of these patients to Level III facilities which can be heavily burdened. In addition, the transport of these patients are almost always by helicopter in the current war and these flights are costly and not without risk.

If a patient is brought to a Level IIb facility, operations such as irrigation and debridement of open fractures can serve a purpose as these types of procedures can be easily performed by a general surgeon and the operation can serve the purpose of downgrading the casualty transport from urgent or priority status to routine. When flying out on routine status, the casualty is placed on a helicopter that is flying into the facility on a daily supply transport rather than an unscheduled flight. When MEDEVAC flights are called for on an urgent or priority basis, they usually always fly in pairs with a gunship and the cost of this transport is obviously higher and more dangerous. Great tactical judgment is required when operating but more is required when deciding when NOT to operate. Care should be tailored to each casualty, their unit, and what is best for the casualty and mission. For example, in a scenario of multiple casualties one undergoes tactical damage control, then these casualties need to be sent out urgently or under priority status. In this case since a MEDEVAC has been called for, other cases that could be easily performed at the Level II facility such as a simple washout of an open fracture probably should not be performed and the casualty are flown out with the urgent case. This will not delay the urgent MEDEVAC and obviate the need for a second or third flight.

The benefit of the Level IIb surgical facilities is their mobility, which also is their downfall. The main disadvantages of performing surgery at a Level IIb facility is the lack of certain subspecialties such as neurosurgery, blood banking capabilities, blood components (FFP, croprecipitate, and platelets), sophisticated radiographic capabilities (CT scan), and any ability to perform long-term ICU care. Thus, some of the surgery performed at the Level IIb setting is staged tactical damage control surgery and this has the disadvantage of possibly requiring multiple anesthetics and operations. While most of the operations performed at the Level IIb should be staged or tactical damage control surgeries, if the patient can tolerate a definitive operation, it can be performed. It must be stressed that all procedures started at Level IIb setting should be started with the tactical damage control mind frame. Simpler, definitive cases performed at the Level IIb facility also serve an important role of decompressing the Level III facility in cases of mass casualty. If all cases are referred to a Level III at all times, they can be unnecessarily inundated with the heavy caseload. This scenario in many ways is no different than the civilian trauma care system. Trauma patients are not taken to clinics (BAS) and are taken to trauma centers. Not every trauma patient should be taken to a civilian Level I trauma center as they can be overburdened. The severe casualties should be taken directly to the highest level of trauma care available unless they cannot afford the delay in transport.

As in the past, all three services have manned a forward surgical capability. While these units serve a specific purpose during maneuver warfare, the problem has arisen in that the line commanders have become accustomed to having surgical support with these teams due to their small size. The smaller size is of significant benefit as the footprint of these units is multitudes smaller than traditionally large Level III support. Thus, the services that can be provided are minimal and this does not always equate to the best care, especially when in close proximity to a Level III facility. These small units sometime do have orthopedic surgeons assigned to them depending on the service but the capability of doing definitive orthopedic surgery is lacking. They, by design, do have portable ultrasound capability, and some limited blood bank capability as they do carry packed red blood cells.

*Reserves:* The reserves are probably comparable to the active duty forces in terms of capability but one very important issue must be stressed. As a whole while the average capability may be similar, the range of capabilities are much broader on both ends. The reserves include the national guards. The difference between the reserves and the National Guard is that the latter is controlled and funded by states rather than the federal level. The experience and training in the reserves can be excellent as they have personnel that work at Level I trauma centers but, on the other hand, the medical personnel sometimes have no background in medicine or have been performing rural nonemergent medical care and trauma experience from a large volume trauma center is more the exception.[49] In the active duty population, trauma experience is systematically lacking as only a few military facilities treat trauma patients on a daily basis.[50] While experience during residency is available for some physicians, others such as nursing, ancillary care, corpsman or medic rarely have any trauma experience. To solve this issue, all of the three services have a training center at high-volume civilian trauma centers but the majority of those being deployed have not been through the training. Currently, the Army has a training center in Miami and New York, the Air Force in Baltimore, Cincinnati, and St Louis, and the Navy in Los Angeles.

## COMBAT CASUALTY CARE

*Fluid Resuscitation:* The COTCCC currently recommends the use of "permissive hypotension." This means that hypotension is permissible and resuscitation to normal blood pressure is not the goal. The rationale includes several points including the possibility that fluid infusion can increase uncontrolled hemorrhage and eventually lead to dilutional coagulopathy.[51–53] Clinical studies examining the use of fluids in the prehospital phase has not been able to show any benefit in both blunt and penetrating trauma[54–59] and one

study showed potential worse outcome with patients with penetrating torso trauma.[6] The decreased emphasis on fluid resuscitation in the field serves a multitude of purposes. The emphasis is to stop external bleeding if possible and to transport seriously injured casualties to the nearest surgical facility; thus, minimizing time spent resuscitating in the field. Since resuscitation is only required in bleeding casualties and because the majority of casualties do not require any fluid resuscitation and the automatic response of giving every casualty intravenous crystalloids can be minimized. It must be understood that only a small minority of casualties are hypotensive due to blood loss.[61] This also minimizes the logistical burden of carrying fluids in the field and the difficulties associated with transporting a casualty with intravenous lines in place.

Lessons learned during the Vietnam conflict included the aggressive use of fluid resuscitation. This lesson was transferred to the civilian sector and currently advanced trauma life support (ATLS) program recommends two large bore IVs and two liters of fluid resuscitation with lactated Ringer's solution in all trauma patients. However, research has shown us that this may have negative impact if fluid resuscitation is too aggressive. In addition, lactated Ringer's solution has been demonstrated to have immunological consequences when infused in large volumes compared to other fluids.[62–66] Basic scientific research has demonstrated that lactated Ringer's solution was made with the racemic form of lactate (D and L isomers of lactate) and that eliminating the D-isomer may be beneficial.[67–70] The Office of Navy Research (ONR) requested that the Institute of Medicine (IOM) review the issue of fluid resuscitation and in their report titled *Fluid resuscitation: State of the science for treating combat casualties and civilian injuries* they made a series of recommendations which includes the reduction of lactate in resuscitation fluids and development of novel resuscitation.[71] As a result, Baxter Corp. manufactures lactated Ringer's with only the L-isomer. Currently, the trend in civilian trauma care in some sectors is to practice permissive hypotension which is to allow for less than optimal restoration of blood pressure with fluids if the casualty does not have traumatic brain injury and is conscious. Interestingly, there has been reports that once common complications such as adult respiratory distress syndrome (ARDS) and multiple organ dysfunction syndrome has been decreasing in trauma patients.[72,73]

The choice of fluid to be used on casualties has also changed. The COTCCC currently recommends the use of small volume colloid as similar resuscitation can be achieved with only one-third the weight and cube compared to crystalloid. Colloids provide the logistical advantage that is of importance in the field that civilian trauma does not face. Up to one liter of a colloid is recommended in two 500cc boluses. Another reason for the recommendation of colloid use is that the review of literature from civilian trauma has shown minimal differences in outcome between the traditional crystalloid resuscitation and the colloid resuscitation.[74–78] Although the IOM report published in 1999 as well as several military consensus panels recommended the use of 7.5% hypertonic saline, the COTCCC could not recommend this at the current time since this solution is not readily manufactured in the United States. However, an alternative is to use 5% or 3% hypertonic saline which also offers logistical benefits with out sequelea,[79] and can also potentially modulate the immune response following injury.

Thus, the recommendation has been to obtain IV access (heparin lock) on all casualties but not to give fluids unless it is required. To determine who should and should not be infused with resuscitation fluids, it is recommended that the casualties' mental status and pulse character are reliable means to determine their status and should be used as a deciding factor for initiating resuscitation. For most casualties, the pulse character and mental status will be normal.[80] In this instance, oral hydration is recommended. Although in civilian trauma care oral fluids are condemned in trauma, this does not apply in the military. In civilian trauma, care of the casualties may need general anesthesia for wound or orthopedic care. Therefore, the thought traditionally had been to keep the stomachs empty to reduce the risk of aspiration. However, we have learned that emergent surgery in trauma is always done with full stomachs and aspiration during rapid sequence intubation is very rare. Therefore, the encouragement of oral hydration is not necessarily detrimental and there is no proof that the use of oral fluids will harm the patient. If the casualty has minor injuries and is alert enough to want fluids, this is an option that is now promoted as the majority of these casualties will not need general anesthesia. However, it is important to note is that there is a difference between oral hydration and oral resuscitation.

*Blood transfusions:* Blood is typically reserved for patients who have lost 30–40% of their blood volume. However, it is probably wise to start blood transfusion with packed red blood cells (PRBCs) on any hypotensive patient with obvious external blood loss. PRBC are readily available in the theater of operations. In Level II surgical facilities, component therapy other than PRBCs are not available except for the walking blood bank. Any surgeon who has had the opportunity to use fresh whole blood will testify to the advantages. The sight of soldiers lined up as far as the eye can see at any time of the day at a moment's notice is truly emotional. Fresh whole blood from the donor may be the best source of such components (especially platelets) despite a potentially greater risk for immunologic reactions than packed cells. Because fresh whole blood is not feasible in civilian trauma, confirming data to the wonders of its use is absent.

The equipment required is minimal and blood recipient bags are available in the field but a special bag is not necessary and any emptied sterile fluid bag will suffice. Collecting it with citrate phosphate dextrose (CPD) allows it to be held in the refrigerator for up to three weeks. However, storage of whole blood for later administration can be kept at room temperature no longer than 24 hours. Blood stored warm for more than 24 hours has a significant risk of bacterial growth and clotting factors will be lost. Platelets will not work in blood stored cold (4°C) for greater than 24 hours, losing one of the main benefits of fresh whole blood; however the plasma in whole blood is still very useful even if all the coagulation factors are not optimal. It is also important to keep a record of donors and patients transfused so they can be tested upon return to stateside. Once the casualty has been stabilized and is in an ICU setting, literature does support minimizing transfusion of packed RBC.[81]

There are some cautions worth mentioning such as the fact that the field conditions increases the risk of bacterial contamination, and definitive testing of blood from transfusion virus disease is not yet available. However, since the military population is heavily screened, this practice in the field is different than what can be expected if one were to try this at civilian trauma centers. The "Dog tag" blood typing can be wrong 2–11% of the time and prescreening helps efficiency of its use. Donation does affect field

endurance, stamina, and performance and one needs to assess if massive donations could affect unit effectiveness. The donation should only be done once a month and women should ideally be placed on iron supplementation before/after donation. In Camp Ramadi (Level IIb surgical facility), fresh whole blood was typically available within 20 minutes from arrival of casualty (Fig. 55-13) Typically the first unit was donated by a member of the medical unit. Prescreened donor roster avoids having to type at the time of donation. Whole blood crossmatching is easily performed using the white tile method where a drop of the donor blood is mixed with the recipient serum on a white ceramic tile and is examined in four minutes: if no agglutination occurs, the blood is suitable for transfusion into that recipient (a hand lens may be useful).

Autotransfusion is an often underutilized approach. Blood collected into sterile containers (suction, chest tube, etc.) may be returned to the patient through a blood filter and is probably the only thing better than fresh whole blood from a donor. Blood from sterile cavities, such as the chest or abdomen without visceral injuries is preferred. Blood from contaminated abdominal wounds can be used but does increase risk of systemic infection. Blood may be filtered through sterile gauze as a field expedient method. One example of intra-abdominal field auto transfusion is in case of vascular or solid organ injury. To do this, sponges can be wrung out into buckets, mixed with CPD and filtered when transfused. Another alternative, if time allows, is to set up a chest tube auto transfuser attached to a suction tip (yankaur) instead of a chest tube and use it for collection and autotransfusion.

*Blood subsitutes:* The future of blood transfusion may include the use of hemoglobin substitutes.[82] Since the definition of shock is inadequate oxygenation at the cellular level, the most ideal fluid would provide volume expansion and oxygen carrying capacity. For this fluid to be useful in deployed settings it needs to be stable at a variety of temperatures and have a low-risk profile. Hemoglobin-based oxygen carrying compounds (HBOCs) currently under investigation may be an attractive future alternative. There are HBOCs derived from either bovine[83–88] or human[89–94] sources that require no refrigeration, have a shelf life of up to three years, are disease free, and require no crossmatching. There is promising

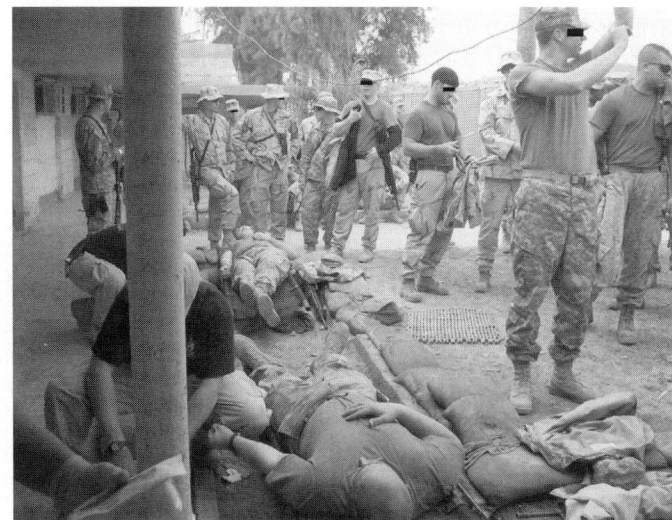

**FIGURE 55-13.** Walking blood bank in action. Soldiers urgently volunteering to donate blood.

research ongoing in field trials for resuscitation of trauma victims with HBOC. The Office of Naval Research has funded a multicenter randomized, prospective trail in civilian human trauma patients.

*Hemostatics in the battlefield:*    Systemic and local hemostatics[95] are relatively new to the trauma community and their exact role is yet to be determined. However, this is an exciting new concept that is being tested in the field today. Through much funding and research, both systemic and local hemostatics have been developed for use in trauma. Recombinant Factor VIIa (rFVIIa) is a relatively new product originally used for hemophiliacs. The uses of this product soon made its way into the trauma setting. Case reports,[96,97] in trauma were followed by case series[98,99] and animal experimentation[100–103] which showed its potential for use in trauma. Currently, there is only one prospective trial that has shown its usefulness.[104] This trial demonstrated that while survival rate was improved when rFVIIa was used, it was not statistically significant. However, it did show a decrease usage of PRBC transfusions in patients that received rFVIIa. For this product to live up to its tremendous potential in trauma, it must be shown that it is efficacious and safe. The product works with tissue factor and platelets to promote clot formation and thus decreased bleeding only at the injured site. Thus, a dose given systemically goes to the injured vessels and only stops bleeding where there is tissue injury. Tissue factor which is ubiquitous in blood vessels are released at injured endothelium of vessels; thus, it is seemingly ideal. Current literature seems to show that the drug is very safe and only occasional expected complications occur. Since atherosclerotic plaques have increased tissue factor there are potentially grave side effects. There are currently 185 reported thromboembolic events such as cerebrovascular accidents, myocardial infarctions, arterial thrombosis, pulmonary embolism, and other venous thromboembolism possibly due to the administration of rFVIIa.[105] However, since the military is a relatively younger population, this may not be as much of a factor.[106] In addition, the reported doses of this drug is over several hundreds of thousands. A recent report published in the *New England Journal of Medicine* has demonstrated efficacy in acute intracerebral hemorrhage.[107] They showed smaller growth of the hematoma size, decreased disability and mortality. While the benefit of using rFVIIa has not been definitively shown, the belief of most surgeons in theater that have used it is that it is a useful tool for coagulopathic casualties. Although rFVIIa does not have a label for use in trauma at this current time, over 700 doses were used at various levels of care in Iraq.[108] Civilian research is currently under plans but it may be several years before its clinical efficacy can be proven. This drug can also be used in various ways. It can

be used as a systemic hemostat to control traumatic bleeding, or it can be used to treat coagulopathy. This is a subtle difference and in most centers it is used to treat refractory coagulopathy. The main reason for this indication is that the cost of the drug is high ($1/µg, average dose is approximately $7–8,000). RFVIIa has been used at the Balad surgical hospital and they have found that a thromboelastogram has been extremely useful to guide the treatment of coagulopathy.

*Local hemostatics:*    This is an exciting area of interest and the lessons learned from the military may eventually be transferred to the civilian sector. Since the main cause of possibly preventable deaths (60%) during the Vietnam conflict was hemorrhage,[109,110] efforts were under way to find, develop, and field local hemostatics that could be used in the field by medics, corpsman, and soldiers when the war in Iraq started. Although there have been many local hemostatic developed,[111,112] two have been recommended by the COTCCC. Both were available in the field during the Iraq war. The first product is chitosan (HemCon® which is a product made from shrimp shells (Fig. 55-14). This product can be safely used on all personnel including those with allergies to shell fish. HemCon is approved by the Food and Drug Administration (FDA) and is composed of poly-N-acetyl glucosamine, also known as chitosan. It does not require refrigeration or any other special conditions. The primary mechanism of action is by adhesion. This product comes in a sealed package containing one 4 × 4 inch dressing with a backing. It is relatively firm and thus is sometimes difficult to mold and pack into a small cavity. In these circumstances, it may be broken up or cut into the appropriate shape and size. The recommended method of use is to wipe the excess blood from the wound and then place it on the bleeding tissue and hold firm pressure for five minutes. Adherence to the tissues can stop bleeding. Since this product is relatively safe, it can be used for minor or major wounds. In animal models of severe uncontrolled hemorrhage, it has been shown to be effective in a variety of circumstances including lacerations to the aorta.[113] The Army has distributed HemCon for use and the first report of its use demonstrated high efficacy in both the field and at treatment facilities.[114]

The second product which was also recommended by the COTCCC is QuikClot[115] (Fig. 55-15). This is also an FDA-approved product and is basically a zeolite mineral that absorbs water molecules and thus concentrates the coagulation factors at the site of bleeding.[116] The mineral is inert, but during the absorption phase an exothermic reaction occurs, which generates heat.[117] Since the heat generated can be significant, initial impression is that it is the main mechanism of action. However, testing of QuikClot with various zeolites with increased residual moisture

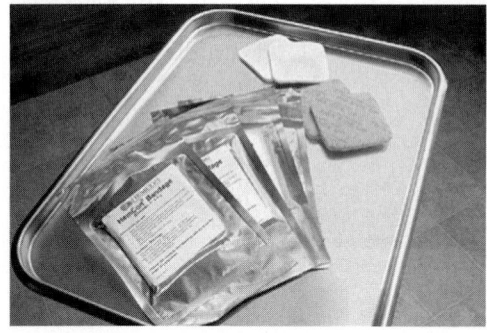
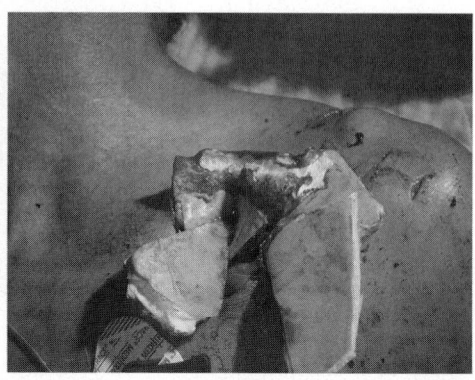

**FIGURE 55-14.**  HemCon cut up and used in the chest wall.

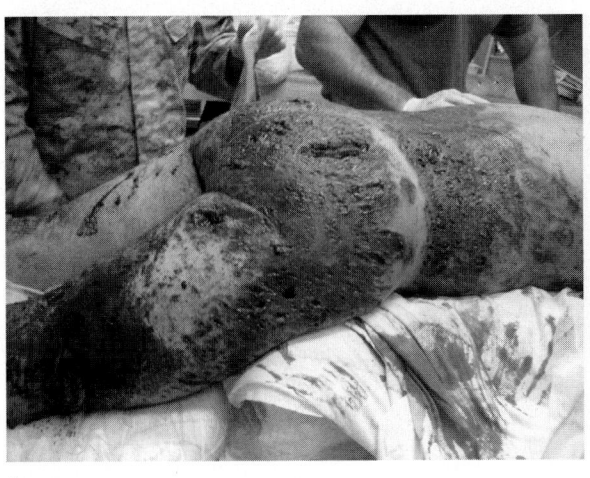
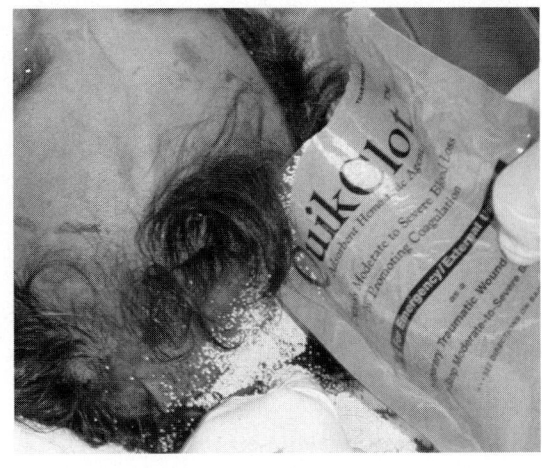

**FIGURE 55-15.** **(A)** Quikclot applied in the field to the buttock wound following IED injury. **(B)** Quickclot application into bleeding scalp injury.

demonstrated decreased effectiveness even though the heat generated was the same.[118] Therefore, it is not a field-cauterizing tool.

There has been worldwide distribution of QuikClot, not only to the US Marines but to several other countries as well. Law enforcement and emergency medical systems in the United States have purchased QuikClot for use in civilian trauma and for disaster preparation. The advantage of this product is that it is effective and cheap (cost to US Military is under $10.00). The disadvantage is the heat generated and the consistency which resembles sand or kitty liter. Thus the application of this product into certain wounds and the removal of the material from tissues is not always easy. Although the material is inert and does cause a foreign body reaction, minimal, long-term consequences are yet to be reported. The manufacturer has recently developed and distributed QuikClot in small tea bag type package so that the granules are not as difficult to remove, if used. There is a clinical case series describing its use in humans and it has been used in both civilian and military personnel externally as well as internally.[119] However, it is important to note that internal use is not recommended by the manufacturers for either HemCon or QuikClot. Although there are over 100 documented uses in the granular form, the experience with the bagged format is few.[120] The method of use is to remove excess blood, apply QuikClot, and apply pressure.

The recommendation for use of the local hemostatics by the COTCCC is that if pressure dressing fails then HemCon should be applied. If the HemCon does not control hemorrhage then it should be removed and QuikClot applied. Both products can be highly effective but in penetrating wounds where the source of bleeding is deep within the wound, superficial application of either product can fail. While seemingly obvious, since the products are distributed for use by first responders as well, training is essential.

*Tourniquets:* This life-saving tool has good and bad aspects. Although it had fallen out of favor, it is making a resurgence in combat casualty care. The classic teaching was that once placed that it should never be removed except by a medical officer. This led to delays in removal and often meant an amputation. Due to the potential prolonged access to surgical care in the military, the COTCCC has re-examined the use of the tourniquet and has made a set of refined recommendations for its use. The COTCCC has

recommended that tourniquet be the first line of therapy rather than the last when under direct fire. During the tactical care phase when you are no longer under fire, the tourniquet should be removed and an attempt at stopping the bleeding with pressure dressing is recommended. If pressure dressings and local hemostatics are not effective then the tourniquet can always be reapplied. Not checking to determine the need for the applied tourniquet will increase the need for amputation. The rationale for the set of recommendation are that when you are under fire, the most assured method of controlling hemorrhage is with the use of a one-handed tourniquet which would also allow one to stay engaged in the fight. Tourniquets also have the advantage over pressure dressings and other local hemostatics which often requires the use of two hands. The military has tested numerous one-handed tourniquets. While there are many variants of the one-handed tourniquet, most are similar in efficacy and the choice is user preference, trainability, costs, and transportability[121] (Fig. 55-16).

The overall experience so far is that while most of the tourniquet uses have been inappropriate or less than satisfactory application, there has been minimal downfall to the usage.[122] In addition, there have been numerous cases where surgeons at all levels of care have felt that they have been used successfully and have saved lives. The main issue with tourniquets is continual training on proper usage to all who have access to them. Since exsanguination from extremity trauma is a rare event in most civilian settings, it may not be applicable in the rural setting.

*Tactical Damage Control Surgery:* As opposed to the civilian damage control surgery, tactical damage control surgery is somewhat different. In civilian terminology, it refers to an abbreviated surgery due to physiologic exhaustion where as the military procedure takes into account the tactical scenario, the resources and best treatment for the casualty at that particular instance.

Trauma surgery has four steps: control of hemorrhage, control of contamination, diagnosis, and reconstruction. It has been recognized that not all of these steps need to be performed in the initial operation. Tactical Damage Control surgery is not a specific procedure but refers to a state of mind. Speed and efficiency during the procedure is vital. All efforts should be made to abbreviate the surgery and anticipate additional casualties. There will

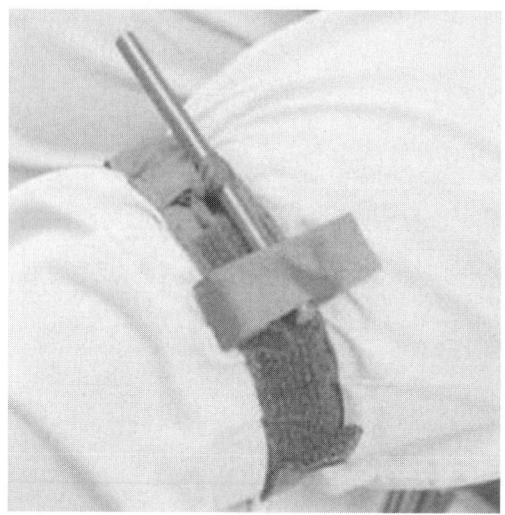
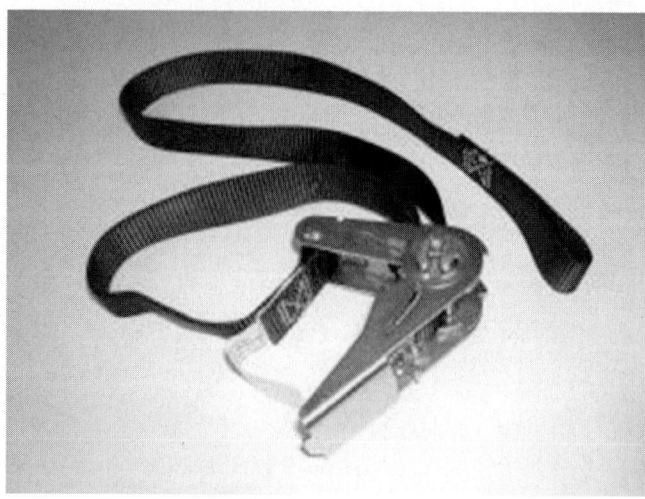
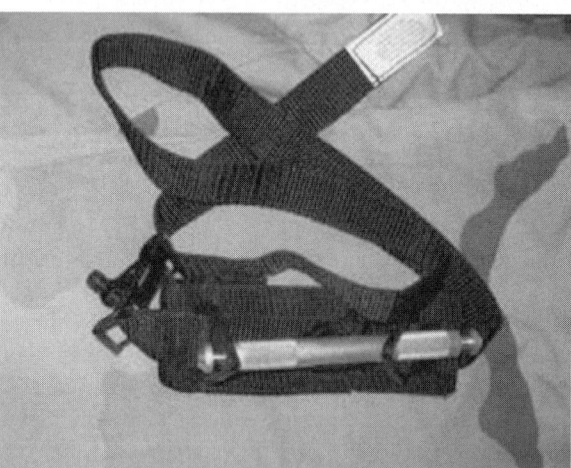
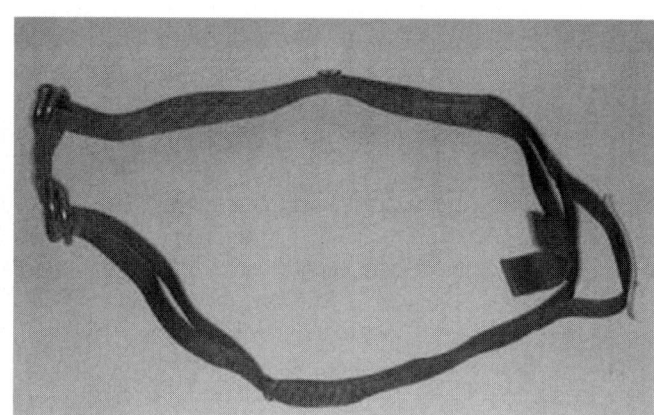

**FIGURE 55-16.**  Various one handed tourniquets.

be circumstances where simple reconstruction should be deferred to the next echelon of care even when the patients' physiologic status could tolerate the definitive procedure for the sake of time or to take advantage of the flights of opportunity. There will be other scenarios where definitive surgery will be in the casualty's best interest as long as they are stable and other casualties do not suffer from the use of time and resources. Vascular shunting is an example (Fig. 55-17). With transected vessels, shunting the artery and/or vein should be the initial approach.[123,124] When placing the shunt minimal resection of the artery should be performed. Rather the injured vessel is tied over the shunt and the ligature is then tied to the shunt. This is performed at both ends to prevent dislodgment of the shunt. After this has been done, if the scenario allows for reconstruction, then it would be better in most circumstances for the reconstruction to be performed at the initial operation. However, if the circumstance dictates that the casualty can tolerate transfer to a higher level of care and that the reconstruction is better performed at the next level of care, then the casualty should be flown out. This decision as to when to send and when to keep are too numerous to list. Additional factors will include concomitant orthopedic injuries which often accompany these casualties. When to wash out the wounds, when to stabilize with splints or external fixators are all factors that must be weighed into

consideration before making the final decision of what to do, when, and where.

## Tactical Damage Control Celiotomy

Current concepts in "damage control" abdominal surgery had been described for decades and is now commonly used in civilian trauma.[125–131] This has also been transferred to casualty care and is the initial mind frame when performing celiotomy in the battlefield. Celiotomy in the combat setting requires speed and experience. When a casualty is deemed to require surgery, no time should be wasted and the ultimate goal is to visualize the peritoneal contents to find the bleeding source. If the casualty is hemodynamically normal and stable, that should not lead to a false sense of security that the casualty is still not bleeding as patients with peritonitis often have ongoing bleeding and this must be assumed.[132] Since the vast majority of casualties undergoing an abdominal operation are for penetrating injuries, the control of hemorrhage and contamination is paramount. Since penetrating trauma celiotomy does have subtle but important differences in approach compared to blunt trauma celiotomy, training and experience prior to the deployment would be beneficial. Due to the high energy associated with battlefield penetrating injuries, bleeding from the abdominal wall can be massive.

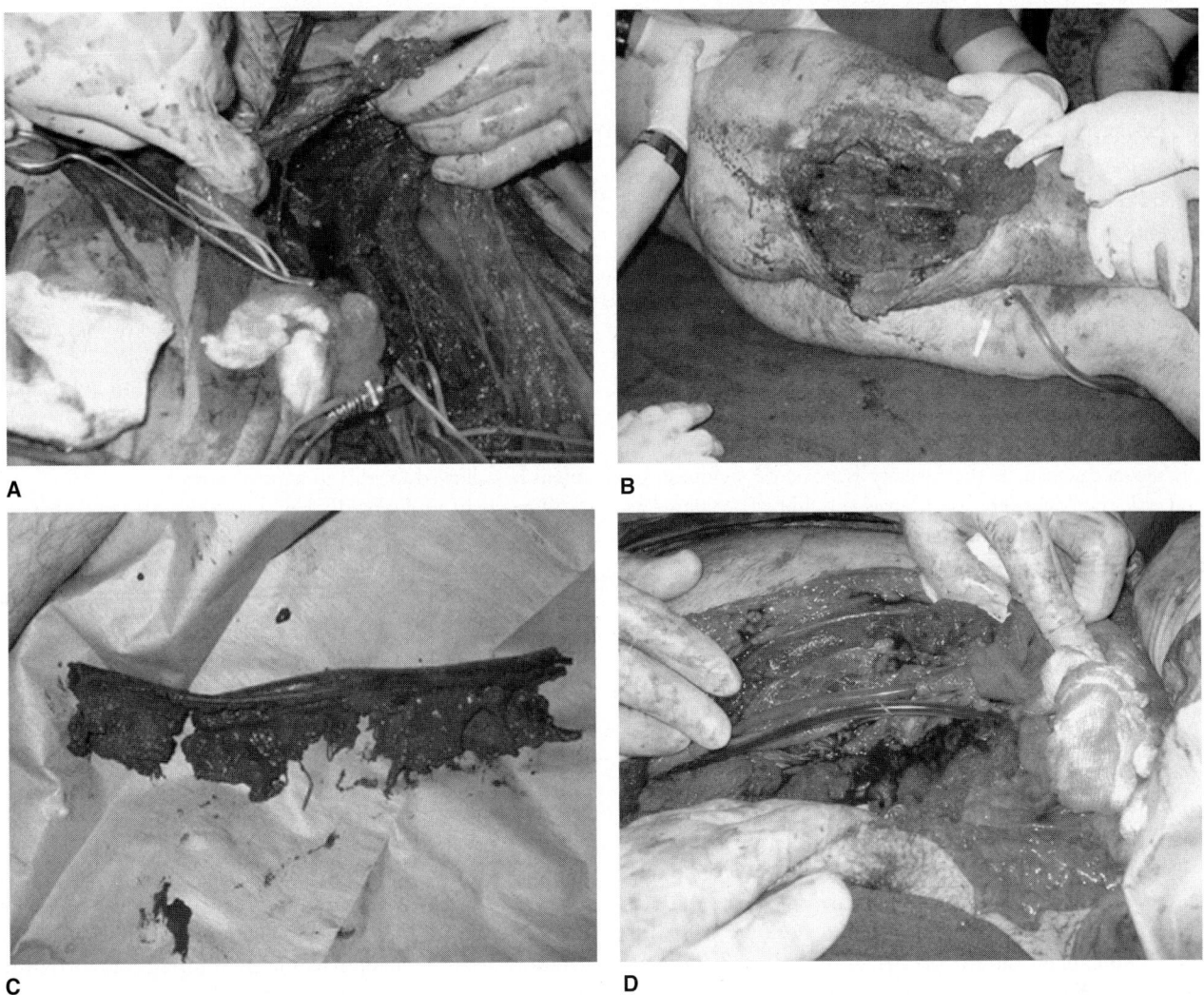

**FIGURE 55-17.** **(A)** Picture of right groin wound from IED attack. **(B)** Back of wounded leg. **(C)** Weather stripping from the vehicle which was removed from the groin wound. **(D)** Superficial femoral artery and vein with vascular shunts in place. *(Pictures courtesy of L.W. Chambers.)*

Not only is it essential to control bleeding from these wounds, they usually require subsequent surgery for re-exploration, washouts, and debriedment. This should be kept in mind at the initial operation.

Packing of the abdomen in penetrating injury is different than blunt trauma. Packing in patients with hemoperitoneum is done in order to soak up and remove the blood quickly so the source of hemorrhage can be addressed. It does not create significant tamponade in the abdomen and only reduces some venous and capillary bleeding. This must be realized as some surgeons may get a false sense of security that the bleeding has stopped when the bleeding has only been masked. Placement of packs so that "anesthesia can catch up" without knowing the source of bleeding can be a fatal mistake. In most circumstances the source of hemorrhage in penetrating trauma needs to be addressed immediately and this cannot be efficiently performed unless the surgeon can see and the surgeon cannot see through blood or packs. Abdominal packing gained popularity with liver injuries following blunt trauma. In these cases where the patient had the abdomen explored for hemoperiotoneum, abdominal packs were used to pack all four quadrants. It was found that following packing, the bleeding seemed to have stopped. As we now know, most of the liver injuries stop bleeding spontaneously as long as the fluids are not given too aggressively than required. This has been extrapolated to that packing stops all bleeding and this is not always true. Other than slowing venous and capillary bleeding in the liver and spleen it does not stop bleeding anywhere else as there are no real organs or sources of hemorrhage in the lower quadrants. The main sources of hemorrhage in penetrating trauma are from the solid organs, and midline vascular structures including the mesentery and the pelvis. The abdominal wall and psoas region are sources of injury and packing the missile tract or cavity does have definite merit. If the addressing of hemorrhage causes massive hemorrhage and the casualty is exsanguinating, a fine balance in judgment will be required as to how much blood is infused while the bleeding is addressed. Waiting for complete refilling of the blood volume deficits before attempting hemorrhage control has negative aspects and most experienced trauma surgeons prefer to address the hemorrhage while the blood pressure is less than optimal in order to minimize blood lost. The infusion of blood and fluids while controlling bleeding is a fine art.

The handling of hollow viscous injuries is control of contamination. This can be done in several ways, but the common denominator should be that it is done quickly. Options include GIA stapling, tying off the ends of bowel with heavy ties or umbilical tape (hog tying), or clamping and leaving the clamps in place. During this phase careful dissection is avoided and speedy exploration is rather preferred. Dissection into the pelvis to determine the exact extent of injuries can be time consuming and can lead to additional bleeding, especially if the casualty becomes coagulopathic. If the casualty is stable at this point the surgeon needs to take a step back and get a picture of the overall situation. He needs to take into account how the casualty is doing, what the other priorities are in this casualty, the other associated injuries, the number of other casualties, time of day, weather, units of blood available, MEDEVAC status, and all the other variables that are too numerous to list. The variables will determine whether the surgeon should then proceed with the next phase which is reconstruction. If the casualty is not cold, acidotic, or coagulopathic then anastamosis of bowel should be considered as this is the optimal time for reconstruction. Reanastamosis can be delayed but can be more technically difficult if performed at the second look operation with swollen bowel. While staged abdominal celiotomy has a role, opportunities should be taken to perform definitive surgery when appropriate as multiple surgeries are associated with increased complications.[133]

Closure.    Closure of the abdomen has multiple variations in damage control surgery. If subsequent exploration is needed, the fascia should not be closed until after the last look or washout. Packs may be left in the abdomen to create local tamponade and aid in hemorrhage control but an abundance of packs left in the abdomen is not always necessary. To close the abdomen, some prefer to use a bag system (bogata bag) but one option is to close the skin with running monofilament suture as this is readily available and efficient. Closing the skin prevents: retraction of the fascia, heat loss, and fluid loss from evaporation. In addition, the skin creates enough tension so that there is a mild tamponade effect to aid in hemostasis. Fluid management in these casualties is a fine art as underresuscitation is obviously undesirable and overresuscitation can lead to complications including ARDS, abdominal compartment syndrome, and swelling of the bowel.[134,135]

The triad of coagulopathy, hypothermia, and acidosis is associated with increased mortality. This is obvious as these three factors are associated with uncontrolled hemorrhage. Bleeding obviously leads to increased mortality. Hemorrhagic shock where there is inadequate tissue perfusion equates to a decreased cellular activity as the ingredients for cellular activity is not circulated. This leads to inadequate heat generation and acidosis. The process of bleeding and resuscitation also leads to coagulopathy. The hypothermic state contributes to the coagulopathy as the enzymes in the coagulation cascade are not efficient below normal body temperature. The coagulopathic state contributes to persistent blood loss. The best method to break this cycle is to attend to the fundamental cause of this triad which is bleeding. If the bleeding was pinpointed, such as a vascular source, then the process reverses itself without much effort. However, for multiple massive sources of hemorrhage such as multiple fractures, pelvic fractures and large wounds, the hypothermia and coagulopathy should be independently addressed. It must also be noted that the red cell surface availability which is directly related to the hematocrit and hemoglobin level affects the ability of the platelets to

form clot. Although in the ICU setting a lower threshold is associated with better outcome, in the field, if fresh whole blood is available, the customary lower hemoglobin levels should not be accepted. Transportation of these casualties will decrease core body temperature as the MEDEVAC flights by helicopter causes significant evaporative losses if prevention measures are not taken.

*Air Evacuation and Transport:*    This has to be one of the most vastly improved aspects of modern military medicine. Previously casualties were kept in theater and transported only when they were in a stable condition and did not need critical care support. The difference is that we now have the technological capability to transport critically injured casualties half-way around the world in just a few days. We probably were capable of doing this previously but our confidence in capability, and some improvement in equipment has allowed for this to become a reality.[136]

The credit undoubtedly belongs to the Air Force that is vastly responsible for this feat. In the war in Iraq and Afghanistan, the US military does have the luxury of air superiority and can fly without opposition from the air. The Army and Marines transport the critically injured with an "en route" care nurse to one of the several Level III facilities. Eventually, the casualty is then routed through Landstul Regional Medical Center (LRMC) in Germany back to the United States. The mission of transporting casualties from Iraq to LMRC and then to the United States is performed by the Critical Care Air Transport Team (CCATT). This team composition and function in listed in Table 55-6. A four-person burn transport team can augment a CCATT team as required for inhalation injury and/or severe burns. These teams have all the equipment necessary to turn any austere mode of transportation into an ICU. CCATT care includes mechanical ventilation, resuscitation, invasive hemodynamic monitoring, blood transfusion, and monitoring of critical lab values. This concept of critical care in the air did not exist in previous eras and has redefined the need for long-term care on the ground in combat theater of operations. To date, more than 25,000 AE missions and 3000 CCATT missions have been completed; mortality associated with this modality of care in the air approaches zero.

There are some general considerations prior to transport that should be considered. Due to altitude effects, limited mobility, decreased staffing en route, and unpredictable evacuation times, the referring physician should tailor vital signs monitoring

---

**TABLE 55-6**

**Composition of Three-Member CCAT Team Description**

1. Intensivist physician
   Capable of providing short term life-support, including advanced airway management, ventilator management, and limited invasive (non-operative) procedures
   Trained in critical care medicine, anesthesiology, or emergency medicine
2. Critical care or emergency medicine nurse
   Experienced in managing patients requiring mechanical ventilation, invasive monitoring, hemodynamic support
3. Cardiopulmonary technician
   Experienced in management of patients requiring mechanical ventilation, invasive monitoring
   Experienced in troubleshooting ventilatory support and monitoring systems

requirements (including temperature), and wound and neurovascular checks frequency to maximally acceptable intervals. Some therapies that might not be used in a fixed MTF are appropriate for AE. For example, patients with significant medical or surgical conditions should have Foley catheters, NG tubes, and provisions for IV pain medications and extended half-life IV antibiotics. Several prophylactic measures should also be considered, including liberal use of fasciotomies/escharotomies and airway protection with prophylactic intubations, chest tubes for potential pnemothorax, bivalving, and creating windows over surgical wounds in casts.

During air transport, the anticipated decrease in barometric pressure should be considered. The diameter of a gas bubble in liquid doubles at 5000 feet above sea level, doubles again at 8000 feet, and doubles again at 18,000 feet. Cabin pressures in most military aircraft are maintained at altitudes between 8000 and 10,000 feet. If an aircraft has the capability, the cabin altitude can be maintained at lower levels, with increased flight time and fuel. Such Cabin Altitude Restriction (CAR) for: penetrating eye injuries with intraocular air; free air in any body cavity; severe pulmonary disease; decompression sickness and arterial gas embolism requires CAR at origination field altitude. Destination altitude should not be higher than origination altitude and patient should be transported on 100% oxygen (by aviator's mask, if available). Air splints should not be used if alternate devices are available. As air expands at altitude, air splints require close observation and adjustments during flight. Ostomy patients require venting of collection bags to avoid excess gas dislodging the bag from the stoma wafer. Using a straight pin, two holes can be made in the bag above the wafer ring.

*Decreased Partial Pressure of Oxygen:* Ambient partial pressure of oxygen decreases with increasing altitude. At sea level, a healthy person has an oxygen saturation of 98–100%. At a cabin altitude of 8000 feet, this drops to 90%, which then corrects to 98–100% with 2 L/min $O_2$. Since hypoxia may worsen neurological injury, the ventilator settings should be adjusted to meet increased oxygen demands at altitude. Similarly, gravitational stress affects traumatic brain injury patients through transient marked increases in intracranial pressure during take-off or landing. Patient positioning on-board the aircraft helps minimize this risk (head forward on take-off, head rearward on landing). Plans should be made for cabin temperature changes from 15°C (59°F) to 25°C (77°F) on winter missions, and 20°C (68°F) to 35°C (95°F) on summer missions. Finally, exposure to noise can produce problems with communication, patient evaluation, and fatigue. Because auscultation is impossible, blood pressure should be monitored with either a noninvasive blood pressure device or arterial line. Hearing protection should be provided for all patients, including those who are intubated/sedated. It should also be kept in mind that audible medical equipment alarms are useless, hence great caution must be taken to remain vigilant for equipment malfunction or patient status changes. Lastly, the humidity is decreased in military transport airplanes as they have very low cabin humidity at altitude. Evaporative losses will increase; therefore patients will require additional fluids, especially those with large burns, and intubated patients are at risk for mucous plugging. Frequently, standard maintenance fluids should be increased 25–50% for patients unable to take in oral hydration.

## SPECIALTY CARE

### Traumatic Brain Injury

In current operations, it is not unusual to care for casualties with significant penetrating brain injury. Primary injury and prevention of additional secondary injury by avoidance of hypoxia and hypotension are the same as in civilian trauma management. Two unique aspects appear to be emerging: fragmentation injury to the brain is dissimilar to small arms fire injury and burr holes have a role in the military environment. Several neurosurgeons with experience in current theater of operations attest to the survivability of fragmentation injury despite low GCS upon arrival (personal communication, Lennarson, Warren, Grant, Ecklund, and Poffenbarger). Not enough information is yet available to make strong recommendations; suffice it to say, for even those casualties presenting with GCS 3 after fragmentation injury to the brain aggressive management should include appropriate volume resuscitation, full diagnostic evaluation, and operative intervention. Cranial burr holes may not only be diagnostic but also therapeutic for patients with TBI in the field environment. In many austere locations, no CT is available, thus the clinician relies on physical exam, mechanism of injury, and high index of suspicion related to TBI. One key component is the ability to perform cranial burr holes. This procedure is reserved for the most austere of situations when the casualty is demonstrating clinical signs of herniation, no neurosurgeon is available, and safe transport of the casualty to the nearest neurosurgeon is not possible. The burr hole should be done in cases of penetrating injury near, but not through, the site of the injury. For blunt trauma, temporal burr holes should be done first, on the side ipsilateral to the larger pupil or, in case of equal pupils, on the side demonstrating external signs of injury (bruising, fracture, etc.).[137]

### Facial Injury Management

There is something unique to facial injury management in the injured combatant as compared to civilian experience. Although noninvasive diagnostic evaluations become the norm in the civilian sector,[138] there is little role for nonoperative approach in the combat zone. Not only are high-resolution multidetector CT scanners unavailable, the patient will not be under the observation and care of the surgeon once the casualty enters the air evacuation system. Unlike soft tissue management in other areas of the body, only minimal debridement is required in the face and neck due to the high resiliency against infection in this highly vascular region. Also, facial injury in the combat zone can be safely closed at the initial operation if adequate debridement and irrigation have been accomplished. Patients should be maintained on antibiotic therapy for 7–10 days postinjury with antibiotics to cover anaerobic oral flora (clindamycin). Fortunately, relatively few (<5%) soldiers sustain eye injury,[139] thanks to protective eyewear mandated for wear by troops in combat. These ballistic proof lenses deflect many fragments, thus protecting the eye from severe injury.

### Burn Wound Care

Burn wound care is not substantially different in the military field environment except in cases of significant associated blast injury.

There appears to be a propensity for malignant edema formation in some casualties treated with usual IV fluid replacement algorithms. There may also be a component of AE transport and the physiology of the casualty under the stresses of flight that have yet to be elucidated. Suffice it to say, very close scrutiny must be done to resuscitation of the burned victim in the field environment. Careful documentation of BSA burned, amount of fluid administered, and urine output are very important factors as the patient traverses the echelons of care. Very strict fluid management is currently in practice, so is moving to colloid-base resuscitation earlier. The patient must be very carefully monitored for the development of compartment syndrome, both of the extremity and of the abdomen, especially during AE transport.

## Orthopedic Care

Damage control orthopedics learned from civilian trauma care is also the initial mode of therapy in the field.[140] External fixation of fracture predominates in the current conflict due to the proliferation of a field-expedient external frame system The use of these devices has been extremely helpful in a variety of ways. One is that it can downgrade the urgency of the MEDEVAC system. By being able to take the casualty to the OR and washing out a fracture and providing temporary stabilization, the casualty can be recovered and sent with less urgency. Also, during the transport, the casualty has tremendous improvement in pain relief. Upon arrival to the next echelon facility, the urgency to rush them to the OR has now been obviated. The final fixation can either occur in country or once the casualty has been flown back to the echelon IV facility in the United States. The use of external fixators are also high when a vascular repair or shunt needs to be stabilized more effectively than external splinting. Since not all Level II surgical facilities have access to orthopedic surgeons, it is imperative that general surgeons be adequately trained to perform these procedures which are relatively simple to do once familiarization of the equipment has been made. Another scenario where external fixators have been found to be of use was on Iraqi personnel who may not be able to stay in the US coalition forces system and they will be inserted back into the Iraqi civilian trauma system. The civilian trauma system in Iraq is in extreme need of assistance and the level of care is not what we are accustomed to in the Western culture due to the war. In many cases, the external fixator is the definitive care and this care.[141] However, there is some caution to be heard as the long-term effects of what we think is beneficial now may not be the case in the future. This may be especially true when general surgeons are sometimes doing this procedure.[142] Precise indications for external fixator use versus casting have not been established. Other indications for external fixator use are when the soft tissues need to be evaluated while en route, when other injuries make use of casting impractical, such as with a femur fracture and abdominal injury, or patients with extensive burns.

The choice of initial fracture stabilization for a particular fracture should be based on the surgeons experience, materials available, and the patients' condition. Advantages of external fixation are that it allows for soft tissue access, can be used for polytrauma patients, and has a minimal physiologic impact on the patient. Disadvantages are the potential for pin site sepsis or colonization and less soft tissue support than casts. Advantages for transportation casts are that they preserve the maximum number of options for

the receiving surgeon, the soft tissues are well supported, and are relatively low tech. Disadvantages are that casts cover soft tissues, may not be suitable for polytrauma patients, and require more weight and cubic space to carry/deliver than external fixators.

Though standard in civilian trauma centers, intramedullary nailing of major long-bone fractures is contraindicated in combat zone hospitals because of a variety of logistical and physiologic constraints. This method may be used once a patient reaches a rear echelon site where more definitive care can be provided.

## Pediatric Injury

This bears mentioning, not from injury management perspective but from a logistics standpoint. Modern military MTFs are often not outfitted with any pediatric-specific equipment (endotracheal tubes, chest tubes, etc.). Unfortunately, children are often "caught in the crossfire" in urban warfare and require treatment. Every surgeon must know the capabilities of the facility as well as the expected casualty demographics. In this case, if there is any likelihood of receiving pediatric injured patients, appropriate equipment and training need to be obtained.

## NEW TECHNOLOGY UTILIZED IN THIS WAR

There are a variety of technological advances being made in a coordinated fashion by the three forces. While some of the technology described below is not necessarily new, it is relatively new to the military medicine. While there are many advances that have been made, there is much that still needs improvement. In the field there is a constant need for all the devices to be compact, portable, quiet, efficient, and wireless.

## Casualty Transporters

Casualty stretchers have been enhanced by light weight and easily mobile carriage systems. For the stretchers, multiple components are available that allow for movement over austere terrain. In addition to low-tech developments that have been made, there are high-tech stretchers or patient carriers that have high potential for the care of casualties in the field. These stretchers are portable ICU beds with built-in oxygen supply, ventilator, monitoring equipment, suction, fluid infusers, and point of care laboratory capability. The weight and cube has been designed to withstand the rigors of travel within the military air transport system, but these requirements have also made them too heavy and expensive. While the high-tech intensive care system has not yet made its way into the war, continued efforts to make these systems more portable and cost effective are underway.

## Monitoring Equipment

At the current time the equipment used in the field are off-the-shelf portable devices that are designed for use in the civilian sector. While these products have made advances in the medical field there is a continued need for specific devices that are dependable, portable, and field usable. One such effort is the development of wireless vital signs (WVS) monitoring devices. Current transport devices are still bulky, heavy, and expensive. With currently available computer technology it is completely possible to develop a system that uses off-the-shelf technology to repackage the monitoring equipment for easy use and transport. The Office of Naval Research (ONR) has invested into this arena and has developed a noninvasive blood pressure cuff that is battery operated and provides vital signs such as intermittent blood pressure, heart rate rhythm, and oxygen saturation with only two attachments emitting from the blood pressure cuff. This data is then transmitted via Wi-Fi technology to portable computers such as handheld PDAs. When the PDA is docked to recharge the battery, it can display onto extremely inexpensive LCD displayers that are used for computers. The provider can then see the recent vital signs of all patients by merely asking the PDA to display the patient's vital signs by picking the patient. The hope is that this device can eventually transmit the vital signs via network servers to anyone who so wishes to see them. Eventually, this information can also be transmitted to eye protection devices so that the vital signs are seen as a heads-up display format. The absence of attaching wires to portable monitors makes the transport of the patient easy as the devices do not have to be detached and reattached when the patient goes from the treatment area to the OR, or during transport in ambulances or helicopters. While much research is being dedicated to monitoring of soldiers in the field, this work being performed by the ONR is to merely make the current monitoring of only injured casualties which is an important distinction.

## Portable Labs

Laboratory results are not mandatory in the field of combat casualty care. However, the continual improvement in equipment has made point-of-care laboratory values available and extremely useful. Hematocrit and hemoglobin values have been traditionally taught that they are highly unreliable in trauma care. If the patient is bleeding quickly the H and H value can be misleading, as they can be normal, it has been found that in both civilian and in combat casualty care there are many circumstances where the rapid fall in H and H occur, and this information can be helpful and reliable. There are many tools that are fielded during the Iraq war such as the use of ISTAT which makes a host of laboratory values available in printed form from a handheld machine that provides many laboratory values such as the arterial blood gases and chemistries that helps guide care. This lesson should be translated to the civilian sector and point-of-care should be available in the resuscitation bays of all trauma facilities and the arguments against it are often political, and cost related.

## Ultrasound

This has become an integral part of trauma. The focused abdominal sonogram for trauma (FAST) is also of value in the field.[143,144] Portable ultrasound does not offer the quality of many machines in civilian trauma centers but is still good enough to provide valuable information. With limited diagnostic capabilities in the field a positive finding indicative of blood in the pericardium or the peritoneal cavity can help with decision making. It can also be used to detect pnemothorax and hemothorax but depends highly on the training and experience of the user. Just as in civilian trauma, it must be stressed that the sensitivity and specificity of FAST is

approximately 75% and 95%, respectively. This means that a negative FAST does not exclude peritoneal penetration nor the absence of blood in the peritoneal cavity. The scenario that is the most helpful in trauma is when the patient is hypotensive and the FAST is positive for fluid. This guides the surgeon to the proper cavity for exploration with the goal of hemorrhage control. When examining the pericardium, the FAST is extremely accurate to rule in or rule out pericardial fluid. It should also be remembered that penetration into the abdominal cavity may result in injury to hollow viscous organs and this does not always lead to bleeding but is usually an indication for exploration.

## Digital Radiographs

This capability is available at Level II facilities and higher. The film can be processed expeditiously and displayed on portable laptop computers. The image is of reasonable quality and there are many images that cannot be obtained. However, it is useful for finding foreign bodies and identifying simple fractures. This is revolutionary in combat casualty care, and has been found to be very useful. Some of the main advantages includes the ability to digitally manipulate the film, enlarging and changing contrast quickly allows for improved effectiveness. The images can easily be stored in a variety of formats including CDs, which can be easily and quickly made so that the casualty may travel with the electronic copy of the films. The images can also be sent to anywhere in the world for rapid consultations. There is much room for improvement in the entire field of digital radiography, but we have taken the first step to make this a better process. It will only get better. While the mechanism to deposit the data to a repository server that can be accessed by all providers is not yet widely available, it will only be a matter of time. Level I and II facilities do not have radiographers and the providers of all level must be familiar with reading the films without the aid of radiologists.

## Oxygen Generators

Technology has made the generation of oxygen available in the forward scenario. This is an important aspect of medical care advancement as this capability has reduced the logistics of oxygen availability. Previously oxygen had to be made at larger facilities which required large machinery and then tanks were filled for portability. The fact that oxygen tanks no longer have to be transported is not a minor feat. These oxygen tanks are often thought of by the transporters as bombs as they can explode easily and cause fire when the tanks are damaged. Some important aspects of oxygen in the field must be mentioned in that the portable oxygen generators (POG) are not yet capable of making 100% oxygen and the highest concentration is usually about 80%. Since oxygen supply is limited and not without costs in the field, it is more important to point out that not all combat casualties need oxygen. In civilian trauma, where oxygen is freely available from a port on the wall, the recommendation for the use of oxygen on all trauma patients does make sense. However due to the availability and difficulty in providing oxygen during transport, it is recommended that oxygen be utilized only on patients who need it. This can be for those with traumatic brain injury, those who are hypotensive, and for patients who demonstrate hypoxia on the pulse oxymetric monitor. Preserving oxygen specifically for those who require it is not a minor point. Transports are also notoriously difficult and not having to transport patients with supplemental oxygen is extremely helpful.

## Portable Equipment

Multiple monitoring and surgical equipment has been made for portability. However, they can and should be continually modified to achieve the least amount of weight and cube. Portable suction devices can be notoriously loud making the use of suction an unpleasant matter. Further development should concentrate on making as much of the gear as portable and lightweight as possible.

# LESSONS LEARNED/WHAT WORKED AND IMPROVEMENTS NEEDED

## Ingredients for Success

The standard of trauma care has been elevated in the United States in recent decades. The current system that we enjoy is far from optimal but is arguably the best in civilization. The main problem in military medicine is that we have enjoyed many decades of peace where we have been less than progressive and not as diligent as the civilian sector in keeping up with their progress. This war has quickly brought us up to similar standards and the better news is that we have also been able to make progress in terms of new methodology and usage of new products in the field.

There are five ingredients for success (Table 55-7) and this includes a trauma system with coordination across all services. The second is proper training for all those who will be caring for the wounded. The third is resources and this should be available in the right place at the right time. This includes equipment, supplies, and people. The fourth is communication. Capability is needed, so those caring for the wounded can talk to others in various levels of care. Finally, the fifth ingredient is data. We need to be able to accurately collect and analyze data so that we can make proper decisions.

Trauma systems concept is relatively new to the three services. Although marked amount of progress has been made to form a Joint Trauma Directors position in theater, this does not necessarily mean that they have jurisdiction among the medical assets in theater nor does it mean that they have authority to make decisions among the three services. This trauma director position is an advisory role. While the exact role of this position still needs to evolve, it is a giant leap toward the right direction as the military now for the first time recognizes the specialty of trauma surgery. The optimal capability of this position would be able to make a decision on

**TABLE 55-7**

| Ingredients for Success |
|---|
| 1. Trauma system |
| 2. Training |
| 3. Resources |
| 4. Communication |
| 5. Data |

the type and number of assets and their location in order to optimize flow and treatment.

Training is a major issue in the military across the three services. For decades during relative peace time since the Vietnam conflict, trauma training has not kept up with the civilian sector. This is because the civilian sector continued to make strides in progress of caring for the injured. However, in the military, since trauma care is only practiced at very few select military hospitals, trauma training is mostly all didactic. The lack of trauma training is problematic at all levels but those who need the training the most are first responders. They rarely have seen severely injured personnel and the first time that they treat a casualty in battle should not be the time to learn. This is an injustice to those who put their lives in harm's way for the service to our country. In order to provide care at the level we are accustomed to in the United States, the military providers need to be trained and given the opportunity to have trauma experience. While the standards of a civilian Level I trauma center is not always attainable, we should make all attempts to reach that level when possible. The three services have a trauma training program set up with collaborative civilian trauma centers. The Air Force is located in Baltimore, Maryland, at the Cowley Shock Trauma Center, the Army at the Ryder trauma center, and the Navy at the Los Angeles County Medical Center. The programs are roughly the same and provide real hands-on experience prior to deployment. The Air Force has two additional centers that are colocated at smaller trauma centers to provide specific training such as en route critical care training. While the training program still suffers from many logistical issues, the acceptance that trauma training is growing is a step in the right direction.[145]

The third issue is resources. As far as the equipment and supply, most will confirm that we do have most things that are essential. Given the difficulty of having a war on the opposite side of the globe, the materials are relatively ample. The things that are needed are better gear. While most of all the gear out there is sufficient, they can always be made better: smaller, rugged, and portable. The research and development has provided many new useful products. The real problematic area is the personnel. This is especially true for the surgical community. The attrition of surgeons is more than bearable and it will be interesting to see what will happen at the current pace. With dwindling number of deployable surgeons, those who are capable of deploying are having to do so more and more frequently than their family will tolerate. As a result, many continue to leave the service which puts the burden on the remaining surgeons even more problematic. There has been much discussion on making a large reserve component of civilian trauma surgeons deployable but changes to the system of this magnitude will take many years.

The fourth issue of communication is problematic though there is tremendous capability in existence. In Iraq, there are some locations where communication is very robust, with surgeons having cell phones and computer access. However, in some remote locations where the casualties are generated, communications can be very poor. Consistency is problematic. There are also issues within the medical system such as the MEDEVAC system. This system uses the traditional "9-line," which is a series of bare essential information that helicopters need in order to arrange transportation. Because the medical system must use the communication system allowed by the fighting forces, changes to this system is difficult at best. However, the optimal method of providing casualty information with injuries and physiologic status allows for the transport of the casualty to the right location in the correct priority. Although the system does not yet exist, the services are heading toward putting together a digital communication system that will allow for collection of casualty data so that it can impact casualty care. Problems with security will always hamper progress in the military but we are headed in the right direction. The hope from the lessons learned is that we will be able to capture information easily and with off-the-shelf equipment such as digital cameras which allows for photography of the casualty at presentation, videos of the injuries, videos of the surgery including dictations, placement of digital radiographs onto the same file for the casualty, and the capture of the written documents by simply taking a picture of the files. This can either be transferred on to a variety of digital storing equipment or the memory chip from the camera itself can be attached to the casualty as an electronic dog tag and medical record.

The final ingredient toward success is data. A joint trauma registry has been initiated which, by design, has many of the data fields that are believed to be vital for providing meaningful information. The problem is that this system is in its infancy and will probably not be able to make an impact until the next war. However, this is an important step that was achieved, and is only a step in the right direction. Currently, the system does have to get used to the fact that a trauma registry record needs to be filled out at all levels and this will indeed take time. This is a valuable lesson learned from the civilian sector and will take time to mature.

There are many aspects of war that is too familiar to those who have experienced war before. Loss of life is always tragic. Loss of life for causes some may not understand or believe in is difficult. The wounds seen on young healthy soldiers that are devastating are hard to accept despite any experience level. If your heart is not affected by the wounds caused by war, then you have no heart. To see innocent civilians pay the price for war is frustrating. These things are common among all wars. However, there has been much progress made in military medicine. Most all of it is directly due to the progress made during peace time and translation from the civilian sector into the military. The "new" way we handle casualties are indeed new and very exciting. This is especially true as we see the survivability increase for the first time in over a century. We have the capability to bring the heroes back home within days of wounding from the other side of the planet. These are not small tasks and are revolutionary. In all, we have made progress and that progress is good.

## REFERENCES

1. DeBakey ME: History, the torch that illuminates: Lessons from military medicine. *Mil Med* 161:711, 1996.
2. Winkenwerder WJ: *Coordination of policy to establish a joint theater trauma registry.* Washington, D.C.: Health Affairs, Department of Defense, 22 Dec 2004.
3. Bellamy RF: *Combat trauma overview. Textbook of military medicine: Anesthesia and pre-operative care of the combat casualty.* Washington, D.C.: Department of the Army, Office of the Surgeon General, Borden Institute; 1994, p. 1.
4. Battle injury, active duty Army personnel, Vietnam origin, 1961–1979. In *US Army Patient Administration Systems and Biostatistics Activity.* Fort Sam Houston, TX: AMEDD Center and School, Department of the Army; 28 June 1984 (Unpublished data).
5. Wound Data and Munitions Effectiveness Team: The WDMET Study. Original data from the Uniformed Services University of the Health Sciences, Bethesda, MD 20814-4799; summary volumes available from: Defense Documentation Center, Cameron Station, Alexandria VA 22304–6145; 1970.
6. Bellamy RF, Zajtchuk R: Assessing the effectiveness of conventional weapons. In Bellamy RF, Zajtchuk R, eds. *Textbook of Military Medicine: Conventional Warfare: Ballistic, Blast, and Burn Injuries.* Washington, D.C.: Department of the Army, Office of the Surgeon General, Borden Institute, 1991, p. 53.
7. Champion HR, Bellamy RF, Roberts CP, et al.: A profile of combat injury. *J Trauma* 54:S13, 2003.
8. Mabry RL, Holcomb JB, Baker AM, et al.: United States Army Rangers in Somalia: An analysis of combat casualties on an urban battlefield. *J Trauma* 49:515, 2000.
9. Patel TH, Wenner KA, Price SA, et al.: A U.S. Army Forward Surgical Team's experience in Operation Iraqi Freedom. *J Trauma* 57:201, 2004.
10. Chambers LW, Rhee P, Baker B, et al.: Initial experience of US Marine Corps' Forward Resuscitative Surgical System during Operation Iraqi Freedom. *Arch Surg* 140:26, 2005.
11. Hinsley DE, Rosell PA, Rowlands TK, et al.: Penetrating missile injuries during asymmetric warfare in the 2003 Gulf conflict. *Br J Surg* 92:637, 2005.
12. Lakstein D, Blumenfeld A: Israeli Army casualties in the second Palestinian uprising. *Mil Med* 170:427, 2005.
13. Kluger Y, Peleg K, Daniel-Aharonson L, et al.: Israeli Trauma Group. The special injury pattern in terrorist bombings. *J Am Coll Surg* 199:875, 2004.
14. Rodoplu U, Arnold JL, Yucel T, et al.: Impact of the terrorist bombings of the Hong Kong Shanghai Bank Corporation headquarters and the British Consulate on two hospitals in Istanbul, Turkey, in November 2003. *J Trauma* 59:195, 2005.
15. Ramalingam T: Extremity injuries remain a high surgical workload in a conflict zone: Experiences of a British Field Hospital in Iraq, 2003. *J R Army Med Corps* 150:187, 2004.
16. Peleg K, Aharonson-Daniel L, Stein M, et al.: Gunshot and explosion injuries: Characteristics, outcomes, and implications for care of terror-related injuries in Israel. *Ann Surg* 239:311, 2004.
17. de Ceballos JP, Turegano-Fuentes F, Perez-Diaz D, et al.: 11 March 2004: The terrorist bomb explosions in Madrid, Spain–an analysis of the logistics, injuries sustained and clinical management of casualties treated at the closest hospital. *Crit Care* 9:104, 2005.
18. Leibovici D, Gofrit ON, Stein M, et al.: Blast injuries: Bus versus open-air bombings–a comparative study of injuries in survivors of open-air versus confined-space explosions. *J Trauma* 41:1030, 1996.
19. Thompson D, Brown S, Mallonee S, et al.: Fatal and non-fatal injuries among U.S. Air Force personnel resulting from the terrorist bombing of the Khobar Towers. *J Trauma* 57:208, 2004.
20. Kluger Y, Mayo A, Hiss J, et al.: Medical consequences of terrorist bombs containing spherical metal pellets: Analysis of a suicide terrorism event. *Eur J Emerg Med* 12:19, 2005.
21. *Emergency War Surgery.* Third United States Revision. Chapter 1. Weapons Effects and Parachute Injuries. Bordens Institute, 2004.
22. Gondusky JS, Reiter MP: Protecting military convoys in Iraq: An examination of battle injuries sustained by a mechanized battalion during Operation Iraqi Freedom II. *Mil Med* 170:546, 2005.
23. Nelson TJ, Wall DB, Stedje-Larsen ET, et al.: Predictors of mortality in close proximity blast injuries during Operation Iraqi Freedom. *J Am Coll Surg* 202:418, 2006.
24. Arnold JL, Halpern P, Tsai MC, et al.: Mass casualty terrorist bombings: A comparison of outcomes by bombing type. *Ann Emerg Med* 43:263, 2004.
25. Thach AB, Ward TP, Dick JS, II, et al.: Intraocular foreign body injuries during Operation Iraqi Freedom. *Ophthalmology* 112:1829, 2005.
26. Mader TH, Carroll RD, Slade CS, et al.: Ocular war injuries of the Iraqi insurgency, January–September 2004. *Ophthalmology* 113:97, 2006.
27. Brennan J: Experience of first deployed otolaryngology team in Operation Iraqi Freedom: The changing face of combat injuries. *Otolaryngol Head Neck Surg* 134:100, 2006.
28. Almogy G, Belzberg H, Mintz Y, et al.: Suicide bombing attacks: Update and modifications to the protocol. *Ann Surg* 239:295, 2004.
29. Zafar H, Rehmani R, Chawla T, et al.: Suicidal bus bombing of French Nationals in Pakistan: Physical injuries and management of survivors. *Eur J Emerg Med* 12:163, 2005.
30. Peleg K, Aharonson-Daniel L, Michael M, et al.: Israel Trauma Group. Patterns of injury in hospitalized terrorist victims. *Am J Emerg Med* 21:258, 2003.
31. Nixon RG, Stewart CE: Recognizing imminent danger: Characteristics of a suicide bomber. *Emerg Med Serv* 34:74, 2005.
32. Hiss J, Kahana T: Trauma and identification of victims of suicidal terrorism in Israel. *Mil Med* 165:889, 2000.
33. Rodoplu U, Arnold JL, Tokyay R, et al.: Mass-casualty terrorist bombings in Istanbul, Turkey, November 2003: Report of the events and the prehospital emergency response. *Prehospital Disaster Med* 19:133, 2004.
34. Arnold JL, Tsai MC, Halpern P, et al.: Mass-casualty, terrorist bombings: Epidemiological outcomes, resource utilization, and time course of emergency needs (Part I). *Prehospital Disaster Med* 18:220, 2003.
35. *Emergency War Surgery.* Third United States Revision. Chapter 3. Triage. Bordens Institute, 2004.

36. Lein B, Holcomb J, Brill S, et al.: Removal of unexploded ordnance from patients: A 50-year military experience and current recommendations. *Mil Med* 164:163, 1999.

37. McSwain M, Frame S, Salomone J: *Military Medicine.* Prehospital advanced life support. 5th ed. St Louis: Mosby, 2003.

38. Beekley AC, Watts DM: Combat trauma experience with the United States Army 102nd Forward Surgical Team in Afghanistan. *Am J Surg* 187:652, 2004.

39. Place RJ, Rush RM Jr, Arrington ED: Forward surgical team (FST) workload in a special operations environment: The 250th FST in Operation ENDUR-ING FREEDOM. *Curr Surg* 60:418, 2003.

40. Patel TH, Wenner KA, Price SA, et al.: A U.S. Army Forward Surgical Team's experience in Operation Iraqi Freedom. *J Trauma* 57:201, 2004.

41. Stevens RA, Bohman HR, Baker BC, et al.: The U.S. Navy's forward resuscitative surgery system during Operation Iraqi Freedom. *Mil Med* 170:297, 2005.

42. Peoples GE, Gerlinger T, Craig R, et al.: The 274th Forward Surgical Team experience during Operation Enduring Freedom. *Mil Med* 170:451, 2005.

43. Marshall TJ Jr: Combat casualty care: The Alpha Surgical Company experience during Operation Iraqi Freedom. *Mil Med* 170:469, 2005.

44. Cho JM, Jatoi I, Alarcon AS, et al.: Operation Iraqi Freedom: Surgical experience of the 212th Mobile Army Surgical Hospital. *Mil Med* 170:268, 2005.

45. Montgomery SP, Swiecki CW, Shriver CD: The evaluation of casualties from Operation Iraqi Freedom on return to the continental United States from March to June 2003. *J Am Coll Surg* 201:7, 2005.

46. Jenkins D, Eastridge B, Schiller H, et al.: Trauma system development in a theater of war: Experiences from Operation Iraqi Freedom. *J Trauma* 59:524, 2005.

47. van Geertruyden PH, Soltis CB: Instituting preventive health programs at a level I aid station in a combat environment. *Mil Med* 170:528, 2005.

48. Murray CK, Reynolds JC, Schroeder JM, et al.: Spectrum of care provided at an echelon II Medical Unit during Operation Iraqi Freedom. *Mil Med* 170:516, 2005.

49. Ben-Abraham R, Paret G, Kluger Y, et al.: Primary trauma care experience of army reserve combat medics: Is a new approach needed? *Mil Med* 164:48, 1999.

50. Wojcik BF, Stein CR, Devore RB Jr, et al.: Status of Trauma Care in U.S. Army Hospitals. *Mil Med* 170:141, 2005.

51. Kowalenko T, Stern SA, Dronen SC, et al.: Improved outcome with hypotensive resuscitation of uncontrolled hemorrhagic shock in a swine model. *J Trauma* 33:349, 1992.

52. Stern SA, Dronen SC, Birrer P, et al.: The effect of blood pressure on hemorrhage volume and survival in a near-fatal hemorrhage model incorporating a vascular injury. *Ann Emerg Med* 22:155, 1993.

53. Burris D, Rhee P, Kaufmann C, et al.: Controlled resuscitation for uncontrolled hemorrhagic shock. *J Trauma* 46:216, 1998.

54. Kaweski SM, Sise MJ, Virgilio RW: The effect of prehospital fluids on survival in trauma patients. *J Trauma* 30:1215, 1990.

55. Turner J, Nicholl J, Webber L, et al.: A randomized controlled trial of prehospital intravenous fluid replacement therapy in serious trauma. *Health Technol Assess* 19:160, 2000.

56. Kwan I, Bunn F, Roberts I: WHO Pre-Hospital Trauma Care Steering Committee: Timing and volume of fluid administration for patients with bleeding following trauma. *Cochrane Database Syst Rev* 1:CD003345, 2001.

57. Dula DJ, Wood GC, Rejmer AR, et al.: Use of prehospital fluids in hypotensive blunt trauma patients. *Prehosp Emerg Care* 6:417, 2002.

58. Greaves I, Porter KM, Revell MP: Fluid resuscitation in pre-hospital trauma care: A consensus view. *J R Coll Surg Edinb* 47:451, 2002.

59. Dutton RP, Mackenzie CF, Scalea TM: Hypotensive resuscitation during active hemorrhage: Impact on in-hospital mortality. *J Trauma* 52:1141, 2002.

60. Bickell WH, Wall MJ, Pepe PE, et al.: Immediate versus delayed fluid resuscitation for hypotensive patients with penetrating torso injuries. *NEJM* 331:1105, 1994.

61. Victorino GP, Battistella FD, Wisner DH: Does tachycardia correlate with hypotension after trauma? *J Am Coll Surg* 196:679, 2003.

62. Rhee P, Wang D, Ruff P, et al.: Human neutrophil activation and increased adhesion by various resuscitation fluids. *Crit Care Med* 28:74, 2000.

63. Alam HB, Stanton K, Koustova E, et al.: Effect of Different Resuscitation Strategies on Neutrophil Activation in a Swine Model of Hemorrhagic Shock. *Resuscitation* 60:91, 2004.

64. Rhee P, Wang D, Ruff P, et al.: Human neutrophil activation and increased adhesion by various resuscitation fluids. *Crit Care Med* 28:74, 2000.

65. Shires TG, Browder LK, Steljes TPV, et al.: The effect of shock resuscitation fluids on apoptosis. *Am J Surg* 189:85, 2005.

66. Coimbra R, Porcides R, Loomis W, et al.: HSPTX protects against hemorrhagic shock resuscitation-induced tissue injury: An attractive alternative to Ringer's lactate. *J Trauma* 60:41, 2006.

67. Jaskille A, Alam HB, Rhee P, et al.: D-Lactate increases pulmonary apoptosis by restricting phosphorylation of Bad and eNOS in a rat model of hemorrhagic shock. *J Trauma* 57:262, 2004.

68. Jaskille A, Koustova E, Rhee P, et al.: Hepatic apoptosis after hemorrhagic shock in rats can be reduced through modifications of conventional Ringer's solution. *J Am Coll Surgeons* 202:25, 2006.

69. Koustova E, Stanton K, Gushchin V, et al.: Effects of lactated Ringer's solutions on human leukocytes. *J Trauma* 52:872, 2002.

70. Ayuste EC, Chen H, Koustova E, et al.: Hepatic and pulmonary apoptosis after hemorrhagic shock in swine can be reduced through modifications of conventional ringer's solution. *J Trauma* 60:52, 2006.

71. Committee on fluid resuscitation for combat casualties: *Fluid resuscitation: State of the science for treating combat casualties and civilian injuries.* Report of the Institute of Medicine. National Academy Press, Washington, D.C., 1999.

72. Martin M, Salim A, Murray J, et al.: The decreasing incidence and mortality of acute respiratory distress syndrome after injury: A 5-year observational study. *J Trauma* 59:1107, 2005.

73. Ciesla DJ, Moore EE, Johnson JL, et al.: A 12-year prospective study of postinjury multiple organ failure: Has anything changed? *Arch Surg* 140:432, 2005.

74. Wade CE, Grady JJ, Kramer GC, et al.: Individual patient cohort analysis of the efficacy of hypertonic saline/dextran in patients with traumatic brain injury and hypotension. *J Trauma* 42:61S, 1997.

75. Junger WG, Coimbra R, Liu FC, et al.: Hypertonic saline resuscitation: A tool to modulate immune function in trauma patients? *Shock* 8:235, 1997. Review.

76. Bunn F, Alderson P, Hawkins V: Colloid solutions for fluid resuscitation. *Cochrane Database Syst Rev* 1:CD001319, 2003.

77. Moretti EW, Robertson KM, El-Moalem H, et al.: Intraoperative colloid administration reduces postoperative nausea and vomiting and improves outcomes compared with crystalloid administration. *Anesth Analg* 96:611, 2003.

78. Alderson P, Schierhout G, Roberts I, et al.: Colloid versus crystalloids for fluid resuscitation in critically ill patients. *Cochrane Database Syst Rev* 2:CD000567, 2000.

79. Cooper DJ, Myles PS, McDermott FT, et al.: Prehospital Hypertonic Saline Resuscitation of Patients With Hypotension and Severe Traumatic Brain Injury: A Randomized Controlled Trial. *JAMA* 291:1350, 2004.

80. Rhee P, Koustova E, Alam HB: Searching for the optimal resuscitation method: Recommendations for the initial fluid resuscitation of combat casualties. *J Trauma* 54:S52, 2003.

81. Hebert PC, Wells G, Blajchman MA, et al.: A multicenter randomized, controlled clinical trial of transfusion requirements in critical care. *N Engl J Med* 340:409–417, 1999.

82. Sloan EP, Koenigsberg M, Gens D, et al.: Diaspirin Cross-Linked Hemoglobin (DCLHb) in the treatment of severe traumatic hemorrhagic shock, a randomized controlled efficacy trial. *JAMA* 282:1857, 1999.

83. Arnaud F, Hammett M, Asher L, et al.: Effects of bovine polymerized hemoglobin on coagulation in controlled hemorrhagic shock in swine. *Shock* 24:145, 2005.

84. Driessen B, Jahr JS, Lurie F, et al.: Arterial oxygenation and oxygen delivery after hemoglobin-based oxygen carrier infusion in canine hypovolemic shock: A dose-response study. *Crit Care Med* 31:1771, 2003.

85. Gurney J, Philbin N, Rice J, et al.: A hemoglobin based oxygen carrier, bovine polymerized hemoglobin (HBOC-201) versus hetastarch (HEX) in an uncontrolled liver injury hemorrhagic shock swine model with delayed evacuation. *J Trauma* 57:726, 2004.

86. Fitzpatrick CM, Savage SA, Kerby JD, et al.: Resuscitation with a blood substitute causes vasoconstriction without oxide scavenging in a model of arterial hemorrhage. *J Am Coll Surg* 199:693, 2004.

87. York GB, Eggers JS, Smith DL, et al.: Low-volume resuscitation with a polymerized bovine hemoglobin-based oxygen-carrying solution (HBOC-201) provides adequate tissue oxygenation for survival in a porcine model of controlled hemorrhage. *J Trauma, Injury, Infect Crit Care* 55:873, 2003.

88. Kim HW, Greenburg AG: Artificial oxygen carriers as red blood cell substitutes: A selected review and current status. *Artificial Organs* 28:813, 2004.

89. Gould SA, Moore EE, Hoyt DB, et al.: The life-sustaining capacity of human polymerized hemoglobin when red cells might be unavailable. *J Am Coll Surg* 195:445, 2002.

90. Thyes C, Spahn DR: Current Status of Artificial O(2) Carriers. *Anesthesiol Clin North Am* 23:373, 2005.

91. Silliman CC, Moore EE, Johnson JL, et al.: Transfusion of the injured patient: Proceed with caution. *Shock* 21:291, 2004.

92. Cothren C, Moore EE, Offner PJ, et al.: Blood substitute and erythropoietin therapy in a severely injured Jehovah's witness. *N Engl J Med* 4;346:1097, 2002.

93. Moore FA, McKinley BA, Moore EE: The next generation in shock resuscitation. *Lancet* 12:363, 2004.

94. Johnson JL, Moore EE, Gonzalez RJ, et al.: Alteration of the postinjury hyperinflammatory response by means of resuscitation with a red cell substitute. *J Trauma* 54:133, 2003.

95. Pusateri AE, Modrow HE, Harris RA, et al.: Advanced hemostatic dressing development program: Animal model selection criteria and results of a study of nine hemostatic dressings in a model of severe large venous hemorrhage and hepatic injury in swine. *J Trauma* 55:18, 2003.

96. O'Neill PA, Bluth M, Gloster ES, et al.: Successful use of recombinant activated factor VII for trauma-associated hemorrhage in a patient without pre-existing coagulopathy. *J Trauma* 52:400, 2002.

97. Kenet G, Walden R, Eldad A, et al.: Treatment of traumatic bleeding with recombinant factor VIIa. *Lancet* 27:354, 1999.

98. Harrison TD, Laskosky J, Jazaeri O, et al.: "Low-dose" recombinant activated factor VII results in less blood and blood product use in traumatic hemorrhage. *J Trauma* 59:150, 2005.

99. Dutton RP, Hess JR, Scalea TM: Recombinant factor VIIa for control of hemorrhage: Early experience in critically ill trauma patients. *J Clin Anesth* 15:184, 2003.

100. Schreiber MA, Holcomb JB, Hedner U, et al.: The effect of recombinant factor VIIa on coagulopathic pigs with grade V liver injuries. *J Trauma* 53:252, 2002.

101. Martinowitz U, Holcomb JB, Pusateri AE, et al.: Intravenous rFVIIa administered for hemorrhage control in hypothermic coagulopathic swine with grade V liver injuries. *J Trauma* 50:721, 2001.

102. Klemcke HG, Delgado A, Holcomb JB, et al.: Effect of recombinant FVIIa in hypothermic, coagulopathic pigs with liver injuries. *J Trauma* 59:155, 2005.

103. Jeroukhimov I, Jewelewicz D, Zaias J, et al.: Early injection of high-dose recombinant factor VIIa decreases blood loss and prolongs time from injury to death in experimental liver injury. *J Trauma* 53:1053, 2002.

104. Boffard KD, Riou B, Warren B, et al.: Recombinant factor VIIa as adjunctive therapy for bleeding control in severely injured trauma patients: Two parallel randomized, placebo-controlled, double-blind clinical trials. *J Trauma* 59:8, 2005.

105. O'Connel KA, Wood JJ, Wise RP, et al.: Thromboembolic adverse events after use of recombinant human coagulation factor VIIa. *JAMA* 295:293, 2006.

106. Martinowitz U, Zaarur M, Yaron BL, et al.: Treating traumatic bleeding in a combat setting: Possible role of recombinant activated factor VII. *Mil Med* 169:16, 2004.

107. Mayer SA, Brun NC, Begtrup K, et al.: Recombinant Activated Factor VII Intracerebral Hemorrhage Trial Investigators. Recombinant activated factor VII for acute intracerebral hemorrhage. *N Engl J Med* 24:777, 2005.

108. Williams DJ, Thomas GO, Pambakian S, Parker PJ: First military use of activated Factor VII in an APC-III pelvic fracture. *Injury* 36:395, 2005.

109. Maughon JS: An inquiry into the nature of wounds resulting in killed in action in Vietnam, *Mil Med* 135:8, 1970.

110. Clifford CC: Treating traumatic bleeding in a combat setting. *Mil Med* 169:8, 2004.

111. Sondeen JL, Pusateri AE, Coppes VG, et al.: Comparison of 10 different hemostatic dressings in an aortic injury. *J Trauma* 54:280, 2003

112. King DR, Cohn SM, Proctor KG; Miami Clinical Trials Group: Modified rapid deployment hemostat bandage terminates bleeding in coagulopathic patients with severe visceral injuries. *J Trauma* 57:756, 2004.

113. Pusateri AE, McCarthy SJ, Gregory KW, et al.: Effect of a Chitosan-based Hemostatic Dressing on Blood Loss and Survival in a Model of Severe Venous Hemorrhage and Hepatic Injury in Swine. *J Trauma* 54:177, 2003.

114. Wedmore I, McManus JG, Pusateri AE, et al.: A special report on the chitosan-based hemostatic dressing: Experience in current combat operations. *J Trauma* 60:655, 2006.

115. Alam HB, Burris D, DaCorta JA, et al.: Hemorrhage control in the battlefield: Role of new hemostatic agents. *Mil Med* 170:63, 2005.

116. Alam HB, Uy GB, Miller D, et al.: Comparative Analysis of Hemostatic Agents in a Swine Model of Lethal Groin Injury. *J Trauma* 54:1077, 2003.

117. Wright JK, Kalns J, Wolf EA, et al.: Thermal injury resulting from application of a granular mineral hemostatic agent. *J Trauma* 57:224, 2004.

118. Alam HB, Chen Z, Jaskille A, et al.: Application of a zeolite hemostatic agent achieves 100% survival in a lethal model of complex groin injury in swine. *J Trauma* 56:974, 2004.

119. Wright FL, Hua HT, Velmahos G, et al.: Intracorporeal use of the hemostatic agent Quikclot in a coagulopathic patient with combined thoracoabdominal penetrating trauma. *J Trauma* 56:205, 2004.

120. Rhee P, Alam H: 100 documented use of QuikClot®. Submitted for publication.

121. Calkins MD, Snow C, Costello M, et al.: Evaluation of possible battlefield tourniquet systems for the far-forward setting. *Mil Med* 165:379, 2000.

122. Lakstein D, Blumenfeld A, Sokolov T, et al.: Tourniquets for hemorrhage control in the battlefield: A four year accumulated experience, *J Trauma* 54:S221, 2003.

123. Starnes BW, Beekley AC, Sebesta JA, et al.: Extremity vascular injuries on the battlefield: Tips for surgeons deploying to war. *J Trauma* 60:432, 2006.

124. Fox CJ, Gillespie DL, O'Donnell SD, et al.: Contemporary management of wartime vascular trauma. *J Vasc Surg* 41:638, 2005.

125. Carmona RH, Peck DZ, Lim RC Jr: The role of packing and planned reoperation in severe hepatic trauma. *J Trauma* 24:779, 1984.

126. Feliciano DV, Mattox KL, Burch JM, et al.: Packing for control of hepatic hemorrhage. *J Trauma* 26:738, 1986.

127. Saifi J, Fortune JB, Graca L, et al.: Benefits of intra-abdominal pack placement for the management of nonmechanical hemorrhage. *Arch Surg* 125:119, 1990.

128. Sharp KW, Locicero RJ: Abdominal packing for surgically uncontrollable hemorrhage. *Ann Surg* 215:467, 1992.

129. Burch JM, Ortiz VB, Richardson RJ, et al.: Abbreviated laparotomy and planned reoperation for critically injured patients. Ann Surg 215:476, 1992.

130. Talbert S, Trooskin SZ, Scalea T, et al.: Packing and re-exploration for patients with nonhepatic injuries. *J Trauma* 33:121, 1992.

131. Rotondo MF, Schwab CW, McGonigal MD, et al.: 'Damage control': An approach for improved survival in exsanguinating penetrating abdominal injury. *J Trauma* 35:375, 1993.

132. Brown CV, Velmahos GC, Neville AL, et al.: Hemodynamically "stable" patients with peritonitis after penetrating abdominal trauma: Identifying those who are bleeding. *Arch Surg* 140:767, 2005.

133. Nicholas JM, Rix EP, Easley KA, et al.: Changing patterns in the management of penetrating abdominal trauma: The more things change, the more they stay the same. *J Trauma* 55:1095, 2003.

134. Hashim R, Frankel H, Tandom M, et al.: Fluid resuscitation-induced cardiac tamponade. *J Trauma* 53:1183, 2002.

135. Balogh Z, McKinley BA, Cocanour CS, et al.: Secondary abdominal compartment syndrome is an elusive early complication of traumatic shock resuscitation. *Am J Surg* 184:538, 2002.

136. Harman DR, Hooper TI, Gackstetter GD: Aeromedical evacuations from Operation Iraqi Freedom: A descriptive study. *Mil Med* 170:521, 2005.

137. Donovan DJ, Moquin RR, Ecklund JM: Cranial burr holes and emergency craniotomy: Review of indications and technique. *Mil Med* 171:12, 2006.

138. Mazolewski P, Curry JD, Browder T, Fildes: Computed tomographic scan can be used for surgical decision making in Zone II penetrating neck injuries. *J Trauma* 51:315, 2001.

139. Zouris J, Walker G, Dye J, et al.: Wounding patterns for U S marines and sailors during Operation Iraqi Freedom, major combat phase. *Mil Med* 171:246, 2006.

140. Taeger G, Ruchholtz S, Waydhas C, et al.: Damage control orthopedics in patients with multiple injuries is effective, time saving, and safe. *J Trauma* 59:409, 2005.

141. Scalea TM, Boswell SA, Scott JD, et al.: External fixation as a bridge to intramedullary nailing for patients with multiple injuries and with femur fractures: Damage control orthopedics. *J Trauma* 48:613, 2000.

142. Clasper JC, Phillips SL: Early failure of external fixation in the management of war injuries. *J R Army Med Corps* 151:81, 2005.

143. Brooks AJ, Price V, Simms M: FAST on operational military deployment. *Emerg Med J* 22:263, 2005.

144. Rozanski TA, Edmondson JM, Jones SB: Ultrasonography in a forward-deployed military hospital. *Mil Med* 170:99, 2005.

145. Peoples GE, Gerlinger T, Budinich C, et al.: The most frequently requested precombat refresher training by the Special Forces medics during Operation Enduring Freedom. *Mil Med* 170:31, 2005.

# Commentary ■ ARI LEPPÄNIEMI

This chapter written by well-known clinical, academic, and military surgeons aims to summarize the current experience of the US military from the recent conflicts in Iraq and Afghanistan, and to incorporate that experience to our common knowledge of combat casualty care based on previous conflicts. Although the perspective is very much that of a dominant military power with air superiority and use of relatively small force in the rapid and nonlinear battlefield facing an enemy embedded with the civilian population and utilizing unconventional military and guerrilla tactics, the lessons learned are more widely applicable to modern warfare and peace-keeping operations facing the European Union and other regional, transnational forces, especially in their rapid deployment mode.

Compared with previous knowledge of combat casualty care and my personal experience from the civil wars in Cambodia, southern Sudan, and Afghanistan in the 1980s and 1990s treating war wounded soldiers and civilians in the field hospitals of the International Committee of the Red Cross (ICRC), the authors present several new or modified concepts of modern combat casualty care that could affect the way wounded war victims are treated in future conflicts.

Although the initial wound care including aggressive removal of all dead tissue and leaving the wound open remains the same, the main difference is in the wound management after initial surgery. The standard practice in the past was to cover the debrided wound with a dressing left untouched for 3–7 days (if not soaking in pus or having a sweet smell indicative of infection in contrast to a bitter smell on a dried surface dressing with absorbed tissue secretions indicating well-progressing healing) followed by delayed primary closure. The authors recommend that the debrided wounds should go a planned second debridement and irrigation in 24–72 hours,

and subsequent procedures until a clean wound is achieved. This practice is justified with better demarcation of nonviable tissue or easier identification of the development of infection between procedures. Although the authors refer to delayed primary closure at 3–5 days of clean wounds that can be closed without tension, the repetitive wound inspection and excision results, in effect, in healing by secondary intention, whether negative pressure dressings are used or not. Undoubtedly, their recommendation is based on their vast experience in treating modern, devastating wounds seen in these conflicts, but whether they are universally applicable to all war wounds remains to be seen. Hopefully, the extraordinary data collected and analyzed from these conflicts will help to establish the best practices of modern combat wound care.

The other new concepts presented in this chapter reflect the recent developments in the civilian trauma experience including the use of limited fluid resuscitation, local and systemic hemostatic agents, and principles of damage control surgery, albeit used more in a tactical fashion. In addition, the authors bring forward some new concepts and practices, such as priorities of care under fire, modern triage principles of evaluating two to four patients as they arrive with transferring of critical patients directly to the operation room without spending time in the resuscitation area, use of oral fluids, whole blood, tourniquets, and sophisticated air evacuation. Finally, some of the established principles including external fixation of complex fractures and early soft tissue coverage of bones and vascular repairs are re-emphasized.

As the authors state, well-trained surgeons who can rely on their clinical skills are still the backbone of combat casualty care. This chapter deserves major credit in advancing and updating the knowledge on which the clinical and judgment skills depend on.

# Weapons of Mass Destruction

*David L. Ciraulo*

## TERRORISM

"The unlawful use of force and violence against persons or property to intimidate or coerce a government, the civilian population, or any segment thereof, in furtherance of political or social objectives."

## FEDERAL BUREAU OF INVESTIGATION[1]

A pre-9/11 assessment of the Eastern Association for the Surgery of Trauma's (EAST) membership revealed that the surgical community was ill-prepared to meet the medical challenges of injury from weapons of mass destruction.[2] The Defense Against Weapons of Mass Destruction Act of 1996 public law, 104–201 (09/23/96) title XIV, defines weapons of mass destructions (WMD) as any weapon or device that is intended or has the capability to cause death or serious bodily injury to a significant number of people through the release, dissemination, or impact of (a) toxic or poisonous chemicals or their precursors; (b) disease organism; and (c) radiation or radioactivity.[3] In broader terms, the acronym BNICE weapons is more consistent in scope and depth with contemporary threat as defined: B-biological, N-nuclear, I-incendiary, C-chemical, and E-explosive.

In response to the validated need for education and training[4] EAST, the American Association for the Surgery of Trauma (AAST), and the American College of Surgeons' Committee on Trauma (ACS-COT) have offered programs to strengthen surgeons' preparedness to respond to injury from WMD. The Disaster Subcommittee of EAST has offered a position statement summarizing the roles of the trauma/critical care surgeon in response to disasters, mass casualty incidents, and WMD. This position statement defines the active role of the trauma/critical care surgeon emphasizing not only their surgical skills but also calling upon their management skills in triage and mass casualty incident

management. With limitations in the number of board certified critical care physicians, the importance of the surgeon's critical care skills and the ability to manage intensive care unit (ICU) patients exposed to chemical, radiation, and biological agents is imperative.

### Blast

Explosive and incendiary devices have historically dominated terrorist activity in this country as well as abroad. The attractiveness of explosives and incendiary devices is related to the availability of precursor materials for making bombs, as well as the potential opportunities for utilizing pre-existing commercial resources as explosive devices.

### Blast Physiology

Blast injury has been defined and broken into four distinct categories reflecting the mechanism of tissue injury and physical tissue damage that occurs as a result of the blast phenomenon: primary, secondary, tertiary, and quaternary blast injury.[5]

The primary blast injury is a result of the physical properties of the blast wave. The blast wave occurs as a function of an increase in atmospheric pressure over time, referred to as blast over preassure.[6] The measure of over pressure is dependent upon the energy of the explosion, the distance from detonation, and the elapsed time from explosion.[6] Molecules in air are constantly in a state of motion which possess intrinsic properties of pressure, temperature, and density and is referred to as the state of the gas.[6] When this state of the gas is disturbed from normal conditions resulting in an escalation of molecular speed and an increase in the number of molecules occupying a defined space, the density, pressure, and temperature of the gas will increase.[6] As a result of this physical change, a shock wave, or blast wave, develops moving at supersonic speeds at velocities of 3000 to 8000 m/second, but loses its pressure and velocity as distance increases.[7] The blast front, the

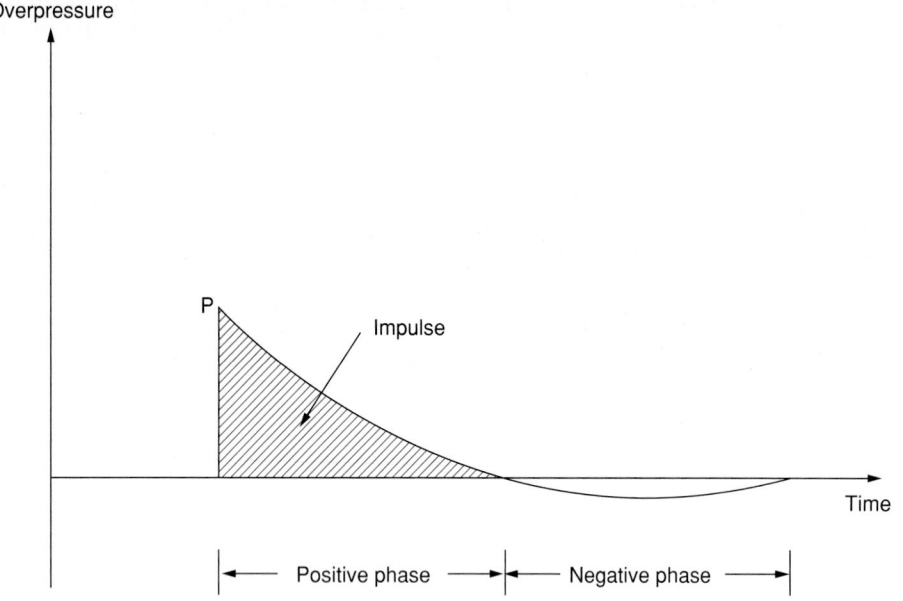

**FIGURE 56-1.** Pressure–time graph of air blast. This graph illustrates the ideal pressure–time history of an air blast in an undisturbed, free-field environment (a Friedlander waveform). The impulse is the integral of pressure over time. P is the peak overpressure.
*(Reproduced with permission from Walter Reed Army Institute of Research, Stuhmiller JH, Phillips YY, Richmond DR. The physics and mechanism of primary blast injury. In Bellamy RF, Jenkins DP, Zajtcjuk JT, et al., eds. Conventional warfare: ballistic, blast, and burn injuries. Washington D.C.: Office of Surgeon General at TMM Publications. 1991,241 Textbook Military Med Series.)*

leading edge of the blast wave, passes through space creating a high-pressure region, or positive phase, called blast wind.[6] From the blast location, as the wave moves forward, a negative-pressure wave propagates from the blast creating a region of low atmospheric pressure.[6] The positive component of the wave peaks instantaneously and exponentially decays to below baseline. The negative component reverses the movement of gas back toward the point of detonation as a result of a vacuum effect (Fig. 56-1). Injury and property damage can occur from both positive and negative phases of the blast wave. In a nuclear blast, an additional component known as the precursor shock wave is observed. This is a shock front near the ground of heated air and moves ahead of the blast wave.[6]

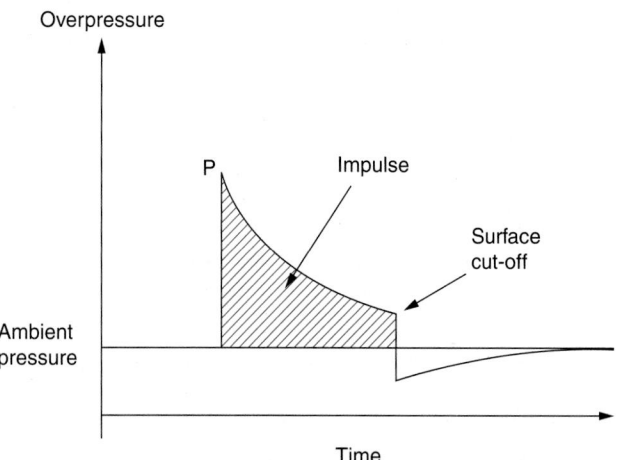

**FIGURE 56-2.** Pressure–time graph of water blast. An underwater blast wave is depicted as measured near the surface. There is a nearly instantaneous rise in pressure, with an exponential decay much like that in air blast (Fig. 56-1). The incident compression wave is reflected from the surface as a tension wave, which interacts with the positive-pressure shock, effectively canceling or cutting it off.
*(Reproduced with permission from Stuhmiller JH, Phillips YY, Richmond DR. The physics and mechanism of primary blast injury. In Bellamy RF, Jenkins DP, Zajtcjuk JT, et al., eds. Conventional warfare: ballistic, blast, and burn injuries. Washington D.C.: Office of Surgeon General at TMM Publications. 1991,241 Textbook Military Med Series.)*

In comparison, an explosion under water produces a large volume of gaseous byproducts resulting in an underwater shock wave.[6,8] As it reaches the surface, the shock wave sends out tiny water droplets referred to as spalling, creating a characteristic dome around a large gas bubble which opens into a spray plume at the surface.[6] The overpressure grafts defines this phase as the cut-off wave, which is a downward reflection from the surface that cancels out the blast wave abruptly (Fig. 56-2). Because water is less compressible, blast wave propagates at high speeds and loses energy less quickly over longer distance.[7]

In general, victim positioning relative to the primary wave or reflective wave results in variation in biological damage. Those that are positioned in a perpendicular fashion to the blast wave, both on land and in water, will experience the greatest amount of impact and injury as compared to those who present in a more horizontal fashion to the blast wave, thus providing less direct surface contact for the impact of the wave on to the person's body.[6] With regard to underwater detonations, the force of the blast wave is greatest at the deepest depths in the water and begins to dissipate as the blast wave approaches the surface. In response to an underwater detonation, the safest location is in a position floating on the surface of the water where maximum dissipation of the explosive energy occurs.[6,8]

## BLAST INJURY

Destructive capacity of this blast wave is due to the mathematically calculated force, which is referred to as blast loading as measured in force per unit area.[6] It is this blast-loading phenomenon that is responsible for the subsequent injury referred to as primary blast injury. Primary blast injury is the first pattern of injury that affects the victim as a result of the blast wave passing through the body. A blast wave has two damaging components, the stress wave which causes damage in relation to the wave's peak of intensity and the sheer wave that is related to the peak velocity strain force of the initiating explosion.[9] These waves have little or no effect on solid or fluid-filled organs;, however, the targets of maximal destruction are air-containing organs.

Perforation of the eardrums and pneumothoraces are hallmarks of primary blast injury. Eardrum perforation occurs at a low peak overpressure of 15–50 psi, with a 50% predictive finding of eardrum perforation at that level.[9] With an overpressure of 50–100 psi, there is a 50% chance of lung injury and lung damage. Therefore, the findings of perforated eardrums are a good indicator for potential life-threatening lung injury necessitating life support and emergency intervention for blunt pulmonary injury.[9–11] The importance of eardrum rupture as a predictor of blast pulmonary injury is exemplified by the Madrid bombing in 2005, where concomitant injury to the ear and lungs were found in a high percentage of those suffering pulmonary blast injury.[12,13] Kruger reports from the Israeli experience that lung injury with a 1% mortality rate is observed with an overpressure of 35 psi but that at a psi of 65, the fatality rate approaches 99%.[9] Factors potentiating the outcome to blast injuries are multiple, relating to magnitude of the explosion, potential building collapse, and the confines of the location of the explosion, that being open air versus enclosed space.[14] As a result of these multifactorial phenomena, the term multidimensional injury has been coined to define of insult to multiple sites as well as to multiple organ systems.[15] In a meta-analysis conducted by Arnold et al., a six-fold increase was observed in pulmonary blasts injuries when the detonation occurred in a confined space.[16–18] Other pathognomonic findings from blast injury are the presence of air emboli that fill the pulmonary vessels and coronary vessels representing the leading cause of death in victims of pulmonary blast injury.[9] Other organs at risk include hollow viscus, which may present early as free air or in a delayed fashion as ischemic injury.[9] Standard surgical intervention as warranted should be implemented with consideration given to a second look for purposes of delayed ischemic complication. Management of the pulmonary injury is supported with mechanical ventilation and surveillance for pneumonic infections and complications.

Secondary blast injury pattern is a result of projectiles resulting in penetrating injury. The interface of debris with skin creates a characteristic skin pattern called spalling.[6] These blast particles may be inert from inanimate objects or they may be biological from dismemberment and fragmentation of victims in and around the primary blast area. Multiple case reports in the literature report allogenic injuries dating back from to the Vietnam conflict to more contemporary times with the frequent bombings that have occurred in Israel and Iraq.[16–18] Of concern, in addition to the penetrating damage that occurs from these projectiles, is the potential for blood-borne pathogen transmission.[17] Several case studies have reported the transmission of hepatitis B and/or found fragments of bone that have tested positive.[17] This has led to the administration of acted hepatitis B vaccines to survivors of penetrating allogeneic tissue.[19,20]

Tertiary blast injury is inclusive of injuries caused from deceleration and structural collapse.[6] These subsequent injuries are consistent with blunt traumatic injury and should be handled accordingly. In addition to the blunt injury, the time delay to recovery and weight of falling debris will cause victims to incur crush injuries.

Quaternary blast injury refers to injuries related to the primary explosion as a result of the byproducts of that explosion, to including burns, and chemical, and radiological exposure.[5] Quaternary blast injury describes the sequela of the reflective of dirty bomb in which chemical or radiologic-laden detonations may occur.

## SPECIAL CONSIDERATIONS IN PREGNANCY

The fetus' hollow organs are void of air, thereby offering protection from primary blast injury. However, the fetus' protective aqueous surroundings, the amniotic fluid, potentially amplifies three-fold the blast wave, three-fold as in underwater detonations bringing concern of potential maternal–fetal injury. The secondary component of blast injury, being that of penetrating shrapnel, heightens the concern for possible fetal injury. As a function of uterine abdominal domain, the closer to term the greater is the potential for penetrating fetal injury. Tertiary blast effects of deceleration should be managed consistent with blunt trauma in pregnancy. Women with previous history of C-sections are at greater risk for uterine rupture following trauma.[21] Women suffering severe trauma should be evaluated by ultrasound with a risk of 40–50% for abruptio placenta.[21] Fetal–maternal hemorrhage may be assessed by the Kleihauer–Betke test and the mother treated accordingly for Rh-isoimmunization.[21] The quaternary effects of blast injury due to contaminants will be addressed in the chemical and radiological discussion of this section. The best chance for fetal survival is that of the stability of the mother suffering traumatic injury.

## CRUSH INJURY

Throughout history, crush injuries have been well-appreciated in both natural and terrorist types of disasters. Crush injuries and crush syndrome were first described by Bywaters in 1941, after many patients who had been trapped under rubble of buildings during the bombing in the Blitz subsequently died of acute renal failure.[22] Crush syndrome or traumatic rhabdomyolysis results when muscle reperfusion injury occurs as a result of the release of compressive forces on the tissues. Following crush injury to the muscle tissue, myoglobin, potassium, and phosphorus leach into the circulation.[23] Clinically, compression of large skeletal muscle is necessary for this syndrome to occur. As a result of compression, the limbs become tense and edematous leading to neurologic and vascular compromise.[24] Vascular compromise is a late sign, resulting in significant delay to treatment and risk for potential failure at limb salvage. This condition, reflective of ischemia, along with elevated tissue pressures in the extremity, is referred to as compartment syndrome.

The physiologic outcome of compartment syndrome is traumatic rhabdomyolysis, which at the cellular level is the loss of capillary integrity of the sarcolemma membrane caused by pressure or stretching of muscle tissues. As this membrane is stretched, sodium, calcium, and water leak into the sarcoplasm trapping extracellular fluid inside the muscle cells.[24]

### Pathophysiology of Renal Injury

Almost 33% of the patients with rhabdomyolysis will develop acute renal failure. This is associated with a mortality rate of 30–50%.[25,26] The mechanisms of renal failure are decreased renal

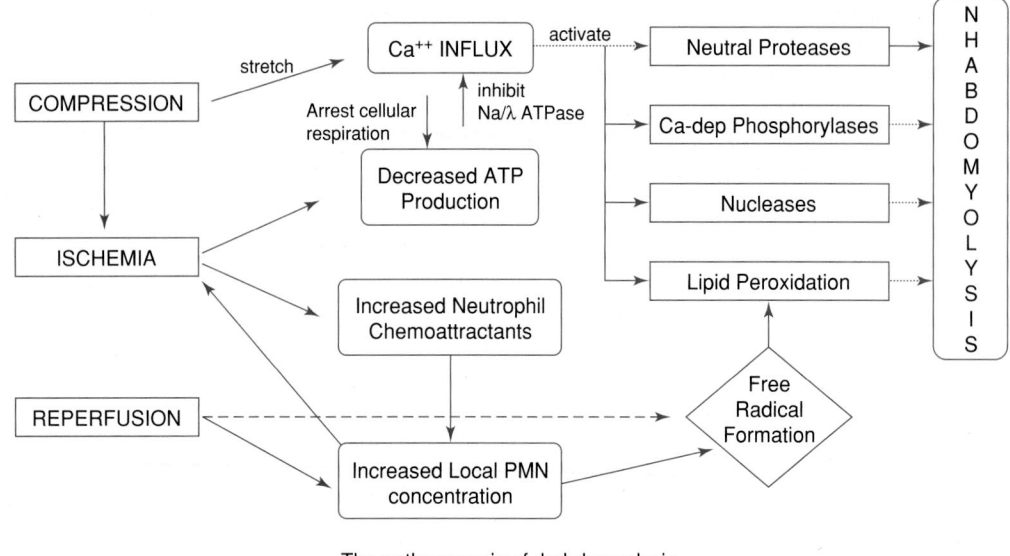

The pathogenesis of rhabdomyolysis.

**FIGURE 56-3.** The pathogenesis of rhabdomyolysis. *(Reproduced with permission from Malinoski PJ, Slater MS, Mullins RJ. Crush injury and rhabdomyolysis. Critical Care Clinics 20:171, 2004.)*

perfusion, cast formation with tubular obstruction, and the direct toxic effects of myoglobin on the renal tubules (Fig. 56-3).[27]

## Diagnosis of Rhabdomyolysis

Rhabdomyolysis is suggested by the presence of dark tea-colored urine, which is dipstick positive for blood despite the absence of red blood cells on the microscopic evaluation following compressive injury. Elevated laboratory findings of creatine kinase (CK) enzymes with typical elevation being greater than 10,000 IU/L are indicative of rhabdomyolysis.[23]

## Management

Early recognition of compartment syndrome as a result of crushed extremities should warrant immediate and expedited intervention. The initial management of these victims is volume resuscitation to maintain a euvolemic state with brisk urine output. To help augment the diuresis, the use of Mannitol, a nonosmotic diuretic, is routinely utilized enhancing the wash out of tubular myoglobin that accumulates in the nephrons. In addition, Mannitol is an effective radical scavenger that may protect the kidney from oxidant injury.[28,29] The use of bicarbonate in the alkalization of the urine serves well to decrease cast formation and lessen the direct toxic effects of myoglobin upon nephrons.[30] Renal toxicity resulting in life-threatening conditions of hyperkalemia, severe acidosis, and hypervolemia should be managed by continuous renal replacement therapy or standard.[31]

Decompressive fasciotomies have been the classic approach to the management of crushes injuries that develop compartment syndrome. If decompressive fasciotomy is not completed within six hours of crush injury, the benefits for limb salvage are negligible due to the irreversible muscle and nerve damage.[32] Direct measurement of the compartments utilizing a pressure device created by Stryker Corporation, Kalamazoo, Michigan (Stryker SCIC device), is complementary to the physical exam. The normal compartment pressure range is from 0 to 15 mm Hg. Pressure exceeding 30–50 mm Hg produce clinically significant muscle ischemia warranting intervention.[32–35] Controversy over the timing and

performing of fasciotomies exists as a result of increased reports of sepsis following decompression.[36–40] The use of adjunct hyperbaric oxygen likewise has been somewhat controversial in its utilization and indications.

## Chemical Terrorism

The use of chemicals in the augmentation of war is perhaps as old as history itself—dating back to 1000 BC with the Chinese use of arsenic-laden smoke as a weapon.[41] Despite diplomatic attempts to curtail chemical warfare, between 1915 and 1917, the modern era of chemical warfare was born with the Germans' use of choline, phosgene, and sulfur mustards against Allied Forces during World War I with devastating effects.[42,43] Mustard agents have repeatedly been used throughout history, including in the 1960s against Yemen and in the 1980s by the Iraqis against the Iranians and the Kurds.[43] Nerve agents were never used in the battlefield until 1984 when the Iraqis used chemicals in the conflict with Iran. From 1984 through 1987, Iraqi's used sulfur mustard, as well as the nerve agents Sarin and Tabun, against the Iranian soldiers and then later against the Iranian civilians resulting in 45,000 to 100,000 Iranian chemical casualties in the war.[44–47] Chemical weapons have been used in several recent events, including the dispersal of Sarin release by the Aum-Shinrikyo Religious Cult (divine truth) in two public attacks with dispersal of Sarin.

The following section will review the five classes of chemical agents with special attention given to agents with high-threat potential (Table 56-1).[48]

## NERVE AGENTS

The nerve agents are perhaps the deadliest of chemical warfare weapons. Nerve agents are known by their NATO codes, which have been internationally accepted as one or two letter abbreviations. The most well-known nerve agents are GA (tabun), GB (sarin), GD (soman), and VX. The NATO code names starting with the letter 'G' are named for those of German origin; the VX

**TABLE 56-1**

## A Quick Reference for Chemical Weapons

| AGENT | SOURCE[a] | ONSET | INITIAL SYMPTOMS | INITIAL MEDICAL MANAGEMENT | CONTACT RISK | PRECAUTIONS |
|---|---|---|---|---|---|---|
| **Nerve agents—** Sarin (GB), soman (GD), tabun (GA), VX (liquid, vapor, aerosol) | WMD | Vapor/aerosol—seconds to minutes Liquid—minutes to hours | Miosis, salivation, rhinorrhea, sweating, wheezing and chest tightness, dyspnea, abdominal cramping, diarrhea, muscle fasciculations, spasms, twitching, paralysis, coma, seizures | **Atropine** 2–6 mg (peds[b] 0.02 µg/kg) IM/IV + **pralidoxime Cl (2-PAMCL)** 600–2000 mg (peds 20 mg/kg) IM/IV[c], repeat atropine 2–4 mg and 2-PAMCL 600–1000 mg Q2–5 min PRN; **Diazepam** 10 mg (peds 0.1–0.3 mg/kg) slow IVP prn seizure mechanical ventilator prn; remove any residual agent from skin with soap and water or one part bleach in nine parts water | High.[d] Avoid contact with residual liquid agent, or inhalation of fumes trapped in patient clothing. | Maximum available protection,[d] including respirator[e] |
| **Vesicants—** mustard, lewisite, phosgene oxime (vapor, liquid) | WMD, I/M | Minutes to hours | Burning/itching/stinging of skin W/erythema and blisters; redness, tearing and burning of eyes, lid spasm, photophobia; nasal irritation and bleeding, sore throat, laryngitis, productive cough | Remove residual agent with one part bleach in nine parts water and rinse with copious water. Supportive care. In **lewisite use BAL** in oil 4 mg deep IM Q4h × 3 doses (Q2h in severe poisoning). **Limit IV fluids.** Systemic analgesics. Treatment of blisters and skin lesions as in thermal burns. | Low. Avoid contact with agent or inhalation of fumes. | Maximum available protection,[d] respirator[e] |
| **Pulmonary agents—** chlorine, phosgene, diphosgene, PFIB (gas) | WMD, I/M | Minutes to hours | Eye, nasal, and oral pain and irritation, tearing, cough, substernal ache and/or pressure. Progresses to dyspnea, choking, rales, hemophysis, pulmonary edema | Supportive with IV fluids, O$_2$, manage airway secretions, intubation, PEEP, observation for at least 24 hour. | Low to none | Standard[f] |
| **Lacrimators (tear gas)—CN, CR, CS** (Particulate solid, mist, smoke) | WMD | Seconds | Eye tearing, redness and lid spasm; burning and pain of eyes, nose, mouth, and throat; sneezing, salivation, chest tightness, and cough. **Unlike pulmonary agents and vesicants, onset is immediate and symptoms improve over 15–30 min following termination of exposure.** | No specific treatment is required. Patients should be decontaminated with one part bleach in nine parts water, or soap and water. Flush eyes with saline or water. | Low | Standard[f] |
| **Cyanide—** hydrogen cyanide, cyanogens (vapor, liquid) | WMD, I/M | Seconds to minutes | Flushing, giddiness, sweating, headache, confusion, gasping, seizure, coma, respiratory arrest, cardiac arrest. Cyanosis is rare. | **100% O$_2$,** CPR, intubation, and mechanical ventilation, **amyl nitrite** via inhalation Q3 min until IV access, then **3% sodium nitrite** 10 ml (peds 0.2 mg/kg in 3% solution) IV over 5 min, followed by **25% Na sodium thiosulfate** 50 ml (peds 1.65 mg/kg in 25% solution) IV over 10 min. Inject each over 3–5 min. May repeat $1/2$ dose of each in 30 min, if needed. | Low to none. Avoid contact with victim's wet clothing.[d] | Standard[f] |
| **Arsine** (AsH$_2$) (gas) | I/M | 2–24 hr | Nausea, vomiting, crampy abdominal pain, malaise, dizziness, headache, dyspnea, RBC, hemolysis, anemia, ↑K, ↓Ca, hypotension, hemoglobinuria, renal, failure. Occasionally delirium. | No specific treatment or antidote. Chelation does not help. Avoid fluid overload in case of renal failure. Consider exchange transfusion. | low to none | Standard[f] |

*(continued)*

**TABLE 56-1    (Continued)**

**A Quick Reference for Chemical Weapons**

| AGENT | SOURCE[a] | ONSET | INITIAL SYMPTOMS | INITIAL MEDICAL MANAGEMENT | CONTACT RISK | PRECAUTIONS |
|---|---|---|---|---|---|---|
| **Anhydrous ammonia** ($NH_3$), **hydrochloric acid** (HCl), **sulfur dioxide** ($SO_2$) [gas, mist, liquid] | I/M, A | Seconds to minutes | Eye, nasal, oral, and upper airway irritation/burns; pain, hoarseness; possible stridor, cough, and wheezing; ↑concentration and/or ↑exposure can act like pulmonary agents | Supportive care; thoroughly rinse victim if not already done, stabilize/protect airway and manage secretions; $O_2$; early intubation if needed, mechanical ventilation and PEEP if necessary; observation for at least 24 hr after exposure | Low to none. Avoid contact with residual liquid. | Standard[f] |
| **Hydrofluoric acid** (HF) [liquid, vapor, aerosol] | I/M | Seconds to days | Initial same as anhydrous ammonia, plus later deep skin burns, ↓Ca, ↓Mg, ↑K, tetany, arrhythmias, CHF, shock death (serious systemic effects may take days to occur) | Supportive care; rapid decontamination ($H_2O$) if not already done; stabilize/protect airway and manage secretions; $O_2$; closely follow and correct lyte imbalances; cover with residual burns W/**2.5 gms Ca gluconate in 100 ml K-Y Jelly**. Avoid emesis. **1.5 ml of 10% Ca gluconate in 4.5 ml NS** via nebulizer inhalation. | Low. Avoid contact with residual liquid or contaminated clothing | Standard,[f] double glove and eye protection if residual liquid |
| **Hydrogen sulfide** ($H_2S$) [gas] | I/M | Minutes | Eye, nasal, oral, and upper airway irritation and pain skin erythema, flushing, sweating, headache, nausea, vomiting, gasping, tachypnea, possible wheezing, rales, and pulmonary edema. High doses rapid apnea, coma, death | **100% $O_2$, CPR**, intubation and mechanical ventilation if needed. **Sodium bicarbonate** ($NaHCO_3$) by IV infusion may be helpful. **Sodium Nitrite** 10 ml (peds 0.2 mg/kg in 3% solution) IV over 5 min. | Low to none | Standard[f] |

[a]Sources of agents. I/M = Industrial/manufacturing. A = Agriculture, WMD = weapon of mass destruction

[b]peds = pediatric medication dosage

[c]Each military **Mark 1** kit contains atropine 2 mg and 2-PAMCl 600 mg in separate autoinjectors.

[d]Assumes absent or incomplete decontamination prior to hospital. In fully decontaminated patients, use only standard precautions.

[e]Respirator: full face with organic vapor filters, PAPR or self-contained breathing apparatus

[f]Standard precautions: gloves and frequent hand washing. For possibility of splashes of fluids, wear gown, mask, and eye protection

(Reproduced with permission from Weinstein RS, Alibek K. Biological and Chemical Terrorism. Thieme: New York, 2003.)

chemical was made in Britain during World War II. Nerve agents are liquids at standard temperatures and pressures, making the term "nerve gas" a misnomer. The G agents have the same density as water and evaporate at about the same rate, making them a nonpersistent chemical given that they disappear within approximately 24 hours in normal environmental situations.[49,50] VX, by contrast, is oily with a consistency similar to motor oil and evaporates very slowly. It possesses fewer vapor hazards than G agents and persists for a longer period of time.[49]

Nerve agents physiologically act similar to organophosphate insecticides.[49] Both interfere with the downregulation of acetylcholine at the postsynaptic membrane by inhibiting acetylcholinesterase (AChE). Once the AChE molecule is inhibited by a nerve agent, the bond must be broken by administration of an oxime, a specific reactivator of the AChE.[49]

The direct effects of a nerve agent due to vaporous molecules penetrating the cornea are pathonomonically represented by changes in the pupillary muscle resulting in myosis. To military medics, this is pathognomonic of a nerve agent exposure. The next most accessible cholinergic dependent organ is the nerve of the exocrine glands in the mouth, which results in rhinorrhea and salivation. Once the victim inhales the nerve agent, the exocrine glands of the respiratory passage will begin to pour excessive secretions into the airway, termed bronchorrhea. Simultaneously, the smooth muscle respiratory passages constrict, resulting in bronchoconstriction and resultant respiratory distress.[49,50] Upon reaching the respiratory tree, the nerve agents pass into the blood stream, resulting in gastrointestinal symptomatology via parasympathetic hyperstimulation leading to abdominal cramping, abdominal pain, nausea, vomiting, diarrhea, and increased bowel movements.[49] Once in the systemic circulation, nerve agents bring about cholinergic overstimulation of the heart and brain. The neuromuscular junctions become overstimulated, resulting in fasciculation and frank twitching, and presenting to the observer as a grand mal type seizure.[49,50] The nerve agent exposure to the brain as a result of the cholinergic overload will elicit result in almost certain unconsciousness and seizure activity. Death from exposure is primarily a result of respiratory failure from a combination of bronchorrhea and bronchospasm, essential apnea stemming from chemical effects upon the brain, and paralysis of the muscles of respiratory system, primarily the diaphragm.[49] The pneumonic SLUDGEM represents the aforementioned symptomatology: S-Salivation, L-Lacrimation, U-Urination, D-Defecation, G-Gastric Distress, E-Emesis, and M-Miosis.

Like nerve agents, cyanide poisoning causes a person to suddenly fall, lose consciousness, and seize. The presence of cyanide poisoning does not present with myosis, however, and although both nerve agents and cyanide can cause seizure, cyanide does not usually cause increase in secretions such as that which occurs with nerve agent exposure.[49]

The major principles for management of nerve agent exposure include (1) decontamination, (2) supportive care with emphasis on respiratory support, and (3) administration of antidotes to include anticholinergic, oxime therapy, and anticonvulsant therapy.[43]

## Antidote Therapy

Antidote therapy for nerve agent and organophosphate exposure is a two-pronged approach administered via Mark I kit auto injectors in the field. First is the administration of Atropine, an anticholinergic drug. It competes with acetylcholine for the postsynaptic muscarinic receptors. Adequate quantities of Aatropine reduce the cholinergic crisis, binding with postsynaptic muscarinic receptors. This is a life-saving antidote controlling the effects of muscarinic receptors on bronchial smooth muscles, exocrine neuro glandular synapsipsis, and the vagus nerve. The adult dose per Mark I intramuscular auto jet injector is 2 mg of atropine.[51] The recommended adult dose is 6 mg to start and then retreat every 5–10 minutes. Mark I auto injector kits, although designed for adults, can be used in children aged three years or older.[48] For children less than three, weight-based dosing is used: Aatropine 0.05–0.1 mg/kg IV or IM repeated every 2–5 minutes to a maximum of 5 mg.[52]

Oximes are a class of drugs that react with the bond between the acetylcholine esterase and the nerve agent. The resulting action cleaves the bond and fragments the nerve agent which is rapidly metabolized, restoring the individual to normal physiologic state.[49] The use of Pralidoxime chloride (2-PAMCl) is to complement Aatropine in the Mark I kit. Each injection delivers 600 mg of 2-PAMCl. As a result of hypertensive effects of 2-PAMCl at 2000 mg or greater, the recommended limitation on the quantity of drug administered per hour is 1800 mg.[53] The adult dosing is appropriate for three years of age and older; for younger children, 2-PAMCl dosing is weight based: 25–50 mg/kg IV or IM to maximum 1 g IV or 2 g IM.[52] Seizure activity secondary to nerve agent exposure is prevalent and more severe than that of status epilepticus. The drug of choice for intervention of nerve agent-induced seizures is Diazepam. However, the Israeli's experience points to propose that Midazolam is a more effective and efficient medication to curtail nerve agent seizures.[54]

## BLOOD AGENTS

### Cyanide

Cyanide exists in two forms: hydrogen cyanide (hydrocyanic acid, AC) and cyanogen, (cyanogen chloride, CK). Hydrogen cyanide has the odor of bitter almonds while cyanogen chloride has a very strong odor that is sometimes described as being sour. The chemical can be absorbed by inhalation, ingestion, or percutaneously into the circulatory system.[42,43] Cyanide ion is a readily available resource in the seeds and pits of many plants, including cherries, peaches, almonds, and lima beans. Cyanides are widely found in the chemical industries in electroplating, mineral extraction, dyeing, printing, photography, and agriculture, and in the manufacture of paper, textiles, and plastics.[43] Cyanide, in general, is an attractive weapon of opportunity for the following reasons: is plentiful and readily available; does not require special knowledge to use as chemical weapon; is capable of causing mass incapacitation and casualties; is capable of causing mass confusion, panic, and social disruption; and requires large quantities of specific resources to combat its dissemination, including the availability of antidotal therapy.[55]

Cyanide is absorbed through the body in via many routes. It can be ingested, absorbed, or inhaled, the last resulting in the most devastating impact. Inhalation of high concentrations of cyanide will quickly find its way to the plasma, the erythrocytes, and in the heart, lungs, and brain. Cyanide combines with iron at cytochrome a3 of the cytochrome oxidase complex, inhibiting oxygen utilization at the cellular level resulting in anaerobic metabolism creating excess lactate and metabolic acidosis and subsequent cellular death.[43]

The signs and symptoms of acute cyanide toxicity occur within seconds of exposure and are concentration dependent. Clinically, the victim begins to have gasping breaths, tachypnea, hypertension, tachycardia, flushing, vomiting, confusion, agitation, and heart palpitations.[43] Symptoms will gradually progress to respiratory failure and arrhythmias. Death from respiratory arrest follows within six to eight minutes. Victims of cyanide toxicity present with cherry red appearance of the skin and venous blood due to the failure of the tissues to be able to extract oxygen secondary to the disruption of the oxidation phosphorylation cascade.[42,43]

Cyanide levels can be directly measured. Cyanide concentrations in the body of 0.5–1 mcg/mL will result in mild effects, whereas concentrations greater than 2.5 mcg per mL are fatal. Venous blood oxygen concentrations are high as a result of cells' inability to extract and utilize oxygen, thereby making use of pulse oximetry futile.[43]

Cyanide also has an affinity for ferric iron in methemoglobin, providing a mechanism for extraction.[43] Recognizing this affinity to ferric iron has led to the treatment protocols for chemical reversal of cyanide exposure. In the field, amyl nitrite pearls can be administered via inhalation to help stabilize the victims until sodium nitrite, the intravenous form of the nitrite antidote, can be administered. These antidotes potentiate the formation of methemoglobin, which possesses a ferric ion. Cyanide has a higher affinity for the ferric ion than does cytochrome a3, thereby causing a dissociation of the cyanide–cytochrome a3 bond, releasing it to form ATP.[42,55]

The second step transforms the cyanide to thiocyanate by the donation of a sulfa group from the infusion of sodium thiosulfate. This reaction creates thiocyanate and sulfite, both of which are easily excreted in the urine.[56]

Treatment should be initiated immediately upon recognition of cyanide poisoning. It should begin with 0.3 mL ampules of amyl nitrite or 3% sodium nitrite (300 mg) IV over three minutes, followed by a dose of 50 cc of 25% of sodium thiosulfate (12.5 g) IV. Pediatric dosing of sodium nitrite is 0.15–0.33 cc per kg of a 3% solution. For sodium thiosulfate, the dosing is 1.65 cc per kg of 50% solution. Treatment may cause hypotension requiring hemodynamic support.[57]

## PULMONARY AGENTS

### Chlorine

Chlorine as a gas is heavier than air and therefore potentiates its exposure time with victims. Chlorine is greenish–yellow in color with a strong characteristic odor.[58] Chlorine is readily available and used in the bleaching of paper and wood pulp and as a disinfectant agent for drinking water and sewage.[59]

The toxicity of chlorine gas is related to the concentration of gas, the duration of exposure, and the water content of the tissues exposed. Chlorine will react with water to form hypochlorite and

hydrochloric acid, which is extremely caustic to the respiratory tissue. Cutaneous burning, occular injury, and aero-respiratory irritation occur acutely following exposure. Exposure to this toxic gas results in upper airway irritation, pulmonary edema with subsequent hypoxemia, and respiratory failure.[60] Symptoms of exposure include shortness of breath, frothy secretions, chest pain, cough, and radiographical infiltration on chest x-ray.

Management of exposure is supportive. Remove the victim from ongoing contamination; decontaminate the victims as soon as possible. Management of respiratory insufficiency may require mechanical support. No antidote therapy exists in the management of this exposure.

### Phosgene

Phosgene characteristically has a smell similar to corn or fresh cut hay. As with chlorine, phosgene is heavier than air, therefore it persists in confined spaces and lower to the ground. Commercially, phosgene is used in the manufacturing of dyestuff and pharmaceuticals.[58] The combustion of polyurethane may produce phosgene, thereby making it a real threat to firefighters. Other industrial risk evolves around chlorinated solvents used in welding and degreasers.

Phosgene, which is relatively insoluble in water, results in only minor upper respiratory irritation. Several hours following phosgene exposure, hydrolysis to hypochloric acid and carbon dioxide occurs in the distal airways increasing capillary permeability.[61] This delayed onset of clinical symptoms is pathognomonic of phosgene.

Given the delay of onset of symptoms, exposure mandates monitoring for at least a period of 12–24 hours with attention to clinical/physical as well as radiographic findings. As with other pulmonary agents, management of respiratory insufficiency acutely and, in severe cases, bacterial pneumonia which may occur within three to five days as a result of damage to the protective lining of the respiratory tree is the focus of patient care.[62]

### Vesicants

*Mustard Agents.*   Mustard agents, as opposed to nerve agents and the cyanides, have low volatility and persist as liquids for prolonged periods of time. The most affected sites are the skin, with the formation of erythema and vesicles; the eyes, with resultant mild conjunctivitis to severe eye damage; and the airways, with mild eruption of the upper respiratory tract, and bronchial damage leading to necrosis and hemorrhage of the airway mucosa and musculature. Prolonged exposure to mustard agents damages precursor cells of the bone marrow, leading to pancytopenia and inability to fight infection.[43] Mustard agents are oily liquids with the smell of garlic, onion, or mustard.[44] The vapors and liquid readily penetrate thin layers of fabrics and begin to penetrate the skin rapidly. Cellular damage results from the DNA alkylation and cross-linking augmentation in rapidly dividing cells. The primary cause of death from vesicant exposure is respiratory failure.

The most immediate intervention for exposure to mustard agents is rapid decontamination of the patient. The patient should be removed from any ongoing contamination or exposure point. The cutaneous lesions should be debrided and managed as burns. Respiratory management is critical and aggressive evaluation and intervention is a top priority. Early intubation should be considered due to potential for laryngeal edema and obstruction. Signs of bone marrow suppression should be monitored, for with intervention as warranted to include antibiotic coverage, bone marrow stimulation, and GI tract sterilization.[43]

## Lewisite

Lewisite's presentation and injury capabilities are similar to those of the mustard agents, vesicant to skin and airway upon contact. It also has the capability to cause increased permeability with the production of hypovolemia shock and organ damage.[43] The presence of the chemical has been likened to the smell of geraniums.

Clinical effects of lewisite vapor or liquid are immediate pain or irritation upon contact. After 5 minutes of contact, the area of the affected skin will develop a grayish area of dead epithelium; erythema and blister formation will follow. Theses lesions are more prone to tissue necrosis and sloughing in comparison to mustard agents. The primary location for significant life-threatening damage is the respiratory mucosa, with sloughing, necrosis, and pseudomembrane formation resulting in airway obstruction.[43] British anti-lewisite, an antidote, will reduce the systemic effects of lewisite. It may have side-effects and toxicities associated with its utilization. British antilewisite skin and ophthalmic ointments are also available for usage as antidotes.[43]

## Riot Control Agents

These compounds cause lacrimation and sneezing. These agents are termed tear gas, which is notably incorrect given that the substrates are in solid form. Among these agents are the following: CS (O-Chlorobenzylidene malononitrile), CA (bromobenzylcyanide), CN (chloroacetophenone), and CR (dibenzoxazepine). All act as lacrimator and irritants; diphenylaminearsine is both an irritant and a vomiting agent; and CS, CN, and DM[63] can cause dermatitis and occular injuries.

Victims of CS may develop a rapid heart rate, respiratory insufficiency, and cutaneous and sensatory changes. These occasionally, in combination with DM, have been reported to cause death. This is usually worse in people who have pre-existing medical conditions that compromise them, or as a result of their refusal to leave confined spaces, leading to a significant exposure. Post-mortem findings in animals exposed to riot agents, identify respiratory damage as the cause of death.[43] The metabolism of CS in animal studies have shown an increase in blood cyanide concentration hours later, indicating that the malononitrile portion of CS has been metabolized to cyanide. Again, at post-mortem it was found that respiratory damage was the cause of death from prolonged exposure and not cyanide toxicity.[43]

Management of these patients is often supportive as the insult is self-limiting, resolving within 15 minutes. Standard decontamination prevents re-exposure of victims and health care providers. In some cases, respiratory irritation will warrant observation of the patient and use of bronchodilators.[43]

## SPECIAL CONSIDERATIONS IN PREGNANCY

Industrial chemical accidents have allowed for some insight into the effects of chemical toxicity in pregnancy. The Bhopal disaster resulted in a significant number of adverse pregnancy outcomes in women who were exposed to isocyanide from an explosion in a chemical factory.[64] The findings demonstrated that 24% of pregnant women exposed to the explosion had spontaneous abortions compared to about 6% in a comparison group. A four-fold increase in the rate of abortion is a result of the exposure to isocyanide. Although no teratogenic changes were noted in the fetuses of those exposed, the placentas of the exposed mothers weighed less than the placentas of mothers who were not exposed.[65,66] In general, there is suggestive evidence that chemicals may traverse the maternal fetal blood barrier through the placenta and at a minimum have adverse effects on the placenta structure itself. Further investigation and research on the effects of chemical exposure in pregnancies appears to be warranted.

## Biological Terrorism

The presence of a biological event and the temporal timing of the identification of such an event are elusive, to say the least. The initiation of a biological terrorist attack may go unrecognized until the first clinical index case or syndromic trends in case presentations seeking medical care are recognized. Early identification of a biological event requires the implementation of a concept referred to as syndromic surveillance. In collaboration with the CDC, states and municipalities have been able to share information leading to the early identification of pathogens in the propagation of disease. This system monitors such things as absenteeism from school, 911 calls within the community, variations in commercial sales of various over-the-counter pharmaceuticals, and the voluntarily reporting by medical groups to the public health community variances and disease presentation to their practices.

## Classification of Biological Agents

Biological terrorism by definition is the use or threatened use of biological agents against a person, group, or large population to create fear or illness for the purpose of intimidation, gaining an advantage, and interruption of normal activities or ideological activities.[48] The CDC has divided the biological threats into three groups referred to as A, B, and C based upon the ease of dissemination or transmission from person to person, potential for high mortality with potential for public health impact, potential to cause public panic and social disruption, and need for special action for public health preparation.[48]

The remainder of this chapter will be dedicated to the review of the category A pathogens that have the potential to be used in weaponized form. Table 56-2 will provide a quick reference of these pathogens and others considered to having the greatest potential for utilization.[48]

## Anthrax (Bacillus anthracis)

Anthrax exists as spores and remains stable for several decades. It is resistant to drying, heat, ultraviolet light, gamma radiation, and many disinfectants.[67,68] Anthrax causes infection in man by three main routes: inhalational, cutaneous, or gastrointestinal.[69]

Clinically, the presentation of inhalational anthrax occurs within 2–100 days. This infectious process of the lymph nodes

**TABLE 56-2**

**A Quick Reference for Potential Biological Weapons**

| DISEASE/AGENT | INCUBATION | INITIAL SYMPTOMS | MEDICAL MANAGEMENT | CONTAGION RISK | INFECTION PRECAUTIONS |
|---|---|---|---|---|---|
| **Anthrax (inhalational)** (Bacillus anthracis) | 1–6 days | FIL[a] (includes fever or history of fever) with chest discomfort, often widened mediastinum and pleural effusions on CXR. Malaise may be profound. Followed by high fever, dry cough, severe respiratory distress, cyanosis, septicemia, and death | **Prophylaxis:** Doxy 100 mg Q12h PO **or** cipro 500 mg bid PO. **Treatment:** Doxy 100 mg Q12h IV **or** cipro 400 mg Q12h IV (levofloxacin may be substituted) **plus** rifampin 600 mg PO qid **or** clinda 900 mg IV Q6h **or** vanco 1 g IV Q12h **or** Biaxin 500 mg PO bid **or** imipenem 500 mg IM/IV Q6h **or** ampi 500 mg IV/PO Q6h. Same drug choices in children and pregnancy, but use peds dosing in children (MMWR 10-26-01) | Very low (cutaneous only) | Standard[b] |
| **Botulinum toxin** (Clostridium botulinum) | 12–36 hr | Diplopia, photophobia, ptosis, hoarseness, slurred speech; progresses to total paralysis | Early administration of botulinum antitoxin is critical; supportive care including mechanical ventilation | None | Standard[b] |
| **Brucellosis** (Brucella suis and melitensis) | Days–months | FIL,[a] back pain, arthralgias. Pneumonia or nodules on CXR | Treat PO with doxy 100 mg Q12h **plus** rifampin 600 mg qid PO for bioterrorism attack | None | Standard[b] |
| **Cholera** (Vibrio cholerae) | 4 hr–5 days | Severe rice water diarrhea, nausea, vomiting, collapse | IV replacement of fluids and lytes. Tetracyline 500 mg Q6h, **or** doxy 100 mg Q12h, **or** cipro 500 mg Q12h. RX × 3 days | Very low | Standard[b] |
| **Ebola and Marburg** viral hemorrhagic fevers | 3–14 days | FIL,[a] stomach pain, diarrhea, rash, weakness, bleeding, shock | No specific treatment. Supportive care, oxygen, replace fluids, management of coagulopathy | **Moderate** | Airborne[d] |
| **Glanders** (Burkholderia mallei) | 3–14 days | Sudden onset of FIL,[a] chest pain, photophobia, diarrhea, splenomegaly, pneumonia | **Prophylaxis:** TMP-SMX DS Q12h may help. **Treatment:** Severe →ceftazidime 2 g IV Q8h TMP-SMX (2 mg/kg–10mg/kg) IV qid **or** sulfadiazine 25 mg/kg Q6h for 2 wks, then switch to PO TMP-SMX. Localized (including pulmonary) → amox-clav 20 mg/kg PO tid **or** tetracycline 13 mg/kg PO tid **or** sulfadiazine 25 mg/kg PO Q6h or TMP 2 mg/kg–SMX 10 mg/kg PO bid for 60–150 days based on clinical response | Low | Droplet[c] |
| **Hantavirus pulmonary syndrome** | 1–5 weeks | FIL,[a] dyspnea, headache, GI symptoms. Later rales and ARDS | Supportive care, mechanical ventilation. No specific treatment | Very low | Standard[b] |
| **Lassa virus and the South American viral hemorrhagic fevers** | 3–19 days | Fever, malaise, myalgias, back, chest, and abdominal pain, dysesthesia, cough, vomiting, ↓BP, oliguria, hemorrhages | Supportive care with IV fluids, colloids, and management of coagulopathy. Ribavirin IV 30 mg/kg loading dose, then 15 mg/kg Q6h for 4 days, then 7.5 mg/kg Q8h for 6 days | **Moderate** | Airborne[d] |
| **Plague (pneumonic)** (Yersinia pestis) | 1–6 days | FIL[a] with high fever, possible hemoptysis, patchy pneumonia | Streptomycin 15 mg/kg/q12h IV (gent may be used instead) **or** doxy 100 mg Q12h IV **or** cipro 400 mg Q12h IV | **Moderate to High** | Droplet[c] |
| **Q fever** (Coxiella burnetii) | 2–14 days | FIL,[a] may progress to atypical pneumonia and/or hepatitis | Doxy 100 mg Q12h IV **or** tetra 500 mg Q6h PO. Cipro 500 mg Q12h IV may also be useful | Low | Standard[b] |
| **Ricin** (castor bean extract) and **Abrin** (rosary pea extract) | 4–8 hr | Fever, dyspnea, cough, nausea, chest tightness, arthralgias, airway necrosis and or ARDS | Supportive only: wash skin with soap and water, respiratory support/mechanical ventilator, gastric lavage, activated charcoal and mg citrate if ingested | Very low | Standard[b] |
| **Smallpox** (Variola major) | 3–19 days | FIL[a] with backache, possible delirium, chickenpox-like rash starting on arms. | Vaccine prior to onset of illness (3–7 days); otherwise supportive care, isolation, or home quarantine | **Very high** | Airborne[d] and contact[e] |

| | | | | | |
|---|---|---|---|---|---|
| **Staphylococcal enterotoxin B** | 3–12 hr | FLI[a] with high fever and prostration. Severe cases produce dyspnea, chest pain, GI symptoms | Symptomatic and supportive care with IV fluids, oxygen, and, if necessary, intubation, mechanical ventilation, PEEP | Very low | Standard[b] |
| **T-2 (trichothecene) mycotoxins** (multiple fungi) | Minutes | Eye/skin pain, burning, redness and blisters, dyspnea, wheezing, cough, N/V, bloody stools, cramping | Supportive; wash patient (soap and water) and remove clothes to remove toxin residue (yellow or greenish oily liquid) | Direct contact only | Standard[b] |
| **Tularemia** (pneumonic) (Francisella tularensis) | 1–21 days | FLI[a] with prostration, chest pain, and hemoptysis | Gent 1 mg/kg/Q8h IV **or** Cipro 400 mg Q12h IV **or** Cipro 750 mg Q12h IV **or** streptomycin 7.5–10 mg/kg/Q12h IM | Low | Standard[b] |

[a]FLI = Flulike illness (fever, chills, cough, malaise, headache, sore throat, and/or myalgias)

[b]Standard precautions: gloves and frequent hand washing. For possibility of splashes of body fluid, wear gown, mask, and eye protection.

[c]Droplet precautions: standard precautions plus surgical or HEPA-filter (or equivalent) mask.

[d]Airborne precautions: isolation, negative pressure room, gloves, gown, HEPA-filter or equivalent mask, frequent hand washing.

[e]Contact precautions: standard precautions plus private room or cohorting of patients, gown, gloves, dedicated noncritical patient care equipment.

(Reproduced with permission from Weinstein RS, Alibek K. Biological and Chemical Terrorism. Thieme: New York, 2003.)

results in hemorrhagic mediastinal lymphadenitis with development of pleural effusions and inflammatory infiltration of the lung parenchyma resulting in respiratory failure.[70,71]

Cutaneous anthrax is a naturally occurring disease that is far more common than inhalational disease processes. Anthrax is an enzootic and epizootic disease, which occurs in wild animals as well as domestic animals. Humans can develop respiratory and cutaneous anthrax from these animals, and it is a somewhat of a common occurrence in those people involved in the processing of wool and hides in the textile manufacturing industry.[67] Cutaneous anthrax is characterized by eschar formation. Characteristic of its presentation, the term anthrax comes from the Greek word which means "coal," which is consistent with the coal black scab or eschar that forms from cutaneous anthrax.[72] If penetration extends into the dermis, a progression will follow through to necrosis, edema, hemorrhage, and perivascular infiltration and vasculitis. Lymph node drainage tracts eventually become enlarged and develop necrosis and hemorrhage.[71]

Gastrointestinal anthrax is rare and occurs as a result of ingesting insufficiently cooked meat from infected animals.[72] It may develop into a systemic illness and/or sepsis as a result of the aggressive nature of this form of anthrax.

Accurate and timely diagnosis of anthrax is essential. This can be accomplished through gram stain, which will identify the bacillus anthracis organism. However, the preferred method of diagnosis is polymerized chain reaction (PCR). This technology can amplify specific markers, making the diagnosis more accurate and timely.[73]

Historically, the treatment of choice for anthrax has been penicillin. Recently, the CDC has advised that the initial therapy should begin with doxycycline or ciprofloxacin and then switch to penicillin as sensitivity allows.[67,74,75] If exposure is suspected, it is recommended that prophylaxis with ciprofloxacin and/or doxycycline be initiated for persons who are characterized as being potentially high risk due to contact.[67,74]

## Botulism (Clostridium botulinum Toxin)

An anaerobic gram-positive bacillus, Clostridium botulinum, produces botulinum toxin. It is one of the deadliest substances known to man, with a single gram of toxin being able to kill more than 1 million people. It is 1500 times more lethal than the highly potent chemical agent VX and 100,000 times more potent than the lethal agent Sarin.[76,77]

Historically, botulinum has been transmitted as food-borne illness and contracted as wound infection. Seven distinct types of toxin exist and have been referred to as type A through G with type A, B, and E being responsible for most human disease.[72] During the Gulf War, Iraqis produced 20,000 liters of botulinum toxin, 12 liters of which were used in field-testing and to fill war heads.[78]

Clinically, botulinum toxin binds with receptors of the presynaptic terminals of cholinergic synapses. It impairs acetylcholine release, resulting in cranial nerve deficits and descending bilateral paralysis, which are the hallmarks of botulinum toxicity.[76,79–81] Because the toxin does not penetrate the blood brain barrier, mental status changes are usually not a hallmark of this descending paralytic process.[76]

The diagnosis of botulinum toxicity is primarily clinical. No routine laboratory test will aid in a diagnosis of this disease process.[72,76] After exposure to the toxin, signs and symptoms should begin to show in six to seven days.[70]

Treatment of the patient with botulinum toxin poisoning centers upon ventilator support and it may take weeks to months before the patient clinically improves. Available from the CDC is a trivalent equine antitoxin, which is active against types A, B, and E. Although this treatment is unable to reverse existing symptoms, the antitoxin may be able to stabilize and stop progression of the disease if administered early.[82,83]

## VIRAL HEMORRHAGIC FEVERS

Viral hemorrhagic fevers are caused by a group of ribonucleic acids (RNA) viruses in four separate families: the Arenaviridae (Argentinian, Bolivian, Venezuelan, Lassa, and Sabia fevers); the Bunyaviridae (Crimean-Congo fever, Rift Valley fever, and Hantavirus fever); the Filoviridae (Ebola and Marburg fever); and Flaviviridae (Yellow fever, Dengue fever, Kyasanur Forest disease, Omsk fever).[79] These viruses are geographically limited in their natural occurring presentations but are highly infectious by way of aerosolized routes, and believed to have an animal reservoir in the arthropod.[72]

These diseases are transmitted via aerosolization of animal excrement, bites, contact with animals, or insect vectors, or contacts with bodily fluids of infected individuals.[79] After exposure, individuals present with fever, myalgias, and prostration.[79] An acute infection then rapidly progresses to fever, systematic inflammatory response, petechiae, and bleeding, with subsequent shock and death. These disease entities have a high mortality rate of 50% with the Ebola virus being considered uniformly fatal.[70] High rates of transmission from human to human make this virus highly contagious. The incubation period is 5–10 days with the onset of symptoms to include fever, malaise, and headaches.[72,84]

The bioterrorism scenario of aerosolized dissemination of this viral pathogen would be devastating as a result of its highly contagious nature. The diagnosis of such a disease entity relies upon the ELISA detection of antiviral IgM antibodies or direct culture of the virus from blood or tissue samples.[72] All body fluids should be considered contagious; normal barrier precautions should be utilized by the staff, as well as negative pressure rooms.[72,84] In the management of hemorrhagic fevers, no specific therapy has demonstrated any significant improvement in outcome; therefore treatment is limited to supportive care. The use of ribavirin is under investigational trials and shows some promise in the treatment of Congo–Crimean hemorrhagic fever, Hantavirus, and Lassa fever infections.[85] The development of vaccines for viral hemorrhagic fevers at present is in the early stages.

## Plague (Yersinia pestis)

Yersinia pestis is one of the oldest forms of biological terrorism used in history. The biological warfare efforts of Tatar warriors included catapulting corpses of plague victims into the city of their adversaries.[79] The medieval Black Death pandemic, so named because of the massive ecchymosis and odor of necrotic flesh, claimed 50 million lives in Europe between 1347–1350.[72,75] If plague is utilized as a weapon of mass destruction in contemporary times, it most likely will be disseminated through an aerosolized approach.[79]

Yersinia is a gram-negative bacillus normally existing in the rodent population and is transmitted to humans by the fleas of the rodents.[67,70,72,75,79,83] This gram-negative organism is nonmotile; it is facultative, anaerobic, and nonspore forming coccobacillus. The bacteria have a safety pin appearance under the microscope.[67] Plague relies upon a complex interaction between rodents, fleas, and humans in order to propagate the cycle of pathogenesis and contagion. Other animals, including mites, gerbils, ground squirrels, chipmunks, and prairie dogs, have also been associated as carriers of plague.[86] Plague is considered to be a high-risk potential weapon for bioterrorism given its high affinity for the respiratory tract. Aerosolized bacteria are easily propagated person-to-person and produce severe clinical symptoms. As a result of the contagion potential, the plague has a high psychological impact factor upon the community out of fear of infection.[67]

*Yersinia pestis* infections can be characterized in three different clinical presentations. Bubonic plague naturally occurs after cutaneous inoculation from the bite of an infected flea. Local proliferation of the inoculation spreads to regional lymph nodes, resulting in a large inflammatory response within seven to eight days. This inflammatory response results in swollen and tender regional lymph nodes (referred to as buboes) of the neck, axilla, and inguinal area. Skin necrosis may occur with the buboes eventually rupturing and draining. Untreated bubonic plague carries a mortality rate of 50%.[70,72] A second characteristic presentation is that of primary septic plague. With the development of lymphadenopathy, the bubonic phase may be bypassed to a more aggressive bacteremia, which leads to disseminated intervascular coagulation problems, purpuric lesions, and even digital necrosis.[70] Bubonic plague, if left untreated, will progress to bacteremic/septicemic plague with a mortality rate approaching that of 60%.[75] The third form, pneumonic plague, has high potential as a weapon of terrorism because of its high contagion with dissemination via aerosolization of bacteria by coughing which becomes the main mode of transmission from human to human. Primarily, pneumonic plague is virulent and leads to 100% mortality rate without therapy.[70,75]

Direct fluorescent antibody staining makes the diagnosis of *Yersinia pestis*. The specimens for this analysis can come from the buboes by direct aspiration with a small-gauge needle. Bipolar safety pin morphology will usually be evident.[72]

Medical management of patients with bubonic plague requires body fluid precaution and segregation from others for at least three days. Historically, the antibiotic of choice for the treatment of plague has been intramuscular streptomycin. Gentamicin and chloramphenicol combinations are acceptable alternative treatments, as are doxycycline and fluoroquinolone.[70,72] Postexposure antibiotic therapy, given the highly contagious and highly fatal origin of plague, should be provided for at least seven days. These postexposure contacts should be treated with oral doxycycline, tetracycline, or trimethoprim/sulfamethoxazole. The plague vaccine has been shown to be effective against bubonic plague but it is unknown if protection is provided against pneumonic plague.[79]

## Smallpox (Variola Virus: Orthopoxvirus)

Smallpox was declared eradicated in 1980 by the World Health Organization. Concerns regarding it as a potential weapon of mass destruction have renewed significant interest in this country; hence, an aggressive program was instituted in 2003 to vaccinate a core group of health care workers and military personnel.[87] After the eradication of smallpox, two laboratories continue to maintain stocks of the virus for potential future vaccine manufacturing needs. These locations include the Institute of Virus Preparation in Moscow and The Center for Disease Control and Prevention (CDC) in Atlanta. Alibek, and Handelman reported that although the world stopped the vaccination program, the former Soviet Union continued to produce smallpox virus for the purpose of biological weaponry in the forms of bombs and missiles. They also reported research efforts to create recombinant strains that would have even greater virulence. With the known existence of smallpox virus availability, grave concerns emerged.[88]

As a biological weapon, smallpox was determined to be a high priority as a result based on the following: the population at large lacked immunity, vaccines will be in short supply, the virus can be delivered in large quantities by aerosol, inoculum would most likely cause infection, and human-to-human transmission would be rampant.

A member of the Poxviridae family, smallpox is an acute and highly contagious disease. The smallpox virus (variola virus) is a DNA virus. There is no human reservoir for this smallpox and no human carriers are known.[72] There are two forms of smallpox, the variola major with a 20–40% mortality rate in unvaccinated people and the variola minor with a 1% mortality rate in unvaccinated people.[89,90] Other pox viruses exist, but only small pox is felt to have the capability to be transmitted from human to human.[72,89]

The smallpox virus is readily transmitted from person to person by way of respiratory particles. These virus can remain viable for up to one week.[71,72,76,83,87] The initial symptoms usually present approximately 7–17 days after the initial exposure with the acute onset of fever, rigors, headache, back pain, and malaise.[72,77] This prodrome phase can last for two to three days. A rash typically develops in approximately 48 hours and begins on the mouth, tongue, and oropharynx preceding the cutaneous component of this presentation by approximately 24 hours.[72,77] The rash then rapidly spreads to the hands and the forearms, followed by legs and trunk; it spreads centrally first as a maculopapular rash, and then progressing to vesicles and pustules, followed by scabs and crusts, and ending as a pitted scar.[71,83] Some forms of smallpox may result in significant secondary infections and organ failure of the intestinal tract with GI bleeding, pneumonia and bronchial pneumonias, renal failure, and even encephalitis.[89] Death usually occurs late in the first week or during the second week of the illness as a result of toxemia from overwhelming viral infection. The greatest period of contagion in smallpox victims occurs during the first week in which the patient becomes symptomatic. From this point until all the scabs have separated, the smallpox victim is considered to be contagious.[77,89] When potential outbreaks occur, individuals should be isolated if exposure is anticipated in order to prevent contagion.

During the vesicular phase, the rash can resemble that of chicken pox but there are two important distinctions. The rash of smallpox develops synchronously in contrast to asynchronously in varicella (chicken pox); second, the rash of smallpox rash is concentrated on the face and extremities as opposed to the trunk in chicken pox. The pustules of smallpox are also known for the characteristic central umbilication presentation.[91] Upon suspicion, immediate notification of public health is warranted as this is considered an international public health emergency.

Although treatment for smallpox is supportive, there is no Food and Drug Administration (FDA) approved treatment. Several studies have indicated that cidofovir has shown promise in the prevention of related orthopoxviruses.[92,93] Smallpox vaccination is also recommended within the first week of exposure.[70] In the event of a smallpox epidemic, personnel providing care in hospitals should immediately be vaccinated; patients should be managed in negative pressure rooms, with standard gloves, gown, and mask precautions. Isolation and the prevention of contagion are key to the management of such an epidemic.[70]

## Tularemia (*Francisella tularensis*)

Tularemia has been recognized as a category A agent because due to its ease of dissemination, high infectivity, and capacity to cause serious illness and death.[67] The most likely presentation of this exposure would be pneumonic and typhoidal tularemia.[67] Similar to anthrax and plague, tularemia is zoonosis. Likewise similar to the plague, arthropod vectors transmit the disease among natural reservoirs including rabbits, deer, squirrels, mice, and beavers. Human infections occur by contact with contaminated animal products or by insect bites, primarily from ticks and deer flies during summertime.[67,72] Human-to-human spread of tularemia is uncommon. Respiratory isolation is not necessary.[83]

*Francisella tularensis*, the causative agent of tularemia, is a small aerobic nonmotile gram-negative coccobacillus.[67] It possesses a strong bacterial capsule that protects the organism from natural barriers and immunological destruction in the respiratory tree. Many forms of tularemia exist based upon the route of inoculation with varying degrees of mortality. Typhoidal tularemia accounts for 5–15% of acquired cases and it mainly occurs as a result of inhalation of infectious aerosols. This is a mechanism that would most likely deliver a WMD for biological terrorism. The ensuing pneumonia may be severe in other forms of tularemia as well. Mediastinal lymphadenopathy is the most common with typhoidal disease. Fatality rate, left untreated, is approximately 35%.[72]

From the weaponization of tularemia, one would expect to see a large populous of patients presenting with nonproductive cough and pneumonia.[72] The mainstay of the diagnosis rests upon serological testing with the ELISA, microagglutinin, hemoagglutinin, and tuber agglutinin assays when available.[67]

The classic treatment for tularemia is gentamicin but other alternative drugs should be considered. An additional concern is the known fact that in the 1950s a biologically engineered avirulent streptomycin-resistant strain of *Francisella tularemias* was developed by the United States; and it is presumed that other countries may be in possession of this bacterial weapon.[72] Therefore, it is recommended that the initial therapy for tularemia exposure include intravenous gentamicin or ciprofloxacin. Recognizing the potential for relapse, a treatment course of at least 10 days is warranted.[72] At present, the United States does not have a licensed tularemia vaccine; however, a live investigational product is available to the US Army Material Research Command at Fort Detrick.[79] Additional guidance for antibiotic dosing in children can be found in Markenson and Redlener's article *Pediatric Terrorism Preparedness National Guidelines Act. Recommendations: Findings of an Evidence-based Consensus Process.*[52]

## SPECIAL CONSIDERATION IN PREGNANCY

Pregnancy, in order to protect the fetus, results in immunosuppression of hormonal, cellular, and humeral precursors. In addition, high circulating levels of steroids inhibit normal humeral response.[94] Although circulating white blood cell counts in pregnancy are increased, there are significant changes resulting in a decrease in immunological response and capabilities. These are neutrophil chemotaxis and adherence, suppression, cell-mediated immunity, and reduction and decrease in natural killer cell activity. These changes are normal, but the end-result overall is a lowering of the woman's defense mechanism and making her more susceptible to potential circulating pathogens. The biological threat of terrorism and the vulnerability of the obstetrical patient as a result of her immunological augmentation places her at somewhat at higher risk, significantly increasing morbidity and mortality maternally and producing an unknown risk to the fetus.[22]

The CDC, in collaboration with the Department of Defense and FDA, is monitoring the outcomes of pregnancy in women exposed to smallpox vaccines. Historically, if a woman is infected with smallpox during pregnancy her mortality approaches 50% compared to 30% for men and nonpregnant women.[95] If infection occurs during the first trimester, it results in a high rate of fetal loss. If the infection results in the latter half of pregnancy, it is associated with significant increase in prematurity of the fetus.[94] It is not recommended to immunize women during pregnancy because smallpox vaccine is a live virus; however, if a high-risk situation develops, vaccination should proceed.

Viral hemorrhagic fevers represent several families of viruses, resulting in clinical disease of high fever and bleeding diaphysis leading to higher maternal mortality rates.[96] Two women, one in Iran and one in India, contracted *Bacillus anthracis* during pregnancy. Their exposure was from eating contaminated meat. Both women died as a result of overwhelming peritonitis.[97,98] No documented maternal to fetal transmissions of anthrax has been documented. As a result of the events of 2001, the American College of Obstetrics and Gynecology and the CDC have recommended that pregnant women who have risk of environmental exposures should receive prophylaxis for anthrax due to its fatal potential.[99,100] Other potential biologic agents of terrorism have been reviewed in relation to their implication in pregnancy, some of which have been *Clostridium botulinum*, *Francisella tularemia*, and *Yersinia pestis*. If contracted by the obstetrical patient, all of these agents should be treated according to standards of the nonpregnant patient as a result of their high mortality and morbidity. If contracted by the obstetrical patient, it should be treated according to standards of the nonpregnant patient.

## RADIOLOGIC TERRORISM

Many physicians and health care providers are unfamiliar with nuclear and radiologic weapons and the medical treatment of radiologic casualties.[101] The availability of nuclear material on the black market, through reappropriation of nuclear products from developed and underdeveloped countries, makes the threat of nuclear terrorism a possibility.

A nuclear bomb created by terrorists would probably yield 0.01–10 kilotons of explosive potential.[102] A more sophisticated compact yield device constructed by purchasing or stealing stockpiles of nuclear material may yield a 10-kiloton explosion—a near equivalent to the bombing of Hiroshima. The International Atomic Energy Agency has recorded 540 incidents of illicit trafficking of nuclear and radioactive material during the past 10 years. This material, although not bomb grade, could be utilized in crude radiologic dispersal devices.[103]

Adding to the concerns, in September 1997, General Alexander Lebed, Secretary of the Russian Security Council, made international headlines with his allegations that more than 100 small nuclear weapons were missing from the Russian arsenal.[104] Dr. Alexey Yablokov also gave testimony to the House Committee for National Security corroborating General Lebed's claim of errant suitcase nuclear weapons.[105] Given the aforementioned and the presumed credible testimony of these individuals, it is of concern that a limited nuclear detonation could occur not only internationally, but also within the confines of the United States.

## Radiological Release

*Radiologic Detonation.*   The air blast effect of a nuclear detonation is referred to as the shock wave, which travels outward from the point of detonation and is associated with strong winds causing personal injuries as a result of airborne projectiles. From the fireball of the explosion, thermal radiation projects heat over long distances, causing significant thermal burn and blindness. The initial radiation is from the pulse of the explosion, with the release of primarily of gamma rays and neutrons. Residual radiation results from radioactive decay over the first minute following detonation and is found in radioactive fallout. Following detonation, a crater will form, its size depending upon the weight of the bomb and the characteristics of the terrain. Physical properties of ground shock cause extensive damage to structures as well as infrastructure.[102]

## RADIOLOGIC DISPERSAL DEVICES (RDDS)

A radiological dispersal device is one that will release radiation without nuclear explosion. The blast effect of the RDD is limited to the explosive potential of the material being utilized to disperse the radionucleotides. Their greatest impacts in general are the fear and social disruption that they cause. The term "Dirty Bomb" is often used to describe this type of weapon. An alternative type of RDD attack would be the dispersal of a liquid in public water supplies, in which the individual exposure would be exceedingly low, but the social impact would be significant.[102] In comparison to industrial sources, medical radioactive materials are of insufficient potential to cause significant radiology damage to individuals in comparison to industrial sources.[102]

## FIELD SOURCE RADIATION OR PASSIVE EMISSION

This process involves the placement of a container of radioactive material in an area of high traffic. Radiation is emitted over a period of time to that population in direct contact with the emitting source. The dose rate from this source is a function of distance and time in proximity to the source and potential emission from the source.[106,107]

## TYPES OF RADIATION

In order to understand the potential risk of ionizing radiation, a basic understanding of the types is necessary.

Alpha particles are massive charged particles, four times the mass of neutrons, containing two protons and two neutrons positively charged. The large alpha particles cannot travel far and cannot penetrate clothes or epithelium of the skin.[102,106,108] Particles are of minimal external hazard, but when they are emitted from an internalized radionucleotide source, they can cause significant cellular damage in the region immediately adjacent to their physical location.[102,108] Particles may be contained in fallout material.

Beta particles are very light, found primarily in fallout radiation. These small, negatively charged particles are electrons that are released from the decaying nucleus of a radioactive substance.[107] These particles travel short distances in tissue and, in large enough quantities, can cause damage to the basal stratum of skin. Injuries, are classically referred to as "beta burn," and appear similar to that of a normal thermal burn. These particles are fixed to the fallout debris in the air. Besides the obvious impact on skin being at risk, the lens of the eye is vulnerable to cataract formation, and risk exists for open wounds and absorption through ingestion.[107,108] Potential carcinogenesis results within internal organs if contamination is internal.[107,108]

Gamma rays are an energetic form of electromagnetic radiation that passes through body tissue and deposits energy in the tissue as it travels. This uncharged type of radiation is similar to x-ray. Because of its high permeability, the whole body is at risk for exposure. This radiation can travel kilometers in the air at the speed of light.[107]

Neutrons are uncharged particles that pass through body tissue, and depositing their energy in the tissue, and travelling through air several meters. As a result of their mass, they can cause significant biological damage, up to 20 times the damage caused by gamma radiation.[107]

Physiologically, radiation interacts with atoms in the body and with energy is deposited, resulting in ionization (electron excitation).[102,108] Radiation effects cause injury to cells directly by altering the atom or molecule of the cell, leading to in irreparable damage. This results in cellular death and/or malfunction. Radiation will cause damage to the cell indirectly by interacting with water molecules. This results in the formation of hyper oxides, leading to cellular damage.[108]

## UNITS OF RADIATION

The radiation-absorbed dose (RAD) is the measure of the energy deposited in matter by ionizing radiation. The international system of skin absorption dose is referred to as a Gray unit (Gy), 1 Gy equals 100 rads, 10 mGy equals 1 rad.[108] Differences in types of radiation are adjusted by a quality factor in assessing risk.[108] The dose in rads times multiplied by a quality factor yields the radiation equivalent man (REM). The international unit for this REM is sievert, used in assessing long-term risks.[108]

$$100 \text{ rad} = 100 \text{ cGy} = 1000 \text{ mGy} = 1 \text{ Gy} = 1 \text{ Sv} = 100 \text{ rem}.$$

## Sample Collection for Cytogenic Analysis

An analysis of blood specimen may add insight as to the degree of exposure. Twenty-four hours within initial radiation, 10 cc of peripheral blood should be collected via lithium heparin blood collection tube or an EDTA tube, kept cool at a temperature of 4°C, and transported to a cytogenic lab. Growing the lymphocytes in culture via stimulation, and then stopping their growth in the first metaphase, and assessment of the radiation dose, can predict exposure utilizing a dose response curve. This may have some value in outcome predictions directing therapeutic maneuvers.[108]

## RADIATION TIME PROFILE

Acute radiation syndrome is a sequence of phased symptoms that occur after exposure in reference to the radiation sensitivity of the individual, the type of radiation, and the radiation dose absorbed. As symptoms worsen, the duration of each phase will shorten with increasing radiation dose.[108]

## Prodrome Phase

Appetite loss, nausea, vomiting, fatigue, diarrhea, prostration, fever, respiratory difficulty, and increased excitability may be present depending on the dose of radiation the person received. Of all the phases, the prodrome period is perhaps the most critical in that the timing and onset of symptoms are predictive of the degree of radiation exposure as well as outcome. The more aggressive exposure resolves in earlier onset of symptoms. In general, hemopoietic changes as the only presenting initial symptoms have a much better prognosis than early presentation of cardiovascular or central nervous system dysfunction following radiation exposure (Table 56-3).[101]

## Latent Phase

Following recovery from the prodrome phase, the exposed individual will be relatively symptom free. The shorter the latent phase, the worse the prognosis and greater the exposure. A reduced lymphocyte count of less than 300 occurring during the first 48 hours is an indicator of critical condition.[107]

## Manifest Illness Phase

This phase is noted by the presentation of injury by the organ system most affected by the radiation exposure.

Exposure to greater than 10 Gy units or 1000 rads will generally be fatal, whereas casualties exposed to less than 4 Gy units or

**TABLE 56-3**

### Findings of the Prodromal Phase of Acute Radiation Syndrome

| SYMPTOMS AND MEDICAL RESPONSE | ARS DEGREE AND THE APPROXIMATE DOSE OF ACUTE WBE, Gy | | | | |
|---|---|---|---|---|---|
| | Mild (1–2 Gy) | Moderate (2–4 Gy) | Severe (4–6 Gy) | Very Severe (6–8 Gy) | Lethal (>8 Gy)[a] |
| **Vomiting** | | | | | |
| Onset | 2 h after exposure or later | 1–2 h after exposure | Earlier than 1 h after exposure | Earlier than 30 min after exposure | Earlier than 10 min after exposure |
| Incidence, % | 10–50 | 70–90 | 100 | 100 | 100 |
| **Diarrhea** | None | None | Mild | Heavy | Heavy |
| Onset | | | 3–8 h | 1–3 h | Within minutes or 1 h |
| Incidence, % | | | <10 | >10 | Almost 100 |
| **Headache** | Slight | Mild | Moderate | Severe | Severe |
| Onset | | | 4–24 h | 3–4 h | 1–2 h |
| Incidence, % | | | 50 | 80 | 80–90 |
| **Consciousness** | Unaffected | Unaffected | Unaffected | May be altered | Unconsciousness (may last seconds/minutes) |
| Onset | | | | | Seconds/minutes |
| Incidence, % | | | | | 100 (at >50 Gy) |
| **Body temperature** | Normal | Increased | Fever | High fever | High fever |
| Onset | | 1–3 h | 1–2 h | <1 h | <1 h |
| Incidence, % | | 10–80 | 80–100 | 100 | 100 |
| **Medical response** | Outpatient observation | Observation in general hospital, treatment in specialized hospital if needed | Treatment in specialized hospital | Treatment in specialized hospital | Palliative treatment (symptomatic only) |

ARS, Acute radiation syndrome; WBE, whole-body exposure.

[a]With appropriate supportive and marrow resuscitative therapy, individuals may survive for 6 to 12 months with whole-body doses as high as 12 Gy. Adapted from International Atomic Energy Agency, Diagnosis and Treatment of Radiation Injuries, Safety Report Series No. 2. Vienna; 1998.

*(Reproduced with permission from Koenig KL, Goans RE, Hatchett RJ, et al. Medical Treatment of Radiological Casualties: Current Concepts. Ann of Emerg Med 45:643, 2005.)*

400 rads will generally recover given effective hemopoietic stimulation and antibiotic prophalaxis.[107]

## ACUTE RADIATION SYNDROME

Following the whole body radiation, rapidly dividing cells, such as those of the intestinal mucosa and bone marrow, are found to be the most sensitive to cell killing and/or alteration. A radiation dose of less than 1 Gy unit, 100 rads, results in modest injury. The majority of cells will survive; however, the potential for malignant transformation does exist.[109] The patients receiving dosing of 0.7–4 Gy units will have depressed bone marrow function leading to pancytopenia. Lymphocytes will be decreased most rapidly and will function as the best indicator of cellular damage.[108] As a result of hemopoietic suppression, anemia will develop within 10 days. A 50% drop in the lymphocyte count in 24 hours is indicative of a significant radiation injury.

Bone marrow suppression is complex, altering the production of erythrocytes (red cells), myelopoietic cells (white cells), and thrombopoietic cells (platelets).[108] These cells originate from a single stem cell line but have different sensitivities to the effects of radiation. The erythropoietic system is the most robust as the first system to rebound after radiation; therefore, anemia should not be recognized as a poor prognostic indicator of a radiation exposure. The function of the myelopoietic cell is to produce mature granulocytes, (neutrophils, eosinophils, and basophils), and recovers rapidly, returning granulocytes into the circulation within two to four days after whole body radiation.[108] The effect of radiation on megakaryocytes is minimal and mature megakaryocytes are relatively radioresistant. Thrombocytopenia usually recovers after three to four weeks.

A single dose of gamma radiation in the order of 6–8 Gy units results in gastrointestinal symptomatology. This will almost always be accompanied by bone marrow suppression, severe fluid loss, hemorrhage, and diarrhea. This occurs following injury to the luminal epithelium and fine vasculature of the submucosal due to loss of intestinal mucosal integrity.[108] Small intestines appear to be among the most vulnerable. Aggressive intervention in this high-risk group is warranted to include maintaining hemodynamic stability, correction of fluid and electrolyte imbalance, control of hemorrhage from devitalized GI tract, and prevention of systemic infection as a result of translocation due to damaged mucosal barriers.

The presence of neurovascular symptoms indicates a 20–40 Gy unit of exposure. This usually results in hypotension, whose presentation varies from that of several hours to 1–3 days with steady deterioration into seizures, coma, and death.[108] In patients presenting with early onset of neurological symptomatology, the outcome is uniformly fatal.[101]

### Management of Acute Radiation Exposure

Nuclear detonation is less likely in today's political arena in comparison to the Cold War era. However, based upon the potential threats of missing weapons grade material as stated previously, preparedness for the worst scenario is imperative. From a nuclear detonation, the spectrum of acute and long-term injury will be all-encompassing to include blast, thermal, blunt, and penetrating trauma to acute and long-term sequela of radiation illness.

Unlike a nuclear detonation with significant Gray units of exposure, the radiological dispersal devices are not likely to result in significant contamination or precipitate acute radiation illness.[101] With RDD detonations, patients are subjected to the sequela of blast injury with concomitant radioisotopes as projectiles. Management of these victims should follow standard guidelines of practice for blunt and penetrating trauma. Operative verses nonoperative management of these penetrating injuries should be assessed in conjunction with risk of ongoing exposure to the emission of the impaled radioisotopes.[108] Patient outcomes with combination injury—radiation and physical trauma—are worse than for those with radiation or trauma in isolation.[106] Thermal burns from radiation exposure have a worse prognosis than conventional burns.[106]

In the aforementioned scenarios of exposure, the application of standard decontamination protocols should be instituted during and/or following stabilization of the victims. The extent and invasiveness of the decontamination is dependent upon physical properties of the emitting source, presence of wounds, and potential for ongoing external and internal exposure. As a general rule, removal of the outer clothing and shoes should reduce the external contamination by 90%. Passing a handheld radiation detector over the patient could assess any residual contamination. Decontamination should reduce the level of radiologic contamination to less than two times the background radiation as it exists in the environment.[106] The radiological risk to health care providers is removed with appropriate decontamination: "the patient does not emit radiation." With exception to the aforementioned, if internal contamination or projectiles of radioactive material exist, precautions should be used in conducting internal decontamination and removal of projectiles as instructed by radiation safety officers of the medical institution. Addressing internal contamination, the provision of gastrointestinal cathartics and bronchoalveolar lavage will help to mitigate any ongoing radiation emitting particles that may have been digested or inhaled.

Following decontamination, attention should be given to wounds and burns. The exposure of burns and wounds to radioactive material carries a much greater risk for morbidity and mortality; and cleansing should be done with debridement. The decision whether to close wounds or leave them open is a controversial issue based upon the risk benefit of delayed healing verses closed space infection in the immunocompromised patient.[102,108]

## MANAGEMENT OF THE NEUTROPENIC FEVER

Patients who have profound neutropenia (less than $0.1 \times 10^9$ cells per liter or an absolute neutrophil count of less than 100 cells /microliter) are at greatest risk for developing infection. Infections arise not only from opportunistic bacteria but also from invasive mycosis.[108] Management of these patients is akin to the management of the neutropenic patient who is receiving chemotherapy. To the broadest degree possible, an empiric regimen of broad-spectrum antibiotics should be instituted, providing coverage for gram-negative bacterial infections as well as gram-positive infections to the broadest degree possible. Antifungal and antiviral prophylaxis should be considered.[108] Colony-stimulating factors should be considered to induce bone marrow hematopoietic cell proliferation and maturation.

**TABLE 56-4**

## Radionuclides Produced After Radiological Terrorism or Disaster–Internal Contamination, toxicity, and Treatment

| ELEMENT | RESPIRATORY ABSORPTION | GI ABSORPTION | SKIN WOUND ABSORPTION | PRIMARY TOXICITY | TREATMENT |
|---|---|---|---|---|---|
| Americium | 75% | Minimal | Rapid | Skeletal deposition Marrow Suppression, hepatic deposition | Chelation with DTPA or EDTA |
| Cesium | Complete | Complete | Complete | Whole body irradiation | Prussian blue |
| Cobalt | High | <5% | Unknown | Whole body irradiation | Supportive |
| Iodine | High | High | High | Thyroid ablation, carcinoma | Potassium iodide |
| Phosphorus | High | High | High | Bone, rapidly replicating cells | Aluminum hydroxide |
| Plutonium | High | Minimal | Limited, may form nodules | Lung, bone, liver | Chelation with DTPA or EDTA |
| Radium | Unknown | 30% | Unknown | Bone, marrow suppression, sarcoma | Magnesium sulfate lavage |
| Strontium | Limited | Moderate | Unknown | Bone | Supportive |
| Tritium | Minimal | Minimal | Complete | Panmyelocytopenia | Dilution with controlled water intake, diuresis |
| Tritiated water | Complete | Complete | Complete | Panmyelocytopenia | Dilution with controlled water intake, diuresis |
| Uranium | High | High to moderate | High absorption, skin irritant | Pulmonary, nephrotoxic | Chelation with DTPA or EDTA, NaHCO$_3$ to alkalinize urine |

*(Reproduced with permission from . Pediatric Terrorism Preparedness National Guidelines Act. Recommendations: Findings of an Evidence-based Consensus Process. Biosecurity and Bioterrorism: Biodefence Strategy, Practice, and Science 2:301, 2004.)*

Reverse isolation measures should be instituted due to the introduction of opportunistic pathogens from health care providers.

Medical counter measures to radiation fall in to three broad classes: the radioprotectants that prevent radiation-induced cell and molecular damage; radiation mitigators are drugs that accelerate recovery or repair after radiation injury; and radionucleotide eliminators are drugs that discorporate or block absorption of internalized radionucleotides.[101]

The radioprotectants currently licensed or under investigation include the phosphorylated-aminothiol, amifostine and phosphonol; templl and other membrane permeable nitroxides; keratinocyte growth factor; the angiotensin converting enzyme inhibitor captopril; the isoflavone genistein; androstenediol; and vitamin E analog alpha-tocopherol succinate.[101]

Amifostine was approved by the FDA in 1999 as the first radioprotectant agent to reduce toxicity associated with certain cancer chemotherapies and radiotherapies. This radioprotectant appears to enhance the chemical and enzymatic repair of damaged DNA.[101]

Radiation mitigators currently under investigation include colony stimulating factor, androgenic steroid androstenediol, glutamine, and pentoxifylline.[101] Colony-stimulating factors are endogenous glycoproteins that induce bone marrow and hemopoietic progenitor cells, to proliferate and differentiate into mature blood cells. Three recombinant colony stimulating factors exist: filgrastim, pegfilgrastim, and sargramostim.[110] Filgrastim and sargramostim appear to hasten recovery of neutrophil counts. Hemopoietic growth factor filgrastim (neupogen) is a granulocytic colony-stimulating factor (G-CSF) and pegfilgrastim (Neulasta) and sargramostim (Leukine) are granulocytic macrophage colony stimulating factors.[101]

Radionuclide eliminators currently licensed include potassium iodine, ferric hexacyanoferrate (Prussian blue), calcium and zinc diethylenetriamine pentaacetate (Ca and Zn-DTPA), bicarbonate, barium sulfate, calcium gluconate, penicillamine, aluminum antacids, and sodium alginate (Table 56-4).[52] Potassium iodine is a drug of choice, which prevents thyroid uptake of radioiodine external irradiation. Children are more sensitive than adults,[111] and therefore should thus be treated as priority. This therapy offers no systemic protection other than direct protection of the thyroid gland and tissue. Prussian blue is an insoluble dye, which orally enhances fecal excretion of cesium and thallium from the body by means of ion exchange. Cesium is considered to be an ideal terrorist weapon given thanin is plentifully available as a result of its commercial and medical applications. Internal decontamination for cesium is not indicated unless one annual limit of intake has exceeded 100 uCi for inhalation and 100 uCi from ingestion.[112] Calcium and Zinc DTPA agents are used to treat contamination of plutonium, americium, and curium.[113] The agents react with the isotope to result in stable ionic complexes that can be excreted in the urine. Care should be taken in administration of these agents as well as other minerals such as zinc, magnesium, and manganese.[101]

## Carcinogenesis

It is estimated that radiation-induced cancer in individuals exposed to 100 mGy of gamma radiation, which is two times the US occupational annual limit of 0.05 Gy, causes a 0.8% increase of lifetime risk of death from cancer.[108] The general US population has an annual lifetime risk of 20%.

## PREGNANCY AND RADIATION

Ionizing radiation is a potential teratogen whose dose-dependent action has not been well defined. The effect of ionizing and radiation in pregnancy, for the most part, is dependent upon gestational age at the time of the exposure, as well as the fetal dose of absorption.[114] The preimplant period of embryo is less radiosensitive than other periods of pregnancy.[115,116] During the first 14 days of conception, the radiation upon the embryo is demonstrated as an increased rate of early abortion and failure of embryo implantation.[117,118] The period between the second and eighth week, primarily the first trimester, is extremely sensitive to teratogenic effects of ionizing radiation. At significant risk is the central nervous system, whose formation and development occurs during the 8th or 15th week of pregnancy.[119] During these weeks of development, the neural stem cells are subjected to mitotic activity and proliferation of the cerebral cortex.[120] However, after the 25th week the central nervous system becomes relatively radioresistant, making fetal malformations highly improbable.[121–124] Other ill effects due to radiation exposure during pregnancy is related to the low birth weight children.[52]

## SUMMARY

This abbreviated presentation of WMD is but an orientation to the broad atypical threat and subsequent injury potential of victims challenging the surgeons today. It is meant to encourage further study and training to strengthen the surgical response to future mass casualty incidents. Recognition of the importance of the surgical intensivist in the management of nonoperative injury from chemical, biological, and radiological agents represents a significant portion of the contemporary surgeons' contribution to Homeland Security Preparedness.

## ACKNOWLEDGMENTS

Special thanks to Christy Westmoreland, RN, for her editorial assistance and to Susan Bourgoine for her administrative and secretarial support.

## REFERENCES

1. Counterterrorism Threat Assessment and Warning Unit, National Security Division, FBI, Terrorism in the United States 1999: 30 Years of Terrorism — A Special Retrospective Edition, Washington, D.C.: United States Department of Justice, 1999, p. i. Online at http://www.fbi.gov/publications/terror/terror99.pdf.
2. Ciraulo DL, Frykberg ER, Feliciano DV, et al.: A survey assessment of the level of preparedness for domestic and mass casualty incidents among Eastern Association for the Surgery of Trauma members. J Trauma 56:1033, 2004.
3. Defense Against Weapons of Mass Destruction: Act of 1996 Public Law: 104-201 (09/23/96) http://www.fas.org/spp/starwars/congress/1996/1104-201-xvi.html.
4. Frykberg ER: Disaster and mass casualty management: A commentary on the American College of Surgeons position statement. JACS 197:5857, 2003.
5. DePalma RG, Burris DG, Champion H, et al.: Current concepts; blast injuries. NEJM 352:1335, 2005.
6. Stuhmiller JH, Phillips YY, Richmond DR: The physics and mechanism of primary blast injury. In Bellamy RF, Jenkins DP, Zajtcjuk JT, et al. Conventional warfare: Ballistic, Blast, and Burn Injuries. Washington DC: Office of Surgeon General at TMM Publications, 1991, p. 241.
7. Phillips YY: Primary blast injury. Ann Emerg Med 18:446, 1986.
8. Landsberg PG: Underwater blast injuries. http://www.scubadoc.com/uwblast.html.
9. Kluger Y: Bomb explosions in acts of terrorism-detonation, wound ballistics, triage, and medical concerns. IMAJ 5:235, 2003.
10. Ryan J, Montgomery H: The London attacks-preparedness: Terrorism and the medical response. N Engl J Med 353:543, 2005.
11. Almogy G, Luria J, Richter E, et al.: Can external signs of trauma guide management? Arch Surg 140:390, 2005.
12. Gutierrez de Ceballos JP, Fuentes I, Diaz DP, et al.: Casualties treated at the closest hospital in the Madrid, March 11 terrorist bombing. Crit Care Med 33:5107, 2005.
13. Gutierrez de Cevallos JP, Turegano-Fuentes F, Perez-Diaz D, et al.: 11 March 2004: The terrorist bomb explosions in Madrid, Spain — an analysis of the logistics, injuries sustained and clinical management of casualties treated at the closest hospital. Crit Care 9:104, 2005.
14. Kluger Y, Peleg K, Daniel-Aharonson L, et al.: The special injury pattern in terrorist bombings. J Am Coll Surg 199:875, 2004.
15. Arnold JL, Halpern P, Tsai M, et al.: Mass casualty terrorist bombing: A comparison of outcomes by bombing type. Ann Emerg Med 43:263, 2004.
16. Leibner ED, Weil Y, Gross E, et al.: A broken bone without a fracture: Traumatic foreign bone implantation resulting from mass casualty bombing. J Trauma 58:388, 2005.
17. Braverman I, Wexler D, Oren M: A novel mode of infection with hepatitis B: Penetrating bone fragments due to the explosion of a suicide bomber. Isr Med Assoc J 4:528, 2002.
18. Eshkol Z, Krtz K: Injuries from biologic material of suicide bombers. Injury, Int J Care Injured 36:271, 2005.
19. Hepatitis B Vaccination Protocol in Survivors of Mass Casualty Bombings. Ministry of Health Medical Guidelines; 2001. (35)/2/13(Communiqué 57/2001).
20. Hepatitis B Vaccination Protocol in Survivors of Mass Casualty Bombings—Revision. Ministry of Health Medical Guidelines; 2001. (35)/2/13(Communiqué 72/2001).
21. Janes DC: Terrorism and the pregnant women. J Perinat Neonat Nurs 19:226, 2005.
22. Bywaters EGL, Beall D: Crush injuries with impairment of renal function. BMJ 1:427, 1941.
23. Better OS: Rescue and salvage of casualties suffering from the crush syndrome after mass disasters. Mil Med 164:366, 1999.
24. Greaves I, Porter K, Smith JE: Consensus statement on the early management of crush injury and prevention of crush syndromes. JR Army Med Corps 149:255, 2003.
25. Slater M, Mullins R: Rhabdomyolysis and myoglobinuric renal failure in trauma and surgical patients: A review. J Am Coll Surg 186:693, 1998.
26. Ward MM: Factors predictive of acute renal failure in rhabdomyolysis. Arch Intern Med 148:1553, 1988.
27. Malinoski PJ, Slater MS, Mullins RJ: Crush injury and rhabdomyolysis. Crit Care Clin 20:171, 2004.
28. Better OS, Zinman C, Reis DN, et al.: Hypertonic mannitol ameliorates intracompartmental tamponade in model compartment syndrome in the dog. Nephron 58:344, 1991.
29. Zager RA: Combined mannitol and deferoxamine therapy for myohemoglobinuric renal injury and oxidant tubular stress. Mechanistic and therapeutic implications. J Clin Invest 90:711, 1992.
30. Zager RA: Studies of mechanisms and protective maneuvers in myoglobinuric acute renal injury. Lab Invest 60:619, 1989.
31. Singh D, Chopra K: Rhabdomyolysis. Methods find. Exp Clin Pharmacol 27:39, 2005.
32. Whitesides T, Heckman M: Acute compartment syndrome: Update on diagnosis and treatment. J Am Acad Orthop Surg 4:209, 1996.
33. Whitesides TE, Haney TC, Morimoto K, et al.: Tissue pressure measurements as a determinant for the need of fasciotomy. Clinical Orthop 113:43, 1975.
34. Matsen III FA, Krugmire Jr RB: Compartmental syndromes. Surg Gynecol Obstet 147:943, 1978.
35. Paton DF: The anterior/tibial/syndrome. Practitioner 225:151, 1981.
36. Sever SM, Erek E, Vanholder R, et al.: Clinical findings in the renal victims of a catastrophic disaster: The Marmara earthquake. Nephrol Dial Transplant 17:1942, 2002.
37. Nadjafi I, Atef MR, Broumand B, et al.: Suggested guidelines for treatment of acute renal failure in earthquake victims. Ren Fail 19:655, 1997.
38. Tetsuya M, Toshiharu Y, Hiroshi T, et al.: Long term physical outcome of patients who suffered crush syndrome after the 1995 Hanshin-Awaji earthquake: Prognostic indicators in retrospect. J Trauma 52:33, 2002.
39. Gunal AI, Celiker H, Dogukan A, et al.: Early and vigorous fluid resuscitation prevents acute renal failure in the crush victims of catastrophic earthquakes. J Am Soc Nephrol 15:1862, 2004.
40. Huang KC, Lee TS, Lin YM, et al.: Clinical features and outcome of crush syndrome caused by the Chi-Chi earthquake. J Formos Med Assoc 101:249, 2002.
41. Hersch SM: Chemical and Biological Warfare: America's Hidden Arsenal. Indianapolis: Bobbs-Merrill Company, 1968.
42. Schecter WP, Fry DE: The Governor's Committee on Blood Borne Infection and Environmental Risk of American College of Surgeons. The Surgeons and Act of Civilian Terrorism: Chemical Agents. J Am Coll Surg 200:128, 2005.
43. US Army Medical Research Institute of Chemical Defense (USAM RICD) Medical Management of Chemical Casualties Handbook, 3rd ed. 2000.
44. Pelletiere SC, Johnson DV: Lessons Learned: The Iran-Iraq War. Carlisle Barracks, PA: Strategic Studies Institute, US Army War College, 1991.

45. Cordesman AH, Wagner AP: *The Lessons of Modern War*, Volume II: The Iran-Iraq War. Boulder, CO: Westview Press, 1990.

46. Dingeman A, Jupa R: Chemical warfare in the Iran-Iraq conflict. *Strategy Tactics* 113:51, 1987.

47. Barnaby F: Iran-Iraq War: The use of chemical weapons against the Kurds. *Ambio* 17:407, 1988.

48. Weinstein RS, Alibek K: *Biological and Chemical Terrorism*. New York: Thieme, 2003.

49. Newmark J: Nerve Agents: Pathophysiology and treatment of poisoning. *Seminars in Necrology* 24:185, 2004.

50. Lee EC: Clinical Manifestations of Sarin nerve gas exposure. *JAMA* 290:659, 2003.

51. Rotenberg JS, Newmark J: Nerve agent attacks on children: Diagnosis and management. *Pediatrics* 112:648, 2003.

52. Markenson D, Redlener I: Pediatric Terrorism Preparedness National Guidelines Act. Recommendations: Findings of an Evidence-based Consensus Process. *Biosecurity and Bioterrorism: Biodefence Strategy, Practice, and Science* 2:301, 2004.

53. Sidell FR: Clinical considerations in nerve agent intoxication. In Somani SM, ed. *Chemical Warfare Agents*. New York: Academic Press, 1992, p. 156.

54. McDonough J, McMonagle J, Copeland T, et al.: Comparative evaluation of benzodiazepines for control of soman-induced seizures. *Arch Toxicol* 73:473, 1999.

55. Eckstein M: Cyanide as a chemical terrorism. *JEMS* 85:1, 2004.

56. Marrs TC: Antidotal treatment of acute cyanide poisoning. *Adverse Drug React Acute Poisoning Rev* 7:179, 1984.

57. Baker D: Critical care requirements after mass toxic agent release. *Crit Care Med* 33:566, 2005.

58. Harrison R: Occupational toxicologic emergencies. In Kravis TC, Warner CG, Jacobs LM, eds. *Emergency Medicine: A Comprehensive Review*. New York: Raven Press, 3rd ed. 1993, p. 761.

59. Key M, Henschel A, Butler J, et al.: *Occupational Disease: A Guide to Their Recognition*. DHEW Publication No. 77, 1978.

60. Kaufman J, Burkons D: Clinical, roentgenographic, and physiologic effects of acute chlorine exposure. *Arch Environ Health* 23:29, 1971.

61. Guo YL, Kennedy TP, Michael JR, et al.: Mechanism of phosgene-induced lung toxicity: Role of arachidonate mediators . *J Appl Physiol* 69:1615, 1990.

62. Urbanetti JS: Toxic inhalation injury. In Sidell FR, Takafuji ET, Franz DR, eds. *Medical Aspects of Chemical and Biological Warfare*. Washington, D.C.: Office of the Surgeon General at TMM Publications, Borden Institute, Walter Reed Army Medical Center, 1997, p. 247.

63. Szincz L: History of chemical and biological warfare agents. *Toxicology* 6:1, 2005.

64. Bhandari NR, Syal AK, Kambo I, et al.: Pregnancy outcome in women exposed to toxic gas at Bhopal. *Indian J Med Res* 92:28, 1990.

65. Goswami HK, Chandorkai M, Bhattacharya K, et al.: Search for chromosomal variations among gas-exposed persons in Bhopal. *Hum Genet* 84:172, 1990.

66. Daniel CS, Singh AK, Siddiqui P, et al.: Preliminary report on the spermatogenesis function of male subjects exposed to gas at Bhopal. *Indian J Med Res* 86:83, 1987.

67. Greenfield RA, Drevets DA, Machado LV, et al.: Bacterial pathogens as biological weapons and agents of bioterrorism. *Am J Med Sci* 323:299, 2002.

68. Jernigan JA, Stephens DS, Ashford DA, et al.: Bioterrorism-related inhalation anthrax: The first 10 cases reported in the United States. *Emerg Infect Dis* 7:933, 2001.

69. Inglesby TB, Henderson DA, Bartlett JG, et al.: Anthrax as a biological weapon. *JAMA* 281:1735, 1999.

70. Fry PE, Schecter WP, Parker JS: The surgeon and acts of civilian terrorism: Biologic agents. *J Am College of Surgeons* 200:291, 2005.

71. Nolte KB, Hanzlick RL, Payne DC, et al.: Medical Examiners, Coroners and Biological Terrorism. A guidebook for Surveillance and Case Management. *Morb Mortal Wkly Rep MMWR* 531:8. 108, 2004.

72. Darling RG, Catlett CL, Huebner KP, et al.: The threats of bioterrorism I: CDC category A agents. *Emerg Med N Am* 20:273, 2002.

73. Makino SI, Cheun III, Watatai M, et al.: Detection of anthrax spores from the air by real-time PCR. *Lett Appl Microbiol* 33:237, 2001.

74. Oncu S, Oncu S, Sakarya S: Anthrax-an overview. *Med Sci Monit* 9:276, 2003.

75. Horn J: Bacterial agents used for bioterrorism. *Surgical Infections* 4:281, 2003.

76. Osterbaure PJ, Dobbs MR: Neurobiological weapons. *Neurol Clin* 23:599, 2005.

77. Alibek K: *Biohazard*. New York: Random House, 1999.

78. Zilinskas RA: Iraq's biological weapons, the past as future? *JAMA* 278:418, 1997.

79. Ales NC, Katial RK: Vaccines against biologic agents: Uses and developments. *Respir Care Clin* 10:123, 2004.

80. Arnon SS, Schechter R, Inglesby TV, et al.: Botulinum toxin as a biological weapon: Medical and public health management. *JAMA* 285:1059, 2001.

81. Middlebrook JL, Franz DR: Botulism. In Sidell FR, Takafuji ET, Franz DR, eds. *Medical Management of Biological Casualties*. 3rd ed. Washington, D.C.: TMM Publications, 1998, p. 86.

82. Martin CO, Adams HP: Neurological aspects of biological and chemical terrorism: A review for neurologists. *Arch Neurol* 60:21, 2003.

83. Bozeran WP, Dilbero D, Schauben JL: Biologic and chemical weapons of mass destruction. *Emerg Med Clin N Am* 20:975, 2002.

84. Polesky A, Bhatia G: Ebola hemorrhagic fever in the era of bioterrorism. *Seminars in Respiratory Infections* 18:206, 2003.

85. Centers for Disease Control and Prevention: Management of patients with suspected viral hemorrhagic fever. *Morb Mortal Wkly Rep MMWR* 37:1, 1988.

86. Perry RD, Fetherston JD: Yersinia pestis: Etiologic agent of plague. *Clin Microbiol Rev* 10:35, 1997.

87. Wortmann G: Pulmonary manifestations of other agents: Brucella, Q fever, tularemia, and smallpox. *Respir Care Clin* 10:99, 2004.

88. Alibek K, Hardelman S: *Biohazard*. New York: Random House, 1999.

89. Henderson DA, Inglesby TV, Bartlett JG, et al.: Smallpox as a biological weapon: Medical and public health management. *JAMA* 281:2127, 1999.

90. McClain DJ: Smallpox. In Sidell FR, Takafuji ET, Franz DR, eds. *Medical Management of Biological Casualties*. 3rd ed. Washington, D.C.: TMM Publications, 1998, p. 58.

91. Henderson DA: Smallpox: Clinical and epidemiologic features. *Emerg Inf Dis* 5:537, 1999.

92. Bray M, Martinez M, Smee DF, et al.: Cidofovir protects mice against lethal aerosol or intranasal cowpox virus challenge. *J Infect Dis* 181:10, 2000.

93. Smee DF, Bailey KW, Sidwell RW: Treatment of lethal vaccinia virus respiratory infections in mice with cidofovir. *Antivir Chem Chemother* 12:71, 2001.

94. White SR, Henretig FM, Dukes RG: Medical management of vulnerable populations and co-morbid conditions of victims of bioterrorism. *Emerg Med Clin North Am* 20:365, 2002.

95. Blair DC: A week in the life of a travel clinic. *Clin Microb Rev* 10:650, 1997.

96. Jamieson DJ, Jernigan DB, Ellis JE, et al.: Emerging infections and pregnancy: West Nile virus, monkeypox, severe acute respiratory syndrome, and bioterrorism. *Clin Perinatal* 32:765, 2005.

97. Handjani AM: Case records of the Pahlavi hospitals. *Pahlavi Med J* 7:147, 1976.

98. Sujatha S, Parija SC, Bhattacharya S, et al.: Anthrax peritonitis. *Top Doct* 32:247, 2002.

99. Centers for Disease Control and Prevention: Updated recommendations for ant microbial prophylaxis among asymptomatic pregnant women after exposure to Bacillus anthracis. *Morb Mortal Wkly Rep MMWR* 50:960, 2001.

100. Committee ACOG: Opinion number 268, February 2002. Management of asymptomatic pregnant or lactating women exposed to anthrax. American College of Obstetricians and Gynecologists. *Obstet Gynecol* 99:366, 2002.

101. Koenig KL, Goans RE, Hatchett RJ, et al.: Medical treatment of radiological casualties: Current concepts. *Ann Emerg Med* 45:643, 2005.

102. Timins JK, Lipoti JA: Radiological terrorism. *Supplement to New Jersey Medicine* 101:66, 2004.

103. International Atomic Energy Agency: *IAEA Illicit Trafficking Database*. Vienna: IAEA, 2003.

104. House Committee of National Security Allegations of Russia's Missing Suitcase Bombs: http://www.ransac.org/new-web-site/related/congress/hearings/suitcasebombs.html.

105. Yablokov A: Do "backpack" nuclear weapons exist? http://www.pbs.org/wgbh//pages/frontline/shows/russia/suitcase/comments.html.

106. Blard SA: Mass Casualty management for radiological and nuclear incidents. *JR Army Med Corps* 150:27, 2004.

107. Briggs SM, Brinsfield KH: *Advanced Disaster Medical Response*. Boston: Harvard Medical International Trauma & Disaster Institute, 2003.

108. Military Medical Operation Armed Forces Radiobiology, Research Institute (AFRRI). *Medical Management of Radiological Casualties*. 2nd ed, 2003.

109. Fajardo LF, Berthrong M, Anderson RE: *Radiation Pathology*. New York, NY: Oxford University Press, 2001.

110. Farese AM, Hunt P, Grab LB, et al.: Combined administration of recombinant human megakaryocyte growth and development factor and gametocyte colony-stimulating factor enhances multilineage hematopoietic reconstitution in nonhuman primates after radiation-induced marrow aplasia. *J Clin Invest* 97:2145, 1996.

111. Committee to Assess the Distribution and Administration of Potassium Iodide in the Event of a Nuclear Incident: *Distribution and Administration of potassium Iodide in the Event of a Nuclear Incident*. Washington, D.C.: National Academies Press, 2003, p. 114.

112. Brandao-Mello CE, Oliveira AR, Valverde NJ, et al.: Clinical and hematological aspects of $^{137}$Cs: The Goiania radiation accident. *Health Phys* 60:31, 1991.

113. US Food and Drug Administration, Center for Drug Evaluation and Research: Questions and answers on Calcium-DTPA and Zinc-DTPA (updated). Available at: http://www.fda.gov/cder/druginfopage/DTPA/OandADTPA.htm. Accessed March 10, 2005.

114. DeSantis M, DiGianantonio E, Straface G, Caurliere DF, et al.: Ionizing radiation in pregnancy and teratogenesis: A review of literature. *Reproductive Toxicol* 20:323, 2005.

115. Brent RL, Bolden BT: The indirect effect of irradiation on embryonic development. The contribution of ovarian irradiation, uterine irradiation, oviduct irradiation, and zygote irradiation to fetal mortality and growth retardation in the rat. *Radiat Res* 30:759, 1967.

116. Russel LB, Badgett SK, Saylors CL: *Comparison of the Effects of Acute, Continuous and Fractionated Irradiation During Embryonic Development.* Conference in Venice. London, UK: Taylor & Francis, 1959, p. 343.

117. ICRP Publication 73. Radiological protection and safety in medicine. *Ann ICRP* 26:1, 1997.

118. Jankowski CB: Radiation and pregnancy. Putting the risks in proportion. *Am J Nurs* 86:260, 1986.

119. Mole RH: Detriment in humans after irradiation in utero. *Int J Radiat Biol* 60:561, 1991.

120. Timins JK: Radiation during pregnancy. *N J Med* 98:29, 2001.

121. International Commission on Radiological Protection: 1990 Recommendations of the International Commission on Radiological Protection. *Ann ICRP* 21:1, 1991.

122. International Commission on Radiological Protection: Doses to the embryo and fetus from intakes of radionuclides by the mother. A report of The International Commission on Radiological Protection. *Ann ICRP* 31:19, 2001.

123. Rakic P: Cell migration and neuronal ectopias in the brain. *Birth Defects Orig Artic Ser* 11:95, 1975.

124. Streffer C, Shore R, Konermann G, et al.: Biological effects after prenatal irradiation (embryo and fetus). A report of the International Commission on Radiological Protection. *Ann ICRP* 33:5, 2003.

# Commentary ■ M. GAGE OCHSNER, JR.

Although the management of patients exposed to weapons of mass destruction (WMD) has been, and still is, taught to physicians serving in the Armed Forces, the increase in global terrorism has expanded the potential for surgeons in civilian communities to encounter victims from chemical, biological, and nuclear weapons. In addition, terrorists are capable of using high-yield explosive devices that result in blast injury. Most of us, even those with military experience, have never encountered patients exposed to these weapons and are ill-prepared to treat them. Combine this fact with the high probability that large numbers of casualties would be created; it is safe to predict that our acute care capabilities would rapidly be overwhelmed.

In this well written, comprehensive chapter Dr Ciraulo addresses the key elements for managing victims of WMD. The sections on diagnosis and management of patients exposed to chemical, biological, and nuclear weapons are concise, thorough, and serve as an excellent reference. In addition, he clearly outlines the basic principles of caring for patients with blast injury. This chapter contains updated information obtained from increasing experience with blast injury from recent terrorist attacks in London and Madrid. Also, the frequent use of improvised explosive devices (IEDs) by insurgents in Iraq continues to add to our clinical experience, particularly with primary blast injury, which until recently, was based on limited historical data.

This chapter also addresses the management of crush injury, emphasizing early diagnosis of compartment syndrome and liberal use of fasciotomy. The diagnosis and treatment of rhabdomyolysis is critical in reducing morbidity and mortality from renal failure. The use of mannitol as an osmotic diuretic and sodium bicarbonate to alkalinize the urine, although supporting my personal bias, is somewhat controversial. The key principle of euvolemia and maintenance of high urine outputs of up to 100 cc per hour is critical, however, and appropriately emphasized.

A truly unique and valuable aspect of this chapter is the inclusion of the management of the pediatric and pregnant patient exposed to WMDs. As these patients could be among those injured in a terrorist mass casualty event, Dr Ciraulo serves us well by drawing our attention to the fact that we will need to be prepared to treat these subsets of patients.

Perhaps the most important observation made by Dr Ciraulo in this chapter is the lack of an effective infrastructure, at the local, state, and national levels capable of dealing with the mass casualties that would be generated by weapons of mass destruction. Many of the national organizations representing trauma surgeons and emergency physicians have recognized the need for better preparedness for mass casualty events and disaster management. Several have even developed programs to teach surgeons how to be better prepared to respond to injury from WMD. The Institute of Medicine's Committee on the Future of Emergency Care in the United States Health System was convened in 2003 and charged to examine the state of emergency care in the Unites States and create a vision for the future of emergency care with recommendations on how to achieve that vision. The results were published recently in three reports: *Hospital Based Emergency Care: At the Breaking Point,*[1] *Emergency Medical Services at the Crossroads,*[2] and *Emergency Care for Children: Growing Pains.*[3] One conclusion from the committee is that the emergency care system is ill prepared to handle surges from disasters, such as hurricanes, terrorist attacks, or disease outbreaks. Trauma surgeons as well as critical surgical specialties should read these reports and be familiar with the recommendations contained within. Well-designed trauma systems remain the best infrastructure for dealing with patients injured by WMDs, yet these systems do not exist in many parts of our country, including some with attractive terrorist targets.

According to most experts, it is not a question of "if" we will have a major terrorist incident in the United States but rather "when" will it occur. This emphasizes the urgency for developing an effective infrastructure now, to mitigate the consequences of a likely terrorist attack with WMDs.

## References

1. Institute of Medicine, Committee on the future of Emergency Care in the United States Health System: *Hospital-Based Emergency Care: At the Breaking Point.* Washington, D.C.: National Academies Press, 2006.

2. Institute of Medicine, Committee on the future of Emergency Care in the United States Health System: *Emergency Medical Services: At the Crossroads.* Washington, D.C.: National Academies Press, 2006.

3. Institute of Medicine, Committee on the future of Emergency Care in the United States Health System: *Emergency Care for Children: Growing Pains.* Washington, D.C.: National Academies Press, 2006.

# Genetic Influence on Response and Outcome

*Grant E O'Keefe*

## INTRODUCTION

Variability is a hallmark of clinical medicine. This variability is possibly more evident in the fields of trauma and intensive care than in any other aspect of surgery. Why do patients with seemingly similar injuries, receiving comparable and appropriate treatment often follow different trajectories or paths — one patient recovering uneventfully from massive transfusion for hemorrhagic shock and another following a prolonged course complicated by nosocomial pneumonia and organ failure? Also, consider the seemingly simpler task of how to adequately prevent and treat deep venous thromboembolic disease. Despite our understanding of the biology of coagulation and related processes and despite seemingly rational pharmacotherapeutic and preventative strategies, patients continue to develop deep vein thrombosis and die from pulmonary emboli.

Numerous clinical (environmental) and genetic factors doubtless contribute to this variability. The role of heritable or genetic factors is now the subject of increased interest and intense study for a number of reasons. First, with the completion of the Human Genome Project, we have knowledge of the entire human genetic sequence.[1] Second, there is marked and variability in this sequence between individuals, which is relatively easily measured and recorded. This variability has been used to begin to establish genotype–phenotype associations for common diseases, such as sepsis. The goals of "Genomic Medicine" is to use this genetic variability to help understand the biology of these diseases and to better direct therapy (such as drug selection and dosing).[2]

Critical illness, including that experienced by the severely injured patient may be greatly influenced by genetic differences in a variety of ways. Two illustrative examples which this chapter will focus on are: (1) how genetic differences in drug response and metabolism (pharmacogenomics) can be used to improve patient care and (2) our understanding of the biology of sepsis and whether genetic differences are important determinants of outcome.

## A REVIEW OF GENETIC CONCEPTS

Since the discovery and publication of the molecular structure of nucleic acids by Watson and Crick in 1954, the genetic basis for many conditions has been determined.[3–5] However, misconceptions remain regarding the role of genetics and the more recently coined term of "genomics" in clinical medicine. Despite the commonly held notion that genetics had little influence on clinical medicine in the past and now has a widespread role, genetics has, in fact, played an important role in the health of albeit few patients for many years. We may now be entering a period of transition to a time when knowledge of genetics will influence the care and health of the majority of us.[6] In order for clinicians to understand and participate in these advances, we must become "literate" in the language of genetics and genomic medicine. Box 57-1 includes some important definitions helpful to a basic understanding of genetic concepts for clinicians. This list is not exhaustive and some of the concepts are elaborated more completely in the following paragraphs.

Much is known, yet a great deal remains unknown about the human genome. We know that the minority of the three gigabases of DNA sequence codes for proteins. It is estimated that approximately 2% of our DNA sequence codes for approximately 30,000 unique proteins. The function of the remaining majority is perhaps the most fascinating aspect of genomics. Figure 57-1 illustrates the general structure of a typical gene. The 5' control region, often termed "promoter," includes DNA sequences that recognized and bound by proteins called transcription factors lead to changes in the shape of the DNA molecule and control access to the coding region by transcriptional proteins. The start code is a series of nucleotide sequences that are recognized by this transcriptional machinery and provide the starting point for transcribing the DNA coding sequence into messenger RNA (mRNA). Not all of this sequence encodes for protein. *Exons* are the regions of DNA that contain the amino acid coding sequences. In most genes, multiple

## Box 57-1: Definitions

**Allele**: One version of a gene at a given location (locus) along a chromosome.

**Allelic heterogeneity**: Different mutations in the same gene at the same chromosomal locus that cause a single phenotype.

**Coding region**: All exons of a gene that contribute to the protein product(s) of that gene.

**Exon**: DNA coding sequences present in mature messenger RNA.

**Frameshift mutation**: An insertion or deletion involving a number of base pairs that is not a multiple of three and consequently disrupts the triplet reading frame, usually leading to the creation of a premature termination (stop) codon and resulting in a truncated protein product.

**Gene**: The basic unit of heredity, consisting of a segment of DNA arranged in a linear manner along a chromosome. A gene codes for a specific protein or segment of protein leading to a particular characteristic or function.

**Genetic predisposition**: Increased susceptibility to a particular disease due to the presence of one or more gene mutations associated with an increased risk for the disease and/or a family history that indicates an increased risk for the disease.

**Genomics**: The study of the functions and interactions of all genes in the genome.

**Genotype**: The genetic constitution of an organism or cell; also refers to the specific set of alleles inherited in a gene region.

**Genotype–phenotype association**: The association between the presence of a certain mutation or mutations (genotype) and the resulting pattern of abnormalities (phenotype).

**Intron**: Noncoding sequence of DNA removed from mature messenger RNA prior to translation into a protein.

**Molecular genetic testing (DNA-based testing)**: Testing that involves the direct analysis of DNA, either through sequencing, or one of several methods of mutation detection.

**Mutation**: Any alteration in a gene from its natural state; may be disease-causing or a benign, silent variant.

**Pharmacogenomics**: The branch of pharmacology which deals with the influence of genetic variation on drug response in patients by correlating gene expression or single-nucleotide polymorphisms with a drug's efficacy or toxicity. By doing so, pharmacogenomics aims to develop rational means to optimize drug therapy, with respect to the patients' genotype, to ensure maximum efficacy with minimal adverse effects.

**Phenotype**: The observable physical and/or biochemical characteristics of the expression of a gene; the clinical presentation of an individual with a particular genotype.

**Phenotyping**: Diagnostic testing and inference of a particular genotype based on clinical or biochemical presentation (phenotype) of the individual, such as measurement of alpha-1-antitrypsin level. With the advent of DNA-based testing, direct mutation analysis (genotyping) is becoming more widely available for many disorders.

**Polymerase chain reaction (PCR)**: A procedure that produces millions of copies of a short segment of DNA through repeated cycles of: (1) denaturation, (2) annealing, and (3) elongation; PCR is a very common procedure in molecular genetic testing and may be used to: (1) generate a sufficient quantity of DNA to perform a test (e.g., sequence analysis, mutation scanning), or (2) may be a test in and of itself.

**Ribonucleic acid (RNA)**: The molecule synthesized from the DNA template; contains the sugar ribose instead of deoxyribose, which is present in DNA; three types of RNA exist, messenger RNA (mRNA), transfer RNA (tRNA), and ribosomal RNA (rRNA)

**Single nucleotide polymorphism (SNP)**: An alteration in DNA sequence caused by a single nucleotide base change. SNPs are the most common type of variation in the human genome. By common use, SNP refers to polymorphisms with greater than 1% frequency in a selected population and excludes "personal" mutations.

### Sections within a typical gene

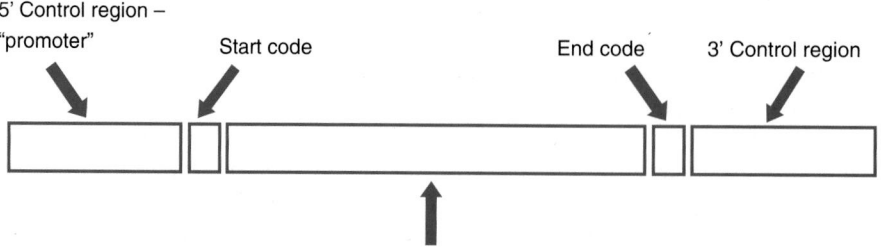

**FIGURE 57-1.** The general structure of a typical gene.

exons are separated by *introns*, which are DNA sequences that are transcribed into the RNA sequence, but then removed or spliced out before translation into protein. The end of transcription is signaled by a nucleotide code at the end of the coding sequence, referred to as a "stop codon." The DNA sequence after this end code, termed the 3" control region can also influence the rate of gene transcription and may affect the stability of the mRNA sequence and its translation into protein. The extent of these noncoding regions within the genome is uncertain. Although introns are located within the known boundaries of a gene (they are interspersed between the exons), promoters and enhancers may be found some distance from the gene whose transcription they affect. Finally, approximately 50% of the genome consists of repetitive sequences, previously and likely incorrectly referred to as "junk DNA," whose function is poorly understood.

Despite our limited knowledge of the function of much of the genome, our knowledge of the genetic basis for disease is, in fact, extensive. Basic research and clinical observation have elucidated the inheritance of single-gene, mendelian disorders (transmitted according to Mendel's laws of inheritance). Most of these are uncommon, and taken together, the most prevalent (cystic fibrosis, hemochromatosis, for example) affect no more than one in several hundred people. However, their effect on individual patients is substantial. Furthermore, understanding the mechanisms underlying many monogenic disorders has provided pathophysiological information about related disorders that occur with far greater frequency than do these genetic disorders. For instance, we have learned a great deal about the pathophysiology of cardiovascular disease from discoveries related to familial hypercholesterolemia, a rare genetic disorder leading to premature atherosclerosis.

In recent years, attention has been redirected toward sequence variation within our genome and understanding how it may influence health and disease. The most common type of variation is single-base substitutions termed single nucleotide polymorphisms or (SNPs). As naturally occurring sequence variations, SNPs have emerged as powerful genetic markers for studying multifactorial diseases.[7] Comprising approximately 90% of human DNA variation, SNPs are single base pair positions in genomic DNA in which different sequence alternatives (alleles) exist in normal individuals. By strict definition, SNP refers to single base pair positions in genomic DNA in which sequence alternatives exist with a frequency of >1%.[8] Therefore, the term SNP does not include numerous other single base substitutions in which the least common allele is present at a frequency of ≤1% (such as "personal mutations" that may be limited to one family), nor does the term encompass other variations such as insertion/deletion polymorphisms. Importantly, SNPs should be distinguished from disease "causing" mutations, which are generally much less common, but have higher penetrance (e.g., sickle cell anemia). Therefore, SNPs do not cause disease but may influence the risk for developing a disease (e.g., diabetes mellitus, asthma) or the outcome from a disease or condition (e.g., death from sepsis, rate of atherosclerosis in recipients of cardiac transplants).[9,10] SNPs that exist in mRNA-coding regions (exons) of DNA can lead to amino acid substitutions and therefore may change the structure of the resultant protein. This type of variant potentially has the most profound impact on protein function; however, this type of SNP is the least common.[11] SNPs in the regulatory (promoter) region of a gene may influence (increase or, more often decrease) transcription of that gene, and

therefore may influence the amount of protein available.[12] Yet other SNPs may not directly alter protein abundance or function, but may be important markers for other (unidentified) functional variants — a concept known as linkage.[13] The analysis of SNPs has been facilitated by two recent and related developments: (1) the establishment of large data repositories of SNPs and (2) the availability of relatively affordable "high-throughput" methods for genotyping. Recent techniques have identified at least 10 million SNPs interspersed throughout the human genome, at a frequency of one SNP per ~300 base-pairs.[14,15] Their role in critical illness, both as risk factors and in determining treatment response, has been investigated for several candidate genes.[16] It is hoped that these studies will contribute to the understanding of the biology of critical illness and toward characterizing patient risk, treatment response, and outcome.

Microsatellite and insertion(deletion polymorphisms represent other genetic variation that may be used to characterize an individual's risk for disease and response to therapy. Microsatellite or simple sequence repeat (SSR) polymorphisms are created by the presence of short sequences (generally 2–4 base pairs) repeated multiple times in tandem. Insertion(deletion polymorphisms are characterized by the presence or absence of a single base in some cases or a longer fragment in others. Microsatellite and insertion(deletion polymorphisms are generally considered to be markers for other functional variants and not themselves functional, but in some cases may directly alter gene activity.[17–19] Typically, they occur in nonfunctional regions or in gene regulatory regions and not in coding regions as they would likely lead to a truncated, completely nonfunctional protein.

## VENOUS THROMBOEMBOLISM: GENETIC RISK FACTORS AND PHARMACOGENOMICS

The human body maintains a delicate balance of procoagulant and anticoagulant processes through a complex system of cofactors and inhibitors, using an elaborate feedback mechanism to maintain equilibrium.[20] When this balance is disrupted, abnormal bleeding or clotting may ensue. Both are familiar to surgeons and intensivists caring for trauma patients. Thrombophilia is the term used to describe the tendency to form abnormal blood clots. The clinical consequences of which are deep vein thrombosis (DVT) and pulmonary embolism (PE), which can both cause considerable suffering and death. Approximately 200,000 new cases of venous thrombosis are diagnosed annually in the United States. An estimated 60,000 deaths occur each year are due to venous thromboembolism (VTE).

There are five established genetic defects considered as risk factors for venous thrombosis (see Table 57-1). Deficiencies in protein C, protein S, and antithrombin III lead to defects in the anticoagulant pathways of blood coagulation and together are found in ~15% of people with familial thrombophilia.[21] The factor V Leiden mutation and increased prothrombin associated with the prothrombin 20210 A allele, are much more prevalent and together may account for >60% of familial thrombophilia. Protein C, protein S, and antithrombin deficiencies all involve defects in anticoagulant pathways, whereas the factor V Leiden mutation and the prothrombin gene mutation involve procoagulant factors. In all cases the expected result of the genetic defect is an enhanced thrombin generation. Multiple genetic defects are responsible for protein C,

**TABLE 57-1**

**Genetic "Causes" of Venous Thrombosis (Adapted from Reference 7)**

|  | PREVALENCE% | MUTATIONS |
|---|---|---|
| Antithrombin deficiency | 4.3 | >79 |
| Protein C deficiency | 5.7 | >160 |
| Protein S deficiency | 5.7 | >69 |
| APC resistance | 45 | 1 |
| Increased prothrombin | 18 | 1 |

protein S, and antithrombin deficiencies whereas both the factor V Leiden and prothrombin defects are caused by single mutations. These mutations are particularly relevant in patients with VTE occurring in the absence of a clear risk factor such as traumatic injury. Up to 50% of such individuals have an underlying defect including these genetic causes.

Ultimately, the development of a thrombotic event is the result of multiple interactions between different genetic and environmental components.[22] Traumatic injury represents an important example of an "environmental" risk for DVT and PE, with incidence rates >50%.[23] Interactions between injury-related risk factors and genetic predisposition to thrombophilia are of potential importance in improving our ability to clinically assess risk. Perhaps of greatest relevance is whether and how genetic factors contribute to failure of prophylaxis. For example, approximately 30% of trauma patients receiving low molecular weight heparin prophylaxis still develop venographic evidence of DVT (approximately one-fifth of these extend proximal to the knee).[24] Although it is likely that traumatic injury, particularly extremity fractures and spinal cord injury, in the absence of prophylaxis, are sufficient to lead to VTE, it is possible that failure of prophylaxis may be, in part, due to the aforementioned genetic variants. Nevertheless, it is presently not recommended that patients with the so-called provoked VTE undergo screening for these genetic variants. The rationale is, in part, due to the notion that treatment will not be affected by the presence of these mutations.[25] However, if the risk of failure of conventional prevention strategies is related to mutations causing thrombophilia, it may be possible to provide more aggressive prophylaxis to those at greatest risk for failure.

For most patients, treatment for established VTE transitions from heparin-based therapy to warfarin-based therapy. The marked interindividual variability in response and a narrow therapeutic window leading to serious bleeding make safe and effective dosing of warfarin a challenge. Variability in drug response can be due to genetic differences at a number of steps along the pathway of a drug's journey. In the case of warfarin and many other drugs used in trauma patients, hepatic catabolism is highly dependent on the cytochrome P450 (CYP) enzyme system. Not only is this system sensitive to influences of diet, and medications, genetic differences exist in many of the cytochrome subfamilies, possibly altering pharmacological responses. Cytochrome P450 2C is the subfamily responsible for the metabolism of many drugs and the CYP2C9 isoform is responsible for warfarin catabolism.[26] Warfarin acts through the interference with Vitamin K epoxide reductase, leading to secretion of inactive Vitamin K-dependent clotting factors.[27] Vitamin K epoxide reductase is encoded by the VKORC1 gene. It is now

well recognized that the CYP2C9 genotype, when combined with the VKORC1 genotype, is predictive of dose requirement for oral anticoagulants, a fact that is likely to have clinical utility. In addition to variation in these two genes, which are estimated to contribute to ~60% of the variation in effective warfarin dose, variation in eight additional genes seem to influence warfarin does, albeit to a lesser degree.[28]

The notion that knowledge of a person's genetic makeup may facilitate effective treatment and avoid adverse drug reactions through optimal dosing is likely to have implications for critically ill trauma patients beyond treatment for VTE. Another less well-developed, but potentially important example is vascular responsiveness to β-adrenergic receptor stimulation. Hypotension exits with sepsis (septic shock) despite maximal endogenous adrenergic stimulation. It appears that certain polymorphisms in the β2-adrenergic receptor are associated with more rapid and extensive desensitization to the vasoconstrictor effects of epinephrine.[29] It is possible that β2-receptor gene polymorphisms might identify patients with sepsis who are at risk of developing vascular collapse.

## GENETIC RISK FACTORS FOR SEPSIS AND ORGAN FAILURE: TARGETING THERAPY IN THE FUTURE

Early evidence favoring a role for genetic differences in infection risk and outcome comes from an epidemiological study of adoptees and their biologic and adoptive parents. A strong association between death from infection in adoptees and their biologic, but not adoptive, parents suggested a genetic influence on the risk for and outcome from infection.[30] More recently, investigators demonstrated that the family members of patients who died from meningococcal infection had a profoundly different blood inflammatory response than did family members of meningococcal sepsis survivors.[31] Although they did not identify a particular genetic difference, their evidence supports the notion that there is a strong familial component determining outcome from severe bacterial infection. Subsequent to these initial observations, numerous studies have identified associations between specific SNPs and sepsis (reviewed in Reference 32). In support of these observed association, molecular mechanisms underlying the risk for acquiring severe infection, such as meningococcal infection, community acquired pneumonia, or septic shock have been identified.[10,33,34]

Sepsis and accompanying multiple organ failure (MOF) are leading contributors to mortality in critically ill trauma victims. While traumatic brain injury and uncontrolled hemorrhage remain the leading causes of death after trauma, patients dying days to weeks after their injuries often die from severe nosocomial infection. Moreover, posttraumatic nosocomial infection and MOF contribute directly to prolonged and costly hospitalization.[35] In severe cases, involving organ dysfunction and shock, sepsis carries a high mortality rate ranging from 30–50%; accounting for 9.3% of all deaths in reported in the United States in 1995.[36,37] Recent developments in supportive care have improved outcomes in certain patient subgroups with sepsis-induced organ failure.[38–42] Nevertheless, the rate of adverse outcomes remains high.

Specific "antimediator" therapies, often observed to be beneficial in preclinical and small clinical trials, have not improved outcomes in Phase III clinical trials.[43–45] This may reflect one of the two general circumstances. First, our understanding of the relevant biology of sepsis and the response to infection may be incomplete. Second, genetic variability creates sufficient background "noise" above which it may be difficult to discern true treatment effects. Empiric evidence suggests both of these circumstances exist. First, new discoveries continue to refine our understanding of the pathways involved in the response to infection and inflammation, improving our understanding of human inflammation and sepsis.[46,47] Second, it has been observed, for example, that anti-inflammatory therapies improve outcomes in subgroups of patients, suggesting that better risk stratification (by clinical and possibly genetic factors) might allow us to better direct our therapies toward patients most likely to benefit.[48] Variation in susceptibility and outcomes among critically ill patients with sepsis is still poorly estimated by current clinical scoring systems. Whether the identification of important genetic risk factors might help us improve our predictions is an important area of future investigation. It is perhaps possible that genetic variability has limited our ability to identify those aspects of the inflammatory response which are the true determinants of risk and outcome. More importantly, such variation may have led to the abandonment of truly efficacious treatments because of the inability to discern treatment effects due to background genetic variation.

Much of our understanding of the biology of inflammation comes from those observations from highly controlled models systems. Examples include the discovery of the nature and the role of tumor necrosis factor-α (TNF-α) and toll-like receptor-4 (TLR4) in the inflammatory response.[49,50] More recently, studies have begun to capitalize on our knowledge of natural genetic variation in these and in other genes, in an attempt to determine how individuals respond differently to infectious or traumatic insults.

TNF-α is an important and extensively studied inflammatory mediator. Multiple SNPs have been identified in the human TNF-α promoter. One has been closely studied and involves the replacement of guanine with cytosine at the -308 position (G-308A). The two alleles have been termed TNF1 (-308G) and TNF2 (-308A) alleles. The TNF2 allele has been linked to elevated TNF-α production, presumably through enhanced promoter activity.[12] The importance of the TNF2 and susceptibility to sepsis and outcome from sepsis is most evident for meningococcal disease.[33] Data are less clear for bacterial sepsis in general.[51] However, at least two studies have implicated TNF2 with outcomes of septic shock.[10,52]

The strongest evidence suggesting a role for SNPs as markers of sepsis severity and outcome comes from a report concerning patients with septic shock from a variety of etiologies, including trauma, treated at seven intensive care units (ICUs) in France. The G-308A SNP was associated with septic shock and death in those with septic shock, compared to healthy blood donors.[10] We have reported a similar association in a study of 152 patients with moderate to severe traumatic injuries. Patients who carried at least one copy of the -308 A-allele had a 2.5-fold (95% CI=1.5–4.3) increased risk for severe sepsis (sepsis complicated by organ failure or shock) than GG homozygotes. Although few patients died (13%), death was more common (relative risk=2.1, 95% CI=0.6–7.3) in the A-allele carriers.[53] Other studies have examined SNPs in the promoter regions of TNF-α and CD14 (LPS receptor) and the first intron of the TNF-β gene. Of these other SNPs, the strongest association with severe posttraumatic sepsis was

seen with the intronic TNFβ SNP in a cohort of 110 patients. Those homozygous for what is termed the "TNFB2" allele were at higher risk for severe sepsis than the nonhomozygotes (OR=3.1, $p$=0.004).[13] Taken together, these data suggest that the severity of posttraumatic nosocomial infection is, in part, influenced by polymorphism in genes considered important in the inflammatory and immune response.

Two relatively common cosegregating SNPs exist in the coding region of the TLR4 gene. One of these alters the extracellular domain of the receptor, seemingly attenuating responsiveness to inhaled endotoxin exposure.[11] These observations implicate the crucial nature of tertiary structure of the TLR4 protein in endotoxin signaling and suggest that SNPs altering protein structure may have clinical implications.

The TLR4 gene encodes a highly conserved transmembrane receptor which is crucial to endotoxin detection and initiation of many of the responses observed in sepsis. Therefore, it is reasonable to consider that nonsynonymous coding region polymorphisms might have a profound effect on the function of this protein. Studies have focused on several candidate polymorphisms at the TLR4 locus including two missense SNPs which confer alterations in the extracellular domain of the receptor. The first represents an A to G base transition at position +896, resulting in an aspartic acid to glycine exchange at position 299 in the amino acid sequence (referred to as Asp299Gly or A+896G). The second often cosegregating SNP involves a C-T transition at position +1196, replacing threonine with isoleucine at position 399 (referred as Thr399Ile or C+11996T).

There is some evidence regarding the role of these variants in the clinical setting of infectious disease. Two groups have observed associations among the TLR4 +896G variant and the incidence of gram-negative infections and septic shock in ICU patients.[54,55] However, other clinical and experimental investigations have failed to reproducibly demonstrate a role for TLR4 variation in altering the inflammatory response.[56–58] As is the case with SNPs in the TNF-α gene, evidence of a functional effect for TLR4 variants, particularly the +896 SNP, has not been reproducibly translated into strong evidence of clinical genotype-phenotype association.

Despite a series of positive studies, many significant challenges remain to be addressed before SNPs can be used in the clinical setting. Most importantly, the usefulness of individual SNPs to predict predisposition and response has been questioned, in light of evidence indicating that many SNP–disease associations are often not reproduced in subsequent studies.[59,60] Table 57-2 summarizes a series of studies and the relevant genetic variants that were studied in relation to the risk for sepsis and outcome from sepsis that may be of relevance to the care of trauma victims.

Even for those few SNP associations that do appear reliable, it has not yet been determined which and even how many SNPs will be needed to provide a reliable estimate of an individual's risk for sepsis or death after injury. Once the predictive SNPs have been identified, it will be necessary to determine whether directing interventions to particular ("high-risk") patients improves outcomes.

An additional concept of likely importance is that SNPs exist in nonrandom patterns, termed haplotypes (variant alleles located together along portions of individual chromosomes that

**TABLE 57-2**

| Selected Gene Polymorphisms Associated with Functional and Clinical Outcomes in Critically Ill Patients | | | |
|---|---|---|---|
| GENE | VARIANT | CLINICAL ASSOCIATION | REFERENCE |
| Tumor necrosis factor-α | G-308A. Located in 5' regulatory region. May influence rate of gene transcription or may simply be a marker for another functional SNP. | Septic shock, death from septic shock. Severe sepsis after trauma | 37,39 |
| Toll-like receptor (TLR)-4 | A+896G. Nonsynonymous coding SNP. Changes amino acid sequence and likely TLR4's signaling capacity. | Risk of gram-negative sepsis. | 2 |
| Plasminogen activator inhibitor-1 (PAI-1) | Insertion-deletion polymorphism (4G/5G) in the PAI-1 promoter. The 4G (deletion) allele increases gene transcription. | Increased plasminogen levels and risk of death after trauma | 14,35 |

appear to be inherited together in "blocks"). It has been hypothesized that these SNP haplotypes, rather than individual SNPs may be more useful, as haplotypes may more accurately account for the effect of multiple SNPs interacting to influence risk or outcome. Haplotypes are known to exist in inflammation-related genes.[61] Some have been shown to determine in vivo responses in pathways important to inflammation, such as IL10 responses to endotoxin and the β2-receptor signaling pathway.[61–63] While most common haplotypes (those with ≥ 5% frequency) can often be characterized by a relatively small number of SNPs (termed "haplotype tagging" SNPs), controversy exists regarding whether focusing on these more common haplotypes will identify genotype–phenotype associations. Haplotypes are defined without particular regard to the potential functional effect of the haplotype tagging SNPs and consider that a particular haplotype may simply be a marker for another unidentified, but functional SNP. An alternative approach has been proposed in which SNPs most likely to be functional — specifically those in the coding region that result in a change in the amino acid sequence — are identified (The previously discussed TLR4 mutations are an example of this concept). As indicated above, these are the rarest type of SNP, but may confer the greatest risk for adverse outcomes.[64]

In sepsis and shock, like most common diseases, including heart disease, diabetes, hypertension, and cancer, multiple genetic and environmental factors influence an individual's risk and clinical course. Within infectious and inflammatory disorders, patient factors, such as age and comorbidity, and disease factors, such as infectious strain, exposure, and concomitant injury, contribute to disease risk and severity making the study of genetic risk factors particularly challenging.

## SUMMARY AND IMPLICATIONS FOR CLINICAL PRACTICE

A growing body of information indicates that genomic data will enhance our understanding of common diseases including sepsis and organ failure.[65,66] Similarly, genetic influences on many biological responses, such as drug metabolism, contribute to clinically important differences in treatment response. The successful integration of genomics into health care in general and into caring for critically ill and injured patients in particular demands

that clinicians become genomically literate.[1] This chapter provides a framework in which to begin that process. The critical care environment, in which biological and pharmacological responses are numerous and complex, will challenge us to understand and apply genetic and genomic principles concerning disease risk factors and drug responses. Despite this challenge, the stakes are truly great given the morbidity and mortality that we may be able to avert.

## REFERENCES

1. Guttmacher AE, Collins FS: Realizing the promise of genomics in biomedical research. *JAMA* 294:1399, 2005.
2. Collins FS, Green ED, Guttmacher AE, et al.: A vision for the future of genomics research. *Nature* 422:835, 2003.
3. Watson JD, Crick FH: Genetical implications of the structure of deoxyribonucleic acid. *Nature* 171:964, 1953.
4. Watson JD, Crick FH: Molecular structure of nucleic acids; a structure for deoxyribose nucleic acid. *Nature* 171:737, 1953.
5. Watson JD, Crick FH: A structure for deoxyribose nucleic acid. 1953. *Nature* 421:397, 2003.
6. Guttmacher AE and Collins FS Genomic medicine—a primer. *N Engl J Med* 347:1512, 2002.
7. Cardon LR, Bell JI: Association study designs for complex diseases. *Nature Rev Genet* 2:91, 2001.
8. Brookes AJ: The essence of SNPs. *Gene* 234:177, 1999.
9. Fernandez-Real JM, Broch M, Vendrell J, et al.: Interleukin-6 gene polymorphism and insulin sensitivity. *Diabetes* 49:517, 2000.
10. Mira JP, Cariou A, Grall F, et al.: Association of TNF2, a TNF-alpha promoter polymorphism, with septic shock susceptibility and mortality: A multicenter study. *JAMA* 282:561, 1999.
11. Arbour NC, Lorenz E, Schutte BC, et al.: TLR4 mutations are associated with endotoxin hyporesponsiveness in humans. *Nat Genet* 25:187, 2000.
12. Wilson AG, Symons JA, McDowell TL, et al.: Effects of a polymorphism in the human tumor necrosis factor alpha promoter on transcriptional activation. *Proc Natl Acad Sci USA* 94:3195, 1997.
13. Majetschak M, Flohe S, Obertacke U, et al.: Relation of a TNF gene polymorphism to severe sepsis in trauma patients. *Ann Surg* 230:207, 1999.
14. Altshuler D, Pollara VJ, Cowles CR, et al.: An SNP map of the human genome generated by reduced representation shotgun sequencing. *Nature* 407:513, 2000.
15. Palmer LJ, Cardon LR: Shaking the tree: Mapping complex disease genes with linkage disequilibrium. *Lancet* 366:1223, 2005.
16. Holmes CL, Russell JA, Walley KR: Genetic polymorphisms in sepsis and septic shock: Role in prognosis and potential for therapy. *Chest* 124:1103, 2003.
17. Marshall RP, Webb S, Bellingan GJ, et al.: Angiotensin converting enzyme insertion/deletion polymorphism is associated with susceptibility and outcome in acute respiratory distress syndrome. *Am J Respir Crit Care Med* 166:646, 2002.
18. Menges T, Hermans PW, Little SG, et al.: Plasminogen-activator-inhibitor-1 4G/5G promoter polymorphism and prognosis of severely injured patients. *Lancet* 357:1096, 2001.
19. Stassen NA, Leslie-Norfleet LA, Robertson AM, et al.: Interferon-gamma gene polymorphisms and the development of sepsis in patients with trauma. *Surgery* 132:289, 2002.

20. Majerus PW: Human genetics. Bad blood by mutation. *Nature* 369:14, 1994.
21. Bertina RM: Factor V Leiden and other coagulation factor mutations affecting thrombotic risk. *Clin Chem* 43:1678, 1997.
22. Podgoreanu MV, Schwinn DA: New paradigms in cardiovascular medicine: Emerging technologies and practices: perioperative genomics. *J Am Coll Cardiol* 46:1965, 2005.
23. Geerts WH, Code KI, Jay RM, et al.: A prospective study of venous thromboembolism after major trauma. *N Engl J Med* 331:1601, 1994.
24. Geerts WH, Jay RM, Code KI, et al.: A comparison of low-dose heparin with low-molecular-weight heparin as prophylaxis against venous thromboembolism after major trauma. *N Engl J Med* 335:701, 1996.
25. Weitz JI, Middeldorp S, Geerts W, et al.: Thrombophilia and new anticoagulant drugs. Hematology. *Am Soc Hematol Educ Program* 424, 2004.
26. Kumar V, Wahlstrom JL, Rock DA, et al.: CYP2C9 inhibition: Impact of probe selection and pharmacogenetics on in vitro inhibition profiles. *Drug Metab Dispos* 34:1966, 2006.
27. Wadelius M and Pirmohamed M Pharmacogenetics of warfarin: Current status and future challenges. *Pharmacogenomics J* 2006.
28. Wadelius M, Chen LY, Eriksson N, et al.: Association of warfarin dose with genes involved in its action and metabolism. *Hum Genet* 2006.
29. Dishy V, Sofowora GG, Xie HG, et al.: The effect of common polymorphisms of the beta2-adrenergic receptor on agonist-mediated vascular desensitization. *N Engl J Med* 345:1030, 2001.
30. Sorensen TI, Nielsen GG, Andersen PK, et al.: Genetic and environmental influences on premature death in adult adoptees. *N Engl J Med* 318:727, 1988.
31. Westendorp RG, Langermans JA, Huizinga TW, et al.: Genetic influence on cytokine production and fatal meningococcal disease. *Lancet* 349:170, 1997.
32. Lin MT, Albertson TE: Genomic polymorphisms in sepsis. *Crit Care Med* 32:569, 2004.
33. Nadel S, Newport MJ, Booy R, et al.: Variation in the tumor necrosis factor-alpha gene promoter region may be associated with death from meningococcal disease. *J Infect Dis* 174:878, 1996.
34. Waterer GW, Quasney MW, Cantor RM, et al.: Septic shock and respiratory failure in community-acquired pneumonia have different TNF polymorphism associations. *Am J Respir Crit Care Med* 163:1599, 2001.
35. O'Keefe GE, Maier RV, Diehr P, et al.: The complications of trauma and their associated costs in a level I trauma center. *Arch Surg* 132:920, 1997.
36. Bernard GR, Vincent JL, Laterre PF, et al.: Efficacy and safety of recombinant human activated protein C for severe sepsis. *N Engl J Med* 344:699, 2001.
37. Martin GS, Mannino DM, Eaton S, et al.: The epidemiology of sepsis in the United States from 1979 through 2000. *N Engl J Med* 348:1546, 2003.
38. Ventilation with lower tidal volumes as compared with traditional tidal volumes for acute lung injury and the acute respiratory distress syndrome. The Acute Respiratory Distress Syndrome Network. *N Engl J Med* 342:1301, 2000.
39. Milberg JA, Davis DR, Steinberg KP, et al.: Improved survival of patients with acute respiratory distress syndrome (ARDS): 1983–1993. *JAMA* 273:306, 1995.
40. Rangel-Frausto MS, Pittet D, Costigan M, et al.: The natural history of the systemic inflammatory response syndrome (SIRS). A prospective study. *JAMA* 273:117, 1995.
41. Rivers E, Nguyen B, Havstad S, et al.: Early goal-directed therapy in the treatment of severe sepsis and septic shock. *N Engl J Med* 345:1368, 2001.
42. van den, Berghe G, Wouters P, Weekers F, et al.: Intensive insulin therapy in the critically ill patients. *N Engl J Med* 345:1359, 2001.
43. Opal SM, Cross AS: Clinical trials for severe sepsis. Past failures, and future hopes. *Infect Dis Clin North Am* 13:285, 1999.
44. Vincent JL, Sun Q, Dubois MJ: Clinical trials of immunomodulatory therapies in severe sepsis and septic shock. *Clin Infect Dis* 34:1084, 2002.
45. Zeni F, Freeman B, Natanson C: Anti-inflammatory therapies to treat sepsis and septic shock: A reassessment. *Crit Care Med* 25:1095, 1997.
46. Riewald M, Petrovan RJ, Donner A, et al.: Activation of endothelial cell protease activated receptor 1 by the protein C pathway. *Science* 296:1880, 2002.
47. Yang H, Ochani M, Li J, et al.: Reversing established sepsis with antagonists of endogenous high-mobility group box 1. *Proc Natl Acad Sci USA* 101:296, 2004.
48. Bernard GR, Wheeler AP, Russell JA, et al.: The effects of ibuprofen on the physiology and survival of patients with sepsis. The Ibuprofen in Sepsis Study Group. *N Engl J Med* 336:912, 1997.
49. Beutler B, Poltorak A: Positional cloning of Lps, and the general role of toll-like receptors in the innate immune response. *Eur Cytokine Netw* 11:143, 2000.
50. Tracey KJ, Fong Y, Hesse DG, et al.: Anti-cachectin/TNF monoclonal antibodies prevent septic shock during lethal bacteraemia. *Nature* 330:662, 1987.
51. Stuber F, Udalova IA, Book M, et al.: -308 tumor necrosis factor (TNF) polymorphism is not associated with survival in severe sepsis and is unrelated to lipopolysaccharide inducibility of the human TNF promoter. *J Inflamm* 46:42, 1995.
52. Tang GJ, Huang SL, Yien HW, et al.: Tumor necrosis factor gene polymorphism and septic shock in surgical infection. *Crit Care Med* 28:2733, 2000.
53. O'Keefe GE, Hybki DL, Munford RS: The G→A single nucleotide polymorphism at the -308 position in the tumor necrosis factor-alpha promoter increases the risk for severe sepsis after trauma. *J Trauma* 52:817, 2002.
54. Agnese DM, Calvano JE, Hahm SJ, et al.: Human toll-like receptor 4 mutations but not CD14 polymorphisms are associated with an increased risk of gram-negative infections. *J Infect Dis* 186:1522, 2002.
55. Lorenz E, Mira JP, Frees KL, et al.: Relevance of mutations in the TLR4 receptor in patients with gram-negative septic shock. *Arch Intern Med* 162:1028, 2002.
56. Erridge C, Stewart J, Poxton IR: Monocytes heterozygous for the Asp299Gly and Thr399Ile mutations in the Toll-like receptor 4 gene show no deficit in lipopolysaccharide signalling. *J Experi Medicine* 197:1787, 2003.
57. Imahara SD, Jelacic S, Junker CE, et al.: The TLR4 +896 polymorphism is not associated with lipopolysaccharide hypo-responsiveness in leukocytes. *Genes Immun* 6:37, 2005.
58. Read RC, Pullin J, Gregory S, et al.: A functional polymorphism of toll-like receptor 4 is not associated with likelihood or severity of meningococcal disease. *J Infect Dis* 184:640, 2001.
59. Hirschhorn JN, Lohmueller K, Byrne E, et al.: A comprehensive review of genetic association studies. *Genet Med* 4:45, 2002.
60. Lohmueller KE, Pearce CL, Pike M, et al.: Meta-analysis of genetic association studies supports a contribution of common variants to susceptibility to common disease. *Nat Genet* 33:177, 2003.
61. Terry CF, Loukaci V, Green FR: Cooperative influence of genetic polymorphisms on interleukin 6 transcriptional regulation. *J Bioll Chem* 275:18138, 2000.
62. Eskdale J, Gallagher G, Verweij CL, et al.: Interleukin 10 secretion in relation to human IL-10 locus haplotypes. *Proc Natl Acad Sci USA* 95:9465, 1998.
63. Fishman D, Faulds G, Jeffery R, et al.: The effect of novel polymorphisms in the interleukin-6 (IL-6) gene on IL-6 transcription and plasma IL-6 levels, and an association with systemic-onset juvenile chronic arthritis. *J Clin Investigation* 102:1369, 1998.
64. Smirnova I, Hamblin MT, McBride C, et al.: Excess of rare amino acid polymorphisms in the Toll-like receptor 4 in humans. *Genetics* 158:1657, 2001.
65. Calvano SE, Xiao W, Richards DR, et al.: A network-based analysis of systemic inflammation in humans. *Nature* 437:1032, 2005.
66. Cobb JP, O'Keefe GE: Injury research in the genomic era. *Lancet* 363:2076, 2004.
67. Dawson SJ, Wiman B, Hamsten A, et al.: The two allele sequences of a common polymorphism in the promoter of the plasminogen activator inhibitor-1 (PAI-1) gene respond differently to interleukin-1 in HepG2 cells. *J Biol Chem* 268:10739, 1993.

# Commentary ■ BRADLEY D. FREEMAN

Genetic technology has potential to impact virtually every facet of medicine. Genetic assays for over 1200 heritable conditions are currently available in numerous U.S.laboratories. The number of genetic variants of undetermined clinical significance that are reported from a variety of resources (such as the Human Genome Project, the HapMap Project, Pharmacogenetics Research Network, and numerous publicly accessible databases) is increasing rapidly. In this chapter, Dr. O'Keefe succinctly summarizes many aspects of genetic technology that pertain to the care of the acutely ill or injured patient. Specifically, that possession of a distinct genotype might predispose to common complications following injury (such as venous thromboembolism) or partly explain interindividual variation in drug effect (for example, excessive anticoagulation in response to standard doses of warfarin). Further, Dr. O'Keefe alludes to recent technological advances that have rendered the ability to collect and interpret high-density genetic data (genome-wide scans) feasible and affordable. The question for the critical care practitioner is what are the implications and challenges of this technology for the foreseeable future?

In the next several years, collection and interpretation of genetic data in the setting of acute illness will occur largely in the context of clinical investigation, and may become a common component of pharmaceutical trials conducted in critically ill patients. As highlighted by Dr. O'Keefe, the results of numerous gene association studies reported to date have been difficult to replicate. This phenomenon appears in part due to the poor methodological quality of many of these investigations. Clark et al. systematically evaluated published studies examining the relationship between genetic variation and sepsis according to established epidemiological guidelines.[1] The majority of the 76 studies reviewed were judged to be of low to intermediate quality. A large number of these studies used inappropriate control groups, reported genotypic data that was not adequately verified, and were grossly underpowered. Using Bayesian analysis, Clark et al. estimated that the majority of studies demonstrating a significant genotypic-phenotypic relationship probably represent a false-positive finding. Thus, one challenge facing the implementation of genetic technology in the critical care environment is that future trials be performed with sufficient methodological rigor so as to yield interpretable findings.

A second challenge centers around societal perceptions of genetic data itself. Many consider genetic data as unique, requiring special protection relative to other types of clinical information.[2] Reasons underlying this *genetic exceptionalism* include the possibility that genetic information is predictive and might recategorize an individual from healthy to at risk of disease, infer information about family members, result in economic discrimination or stigmatization, or produce psychological harm.[2] Collection

of genetic data from patients admitted to ICUs poses unique challenges not encountered in other settings. Conditions prompting ICU admission are frequently precipitous and life threatening and the care provided is highly technological. Typically, neither patients nor family members have had prior opportunity for education regarding the nature of the disease process, expected outcome, or possible treatments. Further, patients in ICUs are frequently nondecisional and unable to personally provide informed consent permitting medical intervention or research participation. Finally, many therapies, such as for sepsis, must be administered quickly following diagnosis. If critically ill patients are to be enrolled in studies in which genetic material is collected, or are to undergo genotyping to direct therapy, permission must frequently be obtained in a timely fashion from proxy or surrogate decision makers, many of whom are being confronted with complex and serious medical issues for the first time.

We examined attitudes of proxy or surrogate decision makers for critically ill patients in four key areas related to collection of genetic information: willingness to permit specimen collection, disclosure of information, confidentiality of results, and trust in organizations to conduct research.[3] These individuals were willing to permit genetic testing to aid diagnosis, guide drug prescription, and to explain familial or ethnic disease predisposition. Further, inclusion of genetic testing did not appear to affect receptiveness to participation in a clinic trial. In contrast, respondents were less likely to participate in research if genetic data were not anonymized, less likely to undergo genetic testing if employers or insurers could access results, and distrustful of federal agencies and pharmaceutical companies relative to universities and nonprofit organizations to conduct genetic research. This undercurrent of concern regarding genomic technology may impact clinical studies that entail collection of genetic material and implementation of this technology in the critical care environment. Gaining greater insight into these concerns and insuring that collection and utilization of genetic information occurs in the most transparent manner possible will be essential to studying and implementing genetic technology in the ICU in an informed and ethical manner.

## References

1. Clark MF, Baudouin SV: A systematic review of the quality of genetic association studies in human sepsis. *Intensive Care Med* 32:1706, 2006.
2. Green MJ, Botkin JR: "Genetic Exceptionalism" in medicine: Clarifying the differences between genetic and non-genetic tests. *Ann Int Med* 138:571, 2003.
3. Freeman BD, Kennedy CR, Coopersmith CM, et al.: Genetic testing and research in critical care: Surrogates' perspective. *Crit Care Med* 34:986, 2006.

# The Convergence of Trauma, Medicine, and the Law

*Anna M. Ledgerwood* ■ *Kathryn A. Lucas* ■ *Charles E. Lucas*

## INTRODUCTION

A society brings together many individuals with varied and often divergent goals. Ideally, each member strives in a synergistic manner to optimize the attainment of all societal objectives. Success reflects the willingness of each participant. The law and medicine are two major societal disciplines. The law, be it by dictatorial fiat, by legislative resolve, or by clannish anarchy, is the higher societal institution; the law defines the framework in which other societal disciplines, such as medicine, can function.

Historically, our great democracy, the United States of America, has stressed health care from the time that our Continental Army fought the War of Independence until the present day. Indeed, the first initiatives in health care by our Continental Congress addressed trauma care in our injured soldiers.[1] The issues were simple. Soldiers had to be attended to on the front line, evacuated, and treated. Field supplies, temporary aide stations, and hospitals were established.[1] Physicians, nurses, and a corps of volunteers were mobilized. These measures were implemented to the extent that the resources required for the greater good, namely, defeating the English troops in our new land, were not compromised. Similar treatment guidelines were established for prisoners of war.[1]

Put in this perspective, one realizes that health care is a societal luxury made available by the successes of the other segments of our society. Fortunately, our society has prospered; consequently, the "luxury" of health care has expanded to the extent that many consider it a "human right" with the expectation of high quality care.[2,3] Although this expectation extends throughout the spectrum of health care, this chapter focuses on some of the more common issues that interdigitate with the law in the treatment of injured patients. The narrative flow is designed to approach issues sequentially from the time of injury until full recovery after definitive therapy.

## ACCESS TO THE INJURED

During the Revolutionary War, the Old World and New World combatants exhibited humanistic traits during the heat of battle when such actions would not have an immediate effect on the military outcome.[1] Temporary truces were arranged to allow for the slain and wounded troops to be removed for burial or medical care. This pattern was repeated during our Civil War and during the two great wars in Europe; hopefully, future conflicts will see the same consideration for wounded soldiers.[2,3] Through these campaigns, great strides were made to provide prompt front line health care and evacuation to more secure facilities. Many of the important facets of this acute care are well presented in the more serious scenes of the movie "M*A*S*H."

Initial front line care by the medics prepares troops for rapid transport, sometimes by helicopter, to M*A*S*H units from which further transport is available to area hospitals near the front lines or to remote hospitals within the United States or other allied countries for long-term care. Definitive transoceanic care is now routine for the severely burned patient, the patient with acute spinal cord injury, and the patient with severe traumatic brain injury. The lessons learned from these endeavors have been applied to civilian injuries not only in urban areas, but also in remote rural areas where natural barriers such as mountains, rivers, or heavy snows impede extrication and transportation. Thus, the trauma system developed within the military from our early years has evolved and serves as the model for trauma system implementation in a civilian setting.[4]

## TRAUMA SYSTEMS AND THE LAW

The implementation of civilian trauma systems dates back to the 19th century when hospitals used their own horse-driven ambulances for proprietary purposes. The continued development has relied on both legislative support and volunteerism. The training of each team member and the equipment for each of the emergency medical services (EMS) rigs have usually been defined in the system guidelines or regulations.[4] These guidelines and regulations may be voluntarily followed while the trauma system is evolving; once fully operational, mandatory adherence to regulations is ensured by the appropriate municipal, county, or state legislative support. Deviation from such guidelines triggers a potential liability for the program. For example, an inability to monitor blood gases by pulse oximetry and end-tidal carbon dioxide determination would be a potential liability for EMS teams having the skills and authority to intubate in the prehospital setting. Thus, the medical directors of EMS teams must work closely with those responsible for management and upgrading of both personnel and equipment to meet published guidelines for care in the prehospital setting.

## THE GOOD SAMARITAN

Occasionally, an injury occurs in proximity to a nurse or physician who is knowledgeable in the care of the injured. This serendipitous event allows the health care professional to initiate care prior to EMS team arrival and, if desired, help provide continuing care by assisting the EMS team. The physician providing help in this setting is sometimes referred to as the "Good Samaritan." One of the early conflicts between the health care industry and the law dealt with the potential liability of the Good Samaritan. If the Good Samaritan were placed in financial jeopardy from alleged malpractice, there would be conflict between the instinctual desire to help a fellow citizen and the need to protect the fiscal security of loved ones. Both the health care industry and the legal profession recognized the greater good for all citizens; fiscal protection of the Good Samaritan outweighed the individual rights of one injured citizen thought to have been harmed by treatment provided by the Good Samaritan.[5,6] Thus, Good Samaritan laws were promoted by both the medical profession and the legal profession and have become universal.[7–11] One state, Vermont, has gone one step further by statutorily mandating a "duty to rescue," in order to provide more motivation than mere instinctual altruism might alone engender.[12] The Vermont code states that a "person who knows that another is exposed to grave physical harm shall, to the extent that the same can be rendered without danger or peril to himself or without interference with important duties owed to others, give reasonable assistance to the exposed person unless that assistance or care is being provided by others."

The other 49 states, however, prefer to preserve personal choice, but like Vermont, have acknowledged the need for greater incentive than mere altruism. Protection, however, may not be absolute. While some states absolve the Good Samaritan of all liability, others absolve him only of liability of mere negligence—not of liability based on gross negligence or wanton and willful conduct. In addition, all states require, as a condition of freedom from liability, that the Good Samaritan not bill or expect reimbursement for the services provided.[5,6,13]

## DELIVERY

The means for conveying the injured patient to intermediate and/or definitive care have evolved commensurate with over two centuries of prosperity in America. During the Revolutionary War,

stretcher bearers sometimes had to walk long distances to either a treatment site or a location where an available wagon, not needed for the immediate war effort, could be used for transportation to the closest care facility.[1] During the 19th century, specialized horse-driven ambulances were provided for the military and later for civilian use, especially in largely populated areas. Volunteers provided most of this transportation; some hospitals had their own ambulance crews staffed by hospital employees. The advent of the automobile and consequent improvement to infrastructure increased the flexibility for delivering injured civilians to specialized trauma hospitals.

The American technological revolution, occurring during the first half of the 20th century, greatly enhanced efficient delivery of injured soldiers to definitive care.[4] The authors recall when a hearse or a police van was the prime mode of transportation. Some surgeons regaled their colleagues with stories about a hearse being driven slowly so that a specific funeral home might have another client. Other surgeons talked about police brutality, which decreased the likelihood that the injured patient would make it to the hospital alive. Such stories did not represent the overwhelming goodness and generosity of the American citizenry, including funeral home directors and police officers, but did highlight the need for a revolution in the delivery system. This led to the creation of city, county and/or state EMS agencies, which slowly but inevitably established our current EMS system. Knowledgeable dispatchers may call on basic life support (BLS), advanced life support (ALS), and mobile intensive care unit (MICU) teams for care and transport to appropriate facilities.[14] This achievement required the cooperative support of the health care industry and the legal profession. Their combined efforts are needed to influence local, state, and national legislators to implement programs rooted in the best health care available within specific fiscal restraints. These efforts have had the desired results, and the public now considers anything less than optimal care to be illegal. Medical directors and institutional sponsors of EMS teams and systems must recognize the potential liability inherent in lack of compliance with published guidelines for EMS training and vehicular equipment.[15]

## DESTINATION

Many medical and legal challenges continually surface in the process of defining where the injured patient should be treated.[2,3] Cooperative solutions base their priority on optimal care of injured patients. Intuitively, some citizens think that the injured patient should be taken to the nearest hospital. In the past, this led to disastrous results. Some psychiatric centers have had to provide roadside signage stressing the facilities' inability to treat emergencies. A far greater hazard arises when a hospital accepts patients for fiscal reasons, but its resources are too limited to provide care for some injuries. Just such a situation occurred in *Nevarez v. New York City Health and Hospitals Corp.* when a woman in her seventh month of pregnancy arrived at a hospital complaining of labor pains. The woman's physician, informed by telephone of her arrival, relayed to a hospital staff worker that he was with a patient and that the woman should wait for him. When finally examined, she was told to go to another hospital because the present hospital did not have the proper facilities to deal with a seven-month premature birth.

Only after another two-and-a-half hours was an ambulance summoned. The over seven-hour delay between the time she presented at the first hospital and the time she delivered at the second resulted in fetal hypoxia, which caused her infant to be born with cerebral palsy, severe retardation, and blindness. A jury found the first hospital liable for not providing an initial examination sooner and for not arranging emergency transportation to a better equipped hospital in a timely manner. This example of inappropriate care identifies the need for a trauma system, thus ensuring appropriate care without inordinate delay.

There are many medical and legal challenges inherent in identifying the appropriate site for trauma care within a geopolitical area. These challenges vary for a system evolving in a city, county, region, or state geographic area; they also vary in regards to population base and natural barriers such as mountains. Individual states invariably have statutes regulating the provision of EMS. Some of these states' statutes are directed mainly toward licensure and standardization of training among health care providers, including EMTs and first responders, leaving the specifics of trauma system implementation to the purview of state agencies or committees, which promulgate regulations. The purpose for this separation of powers between the legislature and the executive branch (which appoints the relevant agency heads and committee members) is that the executive branch is generally better able to respond quickly to, and rectify, observed deficiencies in the provision of emergency medical services. Other states have more proactive legislatures; these states' statutes are very specific as to precisely how EMS are to be rendered, leaving little to the discretion of agency regulations and/or local authority.

The City of Detroit, in consultation with the US Department of Transportation, implemented a trauma system in 1975. The selection of four trauma centers, without detailed reference to specific resources, was based upon geographic location, hospital commitment, and attending physician interest in providing trauma care. Representatives from all segments of the city provided input toward the final product. Initially, representatives of hospitals not designated as trauma centers baulked at the loss of revenue their facilities would suffer if, as per the guidelines of the trauma system, a patient were taken to a trauma center in lieu of these nontrauma hospitals. Their concerns were mitigated by a compromise that allowed an EMS team to bypass the nearest designated trauma center according to patient or family directive. This resulted in bad care, leading to the involvement of the legal profession as agents for the patient, the hospital, and the EMS system. These conflicts resulted in the establishment of a policy that patients with "Code-1" life-threatening injuries must be taken to the closest available designated trauma center. Thus, the legal profession facilitated the evolution of a stronger system. Implementation of this trauma system required the cooperative efforts of the Mayor, the City Council, representatives from the trauma centers, agents from the county and state governments, union officials, the Detroit Police Department, the Detroit Fire Department (which supervised the EMS component), and finally the city legal department. Each segment of this multidisciplinary task force relied upon extensive legal expertise. The final trauma system implementation flows from the budgetary support provided, in this instance, by the City Council. Such support is generated from the tax base; this source of payment, in turn, increases the citizens' expectations for prompt and excellent trauma care. These expectations have legal implications. How these expectations will change when a city loses its tax revenue and is no longer able to meet the same commitment, remains to be seen; one can be certain that there will be many legal ramifications.

There has been a significant maturation in trauma system development with designation of trauma centers based on hospital resources providing care to injured patients and supported by well-defined transfer criteria for expeditiously getting a patient to a higher level of care. Trauma systems have evolved only because of the synergistic efforts of the medical and legal communities. For several years, the Commonwealth of Massachusetts voluntarily defined five regions, each with an EMS agency that directs patient delivery to those centers meeting American College of Surgeons Committee on Trauma (ACSCOT) criteria for verification. This voluntary leadership has paved the way for implementation of a legislated trauma system for the Commonwealth.

The larger and more populated areas have more complicated medical and legal issues, which must be resolved. The greater number of hospitals with potential ability to manage injured patients requires agreements as to which hospitals will participate as trauma centers, delineation of level of care that will be available at each center, and prioritization regarding bypass of one center in order to receive a higher level of care for specific injuries or transfer of patients to a higher level of care. Each center, in turn, must put in place appropriate policies for protection against claims of "dumping" uninsured patients or treating insured patients despite insufficient resources. Likewise, evolutionary changes in the definition of designation criteria mandate a close working relationship between the health care industry, the legal profession, and legislative bodies.

Transfer guidelines also involve insurance carriers and account for patient age; decisions regarding these factors must be well coordinated to prevent inappropriate patient care, as illustrated by the following scenario. A 16-year-old boy was involved in a motor vehicle crash prior to being transported to the Detroit Receiving Hospital (DRH), a verified Level I trauma center. He was stable; his injuries were a femur fracture, humerus fracture, and distal radius fracture, all of which were splinted. His insurance carrier allowed for treatment at a nearby verified Level I trauma center, and plans were made for transfer. Unknown to either trauma team, the patient was transferred to a pediatrician working in a suburban hospital not equipped for trauma; this transfer was based on the insurance carrier transfer system guidelines at the nearby Level I trauma center, which does not care for injured children. The pediatrician promptly arranged for the young man to be transferred to the Children's Hospital of Michigan (CHM), a verified Level I pediatric trauma center, which abuts and is connected by tunnel to DRH. The trauma service at CHM quickly recognized the patient as postpubertal and transferred him through the tunnel to DRH. His definitive surgical repair was delayed for 48 hours; fortunately, his outcome was excellent. The Detroit trauma system failed this young man in many ways: (1) the DRH team failed to confirm that the transfer was to the nearby trauma center; (2) the nearby trauma center coordinator did not know that trauma system patients are to stay within the system regardless of carrier; (3) the suburban team failed to prevent the transfer to a pediatrician who has no experience in trauma care; and (4) the CHM team failed to inform the suburban hospital team that all postpubertal injured patients are, by protocol, treated at DRH. Needless to say, had the outcome not been excellent, many concerns about liability could have been raised.

Sometimes a breakdown in the transfer system leads to a bad outcome as shown in the following scenario. An 80-year-old man was admitted to DRH with a intertrochanteric hip fracture after he fell down a flight of stairs. Significant comorbidity included hypertension, diabetes melitis, and chronic renal failure for which he was undergoing intermittent hemodialysis. He was admitted to the surgical ICU, cleared by cardiology for operation, and scheduled by the orthopedic service for operative reduction and internal fixation (ORIF) the next morning. His primary insurance carrier was Medicare, whereas his secondary coverage was by a carrier that would provide reimbursement in stable injured patients, but only if the definitive procedures were performed at a nearby Level I trauma center. Accordingly, planned operation the next morning was canceled, and the patient was prepared for transfer. Later that day, it was reported that no critical bed was available, so the transfer was deferred until hospital day two; meanwhile, the orthopedic service at DRH had "signed off." The transfer was again delayed on hospital day two; the DRH team reminded the nearby center that care was being compromised, at which point DRH was granted "permission" to operate. ORIF was performed 84 hours after admission. This delay contributed to pneumonia and sacral decubitus directly related to his impaired mobility from hip pain. Antimicrobial therapy and multiple surgical debridements were unsuccessful, and he died on hospital day 23. The peer review committee concluded that this was a preventable death caused by the inordinate delay of ORIF in a high-risk patient.

The lack of well-defined guidelines for transfer, based on third-party carrier, between two cooperative trauma centers, allowed several decisions to be made that could potentially have led to legal liability. The authors recommend that medical and legal experts implement the following policies. First, the time from request for transfer to acceptance should be short (one hour) and not contingent on finding an available bed or specialist physician. Second, the definition of "stable for transfer" should be tailored to include comorbidities; timing of ORIF in an octogenarian requiring cardiac clearance and hemodialysis is far more complicated than ORIF in a younger patient with no comorbidities. In retrospect, the DRH team should have stated on day one that this patient was not "stable for transfer"; this decision would be much easier in the future if better definitions of "stability" are developed within a trauma system. Had the patient been treated by ORIF at DRH the morning after injury, Medicare, the primary carrier, would have reimbursed DRH; the reimbursement by the secondary carrier could have been contentious, but the patient would have received the best care. In the future, improvements in the fine-tuning of trauma system guidelines for transfers, supported by legal decision, will enhance the opportunity for all trauma centers to provide the best care.

## THE OBLIGATION TO TREAT

The legal maze surrounding the potential conflict between trauma center finances, health care interests, and patient needs has created a multitude of legislative actions, which have stimulated congressional implementation of federal mandates designed to protect the injured patient. The Emergency Medical Treatment and Active Labor Act (EMTALA) defines the obligation of trauma centers to provide treatment independent of a patient's fiscal resources.[2,3]

EMTALA mandates, in relevant part, that a hospital with an emergency department (ED) provide medical screening to any patient who comes to the ED and assess whether the patient has an emergency medical condition.[17] If the screening discloses an emergency medical condition, the hospital is obligated to provide further medical examination or treatment "as may be required to stabilize the medical condition" before any transfer can be made.[18] If a hospital transfers an unstabilized patient, it must be because the transfer was medically necessary, given the limitations in resources at the transferring hospital and the greater ability of the receiving hospital to address the patient's needs.[14,19] Although this law applies to all emergencies, most attention has focused on injured patients. Legislative designation that a hospital is a trauma center meeting specific published patient care criteria has far-reaching legal implications. The hospital administration, nurses, and physicians must be available to initiate treatment at the level defined by the designation process or to resuscitate and prepare for transport to a facility with greater resources as the need demands.[20] The "wallet biopsy" as a measure of transfer status has been eliminated. Delay in implementing transfer to a higher level of care can be legally actionable conduct, as was noted above in *Nevarez v. New York City Health and Hospitals Corp.* This principle has been reinforced many times.

Bitterman has clearly presented the legal requirements for such transfers.[14] The sending hospital and physician team must certify that the patient would be better served at the receiving hospital despite the risks inherent in the process of transfer.[19] This certification is much more easily accomplished when predefined transfer arrangements have been established between the sending and receiving trauma centers. These arrangements may be part of a multihospital trauma system protocol. Successful transfer arrangements represent successful conflict resolution among care providers, third-party payers, hospital officials, and their legal representatives. The sending center must certify in writing that the patient or patient representative was informed of the hospital EMTALA obligations and that the risks of transfer were less than the risks of remaining at the sending center.[19] When unavoidable delay in transfer occurs, a re-examination of patient condition is needed to reassure everyone that the transfer is still indicated.[15]

A different problem arises when patients arrive under their own power or are brought to the emergency center by third parties. Ordinary citizens have no way of knowing what resources a trauma center has or does not have at its disposal; valuable time may be lost when the injured patient is brought to a facility understaffed or otherwise unable to properly diagnose or treat the patient.[22,23] California, among other states, has attempted to deal with this problem by legislating when a facility may use the word "emergency" in its name or advertising.[20] A person or public agency cannot use that word—or any words suggesting that it can handle emergency medical services—unless it meets certain minimum standards including: having diagnostic radiology and clinical laboratory services provided by personnel on duty or on call and immediately available to the facility[4]; maintaining a roster of specialty physicians available for referral, consultation, and specialty services; and having transfer arrangements with one or more general acute care hospitals, by which patients in need of more definitive care can be expeditiously transferred to receive that care.[4] When the transfer is medically indicated, the sending center is presumed not to have the requisite personnel or equipment resources to provide indicated therapy. Otherwise, the sending center would be in violation of

EMTALA.[19] This, of course, creates potential liability when the sending center has been designated as having the resources for treating injuries that must subsequently be treated at the receiving center.[14,21] For example, the trauma center holding itself out to the public as being capable of caring for traumatic brain injury must have a neurosurgical response when such a patient arrives for emergency resuscitation and definitive treatment.[22,24–26] When such capabilities are temporarily absent, the trauma center would be well advised to develop a prehospital diversion plan to avoid potential legal liability. This might reduce income generated from a small number of diverted patients, but is in the best interest of the patient and, in the long run, is fiscally sound.

After confirming that transfer is best for the patient and informed consent has been obtained, the actual transfer can occur. It is imperative that the sending hospital optimally stabilize the patient and arrange for the receiving hospital to accept. When the preliminary examination identifies injuries that are clearly beyond the sending hospital's resources, emphasis should be placed on stabilization and expeditious transfer rather than on detailed and time-consuming diagnostic studies. A CAT scan of the head has little value in diagnosing the cause of a severe brain injury when the center has no neurosurgeon; likewise, detailed films of the pelvis, designed to identify the intricacies of a complex acetabular fracture, have little value when the center lacks major orthopedic surgery resources. When a patient cannot be stabilized at the sending hospital, transfer to a higher level of care is permitted when the considered risk of not transferring outweighs the risk of transfer.[14,19]

When these conditions are met, the sending hospital will be protected from liability should the patient refuse transfer.[27,28] The Maryland court of appeals noted as much in *Davis v. Johns Hopkins*, 585 A.2d 841 (Md. App. 1991) aff'd in part, reversed in part on other grounds, 662 A.2d 128. The facts of this case were as follows: the parents of an infant, who had previously been treated at Johns Hopkins for an emergency condition, wanted to bring the infant back to Johns Hopkins when he subsequently redeveloped the condition. The hospital was on "fly by" status, however, and consequently directed the emergency transport helicopter carrying the infant to divert to another hospital of comparable ability. The parents refused the diversion and insisted that their child be treated at Johns Hopkins. In order to accommodate their request, the hospital had to move several emergency room (ER) patients to other areas of the hospital to make available the emergency facilities needed to treat the infant. The delay, the parents alleged in their complaint, caused serious neurological complications to the child. The court, however, rewarded Johns Hopkins for recognizing that it could not care for emergency patients at the time and for arranging alternative treatment at a comparable hospital, by ruling that while there generally is a duty on the part of a hospital to provide emergency care to those patients who present in an emergent condition, there is no obligation that a hospital provide such care when no appropriate facilities are available to do so.

The final step in arranging a proper transfer is identifying a receiving hospital to accept the patient. Even a large urban trauma center may be temporarily overextended in one specialty and unable to accept a patient with specific injuries.[19] Although EMTALA permits transfers to be accepted by nonphysician representatives of the hospital, the specialties that will provide definitive care should be informed of the incoming patient. Thus, the receiving hospital would be advised to establish transfer in arrangements that insure availability of all the appropriate surgical specialists and its operating suite or critical care units.[27]

## TRANSFER ARRANGEMENTS

The decision to transfer from one trauma center to another involves multidisciplinary input from physicians, hospital administrators, representatives of the local EMS agency, and legislators from the geographic area. In crafting transfer guidelines, all parties must remember that the ultimate goal is to safeguard the welfare of patients. Arrangements for transfer between institutions must be defined ahead of time to avoid the scenario in which a sending hospital finds itself "short on resources" to treat a particular injury—conveniently enough—only when the injured patient is uninsured or only between the hours of 1:00 and 6:00 a.m. Ideally, if suspicion arises on the part of the receiving hospital regarding a transfer executed for reasons other than medical necessity, the tremendous advances made in digital communications and resultant hospital registries will provide the means to either confirm or dispel that suspicion; the receiving hospital will be able to simply access the sending hospital's registry program and assure that the transfer was grounded in patient need, not financial interest. Interhospital access to such records requires mutual trust and a close working relationship between the sending and receiving hospitals. Of course, EMTALA provides a federal mandate providing absolute access to such records, if the sending and receiving hospitals cannot work out their concerns in an amicable manner.

Once the definition as to which patients will be transferred is agreed upon, the actual transfer should take place under well-established guidelines. Communication between the two hospitals should insure that all appropriate medical records, including findings and treatments, accompany the patient. The material present on the transfer form should include: patient demographics; history and type of injury; time of injury; vital signs; revised trauma score; Glasgow Coma Scale score; history of medicines and allergies; injuries identified; resuscitation provided, and any treatments given. Conveying this information should become easier as more and more trauma centers institute the use of digital imaging and can simply pass along a disk containing all the necessary patient data as part of the transfer protocol. EMTALA instructs that

> an appropriate transfer to a medical facility is a transfer . . . (C) in which the transferring hospital sends to the receiving facility all medical records (or copies thereof) related to the emergency condition for which the [patient] has presented, available at the time of transfer, including records related to the individual's emergency medical condition, observations of signs or symptoms, preliminary diagnosis, treatment provided, results of any tests and the informed written consent or certification (or copy thereof) provided under paragraph (1) (A), and the name and address of any on-call physician . . . who has refused or failed to appear within a reasonable time to provide necessary stabilizing treatment[.][15]

The enforcement provision of EMTALA also allows any medical facility that has suffered a financial loss due to another hospital's violation of EMTALA to recover compensation for that loss in a civil action against the violating hospital. The potential for conflict grows as health care providers and hospital administrators exert pressure based on fiscal needs as to where and when a patient may be transferred. The expanded potential for conflict creates a legal maze, which is best resolved when everybody tries to employ common sense and recognize that the primary concern is for the injured patients. The policy, which ultimately is best for all parties, is most easily followed within the framework of a trauma system.[4]

## CONSENT FOR THERAPY

Obtaining an informed consent seems like a straightforward, easily achievable objective. Nothing could be further from the truth. This objective has probably been the most time-consuming issue for medical and legal resolution over the past 30 years.[30] Ideally, the patient should be maximally informed about the specific plans for therapy and the expected outcome and potential outcome, be they good or bad. In practice, the specifics of this seemingly simple directive are not always easily defined.

There is guidance available, however, from state legislation regarding the proper scope of the physician's discussion of consent with her patient. Many state legislatures have specifically defined what should be divulged before a physician performs an invasive test or procedure or initiates a course of treatment. A physician know the requirements of his state's informed consent statute—not to mention the rest of its public health laws—and keep abreast of any changes or additions made to the wording of the law. All states post their statutes online, and one can quickly link to a searchable database of each state's code by first visiting FindLaw.com. For instance, Oregon's informed consent statute mandates that as a precondition to a procedure or treatment, a physician "shall explain the following: (a) in general terms the procedure or treatment to be undertaken; (b) that there may be alternative procedures or methods of treatment, if any, and (c) that there are risks, if any, to the procedure or treatment."[22] The statute then states that, after giving that information, the physician must ask the patient whether he desires a fuller explanation. If so, the physician must "disclose in substantial detail the procedure, the viable alternatives and the material risks unless to do so would be materially detrimental to the patient."[22] As guidance in deciding whether a particular disclosure would be detrimental to the patient, the physician is advised to consider what fellow, reasonable physicians would do in the same or similar circumstances.

New York's legislature has taken a more proactive approach to the issue of informed consent by mandating a much more thorough discussion of the risks and benefits to treatment without regard to whether the patient requests the additional information.[14,15] New York defines "lack of informed consent" to mean "the failure of the person providing the professional treatment or diagnosis to disclose to the patient such alternatives thereto and the reasonably foreseeable risks and benefits involved as a reasonable medical, dental or podiatric practitioner under similar circumstances would have disclosed, in a manner permitting the patient to make a knowledgeable evaluation." In addition to requiring all risk/benefit information to be disclosed upfront, the statute also requires more of the plaintiff to prove lack of informed consent in a cause of action against the physician. The plaintiff must "establish that a reasonably prudent person in the patient's position would not have undergone the treatment or diagnosis if he had been fully informed

and that the lack of informed consent or diagnosis is a proximate cause of the injury or condition for which recovery is sought." The statute then enumerates the physician's available defenses, which include: the risk was so well known to the population at large as to make disclosure unnecessary; the patient assured the physician that he would undergo treatment no matter what the risks; consent was not reasonably possible, or the physician determined that it was not in the patient's best interest to be informed of the risks since it would "adversely and substantially affect the patient's condition."

Full adherence to this policy prior to a major elective operative procedure would involve a thorough explanation of the anatomy, physiology, pathology, and complications of operation. Clearly, this level of informed consent is a paradigm that is never achieved. The acceptable consent, therefore, is based on less than complete information. Even the physician with years of training in a non-surgical specialty does not really understand all of the potential risks of a complicated operation. The legal requirements, therefore, focus on important or material risk of therapy; the definition of a complicated operation, however, is a moving target.[30] Add to this the obstacle of obtaining an informed consent from an injured patient who may be in shock, and the difficulty is magnified many times over.

Bitterman provides an excellent review of these legal dilemmas.[30] As indicated above, the consent has four elements; it should identify the patient's problem, define the proposed solution, explain less beneficial alternatives and summarize the potential risks of therapy or the withholding of therapy.[31,32] When the friend or family member is requested to sign a consent form—which may not be valid anyway—the surgeon is faced with the dilemma to provide immediate care or risk harming the injured patient because of delay.[33,34] Indeed, delaying urgently needed therapy to obtain an informed consent is, in itself, a potential trigger for legal libaility.[33]

Elderly patients or incapacitated patients residing in nursing homes may have delegated the "power of attorney" to specific individuals or may have documents indicating that there should be no cardiopulmonary resuscitation in the event that they suffer cardiac or pulmonary collapse. Even these guidelines become useless when one of these patients is acutely injured and a new set of guidelines becomes operative.[30] This is true, for instance, if the patient receives a gunshot wound that is life-threatening if not immediately treated. The responsible surgeon must attend to the life-threatening injuries, which have occurred as a separate incident; the conditions that stimulated the appointment of someone with power of attorney are no longer operative. Likewise, the psychotic patient with life-threatening injury must receive life-saving therapy even when the patient refuses operative intervention. Clearly, the surgeon will feel more secure when the hospital attorney concurs.

Courts are reluctant to find that a patient was truly informed when litigation hinges on a standardized consent form with boiler-plate language that is neither understood by, nor explained to, the patient. Thus, a patient who had to sign an arbitration agreement before she could receive treatment from a medical clinic was held not to have consented to arbitration because the clinic's policy was merely to answer a patient's questions regarding the agreement—not to volunteer that information. Similarly, when a thoracic surgeon's standard practice was to inform a patient that, with every procedure, "there is a morbidity . . . and there is a mortality," but not to apply the specific facts of the procedure to an explanation of those terms, a court held that the surgeon had not provided his patient with enough information for her to give an informed consent to a pericardiocentesis.

The principle of "implied" legal consent applies when delay in therapy to obtain formal consent would harm the patient, although the courts may not always agree on the definition of an "emergency."[15,23] In the case of an acutely injured patient who lacks the legal capacity to consent or deny treatment because he is a minor, mentally incapacitated, or whose interests, in the opinion of the surgeon and the hospital, are not being served by those who have been designated to represent his legal rights, solutions should focus on what will prolong the patient's life. However, each mentated patient has the legal right to refuse treatment.[35,36] When documenting the refusal of life-saving medical therapy, the surgeon should know that the patient is competent and not under the influence of mind-altering medications or illegal substances.[37–39] The patient must be informed about the risks of therapy versus withdrawal of therapy, and this should be documented. Ideally, the patient will sign a form indicating refusal of therapy, although the patient more often refuses to sign anything. Confirmation of this refusal with friends or family members helps if any legal challenge arises in the future. Thus, the patient who has a suspected blunt rupture of the intestine may be legally competent to refuse operative intervention until the time that severe sepsis impairs further cognitive decisions; operative intervention at that time could be undertaken, although both the operative and legal risks are great. A more complicated situation occurs when the mentated patient refuses treatment, such as maintaining digital control and then surgical repair of active external bleeding from a stab wound to the femoral artery. When faced with this dilemma in a fully mentated patient with active bleeding, one of the authors (CEL) removed digital pressure and the patient rebled into hemorrhagic shock; he was taken directly to the operating room without further resuscitation until he was fully anesthetized. This decision was based on the presumption that the patient had, by this time, changed his mind about having the life-saving operation. All patients treated in this manner over the years have expressed gratitude in the postoperative period. No legal sequelae have ensued. When faced with a severely injured patient who is unable to provide a truly informed consent, the multidisciplinary trauma team needs to follow the principles outlined in the "Golden Rule" whereby you do for the patient what you would want someone to do for you in the same circumstances.[41,42] The principle applies to the unaccompanied minor, the minor with a recalcitrant guardian impeding life-saving therapy, and the incapacitated or incompetent adult.[34,35] The role that substance abuse plays in causing the incompetency should be considered in this assessment. Prisoners, too, have the right to refuse operation or any other treatment, even though other rights have been suspended during the period of incarceration.[43]

A more difficult problem arises when a patient compromises ideal therapy for religious reasons by refusing blood or blood products. The authors have honored these beliefs in the elective surgical arena by performing anatomical right hepatic resection for metastatic colon cancer with preoperative hemoglobin of 11 gm/dl in one patient and splenectomy for idiopathic thrombocytopenia purpura with a preoperative hemoglobin of 5.5 gm/dl and a platelet count of 10,000/ml in another patient. Courts have traditionally upheld the patient's right to refuse treatment, particularly when that refusal rests on religious beliefs. Hence, it was ruled that a patient who was a Jehovah's Witness had the right to refuse a blood transfusion and that the court order that her physician obtained to countermand her wishes should not have been issued.[36]

Compliance with these religious tenets does not continue when the patient has a mind-altering substance on board or injury results from an attempted suicide.[30] When the injured patient is mentally incapacitated but is known from history to belong to a religious sect that traditionally refuses blood and blood products, the administration of such would be according to the patient's medical needs.[40,41] When a patient has a wallet card prohibiting blood products, such therapy should be avoided.[42] Although state laws may vary, the presence of this type of card, which is dated and appropriately witnessed or countersigned, statutorily prohibits blood administration in Michigan. Physicians have been found liable for failure to follow those implied wishes.[42] Moreover, physicians have not been found liable for adhering to implied patient wishes by withholding unwanted blood therapy. The most problematic issue regarding treatment of a minor occurs when the withholding of needed blood and blood products is based on the verbal and written wishes of the parents. When faced with this situation, the physician should institute all required therapy including blood products since most, if not all, states do not allow the parental authority to prevent needed therapy for a minor.[35,41] When time permits, one should obtain a formal court decision to overrule parental authority. When the injury is immediately life-threatening, the surgeon and emergency physician should document the critical need for urgent therapy and implement this therapy. The trauma team providing optimal medical therapy in this setting will not be exposed to legal liability.

## CONFIDENTIALITY

More and more emphasis has been placed on protection of individual patient rights as they relate to confidentiality. Privacy concerns have stimulated implementation of state laws that define the extent to which a patient's medical records may be disclosed in order to effectuate proper treatment, while at the same time avoiding breach of patient confidentiality. Illinois, for instance, cautions that "no member of a hospital's medical staff and no agent or employee of a hospital shall disclose the nature or details of services provided to patients,"[44] but makes numerous exceptions, such as for the patient's—or the patient's representative's—information regarding treatment, and for those parties providing treatment to the patient, processing payment for that treatment, instituting peer review or risk management, or defending a claim against the hospital regarding that treatment. The prudent physician would be wise to review his/her own state's confidentiality statute. He/she should not assume that Illinois law is representative of all states' laws on the subject. Illinois law is merely presented here as one example of the many ways in which a state can legislate the scope of patient confidentiality rights and permissible disclosure of medical records.[44] There are also mandated disclosures under the Abused and Neglected Child Reporting Act, the Illinois Sexually Transmitted Disease Control Act, or "where otherwise authorized or required by law." At the federal level, EMTALA mandates that when an injured patient is being transferred to another trauma center for a higher level of care, the patient records, which will be needed by the receiving team, must also be transferred.[29] Records that are not specifically transferred with the patient, but are sent at a later time, should not be transmitted by e-mail which is accessible to uninterested parties. Such information needs to be sent by facsimile after appropriate permission is obtained from the patient or patient representative.

Safeguards must be enhanced when dealing with public figures who stimulate interest from news media more intent on pursuing a story than on protecting an individual's right to privacy. This extends to trauma conference rounds whereby the trauma director and other key members of the trauma team review patient progress on a weekly basis. Such conferences will, in the near future, include only an identifying number without actually identifying a patient by name. This is also true for the trauma peer review performance improvement committee meetings. This restriction may be problematic and possibly interfere with patient care since we know our patients by name rather than number. Hopefully, this issue will evolve in such a way that confidential minutes from peer review meetings can achieve overall trauma care enhancement without violating a patient's confidentiality.

While protecting confidentiality, the trauma team must respect laws of mandatory reporting, particularly those related to possible child abuse and spousal abuse. Included within the framework is the need to protect all potential evidence, such as might be present following a physical assault or rape. Likewise, one has to protect the evidence chain as it relates to foreign bodies, particularly bullets or dildos which are removed from the injured patient.[22] The system of tracking for this type of evidence should be based on trauma center guidelines since many people are involved in the later identification of these objects. Throughout all of this the trauma surgeon should be continually reminded that when in doubt, do what is best for the patient.

## THE MALPRACTICE CHALLENGE

Injury is not planned. There is no preoperative discussion between surgeon and patient in a private, sedate office setting. Amidst the hustle and noise of the ED, an informed consent is obtained. Does the acutely injured patient in this setting remember the details of this discussion?[30] No wonder then that many surgeons avoid trauma call which, in their minds, is likely to lead to litigation. Thal, in 1993, dispelled this myth.[45] He noted in his Scudder Oration that the likelihood for malpractice litigation arising out of trauma care is no greater and possibly less than that which evolves after elective surgery. There are, however, some pitfalls to be avoided if malpractice litigation after trauma care is to be reduced.

Nothing creates greater frustration and anger for the surgeon than the formal accusation of malpractice. The most common misconception about malpractice in the nonmedical community is the notion that a "bad result" must be due to malpractice.[14,30] Ideally, the medical team provides prudent and skillful care, which fully returns the injured patient to the preinjury condition. The very nature of injury, however, creates many variables that compromise this desired result even when the care is excellent. Unfortunately, the ability to convince a jury of one's peers that the undesired result is the result of malpractice all too frequently reflects the skill of the plaintiff attorney and expert witnesses who, in turn, often have little

experience with treatment of the patient's injuries.[46] Many trauma surgeons have found themselves assisting their defense attorneys against expert plaintiff testimony that is clearly the product of a creative mind and has no bearing on the physiology of injury. Unless this testimony can be successfully exposed as such to the jurors, a bad decision may result.[46,47]

The presence of trauma protocols, which serve as a good guideline for treating specific injuries, is one factor that can obfuscate malpractice litigations in trauma patients, but is not a treatment standard. The trauma community must educate defense attorneys that these guidelines must be violated when the trauma team working on the front lines determines that adherence to such guidelines would be detrimental to a patient's outcome. Guidelines are aids to treatment choices, but each patient may present with a slightly different variation of an injury resulting in care choices that may run counter to written guidelines. This highlights one important difference between the health care profession and the legal profession: the law is structured to identify standards for the group, whereas medicine, particularly after injury, is structured to identify the treatment needs of a specific patient.

Another area of concern within the malpractice arena relates to the trauma surgeon providing treatment for many different organ systems. Such treatment is not beyond the realm of his discipline. The trauma community must educate the legal profession about the multidisciplinary training and practice most trauma surgeons receive. The multiple organ dysfunctions subsequent to severe injury and shock are often different from that which occur after elective surgery.[46,47] Trauma surgeons routinely serve as "captains of the ship," responsible for treating the cardiovascular changes, renal needs, fluid replacement needs, and antibiotic therapies that are unique for injury. Recommendations that might be made by a specialist who treats illnesses of these organs in noninjured patients are often inferior to the treatment recommended by the trauma surgeon who has no formal certification in specialty areas, such as neurology, cardiology, and infectious disease. When consultations lead to recommendations that would be injurious to the patient, the trauma surgeon must ignore them and implement the most effective therapy.

There are many examples of controversy arising when trauma surgeons with critical care experience have disagreed with treatment recommendations made by critical care specialists unaccustomed to seeing injured patients. Some examples include the use of colloid supplementation for resuscitation from shock, the use of loop diuretics in patients who have marked extravascular fluid expansion during the post-resuscitation period, and the use of antibiotics for patients with respiratory dysfunction and positive tracheostomy stoma cultures. Many other examples could be given. The trauma surgeon must implement optimal care even when this care conflicts with the recommendations of other specialists.

Record keeping is an important part of the medical defense against malpractice litigation.[14,30] The trauma surgeon, however, must emphasize to all concerned that the prime purpose of the medical record is to benefit the patient and to convey information among treating team members and consulting physicians. The importance of accuracy, brevity and, most of all, timing cannot be overemphasized. When a change is made in the record because of an error caused by writing a note on the wrong patient, the reason for the change should be noted and timed by the responsible physician. Records are never "complete," but should be designed to serve the patient and not serve the legal profession on either the plaintiff or defense side of a subsequent litigation.

This great nation needs a reassessment of conflict resolution as regards medical malpractice.[46] The traditional sparring contests between plaintiff and defense teams often result in judgments that are unjust to either the plaintiff or defense positions. Contrary to claims made by the Institute of Medicine regarding health care, general trauma centers in America have developed outstanding peer review processes.[47,48] Indeed, an effective multidisciplinary peer review program is a criterion for trauma center verification or designation by many of the state trauma systems.[4] The peer review committee meeting minutes succinctly identify poor patient care decisions and what action should be taken to reduce the likelihood of repetition. The current competitive posturing in a "jungle-like" courtroom combat environment impedes these excellent discussions and resolutions from being broadly propagated.[46]

The medical and legal professions should join forces so that the fruits of these meetings can be used to compensate those injured patients who sustain uncalled-for complications because of preventable mistakes and to exonerate trauma teams that provide good care but have bad results. Since most of the investigation about postinjury morbidity and mortality would flow from the peer review process, legal fees could be minimized, injured patients would be compensated, and trauma teams in the vast majority of cases would be exonerated. As stated by Ledgerwood in the 1996 Scudder Oration, trauma surgeons should follow the philosophy of the great poet Robert Frost and lead the nation to take "the road less traveled."[46]

## FUTILE CARE OF THE TRAUMA PATIENT

All trauma surgeons are faced with the problem of providing futile care for the severely injured patient. The issue is less complicated in an adult patient who has sustained a traumatic cardiopulmonary arrest after blunt trauma.[49–51] The pulseless and apneic patient in the prehospital setting, typically, will not be resuscitated. Likewise, the pulseless and apneic patient who has sustained penetrating injury will not be resuscitated if no other signs of life, such as pupillary reaction, exist.[52] This decision, in the prehospital setting, becomes more difficult if the patient is a child or if the insult is caused by electrocution or drowning.

When the patient arrives in the ED, the "Golden Rule" should apply as the trauma team members honor the rights of the patient and recommend that the patient be treated as they would want to be treated in the same circumstance. The two areas where futility-of-care issues commonly arise with inpatients are traumatic brain injury and multiple organ failure. Trauma surgeons need to communicate with family members about expected outcomes so that there is mutual input into the final decision. Often family members are not receptive to this discussion early after injury since the patient was probably normal before injury; continued discussion between surgeon and family will help overcome this reticence. The hospital's ethics committee and the chaplaincy service are excellent adjuncts. Identification of the appropriate patient code status is vital in these circumstances.

The legal profession becomes more acutely involved in futile care when the trauma team members threaten euthanasia. Implementation of a "do not resuscitate" order should only be instituted after full discussion with the family. When one does not implement appropriate care to preserve life, this becomes criminal.

Even when the patient has an advanced directive or a living will decrying cardiopulmonary resuscitation or prolonged intubation and ventilatory support, the acute injury may nullify these guidelines. Redefinition with family support is essential. Physicians treating patients with traumatic brain injury all too often have a live patient in a vegetative state. The futility of care becomes obvious, and the family is so advised. When a family insists that its loved one be "full code," consultation with the ethics team is needed! When all else fails, the trauma team must take the less aggressive treatment regimen when more than one option is available; this pathway slowly leads to the inevitable end, namely, death.

Such passivity, however, must be implemented within the confines of the law. Trauma team members must not "lay down the gauntlet" to society in general and to the legal profession specifically by instituting euthanasia. The medical and legal professions are continually striving to resolve the futility of care issues when family members wish a "full code" status. Euthanasia is a direct challenge to the legal profession; this practice by Dr. Kevorkian in Michigan led to a jury conviction of murder.

The trauma surgeon may be less inclined to give up when the patient has been miraculously brought through horrendous injuries, but progresses to a steady state of multiple organ failure. A consult from a dispassionate surgical coworker may help put the overall picture in proper perspective. Often there is no clear-cut definition of "futility" in this setting. In theory, futility means that one is certain of a negative result regardless of what therapeutic action is taken. The law, however, is designed for the protection of the citizenry, whereas medicine is designed to provide the best care for the individual. In trying to provide optimal care in this setting while avoiding litigation, the trauma surgeon should do "what a reasonable, ordinary, prudent physician would do in the same or similar circumstance." Applying this guideline will help the trauma surgeon avoid being accused of abandonment.

The act of malpractice, which may result from negligent care, has four elements, namely, physician duty, violation of a standard of care, approximate causation resulting from lack of providing a standard of care, and subsequent patient injury or damages. When it is in the judgment of the trauma team that further treatment is futile, then there is no proximate causation or damages brought about by lack of treatment. The patient–physician relationship will help with the identification of optimal code status and in the subsequent discussion on organ donation.

## INITIATING LEGISLATIVE CHANGES

A democracy allows for all views to be promoted by interested citizens to legislative bodies. Thus, no project is left without representation. However, each project must compete with many other projects to achieve enactment into law. By tradition, the identification of problems and proposed solutions within the trauma community flows from frank and honest discussions at peer review meetings where preventable morbidity and mortality issues are identified and properly resolved. This efficient resolution leads to better patient care within a trauma center or even a trauma system, but has little impact on resolving state or national trauma issues. Once a new therapeutic procedure is identified, such as decompression laparotomy for the abdominal compartment syndrome, it is quickly tested at many centers and then is disseminated widely. The success of this process reflects ongoing conversations with peers who have encountered the same clinical difficulties.

The same technique fails miserably when a legislative solution is needed. The physician teams, especially the surgical specialists and emergency medicine specialists, must work with regional hospital administrators and prehospital providers to promote their solutions to civic leaders, labor representatives, and all segments of the citizenry, the ultimate consumer. This multidisciplinary group can often benefit from the expertise and political savvy of an "agent" or lobbyist who can bring the defined issues to legislative bodies. The lobbyist is able to define the beneficial effects for each segment of society and hopefully downplay potential negative effects. This process filters out many of the distracting but unimportant issues in preparation for promoting the solution to the legislative body. Often a legislator will have a special interest in the program being proposed and serve as a sponsor for the desired legislation. In turn, that legislator will need to be recognized for this support in order to foster reelection and continued support for the program at a later date.

## AUTHORIZATION AND FUNDING

Successful enactment of legislative goals varies directly with diversity of support and inversely with the cost. Careful preparation is essential. Conflicts among different supporting groups need to be resolved. Support by neutral legislators is essential; antagonizing key members of this neutral group is fatal. Our system of government is based on compromise, a process abhorrent to the trauma surgeon. The trauma system, begun in Detroit over 30 years ago, would have floundered without union concessions and support. The federal legislative process is much more complicated. Both the House of Representatives and the Senate must join together in support of each issue. When more than one legislative body has the authority to enact laws, the difference between the two bodies must be diffused in a collegial manner. Once legislated, executive approval is required.

There are many steps before a proposal becomes law. The sponsoring legislator will introduce the program to his colleagues. The legislative body will identify a committee and/or subcommittee for discussion. The sponsor will drum up support among his colleagues. At the federal level, a bill often has an identified author or coauthor in addition to sponsors. Once the bill is introduced, the formal assignment to a specific committee occurs. The supporters, or "champions," attempt to engender further support of colleagues and committee members. Once successfully through committee, the bill is proposed to the full legislative body. Full consideration ensues following the rules of discussion, which may vary according to city, county, state, or federal government. This may be a "stand alone" bill or included as part of a larger bill. For example, the Trauma Care Systems Planning and Development Act was passed as a "stand alone" law, whereas the Access to Emergency Medical Services Act was part of the Balanced Budget Act of 1997. Once passed, the bill is forwarded to the executive (mayor, governor, or president) who may sign the bill into law or veto the proposed legislation. The local and federal systems of government provide a mechanism for overriding the executive's rejection, but the practical

approach is to modify the trauma legislation so that it is acceptable to both the legislative bodies and the executive body. Finally, the multidisciplinary team must continue to promote enacted laws since all legislative efforts are in competition with many other projects and resources are limited. Furthermore, the sponsoring group needs to demonstrate the benefit of enacted legislation by documenting decreased morbidity and mortality, hopefully at a reduced cost to society.

Enacted trauma legislation has little benefit unless it is funded. The appropriation of funding for specific projects must follow the same steps within the legislative bodies and again face the same challenges from those legislators who represent competing interests. Often, fiscal appropriation in support of trauma legislation must be apportioned within a zero–sum game, which means that funds have to be removed from other projects that may be equally deserving. Legislative enactments fall into two broad categories, namely, mandatory (entitlement) programs and discretionary programs. Legislation is defined as mandatory when a citizen has a right (entitlement) to the benefits of a program. The Medicare and Medicaid programs are examples of mandatory programs. Legislation may be defined as a discretionary program when the citizen would benefit from the program, but the extent of benefit varies with competing societal needs, which are met by other programs. The National Institute of Health (NIH) is an example of a discretionary program.

## SUCCESSFUL TRAUMA LEGISLATION

There are many examples where governments, both local and national, have responded to citizenry by enacting trauma legislation. The specific federal committees that deal with most proposed trauma legislation include the House and Senate Appropriation Committees, the House Judiciary Committee, the House Ways and Means Committee, and the Senate Finance Committee. These committees have worked synergistically to enact trauma programs. The Federal Highway Safety Act of 1956 provided the impetus for identifying projects that might improve highway safety. This led to the National Highway Traffic Safety Administration (NHTSA), which continues to be a major force in identifying safety problems and implementing solutions. The National Academy of Sciences in 1966 published *Accidental Death and Disability: The Neglected Disease of Modern Society*. This widely quoted report covered many objectives related to injury including problems with prevention, delay in access, and implementation of definitive care. Urban centers benefited from this report when Congress promoted the development of EMS systems. This Congressional program was funded from 1974 through 1981. The Detroit system was implemented during the first year of funding support with guidance from the federal Department of Transportation. Many similar federal programs have been successfully implemented over the past 30 years. Once funded, interested citizenry, particularly the trauma community, need to continually gather data supporting the conclusion that the accompanying appropriations have reduced morbidity and mortality after injury. The acquisition and interpretation of such data will be fostered by the National Trauma Data Bank and the future activities of trauma systems. Knowledge is power; these sources of accurate data are vital to ensuring continued local and federal support of effective and cost-effective trauma programs.

# REFERENCES

1. McCullough, David: *John Adams*, New York, Simon & Schuster, 2001, p. 141.
2. 42 U.S.C. Sec. 1395 dd(a) (2005).
3. 42 U.S.C. Sec. 1395 dd(b) (2005).
4. American College of Surgeons: *Resources for Optimal Care of the Injured Patient*, 1999, p. 5.
5. Cal. Civ. Code Sec. 1714.2(b) 2005).
6. Mich. Comp. Laws Sec. 691.1501(1) (2005).
7. 42 U.S.C. Sec. 238q (2005).
8. Lazar, RA: Are you prepared for a medical emergency? *Bus H* 15:55, 1997.
9. Sorelle R: States said to pass laws limiting liability for lay users of automated external defibrillators. *Circulation* 99:2606, 1999.
10. Takata TS, Page RL, Joglar JA: Automated external defibrillators: Technical considerations and clinical promise. *Ann Intern Med* 135:990, 2001.
11. Weaver WD, Hill D, Fahrenbruch CE, et al.: Use of automated external defibrillator in the management of out-of-hospital cardiac arrest. *N Engl J Med* 319:666, 1988.
12. 12 Vt. Stats. Ann. Sec. 519(a) (2005).
13. Off. Code Ga. Ann. Sec. 51-1-29 (2005).
14. Bitterman RA: *Legal Requirements for Transferring Trauma Patients, in Trauma Management: An Emergency Medicine Approach.* St. Louis: Mosby, Inc., 2001, p. 644.
15. 42 U.S.C. Sec. 1395 dd(c)(1)(A)(ii) (2005).
16. Nevarez v. New York City Health and Hospitals Corp., 670 N.Y.S.2d 486 (N.Y. App. Div. 1st Dept. 1998).
17. 42 U.S.C. Sec. 1395 dd(a) (2005).
18. Rogers FB, Shackford SR, Hoyt DB, et al.: Trauma deaths in a mature urban v. rural trauma system. *Arch Surg* 1997.
19. 42 U.S.C. 1395 dd(c)(1) (2005).
20. Mitchiner JC, Yeh CS: The Emergency Medical Treatment and Active Labor Act: What emergency nurses need to know. *Nurs Clin N Am* 37:19, 2002.
21. Frew SA: Clarifications, examples of how hospital can violate COBRA. *Med Malprac Law Strategy* 1:5, 1994.
22. Fields WW, Asplin BR, Larkin GL, et al.: The Emergency Medical Treatment and Active Labor Act as a Federal Health Care Safety Net Program. *Acad Emerg Med* 8:1064, 2001.
23. Velianoff GD: Overcrowding and diversion in the emergency department: The health care safety net unravels. *Nurs Clin N Am* 37:59, 2002.
24. Allen J: *ER Overcrowding Spreads into Crisis Territory.* Los Angeles Times, May 1, 2001.
25. Taylor TD: Emergency services crisis of 2000 – the Arizona experience. *Acad Emerg Med* 8:1107, 2000.
26. Matthews P, Fehr-Snyder K: A tragedy waiting to happen? Arizona Republic, January 13, 2001, p. A19.
27. Davis v. Johns Hopkins, 622 A.2d 128 (Md. App. 1993).
28. 42 C.F.R. 489.24(b) (2006).
29. 42 U.S.C. Sec. 1395 dd (2005).
30. Bitterman RA: *Legal Issues Concerning Informed Consent in Trauma Care, in Trauma Management: An Emergency Medicine Approach.* St. Louis: Mosby, Inc., 2001, p. 671.
31. Percle v. St. Paul Fire and Marine Ins. Co., 349 So.2d 1289 (1977).
32. Iowa Code Sec. 147.137 (2004).
33. Wheeler v. Barker, 208 P.2d 6068 (Cal. App. 1949).
34. Holder A: Minors' right to consent to medical care. *JAMA* 257:3400, 1987.
35. Goldstein J: Medical care for the child at risk: State supervision of parental authority. *Yale Law J* 86:645, 1977.
36. Cruzan v. Director, Missouri Department of Health, 497 U.S. 261, 279 (1990).
37. Miller v. Rhode Island Hospital, 625 A.2d 778 (R.I. 1993).
38. Siegel DM: Consent and refusal of treatment. *Emerg Med Clin N Am* 11:833, 1993.
39. Etherington JM: Emergency management of acute alcohol problems. *Can Fam Physician* 42:2423, 1996.
40. University of Cincinnati Hospital v. Edmond, 506 N.E.2d 299 (Ohio1986).
41. Werth v. Taylor, 475 N.W.2d 426 (Mich. App. 1991).
42. Rodriguez v. Pinol: Suing health care providers for saving lives: Liability for providing unwanted life-saving treatment. *J Leg Med* 20:1, 1999.
43. Commissioner of Corrections v. Myers, 399 N.E.2d 452 (Mass. 1979).
44. Sullivan DJ: Patient discharge against medical advice. *Emerg Depart L L* 7:91, 1996.
45. Thal ER: Out of apathy. *Bull Am Coll Surg* 78:6, 1983.
46. Ledgerwood AM: With liberty and justice for all. *Bull Am Coll Surg* 82:17, 1997.
47. Inglehart JK: Congress moves to bolster peer review: The Health Care Quality Improvement Act of 1986. *N Engl J Med* 316:960, 1987.
48. Lozen YM, Cassin BJ, Ledgerwood AM, et al.: The value of the medical examiner as a member of the multidisciplinary trauma morbidity/mortality committee. *J Trauma* 39:1054, 1995.
49. Gmoremurgy AS, Norris PA, Olson SM, et al.: Pre-hospital traumatic arrest: The cost of futility. *J Trauma* 35:468, 1993.
50. Marjolin DA, Johan DJ, Fallon WF: Response after out-of-hospital cardiac arrest in the trauma patient should determine aeromedical transport to a trauma center. *J Trauma* 41:721, 1996.
51. Shimazu S, Shatney CH: Outcomes of trauma patients with no vital signs on hospital admission. *J Trauma* 23:213, 1983.
52. Battistella FD, Nugent W, Owings JT, et al.: Field triage of pulseless trauma patients. *Arch Surg* 134:742, 1999.

# Commentary ■ ROCHELLE A. DICKER

Consummate health care is a cornerstone of any prosperous and productive society. Physicians and nurses, as well as politicians and the public, share a vested interest in the preservation and improvement of our nation's health care delivery. However, the eyes through which these vested parties imagine the working structure and its execution often lead to divergent visions. The current heightened interest in reforming critical aspects of health care in our country is well founded when one considers the context: American mores regarding health care call for uncompromising treatment at any time, often urgently, in fact. However, there exist critical challenges: Health care policy and delivery is mired in the complicating factors of having 46 million uninsured individuals, shrinking numbers of general surgeons paradoxically in an aging nation, strict interpretations of the Uniform Accident and Sickness Policy Provision Law and the implications of the EMTALA.

The authors of this chapter, two surgeons and one lawyer, bring a wealth of practical experience and mature insight into the interactions of medicine, policy, and law. The wisdom and depth of information they provide regarding legal and political issues in trauma systems, confidentiality, consent, malpractice, and futility of care, impart readers with material vital to those of us caring for patients in today's charged environment. It is only through the insights of experienced and thoughtful practitioners such as these authors that we can begin to participate in efforts to reverse the political and legal underpinnings of our impending shortage of surgeons attending to the injured and the acutely ill.

The authors eloquently highlight the importance of a well-choreographed trauma system by imparting convincing examples of what can happen when that system breaks down. Unfortunately, at a time when the Institute of Medicine recognizes the importance of "reducing the burden of injury", only one-fourth of our nation's population lives within the safety net of a trauma care system. The federal Trauma Care Systems Planning and Development Act allowed for allocation of a significant amount of funding in the past; however, in the current budget cycle, the funds are yet to be authorized, greatly hindering progress in covering more of our citizens.

Trauma systems are highly dependent upon the expertise and availability of acute care surgeons and other surgical specialists. Recognition of the need for appropriate expertise can be found within the details of the legislation charged with providing it: EMTALA. The ethical and moral motivations behind the drafting and implementation of EMTALA were honorable but there are shortcomings; in some centers, it is a safeguard of expertise, at the expense of availability. Shrinking Medicare reimbursements, fear of lawsuits from patients first seen in EDs, and the onerous reputation of night call, has led to critical shortages in call coverage. This situation exists on the back of an already insufficient number of trained general surgeons and specialists in light of our aging baby boomer population. As the authors of this chapter point out, even a regional trauma center should go on temporary divert if the resources do not exist at a given point in time, to the extent expected of its certified level of care.

As trauma and acute care surgeons, we are critical stakeholders in protecting emergent surgical care for our patients. It is only through our understanding and involvement in the process of tort reform regarding frivolous lawsuits, recruitment of our trainees to the fields of trauma and acute care surgery, and advocacy for trauma system funding that we can begin to turn the tides for our trauma centers. Media advocacy and carrying our message to our legislators bear with it the "white coat effect" which continues to have a tremendous impact.

One large subsection of this chapter is dedicated to the discussion of futile care. The context in which futile care may exist in our population of trauma patients is quite distinct from futile care in the chronically ill. Paralleling the disease of trauma itself, discussions of futile care in this population often occur abruptly and on the heels of an unexpected single event affecting a previously spirited and productive life. Next of kin may be unable to articulate the wishes, on a loved one's behalf, when asked the critical questions germane to discussions of futility of care.

The issue of futility of care may manifest itself in another distinct way in acute care. Our field is one in which we must often push at "full tilt" determination to save a life, particularly in the first several hours, and then again as multiple organ failure advances. On occasion, perspective about pushing beyond any hope of a favorable outcome may be lost. The fresh judgment of an objective colleague may bring us back to a place where we are able to consider the utility or the futility of persevering. When discussions with family regarding organ donation are appropriate, "decoupling" from the health care team by having the Organ and Tissue Donation Network facilitate the conversations is extremely valuable and leaves little room for conflict of interest issues.

Improvements in trauma care over the last several decades have come through tremendous efforts in research and practice at the basic science level and at the bedside. Improvements have also come through work in prevention and policy change. We understand the issues because they directly affect our patients and our livelihood. Our involvement in the legislative process will bring continued advancements in topics as diverse as implementation of trauma systems, injury prevention strategies and the creation of ballot measures that maintain the vital infrastructure of our trauma centers.

# Acute Care Surgery

*Gregory J. Jurkovich*

Training in trauma surgery is deeply rooted in all branches of surgery, but is perhaps most recognized today as a component of general surgery. The forerunner of today's Committee on Trauma of the American College of Surgeons was known as the Committee on Fractures, and was founded in 1922 with 22 fellows, chaired by Charles L. Scudder, a general surgeon from Boston who had a strong academic interest in fracture management. As the results of physical force injury from wars, motor vehicle crashes, and interpersonal violence fostered the training of "trauma care" during the mid-20th century, the scope of the trauma surgeon encompassed more than fracture management. In 1950 the Regents of the College authorized the current title — the Committee on Trauma — to emphasize this expanding scope of practice.[1]

Further advancement of a surgical disciplines uniquely dedicated to the care of the injured patient in the United States began in the 1960s with the establishment of civilian trauma centers within city–county hospitals such as Chicago, Dallas, and San Francisco and was rapidly spread by devotees of these charismatic leaders.[2] During the ensuing two decades, trauma surgery became an attractive career based largely on the mentorship of trauma surgeons in urban city–county hospitals who epitomized the master technician, and who developed an academically productive career based on the physiology of the injured patient. These proclaimed trauma surgeons operated confidently and effectively in all body cavities, and perhaps were the last of the "master surgeons" that once were the hallmark of general surgery. Operating primarily in large volume public, city–county hospitals, these surgeons were also typically referred the most challenging surgical problems not only in their own institution, but from the surrounding city or region, particularly if there was a financial disincentive to providing care in a private for-profit hospital. As a result, the city–county or "safety net" hospital trauma surgeons developed an active elective surgical practice while providing trauma coverage.[3]

Yet the attractiveness of this career, and indeed this type of practice, has been challenged and changed by a number of forces. The trauma surgeon is no longer the "renaissance surgeon" of the urban/county hospitals of the 1970s. The academic success of these leading trauma surgeons (Blaisdell, Carrico, Davis, Freeark, Lucas, Ledgerwood, Mattox, Moore, Shires, Feliciano) fostered their incorporation into university hospitals, and the economic viability of civilian blunt trauma care, particularly in no-fault auto insurance states, led to an expansion of trauma programs out of the safety net hospitals and into private hospitals. The American College of Surgeons contributed to the wide-spread adoption of trauma programs by the remarkably successful and innovated activities of the Committee on Trauma, including hospital verification, the advanced trauma life support (ATLS) course, and the National Trauma Data Bank (NTDB). The federal government fostered the "inclusive trauma system" concept and encouraged the widespread development of trauma centers, in large part by reports of high preventable death rates in nontrauma hospitals, and by publications from the prestigious and influential National Research Council which characterized trauma as "the neglected disease" of modern society.[4] The result is that today there are over 1100 trauma centers in the United States, including 190 Level I centers and 260+ Level II centers,[5] with 84% of the population within one hour of a Level I or II trauma center.[6] This remarkable adaptation of regionalized medical care is nearly unique to trauma, and has been fostered by the recognition of the specialty of its care model and the evidence of is survival benefit.[7]

Yet this success may in and of itself have paradoxically led to a declining interest and commitment to the practice of trauma and emergency surgery. The requirement of a surgical presence for the resuscitation and early decision-making was interpreted by many hospitals (and surgeons) as a preclusion to developing a competitive elective practice, thereby discouraging technically proficient and talented clinicians from accepting such positions. Yet perhaps most importantly, as pointed out in an essay by Gene Moore and his "senior active trauma surgeon" colleagues, the rise and fall of trauma surgery has been influenced by the loss of operative practice due to a number of factors: the nonoperative management of solid organ injuries; effective injury prevention strategies; the emergence of surgical specialties diverting thoracic and vascular injuries away from trauma surgeons; the explosion of technical capabilities of interventional radiology; and the emergence of surgical critical care as a part and parcel of trauma care.[8] These forces have challenged the viability of a career in trauma surgery, with perhaps the most pressing concern being the lack of interest in a trauma by current residents and students. The 2006 collective review by Esposito and colleagues highlight some of the statistics that support this contention: declining interest in surgical careers by medical students (somewhat abated by the 80-hour work restriction); unfilled Accreditation Council for Graduate Medical Education (ACGME)-approved surgical critical care fellowship positions; the aging of the trauma surgeon work force (mean age: 54 years); disinterest in emergency on-call (50%) and trauma care (26%) among surgeons. This supports the observations made by Richardson and Miller in 1992 that only 8% of surgical residents were interested in a trauma fellowship, yet 18% considered trauma as a career track. This mimics the results of an unpublished survey of surgical residents by the Eastern Association for the Surgery of Trauma (Reilly P, unpublished data, August, 2003) that found 17% of residents planned a post-general surgical training fellowship in trauma/critical care.

Residents and students largely perceive trauma surgery as a nonoperative field. Trauma surgeons themselves share this concern. A survey of the operative experience of surgeons practicing in Level I and II ACS-verified trauma centers revealed that over one-half of the trauma directors at 79 Level I facilities performed fewer than 50 operations per year, and more than 70% of the other trauma panel surgeons did fewer than 50 operations per year.[9] The lack of operative experience is even more dramatic at Level II centers, where 70% of trauma surgeons did fewer than 20 operations per year. Fakhry et al. have estimated that surgical residents have to provide nonoperative care to 500 blunt trauma patients for every splenectomy or liver-injury repair. The rates for trauma laparotomy have fallen to 39 per 1000 trauma admissions for high blunt-trauma volume institutions.[10] The majority of patients cared for by trauma surgeons have never had an abdominal or thoracic operation, but most have had an operation by another surgical specialist, notably an orthopedist or neurosurgeon. Trauma surgeons are often seen as resuscitation doctors who provide important decision making during the resuscitation and critical care, yet often have no operative intervention. Remuneration for this effort is significantly less than that received by the operating surgeons, particularly considering the time involved.[11,12] Added to this are the largely unrewarding jobs of interdisciplinary coordination, communication and discharge planning. This is a far cry from the "golden age of trauma surgery," nostalgically describe by Dr. Gene Moore as a time when trauma surgeons were considered "master surgeons" who operated on the neck, chest, abdomen, and any injured vessel, and nonoperative management was unusual.[13]

Equally pressing has been the continued and unabated spread of specialty training beyond core general surgery training. This is a universal trend in medicine as evidenced by the 96 subspecialty certificates are awarded by the 24 member boards of the American Board of Medical Specialties. The exodus of general surgery trainees into surgical subspecialties has created a void of general surgeons with broad-based training who are capable of providing the expertise needed continue the type of practice once common in city–county hospitals as well as in many rural communities. Many general surgeons, particularly those in group practices, will "subspecialize" within their group by virtue of additional training. Increasingly, surgical subspecialists exhibit less interest in providing emergency and trauma on-call coverage, often concluding that they "aren't comfortable" or "don't feel qualified" to do so. Lifestyle interests and an elective practice volume that does not require taking emergency room call to enhance billing often fuel this attitude. This is a reflection of both a demand in surgical manpower that has not yet been addressed and a tendency of hospitals and surgical departments to acquiesce to this demand in order to attract and retain these lucrative and desirable elective clinical practices.

Stitzenberg and Sheldon report that 70% of trainees who complete general surgery residencies pursue further training.[14] The greatest interest has been in newer subspecialties, particularly surgical oncology (including breast surgery), endocrine surgery, and "minimally invasive surgery," which usually include gastrointestinal and bariatric diseases. In contrast, cardiothoracic surgery, vascular surgery, and surgical critical care have experienced a decline in interest as evidenced by the marked reduction of applicants to fellowships in these areas and a high number of vacant positions in the match. Each of these specialties has had a decline in traditional open operative caseload primarily because of technological advances. Vascular surgeons have responded to this challenge by adding required training in endovascular techniques to their fellowship programs. Cardiothoracic surgery has chosen to increase its focus on thoracic surgical procedures. Surgical critical care is a nonoperative specialty by design. Only 48% of offered positions in surgical critical care were filled in the 2005 match while 98% of pulmonary critical care positions filled. There is a common thread here. Specialties that have declining operative caseloads are not as attractive to those interested in a career in surgery.[15]

The recent survey of membership of the major trauma societies of the United States has documented the extent to which these factors influence the thinking of current trauma surgeons.[16] Only 54% of the respondents practiced in a Level I university program, so the survey was not that of solely academicians. The average workweek was 80 hours, with half reporting mandatory in-house night call. Two-thirds (67%) of the respondents care for trauma, surgical critical care, and emergency general surgery while on call. Widely valued and enjoyed were the intellectual challenges and the diverse aspect of a trauma career, but the major disincentives to participating in trauma care were the disproportionately poor income, irregular-hour time demands, and an inadequate trauma operative practice spurred by a preponderance of blunt trauma and interference or prohibition from developing an elective general surgical practice. These practicing trauma surgeons largely felt the best current model of trauma care was a training and practice paradigm that included trauma, surgical critical care, and emergency general surgery, also allowed the option of an elective surgical practice, if desired. They generally endorse an option to include limited orthopedic and neurosurgical skills such as external fixation of uncomplicated long-bone fractures and intracranial pressure (ICP) monitoring, but only if such specialty coverage was unavailable. They envision the ideal practice model as one involving a group practice at a designated trauma center, supported financially by the hospital and regionalized care. They would not mind mandatory in-house night call if such call was necessary for good care, limited in its frequency, predictable, compensated, and earns the next day off.

The future training of trauma surgeons must take into account these social, economic, and lifestyle preferences forces that are influencing all of medical practice. In response to this demand, a joint meeting of the leadership of the American College of Surgeons and the Association for the Surgery of Trauma (AAST), Eastern Association for the Surgery of Trauma, and Western Trauma Association was held in March 2003, with the AAST taking the lead in considering how to restructure the training and practice of trauma surgery to make it a viable, attractive, and sustainable career, in the best interest of patient care, and importantly, to keep trauma a surgical care disease. The result was the formation of a working group within the AAST to develop a surgical training curriculum that would be attractive to new trainees, and provide the training for a practice that would be viable, sustainable, and importantly, in the best interest of the patients.[17]

The AAST Committee on Acute Care Surgery has resulted in the development of training curriculum for a specialist that has broad training in elective and emergency general surgery, trauma surgery, and surgical critical care.[17] As reflected by the name of this committee, this proposed new surgical specialist has been called the Acute Care Surgeon. A graduate of this proposed fellowship training paradigm would be trained for a career in managing acute general surgical problems, providing surgical critical care, and managing acute trauma. This surgical specialist could do "shift" work, not unlike the emergency physicians, if local practice patterns support this approach. The training of this surgical specialist would require core general surgery training, as well as advanced thoracic, vascular, and G-I surgery, so as to not just allow, but to encourage the development of a diverse elective surgical practice, again, as local practice patterns permit. It has also been proposed that the Acute Care Surgeon specialist could also perform selected and limited neurosurgical and orthopedic procedures, with national and local support from these fellow surgical specialists, and when such subspecialty coverage is not immediately available. While there has been considerable resistance to this part of the proposal, the fact that many hospitals are having difficulty with surgical emergency coverage argues for its addition.[18]

Current practicing trauma surgeons find that this new specialty makes sense. The broadened training in thoracic, vascular, and GI operative skills and techniques make this a more desirable surgical specialty. Further training in these areas is required given the shrinking training time brought on by the limited workweek and the siphoning of advanced operative cases by other fellowship trainees. The option of working on a preset schedule allows for a more controllable lifestyle, and potentially makes this specialty more attractive to surgeon who wishes to take a more active part in childrearing or other family activities. This is more than a "surgical hospitalist" who would only cover the on-call window or take care of the patients of other physicians during undesirable hours, rather, the Acute Care Surgeon could well seen as the most experienced surgeon for most circumstances in most hospitals, a resource for all the medical staff. Also, since this surgical specialist will most commonly be "in-house" 24-hours a day, the likelihood of significant complications due to lack of an experienced surgeon at night and on weekends will be reduced; thus, the cost of care is likely to be reduced. Finally, in academic centers, the ready availability of an in-house surgical specialist will increase the exposure of medical students and residents to surgical attendings. The Acute Care Surgeon specialist will be filling a niche, which now might be termed a void in our provision of acute surgical care to the American public. This void needs to be filled as many of our surgical specialty brethren are increasingly refusing to participate in the surgical call schedule. Although the field of trauma surgery would benefit from these changes, those who will benefit most are our patients. With this in mind, these changes should be welcome in the future of trauma surgery.[8]

The Acute Care Surgery fellowship is also designed to have the flexibility to adapt to the possible shortening of core general surgery training to four years. Early specialization, or limiting core general surgery to three to four years, followed by some self-selected area of concentration is a concept that continues to be discussed and considered, even in the face of shrinking training hours.[19] The training paradigm of the Acute Care Surgeon would fit well within this construct, with core general surgery followed by two to three years of trauma, surgical critical care, and advanced general surgical procedures, as envisioned by some members of the American Surgical Association committee on the future of surgical training in 2004 and modified in Fig. 59-1.[20] This concept of abbreviated core training followed by specialty training ultimately leading to board certification in both general surgery and the specialty of choice is being considered and trialed or considered at this time by thoracic, vascular, and plastic surgery. The American Board of Surgery (ABS) has recently added four new advisory councils, including one in trauma, burns, and critical care, along with advisory councils in surgical oncology (including breast and endocrine), transplantation, and gastrointestinal

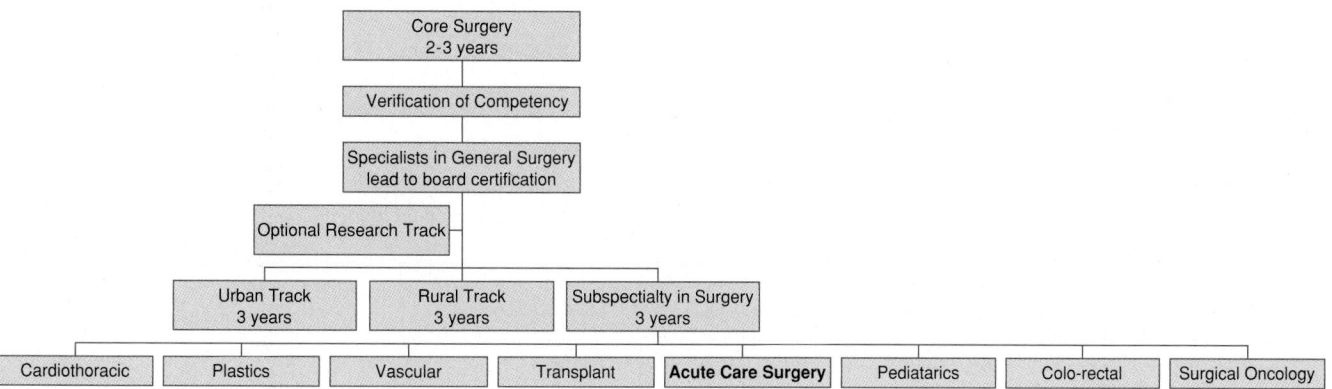

**FIGURE 59-1.** Proposal for restructured surgical residency training.

surgery (including endocscopy, hepatobiliary, and bariatric surgery) to provide advise and guidance from these specialty areas,[21] and in 2006 the ABS hired Dr. Richard H. Bell, Jr. MD, for a newly created administrative leadership role of assistant executive director to specifically facilitate the development of a standardized surgery residency curriculum.[22]

At the current time the proposed curriculum for Acute Care Surgical training is 24 months. The outline of this curriculum is presented in Table 59-1. The curriculum includes a dedicated nine months of surgical critical care, as mandated for Residency Review Committee (RRC) approved surgical critical care fellowships. The remaining 15 months are focused on operative rotations in emergency and elective surgery, with the expectation that there will be at least 12 months of acute care surgical on-call experience. The 15 months of operative rotations have as their foundation 4–6 months on an intact, functioning, active acute care surgical service. This is supplemented by three core rotations in thoracic, vascular, and hepatobiliary-pancreatic surgery, with the knowledge that these rotations must be able to provide adequate exposure to advanced surgical skills and patient care challenges that might be lacking in core general surgery training. Limited time is required on orthopedics and neurosurgical services, with additional elective time to be allocated to meet the needs of the trainee. The expectation is that trainees will be competent in the management of a wide spectrum of acute care surgical needs, and have specific operative competency in the procedures listed in Table 59-2. Essential elements of the training program will be the operative experience, the presence of an RRC-approved surgical critical care fellowship, and the commitment of the hospital and surgical colleagues to support this new paradigm. The curriculum will meet the American Council on Graduate Medical Education (ACGME) requirements for competency-based training, and the evaluation of the fellows' performance will reflect that expectation. The ABS, along with the Residency Review Committee and the ACGME will be considering how all of surgical training might be evolving over this time as well, and specifically how acute care surgery meets the needs of patients, the populations, and trainees.

The timeline for implementation of this fellowship has finalization of the curriculum occurring in 2006, with training site visits and site selections in 2007, with enrollees entering a limited number of acute care surgical training approved sites in 2008. The American Association for the Surgery of Trauma plans on conducting site visits to select training programs, and will oversee the development of competency-based evaluations and tests. It is anticipated that some of the training requirements will be met by simulated training, such as occurs in the ATLS course, and the newer courses that stress advanced surgical operative skills required in trauma care, such as the advanced trauma operative management (ATOM) or Definitive Surgical Trauma Course (DSTC) courses or the military extremity war surgery course, formerly known as Trauma Refresher Course for Surgeons.[23,24] Additional roles for simulator training in endoscope skills, and resuscitation skills will be inevitable as these simulation models develop more sophistication.

### TABLE 59-1

| Curriculum: 24-Month Curriculum | |
| --- | --- |
| **REQUIRED CLINICAL ROTATION** | **LENGTH** |
| Surgical Critical Care: | |
| • Trauma/Critical Care (resuscitative and post-op management of complex surgical illness related to general surgery and trauma) | 6 months |
| • Electives in Critical Care (management of complex critical illness such as pediatric surgical critical care, neuro critical care, burns, etc.) | 3 months |
| Emergency and Elective Surgery | 15 months |
| **Total** | **24 months** |

| Suggested Rotations During Emergency and Elective Surgical Experience | |
| --- | --- |
| **SUGGESTED CLINICAL ROTATIONS** | **LENGTH** |
| • Acute Care Surgery | 4–6 months |
| • Thoracic | 1–3 months |
| • Transplant/Hepatobiliary/Pancreatic | 1–3 months |
| • Vascular/Interventional Radiology | 1–3 months |
| • Orthopaedic Surgery | 1 month |
| • Neurological Surgery | 1 month |
| • Electives (Burn Surgery and Pediatric Surgery recommended; others would include: Endoscopy, Imaging, Plastic Surgery, etc.) | 1–3 months |
| • Or: maximize time in above rotations | |
| **Total** | **15 months** |

Notes:
1. It is a requirement that over the 2-year fellowship, trainees participate in Acute Care Surgery call for no less than 12 months.
2. Flexibility in the timing of these rotations, and the structure of the 24-month training should be utilized to optimize the training of the fellow.
3. Rational for out of system rotations for key portions of the training must be based on educational value to the fellow.
4. Acute Care Surgery fellowship sites must have RRC-approval for Surgical Critical Care training.
5. Experience in elective surgery is an essential component of fellowship training.
6. An academic environment is mandatory and fellows should be trained to teach others and conduct research in Acute Care Surgery.

**TABLE 59-2**

## Operative Management Principles Technical Procedures Requirements & Minimums

Principles:

- Required experience should consider the feasibility and practicality of maintaining operative proficiency in a given area.
- Required experience should be sufficiently broad as to allow a wide range of practice patterns in a variety of communities.
- In consideration of local program constraints, there may be a need for flexibility with respect to strict "required minimums," across the board, for some procedures.
- Requirements should reflect the need, based on timeliness and good patient care, for proficiency in certain operative procedures rather than be bound by strict or traditional disciplinary boundaries. (i.e., this is not "trespassing")
- Requirements should consider the difference between high-risk, volume-sensitive cases and lower risk, volume-insensitive cases.
- It is assumed that the fellow is capable of performing all essential procedures in the acute setting.
- Operations listed in the "Desirable" category provide valuable experience in operative exposure and related surgical techniques. It also emphasizes that an elective general surgical practice is a foundation for the discipline.

| AREA / PROCEDURE | ESSENTIAL | DESIRABLE |
|---|---|---|
| **AIRWAY** | | |
| Tracheostomy, open and percutaneous | X | |
| Cricothyroidotomy | X | |
| Nasal and oral endotracheal intubation including rapid sequence induction | X | |
| **HEAD/FACE:** | | |
| Nasal packing | X | |
| ICP monitor | | X |
| Ventriculostomy | | X |
| Lateral canthotomy | | X |
| **NECK:** | | |
| Exposure & definitive management of vascular and aerodigestive injuries | X | |
| Thyroidectomy | | X |
| Parathyroidectomy | | X |
| **CHEST:** | | |
| Exposure & definitive management of cardiac injury, pericardial tamponade | X | |
| Exposure & definitive management or thoracic vascular injury | X | |
| Repair blunt thoracic aortic injury | | X |
| Partial left heart bypass | | X |
| Elective pulmonary resections | | X |
| Exposure & definitive management of tracheo-bronchial & lung injuries | X | |
| Diaphragm injury, repair | X | |
| Definitive management of empyema: decortication (open and VATS) | X | |
| Video-assisted thoracic surgery (VATS) for management of injury and infection | X | |
| Bronchoscopy: diagnostic and therapeutic for injury, infection and foreign body removal | X | |
| Exposure & definitive management of esophageal injuries & perforations | X | |
| Spine exposure, thoracic & thoraco-abdominal | X | |
| Advanced thoracoscopic techniques as they pertain to the above conditions | X | |
| Damage control techniques | X | |

*(continued)*

**TABLE 59-2**   *(Continued)*

## Operative Management Principles Technical Procedures Requirements & Minimums

| AREA / PROCEDURE | ESSENTIAL | DESIRABLE |
|---|:---:|:---:|
| **ABDOMEN & PELVIS** | | |
| Exposure & definitive management of gastric, small intestine and colon injuries. | X | |
| Exposure & definitive management of gastric, small intestine,and colon inflammation, bleeding, perforation & obstructions. | X | |
| Gastrostomies (open and percutaneous) and jejunostomies | X | |
| Exposure & definitive management of duodenal injury | X | |
| Management of rectal injury | X | |
| Management of severe liver injury | X | |
| Elective hepatic resection & organ harvesting | | X |
| Management of severe splenic injury, infection, inflammation, or diseases | X | |
| Management of pancreatic injury, infection, and inflammation | X | |
| Elective pancreatic resection | | X |
| Management of renal, ureteral and bladder injury | X | |
| Management of injuries to the female reproductive tract | | X |
| Management of acute operative conditions in the pregnant patient | | X |
| Management of abdominal compartment syndrome | X | |
| Damage control techniques | X | |
| Abdominal wall reconstruction | X | |
| Radical soft tissue debridement for necrotizing infection | X | |
| Spine exposure | | X |
| Advanced laparoscopic techniques as they pertain to the above procedures | X | |
| Exposure & definitive management of major abdominal and pelvic vascular injury | X | |
| Exposure & definitive management of major abdominal and pelvic vascular rupture or acute occlusion | | X |
| Place IVC filter | | X |
| **EXTREMITIES** | | |
| On-table arteriography | X | |
| Exposure and management of upper extremity vascular injuries | X | |
| Exposure and management of lower extremity vascular injuries | X | |
| Damage control techniques in the management of extremity vascular injuries, including temporary shunts | X | |
| Acute thromboembolectomy | | X |
| Hemodialysis access, permanent | | X |
| Fasciotomy, upper extremity | | X |
| Fasciotomy, lower extremity | X | |
| Amputations, lower extremity (Hip disartic., AKA, BKA, Trans-met.) | X | |
| Reducing dislocations | X | |
| Splinting fractures | X | |
| Applying femoral/tibial traction | | X |
| **OTHER PROCEDURES** | | |
| Split thickness, full thickness skin grafting | X | |
| Multicavity organ harvest | | X |
| Operative management of burn injuries | | X |
| Upper GI endoscopy | | X |
| Colonoscopy | | X |
| Core rewarming (CAVR, CVVR) | X | |
| Diagnostic and therapeutic ultrasound | X | |
| Other procedures required by RRC for Surgical Critical Care | X | |

The AAST Acute Care Surgery committee had considered three other options for the future of trauma surgery: (1) deemphasize the field from surgery; i.e., encourage nonsurgeons to assume responsibility for initial care and surgical intensive care unit (SICU) management (United Kingdom model), (2) expand the discipline of trauma surgery to include more orthopedics (European model), and (3) maintain status quo. The vast majority of current trauma surgeons find the status quo untenable, and are unwilling to abandon trauma care to nonsurgical disciplines.[16,25] Others, exampled by the writing of Richardson and Malangoni, have argued that the acute care surgeon *is* a general surgeon, and that trauma training and practice is part of the broader practice of general surgery.[15,26–28] Yet the Louisville group practice of trauma care has closely exemplified the Acute Care Surgeon model being proposed, in that their trauma service is designed to include all emergency operations and inpatient consults, and indeed is referred to as "*the crucible*, where high-volume, high-intensity, results matter, life or death decisions are made, and treatment is provided."[29] Additionally, all (trauma) surgeons have been encouraged (and supported) to pursue an elective surgical practice. The proposed Acute Care Surgery paradigm is exactly that, where trauma and general surgery together create a specialist that has broad training in elective and emergency surgery, trauma surgery, and surgical critical care.[7] In fact, a number of academic urban trauma centers, mostly safety net hospitals, have always employed this model to ensure optimal care of the injured patient — convinced that emergent torso trauma surgery and elective general surgery are inseparable.[30] Moreover, this has always been the scope of practice for rural trauma surgeons, and the possibility of Acute Care Surgery fellowship training that is tailored to the rural trauma surgeon has great appeal.[31–33] Likewise, the training of modern military surgeons seems ideally suited to the Acute Care Surgeon model, as exemplified by the incorporation of military surgeons into urban trauma center hospital staff to expand their clinical operative experience.

The options of including surgical skills and patients with some orthopedic and neurological injuries with the domain of the acute care surgeons (Option 2 above) has been challenged by the leadership of neurosurgical societies and the Orthopedic Trauma Association. The initial proposals ranged as far as including decompressive craniotomies for mass lesions from bleeding and open reduction internal fixation (ORIF) of all long-bone fractures, to as little as splinting simple fractures, reducing dislocations and placing ICP monitors. All have been met with significant resistance, which seems incongruous given the data on lack of specialty coverage from many hospitals for exactly this type of care.[25,34] While this represents the model of much of European trauma care,[35,36] without the support of these leading organizations, the lack of neurosurgical and orthopedic emergency surgical coverage affecting many hospitals will not be solved by acute care surgeons.

The name Acute Care Surgery was chosen carefully. The term surgical hospitalist, no doubt appealing to hospital administrators, was rejected because of the connotation of primarily providing surgical care deemed burdensome and undesirable to other surgical disciplines. Emergency Surgery is a recent discipline championed in Europe, including a new *World Journal of Emergency Surgery*. This name, however, was viewed as suboptimal because of the implication that acute surgical care can be relegated to shift work and is limited to patients seen in the emergency department (ED). Acute Care Surgery, as with existing trauma surgery, must provide comprehensive patient management from ED arrival to hospital discharge and seamless 24/7 services.

In some ways current trauma surgeons are responding to the stresses of health care that are external to the discipline of surgery, and are affecting a change in all of medicine. The public, payers, and legislators are expecting improvements in both the process and outcome of care. The expectation of a continuous in-house physician is no longer confined to the emergency room, but extends to the ICU, the trauma team, and the in-patient floors. Yet this expectation of continuous presence is challenged by equally strong expectations of a limited workweek, and a nonsustainable health care budget. The demographics of medicine are changing as well, with more women entering higher education, medical school, and surgery. This changing demographic will inevitably impact the future of surgery. Acute Care Surgery is part of this evolution.

## REFERENCES

1. *A guide to organization, objectives and activities of the Committee on Trauma.* http://www.facs.org/trauma/publications/bluebook2005.pdf. Accessed July 1, 2006. American College of Surgeons; Chicago, 2005.
2. Blaisdell FW: Development of the city-county (public) hospital. *Arch Surg* 129:760, 1994.
3. Moore EE: Acute Care Surgery: The safety-net hospital model. *Surgery* 141:297, 2007.
4. Committee on Trauma and Shock of the Division of Medical Sciences. *Accidental Death and Disability: The Neglected Disease of Modern Society.* Washington, D.C.: National Academy of Sciences, 1966.
5. MacKenzie E, Hoyt D, Sacra J, et al.: National inventory of hospital trauma centers. *JAMA* 289:1566, 2003.
6. Branas C, MacKenzie E, Williams J, et al.: Access to trauma centers in the United States. *JAMA* 293:2626, 2005.
7. MacKenzie EJ, Rivara FP, Jurkovich GJ, et al.: A national evaluation of the effect of trauma-center care on mortality. *N Engl J Med* 354:366, 2006.
8. Moore EE, Maier RV, Hoyt DB, et al.: Acute care surgery: Eraritjaritjaka. *J Am Coll Surg* 202:698, 2006.
9. Meredith J, Miller P, Chang M: Operative experience at ACS verified Level I trauma centers. Paper presented at: Halstead Society, Cashiers, North Carolina, 2002.
10. Fakhry S, Watts D, Michette C, et al.: The resident experience on trauma: Declining surgical opportunities and career incentives? Analysis of data from a large multi-institutional study. *J Trauma* 54:1, 2003.
11. Aucar J, Hicks L: Economic modeling comparing trauma and general surgery reimbursement. *Am J Surg* 190:932, 2005.
12. Esposito TJ, Kuby AM, Unfred C, et al.: Perception of differences between trauma care and other surgical emergencies: Results from a national survey of surgeons. *J Trauma* 37:996, 1994.
13. Moore E: Trauma surgery: Is it time for a facelift? *Ann Surg* 240:563, 2004.
14. Stitzenberg KB, Sheldon GF: Progressive specialization within general surgery: Adding to the complexity of workforce planning. *J Am Coll Surg* 201:925, 2005.
15. Malangoni M: Acute Care Surgery: The challenges ahead. *Surgery* 141:324, 2007.
16. Esposito T, Leon L, Jurkovich G: The shape of things to come: Results from a national survey of trauma surgeons on issues concerning their future. *J Trauma* 60:8, 2006.
17. Acute care surgery: Trauma, critical care, and emergency surgery. *J Trauma* 58:614, 2005.
18. Gore L, Huges C: Two-thirds of emergency department directors report on-call specialty coverage problems. http://www.acep.org/webportal/Newsroom/NR/general/2004/TwoThirdsofEmergencyDepartmentDirectorsReportOnCallSpecialtyCoverageProblems.htm. Accessed February 16, 2006.
19. Lewis FJ: The American Board of Surgery. *Bulletin ACS* 69:52, 2004.
20. Pellegrini CA, Warshaw AL, Debas HT: Residency training in surgery in the 21st century: A new paradigm. *Surgery* 136:953, 2004.
21. ABS New Letter: http://home.absurgery.org/default.jsp?newsletter&ref=news. Accessed February 16, 2006.
22. American Board of Surgery news. Philadelphia: American Board of Surgery; 2006. http://home.absurgery.org/default.jsp?newsdrbell. Accessed July 1, 2006.

23. Jacobs LM, Burns KJ, Luk SS, et al.: Follow-up survey of participants attending the Advanced Trauma Operative Management (ATOM) Course. *J Trauma* 58:1140, 2005.

24. Jacobs LM, Lorenzo C, Brautigam RT: Definitive surgical trauma care live porcine session: A technique for training in trauma surgery. *Conn Med* 65:265, 2001.

25. Esposito TJ, Rotondo M, Barie PS, et al.: Making the case for a paradigm shift in trauma surgery. *J Am Coll Surg* 202:655, 2006.

26. Cheadle WG, Franklin GA, Richardson JD, et al.: Broad-based general surgery training is a model of continued utility for the future. *Ann Surg* 239:627, (discussion 632), 2004.

27. Richardson JD: Training surgeons to care for the injured: The general surgery model. *Bull Am Coll Surg* 79:31, 1994.

28. Richardson JD, Miller FB: Is there an ideal model for training the trauma surgeons of the future? *J Trauma* 54:795, 2003.

29. Richardson JD: Trauma centers and trauma surgeons: Have we become too specialized? *J Trauma* 48:1, 2000.

30. Ciesla DJ, Moore EE, Moore JB, et al.: The academic trauma center is a model for the future trauma and acute care surgeon. *J Trauma* 58:657 (discussion 661), 2005.

31. Finlayson SR: Surgery in rural America. *Surg Innov* 12:299, 2005.

32. Hunter J, Deveny K: Training the rural surgeon. *Bull Am Coll Surg* 88:13, 2003.

33. Cogbill T: What is a Career in Trauma. *J Trauma* 41:203, 1996.

34. Esposito TJ, Reed RL II, Gamelli RL, et al.: Neurosurgical coverage: Essential, desired, or irrelevant for good patient care and trauma center status. *Ann Surg* 242:364 (discussion 370), 2005.

35. Gosling JC, Ponsen KJ, Luitse JS, et al.: Trauma surgery in the era of nonoperative management: The Dutch model. *J Trauma* 61:111, 2006.

36. Allgower M: Trauma systems in Europe. *Am J Surg* 161:226, 1991.

# Commentary ■ RUSSELL J. NAUTA

Who can argue with the desirability of a specialist broadly trained in elective and emergency general surgery, trauma surgery, and surgical critical care — particularly one capable of leading a team, with both citizenship and pedagogical prowess? Many general surgeons recognize themselves in Dr. Jurkovich's description of the acute care surgeon.

Reading the American Board of Surgery's requirements for certification, general surgical residents finishing their training find that they are required to produce evidence that they had been trained to render longitudinal care for all abdominal conditions, most cancer, trauma and endocrine surgery patients, and patients in an ICU; current requirements also require that they be familiar with open, endoscopic, and minimally invasive techniques. Thus, board-certified general surgeons, led to believe by their Board that these are core competencies, already consider themselves to be acute care surgeons by Jurkovich's definition.

The acute care surgeon model would place the ICU in the stewardship of the acute care surgeon trained in trauma. However, not all would concede that critical care is the sole province of the trauma surgeon. For example, those surgeons who have differentiated in a direction wherein they render care to postoperative pancreatectomies, vascular patients, or abdominoperineal resections, might reasonably consider their care of elderly patients with multiple comorbidities to be as sophisticated as that rendered to trauma victims.

The acute care model, as currently proposed, is poised to divide general surgery; with minor modifications, however, it could contribute to the standardization of general surgical training and the strengthening of general surgery. But first, the two elephants in the surgical living room — the general surgical program directors' difficulty in coping with the ACGME mandates, and the proliferation of fellowships, would have to be acknowledged.

The ACGME mandates related to work hours are squarely and selectively directed at surgical programs, as nonsurgical residency programs would have to assemble several trainees to account for 80 hours of work in a given week. The mandates in surgical programs have become like the emperor's clothes in the Andersen fairytale, with surgeons publicly acknowledging their finery, but privately grousing about the mathematical impossibility of reducing the faculty's "face time" with residents by as much as one-third (from 120 hours per week to 80) and claiming to retain the desirable mentorship, continuity of care, collegiality, and involvement with sophisticated cases at off hours. Neither trainees nor their faculty believe that this is happening or is possible. In fact, cynics view some fellowships as a hedge on the ACGME regulations, in that fellowships are a largely unregulated industry not as tightly scrutinized as residency programs for compliance with ACGME work hour regulations.

While we all welcome someone of our own to mentor, we all consider what we have to teach special (or specialized). Someone to "carry the clubs" is nice, but not all such arrangements are "value added" to the trainee or the surgical community. Fellowships have proliferated with little regard for whether they adversely impact general surgical training; even the vascular surgeons, who once affirmed that their training fellowships would exist only alongside general surgical programs large enough so that they would not encroach upon general surgical vascular case volume for open procedures, can no longer make the claim that they do not do so. The trainees themselves, less confident that they will have a practice "niche" have lost confidence in their five-year programs' ability to confer broad self-sufficiency even as EDs and small communities struggle with their surgical staffing. Hospitals in some cases are receiving new surgeons with fewer numbers of cases than in years past, and little additional operating in their fellowships.

Despite its open general surgical heritage, vascular surgery is becoming an increasingly catheter-based specialty. It may well be that breast surgery is so multidisciplinary that those restricting themselves to breast surgery would not require the breadth of training currently in the 5-year general surgery curriculum. Cardiac surgery discussions have also highlighted the evolving differences between the two disciplines and questioned the need for lengthy general surgical training before beginning a cardiac surgical residency.

The discourse around cardiac, vascular, and breast surgery are thus framed around their practitioners' assertion that major differences from general surgery have evolved. If true, there is less of a need to certify them in general surgery and less of a need for the general surgical trainee to spend service time on those services. If the general surgical trainees' service obligation to these disciplines is thereby reduced, it may well be possible to augment the general surgical trainee's experience not only in trauma and critical care, but in surgical oncology, hepatobiliary surgery, noncardiac thoracic surgery, minimally invasive surgery, and endocrine surgery.

The designers of the acute care surgical curriculum have held to the architects' dictum of form following function. They are poised to defend the curriculum in terms of content, rigor, and time commitment in the interest of turning out a competent, confident trainee. Supported conceptually by an American Surgical Association taskforce convened to study trends in surgical education, the curriculum stands in stark counterpoint to an uncharacteristic surgical passivity which has placed acceptance of ACGME governance ahead of the traditional core values taught by Jurkovich's giants of trauma surgery.

What is now discussed as an "acute care" surgical curriculum, with minimal modification, has the potential to define a meld of trauma surgery, endocrine surgery, hepatobiliary surgery, surgical oncology, minimally invasive surgery, and current general surgery in a way which reflects the growth, richness, and sophistication of the broad-based, board-certified general surgery. As documented in past reviews of ABS recertification data, individuals board-certified in general surgery may in time choose to limit their practice to one or another narrow area of this rich field, but they would do so from the legitimate position of having undergone comprehensive training. Specialties whose structure no longer bears a strong resemblance to this training would exit it early, as proposed most recently in vascular surgery.

Acute care surgery is not such a specialty; particularly in its augmented form, with a new curriculum, it is too much like general surgery to gain wide acceptance. The acute care surgery proposal is, in fact, general surgery energized, with an acknowledgment of its depth and breadth, and the mathematical impossibility of general surgical training programs delivering the ABS brochure's product in less time without curricular modification. The implementation of such reform may involve difficult choices, such as the closure of surgical residencies incapable of delivering such broadbased training, the rejection of ACGME reforms, or the rejection of ACGME governance itself. Those working on acute care surgery have the opportunity to seize the academic high ground, rather than self-anoint as another poorly defined general surgery specialty. In turn, they should be engaged as thoughtful academic leaders and program directors in general surgery as acknowledgment of their head-on engagement of these complex training issues.

# MANAGEMENT OF COMPLICATIONS AFTER TRAUMA

# Principles of Critical Care

*Robert C. Mackersie* ■ *Jean Francois Pittet* ■ *Rochelle A. Dicker*

The term *critical care* pertains to care given as part of the crisis or turning point of a disease, condition, or injury. While initial operative management of traumatic injury has historically been regarded as the live-or-die turning point, this literal definition reflects the importance of postoperative management of the trauma patient. Critical care may be defined loosely as the process of high-intensity physiologic monitoring coupled with short-response-time pharmacologic, ventilatory, and procedural interventions. This activity is designed to reestablish normal homeostasis and minimize complications of primary, secondary, and iatrogenic injury. Surgical critical care is inherently different from medical intensive care insofar as surgical patients, and particularly trauma patients, require intensive care as the result of an acute surgical intervention or injury and not as part of the (often inexorable) progression or exacerbation of chronic disease. This fundamental difference affects a multitude of patient management practices and decisions.

Due to the severity of injury in many trauma patients, basic critical care begins in the prehospital setting and intensifies upon hospital arrival. Critical care is perhaps more closely linked to the care of severely injured patients than to any other surgical patient population. As our ability to resuscitate patients with injuries that previously would have been fatal improves, so does our reliance on the functions of critical care. In the "trimodal" mortality curve (see Chap. 2) that has been described,[1] most of the postresuscitation trauma deaths and possibly a significant percentage of the early deaths may prove to be ultimately preventable through improvements in critical care treatment.[2] Secondary brain injury caused by uncontrolled cerebral edema and resultant intracranial pressure (see Chap. 20); nonspecific amplification of the inflammatory response, producing multiple-organ dysfunction syndromes (see Chap, 68); and late sepsis, related to the original injury or subsequent interventions and amplified by delayed immunosuppression (see Chap. 67), are all examples of late and potentially treatable causes of trauma mortality. The inherent integration between surgical critical care and the management of severe traumatic injury is reflected by the organization and content of this textbook, where the related aspects of critical care are discussed in the context of the management of specific injuries. This chapter focuses on elements of critical care essential to the management of the acutely injured patient and briefly reviews some of the more recent developments in the management of specific organ-system dysfunction.

## HISTORICAL PERSPECTIVES

The modern critical care unit (CCU) saw its beginnings in the postanesthesia, postoperative recovery room. As more complex surgical procedures developed following the turn of the century and the need for specialized postanesthetic monitoring also developed, specialized facilities for the short-term monitoring of these patients also began to appear. The first critical care unit, developed at Johns Hopkins Hospital in 1923, was designed for the care of postoperative neurosurgical patients. Following the growing practice of managing high-risk surgery patients in postoperative CCUs, the polio epidemic spurred the development of respiratory care units and stimulated the further development of automated machines capable of intermittent positive pressure ventilation, the precursor of the modern ventilator. Improvements in continuous electrocardiographic (ECG) monitoring and the development of external defibrillators around 1956 fostered the development of specialized coronary care units. By the 1960s, additional growth in medical technology and the increasing severity of illness further stimulated the development of specialized expertise in critical care and led to the creation of the modern model for intensive care in the United States. By the end of the 1960s, roughly 95% of all acute care hospitals in the United States had some form of CCU. Expansion of critical care services was facilitated in 1965, when federal Medicare and Medicaid programs provided funding for a broad range of health services, including critical care, for the poor and elderly. CCUs in the 1980s were developed around specific patient populations: those with demonstrated and ongoing organ-system instability and those at risk for the development of physiologic or organ-system decompensation. Many hospitals developed separate units for respiratory, neurological, cardiac, and surgical patients. In the 1990s, cost and staffing considerations associated with multiple independent CCUs led to greater centralization of critical care, often in separate sections of a larger unit. In addition, most institutions have developed intermediate or "step-down" units in order to improve resource utilization of the more expensive CCU. In the last several years, increasing emphasis has been placed on quality of care indicators and physician staffing models for CCUs.

## ORGANIZATION OF THE CRITICAL CARE UNIT

From a provider's standpoint, the growing number and complexity of CCU patients often exceeded the availability of adequately trained physicians in past years. The medical community responded to this deficit by the development of subspecialty credentialing in critical care. Currently, the American boards of internal medicine, surgery, pediatrics, anesthesiology, and neurosurgery offer subspecialty critical care boards. With increasing multidisciplinary specialization in critical care, there has also developed more formal administrative links to clinical departments, although a wide variety of patterns appears to exist. In a study of approximately 1700 hospitals, Groeger and colleagues found that 36% of units were run within departments of medicine, with 23% having no individual department affiliation. Surgeons served as directors of most "pure" surgical CCUs and as directors in 21% of mixed units.[3]

Given the wide variety of clinical expertise and patient populations, several patterns of CCU physician organization have developed. The first is the "closed" unit that relies almost exclusively on a critical care team (or attending intensivist) for primary patient management. Under this scheme, comprehensive management is assumed by the CCU team along with responsibility for all orders and procedures, with other services providing care as consultants on an as-needed basis. Most medical CCUs are staffed in this manner along with some surgical CCUs where the CCU team is directed by another surgeon.

In an alternative model, the "open" unit, there may or may not be a designated CCU director, a separate CCU team, or even an intensivist immediately available to the CCU. Under this system, individual physicians manage and direct intensive care for their respective patients, depending on their institutional privileges, with or without house staff. Consultative involvement of a board certified intensivist is at the discretion of each primary attending physician, and is neither required nor necessarily expected.

Many larger surgical CCUs have a "semi-open" or transitional unit plan of practice whereby the CCU is staffed, 24 hours a day, seven days a week, with dedicated on-site CCU physicians. On-call physicians are often attending-supervised house staff in larger teaching centers, and responsibility for care is shared between the CCU team and the primary specialty service. With the 24/7 in-unit staffing in the semi-open model, critical care team involvement in each patient is typically either mandatory or expected. There are often specific areas of designated critical care autonomy, such as the management of mechanical ventilators, invasive hemodynamic monitoring, pain management, and conscious sedation. In these units, the ultimate responsibility for the patient remains with the primary team, but patient care is a collaborative effort. This semi-open model combines the advantages of maintaining a separate in-house critical care team 24 hours/day while maintaining primary surgical service responsibility for overall patient management. This arrangement is consistent with Accreditation Council for Graduate Medical Education (ACGME) program requirements for general surgery training programs as well as guidelines for the optimal care of the injured patient suggested by the American College of Surgeons Committee on Trauma for Level 1 Trauma Centers.[4] There is now a growing body of work examining the relationship between CCU staffing models and patient outcome. For these purposes, rather than trying to compare various models of care, a distinction has been made between "high intensity" and "low intensity" physician staffing models. Loosely translated, a "high intensity" model involves 24/7 dedicated CCU physician staffing and mandatory CCU team involvement with patient management. This includes all closed units and most semi-open units (as previously defined). The remaining 'open' units typically involve "low intensity" CCU physician staffing. The principal hypothesis is that dedicated, higher intensity intensivist staffing for CCU patients will ultimately improve outcome from a variety of conditions and illnesses.

In a meta-analysis of 26 pooled studies, Pronovost et al. found a relative risk of 0.71 (95% CI = 0.62–0.82) for hospital mortality and 0.61 (95% CI = 0.5–0.75) for CCU mortality associated with high intensity CCU staffing for adults and children.[5] This validated previous work done by the same author.[6,7] Similar results were found by Nathens et al. who specifically examined the effect of high intensity staffing on outcome from major trauma.[8] Utilizing prospective cohort data from 68 trauma centers, the authors reported a relative risk reduction of 0.78 (95% CI = 0.58–1.04) for CCUs whose patients were either managed (closed unit) or comanaged (semi-open) by board certified intensivists. The effect of dedicated intensivist involvement seems to extend also to neurology and neurosurgical patients, with reports demonstrating improved overall mortality and length of stay.[9,10]

These and other observations have led to attempts to improve patient safety in the CCU. In 2000, a group of Fortune 500 companies and large public and private health care purchasers formed the Leapfrog Group for the purpose of identifying and creating incentives for sustained patient safety measures in acute care hospitals. This group has identified standards for physician staffing the CCU which involves the presence of experienced intensivists providing daytime care and response requirements for off-hours care.[11] The intent of the Leapfrog initiative is to provide market incentives designed to stimulate preferential use of institutions adhering to these types of guidelines.

Another component of CCU organization is the designation and support of a medical CCU director. Designated directors function in both closed and semi-open models of CCU care and are a standard element in CCUs at larger institutions.[3] The precise role of the medical director will vary according to institutional practice patterns, staffing, and the model utilized but generally includes oversight responsibility for house staff supervision and teaching, call scheduling, quality assurance, and unit resource utilization. Additional responsibilities of surgical CCU directors may include (a) practice protocols and guideline development, (b) unit and institutional policymaking, (c) administrative supervision of ancillary staff (e.g., respiratory therapy), (d) CCU information system development, (f) professional billing oversight and compliance with

Health Care Financing Administration (HCFA) guidelines, (g) oversight of critical care research and development of investigational protocols, and (h) collaborative program development (e.g., spinal cord injury center, extracorporeal membrane oxygenation).

Hospitals specifically designated as trauma centers, to be eligible for verification through the American College of Surgeons Committee on Trauma (ACSCOT), must also comply with established guidelines for critical care.[4] The requirements for Level I centers include the provision of 24-hour in-house physician coverage for critical care and stipulate that administrative direction for the CCU include a surgeon involved with the care of trauma patients. In addition, these guidelines specify that the surgeon should remain primarily responsible for the patient, regardless of admission to a CCU.

## PERFORMANCE IMPROVEMENT AND RESOURCE UTILIZATION

The dictum that high-quality care constitutes cost-effective care reflects the fact that errors and mishaps in critical care are usually expensive. Performance improvement and resource utilization monitoring are complementary activities in the CCU. The total annual cost of health care in the United States comprises a substantial proportion of the gross domestic product and is anticipated to continue to rise, particularly in the face of an ageing population. Critical care has, in recent years, accounted for as much as 10% of annual health care costs[12] and from 20% to 28% of all acute care hospital costs.[13] The enormity of these critical care costs raises the obvious question regarding cost-effectiveness and overall utility. A number of reports suggest that for trauma and surgical patients, the outcome from critical illness in many cases is good, with age, severity of injury, and pre-injury comorbidity affecting outcome.[14,15] More recent studies have identified the problem of diminished neurocognitive function affecting long-term recovery.[16]

Quality assurance and performance improvement in a surgical CCU are complex processes requiring the ongoing identification of outcome measures or performance indicators, data collection and analysis, and the development of action plans to correct deficiencies and subsequent monitoring of the performance (outcome) measures. The underlying goal of delivering high-quality care also depends, to a significant degree, on specialization (critical care specialists), provider education and training, and good communication and collaborative interaction between specialty and ancillary services. Existing critical care quality assurance programs have used a variety of clinical indicators or "filters" as a measure of the quality of care. These indicators may reflect process measures (e.g., percentage of eligible patients receiving deep venous thrombosis prophylaxis in a timely manner), and outcome measures (complicate rate [%] for central venous line sepsis) (Table 60-1). Illness severity indices, discussed in the following section, have been developed for the purpose of predicting outcome of critically ill patients and are being increasingly used as benchmarking tools, allowing participating units, through the use of statistical comparisons, to compare their outcomes with those predicted by the various indices. These performance measurement systems will become increasingly important in allowing managed care organizations to assess program performance. In addition to improved instruments for assessing critical care outcome, the development and implementation of

**TABLE 60-1**

| Typical Indicators Used to Assess CCU Quality of Care |
|---|
| **PROCESS MEASURES** |
| Delayed diagnosis |
| Delayed treatment |
| DVT prophylaxis |
| Implementation of timely nutritional support |
| Inappropriate admissions or delayed discharges |
| Unplanned readmission to the CCU |
| Compliance with traumatic brain injury protocol |
| **OUTCOME MEASURES** |
| Infection rates: ventilator-associated pneumonia, central venous catheters, etc |
| Risk-adjusted mortality, mortality review (all cases) |
| Iatrogenic pneumothorax following central line placement |
| Unplanned extubations |
| Medication errors requiring intervention |
| Opiate or benzodiazepine withdrawal |
| Iatrogenic soft tissue infections |
| Donor organ procurement rates (eligible patients) |

clinical protocols and clinical management guidelines (CMGs)[17,18] directed at reducing undesirable treatment variability will be linked to CCU performance improvement. Protocols and guidelines, once developed and implemented, can later be analyzed in terms of their clinical efficacy and cost-effectiveness and can be subsequently modified and further developed as part of the overall programs in performance improvement and cost control.

The effectiveness of protocols and CMGs has been demonstrated for a variety of problems and conditions including ventilator weaning, pneumonia, nutrition, and sedation.[19–25] The difficulties that most institutions experience, however, relate more to the implementation of CMGs rather than to their development. Current methods of improving implementation of and compliance with CMGs include ongoing education, standing (preprinted) order forms, the assignment of some management responsibilities to specialized teams (e.g., nutrition, respiratory therapy), and the use of advance practice staff (nurse practitioners, physician's assistants).

## PHYSIOLOGIC MONITORING IN THE CRITICAL CARE UNIT

For every patient, based on the type and severity of injury, age, underlying chronic disease, and response to therapy, there is an anticipated or even optimal clinical "trajectory." Experienced clinicians, within the bounds governed by the complexities of human biology, have certain clinical expectations and can anticipate the clinical behavior and specific complications that are reasonably likely to occur following major injury. The majority of the practice of critical care medicine for the trauma patient involves the monitoring of this clinical trajectory, and the remainder involves prophylactic and therapeutic interventions designed to keep patients from deviating or falling off this trajectory. The questions that must be addressed with any form of monitoring involve "when?" (indications and timing), "what?" or "how much?" (which specific monitoring tools or techniques), and "why?" (an analysis of the associated risks and benefits).

## HEMODYNAMIC MONITORING

Hemodynamic monitoring is directed at assessing the results of resuscitation and as a guide to reestablishing and maintaining adequate tissue and end-organ perfusion (see Chap. 62). The general principle applicable to this monitoring is that maintenance of "optimal" parameters ensures adequate tissue perfusion, avoids ischemia, and thereby preserves organ function and decreases the incidence and severity of postinjury inflammatory response syndromes (see Chap. 68). Insofar as methods for measuring perfusion/oxygenation at the cellular level are not yet applicable to the bedside environment, clinicians continue to rely on relatively crude, global physiologic measurements that may or may not accurately reflect events at the tissue level.

### Arterial Pressure Monitoring

The most frequent type of blood pressure monitoring device utilized in hospitals is the "Dynamap" or other automated cuff. While these instruments are generally accurate in measurement of the mean arterial pressure, they are not as reliable and practical for systolic, diastolic, and continuous monitoring purposes. The arterial line is the more accurate alternative. Additionally, arterial lines can be "space saving" in a patient without a lot of body surface area (i.e., those with burns and extremity fractures) to place a large cuff. Arterial line monitoring provides continuous readings of systolic, diastolic, and mean arterial pressures, and are indicated for a wide variety of situations encountered in major trauma (Table 60-2). Lines may be inserted in the radial (after assessment of collateral perfusion through an Allen's test) or femoral artery. Reported line infection rates are low,[26] although thrombotic complications occur at rates of as high as 30–40%. Digital ischemia, particularly in association with high-dose vasoactive agents, can occur. Damped line tracing, inability to withdraw blood specimens, and any evidence of infection (pus, erythema) or digital ischemia are indications for removal and site change. Although arterial line infections remain rare, sterile technique should be employed with lines that may be used for several days.

### Central Venous Pressure Monitoring

If cardiac output can be used as a surrogate to global perfusion, then its principal determinants are preload, afterload, and contractility. Right-sided ventricular volume (preload) may be measured directly, as discussed in the sections that follow, or estimated through the use of a surrogate pressure measurement, the central venous pressure (CVP). "Central" refers to placement of the catheter tip in a location where pressure will accurately reflect right atrial pressures. This requires an intrathoracic position so that negative or positive pleural pressures are accounted for. Ideal placement is the distal superior vena cava, at the junction with the right atrium, with confirmation based on the presence of a typical CVP waveform. Short, large-bore femoral lines, while useful for fluid and blood administration, should not be used for measuring or monitoring "CVP" due to inaccuracies produced by abdominal pressure.[27]

Choosing a site for central venous line placement is often a matter of physician preference. Regardless of the site chosen, sterile technique should be employed with full gowning and gloving. The subclavian vein is more readily available in the injured patient with a cervical-spine collar in place, and it is often preferred in the

**TABLE 60-2**

**Indications (Suggested) for Hemodynamic Monitoring**

**ARTERIAL LINE MONITORING**
Shock states (any)
  Cardiac
  Septic
  Neurogenic
  Hypovolemia/hemorrhage
  Monitoring intraoperatively/postoperatively
Head Injury
Serial monitoring of ABG
Labile Hemodynamic Status
Respiratory Failure
Hypertensive crisis
Vasoactive drug infusions
High risk or elderly trauma patient

**CENTRAL VENOUS PRESSURE MONITORING**
Volume status in acute head injury
Complex trauma/pelvic fracture
Shock states
Hypovolemia
Acute renal failure
Vasoactive drug infusions
Monitoring during acute ICU hemodialysis
Cardiac pacing
Elderly trauma patient
Massive transfusion
Pulmonary contusions

**PA CATHETER MONITORING**
Refractory septic and cardiogenic shock states
Severe hypoxemia, pulmonary edema/embolism ARDS
High risk intraoperative monitoring
Barbiturate coma (iatrogenic myocardial depression)
Monitoring of mixed venous $O_2$ ($SVO_2$)
Diagnosis: unexplained shock, hypoxia, renal failure

head-injured patient. This leaves sites available for jugular venous saturation monitoring. The subclavian line has a slightly lower infectious rate (discussed in a later section), and the internal jugular site has a slightly lower pneumothorax rate. The need to assess and monitor right-sided filling pressure is generally based on patient risk and the intensity of intervention (see Table 60-2). High-risk patients include those particularly susceptible to complications related to too much or too little volume. This category includes the elderly patient with major injuries, traumatic brain injuries, pulmonary contusions, etc. High-intensity intervention might include massive transfusion, vasoactive drugs, or the need for emergent operation or procedures to control hemorrhage, including arteriographic embolization.

Interpreting CVP in patients receiving higher pressure mechanical ventilation warrants special consideration. CVP should ideally be recorded when the patient is temporarily removed from positive expiratory pressure. Alternatively, the CVP may be *approximated* by subtracting the level of positive end-expiratory pressure (PEEP) exceeding 5 cm $H_2O$. Estimation of right or left ventricular preload may be very difficult in patients receiving high PEEP with low pulmonary compliance, as exists in acute respiratory distress syndrome (ARDS).

The most critical element in utilizing the CVP for management of resuscitation is to consider it in the context of the particular individual's requirements for end-organ perfusion, as part of the equation in the endpoints of resuscitation. Particular attention to base deficit, urine output, and mental status, along with a knowledge of the estimated preload can help tailor volume resuscitation or aid in the consideration for inotropic therapy when appropriate.

## Pulmonary Artery Catheters

Pulmonary artery (PA) catheters, placed via a subclavian or internal jugular venous approach by literally floating a partially inflated balloon, using blood flow direction, into a branch of the pulmonary artery, have become a mainstay of hemodynamic monitoring since their introduction over 25 years ago. By measuring PA back pressure with the catheter-tip balloon "wedged" in a PA branch, a surrogate for left atrial filling pressure can be obtained. Cardiac output, measured and calculated by exponential thermodilution washout data, is used to direct therapy aimed at the restoration or maintenance of tissue perfusion. PA catheters may be used to measure or calculate several physiologic parameters useful in the diagnosis and management of a number of conditions or disease states (Table 60-3). Suggested indications for PA catheters include unexplained shock, hypoxemia, renal failure, and peri-injury monitoring in high-risk patients (see Table 60-2). Prior to 1996 there had been general acceptance and widespread use of PA catheters. A number of subsequent reports, however, questioned their utility, and a study by Connors et al.[28] concluded that PA catheters were associated with increased mortality and increased utilization of resources. This perspective has not been supported by more recent studies which have not demonstrated major adverse sequelae associated with the use of PA catheters.[29] The use of PA catheters in surgical patients may be different than that in medical patients is suggested by additional reports of benefits associated with the use of PA catheter monitoring in a more select patients population.[30,31]

Recognition that a clinician's ability to obtain and interpret PA catheter data and intervene appropriately based on it is a large determinant of outcome was an important component of a National Institutes of Health (NIH) consensus statement and workshop on the use of PA lines.[32]

The fundamental principle behind invasive hemodynamic monitoring in the surgical patient derives from the observation that an adverse hemodynamic response to the stress of surgery, injury, or sepsis has been associated with a significantly higher mortality. The assumption is that if PA catheter use changes therapy and acts to correct physiologic defects, mortality/morbidity can be reduced. With respect to changing therapy in surgical patients, based on available information, it appears that monitoring data obtained through the use of a PA catheter results in therapeutic changes in 30–60% of cases. Of these, it has been estimated that between 25% and 35% are major therapeutic changes.

*Special-Use Pulmonary Artery Catheters.* Modified PA catheters with implanted rapid-response thermistors allowed assessment of right heart function beginning in the early 1990s. Through the use of beat-to-beat analysis of thermal signs and ECG timing of the PR interval, right heart ejection fraction could be calculated. The technique has been verified both in vitro and in clinical studies.[33,34] Since many severe septic states and ARDS are often associated with increases in PA pressures and resultant degrees of right heart failure, these catheters may have utility for the monitoring of ejection fraction (EF) in these settings.

A more common situation arises where right heart EF catheters are useful. In the setting of high intrathoracic pressures, most commonly associated with ARDS, the accuracy of the CVP and/or pulmonary artery occlusion pressures (PaOP) as a surrogate for right and left ventricular preload (respectively) is substantially degraded. In this setting, often with high PEEP and plateau (inspiratory) pressures, CVP and PaOP are not accurate reflections of preload and management cannot be reliably guided by these parameters. The advantage of right heart EF catheters is that they allow actual right heart end-diastolic volume index (normalized preload) to be calculated through the equation:

$$RVEDVi = SVi / EF_{(measured)}$$

where

$$SVi = C.I._{(measured)} / heart\ rate_{(measured)}$$

The clinical issue in this question is: is RVEDVi more accurate than PaOP in predicting preload-recruitable increases in CI (with volume loading) at higher intrathoracic pressures? Prospective studies suggest that RVEDVi, as an actual preload volume, versus a pressure surrogate, is a better indicator of RV preload over a range of end-expiratory pressures up to 50 cm $H_2O$.[35,36] Additional reports suggest that underresuscitation, based on an RVEDVi of <100 mL/m$^2$ may have an associated increase in organ dysfunction.[37]

In an era in which there is good data to support early goal directed therapy for sepsis, it is likely prudent to be aggressive and timely in line placement and accrual of data in order to guide restoration of end-organ perfusion in trauma.

## TRANSESOPHAGEAL ECHOCARDIOGRAPHY

Transesophageal echocardiography (TEE) has been used for a number of years as an intraoperative monitor for high-risk cardiovascular patients and has more recently been evaluated as a means of diagnosing blunt aortic rupture (see Chap. 30). The evolution of transesophageal echocardiography have increased the accessibility of this method of monitoring and expanded its use in the CCU. Recent studies suggest that TEE may supplant the PA catheter for

**TABLE 60-3**

### Clinical Information that may be Obtained Through the use of a PA Catheter

| MEASUREMENT/CALCULATION | ASSOCIATED CONDITIONS |
| --- | --- |
| Pulmonary artery pressures, pulm. vascular resistance | Pulmonary hypertension, P.E., right heart failure |
| Systemic vascular resistance | Sepsis, need for afterload reduction |
| Cardiac output, cardiac index | Assessment and correction of global perfusion/malperfusion, assessment of myocardial performance |
| Left ventricular stroke work index | Assessment and optimization of myocardial contractility through volume loading or adjustment. |
| Right heart ejection fraction | Right heart failure, P.E. |
| Oxygen delivery/consumption | Resuscitation endpoints |
| Mixed venous saturation | Oxygen delivery/consumption. |

hemodynamic monitoring and predicting changes in preload with volume resuscitation, and for use in the early resuscitation of the trauma patient.[38,39] Doppler capabilities allow for accurate measure of blood cell velocity. Stroke volume can then be determined by multiplying velocity by cross-sectional area of the blood vessel (the aorta in this case). While it is reasonably likely that TEE will be adapted for use as a routine monitoring device in the CCU, the devices are not quite to the point where they are "user friendly" in this setting.

## ARTERIAL BASE DEFICIT

The base deficit (BD) is a number calculated using the Henderson–Hasselbalch relationship (see following section) between pH, $PaCO_2$, and serum bicarbonate, which represents the stoichiometric equivalent of base that has to be added to the pH to return the patient to a normal pH of 7.40. Arterial BD is routinely calculated by blood gas analyzers and provides perhaps the best accessible metabolic indicator of shock states in the setting of major hemorrhage. It has been shown to be superior, as an indicator of hemorrhagic shock, to other parameters such as blood pressure, pulse, and urine output.[40,41] A rising base deficit in the setting of resuscitation indicates increasing metabolic acidosis; it has been correlated with the amount of blood transfused and occult abdominal injury and may stratify mortality in patients after major trauma.[41,42] In more recent studies, failure to clear a base deficit, defined as a persistent BD of <6, has been associated with increased incidence of ARDS, multiple-organ failure, and mortality.[43] Normalization of BD should, in the setting of major hemorrhage, be a primary goal of resuscitation in the operating room or CCU. Despite its utility as an indicator of hemorrhagic shock, BD is a nonspecific indicator of metabolic acidosis and may be elevated with ethanol, cocaine, and methamphetamine ingestion as well as seizures. Interpretation may be difficult under these circumstances and should be used carefully as a guide to volume resuscitation.[44]

## GASTRIC TONOMETRY

Gastric tonometry represents one of the first attempts at utilizing a measurement of specific organ perfusion as an endpoint to resuscitation. The rationale for monitoring gastrointestinal (GI) mucosal perfusion is based on the observation that splanchnic perfusion is often impaired, even in the setting of adequate blood pressure and cardiac output, and the increasing evidence pointing to impaired GI mucosal barrier function as an inciting factor in the development of multiple-organ dysfunction (see Chap. 68). At this time, however, the comparisons of gastric tonometry data to conventional resuscitation indices have not demonstrated a clear advantage of tonometry in detecting earlier or clinically significant malperfusion, and its use has not been widely adopted.[45,46]

## ERYTHROPOIETIN IN THE INTENSIVE CARE UNIT

There is mounting evidence that blood transfusions, independent of shock, or injury/disease severity, are associated with worsened outcomes in a variety of settings. Rates of infection, the incidence of multiple organ dysfunction, and even mortality appear to be correlated to the amount of blood transfused and the age of the banked blood. The need for blood transfusion in critically ill patients is substantial, with 40–45% of patients receiving on average 5 units of packed red blood cells. In addition, for patients with ICU stays longer than 13 days, that number increases to 85%.[47,48] These observations have led to attempts to reduce blood transfusion requirements in the CCU through the administration of exogenous erythropoietin, hoping to both stimulate new red cell production and offset the cytokine-related depression of erythropoietin production that occurs in many of these patients. In a study of this approach, Corwin, Gettinger et al.[49] conducted a Phase III randomized controlled trial of 1302 patients at 65 centers and found that the cohort receiving erythropoietin had a reduced need for red cell transfusion from 60.4% in the placebo group to 50.5%. Despite this reduction in units transfused, no significant differences were found between the two groups regarding mortality, lengths of stay, organ failure, or ventilator-free days. In a more recent randomized study by Silver et al.[50] 40,000 units of erythropoietin alfa was given to the experimental group of patients who were deemed "chronically" critically ill. In this subset, results again demonstrated reduced exposure to red cells but no difference in clinical outcomes. These studies suggest that the benefit of exogenously administered erythropoietin relate more to reductions in blood utilization rather than a clear improvement in outcomes.

## NEUROLOGICAL MONITORING

Neurological monitoring in the CCU has two goals: (a) the early detection of cerebral edema and/or expanding intracranial hematoma and (b) the avoidance of secondary brain injury by maintenance of adequate oxygenation and cerebral perfusion (see Chap. 20). The neurologic exam remains a mainstay for monitoring the multiply injured patient. Within this framework is the Glasgow Coma Scale (GCS) for assessment of verbal, motor, and occular response. For comatose patients and patients requiring mechanical ventilation, assessment of brain stem reflexes is imperative. Frequent reassessment of the neurologic exam is critical since even subtle changes may reflect early increases in intracranial pressure caused by cerebral edema or intracranial hemorrhage.

### Intracranial Pressure Monitoring

Intracranial pressure (ICP) monitoring with either a ventriculostomy catheter or subdural bolts has become the standard practice in most major centers for patients whose neurologic exams are unreliable, unavailable, or sufficiently depressed following head trauma. Latest guidelines published by the Brain Trauma Foundation call for early and aggressive monitoring of ICP and calculated cerebral perfusion pressure (CPP), the difference between mean arterial pressure and ICP.[51] The goal in ICP/CPP monitoring is to guide therapy (vasopressors, drainage, etc.) and provide surveillance for recurrent intracranial bleeding. The efficacy of ICP monitoring in a large population was the subject of a report by Thomason and Rutledge, who found a 51% versus 35% survival in patients with and without ICP monitoring despite a higher severity of injury in the monitored group.[52]

## JUGULAR VENOUS SATURATION MONITORING AND BRAIN TISSUE OXYGEN MONITORING

Several other monitoring devices continue to evolve in an attempt to understand and treat acute changes in oxygenation and perfusion, both globally and locally, in the injured brain. Jugular venous saturation monitoring reflects a ratio between cerebral blood flow and the cerebral metabolic rate for oxygen. The jugular venous saturation catheter provides a method of monitoring cerebral metabolism in the clinical setting. Saturation monitoring reflects a ratio between cerebral blood flow (CBF) and cerebral metabolic rate for oxygen ($CMRO_2$). To measure the saturation, one of three techniques are used: the standard intravascular technique for intermittent monitoring, fiberoptic oximetry (continuous measurement), or fiberoptic probes (continuous $PO_2$ monitoring). The catheter is used to determine oxygen saturation through the use of the Fick equation to estimate $CMRO_2$. The $C(a - jb)O_2$ calculation is the difference in arterial and jugular bulb venous oxygen content (jb = jugular bulb; CBF = cerebral blood flow).

The average saturation of jugular vein in the normal patient is 62%, with a range of 55–71%. For patients with severe head injury, the range of what is acceptable saturation varies more widely. Most investigators have used sustained desaturations of less than 50–55% to identify patients that need aggressive evaluation to exclude new pathology.[53–56]. If the catheter has a consistent reading below the 50% level, then trouble-shooting procedures should be used to ascertain whether there is a technical problem with the monitor.

The limitations of $SJO_2$ monitoring relate to its inability to identify regional brain ischemia, specifically in the "penumbra" of injured brain with impaired autoregulation at risk for secondary injury.

One of the most recent devices creating enthusiasm in the field is the use of brain tissue oxygen probes ($PtiO_2$). $PtiO_2$ is being used to measure the balance between oxygen supply and utilization. Low $PtiO_2$ measures are used to represent reduced levels of oxygen supply.[57] Thus far, $PtiO_2$ appears to correlate well with cerebral blood flow but is only considered "fair" in its ability to detect brain ischemia. A $PtiO_2$ measure of <20 mm Hg is considered a marker for brain ischemia.[58] In a recent study by Jaeger and colleagues, the $PtiO_2$ value seemed to act more as a cerebral blood flow monitor than as a measure of cerebral oxygen utilization.[59] $PtiO_2$, therefore is likely to be a rough measure of that balance between supply and demand more than a clear measure of utilization. In addition, $PtiO_2$ is likely to be affected by the state of cerebral autoregulation in the injured brain. Whether or not changes in the therapy for traumatic brain injury, guided by $PtiO_2$ will confer any survival or functional outcome benefit remains to be determined.

## NUTRITIONAL MONITORING

Nutritional assessment and monitoring in the critical care patient should begin shortly after CCU admission (see Chap. 66). Enteral alimentation, for simplicity and to minimize alterations in gut mucosal barrier function, is the preferred approach. Nutritional monitoring should begin with an assessment of the degree of preinjury malnutrition as well as current needs.

The calculation of nitrogen balance provides a more quantitative estimate of daily caloric requirements and should be assessed once weekly in the critically ill trauma patient. The calculation takes the difference from excreted nitrogen (calculated from 24-hour urine urea nitrogen) and the infused or ingested nitrogen. The overall goal is to have the patient at a 2- to 4-g positive nitrogen balance, if possible.[60] Indirect calorimetry (metabolic cart) provides the only online assessment of caloric requirements and metabolic rate. The technique uses the rate that gases are produced in the intubated patient to estimate the caloric expenditure. The basic principle is that $O_2$ ($\dot{V}O_2$) is consumed and $CO_2$ ($\dot{V}O_2$) is produced with nitrogenous waste and water. The metabolic cart measures $\dot{V}O_2$ and $CO_2$ for a period of time. When the RQ is known, energy estimated can be extrapolated to 24 hours. The RQ can vary from 0.7 to 1.2, depending on the metabolic substrate the whole body is consuming. Measurements are typically made several times a day or continuously to estimate the caloric needs over a 24-hour period.

## TIGHT GLYCEMIC CONTROL IN THE INTENSIVE CARE UNIT

Hyperglycemia with or without insulin resistance appears to be a common phenomenon in the critically ill. Based on the literature on diabetics who have improved long-term outcomes if their blood sugars are maintained below 215 mg/dL, Van den Berghe and colleagues hypothesized that hyperglycemia, or perhaps insulin deficiency leads to worse outcomes in the critically ill population.[61] In their prospective randomized controlled trial, they demonstrated that normalizing blood glucose levels (at or below 110 mg/dL) with intensive insulin therapy, improved mortality, such as infection rate, multiple organ failure rate and ventilator days, and morbidity.

Specifically addressing the effect of glycemic control in trauma patients who are critically ill, Vogelzang et al. retrospectively reviewed 12 years of data on trauma and nontrauma patients and found that hyperglycemia in the trauma patient correlated with an even worse mortality rate than in other surgical patients.[62]

These results have led to additional studies attempting to determine whether the effect on mortality in intensive insulin therapy for glycemic control is due to normalizing blood glucose or in the delivery of exogenous insulin. Preliminary reports suggest that lower levels of glucose confers most of the survival benefit based on observations that increased insulin administration was associated with increased mortality in the ICU, regardless of blood glucose levels.[63]

## ADRENAL INSUFFICIENCY IN THE CRITICALLY ILL

Increased levels of tissue corticosteroids during critical illness are likely a necessary part of the normal response to physiological stress. The normal corticosteroid response can be impaired however, in a variety of conditions including sepsis, SIRS, and traumatic brain injury. Failure to diagnosis and treat adrenal insufficiency has been associated with increased mortality.[64] Any patient with more severe sepsis, SIRS, prolonged respiratory failure, or unexplained hypotension or blood pressure lability should be considered high risk.

There is no uniform standard for the diagnosis of acute adrenal insufficiency in the critically ill patient. Random cortisol sampling may be helpful in screening patients, followed by treatment for low values ($<15$ $\mu$g/dL), or a corticotrophin stimulation test for intermediate values (15–34 mg/dL). Patients with abnormal stimulation tests (increases $<9$ mg/dL) require corticosteroid supplementation.[65]

Other approaches utilize serum-free cortisol for screening, thereby reducing the incidence of false-positive test related to hypoproteinemia effects on random cortisol levels (90% of total cortisol is protein-bound).[66]

## INFECTIOUS MONITORING AND SURVEILLANCE

Infectious sequelae of major injury (see Chap. 19) may occur as a result of the injury itself (e.g., open fractures), as a result of complications of treatment (e.g., anastomotic leak), or as iatrogenic complications of critical care management (e.g., ventilator-associated pneumonia). Specific monitoring for infections will depend on the injury type and severity, the types of interventions, and the duration of postinjury critical illness (Table 60-4). Monitoring for infection in the CCU can be complicated and must begin with vigilance. Mortality in the CCU is often attributed to infection and is thought to contribute to more than 88,000 deaths.[67] In a study using multiple regression analysis, the most important variables for infection were found to be central venous catheters, mechanical ventilation, pleural drainage, and trauma with open fractures.[68]

Patients at risk for infectious sequelae should be routinely tested by culture and examined for clinical indications such as hyperpyrexia, leukocytosis, related change in physical examination, pyuria, the development of purulent sputum, or a new infiltrate on chest x-ray.

The decision to institute presumptive (empiric) antibiotics should be based on risk factors, the expected sequelae of injury, and previous infections. Presumptive treatment should be started, if indicated, with a defined endpoint for culture-negative patients or a planned review with sensitivity and spectrum-based adjustment when culture information becomes available. All critically injured trauma patients with unexplained febrile episodes do not a priori require the administration of antibiotics. Persistently febrile, culture-negative patients often present a difficult diagnostic and therapeutic challenge. Fever in these patients may have noninfectious

**TABLE 60-4**

| Potential Sources of Infection in Critical Illness |
| --- |
| Nosocomial pneumonia |
| Line infection, thrombophlebitis |
| Urinary tract |
| Pseudomembranous/antibx.-associated colitis |
| Soft tissue wound infections |
| Site of injury infections: |
|    Chest, abdomen, mediastinum, neck, retroperitoneum |
| Intra-abdominal abscess/peritonitis |
| Acalculus cholecystitis/cholangitis/hepatitis |
| Perirectal/perianal abscess |
| Decubitis ulcer |
| Osteomyelitis |
| Endocarditis/pericarditis |
| Sinusitis |
| Mennigitis/ICP catheter infections |
| Otitis media |

**TABLE 60-5**

| Noninfectious Sources of Fever in Critical Illness |
| --- |
| Rhabdomyolysis |
| SIRS/sepsis syndrome |
| Adrenal cortical insufficiency |
| Pheochromocytoma (rare) |
| Drug fevers |
| Transfusion reaction |
| Malignant hyperthermia |
| Pancreatitis |
| Burn injury |
| Pulmonary embolism/DVT |
| Alcohol and drug withdrawal |
| CNS hemorrhage |

etiology (Table 60-5) or be due to occult infection that has either not been considered, not been successfully cultured, or has been present with no referable signs or symptoms. Low-grade culture-negative fungal sepsis should be considered in patients with prolonged CCU hospitalization, previous antibiotic treatment, and some degree of immunosuppression.

## MECHANICAL VENTILATION

The principal focus of a great deal of critical care is the management of mechanical ventilation and monitoring of mechanical ventilation (see Chap. 63). Ventilatory monitoring involves five areas: (a) gas exchange (the level of arterial oxygenation and the ability of the lungs to oxygenate the blood), (b) ventilation (the ability of the lungs to exchange $CO_2$), (c) lung mechanics (the elastic and resistive properties of the lungs), (d) inspiratory/expiratory pressures (the degree of positive pressure applied to the lungs during mechanical ventilation), and (e) the ventilatory capacity of the patient. Ventilatory and hemodynamic monitoring are inextricably linked due to the ability of transmitted mean intrathoracic pressures to impair cardiac output and the effect of cardiac output on dead space ratios, shunt fraction, and arterial oxygenation.

## MONITORING OF GAS EXCHANGE

Arterial oxygen tension ($PaO_2$) has long been the standard for assessment of oxygenation. More recently, the widespread use of pulse oximetry, which provides a continuous reading, has replaced much of the need for frequent blood gas sampling to assess oxygenation. Oximetry has limited use, however, in severe shock states, hypothermia, severe anemia, or in the measurement of other hemoglobin saturations (e.g., methemogloblin and carboxyhemoglobin).

Indices of the pulmonary oxygenating capacity include the (calculated) alveolar arterial oxygen gradient, the (calculated) intrapulmonary shunt fraction, and the ratio between the $PaO_2$ and $FIO_2$. This P/F ratio constitutes one of the basic criteria for defining acute lung injury (ALI) and ARDS (see Chap. 63). It provides a simple, direct, and highly useful bedside measure of gas exchange and avoids the extensive calculations required for both A-a gradient and shunt fractions.

## MONITORING OF VENTILATION

Arterial $CO_2$ tension remains the most accurate means of assessing ventilation. The development of infrared measurement of $CO_2$ allows continuous on-line determination of the end-expiratory $P_{CO_2}$ as an indirect reflection of $Pa_{CO_2}$. The critical issue in the use of end-tidal $CO_2$ ($ET_{CO_2}$) monitoring is the alveolar–arterial $CO_2$ gradient. In healthy patients with normal lungs, this gradient is typically 2–3 mm Hg. In selected populations of acutely injured trauma patients, the gradient appears to be low and allows, in effect, rapid, early, and continuous $Pa_{CO_2}$ monitoring.[69] There are a number of potential problems, however, with the routine use of $ET_{CO_2}$ in the intensive care population. The accuracy of the technique over time depends on a constant alveolar–arterial $CO_2$ gradient. This gradient is known to vary considerably with cardiac output, dead space ratios, airway resistance, and metabolic rate. As a result, longer-term $ET_{CO_2}$ monitoring in patients with more severe cardiac or pulmonary insufficiency is not recommended.

Measurement of dead space, a combination of both anatomic and physiologic dead space in the ventilator–lung circuit, may be calculated through the following equation:

$$V_D / V_T = (Pe_{CO_2} - Pa_{CO_2}) / Pa_{CO_2}$$

where $Pe_{CO_2}$ is the $CO_2$ of a multibreath sample. Dead space is dependent on a variety of factors, including cardiac output, ventilation–perfusion matching, breathing circuit dead space, and the presence of ALI or chronic obstructive pulmonary disease, and is an important determinant of minute volume requirements and ventilator weaning. The range of potential etiologies of hypercapnia in the trauma patient can be very broad. Increased $CO_2$ production may result from hypermetabolism in the multiply injured patient, the burn patient, or the septic patient. Hypoventilation from severe CNS injury or sedative/narcotics may be another source. Attention must also be given to the possibility of increased dead space resulting from ALI/ARDS or, more acutely, pulmonary embolism.

## ASSESSMENT OF LUNG MECHANICS AND INSPIRATORY/EXPIRATORY PRESSURES

The most important parameters used in assessing the mechanical properties of the airways and lungs are static and dynamic compliance. Compliance, the change in volume produced by a given change in pressure, is typically calculated from measured intratracheal (or ventilator circuit) pressures, and includes both lung and chest wall compliance. Compliance may be calculated based on peak inspiratory pressures (PIP) and incorporates any tube, airway, or bronchial resistance (dynamic compliance), or on the basis of inspiratory hold pressures (static compliance). Compliance is nonlinear and is increased at very low and very high lung volumes. The normal compliance of the lung and the chest wall (static) is approximately 100 mL/cm $H_2O$. Compliance is an important indicator of ALI and other disease states and is often a reflection of intra-alveolar injury (see Chap. 63). The measured difference between static and dynamic compliance is a reflection of airway resistance and may be increased with tracheal tube kinking or narrowing, cuff balloon occlusions, or bronchospasm. Large static–dynamic compliance gradients should provoke a search for a cause of high airway resistances.

The importance of inspiratory/expiratory pressure monitoring is related to the effect of these pressures on alveolar recruitment and gas exchange, as well as barotrauma/volutrauma (ventilator-induced lung injury). In acute respiratory failure, and particularly with ARDS or pulmonary edema, mean airway pressure is probably the most important determinant of alveolar recruitment and decreases in intrapulmonary shunt. Mean airway pressure may be increased through a number of ventilator settings including increased PEEP, increased PIP, increased intrinsic PEEP (planned or unplanned air trapping), and increased inspiratory:expiratory times (I:E ratio). While important for gas exchange in more severe lung injury, increased airway pressures have been linked to ventilator-induced lung injury (see "Mechanical Ventilation," above) and barotrauma.

Assessment of the pressure-volume curve in patients with more advanced acute lung injury has been utilized in an attempt to determine the mean critical pressure needed to reopen collapsed alveolar units.[70] This point corresponding to the transition between the flat portion and linear portion of the curve has been termed the lower inflection point (LIP) or Pflex. The steep part of the curve, between the LIP and the upper inflection point, may represent the zone of optimal ventilation, the physiologic space whereby alveolar recruitment is maintained and overdistention of alveoli is avoided (Fig. 60-1).[71]

There is concern on the part of some investigators that Pflex may not coincide with the mathematical point of maximum increased compliance, and interpretation may be further confounded by intra- and interobserver variability. More work needs to be done to better understand the relationships of the P–V curve and its application in the ventilation of patients with ALI/ARDS.

## VENTILATORY CAPACITY

In patients recovering from a variety of injuries associated with decreased ventilatory capacity—such as spinal cord injury, flail chest/rib fractures, and critical illness polyneuropathy (see section in this chapter, below)—it is important to assess ventilatory capacity regularly for purposes of both following clinical improvement

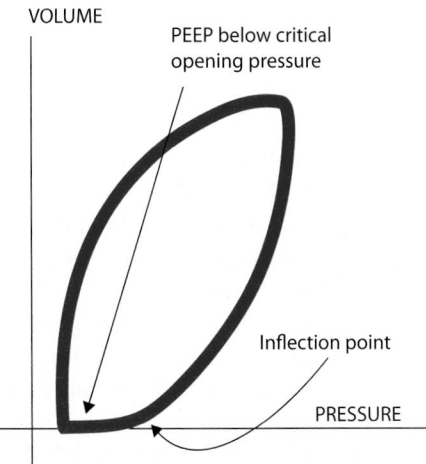

**FIGURE 60-1.** Typical IMV time/pressure tracing. Spontaneous breaths occur in between synchronized ventilator breaths.

and predicting tolerance of extubation. The most frequently measured indices of ventilatory capacity are voluntary vital capacity and maximum inspiratory pressure. Normally, vital capacity is between 65 and 75 mL/kg; a value of 10–15 mL/kg is typically used as a rough predictor of weaning outcome.

Maximum inspiratory pressure has been used by some clinicians as an indicator of weaning outcome, but it has not been accurate because of the dependency of this measurement on patient cooperation. A modified technique has been developed to make it more accurate.[72] This method uses a one-way valve to the airway to ensure that inspiratory efforts are made at low lung volume and the valve is occluded for a period of 20 seconds. A value of –30 cm $H_2O$ has been used as a predictor of weaning success. Tobin and Yang analyzed predictors of weaning and found the ratio of respiratory frequency to tidal volume (f/TV) to be the best predictor of weaning failure and weaning success in a group of medical CCU patients.[73]

## GENERAL MANAGEMENT OF MECHANICAL VENTILATION

Acute respiratory failure constitutes the most common indication for admission to many surgical CCUs and is a common sequela of major injury. As such, the use of mechanical ventilators is central to the function of posttrauma critical care. With the increase in the severity and duration of respiratory failure seen in many units today, management of mechanical ventilation is often conducted on a minute-to-minute, hour-to-hour basis. The need for constant attention to both ventilatory management and weaning constitutes the principal reason for independent, in-unit teams of physicians dedicated to the management of critically ill patients.

The institution of endotracheal intubation and mechanical ventilation often begins during the early resuscitative phase of treatment. Principal indications for endotracheal intubation and mechanical ventilation include the following:

1. The need to establish and maintain a secure airway
2. The need to assume the function of the ventilatory pump, moving gas in and out of the alveolar spaces (ventilation)
3. The need to provide increased $FIO_2$ and expiratory pressure to compensate for diminished gas exchange (oxygenation)
4. The need to prevent secondary injury to the brain by controlling $PaO_2$, $PaCO_2$ (and pH)
5. Prophylactic intubation in patients with anticipated (because of shock) neurologic injury, debility, chest wall/lung injury, large-volume fluid resuscitation, or possible inhalation injury to eventually require mechanical ventilation

The complexity of mechanical ventilators themselves has increased enormously since the first generation of simple volume cycle ventilators used prior to the mid-1960s. The development and increasing utilization of PEEP to maintain functional residual capacity and prevent deterioration of gas exchange was followed by development of modes using partial ventilatory support such as intermittent mandatory ventilation (IMV) in the early 1970s. Increasing utilization of microprocessors permitted additional modes of mechanical ventilation and led to the development of pressure support ventilation (PSV), time-cycled pressure-control ventilation (PCV), and inverse ratio ventilation over the last 10–15 years. Newer ventilators, equipped with waveform analyzers, allow continuous evaluation of breath-by-breath pressure-flow curves and calculation of machine work of breathing. In addition to the more conventional modes of ventilation, a number of alternatives have gained some popularity in adults over the last 5–10 years; high-frequency oscillation, pressure-regulated volume control (PRVC), and airway pressure-release ventilation (APRV). All of these modes alongside therapies such as prone ventilation, nitric oxide, and prostacycline represent attempts to limit lung injury, alleviate hypoxia, and improve comfort in the ventilated patient. (For a more complete review of the pathophysiology and treatment of acute lung injury see Chap. 63.)

## VENTILATOR-INDUCED LUNG INJURY

The need for prolonged, high-pressure mechanical ventilation has been increasing along with the severity and survivability of patients with severe ARDS. Barotrauma, most commonly heralded by spontaneous pneumothorax or persistent bronchopleural fistula, has historically been a common problem with the past use of high-pressure mechanical ventilation.

In addition to barotrauma, high-pressure ventilation may produce impairment of cardiac output through transmitted intrathoracic pressure, pulmonary edema (possibly through direct injury to the terminal airways), and further decreases in lung compliance.[74] Ventilator factors implicated in induced lung injury include peak, mean, and end-expiratory pressures, use of excessive tidal volumes and inspiratory flow rates, and high concentration of inspired oxygen. Limitation of high pressures and high volumes may be facilitated through the use of pressure-control ventilation, pressure support ventilation in eligible patients, and permissive hypercapnia. Permissive hypercapnia refers to "permitted" increases in $PaCO_2$ through reduced tidal volumes, airway pressures, and alveolar ventilation, and is thought to be useful in limiting ventilator-induced lung injury in patients with severe alterations in lung mechanics (see Chap. 63).

The use of specific ventilatory modes to achieve lower airway pressures and the outcome utility of doing so has been the subject of several earlier reports of promising results.[75–77] Against this background, the NIH initiated a network of critical care centers in 1994 for the purposes of multi-institutional trials for ARDS interventions. In 1996, the ARDS network began a multi-institutional study comparing outcomes of two ventilation strategies using larger (12 mg/kg ideal body weight) and small (6 mg/kg ideal body weight) tidal volume breaths in patients with acute lung injury. This study was discontinued in 1999 after recruiting 861 patients as the result of significant decreased mortality in the low tidal volume group (31.0% vs. 39.8%, $p=0.007$) and increased number of ventilator-free days during the first month ($12\pm11$ vs. $10\pm11$; $p=0.007$). There were also fewer disease-related complications.[78] The results of this RCT have substantially altered the approach to ventilator management in the setting of acute lung injury, justifying the routine use of lower tidal volume ventilation with or without the use of permissive hypercapnia. More recent reports suggest that higher tidal volumes at the initiation of mechanical ventilation may play a role in the induction of ventilator-associated lung injury, even prior to the onset of ARDS.[79] This supports the increasing use of "preemptive" low tidal volume ventilation in patients deemed to be at higher risk for the development of ARDS.

Preliminary clinical and experiment observations have suggested a relationship between ventilator-induced lung injury and lower end-expiratory volumes, possibly caused by the mechanical forces associated with recurrent opening and closing of distal bronchi and alveoli. This led to a subsequent network study examining the effects of higher PEEP, lower $FIO_2$ versus lower PEEP, higher $FIO_2$ on patients with acute lung injury. This report, involving the randomized study of 549 patients, showed similar outcomes in the treatment (high PEEP) and control groups.[80] A more recent, albeit smaller randomized clinical trial refuted these results when PEEP was adjusted based on the pressure–volume inflection point. Villar et al. showed improved outcomes, including ICU mortality (53 vs. 32% $p = 0.04$), hospital mortality, and ventilator-free days.[81] These conflicting results suggest that higher PEEP may have some advantages in a more selected subset of patients.

## VENTILATORY MODES

The principal physiologic effect produced by mechanical ventilation is related to positive versus negative airway pressures, as is the case during spontaneous ventilation. Positive pressure has a number of salutary effects on gas exchange, produced mainly by the recruitment of marginal alveolar air spaces, increasing functional residual capacity, improving ventilation/perfusion matching, and decreasing intrapulmonary shunt. Adverse effects of positive pressure relate to its ability to produce barotrauma and ventilator-induced lung injury through the use of either excessive inflation volumes or inflation pressures and the potential for impairment of cardiac output produced by increases in mean intrathoracic pressure. In general, some degree of both salutary and adverse effects of mechanical ventilation is common to all modes of mechanical ventilation since they all utilize, to varying degrees, positive insufflation pressures.

## CONTROL-MODE AND ASSIST/CONTROL-MODE VENTILATION

Control-mode (CV) and assist/control-mode ventilation (ACV) are volume-cycled modes that deliver a preset tidal volume at a minimum set respiratory rate and inspiratory flow rate, regardless of the patient's own ventilatory efforts. In CV, the ventilator will not trigger with patient effort, and no additional breaths will be administered despite additional patient-derived ventilatory effort. Given the safety and comfort of other ventilatory modes, CV should generally not be used as a routine setting.

ACV allows a patient, through his or her own inspiratory efforts, to trigger the ventilator and receive a single, preset breath. Depending on the patient's condition and the sensitivity and type (flow vs. pressure) of inspiratory trigger, this mode allows the patient to preset his or her own rate of tidal volume (with set ventilator rate acting as a backup minimum). ACV is typically used in patients with paralytic conditions (e.g., chemical paralysis, paralytic neuromuscular disease), or those requiring large amounts of conscious sedation who are not necessarily capable of triggering the ventilator or breathing spontaneously on PSV or IMV mode. ACV may also be used to minimize patient-derived work of breathing (WOB) by setting a sufficiently high rate so as to prevent more than minimal triggering of the ventilator. Excessive ventilator triggering has been associated with

substantial increases in patient WOB. However, the inspiratory trigger must be sufficiently sensitive as to not require, independently, large amounts of inspiratory force, thereby increasing work of breathing.[82]

## PRESSURE–REGULATED VOLUME-CONTROLLED VENTILATION (PRVC)

PRVC was developed as a means of delivering volume-controlled ventilation that was not as subject to excessive peak airway pressures and associated alveolar overdistention as conventional volume-control modes. The PRVC mode utilizes a regulated, decelerating inspiratory flow pattern that limits peak inspiratory pressures but still delivers a preset tidal volume, unlike pressure-controlled modes. Although there are theoretical advantages with PRVC, preliminary randomized studies have been unable to demonstrate clear salutary effects with the exception of reduced peak inspiratory pressures.[83]

## INTERMITTENT MANDATORY VENTILATION

IMV was developed in the early 1970s in order to allow spontaneous patient ventilation in addition to that provided by a preset minimum ventilator rate and tidal volume (Fig. 60-2). This mode was developed initially as a method of weaning patients from mechanic ventilation, allowing a smoother transition than the classic "T-piece trials" generally in use at the time. Synchronized IMV (SIMV) was developed to avoid "stacking" ventilatory breath on top of a spontaneous patient breath at end-inspiration.

SIMV continues to be widely used as a weaning mode and has the advantage of allowing stepwise decreases in machine work versus patient work. In patients with a low compliance, however, IMV may not allow sufficient spontaneous tidal volumes due to extremely limited patient inspiratory capacity. In this setting, pressure support may be used to support each IMV breath, thereby increasing patient-initiated tidal volume and decreasing incremental patient-derived work.

## PRESSURE SUPPORT VENTILATION

PSV was developed in the 1980s as a patient-triggered pressure-limited flow-cycled ventilatory mode. Each PS ventilator breath is triggered spontaneously by the patient and provides a pressure-limited ventilatory assist, typically with high maximum inspiratory

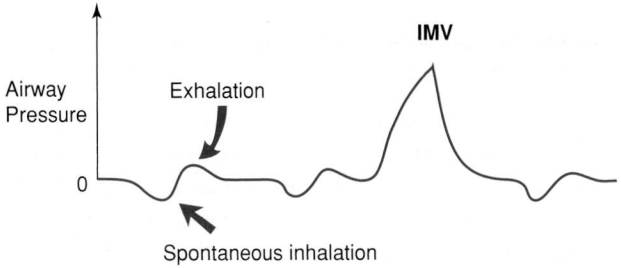

**FIGURE 60-2.** Typical IMV time/pressure tracing. Spontaneous breaths occur in between synchronized ventilator breaths.

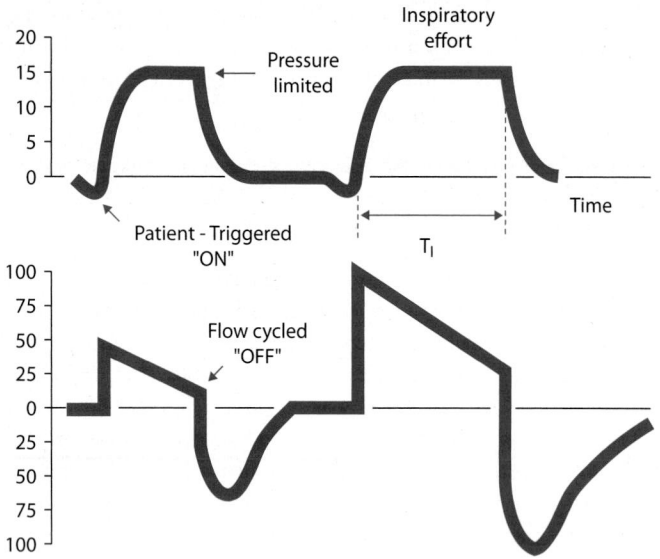

FIGURE 60-3. Pressure support ventilation. Pressure limitation (15 mmHg.) is shown in upper tracing. As tidal volume approaches maximum, inspiratory flow decreases, terminating the pressure assist. In the second wave-form, increased patient-derived inspiratory effort results in higher flow rates and larger tidal volumes.

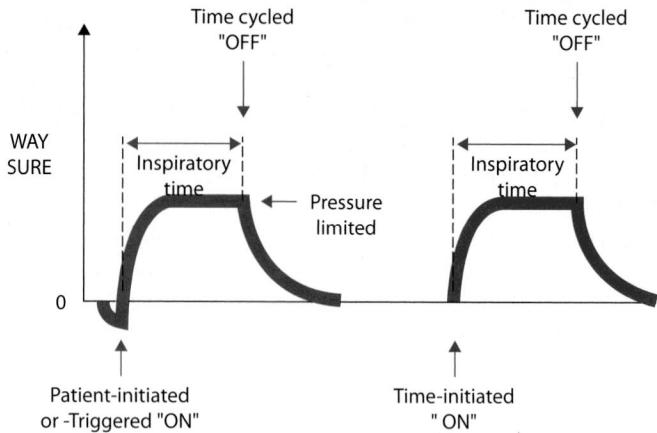

FIGURE 60-4. Time-cycled, pressure control ventilation. Fixed time-cycled breath with pressure limitation may be driven by minimum set rate ± patient triggered breaths.

flow rates during inspiration. Termination of this ventilatory assist occurs when the patient's own inspiratory flow demand decreases below a preset limit, allowing spontaneous expiration. This produces a flow-cycled as opposed to pressure volume-cycled ventilatory breath (Fig. 60-3). Pressure support ventilation does not rely on a mandatory preset ventilatory rate and each breath must be patient triggered. This makes PSV unusable in patients with neuromuscular disease, chemical paralysis, or heavy conscious sedation.

PSV has a number of inherent advantages, including improved patient–ventilator synchrony due to spontaneous triggering. PSV may be used at low levels of support to provide minimal ventilatory support just prior to extubation or at high levels (20 to 40 cm H$_2$O) as a means of providing a full mechanical ventilatory support with relatively small patient-derived WOB. As a weaning mode, pressure support may be used in conjunction with intermittent mandatory ventilation as previously described, or as a stand-alone mode with a preset level of inspiratory pressure being gradually reduced to allow the patient to assume more of his or her own WOB. In patients with weak ventilatory reserve, however, inappropriately low levels of pressure support may provide grossly inadequate minute ventilation, and the use of this mode requires careful monitoring of rate and tidal volume.

## TIME-CYCLED PRESSURE-CONTROL VENTILATION

Volume-cycled ventilation, particularly in the setting of severe acute lung injury (ARDS) and poor lung compliance, may lead to excessive PIP and/or high inflation volumes in some pulmonary segments, causing secondary ventilator-induced lung injury. This recognition has led to the increased use of time-cycled pressure-control ventilation. In this ventilatory mode, inspired gas is delivered at a present inspiratory flow rate up to a preset pressure (Fig. 60-4). The ventilator breath is terminated on the basis of set cycle time, not on the basis of flow, as is the case with pressure control. Pressure-control ventilation has the advantage of providing a continuous limit to PIP, despite changes in lung and chest wall compliance or patient dyssynchrony. As such, it is a useful and perhaps safer ventilatory mode in the setting of low-compliance lung injury typically seen with ARDS. PCV, however, is not uniformly well tolerated by awake patients and often requires appropriately titrated conscious sedation.

Inverse ratio ventilation (IRV)[84–86] may be a variation of either volume-control or pressure-control ventilation but is most commonly used in conjunction with PCV. IRV is a modern adaptation of the older practice of using prolonged inspiratory "holds" introduced in the early 1970s, associated with improved functional residual capacity and gas exchange in some patients. Conventional mechanical ventilation uses I:E ratios of 1:2 to 1:1.2, allowing a relatively long expiratory phase, thereby minimizing mean airway pressures. IRV, typically used with I:E ratios of 1.1:1 to 2:1, may be achieved by using relatively rapid inspiratory flow rates and decelerating flow patterns to maintain a designated pressure during the inspiratory ventilatory phase (see Fig. 60-4).

There are two principal effects of IRV: (a) prolonged inspiratory time acts to increase MAP and recruit marginal alveolar airspaces, similar to the effect produced by increases in set PEEP, and (b) in more severe airway disease, as a result of peribronchial narrowing in the terminal airways, there is slower equilibration of intrapulmonary pressures with each tidal volume, leading to differential alveolar ventilation. This unequal ventilation may deprive perfused alveoli of adequate gas exchange, leading to increased intrapulmonary shunt. Through the careful application of IRV, a desired amount of gas trapping, reflected by auto- or intrinsic PEEP, may be produced, thereby selectively increasing intra-alveolar pressure in these smaller, narrowed airspaces. This effect may be associated with improved shunt and oxygenation. Intrinsic PEEP must be carefully measured, however, to avoid progressive gas-trapping alveolar overdistention and secondary ventilator-induced lung injury. The utility of IRV in this setting, however, is controversial, and is discussed more completely in Chap. 63.

Despite the attractiveness of the ability to selectively deliver PEEP with IRV, there is some question as to whether this effect adds anything to the simpler effect of increasing mean airway pressures.

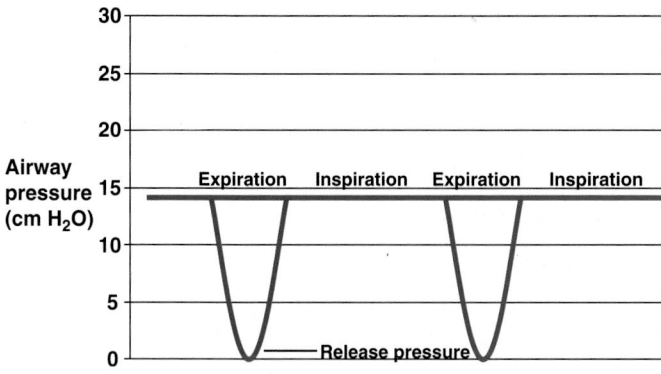

**FIGURE 60-5.** Airway pressure patterns in APRV.

Studies such as the one by Lessard[87] suggest that although pressure control may be used to reduce peak inspiratory pressures, no significant benefit of PCV or PCIRV versus conventional volume ventilation with additional PEEP could be demonstrated in patients with acute respiratory failure. This point of view is also further developed by Shanholtz and Brower, who questioned the utility of IRV in the treatment of ARDS.[88]

## AIRWAY-PRESSURE-RELEASE VENTILATION

APRV is fundamentally a high-level continuous positive airway pressure (CPAP) mode (Fig. 60-5). The short release period allows for carbon dioxide to be cleared. The patient is able to breath spontaneously throughout all phases of the cycle. The theoretical advantages in APRV include lower airway pressures and minute ventilation, improved alveolar recruitment, improved patient comfort with spontaneous breathing, and minimal hemodynamic effects. Since the patient is able to breathe spontaneously through an open and floating expiratory valve, this mode may be more tolerable, particularly in patients being actively weaned from sedation or showing signs of clinical improvement after head injury. Early work with this mode of ventilation reveals improvement in hemodynamics, attributed to improved alveolar recruitment. Additionally, there is some evidence that providing a mode that allows for spontaneous breathing throughout decreases sedation requirements.[89]

## HIGH-FREQUENCY OSCILLATORY VENTILATION

Interest in HFOV in adults with respiratory failure evolved out of the concern that conventional ventilation may induce further lung injury due to the shear forces generated by repetitive opening and closing of airways. In HFOV, a relatively higher mean airway pressure is set and small tidal volumes at very high rates are delivered. The objective, therefore, is to achieve and maintain lung recruitment and avoid large shear forces to the alveoli.

Most experience in the literature with this mode of ventilation is seen in the neonatal and pediatric populations. In a recently published study by Mehta et al., 24 adults with ARDS with a variety of etiologies were enrolled in a prospective trial to receive HFOV as "rescue therapy."[90] Of these patients, 42% showed improvement in oxygenation and were able to be weaned back to conventional ventilation. The barotrauma rate was similar to that of other ARDS populations. Finally, survivors tended to have fewer ventilator days prior to placement on HFOV than nonsurvivors. More investigation needs to be conducted to shed light on its suspected high efficacy in patients with early ARDS or inhalational injuries.

## ADJUVANT THERAPIES IN RESPIRATORY FAILURE

Developments in the laboratory and at the bedside over the last several years have expanded the armamentarium available for the treatment of patients with respiratory failure. Mechanical and pharmaceutical therapies have been combined with conventional mechanical ventilation in an effort to improve outcomes in this patient population (see Chap. 63). The use of prone positioning to effect improvement in gas exchange appears to be based on the more uniform distribution of gas within the lungs and associated improvement in shunt fraction, associated with the supine position of the relatively larger dorsal components of the lung. Randomized clinical trials to date have failed to demonstrate a survival benefit, but reports of improved oxygenation have been relatively consistent.[91–94] In addition, there is suggestion that an earlier application of prone ventilation to patients prior to developing low-compliance acute lung injury may have durable benefit.[91,92]

Inhalational agents designed to improve gas exchange include nitric oxide (NO) and the prostaglandins $PGE_1$ and $PGI_2$. While not definitively worked out, the mechanism of actions of these agents appears to be related to their ability to reverse, to some degree, the adverse effects of acute lung injury on normal hypoxic vasoconstrictive reflexes in the lung. By relaxing vascular smooth muscle in the lung, shunt fraction is improved by allowing improved circulation to ventilated alveoli. The effect of NO appears to be more pronounced in patients with high pulmonary vascular resistance, suggesting altered or excessive HPV. Unfortunately, clinical trials of inhalational agents have shown early improvement in gas exchange but have not been able to demonstrate any overall improvement in outcome from acute lung injury.[95–97]

The potential for combination therapy to produce synergistic effects in the setting of acute lung injury has generated several reports. Almitrine, a peripheral chemoreceptor stimulant and selective pulmonary vasoconstrictor, has been combined with NO to produce improvement in P/F ratios and vascular pressures.[98] Combining prone positioning and inhaled nitric oxide in patients with ARDS has also been associated with improvement in gas exchange, with an apparent synergistic effect.[99] As has been a recurring theme with adjuvant therapies, however, sustainable positive effects and improvements in outcome have yet to be proven.

## WEANING FROM MECHANICAL VENTILATION

One of the primary and unique functions of a critical care team, and one that often occupies considerable time and effort, is the management of weaning from mechanical ventilation. Ventilator weaning is the transition process by which the patient, as opposed to the mechanical ventilator, assumes the function of the ventilatory pump—moving air in and out of the lungs. Most of this process is dedicated to improving ventilatory strength and endurance sufficient to allow discontinuation of mechanical ventilation. This program of ventilatory strength and endurance training constitutes ventilatory reconditioning. Ventilatory reconditioning should not necessarily be equated with extubation, although there is frequently a strong temporal association in the course of critical illness. The reconditioning process should also not necessarily be delayed or deferred due to contraindications to extubation.

For the majority of postinjury patients requiring mechanical ventilation, the reconditioning process is relatively short and straightforward. In patients with short-term ventilatory requirements who have no decreases in ventilatory capacity or increases in their work of breathing (e.g., patients undergoing elective surgery), the process is limited to the reversal of chemical paralysis and anesthetic agents, perhaps a brief trial of spontaneous "T-piece" ventilation, and extubation. For patients with more prolonged but transient decreases in ventilatory capacity and increases in ventilatory work, such as patients requiring large-volume resuscitation or patients with moderate head injuries, weaning from mechanical ventilation does not usually require ventilatory strength and endurance conditioning and can be satisfactorily achieved by reductions in ventilatory support commensurate with the patient's recovery. In this setting, stepwise ("staircase") reductions in either IMV rate or set pressure support level result in progressive reductions in machine WOB to the extent it is tolerated by the patient and allow extubation at or near a time at which the patient has normalized his or her own ventilatory capacity and ventilatory work.

The group of patients that require prolonged, directed efforts at reconditioning from mechanical ventilation are those with longer-term/permanent decreases in ventilatory work or longer-term/permanent decreases in ventilatory capacity. This group might include patients with high spinal cord injury, those with post-ARDS pulmonary fibrosis, and elderly patients recovering from prolonged respiratory failure/malnutrition. In many cases, this patient population is distinguished by their need for some sort of respiratory muscle strength and conditioning to compensate for chronically increased ventilatory work or decreased capacity.

Under normal circumstances, it is thought that the ratio of resting ventilatory reserve compared to normal ventilatory work is approximately 10:1, creating a large margin of safety in most patients. Ventilatory failure, a failure of the ventilatory pump, occurs when this safety margin is overcome and ventilatory capacity is exceeded by the work requirements. In analyzing the treatable causes of ventilatory failure as part of the weaning process, it is useful to separate the various causes into those acting to increase ventilatory work and those acting to reduce ventilatory capacity (Table 60-6). Efforts at ventilatory weaning should be directed at reversing or decreasing injury and iatrogenically related increases in WOB and instituting measures that will improve the patient's individual ventilatory capacity.

## WEANING AND WORK OF BREATHING

The ventilatory WOB is roughly a function of pressure or force required to expand the lungs and chest wall and the total volume (minute volume) required to meet physiologic demands. Ventilatory "horsepower" requirements, therefore, equate roughly to pressure (force) × volume (distance)/time (minutes). Factors acting to increase ventilatory work include any that will produce decreased thoracoabdominal compliance, including increased chest wall

edema or hematoma, abdominal distention, endobronchial hemorrhage or pulmonary contusion, and disruption of the surfactant monolayer as well as post-ARDS pulmonary fibrosis. Increased airway resistance may also interfere with the weaning process by increasing ventilatory work. In patients intubated with smaller sized (<7 mm) endotracheal tubes, there may be significant additional imposed work due to flow restriction, particularly in the face of higher minute volumes or narrowing of the tube caused by inspissated secretions. The use of pressure support during the weaning process and prior to extubation is one method, short of exchanging the endotracheal tube, for counteracting this added resistive work.[100] There is preliminary evidence suggesting that certain ventilatory strategies such as the use of decelerating inspiratory flow rates and periodic hyperinflation may minimize WOB.[101,102]

Volume- and time-related factors are those that act to increase minute ventilation (tidal volume × rate). These factors include increased physiologic or anatomic dead space such that occurs following lung injury, decreased cardiac output, and shock states, which act to increase physiologic dead space and increases in anatomic dead space associated with endotracheal intubation. Increased $CO_2$ productions from fever or overfeeding will also increase minute volume requirements (for a set pH) and increase ventilatory work.

## WEANING AND VENTILATORY CAPACITY

Ventilatory capacity is a function of respiratory muscle (diaphragm, intercostals, abdominals, accessories) strength and endurance, muscle innervation, and the adequate delivery of nutritional substrates and oxygen. Prior to beginning the weaning process, all these factors should be considered and deficiencies corrected to the extent possible. Ultimately, improvement in ventilatory capacity may require a program of respiratory muscle conditioning as described below.

Factors such as severe hypophosphatemia are an easily reversible cause of muscular weakness (see Table 60-6). Malnutrition and critical illness polyneuropathy may also produce deficits in muscle strength and endurance, and typically take longer to correct. Diminished cardiac reserve, particularly in association with high WOB requirements, may affect respiratory muscle blood flow and retard the weaning process. Spinal cord injuries may start to produce changes in ventilatory capacity as low as the T10 level by decreasing abdominal muscle tone and interfering with diaphragmatic contour, thereby reducing inspiratory force.

Impairment of ventilatory capacity secondary to chest wall injury, pain, and even the dyssynchrony that occurs frequently after abdominal surgery may also be important factors to consider when beginning the weaning process, particularly in patients with increased ventilatory work.

## WEANING VERSUS EXTUBATION

A clear distinction should be made between weaning from mechanical ventilation (stepwise reduction machine-related ventilatory work) to actual removal of the *artificial airway* (extubation). Often, the two are equated and confused, leading to delays in the actual reconditioning and weaning process. In most circumstances, the weaning process should begin as soon as actual or anticipated

**TABLE 60-6**

**Factors Pertaining to Ventilatory Capacity and Work of Breathing**

| DECREASED VENT. CAPACITY | CAUSE | TREATMENT |
|---|---|---|
| Malnutrition | Chronic respiratory muscle weakness caused by protein-calorie insufficiency and catabolism | Establish anabolic state. Ensure adequate nutrition. Recovery may be prolonged. |
| Metabolic Derangements: PO4, Mg++, Ca++ etc. | Typically associated with hyperalimentation and inadequate replacement. | Replenishment. Adjustment of hyper/enteral alimentation. Evaluate other causes. |
| Cardiac Insufficiency | Underlying disease, myocardial infarction, blunt myocardial injury | Establish diagnosis & appropriate monitoring to evaluate function & volume status. Treat underlying cause of myocardial insufficiency. May require inotropic agents |
| Spinal Cord Injury | Primary injury | Abdominal binding to improve function & tussive capacity. Upright posture. Establish program for respiratory muscle conditioning. |
| Chest Wall Injury, thoracotomy incision/pain. | Dysfunctional respiratory patterns caused by pain, splinting or mechanical instability of the chest wall | Directed analgesia: epidural opiates ± bipuvacaine or other methods. [surgical stabilization of chest wall – very selected cases] |
| Abdominal Injury/Laparotomy | Dys-synchronous respiratory pattern associated with laparotomy ± opiate agents. | Pain control. Ambulation (if possible). Early respiratory muscle exercise (e.g. incentive spirometry) |
| Critical illness polyneuropathy | May be associated with prolonged use of paralytic agents and steroids. Nonspecific. | Confirm diagnosis & exclude other causes. Limit/discontinue use of paralytic agents ± steroids. Establish program for respiratory muscle conditioning. Expectant. |
| Decreased muscle strength/atrophy | Nonspecific. Dis-use atrophy associated with prolonged mechanical ventilation, prolonged critical illness, prolonged catabolic state. | Exclude other causes. Treat other reversible causes of decr. vent. Capacity or increase WOB. EARLY establishment of program for respiratory muscle conditioning. |
| Functional limitation: fear/anxiety, lack of motivation, lack of understanding. | Lack of understanding process & goals. Poor tolerance of decrease tidal volumes/rate. | Reassurance, encouragement, "coaching", careful use of anxiolytics. Use of different weaning ventilatory modes. |
| **INCREASED VENTILATORY WORK** | | |
| Decreased pulmonary & chest wall compliance. | Surfactant depletion/sepsis/ARDS, chronic/acute pulmonary fibrosis, endo-bronchial hemorrhage, massive fluid resuscitation and chest wall edema, high FRC ventilation/overdistention | Restrict high pressure/volume ventilation. Assess PEEP/TV compliance grid. Active or passive diuresis. |
| Decreased abdominal compliance. | Ileus/abdominal distention, intra-abd compart. syndrome (IACS), ascites | NG decompression. Restriction of enteral alimentation temporarily. Dx./rx. IACS, fluid/salt restriction, diruesis as needed. |
| Increased airway resistance | Endotracheal tube size/obstruction/narrowing. Bronchospasm, bronchial mucus plugging | Consider up-sizing ETT. Wean with pressure support sufficient to overcome tube resistance. Bronchodialators as needed. Suctioning & mucolytic agents as needed. [bronchoscopy] |
| Increased minute volume requirements: increases in physiologic/anatomic deadspace. | Acute lung injury, barotrauma, emphysema, decreased cardiac output, excessive breathing circuit deadspace. | Restrict high pressure/volume ventilation. Rx. Myocardial dysfunction as above. [tracheostomy] |
| Increased minute volume requirements: CO2 production, metabolic acidosis. | Infection, SIRS, high carbohydrate substrates, excessive hyper or enter alimentation | Rx. Infection. Pyrolytics. Alter nutritional substrate to higher lipid content. Adjust hyper/enteral alimentation. |

organ-system instability has resolved. In a recent consensus report, several criteria for the consideration of discontinuation of mechanical ventilation were suggested[103]:

1. Evidence of reversal of underlying cause for respiratory failure

2. Adequate oxygenation (P/F ratio >150–200 with PEEP less than 5–8, $FIO_2 < 0.4$–0.5, and pH>7.25)

3. Hemodynamic stability (absence of shock states with adequate cardiac function)

4. The capacity to initiate an inspiratory effort

Further factors entering into the decision to discontinue endotracheal intubation, in addition to ventilatory capacity and demands, include airway protection, tussive capacity, the extent of mucous secretions, and anticipated organ-system stability (Table 60-7). Assessment of capacity for airway protection in the trauma patient can be broken into two categories: evaluation of suspected anatomic compromise and neurologic fitness.

In order to assess subglottic airway patency, deflation of the cuff slowly and listening for the pressure at which a "leak" can be detected can give valuable information. Pressures higher than

**TABLE 60-7**

**Suggested Criteria for Extubation**

| CRITERIA FOR EXTUBATION (ALL MUST BE MET) | ASSOCIATED (SUGGESTED) PHYSIOLOGICAL PARAMETERS OR PHYSICAL FINDINGS |
|---|---|
| Ability to maintain & protect airway | • Adequate laryngeal function<br>• Intact gag and swallowing reflexes<br>• Adequate leak around deflated ETT balloon<br>• No evidence for cord/laryngeal edema<br>• Exclusion of possible cord/laryngeal function/edema by laryngoscopy as needed.<br>• Mental status commensurate w/ airway protection |
| Ability to maintain adequate oxygenation | • $FiO_2 \leq 0.4$ & adequate $O_2$ saturation ($>97\%$)<br>• No requirement for PEEP<br>• Adequate independent ventilation |
| Ability to maintain adequate ventilatiion | • Minute ventilation $<10–12$ Liters/min<br>• RR $<30\text{-}35$<br>• MIF $> -30$, VC $> 12–15$ cc/kg.<br>• Toleration of minimal ventilator support of t-piece without clinical evidence of ventilatory fatigue |
| Ability to clear secretions | • Adequate tussive capacity (subjective)<br>• No significant impairment of mucocilliary function<br>• Secretions not excessive<br>• Postextubation tracheal suctioning not difficult and suctioning requirements not excessive. |
| No expected deterioration in relevant organ system function (re-intubation not anticipated) | • No developing major infection, sepsis etc.<br>• Adequate cardiac reserve<br>• No anticipated deterioration in neurological, pulmonary, or cardiac function.<br>• No short-term need for re-operation. |

10 cm $H_2O$ are associated with increased risk for airway compromise. This test can be difficult to reproduce without a large margin of error, however. In a compliant patient, deflating the cuff and assessing the ability to breath around the tracheal tube can be helpful. Evaluating the airway and supraglottic structures in higher-risk patients may be accomplished using a fiberoptic scope. Additionally, direct laryngoscopy can be used to assess the characteristics of the soft tissues in the hypopharynx and of the true vocal cords.

Precise guidelines for extubation of the head-injured patient have been very difficult to establish. Somewhat arbitrary guidelines such as spontaneous eye opening have been used to determine eligibility for weaning. A recent study by Namen et al. looked at the association of GCS with success of extubation.[104] They found that a GCS of 8 or greater was associated with success 75% of the time, versus 33% for a GCS <8. The group's recommendations centered on incorporating information from a rigorous neurologic assessment into standard guidelines for weaning when making ventilator decisions in this population.

## THE WEANING PROCESS

A weaning method consists of the application of a specific ventilatory mode with the goal of reduction and eventual removal of mechanical ventilatory support. A weaning ventilatory mode is typically one that allows stepwise decrements in the amount of machine support of the WOB (e.g., IMV, pressure support, or a combination). The mode of ventilation used for the weaning process is probably less critical than the method used. The critical distinction is between those weaning methods that incorporate a conditioning regimen for respiratory musculature and those that do not. The muscles of ventilation (diaphragm, intercostals, etc.) are skeletal muscles and would be expected to respond to a conditioning program in a manner similar to all skeletal muscle. Most conditioning programs involve the common elements of periods of vigorous muscle work separated by periods of complete muscle rest. There is considerable literature supporting the concept of inspiratory (respiratory) muscle strength and endurance conditioning, which is consistent with endurance training in older studies of skeletal muscle.[105–107] There is additional evidence that suggests that ventilatory muscle performance may be enhanced by this type of conditioning.[108] In addition, it appears that the muscles of respiration may be conditioned separately for either strength or endurance,[109] although the clinical relevance of such focused conditioning is questionable. The most commonly used weaning method has traditionally been one that involves a continuous or "staircase" progression of decreasing IMV and/or pressure-support ventilation to the point of allowing independent patient ventilation. This method generally does not utilize either periods of vigorous respiratory exercise or periods of ventilatory rest. While probably successful in the majority of low-work, high-capacity patients, these staircase methods have the disadvantage of either underworking the patient, leading to delayed extubation, or overworking the patient, leading to a state of chronic fatigue from which further weaning, in the absence of a substantial period of rest, will be impossible.

One of the first comparative studies of ventilatory weaning was performed by Brochard and colleagues.[110] In this randomized study, three methods of weaning were compared: T-piece trials, synchronized IMV, and pressure-support ventilation. The study found pressure-support weaning in a staircase manner to be associated with a shorter period of mechanical ventilation. The criteria for extubation in this study were different, however, and the numbers were relatively small (n = 109). In a subsequent, much larger randomized prospective study, Esteban and coworkers, in a multi-institutional setting, compared four different methods of weaning from mechanical ventilation.[111] In this study, two continuous or staircase methods using intermittent mandatory ventilation and pressure-support ventilation were compared to two intermittent methods, one using a once-daily trial of spontaneous breathing and one using multiple daily trials of spontaneous breathing. The study found that both intermittent methods led to extubation significantly more rapidly than either of the continuous (staircase) methods. Although based on indirect evidence, this study supports the use of respiratory muscle conditioning through a weaning protocol involving exercise and rest periods and suggests that this is a superior means of reconditioning weakened respiratory muscles following prolonged critical illness. These results are also consistent with previous observations that adaptive changes of skeletal/respiratory musculature are best produced by specific conditioning programs involving elements of relatively strenuous work and periods of complete rest.[112,113]

The utility of a program of muscle conditioning using progressive resistive exercise protocols in high quadriplegics was further supported in a report by Lerman and Weiss in a 1987 study examining the use of such a protocol in a small series of quadriplegics. The authors concluded that specific focused diaphragmatic training is useful in weaning high-level quadriplegics with chronic decreases in ventilatory capacity from mechanical ventilation.[114] Validation of the concept of inspiratory muscle strength conditioning for ventilator weaning has been more recently provided.[115]

The randomized studies of weaning methods have tended to use intermittent T-piece breathing as the means for providing respiratory muscle exercise and conditioning. Many patients, however, particularly elderly patients with prolonged critical illness and ventilatory muscle deconditioning, may not tolerate even short periods of T-piece (or low-pressure CPAP) breathing. For these patients, a ventilatory workload sufficient to produce ventilatory muscle conditioning may be achieved by significantly lower levels of patient versus machine ventilatory work. It is often necessary to use intermittent pressure-support breathing with or without IMV for these weaning "sprints." Ventilatory rest may be accomplished by the use of several modes but is most easily accomplished through the use of assist control with a rate set just slightly lower than the patient's demand rate.

## THERAPIST-DRIVEN PROTOCOLS FOR WEANING MECHANICAL VENTILATION

The large-scale implementation of respiratory therapist-driven ventilator weaning protocols began several years ago, particularly in medical ICUs.[116] Since the original publications, many investigators have duplicated the outcomes demonstrating more ventilator free days when compared to physician-dictated weaning strategies.[117]

Investigators more recently have taken protocol-driven weaning to the next level: Computer-driven weaning protocols. In this model, a closed-loop knowledge based algorithm introduced in a ventilator implemented an automatic gradual reduction in pressure support and automatic spontaneous breathing trials. Results indicated that this model reduces time to extubation, reduced critical care lengths of stay, and did not lead to higher reintubation rates.[118]

The experience of protocol-driven ventilator weaning in surgical patients has not been as extensive as in medical ICUs, although efforts are underway to test the implementation of these protocols in the broader population. A recent review of protocol-driven weaning, when applied to injured and other surgical patients, reflected similar results to that of medical patients: Protocol implementation lead to more ventilator-free days and lower rates of ventilator associated pneumonia. Prospective trials in the surgical population are now underway.[119]

## TRACHEOSTOMY: TIMING AND METHODS

The utility of a "surgical" airway as an adjunct in the management of acute respiratory failure has yet to be completed determined. Ease of oral care and pulmonary toilet, as well as patient comfort, remain the strongest considerations in advocating for early tracheostomy. The relative benefits of decreased anatomic dead space, ease of pulmonary toilet, and reduced risks associated with reintubation must be weighed against the risks and complications of a surgical procedure. In a cohort comparison by Rodriguez and colleagues, the investigators found that early tracheostomy was associated with shorter ventilator, CCU, and hospital days, but they were unable to correlate this finding to any specific salutary effects of early tracheostomy.[120] An early randomized study by El-Naggar found an eightfold increase in airway contamination with tracheostomy.[121] Sugerman and colleagues, in a study of surgical patients, found no differences in length of intubation or CCU stay, incidence of pneumonia, or mortality.[122]

In a recent study of medical patients, Rumbak et al.[123] showed both a survival benefit (31.7% vs. 61.7%) to "early" (48 hours.) vs. "late" (14–16 days) tracheostomy, as well as a decreased incidence of pneumonia and fewer ventilator days. These results however, were not reproduced in a randomized study of trauma patients by Barquist et al., who found no benefit to early (eight postinjury days) versus late (≥28 postinjury days) tracheostomy.[124]

The use of percutaneous tracheostomy (PcT), often performed at the bedside in the CCU, continues to gain popularity since 1985. In several recent randomized clinical trials, PcT was found to require less resources and have a similar rate of complications when compared to open tracheostomy.[125,126] Other reports cite a high incidence of subglottic stenosis and other complications.[127,128] A more recent randomized trial with a one-year follow-up suggested less bleeding with PcT, but failed to show any improvement in the incidence of postoperative complications or longer term quality of life.[129]

## ANALGESIA AND CONSCIOUS SEDATION

During the last decade, there has been a fundamental change in the perception of the role of and anxiety in the outcome of critically ill patients. These patients have historically been perceived as being at risk primarily from the adverse effects associated with treatment. More recently, the contribution of pain and anxiety to morbidity and possibly even mortality is better appreciated, particularly in the CCU. The development of improved analgesic and sedative agents and the expanding use of regional anesthetic techniques have led to greater efforts to develop uniform approaches to the management of conscious sedation and post injury pain. Consensus recommendations to guide analgesic and sedative therapy in the CCU are available.[130,131] It is now recognized that analgesia and sedation are important components of quality critical care.

Trauma patients present special analgesia and sedation challenges for the CCU physician for a variety of reasons:

1. Traumatic injuries may be particularly painful, requiring directed analgesic therapy.

2. Highly severe injuries often lead to prolonged critical illness, mechanical ventilation, and the need for long-term conscious sedation.

3. Trauma patients frequently have a history of active substance use and are therefore at risk for potentially serious problems such as acute withdrawal syndromes and opioid and benzodiazepine tolerance.

## CHOICE OF PARENTERAL OPIOID FOR ANALGESIA IN CRITICALLY ILL ADULTS

The provision of adequate analgesia is of paramount importance in the treatment of CCU patients, and parenteral opioids have a long history of efficacy and safety for this indication. Since bioavailability is variable in this patient population, the intravenous route should be used whenever possible; the intramuscular and subcutaneous routes should be avoided because extremely variable serum levels have been demonstrated.[132] Furthermore, patient-controlled analgesia (PCA) may be of great benefit in carefully selected adult CCU patients because of the increased sense of control that this modality affords. An executive panel has published recommendations regarding preferred parenteral opioid agents in the treatment of pain in adult CCU patients.[130] This analysis, based on an exhaustive review of the literature, supports the use of parenteral morphine, fentanyl, and hydromorphone as agents of choice for the treatment of pain in the CCU (Table 60-8).

### Morphine

Morphine remains the most commonly used opioid analgesic in the CCU setting because most clinicians are familiar with its pharmacokinetic and pharmacodynamic properties, and it is inexpensive. As the result of its high water-solubility, morphine penetrates

the blood–brain barrier slowly. The result is a delayed peak but prolonged effect compared to the more lipid-soluble agent fentanyl. Although morphine has no direct inotropic effects, it has predictable hemodynamic effects, including both arteriolar and venous dilatation. Morphine increases venous capacitance to a greater extent than arteriolar capacitance and also decreases heart rate through both central sympatholysis and direct sinoatrial node effects. These hemodynamic properties suggest that morphine may be an advantageous agent in the hemodynamically stable (or hypertensive) patient with myocardial ischemia or cardiogenic pulmonary edema. Morphine is recommended as the first-line opioid analgesic for parenteral use in the CCU.[130]

The primary disadvantages of morphine (and other opioid agonists) are their opioid receptor-associated side effects, the most serious of which is centrally mediated respiratory depression. Most of the receptor-associated side effects (respiratory depression, sedation, nausea, sphincter of Oddi spasm) can be reversed with the careful titration of the opioid receptor antagonist naloxone. Careful titration of naloxone may also allow the reversal of side effects without complete reversal of analgesia. However, naloxone must be administered with care, as undesirable hemodynamic effects (hypertension, tachycardia, and myocardial ischemia) and acute pulmonary edema can occur with reversal of opioid effects. The primary nonreceptor-associated side effect of morphine is release of histamine, which can result in undesired hypotension, tachycardia, and a theoretical risk of exacerbating bronchospasm in patients with reactive airways. In addition, morphine-6-glucuronide, a morphine metabolite, accumulates in critically ill patients with impaired renal function and may cause a prolonged sedative effect.

### Fentanyl

Fentanyl is a potent, lipid-soluble synthetic opioid having a more rapid onset of action than morphine. Like morphine, it is also quite inexpensive. When small doses are administered, the duration of action is short due to redistribution. When large, cumulative doses are administered, especially by continuous infusion, termination of effect requires elimination, presumably due to the saturation of poorly perfused adipose tissue. The pharmacokinetics of fentanyl are not significantly altered in the presence of cirrhosis, and clearance appears to remain normal in renal failure. Hemodynamically, fentanyl maintains cardiovascular stability and does not effect an inotropic state. In the presence of high sympathetic tone, fentanyl may decrease blood pressure indirectly by decreasing central sympathetic output. Fentanyl also predictably causes a decrease in heart rate via a central vagotonic effect.

**TABLE 60-8**

| Suggested Intravenous Opioid Doses for Adult ICU Patients | | | | | | | | |
|---|---|---|---|---|---|---|---|---|
| | | | | **SUGGESTED DOSES** | | | | |
| | Distribution Half-Life (min) | Elimination Half-Life (h) | Peak Effect (min) | Approx. Equi-Analgesic Dose (mg) | Bolus | Infusion | PCA Bolus | PCA Infusion |
| Morphine | 20 | 2–4 | 30 | 10 | 2–5.0 mg | 2–10 mg/h | 0.5–1.0 μg | 2–10 mg/h |
| Fentanyl | 3 | 2–5 | 4 | 0.1 | 25–100 μg | 25–100 μg/h | 10–50 μg | 25–100 μg/h |
| Hydromorphone | 15 | 2–4 | 20 | 2 | 0.5–1.0 mg | 0.5–2.0 mg/h | 0.2–0.3 mg | 0.4–2.0 mg/h |

The receptor-associated side effects of fentanyl and their management are the same as described for morphine. However, fentanyl is 80–100 times more potent than morphine and has a more rapid onset of action, requiring vigilance with its use. Unlike morphine, fentanyl does not release histamine and therefore may be a better analgesic choice for patients who are hemodynamically unstable or have significant reactive airway disease. For critically ill patients, fentanyl has been recommended as an alternative to morphine in situations of hemodynamic instability, known allergy to morphine, or previous histamine release with morphine.[130]

## Hydromorphone

Hydromorphone is a semisynthetic opioid agent which is lipophilic and five- to tenfold more potent than morphine. Time to clinical onset and duration of action is similar to that of morphine, and hydromorphone's terminal half-life is 184 minutes. Surprisingly, little information is available regarding its hemodynamic properties: a study has demonstrated that hydromorphone 0.1 mg/kg has minimal hemodynamic effect and does not result in the release of histamine. Based on this profile, hydromorphone has been recommended as the third-line parenteral opioid agent (after morphine and fentanyl) for analgesia in CCU patients.[136] Like morphine and fentanyl, hydromorphone is inexpensive.

## PARENTERAL AGENTS FOR THE TREATMENT OF ANXIETY IN ADULT CRITICAL CARE UNIT PATIENTS

The benzodiazepines (midazolam, lorazepam, and diazepam) have been the cornerstone of anxiolytic, amnestic, and sedative therapy for adult CCU patients, but the introduction of propofol has expanded the number of agents available for this indication. The provision of anxiolysis and amnesia are of major importance for CCU patients undergoing (a) intermittent painful procedures and (b) mechanical ventilation, especially when neuromuscular blockade is used. In fact, a survey has demonstrated that the majority of patients surviving prolonged mechanical ventilation found memory of the experience unpleasant.[133–135] Recent recommendations suggest the use of propofol or midazolam for routine short-term CCU sedation and lorazepam for long-term sedation.[130] Due to its potential to form active metabolites with prolonged duration of action, diazepam is not recommended for routine use in critically ill adults. Recommended starting doses for the commonly used benzodiazepines are listed in Table 60-9.

## Midazolam

Midazolam has a rapid onset of action and relatively short elimination half-life (2–2.5 hours). In critically ill patients, particularly those with impaired hepatic metabolism, its elimination half-life may be prolonged (4–12 hours). Additionally, midazolam may cause hypotension, particularly in the presence of hypovolemia.[130,136] Respiratory depression is an expected side effect, but infusions of midazolam need not be withdrawn to wean patients successfully from mechanical ventilation. Midazolam is metabolized to compounds known as hydroxymidazolams, which have minimal intrinsic benzodiazepine activity. A critical care task force has recently recommended midazolam as the first-line benzodiazepine for short-term (<24 hours) sedation and anxiolysis in the critical care setting.[130]

## Lorazepam

Lorazepam is a potent benzodiazepine having lower lipid solubility than either diazepam or midazolam, but higher receptor specificity. Its lower lipid solubility delays penetration of the blood–brain barrier, resulting in a longer time to peak effect despite a short distribution half-life. Duration of clinical effect from a single bolus dose is also longer than that obtained with single bolus of midazolam or diazepam. Lorazepam has an intermediate terminal half-life of 10–20 hours and is metabolized to compounds with no intrinsic benzodiazepine activity. Theoretically, lorazepam's lower lipid solubility and inactive metabolites decrease the likelihood of prolonged sedation after large cumulative doses, relative to midazolam and diazepam. Although there is no randomized, controlled trial comparing the benefits of the benzodiazepines as long-term sedatives in the CCU, lorazepam has recently been recommended as the first-line benzodiazepine for sedation and anxiolysis in CCU patients requiring treatment for medium term (<24 hours).[130] Due to its water insolubility, lorazepam is packaged in a glycol-containing solution that may cause phlebitis or intravascular catheter infiltration on injection. Lorazepam is inexpensive in comparison to midazolam.

## Propofol

Propofol is a lipid-soluble alkylphenol intravenous anesthetic that is insoluble in water and formulated in a lipid emulsion. Although propofol has hypnotic, amnestic, and antiemetic properties, it is devoid of analgesic properties. At low doses, it produces sedation. Propofol has minimal cumulative properties, even with repeated administration: in critically ill patients sedated with continuous infusions of propofol for a mean of 86 hours, serum levels declined by 50% 10 minutes after termination of the infusion.

**TABLE 60-9**

| Pharmacology of Intravenous Benzodiazepines | | | | | | | |
|---|---|---|---|---|---|---|---|
| | DISTRIBUTION HALF-LIFE (MIN) | ELIMINATION HALF-LIFE (H) | PEAK EFFECT (MIN) | EQUIPOTENT DOSE | BOLUS (MG) | INFUSION (MG/KG/H) | ACTIVE METABOLITES |
| Diazepam | 10–15 | 20–40 | 3–5 | 5 | 5-10 | N/a | Yes[a] |
| Midazolam | 7–10 | 2.0–2.5 | 2–5 | 3 | 0.5-2.0 | 0.01–0.2 | Possibly[b] |
| Lorazepam | 3–10 | 10–20 | 15–30 | 1 | 0.5-2.0 | 0.01–0.1 | No |

[a]Desmethyldiazepam and oxazepam have intrinsic benzodiazepine activity and prolonged half-lives (96 hours).

[b]Hydroxymidazolams have minimal benzodiazepine activity.

*(Reproduced with permission from Philip B. Pharmacology of intravenous sedative agents. In Rogers M, ed. Principles and Practice of Anesthesia. St. Louis: Mosby; 1993.)*

There are a number of controlled trials of propofol administration at subanesthetic doses for sedation in critically ill patients requiring mechanical ventilation. These studies, which include primarily postoperative cardiac surgery patients but also surgical and medical CCU patients, have shown that doses of 17–50 µg/kg/minute of propofol effectively sedate most critically ill patients. Generally, rapid and predictable levels of sedation are achieved, and recovery occurs quickly when the infusion is terminated. Additionally, prolonged administration does not appear to extend recovery time. When administered at an average infusion rate of 47.5 µg/kg/minute for four days, recovery times were not delayed and plasma concentrations were similar each day, indicating a lack of cumulative effects. In two similar trials comparing propofol to midazolam for sedation in CCU patients, the time to wake-up and to tracheal extubation were significantly shorter for the group sedated with propofol.[137,138] Two other trials have shown no significant difference in time to wakefulness when propofol and midazolam were compared in postoperative cardiac surgery patients, but these patients generally were sedated for less than 24 hours.[139,140]

In one study comparing propofol to midazolam, cardiovascular depression limited the use of propofol in 23% of patients and the use of midazolam in 24%.[141] In both groups, hypotension responded to increases in intravenous fluid. A recent study demonstrated a significantly higher incidence of hypotension in CCU patients administered a loading dose of propofol when compared to those patients treated with midazolam.[140] Propofol has predictable hemodynamic effects, including arterial and venous dilation, decreased inotropy, and a decrease in systolic blood pressure of 20 to 30% in anesthetized patients. Propofol (in response to a loading dose) will cause profound ventilatory depression. For this reason, it is used only in mechanically ventilated patients in our CCU.

Propofol has been recommended as an agent for short-term (<24 hours) sedation in the CCU.[130] The impressively rapid time to wake-up for patients receiving long-term infusions of propofol compared to midazolam (1 vs. 37 hours) demonstrated by Carrasco and coworkers[142] and the equally impressive time to extubation (2 vs. 55 hours) suggest that propofol may be useful for sedating critically ill patients longer than 24 hours if practitioners remain vigilant for potential toxicities. Propofol is expensive in comparison to midazolam.

Hypertriglyceridemia and lipid-induced pancreatitis have been reported during prolonged infusion in the CCU, suggesting that serum triglyceride levels should be monitored in these patients. In a mechanically ventilated CCU patient requiring prolonged high-dose propofol (200 µg/kg/minute), hypercarbia was noted despite increases in minute ventilation. In this case, the hypercarbia was assumed to have been caused by increased $CO_2$ production secondary to excessive lipid delivery (>2 L/day) necessitated by the high propofol infusion rate. The lipid solution of propofol also supports rapid bacterial growth at room temperature, and a number of postoperative bacteremias have been linked to poor administration technique.[138]

## Dexmedetomidine

Dexmedetomidine, an imidazole compound, is the most recently developed and released agent for use as sedative/analgesic agent in the CCU. Dexmedetomidine is a member of α2-adrenergic agonists. It is a highly selective agonist of the α2-adrenergic receptor that has an eight times greater affinity for the receptor than clonidine. It is also shorter-acting than clonidine. This characteristic

allows its use as an intravenous infusion. It was initially evaluated as an anesthetic but was associated with excessive bradycardia and hypotension. In late 1999, dexmedetomidine was approved for the adult CCU as a sedative infusion for less than 24 hours. Most of the clinical experience with dexmedetomidine has been with surgical patients undergoing cardiac and vascular procedures.[143] Patient selection and proper drug infusion are needed to avoid deleterious hemodynamic effects. For example, slower bolus loading over 20 minutes results in minimal hemodynamic effects. Interestingly, continuous infusion causes sedation but easy arousal, an analgesic-sparing effect, and minimal depression of the respiratory drive. These initial observations indicate that dexmedetomidine may be of benefit for selected CCU patients.[144] The characteristics of sedation with dexmedetomidine are unique in that patients appear to be sedated while receiving it but are readily roused and interactive when stimulated. However, more clinical experience is needed before conclusions can be drawn about the drug's potential for wider application and its long-term safety in CCU patients.

## MONITORING AND THE DAILY INTERRUPTION OF SEDATION IN CRITICAL CARE UNIT PATIENTS

The Ramsay scale is a six-point scale developed to monitor the level of sedation in critically ill patients (Table 60-10) and is widely used for this purpose.[145] A Ramsay score of 2 or 3 is optimal. In the absence of organic or structural causes of obtundation (e.g., central nervous system pathology), a Ramsay score of 5 or 6 represents oversedation. Conversely, a score of 1 represents an inadequate level of anxiolysis. A major limitation of this scale is that it is not applicable to patients who are being treated with neuromuscular blocking agents or who have head injuries. A major advantage is that a high degree of patient cooperation is not critical to its successful use.

Respective, controlled studies conducted in mechanically ventilated patients receiving continuous I.V. sedation demonstrated that a daily interruption in the sedation until the patient was awake, decreased the duration of mechanical ventilation and ICU length of stay.[146,147] The daily interruption and awakenings allowed for titration of sedation, making de facto the dosing intermittent. The bispectral index (BIS) is an objective assessment tool for the monitoring of sedation in the CCU. Until now, sedation assessment has been primarily guided by vital signs or subjective assessment scales. These approaches may not be sufficient to achieve optimal patient assessment. In a study by Kaplan and Bailey, more than 69% of patients in a CCU were found to be inappropriately sedated.[148] Of those, 15% were undersedated, leading to fear, anxiety and agitation; unpleasant recall;

**TABLE 60-10**

| Ramsay Scale to Assess Level of Sedation | |
|---|---|
| LEVEL | RESPONSE |
| 1 | Anxious and agitated, or restless or both |
| 2 | Cooperative, oriented and tranquil |
| 3 | Responding to commands |
| 4 | Brisk response to stimulus[a] |
| 5 | Sluggish response to stimulus[a] |
| 6 | No response to stimulus[a] |

[a]Light glabellar tap or loud auditory stimulus.

medical device removal; this outcome led to additional costs and increased nursing time. Oversedation was around 54%, leading to increased time on mechanical ventilation, increased length of stay in the CCU, additional cost of care, an increased risk of complications, as well as a need for additional diagnostic testing to rule out neurologic problems versus slow return to consciousness due to prolonged sedation or oversedation. Now, with an objective way to assess sedation, the BIS monitor can help to determine patients' level of sedation and enable informed decisions about the titration of sedative drugs. The BIS is especially useful for sedation assessment during mechanical ventilation, neuromuscular blockade, barbiturate coma, and bedside procedures. Raw electroencephalographic (EEG) information is obtained through a sensor placed on the forehead. The BIS system processes the EEG information and calculates a number between 0 and 100, which provides a direct measure of the patient's level of consciousness and response to sedation. A BIS value of 100 indicates that a patient is fully awake, and a BIS level of 0 indicates the absence of electrical brain activity. Sedation may be titrated to a variety of BIS values depending on the goals for each patient. The BIS values correlate directly with commonly used sedation scales.[149]

## THE USE OF INTRAVENOUS HALOPERIDOL IN CRITICAL CARE UNIT

The butyrophenone haloperidol has been recommended for use in the CCU setting for the treatment of acute delirium[130] and is effective for this indication. Haloperidol induces a disassociative state of apathy and general detachment in which patients may appear calm. When later interviewed, however, they report having felt apprehensive. This complication appears to be reduced by combining this agent with a benzodiazepine. When delirium occurs in the CCU, treatable etiologies such as hypoxemia, hypoglycemia, hypercapnia, electrolyte abnormalities, and central nervous system lesions must be sought first, because treatment with a major tranquilizer may mask important clinical signs of end-organ pathology.

Peak plasma levels of haloperidol are reached 11 minutes after intravenous injection, and the half-life of the drug is 10–24 hours. The dose of haloperidol required to control agitation in critically ill patients varies markedly. One recommended approach is to administer an intravenous injection of 2.5–5.0 mg every 30 minute until agitation ceases. Doses of haloperidol as high as 1200 mg/day have been reported to have been safely administered. Continuous infusion of haloperidol for delirium has been described. A retrospective comparison of continuous infusion of haloperidol with intermittent bolus administration in patients refractory to bolus therapy demonstrated excellent control of delirium in the infusion group, although mean dosage was high (269 mg/day). Although haloperidol has a reputation for safety, several issues bear discussion. Haloperidol reduces seizure threshold and must be used with caution in patients with seizure disorders or who are otherwise at risk for seizures. Also, butyrophenones may precipitate extrapyramidal reactions (dyskinesia) and laryngeal dystonia. Interestingly, the incidence of dystonia is reduced if haloperidol is administered intravenously rather than orally.

Haloperidol prolongs the QT interval (through an unclear mechanism) and has resulted in a number of episodes of torsades de pointes (TDP). Potentially confounding conditions (cardiomyopathy, ischemic heart disease, electrolyte abnormalities, and coadministered medications) existed in most patients reported to have had TDP while receiving intravenous haloperidol, making conclusions regarding its causative effect difficult. Nevertheless, high-dose intravenous haloperidol should be used only in a monitored critical care setting, and serial electrocardiograms should be obtained in order to follow the duration of the QT interval, which may provide an early indication of those patients at risk for TDP.

## UTILITY OF REGIONAL ANALGESIA AND ANESTHESIA IN THE SETTING OF BLUNT TRAUMA

There is always a respiratory deficit following upper abdominal and thoracic surgery or blunt thoracic trauma (see Chap. 15). Systemic administration of narcotics may exacerbate this deficit by inducing significant respiratory depression, a particularly undesirable effect in critically ill patients. Regional techniques generally do not induce respiratory depression but may fail to restore respiratory function to preoperative levels. Multiple studies have demonstrated the effectiveness of regional analgesia in improving lung volumes and oxygenation and decreasing pulmonary complications following blunt thoracic trauma.[150–154] Epidural analgesia has become a well-accepted modality for the treatment of rib fracture pain and the restoration of ventilatory function, although not all studies have reproduced these results. Even with complete relief of pain, the epidural methods may only partially restore forced vital capacity and forced expiratory volume, minimally improve functional residual capacity, and modestly increase oxygenation. Thus, pain is only one of several factors leading to a restrictive pulmonary pattern postoperatively. Diaphragmatic dysfunction has been suggested as a contributor to the decreased lung volumes observed after blunt thoracic trauma. This diaphragmatic dysfunction has been attributed to a visceral or somatic reflex decreasing phrenic nerve activity. Spasm and splinting of the abdominal and intercostal muscles may also be involved. Thoracic epidural local anesthesia decreases diaphragmatic dysfunction, increases tidal volume, and decreases respiratory frequency, while spinal opiates do not. These effects of epidural local anesthesia may be direct or indirect.

In summary, pain is a significant problem after trauma, and its relief is necessary not only for patient comfort but also for efficient respiratory therapy. However, pain does not appear to be the sole mechanism underlying respiratory muscle dysfunction. Inhibitory reflexes of the phrenic nerve are involved and do not appear to be blocked by spinal opiates; they are, however, partially blocked by thoracic epidural local anesthetics. Nevertheless, the analgesia provided by spinally administered opiates or local anesthetic solutions improves respiratory function more than systemically delivered narcotics and can be expected to reduce morbidity in some situations.

## COMPLICATIONS OF CRITICAL CARE

Critical illness complications impose a substantial cost burden to any institution, in addition to being an important cause of patient morbidity/mortality. The continuing evolution of managed care markets will provide a strong financial impetus for high-risk/high-cost areas of hospitals to develop cost-effective management guidelines.

The emphasis of many of these guidelines will be on prophylaxis, particularly with respect to complications of critical illness. It will also be important that any such management guidelines for critical care, to a greater degree than resuscitation or operative management guidelines, take into account the individual and sometimes unique conditions and practices that exist in a given unit. For example, guidelines governing central venous catheter infections must consider individual unit microbial ecology, line usage type (monitoring, infusion, multiport), and nursing management practices. A complete discussion of critical illness complications is well beyond the scope of this chapter. Selected complications either unique to critical care or of particular importance as causes of morbidity are included. Specific organ-system complications are discussed more completely in other chapters in this section.

## VENTILATOR-ASSOCIATED PNEUMONIA

Although a variety of nosocomial infections occur in the critical care setting following major injury (see Chap. 19), two of the most troublesome and expensive are central venous catheter-related infections and ventilator-associated pneumonias (VAPs). One of the principal questions regarding VAP is its overall impact on the outcome from major injury. There is evidence that pneumonia may exacerbate multiple organ failure and ARDS[155] and should presumably be associated with increased mortality, as has been found in other studies.[156,157] Sepsis from pneumonic sources, as a second hit-inducing factor, might also be expected to substantially worsen outcome. Unfortunately, despite this intuitive causal link, most studies (see below) demonstrating the efficacy of a prophylactic regimen have failed to demonstrate associated reductions in mortality, although many of these studies have been conducted in mixed medical/surgical populations.[158] More recent reports have shown a survival benefit, but these effects may be related, in part, to a low rates of resistant organisms.[159] Risk factors for VAP include coma/head injury, prolonged ventilatory support, APACHE II greater than 16, impaired airway reflexes, shock on admission, and surgery involving the head and chest.[160,161]

Probable pathophysiology of colonization/infection in this group of patients involves a number of postinjury as well as iatrogenic factors. Endotracheal intubation per se constitutes a risk factor insofar as a majority of patients have respiratory tract colonization at 10 days. While endotracheal tube cuffs prevent large-volume aspiration, aspiration of heavily contaminated fluids that lie adjacent to the top of the endotracheal tube cuff probably occurs frequently with cuff manipulations. The establishment of bacterial reservoirs promoting this type of colonization probably occurs first in the stomach, and has been attributed to the widespread use of $H_2$-blocking agents for stress ulcer prophylaxis. Neutralization of gastric acid results in heavily colonized gastric contents ($>10^6$ organisms) after four to five days. The common use of nasogastric tubes for gastric decompression further provides a "wick" that may further promote lower esophageal sphincter incompetence, leading to colonization of the oropharynx. Bacterial overgrowth in the oropharanx may have direct access to the upper respiratory tree via an indwelling tracheal tube. Patient-related factors such as chemical paralysis, absence of vigorous pulmonary toilet (such as exist in severe head injuries), and impaired mucociliary clearance further conspire to promote pooling of secretions. For the many patients, the conventional clinical criteria of fever, leukocytosis, new chest x-ray infiltrates, and increased sputum neutrophils are sufficient for the diagnosis of VAP. More sophisticated clinical scores such as the clinical pulmonary infection score (CPIS) and the National Nosocomial Infection Surveillance System (NNISS) have relatively good specificity and sensitivity when compared to the basic clinical criteria, and their use may improve diagnostic accuracy and better guide treatment.[162]

For patients with established ARDS or those requiring prolonged mechanical ventilation with upper respiratory colonization, reliance on simple tracheal aspirates may be misleading. Two methods, protected specimen breaths (PSBs) and broncheoalveolar lavage (BAL), have been used successfully to identify lower respiratory infection. A metaanalysis of 23 studies reported a mean sensitivity of 73% and specificity of 82% for bronchoscopic lavage.[163] Less invasive nonbronchoscopic lavage methods improve the ease of specimen procurement and may help facilitate earlier treatment. Experience with these methods suggest that blind sampling methods may be a viable alternative to more invasive bronchoscopic sampling techniques.[164,165]

Prophylactic regimens for VAP have focused on decreasing bacterial colonization in the stomach, oropharanyx, and trachea through a regimen of selective decontamination. Additional factors that may be related to the development of VAP include the frequency of ventilator circuit changes and the type of endotracheal suction systems, heated humidifiers, and so forth. In a study by Cook and colleagues, the investigators reviewed the influence of airway management on VAP. They found that the frequency of ventilator circuit changes and types of suction systems do not appear to influence the incidence of VAP.[166] In a meta-analysis by Dezfulian et al.[167], the authors used five randomized trials comparing subglottic secretion drainage and conventional endotracheal tubes. The former permit suctioning of the subglottic fluid collections that occurs at the balloon cuff and thought to be associated with a significantly decreased incidence of VAP. The results of the meta-analysis suggest that subglottic suctioning may be effective in preventing early-onset VAP in patients requiring prolonged mechanical ventilation. These conclusions however, have not been universally accepted, with continued concerns regarding the adverse effects of suctioning and the increased tube diameters required for this technique.[168] Various other reports have suggested other factors that may be important in the etiology of VAP, including the use of heated humidifiers, oral versus nasal intubation, suction methods, and kinetic versus conventional beds. Clearly, there are a number of airway management factors that must be considered in each individual CCU as management guidelines are developed in an effort to reduce the incidence of VAP.

## UNPLANNED EXTUBATIONS

Unplanned extubations are potentially serious complications and constitute a commonly utilized clinical indicator in critical care quality-assurance programs. The reported incidence, depending on the population studied, varies between 4% and 14 %.[169–171] The mortality for such events is approximately 2%, making it an important cause of preventable death for this select group of patients. Unplanned extubations have been linked to inadequate sedation or inadequate restraints in agitated patients. Inadequate fixation of the tracheal tube and the use of oral versus nasal intubation route were also significant factors associated with unplanned extubations.[172] Patient-initiated extubation often occurs during weaning from mechanical ventilation and is often well tolerated. Predictors for reintubation have been reported to include a GCS score of less than 11, accidental versus patient-initiated extubations, and hypoxia, with a $PaO_2/FIO_2$ ratio of less than 200 hours, and age.[169,171] Careful attention to adequate conscious sedation, avoidance of hypoxia or underventilation in lightly sedated patients, proper fixation of the oral tracheal tube, and care in handling of the endotracheal tube during patient transfers are essential to avoiding this preventable complication. Reintubation, particularly in high-risk patients in accidental settings may be difficult and should mandate the presence of individuals with well-developed airway management skills immediately at the bedside. Unplanned intubations should be monitored and reviewed on a regular basis by the CCU team as part of the quality assurance and/or teaching programs.

## CENTRAL VENOUS CATHETER INFECTIONS

In the United States, it has been estimated that between 35,000 and 50,000 patients are affected annually by central venous catheter (CVC) bacteremia, representing roughly 2–9 % of all catheters. Some of the variability in incidence is related to a lack of consistent definitions of catheter-related sepsis or catheter-related infections. A CVC infection may be diagnosed on the basis of the presence of clinical sepsis, the presence of an indwelling CVC, and identical organisms isolated from peripheral cultures and catheter tips.

Migratory skin colonization, hub colonization, contaminated insertion, and bacteremic seeding are all mechanisms whereby organisms gain access to indwelling catheters. Coupled with this variable route of colonization are a large number of factors that influence infection rates (Table 60-11). Depending on patient population, CCU practices, severity of illness, and protocols for placement and maintenance of CVCs, variable rates of infection and different sites of colonization have been reported. This inherent heterogeneity has acted to perpetuate the substantial confusion that exists in many CCUs with respect to developing "optimal" management protocols for CVCs.

Against the background of this considerable clinical variability, a number of studies have defined interventions that may be effective in reducing overall catheter-related sepsis rates (see Table 60-11). That strict adherence to line insertion technique is associated with a lower incidence of catheter-related infection (CRI) should not come as much of a surprise and was recently validated in a randomized series of 343 patients.[173] Even the type of site-preparation agent may have an impact on catheter infection rates, as one recent study demonstrated.[174] Occlusive dressings probably cause an overgrowth of yeast and gram-negative organisms, and although previous studies suggest equal colonization rates, a more recent meta-analysis of 14 separate studies demonstrated a significantly increased risk of catheter-tip infection in the use of transparent dressings.[175] Triple-lumen catheters, as opposed to single-lumen catheters, have been implicated in a higher rate of CRI, which may be related either to more frequent manipulation, breaches in line integrity, or the actual catheter material. In one older study,

**TABLE 60-11**

**Factors Associated with Central Catheter Infections**

| LEVEL | RESPONSE |
|---|---|
| Line insertion technique | Strict aseptic technique: caps, masks, gloves, wide draping. Early removal for emergency lines. |
| Insertion site preparation | Chlorhexidine 2% |
| Insertion site dressing | Avoid use of transparent occlusive dressings |
| Multi-use lines/single v. triple lumen catheters | Dedicated, single-lumen for high-risk lines. |
| TPN v. non-TPN line | Utilize enteral nutrition |
| Frequent catheter hub manipulations | Maintain line integrity: limit disconnects |
| Catheter material | Use silastic catheters when available |
| Antimicrobial impregnation, heparin infusion | Probably indicated for high-risk lines |
| Duration of catheter | Limit duration for high-risk lines |
| Age >60, >12 months severe illness. Open wounds. | Risk factors for high risk lines |
| Inconsistent approach to line monitoring & management | Utilize intravenous therapy team wherever feasible. |

catheter material played an important role in the subsequent incidence of CRI, with Silastic catheters having roughly an eightfold lower CRI rate.[176] Total parenteral nutrition (TPN) solutions, particularly those containing emulsified lipid, also predispose to higher rates of infection.

The ability to bond antibiotics and other anti-mircobial agents directly to catheters appears a promising approach. Several prospective, randomized trials have reported favorable results with this approach, finding reductions in catheter colonization and reductions in the incidence of CVC-related bacteremias.[176–188] Protocols governing the management of CVC and CRI are helpful in standardizing and optimizing management. These protocols and CMGs must be tailored to each individual CCU, and take into account the individual CCU microbial ecology and the types and durations of CVC catheters that are used. This will also determine the indications for CVC catheter removal or exchange for suspected infection. The practice of routine CVC replacement has been abandoned, based on recent literature, in favor of removal/replacement based on clinical indications.[189]

## MICROBIAL RESISTANCE IN THE CRITICAL CARE UNIT

Although not necessarily considered a complication of critical illness, the emerging number of multiply drug-resistant organisms present in the CCU has become an increasingly serious problem. Therapeutic failure may occur in approximately 50% of patients who develop bacterial resistance in the course of antibiotic treatment. The most important source of resistance for many antimicrobials used in the CCU is beta-lactamase production by a wide variety of bacteria. *Enterobacter, Serratia,* and *Pseudomonas* species possess inducible beta-lactamases which may bind, rather than hydrolyze, the newer beta-lactam agents. *Escherichia coli* and *Klebsiella* species have been found to produce an extended-spectrum cephalosporinase. Plasmid-encoded TEM- and

SHV-type beta-lactamases may be transferred between bacteria. Methicillin-resistant staphylococcal infections continue to pose problems, and a staphylococcal species with reduced susceptibility to vancomycin has been reported. The results of these developments are the emergence of resistance that may occur and be induced during a course of even newer-generation cephalosporins, ureidopenicillins, or monobactam agents. The systematic overuse of antimicrobials in the CCU has led, in part, to the more frequent induction of these resistant organisms, and if allowed to continue unchecked, may produce only more of the same in the future. The adherence to guidelines for antibiotic management in the CCU may, in the meantime, help reduce the prevalence of these organisms. Such guidelines might include the following:

- Limit prophylactic treatment to those regimens consistent with established guidelines or CCU management protocols.
- Tailor presumptive antibiotic treatment to risk factors for resistant organisms and individual CCU microbial ecology.
- Perform surveillance cultures for specific and proper indications (e.g., temperature spikes, worsening leukocytosis, chest x-ray findings, etc.).
- Treat for identified specific infections for a defined period. Do not predicate duration of antibiotic course on nonspecific indicators (e.g., continued fevers, leukocytosis).
- Limit presumptive treatment: if cultures, physical findings, and lab x-ray studies do not indicate a specific infection, STOP antibiotics and reculture as indicated.
- Monitor microbial sensitivity for developing resistance and utilize updated institutional microbial sensitivity data.

Strategies for combating antibiotic resistance include the development of new agents, the use of combination therapy to reduce induction pressure on existing organisms, and protocols for planned individual unit or institutional rotation of presumptive treatment and "drug of choice." Scheduled antibiotic formulary rotation has been proposed as a means of reducing mutation pressure and the incidence of resistant organisms in a given unit of institution. To date, however, results with this approach have been disappointing[190] prompting some authors to suggest a broadened formulary rather than a restricted one.[191]

## CRITICAL ILLNESS POLYNEUROPATHY

Prolonged neuromuscular weakness associated with critical illness, reported as early as the 1950s, has more recently been the focus of several descriptive reports.[192–194] Found to be associated with sepsis, hypotension, or multiple organ dysfunction, critical illness polyneuropathy (CIP) may prolong weaning from mechanical ventilation, delay return to ambulation, and significantly affect overall recovery from posttraumatic critical illness.

The syndrome is characterized by the development of diffuse neurogenic muscle weakness, developing typically over a several-week course of severe critical illness. The neurologic manifestations may include unexplained failure to wean from mechanical ventilation, decreased/absent deep tendon reflexes, tetraparesis, muscle atrophy, and decreased fibrillations and compound muscle action potentials, and evidence for axonal damage found on electrophysiologic testing. Nerve conduction velocities are near normal, and

histologic evaluation of peripheral nerves has shown acute, diffuse, neurogenic atrophy in muscles and axonal degeneration in nerve tissue. CIP may be far more common than is currently recognized and may commonly affect ventilator weaning and functional recovery.[194,195] CIP should be considered as a cause of unexplained weaning failures or generalized weakness in the setting of prolonged critical illness. Electrophysiologic evaluation of muscle and nerve function is important for the diagnosis. Although not conclusive, available data suggest that the avoidance of long-term paralytic agents, particularly in combination with corticosteroids or aminoglycoside antibiotics, may be an important preventative measure. Several factors contributing to CIP have been identified and include the long-term use of neuromuscular blocking agents (e.g., pancuronium, vecuronium) and aminoglycoside antibiotics. The combination of neuromuscular blocking agents and high-dose corticosteroids may be a particularly important cause. Recovery from CIP, although prolonged, may be nearly complete from a clinical standpoint. Follow-up electromyographic studies have shown changes consistent with chronic neurogenic damage, however.

## ETHICAL ISSUES IN CRITICAL CARE

Ethics may be regarded, in part, as a series of societal formulations predicated on moral values designed to produce a theoretical "optimal good." With the ability of modern CCUs to maintain physiologic support and homeostasis well beyond the bounds of reasonable sentient existence, physicians are increasingly called on to participate in sometimes difficult live-or-die, withdraw/withhold support decisions. While CCU ethics also include other considerations, such as consent issues and donor organ procurement (see Chap. 58), this section focuses on the withdrawal/withholding of physiologic support, including the application of do not resuscitate (DNR) orders in the surgical CCU.

## ETHICAL PRINCIPLES APPLICABLE TO MEDICAL DECISION MAKING

Ethical decision making should involve the careful, considered application of established principles. The temptation to apply one's individual value system to the decision-making process is strong, but the personal values of the patient are paramount, and the personal judgments of both family members and physicians must be considered in the context of the ethical principles involved. With the possible exception of the principle of distributive justice, each of the following principles should be applied in any given decision-making process:

*Beneficence:* The principle of "doing good" as applies to a particular patient, individual, or situation.

*Nonmalfeasance:* The principle of avoiding harm or wrongdoing, as applied to a particular situation or individual patient.

*Autonomy:* Perhaps the most important operative principle in critical care ethics is the right of self-determination—the inherent right of individuals to make decisions regarding their own treatment options (or withholding thereof) and ultimately to make decisions that will impact their survival.

*Full disclosure:* The principle of accurate communication of information that will allow individuals (or their surrogates) to exercise autonomy or surrogate decision making.

*Social (distributive) justice:* The principle whereby benefits to an individual, if associated with burdens to another individual or individuals, must be weighed in terms of the most "good" done to the society or group as a whole.

This last principle typically involves decisions regarding the distribution of scarce resources to allow the "optimum" treatment of not a single individual, but a population of individuals (society). Such a principle may apply during wartime casualty triage or civilian mass-casualty triage. With respect to CCUs in the United States, it is uncommon, within a given municipality or region, that critical care resources are sufficiently scarce so as to result in a denial of treatment opportunities, regardless of the medical conditions involved.

## WITHDRAW/WITHHOLD SUPPORT DECISIONS

Modern CCUs have developed the increasing technical capability of supporting homeostasis, even in the face of what would otherwise be overwhelming disease. Increasingly in the trauma population of CCU patients, patient demise is the result of a decision to withdraw or withhold life support. The consequences and irreversibility of such withdraw/withhold decisions in the CCU mandate that they be considered very carefully and predicted on the careful application of ethical and legal principles. Physicians often assume that withdrawing and withholding support are fundamentally different actions that require different thresholds and criteria and potentially have different legal consequences. Case law has served to clarify this issue, beginning with *Barber v. Santa Barbara Superior Court.*[196] In this case, the court considered withdrawal of support to be the equivalent of withholding, equating each milligram of drug infusion or each ventilator breath as an active intervention. That withdrawal of this type of intervention required an additional order was immaterial and still considered a passive (vs. active) act equivalent to withholding. This concept has been further supported by the President's Commission[197] and critical care consensus panels.[198] This critical legal precedent, generally upheld since that time, had the effect of making the withdrawal of support for critical illness the equivalent of withholding support, and thereby not subjecting health care providers to subsequent legal action regarding active (vs. passive) interventions acting to hasten demise.

The importance and impact of withdraw/withhold decisions is considerable. In a review of such decision, Smedira and associates found that in a mixed population of surgical and medical CCU patients, support was withheld in 1% and withdrawn in 5%. The resultant deaths accounted for 45 % of all CCU deaths in the two institutions under study.[199]

The general setting under which withdraw/withhold decisions are made is poor prognosis, which would include a low chance of survival and high likelihood of poor cognitive function.[200] Specific criteria that may allow withdrawal/withholding include the following:

1. Provision of further treatment is considered medically futile with respect to achieving well-defined therapeutic goals.

2. The patient with decision-making capacity (DMC), in exercising his or her autonomy, chooses to have support withdrawn/withheld.

3. A legal surrogate decision maker (legal guardian or durable power of attorney) chooses to have support withdrawn/withheld under medically appropriate circumstances.

4. The decision is made on the basis of a prior written medical directive stipulating circumstances under which support may be withdrawn/withheld.

5. The physician, acting as a surrogate decision maker in conjunction with next of kin, other consultants, and possibly an ethics committee, elects to withdraw/withhold support. The decision should be based on the following considerations:

*Information regarding the patient's wishes:* What the patient would be likely to decide if he or she had DMC. This may be obtained from family, friends, or other providers with a history of relevant contact with the patient.

*The benefits/burdens test:* The benefits of continued treatment are outweighed by the burdens to the patient of such treatment in accomplishing the defined therapeutic goals.

*Substituted judgment:* The "reasonable person test." In the absence of other available information regarding a patient's wishes, a withdraw/withhold decision should be regarded as one likely to be made by any "reasonable person."

*Best interests test:* The decision to withdraw/withhold must be medically appropriate and should not significantly diminish opportunity for recovery within the bounds of benefits/burdens.

## FUTILITY

The concept of futility, derived from the word *futilis,* meaning "to leak" (as in Greek mythology), refers to the inability to accomplish a therapeutic goal through medical interventions regardless of the duration of such interventions or the frequency with which they are repeated.[201–203] The concept of futility is central to initial withdraw/withhold support decisions. Determination of futility requires two elements: (a) the establishment of an agreed-upon therapeutic goal and (b) determination of the probability, given the application of medical therapy, of reaching these therapeutic goals. Therapeutic goals should be outlined as specifically as possible and may incorporate elements of both physical and cognitive function. Patients with DMC must be allowed to define their own therapeutic goals, regardless of how "unreasonable" or stringent these goals may seem. The determination of the probability of medical therapy in achieving those goals should be left to the team of treating physicians.

Schneiderman and colleagues have suggested a numerical definition of futility corresponding to a 1% probability.[204] This would imply that medical care was futile if, in the experience of a provider or that reported in the literature, the intervention failed to achieve therapeutic goals in the last 100 cases in which it was applied. Although not all providers may adhere to such rigorous quantitative definitions, the general concept of futility is well recognized and broadly applied in such settings. Futility must always be judged, however, based on defined therapeutic goals. Once a given treatment or treatments are deemed to be futile, based on established therapeutic goals, the physician is under no legal or ethical obligation to provide such treatment. Current writing in medical ethics, public policy, and more recently by case law has supported this perspective, although some ethicists do not support this medical prerogative. Individual circumstances, however, particularly in regard to family considerations and consistent with the principle of beneficence, may occasionally be indications for short-term delivery of what otherwise would be considered medically futile care.

## DECISION-MAKING CAPACITY AND THE EXERCISE OF AUTONOMY

*Decision-making capacity*, which has different implications than the legal term *competent*, requires the following:

1. The patient must be able to comprehend and communicate information relevant to making a decision.

2. The patient must be able to comprehend his or her alternatives and the benefits and burdens (risks) associated with each.

3. The patient must be able to reason and deliberate about these alternatives against a background of stable personal values.

The determination of DMC may generally be made by the primary physician or team, but occasionally, particularly in the presence of underlying psychiatric illness, psychiatric consultation may be of benefit in making this determination. The exercise of autonomy is best accomplished by allowing any patient with DMC to participate in withdraw/withhold or DNR decisions. In many cases, a patient's specific wishes may not be known and legal surrogates or medical directives may be unavailable. With careful adjustment (lightening to the extent possible) of any conscious sedation and directed efforts made in communicating the alternatives (full disclosure), many patients can make decisions or at least provide valuable information allowing surrogates to do so.

The written medical directive provides an alternative means by which a patient may exercise autonomy. Medical directives may be structured in a variety of ways—depending on known medical conditions, age of the patient, and so forth—but it typically contains language stipulating preferences (or not) for life-sustaining treatment as a function of expected physical and cognitive outcomes.

## DECISION MAKING IN THE ABSENCE OF DECISION-MAKING CAPACITY

In situations where the patient does not have DMC and no specific medical directive is available, a surrogate decision-making process is utilized. Participants in the surrogate decision-making process may include family members, friends, other health care providers, clergy, and members of the institutional ethics committee. Family members invested with durable power of attorney may make clinically appropriate decisions independently on behalf of the patient. (*Durable* refers to power of attorney, including instances in which the patient is incapacitated.) Surrogate decision making should involve close collaboration between health care providers and the family to the extent possible. The specific role of the family, however, in the absence of durable power, is not to actually make withdraw/withhold decisions but to provide information allowing providers to best formulate decisions consistent with what the patient's desires would be. This information may include a knowledge of the patient's values, goals, religious or philosophical beliefs, or previously expressed wishes with respect to medical care. The

importance of this information should not be underestimated. But in the absence of durable power of attorney, family members have no recognized legal authority to dictate care or to make demands that are medically or ethically inappropriate. Health care providers also have a primary responsibility to act in what they perceive to be the best interests of the patient, which may occasionally be in conflict with wishes expressed by the family or, on rare occasion, wishes expressed by a durable power agent.

In the absence of any information pertaining to the presumptive wishes of the patient, substituted judgment may be applied based on several considerations:

1. What would a "reasonable" person want under similar circumstances? Physicians should rarely be making this judgment independently, and the involvement of colleagues or a formal ethics committee consultation may be appropriate.

2. What would the likely benefits of continued treatment be (treatment outcome), weighed against the burdens imposed by both the treatment and the treatment outcome? The anticipated degree of functional recovery and resultant quality of life are important factors in this consideration. Therapeutic intervention designed to prolong life in a setting in which the quality of that life—because of severity of pain, lack of cognitive function, and so forth—is regarded as being excessively burdensome to an individual may not be medically appropriate.

3. What would, overall, be in the patient's best interests? In many cases, the outcome from a critical illness and specific degree of disability, at a given point in time, cannot be predicted with any degree of certainty. The best-interests test prevents premature withdraw/withhold decisions from being made that might deprive a patient of an opportunity for satisfactory recovery.

Substituted judgment involves subjective analysis and is associated with a significant amount of uncertainty. Although the strong tendency may be to continue treatment when therapeutic goals or the patient's wishes are not known, this course of action may also be inappropriate. Additional professional consultation, including the institutional ethics committee, may help resolve the more difficult cases.

## CONFLICT RESOLUTION

With good ongoing communication, full disclosure of relevant information and prognosis, and a sensitivity to patient/family dynamics, withdraw/withhold support decisions can generally be made smoothly. Protocols or guidelines for the withdrawal process may be of use also.[205] The liberal use of consultants, particularly those involving the neurosciences, may be a valuable adjunct under such circumstances. Ethics consultation services have also been shown to affect management outcome when they are made available.[206,207] Conflicts may arise, however, over issues of futility, therapeutic goals, and the conduct of surrogate decision making. These conflicts are often based on misunderstanding or mistrust and exacerbated by the lack of good communication.

In situations in which conflict between care providers and family members appears to be irreconcilable, even with ethics committee and institutional risk management/legal consultation, a number of alternatives should be offered to the family. These alternatives may include the following: (a) procurement of additional intra- or extramural medical, religious, or ethical consultations;

(b) transferring the care of the patient to another provider within the institution; (c) transfer of the patient to another institution, under the care of another provider; and (d) procurement of a court order mandating a course of treatment.

In most cases, careful collaboration with next of kin and extensive consultation with subspecialty services and/or ethics committee usually will serve to clarify issues surrounding the withdrawal/withholding of support and allow reasonable decisions to be made.

## DO NOT RESUSCITATE ORDERS

The institution of do not resuscitate (DNR) medical directives has been primarily based on the desire to avoid the indignity of futile cardiopulmonary resuscitation in the setting of inexorable progression of underlying known disease processes. Such orders are frequently applied to patients with long-standing terminal disease (e.g., cancer, end-stage acquired immune deficiency syndrome [AIDS], irreversible multiple-organ failure, etc.). DNR orders are implicitly coupled to futility judgments about the benefit of cardiopulmonary resuscitation to achieve prospectively defined therapeutic goals. Under such circumstances, these orders are entirely appropriate and quite desirable in the variety of clinical disease states. The practice of DNR suspension has occurred most frequently in the operating room, where the intensity of therapeutic intervention frequently results in iatrogenic complications. Most physicians and ethicists believe these complications should be treated, since they generally do not constitute inexorable progression of a known disease process, for which the DNR order was originally designed. In the CCU, particularly the surgical CCU, similar situations may exist. The intensity of critical care interventions with mechanical ventilators and the use of complex drug regimens, including vasoactive drugs, may lead to unexpected (iatrogenic) complications unrelated directly to the underlying disease process for which a DNR order may have been originally placed. In addition, the critical illness being treated in the surgical CCU, particularly for trauma patients, results from a discrete event (surgery or injury) as opposed to complications or exacerbations of chronic disease, as is often the case for medical patients. The presumed reversibility of the physiologic sequelae constitutes the basis for CCU treatment of the trauma patient. As such, DNR orders for the trauma patient should be applied very carefully to expected complications, or physiologic changes due to inexorable progression of known underlying disease, as opposed to unexpected and very reversible iatrogenic complications.

DNR orders for trauma patients may be more appropriately linked to withdraw/withhold support conditions than more generally applied to patients with a poor but potentially reversible prognosis. The variability with which DNR orders are interpreted and the "message" such orders send to providers also raise concerns about their applicability for trauma patients. A study by Clemency and Thompson suggests a wide variability in the perception of DNR orders in the perioperative period.[208] This variability conceivably would apply to the "periinjury" period as well. In addition to the potential for the inappropriate application of DNR orders in a CCU, such application may result in less aggressive care on the part of ancillary health care providers.[209,210] DNR orders constitute the prospective application of a specific "withhold support" decision and should be made with the same care and consideration, as described in the section above, as any decision involving the limitation of critical care.

## REFERENCES

1. Trunkey DD: Trauma. Accidental and intentional injuries account for more years of life lost in the U.S. than cancer and heart disease. *Sci Am* 249:28, 1983.
2. Shackford SR, Mackersie RC, Holbrook TL, et al.: The epidemiology of traumatic death: A population-based analysis. *Arch Surg* 128:571, 1993.
3. Groeger JS, Strosberg MA, Halpern NA, et al.: Descriptive analyses of critical care units in the United States. *Crit Care Med* 20:846, 1992.
4. *Resources for Optimal Care of the Injured Patient.* American College of Surgeons, 2006.
5. Pronovost PJ, Angus DC, Dorman T, et al.: Physician staffing patterns and clinical outcomes in critically ill patients: A systematic review. *JAMA* 288:2151, 2002.
6. Pronovost PJ, Jenckes MW, Dorman T, et al.: Organizational characteristics of intensive care units related to outcomes of abdominal aortic surgery. *JAMA* 281:1310, 1999.
7. Pronovost PJ, Young T, Dorman T, et al.: Association between CCU physician staffing and outcomes: A systematic review. *Crit Care Med* 27:A43, 1999.
8. Nathens AB, Rivara FP, MacKenzie EJ, et al.: The impact of an intensivist-model ICU on trauma-related mortality. *Ann Surg* 244:545, 2006.
9. Suarez JI, Zaidat OO, Suri MF, et al.: Length of stay and mortality in neuro-critically ill patients: Impact of a specialized neurocritical care team. *Crit Care Med* 32:2311, 2004.
10. Varelas PN, Conti MM, Spanaki MV: The impact of a neurointensivist-led team on a semiclosed neurosciences intensive care unit. *Crit Care Med* 32:2191, 2004.
11. Internet website: www.leapfroggroup.org.
12. Hoyt JW, Leisifer DJ, Rafkin HS: Critical care units. In Wenzel R, ed. *Assessing Quality Health Care: Perspectives for Clinicians.* Baltimore: Williams & Wilkins, 1992.
13. Calvin JE: Balancing cost considerations and quality of care. In Parriloje JE, Bone RC, eds. *Critical Care Medicine: Principles of Diagnoses and Management.* St Louis: Mosby, 1995.
14. Fakhry SM, Kercher KW, Rutledge R: Survival, quality of life, and changes in critically ill surgical patients requiring prolonged CCU stays. *J Trauma* 41:999, 1996.
15. Goins WA, Reynolds HN, Nyanjom D, et al.: Outcome following prolonged intensive care unit stay in multiple trauma patients. *Crit Care Med* 19:339, 1991.
16. Hopkins RO, Jackson JC: Long-term neurocognitive function after critical illness. *Chest* 130:869, 2006.
17. Agency for Health Care Policy and Research: *Interim Manual Clinical Practice Guideline Development.* Rockville, MD: Agency for Health Care Policy and Research, May 1991.
18. Hammond JJ: Protocols and guidelines in critical care: Development and implementation. *Curr Opin Crit Care* 7:464, 2001.
19. Cocanour CS, Peninger M, Domonoske BD, et al.: Decreasing ventilator-associated pneumonia in a trauma ICU. *J Trauma* 61:122, 2006.
20. McLean SE, Jensen LA, Schroeder DG, et al.: Improving adherence to a mechanical ventilation weaning protocol for critically ill adults: Outcomes after an implementation program. *Am J Crit Care* 15:299, 2006.
21. Aboutanos SZ, Duane TM, Malhotra AK, et al.: Prospective evaluation of an extubation protocol in a trauma intensive care unit population. *Am Surg* 72:393, 2006.
22. Keroack MA, Cerese J, Cuny J, et al.: The relationship between evidence-based practices and survival in patients requiring prolonged mechanical ventilation in academic medical centers. *Am J Med Qual* 21:91, 2006.
23. Curtis JR, Cook DJ, Wall RJ, et al.: Intensive care unit quality improvement: A "how-to" guide for the interdisciplinary team. *Crit Care Med* 34:211, 2006.
24. Kennedy JF, Nightingale JM: Cost savings of an adult hospital nutrition support team. *Nutrition* 21:1127, 2005.
25. Pun BT, Gordon SM, Peterson JF, et al.: Large-scale implementation of sedation and delirium monitoring in the intensive care unit: A report from two medical centers. *Crit Care Med* 33:1199, 2005.
26. Frezza EE, Mezghebe H: Indications and complications of arterial catheter use in surgical or medical intensive care units: Analysis of 4,932 patients. *Am Surg* 64:127, 1998.
27. Dillon PJ, et al.: Comparison of superior vena cava and femoral-iliac venous pressure measurements during normal and inverse ratio ventilation. *Crit Care Med* 29:37, 2001.
28. Connors AR, Speroff T, Dawson NV, et al.: The effectiveness of right heart catheterization in the initial care of critically ill patients. *JAMA* 276:889, 1996.
29. Ivanov R, Allen J, Calvin JE: The incidence of major morbidity in critically ill patients managed with pulmonary artery catheters: A meta-analysis. *Crit Care Med* 28:615, 2000.
30. Scalea TM, Simon HM, Duncan AO, et al.: Geriatric blunt multiple trauma: Improved survival with early invasive monitoring. *J Trauma* 30:129, 1990.
31. Friese RS, Shafi S, Gentilello LM: Pulmonary artery catheter use is associated with reduced mortality in severely injured patients: A National Trauma Data Bank analysis of 53,312 patients. *Crit Care Med* 34:1597, 2006.

32. Bernard GR, Sopko G, Cerra F, et al.: Pulmonary artery catheterization and clinical outcomes: National Heart, Lung, and Blood Institute and Food and Drug Administration Workshop Report. Consensus Statement. *JAMA* 283:2568, 2000.

33. Urban P, Scheidegger D, Gabathuler J, et al.: Thermodilution measurement of the right ventricular ejection fraction: A comparison with biplane angiography. *Crit Care Med* 15:652, 1987.

34. Jardin F, Brun-Ney D, Hardy A, et al.: Combined thermodilution and two-dimensional echocardiographic evaluation of right ventricular function during respiratory support with PEEP. *Chest* 99:162, 1991.

35. Cheatham ML, et al.: Right ventricular end-diastolic volume index as a predictor of preload status in patients on positive end-expiratory pressure *Crit Care Med* 26:1801, 1998.

36. Guy JS, et al.: Right ventricular end-diastolic volume index is not affected by increases in PEEP. *J Trauma* 45:1117, 1998.

37. Chang MC, Meredith JW: Cardiac preload, splanchnic perfusion and their relationship during resuscitation in trauma patients. *J Trauma* 42:577, 1997.

38. Burns JM, Sing RF, Mostafa G, et al.: The role of transesophageal echocardiography in optimizing resuscitation in acutely injured patients. *J Trauma* 59:36, 2005.

39. Price S, Nicol E, Gibson DG, et al.: Echocardiography in the critically ill: Current and potential roles. *Intensive Care Med* 32:48, 2006; Epub November 16, 2005.

40. Davis JW, Mackersie RC, Holbrook TI, et al.: Base deficit as an indicator of significant abdominal injury. *Ann Emerg Med* 20:842, 1991.

41. Davis JW, Shackford SR, Mackersie RC, et al.: Base deficit as a guide to volume resuscitation. *J Trauma* 28:146, 1988.

42. Rutherford EJ, Morris JA Jr, Reed GW, et al.: Base deficit stratifies mortality and determines therapy. *J Trauma* 33:417, 1992.

43. Davis JW, Kaups KL, Parks SN: Base deficit is superior to pH in evaluating clearance of acidosis after traumatic shock. *J Trauma* 44:114, 1998.

44. Davis JW, Kaups KL, Parks SN: Effect of alcohol on the utility of base deficit in trauma. *J Trauma* 43:3507, 1997.

45. Miami Trauma Clinical Trials Group: Splanchnic hypoperfusion-directed therapies in trauma: A prospective, randomized trial. *Am Surg* 71:252, 2005.

46. Gomersall CD, Joynt GM, Freebairn RC, et al.: Resuscitation of critically ill patients based on the results of gastric tonometry: A prospective, randomized, controlled trial. *Crit Care Med* 28:607, 2000.

47. Vincent JL, Baron J-F, Reinhart K, et al.: Anemia and blood transfusion in critically ill patients. *JAMA* 288:1499, 2002.

48. Corwin HL, Gettinger A, Pearl RG, et al.: The CRIT study: Anemia and blood transfusion in the critically ill: Current clinical practice in the United States. *Crit Care Med* 32:39, 2004.

49. Corwin HL, Gettinger A, Pearl RG, et al.: Efficacy of recombinant human erythropoietin in critically ill patients: A randomized controlled trial. *JAMA* 288:2827, 2002.

50. Silver M, Corwin MJ, Bazan A, et al.: Efficacy of recombinant human erythropoietin in critically ill patients admitted to a long-term acute care facility: A randomized, double-blind placebo-controlled trial. *Crit Care Med* 34:2310, 2006.

51. Brain Trauma Foundation, American Association of Neurological Surgeons, Joint Section on Neurotrauma and Critical Care: Guidelines for the management of severe head injury. *J Neurotrauma* 13:641, 1996.

52. Thomason MH, Rutledge R: A statewide analysis of the use of intracranial pressure monitoring with the outcome of severe head injury in 1,563 patients (abstr). *J Trauma* 45:192, 1998.

53. Sheinberg M, Kanter MJ, Robertson CS, et al.: Continuous monitoring or jugular venous oxygen saturation in head injured patients. *J Neurosurg* 76:212, 1992.

54. Cruz J: On-line monitoring of global cerebral hypoxia in acute brain injury. Relationship to intracranial hypertension. *J Neurosurg* 79:228, 1993.

55. Chan MT, Ng SC, Lam JM, et al.: Re-defining the ischemic threshold for jugular venous oxygen saturation–a microdialysis study in patients with severe head injury. *Acta Neurochir Suppl* 95:63, 2005.

56. Robertson CS, Valadka AB, Hannay HJ, et al.: Prevention of secondary ischemic insults after severe head injury. *Crit Care Med* 27:2086, 1999.

57. Dohmen C, Bosche B, Graf R, et al.: Prediction of malignant course in MCA infarction by PET and microdialysis. *Stroke* 34:2152, 2003.

58. Palmer S, Bader MK: Brain tissue oxygenation in brain death. *Neurocrit Care* 2:17, 2005.

59. Jaeger M, Schuhrmann M, Soehle M: Continuous assessment of cerebrovascular autoregulation after traumatic brain injury using brain tissue oxygen pressure reactivity. *Crit Care Med* 34:1783, 2006.

60. Christman JM, McClain RW: Sensible approach to the nutritional support of mechanically ventilated patients. *Intens Care Med* 19:129, 1992.

61. Van den Berghe G, Wouters P, et al.: Intensive insulin therapy in the surgical intensive care unit. *N Engl J Med* 345:1355, 2001.

62. Voeglzang M, Nijboer JMM, van der Horst ICC, et al.: Hyperglycemia has a stronger relation with outcome in trauma patients than in other critically ill patients. *J Trauma* 60:873, 2006.

63. Finney SJ, Zekveld C, et al.: Glucose control and mortality in critically ill patients. *JAMA* 290:2041, 2003.

64. Annane D, Sebille V, Charpentier C, et al.: Effect of treatment with low doses of hydrocortisone and fludrocortisone on mortality in patients with septic shock. *JAMA* 288:862, 2002.

65. Cooper MS, Stewart PM: Corticosteroid insufficiency in acutely ill patients. *N Engl J Med* 348:727, 2003.

66. Hamrahian AH, Tawakalitu S, Oseni MD, et al.: Measurements of serum free cortisol in critically ill patients. *N Engl J Med* 350:1629, 2004.

67. Reed RL: Contemporary issues with bacterial infection in the intensive care unit. *Surg Clin North Am* 3:895, 2000.

68. Appelgren P, Hellstrom I, Weitzberg E, et al.: Risk factors for nosocomial intensive care unit infection: A long-term prospective analysis. *Acta Anaesthesiol Scand* 45:710, 2001.

69. Mackersie RC, Karagianes TG, York J: End-tidal PCO2 monitoring during resuscitation of severe head injuries. *Crit Care Med* 18:764, 1990.

70. Karason S, Sondergaard S, Lundin S, et al.: Continuous on-line measurements of respiratory system, lung and chest wall mechanics during mechanic ventilation. *Intens Care Med* 27:1328, 2001.

71. Maggiore SM, Brouchard L: Pressure-volume curve in the critically ill. *Curr Opin Crit Care* 6:1, 2000.

72. Marini JJ, Rodriguez RM, Lamb V: The inspiratory work load of patient-initiated mechanical ventilation. *Am Rev Respir Dis* 134:902, 1986.

73. Yang KL, Tobin MJ: A prospective study of indexes predicting the outcome of trials of weaning from mechanical ventilation. *N Engl J Med* 324:1445, 1991.

74. Parker JC, Hernandez LA, Peevy KJ: Mechanisms of ventilator-induced lung injury. *Crit Care Med* 21:131, 1993.

75. Sternberg R, Sahebjami H: Hemodynamic and oxygen transport characteristics of common ventilatory modes. *Chest* 105:1798, 1994.

76. Rappaport SH, Shpiner R, Yoshihara G, et al.: Randomized, prospective trial of pressure-limited versus volume-controlled ventilation in severe respiratory failure. *Crit Care Med* 22:22, 1994.

77. Hickling KG, Walsh J, Henderson S, et al.: Low mortality rate in adult respiratory distress syndrome using low-volume, pressure-limited ventilation with permissive hyper-capnia: A prospective study. *Crit Care Med* 22:1568, 1994.

78. The Acute Respiratory Distress Syndrome Network: Ventilation with lower tidal volumes as compared with traditional tidal volumes for acute lung injury and the acute respiratory distress syndrome. *N Engl J Med* 342:1301, 2000.

79. Gajic O, Dara SI, Mendez JL, et al.: Ventilator-associated lung injury in patients without acute lung injury at the onset of mechanical ventilation. *Crit Care Med* 32:1817, 2004.

80. Brower RG, Lanken PN, MacIntyre N, et al.: Higher versus lower positive end-expiratory pressures in patients with the acute respiratory distress syndrome. *N Engl J Med* 351:327, 2004.

81. Villar J, Kacmarek RM, Perez-Mendez L, et al.: A high positive end-expiratory pressure, low tidal volume ventilatory strategy improves outcome in persistent acute respiratory distress syndrome: A randomized, controlled trial. *Crit Care Med* 34:1311, 2006.

82. Hinson JR, Marini JJ: Principles of mechanical ventilator use in respiratory failure. *Annu Rev Med* 43:341, 1992.

83. Guldager H, Nielsen SL, Carl P, et al.: A comparison of volume control and pressure-regulated volume control ventilation in acute respiratory failure. *Crit Care (Lond)* 1:75, 1997.

84. Marcy TW, Marini JJ: Inverse ratio ventilation in ARDS. Rationale and implementation. *Chest* 100:494, 1991.

85. Chan K, Abraham E: Effects of inverse ratio ventilation on cardiorespiratory parameters in severe respiratory failure. *Chest* 102:1556, 1992.

86. Armstrong BW Jr, MacIntyre NR: Pressure-controlled, inverse ratio ventilation that avoids air trapping in the adult respiratory distress syndrome. *Crit Care Med* 23:279, 1995.

87. Lessard MR, Guerot E, Lorino H, et al.: Effects of pressure-controlled with different I:E ratios versus volume-controlled ventilation on respiratory mechanics, gas exchange, and hemodynamics in patients with adult respiratory distress syndrome. *Anesthesiology* 80:983, 1994.

88. Shanholtz C, Brower R: Should inverse ratio ventilation be used in adult respiratory distress syndrome? *Am J Respir Crit Care Med* 149:1354, 1994.

89. Kaplan LJ, et al.: Airway pressure release ventilation increases cardiac performance in patients with acute lung injury/adult respiratory distress syndrome. *Crit Care* 5:221, 2001.

90. Mehta S, Lapinsky SE, Hallett DC, et. al.: Prospective trial of high-frequency oscillation in adults with acute respiratory distress syndrome *Crit Care Med* 29:1360, 2001.

91. Lee DL, Chiang HT, Lin SL, et al.: Prone-position ventilation induces sustained improvement in oxygenation in patients with acute respiratory distress syndrome who have a large shunt. *Crit Care Med* 30:1446, 2002.

92. Beuret P, Carton MJ, Nourdine K, et al.: Prone position as prevention of lung injury in comatose patients: A prospective, randomized, controlled study. *Intens Care Med* 28:564, 2002.

93. Gattinoni L, Tognoni G, Pesenti A: Effect of prone positioning on the survival of patients with acute respiratory failure. *N Engl J Med* 345:568, 2001.

94. Voggenreiter G, Aufmkolk M, Stiletto RJ, et al.: Prone positioning improves oxygenation in post-traumatic lung injury: a prospective randomized trial. *J Trauma* 59:333, 2005.

95. Taylor RW, Zimmerman JL, Dellinger RP: Low-dose inhaled nitric oxide in patients with acute lung injury: A randomized controlled trial. *JAMA* 291:1603, 2004.

96. Michael JR, Barton RG, Saffle JR, et al.: Inhaled nitric oxide versus conventional therapy: Effect on oxygenation in ARDS. *Am J Respir Crit Care Med* 157:1372, 1998.

97. Putensen C, et al.: Cardiopulmonary effects of aerosolized prostaglandin E1 and nitric oxide inhalation in patients with acute respiratory distress syndrome. *Am J Respir Crit Care Med* 157:1743, 1998.

98. Gallart L, et al.: Intravenous almitrine combined with inhaled nitric oxide for acute respiratory distress. *Am J Respir Crit Care Med* 158:1770, 1998.

99. Johannigman JA, et al.: Prone positioning and inhaled nitric oxide: Synergistic therapies for acute respiratory distress syndrome. *J Trauma* 50:589, 2001.

100. Shapiro M, Wilson K, Casar G, et al.: Work of breathing through different sized endotracheal tubes. *Crit Care Med* 14:1028, 1986.

101. Wong PW, et al.: The effect of varying inspiratory flow waveforms on pulmonary mechanics in critically ill patients. *J Crit Care* 15:133, 2000.

102. Pelosi P, et al.: Effects of different continuous positive airway pressure devices and periodic hyperinflations on respiratory function. *Crit Care Med* 29:1683, 2001.

103. Collective Task Force: Evidence-based guidelines for weaning and discontinuing ventilatory support. *Chest* 6:375s, 2001.

104. Namen AM, et al.: Predictors of successful extubation in neurosurgical patients. *Am J Respir Crit Care Med* 163:658, 2001.

105. Aldrich TK, Karpel JP: Inspiratory muscle resistive training in respiratory failure. *Am Rev Respir Dis* 131:461, 1985.

106. Anderson T, Kearney JT: Effects of three resistance training programs on muscular strength and absolute and relative endurance. *Res Q Exerc Sport Med* 53:1, 1982.

107. DeLateur BJ, Lehmann JF, Giaconi R: Mechanical work and fatigue: Their roles in the development of muscle work capacity. *Arch Phys Med Rehabil* 57:319, 1976.

108. Clanton TL, Dixon G, Drake J, et al.: Inspiratory muscle conditioning using a threshold loading device. *Chest* 87:62, 1985.

109. Leith DE, Bradley M: Ventilatory muscle strength and endurance training. *J Appl Physiol* 41:508, 1976.

110. Brochard L, Rauss A, Benito S, et al.: Comparison of three methods of gradual withdrawal from ventilatory support during weaning from mechanical ventilation. *Am J Respir Crit Care Med* 150:896, 1994.

111. Esteban A, Frutos F, Tobin MJ, et al.: A comparison of four methods of weaning patients from mechanical ventilation. Spanish Lung Failure Collaborative Group. *N Engl J Med* 332:345, 1995.

112. Faulkner JA: Structural and functional adaptations of skeletal muscle. In Roussos C, Macklem PT, eds. *Lung Biology in Health and Disease: The Thorax.* Part B, Vol 29. New York: Marcel Dekker, 1985, p. 1329.

113. Rochester DF: Does respiratory muscle rest relieve fatigue or incipient fatigue? *Am Rev Respir Dis* 138:516, 1988.

114. Lerman RM, Weiss MS: Progressive resistive exercise in weaning high quadriplegics from the ventilator. *Paraplegia* 25:130, 1987.

115. Martin AD, Davenport PD, Franceschi AC, et al.: Use of inspiratory muscle strength training to facilitate ventilator weaning: A series of 10 consecutive patients. *Chest* 122:192, 2002.

116. Ely EW, Meade MO, Haponik EF, et al.: Mechanical ventilator weaning protocols driven by non-physician health-care professionals: Evidence-based clinical practice guidelines. *Chest* 120:454S, 2001.

117. Scheinhorn DJ, Chao DC, Stearn-Hassenpflug M: Liberation from prolonged mechanical ventilation. *Crit Care Clin* 18:569, 2002.

118. Lellouche F, Mancebo J, Jolliet P, et al.: A multicenter randomized trial of computer-driven protocolized weaning from mechanical ventilation. *Am J Respir Crit Care Med* 174:894, 2006.

119. Dries DJ, McGonigal MD, Malian MS: Protocol-driven ventilator weaning reduces use of mechanical ventilation, rate of early reintubation, and ventilator-associated pneumonia. *J Trauma* 56:943, 2004.

120. Rodriguez JL, Steinberg SM, Luchetti FA, et al.: Early tracheostomy for primary airway management in the surgical critical care setting. *Surgery* 108:655, 1990.

121. El-Naggar M, Sadagopan S, Levine H, et al.: Factors influencing choice between tracheostomy and prolonged translaryngeal intubation in acute respiratory failure: A prospective study. *Anesth Analg* 55:195, 1976.

122. Sugerman HJ, Wolfe L, Pasquale MD, et al.: Multicenter, randomized, prospective trial of early tracheostomy. *J Trauma* 43:741, 1997.

123. Rumbak MJ, Newton M, Truncale T, et al.: A prospective, randomized, study comparing early percutaneous dilational tracheotomy to prolonged translaryngeal intubation (delayed tracheotomy) in critically ill medical patients. *Crit Care Med* 32:1689, 2004. Erratum in: *Crit Care Med* 32:2566, 2004.

124. Barquist ES, Amorteegui J, Hallal A, et al.: Tracheostomy in ventilator dependent trauma patients: A prospective, randomized intention-to-treat study. *J Trauma* 60:91, 2006.

125. Gysin C, Dulguerov P, Guyot JP, et al.: Percutaneous versus surgical tracheostomy: A double-blind randomized trial. *Ann Surg* 230:708, 1999.

126. Freeman BD, Isabella K, Cobb JP, et al.: A prospective, randomized study comparing percutaneous with surgical tracheostomy in critically ill patients. *Crit Care Med* 29:926, 2001.

127. Melloni G, Muttini S, Gallioli G, et al.: Surgical tracheostomy versus percutaneous dilatational tracheostomy. A prospective-randomized study with long-term follow-up. *J Cardiovasc Surg (Torino)* 43:113, 2002.

128. Norwood S, Vallina VL, Short K, et al.: Incidence of tracheal stenosis and other late complications after percutaneous tracheostomy. *Ann Surg* 232:233, 2000.

129. Antonelli M, Michetti V, Di Palma A, et al.: Percutaneous translaryngeal versus surgical tracheostomy: A randomized trial with 1-yr double-blind follow-up. *Crit Care Med* 33:1015, 2005.

130. Jacobi J, Fraser GL, Coursin DB, et al.: Clinical practice guidelines for the sustained use of sedatives and analgesics in the critically ill adult. *Crit Care Med* 30:119, 2002.

131. Vender JS, Szokol JW, Murphy GS, et al.: Sedation, analgesia, and neuromuscular blockade in sepsis: An evidence-based review. *Crit Care Med* 32:S554, 2004.

132. Austin KL, Stapleton JV, Mather LE: Relationship between blood meperidine concentrations and analgesic response. *Anesthesiology* 53:460, 1980.

133. Bergbom-Engberg I, Haljamae H: Assessment of patient's experience of discomforts during respirator therapy. *Crit Care Med* 17:1068, 1989.

134. van de Leur JP, van der Schans CP, Loef BG, et al.: Discomfort and factual recollection in intensive care unit patients. *Crit Care Med* 8:R467, 2004.

135. Rotondi AJ, Chelluri L, Sirio C, et al.: Patients' recollections of stressful experiences while receiving prolonged mechanical ventilation in an intensive care unit. *Crit Care Med* 30:746, 2002.

136. Adams P, Gelman S, Reeves JG, et al.: Midazolam pharmacodynamics and pharmacokinetics during acute hypovolemia. *Anesthesiology* 63:140, 1985.

137. Barrientos-Vega R, Sanchez-Soria M, Morales-Garcia C, et al.: Prolonged sedation of critically ill patients with midazolam or propofol: Impact on weaning and costs. *Crit Care Med* 25:33, 1997.

138. De Cosmo G, Congedo E, Clemente A, et al.: Sedation in PACU: The role of propofol. *Curr Drug Targets* 6:741, 2005.

139. Snellen F, Lauwers P, Demeyere R, et al.: The use of midazolam versus propofol for short-term sedation following coronary artery bypass grafting. *Intens Care Med* 16:312, 1990.

140. Higgins T, Vared J, Estafanous F, et al.: Propofol vs midazolam for intensive care unit sedation after coronary artery bypass grafting. *Crit Care Med* 22:1415, 1994.

141. Aitkenhead AR, Willatts SM, Parks GR, et al.: Comparison of propofol and midazolam for sedation in critically ill patients. *Lancet* 2:704, 1989.

142. Carrasco G, Molina R, Costa J, et al.: Propofol vs midazolam in short-, medium-, and long-term sedation of critically ill patients: A cost-benefit analysis. *Chest* 103:557, 1993.

143. Coursin DB, Coursin DB, Macciolo GA: Dexmedetomidine. *Curr Opin Crit Care* 7:221, 2001.

144. Siobal M, Kallet R, Divett V, et al.: Use of dexmedetomidine to facilitate extubation in surgical ICU patients that failed previous weaning attempts following prolonged mechanical ventilation. *Resp Care* 51:492, 2006.

145. Ramsay MAE, Savege TM, Simpson BRJ, et al.: Controlled sedation with alphaxalone-alphadolone. *BMJ* 2:656, 1974.

146. Kress JP, Pohlman AS, O'Connor MF, et al.: Daily interruption of sedative infusions in critically ill patients undergoing mechanical ventilation. *N Engl J Med* 342:1471, 2000.

147. Kress JP, Gehlbach B, Lacy M, et al.: The long-term psychological effects of daily sedative interruption on critically ill patients. *Am J Respir Crit Care Med* 168:1457, 2003.

148. Kaplan LJ, Bailey H: Bispectral index (BIS) monitoring of ICU patients on continuous infusion of sedatives and paralytics reduces sedative drug utilization and cost. *Crit Care Med* 4:S110, 2000.

149. Simmons L, Riker R, Prato S, et al.: Assessing sedation during intensive care unit mechanical ventilation with the bispectral index and the sedation-agitation scale. *Crit Care Med* 27:1499, 1999.

150. Dittmann M, Wolff GA: A rationale for epidural analgesia in the treatment of multiple rib fractures. *Intens Care Med* 4:192, 1978.

151. Mackersie RC, Shackford SR, Hoyt DB, et al.: Continuous epidural fentanyl analgesia: Ventilatory function improvement with routine use in treatment of blunt chest trauma. *J Trauma* 27:1207, 1987.

152. Mackersie R, Karagianes T, Hoyt D, et al.: Prospective evaluation of epidural and intravenous administration of fentanyl for pain control and restoration of ventilatory function following multiple rib fractures. *J Trauma* 31:443, 1991.

153. Bolliger CT, VanEeden SF: Treatment of multiple rib fractures: Randomized controlled trial comparing ventilatory with nonventilatory management. *Chest* 97:943, 1990.

154. Wisner DH: A stepwise logistic regression analysis of factors affecting morbidity and mortality after thoracic trauma: Effect of epidural analgesia. *J Trauma* 30:799, 1990.

155. Sauaia A, Moore FA, Moore EE, et al.: Pneumonia: Cause or symptom of postinjury multiple organ failure? *Am J Surg* 166:606, 1993.

156. Warren DK, Shukla SJ, Olsen MA, et al.: Outcome and attributable cost of ventilator-associated pneumonia among intensive care unit patients in a suburban medical center. *Crit Care Med* 31:1312, 2003.

157. Rello J, Ollendorf DA, Oster G, et al.: Epidemiology and outcomes of ventilator-associated pneumonia in a large US database. *Chest* 122:2115, 2002.

158. Pineda LA, Saliba RG, El Solh AA, et al.: Effect of oral decontamination with chlorhexidine on the incidence of nosocomial pneumonia: A meta-analysis. *Crit Care* 10:R35, 2006.

159. Koeman M, van der Ven AJ, Hak E, et al.: Oral decontamination with chlorhexidine reduces the incidence of ventilator-associated pneumonia. *Am J Respir Crit Care Med* 173:1348, 2006; Epub April 7, 2006.

160. Hoyt DB, Simons RK, Winchell RJ, et al.: A risk analysis of pulmonary complications following major trauma. *J Trauma* 35:524, 1993.

161. Chevret S, Hemmer M, Carlet J, et al.: Incidence and risk factors of pneumonia acquired in intensive care units. Results from a multicenter prospective study on 996 patients. European Cooperative Group on Nosocomial Pneumonia. *Intens Care Med* 19:256, 1993.

162. Porzecanski I, Bowton DL: Diagnosis and treatment of ventilator-associated pneumonia. *Chest* 130:597, 2006.

163. Torres A, El-Ebiary M: Bronchoscopic BAL in the diagnosis of ventilator-associated pneumonia. *Chest* 117:198S, 2000.

164. Mentec H, May-Michelangeli L, Rabbat A, et al.: Blind and bronchoscopic sampling methods in suspected ventilator-associated pneumonia. A multicentre prospective study. *Intensive Care Med* 30:1319, 2004; Epub April 20, 2004.

165. Wood AY, Davit AJ II, Ciraulo DL, et al.: A prospective assessment of diagnostic efficacy of blind protective bronchial brushings compared to bronchoscope-assisted lavage, bronchoscope-directed brushings, and blind endotracheal aspirates in ventilator-associated pneumonia. *J Trauma* 55:825, 2003.

166. Cook D, DeJonghe B, Brochard L, et al.: Influence of airway management on ventilator-associated pneumonia: Evidence from randomized trials. *JAMA* 279:781, 1998.

167. Dezfulian C, Shojania K, Collard HR, et al.: Subglottic secretion drainage for preventing ventilator-associated pneumonia a meta-analysis. *Am J Med* 118:11, 2005.

168. Van Saene HKF, Ashworth M, Petros AJ, et al.: Do not suction above the cuff, *Crit Care Med* 32:2160, 2004.

169. Chevron V, Menard JF, Richard JC, et al.: Unplanned extubation: Risk factors of development and predictive criteria for reintubation. *Crit Care Med* 26:1049, 1998.

170. Boulain T: Unplanned extubations in the adult intensive care unit: A prospective multicenter study. *Am J Resp Crit Care Med* 157:1131, 1998.

171. Krinsley JS, Barone JE: The drive to survive: Unplanned extubation in the ICU. *Chest* 128:560, 2005.

172. Mort TC: Unplanned tracheal extubation outside the operating room: A quality improvement audit of hemodynamic and tracheal airway complications associated with emergency tracheal reintubation. *Anesth Analg* 86:1171, 1998.

173. Raad IL, Hohn DC, Gilbreath BJ, et al.: Prevention of central venous catheter-related infections by using maximal sterile barrier precautions during insertion. *Infect Control Hosp Epidemiol* 15:231, 1994.

174. Maki DG, Ringer M, Alvarado CJ: Prospective randomised trial of povidone-iodine, alcohol, and chlorhexidine for prevention of infection associated with central venous and arterial catheters. *Lancet* 338:339, 1991.

175. Hoffmann KK, Weber DJ, Samsa GP, et al.: Transparent polyurethane film as an intravenous catheter dressing. A meta-analysis of the infection risks. *JAMA* 267:2072, 1992.

176. Welch GW, McKeel DW Jr, Silverstein P, et al.: The role of catheter composition in the development of thrombophlebitis. *Surg Gynecol Obstet* 138:421, 1974.

177. Kamal GD, Pfaller MA, Rempe LE, et al.: Reduced intravascular catheter infection by antibiotic bonding. A prospective, randomized, controlled trial. *JAMA* 265:2364, 1991.

178. Bach A, Bohrer H, Motsch J, et al.: Prevention of bacterial colonization of intravenous catheters by antiseptic impregnation of polyurethane polymers. *J Antimicrob Chemother* 33:969, 1994.

179. Heard SO, Wagle M, Vijayakumar E, et al.: Influence of triple-lumen central venous catheters coated with chlorhexidine and silver sulfadiazine on the incidence of catheter-related bacteremia. *Arch Intern Med* 158:81, 1998.

180. Tennenberg S, Lieser M, McCurdy B, et al.: A prospective randomized trial of an antibiotic- and antiseptic-coated central venous catheter in the prevention of catheter-related infections. *Arch Surg* 132:1348, 1997.

181. Maki DG, Stolz SM, Wheeler S, et al.: Prevention of central venous catheter-related bloodstream infection by use of an antiseptic-impregnated catheter. A randomized, controlled trial (see comments). *Ann Intern Med* 127:257, 1997.

182. Kamal GD, Divishek D, Kumar GC, et al.: Reduced intravascular catheter-related infection by routine use of antibiotic-bonded catheters in a surgical intensive care unit. *Diagn Microbiol Infect Dis* 30:145, 1998.

183. Raad I, Darouiche R, Dupuis J, et al.: Central venous catheters coated with minocycline and rifampin for the prevention of catheter-related colonization and bloodstream infections. A randomized, double-blind trial. *Ann Intern Med* 127:267, 1997.

184. Kowalewska-Grochowska K, Richards R, Moysa GL, et al.: Guidewire catheter change in central venous catheter biofilm formation in a burn population. *Chest* 100:1090, 1991.

185. Eyer S, Brummitt C, Crossley K, et al.: Catheter-related sepsis: Prospective, randomized study of three methods of long-term catheter maintenance. *Crit Care Med* 18:1073, 1990.

186. Cobb DK, High KP, Sawyer RG, et al.: A controlled trial of scheduled replacement of central venous and pulmonary-artery catheters. *N Engl J Med* 327:1062, 1992.

187. Raymond DP, Pelletier SJ, Crabtree TD, et al.: Impact of a rotating empiric antibiotic schedule on infectious mortality in an intensive care unit. *Crit Care Med* 29:1101, 2001.

188. Gruson D, Hilbert G, Vargas F, et al.: Rotation and restricted use of antibiotics in a medical intensive care unit. Impact on the incidence of ventilator-associated pneumonia caused by antibiotic-resistant gram-negative bacteria. *Am J Respir Crit Care Med* 162:837, 2000.

189. Timsit JF: Scheduled replacement of central venous catheters is not necessary. *Infect Control Hosp Epidemiol* 21:371, 2000.

190. Warren DK, Hill HA, Merz LR, et al.: Cycling empirical antimicrobial agents to prevent emergence of antimicrobial-resistant Gram-negative bacteria among intensive care unit patients. *Crit Care Med* 32:2450, 2004.

191. Kollef MH: Is antibiotic cycling the answer to preventing the emergence of bacterial resistance in the intensive care unit? *Clin Infect Dis* 43:S82, 2006.

192. Bolton CF, Gilbert JJ, Hahn AF, et al.: Polyneuropathy in critically ill patients. *J Neurol Neurosurg Psychiatry* 47:1223, 1984.

193. Witt NJ, Zochodne DW, Bolton CF, et al.: Peripheral nerve function in sepsis and multiple organ failure. *Chest* 99:176, 1991.

194. Hund EF, Forgel W, Krieger D, et al.: Critical illness polyneuropathy: Clinical findings and outcomes of a frequent cause of neuromuscular weaning failure. *Crit Care Med* 24:1328, 1996.

195. Coakley JH, Nagendran K, Ormerod IE, et al.: Prolonged neurogenic weakness in patients requiring mechanical ventilation for acute airflow limitation. *Chest* 101:1413, 1992.

196. Luce JM: Withholding and withdrawing life support from the critically ill: How does it work in clinical practice? *Respir Care* 36:417, 1991.

197. President's Commission for the Study of Ethical Problems in Medicine and Biomedical and Behavioral Research: Making health care decisions: The ethical and legal implications of informed consent in the patient–practitioner relationship. Informed Consent as Active, Shared Decision Making. Vol 1. Washington, DC: US Government Printing Office, 1982.

198. AACP/SCCM Consensus Panel: Ethical and moral guidelines for the initiation, continuation, and withdrawal of intensive care. *Chest* 97:949, 1990.

199. Smedira NG, Evans BH, Grais LS: Withholding and withdrawal of life support from the critically ill. *N Engl J Med* 322:309, 1990.

200. Cook D, Rocker G, Marshall J, et al.: Withdrawal of mechanical ventilation in anticipation of death in the intensive care unit. *N Engl J Med* 349:1123, 2003.

201. Schneiderman LJ, Faber-Langendoen K, Jecker NS: Beyond futility to an ethic of care. *Am J Med* 96:110, 1994.

202. Baker R: The ethics of medical futility. *Crit Care Clin* 9:575, 1993.

203. Lantos JD, Singer PA, Walker RM, et al.: The illusion of futility in clinical practice. *Am J Med* 87:81, 1989.

204. Schneiderman LJ, Jecker NS, Jonsen AR: Medical futility: Its meaning and ethical implications. *Ann Intern Med* 112:949, 1990.

205. Hall RI, Rocker GM, Murray D: Simple changes can improve conduct of end-of-life care in the intensive care unit. *Can J Anaesth* 51:631, 2004.

206. Perkins HS, Bunnie S, Saathoff BA: Impact of medical ethics consultations on physicians: An exploratory study. *Am J Med* 85:761, 1988.

207. LaPuma J, Stocking CB, Silverstein MD, et al.: An ethics consultation service in a teaching hospital. *JAMA* 260:808, 1988.

208. Clemency MV, Thompson NJ: "Do not resuscitate" (DNR) orders in the perioperative period—A comparison of the perspectives of anesthesiologists, internists, and surgeons. *Anesth Analg* 78:651, 1994.

209. Sherman DA, Branum K: Critical care nurses' perceptions of appropriate care of the patient with orders not to resuscitate. *Heart Lung* 24:321, 1995.

210. Azoulay E, Pochard F, Garrouste-Orgeas M, et al.: Decisions to forgo life-sustaining therapy in ICU patients independently predict hospital death. *Intensive Care Med* 29:1895, 2003; Epub October 7, 2003.

# Commentary ■ ANDREW J. PATTERSON ■ DAVID A. SPAIN

In this chapter, Mackersie and colleagues provide a comprehensive review of surgical critical care. They describe its evolution, the tools that make it possible, and the approaches to utilizing these tools. The authors also discuss some of the financial issues that influenced the development of critical care during the past 30 years. We would like to expound upon this topic. We believe that financial constraints will soon lead to major cost cutting in surgical intensive care units and force dramatic changes in how we practice critical care medicine.

As the age and acuity of our patients increase, the challenge for intensivists will be to transform surgical critical care so we can manage larger numbers of sicker patients with fewer resources while achieving better outcomes. There are several tools that may allow us to accomplish this goal. We would like to highlight four of them: (1) point-of-service devices that will allow intensivists to make rapid and accurate diagnoses; (2) tissue perfusion based hemodynamic monitoring that will provide better assessment of the health of vital organs; (3) gGene and protein array research that is already enhancing our understanding of inflammatory states and how they might be regulated and (4) integrated health care networks that utilize advancements in informatics, communication, and transportation to link the sickest patients to physicians with the best equipment and training for managing the critically ill.

Point-of-service devices are already becoming more common in the ICU. Blood glucose levels, arterial blood gas values, even serum lactic acid concentrations can now be measured at the bedside. However, complex analyses such as those for pathogen detection and characterization have been limited by expense, complexity, and lack of reliability. Nanoparticle-based diagnostic devices may soon solve these problems. For example, nanoparticle instruments are now being developed with the capacity to detect pathogens in droplet-sized body fluid samples. These devices are small enough and simple enough for clinicians to use at the bedside. Further, they may soon allow not only the detection of pathogens, but speciation and identification of antibiotic resistance patterns. The days of broad-spectrum antibiotics with their numerous side effects and risk of selecting for drug resistant organisms may soon be over. In the near future, surgical ICU patients may expeditiously receive antibiotics based on a combination of efficacy and cost.

For the past 60 years assessment of systemic arterial blood pressure, central venous pressure, and(or pulmonary artery pressure has been the focus of hemodynamic monitoring for the critically ill. However, it is now widely recognized that in many instances pressure monitoring does not accurately reflect cardiac performance or vital organ perfusion. Advances in hemodynamic monitoring such as echocardiography, central venous oximetry, and measurement of metabolic indicators of tissue perfusion are

first attempts at providing more relevant hemodynamic data. In the not-so-distant future a new generation of technology promises to bring real-time vital organ tissue perfusion data to the ICU. For example, noninvasive near-infrared spectrophotometry may soon allow clinicians to assess microcirculatory perfusion and/or impairment of oxygen utilization in the hepatosplanchnic organs (a potentially important breakthrough in the treatment of sepsis-induced organ failure). Whether technology like near-infrared spectrophotometry will improve outcomes and reduce costs in surgical ICUs remains to be seen. However, it stands to reason that measuring more relevant parameters of hemodynamic function will improve the intensivist's ability to more effectively choose appropriate fluid resuscitation strategies and hemodynamic pharmaceuticals.

Gene and protein expression research is now demonstrating that immune system activation links seemingly unrelated processes like perioperative myocardial infarction, postoperative wound healing, and immune response to infectious pathogens. This research is also providing insight into inflammatory states and how they might be regulated in order to prevent costly disease processes in the critically ill. One example of this applied basic science research is the use of white blood cell microarray gene expression pattern analysis for early detection of sepsis. In the near future, intensivists may be able to use white blood cell gene expression surveillance to rapidly and accurately diagnose sepsis before it causes hemodynamic deterioration and multiorgan dysfunction. Eradication of the infection source and institution of appropriate antibiotic therapy may be possible before clinical symptoms of sepsis are ever observed. This strategy promises to significantly reduce costs of surgical critical care while improving outcomes.

Finally, integrated health care networks that utilize advancements in informatics, communication, and transportation may improve surgical critical care in many ways. Like trauma networks, these systems may reduce the need to duplicate expensive patient care services by creating more expansive areas from which ICUs may draw patients. As health care information networks develop, the highly trained physicians who staff these units may gain access to more information regarding the patients in their networks, allowing them to make better decisions with less duplication of diagnostic procedures. If adequate resources can be provided, fewer ICUs might provide service to more patients at lower cost while achieving better outcomes.

Despite the considerable challenges that lie ahead, surgical critical care has a bright future. Innovation will lead to significant changes in the tools we use and how we manage patients during next decade. As a consequence, Americans are likely to receive better health care than ever before.

# Bleeding and Coagulation Complications

*Samir M. Fakhry* ■ *Christopher P. Michetti*

Bleeding is a leading cause of death after injury, and control of hemorrhage continues to be a major priority in trauma care (see Chap. 13). Paradoxically, trauma patients who survive the threat of bleeding in the early phases of injury go on to face the dangers of the hypercoagulable state that follows. An understanding of the current state of scientific knowledge relating to the physiologic processes of hemostasis and coagulation will allow the practicing trauma surgeon to address these competing forces in the patient with injury. In this chapter, we review the basic principles of primary and secondary hemostasis, fibrinolysis, and the altered hemostasis that accompanies shock and massive transfusion. To assist in the diagnosis and management of bleeding and coagulation disorders, a review of congenital and acquired bleeding conditions and methods for the evaluation of bleeding and coagulation disorders is provided. Finally, the evolving understanding of the relationship between altered coagulation and sepsis is discussed.

## HEMOSTASIS

Physiologic cessation of bleeding ("hemostasis") is complex and involves many interrelated events. Hemostasis can be divided into primary and secondary phases. Primary hemostasis involves the initial formation of clot, characterized by the adherence of platelets to the damaged vessel wall. Secondary hemostasis involves thrombin generation through the "coagulation cascade," with the ultimate deposition and cross-linking of fibrin. The combination of platelet aggregation, fibrin deposition, and cross-linking results in the clinically observed stable clot. Without platelets, the fibrin mesh is weak and conversely, without the cross-linked fibrin scaffolding, platelets alone cannot provide adequate hemostasis. This complementary relationship is clearly evident in clinical cases of deficiency of either platelets (thrombocytopenia with normal coagulation factor levels) or the process of thrombin generation and deposition of fibrin (coagulation factor disorders such as hemophilia without platelet abnormalities).

## PRIMARY HEMOSTASIS

The components of primary hemostasis are platelets and endothelial cells. Platelets are 1.5–3.5 μm discoid blood cells without nuclei or DNA that are formed from bone marrow megakaryocytes. They contain secretory granules enclosed in a contractile cytoskeleton and outer proteoglycan coat containing membrane receptors.[1] Two types of intracellular granules are identified: alpha granules and dense granules (or dense bodies). Alpha granules contain platelet thrombospondin, fibrinogen, fibronectin, platelet factor 4, von Willebrand factor (vWf), platelet-derived growth factor (PDGF), factors V, VIII, and X, and many other proteins. Dense granules contain ATP, ADP, GTP, GDP, other phosphates, calcium, and serotonin. With platelet activation, the contents of the granules are released; thus the presence of platelet-specific proteins in the serum is an indication of platelet activation.

The endothelium is now recognized as a metabolically active tissue with a prominent role in coagulation and inflammation (see Chap. 67). The endothelium maintains a nonthrombogenic surface in normal blood vessels, allowing an equilibrium between the continuous processes of coagulation and fibrinolysis. While the normal endothelium is nonthrombogenic, it secretes a subendothelial matrix which, when exposed to the plasma, is highly thrombogenic. The endothelium produces vWf, also a product of megakaryocytes. When the endothelium is damaged, it releases its stores of vWf. This initiates platelet adhesion, leading to degranulation and further adhesion. Vasoconstriction in small vessels enhances hemostasis by reducing vessel diameter and slowing regional blood flow.

The initial step in primary hemostasis is adhesion of circulating platelets to exposed subendothelial collagen in the damaged vessel wall. Adhesion initially depends on the binding of subendothelial vWf to the platelet glycoprotein (GP) Ib-alpha receptor, part of the Ib-IX-V complex, its principal receptor.[2] The initial binding of vWf to the GP complex does not irreversibly tether the platelets to the endothelium.[3] Definitive adhesion depends on subsequent binding of integrin receptors. The bleeding disorders resulting from deficiency of GPIb-IX-V (Bernard-Soulier disease) and vWf (von Willebrand disease) demonstrate the critical role of these processes in platelet adhesion and hemostasis. The adherent platelets are then activated by exposure to collagen and other components of the damaged vessel wall. Mediators of activation include thrombin, ADP, epinephrine, and thromboxane $A_2$. Thrombin is the most potent physiologic platelet agonist.[4] It causes degranulation and activates phospholipase $A_2$, which acts on cell membrane phospholipids to produce arachidonic acid (AA). Cyclooxygenase converts AA to prostaglandins $G_2$ and $H_2$, and then to thromboxane $A_2$ ($TXA_2$). All are released from platelets and cause vasoconstriction and further platelet aggregation.

Platelet activation also causes degranulation, with platelets releasing the contents of their alpha and dense granules. Adenosine diphosphate (ADP) is released and induces further platelet deformation and aggregation. Growth factors such as platelet-derived growth factor (PDGF) and transforming growth factor-beta (TGF-$\beta$) are released and induce tissue growth and repair. Clotting factors are released to aid in secondary hemostasis. Approximately 20% of factor V is normally contained within platelets, and this portion may be more important to the clotting mechanism than serum factor V.[5] Thromboxane $A_2$ and other products of AA metabolism are released during degranulation and promote vasoconstriction and further aggregation to enhance primary hemostasis.

As platelets are reversibly bound and activated, cohesion and aggregation occur, with formation of a platelet plug and stronger binding to the vessel wall. This process involves binding of various agonists to platelet surface membrane receptors. First identified was ADP, whose central role has resulted in the development of new ADP antagonist drugs used to prevent thrombosis.[5] These agonists continue to activate the platelets and allow binding of the GPIIbIIIa integrin in the platelet wall to ligands such as vWf and fibrinogen.[6] This step is required for thrombus formation, since it immobilizes the clot on the vessel wall. Fibrinogen is the major ligand for GPIIbIIIa,[7] which it binds on activated platelets only.[8] By binding fibrinogen or vWf, platelets are joined to form a thrombus. These aggregated platelets then provide a surface for the enzymatic reactions of the coagulation system and the formation of fibrin.

## SECONDARY HEMOSTASIS

Following the initiation of the hemostatic process by the interaction of platelets and the vessel wall, the "coagulation cascade" is activated, which ultimately leads to formation of a stable fibrin clot. Inactive precursors are sequentially converted to their active forms, leading to a cascade effect with progressively larger amounts of coagulation factors produced. Fibrin monomers are generated as the final product of the cascade and are cross-linked to form the final stable clot. Normal coagulation involves the interaction of many elements and is limited to the locale of the vessel wall injury under normal conditions through a complex series of inhibitory and regulatory substances, feedback loops, and the diluting effect of the blood flowing through the affected area.

Until recently, coagulation was understood to involve two "pathways": intrinsic and extrinsic (Fig. 61-1). The intrinsic

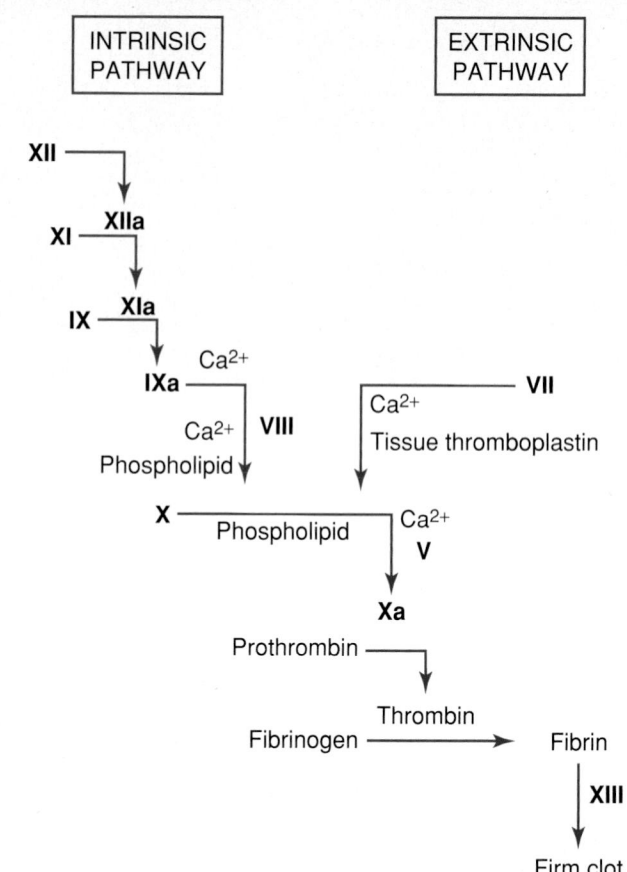

**FIGURE 61-1.** Classical depiction of the blood coagulation cascade.

pathway did not require interaction with the injured vessel wall and posited the activation of factor XII as the initiating event for coagulation. Activated factor XII then activated factor XI, in turn activating factor IX. A complex of activated factors VIII and IX with calcium and phospholipid then activated factor X. Activated factor X then converted prothrombin to thrombin, which, in turn, converted fibrinogen to fibrin. Factor XIII converted the fibrin monomers into a cross-linked fibrin clot in the presence of calcium. In the extrinsic pathway, coagulation is initiated when circulating factor VII interacts with subendothelial tissue factor (TF) in the presence of calcium. Subendothelial TF is exposed to the circulation as a result of endothelial injury. The factor VII–TF complex activates factor X to factor Xa. Activated factor Xa then converts prothrombin to thrombin, and the reaction proceeds as described previously to generate a stable fibrin clot.

It is not clear that the intrinsic pathway plays a major role in vivo. Inadequate levels of some of its key components do not routinely result in a clinically significant bleeding disorder, while rendering standard coagulation tests abnormal. This inconsistency is exemplified by deficiency of factor XII, which is not associated with a bleeding tendency in humans, while deficiencies of factor VIII or IX exhibit the pronounced bleeding disorders known as hemophilia A and B. On the other hand, the importance the TF pathway as the predominant mechanism for in vivo coagulation is supported by recent work.[9,10] The distribution of TF in the subendothelial layer, the epidermis, and the myoepithelial cells constitutes a "hemostatic envelope." Injury puts TF into contact with factor VII, thus initiating coagulation. As mentioned above, the TF-factor VIIa complex catalyzes the activation of factor IX to factor IXa. In addition, the

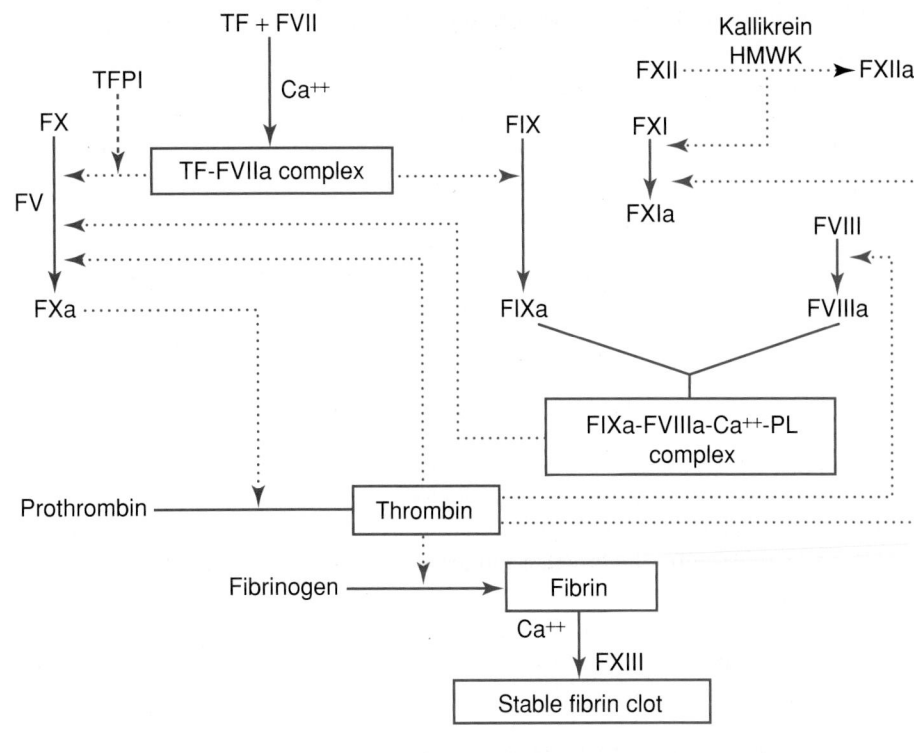

**FIGURE 61-2.** Contemporary depiction of the blood coagulation cascade.

TF-factor VIIa complex can directly convert factor X to factor Xa, converting prothrombin to thrombin. The relatively small amounts of thrombin formed by the direct activation of factor X to factor Xa cannot account for observed hemostatic effects. Although rapid inactivation of the TF-factor VIIa–factor Xa complex by TF pathway inhibitor (TFPI) occurs locally, there is sufficient activity of the complex to activate factors VIII and IX, thereby perpetuating the cascade. Factor IXa creates a complex with factor VIIIa, calcium, and phospholipid. This complex activates factor X to factor Xa and produces large amounts of thrombin, which, in turn, catalyzes the production of significant fibrin from fibrinogen. The activation of factor X to factor Xa by the factor VIII–factor IX–phospholipid complex appears to be the predominant mechanism for generation of thrombin in vivo (Fig. 61-2). Thrombin then cleaves fibrinogen to fibrin while activating factor XIII. The activated factor XIII cross-links fibrin, resulting in a stable clot. Thrombin also contributes to the initiation of fibrinolysis, as is discussed further on. This concept of a single coagulation pathway (TF pathway) is most consistent with current data and observed clinical syndromes and should replace the older concept of two pathways.

## FIBRINOLYSIS AND REGULATION OF THROMBOSIS

The fibrinolytic system acts to break down fibrin and dissolve thrombus, allowing wound healing. It provides a balance to the thrombotic mechanism and maintains a level of homeostasis within the hemostatic system. Therefore abnormalities of the fibrinolytic system can result in hemorrhage from excess fibrinolysis and thrombosis from inadequate fibrinolysis. The main mechanism of fibrinolysis is the breakdown of fibrin into soluble fragments by the proteolytic enzyme plasmin. Plasminogen is the precursor to plasmin. It is converted to plasmin by tissue plasminogen activator (tPA), which is released from endothelial cells near the site of injury. While this reaction is inefficient in the general circulation, it is rapid in the presence of a fibrin clot. Thus, fibrin is both the substrate and regulator of its own destruction. Urokinase, eponymously named due to its high concentration in the urine, is a plasminogen activator that is not fibrin specific. That is, it converts plasminogen to plasmin in the circulation and not just on the clot. It is also the main activator of fibrinolysis in the extravascular space.[8] Urokinase is formed from the single-chain urokinase plasminogen activator (scuPA) precursor.

Plasmin binds fibrin and degrades it by cleaving it at multiple sites, resulting in fibrin split products (FSPs). When two FSPs are cross-linked by factor XIIIa, the result is the D-dimer. Carboxy-terminal lysine residues are generated after the initial fibrinolysis, and these residues are bound by plasminogen also, further accelerating fibrinolysis.

Alpha$_2$-antiplasmin (alpha$_2$-AP) is the main inhibitor of plasmin, but it can also bind plasminogen. Plasmin is inhibited by alpha$_2$-AP when in the circulation, but its degradation is prevented when bound to the fibrin clot. This ensures localized and not systemic fibrinolysis. However, fibrin's protective effect on plasmin is partly balanced by the binding of alpha$_2$-AP to fibrin during cross-linking. In this manner, alpha$_2$-AP is also protected from degradation.

Fibrinolysis is kept in check by several inhibitors of plasminogen activation. Plasminogen activator inhibitor (PAI) -1 is the foremost of these. The main pool for PAI-1 is within platelets, with only low concentration in the plasma. Levels of PAI-1 are about five times greater than tPA, so that most of the tPA in circulation is bound to PAI-1. In response to certain stressors however, tPA is released from the endothelium and is available to activate plasminogen.[11] PAI-2 is secreted by monocytes and the placenta but is not normally present in the plasma except during pregnancy.

Thrombin-activatable fibrinolysis inhibitor (TAFI) is a recently discovered inhibitor of fibrinolysis. TAFI removes the carboxy-terminal lysine residues that remain on partially degraded fibrin, preventing their binding by plasminogen and slowing the process of fibrinolysis.[12]

Other processes also contribute to the autoregulation of thrombosis. After fibrin is formed by thrombin, thrombin binds to thrombomodulin on the endothelium, and thrombin's procoagulant activity is lost due to inactivation by antithrombin and protein C inhibitor.[13] The thrombin–thrombomodulin complex greatly accelerates the activation of protein C, which, with protein S as a cofactor, inhibits activated factors 5 and 8, thus inhibiting thrombin formation.

## BLEEDING PROBLEMS WITH MASSIVE TRANSFUSION

Trauma surgeons are frequently faced with patients requiring massive transfusion as a result of hemorrhagic shock (see Chap. 13). These patients sustain bleeding and coagulation abnormalities secondary to the shock insult as well as from the infusion of cold, packed RBCs (see Chap. 51). Massive transfusion may be described in a number of ways, including replacement of a patient's entire blood volume with stored RBCs in 24 hours or as the transfusion of more than 10 units of blood over three to four hours. Massive transfusion can create significant changes in the patient's metabolic status because of the infusion of large volumes of cold citrate-containing blood that has undergone changes during storage.[14] When blood is stored at 1°C to 6°C, changes occur over time, including leakage of intracellular potassium; decrease in pH; reduced levels of intracellular adenosine triphosphate and 2, 3-DPG in the RBCs, with increased affinity of hemoglobin for oxygen; degeneration of functional granulocytes and platelets; and deterioration of clotting factors V and VIII. Thus, if a large volume of stored blood is infused rapidly, significant effects may be seen in the recipient, depending on his or her metabolic state. Many of the expected changes can be reversed after transfusion or may produce different metabolic patterns than predicted. Consequently, the use of standard formulas for the infusion of fresh frozen plasma (FFP), platelets, calcium, bicarbonate, and other substances for a specific number of units of packed RBCs transfused is contraindicated and may add risk for the patient.

## THERMAL LOAD

Significant degrees of hypothermia occur with rapid transfusion of large volumes of cold blood products. This is exacerbated in patients who have an open thoracic or abdominal cavity, which accelerates heat loss (see Chap. 51). Hypothermia increases the affinity of hemoglobin for oxygen, as do alkalosis and reduced 2,3-DPG in the transfused RBCs. Hypothermia impairs the function of platelets.[15,16] The blood of patients who have a core temperature below 34°C does not clot normally, even if the levels of clotting factors and platelets are normal. Low temperature also increases the potential for hypocalcemia, because the cold liver does not metabolize citrate as well, an effect exacerbated by shock. If the blood is being rapidly infused through a central line with its tip near the sinoatrial node, fatal dysrhythmias can result. Hypothermia can be ameliorated by warming intravenous fluids before they are given. However, care must be taken to not heat RBCs above 40°C, because shortened survival or acute hemolysis can result.

## ACID-BASE CHANGES

Even though stored RBCs and whole blood have an acid pH (about 6.3), alkalosis is the usual result of massive transfusion. Sodium citrate, the anticoagulant in blood products, is converted to sodium bicarbonate in the liver. The alkalosis initially increases the oxygen affinity of hemoglobin. However, because it stimulates enzymes in the Embden–Meyerhof pathway of glycolysis, the net effects of alkalosis are to increase intracellular 2,3-DPG and restore RBC transport of oxygen. The posttransfusion pH may range from 7.48 to 7.50 and is associated with an increased excretion of potassium. The routine administration of bicarbonate with large transfusion volumes causes more severe alkalosis in the patient, with undesirable effects on myocardial contractility and greater affinity of hemoglobin for oxygen, so that less oxygen is released to tissues (see Chap. 12).

## CHANGES DUE TO CITRATE

Massive transfusion of citrated blood products can lead to transiently decreased levels of ionized calcium (see Chap. 14). The effects of hypocalcemia include hypotension, narrowed pulse pressure, and elevated left ventricular end-diastolic, pulmonary artery, and central venous pressures. Electrocardiographic abnormalities (e.g., prolonged QT intervals) also occur. Commercially available electrodes can determine ionized calcium. Most normothermic adults who are not in shock can withstand the infusion of 1 unit of RBCs every five minutes without requiring calcium supplementation. Indiscriminate administration of calcium can produce transient hypercalcemia and should be avoided.

## CHANGES IN POTASSIUM

Hyperkalemia is theoretically possible with massive blood transfusion because stored blood commonly has elevated potassium concentrations, as high as 30–40 mEq/L by three weeks of storage. However, unless the transfusion rate exceeds 100–150 mL/minute, clinical problems associated with potassium are rare. Most patients requiring rapid transfusion are in shock and have an increase in aldosterone, antidiuretic hormone, and the permissive steroid hormones. Therefore, most massively transfused patients are hypokalemic unless renal function ceases. Hyperkalemia may cause peaked T waves on the electrocardiogram. Hyperkalemia, especially if associated with hypocalcemia, may significantly alter cardiac function.

## CHANGES IN 2,3-DIPHOSPHOGLYCERATE

Because 2,3-DPG is greatly reduced in RBCs after about three weeks of storage, massive transfusion of a patient with blood near the end of its storage life may decrease oxygen off-loading (see Chap. 13). Rapid correction occurs in most cases after the RBCs are transfused and rewarmed. If the patient's hematocrit is low with depressed cardiac function, as in the case of elderly persons with atherosclerosis, the reduced level of 2,3-DPG may be detrimental.

## HEMOSTASIS

Dilutional thrombocytopenia may occur in a patient who is massively transfused because the number of viable platelets is almost nil in blood stored for 24 hours at 1°C to 6°C. The decrease is often less than one would expect on the basis of simple dilution, and this effect is not completely understood. Release of platelets from the spleen and the bone marrow may account for part of this difference. Despite the fact that platelet counts may fall with massive transfusion, dilutional thrombocytopenia alone usually does not account for microvascular bleeding.[14] Prophylactic use of platelet concentrate in the massively transfused patient is not justified without evidence of microvascular bleeding.[15,17] Platelet concentrate contains significant amounts of all clotting factors except factor VIII, a factor often increased in shock victims. Patients receiving large-volume blood transfusion who are experiencing microvascular bleeding unrelated to hypothermia are best treated with platelet concentrate, which provides clotting factors in addition to platelets (see Chap. 14). The PT and aPTT provide a reliable indicator for the need for FFP and factor replacement. The prophylactic use of FFP along with transfusion of RBCs is no longer acceptable in light of convincing data from several studies and the added risk of transfusion.[14,19] In patients who develop disseminated intravascular coagulation (DIC), large doses of platelet concentrate, FFP, and cryoprecipitate may be required.

The expected hematologic changes in the patient undergoing massive transfusion for hemorrhagic shock are not those predicted based on the known properties of stored, citrated packed RBCs. In trauma patients requiring massive transfusion, packed RBCs should be transfused as needed to replace lost oxygen-carrying capacity; platelets should be administered when microvascular bleeding is encountered in a normothermic patient; and crystalloid solution infused per accepted standards for volume re-expansion (see Chap. 14). The majority of patients will not benefit from (and may in fact be harmed by) the administration of bicarbonate or calcium and the prophylactic transfusion of FFP.

## ACQUIRED DISORDERS OF BLEEDING AND COAGULATION

### Vitamin K Deficiency

Vitamin K is a necessary cofactor in the gamma-carboxylation of glutamate residues of factors II, VII, IX, X, protein C, and protein S. These factors are referred to as the vitamin K-dependent factors. Without vitamin K, these coagulants cannot bind calcium properly and thus are inactive. The causes of vitamin K deficiency are many. Dietary intake may be poor, or the intake may be adequate but malabsorbed (see Chap. 66). Vitamin K is a fat-soluble vitamin, so any factor that causes decreased fat emulsification by bile salts can lead to malabsorption (e.g., biliary obstruction, decreased bile salt formation, cholestasis, biliary fistula). Antibiotic causes include oral antibiotics that can destroy vitamin K-producing bacteria in the gut or cephalosporin antibiotics containing the *N*-methylthiotetrazole side chain (e.g., cefoperazone, cefotaxime, cefamandole, moxalactam). Other etiologies include parenteral alimentation without vitamin K supplementation, renal insufficiency, or hepatic dysfunction.

Vitamin K may be given orally or parenterally to correct coagulopathy from deficiency or to reverse the effects of warfarin.

### Anticoagulant Drugs

Drugs that affect hemostasis are abundant and increase each year (Table 61-1). More detailed information on hemoactive drugs can be found further on in this chapter.

### Thrombocytopenia

Thrombocytopenia is generally defined as a platelet count <100,000/mm³. Bleeding is more common after surgery or injury, with counts from 50,000 to 100,000. However, spontaneous bleeding usually does not occur until the count drops below 20,000 and is common with counts below 10,000. The etiology of thrombocytopenia may be (a) decreased production of platelets; (b) increased use, consumption, or sequestration of platelets; or (c) dilution. Decreased production may occur with various oncologic disorders or after chemotherapy. Consumption of

**TABLE 61-1**

**Hemoactive Drugs**

| COAGULATION CASCADE | PLATELETS | FIBRINOLYTICS/ THROMBOLYTICS |
|---|---|---|
| Heparin | Aspirin | Urokinase (Abbokinase) |
| Warfarin (Coumadin) | Ibuprofen | Streptokinase (Kabikinase, Streptase) |
| Enoxaparin (Lovenox) | Tirofiban (Aggrastat) | Alteplase (Activase) |
| Dalteparin (Fragmin) | Anagrelide (Agrylin) | Bivalirudin (Angiomax) |
| Danaparoid (Organan) | Dipyridamole (Persantine) | Anistreplase (Eminase) |
| Lepirudin (Refludan) | Eptifibatide (Integrilin) | Retaplase (Retavase) |
| Antithrombin III (Atnativ, Thrombate III) | Clopidogrel (Plavix) | Tenectaplase (TNKase) |
| | Cilostazol (Pletal) | Alteplase (tPA) |
| | Abciximab (Reopro) | |
| | Ticlopidine (Ticlid) | |

platelets may occur in sepsis, DIC, or TTP, and sequestration can occur in the spleen. Dilutional thrombocytopenia is theoretically possible after massive transfusion. In addition, many drugs can cause thrombocytopenia through an immune mechanism, whereby antibodies to platelet glycoproteins are formed.[20] Examples of such drugs are quinidine, sulfa drugs, $H_2$ antagonists, oral hypoglycemics, gold salts, rifampin, and heparin. The most common of these is heparin. Chronic alcohol consumption may lead to alcohol-induced thrombocytopenia.

Clinical manifestations of thrombocytopenia include cutaneous petechiae or purpura, mucosal bleeding, easy bruising, and excessive bleeding after surgery or injury. Management involves correcting or reversing the underlying cause if one is found. Transfusion of platelet concentrates is indicated for active bleeding associated with thrombocytopenia and to keep platelet counts above 10,000–20,000/mm$^3$. If an invasive procedure or surgery is necessary in a thrombocytopenic patient, transfusion is most beneficial in providing hemostasis when given just before or during the procedure. Multiple platelet transfusions often lead to formation of alloantibodies, thus decreasing the efficacy of repeated administration. As noted above, platelet transfusion is not indicated for empiric or prophylactic treatment during massive transfusion or resuscitation unless there is clinical evidence of microvascular bleeding or a prolonged bleeding time.

## Hypothermia

Hypothermia is a common but often overlooked cause of coagulopathy in surgical patients that is very frequently associated with shock and massive transfusion (see Chap. 51). As body temperature decreases, the rate of all biological enzymatic reactions slows. Since the coagulation cascade consists of a series of proteolytic enzymes, hypothermia slows the process of coagulation. As a result, clotting is significantly slowed. Coagulation, enzyme activity, and platelet function are significantly altered in trauma patients with a core temperature <34°C compared to those above 34°C.[21] This defect is not detected by the PT/PTT, because blood samples are warmed to 37°C prior to testing. Hypothermia also causes decreased thromboxane production, resulting in platelet dysfunction, microvascular bleeding, and a prolonged bleeding time (Table 61-2).[22]

Typically, coagulopathy from hypothermia occurs in the perioperative setting, when patients receive large volumes of fluid during prolonged procedures, or in patients with hemorrhagic shock receiving massive resuscitation. The result is diffuse nonmechanical or "nonsurgical" bleeding, for which the only treatment is rapid rewarming of the patient. Transfusion of FFP and platelets in an attempt to stop bleeding usually worsens the hypothermia and exacerbates the coagulopathy. Management usually requires rapid completion or abbreviation of the procedure without definitive treatment, packing of bleeding areas, and transport to the intensive care unit for rewarming (see Chap. 41). This "damage control" technique is commonly used in exsanguinating trauma patients in whom core temperatures less than 32°C are usually associated with death.[23,24] Patients are returned to the operating room for definitive care after rewarming and resuscitation are complete.

## Consumptive Coagulopathy

In certain conditions, bleeding is caused by a decrease in platelets and/or coagulation factors due to their consumption in the

**TABLE 61-2**

| Physiologic Changes in Hypothermia | | |
| --- | --- | --- |
| LEVEL | TEMPERATURE | PHYSIOLOGIC EFFECT |
| Mild | 36.9–33.0°C | Catecholamine release |
| | | Increased heart rate |
| | | Vasoconstriction |
| | | Increased respiratory rate |
| | | Mild respiratery alkalosis |
| | | Cold-induced diuresis |
| | | Increased hematocrit |
| | | Confusion, faulty judgment |
| | | Shivering |
| | | Hyperreflexia |
| Moderate | 32.9–28.0°C | Decreased metabolic rate |
| | | Decreased oxygen consumption |
| | | Enzyme suppression |
| | | Sympathetic nervous "switch-off" |
| | | Decreased insulin release |
| | | Sinus bradycardia, atrial fibrillation and flutter |
| | | Prolonged PR, QRS, QT, on ECG |
| | | Decreased respiratory rate |
| | | Decreased cough reflex |
| | | Decreased lung compliance |
| | | Oxyhemoglobin dissociation curve shifts left |
| | | Continued decreased in LOC |
| | | Hyporeflexia |
| | | Coagulopathies |
| | | Increased fibrin split products |
| | | Mild Ileus |
| Severe | 27.9–20.0°C | Metabolic acidosis |
| | | Increased ventricular irritability/fibrillation |
| | | Hypotension |
| | | Decreased myocardial contractility and cardiac output |
| | | Severely decreased blood pressure |
| | | Osborne wave |
| | | Profoundly decreased or absent respirations |
| | | Inactivation of hypothalamic thermoregulation |
| | | Hyperkalemia |
| | | Unconsciousness |
| Profound | <20°C | Asystole |
| | | Isoelectric electroencephalogram |
| | | Cell death |

*Source:* Adapted from Britt L. Dascombe W, Rodriguez A: New horizons in management of hypothermia and frosbite injury. Surg Clin North Am 71:345-370, 1991, and Fritsch D: Hypothermia in the trauma patient. AACN Clin Issues 6:196-211, 1995. With permission.

microvasculature. This process is referred to as *consumptive coagulopathy*. Accelerated fibrin deposition occurs, decreasing the fibrinogen level, and platelets become trapped, causing thrombocytopenia. Hypofibrinogenemia concurrent with thrombocytopenia in a bleeding patient is good evidence for a consumptive coagulopathy. Fibrinolysis is induced, resulting in increased fibrin degradation products in the blood.

There are many etiologies of consumptive coagulopathy, the principal example being the syndrome of Disseminated Intravascular

*Coagulation (DIC).* The distinction between DIC and the other conditions listed is ill defined, and one or more of the processes may be overlapping.

*Sepsis or Infection.* These are a common cause of postoperative thrombocytopenia. The mechanism is unclear but may in part be due to endotoxin-induced aggregation and destruction of platelets in the microvasculature or by direct activation of the coagulation cascade (see Chap. 19). Also, activated protein C is deficient; therefore formation of microthrombi is not inhibited.

*Shock, Trauma, Burns, Pancreatitis.* These conditions cause release of thromboplastic substances that increase thrombin formation and consumption of coagulation factors (see Chap. 50). They can also lead to thrombocytopenia. In addition, inadequate tissue perfusion incites the inflammatory response, which leads to coagulopathy.

*Traumatic Brain Injury.* Injured brain tissue releases its rich stores of thromboplastin, which leads to hypercoagulability by accelerating fibrin formation and microvascular thrombosis (see Chap. 20). Coagulation substrates are consumed and further clotting is impaired.

*Obstetric Emergencies.* Placental abruption, amniotic fluid embolism, dead fetus, eclampsia, septic abortion, and hydatidiform mole can all cause release of thromboplastic substances that increase thrombin formation and consumption of coagulation factors (see Chap. 40).

*Disseminated Intravascular Coagulation (DIC).* DIC is an acquired coagulation disorder involving diffuse activation of the coagulation system, with fibrin deposition in the microvasculature, platelet aggregation, and thrombosis. Its severity ranges from subclinical or low grade to severe and life threatening. Clinically, DIC is manifest by generalized bleeding, and end-organ failure results from the diffuse microvascular thrombosis. The more severe form can lead to multiple organ system failure and death (see Chap. 68). Mortality is increased in septic or severely injured patients with DIC.[25]

A variety of clinical conditions are associated with DIC. In addition to all of the processes listed above, DIC may be associated with massive transfusion, hemolysis, liver disease, and malignancy (including leukemia). The pathophysiologic process in DIC is initiated through inflammatory mechanisms and cytokines, especially interleukin-6.[26] The systemic formation of fibrin results from three mechanisms.[27] First, tissue factor (TF) activates factor VII, and the TF-factorVIIa complex mediates formation of thrombin, with subsequent conversion of fibrinogen to fibrin and activation of platelets. Second, the natural anticoagulant mechanisms—via ATIII, protein C, and TF-pathway inhibitor—are all impaired in DIC. This leads to a shift in the hemostatic balance toward thrombosis. Finally, fibrin clearance is decreased due to a relative excess of PAI-1, which inhibits plasmin formation and fibrinolysis.

Diagnosis of DIC is made by the combination of clinical findings and certain supportive laboratory tests. There is no specific test that confirms or rules out the diagnosis. Clinically one suspects DIC in patients with a generalized coagulopathy, bleeding, and the presence of an inciting factor or disease associated with DIC. The patient usually has a low or decreasing platelet count and prolonged PT/PTT. Fibrin split products may be present in the plasma, and coagulation inhibitors such as ATIII may be deficient. Fibrinogen levels may be low in severe DIC, but since fibrinogen is an acute-phase reactant, its production is increased as part of the stress response, and levels may be normal. The D-dimer assay is the most sensitive test for DIC, being abnormal in up to 94% of patients with a diagnosis of DIC.[28] In many patients with coagulopathy who are suspected of having DIC, hypothermia must be considered as the primary etiology of the bleeding disorder, especially if sepsis is not present.

Treatment of DIC centers around treatment of the underlying disease process. Symptomatic treatment is generally futile if the proinflammatory impetus is not addressed concomitantly. Several strategies have been investigated as specific therapy for DIC.

Anticoagulation has been used as an attempt to halt the underlying hypercoagulation in DIC. Currently, there have been no controlled studies showing any benefit of unfractionated or low-molecular-weight heparin (LMWH) in DIC. One randomized, double-blind, placebo-controlled trial in healthy humans showed that unfractionated heparin and LMWH can improve laboratory measures of coagulation in endotoxin-induced coagulation in humans.[29] This has not been confirmed in patients with DIC. ATIII-independent thrombin inhibitors such as desirudin are currently being studied. The transfusion of platelets and fresh frozen plasma has no benefit when used prophylactically in patients with DIC. However, benefit exists for patients with active bleeding and those undergoing invasive procedures. In the latter case, such transfusions are best given just prior to or during the procedure to maximize the chances of hemostasis before the platelets and coagulation factors are consumed.

As mentioned previously, ATIII levels are low in DIC patients. Administration of high doses of ATIII has shown some efficacy in the subgroup of patients with septic shock, with improvement in symptoms of DIC, organ function, and mortality.[31,32] This therapy may hold promise for the future. Antifibrinolytics such as epsilon-aminocaproic acid have improved bleeding in specific oncologic disorders and fibrinolytic syndromes but not DIC. Their use cannot be recommended in DIC.

## Hepatic Failure

The liver is the site of synthesis for all coagulation factors except factor VIII; therefore, in hepatic failure, synthesis of these and other proteins is decreased (see Chap. 65). Cirrhotics produce less fibrinogen but also make an abnormal form of fibrinogen with impaired clotting ability.[32] Poor oral intake, malabsorption, or biliary obstruction may lead to vitamin K deficiency and impaired synthesis of the vitamin K-dependent factors by the liver. These patients usually have a prolonged PT, normal to slightly elevated PTT, and low fibrinogen levels (demonstrated by prolonged thrombin time). Correction of the coagulopathy may be effected by administration of desmopressin (DDAVP) in cirrhotics,[33] transfusion of FFP, or replacement of vitamin K, as the situation dictates.

## Liver Trauma

Severe liver injury can cause coagulopathy through several mechanisms (see Chap. 32). Massive transfusion is often required, leading to hypothermia and consumptive coagulopathy. If a large portion of the liver is damaged, production of coagulation factors may be decreased and clearance of profibrinolytic substances is reduced, impairing coagulation.

## Renal Failure

Renal failure (see Chap. 65) causes a qualitative platelet defect attributable to decreased platelet adhesiveness and aggregation.[34] The mechanism of this dysfunction is not known, but the effects can be reversed with dialysis (most effective), DDAVP, cryoprecipitate, and conjugated estrogens. DDAVP reduces bleeding complications after a number of procedures in renal failure patients.[35] It can be given intravenously in a dose of 0.3 μg/kg in uremic patients and can help to decrease the bleeding time, as do cryoprecipitate and conjugated estrogens. Conversely, dialysis patients with chronic renal failure can have a defect in fibrinolysis that correlates with the severity of the renal dysfunction,[36] leading to thrombotic complications.

## CONGENITAL DISORDERS OF BLEEDING AND COAGULATION

### Hemophilia A

Hemophilia A is an X-linked recessive disorder resulting from factor VIII deficiency and is a relatively common congenital bleeding disorder. Its pattern of inheritance makes it almost universally a disease in males, occurring in about 1 in 10,000 male births, and a carrier state in females. Bleeding tendency correlates inversely with factor VIII levels. Spontaneous bleeding may occur with levels <5%, and those with higher levels (mild disease) tend to bleed abnormally after surgery or injury. Carriers generally have levels >50% and do not have clinical manifestation of the disease. A factor VIII level of at least 30% is needed for surgical hemostasis.[37] Patients with hemophilia A will have a prolonged PTT and decreased factor VIII levels. The PT and bleeding time are normal. Normal vWF levels distinguish hemophilia from vWD, since both have low-factor VIII levels.

Treatment of bleeding is with factor VIII replacement. Although FFP and cryoprecipitate both contain factor VIII in low levels (5–10 times higher in cryoprecipitate vs. FFP), the preferred treatment is transfusion of pooled factor VIII concentrate. Since 1984, factor VIII concentrates have been treated to inactivate HIV, hepatitis, and other viruses, making viral infection unlikely. DDAVP may temporarily raise factor VIII levels in patients with mild hemophilia A. About 10–20% of hemophiliacs develop inhibitors (IgG antibodies) to factor VIII, usually in response to factor VIII infusions.[38] Treatment can be complicated, and detection of such inhibitors requires a mixing study.

### Hemophilia B

Hemophilia B, or Christmas disease, is an X-linked disorder of factor IX deficiency. Clinical manifestations are similar to those in patients with hemophilia A, and the severity of symptoms correlates inversely with factor IX levels. Laboratory studies reveal an abnormal PTT and low factor IX levels, with a normal PT and bleeding time. Treatment is with factor IX concentrates, aimed at increasing levels up to 50% of normal, since higher levels may actually cause arterial and venous thromboses. As in the case of hemophilia A, inhibitors may develop; they can be detected with a mixing study.

## VON WILLEBRAND DISEASE

Von Willebrand disease (vWD) is an inherited bleeding disorder caused by deficiency or dysfunction of von Willebrand factor (vWf), which facilitates platelet adhesion to damaged endothelium and also stabilizes factor VIII in the blood.[34] It is the most common congenital bleeding disorder. There are three types of vWD. Type 1 is characterized by a partial deficiency in levels of vWf, and type 3 involves the complete absence of vWf. Type 2 vWD has several subtypes, but all are due to a qualitative defect in vWf, which is present in normal quantity. vWD is generally characterized by low levels of factor VIII coagulant activity and a prolonged bleeding time. Symptoms are similar to those caused by platelet dysfunction and include mucosal bleeding, epistaxis, petechial hemorrhage, menorrhagia, and prolonged bleeding after surgery.

Diagnosis may be difficult due to the lack of any one test with sufficient sensitivity and specificity. The PT/PTT and bleeding time may be prolonged. Types 1 and 3 vWD have reduced levels of factor VIII:c and vWf antigen. Factor VIII:c is reduced because vWf is the major serum carrier for circulating factor VIII. Other tests include vWf ristocetin cofactor assay, which measures the ability of vWf to aggregate platelets in the presence of the antibiotic ristocetin, or the vWf collagen binding activity (vWf:CBA) assay.

Treatment of vWD varies according to the specific subtype. DDAVP, a synthetic vasopressin analogue, causes release of factor VIII and vWf into the plasma and can cause correction of abnormal bleeding times and levels of vWf and factor VIII.[39] Since endothelial stores of vWf may take up to 48 hours to reaccumulate, repeated doses of DDAVP are sometimes less effective, though this problem is less frequent in patients with type 1 vWD.[40] DDAVP is ineffective in type 3 vWD due to absence of significant stores of vWf, and it is contraindicated in type 2 vWD because it can cause thrombocytopenia and increase bleeding.

Transfusion of cryoprecipitate can be used to treat or prevent bleeding associated with all types of vWD. Fresh frozen plasma contains 5–10 times less vWf and factor VIII than cryoprecipitate, and therefore is not effective unless given in large volumes. Factor VIII-vWf concentrates are also available for bleeding patients with vWD who are unresponsive to DDAVP. These, unlike cryoprecipitate, are virus-inactivated, and risk of infection transmission is less of a concern. Factor VIII-vWf concentrates are believed by some to be the treatment of choice for types 2 and 3 vWD.[41] Adjunctive therapy can also be given with the antifibrinolytic agents epsilon aminocaproic acid (50–60 mg/kg every four to 6 hours) and tanexamic acid (20–25 mg/kg every 8–12 hours).[41]

## OTHER CONGENITAL DEFICIENCIES

Several other rare congenital deficiencies exist, including deficiencies of factors V, VII, X, XI, XII, XIII, prekallikrein, high-molecular-weight kininogen (HMWK), and proteins C and S. Most are autosomal recessive and heterogeneous in their phenotypic expression. Protein C and S deficiencies and activated protein C resistance (associated with the factor V Leiden mutation) predispose to venous thrombosis.

## EVALUATION OF BLEEDING AND COAGULATION

### Preoperative Period

Although it is not always possible in the setting of trauma, patients who are to have surgery should undergo screening for bleeding abnormalities as part of their history and physical examination. Diagnosis of most disorders is made predominately by clinical evaluation, with laboratory studies used only in certain circumstances. The patient should be questioned about his or her bleeding history including known bleeding disorders, bruising tendency, excessive bleeding during medical or dental procedures, prolonged menorrhea, GI bleeding, or repeated or severe epistaxis. Primary hemostatic defects (platelets) manifest as excessive bleeding from cuts, mucosal surfaces, or easy bruising. Secondary defects (factor deficiencies) are usually associated with hemarthroses or intramuscular hematomas.

A medication history should always be obtained, to determine the use of oral anticoagulants such as warfarin (Coumadin) or aspirin and other nonsteroidal anti-inflammatory drugs (NSAIDs), among others. One should specifically ask if the patient is taking these drugs or any over-the-counter products, since many patients may not consider agents such as aspirin or "health supplements" to be medications and may fail to mention them. Finally, one should ask about medical conditions that may affect hemostasis, such as alcohol abuse, liver or kidney dysfunction, or a family history of hemophilia or other disorder.

Physical examination may reveal bruising, joint abnormalities, petechiae, purpura, ecchymosis, telangiectasia, hepatosplenomegaly, or malnutrition. These findings would increase suspicion of an underlying coagulation disorder.

Laboratory testing should not be done routinely on patients with a normal hematologic history and physical examination. Current data do not support routine screening laboratory evaluation preoperatively in patients without a history of abnormal bleeding or clinical indications of a bleeding disorder.[42–45] In addition, the PT, PTT, and bleeding time have a low yield in revealing occult bleeding disorders or in predicting clinically significant perioperative bleeding and may give false-positive results. Indications for specific tests should be based on the history and physical examination and the existence of other processes that may alter hemostasis, such as the systemic inflammatory response syndrome, sepsis, malnutrition, or organ failure.

Following is a listing and descriptions of the laboratory tests most commonly used in the investigation of bleeding abnormalities:

*Prothrombin Time (PT).*    This test is done by adding a thromboplastin, containing tissue factor, phospholipid, and calcium, to citrated plasma and measuring the time in seconds until a fibrin clot is formed compared to a control. The PT measures the activity of the extrinsic pathway (factor VII) and the common pathway (fibrinogen, factors II, IX, and X). It is used to monitor warfarin therapy and affected by depletion of the vitamin K-dependent factors (factors II, VII, IX, and X, and proteins C and S).

*International Normalized Ratio (INR).*    The INR is used to adjust for individual laboratory variation in the PT, using the formula INR = (log patient PT/log control PT) to the power of "c," where c is the international sensitivity index (ISI). The thromboplastin used in individual laboratories is thus calibrated against a reference thromboplastin.

*Partial Thromboplastin Time (PTT).*    The PTT is done by adding a partial thromboplastin (mixture of phospholipids), an activating substance, and calcium chloride to citrated plasma. It measures the activity of the intrinsic pathway (HMWK, prekallikrein, and factors VIII, IX, XI, and XII) and the common pathway (fibrinogen, factors II, IX, and X). Only factor VII is not measured by the PTT. It is used to monitor heparin therapy, since heparin affects the intrinsic pathway but not factor VII of the extrinsic pathway.

*Platelet Count.*    This is a quantitative measure of circulating platelets. Counts $<50,000/mm^3$ increase bleeding from cut surfaces, and counts $<20,000/mm^3$ may be associated with spontaneous bleeding.

*Bleeding Time.*    The bleeding time is the only test that measures platelet function and primary hemostasis. However, due to variation in the performance of the test and the methods used, it is relatively insensitive and nonspecific in identifying platelet function abnormalities.[46] In addition, the test may not predict surgical bleeding.[47]

*Thrombin Time (TT).*    The TT is done by adding thrombin to citrated plasma ± calcium. The TT measures the time for conversion of fibrinogen to fibrin, which is induced by thrombin. It is prolonged when fibrinogen is deficient ($<100$ mg/dL) or abnormal, in the presence of circulating anticoagulants, including FSPs and heparin, and during excessive fibrinolysis. Its high sensitivity to exogenous anticoagulants such as heparin limit its usefulness in hospitalized patients, but it can be used to detect low levels of circulating heparin, which do not cause changes in the PTT.

*Fibrinogen.*    Fibrinogen is a large protein that is cleaved by thrombin to produce fibrin monomers. These then cross-link to form a fibrin clot in the presence of factor XIII. Thus, as clotting increases (i.e., fibrin is formed) the fibrinogen level decreases. Low levels may be seen with consumptive conditions such as DIC, sepsis, severe traumatic brain injury, and obstetric emergencies or with overanticoagulation by thrombolytic agents. However, fibrinogen is an acute-phase reactant that may be elevated in response to physiologic stress, producing normal levels even while its consumption is accelerated.

*Thrombelastography (TEG).*    TEG analyzes various characteristics of clot formation in a sample of whole blood and converts these data to graphic form by computer analysis. A unique thromboelastogram tracing is depicted based on the rate of clot formation, fibrin cross-linking, and platelet-fibrin interaction. By measuring various parameters of the tracing, TEG provides an assessment of platelet function, coagulation enzyme activity, and the overall degree of coagulability. It can also identify primary fibrinolysis, consumptive coagulopathy, anticoagulant therapy, and even the effect of hypothermia on clotting. TEG is used frequently during cardiopulmonary bypass, liver transplantation, and in intensive care settings due to its rapid availability and ability to assess the components of coagulation in an integrated fashion.

*Fibrin Split Products (FSPs).*   FSPs are fragments of the fibrin molecule that result from breakdown of fibrin by plasmin during fibrinolysis. The presence of FSPs is not diagnostic in and of itself but when added to the clinical scenario can provide evidence of a consumptive process such as DIC. The D-dimer is a specific form of FSP that is most closely associated with DIC.

*Factor Assays.*   Specific coagulation factor levels can be used to diagnose specific diseases or deficiencies. The PT/PTT is not altered until factor levels are significantly depleted. The more common assays are factor VIII for hemophilia A and factor IX for hemophilia B. Other assays may detect deficiencies in factors V, VII, X, XI, and XII (Hagemann factor), prekallikrein, and HMWK. All are very rare disorders.

## Intraoperative Period

*Surgical vs. Nonsurgical Bleeding.*   During surgery, bleeding may arise from direct injury to tissues and transection of vessels; this is known as *surgical bleeding* because the cause and remedy are surgical in nature (see Chap. 41). When encountered in the trauma patient, such bleeding should be controlled by direct approaches (suture, coagulation, etc.). Nonsurgical bleeding, also referred to as *microvascular bleeding*, arises from a disturbance in the clotting mechanism and is diagnosed clinically by the observation of diffuse oozing of blood from all damaged tissues, including areas that may not have been directly cut or injured. The most common nonsurgical causes of intraoperative bleeding are hypothermia and thrombocytopenia. DIC is rarely the cause of intraoperative microvascular bleeding in the early management of the trauma patient.[34] Treatment is directed at the cause of the coagulopathy, which should prompt serious consideration for termination of the operative procedure.

*Postoperative Period.*   Postoperative hemorrhage must be evaluated in a systematic fashion designed to detect the cause and direct the treatment of the bleeding. Evaluation should always begin with a detailed history. One should review the operative note for the exact procedure performed and any details pertinent to the current situation. Pre- and postoperative medications should be reviewed for drugs that may affect coagulation as well as any medical conditions that may influence hemostasis (see above). Physical examination should be directed toward localizing the source of the bleeding if possible (e.g., a wound hematoma, fresh blood from a drain) but also toward other signs that may indicate the cause. For example, bleeding from all cut surfaces, intravenous sites, and needle puncture sites may indicate a coagulation disorder, as opposed to a purely technical problem such as a slipped ligature. Petechiae indicate platelet deficiency or dysfunction. Fever, tachycardia, and tachypnea may point toward infection or sepsis as the cause of consumptive coagulopathy.

Laboratory tests may be helpful in the diagnosis of the cause of the coagulopathy. Platelet count, bleeding time, PT, and PTT help to differentiate primary versus secondary hemostatic problems, and low fibrinogen levels may indicate a consumptive coagulopathy. Note that a hematocrit level does not help in determining the presence of acute bleeding. The intravascular space must first be diluted with either fluid shifted from the interstitial space or by intravenous administration before the hematocrit will fall. This often takes several hours, by which time the presence of bleeding should be clinically obvious.

The etiology of postoperative bleeding may fall into one of the following broad categories: loss of surgical hemostasis or coagulation disorders. Loss of surgical hemostasis refers to bleeding from the operative site. This may be due to a technical failure, such as a slipped ligature or disruption of a vascular anastomosis, or inadequate hemostasis during the procedure. The problem may stem from cut surfaces that did not bleed intraoperatively due to vasoconstriction but bled postoperatively when the patient was warmed and fluid-resuscitated. Loss of surgical hemostasis usually requires a return to the operating room for definitive control. The diagnosis is often made by observing signs and symptoms of hypovolemia, such as tachycardia, restlessness, anxiety, pallor, oliguria, and hypotension. An anxious, agitated surgical patient should never be sedated without a thorough evaluation for the causes of this deceptive clinical presentation. It is also important to remember that a normal blood pressure does not exclude hemorrhage, since up to 30% of the normal blood volume may be lost before hypotension occurs.

Coagulation disorders may arise from a congenital or acquired defect in primary or secondary hemostasis. *Primary hemostatic failure* denotes a problem with formation of the initial platelet plug. This may be due to a qualitative or quantitative platelet defect. Qualitative defects in platelet dysfunction can be caused by drugs, hypothermia, acute renal failure, or congenital diseases such as von Willebrand disease. Quantitative abnormalities (thrombocytopenia) can accompany massive transfusion, sepsis, or major infection, consumptive coagulopathy, chemotherapy, radiation, hemolytic-uremic syndrome, thrombotic thrombocytopenic purpura, idiopathic or immune thrombocytopenic purpura, posttransfusion purpura, or drug-induced immune thrombocytopenia (e.g., quinine).

*Secondary hemostatic failure* refers to problems in the coagulation cascade, which may arise from either qualitative or quantitative abnormalities. Decreased production of factors may result from liver failure, or there may be decreased availability of activated factors due to vitamin K deficiency. Existing factors may function abnormally, as with hypothermia, or be inhibited by drugs, as with warfarin and heparin use. The effects of heparin can be reversed with protamine, as described further on in this chapter. Note that while administration of FFP will correct prolongation of the PT, it will not correct bleeding due to unfractionated heparin, which prolongs the PTT, or LMWH. Increased destruction of factors can result from consumptive coagulopathy. Dilution of coagulation proteins by massive fluid or plasma infusion rarely occurs. There is no need to replace factors based solely on the volume of fluids or blood infused.[34]

## Fibrinolysis

No single test confirms fibrinolysis, but the process can be inferred by laboratory evaluation of several factors along with the clinical scenario. One can measure levels of fibrinogen, fibrin split products, plasminogen, plasminogen activators, and plasmin inhibitors. Thromboelastography can also be useful. The thrombin time (TT) is prolonged in fibrinolysis, and is useful in monitoring the fibrinolytic state during fibrinolytic therapy. Bleeding complications from such therapy are more common when the fibrinogen level is less than 100 mg/dL, and when FSPs are greater than 100 U/dL. Fresh frozen plasma (FFP) can be used to replenish fibrinogen levels and reduce coagulopathy in such situations.

## TREATMENT WITH HEMOACTIVE DRUGS

## Anticoagulants

*Unfractionated Heparin (UFH).*    UFH is a glycosaminoglycan that exerts its anticoagulant effect through binding and potentiation of ATIII. ATIII inactivates factors IIa, IXa, and Xa and inhibits the prothrombinase complex, which consists of factors Xa and Va assembling in the presence of calcium on a phospholipid membrane. Therapy with UFH is gauged by the PTT, which is prolonged by inhibition of the above-named factors. UFH is not absorbed orally, so it must be given intravenously or subcutaneously. The half-life is about 1 hour. UFH can be reversed by protamine sulfate (see below), which binds and neutralizes the heparin molecule.

Major adverse reactions with UFH include bleeding, thrombocytopenia, and osteoporosis. Heparin may cause a thrombocytopenia that reverses spontaneously, even with continued use of heparin. Heparin-induced thrombocytopenia (HIT), however, is an IgG-mediated immune disorder that can have severe sequelae in a small percentage of patients.[48] In addition to the low platelet count, HIT can lead to paradoxical arterial or venous thrombosis, with their resultant problems. Diagnosis is made with the appropriate clinical scenario plus the presence of heparin antibodies in the serum. Discontinuation of the heparin is mandatory in such cases. If continued anticoagulation is required and warfarin use is not feasible, danaparoid sodium may be used. Lepirudin, a hirudin derivative, is the only drug approved by the U.S. Food and Drug Administration (FDA) to treat HIT-related thromboses.

*Low-Molecular-Weight Heparin (LMWH).*    LMWH is produced by fragmentation of heparin molecules to produce smaller molecules (4000–5000 kDa vs. 5000–30,000 kDa). LMWH has reduced binding ability, longer half-life, and more efficient bioavailability than UFH, accounting for different physiologic effects. Less binding to plasma proteins leads to a predictable anticoagulant response,[49] which permits therapy without monitoring coagulation tests. Decreased binding to platelets may result in a lower incidence of HIT.[50] The mechanism of action, like that of UFH, is activation of ATIII. While UFH affects factors IIa and Xa equally, LMWH's inhibition of factor Xa is two to five times greater than that for factor IIa.

Complications include bleeding but a lower incidence of HIT and osteoporosis compared to UFH. It may be used for prophylaxis (40 mg SQ daily for perioperative elective general surgery; 30 mg SQ bid for major trauma and orthopedic procedures) or treatment. The treatment dose is based on patient weight (1mg/kg SQ bid).

*Warfarin.*    Warfarin is the most commonly used oral anticoagulant in North America. Its mechanism of action is inhibition of thrombin formation by interfering with the activation and conformational change of the vitamin K-dependent coagulation factors (II, VII, IX, and X). Vitamin K is oxidized and reduced in cyclic fashion while acting as a cofactor for the gamma-carboxylation of glutamate residues on the vitamin K-dependent proteins. Warfarin inhibits the enzymes vitamin K epoxide reductase and vitamin K reductase, which are necessary for these reactions, thus decreasing the activation of the vitamin K-dependent factors.

Warfarin also inhibits the natural anticoagulants protein C and protein S through the same mechanism. Since these proteins have shorter half-lives than II, VII, IX, and X, warfarin theoretically causes an initial hypercoagulable state. Although clinical manifestations of this hypercoagulable state are rare in patients without factor deficiencies, this is the rationale for initiating therapeutic levels of anticoagulation with heparin prior to starting warfarin.

Therapy is gauged by the PT and INR. Factor VII has the shortest half-life of the vitamin K-dependent factors (about 6 hours), so prolongation of the PT in the first two to three days after initiation of warfarin may reflect factor VII inhibition and not full anticoagulation.

Many drugs affect warfarin therapy by reducing its absorption, altering its metabolism in the liver, or changing its clearance. Adverse reactions include bleeding and skin necrosis. The latter has an unknown mechanism and may be more common with concomitant protein C or S deficiency.[51]

*Hirudin.*    Hirudin is a direct thrombin inhibitor originally isolated from the leech *Hirudo medicinalis* but now genetically engineered. It binds and inactivates thrombin independent of ATIII. Lepirudin is the only hirudin currently approved in the United States. It is indicated for use mainly in patients with HIT. Like heparin, it causes prolongation of the PTT.

## Antiplatelet Agents

*Aspirin.*    Aspirin is the classic platelet antagonist. It permanently and irreversibly acetylates the enzyme cyclooxygenase (COX), preventing its binding to AA and subsequent metabolism of AA to TXA2, thus inhibiting platelet aggregation and plug formation. Since platelets are anucleic and cannot resynthesize COX, new platelets are required before normal platelet function returns. Thus, aspirin must be discontinued (e.g., before surgery) for the 8- to 12-day life span of the platelet for its effects to vanish.

*ADP Inhibitors.*    Ticlopidine and clopidogrel are inhibitors of ADP-mediated platelet activation and aggregation. They are used primarily in prevention of thrombosis in patients with vascular disease, such as stroke or myocardial infarction. Clopidogrel may be preferred due to its decreased incidence of side effects compared to ticlopidine.[7]

*GPIIb/IIIa Antagonists.*   Abciximab is the Fab fragment of a monoclonal antibody; it binds to the GPIIb/IIIa receptor on activated platelets, thereby inhibiting platelet aggregation and plug formation. It is used in the acute setting to prevent thrombosis associated with percutaneous coronary procedures and refractory unstable angina.[7] Its main adverse effect is thrombocytopenia. Eptifibatide and tirofiban are two newer drugs that reversibly inhibit platelet aggregation. Their effects are reversed within a few hours of discontinuation of the infusion. They are indicated for treatment of unstable angina or non-Q-wave MI, with an additional indication for eptifibatide for patients undergoing percutaneous coronary procedures.

*Phosphodiesterase (PDE) Inhibitors.*   Inhibition of PDE results in higher concentrations of cAMP within platelets. This, in turn, inhibits phospholipase and COX, thus inhibiting thromboxane production and platelet aggregation. Dipyridamole is one such agent with efficacy in the prevention of stroke, especially when combined with aspirin. It also has coronary vasodilatory effects, which is the basis for its use in nuclear imaging of the heart. Pentoxifylline was the first agent approved for treatment of claudication. Its exact mechanism of action remains unclear, but it is reported to increase red blood cell deformability and to decrease blood viscosity. Cilostazol is only the second agent that is FDA-approved for treatment of claudication. It inhibits $PGE_3$, which is the predominant form of PDE within platelets,[52] and selectively inhibits cAMP-phosphodiesterase.

## Nonsteroidal Anti-inflammatory Drugs (NSAIDs)

*Ibuprofen.*   Ibuprofen blocks prostaglandin metabolism temporarily by reversibly binding to COX. Its inhibition lasts about three to four days.

*COX-2 Inhibitors.*   It has recently been recognized that there are two forms of the COX enzyme. COX-1, which is constitutively expressed in most tissues, is the catalyst for TXA2 synthesis and for prostaglandins in the gastrointestinal tract. Inhibition of COX-1 is thought to be responsible for the GI side effects of aspirin and NSAIDS. Aspirin inhibits COX-1 more than COX-2.

COX-2 is not detectable in most tissues but is rapidly upregulated in response to inflammatory and other stimuli. COX-2 is mainly involved in synthesis of prostacyclin.[53] Selective COX-2 inhibitors, such as celecoxib and rofecoxib, retain anti-inflammatory and analgesic properties while sparing most of the GI and bleeding side effects of the COX-1 enzyme.

Shortly after their introduction in 1999, these agents became some of the most widely prescribed medications in the United States. However, the COX-2 inhibitors can have undesirable renal and cardiovascular side effects, similar to traditional NSAIDs, and they should be used with caution in certain patient populations.[54,55] Also, since COX-2 inhibitors prevent prostacyclin synthesis while preserving TXA2, there is a theoretical risk of increased thrombosis. However, this has not yet been proven clinically.

## Thrombolytics

*Streptokinase.*   Streptokinase is not an enzyme per se but a glycoprotein produced by beta-hemolytic streptococcal bacteria. It binds to plasminogen both on the fibrin clot and systemically, and then this streptokinase–plasminogen complex activates other plasminogen molecules to form plasmin. Due to its bacterial derivation, it is highly immunogenic and so cannot be used repeatedly in the same patient.

*Urokinase.*   Urokinase is a plasminogen activator found in urine and converts plasminogen to plasmin. Like streptokinase, urokinase acts systemically and therefore poses a higher risk of bleeding complications.

*Tissue Plasminogen Activator (tPA).*   tPA binds to fibrin; there it cleaves fibrin-bound plasminogen to plasmin. It has little effect on plasminogen in the systemic circulation but still poses significant systemic bleeding risks. The original human tPA has been produced in a recombinant form (rtPA) that is not antigenic and does not produce allergic reactions, like the nonsynthetic form.[56] Other thrombolytic agents include the second-generation agent anistreplase (anisoylated plasminogen streptokinase activator complex) and the third-generation drug reteplase. Bioengineering techniques have improved many features of the newer thrombolytics, but a major goal continues to be development of a drug that has high clot specificity with few systemic effects and little bleeding risk.

## Procoagulants

*DDAVP (Desmopressin).*   DDAVP is a synthetic vasopressin analogue that causes release of factor VIII and vWF from the endothelium into the plasma and can cause correction of abnormal bleeding times as well as levels of vWF and factor VIII.[39] It is used to treat bleeding complications associated with type I vWD and platelet dysfunction due to renal failure.

*Epsilon Aminocaproic Acid (EACA).*   EACA is an antifibrinolytic agent that inhibits lysis of clots. It binds plasminogen, preventing its adherence to fibrin and conversion to plasmin. It is used in surgical patients mainly to reverse the effects of thrombolytic drugs and in cardiac surgery to reduce bleeding after cardiopulmonary bypass.

*Aprotinin.*   Aprotinin is a serine protease inhibitor that improves platelet function and promotes antifibrinolysis, and may also have complex antiinflammatory effects.[57] Like EACA, it is used for hemostasis during and after cardiopulmonary bypass.

*Protamine Sulfate.*   Protamine is a protein that binds to heparin and neutralizes its anticoagulant effects. The dose is 1 mg of protamine for each 100 units of heparin given. The half-life of heparin must be taken into account when calculating the protamine dose, such that the dose of heparin must be halved for each hour since its injection. So for example, a 5000-unit bolus of heparin given three hours ago would require 6.25 mg of protamine (sequentially halve 5000 three times to get 625, then divide 625 by 100 to get 6.25). Adverse reactions include hypotension, which may be avoided by slow injection over 10 minutes, and a 1% risk[58] of anaphylaxis in patients who have had previous exposure to protamine or NPH insulin. Protamine has also been reported rarely to cause a hypercoagulable state.[59]

*Estrogen.* Estrogen is used frequently for hormone replacement therapy in postmenopausal women. It has been reported to have cardioprotective effects but also prothrom-botic effects in the venous system. The exact mechanism of the increased risk of venous thrombosis is not clear, but proposed mechanisms are inhibition of fibrinolysis, decreases in natural anticoagulants such as antithrombin III and protein S,[60] or increases in coagulation factors.

## Coagulation and Sepsis

Sepsis is the coexistence of the systemic inflammatory response syndrome (SIRS) with a known or presumed infectious source. Severe sepsis is defined as sepsis with failure of one or more organ systems. There is increasing evidence of the interrelation of the coagulation system with the inflammatory response. Acute inflammation causes expression of tissue factor (TF), which activates the coagulation cascade, increases fibrin formation, and increases expression of adhesion molecules, which promote inflammation directly.[20]

Thrombin binds to TM and this complex activates protein C. Activated protein C (APC) then causes feedback inhibition of thrombin formation by inhibiting FVa and FVIIIa. In addition, APC inhibits TF and thus downregulates the coagulation cascade. APC also enhances fibrinolysis by inactivating PAI-1, and preventing activation of TAFI.[61] APC is found in the highest concentrations in the microcirculation,[62] where it functions to quickly clear the capillary bed of thromboses. APC activity is decreased in up to 85% of patients with severe sepsis.[63] As a result, microvascular thrombosis occurs, leading to end-organ congestion and eventually failure. APC also has more direct anti-inflammatory effects, such as inhibition of nuclear factor-kappa B,[64] tumor necrosis factor,[65] and leukocyte adhesion molecules.[66]

Given the role of APC in modulation of the coagulation and inflammation involved in sepsis, it is now evident that a subclinical coagulopathy plays a more important role in sepsis than had previously been thought. Indeed, administration of recombinant human APC has been shown to reduce mortality in severely septic patients.[67] Activated protein C has received FDA approval in the United States for the treatment of severe sepsis. In light of the very high cost of the medication, it appears prudent to utilize APC as part of an organized approach to the care of the septic patient. Ongoing data collection and analysis are needed to provide feedback on the drug's efficacy, safety, and cost-benefit ratio.

## Venous Thromboembolism in Trauma

Venous thromboembolism (VTE) is a common problem in trauma patients and a source of significant morbidity and mortality.[68,69] VTE encompasses deep vein thrombosis (DVT) and pulmonary embolism (PE). Major trauma often precipitates one or all of the risk factors in Virchow's Triad of hypercoagulability, endothelial injury, and venous stasis. Trauma patients may become hypercoagulable from diminished levels of antithrombin III,[70,71] suppression of fibrinolysis,[72,73] or other alterations of the coagulation system. Direct injury to blood vessels can cause intimal damage leading to thrombosis. Prolonged bed rest, immobilization, hypoperfusion, and paralysis all promote venous stasis. These elements all contribute to the occurrence of VTE in the trauma population.

Prevention of VTE in patients who are simultaneously at high risk for thrombosis and bleeding poses a formidable challenge. The difficulty is magnified by the fact that more than 60% of DVTs are clinically occult.[74,75] In addition, although methods of prophylaxis and detection continue to improve, a significant proportion of patients develop VTE despite our best efforts. In fact, PE is the third most common cause of death in trauma patients who survive past the first day.[76] A recent comprehensive literature review has shed additional light on this subject.[77]

### Risk Factors

Numerous factors have been variably cited in the literature as posing a high risk for VTE in trauma patients. However, most of these factors are supported only by indirect evidence, single-institution studies, and retrospective analysis. Traditionally, pelvic and lower extremity fractures, head injury, and prolonged immobilization have been considered risk factors for VTE.[69,78–80] In addition, high-volume blood transfusions have shown correlation with the development of VTE.[69,75,79] It is unclear whether risk is increased by transfusion itself or if the administration of blood products is just a marker of severe injury.

Certain factors may increase one's risk when considered in combination rather than separately. A risk assessment profile (RAP) score developed by Greenfield et al.,[81] and later validated by Gearhart et al.,[75] takes into account the possible synergistic effect of multiple factors on VTE risk. By assigning points for injury-related and iatrogenic factors, age, and underlying conditions and adding the points as they apply to each patient, a RAP score ≥5 identified patients at increased risk for DVT. Its use as part of an algorithm to identify patients for VTE prophylaxis is shown in Fig. 61-3.

Current evidence clearly implicates spinal cord injury and spinal fractures as risk factors for VTE.[82] In general, older age also increases risk. The specific age at which risk increases is unclear; various studies have cited ages from 30[80,83] to 60[84] as the transition point. However, no cause-and-effect relationship has been shown between traditionally cited factors—such as head injury, pelvic and long-bone fractures, immobilization, high Injury Severity Score (ISS), and high-volume transfusion—and development of VTE. These conditions may indeed increase risk, but further research is needed to clarify their degree of influence.

VTE can also result from iatrogenic interventions. Placement of femoral venous catheters, a frequent practice in severely injured and critically ill patients, correlates with development of DVT at the insertion site. Meredith et al.[85] reported a 12% (9 of 76 patients) incidence of ipsilateral iliofemoral DVT in patients who had placement of 8.5 Fr introducer catheters into the femoral vein, compared to 2.6% (2 of 76) in the contralateral uncannulated side ($p < 0.05$). Remarkably, all of these were clinically silent. Merrer et al.[86] noted a 21.5% incidence of thrombotic complications with the use of standard central venous catheters in the femoral vein, compared to 1.9% at the subclavian site. Complete vessel thrombosis occurred in 6% of femoral sites versus zero at the subclavian site.

### Diagnosis

Diagnosis of DVT or PE is hindered by their insidious onset, frequent absence of clinical signs or symptoms, and nonspecific

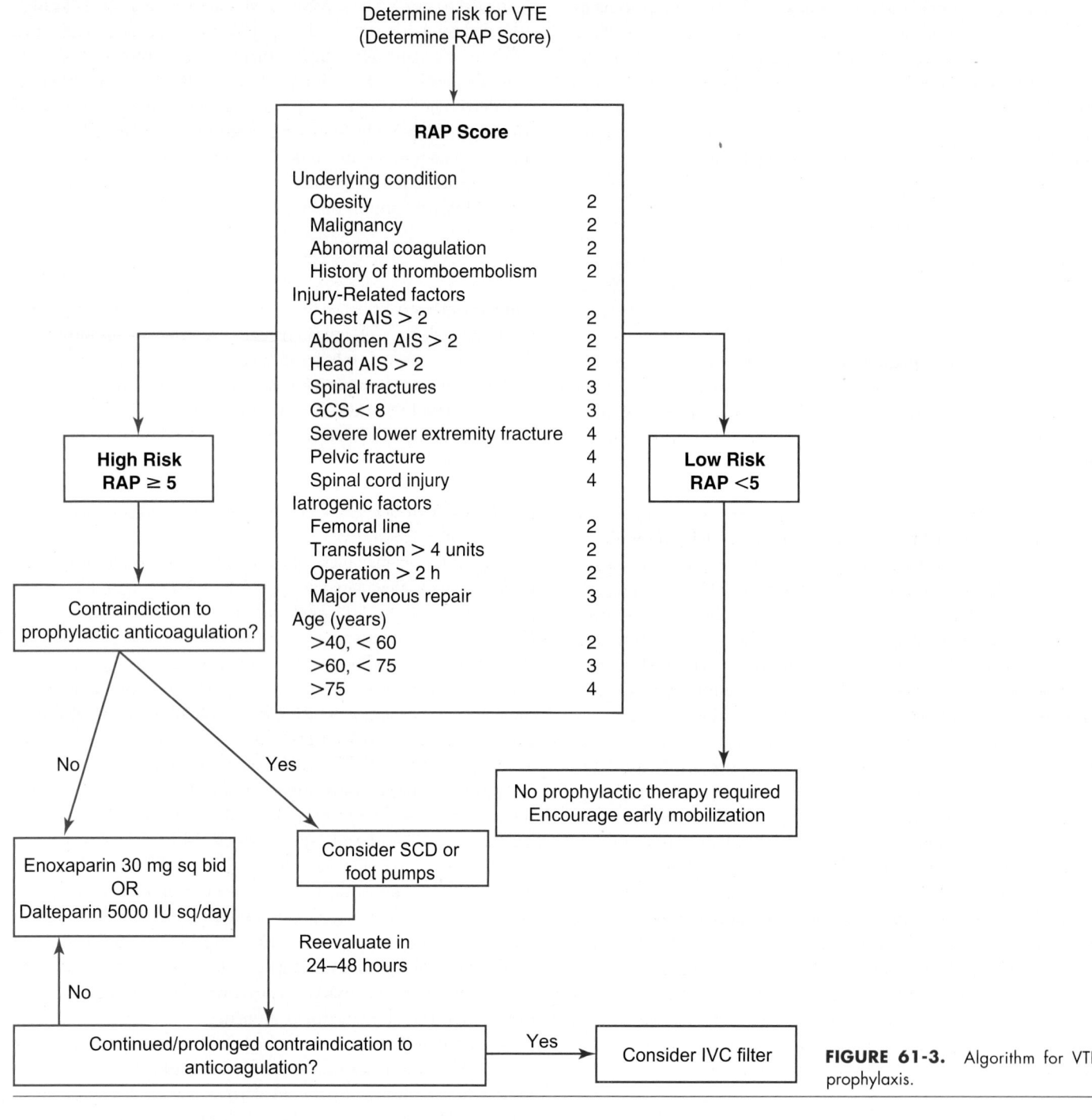

**FIGURE 61-3.** Algorithm for VTE prophylaxis.

presentation when signs and symptoms do occur. Considering the risks of indiscriminate anticoagulation for VTE, especially in the injured population, objective methods must be used to solidify the diagnosis prior to long-term treatment.

DVTs in trauma patients are overwhelmingly asymptomatic. In one large prospective study, only 2% of patients with venographically detected DVT had clinical features suggestive of the diagnosis.[69] Physical examination is clearly unreliable for this diagnosis. Venography is the most accurate test for DVT. However, it is not commonly used, owing to its invasive and sometimes painful nature, risk of allergic reactions, nonportability, and limited availability.

Duplex scanning, which combines ultrasound imaging with Doppler measurement of flow velocity, is a widely used noninvasive

method for screening and diagnosis of DVT. Unfortunately, duplex has low sensitivity in asymptomatic patients.[87,88] Its use is limited further by the frequent presence of lower extremity splints or dressings in the trauma population and its inability to adequately visualize the pelvic veins. Impedance plethysmography (IPG) and fibrinogen leg scanning are other methods of screening. IPG is a noninvasive modality that uses measurements of venous capacitance and outflow, obtained by inflating and deflating a cuff around the thigh, to infer presence of a DVT. Fibrinogen scanning uses iodine 125 to measure local fibrinogen activity to detect newly formed thrombi. Both IPG and fibrinogen scanning suffer from poor sensitivity and specificity, which limit their usefulness.

PE presentation may range from clinically silent to immediately fatal. Tachypnea is the most common sign. Arterial blood gas (ABG) analysis may show hypocarbia (due to tachypnea) and hypoxemia (from ventilation/perfusion mismatch). Chest x-ray is useful only in detecting other causes for respiratory distress, not in diagnosing PE. Unfortunately, no constellation of signs, symptoms, or laboratory tests is adequate to diagnose or exclude PE. Therefore, clinical suspicion should prompt further diagnostic testing.

The "gold standard" for diagnosis of PE is the pulmonary arteriogram. While this is an invasive test with potential for complications, it has advantages. It can definitively confirm or refute the clinical diagnosis of PE in most cases and may also offer a therapeutic opportunity in cases of massive emboli with hemodynamic consequences by means of mechanical or chemical clot lysis.

The ventilation/perfusion $\dot{V}/\dot{Q}$ scan is a common screening test for PE. Results should be coupled with clinical index of suspicion to increase the predictability of the scan. Disadvantages to $\dot{V}/\dot{Q}$ scan are duration of the study, limited availability at night, and limited ability to interpret the results when pulmonary abnormalities are present on the chest radiograph. The PIOPED[89] study was a landmark investigation of the value of the $\dot{V}/\dot{Q}$ scan. It showed that a high-likelihood clinical assessment associated with a high-probability scan diagnoses PE, while a low-probability scan plus a low-likelihood clinical assessment may exclude PE. However, the incidence of PE on angiogram for indeterminate/intermediate, low-probability, and normal $\dot{V}/\dot{Q}$ scans was 33%, 16%, and 9%, respectively. Therefore $\dot{V}/\dot{Q}$ is useful only in a minority of patients—those in whom the clinical and scan findings are, in the words of the authors, clear and concordant.

Spiral chest computed tomography (CT) has been advocated recently for investigation of PE. Prospective studies have shown a variation in sensitivity from 53 to 100% and in specificity from 81 to 100%.[90] Since current spiral CT resolution is often inadequate to identify segmental and subsegmental emboli, a negative CT does not exclude the diagnosis of PE. Therefore a negative CT should not be used as a diagnostic endpoint. A positive CT, however, is sufficient to confirm the diagnosis. The greater rapidity and availability of CT compared to $\dot{V}/\dot{Q}$ scan makes it a better option for screening in most situations. In patients for whom a strong clinical suspicion of PE exists, a negative CT should be followed by a pulmonary arteriogram to establish or exclude the diagnosis. As CT technology improves, the utility of spiral CT scan in the work-up of PE will likely increase.

## Screening

Ideally, screening for DVT would reveal occult thrombi, allowing earlier institution of therapy and thereby preventing PE and postphlebitic syndrome. Many groups use duplex for this purpose. When one considers the inadequacy of duplex in asymptomatic patients, the cost of implementing routine screening, and the lack of evidence for a lower PE rate with surveillance, this practice does not appear to be justified. Meyer et al. estimated that if surveillance duplex scans were done on all trauma patients in the intensive care unit, the annual expense would be $300,000,000 nationwide.[91] Some reports showing a benefit of screening duplex have used ineffective methods of VTE prophylaxis,[92,93] making it difficult to draw firm conclusions. It appears that implementation of an evidence-based guideline for VTE prophylaxis is more likely to reduce incidence and complications from VTE than screening duplex.[94,95]

## Methods of Prophylaxis

Most methods of VTE prophylaxis that are effective in nontrauma patients are ineffective for multiply injured patients. Interpretation of research in this area is distorted by the fact that most studies compare ineffective methods to each other, lack a control group, or use inaccurate diagnostic tests to measure the effectiveness of their prophylactic regimens.

Serial compression devices (SCDs), or intermittent pneumatic compression, affect thrombosis by increasing venous flow through the extremity and activating the fibrinolytic system. Despite their benefit in general surgical patients, SCDs do not prevent VTE in major trauma patients, offering no benefit over no prophylaxis in several studies.[80,92,96] Likewise, elastic stockings have not been shown to be effective prophylaxis in trauma patients. SCDs may be useful initially in patients with traumatic brain injury, until it is safe to give anticoagulants. Venous foot pumps fare even worse than SCDs, allowing three times the number of DVTs when compared with SCDs in one trial[97] and a 57% DVT rate by venography when used as prophylaxis in another trial.[76] Unfractionated heparin (UFH), commonly used subcutaneously for DVT prophylaxis, also has not been shown to decrease the incidence of DVT in multitrauma patients when compared to SCDs and elastic stockings[79] or to no prophylaxis.[80,98]

Low-molecular-weight heparin (LMWH) has emerged in the late 1990s as the most (or only) effective method of DVT prophylaxis in trauma patients. In a randomized, double-blind trial by Geerts et al.[99] comparing the LMWH enoxaparin to UFH in trauma patients, LMWH reduced the overall DVT rate (as diagnosed by venography) by 30% and reduced the proximal DVT rate by 58%. Bleeding complications were similar between the groups. The safety and superior efficacy of LMWH over SCDs and foot pumps has also been shown in trauma patients[100] and versus placebo in patients with leg fractures requiring immoblization.[101]

## Vena Cava Filters

Certain injuries pose such a high risk of VTE, such as spinal cord injury with paralysis and severe pelvic fractures, that one may consider placement of an inferior vena cava (IVC) filter prophylactically to prevent PE. This topic is controversial, with some authors showing a decrease in the incidence of PE versus historical controls,[102,103] while others cite no change in PE rate,[104] persistence of morbidity from DVT,[105,106] or no change in long-term outcome.[105] Liberal use of IVC filters in trauma patients is associated with extraordinary costs, and the filters may have both acute and long-term complications.[72] It is important, however, to continue VTE prophylaxis with LMWH (unless contraindicated) in patients receiving IVC filters, since they continue at high risk for DVT, which has its own risk of morbidity if left untreated.

## VTE State of the Art

The state-of-the-art approach to patients with injury must consider the need for VTE prophylaxis, and the ongoing management of these patients involves constant attention to the possibility of a VTE. As demonstrated in the expanding body of literature on this subject,[107] the hypercoagulable trauma patient presents challenges that may be no less daunting than those posed by the patient with coagulopathy. After the early stages of trauma care, concerns for VTE may, in fact, outweigh those for bleeding. All patients who are managed by a trauma service must be considered for VTE prophylaxis and monitored for the possible development of these conditions. Although far from perfect, currently available techniques have improved our ability to protect our patients from these conditions. The many unanswered questions that remain should be fertile ground for investigation.

## FUTURE DIRECTIONS

### Recombinant Activated Factor VII

Recombinant activated coagulation factor VII (rFVIIa, NovoSeven, Novo Nordisk, Bagsvaerd, Denmark) is a preparation that is currently receiving significant attention in trauma care as a systemically administered therapy for uncontrolled hemorrhage and coagulopathy. The drug is approved in the United States for use in hemophilia patients with inhibitors. It is approved in Europe for additional indications such as factor VII deficiency and Glanzmann's thrombasthenia. The drug has a rapid onset and a short half life. Its mechanism of action is controversial.[108–110] It appears to act, at least in part, at the site of injury in the presence of activated platelets to promote a burst of thrombin formation thus promoting coagulation. Because it promotes coagulation by binding exposed TF and/or activated platelets at the site of injury, its effects are local and, at least in theory, systemic effects are absent.

Enthusiastic early reports of dramatic cessation of bleeding in damage-control scenarios first focused attention on the potential role of FVIIa in severe traumatic hemorrhage.[111,112] A randomized, placebo-controlled, double-blind clinical trial in patients with blunt or penetrating trauma to assess the role and safety of rFVIIa in the management of severe hemorrhage was published in 2005. In this trial, Boffard et al. enrolled 277 patients with blunt and penetrating injury from 32 centers in eight countries.[113] Patients aged 16–65 years who required 6 units of pRBCs in the first four hours after admission were eligible for enrollment. Severe traumatic brain injury and catastrophic pre-hospital physiology (e.g., cardiac arrest, pH <7) were exclusion criteria. Enrolled patients received the first dose of rFVIIa (200 μg/kg) after the eighth unit of RBC transfusion followed by additional doses (100 μg/kg) one and three hours later. The primary endpoint was the number of units of RBCs transfused in the first 48 hours. Of 301 patients randomized, 143 with blunt and 134 with penetrating trauma were analyzed. In blunt trauma patients, the authors reported a reduction in RBC requirements of 2.6 units by Hodges-Lehmann estimate ($p = 0.02$). There was no statistically significant reduction in RBC transfusion in patients with penetrating trauma. No safety issues were noted; in particular there was no increase in thromboembolic events reported. As a result of this phase 2 trial and the preliminary data available, the manufacturer is currently sponsoring a large, blinded, randomized, placebo-controlled trial to further define the efficacy and safety of rFVIIa in patients with severe hemorrhagic shock from torso trauma.

In addition to its use in trauma, patients with conditions besides trauma have been treated with rFVIIa.[114–116] Although not approved by the FDA for such indications, the drug has shown promise. In view of the enthusiasm for its use coupled with its high cost, guidelines for use have been developed in hospitals and by organizations.[117,118] The recommended dosage for the reversal of urgent anticoagulant effects is 20–40 μg/kg. The recommended dosage for all other patients is 40–90 μg/kg. Doses utilized for trauma patients with uncontrollable hemorrhage have been as high as 200 μg/kg. Some patients with hemophilia and high titers of inhibitors have received 300 μg/kg. At this time, it is not entirely clear what the optimal dose should be for trauma patients.

In 2005, Mayer et al. reported the results of a phase 2B study designed to test the utility of FVIIa in reducing hematoma expansion in patients with acute intracerebral hemorrhage without coagulopathy. This multicenter, prospective, randomized, blinded study compared three doses of FVIIa (40, 80, or 160 μg/kg) given within four hours of symptom onset. The highest dose was associated with a significantly smaller increase in hematoma size when compared to placebo. In addition, the functional outcomes and mortality at three months were lower in the combined group of patients receiving the drug compared to the placebo group. Also reported was a significantly higher rate of serious thromboembolic complications in the study group compared to the control group (7% vs 2%).

Concerns have been raised with regards to the safety of rFVIIa. In a report from the FDA's Adverse Event Reporting System (AERS), O'Connell et al. cited 168 reports describing 185 thromboembolic events.[119] The vast majority were in patients receiving the drug for "unlabeled" indications with active bleeding being the most common. Among the adverse reports were serious thromboembolic events such as cerebrovascular accidents, myocardial infarctions, pulmonary embolism, and DVT. There were 50 deaths reported and in 72% of these deaths the thromboembolic event was listed as the probable cause of death. These data should be interpreted very cautiously since these are self-reports, the denominator cannot be determined and this is a patient population with very high rates of baseline thromboembolism.

A more rigorous analysis by Levy et al. of data from double-blind controlled studies of rFVIIa showed no difference in rates of thromboembolism between patients treated with rFVIIa and those treated with placebo.[120] The authors reviewed data from 13 studies sponsored by Novo Nordisk, the drug's manufacturer. They found an incidence of thrombotic events of 5.3% (23/430) in placebo-treated patients and 6.0% (45/748) in patients receiving rFVIIa, a nonsignificant difference ($p=0.57$).[120]

At present, FVIIa remains a very promising drug with great potential to affect the outcome of patients with severe hemorrhagic shock and coagulopathy. Ongoing and future studies will better define its role, the optimal dosage for bleeding, and any thromboembolic complications.

### Topical Hemostatic Agents

Topical hemostatic agents are products that promote blood coagulation when applied directly to bleeding surfaces. These agents are usually used for generalized oozing from raw surfaces after larger bleeding vessels have been ligated, on delicate tissues that are not amenable to suturing or cautery, or in deeper spaces that are less accessible to direct control of bleeding. Although a few products have been in use for many decades, many more have become available in the last two (see Table 61-3).

**TABLE 61-3**

**Topical Hemostatic Agents**

| BRAND NAME | TYPE OF AGENT | MANUFACTURER |
|---|---|---|
| Tisseel VH | Fibrin sealant (bovine) | Baxter Healthcare |
| Evicel | Fibrin sealant (human) | Johnson & Johnson |
| Surgicel | Oxidized cellulose | Johnson & Johnson |
| Gelfoam | Porcine gelatin sponge | Pharmacia & Upjohn |
| Surgifoam | Porcine gelatin sponge | Johnson & Johnson |
| Actifoam | Bovine collagen | CR Bard |
| Avitene | Bovine collagen | Davol |
| Instat | Bovine collagen | Johnson & Johnson |
| Helistat | Bovine collagen | Integra LifeSciences |
| Helitene | Bovine collagen | Integra LifeSciences |
| Thrombin JMI | Bovine thrombin | Jones Pharma |
| CoStasis | Bovine collagen & bovine thrombin combined with autologous platelets | Cohesion Technologies |
| FloSeal | Bovine gelatin matrix & human thrombin | Baxter Healthcare |

## Fibrin Sealants

Fibrin sealants are liquids that are dripped or sprayed onto bleeding surfaces, and cause hemostasis by initiating the latter steps of the coagulation pathway. Those in current use are virus-inactivated products derived from human plasma. The agents contain thrombin (along with ionic calcium) and fibrinogen (with factor XIII), which mix together during application resulting in formation of fibrin monomers that polymerize and form a fibrin clot. Calcium activates factor XIII, which promotes cross-linking of fibrin into a stable clot. After application the products quickly congeal into a gel-like consistency.

Two fibrin sealant products are currently available in the United States: Tisseel VH Fibrin Sealant (Baxter Healthcare Corp) and Evicel Fibrin Sealant (Human) (Johnson & Johnson Wound Management, a division of Ethicon, Inc.). Evicel has recently replaced Crosseal, a previous fibrin sealant from Johnson & Johnson. Both Tisseel and Crosseal contain antifibrinolytic agents intended to prevent dissolution of clot; Tisseel contains bovine-derived aprotinin, and Crosseal contains tranexamic acid. Crosseal was contraindicated for use with possible contact with dura mater or cerebrospinal fluid, because tranexamic acid may cause severe convulsions when applied to central nervous system tissues.[121] Evicel does not contain tranexamic acid, and has been FDA approved without the above contraindication. Aprotinin has been associated with allergic and anaphylactic reactions in rare cases. Although each product is licensed for use in specific surgical conditions, both have had broad off-label use. Intravascular use is contraindicated for both.

Large, prospective randomized data on use of fibrin sealants in human trauma patients is scarce, but a mounting body of literature in various other surgical specialties[121] and in animal models of severe traumatic liver injury[122] suggest that these products may provide a considerable benefit in achieving hemostasis. Fibrin sealants have been used extensively in elective liver resection, and may improve hemostasis compared to standard topical hemostats.[123] Fibrin sealants also have shown benefit in reducing postoperative blood loss and perioperative allogeneic blood transfusion in elective surgery.[124]

## Absorbable Hemostatic Agents

Local absorbable hemostatic agents work by contact activation (cellulose or gelatin-based products: Surgicel, Gelfoam, Surgifoam), both contact activation and platelet aggregation (collagen-based products: Avitene, Instat, Helistat, Helitene), or direct activation of platelets and coagulation proteins (Thrombin). Most topical absorbable agents require a near-dry field, and are best used in conjunction with local pressure to stop bleeding, as opposed to fibrin sealants which can be applied to actively bleeding areas. Absorption may be variable, depending on the amount used, and although agents may dissolve to some extent, they may not entirely disappear. The agents may be seen postoperatively on radiologic studies such as CT and MR, and may sometimes be difficult to differentiate from tissue, hematoma, or abscess.[125]

Adverse effects have been reported with many of these products,[126] and clinicians using them should be knowledgeable in their proper use and administration. Absorbable hemostaticss may slightly increase the chance of local infection, and possibly interfere with wound healing. Antigenicity and allergic reactions remain a concern with bovine-derived products such as thrombin and the collagen-based agents. When antibody formation to thrombin occurs, it may paradoxically result in a severe coagulopathy. Injection of topical thrombin is contraindicated, and adverse reactions may occur with intravascular administration of many products intended for topical use. Overall, the risk of side effects is low, and there are many direct benefits attributable to use of topical hemostatic agents. Reducing blood loss and therefore avoiding additional blood transfusion and shortening operating time not only provide an advantage to patients, but result in indirect economic benefits as well. Given the central role that achieving hemostasis plays in surgery in general, and trauma specifically, the development and use of topical hemostatic agents is likely to advance at a rapid pace.

## Platelet Function Assays

As the population has aged and more individuals are receiving antiplatelet therapies for a variety of medical conditions, the trauma surgeon is increasingly likely to encounter injured patients who are bleeding or at high risk for bleeding with abnormal platelet function.

Several tests of platelet function are available although there is no single test that is currently recommended by a majority of authorities in the field. Some tests of platelet function are maintained in a central hospital laboratory and others are available as point-of-care tests. The bleeding time is longer considered a reliable test and should not be used to guide platelet therapy in trauma patients.[43–47,126] Our hospital has abandoned the bleeding time in favor of the PFA-100 (Platelet Function Analyzer, Dade-Behring).[127–128] The PFA-100 measures platelet function by the time it takes whole blood to occlude an aperture in a filter treated with either collagen and epinephrine (CEPI) or collagen and ADP (CADP). The blood is passed through the aperture at high shear rates to simulate the conditions platelets encounter at damaged vessel walls. The time it takes for the hole to become occluded is termed the "closure time" and is reported in seconds. The test ends at a maximum of 300 seconds. It is a global test of primary hemostasis that may detect platelet dysfunction due to certain disorders or medications as well as congenital diseases such as vWD. It is important to note that its role has not yet been completely defined. Results from the PFA-100 are dependent on a number of variables (such as vWF binding to the platelet membrane) and each laboratory needs to establish its own reference ranges and quality controls.[129] A recent communication from a professional organization recommended further investigation and noted that additional studies were needed before the PFA-100 can be widely adopted.[129]

Other tests are available measure the percentage of platelets that are working normally and to determine the functional platelet count. Many have been used in the cardiac surgery setting.[128,130] These include point-of-care tests to evaluate platelet inhibition by drugs such as aspirin or GPIIb/IIIa inhibitors as well as tests of platelet aggregation in response to a variety of agonists. Platelet aggregation is likely the "gold standard" test but takes hours to perform and requires specialized equipment and training, making it less useful for the management of patients with acute coagulopathy.

# REFERENCES

1. Scott-Conner CEH, Rigdon EE, Rock WA Jr, et al.: Hematology. In O'Leary JP, Capote LR, eds. *The Physiologic Basis of Surgery*, 2d ed. Baltimore: Williams & Wilkins, 1996, p 479.
2. Andrews RK, Shen Y, Gardiner EE, et al.: The glycoprotein Ib-IX-V complex in platelet adhesion and signalling. *Thromb Haemost* 82:357, 1999.
3. Ruggeri ZM: Role of von Willebrand factor in platelet thrombus formation. *Ann Med* 32:2, 2000.
4. Ofosu FA, Nyarko KA: Human platelet thrombin receptors: Roles in platelet activation. *Hematol Oncol Clin North Am* 14:1185, 2000.
5. Gachet C: Platelet activation by ADP: The role of ADP antagonists. *Ann Med* 3232:15, 2000.
6. Bennett JS: Structural biology of glycoprotein IIb-IIa. *Trends Cardiovasc Med* 16:31, 1996.
7. Bennett JS: Novel platelet inhibitors. *Annu Rev Med* 52:161, 2001.
8. Owings JT, Gosselin RC: Bleeding and transfusion. In Wilmore DW, Cheung LY, Harken AH, et al. eds. *ACS Surgery: Principles & Practice*. New York: WebMD, 2003, p. 75.
9. Broze GJ: The role of tissue factor pathway inhibitor in a revised coagulation cascade. *Semin Hematol* 29:159, 1992.
10. McVey JH: Tissue factor pathway. *Baillieres Clin Haematol* 7:469, 1994.
11. Booth NA: Fibrinolysis and thrombosis. *Best Pract Res Clin Haematol* 12:423, 1999.
12. Rijken DC, Sakharov DV: Basic principles in thrombolysis: Regulatory role of plasminogen. *Thromb Res* 103:S41, 2001.
13. Esmon CT: Protein C anticoagulation pathway and its role in controlling microvascular thrombosis and inflammation. *Crit Care Med* 29:S48, 2001.
14. Rutledge R, Sheldon GF, Collins ML: Massive transfusion. *Crit Care Clin* 2:791, 1986.
15. Valeri CR, Cassidy G, Khuri S, et al.: Hypothermia induced reversible platelet dysfunction. *Ann Surg* 205:175, 1987.
16. Oung CM, Li MS, Shum Tim D, et al.: In vivo study of bleeding time and arterial hemorrhage in hypothermic versus normothermic animals. *J Trauma* 35:251, 1993.
17. Harrigan C, Lucas CE, Ledgerwood AN, et al.: Serial changes in primary hemostasis after massive transfusion. *Surgery* 98:836, 1985.
18. Ciavarella D, Reed RL, Counts RB, et al.: Clotting factor levels and the risk of diffuse microvascular bleeding in the massively transfused patient. *Br J Haematol* 67:365, 1987.
19. Reed RL, Ciavarella D, Heimbach DM, et al.: Prophylactic platelet transfusion during massive transfusion: A prospective double-blind clinical study. *Ann Surg* 203:40, 1986.
20. Lorant DE, Topham MK, Whatley RE, et al.: Inflammatory roles of P-selectin. *J Clin Invest* 92:559, 1993.
21. Watts DD, Trask A, Soeken K, et al.: Hypothermic coagulopathy in trauma: Effect of varying levels of hypothermia on enzyme speed, platelet function, and fibrinolytic activity. *J Trauma* 44:846, 1998.
22. Valeri CR, Feingold H, Cassidy G, et al.: Hypothermia-induced reversible platelet dysfunction. *Ann Surg* 205:175, 1987.
23. Shapiro MB, Jenkins DH, Schwab CW, et al.: Damage control: Collective review. *J Trauma* 45:969, 2000.
24. Jurkovich G, Greiser W, Luterman A, et al.: Hypothermia in trauma victims: An ominous predictor of survival. *J Trauma* 27:1019, 1987.
25. Levi M: Pathogenesis and treatment of disseminated intravascular coagulation in the septic patient. *J Crit Care* 16:167, 2001.
26. Levi M, van der Poll T, ten Cate H, et al.: The cytokine-mediated imbalance between coagulant and anticoagulant mechanisms in sepsis and endotoxaemia. *Eur J Clin Invest* 27:3, 1997.
27. Levi M, ten Cate H: Disseminated intravascular coagulation. *N Engl J Med* 341:586, 1999.
28. Bick RL, Baker WF: Diagnostic efficacy of the D-dimer assay in disseminated intravascular coagulation (DIC). *Thromb Res* 65:785, 1992.
29. Pernerstorfer T, Hollenstein U, Hansen J-B, et al.: Heparin blunts endotoxin-induced coagulation activation. *Circulation* 100:2485, 1999.
30. Fourrier F, Chopin C, Huart JJ, et al.: Double-blind, placebo-controlled trial of antithrombin III concentrates in septic shock with disseminated intravascular coagulation. *Chest* 104:882, 1993.
31. Eisele B, Lamy M, Thijs LG, et al.: Antithrombin III in patients with severe sepsis: A randomized, placebo-controlled, double-blind multicenter trial plus a meta-analysis on all randomized, placebo-controlled, double-blind trials with antithrombin III in severe sepsis. *Intensive Care Med* 24:663, 1998.
32. Francis JL, Armstrong DJ: Acquired dysfibrinogenemia in liver disease. *J Clin Pathol* 35:667, 1982.
33. Lethagen S: Desmopressin (DDAVP) and hemostasis. *Ann Hematol* 69:173, 1994.
34. Fakhry SM, Rutherford EJ, Sheldon GF: Hematologic principles in surgery. In Townsend CM, Beauchamp RD, Evers BM, Mattox KL, eds. *Textbook of Surgery: The Biological Basis of Modern Surgical Practice*, 16th ed. Philadelphia: Saunders, 2001; p 68.
35. Lethagen S: Desmopressin (DDAVP) and hemostasis. *Ann Hematol* 69:173, 1994.
36. Opatrny K Jr: Hemostasis disorders in chronic renal failure. *Kidney Int Suppl* 62:S87, 1997.
37. Rose EH, Aledort LM: Nasal spray desmopressin (DDAVP) for mild hemophilia and von Willebrand disease. *Ann Intern Med* 114:563, 1991.
38. Kasper CK: Treatment of factor VIII inhibitors. *Prog Hemost Thromb* 9:57, 1989.
39. Mannucci PM, Canciani MT, Rota L, et al.: Response of factor VIII/von Willebrand factor to DDAVP in healthy subjects and patients with haemophilia A and von Willebrand disease. *Br J Haematol* 47:283, 1981.
40. Mannucci PM, Bettega D, Cattaneo M: Patterns of development of tachyphylaxis in patients with haemophilia and von Willebrand disease after repeated doses of desmopressin (DDAVP). *Br J Haematol* 82:87, 1992.
41. Mannucci PM: How I treat patients with von Willebrand disease. *Blood* 97:1915, 2001.
42. Eisenberg JM, Clarke JR, Sussman SA: Prothrombin and partial thromboplastin times as preoperative screening tests. *Arch Surg* 117:48, 1982.
43. Gewirtz AS, Kottke-Marchant K, Miller ML: The preoperative bleeding time test: Assessing its clinical usefulness. *Cleve Clin J Med* 62:379, 1995.
44. Gewirtz AS, Miller ML, Keys TF: The clinical usefulness of the preoperative bleeding time. *Arch Pathol Lab Med* 120:353, 1996.
45. Klopfenstein CE: Preoperative clinical assessment of hemostatic function in patients scheduled for a cardiac operation. *Ann Thorac Surg* 62:1918, 1996.
46. Rodgers RPC, Levin J: A critical reappraisal of the bleeding time. *Semin Thromb Haemost* 16:1, 1990.
47. Lind SE: The bleeding time does not predict surgical bleeding. *Blood* 77:2547, 1991.
48. Hirsh J, Warkentin E, Raschke R, et al.: Heparin and low-molecular-weight heparin: Mechanisms of action, pharmacokinetics, dosing considerations, monitoring, efficacy, and safety. *Chest* 114:489S, 1998.
49. Young E, Wells P, Holloway S, et al.: Ex-vivo and in-vitro evidence that low molecular weight heparins exhibit less binding to plasma proteins than unfractionated heparin. *Thromb Haemost* 71:300, 1994.
50. Warkentin TE, Levine MN, Hirsh J, et al.: Heparin-induced thrombocytopenia in patients treated with low-molecular-weight heparin or unfractionated heparin. *N Engl J Med* 332:1330, 1995.
51. Hirsh J, Dalen JE, Anderson DR, et al.: Oral anticoagulants: Mechanism of action, clinical effectiveness, and optimal therapeutic range. *Chest* 114:445S, 1998.
52. Ikeda Y: Antiplatelet therapy using cilostazol, a specific PDE3 inhibitor. *Thromb Haemost* 82:435, 1999.
53. McAdam BF, Catella-Lawson F, Mardini I, et al.: Systemic biosynthesis of prostacyclin by cyclooxygenase (COX)-2: The human pharmacology of a selective inhibitor of COX-2. *Proc Natl Acad Sci USA* 96:272, 1999.
54. Mukherjee D, Nissen SE, Topol EJ: Risk of cardiovascular events associated with selective COX-2 inhibitors. *JAMA* 286:954, 2001.
55. Komers R, Anderson S, Epstein M: Renal and cardiovascular effects of selective cyclooxygenase-2 inhibitors. *Am J Kidney Dis* 38:1145, 2001.
56. Frangos SG, Chen AH, Sumpio B: Vascular drugs in the new millennium. *J Am Coll Surg* 191:76, 2000.

57. Landis RC, Asimakopoulos G, Poullis M, et al.: The antithrombotic and anti-inflammatory mechanisms of action of aprotinin. *Ann Thorac Surg* 72:2169, 2001.

58. Majerus PW, Tollefsen DM: Anticoagulant, thrombolytic, and antiplatelet drugs. In Hardman JG, Limbird LE, Gilman AG, eds. *Goodman & Gilman's The Pharmacological Basis of Therapeutics,* 10th ed. New York: McGraw-Hill, 2001, p 1025.

59. Levy JH, Schwieger IM, Zaidan JR, et al.: Evaluation of patients at risk for protamine reactions. *J Thorac Cardiovasc Surg* 98:200, 1989.

60. Gottsater A, Berg A, Centergard J, et al.: Clinically suspected pulmonary embolism: Is it safe to withhold anticoagulation after a negative spiral CT? *J Intern Med* 249:237, 2001.

61. Grinnell BW, Joyce D: Recombinant human activated protein C: A system modulator of vascular function for treatment of severe sepsis. *Crit Care Med* 29:S53, 2001.

62. Esmon CT: The roles of protein C and thrombomodulin in the regulation of blood coagulation. *J Biol Chem* 264:4743, 1989.

63. Matthay MA: Severe sepsis—A new treatment with both anticoagulant and antiinflammatory properties. *N Engl J Med* 344:759, 2001.

64. Murakami K, Okajima K, Uchida M, et al.: Activated protein C prevents LPS-induced pulmonary vascular injury by inhibiting cytokine production. *Am J Physiol* 272:L197, 1997.

65. Taylor FB, Chang A, Esmon CT, et al.: Protein C prevents the coagulopathic and lethal effects of *Escherichia coli* infusion in the baboon. *J Clin Invest* 79:918, 1987.

66. Grinnell BW, Hermann RB, Yan SB: Human protein C inhibits selectin-mediated cell adhesion: Role of unique fucosylated oligosaccharide. *Glycobiology* 4:221, 1994.

67. Bernard GR, Vincent JL, Laterre PF, et al.: Efficacy and safety of recombinant human activated protein C for severe sepsis. *N Engl J Med* 344:699, 2001.

68. Shackford SR, Mackersie RC, Holbrook TL, et al.: The epidemiology of traumatic death: A population-based analysis. *Arch Surg* 128:571, 1993.

69. Geerts WH, Code KI, Jay RM, et al.: A prospective study of venous thromboembolism after major trauma. *N Engl J Med* 331:1601, 1994.

70. Seyfer AE, Saeber AV, Dombrose FA, et al.: Coagulation changes in elective surgery and trauma. *Ann Surg* 193:210, 1981.

71. Owings JT, Bagley M, Gosselin R, et al.: Effect of critical injury on plasma antithrombin activity: Low antithrombin levels are associated with thromboembolic complications. *J Trauma* 41:396, 1996.

72. Attar S, Boyd D, Layne E, et al.: Alterations in coagulation and fibrinolytic system in acute trauma. *J Trauma* 9:939, 1969.

73. Enderson BL, Chen JP, Robinson R, et al.: Fibrinolysis in multisystem trauma patients. *J Trauma* 31:1240, 1991.

74. Kudsk KA, Fabian T, Baum S, et al.: Silent deep venous thrombosis in immobilized multiple trauma patients. *Am J Surg* 158:515, 1989.

75. Gearhart MM, Luchette FA, Proctor MC, et al.: The risk assessment profile score identifies trauma patients at risk for deep vein thrombosis. *Surgery* 128:631, 2000.

76. Geerts WH, Heit JA, Clagett GP, et al.: Prevention of venous thromboembolism. *Chest* 119(Suppl):132S, 2001.

77. Pasquale M, Fabian TC, the EAST Ad Hoc Committee on Practice Management Guideline Development: Practice management guidelines for trauma from the Eastern Association for the Surgery of Trauma. *J Trauma* 44:941, 1998.

78. Shackford DR, Davis JW, Hollingsworth-Fridlund P, et al.: Venous thromboembolism in patients with major trauma. *Am J Surg* 159:365, 1990.

79. Knudson MM, Collins JA, Goodman SB, et al.: Thromboembolism following multiple trauma. *J Trauma* 32:2, 1992.

80. Knudson MM, Lewis FR, Clinton A, et al.: Prevention of venous thromboembolism in trauma patients. *J Trauma* 37:480, 1994.

81. Greenfield LJ, Proctor MC, Rodriquez JL, et al.: Posttrauma thromboembolism prophylaxis. *J Trauma* 42:100, 1997.

82. Velmahos GC, Kern J, Chan LS, et al.: Prevention of venous thromboembolism after injury: An evidence-based report—Part II: Analysis of risk factors and evaluation of the role of vena cava filters. *J Trauma* 49:140, 2000.

83. Spannagel U, Kujath P: Low molecular weight heparin for the prevention of thromboembolism in outpatients immobilized by plaster cast. *Semin Thromb Hemost* 19:131, 1993.

84. Abelseth G, Buckley RE, Pineo GE, et al.: Incidence of deep vein thrombosis in patients with fractures of the lower extremity distal to the hip. *J Orthop Trauma* 10:230, 1996.

85. Meredith JW, Young JS, O'Neil EA, et al.: Femoral catheters and deep venous thrombosis: A prospective evaluation with venous duplex sonography. *J Trauma* 35:187, 1993.

86. Merrer J, DeJonghe B, Golliot F, et al.: Complications of femoral and subclavian venous catheterization in critically ill patients: A randomized controlled trial. *JAMA* 286:700, 2001.

87. Davidson BL, Elliot CG, Lensing AW, et al.: Low accuracy of color Doppler ultrasound in the detection of proximal leg vein thrombosis in asymptomatic high-risk patients. *Ann Intern Med* 117:735, 1992.

88. Kearon C, Julian JA, Newman TE, et al.: Noninvasive diagnosis of deep venous thrombosis. *Ann Intern Med* 128:663, 1998.

89. The PIOPED Investigators: Value of the ventilation/perfusion scan in acute pulmonary embolism. Results of the prospective investigation of pulmonary embolism diagnosis (PIOPED). *JAMA* 263:2753, 1990.

90. Rathbun SW, Raskob GE, Whitsett TL: Sensitivity and specificity of helical computed tomography in the diagnosis of pulmonary embolism: A systematic review. *Ann Intern Med* 132:227, 2000.

91. Meyer CS, Blebea J, Davis K Jr, et al.: Surveillance venous scans for deep venous thrombosis in multiple trauma patients. *Ann Vasc Surg* 9:109, 1995.

92. Napolitano LM, Garlapati VS, Heard SO, et al.: Asymptomatic deep venous thrombosis in the trauma patient: Is an aggressive screening protocol justified? *J Trauma* 39:651, 1995.

93. Piotrowski JJ, Alexander JJ, Brandt CP, et al.: Is deep vein thrombosis surveillance warranted in high-risk trauma patients? *Am J Surg* 172:210, 1996.

94. Schwarcz TH, Quick RC, Minion DJ, et al.: Enoxaparin treatment in high-risk trauma patients limits the utility of surveillance venous duplex scanning. *J Vasc Surg* 34:447, 2001.

95. Cipolle MD, Wojcik R, Seislove E, et al.: The role of surveillance duplex scanning in preventing venous thromboembolism in trauma patients. *J Trauma* 52:453, 2002.

96. Fisher CG, Blachut PA, Salvain AJ, et al.: Effectiveness of pneumatic leg compression devices for the prevention of thromboembolic disease in orthopaedic trauma patients: A prospective, randomized study of compression alone versus no prophylaxis. *J Orthop Trauma* 9:1, 1995.

97. Elliot CG, Dudney TM, Egger M, et al.: Calf-thigh sequential pneumatic compression compared with plantar venous pneumatic compression to prevent deep-vein thrombosis after non-lower extremity trauma. *J Trauma* 47:25, 1999.

98. Upchurch GR, Demling RG, Davies J, et al.: Efficacy of subcutaneous heparin in prevention of venous thromboembolic events in trauma patients. *Am Surg* 61:749, 1995.

99. Geerts WH, Jay RM, Code KI, et al.: A comparison of low-dose heparin with low-molecular-weight heparin as prophylaxis against venous thromboembolism after major trauma. *N Engl J Med* 335:701, 1996.

100. Knudson MM, Morabito D, Paiement GD, et al.: Use of low molecular weight heparin in preventing thromboembolism in trauma patients. *J Trauma* 41:446, 1996.

101. Lassen MR, Borris LC, Nakov RL: Use of the low-molecular-weight heparin reviparin to prevent deep-vein thrombosis after leg injury requirin immobilization. *N Engl J Med* 347:726, 2002.

102. Rogers FB, Shackford SR, Ricci MA, et al.: Routine prophylactic vena cava filter insertion in severely injured trauma patients decreases the incidence of pulmonary embolism. *J Am Coll Surg* 180:641, 1995.

103. Carlin AM, Tyburski JG, Wilson RF, et al.: Prophylactic and therapeutic inferior vena cava filters to prevent pulmonary emboli in trauma patients. *Arch Surg* 137:521, 2002.

104. McMurtry AL, Owings JT, Anderson JT, et al.: Increased use of prophylactic vena cava filters in trauma patients failed to decrease overall incidence of pulmonary embolism. *J Am Coll Surg* 189:314, 1999.

105. Decousus H, Leizorovicz A, Parent F, et al.: A clinical trial of vena caval filters in the prevention of pulmonary embolism in patients with proximal deep-vein thrombosis. *N Engl J Med* 338:409, 1998.

106. Rodriquez JL, Lopez JM, Proctor MC, et al.: Early placement of prophylactic vena caval filters in injured patients at high risk for pulmonary embolism. *J Trauma* 40:779, 1996.

107. Rogers FB. Venous thromboembolism in trauma patient: A review. *Surgery* 130:1, 2001.

108. Roberts HR, Monroe DM, White GC: The use of recombinant factor VIIa in the treatment of bleeding disorders. *Blood* 104:3858, 2004.

109. Hoffman M, Monroe DM, Roberts HR: Activated factor VII activates factors IX and X on the surface of activated platelets: Thoughts on the mechanism of action of high-dose activated factor VII. *Blood Coagul Fibrinolysis* 9:S61, 1998.

110. Monroe DM, Hoffman M, Oliver JA, et al.: Platelet activity of high-dose factor VIIa is independent of tissue factor. *Br J Haematol* 99:542, 1997.

111. Kenet G, Walden R, Eldad A, et al.: Treatment of Traumatic Bleeding with Recombinant Factor VIIa. *The Lancet* 354:1879, 1999.

112. O'Neill PA, Bluth M, Gloster ES: Successful use of recombinant activated factor vii for trauma-associated hemorrhage in a patient without preexisting coagulopathy. *J Trauma* 52:400, 2002.

113. Boffard KD, Riou B, Warren B, et al.: Recombinant Factor VIIa as adjunctive therapy for bleeding control in severely injured trauma patients: Two parallel randomized, placebo-controlled, double-blind clinical trials. *J Trauma* 59:8, 2005.

114. Holcomb JB: Use of recombinant activated Factor VII to treat the acquired coagulopathy of trauma. *J Trauma* 58:1298, 2005.

115. Barletta JF, Ahrens CL, Tyburski JG, et al.: A review of recombinant factor VII for refractory bleeding in nonhemophiliac trauma patients. *J Trauma* 58:646, 2005.

116. Hedner U, Erhardtsen E: Potential role for rFVIIa in transfusion medicine. *Transfusion* 42:114, 2002.
117. Goodnough LT, Lublin DM, Zhang L, et al.: Transfusion medicine service policies for recombinant factor VIIa administration. *Transfusion* 44:1325, 2004.
118. Shander A, Goodnough LT, Ratko T, et al.: Consensus recommendations for the off-label use of recombinant human factor VIIa (Novoseven) therapy. *Pharmacy and Therapeutics* 30:644, 2005.
119. O'Connell KA, Wood JJ, Wise RP, et al.: Thromboembolic Adverse Events After Use of Recombinant Human Coagulation Factor VIIa. *JAMA* 295:293, 2006.
120. Levy JH, Fingerhut A, Brott T, et al.: Recombinant factor VIIa in patients with coagulopathy secondary to anticoagulant therapy, cirrhosis, or severe traumatic injury: Review of safety profile. *Transfusion* 46:919, 2006.
121. Albala DM, Lawson JH: Recent clinical and investigational applications of fibrin sealant in selected surgical specialties. *J Am Coll Surg* 202:685, 2006.
122. Cohn SM, Cross JH, Ivy ME, et al.: Fibrin glue terminates massive bleeding after complex hepatic injury. *J Trauma* 45:666, 1998.
123. Schwartz M, Madariaga J, Hirose R, et al.: Comparison of a new fibrin sealant with standard topical hemostatic agents. *Arch Surg* 139:1148, 2004.
124. Carless PA, Henry DA, Anthony DM: Fibrin sealant use for minimizing perioperative allogeneic blood transfusion. *Cochrane Database Syst Rev* 2: CD004171, 2003.
125. Tomizawa Y: Clinical benefits and risk analysis of topical hemostats: A review. *J Artif Organs* 8:137, 2005.
126. Gabay M: Absorbable hemostatic agents. *Am J Health-Syst Pharm* 63:1244, 2006.
127. Rodgers RP, Levin J: A critical reappraisal of the bleeding time. *Semin Thromb Hemost* 16:1, 1990.
128. Michelson AD: Platelet function testing in cardiovascular diseases. *Hematology* 10:132, 2005.
129. Platelet Function Analyzer (PFA-100) Closure time in the evaluation of platelet disorders and platelet function. *J Thromb Haemost* 4:312, 2006.
130. Quantifying the effect of antiplatelet therapy. *Anesthesiology* 105:676, 2006.

## Commentary ■ ERNEST F. J. BLOCK

Drs. Fakhry and Michetti have provided the readers with a thorough and highly readable review of the current love-hate relationship between traumatologist and the patient's coagulation state. When the acutely injured and bleeding patient is coagulopathic, the surgeon is focused on resuscitative strategies to cause clot to form. After stabilization, the same surgeon initiates anticoagulation as prophylaxis against venous thromboembolic complications! This relationship reminds us of Aristotle's observation that mankind is never satisfied with what it has, a classical view of "buyer's remorse."

A comprehensive regurgitation of the coagulation cascade is rarely of clinical value at the bedside. However, as industry produces potential solutions for complications for the coagulation system, a reputable source like the initial portion of this chapter is essential to plan institutional protocols for care. The mechanisms responsible for failure of the coagulation system require recognition and appreciation in order to develop proactive strategies to prevent and treat them. This knowledge is critical to the management of specific new scenarios in coagulation disorders in trauma.

Recombinant factor VIIa is currently being scrutinized for its adjunctive role in control of hemorrhage following injury. Its role in massive hemorrhage as a life-saving strategy is under debate. Due to the high mortality of the patient group in whom this drug is used as salvage therapy, the noise-to-signal ratio from death may be too high to detect benefit. However, Boffard's study showed a reduction in units transfused suggesting that a greater effect may exist if a valid patient population can be identified for study. More interest may be seen in patient populations where any control of bleeding may be beneficial, such as Mayer's work in intracerebral hemorrhage following stroke cited in the chapter. Although the study group appeared to have less expansion of bleed and better early mortality, the study group experienced more thromboembolic complications. Which of these competing complications shall we accept? Additional questions remain in terms of long-term survival and function since survival of a vegetative patient who may have otherwise succumbed may not be seen as optimal outcome. Application to the trauma population is fertile grounds for study.

Correction of medical coagulopathy is of increasing importance to the traumatologist. As the profession morphs into the Acute Care Surgeon who deals with many surgical emergencies, the dilemma of operating in the face of complete and intentional anticoagulation increases in frequency. Correction with use of fresh frozen plasma other than for life-threatening bleeding exposes the patient to the transfusion risks and uses a product that depends on volunteer donors that are in limited supply. Patients on warfarin often need not be corrected with high doses of vitamin K; as they will likely needre-anticoagulation in the postoperative phase. An alternative is partial correction with small doses of vitamin K via intravenous route (0.5–1 mg) that reduces the risk of bleeding complications while limiting the thromboembolic disease state for which they were originally treated. Certainly intracranial hemorrhage and major multisystem trauma may warrant use of FFP.

In the hypercoagulable phase of recovery, trauma patients warrant prophylaxis. The authors detail current status of dealing with a difficult clinical conundrum and describe the relative values of the available options. At what time do the risks of venous thromboembolic events overshadow those of further bleeding? Experienced traumatologists have all faced the patient who early on manifested VTE but are similarly daunted by those patients whose bleed worsened after initiation of anticoagulant prophylaxis.

Finally, trauma providers as critical care specialists, use recombinant activated protein C for treatment of severe sepsis. The understanding that microthrombi in sepsis may be responsible for organ dysfunction and death underscores the importance of mastering the coagulation cascade at various levels. Treatment with this novel agent again challenges the trauma team with balancing the benefit of therapy with the possibility of bleeding complications.

Here we sit with the diametrically opposed concerns, two primal competing but complementary forces, the Yin and Yang of the coagulation cascade. In Aristotle's solution to his observation, our desire and passion must be regulated to find the ultimate end in itself, the one good that can be achieved in life. Trauma care providers must deal rationally and objectively with these competing interests of correcting coagulopathy and later preventing the hypercoagulable state. The readers of this chapter are better armed to deal with the difficult dilemma with which they are faced on a daily basis.

# Cardiovascular Failure

*Ankush Gosain* ▪ *John Santaniello* ▪ *Fred Luchette*

## INTRODUCTION

Cardiovascular failure can be either the end result of multi system organ failure (MSOF) or a precursor to shock and MSOF (see Chap. 68). Most often cardiovascular collapse will manifest itself with clinical signs and symptoms of cardiac failure. In trauma, the most common cause of shock is acute blood loss (hypovolemia), which results in decreased preload or decreased right heart filling volumes and manifests as tachycardia and hypotension (see Chap. 13). Although this is the most common type of shock occurring after injury, cardiogenic shock, resulting from impaired myocardial contractility, and septic shock, characterized by failure of the heart to overcome decreased vascular tone and failure of end organ utilization of delivered oxygen, are also seen. Therapy to support the failing cardiovascular system is directed at the etiology of the shock state and includes fluid resuscitation (preload) as well as pharmacologic modulation of vascular tone (afterload), contractility (with inotropes), and heart rate (with chronotropes) (Fig. 62-1).

## DETERMINANTS OF CARDIAC OUTPUT

Cardiac output is defined as the quantity of blood ejected into the aorta by the heart each minute and is calculated as heart rate multiplied by stroke volume ($CO = HR \times SV$). This is the quantity of blood that flows through the circulation and is responsible for oxygen and nutrient transport to the tissues. The primary determinants of cardiac output are preload (the venous return to the heart), afterload (the resistance against which the heart must pump), contractility (the extent to which the myocardial cells can contract), and heart rate. As will be detailed below, the primary determinant of cardiac output is the filling of the heart and the ability to pump that volume effectively. Accordingly, the majority

of therapeutic modalities aimed at augmenting cardiac output focus on restoring filling pressures and augmenting ineffective contractility.

Multiple studies and textbooks cite 5.6 L/minute as a "normal" resting cardiac output as measured in young, healthy males. However, cardiac output varies with the level of activity of the body, and is influenced by level of metabolism, exercise state, age, size of the individual, and other factors. Accordingly, cardiac output in women is generally stated as being 10–20% lower than in men. Additionally, when factoring in age, the average cardiac output for adults is approximated as 5 L/minute. Laboratory and clinical research have demonstrated that cardiac output increases in proportion to increasing body surface area. Therefore, to standardize cardiac output measurements between individuals, the parameter of cardiac index (defined as cardiac output divided by body surface area in m$^2$) is employed.

### Preload

In the discussion of cardiovascular physiology, *preload* is the force that stretches myocardium prior to contraction. The concept of preload is derived from laboratory experiments in which strips of muscle are stretched by small weights (preload) prior to initiating contraction. In these experiments, contraction is triggered by electrical stimulation and a transducer determines the resultant force. Both in vitro experiments and in vivo correlates have revealed that increasing sarcomere length to a maximum of 0.2 μm by the addition of weights results in increased force of contraction. Once stretched beyond this length, the contractility of the muscle decreases. This relationship, the Frank–Starling relationship, was described in amphibian hearts by Otto Frank in 1884 and extended to mammalian hearts by Ernest Starling in 1914. The mechanisms linking preload and contractile force are incompletely understood. While it was initially thought that increased myocardial stretch optimized the overlap of contractile actin and myosin

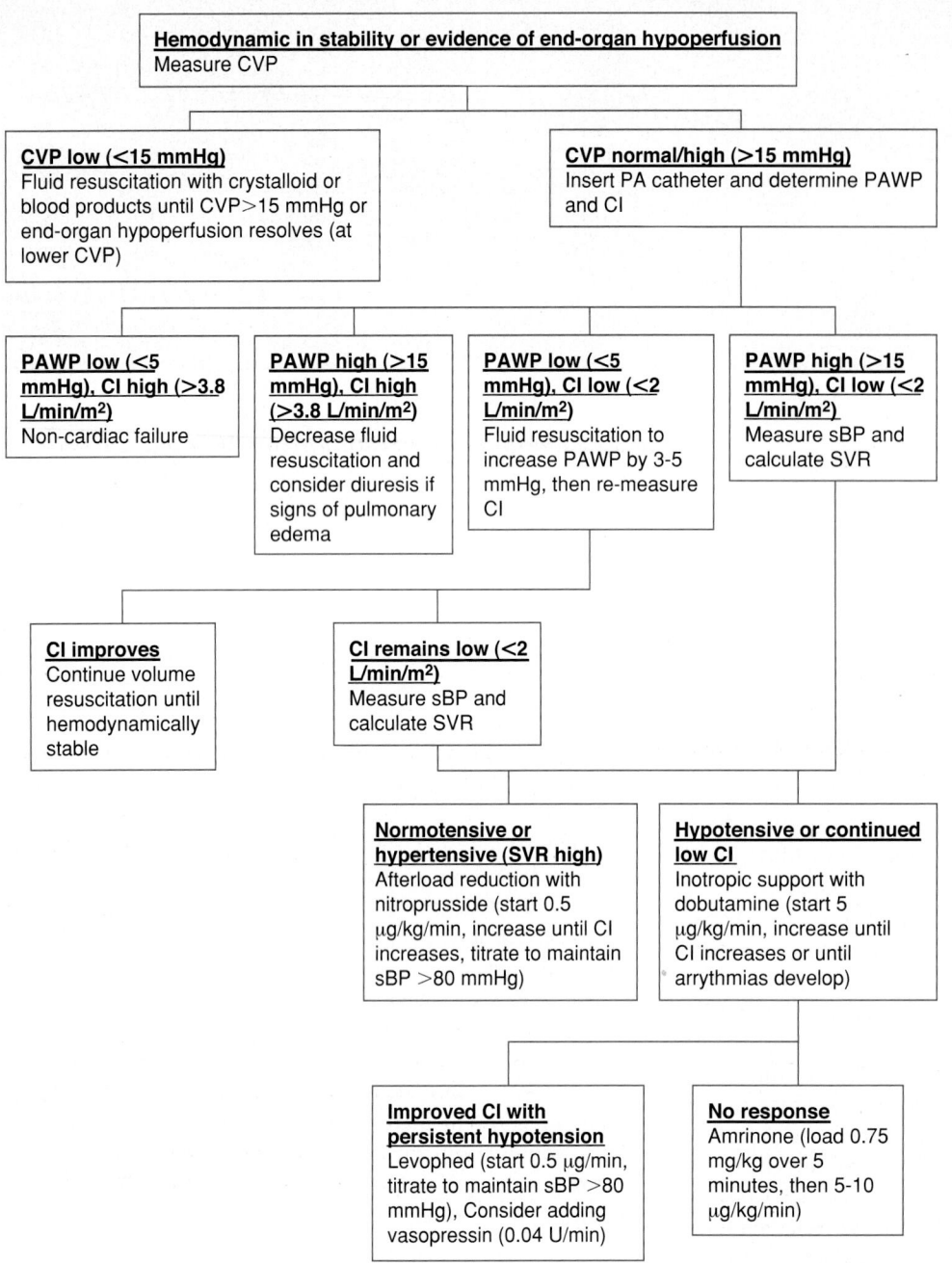

**FIGURE 62-1.** Clinical decision tree for the diagnosis and management of cardiovascular failure.

leading to increased force of contraction, more recent research indicates that contractile force is also dependent on sensitivity of the myocyte to ionized calcium gradients, as determined by sarcomere length.[1]

The Frank–Starling relationship provides a paradigm by which the cardiovascular system and its derangements can be approached. Hypovolemia, or decreased preload, is the result of hemorrhage or contraction of the intravascular space due to internal or external fluid losses. Additionally, venous return to the heart depends on the vascular tone of the venous system. As will be discussed in the pharmacology portion of this chapter, changes in venous capacitance are often unwanted side effects of pharmacologic agents used in treating the injured patient.

Taken together, intravascular volume and venous return determine left ventricular end-diastolic volume (LVEDV), which determines the force of ventricular contraction. The Swan–Ganz catheter is used to measure the pulmonary arterial wedge pressure (PAWP), which approximates left ventricular end-diastolic pressure (LVEDP). Assuming unaltered ventricular compliance, LVEDP theoretically approximates the LVEDV. Unfortunately, in the setting of critically ill trauma patients, factors such as myocardial ischemia, heart failure, myocardial edema, endotoxemia, cardiac hypertrophy, and circulating tumor necrosis factor (TNF) can decrease ventricular compliance, rendering measurement of PAWP as a surrogate for LVEDV unreliable. In these situations, normal or elevated PAWP may not eliminate inadequate preload as a cause of low cardiac output.

Besides changes in venous capacitance, venous return to the heart can be compromised by increased intrathoracic or intra-abdominal pressure, as seen in abdominal compartment syndrome and pregnancy (see Chap. 41). This is most evident with tension pneumothorax, when the shock state is immediately reversed by decompression of the pleural space. Additionally, in the mechanically ventilated patient, the use of positive-pressure ventilation coupled with positive end-expiratory pressure (PEEP) may impair venous return to the heart (see Chap. 63). In this patient population, when intravascular volume is low, the adverse effects of increased intrathoracic pressure on preload predominate and cardiac output is diminished. Importantly, when an under-resuscitated patient is placed on positive-pressure ventilation, this situation may lead to cardiovascular collapse. However, in the reverse scenario, patients with normal to high intravascular volume may benefit from the afterload-reducing effects of elevated intrathoracic pressure seen with positive-pressure ventilation. Indeed, synchronization of positive-pressure ventilation with the cardiac cycle has been described as a method of afterload reduction and cardiac output augmentation.[2] It should be noted that patients in cardiogenic shock could demonstrate sudden cardiovascular collapse upon removal of ventilatory support. It is important to note that the net result of these physiologic changes may be hard to predict in clinical practice, but a thorough knowledge of the underlying physiology is the key to prompt diagnosis and management.

## Afterload

Cardiovascular failure due to a reduction in afterload is referred to as distributive shock, and has multiple etiologies: septic shock, neurogenic shock, and anaphylactic shock. Afterload is the force that opposes ventricular contraction. Similar to preload, the concept of afterload is derived from in vitro experiments using strips of cardiac muscle. In these experiments, length is held constant while the muscle is given a variable load that must be moved (afterload). These studies have established that increasing afterload decreases the speed and force of contraction. Clinically, vascular input impedance appears to be the best in vivo correlate of ventricular afterload. Unfortunately, vascular input impedance is not a readily assessed clinical quantity, and therefore the clinician must rely on systemic vascular resistance (SVR) as a surrogate. SVR is calculated using the hemodynamic equivalent of Ohm's law:

$$SVR = (MAP - CVP) / CO$$

In this equation, MAP is the mean arterial blood pressure, CVP is the central venous pressure, and CO is the cardiac output. This equation provides an approximation of vascular impedance with the assumption of nonpulsatile flow. Therefore, it is important to realize that the clinical practice of "measuring" afterload or SVR with data from the Swan–Ganz catheter actually provides a calculated value. Finally, because SVR is inversely proportional to cardiac output, rather than directly treating an abnormally high SVR, one should first treat the low cardiac output with fluid administration to maximize preload, which will serve to increase CO and decrease SVR.

## Contractility

Contractility, also known as inotropic state, is the force with which the myocardium contracts. The inotropic state of the myocardium, and the stroke work performed, can be visualized by the construction of a left ventricular pressure-volume loop (Fig. 62-2). This loop is bounded by the four phases of the cardiac cycle: isovolemic relax-

ation, diastolic filling, isovolemic contraction, and systolic ejection. Stroke work is defined as the area bounded by this loop.

Instantaneous pressure-volume curves also provide a method to determine both external (stroke work) and internal (loss as heat) work performed by the heart during the cardiac cycle. As described above, the area bounded by the pressure-volume loop defines the external, or stroke work performed by the myocardium. The internal work is defined as the area of the triangle determined graphically by three lines: an extrapolation of the elastance line to the x-intercept, the isovolemic relaxation portion of the pressure-volume loop, and the diastolic filling portion of the pressure-volume loop (Fig. 62-3). Under this system, the failing heart with low contractility will demonstrate a shallow elastance line which translates to low efficiency (more internal work performed for the same external work). Clinically, this points toward manipulation of contractility to balance myocardial oxygen demand and delivery. Finally, the strong influence of changes in afterload are readily appreciated under this model, as increasing afterload at a given stroke volume results in increased external work performed by the heart.

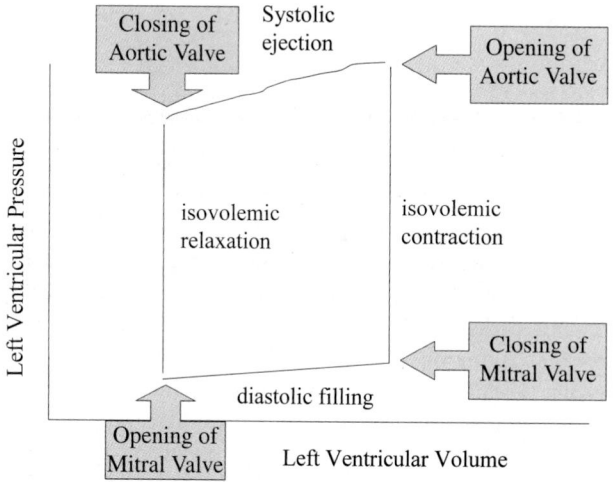

**FIGURE 62-2.** The relationship between left ventricular pressure and left ventricular volume during a stylized cardiac cycle.

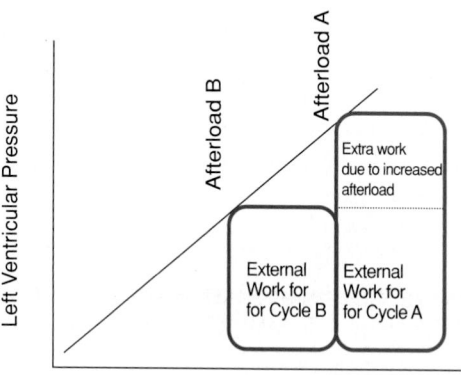

**FIGURE 62-3.** The effect of changes in afterload on (external) ventricular stroke work at constant stroke volume. The areas inscribed by the heavy lines represent the external stroke work performed during two representative cardiac cycles. Decreasing afterload (from A to B) decreases stroke work.

Presently, the use of pressure-volume curves in patient care is limited to centers using newer generation pulmonary artery catheters that measure ventricular volume as well as pressure.[3] More commonly, clinicians rely on Frank–Starling curves to determine myocardial performance and estimate contractility. Finally, contractility can be estimated by angiographic or echocardiographic determination of ventricular ejection fraction, but this method is highly sensitive to changes in afterload, and may be less reliable.

## Heart Rate

Heart rate is a key determinant of cardiac output. In the setting of constant stroke volume, increasing the number of cardiac ejections per unit time results in increased cardiac output. In addition, increasing the heart rate increases contractility, a phenomenon known as the Bowditch effect. However, in the setting of myocardial failure, it is not uncommon to observe heart rates high enough that ventricular filling is compromised, resulting in decreased cardiac output. Rapid ventricular rates that impair cardiac filling are most commonly seen in patients with pre-existing or evolving myocardial ischemia. In this setting, rate control becomes paramount in ensuring matched oxygen delivery and utilization.

## MYOCARDIAL DYSFUNCTION

Myocardial dysfunction can be defined on the basis of perturbed preload, afterload, contractility, or heart rate. Systemic hypovolemia (e.g., inadequate preload), secondary to hemorrhage or third space losses, is the most common etiology in the postsurgical or trauma patient. Other causes of decreased cardiac output may arise from failing or decreased contractile function of the heart. Evolving ischemia can lead to areas of heart muscle that lose their ability to contract, leading to decreased cardiac output. The contractility of heart muscle can also become altered following any insult that results in intrinsic metabolic derangements at the cellular level. This typically occurs in the settings of sepsis, postcardiac arrest, or postcardiopulmonary bypass. Direct physical injury to the myocardium, as occurs following blunt chest injury, may produce contused cardiac muscle, which can lead to contractile dysfunction and decreased cardiac output.

The optimal modalities to diagnose myocardial dysfunction in critically ill patients are poorly established. In this chapter we discuss the evaluation of cardiac function, focusing on measurement of central venous pressure (CVP), the use of pulmonary artery (Swan-Ganz) catheters, echocardiography, and noninvasive techniques (see Chap. 13).

## MANAGEMENT OF MYOCARDIAL DYSFUNCTION

### Preload Augmentation and Rewarming

Myocardial dysfunction secondary to hypovolemia may be caused by hemorrhage or other causes of intravascular volume loss. Prior to the development of hypotension, most adult patients will demonstrate a decrease in urine output, indicative of end-organ hypoperfusion. Augmentation of preload, or restoration of intravascular volume, will reverse this dysfunction if instituted promptly. Depending on the degree of volume loss, most patients respond to simple crystalloid solutions. However, if severe or ongoing hemorrhage is present, and the patient is not responding to crystalloid administration, transfusion of blood products may be necessary. Normalization of heart rate and blood pressure, along with adequate urine output are simple and effective measurements of adequate volume restoration.

During the period of volume replacement, attention must be given to the temperature status of the patient (see Chap. 51). Multiple studies have clearly demonstrated that hypothermia induces a significant depression of both systolic and diastolic left ventricular function.[4] The use of warmed fluids during resuscitation results in rapid restoration of left ventricular diastolic function, while recovery of systolic function is prolonged.[5] This is likely due to long-lasting effects of hypothermia on the excitation–contraction coupling of the actin–myosin complex.

## Pharmacologic

A multitude of pharmacologic agents are available for the management of myocardial dysfunction. Selection of the appropriate agent (or agents) should be tailored to the specific clinical situation. Broadly, the agents can be classified into those that act directly on the vascular system (vasodilatation or constriction) and those that augment cardiac contractility. Selected agents have multiple mechanisms of action (Table 62-1).

### Dopamine

Dopamine is a naturally occurring catecholamine that has several cardiovascular effects, including increased heart rate, increased contractility, and peripheral vasoconstriction. It is used primarily for inotropic support in order to maintain brain, heart, and kidney perfusion. Dopamine acts on $\alpha$- and $\beta$-adrenoreceptors as well as DA1 and DA2 dopamine receptors, and its actions can be classified based on dose. At moderate doses (3–5 $\mu$g/kg/minute), dopamine stimulates primarily cardiac $\beta$-adrenoreceptors, increasing contractility and thus cardiac output.

It has long been thought that low dose dopamine (1–3 $\mu$g/kg/minute), also referred to as "renal-dose" dopamine, increases renal blood flow and maintains diuresis via the DA1 and DA2 receptors.[6] Recent investigation has revealed that individual variation in the pharmacokinetics of dopamine typically results in poor correlation between blood levels and administered dose. Low-dose dopamine acts as a proximal tubule diuretic by increasing sodium delivery to tubular cells, increasing their oxygen demands, and causing naturesis. Finally, two meta-analyses and a large prospective, double-blinded randomized controlled trial have failed to demonstrate that dopamine protects the kidney in critically ill patients with acute renal failure.[7–9] For these reasons, there is insufficient evidence to support the use of low-dose dopamine to maintain renal perfusion in an effort to reduce the incidence of acute renal failure (see Chap. 65).

At higher doses of dopamine (10 $\mu$g/kg/minute), peripheral vasoconstrictive effects from stimulation of $\alpha$-adrenergic receptors predominate. This can result in significant coronary vasoconstriction resulting in angina, vasospasm, and increased PAWP.[10] Additionally,

**TABLE 62-1**

**Dosage, Mechanism, and Actions of Pharmacologic Agents Commonly used in the Treatment of Cardiovascular Failure**

| AGENT | TYPICAL DOSAGE | HR | MAP | CO | SVR | $\alpha_1$ | $\beta_1$ | $\beta_2$ | DA1 | DA2 |
|---|---|---|---|---|---|---|---|---|---|---|
| Catecholamines: | | | | | | | | | | |
| Dopamine | 3–5 mcg/kg/min | + | + | ++ | | | ++ | | + | + |
| | 10–20 mcg/kg/min | ++ | ++ | + | +++ | ++ | + | | + | + |
| Dobutamine | 2–20 mcg/kg/min | + | +/− | ++ | − | | ++ | + | | |
| Epinephrine | 0.5–2 mcg/min | ++ | + | + | − | | ++ | ++ | | |
| | 2–10 mcg/min | ++ | ++ | + | ++ | ++ | ++ | + | | |
| Norepinephrine | 0.5–30 mcg/min | + | ++ | + | ++ | ++ | + | | | |
| Vasopressin | 0.01–0.04 U/min | − | ++ | | ++ | | | | | |
| Phosphodiesterase Inhibitors: | | | | | | | | | | |
| Amrinone | 5–10 | | | ++ | − | | | | | |
| Milrinone | 0.3–1.5 | | | +++ | − | | | | | |
| Nitrovasodilators: | | | | | | | | | | |
| Sodium Nitroprusside | 0.1–5 mcg/kg/min | | | + | − | | | | | |
| Nitroglycerin | 10–20 mcg/min | − | | + | − | | | | | |

increasing afterload from vasoconstriction coupled with an increased heart rate seen at this dose, results in increased myocardial oxygen consumption and demand.

Tachycardia can occur with any dose of dopamine, particularly in the hypovolemic patient. When excessive, the increased heart rate will increase myocardial oxygen demand and worsen cardiovascular failure. Due to the variable effects of dopamine, the dosage ranges used to define which receptors it affects are to be used as broad guidelines only, with the awareness that "low-dose" (1–3 μg/kg/minute) dopamine may have the unwanted effects of "medium-" (3–5 μg/kg/minute) or "high-dose" (>10 μg/kg/minute) dopamine on an individual patient.

## Dobutamine

Dobutamine is a synthetic catecholamine with primarily β-adrenegic effects, although it does possess some $\alpha_1$-adrenergic properties. It is primarily an inotrope, increasing contractility, while exerting minimal effects on heart rate. Dobutamine also possesses mild β2-adrenoreceptor activity, producing peripheral vasodilatation. This combination of increased contractility and reduced afterload result in improved left ventricular function. Importantly, the increase in cardiac output occurs without an increase in myocardial oxygen consumption.[11] Because of the vasodilatory effects, dobutamine may reduce blood pressure and is ideally suited for use in low-output cardiac states. For these reasons, dobutamine should be considered the first-choice inotrope for patients with low cardiac output in the presence of adequate preload.[12] However, two large prospective trials in critically ill patients failed to demonstrate a benefit to raising oxygen delivery to supra-normal levels with the use of dobutamine,[13,14] likely due to an inability of the peripheral tissues to utilize the additional oxygen delivered.

## Epinephrine

Epinephrine is an endogenous catecholamine with α- and β-adrenergic activity. At low doses, epinephrine exerts primarily β-adrenergic effects, increasing contractility and reducing systemic vascular resistance. Despite this, there is little evidence that epinephrine is superior to dobutamine in the treatment of low-output states (e.g., myocardial infarction). The increases in stroke volume and cardiac output seen with epinephrine have the potential of decreasing blood pressure in patients with inadequate preload. In patients with septic shock that have been adequately fluid resuscitated, epinephrine increases heart rate and stroke volume (and therefore cardiac output) and systemic oxygen delivery without altering vascular tone.[15] At higher rates of infusion, epinephrine exerts primarily α-adrenergic effects, increasing systemic vascular resistance and blood pressure. It is indicated for patients with ventricular dysfunction refractory to dopamine or dobutamine.

Care must be taken when using epinephrine, as renal vasoconstriction, cardiac arrythmias, and increased myocardial oxygen consumption and demand may result. Additionally, metabolic abnormalities are common, including dyskalemias, hyperglycemia, and ketoacidosis. Finally, epinephrine increases blood lactate levels in patients recovering from cardiopulmonary bypass or those with septic shock, likely through increases in tissue oxygen extraction in the absence of adequate delivery.[16–18]

## Norepinephrine

Norepinephrine is an endogenous sympathetic neurotransmitter with α- and β-adrenergic effects. At high doses, α-adrenergic effects predominate and increased systemic vascular resistance and increased blood pressure result. Because of this potent vasoconstriction, norepinephrine is generally reserved for patients that are refractory to both volume resuscitation and other inotropic agents.[19,20] However, at low doses, the β-adrenergic actions of norepinephrine predominate, resulting in increased heart rate and contractility. Specifically, in the setting of right ventricular failure, low-dose norepinephrine improves cardiac function without adversely affecting visceral perfusion.[21] Additionally, norepinephrine is widely used in the care of the head-injured patient in shock because its vasoconstrictive effects do not extend to the cerebral vasculature, making it an ideal agent for maintaining cerebral perfusion pressure.[22]

## Amrinone and Milrinone

Amrinone and milrinone are synthetic bipyridines that belong to the phosphodiesterase inhibitor class, demonstrating both positive inotropic and vasodilatory actions. While these agents inhibit phosphodiesterase III, leading to increased intracellular cAMP, their positive inotropic effects are likely related to downstream increases in intracellular calcium.[23]

These unique cardiac drugs have the theoretical advantage of dual mechanisms of action-augmenting cardiac output while reducing cardiac work by positive inotropic actions and peripheral vasodilatation.[23] Both have demonstrated clinical utility in multiple low cardiac output states, however, as single-agent therapy, neither has been proven superior to single inotropes (e.g., dobutamine) in improving ventricular performance. Additionally, the longer half-lives of amrinone and milrinone as compared to that of dobutamine do not permit minute-to-minute titration of their cardiovascular effects.

In selected situations, an additive effect in myocardial function is observed when dobutamine and amrinone/milrinone are combined. The phosphodiesterase inhibitors may be used as single-agent therapy in patients with isolated systolic heart failure but are more commonly employed as secondary agents (in addition to dobutamine) in cases of refractory heart failure. In this scenario, the beneficial effects on cardiac output are additive as amrinone and milrinone do not act via the adrenergic receptors. The potent vasodilatory effect of the bypyridines requires careful attention from the clinician to avoid hypotension in hypovolemic patients.

## Vasopressin

Arginine vasopressin, or vasopressin, is a potent vasoconstrictor. This natural hormone produced by the posterior pituitary has gained widespread acceptance as a treatment for septic shock refractory to volume resuscitation and conventional pressor agents. During septic shock, the supply of endogenous vasopressin is quickly depleted, and restoration of this deficiency has shown benefits in the weaning of norepinephrine and other pressor agents and also imparts a short-term survival benefit in this group of patients. When vasopressin is combined with norepinephrine, outcomes in the treatment of catecholamine resistant cardiovascular failure in septic shock are superior to therapy with norepinephrine alone.[24]

Vasopressin has also emerged as a therapy for cardiac arrest and acute resuscitation.[25] Current guidelines for cardiopulmonary resuscitation recommend vasopressin as an alternative to epinephrine for shock resistant ventricular fibrillation. Vasopressin is a superior agent to epinephrine in asystolic patients but is similar to epinephrine alone in the treatment of ventricular fibrillation and pulseless electrical activity.[26] In the postoperative cardiotomy patient, vasopressin significantly reduces heart rate and the need for both pressor and inotropic support, with no adverse effect on the heart. A significant reduction in cardiac enzymes and cardioversion of arrythmias into sinus rhythm has also been demonstrated with the use of vasopressin in these patients.[27] Patients undergoing cardiopulmonary bypass often experience hemodynamic disturbances similar to those seen in septic patients, with characteristics of peripheral vasodilatation causing hypotension, and diminished response to conventional pressor agents. Vasopressin has been shown to correct vasodilatory shock following cardiopulmonary bypass regardless of normal circulating vasopressin levels.[28]

## Nitrovasodilators

The nitrovasodilators are useful agents for reducing vascular tone, allowing manipulation of both preload and afterload. The most common scenario for their use is in states of elevated systemic vascular resistance. Sodium nitroprusside acts primarily on arteriolar smooth muscle, reducing afterload. The onset of action of sodium nitroprusside is rapid, and its effects cease within minutes once the infusion is discontinued. When titrating the dose of sodium nitroprusside, systemic vascular resistance should be decreased with a concomitant increase in cardiac output, thereby maintaining a relatively constant systemic arterial pressure. While the effects of sodium nitroprusside favor arterial dilatation, it does have mild venous dilatory effects that can lead to an increase in venous capacitance and decreased preload.

Care must be taken when using sodium nitroprusside, as cyanide toxicity is a known side effect. Briefly, the ferrous iron contained in sodium nitroprusside reacts with sulfhydryl-containing compounds in erythrocytes, producing cyanide. Toxicity results when the rate of production exceeds the capacity of the liver to metabolize cyanide to thiocyanate. This is generally seen with infusion rates in excess of 10 μg/kg/minute or with prolonged therapy (several days). Toxicity manifests as an unexplained rise in mixed venous oxygen tension as a result of reduced oxygen consumption. Treatment is with sodium nitrite and is aimed at providing an alternate substrate for the cyanide ion. Sodium nitrite also converts hemoglobin to methemoglobin, producing a ferric ion that competes with the ferric ion in the cytochrome system for the cyanide ion. Methylene blue can be administered to treat the methemoglobinemia that results from sodium nitrite treatment.

Nitroglycerin, a potent arteriolar and venous smooth muscle dilator, is a useful agent when both preload and afterload are elevated. The cardiovascular effects are dose-dependent, with low doses (5–20 μg/minute) primarily increasing venous capacitance and higher doses (>20 μg/minute) relaxing arterial tone. Side effects are generally the result of an overly rapid reduction in venous or arterial tone, and are readily reversed by cessation of the medication.

Phosphodiesterase type 5 inhibitors, such as sildenafil, have been used with success to treat primary pulmonary hypertension[29]; however their use in pulmonary hypertension secondary to ARDS or in the acute setting has not been studied adequately to draw conclusions on its benefit in this setting. Further studies in this specific subset of patients with secondary or acute pulmonary hypertension are warranted.

## Steroids

The use of steroids as replacement therapy for insufficient adrenal production and release of corticosteroids has been proven to be a life-saving intervention. Their role in septic shock, however, is less clear. The use of steroids in cardiovascular collapse secondary to sepsis has gained renewed interest, with new data suggesting that in adrenal-insufficient patients, low dose glucocorticoid replacement therapy is beneficial.[30] However, no survival benefit is seen in patients who are not adrenal-insufficient given the same therapy.

In addition to their use as a replacement therapy, steroids are known anti-inflammatory agents. Cardiopulmonary bypass produces a brisk inflammatory response, including the production oxygen free radicals, resulting in hypotension and arrythmias. The use of steroids to temper the production of free radicals in post-bypass patients has been studied. In a prospective, randomized trial there was no improvement in the incidence of cardiac arrythmias.[31] Therefore, the use of steroids in the treatment of cardiovascular failure secondary to sepsis in nonadrenal insufficient patients, or as an anti-inflammatory agent in cardiopulmonary bypass patients cannot be recommended.

## Intra-aortic Balloon Pump Counterpulsation

When myocardial failure has an underlying, surgically correctable, anatomic cause (e.g., acute mitral regurgitation, intraventricular septal defect, high-grade coronary artery stenosis) and pharmacologic methods have been ineffective in augmenting cardiac output, the use of intra-aortic balloon counterpulsation (IABP) is indicated. IABP involves placement of a balloon catheter into the proximal descending aorta (distal to the origin of the left subclavian artery) via a femoral arterial approach. The balloon catheter is connected to a pumping device that, in synchrony with the electrocardiogram, inflates the balloon during cardiac diastole and deflates it during systole. By filling during diastole, the balloon displaces ~40 cc of blood retrograde into the coronary arterial circulation and antegrade into the descending aorta. The balloon is abruptly deflated at the beginning of systole, allowing the left ventricle to eject its stroke volume. These dual functions augment coronary arterial flow while decreasing afterload, thereby reducing myocardial oxygen consumption. While IABP technology has improved and the risk of complications in cardiac surgical patients has decreased dramatically over the last decade,[32] the utility of balloon counterpulsation in trauma patients remains unclear. One study demonstrated improved left ventricular function in dogs sustaining blunt cardiac injury,[33] but studies in humans have been limited to case reports. Clinical evaluation of IABP in penetrating trauma is even more limited.[34] This device should be reserved as a method of last resort in treating myocardial failure.

# EVALUATION OF CARDIAC FUNCTION

## Central Venous Pressure (CVP)

Central venous pressure monitoring has been used for over four decades as a measurement of preload. In the young trauma patient with a normal functioning heart, the CVP monitor provides an adequate assessment of right-sided filling pressure or preload. Usually placed percutaneously into the superior vena cava, adequate assessment of volume status is achieved, and fluid resuscitation guided. Normal CVP is between 0 and 4 mm Hg; however, response to fluid is more useful than an absolute number. A low CVP usually indicates hypovolemia whereas an elevated CVP may be evidence of volume overload. Increases or decreases in cardiac output/index may be further used in conjunction with CVP to assess volume status as evidenced by the Frank–Starling curve. CVP and PAWP correlate well in the normal functioning heart (EF >50%), but this correlation is not maintained in patients with cardiac impairment (EF <40%).[35] Central venous pressure measurement has its limitations and is affected by multiple variables, which may cause an inadequate assessment of true volume status. Misplacement of the catheter, congestive heart failure (right- or left-sided), pneumothorax, venomotor tone, pulmonary embolus, cardiac tamponade, increased intrathoracic and or intra-abdominal pressure may all lead to increases in CVP not reflecting true overall volume status.

## Pulmonary Artery Catheters (PAC)

Pulmonary artery catheters or Swan-Ganz catheters, first introduced for human use in 1970, have been widely accepted as the standard for invasive monitoring of not only volume status but also of cardiac function by measurement and approximation of left-sided cardiac pressures. Continuous monitoring of cardiac output/index along with other information provided by newer PACs may help identify cardiovascular failure early and allow treatment to be adjusted accordingly. Measurement of the PAWP is used as an indirect measurement of LVEDP and LVEDV; however, these measurements often show poor correlation.[36] Commercially available PACs currently incorporate multiple calculations to derive other indices of cardiac function and tissue perfusion such as mixed venous oxygen saturation ($S_vO_2$), systemic vascular resistance, oxygen delivery ($DO_2$), and consumption ($VO_2$).[37]

## Echocardiography

Echocardiography, trans-thoracic and trans-esophageal, has gained wide acceptance in the monitoring of cardiac function and has emerged as an effective tool in the intensive care unit (ICU) as a guide to resuscitation and fluid status. In addition, information about structural abnormalities of the heart, aorta, and main pulmonary arteries can be obtained by this method, along with assessment of ventricular dysfunction, ventricular filling, valvular abnormalities, ventricular hypertrophy, and pulmonary embolus. Trans-esophageal echocardiography can give accurate measurements of both right- and left-sided filling volumes of the heart and may provide a better assessment of myocardial preload when compared to CVP or PA catheter measurements.[38] Placed in the esophagus, Doppler probes can accurately predict cardiac output using the diameter of the aorta and measurements of blood flow velocity. These devices can provide invaluable information in the multiply injured patient with comorbidities that make readings from the PAC difficult to interpret.

## Mixed Venous Oxygen Saturation ($S_vO_2$)

Mixed venous oxygen saturation ($S_vO_2$) is a measurement of the oxygen saturation in the venous return to the heart and therefore an indirect measurement of oxygen utilization by the end organs. Normal values are approximately 75–80% and are calculated by taking the difference between measured oxygen delivery and oxygen consumption. During the septic state, the cell's inability to utilize delivered oxygen may increase $S_vO_2$. Cellular destruction from prolonged ischemia or cellular metabolic poisoning following carbon monoxide inhalation often yield normal or increased $S_vO_2$ despite inadequate end-organ perfusion because of an inability to utilize the oxygen delivered.

## Lactate and Base Deficit

Elevated serum lactate, or lactic acidosis, may be an indicator of cellular hypoxia or shock. When cells can no longer function normally due to hypoxia or decreased blood flow, the normal mechanism of ATP generation by aerobic metabolism is shifted to anaerobic metabolism. This inefficient method of ATP production yields increased amounts of pyruvate, which is converted to lactate. Therefore, increased levels of lactate may be a reflection of ongoing tissue hypoxia. Hepatic dysfunction may increase serum lactate levels due to inability of the liver to transform lactate to carbon dioxide. The use of serum lactate measurements as a guide to resuscitation is limited due to the time necessary for lab results to return. However, in critically ill patients past the acute resuscitation phase of treatment, serum lactate levels may be useful in determining the onset of organ dysfunction.[39] In clinical practice, multiple other factors may also affect lactate production. Following severe injury, increased circulating epinephrine may cause an increase in lactate production by anaerobic glycolysis in response to increased activity of the $Na^+/K^+$-ATPase despite adequate tissue perfusion.[40]

The base deficit is the difference between the standard value of 24 mEq/L and the serum bicarbonate level. This value is typically negative in hemorrhagic shock and therefore the term base deficit is widely used. The magnitude of the base deficit has been used to quantify the magnitude of acidosis, with mild acidosis having a base deficit of $-2$ to $-5$ mEq/L, moderate acidosis $-5$ to $-15$ mEq/L, and severe acidosis less than $-15$ mEq/L. As the magnitude of the base deficit increases, the resuscitation volumes of both blood and fluid increases, as does mortality.[41] Patients that are able to clear their base deficits in less than 48 hours have decreased mortality when compared to patients whose base deficits persist beyond this time frame.[42] Persistent base deficits despite normal vital signs may be a signal of compensated shock requiring further resuscitation, and if left untreated may lead to multisystem organ failure and increased morbidity and mortality. New onset lactic acidosis and increasing base deficit in the critically ill patient may be early signs of a low flow state, cellular hypoxia, and/or end-organ injury, therefore every effort should be made to find the cause and address it as quickly as possible.

## Capnography

Defined as the measurement of carbon dioxide, capnography is most commonly used during endotracheal intubation to insure proper placement of the endotracheal tube. Recent studies have reported its use to predict prognosis following cardiopulmonary arrest, to assess resuscitation efforts, to detect alveolar dead space changes, and to monitor sedation and paralytic therapy.[43,44] Under normal conditions, exhaled carbon dioxide closely correlates with arterial blood $CO_2$ levels. Due to unmatched areas of ventilation and perfusion in the lungs, the arterial $PaCO_2$ will usually be slightly higher than the exhaled $CO_2$.

End-tidal $CO_2$ has been shown to predict resuscitation efforts during cardiopulmonary arrest.[43] In one study higher ET-$CO_2$ levels correlated with increased survival after cardiac arrest.[45] Nonsurvivors with prehospital arrests after 20 minutes of ACLS, were found to have an average ET-$CO_2$ of 3.9 mm Hg while survivors had ET-$CO_2$ values of 31 mm Hg.[46] An ET-$CO_2$ value of 10 mm Hg has been determined to provide a 100% sensitivity to predict return of spontaneous circulation.[47]

Studies have shown that sublingual $CO_2$ (SL$CO_2$) is a reliable marker of tissue perfusion, with impaired circulatory blood flow correlating with high levels of SL$CO_2$.[48] In a prospective observational cohort study, SL$CO_2$ correlated with blood loss in penetrating trauma patients.[49] While gastric tonometry and measurement of submucosal pH has its merits in determining ongoing tissue hypoxia in the ICU setting, it has not gained wide use in the initial assessment of patients due to the need for serum $HCO_3$ measurement with each tonometric reading.

## MANAGEMENT OF RIGHT AND LEFT HEART AIR EMBOLUS

Air embolism most commonly occurs as a consequence of iatrogenic introduction of air into the right heart during central venous access procedures. The ensuing right heart failure leads to hypotension and death if not diagnosed and treated promptly. Patients with right heart air embolism should be placed on 100% oxygen, positioned head down (Trendelenburg), and in a left lateral decubitus position to prevent migration of the air into the pulmonary circulation. Attempts should then be made to aspirate the air using a central line advanced into the right atrium. Echocardiography is very useful in these instances, to both identify the air embolus in the right ventricle and also to guide positioning of the catheter for aspiration.

Left-sided air embolism or systemic air embolism is seen following penetrating chest and lung injuries (see Chaps.15 and 26). Left-sided air embolism can occur with a smaller volume of air than that needed to produce a right-sided air embolism. Air gains access to the left heart and the systemic circulation via communication between the alveoli and the pulmonary veins of the injured lung. This process is often accelerated with the institution of endotracheal intubation and positive pressure ventilation. Cross clamping the hilum of the injured lung to prevent further air access may be a life-saving maneuver. If air progresses to the coronary circulation, sudden cardiac collapse ensues. If air reaches the cerebral circulation, a new neurologic deficit will manifest.[50] In patients who survive the initial insult of a left-sided air embolism, hyperbaric oxygen therapy has shown some benefit in reversing neurologic deficits.[51]

## MYOCARDIAL PROTECTION

Patients at high risk for cardiac events during noncardiac surgery have been the topic of discussion for years due to the increased mortality from perioperative arrythmias and myocardial infarction. Myocardial infarction or cardiac death occurs in 1–5% of unselected patients undergoing noncardiac surgery and is the most common reason for preoperative evaluation.[52] The pathophysiology of myocardial infarction in the perioperative setting differs from that seen in nonsurgical patients. In the nonsurgical setting, myocardial infarction usually follows rupture of atherosclerotic plaques in the coronary arteries leading to platelet aggregation and thrombus formation.[53] Myocardial infarction in the perioperative setting is due to plaque rupture approximately 50% of the time, with the remainder resulting from myocardial ischemia from decreased myocardial oxygen supply and increased demand in the face of atherosclerotic coronary artery disease. These demands are usually exacerbated by anemia, hypotension, hypoxia, hypertension, and tachycardia. Shifts in intravascular volume, withdrawal of anesthesia, and postoperative pain are all factors that may contribute to the increased demand of oxygen in the perioperative setting. Postoperative tachycardia, arrhythmias, and myocardial infarction most commonly occur three days after an operation, when fluid shifts are at their greatest.[54] Until recently, reduction in the occurrence of these events centered on preoperative risk assessment with clinical recommendations and often cancellation or postponement of procedures.[55] Medical strategies have been proposed to reduce perioperative ischemia, as this has been linked to postoperative myocardial infarction with a 21-fold increase in risk.[56] Mixed results have been obtained in studies using intraoperative calcium channel blockers[57] and nitroglycerin.[58] Two randomized controlled trials have shown that β-blocker therapy reduces perioperative cardiac complications.[59,60] Mangano and colleagues performed a randomized, double-blinded, placebo-controlled trial using atenolol in 200 patients with known coronary artery disease and/or risk factors for atherosclerosis who underwent noncardiac surgery. While acute perioperative mortality did not differ between the two groups at six months, eight deaths occurred in the placebo group and none in the atenolol group ($p < 0.001$), with the difference being sustained at the two-year follow-up period. In another study, patients with clinical risk factors and ischemia demonstrated by dobutamine stress echo who were to undergo major vascular procedures were randomly assigned to bisoprolol or placebo.[60] The study was terminated early when investigators noted that bisoprolol markedly reduced perioperative mortality (17% vs. 3.4%; $p = 0.02$) and myocardial infarction (17% vs. 0%; $p < 0.001$). A recent meta-analysis of randomized, controlled trials concluded that β-blockade may be beneficial in preventing perioperative cardiac morbidity despite the heterogeneity of the trials.[61] Therefore, it seems that β-blockade reduces the risk of perioperative morbidity and mortality in patients at increased risk and is effective in patients with inducible ischemia by dobutamine stress echo.[62]

## CURRENT TREATMENT OF ACUTE MYOCARDIAL INFARCTION

The definition of acute myocardial infarction (MI) encompasses a range of clinical entities ranging from non-ST-segment elevation MI (also known as acute coronary syndromes [ACS] or unstable angina) to acute ST-segment elevation MI. The pathophysiology for ACS differs from that of ST segment elevation MI, as does the treatment. Whereas ACS are commonly due to a partial occlusion of the coronary arteries or transient ischemia (due to plaque rupture with platelet aggregation), in the surgical patient ACS is more commonly secondary to decreased oxygen supply or increased demand due to anemia, tachycardia, intravascular fluid shifts, hypotension, or arrhythmias. Acute ST segment elevation MI refers to complete occlusion of the coronary arteries with myocardial injury. The scope of this discussion centers on the treatment of acute ST segment elevation MI.

Despite marked advances in diagnosis and treatment, there is still a 10% mortality associated with acute MI.[63] Reduced mortality has been shown to result from adherence to three basic tenets of treatment for acute MI: (1) prompt diagnosis, (2) immediate aspirin therapy, and (3) rapid restitution of blood flow to the infarcted myocardium. Whereas prompt diagnosis and institution of aspirin therapy are relatively straight forward, the re-establishment of blood flow to the affected myocardium has evolved into two primary therapies, pharmacologic therapy with thrombolytics and interventional therapy with percutaneous angioplasty (PTCA). With its ease of administration, early studies on the use of thrombolytic therapy consistently showed decreased mortality and improved myocardial performance compared with placebo.[64] However, thrombolytic therapy has well documented limitations and contraindications. Intracranial bleeding resulting in death or stroke occurs in 0.6–1.4% of patients who receive thrombolytic therapy.[64] Thrombolytic therapy is also associated with a re-occlusion

rate of 30%, resulting in re-infarction of the affected area within three months.[65] In the multiply injured patient with an increased risk of bleeding, head injury, or multi-vessel disease, thrombolytic therapy is contraindicated.

Patients who are not candidates for thrombolytic therapy have been shown to benefit from PTCA.[66] This invasive therapy has been shown to result in better clinical outcomes when compared to thrombolysis.[67] In addition to improved outcomes, PTCA offers direct visualization of the affected anatomy, gives specific hemodynamic and functional data that can be used to guide further therapy. It can also quickly identify those patients who should not undergo reperfusion therapy, which include patients with minimal residual stenosis, spontaneous reperfusion, coronary vasospasm, myocarditis, and aortic dissection involving the ostia.[68] Unfortunately, PTCA is not available in all medical centers. Complications from PTCA include major bleeding (7%), vascular complications that require surgical repair (2%), and renal failure (13%). The incidence of renal failure rises with increasing age, volume of contrast material, decreased baseline renal function, and hypovolemia. When comparing thrombolytic therapy to PTCA, primary PTCA had been found to be more effective in reducing both short and long term outcomes, including death.[68] Recent trials of PTCA with or without stent placement show no difference in mortality but stented vessels had a decreased rate of re-stenosis and re-occlusion over six months. The use of platelet glycoprotein (GP) IIb/IIIa inhibitors (e.g., abciximab) at the time of PTCA reduces the rates of subacute thrombosis, recurrent ischemia, and need for repeat revascularization procedures during the first month after PTCA with or without stents.[69] However, clinical outcomes do not differ at six-month follow-up. Despite the heterogeneity of these trials, including whether stents were used or not and the use of platelet GP IIb/IIIa inhibitors versus the various thrombolytic agents, the accumulated data appears to favor primary PTCA in the treatment of acute ST segment MI.

## MANAGEMENT OF DIASTOLIC DYSFUNCTION

The syndrome of congestive heart failure (CHF) typically brings to mind an enlarged heart and decreased systolic function. However when systolic function is normal or near normal, as is the case in nearly 50% of patients diagnosed with CHF, and the other clinical manifestations of CHF exist, such as orthopnea, dyspnea, increased jugular venous pressure, and abnormal heart sounds on auscultation, the diagnosis of diastolic dysfunction or, more accurately, diastolic heart failure is made. Diastolic dysfunction (DD) should be described as CHF with increased resistance to diastolic filling. The causes of DD can be divided into myocardial, which include impaired relaxation or increased passive stiffness, endocardial, epicardial/pericardial, coronary microcirculation, and other. With hypertension being the primary predisposing factor for CHF, neurohormonal regulation has also been shown to play a role in CHF and DD. The renin-angiotensin system influences CHF indirectly by causing hypertension and left ventricular hypertrophy (LVH), and directly by both angiotensin II and endothelin contributing to LVH and impaired myocardial relaxation.[70,71] The diagnosis of DD is generally made clinically and is often one of exclusion. Objective testing should include echocardiography or cardiac catheterization. Because the normal ejection fraction is not a standardized number, and given that systolic dysfunction often accompanies DD, the diagnosis of diastolic dysfunction is often not clear-cut. Therefore, the diagnostic "gold standard" for diastolic dysfunction is cardiac catheterization demonstrating increased ventricular diastolic pressure with normal systolic function and volumes. Echocardiography, being noninvasive and practical, can be used to exclude systolic dysfunction. While the majority of clinical studies focus on systolic dysfunction, few exist which specifically target diastolic dysfunction.

Treatment of DD is geared toward modification of the primary pathophysiology. Volume overload can be reduced with diuretics or renal replacement therapy in renal failure patients. In DD, the use of β-adrenergic blockade or calcium channel blockade to reduce heart rate and increase left ventricular filling time reduces mortality.[72] Digoxin decreases hospitalization of patients with CHF with and without systolic dysfunction; however, since digoxin is a negative chronotrope the benefit may be due to the rate lowering effect of the drug rather than to its other properties.[73] Patients with rate-altering arrhythmias such as atrial flutter or fibrillation show increased filling times once normal sinus rhythm is restored and may also benefit from rate control. Blockade of the rennin–angiotensin system improves diastolic distensibility in both human and animal studies.[71] Aldosterone has also been shown to contribute to CHF with detrimental effects on endothelial function as well as inducing a vasculopathy.[74] Infusion of aldosterone into healthy volunteers for one-hour results in endothelial dysfunction with a notably reduced vascular response to acetylcholine. Patients with mild CHF treated with β-blocker therapy, ACE inhibitors, and statins show an improvement in acetylcholine-mediated endothelium-dependent vasodilatation.[75] Therefore, the general treatment principles for patients diagnosed with DD include reduction of volume overload, decreasing heart rate, antihypertensive therapy and reduction of ischemia.

# REFERENCES

1. McDonald KS, Field LJ, Parmacek MS, et al.: Length dependence of Ca2+ sensitivity of tension in mouse cardiac myocytes expressing skeletal troponin C. *J Physiol* 483:131, 1995.
2. Pinsky MR, Marquez J, Martin D, et al.: Ventricular assist by cardiac cycle-specific increases in intrathoracic pressure. *Chest* 91:709, 1987.
3. Chang MC, Mondy JS III, Meredith JW, et al.: Clinical application of ventricular end-systolic elastance and the ventricular pressure-volume diagram. *Shock* 7:413, 1997.
4. Fischer UM, Cox CS, Laine GA, et al.: Mild hypothermia impairs left ventricular diastolic but not systolic function. *J Invest Surg* 18:291, 2005.
5. Tveita T, Ytrehus K, Myhre ES, et al.: Left ventricular dysfunction following rewarming from experimental hypothermia. *J Appl Physiol* 85:2135, 1998.
6. McDonald RH Jr, Goldberg LI, McNay JL, et al.: Effect of dopamine in man: Augmentation of sodium excretion, glomerular filtration rate, and renal plasma flow. *J Clin Invest* 43:1116, 1964.
7. Bellomo R, Chapman M, Finfer S, et al.: Low-dose dopamine in patients with early renal dysfunction: A placebo-controlled randomised trial. Australian and New Zealand Intensive Care Society (ANZICS) Clinical Trials Group. *Lancet* 356:2139, 2000.
8. Kellum JA, Decker JM: Use of dopamine in acute renal failure: A meta-analysis. *Crit Care Med* 29:1526, 2001.
9. Marik PE: Low-dose dopamine: A systematic review. *Intensive Care Med* 28:877, 2002.
10. Crea F, Chierchia S, Kaski JC, et al.: Provocation of coronary spasm by dopamine in patients with active variant angina pectoris. *Circulation* 74:262, 1986.
11. Ko W, Zelano JA, Fahey AL, et al.: The effects of amrinone versus dobutamine on myocardial mechanics and energetics after hypothermic global ischemia. *J Thorac Cardiovasc Surg* 105:1015, 1993.
12. Dellinger RP, Carlet JM, Masur H, et al.: Surviving Sepsis Campaign guidelines for management of severe sepsis and septic shock. *Crit Care Med* 32:858, 2004.
13. Gattinoni L, Brazzi L, Pelosi P, et al.: A trial of goal-oriented hemodynamic therapy in critically ill patients. SvO2 Collaborative Group. *N Engl J Med* 333:1025, 1995.
14. Hayes MA, Timmins AC, Yau EH, et al.: Elevation of systemic oxygen delivery in the treatment of critically ill patients. *N Engl J Med* 330:1717, 1994.
15. Moran JL, O'Fathartaigh MS, Peisach AR, et al.: Epinephrine as an inotropic agent in septic shock: A dose-profile analysis. *Crit Care Med* 21:70, 1993.
16. Bourgoin A, Leone M, Delmas A, et al.: Increasing mean arterial pressure in patients with septic shock: effects on oxygen variables and renal function. *Crit Care Med* 33:780, 2005.
17. Meier A-Hellmann, Reinhart K, Bredle DL, et al.: Epinephrine impairs splanchnic perfusion in septic shock. *Crit Care Med* 25:399, 1997.
18. Totaro RJ, Raper RF: Epinephrine-induced lactic acidosis following cardiopulmonary bypass. *Crit Care Med* 25:1693, 1997.
19. Martin C, Papazian L, Perrin G, et al.: Norepinephrine or dopamine for the treatment of hyperdynamic septic shock? *Chest* 103:1826, 1993.
20. Levy B, Bollaert PE, Charpentier C, et al.: Comparison of norepinephrine and dobutamine to epinephrine for hemodynamics, lactate metabolism, and gastric tonometric variables in septic shock: A prospective, randomized study. *Intensive Care Med* 23:282, 1997.
21. Angle MR, Molloy DW, Penner B, et al.: The cardiopulmonary and renal hemodynamic effects of norepinephrine in canine pulmonary embolism. *Chest* 95:1333, 1989.
22. Steiner LA, Johnston AJ, Czosnyka M, et al.: Direct comparison of cerebrovascular effects of norepinephrine and dopamine in head-injured patients. *Crit Care Med* 32:1049, 2004.
23. Alousi AA, Johnson DC: Pharmacology of the bipyridines: amrinone and milrinone. *Circulation* 73:III10, 1986.
24. Dunser MW, Mayr AJ, Ulmer H, et al.: Arginine vasopressin in advanced vasodilatory shock: A prospective, randomized, controlled study. *Circulation* 107:2313, 2003.
25. Guidelines 2000 for Cardiopulmonary Resuscitation and Emergency Cardiovascular Care. Part 6: advanced cardiovascular life support: section 1: Introduction to ACLS 2000: overview of recommended changes in ACLS from the guidelines 2000 conference. The American Heart Association in collaboration with the International Liaison Committee on Resuscitation. *Circulation* 102:I86, 2000.
26. Wenzel V, Krismer AC, Arntz HR, et al.: A comparison of vasopressin and epinephrine for out-of-hospital cardiopulmonary resuscitation. *N Engl J Med* 350:105, 2004.
27. Dunser MW, Mayr AJ, Stallinger A, et al.: Cardiac performance during vasopressin infusion in postcardiotomy shock. *Intensive Care Med* 28:746, 2002.
28. Forrest P: Vasopressin and shock. *Anaesth Intensive Care* 29:463, 2001.
29. Sastry BK, Narasimhan C, Reddy NK, et al.: Clinical efficacy of sildenafil in primary pulmonary hypertension: A randomized, placebo-controlled, double-blind, crossover study. *J Am Coll Cardiol* 43:1149, 2004.
30. Annane D, Sebille V, Charpentier C, et al.: Effect of treatment with low doses of hydrocortisone and fludrocortisone on mortality in patients with septic shock. *Jama* 288:862, 2002.
31. Volk T, Schmutzler M, Engelhardt L, et al.: Effects of different steroid treatment on reperfusion-associated production of reactive oxygen species and arrhythmias during coronary surgery. *Acta Anaesthesiol Scand* 47:667, 2003.
32. Elahi MM, Chetty GK, Kirke R, et al.: Complications related to intra-aortic balloon pump in cardiac surgery: A decade later. *Eur J Vasc Endovasc Surg* 29:591, 2005.
33. Saunders CR, Doty DB: Myocardial contusion: Effect of intra-aortic balloon counterpulsation on cardiac output. *J Trauma* 18:706, 1978.
34. Jacobs JP, Horowitz MD, Ladden DA, et al.: Intra-aortic balloon counterpulsation in penetrating cardiac trauma. *J Cardiovasc Surg* (*Torino*) 33:38, 1992.
35. Mangano DT: Monitoring pulmonary arterial pressure in coronary-artery disease. *Anesthesiology* 53:364, 1980.
36. Raper R, Sibbald WJ: Misled by the wedge? The Swan-Ganz catheter and left ventricular preload. *Chest* 89:427, 1986.
37. Girolami A, Little RA, Foex BA, et al.: Hemodynamic responses to fluid resuscitation after blunt trauma. *Crit Care Med* 30:385, 2002.
38. Madan AK, UyBarreta VV, Aliabadi S-Wahle, et al.: Esophageal Doppler ultrasound monitor versus pulmonary artery catheter in the hemodynamic management of critically ill surgical patients. *J Trauma* 46:607, 1999.
39. Benedict CR, Rose JA: Arterial norepinephrine changes in patients with septic shock. *Circ Shock* 38:165, 1992.
40. Luchette FA, Jenkins WA, Friend LA, et al.: Hypoxia is not the sole cause of lactate production during shock. *J Trauma* 52:415, 2002.
41. Moomey CB Jr, Melton SM, Croce MA, et al.: Prognostic value of blood lactate, base deficit, and oxygen-derived variables in an LD50 model of penetrating trauma. *Crit Care Med* 27:154, 1999.
42. Davis JW, Shackford SR, Mackersie RC, et al.: Base deficit as a guide to volume resuscitation. *J Trauma* 28:1464, 1988.

43. Ahrens T, Schallom L, Bettorf K, et al.: End-tidal carbon dioxide measurements as a prognostic indicator of outcome in cardiac arrest. *Am J Crit Care* 10:391, 2001.
44. Bilkovski RN, Rivers EP, Horst HM: Targeted resuscitation strategies after injury. *Curr Opin Crit Care* 10:529, 2004.
45. Sanders AB, Kern KB, Otto CW, et al.: End-tidal carbon dioxide monitoring during cardiopulmonary resuscitation. A prognostic indicator for survival. *Jama* 262:1347, 1989.
46. Wayne MA, Levine RL, Miller CC: Use of end-tidal carbon dioxide to predict outcome in prehospital cardiac arrest. *Ann Emerg Med* 25:762, 1995.
47. Cantineau JP, Lambert Y, Merckx P, et al.: End-tidal carbon dioxide during cardiopulmonary resuscitation in humans presenting mostly with asystole: A predictor of outcome. *Crit Care Med* 24:791, 1996.
48. Rackow EC, O'Neil P, Astiz ME, et al.: Sublingual capnometry and indexes of tissue perfusion in patients with circulatory failure. *Chest* 120:1633, 2001.
49. Baron BJ, Sinert R, Zehtabchi S, et al.: Diagnostic utility of sublingual PCO2 for detecting hemorrhage in penetrating trauma patients. *J Trauma* 57:69, 2004.
50. Heckmann JG, Lang CJ, Kindler K, et al.: Neurologic manifestations of cerebral air embolism as a complication of central venous catheterization. *Crit Care Med* 28:1621, 2000.
51. van Hulst RA, Haitsma JJ, Lameris TW, et al.: Hyperventilation impairs brain function in acute cerebral air embolism in pigs. *Intensive Care Med* 30:944, 2004.
52. Khuri SF, Daley J, Henderson W, et al.: The National Veterans Administration Surgical Risk Study: Risk adjustment for the comparative assessment of the quality of surgical care. *J Am Coll Surg* 180:519, 1995.
53. Fuster V, Badimon L, Badimon JJ, et al.: The pathogenesis of coronary artery disease and the acute coronary syndromes (1). *N Engl J Med* 326:242, 1992.
54. Raby KE, Barry J, Creager MA, et al.: Detection and significance of intraoperative and postoperative myocardial ischemia in peripheral vascular surgery. *JAMA* 268:222, 1992.
55. Guidelines for assessing and managing the perioperative risk from coronary artery disease associated with major noncardiac surgery. American College of Physicians. *Ann Intern Med* 127:309, 1997.
56. Landesberg G, Luria MH, Cotev S, et al.: Importance of long-duration postoperative ST-segment depression in cardiac morbidity after vascular surgery. *Lancet* 341:715, 1993.
57. Godet G, Coriat P, Baron JF, et al.: Prevention of intraoperative myocardial ischemia during noncardiac surgery with intravenous diltiazem: A randomized trial versus placebo. *Anesthesiology* 66:241, 1987.
58. Coriat P: Intravenous nitroglycerin dosage to prevent intraoperative myocardial ischemia during noncardiac surgery. *Anesthesiology* 64:409, 1986.
59. Mangano DT, Layug EL, Wallace A, et al.: Effect of atenolol on mortality and cardiovascular morbidity after noncardiac surgery. Multicenter Study of Perioperative Ischemia Research Group. *N Engl J Med* 335:1713, 1996.
60. Poldermans D, Boersma E, Bax JJ, et al.: The effect of bisoprolol on perioperative mortality and myocardial infarction in high-risk patients undergoing vascular surgery. Dutch Echocardiographic Cardiac Risk Evaluation Applying Stress Echocardiography Study Group. *N Engl J Med* 341:1789, 1999.
61. Auerbach AD, Goldman L: beta-Blockers and reduction of cardiac events in noncardiac surgery: Scientific review. *JAMA* 287:1435, 2002.
62. Grayburn PA, Hillis LD: Cardiac events in patients undergoing noncardiac surgery: Shifting the paradigm from noninvasive risk stratification to therapy. *Ann Intern Med* 138:506, 2003.
63. Rogers WJ, Canto JG, Lambrew CT, et al.: Temporal trends in the treatment of over 1.5 million patients with myocardial infarction in the US from 1990 through 1999: The National Registry of Myocardial Infarction 1, 2 and 3. *J Am Coll Cardiol* 36:2056, 2000.
64. Indications for fibrinolytic therapy in suspected acute myocardial infarction: collaborative overview of early mortality and major morbidity results from all randomised trials of more than 1000 patients. Fibrinolytic Therapy Trialists' (FTT) Collaborative Group. *Lancet* 343:311, 1994.
65. Gibson CM, Karha J, Murphy SA, et al.: Early and long-term clinical outcomes associated with reinfarction following fibrinolytic administration in the thrombolysis in myocardial infarction trials. *J Am Coll Cardiol* 42:7, 2003.
66. Grzybowski M, Clements EA, Parsons L, et al.: Mortality benefit of immediate revascularization of acute ST-segment elevation myocardial infarction in patients with contraindications to thrombolytic therapy: A propensity analysis. *Jama* 290:1891, 2003.
67. Keeley EC, Boura JA, Grines CL: Primary angioplasty versus intravenous thrombolytic therapy for acute myocardial infarction: A quantitative review of 23 randomised trials. *Lancet* 361:13, 2003.
68. Keeley EC, Grines CL: Primary coronary intervention for acute myocardial infarction. *JAMA* 291:736, 2004.
69. Dangas G, Aymong ED, Mehran R, et al.: Predictors of and outcomes of early thrombosis following balloon angioplasty versus primary stenting in acute myocardial infarction and usefulness of abciximab (the CADILLAC trial). *Am J Cardiol* 94:983, 2004.
70. Flesch M, Schiffer F, Zolk O, et al.: Angiotensin receptor antagonism and angiotensin converting enzyme inhibition improve diastolic dysfunction and Ca (2+)-ATPase expression in the sarcoplasmic reticulum in hypertensive cardiomyopathy. *J Hypertens* 15:1001, 1997.
71. Friedrich SP, Lorell BH, Rousseau MF, et al.: Intracardiac angiotensin-converting enzyme inhibition improves diastolic function in patients with left ventricular hypertrophy due to aortic stenosis. *Circulation* 90:2761, 1994.
72. Banerjee P, Banerjee T, Khand A, et al.: Diastolic heart failure: Neglected or misdiagnosed? *J Am Coll Cardiol* 39:138, 2002.
73. The effect of digoxin on mortality and morbidity in patients with heart failure. The Digitalis Investigation Group. *N Engl J Med* 336:525, 1997.
74. Struthers AD: Aldosterone: Cardiovascular assault. *Am Heart J* 144:S2, 2002.
75. Farquharson CA, Struthers AD: Aldosterone induces acute endothelial dysfunction in vivo in humans: Evidence for an aldosterone-induced vasculopathy. *Clin Sci (Lond)* 103:425, 2002.

## Commentary ■ ROBERT D. BARRACO ■ MICHAEL PASQUALE

In this chapter on cardiovascular failure, Drs. Gosain, Santaniello, and Luchette quite nicely summarize cardiovascular physiology. In this era of increased prevalence of morbid obesity, the use of indices to standardize cardiac output measurements is especially useful and their caution on interpretation of pulmonary artery catheter (PAC) measurements is well taken.

Many causes of unreliability in the pulmonary artery wedge pressure (PAWP) as a proxy for left ventricular end diastolic volume (LVEDV) are listed in the chapter. However, it is paramount that we be familiar with the assumptions made in this approximation. The first assumption is that the left ventricular end diastolic pressure (LVEDP) approximates LVEDV. This relationship can be altered by myocardial ischemia, ventricular outflow obstruction, mitral regurgitation, vasodilator therapy, or severe heart failure. The second assumption is that left atrial pressure (LAP) approximates LVEDP through an open mitral valve during

end-diastole; however, mitral stenosis or aortic regurgitation can cause a pressure gradient during diastole. Thirdly, approximation of LAP to PAWP presumes a continuous column of blood from the tip of the Swan–Ganz catheter to the left atrium. This may not be the case if alveolar pressure is greater than pulmonary artery pressure (West's Zone I) or in cases where pulmonary venous pressure is reduced (hypovolemia or sepsis). Pulmonary compliance may affect PAWP and by convention, each 5 cm $H_2O$ of PEEP results in an increase of the PAWP by 1 mm Hg, although this is not always consistent. Lastly, lung recruitment strategies that utilize high mean airway pressures may falsely elevate the PAWP, particularly in noncompliant lungs. In such cases, however, the trending of the PAWP can be useful in making treatment decisions.

One practical method of determining the adequacy of preload may be the timed-fluid challenge. A plot is made of the PAWP,

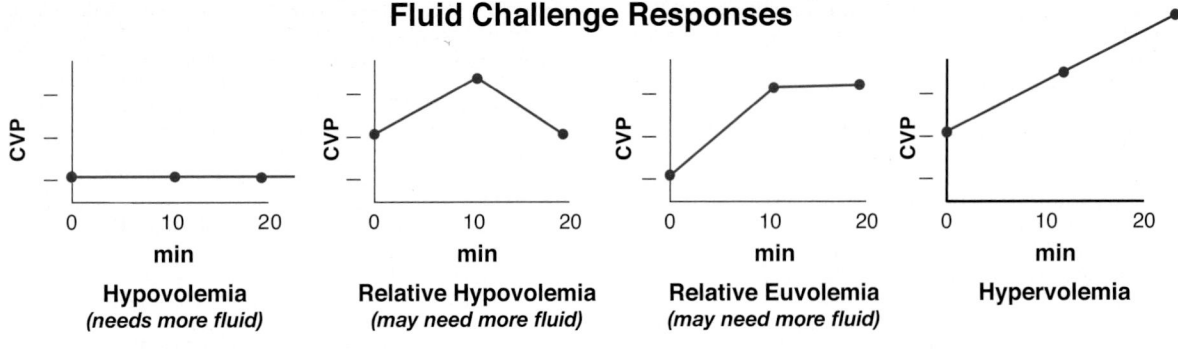

**Fluid Challenge Responses**

CVP = Central Venous Pressure

**FIGURE 1.**  Fluid challenge responses.

cardiac index, or central venous pressure versus time prior to and 10 and 20 minutes after the challenge. The shape of the resulting graph can guide your fluid management (Fig. 1). This method of rapid alteration of intravascular volume has been referred to in principle in various critical care texts and handbooks.[1,2] Also worth mentioning is the recent Cochrane review published in 2006 which examines the effect of PAC utilization on mortality and cost in the adult ICU.[3] Twelve studies were identified and analyzed showing no difference in mortality in high-risk surgery patients. Additionally, pulmonary artery catheterization did not affect ICU or hospital length of stay and costs were, on average, higher in the PAC groups. Further multicenter studies are obviously needed in this area.

With respect to myocardial dysfunction and its management, volume restoration is key and global indicators of resuscitation, namely, clearance of base deficit and lactatemia are vital. This is extremely important in assessing ongoing resuscitation. These endpoints are especially useful in elderly trauma patients, where a base deficit of 6 or more portends a 66% mortality rate.[4] According to a Level III recommendation in the EAST practice management guideline, attempts should be made to optimize cardiac index in this elderly trauma population which contradicts the nontrauma literature presented in the chapter.[4] Recognition of a role for the intra-aortic balloon pump in cases of refractory cardiac failure is an important part of the updated chapter.

The two areas of interest in the monitoring section of the chapter are the use of echocardiography and capnography. Formal echocardiography can assist in the evaluation of patients with unreliable PAC values and esophageal duplex monitor (EDM) technology

is recommended for this purpose. Dark and Singer performed a meta-analysis of the validity data comparing PAC to EDM and found no bias and high clinical agreement between the two technologies.[5] There are two modalities of capnography: (1) end-tidal and (2) sublingual. The former may be useful as a predictor of resuscitative efforts but has not been useful in monitoring ongoing resuscitation. There have been no randomized prospective trials to date or an evidence-based review on the sublingual capnography. However, the studies seem to agree that sublingual capnometry may a useful noninvasive means of evaluating tissue perfusion during an ongoing resuscitation.

It is important that the reader understand that the diagnostic adjuncts mentioned must be used in concert with the clinical exam and indicators (i.e., vital signs, urine output). Only through such a detailed evaluation can the best outcomes be achieved. The pharmacologic section is extremely well written. The authors of this chapter are to be commended for the depth and breadth of their review of cardiovascular failure.

## References

1. Civetta, Taylor, Kirby JB: Lippincott Company: *Critical Care*, 2:255, 1992.
2. Lanken, Hansen, Manaker: *The Intensive Care Unit Manual*, W.B. Saunders Company, 2001, p. 66.
3. Harvey S, Young D, Brampton W, et al.: Pulmonary artery catheters for adult patients in intensive care. *Cochrane Database of Systematic Reviews* 2006, Issue 3. Art. No.: CD003408. DOI: 10.1002/14651858.CD003408.pub2.
4. Practice Management Guidelines for Geriatric Trauma, http://www.east.org/tpg/geriatric.pdf
5. Dark PM, Singer M: The validity of trans-esophageal Doppler ultrasonography as a measure of cardiac output in critically ill adults. *Intensive Care Med* 30:2060, 2004.

# Respiratory Insufficiency

*Jeffrey L. Johnson* ■ *James B. Haenel*

The maintenance of eucapnia and normoxia may be tenuous in the injured patient because of dysfunction in three key elements of the respiratory system. First, the central nervous system (CNS) may be impaired, resulting in inadequate respiratory drive, or inability to maintain patent proximal airways. Second, injury to the torso can produce changes in compliance, ineffective respiratory effort, and pain that impact the patient's ability to complete the work of breathing. Third, primary and secondary insults to the lung result in ineffective gas exchange.

In practice, it is common for patients to suffer simultaneous insults, affecting all three elements. Impaired airway patency (e.g., CNS injury), increased work of breathing (e.g., multiple rib fractures), and impaired gas exchange (e.g., pulmonary contusion, fat emboli syndrome) often coexist in the same patient. Respiratory failure which relates primarily to CNS injury is discussed at length in other chapters and will not be extensively covered here. This chapter will focus on insults that affect work of breathing and gas exchange. The syndrome of postinjury acute respiratory distress syndrome (ARDS) will be a major focus.

## HYPERCAPNIC PULMONARY FAILURE

The neurohormonal response to injury (see Chap. 67) results in a remarkable increase in cellular metabolism. This creates a substantial increase in $CO_2$ production that must be effectively matched by increased excretion from the lungs. While a resting adult must eliminate 200 cc/kg/minute of $CO_2$, postinjury hypermatabolism results in $CO_2$ production in the range of 425 cc/kg/minute.[1] Thus, the minute ventilation required to maintain eucapnia may rise from a resting rate of approximately 5 L/minute to about 10 L/minute. This represents a 100% increase in the work of breathing simply to meet metabolic demands.

Additionally, injured patients typically have an increase in physiologic and anatomic dead space — ventilated regions that do not participate in gas exchange. In a normal adult, the proportion of each breath that is dead space ($V_d/V_t$) is approximately 0.35. In the intubated, ventilated patient, the $V_d/V_t$ can be calculated by a number of techniques including the Bohr–Enghoff method [$V_d/V_t = ((PaCO_2 - \text{Mean Expired } CO_2)/PaCO_2)$].[2] For practical purposes (since mean expired $CO_2$ is not commonly measured), this is a reflection of the minute volume required to achieve a given $PaCO_2$. In ventilated patients with pulmonary failure, the $V_d/V_t$ often exceeds 0.6. Simply put, this extra dead space is a burden because each breath is less effective at eliminating $CO_2$, and therefore minute ventilation requirements in the 12–20 L/minute range are not uncommon in an intensive care unit (ICU) setting.

The above increase in respiratory demand might be met by a healthy adult; however, the injured patient faces several challenges in completing this additional work. CNS dysfunction from injury impairs respiratory drive, as do many medications routinely used for sedation and analgesia. Decreased thoracic compliance from abdominal distension (e.g., as part of the abdominal compartment syndrome; see Chap. 41), chest wall edema, and recumbent positioning increases the energy required to complete a respiratory cycle. Decreased pulmonary compliance from an increase in extravascular lung water, and pleural collections (effusions/hemothorax) also contribute. Muscular weakness from impaired energetics (acidosis, hemodynamic insufficiency, mitochondrial dysfunction, oxidant stress) or fatigue may be an insurmountable challenge. Finally, pain from torso injuries or operative interventions make the increased ventilatory demand a substantial burden to the patient.

The net effect of increased demand and diminished capacity to execute the work of breathing is hypercapnic respiratory failure. Patients present with respiratory acidosis, or more commonly a mixed acid-base picture where ventilation is inadequate to maintain physiologic pH in the face of a metabolic acidosis. While efforts to diminish the work of breathing should be routine, most patients with hypercapnic failure require some form of mechanical ventilation to meet their demands (see Chap. 60).

One approach to addressing the challenge of increased $CO_2$ production in the injured patient might be to diminish the hypermetabolic response. Despite being intuitively attractive, simple maneuvers like maintenance of euthermia, delivery of nutrition, and minimizing pain-induced stress do not appear to affect the incidence or outcome of hypercapnic respiratory failure. A more novel approach is delivery of beta adrenergic blockade, which in a retrospective analysis, improves outcomes in injured patients. There is reasonably compelling data in the pediatric burn population and the acutely brain injured that blunting of hypermetbolism is beneficial.[3] A prospective safety and efficacy evaluation of this approach in injured adults is needed before it can be recommended as routine practice.

Two injury patterns that precipitate hypercapnic respiratory failure are worthy of special mention: spinal cord injury and flail chest/pulmonary contusion. In spinal cord injury, conventional wisdom asserts that lesions below C5 should not result in pulmonary failure, because innervation to the diaphragm remains intact. In practice, however, most complete cord lesions in the cervical and upper thoracic regions result in failure requiring mechanical ventilation.[4,5] The genesis of this is likely multifactorial, including delays in patient mobilization, ineffective cough due to loss of innervation of intercostal and abdominal musculature, pneumonia in the setting of multiple injuries, and aspiration at the time of the initial insult. This patient population requires aggressive mobilization and pulmonary care as recurrent lobar collapse and pneumonia are the rule. Early operative stabilization of the spine can be recommended as it has been shown to decrease the need for mechanical ventilation and ICU stay.[6-8] Other adjuncts such as noninvasive ventilation, bronchodilators, mucolytics, and percussion should be considered, though most of these have not been studied in a fashion that permits a firm recommendation. While diaphragmatic pacing may be of benefit in select patients,[9] its role in the acute setting remains to be defined.

Flail chest and pulmonary contusion can be thought of as a single entity. This is a challenging injury pattern, because it impacts both the patients' ability to execute the work of breathing (from pain and mechanical instability of the thoracic) and gas exchange (from the pulmonary contusion). Isolated pulmonary contusion rarely requires mechanical ventilation; since this is now frequently identified by computed tomography (CT), it is important to realize that this tends to take a relatively benign course (see Chap. 26). In contradistinction, it is clear that number of rib fractures is strongly associated with pulmonary failure, ARDS, and mortality, and that this effect is more dramatic in the elderly population.[10,11] Early pain control, preferably beginning in the emergency department with regional anesthesia, has been shown to be effective in reducing the impact of multiple rib fractures and should be routinely applied. A common pitfall is to underestimate the degree of hypoventilation in the patient with chest wall injury. Because oxygenation is routinely measured and maintained — the tendency is to intervene too late, only after the patient has developed hypercapnic pulmonary failure. One helpful adjunct is the routine measurement of bedside incentive spirometry values — as a surrogate for pain control and ventilatory capacity. A recent study demonstrated that early aggressive care of patients >45 years of age with multiple rib fractures could decrease ICU length of stay, infectious complications, and mortality.[12]

## HYPOXIC PULMONARY FAILURE

In addition to hypercapnic pulmonary failure, hypoxic pulmonary failure is a substantial contributor in the trauma setting. The etiologies are diverse including aspiration pneumonitis, pneumonia, pulmonary embolism, acute lung injury (ALI), and acute respiratory distress syndrome (ARDS). Most of these entitites are discussed in other chapters — ALI and ARDS will be the focus of this chapter. Indeed, the mechanisms at work in ALI and ARDS share many common features with these other processes that affect the alveolar–capillary interface.

## ALI AND ARDS

ALI and ARDS are clinical syndromes of inflammatory lung injury that represent a single final pathway of what are, in fact, diverse systemic processes. Its pathophysiology is complex, variable, and incompletely understood. A standard definition of ALI and ARDS has improved our ability to characterize and study the syndrome; however, the working definition is arguably arbitrary and imposes a single set of criteria for multiple etiologies of disease. This continues to make outcome studies, treatment, and assessment of ARDS difficult.

Formerly termed *"adult" respiratory distress syndrome,* the term "acute" is preferred, recognizing that ARDS is not limited to adults.[13] In fact, one of the patients reported in the seminal description of this syndrome by Ashbaugh and colleagues in 1967 was 11 years old.[14] Since its original description, the diagnosis and management of ARDS has become increasingly important. This is due in part to improvements in technology and critical care that have allowed severely injured patients to survive the initial insult. The mortality related to ARDS is reported to be in the range of 25–60%.[15,16] In the last few years, however, multiinstitutional studies have revealed management strategies that result in a mortality approaching 30%.[17] Indeed, while trauma is a common precipitating factor, ARDS mortality in this group of patients is thought to be substantially lower (24%) than for those, for example, with severe sepsis of pulmonary origin (41%).[18] A 2006 study[19] strongly suggests that while the diagnosis of ARDS is associated with substantial morbidity, it is not independently associated with death in the trauma setting. Further, with optimal ICU care, postinjury lung dysfunction may progress less frequently to lung and other organ failure.[20]

## CURRENT DEFINITIONS AND THEIR LIMITATIONS

The recognition of ARDS as a distinct clinical entity resulted from the description by Ashbaugh and Petty in 1967. Subsequent descriptions have included five principle criteria: (1) hypoxemia refractory to oxygen administration; (2) diffuse, bilateral infiltrates on chest radiograph; (3) low static lung compliance; (4) absence of congestive heart failure; and (5) presence of an appropriate at-risk diagnosis.

The most common standard definition of ARDS was developed in 1994, after a Consensus Conference of American and European investigators (AECC) agreed that ARDS should be viewed as the most severe end of the spectrum ALI. It also recommended diagnostic criteria for acute lung injury and ARDS (Table 63-1). The diagnostic criteria for ARDS include acute onset, the $PaO_2/FIO_2$ 200 mm Hg or less (<300 for ALI), bilateral infiltrates on chest radiograph, and no evidence of left arterial hypertension (either clinical or with pulmonary artery catheter measurement). Moreover, the committee recognized that ARDS is most often associated with sepsis syndrome, aspiration, primary pneumonia, trauma, cardiopulmonary bypass, multiple blood transfusions, fat embolism, and pancreatitis. Although debate exists as to the usefulness of the AECC diagnostic criteria, they have promoted study of reasonably homogeneous populations, are largely accepted by clinical investigators, and are likely to be used for some time.[21]

Despite the research utility of a standard definition, there are substantial limitations to its application at the bedside. For example, transient hypoxemia from mucus plugging is common in an ICU setting, and it is unclear that a patient who only transiently meets *P/F* criteria should be grouped with patients who have ongoing poor oxygenation. Additionally, recruitment of collapsed alveoli may result in a remarkable improvement in *P/F* ratio in a short period of time — does this patient no longer have ARDS? Lastly, while the AECC definition excludes patients with left atrial pressure (LAP) >18, Ferguson et al.[22] showed that patients with no risk factors for congestive heart failure commonly had LAP>18 during a clinical course consistent with ARDS.

Whether the current definition is too broad also remains a matter of debate. In favor of that argument is a 2004 study comparing postmortem analysis of lung tissue with the AECC definition. This investigation found the latter to be only 84% specific and 75% sensitive for the pathologic lung lesions characteristic of ARDS.[23] It is clear, then, that the AECC definition, while useful for studies of populations, should be applied with caution to individual patients. While it has clearly been helpful to have the standardized AECC definition, it is worthwhile to know its limitations and consider some alternative methods for objectively assessing lung injury. The Murray Lung Injury Score (LIS) was proposed in 1988 and is based on four components: chest radiograph, hypoxemia, positive end-expiratory pressure (PEEP), and respiratory system compliance (Table 63-2).[24] The chest radiograph and hypoxemia criteria must be available in all patients. Each component is scored from 0 to 4. The LIS is calculated by summing the scores of the available components and dividing by the number of components used. ARDS (or severe lung injury) is defined as a LIS greater than 2.5. Zero represents no lung injury and 0.1 to 2.5 represents mild to moderate lung injury.

## TABLE 63-1

### American-European Consensus Conference Definitions of Acute Lung Injury and Acute Respiratory Distress Syndrome

**Acute Lung Injury Criteria**

Timing: acute onset

Oxygenation: $PaO_2/FIO_2$ ≤300 mm Hg (regardless of positive end-expiratory pressure)

Chest radiograph: bilateral infiltrates on anteroposterior chest radiograph

Pulmonary artery occlusion pressure: ≤18 mm Hg or no clinical evidence of left atrial hypertension

**ARDS Criteria**

Same as acute lung injury except:

Oxygenation: $PaO_2/FIO_2$ ≤200 mm Hg (regardless of positive end-expiratory pressure)

## TABLE 63-2

### Lung Injury Score[a]

| Chest Radiograph Score | |
|---|---|
| No alveolar consolidation | 0 |
| Alveolar consolidation confined to one quadrant | 1 |
| Alveolar consolidation confined to two quadrants | 2 |
| Alveolar consolidation confined to three quadrants | 3 |
| Alveolar consolidation confined to four quadrants | 4 |
| **Hypoxemia Score** | |
| $PaO_2/FIO_2$ ≥300 | 0 |
| $PaO_2/FIO_2$ 225–299 | 1 |
| $PaO_2/FIO_2$ 175–224 | 2 |
| $PaO_2/FIO_2$ 100–174 | 3 |
| $PaO_2/FIO_2$ <100 | 4 |
| **PEEP Score (When Ventilated)** | |
| PEEP ≥5 cmH$_2$O | 0 |
| PEEP 6–8 cmH$_2$O | 1 |
| PEEP 9–11 cmH$_2$O | 2 |
| PEEP 12–14 cmH$_2$O | 3 |
| PEEP ≥15 cmH$_2$O | 4 |
| **Respiratory System Compliance Score (When Available)** | |
| Compliance ≥80 mL/cmH$_2$O | 0 |
| Compliance 60–79 mL/cmH$_2$O | 1 |
| Compliance 40–59 mL/cmH$_2$O | 2 |
| Compliance 20–39 mL/cmH$_2$O | 3 |
| Compliance ≤19 mL/cmH$_2$O | 4 |

[a]The final value is obtained by dividing the aggregate sum by the number of components that were used: no lung injury, 0; mild to moderate lung injury, 0.1–2.5; severe lung injury (ARDS), .2.5.

*Source: Murray JF, Matthay MA, Luce JM, Flick MR: Pulmonary perspectives: An expanded definition of the adult respiratory distress syndrome. Am Rev Respir Dis 134:720, 1988. Official Journal of the American Thoracic Society. Copyright © American Lung Association. With permission.*

## TABLE 63-3

### The "DELPHI" Definition of ARDS

Timing: acute onset

Oxygenation: $PaO_2/FIO_2$ ≤200 with PEEP ≥10

Chest radiograph: bilateral infiltrates

Absence of CHF *OR* presence of recognized risk factor for ARDS

A more recent definition developed by clinicians using the Delphi process makes a simple adjustment of the ARDS definition which appears to approve diagnostic accuracy when compared to pathologic lesions found at autopsy (Table 63-3).[25] Briefly, the authors include PEEP in the consideration of hypoxia and require either the absence of CHF *or* the presence of a recognized risk factor for ARDS. The degree of hypoxia required is a *P/F* less than 200 with PEEP≥10; therefore it excludes patients who are hypoxic purely because of de-recruitment or suboptimal PEEP. By allowing patients with high filling pressures in the presence of a recognized ARDS risk factor, the definition recognizes the prevalence of high left atrial pressures during the course of ARDS and includes patients with concomitant CHF and ARDS. This is an attractive definition that deserves further prospective evaluation.

## EPIDEMIOLOGY AND RISK FACTORS

The 1972 report of the National Heart and Lung Institute Task Force of Respiratory Diseases reported that there were approximately 150,000 cases of ARDS per year (60 to 71 cases per 100,000 person-years).[26] This figure was based on a consensus panel estimate derived from cross-sectional survey data. In this widely cited study, no operational definition of ARDS was specified. Since the adoption of the AECC definition, reports that are methodologically more sound estimate the incidence of ARDS on the order of 15–60 cases per 100,000 person-years.[27–32] Each of these studies is a population-based, prospective cohort study.

## RISK FACTORS

Several studies demonstrate that age is a risk factor for ARDS. Hudson and coworkers documented an increasing incidence of ARDS with increasing age. Subgroup analysis, however, showed that age was not a risk factor when sepsis syndrome or drug overdose/aspiration was the inciting event. In contrast, patients who developed postinjury ARDS were significantly older (44 years vs. 36 years).[33] These authors also observed that a higher Injury Severity Score (ISS) was a risk factor for ARDS.

Clinical risk factors for ARDS can be broadly categorized into direct and indirect groups (Table 63-4). Direct factors are those primarily associated with local pulmonary parenchymal injury and include pulmonary contusion, aspiration, and pulmonary infection. Indirect factors are those thought to be associated with systemic inflammation and resultant lung injury. These include severe sepsis, transfusion of banked red cells, and multiple long-bone fractures. Unless shock is associated with significant tissue injury or other known risk factors, it has not been shown to result in ARDS.[34] The time from identification of risk to onset of ARDS varies depending on the risk factor. In general, onset of ARDS is slower in trauma patients compared to those with sepsis. Following diagnosis of sepsis, 32% and 54% of patients who developed ARDS did so by 12 hours and 24 hours, respectively. Of patients who developed postinjury ARDS, 16% did so within 12 hours and 29% by 24 hours. ARDS developed in 80% or more by 72 hours in patients with either sepsis or trauma.

**TABLE 63-4**

| Clinical Risk Factors for ARDS | |
| --- | --- |
| RISK FACTOR | FREQUENCY OF ARDS (%) |
| **DIRECT** | |
| Aspiration | 12–36 |
| Pneumonia | 12–31 |
| Pulmonary contusion | 5–22 |
| Toxic inhalation | 2–17 |
| **INDIRECT** | |
| Sepsis syndrome | 11–80 |
| Multiple transfusions | 5–36 |
| Multiple fractures | 2–21 |
| Pancreatitis | 7–18 |
| Disseminated intravascular coagulation | 23 |

Genetic variability between patients may also contribute to risk for ARDS (for a discussion of genomics relevant to trauma, see Chap. 57). One candidate gene of interest is the angiotensin converting enzyme (ACE) gene. ACE levels are often reduced in patients with ARDS, but there is considerable variability between individuals.[35] One potential source of this variability is a common noncoding deletion in the gene (D allele), which is associated with lower circulating ACE activity. Marshall et al. have recently demonstrated that patients with ARDS were much more likely to have the DD genotype.[36] Furthermore, outcome of lung injury in medical patients has been associated with the I/D genotype.[37] Other candidate genes include Interleukin-10 and the Pre-B-Cell Colony Enhancing Factor.[38,39]

## PATHOLOGY

The current paradigm of systemic inflammation leading to ALI and ARDS posits that a variety of insults, both infectious and noninfectious, can result in an unbridled hyperinflammatory response. This leads to organ injury from indiscriminate activation of effector cells that subsequently release oxidants, proteinases, and other potentially autotoxic compounds. If the initial insult is severe enough, early organ dysfunction results ("one-hit" or single insult model). More often, a less severe insult results in a systemic inflammatory response that is not by itself injurious. These patients appear, however, to be primed such that they have an exaggerated response to a second insult, which leads to an augmented/amplified systemic inflammatory response and multiple-organ dysfunction ("two-hit" or sequential insult model, see Chap. 68).[40]

Inflammatory models provide a unifying hypothesis for ARDS and multiple organ failure (MOF); however, the precise relationship between ARDS and MOF remains to be defined. MOF is a frequent occurrence and the most common cause of mortality in patients with ARDS.[41] It is possible that ARDS is an early indicator of MOF because the lungs are most sensitive to the actions of inflammatory cells; alternatively, it may be that lung dysfunction is more easily measured than other organ dysfunction. Indeed, postinjury ARDS appears to be an obligate precursor of other organ failure.[42] This may be because the lung is a primary target of the inflammatory process, or that the resultant pulmonary damage impairs the lung's ability to metabolize inflammatory mediators and control cellular effectors of injury.[43] It is also now clear that ventilator strategies which inadvertently promote lung injury, may produce systemic inflammation, perhaps leading to other organ failures.[44]

Inflammatory lung injury leads to the pathologic lesion of diffuse alveolar damage. This prototypic lesion of ARDS is at the alveolocapillary interface, which results in epithelial and endothelial damage as well as high permeability pulmonary edema. The histologic appearance of this lesion can be divided into three overlapping phases: (1) the exudative phase, with edema and hemorrhage; (2) the proliferative phase, with organization and repair; and (3) the fibrotic phase.[45]

The exudative phase generally encompasses the first 3–5 days but may last up to a week. The initial histologic changes include interstitial edema, proteinaceous alveolar edema, and intra-alveolar hemorrhage. The exudative phase is characterized by the appearance of hyaline membranes, which are composed of plasma proteins mixed with cellular debris. Electron microscopy reveals endothelial injury with cell swelling, widening intercellular junctions, and increased pinocytotic vesicles. In addition, there is disruption of the basement membrane. The alveolar epithelium usually exhibits extensive necrosis of type I cells, which slough and leave a denuded basement membrane. Type II pneumocytes also undergo necrosis but are, in general, less susceptible to injury than type I cells. This loss of the alveolar epithelial barrier results in alveolar edema. The cellular infiltrate may be sparse or predominantly neutrophils.[46,47]

During the proliferative phase, type II cells divide and cover the denuded basement membrane along the alveolar wall. This process may be seen as early as three days after the onset of clinical ARDS. Type II cells are also capable of differentiating into type I epithelial cells. Fibroblasts and myofibroblasts proliferate and migrate into the alveolar space in the third phase. Fibroblasts change the alveolar exudate into granulation tissue, which subsequently organizes and forms dense fibrous tissue. Eventually, epithelial cells cover the granulation tissue. This whole process is called fibrosis by accretion and is important in lung remodeling. Septal collagen deposition by fibroblasts and "collapse induration" also contribute to fibrous remodeling of the lung in ARDS. During this phase, the neutrophilic infiltrate becomes predominantly mononuclear.[48]

The fibrotic stage is characterized by thickened, collagenous connective tissue in the alveolar septa and walls. Pulmonary vascular changes occur as well, with intimal thickening and medial hypertrophy of the pulmonary arterioles. Complete obliteration of portions of the pulmonary vascular bed is the end result.

## PATHOGENESIS

Lung injury in ARDS involves components of inflammation, coagulation, vasomotor tone, and other systems (see Chap. 67). The pivotal cellular mediators appear to be leukocytes, with both local and humoral mediators orchestrating their function. Activation of these leukocytes results in release or activation of multiple cytokines, chemokines, oxidants, and proteases that result in the final common pathway of tissue injury in ARDS.

## LEUKOCYTES AND PULMONARY EPITHELIUM

A consistent histopathologic feature of ARDS is neutrophil infiltration of the pulmonary microvasculature, interstitium, and alveoli. In a way, neutrophils are uniquely equipped to cause damage through the release of reactive oxygen species and proteases.[49,50] Furthermore, neutrophils may be an important source of proinflammatory cytokines.[51,52] Persistence of neutrophils in serial bronchoalveolar lavage (BAL) fluid samples from patients with ARDS suggests unbridled inflammation and portends poor prognosis.[48] In animal models, neutrophil depletion prior to an insult markedly attenuates resulting lung injury.[53] ARDS is known to occur in neutropenic patients, however, suggesting alternative mechanisms can be involved. The lung normally contains a significant number of sequestered neutrophils, and their mere presence is not sufficient to cause tissue injury. A long-standing model suggests that after a "priming" stimulus, neutrophils firmly adhere to endothelium and accumu-

late in the lungs; however, lung injury does not occur unless a second activating stimulus is applied.[54] Thus, for neutrophils to cause tissue damage, there must be adherence to the endothelium, transmigration to the interstitium, and subsequent activation with release of mediators. This adherence and transmigration creates a toxic microenvironment that is protected from endogenous antioxidants and antiproteases normally present in the plasma.

Both cellular biomechanical and adhesive mechanisms are operative in the process of neutrophil sequestration. The initial phase probably results from a change in the cytoskeleton of the neutrophil which increases rigidity. This change impedes flow through the pulmonary microvasculature.[55] A second, more prolonged phase is related to increased adhesive forces between neutrophils and endothelial cells. Initially, neutrophils "roll" along the endothelium as a result of the interaction of L-selection on the neutrophil with its counter-ligand (sialyl-x) on the endothelium or P- or F-selectin with sialyl-x on the neutrophil.[56] This is followed by firm adhesion, which is mediated by $\beta_2$ integrins on the neutrophil and intracellular adhesion molecule-1 (ICAM-1) on the endothelium.[57] Blocking antibodies to $\beta_2$ integrins, ICAM-1, and selectins have decreased lung injury in various experimental models.[57–60] Endothelial transmigration occurs even in the absence of endothelial cell injury and appears to be mediated by platelet–endothelial cell adhesion molecule-1 (PECAM-1).[61]

## MACROPHAGES

The lung contains large numbers of fixed tissue macrophages that are a critical component of the inflammatory response in acute lung injury. Activated macrophages can cause tissue injury by releasing the same toxic mediators as neutrophils (reactive oxygen species and proteases). Probably more important is the macrophage capability to synthesize multiple proinflammatory mediators, such as complement fragments, cytokines (tumor necrosis factor [TNF]; interleukin-1, -6, -8 [IL-1, IL-6, IL-8]), platelet-activating factor, and eicosanoids. Thus, macrophages are thought to have a major role in amplifying and perpetuating the inflammatory response. This is exacerbated by the long half-life of the macrophage, which is measured in days rather than hours as in the neutrophil. The alveolar macrophage has two additional key functions: control of local infection and modulation of fibrosis.[62] Alveolar macrophage from ARDS patients demonstrate defective phagocytosis and bacterial killing, reflecting an increased risk for infection in these patients.

## ENDOTHELIUM

The pulmonary endothelium is not a passive bystander in the pathogenesis of ARDS, but actively participates in initiating and perpetuating the inflammatory response. Endothelial cells increase the expression of adhesion molecules (ICAM-1, ICAM-3, and selectins) following exposure to an activating stimulus. These ligands serve as tethering and signaling molecules by binding to their cognate leukocyte membrane proteins. Thus, the endothelial cell actively coordinates trafficking, firm and adhesion, and transmigration. In the setting of systemic inflammation, inappropriate endothelial cell activation may lead to indiscriminate leukocyte recruitment and parenchymal inflammation. Moreover, endothelial cells produce and release vasoactive substances, such as prostacyclin, nitric oxide, and endothelins. These substances may mediate much of the pulmonary vascular dysfunction characteristic of ARDS. Activated endothelium also expresses procoagulant activity, which contributes to intravascular coagulation and microvascular dysfunction.[63] Thrombin, in turn, has proinflammatory effects on leukocytes. Endothelial injury, then, may be both a proximate cause and a marker for acute lung injury.[43]

## HUMORAL MEDIATORS

Systemic complement activation secondary to trauma or sepsis is considered a major early factor in ARDS.[64,65] C5a, a product of complement activation, is a powerful neutrophil chemoattractant. Moreover, C5a induces neutrophil aggregation and activation leading to pulmonary neutrophil sequestration and lung injury. Clinically, plasma and bronchoalveolar C3a levels correlate with the development of ARDS.[66,67]

## CYTOKINES

Increased levels of proinflammatory cytokines have been observed in the plasma and BAL fluid of patients with ARDS. As such, cytokines are generally accepted to play a significant role in the development of ALI.[68,69] It is also recognized that cytokines are part of a complex network with both protective and potentially damaging effects.[70] The balance between proinflammatory and anti-inflammatory processes may be more important than either component alone.[71,72]

## LIPID MEDIATORS

Phospholipids are potent inflammatory mediators that are formed by the action of phospholipase $A_2(PLA_2)$ on membrane phospholipids. $PLA_2$ contributes to the inflammatory response by two separate pathways, catalyzing the production of both platelet-activating factor (PAF) and arachidonic acid. Arachidonic acid metabolism results in release of eicosanoids such as leukotrienes, thromboxane, and prostaglandins. Each of these is an important mediator in the inflammatory cascade and has been implicated in the pathogenesis of ARDS.[73,74]

Platelet activating factor is a phospholipid with potent vasoactive and inflammatory properties. It is produced by a number of cell types including macrophages, neutrophils, endothelial cells, and type II pneumocytes. PAF production is stimulated by endotoxin, TNF, and leukotrienes, and exerts diverse biologic actions, including neutrophil activation and adherence, platelet aggregation and degranulation, and macrophage production of inflammatory mediators.[75] Infusion of PAF in animals results in increased vascular permeability and neutrophil-mediated acute lung injury.[76]

Lysophosphatidyl cholines are another class of bioactive lipids that may play a significant role in lung injury after trauma. These compounds accumulate during routine storage of packed red blood cells and have been shown to cause lung injury in isolated perfused

rodent lungs.[77] These or related compounds from transfusion of banked red cells may provide a second insult leading to inflammatory organ injury in the injured patient.

## THE GUT LYMPH HYPOTHESIS

It has long been understood that reperfusion of the ischemic gut can lead to lung injury.[78] Because gut ischemia/reperfusion is an established phenomenon in the injured patient with hemorrhagic shock, this remains a tantalizing hypothesis for the development of inflammatory injury to the lung. Curiously, however, convincing evidence of inflammatory mediators leaving the gut into the portal circulation has been lacking in humans. This led Deitch[79] to hypothesize that the egress of proinflammatory substances from the gut may be via lymph, not venous blood. This intriguing hypothesis has substantial support in animal models, including the finding that diversion of gut lymph abrogates lung injury. While the precise mediators of this phenomenon are as yet unknown, changes in posthemorrhagic shock lymph flow, lipid content, and protein content are an active area of investigation.[80,81]

## BIOLOGICAL MARKERS OF ACUTE RESPIRATORY DISTRESS SYNDROME

In addition to clinical risk factors, laboratory predictors of ARDS have been intensely studied. Biological markers of ARDS are potentially important for several reasons. They may further improve prediction of ARDS in patients with any of the aforementioned clinical risk factors. Moreover, they may provide much needed insight into the pathogenetic mechanisms of ALI. Finally, they may facilitate outcome predictions in patients with established ARDS. Biological markers can be measured in either plasma or distal airways (using BAL or directly sampling pulmonary edema fluid). These can be broadly categorized as protein measurements, cell-specific markers of acute lung injury, and markers of acute inflammation.[82]

The pulmonary endothelium is recognized as an active participant in the development of ALI. As such, markers of endothelial activation or injury have been investigated as predictors of the development of ARDS. von Willebrand factor antigen (vWF:Ag) has been studied fairly extensively as a marker of endothelial dysfunction. vWF:Ag is synthesized largely by vascular endothelial cells and has been shown to be a sensitive marker of endothelial injury or activation.[83] Carvallo and colleagues noted a five-fold increase in plasma vWF:Ag in 100 patients with ALI compared to normal subjects.[84] This antigen was studied prospectively in 45 patients to determine whether elevated levels of vWF:Ag are predictive for the development of ALI.[85] Only patients with nonpulmonary sepsis were included, and one-third developed ALI. Elevated plasma levels of vWF:AG (>45% above controls) were 87% sensitive and 77% specific for development of ALI. Positive predictive value was 65%. Moss and coworkers studied a more heterogeneous group of patients at risk for ARDS and concluded that although vWF:Ag levels are elevated in at-risk patients, they were not helpful in predicting progression to ARDS.[86] Following activation, endothelial expression of adhesion molecules, including ICAM-1, VCAM-1,

E-selectin, and P-selectin, is upregulated. These compounds are susceptible to proteolytic cleavage and may exist in the circulation in a soluble form.[87] Therefore, these molecules represent a measure of endothelial activation or damage. We and others have demonstrated elevated ICAM-1 levels in severely injured patients who subsequently developed MOF.[88,89] In contrast, plasma levels of soluble E- and P-selectins measured at admission were not useful in predicting ALI.[87] Moss and coworkers measured soluble E-selectin and ICAM-1 levels in patients at risk for ARDS (including both sepsis and trauma patients).[90] E-selectin and ICAM-1 levels were significantly higher in the septic patients than in the trauma patients. Moreover, the levels in the trauma patients were not different from healthy volunteers. This difference between trauma and sepsis patients was maintained at onset of ARDS.

It has been suggested that the permeability defect in ARDS is generalized and not confined to the pulmonary vasculature. The relationship between posttraumatic lung dysfunction and systemic capillary permeability has been investigated. Gosling and associates found that all trauma patients admitted to their trauma center had an early postinjury increase in microalbuminuria. In most patients, this rapidly returned to normal; however, there was a strong association between pulmonary dysfunction and sustained elevated urinary albumin excretion.[91] Subsequently, it was observed that the urinary albumin excretion rate detected the capillary leak of posttraumatic acute lung injury within eight hours of admission. Moreover, the albumin excretion rate predicted the development of pulmonary dysfunction and ARDS with reasonable accuracy.[92] An albumin excretion rate of greater than 130 $\mu$g/minute had positive and negative predictive values of 85% and 95%, respectively.

The importance of the lung epithelial barrier in ALI is well recognized.[93] The maintenance of a functioning alveolar epithelium is important for recovery from ALI.[94] Unlike the endothelium, there is a lack of specific histological markers of alveolar epithelial injury. Surfactant abnormalities have been noted in the earliest reports of ARDS.[14] Surfactant lipids and proteins are synthesized and released by alveolar epithelial type II cells. The surfactant associated proteins SP-A and SP-B are decreased in BAL fluid from patients with ARDS and at risk for ARDS.[95] The lungs also contain a large population of alveolar and interstitial macrophages. These cells are an important source of proinflammatory cytokines. A recent study observed several changes in BAL fluid cell populations in patients with ARDS. The evolution from BAL fluid neutrophilia to a larger proportion of macrophages is associated with resolution of lung injury and better outcome.[48]

It is generally accepted that neutrophils are important in the pathogenesis of ARDS.[96] Neutrophils cause tissue injury by two mechanisms: release of proteases, such as elastase, and production of reactive oxygen species.[97] Each of these has been measured in plasma and BAL fluid of patients in an attempt to predict development of ARDS. Gorden and associates noted markedly elevated plasma elastase levels very early after multisystem trauma.[98] These investigators subsequently demonstrated that plasma elastase levels were significantly elevated in patients who later developed ARDS compared to those who did not.[99] There was, however, considerable overlap in plasma elastase levels between the two groups. Neutrophil adhesion molecules are also possible markers for the development of ARDS. Initial plasma concentrations of soluble

L-selectin were significantly lower in patients who developed ARDS compared to those who did not; as with elastase levels, however, there was considerable overlap.

Increased expression of the CD11/CD18 receptor, a beta$_2$ integrin, was observed on the surface of circulating pulmonary artery neutrophils in patients at risk for postinjury ARDS.[100] Although early tissue sequestration of neutrophil and decreasing circulating neutrophil counts have been observed in patients who develop postinjury MOF, peripheral white blood cell, and neutrophil counts have not proven useful in predicting development of ARDS.[101,102] Similarly, thrombocytopenia has been associated with ARDS; however, it has not proven to be a reliable or specific predictor for development of lung injury.[82,103]

Circulating and BAL fluid levels of cytokines are also inherently attractive as predictors of ARDS. Cytokines are polypeptide molecules with diverse biologic functions, many of which have been implicated in the inflammatory process. Tumor necrosis factor-alpha (TNF-$\alpha$), interleukin-I$\beta$ (IL-1$\beta$), Interleukin-6, and Interleukin-8 have been the most intensely investigated in relation to the development of ARDS. Studies examining the predictive value of cytokines central to sepsis (TNF-$\alpha$ IL-1$\beta$) levels in ARDS have had negative or mixed results.[104-107] IL-8 is a neutrophil chemoattractant that has been studied both in plasma and BAL fluid. IL-8 is elevated in the plasma following injury but does not appear to consistently predict development of ARDS.[107,108] Plasma IL-8 measurements, however, are difficult to interpret because of red blood cell binding of IL-8.[109,110] Donnelly and colleagues studied 29 patients at risk for developing ARDS and observed that IL-8 levels in BAL fluid were significantly higher in patients who later progressed to ARDS.[111]

As discussed earlier, the complement system has also been studied as both a cause and a predictor of ARDS. Complement activation leads to neutrophil accumulation in the lung and has been highly associated with ARDS.[112,113]

Lipid mediators, such as PAF and leukotrienes, are potent inflammatory stimuli that have been associated with ARDS.[114] Whether these mediators are reliable and accurate predictors of ARDS in at-risk patients, however, remains to be determined.[115,116] Reactive oxygen species (ROS) and closely related reactive nitrogen species (RNS) released by activated neutrophils and macrophages are believed to be major contributors to ARDS. Because these radicals are unstable, investigators have focused on measurement of hydrogen peroxide, nitrosylated compounds, and antioxidant levels in various biological fluids. Catalase and manganese superoxide dismutase are elevated in the serum of patients at high risk for developing ARDS.[117]

## PATHOPHYSIOLOGY

ARDS is characterized by diffuse, patchy, panlobar pulmonary infiltrates on plain chest radiograph (Fig. 63-1). Computed tomography of the chest will demonstrate that the parenchymal changes are inhomogeneous with the dependent lung regions most affected (Fig. 63-2).[118-120] The inhomogeneous distribution of parenchymal densities led to the concept of a three-compartment model of the lung in ARDS.[121] One compartment is substantially normal (healthy zone); one is fully diseased without any possibility of recruitment (diseased zone); and, finally, the third compartment is composed of collapsed alveoli potentially

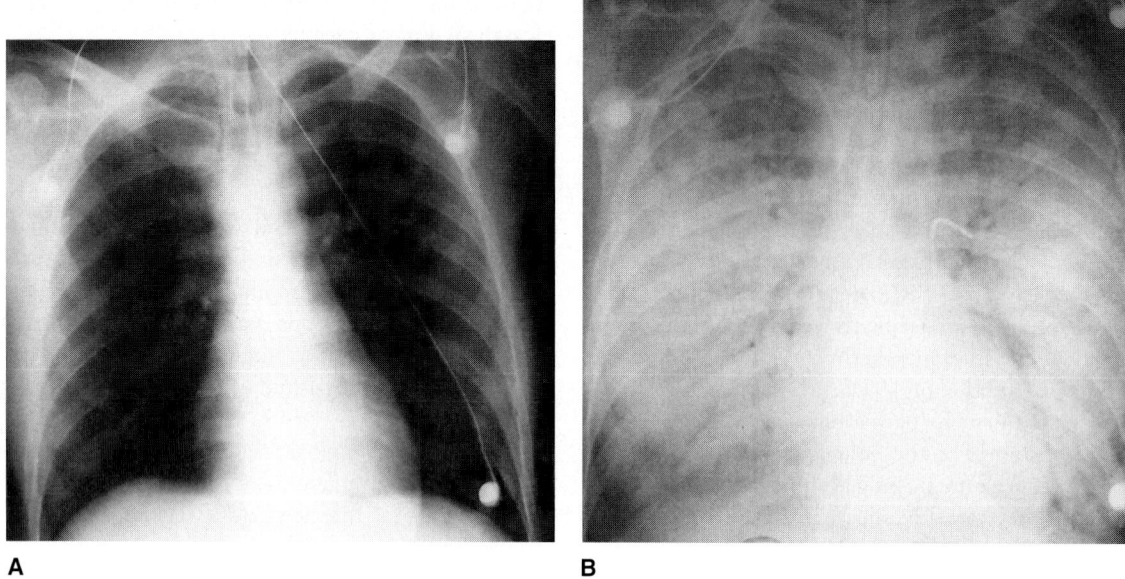

**FIGURE 63-1.** **(A)** Normal admission chest x-ray in a 27-year-old trauma patient with multiple lower extremity fractures. **(B)** Chest x-ray from the same patient following onset of respiratory insufficiency. Note the bilateral, dense pulmonary infiltrates consistent with severe ARDS.

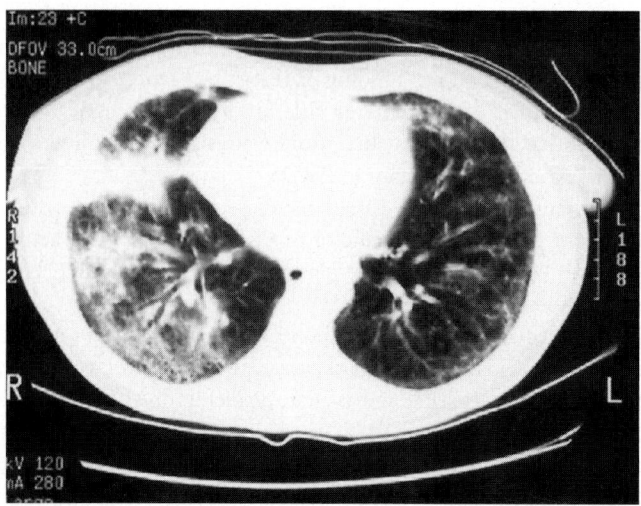

**FIGURE 63-2.** Chest CT scan of a patient with ARDS shows marked inhomogeneity of the process with areas of dense consolidation and essentially normal intervening pulmonary parenchyma.

**FIGURE 63-3.** Idealized static pressure-volume curve of the lungs in ARDS. At low pressures and volumes, derecruitment, atelectasis and lung injury from repetitive opening and closing of gas exchange units are a concern. At high pressures and volumes, overdistention, increased shunt and lung injury from excessive stretch predominate. Inbetween these two extremes is the optimal zone where lung stays recruited but is not overstretched.

recruitable with increasing pressure (recruitable zone). Using regional CT analysis, however, Pelosi observed that the lung parenchyma was homogeneously diseased, with an even distribution of edema throughout the lung.[122] This suggests that the vascular permeability defect in ARDS is evenly distributed as well, which has recently been demonstrated using nuclear imaging techniques.[123]

If the disease process is, in fact, homogeneous, how does one explain the inhomogeneous distribution of parenchymal densities? The "lung weight hypothesis" has suggested that the lung progressively collapses under its own weight (which is more than twice of that normal lung).[124] Increased airway pressure is necessary to recruit collapsed alveoli; however, this may result in overdistention of the open alveoli. This ventilator-induced lung injury may be

responsible for severe protracted ARDS, as well as perpetuation of systemic inflammation and MOF.[125,126]

A standard method used to describe the mechanical properties of the lung is to determine the static pressure–volume curve during inflation and deflation (Fig. 63-3). In early ARDS, the lower inflection point represents the airway pressure at which considerable alveolar recruitment occurs. The upper inflection point is where near maximal inflation occurs such that further increases in airway pressure result in alveolar overdistension and little change in volume. The "open lung approach" to mechanical ventilation in ARDS advocates setting PEEP at or just above the lower inflection point to avoid repetitive alveolar recruitment and collapse with each breath. In practice, however, inflection points in individual patients have been difficult to consistently measure.

## Pulmonary Edema

Increased pulmonary capillary permeability is a consistent feature. Increased permeability promotes alveolar flooding with protein-rich edema fluid, as well as release of proteins generally confined to the lung into the systemic circulation. Multiple studies have documented elevated total protein concentrations in BAL fluid from patients with established ARDS.[127–128] One study observed higher BAL fluid protein concentrations in nonsurvivors, suggesting that more severe lung injury is associated with greater endothelial and epithelial permeability.[129] Surfactant protein-A is normally found in appreciable quantities only in the lung; however, serum levels have been observed to be elevated in patients with ARDS compared to healthy controls.[130,131]

## GAS EXCHANGE

Hypoxemia in ARDS results from ventilation–perfusion mismatching and intrapulmonary shunting of blood flow. Shunting results from blood that passes through the systemic venous to pulmonary arterial system without going through the normal gas exchange units in the lung (i.e., right-left shunt). Normally, the shunt fraction is less than 5%; however, in ARDS, it may exceed 25%. Because blood flowing through a shunt is not exposed to alveoli participating in gas exchange, supplemental oxygen is ineffective in increasing arterial oxygen concentration. Other techniques designed to restore ventilation to nonventilated lung regions, such as PEEP or continuous positive airway pressure (CPAP), are thus necessary to improve oxygenation. Hypoxic pulmonary vasoconstriction is a protective mechanism that limits perfusion to poorly ventilated alveoli and minimizes shunting. In ARDS, hypoxic pulmonary constriction is impaired, resulting in greater intrapulmonary shunt. Multiple factors may contribute to loss of hypoxic pulmonary vasoconstriction in ALI, including local prostaglandin or nitric oxide production.[132–134]

In early ARDS, most patients are tachypneic from hypoxemia and are secondarily hypocapneic. With disease progression, hypercapnia may become a prominent feature because of physiologic deadspace and carbon dioxide ($CO_2$) production. Increased deadspace ventilation is invariably present. As discussed earlier, the normal deadspace to tidal volume ratio is approximately 35%; but in ARDS, it can approach 60%.

## PULMONARY MECHANICS

Lung compliance is defined as the change in lung volume per change in transpulmonary pressure. Normal lung compliance in a mechanically ventilated patient ranges from 60 to 80 mL/cm $H_2O$. With ARDS, it is not unusual to see greatly diminished lung compliance on the order of 10 to 30 mL/cm $H_2O$. Initially, reduced compliance is the result of interstitial and alveolar edema with alveolar flooding. Surfactant dysfunction and terminal bronchiolar spasm contribute to loss of ventilated alveoli. In later ARDS, interstitial fibrosis and parenchymal loss further reduce pulmonary compliance.

## CARDIOPULMONARY HEMODYNAMICS

Pulmonary hypertension is a frequent finding in patients with ARDS and can lead to increased interstitial pulmonary edema, right ventricular dysfunction, and impaired cardiac output. When severe, pulmonary hypertension has been observed to be a marker of poor outcome.[135] The etiology of pulmonary hypertension in ARDS is multifactorial. Early in ARDS, the predominant mechanism is most likely impaired vasorelaxation related to hypoxemia, acidosis, and vasoactive mediators, in concert with obstruction from microvascular coagulation. In late ARDS, fibrosis and obliteration of the pulmonary vascular bed are most likely responsible. Steltzer and coworkers noted markedly depressed right ventricular function in nonsurvivors of ARDS.[136] The authors related this to reduced myocardial contractility and not to pulmonary hypertension. They also noted that oxygen delivery was more related to cardiac performance than to pulmonary gas exchange.

## PRESENTATION

The diagnosis of ARDS is based on the criteria used to define the syndrome and can be divided into four clinical phases with radiographic, clinical, physiologic, and pathologic correlates (Table 63-5). In the initial phase, dyspnea and tachypnea are evident, with a remarkably normal chest examination (radiographically and clinically). Arterial oxygen saturation is preserved, and hypocapnia from hyperventilation is frequently noted.

The second phase quickly follows (12 to 24 hours), with physiologic and pathologic evidence of lung injury. The chest x-ray now shows bilateral patchy alveolar infiltrates with hypoxemia evident on arterial blood gas (ABG) determination. Heart size is normal, with a lack of perivascular cuffing unless the patient has concomitant cardiac disease or has received overly vigorous volume resuscitation.

If ARDS persists and progresses, the third clinical phase becomes evident. Acute respiratory failure necessitates mechanical ventilation with increasing inspired oxygen concentrations. There is an increase in physiologic deadspace and rising minute ventilation. Patients at this point may develop sepsis syndrome with a hyperdynamic hemodynamic pattern. The radiographic picture worsens with more diffuse infiltrates, consolidation, and air bronchograms.

Without resolution, progressive pulmonary failure and fibrosis characterize the fourth phase. Pneumonia, often recurrent, is frequent (see Chap. 18). Hypercapnia may worsen and become more difficult to control. MOF commonly develops and is the most common cause of death (see Chap. 68).

## MANAGEMENT

Because there is no proven specific treatment for ARDS, therapy primarily involves supportive measures to maintain life while the lung injury resolves. Such measures include identifying and treating predisposing conditions, mechanical ventilatory support with oxygen, nutritional support, nonpulmonary organ support, and hemodynamic monitoring as necessary. Attention to detail is necessary to avoid nosocomial infection and iatrogenic complications.

**TABLE 63-5**

## Pathophysiologic Changes of Modern Adult Respiratory Distress Syndrome (Low-Pressure Pulmonary Edema)

| RADIOGRAPHIC CHANGE | CLINICAL FINDING | PHYSIOLOGIC CHANGE | PATHOLOGIC CHANGE |
|---|---|---|---|
| **Phase 1 (Early Change)** | | | |
| Normal radiograph | Dyspnea, tachypnea, normal chest examination | Mild pulmonary hypertension, normoxemic or mild hypoxemia hypocarbia | Neutrophil sequestration, no clear tissue damage |
| **Phase 2 (Onset of Parenchymal Changes)[a]** | | | |
| Patchy alveolar infiltrates begining in dependent lung | Dyspnea, tachypnea, cyanosis, tachycardia, coarse rales | Pulmonary hypertension, normal wedge pressure, increased lung permeability, increased lung increasing shunt, progressive decrease in compliance, moderate-to-serve hypoxemia | Neutrophil infiltration, vascular congestion, fibrin strands, platelet clumps, alveolar septal edema, intraalveolar protein, white cells, type 1 epithelial damage |
| No perivascular cuffs (unless a component of water, high-pressure edema is present) | | | |
| Normal heart size | | | |
| **Phase 3 (Acute Respiratory Failure with Progression, 2–10 Days)** | | | |
| Diffuse alveolar infiltrates | Tachypnea, tachycardia, hyperdynamic state, sepsis syndrome, signs of consolidation, diffuse rhonchi | Phase 2 changes persist, progression of symptoms, increasing shunt fraction, further decrease in compliance, increased minute ventilation, impaired oxygen extraction of hemoglobin | Increased interstitial and alveolar inflammatory exudate with neutrophil and mononuclear cells, type II cell proliferation, beginning fibroblast proliferation, thromboembolic occlusion |
| Air bronchograms | | | |
| Decreased lung volume | | | |
| No bronchovascular cuffs | | | |
| Normal heart size | | | |
| **Phase 4 (Pulmonary Fibrosis-Pneumonia with Progression, >10 Days)[b]** | | | |
| Persistent diffuse infiltrates | Symptoms as above, recurrent sepsis, evidence of multiple-system organ failure | Phase 3 changes persist, recurrent pneumonia, progressive lung restriction, impaired tissue oxygenation, impaired oxygen extraction, multiple-system organ failure | Type II cell hyperplasia, interstitial thickening, infiltration of lymphocytes, macrophages, fibroblasts, loculated pneumonia and/or interstitial fibrosis, medial thickening and remodeling of arterioles |
| Superimposed new pneumonic infiltrates | | | |
| Recurrent pneumothorax | | | |
| Normal heart size | | | |
| Enlargement with pulmonale | | | |

[a]Process readily reversible at this stage if initiating factor controlled.

[b]Multiple-system organ failure common mortality rate > 80% at this stage, as resolution is more difficult.

*Source: From Demling RH: Adult respiratory distress syndrome: Current concepts. New Horiz 1:388, 1993.*

## FLUID MANAGEMENT AND HEMODYNAMIC SUPPORT

Given the central role of alveolar flooding in ARDS, the appropriate use of fluids and diuretics in managing patients has been a matter of debate since the description of this syndrome. In large part, the discussion centers on whether hydrostatic forces, or changes in membrane permeability are the prime contributors to capillary leak.

Some investigators believe that hydrostatic intravascular forces contribute significantly to pulmonary edema in ARDS and favor early diuresis and fluid restriction to minimize interstitial and alveolar edema.[137,138] With this approach, pulmonary capillary wedge pressure (PCWP) is maintained at 5 to 8 mm Hg; if necessary, cardiac output and blood pressure are supported with vasopressors. Potential problems with this approach include decreased end-organ perfusion with precipitation of MOF, and an increased shunt fraction. One study has observed that increased extravascular lung water did not correlate with oxygenation or outcome in ARDS patients, and calls into question the physiologic basis for this approach.[139] Because hypovolemia may be uniquely dangerous in the resuscitation of the injured patient, caution should be exercised before adopting such an approach.

Two landmark trials published by the ARDS network in 2006 attempted to address appropriate fluid management in this group of patients. In one study, a total of 1000 patients was randomized to either liberal or conservative fluid strategies over a period of seven days.[140] The conservative group received approximately a net one liter less per day, and spent 2.5 fewer days on the ventilator. There was no mortality difference and no increase in other organ failures in the conservative group. In the second study, care was based on either CVP measurements or pulmonary artery catheter measurements. This study also showed no difference in mortality. Overall, these studies do not show a profound effect of a specific invasive monitor or the amount of fluid administered. It may be that the uniform application of pressure-limited ventilation trumps any major effect of fluid balance in this patient population.

With respect to colloids, there is no evidence that their use for acute resuscitation improves outcome. It has been well documented that patients with ALI leak albumin and other large-molecular-weight proteins into the alveolar space.[141] Thus, colloids administered early in ARDS are likely to leak into the pulmonary interstitium and are unlikely to reduce tissue edema more than transiently. Theoretically, this increase in interstitial tissue albumin could actually delay the resolution of pulmonary edema. The use of colloids later in ARDS (when the capillary permeability has been restored) has not been well studied. A recent study in hypoproteinemic patients suggests that gas exchange can be improved in late ALI by using colloid in concert with diuretics to mobilize interstitial fluid and promote diuresis.[142] A 2006 randomized study also suggested that critically ill patients with profound hypoproteinemia have fewer organ failures (by SOFA score) when given colloid therapy.[143] Short-term improvement in physiology is not, however, accompanied by an improved outcome in these investigations. The very large Australian SAFE study suggests that routine use of albumin cannot be supported.[144] Thus, outside of the profoundly hypoproteinemic patient, it is difficult to argue that colloids are of any benefit.

## MECHANICAL VENTILATION

Respiratory support with a mechanical ventilator is a cornerstone in the supportive management of patients with or at risk for ARDS. It has become increasingly clear, however, that mechanical ventilation can perpetuate or worsen lung injury, as well as result in more readily recognized forms of barotrauma (mediastinal emphysema, pneumothorax, etc.). This recognition has led to the concept of lung protective strategies in mechanical ventilation.[145]

Most patients with ARDS require endotracheal intubation for mechanical ventilation. Patients with mild ALI may occasionally be managed initially with noninvasive positive pressure mask ventilation. This technique reduces shunt physiology and administers high concentrations of oxygen. It requires an alert and cooperative patient to tolerate the tight-fitting mask and avoid complications (in particular, vomiting and aspiration). Patients with multisystem injuries are frequently poor candidates for this approach. Emergent intubation is associated with significantly higher morbidity and mortality. Accordingly, early elective intubation should be considered in all patients with deteriorating gas exchange or mental status. Initially, oral endotracheal intubation is the preferred route. Although nasotracheal intubation is feasible, this route is associated with frequent sinusitis (87% in patients intubated more than six days)[146] and often limits the size of the endotracheal tube to 7.5 or less. This reduction in tube size may limit the ability to safely perform diagnostic and therapeutic bronchoscopy. Moreover, airway resistance and peak airway pressure are increased, potentially interfering with ventilation and resulting in auto-PEEP.

Traditional ventilation strategies used in the ICU have evolved directly from anesthetic and surgical applications.[147] In the past, relatively large tidal volumes (10 to 15 mL/kg) were used to achieve normal gas exchange while avoiding microatelectasis and patient discomfort. With little modification and the addition of PEEP, this approach was applied as the standard for most critically ill patients. In the setting of ARDS, the conventional goals of mechanical ventilation have been to achieve adequate oxygenation using the least PEEP possible and a nontoxic $FIO_2$ while at the same time maintaining normocarbia. This strategy was intended to minimize or avoid hyperoxic lung injury and the adverse effects of PEEP. The primary priority has shifted from maximizing tissue oxygen delivery to ensuring adequate lung protection (Table 63-6).

## POSITIVE END-EXPIRATORY PRESSURE

PEEP is one of several methods of increasing mean airway pressure and improving oxygenation. Ashbaugh and colleagues first recommended its use in the ventilatory management of ARDS in 1967.[14] Since then, PEEP has become a key element of all ventilator management strategies for ARDS. PEEP improves oxygenation by enhancing lung volume, and increasing functional residual capacity (FRC) through recruitment of collapsed alveoli. Moreover, extravascular lung water is redistributed from the alveolar to the interstitial space. The net effect is an increase in total alveolar sur-

**TABLE 63-6**

| Ventilatory Strategies in ARDS | | |
| --- | --- | --- |
| | **CONVENTIONAL** | **LUNG PROTECTIVE** |
| Goals | Normal arterial blood gases | Acceptable arterial blood gases |
| | Nontoxic $FIO_2$ ($\leq 0.50$) | Prevent alveolar damage |
| | Adequate $O_2$ delivery | Facilitate healing |
| | | Nontoxic $FIO_2$ ($\leq 0.50$) |
| Ventilator mode | Volume-cycled | Pressure-limited |
| Settings | | |
| Tidal volume | 10–15 mL/kg | 4–8 mL/kg/IBW |
| PEEP | 5–20 $cmH_2O$ as needed | Sufficient to prevent tidal recruitment/derecruitment |
| | | Achieve acceptable $PaO_2/FIO_2$ ratio |
| I:E ratio | 1:2 to 1:4 | 1:1 to 1:4 |
| Plateau airway pressure | As required by PEEP and tidal volume | < 30 $cmH_2O$ |

face available for gas exchange and a decrease in the shunt fraction. Lung compliance may also be improved. The use of PEEP in patients with ARDS has two primary goals: adequate tissue oxygen delivery and the reduction of $FIO_2$ to nontoxic (generally below 0.6) levels. Increasing PEEP above a certain level, however, may have significant adverse effects. By raising intrathoracic pressure, PEEP may significantly reduce venous return and cardiac output.[148] This may result in decreased tissue oxygen delivery despite improvement in arterial oxygen saturation. This effect is accentuated in the hypovolemic patient, and can usually be reversed with intravascular volume expansion. Cardiac depression is rarely seen with PEEP levels less than or equal to 10 cm $H_2O$. IF PEEP >10 cm $H_2O$ is required, pulmonary artery catheterization should be considered to help assess preload and monitor the effects of PEEP on oxygen delivery. It is important to remember that PEEP may elevate the measured PCWP because some of the elevation in mean airway pressure produced by PEEP is transmitted to the intravascular space (see Chap. 62). Measurement of right ventricular end-diastolic volume index may be a more accurate indicator of preload in this setting.[149,150]

PEEP may also result in alveolar overdistention with compression and obliteration of surrounding pulmonary capillaries. This alveolar overdistention may actually worsen oxygenation by increasing the shunt fraction. Moreover, deadspace ventilation may be increased, resulting in a higher minute ventilation requirement. Finally, PEEP may cause a maldistribution of tidal volumes and pressures, creating overdistension of normally aerated lung regions. This hyperinflated form of lung injury may result in barotrauma referred to as "volutrauma."

The optimal approach to PEEP for ARDS remains a matter of debate. Several strategies have been proposed for determining optimal PEEP.[151] "Best PEEP" is that PEEP level where static lung compliance is greatest. "Optimal" PEEP is directed toward achieving the lowest shunt fraction. In "preferred" PEEP, the goal is maximal oxygen delivery. The most conservative approach is the use of "least" PEEP, in which the lowest amount of PEEP is used to reduce the $FIO_2$ to a nontoxic level (0.5 to 0.6) while maintaining adequate arterial oxygenation. In the ARDS-net trial comparing high to low PEEP in a low tidal volume strategy, there was no clear difference in outcomes.[152]

Given the potential adverse effects, the application of PEEP needs to be balanced between providing a sufficient inspiratory plateau pressure (peak alveolar pressure) thus maintaining adequate oxygenation while at the same time avoiding derecruitment of the alveoli during exhalation. Figure 63-3 demonstrates the area on the pressure-volume curve where optimal ventilation occurs. In the early management of patients with acute lung injury, a formal PEEP trial should be performed. During a PEEP trial, blood gas and hemodynamic measurements are made at baseline and after incremental increases in PEEP. PEEP is usually increased in 5 cm $H_2O$ increments, and effects (such as $PaCO_2$, arterial oxygen saturation, airway pressures, cardiac output, etc.) are measured 15 to 30 minutes later.

With recent ventilatory strategies emphasizing pressure-limiting techniques, the "least" PEEP method seems logical. This approach has been associated with less barotrauma and cardiac compromise.[153] The use of minimal PEEP, however, does not address the potential damage from repeated alveolar opening and collapse with each breath.[154] This forms the basis for the "open lung" ventilation strategy. Static pressure-volume curves are used to select a PEEP level above the lower infection point to prevent alveolar end-expiratory collapse. Although this approach is intriguing, static pressure-volume curves can be difficult to obtain as well as to implement.

Practically speaking, bedside PEEP trials are frequently initiated in response to worsening hypoxemia. We identify the optimal or least PEEP in the following manner. Baseline PEEP is set at 10 cm $H_2O$, with a $V_t$ of 6 mL/kg ideal body weight. If the patient desaturates then the patient is recruited for two minutes using pressure controlled ventilation with a PIP of 20 cm $H_2O$, a respiratory rate of 10 breaths per minute and an I:E of 1:1 with PEEP raised to 25–40 cm $H_2O$ for approximately two minutes. The patient is monitored for cardiopulmonary instability during recruitment because this maneuver may result in substantial hypoventilation for the period of recruitment. The patient is returned to his/her previous settings and if desaturation reoccurs the recruitment maneuver is repeated for two minutes and the patient is returned to their previous ventilator settings except the PEEP is increased by 2.5 to 5 cm $H_2O$. This process is repeated as need until oxygen saturation remains stable.

With improvement in the patient's lung injury, PEEP should be withdrawn as the pulmonary compliance, shunt fraction and dead space ventilation improves. Premature attempts at PEEP reduction, however, will only delay resolution of lung injury and prolong the need for ventilatory support. PEEP weaning should be performed in an orderly fashion. PEEP is reduced slowly in 2.5 to 5 cm $H_2O$ increments, with serial monitoring of arterial oxygen saturation using ABG or oximetry. In general, tidal volumes should be increased to both maintain mean airway pressure and allow respiratory rates associated with greater patient comfort. A significant decrease in $PaO_2$ should prompt a quick return to previous levels of PEEP. Once alveolar collapse and loss of FRC occur, higher levels of PEEP for more prolonged periods may be needed. Generally, PEEP should not be reduced by more than 3 to 5 cm $H_2O$ in a 12-hour period.

## PRESSURE-LIMITED VENTILATORY SUPPORT

In patients with ARDS, the aerated lung volume able to participate in gas exchange is markedly reduced to one-third of the original volume.[155] Thus, in nonfibrotic stages of ARDS, the lungs may be thought of as small rather than stiff. There is accumulating evidence that pulmonary gas exchange may be essentially normal in the aerated portion of the injured lung.[156] The use of conventional tidal volumes in this setting would be expected to result in alveolar overdistention with further impairment of gas exchange, frequent barotrauma, and ventilator-induced lung injury.

One approach is to reduce tidal volume in order to limit airway pressures while maintaining adequate alveolar ventilation with an increased respiratory rate. While the safe upper limit of airway pressure is not precisely known, pressure in excess of 35 to 40 cm $H_2O$ are associated with lung injury in animal models.[157] A benchmark clinical trials of low volume, pressure-limited ventilation in established ARDS is now complete.[158] In this study, patients ventilated using smaller (6 cc/kg) tidal volume had a mortality of 31% versus a 40% mortality in a group ventilated with a larger (12 cc/kg) tidal volumes. This study has solidified the basis for "low stretch" strategies which are thought to diminish both local and systemic inflammation.

## PERMISSIVE HYPERCAPNIA

Now that the importance of defending airway pressures has been highlighted in the survival advantage of low versus high tidal volume, the maintenance of eucapnia is no longer stressed. This goal can be difficult to meet with the increased physiologic deadspace and hypermetabolism frequently associated with ARDS. Moreover, pressure-limited ventilatory strategies may lead to decreased minute ventilation and hypercapnia. Controlled hypoventilation with increased $PaCO_2$ is referred to as permissive hypercapnia.[159] Gradual increases in $PaCO_2$ are usually well tolerated, provided renal compensation is adequate (see Chap. 65) and severe acidosis (pH <7.1) does not occur.

Respiratory acidosis has a myriad of physiologic effects that may be relevant to the critical care physician. Because $CO_2$ diffuses freely across cell membranes, an increase in extracellular $PCO_2$ will result in intracellular acidosis.[160] The decrease in intracellular pH may occur rapidly because of the abundance of cytosolic carbonic anhydrase.[161] The cellular effects of hypercapnia are related to the severity and regulation of intracellular acidosis. Cytosolic pH is normally tightly regulated between 6.9 and 7.2.[162] Three mechanisms are responsible for this regulation: (1) physiochemical buffering, mainly due to proteins and phosphates; (2) reduced intracellular generation of protons; and (3) changes in transmembrane ion exchange. Physiochemical buffering is immediate, while the other mechanisms require one to three hours.[163] These regulatory mechanisms are remarkably powerful and efficient. As a result, normoxic hypercapnia has only limited potential for resulting in intracellular acidosis.

Hypercapnia has multiple cardiovascular effects. Acute respiratory acidosis results in reversible impairment of myocardial contractility. The principal mechanism for this decrease in cardiac contractility is intracellular acidosis, which interferes with myofilament responsiveness to activator calcium.[164] Hypercapnia may lead to a substantial increase in coronary flow and a rise in coronary sinus oxygen tension. The overall hemodynamic response to acute hypercapnia in human experiments is increased cardiac output, heart rate, and stroke volume, with decreased systemic vascular resistance. This reflects the net result of the myocardial depressive effects of $CO_2$, as well as indirect effects with stimulation of the sympathetic nervous system and catecholamine release.[165,166] Hypercapnia may adversely affect right ventricular function. It results in pulmonary vasoconstriction and may lead to pulmonary hypertension with right ventricular dysfunction.[167]

Increased $PCO_2$ produces a rightward shift of the oxygen–hemoglobin dissociation curve by two mechanisms. The major mechanism is related to $CO_2$ hydration to carbonic acid with increased hydrogen ion concentration. The other involves the formation of carbamino compounds from $CO_2$ reacting with amino acids on the hemoglobin molecule. This rightward shift of the curve increases the P50 and facilitates unloading of oxygen at the tissue level. This decreased affinity, however, may compromise oxygen loading at the alveolar level. Thus, with hypoxemia, severe hypercapnia may produce a dramatic decrease in arterial oxygen saturation.

Hypercapnia has multiple effects on the CNS. Similar acid-base changes to those described above also occur in the brain. Preliminary studies suggest a decrease in the oxygen demand of the brain.[168] It has long been recognized that hypercarbia increases cerebral blood flow and intracranial pressure. Increased intracranial pressure results from enlargement of cerebral blood volume secondary to diminished vascular tone.

Other miscellaneous effects of hypercarbia include release of epinephrine and norepinephrine from adrenal medulla stimulation and increased secretion of adrenocorticotropic hormone, cortisol, aldosterone, and antidiuretic hormone.[163]

Contraindications to permissive hypercapnia include increased intracranial pressure or other cerebral disorders in which intracranial hypertension may be detrimental. Uncorrected hypovolemia and significant cardiac disease are relative contraindications due to the negative inotropic effects of permissive hypercarbia.

Several reports document that permissive hypercapnia in the setting of ARDS is remarkably well tolerated.[159,169,170] Ideally, this strategy should be implemented slowly over several hours to allow compensatory mechanisms to act. The role of sodium bicarbonate infusion is unclear. In most institutions, sodium bicarbonate would not be administered unless the pH was less than 7.2. With increased experience, however, many centers reserve bicarbonate infusion for pH less than 7.0.[162] Sedation is mandatory with permissive hypercapnia in mechanically ventilated patients in order to control respiratory drive and prevent discomfort. Even with heavy sedation, however, respiratory drive may be insufficiently suppressed, resulting in patient–ventilator dyssynchrony. Neuromuscular blockade is often necessary in these patients.

## PRESSURE CONTROL AND INVERSE RATIO VENTILATION

Pressure-control ventilation uses a fixed, preset pressure applied to the airway for a defined time period or a percentage of the respiratory cycle. As such, the delivered tidal volume depends on the lung compliance and will vary if airway resistance or lung compliance changes. Inverse ratio ventilation (IRV) is an alternative ventilatory strategy in which the inspiratory time is greater than the expiratory time; in other words, the I:E ratio is greater than 1.[171] This results in sustained elevation of mean air pressure and reduced peak airway pressure. It is theorized that the sustained elevation in mean

airway pressure recruits collapsed alveoli. The salutary effects of IRV on gas exchange can be explained by a lung model in which different regions of the lung have different time constants (determined by regional airway resistance and lung compliance). "Slow" lung compartments have high airway resistance and low compliance. Thus, alveolar opening and gas equilibration occur more slowly. Deliberately lengthening the inspiratory time and the I:E ratio allows these slower alveolar compartments to be recruited and more time for gas exchange. Moreover, regional air trapping or auto-PEEP keeps the compartments open throughout the respiratory cycle. External PEEP is still necessary to prevent tidal collapse of fast lung compartments. Therefore, the combination of external PEEP and IRV (with auto-PEEP) may improve the gas exchange by improving ventilation–perfusion matching in the setting of heterogeneous lung injury (in which time constants vary considerably within the lung).

IRV can be accomplished using either volume-control or pressure-control ventilation. In volume-control IRV, low inspiratory flow rates, an inspiratory pause, or a decelerating flow pattern may be used alone or in combination. In this model, airflow and tidal volume are set, while airway pressure is allowed to vary. In pressure-control IRV, a pressure limit is set with a square wave airway pressure pattern and a decelerating flow pattern. Therefore, tidal volume and airflow may vary depending on airway resistance and lung compliance. The advantages of volume-control IRV are its availability on all standard ventilators, similarity to conventional volume-control ventilation and delivery of a guaranteed tidal volume. The major advantage of pressure-control IRV is the ability to limit peak airway pressure to a predetermined level. The rapid inspiratory flow and pressure rise may recruit more alveoli and allow time for equilibration of gas exchange. The lack of guaranteed tidal volume, however, demands close observation.

This mode of ventilation is rarely used today; we prefer to utilize frequent recruitment maneuvers and extrinsic PEEP. IRV is not a physiologic mode of ventilation and patients almost universally require neuromuscular blockade and sedation to facilitate patient–ventilator synchrony. Auto-PEEP can have the same detrimental effects as extrinsic PEEP and needs careful monitoring during IRV. Finally, recruitment of collapsed alveoli with IRV can take several hours to occur. Thus, clinical improvement may be delayed as well.[172]

## PRONE VENTILATION

Recently, there has been growing interest in mechanical ventilation of ARDS patients in the prone position. Bryan described the beneficial effects of the prone position on arterial oxygenation more than 30 years ago.[173] Other investigators subsequently confirmed these findings.[174–176] Although large controlled studies are lacking, it appears that at least 50% of patients show improved oxygenation with prone positioning.[176–179] Although these initial reports did not explore the mechanisms by which oxygenation is improved, several potential explanations were suggested. These include improved removal of secretions, increased FRC, a change in regional diaphragm motion, and redistribution of perfusion along a gravitational gradient to less injured lung regions.

Pappert and colleagues used the multiple inert gas elimination technique and showed that the improvement in oxygenation was the result of decreased intrapulmonary shunt fraction.[177] Albert and coworkers have investigated the mechanism of prone ventilation in a canine oleic acid model of ARDS.[180] The prone position consistently reduced shunt fraction compared with the supine position. The improvement in gas exchange was independent of changes in cardiac output or FRC between the two positions. Subsequently, pulmonary blood flow was shown to be distributed preferentially to dorsal lung regions in the supine and prone positions.[181] In supine animals, pleural pressure increases from nondependent to dependent regions. This may lead to dependent atelectasis in the highly perfused dorsal lung regions, resulting in intrapulmonary shunt and hypoxemia. In the prone position, the pleural pressure gradient is less, and the dorsal (now nondependent) regions are exposed to a lower pleural pressure. This results in opening of previously atelectatic alveoli. Intrapulmonary shunting is reduced because perfusion of the dorsal lung regions is maintained. Lamm and colleagues recently confirmed this mechanism in a canine oleic acid lung injury model.[182] The investigators used single photon emission computed tomography (SPECT) scanning to quantitate regional ventilation and perfusion. Supine animals had markedly reduced or absent ventilation to the dorsal lung regions while maintaining perfusion to those areas. With prone positioning, ventilation of dorsal regions improved significantly and perfusion was maintained. Using chest CT, Gattinoni and colleagues showed that in the supine position, gasless lung was found predominantly in the dorsal regions.[183] With prone positioning, densities redistributed to the ventral areas and dorsal regions were well aerated. Thus, prone positioning results in recruitment of previously atelectatic dorsal lung regions.

Although prone positioning appears to improve oxygenation in many patients with ARDS, a significant number of patients have no response. In a small number of patients, gas exchange actually deteriorates. Currently, responders to prone positioning cannot be reliably predicted while in the supine positions.

Despite early reports documenting improved gas excange in approximately two-thirds of patients it is remarkable that it took 20 years for the first prospective, randomized trial to be performed. The trial, reported by Gattinoni et al.[184] consisted of 152 patients randomized to a prone group and 152 patients to a supine group. Patients randomized to the prone arm were followed for the first 10 days and turned prone for at least six hours each day if they met the necessary criteria. Regrettably, no differences in mortality rates were noted between the two groups after a 10-day period (21.1% vs. 25%). A post hoc analysis revealed that patients with severe hypoxemia, defined as a $P/F$ ratio <90, an APACHE score >49 or having been exposed to high $V_t$ (>12 mL/kg) mortality was significantly lower in the prone group than in the supine group (20.5% vs. 40.00%). Retrospective analysis of these data in a separate report indicated that the best predictor of improved outcome during prone ventilation was a decrease in the $PaCO_2$ and not the response to arterial oxygenation. Since the Gattinoni trial there have been three other randomized trials of prone ventilation. Unfortunately, these studies do not strongly suggest that prone positioning affects survival.[185–187]

Prone positioning must be performed with care to avoid inadvertent extubation or loss of intravenous lines or chest tubes.

Transient hemodynamic instability and desaturation may also occur during repositioning. Cardiopulmonary resuscitation is difficult, if not impossible, in the prone position. Placement of multifunction electrode pads, which allow defibrillation, cardioversion, and pacing, has been recommended to facilitate cardiopulmonary resuscitation in the prone position.[188] Other areas of concern that accompany prone positioning include facial and eyelid edema, peripheral nerve injury, tongue injuries, and skin necrosis.[189] Multiply injured patients may present unique problems due to the presence of incisions, drainage tubes, extremity fractures, cervical spine or facial fractures, and the like. In some challenging patients, we have used a halo to facilitate prone positioning. Other important questions remain regarding the use of prone positioning. In patients who respond, how long should prone positioning be maintained? Some suggest that it be limited to 8 to 12 hours to allow for patient care.[190] It is not clear that this is necessary except for procedures that can only be performed supine (i.e., central line placement). A subset of patients will maintain improved oxygenation when returned to the supine position. Should prone positioning be considered for reasons other than refractory hypoxemia? Should prone positioning be used prophylactically in patients at risk for ARDS or those likely to have prolonged mechanical ventilation? Further investigation is needed to define the role of prone positioning in ARDS.

## TRACHEAL GAS INSUFFLATION

Tracheal gas insufflation (TGI) is a technique used to improve the ventilatory efficiency of mechanical ventilation. This may be necessary for several reasons. Deadspace ventilation is increased significantly in patients with ARDS due to microvascular obliteration. Moreover, positive pressure ventilation may further increase deadspace ventilation by alveolar overdistention and compression of interstitial vascular beds. Pressure-limited ventilation strategies may also decrease minute ventilation and result in hypercarbia. TGI is performed by continuous or phasic insufflation of fresh gas into the central airways. This fresh gas flushes the $CO_2$ accumulated in the anatomic deadspace and enhances gas mixing in the distal airways.[190] Elimination of $CO_2$ during TGI depends on catheter flow rate and position. Higher flow rates flush a greater portion of the proximal deadspace and generate more distal turbulence. Distal catheter placement further enhances this effect.[191] The exact location of the catheter tip is not crucial as long as it is within a few centimeters of the main carina.

TGI increases end-expiratory lung volume in three ways. First, part of the momentum of the gas stream is transmitted to the alveoli. Second, placement of the TGI catheter within the trachea decreases its cross-sectional area, increases expiratory resistance, and delays emptying. Finally, catheter flow through the endotracheal tube and ventilator circuit during expiration can result in back pressure that impedes expiratory flow from the lung. One report on the use of TGI in nine out of 69 trauma patients being treated with permissive hypercapnia for ARDS[192] noted a significant improvement in pH, $PCO_2$, and minute ventilation. Prospective clinical trials are needed to further define the role of TGI in the management of patients with ARDS.

TGI has several potential complications. With high flows delivered into the airways, any obstruction to outflow of gas may overinflate the lungs and result in barotrauma, venous air embolism, or hemodynamic compromise. Monitoring of basic ventilatory parameters is difficult during TGI. Tracheobronchial mucosal damage from the gas stream or catheter tip is another concern. Moreover, inspissation and retention of secretions may occur if there is inadequate humidification of the insufflated gas. Finally, placement of the TGI catheter through the endotracheal tube interferes with tracheal suctioning. Newly designed endotracheal tubes with built-in TGI channels will solve many of these problems and simplify the use of TGI.

## HIGH-FREQUENCY VENTILATION

Recognition of the impact of mechanical ventilation on furthering lung injury has been the leading impetus to focus on newer modes of ventilation such as high frequency modes of ventilation (HFV).

Several modes of high-frequency ventilation are available, including high-frequency jet ventilation, high-frequency positive pressure ventilation, ultra-high-frequency ventilation, and high-frequency oscillatory ventilation. These techniques use very small tidal volumes (1 to 5 mL/kg) delivered at rates of 60 to 3600 cycles/minute. To date there are a number of prospective clinical studies which have failed to demonstrate any meaningful benefit of high-frequency ventilation over conventional modes of positive pressure ventilation in patients with ARDS.[193–195] Although peak airway pressures are reduced compared to conventional modes, mean airway pressures, barotrauma, and hemodynamic compromise appear unchanged. A preliminary report using ultra-high-frequency ventilation showed improved gas exchange and reduced airway pressures both at 1 hour and 24 hours in patients with severe ARDS.[196] Ultra-high-frequency ventilation uses respiratory rates at or near the resonant frequency of the lung. Theoretically, this method takes advantage of the diminished impedance resulting from the resonant frequency ventilation and improves gas exchange.

Over the last ten years, proponents of high-frequency ventilation argue that it provides the ideal approach to lung protective ventilation. By definition, HFV delivers an extremely low tidal volume in concert with a relatively high mean airway pressure using a piston pump. Mean airway pressures of 25–45 cm $H_2O$ are not unusual. Delivery of plateau pressures in this range with tidal volumes that may be just larger than dead space ventilation, perhaps as high as 5 mL/kg may not be equally protective in all settings of lung injury. For example, will ARDS that is caused by a direct pulmonary insult such as aspiration respond the same as an injured lung from a nonpulmonary cause of ARDS such as pancreatitis? In an effort to answer these types of questions recently investigators from the Multicenter Oscillatory Ventilation for Acute Respiratory Distress Syndrome Trial (MOAT) published the results of a randomized, controlled study comparing HFV with a CV arm in adults with early ARDS.[197] One hundred and forty-eight patients were enrolled with 75 randomized to HFV and 73 to CV. The primary study end point was safety and effectiveness of HFV compared to CV. Tidal volume in the CV group was based on actual weight and averaged 10.2 mL/kg, while peak airway pressures were 38 cm $H_2O$. As expected, mean airway pressures were signficantly higher at 29 versus 23 cm $H_2O$ in the HFV group. Oxygenation, as evidenced by the $PaO_2/FIO_2$ ratio, was higher in the initial 16 hours in the HFV group but was subsequently decreased and the *P/F* ratio was no longer significantly different between the two groups. While not statistically significant, there was a clear trend toward a better outcome in the HFV group; mortality was 37% in the HFV group and 52% in the CV group ($p = 0.12$). It is regrettable, however, that this trial failed to provide a lung-protective approach for the CV group. So, until a true, randomized, prospective trial comparing HFV to CV using a lung protective strategy is performed, all we really know is that HFV is safe and effective when compared to CV.

Currently, the primary clinical indications for high-frequency ventilation include treatment of neonatal respiratory distress syndrome, ventilatory support during proximal airway procedures, and significant bronchopleural fistulas (see Chap. 26). Bronchopleural fistulae are frequently present in ARDS patients, either as a result of their underlying disease or as a consequence of their treatment (barotrauma). High-frequency ventilation is theoretically beneficial in patients with a bronchopleural fistula because of decreased airway pressures. Clinical trials to date have shown varied results, ranging from improved air leaks with fistula healing to worsening gas exchange and larger air leaks.[198,199]

## EXTRACORPOREAL LIFE SUPPORT

Extracorporeal life support (ECLS) is the new term for what was previously called extracorporeal membrane oxygenation (ECMO). ECLS also encompasses the technique of extracorporeal carbon dioxide removal ($ECCO_2R$). It is a modified form of cardiopulmonary bypass that allows for oxygenation and $CO_2$ removal while "resting" the lungs. During ECLS, gas exchange occurs independent of the lungs. Therefore, the lungs are not exposed to potential barotrauma from mechanical ventilation or to oxygen toxicity from exposure to toxic $FIO_2$ levels. Theoretically, the lung is better able to heal during this period of rest and support.

A multicenter, prospective trial of ECLS using venoarterial bypass in the late 1970s did not demonstrate improved survival in patients with severe ARDS.[200] In contrast, this modality has achieved success in managing neonates with persistent pulmonary hypertension and is considered the standard of care in this group. The technology has changed considerably and more recent studies in adults with ARDS suggest better survival rates compared to historical controls.[201] The lack of both concurrent control groups and randomization make these studies difficult to interpret. The principal complication of ECLS is hemorrhage due to the need for systemic heparinization and frequent thrombocytopenia. Moreover, ECLS is extremely labor intensive and costly. Technical advancements, such as heparin-bonded circuits may alleviate many of these problems. $ECCO_2R$ is still used in Europe. In the United States, however, no survival benefit was identified in a group of patients with ARDS who were treated with $ECCO_2R$.[202] The intravenous gas exchange catheter (IVOX) is a potentially less invasive option for augmenting gas exchange.[203,204] This device contains a gas-permeable membrane of hollow core fibers that allow $CO_2$ and $O_2$ exchange. It is placed into the inferior vena cava by femoral cutdown and is connected to an $O_2$ source. Significant complications have been associated with this device, including vena cava and hepatic vein obstruction, bleeding, thrombocytopenia, and infection.[205]

## PARTIAL LIQUID VENTILATION

Intratracheal administration of perfluorocarbon, a compound with low surface tension and high solubility for $O_2$ and $CO_2$ has been shown to improve gas exchange and lung compliance in animal models.[206,207] Partial liquid ventilation may improve lung mechanics by two mechanisms. Perfluorocarbon may act as exogenous surfactant and decrease surface tension of the alveoli, thus stabilizing and preserving alveolar patency. In addition, the perfluorocarbon fills the alveoli and physically distends the lung parenchyma.[208,209] Partial liquid ventilation may potentially improve surface tension, recruit alveoli, maintain alveolar recruitment, and improve ventilation–perfusion mismatch. Moreover, it can theoretically provide a cleansing action with removal of debris and bacteria from the alveoli, provide a method of direct delivery for drugs (such as antibiotics), and modulate the alveolar inflammatory response. Hirschl and colleagues reported a randomized study in 2002 which showed positive subgroup trends in a post hoc analysis but also documented complications such as bradycardia and hypercapnia with this approach.[210]

## PHARMACOLOGIC THERAPY

### Inhaled Nitric Oxide

Pulmonary hypertension is a frequent finding in patients with ARDS and can lead to increased interstitial pulmonary edema, right ventricular dysfunction, and impaired cardiac output. When severe, it has been observed to be a marker of poor outcome.[211] Intravenous vasodilators have been used in an attempt to lower pulmonary artery pressure in ARDS; however, they have not proven beneficial. Moreover, their use may be associated with systemic vasodilation and hypotension. Intravenous vasodilators may increase ventilation–perfusion mismatching, leading to worsening hypoxemia and impaired peripheral oxygen delivery. This is due to indiscriminate vasodilation of the entire pulmonary vascular bed, including areas that are not being ventilated.[212]

Nitric oxide (NO) has been identified as endothelium-derived relaxation factor and probably is responsible for regulation of basal vascular tone.[213] When delivered by the inhaled route, nitric oxide is a selective pulmonary vasodilator with no systemic side effects. This is related to its rapid binding and inactivation by hemoglobin.[214] Moreover, delivery of NO by the inhaled route exposes only ventilated alveoli to its vasodilatory effects. Selective vasodilation of pulmonary vessels in ventilated areas diverts blood away from nonventilated areas, improving ventilation–perfusion matching and hypoxemia. NO decreases

mean pulmonary artery pressure, and in doing so, lessens the hydrostatic pressure for pulmonary edema.[215] In a porcine model of endotoxin-induced ALI, inhaled NO was shown to reduce pulmonary hypertension, improve right ventricular ejection fraction, improve ventilation–perfusion matching, and increase arterial oxygen saturation.[216,217] Clinical studies have demonstrated similar results[218–220]; however, the response is highly variable.[221–223] Consistent predictors of who will respond to inhaled NO have not been identified. In certain animal models, the multiple inert gas elimination technique (MIGET) has shown that improvement in oxygenation with inhaled NO is associated with a redistribution of blood flow away from shunt areas.[224] In other animal models of ARDS, in particular the oleic acid model, inhaled NO poorly improves oxygenation.[225] These experimental studies suggest that inhaled NO will be effective only in improving oxygenation in lung injury where blood flow can be diverted away from shunt areas to those that have normal ventilation–perfusion distribution. If low ventilation–perfusion areas are predominantly responsible for hypoxemia, inhaled NO cannot impact oxygenation.

It appears that achieving maximal oxygenation benefit from inhaled NO may require other maneuvers to optimize alveolar recruitment. Such maneuvers could include titration of PEEP, IRV, or prone ventilation.[226–229] The combination of inhaled NO and a selective pulmonary vasoconstrictor has been suggested. Such agents would theoretically enhance pulmonary vasoconstriction in nonventilated lung units and further improve ventilation–perfusion matching with inhaled NO. Lu and colleagues recently reported results using almitrine bimesylate, a selective pulmonary vasoconstrictor, in combination with inhaled NO.[230] They observed that responders to inhaled NO alone had further improvements in oxygenation with the addition of almitrine.

Results of five prospective randomized clinical trials of inhaled NO versus placebo or standard therapy have been reported.[231–235] The results are remarkably similar and not encouraging. The largest trial was a multicenter study and was placebo controlled and blinded (Dellinger, 1998, p. 245). Results from this study used fixed doses of NO at 0,1.25,5, 20, and 40 parts per million were delivered to patients with ARDS from causes other than sepsis. Only at doses at 5 ppm were there decreases (not statistically significant) in the oxygenation index and duration of mechanical ventilation. As a result of this trial, the investigators went on to perform a low dose trial using 5 ppm of NO versus a placebo.[234] The primary endpoints were days alive and off assisted ventilation. Mortality was actually a secondary outcome variable, as was meeting extubation criteria. Not surprisingly, there was a statistically significant increase in $PaO_2$, but this diminished after 48 hours. Unfortunately, inhaled NO at 5 PPM had no substantial effect on duration of mechanical ventilation or mortality. Currently, the role NO should be limited to those patients with severe, refractory hypoxemia, or pulmonary hypertension in which inhaled NO may act as a "bridge" allowing short-term physiologic support. Application of NO in these situations may allow for possible patient survival until other therapies may be employed such as pronation or alternative modes of ventilation. Given the apparent transient effects and rebound phenomenon (discussed below), fixed dosing of NO may not be the optimal approach.[235]

Most studies observe that inhaled NO resulted in only modest improvements in oxygenation that were not sustained beyond

24 hours and frequently did not allow significant reduction in the intensity of ventilatory support. There were no differences in mortality in any of the studies. The multicenter trial also noted no differences in the number of days alive and the number days off mechanical ventilation. Some argue that these results are not surprising given that the minority of ARDS patients die of respiratory failure. Moreover, inhaled NO should be viewed as supportive therapy, much like PEEP and pulmonary artery catheters, and should not be expected to influence mortality.

NO has other effects, however, that are potentially beneficial in postinjury ARDS. It has been shown to inhibit leukocyte adhesion to endothelial cells.[236] We have shown that NO reduces endothelial ICAM-1,[237] as well as attenuates platelet-activating factor priming for elastase release in vitro.[238] Moreover, we demonstrated that inhaled NO prevents endotoxin-induced lung neutrophil accumulation.[239] One report in humans with ARDS suggests that inhaled NO can reduce lung inflammation by downregulating neutrophil oxidative function, $\beta_2$ integrin expression, and cytokine release.[240] In light of the effects of nitric oxide on neutrophil-endothelial cell interaction, it is conceivable that inhaled nitric oxide administered to injured patients at risk for ARDS may limit its incidence and/or severity.

NO is a potentially toxic molecule and its biochemistry is not fully understood. Two decades ago, NO was viewed primarily as a toxic gas that was an important component of air pollution.[241] It has been implicated in the etiology of Silo filler's disease. Moreover, 400 to 600 ppm of NO are generated in tobacco smoke. Toxicity of inhaled NO is most likely related to the formation of reactive products or metabolites. Methemoglobin, nitrogen dioxide, and peroxynitrite have been of most concern. To date, these have not been shown to be clinically relevant concerns. Guidelines for safe usage have been proposed in order to minimize the potential for toxicity. These include careful monitoring of NO, $NO_2$, and methemoglobin levels; scavenging of exhaust gases; and the use of delivery systems that minimize contact time between NO and oxygen.[242,243] A rebound phenomenon has been described, which is characterized by marked pulmonary hypertension and hypoxemia with cessation of NO therapy. This is obviated by gradual weaning of inhaled NO therapy.[244]

## SURFACTANT REPLACEMENT THERAPY

An original observation in ARDS patients by Ashbaugh and colleagues was an increase in the minimum surface tension of surfactant recovered from lung specimens at autopsy.[14] This was the first suggestion that abnormal surfactant function contributes to the pathophysiology of ARDS. Pulmonary surfactant is a complex mixture of phospholipids and associated proteins secreted by alveolar type II cells. Surfactant lines the alveolar surface and is critical for survival.[245,246] The most well characterized function of surfactant is its ability to reduce surface tension at the alveolar air–liquid interface, thus stabilizing alveoli and terminal airways. The surfactant-associated proteins (SP-A, SP-B, SP-C, and SP-D) have a variety of functions in the lung including formation of tubular myelin (SP-A, SP-B)[247] as well as host defense (SP-A, SP-D).[248] Abnormalities in the concentration of surfactant proteins and surfactant phospholipids have been observed in BAL fluid[249,250] and serum[251] of patients with ARDS. There is, however, limited clinical experience with administration of exogenous surfactant to humans with ARDS.

The rationale for giving exogenous surfactant to patients with ARDS is based primarily on clinical data from neonates with respiratory distress syndrome (RDS). In this setting, surfactant replacement is of proven efficacy and is considered standard care. In RDS, the surfactant deficiency is the primary pathophysiologic abnormality. The pathophysiology of ARDS, however, is far more complex, involving a variety of insults and secondary abnormalities in surfactant. Nonetheless, the lungs are acutely inflamed in both processes and lack functional surfactant. Further rationale for exogenous surfactant administration is provided by observations of improved gas exchange and survival in numerous animal models of ALI treated with exogenous surfactant.[252–254]

There are a variety of natural, modified, and synthetic preparations of pulmonary surfactant potentially available for therapeutic use. Synthetic preparations are desirable because they are available in large quantity, inexpensive, and carry no risk of transmitted disease. None of the synthetic preparations contain intact surfactant apoproteins that may be important for improved function, as well as host defense properties. There are reports of preparations that incorporate peptide analogues of hydrophobic proteins, and clinical studies with one such preparation are ongoing.[255,256] Despite substantial experience in the treatment of infant RDS with exogenous surfactant, direct clinical comparison of the efficacy of various surfactant preparations is not available. More importantly, the optimal surfactant preparation for the immature lung may prove to be different from the optimal preparation for the treatment of ARDS. Preliminary experience with the administration of a liquid extract of mammalian surfactant to patients with ARDS suggested that oxygenation and ventilatory requirements could be transiently improved.[257–259] However, the only large, multicenter, randomized, controlled trial of surfactant therapy administered by aerosol to patients with sepsis-induced ARDS showed no effect on 30-day survival.[260] One potential explanation for this was the use of Exosurf (Glaxo Wellcome, Research Triangle Park, NC). Exosurf is a preparation of dipalmitoylphosphatidylcholine with tyloxapol and hexadecanol as emulsifiers and spreading agents. It contains no surfactant-associated proteins (which may be important in the treatment of ARDS) and is effective in only about 50% of neonates with RDS.[261] In addition, the Exosurf was administered via nebulization, in which less than 5% of the surfactant reaches the lungs and is deposited only in the better-ventilated alveoli.

A recent trial of surfactant therapy in pediatric pulmonary failure showed encouraging results,[262] however, results in the most recent adult trial of ARDS failed to show an improvement in survival. Like many other adjuncts that have been described for the treatment of ALI and ARDS, some surrogate outcomes, such as short-term oxygenation, were better in this trial, but ventilator-free days and hospital mortality were unchanged.[263] Surfactant therapy cannot be routinely recommended for adults with ARDS.

## CORTICOSTEROIDS

The ability of corticosteroids to attenuate the inflammatory response would seem to make them ideal treatment for ARDS. From the first description of ARDS, corticosteroids were suggested as possible therapeutic agents.[14] Large prospective clinical trials, however, showed no survival benefit with high-dose steroids in early ARDS.[264-266] These initial studies focused only on early ARDS and utilized a short course (less than 48 hours) of high-dose steroids. It has become increasingly clear that pathogenetic mechanisms initiating ARDS are different from those that perpetuate late ARDS. The fibroproliferative phase of ARDS is particularly critical. Why lung injury completely resolves in one patient and extensive fibrosis develops in another is unknown. The extent of initial injury, especially the amount of basement membrane disruption, may be an important factor.[267] Another important factor is ongoing injury or inflammation. Histologic evidence of continued endothelial injury has been described in patients with advanced fibroproliferation.[268] Meduri and associates provide evidence suggesting a link between ongoing fibroproliferation and persistent inflammation.[269] The authors measured plasma and BAL fluid cytokine levels following initiation of steroid rescue treatment in patients with late ARDS. They noted a significant reduction in plasma TNF-$\alpha$ and IL-6 levels in patients who responded compared to those who did not.

Several anecdotal reports support the use of steroids in late ARDS.[269-272] Most of these investigators used methylprednisolone (or its equivalent) in doses ranging from 2 to 8 mg/kg/day for at least two weeks. Survival ranged from 76 to 83%, well exceeding that expected in this group of patients. Meduri and associates reported results from a prospective, randomized trial of steroids in late ARDS.[273] Twenty-four patients were randomized to receive methylprednisolone 2 mg/kg/day for 32 days or placebo. Patients treated with steroids had reduced lung injury scores, increased $PaO_2$ to $FIO_2$ ratios and greater extubation success 10 days after treatment. ICU and hospital mortality were significantly reduced (0% vs. 62% and 12% vs. 62%, respectively). This study can be criticized for the small number of control patients ($n = 8$) and the crossover of patients from the placebo group to the steroid group (4 out of 8). A subsequent publication demonstrated that patients treated with methylprednisolone have a rapid reduction in the proinflammatory cytokines IL-1, IL-6, and TNF,[274] supporting the hypothesis that ongoing ARDS represents a pathologically persistent inflammatory state.

Recently, the NIH ARDS Clinical Trials Network reported the results of a multicenter, randomized, controlled trial of corticosteroids in patients with persistent ARDS.[275] One hundred and eighty patients with ARDS of at least seven days duration were assigned either methylprednisolone or placebo. The primary endpoint was 60-day mortality, and secondary endpoints were ventilator free days, organ failure, and various biomarkers. There was no difference in 60-day mortality except in those patients who received methylprednisolone after ARDS day 14, then mortality significantly *increased*. Methylprednisolone did increase the number of ventilator-free days, improved oxygenation, respiratory compliance, and resulted in less vasopressor use. Interestingly, the rate of infectious complications was no different between the groups, but the methylprednisolone group had a higher incidence of neuromuscular weakness. Given the challenges of this patient group, any use of steroids for late ARDS must be individualized and, optimally, delivered before disease day 14.

## Nutritional Support

Overfeeding patients or administering excess carbohydrates can lead to excess production of $CO_2$. In the setting of marginal abilty to execute work of breathing, this may, in theory, precipitate or prolong hypercapnic pulmonary failure. Careful monitoring of nutritional support may be necessary in patients with tenuous respiratory status. An indirect calorimeter can be helpful in providing estimates of $CO_2$ production and the respiratory quotient. The respiratory quotient should be kept below 0.9 by appropriate adjustment of the proportion of lipid and total calories administered. Our goals for nutritional support are to deliver 21 to 25 nonprotein calories/kg/day and 0.25 to 0.30 g of nitrogen/kg/day. The primary goal of carbohydrate administration should be a rate of less than 5 mg/kg/minute.

## INFECTION SURVEILLANCE AND MANAGEMENT

Sepsis is a predominant risk factor for ARDS. Moreover, nosocomial infections, in particular pneumonia, frequently complicate the course of ARDS due to immune suppression in critically injured patients (see Chap. 19). In patients with ARDS, the frequency of ventilator-associated pneumonia is as high as 70%. The diagnosis of pneumonia in ARDS is difficult and frequently not recognized ante mortem. Traditional criteria for the diagnosis of pneumonia include the radiographic appearance of a new or progressive infiltrate, fever, leukocytosis, and purulent tracheobronchial secretions. Because ARDS is due to a systemic inflammatory process, leukocytosis and fever are nonspecific and frequently present in the absence of documented infection. New or progressive infiltrates on chest radiographs can be difficult to discern due to the radiographic changes present in ARDS.

One approach to diagnosis of pneumonia is the use of quantitative scoring systems such as the clinical pulmonary infection score (CPIS). While its diagnostic accuracy remains in question, particularly in the trauma setting, it has some utility for guiding therapy. For example, a score can be used as trigger for an invasive diagnostic maneuver bronchoalveolar lavage (BAL) and can be used to guide the aggressiveness of empiric antibiotic therapy.

Sputum cultures may be helpful if they show a predominant organism in association with neutrophils. Most ARDS patients are intubated and secretions are sampled via the endotracheal tube. Several studies document the inaccuracy of tracheal aspirates obtained through endotracheal or tracheostomy tubes.[277-279] Bronchoscopic-guided techniques have become the standard in many centers. These include protected specimen brushing BAL, and mini-BAL. We have found BAL to be useful and generally well tolerated in this critically ill group of patients. Pneumonia is generally diagnosed with greater than $10^4$ colony-forming units/mL. It is important to recognize that antibiotics may alter this threshold such that greater than $10^3$ colony-forming units/mL is considered diagnostic for pneumonia. Ideally, empiric antibiotics should be stopped for 48 hours prior to the BAL. This, of course, depends on the clinical situation and the patient's stability. Due to the critical condition of patients with ARDS, presumptive broad-spectrum antibiotic coverage may be indicated initially. Antibiotics can be subsequently tailored or stopped when culture results are available.

## OUTCOME

Mortality associated with ARDS has historically ranged from 30 to 60%. The majority of deaths are related to sepsis and MOF (see Chap. 68). Respiratory failure is a cause of death in only 15% of patients.[280] The principal therapy that improves outcome in patients with ARDS is low-tidal volume ventilation; protocolized adherence to this regimen is strongly encouraged.

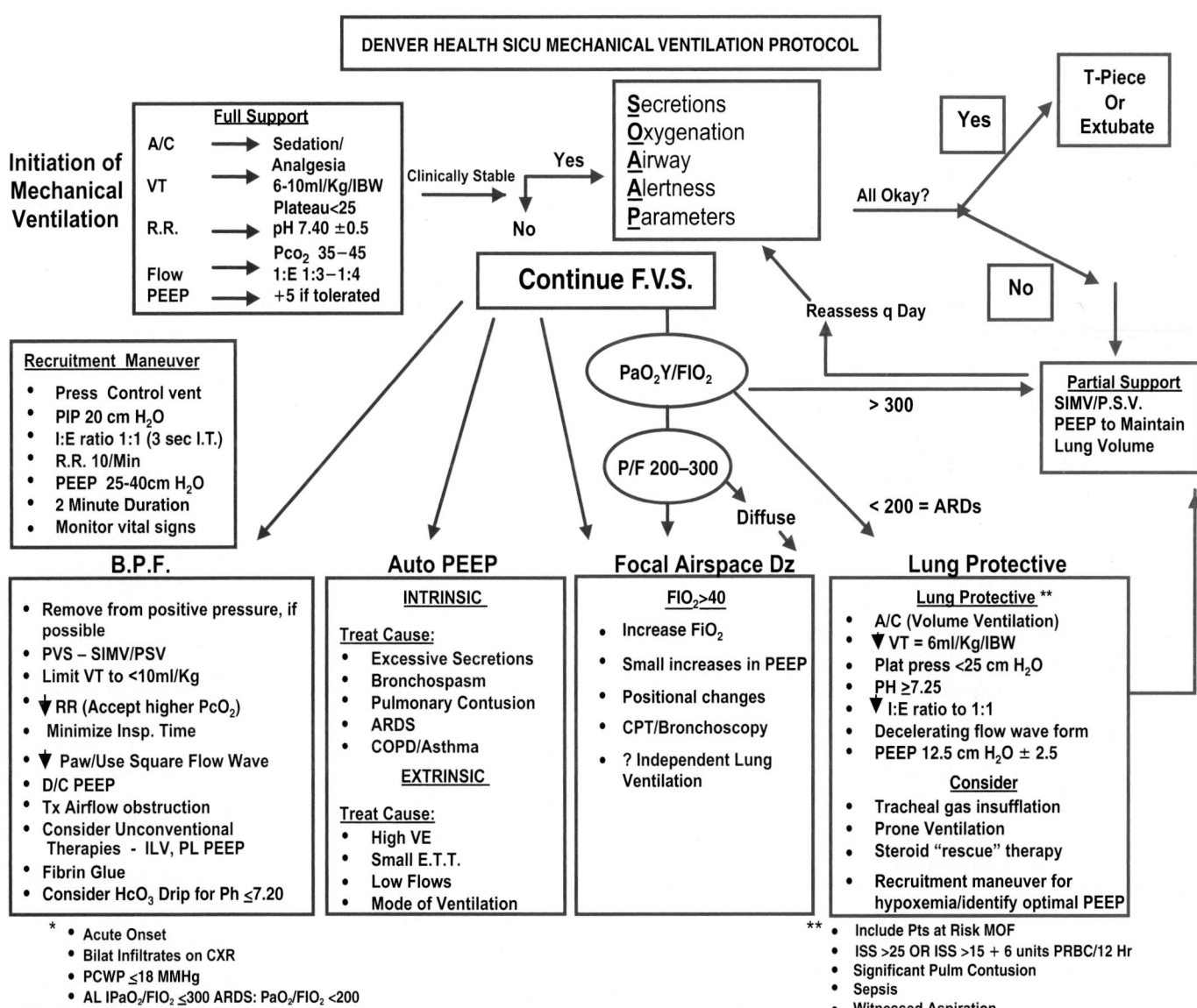

DENVER HEALTH SICU MECHANICAL VENTILATION PROTOCOL

**Initiation of Mechanical Ventilation**

**Full Support**
A/C → Sedation/ Analgesia
VT → 6-10ml/Kg/IBW Plateau<25
R.R. → pH 7.40 ±0.5
Flow → Pco₂ 35–45
PEEP → 1:E 1:3–1:4
+5 if tolerated

Clinically Stable — Yes → **S**ecretions **O**xygenation **A**irway **A**lertness **P**arameters

No → **Continue F.V.S.**

All Okay? — Yes → T-Piece Or Extubate
No

Reassess q Day

PaO₂Y/FIO₂ — > 300 → Partial Support SIMV/P.S.V. PEEP to Maintain Lung Volume

P/F 200–300

Diffuse

< 200 = ARDs

**Recruitment Maneuver**
• Press Control vent
• PIP 20 cm H₂O
• I:E ratio 1:1 (3 sec I.T.)
• R.R. 10/Min
• PEEP 25-40cm H₂O
• 2 Minute Duration
• Monitor vital signs

**B.P.F.**
• Remove from positive pressure, if possible
• PVS – SIMV/PSV
• Limit VT to <10ml/Kg
• ▼RR (Accept higher PcO₂)
• Minimize Insp. Time
• ▼Paw/Use Square Flow Wave
• D/C PEEP
• Tx Airflow obstruction
• Consider Unconventional Therapies - ILV, PL PEEP
• Fibrin Glue
• Consider HcO₃ Drip for Ph ≤7.20

**Auto PEEP**
INTRINSIC
Treat Cause:
• Excessive Secretions
• Bronchospasm
• Pulmonary Contusion
• ARDS
• COPD/Asthma
EXTRINSIC
Treat Cause:
• High VE
• Small E.T.T.
• Low Flows
• Mode of Ventilation

**Focal Airspace Dz**
FIO₂>40
• Increase FiO₂
• Small increases in PEEP
• Positional changes
• CPT/Bronchoscopy
• ? Independent Lung Ventilation

**Lung Protective**
Lung Protective **
• A/C (Volume Ventilation)
• ▼VT = 6ml/Kg/IBW
• Plat press <25 cm H₂O
• PH ≥7.25
• ▼I:E ratio to 1:1
• Decelerating flow wave form
• PEEP 12.5 cm H₂O ± 2.5
Consider
• Tracheal gas insufflation
• Prone Ventilation
• Steroid "rescue" therapy
• Recruitment maneuver for hypoxemia/identify optimal PEEP

\*
• Acute Onset
• Bilat Infiltrates on CXR
• PCWP ≤18 MMHg
• AL IPaO₂/FIO₂ ≤300 ARDS: PaO₂/FIO₂ <200

\*\*
• Include Pts at Risk MOF
• ISS >25 OR ISS >15 + 6 units PRBC/12 Hr
• Significant Pulm Contusion
• Sepsis
• Witnessed Aspiration

*Abbreviation*
ALI; Acute Lung Injury; A/C: Assist/Control; ARDS: Acute Respiratory Distress Syndrome; BPF: Bronchopleural Fistula; CPT: Chest Physical Therapy; E.T.T.: Endotracheal Tube; FIO₂: Fraction of Inspired Oxygen; FVS: Full Ventilatory Support; IE: Inspiratory to Expiratory Ratio; ILV: Independent Lung Ventilation; PAW: Peak Airway Pressure; PEEP: Positive End Expiratory Pressure; PIP: Peak Inspiratory Pressure; PLAT PRESS: Plateau Pressure; PL PEEP: Pleural Positive End Expiratory Pressure; PVS: Partial Ventilator Support; R.R.: Respiratory Rate; SIMV: Synchronized Intermittent Mandatory Ventilation; Vt: Tidal Volume.

## REFERENCES

1. Uehara M, Plank LD, Hill GL: Components of energy expenditure in patients with severe sepsis and major trauma: A basis for clinic care. *Crit Care Med* 27:1295, 1999.
2. Tang Y, Turnery MJ, Baker AB: A new equal area method to calculate and represent physiologic, anatomical and alveolar dead spaces. *Anesthesiology* 104:696, 2006.
3. Herndon DN, Hart DW, Wolfe SE, et al.: Reversal of catabolism by beta-blockade after severe burns. *N Engl J Med* 345:1223, 2001.
4. Como JJ, Sutton ER, McCunn M, et al.: Characterizing the need for mechanical ventilation following cervical spinal cord injury with neurologic deficit. *J Trauma* 59:912, 2005.
5. Harrop JS, Sharan AD, Scheid EH Jr, et al.: Tracheostomy placement in patients with complete cervical spinal cord injuries: American spinal injury association grade A. *J Neurosurg* 100:20, 2004.
6. McHenry TP, Mirza SK, Wang J, et al.: Risk factors for respiratory failure following operative stabilization of thoracic and lumbar spine fractures. *J Bone Joint Surg Am* 88:997, 2006.
7. Kerwin AJ, Frykberg ER, Schinco MA, et al.: The effect of early spine fixation on non-neurologic outcome. *J Trauma* 58:15, 2005.
8. Schinkel C, Frangen TM, Kmetic A, et al.: Timing of thoracic spine stabilization in trauma patients: Impact on clinical course and outcome. *J Trauma* 61:156, 2006.
9. DiMarco AF, Onders RP, Ignagni A, et al.: Phrenic nerve pacing via intramuscular diaphragm electrodes in tetraplegic subjects. *Chest* 127:671, 2005.
10. Bulger EM, Arneson MA, Mock CN, et al.: Rib fractures in the elderly. *J Trauma* 48:1040, 200.
11. Flagel BT, Luchette FA, Reed RL, et al.: Half-a-dozen ribs: The breakpoint for mortality. *Surgery* 138:717, 2005.
12. Todd SR, McNally MM, Holcomb JB, et al.: A multidisciplinary clinical pathway decreases rib fracture-associated infectious morbidity and mortality in high-risk trauma patients. *Am J Surg* 192:806, 2006.

13. Bernard GR, Artigas A, Brigham KL: The American-European Consensus Conference on ARDS. Definitions, mechanisms, relevant outcomes, and clinical trial coordination. *Am J Respir Crit Care Med* 149:818, 1994.

14. Ashbaugh DG, Bigelow DB, Petty TL: Acute respiratory distress in adults. *Lancet* 2:319, 1967.

15. Hyers TM: Prediction of survival and mortality in patients with adult respiratory distress syndrome. *New Horiz* 1:466, 1993.

16. Montgomery AB, Stager MA, Carrico CJ: Causes of mortality in patients with the adult respiratory distress syndrome. *Am Rev Respir Distress* 132:485, 1985.

17. ARDSnet: Ventilation with lower tidal volumes as compared with traditional tidal volumes for acute lung injury and the acute respiratory distress syndrome. The Acute Respiratory Distress Syndrome Network. *N Engl J Med* 342:1301, 2000.

18. Rubenfeld GD, Caldwell E, Peabody E, et al.: Incidence and outcomes of acute lung injury. *N Engl J Med* 353:1685, 2005.

19. Salim A, Marint M, Constantinou C, et al.: Acute respiratory distress syndrome in the trauma intensive care unit: Morbid but not mortal. *Arch Surg* 141:655, 2006.

20. Ciesla DJ, Moore EE, Johnson JL, et al.: Decreased progression of postinjury lung dysfunction to the acute respiratory distress syndrome and multiple organ failure. *Surgery* 140:640, 2006.

21. Luce JM: Acute lung injury and the acute respiratory distress syndrome. *Crit Care Med* 26:369, 1998.

22. Ferguson ND, Meade MO, Hallett DC, et al.: High values of the pulmonary artery wedge pressure in patients with acute lung injury and acute respiratory distress syndrome. *Int Care Med* 28:1073, 2002.

23. Esteban A, Fernandez-Segovia P, Frutos-Vivar F, et al.: Com parison of clinical criteria for the acute respiratory distress syndrome with autopsy findings. *Ann Intern Med* 141:440, 2004.

24. Murray JF, Matthay MA, Luce JM, et al.: An expanded definition of the adult respiratory distress syndrome. *Am Rev Respir Dis* 138:720, 1988.

25. Ferguson ND, Frutos-Vivar F, Esteban A, et al.: Acute respiratory distress syndrome: Underrecognition by clinicians and diagnostic accuracy of three clinical definitions. *Crit Care Med* 33:2228, 2005.

26. Villar J, Slutsky AS: The incidence of the adult respiratory distress syndrome. *Am Rev Respir Distress* 140:814, 1989.

27. Frutos-vivar F, Ferguson ND, Esteban A: Epidemiology of Acute lung injury and acute respiratory distress syndrome. *Sem Respir Crit Care Med* 27:327, 2006.

28. Avecillas JF, Freire AX, Arroliga AC: Clinical epidemiology of acute lung injury and acute respiratory distress syndrome: Incidence, diagnosis and outcomes. *Clin Chest Med* 27:549, 2006.

29. Luhr OR, Antonsen K, Karlsson M, et al.: Incidence and mortality after acute respiratory failure and acute respiratory distress syndrome in Sweden. *Am J Respir Crit Care Med* 156:1849, 1999.

30. Arroliga AC, Ghamra ZW, Perez Trepichio A, et al.: Incidence of ARDS in an adult population of north-east Ohio. *Chest* 121:1972, 2002.

31. Goss CH, Brower RG, Hudson LD, et al.: Incidence of acute lung injury in the United States. *Crit Care Med* 31:1607, 2003.

32. Hughes M, MacKirdy FN, Ross J, et al.: Acute respiratory distress syndrome: An audit of incidence and outcome in Scottish intensive care units. *Anaesthesia* 58:838, 2003.

33. Hudson LD, Milberg JA, Anardi D: Clinical risks for development of the acute respiratory distress syndrome. *Am J Respir Crit Care Med* 151:293, 1995.

34. Norwood SH, Civetta JM: The adult respiratory syndrome. *Surg Gynecol Obstet* 161:497, 1985.

35. Fourrier F, Chopin C, Wallaert B, et al.: Compared evolution of plasma fibronectin and angiotensin-converting enzyme levels in septic ARDS. *Chest* 87:191, 1985.

36. Marshall RP, Webb S, Bellingan GJ, et al.: Angiotensin converting enzyme insertion/deletion polymorphism is associated with susceptibility and outcome in acute respiratory distress syndrome. *Am J Respir Crit Care Med* 166:646, 2002.

37. Jerng JS, Yu CJ, Wang HC, et al.: Polymorphism of the angiontensin-converting enzyme gene affects the outcome of acute respiratory distress syndrome. *Crit Care Med* 34:1001, 2006.

38. Gong MN, Thompson BT, Williams PL, et al.: Interleukin-10 polymorphism in position -1082 and acute respiratory distress syndrome. *Eur Respir J* 27:674, 2006.

39. Ye SQ, Simon BA, Maloney JP, et al.: Pre-B-cell colony enhancing factor as a potential novel biomarker in acute lung injury. *Am J Respir Crit Care Med* 171:361, 2005.

40. Moore EE, Moore FA, Harken AH, et al.: The two-event construct of postinjury multiple organ failure. *Shock* 24 (Suppl 1):71, 2005.

41. Stapleton RD, Wang BM, Hudson LD, et al.: Causes and timing of death in patients with ARDS. *Chest* 128:525, 2005.

42. Ciesla DJ, Moore EE, Johnson JL, et al.: The role of the lung in postinjury multiple organ failure. *Surgery* 138:749, 2005.

43. Wiedemann HP, Matthay MA, Gillis CN: Pulmonary endothelial cell injury and altered lung metabolic function. Early detection of the adult respiratory distress syndrome and possible functional significance. *Clin Chest Med* 11:723, 1990.

44. Tremblay LN, Slutsky AS: Ventilator-induced lung injury: From bench to the bedside. *Intensive Care Med* 32:24, 2006.

45. Tomashefski JF Jr: Pulmonary pathology of the adult respiratory distress syndrome. *Clin Chest Med* 11:593, 1990.

46. Mendez JL, Hubmayr RD: New insights into the pathology of acute respiratory failure. *Curr Opin Crit Care* 11:29, 2005.

47. Ware LB: Pathophysiology of acute lung injury and the acute respiratory distress syndrome. *Semin Respir Crit Care Med* 27:337, 2006.

48. Steinberg KP, Milberg JA, Martin TR, et al.: Evolution of bronchoalveolar cell populations in the adult respiratory distress syndrome. *Am J Respir Crit Care Med* 150:113, 1994.

49. Tate RM, Repine JE: Neutrophils and the adult respiratory distress syndrome. *Am Rev Respir Dis* 128:552, 1983.

50. Sibille Y, Reynolds HY: Macrophages and polymorphonuclear neutrophils in lung defense and injury. *Am Rev Respir Dis* 141:471, 1990.

51. Cassatella MA, Bazzoni F, Ceska M, et al.: IL-8 production by human polymorphonuclear leukocytes. The chemoattractant formyl-methionyl-leucyl-phenylalanine induces the gene expression and release of IL-8 through a pertussis toxin-sensitive pathway. *J Immunol* 148:3216, 1992.

52. Zallen G, Moore EE, Johnson JL, et al.: Circulating postinjury neutrophils are primed for the release of proinflammatory cytokines. *J Trauma* 46:42, 1999.

53. Heflin AC Jr, Brigham KL: Prevention by granulocyte depletion of increased vascular permeability of sheep lung following endotoxemia. *J Clin Invest* 68:1253, 1981.

54. Anderson BO, Bensard DD, Brown JM, et al.: FNLP injures endotoxin-primed rat lung by neutrophil-dependent and -independent mechanisms. *Am J Physiol* 260:R413, 1991.

55. Worthen GS, Schwab B III, Elson EL, et al.: Mechanics of stimulated neutrophils: Cell stiffening induces retention in capillaries. *Science* 245:183, 1989.

56. Strieter RM, Kunkel SL: Acute lung injury: The role of cytokines in the elicitation of neutrophils. *J Invest Med* 42:640, 1994.

57. Albelda SM, Smith CW, Ward PA: Adhesion molecules and inflammatory injury. *FASEB J* 8:504, 1994.

58. Goldman G, Welbourn R, Kobzik L, et al.: Neutrophil adhesion receptor CD18 mediates remote but not localized acid aspiration injury. *Surgery* 117:83, 1995.

59. Lo SK, Everitt J, Gu J, et al.: Tumor necrosis factor mediates experimental pulmonary edema by ICAM-1 and CD18-dependent mechanisms. *J Clin Invest* 89:981, 1992.

60. Ridings PC, Windsor AC, Jutila MA, et al.: A dual-binding antibody to E-and L-selectin attenuates sepsis-induced lung injury. *Am J Respir Crit Care Med* 152:247, 1995.

61. Vaporciyan AA, DeLisser HM, Yan HC, et al.: Involvement of platelet-endothelial cell adhesion molecule-1 in neutrophil recruitment in vivo. *Science* 262:1580, 1993.

62. Demling RH: Adult respiratory distress syndrome: Current concepts. *New Horiz* 1:388, 1993.

63. Idell S, Gonzalez K, Bradford H, et al.: Procoagulant activity in bronchoalveolar lavage in the adult respiratory distress syndrome. Contribution of tissue factor associated with factor VII. *Am Rev Respir Dis* 136:1466, 1987.

64. Duchateau J, Haas M, Schreyen H, et al.: Complement activation in patients at risk of developing the adult respiratory distress syndrome. *Am Rev Respir Dis* 130:1058, 1984.

65. Fosse E, Pillgram-Larsen J, Svennevig JL, et al.: Complement activation in injured patiens occurs immediately and is dependent on the severity of the trauma. *Injury* 29:509, 1998.

66. Zilow G, Joka T, Obertacke U, et al.: Generation of anaphylatoxin C3a in plasma and bronchoalveolar lavage fluid in trauma patients at risk for the adult respiratory distress syndrome. *Crit Care Med* 20:468, 1992.

67. Gama de Abreu M, Kirschfink M, Quintel M, et al.: White blood cell counts and plasma C3a have synergistic predictive value in patients at risk for acute respiratory distress syndrome. *Crit Care Med* 26:1040, 1998.

68. Suter PM, Suter S, Girardin E, et al.: High bronchoalveolar levels of tumor necrosis factor and its inhibitors, interleukin-1, interferon, and elastase, in patients with adult respiratory distress syndrome after trauma, shock, or sepsis. *Am Rev Respir Dis* 145:1016, 1992.

69. Abraham E, Jesmok G, Tuder R, et al.: Contribution of tumor necrosis factor-alpha to pulmonary cytokine expression and lung injury after hemorrhage and resuscitation. *Crit Care Med* 23:1319, 1995.

70. Kim PK, Deutschmann CS: Inflammatory responses and mediators. *Surg Clin North Am* 80:885, 2000.

71. Bone RC: Immunologic dissonance: A continuing evolution in our understanding of the systemic inflammatory response syndrome (SIRS) and the multiple organ dysfunction syndrome (MODS). *Ann Intern Med* 125:680, 1996.

72. Armstrong L, Millar AB: Relative production of tumour necrosis factor alpha and interleukin 10 in adult respiratory distress syndrome. *Thorax* 52:442, 1997.

73. Chang SW, Feddersen CO, Henson PM, et al.: Platelet-activating factor mediates hemodynamic changes and lung injury in endotoxin-treated rats. *J Clin Invest* 79:1498, 1987.

74. Edelson JD, Vadas P, Villar J, et al.: Acute lung injury induced by phospholipase A2. Structural and functional changes. *Am Rev Respir Dis* 143:1102, 1991.

75. Zimmerman GA, McIntyre TM, Prescott SM, et al.: The platelet-activating factor signaling system and its regulators in syndromes of inflammation and thrombosis. *Crit Care Med* 30:S294, 2002.

76. Anderson BO, Bensard DD, Harken AH: The role of platelet activating factor and its antagonists in shock, sepsis and multiple organ failure. *Surg Gynecol Obstet* 172:415, 1991.

77. Silliman CC, Voelkel NF, Allard JD, et al.: Plasma and lipids from stored packed red blood cells cause acute lung injury in an animal model. *J Clin Invest* 101:1458, 1998.

78. Hassoun HT, Kone BC Mercer DW, et al.: Post-injury multiple organ failure: The role of the gut. *Shock* 15:1, 2001.

79. Magnotti LJ, Upperman JS, Xu DZ, et al.: Gut-derived mesenteric lymph but not portal blood increases endothelial cell permeability and promotes lung injury after hemorrhagic shock. *Ann Surg* 228:518, 1998.

80. Gonzalez RJ, Moore EE, Ciesla DJ, et al.: Post-hemorrhagic shock mesenteric lymph activates human pulmonary microvascular endothelium for in vitro neutrophil-mediated injury: The role of intercellular adhesion molecule-1. *J Trauma* 54:219, 2003.

81. Deitch EA, Xu D, Kaise VL: Role of the gut in the development of injury- and shock induced SIRS and MODS: The gut-lymph hypothesis, a review. *Front Biosci* 11:520, 2006.

82. Pittet JF, Mackersie RC, Martin TR, et al.: Biological markers of acute lung injury: Prognostic and pathogenetic significance. *Am J Respir Crit Care Med* 155:1187, 1997.

83. Jones DK, Perry EM, Grosso MA, et al.: Release of von Willebrand factor antigen (vWF:Ag) and eicosanoids during acute injury to the isolated rat lung. *Am Rev Respir Dis* 145:1410, 1992.

84. Carvallo CR, Barbas CS, Medeiros DM, et al.: Temporal hemodynamic effects of permissive hypercapnia associated with ideal PEEP in ARDS. *Am J Respir Crit Care Med* 156:1458, 1997.

85. Rubin DB, Wiener-Kronish JP, Murray JF, et al.: Elevated von Willebrand factor antigen is an early plasma predictor of acute lung injury in nonpulmonary sepsis syndrome. *J Clin Invest* 86:474, 1990.

86. Moss M, Ackerson L, Gillespie MK, et al.: von Willebrand factor antigen levels are not predictive for the adult respiratory distress syndrome. *Am J Respir Crit Care Med* 151:15, 1995.

87. Donnelly SC, Haslett C, Dransfield I, et al.: Role of selectins in development of adult respiratory distress syndrome. *Lancet* 344:215, 1994.

88. Partrick DA, Moore FA, Moore EE: The inflammatory profile of interleukin-6, interleukin-8, and soluble intercellular adhesion molecule-1 in postinjury multiple organ failure. *Am J Surg* 172:425, 1996.

89. Law MM, Cryer HG, Abraham E: Elevated levels of soluble ICAM-1 correlate with the development of multiple organ failure in severely injured trauma patients. *J Trauma* 37:100, 1994.

90. Moss M, Gillespie MK, Ackerson L, et al.: Endothelial cell activity varies in patients at risk for the adult respiratory distress syndrome. *Crit Care Med* 24:1782, 1996.

91. Gosling P, Sanghera K, Dickson G: Generalized vascular permeability and pulmonary function in patients following serious trauma. *J Trauma* 36:477, 1994.

92. Pallister I, Gosling P, Alpar K, et al.: Prediction of posttraumatic adult respiratory distress syndrome by albumin excretion rate eight hours after admission. *J Trauma* 42:1056, 1997.

93. Matthay MA, Folkesson HG, Campagna A, et al.: Alveolar epithelial barrier and acute lung injury. *New Horiz* 1:613, 1993.

94. Matthay MA, Wiener-Kronish JP: Intact epithelial barrier function is critical for the resolution of alveolar edema in humans. *Am Rev Respir Dis* 142:1250, 1990.

95. Gregory TJ, Longmore WJ, Moxley MA, et al.: Surfactant chemical composition and biophysical activity in acute respiratory distress syndrome. *J Clin Invest* 88:1976, 1991.

96. Wortel CH, Doerschuk CM: Neutrophils and neutrophil-endothelial cell adhesion in adult respiratory distress syndrome. *New Horiz* 1:631, 1993.

97. Weiss SJ: Tissue destruction by neutrophils. *N Engl J Med* 320:365, 1989.

98. Gordon MW, Robertson CE, Dawes J: Neutrophil elastase levels and major trauma in man. *Intens Care Med* 15:543, 1989.

99. Donnelly SC, MacGregor I, Zamani A, et al.: Plasma elastase levels and the development of the adult respiratory distress syndrome. *Am J Respir Crit Care Med* 151:1428, 1995.

100. Simms HH, D'Amico R: Increased PMN CD11b/CD18 expression following post-traumatic ARDS. *J Surg Res* 50:362, 1991.

101. Connelly KG, Repine JE: Markers for predicting the development of acute respiratory distress syndrome. *Annu Rev Med* 48:429, 1997.

102. Botha AJ, Moore FA, Moore EE, et al.: Early neutrophil sequestration after injury: A pathogenic mechanism for multiple organ failure. *J Trauma* 39:411, 1995.

103. Bone RC, Francis PB, Pierce AK: Intravascular coagulation associated with the adult respiratory distress syndrome. *Am J Med* 61:585, 1976.

104. Raponi G, Antonelli M, Gaeta A: Tumor necrosis factor in serum and in bronchoalveolar lavage of patients at risk for the adult respiratory distress syndrome. *J Crit Care* 7:183, 1992.

105. Tracey KJ, Lowry SF, Cerami A: Cachectin/TNF-alpha in septic shock and septic adult respiratory distress syndrome. *Am Rev Respir Dis* 138:1377, 1988.

106. Marks JD, Marks CB, Luce JM, et al.: Plasma tumor necrosis factor in patients with septic shock. Mortality rate, incidence of adult respiratory distress syndrome, and effects of methylprednisolone administration. *Am Rev Respir Dis* 141:94, 1990.

107. Donnelly TJ, Meade P, Jagels M, et al.: Cytokine, complement, and endotoxin profiles associated with the development of the adult respiratory distress syndrome after severe injury. *Crit Care Med* 22:768, 1994.

108. Meade P, Shoemaker WC, Donnelly TJ, et al.: Temporal patterns of hemodynamics, oxygen transport, cytokine activity, and complement activity in the development of adult respiratory distress syndrome after severe injury. *J Trauma* 36:651, 1994.

109. Darbonne WC, Rice GC, Mohler MA, et al.: Red blood cells are a sink for interleukin 8, a leukocyte chemotaxin. *J Clin Invest* 88:1362, 1991.

110. de Winter RJ, Manten A, de Jong YP, et al.: Interleukin 8 released after acute myocardial infarction is mainly bound to erythrocytes. *Heart* 78:598, 1997.

111. Donnelly SC, Strieter RM, Kunkel SL: Interleukin-8 and development of adult respiratory distress syndrome in at-risk patient groups. *Lancet* 341:643, 1993.

112. Craddock PR, Fehr J, Dalmasso AP, et al.: Hemodialysis leukopenia: Pulmonary vascular leukostasis resulting from complement activation by dialyzer cellophane membranes. *J Clin Invest* 59:879, 1977.

113. Hammerschmidt DE, Weaver LJ, Hudson LD, et al.: Association of complement activation and elevated plasma-C5a with adult respiratory distress syndrome: Pathophysiological relevance and possible prognostic value. *Lancet* 1:947, 1980.

114. Fink A, Geva D, Zung A, et al.: Adult respiratory distress syndrome: Roles of leukotriene C4 and platelet activating factor. *Crit Care Med* 18:905, 1990.

115. Stephenson AH, Lonigro AJ, Hyers TM, et al.: Increased concentrations of leukotrienes in bronchoalveolar lavage fluid of patients with ARDS or at risk for ARDS. *Am Rev Respir Dis* 138:714, 1988.

116. Davis JM, Meyer JD, Barie PS, et al.: Elevated production of neutrophil leukotriene B4 precedes pulmonary failure in critically ill surgical patients. *Surg Gynecol Obstet* 170:495, 1990.

117. Leff JA, Parsons PE, Day CE, et al.: Serum antioxidants as predictors of adult respiratory distress syndrome in patients with sepsis. *Lancet* 341:777, 1993.

118. Gattinoni L, Mascheroni D, Torresin A, et al.: Morphological response to positive end expiratory pressure in acute respiratory failure: Computerized tomography study. *Intens Care Med* 12:137, 1986.

119. Maunder RJ, Shuman WP, McHugh JW, et al.: Preservation of normal lung regions in the adult respiratory distress syndrome: Analysis by computed tomography. *JAMA* 255:2463, 1986.

120. Gattinoni L, Caironi P, Valenza F, et al.: The role of CT-scan studies for the diagnosis and therapy of acute respiratory distress syndrome. *Clin Chest med* 27:559, 2006.

121. Gattinoni L, Pesenti A, Avalli L, et al.: Pressure-volume curve of total respiratory system in acute respiratory failure: Computed tomographic scan study. *Am Rev Respir Dis* 136:730, 1987.

122. Pelosi P, D'Andrea L, Vitale G, et al.: Vertical gradient of regional lung inflation in adult respiratory distress syndrome. *Am J Respir Crit Care Med* 149:8, 1994.

123. Sandiford P, Province MA, Schuster DP: Distribution of regional density and vascular permeability in the adult respiratory distress syndrome. *Am J Respir Crit Care Med* 151:737, 1995.

124. Pelosi P, Crotti S, Brazzi L, et al.: Computed tomography in adult respiratory distress syndrome: What has it taught us? *Eur Respir J* 9:1055, 1996.

125. Slutsky AS, Tremblay LN: Multiple system organ failure. Is mechanical ventilation a contributing factor? *Am J Respir Crit Care Med* 157:1721, 1998.

126. Finfer S, Rocker G: Alveolar overdistension is an important mechanism of persistent lung damage following severe protracted ARDS. *Anaesth Intens Care* 24:569, 1996.

127. Weiland JE, Davis WB, Holter JF, et al.: Lung neutrophils in the adult respiratory distress syndrome: Clinical and pathophysiologic significance. *Am Rev Respir Dis* 133:218, 1986.

128. Holter JF, Weiland JE, Pacht ER, et al.: Protein permeability in the adult respiratory distress syndrome: Loss of size selectivity of the alveolar epithelium. *J Clin Invest* 78:1513, 1986.

129. Clark JG, Milberg JA, Steinberg KP, et al.: Type III procollagen peptide in the adult respiratory distress syndrome. Association of increased peptide levels in bronchoalveolar lavage fluid with increased risk for death. *Ann Intern Med* 122:17, 1995.

130. Doyle IR, Bersten AD, Nicholas TE: Surfactant proteins-A and -B are elevated in plasma of patients with acute respiratory failure. *Am J Respir Crit Care Med* 156:1217, 1997.

131. Doyle IR, Nicholas TE, Bersten AD: Serum surfactant protein-A levels in patients with acute cardiogenic pulmonary edema and adult respiratory distress syndrome. *Am J Respir Crit Care Med* 152:307, 1995.

132. Leeman M, Delcroix M, Vachiery JL, et al.: Blunted hypoxic vasoconstriction in oleic acid lung injury: Effect of cyclooxygenase inhibitors. *J Appl Physiol* 72:251, 1992.

133. Leeman M, De Beyl VZ, Gilbert E, et al.: Is nitric oxide released in oleic acid lung injury? *J Appl Physiol* 74:650, 1993.

134. Marshall BE, Hanson CW, Frasch F, et al.: Role of hypoxic pulmonary vasoconstriction in pulmonary gas exchange and blood flow distribution. 2. Pathophysiology. *Intens Care Med* 20:379, 1994.

135. Zapol WM, Hurford WE: Inhaled nitric oxide in the adult respiratory distress syndrome and other lung diseases. *New Horiz* 1:638, 1993.

136. Steltzer H, Krafft P, Fridrich P, et al.: Right ventricular function and oxygen transport patterns in patients with acute respiratory distress syndrome. *Anaesthesia* 49:1039, 1994.

137. Schuster DP: The case for and against fluid restriction and occlusion pressure reduction in adult respiratory distress syndrome. *New Horiz* 1:478, 1993.

138. Humphrey H, Hall J, Sznajder I, et al.: Improved survival in ARDS patients associated with a reduction in pulmonary capillary wedge pressure. *Chest* 97:1176, 1990.

139. Brigham KL, Kariman K, Harris TR, et al.: Correlation of oxygenation with vascular permeability–surface area but not with lung water in humans with acute respiratory failure and pulmonary edema. *J Clin Invest* 72:339, 1983.

140. National Heart, Lung and Blood Institute Acute Respiratory Distress Syndrome (ARDS) Clinical Trials Network. Comparison of two fluid-management strategies in acute lung injury. *N Engl J Med* 354:2564, 2006.

141. Sibbald WJ, Short AK, Warshawski FJ, et al.: Thermal dye measurements of extravascular lung water in critically ill patients. Intravascular Starling forces and extravascular lung water in the adult respiratory distress syndrome. *Chest* 87:585, 1985.

142. Martin GS, Moss M, Wheeler AP, et al.: A randomized, controlled trial of furosemide with or without albumin in hypoproteinemic patients with acute lung injury. *Crit Care Med* 183:1681, 2005.

143. Dubois MJ, Orellana-Jimenez C, Melot C, et al.: Albumin administration improves organ function in critically ill hypoalbuminemic patients: A prospective, randomized, controlled pilot study. *Crit Care Med* 34:2536, 2006.

144. Finfer S, Bellomo R, Boyce N, et al.: A comparison of albumin and saline for fluid resuscitation in the intensive care unit. *N Engl J Med* 350:2247, 2004.

145. Marini JJ: New options for the ventilatory management of acute lung injury. *New Horiz* 1:489, 1993.

146. Heffner JE: Airway management in the critically ill patient. *Crit Care Clin* 6:533, 1990.

147. Marini JJ: Evolving concepts in the ventilatory management of acute respiratory distress syndrome. *Clin Chest Med* 17:555, 1996.

148. Van Hook CJ, Carilli AD, Haponik EF: Hemodynamic effects of positive end-expiratory pressure. Historical perspective. *Am J Med* 81:307, 1986.

149. Yu M, Takiguchi S, Takanishi D, et al.: Evaluation of the clinical usefulness of thermodilution volumetric catheters. *Crit Care Med* 23:681, 1995.

150. Martin C, Saux P, Albanese J, et al.: Right ventricular function during positive end-expiratory pressure: Thermodilution evaluation and clinical application. *Chest* 92:999, 1987.

151. Stoller JK, Kacmarek RM: Ventilatory strategies in the management of the adult respiratory distress syndrome. *Clin Chest Med* 11:755, 1990.

152. Brower RG, Lanken PN, MacIntyre N, et al.: Higher versus lower positive end-expiratory pressures in patients with the acute respiratory distress syndrome. *N Engl J Med* 351:327, 2004.

153. Carroll GC, Tuman KJ, Braverman B, et al.: Minimal positive end-expiratory pressure (PEEP) may be "best PEEP." *Chest* 93:1020, 1988.

154. Muscedere JG, Mullen JB, Gan K, et al.: Tidal ventilation at low airway pressures can augment lung injury. *Am J Respir Crit Care Med* 149:1327, 1994.

155. Gattinoni L, D'Andrea L, Pelosi P, et al.: Regional effects and mechanism of positive end-expiratory pressure in early adult respiratory distress syndrome. *JAMA* 269:2122, 1993.

156. Burchardi H: New strategies in mechanical ventilation for acute lung injury. *Eur Respir J* 9:1063, 1996.

157. Dreyfuss D, Saumon G: Ventilator-induced lung injury: Lessons from experimental studies. *Am J Respir Crit Care Med* 157:294, 1998.

158. The Acute Respiratory Distress Syndrome Network: Ventilation with lower tidal volumes as compared with traditional tidal volumes for acute lung injury and the acute respiratory distress syndrome. *N Engl J Med* 342:1301, 2000.

159. Hickling KG, Henderson SJ, Jackson R: Low mortality associated with low-volume pressure-limited ventilation with permissive hypercapnia in severe adult respiratory distress syndrome. *Intens Care Med* 16:372, 1990.

160. Stewart TE, Meade MO, Cook DJ, et al.: Evaluation of a ventilation strategy to prevent barotrauma in patients at high risk for acute respiratory distress syndrome. Pressure- and Volume-Limited Ventilation Strategy Group. *N Engl J Med* 338:355, 1998.

161. Thomas RC: Experimental displacement of intracellular pH and the mechanism of its subsequent recovery. *J Physiol* 354:3P, 1984.

162. Dries DJ: Permissive hypercapnia. *J Trauma* 39:984, 1995.

163. Feihl F, Perret C: Permissive hypercapnia. How permissive should we be? *Am J Respir Crit Care Med* 150:1722, 1994.

164. Orchard CH, Kentish JC: Effects of changes of pH on the contractile function of cardiac muscle. *Am J Physiol* 258:C967, 1990.

165. Walley KR, Lewis TH, Wood LD: Acute respiratory acidosis decreases left ventricular contractility but increases cardiac output in dogs. *Circ Res* 67:628, 1990.

166. Tang WC, Weil MH, Gazmuri RJ, et al.: Reversible impairment of myocardial contractility due to hypercarbic acidosis in the isolated perfused rat heart. *Crit Care Med* 19:218, 1991.

167. Viitanen A, Salmenpera M, Heinonen J: Right ventricular response to hypercarbia after cardiac surgery. *Anesthesiology* 73:393, 1990.

168. Prough DS, Rogers AT, Stump DA, et al.: Hypercarbia depresses cerebral oxygen consumption during cardiopulmonary bypass. *Stroke* 21:1162, 1990.

169. McIntyre RC Jr, Haenel JB, Moore FA, et al.: Cardiopulmonary effects of permissive hypercapnia in the management of adult respiratory distress syndrome. *J Trauma* 37:433, 1994.

170. Simon RJ, Mawilmada S, Ivatury RR: Hypercapnia: Is there a cause for concern? *J Trauma* 37:74, 1994.

171. Marcy TW, Marini JJ: Inverse ratio ventilation in ARDS: Rationale and implementation. *Chest* 100:494, 1991.

172. Chan K, Abraham E: Effects of inverse ratio ventilation on cardiopulmonary parameters of severe respiratory failure. *Chest* 105:646, 1992.

173. Bryan AC: Conference on the scientific basis of respiratory therapy. Pulmonary physiotherapy in the pediatric age group. Comments of a devil's advocate. *Am Rev Respir Dis* 110:143, 1974.

174. Piehl MA, Brown RS: Use of extreme position changes in acute respiratory failure. *Crit Care Med* 4:13, 1976.

175. Douglas WW, Rehder K, Beynen FM, et al.: Improved oxygenation in patients with acute respiratory failure: The prone position. *Am Rev Respir Dis* 115:559, 1977.

176. Langer M, Mascheroni D, Marcolin R, et al.: The prone position in ARDS patients: A clinical study. *Chest* 94:103, 1988.

177. Pappert D, Rossaint R, Slama K, et al.: Influence of positioning on ventilation-perfusion relationships in severe adult respiratory distress syndrome. *Chest* 106:1511, 1994.

178. Stocker R, Neff T, Stein S, et al.: Prone positioning and low-volume pressure-limited ventilation improve survival in patients with severe ARDS. *Chest* 111:1008, 1997.

179. Blanch L, Mancebo J, Perez M, et al.: Short-term effects of prone position in critically ill patients with acute respiratory distress syndrome. *Intens Care Med* 23:1033, 1997.

180. Albert RK, Leasa D, Sanderson M, et al.: The prone position improves arterial oxygenation and reduces shunt in oleic-acid–induced acute lung injury. *Am Rev Respir Dis* 135:628, 1987.

181. Wiener CM, Kirk W, Albert RK: Prone position reverses gravitational distribution of perfusion in dog lungs with oleic acid–induced injury. *J Appl Physiol* 68:1386, 1990.

182. Lamm WJ, Graham MM, Albert RK: Mechanism by which the prone position improves oxygenation in acute lung injury. *Am J Respir Crit Care Med* 150:184, 1994.

183. Gattinoni L, Pelosi P, Vitale G, et al.: Body position changes redistribute lung computed-tomographic density in patients with acute respiratory failure. *Anesthesiology* 74:15, 1991.

184. Gattinoni L, Tognoni G, Pesenti A, et al.: Effect of prone positioning on the survival of patients with acute respiratory failure. *N Engl J Med* 345:568, 2001.

185. Curley MA, Hibbard PL, Fineman LD: Effect of prone positioning on clinical outcomes in children with acute lung injury. A randomized, controlled trial. *JAMA* 294:229, 2005.

186. Guerine E, Gaillard S, Lemasson S, et al.: Effects of systematic prone positioning in hypoxemia acute respiratory failure: A randomized controlled trial. *JAMA* 19:2379, 2004.

187. Mancebo JM, Fernandez R, Blanch L, et al.: A multicenter trial of prolonged prone ventilation in severe acute respiratory distress syndrome. *Am J Resp Crit Care Med* 173:1233, 2006.
188. Marik PE, Iglesias J: A "prone dependent" patient with severe adult respiratory distress syndrome. *Crit Care Med* 25:1085, 1997.
189. Offner PJ, Haenel JB, Moore EE, et al.: Complications of prone ventilation in patients with multisystem trauma with fulminant acute respiratory distress syndrome. *J Trauma* 48:224, 2000.
190. Nahum A, Shapiro R: Adjuncts to mechanical ventilation. *Clin Chest Med* 17:491, 1996.
191. Nahum A, Ravenscraft SA, Nakos G, et al.: Tracheal gas insufflation during pressure-control ventilation. Effect of catheter position, diameter, and flow rate. *Am Rev Respir Dis* 146:1411, 1992.
192. Barnett C, Moore F, Moore E: Tracheal gas insufflation is a useful adjunct in permissive hypercapnic management of acute respiratory distress syndrome. *Am J Surg* 172:518, 1996.
193. Schuster DP, Klain M, Snyder JV: Comparison of high-frequency jet ventilation to conventional ventilation during severe acute respiratory failure in humans. *Crit Care Med* 10:625, 1982.
194. Hurst JM, Branson RD, Davis K Jr, et al.: Comparison of conventional mechanical ventilation and high-frequency ventilation: A prospective, randomized trial in patients with respiratory failure. *Ann Surg* 211:486, 1990.
195. Carlon GC, Howland WS, Ray C, et al.: High-frequency jet ventilation: A prospective randomized evaluation. *Chest* 84:551, 1983.
196. Gluck E, Heard S, Patel C, et al.: Use of ultrahigh-frequency ventilation in patients with ARDS: A preliminary report. *Chest* 103:1413, 1993.
197. Derdak S, Mehta S, Stewart T, et al.: High-frequency oscillatory ventilation for acute respiratory distress syndrome in adults: A randomized, controlled trial. *Am J Respir Crit Care med* 166:801, 2002.
198. Bishop MJ, Benson MS, Sato P, et al.: Comparison of high-frequency jet ventilation with conventional mechanical ventilation for bronchopleural fistula. *Anesth Analg* 66:833, 1987.
199. Carlon GC, Kahn RC, Howland WS, et al.: Clinical experience with high-frequency jet ventilation. *Crit Care Med* 9:1, 1981.
200. Zapol WM, Snider MT, Hill JD, et al.: Extracorporeal membrane oxygenation in severe acute respiratory failure: A randomized prospective study. *JAMA* 242:2193, 1979.
201. Anderson H III, Steimle C, Shapiro M, et al.: Extracorporeal life support for adult cardiorespiratory failure. *Surgery* 114:161, 1993.
202. Morris AH, Wallace CJ, Menlove RL, et al.: Randomized clinical trial of pressure-controlled inverse ratio ventilation and extracorporeal CO$_2$ removal for adult respiratory distress syndrome. *Am J Respir Crit Care Med* 149:295, 1994.
203. Conrad SA, Eggerstedt JM, Grier LR, et al.: Intravenacaval membrane oxygenation and carbon dioxide removal in severe acute respiratory failure. *Chest* 107:1689, 1995.
204. Conrad SA, Eggerstedt JM, Morris VF, et al.: Prolonged intracorporeal support of gas exchange with an intravenacaval oxygenator. *Chest* 103:158, 1993.
205. Gentilello LM, Jurkovich GJ, Gubler KD, et al.: The intravascular oxygenator (IVOX): Preliminary results of a new means of performing extrapulmonary gas exchange. *J Trauma* 35:399, 1993.
206. Tutuncu AS, Faithfull NS, Lachmann B: Comparison of ventilatory support with intratracheal perfluorocarbon administration and conventional mechanical ventilation in animals with acute respiratory failure. *Am Rev Respir Dis* 148:785, 1993.
207. Richman PS, Wolfson MR, Shaffer TH: Lung lavage with oxygenated perfluorochemical liquid in acute lung injury. *Crit Care Med* 21:768, 1993.
208. Fuhrman BP, Paczan PR, DeFrancisis M: Perfluorocarbon-associated gas exchange. *Crit Care Med* 19:712, 1991.
209. Tutuncu AS, Faithfull NS, Lachmann B: Intratracheal perfluorocarbon administration combined with mechanical ventilation in experimental respiratory distress syndrome: Dose-dependent improvement of gas exchange. *Crit Care Med* 21:962, 1993.
210. Hirschl RB, Croce M, Gore D, et al.: Prospective, randomized, controlled pilot study of partial liquid ventilation in adult acute respiratory distress syndrome. *Am J Respir Crit Care Med* 165:781, 2002.
211. Zapol WM, Hurford WE: Inhaled nitric oxide in adult respiratory distress syndrome and other lung diseases. *Adv Pharmacol* 31:513, 1994.
212. Radermacher P, Santak B, Wust HJ, et al.: Prostacyclin and right ventricular function in patients with pulmonary hypertension associated with ARDS. *Intens Care Med* 16:227, 1990.
213. Palmer RM, Ferrige AG, Moncada S: Nitric oxide release accounts for the biological activity of endothelium-derived relaxing factor. *Nature* 327:524, 1987.
214. Edwards AD: The pharmacology of inhaled nitric oxide. *Arch Dis Child Fetal Neonatal Ed* 72:F127, 1995.
215. Benzing A, Brautigam P, Geiger K, et al.: Inhaled nitric oxide reduces pulmonary transvascular albumin flux in patients with acute lung injury. *Anesthesiology* 83:1153, 1995.
216. Ogura H, Cioffi WG Jr, Jordan BS, et al.: The effect of inhaled nitric oxide on smoke inhalation injury in an ovine model. *J Trauma* 37:294, 1994.
217. Offner PJ, Ogura H, Jordan BS, et al.: Effects of inhaled nitric oxide on right ventricular function in endotoxin shock. *J Trauma* 39:179, 1995.
218. Gerlach H, Pappert D, Lewandowski K, et al.: Long-term inhalation with evaluated low doses of nitric oxide for selective improvement of oxygenation in patients with adult respiratory distress syndrome. *Intens Care Med* 19:443, 1993.
219. Fierobe L, Brunet F, Dhainaut JF, et al.: Effect of inhaled nitric oxide on right ventricular function in adult respiratory distress syndrome. *Am J Respir Crit Care Med* 151:1414, 1995.
220. Rossaint R, Slama K, Steudel W, et al.: Effects of inhaled nitric oxide on right ventricular function in severe acute respiratory distress syndrome. *Intens Care Med* 21:197, 1995.
221. McIntyre RC Jr, Moore FA, Moore EE, et al.: Inhaled nitric oxide variably improves oxygenation and pulmonary hypertension in patients with acute respiratory distress syndrome. *J Trauma* 39:418, 1995.
222. Johannigman JA, Davis K Jr, Campbell RS, et al.: Inhaled nitric oxide in acute respiratory distress syndrome. *J Trauma* 43:904, 1997.
223. Rossaint R, Gerlach H, Schmidt-Ruhnke H, et al.: Efficacy of inhaled nitric oxide in patients with severe ARDS. *Chest* 107:1107, 1995.
224. Ogura H, Cioffi WG, Offner PJ, et al.: Effect of inhaled nitric oxide on pulmonary function after sepsis in a swine model. *Surgery* 116:313, 1994.
225. Shah NS, Nakayama DK, Jacob TD, et al.: Efficacy of inhaled nitric oxide in a porcine model of adult respiratory distress syndrome. *Arch Surg* 129:158, 1994.
226. Puybasset L, Rouby JJ, Mourgeon E, et al.: Factors influencing cardiopulmonary effects of inhaled nitric oxide in acute respiratory failure. *Am J Respir Crit Care Med* 152:318, 1995.
227. Levy B, Bollaert PE, Bauer P, et al.: Therapeutic optimization including inhaled nitric oxide in adult respiratory distress syndrome in a polyvalent intensive care unit. *J Trauma* 38:370, 1995.
228. Guinard N, Belsoucif S, Gatecel C, et al.: Interest of a therapeutic optimization strategy in severe ARDS. *Chest* 111:1000, 1997.
229. Jolliet P, Bulpa P, Ritz M, et al.: Additive beneficial effects of the prone position, nitric oxide, and almitrine bismesylate on gas exchange and oxygen transport in acute respiratory distress syndrome. *Crit Care Med* 25:786, 1997.
230. Lu Q, Mourgeon E, Law-Koune JD, et al.: Dose-response curves of inhaled nitric oxide with and without intravenous almitrine in nitric oxide-responding patients with acute respiratory distress syndrome. *Anesthesiology* 83:929, 1995.
231. Michael JR, Barton RG, Saffle JR, et al.: Inhaled nitric oxide versus conventional therapy: Effect on oxygenation in ARDS. *Am J Respir Crit Care Med* 157:1372, 1998.
232. Troncy E, Collet JP, Shapiro S, et al.: Inhaled nitric oxide in acute respiratory distress syndrome: A pilot randomized controlled study. *Am J Respir Crit Care Med* 157:1483, 1998.
233. Dellinger RP, Zimmerman JL, Taylor RW, et al.: Effects of inhaled nitric oxide in patients with acute respiratory distress syndrome: Results of a randomized phase II trial. Inhaled Nitric Oxide in ARDS Study Group. *Crit Care Med* 26:15, 1998.
234. Taylor RW, Zimmerman JL, Dellinger RP, et al.: Low-dose inhaled nitric oxide in patients with acute lung injury: A randomized, controlled trial. *JAMA* 291:1603, 2004.
235. Adhikari N, Granton JT: Inhaled nitric oxide for acute lung injury. *JAMA* 291:1629, 2004.
236. Kubes P, Suzuki M, Granger DN: Nitric oxide: An endogenous modulator of leukocyte adhesion. *Proc Natl Acad Sci USA* 88:4651, 1991.
237. Biffl WL, Moore EE, Moore FA, et al.: Nitric oxide reduces endothelial expression of intercellular adhesion molecule (ICAM)-1. *J Surg Res* 63:328, 1996.
238. Partrick DA, Moore EE, Offner PJ, et al.: Nitric oxide attenuates platelet-activating factor priming for elastase release in human neutrophils via a cyclic guanosine monophosphate-dependent pathway. *Surgery* 122:196, 1997.
239. Friese RS, Fullerton DA, McIntyre RC Jr, et al.: NO prevents neutrophil-mediated pulmonary vasomotor dysfunction in acute lung injury. *J Surg Res* 63:23, 1996.
240. Chollet-Martin S, Gatecel C, Kermarrec N, et al.: Alveolar neutrophil functions and cytokine levels in patients with the adult respiratory distress syndrome during nitric oxide inhalation. *Am J Respir Crit Care Med* 153:985, 1996.
241. Pearl RG: Inhaled nitric oxide: The past, the present, and the future. *Anesthesiology* 78:413, 1993.
242. Young JD, Dyar OJ: Delivery and monitoring of inhaled nitric oxide. *Intens Care Med* 22:77, 1996.
243. Fink MP, Payen D: The role of nitric oxide in sepsis and ARDS: Synopsis of a roundtable conference held in Brussels on 18–20 March 1995. *Intens Care Med* 22:158, 1996.
244. Lavoie A, Hall JB, Olson DM, et al.: Life-threatening effects of discontinuing inhaled nitric oxide in severe respiratory failure. *Am J Respir Crit Care Med* 153:1985, 1996.
245. King RJ, Clements JA: Surface active materials from dog lung: I. Method of isolation. *Am J Physiology* 223:707, 1972.

246. King RJ, Clements JA: Surface active materials from dog lung: II. Composition and physiological correlations. *Am J Physiol* 223:715, 1972.
247. Lewis JF, Jobe AH: Surfactant and the adult respiratory distress syndrome. *Am Rev Respir Dis* 147:218, 1993.
248. Mason RJ, Greene K, Voelker DR: Surfactant protein A and surfactant protein D in health and disease. *Am J Physiol* 275:L1, 1998.
249. Pison U, Obertacke U, Brand M, et al.: Altered pulmonary surfactant in uncomplicated and septicemia-complicated courses of acute respiratory failure. *J Trauma* 30:19, 1990.
250. Pison U, Seeger W, Buchhorn R, et al.: Surfactant abnormalities in patients with respiratory failure after multiple trauma. *Am Rev Respir Dis* 140:1033, 1989.
251. Greene K, Wright J, Wong W: Serial SP-A levels in BAL and serum of patients with ARDS (abstr). *Am J Respir Care Med* 153:A587, 1996.
252. Kerr CL, Ito Y, Manwell SE, et al.: Effects of surfactant distribution and ventilation strategies on efficacy of exogenous surfactant. *J Appl Physiol* 85:676, 1998.
253. Lewis JF, Goffin J, Yue P, et al.: Evaluation of exogenous surfactant treatment strategies in an adult model of acute lung injury. *J Appl Physiol* 80:1156, 1996.
254. Ito Y, Manwell SE, Kerr CL, et al.: Effects of ventilation strategies on the efficacy of exogenous surfactant therapy in a rabbit model of acute lung injury. *Am J Respir Crit Care Med* 157:149, 1998.
255. Revak SD, Merritt TA, Hallman M, et al.: The use of synthetic peptides in the formation of biophysically and biologically active pulmonary surfactants. *Pediatr Res* 29:460, 1991.
256. McLean LR, Krstenansky JL, Jackson RL, et al.: Mixtures of synthetic peptides and dipalmitoylphosphatidylcholine as lung surfactants. *Am J Physiol* 262:L292, 1992.
257. Nosaka S, Sakai T, Yonekura M, et al.: Surfactant for adults with respiratory failure. *Lancet* 336:947, 1990.
258. Spragg RG, Gilliard N, Richman P, et al.: Acute effects of a single dose of porcine surfactant on patients with the adult respiratory distress syndrome. *Chest* 105:195, 1994.
259. Walmrath D, Gunther A, Ghofrani HA, et al.: Bronchoscopic surfactant administration in patients with severe adult respiratory distress syndrome and sepsis. *Am J Respir Crit Care Med* 154:57, 1996.
260. Anzueto A, Baughman RP, Guntupalli KK, et al.: Aerosolized surfactant in adults with sepsis-induced acute respiratory distress syndrome. Exosurf Acute Respiratory Distress Syndrome Sepsis Study Group. *N Engl J Med* 334:1417, 1996.
261. Jobe AH: Surfactant in the perinatal period. *Early Hum Dev* 29:57, 1992.
262. Wilson DF, Thomas NJ, Markovitz BP, et al.: Effect of exogenous surfactant (calfactant) in pediatric acute lung injury: A randomized, controlled trial. *JAMA* 293:470, 2005.
263. Spragg RJ, Lewis JF, Walmrath HD, et al.: Effect of recombinant surfactant protein C-based surfactant on the acute respiratory distress syndrome. *New Engl J Med* 351:884, 2004.
264. Bernard GR, Luce JM, Sprung CL, et al.: High-dose corticosteroids in patients with the adult respiratory distress syndrome. *N Engl J Med* 317:1565, 1987.
265. Bone RC, Fisher CJ Jr, Clemmer TP, et al.: Early methylprednisolone treatment for septic syndrome and the adult respiratory distress syndrome. *Chest* 92:1032, 1987.
266. Luce JM, Montgomery AB, Marks JD, et al.: Ineffectiveness of high-dose methylprednisolone in preventing parenchymal lung injury and improving mortality in patients with septic shock. *Am Rev Respir Dis* 138:62, 1988.
267. Crouch E: Pathobiology of pulmonary fibrosis. *Am J Physiol* 259:L159, 1990.
268. Bachofen A, Weibel E: Alterations of the gas exchange apparatus in adult respiratory insufficiency associated with septicemia. *Am Rev Respir Dis* 116:589, 1977.
269. Meduri GU, Chinn AJ, Leeper KV, et al.: Corticosteroid rescue treatment of progressive fibroproliferation in late ARDS: Patterns of response and predictors of outcome. *Chest* 105:1516, 1994.
270. Ashbaugh DG, Maier RV: Idiopathic pulmonary fibrosis in adult respiratory distress syndrome: Diagnosis and treatment. *Arch Surg* 120:530, 1985.
271. Hooper RG, Kearl RA: Established ARDS treated with a sustained course of adrenocortical steroids. *Chest* 97:138, 1990.
272. Biffl WL, Moore FA, Moore EE, et al.: Are corticosteroids salvage therapy for refractory acute respiratory distress syndrome? *Am J Surg* 170:591, 1995.
273. Meduri GU, Headley AS, Golden E, et al.: Effect of prolonged methylprednisolone therapy in unresolving acute respiratory distress syndrome: A randomized controlled trial. *JAMA* 280:159, 1998.
274. Meduri GU, Tolley EA, Chrousos GP, et al.: Prolonged methylprednisolone treatment suppresses systemic inflammation in patients with unresolving acute respiratory distress syndrome: Evidence for inadequate endogenous glucocorticoid secretion and inflammation-induced immune cell resistance to glucocorticoids. *Am J Respir Crit Care Med* 165:983, 2002.
275. Steinberg KP, Hudson LB, Goodman RB, et al.: Efficacy and safety of corticosteroids for persistent acute respiratory distress syndrome. *New Engl J Med* 354:1671, 2006.
276. Leeper KV Jr: Diagnosis and treatment of pulmonary infections in adult respiratory distress syndrome. *New Horiz* 1:550, 1993.
277. Eason A, Wunderink RG, Meduri GU: Overrepresentation of gram-negative enterics in suspected ventilator-associated pneumonia (abstr). *Chest* 100:36S, 1991.
278. Lambert RS, Vereen LE, George RB: Comparison of tracheal aspirates and protected brush catheter specimens for identifying pathogenic bacteria in mechanically ventilated patients. *Am J Med Sci* 297:377, 1989.
279. Hill JD, Ratliff JL, Parrott JC, et al.: Pulmonary pathology in acute respiratory insufficiency: Lung biopsy as a diagnostic tool. *J Thorac Cardiovasc Surg* 71:64, 1976.
280. Ferring M, Vincent JL: Is outcome from ARDS related to the severity of respiratory failure? *Eur Respir J* 10:1297, 1997.

# Commentary ■ WALTER L. BIFFL

This chapter provides an extensive discussion of respiratory insufficiency primarily as it relates to the acute respiratory distress syndrome (ARDS). The discussion is thorough, and is well referenced and up to date.

As the authors point out, pulmonary insufficiency in the trauma patient is multifactorial and thus there are a few topics worthy of further discussion. First, the need for mechanical ventilation is the primary risk factor for the development of ventilator-associated pneumonia (VAP). Given the high mortality associated with VAP, it is important to consider potential strategies to prevent it. The current bundled initiatives include daily sedation holidays and trials of spontaneous breathing to assess readiness to extubate; elevation of the head of the bed; thromboembolism prophylaxis; and stress ulcer prophylaxis. In addition, intensive glycemic control and aspiration of subglottic secretions are currently under study.

Much has been written about the benefits of early tracheostomy in trauma patients. The Denver group has been performing bedside tracheostomies routinely for over a decade, and could probably provide a useful description of its place in the SICU based on their extensive experience

Overall, the chapter proves a valuable resource for the trauma/critical care surgeon managing patients with respiratory insufficiency.

# Gastrointestinal Failure

*Rosemary A. Kozar* ■ *Norman W. Weisbrodt* ■ *Frederick A. Moore*

## INTRODUCTION

For patients who survive the first 48 hours of intensive care, sepsis related multiple organ failure (MOF) is the leading cause for prolonged ICU stays and deaths. Several lines of clinical evidence convincingly link gut injury and subsequent dysfunction to MOF.[1] First, patients who experience persistent gut hypoperfusion (documented by gastric tonometry) after resuscitation are at high risk for abdominal compartment syndrome (ACS), MOF, and death.[2] Second, epidemiologic studies have consistently shown that the normally sterile proximal gut becomes heavily colonized with a variety of organisms. These same organisms have been identified to be pathogens that cause late nosocomial infections. Thus, the gut has been called the "undrained abscess" of MOF.[3] Third, gut specific therapies (selective gut decontamination, early enteral nutrition, and most recently immune enhancing enteral diets) have been shown to reduce these nosocomial infections.[4–7] The purpose of this chapter will be to first provide a brief overview of why critically injured trauma patients develop gut dysfunction and how gut dysfunction contributes to adverse outcomes. The discussion will then focus on the pathogenesis and clinical monitoring of specific gut dysfunctions. Based on this information, potential therapeutic strategies to prevent and/or treat gut dysfunction to enhance patient outcome will be discussed.

## HOW GUT DYSFUNCTION CONTRIBUTES TO ADVERSE PATIENT OUTCOME

### Multiple Organ Failure

A recent paradigm of postinjury MOF pathogenesis is depicted in Fig. 64-1.[8] MOF occurs as a result of a dysfunctional inflammatory response and in two different patterns (i.e., early vs. late) (see

Chap. 68). After a traumatic insult, patients are resuscitated into a state of systemic hyperinflammation, now referred to as the systemic inflammatory response syndrome (SIRS). The intensity of SIRS is dependent upon (1) inherent host factors, (2) the degree of shock, and (3) the amount of tissue injured. Of the three, shock is the predominant factor.[9] Mild to moderate SIRS is most likely beneficial while severe SIRS can result in early MOF. As time proceeds, negative feedback systems downregulate certain aspects of acute SIRS to restore homeostasis and limit potential autodestructive inflammation (see Chap. 67). This latter response has been dubbed the compensatory anti-inflammatory response syndrome (CARS) and results in delayed immunosuppression.[10] Mild to moderate delayed immunosuppression is clinically insignificant, but severe immunosuppression is associated with late infections. These late infections can worsen early MOF or precipitate late MOF. More recently, it has been hypothesized that SIRS and CARS are present concurrently following injury. With time though, SIRS ceases to exist and CARS is the predominant force.

The gut is believed to be both an instigator and victim of this dysfunctional inflammatory response.[1] Shock is associated with obligatory gut ischemia. With resuscitation, reperfusion results in a local inflammatory response that can injure the gut setting the stage for ACS (see below).[11] Additionally, the reperfused gut releases mediators, including proteins such as cytokines and lipid such as phospholipase A2, via the mesenteric lymph that amplify SIRS.[12–14] Moreover, for patients undergoing laparotomy, bowel manipulation and anesthetics cause further gut dysfunction.[15] Finally, standard ICU therapies (morphine, $H_2$-antagonists, catecholamines, and broad spectrum antibiotics) and intentional disuse (use of total parenteral nutrition rather than enteral nutrition) promote additional gut dysfunction. The end result is progressive dysfunction (Table 64-1) characterized by gastroesophageal reflux, gastroparesis, duodenogastric reflux, gastric alkalinization, decreased mucosal perfusion, impaired intestinal transit, impaired absorptive capacity, increased permeability, decreased mucosal

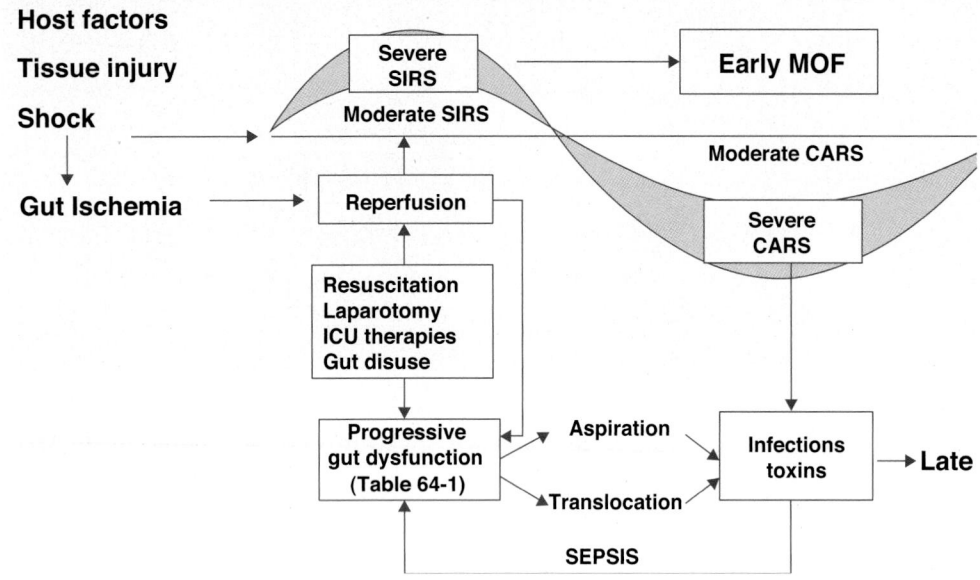

**FIGURE 64-1.** Postinjury multiple organ failure as a result of gut dysfunctions. SIRS, systemic inflammatory response syndrome; ICU, intensive care unit; MOF, multiple organ failure; CARS, counter anti-inflammatory response syndrome.

**TABLE 64-1**

| Progressive Gut Dysfunction in Critically Injured Patients |
| --- |
| Gastroesophageal Reflux |
| Gastroparesis and Duodenogastric Reflux |
| Gastric Alkalinization |
| Decreased Mucosal Perfusion |
| Impaired Intestinal Transit |
| Impaired Gut Absorptive Capacity |
| Increased Gut Permeability |
| Decreased Gut Mucosal Immunity |
| Increased Gut Colonization |
| Gut Edema |

immunity, increased colonization, and gut edema. As time proceeds, the normally sterile upper gut becomes heavily colonized, mucosal permeability increases, and local mucosal immunity decreases.[16] Intraluminal contents (e.g., bacteria and their toxic products) then disseminate by aspiration or translocation to cause systemic sepsis which then promotes further gut dysfunction.[17]

## Abdominal Compartment Syndrome

Intra-abdominal pressure (IAP) is monitored by urinary bladder pressure measurements. When these pressures exceed 25 cm $H_2O$, extra-abdominal organ functions may become impaired (see Chap. 41). By definition, this is ACS. There are two types of ACS: primary (1°) and secondary (2°).[2] Primary ACS occurs in patients with abdominal injuries that typically have undergone "damage control" laparotomy (where obvious bleeding is rapidly controlled and the abdomen is packed) and have entered the "bloody viscus cycle" of coagulapathy, acidosis, and hypothermia which promotes ongoing bleeding (see Chap. 61). Accumulation of blood, worsening bowel edema from resuscitation, and the presence of intra-abdominal packs all contribute to increasing IAP that causes ACS. Secondary ACS occurs when an extra-abdominal injury (e.g., pelvic fracture or mangled extremity) requires massive

resuscitation which causes bowel edema, thus increasing IAP and eventually ACS. Markedly elevated IAP also decreases gut perfusion which may adversely affect a variety of gut functions. Clinical studies have clearly documented the poor outcome of patients developing ACS and the frequent association of ACS and MOF.[18,19]

## Nonocclusive Small Bowel Necrosis (NOBN)

NOBN is a relatively rare, but frequently fatal entity that is associated with the use of enteral nutrition in critically ill patients.[20] Patients typically present with complaints of cramping abdominal pain and progressive abdominal distention associated with SIRS. Computed tomography (CT) may reveal pneumatosis intestinalis or thickened dilated bowel in more advanced stages. For those who progress and require exploratory celiotomy, extensive patchy necrosis of the small bowel is found. Pathologic analysis of the resected specimens yields a spectrum of findings from acute inflammation with mucosal ulceration to transmural necrosis and multiple perforations. The consistent association with enteral nutrition indicates that inappropriate administration of nutrients into a dysfunctional gut plays a pathogenic role. There are three popular hypotheses (Fig. 64-2).[20] First, metabolically compromised enterocytes become ATP depleted as a result of increased energy demands induced by the absorption of intraluminal nutrients, leading to hypoperfusion and subsequent NOBN.[21] The second hypothesis is that when nutrients are delivered into the dysmotile small bowel, fluid shifts into the lumen as a result of the presence of hyperosmolar enteral formula, leading to abdominal distention, which when severe progresses to NOBN. Third, bacterial colonization leads to intraluminal toxin accumulation which can result in mucosal injury and inflammation, and if significant, NOBN.

## SPECIFIC GUT DYSFUNCTIONS

The gut is a complex organ that performs a variety of functions, some of which are vital for ultimate survival of critically ill patients (e.g., barrier function, immune competence, and metabolic regulation).

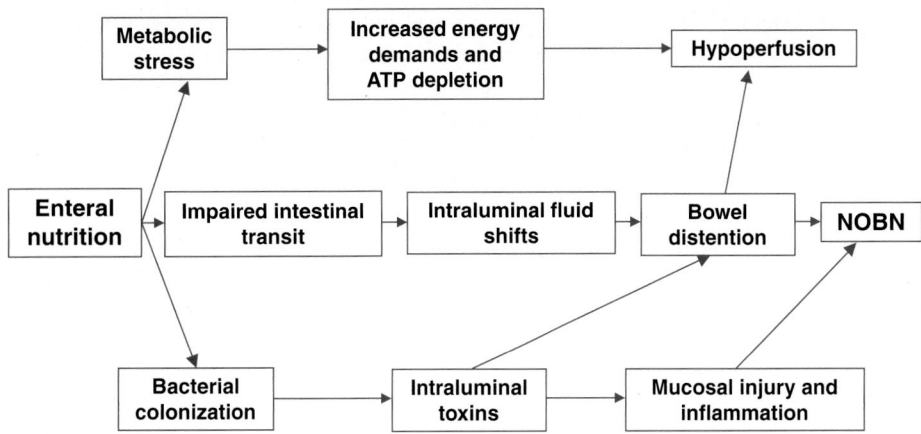

**FIGURE 64-2.** Proposed pathogenesis of nonocclusive bowel necrosis (NOBN).

Unfortunately, gut dysfunction in critically injured patients is poorly characterized and routine monitoring of gut function is crude. Currently, the best parameter of gut function is tolerance to enteral nutrition (see Chap. 66). For several reasons, this is an attractive parameter to monitor and potentially modulate. First, tolerance to enteral nutrition requires integrative gut functioning (e.g., secretion, digestion, motility, and absorption). Second, locally administered nutrients may improve perfusion and optimize the recovery of other vital gut functions (e.g., motility, barrier function, mucosal immunity).[22] Third, tolerance correlates with patient outcome and improving tolerance will likely improve patient outcome. Fourth, refined therapeutic interventions to improve enteral nutrition tolerance will lessen the need to use parenteral nutrition and decrease its associated complications (see Chap. 66).

Parameters of gut dysfunctions are outlined in Table 64-1 and are likely contributors to intolerance to enteral nutrition. A brief overview of the pathogenesis of each of these dysfunctions and how they are monitored clinically will be reviewed to provide the rationale for proposed therapeutic strategies to improve tolerance to enteral nutrition.

## Gastroesophageal Reflux (GER)

GER is an important contributing factor to aspiration of enteral feedings, which is a common cause of pneumonia in ICU patients. Reflux will occur whenever the pressure difference between the stomach and esophagus is great enough to overcome the resistance offered by the lower esophageal sphincter. Increases in gastric pressure can be due to distention with fluids and failure of the stomach to relax to accommodate fluid. Decreases in resistance at the lower esophageal sphincter can be due to relaxation of the sphincter muscle in response to many stimuli including mediators released during injury and resuscitation.[23] Additional contributing factors include: (a) forced supine position, (b) the presence of a nasoenteric tube, (c) hyperglycemia, and (d) morphine.

Commonly used clinical monitors include laboratory testing for presence of glucose in tracheal secretions or by observing blue food dye which has been added to the enteral formula in tracheal aspirates.[24] Detection of glucose lacks specificity. False positive results can occur with high serum glucose levels or presence of blood in tracheal secretions. The use of blue food dye is poorly standardized and lacks sensitivity. More importantly, however,

several reports document absorption of blue food dye in critically ill patients that is associated with death. This is presumably due to a toxic effect that BFD has on mitochondrial function. A recent consensus conference recommended that both these techniques be abandoned.[29] Unfortunately, there are no simple monitors of GER other than observing for vomiting or regurgitation which are not very sensitive. The head of the bed should be elevated 30° to 45° to decrease the risk that when GER occurs that it is less likely to result in pulmonary aspiration (see Chap. 60). Gastric residual volumes should be monitored with the presumption that a distended stomach will lead to higher volume GER (see Chap. 66).

## Gastroparesis and Duodenogastric Reflux

Recent studies have confirmed that gastroparesis is common in ICU patients.[26] Gastroparesis predisposes to increased duodenogastric reflux (a potential contributing factor for gastric alkalinization) and GER (a contributing factor for aspiration). The mechanisms responsible for gastroparesis in critical illness have not been well studied. Potential factors include (a) medications (e.g., morphine, dopamine), (b) sepsis mediators (e.g., nitric oxide), (c) hyperglycemia, and (d) increased intracranial pressure.

The common clinical monitors for gastroparesis are intermittent measurement of gastric residual volumes (GRV) when feeding into the stomach or measurement of continuous suction nasogastric tube output when feeding postpyloric. The practice of using GRV is poorly standardized and is a major obstacle to advancing the rate of enteral nutrition.[27] GRVs appear to correlate poorly with gastric function and GRVs <200 cc generally are well tolerated. GRVs of 200–500 cc should prompt careful clinical assessment and the initiation of a prokinetic agent. With GRVs >500 cc, enteral nutrition should be stopped. After clinical assessment excludes small bowel ileus or obstruction, placement of a post ligament of Treitz feeding tube should be considered (see Chap. 66).

While not well studied in trauma specifically, critically ill patients are known to have a high incidence of gastroduodenal reflux. In a study of antral, duodenal, and proximal jejunal motility, Tournadre et al. demonstrated that postoperative gastroparesis occurs after major abdominal surgery and is associated with discoordinated duodenal contractions of which 20% migrated in a retrograde fashion.[28] Heyland et al. administered radio-labeled enteral formulas through a standard post pyloric naso enteric feeding tube in ventilated ICU patients and documented an 80% rate of radio isotope label reflux into the stomach, 25% reflux rate into the esophagus, and a 4% reflux rate into the lung.[29] Finally, Wilmer et al. reported monitoring bile reflux in the esophagus of ventilated ICU patients using a fiberoptic spectrophotometer that detects and quantifies bilirubin concentration.[30] Endoscopy was performed and documented erosive esophagitis in half of the patients of which 15% had pathologic acid reflux and 100% had pathologic bile reflux. These studies provide convincing evidence that duodenogastric reflux is a common event in ICU patients.

## Gastric Alkalinization

The stomach, through secretion of hydrochloric acid, normally has a pH below 4.0. This acid environment has been correlated with the relatively low bacterial counts found in the stomach. Reviews of several studies have shown that alkalinization of the stomach through the use of antacids, $H_2$ antagonists, and proton pump inhibitors results in gastric colonization by bacteria not normally found in the stomach; and several, but not all, studies have shown that gastric colonization predispose patients to ventilator-associated pneumonia,[31,32] and can increase the risk of community-acquired *C. difficile*-associated disease.[33]

Several animal studies conducted recently by our group have shown that both lipopolysaccharide administration and mesenteric ischemia/reperfusion result in the gastric accumulation of an alkaline fluid.[34] This most likely results from a decrease in gastric acid secretion with continued gastric bicarbonate secretion and the reflux of duodenal contents into the stomach. Even more recently, we have reported that the pH of gastric contents in trauma patients also is elevated, possibly due to similar events.[35] Thus, even without the administration of antacids or inhibitors of acid secretion, gastric alkalinization and bacterial colonization of the stomach are likely in this group of patients. When this is combined with the gastroparesis often seen in these patients (see above), it is easy to envision the stomach becoming a major source of bacteria for ventilator-assisted pneumonia and perhaps translocation to other organs.

## Impaired Mucosal Perfusion

Shock results in disproportionate splanchnic vasoconstriction. The gut mucosa appears to be especially vulnerable to injury during hypoperfusion. The arterioles and venules in the small bowel mucosal villi form "hairpin loops."[36] This anatomic arrangement improves absorptive function, but it also permits a countercurrent exchange of oxygen from the arterioles to the venules in the proximal villus. Under hypoperfused conditions, a proximal "steal" of oxygen is believed to reduce the $pO_2$ at the tip of the villi to zero. The gut mucosa is further injured during reperfusion by reactive oxygen metabolites and recruitment of activated neutrophils (see Chap. 67). This mucosal injury, however, appears to quickly repair. Mucosal blood flow does not always, though, return to baseline with resuscitation and this is in part due to defective vasorelaxation. The gut mucosa is also vulnerable to recurrent episodes of hypoperfusion from ACS, sepsis, and use of vasoactive drugs. Whether recurrent hypoperfusion results in additional

ischemia/reperfusion injury is not known, but it is reasonable to assume that hypoperfusion would decrease gut nutrient absorption and render the patient more susceptible to NOBN.

Monitoring gastric mucosal perfusion in the clinical setting can be done by gastric tonometry. With hypoperfusion, intramucosal $CO_2$ increases due to insufficient clearance of $CO_2$ produced by aerobic metabolism or due to buffering of extra hydrogen ions produced in anaerobic metabolism. As intramucosal $CO_2$ accumulates, it diffuses into the lumen of the stomach. The tonometer measures the $CO_2$ that equilibrates in a saline filled balloon (newer monitor uses air filled balloon) that sits in the stomach. This is the regional $CO_2$ tension ($PrCO_2$) and is assumed to equal the intramucosal $CO_2$ tension. Using this measured $PrCO_2$ and assuming that arterial bicarbonate equals intramucosal bicarbonate, the intramucosal pH (pHi) is calculated by using the Henderson-Hasselbalch equation. Numerous studies have documented that a persistently low pHi (or high $PrCO_2$ level) despite effective systemic resuscitation predicts adverse outcomes[37] and that attempts to resuscitate to correct a low pHi do not favorably influence mortality.[38] Unfortunately, alternative resuscitation strategies have not been able to increase pHi to improve outcome and thus this monitoring tool is in search of a novel application (see Chap. 60).

## Impaired Intestinal Transit

Laboratory models of shock, bowel manipulation, and sepsis demonstrate that small bowel transit is impaired.[15,17,39] In all of these models, cytokines and other mediators are produced by cells in the intestine that impair enteric nerve and/or intestinal smooth muscle function.[17] This impairment in turn is expressed as a decrease in the number and/or force of contractions, or as an abnormal pattern of contractions. Although the results in animal models are convincing, surprisingly, clinical studies indicate that small bowel motility and transit are more often than not well preserved after major elective and emergency laparotomies.[40] This observation coupled with the observation that small bowel absorption of simple nutrients is relatively intact provided the rationale for early jejunal feeding.

Clinical studies have documented that over 85% of critically ill patients tolerate early jejunal feeding.[41,42] In a recent study, severely injured patients had jejunal manometers and feeding tubes placed at secondary laparotomy.[40] Surprisingly, 50% had fasting patterns of motility that included components of the normal migrating motor complexes (MMC). These patients tolerated advancements of enteral nutrition without problems. The other 50% who did not have fasting MMCs did not tolerate early advancement of enteral nutrition. Of note, none of the patients converted to a normal fed pattern of motility once they reached full dose enteral feeding. This could be due to infusion of caloric loads insufficient to bring about conversion. On the other hand, the failure to develop fed activity, a pattern of motility promoting mixing and absorption, might explain why diarrhea is a common problem in this patient group.

Although manometry can be used to monitor motility, it is not practical. Unfortunately, simpler indicators of motility such as the presence of bowel sounds or the passing of flatus are unreliable. Other minimally invasive methods to monitor transit are needed. Contrast studies through the feeding tubes are relatively simple, but not validated.

## Impaired Gut Absorptive Capacity (GAC)

Small bowel absorption of glucose and amino acids is depressed after trauma and sepsis. Multiple factors have been identified including (a) cytosolic calcium overload, (b) ATP depletion, (c) diminished brush border enzyme activity, (d) decreased carrier activity, (e) decreased absorptive epithelial surface area, and (f) hypoalbuminemia. In a recent animal study, intestinal ischemia/reperfusion caused significant mucosal injury and significant depletion of mucosal ATP.[21] When this was combined with exposure of the bowel to a nonmetabolizable nutrient, the damage and ATP depletion were more severe and the absorption of glucose was impaired. In contrast, exposure of the bowel to metabolizable nutrients preserved ATP levels, protected against mucosal injury, and improved GAC.

The clinical significance of these observations remains unclear since most patients tolerate enteral nutrition when delivered into the small bowel. However, decreased GAC may be a cause for diarrhea and may explain why patients commonly experience diarrhea with reinstitution of enteral nutrition after prolonged bowel rest. Unfortunately, there are no easily performed clinical monitors for GAC.

Diarrhea may be indicative of depressed GAC, but there are other causes for diarrhea in the critically ill including impaired transit, bacterial overgrowth (e.g., presence of Clostridium difficile), contaminated enteral formulas, abnormal colonic responses to enteral nutrition (e.g., ascending colon secretion rather than absorption, or impaired distal colon motor activity), and administration of drugs which contain sorbitol (e.g., medication elixirs) or magnesium (e.g., antacids).

## Increased Gut Permeability

Enhanced paracellular permeability represents a type of barrier dysfunction which allows increased passage between viable cells and may induce an inflammatory cascade. The major components of the epithelial barrier are tight junctions, which bind cells together and serve as the gateways to the underlying paracellular spaces. The integrity of the tight junctions is modulated by the actin cytoskeleton. Under conditions of ATP depletion, such as would occur during shock, disruption of the actin cytoskeleton with consequent opening of the tight junctions and loss of the integrity of the permeability barrier can occur.[43]

Intestinal barrier dysfunction has been suggested as a means by which inflammatory cytokines can lead to the systemic inflammatory response syndrome and multiple organ failure.[44] Additionally, increased intestinal permeability has been documented in high-risk patients after burns, sepsis, and shock, in most but not all studies.[45]

## Decreased Gut Mucosal Immunity

During periods of intestinal disuse, critically injured patients are subject to a reduction in gut mucosal immunity. Lack of enteral stimulation (such as during starvation or with use of parenteral nutrition) quickly leads to lack of immunologic protection by mucosal-associated lymphoid tissue, which normally provides protection for both the gastrointestinal and respiratory tracts against microbial flora and infectious pathogens.[16] Kudsk et al. have demonstrated a link between intestinal IgA, intestinal cytokine production, and the vascular endothelium of the GI tract. With enteral stimulation, IL-4, and IL-10 production from the lamina propria of the small intestine stimulate production of IgA on the mucosal surface and inhibit intracellular adhesion molecule-1 (ICAM-1) of the vascular endothelium and subsequent neutrophil-associated inflammation and injury.[46,47]

## Increased Gut Colonization

With progressive gut dysfunction, the normally sterile upper gastrointestinal tract becomes colonized with organisms that become pathogens in nosocomial infections.[3] Gastric alkalinization, paralytic ileus, loss of colonization resistance due to broad spectrum antibiotics, and decreased local gut immunity, have all been proposed mechanisms by which the upper gastrointestinal tract becomes colonized. In an effort to decrease the incidence of infectious complications, selective digestive decontamination (SDD) has been proposed. SDD generally consists of topical nonabsorbed antibiotics along with a short course of parenteral antibiotics. There have been numerous clinical trials and at least six meta-analyses addressing this practice. Most studies have examined the incidence of ventilator associated pneumonias and mortality and, in general, have demonstrated a decrease in both,[48] with benefit greater for surgical than medical ICU patients.[49] Despite rather impressive results of these trials, most of which have been performed in Europe, intensivists in the United States have generally avoided use of SDD due to reports of antimicrobial resistance.[50]

## Gut Edema

Aggressive fluid resuscitation can result in significant bowel edema and altered intestinal function. Both in the laboratory and clinically, significant bowel edema following resuscitation can lead to elevated intraabdominal pressure and potentially to ACS. The precise mechanisms by which bowel edema adversely effects bowel function, however, have not been fully elucidated. Laboratory investigations by Moore-Olufemi et al. have shown that bowel edema alone (not associated with gut ischemia/reperfusion or hemorrhagic shock) is associated with impaired intestinal transit.[51] They subsequently demonstrated that changes in transit are due to alterations in the physical characteristics of the intestine with loss of stiffness and residual stress when edema is present.[52] A number of clinical studies, albeit not in resuscitated trauma patients, have demonstrated the benefit of fluid restriction on postoperative bowel function and complications.[53]

# STRATEGIES TO IMPROVE GUT DYSFUNCTION

## Gut Specific Resuscitation and Monitoring for Abdominal Compartment Syndrome

If shock-induced gut hypoperfusion is assumed to be a prime inciting event for gut dysfunction, then resuscitation protocols need to be devised to optimize early gut perfusion and prevent reperfusion injury. Traditional resuscitation is aimed at optimizing systemic perfusion and the standard of care is to first administer two liters of isotonic crystalloids and then add packed red blood cells to the regimen at a ratio of 3 to 1 crystalloid to blood (see Chap. 13).

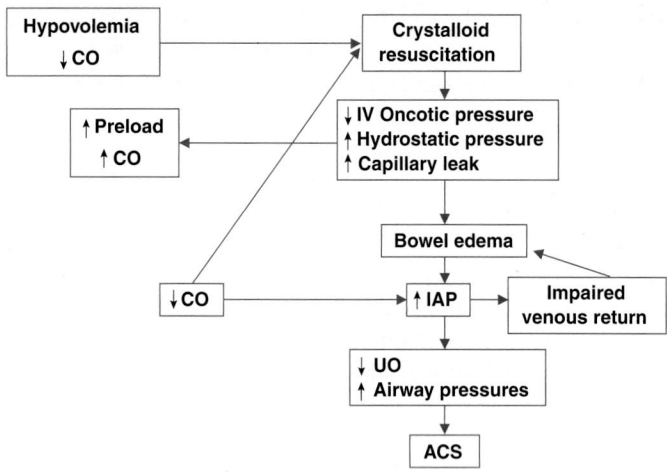

**FIGURE 64-3.** Crystalloid viscious cycle leading to abdominal compartment syndrome. CO, cardiac output; IV, intravenous; IAP, intra-abdominal pressure; UO, urine output; ACS, abdominal compartment syndrome.

While this approach is effective in most patients, it is associated with problematic bowel edema in patients at high risk for MOF. In fact, when at risk patients undergoing standardized shock resuscitation had the endpoint of resuscitation switched from a supranormal to a normal resuscitation goal, less fluid was administered and the incidence of both intra-abdominal hypertension and ACS was decreased as were MOF and mortality.[68]

As edema worsens and intraabdominal pressure increases, bowel perfusion becomes impaired, setting up a vicious cycle that leads to ACS (Fig. 64-3).[54] The hypovolemic trauma patient is volume loaded with crystalloid infusions that decrease intravascular colloid oncotic pressure, increase hydrostatic pressure, and increase capillary leak. Though this intervention can be beneficial in increasing cardiac output through increased preload, it can also have a detrimental effect through increased edema of the reperfused gut. Bowel edema causes intraabdominal pressure to increase, which impairs venous return and may further worsen bowel edema. As abdominal pressures increase, cardiac output is impeded and patients can enter the futile crystalloid preloading cycle, during which further crystalloid infusion worsens bowel edema, and increases intraabdominal pressure until full blown ACS has developed.[55]

Intra-abdominal pressures should be measured routinely in patients in whom significant resuscitation is anticipated as ACS can be predicted early in at risk patients.[2] A high index of suspicion and knowledge of these predictors is warranted. In the past, surgeons have not decompressed the abdomen until clear signs of organ dysfunction were present (e.g., decreased urine output, decreased $PaO_2/F_IO_2$ ratio, decreased cardiac output despite volume loading) in part because of fear of creating an open abdomen with consequent need for planned ventral hernia and delayed reconstruction (see Chap. 41). However, with the advent of vacuum-assisted wound closure of open abdomens this long-term problem is unlikely.[56] As IAP approaches 25 mm Hg, the abdomen is on the steep portion of its compliance curve and additional fluid pushes IAP into pathologic ranges. Thus, based on prediction models,[2] those patients who meet defined high risk criteria and are requiring ongoing aggressive resuscitation may be considered for a "presumptive" decompressive laparotomy.

Alternative resuscitation strategies are under investigation which may lessen bowel edema and therefore reduce the incidence of ACS and may include the earlier use of blood products, more aggressive use of coagulation products, use of blood substitutes, and the use hypertonic saline or colloids in place of isotonic crystalloids.[57,58]

## Analgesics and Sedatives

There are three types of opioid receptors, δ, κ, μ, and all have been identified as having gastrointestinal side effects including delayed gastric emptying and delayed transit time in both the small bowel and colon.[59] One major cause of ileus is stress-related stimulation of opioid receptors. In animal models and humans, both endogenously released and exogenously administered opioids act on receptors in both the central nervous system and in the enteric nervous system to alter intestinal function, especially motility.[60] Although actions at both the central nervous system and enteric nervous system are involved, recent studies indicate that if opioid actions at the enteric nervous system are blocked, ileus may be prevented or resolved without interfering with the desired opioid actions on the central nervous system and other systems. An investigational opioid receptor antagonist that has limited systemic absorption after oral administration and minimal access to the central nervous system has been shown to speed recovery of bowel function and shorten the duration of hospitalization after surgery.[61] There is also a novel, peripherally acting mu receptor antagonist that has recently been shown in a prospective, randomized controlled trial to accelerate time to recovery of gastrointestinal function in patients undergoing elective major abdominal surgery.[62] Both these studies need to be expanded to include patients at high risk for postoperative bowel dysfunction, particularly patients who have undergone major resuscitation from shock.

Ketamine, an antagonist of the *N*-methyl-D-aspartate receptor, combines both analgesic and sedative effects and may represent an alternative to benzodiazapenes for sedation and opioids for pain control in ICU patients. There are reports in burn patients of the opiate-sparing effect of ketamine minimizing prolonged gut dysfunction and ileus.[63] Additionally, both pro-inflammatory cytokines and mediators have been suppressed in laboratory models of sepsis following ketamine administration.[64,65]

## ENTERAL AGENTS

### Benefits of Enteral versus Parenteral Nutrition

Several prospective randomized controlled trials (PRCT) performed in the late 1980s and early 1990s had significant impact on clinical practice in surgical, and particularly trauma ICUs. These single institutional trials all randomized trauma patients to early enteral nutrition or parenteral nutrition and all demonstrated that patients receiving early enteral nutrition had significantly fewer infectious complications (see Chap. 66). A meta-analysis that combined data from eight PRCTs (six published, two not published) was then conducted to assess the nutritional equivalence of enteral nutrition compared to parenteral nutrition in high-risk trauma and/or postoperative patients.[6] Similar to the single institutional trials, fewer infectious complications developed in patients receiving enteral nutrition. Even when patients with catheter-related sepsis were removed from the analysis, a significant difference in infections between groups remained. Taken together, these trials provide convincing evidence that enteral nutrition is preferred to parenteral nutrition in patients sustaining major torso trauma. A recent meta-analysis evaluating the effect of early versus delayed enteral nutrition in acutely ill (medical and surgical) patients also confirmed a decrease in infectious complications in patients receiving early enteral nutrition.[66]

## Modified Enteral Formulas

Recent basic and clinical research suggests that the beneficial effects of enteral nutrition can be amplified by supplementing specific nutrients that exert pharmacologic immune-enhancing effects beyond the prevention of acute protein malnutrition. There are at least 18 PRCT and three meta-analyses[67–69] where an immune-enhancing enteral diet (IED) is compared with a standard enteral diet or no diet and where the patient outcome was a predetermined end point. Of the 18 PRCTs, 11 trials demonstrated improved outcome, four trials were highly suggestive of improved outcome, and three trials did not demonstrate any clinical outcome advantage. The majority of trials are in trauma and cancer patients, though a few trials include mixed ICU and septic ICU patients.

The proposed immune enhancing agents include glutamine, arginine, omega-3 poly unsaturated fats (PUFA), and nucleotides, though the individual contributions of each have not been well investigated. Glutamine is actively absorbed across the intestinal epithelium and then metabolized in the small bowel to ammonia, citrulline, alanine, and proline, and serves as an energy source for the enterocyte. Glutamine is therefore acknowledged to be the preferred fuel of the enterocyte, and stimulates lymphocyte and monocyte function. The demand for glutamine is increased during stressed states and supplementation at pharmacologic doses may be required. Glutamine also promotes protein synthesis, is a precursor for nucleotides as well as glutathione, and is thought to play a role in maintaining gut integrity. In a recent meta-analysis, glutamine (parenteral and enteral) administered to critically ill and surgical patients resulted in a lower mortality, less infectious complications, and shorter hospital stay.[70] High dose and parenteral glutamine had the greatest effect, though the study was not designed to examine these parameters. Additionally, a mixed patient population was included with limited (randomized) studies and clinical endpoints. A randomized trial of glutamine-enriched enteral nutrition in severely injured patients demonstrated a decrease in pneumonia, sepsis, and bacteremia.[71] Laboratory data suggests that enteral glutamine may provide gut protection during periods of gut hypoperfusion through enhanced expression of the anti-inflammatory mediator, peroxisome proliferator activated receptor-gamma.[72]

One proposed mechanism by which enteral nutrients may be beneficial is via prevention or reduction of increased intestinal permeability. Glutamine, in particular, has been suggested as an important nutritional supplement with beneficial effects related to intestinal permeability[73] and although not confirmed by clinical trials may reduce the translocation of bacteria in humans.[74]

Arginine is a semi-essential amino acid that is important for T-cell function and wound healing. Endogenous production is insufficient during periods of metabolic stress (such as illness) and exogenous supplementation is required for maximal function of the immune system. It also is a powerful secretagogue, increasing the production of growth hormone, prolactin, somatostatin, insulin, and glucagon. Additionally, arginine is the chief precursor of nitric oxide and has been shown to increase protein synthesis and improve wound healing.[75] It is the association with nitric oxide production that has led to speculation that arginine may enhance the systemic inflammatory response and therefore be potentially harmful, particularly in the septic patient.[76] Sepsis increases levels of inducible nitric oxide synthetase (iNOS). Arginine is a substrate for iNOS and in its presence, arginine combines with molecular oxygen to produce citrulline and nitric oxide. The resulting nitric oxide could have numerous adverse effects in sepsis including vasodilation, cardiac dysfunction, and direct cytotoxic injury by generating potent reactive oxygen species. Increased mortality has been demonstrated in some critically ill septic patients when receiving an immune enhancing diet, and arginine has been implicated as the causative agent.[77,78] However, Ochou and others have examined arginine metabolism in trauma patients and demonstrated induction of systemic arginase 1, an enzyme which shunts arginine away from the iNOS pathway.[79,80] Though increased arginine at the systemic level does not appear to be problematic for trauma patients, its effects at the gut level are largely unknown.

Although traditional enteral products contain a high proportion of omega-6 polyunsaturated fatty acids (PUFA), diets with a low omega-6 PUFA and high omega-3 PUFA content more favorably alter the fatty acid composition of membrane phospholipids toward reduced inflammation.[81] Finally, nucleotides (purines and pyrimidines) are needed for DNA and RNA synthesis and may be necessary in stressed states to maintain rapid cell proliferation and responsiveness. In the setting of increased demand, most tissues can increase intracellular de novo synthesis of nucleotides. Lymphocytes, macrophages, and enterocytes, however, rely on increased salvage from the extracellular pool that may be depleted during stress.

## Pro-Kinetic Agents

Because gastroparesis and ileus are commonly seen postoperatively and following resuscitation, and because they can complicate initiation of enteral feeding, agents to restore motility have been sought. Evaluation of such pro-kinetic agents is difficult because it is not enough to just stimulate contractions, but contractions at adjacent sites must be coordinated in order for normal digestion, absorption, and transit to take place. Coordinated contractions are under the control of hormonal and neural, both central and peripheral, pathways and it is these pathways that are affected by the cytokines and other mediators that are upregulated following a traumatic insult.[82] Pro-kinetic strategies are aimed at either blocking these mediators or overriding them by stimulating normal pathways.

Agents like erythromycin that act on receptors for motilin, the naturally occurring hormone responsible in part for regulating normal GI motility, have been shown to enhance gastric emptying and intestinal transit in animal models and in some clinical trials. Though clinical studies have documented their effectiveness in promoting gastric emptying[83] their effectiveness in reducing postoperative ileus has been disappointing[84] A promising new peptide, ghrelin, has been shown in a rodent model to not only accelerate gastric emptying and small intestinal transit in unoperated animals but also to reverse postoperative gastric ileus.[85] In a recent clinical trial ghrelin enhanced gastric emptying in patients with diabetic gastroparesis.[86] Additional clinical trials examining the efficacy in postoperative and critically injured patients have yet to be performed.

## Serotonin Antagonists

One of the major transmitters within the enteric nervous system is serotonin. By acting at various serotonin receptors, serotonin can either enhance or inhibit intestinal contractions and transit. In animal and some human studies, motility has been enhanced by 5-HT$_3$ receptor antagonists as well as by 5-HT$_4$ agonists.[87] Although the results were never overwhelmingly convincing or consistent, a few agents have been used in clinical situations. Side effects, however, have resulted in their being removed from the market. This may be an area for future research.

## Antioxidants

The cycle of organ hypoperfusion during shock followed by reperfusion during resuscitation results in the formation of detrimental reactive oxygen species. Thus, it is logical to propose that administration of antioxidants could prove beneficial. In many animal models, administration of agents such as superoxide dismutase, ethyl pyruvate, and melatonin limit damage induced by ischemia/reperfusion.[88,89] In a recent animal study, administration of alpha-melanocyte-stimulating hormone preserved both the function and the structural integrity of the intestine following mesenteric ischemia/reperfusion.[39] A randomized, prospective trial of antioxidant supplementation with Vitamins C and E to critically ill surgical patients, primarily trauma patients, demonstrated a significant reduction in organ failure.[90]

## Probiotics and Prebiotics

A probiotic is defined as a live microbial feed supplement which improves the host's intestinal microbial balance. Commonly utilized probiotics include lactobacilli, bifidobacteria, and saccharomyces. A prebiotic is defined as a nondigestible food ingredient that beneficially affects the host by selectively stimulating the growth and/or activity of specific bacteria in the colon. Probiotics are usually nondigestible oligosaccharides. The most extensively studied are the fructoligosaccharides (FOS) such as oligofructose. FOS are fermented in the colon which promotes the proliferation of bifidobacteria with a reduction in clostridia and fusobacteria. Manipulation of the colonic microflora may reduce the incidence of enteral nutrition-associated diarrhea by suppressing enteropathogens. Results of recent clinical trails employing either probiotics, prebiotics, or a combination, in critically ill and burn patients, however, have been disappointing.[91–93]

In summary, abdominal compartment syndrome and nonocclusive bowel necrosis are two extreme outcomes of gut dysfunction that can directly contribute to multiple organ failure and mortality. Newer modalities to monitor and modulate gut dysfunction need to be developed and appropriate measures taken to reduce its occurrence. The use gut specific resuscitants, opioid antagonists,

alternative sedatives, and early use of enteral nutrients with select supplements such as glutamine or antioxidants, may all assist in preventing the untoward effects of gut dysfunction in critically injured patients.

## REFERENCES

1. Hassoun HH, Mercer DW, Moody FG, et al.: Postinjury multiple organ failure: The role of the gut. *Shock* 15:1, 2001
2. Balogh Z, McKinley BA, Cocanour CS, et al.: Both primary and secondary abdominal compartment syndrome can be predicted early and are harbingers of multiple organ failure. *J Trauma* 54:848, 2003.
3. Marshall JC, Christou NV, Meakins JL: The gastrointestinal tract: The "undrained abscess" of multiple organ failure. *Ann Surg* 218:111, 1993.
4. Heyland DK, Cook DJ, Jaeschke R, et al.: Selective decontamination of the digestive tract: An overview. *Chest* 105:1221, 1994.
5. Moore EE, Jones TN: Benefits of immediate jejunal feeding after major abdominal trauma: A prospective randomized study. *J Trauma* 26:874, 1986.
6. Moore FA, Feliciano DV, Andrassy R, et al.: Enteral feeding reduces postoperative septic complications: A meta-analysis. *Ann Surg* 216:62, 1992.
7. Moore FA: Effects of immune-enhancing diets in infectious morbidity and multiple organ failure. *JPEN* 25:1, 2001.
8. Moore FA, Sauaia A, Moore EE, et al.: Postinjury multiple organ failure: A bimodal phenomenon. *J Trauma* 40:502, 1996.
9. Sauaia A, Moore FA, Moore EE, et al.: Multiple organ failure can be predicted as early as 12 hours postinjury. *J Trauma* 45:291, 1998.
10. Bone RC: Sir Isaac Newton, sepsis, SIRS, and CARS. *Crit Care Med* 24:1125, 1996.
11. Simpson R, Alon R, Kobzik L, et al.: Neutrophil and non-neutrophil-mediated injury in intestinal ischemia/reperfusion. *Ann Surg* 218:444, 1993.
12. Moore EE, Moore FA, Franciose RJ, et al.: Postischemic gut serves as a priming bed for circulating neutrophils that provoke multiple organ failure. *J Trauma* 37:881, 1994.
13. Davidson MT, Deitch EA, Lu Q, et al.: A study of the biologic activity of trauma-hemorrhagic shock mesenteric lymph over time and the relative role of cytokines. *Surgery* 136:32, 2004.
14. Gonzalez RJ, Moore EE, Biffl WL, et al.: The lipid fraction of post-hemorrhagic shock mesenteric lymph (PHSML) inhibits neutrophil apoptosis and enhances cytotoxic potential. *Shock* 14:404, 2000.
15. Schwarz NT, Beer-Stolz D, Simmons RL, et al.: Pathogenesis of paralytic ileus: Intestinal manipulation opens a transient pathway between the intestinal lumen and the leukocytic infiltrate of the jejunal muscularis. *Ann Surg* 235:31, 2002.
16. Sacks GS, Kudsk KA: Maintaining mucosal immunity during parenteral feeding with surrogates to enteral nutrition. *Nutr Clin Pract* 18:483, 2003.
17. Weisbrodt NW, Pressley TA, Li Y-F, et al.: Decreased ileal muscle contractility and increased NOS II expression induced by lipopolysaccharide. *Am J Physiol* 271:G454, 1996.
18. Balogh Z, McKinley BA, Cox CS Jr, et al.: Abdominal compartment syndrome: The cause of effect of postinjury multiple organ failure. *Shock* 20:483, 2003.
19. Raeburn CD, Moore EE, Biffl WL, et al.: The abdominal compartment syndrome is a morbid complication of postinjury damage control surgery. *Am J Surg* 182:542, 2001.
20. Marvin RG, McKinley BA, McQuiggan M, et al.: Nonocclusive bowel necrosis which occurs in critically ill trauma patients receiving enteral nutrition manifests no reliable clinical signs for early detection. *Am J Surg* 179:7, 2000.
21. Kozar RA, Schultz SG, Hassoun HT, et al.: The type of sodium-coupled solute modulates small bowel mucosal injury, transport function and ATP after ischemia/reperfusion injury in rats. *Gastroenterology* 123:810, 2002.
22. Houdijk APJ, Van Leeuwen PAM, Boermeester MA, et al.: Glutamine-enriched enteral diet increases splanchnic blood flow in the rat. *Am J Physiol* 267:G1035, 1994.
23. Fan YP, Chakder S, Gao F, et al.: Inducible and neuronal nitric oxide synthase involvement in lipopolysaccharide-induced sphincteric dysfunction. *Am J Physiol* 280:G32, 2001.
24. Maloney JP, Ryan TA: Detection of aspiration in enterally-fed patients: A requiem for bedside monitors of aspiration. *JPEN* 28:62, 2004.
25. McClave SA, Demeo MT, Delegge MH, et al.: North American Summit on Aspiration in the critically ill patient: Consensus statement. *JPEN* 26:S80, 2002.
26. Ritz MA, Fraser RJ, Edwards N, et al.: Delayed gastric emptying in ventilated critically ill patients: Measurement by 13 C-octanoic acid breath test. *Crit Care Med* 9:1744, 2001.
27. McClave SA, Snider HL: Clinical use of gastric residual volumes as a monitor for patients on enteral tube feeding. *JPEN* 26:S43, 2002.

28. Tournadre JP, Barclay M, Fraser R, et al.: Small intestinal motor patterns in critically ill patients after major abdominal surgery. *Am J Gastroenterol* 96:2418, 2001.

29. Heyland DK, Drover JW, MacDonald S, et al.: Effect of postpyloric feeding on gastroesophageal regurgitation and pulmonary microaspiration: Results of a randomized controlled trial. *Crit Care Med* 29:1495, 2001.

30. Wilmer A, Tack J, Frans E, et al.: Duodenogastroesophageal reflux and esophageal mucosal injury in mechanically ventilated patients. *Gastroenterology* 116:1293, 1999.

31. Heyland D, Mandell LA: Gastric colonization by gram-negative bacilli and nosocomial pneumonia in the intensive care unit patient. Evidence for causation. *Chest* 101:187, 1992.

32. Torres A, El-Ebiary M, Soler N, et al.: Stomach as a source of colonization of the respiratory tract during mechanical ventilation: Association with ventilator-associated pneumonia. *Eur Respir J* 9:1729, 1996.

33. Dial S, Delaney JAC, Barkun AN, et al.: Use of gastric acid-suppressive agents and the risk of community-acquired *Clostridium difficile*-associated disease. *JAMA* 294:2989, 2005.

34. Castaneda A, Vilela R, Chang L, et al.: Effects of intestinal ischemia/reperfusion injury on gastric acid secretion. *J Surg Res* 90:88, 2000.

35. Cocanour CS, Dial ED, Kozar RA, et al.: Gastric alkalinization following major trauma. *J Trauma* 54:211, 2003.

36. Lundgren O, Haglund U: The pathophysiology of the intestinal countercurrent exchanger. *Life Sci* 23:1411, 1978.

37. Levy B, Gawalkiewicz P, Vallet B, et al.: Gastric tonometry with air-automated tonometry predicts outcome in critically ill patients. *Crit Care Med* 31:474, 2003.

38. Miami Trauma Clinical Trials Group: Splanchnic hypoperfusion-directed therapies in trauma: A prospective, randomized trial. *Am Surg* 71:252, 2005.

39. Hassoun HT, Moore FA, Kozar RA, et al.: Alpha-melanocyte stimulating hormone protects against mesenteric ischemia/reperfusion injury. *Am J Physiol* 282:G1059, 2002.

40. Moore FA, Cocanour CS, McKinley BA, et al.: Migrating motility complexes persist after severe traumatic shock in patients who tolerate enteral nutrition. *J Trauma* 51:1075, 2001.

41. Kozar RA, McQuiggan MM, Moore EE, et al.: Postinjury enteral tolerance is reliably achieved by a standardized protocol. *J Surg Res* 104:70, 2002.

42. Cothren CC, Moore EE, Ciesla DJ, et al.: Postinjury abdominal compartment syndrome does not preclude early enteral feeding after definitive closure. *Am J Surg* 188:653, 2004.

43. Sun Z, Wang X, Deng X, et al.: The influence of intestinal ischemia and reperfusion on bi-directional intestinal barrier permeability, cellular membrane integrity, proteinase inhibitors, and cell death in rats. *Shock* 19:203, 1998.

44. Deitch EA, Xy DZ, Franko L, et al.: Evidence favoring the role of the gut as a cytokine-generating organ in rats subjected to hemorrhagic shock. *Shock* 1:141, 1995.

45. Pape HC, Dwenger A, Regel G, et al.: Increased intestinal permeability after multiple trauma. *Br J Trauma* 81:850, 1999.

46. Kudsk KA: Effect of route and type of nutrition on intestine-derived inflammatory responses. *Am J Surg* 185:16, 2003.

47. Ikeda S, Kudsk KA, Fukatsu K, et al.: Enteral feeding preserves mucosal immunity despite in vivo MAdCAM-1 blockade of lymphocyte homing. *Ann Surg* 237:677, 2003.

48. Liberati A, D'Amico R, Pifferi S, et al.: Antibiotic prophylaxis to reduce respiratory tract infections and mortality in adults receiving intensive care. Cochrane Database Syst Rev. (1):CD000022; 2004.

49. Nathens AB, Marshall JC: Selective decontamination of the digestive tract in surgical patients. *Arch Surg* 134:170, 1999.

50. Kollef MH: Selective digestive decontamination should not be routinely employed. *Chest* 123:464S, 2003.

51. Moore-Olufemi SA, Xue H, Attuwaybi BO, et al.: Resuscitation-induced gut edema and intestinal dysfunction. *J Trauma* 58:264, 2005.

52. Radhakrishnan RS, Xue H, Weisbrodt N, et al.: Resuscitation-induced intestinal edema decreases the stiffness and residual stress of the intestine. *Shock* 24:165, 2005.

53. Brandstrup B, Tonnesen H, Beier-Holgersen R, et al.: Danish Study Group on Perioperative Fluid Therapy. Effects of intravenous fluid restriction on postoperative complications: Comparison of two perioperative fluid regimens: A randomized assessor-blinded multicenter trial. *Ann Surg* 238:641, 2003.

54. Balogh Z, McKinley BA, Cocanour CS, et al.: Supra-normal trauma resuscitation causes more cases of abdominal compartment syndrome. *Arch Surg* 138:637, 2003.

55. Balogh Z, McKinley BA, Cocanour CS, et al.: Patients with impending abdominal compartment syndrome do not respond to early volume loading. *Am J Surg* 186:602, 2003.

56. Miller PR, Meredith JW, Johnson JC, et al.: Prospective evaluation of vacuum-assisted fascial closure after open abdomen: Planned ventral hernia rate is substantially reduced. *Ann Surg* 239:608, 2004.

57. Attuwaybi B, Kozar RA, Gates KS, et al.: Hypertonic saline prevents inflammation, injury, and impaired intestinal transit after gut ischemia/reperfusion by inducing heme oxygenase 1 (HO-1) enzyme. *J Trauma* 56:749, 2004.

58. Gonzalez EA, Moore FA, Holcomb JC, et al.: Fresh frozen plasma should be given earlier to patients requiring massive transfusions. *J Trauma* 62:112, 2007.

59. De Schepper HU, Cremonini F, Park MI, et al.: Opioids and the gut: Pharmacology and current clinical experience. *Neurogastroenterol Motil* 16:383, 2004.

60. Bauer AJ, Boeckxstaens GE: Mechanisms of postoperative ileus. *Neurogastroenterol Motil* 16:54, 2004.

61. Taguchi A, Sharma N, Saleem RM, et al.: Selective postoperative inhibition of gastrointestinal opioid receptors. *N Engl J Med* 345:935, 2001.

62. Wolff BG, Michelassi F, Gerkin TM, et al.: Alvimopan, a novel, peripherally acting mu opioid antagonist: Results of a multicenter, randomized, double-blind, placebo-controlled, phase III trial of major abdominal surgery and postoperative ileus. *Ann Surg* 240:728, 2004.

63. Edrich T, Friedrich AD, Eltzschig HK, et al.: Ketamine for long-term sedation and analgesia of a burn patient. *Anesth Analg* 99:393, 2004.

64. Helmer KS, Cui Y, Chang L, et al.: Effects of ketamine/xylazine on expression of TNF-alpha, inducible nitric oxide snythase, and cyclo-oxygenase-2 in rat mucosa during endotoxemia. *Shock* 20:63, 2003.

65. Sun J, Wang XD, Liu H, et al.: Ketamine suppresses endotoxin-induced NF-kappaB activation and cytokines production in the intestine. *Acta Anaesthesiol Scand* 48:317, 2004.

66. Marik PE, Zaloga P: Early enteral nutrition in acutely ill patients: A systematic review. *Crit Care Med* 29:2264, 2002.

67. Heys SD, Walker LG, Smith I, et al.: Enteral nutrition supplementation with key nutrients in patients with critical illness and cancer. *Ann Surg* 229:467, 1999.

68. Beale RJ, Bryg DJ, Bihari DJ: Immunonutrition in the critically ill: A systematic review of clinical outcome. *Crit Care Med* 27:2799, 1999.

69. Heyland DK, Novak F, Drover JW, et al.: Should immuno-nutrition become routine in the critically ill patient? *JAMA* 286:944, 2001.

70. Novak F, Heyland DK, Avenell A, et al.: Glutamine supplementation in serious illness: A systematic review of the evidence. *Crit Care Med* 30:2002, 2002.

71. Houdijk APJ, Rijnsburger ER, Jansen J, et al.: Randomized trial of glutamine-enriched enteral nutrition on infectious morbidity in patients with multiple trauma. *Lancet* 352:772, 1998.

72. Sato N, Moore FA, Kone BC, et al.: Differential induction of PPARgamma by luminal glutamine and iNOS by arginine in the rodent model of post ischemic small bowel. *Am J Physiol* Epub ahead of print Oct 27, 2005.

73. Peng X, Yan H, You Z, et al.: Effects of enteral supplementation with glutamine granules on intestinal mucosal barrier function in severe burns. *Burns* 30:135, 2004.

74. De-Souza DA, Greene LJ: Intestinal permeability and systemic infections in critically ill patients: Effect of glutamine. *Crit Care Med* 33:1125, 2005.

75. Barbul A, Lazarou SA, Efron DT: Arginine enhances wound healing and lymphocyte immune responses in humans. *Surgery* 108:331, 1990.

76. Suchner U, Heyland DK, Peter K: Immune-modulatory actions of arginine in the critically ill. *Br J Nutr* 87:S121, 2002.

77. Bower RH, Cerra FB, Bershadsky B, et al.: Early administration of a formula (Impact) supplemented with arginine, nucleotides, and fish oil in intensive care patients: Results of a multicenter, prospective, clinical trial. *Crit Care Med* 23:834, 2001.

78. Bruzzone R, Radrizzani D: Early enteral immunonutrition in patients with severe sepsis. Results of an interim analysis of a randomized multicenter trial. *Int Surg* 29:834, 2003.

79. Ochoa JB, Bernard AC, O'Brien WE, et al.: Arginase 1 expression and activity in human mononuclear cells after injury. *Ann Surg* 233:393, 2001.

80. Tsuei BJ, Bernard AC, Barksdale AR, et al.: Supplemental enteral arginine is metabolized to ornithine in injured patients. *J Surg Res* 123:17, 2004.

81. De Caterina R, Liao JK, Libby P: Fatty acid modulation of endothelial activation. *Am J Clin Nutr* 71:213S, 2000.

82. Collins SM: The immunomodulation of enteric neuromuscular function: Implications for motility and inflammatory disorders. *Gastroenterology* 111:1683, 1996.

83. Boivin MA, Levy H: Gastric feeding with erythromycin is equivalent to transpyloric feeding in critically ill patients intolerant of nasogastric feeding. *Crit Care Med* 29:1916, 2001.

84. Smith AJ, Missan A, Lanouette NM, et al.: Prokinetic effect of erythromycin after colorectal surgery: Randomized, placebo-controlled, double-blind study. *Dis Colon Rectum* 43:333, 2000.

85. Trudel L, Tomasetto C, Rio MC, et al.: Ghrelin/motilin-related protein is a potent prokinetic to reverse gastric postoperative ileus in rat. *Am J Physiol Gastrointest Liver Physiol* 282:948, 2002.

86. Murray CD, Martin NM, Patterson M, et al.: Ghrelin enhances gastric emptying in diabetic gastroparesis: A double blind, placebo controlled, crossover study. *Gut* 54:1693, 2005.

87. Aros SD, Camilleri M: Small-bowel motility. *Curr Opin Gastroenterol* 17:140, 2001.
88. Kazez A, Demirbag M, Ustundag B, et al.: The role of melatonin in prevention of intestinal ischemia-reperfusion injury in rats. *J Pediatr Surg* 35:1444, 2000.
89. Sims CA, Wattanasirichaigoon S, Menconi MJ, et al.: Ringer's ethyl pyruvate solution ameliorates ischemia/reperfusion-induced intestinal mucosal injury in rats. *Crit Care Med* 29:1513, 2001.
90. Nathens AB, Neff MJ, Jurkovich GJ, et al.: Randomized, prospective trial of antioxidant supplementation in critically ill surgical patients. *Ann Surg* 236:814, 2002.
91. McNaught CE, Woodcock NP, Anderson AD, et al.: A prospective randomized trial of probiotics in critically ill patients. *Clin Nutr* 24:211, 2005.
92. Olguin F, Araya M, Hirsh S, et al.: Prebiotic ingestion does not improve gastrointestinal barrier function in burn patients. *Burns* 31:482, 2005.
93. Jain PK, McNaught CE, Anderson AD, et al.: Influence of synbiotic containing Lactobacillus acidophilus La5, Bifidobacterium lactis Bb 12, Streptococcus thermophilus, Lactobacillus bulgaricus and oligofructose on gut barrier function and sepsis in critically ill patients: A randomized controlled trial. *Clin Nutr* 23:467, 2004.

# Commentary   ■ JEFFREY M. NICHOLAS

The authors have provided an excellent review of gastrointestinal failure illustrating how gut dysfunction contributes to multiple organ failure (MOF), abdominal compartment syndrome (ACS), and nonocclusive bowel necrosis (NOBN). They discuss in detail specific gut dysfunctions that occur in trauma and critical illness and provide strategies to minimize gut dysfunction. One is left with a clear understanding of this problem and the authors are to be congratulated on their comprehensive review of this complex subject.

Enteral nutrition reduces septic complications; however, the authors point out that gastroesophageal reflux, gastroparesis, and duodenogastric reflux limit the ability to successfully feed the stomach. In addition previous aspiration, high gastric residuals, diabetes mellitus, and presence of a nasogastric tube are known risk factors for aspiration, while enteral fat further delays gastric emptying. Patients with head injury have a decreased lower esophageal sphincter tone placing them at increased risk of aspirating gastric feeds. While postpyloric feeding seems preferable, no aspiration difference has been shown when compared to gastric feedings possibly due to duodenogastric reflux.

Jejunal feeding reduces aspiration and improves tolerance when enteral formulas are provided distal to the ligament of Treitz. However, this is not easily accomplished due to the difficulty in timely, nonoperative, placement of feeding tubes distal to the ligament of Treitz. Early jejunal feeding is well tolerated by the critically ill and is superior to total parenteral nutrition (TPN) in reducing septic complications. Additional benefit may be gained from immune enhancing diets containing glutamine, arginine, and omega-3 fatty acids.

We have employed the following strategy quite successfully even in our damage control and open abdominal patient populations. Tube feedings are never considered in patients on alpha agonists or in patients that are not fully resuscitated. Normalization of hemodynamic parameters, urine output, pH, and base deficit can be used to determine resolution of the shock state. Bedside endoscopic placement of a 7-Fr Wilson-Cook nasobiliary drainage catheter distal to the ligament of Treitz is performed as described by Reed when it is deemed appropriate to begin enteral feeds. Our group placed 226 feeding tubes using this technique and found overall placement distal to the ligament of Treitz in 90.3% (95% CI 85.7% to 93.5%) with a 93.8% success rate in trauma patients (95% CI 89.3% to 96.5%). A 59% reduction in the number of patients receiving TPN and a 45% reduction in the number of TPN days was accomplished using this technique including a 68% reduction in the number of trauma patients on TPN and a 71%

decrease in the number of trauma patient TPN days. Enteral feeding is begun with an isotonic immune enhancing formula at 20 cc/hour and advanced 15cc every eight hours to a goal of 25–35 non-protein kcal/kg/day and 1.5 to 2.0 grams of protein/kg/day based on ideal body weight. Ten grams of glutamine is supplemented every eight hours through a nasogastric tube (NGT). Jejunal feedings are not held except for signs of intolerance such as gastric reflux of tube feeds as determined by NGT aspiration, abdominal distension, or diarrhea. Jejunal feeds are also held in patients requiring vasopressors or with new onset acidosis or worsening base deficit suggesting malperfusion. Consideration should be given to changing feeds in septic, hypotensive patients to a formula that does not contain arginine due to the potential for increased production of nitric oxide. We have recently been using a formula containing omega-3 fatty acids, eicosapentaenoic acid, and gamma linolenic acid in our ARDS population for benefits thought to be related to reduction in the proinflammatory mediators generated by arachadonic acid metabolism. All patients are monitored for abdominal distension and bladder pressures are measured routinely in those at risk for ACS. Tube feedings are held in patients with concern for ACS. Patients with diarrhea have their tube feedings held or decreased. They are routinely tested for Clostridium Difficile and their medications are reviewed for sorbitol containing elixirs. Lactobacillus packets may be useful in resolving diarrhea in patients that have been on broad-spectrum antibiotics.

In summary, enteral nutrition may reduce sepsis and prevent gastrointestinal failure and its sequela. It is tolerated in most resuscitated critically ill patients when delivered distal to the ligament of Treitz. An immune enhancing formula should be used in the absence of sepsis and close monitoring of tolerance is critical in all patients. This strategy can be accomplished in a timely manner using an endoscopic approach to placement of jejunal feeding tubes in patients that have not had operatively placed feeding tubes.

## References

1. Saxe JM, Ledgerwood AM, Lucas CE, et al.: Lower esophageal sphincter dysfunction precludes safe gastric feeding after head injury. *J Trauma* 37:581, 1994.
2. Reed RL, Eachempati SR, Russell MK, et al.: Endoscopic placement of jejunal feeding catheters in critically ill patients by a "push" technique. *J Trauma* 45:388, 1998.
3. Nicholas JM, Cornelius MW, Tchorz KM, et al.: A two institution experience with 226 endoscopically placed jejunal feeding tubes in critically ill surgical patients. *Am J Surg* 186:583, 2003.

# Acute Renal Failure

*H. Gill Cryer*

Acute deterioration of renal function often complicates care of trauma patients, increasing morbidity and mortality through effects on nearly all other organ systems (see Chap. 68). Traumatic damage to the kidney or to the renovascular system rarely causes renal dysfunction in the trauma patient. Prerenal azotemia or postrenal (obstructive) uropathy may complicate the immediate postinjury period, manifesting as a sudden drop in urine output. Additional common etiologies of renal dysfunction are renal hypoperfusion and toxin-mediated (radiocontrast, antimicrobials) renal parenchymal injury. This intrinsic renal failure—most often manifesting as acute tubular necrosis—has a more gradual onset, requires more time to resolve, and has greater therapeutic and prognostic implications. This chapter reviews normal renal physiology, the pathophysiology of intrinsic renal failure, management principles, and experimental approaches with emphasis on the pathogenesis and treatment of acute renal failure in trauma patients.

## DEFINITIONS

Acute renal failure (ARF) is abrupt (hours or days) deterioration of renal function with a decrease in glomerular filtration rate (GFR), or renal tubular injury compromising the kidney's ability to maintain fluid or electrolyte homeostasis. Despite the effort devoted to the study of ARF, no consensus definitions of ARF exist. Most commonly, investigators define ARF as (1) an increase in serum creatinine ($P_{Cr}$) of 0.5 mg/dL or greater from baseline, (2) a 50% increase in $P_{Cr}$, (3) a 50% reduction in calculated creatinine clearance ($C_{Cr}$), or (4) a decrease in renal function that warrants dialysis.[1] Consequently, clinical trials assessing various proposed interventions for ARF use disparate entry criteria and outcome measures.[2]

In the absence of a universal definition, a reasonable definition of ARF is an acute and sustained increase in serum creatinine concentration of 44.2 μmol/L if the baseline is less than 221 μmol/L, or an increase in serum creatinine concentration of more than 20% if the baseline is more than 221 μmol/L.[3] The Acute Dialysis Quality Initiative group lately proposed the RIFLE system (Table 65-1), classifying ARF into three severity categories (risk, injury, and failure) and two clinical outcome categories (loss and end-stage renal disease).[4]

Other established definitions include the following. Acute azotemia is any increase in serum blood urea nitrogen (BUN) or creatinine of greater than 50% over baseline in 24 hours. Prerenal azotemia denotes azotemia resulting from decreased renal perfusion in the absence of intrinsic renal dysfunction, while obstructive or postrenal uropathy is a sudden decrease in urine output due to obstruction of the urethra or ureters. Both prerenal azotemia and postrenal uropathy are reversible if identified and treated quickly, but either may damage the renal parenchyma, progressing to intrinsic renal failure if left untreated. While clinicians may presumptively diagnose acute tubular necrosis (ATN) in patients with renal parenchymal damage, ATN is a specific pathologic diagnosis applied to characteristic damage in the tubular structures of the nephron. Classes of intrinsic renal failure other than ATN include acute interstitial nephritis, glomerulonephritis, and vasculitis, but these are uncommon in the trauma patient.

Acute renal failure may or may not include a decrease in urine output. Acute oliguria is typically defined as urine output (UOP) less than 400 mL in any 24-hour period. Accumulation of nitrogenous waste products, or failure to maintain water or electrolyte homeostasis in the face of UOP of 400 to 1,000 mL/day is nonoliguric renal failure. High-output renal failure is renal insufficiency despite maintenance of greater than 1,000 mL of UOP per day. Anuria is any urine volume of less than 50 mL/day. Oliguria associated with ATN rarely progresses to anuria, but it may occur in ATN associated with severe sepsis. Thus, abrupt development of anuria suggests other conditions such as renal vascular occlusion, obstructive uropathy, or severe cortical necrosis.

**TABLE 65-1**

**RIFLE Classification**

| GFR CRITERIA | URINE OUTPUT CRITERIA | |
|---|---|---|
| Risk | Serum creatinine increased 1.5 times | <0.5mL kg$^{-1}$h$^{-1}$ for 6h |
| Injury | Serum creatinine increased 2.0 times | <0.5 mL kg$^{-1}$h$^{-1}$ for 12h |
| Failure | Serum creatinine increase 3.0 times or | <0.3 mL kg$^{-1}$h$^{-1}$ for 24h |
| | Creatinine 355 μmol/L when there was an Acute rise of 44 μmol/L | or anuria for 12h |
| Loss | Persistent acute renal failure; complete Loss of kidney function for longer than 4 weeks | |
| End-stage | End-stage renal disease for longer than 3 months | RENAL DISEASE |

GFR, glomerular filtration rate.

## INCIDENCE AND RISK FACTORS

Advances in evacuation and resuscitation produced declining rates of posttraumatic renal failure in war casualties (42% in World War II, 35% in Korea, 0.17% in Vietnam). This decline in posttraumatic ARF was reproduced in the civilian population: ARF requiring dialysis in trauma patients is rare (<0.1 to 3.7% of all trauma admissions[5]), and incidence appears to be decreasing.[3,4] Overall, ARF is reported in approximately 0.5% of all hospital admissions.[6] The relatively small number of patients progressing to dialysis-dependent ARF reflects rapid transport, early resuscitation, and careful vigilance in the intensive care unit (ICU). On the other hand, renal dysfunction without dialysis dependence remains common, and it may become more common as an older population increasingly survives traumatic insults past initial resuscitation (see Chap. 47).

Primary risk factors for development of ARF include severity and duration of renal hypoperfusion, exposure to nephrotoxins, and pre-existing renal insufficiency. Historical data and clinical observation demonstrate that increasing time from injury until resuscitation increases risk for ARF (see Chap. 11). A recent prospective analysis of high-risk trauma patients found a 31% incidence of ARF in 153 consecutive trauma patients admitted to the ICU. The risk of ARF was increased by age, Injury Severity Score (ISS) >17, hemoperitoneum, shock, hypotensive, bone fractures, acute lung injury repair requiring mechanical ventilation, and Glasgow Coma Score (GCS) < 10. In a logistic model the need for mechanical ventilation with a peep > 6 cm $H_2O$, rhabdomyolysis with CPK > 10,000 IU/1, and hemoperitoneum were the three conditions most strongly associated with ARF.[7] Patients with diabetes, advanced age, or peripheral vascular disease may have sustained progressive loss of functional nephrons, and may also have less effective compensatory and protective mechanisms.

While most hospitalized patients who develop ARF have more than one risk factor, renal ischemia is the central contributor in at least half of these cases.[8] Ischemia can result from low renal blood flow or from altered intrarenal hemodynamics. Many processes decrease renal blood flow: absolute loss of intravascular volume (hemorrhage, gastrointestinal tract losses, etc.), decreased effective intravascular volume (sepsis, peritonitis, rhabdomyolysis, severe soft-tissue injuries, or burns), or diminished cardiac output (congestive heart failure, myocardial ischemia, dysrhythmia). A variety of medications (nonsteroidal anti-inflammatory drugs [NSAIDs], angiotensin-converting enzyme inhibitors, radiocontrast, and amphotericin-B) alter intrarenal hemodynamics, disrupt renal autoregulation, and produce patchy areas of ischemia. After ischemia, toxins account for most cases of ARF. Many agents (aminoglycosides, amphotericin, myoglobin, hemoglobin) are directly toxic to renal parenchymal cells (see Chap. 19). The onset of renal insufficiency days after an injury or operation is often the first sign of the onset of multiple organ dysfunction syndrome (MODS) secondary to sepsis (see Chap. 68). Perhaps most important, multiple insults (e.g., sustained hypotension in a patient receiving radiocontrast) increase the likelihood of renal damage (see Chap. 16). Despite the identification of many well-known risks, predicting which patients will develop ARF remains difficult. However, understanding of the mechanisms underlying these risk factors continues to improve; most of the risk factors identified above have been linked to specific pathophysiologies.

## NORMAL RENAL PHYSIOLOGY

The major aspects of renal function are renal blood flow, glomerular filtration, and tubular excretion and reabsorption. In normal circumstances, renal blood flow (RBF) is the highest per weight of any organ (20 to 25% of cardiac output) and is directed primarily to the renal cortex to optimize glomerular filtration (Fig. 65-1). In contrast, relatively less blood perfuses the renal medulla. Blood flow to the kidney is maintained over a wide range of arterial blood pressure (autoregulation) and is governed by neural, hormonal, and local paracrine effectors. Several mechanisms regulate RBF and GFR including tubuloglomerular feedback (TGF), the renin–angiotensin system, dynamic myogenic response of the renal vasculature, direct innervation by sympathetic fibers,[9] and circulating catecholamines. Local paracrine or autocrine effectors include vasodilators (nitric oxide, prostaglandin $E_2$ [$PGE_2$], and adenosine) and medullary vasoconstrictors (endothelin [ET-1], thromboxane $A_2$, serotonin, and platelet-activating factor [PAF]).[10] The result of interplay among these controllers is maintenance of nearly constant blood flow to the glomerulus despite widely or rapidly ranging perfusion pressures.[10]

An important component of the RBF autoregulatory mechanism is control of the GFR. Tight regulation of glomerular capillary hydraulic pressure ($P_{GC}$) via afferent arteriole dilation and efferent arteriole constriction allows precise control of GFR (Figs. 65-2 and 65-3). The equation governing filtration through the glomerulus is an adaptation of Starling's equation:

$$GFR = L_P \cdot S \cdot [(P_{gc} - P_{bs}) - s(\pi_p - \pi_{bs})]$$

where $L_p$ is porosity of the capillary wall per unit area, $S$ is the filtration surface area, $P_{gc}$ and $P_{bs}$ are hydraulic pressures in the glomerular capillary and in Bowman's space, $\pi_{ps}$ and $\pi_{bs}$ are oncotic pressures in the plasma, and $s$ is the reflection coefficient for proteins.

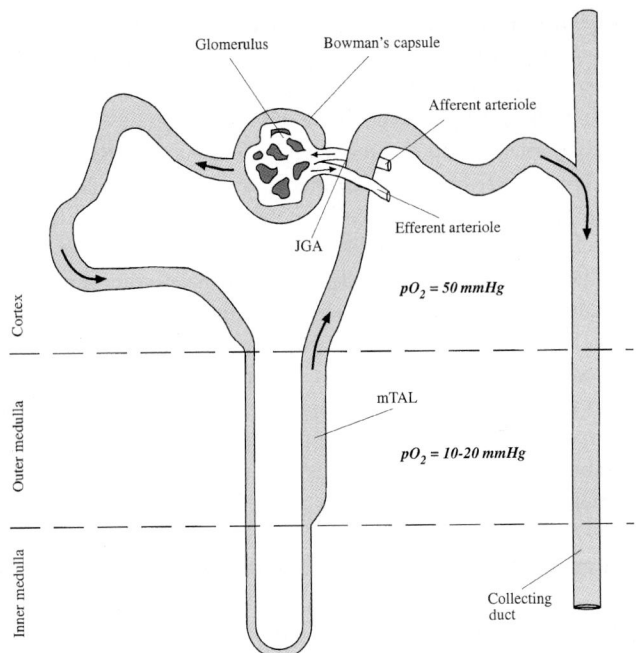

**FIGURE 65-1.** A cartoon of a typical nephron. Around 20% of the total cardiac output goes to the kidneys, entering the nephrons via the afferent arterioles. Most of the filtered fluid, electrolytes, and sugars are reabsorbed in the proximal convoluted tubule. Active transport by Na/K-2Cl adenosine triphosphatases in the medullary thick ascending limb (mTAL) allows further concentration of urine. Counter-current exchange between the loop of Henle and the vasa recta (supplied by the efferent arteriole, not shown) produces low oxygen tension in the outer medulla, leaving the mTAL vulnerable to ischemia if blood flow is compromised or tubular work is increased. Flow through the nephron is carefully regulated by the juxtaglomerular apparatus (JGA), the region where the cells of the macula densa on the distal convoluted tubule appose the renin-secreting juxtaglomerular cells of the afferent arteriole.

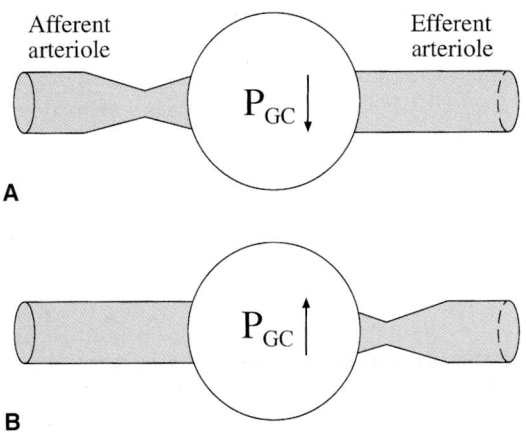

**FIGURE 65-2.** GFR depends directly on the pressure inside the glomerulus ($P_{GC}$). Constriction of the afferent arteriole (**A**) leads to decreased downstream pressures, decreasing both the GFR and renal blood flow. Constriction of the efferent arteriole (**B**) will increase GFR, but still compromises renal blood flow. Substances that dilate both arterioles (like dopamine) will increase renal blood flow, but may have little effect on GFR since $P_{GC}$ remains unchanged.

However, because proteins are generally not filtered, plasma oncotic pressure in Bowman's space approaches 0 and the reflection coefficient becomes 1, leaving

$$GFR = L_p \cdot S \cdot (P_{gc} - P_{bs} - \pi_p)$$

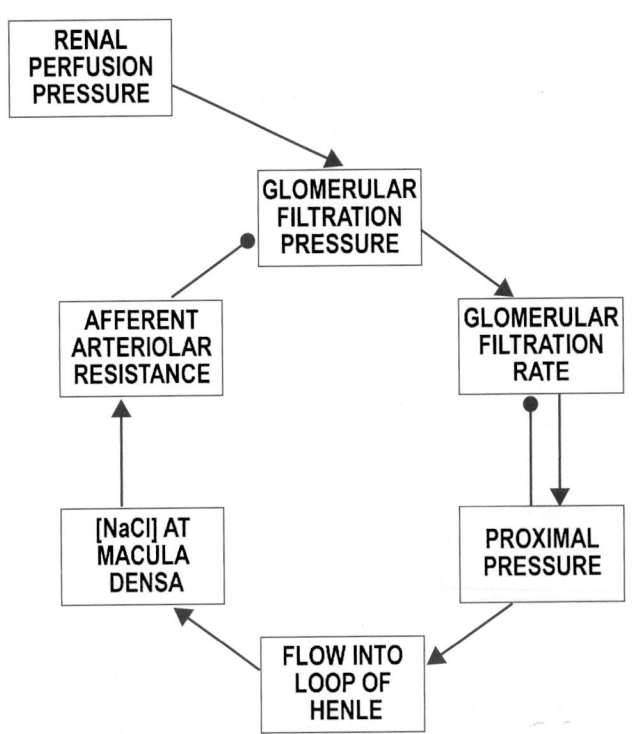

**FIGURE 65-3.** Schematic depiction of tubuloglomerular feedback (TGF). TGF allows the kidney to carefully regulate glomerular filtration by coupling it to salt load seen in the distal convoluted tubule (macula densa). Arrowheads represent positive control, blunt ends represent negative control. Rising flow through the nephron is sensed as increased NaCl at the macula densa. Because the macula densa is directly apposed to the afferent arteriole, it can signal smooth muscle to constrict, raising afferent arteriolar resistance. Increased resistance here causes a fall in glomerular pressure (see Fig. 60-2) and GFR. Falling GFR leads to decreased flow, which, when sensed at the macula densa, leads to dilatation of the afferent arteriole.

Because $L_p$ and $S$ remain nearly constant, and because $P_{bs}$ and $\pi_{ps}$ are small, pressure in the glomerular capillary ($P_{gc}$) is revealed as the most important determinant of GFR.[11]

The primary role of the renal tubules is concentration of the urine via reabsorption of sodium and water. In addition, glucose, potassium, chloride, and phosphate are actively reabsorbed in the tubules. Urea undergoes passive reabsorption in the tubules, depending on tubular flow rates. Up to 70% of urea is excreted during high tubular flow, dropping to only 10 to 20% excretion of filtered urea during low tubular flow rates. In contrast, creatinine, with far less secretion and resorption in the tubules compared to BUN, depends chiefly on GFR for elimination, allowing its use to estimate GFR (see below). Hydrogen and ammonium ions are also both secreted in the proximal and distal tubules, depending on serum and urine pH.

Within the medulla, tubules and vasa recta are arranged in parallel bundles allowing maximum concentrating ability by a countercurrent-exchange system. The medullary thick ascending limb (mTAL) is responsible for the generation of an osmotic gradient by active reabsorption of sodium, a process that generates a large oxygen demand. If medullary blood flow is too high, osmotic gradients established by countercurrent exchange are diminished. If oxygen demand is increased from basal conditions, the cells of the medulla, particularly the cells of thick ascending limbs, are at risk for severe hypoxia. This combination of low regional oxygen delivery and high cellular oxygen consumption creates a tenuous oxygen supply–demand relationship, placing renal tubules at risk for ischemic injury. Analogous vulnerabilities may be found in "watershed" areas of the brain, or in hepatocytes farthest from the hepatic arterioles and porta venules ("zone 3" hepatocytes).[12]

## PATHOPHYSIOLOGY

Etiologies of acute azotemia are typically categorized according to anatomic location (Table 65-2): prerenal azotemia, postrenal azotemia, or intrinsic renal failure. Prerenal azotemia is the most common source of declining urine output and accumulation of nitrogen wastes. Although hemorrhage and surgical losses are easily recognized sources of volume loss, occult losses of intravascular volume from excessive renal or gastrointestinal output may quickly become clinically important if overlooked. Loss of *effective* circulating volume may result from capillary endothelial leak and vasomotor dysfunction producing third-spacing and regional perfusion deficits. Sepsis, pancreatitis, bowel ischemia–reperfusion injury,

**TABLE 65-2**

| Modulators of Renal Oxygen Delivery and Consumption | |
|---|---|
| Decreased delivery | Global |
| | Hypotension |
| | Low $Sao_2$ |
| | Anemia |
| | Hypovolemia |
| | Cardiac failure |
| | Microvascular |
| | Vasoconstrictors |
| | Endothelin |
| | Angiotensin II |
| | Vasopressin |
| | Cyclosporine |
| | Radiocontrast |
| | Heme pigment (myoglobin, hemoglobin) (through binding of nitric oxide) |
| | Vascular injury |
| | Complement |
| | Neutrophils |
| | Nitric oxide (in excess) |
| | Disseminated intravascular coagulation |
| | Calcium? |
| Increased delivery | Microvascular (vasodilators) |
| | Nitric oxide |
| | Prostaglandin $E_2$ |
| | Adenosine |
| | Dopamine? |
| | Dobutamine? |
| | Urodilantin |
| Decrease work | Prostaglandin $E_2$ |
| | Adenosine |
| | Dopamine |
| | Furosemide (and other loop diuretics) |
| | Ouabain |
| Increase work | Hypovolemia |
| | Decreased salt concentration |
| | Increased permeability (e.g., amphotericin) |
| | Back leak (tubular cellular damage) |
| | Radiocontrast |

major burns, soft-tissue injury, or massive rhabdomyolysis may all diminish effective circulating volume and dramatically reduce RBF. Primary cardiac dysfunction may also be overlooked as a source of declining RBF secondary to declining cardiac output (see Chap. 62). In this situation, increased systemic vascular resistance (SVR) may compromise marginal cardiac performance, maintaining mean arterial pressure (MAP) at the expense of mesenteric perfusion and RBF.

As effective circulating volume, mean arterial pressure, and renal blood flow decrease below levels at which renal autoregulation can maintain flow to the glomerulus, GFR declines. In response to hypovolemia, aldosterone and antidiuretic hormone (ADH) are both secreted to conserve sodium and water, respectively. As a result, the kidney produces a small volume of concentrated urine with low sodium content. Due to low urine flow rates, BUN is reabsorbed in the tubules resulting in azotemia. Prompt recognition and rapid treatment usually rapidly reverses prerenal azotemia. While renal tubular cell integrity is maintained in reversible prerenal azotemia, severe and prolonged azotemia can result in tubular cell dysfunction or cell death with acute tubular necrosis.

Postrenal or obstructive renal failure results from blockage of both ureters (or of a single ureter in a patient with only one functioning kidney) or of the urethra. In trauma patients, urethral obstruction or transection can occur in pelvic fractures. Ureteral compression can also occur in the trauma patient secondary to a rapidly expanding retroperitoneal hematoma. Iatrogenic, intraoperative ureteral injury may occur during a difficult celiotomy in the trauma patient. Because sudden anuria is rare in the absence of hemorrhage of fulminate sepsis, obstructive uropathy must be suspected in patients who become anuric soon after presentation.

Although less common than acute obstruction, chronic obstruction of the urinary tract can occur in the trauma patient (as in some forms of neurogenic bladder). Ensuring unimpeded urine flow by Foley catheterization or intermittent catheterization is required to avoid ongoing obstructive uropathy. In the critically ill inpatient, a common source of postrenal anuria may be blockage of a neglected Foley catheter. Prolonged obstruction of urine flow results in increased renal basal vascular tone and reduction in renal blood flow, eventually causing irreversible cortical atrophy and chronic renal failure. Whatever the etiology, prompt recognition and relief of the obstruction grants the best chance of avoiding parenchymal damage and recovering renal function.

## ACUTE INTRINSIC RENAL FAILURE

Intrinsic renal disease resulting in ARF can be categorized according to the primary site of injury within the renal parenchyma (Table 65-2): glomerular disease, interstitial nephritis, vasculopathy, and ATN. Whereas acute glomerular disease can result from drugs or infection, interstitial nephritis may be seen with drug allergies, and vascular injury can occur; these rarely appear as the primary etiology of ARF in trauma patients. Much more common is damage to the tubules, particularly the cells of the ascending limb of the loop of Henle located in the outer renal medulla. These cells are particularly vulnerable to hypoxia and nephrotoxins, and damage to these cells is central to the pathophysiology of ATN.

## PATHOPHYSIOLOGY OF ACUTE TUBULAR NECROSIS

A number of animal models have been developed to investigate the pathophysiology of ischemic and toxic renal failure. Bilateral renal artery clamping or renal artery norepinephrine infusion followed by reperfusion mimics clinical ischemia/reperfusion injury. Contrast injection, indomethacin administration, and other models allow investigation of the mechanisms of toxic ATN. Recent models also include cell culture technique, isolated tubules, and isolated perfused kidneys. Experimental and clinical studies have elucidated several pathophysiologic characteristics common to a variety of experimental models and clinical scenarios.

### Local Ischemia

A unifying theme emerging from these studies is the balance between renal tubule oxygen supply (local blood flow) and oxygen consumption (tubular cell pump work). Renal blood flow is directed primarily to the cortex to optimize glomerular filtration. In contrast, blood flow to the renal medulla must remain low to preserve osmotic gradients and to enhance urinary concentration by countercurrent exchange.[13] Oxygen diffuses from arterial to venous vasa recta, leaving the outer medulla relatively hypoxic (Fig. 65–1). The mTAL generates an osmotic gradient by active sodium reabsorption, an activity that requires high oxygen consumption. The medullary partial pressure of oxygen in the outer medulla is normally in the range of 10 to 20 mm Hg.[12]

A number of defense mechanisms are in place to protect the outer medulla from injury by oxygen imbalances. Cells in the outer medulla display receptors for mediators that govern medullary blood flow and oxygen homeostasis. Vasodilators include $PGE_2$, nitric oxide, and urodilantin. Vasoconstrictors include angiotensin and endothelin.[12–14] Adenosine, released from adenosine triphosphate (ATP) during oxidative stress, is a vasodilator in most systems. In the kidney, adenosine induces cortical vasoconstriction and medullary vasodilation, suggesting a role in attenuating medullary hypoxia. While these mechanisms serve to preserve intrarenal blood flow, severe ischemic stress or direct tubular toxins can exceed compensatory thresholds. When this occurs, some of these same mediators can initiate and amplify renal tubular injury.

Recently, dysregulation of microvascular protective mechanisms has been demonstrated in ischemia/reperfusion injury. Early vascular events include elaboration of intracellular adhesion molecules of the endothelium (ICAM-1), adherence and activation of polymorphonuclear neutrophils, elaboration of PAF, and enhanced production of potent endothelium-derived vasoconstrictors such as endothelin-1 (ET-1).[15] In the established phase of ATN, vascular changes are characterized by increased basal vascular resistance, increased vascular permeability, increased sensitivity to vasoconstricting agents, and decreased or absent response to endothelium-dependent vasodilators. Other factors implicated in postischemic vasoconstriction include increased levels of angiotensin II, increased cytosolic smooth-muscle cell calcium concentration, and increased thromboxane $A_2$.[16] As decreased renal blood flow persists in postischemic ATN, adherent neutrophils and platelets further obstruct capillaries. Thus, the same mediators that preserve normal RBF may instead cause ongoing ischemia with collapse of normal feedback mechanisms. Besides initiating renal injury, these factors may

predispose the kidney to further damage from subsequent episodes of hypotension, toxic drugs, or use of vasoconstricting pressors. Table 65-3 summarizes mediators of renal medullary oxygen balance.

### Tubular Cellular Injury

Morphologic changes in tubular cells following ischemic injury include loss of the brush border, loss of polarity, and loss of integrity of tight junctions of proximal tubular cells. There is a redistribution of Na/K-ATPase from the basal surface with a

**TABLE 65-3**

| Common Etiologies of Acute Oliguria | |
| --- | --- |
| Prerenal | Hypovolemia |
| |     Hemorrhage |
| |     Gastrointestinal fluid loss (nasogastric suction, high-output fistula, diarrhea, etc.) |
| |     Renal loss (excessive diuretic use, diabetes insipidus, diabetes mellitus) |
| |     Surgery |
| |     Burns |
| | Decreased effective vascular volume |
| |     Sepsis |
| |     Hepatic failure |
| |     Anaphylactic shock |
| |     Neurogenic shock |
| |     Vasodilators |
| | Impaired cardiac function |
| |     Myocardial infarction |
| |     Pulmonary embolus |
| |     Cardiac tamponade |
| |     Congestive heart failure |
| |     Mechanical ventilation |
| Renal parenchymal injury dysfunction | Glomerulonephritis |
| |     Poststreptococcal glomerulonephritis |
| |     Systemic lupus erythematosus and other connective tissue disorders |
| |     Scleroderma |
| |     Malignant hypertension |
| |     Eclampsia/preeclampsia |
| |     Others |
| | Vasculitis |
| | Interstitial nephritis |
| |     Drugs (methicillin) |
| |     Infection |
| |     Neoplasm (lymphoma, leukemia, or sarcoidosis) |
| | Acute tubular necrosis |
| |     Ischemia (prerenal events) |
| |     Antibiotics (amphotericin, aminoglycosides) |
| |     Radiocontrast agents |
| |     Pigment load (e.g., myoglobin as in rhabdomyolysis) |
| |     Heavy metals (mercury) |
| |     Solvents (carbon tetrachloride, ethylene glycol) |
| Postrenal/obstructive | Ureteral obstruction |
| |     Stone |
| |     Infection (pyelonephritis) |
| |     Traumatic disruption |
| | Urethral obstruction |
| |     Obstruction of Foley catheter |
| |     Mucus |
| |     Blood clots |

decrease in sodium-transport efficiency.[17] Dead or dying cells slough into the tubular lumen contributing to cast formation. These casts cause increased intratubular pressure and reduce GFR. Loss of epithelial cells and rupture of tight junctions between viable cells leave a denuded basement membrane resulting in back-leakage of glomerular filtrates into the interstitial space.

Ischemia–reperfusion injury leads to a rapid burst of reactive oxygen metabolites. Sources of oxidant formation in the kidney include the xanthine oxidase system, neutrophils, and cyclo-oxygenases. Reactive oxygen species contribute to cellular injury by altering protein structure and forming lipid peroxides in cell membranes. Some animal studies support the use of antioxidants or scavengers of reactive oxygen species in experimental renal failure whereas others do not.[18]

Ischemia leads to depletion of ATP with release of adenosine, inosine, and hypoxanthine, leading to vasoconstriction. Depletion of ATP activates cellular phospholipases, increases arachidonic acid metabolite production, and degrades phospholipids, destabilizing cellular membranes. Some studies have suggested that exogenously administered ATP and magnesium protect against ischemic renal injury in rats.[19]

Depletion of cellular ATP and destabilization of cellular membranes also lead to an increase in cytosolic calcium concentrations in tubular and endothelial cells.[20] As intracellular calcium exceeds the sequestration ability of mitochondria, high tonic levels of calcium produce mitochondrial swelling (permeability transition), uncoupling of oxidative phosphorylation, activation of calcium-dependent proteases and phospholipases, membrane and cytoskeletal disruption, and eventual cell death.[21] In addition, increased cytosolic calcium in vascular smooth muscle cells causes vasoconstriction further exacerbating ischemia. Phospholipase A$_2$ (PLA$_2$) is activated following ischemia-reperfusion which alters the permeability of cell and mitochondrial membranes. Moreover, PLA$_2$ enhances production of arachidonic acid metabolites, mediators with vasoconstrictive and neutrophil chemotactic properties.[22] The dual role of nitric oxide in the pathogenesis of ischaemic ARF was recently summarized by Goligorsky and Rabelink. Acute renal ischemia induces increased expression of inducible nitric oxide synthase; blockade of the enzyme by antisense oligonucleotides affords functional protection, at least in rats. Scavenging of nitric oxide produces peroxynitrite, which causes tubule damage during ischemia.

Inflammation—manifesting as infiltration and activation of neutrophils, activation of complement, and elaboration of cytokines—plays a role in all models of intrinsic renal dysfunction (see Chap. 68). Moreover, inflammatory mediators released by the endothelium after Renal I/R can cause macrophage mediated increases in pulmonary vascular permeability. This increase in pulmonary vascular permeability can be abrogated by inhibiting macrophage activation, but the course of ARF is not.[23] Adherence of neutrophils to the vascular endothelium is mediated by ICAM-1 on endothelial cells binding CD11a/CD18 on neutrophils. Synthesis and display intercellular adhesion molecules are upregulated within minutes following ischemia. After adhesion and activation, neutrophils release reactive oxygen species, proteases, elastase, and myeloperoxidase. Interactions between PMNs and endothelia may lead to endothelial dysfunction and edema, prolonging ischemia. In models of renal, myocardial, and intestinal ischemia, depletion of neutrophils or blockade of neutrophil

adhesion molecules is protective against ischemia–reperfusion injury. Activation of the complement cascade has also been shown to inhibit recovery from ARF in experimental animals,[24] perhaps by prolonging or enhancing leukocyte activation. Cytokines and chemokines, generated locally in response to cellular stressors or systemically as part of the immune response, may magnify renal vasoconstriction and mesangial cell contraction, thereby exacerbating medullary ischemia and diminishing filtration pressure.

Recent animal models of sepsis demonstrate that chemokine transcription and adherence of neutrophils and monocytes to renal microvascular endothelium is associated with the development of ARF. The required development of anuria and elevation of BUN and creatinine in conjunction with marked upregulation of chemokines of the CC and CXC group in this peritonitis model suggests that inflammation itself may play a part in ARF without invoking an I/R mechanism.[25]

Following renal ischemia/reperfusion (I/R) or toxic injury, renal tubular cells progress to one of the three fates: apoptosis (predominantly in cells of the distal nephron segments), necrosis (predominantly in cells of the proximal straight and proximal convoluted tubules), or dedifferentiation and proliferation leading to recovery of tubular function. Current research focuses on intracellular pathways governing these cellular outcomes with hopes of diverting cells from apoptosis or necrosis toward proliferation and repair. In some ways, intracellular molecular events observed in cellular stress resemble the events observed in cells exposed to various growth factors (e.g., rapid, brief expression of immediate early [IE] genes).[26] IE gene products include transcription factors c-fos and c-jun and cytokines such as interleukin-10 (IL-10). Activation of c-jun transcription is dependent on phosphorylation by stress-activated protein kinases (SAPKs).[27] SAPK activation during the IE response is usually antiproliferative. SAPKs are activated by oxidative and hypertonic stress as well as by tumor necrosis factor-alpha (TNF-α) and lipopolysaccharide (LPS).[28] Additionally, oxidative stress promotes cyclin-dependent kinase (CDK) inhibitors which block normal cell cycle progression and lead to apoptosis.[29] In contrast, IE gene activation by growth factors is mediated by extracellular regulated kinases (ERKs), which drive the cell toward proliferation.[30] The antioxidant N-acetylcysteine (NAC) blocks SAPKs and CDK inhibitors which are normally activated by oxidative stress.[29] Experimentally, NAC administration prior to or immediately after renal ischemia inhibits IE gene activation and enhances renal recovery.[31]

Renal I/R models also demonstrate endonuclease activation with deoxyribonucleic acid (DNA) fragmentation and apoptosis. Endonuclease activation is believed to be an early event at least partially responsible for cell death following I/R, whether cells die by apoptosis or by necrosis. Activation of proto-oncogenes such as c-myc is seen in renal tubular cells following a variety of experimental stressors and is known to render cells more susceptible to endonuclease activity and apoptosis. Bcl-2, presumably via an anti-apoptotic mechanism, has been shown to be protective of renal tubular cells in experimental ARF.[30] However, the precise role of proto-oncogenes and endonuclease activation in ATN remains undetermined. As further differences in molecular responses to I/R and toxic stress are understood, these pathways may reveal opportunities to prevent cell injury or enhance cell recovery.

Unlike most other organs, the kidney can completely regenerate normal structure and restore full function after injury. Growth factors produced in the kidney play a role in proliferation, may inhibit apoptosis, and may initiate or promote protein and lipid biosynthesis. Growth factors produced in response to acute injury include heparin-binding epidermal growth factor (HB-EGF), hepatocyte growth factor (HGF), insulin-like growth factor-1 (IGF-1), and transforming growth factor-beta (TGF-β). Another potential role for growth factors following renal injury is to increase regional blood flow, as demonstrated experimentally with IGF-1.[32] Epidermal growth factor, hepatocyte growth factor, and IGF-1, when administered to animals subjected to renal ischemia, reduce the severity of renal dysfunction and accelerate renal recovery.[28,33,34] Exogenous IGF-1 enhances renal recovery in the rat following I/R injury by enhancing proliferation of tubular epithelium, augmenting renal blood flow and GFR.[35] IGF-1 has recently been shown to protect patients from renal insufficiency following suprarenal aortic surgery.[36]

## REPAIR OF RENAL INJURY

Proximal tubules can undergo repair, regeneration, and proliferation after damage. In the outer cortex, most of the cells are not lethally injured and undergo repair after adequate reperfusion.[3] The first phase of this regeneration process consists of the death and exfoliation of the proximal tubular cells and is characterized by expression of stress response genes and the accumulation of mononuclear cells. Shortly after the experimental induction of ARF, many normally quiescent kidney cells enter the cell cycle. The cell undergoing these changes can either check the progression of the cycle and repair damage before proceeding or entering a pathway destined to cell death. This decision point is carefully regulated, and cyclin-dependent kinase inhibitors, especially p21, are important in the regulation. Investigation of the effects on ARF of selected gene knockouts in mice has contributed to the recognition of many previously unappreciated molecular pathways. The interface between the repair pathways and the cell-death pathways is emerging, but phosphorylation events crucial to cell function reside in the cyclindependent kinases and the kinases, phosphatases, inhibitors, and activators that regulate their activities.[37] Growth factors could play a part in determining the fate of the epithelial cells and might contribute to the generation of signals that result in neutrophil and monocyte infiltration. In the second phase, poorly differentiated epithelial cells appear; they are thought to represent a population of stem cells residing in the kidney. This stage is therefore a dedifferentiation stage. In the third phase, there is a pronounced increase in proliferation of the surviving proximal tubule cells, and growth factors could have an important role in this response. In this last phase, the regenerative tubular cells regain their differentiated character and produce a normal proximal-tubule epithelium. Stem-cell research has shown that haemopoietic and other tissue-specific stem cells can cross tissue and even germ-line barriers and give rise to a wide range of cell types.[38]

Therefore, stem cells could be useful in therapeutic strategies designed to improve tissue regeneration after severe organ injury. Experiments with transplantation of whole bone marrow showed that bone-marrow-derived stem cells could populate the renal tubular epithelium. Injection of mesenchymal stem cells derived from male bone marrow protected cisplatintreated syngeneic female mice from renal functional impairment and severe tubular injury.[39] Unfortunately, however, mobilization of haemopoietic stem cells is also associated with granulocytosis, which can worsen ARF.[40]

## ACUTE RENAL FAILURE SYNDROMES

Sepsis is considered the most common cause of ARF in today's ICU setting. In ICUs, 35–50% of cases of acute tubular necrosis can be attributed to sepsis.[41] The disorder is increasingly recognized in the context of multiple organ failure, especially in critically ill patients; only a minority of cases in ICUs occur without failure of another organ. Acute tubular necrosis after surgery accounts for 20–25% of all cases of hospital-acquired ARF; many of them have prerenal causes. Groups at risk include patients with pre-existing renal impairment, hypertension, cardiac disease, peripheral vascular disease, diabetes mellitus, jaundice, and advanced age. New forms of postsurgery acute tubular necrosis, such as those following liver and cardiac transplantation, reflect changes in types of surgical interventions.[3] Acute radiocontrast nephropathy is the third commonest cause of acute tubular necrosis in patients admitted to hospital,[3] and up to 7% need temporary dialysis or progress to end-stage renal disease. The occurrence of radiocontrast nephropathy is associated with increased risk of death and leads to an extended hospital stay and increased health-care costs.[42] Several classes of antibacterial, antifungal, antiviral, and antineoplastic 49 agents are nephrotoxic.

## AMINOGLYCOSIDES

Aminoglycoside nephrotoxicity remains the single most common drug class implicated in drug toxicity-induced ATN (see Chap. 17). An estimated 10–25% of patients treated with aminoglycosides develop some degree of renal insufficiency.[43,44] Aminoglycosides such as gentamicin are directly toxic to renal proximal tubular cells. After glomerular filtration, aminoglycosides are reabsorbed and concentrated in proximal tubular epithelial cells' lysosomes. Precisely how aminoglycosides damage cells once in lysosomes is unclear; proposed mechanisms of toxicity include mitochondrial damage, cell membrane destruction, phospholipase activation, or alteration of lysosomes. Additionally, vasoconstriction within the renal microcirculation contributes to toxicity by diminishing RBF.

Absolute or effective volume contraction further concentrates aminoglycosides within proximal tubular cells. Risk factors for development of aminoglycoside nephrotoxicity include prolonged exposure to aminoglycosides (high serum trough levels), volume depletion, sepsis, and advanced patient age. Synergistic toxicity may also occur with other drugs, such as amphotericin B, NSAIDs, cyclosporine, radiographic contrast, and antimicrobials such as cephalosporins and vancomycin. Because nephrotoxicity is more closely related to trough concentrations, whereas antimicrobial efficacy varies with peak concentrations of the drugs, once-a-day dosing of aminoglycosides may be less nephrotoxic with equal efficacy in patients with normal renal function.[45] Unfortunately, following serum trough level does not ensure protection against nephrotoxicity: A rising trough level indicates that toxicity has already occurred. Toxicity rarely occurs when the duration of therapy is less than five days.

Because aminoglycosides are predominantly tubular toxins, GFR may be preserved early in the course of aminoglycoside nephrotoxicity. Thus, loss of urinary concentrating capacity (isothenuria) is often the earliest and most sensitive indicator of the onset of intrinsic renal damage.[46] Clinically, the isothenuric patient will exhibit relatively dilute polyuria with only a mild-to-moderate reduction in GFR. Failure to recognize this syndrome may lead to progressive tubular damage and renal failure.

## POLYENE MACROLIDES

Polyene antimicrobials such as amphotericin are particularly nephrotoxic. Amphotericin B damages cellular membranes increasing membrane permeability, and the resulting ion back-leak drives increased sodium pump activity, thereby increasing oxygen requirements. Polyene antimicrobials also have direct lytic effects on lysosomal membranes. Amphotericin compounds these insults by producing profound renal vasoconstriction, diminishing flow to the mTALs, and exacerbating the disparity between oxygen supply and demand. The contribution of increased tubular work can be demonstrated in isolated perfused kidneys, where polyene toxicity is prevented by inhibiting active sodium pumps with ouabain.[47] Amphotericin can also cause a distal renal tubular acidosis with resultant metabolic acidosis, potassium wasting, and magnesium wasting. Amphotericin toxicity depends on *total* dose: less than 600 mg rarely produces important alterations in renal function, whereas cumulative doses exceeding 3 g cause significant renal toxicity in over 80% of patients. Maintaining adequate hydration with intravenous saline over the course of treatment is the most effective means of reducing this dose-dependent toxicity.[47] Experimental preparations of lipid-encapsulated amphotericin promise reduced toxicity in the future.

## CONTRAST-INDUCED NEPHROPATHY

Acute radiocontrast nephropathy is the third commonest cause of acute tubular necrosis in patients admitted to hospital,[39] and up to 7% need temporary dialysis or progress to end-stage renal disease. The occurrence of radiocontrast nephropathy is associated with increased risk of death and leads to an extended hospital stay and increased health-care costs.[42]

Several factors are known to heighten the risk of contrast.[48] Chief among these is pre-existing renal insufficiency which increases the incidence of renal failure after contrast from 2 to 33%.[49] As baseline serum creatinine increases about 1.5 mg/dL, the incidence of ARF following radiocontrast administration rises exponentially. This risk particularly affects in patients with diabetes mellitus, where incidence of ARF can climb to 80% if baseline creatinine is greater than 4 mg/dL.[48] Depletion of extracellular volume accentuates nephrotoxicity of radiocontrast agents in all patients.

Radiological contrast agents exacerbate mTAL hypoxia. After an initial increase, total renal blood flow declines into a sustained hypoperfusion where return of RBF lags by hours after dosing. Radiocontrast agents produce local (medullary) ischemia related to endothelin release and depressed nitric oxide (NO)-mediated vasodilatation. Meanwhile, outer medullary oxygen requirements increase due to the osmotic effect that enhances solute delivery to the distal nephron. Worse, radiocontrast agents commonly compromise global oxygen delivery by reducing cardiac output, producing pulmonary ventilation–perfusion mismatch, shifting the oxygen hemoglobin dissociation curve leftward, and altering blood rheologic properties. The net effect is aggravation of medullary hypoxia.[50]

Contrast-induced renal failure can be ameliorated by pre- and post-imaging saline and volume loading. A recent prospective randomized comparison of two hydration regimens in preventing contrast media-associated nephropathy, convincingly showed that isotonic hydration was superior to half-isotonic hydration especially in patients with diabetes, and those receiving more than 250 mL of contrast.[51] Other therapeutic strategies include using the smallest effective amount of contrast or avoiding contrast studies altogether, if possible, in patients at risk by utilizing alternative imaging modalities (such as magnetic resonance angiography). Loop diuretics and mannitol have been proposed but not proven as useful prophylaxis. Indeed, mannitol appears to increase the risk for contrast nephropathy in diabetic patients with pre-existing renal disease.[52] Calcium channel blockers, by decreasing vasoconstriction associated with radiocontrast agents, have been shown to be effective prophylaxis for preventing contrast-induced nephrotoxicity in a prospective randomized trial.[53] There is no convincing evidence that nonionic or low-molecular-weight contrast material is less nephrotoxic in the low-risk patient.[54]

Fortunately, the clinical course of contrast nephropathy is usually self-limited. Oliguria is rare, and serum creatinine usually peaks within 72 hours after administration. The majority of patients return to baseline renal function by 7 to 10 days. However, up to 30% of patients, especially those with the known risks described above, sustain permanent functional loss.[55] In any case, adequate saline fluid loading before infusion of radiocontrast remains the mainstay of prophylaxis against damage by radiocontrast.

## PIGMENT-INDUCED NEPHROPATHY

Many injuries can set the stage for pigment-induced renal injuries. Rhabdomyolysis is the release of free myoglobin from skeletal muscle after muscle necrosis. Besides major crush injuries and prolonged limb ischemia, seizures, drugs (heroin, cocaine, amphetamines, propofol), toxins (isopropyl alcohol, ethylene glycol), streptococcal infections, and myositis can cause rhabdomyolysis. Massive hemoglobinuria usually occurs in the setting of extensive hemolysis from transfusion reactions (see Chap. 14). When myoglobin or hemoglobin are released in small amounts, haptoglobin binds these pigments, preventing their filtration through the glomerulus. If the binding capacity of haptoglobin is exceeded, free myoglobin or hemoglobin will be filtered by the glomerulus.

The pathophysiology of myoglobinuric ARF has been studied extensively in the animal model of glycerol-induced ARF. The main pathophysiologic mechanisms include renal vasoconstriction, intraluminalcast formation, and direct heme protein induced cytotoxicity.[56] Myoglobin is easily filtered through the glomerular basement membrane. Water is progressively reabsorbed in the tubules, and the concentration of myoglobin rises proportionally, until it precipitates and causes obstructive cast formation. Dehydration and renal vasoconstriction, which decrease tubular flow and enhance water reabsorption, favor this process. The high rates of generation and urinary excretion of uric acid further contribute to tubular obstruction by uric acid casts. Another factor favoring precipitation of myoglobin and uric acid is a low pH of tubular urine, which is common because of underlying acidosis. The degradation of intratubular myoglobin results in the release of free iron, which catalyzes free radical production and further enhances ischemic damage. Even without invoking release of free iron, the heme center of myoglobin will initiate lipid peroxidation and renal injury.[57] Alkaline conditions prevent this effect by stabilizing the reactive ferryl myoglobin complex.

In addition to tubular obstruction, renal juxtamedullary vasoconstriction (believed to be in part due to binding of NO by hemoglobin and myoglobin[58]) occurs, resulting in deterioration of medullary oxygenation.[59] Compounding these effects, massive sequestration of fluid in rhabdomyolysis diminishes circulating volume, compounding the local toxic effects with global hypoperfusion. Finally, myoglobinuria and shock have synergistic nephrotoxicity[17]; each is known to lead to renal tubular loss of ATP following hypoxic insult.[59]

Diagnosis is secured by the finding of heme pigment in the urine in the absence of red blood cells, and an elevated serum creatinine phosphokinase in patients with clinical findings consistent with rhabdomyolysis or hemoglobinuria. Severe hyperkalemia often also rapidly develops in the presence of massive muscle destruction or I/R. The diagnosis can be suspected by the appearance of dark (cola-colored) urine containing dark brown granular casts.

Several recent natural disasters have allowed the characterization of multiple casualties with ARF complicating muscle crush injury following large earthquakes. The syndrome is initially associated with profound hypovolemic and hypocalcemic shock and hyperkalemia followed by myoglubinuric ARF.[58] The mainstay of treatment in these studies was intravenous fluid infusion, diuretics including manitol, and alkalinization of the urine; and dialysis.[60,61] The most recent study evaluated 639 patients admitted to 35 Turkish hospitals with ARF due to crush syndrome after the Marmara earthquake. Seventy-five percent required dialysis and 15% died. Death was usually due to complication of ARF, ARDS, and sepsis. The prime therapeutic principle is the interruption of the pathophysiologic cascade leading to ARF, i.e., volume depletion, tubular obstruction, aciduria, and free radical release.[57] The ideal fluid regimen for patients with rhabdomyolysis consists of half isotonic saline (0.45%, or 77 mmol/L sodium), to which 75 mmol/L sodium bicarbonate is added. Alkali prevents the acidification of the urine, which promotes tubular precipitation of myoglobin. Alkali also reduces the risk of hyperkalemia, caused by leakage of potassium from damaged muscle cells.[60] This combination may be complemented by 10 mL/hour of 15% mannitol if patient continues to have a diuresis. Mannitol is a renal vasodilator. It increases the glomerular pressure, attracts fluid from the muscular and interstitial compartments, increases urine flow, prevents tubular obstruction by myoglobin deposits, and acts as a free-radical scavenger. Mannitol, should, however, be withheld if the patient develops oligoanuria. Once overt renal failure has developed, the only reliable therapeutic modality is dialysis.

## NONSTEROIDAL ANTI-INFLAMMATORY DRUGS

Inactivation of renal prostaglandin production by NSAIDs may compromise medullary oxygen balance through two mechanisms: regional hypoperfusion and increased tubular reabsorption. Acute renal insufficiency secondary to NSAIDs is usually reversible by stopping the offending drug. Long-term exposure to NSAIDs can cause analgesic nephropathy and medullary necrosis. Because they predispose patients (particularly those with other risk factors) to ARF, NSAIDs have no role in the treatment of the critically ill patient.

## ABDOMINAL COMPARTMENT SYNDROME

The abdominal compartment syndrome (ACS) may be an overlooked cause of oliguria and ARF in trauma patients (see Chap. 37). ACS is described as intra-abdominal pressure greater than 25 cm $H_2O$ (around 18 mm Hg) associated with rapidly increasing $PCO_2$, decreased cardiac output, and decreased UOP. Intra-abdominal pressure may be increased by hemorrhage, ascites, bowel edema, or intra-abdominal packing. Furthermore, compromise in renal function has been described during laparoscopy with intra-abdominal pressures as low as 12 mm Hg (approximately 16 cm $H_2O$).[62] High intra-abdominal pressure probably limits renal perfusion at least two ways. First, increased abdominal pressure may compromise cardiac output by decreasing venous return from the inferior vena cava. Second, and more importantly, increased abdominal pressure may exceed the critical closing pressure of renal arterioles (approximately 20 to 30 mm Hg), inhibiting flow by increasing intrarenal resistance (Starling resistor).[63] Critically ill patients are frequently unable to generate a MAP high enough to overcome this increased intrarenal resistance. Both of these processes decrease RGF and GFR. Because volume loading and inotropes rarely restore renal blood flow in ACS, only prompt decompression of the abdominal cavity is likely to restore renal function; indeed, failure to recognize and treat ACS is inevitably fatal.[64] In contrast, abdominal decompression quickly leads to improved cardiac index, decreased $PCO_2$, and resumption of urinary flow.[64]

## SEPSIS

Sepsis is considered the most common cause of ARF in today's ICU setting. In ICUs, 35–50% of cases of acute tubular necrosis can be attributed to sepsis.[41] The disorder is increasingly recognized in the context of multiple organ failure, especially in critically ill patients. Only a minority of cases in ICUs occur without failure of another organ.

Systemic hemodynamic derangements, intrarenal perfusion deficits, specific local inflammatory mediators, and iatrogenic interventions combine to make ARF common in sepsis. Oliguria is often the first clinical sign of MODS in sepsis (see Chap. 68). ARF can occur without arterial hypotension in the septic patient.[65] Decreased effective intravascular volume, hypotension, and alpha-adrenergic agents (which may maintain blood pressure at the expense of mesenteric and renal flow) all reduce flow to the kidneys. Additionally, altered intrarenal hemodynamics, particularly increased renal vascular resistance, further reduces renal plasma flow and GFR.[65] Many of the substances implicated in pathologic intrarenal vascular vasoconstriction also provoke an intense inflammatory response within the kidney and cause endothelial cell damage and microvascular hypercoagulability.[66] These mediators include endotoxin, cytokines such as IL-1 and TNF-α, chemokines[67] and vasoconstrictors such as ET-1.

Clinically, patients may or may not have signs of overwhelming sepsis. Soft signs of sepsis may be the only clues to the diagnosis: thrombocytopenia, change in mental status, unexplained respiratory alkalosis, or subtle alteration of liver function tests.[8] Oliguria or azotemia in this setting should be considered occult septicemia and clinicians should diligently search for any treatable septic focus (see Chap. 18). However, many patients who clinically appear "septic" may not have an identifiable septic focus, especially those who have sustained I/R injury to the gut. Regardless of septic etiology, support of renal function consists of optimization of oxygen delivery primarily through maintenance of intravascular volume and cardiac output. Meanwhile, it is imperative to minimize additional renal insults such as prolonged hypoperfusion, nephrotoxic drugs, contrast dye loads, or failure to promptly recognize and drain a septic focus.

## EFFECTS ON OTHER ORGAN SYSTEMS

Few organ systems escape the effects of ARF. If ARF produces increased free water and sodium load, volume complications can occur, including congestive heart failure, pulmonary edema, and hypertension. Arrhythmias occur in 10–30% of patients and can be exacerbated during intermittent hemodialysis. Pericarditis may occur in severe uremia. Gastrointestinal complications of uremia include anorexia, nausea, emesis, and ileus. Gastrointestinal bleeding can occur in up to 30% of patients with ARF, particularly as BUN levels exceed 80 mg/dL and platelet dysfunction ensues. Neurologic changes occurring in patients with uremia include confusion, asterixis, somnolence, and seizures. Neurologic manifestations are sometimes exacerbated by electrolyte shifts during intermittent hemodialysis. Conversely, such symptoms can be improved following dialysis therapy.

Infections often complicate ARF. While many infections are iatrogenic (e.g., central line infections or urinary tract infections from the indwelling Foley catheters), patients in ARF are prone to pneumonia and other infections. Impaired host defenses and inappropriate use of antibiotics have been implicated in the high degree of infections at remote sites in renal failure patients. Sepsis syndrome stemming from these infections not only exacerbates renal impairment, but also dramatically increases mortality.

Uremia also produces hematological abnormalities. Increased hemolysis in uremia leads to anemia compounded by decreased erythropoiesis as renal secretion of erythropoietin falls. While some advocate administration of recombinant erythropoietin, transfusion of packed red blood cells is clearly the better choice for correction of anemia in the trauma patient. Platelet dysfunction producing risk of clinically important bleeding occurs as BUN rises above 60 to 80 mg/dL. Because this dysfunction is not corrected by platelet infusion, desmopressin or dialysis may be required to treat significant hemorrhage from the gastrointestinal tract or intracranial bleeds.

## DIAGNOSIS AND MANAGEMENT

### Prevention

The most important therapeutic modality in the management of ARF is prevention: maintenance of intravascular volume, avoidance of hypotensive episodes, minimization of toxic exposures, aggressive treatment of infection, and early intervention. Because diminished renal perfusion secondary to absolute or effective volume loss is the most common contributor to ATN in postoperative trauma patients, preservation of intravascular volume is essential to maintain adequate renal perfusion (see Chap. 62). Since renal autoregulation fails when MAP reaches 65 to 80 mm Hg, periods of hypotension (MAP < 80 mm Hg) must be avoided to maintain regulated RBF. In vulnerable patients, nephrotoxins should be avoided or steps should be taken to attenuate their effects (e.g., daily dosing of aminoglycosides as described earlier). The contribution of infection and sepsis to ARF was described earlier. Septic foci should never be allowed to smolder. Finally, treatment of underlying pathologies as soon as any renal dysfunction is detected affords the best chance of avoiding ARF.

A general algorithm for diagnosis and management of acute renal dysfunction is shown in Fig. 65-4. In general, the objectives of ARF management include early identification of renal dysfunction, elimination of obstruction as a source of compromise, identification, and treatment of prerenal failure, laboratory confirmation of renal parenchymal damage, optimization of intravascular volume and of oxygen delivery, trial of loop diuretics, elimination of nephrotoxins, correction of associated metabolic abnormalities, institution of renal replacement therapies if indicated, provision of adequate nutrition, and adjustment of drugs to account for decreased clearance.

## EARLY DETECTION OF RENAL DYSFUNCTION

Most commonly, the clinician will suspect renal dysfunction after a sudden drop in urine output or a rise in a daily creatinine level. More specifically, intervention is indicated if the urine output drops below 0.5 mL/kg/hour for four hours. While the classical definition of oliguria is less than 400 mL of urine production in 24 hours, the physician treating patients in the ICU should recognize an acute decrease in urine output more quickly. Even at maximal concentration, at least 0.5 mL/kg/hr of urine is required to clear nitrogen wastes and other solutes. Smaller volumes and sudden decreases in urine flow imply decreased renal function. Alternatively, a rise in creatinine of 0.25 mg/dL in a day should prompt examination of renal function. Assuming a normal creatinine (approximately 1.0 mg/dL) at baseline and unchanged protein metabolism, a rise in creatinine to 1.5 mg/dL may represent a 50% decrease in GFR. Indeed, the loss of functioning nephrons may be greater since remaining units have partially compensated for the loss.

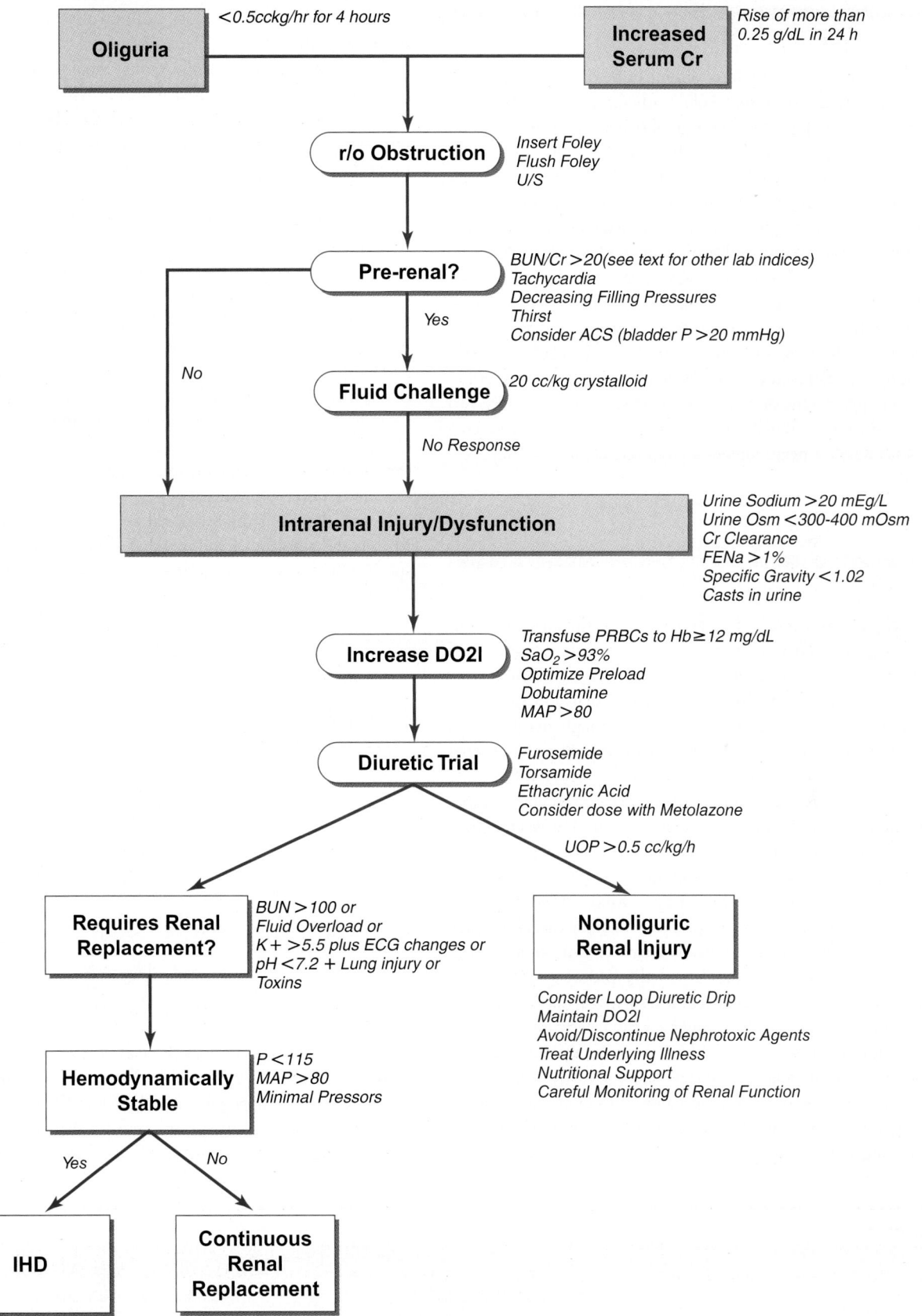

**FIGURE 65-4.** General algorithm for diagnosis and treatment of oliguria and azotemia. See text for details.

## RULE OUT OBSTRUCTION

Obstructive (or postrenal) failure often can be diagnosed and corrected simply by insertion of a Foley catheter. However, the presence of a catheter does not rule out obstruction—mucus, blood clots, or stones may clog catheters left in place for long periods. In addition, the catheter may become dislodged, although appearing to remain in place on cursory examination, especially in women or the obese. If a catheter's position is confirmed, obstruction of the catheter itself may be corrected by flushing with sterile saline or by changing to a new catheter. If obstructive uropathy is still suspected, renal ultrasonography is diagnostic with a sensitivity of approximately 80%.[1] In the severely hypovolemic patient, or immediately following ureteral or urethral obstruction, ultrasonography may fail to reveal an obstruction. In these cases, either intravenous pyelogram or retrograde studies may be required to secure the diagnosis. Rarely, these problems may need to be corrected with either a percutaneous suprapubic catheter or nephrostomy tubes.

## RULE OUT PRERENAL DYSFUNCTION

In surgical patients, decreased renal perfusion is the most common cause of oliguria. Left uncorrected, the combination of increased renal work (increased oxygen consumption) combined with decreasing renal perfusion (decreased oxygen delivery) will cause renal parenchymal injury, usually ATN. Although many factors affect end-organ oxygen delivery, the most common cause of renal hypoperfusion is hypovolemia (see Chap. 62). Although no single test gives an absolute indication of adequate intravascular volume, the clinician can build an accurate picture by noting several clinical clues in the history and physical. The hypovolemic patient will be tachycardic and may complain of thirst. Invasive monitoring (pulmonary artery catheter) should be considered early for any patient with dependence on inotropes, poor baseline cardiac output, or evidence of large volume shifts. If central monitoring (central venous pressure, pulmonary capillary wedge pressure, and/or end-diastolic volume index) is employed, a downward trend in cardiac filling pressures or volumes accompanied by a decrease in cardiac output indicates hypovolemia. As the kidney attempts to compensate for this hypovolemia, aldosterone and ADH will change the urine composition by increasing the action of sodium pumps in the ascending limb of the loop of Henle and opening water channels in the collecting ducts of the nephron. The result is a concentrated

(specific gravity > 1.020), low sodium (urine sodium <20 mEq/L) urine (see Table 65-4).

The increased work of the kidney may manifest in changes in serum chemistries. Decreased filtration will cause both creatinine (Cr) and BUN to rise. Increasing tubular absorption will further raise serum BUN levels. Because Cr is not reabsorbed, Cr levels rise more slowly during low tubular flow rates. As a result, serum BUN rises more quickly than serum Cr. A ratio of BUN to Cr greater than 15 implies renal hypoperfusion. BUN is markedly influenced in terms of production by the patient's metabolic state. During times of catabolism, a marked increase in production of nitrogenous waste occurs while skeletal muscle is recruited for energy. Massive gastrointestinal hemorrhage or reabsorption of any large hematoma will markedly enhance BUN production. BUN can also be elevated in the absence of intrinsic renal dysfunction by excessive protein–calorie intake or the administration of steroids. Despite these limitations, BUN and creatinine are widely used as clinical assessments of renal function, and changes in their values can yield important clues as to change in clinical status.

Another method to distinguish prerenal dysfunction from other causes of oliguria is the fractional excretion of sodium ($FE_{Na}$). The $FE_{Na}$ is the amount of sodium that is filtered and excreted. More specifically, it is the ratio of the sodium clearance to the creatinine clearance:

$$FE_{Na} = \frac{C_{Na}}{C_{Cr}}$$

By applying the generic equation for renal clearance of any substance we have:

$$FE_{Na} = \frac{\dfrac{U_{Na} \times V}{P_{Na}}}{\dfrac{U_{Cr} \times V}{P_{Cr}}}$$

Then, simplifying leaves the final equation:

$$FE_{Na} = \frac{U_{Na} \times P_{Cr}}{P_{Na} \times U_{Cr}}$$

Because the urine volumes ($V$) cancel, a 24-hour collection is not needed. A value for $FE_{Na}$ less than 1% implies enhanced concentration in response to hypovolemia (oliguria, in this case, has been called "renal success"). In contrast, $FE_{Na}$ greater than 2% may be seen in patients unable to concentrate urine as a result of injury to the

## TABLE 65-4

### Laboratory Indices of Intrinsic Renal Dysfunction and Prerenal Azotemia/Oliguria[a]

|  | PRERENAL AZOTEMIA | RENAL DYSFUNCTION |
|---|---|---|
| Plasma BUN:Cr | >20 | <10 |
| Urine osmolality | >500 mOsm/L or > 100 over plasma | <350 mOsm/L or < plasma |
| Urine specific gravity | >1.020 | <1.010 |
| Urine sodium | <20 mEq/L | >30 mEq/L |
| Fractional excretion of sodium | <1% | 2% |
| $U_{Cr}/P_{Cr}$ | >40 | <20 |

[a]Laboratory values unreliably distinguish between intrarenal and obstructive pathology.

tubules (ATN). Although more accurate than simple urine sodium, there are limitations to the use of $FE_{Na}$. The diagnostic accuracy of $FE_{Na}$ is diminished in patients with pre-existing renal insufficiency or recent diuretic use, and in elderly patients. Early in the course of ATN caused by pigment or radiocontrast nephropathy, $FE_{Na}$ may remain below 1%. Also, administration of loop diuretics will confuse the relationship between sodium excretion and loop function.

If renal hypoperfusion is suspected, an empiric fluid challenge of isotonic crystalloid (20 mL/kg bolus of normal saline or Ringer's lactate) should be tried. An increase in urine output combined with improvement in hemodynamic values (decreased tachycardia, increased cardiac filling indices) is diagnostic. Failure to respond to a fluid challenge should prompt a search for evidence of renal injury.

## DIAGNOSE RENAL PARENCHYMAL INJURY

The best measure of proportion of functional nephrons is the glomerular filtration rate. Creatinine is filtered but not reabsorbed or metabolized in the kidney, making it a good marker for filtration through the glomerulus. While a small amount of creatinine is secreted from the distal tubule, an overestimate of GFR is offset by errors in measurement of plasma creatinine ($P_{Cr}$). GFR (mL/minute) can be estimated by the creatinine clearance:

$$C_{Cr} = \frac{U_{Cr} \times V}{P_{Cr}}$$

where $U_{Cr}$ is urine creatinine concentration (mg/dL), $V$ is volume of urine (mL/minute or mL/day ÷ 1,440 minute/day), and $P_{Cr}$ (mg/dL). While a 24-hour collection gives more reliable results, creatinine clearance can be checked by four-hour collections to approximate GFR. An immediate approximation of GFR can be derived from the following equation:

$$C_{Cr} = \frac{(140 - age) \times kg}{P_{Cr} \times 72}$$

In women, this value is multiplied by 0.85. Besides being quicker than the previous calculation, this equation has the additional advantage of accounting for errors produced by differences in body weight, age, and sex (all of which change the amount of muscle mass, the chief determinant of creatinine production aside from dietary intake).

GFR may be overestimated by creatinine clearance in the early stages of renal dysfunction. As GFR falls, rises in plasma creatinine may be partially offset by increased secretion of creatinine leading to a normal-appearing GFR in up to half of patients with a true GFR less than 70 mL/minute. Additionally, the chemical assay method for measuring serum creatinine can be rendered inaccurate by commonly used drugs, including cefoxitin, cimetidine, and trimethoprim. Therefore, creatinine clearance should be regarded as an *upper* estimate of the true GFR. Normal values for creatinine clearance are $95 \pm 20$ mL/minute in women, and $120 \pm 25$ mL/minute in men.[13]

Changes in GFR may be reflected as changes in $P_{Cr}$. Because many variables contribute to serum $P_{Cr}$, and because there is a non-linear relationship between the degree of rise of $P_{Cr}$ and GFR, $P_{Cr}$ is not a perfect indicator of GFR. In some cases, a large decrease in GFR may be sustained but not reflected as an abnormal $P_{Cr}$. Alternatively, a patient with increased protein catabolism (as might be seen in a patient reabsorbing a large hematoma) may have abnormally high $P_{Cr}$ but have normal renal function. Like most chemistries, $P_{Cr}$ has little value outside clinical context.

Examination of the urine may aid diagnosis of intrarenal injury. Urine sodium less than 20 mEq/L generally indicates prerenal failure, whereas value greater than 40 mEq/L imply intrarenal injury. Urinary sediment analysis may allow identification of the etiology of deteriorating renal function. In prerenal azotemia a few hyaline casts may be present. Dirty brown sediment with tubular epithelial cells and granular casts suggests ATN from an ischemic or toxic etiology. White cell casts are common in interstitial nephritis, while red cell casts are consistent with glomerulonephritis. The presence of heme pigment in the absence of red cells strongly suggests rhabdomyolysis.

## OPTIMIZE RENAL PERFUSION/OXYGEN DELIVERY

Insufficient renal perfusion is the most common cause of both oliguria and renal parenchymal injury. Ensuring that the kidneys receive enough blood flow prevents further injury and allows the kidneys to begin to heal. Recent interest in goal directed therapy particularly for patients with sepsis and septic shock has resulted in a number of clinical trials.[68]

It seems intuitive that rapidly correcting haemodynamic derangement in patients with sepsis to normal or supra-normal physiological values is likely to result in a better outcome. Surprisingly, initial controlled trials of such interventions in patients with established sepsis not only failed to reduce mortality, but also seemed to be associated with increased mortality. In a more recent study, patients who arrived at an urban emergency department with SIRS were randomized to receive either six hours of early goal-directed therapy or standard care, before admission to the ICU.[69] All patients received arterial and central venous catheterization (capable of measuring central venous oxygen saturation in the goal-directed group). Goal-directed therapy aimed at optimizing cardiac preload, afterload, and contractility using an algorithm to achieve a target central venous pressure (using crystalloid or colloid), mean arterial pressure (using vasoactive agents), and central venous oxygen saturation (using blood transfusions and inotropic agents). Deaths in hospital were significantly fewer in the group assigned to early goal-directed therapy than in the group receiving standard therapy (30.5% vs 46.5% $P = 0.009$). Furthermore, at 72 hours patients in the early goal-directed group had improved levels of cellular oxygen use, lower lactate concentrations, were less acidotic, and had lower organ-dysfunction scores than those assigned to standard therapy. The contrast between this result and those from earlier studies may be explained by the very short interval between the initial hospital assessment and intervention before the critical illness was established. Goal-directed therapy should be initiated as early as possible in patients who present with sepsis or sepsis like syndromes

Regarding the most appropriate fluid to use for volume replacement a recent. large double-blind randomized controlled trial of albumin versus saline for fluid resuscitation of critically ill patients in the ICU showed that there was no difference in 28-day outcome when either 4% albumin or normal saline was used for fluid resuscitation in the ICU.[70] While maintenance of intravascular volume is chief among the methods of maximizing oxygen delivery, other interventions are important. From the oxygen delivery equation, there are seven variables that govern oxygen delivery to organs: hemoglobin, arterial oxygen saturation, end-diastolic volume (preload), heart rate, ejection fraction, SVR (afterload), and MAP (see Chap. 62). Besides intravascular volume, hemoglobin (Hb) and MAP are the most important determinants of renal perfusion and function. Importantly, pulmonary artery catheter placement is indicated in any patient with persistent oliguria resistant to fluid boluses.

Transfusion potentially boosts oxygen delivery in patients with Hb of less than 12 mg/dL. For example, if all other values remain constant, increasing Hb from 9 to 12 mg/dL produces a 33% increase in oxygen delivery. On the other hand, there are significant risks associated with blood transfusion. A recent multicenter randomized controlled clinical trial (nejm) demonstrated improved outcome in patients randomized to a restrictive blood transfusion target of 7 mg/dL. However, ARF was not specifically mentioned in this study. A recent study[71] clearly showed that patients with ARF have worse survival if their Hg is less than 9 mg/dL. In addition, patients in renal failure, because of diminished synthesis of erythropoietin, may have increased need for transfusion compared to other critically ill patients. For these reasons, transfusion should be considered in any critically ill patient with Hb of less than 9 mg/dL, especially if renal dysfunction has already manifested.

MAP is another key determinant of renal perfusion and of the GFR. Blood flow ($Q$) to any body compartment $C$ is determined largely by the perfusion pressure of that compartment ($PPc$):

$$Q_c = \frac{PP_c}{R}$$

where $R$ is the total resistance of flow to the body compartment. $PPc$ is determined by:

$$PP_c = \text{MAP} - IP_c$$

where $IPc$ is the internal pressure of the compartment. Because pressure inside any body compartment and resistance to flow within that compartment are both usually small, MAP governs flow to that compartment. An exception to this case, of course, is compartment syndrome, where pressure inside a body compartment becomes large compared to MAP. Interestingly, a type of intrarenal compartment syndrome has been proposed for the kidney in which renal edema accompanies severe global edema, as commonly seen in resuscitation of patients with septic or traumatic shock. Because the fibrous renal capsule cannot expand outward, renal edema quickly leads to increased intrarenal pressure and decreased renal flow. This provocative hypothesis awaits further study.

Glomerular filtration also depends directly on MAP. The importance of maintaining adequate perfusion pressure (approximately 80 mm Hg) is clear. In healthy individuals, renal blood flow drops by approximately 30% as MAP drops from 80 to 60 mm Hg. In septic patients with altered intrarenal hemodynamics, the same drop in renal perfusion pressure may produce much deeper reductions in RBF and medullary oxygen tension. If fluid boluses and transfusion fail to maintain renal perfusion pressure, pressors should be employed. While many aspects of the use of pressors remain controversial, general principles regarding their use are clear. First, the *fewest number* of different drugs should be used to

maintain adequate MAP. Second, the *minimal effective dose* should be used. Third, pressors should be *discontinued as soon as possible*. Finally, pressors should *never be allowed to substitute for adequate intravascular volume and hemoglobin.*

Dopamine is the most commonly used pressor in renal dysfunction. Because changes in renal blood flow are a feature common to most forms of ARF, there has been significant interest in the use of renal vasodilators to improve the outcome of ARF. Low-dose or "renal-dose" dopamine has been extensively utilized for this purpose. Despite its numerous[72–74] theoretic advantages clinical efficacy of low-dose dopamine has not been established in humans. Prophylactic use of low-dose dopamine after major cardiovascular surgery,[75] abdominal aortic surgery,[76] or surgery for obstructive jaundice[77] failed to demonstrate an increase in urine output or a decrease in serum creatinine,[75] decreased creatinine,[76] or increased GFR or urine output.[77] Recently, a large prospective randomized controlled clinical trial showed no benefit from low-dose dopamine in ICU patients with SIRS, oliguria, and renal impairment in either renal function, need for dialysis, mortality, or length of stay.[78] A similar randomized, prospective study of dopamine in 48 patients after liver transplant found no change in BUN or creatinine postoperatively or GFR one month postoperatively.[79] Taken together, these data do not justify prophylactic low-dose dopamine treatment in high-risk patients or in patients with established ARF.

Dobutamine enhances renal perfusion by increasing myocardial contractility and decreasing systemic vascular resistance. In one trial,[80] low-dose (5 μg/kg/minute) dobutamine protected critically ill patients from renal failure, while low-dose dopamine was ineffective. These interesting results await confirmation.

Epinephrine and norepinephrine are usually administered in combination with other pressors to maintain MAP in patients in shock. While effective in raising MAP, these drugs may result in decreased organ perfusion secondary to distal arteriole vasoconstriction.[81] The treatment of vasodilatory shock with help of norepinephrine has been feared to contribute to ARF in humans, since animal experiments have indicated that ARF can be produced by administering high-dose norepinephrine directly in the renal artery. This fear has not been substantiated for intravenous doses in humans, provided that euvolemia is present.[82] As for patients with sepsis and shock, Morimatsu et al.[83] report that norepinephrine treatment does not have adverse effects on the kidney in patients after cardiac surgery with vasodilatory shock; however, this was a retrospective observational study only, and a beneficial effect of maintaining arterial blood pressure with norepinephrine was not confirmed. In the absence of clear data, the best strategy is to employ these drugs according to the principles outlined above.

## DIURETICS

Loop diuretics such as furosemide (Lasix) and bumetanide (Bumex) are commonly used in the management of ARF. Loop diuretics act primarily by inhibiting active sodium transport (Na/K-2Cl ATPase) in the mTAL. Loop diuretics (and ouabain) have been shown to increase medullary oxygen tension from 15 to 35 mm Hg[14] by reducing pumping activity of these ATPases. In this way, reducing oxygen demand is thought to prevent cellular anoxia and subsequent injury. Additionally, by increasing tubular flow, tubular debris may be cleared and back pressure may be decreased, enhancing GFR. While experimental animal data suggests loop diuretics may attenuate renal damage early in the course of ATN, clinical data is mixed at best. An early, uncontrolled report demonstrated the ability of high-dose furosemide to maintain a high-urine output in patients at risk for development of an oliguric ATN.[84] A subsequent prospective, randomized report of high-dose continuous furosemide infusion demonstrated successful conversion of 24 of 28 patients from oliguric to nonoliguric ATN; however, there was no difference in the duration of renal failure or mortality.[85] Furosemide has also been studied as prophylaxis for contrast nephropathy. Several prospective reports[86–88] showed that the prophylactic use of furosemide was associated with significant worsening of renal outcome compared to placebo in patients undergoing cardiac surgery or contrast studies. Similarly, in a double-blind trial patients with oliguric ARF not responsive to correction of hypovolemia randomized to a continuous infusion of a loop diuretic or placebo, there was no difference in renal recovery, need for dialysis, or death between groups.[89]

Other controlled studies have also not demonstrated an improvement in the severity or duration of renal failure or patient outcome with the use of either bolus or continuous loop diuretic therapy in ATN.[74,85,90] Nevertheless, achieving some level of urine flow in critically ill patients does simplify care. Fluid overload can be avoided, hyperkalemia can be treated, and some level of solute clearance can be maintained. Therefore, a trial of loop diuretics in the early stages of renal dysfunction to convert oliguric to nonoliguric ARF may be warranted. A diuretic drip can be considered in those who respond. However, these patients must be carefully monitored; hypovolemia may convert the patient from a recoverable to an unrecoverable renal injury.

Mannitol was the first pharmacological agent to be used in ARF. Besides its ability to increase UOP, the capacity of mannitol to reduce proximal tubular sodium reabsorption implies reduced oxygen consumption in vulnerable medullary tubules. It also decreases renin secretion, acts as a reactive oxygen metabolite scavenger, and improves GFR in experimental models. Mannitol also reduces tubular cell swelling in experimental models, increasing intratubular flow and relieving intratubular obstruction. Nevertheless, while these features make mannitol theoretically attractive, clinical trials in humans point to a limited role for mannitol in the treatment of ARF. Moreover, these are a few clinical reports of mannitol actually causing ARF.[91]

Early uncontrolled studies generally report a positive effect of mannitol used prophylactically in surgery and in radiocontrast-exposed patients.[45] Later, prospective studies of mannitol with retrospective controls had mixed results. Recently, a prospective controlled study of the prophylactic use of mannitol in patients at risk for contrast nephropathy found no benefit. Instead, mannitol increased the risk of renal insufficiency in diabetics with pre-existing renal disease.[52] Four other prospective controlled studies examined prophylactic use of mannitol in high-risk patients. A study in vascular surgery and one in biliary tract surgery found neither improvement in GFR or patient survival.[92,93] Only in renal transplantation has mannitol demonstrated beneficial prophylactic effects.[94,95] There are no prospective controlled studies on the effects of mannitol in early or established ARF. Whereas in animal models mannitol (administered between one hour prior to ischemic insult and up to 15 minutes after an acute ischemic insult) has been shown to attenuate or even prevent ARF, this finding has not been replicated in humans.[96] Besides renal transplantation, pigment-induced nephropathy is the only other

indication for mannitol in ARF, but only in combination with vigorous volume replacement.[97]

## ELIMINATE OR MINIMIZE ALL NEPHROTOXIC AGENTS

Because of the additive effect of nephrotoxic agents on renal injury, they should be minimized or eliminated to the extent possible. Radiological studies using contrast should be reconsidered or attempted without contrast. Amphotericin should not be used if fluconazole will suffice. Alternatively, amphotericin delivered in lipozomal micelles, markedly reduces but does not eliminate its nephrotoxic potential (see Chap. 17). Aminoglycosides should be replaced by other antibiotics to which infecting organisms are sensitive, if possible. Adjustment of the dosing interval to once-a-day or less frequently has been shown to decrease nephrotoxicity in some studies[89] but not others.[98] The use of NSAIDs to supplement pain control should be avoided in patients at risk for or with established ARF.

## Correct Metabolic Abnormalities Hyperkalemia

Hyperkalemia is the most common life-threatening electrolyte abnormality occurring in ARF. Hyperkalemia can develop rapidly during conditions of net potassium flux from tissues (rhabdomyolysis, compartment syndrome, transfusion reactions, or hypercatabolism). Acidosis or succinylcholine drive potassium from the cytoplasm into extracellular space. Several medications (e.g., potassium penicillin) have substantial potassium loads. Mild-to-moderate hyperkalemia can be treated by limiting potassium intake and with medical therapy such as potassium binder therapy, particularly in nonoliguric ARF. Marked hyperkalemia ($K^+ > 6$ mEq/L) associated with electrocardiographic changes requires urgent treatment. First, if electrocardiographic changes or cardiac conduction abnormalities occur, intravenous (IV) calcium chloride (10 mg) or calcium gluconate (1 g) may stabilize cardiac conduction while other measures are applied. Next, potassium can be driven from circulation into cells with IV boluses of glucose (dextrose 50) plus insulin (10 units). Decreasing acidosis with IV bicarbonate and/or hyperventilation enhances movement of K into cells (extracellular K is exchanged for intracellular H as the hydrogen ions flow from the cells into the relatively basic extracellular space). Importantly, these temporizing measures do not correct the actual K excess. Ultimately, excess potassium must be treated by enhancing elimination of potassium. Potassium elimination can be accomplished by potassium-binding resins (Kayexelate given orally or rectally) or loop diuretics (i.e., furosemide accompanied by saline boluses). If these medications are ineffective, life-threatening hyperkalemia may require emergent dialysis.

## Hypocalcemia

Hypocalcemia is another common electrolyte abnormality in critically injured patients with ARF. Severe hypocalcemia may accompany conditions such as rhabdomyolysis and pancreatitis, or occur as a consequence of multiple rapid red blood cell transfusions (citrate anticoagulant binds ionized calcium). Alternatively, the patient with ARF may become hypocalcemic without a recognizable etiology. Hypocalcemia compromises myocardial contractility and potentiates conduction disturbances seen in hyperkalemia. Clinically, patients may exhibit decreased cardiac contractility, increased skeletal muscle spasticity (as demonstrated by Trousseau's or Chvostek's signs), or sensations of numbness or tingling in the face and extremities. Correction is with intravenous calcium chloride or calcium gluconate. As a practical matter, some clinicians prefer to use only calcium gluconate because it does not cause the same degree of muscle necrosis if it infiltrates during administration. Finally, clinicians should watch for hyperphosphatemia which can occur in hypocalcemia, especially if GFR falls below 30% of normal.

## Sodium

Hypernatremia and hyponatremia should be understood not as disorders of sodium, but of disorders of sodium and free water. In each case, the clinician must first assess extracellular volume status (hypovolemic, isovolemic, or hypervolemic). The specific treatment in each case will be careful correction of excess or depletion of sodium or free water.

Although uncommon as a direct effect of ARF, hypernatremia (serum sodium > 145 mEq/L) is common in the ICU. The chief danger of hypernatremia is metabolic encephalopathy stemming from hypertonic cellular dehydration in the central nervous system. Although mortality can approach 50%, hasty correction will endanger the patient. In hypovolemic hypernatremia, the defect is loss of hypotonic body fluids (nasogastric suction, diarrhea, excessive diuresis). In this case, patients are more threatened by hypovolemia than by the hypernatremia as hypotension produces hypoperfusion to kidney, gut, and other organs. Therefore, the first goal of treatment is to restore intravascular volume with volume expanders such as albumin or hetastarch. Then the patient's free-water deficit can be corrected (see below).

When hypotonic body fluids are lost and replaced 1:1 with normal saline, the result may be normovolemic hypernatremia. Since the defect is a loss of free water (essentially an exchange of free water for water plus sodium), the treatment is slow replacement of the free water deficit. Diabetes insipidus (DI) treated with normal saline will produce this clinical picture. DI is a failure of the kidneys to conserve water because of a failure of the action of

ADH. In the context of a progressive increase in serum sodium, a urine osmolality of less than 100 mOsm is diagnostic of DI. Without the action of ADH, the water channels of the collecting duct remain open, yielding urine that is nearly water—very low sodium and very low specific gravity. Central DI is a failure of release of ADH from the posterior pituitary as may occur in closed head injury, anoxic brain injury, or meningitis (see Chap. 20). Besides correction of free water deficit, vasopressin (5 to 10 units subcutaneously q6 to 8 hours) can prevent ongoing free water losses. Nephrogenic DI is failure of the kidney to respond to ADH. It may be caused by aminoglycosides, amphotericin, or radiocontrast, or may occur in the early (polyuric) phase of ATN. Vasopressin will have no effect in nephrogenic DI.

In contrast to these conditions, hypervolemic hypernatremia is actual sodium overload. This condition is almost always iatrogenic, stemming from (over) use of sodium bicarbonate or hypertonic saline in patients with renal insufficiency. In this case, treatment consists of induction of a sodium diuresis with a loop diuretic, plus gentle free-water replacement with hypotonic fluids. Because the maximum urine concentration achievable with loop diuretics is still hypotonic compared to plasma (i.e., 75 mEq/L vs. > 140 mEq/L), loop diuretics alone produce a net loss of free water, exacerbating hypernatremia. Instead, water and sodium (urine) must be exchanged for water alone.

The equation for calculation of free-water deficit is:

$$FWD = Wt\,(kg) * 0.5 * \left(1 - \frac{140}{[Na]_p}\right)$$

where $Wt$ is the patient's lean body weight, and $[Na]p$ is plasma sodium concentration. Substitute 0.6 in place of 0.5 for women. Rapid infusion of large volumes of free water can cause cerebral edema leading to altered mental status, permanent neurologic deficits, or death. Therefore, free water should be replaced over 48 to 72 hours.

Low serum sodium concentration produces cerebral edema, increased intracranial pressure, coma, and even death. Hyponatremia (serum sodium < 135 mEq/L) is more commonly a free-water problem than a sodium problem. Like hypernatremia, identifying the etiology is essential to safe and effective correction (Fig. 65-5).

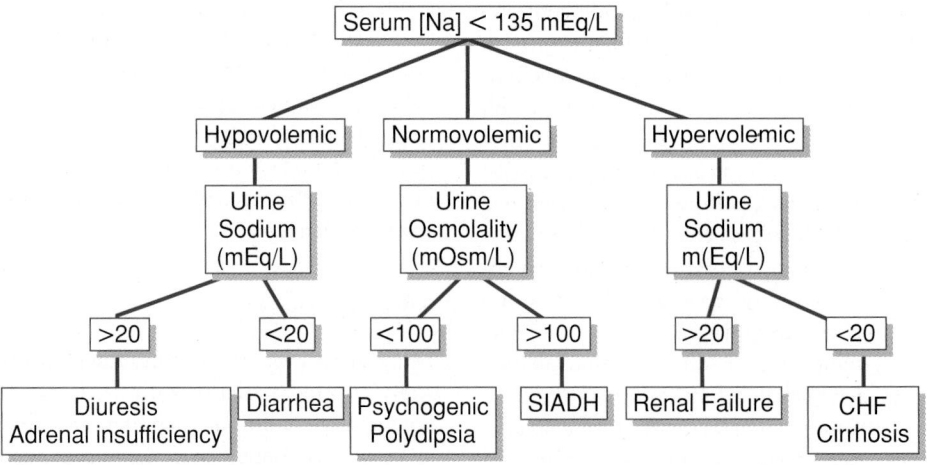

**FIGURE 65-5.**  Algorithm for diagnosis of hyponatremia.

Hypovolemic hyponatremia results when fluid losses are partially replaced by relatively hypotonic fluids, such as a patient with diarrhea who drinks large volumes of tap water. Isovolemic hyponatremia may be seen in the syndrome of inappropriate antidiuretic hormone (SIADH), which may occur in posttraumatic, postsurgical, or other stressed patients. The severe hyponatremia (< 120 mEq/L) resulting from this excess of ADH produces a very concentrated urine (urine sodium > 20 mEq/L, urine osmolality >100 mOsm/L), but only a small overload of free water. Finally, various organ failures (see Chap. 68), including ARF, can lead to both sodium and water overload, with relatively more water than sodium retained.

Treatment goals for hyponatremia include correction of both water and sodium problems. Like hypernatremia, hyponatremia must be corrected slowly. Rapid correction of hyponatremia can produce diffuse demyelinating CNS lesions such as central pontine myelinosis, pituitary damage, or oculomotor nerve palsies. To avoid these complications, the rate of rise of serum sodium concentration should be less than 0.5 mEq/L/hour, and the plasma sodium should not rise above 130 mEq/L. Hypertonic saline (3% NaCl or "hot salt") should be reserved for use in symptomatic hypo- or isovolemic hyponatremia. (Note that, because the rate of sodium replenishment must remain slow, the only advantage of 3% NaCl solutions may be smaller total volume infusion; i.e., less water accompanies the salt.) Asymptomatic patients can be treated with isotonic saline. Patients with hypervolemic hyponatremia are treated with a loop diuretic.

The equation for sodium deficit (assuming 130 mEq/L as the therapeutic endpoint) is:

$$\text{Sodium deficit (mEq)} = \text{Wt (kg)} * 0.5 * (130 - [\text{Na}]_p)$$

where the variables are the same as in the free-water deficit equation and 0.5 is also replaced by 0.6 in men.

## Acid-base Abnormalities

Metabolic acidosis occurs commonly in ARF. As hydrogen secretion by the tubules is impaired, a nonanion gap acidosis occurs. Later, as GFR falls and organic acids accumulate, an anion gap acidosis may also occur. Metabolic acidosis develops more rapidly during any condition stemming from increased lactate production (e.g., septic shock or I/R injury). Untreated metabolic acidosis can lead to decreased cardiac output, cardiac arrhythmias, lack of cardiac response to inotropic support, or cardiac arrest (see Chap. 62). Life-threatening metabolic acidosis can be temporized with IV sodium bicarbonate or hyperventilation (in ventilated patients). However, bicarbonate is of limited value, and it may even harm patients who have both metabolic and respiratory acidosis: in the absence of effective carbon dioxide ($CO_2$) elimination by ventilation (as in ARDS), adding bicarbonate may actually worsen acidosis.[99,100] In general, hyperventilation is a more physiologic and rapid temporizing measure for life-threatening acidosis. In any case, the specific cause of the acidosis must be addressed. For example, prolonged or worsening metabolic acidosis implies ongoing global hypoperfusion; increasing oxygen delivery often corrects the acidosis. However, severely acidotic (pH < 7.2) patients in oliguric or anuric ARF may also require dialysis.

Metabolic alkalosis is also a common finding in ICU patients, including those with ARF, particularly when large nasogastric

losses of hydrogen ions combine with volume contraction. Similarly, loop diuretics increase renal H loss, and will also lead to metabolic alkalosis, if excess diuresis causes hypovolemia. Increased serum pH may produce cardiac dysrhythmias, decreased oxygen delivery, hypotension, hypoventilation, impaired mentation, hypocalcemia, and hypokalemia. Repletion of volume and chloride deficits (allowing improved elimination of bicarbonate in the urine) usually corrects pH in these patients. Additionally, administration of $H_2$ blockers or $H^+$ pump inhibitors (e.g., omeprazole) will cut nasogastric tube losses. Occasionally, patients in ARF require intravenous hydrochloride or dialysis with a low-buffer dialysis solution.

## RENAL REPLACEMENT

Despite decades of use, no consensus indications for the initiation or dosing (frequency and duration) of renal replacement therapy have been accepted, and aspects of its use are controversial. Debate continues whether to adopt an early, aggressive approach to patients with renal dysfunction. Advocates argue that early dialysis may avoid uremic complications, simplify fluid management, and facilitate nutrition delivery.[101] Detractors point up the lack of data demonstrating improved outcome with early dialysis. However, a recent retrospective analysis of patients with posttraumatic ARF showed that survival rate was significantly increased (39 vs. 20%, $p < .05$) when continuous renal replacement therapy was started early (BUN < 60 mg/DL).[102] On the other hand, hemodialysis is not a benign procedure: Patients routinely experience hypotension requiring increased pressor support, cardiac arrhythmias, hypoxemia, bleeding complications, and infections at dialysis catheter sites.[103] Despite these arguments, dialysis has some clear indications.

Renal replacement therapy is indicated for any one of several life-threatening metabolic derangements: fluid overload, severe uremia, critical electrolyte abnormalities, metabolic acidosis that cannot be compensated by hyperventilation, and some toxins. Dialysis for clinical volume overload should be approached with care; in the trauma population, hypovolemia is more common and far more dangerous than fluid overload. As BUN approaches 100 mg/dL, patients exhibit mental status changes and coagulopathy secondary to platelet dysfunction. Some clinicians advocate earlier initiation of dialysis, for example, when BUN reaches 60 mg/dL in order to avoid complications of azotemia. The most common electrolyte abnormality treated with dialysis is hyperkalemia. Critical values are usually regarded as greater than 7 mEq/dL, but any value above normal accompanied by electrocardiographic changes is an emergency. Metabolic acidosis is best addressed by remedying the underlying cause of the acidosis. Importantly, hyperventilation and sodium bicarbonate may be ineffective or dangerous in patients unable to increase respiratory $CO_2$ elimination, such as patients with acute respiratory distress syndrome (ARDS) or pulmonary contusion. In these situations, if medical approaches fail to correct progressive acidosis, dialysis is indicated for pH of less than 7.2 (the point at which many enzymes and drugs such as inotropes fail). In general, timing and frequency of hemodialysis are best decided within daily clinical context rather than simply by strict biochemical criteria.

Once dialysis has been initiated, the length of time that patients continue to require dialysis varies from a single treatment to progression to chronic dialysis depending on the indication and severity of insult. For example, a patient with severe alcohol toxicity may require only a single treatment, whereas a diabetic patient who survives septic shock and MODS may never recover adequate renal capability. In general, however, most patients eventually re-establish renal function and will do so within four to six weeks (although recovery after longer periods has been reported). In any case, continuation of renal replacement must be considered within the context of overall prognosis: Withdrawal of dialysis is appropriate if there is no likelihood of patient recovery.

Three forms of renal replacement therapy are commonly used in hospitals today: peritoneal dialysis, intermittent hemodialysis, and continuous renal replacement. Peritoneal dialysis (PD) is a poor choice to treat ARF in trauma patients for several reasons. First, PD is obviously contraindicated in ARF associated with intra-abdominal abscesses or recent abdominal surgery because of the increased risk of peritonitis. Moreover, PD is relatively inefficient with regard to volume or solute removal, rendering it unhelpful in emergencies. Finally, infusion of intraperitoneal volume reduces diaphragmatic compliance, compromising ventilation. Because of these weaknesses, PD is rarely if ever used in posttraumatic ARF.

Established efficacy has made intermittent hemodialysis (IHD) the standard therapy for ARF. Besides ready availability in most hospitals, IHD rapidly removes fluid, solutes, and toxins. IHD may also be used to rapidly replace red cells or to quickly correct electrolyte imbalance. IHD removes small, nonprotein-bound solutes more efficiently than other methods of renal replacement. These advantages are tempered by dangers. Due to rapid volume solute shifts, intermittent dialysis in the critically ill ICU patient is associated with episodes of hypotension, hypoxemia, hemolysis, and cardiac arrhythmias.[88] Rapid solute shifts have also been associated with worsening of cerebral edema. Recent reports also document a decrease in cardiac index and an increase in oxygen consumption during IDH.[104,105] Additionally, in inotrope-dependent critically ill patients with multiple organ dysfunction syndrome, intermittent dialysis increases inotropic support requirements to maintain blood pressure and cardiac index (see Chap. 68). Moreover, IHD is associated with increased oxygen consumption and decreased oxygen delivery, leading to intestinal mucosal acidosis that persists after the procedure.[106] Finally, hemodialysis activates the systemic inflammatory reaction by priming neutrophils, activating the complement system, causing generation of reactive oxygen species, and increasing release of leukotrienes and proinflammatory cytokines.[107]

The combination of renal hypoperfusion and systemic inflammation may explain clinical observations that many patients become oliguric or anuric shortly after initiation of IHD.[108] A prospective, randomized study of two different levels of IHD intensity demonstrated a trend toward increased mortality in the group of patients dialyzed more frequently, suggesting that intensive intermittent hemodialysis may have a deleterious effect.[103] Other investigators have reported that intermittent hemodialysis may delay recovery from ARF.[108] Suffice it to say the optimal dose of dialysis in ARF has not been determined. However, a recent randomized trial comparing daily with alternate-day haemodialysis in 160 patients with ARF in the medical and surgical ICUs of a German hospital, daily treatment was associated with better biochemical control, fewer hypotensive episodes during haemodialysis, more rapid recovery of renal function, and improved survival (28% vs. 46%)[109]

The authors proposed that alternate-day haemodialysis should no longer be considered adequate for critically ill patients with ARF.

## Biocompatible Membranes

Because of suspicion that the cuprophane (cellulose-based) membranes normally used in IHD provoke hazardous inflammation, some investigators have turned to "biocompatible" IHD membranes that do not exhibit proinflammatory effect. Several reports have compared outcomes using biocompatible membranes compared to cuprophane membranes in IHD for ARF. Biocompatible membranes are associated with less hypotension, decreased reliance on pressors, decreased activation of complement (C3a), decreased lethal sepsis, quicker recovery of renal function, and overall lower mortality.[109,110] A prospective study using cuprophane versus polymethylmethacrylate biocompatible membrane showed a significant increase in the number of patients who recovered renal function (62% vs. 37%), a shorter duration of dialysis dependence (11 days vs. 33 days), and a trend toward improved survival in the biocompatible membrane group (57% vs. 37%).[107] Another study comparing biocompatible versus cellulosic membranes documented a significant decrease in mortality, an increased return of renal function, and a shorter time to recovery of renal function in patients treated with biocompatible membranes.[111] Additionally, fewer nonoliguric patients became oliguric while being treated with biocompatible membranes compared to traditional cellulosic membranes (44% vs. 70%). In this study, the advantages of decreased mortality, increased renal function, and decreased duration of ARF were all confined to the subset of patients who were nonoliguric at the initiation of dialysis. Meta-analyses have further shown that the use of biocompatible membranes might influence survival positively, however, without effect on recovery of renalfunction.[113-114]

## Continuous Renal Replacement Techniques

Even with biocompatible membranes, many patients are too unstable to tolerate IHD. The application of dialysis is different from its use in chronic kidney disease, because the patients are often haemodynamically unstable, hypercatabolic, require nutritional support and receive large volumes of fluid. Different RRT methods have been used and include intermittent haemodialysis, peritoneal dialysis, continuous RRT, e.g., continuous veno-venous haemofiltration (CVVH, most commonly used in ICUs) and an emerging technique termed 'slow low-efficient daily dialysis.'[115] The choice of RRT usually depends on technical expertise, equipment availability, and local experience or practice. The most common indication for continuous RRT such as CVVH is the presence of haemodynamic instability. The gradual removal of solute and plasma water over a 24-hour period is thought to induce less haemodynamic stress than with rapid solute and fluid removal by intermittent haemodialysis over four hours. Other theoretical advantages include better correction of acidosis and malnutrition, and better removal of cytokines. A potential disadvantage of continuous RRT in patients with bleeding tendencies is the need for continuous anticoagulation to prevent the extracorporeal circuit from clotting. Despite the theoretical advantages of continuous RRT in treating severe ARF, no prospective controlled studies have shown better patient survival with this technique than with intermittent haemodialysis.[114] A recent meta-analysis of all previous trials and observational studies comparing continuous RRT with intermittent haemodialysis showed no difference in mortality between them.[114] In specific conditions, however, one of the dialysis modalities is an absolute preference: for example, continuous therapy in patients with cerebral oedema or liver failure, or intermittent haemodialysis in patients with increased bleeding risk.

In addition, a recent study underscored the importance of the dose of dialysis in continuous renal replacement therapy.[116] Patients' undergoing continuous venovenous haemofiltration had better outcomes with filtration rates of 35 mL kg$^{-1}$ h$^{-1}$ or 45 mL kg$^{-1}$ h$^{-1}$ than those treated at the lower rate of 20 mL kg$^{-1}$ h$^{-1}$. Although no comparable study has been done in intermittent haemodialysis,[116] daily dialysis resulted in better control of uraemia, fewer hypotensive episodes during dialysis, and more rapid resolution of ARF.[109]

To provide renal replacement to these patients, various continuous, low-flow replacement therapies have been devised. These methods differ essentially in terms of the driving force for blood flow through the device and of the mechanism of solute removal. Arteriovenous (AV) circuits use MAP as the driving force. Venovenous (VV) circuits use an external pump as the driving force and generally permit better control and higher blood flow rates. Arteriovenous systems (e.g., continuous arteriovenous hemofiltration, or CAVH) are the simplest and least expensive systems, but require more risky arterial access and depend on a MAP of greater than 80 for effective flow. VV systems, utilizing external pumps, add complexity and cost but are generally more efficient. Each system requires anticoagulation of the external system via citrate or heparin (Fig. 65-6).

Continuous renal replacement techniques (CRRT) use highly permeable, biocompatible, synthetic membranes that allow gradual, continuous removal of fluids and solutes. Solute removal by these techniques is achieved by convection, diffusion, or a combination of these. Convection techniques include ultrafiltration and hemofiltration. Solute removal occurs by solvent drag, which is effective for molecules up to 20,000 daltons. In hemofiltration, there is partial or complete replacement of volume loss with continuous infusion of a replacement fluid with electrolytes in a composition similar to plasma. The diffusion techniques add a countercurrent dialyzate flow and utilize a solute gradient between blood and a dialyzate fluid to increase the efficiency of clearance of small solutes. In contrast to IHD, the dialyzate flow rates of CRRT are significantly lower than blood flow rates. Small molecules are preferentially removed by diffusion-based (dialyzate) methods. If both convection and diffusion techniques are used in the same technique, the process is termed hemodiafiltration (HDF). In this system, both a dialyzate and replacement fluid are used and clearance is efficient for both large and small molecules. Systems which incorporate hemofiltration or HDF clear larger molecules than dialysis-based techniques, readily clearing heparin, insulin, vancomycin, and cytokines.

A principal advantage of these methods is the ability to directly control fluid balance and allow continuous fine-tuning of intravascular and electrolyte status. Despite slower flow rates, due to continuous operation, weekly clearance of solute may equal or exceed clearance achievable with IHD. On the other hand, the very slow flow of CAVH, the oldest and simplest of the techniques, may not provide enough power to clear small solutes in hypercatabolic patients with high rates of urea generation. In this

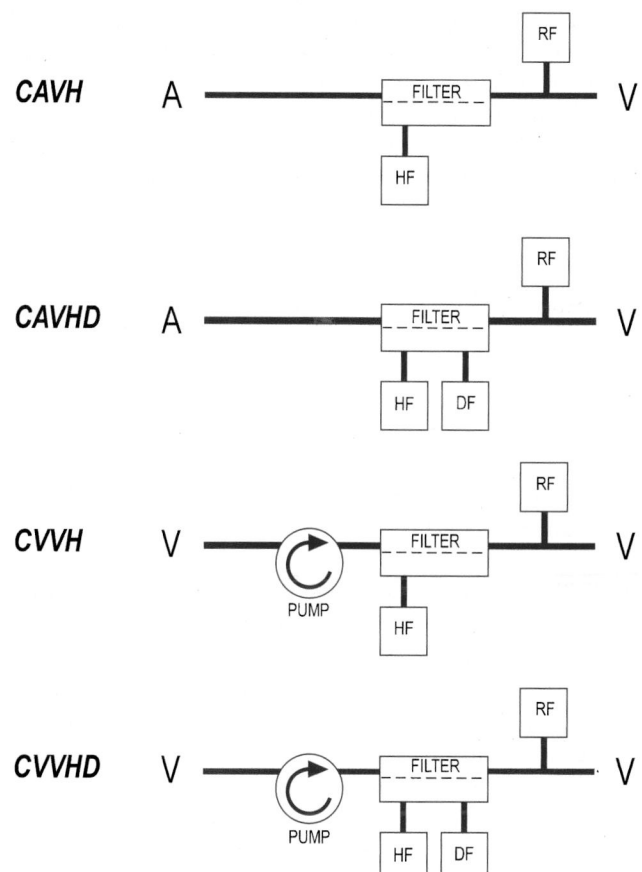

**FIGURE 65-6.** Schematic depiction of various methods of continuous renal replacement. Flow is from left to right. CAVH, continuous arteriovenous hemofiltration; CAVHD, continuous arteriovenous hemodialysis; CVVH, continuous venovenous hemofiltration; CVVHD, continuous venovenous hemodialysis; UF, ultrafiltrate; DF, dialysis fluid; RF, replacement fluid.

circumstance, CAVHD or CVVH may be a better choice, each of which is actually more effective than IHD in terms of ability to clear nitrogenous wastes.[117,118] Moreover, all the continuous techniques have such advantages as the ability to provide nutrition without risk of volume overload, decreased incidence of cardiac arrhythmias, and decreased exacerbation of cerebral edema in closed-head injury patients.

CRRT may be preferred over IHD for critically ill patients who demonstrate hemodynamic instability or who have systemic inflammatory response syndrome with multiple organ failure. A decrease in the number of hypotensive episodes has been shown using CRRT versus IHD.[118] Other investigators have demonstrated the ability of CVVHD to clear cytokines from the circulation of septic patients.[117] A decreased number of hypotensive episodes and clearance rather than exacerbation of inflammatory mediators might be expected to improve renal or patient outcome using these methods for critically ill patients. However, useful convective removal of mediators from the human septic circulation has not been achieved to date, although many cytokines have a molecular weight below the theoretical cutoff point of commercial membranes currently in use.[119] Studies examining this question are ongoing. Further indications might exist for CRRT beyond solely renal support. CRRT provides a degree of cytokine removal via filtration and adsorption.[120] However, the clinical significance of such removal is still undetermined since multiple studies show that the plasma levels of these mediators remain unchanged, probably due to excessive production and saturation at the cellular level. In a randomized controlled clinical trial using CVVH versus no CVVH in early sepsis, Cole et al. demonstrated that the early use of CVVH at 2000 mL/hour did not reduce circulating cytokine concentrations, anaphylatoxins, or organ dysfunction that followed severe sepsis.[121] There is some evidence, however, of an immunomodulatory effect of CVVH in the porcine model of sepsis[121] and in human studies[122,123] Diffusion of suppressive "uremic toxins" may be important in acutely uremic patients. In agreement with this contention, a study in 12 critically ill patients with ARF comparing low-volume CVVH (1500 mL/hour) with a diffusive technique was performed in a nonrandomized, comparative fashion.[122] High-flux bicarbonate dialysis amounting to 4200 mL/hour was used, and the effect on monocyte responsiveness (ex-vivo endotoxin-stimulated TNF-production) was studied. Both techniques resulted in early improvement, but only the diffusive technique displayed persistent effects. Ultrafiltrate contained monocyte suppressive activity only with high-flux dialysis.[122,123]

Selection bias in earlier reviews, in which only the sickest patients received CRRT, probably obscured advantages of CRRT. Because mortality remains high in these critically ill patients, recovery of renal function may be a more realistic endpoint when comparing these techniques. Randomized, prospective trials are pending. In the meantime, CRRT remains a useful option in patients unable to tolerate IHD but who nevertheless have clear indications for dialysis.

Another alternative is to attain higher removal rates of middle molecular weight molecules using membranes with a larger pore size. Animal data[124] as well as preliminary clinical data[125] showed that the goal of attaining higher removal rates of selected cytokines could indeed be reached. The pursuit of ultra-high-efficiency clearance has led to rediscovery of plasma exchange in the form of plasma filters. There appears to be little benefit from plasma filtration; however, according to a recent clinical trial[126] both high costs from excessive plasma substitution fluids and unregulated losses of beneficial plasma constituents may also be limits to this modality of treatment. These limitations have produced new enthusiasm for adsorbent technology.[127] Uncoated adsorbents (i.e., maximizing their adsorptive ability) could, in fact, allow the regeneration of ultrafiltrate or plasma, which would then be used as reinfusion fluids without the need for exogenous supplementation. In summary, while much needs to be done, CRRT appears to be the preferred extracorporeal treatment once ARF develops as part of MOF. It has been demonstrated that CRRT has many benefits over intermittent therapies but to date, no suitably powered randomized, controlled trials have been conducted to test whether CRRT decreases mortality.

## NUTRITION

The goal of nutritional support in ARF is to provide enough calorie and protein substrates to minimize catabolism, allow wound healing, and sustain immune function (see Chap. 66).

A common mistake in treating patients with renal dysfunction is withholding of protein calories for fear of driving serum nitrogen levels upward. Because trauma and surgical patients with ARF are usually catabolic from injuries or from sepsis, withholding protein calories can exacerbate protein wasting in skeletal muscle (including respiratory musculature), heart, and liver. These deficits may decrease ability to clot, fight infection, wean from the ventilator, and so forth. Both the rate of protein catabolism and caloric requirements vary depending on the etiology of ARF. In mild ARF without other organ system involvement, metabolic rate and catabolism may not be greatly increased; however, patients with comorbid illnesses or MOF may have net protein catabolism of 150 g/day or more.[128] There are few prospective, randomized clinical trials assessing the effect of parenteral nutrition on morbidity and mortality in ARF.[128] Most of these were unable to demonstrate any protective benefit of parenteral nutrition; however, small patient numbers may mask differences between outcomes. More importantly, any benefits of parenteral nutrition could easily be obscured by other factors (such as underlying etiology), which govern outcomes from ARF. There are no randomized clinical trials assessing the benefit of enteral nutrition in ARF. Nevertheless, because nutritional support has clear benefits in other critical illness, most clinicians accept the need for aggressive nutritional support in highly catabolic ARF patients, particularly if illness is likely to be prolonged. Suppression of catabolism by provision of adequate nutrition decreases urea and potassium production of the catabolic patient, reducing solute load for struggling kidneys. Nutritional support should take precedence over withholding renal replacement therapy.

Calculation of nitrogen balance aids estimation of protein and energy requirements. Total protein goals should be established to achieve positive nitrogen balance, although this is often difficult to achieve in clinical practice. Losses of unbound amino acid in dialyzate are on the order of 13 g/dialysis in patients on IV nutrition. Free amino acid losses also occur in continuous renal replacement therapy related to the permeability of the filter, flow rates, and plasma amino acid levels, on the order of 4 to 7 g/day. Although these losses can be attenuated by adding free amino acid to dialyzate,[129] protein requirements may still be as high as 2.5 g/kg/day. In addition, CRRT causes significant loss of magnesium and calcium necessitating administration of more magnesium and calcium than is provided in standard parenteral nutrition formulas.[130] As a final practical note, in hemodiafiltration, the hemodialyzate is 0.5 to 0.25% glucose, adding 150 to 270 g of carbohydrate per day, an amount that needs to be included in energy calculations.

Finally, enteral nutrition is the preferred method of nutritional support whenever possible in critically ill patients (see Chap. 66). Enteral feeding maintains gastrointestinal integrity and bolsters immune function. Compared to parenteral nutrition, enteral feeds are associated with decreased risk of infections, lower incidence of hepatic dysfunction, and less prevalent stress gastritis. Costs are also reduced with enteral formulations. Intolerance of enteral feeds usually manifests as diarrhea, but other patients may have an ileus precluding enteral feeding. If the patient does not tolerate enteral feeds, parenteral nutritional support should be used until enteral nutrition is possible.

# DRUG–KIDNEY INTERACTIONS

Because most drugs and their metabolites are at least partly metabolized and excreted by the kidney, pharmacokinetics of most drugs can be drastically altered in ARF. The following mechanisms are important in altering available drug levels during ARF. These include the following:

1. *Decreased filtration.* Most nonprotein-bound drugs and metabolites undergo glomerular filtration. As GFR decreases, drugs such as digoxin, aminoglycosides, and several antihypertensives may accumulate unless dosages are adjusted.

2. *Decreased tubular secretion.* Cephalosporins, histamine antagonists, procainamide, and morphine are examples of drugs that undergo tubular secretion and hence accumulate in the presence of acute tubular injury.

3. *Decreased tubular reabsorption.* Decreased tubular reabsorption of salicylates and sulfonamide derivatives is impaired in acute tubular injury.

4. *Altered volume of distribution.* Volume resuscitation and extracellular space expansion may affect a drug's volume of distribution, as can changes in serum pH and changes in protein binding. The accumulation of organic acids in patients with severely compromised GFR can displace drugs from albumin binding sites and increase their activity or toxicity.

Drug therapy should be designed specifically for each patient in ARF. Dosing tables or the hospital pharmacist should be consulted for a dosing regimen. Many drugs are best avoided in the setting of ARF. For example, aminoglycosides and amphotericin B may precipitate or aggravate renal dysfunction. Other drugs have active metabolites that accumulate to toxic levels in renal failure. For example, normeperidine, the renally excreted active metabolite of meperidine, can rapidly accumulate in ARF and cause neurotoxicity, including seizures.[131] Morphine is a preferred analgesic in ARF, but it should also be used with caution; decreased protein binding in ARF increases the bioavailability of a given dose of morphine. As with meperidine, metabolites of diazepam can accumulate and cause prolonged sedation in patients with ARF. Other drugs carry large electrolyte loads, potentially exacerbating electrolyte disorders in ARF. Examples include carbenicillin and ticarcillin (sodium) loads, potassium penicillin (potassium), and many antacids (magnesium). Hemodialysis also affects drug dosing. Typically, drugs with a molecular size less than 500 daltons are readily removed by hemodialysis unless they are largely protein bound (Table 65-5). For example, hemodialysis removes gentamicin but not vancomycin (molecular weight of vancomycin is 1140 daltons). Postdialysis dosing is recommended for drugs that are cleared during dialysis (see Chap. 16).

# EXPERIMENTAL APPROACHES

Several agents have been found effective in treatment or prevention of ARF in animals, and a few have been tested in clinical trials. In general, these treatments are directed toward recognized derangements in ARF; all act by protecting renal blood flow, attenuating postischemic inflammation, or facilitating recovery

**TABLE 65-5**

## Dialyzable and Nondialyzable Drugs

### NEGLIGIBLE CLEARANCE BY IHD

| Antibiotics | Cardiovascular Agents | Miscellaneous |
|---|---|---|
| Amphotericin B | Amiodarone | Benzodiazepines |
| Azidothymidine | Digoxin | Cimetidine |
| Cefotetan | Diltiazem | Cyclosporine |
| Ciprofloxacin | Disopyramide | Famotidine |
| Clindamycin | Esmolol | Morphine |
| Cloxacillin | Labetalol | Omeprazole |
| Doxycycline | Metoprolol | Phenytoin |
| Erythromycin | Propafenone | Prednisone |
| Itraconazole | | Propoxyphene |
| Ketoconazole | | |
| Nafcillin | | |
| Vancomycin | | |

### SIGNIFICANT CLEARANCE BY IHD

| Antibiotics | Miscellaneous |
|---|---|
| Acyclovir | Allopurinol |
| Aminoglycosides | Atenolol |
| Ampicillin | Captopril |
| Aztreonam | Cyclophosphamide |
| Trimethoprim–sulfamethoxazole | N-acetylprocainamide |
| Flucytosine | Ranitidine |
| Ganciclovir | Sotalol |
| Imipenem | |
| Isoniazid | |
| Metronidazole | |
| Most cephalosporins | |
| Piperacillin | |

of tubular epithelium (see Chap. 67). A number of agents have been proposed to improve renal blood flow and GFR. Because patients in septic shock were shown to produce increased amounts of the vasodilator NO, some investigators tried using nonspecific inhibitors of nitric oxide synthase (NOS) as a pressor. Early results have been disappointing, however, with most studies showing either no effects or adverse effects on end-organ perfusion. In particular, inhibition of NO augments renal injury in rats.[132] The role of NO in regulation of renal blood flow is complex (see previous sections) and so this type of intervention awaits clarification and more specific inhibitors. Vasopressin may be useful to improve MAP in severely septic patients. Occasionally, patients with severe sepsis are unable to respond to alpha-adrenergic stimulation. In these patients, case reports have suggested that a vasopressin drip leads to significant improvement in MAP. The effect of vasopressin on renal perfusion and on overall mortality has not been tested.[133] Prostaglandins (in particular $PGE_2$) have been used with some success to treat renal dysfunction in some patients. $PGE_2$ selectively dilates the afferent renal arteriole, improving flow. $PGE_2$ may be most effective in selected patients, especially morbidly obese patients. Misoprostol, a prostaglandin $E_1$ analog, is protective against ischemic and toxic injury to the kidneys in experimental models.[134] Neither the exact physiologic reasons for this beneficial effect nor the ultimate effect on outcomes has been determined.

Identification of increased cytosolic calcium as a contributor to tubular cell injury prompted consideration of calcium channel blockers as prophylaxis or therapy for ARF. Besides modulating intracellular events, calcium channel blockers may protect against tubular hypoxia by dilatation of afferent arterioles and producing a solute diuresis. Increased GFR can be demonstrated in animal models of I/R, if calcium channel blockers are administered prior to insult.[135] In human trials, diltiazem was found to be protective in preventing ATN and delayed graft function in renal transplant patients in prospective, randomized trials.[136,137] In this setting, calcium channel blockers may exert their effect by antagonism of cyclosporine-mediated renal vasoconstriction. There are no randomized reports utilizing calcium channel blockers early in the course of ARF from other etiologies. Intrarenal verapamil combined with IV furosemide improved GFR better than furosemide alone in malaria- or leptospirosis-related ARF, but this observation has not been linked to better outcomes or applied to other etiologies of ARF.[138] Calcium channel blockers may also prevent vasoconstriction caused by radiocontrast agents.[53] However, since calcium antagonists may cause hypotension and diminished cardiac contractility, use of calcium channel blockers is probably not justified in most forms of postischemic ARF encountered in trauma patients.

Atrial natriuretic peptide (ANP) has many properties suggesting that it could be useful to treat ARF. ANP has been shown to increase renal blood flow in several forms of experimental renal failure. ANP increases GFR in experimental models by dilating afferent and constricting efferent glomerular arterioles. By blocking tubular reabsorption of sodium and chloride and reversing endothelin-induced vasoconstriction, ANP protects against medullary hypoxia. In animal models, ANP is shown to be effective in both preventing ARF and improving recovery from established ARF.[139,140] Clinical utility of ANP, however, has not been demonstrated. A prospective, nonrandomized study of patients with established ATN treated with ANP demonstrated increased creatinine clearance, decreased progression to dialysis (23% vs. 52%), and decreased mortality (17% vs. 35%) compared to patients not treated with ANP.[140] Unfortunately, as the authors themselves pointed out, these promising results were tempered by study design flaws including lack of randomization, lack of blinding, administration protocols that changed midway through the study, and lack of a protocol for administration of diuretics.[141] The subsequent multicenter, prospective, randomized, blinded placebo controlled trial of anaritide (a synthetic homologue of ANP) demonstrated no overall difference in dialysis-free survival among 504 patients with established ATN from various etiologies.[142] However, a subgroup analysis revealed interesting differences. In the subgroup of oliguric patients, anaritide increased dialysis-free survival (8% vs. 27%). Oliguric patients at the beginning of treatment who converted to nonoliguric ARF during treatment benefited the most from anaritide. However, among nonoliguric patients, anaritide significantly *worsened* dialysis-free survival compared to placebo (59% vs. 48%, $p = 0.03$).[141] In this study, ANP appeared to be of benefit in oliguric patients but had a deleterious effect in nonoliguric patients. No clear recommendations for the use of ANP emerge from these observations.

Sustained vasoconstriction of intrarenal blood flow, mediated by potent vasoconstrictors such as endothelin-1, is known to be an important component of the pathophysiology of ATN.[17] In animal models of ischemic ARF, administration of anti-endothelin antibodies or endothelin-receptor antagonist protects the kidney against ARF.[143,144]

Because reactive oxygen metabolites contribute to I/R injury in the kidney and other organs, antioxidants have been examined. Reactive oxygen species contribute to cellular injury by altering protein structure, forming lipid peroxides in cell membranes, recruiting activated neutrophils, and promoting subsequent inflammatory events. The antioxidant (hydroxyl radical scavenger) properties of mannitol have been proposed as a possible mechanism of its beneficial effects. Oxygen radical scavengers such as glutathione, superoxide dismutase, and allopurinol have shown mixed results in experimental models of ARF.[134,145] N-acetylcysteine (NAC), an oxygen-radical scavenger commonly used to attenuate liver damage in acetaminophen toxicity, markedly increases GFR in a rat model of renal I/R.[15] Besides its direct antioxidant actions, NAC has other actions with potential benefit in ARF: prevention of tolerance to NO-induced vasodilation; inhibition of stress-activated protein kinases; inhibition of NFB-controlled cytokines (IL-6, IL-8, MCP-1, etc.). NAC has now undergone numerous clinical trials and a recent meta-analysis shows that it appears to have some protective benefit compared to placebo especially in patients with chronic renal failure undergoing contrast studies.[146] Future studies are needed to determine long-term effects and effects in other etiologies of AFR than contrast-induced nephropathy.

Another anti-inflammatory strategy targets ICAM-1. Activated neutrophils play a central role in the intense inflammation thought to initiate and extend cellular damage in severe ATN (see Chap. 63). Neutrophil binding to ICAM-1 is crucial for direction of neutrophils to damaged tissue. ICAM-1 is strongly upregulated in hypoxic medullary endothelium, allowing neutrophils to invade hypoxic parenchyma where they release cytokines, oxygen radicals, and proteases.[147] Antibodies to ICAM-1 protect the kidney against ischemic injury in experimental models.[148] ICAM-1-deficient mice are protected against both renal failure and death following renal ischemia reperfusion.[149] In a phase 1 clinical trial, anti-ICAM-1 antibody protected high-risk cadaveric donor renal allografts against both delayed graft function and primary nonfunction of the allografts.[150] These and other observations implicate the neutrophil infiltration as a major contributor to hypoxic renal parenchymal damage, making ICAM-1 an attractive target for clinical manipulation in ARF.

Platelet-activating factor (PAF) is produced in the postischemic kidney, and it plays a role in recruitment of inflammatory cells in amplification of the inflammatory cascade. PAF antagonists are protective in models of experimental renal I/R injury.[149] None of these antagonists are available to treat renal failure in humans. Adenosine has been shown to enhance healing of damaged tubular epithelium. Ischemia depletes ATP in tubular cells, causing accumulation of metabolites of this nucleotide (inosine and hypoxanthine) and leading to vasconstriction and formation of reactive oxygen species. Adenine nucleotides (ATP, ADP, and ANP) have a protective effect in experimental models of both ischemic and toxic ARF, even if administered several hours after the renal insult.[151,152] The fate of renal tubular cells following ischemic injury is influenced by locally produced growth factors. Growth factors likely influence proliferation, inhibit apoptosis, initiate protein and lipid biosynthesis, and augment local renal blood flow.[36] Epidermal growth factor (EGF), hepatocyte growth factor (HGF), and insulin-like growth factor-1 (IGF-1) reduce renal injury and accelerate renal recovery in experimental renal ischemia. IGF-1 protects against renal insufficiency in patients following suprarenal aortic and renal artery surgery when given postoperatively versus controls in a double-blind, randomized, placebo-controlled trial.[153] Two subsequent prospective randomized trials have had negative results.[154–155]

## OUTCOMES

Most patients with renal dysfunction can be managed without dialysis if treated early. Allowed to progress, ARF contributes significantly to morbidity and mortality.[2] Overall, reported mortality ranges from 7% to as high as 80%. Mortality is not strongly correlated with Acute Physiology and Chronic Health Evaluation System (APACHE II) scores, although higher APACHE II scores are associated with higher incidence of ARF. Greater age and a higher number of dysfunctional organ systems have the strongest association with mortality in ARF.[156] Higher mortality is also seen in ARF secondary to ischemic ATN than from other etiologies. Finally, patients with oliguric ARF have an eight-fold increased risk of requiring dialysis and a correspondingly worse prognosis than nonoliguric patients. Pharmacologic attempts to convert oliguric to nonoliguric renal failure have not conferred similar advantages in outcome. Unfortunately, mortality from ARF has apparently not improved despite routine availability of dialysis and advances in critical care.[157] A recent study found that once ARF is severe enough to require dialysis in the ICU setting mortality exceeds 50% and if it is associated with multiple organ failure exceeds 85%.[158]

On the other hand, advances may have been obscured in an older, sicker ICU population. Some investigators have recently found improvement in outcome when data is corrected for comorbidities.[159]

Still, of patients who survive initiation of dialysis, fewer than 25% will require chronic dialysis, demonstrating the capability of the kidney to recover from severe injury with time. Most survivors regain nearly normal renal function within 30 days. One large series reported that almost all of the 97% of survivors regained renal function within 30 days.[160] Even among patients with severe ARF secondary to sepsis or trauma, who may take longer to recover even partial renal function, few survivors remain dialysis dependent. Currently, there are no specific agents available to enhance the rate or completeness of recovery, but experimental studies support a possible role for growth factors in the future.[2]

## REFERENCES

1. Thadhani R, Pascua M, Bonventre J: Acute renal failure. *N Engl J Med* 334:1448, 1996.
2. Mehta R: Acute renal failure in the intensive care unit: Which outcomes should we measure? *Am J Kidney Dis* 28:S74, 1996.
3. Lameire N, Van Biesen W, Vanholder R: Acute renal failure. *Lancet* 365:417, 2005.
4. Bellomo R, Ronco C, Kellum JA, et al., and the ADQI workgroup: Acute renal failure-definition, outcome measures, animal models, fluid therapy and information technology needs: the Second International Consensus Conference of the Acute Dialysis Quality Initiative (ADQI) Group. *Crit Care* 8:R204, 2004.
5. Morris JJ, et al.: Acute posttraumatic renal failure: A multicenter perspective. *J Trauma* 31:1584, 1991.
6. Nadvi SS, Mokena T, Gouws E, et al.: Prognosis in posttraumatic acute renal failure is adversely influenced by hypotension and hyperkalaemia. *Eur J Surg* 162:121, 1996.
7. Regel G, Lobenhoffer P, Grotz M, et al.: Treatment results of patients with multiple trauma: An analysis of 3406 cases treated between 1972 and 1991 at a German Level I trauma center. *J Trauma* 38:70, 1995.
8. Barretti P, Soares VA: Acute renal failure: Clinical outcome and causes of death. *Renal Failure* 19:253, 1997.
9. Vivino G, Antonelli M, Moro ML, et al.: Risk Factors for acute renal failure in trauma patients. *Intensive Care Med* 24:808, 1998.
10. Rasmussen H, Ibels L: Acute renal failure: Multivariate analysis of causes and risk factors. *Am J Med* 73:211, 1982.
11. Navar G: Integrating multiple paracrine regulators of renal microvascular dynamics. *Am J Phys* 274:F433, 1998.
12. Holstein-Rathlou NH, Marsh DJ: Renal blood flow regulation and arterial pressure fluctuations: A case study in nonlinear dynamics. *Physiol Rev* 74:637, 1994.
13. Rose BD: *Clinical Physiology of Acid–Base and Electrolyte Disorders*, 4th ed.. New York: McGraw-Hill, 1994, p. 916.
14. Brezis M, Rosen S: Hypoxia of the renal medulla—Its implications for disease. *N Engl J Med* 332:647, 1995.
15. Brezis M, Heyman SN, Dinour D, et al.: Role of nitric oxide in renal medullary oxygenation: Studies in isolated and intact rat kidneys. *J Clin Invest* 88:390, 1991.
16. MacCumber M, Ross CA, Glaser BM, et al.: Endothelin: Visualization of mRNAs by in situ hybridization provides evidence for local action. *Proc Natl Acad Sci* 86:7285, 1989.
17. Hunley TE, Kon V: Endothelin in ischemic acute renal failure. *Curr Opin Nephrol Hypertens* 6:394, 1997.
18. Conger J, Falk S, Robinette J: Cytosolic smooth muscle calcium: Kinetics in the 48-hour post-ischemic renal vasculature. *J Am Soc Nephrol* 5:895, 1994.
19. Mlitoris B, Dahl R, Geerdes A: Cytoskeletal disruption of proximal tubule NaK-ATPase during ischemia. *Am J Physiol* 263:F971, 1992.
20. Bonventre JV: Mechanisms of ischemic acute renal failure. *Kidney Intl* 43:1160, 1993.
21. Dowd TL, Gupta RK: NMR studies of the effect of Mg$_2$ on post-ischemic recovery of ATP and intracellular sodium in perfused kidney. *Biochim Biophys Acta* 1272:133, 1995.
22. Snowdowne K, Borle A: Effects of low extracellular sodium on cytosolic ionized calcium: Na-Ca2- exchange as a major calcium influx pathway in kidney cells. *J Biol Chem* 260:14998, 1985.
23. Venkatachalam M, Weinberg J: Mechanisms of cell injury in ATP-depleted proximal tubules: Role of glycine, calcium, and phosphoinositides. *Nephrol Dial Transplant* 9:15, 1994.
24. Klausner J, Paterson IS, Goldman G, et al.: Postischemic renal injury is mediated by neutrophils and leukotrienes. *Am J Physiol* 256:F794, 1989.
25. Golikorsky MS, Rabelink T: Meeting report: ISN forefronts in nephrology on endothelial biology and renal disease: From bench to prevention. *Kidney Intl* 70:258,2006.
26. Kramer AA, Salhab KF, Shafi AE, et al.: Renal ischemia/reperfusion leads to macrophage-mediated increase in pulmonary vascular permeability. *Kidney Intl* 55:2362, 1999.
27. Schulman G, Folgo A, Gung A, et al.: Complement activation retards resolution of acute ischemic renal failure in the rat. *Kidney Intl* 40:1069, 1991.
28. Maier S, Emmanulidis K, Entleuter M, et al.: Massive chemokine transcription in acute renal failure due to polymicrobial sepsis. *Shock* 14:187, 2000.
29. Kyriakis J, Avruch J: Sounding the alarm: Protein kinase cascades activated by stress and inflammation. *J Biol Chem* 271:24313, 1997.
30. Derijard B, Raingeaud J, Barrett T, et al.: Independent human MAP kinase signal transduction pathways defined by MEK and MKK isoforms. *Science* 267:682,1995.
31. Safirstein R: Renal stress response and acute renal failure. *Adv Renal Repl Ther* 4:38, 1997.
32. Devary Y, Gottlieb RA, Smeal T, et al.: The mammalian ultraviolet response is triggered by activation of Src tyrosine kinases. *Cell* 71:1081, 1992.
33. Ueda N, Kaushal G, Shah V: Recent advances in understanding mechanisms of renal tubular injury. *Adv Renal Repl Ther* 4:17, 1997.
34. DiMari J, Megyesi J, et al.: N-acetyl cysteine ameliorates ischemic renal failure. *J Am Physiol* 272:F292, 1997.
35. Haylor J, Singh I, el Nahas A: Nitric oxide synthesis inhibitor prevents vasodilation by insulin-like growth factor 1. *Kidney Int* 39:333, 1991.
36. Harris R: Growth factors and cytokines in acute renal failure. *Adv Renal Repl Ther* 4:43, 1997.
37. Price PM, Megyesi J, Saf Irstein RL: Cell cycle regulation: Repair and regeneration in acute renal failure. *Kidney Int* 66:509, 2004.
38. Rookmaaker MB, Verhaar MC, Van Zonneveld AJ, Rabelink TJ: Progenitor cells in the kidney: Biology and therapeutic perspectives. *Kidney Intl* 66:518, 2004.
39. Morigi M, Imberti B, Zoja C, et al.: Mesenchymal stem cells are renotropic, helping to repair the kidney and improve function in acute renal failure. *J Am Soc Nephrol* 15:1794, 2004.

40. Togel F, Isaac J, Westenfelder C: Hematopoietic stem cell mobilization-associated granulocytosis severely worsens acute renal failure. *J Am Soc Nephrol* 15:1261, 2004.

41. Hoste EA, Lameire NH, Vanholder RC, et al.: Acute renal failure in patients with sepsis in a surgical ICU: Predictive factors, incidence, comorbidity, and outcome. *J Am Soc Nephrol* 14:1022, 2003.

42. Gruber SJ, Shapiro CJ: Nephropathy induced by contrast medium. *N Engl J Med* 348:2257, 2003.

43. Smith C, Lipsky JJ, Laskin OL, et al.: Double-blind comparison of the nephrotoxicity and auditory toxicity of gentamicin and tobramycin. *N Engl J Med* 302:1106, 1980.

44. Smith C, Baughman KL, Edwards CQ, et al.: Controlled comparison of amikacin and gentamicin. *N Engl J Med* 296:349, 1977.

45. Gilbert D: Minireview: Once-daily aminoglycoside therapy. *Antimicrob Agents Chemother* 35:399, 1991.

46. Miller T, Anderson RJ, Linas SL, et al.: Urinary diagnostic indices in acute renal failure: A prospective study. *Ann Intern Med* 89:47, 1978.

47. Branch R: Prevention of amphotericin B induced renal impairment: A review on the use of sodium supplementation. *Arch Int Med* 148:2389, 1988.

48. Parfrey P, Vavasour H, Bullock M, et al.: Contrast material induced renal failure in patients with diabetes mellitus, renal insufficiency, or both. *N Engl J Med* 320:143, 1989.

49. D'Elia J, Gleason RE, Alday M, et al.: Nephrotoxicity from angiographic contrast material. *Am J Med* 72:719, 1982.

50. Heyman S, Brezis M, Epstein FH, et al.: Early renal medullary hypoxic injury from radiocontrast and indomethacin. *Kidney Intl* 40:632, 1991.

51. Mueller C, Buerkle G, Buettner HJ, et al.: Prevention of contrast media-associated nephropathy: Randomized comparison of 2 hydration regimens in 1620 patients undergoing coronary angioplasty. *Arch Intern Med* 11:329, 2002.

52. Weisberg L, Kurnik P, Kurnik B: Risk of radiocontrast nephropathy in patients with and without diabetes. *Kidney Intl* 45:259, 1994.

53. Neumayer HH, Jung W, Kufner A, et al.: Prevention of radiocontrast-induced nephrotoxicity by the calcium channel blocker nitrendipine: A prospective randomized clinical trial. *Nephrol Dial Transplant* 4:1030, 1989.

54. Scwab S, Hlatky MA, Pieper KS, et al.: Contrast nephrotoxicity: A randomized controlled trial of a nonionic an an ionic radiographic contrast agent. *N Engl J Med* 320:149, 1989.

55. Mudge G: Nephrotoxicity of urographic contrast drugs. *Kidney Intl* 18:540, 1980.

56. Zager RA: Rhabdomyolysis and myohemoglobinuric acute renal failure. *Kidney Intl* 49:314, 1996.

57. Singh D, Chander, Chopra K: Rhabdomyolysis. *Methods Find Exp Clin Pharmacol* 27:39, 2005.

58. Abassi ZA, Hoffman A, Better OS: Acute renal failure complicating muscle crush injury. *Semin Nephrol* 18:558, 1998.

59. Zager R, Foerder C: Effects of inorganic iron in myoglobin on in vitro proximal tubular lipid peroxidation and cytotoxicity. *J Clin Invest* 89:989, 1992.

60. Better OS, Rubinstein I: Management of shock and acute renal failure in casualties suffering from the crush syndrome. *Renal Failure* 19:647, 1997.

61. Oda Y, Shindoh M, et al.: Crush syndrome sustained in the 1995 Kobe, Japan earthquake:treatment and outcome. *Ann Emerg Med* 30:507, 1997.

62. Iwase K, et al.: Serial changes in renal function during laparoscopic cholecystectomy. *Eur Surg Res* 25:203, 1993.

63. Harman P, et al.: Elevated intra-abdominal pressure and renal function. *J Surg Res* 196:594, 1982.

64. Meldrum D, et al.: Prospective characterization and selective management of the abdominal compartment syndrome. *Am J Surg* 174:667, 1997.

65. Johnson JP, Rokaw MD: Sepsis or ischemia in experimental acute renal failure: What have we learned? *New Horiz* 3:608, 1995.

66. Garcia-Fernandez N, Montes R, Purroy A, et al.: Hemostatic disturbances in patients with systemic inflammatory response syndrome (SIRS) and associated acute renal failure (ARF). *Thromb Res* 100:19, 2000.

67. Molitoris BA, Sandoval R, Sutton TA: Endothelial injury and dysfunction in ischemicacute renal failure. *Crit Care Med* 30:S235, 2002.

68. Dudley C: Maximizing renal preservation in acute renal failure. *BJU international* 94:1202.

69. Rivers E, Nguyen B, Havstad S, et al.: Early goal-directed therapy in the treatment of severe sepsis and septic shock. *N Engl J Med* 345:1368.

70. The SAFE Study Investigators: A comparison of albumin and saline for fluid resuscitation in the intensive care unit. *N Engl J Med* 350:2247, 2004.

71. du Cheyron D, Bouchet B, Parienti JJ, et al.: The attributable mortality of acute renal failure in critically ill patients with liver cirrhosis. *Intensive Care Med* 31:1693, 2005; Epub October 22, 2005.

72. Denton M, Chertow G, Brady H: "Renal-dose" dopamine for the treatment of acute renal failure: Scientific rationale, experimental studies, and clinical trials. *Kidney Intl* 49:4, 1996.

73. Felder C, et al.: Dopamine receptor subtypes in renal brush border and basolateral membranes. *Kidney Intl* 36:183, 1989.

74. Conger JD: Interventions in clinical acute renal failure: What are the data? *Am J Kidney Dis* 26:565, 1995.

75. Myles P, Buckland MR, Schenk NJ, et al.: Effect of "renal dose" dopamine on renal function following cardiac surgery. *Aneasth Intens Care* 21:56, 1993.

76. Baldwin L, Henderson A, Hickman P: Effect of postoperative low-dose dopamine on renal function after elective major vascular surgery. *Ann Intern Med* 120:744, 1994.

77. Parks R, Diamond T, McCrory DC, et al.: Prospective study of postoperative renal function in obstructive jaundice and the effect of perioperative dopamine. *Br J Surg* 81:437, 1994.

78. Bellomo R, Chapman M, Finfer S, for the Australian and New Zealand Intensive Care Society (ANZICS) Clinical Trials Group: Low-dose dopamine in patients with early renal dysfunction: a placebo controlled randomized trial. *Lancet* 356:2139, 2000.

79. Swygert TH, et al.: Effect of intraoperative low-dose dopamine on renal function in liver transplant recipients. *Anesthesiology* 75:571, 1991.

80. Duke GJ, Briedis JH, Weaver RA: Renal support in critically ill patients: Low-dose dopamine or low-dose dobutamine? [see comments]. *Crit Care Med* 22:1919, 1994.

81. Hellman-Meier A, et al.: Epinephrine impairs splanchnic perfusion in septic shock. *Crit Care Med* 27:399, 1997.

82. Abraham E, Diamond T, McCrory DC, et al.: *Intensive Care Med* 30:1266, 2004.

83. Morimatsu, Uchino S, Chung J, et al.: *Intensive care med* 29:1121, 2003.

84. Brown R: Renal dysfunction in the surgical patient: Maintenance of the high-output state with furosemide. *Crit Care Med* 7:63, 1979.

85. Brown C, Ogg C, Cameron J: High dose furosemide in acute renal failure: A controlled trial. *Clin Nephrol* 15:90, 1981.

86. Uchino S, Doig GS, Bellomo R, et al.: Diuretics and mortality in acute renal failure. *Crit Care Med* 32:1669, 2004.

87. Weinstein J, Heyman S, Brezis M: Potential deleterious effect of furosemide in radiocontrast nephropathy. *Nephron* 62:413, 1992.

88. Solomon R, et al.: Effects of saline, mannitol, and furosemide on acute decreases in renal function induced by radiocontrast agents. *N Engl J Med* 331:1416, 1994.

89. Shilliday IR, Quinn KJ, Allison ME: Loop diuretics in the management of acute renal failure: A prospective, double-blind, placebo-controlled randomized study. *Nephrol Dial Transplant* 12:2592, 1997.

90. Lassnigg A, Donner E, Grubhoffer G, et al.: Lack of renoprotective effects of dopamine and furosemide during cardiac surgery. *J Am Soc Nephrol* 11:97, 2000.

91. Visweswaran P, Massin EK, Dubose TD Jr: Mannitol-induced acute renal failure. *J Am Soc Nephrol* 6:1028, 1997.

92. Beall A, Hall CW, Morris GC, et al.: Mannitol-induced osmotic diuresis during vascular surgery. *Arch Surg* 86:34, 1963.

93. Gubern J, Sancho JJ, Simo J, et al.: A randomized trial on the effect of mannitol on postoperative renal function in patients with obstructive jaundice. *Surgery* 103:39, 1988.

94. Van Valenberg P, Hoitsma A, Tiggeler R: Mannitol as an indispensible constituent of an intraoperative protocol for the prevention of acute renal failure after cadaveric transplantation. *Transplantation* 44:784, 1987.

95. Grino J, Miravitlles R, Castelao A: Flush solution with mannitol in the prevention of post-transplant renal failure. *Transplant Proc* 19:4140, 1987.

96. Teschan P, Lawson N: Studies in acute renal failure—Prevention by osmotic diuresis, and observations on the effects of plasma and extracellular volume expansion. *Nephron* 3:1, 1966.

97. Better O, Stein J: Early management of shock and prophylaxis of renal failure in traumatic rhabdomyolysis. *N Engl J Med* 322:825, 1990.

98. Hatala R, Dinh TT, Cook DJ: Single daily dosing of aminoglycosides in immunocompromised adults: A systematic review. *Clin Infect Dis* 24:810, 1997.

99. Graf H, Leach W, Arieff A: Evidence for a detrimental effect of bicarbonate therapy in hypoxic lactic acidosis. *Science* 227:754, 1985.

100. Stacpoole P: Lactic acidosis: The case against bicarbonate therapy. *Ann Int Med* 105:276, 1986.

101. Makua L, Latimer R: Acute hemodialysis in the surgical intensive care unit. *Am Surg* 54:548, 1988.

102. Gettings LG, Reynolds HN, Scalea T: Outcome in post-traumatic acute renal failure when continuos renal replacement therapy is applies early vs. late. *Intensive Care Med* 25:805, 1999.

103. Gillum D, Dixon BS, Yanowver MJ, et al.: The role of intensive dialysis in acute renal failure. *Clin Nephrol* 25:249, 1986.

104. Bouffard Y, Viale JP, Annat G, et al.: Pulmonary gas exchange during hemodialysis. *Kidney Intl* 30:920, 1986.

105. Huyghebaert M, Dhainaut JF, Monsallier JF, et al.: Bicarbonate hemodialysis of patients with acute renal failure and severe sepsis. *Crit Care Med* 13:840, 1985.

106. Van der Shueren G, et al.: Intermittent hemodialysis in critically ill patients with multiple organ dysfunction syndrome is associated with intestinal intramucosal acidosis. *Intensive Care Med* 22:747, 1996.

107. Hakim R, Wingard R, Parker R: Effect of the dialysis membrane in the treatment of patients with acute renal failure. *N Engl J Med* 331:1338, 1994.

108. Conger J: Does hemodialysis delay recovery from acute renal failure? *Am J Nephrol* 7:8, 1990.

109. Schiffl H, Lang S, Fischer R: Daily haemodialysis and the outcome of acute renal failure. *N Engl J Med* 346:305, 2002.

110. Mehta R, et al.: Continuous v. intermittent dialysis for acute renal failure in the ICU: Results from a randomized multicenter trial (abstract). *J Am Soc Nephrol* 7:1456, 1996.

111. Himmelfarb J, Tolkoff RN, Chandran P, et al.: A multicenter comparison of dialysis membranes in the treatment of acute renal failure requiring dialysis. *J Am Soc Nephrol* 9:257, 1998.

112. John S, Griesbach D, Baumgartel M, et al.: Effects of continuous haemofiltration vs intermittent haemodialysis on systemic haemodynamics and splanchnic regional perfusion in septic shock patients: a prospective, randomized clinical trial. *Nephrol Dial Transplant* 16:320, 2001.

113. Manns B, Doig CJ, Lee H, et al.: Cost of acute renal failure requiring dialysis in the intensive care unit: clinical and resource implications of renal recovery. *Crit Care Med* 31:449, 2003.

114. Mehta RL, McDonald B, Gabbai FB, et al.: A randomized clinical trial of continuous versus intermittent dialysis for acute renal failure. *Kidney Int* 60:1154, 2001.

115. Vanholder R, Van Biesen W, Lamiere N: What is the renal replacement method of first choice for intensive care patients? *J Am Soc Nephrol* 12:S40, 2001.

116. Ronco C, Bellomo R, Homel P, et al.: Effects of different doses in continuous veno-venous haemofiltration on outcomes of acute renal failure: A prospective randomised trial. *Lancet* 356:26, 2000.

117. Bellomo R, Tipping P, Boyce N: Continuous veno-venous hemofiltration with dialysis removes cytokines from the circulation of septic patients. *Crit Care Med* 21:522, 1993.

118. Clark W, et al.: Continuous arteriovenous hemo-filtration for acute renal failure: Workshop summary. *Trans Am Soc Artif Intern Organs* 34:67, 1992.

119. Schetz M: Evidence-based analysis of the use of hemo-filtration in sepsis and MODS. *Curr Opin Intens Care* 3:434, 1997.

120. Silvester W: Mediator removal with CRRT: Complement and cytokines. *Am J Kidney Dis* 30:S38, 1997.

121. Cole L, Bellomo R, Hart G, et al.: A phase II randomized controlled trial of continuous hemofiltration in sepsis. *Crit Care Med* 30:100, 2002.

122. Lonnemann G, Bechstein M, Linnenweber S, et al.: Tumor necrosis factor-alpha during continuous high-flux hemodialysis in sepsis with acute renal failure. *Kidney Intl* 56:S-84, 1999.

123. Ronco C, Brendolan A, Lonnemann G, et al.: A pilot study on coupled plasma filtration with adsorption in septic shock. *Crit Care Med* 30:1250, 2002.

124. Lee PA, Weger G, Pryor RW, et al.: Effects of filter pore size on efficacy of continuous arteriovenous hemofiltration therapy for staphylococcus aureus-induced septicemia in immature swine. *Crit Care Med* 26:730, 1998.

125. Morgera S, Buder W, Lehmann C, et al.: High cut off membrane haemofiltration in septic patients with multiorgan failure. A preliminary report. *Blood Purif* 18:61(abstract), 2000.

126. Reeves JH, Butt WW, Shann F, et al.: Continuous plasmafiltration in sepsis syndrome. Plasmafiltration in sepsis study group. *Crit Care Med* 27:2096, 1999.

127. Lameire NH, De Vriese AS: Adsorption techniques and the use of sorbents. *Contrib Nephrol* (133):140–53, 2001***.76. Ronco C, Bordoni V, Levin NW. Adsorbents: from basic structure to clinical application. *Contrib Nephrol* 2002;137:158–64.

128. Kopple J: The nutrition management of patients with acute renal failure. *Parenteral Enteral Nutr* 20:3, 1995.

129. Chazot C, et al.: Provision of amino acids by dialysis during maintenance hemodialysis (MHD) (abstract). *J Am Soc Nephrol* 6:1010, 1995.

130. Klein CJ, moser-Veillon PB, Schweitzer A, et al.: Magnesium, calcium, zinc, and nitrogen loss in trauma patients during continuous renal replacement therapy. *JPEN J Parenter Enteral Nutr* 26:77, 2002.

131. Szeto H, Inturrisi CE, Houde R, et al.: Accumulation of normoperidine, an active metabolite of, meperidine in patients with renal failure or cancer. *Ann Intern Med* 86:738, 1977.

132. Schramm L, Heidbreder E, Schaar J, et al.: Role of l-arginine derived nitric oxide in ischemic acute renal failure in the rat. *Renal Failure* 16:555, 1994.

133. Landry D, Levin HR, Gallant EM, et al.: Vasopressin pressor hypersensitivity in vasodilatory septic shock. *Crit Care Med* 25:1279, 1997.

134. Paller M, Manivel J: Prostaglandins protect kidneys against ischemic and toxic injury by a cellular effect. *Kidney Intl* 42:1345, 1992.

135. Malis C, C JY, Leaf A: Effects of verapamil in models of ischemic acute renal failure in the rat. *Am J Physiol* 245:F735, 1983.

136. Wagner K, Albrecht S, Neumayer H: Prevention of posttransplant acute tubular necrosis by the calcium antagonist diltiazem: A prospective randomized study. *Am J Nephrol* 7:287, 1987.

137. Neumayer H, Wagner K: Prevention of delayed graft function in cadaver kidney transplants by diltiazem: Outcome of two prospective, randomized clinical trials. *J Cardiovasc Pharm* 10:S170, 1987.

138. Lumlertgul D, Hutgadoon P, Sirivnichai C: Beneficial effect of intrarenal verapamil in human acute renal failure. *Renal Failure* 11:201, 1989.

139. Conger J, Falk S, Yuan B: Atrial natriuretic peptide and dopamine in a rat model of ischemic acute renal failure. *Kidney Intl* 35:1126, 1989.

140. Conger J, Falk S, Hammond W: Atrial natriuretic peptide and dopamine in established acute renal failure. *Kidney Intl* 35:1126, 1989.

141. Rahman N, et al.: Effects of atrial natriuretic peptide in clinical acute renal failure. *Kidney Intl* 45:1731, 1994.

142. Allgren RL, et al.: Anaritide in acute tubular necrosis. Auriculin Anaritide Acute Renal Failure Study Group [see comments]. *N Engl J Med* 336:828, 1997.

143. Kon V, Yoshioka T, Yared A, et al.: Glomerular actions of endothelin in vivo. *J Clin Invest* 83:1762, 1989.

144. Chan L, Chittinandana A, Shapiro JL, et al.: Effect of an endothelin-receptor antagonist on ischemic acute renal failure. *Am J Physiol* 266:F135, 1994.

145. Paller M, Hoidal J, Ferris T: Oxygen free radicals in ischemic acute renal failure in the rat. *J Clin Invest* 74:1156, 1984.

146. Liu R, Nasir D, Ix J, et al.: N-Acetylcysteine for the prevention of contrast induced nephropathy: A systematic review and meta-analysis. *J Gen Intern Med* 20:193, 2005.

147. Springer T: Traffic signals for lymphocyte recirculation and leukocyte emigration: The multistep paradigm. *Cell* 76:301, 1994.

148. Kelly K, Williams WW, Colvin RB, et al.: Antibody to intercellular adhesion molecule 1 protects the kidney against ischemic injury. *Proc Natl Acad Sci* 91:812, 1994.

149. Kelly K, Williams WW, Colvin RB, et al.: Intercellular adhesion molecule-1-deficient mice are protected against ischemic renal injury. *J Clin Invest* 97:1056, 1996.

150. Haug C, Colvin RB, Delmonico FL, et al.: A phase-I trial of immunosuppression with anti-ICAM-I (CD54) mAB in renal allograft recipients. *Transplantation* 55:766, 1993.

151. Wagener OE, Lieske JC, Toback FG: Molecular and cell biology of acute renal failure: New therapeutic strategies. *New Horiz* 3:634, 1995.

152. Gould J, Bowmer CJ, Yates MS: Renal haemodynamic responses to adenosine in acute renal failure. *Nephron* 71:184, 1995.

153. Wang S, Hirschberg R: Role of growth factors in acute renal failure (editorial). *Nephrol Dial Transplant* 12:1560, 1997.

154. Hirschberg R, Kopple J, Lipsett P, et al.: Multicenter clinical trial of recombinant human insulin-like growth factor I in patients with acute renal failure. *Kidney Intl* 55:2423, 1999.

155. Hladunewich MA, Corrigan G, Derby GC, et al.: A randomized, placebo-controlled trial of IGF-1 for delayed graft function: A human model to study postischemic ARF. *Kidney Intl* 64:593, 2003.

156. Schwilk B, Wiedeck H, Stein B, et al.: Epidemiology of acute renal failure and outcome of haemodiafiltration in intensive care. *Intensive Care Med* 23:1204, 1997.

157. Chertow G, Christiansen C, et al.: Prognostic stratification in critically ill patients with acute renal failure requiring dialysis. *Arch Intern Med* 155:1505, 1995.

158. d'Avila DO, Cendoroglo NM, dos Santos OF, et al.: Acute renal failure needing dialysis in the intensive care unit and prognostic scores. *Ren Fail* 26:59, 2004.

159. Forni L, Wright DA, Hilton PJ, et al.: Prognostic Stratification in Acute Renal Failure. *Arch Intern Med* 156:1023, 1996.

160. Kjellstrand C, Gormick C, Davin T: Recovery from acute renal failure. *Clin Exp Dial Apheresis*, 5:143, 1981.

# Commentary ■ CHRISTOPHER J. DENTE

Acute renal failure (ARF) remains a morbid and costly complication of severe trauma. Despite advances in our understanding of the disease's pathophysiology, treatment algorithms have not changed drastically in the last several decades. While not terribly common in trauma patients, mortality rates range from 30% with isolated nephrotoxic renal failure to as high as 90% when ARF is part of multiple organ failure.[1]

Cryer's chapter is a comprehensive overview of the topic as it relates to the critically ill trauma patient and includes a broad discussion of the kidney's normal physiology as well as a summary of the extensive clinical and basic science research into the pathophysiology of ARF. This leads to a strong foundation for his emphasis on several key concepts as follows:

1. Studies relating to ARF are sometimes difficult to interpret because there is no clear consensus definition. While anuria, oliguria, and high output renal failure are well defined, different studies on ARF use different inclusion criteria and therefore all must be read and digested carefully.

2. While ARF has become less common with more precise resuscitative techniques, certain groups remain at high risk, including those with pre-existing renal disease and those who have prolonged renal hypoperfusion.

3. While the best modality is prevention, management strategies begin with early detection, separation of intrinsic renal failure from pre- or post-renal failure, and the optimization of oxygen delivery to the kidney. The management algorithm listed in Fig. 65-4 is a simple, yet excellent organizational chart for the physician dealing with ARF.

4. Conversion of oliguric renal failure to nonoliguric renal failure, while not proven to change outcome or duration of renal failure, is worthwhile to consider in that it may simplify fluid management.

5. Early aggressive use of renal replacement therapy is warranted, even though it has failed to definitively show improvements in overall mortality. With the advent and popularization of continuous renal replacement therapy (CRRT),[2] even patients with marginal hemodynamics are now candidates for dialysis.

In this author's experience, ARF in the ICU remains a difficult problem. In our institution, like many others, the most common clinical scenario associated with ARF is the patient with severe sepsis or septic shock. Fortunately, early goal-directed therapy, as described in this chapter, has helped to ameliorate the problem. In addition, of the other potent nephrotoxins listed in this chapter, intravenous contrast and pigment-induced ARF have been the most problematic in our recent experience. Single daily dosing of aminoglycosides, in combination with careful monitoring of trough levels by our very active pharmacy service have limited recent cases of aminoglycoside nephrotoxicity. Also, the lipophilic preparations of Amphotericin B seem to be better tolerated from a renal standpoint than older formulations.

Finally, this chapter mentions the two most common difficulties this author has encountered in treating patients with renal failure and both should be re-emphasized. First, these patients should be managed with aggressive renal replacement therapy. In the hypermetabolic, multiply injured patient, every other day hemodialysis (HD) is likely not enough. Nephrology services should be pushed to provide gentler, more frequent HD in order to minimize rapid fluid shifts and hypotensive episodes in critically ill patients. Continuous renal replacement therapy is the logical endpoint to this philosophy and, hopefully, more and more centers will establish CRRT programs. Second, nutritional support in patients with ARF should be aggressive, especially with regards to protein requirements. Withholding protein calories to avoid HD will exacerbate muscle wasting and weaken the immune system in these highly catabolic patients.

All in all, the author has compiled a comprehensive chapter on ARF, covering normal physiology, pathophysiology, diagnosis, and management of this morbid disease. With careful attention to prevention as well as with early, aggressive treatment, the systemic sequelae of ARF can be minimized and most patients will experience a significant return of renal function, thus avoiding the need for chronic HD.

## References

1. Mehta, RL: Therapeutic alternatives to renal replacement for critically ill patients with acute renal failure. *Semin Nephrol* 14:64, 1994.
2. Forni LG, Hilton PJ: Continuous hemofiltration in the treatment of acute renal failure. *N Eng J Med* 336:1303, 1997.

# Nutritional Support and Electrolyte Management

*Kenneth A. Kudsk* ■ *Gordon S. Sacks*

Nutritional therapy is an integral part of the management of severely injured patients. Although malnutrition is a frequent comorbid factor in general hospitalized patients,[1] most trauma patients are young and well nourished. Their nutritional risk is not from pre-existing defects in protein stores but due to a hypermetabolic response to injury, inflammation, and sepsis (see Chap. 67). Rapid mobilization of protein from muscle supports healing, the acute-phase response, and systemic and local host barriers to infection. While tolerated for a limited time, complications during healing, sepsis, and multiple organ dysfunction syndrome (MODS) (see Chap. 68) progressively drain the ability to maintain defenses and heal wounds. This chapter focuses on the role of enteral and parenteral nutritional support in reducing complications in critically injured patients with particular attention to the identification, institution, and successful management of enteral feeding.

## POSTINJURY HYPERMETABOLISM

The response to the stress of injury has been classified into "ebb" and "flow" phases, which are influenced by the magnitude of injury.[2] Changes in oxygen consumption, hyperglycemia, and increased vascular tone characterize the "ebb" phase. Epinephrine, norepinephrine, cortisol, aldosterone, and antidiuretic hormone release exert their central and peripheral effects. Energy expenditure and body temperature are influenced possibly through regulatory changes within the hypothalamus.[3]

Oxygen consumption and delivery and body temperature increase during the "flow" phase, as amino acids are mobilized into the amino acid pool from peripheral tissues for redistribution for gluconeogenesis, acute-phase protein production, immunologic proliferation, red blood cell production, and fibroblast proliferation. The magnitude of the flow phase correlates with the magnitude and severity of injury but gradually resolves unless a complication intervenes (see Chap. 67). In uncomplicated cases, diuresis of retained intracellular and extracellular water reflects resolution of this hypermetabolism as stress hormone levels drop. Appetite and gastrointestinal (GI) function return and positive nitrogen balance reappears with repletion of fat and lean body mass.

During this hypermetabolism, patients are usually immobilized and restricted by injuries and the medical therapy. Exercise is a fundamental determinant of muscle mass[4] and immobilization of uninjured patients results in negative nitrogen balance for approximately three to four weeks despite adequate nutrition. Except on a very temporary basis, "positive nitrogen balance" cannot be achieved in immobilized injured patients during the first three weeks of hospitalization, and attempts to overfeed the negative nitrogen balance must be avoided.

## THE ENDOCRINE RESPONSE TO STRESS AND INJURY

The hypercatabolism of injury, stress, and sepsis differs from that of starvation where inadequate substrate is available to meet metabolic demands; a comparison is shown in Table 66-1.[5] Starvation is characterized by a decrease in metabolic rate, lethargy, a decrease in cardiac output, and a transition to ketone bodies as a major energy source.[5] Within 18 to 24 hours, glycogen stores are depleted and amino acids provide the substrate for gluconeogenesis. As serum insulin levels drop, fatty acids, ketones, and glycerol become the primary substrate in tissues over 7 to 10 days. Ketone bodies can meet 70% of the energy requirements of the brain, normally an obligate glucose requiring tissue. Even at full adaptation, some tissues require glucose for function. This adaptation preserves lean tissue, since amino acid demand drops and protein synthesis and catabolism decrease compared to the fed state. The respiratory quotient ([RQ], the ratio of carbon dioxide production to oxygen consumed) is approximately 0.6 to 0.7 in starvation, indicative of utilization of fat as a primary fuel.[6]

**TABLE 66-1**

## Starvation vs. Severe Stress Hypercatabolism

| | STARVATION ←CONTINUUM→ | STRESS |
|---|---|---|
| Resting energy expenditure | ↓ | ↑↑ |
| Respiratory quotient | Low (0.65) | High (0.85) |
| Counterregulatory hormones | − | ↑↑↑ |
| Primary fuel | Fat | Fat + amino acids |
| Proteolysis | + | +++ |
| Branched-chain oxidation | + | +++ |
| Hepatic protein synthesis | + | +++ |
| Acute-phase protein production | − | +++ |
| Constitutive protein production | ↓ | ↓↓↓ |
| Urinary nitrogen losses | + | +++ |
| Gluconeogenesis | + | +++ |
| Ketone body production | ++++ | + |

During hypermetabolism, the RQ ranges between 0.80 and 0.85. Hyperglycemia and glucose intolerance characterize this condition. Hyperglycemia is due to elevated catecholamines, which induce hepatic glycogenolysis and gluconeogenesis while inhibiting insulin secretion. Elevated cortisol stimulates glycogenolysis, muscle proteolysis, and gluconeogenesis and induces a peripheral insulin resistance to limit glucose uptake. Cortisol also inhibits gluconeogenic enzymes, potentiates hepatic effects of epinephrine and glucagon, and stimulates muscle proteolysis.[7,8] Overall, the circulating insulin level drops and its anabolic effects are lost, resulting in increased lipolysis, fat oxidation glucose production,[9] and dependence on amino acids for glucose production.

Other hormones released with injury include glucagon and arginine vasopressin (AVP) (formerly antidiuretic hormone). Glucagon increases gluconeogenesis, glycolysis, and lipolysis, partly by reducing the insulin to glucagon ratio. AVP stimulates hepatic glycogenolysis and gluconeogenesis.[10] Growth hormone (GH) is normally anabolic and increases glycogen deposition and protein synthesis while mobilizing fatty acids. It is inhibited following injury and during stress, as is insulin-like growth factor I (IGF-I), which is produced by the liver in response to growth hormone. The overall effect is an imbalance in the direction of the counterregulatory hormones, a reduction in the anabolic hormones, and an accelerated loss in lean tissue. If the hypermetabolism remains unchecked, peripheral tissues become incapable of amino acid mobilization for gluconeogenosis or protein synthesis.

## CHANGES IN INTERMEDIARY METABOLISM WITH STRESS AND SEPSIS

### Protein Metabolism

Both protein synthesis and catabolism increase after severe trauma. Starvation, immobilization, and the hormonal and cytokine milieu

factor in this response.[11,12] Release of 3-methyl-histidine, an amino acid derived from actin and myosin metabolism in damaged and undamaged tissue, increases.[13] Essential amino acid levels, especially branched-chain amino acids (BCAA), increase within the cell and levels of nonessential amino acids decrease, primarily through a 50% reduction in intracellular glutamine. Up to 70% of the amino acids released by skeletal muscle are alanine and glutamine, although they constitute 10–15% of muscle composition. The production and metabolism of these amino acids have been studied extensively.[14,15] During stress, skeletal muscle is capable of utilizing the BCAAs, valine, isoleucine, and leucine. While the non-BCAAs are released into the systemic amino acid pool, waste nitrogen of BCAA is disposed in two ways. In the cell, glucose is metabolized to pyruvate, which accepts a nitrogen molecule from the BCAA via transamination to create alanine. Alanine is released, cleared by the liver, deaminated, and recycled to glucose. The nitrogen is converted to urea. Additional pyruvate is converted to acetyl CoA for entry into the Krebs cycle. The transamination of nitrogen from BCAA onto alpha-ketoglutarate in the Krebs cycle produces glutamate. Transamination of a second nitrogen completes the synthesis of glutamine (GLN). GLN is released and functions as a primary fuel for enterocytes, various immunologic cells (especially T-lymphocytes), and for conversion to glucose by the kidney. GLN is converted by the gut-associated lymphoid tissue (GALT) and splanchnic tissue to ammonia, ornithine, citrulline, and alanine and released into the portal circulation. Hepatic uptake clears these byproducts for entry into appropriate metabolic cycles. Although serum and intracellular levels of GLN drop, overall production is increased. Waste nitrogen in the kidney is excreted as ammonia into the tubules binding hydrogen ion for elimination.

Skeletal muscle protein catabolism exceeds synthesis but there are net increases in hepatic protein production and gluconeogenesis in the liver.[16,17] Synthesis of constitutive transport proteins (e.g., albumin and prealbumin) is depressed while synthesis of acute phase proteins (e.g., c-reactive protein and $\alpha_2$ acid-glycoprotein) is increased. This catabolism is tolerated by well-nourished patients for a limited period, but prolonged body protein loss is associated with pulmonary, cardiovascular, metabolic, and immunologic system failure.

### Glucose Metabolism

Hepatic gluconeogenesis remains elevated despite hyperglycemia. After glycogen depletion, protein provides the substrate since fat cannot be converted into glucose. Glucose infusions do not inhibit this accelerated gluconeogenesis.[18,19] Alanine, GLN, increased lactate levels released by hypoxic tissues, and glycerol released from adipose tissue can be converted into glucose. Alanine levels increase by 40% while glycerol and lactate increase by as much as 100% in trauma patients.[11] Recent work in burn patients[20] suggests that glucose production is controlled by the liver, at least in burn patients, since lowering of insulin and glucagon concentrations by somatostatin reduces hepatic glucose production despite elevated levels of substrate appropriate for gluconeogenesis.

There is evidence of less efficient glucose oxidation in both septic and trauma patients[21] which may be secondary to intracellular derangements in control pathways caused by low pyruvate dehydrogenase levels. It is unlikely that reduced glucose oxidation is due only to insulin resistance, since glucose clearance from plasma is unrelated to glucose oxidation.[22] This mobilization of glucose may be protective since experimental infusion of hypertonic glucose following hemorrhage reduces mortality in pigs and increases blood pressure clinically.[23,24] Some effect may be due to fluid shifts due to hyperglycemia, but a positive pressor effect from increased myocardial glucose uptake has been postulated.

## Fat Metabolism

Fat is the primary fuel during stress and sepsis. Increased levels of epinephrine, glucagon, cortisol, and perhaps growth hormone enhance lipolysis following injury[25] despite increased levels of plasma insulin. Plasma free fatty acid levels do not correlate with the degree of trauma,[26] perhaps from shunting of blood from adipose tissue or drops in serum albumin since it is a transport molecule for free fatty acids. Lactic acidosis lowers free fatty acids by augmenting reesterification.[27] The contribution of fat is evident by the depressed RQ in septic patients.[28] As the patient recovers, the RQ increases from 0.7 of fat to that of carbohydrate with an RQ of 1.0, but the RQ remains depressed in septic patients.

The type of fat administered influences cellular responses. All forms of intravenous fat currently available in the United States are omega-6 fatty acids derived from vegetable oils. The omega-6 polyunsaturated fatty acid (PUFA) linoleic acid, is subsequently incorporated into membranes of both immune and nonimmune cells as arachadonic acid.[29] During stress, increased intracellular calcium releases the fatty acids by activating phospholipase $A_2$. The products are acted upon by cyclooxygenase and lipoxygenase to produce the prostanoid $PGE_2$, a vasodilator prostanoid, while lipoxygenase produces leukotriene B4 and 5-hydroxy-6,8,11, 14-eicosatetraenoic acid (5-hete).[30] At high concentrations $PGE_2$ is immunosuppressive and reduces T-cell function and migration and generation of cytotoxic cells. Leukotrienes are powerful chemoattractants which stimulate aggregation and adherence of leukocytes and natural killer cell activity. Most contemporary enteral formulas contain omega-3 fatty acids from fish and canola oil. After their subsequent release, intracellular enzymes produce prostaglandins of the 3 series ($PGE_3$) and leukotrienes of the 5 series, which are less immunosuppressive and not as proinflammatory as the omega-6 products. Clinically, these cell membrane increases are measurable within a few days of administration.[31]

## Current Issues

Nutritional support is but one very important aspect in the overall management of the trauma patient. Most trauma patients are well nourished, although geriatric patients and younger patients with histories of substance abuse may have varying degrees of malnutrition. Debridement, drainage, resection of infected tissue, stabilization of fractures, adequate resuscitation, etc., are the priorities in early management, because early control will influence the subsequent metabolic response (see Chap. 67). If sources of inflammatory mediators are not controlled, nutrition support will not preserve catabolic lean tissue. With control, nutritional support can maintain host defenses, preserve lean body mass, improve patient outcome, and, if administered early via the GI tract, reduce infections.

Aggressive nutrition support in critically injured patients is an invasive form of therapy with risks and benefits that cannot be approached casually. In elective surgical patients undergoing general surgical procedures, the risks of therapy can, in some circumstances, outweigh benefits.[32] However, in patients who are malnourished or at risk of becoming so, the benefits outweigh the risks if nutritional support is carefully instituted and monitored. There are significant clinical data demonstrating that after gaining hemodynamic stability, *severely* injured patients who are fed early via the GI tract have a reduced risk of septic complications and, in some circumstances, MODS.[33–38] The availability of effective tools to quantitate the magnitude of injury and likelihood of subsequent septic complication allows surgeons to identify patients for whom enteral access is warranted at the time of initial celiotomy (see Chap. 64).

Not all patients can be fed enterally, particularly if enteral access is not obtained at the initial laparotomy. In these situations, intravenous nutrition should be instituted on the fifth day, since there is no evidence that *early* intravenous nutrition significantly improves clinical outcome. However, when it is clear that the GI tract is not functioning or will not function, parenteral nutrition (PN) is indicated.

## ENTERAL VERSUS PARENTERAL FEEDING: THE CLINICAL ARGUMENT

The preponderance of evidence demonstrates benefits with enteral feeding. The most compelling data exist in randomized, prospective clinical studies[33–37] of victims of blunt and/or penetrating trauma. With the first clinical data of improved outcome shown in pediatric burn patients,[39] subsequent trauma and burn studies compared various enteral products to either no feeding or intravenous feeding and showed reductions in intraabdominal abscess and pneumonia in the enterally fed group. Moore et al. in Denver randomized patients with an abdominal trauma index (ATI) between 15 and 40 to early feeding with a defined formula diet or no early feeding and showed a three-fold reduction in sepsis (primarily intraabdominal abscess) with enteral feeding.[34] Subsequently, they showed a significant reduction in pneumonia with enteral feeding compared to IV PN,[35] consistent with Border's[40] work, which showed lower septic rate in patients who received the majority of their nutrition enterally.

Later work from our group at the University of Tennessee[33] showed that enteral feeding significantly reduced pneumonia (11.8% vs. PN 31%), intraabdominal abscess (1.9 % vs. PN 13.3 %), and line sepsis (1.9% vs. PN 13.3%). Severity of injury induced the efforts, since the reduced infection rate occurred in patients with an Injury Severity Score (ISS) > 20, and an ATI > 24, where PN increased infectious rates by 6.3 and 7.3, respectively.

A few studies have produced conflicting data. One group found similar rates of infection in trauma patients receiving intravenous feeding or enteral nutrition.[41] The diagnosis of pneumonia and intraabdominal infection was comparable between the two groups, suggesting no benefit in early enteral feeding. However, there were nearly twice as many head injuries, three times as many severe thoracic injuries, and three times as many pelvic fractures in the patients randomized to enteral feeding. There were also six times as many soft tissue injuries. The increased incidence of severe chest injuries in the enteral group made the diagnosis of pneumonia suspect, since pneumonia was diagnosed using the standard criteria of fever, leukocytosis, and a new or changing infiltrate on chest x-ray, which overdiagnoses pneumonia in two-thirds to three-quarters of the cases.[42]

Another study randomized patients with blunt trauma that require intensive care unit (ICU) care to either early (<24 hours) or late (>72 hours) enteral feeding.[43] Total infectious complications—ranging from pneumonia to an eye infection—were significantly greater in the early-fed group. There was a very high dropout rate, and the early-fed patients had more severe injury, as measured by the $PA_{O_2}/FI_{O_2}$ ratio. Eleven of the 19 patients in the early group had a $PA_{O_2}/FI_{O_2}$ ratio <150, whereas, only 4 of 19 patients in the late group had such severe pulmonary dysfunction. Pneumonia was present in twice as many early-fed patients, but results were confounded by the increased chest trauma.

## DETERMINING INDICATORS FOR ENTERAL (POSTPYLORIC) ACCESS DURING CELIOTOMY FOR TRAUMA

The ATI (Table 66-2) can be rapidly tabulated at the operating table to determine the need for direct small bowel access.[44] Patients with an ATI ≥ 25 appear to benefit from early enteral nutrition once they are hemodynamically stable. Patients with insignificant intraabdominal injuries at celiotomy will benefit from early feeding if they sustain significant extraabdominal injuries such as a severe pulmonary contusion; multiple rib fractures; a closed-head injury with a Glasgow Coma Scale (GCS) score ≤ 8; a spinal injury; a major soft tissue injury requiring repeated irrigation, debridement, and skin grafts; or multiple extremity fractures necessitating later surgery. In addition, geriatric patients with multiple chronic diseases or patients who will require prolonged ventilator support or have delayed resumption of oral intake are appropriate candidates. Most patients with these criteria have an ISS > 20 and benefit from the early enteral feeding (Fig. 66-1). Although certain intraabdominal injuries (colon, pancreas, liver, or duodenum) increase the risk of septic complications, enteral access is usually unnecessary with relatively minor, isolated injuries to these organs.

### Patients with Closed Head Injury

There is little evidence that early enteral or parenteral feeding reduces sepsis or improves outcome after severe head injuries. Our policy has been to wait until GI tract function returns and gastroparesis resolves (generally within three days) before the institution of intragastric feeding. With prolonged gastroparesis (>6 days) unresponsive to gastric motility agents, a tube should be advanced into the distal duodenum and ideally beyond the ligament of Treitz using endoscopic or fluoroscopic techniques. Intravenous nutrition should start if these techniques are not possible.

This approach stems from a critical review of the head-injury studies. Rapp et al.[45] randomized 38 patients to PN or delayed enteral feeding (>1 week) once gastroparesis resolved. Initial work suggested an improved GCS score at three months with early PN, but differences disappeared later. This result was not confirmed in a follow-up study by these authors.[46] Grahm et al.[47] randomized head-injured patients to enteral feeding via nasojejunal tube placed fluoroscopically within 36 hours of injury or via a gastrostomy tube

once gastric atony resolved, usually within five days. A significant reduction in bacterial infections and the number of ICU days followed early enteral feeding. However, bronchitis was the major diagnostic category separating the groups, rather than established infections such as pneumonia or abscess. Borzotta et al.[48] randomized patients with severe head injuries to early enteral feeding with a nasojejunal tube or delayed enteral feeding and demonstrated no reduction in infections and a slight, perhaps clinically insignificant improvement in neurologic outcome with early feeding. Our study[49] found no difference between an early placement of a tube beyond the ligament of Treitz versus intragastric feeding. There was no dramatic improvement in GCS scores, no reduction in infectious complications, and no obvious benefit with early feeding.

The failure of enteral nutrition to reduce infections in head-injured patients appears contradictory to multiple trauma results, but the groups differ significantly. Prolonged intubation and pneumonia may be unavoidable after severe closed-head injury, since patients with such injuries often remain intubated for weeks, while many multiple trauma patients require support only for several days.

### Burn Patients

Early enteral feeding in burn patients is well established. Alexander et al.[39] randomized severely burned children to either a standard enteral diet or a protein-supplemented diet. Patients receiving the high-protein diet had a higher survival rate and a lower sepsis rate but received significantly less PN than control patients. Herndon et al.[50] randomized 39 patients with 50% or greater total body burn to early IV or enteral feeding and measured significant decreases in natural killer cell activity and the T-helper/suppressor ratio with PN. Since higher survival rates occurred with enteral feedings, they concluded that PN should be used only with total enteral failure.

We start intragastric feeding within 12 hours of burn, since this approach reduces the incidence of gastroparesis.[51] Gastroparesis occurs in 45% of patients with intragastric feeding delayed for 18 hours, but it occurs less than 5% if feeding is instituted within 8 hours of burn. Laboratory suggests a blunting of the hypermetabolic response after burn by reducing levels of cortisol and catecholamines.[52]

## INFLUENCE OF THE TYPE OF ENTERAL FEEDING ON INFECTIOUS COMPLICATIONS

### Specialty "Immune-Enhancing" Diets

The concept that some nutrients became "conditionally-essentially" during stress and sepsis (e.g., glutamine) or that other substrates such as omega-6 fatty acids could potentially aggravate inflammation through production of proinflammatory products led to the creation of a family of immune-enhancing diets (IEDs). These IEDs contain various combinations of glutamine (GLN), arginine, omega-3 fatty aids, beta carotene, and nucleotides. Liquid diets cannot be supplemented with glutamine as a free amino acid because of its propensity to degrade into the toxic products pyroglutamate and ammonia after heat sterilization. Free GLN is

**TABLE 66-2**

## Calculated Risk of Sepsis by the Abdominal Trauma Index

| ORGAN INJURED | RISK FACTOR | SCORING | ORGAN INJURED | RISK FACTOR | SCORING |
|---|---|---|---|---|---|
| **HIGH RISK** | | | **LOW RISK** | | |
| Pancreas | (5) | 1. Tangential<br>2. Through-and-through (duct intact)<br>3. Major debridement or distal duct injury<br>4. Proximal duct injury<br>5. Pancreaticoduodenectomy | Kidney | (2) | 1. Nonbleeding<br>2. Minor debridement or suturing<br>3. Major debridement<br>4. Pedicle or major calyceal<br>5. Nephrectomy |
| Large intestine | (5) | 1. Serosal<br>2. Single wall<br>3. ≤ 25% wall<br>4. > 25% wall<br>5. Colon wall and blood supply | Ureter | (2) | 1. Contusion<br>2. Laceration<br>3. Minor debridement<br>4. Segmental resection<br>5. Reconstruction |
| Major vascular | (5) | 1. ≤ 25% wall<br>2. > 25% wall<br>3. Complete transection<br>4. Interposition grafting or bypass<br>5. Ligation | Bladder | (1) | 1. Single wall<br>2. Through-and-through<br>3. Debridement<br>4. Wedge resection<br>5. Reconstruction |
| **MODERATELY HIGH RISK** | | | | | |
| Duodenum | (4) | 1. Single wall<br>2. ≤ 25% wall<br>3. > 5% wall<br>4. Duodenal wall and blood supply<br>5. Pancreaticoduodenectomy | Extrahepatic Biliary | (1) | 1. Contusion<br>2. Cholecystectomy<br>3. ≤ 25% wall<br>4. > 25% wall<br>5. Biliary enteric reconstruction |
| Liver | (4) | 1. Nonbleeding peripheral<br>2. Bleeding, central, or minor debridement<br>3. Major debridement or hepatic artery ligation<br>4. Lobectomy<br>5. Lobectomy with caval repair or extensive bilobar debridement | Bone | (1) | 1. Periosteum<br>2. Cortex<br>3. Through-and-through<br>4. Intra-articular<br>5. Major bone loss |
| **MODERATE RISK** | | | | | |
| Stomach | (3) | 1. Single wall<br>2. Through-and-through<br>3. Minor debridement<br>4. Wedge resection<br>5. > 35% resection | Small bowel | (1) | 1. Single wall<br>2. Through-and-through<br>3. ≤ 25% wall<br>4. > 25% wall<br>5. Wall and blood supply or > 5 injuries |
| Spleen | (3) | 1. Nonbleeding<br>2. Cautery or hemostatic agent<br>3. Minor debridement or suturing<br>4. Partial resection<br>5. Splenectomy | Minor vascular | (1) | 1. Nonbleeding small hematoma<br>2. Nonbleeding large hematoma<br>3. Suturing<br>4. Ligation of isolated vessels<br>5. Ligation of named vessels |

*Source: Adapted from Moore EE, Dunn EL, Moore JB, et al: Penetrating abdominal trauma index. J Trauma 21:440, 1981; and Borlase BC, Moore EE, Moore FA: The abdominal trauma index—A critical reassessment and validation. J Trauma 30:1341, 1990. With permission, from Lippincott Williams & Wilkins.*

found only in dry, powdered diets, which require reformulation prior to administration. These diets can be administered via transgastric jejunostomies, large-bore (12 to 18 Fr) jejunostomies and 7-Fr needle catheter jejunostomies (NCJs), but they tend to clog 5-Fr NCJs.

The rationale for these specific nutrient supplementations has been partly discussed above. Although skeletal muscle production of GLN increases during stress and sepsis, serum and intracellular levels decrease. GLN is a substrate for various immunologic cells and for enterocytes in the unfed state.[14–16] Arginine promotes proliferating T-cells after mitogen or cytokine stimulation in vitro and increases natural killer cell cytotoxicity, specific cytolytic T-cell activity, and macrophage tumor cytotoxicity.[53] Arginine also exerts a positive effect on wound healing; stimulates pituitary growth

hormone, prolactin, insulin, and insulin-like growth factor I, and acts as a precursor for nitric oxide, nitrites, and nitrates as well as the growth substances putrescine, spermine, and spermidine, which may be involved in GI tract integrity. Omega-3 polyunsaturated fatty acids (PUFAs) from fish or canola oil can replace omega-6 polyunsaturated fatty acids, such as linoleic acid, found mainly in vegetable oils. Omega-6 fatty acids inhibit killer cell activity, antibody formation, and cell-mediated immune response due to the inhibitory nature of their metabolic end products.[30] Animal studies have shown that omega-3 supplementation reduces mortality after burn injury, reduces bacterial translocation compared with other lipids, promotes cell-mediated immunity, increases resistance to infection, reduces inflammation, and reduces

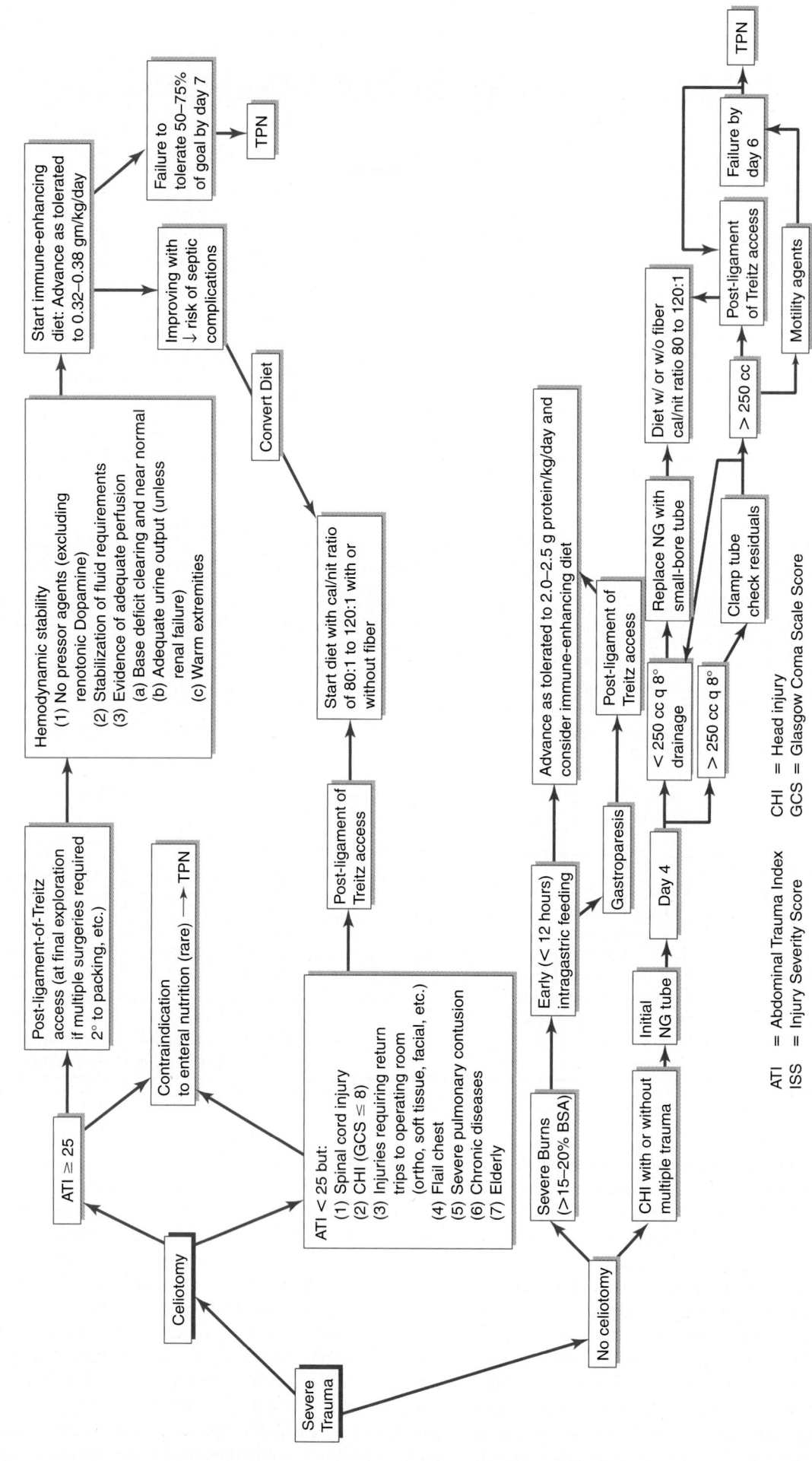

**FIGURE 66-1.** Protocol for nutrition support at the Elvis Presley Trauma Center, University of Tennessee, Memphis.

1322

mortality following bacterial peritonitis.[54] The administration of RNA via nucleotides improves survival to a septic challenge with *Candida albicans,* and malnourished animals provided RNA during refeeding from a malnourished state had more rapid improvement in immune function.[55] Nucleotide deprivation suppresses helper T-cell and interleukin-2 (IL-2) production, largely due to uracil, since adenine does not prevent this immunosuppression. Clinically, various combinations of these nutrients have been made available in specialty nutrient diets. The majority of clinical studies carried out in critically ill patients, general surgical patient populations, trauma patients, and burn patients suggest an additional benefit with the IEDs over unsupplemented diets.[37,38,56,57]

Gottschlich and Alexander[58] randomized 50 pediatric and adult patients with burns over 10–89% of their body surface area to diets including a modular feeding supplemented with arginine, cysteine, histidine, and omega-3 fatty acids. A significant reduction in wound infection, length of stay per percent body burn, and total number of infectious complications occurred in this group, with a trend ($p = 0.06$) toward reduced pneumonia. More inhalation injuries in the control group as well as more fat and less carbohydrates in the control formula were confounding variables.

Patients with an ATI between 18 and 40 randomized to an IED or a chemically defined diet generated significant increases in total lymphocyte count and T-lymphocyte and T-helper cell numbers as well as fewer intra-abdominal abscesses and less multiple organ failure with the supplemented diet.[38] A confounding variable in this study was the higher nitrogen content in the IED. In a study of patients with an ATI >25 or an ISS >20, the subjects received an IED or an isonitrogenous, isocaloric diet.[37] Unfed cohorts, eligible for the trial entry but without enteral access, were also prospectively followed. The IED resulted in fewer major septic complications, fewer therapeutic antibiotics, and a shorter hospital stay than in the unfed group or those receiving the control diet. The incidence of intra-abdominal abscess, pneumonia, bacteremia, major wound infections, or any major complication was highest in the unfed population. Complications and antibiotic use with the control diet were between the unfed and IED groups. Administration of a GLN-supplemented enteral diet has also been shown to reduce pneumonia, bacteremia, and sepsis.[59] Potential negative effects may also occur with these diets. One study noted an increase in respiratory failure with an IED.[60] An increased incidence of respiratory failure in the treatment group at baseline limits the ability to implicate the diet, however.

We institute an IED in patients with an ATI >25 or an ISS >20 (Fig. 66-1) and convert to a standard high-protein enteral diet once the patients are less vulnerable to septic complications, usually within 7 to 10 days. Patients with less severe injuries receive a high-protein diet.

## POSSIBLE DELETERIOUS AFFECTS OF IMMUNONUTRITION IN THE CRITICALLY ILL

Recently published Canadian practice guidelines for nutrition support in mechanically ventilated critically ill patients recommended that arginine containing diets (oral immunonutrition that contains arginine supplementation) should not be used in critically ill ICU patients.[61] The conclusion was reached despite significantly

reduced hospital stays and trends toward reduced ventilator days and ICU days noted with these diets in trials. This meta-analysis based these recommendations on three studies. One trial studied trauma, surgical, and medical ICU patients randomized to a diet enriched in arginine, omega-3 fatty acids, and nucleotides.[62] Patients tolerating more than 821 mL/day benefited clinically in a post hoc analysis, but septic patients randomized to the arginine-containing diet sustained an increased mortality while mortality in all recruited critically ill patients was not affected. In a second randomized, as yet unpublished prospective study conducted in 1996,[63] critically ill patients were randomized to a specialized diet containing moderate amounts of arginine and omega-3 fatty acids. Mortality with the specialty diet increased in elderly male patients admitted with sepsis and pneumonia. However, significantly more patients with pneumonia were randomized to the specialty diet due to a randomization breakdown. Most patients who died received either less than three days of feeding or died after study completion but not while receiving the specialty diet. In the third study,[64] septic patients requiring more than four days of nutrition support and a 'higher level of care' were randomized to PN or an omega-3 fatty acid/arginine-supplemented enteral diet. Increased mortality occurred in this group. The majority of patients who died were septic with pneumonia similar to the Heyland/Dent trial.

Although there are significant reservations regarding the design and implementation of these three trials, septic patients—particularly if septic with pneumonia—may have a poorer outcome with immunonutrition for unknown reasons. Unfortunately, these studies are flawed and the patients are poorly defined. Two trials noted no increase in mortality with sepsis using similar diets.[65,66] With the clinical evidence demonstrating significant improvement in trauma patients, there is no evidence to suggest this population has increased risks with administration of these specialty diets.

## POTENTIAL REASONS FOR IMPROVED OUTCOME WITH ENTERAL FEEDING

The unfed GI tract has altered function and architecture (see Chap. 64). Decreases in villus height occur in unfed human patients,[67] but to a lesser extent than in rat models of starvation or intravenous feeding,[68] where 40–50% of villus height is lost in the proximal intestine. Changes occur quickly in the GI tract following shock and stress, with rapid decreases in enzymes and motility and temporary increases in permeability. The reduced motility (i.e., ileus) occurs in the stomach and colon, allowing absorption of nutrients delivered into the small intestine.[69]

Shock, trauma, and sepsis increase gut permeability,[70] which increases bacterial translocation to mesenteric lymph nodes in animal models and under certain clinical conditions, such as bowel obstruction, inflammatory bowel disease, and shock.[71] This does not appear to be clinically relevant following trauma.[72] Increased permeability in trauma patients is unrelated to the magnitude of trauma but does correlate with the IL-6 and acute-phase protein response of severely injured patients.[70] The level of permeability returns to baseline within a week.

The well-fed intestine is a metabolically and immunologically active organ that passively and actively maintains a bacterial barrier through peristalsis, IgA, mucin, and mucosal cell integrity.

Experimentally, these systems fail in starvation, shock, and sepsis. Approximately 75% of the body's immunoglobulin-producing cells line the GI and respiratory tracts to produce 70–80% of the immunoglobulin as secretory IgA (SIgA), which is transported across the mucosa.[73] The gut-associated lymphoid tissue (GALT) is affected by parenteral nutrition, producing decreases in GALT mass and reductions in intestinal and respiratory IgA.[74] Normally, the IgA coating the surface of the epithelium binds and neutralizes viruses, bacteria, and other pathogenic antigens by trapping them in the mucin layer. As a result, these infective agents cannot attach to the mucosa, a prerequisite to invasive infection.[75] GALT function is preserved if IV-PN is supplemented with GLN or the neuropeptide bombesin.[76] Bombesin is analogous to gastrin-releasing peptide in humans. Experimentally, PN-fed animals lose established antibacterial and antiviral immunity,[77] which can be partially preserved with glutamine supplementation and completely preserved with bombesin supplementation.

Intraperitoneal protection can also be explained by similar mechanisms. Enteral feeding significantly improves the survival of malnourished or well-nourished animals with septic peritonitis. Animals fed enterally inhibit bacterial proliferation and increase intraperitoneal tumor necrosis factor (TNF) response, resulting in less systemic cytokine response and bacteremia compared to animals fed intravenously.[78] A differential cytokine response has also been confirmed in patients. Normal volunteers administered PN increase production of TNF compared with enterally fed patients following intravenous injection of endotoxin.[79] Since TNF has been considered one of the precipitating stimuli for the subsequent proinflammatory cytokine response, this may be clinically relevant (see Chap. 67).

Exposure of the systemic circulation to bacterial products has been postulated to be a driving force in the development of MODS.[80] Enteral stimulation maintains a normal gut cytokine response with high levels of IL-4 and IL-10.[81] These cytokines upregulate IgA production from mucosal protection and downregulate adhesion molecule expression on the vascular endothelium. Parenteral feeding reduces these cytokines, leading to an upregulation of vascular adhesion molecules and accumulation of neutrophils within the intestine and priming of these neutrophils to subsequent ischemic events.[82] Ischemic events within the gut have been previously related to neutrophil priming as an initial step in MODS development.[83] These experimental data are consistent with the reduction in MODS in trauma patients fed enterally.[38,84]

## THE NUTRIENT PRESCRIPTION: ISSUES COMMON TO ENTERAL OR PARENTERAL FEEDING

There are a number of issues common to both enteral and parenteral feeding related to the amount and type of nutrition administered to trauma patients. In the past, calculation of nutrient needs used standard equations, such as the Harris–Benedict equation, multiplied by correction factors. Indirect calorimetry has shown that these correction factors for stress and activity tend to overestimate nutrient needs. Overfeeding leads to increased oxygen consumption, increased $CO_2$ production, hepatic lipogenesis, potential immune suppression secondary to hyperglycemia, and other negative effects without reducing weight loss or lean tissue catabolism.

## ESTIMATING NUTRITIONAL NEEDS

The most common calculation used to determine basal energy expenditure is the Harris–Benedict formula, defined as follows:

For males: BEE = 66 + (13.8 × W) + (5 × H) − (6.8 × A)
For females: 665 + (9.6 × W) + (1.8 × H) − (4.7 × A)

where W is the weight in kilograms, H is the height in centimeters, and A the age in years. These calculated values have been increased by a stress factor (ranging from 1.25 to 2) and an activity factor to account for the increases in metabolic rate by injury and stress.

Indirect calorimetry measures metabolic needs using expired gas analysis to determine overall resting energy expenditure (REE). Carbon dioxide production ($\dot{V}_{CO2}$) and oxygen consumption ($\dot{V}_{O2}$) are used to calculate the respiratory quotient. When $\dot{V}_{O2}$ and $\dot{V}_{CO2}$ are applied to the Weir equation, REE can be determined. There is an RQ characteristic for each fuel utilized: e.g., fat is 0.7, glucose is 1.0, and protein 0.8. Since fat deposition with overfeeding has an RQ value of approximately 8, an RQ value greater than 1.0 generally means that lipogenesis and overfeeding are occurring. In studies of patients in surgical ICUs, metabolic cart measurements were generally within 5–10% of the energy requirements calculated by the Harris–Benedict equation; addition of stress factors led to unnecessary administration of nutrients.[85,86]

There are drawbacks to indirect calorimetry. Since $\dot{V}_{O2}$ is an integral part of the measurement, there is loss of accuracy as the $FI_{O2}$ increases because of the errors between the inspired and expired oxygen consum ption. With an $FI_{O2}$ of 0.8, a 1% error in measurement of the inspired or expired $\dot{V}_{O2}$ leads to 100 % error in $\dot{V}_{O2}$ calculation. Since any air leaks are interpreted as increases in oxygen consumption, critically ill patients requiring a high $FI_{O2}$ and high positive end-expiratory pressure are most likely to have inaccurate measurements. In addition, these calculations are labor-intensive and results are most reliable when protocols defined by trained technicians are used.[87] Indirect calorimetry measurements only reflect caloric needs over a 20- to 30-minute period when the patients are turned, suctioned, or receiving physical therapy, and those measurements may not represent total energy expenditure. For these reasons, many practitioners increase the REE by 10 to 15% to calculate total energy expenditure. Because of the expenses necessary to avoid the pitfalls of indirect calorimetry, its routine use is not recommended. However, data obtained from sites proficient in the technique have provided valuable guidelines to avoid overfeeding, especially in cases of obesity, amputation, or quadriplegia, where traditional calculations are not reliable.

Current recommendations for caloric support range between 25 to 30 total kcal/kg/day.[88] While some studies have recommended other values, if 30 kcal/kg is provided, 90% of patients will reach their energy requirement with overfeeding in approximately 15 to 20% of patients.[86] To avoid complications of overfeeding (Fig. 66-2), we administer approximately 25 to 30 total kcal/kg/day to multiply injured patients initially and decrease this to 22 to 25 kcal/kg as they improve clinically, with diuresis, ventilator weaning, and discontinuation of antibiotics. Presumed body weight is obtained from family members or the patient, when possible, to avoid overfeeding based on false elevations due to edema from resuscitation. As diuresis occurs, weight is rechecked with appropriate adjustments in total caloric load. With this approach,

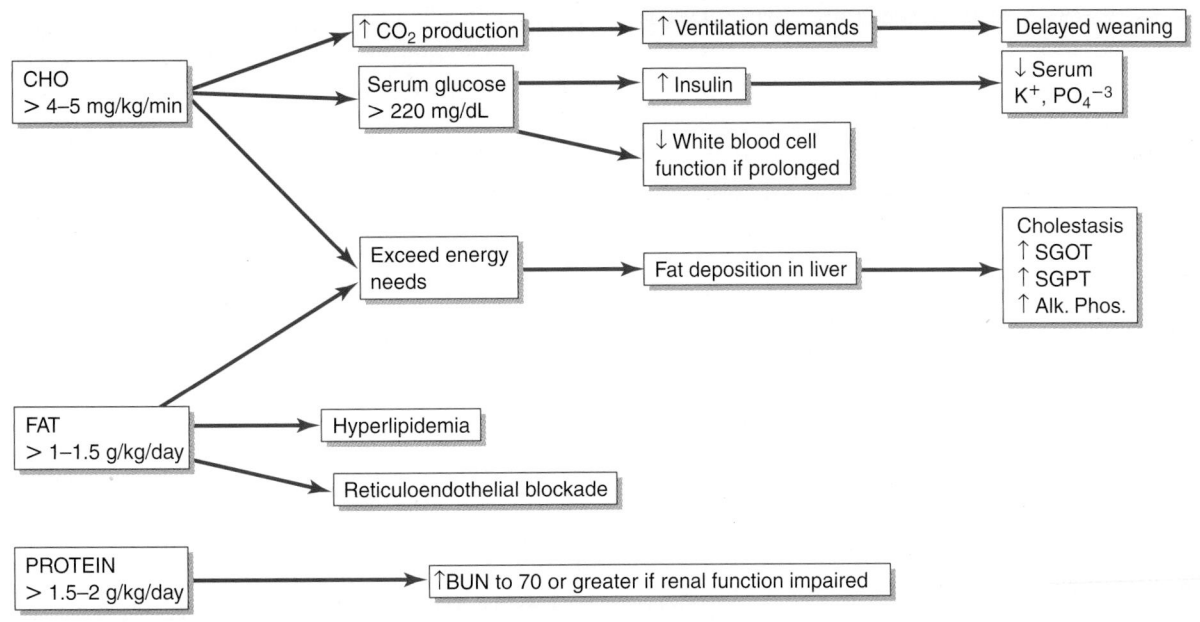

**FIGURE 66-2.** Complications of overfeeding.
*(Reproduced with permission from Frankel WL, Evans NJ, Rombeau JL: Scientific rationale and clinical application of parenteral nutrition in critically ill patients. In Rombeau JL, Caldwell MD, (eds): Clinical Nutrition. Vol. 2. Parenteral Nutrition, 2nd ed. Philadelphia: Saunders, 1993; p. 597.)*

hyperglycemia rarely exceeds 175 to 200 mg/dL except with severe stress, diabetes, or catecholamine infusions at levels necessary to maintain hemodynamic stability. In general, we withhold nutrition in patients requiring high rates of catecholamine infusion, since there is no evidence that administered glucose or protein (or amino acids) slow lean body tissue mobilization or the rate of gluconeogenesis.

Stress induces an increase in both glucose utilization and gluconeogenesis with significant recycling of glucose from lactate (the Cori cycle) and alanine. Lactic acid is produced in the periphery when pyruvate cannot enter the Krebs cycle. As NADPH is converted to NADP+, hydrogen ion is transferred to pyruvate creating lactate, which is then released, transported back to the liver, and converted to glucose. Alanine is formed by transamination of pyruvate during branched-chain amino acid metabolism in skeletal muscle and released for conversion back to pyruvate and glucose by the liver. Hyperglycemia occurs as hepatic gluconeogenesis increases from 2.0 to 2.5 mg/kg/minute under the normal condition to 4 to 5 mg/kg/minute in the stressed or septic patient.[89] Given these conditions, high levels of infused glucose aggravate hyperglycemia causing glucosuria, hepatic fatty deposition, increased $CO_2$ production (rarely a significant clinical problem in young trauma victims), and potentially an increased infection rate. Since the maximal rate of glucose oxidation is 5 mg/kg/minute or approximately 7.2 g/kg/day, cumulative glucose administration including enteral and parenteral products as well as intravenous fluids should not exceed these levels.[90,91] In a 70-kg man, this is 500 g of glucose at maximum, which is almost completely met by 2 L of a 25% dextrose PN solution. Ideally, blood sugars should be maintained below 150 mg/dL. With insulin, it is usually possible to keep blood sugars below 150 mg/dL except in trauma patients with insulin-dependent diabetes mellitus or those with steroid or high catecholamine needs (see Chap. 60).

## ENERGY REQUIREMENTS AND FEEDING RECOMMENDATIONS IN THE MORBIDLY OBESE

Current feeding recommendations for morbidly obese trauma or surgical ICU patients are for 20 to 22 total kcal/kg ideal body weight and 2 g of protein/kg ideal body weight. This is based on observations that nitrogen retention increases as caloric intake increases until caloric intake approaches 50–60% of total energy expenditure.[92] Additional energy further improves nitrogen retention but less efficiently. Although weight loss occurs, this is primarily due to fat loss.[93]

In a two-week study of enteral feeding,[94] this population received 1.5–1.9 g/kg ideal body weight/day of protein with either 19 kcal/kg actual body weight/day (30 total kcal/kg ideal body weight/day) or 11 total kcal/kg actual body weight/day (hypocaloric group: 22 total kcal/kg ideal body weight/day). Prealbumin increases were similar in the two groups. Both had negative nitrogen balance due to catabolism, but the hypocaloric group had a shorter ICU stay, fewer antibiotic days, and a trend to reduced ventilator days ($p < 0.09$).

Hypocaloric, parenteral high-protein feeding of postoperative obese patients with 2.1 g of protein and 20 total/kcal ideal body weight resulted in 1.7 kg/week of weight loss, net protein anabolism (improved serum protein concentration and positive nitrogen balance), and successful wound healing.[95] Two other randomized double blind studies of obese patients compared hypocaloric feeding to higher caloric regimens.[96] In the first, both groups received 2 g/kg ideal body weight per day but calories were administered at 100% or 50% of the measured energy expenditure. Nitrogen balances were similar. In the second, hypocaloric or higher calorie parenteral regimens (14±3 vs. 22±5 total kcal/kg actual weight/day) were given for up to 14 days with both groups receiving 2 g/kg ideal body weight of protein. Nitrogen balances were similar but, glucose control was improved and less exogenous insulin was necessary with the hypocaloric regimen.[97,98]

## FAT REQUIREMENTS

Free fatty acids are the primary energy source utilized during stress and sepsis. Lipolysis and mobilization of free fatty acids is enhanced by beta-adrenergic stimulation of lipases and hormone-sensitive tissues as fatty acid oxidation increases. The administration of glucose as calculated above can provide approximately 50 to 60% of total caloric requirements; the balance of nonprotein calories (20 to 30% of total calories) can be met by fat at a dose of 1 g/kg/day. Although the maximum adult dose of intravenous lipid is 2.5 g/kg/day,[99] this is rarely used and virtually never given in critically ill patients. In patients in whom and ventilator weaning is an important issue, administration of fat as total calories up to 50% may be beneficial in selected patients. Increased $CO_2$ production is rarely a cause of weaning problems in trauma patients except, perhaps, in geriatric patients following flail chest injuries or those with prolonged recovery. Trauma patients with moderate to severe chronic obstructive pulmonary disease (COPD) who have trouble weaning from the ventilator may benefit from a diet higher in fat. If overfeeding is suspected, reduction in total calories administered is the most appropriate intervention.[100] Higher doses of fat may also be useful in hyperglycemic patients as a result of diabetes or corticosteroid administration. This may cause hyperlipidemia, cholestasis, increased risk of infection, and perhaps immunosuppression.[101] All lipid emulsions available in the United States are vegetable oils, which provide mainly omega-6 long-chain PUFAs; these may increase production of immunosuppressive prostaglandins and leukotrienes. Currently, structured lipids containing both omega-6 and medium-chain triglycerides as their primary fatty acid side chains are being tested as are intravenous fats with omega-3 fatty acids. Additional immunosuppression may come from blockade of the reticuloendothelial system by lipid particles. Omega-3 fatty acids from canola or fish oil are found in most enteral products; these can be metabolized to the less immunosuppressive 3 or 5 series of prostaglandins. Omega-3 polyunsaturated fatty acids may increase the production of lipid peroxidases and inhibit platelet aggregation, but these concerns have not appeared to be of clinical significance.

Several investigators have determined the maximum hydrolysis rate for intravenous lipids by LPL in normal adults to be approximately 0.12 g/kg/h (2.9 g/kg/day); above this infusion rate emulsion triglyceride particles begin to accumulate.[102] Intravenous lipid emulsion in the critically ill adult below this infusion rate is recommended in order to avoid elevated triglyceride concentrations and other metabolic complications. Doses of intravenous lipids should be limited to the provision of essential fatty acids (e.g., 250 mL of 20% lipid emulsion once or twice weekly) when triglyceride concentrations rise above 400 mg/dL. Withholding intravenous lipids must be considered when triglyceride concentrations are greater than 500 mg/dL or in the presence of lipemic serum.

## PROTEIN REQUIREMENTS

Skeletal muscle loses considerable mass as amino acids are redistributed for healing wounds, acute-phase proteins, and substrate for lymphoid tissue and the GI tract. Overall, nitrogen is lost through ureagenesis by the liver and ammonia synthesis by the kidney. Immobilization aggravates the loss. Total protein catabolism exceeds synthesis, which leads to loss of function and potential morbidity and mortality. Unfortunately, this hypercatabolism and lean tissue loss is not blunted by the administration of exogenous calories or amino acids.[103,104]

In general, the recommended dose of amino acid protein for stressed or septic patients without renal dysfunction is 1.5 to 2 g/kg/day. Although blood urea nitrogen (BUN) may increase to approximately 40 mg/dL, these levels cause no metabolic complications and BUN generally stabilizes at that level. If urea levels climb to greater than 100 mg/dL, protein administration must be reduced. If creatinine levels are low, i.e., no evidence of acute renal failure, and elevated BUN appears due to excessive protein (or amino acid) administration, protein should be decreased to 1.3 to 1.5 g/ kg/day. As the stress phase resolves, 1 to 1.5 g/kg/day of protein meets nutrient requirements in most patients. In burn patients, administration of 2 to 2.5 g/kg/day is desirable due to excessive urinary losses and the inability to accurately assess wound losses of nitrogen.

Patients who develop acute renal failure secondary to injury/hypotension still require high doses of protein for wound repair; however, it is practical to provide only 0.8 to 1.0 g/kg/day of protein until a decision on initiation of dialysis is made. Once dialysis has been initiated, the type and frequency will dictate how much the protein dose can be liberalized. Generally, 1.2 to 1.5 g/kg/day can be administered to a patient receiving hemodialysis three times a week (assuming that the hemodialysis is effective). Patients who cannot tolerate hemodialysis secondary to hypotension may receive continuous arterial venous hemodialysis (CAVHD) or continuous venovenous hemodialysis (CVVHD). These methods of dialysis provide the critical care practitioner volume to administer PN with nonconcentrated formulas, and protein can usually be administered as high as 2.5 g/kg/day if indicated.

## THE FORMULA

### Calorie-to-Nitrogen Ratio

Caloric density for nutrients are as follows: 1 g protein equals 4 kcal, 1 g of hydrated glucose equals 3.4 kcal, and 1 g of fat (as an enteral form) equals 9.1 kcal, but 1 g of lipid emulsion contains 10 kcal/g because of glycerol contained within the emulsion. In patients who are not critically ill or septic but at risk of developing starvation-induced malnutrition if not fed (e.g., small bowel obstruction, prolonged intestinal paresis, multiple small bowel fistulas, etc.), a calorie:nitrogen ratio between 130 to 160:1 is appropriate, and protein should be administered at a dose of 1 to 1.5 g/kg/day. In patients who are stressed or septic, however, the calorie:nitrogen ratio should drop to 80:1 to 120:1. The goal in the stressed or septic patient is approximately 30 kcal/kg total with 1.5 to 2 g/kg/day of protein. In burn patients, protein is administered with approximately the same low calorie:nitrogen ratio, providing 35 to 40 kcal/kg/day total and 2 to 2.5 g/kg/day of protein. Refer to Fig. 66-3 for sample calculations of a PN formulation involving a 70-kg trauma patient.

Fat can be used to displace glucose calories and, in fact, should meet 20–30% of total calories. Figure 66-3 illustrates how intravenous fat would be incorporated into PN formulation for

Example: 70-kg man sustaining severe multiple long-bone fractures

Estimated kcal: 30 kcal/kg/day × 70 kg = 2100 kcal/day

Protein: 1.5 g/kg/day × 70 kg = 105 g/day

For 2-in-1 (dextrose/amino acid) formulation:

$$\frac{70 \text{ kg} \times 5 \text{ mg/kg/min} \times 1440 \text{ min/day}}{1000 \text{ mg/g}}$$

$$= 504 \text{ g or } \sim 500 \text{ g dextrose per day}$$

Using a 70% dextrose (D70W) stock solution for compounding:

$$\frac{70 \text{ g}}{100 \text{ ml}} = \frac{500 \text{ g}}{x}$$

Solving for x yields approximately 714 mL of $D_{70}W$

Using a 10% amino acid (AA10) stock solution for compounding:

$$\frac{10 \text{ g}}{100 \text{ mL}} = \frac{105 \text{ g}}{x}$$

Solving for x yields 1050 mL of AA10%

Total kcal from regimen: 500 g × 3.4 kcal/g + 105 g × 4 kcal/g

$$= 1700 + 420 = 2120 \text{ kcal}$$

Calculation of administration rate: 714 mL dextrose + 1050 mL AA

$$= 1764 \text{ mL/day} + 50 \text{ mL for additives} = 1814 \text{ mL/day}$$

$$\frac{1814 \text{ mL}}{24 \text{ hr}} = 75 \text{ mL/h for 2-in-1 solution}$$

OR using final concentrations

30 mL/kg/day × 70 kg = 2100 mL/day to meet maintenance IV fluid requirements

Dextrose calculation:

$$\frac{500 \text{ g}}{2100 \text{ mL}} = \frac{x}{100 \text{ mL}}$$

Solving for x yields 23.8% or approximately 25% dextrose.

Protein calculation:

$$\frac{105 \text{ g}}{2100 \text{ mL}} = 50 \text{ g/L or AA5\%}$$

For 3-in-1 (dextrose, amino acid, lipid) formulation:

Estimated kcal: 30 kcal/kg/day × 70 kg = 2100 kcal/day

Lipid provision = 20% total kcal = 0.2 × (2100-2450) = 420–490 kcal/day

Using a 20% lipid emulsion (which provides 2 kcal/mL):

$$\frac{420 \text{ kcal}}{2 \text{ kcal/mL}} = 210 \text{ mL of 20\% lipid emulsion}$$

Solving for total grams of lipid:

$$\frac{20 \text{ g}}{100 \text{ mL}} = \frac{x}{210 \text{ mL}}$$

Solving for x yields 42 g lipid emulsion

Using final concentrations:

$$\frac{42 \text{ g}}{2100 \text{ mL}} = 20 \text{ g/L or 2\% lipid}$$

**FIGURE 66-3.** Calculation of PN formulation.

the 70-kg trauma patient used in the first example. The issues are much simpler with enteral formulas, since labels contain the calorie:nitrogen ratio, allowing clinicians to determine the appropriate patient population for use. Enteral products with a calorie:nitrogen ratio between approximately 130:1 and 170:1 should be used in nonstressed patients who are malnourished or at risk of becoming malnourished, while solutions with a calorie:nitrogen ratio of 80:1 to 110:1 should be used in stressed or septic patients. Particular care should be taken, however, with the immune-enhancing diets, which, because of their supplemental glutamine and/or arginine and/or branched-chain amino acids, have a much lower calorie:nitrogen ratio, in the range of 55:1 to 60:1. Although this would seem to provide either too few total calories or too much nitrogen for the stressed patient, the additional benefits that are gained in severely injured trauma patients with these formulas would warrant their administration in select cases. In these situations, patients are usually provided 2 to 2.2 g/kg of protein or amino acid (0.32 to 0.35 g/kg/day of nitrogen), with nonprotein calories of approximately 20 kcal. Using these formulations, BUN often rises to 50 mg/dL but rarely higher unless there is compromised renal function.

## Renal Failure

In some patients with climbing BUN and creatinine levels, it is unclear whether the changes are due to volume deficits or renal dysfunction (see Chap. 65). Acute renal failure can be confirmed by calculating the fractional excretion of sodium (FeNa) obtained from a urine specimen in the following equation:

$$\text{FeNa } (\textit{percent}) = [U_{Na} \times V/P_{Na} \times (U_{cr} \times V/P_{cr} \, 0] \times 100$$
$$= [U_{N\hat{a}} \times P_{cr}/P_{Na} \times U_{cr}] \times 100$$

where $U_{Na}$ is the urine sodium concentration, $V$ is the urine volume, $P_{Na}$ is the plasma sodium concentration, $U_{cr}$ is a urinary creatinine concentration, and $P_{cr}$ is the serum creatinine concentration.[105] A FeNa less than 1% reflects a reabsorption of sodium of more than 99%, suggesting an adequate renal response to hypovolemia, renal hypoperfusion, and other nontubular disorders. Damage to the renal tubules reduces the ability of the kidney to resorb sodium, and the FeNa is then usually 2 to 3% or greater. Calculation of the FeNa minimizes affects of inappropriate ADH, hypovolemia, or low flow states such as congestive heart failure on variability in water and sodium absorption not due to renal dysfunction. In patients with *chronic* renal failure, protein-restricted diets (0.6 to 0.8 g/kg/day) can slow the progression of renal dysfunction and delay the need for dialysis. Because of associated injuries, the hormonal milieu, and immobilization, the rate of urea accumulation is increased in these patients, compared to those suffering from chronic renal disease. A convenient method to determine urea loads, the urea nitrogen appearance (UNA), can be calculated by the following equations:

$$\text{UNA (g/day)} = \text{urinary urea nitrogen (g/day)}$$
$$+ \text{change in body urea nitrogen (g/day)}$$

$$\text{Change in body urea nitrogen (g/day)} = \text{SUN}_f \times \text{BW}_f$$
$$\times 0.8 \text{ L/kg} - \text{SUN}_i \text{ (g/L)} \times \text{BW}_i/\text{kg/day} \times 0.8 \text{ L/kg}$$

where i and f are the initial and final values for the period of measurement and SUN is the serum urea nitrogen in grams per liter.

BW is body weight in kilograms, and although 0.6 is the usual number to estimate the fraction of body weight that is body water in health, following trauma, body water compartments are expanded and as much as 80% can be total body water.[106] When dialysis is started,

$$UNA \ (g/day) = urinary \ urea \ nitrogen \ (g/day)$$
$$+ \ dialysis \ urea \ nitrogen \ (g/day)$$
$$+ \ change \ in \ body \ urea \ nitrogen \ (g/day)$$

In contrast, no benefit has been shown from protein restriction in acute renal failure and prolonged delivery of such regimens may actually increase skeletal muscle protein breakdown. Before dialysis is started, patients should receive a normal dose of total calories and a protein dose ranging from 0.8 to 1 g/kg/day. Specialized, essential amino acid solutions have not been shown to be of benefit, and a standard mixture of amino acids can be used.[107] Often both serum potassium and phosphate concentrations drop from abnormal or high normal ranges into normal ranges with the institution of PN; potassium, phosphorus, and magnesium should not be added to PN initially but supplemented as necessary over time. If the acute renal failure is short lived, this therapy may avoid dialysis completely, particularly if the renal failure is nonoliguric. At approximately 90 mg/dL, urea exerts toxic effects on platelets. After hemodialysis is started, protein administration can be increased to 1.2 to 1.5 g/kg/day. Alternative renal replacement therapies such as continuous venovenous hemofiltration (CVVH), continuous venovenous hemodialysis (CVVHD), and continuous venovenous hemodiafiltration (CVVHDF), usually necessitates a higher protein intake (1.5 to 2.5 g/kg/day) due to considerable loss of amino acids with the dialysate.

As the kidneys recover, 3 to 5 L of urine per day may be excreted, and urinary output should be replaced with appropriate fluids. With resolving acute renal failure, urine has 70 to 80 mEq of sodium per liter, and the most commonly used fluid for replacement is 0.45 % saline. A urine sample should be sent for electrolyte analysis. As Serum Urea Nitrogen (SUN) drops to 60 mg/dL or less, urinary replacement can be stopped. The urea has little osmotic effect and renal function has usually recovered adequately. Higher levels of SUN (i.e., greater than 80 mg/dL) act as an osmotic drag and, without fluid replacement, cause hypovolemia and recurrence of oliguric renal failure.

## PULMONARY FAILURE

Although considerable attention has been drawn to avoiding overfeeding of patients with pulmonary dysfunction,[108] overfeeding and lipogenesis with increased $CO_2$ production rarely poses clinically significant problems in trauma patients (see Chap. 63). Usually, multiple rib fractures, pulmonary contusion, pneumonia, closed-head injury, or spinal cord injuries delay weaning. Selected patients, who have been chronically intubated but require a low rate of ventilator support may benefit by increasing fat as a percentage of total calories. A typical example is a geriatric patient with multiple injuries and chest trauma who has been weaned to a rate of 2 to 4 over several weeks but cannot tolerate prolonged continuous positive airway pressure or tracheostomy collar. Usually

GI function is normal and transitioning to a high-fat enteral formula providing 1 g/kg/day of protein and a calorie:nitrogen ratio of approximately 120:1 with 40 to 50% of the calories as of fat may help. Since scant clinical data demonstrate improved outcome with pulmonary specific formulas, it is difficult to recommend their routine use in intubated patients.

## HEPATIC FAILURE

Following trauma, the onset of hepatic failure with MODS carries a dismal prognosis (see Chap. 68). Very few nutritional manipulations influence outcome. Excessive protein restriction should be avoided. Intravenous amino acid solutions are better tolerated (e.g., 1 to 1.5 g/kg/day) than the enteral protein, and high levels of glucose should be avoided. The onset of hypoglycemia with severe hepatic failure represents final stages of systemic failure. Although high branched-chain formulas specific for hepatic dysfunction are commercially available, the desperate clinical situation of severe hepatic failure usually does not warrant their usage. Unless some etiologic cause—such as sepsis, acalculous cholecystitis, or obstructive biliary pathology—can be identified and successfully treated, nutritional support probably has little bearing on the outcome from hepatic failure in trauma patients.

## FLUID AND ELECTROLYTES

In the first 48 hours, lactated Ringer's solution is the principal fluid given in the ICU. Initial expansion of both intracellular and extracellular water occurs as part of the neuroendocrine response to injury. During the hypercatabolic phase, the intracellular water and associated electrolytes (in particular potassium, magnesium, and phosphorus) associated with catabolism of protein are released into the extracellular space. As the catabolic phase improves and cells regain the ability to respond to exogenous nutrients, intracellular electrolytes associated with cytosolic fluid expansion must also be replaced or cell growth does not occur[109] and a "refeeding syndrome" develops, which severely depresses serum potassium, phosphate, and magnesium levels. Since many of these severely injured trauma patients are intubated, respiratory muscle weakness may not be noted, but hypokalemia can reduce the effectiveness or increase the toxicity of various cardiac medications. Severe problems rarely develop if electrolytes are closely monitored and can be treated quickly if they occur (see Chap. 62).

### Sodium

The most common electrolyte problems noted in trauma patients are derangements in sodium. While diabetes insipidus or inappropriate ADH may occur with head injuries, producing hyper- and hyponatremia (see Chap. 20), respectively, the most common cause for abnormalities in sodium levels are either an excess in sodium administration, fluid restriction in closed-head injury patients, or administration of large volumes of fluid containing low sodium. In the first case, prolonged use of normal saline or lactated Ringer's as a maintenance fluid in association with other hidden sources of sodium administered through multiple antibiotics, $H_2$ blockers, etc., in saline produce a gradual and progressive hypernatremia. Many antibiotics contain large amounts of sodium, and since specific admixtures for medications are rarely ordered, intravenous "piggybacks" can reach 2 to 2.5 L/day in some patients. If this is administered in normal saline, hypernatremia develops. Likewise, if medications are mixed in 5% dextrose and water, significant hyponatremia develops (probably the most common etiology of hyponatremia in our ICU).

Assessment of volume status in concert with the low serum sodium concentration will usually identify the patient as hypovolemic, isovolemic, or hypervolemic. Hypovolemic patients usually respond to normal saline or lactated Ringer's infusions. If losses of fluid are chronic and similar to serum (e.g., ileostomy losses), additional sodium may be needed in the nutrient solutions. Isovolemic, hyponatremic patients often need little treatment beyond increasing the sodium content in intravenous fluids. In severe cases where urine sodium is elevated at 100 to 200 mEq/L, restriction of free water is necessary by decreasing fluid administration and concentrating the nutrient solution. This problem is most commonly seen with severe head injury or pneumonia and resolves as the patient recovers. Hypervolemic, hyponatremia patients should have nutrient formulas concentrated as much as possible. Other therapy such as diuretics may occasionally be needed.

A less common cause of hyponatremia after trauma is inappropriate ADH secretion (see Chap. 20). It is usually associated with central nervous system (CNS) effects induced by head injury, meningitis, subarachnoid hemorrhage, anesthetics, meperidine, carbamazepine, or tricyclic drugs. In addition, a decrease in the vascular volume, secondary to use of diuretics in patients who are on high levels of PEEP or have large fluid losses from the GI tract, open abdominal wounds, etc., can also lead to increased ADH secretion and increased sodium loss. Typically, serum chloride concentrations decrease with the hyponatremia, and a hypokalemic metabolic alkalosis with a high serum bicarbonate occurs, especially when diuretic-induced. The diagnosis of inappropriate ADH is made by a combination of hyponatremia, a decrease in serum osmolality, a urine osmolality which is elevated relative to serum osmolality, a urine sodium greater than 20, and if measured, an increase in ADH. Because of the effect of ADH on the kidney, water is absorbed without sodium so that urine sodium and tonicity are high relative to serum. The appropriate therapy is water restriction.

Hypernatremia is also relatively common in the critically ill trauma patient, especially in patients with severe head injury, where a mild hyperosmolar state is often used to decrease intracranial pressure (see Chap. 20). After bedside assessment, most of these patients can be categorized as either hypovolemic, isovolemic, or hypervolemic. Patients with hypovolemic hypernatremia are usually treated with lactated Ringer's solution first to ensure adequate organ perfusion, and then with solutions containing substantial free water (e.g., D5W, 0.22 or 0.45% sodium chloride injection). During free water administration, it is appropriate for the sodium to be reduced in the nutrient solution. Patients with isovolemic hypernatremia usually need free water and sodium should be removed from the PN. Patients with hypervolemic hypernatremia should have intake minimized by concentrating the nutrient formula. Exogenous sodium should be eliminated from PN, medications, and other infusions to the extent possible.

## Potassium

Hypokalemia is very common after trauma, especially in patients with normal renal function who require aggressive resuscitation with crystalloid. Loss of gastrointestinal fluids rich in hydrogen and chloride aggravate this hypokalemia. Patients with prolonged nasogastric suction will lose considerable HCl resulting in metabolic alkalosis and substantial renal wasting of potassium. Drug therapy with loop diuretics, amphotericin B, antipseudomonal penicillins, and corticosteroids have all been reported to aggravate renal wasting of potassium. Other drugs, such as inhaled beta agonists (e.g., albuterol) and insulin, drive potassium into the cell also resulting in hypokalemia in some patients. All the above conditions will require additional potassium added to the nutrient solution above the standard of 30 to 40 mEq/L that is commonly used in PN or present in enteral formulas. Occasionally up to 120 mEq of potassium per liter must be added to nutrient solutions of patients who were receiving three or four of the above-mentioned drugs to keep them in potassium balance.

Body potassium needs are not proportionate to serum levels. Each 0.25-mEq drop in serum potassium levels between 3.0 and 4.0 mEq/L represents a 25- to 50-mEq deficit in total body potassium. Between 2.5 and 3.0 mEq/L, each 0.25-mEq drop represents an additional 100 to 200 mEq deficit, which must be replaced to avoid precipitous drops with refeeding.[110]

Hyperkalemia is less common than hypokalemia after trauma, and is usually associated with compromise in renal function. In general, hyperkalemia from acute renal failure (ARF) warrants potassium removal from the nutrient solution. Once levels have decreased to 4.0 mEq/L, potassium should be added back in modest doses (e.g., 10 mEq/L). Other causes of hyperkalemia are hemolysis of the blood sample and drugs known to cause this disorder, even when renal function is normal. Most laboratories will identify hemolyzed samples that do not require treatment other than repeat analysis. Heparin and trimethoprim have been reported to cause hyperkalemia in patients.[111,112] Heparin is an aldosterone antagonist which causes sodium wasting and potassium retention. This drug-nutrient interaction occurs with both systemic and low-dose heparin, especially in patients with diabetes and chronic renal dysfunction. Trimethoprim is a component of the combination product of trimethoprim/ sulfamethoxazole used frequently for gram-negative systemic infections. It is a weak diuretic with potassium-sparing activities. Patients who experience these interactions should have potassium decreased in the nutrient solution, event when renal function is normal.

## Phosphorus

Hypophosphatemia is a common metabolic complication of critically ill patients receiving nutritional support. While most practitioners add phosphorus to PN solutions routinely, several patient populations require greater amounts, including patients with a history of alcohol abuse, poor nutritional status preinjury, or chronic use of antacids or sucralfate. Even when serum phosphorus concentrations are monitored closely, hypophosphatemia occurs in approximately 30% of patients receiving PN.[113] Treatment of hypophosphatemia is dictated by the severity, and intravenous replacement doses are most frequently used. The enteral route should be considered in mild cases of hypophosphatemia by adding

5 to 10 mL of Fleet's phosphosoda to each liter of the enteral formula in patients requiring additional phosphate. In patients requiring both potassium and phosphate, potassium phosphate (usually 15 to 22.5 mmol/L) can be added to the formula. For isolated potassium depression, potassium chloride can be added either to the enteral. We have developed a graduated dosing scheme for replacement of phosphorus in patients receiving specialized nutrition support (i.e., either parenteral nutrition, enteral nutrition, or both) based on the serum phosphorus concentration of the patient[114]:

| SERUM PHOSPHORUS CONCENTRATION[a] | PHOSPHORUS DOSE |
|---|---|
| 2.3 to 3.0 mg/dL | 0.16 mmol/kg over 4 h |
| 1.6 to 2.2 mg/dL | 0.32 mmol/kg over 4 to 6 h |
| <1.5 mg/dL | 0.64 mmol/kg over 8 h |

[a]Normal phosphorus concentration is mg/dL.

Additional phosphorus can be added to the PN or enteral formula following correction of initial hypophosphatemia.

Hyperphosphatemia is much less prevalent than hypophosphatemia in trauma patients and is usually associated with renal compromise when it does occur (see Chap. 65). Phosphorus should be decreased or removed from the nutrient solution.

## Magnesium

The development of hypomagnesemia is underappreciated. Magnesium is rapidly depleted in stress, particularly when diuretics and antibiotics such as aminoglycosides are administered. Dysrhythmias, hypocalcemia (an unusual problem in trauma patients), and irritability are avoided with magnesium monitoring and appropriate treatment. Patients with a history of alcohol abuse or lower gastrointestinal losses, such as diarrhea, are particularly prone to develop hypomagnesemia. Amphotericin B, aminoglycosides, and loop diuretics (and in addition cisplatin and cyclosporine) have all been reported to cause renal wasting of magnesium. Intravenous magnesium replacement therapy is usually necessary in patients with moderate to severe magnesium deficiency due to poor absorption of oral magnesium salts. Magnesium has a renal tubular threshold similar to glucose, so rapid administration over a short period of time will invariably result in high urinary losses. We have developed a weight-based dosing regimen for magnesium deficiency in which intravenous doses are infused slowly over 12 to 24 hours to facilitate better retention:

| SERUM MAGNESIUM CONCENTRATION[a] | MAGNESIUM DOSE |
|---|---|
| 1.5 to 1.8 mg/dL | 0.5 mEq/kg over 12 h |
| 1.1 to 1.4 | 1 mEq/kg over 24 h |
| ≤1 | 1.5 mEq/kg over 24 h |

[a]Normal magnesium concentration is 1.7 to 2.3 mg/dL.

Magnesium status should also be considered in evaluating a hypokalemic patient, as magnesium is an important cofactor for the Na-K ATPase pump. We often administer magnesium replacement therapy for low-normal serum magnesium concentrations in the presence of hypokalemia, because magnesium is an intracellular cation and serum concentrations may not accurately reflect intracellular status. Our standard magnesium concentration in PN

solutions is 12 mEq/L; however, some patients as described above need increased doses. We have safely administered as high as 28 mEq/L via PN in selected patients. Hypermagnesemia usually occurs in association with renal dysfunction or failure. Magnesium should be removed from the PN of these patients.

## Electrolyte Management in Severely Injured Trauma Patients

Table 66-3 shows the composition of the various gastrointestinal secretions that must be considered in fluid and electrolyte balance of patients. Two values are given for potassium in gastric drainage, 10 and 40 mEq; NG drainage contains approximately 10 mEq/L, but because of hydrogen loss, gastric loss should be calculated as 40 mEq/L because of increased renal potassium excretion. In the overall management of critically injured patients, unusual fluid losses in significant quantity (>500 mL/day) through such sources as duodenal fistulas, pancreatic fistulas, or high small bowel fistulas should be sent for electrolyte analysis and appropriate adjustments made in intravenous nutrition to account for the excessive losses. It is often helpful to calculate sodium balance by comparing losses versus administered intake considering all intravenous solutions and admixtures. Most cases of hyponatremia are due to significant discrepancies (often 600 to 800 mEq/day) between the sodium administered and the sodium lost. There are several rules of thumb in fluid management of complex trauma patients. Gastric drainage should be replaced with 0.45 saline with 40 mEq of potassium chloride to avoid hypokalemia, hypochloremia with metabolic alkalosis. Fluid losses from the gastrointestinal tract distal to the pylorus, including the liver and pancreas, have a sodium of approximately 130 to 140 mEq/L. Losses of associated bicarbonate and chloride vary, depending on the organ. Bicarbonate is equivalent to serum in bile and small bowel fluids, and the appropriate replacement fluid for them is lactated Ringer's. High-output pancreatic fistulas produce bicarbonate loss (80 to 90 mEq/L) and an appropriate replacement fluid (greater than 300 mL/day) is 0.2 sodium chloride with two ampules of sodium bicarbonate.

Standard adult electrolyte requirements for parenteral nutrition are provided in Table 66-4 with adjustments as necessary, depending upon unusual losses. Sodium can be administered as the chloride, acetate, or phosphate salt depending on needs. Generally, chloride salts are used for patients with metabolic alkalosis and acetate salts for metabolic acidosis. Patients with severe edema or anasarca generally should receive a sodium-free PN solution. Most enteral formulas have

**TABLE 66-3**

**Electrolyte Composition of Gastrointestinal Secretions: Average (Range)**

| SECRETION | Na⁺ (mEq/L) | K⁺ (mEq/L) | Cl⁻ (mEq/L) | HCO₃⁻ (mEq/L) |
|---|---|---|---|---|
| Gastric | 70(60–90) | 10(4–12) 40[b] | 90(50–150)[a] | 0 |
| Pancreatic fistula | 140(135–155) | 5(4–6) | 75(60–110) | 80(70–90) |
| Bile | 140(135–145) | 5(4–6) | 100(90–110) | 35(30–40) |
| New Ileostomy | 130(120–140) | 5(4–10) | 105(60–125) | 35(30–40) |

[a]Lower in achlorhydria.
[b]Includes renal losses.

**TABLE 66-4**

**Electrolytes in Total Parenteral Nutrition**

| ELECTROLYTE | USUAL REQUIREMENT PER DAY | STANDARD TPN CONDENTRATION/L |
|---|---|---|
| Sodium | 100–150 mEq | 40–60 mEq/L |
| Potassium | 80–100 mEq (more if anabolic) | 20 mEq/L as phosphate 20 mEq/L as acetate |
| Magnesium | 8–30 mEq | 8 mEq/L as sulfate |
| Calcium | 10–15 mEq | 5 mEq/L as gluconate |
| Phosphorus | 20–40 mmole | 15 mmole/L as K$^+$ salt or Na$^+$ salt |

**TABLE 66-5**

**Principles of Enteral Feeding Access**

Determine appropriateness of patient
Choose the tube appropriate for expected needs:
- Needle catheter: 3–4 weeks
- Large-bore tube: Chronic needs
- Transgastric jejunostomy: If there is a contraindication to direct small bowel access or for simultaneous gastric drain. Read the instructions provided!

Obtain safe postpyloric access:
- Position jejunostomy to avoid afferent loop tension if distention occurs.
- Create lax Witzel tunnel.
- Suture 6–10 cm of jejunum to the anterior abdominal wall with 4–5 sutures.
- Position at the lateral aspect of the rectus sheath away from the midline.
- Examine patient daily with all dressings off prior to advancing feeding rate.

30 to 40 mEq of sodium per liter (i.e., approximately 0.2 saline) which should be considered in the overall fluid management. Like sodium, potassium is available as the chloride, acetate, or phosphate salts. Calcium is usually administered as the gluconate salt in PN because it is more stable and less likely to precipitate with phosphorus. Magnesium is generally given as the sulfate salt in PN. Significant fluid and electrolyte disorders are unusual unless supplemental fluids administered through admixtures to drugs are ignored.

## ISSUES OF RELEVANCE TO ENTERAL FEEDING

### Patients Requiring Celiotomy

Early enteral feeding of severely injured patients reduces septic complications compared with starvation or PN, but several principles (Table 66-5) must be appreciated to avoid unacceptably high complication rates. First, ISS and ATI can identify patients benefiting from early feeding using the previously noted algorithm. Second, safe effective access should be obtained beyond the ligament of Treitz, using a needle catheter jejunostomy (NCJ), transgastric jejunostomy (TGJ), or nasoenteric tube advanced during celiotomy. While direct small bowel access is usually successful, two recent studies showed an unusually high incidence of complications.[115,116] This section details techniques to avoid these complications. Third, an appropriate nutritional regimen should be instituted. Fourth, early small bowel feeding should be started only in hemodynamically stable patients. Finally, close monitoring and gradual advancement is paramount.

Multiple tubes are available. In general, a 5- or 7-Fr NCJ can be placed in most patients, but the life span of these devices is only about three to four weeks; therefore their use should be limited to short-term enteral support. For more "permanent" access, (e.g., severely injured geriatric or patients with severe closed-head injury), placement of a larger (14, 16, or 18 Fr) catheter is advisable, since it can be replaced after five to seven days, if necessary. Finally, a TGJ is helpful in patients requiring prolonged gastric drainage as well as small bowel feedings. They are also useful when surgeons prefer not to cannulate the small bowel directly.

Certain instances mandate specific tubes. The 5-Fr NCJ tube tolerates most standard enteral products, including those containing fiber,[117] and their use need not be limited to defined formula elemental diets. Fiber reduces diarrhea in critically ill patients. Bacteria metabolize soluble fiber to short-chain fatty acids which provide energy to the colonocyte for sodium and water reabsorption. 5-Fr NCJ tubes clog if protein supplements are added to standard enteral formulas or when immune-enhancing diets (IEDs) are used. For these circumstances, a 7-French NCJ or larger diameter catheter should be used. Medications should not be administered via NCJs, since the elixirs containing medication such as theophylline, potassium chloride, etc., coagulate the tube feedings to produce early tube loss. In general, an NCJ should be used only for the enteral formula.

Placement of jejunostomies is critically important. A site should be chosen with a long mesenteric loop to avoid traction by the afferent limb from the fixed ligament of Treitz, should distention occur. In all circumstances, we recommend creating a Witzel tunnel around the tube with five 3-0 silk sutures placed approximately 1 cm apart, leaving the needle on the first, third, or fifth suture. The sutures creating the Witzel tunnel should loosely approximate the bowel around the tube to prevent tearing if significant edema occurs in the bowel wall. If the bowel is too edematous or indurated to create a lax Witzel tunnel around a 16- or 18-Fr tube, an NCJ can be used. Another form of access should be chosen if bowel is too indurated to create a Witzel tunnel around an NCJ. The Witzel tunnel eliminates dislodgment of the tube into the peritoneal cavity. The jejunostomy should exit the peritoneal cavity at the lateral aspect of the rectus sheath. Placement at or lateral to the rectus sheath—most commonly on the left side, but acceptable on the right side if a stoma is necessary in the left upper quadrant—minimizes the chance of volvulus of intestine over the attachment point. Placement near the midline incision also interferes with re-exploration. Finally, the jejunostomy itself, particularly an NCJ, should not be brought out at a 90° angle through the abdominal wall to avoid kinking the tube as it exits the fascia. The externalized jejunostomy tube should be kept short, less than 3 to 4 cm, and anchored securely to the anterior abdominal wall. A transparent dressing over the catheter prevents disoriented patients from pulling and dislodging the jejunostomy.

If prolonged gastric drainage is likely, TGJ allows gastric decompression and direct small bowel feeding. The distal limb of the TGJ should lie beyond the ligament of Treitz and not in the duodenum. Intraduodenal feeding with shorter tubes stimulates pancreaticoduodenal and gastric secretions, which can result in fluid and electrolyte problems. Nutrients introduced beyond the ligament of Treitz do not stimulate significant upper GI secretion.[118] A note of caution with TGJs is in order. The gastroesophageal junction is the most dependent part of the stomach in supine patients and the stomach should be decompressed with an NG tube until the patient can be elevated to 30 to 40° to avoid reflux and aspiration.

As a final technique for small bowel access, long tubes can be advanced through the nose or mouth into the proximal small intestine at celiotomy. Although some institutions successfully use this technique, it requires close vigilance by nursing staff during routine patient care, transport, or ambulation.

## DIET CHOICE BY THE ENTERAL ROUTE

Several clinical trials support the use of an IED in patients at high risk of developing sepsis (ATI ≥ 25, ISS >20; Fig. 66-1). Some powdered diets, such as Immunaid, contain free L-glutamine in addition to omega-3 fatty acids, nucleotides, BCAAs, and arginine. Liquid diets such as Perative do not contain such free glutamine because of the instability of that amino acid in liquid form. A recently introduced enteral liquid product has higher levels of GLN in the protein component. Liquid diets may contain soluble fiber, which serves as an energy source for enterocytes after metabolism by endogenous bacteria to the short-chain fatty acids, acetoacetate, butyrate, and propionate. In our experience, the IEDs should be administered through larger-bore catheters, such as the 7-Fr or larger NCJ, since increased clogging occurs in the 5-Fr NCJs.

In less severely injured patients, a nonprotein calorie:nitrogen (NCP:N) ratio of approximately 80:1 to 120:1 increases the protein loading without a high NPC:N load. Chemically defined diets are not mandatory, although they are still frequently used and provide an adequate nutritional substrate. Chemically defined diets are often associated with a higher incidence of diarrhea due to their high osmolarity and lack of soluble fiber. Fiber-containing diets are not contraindicated in critically ill patients; in our experience, diarrhea is reduced by their use, although impaction may occasionally mimic bowel obstruction. Typically, if intragastric feedings are being given, impaction presents as distention without high gastric residuals. The diagnosis is made by recognizing colonic distention in an x-ray. Most patients respond to colonic stimulation with enemas or suppositories. Recent reports suggest neostigmine to stimulate colonic motility but bradycardia and hypotension may occur.

If the patient improves but continued enteral feeding is necessary due to prolonged inability to take an ad libitum diet, the NPC:N should be increased to 130:1 to 160:1 and protein administration reduced to 1.2 to 1.5 g/kg. Total calories are given in the range of 20 to 25 kcal/kg/day. In diabetic patients, a formula with a higher percentage of fat may reduce hyperglycemia if hypertriglyceridemia is not a problem. In the occasional, rare patient who cannot be weaned from low levels of ventilator support, transition to a higher-fat diet may improve weaning, although this scenario is very uncommon in young trauma patients.

## DIET PROGRESSION

Diet advancement requires close monitoring. Direct small intestinal feeding should be delayed if multiple blood transfusions, fluid boluses, or pressor agents (other than low-dose dopamine) are

### TABLE 66-6

**Protocol for Advancement of Chemically Defined Diet by Jones and Moore**

| STRENGTH | RATE | DURATION |
|---|---|---|
| 1/4 | 50 mL/h | 8 h |
| 1/4 | 75 mL/h | 8 h |
| 1/4 | 100 mL/h | 8 h |
| 1/2 | 100 mL/h | 8 h |
| 3/4 | 100 mL/h | 8 h |
| Full | 100 mL/h | 8 h |
| Full | 125 mL/h[a] | |

[a]If required.

required to maintain hemodynamic stability. Enteral feeding increases splanchnic blood flow and increases splanchnic metabolic rate. Shock, sepsis, and hemodynamic instability shunt blood away from the GI tract, and it is presumed that inability to shunt blood to the mucosa may be the cause of feeding-related small bowel necrosis. Evidence of adequate splanchnic perfusion includes adequate urine output, hemodynamic stability, warm peripheral extremities, etc.

Progression is determined by the type of formula. Protocols have been defined for progression of defined-formula diets (Table 66-6). More complex diets should be started at 15 mL/hour for the first six to eight hours in patients who were previously unstable or in shock. Diets can be advanced after six to eight hours to 25 mL/hour and at increments of 25 mL/hour/day increments depending on tolerance.

Moore et al.[34] advanced patients with less severe injuries (i.e., an ATI >40 and no bowel injury) to goal rate within 48 hours following institution of a chemically defined diet. Patients with an ATI >40 or bowel injuries had increased bloating, cramps, and general intolerance when advanced this quickly[119] and should be advanced more slowly, generally by 25 mL/hour/day, up to the calculated goal rate, while being observed for intolerance. In our experience, approximately 50% of severely injured patients can be advanced up to or close to the goal rate within three to four days with few if any problems. Approximately 10% of patients do not tolerate feedings at all, with intolerance manifest by reflux of feedings into the stomach (which necessitates the immediate discontinuation of direct small bowel feedings), significant bloating, or complaints of cramps. The remaining 40% of patients generally tolerate feedings to approximately 50 to 75% of goal but develop temporary (two to three days) intolerance, such as discomfort or diarrhea, at higher rates. Tube feedings should be slowed to the tolerated rate for 24 to 48 hours and then advanced. If patients tolerate at least 50% of goal rate, we do not add PN. In the minority of patients with complete tolerance, however, PN should be instituted by the fourth or fifth day, with transition to enteral feedings as soon as possible. Once PN is started, it is not weaned until patients tolerate at least 50% of the goal enteral rate and feedings are being advanced to 75% of the calculated rate.

## PROKINETIC AGENTS

Gastroparesis is manifested by high aspirated residual volume (>150 mL) and is one of the more troublesome GI complications (see Chap. 64). The nurse should check gastric residuals every four to six hours to assure that gastric residuals remain low. Acutely elevated residuals in patients who previously tolerated a high rate indicates ileus from a septic process or acute stress ulceration. Evidence of upper GI bleeding (coffee-grounds aspirate or obvious bleeding) warrants early endoscopy because of a high rate of duodenal or gastric ulceration, especially following spinal cord injuries, severe head injuries, or burns.

With gastroparesis persistent beyond three to four days, most practitioners use a prokinetic agent to enhance gastric emptying.[120,121] The three drugs used most commonly in the critical care setting are metoclopramide, cisapride, and erythromycin. Metoclopramide is available as a tablet, syrup, or intravenous solution in the United States and is a selective dopamine-2 agonist which enhances peristalsis contractility of the esophagus, gastric antrum, and small intestine. Metoclopramide enhanced gastric emptying of acetaminophen in trauma patients and reduced time to maximal plasma concentration compared with erythromycin or placebo.[122] Cisapride is no longer available in the United States because it was associated with events of cardiac arrhythmia.

Erythromycin is available as a capsule, suspension, or intravenous solution acting locally to enhance motilin release from enterochromaffin cells of the duodenum. Motilin enhances contractile activity of the gastric antrum and duodenum. Compared to placebo, erythromycin significantly increased the frequency of gastric contractions, amplitude of contractions, and the motility index. The time to reach the maximal concentration of acetaminophen (gastric emptying marker) was also shortened when compared to the placebo group in this one-dose study involving 10 critically ill patients receiving mechanical ventilation.[120] In healthy volunteers, both total gastric volume and gastric volume of a continuous liquid meal decreased by 22% in patients receiving erythromycin versus placebo.[123]

## DRUG-NUTRIENT INTERACTIONS

Critically ill trauma patients receive a large number of pharmacological agents. A few agents influence the designing of the nutritional formula. Propofol, commonly used for sedation, is manufactured in a lipid emulsion that provides 1.1 kcal/mL. The caloric contribution from the lipid vehicle is negligible in small doses; however, it becomes very important with higher rates of infusion. The nutritional prescription should be modified by decreasing or eliminating lipids from the parenteral solution or by using a high-protein enteral formula with added protein powder to provide an appropriate mix of carbohydrate, fat, and protein.

Enteral nutrition influences effectiveness of drugs such as the antiepileptics, phenytoin, or carbamazepine, when given via the GI tract. Phenytoin interacts with calcium or the caseinates within the formula to decrease drug absorption. Recommendations for phenytoin administration include discontinuation of tube feedings for 2 hours before and after the drug dose, dilution of phenytoin, irrigation of the tube with 60-mL flushes, and increases in the phenytoin dosage as necessary.[124] Serum levels should be monitored during initiation of therapy or with changes in enteral nutrition. Carbamazepine absorption is slower with continuous enteral feeding and monitoring of serum levels is appropriate.[125]

**TABLE 66-7**

| Medications Incompatible with Enteral Formulation | |
| --- | --- |
| Dimetapp Elixir | Feosol Elixir |
| Dimetane Elixir | Robitussin Expectorant |
| Sudafed Syrup | Mellaril Oral Solution |
| Thorazine Concentrate | |

*Adapted from Cutie AJ, Altman E, Lenkel L. Compatibility of Enteral Products with Commonly Employed Drug Additives. JPEN J Parenter Enteral Nutr. 1983;7;186–191, with permission from the American Society for Parenteral and Enteral Nutrition (A.S.P.E.N.). A.S.P.E.N. does not endorse the use of this material in any form other than its entirety.*

Warfarin is commonly used in the treatment of deep venous thrombosis (DVT) prophylaxis, but enteral products can interfere due to the vitamin K in the formula or through physical/chemical interaction, which impairs drug absorption.[126] Hydralazine,[127] ciprofloxacin,[128] and itraconazole[129] are affected by enteral administration when tube feedings are in progress and necessitate close monitoring.

Addition of drugs to the enteral formula can affect stability of the fat, alter viscosity, and change the consistency and particulate size of the formula. Calcium, zinc, and iron produce jelling or curdling and a number of drug products increase clumping and change viscosity due to their acidic nature. Drugs incompatible with enteral products are listed in Table 66-7.[130]

## COMPLICATIONS OF ENTERAL FEEDING

### Distention

Patients should be examined six hours following institution of their feedings and when cramping or diarrhea occurs. Mild abdominal distention is common in fed and unfed trauma patients and discontinuation of the tube feedings for minimal symptoms is not necessary. If, however, alert patients complain of severe discomfort, the rate should be reduced if the pain is not incisional. Colonic distension secondary to constipation or impaction is likely in patients receiving intragastric feeding even with low residuals; it responds to suppositories and/or enemas. The institution and advancement of early enteral feedings into the small bowel requires that patients be examined approximately six hours following institution of their feedings as well as if there are any complaints of significant cramping or diarrhea.

### Diarrhea

Diarrhea occurs commonly in fed and unfed critically ill patients. In tube-fed patients, diarrhea occurs from 5 to 25% depending on the definition of diarrhea.[131] Five to six formed or semiformed stools per day are not diarrhea. However, watery stools that constantly soil the patient during turning eventually cause irritation and skin breakdown. While tube feedings are often implicated, diarrhea is more commonly caused by medications.[132] Twenty percent of severely injured trauma patients administered a chemically defined diet developed significant diarrhea in our study,[33] which decreased to 4% with a fiber-containing diet. Diarrhea occurred in

**TABLE 66-8**

**Sorbitol Content of Oral Medications**

| DRUG g/DAY | SORBITOL g/5 mL | Average |
|---|---|---|
| Acetaminophen Elixir (Roxane) | 1.8 | 29.25 g/2600 mg |
| Acetaminophen Suspension (McNeil Children's) | <0.84 | 13.7 g/2600 mg |
| Acetaminophen Liquid (McNeil Adult) | <0.4 | 6.2 g/2600 mg |
| Maalox | 0.225 | 5.4 g/120 mL |
| Calcium Carbonate Suspension (Roxane) | 1.4 | 4.2 g/3750 mg |
| Tagamet Liquid (SK Beecham) | 2.52 | 10 g/1200 mg |
| Diphenoxylate and Atropine (Lomotil Searle) | 1.05 | 8.4 g |
| Diphenoxylate and atropine (Roxane) | 2.3 | 18.4 g |
| Metoclopramide (Reglan Robbins) | 2.25 | 18 g |
| Theophylline (Rorer) | 2.02 | 30.2 g |
| Bactrim (Roche) | 0.35 | 2.8 g/40 mL |

*Source: Lutomski DM, Gora ML, Wright SM, Martin JE: Sorbitol content of selected oral liquids. Ann pharmacother 27:269, 1993. With permission.*

two of 71 patients administered a chemically defined diet in another study of patients sustaining major trauma.[119]

Approximately three-quarters of cases of diarrhea are caused by antibiotic-induced pseudomembranous enterocolitis (see Chap. 19), magnesium medications, or sorbitol.[133] Sorbitol is used for sweetness or as a solubilizing agent replacing alcohol. Surprisingly large amounts of sorbitol are present in commonly administered medication (Table 66-8) such as potassium chloride, theophylline medications, phenytoin, and even antidiarrheal drugs. On occasion, prokinetic drugs successfully instituted for gastroparesis cause diarrhea which stops after discontinuation.

Multiple antibiotics generate bacterial overgrowth and rarely pseudomembranous colitis. Proctosigmoidoscopy should be performed for suspected *Clostridium difficile*, particularly in guaiac-positive patients. Specimens should be sent for fecal leukocytes and the mucosa observed for pseudomembranes. In patients receiving antibiotics and enteral nutrition, *C. difficile* was present in over 50% of patients with diarrhea.[134]

Patients with diarrhea should receive an isotonic formula with soluble fiber. Prokinetic agents and enteral medications are immediately discontinued and the rate of feeding reduced to 50% of the current rate. Diarrhea commonly persists for another 12 hours as the GI tract eliminates the fluid. Sigmoidoscopy is performed and stool for *C. difficile* is sent, if clinically appropriate. If positive, appropriate therapy is started (see Chap. 19).

Although hypoalbuminemia was implicated as an important cause of diarrhea in critically ill patients, a prospective study using peptide formulas (promoted as a benefit in hypoalbuminemic patients) in standard isotonic formulas produced no benefit in hypoalbuminemic patients[135] compared to an intact protein diet. In a very small percentage of patients, many of whom are not being fed, diarrhea persists, and administration of *Lactobacillus acidophilus* has been successful on occasion. *L. acidophilus,* however, is sensitive to erythromycin.[134] Antidiarrheal medicines, such as tincture of opium or loperamide, are used only as a last resort.

## PNEUMATOSIS INTESTINALIS AND NECROSIS

Necrosis secondary to direct small bowel feedings seems to occur in hemodynamically unstable patients often on pressor. Tachycardia (≥ 160/minute), a temperature spike to 103°F and rapid abdominal distention are hallmarks of this devastating complication. Although the mechanism for necrosis is unclear, potential explanations include bacterial invasion of the bowel wall with mucosal necrosis, abnormal carbohydrate metabolism, or ischemia secondary to low GI blood flow. While spontaneous necrosis has occurred in unfed critically ill patients, enteral feedings are an important factor as shown by the report of necrosis following radical cytectomy and jejunostomy feeding. Necrosis of the entire small intestine developed except for the isolated ileoconduit.[136]

Pneumatosis intestinalis occurs both in fed and unfed ICU patients and if diagnosed necessitates immediate discontinuation of tube feedings and initiation of antibiotic therapy against both aerobic and anaerobic organisms. The use of antibiotics are debatable but probably should be instituted. Surgery is necessary in rare cases, but if necrosis is found at exploration, immediate anastomosis should be delayed for 24 hours to eliminate progressive necrosis not initially recognized.

Tube feedings should never be administered to patients with an obstruction or immediately after release of the obstruction because of the potential for necrosis. Postoperative diuresis and resolution of abdominal distention should be complete prior to instituting enteral nutrition.

## ASPIRATION

Aspiration occurs in 1–70% of patients who are enterally fed[137]; in our experience, it is uncommon in trauma patients. While some protection is probably provided by direct small bowel feeding, gastric decompression should be continued until gastric residuals drop since mortality with aspiration can be 50% or greater. Tracheostomy or endotracheal intubation with an inflated cuff does not completely protect against lethal aspiration in ventilated patients.

Monitoring of residual gastric volumes is the major watchdog to minimize aspiration with intragastric feeding. Unfortunately, the tip of the feeding tube may not lie in the pool of residual tube feeding and the gastroesophageal junction becomes the most dependent area of the stomach in the supine position. In critically ill patients, residual volumes of 50 mL in patients with nasogastric tubes and 100 mL volumes in patients with gastrostomy tubes create concern of impending intolerance and reflux.[138] If a single residual is high, feedings can be replaced into the stomach and residuals checked in two hours. If they remain high, feedings should not be restarted. A prokinetic agent should be started if appropriate. Critically ill patients tolerating successful intragastric feeding at goal or near goal rates who suddenly develop high residual volumes may have impending sepsis or have a pyloric channel or duodenal ulcer. This is particularly common in patients with spinal cord injuries, severe closed-head injuries, or burns. If the NG aspirate is guaiac-positive, upper endoscopy is warranted, particularly if there is an unexplained drop in hematocrit. More commonly, gastroparesis signals the early onset of sepsis from either pneumonia, intraabdominal abscess, or another cause of sepsis (see Chap. 64). Patients with direct small bowel access do not need residual volumes checked, but reflux of tube feeding into the stomach require that feeding be discontinued immediately since this is a reliable marker of distal bowel obstruction or significant intolerance.

## MECHANICAL COMPLICATIONS

Jejunostomy tube dislodgement into the peritoneal cavity or volvulus at the jejunostomy site are avoided by the surgical techniques described earlier. Complete dislodgment can be avoided by secure suture of the tube at the anterior abdominal wall and by keeping the external segment short and covered with an occlusive dressing. While complete dislodgment of a large-bore red rubber feeding tube is considered a minor inconvenience if replaced promptly with an appropriately sized catheter, dislodgment of an NCJ loses the portal for direct small bowel access. Large-bore tubes in place for at least a week can be replaced with a tube of a smaller or similar size.

Occlusion of feeding tubes is common, but this is of little significance with a 14- or 16-Fr tube, since it can be replaced. Occlusion may necessitate removal of a 5- or 7-Fr NCJ. If NCJs occlude within the first 24 to 48 hours, the cause is a kink at the point where the NCJ tube pierces the fascia and enters the bowel. By applying pressure with a 10-mL saline-filled syringe while gently withdrawing the catheter, the flow restarts as soon as the kink is straightened. The catheter should be withdrawn 5 or 6 cm until the catheter can be divided beyond the kink and reattached. This rarely occurs a second time. If an NCJ occludes after two to three weeks, flushing may temporarily open the tube, but the life span of the NCJ is limited. Fortunately, since most patients tolerate direct intragastric feeding by this time, the NCJ has served its function. No medications are permitted via an NCJ because elixirs used to solubilize medications coagulate feedings and occlude the tube. Medications given through a larger-bore catheter should be flushed with 15 to 20 mL fluid prior and another 40 to 50 mL water or saline after administering the medication. Use of a guidewire to disimpact a tube is not advisable, since it can perforate the tube or the intestine.[139] Special devices are marketed that can be inserted into clogged tubes. Such a device usually consists of a small catheter fitted with an adapter for connection of a syringe. Water or declogging powder can be instilled by the syringe for irrigation. Although a variety of agents (i.e., carbonated beverages, acidic juices, meat tenderizer) have been tried to restore patency to occluded tubes, a combination of pancreatic enzymes and sodium bicarbonate appears to produce the best results.[140]

Other devices resembling soft, threaded screws have been inserted inside a large-bore gastrostomy or jejunostomy tube and rotated to bore through a clog.

## PARENTERAL FEEDING

### Access and Monitoring of Lines

The critically ill trauma patient will require reliable venous access at all times. Therefore most patients who are hospitalized in the ICU will already have central vein access when the decision to start PN is made. This allows for the administration of central PN, which usually includes very hyperosmolar formulas that must be diluted quickly in the vasculature. Peripheral PN has been used with some success in hospitalized patients; however, it is not frequently administered to critically ill trauma patients because of fluid considerations and the resulting thrombophlebitis necessitating frequent vein rotation to maintain the infusion. To administer adequate nonprotein energy with peripheral PN, greater than 50% of energy calories is usually give as intravenous lipid. This may result in a mixture of nutritional substrates that is not optimal for the critically ill patient.

The percutaneous subclavian vein approach is the procedure of choice for obtaining central vein access in critically ill trauma patients. Alternative methods, though less desirable, include the internal jugular vein approach and the femoral vein approach. There is an increased rate of catheter sepsis with each of these techniques and a potential risk of DVT with femoral lines. When the decision to start central PN has been made, the critical care practitioner is faced with several choices regarding access: (a) use the current central line for the provision of PN (e.g., triple-lumen catheter, Swan–Ganz catheter), (b) change the present catheter to a new triple-lumen catheter using the modified Seldinger technique with a flexible guide wire, or (c) place an entirely new central line with a triple-lumen catheter dedicating one port for the provision of PN. The method used will depend on the patient's hemodynamic stability, the length of time the existing catheter has been in place, the condition of the site where the existing central catheter was placed (e.g., redness, swelling, gross pus), and the other fluid requirements of the patient including intravenous fluid, continuous medication drips, electrolyte boluses, and other medications and blood. An open port on the Swan–Ganz catheter can be used for PN in patients who are hemodynamically unstable. This obviates the need to subject the critically ill patient to another procedure, especially one who may have a coagulopathy. Once hemodynamic stability is achieved, the Swan–Ganz catheter should be "changed out" to a triple-lumen catheter using the modified Seldinger technique with a sterile guidewire. If there is purulence present at the central vein site or a high index of suspicion that the present catheter is infected, access at an alternative site (e.g., the opposite subclavian vein) should be strongly considered.

Placement of an indwelling central catheter does include some short-term and long-term risks (see Chap. 60). Pneumothorax, hemothorax, aneurysms, arterial puncture, and nerve injury may all occur during attempted cannulation of a central vein. Subclavian thrombosis and catheter-related sepsis are major problems that occur after placement of a central vein catheter. Patients with subclavian central catheters should be observed frequently for neck swelling or complaints of stiffness to aid in the diagnosis of subclavian thrombosis. Subclavian vein thrombosis may require removal of the catheter and anticoagulation. Also, the use of catheters made of silicone or polyurethane elastomers result in less thrombogenicity than ones made of polyvinyl or polyethylene. Catheter-related thrombotic occlusions frequently complicate the care of central venous catheters. Catheter occlusion may occur in the form of thrombotic and nonthrombotic causes. Types of thrombotic catheter occlusions include (a) intraluminal thrombus, (b) mural thrombus, (c) fibrin sheath, and (d) and fibrin tail.[141] Intraluminal thrombus development is characterized as occurring within the lumen of the catheter. This usually presents as resistance to infusion or blood aspiration from the catheter. Inadequate flushing or blood reflux may account for this type of occlusion. A mural thrombus refers to the formation of fibrin from vessel wall injury that extends to the surface of the catheter. Clinical symptoms consistent with vascular obstruction, such as neck vein distention, edema, and pain over the ipsilateral neck may signify the presence of this type of occlusion. Fibrin sheath formation can encase the catheter and occlude the distal tip, whereas a fibrin tail refers to an accumulation of fibrin that surrounds the end of the catheter. Thrombolytic therapy is recommended for all of the preceding types of catheter occlusion that are thrombotic in nature. Due to the unavailability of urokinase, t-PA is now the recommended agent for thrombosed catheters. A 2-mg dose of t-PA administered with a 30-minute to 2-hour dwell time has been shown to restore patency to occluded catheters.[142] Nonthrombotic causes of occlusion can arise from precipitation of drugs, intravenous lipids, and calcium-phosphate complexes. If drug or mineral deposits are suspected, 1 to 3 mL of 0.1 N HCl is recommended for clearance.[131] On the other hand, if waxy lipid deposits are thought to be responsible for impaired catheter flow, 1 to 3 mL of 70% ethanol can restore patency.[143]

Other problems such as air embolism may occur at anytime if there is a central catheter present. Catheter-related infection/sepsis is always a possibility for the critically ill patient with a central vein catheter. Hyperthermia, tachypnea, tachycardia, leukocytosis with "left shift," and the presence of shaking and chills all may occur in patients who have catheter-related sepsis. With the presence of the above signs, most practitioners would "change out" the central catheter using a sterile guidewire and culture the tip of the removed catheter, as well as a central and peripheral blood culture for definitive diagnosis. If the catheter tip grows a pathologic organism with >15 colony-forming units, the replaced catheter should be removed after obtaining central access at a new site. If catheter removal is undesirable because of limited vascular access, recommendations from the Centers for Disease Control (CDC) are available for quantitative blood culturing techniques to assist the clinical in diagnosis of a catheter-related bloodstream infection (CR-BSI).[144] Testing of paired blood samples is required. Criteria for the presence of a CR-BSI is met if the colony count obtained via the central catheter is five-to ten-fold greater than the sample obtained from the peripheral vein.

## FORMULA PREPARATION

### Components

The PN admixture is made from a complex combination of macronutrients (dextrose, amino acids, and fat emulsion), micronutrients (electrolytes, vitamins, trace elements), and water. Hydrated dextrose is the most frequently used parenteral carbohydrate in the world for the preparation of PN. Fructose, sorbitol, and xylitol are other carbohydrates that have been used with varying success in PN. Each gram of hydrated dextrose yields 3.4 kcal. Stock solutions of dextrose for the preparation of PN come in strengths varying from $D_{10}W$ to $D_{70}W$. Many institutions that make PN solutions with an automated compounder stock only $D_{70}W$ because it can be diluted with sterile water for injection to make many different final concentrations of dextrose, even odd

**TABLE 66-9**

**Available Intravenous Fat Emulsions in the United States**

| TRADE NAME | SOURCE | STRENGTH | KCAL/ML | GLYCERIN (%) | EGG PHOS (%) |
|---|---|---|---|---|---|
| Intralipid | Soybean | 10% | 1.1 | 2.25 | 1.2 |
|  |  | 20% | 2.0 | 2.25 | 1.2 |
|  |  | 30% | 3.0 | 2.25 | 1.2 |
| Liposyn II | Soybean/ safflower | 10% | 1.1 | 2.5 | 1.2 |
|  |  | 20% | 2.0 | 2.5 | 1.2 |
| Liposyn III | Soybean | 10% | 1.1 | 2.5 | 1.2 |
|  |  | 20% | 2.0 | 2.5 | 1.2 |

strengths such as $D_{17}W$. As previously mentioned, dextrose administration in PN should not exceed 5 mg/kg/minute (approximately 25 kcal/kg/day).[22] Many critical care practitioners administer dextrose at a slightly lower dose routinely (e.g., 3 to 4 mg/kg/minute) to minimize $CO_2$ production, lipogenesis, and hyperglycemia.

Intravenous fat emulsions (IVFE) are used in PN to provide essential fatty acids and to provide another source of nonprotein calories. The commercially available IVFE in the United States are either soybean oil emulsions or a combination of soybean/safflower oil emulsions. The current products and their pertinent characteristics are listed in Table 66-9. These products are available as 10, 20, and 30% IVFE. The 10 and 20% IVFE may be infused directly into a patient's vein or added to dextrose and amino acids to make a total nutrient admixture (TNA). The 30% IVFE can only be used as part of a TNA in the United States; however, it is approved for direct vein infusion in Europe. Fat is a concentrated calorie source by providing 9 kcal/g. The maximum dose of IVFE in adults is 2.5 g/kg/day; however, most clinicians caring for critically ill patients administer approximately 1 g/kg/day as either a continuous infusion or as part of a TNA administered over 24 hours in each case. Considerable controversy exists regarding the effects of IVFE on immune function. Bactericidal and migratory functions of polymorphonuclear cells and decreased bacterial clearance have been demonstrated in patients who have received excessively high or rapidly infused doses of IVFE. To date, these changes have not demonstrated significant effects on patient outcome; however, clinicians are usually cautious with the infusion of IVFE in critically ill patients. Patients who have acute respiratory distress syndrome (ARDS) should have IVFE given in lower doses (0.5 to 1 g/kg/day as a continuous infusion) because problems with oxygenation have been reported when rapid infusions (3 mg/kg/minute) have been given.[145] Currently available forms of IVFE contain mainly omega-6 fatty acids, which result in products that can induce inflammation and immunosuppression. Again, cautious administration of IVFE appears to be safe and efficacious in critically ill trauma patients.

Vitamins are necessary for normal metabolism and cellular function. There are currently 13 known vitamins, with vitamin $B_{12}$ being the last one isolated, in 1948. Trauma patients receiving PN should receive a parenteral multivitamin preparation daily. Most commercially available products for adults contain 12 of the 13 known vitamins (all except vitamin K). In April 2000, the U.S. Food and Drug Administration (FDA) amended requirements for marketing of an "effective" adult parenteral multivitamin formulation and recommended changes to the 12-vitamin formulation that has

**TABLE 66-10**

| Parenteral Vitamins Recommended By New FDA Guidelines | |
|---|---|
| **VITAMIN** | **DOSE** |
| Vitamin A | 3300 International Units (1mg retinol) |
| Vitamin $D_2$ | 200 International Units (5 $\mu$g cholecalciferol) |
| Vitamin E | 10 mg (alpha-tocopherol) |
| Thiamin | 6 mg |
| Riboflavin($B_2$) | 3.6 mg |
| Pyridoxine($B_6$) | 6 mg |
| Niacin | 40 mg |
| Pantothenate | 15 mg |
| Biotin | 60 $\mu$g |
| Folate | 600 $\mu$g |
| Cyanocobalamin ($B_{12}$) | 5 $\mu$g |
| Ascorbic acid (C) | 200 mg |

been available for over 20 years.[146] The new requirements for increased dosages of vitamins $B_1$, $B_6$, C, and folic acid as well as addition of vitamin K are based upon the recommendations from a 1985 workshop sponsored jointly by the American Medical Association's (AMA) Division of Personal and Public Health Policy and the FDA's Division of Metabolic and Endocrine Drug Products. Specific modifications of the previous formulation include increasing the provision of ascorbic acid (vitamin C) from 100 to 200 mg/day, pyridoxine (vitamin $B_6$) from 4 to 6 mg/day, thiamine (vitamin $B_1$) from 3 to 6 mg/day, folic acid from 400 to 600 $\mu$g/day, and addition of phylloquinone (vitamin K) 150 $\mu$g/day (Table 66–10). When the 12-vitamin formulation is being used, vitamin K can be given individually as a daily dose (0.5 to 1 mg) or a weekly dose (5 to 10 mg given once weekly). Patients who are to receive warfarin should be monitored more closely when receiving vitamin K to ensure the appropriate level of anticoagulation is maintained. It is reasonable to supplement the PN with thiamine (25 to 50 mg/day) in trauma patients who have a history of alcohol abuse, especially when they did not receive thiamine at admission, or in times of parenteral multivitamin shortages (common in the United States in the 1990s).

The United States has been plagued with two periods of short supply of multiple vitamin products in the 1990s. This has resulted in vitamin deficiencies in patients receiving PN without parenteral vitamins. Several recommendations emanated from the American Society for Parenteral and Enteral Nutrition (ASPEN) following the latest parenteral vitamin shortage, which began in 1996: (a) the use of oral multivitamins when possible, especially liquid multivitamins via feeding tubes; (b) restriction of the use of multivitamin products in PN during periods of short supply, such as one infusion three times per week; (3) administration of thiamine, ascorbate, niacin, pyridoxine, and folic acid daily as individual entities in the PN during periods of short supply; and (4) administration of vitamin $B_{12}$ at least once per month during periods of short supply. The shortage in 1996–1998 was caused by one manufacturer that stopped making its multivitamin product and another that was unable to meet the national demand because of manufacturing difficulties.

Trace elements are usually provided daily during PN in trauma patients as a cocktail of four or five separate metals. Trace element cocktails providing zinc, copper, manganese, chromium, and selenium should be given daily to most trauma patients receiving PN. Patients who have sustained small bowel or large bowel fluid losses should receive supplemental zinc (5 to 10 mg/day) in addition to the amount in the trace element cocktail (3 to 5 mg/day). Provision of large intakes of trace elements to thermal injury patients may facilitate wound healing and decrease length of hospital stay. Based upon exudative losses from burn wounds, one group of investigators increased daily intakes of copper (4.5 mg), selenium (187 $\mu$g), and zinc (39 mg). A reduction in grafting requirements and total hospital days (45 $\pm$ 16 days vs. 57 $\pm$ 27 days, $p < 0.05$) was observed in the supplemented group versus the group receiving standard trace element intakes.[147] Patients who have hepatic cholestasis should have copper and manganese withheld from the PN solution because these trace elements are excreted in the bile. Neurologic damage from deposition of manganese in the basal ganglia has been reported in PN patients with chronic liver disease or cholestasis.[148] Parenteral molybdenum and iodine are also available; however, these trace elements are usually reserved for long-term PN patients if they are used at all.

Water is a vital component for life and an important part of the PN formula. Trauma patients who require PN will vary considerably in their water requirements. Fluid balance should be assessed by intake and output and hemodynamic monitoring as appropriate. In many cases the trauma patient is septic and has difficulty in mobilizing fluid from third spaces. This results in edema and fluid overload. The PN prescription for these patients should be maximally concentrated and be void of free water if possible. This can be accomplished by using only the most concentrated macronutrients (e.g., D70W, 15% amino acids, 30% IVFE) for the preparation of the PN formula. Other patients, such as those with multiple GI drains or fistulas, may have water and salt requirements that exceed that provided by standard PN solutions that can meet nutritional needs. In this case, an additional intravenous fluid such as 0.45% sodium chloride injection will need to be used as a fluid supplement to keep the patient in proper water and sodium balance.

## Examples of PN Formulas

There are several ways in which to prescribe PN formulas. Each institution or health care system will usually have a single method that is preferable for the respective pharmacy. Many health care systems use a preprinted order form to minimize confusion for the prescriber, especially where there are multiple prescribers. The examples used in this chapter are expressed in final concentrations of the respective macronutrients. This appears to be an effective

**TABLE 66-11**

| Examples of TPN Formulas Used in Trauma Patients | | | |
|---|---|---|---|
| **TYPE** | **CARBOHYDRATE** | **PROTEIN** | **FAT** |
| Standard #1 | $D_{20}W$ | $AA^a$ 5% | Lipids 2% |
| Standard #2 | $D_{15}W$ | AA 5% | Lipids 3% |
| Concentrated | $D_{30}W$ | AA 6% | Lipids 4% |
| $ARF^b$-no dialysis | $D_{30}W$ | AA 2% | Lipids 2% |
| $ARF^b$- dialysis | $D_{30}W$ | AA 4% | Lipids 2% |

$^a$Amino acids.
$^b$Acute renal failure.

way of teaching these concepts in systems with multiple pre-scribers or where there are a few prescribers who change services every month. Table 66-11 lists several PN formulas that have been used for critically ill trauma patients. PN formulas containing between $D_{15}W$–$D_{25}W$, 4 to 5% amino acids, and 2 to 3% lipids are usually suitable for trauma patients with normal organ function and relatively normal fluid balance. Electrolyte components of PN may vary considerably in these types of patients depending on serum concentrations, concomitant drug therapy, acid-base status, preinjury nutritional status, and extrarenal losses of fluid and electrolytes.

## INSTITUTION OF THERAPY

Most patients can be started on PN and advanced to a desired goal over two to three days. A reasonable initiation rate is 25 to 50 mL/hour for 12 to 24 hour. If glucose homeostasis is reasonable, the PN rate can be advanced by 25 to 40 mL/hour/day until the desired goal is reached. For example, an 80-kg critically ill trauma patient with normal organ function and serum electrolyte concentrations may have a PN formula ($D_{15}W$, amino acids 5%, lipids 2%) started at 50 mL/hour, advanced to 85 mL/hour on day 2, and then advanced to the desired goal of 115 mL/hour on day 3. A different approach would be taken for the fluid-over-loaded, hyperglycemic, septic trauma patient with normal renal function. The PN would be concentrated ($D_{30}W$, amino acids 6%, lipids 4%), undoubtedly have regular insulin added to it (or coinfused with an infusion of insulin), and initiated at a low rate such as 15 to 25 mL/hour. This PN formula would be advanced slowly (e.g., 25 mL/hour/day) based on patient clinical status, glucose tolerance, and fluid balance.

## COMPLICATIONS OF PARENTERAL NUTRITION AND THEIR TREATMENT

The complications of PN are often divided into three broad categories: mechanical, metabolic, and infectious. The major mechanical and infectious complications are covered in the section on access and monitoring lines, above, and are therefore not repeated here.

### Glucose

The most common metabolic complication of PN is glucose homeostasis. Hyperglycemia is a common finding in critically ill patients receiving PN not only because of the administered dextrose, but because of the accompanying stress associated with injury (e.g., increased corticosteroids, cytokines), dextrose administration from intravenous fluids and medications, chronic diseases such as diabetes, and coadministration of drugs which can exacerbate glucose homeostasis such as glucocorticosteroids. One recent study reported that patients receiving PN with higher glucose doses demonstrated hyperglycemia and complications associated with this disorder.[149] A landmark trial has shown benefits from strict glycemic control in ICU patients receiving specialized nutrition support (i.e., PN and EN). Intensive insulin therapy which

### TABLE 66-12

| Algorithm for Regular Insulin Administration | | | |
|---|---|---|---|
| PLASMA GLUCOSE, MG/DL | SQ INSULIN DOSE, UNITS[a] | IV BOLUS INSULIN DOSE, UNITS[b] | INSULIN INFUSION RATE, UNITS/h |
| <79[c] | 1 ampule $D_{50}W$ | 1 ampule $D_{50}W$ | 1 ampule $D_{50}W$ |
| 80–99 | No treatment | No treatment | Discontinue |
| 101–120 | No treatment | No treatment | Discontinue |
| 121–150 | No treatment | No treatment | 1 |
| 151–200 | 2 | 2 | 2 |
| 201–250 | 4 | 4 | 4 |
| 251–300 | 8 | 6 | 6 |
| 301–350 | 12 | 8 | 8 |
| 351–400 | 16 | 10 | 10 |
| >400[c] | 20 | 12 | 12 |

[a]SQ administration of regular insulin should not be more often than every 4 h.
[b]IV administration of regular insulin should not be more often than every 1 h.
[c]Notify the physician and order a stat serum glucose.

maintained serum glucose levels between 80–110 mg/dL were compared to conventional treatment which maintained glucose between 180–200 mg/dL). Intensive therapy reduced mortality from 8% to 4.6% ($p < 0.04$), primarily in the cardiac patients. The mean glucose concentrations would not appear to be different enough to be clinically significant (intensive insulin therapy group: 103 ± 19 mg/dL vs. conventional treatment group: 153 ± 33 mg/dL). However, in addition to survival benefits, other positive clinical outcomes included a 46% reduction in bloodstream infections, a 41% reduction in acute renal failure requiring hemodialysis or hemofiltration, and a 44% reduction in critical-illness polyneuropathy. As a result, many clinicians have changed their clinical practice to initiate insulin therapy when serum glucose concentrations exceed 150 mg/dL rather than 200 mg/dL.[150]

There are several options to treat hyperglycemia and glucosuria during PN in the critically ill trauma patient. We administer regular insulin intravenously or subcutaneously when the glucose values exceed 150 mg/dL or glucosuria becomes moderate to severe (500 mg/dL or greater).[151] Table 66-12 contains an algorithm for intravenous or subcutaneous administration of regular insulin. While fingersticks for glucose are routinely checked every six hours in most patients, it can be increased to every three or four hours in patients that need better control. If regular human insulin is added directly to the PN solution, usually begin with 0.1 unit of insulin per gram of dextrose (i.e., 15 units/liter of 15% dextrose, 20 units/liter of 20% dextrose). A continuous insulin infusion of regular human insulin is used in patients who continue to be intolerant with the above interventions (see Table 66-13). Strategies other than insulin drips have been recommended for optimizing glycemic control in patients receiving PN.[152] Avoiding overfeeding

### TABLE 66-13

| Equation for Calculating Nitrogen Balance |
|---|

$$\text{Nitrogen balance (g)} = \frac{\text{protein intake (g)}}{6.25 \text{ (conversion factor)}} - \begin{bmatrix} \text{urinary excretion} \\ \text{of urea nitrogen (g)} + 4 \end{bmatrix}$$

Note: The 4 g in this equation is used as a "fudge factor" to account for skin, fecal, and non—urea nitrogen losses. The conversion factor for 6.25 g of protein = 1 g nitrogen.)

with hypocaloric regimens for obese patients and limiting caloric goals to 25 total kcal/kg/day for nonobese individuals have been effective. Dextrose should be restricted to less than 200 g on day 1 of PN, with patients at high risk for hyperglycemia (i.e., history of diabetes, corticosteroid use, etc.) receiving no more than 100 g/day. When baseline serum glucose concentrations exceed 300 mg/dL, PN should be instituted when serum glucose concentrations are below 200 mg/dL. Daily intake of dextrose calories should be advanced toward goal only when serum glucose concentrations can be maintained under this level.

Patients who have experienced significant glucosuria resulting in an osmotic diuresis will often need to be supplemented with intravenous fluid to prevent dehydration. Intravenous solutions like 0.45% sodium chloride or 0.22% sodium chloride injection are very effective in these situations.

## Essential Fatty Acid Deficiency

As long as at least 2–4% of total calories from PN are given as essential fatty acids (i.e., linoleic acid and linolenic acid), essential fatty acid deficiency (EFAD) should be prevented. Most trauma patients will receive from 15 to 25% of total calories as intravenous fat emulsion (IVFE) during PN, which easily prevents EFAD and also provides a source of nonprotein calories. Occasionally, a critically ill patient who is receiving PN will have sustained hypertriglyceridemia (e.g., >500 mg/dL). Most practitioners would withhold intravenous lipid in this situation until the serum triglyceride concentration falls below 400 mg/dL. After two weeks of fat-free PN in the adult, biochemical evidence of EFAD occurs, with symptoms following as early as one week later. Some practitioners have administered small doses of intravenous lipid cautiously to prevent EFAD during hypertriglyceridemia, while others have attempted to give essential fatty acids with the topical administration of safflower or sunflower oil.

## Micronutrient Deficiencies

Zinc is a trace element that is concentrated in small and large bowel fluids. Patients who have substantial ostomy losses are prone to develop zinc deficiency and should be supplemented with extra zinc in the PN solution. The stress of injury will cause enhanced urinary excretion of zinc so the recommendation is to give at least 5 mg/day during PN administration in trauma patients. Trauma patients with a history of alcohol abuse who are to receive PN often need supplemental thiamine and folic acid added to the solution over and above standard vitamin additives. Although not widely appreciated, thermal injury patients experience high rates of postburn bone disease. Klein and colleagues recently found that a defect in the skin conversion of 7-dehydrocholesterol into previtamin D3.[153] In children with a mean time of 14 months after their burn injury, skin 7-dehydrocholesterol was significantly lower in the burn scar than in unburned controls, and previtamin D3 was significantly lower than controls in both burn scar and unburned skin adjacent to the scar. Low serum 25-hydroxyvitamin D concentrations were also found. Obviously, adults are at risk for developing postburn bone disease, especially in women after menopause and as both men and women attain ages beyond 50 years old. These findings also suggest that vitamin D supplementation should be encouraged to prevent bone disease in this particular population of patients.

## TRANSITION TO ENTERAL NUTRITION

Most trauma patients who receive PN have a GI tract that becomes functional with recovery. Nasogastric tubes for suction can be removed as the patient regains bowel function. As oral nutrition is introduced and progressed, weaning of the PN solution becomes an important issue. Generally, weaning of PN only begins when the trauma patient has demonstrated tolerance to at least a full liquid diet (i.e., one that can be nutritionally complete). Once the patient is ingesting at least one-half a nutritionally complete diet, the PN can be decreased to a lower rate. As the patient approaches an intake of two-thirds to three-fourths of the diet, the PN can be discontinued.

Many trauma patients will be unable to or will not eat orally when the GI tract is recovering. These patients become excellent candidates for enteral tube feeding, either temporarily until oral intake is established or permanently in the patient in a chronic vegetative state where the decision has been made to provide adequate nutrition. Generally, the PN solution is weaned as the rate of enteral tube feeding is increased. This way the patient continues to receive adequate nutrition during the transition to nutritional support via the GI tract. Once patients are receiving three-fourths to complete enteral nutrition, the PN can be discontinued. Most trauma patients eventually progress to an oral diet and ingest sufficient amounts so that the enteral tube feeding can be discontinued as well.

## MONITORING THERAPY

The fluid administered during PN in critically ill patients provides anywhere from 50 to 95% of the patient's intake once the goal rate is attained. Therefore, all general monitoring measurements become exceedingly important to the critical care practitioner responsible for prescribing the administration of PN. Fluid status and fluid balance should be assessed each day in critically ill trauma patients. The PN formula should be concentrated and reduced in sodium for the overloaded patients. Patients who are euvolemic but require large volumes of fluid can have the PN solution administered with addition of IVF to keep the patient in proper water balance. Laboratory measurements for glucose, sodium, potassium, acid/base status, and renal function should be done daily in the critically ill trauma patient. Laboratory measurements for calcium, phosphorus, magnesium should be performed at least three times a week, while triglyceride concentrations should be assessed weekly during the acute phase of injury in this patient population.

After collection of a 24-hour urine for volume and urea nitrogen, nitrogen balance can be calculated by finding the difference between nitrogen intake from PN (and enteral tube feeding or oral intake if applicable)[154] and nitrogen output (see Table 66-13). Generally, nitrogen equilibrium in the young, stressed, previously healthy trauma patient is an appropriate goal. Patients who have spinal cord or severe head injuries will remain in negative nitrogen balance even when a dose of protein of 2 g/kg/day is given because of disuse atrophy. Nitrogen equilibrium usually can be attained three to four weeks after injury in these cases.

Other practitioners favor the serial monitoring of serum proteins during administration of PN. Serum albumin concentration is usually depressed following trauma mainly due to redistribution from the intravascular space to the interstitial space. It takes several months for this protein to normalize, so it is not a good marker of nutrition support efficacy. Serum proteins with short half-lives like prealbumin (two days) and transferrin (seven days) have the potential of rising acutely with adequate nutritional support. They are also very sensitive to the clinical course of the patient and will rise and fall independently of nutrition intake when the patient is recovering or decompensating, respectively. Assessment of C-reactive protein (CRP) will help determine whether the decline in short-term serum proteins (i.e., prealbumin) is associated with an acute-phase response or nutritional deficiency. CRP is recognized as a positive acute-phase protein, defined as one whose plasma concentration increases by at least 25% during inflammatory disorders. If CRP is elevated and prealbumin has fallen, this is more indicative of the systemic response to inflammation.[155] However, a falling prealbumin with a concurrent low CRP concentration may represent an inadequate intake of energy or protein. Use of these basic principles can assist the clinician in determining the appropriate time to alter a patient's nutritional regimen.

## ANABOLIC AGENTS IN TRAUMA PATIENTS

It is recognized that standard nutritional support in patients subjected to severe trauma rarely allows them to attain nitrogen equilibrium during the first two weeks following injury. In fact, some severely injured patients may lose up to 30 to 40 g of nitrogen per day during the early flow phase of injury. Because there are toxicities associated with excessive administration of specialized nutrition support, anabolic agents as adjunctive therapy with parenteral or enteral nutrition to enhance recovery have been considered. There are some data supporting the administration of growth hormone, IGF-I, or anabolic steroids to patients with polytrauma. Petersen et al. reported significantly improved nitrogen balance and whole body protein synthesis following the administration of growth hormone with parenteral nutrition when compared to a group receiving parenteral nutrition alone.[156] Our work has shown that growth hormone affects visceral protein status and increases serum albumin in critically injured patients but has relatively little effect upon nitrogen retention in severely immobilized patients.[157,158] Unfortunately, patients receiving growth hormone tended to be hyperglycemic, particularly if there were infectious complications. The safety of growth hormone therapy use has been further questioned based upon two well-designed multicenter trials conducted in Europe, which reported an increase in mortality among critically ill patients treated with growth hormone. These two independent, prospective, double-blind, randomized trials were conducted in parallel involving 247 Finnish patients and 285 patients from other European countries, and the results were published as one report in the *New England Journal of Medicine*. A total of 532 critically ill patients received high-dose growth hormone ($0.1 \pm 0.02$ mg/kg/day) or placebo until discharge from the ICU or for a maximum of 21 days. In the Finnish study, mortality rate was significantly higher in the growth hormone group as compared with the placebo group (39% vs. 20%, $p < 0.001$).[159] A similar finding was observed in the multinational study conducted in other European countries, with a 44% mortality rate in the treatment group versus 18% in the placebo group. Previous trials in ICU patients and thermal injury patients demonstrated

improvements in lean tissue mass accretion or wound healing and none demonstrated a decrease in survival. Herndon et al. have demonstrated improved healing of donor sites and shorter length of stay/ percent burn in thermally injured children who received recombinant growth hormone as adjunctive therapy to nutrition support.[160] However, the Finnish and multinational studies excluded patients with burns or septic shock and trauma patients accounted for less than 10% of the total population. Demographic data also revealed that 95% of patients from both trials combined had respiratory failure on enrollment and the average age of patients was 60 years. Despite these differences in patient characteristics and study methodology, these results sharply diminished the enthusiasm of practitioners to use recombinant growth hormone therapy in adult trauma patients.

Much of the effects of growth hormone occur because of IGF-I. IGF-I is produced by the liver in response to growth hormone but does not have the hyperglycemic effects induced by direct growth hormone administration. In a phase II safety and efficacy trial using IGF-I in patients with moderate or severe head injury, Hatton et al.[161] reported that patients receiving the hormone had significantly decreased nitrogen excretion. A subset of patients with Glasgow Coma Scale scores of 5 to 7 who received IGF-I demonstrated improved neurologic outcome at six months postinjury.[162] Administration of the anabolic steroid nandrolone decanoate has been shown to decrease nitrogen excretion in trauma patients.[163] One group of investigators has published several positive studies evaluating the use of oxandrolone, a newer anabolic agent, in thermal injury patients.[163] Reductions in weight loss and net nitrogen loss accompanied by increases in donor site wound healing and rates of weight restoration in the recovery phase have been observed in burn patients (total body surface area burns of 40–70%) receiving oxandrolone 20 mg/day. One study[164] evaluated oxandrolone in multiple trauma patients and showed no significant differences in length of hospital stay, length of ICU stay, body cell mass, nor infectious complications between oxandrolone 20 mg/day or placebo. Thus, more clinical research with IGF-I and anabolic steroids is needed in trauma patients.

## REFERENCES

1. Detsky AS, Smalley PS, Chang J: Is this patient malnourished? *JAMA* 271:54, 1994.
2. Cuthbertson DP: The metabolic response to injury and its nutritional implications: Retrospect and prospect. *JPEN* 3:108, 1979.
3. McClave SA, Snider HL: Understanding the metabolic response to critical illness: Factors that cause patients to deviate from the expected pattern of hypermetabolism. *New Horiz* 2:139, 1994.
4. Deitrick JE, Whedon GD, Shorr E: Effects of immobilization upon various metabolic and physiologic functions of normal men. *Am J Med* 4:3, 1948.
5. Cerra FB: Metabolic and nutritional support. In Mattox KL, Feliciano DV, Moore EE, eds. *Trauma*, 3rd ed. Stamford, CT: Appleton & Lange, 1996, p. 1155.
6. Shaw-Delanty SN, Elwyn DH, Askanazi J, et al.: Resting energy expenditure in injured, septic, and malnourished adult patients on intravenous diets. *Clin Nutr* 9:305, 1990.
7. Frankel WL, Evans NJ, Rombeau JL: Scientific rationale and clinical application of parenteral nutrition in critically ill patients. In Rombeau JL, Caldwell MD, eds. *Clinical Nutrition: Vol 2. Parenteral Nutrition*, 2nd ed. Philadelphia: Saunders, 1993, p. 597.
8. Hershey SD, Moore EE, Jones TN: Nutritional care of the acutely injured. In Maul KI, ed. *Advances in Trauma*. Chicago: Year Book, 1986, p. 21.
9. Moore FD: Bodily changes during surgical convalescence. *Ann Surg* 137:289, 1953.

10. Gann DS, Foster AH: Endocrine and metabolic responses to injury. In Schwartz SI, Shires GT, Spencer FC, et al., eds. *Principles of Surgery*, 6th ed. New York: McGraw-Hill, 1994, p. 3.

11. Shaw JHF, Wolfe RR: An integrated analysis of glucose, fat and protein metabolism in severely traumatized patients: Studies in the basal state and the response to intravenous nutrition. *Ann Surg* 207:63, 1989.

12. Shaw JHF, Klein S, Wolfe RR: Assessment of alanine, urea and glucose inter-relationships in normal subjects and in patients with sepsis with stable isotopic tracers. *Surgery* 97:557, 1985.

13. Threlfall CJ, Maxwell AR, Stoner HB: Post-traumatic creatinuria. *J Trauma* 24:516, 1984.

14. Wilmore DW, Smith RJ, O'Dwyer ST, et al.: The gut: A central organ following surgical stress. *Surgery* 104:917, 1988.

15. Souba WW: Glutamine: A key substrate for the splanchnic bed. *Ann Rev Nutr* 11:285, 1991.

16. Windmueller HG, Spaeth AE: Uptake and metabolism of plasma glutamine by the small intestine. *J Biol Chem* 249:5070, 1974.

17. Van Gool J, Boers W, Ladiges NCJ: Glucocorticoids and catecholamines as mediators of acute-phase proteins, especially rat alpha-macrofoetoprotein. *Biochem J* 220:125, 1984.

18. Long CL, Kinney JM, Geiger JW: Nonsuppressibility of gluconeogenesis by glucose in septic patients. *Metabolism* 25:193, 1976.

19. Shaw JHF, Wolfe RR: Determination of glucose turnover and oxidation in normal volunteers and septic patients using stable and radioisotopes: The response of glucose infusion and total parenteral nutrition. *Aust N Z J Surg* 56:785, 1986.

20. Jahoor F, Herndon DN, Wolfe RR: Role of insulin and glucose in the response of glucose and alanine kinetics in burn injured patients. *J Clin Invest* 78:807, 1986.

21. Shaw JHF, Wolfe RR: Energy and protein metabolism in sepsis and trauma. *Aust N Z J Surg* 57:41, 1987.

22. Wolfe R, O'Donnell T, Stone M, et al.: Investigation of factors determining the optimal glucose infusion rate in total parenteral nutrition. *Metabolism* 29:892, 1980.

23. Stremple JF, Thomas H, Sakach V, et al.: Myocardial utilization of hypertonic glucose during haemorrhagic shock. *Surgery* 80:4, 1976.

24. McNamara JJ, Molot MD, Dunn RA, et al.: Effect of hypertonic glucose in hypovolemic shock in man. *Ann Surg* 176:247, 1972.

25. Frayn KN: Substrate turnover after injury. *Br Med Bull* 41:232, 1985.

26. Stoner HB, Frayn KN, Barton RN, et al.: The relationship between plasma substrates and hormone and the severity of injury in 277 recently injured patients. *Clin Sci* 56:563, 1979.

27. Miller HI, Issekutz B Jr, Paul P: Effect of lactic acid on plasma free fatty acids in pancreatectomized dogs. *Am J Physiol* 3:857, 1967.

28. Nanni G, Siegel JH, Coleman B, et al.: Increased lipid fuel dependence in the critically ill septic patient. *J Trauma* 24:14, 1984.

29. Kinsella JE, Lokesh B, Broughton S, et al.: Dietary polyunsaturated fatty acids and eicosanoids: Potential effect on the modulation of inflammatory and immune cells: An overview. *Nutrition* 6:24, 1990.

30. Gurr MI: The role of lipids in the regulation of the immune system. *Prog Lipid Res* 22:257, 1983.

31. Kenler AS, Swails WS, Driscoll DF, et al.: Early enteral feeding in postsurgical cancer patients: Fish oil structured lipid-based polymeric formula versus a standard polymeric formula. *Ann Surg* 223:316, 1996.

32. The Veteran Affairs Total Parenteral Nutrition Cooperative Study Group: Perioperative total parenteral nutrition in surgical patients. *N Engl J Med* 325:525, 1991.

33. Kudsk KA, Croce MA, Fabian TC, et al.: Enteral vs. parenteral feeding: Effects on septic morbidity following blunt and penetrating abdominal trauma. *Ann Surg* 215:503, 1992.

34. Moore FA, Moore EE, Jones TN: Benefits of immediate jejunostomy feeding after major abdominal trauma—A prospective randomized study. *J Trauma* 26:874, 1986.

35. Moore FA, Moore EE, Jones TN, et al.: TEN vs. PN following major abdominal trauma—reduced septic morbidity. *J Trauma* 29:916, 1989.

36. Moore FA, Feliciano DV, Andrassy RJ, et al.: Early enteral feeding, compared with parenteral, reduces postoperative septic complications: The results of a meta-analysis. *Ann Surg* 216:172, 1992.

37. Kudsk KA, Minard G, Croce MA: A randomized trial of isonitrogenous enteral diets following severe trauma: An immune-enhancing diet (IED) reduces septic complications. *Ann Surg* 224:531, 1996.

38. Moore FA, Moore EE, Kudsk KA, et al.: Clinical benefits of an immune-enhancing diet for early postinjury enteral feeding. *J Trauma* 37:607, 1994.

39. Alexander JW, Macmillan BG, Stinnett JD, et al.: Beneficial effects of aggressive protein feeding in severely burned children. *Ann Surg* 192:505, 1980.

40. Border JR, Hassett J, LaDuca J, et al.: The gut origin septic states in blunt multiple trauma (ISS=40) in the ICU. *Ann Surg* 206:427, 1987.

41. Adams S, Dellinger EP, Wertz MJ, et al.: Enteral versus parenteral nutritional support following laparotomy for trauma: A randomized prospective trial. *J Trauma* 26:882, 1986.

42. Fagon JY, Chastre J, Domart Y, et al.: Nosocomial pneumonia in patients receiving continuous mechanical ventilation: Prospective analysis of 52 episodes with use of a protected specimen brush and quantitative culture techniques. *Am Rev Respir Dis* 139:877, 1989.

43. Eyer SD, Micon LT, Konstantinides FN, et al.: Early enteral feeding does not attenuate metabolic response after blunt trauma. *J Trauma* 34:639, 1993.

44. Borlase BC, Moore EE, Moore FA: The Abdominal Trauma Index—A critical reassessment and validation. *J Trauma* 30:1340, 1990.

45. Rapp RP, Young B, Twymand D, et al.: The favorable effect of early parenteral feeding on survival in head injured patients. *J Neurosurg* 58:906, 1983.

46. Young B, Ott L, Twyman D, et al.: The effect of nutritional support on outcome from severe head injury. *J Neurosurg* 67:668, 1987.

47. Grahm TW, Zadrozny DB, Harrington T: The benefits of early jejunal hyperalimentation in the head-injured patient. *Neurosurgery* 25:729, 1989.

48. Borzotta AP, Pennings J, Papasadero B, et al.: Enteral versus parenteral nutrition after severe closed head injury. *J Trauma* 37:459, 1994.

49. Minard G, Kudsk KA, Melton S, et al.: Early versus delayed feeding with an immune-enhancing diet in patients with severe head injuries. *JPEN* 24:145, 2000.

50. Herndon DN, Barrow RE, Stein M, et al.: Increased mortality with intravenous supplemental feeding in severely burned patients. *J Burn Care Rehabil* 10:309, 1989.

51. McDonald WS, Sharp CW Jr, Deitch EA: Immediate enteral feeding in burn patients is safe and effective. *Ann Surg* 213:177, 1991.

52. Saito H, Trocki O, Alexander JW, et al.: The effect of route of nutrient administration of the nutritional state, catabolic hormone secretion, and gut mucosal integrity after burn injury. *JPEN* 11:1, 1987.

53. Kirk SJ, Barbul A: Role of arginine in trauma, sepsis, and immunity. *JPEN* 14:226S, 1990.

54. Cerra FB, Aldon PA, Negro F, et al.: Clinical sepsis, endogenous and exogenous lipid modulation. *JPEN* 12:63S, 1988.

55. Kulkarni AD, Fanslow WC, Drath DB, et al.: Influence of dietary nucleotide restriction on bacterial sepsis and phagocytic cell function in mice. *Arch Surg* 121:169, 1986.

56. Daly JM, Lieberman MD, Goldfine J, et al.: Enteral nutrition with supplemental arginine, RNA, and omega-3 fatty acids in patients after operation: Immunologic, metabolic, and clinical outcome. *Surgery* 112:56, 1992.

57. Bower RH, Cerra FB, Bershadsky B, et al.: Early enteral administration of a formula supplemented with arginine, nucleotides, and fish oil in intensive care unit patients: Results of a multicenter prospective, randomized, clinical trial. *Crit Care Med* 23:436, 1995.

58. Gottschlich MM, Jenkins M, Warden GD, et al.: Differential effects of three enteral dietary regimens on selected outcome variables in burn patients. *JPEN* 14:225, 1990.

59. Houdijk AP, Rijnsburger ER, Jansen J, et al.: Randomised trial of glutamine-enriched nutrition on infectious morbidity in patients with multiple trauma. *Lancet* 352:772, 1998.

60. Mendez C, Jurkovich GJ, Garcia I, et al.: Effects of an immune-enhancing diet in critically injured patients. *J Trauma* 42:933, 1997.

61. Heyland DK, Dhaliwal R, Drover JW, et al.: Canadian Clinical Practice Guidelines for nutrition support in mechanically ventilated, critically ill adult patients. *JPEN* 27:355, 2003.

62. Bower RH, Cerra FB, Bershadsky B, et al.: Early enteral administration of a formula supplemented with arginine, nucleotides, and fish oil in intensive care unit patients: Results of a multicenter prospective, randomized, clinical trial. *Crit Care Med* 23:436, 1995.

63. Dent DL, Heyland DK, Levy H, et al.: Immunonutrition may increase mortality in critically ill patients with pneumonia: Results of a randomized trial. *Crit Care Med* 30:17, 2003 (Abstract).

64. Bertolini G, Lapichino G, Radrizzani D, et al.: Early immunonutrition in patients with severe sepsis: Results of as interim analysis of a randomized multicenter clinical trial. *Int Care Med* 29:834, 2003.

65. Galban C, Montejo JC, Mesejo A, et al.: An immune-enhancing enteral diet reduces mortality rate and episodes of bacteremia in septic intensive care unit patients. *Cri Care Med.* 28:643, 2000.

66. Atkinson S, Sieffert E, Bihari D: A prospective randomized, double-blind controlled clinical trial of enteral immunonutrition in the critically ill. *Crit Care Med* 26:1164, 1998.

67. van der Hulst RRWJ, von Meyenfeldt MF, van Kreel BK, et al.: Glutamine and the preservation of gut integrity. *Lancet* 341:1363, 1993.

68. Johnson LR, Copeland EM, Dudrick SJ, et al.: Structural and hormonal alterations in the gastrointestinal tract of parenteral fed rats. *Gastroenterology* 68:1177, 1975.

69. Tinckler LF: Surgery and intestinal motility. *Br J Surg* 52:140, 1965.

70. Janu P, Li J, Minard G, et al.: Systemic interleukin-6 (IL-6) correlates with intestinal permeability. *Surg Forum* 47:7, 1996.

71. Deitch EA: Does the gut protect or injure patients in the ICU? *Perspect Crit Care* 1:1, 1988.

72. Moore FA, Moore EE, Poggetti R, et al.: Gut bacterial translocation via the portal vein: A clinical perspective with major torso trauma. *Trauma* 31:629, 1991.

73. Brandgtzaeg P, Halstensen TS, Kett K, et al.: Immunobiology and immunopathology of human gut mucosa: Humoral immunity and intraepithelial lymphocytes. *Gastroenterology* 97:1562, 1989.

74. Li J, Gocinski B, Henken B, et al.: Effects of parenteral nutrition on gut-associated lymphoid tissue. *J Trauma* 39:44, 1995.

75. Svanborg C: Bacterial adherence and mucosal immunity. In Ogra PL, Lamm ME, McGhee JR, et al., eds. *Handbook of Mucosal Immunology*. San Diego, CA: Academic Press, 1974, p. 71.

76. Li J, Kudsk KA, Hamidian M, et al.: Bombesin affects mucosal immunity and gut-associated lymphoid tissue in IV-fed mice. *Arch Surg* 130:1164, 1995.

77. Kudsk KA, Li J, Renegar KB: Loss of upper respiratory tract immunity with parenteral feeding. *Ann Surg* 223:629, 1996.

78. Lin M-T, Saito H, Fukushima R, et al.: Route of nutritional supply influences local, systemic, and remote organ responses to intraperitoneal bacterial challenge. *Ann Surg* 223:84, 1996.

79. Fong Y, Marano MA, Barber E, et al.: Total parenteral nutrition and bowel rest modify the metabolic response to endotoxin in humans. *Ann Surg* 210:449, 1989.

80. Marshall JC, Christou NV, Horn R, et al.: The microbiology of multiple organ failure: The proximal gastrointestinal tract as an occult reservoir of pathogens. *Arch Surg* 123:309, 1988.

81. Wu Y, Kudsk KA, DeWitt RC, et al.: Route and type of nutrition influence IgA-mediating intestinal cytokines. *Ann Surg* 229:662, 1999.

82. Fakatsu K, Zarzaur BL, Johnson CD, et al.: Enteral nutrition prevents remote organ injury and death after gut ischemic insult. *Ann Surg* 233:660, 2001.

83. Moore EE, Moore FA, Franciose RJ, et al.: The postischemic gut serves as a priming bed for circulating neutrophils that provoke multiple organ failure. *J Trauma* 37:881, 1994.

84. Kompan L, Kremzar B, Gadzijev E, et al.: Effects of early enteral nutrition on intestinal permeability and the development of multiple organ failure after multiple injury. *Intens Care Med* 25:157, 1999.

85. Hunter DC, Jaksik T, Lewis D, et al.: Resting energy expenditure in the critically ill: Estimations versus measurement. *Br J Surg* 75:875, 1988.

86. Hwang T-L, Hwang S-L, Chen M-F: The use of indirect colorimetry in critically ill patients—Relationship with measured energy expenditure to injury severity score, a septic severity score, and Apache II score. *J Trauma* 34:247, 1993.

87. Campbell SM, Kudsk KA: "High tech" metabolic measurements: Useful in daily clinical practice? *JPEN* 12:610, 1988.

88. Roulet M, Detsky AS, Marliss EB, et al.: A controlled trial of the effect of parenteral nutritional support on patients with respiratory failure and sepsis. *Clin Nutr* 2:97, 1983.

89. Long CL, Schaffel N, Geiger JW, et al.: Metabolic response to injury and illness: Estimation of energy and protein needs from indirect calorimetry and nitrogen balance. *JPEN* 3:452, 1979.

90. Wolfe R, Allsop J, Burke J: Glucose metabolism in man: Responses to intravenous glucose infusion. *Metabolism* 28:210, 1979.

91. Wolfe RR, Shaw JHF: Glucose and FFA in kinetics in sepsis: Role of glucagon and sympathetic nervous system activity. *Am J Physiol* 248:E236, 1985.

92. Shaw SN, Elwyn DH, Askanazi J, et al.: Effects of increasing nitrogen inrtake on nitrogen balance and enery expenditure in nutritionally depleted adult patients receiving parenteral nutrition. *Am J Clin Nutr* 37:930, 1983.

93. Dickerson RN, Rosato EF, Mullen JL: Net protein anabolism with hypocaloric parenteral nutrition in obese stressed patients. *Am J Clin Nutr* 44:747, 1986.

94. Dickerson RN, Boschert KJ, Kudsk KA, et al.: Hypocaloric enteral tube feeding in critically ill obese patients. *Nutrition* 18:241, 2002.

95. Dickerson RN: Specialized nutrition support in the hospitalized obese patient. *Nutr Clin Pract* 19:245, 2004.

96. Choban PS, Burge JC, Scales D, et al.: Hypoenergetic nutrition support in hospitalized obese patients: A simplified method for clinical application. *Am J Clin Nutr* 66L:546, 1997.

97. Burge JC, Goon A, Choban PS, et al.: Efficacy of hypocaloric total parenteral nutrition in hospitalized obese patients: A prospective, double-blind randomized trial JPEN 18:203, 1994.

98. Liu KJ, Cho MJ, Atten MJ, et al.: Huypocaloric parenteral nutrition support in elderly obese patients. *Am Surg* 66:394, 2000.

99. Pelham LD: Rational use of intravenous fat emulsions. *Am J Hosp Pharm* 38:198, 1981.

100. Talpers SS, Romberger DJ, Dunce SB, et al.: Nutritionally associated increased carbon dioxide production. Excess calories vs. high proportion of carbohydrate calories. *Chest* 102:551, 1992.

101. Allardyce DB: Cholestasis caused by lipid emulsions. *Surg Gynecol Obstet* 154:641, 1982.

102. Carpentier YA, Kinney JM, Siderova VS, et al.: Hypertriglyceridemic clamp: A new model for studying lipid metabolism. *Clin Nutr* 9:1, 1990.

103. Shaw JHF, Widbone M, Wolfe RR: Whole body protein kinetics in severely septic patients. *Ann Surg* 205:288, 1987.

104. Long CL, Jeevanaudan M, Kinney JM: Whole body protein synthesis and catabolism in septic man. *Am J Clin Nutr* 30:1340, 1977.

105. Kellen M, Aronson S, Roizen MF, et al.: Predictive and diagnostic tests of renal failure: A review. *Anesth Analg* 78:134, 1994.

106. Roos AN, Westendorp RG, Frolich M, et al.: Weight changes in critically ill patients evaluated by fluid balances and impedance measurements. *Crit Care Med* 21:871, 1993.

107. Mirtallo JM, Kudsk KA, Ebbert ML: Nutritional support of patients with renal disease. *Clin Pharm* 3:253, 1984.

108. Askanazi J, Elwyn DH, Silverberg BS, et al.: Respiratory distress secondary to a high carbohydrate load: A case report. *JAMA* 243:1444, 1980.

109. Rudman D, Millikan WJ, Richardson TJ, et al.: Elemental balances during intravenous hyperalimentation of underweight adult subjects. *J Clin Invest* 55:99, 1975.

110. Pemberton LB, Pemberton DA (eds): *Treatment of Water, Electrolyte, and Acid-Base Disorders in the Surgical Patient*. New York, McGraw-Hill, 1994, p. 176.

111. Oster JR, Singer I, Fishman LM: Heparin-induced aldosterone suppression and hyperkalemia. *Am J Med* 98:575, 1995.

112. Greenberg S, Reiser IW, Chou SY, et al.: Trimethoprim-sulfamethoxazole induces reversible hyperkalemia. *Ann Intern Med* 119:291, 1993.

113. Sacks GS, Walker J, Dickerson RN, et al.: Observations of hypophosphatemia and its management in nutrition support. *Nutr Clin Pract* 9:105, 1994.

114. Clark CL, Sacks GS, Dickerson RN, et al.: Treatment of hypophosphatemia in patients receiving specialized nutrition support using a graduated dosing scheme: Results from a prospective trial. *Crit Care Med* 23:1504, 1995.

115. Eddy VA, Snell JE, Morris JA: Analysis of complications and long term outcome of trauma patients with needle catheter jejunostomy. *Am Surg* 62:40, 1996.

116. Holmes JH IV, Brundage SI, Yuen P, et al.: Complications of surgical feeding jejunostomy in trauma patients. *J Trauma* 47:1009, 1999.

117. Collier P, Kudsk KA, Glezer J, et al.: Fiber-containing formula and needle catheter jejunostomies: A clinical evaluation. *Nutr Clin Pract* 9:101, 1994.

118. Bodoky G, Harsanyi L, Pap A, et al.: Effect of enteral nutrition on exocrine pancreatic function. *Am J Surg* 161:144, 1991.

119. Jones TN, Moore FA, Moore EE, et al.: Gastrointestinal symptoms attributed to jejunostomy feeding after major abdominal trauma—A critical analysis. *Crit Care Med* 17:1146, 1989.

120. Dive A, Miesse C, Galanti L, et al.: Effect of erythromycin on gastric motility in mechanically ventilated critically ill patients: A double-blind, randomized, placebo-controlled study. *Crit Care Med* 23:1356, 1995.

121. Heyland DK, Tougas G, Cook DJ, et al.: Cisapride improves gastric emptying in mechanically ventilated, critically ill patients. A randomized, double-blind trial. *Am J Respir Crit Care Med* 154:1678, 1996.

122. MacLaren R, Kuhl DA, Gervasio JM, et al.: Sequential single doses of cisapride, erythromycin, and metoclopramide in critically ill patients intolerant to enteral nutrition: A randomized, placebo-controlled, crossover study. *Crit Care Med* 28:438, 2000.

123. Landry C, Vidon N, Sogni P, et al.: Could erythromycin optimize high energy continuous enteral nutrition? *Aliment Pharmacol Ther* 10:967, 1996.

124. Pugh CB: Phenytoin and enteral feedings: A clinically significant interaction. *Hosp Pharm* 24:562, 1989.

125. Bass J, Miles MV, Tennison MB, et al.: Effects of enteral tube feeding on the absorption and pharmacokinetic profile of carbamazepine suspension. *Epilepsia* 30:364, 1989.

126. Martin JE, Lutomski DM: Warfarin resistance and enteral feedings. *JPEN* 13:206, 1989.

127. Semple HA, Koo W, Tam YK, et al.: Interactions between hydralazine and oral nutrients in humans. *Ther Drug Monit* 13:304, 1991.

128. Yuk JH, Nightingale CH, Quintiliani R, et al.: Absorption of ciprofloxacin administered through a nasogastric or a nasoduodenal tube in volunteers and patients receiving enteral nutrition. *Diagn Microbiol Infect Dis* 13:99, 1990.

129. Kintzel PE, Rollins CJ, Yee WJ, et al.: Low itraconazole serum concentrations following administration of itraconazole suspension to critically ill allogeneic bone marrow transplant recipients. *Ann Pharmacother* 29:140, 1995.

130. Cutie AJ, Altman E, Lenkel L: Compatibility of enteral products with commonly employed drug additives. *JPEN* 7:186, 1983.

131. Edes TE, Walk BE, Austin JL: Diarrhea in tube-fed patients: Feeding formula not necessarily the cause. *Am J Med* 88:91, 1990.

132. Eisenberg PG: Causes of diarrhea in tube-fed patients: A comprehensive approach to diagnosis and management. *Nutr Clin Pract* 8:119, 1993.

133. Lutomski DM, Gora ML, Wright SM, et al.: Sorbitol content of selected oral liquids. *Ann Pharmacother* 27:269, 1993.

134. Guenter PA, Settle RG, Perlmutter S, et al.: Tube feeding-related diarrhea in acutely ill patients. *JPEN* 15:277, 1991.

135. Mowatt-Larssen CA, Brown RO, Wojtysiak SL, et al.: Comparison of tolerance and nutritional outcome between a peptide and a standard enteral formula in critically ill, hypo-albuminemic patients. *JPEN* 16:20, 1992.

136. Brenner DW, Schellhammer PF: Mortality associated with feeding catheter jejunostomy after radical cystectomy. *Urology* 30:337, 1987.

137. Mullan H, Roubenoff RA, Roubenoff R: Risk of pulmonary aspiration among patients receiving enteral nutrition support. *JPEN* 16:160, 1992.

138. McClave SA, Snider HL, Lowen CC, et al.: Use of residual volume as a marker for enteral feeding intolerance: Prospective blinded comparison with physical examination and radiographic findings. *JPEN* 16:99, 1992.

139. Frankel EH, Enow NB, Jackson KC, et al.: Methods of restoring patency to occluded feeding tubes. *Nutr Clin Pract* 13:129, 1998.

140. Marcuard SP, Stegall KL, Trogdon S: Clearing obstructed feeding tubes. *JPEN* 13:81, 1989.

141. Herbst SL, Kaplan LK, McKinnon BT: Vascular access devices: Managing occlusions and related complications in home infusion. *Infusion* 4:S1, 1998.

142. Haire WD, Atkinson JB, Stephens LC: Urokinase versus recombinant tissue plasminogen activator in thrombosed central venous catheters: A double-blinded, randomized trial. *Thromb Haemost* 72:543, 1994.

143. Werlin SL, Lausten T, Jessen S, et al.: Treatment of central venous catheter occlusions with ethanol and hydrochloric acid. *JPEN* 19:416, 1995.

144. Pearson M: Guidelines for prevention of intravascular device-related infections, Hospital Infection Control Practices Advisory Committee, Centers for Disease Control and Prevention. *Infect Control Hosp Epidemiol* 17:438, 1996.

145. Venus B, Smith RA, Patel CB, et al.: Hemodynamic and gas exchange alterations during Intralipid infusion in patients with adult respiratory distress syndrome. *Chest* 95:1278, 1989.

146. Department of Health and Human Services, Food and Drug Administration. Parenteral Multivitamin products, drugs for human use–drug efficacy study implementation amendment. *Federal Register* April 20, 2000 (Volume 65, Number 77).

147. Berger MM, Cavadini C, Chiolero R, et al.: Influence of large intakes of trace elements on recovery after major burns. *Nutrition* 10:327, 1994.

148. Fitzgerald K, Mikalunas V, Rubin H, et al.: Hypermanaganesemia in patients receiving total parenteral nutrition. *JPEN* 23:333, 1999.

149. Rosmarin DK, Wardlaw GM, Mirtallo J: Hyperglycemia associated with high, continuous infusion rates of total parenteral nutrition dextrose. *Nutr Clin Prac* 11:151, 1996.

150. Van den Berghe G, Wouters P, Weekers F, et al. Intensive insulin therapy in critically ill patients. *N Engl J Med* 345:1359, 2001.

151. Dickerson RN: Management of hyperglycemia in patients receiving specialized nutritional support. *Hosp Pharm* 38:702, 2003.

152. McCowen KC, Malhotra A, Bistrian BR: Stress-induced hyperglycemia. *Crit Care Clin* 17:107, 2001.

153. Klein GL, Chen TC, Hollick MF, et al.: Synthesis of vitamin D in skin after burns. *Lancet* 363:291, 2004.

154. Miller SJ: The nitrogen balance revisited. *Hosp Pharm* 25:61, 1990.

155. Gabay C, Kushner I: Acute-phase proteins and other systemic responses to inflammation. *N Engl J Med* 340:448, 1999.

156. Petersen SR, Holaday NJ, Jeevanandam M: Enhancement of protein synthesis efficiency in parenteral fed trauma victims by adjuvant recombinant human growth hormone. *J Trauma* 36:726, 1994.

157. Behrman SW, Wojtysiak S, Brown RO, et al.: The effect of growth hormone on nutritional markers in enterally fed, immobilized trauma patients. *Surg Forum* 41:20, 1990.

158. Behrman SW, Kudsk KA, Brown RO, et al.: The effect of growth hormone on nutritional markers in enterally fed immobilized trauma patents. *JPEN* 19:41, 1995.

159. Takala J, Ruokonen E, Webster NR, et al.: Increased mortality associated with growth hormone treatment in critically ill adults. *N Engl J Med* 341:785, 1999.

160. Herndon DN, Barrow RE, Kunkel KR, et al.: Effects of recombinant human growth hormone on donor-site healing in severely burned children. *Ann Surg* 212:424, 1990.

161. Hatton J, Rapp RP, Kudsk KA, et al.: Intravenous insulin-like growth factor-I (IGF-1) in moderate-to-severe head injury: A phase II safety and efficacy trial. *J Neurosurg* 86:779, 1997.

162. Hausmann DF, Nutz V, Rommelsheim K, et al.: Anabolic steroids in polytrauma patients. Influence on renal nitrogen and amino acid losses: A double-blind study. *JPEN* 14:111, 1990.

163. Demling RH, DeSanti L: Oxandrolone, and anabolic steroid, significantly increases the rate of weight gain in the recovery phase after major burns. *J Trauma* 43:47, 1997.

164. Gervasio JM, Dickerson RN, Swearingen J, et al.: Oxandrolone in trauma patients. *Pharmacotherapy* 20:1328, 2000.

# Commentary ■ JEFFRY L. KASHUK ■ JOHN B. MOORE

Surgical critical care has now been firmly established as an integral arm of acute care surgery and trauma. Furthermore, improved understanding of these topics has recently led to important advances, such as intensive glucose monitoring and adrenal axis evaluation, which have greatly impacted the morbidity and mortality of our critically ill patients. Accordingly, nutritional support and electrolyte management demands a thorough knowledge and understanding.

This well-written chapter by Kudsk and Sacks, known experts in the field, offers a comprehensive overview of the subject. The authors initially present a thorough summary of the physiological basis for postinjury hypermetabolism which is essential prior to diagnosis and treatment of the various disorders. With appropriate explanations of the endocrine response to injury, stress, and sepsis, and a nice review of the biochemistry of glucose metabolism, amino acid mobilization, glycogenolysis, muscle proteolysis, starvation states, and obesity, the reader is well prepared to understand current concepts of nutritional support.

The principles outlined in this chapter, emphasizing the importance of enteral nutrition in the surgical patient as the preferred route whenever possible, is a central tenet of therapy and reflects our experience and practice in Denver over the past 25 years. As the authors aptly state: "The well-fed intestine is a metabolically and immunologically active organ...."

Although differences exist as to the timing and route of administration of enteral support, the overriding concept is "enterocyte happiness." In trauma patients, based upon severity of injury, this is most often accomplished with the needle catheter jejunostomy. With careful attention to technique and detail, as outlined by the authors, complication rates have been quite low. In damage control operations with the open abdomen, we will often delay catheter placement until abdominal closure, as multiple trips to the operating room for washouts often preclude safe positioning. In other patients with a prolonged course, we have been reluctant to place feeding tube access, due to concerns of fistula formation. For similar reasons, we try to position the exit site far from the midline wound.

In other patients in whom the operating surgeon believes there may be reasons for avoidance of surgically placed enteral access, we will ask the anesthesiologists to pass a nasal–jejunal (dobhoff) tube intraoperatively for later use.

Although parenteral nutritional support has seen a dramatic decrease in use due to the preferred enteral route, we agree with the authors that there remain certain situations in which parenteral support is required. In such situations, prior establishment of enteral access serves as an "insurance policy" for later use, if needed. Once shock, sepsis, or hemodynamic instability have resolved, the gut should be used as a preferred route.

Indeed, the tolerance of enteral nutrition by critically ill patients is often a marker of the impending resolution of sepsis. In contrast, as pointed out by the authors, "Critically ill patients tolerating … feeding who suddenly develop high residual volumes may have impending sepsis…" In critically ill patients in whom reduced splanchnic flow prevents enteral feeding, we initiate parenteral support early in an effort to counter progressive negative nitrogen balance, transitioning to the enteral route when feasible.

The arguments for "immune enhancing diets" as presented by the authors, have a sound physiologic basis, and current clinical studies support their additional benefit over unsupplemented diets.

Despite this, there are cost concerns, and our group has had difficulty identifying appropriate patients for these regimens. In addition, the authors have pointed out that care should be taken with these diets, because supplemental glutamine, arginine, or branched chain amino acids have a lower calorie to nitrogen ratio than standard formulas.

In sum, this chapter is an excellent overview of current concepts of nutritional support and electrolyte management in surgical critical care patients. With the growth of the acute care surgery paradigm and the aging population, increased numbers of surgical critical care patients are likely to require expert nutritional support in the coming years.

# The Immune Response

*Eugen Faist* ■ *Heiko Trentzsch*

Major trauma is associated with severe hemorrhage, shock, low-flow conditions, impaired oxygen delivery, tissue destruction, and release of debris, as well as gut bacterial translocation. These factors provide the mechanistic rationale for substantial dyshomeostasis that ultimately leads to organ dysfunction (see Chap. 68). The subsequent dysfunction of the immune system is characterized by a massive inflammatory response (Fig. 67-1). The magnitude of this response depends on the type of injury and its severity but moreover, it is determined by intrinsic factors such as age, sex, comorbidities, and even genetic predisposition. Comprehension of the biologic response to injury however will help to understand clinical problems associated with severe trauma, like increased susceptibility to infection, (see Chap. 19) increased risk for sepsis, and development of multiple organ failure (MOF).

In a large epidemiologic study including 14,364 ICU-patients Alberti et al. found 17% of those patients admitted for trauma to have proven infection (9% community-acquired and 8% hospital-acquired).[1] Bochicchio et al. found that one-third of blunt trauma patients with an Injury Severity Score (ISS) >16 suffer invasive infection.[2] In 25% of trauma patients MOF is observed and one-third of these patients will die. This represents 51% of all trauma-related deaths.[3] In patients with multiple trauma, acute respiratory distress syndrome (ARDS) is encountered depending on injury-pattern and injury severity. In an epidemiologic mono-center study including 7192 patients, posttraumatic ARDS was observed in 3% if laparotomy was required for surgical intervention and in up to 10% if three or more body regions sustained injury. Patients with an ISS 16–24 had an eightfold increased risk for developing ARDS.[4]

Incidence of organ dysfunction and mortality from late onset MOF correlate with the magnitude of the initial inflammatory response.[5] The underlying complex network of cellular function and humoral mediators that define the inflammatory response alternating immune function and subsequently leaving patients prone to complications is the focus of this chapter.

## TRAUMATIC INJURY AND SYSTEMIC INFLAMMATORY RESPONSE

The inflammatory response is a physiologic mechanism to control injury, to protect against invasion of microbes after the collapse of physiologic barriers, and to initiate healing. This systemic inflammatory response syndrome (SIRS) ranging from mild local inflammation to a likewise malignant systemic spillover may escalate and lead to critical illness featuring severe sepsis with organ dysfunction and MOF[6,7] (see Chap. 68).

SIRS has been defined by the Consensus Conference of the American College of Chest Physicians (ACCP) and the Society of Critical Care Medicine (SCCM) in 1991 under the presidency of Roger C. Bone (1941–1997), in order to provide a conceptual and a practical framework for describing the systemic inflammatory response to infection.[8] Since then, SIRS has been defined as the presence of at least two or more of the following clinical findings: body temperature >38°C or <36°C, heart rate >90/minutes, hyperventilation evidenced by a respiratory rate of >20/minutes or a $PaCO_2$ <32 mm Hg, and a white blood cell count >12.000 cells/μL or <4.000 cells/μL.[8] However, SIRS is not restricted to patients suffering from infection (Fig. 67-2). It can and does occur in the absence of infection in patients with sterile inflammatory process such as acute pancreatitis, trauma, tissue-injury caused by major surgical intervention, burns, ischemia, hemorrhagic shock, immune-mediated organ injury, and the exogenous administration of putative pro-inflammatory mediators such as tumor necrosis factor alpha (TNF-α).[8,9] Studies have revealed that this physiologic response may progress to kill the patient, even when at autopsy no infectious focus can be demonstrated.[10] In 2001, the definition of SIRS was revisited during the International Sepsis Definitions Conference. It was agreed that the 1991 criteria were globally adopted by clinicians and investigators, but that they were too oversensitive and nonspecific to diagnose a cause for the syndrome or to identify a distinct pattern in the response to heterogeneous insults. However,

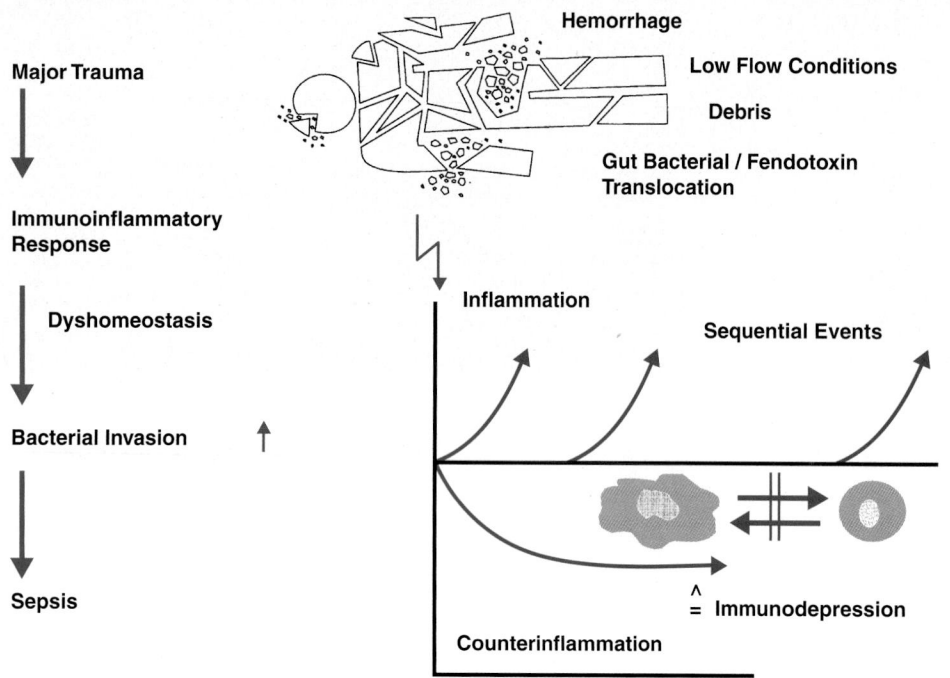

**Major Trauma**

**Immunoinflammatory Response**

Dyshomeostasis

**Bacterial Invasion**

**Sepsis**

Hemorrhage

Low Flow Conditions

Debris

Gut Bacterial / Fendotoxin Translocation

Inflammation

Sequential Events

^ = **Immunodepression**

Counterinflammation

**FIGURE 67-1.** Major trauma induces a massive dyshomeostasis of the immunoinflammatory response. This response is characterized through events of profound inflammation and anti-inflammatory immunodepression. These immunomechanistic interactions result in disturbance of immune cell function and may lead to the onset of sepsis.

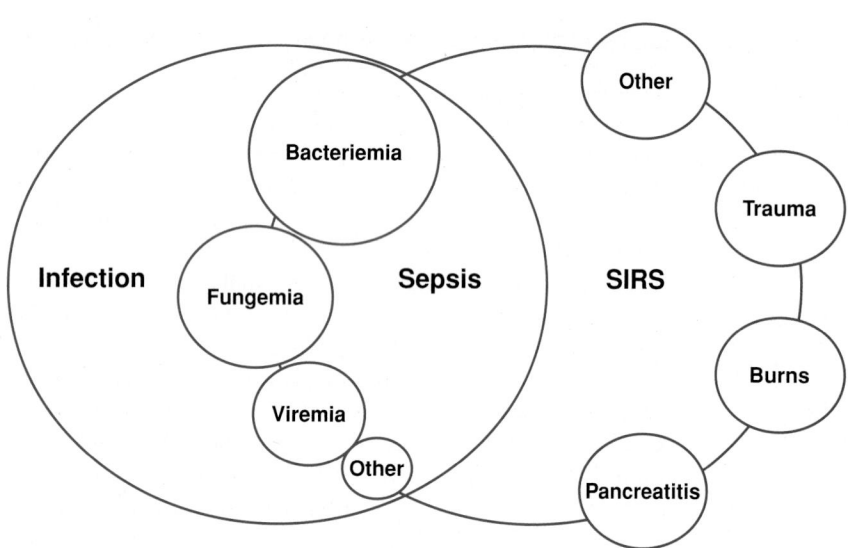

**FIGURE 67-2.** Relation between infection, sepsis, and the systemic inflammatory response syndrome (SIRS). A systemic inflammatory response may follow a variety of infectious and noninfectious insults. SIRS is not restricted to patients suffering infection. It can and does occur in the absence of infection in patients with sterile inflammatory process. Only when it occurs as a result of infection is it referred to as sepsis. *(Reproduced with permission from Nathens AB, Marshall JC: Sepsis, SIRS, and MODS: What's in a name? World J Surg 20:386, 1996.)*

no consensus has yet been reached for the use of biomarkers that would give a better definition.[11]

As a matter of fact, about one-third of trauma patients show signs of SIRS on admission.[2,12,13] Moreover, SIRS predicts increased mortality and prolonged length of hospital stay depending on ISS.[12] In trauma patients with SIRS and ISS >16, incidence of ARDS is up to over 50% and the incidence of multiple organ failure syndrome (MODS) is about 88%.[13] SIRS on admission predicts risk of infection.[2] However, SIRS is too unspecific to be used as a tool of risk assessment.

## MECHANISMS OF INFLAMMATION

Since the early 1st century, when Aulus Cornelius Celsus first described the cardinal symptoms of acute inflammation, it has been characterized by the classic findings of rubor (redness), calor

(heat), dolor (pain), and tumor (swelling). Based on a modern understanding, however, acute inflammation is characterized by vasodilatation, edema from exudation of protein-rich fluid and leukocyte infiltration. Moreover, acute inflammation involves a number of complex systems such as the innate and adaptive immune system, the coagulation cascade, and the complement system. Regardless of the underlying cause, the molecular mechanisms of the inflammatory response share a number of mutual, indeed essential features.[14]

Vasodilatation is clinically characterized by redness and warmth at the site of injury. It is primarily mediated by nitric oxide (NO) and vasodilatatory prostaglandins. NO is produced by nitric oxide synthase (NOS), which constitutively is located on endothelial cells (eNOS) and neuronal cells (nNOS). Moreover, activated leukocytes produce inducible NOS (iNOS). The purpose of vasodilatation may be to facilitate local delivery of soluble inflammatory mediators and cells. However, in cases of severe systemic inflammation, widespread vasodilatation can cause systemic hypotension consequently producing the clinical picture of septic shock. Secondary to vasodilatation and increased cardiac output patients will manifest as "warm" shock with pink, dry skin.

Formation of edema is caused by transvascular flux of protein-rich fluid from the intravasal compartment into the interstitium as a result of the actions of histamine, bradykinin, leukotrienes, complement components, substance P, and platelet-activated factor (PAF). These factors alter the function of physiological barriers. Increased vascular permeability in combination with increased hydrostatic capillary pressure and fall of intravasal oncotic pressure will promote flux of fluid and protein into the inflamed tissue. This alteration presumably allows delivery of soluble antibodies and acute phase proteins to the site of injury. Clinically, capillary leakage evolving with fluid collection in the lung is the mechanism behind ARDS.

The most abundant leukocyte to be found in inflamed tissue are neutrophil granulocytes (PMN). These cells transmigrate from the blood stream, a complex process that is divided into several steps and which is mediated by several endothelial cell adhesion molecules. Chemoattractants guide PMNs to move from the central blood stream to the periphery of the vessel. Upon margination, weak adhesive interaction with the endothelium cause rolling of PMNs as their ligands bind to endothelial selectins (E-selectin). Integrins mediate adherence of PMNs to the endothelium. Neutrophils bear beta-2 integrins (composed of CD11 subunits and CD18) that ligate to endothelial molecules, in particular to intercellular adhesion molecule-1 (ICAM-1). Diapedesis, the movement of PMNs through the endothelium and its basement membrane, is facilitated by additional adhesion molecules such as platelet-endothelial cell adhesion molecule-1 (PECAM-1). Chemotaxis leads the cells to the inflammatory focus. There are at least four families of chemokines, two of which that have been extensively described are alpha and beta chemokines. Alpha chemokines include Interleukin 8 (IL-8), which is a potent chemoattractant. Beta chemokines attract a variety of leucocytes including basophils, monocytes, eosinophils, and lymphocytes.

Inflammation and coagulation are intimately intertwined. In response to pro-inflammatory cytokines like TNF-α, IL-1, and IL-6 or acute phase reactants like C-reactive protein (CRP), endothelial cells, and monocytes exhibit tissue-factor on their cell-surface. Tissue-factor (TF) induces activation of Factor VII which mounts thrombin-formation through the cascade of the extrinsic pathway of the clotting cascade (see Chap. 61). Vice versa, thrombin, activated Factor X, and TF-FVIIa complex have been shown to induce pro-inflammatory activities. Simultaneously, activation of the clotting cascade during inflammation is limited by inhibitory proteases like anti-thrombin, the protein C system, and tissue factor pathway inhibitor (TFPI).

The complement system consists of a series of proteins that also promote inflammation and microbial destruction. In acute inflammation, this cascade is activated in three ways: first, the classical pathway, i.e., opsonising IgM or IgG antibodies that label microbes or other target structures; second, the alternative pathway is triggered by direct activation of complement component C3; and third, the lectin pathway activated by mannose-binding lectins which interact with microbial glycoproteins and glycolipids. Complement components form membrane attacking complexes that disrupt microbial cell membranes and subsequently destroy them. Moreover, complement components also function as chemoattracting factors for PMN migration and alteration of vascular permeability.

The initial response during inflammation however, is mounted by cells of the innate immune system. Its primarily cellular components are macrophages, dendritic cells, natural killer cells, and PMNs. Macrophages are the classic cytokine-secreting cells of the innate immune system. The magnitude of the innate response is defined by the activity of cytokines (i.e., TNF-α, IL-1, IL-6, IL-8, IFN-γ, IL-12, IL-10, G-CSF) and a vast number of other noncytokine mediators (i.e., PAF, eicosanoids, leukotriens, thromboxane A2 etc.). The activities of the innate immune system aim at clearance of the inflammatory focus by phagocytosis and respiratory burst. It also activates and amplifies the acquired immune system, primarily by presenting antigen to CD4+ and CD8+ T-cells but also by release of cytokines such as IL-1 or IL-12. T-cells represent antigen-specific immunity and control the function of immunoglobulin-producing B-cells and clonal expansion of memory cells (CD45 R0+). CD4+ T-cells can be divided into functionally distinct subsets, i.e., Th1 and Th2 cells. While IFN-γ promotes differentiation of naïve T-cells into Th1 cells, IL-4 induces differentiation of Th2 cells. T-helper cell subsets are defined by the cytokines they secrete: Th1 cells produce IL-2, IL-12, INF-γ, and TNF-β, while Th2 cells preferentially produce IL-4, IL-5, IL-10, IL-13, and TNF-α. Moreover, the two subsets represent functionally distinct arms of the T-cell response. Th1 cells promote phagocyte-mediated antimicrobial immunity and stimulation of cytotoxic CD8+ T-cells. Humoral immunity is primary function of Th2 cells. They also play a central role in the facilitation of asthma and allergic reaction. Moreover, IL-10 and IL-13 from Th2 cells suppresses macrophage activity.

Another important subset of T-cells are CD8+ cells. Just like CD4+ cells, CD8+ lymphocytes can be divided into Th1-like (cytotoxic T-cells) and Th2-like (suppressor T-cells) subpopulations according to their cytokines-profiles. Two additional subsets of T-cells have been observed, Th3 and T-regulatory I (TrI) cells, which secrete TGF-β and IL-10 and thus promote the development of immune tolerance and suppress Th1 and Th2 cell activity.[14]

## DYNAMIC STAGES IN THE IMMUNE RESPONSE TO TRAUMA

Regarding the pathogenesis of the systemic inflammatory response syndrome, Bone proposed a phased model divided into three stages[7] (Fig. 67-3). In stage 1, a local inflammatory response helps to promote wound repair and recruitment of immune cells as described above. During stage 2, small amounts of inflammatory mediators are released into the circulation and initiate an acute phase response. This stage must not be thought as pathologic or abnormal. It rather represents the body's main line of defense. Tight control occurs from a network of mediators that usually functions effectively to limit the response to the site of action. Anti-inflammatory mediators such as IL-10, TGF-β, certain prostaglandins, and G-CSF but also soluble antagonists such as sTNF-R and IL-1Ra normally balance the inflammatory response.[14] It is important to understand that these events do not

| Stage 1:<br>Local Inflammatory Response | |
|---|---|
| Stage 2:<br>Systemic "Spill-Over" of Mediators | Laboratory: Detectable Response<br>Clinic: "Bone-Criteria" |
| Stage 3:<br>Massive Systemic Inflammation<br>SIRS | Massive Dyshomeostasis<br>"Dirty Serum Environment" |
| Stage 4:<br>Systemic Hyperresponsiveness<br>Systemic Immunosupression | Multiple Organ Failure |

**FIGURE 67-3.** Dynamic stages in the immune response to trauma. Based on a proposal by R.C. Bone,[7] the inflammatory response initiated by trauma escalates within stages that dynamically evolve one after the other. Depending on the particular stage, patients will show clinically assessable changes.

happen sequentially, but commence simultaneously. Pro- and anti-inflammatory mediators can both be detected at time points as early as minutes after the injury.[15–18]

Under normal circumstances, wounds heal, infections are fought off, and homeostasis is restored. If, however, dyshomeostasis persists, massive systemic reaction begins in stage 3 as the onset of SIRS is entered. In the sequel, overrepresentation of either pro-inflammatory or anti-inflammatory activities and repeated disturbance of the homeostatic equilibrium by secondary insults such as secondary surgical procedures, infectious complications, or additional immune stress from transfusion of blood products increase the risk for MOT[6] (Fig. 67-4).

## TRAUMA-INDUCED CHANGES IN IMMUNE FUNCTION

Repair and healing or perpetuation of acute inflammation is characterized by a complex network of interacting cellular and humoral defense mechanisms. The above described mechanisms of inflammation produce changes and abnormalities in the function of immune cells that characterize the immune response after trauma:

## POLYMORPHONUCLEAR NEUTROPHIL ABNORMALITIES

Functional abnormalities of polymorphonuclear neutrophil granulocytes (PMN) after serious injury have been interpreted by some as signs of unresponsiveness, whereas others have demonstrated evidence for PMN hyperactivation.[19] These apparently contradictory findings, however, may be time-dependent, that is, early postinjury (<6 hours) versus delayed (>48 hours). Several laboratories have found a significant correlation between the degree of PMN dysfunction and morbidity of the patient.[20] A decrease in PMN phagocytic activity[21,22] reduction of intracellular bacterial killing,[23] and a large number of cellular parameters were found to be altered. Those include a decrease of glucose oxidation and oxygen consumption, reduced hydrogen peroxide ($H_2O_2$) production, alterations of phagolysosomal acidification, and a loss of or defect in lysosoma enzymes.[24–28] Koller et al. reported lowered leukotriene (LT), including $LTB_4$ generation from PMNs of severely burned patients,[29,30] which could account for some of the chemotactic and chemokinetic alterations reported by others.

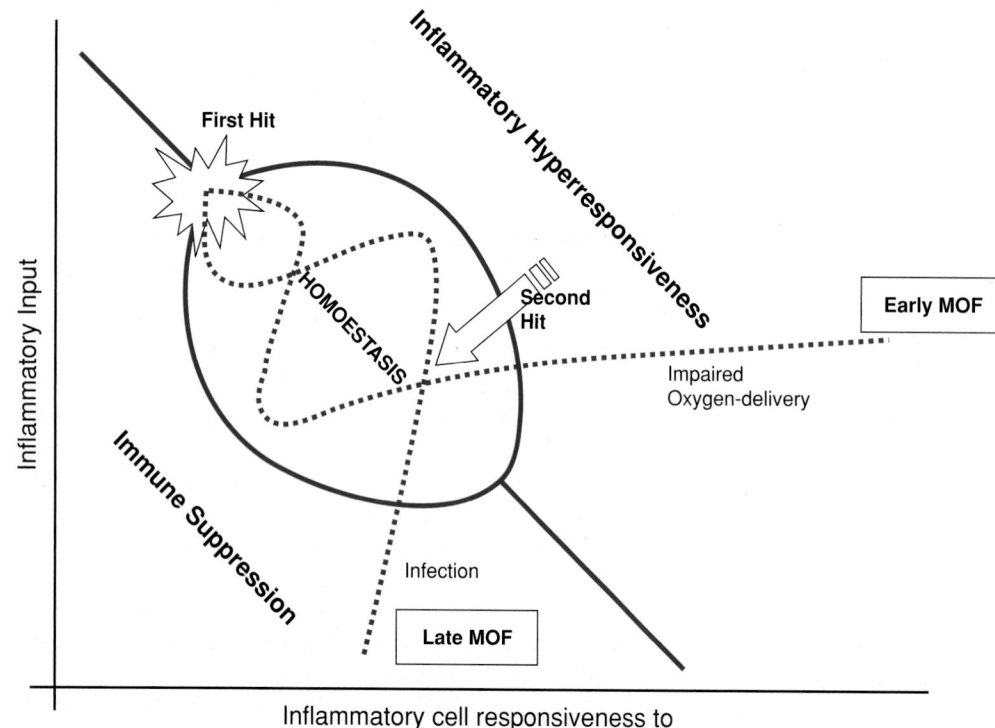

**FIGURE 67-4.** Following a traumatic insult (first hit) the immune system will respond with a delicately balanced response composed of pro- and anti-inflammatory facets. Homeostasis will be maintained by keeping the global system to midline functionality. If, however, dyshomeostasis persists due to the severity of the first hit or as a result of a second hit, massive systemic reaction begins and the balance collapses. As indicated by the dotted lines one may observe either increased inflammatory responsiveness with impaired oxygen-delivery that will ultimately result in direct organ damage ("early MOF") or, on the other hand, will lead into severe immune depression that increases susceptibility to infection with concomitant organ failure ("late MOF"). (Reproduced with permission from Moore FA, Sauaia A, Moore EE, et al.: Postinjury multiple organ failure: A bimodal phenomenon. J Trauma 40:501, 1996.); and Cobb JP O'Keefe GE: Injury research in the genomic era. Lancet 363:2076, 2004.)

Babcock and colleagues found PMN dysfunction in circulating blood within 72 hours after trauma; 70% of all PMNs had down-regulated or nonexistent beta-2 integrins.[31,32] These cells did not phagocytose, had reduced respiratory bursts, and appeared to be completely degranulated. Others report, however, that stress increased expression of CR3 receptors (CD11, CD18 complex) on circulating PMNs,[33] which increases the ability of these cells to adhere to intercellular adhesion molecules.

Of the numerous inflammatory mediators, the proteolytic lyso-somal enzyme PMN elastase is highly destructive when released extracellularly, thus contributing to organ dysfunction after injury. Clinical studies found significant increase in plasma elastase following major trauma and demonstrate a correlation between elevated elastase levels on hospital arrival and the development of organ failure.[34-36] Pacher and coworkers could predict the onset of organ failure with a sensitivity of 88% and a specificity of 83% by elevated elastase levels after injury.[37]

## MONOCYTES AND MACROPHAGES

Macrophages and monocytes, their blood-borne precursor cells feature two classic changes following trauma — one is hyporesponsiveness to additional stimuli, the other one is diminished capability to present antigen.

Following the rather short-lived hyperactivation with release of inflammatory mediators, such as TNF-a or IL-1, these cells become hyporesponsive, which is documented by the fact that ex vivo attempts to restimulate monocytes taken from traumatized individuals demonstrate exhaustion, manifest as tolerance of these cells to become activated when stimulated in vitro with bacteria or endotoxin, i.e., lipopolysaccharide (LPS).[38,39] Monocytic deactivation is understood to lead to immunologic paralysis, which is only partially compensated after three to five days due to the influx of new and immature monocytes/macrophages.[40] Under stressful conditions, these cells release prostaglandin $E_2$ (PGE$_2$), which is a powerful endogenous immune suppressant. PGE$_2$ has been demonstrated to be uniformly unregulated for as long as 21 days after trauma.[41] PGE$_2$ is an inhibitor of T-cell mitogenesis, IL-2 production, IL-2 receptor (IL-2R) expression, and IgM antibody synthesis by B cells.[41] PGE$_2$ negatively controls synthesis of TNF-$\alpha$ and IL-1 in monocytes. We have demonstrated in the past that therapeutic administration of the cyclooxygenase inhibitor indomethacin could partially restore adequate monocyte function in patients undergoing cardiac surgery.[42] Besides PGE2, transforming growth factor-beta (TGF-$\beta$), IL-10, IL-4, nitric oxide, and many other mediators also promote sustained depression of the antigen-presenting cell function.[43,44] This functional impairment has been shown to persist for up to seven days, depending on the severity of the injury. It is then overcome with newly recruited, possibly yet immature monocytes that may lack the full spectrum of activity as compared to their predecessors.[40,44]

Antigen presentation is defined as a process whereby a cell expresses antigen on its surface in a form capable of being recognized by T-cells. After degradation and processing, macrophages present phagocytosed antigen via membrane-located molecules, the major histocompatibility complex (MHC). Peptides presented in association with MHC Class II are exposed to CD4+ T-helper cells. Those displayed in association with MHC I become target for

CD8+ cytotoxic T lymphocytes.[43] However, for competent antigen presentation to take place, the antigen-presenting macrophage must provide costimulatory signal in form of B7, a membrane factor that interact with CD3, the T-cell receptor (TCR). Impaired monocyte function and disruption of monocyte/T-cell interaction have been shown to be crucial.

HLA-DR is a MHC II molecule easily detectable on the cell surface of monocytes from perhipheral blood by use of flow cytometry and fluorescence activated cell sorting (FACS). Several studies have shown that HLA-DR expression on monocytes decreases after major injury and that prolonged depression was associated with increased rate of infections and septic complications.[15,45-47] Reduced HLA-DR expression may be a consequence of IL-10 released during the inflammatory response.[48-50]

It should be noted that a normal or enhanced capacity of peripheral blood monocytes to present bacterial superantigens and to stimulate T-cell proliferation after surgery has been found despite decreased HLA-DR antigen presentation.[51] Those changes were evident despite a significant loss of cell surface HLA-DR molecules. Thus, the level of MHC-II protein expression does not necessarily predict the antigen-presenting capacity of monocytes.

Monocytes can be divide into functionally different subpopulations by the presence of Fc receptors (FcR).[52-54] A significant shift toward FcR+ monocyte subsets (CD16+) can be found in patients with severe sepsis.[55] This subpopulation has previously been referred to as "angry macrophages," which are characterized by high pro-inflammatory cytokine production, release of prostaglandin E2 (PGE2), and impaired antigen presentation.[56]

With the irreversible loss of their function as antigen presenting cells (APC), these changes do cause failure of the nonspecific (innate) cellular immunity and moreover, result in impairment of the antigene specific immunity by profound disturbance of an adequate monocyte/T-cell interaction.[40,44]

## T-CELL FUNCTION AND POLARIZATION OF THE ADAPTIVE IMMUNE RESPONSE

T-helper cells (CD4+) interact with monocytes upon cell-to-cell contact via MHC-II, such as HLA-DR (Fig. 67-5). According to the concept derived from murine models by Mosmann et al., T-helper cells can functionally be divided into two distinct types, Th1 and Th2.[57] Th1 cells predominantly produce pro-inflammatory cytokines, such as IL-2, IFN-$\gamma$, and TNF-$\beta$. They are responsible for macrophage activation and delayed-type hypersensitivity reaction (DTH). Moreover, they participate in the production of opsonizing and complement-fixing antibodies of the immunoglobulin G2a class (IgG2a). Th2 cells are defined by the production of mainly anti-inflammatory cytokines such as IL-4, IL-10, IL-13 but also IL-5, IL-6, TNF-$\alpha$, and granulocyte-macrophage colony stimulating factor (GM-CSF). However, the latter cytokines are not as tightly restricted to a sole subset as observed in T-cells from mice. Th2 cells were originally defined as predominant helpers of B-cell response, including IgE and IgG1 isotype switching, mucosal immunity, and differentiation of IgA synthesis. Moreover, several macrophage functions are inhibited by Th2 derived IL-4, IL-10, and IL-13.[58]

It is important to understand that Th1 and Th2 clones are reciprocally regulated by their secreted cytokines and that monocyte

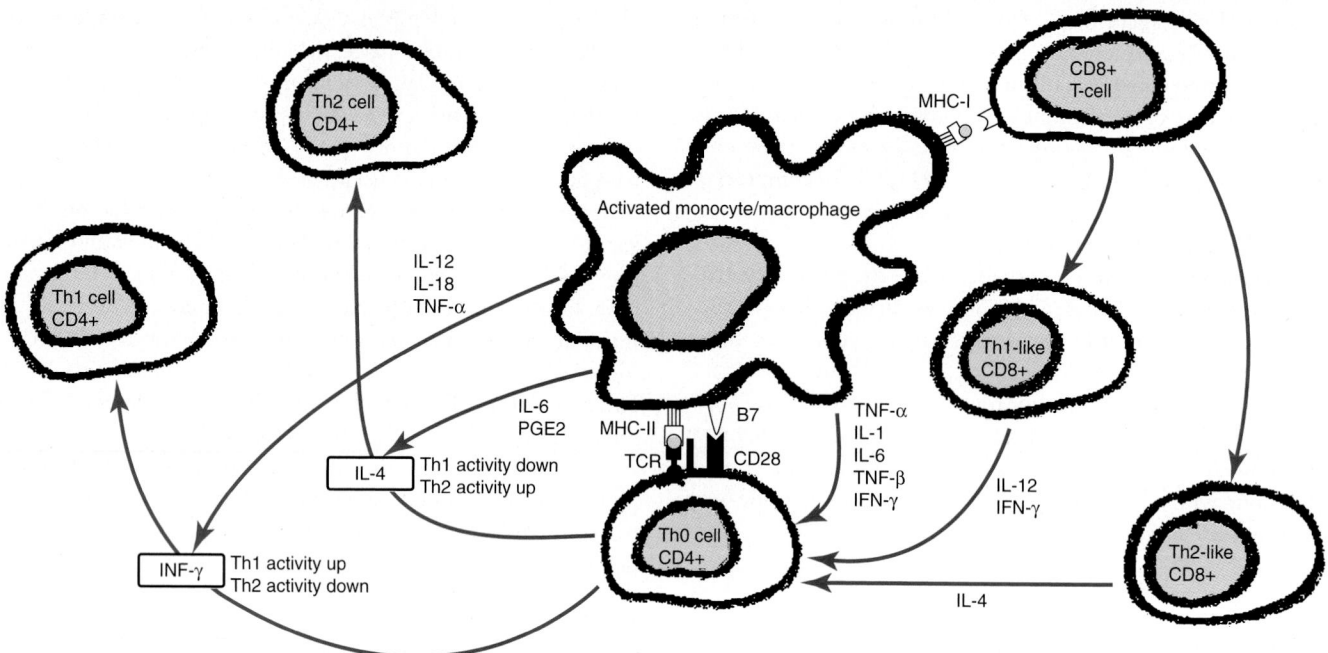

**FIGURE 67-5.** The complex interaction of antigen-presenting-cells and T-cells. For a better understanding of the complex interaction this figure illustrates the relationship between antigen-presenting cells such as monocytes and macrophages and the role of cytokines in the polarization of T-cell function.

activation is influenced by Th1 and Th2 cell activity: INF-γ inhibits the proliferation of Th2 clones whereas IL-10 shuts down proliferation of Th1 clones.[59] IFN-γ from Th1 cells activates monocytes and depresses Th2 cells, while Th2 cells are suppressor–active toward Th1 cells and monocytes via IL-4 and IL-10 secretion.[40] At the same time, antigen presenting cells (APCs), such as macrophages or dendritic cells activated monocytes, promotes Th1 differentiation via IL-12, a powerful inducer of INF-γ. Besides these two, IFN-α, TGF-β, IL-1, and IL-18 also induce Th1 differentiation.[40,58]

Surgical interventions are associated with a significant decrease in total systemic lymphocyte counts, including both CD4+ and CD8+ cells.[60,61] Patients who develop septic complications, however, display a predominant decrease in CD4+ cells.[62] After trauma, lymphocyte function is altered. For example, T lymphocytes do not proliferate in respond to mitogenic activation with concanavalin A (Con A) and phytohemagglutinin (PHA).[63,64] Patients after major trauma lack DTH reaction to recall antigens and impaired production of Th1 lymphokines such as IL-2 and IFN-γ can be observed.[40,43] Hensler et al. have shown a severe defect of T-lymphocyte proliferation and cytokine secretion in vitro following major surgery. In those studies, reduced cytokine secretion by T-lymphocytes was observed for IL-2, IFN-γ, and TNF-α during the early postoperative course.[51]

These observations suggest loss of Th1 function.[40] It seemed appropriate to look for increased Th2 activity in states of traumatic and septic stress in patients and relevant animal models.[19]

In search for trauma-induced mechanism the shift of polarization in the T-helper cell population may be secondary to PGE2 release from monocytes. PGE$_2$ profoundly decrease Th1 subset production of IL-2 and IFN-γ.[65] Interleukin 6 can induce the production of IL-4 from naïve T-cells. IL-4 has been proposed to be the predominant cytokine in polarization towards Th2.[40,58]

However, the actual source of IL-4 is not clearly identified. Mast cells and autocrine mechanism have been proposed as a possible source of significant amounts of IL-4. However, experimental data indicates CD8+ T-cells as another source of IL-4. Interestingly, the release of IL-4 from these cells has been found to correlate with mortality after burn trauma.[66,67] Although the absolute number of those cells isolated from peripheral blood is relatively low, their biologic importance must not be underestimated. Cytokines are potent mediators. Like hormones they can induce large effect even in small doses in a paracrine fashion. Consequently, even small numbers of cells can create significant effect since these cells circulate the systemic blood stream and thus contribute to systemic spread of anti-inflammatory cytokines.

Downregulation of IL-12 may also be of importance in T-cell polarization in the inflammatory response to injury.[68] For example, thrombin is generated upon tissue damage or as a result of proinflammatory cytokines, it downregulates IL-12 production at protein and mRNA level in human PBMC. The inhibition of IL-12 production was accompanied by an enhanced release of IL-10, which inhibits Th1-related processes and promotes Th2-type responses.[69]

Apparently changes in T-cell function reflect severity of tissue damage. Comparing open cholecystectomy to laparoscopic cholecytectomy, it seems as if the more invasive the procedure, the more significant the shift.[70]

From the wide spectrum of available data, we believe that a shift in T-cell function toward Th2 plays a key role in cell-mediated immune dysfunction after trauma and critical illness.[40,44,71] Analysis of T-cell function indicates depression of Th1 activity along with upregulation of Th2 cell activity or at least a relative increased of Th2 function due to the loss of Th1 activity after trauma,[70] burns,[68] surgery,[72] and abdominal sepsis.[73]

This shift promotes loss of antigen-presenting capacity of monocytes, reduction of monocyte activation, and a lack of antigen-specific cellular immunity.[16,44,68] This change in function of the adaptive immune response has been found to be associated with decreased resistance to infection.[68] Depressed delayed type hypersensitivity (DTH) reaction indicates increased risk for infectious complications following surgery and is associated with worsen outcome.[74]

## CYTOKINES AND SOLUBLE MEDIATORS

Patients with multiple injuries have alterations in hemodynamic, metabolic, and immune responses that largely are orchestrated by endogenous mediators referred to as cytokines.[75]

Cytokines are pleotropic polypeptides that are produced by immune cells in response to tissue injury or infection. Given a size of 8 to 50.000 Dalton, they are rather small molecules. Derived by their primary source of production they once have been classified as monokines or lymphkines. However, as a matter of fact, cytokines can be produced by almost every core-bearing cell. Consequently, a more common classification is by effect: pro-inflammatory cytokines are IL-1, IL-6, IL-8, interferon gamma (IFN-γ), and tumor necrosis factor alpha (TNF-α). Anti-inflammatory cytokines such IL-4, IL-10, IL-13, and tissue growth factor beta (TGF-β) counterregulate the pro-inflammatory response. A third group of closely related mediators with central regulatory role are endogenous receptor-antagonists or soluble cytokine receptors like sTNF-RI (p55), sTNF-RII (p75), or IL-1 receptor antagonist (IL-1Ra). Any imbalance of pro- versus anti-inflammation causes either a hyper-inflammatory or severe immunosuppressive state, neither of which is conducive to longevity.[75]

As the following data will illustrate, cytokine levels correlate with the degree of tissue damage. Consequently, extent of an injury plays a major role in determining the release of inflammatory mediators. Patients suffering blunt or penetrating trauma represent a rather heterogeneous group, not only in terms of extent of injury. Apart from animal studies, a large body of evidence on the inflammatory response to better defined insults like elective surgery[76,77] and in septic patients,[78] has been generated. This data suggests that cytokine release patterns are closely related. In this chapter however, we will try to primarily focus on the population of trauma patients.

While the above described changes in cellular function reflect aggravated clinical course and increased risk of complications, their assessment requires costly laboratory equipment and experienced laboratory personnel. Soluble mediators such as cytokines and acute phase reactants, however, can quickly be obtained from the hospitals' clinical laboratory without too much of sample-processing, within a reasonable time-frame, and at affordable price. The following mediators have been proposed to be good markers of magnitude and severity of the inflammatory response after trauma:

## TNF-α, INTERLEUKIN-1, AND THEIR NATURAL ANTAGONISTS

There is strong evidence suggesting that one of the most important initiating events in the posttraumatic inflammation is the overproduction of TNF-α and IL-1. These cytokines induce biochemical changes including increased synthesis of nitric oxide (NO), activation

of cyclooxygenase (COX), and lipooxygenase pathways with generation of thromboxanes and prostaglandins, production of PAF, intracellular adhesion molecules (iCAM), and selectins that enhance blood coagulation. However, experimental data is contradictive and due to their rather short plasma half-life these two cytokines do not qualify for parameters to assess the inflammatory response after trauma despite their important biological role in initiating inflammation.[75] Moreover, soluble molecules that antagonize their effects were found to be more stable and more predictable for outcome and end-organ failure. Interleukin-1 receptor antagonist (IL-1Ra) competitively binds to the IL-1 receptor and thus blocks IL-1 activities. Soluble TNF receptor I and II (sTNF-RI and RII) can be found in the circulation where they bind biological active TNF and thus antagonize its effect.[76] In trauma patients, high plasma levels of IL-1Ra and sTNF-RI and -RII predicted lethal outcome and correlate with ISS.[75,79]

### Interleukin-6 (IL-6)

This cytokine is considered a very sensitive marker for the degree of tissue injury. There is a broad variety of cell types being able to produce IL-6. Not only immune cells like monocytes, macrophages, neutrophils, T-cells, and B-cells but also endothelial cells, smooth muscle cells, fibroblasts, and many more cell types can produce IL-6. A broad variety of factors increasing IL-6 expression is known, bradykinin, TGF-β, platelet derived growth, but also pro-inflammatory cytokines like TNF-α and IL-1. It has been well described to be elevated in correlation with tissue injury during elective surgery, percent total body surface area burns in thermal injury and injury severity after major trauma.[18,80] Interleukin-6 levels peak early after injury and can be detected as early as 70 minutes after trauma.[18] During the first 24 hours major peaks can be found, that decline back to normal over time. Increased IL-6 levels reflect risk and fatal outcome from organ failure after trauma.[5,81] Systemic levels of IL-6 have been correlated with the likelihood of developing ARDS and MOF. Moreover, IL-6 became appreciated as a biologic marker for risk assessment in surgical decision making. Patients with initial high levels of IL-6 after injury are prone to MOF and are recommended to undergo secondary surgery not earlier than five days after trauma.[82] Its biologic significance lies in induction of the acute phase response. In the liver, IL-6 induces the synthesis of acute phase proteins such as fibrinogen, complement factors, α1-antithrypsin, and C reactive protein (CRP).[76] About 12 hours after systemic detection of IL-6, increased CRP serum-levels can be detected. Those levels were found to correlate with previously detected IL-6 levels.[18,75] CRP has been well established as a marker of states with increased inflammation and found to be predictive for adverse outcome from in terms of organ failure following secondary surgery.[82] Consequently, IL-6 can be considered equivalent in clinical importance however, it can be detected at an early time-point, i.e., that CRP is lagging IL-6. There is also evidence that IL-6 promotes anti-inflammatory activities by inhibiting certain proteases in the acute phase response,[75] reduction of TNF and IL-1 synthesis, and release of immunosuppressive glucocorticoids.[83] Interestingly, IL-6 also promotes the release of IL-1Ra and sTNF-Rs.[76]

### Interleukin-8 (IL-8)

After traumatic injury plasma levels of IL-8 show similar kinetic as IL-6 levels. There is a peak within the first 24 hours after injury which decline over time. However, prolonged elevation of IL-8 levels has been correlated with onset of MOF and mortality.[5,81] Interleukin-8 is secreted by monocytes, macrophages, neutrophils, and endothelial cells. It functions to recruit inflammatory cells to the site of injury. Interleukin-8 is an alpha chemokine and is considered the most important chemoattractant for PMNs. It plays a central role in the pathogenesis of ARDS. In patients who develop early posttraumatic ARDS, IL-8 is produced rapidly within the lung. Pulmonary macrocphages are likely to be the source of this rapid IL-8 production induced by local hypoxia. Circulating PMNs will migrate in response to IL-8 and lead to massive infiltration into the lungs of patients who will develop ARDS as an early organ failure resulting from a massive first hit.[84,85]

## Interleukin-10 (IL-10)

Interleukin-10 is a cytokine with strong anti-inflammatory properties. Its major sources are T-cells and monocytes.[75] IL-10 directly inhibits the synthesis of pro-inflammatory cytokines like IL-1 and TNF-α in human monocytes at mRNA level.[50,86] Moreover, a number of features observed in the immune response to trauma is explained through IL-10 activities. For example, IL-10 is responsible for reduction of class II major histocompartibilitiy complex on monocytes.[48-50]

ISS correlates with IL-10 levels after blunt trauma. Systemic levels of IL-10 have been correlated with the risk of developing serious septic complications.[15]

In a prospective study enrolling 417 patients sustaining multiple trauma and who presented with at least two SIRS-criteria on admission, Neidhart et al. observed increased IL-10 levels throughout the period of 21 days as compared to healthy controls. In these patients, IL-10 plasma-levels reflected injury severity and were markedly increased in patients who later on developed sepsis, MODS, or ARDS. Moreover, nonsurvivors had higher IL-10 plasma level than survivors.[16]

It has been shown that reamed femoral nailing increases IL-10 release significantly as compared to unreamed femoral nailing. Assuming reaming to produce greater tissue damage, this finding suggests that more invasive surgical procedures can augment IL-10 levels. These patients were also found to have decreasing HLA-DR expression. Thus, surgical treatment contributes not only to the systemic burden caused by the initial injury but also promotes immune suppression.[17]

## CLINICAL IMPLICATIONS IN MONITORING THE IMMUNE RESPONSE TO INJURY

Damage control strategies propose restriction of early total care to a minimum if the patient appears unstable (see Chap. 41). After initial stabilization, the patient should be taken to the intensive care unit (ICU) in order to recover from the injury itself but furthermore to recover from dyshomeostasis caused by the systemic inflammatory response. Later on, secondary surgery can be performed safely in order to treat non life-threatening injuries or for definitive repair of injuries that were just stabilized within the first (damage controlling) approach.[87-89] The immune response to trauma can be quantified by measurement of soluble inflammatory

mediators or cellular markers in order to assess the actual deviation of the system from the homeostatic midline. These markers reflect the systemic burden created by injury. As a matter of fact, operating on a trauma patient contributes to the inflammatory burden created by the initial injury.[82,90] Tissue damage from surgery increases the amount of circulating "danger signals" that subsist dyshomeostasis. Duration of surgery, type of procedure, and the time-point scheduled for surgery influence the inflammatory response and define the burden, which is laid on the system (Fig. 67-6). For example, studies revealed that early secondary surgery (within two to four days) not only increases IL-6 plasma levels, but also increases the risk for ARDS and organ dysfunction as compared to patients who underwent secondary surgery five to eight days after the initial trauma.[82] Operative procedures exceeding 6 hours are associated with prolonged ventilator therapy, increased overall mortality, and increased lethality secondary to MOF.[91] Staged surgical therapy by the use of initial stabilization with external fixation and than secondary femoral nailing was accompanied with less systemic IL-6 and IL-8 plasma levels as opposed to early total care with immediate femoral nailing. While early nailing further enhanced the systemic load with IL-6 and IL-8, basically the same procedure (i.e., femoral nailing) produced significantly less systemic deterioration in terms of a much lower IL-6 and IL-8 levels.[92] Although the authors found no difference in outcome or incidence of ARDS, sepsis, or MOF, this study demonstrates how a surgical procedure contributes to the systemic response following injury.

Secondary surgery during phases of increased inflammation maintains dyshomeostasis and promotes complications in the clinical course.[34] Consequently, surgical procedures that do not aim at clearing a focus of sepsis or that have to be considered ultimately life saving shall be postponed until inflammation returns back to normal in the consciousness that at least no further harm will be done. Even though clinical findings such as urine out-put,

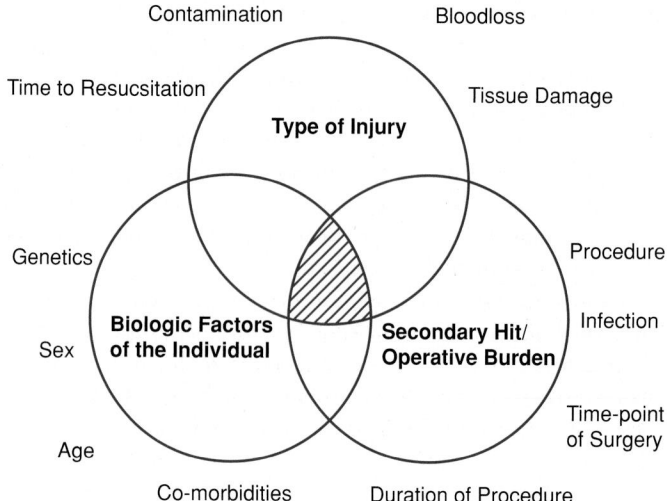

**FIGURE 67-6.** Modulators of the inflammatory response after trauma. The inflammatory response can be quantified by the use of plasma cytokine levels, soluble mediators, or by assessment of cellular dysfunction. In the figure, this response is resembled by the intersection of three circles, each one representing modulators that determine the magnitude of the response. Controlling these factors as well as possible allows control of the inflammatory response and thus may reduce associated morbidity.

SaO2/FiO2-Quotient, blood pressure, heart-rate, lactate levels, and coagulation parameters may suggest stable conditions and seem to guarantee operability, the inflammatory response may not yet be overcome. Patients who seem to be perfectly stable based on clinical parameters but than rapidly succumb to septic complications and organ failure after extensive surgical procedure have been classified as "borderline" patients,[93,94] Biomarkers of the immune response to injury seem to be helpful in identifying patients at risk. Monitoring the inflammatory response and immune cellular dysfunction may be helpful to decide if a patient can be taken to the operating room (OR) for secondary surgical procedures or better stays in the ICU for further stabilization.[33]

Clinical data shows that such markers can help determine the right moment to operate on the patient and thus become a tool of surgical decision making. Inflammatory markers that may indicate operability in trauma patients were proposed by Waydhas et al. Patient should have declining C-reactive protein (CRP) or CRP <11 mg/dL, IL-6 <500–1000 pg/dL, and white blood cell count >2000 and <12.000/μL. Moreover, patients should not have clinical suspicion of severe sepsis except from those in which the procedure aims at clearing an infectious focus.[95]

Furthermore, immune-monitoring seems to be the key to decide type of regimen (pro- vs. anti-inflammatory) and time-point of intervention for immuno-modulatory therapies.

# RATIONALE FOR THERAPEUTIC INTERVENTION AND SUITABLE CONCEPTS

Although conventional treatment for trauma patients consists of reversing blood loss, limiting hypoperfusion, timely surgery, and debridement of devitalized tissue, the complex mechanisms of the inflammatory response offer a broad variety of targets for therapeutic interventions in order to establish homeostasis. Trauma not only alters the specific performance of various cell types but promotes loss of regulatory function. Downregulation of cellular integrity through a "dirty serum environment" (i.e., release of cytokines and danger signals) in the aftermath of trauma leads to irreversible monocytic deactivation. Modulation of single mediator pathways within this complex network in the sense of "small spectrum" functional corrections in mononuclear leukocytes does not represent the right approach. It is not the correction of individual functional areas of the immuno-inflammatory response but rather the shifting back of the global system to midline functionality. Immunomodulation does not aim at the inflammatory response itself, which is a physiologic and indispensable reaction to protect the systems. In fact the goal is to restore homeostasis. This goal, however, cannot be achieved by completely shutting down either pro- or anti-inflammatory pathways. And that is probably why at first glance a number of successful therapeutic concepts in ICU-management appear not to address an immuno-mechanistic approach at all.

## Immunonutrition

This strategy has been developed very aggressively over the past years (see Chap. 66). It has been accepted that enteral nutrition has clear advantages over parenteral nutrition.[96] In order to protect bowel integrity, continuous enteral nutrition should begin as soon as possible, using a nasoenteric tube or a catheter jejunostomy. Preferably, enteral nutritional substrates should contain fiber, pectins, probiotic bacteria, polyphenol antioxidants, arginine, omega-3 unsaturated fatty acids, and nucleotides.[97,98] In addition, substantial amounts of glutamine should be administered.[99]

## Intensive Insulin Therapy

Van den Berge et al. showed in a prospective, randomized controlled study that hyperglycemia increases mortality of critically ill patients in the setting of a surgical ICU (see Chap. 60). Best outcomes were observed in patients with tight blood glucose levels of 80 to 110 mg/dL.[100] The effect was independent of the insulin dosage but strictly associated with blood glucose levels.[101] Hyperglycemia induces oxidative stress, promotes coagulation and phagocyte dysfunction. In addition, hyperglycemia enhances the formation of "advanced glycation end-products," which can initiate inflammation by binding to their specific ligands, receptors for advanced glycation end-prodcts (RAGE). Insulin itself has anabolic, anti-inflammatory, and anti-apoptotic effects.[78] Insulin therapy in children with burns showed reduction of the pro-inflammatory mediators and the acute phase response.[102]

## Activated Protein C (apC, *Drotrecogin alfa*)

Activated protein C (apC) is a physiologic substance that inactivates factor Va and VIIIa of the coagulatory cascade and thus reduces thrombin formation (see Chap. 19). Thrombin acts as a strong pro-inflammatory stimulus on human monocytes via protease activated receptor 1 (PAR-1).[69,103] Moreover, apC stimulates anti-inflammatory pathways directly through interaction with PAR-1. The anti-inflammatory properties of apC have been addressed to explain reduced IL-6 levels observed in apC treated patients enrolled into the PROWESS-trial. In this large multicenter study, Bernard et al. found that apC-treatment of critically ill patients suffering from severe sepsis significantly reduced mortality rates by 6%.[104] As a side-effect, an increased incidence of serious bleeding was observed as compared to placebo-treated controls, from 2% with placebo to 3.5% with apC treatment. This finding leads to controversial discussions, whether an anti-coagualant protease should be used for the treatment of surgical patients at all. In patients with severe sepsis following abdominal surgery, apC reduced mortality by 9% and by 18% if APACHE II score was >25, respectively. There was no difference in episodes of bleeding as compared to the non-surgical group. Treatment however did not start earlier than 12 hours from the end of the procedure. In summary, the retrospective subgroup analysis of the PROWESS data recognized a favorable risk/benefit profile of *Drotrecogin alfa* in surgical patients.[105]

However, there are a number of experimental concepts. We will discuss some examples to show how the field is developing:

## Interferon Gamma (IFN-γ)

In vitro studies suggest that administration of IFN-γ to trauma patients might help to overcome paralysis of peripheral mononucleated blood cells (PBMC).[106–109] However, clinical studies demonstrate only minimal effect on outcome or reduction of infection related deaths.[106,108,110] Experimental studies have demonstrated the ability of recombinant IFN-γ to upregulate the expression of

MHC-I and MHC-II.[107,109] Moreover, IFN-γ directly promotes the polarization of T-cells towards a Th1 response while inhibiting proliferation of Th2 cells. It has profound effects on activation of CD4+ T-cells and also promotes Th1-like differentiation of CD8+ T-cells.[111] It produces a strong pro-inflammatory effect by triggering the release of TNF-α, IL-1, and its own promoting cytokine, IL-12.[112] Although administration of IFN-γ to patients with cellular dysfunction after major injury restored functional parameters such as cytokine release upon ex vivo stimulation or HLA-DR expression on monocytes, beneficial effects such as improved outcome and decreased susceptibility to infectious complications have yet to be established.[111] Perioperative treatment of patients undergoing elective surgery showed that treatment with rhIFN-γ is capable to partially avoid the functional shift of T-cells towards Th2 response. Significant upregulation of PHA-induced IL-4 was observed in untreated controls while IFN-γ treatment maintained preoperative baseline levels.[113] Experimental data in PBMC indicate that rhIFN-γ therapy in humans can restore monocyte function and strengthen Th1 cytokine production in surgical patients.[112,113]

## Human Recombinant Granulocyte Colony Stimulating Factor (rh-G-CSF, Molgramostim)

This potent physiologic growth factor has been evaluated as an adjuvant to supply the biological system with sufficient quantity of functionally mature leukocytes that allow a timely normalization of the immuno-inflammatory performance. Rh-G-CSF stimulates proliferation and release of immune cells from the bone marrow. In a randomized, placebo-controlled clinical study, perioperatively administered rh-G-CSF attenuated acute-phase response and preserved an adequate Th1/Th2 balance. Monocytes from rh-G-CSF-treated patients showed intact monocytic cytokine response and HLA-DR expression.[114]

## Cyclooxygenase-Inhibitors

Studying the effectiveness of ibuprofen in human sepsis showed improved circulatory function and oxygen consumption; however, the treatment had no effect on survival.[115] With the discovery of two isoforms of cyclooxygenase (COX)[116] new aspects in immuno-modulation via PGE2-reduction was anticipated. Animal models show that PGE2-reduction by use of COX-2 inhibitors improves survival after burn injury followed by abdominal sepsis,[117] peritoneal infection with Pseudomonas aerogenosa,[118] and after-trauma hemorrhage followed by abdominal sepsis.[119] However, data from the VIGOR[120] and the APPROVe-trial,[121] show increased risk for cardiovascular side effects with potentially lethal consequences, thus leading to the withdrawal of the two most renowned COX-2 inhibitors, Rofecoxib (Vioxx™) and Valdecoxib (Bextra™).

## Sex Steroids

Based on sex-specific differences in the inflammatory response observed in animal models,[122] sexsteroids have been proposed as immune-modulators. It has been hypothesized that male sex steroids may have adverse effects on the immune function associated with increased risk for infection and worse outcome whereas female sex steroids might be protective. Sex hormones function as steroidal hormones that obviously exert potent effect on immune cells. However, clinical trials on their use and effectiveness as immune-modulators are missing, maybe because the question of sex differences in humans and their significant impact remains undecided. A number of studies look for sex-specific differences in outcome, susceptibility to infection, and development of organ failure. Some are in favor of male gender as a risk-factor for adverse outcome,[123–125] others find no difference between sexes.[126–129] Interestingly, Napolitano et al. report female trauma victims to have higher mortality from pneumonia although males had higher incidence of this complication.[126] Experimental data suggests that immune-modulatory capacity of sex steroids and its effects on outcome may be dependent not only on the type of injury but moreover on intrinsic factors that vary with the individual, such as genetic diversity.[130,131]

In summary, the development of highly efficient immune-modualatory therapies is constantly evolving. Establishment of validated, nonexpensive, and easy-to-use parameters for immune monitoring is mandatory to provide the basis for high quality studies to evaluate proposed and future therapeutic regimen.

## GENETIC CONTRIBUTION TO INFLAMMATION AND IMMUNE FUNCTION

New technologies such as gene chip arrays, high throughput genotyping, and analysis of complex systems has given entirely new insights into the immune response (see Chap. 57). Polymorphisms in genes encoding for mediators of the inflammatory response have been evaluated as risk-factors for adverse outcome.[132] However, these trials are small in sample size and have controversial results.

A large scale project founded by the German Research Society (DFG) investigates whether specific genotypes (single nucleotide polymorphisms, SNPs) and genetic markers are associated with adverse outcome in trauma patients. In this multicenter trial a panel of well-defined 200 candidate markers in 50 genes will be genotyped in a large cohort of 1000 trauma patients with a injury severity score (ISS) >16 treated at 17 trauma centers engaged within the German trauma registry.[133]

The use of outcome–prediction and risk-assessment for septic complications or organ failure based on genetic information may lead to an ethical debate (see Chap. 58); however this knowledge can also help to improve therapeutic approach to a difficult-to-treat critical condition endangering thousands of lives worldwide every year. Pharmacogenomics may play an important role in the future. Thus, genetic markers may be useful to stratify patients in clinical trials. An animal model on the impact of variable genetic background of the individual during endotoxic shock clearly demonstrates that improved survival by testosterone depletion is restricted to individuals with a defined genetic disposition which is inherited on the X chromosome.[130] Consequently, individuals identified for carrying a particular genetic trait will qualify for additional therapies that may not be effective within the entire population of patients.

Gene expression profiling by the use of mRNA gene chip arrays allow genome-wide analysis of transcriptional activities. Measuring gene expression profiles of human-derived dendritic cells in response to Escherichia coli, Candida albicans, and Influenza virus shows a number of commonly regulated genes for each stimulus whereas some genes are regulated for a specific pathogen only.[134] Apparently, immune cells sense diverse pathogens and elicit tailored pathogen-specific immune responses. These findings support the idea of common clusters in response to infection and provide proof-of-concept that leukocyte expression profiles may be eligible to allow differentiation of sterile inflammation from invasive infection (see Chap. 19).

Pattern recognition in gene expression of peripheral monocytes isolated from multiple injured patients has been suggested for outcome prediction after severe blunt trauma.[135] Given the small sample size, these findings however, have to be considered preliminary and will need to be determined in large scale in prospective, well-designed multicenter trials.

However, less than half of the changes at the mRNA level are translated into the protein level in the majority of systems.[136] Thus, proteomics are advocated by those who believe that evaluating protein formation will be necessary to confirm biological relevance. The use of gene and protein expression profiling is in the focus of The Inflammation and the Host Response to Injury Large-Scale collaborative Research Program by the National Institute of General Medical Sciences (NIGMS).[137,138] Such efforts in genetics, genomics, and proteomics will ultimately expand our current understanding of the immune response after trauma in the future and will help us to better understand the biological basis for its complex pathophysiology (see Chap. 57).

## REFERENCES

1. Alberti C, Brun-Buisson C, Burchardi H, et al.: Epidemiology of sepsis and infection in ICU patients from an international multicentre cohort study. *Intensive Care Med* 28:108, 2002.
2. Bochicchio GV, Napolitano LM, Joshi M, et al.: Systemic inflammatory response syndrome score at admission independently predicts infection in blunt trauma patients. *J Trauma* 50:817, 2001.
3. Ciesla DJ, Moore EE, Johnson JL, et al.: A 12-year prospective study of postinjury multiple organ failure: Has anything changed? *Arch Surg* 140:432, 2005.
4. White TO, Jenkins PJ, Smith RD, et al.: The epidemiology of posttraumatic adult respiratory distress syndrome. *J Bone Joint Surg Am* 86-A:2366, 2004.
5. Nast-Kolb D, Waydhas C, Gippner-Steppert C, et al.: Indicators of the posttraumatic inflammatory response correlate with organ failure in patients with multiple injuries. *J Trauma* 42:446, 1997.
6. Moore FA, Sauaia A, Moore EE, et al.: Postinjury multiple organ failure: A bimodal phenomenon. *J Trauma* 40:501, 1996.
7. Bone RC: Toward a theory regarding the pathogenesis of the systemic inflammatory response syndrome: What we do and do not know about cytokine regulation. *Crit Care Med* 24:163, 1996.
8. Bone RC, Balk RA, Cerra FB, et al.: Definitions for sepsis and organ failure and guidelines for the use of innovative therapies in sepsis. The ACCP/SCCM Consensus Conference Committee. American College of Chest Physicians/Society of Critical Care Medicine. *Chest* 101:1644, 1992.
9. Nathens AB, Marshall JC: Sepsis, SIRS, and MODS: What's in a name? *World J Surg* 20:386, 1996.
10. Nuytinck HK, Offermans XJ, Kubat K, et al.: Whole-body inflammation in trauma patients. An autopsy study. *Arch Surg* 123:1519, 1988.
11. Levy MM, Fink MP, Marshall JC, et al.: 2001 SCCM/ESICM/ACCP/ATS/SIS International Sepsis Definitions Conference. *Crit Care Med* 31:1250, 2003.
12. Napolitano LM, Ferrer T, McCarter RJ Jr, et al.: Systemic inflammatory response syndrome score at admission independently predicts mortality and length of stay in trauma patients. *J Trauma* 49:647, 2000.
13. Ertel W, Keel M, Marty D, et al.: Significance of systemic inflammation in 1,278 trauma patients. *Unfallchirurg* 101:520, 1998.
14. Sherwood ER, Toliver-Kinsky T: Mechanisms of the inflammatory response. *Best Pract Res Clin Anaesthesiol* 18:385, 2004.
15. Giannoudis PV, Smith RM, Perry SL, et al.: Immediate IL-10 expression following major orthopaedic trauma: Relationship to anti-inflammatory response and subsequent development of sepsis. *Intensive Care Med* 26:1076, 2000.
16. Neidhardt R, Keel M, Steckholzer U, et al.: Relationship of interleukin-10 plasma levels to severity of injury and clinical outcome in injured patients. *J Trauma* 42:863, 1997.
17. Smith RM, Giannoudis PV, Bellamy MC, et al.: Interleukin-10 release and monocyte human leukocyte antigen-DR expression during femoral nailing. *Clin Orthop Relat Res* 233, 2000.
18. Gebhard F, Pfetsch H, Steinbach G, et al.: Is interleukin 6 an early marker of injury severity following major trauma in humans? *Arch Surg* 135:291, 2000.
19. Mannick J: Trauma, sepsis and immune defects. In Faist E, Meakins J, Schildberg FW, eds. *Host Defense in Trauma, Shock and Sepsis: Mechanisms and Therapeutic Approches*, New York: Springer-Verlag, 1993, p. 15.
20. Babcock GF, White-Owen CL, Alexander JW, et al.: Characteristics of neutrophil dysfunction. In Faist E, Meakins J, Schildberg FW, eds. *Host Defense in Trauma, Shock and Sepsis: Mechanisms and Therapeutic Approches*. New York, Springer-Verlag, 1993, p. 95.
21. Grogan JB: Altered neutrophil phagocytic function in burn patients. *J Trauma* 16:734, 1976.
22. Heck E, Edgar MA, Hunt JL, et al.: A comparison of leukocyte function and burn mortality. *J Trauma* 20:75, 1980.
23. Bjerknes R, Vindenes H, Pitkanen J, et al.: Altered polymorphonuclear neutrophilic granulocyte functions in patients with large burns. *J Trauma* 29:847, 1989.
24. Heck EL, Browne L, Curreri PW, et al.: Evaluation of leukocyte function in burned individuals by in vitro oxygen consumption. *J Trauma* 15:486, 1975.
25. Duque RE, Phan SH, Hudson JL, et al.: Functional defects in phagocytic cells following thermal injury. Application of flow cytometric analysis. *Am J Pathol* 118:116, 1985.
26. Gadd MA, Hansbrough JF: The effect of thermal injury on murine neutrophil oxidative metabolism. *J Burn Care Rehabil* 10:125, 1989.
27. Bjerknes R, Vindenes H: Neutrophil dysfunction after thermal injury: Alteration of phagolysosomal acidification in patients with large burns. *Burns* 15:77, 1989.
28. Gallin JI: Neutrophil specific granule deficiency. *Annu Rev Med* 36:263, 1985.
29. Koller M, Wick M, Muhr G: Decreased leukotriene release from neutrophils after severe trauma: Role of immature cells. *Inflammation* 25:53, 2001.
30. Koller M, Konig W, Brom J, et al.: Studies on the mechanisms of granulocyte dysfunctions in severely burned patients–evidence for altered leukotriene generation. *J Trauma* 29:435, 1989.
31. White-Owen C, Alexander JW, Babcock GF: Reduced expression of neutrophil CD11b and CD16 after severe traumatic injury. *J Surg Res* 52:22, 1992.
32. Babcock GF, Alexander JW, Warden GD: Flow cytometric analysis of neutrophil subsets in thermally injured patients developing infection. *Clin Immunol Immunopathol* 54:117, 1990.
33. Botha AJ, Moore FA, Moore EE, et al.: Postinjury neutrophil priming and activation states: Therapeutic challenges. *Shock* 3:157, 1995.
34. Waydhas C, Nast-Kolb D, Trupka A, et al.: Posttraumatic inflammatory response, secondary operations, and late multiple organ failure. *J Trauma* 40:624, 1996.
35. Nast-Kolb D, Waydhas C, Jochum M, et al.: Biochemical factors as objective parameters for assessing the prognosis in polytrauma. *Unfallchirurg* 95:59, 1992.
36. Dittmer H, Jochum M, Fritz H: Release of granulocyte elastase and plasma protein changes in traumatic hemorrhagic shock. *Unfallchirurg* 89:160, 1986.
37. Pacher R, Redl H, Frass M, et al.: Relationship between neopterin and granulocyte elastase plasma levels and the severity of multiple organ failure. *Crit Care Med* 17:221, 1989.
38. Haupt W, Riese J, Mehler C, et al.: Monocyte function before and after surgical trauma. *Dig Surg* 15:102, 1998.
39. Faist E, Mewes A, Strasser T, et al.: Alteration of monocyte function following major injury. *Arch Surg* 123:287, 1988.
40. Faist E, Schinkel C, Zimmer S: Update on the mechanisms of immune suppression of injury and immune modulation. *World J Surg* 20:454, 1996.
41. Faist E, Mewes A, Baker CC, et al.: Prostaglandin E2 (PGE2)-dependent suppression of interleukin alpha (IL-2) production in patients with major trauma. *J Trauma* 27:837, 1987.
42. Faist E, Ertel W, Cohnert T, et al.: Immunoprotective effects of cyclooxygenase inhibition in patients with major surgical trauma. *J Trauma* 30:8, 1990.
43. Ayala A, Ertel W, Chaudry IH: Trauma-induced suppression of antigen presentation and expression of major histocompatibility class II antigen complex in leukocytes. *Shock* 5:79, 1996.
44. Faist E, Angele MK: Immunosupression with injury and operation and increased susceptibility to infection. In Baue AE, Faist E, Fry DE, eds. *Multipe Organ Failure - Pathophysiology, Prevention, and Therapy*. New York: Springer Verlag, 2000, p. 134.
45. Hershman MJ, Cheadle WG, Wellhausen SR, et al.: Monocyte HLA-DR antigen expression characterizes clinical outcome in the trauma patient. *Br J Surg* 77:204, 1990.

46. Livingston DH, Appel SH, Wellhausen SR, et al.: Depressed interferon gamma production and monocyte HLA-DR expression after severe injury. *Arch Surg* 123:1309, 1988.
47. Ditschkowski M, Kreuzfelder E, Rebmann V, et al.: HLA-DR expression and soluble HLA-DR levels in septic patients after trauma. *Ann Surg* 229:246, 1999.
48. Koppelman B, Neefjes JJ, de Vries JE, et al.: Interleukin-10 down-regulates MHC class II alphabeta peptide complexes at the plasma membrane of monocytes by affecting arrival and recycling. *Immunity* 7:861, 1997.
49. de Waal Malefyt R, Haanen J, Spits H, et al.: Interleukin 10 (IL-10) and viral IL-10 strongly reduce antigen-specific human T cell proliferation by diminishing the antigen-presenting capacity of monocytes via downregulation of class II major histocompatibility complex expression. *J Exp Med* 174:915, 1991.
50. de Waal Malefyt R, Abrams J, Bennett B, et al.: Interleukin 10(IL-10) inhibits cytokine synthesis by human monocytes: An autoregulatory role of IL-10 produced by monocytes. *J Exp Med* 174:1209, 1991.
51. Hensler T, Hecker H, Heeg K, et al.: Distinct mechanisms of immunosuppression as a consequence of major surgery. *Infect Immun* 65:2283, 1997.
52. Ohkawa S, Martin LN, Fukunishi Y, et al.: Regulatory role of FcR+ and FcR- monocyte subsets in Mycobacterium leprae-induced lymphoproliferative response in vitro. *Clin Exp Immunol* 67:43, 1987.
53. Miller-Graziano CL, Szabo G, Kodys K, et al.: Aberrations in post-trauma monocyte (MO) subpopulation: Role in septic shock syndrome. *J Trauma* 30:S86, 1990.
54. Zembala M, Uracz W, Ruggiero I, et al.: Isolation of human monocytes by rosetting with antibody coated human erythrocytes and isopycnic gradient centrifugation. *Clin Exp Immunol* 49:225, 1982.
55. Schinkel C, Sendtner R, Zimmer S, et al.: Functional analysis of monocyte subsets in surgical sepsis. *J Trauma* 44:743, 1998.
56. Maier RV: The "angry" macrophage and its impact on host response mechanisms. In Faist E, Meakins J, Schildberg FW, eds. *Host Defense Dysfunction in Trauma, Shock and Sepsis.* Heidelberg: Springer Verlag, 1993, p. 191.
57. Mosmann TR, Coffman RL: TH1 and TH2 cells: Different patterns of lymphokine secretion lead to different functional properties. *Annu Rev Immunol* 7:145, 1989.
58. Zedler S, Faist E: Pathophysiologic and clinical importance of stress-induced Th1/Th2 T cell shifts. In Baue AE, Faist E, Fry DE, eds. *Multipe Organ Failure - Pathophysiology, Prevention, and Therapy.* New York: Springer Verlag, 2000, p. 524.
59. Giron-Gonzalez JA, Moral FJ, Elvira J, et al.: Consistent production of a higher TH1:TH2 cytokine ratio by stimulated T cells in men compared with women. *Eur J Endocrinol* 143:31, 2000.
60. Feeney C, Bryzman S, Kong L, et al.: T-lymphocyte subsets in acute illness. *Crit Care Med* 23:1680, 1995.
61. Dietz A, Heimlich F, Daniel V, et al.: Immunomodulating effects of surgical intervention in tumors of the head and neck. *Otolaryngol Head Neck Surg* 123:132, 2000.
62. O'Mahony JB, Wood JJ, Rodrick ML, et al.: Changes in T lymphocyte subsets following injury. Assessment by flow cytometry and relationship to sepsis. *Ann Surg* 202:580, 1985.
63. Stephan RN, Kupper TS, Geha AS, et al.: Hemorrhage without tissue trauma produces immunosuppression and enhances susceptibility to sepsis. *Arch Surg* 122:62, 1987.
64. O'Mahony JB, Palder SB, Wood JJ, et al.: Depression of cellular immunity after multiple trauma in the absence of sepsis. *J Trauma* 24:869, 1984.
65. Harris SG, Padilla J, Koumas L, et al.: Prostaglandins as modulators of immunity. *Trends Immunol* 23:144, 2002.
66. Zedler S, Bone RC, Baue AE, et al.: T-cell reactivity and its predictive role in immunosuppression after burns. *Crit Care Med* 27:66, 1999.
67. Zedler S, Faist E, Ostermeier B, et al.: Postburn constitutional changes in T-cell reactivity occur in CD8+ rather than in CD4+ cells. *J Trauma* 42:872, 1997.
68. O'Sullivan ST, Lederer JA, Horgan AF, et al.: Major injury leads to predominance of the T helper-2 lymphocyte phenotype and diminished interleukin-12 production associated with decreased resistance to infection. *Ann Surg* 222:482, 1995.
69. Naldini A, Aarden L, Pucci A, et al.: Inhibition of interleukin-12 expression by alpha-thrombin in human peripheral blood mononuclear cells: A potential mechanism for modulating Th1/Th2 responses. *Br J Pharmacol* 140:980, 2003.
70. Decker D, Schondorf M, Bidlingmaier F, et al.: Surgical stress induces a shift in the type-1/type-2 T-helper cell balance, suggesting down-regulation of cell-mediated and up-regulation of antibody-mediated immunity commensurate to the trauma. *Surgery* 119:316, 1996.
71. Hotchkiss RS, Karl IE: The pathophysiology and treatment of sepsis. *N Engl J Med* 348:138, 2003.
72. Berguer R, Bravo N, Bowyer M, et al.: Major surgery suppresses maximal production of helper T-cell type 1 cytokines without potentiating the release of helper T-cell type 2 cytokines. *Arch Surg* 134:540, 1999.

73. Heidecke CD, Weighardt H, Hensler T, et al.: Immune paralysis of T-lymphocytes and monocytes in postoperative abdominal sepsis. Correlation of immune function with survival. *Chirurg* 71:159, 2000.
74. Christou NV, Meakins JL, Gordon J, et al.: The delayed hypersensitivity response and host resistance in surgical patients 20 years later. *Ann Surg* 222:534, 1995.
75. DeLong WG Jr, Born CT: Cytokines in patients with polytrauma. *Clin Orthop Relat Res* 57, 2004.
76. Lin E, Calvano SE, Lowry SF: Inflammatory cytokines and cell response in surgery. *Surgery* 127:117, 2000.
77. Menger MD, Vollmar B: Surgical trauma: Hyperinflammation versus immunosuppression? *Langenbecks Arch Surg* 389:475, 2004.
78. Weigand MA, Horner C, Bardenheuer HJ, et al.: The systemic inflammatory response syndrome. *Best Pract Res Clin Anaesthesiol* 18:455, 2004.
79. Ertel W, Keel M, Bonaccio M, et al.: Release of anti-inflammatory mediators after mechanical trauma correlates with severity of injury and clinical outcome. *J Trauma* 39:879, 1995.
80. Biffl WL, Moore EE, Moore FA, et al.: Interleukin-6 in the injured patient. Marker of injury or mediator of inflammation? *Ann Surg* 224:647, 1996.
81. Partrick DA, Moore FA, Moore EE, et al.: Jack A. Barney Resident Research Award winner. The inflammatory profile of interleukin-6, interleukin-8, and soluble intercellular adhesion molecule-1 in postinjury multiple organ failure. *Am J Surg* 172:425, 1996.
82. Pape HC, van Griensven M, Rice J, et al.: Major secondary surgery in blunt trauma patients and perioperative cytokine liberation: Determination of the clinical relevance of biochemical markers. *J Trauma* 50:989, 2001.
83. Opal SM, DePalo VA: Anti-inflammatory cytokines. *Chest* 117:1162, 2000.
84. Pallister I, Empson K: The effects of surgical fracture fixation on the systemic inflammatory response to major trauma. *J Am Acad Orthop Surg* 13:93, 2005.
85. Pallister I, Dent C, Topley N: Increased neutrophil migratory activity after major trauma: A factor in the etiology of acute respiratory distress syndrome? *Crit Care Med* 30:1717, 2002.
86. Oswald IP, Wynn TA, Sher A, et al.: Interleukin 10 inhibits macrophage microbicidal activity by blocking the endogenous production of tumor necrosis factor alpha required as a costimulatory factor for interferon gamma-induced activation. *Proc Natl Acad Sci U S A* 89:8676, 1992.
87. Rotondo MF, Zonies DH: The damage control sequence and underlying logic. *Surg Clin North Am* 77:761, 1997.
88. Feliciano DV, Mattox KL, Burch JM, et al.: Packing for control of hepatic hemorrhage. *J Trauma* 26:738, 1986.
89. Scalea TM, Boswell SA, Scott JD, et al.: External fixation as a bridge to intramedullary nailing for patients with multiple injuries and with femur fractures: Damage control orthopedics. *J Trauma* 48:613, 2000.
90. Giannoudis PV, Smith RM, Bellamy MC, et al.: Stimulation of the inflammatory system by reamed and unreamed nailing of femoral fractures. An analysis of the second hit. *J Bone Joint Surg Br* 81:356, 1999.
91. Pape H, Stalp M, Dahlweid M, et al.: Optimal duration of primary surgery with regards to a "Borderline"-situation in polytrauma patients. Arbeitsgemeinschaft "Polytrauma" der Deutschen Gesellschaft fur Unfallchirurgie. *Unfallchirurg* 102:861, 1999.
92. Pape HC, Grimme K, Van Griensven M, et al.: Impact of intramedullary instrumentation versus damage control for femoral fractures on immunoinflammatory parameters: Prospective randomized analysis by the EPOFF Study Group. *J Trauma* 55:7, 2003.
93. Pape HC, Giannoudis PV, Krettek C, et al.: Timing of fixation of major fractures in blunt polytrauma: Role of conventional indicators in clinical decision making. *J Orthop Trauma* 19:551, 2005.
94. Hildebrand F, Giannoudis P, Kretteck C, et al.: Damage control: Extremities. *Injury* 35:678, 2004.
95. Waydhas C, Flohe S: Criteria for secondary operations in patients with multiple injuries. *Unfallchirurg* 108:866, 2005.
96. Fong YM, Marano MA, Barber A, et al.: Total parenteral nutrition and bowel rest modify the metabolic response to endotoxin in humans. *Ann Surg* 210:449, 1989.
97. Gianotti L, Braga M, Vignali A, et al.: Effect of route of delivery and formulation of postoperative nutritional support in patients undergoing major operations for malignant neoplasms. *Arch Surg* 132:1222, 1997.
98. Bengmark S, Andersson R, Mangiante G: Uninterrupted perioperative enteral nutrition. *Clin Nutr* 20:11, 2001.
99. van Acker BA, von Meyenfeldt MF, van der Hulst RR, et al.: Glutamine: The pivot of our nitrogen economy? *JPEN J Parenter Enteral Nutr* 23:S45, 1999.
100. van den Berghe G, Wouters P, Weekers F, et al.: Intensive insulin therapy in the critically ill patients. *N Engl J Med* 345:1359, 2001.
101. Van den Berghe G, Wouters PJ, Bouillon R, et al.: Outcome benefit of intensive insulin therapy in the critically ill: Insulin dose versus glycemic control. *Crit Care Med* 31:359, 2003.
102. Jeschke MG, Klein D, Herndon DN: Insulin treatment improves the systemic inflammatory reaction to severe trauma. *Ann Surg* 239:553, 2004.

103. Naldini A, Pucci A, Carney DH, et al.: Thrombin enhancement of interleukin-1 expression in mononuclear cells: Involvement of proteinase-activated receptor-1. *Cytokine* 20:191, 2002.

104. Bernard GR, Vincent JL, Laterre PF, et al.: Efficacy and safety of recombinant human activated protein C for severe sepsis. *N Engl J Med* 344:699, 2001.

105. Barie PS, Williams MD, McCollam JS, et al.: Benefit/risk profile of drotrecogin alfa (activated) in surgical patients with severe sepsis. *Am J Surg* 188:212, 2004.

106. Polk HC Jr., Cheadle WG, Livingston DH, et al.: A randomized prospective clinical trial to determine the efficacy of interferon-gamma in severely injured patients. *Am J Surg* 163:191, 1992.

107. Ertel W, Morrison MH, Ayala A, et al.: Interferon-gamma attenuates hemorrhage-induced suppression of macrophage and splenocyte functions and decreases susceptibility to sepsis. *Surgery* 111:177, 1992.

108. Dries DJ, Jurkovich GJ, Maier RV, et al.: Effect of interferon gamma on infection-related death in patients with severe injuries. A randomized, double-blind, placebo-controlled trial. *Arch Surg* 129:1031, 1994.

109. Hershman MJ, Appel SH, Wellhausen SR, et al.: Interferon-gamma treatment increases HLA-DR expression on monocytes in severely injured patients. *Clin Exp Immunol* 77:67, 1989.

110. Wasserman D, Ioannovich JD, Hinzmann RD, et al.: Interferon-gamma in the prevention of severe burn-related infections: A European phase III multicenter trial. The Severe Burns Study Group. *Crit Care Med* 26:434, 1998.

111. Faist E, Schinkel C, Kim C: Pathophysiologic and clinical role of interferone-γ and its release triggering cytokines IL-12 and IL-18. In Baue AE, Faist E, Fry DE, eds. *Multiple Organ Failure - Pathophysiology, Prevention, and Therapy.* New York: Springer Verlag, 2000, p. 531.

112. Schinkel C, Licht K, Zedler S, et al.: Interferon-gamma modifies cytokine release in vitro by monocytes from surgical patients. *J Trauma* 50:321, 2001.

113. Licht AK, Schinkel C, Zedler S, et al.: Effects of perioperative recombinant human IFN-gamma (rHuIFN-gamma) application in vivo on T cell response. *J Interferon Cytokine Res* 23:149, 2003.

114. Schneider C, von Aulock S, Zedler S, et al.: Perioperative recombinant human granulocyte colony-stimulating factor (Filgrastim) treatment prevents immunoinflammatory dysfunction associated with major surgery. *Ann Surg* 239:75, 2004.

115. Bernard GR, Wheeler AP, Russell JA, et al.: The effects of ibuprofen on the physiology and survival of patients with sepsis. The Ibuprofen in Sepsis Study Group. *N Engl J Med* 336:912, 1997.

116. Smith WL, Garavito RM, DeWitt DL: Prostaglandin endoperoxide H synthases (cyclooxygenases)-1 and -2. *J Biol Chem* 271:33157, 1996.

117. Schwacha MG, Chung CS, Ayala A, et al.: Cyclooxygenase 2-mediated suppression of macrophage interleukin-12 production after thermal injury. *Am J Physiol Cell Physiol* 282:C263, 2002.

118. Strong VE, Mackrell PJ, Concannon EM, et al.: Blocking prostaglandin E2 after trauma attenuates pro-inflammatory cytokines and improves survival. *Shock* 14:374, 2000.

119. Shoup M, He LK, Liu H, et al.: Cyclooxygenase-2 inhibitor NS-398 improves survival and restores leukocyte counts in burn infection. *J Trauma* 45:215, 1998.

120. Juni P, Nartey L, Reichenbach S, et al.: Risk of cardiovascular events and rofecoxib: Cumulative meta-analysis. *Lancet* 364:2021, 2004.

121. Bresalier RS, Sandler RS, Quan H, et al.: Cardiovascular events associated with rofecoxib in a colorectal adenoma chemoprevention trial. *N Engl J Med* 352:1092, 2005.

122. Angele MK, Schwacha MG, Ayala A, et al.: Effect of gender and sex hormones on immune responses following shock. *Shock* 14:81, 2000.

123. Mostafa G, Huynh T, Sing RF, et al.: Gender-related outcomes in trauma. *J Trauma* 53:430, 2002.

124. Offner PJ, Moore EE, Biffl WL: Male gender is a risk factor for major infections after surgery. *Arch Surg* 134:935, 1999.

125. Oberholzer A, Keel M, Zellweger R, et al.: Incidence of septic complications and multiple organ failure in severely injured patients is sex specific. *J Trauma* 48:932, 2000.

126. Napolitano LM, Greco ME, Rodriguez A, et al.: Gender differences in adverse outcomes after blunt trauma. *J Trauma* 50:274, 2001.

127. Rappold JF, Coimbra R, Hoyt DB, et al.: Female gender does not protect blunt trauma patients from complications and mortality. *J Trauma* 53:436, 2002.

128. Coimbra R, Hoyt DB, Potenza BM, et al.: Does sexual dimorphism influence outcome of traumatic brain injury patients? The answer is no! *J Trauma* 54:689, 2003.

129. Gannon CJ, Napolitano LM, Pasquale M, et al.: A statewide population-based study of gender differences in trauma: Validation of a prior single-institution study. *J Am Coll Surg* 195:11, 2002.

130. Torres MB, Trentzsch H, Stewart D, et al.: Protection from lethal endotoxic shock after testosterone depletion is linked to chromosome X. *Shock* 24:318, 2005.

131. Trentzsch H, Stewart D, De Maio A: Genetic background conditions the effect of sex steroids on the inflammatory response during endotoxic shock. *Crit Care Med* 31:232, 2003.

132. Tabrizi AR, Zehnbauer BA, Freeman BD, et al.: Genetic markers in sepsis. *J Am Coll Surg* 192:106, 2001.

133. Schewe JC, Stueber F: Genetic predisposition for adverse outcomes in trauma patients. 2003, http://www.uniklinik-bonn.de/42256BC8002AF3E7/vwWebPagesByID/ 2432D6BF0360A01FC125705800262364. Accessed January 21, 2006.

134. Huang Q, Liu D, Majewski P, et al.: The plasticity of dendritic cell responses to pathogens and their components. *Science* 294:870, 2001.

135. Biberthaler P, Bogner V, Baker HV, et al.: Genome-wide monocytic mRNA expression in polytrauma patients for identification of clinical outcome. *Shock* 24:11, 2005.

136. Cobb JP, O'Keefe GE: Injury research in the genomic era. *Lancet* 363:2076, 2004.

137. Calvano SE, Xiao W, Richards DR, et al.: A network-based analysis of systemic inflammation in humans. *Nature* 437:1032, 2005.

138. Cobb JP, Mindrinos MN, Miller-Graziano C, et al.: Application of genome-wide expression analysis to human health and disease. *Proc Natl Acad Sci U S A* 102:4801, 2005.

# Commentary ■ MICHAEL A. WEST

Sepsis and multiple organ failure (MOF) are major factor associated with a significant share of trauma deaths, particularly with respect to deaths occurring in the hospital. Dr. Faist points out that as many as 25% of severely injured trauma patients develop MOF and one-third of these patients will die. It is well for surgeons to consider that even elective surgery MOF really represents one end of a continuous spectrum of "traumatic injury." Whereas elective surgery is a "controlled" traumatic insult, the same inflammatory responses discussed herein by Dr. Faist, occur to a lesser extent with *all* surgical interventions. Thus, understanding the information in this chapter is important for all surgeons.

Currently, our ability to *understand* the inflammatory response may be hindered by limitations in our taxonomy and classification systems. As reviewed by Dr. Faist, the existing paradigm emphasizes the construct initially proposed by Bone (shown in Fig. 67-3) that divides acute inflammation into three initial stages. Dr. Faist proposes that "tight control of the mediators responsible for the inflammatory response" usually limits the responses to the site of injury or infection. While his concepts absolutely pertain in controlled in vivo and in vitro model systems, it is not clear whether similar, "tight" controls really operate in the more complex in vivo clinical situation.

At a minimum the extent to which these various stages or processes are regulated are not completely understood. As part of this conceptional construct, Dr. Faist emphasizes that pro- and anti- inflammatory processes are initiated *simultaneously*. Thus, whereas Fig. 67-3 depicts a "sequential" inflammatory response that progresses to the hypo-responsive state seen at the bottom of the figure, it may be misleading. More to the point, it may be that the fundamental alterations responsible for the "progression" to organ failure, SIRS, or severe sepsis, is an *imbalance* of these simultaneous pro- and anti- inflammatory processes. The chapter also notes that the temporal sequence of these events undoubtedly varies depending on the initiating stimulus, pre-existing factors, the genetic background of the patient, and therapeutic interventions. Although clinicians have a strong desire to classify and characterize biologic processes that are incompletely understood we must recognize that in doing so we may hinder, rather than aid, our understanding of the underlying processes.

One of the increasingly well-characterized aspects of the innate immune response is the alteration and the function of monocytes and macrophages that occurs after response to inflammatory stimuli. Dr. Faist states that these cells become "hypo-responsive" and "exhaustion" manifests as tolerance of these cells to restimulation with prototypic inflammatory stimuli such as bacterial lipopolysaccharide (LPS). Depending on what cellular processes are examined, macrophages and monocytes are indeed hypo-responsive to restimulation, a process most widely termed "endotoxin tolerance." However, this characterization of the cells as being "hypo-responsive" or "exhausted" is at best incomplete. At the same time, other cellular functions are simultaneously increased (i.e., $PGE_2$ production, nitric oxide synthase activity, and secretion of IL-10 or TGFβ). Thus, whereas endotoxin tolerance is the term most widely used to describe alterations in these cells other investigators call these responses macrophage "reprogramming" or "dysregulation."

Having described the current state of analytic characterization of altered, innate, and adaptive immune cellular function, Dr. Faist points out that these studies are clinically inaccessible as biomarkers. In contrast, soluble mediators such as cytokines and acute phase reactants may be clinically accessible biomarkers. He proposes that interleukin-6, a compound that stimulates acute phase proteins, and C-reactive protein (CRP) which is an acute phase protein, may be much more useful as biomarkers of the inflammatory process. Recent evidence suggests that some of the acute phase proteins, especially heat shock proteins (HSPs) may amplify the immune response by interacting with toll-like receptors (e.g., TLR4). So-called endogenous "danger signal" ligands (e.g., HSP, HMGB1, etc.) may explain how and why the inflammatory response is activated with severe injury and/or trauma. Clearly, there is a need to obtain better biomarkers of the inflammatory response.

There is increasing recognition that secondary injury, or exacerbation of the primary injury, can occur by inappropriate application of surgical interventions in the early postinjury phase. We now recognize that a number of "therapeutic interventions" (i.e., ventilatory support, high $F_iO_2$, blood transfusion, vasopressors, etc.) may be deleterious to patients. Dr. Faist proposes that biomarkers may allow us to determine if/when the inflammatory response has been reset and thereby identify when surgical interventions will not exacerbate the acute inflammatory response. On the surface this seems to conflict with patient care needs, but we should not be complacent about the impact of our therapeutic interventions. For example, we would not be sanguine about the immune consequences of subjecting a motor vehicle collision victim to a second collision 2–4 days after admission, yet be relatively blasé about the inflammatory insult arising from a major surgical intervention 2–4 days after injury.

And what about the frontiers of biomarkers? Both the German Research Society and the NIGMS Glue Grant are attempting to identify genomic and proteomic markers of inflammatory responses and outcome. Future studies may indeed identify much better, clinically accessible markers that will permit clinicians to tailor therapy, institute or discontinue therapy at the appropriate time, and generally optimize care of the critically ill traumatized patient. Understanding the inflammatory and immune response to trauma and injury will help us to better care for these patients.

# Multiple Organ Failure

*David J. Ciesla* ■ *Frederick A. Moore* ■ *Ernest E. Moore*

## INTRODUCTION

Multiple organ failure (MOF) emerged as clinical entity from our ability to keep critically ill or injured patients alive through advanced technology.[1–3] Despite intensive study, postinjury MOF continues to be a major cause of death in the surgical intensive care unit (ICU).[4,5] The epidemiology has changed over the last three decades and will certainly continue to change as we develop further advances in postinjury care. This chapter provides a historical perspective, clarifies definitions, discusses epidemiology and pathophysiology, and reviews recent changes in patient outcome. A brief discussion of clinical implications and relevant patient care protocols is included.

## HISTORICAL PERSPECTIVE

Failure of vital organs has long been the major cause of postinjury deaths. In World War I, soldiers died on the battlefield of profound cardiac failure presumed to be a result of wound toxins (Table 68-1). By the 1930s however, reduced circulating blood volume was recognized as the cause of shock. Casualties in World War II and later Korea were resuscitated with blood and plasma until blood pressure returned to normal. In addition to rapid transport for definitive care in field medical units, blood and plasma resuscitation improved battlefield survival but late deaths due to oliguric renal failure became more common. In the 1960s Shires and associates proposed that extracellular fluid deficits (third space losses) compounded traumatic shock and were best replenished with balanced salt solutions (see Chap. 13). Consequently, crystalloid resuscitation was added to blood and plasma resuscitation in the Vietnam war and resuscitation endpoints focused on maintaining adequate urine output at that time. Helicopter evacuation also enabled rapid transport of casualties and the overall mortality rate decreased. Although late deaths from renal failure also decreased, a new entity

termed "shock lung" emerged as the primary cause of late deaths. This new disorder was recognized in civilian trauma centers as the adult respiratory distress syndrome (ARDS) (see Chap. 63). In the 1970s, subsequent improvements in advanced organ support such as mechanical ventilation, vasoactive drugs, total parenteral nutrition, and hemodialysis, armed physicians with better treatment to sustain the critically ill. Death from isolated pulmonary failure became rare, and a new syndrome of progressive multiple organ failure became the leading cause of late postinjury deaths.

Eiseman and associates in Denver introduced the term *multiple organ failure* in 1977 to describe the clinical course of 42 patients with progressive organ failure. Half of these patients had an abdominal infection implicated as the inciting event and thus, abdominal sepsis became viewed as a dominant risk factor for MOF.[6] Subsequently, Fry and colleagues reviewed 553 patients who required emergency operations, two-thirds of whom had sustained major trauma.[7] Thirty-eight patients (7%) developed MOF, and 90% of these patients were septic, half with abdominal infection. Consequently, the investigators proposed that MOF was a "fatal expression of uncontrolled infection." These seminal reviews as well as other clinical reports in the late 1970s and early 1980s appeared to identify consistent epidemiologic relationships between the initial traumatic event, subsequent infection, and the development of ARDS and MOF.[8–12] Further research interests from 1977 to 1987 focused on determining the relationship between the initial traumatic insult and the development of infection and how infection contributed to the development of ARDS and MOF.

While infection remained a frequent cause of organ failure, by the mid-1980s it was convincingly shown that organ failure often occurred in the absence of infection. In 1973, Tilney and coworkers first described sequential failure of multiple organs in 18 consecutive patients with ruptured abdominal aortic aneurysms who required postoperative hemodialysis. These investigators concluded that MOF syndrome was the result of a combination of pre-existing disease and hemorrhagic shock.[2] In a 1976 report from Denver, two

**TABLE 68-1**

## Historical Perspective of Postinjury Multiple Organ Failure

| TIME PERIOD | PROPOSED EIITIOLOGY | INTERVENTIONS | CLINICAL PATTERNS |
|---|---|---|---|
| World War I | Wound toxins | Undefined | Cardiac failure |
| World War II | ↓ Blood volume | Resuscitate to normal SBP | Renal failure |
| Korean Conflict | ↓ Blood volume | | |
| Viet Nam War | ↓ Blood volume | Resuscitate to normal urine output | Respiratory failure |
| | ↓ Extracellular fluid | Crystalloid resuscitation | |
| Mid 1970's | Shock | Advanced organ support | Sequential multiple organ failure |
| | Advanced age Sepsis | | |
| Early 1880's | Uncontrolled infection | Prevent and treat septic complications | Infectious models |
| Late 1980's | Systemic inflammation | Control inciting event | Inflammatory models |
| | Bacterial translocation | Attenuate early inflammation | |
| 1990's | SIRS/CARS | Improved resuscitation endpoints | Dysfunctional inflammation |
| | | Avoid secondary events | |
| 2000 to present | Cellular and subcellular signaling | Immunomoduladion | Decreased MOF incidence and severity |

patterns of postinjury ARDS were recognized; early onset within 12 hours of injury, and late onset more than five days after injury which was associated death from unremitting sepsis.[11] This was consistent with a 1983 study by Faist and associates from Munich, who described two distinct patterns: rapid single-phase MOF due to massive tissue injury and shock, or delayed two-phase MOF due to moderate trauma and shock followed by delayed sepsis.[12] A 1985 report from the Netherlands, confirmed bacterial sepsis in only 33% of patients with trauma related MOF compared to 65% of patients with nontrauma related MOF.[13] Waydhas and colleagues observed that virtually all of the patients with early MOF and half of the patients with late MOF had signs of organ failure before developing evidence of infection.[14]

Thus, early studies correctly observed that infection with systemic sepsis can produce MOF, but more recent clinical observations suggested that MOF frequently occurs in the absence of infection. As a result, noninfectious inflammatory models of MOF became the focus.[15] In this conceptual framework, patients are

resuscitated into a state of early systemic hyperinflammation, now referred to as the systemic inflammation response syndrome (SIRS) (Fig. 68-1). A mild response is presumed to be beneficial and resolves in most patients as they recover. In the "one-event" model, a massive traumatic insult overwhelms the capacity of the patient to respond to resuscitation and precipitates severe SIRS and early organ failure. In the alternative "two-event" model, patients who are initially resuscitated to a mild or moderate response (primed) are vulnerable to a second (activating) event that can also precipitate hyperinflammation leading to early organ failure. Patients that escape early MOF become susceptible to infection during the later compensatory anti-inflammatory response syndrome (CARS).[16] If infected during this window, patients are at risk of developing late MOF. This inflammatory construct evolved from clinical observations and experimental studies at the bench level, and is the foundation of contemporary MOF research.

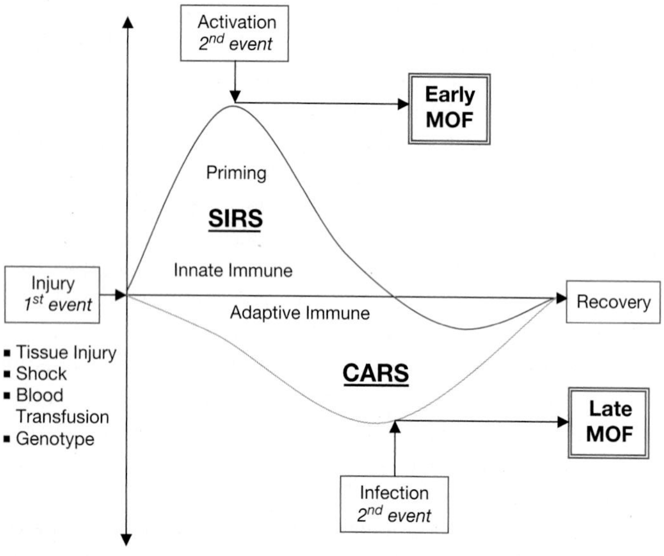

Parallel to exploring MOF pathophysiology, research is progressing toward therapeutic targets. Pharmacologic products to interrupt inflammatory signaling at the cellular and subcellular levels have been developed. New strategies to attenuate the inflammatory response in the early postinjury period and during the ICU recovery phase have also been implemented. Additionally, emerging clinical situations such as abdominal compartment syndrome have also been recognized as potential triggers for MOF.[17–19]As a result, the presentation and outcome of postinjury MOF has changed considerably over the past 15 years. It remains to be seen if a new clinical entity will emerge as we control MOF-related morbidity and mortality. For the present, postinjury MOF remains the most significant cause of postinjury morbidity and resource utilization in the ICU.[4,5]

**FIGURE 68-1.** Postinjury inflammatory profile.

## DEFINITIONS

### Systemic Inflammatory Response Syndrome (SIRS)

Recognizing the fact that a number of noninfectious and infectious insults can provoke a similar physiologic response, the term systemic inflammatory response syndrome (SIRS) was coined.[20] SIRS is defined as two or more of the following conditions: (a) temperature above 38°C or below 36°C, (b) heart rate greater than 90 beats per minute, (c) respiratory rate greater than 20 breaths per minute or a $pCO_2$ less than 32 mm Hg, and (d) white blood cell count greater than 12,000 or less than 4000, or greater than 10% immature forms (bands). Additionally, the term sepsis was reserved for conditions where SIRS was a result of an identifiable infectious source. Although this terminology was a step forward in that it emphasized that both infectious and noninfectious insults can provoke the same physiologic response, it is too sensitive to differentiate patients who are at risk for postinjury multiple organ failure and death from those who are not. Therefore, when we employ the nomenclature in our discussion, we further attempt to quantify SIRS by the descriptive terms mild, moderate, and severe.

## Multiple Organ Failure (MOF)

MOF was first described as a syndrome of sequential progressive organ dysfunction involving the lungs, kidneys, liver, gastrointestinal tract, and coagulation cascade.[6] Later reports included heart, hematologic, central nervous system, and metabolic dysfunctions in the description of MOF. These proposed definitions however lacked uniformity. Indeed, there have been wide variations on the terms labeling the clinical syndrome itself including *progressive* or *sequential organ failure, multiple systems organ failure, multiple organ dysfunction syndrome,* and *multiple organ failure.*[21] Consequently, disparate descriptions made direct comparison of clinical studies difficult. Despite this, investigators were describing a common series of progressive physiologic derangements with a variety of

etiologic factors that led to failure of two or more interrelated organ systems and conferred a high risk of death. Growing interest in research warranted a useful definition based on readily available objective clinical data.

In 1987 we developed the Denver MOF Score as a descriptive endpoint for clinical studies. This score originally included eight organ systems (pulmonary, renal, hepatic, gastrointestinal, hematologic, central nervous system [CNS], and metabolic).[22] Each system was assigned a failure grade of 0 to 3 to reflect a continuum of physiologic dysfunction and a daily sum score calculated. After several years of study however, the score was revised after evaluating this score in a multicenter trial. Gastrointestinal, hematologic, CNS, and metabolic failure were dropped from the score because their grading was largely subjective and their presence did not improve the characterization of MOF. The definitions of pulmonary, cardiac, hepatic, and renal failure were revised based on consensus with other investigators to facilitate consistent application in multicenter trials. The pulmonary score has subsequently been modified to assign a dysfunction grade based on the $PaO_2$ to $FiO_2$ ratio.[23] This simplifies calculation of the pulmonary score and better predicts mortality than the earlier more complex and therapy dependent scoring method.[24]

The current Denver MOF scoring system is depicted in Table 68-2.[25] A daily dysfunction grade is assigned to each of the pulmonary, cardiac, hepatic, and renal systems. Individual organ failure is defined as a dysfunction score of two or more, while MOF is defined as a sum of the simultaneously obtained organ dysfunction grades of four or more. Organ failure scores obtained within 48 hours of injury are not used to define MOF because transient

**TABLE 68-2**

**Denver Postinjury Multiple Organ Failure Score. MOF Score = A + B + C + D not Owing to Chronic Disease. Pulmonary Score is Based on $PaO_2$ to $FiO_2$ Ratio in Conjunction with Bilateral Pulmonary Infiltrates**

| DYSFUNCTION | GRADE 0 | GRADE 1 | GRADE 2 | GRADE 3 |
|---|---|---|---|---|
| **A. Pulmonary** | | | | |
| P/F ratio | $X > 250$ | $250 \geq X > 200$ | $200 \geq X > 100$ | $X \leq 100$ |
| **B. Renal** | | | | |
| Creatinine (mg/dL) | $X \leq 1.8$ | $1.8 < X \leq 2.5$ | $2.5 < X \leq 5.0$ | $X > 5.0$ |
| **C. Hepatic** | | | | |
| T Bilirubin (mg/dL) | $X \leq 2.0$ | $2.0 < X \leq 4.0$ | $4.0 < X \leq 8.0$ | $X > 8.0$ |
| **D. Cardiac** | No Inotropes | Minimal Inotropes | Moderate Inotropes | High Inotropes |

MOF = MOF score >3.

Cardiac Score:

Inotrope Dose

| AGENT | SMALL | MODERATE | LARGE |
|---|---|---|---|
| Dopamine (μg/kg/min) | < 6.0 | (6.0–15.0) | > 15.0 |
| Dobutamine (μg/kg/min) | < 6.0 | (6.0–15.0) | > 15.0 |
| Epinephrine (μg/kg/min) | < 0.06 | (0.06–0.25) | > 0.25 |
| Norepinephrine (μg/kg/min) | < 0.11 | (0.11–0.50) | > 0.50 |
| Phenylephrine (μg/kg/min) | < 0.6 | (0.60–3.0) | > 3.0 |
| Milrinone (μg/kg/min) | < 0.4 | (0.4–0.7) | > 0.7 |
| Vasopressin (units/min) | < 0.03 | (0.03–0.07) | > 0.07 |

Single agent

| DOSE | SMALL | MODERATE | LARGE |
|---|---|---|---|
| Cardiac Score | 1 | 2 | 3 |

Two Agents

| DOSE | (S,S) | (S,M) | (M,M) | ANY L |
|---|---|---|---|---|
| Cardiac Score | 2 | 2 | 3 | 3 |

Three or more agents: Cardiac Score = 3

organ dysfunction can be reflective of the initial insult or the host response to resuscitation and does not invariably progress to MOF.[26] MOF is defined as "early" if the MOF score on postinjury day three is four or more, and "late" if the first MOF score of four or more occurs after postinjury day three. Scores are determined serially so that the intensity and duration of MOF can be quantified.

Although alternative MOF scores have been proposed (Table 68-3), a consensus definition has not emerged as the gold standard.[7,12,13,27–34] Development of such a score is complicated by the periodic changing presentation and outcome of organ dysfunction. Most scores include assessments of lung, heart, liver, and kidney function based on readily available objective clinical data. Ideally, any MOF score should be easily calculated from data routinely collected in the care of the severely injured; reflect the severity of organ dysfunction as a continuum from mild to severe disease; obtained serially to describe disease presentation and resolution; and predict a definable outcome such as death, need for advanced organ support, or ICU length of stay.[30] Other crucial elements are that the data used to calculate the score should be independent of patient or injury mechanism and should not be directly altered by therapeutic intervention.[35] Additionally, a scoring system should be flexible to allow modification over time as more information about the epidemiology and pathophysiology is brought to light. That being stated, a more sophisticated score that incorporates biochemical markers of inflammation (see Chap. 67) or gene expression profiles (see Chap. 57) may be required to conduct interventional trials in the ICU.[36–39]

## PROSPECTIVE STUDY OF PATIENTS AT RISK FOR MOF

Constructive interpretation of studies in the 1980s and 1990s has been difficult due to small, disparate patient populations and varying definitions of organ dysfunction. Based on a literature review and a retrospective study in our SICU, we identified the patient population at risk and the pertinent clinical data that needed to be collected. Standard definitions of clinical variables and outcomes were also defined. In 1992 we established a prospective clinical database for the study of patients at risk for postinjury MOF.[40,41] Inclusion criteria were an Injury Severity Score (ISS) greater than 15, survival longer than 48 hours from injury, admission to the SICU within 24 hours of injury, and age greater than 15 years. Patients with isolated head injuries and head injuries with an extracranial abbreviated injury score (AIS) less than two were excluded because the primary determinant of outcome in this group is the severity of the initial head injury. Although MOF does occur in this group, it is a result of nosocomial infection and usually does not contribute to mortality of prolonged hospital stay.[42]

Patient characteristics were recorded at the time of hospital admission and daily physiologic and laboratory data were collected through SICU day 28. Clinical events were recorded on all patients thereafter until death or hospital discharge. The data collection and storage processes were made compliant with HIPAA regulations and were approved by our Institutional Review Board. By 2004, data from over 1500 patients had been entered into the database with an overall MOF incidence of 25%.

Development and maintenance of this database enabled a detailed longitudinal study of a uniform patient population over time.[43] An early priority was to identify MOF risk factors and validate definitions of organ dysfunction.[44] Prospective study permitted the development of predictive models that were used to assess new therapeutic interventions.[40,45] Identification of risk factors also suggested underlying pathophysiology and sparked several line of scientific investigation including optimal methods of resuscitation,[46,47] the effects of stored blood,[48] and the manifestations of the systemic inflammatory response.[49] A better understanding of the inflammatory pathophysiology in turn pointed to therapeutic strategies targeting the postinjury inflammatory response. Equally important is the longitudinal nature of the study which has tracked changes in risk factors and documented a dramatic decrease in the incidence and severity of postinjury MOF and the MOF-related mortality over the last 13 years.[43] The importance of these data was recently emphasized during the renewal of our NIH funded Trauma Center Research grant. The MOF database is the keystone of the human subject's core section of the grant which is designed to link clinical physiologic data with mechanistic basic science research on patient tissue. It has thus become vital to translational research from bedside to bench and back, and serves as a model investigative tool for a variety of disease states.

## EPIDEMIOLOGY

### Risk Factors

A study 457 patients over a four-year period revealed several independent risk factors for postinjury MOF.[44] Host factors, tissue injury indices, and the clinical indicators of shock for patients that did and did not develop MOF were identified. While MOF patients were older, the incidence of pre-existing diseases was low and not significantly associated with MOF. Injury severity, number of units of red blood cells (RBCs) transfused, base deficit, and lactate levels were all associated with MOF. (Table 68-4) Others have also found these early risk factors to be reliable predictors of MOF.[50]

More recent study has also identified obesity as an independent risk factor for postinjury MOF. Obese patients are known to be at increased risk of postinjury morbidity and mortality. In a study of 716 at risk patients, we observed 37% of obese patients developed MOF compared to 22% of nonobese patients. After adjusting for patient age, injury severity, and blood transfused during resuscitation, obesity was associated with an 80% increased risk of MOF (Fig. 68-2). Obese patients were also more likely to develop MOF within 72 hours of injury compared to nonobese patients. Since early MOF is thought to reflect the effects of unbridled postinjury hyperinflammation as opposed to uncontrolled infection, this observation supports the proinflammatory nature of the obese state. Alternatively, early organ dysfunction could represent decreased physiologic reserve of these patients. These findings in conjunction with evidence for an altered inflammatory potential in obese patients may point to therapeutic targets to improve outcomes in both obese and nonobese patients. Ongoing study will likely uncover previously unrecognized risk factors as the disease and treatment change over time.

**TABLE 68-3**

**Postinjury MOF Definitions**

| AUTHOR | LUNGS | KIDNEYS | LIVER | HEART | GASTROINTESTINAL | HEMATOLOGIC | CNS | METABOLIC |
|---|---|---|---|---|---|---|---|---|
| Fry (1980) | Hypoxia +5 d MV | Cr >2mg/dL or 2x preinjury | T.B. > 2.0 mg/dl + SGOT + LDH > 2x normal | — | UGI Bleed > 2 units/24 h | — | — | — |
| Faist (1983) | $FiO_2$ = 40% or PEEP ≥ 72 h | Cr ≥2.0 mg/dL | T.B. > 3.0 mg/dl + LDH > 2x normal | High Filling pressures, autopsy findings | UGI Bleed > 2 units/24 h | Plt < 60 K | — | — |
| Goris (1985) | Grade 1 = MV + PEEP 0–10 cmH2O +$FiO_2$ = 40% Grade 2 = MV + PEEP >10 +$FiO_2$ > 40% | Grade 1 = Cr ≥ 2.0 mg/dL Grade 2 = dialysis | Grade 1 = T.B. ≥ 2.0 mg/dL Grade 2 = dialysis | Grade 1 = BP<100 + dopamine < 10 µg/kg/minor NTG <20 µg/min Grade 2 = BP<100 + dopamine > 10 µg/kg/minor NTG > 20 µg/min | Grade 1 = Acalculus chlecystitis or ulcer Grade 2 = UGI Bleed > 2 units/24 h, NEC, Pancratitis, Gall Bladder Perf | Grade 1 = Plt < 50 K or WBC < 30 K Grade 2 = Hemorrhagic diathesis or WBC ≥ 60 K, ≤ 2.5 K | Grade 1 = decreased response Grade 2 = severely decreased response, diffuse neuropathy | — |
| Knaus (1985) | RR ≤5 or ≥>=49 $PaO_2$ ≥50 or A-aDo2 ≥350 mm hg | UO ≤ 479 mL/24 h or < 159 mL/8 h or BUN ≥ 100 mg/mL or Cr ≥3.5 | — | HR ≤ 54 or MAP ≤ 49 or Vtach or Vfib or pH ≤ 7.24 or $PaO_2$ ≤ 49 mm Hg | — | WBC ≤ 1 K or Plt ≤ 20 K or Hct ≤ 20% | GCS ≤ 6 | — |
| Marshall (1988) | Grade 1 = MV+ $FiO_2$ ≤40% > 5 d Grade 2= MV+ $FiO_2$ > 40% > 3 d | Grade 1 = Cr ≤2.4 or chronic renal failure, Grade 2 = Cr > 2.4 mg/dL | Grade 1 = T.B. <2.0 or Alb > 2.5 g/dL, Grade 2 = T.B. ≥ 2.0 mg/dL or Alb ≤ 2.0 g/dL | Grade 1 = C.O. > 7.0 or PACW ≥ 20 cm $H_2O$ Grade 2 = Inotropes | — | Grade 1 = Plt ≤ 99 K Grade 2 = Plt ≤ 60 K | Grade 1 = GCS <14 Grade 2 = GCS < 10 | Grade 1 = Insulin < 4U Grade 2 = Insulin ≥ 4U to keep Gluc ≤220 mg/dL |
| Deitch (1992) | Dysfunction = hypoxia + MV>3 d Failure = ARDS with PEEP >10cm $H_2O$ +$FiO_2$>50% | Dysfunction = UO ≤ 479 mL/24 h or Cr ≥2.0 mg/dL Failure = Dialysis | Dysfunction = T.N. >2.0 mg/dL, LFT's > 2x normal, Failure= T.B. >8.0 mg/dl | — | Dysfunction = Ileus + tube feed intolerance > 5 d Failure = UGI bleed, acalculus cholecystitis | Dysfunction = PT + PTT > 25%, Plt <50 K Failure = DIC | Dysfunciton = Confusion Failure = Progressive Coma | — |
| Marshall (1995) | Grade 0–4 based on $PaO_2/FiO_2$ | Grade 0–4 based on Cr and OU | Grade 0–4 based on T.B. | Grade 0–4 based on Pressure adjusted heart rate (PAR) | — | Grade 0–4 based on Plt | Grade 0–4 based on GCS | — |
| Vincint (1996) | Grade 0–4 based on $PaO_2/FiO_2$ and MV | Grade 0–4 based on Cr and OU | Grade 0–4 based on T.B. | Grade 0–4 based on MAP and Inotrop dosing | — | Grade 0–4 based on WBC | Grade 0–4 based on GCS | — |

## TABLE 68-4

| Risk Factors for MOF |
| --- |
| Age |
| Age > 55 |
| Injury Severity Score |
| ISS > 25 |
| 0–12 h Blood Transfusion |
| > 6 U PRBC |
| 0–12 h Base Deficit |
| BD > 8.0 mEq/L |
| 0–12 h lactate |
| > 2.5 mmol/L |
| 13–24 h base deficit |
| BD > 8.0 mEq/L |
| 13–24 h lactate |
| > 2.5 mmol/L |

## TABLE 68-5

| Independent Predictors of Subsequent Multiple Organ Failure According to Postinjury Time Window | | | | |
| --- | --- | --- | --- | --- |
| | ADMISSION | 0–12H | 0–24H | 0–48H |
| Age > 45 | + | + | + | + |
| Injury Severity | | | | |
| ISS > 40 | + | + | + | + |
| Shock | | | | |
| RBC > 6 units | + | + | + | + |
| Lactate > 4 mmol | | | + | |
| Inotropes | | + | + | + |
| Platelets < 80 K | | | + | |
| APS-APACHE III 25–48 h | | | | + |

## Prediction

The next step in improving study design was to develop prediction models that identify patients likely to develop postinjury MOF who would most likely benefit from early intervention. Systemic innate immunologic priming occurs within three hours and is maximally established within 12 hours of injury.[51] Therefore, we sought to determine the earliest point at which we could reliably predict MOF. Specifically, predictive models were developed at four sequential time points — admission, 12 hours, 24 hours, and 48 hours postinjury — and goodness-of-fit measures were compared to determine the relative ability to predict MOF at the various time points.[45] The predictive models were built by sequentially adding the prospectively collected patient data obtained at the subsequent time window while keeping the significant variables obtained in the previous time window. We found that the injury severity score, RBC transfusions, age, and platelet count remained significant predictors in all four models; the need for inotropes was a strong predictor in the 0- to 12-hour, 0- to 24-hour, and 0- to 48-hour models; failure to normalize lactate by 13 to 24 hours was a powerful predictor in the 0- to 24-hour and 0- to 48-hour models. The Acute Physiology Score–Acute Physiology And Chronic Health Evaluation (APS-APACHE III) emerged only as an independent predictor in the 0- to 48-hour model. (Table 68-5) Using goodness-of-fit measurements, we found that our ability to predict

MOF improved in the later time windows but all of the models were consistently more specific than sensitive. Having thus developed prediction models using readily available clinical data, we could formulate a basis to evaluate changes in postinjury MOF presentation and outcome over time, and evaluate the effect of new management strategies adopted in the care of the injured patient.

## Presentation

Clinicians have recognized changes in MOF presentation and disease progression since the syndrome was originally described. Reports identified patterns of early and late MOF as well as differing patterns of organ involvement, degree of dysfunction, and the incidence of sepsis. Subsequent investigations defined early and late MOF as distinct clinical entities with separate risk factors and outcome but with common pathophysiology.[41] This bimodal disease presentation (Fig. 68-3) has withstood the test of time[25] and is consistent with the two event inflammatory model.

Organ dysfunction during resuscitation is a common occurrence following major trauma. Patients often require mechanical ventilation for impaired oxygenation and inotropic agents to support cardiac function to deliver oxygen. Transient acute renal dysfunction is also occasionally seen following severe injury requiring aggressive shock resuscitation. However, these early organ dysfunctions do not invariably progress to durable MOF beyond the resuscitation period.[26] Organ dysfunction within 48 hours of injury resolves in approximately half of patients. These alterations in physiology represent the host response to injury and resuscitation and are not self-perpetuating processes that eventuate in

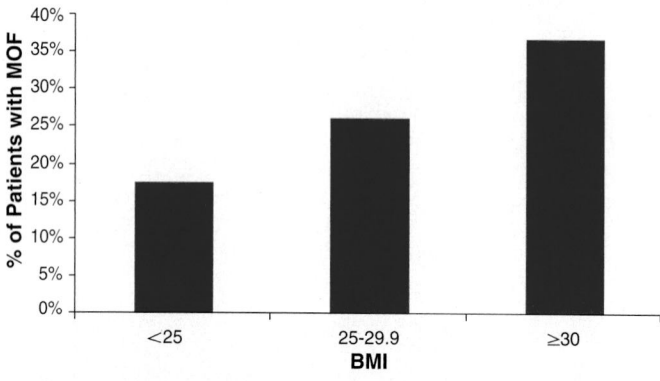

**FIGURE 68-2.** Proportion of patients that developed postinjury MOF stratified by Body Mass Index (BMI).

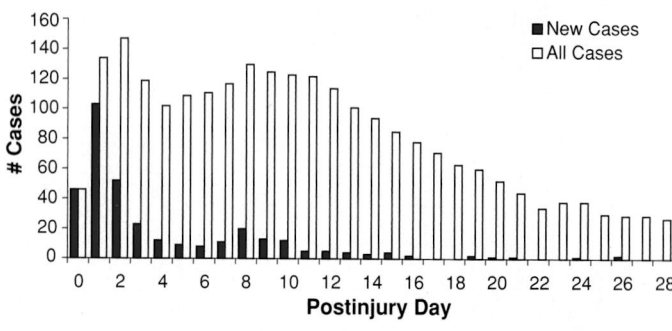

**FIGURE 68-3.** Temporal distribution of postinjury MOF.

**TABLE 68-6**

| Classification of Major Infection in Early and Late MOF | | | | |
|---|---|---|---|---|
| **32 MAJOR INFECTIONS / 23 PATIENTS (85%)** | | | | |
| **Early MOF (n=27)** | **Not Related** | **Trigger** | **Worsen** | **Symptom** |
| Pneumonia | 2(6%) | 1(3%) | 3(9%) | 14(44%) |
| Abdominal abscess | | | 2(6%) | 2(6%) |
| Wound infection | | 1(3%) | | 4(6%) |
| Other infections | | | | 3(9%) |
| Total | 2(6%) | 2(6%)ᵃ | 5(16%) | 23(72%) |
| **59 MAJOR INFECTIONS / 38 PATIENTS (88%)** | | | | |
| **Late MOF (n=43)** | **Not Related** | **Trigger** | **Worsen** | **Symptom** |
| Pneumonia | 15(25%) | 11(19%) | 1(2%) | 13(22%) |
| Empyema/abscess | 1(2%) | | | 1(2%) |
| Abdominal abscess | 2(3%) | 3(5%) | 1(2%) | 3(5%) |
| Wound infection | | 2(2%) | 1(2%) | 3(7%) |
| Other | 1(2%) | | | 1(3%) |
| Total | 19 (32%) | 16(27%)ᵃ | 3(5%) | 21(36%) |

ᵃp=0.025 number of major infections serving as "triggers" for early MOF compared to late MOF.

definable organ failure. Furthermore, approximately half of the patients that develop MOF will do so more than 72 hours after injury.[26,41] For these reasons, transient organ dysfunction that occurs within 48 hours of injury is not considered MOF. To investigate the inciting mechanisms, MOF that is present on day three is considered early; MOF that occurs after day three is considered late.

Early MOF begins shortly after injury as an overwhelming inflammatory response to massive tissue injury and shock (one event model). In such cases, metabolic collapse ensues as a result of irreversible shock. Alternatively, patients in the primed state (usually within 12 to 36 hours of injury) who suffer a second event develop MOF following the second stimulus. Organ dysfunction is usually evident within 48 hours and is established within 72 hours of injury.[50] The risk factors for early MOF include an ISS greater than 24, emergency department systolic blood pressure less than 90 mm Hg, blood transfusion of more than 6 units within 12 hours of injury, and a lactate level of more than 2.5 nmol/L measured between 12 and 24 hours after injury.[41] Major infections are more likely to be a symptom that follows or worsens organ dysfunction than a trigger that precipitates early MOF (Table 68-6). Early MOF is typically associated with a higher incidence of heart failure and death (34%) than late MOF.

Late MOF occurs more than 72 hours following injury. Consistent with the two event construct, MOF patients develop a state of relative immunosupression between 24 and 48 hours after the initial SIRS resolves. These patients are at increased risk of infection and systemic sepsis which, in turn, can lead to MOF. Independent risk factors for late MOF include age over 55 years, blood transfusion more than 6 units within 12 hours of injury, early base deficit more than 8 mEq/L in the first 12 hours postinjury, and a lactate level greater than 2.5 nmol/L measured between 12 and 24 hours postinjury. Although the risk factors for both early and late MOF included blood transfusion, base excess, and lactate levels, the shock indices were stronger risk factors for early MOF; whereas, major infections were more frequently classified as triggers in

patients that developed late MOF. Patients with late MOF also had a higher incidence of liver failure but a lower mortality (16%) than early MOF patients.

The lung is virtually always the first organ to show evidence of dysfunction in the absence of pre-existing disease.[25] Lung dysfunction precedes heart dysfunction by an average of $0.6 \pm 0.2$ days, liver dysfunction by $4.8 \pm 0.2$ days, and kidney dysfunction by $5.5 \pm 0.5$ days (Fig. 68-4). The number of involved organs and the severity of other organ dysfunction are also dependent on the severity of lung impairment. This prompted some to conclude that the lung is the motor that drives postinjury MOF and that MOF is really just a severe case of ARDS. The overall incidence of MOF has been reported to as low as 7% and as high as 66%.[5,7,45,52] The true incidence is difficult to estimate because of disparate study populations reported in the literature and varying definitions of organ failure. Similarly, overall mortality from MOF has been reported to be as high as 80% but has gradually decreased over time.[5,43] MOF-related mortality increases with the severity of organ dysfunction and with the number of organ systems involved.[30,25,53]

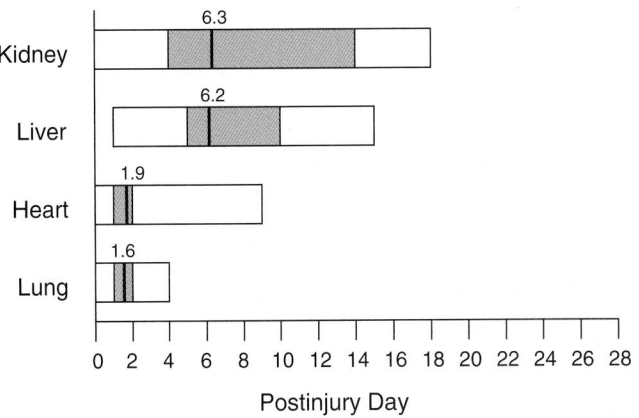

**FIGURE 68-4.** Sequence of organ failure onset. Mean time of onset is listed for each organ, the interquartile range is shaded, the 95th percentile is open.

## Changes in MOF over Time

Care of the injured patient has evolved significantly during the past 15 years. It has been suggested that MOF is disappearing due to advances in trauma and critical care[54,55]; however, recent reports have not demonstrated a consistent change in the either the incidence or the mortality associated with postinjury MOF. Some groups have reported no change in the incidence but a decreased mortality[5] while others have reported both decreased incidence and mortality compared to historic controls.[56,57] Again, the disparity reported in the literature is in part due to different populations studied over relatively short observation intervals.

We reviewed prospective data on 1244 patients collected over 12 years applying a uniform definition of postinjury MOF.[43] We found that the unadjusted MOF rate did not change significantly between 1991 and 2002. However, we observed a significant increase in patient age and injury severity concomitant with a decrease in the amount of blood transfused during resuscitation (Fig. 68-5). Subsequently, multiple logistic regression models demonstrated a significant reduction in the incidence of MOF after adjusting for these factors. In addition to reduced incidence, the severity, duration, and death attributed to MOF decreased significantly over the same time period. By comparing data on patients admitted during the first five years of the study to those admitted during the last five years of the study, we found that influence of the previously identified risk factors on the probability of developing MOF had changed over time (Table 68-7). Age and injury severity became less important risk factors while blood transfusion became a more important risk factor. Since blood transfusion was the only risk factor observed to decrease during the study, we concluded that the decrease in MOF was due at least in part to judicious use of blood during the resuscitation period.

In a more focused study, we reviewed data collected on 897 patients since 1997.[57a] In agreement with our previous report, we found that the incidence of postinjury MOF decreased significantly from 33% in 1997 to 12% in 2004, and the incidence of early MOF decreased from 22% in 1997 to 7% in 2004 (Fig. 68-6). There was a concurrent decrease in the incidence of postinjury ARDS from 43% in 1997 to 25% in 2004. We were surprised to find, however, that the incidence of lung dysfunction (measured as the $PaO_2$ to $FiO_2$ ratio recorded at 72 hours postinjury, and the lowest ratio

### TABLE 68-7

**Changes in the Influence of Independent MOF Risk Factors Over Time**

| Risk Factor | 1992–1996 OR (95% CI) | 1997–2003 OR (95% CI) |
|---|---|---|
| Age>55 | 3.09 (1.63–5.85) | 2.88 (1.93–4.31) |
| ISS ≥25 | 2.76 (1.69–4.50) | 1.66 (1.13–2.44) |
| 12 h RBC > 6 | 3.62 (2.28–5.72) | 4 .00 (2.73–5.85) |

recorded within 28 days of injury) did not change significantly over the same time period. This study strongly suggests a decrease in the progression of postinjury lung dysfunction to ARDS and MOF over time.

We interpreted these findings to represent a decrease in activation of the postinjury inflammatory response despite a constant rate of priming.[58,59] Clinically, priming is characterized by alterations in body temperature, white blood cell count, respiratory dysfunction, and a hyperdynamic state.[20] We found no change in early lung function, heart rate, temperature, and WBC count measured at 24 hours postinjury. This is not surprising in that identifying the primed state based on routine clinical indicators is virtually impossible. The causes of postinjury SIRS are multifactorial and its criteria are not specific for priming. Moreover, systemic priming is present to some degree in all trauma patients because the priming event is the initial injury itself. Since priming is established within three hours of injury,[51] interventions to decrease its magnitude are limited to the period immediately following injury.

Conversely, unbridled activation of the innate immune system is a destructive process clinically manifested by ARDS and MOF. Of particular interest with respect to the activating event was an observed decreased incidence of early MOF which is more representative of an activated inflammatory response. While impaired oxygen exchange itself could represent a multitude of underlying conditions, the diffuse bilateral infiltrates in the absence of heart failure observed on chest x-ray define ARDS and a hallmark of inflammatory mediated pulmonary edema. Thus, a decreased incidence of ARDS and MOF over time relative to postinjury SIRS suggests a decrease in activation relative to priming. As discussed below, this effect can be attributed to

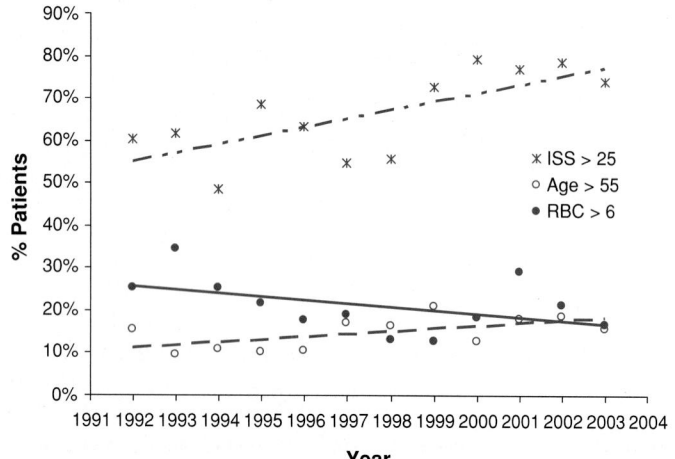

**FIGURE 68-5.**  Changes in MOF risk factors from 1992 to 2003.

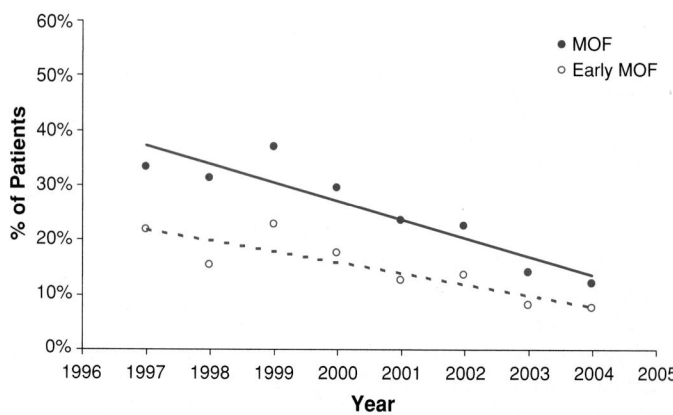

**FIGURE 68-6.**  Decreased incidence of MOF and early MOF since 1997.

several recent advances in postinjury care adopted over the last decade.

The longitudinal study of a discrete population using uniform definitions has enabled evaluation of pathophysiologic models based on clinical observations and refined by experimental data, permitted a global assessment of advances in postinjury care over time, and generated new hypotheses for further clinical and basic research.

## PATHOPHYSIOLOGY: A UNIFIED INFLAMMATORY CONSTRUCT

The inflammatory model of postinjury MOF was developed from epidemiologic studies, predictive models, and basic investigations using in vivo and in vitro models. As mentioned above, severe trauma patients are resuscitated into an early state of systemic hyperinflammation (i.e., SIRS). The initial intensity of SIRS is dependent on the amount of tissue injury, the degree of shock, and the presence of host factors (such as gene expression, age and comorbid disease, and blood transfusion). Mild to moderate SIRS is presumed to be beneficial (i.e., it is the stress response to injury) and resolves as the host recovers. However, if the initial insult is massive (one-hit model), the resulting severe SIRS can precipitate early MOF. Alternatively, early MOF can occur when patients are initially resuscitated into moderate SIRS (the "primed" state) then exposed to early secondary inflammatory insults (two-hit model). Examples include delayed hemorrhage, hypoxic events, secondary operations, skeletal fracture fixation, abdominal compartment syndrome, and aspiration. At the same time, negative feedback systems (i.e., compensatory anti-inflammatory response syndrome [CARS]) attempt to limit certain components of SIRS so that it does not become an autodestructive process (see Chap. 67).[16,60,61] This results in delayed immunosuppression. While mild to moderate delayed immunosuppression may be beneficial, when severe, it is associated with major infectious complications (principally pneumonia) and late MOF. Ultimately, the predominant mechanism responsible for early or late MOF may be the balance between proinflammatory and counter-inflammatory states.

Although the effects of the inflammatory process are realized at the systemic level, the mechanisms originate at the cellular and subcellular level. A comprehensive discussion of such mechanisms is beyond the scope of this chapter and many are discussed elsewhere in this book. Therefore, the following review focuses on those mechanisms that are consistent with the above construct.

### Ischemia and Reperfusion

Ischemia in the absence of direct tissue injury also elicits a systemic inflammatory response. Extended periods of ischemia will produce cell death as energy stores are depleted. (see Chap. 13) Upon restoration of blood flow, dead tissue will incite an inflammatory response. Additionally, ischemic but viable tissue in a variety of organs is vulnerable to xanthine oxidase (XO) mediated reperfusion injury.[62] XO has been found in vascular endothelium as well as the gut epithelium. Under normal conditions, XO exists predominantly as xanthine dehydrogenase (XD) and the cell has an ample supply of adenosine triphosphate (ATP). With ischemia, ATP breaks down to adenosine diphosphate (ADP), which further breaks down to adenosine monophosphate (AMP), adenosine, and hypoxanthine. During the same ischemic period, XD is converted to XO. With reperfusion, oxygen becomes available, and XO catalyzes the oxidation of hypoxanthine to uric acid with a concomitant burst of superoxide ($O_2^-$) production, which is converted into more toxic ROMs (see Chap. 67). Reperfusion also impairs endothelium-dependent vasodilation in arterioles by altering the balance of nitric oxide (NO) and $O_2^-$ in the endothelial cells (EC).[63] Under normal conditions, NO production greatly exceeds $O_2^-$ production in the EC. However, with reperfusion, the balance between NO and $O_2^-$ shifts in favor of $O_2^-$. The relatively low level of NO by constitutive endothelial nitric oxide synthase (NOS-I) reacts with the now abundant $O_2^-$ to generate peroxynitrites, leaving little NO available to reduce arteriolar tone (via guanylate cyclase activation in smooth muscle), prevent platelet aggregation, and minimize PMN adhesion to the EC.[64] ROMs also promote PMN binding to endothelial cells by upregulating endothelial adhesion molecule expression.[65]

### Tissue Destruction

Direct tissue destruction results in localized cellular death, microvascular thrombosis, tissue ischemia, secondary cell death, and a localized inflammatory reaction. The effect is to restore or maintain function of the tissues while eradicating or repairing dysfunctional cells. The local effects are mediated primarily by cytokines generated and released by endothelial cells in a paracrine fashion through binding to specific cell surface receptors and activation of intracellular signaling pathways. Leukocytes, primarily neutrophils, are also recruited to the injury site by the chemoattractant properties of several cytokines and stimulated to clear cellular debris and foreign material.[66,67] More recently it has become apparent that cellular breakdown products themselves (e.g., actin, RNAse, DNAse, HMGB, etc.) may also act as inflammatory mediators.

### Blood Transfusion

The available literature incriminates early blood transfusion to be a consistent predictor of infection, ARDS, MOF, and death following major trauma. While it has been assumed that the need for blood transfusion reflects the presence of shock, the popular alternative explanation is that blood transfusions are immunoactive and thus contribute to infectious complications that cause late MOF.[68] More recently, it has been recognized that stored blood also contains proinflammatory mediators (Lysi-PC, PAF, IL-6, IL-8, and IL-18) that may amplify early SIRS and thus cause early MOF.[69–71] The hypothesis that blood transfusions are immunosuppressive and thus responsible for the major septic morbidity that causes late MOF was first suggested by the transplantation literature of the late 1970s.[72] It was clearly demonstrated that kidney transplants were less likely to be rejected if the patient received preoperative blood transfusions. Soon thereafter, in the surgical oncology literature, it was shown that perioperative blood transfusions were associated with tumor recurrence. The inflammatory effects of blood transfusion itself are well represented by transfusion related lung injury (TRALI).[73–75] In this syndrome, blood transfusion can serve as either a first or second event that triggers lung dysfunction in a neutrophil mediated mechanism. In the trauma literature, blood transfusions have been shown to independently correlate with major infections, MOF, increased ICU length of stay, and mortality.[68,76–78] In addition to the inflammatory potential in the early postinjury period, late blood transfusion could exacerbate delayed immunosupression and increase the risk of late infections.[79]

Our interest in this topic was prompted by the finding that early blood transfusion is the most powerful independent risk factor for postinjury MOF[48] and that stored blood primes PMNs for enhanced cytotoxicity. Further investigation demonstrated that the age of the blood transfused was independently associated with increased postinjury MOF.[80] The mechanism was believed due to the generation of proinflammatory agents during RBC storage initially thought to be PAF, IL-6, and IL-8.[69–71,81] Later studies found that additional biologically active cytokines and lipid mediators (lysophosphatidylcholines) accumulate in stored blood and are capable of PMN priming.[69,82–84] "Passenger leukocytes" present in stored blood have been implicated as pivotal components by the finding that prestorage leukoreduction decreases the PMN priming and transfusion mediated lung injury in animal models.[85]

The above clinical and laboratory studies suggest that residual leukocytes remaining in packed red blood cell units after standard processing generate proinflammatory agents which accumulate over time. These neutrophils and neutrophil degradation products act on cell membrane fragments to produce proinflammatory lipids. Together, these agents can either prime or activate the inflammatory response in the early postinjury period. In the late postinjury period, blood transfusion is associated with a relatively immunosupressed state and an increased risk of major infection. This growing body of evidence underscores the immunomodulatory effects of blood transfusion and contributes to postinjury morbidity.

## Secondary Operation

Among the early observations in postinjury MOF was the clinical deterioration of a trauma patient that was initially resuscitated, but then quickly developed severe MOF following an otherwise routine second operation.[86] In one sense, the second operation can be considered a controlled traumatic event where surgical trauma takes the place of the initial injury; there is a certain degree of tissue destruction, tissue ischemia, and stimulation of the systemic inflammatory response. Additional stresses of secondary operations include higher intraoperative fluid consumption, hypothermia, hypotension, tissue hypoxia, and intraoperative blood loss. Indeed, several manifestations of SIRS are evident following a variety of elective operations.[87–90] The effects of a second operation in a patient whose inflammatory response is already primed can be overwhelming. Since the second operation would not normally be expected to provoke MOF, clinical investigation has focused on the timing between the initial trauma and secondary operations.

The timing of the second operation has been variously studied over the last decade mostly as related to operative fracture fixation. While early definitive fracture fixation decreases postinjury morbidity and improves recovery,[91–93] it is not without consequences in the multiply injured patient when performed within the priming window. Patients with severe chest trauma were found to have a higher incidence of postinjury ARDS and death when intramedullary femur fracture fixation was performed within 24 hours of injury.[94] Study of the inflammatory profile patients undergoing operative fixation of femoral shaft fractures demonstrated postsurgical increases in several inflammatory cytokines including IL-6 and TNFa.[95] Further study demonstrated that patients undergoing intramedullary fixation of femoral shaft fractures had a higher incidence of postoperative organ dysfunction if the preoperative IL-6 levels were greater than 500pg/dL,[96] and that early external fixation followed by delayed conversion to intramedullary instrumentation was associated with a decreased inflammatory response to the operative fixation.[97] These findings strongly suggest that an additional inflammatory insult, in this case secondary operation, can amplify the postinjury inflammatory response and thus has the potential to precipitate MOF.

## Abdominal Compartment Syndrome

A hallmark of the postinjury inflammatory state is generalized capillary leak and associated tissue edema. Historically, peripheral edema was considered to be minimally significant consequence of fluid resuscitation. This view has changed with the resurgent interest in intra-abdominal hypertension that has accompanied the recent widespread application of damage control procedures. It is now recognized that increased intra-abdominal pressures are accompanied by a host of physiologic derangements that include high ventilator pressures, decreased cardiac output, and impaired renal function termed the abdominal compartment syndrome (ACS).[98] Usually associated with abdominal injuries (primary ACS), these effects can also be observed following extra-abdominal injury or following large volume resuscitation for nontraumatic or nonsurgical conditions (secondary ACS).[99,100] The common feature of secondary ACS is the presence of shock requiring massive crystalloid resuscitation.

The clinical manifestations are the same for primary and secondary ACS and include reduced cardiac output despite adequate measured preload, increased ventilatory pressures and decreased compliance, oliguria, and increased intracranial pressure. The incidence of ACS varies greatly according to the resuscitation strategy but is primarily dependent on the severity of injury and the degree of shock. Global capillary leak following ischemia and reperfusion leads to generalized tissue edema. The bowel is particularly susceptible to the effects of low arterial flow states. Mesenteric ischemia reperfusion increases microvascular permeability causing bowel wall edema which can directly cause decreased bowel motility, decreased barrier function, and further capillary leak. Splanchnic hypoperfusion during shock is compounded by even mild increases in intra-abdominal pressure (which can reduce the abdominal perfusion pressure) and decreased plasma oncotic pressure from crystalloid resuscitation (which worsens edema).[19,101] As with any compartment syndrome, the increased pressure within the compartment rises above postcapillary pressure causing a functional venous and lymphatic obstruction. Under conditions of acute mesenteric venous congestion, the microvili of the intestinal epithelium secrete fluid into the gut lumen. Transudation of free fluid into the peritoneal space also contributes to further increases in intra-abdominal pressure. The net result of bowel wall edema, intraluminal secretion of fluid, and accumulation of fluid in the peritoneal cavity further increases intra-abdominal pressure. The cycle of capillary leak, obstruction, ischemia, and further inflammation is self reinforcing and ultimately results in the physiologic changes mentioned above.

Additionally, gut ischemia has profound effects on the inflammatory response (see Chap. 64). Gut ischemia alone increases vascular permeability in the lung.[102] The postischemic gut serves a priming bed for circulating neutrophils and generates inflammatory mediators that are released into the mesenteric lymph.[103] In fact, gut ischemia alone is sufficient to cause multiple organ failure. This has been demonstrated in animal models and is clinically observed following mesenteric vascular occlusion. While the physiologic effects of ACS are usually reversed upon decompression, the immunoimodulatory effects persist and often trigger multiple organ failure.[17,104,105]

## Ventilator Induced Lung Injury

The lung plays a central role in the pathogenesis of postinjury MOF. The lung is almost always the first organ to show signs of dysfunction and other organ failure is dependent on the presence of lung failure.[25] In addition to direct injury and secondary inflammatory mediated injury discussed below, the lung is also subject to ventilator induced lung injury (see Chap. 63). While the mechanical ventilator is an indispensable therapy for lung failure, the administration of positive pressure ventilation can result in lung injury that is functionally and histologically identical to that seen in ARDS.[106] Conversion from negative pressure ventilation to positive pressure ventilation is associated with unequal distribution of tidal volumes to the heterogeneously involved lung parenchyma. Areas of low compliance (as seen in pulmonary contusion, edema, or infection) force tidal volumes to areas of high compliance resulting in increased alveolar pressures, over distension, and injury to uninvolved lung tissue.[107] Barotrauma describes a mechanism whereby increased transpulmonary pressures allow air into the bronchovesicular sheath that tracks to the mediastinum. Volutrauma refers to over distension of the alveoli and stretching of the pulmonary epithelium and vascular bed leading to mechanical injury of the lung parenchyma. Atelectrauma implicates shear stresses generated on the opposing epithelial cell membranes during collapse and opening of the alveoli at low tidal volumes. The membrane shear causes additional mechanical damage to the cell. These mechanical injuries to the lung initiate a local inflammatory reaction and biotrauma; where inflammatory mediators released from damaged cells provoke a local inflammatory reaction mediated by circulating leukocytes.[108] There is also evidence for mechanotransduction signaling whereby mechanical stresses on the living cell are translated into intracellular inflammatory signal transduction.[109,110] Recruitment of PMNs to the site of injury results in further nonspecific cell damage as described below. The combination of mechanical damage from positive pressure ventilation and the inflammatory mediated parenchyma damage furthers pulmonary dysfunction.

The effects of ventilator-induced lung injury extend beyond the lung. Impaired oxygen delivery amplifies posttraumatic ischemia/reperfusion injury. Mechanical disruption of normal lung defense mechanisms increases the infectious potential and the risk of pulmonary sepsis. Inflammatory cytokines generated in the lung spill over into the systemic circulation and have the capacity to increase the inflammatory state (priming) and promote remote

organ dysfunction via direct cell signaling (activation). Lung tissue that has undergone a prior stress such as direct injury or ischemia/reperfusion is particularly sensitive to further ventilator-induced lung injury.[111]

Clinical evidence of the contributing effects of mechanical ventilation on the incidence of MOF was demonstrated in the ARDS network lung protective ventilation trails.[112] The ARDS network study demonstrated less barotrauma, a greater reduction in plasma IL-6 levels and fewer days of other organ failure, and decreased mortality in the patients treated with a lung protective ventilation strategy. Lung protective ventilation has recently been associated with a more rapid decrease in plasma IL-6 and IL-8 levels.[113] These studies represent a growing body of evidence that establishes ventilator induced lung injury as an important factor in critical illness morbidity and mortality. As a result, lung protective strategies have become the standard therapy for respiratory support of patients at risk for ARDS.[114]

## Pharmacologic Agents

One area of great potential influence is the effect of pharmacologic agents used during acute resuscitation on the postinjury inflammatory response. Severely injured patients are routinely exposed to a variety of drugs that include resuscitation fluids, sedatives, analgesics, anesthetics, paralytics, inotropes, and contrast media, the immunomodulatory effects of which are only recently acknowledged. Research on resuscitation fluids has historically focused on efficacy of restoring intravascular volume and reaching physiologic endpoints. It is now recognized that different resuscitation fluids have widely disparate effects on PMN function.[115–118] Benzodiazapines are also known to decrease inflammation through a mechanism involving cytokine and nitric oxide (NO) production.[119–121] Ketamine also decreases cytokine production following cardiac surgery[122] and animal models of septic shock,[123] and protects the gut from ischemia/reperfusion injury.[124] Conversely, etomidate may induce a state of relative adrenal insufficiency which is associated with an increased inflammatory potential.[125–127] In addition to hemodynamic effects, opiate based analgesic agents may increase the inflammatory potential by increasing TNF-a and IL-1b expression in lung tissue[128] and peripheral leukocytes.[129] Adrenergic receptors also have differential roles in modulating the inflammatory response.[130] Beta-adrenergic stimulation decreases some PMN cytotoxic functions[131–133] while beta-adrenergic blockade increases PMN mediated tissue edema.[134] Radiographic contrast has a multitude of effects on PMNs, platelets, and endothelial cells.[135–137] These represent only a fraction of the agents commonly used in the routine care of the severely injured patient. As more is learned about the immunomodulatory effects of these and other drugs, further clinical study will determine if these effects are important contributors to inflammatory mediated complications.

## Infection

Early reports identified a strong and consistent association between "sepsis" and MOF. Thus, in the early 1980s, MOF was considered to be "a fatal expression of uncontrolled infection" and intraabdominal abscess (IAA) was identified to be the inciting event in half of the cases. As a result, trauma surgeons focused their research interest on identifying methods to reduce IAA in patients requiring emergency trauma laparotomy. Basic laboratory studies established that if injured tissue is contaminated with bacteria, it could serve as a later nidus of infection, and that the rate of infection can be reduced by prophylactic administration of antibiotics.[138–140] This prompted a series of studies to define the appropriate use of presumptive antibiotics in patients sustaining abdominal trauma (see Chap. 19). Other areas of clinical research to reduce IAA included the avoidance of delayed diagnosis of hollow-viscus injury (see Chap. 30). As a result of these efforts, the incidence of postinjury IAA has decreased, and those that do occur seldom precipitate or worsen MOF. The epidemiology of postinjury infections has changed; nosocomial pneumonia is now the principal infection associated with MOF.[41]

Early pneumonias are difficult to diagnose and can trigger MOF. The pathogenic implications of late MOF-associated pneumonia are not as clear. They appear to occur in patients with acquired impairment in host defense. The exact cause of this generalized immunosuppression is not clear and undoubtedly multifactorial (see Chap. 67).[141–145]

From a teleologic standpoint, this may reflect dysfunctional regulation of inflammation. Following a traumatic insult, nonspecific inflammation, which is primarily mediated by neutrophils and tissue macrophages, targets devitalized tissue and invading bacteria until specific immune responses can be brought into play. This is generally a localized process; however, with extensive insults, this early hyperinflammation becomes systemic. Its amplitude and duration (generally three to five days) are dependent on the magnitude of the initial insult. Both nonspecific and specific immunity have negative feedback mechanisms. Monocytes/macrophages and suppressor T-lymphocytes have been implicated to be key modulators that downregulate a host of immune functions (e.g., decrease granulopoiesis, decrease PMN numbers and function, decrease lymphocyte proliferation, decrease CD4/CD8 ratio, decrease IL-2 and IL-2 receptors, Th1 to Th2 shift, immunoglobulin M to immunoglobulin G (IgM to IgG) shift) (see Chap. 67). This downregulation of early hyperinflammation may be protective because it limits unnecessary (potentially autodestructive) inflammation. However, following a massive insult, this downregulation persists inappropriately and creates an immunocompromised host who cannot respond well to later infectious challenges. Recognition that major trauma induces a delayed immunosuppression that contributes to late MOF-associated infections has focused research efforts over the past decade to identify pharmacologic interventions that maintain or enhance immune responsiveness. While a number of interventions (e.g., cyclooxygenase inhibition, thymomimetic agents, interferon-gamma, PGG-glucan, levamisole, hematopoietic stimulating factors [G-CSF, GM-CSF], pentoxyfylline, immunonutrition) have been shown to be beneficial in basic laboratory models, it has been difficult to document outcome advantages in subsequent clinical trials. The most promising approach to date is the administration of "immune-enhancing" nutrients via the enteral route.

Another area of research interest has been the potential role of persistent hypercatabolism in the development of infections[146,147] (Fig. 68-8). Traditionally, the injury stress response was viewed as a neuroendocrine reflex mediated via counterregulatory hormones (cortisol, glucagon, and epinephrine) that alter substrate metabolism while the body is in a state of repair. More recently, it has been convincingly demonstrated that a host of inflammatory mediators (similar to those seen with infection and systemic sepsis) are also involved. Although energy expenditure can increase dramatically following injury, the associated hypercatabolism is emphasized to

be the critical metabolic alteration. If not supported by exogenous nutrients, the consequent obligatory protein turnover quickly erodes somatic protein stores and then the critical visceral mass. The resulting acute protein malnutrition causes well-documented adverse immunologic consequences and is a recognized cofactor for the development of postinjury infection. Thus, nutritional support for highly stressed patients is a standard of care (see Chap. 66).

Predicated on the consistent epidemiologic observation that infection was associated with MOF, there was an era of intense basic animal investigation to elucidate how remote infection might produce MOF. Because ARDS was observed to invariably be the first organ dysfunction in the MOF cascade, basic researchers focused on acute lung injury (ALI) models. ALI was induced in animal models by creating a remote infection (e.g., cecal ligation and puncture), infusing live bacteria or endotoxin (lipopolysaccharide [LPS]), infusing a known secondary mediator of bacterial sepsis (e.g., TNF), or activating complement.[148–151] A popular laboratory model was the chronically instrumented unanesthetized sheep. LPS infusion in this model is associated with the rapid onset of ALI characterized by (a) bronchospasm, (b) pulmonary hypertension, and (c) increased pulmonary vascular permeability with protein-rich interstitial edema despite normal left atrial pressure. The latter endothelial leak is believed to be the hallmark of early ARDS. This standard sheep model as well as other septic animal models have implicated a variety of effector cells (neutrophils, endothelial cells, macrophages, platelets) and circulating mediators (complement fragments, cytokines, lipid mediators) to be mechanistically involved in producing similar types of acute lung leak. Moreover, in animal models of sepsis-induced ALI, a variety of interventions (e.g., corticosteroids, antiendotoxin and anti-TNF antibodies, soluble TNF receptors, IL-1 receptor antagonists, cyclooxygenase inhibition, PAF receptor antagonist, naloxone, bradykinin antagonist, adhesion receptor blockade) have been shown to be effective in preventing or ameliorating ALI.[152,153] In the clinical arena, many of these same mechanisms have been temporally associated with early ARDS, but it is unclear whether the presence of a specific mediator is an epiphenomenon or causally related. As with the previously described trials aimed at enhancing immune responsiveness, clinical trials testing anti-inflammatory interventions to decrease sepsis-induced SIRS have failed to document improved outcome.[152–154] In sum, these basic studies convincingly support the clinical observation that infection with systemic sepsis can provoke ARDS and MOF.

## The Role of the Neutrophil

In massive tissue injury, the local inflammatory response can have systemic effects as locally derived inflammatory mediators are released in the circulatory system extending the paracrine function of cytokines to an endocrine function. Distal organ effects are similar to local effects, and include changes in vascular permeability, upregulation of endothelial adhesion molecules, altered metabolism, gene transcription, and impaired cellular function. Circulating neutrophils also exhibit increased adhesion molecule expression and become sequestered in capillary beds via endothelial cell binding. As a key component to the nonspecific innate immune system, neutrophils play a central role in postinjury organ dysfunction through indiscriminate secondary tissue destruction and generation of soluble inflammatory mediators (Fig. 68-7). While many leukocyte types are involved in the local

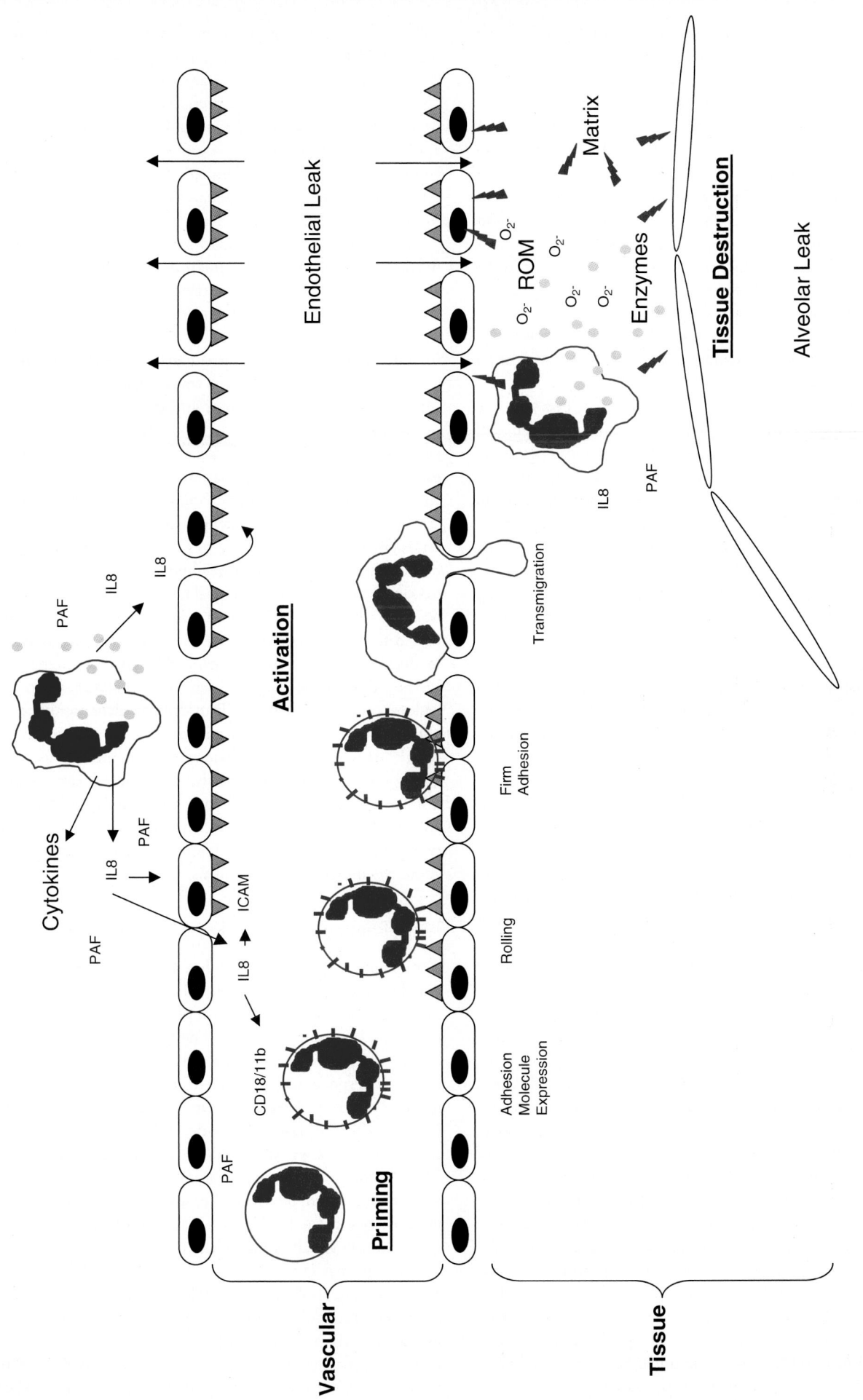

**FIGURE 68-7.** Tissue destruction by PMNs.

and systemic inflammatory responses, the neutrophil is the most conspicuous and acts directly on host tissues.

Adherence to the endothelium is a necessary step in PMN-mediated tissue injury. The regulated adhesion and migration through endothelium are crucial steps in acute inflammation. A complex series of events includes (a) rolling, (b) firm adhesion, and (c) emigration. Induction and control of these events involve the expression and interaction of adhesion molecules on both endothelium and PMNs.[155–157] Neutrophil rolling is dependent on the selectin family of adhesion molecules. L-selectin is constitutively expressed on the surface of neutrophils and appears to be essential for the ability of neutrophils to initiate rolling in the microcirculation. Two other selectins, P-selectin (induced in minutes) and E-selectin (four to six hours for maximal induction) expressed on activated endothelium also contribute significantly to the rolling event.

The second step involves the tight adhesion between the endothelium and the PMN.[158,159] This is predominantly mediated by $\beta_2$ integrins on the PMN and members of the immunoglobulin superfamily (e.g., ICAM-1) on the endothelium. Adherent cells then transmigrate through the junctions of endothelial cells, an event that requires a chemotactic gradient. Another adhesion molecule, platelet–endothelial cell adhesion molecule-1 (PECAM-1), has been implicated in PMN transmigration. In basic laboratory models of burns, hemorrhage, and ischemic/reperfusion, blocking integrin–ICAM-1 interactions by administering specific monoclonal antibodies prevents PMN-mediated endothelial cell injury and improves organ function.

The establishment of adhesive interactions between PMNs and endothelium not only allows these phagocytic cells to marginate and extravasate to sites of inflammation but, when excessive adhesion occurs, the cytotoxic arsenal of PMNs is focused on the endothelial or parenchymal cell. Upon PMN activation, preformed granules fuse with the phagosome or plasma membrane by regulated exocytosis.[160] Different granule types have been characterized in neutrophils that differ in their content, membrane proteins, and propensity to be secreted. Azurophilic (primary) granules contain lysosomal hydrolases, myeloperoxidase, and defensins. Peroxidase negative (nonazurophilic) granules are divided into specific (secondary) granules, gelatinase granules, and secretory vesicles[161,162] which contain proteolytic enzymes, lipases, and membrane bound adhesion molecules. PMN activation also leads to "respiratory burst," the assembly of the NADPH oxidase complex on the plasma membrane that, in turn, generates the superoxide anion ($O_2^-$.) which is metabolized to a family of reactive oxygen metabolites that include, hydrogen peroxide ($H_2O_2$), the hydroxyl radical (OH.), and large amount of hypochlorus acid (HOCl), the active ingredient in household bleach. HOCl is an extremely powerful oxidant that rapidly and nonspecifically attacks a wide range of biologically relevant molecules generating longer lived nitrogen chloramines (N-Cl). Once activated, the PMN oxidative machinery produces these reactive oxygen species for up to three hours.

Of the PMN granule constituents, the proteolytic enzymes collagenase elastase, and gelatinase have the greatest potential for nonspecific tissue destruction. These enzymes are rapidly inhibited when released into the circulation by the presence of several proteinase inhibitors (a1-proteinase inhibitor, a2-macroglobulin, etc.). However, when released in the local environment between the adherent PMN-endothelial cell environment or the extracellular space, the enzymatic activity proceeds unchecked. Local inhibitors are further inactivated by chlorinated oxidants generated by the activated PMN. Each of these enzymes target the extracellular matrix once liberated from the PMN. Destruction of the extracellular matrix has profound effects on the structure and function of the parenchyma and is thought to be the key to organ dysfunction. Moreover, the combination of oxidants and proteolytic enzymes has the capacity to directly attack host cells. Although the lung is particularly sensitive to this PMN mediated cell damage,[163] the liver is also at risk.[164]

In addition to the direct cytotoxic effects, PMNs generate significant amounts of proinflammatory mediators including platelet activating factor (PAF), leukotriene-A4 (LTA-4), interleukin-1 (IL-1), interlekin-8 (IL-8), and tumor necrosis factor (TNFa).[165,166] The effects of these cytokines on PMNs are well described and include chemoattraction, upregulation of adhesion molecules, enhancement of endothelial cell transmigration, priming and activation of the respiratory burst, and degranulation. Additionally, proinflammatory cytokines are capable of direct action on the endothelium promoting endothelial cell leak.[167] In the local environment, PMN derived chemoattractant cytokines recruit and prime circulating PMNs to the site of injury. Additionally, inflammatory cytokines released into the systemic circulation have profound effects on distal organ function.

PMNs also interact with neighboring cells to produce inflammatory mediators that neither cell has the machinery to produce in isolation. Inactive metabolites of arachadonic acid (e.g., LTA-4) are passed to nearby platelets where they are converted to active lipid mediators including thromboxane B2 and leukotriene C4.[168,169] PMNs also utilize platelet derived arachadonate to increase leukotriene biosynthesis.[170] Transcellular eicosanoid metabolism also occurs between PMNs and other cells such as endothelial cells,[171] as well as between platelets and pulmonary macrophages, eosiniphils, and natural killer cells.[172] The overall effect is that these cellular interactions alter the nature and quantity of lipid mediators and the behavior of the interacting cells. This offers a potential therapeutic target to modify PMN responses as more is learned about the underlying mechanisms.

## PMN Priming and the "Two-Hit" Hypothesis

The activity of the NADPH oxidase as well as other PMN functions may be augmented by a process called PMN priming.[173–175] Priming is defined as the amplification of a cellular physiologic response to a second unrelated stimulus. The PMN priming agent does not, by itself, activate the respiratory burst but enhances the production of $O_2^-$ in response to a subsequent stimulus. The priming response in the PMN is now recognized to include the upregulation of the CD11/CD18 adhesion molecule and enhanced release of proteases/elastases as well as cytokines (e.g., IL-8) on activation.[176,177] The physiologic purpose of priming is to enhance bacterial killing at sites of infection; however, after severe trauma, the inflammatory response bombards PMNs with a multitude of priming and activating stimuli which can then lead to cytotoxic responses, resulting in tissue injury.

Many biological mediators relevant to postinjury MOF have been demonstrated in vitro to prime PMN responses, including interleukins (IL-1, IL-6, and IL-8), tumor necrosis factor (TNF), PAF, leukotriene $B_4$ (LTB$_4$), lipopolysaccharide (LPS), and complement-derived C5a. To determine the potential clinical

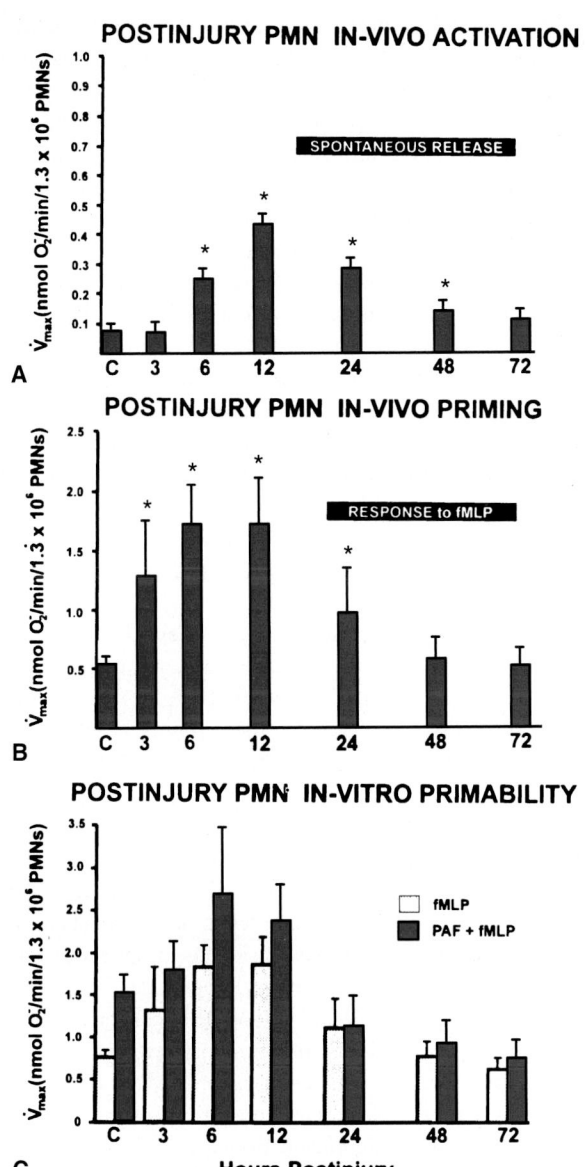

**FIGURE 68-8.** PMN priming responses.
Data represent mean ± SEM. $\dot{V}_{max}$ values for in vitro $O_2^2$ release by unstimulated PMNs from normal adult controls (C) and from trauma patients under various conditions. Denotes data that are significantly different ($p > 0.05$) from control. **(A)** In vitro release of $O_2^2$ by unstimulated PMNs harvested at various times from patients with major torso trauma. **(B)** In vitro release of $O_2^2$ by n-formyl-methyl-leucyl-phenylalanine (fMLP)-activated PMNs harvested at various times from patients with major torso trauma. **(C)** In vitro release of $O_2^2$ after addition of either fMLP or combination of PAF and fMLP to PMNs harvested at various times from patients with major torso trauma. PMN $O_2^2$ release in response to fMLP is indicated for control and trauma patients by white bars. PMN $O_2^2$ release in response to fMLP + PAF combination is depicted by black bars. Increase in $O_2^2$ release in PMNs treated with PAF + fMLP versus fMLP alone (i.e., priming) was statistically significant ($p < 0.05$) only for PMNs harvested from controls.

relevance of PMN priming in the pathogenesis of postinjury MOF, we obtained blood samples at 3, 6, 12, 24, 48, and 72 hours after injury in 17 high-risk trauma patients (ISS > 25) and in 10 healthy donor controls.[51] The PMNs were isolated and the kinetics of extracellular release of $O_2^-$ was quantitated in vitro under three different sets of culture conditions in order to answer three specific questions about the functional in vivo state of circulating

PMNs following trauma. We observed that postinjury PMNs were (a) mildly activated in vivo from 6 to 48 hours after injury (i.e., increased spontaneous $O_2^-$ release compared to controls; see Fig. 68-8A); (b) markedly primed in vivo between three and 24 hours after injury (i.e., increased $O_2^-$ release in response to fMLP activation compared to control; see Fig. 68-8B); and (c) maximally primed in vivo between 3 and 24 hours after injury (i.e., no additional increase in $O_2^-$ release in response to fMLP when re-treated in vitro for five minutes with the priming agent PAF; see Fig. 68-8C). These data indicate that major torso trauma (the first hit) primes circulating PMNs. We next questioned whether the plasma simultaneously obtained from these study patients could "prime" unsuspecting PMNs. PMNs obtained from normal controls were coincubated with the plasma samples. We observed that the plasma samples obtained at 3, 6, 12, and 24 hours after injury primed normal PMNs, but the samples obtained at 48 and 72 hours did not prime. Subsequent work demonstrated that postinjury circulating PMNs were also primed for expression of adhesion molecules, enhanced elastase release (degranulation), increased IL-8 (cytokine) production, and delayed apoptosis.[49,177–180]

PMN priming is not limited to the initial traumatic event. Shock independent of tissue injury is also capable of priming the PMN response.[181] Circulating PMNs isolated 24 hours after femur fracture fixation are also primed for enhanced $O_2^-$ production,[182] and components from stored blood are capable of priming resting PMNs.[183]

In summary, the PMN is considered the key functional cell in the genesis of postinjury MOF. The ability of the PMN to be primed by a variety of stimuli and recruited into the extravascular space places the PMN in position to exacerbate a local inflammatory response. The nonspecific nature of the PMN cytotoxic constituents put the host tissue at risk once the PMN is activated. The ability of the PMN to generate chemokines that further recruit circulating PMNs and cause distant organ dysfunction extends the influence of PMN activation beyond its local environment. Control of these PMN responses may be the solution to attenuation of early postinjury hyperinflammation.

## INTERACTION BETWEEN ORGAN SYSTEMS

The study of complex systems is limited by the knowledge of the component parts. When individual clinical and laboratory investigations are considered together, a broad understanding of the pathogenesis underlying postinjury MOF becomes plausible. In the following global hypotheses, local effects from the initial injury that begin at the cellular level are compounded and amplified to result in distant organ dysfunction and failure of the organism.

The initial tissue destruction and surrounding ischemia provokes a local reaction that releases inflammatory mediators into the systemic circulation. Concurrent shock and visceral ischemia generates proinflammatory lipids in the mesenteric lymph that are also released into the systemic circulation via the thoracic duct. These inflammatory mediators pass through the pulmonary circulation causing capillary leak and endothelial cell adhesion molecule expression. Circulating PMNs primed by passage through the postischemic gut or exposure to soluble inflammatory mediators, are then sequestered in the lung through binding to endothelial cells. The lung is positioned to receive both the mesenteric lymph and circulating PMNs returning from ischemic tissue. Together with the marginating PMNs in the pulmonary vasculature, the circulating PMNs attach to the pulmonary endothelium.

Once activated, the adherent PMNs transmigrate into the pulmonary interstitial space and release their cytotoxic components causing indiscriminate tissue destruction. This local inflammatory reaction is amplified by PMN production of chemoattractant cytokines that further recruit circulating PMNs to the area. The resulting biotrauma to the lung and further generation of systemic inflammatory mediators released into the systemic circulation activates endothelial cells in peripheral vascular beds resulting in endothelial leak. Endothelial activation also promotes PMN binding in the periphery where PMN mediated tissue destruction can also occur. In this chain of events, a variety of stimuli sequentially elevate the inflammatory potential until a threshold of systemic organ dysfunction is reached.

## PREVENTING POSTINJURY MOF

### Resuscitation

Control of the initial inflammatory response (priming) and avoidance of second insults (activation) are the most likely areas to impact the incidence of MOF once the injury has occurred. Clinically, priming is manifested by the systemic inflammatory response syndrome (SIRS) characterized by alterations in body temperature, white blood cell count, respiratory dysfunction, and a hyperdynamic state.[20] Systemic priming is considered to be a nondestructive process that resolves spontaneously if unprovoked. The degree of priming is dependent on the severity of the initial insult, the depth of shock, and the response to early resuscitation. Therefore, changes in the primed state over time would be a reflection of improved resuscitation after adjusting for severity of injury. To determine if the decreased incidence of postinjury MOF observed over the recent decade was due to decreased priming, we examined clinical markers of SIRS in relationship to the incidence of MOF. We characterized the degree of priming by measuring the $PaO_2/FiO_2$ ratio at 24 hours after injury. We observed no change in early lung function over the study period and found no difference in heart rate, temperature, and WBC count measured at 24 hours.(Ciesla, *Surgery*, 2006, in press) This is not surprising in that identifying the primed state based on routine clinical indicators is virtually impossible. The causes of postinjury SIRS are multifactorial and its criteria are not specific for priming. Altered physiology after trauma is not only a result of the injury itself, but also a response to ischemia-reperfusion, resuscitation, and the host response. Therefore, our inability to detect a change in the primed state over time could be a result of our metric's insensitivity. Since we have previously reported an overall increase in injury severity in this patient population over the last decade,[43] it could be that there was no actual change in systemic priming to be observed. Moreover, since priming is established within three hours of injury,[173] interventions to decrease its magnitude are limited to the immediate postinjury period.

Another potential strategy to limit priming is the pharmacologic modulation of the response to injury. Resuscitation strategies not only aim to define ideal endpoints but also determine optimal resuscitation fluids.[115,118] While most clinical studies have failed to demonstrate a clearly superior crystalloid fluid, resurgent interest in hypertonic solutions was sparked by the finding that resuscitation using hypertonic saline improved outcome in patients with head injury and those requiring emergent operation.[184–186] In addition to more efficient volume restoration, the improved outcome was attributed to the influence of hypertonicity on PMN cytotoxic functions. In our laboratory we demonstrated that clinically relevant concentrations of hypertonic saline reversibly attenuated several PMN cytotoxic by interrupting PMN signal transduction.[117,187,188] Others have demonstrated decreased lung injury in animals resuscitated with hypertonic saline following hemorrhagic shock.[116,189,190] However, despite this laboratory and clinical evidence the clinical benefits use of hypertonic saline for acute resuscitation remain to be established.

### Avoiding Second Insults

Since priming is largely dependent on the severity of initial trauma and is established within three hours of injury,[51] interventions to control priming are limited. More effective strategies to avoid MOF may be achieved by limiting the exposure or effects of second (activating) events. Clinical evidence of an activating event includes the development of ARDS and MOF. While impaired oxygen exchange itself could represent a multitude of underlying conditions, the diffuse bilateral infiltrates in the absence of heart failure observed on chest x-ray define ARDS and are hallmark of inflammatory mediated pulmonary edema. As described above, the destructive processes active in ARDS are also responsible for progression of ARDS to MOF. Therefore, progression from SIRS and respiratory dysfunction to ARDS and MOF is clinical evidence for activation of the dysfunctional inflammatory response.

Longitudinal study of patients at risk for MOF demonstrated no change in clinical indicators of postinjury priming or overall lung dysfunction, but a significant decrease in the progression to ARDS and MOF (Fig. 68-9).[57a] Of particular interest with respect to the activating event is the observed decreased incidence of early MOF. In contrast to late MOF, which can be the result of delayed immunosupression and overwhelming infection, early MOF is predominantly inflammatory mediated. The finding that the major infection rate in this population did not change over time further supports the conclusion that the observed reduction in postinjury

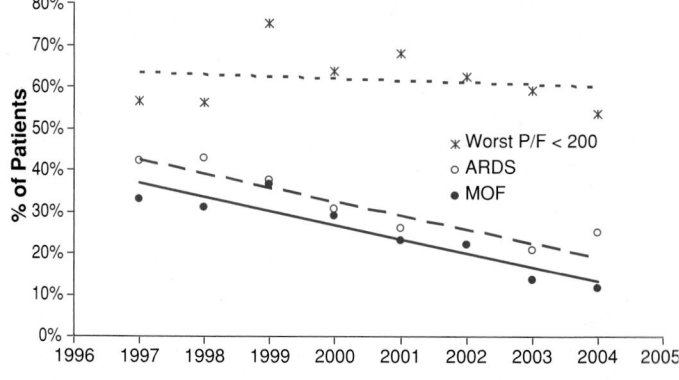

**FIGURE 68-9.** Decreased progression of lung dysfunction to ARDS.

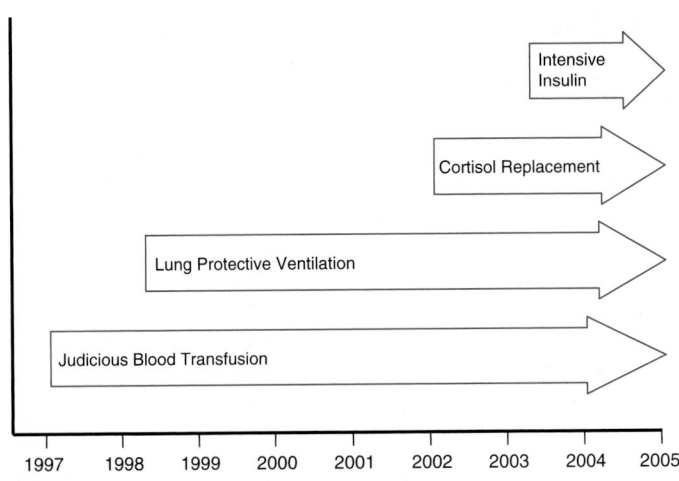

**FIGURE 68-10.**  Implementation of ICU advances.

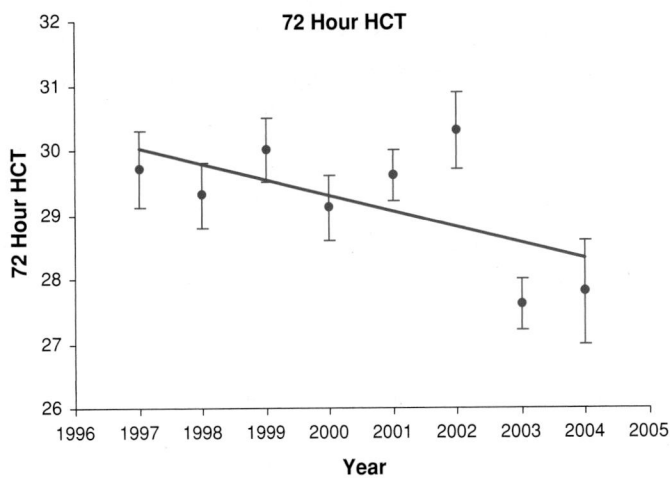

**FIGURE 68-11.**  Decreased 72-hour Hct over time.

MOF was a result of decreased activation of dysfunctional inflammation over time.

This improvement in postinjury morbidity is coincident with implementation of several therapies known to effect postinjury hyperinflammation. While many studies are available that examine the effect of each therapy alone, it is difficult to characterize the combined impact of such therapies on global trauma outcomes. Moreover, it may be that no single treatment but a synergistic combination of new treatments over recent years is responsible for decreasing the postinjury MOF rate to its lowest level since the syndrome was first described. In our own patient population, several therapeutic advances were sequentially adopted over time (Fig. 68-10).

The first consideration was the use of blood transfusion during resuscitation. The realization that blood transfusion itself could serve as an activating stimulus prompted us to adopt an institutional approach to resuscitation based on judicious blood transfusion. Patients arriving in shock were transfused to a target hemoglobin concentration of 10mg/dL. Upon completion of resuscitation, asymptomatic patients were not transfused until hemoglobin concentrations fell below 7mg/dL. Over time this resulted in decreased use of blood transfusion during resuscitation in this study population[43] and is reflected by an observed decreased hematocrit measured 72 hours postinjury over the study period after adjusting for ISS and need for urgent or emergent operation (Fig. 68-11). While not definitive, we noted that among the independent risk factors for postinjury MOF (patient age, injury severity, degree of shock, and blood transfusion) blood transfusion alone decreased, while the others increased over the last decade.

A second consideration is the impact of lung protective ventilation on the systemic inflammatory response. The lung protective strategy is designed to minimize the potential for ventilator induced lung injury.[191] This has important downstream effects in that lung injury is recognized to contribute to remote organ dysfunction through the release of inflammatory mediators generated in the lung to the systemic circulation.[192] A key supporting observation of the ARDS lung protective trials was the decreased incidence of MOF and decreased circulating levels of IL-6 in the lung protective group.[191] We adopted a lung protective ventilator strategy in patients that the ARDS network criteria in 1998. Our study was not designed to evaluate the effect of lung protective ventilation on the development of ARDS so a causative relationship cannot be established. However, we can observe a temporal relationship and the above mentioned mechanistic evidence supports the idea that lung protective ventilation has contributed to attenuation of systemic hyperinflammation.

Intensive insulin therapy has also recently been shown to improve outcome in critically ill patients.[193,194] Further investigation suggests that insulin therapy may attenuate the systemic inflammatory potential.[195–197] We began treating patients receiving mechanical ventilation with intensive intravenous insulin therapy in 2002 to achieve plasma glucose levels between 80 and 110 mg/dL (Fig. 68-6). By 2004 approximately 40% of all the patients in the study had received intensive insulin therapy at some point during their ICU course. This, of course, demands further investigation to determine if protocol implementation was optimal and if protocol goals were met, but previous mechanistic research again provides a reasonable connection between this therapy and improved outcome following injury.

An area still under intense investigation is the diagnosis and treatment of adrenal insufficiency in the critically ill. Adrenal insufficiency is associated with increased circulating inflammatory mediators such as IL-1b, IL-6, and TNF-a.[127] Several groups have reported lower mortality when adrenal insufficiency was recognized and treated in critically ill patients with cortisol replacement therapy.[198,199] There is also evidence that cortisol replacement therapy decreases systemic inflammatory mediators such as IL-6 and IL-8.[200,201] The goal of cortisol replacement therapy is to reestablish a "eucorticoid state" without untoward immunosupression. We began screening for adrenal insufficiency in severely injured trauma patients in 2002. Those patients found to have adrenal insufficiency were treated with cortisol replacement. By 2004, 25% of patients in this study and 100% of patients that met screening criteria were treated with cortisol replacement. Although evaluation of our protocol is in progress, based on the available literature we expect cortisol replacement therapy to be associated with improved outcomes related to postinjury hyperinflammation. It is also encouraging that we did not see an increase in major or minor infections after institution of this protocol.

## Damage Control Orthopedics

The benefits of early definitive fracture stabilization are well described and include early patient mobility, improved pulmonary toilet, decreased systemic inflammation, decreased thromboembolic events, decreased morbidity and mortality, and decreased hospital resource utilization.[93,202–206] However, as discussed above, operative fracture fixation exposes the patient to an additional inflammatory insult that can precipitate MOF if performed in a primed patient. Moreover, not all multiply injured patients are able to tolerate early definitive fixation due to hemodynamic instability, refractory hypoxemia, or uncontrolled intracranial hypertension. In such cases, treatment of fractures by traction or splints increases the risk of pulmonary complications and MOF.[91,92] Consequently, alternative strategies to provide early fracture stabilization while avoiding the risk of early total care have been proposed. The concept of damage control surgery was thus extended to the initial management of major fractures in the severely injured.[207–210] The principle is to provide early fracture stabilization by external fixation as a bridge to definitive fracture care once the patient is more physiologically appropriate. Conversion of external fixation to intramedullary implantation is associated with reduced procedure related inflammatory response compared to early primary femur fracture fixation.[97] When compared to early total care, the damage control approach with delayed conversion to definitive care has been shown to decrease the initial operative time and intraoperative blood loss without increasing the risk of procedure related complications such as infection and nonunion, and may improve overall survival.[209,211] This has prompted some centers to adopt damage control orthopedics as the treatment of choice for the severely injured which has been associated with a general improvement patient outcome and a decreased incidence of postinjury MOF.[212]

## Infection Surveillance

Optimizing host defenses and preventing secondary nosocomial infections are other important aspects of care. For patients who require emergency exploratory laparotomies, a single antibiotic with broad-spectrum coverage of gram-negative aerobes and anaerobes (addition of enterococcal coverage adds questionable benefits) should be administered as soon as possible and continued for 24 hours.[213] Longer dosing is more costly and associated with increased toxicity and emergence of resistance. It should be remembered that the normal recommended dosing may be inadequate in patients with an increased volume of distribution.[214] We recommend repeat dosing in the operating room in patients requiring massive resuscitation. Because the GI tract appears to be the source of pathogens found in late MOF-associated infections, measures used to decrease GI tract colonization with resistant organisms include (a) sucralfate instead of $H_2$ antagonist for stress gastritis prophylaxis, (b) early enteral feeding, and (c) avoidance of prolonged use of antibiotics, particularly those agents that are active against normal anaerobic flora (see Chap. 19). Other important sources of late infections are indwelling devices (e.g., endotracheal tubes, central lines, chest tubes, Foley catheters). Catheter-related sepsis (CRS) is an iatrogenic complication. The incidence of CRS can be dramatically reduced by establishing guidelines for catheter care and a surveillance system that feeds back to the bedside personnel.[215] Pneumonia is the most frequent infection; its prevention demands an aggressive respiratory care protocol to enhance lung volume and clear secretions. Patients should be positioned with the head of the bed (HOB) elevated at 45°.[216] For patients who have evidence of ALI, a ventilatory strategy with low tidal volume and optimized positive end-expiratory pressure (PEEP) should be utilized.[112] Therapeutic bronchoscopy with possible intrabronchial air insufflation may occasionally be needed in patients with refractory lobar collapse. Differentiating pneumonia from SIRS in ventilated trauma patients is difficult. The clinical diagnosis of pneumonia in these patients is notoriously inaccurate.[217,218] This is a dilemma; overtreatment with empiric therapy will promote the emergence of resistant strains while waiting for definite signs in a high-risk patient will increase mortality. Therefore, high-risk patients are treated empirically and invasive diagnostic techniques have been promoted to enhance early diagnosis and direct early antibiotic therapy. There is no ideal antibiotic regimen for ICU pneumonias. Unit-specific resistance patterns and known frequency of specific pathogens are quite helpful in developing guidelines for empiric treatment.

## REFERENCES

1. Baue AE: Multiple, progressive, or sequential systems failure. A syndrome of the 1970s. *Arch Surg* 110:779, 1975.
2. Tilney NL, Bailey GL, Morgan AP: Sequential system failure after rupture of abdominal aortic aneurysms: An unsolved problem in postoperative care. *Ann Surg* 178:117, 1973.
3. Eiseman B, Sloan R, Hansbrough J, et al.: Multiple organ failure: Clinical and experimental. *Am Surg* 46:14, 1980.
4. Sauaia A, Moore FA, Moore EE, et al.: Epidemiology of trauma deaths: A reassessment. *J Trauma* 38:185, 1995.
5. Nast-Kolb D, Aufmkolk M, Rucholtz S, et al.: Multiple organ failure still a major cause of morbidity but not mortality in blunt multiple trauma. *J Trauma* 51:835, 2001.
6. Eiseman B, Beart R, Norton L: Multiple organ failure. *Surg Gynecol Obstet* 144:323, 1977.
7. Fry DE, Pearlstein L, Fulton RL, et al.: Multiple system organ failure. The role of uncontrolled infection. *Arch Surg* 115:136, 1980.
8. Bell RC, Coalson JJ, Smith JD, et al.: Multiple organ system failure and infection in adult respiratory distress syndrome. *Ann Intern Med* 99:293, 1983.
9. Montgomery AB, Stager MA, Carrico CJ, et al.: Causes of mortality in patients with the adult respiratory distress syndrome. *Am Rev Respir Dis* 132:485, 1985.
10. Hudson LD: Multiple systems organ failure (MSOF): Lessons learned from the adult respiratory distress syndrome (ARDS). *Crit Care Clin* 5:697, 1989.
11. Walker L, Eiseman B: The changing pattern of post-traumatic respiratory distress syndrome. *Ann Surg* 181:693, 1975.
12. Faist E, Baue AE, Dittmer H, et al.: Multiple organ failure in polytrauma patients. *J Trauma* 23:775, 1983.
13. Goris RJ, te Boekhorst TP, Nuytinck JK, et al.: Multiple-organ failure. Generalized autodestructive inflammation? *Arch Surg* 120:1109, 1985.
14. Waydhas C, Nast-Kolb D, Jochum M, et al.: Inflammatory mediators, infection, sepsis, and multiple organ failure after severe trauma. *Arch Surg* 127:460, 1992.
15. Moore FA, Moore EE: Evolving concepts in the pathogenesis of postinjury multiple organ failure. *Surg Clin North Am* 75:257, 1995.
16. Bone RC: Sir Isaac Newton, sepsis, SIRS, and CARS. *Crit Care Med* 24:1125, 1996.
17. Raeburn CD, Moore EE, Biffl WL, et al.: The abdominal compartment syndrome is a morbid complication of postinjury damage control surgery. *Am J Surg* 182:542, 2001.
18. Rezende-Neto JB, Moore EE, Masuno T, et al.: The abdominal compartment syndrome as a second insult during systemic neutrophil priming provokes multiple organ injury. *Shock* 20:303, 2003.
19. Balogh Z, McKinley BA, Cox CS Jr, et al.: Abdominal compartment syndrome: The cause or effect of postinjury multiple organ failure. *Shock* 20:483, 2003.
20. American college of chest physicians/society of critical care medicine consensus conference: Definitions for sepsis and organ failure and guidelines for the use of innovative therapies in sepsis. *Crit Care Med* 20:864, 1992.

21. Bone RC, Balk RA, Cerra FB, et al.: Definitions for sepsis and organ failure and guidelines for the use of innovative therapies in sepsis. The ACCP/SCCM consensus conference committee. American College of Chest Physicians/Society of Critical Care Medicine. *Chest* 101:1644, 1992.

22. Moore FA, Moore EE, Poggetti R, et al.: Gut bacterial translocation via the portal vein: A clinical perspective with major torso trauma. *J Trauma* 31:629, 1991.

23. Offner PJ, Moore EE: Lung injury severity scoring in the era of lung protective mechanical ventilation: The PaO$_2$/FiO$_2$ ratio. *J Trauma* 55:285, 2003.

24. Murray JF, Matthay MA, Luce JM, et al.: An expanded definition of the adult respiratory distress syndrome. *Am Rev Respir Dis* 138:720, 1988.

25. Ciesla DJ, Moore EE, Johnson JL, et al.: The role of the lung in postinjury multiple organ failure. *Surgery* 138:749, 2005.

26. Ciesla DJ, Moore EE, Johnson JL, et al.: Multiple organ dysfunction during resuscitation is not postinjury multiple organ failure. *Arch Surg* 139:590, 2004.

27. Knaus WA, Draper EA, Wagner DP, et al.: Prognosis in acute organ-system failure. *Ann Surg* 202:685, 1985.

28. Marshall JC, Christou NV, Horn R, et al.: The microbiology of multiple organ failure. The proximal gastrointestinal tract as an occult reservoir of pathogens. *Arch Surg* 123:309, 1988.

29. Deitch EA: Multiple organ failure. Pathophysiology and potential future therapy. *Ann Surg* 216:117, 1992.

30. Marshall JC, Cook DJ, Christou NV, et al.: Multiple organ dysfunction score: A reliable descriptor of a complex clinical outcome. *Crit Care Med* 23:1638, 1995.

31. Le Gall JR, Klar J, Lemeshow S, et al.: The logistic organ dysfunction system. A new way to assess organ dysfunction in the intensive care unit. Icu scoring group. *JAMA* 276:802, 1996.

32. Bernard A, Lauwerys R: Low-molecular-weight proteins as markers of organ toxicity with special reference to clara cell protein. *Toxicol Lett* 77:145, 1995.

33. Vincent JL, Moreno R, Takala J, et al.: The sofa (sepsis-related organ failure assessment) score to describe organ dysfunction/failure. On behalf of the working group on sepsis-related problems of the european society of intensive care medicine. *Intensive Care Med* 22:707, 1996.

34. Graciano AL, Balko JA, Rahn DS, et al.: The pediatric multiple organ dysfunction score (p-mods): Development and validation of an objective scale to measure the severity of multiple organ dysfunction in critically ill children. *Crit Care Med* 33:1484, 2005.

35. Dicker RA, Morabito DJ, Pittet JF, et al.: Acute respiratory distress syndrome criteria in trauma patients: Why the definitions do not work. *J Trauma* 57:522, 2004.

36. Rixen D, Siegel JH, Friedman HP: "Sepsis/SIRS," Physiologic classification, severity stratification, relation to cytokine elaboration and outcome prediction in posttrauma critical illness. *J Trauma* 41:581, 1996.

37. Oda S, Hirasawa H, Sugai T, et al.: Cellular injury score for multiple organ failure severity scoring system. *J Trauma* 45:304, 1998.

38. Gando S, Nanzaki S, Kemmotsu O: Disseminated intravascular coagulation and sustained systemic inflammatory response syndrome predict organ dysfunctions after trauma: Application of clinical decision analysis. *Ann Surg* 229:121, 1999.

39. Murphy TJ, Paterson HM, Kriynovich S, et al.: Linking the "two-hit" response following injury to enhanced tlr4 reactivity. *J Leukoc Biol* 77:16, 2005.

40. Sauaia A, Moore FA, Moore EE, et al.: Early predictors of postinjury multiple organ failure. *Arch Surg* 129:39, 1994.

41. Moore FA, Sauaia A, Moore EE, et al.: Postinjury multiple organ failure: A bimodal phenomenon. *J Trauma* 40:501, 1996.

42. Sauaia A, Moore FA, Moore EE, et al.: Pneumonia related multiple organ failure is not a primary cause of death in head trauma. *Pan Amer J Trauma* 3:90, 1992.

43. Ciesla DJ, Moore EE, Johnson JL, et al.: A 12-year prospective study of postinjury multiple organ failure: Has anything changed? *Arch Surg* 140:432, 2005.

44. Sauaia A, Moore FA, Moore EE, et al.: Early risk factors for postinjury multiple organ failure. *World J Surg* 20:392, 1996.

45. Sauaia A, Moore FA, Moore EE, et al.: Multiple organ failure can be predicted as early as 12 hours after injury. *J Trauma* 45:291, 1998.

46. Moore FA, McKinley BA, Moore EE: The next generation in shock resuscitation. *Lancet* 363:1988, 2004.

47. Hassoun HT, Kone BC, Mercer DW, et al.: Post-injury multiple organ failure: The role of the gut. *Shock* 15:1, 2001.

48. Moore FA, Moore EE, Sauaia A: Blood transfusion. An independent risk factor for postinjury multiple organ failure. *Arch Surg* 132:620, 1997.

49. Partrick DA, Moore FA, Moore EE, et al.: Neutrophil priming and activation in the pathogenesis of postinjury multiple organ failure. *New Horiz* 4:194, 1996.

50. Cryer HG, Leong K, McArthur DL, et al.: Multiple organ failure: By the time you predict it, it's already there. *J Trauma* 46:597, 1999.

51. Botha AJ, Moore FA, Moore EE, et al.: Postinjury neutrophil priming and activation: An early vulnerable window. *Surgery* 118:358, 1995.

52. Regel G, Lobenhoffer P, Grotz M, et al.: Treatment results of patients with multiple trauma: An analysis of 3406 cases treated between 1972 and 1991 at a German Level I trauma center. *J Trauma* 38:70, 1995.

53. Flaatten H, Gjerde S, Guttormsen AB, et al.: Outcome after acute respiratory failure is more dependent on dysfunction in other vital organs than on the severity of the respiratory failure. *Crit Care* 7:R72, 2003.

54. Baue AE, Durham R, Faist E: Systemic inflammatory response syndrome (SIRS), multiple organ dysfunction syndrome (MODS), multiple organ failure (MOF): Are we winning the battle? *Shock* 10:79, 1998.

55. Levine JH, Durham RM, Moran J, et al.: Multiple organ failure: Is it disappearing? *World J Surg* 20:471, 1996.

56. Durham RM, Moran JJ, Mazuski JE, et al.: Multiple organ failure in trauma patients. *J Trauma* 55:608, 2003.

57. Regel G, Grotz M, Weltner T, et al.: Pattern of organ failure following severe trauma. *World J Surg* 20:422, 1996.

57a. Ciesla DJ, Moore EE, Sauaia A, et al.: Decreased progression of postinjury lung dysfunction to the acute respiratory distress syndrome and multiple organ failure. *Surgery* 140:640, 2006.

58. Roumen RM, Hendriks T, van der Ven-Jongekrijg J, et al.: Cytokine patterns in patients after major vascular surgery, hemorrhagic shock, and severe blunt trauma. Relation with subsequent adult respiratory distress syndrome and multiple organ failure. *Ann Surg* 218:769, 1993.

59. Botha AJ, Moore FA, Moore EE, et al.: Sequential systemic platelet-activating factor and interleukin 8 primes neutrophils in patients with trauma at risk of multiple organ failure. *Br J Surg* 83:1407, 1996.

60. Mannick JA, Rodrick ML, Lederer JA: The immunologic response to injury. *J Am Coll Surg* 193:237, 2001.

61. Angele MK, Chaudry IH: Surgical trauma and immunosuppression: Pathophysiology and potential immunomodulatory approaches. *Langenbecks Arch Surg* 390:333, 2005.

62. Granger DN: Role of xanthine oxidase and granulocytes in ischemia-reperfusion injury. *Am J Physiol* 255:H1269, 1988.

63. Grisham MB, Granger DN, Lefer DJ: Modulation of leukocyte-endothelial interactions by reactive metabolites of oxygen and nitrogen: Relevance to ischemic heart disease. *Free Radic Biol Med* 25:404, 1998.

64. Galkina SI, Dormeneva EV, Bachschmid M, et al.: Endothelium-leukocyte interactions under the influence of the superoxide-nitrogen monoxide system. *Med Sci Monit* 10:BR307, 2004.

65. Ichikawa H, Wolf RE, Aw TY, et al.: Exogenous xanthine promotes neutrophil adherence to cultured endothelial cells. *Am J Physiol* 273:G342, 1997.

66. Tidball JG: Inflammatory cell response to acute muscle injury. *Med Sci Sports Exerc* 27:1022, 1995.

67. Tidball JG: Inflammatory processes in muscle injury and repair. *Am J Physiol Regul Integr Comp Physiol* 288:R345, 2005.

68. Edna TH, Bjerkeset T: Association between blood transfusion and infection in injured patients. *J Trauma* 33:659, 1992.

69. Silliman CC, Clay KL, Thurman GW, et al.: Partial characterization of lipids that develop during the routine storage of blood and prime the neutrophil nadph oxidase. *J Lab Clin Med* 124:684, 1994.

70. Stack G, Snyder EL: Cytokine generation in stored platelet concentrates. *Transfusion* 34:20, 1994.

71. Aiboshi J, Moore EE, Ciesla DJ, et al.: Blood transfusion and the two-insult model of post-injury multiple organ failure. *Shock* 15:302, 2001.

72. Opelz G, Terasaki PI: Improvement of kidney-graft survival with increased numbers of blood transfusions. *N Engl J Med* 299:799, 1978.

73. Silliman CC: Transfusion-related acute lung injury. *Transfus Med Rev* 13:177, 1999.

74. Toy P, Popovsky MA, Abraham E, et al.: Transfusion-related acute lung injury: Definition and review. *Crit Care Med* 33:721, 2005.

75. Silliman CC: The two-event model of transfusion-related acute lung injury. *Crit Care Med* 34:S124, 2006.

76. Dunne JR, Malone DL, Tracy JK, et al.: Allogenic blood transfusion in the first 24 hours after trauma is associated with increased systemic inflammatory response syndrome (SIRS) and death. *Surg Infect (Larchmt)* 5:395, 2004.

77. Silverboard H, Aisiku I, Martin GS, et al.: The role of acute blood transfusion in the development of acute respiratory distress syndrome in patients with severe trauma. *J Trauma* 59:717, 2005.

78. Malone DL, Dunne J, Tracy JK, et al.: Blood transfusion, independent of shock severity, is associated with worse outcome in trauma. *J Trauma* 54:898, 2003.

79. Croce MA, Tolley EA, Claridge JA, et al.: Transfusions result in pulmonary morbidity and death after a moderate degree of injury. *J Trauma* 59:19, 2005.

80. Zallen G, Offner PJ, Moore EE, et al.: Age of transfused blood is an independent risk factor for postinjury multiple organ failure. *Am J Surg* 178:570, 1999.

81. Zallen G, Moore EE, Ciesla DJ, et al.: Stored red blood cells selectively activate human neutrophils to release Il-8 and secretory pla2. *Shock* 13:29, 2000.

82. Shanwell A, Kristiansson M, Remberger M, et al.: Generation of cytokines in red cell concentrates during storage is prevented by prestorage white cell reduction. *Transfusion* 37:678, 1997.

83. Lenahan SE, Domen RE, Silliman CC, et al.: Transfusion-related acute lung injury secondary to biologically active mediators. *Arch Pathol Lab Med* 125:523, 2001.

84. Silliman CC, Elzi DJ, Ambruso DR, et al.: Lysophosphatidylcholines prime the nadph oxidase and stimulate multiple neutrophil functions through changes in cytosolic calcium. *J Leukoc Biol* 73:511, 2003.

85. Silliman CC, Moore EE, Johnson JL, et al.: Transfusion of the injured patient: Proceed with caution. *Shock* 21:291, 2004.

86. Moore EE, Moore FA, Harken AH, et al.: The two-event construct of postinjury multiple organ failure. *Shock* 24 Suppl 1:71, 2005.

87. Haga Y, Beppu T, Doi K, et al.: Systemic inflammatory response syndrome and organ dysfunction following gastrointestinal surgery. *Crit Care Med* 25:1994, 1997.

88. Harwood PJ, Giannoudis PV, van Griensven M, et al.: Alterations in the systemic inflammatory response after early total care and damage control procedures for femoral shaft fracture in severely injured patients. *J Trauma* 58:446, 2005.

89. Takenaka K, Ogawa E, Wada H, et al.: Systemic inflammatory response syndrome and surgical stress in thoracic surgery. *J Crit Care* 21:48, 2006.

90. Ishikawa M, Nishioka M, Hanaki N, et al.: Postoperative metabolic and circulatory responses in patients that express SIRS after major digestive surgery. *Hepatogastroenterology* 53:228, 2006.

91. Seibel R, LaDuca J, Hassett JM, et al.: Blunt multiple trauma (ISS 36), femur traction, and the pulmonary failure-septic state. *Ann Surg* 202:283, 1985.

92. Charash WE, Fabian TC, Croce MA: Delayed surgical fixation of femur fractures is a risk factor for pulmonary failure independent of thoracic trauma. *J Trauma* 37:667, 1994.

93. Brundage SI, McGhan R, Jurkovich GJ, et al.: Timing of femur fracture fixation: Effect on outcome in patients with thoracic and head injuries. *J Trauma* 52:299, 2002.

94. Pape HC, Auf'm'Kolk M, Paffrath T, et al.: Primary intramedullary femur fixation in multiple trauma patients with associated lung contusion—a cause of posttraumatic ARDS? *J Trauma* 34:540, 1993.

95. Pape HC, Schmidt RE, Rice J, et al.: Biochemical changes after trauma and skeletal surgery of the lower extremity: Quantification of the operative burden. *Crit Care Med* 28:3441, 2000.

96. Pape HC, van Griensven M, Rice J, et al.: Major secondary surgery in blunt trauma patients and perioperative cytokine liberation: Determination of the clinical relevance of biochemical markers. *J Trauma* 50:989, 2001.

97. Pape HC, Grimme K, Van Griensven M, et al.: Impact of intramedullary instrumentation versus damage control for femoral fractures on immunoinflammatory parameters: Prospective randomized analysis by the EPOFF study group. *J Trauma* 55:7, 2003.

98. Sugrue M: Abdominal compartment syndrome. *Curr Opin Crit Care* 11:333, 2005.

99. Biffl WL, Moore EE, Burch JM, et al.: Secondary abdominal compartment syndrome is a highly lethal event. *Am J Surg* 182:645, 2001.

100. Kirkpatrick AW, Balogh Z, Ball CG, et al.: The secondary abdominal compartment syndrome: Iatrogenic or unavoidable? *J Am Coll Surg* 202:668, 2006.

101. Balogh Z, McKinley BA, Cocanour CS, et al.: Supranormal trauma resuscitation causes more cases of abdominal compartment syndrome. *Arch Surg* 138:637, 2003.

102. Iglesias JL, LaNoue JL, Rogers TE, et al.: Physiologic basis of pulmonary edema during intestinal reperfusion. *J Surg Res* 80:156, 1998.

103. Moore EE, Moore FA, Franciose RJ, et al.: The postischemic gut serves as a priming bed for circulating neutrophils that provoke multiple organ failure. *J Trauma* 37:881, 1994.

104. Rezende-Neto JB, Moore EE, Melo de Andrade MV, et al.: Systemic inflammatory response secondary to abdominal compartment syndrome: Stage for multiple organ failure. *J Trauma* 53:1121, 2002.

105. Balogh Z, McKinley BA, Holcomb JB, et al.: Both primary and secondary abdominal compartment syndrome can be predicted early and are harbingers of multiple organ failure. *J Trauma* 54:848, 2003.

106. Tsuno K, Miura K, Takeya M, et al.: Histopathologic pulmonary changes from mechanical ventilation at high peak airway pressures. *Am Rev Respir Dis* 143:1115, 1991.

107. Slutsky AS: Lung injury caused by mechanical ventilation. *Chest* 116:9S, 1999.

108. dos Santos CC, Slutsky AS: The contribution of biophysical lung injury to the development of biotrauma. *Annu Rev Physiol* 68:585, 2006.

109. Chen KD, Li YS, Kim M, et al.: Mechanotransduction in response to shear stress. Roles of receptor tyrosine kinases, integrins, and SHC. *J Biol Chem* 274:18393, 1999.

110. Dolinay T, Kaminski N, Felgendreher M, et al.: Gene expression profiling of target genes in ventilator-induced lung injury. *Physiol Genomics* 28:28, 2006.

111. Crimi E, Zhang H, Han RN, et al.: Ischemia and reperfusion increases susceptibility to ventilator-induced lung injury in rats. *Am J Respir Crit Care Med* 27:27, 2006.

112. Ventilation with lower tidal volumes as compared with traditional tidal volumes for acute lung injury and the acute respiratory distress syndrome. The acute respiratory distress syndrome network. *N Engl J Med* 342:1301, 2000.

113. Parsons PE, Eisner MD, Thompson BT, et al.: Lower tidal volume ventilation and plasma cytokine markers of inflammation in patients with acute lung injury. *Crit Care Med* 33:1, 2005.

114. Nathens AB, Johnson JL, Minei JP, et al.: Inflammation and the host response to injury, a large-scale collaborative project: Patient-oriented research core—standard operating procedures for clinical care. I. Guidelines for mechanical ventilation of the trauma patient. *J Trauma* 59:764, 2005.

115. Rhee P, Burris D, Kaufmann C, et al.: Lactated Ringer's solution resuscitation causes neutrophil activation after hemorrhagic shock. *J Trauma* 44:313, 1998.

116. Rizoli SB, Kapus A, Fan J, et al.: Immunomodulatory effects of hypertonic resuscitation on the development of lung inflammation following hemorrhagic shock. *J Immunol* 161:6288, 1998.

117. Ciesla DJ, Moore EE, Gonzalez RJ, et al.: Hypertonic saline inhibits neutrophil (PMN) priming via attenuation of p38 MAPK signaling. *Shock* 14:265, 2000.

118. Rhee P, Koustova E, Alam HB: Searching for the optimal resuscitation method: Recommendations for the initial fluid resuscitation of combat casualties. *J Trauma* 54:S52, 2003.

119. Torres SR, Frode TS, Nardi GM, et al.: Anti-inflammatory effects of peripheral benzodiazepine receptor ligands in two mouse models of inflammation. *Eur J Pharmacol* 408:199, 2000.

120. Fruscella P, Sottocorno M, Di Braccio M, et al.: 1,5-benzodiazepine tricyclic derivatives exerting anti-inflammatory effects in mice by inhibiting interleukin-6 and prostaglandine(2)production. *Pharmacol Res* 43:445, 2001.

121. Lazzarini R, Maiorka PC, Liu J, et al.: Diazepam effects on carrageenan-induced inflammatory paw edema in rats: Role of nitric oxide. *Life Sci* 78:3027, 2006.

122. Bartoc C, Frumento RJ, Jalbout M, et al.: A randomized, double-blind, placebo-controlled study assessing the anti-inflammatory effects of ketamine in cardiac surgical patients. *J Cardiothorac Vasc Anesth* 20:217, 2006.

123. Mazar J, Rogachev B, Shaked G, et al.: Involvement of adenosine in the anti-inflammatory action of ketamine. *Anesthesiology* 102:1174, 2005.

124. Helmer KS, Cui Y, Chang L, et al.: Effects of ketamine/xylazine on expression of tumor necrosis factor-alpha, inducible nitric oxide synthase, and cyclo-oxygenase-2 in rat gastric mucosa during endotoxemia. *Shock* 20:63, 2003.

125. Jackson WL Jr: Should we use etomidate as an induction agent for endotracheal intubation in patients with septic shock?: A critical appraisal. *Chest* 127:1031, 2005.

126. Schenarts CL, Burton JH, Riker RR: Adrenocortical dysfunction following etomidate induction in emergency department patients. *Acad Emerg Med* 8:1, 2001.

127. Papanicolaou DA, Tsigos C, Oldfield EH, et al.: Acute glucocorticoid deficiency is associated with plasma elevations of interleukin-6: Does the latter participate in the symptomatology of the steroid withdrawal syndrome and adrenal insufficiency? *J Clin Endocrinol Metab* 81:2303, 1996.

128. Molina PE, Zambell KL, Zhang P, et al.: Hemodynamic and immune consequences of opiate analgesia after trauma/hemorrhage. *Shock* 21:526, 2004.

129. Brand JM, Frohn C, Luhm J, et al.: Early alterations in the number of circulating lymphocyte subpopulations and enhanced proinflammatory immune response during opioid-based general anesthesia. *Shock* 20:213, 2003.

130. Molina PE: Neurobiology of the stress response: Contribution of the sympathetic nervous system to the neuroimmune axis in traumatic injury. *Shock* 24:3, 2005.

131. Barnett CC Jr, Moore EE, Partrick DA, et al.: Beta-adrenergic stimulation down-regulates neutrophil priming for superoxide generation, but not elastase release. *J Surg Res* 70:166, 1997.

132. van der Poll T, Lowry SF: Lipopolysaccharide-induced interleukin 8 production by human whole blood is enhanced by epinephrine and inhibited by hydrocortisone. *Infect Immun* 65:2378, 1997.

133. Dhingra VK, Uusaro A, Holmes CL, et al.: Attenuation of lung inflammation by adrenergic agonists in murine acute lung injury. *Anesthesiology* 95:947, 2001.

134. Weisdorf DJ, Jacob HS: Beta-adrenergic blockade: Augmentation of neutrophil-mediated inflammation. *J Lab Clin Med* 109:120, 1987.

135. Rasmussen F: The influence of radiographic contrast media on some granulocyte functions. *Acta Radiol Suppl* 419:7, 1998.

136. Laskey WK, Gellman J: Inflammatory markers increase following exposure to radiographic contrast media. *Acta Radiol* 44:498, 2003.

137. Ji Q, Ghaly M, Hjemdahl P, et al.: Contrast medium attenuates platelet activation and platelet-leukocyte cross-talk. *Thromb Haemost* 93:922, 2005.

138. Bartlett JG, Onderdonk AB, Louie T, et al.: A review. Lessons from an animal model of intra-abdominal sepsis. *Arch Surg* 113:853, 1978.

139. Thadepalli H: Principles and practice of antibiotic therapy for post-traumatic abdominal injuries. *Surg Gynecol Obstet* 148:937, 1979.

140. Polk HC Jr, George CD, Wellhausen SR, et al.: A systematic study of host defense processes in badly injured patients. *Ann Surg* 204:282, 1986.

141. Faist E, Mewes A, Baker CC, et al.: Prostaglandin E2 (PGE2)-dependent suppression of interleukin alpha (Il-2) production in patients with major trauma. *J Trauma* 27:837, 1987.

142. Livingston DH, Appel SH, Wellhausen SR, et al.: Depressed interferon gamma production and monocyte HLA-DR expression after severe injury. *Arch Surg* 123:1309, 1988.

143. Moore FA, Peterson VM, Moore EE, et al.: Inadequate granulopoiesis after major torso trauma: A hematopoietic regulatory paradox. *Surgery* 108:667, 1990.

144. Christou NV, Meakins JL, Gordon J, et al.: The delayed hypersensitivity response and host resistance in surgical patients. 20 years later. *Ann Surg* 222:534, 1995.

145. Menges T, Engel J, Welters I, et al.: Changes in blood lymphocyte populations after multiple trauma: Association with posttraumatic complications. *Crit Care Med* 27:733, 1999.

146. Cerra FB, Siegel JH, Coleman B, et al.: Septic autocannibalism. A failure of exogenous nutritional support. *Ann Surg* 192:570, 1980.

147. Wilmore DW: Alterations in protein, carbohydrate, and fat metabolism in injured and septic patients. *J Am Coll Nutr* 2:3, 1983.

148. Brigham KL, Bowers R, Haynes J: Increased sheep lung vascular permeability caused by escherichia coli endotoxin. *Circ Res* 45:292, 1979.

149. Bersten A, Sibbald WJ: Acute lung injury in septic shock. *Crit Care Clin* 5:49, 1989.

150. Henson PM, Larsen GL, Webster RO, et al.: Pulmonary microvascular alterations and injury induced by complement fragments: Synergistic effect of complement activation, neutrophil sequestration, and prostaglandins. *Ann N Y Acad Sci* 384:287, 1982.

151. Stephens KE, Ishizaka A, Larrick JW, et al.: Tumor necrosis factor causes increased pulmonary permeability and edema. Comparison to septic acute lung injury. *Am Rev Respir Dis* 137:1364, 1988.

152. Fisher CJ, Jr, Zheng Y: Potential strategies for inflammatory mediator manipulation: Retrospect and prospect. *World J Surg* 20:447, 1996.

153. Guirao X, Lowry SF: Biologic control of injury and inflammation: Much more than too little or too late. *World J Surg* 20:437, 1996.

154. Cronin L, Cook DJ, Carlet J, et al.: Corticosteroid treatment for sepsis: A critical appraisal and meta-analysis of the literature. *Crit Care Med* 23:1430, 1995.

155. Vedder NB, Fouty BW, Winn RK, et al.: Role of neutrophils in generalized reperfusion injury associated with resuscitation from shock. *Surgery* 106:509, 1989.

156. Mileski WJ, Winn RK, Vedder NB, et al.: Inhibition of CD18-dependent neutrophil adherence reduces organ injury after hemorrhagic shock in primates. *Surgery* 108:206, 1990.

157. Sharar SR, Mihelcic DD, Han KT, et al.: Ischemia reperfusion injury in the rabbit ear is reduced by both immediate and delayed CD18 leukocyte adherence blockade. *J Immunol* 153:2234, 1994.

158. Weiss SJ: Tissue destruction by neutrophils. *N Engl J Med* 320:365, 1989.

159. Ward PA, Varani J: Mechanisms of neutrophil-mediated killing of endothelial cells. *J Leukoc Biol* 48:97, 1990.

160. Tapper H: The secretion of preformed granules by macrophages and neutrophils. *J Leukoc Biol* 59:613, 1996.

161. Borregaard N, Kjeldsen L, Lollike K, et al.: Granules and vesicles of human neutrophils. The role of endomembranes as source of plasma membrane proteins. *Eur J Haematol* 51:318, 1993.

162. Borregaard N, Cowland JB: Granules of the human neutrophilic polymorphonuclear leukocyte. *Blood* 89:3503, 1997.

163. Windsor AC, Mullen PG, Fowler AA, et al.: Role of the neutrophil in adult respiratory distress syndrome. *Br J Surg* 80:10, 1993.

164. Poggetti RS, Moore FA, Moore EE, et al.: Liver injury is a reversible neutrophil-mediated event following gut ischemia. *Arch Surg* 127:175, 1992.

165. Biffl WL, Moore EE, Moore FA, et al.: Interleukin-6 stimulates neutrophil production of platelet-activating factor. *J Leukoc Biol* 59:569, 1996.

166. Cassatella MA: The production of cytokines by polymorphonuclear neutrophils. *Immunol Today* 16:21, 1995.

167. Biffl WL, Moore EE, Moore FA, et al.: Interleukin-8 increases endothelial permeability independent of neutrophils. *J Trauma* 39:98, 1995.

168. Maclouf J, Sala A, Rossoni G, et al.: Consequences of transcellular biosynthesis of leukotriene C4 on organ function. *Haemostasis* 26:28, 1996.

169. de Gaetano G, Cerletti C, Evangelista V: Recent advances in platelet-polymorphonuclear leukocyte interaction. *Haemostasis* 29:41, 1999.

170. Faint RW: Platelet-neutrophil interactions: Their significance. *Blood Rev* 6:83, 1992.

171. Sala A, Zarini S, Folco G, et al.: Differential metabolism of exogenous and endogenous arachidonic acid in human neutrophils. *J Biol Chem* 274:28264, 1999.

172. Maghni K, Carrier J, Cloutier S, et al.: Cell-cell interactions between platelets, macrophages, eosinophils and natural killer cells in thromboxane A2 biosynthesis. *J Lipid Mediat* 6:321, 1993.

173. Botha AJ, Moore FA, Moore EE, et al.: Postinjury neutrophil priming and activation states: Therapeutic challenges. *Shock* 3:157, 1995.

174. Worthen GS, Seccombe JF, Clay KL, et al.: The priming of neutrophils by lipopolysaccharide for production of intracellular platelet-activating factor. Potential role in mediation of enhanced superoxide secretion. *J Immunol* 140:3553, 1988.

175. Gay JC: Mechanism and regulation of neutrophil priming by platelet-activating factor. *J Cell Physiol* 156:189, 1993.

176. Partrick DA, Moore EE, Offner PJ, et al.: Maximal human neutrophil priming for superoxide production and elastase release requires P38 mitogen-activated protein kinase activation. *Arch Surg* 135:219, 2000.

177. Zallen G, Moore EE, Johnson JL, et al.: Circulating postinjury neutrophils are primed for the release of proinflammatory cytokines. *J Trauma* 46:42, 1999.

178. Botha AJ, Moore FA, Moore EE, et al.: Early neutrophil sequestration after injury: A pathogenic mechanism for multiple organ failure. *J Trauma* 39:411, 1995.

179. Johnson JL, Moore EE, Offner PJ, et al.: Resuscitation with a blood substitute abrogates pathologic postinjury neutrophil cytotoxic function. *J Trauma* 50:449, 2001.

180. Biffl WL, West KE, Moore EE, et al.: Neutrophil apoptosis is delayed by trauma patients' plasma via a mechanism involving proinflammatory phospholipids and protein kinase C. *Surg Infect (Larchmt)*. 2:289, 2001.

181. Fan J, Marshall JC, Jimenez M, et al.: Hemorrhagic shock primes for increased expression of cytokine-induced neutrophil chemoattractant in the lung: Role in pulmonary inflammation following lipopolysaccharide. *J Immunol* 161:440, 1998.

182. Gago LA, Moore EE, Partrick DA, et al.: Secretory phospholipase A2 cleavage of intravasated bone marrow primes human neutrophils. *J Trauma* 44:660, 1998.

183. Silliman CC, Thurman GW, Ambruso DR: Stored blood components contain agents that prime the neutrophil nadph oxidase through the platelet-activating-factor receptor. *Vox Sang* 63:133, 1992.

184. Mattox KL, Maningas PA, Moore EE, et al.: Prehospital hypertonic saline/dextran infusion for post-traumatic hypotension. The U.S.A. Multicenter trial. *Ann Surg* 213:482, 1991.

185. Younes RN, Aun F, Accioly CQ, et al.: Hypertonic solutions in the treatment of hypovolemic shock: A prospective, randomized study in patients admitted to the emergency room. *Surgery* 111:380, 1992.

186. Younes RN, Aun F, Ching CT, et al.: Prognostic factors to predict outcome following the administration of hypertonic/hyperoncotic solution in hypovolemic patients. *Shock* 7:79, 1997.

187. Ciesla DJ, Moore EE, Biffl WL, et al.: Hypertonic saline attenuation of the neutrophil cytotoxic response is reversed upon restoration of normotonicity and reestablished by repeated hypertonic challenge. *Surgery* 129:567, 2001.

188. Ciesla DJ, Moore EE, Musters RJ, et al.: Hypertonic saline alteration of the pmn cytoskeleton: Implications for signal transduction and the cytotoxic response. *J Trauma* 50:206, 2001.

189. Corso CO, Okamoto S, Ruttinger D, et al.: Hypertonic saline dextran attenuates leukocyte accumulation in the liver after hemorrhagic shock and resuscitation. *J Trauma* 46:417, 1999.

190. Bahrami S, Zimmermann K, Szelenyi Z, et al.: Small-volume fluid resuscitation with hypertonic saline prevents inflammation but not mortality in a rat model of hemorrhagic shock. *Shock* 25:283, 2006.

191. ARDS, Network. Ventilation with lower tidal volumes as compared with traditional tidal volumes for acute lung injury and the acute respiratory distress syndrome. *N Engl J Med* 342:1301, 2000.

192. Slutsky AS, Tremblay LN: Multiple system organ failure. Is mechanical ventilation a contributing factor? *Am J Respir Crit Care Med* 157:1721, 1998.

193. van den Berghe G, Wouters P, Weekers F, et al.: Intensive insulin therapy in the critically ill patients. *N Engl J Med* 345:1359, 2001.

194. Van den Berghe GH: Role of intravenous insulin therapy in critically ill patients. *Endocr Pract* 10 Suppl 2:17, 2004.

195. Jeschke MG, Einspanier R, Klein D, et al.: Insulin attenuates the systemic inflammatory response to thermal trauma. *Mol Med* 8:443, 2002.

196. Jeschke MG, Klein D, Bolder U, et al.: Insulin attenuates the systemic inflammatory response in endotoxemic rats. *Endocrinology* 145:4084, 2004.

197. Jeschke MG, Klein D, Herndon DN: Insulin treatment improves the systemic inflammatory reaction to severe trauma. *Ann Surg* 239:553, 2004.

198. Marik PE, Zaloga GP: Adrenal insufficiency in the critically ill: A new look at an old problem. *Chest* 122:1784, 2002.

199. Cooper MS, Stewart PM: Corticosteroid insufficiency in acutely ill patients. *N Engl J Med* 348:727, 2003.

200. Keh D, Boehnke T, Weber-Cartens S, et al.: Immunologic and hemodynamic effects of "Low-dose" Hydrocortisone in septic shock: A double-blind, randomized, placebo-controlled, crossover study. *Am J Respir Crit Care Med* 167:512, 2003.

201. Oppert M, Schindler R, Husung C, et al.: Low-dose hydrocortisone improves shock reversal and reduces cytokine levels in early hyperdynamic septic shock. *Crit Care Med* 33:2457, 2005.

202. Riska EB, von Bonsdorff H, Hakkinen S, et al.: Primary operative fixation of long bone fractures in patients with multiple injuries. *J Trauma* 17:111, 1977.
203. Johnson KD, Cadambi A, Seibert GB: Incidence of adult respiratory distress syndrome in patients with multiple musculoskeletal injuries: Effect of early operative stabilization of fractures. *J Trauma* 25:375, 1985.
204. Bone LB, Johnson KD, Weigelt J, et al.: Early versus delayed stabilization of femoral fractures. A prospective randomized study. *J Bone Joint Surg Am* 71:336, 1989.
205. Behrman SW, Fabian TC, Kudsk KA, et al.: Improved outcome with femur fractures: Early vs. delayed fixation. *J Trauma* 30:792, 1990.
206. Croce MA, Bee TK, Pritchard E, et al.: Does optimal timing for spine fracture fixation exist? *Ann Surg* 233:851, 2001.
207. Scalea TM, Scott JD, Brumback RJ, et al.: Early fracture fixation may be "Just fine" After head injury: No difference in central nervous system outcomes. *J Trauma* 46:839, 1999.
208. Nowotarski PJ, Turen CH, Brumback RJ, et al.: Conversion of external fixation to intramedullary nailing for fractures of the shaft of the femur in multiply injured patients. *J Bone Joint Surg Am* 82:781, 2000.
209. Scalea TM, Boswell SA, Scott JD, et al.: External fixation as a bridge to intramedullary nailing for patients with multiple injuries and with femur fractures: Damage control orthopedics. *J Trauma* 48:613, 2000.
210. Pape HC, Giannoudis P, Krettek C: The timing of fracture treatment in polytrauma patients: Relevance of damage control orthopedic surgery. *Am J Surg* 183:622, 2002.
211. Taeger G, Ruchholtz S, Waydhas C, et al.: Damage control orthopedics in patients with multiple injuries is effective, time saving, and safe. *J Trauma* 59:409, 2005.
212. Pape HC, Hildebrand F, Pertschy S, et al.: Changes in the management of femoral shaft fractures in polytrauma patients: From early total care to damage control orthopedic surgery. *J Trauma* 53:452, 2002.
213. Dellinger EP, Wertz MJ, Lennard ES, et al.: Efficacy of short-course antibiotic prophylaxis after penetrating intestinal injury. A prospective randomized trial. *Arch Surg* 121:23, 1986.
214. Ericsson CD, Fischer RP, Rowlands BJ, et al.: Prophylactic antibiotics in trauma: The hazards of underdosing. *J Trauma* 29:1356, 1989.
215. Civetta JM, Hudson-Civetta J, Ball S: Decreasing catheter-related infection and hospital costs by continuous quality improvement. *Crit Care Med* 24:1660, 1996.
216. Drakulovic MB, Torres A, Bauer TT, et al.: Supine body position as a risk factor for nosocomial pneumonia in mechanically ventilated patients: A randomised trial. *Lancet* 354:1851, 1999.
217. Sauaia A, Moore FA, Moore EE, et al.: Diagnosing pneumonia in mechanically ventilated trauma patients: Endotracheal aspirate versus bronchoalveolar lavage. *J Trauma* 35:512, 1993.
218. Croce MA, Fabian TC, Waddle-Smith L, et al.: Utility of gram's stain and efficacy of quantitative cultures for posttraumatic pneumonia: A prospective study. *Ann Surg* 227:743, 1998.

# Commentary ■ MICHAEL CHANG

The preceding chapter by Ciesla et al. provides a comprehensive and up-to-date description of multiple organ failure (MOF), the prevention of which remains the Holy Grail of clinical critical care. As the leading cause of late death in surgical patients for the past 40 years, MOF has been the subject of a tremendous volume of basic, clinical, and translational research. The intent of this invited commentary will be to highlight important points in the evolution of this clinical syndrome, and to attempt to place posttraumatic inflammation, resuscitation, and organ failure in a unified framework to facilitate translation of physiologic concepts into bedside care.

At the first approximation, MOF is the end-result of uncontrolled, dysregulated inflammation due to the persistence of one or more of three basic types of inflammatory stimuli: (1) infection, (2) ischemia/reperfusion injury, and (3) dead or injured tissue. These are the classic pathophysiologic conditions that mandate emergency intervention, and though historically, surgeons may not have been aware of the exact molecular pathways and processes that lead to systemic inflammation and subsequent organ failure, they most certainly understood that surgical pathology involving one or more of these classes of stimuli was, if allowed to persistent, clearly associated with a worse outcome than if these issues were dealt with immediately. Hence the development of the distinction between emergent, urgent, and elective surgical cases.

Failure to identify any one or more of these types of insults in critically injured patients leads to the development of a persistent, pathologic inflammatory state which, if unchecked, will ultimately lead to sequential organ failure and death. Whether this dysfunctional state is upregulation of inflammation in the early phase, or downregulation with subsequent immunosuppression in later stages, timely intervention with achievement of hemostasis, identification of injuries with resection/repair of dead or injured tissue, and aggressive resuscitation will presumably ameliorate this state of dysfunctional inflammation, thus allowing the patient to maintain crucial organ function.

Over recent years, as eloquently described by Ciesla et al., the clinical presentation of MOF has changed, as advances in resuscitation and specific organ support have evolved. Also important in this evolution is the ongoing development and refinement of trauma systems, trauma centers, and trauma-specific patient care protocols. Advances in each of these areas have led to changes in the patterns of organ failure described in these patients. However, though the clinical syndrome may have changed, the problem still remains, as manifest by the inability of clinicians to significantly and durable impact the incidence and mortality of this entity.

Early research in this field was hampered by the lack of a uniform scoring system for MOF. Lack of a reproducible, understandable, and objective scoring system made interpretation of observational studies difficult, and design and implementation of outcome studies impossible. The scoring system created by Moore and Moore et al., outlined in this chapter, represents an important step in toward solving this problem. This scoring system is comprehensive and clinically correlated with outcome and bridges the gap between information learned from laboratory research and clinical observation and outcome. Furthermore, it is designed in such a way that it is adaptable, with definitions that can evolve with changes in the clinical entity that have and will inevitably result from our changing understanding of the disease process and the support needed by patients suffering from this syndrome.

Finally, it is important to understand that MOF is not a disease process, but rather a clinical syndrome that is manifest by critically ill patients as a result of a myriad number of different possible stimuli. While reversal of organ failure is a laudable clinical goal, at the present time the best treatment for this syndrome remains prevention, through rapid transport of critically injured patients to efficient and optimally performing trauma centers, timely identification of life-threatening injuries and achievement of hemostasis, aggressive resuscitation from hemorrhagic shock, and protocol-driven prevention of infection. As trauma care and prevention evolves and develops, so too will the natural history of MOF.

# INDEX

*Note:* Page numbers in **bold** indicate **tables**; those in *italic* indicate *figures*.

# V

V²A steel, 9. *See also* fractures
vaccination
    meningococcal, 372
    anthrax, **370**, 371
    infection prevention aspects, 369–370
    post-splenectomy, **370**
        evidence-based recommendations, 372
        revaccination, 372
        timing aspects, 372
    rabies, **370**, 371
    tetanus, **370**, 371
vacuum assisted closure, 865
vacuum assisted fascial closure, 863
vaginal injuries, 846. *See also* genitourinary injuries; nonpregnant patients trauma
valvular injury, 581. *See also* blunt cardiac injuries
VAP. *See* ventilator associated pneumonia
variability, 1161. *See also* genetic factors
*Variola* virus, 1151–1152. *See also* biological warfare
vascular access, pediatric trauma and, 989
vascular control
    inframesocolic region (ZONE 1) injuries, 745–746
    lateral retroperitoneum (ZONE 2) injuries, 747–748
    pelvic retroperitoneum (ZONE 3) injuries, 749
    porta hepatis injuries, 751
    supramesocolic region (ZONE 1) abdominal vascular injuries, 740–741
vascular injuries. *See also* abdominal vascular injuries; peripheral vascular injuries
    damage control and operative techniques, 857
    intraventricular hemorrhage, 401
    neck, 473–475
    subarachnoid hemorrhage, 401
    thoracic, 593
    upper extremity injuries and, 895
vasodilatation, 1346
vasogenic shock, 213
vasopressin, 1250
vecuronium, 193, 352
vehicle borne improvised explosive devices (VBIED), 1112. *See also* combat trauma
veins. *See also* venous injuries
    iliac, 750
    portal, 751
Velcro-like sheets, 863. *See also* open abdomen
velocity, guns, **108**
vena cava
    filters for VTE, 1239
    infrahepatic inferior, 746–747
    stenting, 651
vena cava injuries
    liver injury, 650–651
    thoracic great vessel injury and, 601
venography, 949. *See also* arteriography
venomous fish, bites and stings by, 1047. *See also* bites
venous injuries. *See also* arterial injuries
    azygos veins, 601
    peripheral vascular injuries, 955, 964–966
    pulmonary veins, 601
    repair
        peripheral vascular injuries, 955
        direct (liver injuries), 650
    subclavian veins, 601
    thoracic vena cava, 601
venous thromboembolism (VTE). *See also* deep vein thrombosis (DVT)
    bleeding and coagulation and, 1237
    diagnosis, 1237–1238
    genetic risk factors, 1163–1164
    pharmacogenomics, 1163–1164
    prophylaxis, 1239
    risk factors, 1237
    state-of-the-art approach, 1239–1240
    vena cava filters for, 1239
ventilation. *See also* airway management; breathing
    ARDS, 1267–1271
    BVM, 204–205

CCU and, 1203–1206, 1209
    mechanical ventilation discontinuation, 1205–1206
    monitoring, 1201
    respiratory failure, adjuvant therapies in, 1205
    WOB discontinuation, 1206
extracorporeal life support (ECLS), 1271
high-frequency ventilation (HFV), 1271
induced lung injury
    critical care unit (CCU), 1202
    MOF and, 1369
inverse ratio ventilation (IRV), 1269
mechanical
    ARDS and, 1267
    critical care unit (CCU), 1200, 1202
    discontinuation, 1205–1206
modes
    airway-pressure-release ventilation (APRV), 1205
    assist/control-mode ventilation (ACV), 1203
    control-mode (CV), 1203
    high-frequency oscillatory ventilation (HFOV), 1205
    intermittent mandatory ventilation (IMV), 1203
    inverse ratio ventilation (IRV), 1204
    mechanical ventilation weaning, 1209
    pressure regulated volume-controlled ventilation (PRVC), 1203
    pressure support ventilation (PSV), 1203, 1204
    time-cycled pressure-control ventilation, 1204
    weaning, 1205–1209
partial liquid, 1272
PEEP, 1267–1268
percutaneous transtracheal (PTV), 130
permissive hypercapnia, 1268–1269
prehospital care aspects, 130
pressure control ventilation, 1269
pressure-limited ventilatory support, 1268
primary survey aspects, 171–174
prone ventilation, 1269
pulmonary dysfunction after chest trauma, management of, 543–544
tracheal gas insufflation (TGI), 1270
tracheostomy and, 1209
ventilatory capacity, 1201–1202, 1206
ventilator associated pneumonia (VAP), 207
    critical care unit (CCU), 1214
    diagnosis, 384
    pathogenesis, 382–383
    prevention, 383
    therapy, 384–387
ventricular injuries, 575. *See also* penetrating cardiac injuries
ventriculography, air, 404. *See also* traumatic brain injury (TBI)
vertebral column. *See also* spinal cord; spine injuries
    anatomy
        cervical, 480–481
        lumbar, 481
        thoracic, 481
    spinal instability injury, 485–487
    spine kinematics, 481–483
vesicants. *See also* chemical warfare
    lewisite, 1147
    mustard agents, 1146
video-assisted thoracoscopic surgery (VATS), 540
Vietnam War, 9, 18, 1109. *See also* combat trauma; trauma care
violence, 1019
    against women, 1020–1021
    domestic/family violence, 51, 1020–1023
    intentional, 1019
    interpersonal, 1019, 1023
    youth violence, 1023–1025
viral hemorrhagic fevers, 1150. *See also* biological warfare
visceral system. *See also* bony system
    anatomy, 441
    evaluation, 444
    management, 448
    secondary repair aspects, 461–462
visual fields, confrontational, 424. *See also* eye injuries
vitamin K deficiency, 1229. *See also* bleeding and coagulation